CLINICAL IMMUNOLOGY

Principles and Practice

Content Strategist: Belinda Kuhn
Content Development Specialist: Rachael Harrison
Content Coordinator: Sam Crowe
Project Manager: Andrew Riley
Design: Stewart Larking
Illustration Manager: Jennifer Rose
Illustrator: Martin Woodward
Marketing Managers (UK/USA): Gaynor Jones & Helena Mutak

CLINICAL IMMUNOLOGY
Principles and Practice

FOURTH EDITION

ROBERT R. RICH MD
Professor of Medicine and Microbiology
University of Alabama at Birmingham
Birmingham, AL
USA

THOMAS A. FLEISHER MD
Fellow, American Academy of Allergy,
Asthma, and Immunology
Chief, Department of Laboratory Medicine
NIH Clinical Center
Adjunct Professor of Pediatrics
Uniformed Services University of the Health Sciences
Bethesda, MD
USA

WILLIAM T. SHEARER MD, PhD
Allergy and Immunology Service
Texas Children's Hospital
Professor of Pediatrics and Immunology
Section of Allergy and Immunology
Department of Pediatrics
Baylor College of Medicine
Houston, TX
USA

HARRY W. SCHROEDER, JR. MD, PhD
Professor of Medicine, Microbiology, and Genetics
Division of Clinical Immunology and Rheumatology
Director, UAB Program in Immunology
University of Alabama at Birmingham
Birmingham, AL
USA

ANTHONY J. FREW MD, FRCP
Professor of Allergy and Respiratory Medicine
Department of Respiratory Medicine
Royal Sussex County Hospital
Brighton
UK

CORNELIA M. WEYAND MD, PhD
Professor of Medicine
Stanford University
Stanford, CA
USA

For additional online content visit
www.expertconsult.com

Expert | CONSULT

ELSEVIER
SAUNDERS

Notices

Knowledge and best practice in this field are constantly changing. As new research and experience broaden our understanding, changes in research methods, professional practices, or medical treatment may become necessary.

Practitioners and researchers must always rely on their own experience and knowledge in evaluating and using any information, methods, compounds, or experiments described herein. In using such information or methods they should be mindful of their own safety and the safety of others, including parties for whom they have a professional responsibility.

With respect to any drug or pharmaceutical products identified, readers are advised to check the most current information provided (i) on procedures featured or (ii) by the manufacturer of each product to be administered, to verify the recommended dose or formula, the method and duration of administration, and contraindications. It is the responsibility of practitioners, relying on their own experience and knowledge of their patients, to make diagnoses, to determine dosages and the best treatment for each individual patient, and to take all appropriate safety precautions.

To the fullest extent of the law, neither the Publisher nor the authors, contributors, or editors, assume any liability for any injury and/or damage to persons or property as a matter of products liability, negligence or otherwise, or from any use or operation of any methods, products, instructions, or ideas contained in the material herein.

Elsevier
British Library Cataloguing in Publication Data
Clinical immunology : principles and practice. — 4th ed.
1. Clinical immunology.
I. Rich, Robert R.
616'.079–dc23

ISBN-13: 978-0-7234-3691-1
Ebook ISBN: 978-0-7234-3710-9

Printed in China

Last digit is the print number: 9 8 7 6 5 4 3 2 1

Contents

PART ONE: Principles of immune response

PART TWO: Host defense mechanisms and inflammation

v

PART SEVEN: Organ-specific inflammatory disease

PART EIGHT: Immunology of neoplasia

PART NINE: Transplantation

PART TEN: Prevention and therapy of immunologic diseases

PART ELEVEN: Diagnostic immunology

Appendices

List of contributors

ROSHINI SARAH ABRAHAM PhD, D(ABMLI)
Associate Professor of Medicine,
Associate Professor of Laboratory Medicine and Pathology,
Consultant
Department of Laboratory Medicine and Pathology
Mayo Clinic
Rochester, MN, USA

CRISTINA ALBANESI BSc, PhD
Senior Investigator
Laboratory of Experimental Immunology
Dermopathic Institute
Istituto Dermopatico dell'Immacolata (IDI)-IRCCS
Rome, Italy

ILIAS ALEVIZOS DMD, MMSc
Assistant Clinical Investigator
National Institute of Dental and Craniofacial Research
National Institutes of Health
Bethesda, MD, USA

JUAN ANGUITA PhD
Associate Professor
Department of Veterinary and Animal Sciences
University of Massachusetts Amherst
Amherst, MA, USA

GREGORY M. ANSTEAD MD, PhD
Associate Professor,
Department of Medicine,
University of Texas Health Science Center at San Antonio,
Director
Immunosuppression and Infectious Diseases Clinics
South Texas Veterans Health Care System
San Antonio, TX, USA

CYNTHIA ARANOW MD
Investigator Clinical Research
Autoimmune and Musculoskeletal Diseases
The Feinstein Institute for Medical Research
Manhasset, NY, USA

HOWARD A. AUSTIN III MD
Senior Clinical Investigator
National Institute of Diabetes and Digestive and Kidney Diseases
National Institutes of Health
Bethesda, MD, USA

SUBASH BABU MBBS, PhD
Scientific Director
International Centers for Excellence in Research
Tuberculosis Research Center
National Institutes of Health India
Chennai, India

MARK C. BALLOW MD
Professor
Department of Pediatrics, Division of Allergy, Immunology
& Pediatric Rheumatology
Women and Children's Hospital of Buffalo
State University of New York at Buffalo
School of Medicine and Biomedical Sciences
Buffalo, NY, USA

JAMES E. BALOW MD
Clinical Director and Chief
Kidney Disease Section
National Institute of Diabetes and Digestive and Kidney Diseases
National Institutes of Health
Bethesda, MD, USA

DAVID R. BARNIDGE PhD
Assistant Professor
Department of Biochemistry and Molecular Biology
Mayo Clinic
Rochester, MN, USA

JOHN W. BELMONT MD, PhD
Professor
Department of Molecular and Human Genetics
Baylor College of Medicine
Houston, TX, USA

GABRIELLE T. BELZ BVBiol, BVSc, DVSc
Professor
Molecular Immunology
The Walter and Eliza Hall Institute
Melbourne, VIC, Australia

DINA BEN-YEHUDA MD
Head
Department of Hematology
Hadassah- Hebrew University Medical Center
Jerusalem, Israel

CLAUDIA BEREK PhD
Group Leader
B Cell Immunology
Deutsches Rheuma-Forschungszentrum Berlin (DRFZ)
Berlin, Germany

TIMOTHY BEUKELMAN MD, MSCE
Assistant Professor of Pediatric Rheumatology
Division of Rheumatology
The University of Alabama at Birmingham
Birmingham, AL, USA

THOMAS BIEBER MD, PhD, MDRA
Professor and Chair
Department of Dermatology and Allergy
University of Bonn
Bonn, Germany

JOHANNES W.J. BIJLSMA MD
Professor
Department of Rheumatology and Clinical Immunology
University Medical Center Utrecht
Utrecht, The Netherlands

JACK J.H. BLEESING MD, PhD
Associate Professor
University of Cincinnati Department of Pediatrics
Cincinnati Children's Hospital Medical Center
Cincinnati, OH, USA

SARAH E. BLUTT PhD
Assistant Professor
Department of Molecular Virology and Microbiology
and Department of Molecular and Cellular Biology
Baylor College of Medicine
Houston, TX, USA

BARBARA BOHLE PhD
Head of the Christian Doppler Laboratory for Immunomodulation
Department of Pathophysiology and Allergy Research
Center for Pathophysiology, Immunology and Infectiology
Medical University of Vienna
Vienna, Austria

ELENA BORZOVA MD, PhD
Clinical Research Fellow
Dermatology Centre
Norfolk and Norwich University Hospital
Norwich, UK

PROSPER N. BOYAKA MD
Professor
Department of Veterinary Biosciences
The Ohio State University
College of Veterinary Medicine
Columbus, OH, USA

KNUT BROCKOW MD
Professor
Department of Dermatology and Allergology (Biederstein)
Technische Universitaet Muenchen
Munich, Germany

JACINTA BUSTAMANTE MD, PhD
Research Associate,
Laboratory of Human Genetics of Infectious Diseases,
Necker Branch,
INSERM U980,
Necker Medical School,
Paris Descartes University,
Paris Sorbonne Cité,
Study Center for Primary Immunodeficiencies
Assistance Publique Hôpitaux de Paris
Necker Hospital
Paris, France

FRANK BUTTGEREIT MD
Deputy Clinical Director,
Professor of Rheumatology
Department of Rheumatology and Clinical Immunology
Charité University of Medicine Berlin
Berlin, Germany

MARY BYRNE PHARMD, BCPS
Assistant Chief Pharmacist
National Institutes of Health Clinical Center
Bethesda, MD, USA

VIRGINIA L. CALDER PhD
Senior Lecturer in Immunology
Department of Molecular Therapy & Genetics
UCL Institute of Ophthalmology
London, UK

MAGDA CARNEIRO-SAMPAIO MD, PhD
Professor of Pediatrics
Faculty of Medicine
University of São Paulo
São Paulo, Brasil

SEBASTIAN CAROTTA PhD
Professor of Molecular Immunology
The Walter and Eliza Hall Institute
Melbourne, VIC, Australia

JEAN-LAURENT CASANOVA MD, PhD
Professor of Pediatrics,
Pediatric Hematology-Immunology Unit,
Necker Hospital,
Assistance Publique Hôpitaux de Paris,
Co-director
Laboratory of Human Genetics of Infectious Diseases
Necker Branch
INSERM U980
Necker Medical School
Paris Descartes University, Paris Sorbonne Cité, France
Director
St Giles Laboratory of Human Genetics of Infectious Diseases
Rockefeller Branch
The Rockefeller University
New York, NY, USA

LISA A. CAVACINI PhD
Assistant Professor
Department of Medicine
Beth Israel Deaconess Medical Center
Harvard Medical School
Boston, MA, USA

EDWIN S.L. CHAN MD, FRCPC
Assistant Professor
Department of Medicine
New York University School of Medicine
New York, NY, USA

JAVIER CHINEN MD, PhD
Assistant Professor
Departments of Pediatrics
Baylor College of Medicine
Houston, TX, USA

TANUJA CHITNIS MD
Assistant Professor of Neurology
Department of Neurology
Brigham and Women's Hospital
Harvard Medical School
Boston, MA, USA

MONIQUE CHO MD, PhD
Clinical Investigator
Kidney Disease Branch
National Institute of Diabetes and Digestive and Kidney Diseases
National Institutes of Health
Bethesda, MD, USA

LISA CHRISTOPHER-STINE MD, MPH
Assistant Professor of Medicine
Co-Director
John Hopkins Mytosis Centre
Johns Hopkins University Bloomberg School of Public Health
Baltimore, MD, USA

ANDREW P. COPE BSc, PhD, MBBS, FRCP, FHEA
Arthritis Research UK Professor of Rheumatology,
Head
Academic Department of Rheumatology
Centre for Molecular and Cellular Biology of Inflammation
Division of Immunology, Infection and Inflammatory Disease
King's College School of Medicine
King's College London
London, UK

DAVID B. CORRY MD
Professor
Departments of Medicine and Pathology & Immunology
Baylor College of Medicine
Houston, TX, USA

TRICIA COTTRELL BA
MD/PhD Candidate
Johns Hopkins University School of Medicine
Baltimore, MD, USA

ANTONIO COUTINHO MD
Professor,
Department of Basic Immunology,
Faculdade de Medicina de Lisboa,
Director
Instituto Gulbenkian de Ciência
Oeiras, Portugal

MARCO CRAVEIRO
Institut de Génétique Moléculaire de Montpellier
Montpellier, France

RANDY Q. CRON MD, PhD
Professor of Pediatrics and Medicine
Children's Hospital of Alabama
University of Alabama at Birmingham
Birmingham, AL, USA

JENNIFER CUELLAR-RODRIGUEZ MD
Staff Clinician
Laboratory of Clinical Infectious Diseases
National Institute of Allergy and Infectious Diseases
National Institutes of Health
Bethesda, MD, USA

MARINOS C. DALAKAS MD, FAAN
Professor
Neuroimmunology Unit
Department of Pathophysiology
National University of Athens Medical School
Athens, Greece

STEPHANIE C. DE BARROS
Institut de Génétique Moléculaire de Montpellier
Montpellier, France

BLYTHE H. DEVLIN PhD
Assistant Professor
Department of Pediatrics
Duke University Medical Center
Durham, NC, USA

BETTY DIAMOND MD
Head,
Center for Autoimmune Diseases and Musculoskeletal Disorders,
Director
Laboratory of Autoimmune Diseases and Musculoskeletal
Disorders
Professor
Department of Microbiology & Immunology and Medicine
(AECOM)
The Feinstein Institute for Medical Research
Manhasset, NY, USA

ANGELA DISPENZIERI MD
Professor
Department of Medicine
Division of Hematology
Department of Laboratory Medicine
Mayo Clinic
Rochester, MN, USA

TERRY W. DU CLOS MD, PhD
Professor of Medicine,
School of Medicine,
University of New Mexico,
Head of Rheumatology
VA Medical Center
Albuquerque, NM, USA

STÉPHANIE DUPUIS-BOISSON PhD
Research Associate
St Giles Laboratory of Human Genetics of
Infectious Diseases
Rockefeller Branch
The Rockefeller University
New York, NY, USA

TODD N. EAGAR PhD
Assistant Professor
Departments of Pathology and Immunology
University of Texas Southwestern Medical Center
Dallas, TX, USA

GEORGE S. EISENBARTH MD, PhD
Executive Director and Professor of Pediatrics and Medicine
University of Colorado
Denver, CO, USA

CRAIG A. ELMETS MD
Professor and Chair,
Department of Dermatology,
Director
UAB Skin Diseases Research Center
University of Alabama at Birmingham
Birmingham, AL, USA

DORUK ERKAN MD
Associate Attending Rheumatologist,
Hospital for Special Surgery,
Associate Professor of Medicine
Weill Cornell Medical College
Associate Physician-Scientist
Barbara Volcker Center for Women and Rheumatic Disease
New York, NY, USA

MARK B. FEINBERG MD, PhD
Vice President and Chief Public Health and Science Officer
Merck Vaccines
Merck & Co., Inc.
West Point, PA, USA

EROL FIKRIG MD
Waldemar Von Zedtwitz Professor of Medicine (Infectious Diseases),
Professor of Epidemiology (Microbial Diseases) and Microbial Pathogenesis
Investigator
Howard Hughes Medical Institute
Section Chief
Division of Infectious Diseases
Yale University
New Haven, CT, USA

THOMAS A. FLEISHER MD
Fellow, American Academy of Allergy, Asthma, and Immunology
Chief, Department of Laboratory Medicine
NIH Clinical Center
Adjunct Professor of Pediatrics
Uniformed Services University of the Health Sciences
Bethesda, MD, USA

ANDREW P. FONTENOT MD
Henry N. Claman Professor of Medicine,
Division Head
Allergy and Clinical Immunology
University of Colorado Denver
Aurora, CO, USA

LUIS M. FRANCO MD
Assistant Professor
Department of Molecular and Human Genetics
Baylor College of Medicine
Houston, TX, USA

ALEXANDRA F. FREEMAN MD
Staff Clinician
Laboratory of Clinical Infectious Diseases
National Institute of Allergy and Infectious Diseases
National Institutes of Health
Bethesda, MD, USA

ANTHONY J. FREW MD, FRCP
Professor of Allergy and Respiratory Medicine
Department of Respiratory Medicine
Royal Sussex County Hospital
Brighton, UK

The late THEA FRIEDMAN PhD
Associate Scientist
The David Joseph Jurist Research Center for Tomorrows Children
Hackensack University Medical Center
Hackensack, NJ, USA

KOHTARO FUJIHASHI DDS, PhD
Professor
Department of Pediatric Dentistry
Immunobiology Vaccine Center
The Institute for Oral Health Research
School of Dentistry
The University of Alabama at Birmingham
Birmingham, AL, USA

MASSIMO GADINA PhD
Director
Office of Science and Technology
National Institute of Arthritis Musculoskeletal and Skin diseases
National Institutes of Health
Bethesda, MD, USA

STEPHEN J. GALLI MD
Chair,
Department of Pathology,
Professor of Pathology and of Microbiology and Immunology
Mary Hewitt Loveless MD Professor
Stanford University School of Medicine
Stanford, CA, USA

H. BOBBY GASPAR PhD, MRCP, MRCPCH
GOSHCC Professor of Paediatrics and Immunology
UCL Institute of Child Health
University College London
London, UK

MOSHE E. GATT MD
Resident
Department of Hematology
Hadassah-Hebrew University Medical Center
Jerusalem, Israel

M. ERIC GERSHWIN MD
Distinguished Professor of Medicine,
Jack and Donald Chi Professor of Medicine,
Chief
Division of Rheumatology, Allergy and Clinical Immunology
University of California Davis Health System
Davis, CA, USA

KAMRAN GHORESCHI MD
Postdoctoral Visiting Fellow
Molecular Immunology and Inflammation Branch
National Institute of Arthritis, Musculoskeletal and Skin Diseases
National Institutes for Health
Bethesda, MD, USA

SUSAN L. GILLESPIE MD, PhD
Associate Professor of Pediatrics
Baylor College of Medicine
Baylor International Pediatric AIDS Initiative (BIPAI)
Texas Children's Health Center for International Adoption
Houston, TX, USA

JÖRG J. GORONZY MD, PhD
Professor of Medicine
Stanford University School of Medicine
Stanford, CA, USA

CLIVE E.H. GRATTAN MD, FRCP
Consultant Dermatologist
Dermatology Centre
Norfolk and Norwich University Hospital
Norwich, UK

NEIL S. GREENSPAN MD, PhD
Professor of Pathology
Case Western Reserve University
Cleveland, OH, USA

EYAL GRUNEBAUM MD
Associate Professor,
Pediatrics,
University of Toronto,
Staff
Division of Allergy and Clinical Immunology
Blood and Marrow Transplantation Unit
Scientist
Developmental and Stem Cell Biology Program
Hospital for Sick Children
Toronto, ON, Canada

GABRIELLE HAEBERLI MD
Department of Medicine
Allergy Station Medical Clinic
Hospital Ziegler
Spitalnetz Bern
Bern, Switzerland

RUSSELL P. HALL III MD
J. Lamar Callaway Professor and Chair
Department of Dermatology
Duke University School of Medicine
Durham, NC, USA

ROBERT G. HAMILTON PhD, D(ABMLI)
Professor
Department of Medicine and Pathology
Johns Hopkins University School of Medicine
Baltimore, MD, USA

GREGORY R. HARRIMAN MD
Research Professor
School of Biomedical Engineering
Science & Health Systems
Drexel University
Philadelphia, PA, USA

SARFARAZ A. HASNI MD
Lawrence Schulman Clinical Research Scholar
National Institute of Arthritis, Musculoskeletal and Skin Diseases
National Institutes for Health
Bethesda, MD, USA

KHALED M. HASSAN MD
Department of Dermatology
Mercy Fitzgerald Hospital
Darby, PA, USA

ARTHUR HELBLING MD
Associate Professor of Allergology and Clinical Immunology
Division of Allergology
University Clinic for Rheumatology
Immunology and Allergology (RIA) Inselspital
Bern, Switzerland

MELANIE HINGORANI MA, MBBS, FRCOphth, MD
Consultant Ophthalmologist
Paediatric Ophthalmology and Strabismus Service
Moorfields Eye Hospital
London, UK

STEVEN M. HOLLAND MD
Chief,
Laboratory of Clinical Infectious Diseases,
Chief,
Immunopathogenesis Section,
Tenured Investigator
National Institute of Allergy and Infectious Diseases
National Institutes of Health
Bethesda, MD, USA

PETR L. HRUZ MD PhD
Resident
Department of Gastroenterology and Hepatology
University Hospital Basel
Basel, Switzerland

GABOR ILLEI MD, PhD, MHS
Head
Sjögren's Syndrome Clinic
Molecular Physiology and Therapeutics Branch
National Institutes of Health
Bethesda, MD, USA

JOHN B. IMBODEN MD
Alice Betts Endowed Chair for Research in Arthritis
Professor of Medicine
Department of Medicine
University of California
San Francisco, CA, USA

SHAI IZRAELI MD
Associate Professor of Pediatrics
Department of Pediatric Hemato-Oncology
Edmond and Lily Safra Children Hospital
Sheba Medical Center and University of Tel-Aviv School of Medicine
Tel-Aviv, Israel

ELAINE S. JAFFE MD
Head, Hematopathology
Laboratory of Pathology
Center for Cancer Research
National Cancer Institute
Bethesda, MD, USA

CAROLINE JAGOBI MD
Medical Assistant and Research Associate
Department of Dermatology and Allergy
University of Bonn
Bonn, Germany

SIRPA JALKANEN MD, PhD
Academy Professor
Center of Excellence
University of Turku
Turku, Finland

PIM JETANALIN MD
Rheumatology Fellow
Division of Rheumatology, Allergy, and Immunology
The University of California at San Diego
La Jolla, CA, USA

EMMANUELLE JOUANGUY PhD
Research Associate
The Rockefeller University
New York, NY, USA

CARL H. JUNE MD
Professor
Department of Pathology and Labratory Medicine
Universtery of Pennsylvania
Philadelphia, PA, USA

AXEL KALLIES PhD
Professor
Molecular Immunology
The Walter and Eliza Hall Institute
Melbourne, VIC, Australia

STEFAN H.E. KAUFMANN PhD, DR. H.C
Director and Professor of Microbiology and Immunology
Max-Planck-Institute for Infection-Biology
Charité Universitätsmedizin Berlin
Berlin, Germany

ARTHUR KAVANAUGH MD, PhD
Professor of Medicine
Director, Center for Innovative Therapy
Division of Rheumatology, Allergy, and Immunology
The University of California at San Diego
La Jolla, CA, USA

SABIHA KHAN MD
Director
RACE Clinic
Division of Rheumatology
Bethesda, MD, USA

FARRAH KHERADMAND MD
Professor of Medicine, Pathology & Immunology
Department of Medicine
Baylor College of Medicine
Houston, TX, USA

SAMIA J. KHOURY MD
Jack, Sadie and David Breakstone Professor of Neurology
Harvard Medical School
Boston, MA, USA

GARY A. KORETZKY MD, PhD
Francis C. Wood Professor of Medicne
University of Pennsylvania Perelman School of Medicine
Philadelphia, PA, USA

ROBERT KORNGOLD PhD
Chairman and Senior Scientist
Department of Research
Hackensack University Medical Center
Hackensack, NJ, USA

ANNA KOVALSZKI MD
Instructor of Medicine
Harvard Medical School
Division of Allergy and Inflammation
Beth Israel Deaconess Medical Center
Brookline, MA, USA

DOUGLAS B. KUHNS PhD
Head
Neutrophil Monitoring Laboratory
Clinical Services Program
SAIC-Frederick, Inc.
NCI Frederick
Frederick, MD, USA

ROBERT A. KYLE MD, MACP
Professor of Medicine
Department of Laboratory Medicine & Pathology
Mayo Clinic
Rochester, MN, USA

IAN R. LANZA PhD
Assistant Professor
Department of Medicine
Mayo Clinic
Rochester, MN, USA

ARIAN LAURENCE PhD
Postdoctoral Fellow
Molecular Immunology and Inflammation Branch
National Institute of Arthritis and Musculoskeletal and skin Diseases
National Institutes of Health
Bethesda, MD, USA

SUSAN J. LEE MD
Assistant Professor,
Division of Rheumatology,
Interdisciplinary Liaison
Clinical Investigation Institute (CII) – Clinical Trials Unit
Co-Investigator for the Center for Innovative Therapy
University of California at San Diego School of Medicine
La Jolla, CA, USA

MICHAEL J. LENARDO MD
Chief,
Molecular Development of the Immune System Section,
Laboratory of Immunology,
National Institute of Allergy and Infectious Diseases,
National Institutes of Health,
Bethesda, MD,
Adjunct Professor of Pathology
Perelman School of Medicine
University of Pennsylvania
Philadelphia, PA, USA

ARNOLD I. LEVINSON MD
Emeritus Professor of Medicine,
Associate Dean for Research
University of Pennsylvania Medical Center
Pulmonary, Allergy & Critical Care Division
Philadelphia, PA, USA

OFER LEVY MD, PhD
Staff Physician,
Division of Infectious Diseases,
Department of Medicine,
Children's Hospital Boston,
Assistant Professor of Pediatrics
Harvard Medical School
Cambridge, MA, USA

DAVID B. LEWIS PhD
Chief,
Stanford Department of Pediatrics,
Division of Immunology and Allergy,
Professor
Stanford University
Department of Pediatrics
Director of the Jeffrey Modell Primary Immunodeficiency Center at Stanford
Standford, CA, USA

DOROTHY E. LEWIS PhD
Professor of Internal Medicine
Division of Infectious Diseases
University of Texas Health Sciences Center
Houston, TX, USA

SUE L. LIGHTMAN PhD, FRCP, FRCOPHTH, FMedSci
Professor of Clinical Ophthalmology
Consultant Ophthalmologist
Department of Clinical Ophthalmology
Moorfields Eye Hospital
London, UK

MICHAEL D. LOCKSHIN MD, MACR
Director,
Barbara Volcker Center for Women and Rheumatic Disease,
Co-Director,
Mary Kirkland Center for Lupus Research,
Hospital for Special Surgery,
Attending Physician,
Hospital for Special Surgery,
Professor of Medicine and Obstetrics-Gynecology
Joan and Sanford Weill College of Medicine of Cornell University
New York, NY, USA

MICHAEL T. LOTZE MD
Professor of Surgery and Bioengineering,
Vice Chair
Department of Surgery
University of Pittsburgh
Hillman Cancer Center
Pittsburgh, PA, USA

AMBER LUONG MD, PhD
Assistant Professor of Otorhinolaryngology – Head and Neck
Surgery and Immunology & Autoimmune Diseases
The University of Texas Health Science Center at Houston
Houston, TX, USA

MEGGAN MACKAY MD
Associate Investigator Clinical Research
Autoimmune and Musculoskeletal Diseases
The Feinstein Institute for Medical Research
Manhasset, NY, USA

JEAN-LUC MALO MD
Professor
Department of Chest Medicine
Université de Montréal and Hôpital du Sacré-Coeur de Montréal
Montréal, Canada

JONATHAN S. MALTZMAN MD, PhD
Assistant Professor
Renal-Electrolyte and Hypertension Division,
Department of Medicine,
University of Pennsylvania,
Philadelphia, PA, USA

PETER J. MANNON MD, MPH
Director,
Gastroenterology/Hepatology Clinical Research Program,
Professor of Medicine
Mucosal HIV and Immunobiology Center
University of Alabama at Birmingham
Birmingham, AL, USA

MICHAEL P. MANNS MD
Professor and Chairman
Department of Gastroenterology, Hepatology and Endocrinology
Hannover Medical School
Hannover, Germany

MARY LOUISE MARKERT MD, PhD
Professor of Pediatrics and Immunology
Duke University Medical Center
Durham, NC, USA

ELIZABETH A. MCCARTHY RN, MSN, CCRP
Associate in Research
Department of Pediatrics
Duke University Medical Center
Durham, NC, USA

DOUGLAS R. MCDONALD MD, PhD
Assistant Professor of Immunology
Departments of Pediatrics and Immunology
Children's Hospital
Boston and Harvard Medical School
Boston, MA, USA

JERRY R. MCGHEE PhD
Adjunct Professor
Department of Pediatric Dentistry, School of Dentistry, The
University of Alabama at Birmingham
Birmingham, AL, USA

PETER C. MELBY MD
Professor of Medicine
Departments of Internal Medicine, Microbiology and
Immunology, and Pathology
University of Texas Medical Branch
Galveston, Texas, USA

DEAN D. METCALFE MD
Chief
Laboratory of Allergic Diseases
Division of Intramural Research
National Institute of Allergy and Infectious Diseases
National Institutes of Health
Bethesda, MD, USA

MARTIN METZ MD
Associate Professor
Department of Dermatology and Allergy
Charité - Universitätsmedizin Berlin
Berlin, Germany

STEPHEN D. MILLER PhD
Professor
Department of Microbiology-Immunology
Northwestern University Medical School
Chicago, IL, USA

ANNA L. MITCHELL MB, BS, BMednsci, MRCP (UK)
Clinical Research Training Fellow
Institute of Genetic Medicine
International Centre for Life
Newcastle University
Newcastle-upon-Tyne, UK

SHRUTI MITTAL MBBS, BSc, MRCS
Resesarch Fellow
Nuffield Department of Surgical Sciences
Oxford Transplant Centre
Churchill Hospital
Oxford, UK

MAKOTO MIYARA MD, PhD
Senior Practitioner
Department of Immunology – Immune Chemistry and
Autoimmunity
Internal Medicine Department
French National Referral Centre for Systemic Lupus
Erythematosus and Antiphospholipid Syndrome
Groupe Hospitalier Pitié-Salpètrière
Paris, France

CAROLYN MOLD PhD
Professor
Department of Molecular Genetics and Microbiology
University of New Mexico School of Medicine
Albuquerque, NM, USA

DAVID R. MOLLER MD
Professor of Medicine
Johns Hopkins University School of Medicine
Baltimore, MD, USA

SCOTT N. MUELLER PhD
Australian Research Council Queen Elizabeth II Research Fellow
Department of Microbiology and Immunology
University of Melbourne
Parkville, VIC, Australia

ULRICH R. MÜLLER MD
Professor
Consultant
Spital Ziegler
Spital Netz Bern
Bern, Switzerland

PHILIP M. MURPHY MD
Chief
Laboratory of Molecular Immunology
National Institute of Allergy and Infectious Diseases
National Institutes of Health
Bethesda, MD, USA

PIERRE NOEL MD
Associate Professor of Medicine
Division of Hematology-Oncology
Mayo College of Medicine
Scottsdale, AZ, USA

LUIGI NOTARANGELO MD
Jeffrey Modell Chair of Pediatric Immunology Research,
Division of Immunology,
Children's Hospital Boston,
Professor of Pediatrics and Pathology
Harvard Medical School
Boston, MA, USA

THOMAS B. NUTMAN MD
Head,
Helminth Immunology Section,
Clinical Parasitology Section
Laboratory of Parasitic Diseases
National Institutes of Health
Bethesda, MD, USA

STEPHEN L. NUTT PhD
Professor
Molecular Immunology
The Walter and Eliza Hall Institute
Melbourne, VIC, Australia

JOÃO B. OLIVEIRA MD, PhD
Assistant Chief,
Immunology Service,
Department of Laboratory Medicine at National Institutes
of Health,
Head
Human Disorders of Lymphocyte Homeostasis Unit
National Institutes of Health
Bethesda, MD, USA

CHRIS M. OLSON, JR. PhD, LT, MSC, USN
Microbiologist
National Naval Medical Center
Microbiology Laboratory
Bethesda, MD, USA

JOHN J. O'SHEA MD
Scientific Director
Molecular Immunology and Inflammation Branch
National Institute of Arthritis and Muscoskeletal and Skin
Diseases
Bethesda, MD, USA

SUNG-YUN PAI MD
Assistant Professor of Pediatrics
Division of Pediatric Hematology-Oncology
Children's Hospital Boston
Department of Pediatric Oncology
Dana-Farber Cancer Institute
Harvard Medical School
Boston, MA, USA

LAVANNYA PANDIT MD
Assistant Professor of Medicine
Department of Medicine, Pulmonary/Critical Care Section
Baylor College of Medicine
Houston, TX, USA

MARY E. PAUL MD
Associate Professor
Department of Pediatrics
Texas Children's Hospital
Houston, TX, USA

SIMON H.S. PEARCE MD, FRCP
Professor of Endocrinology
Institute of Genetic Medicine
International Centre for Life
Newcastle University
Newcastle-upon-Tyne, UK

ERIK J. PETERSON MD
Center for Immunology
Department of Medicine
University of Minnesota
Minneapolis, MN, USA

CAPUCINE PICARD MD, PhD
Director,
Study Center for Primary Immunodeficiencies,
Assistance Publique Hôpitaux de Paris,
Necker Hospital,
Paris,
Research associate
Laboratory of Human Genetics of Infectious Diseases
Necker Branch
INSERM U980
Necker Medical School
Paris Descartes University
Paris Sorbonne Cité, France

WERNER J. PICHLER MD
Professor of Internal Medicine and Immunology,
Head of Allergology
Department of Rheumatology, Clinical Immunology
and Allergology
Inselspital/University Hospital of Bern
Bern, Switzerland

STEFANIA PITTALUGA MD, PhD
Staff Physician
Laboratory of Pathology
National Cancer Institute
National Institutes of Health
Hematopathology Section
Bethesda, MD, USA

ANNE PUEL PhD
Research Associate
Laboratory of Human Genetics of Infectious Diseases
Necker Branch
INSERM U980
Necker Medical School
Paris Descartes University
Paris Sorbonne Cité, France

ANDREAS RADBRUCH PhD
Scientific Director
Deutsches Rheuma-Forschungszentrum Berlin (DRFZ)
Leibniz Institute
Berlin, Germany

STEPHEN T. REECE PhD
Staff Scientist
Department of Immunology
Max-Planck-Institute for Infection Biology
Berlin, Germany

JOHN D. REVEILLE MD
Professor of Medicine
Division of Rheumatology
Department of Medicine
University of Texas Health Science Center at Houston
Houston, TX, USA

ROBERT R. RICH MD
Professor of Medicine and Microbiology
University of Alabama at Birmingham
Birmingham, AL, USA

CHRISTINE RIVAT PhD
Research Associate
Institute of Child Health
Molecular Immunology Unit
London, UK

BRUCE W.S. ROBINSON MBBS, MD, FRACP, FRCP, OTMTH, FCCP
Professor of Respiratory Medicine
University of Western Australia
School of Medicine and Pharmacology
Crawley, WA, Australia

JOHN R. RODGERS PhD
Assistant Professor
Department of Immunology
Baylor College of Medicine
Houston, TX, USA

CHAIM M. ROIFMAN MD, FRCPC
Professor
Department of Paediatrics and Immunology
The Hospital for Sick Children
Toronto, ON, Canada

ANTONY ROSEN MD
Mary Betty Stevens Professor of Medicine,
Professor of Medicine and Pathology
Director
Division of Rheumatology
Johns Hopkins University School of Medicine
Baltimore, MD, USA

JAMES T. ROSENBAUM MD
Edward E. Rosenbaum Professor of Inflammation Research
Departments of Ophthalmology
Medicine and Cell Biology
Oregon Health and Science University
Portland, OR, USA

BARRY T. ROUSE DVM, PhD, DSc
Distinguished Professor
Department of Pathobiology
University of Tennessee
Knoxville, TN, USA

SCOTT D. ROWLEY MD
Chief
Blood and Marrow Transplantation
John Theurer Cancer Center
Hackensack University Medical Center
Hackensack, NJ, USA

SHIMON SAKAGUCHI MD, PhD
Professor and Chair
Department of Experimental Pathology
Insititute for Frontier Medical Sciences
Kyoto University
Kyoto, Japan

MARKO SALMI MD, PhD
Molecular Medicine
Department of Medical Biochemistry and Genetics
University of Turku
Turku, Finland

HARRY W. SCHROEDER, JR. MD, PhD
Professor of Medicine, Microbiology, and Genetics
Division of Clinical Immunology and Rheumatology
Director, UAB Program in Immunology
University of Alabama at Birmingham
Birmingham, AL, USA

MARKUS J.H. SEIBEL MD, PhD, FRACP
Professor of Medicine
Department of Endocrinology and
Bone Research Program
ANZAC Research Institute
The University of Sydney
Concord, NSW, Australia

CARLO SELMI MD
Assistant Professor of Medicine,
Division of Rheumatology,
Allergy and Clinical Immunology,
University of California at Davis,
Davis, CA, USA,
Department of Medicine and Hepatobiliary Immunopathology Unit
IRCCS Istituto Clinico Humanitas
Department of Translational Medicine
University of Milan
Milan, Italy

WILLIAM M. SHAFER PhD
Professor of Microbiology and Immunology,
Department of Microbiology and Immunology,
Emory University School of Medicine,
Atlanta, GA, USA
Laboratories of Bacterial Pathogenesis
VA Medical Center
Research Service
Decatur, GA, USA

PREDIMAN K. SHAH MD
Director,
Division of Cardiology and Oppenheimer Atherosclerosis
Research Center,
Cedars Sinai Heart Institute,
Shapell and Webb Professor of Medicine
Cedars Sinai Medical Center
Los Angeles, CA, USA

SUSHMA SHANKAR BM, BCh, Ba Physiol Sci (Hons), MRCS
Academic Clinical Fellow
Department of Surgery
John Radcliffe Hospital
Oxford, UK

ALAN R. SHAW PhD
Chairman and Chief Scientific Officer
VaxInnate Corporation
Cranbury, NJ, USA

WILLIAM T. SHEARER MD, PhD
Allergy and Immunology Service,
Texas Children's Hospital,
Professor of Pediatrics and Immunology,
Section of Allergy and Immunology
Department of Pediatrics
Baylor College of Medicine
Houston, TX , USA

JAVED SHEIKH MD, FAAAAI
Assistant Professor, Harvard Medical School
Clinical Director
Allergy and Inflammation Division
Beth Israel Deaconess Medical Center
Boston, MA, USA

RICHARD SIEGEL MD, PhD
Chief
Immunoregulation Section
Autoimmunity Branch
NIAMS National Institutes of Health
Bethesda, MD, USA

ANNA SIMON MD, PhD
Associate Professor of Immunodeficiency and Autoinflammation
Department of General Internal Medicine
N4i Centre for Immunodeficiency and Autoinflammation
(NCIA)
Radboud University Nijmegen Medical Centre
Nijmegen, The Netherlands

PHILIP L. SIMONIAN MD
Assistant Professor of Medicine
University of Colorado Denver
Aurora, CO, USA

GIDEON P. SMITH MD, PhD
Director Connective Tissue Diseases
Department of Dermatology
Massachusetts General Hospital of Harvard University
Boston, MA, USA

JUSTINE R. SMITH MBBS, PhD, FRANZCO, FRACS
Associate Professor of Ophthalmology
Casey Eye Institute,
Oregon Health and Science University,
Portland, OR, USA

ANDREW L. SNOW PhD
Assistant Professor
Department of Pharmacology
Uniformed Services University of the Health Sciences
Bethesda, MD, USA

DAVID S. STEPHENS MD
Professor of Medicine, Microbiology & Immunology,
and Epidemiology
Emory University School of Medicine
Vice President for Research
Robert W. Woodruff Health Sciences Center
Emory University
Atlanta, GA, USA

JOHN H. STONE MD, MPH
Associate Professor of Medicine,
Harvard Medical School,
Director of Clinical Rheumatology
Rheumatology Unit
Massachusetts General Hospital
Boston, MA, USA

ALEX STRAUMANN MD
Professor of Gastroenterology
Swiss EoE Research Group
Department of Gastroenterology
University Hospital Basel
Basel, Switzerland

HELEN C. SU MD, PhD
Chief
Human Immunological Diseases Unit
Laboratory of Host Defenses
National Institute of Allergy and Infectious Diseases
National Institutes of Health
Bethesda, MD, USA

LOUISE SWAINSON PhD
Assistant Professional Researcher
Division of Experimental Medicine
University of California at San Francisco
San Francisco, CA, USA

EWA SZYMANSKA-MROCZEK BS
Graduate Student
Department of Microbiology
University of Alabama at Birmingham
Birmingham, AL, USA

NAOMI TAYLOR MD, PhD
Professor (Inserm Research Director)
Institut de Génétique Moléculaire de Montpellier,
Montpellier, France

ADRIAN J. THRASHER PhD, FRCP, FRCPCH, FMedSci
Professor of Paediatric Immunology
UCL Institute of Child Health
University College London
London, UK

LAURA TIMARES PhD
Associate Professor of Dermatology
Department of Dermatology
University of Alabama at Birmingham School of Medicine
Birmingham, AL, USA

RAUL M. TORRES PhD
Associate Professor of Immunology
Integrated Department of Immunology
University of Colorado School of Medicine and
National Jewish Health
Denver, CO, USA

GÜLBÛ UZEL MD
Staff Clinician
Laboratory of Clinical Infectious Diseases, NIAID, NIH
Allergy & Immunology - Clinical & Laboratory Immunology
and Pediatric Rheumatology
National Institute of Allergy and Infectious Diseases
National Institutes of Health
Bethesda, MD, USA

JOS W.M. VAN DER MEER MD, PhD
Professor of Medicine,
Head
Department of General Internal Medicine
Nijmegen Institute for Infection, Inflammation and Immunity
N4i Centre for Immunodeficiency and Autoinflammation
(NCIA)
Radboud University Nijmegen Medical Centre
Nijmegen, The Netherlands

JEROEN C.H. VAN DER HILST MD
Internal Medicine Resident
Department of General Internal Medicine
Radboud University Nijmegen Medical Center
Nijmegen, The Netherlands

JOHN VARGA MD
John and Nancy Hughes Professor of Medicine
Division of Rheumatology
Northwestern University
Feinberg School of Medicine
Chicago, IL, USA

MERYL WALDMAN MD
Senior Clinical Research Fellow
Kidney Disease Section
Kidney Disease Branch
National Institute of Diabetes and Digestive and Kidney Diseases
National Institute of Health
Bethesda, MD, USA

PETER WEISER MD
Assistant Professor of Pediatric Rheumatology
Division of Rheumatology
Department of Pediatrics
The University of Alabama at Birmingham
Birmingham, AL, USA

PETER F. WELLER MD, FACP, FAAAAI
Professor of Medicine,
Harvard Medical School,
Professor of Immunology and Infectious Diseases,
Harvard School of Public Health,
Chief
Allergy and Inflammation Division
Chief
Infectious Diseases Division
Beth Israel Deaconess Medical Center
Boston, MA, USA

CORNELIA M. WEYAND MD, PhD
Professor of Medicine
Stanford University
Stanford, CA, USA

THERESA L. WHITESIDE PhD, ABMLI
Professor of Pathology, Immunology and Otolryngology
University of Pittsburgh School of Medicine
University of Pittsburgh Cancer Institute
Pittsburgh, PA, USA

FREDRICK M. WIGLEY MD
Professor of Medicine
Department of Medicine
Division of Rheumatology
Johns Hopkins University School of Medicine
Baltimore, MD, USA

ROBERT J. WINCHESTER MD
Professor of Medicine
College of Physicians and Surgeons
Columbia University
New York, NY, USA

KAJSA WING PhD
Assistant Professor
Department of Medical Biophysics and Biomedicine
Section of Medical Inflammation Research
Karolinska Institute
Stockholm, Sweden

KATHRYN WOOD DPhil
Professor of Immunology
Nuffield Department of Surgical Sciences
University of Oxford
John Radcliffe Hospital
Oxford, UK

HUI XU MD, PhD
Professor of Dermatology
University of Alabama at Birmingham
Birmingham, AL, USA

SHEN-YING ZHANG MD, PhD
Research associate
St. Giles Laboratory of Human Genetics of Infectious Diseases
Rockefeller Branch
The Rockefeller University
New York, NY, USA

VALÉRIE S. ZIMMERMANN PhD
Assistant Professor
Institut de Génétique Moléculaire de Montpellier
Montpellier, France

Preface to the first edition

Clinical immunology is a discipline with a distinguished history, rooted in the prevention and treatment of infectious diseases in the late nineteenth and early twentieth centuries. The conquest of historical scourges such as smallpox and (substantially) polio and relegation of several other diseases to the category of medical curiosities is often regarded as the most important achievement of medical science of the past fifty years. Nevertheless, the challenges facing immunologists in the efforts to control infectious diseases remain formidable; HIV infection, malaria and tuberculosis are but three examples of diseases of global import that elude control despite major commitments of monetary and intellectual resources.

Although firmly grounded in the study and application of defenses to microbial infection, since the 1960s clinical immunology has emerged as a far broader discipline. Dysfunction of the immune system has been increasingly recognized as a pathogenic mechanism that can lead to an array of specific diseases and failure of virtually every organ system. Pardoxically, although the importance of the immune system in disease pathogenesis is generally appreciated, the place of clinical immunology as a practice discipline has been less clear. As most of the non-infectious diseases if the human immune system lead eventually to failure of other organs, it has been organ-specific subspecialists who have usually dealt with their consequences. Recently, however, the outlook has begun to change as new diagnostic tools increasingly allow the theoretical possibility of intervention much earlier in disease processes, often before irreversible target organ destruction occurs. More importantly, this theoretical possibility is increasingly realized as clinical immunologists find themselves in the vanguard of translating molecular medicine from laboratory bench to patient bedside.

In many settings, clinical immunologists today function as primary care physicians in the management of patients with inmune-deficiency, allergic, and autoimmune diseases. Indeed many influential voices in the clinical disciplines of allergy and rheumatology support increasing coalescence of these traditional subspecialities around their intellectual core of immunology. In addition to his or her role as a primary care physician, the clinical immunologist is increasingly being looked to as a consultant, as scientific and clinical advances enhance his or her expertise. The immunologist with a 'generalist' perspective can be particularly helpful in the application of unifying principles of diagnosis and treatment across the broad spectrum of immunologic diseases.

Clinical Immunology: Principles and Practice has emerged from this concept of the clinical immunologist as both primary care physician and expert consultant in the management of patients with immunologic diseases. It opens in full appreciation of the critical role of fundamental immunology in this rapidly evolving clinical discipline. Authors of basic science chapters were asked, however, to cast their subjects in a context of clinical relevance. We believe the result is a well-balanced exposition of basic immunology for the clinician.

The initial two sections on basic principles of immunology are followed by two sections that focus in detail on the role of the immune system in defenses against infectious organisms. The approach is two-pronged. It begins first with a systematic survey of immune responses to pathogenic agents followed by a detailed treatment of immunologic deficiency syndromes. Pathogenic mechanisms of both congenital and acquired immune deficiency diseases are discussed, as are the infectious complications that characterize these diseases. Befitting its importance, the subject of HIV infection and AIDS receives particular attention, with separate chapters on the problem of infection in the immunocompromised host, HIV infection in children, anti-retroviral therapy and current progress in the development of HIV vaccines.

The classic allergic diseases are the most common immunologic diseases in the population, ranging from atopic disease to drug allergy to organ-specific allergic disease (e.g., of the lungs, eye and skin). They constitute a foundation for the practice of clinical immunology, particularly for those physicians with a practice orientation defined by formal subspecialty training in allergy and immunology. A major section is consequently devoted to these diseases, with an emphasis on pathophysiology as the basis for rational management.

The next two sections deal separately with systemic and organ-specific immunologic diseases. The diseases considered in the first of these sections are generally regarded as the core practice of the clinical immunologist with subdisciplinary emphasis in rheumatology. The second section considers diseases of specific organ failure as consequences of immunologically mediated processes that may involve virtually any organ system. These diseases include as typical examples the demyelinating diseases, insulin-dependent diabetes mellitus, the glomerulonephritides and inflammatory bowel diseases. It is in management of such diseases that the discipline of clinical immunology will have an increasing role as efforts focus on inetervention early in the pathogenic process and involve diagnostic and therapeutic tools of ever-increasing sophistication.

One of the major clinical areas in which the expertise of a clinical immunologist is most frequently sought is that of allogeneic organ transplantation. A full section is devoted to the issue of transplantation of solid organs, with an introductory chapter on general principles of transplantation and management of transplantation rejection followed by separate chapters dealing with the special problems of transplantation of specific organs or organ systems.

Appreciation of both the molecular and clinical features of lymphoid malignancies is important to the clinical immunologist regardless of subspecialty background, notwithstanding the fact that primary responsibility for management of such patients will generally fall to the haematologist/oncologist. A separate section is consequently devoted to the lymphocytic leukemias and lymphomas that constitute the majority of malignancies seen in the context of a clinical immunology practice. The separate issues of immune responses to tumors and immunological strategies to treatment of malignant diseases are subjects of additional chapters.

Another important feature is the attention to therapy of immunologic diseases. This theme is constant throughout the chapters on the allergic and immunologic diseases, and because of the importance the editors attach to clinical immunology as a therapeutic discipline, an extensive section is also devoted specifically to this subject. Subsections are devoted to issues of immunologic reconstitution, with three chapters on treatment of immunodeficiencies, malignancies and metabolic diseases by bone marrow transplantation. Also included is a series of chapters on pharmaceutical agents currently available to clinical immunologists, both as anti-allergic and anti-inflammatory drugs, as well as newer agents with greater specificity for T cell-mediated immune responses. The section concludes with a series of chapters that address established and potential applications of therapeutic agents and approaches that are largely based on the new techniques of molecular medicine. In addition to pharmaceutical agents the section deals in detail with such subjects as apheresis, cytokines, monoclonal antibodies and immunotoxins, gene therapy and new experimental approaches to the treatment of autoimmunity. The book concludes with a section devoted to approaches and specific techniques involved in the diagnosis of immunologic diseases. Use of the diagnostic laboratory in evaluation of complex problems of immunopathogenesis has been a hallmark of the clinical immunologist since inception of the discipline and many clinical immunologists serve as directors of diagnostic immunology laboratories. Critical assessment of the utilization of techniques ranging from lymphocyte cloning to flow cytomeric phenotyping to molecular diagnostics are certain to continue as an important function of the clinical immunologist, particularly in his or her role as expert consultant.

In summary, we have intended to provide the reader with a comprehensive and authoritative treatise on the broad subject of clinical immunology, with particular emphasis on the diagnosis and treatment of immunological diseases. It is anticipated that the book will be used most frequently by the physician specialist practicing clinical immunology, both in his or her role as a primary physician and as a subsequent consultant. It is hoped, however, that the book will also be of considerable utility to the non-immunologist. Many of the diseases discussed authoritatively in the book are diseases commonly encountered by the generalist physician. Indeed, as noted, because clinical immunology involves diseases of virtually all organ systems, competence in the diagnosis and management of immunological diseases is important to virtually all clinicians. The editors would be particularly pleased to see the book among the references readily available to the practicing internist, pediatrician and family physician.

Robert R. Rich
Thomas A. Fleisher
Benjamin D. Schwartz
William T. Shearer
Warren Strober

Preface to the fourth edition

How much has changed since publication of the 3rd edition of *Clinical Immunology* in 2008? Plenty! And we hope that we have successfully captured the essence of those changes with this new edition. Perhaps the most difficult changes to follow relate to continuing refinements in our understanding of the molecular complexities in the pathogenesis of immunologic diseases (how many kinases/interleukins/transcription factors can there possibly be?). Moreover, the complexities aren't limited to molecular pathways; they also extend to the diseases within the purview of clinical immunologists. Clinicians continue to be intrigued by the seemingly paradoxical behavior of immune responses as exemplified by the growing realization of the two-sided coin closeness of immunodeficiency and autoimmunity. Thus, experts in immunodeficiency, allergy and rheumatology now find increasingly common discourse in the evaluation and management of their patients. We further believe that this increasing appreciation of complexity offers additional, and oftentimes more specific, targets for control of immune responses and hence new avenues in the prevention and treatment of diseases of inflammation and immunity.

An obvious new feature of the 4th edition reflects appreciation of how the continuing proliferation of such targets can impact progress in disease management (many of which are, in fact, practice-based rather than molecular). Hence we have challenged chapter contributors to share their specialized expertise in immunologic diseases or mechanisms in order to predict how new opportunities in science or clinical practice might be translated into improved patient care. Many authors happily accepted the challenge, providing a new section of their chapters that is specifically focused on anticipated advances in translational research and accompanied by summary boxes entitled "On the Horizon". We believe that these predictions can fertilize the creativity of translational immunologists, both clinicians and basic scientists. Indeed, reflecting the commonality of mechanisms and pathogenetic pathways across the spectrum of immunologic and inflammatory diseases, we add an editorial prediction—that some of the most useful ideas put forward by authors of one chapter will bear fruit in the minds of translational physicians and scientists working on quite different diseases.

Much of the content of this edition will be familiar to users of previous editions. In one (albeit rather massive) full-colored volume we have again attempted to balance *Principles* with *Practice*. We have emphasized the use of summary boxes in multiple "flavors" to provide a concise summary of essential points in the text. A significant number of new chapters and new authors have been added. In recognition of an increasingly global readership, chapter authorship has become more international. And, in keeping with remarkable advances in innate immunity, readers will notice that broad principles of inflammation and its roles in immune defenses and disease pathogenesis again demand increased attention.

In the tradition of the previous editions, we have pursued the goal of providing a comprehensive overview of disorders of the immune system useful to specialists in clinical immunology and its various organ-based subspecialties. But we have also attempted to anchor our consideration of immunologic diseases in their practical management. To that end, we trust that the book can serve not only as a key resource for clinical immunologists, but also as a useful adjunct to the libraries of generalist physicians. We hope that we have again accomplished that ambitious goal.

Finally, we recognize the essential contributions of numerous individuals in addition to the editors and authors who have made this 4th edition a reality; in particular we thank Ms. Rachael Harrison of Elsevier for her unflagging dedication to both its quality and its timely completion.

Robert R. Rich
Thomas A. Fleisher
William T. Shearer
Harry W. Schroeder, Jr.
Anthony J. Frew
Cornelia M. Weyand

Dedication

To:
Eloise, Harlow and Roscoe Rich and Aidan, Annika and Max Todorov
Sierra, Grady, Jackson and Kenzie Fleisher
Lynn Des Prez and Christine, Mark, Christopher, Martin, John, Jesse and Melissa Shearer
Dixie, Trey & Isabel, Elena and Jeannette Schroeder
Helen, Edward, Sophie, Georgina and Alex Frew
Jörg Goronzy and Dominic and Isabel Weyand Goronzy

PART ONE
Principles of immune response

CHAPTERS

The human immune response | Robert R. Rich

Clinical immunology is a medical subspecialty largely focused on a specific physiologic process, inflammation, that is essential to good health, particularly in defense against pathogenic organisms and recovery from injury. But inflammation, mediated by the cells and soluble products of the immune system, is also a powerful contributor to the pathogenesis of diseases that affect virtually every organ system. A consequent challenge for clinical immunologists, both clinicians and basic scientists, is to reduce a dizzying array of disease descriptions to a systematic approach to disease management or prevention and to translate new discoveries and concepts into more effective treatment or prevention.

This introductory chapter is directed to non-immunologist clinicians and researchers. It is based on the notion that appreciation of fundamental aspects of immune responses will facilitate understanding of immunologic diseases. The chapter is structured as an introduction to the interacting elements of the human immune system and their disordered functions in diseases. The subtleties are described in detail in the chapters that follow.

The host–microbe interaction

The vertebrate immune system is a product of eons of evolutionary struggle between rapidly evolving microbial pathogens and their much less rapidly reproducing, and hence less adaptable, hosts.[1] Unable to win the battle with microbial invaders by rapid mutation and selection, the vertebrate immune system employs a strategy of complexity and redundancy involving both the individual organism and its collective population. Microbes respond by adaptations to particular elements of the immune system that they can turn to their own advantage. Reflecting plasticity of the response, specific defenses differ based upon the nature of the infectious agent and its point of entry and distribution within the body. Regardless of the defense mechanism, an intended outcome is destruction or neutralization of the invading organism. A secondary consequence, however, can be collateral damage to host cells. These cells can be involved in the attack either as sites of microbial residence or as "innocent bystanders." Depending on the site and severity of the host's defensive response, it may be accompanied by local and/or systemic symptoms and signs of inflammation.

Acquired and innate immunity

Immune responses are traditionally classified as acquired (or specific) and innate (or nonspecific) (Table 1.1). The acquired immune system, present uniquely in vertebrates, is specialized for development of an inflammatory response based on recognition of specific "foreign" macromolecules that are predominantly, but not exclusively, proteins, peptides and carbohydrates. Its primary actors are antibodies, B lymphocytes, T lymphocytes, and antigen-presenting cells.

Innate immune responses are phylogenetically far more ancient, being widely represented in multicellular phyla.[2,3] Rather than being based upon exquisitely specific recognition of a diverse array of macromolecules (i.e., antigens), they are focused on recognition of common molecular signatures of potential pathogens.[4] For responses of both types, defense effector mechanisms can involve elaboration of soluble products acting systemically (humoral immunity) or can require direct cell-to-cell contact or the activity of cytokines and chemokines acting in the cellular microenvironment (cell-mediated immunity). And most immune responses include participation of both modes of response. The elements of innate immunity are diverse (Chapter 3). They include physical barriers to pathogen invasion (such as skin, mucous membranes, cilia, and mucus), as well as an array of cellular and soluble factors that can be activated by secreted or cell-surface products of the pathogen. Activation of innate immunity induces an inflammatory response using mechanisms that are broadly shared with those of the specific immune system. These include natural killer (NK) cell-mediated cytotoxicity, activation of granulocytes and other phagocytes, the secretion of inflammatory cytokines and chemokines, and the interactions of the many participants in the complement cascade.

Despite substantial overlap and redundancy between the innate and acquired immune systems,[5] a distinguishing feature of the latter is the need for clonal expansion of individual lymphocytes directly activated by antigen and requiring recognition by antigen-specific, gene-rearranged receptors. Because recognition of pathogens by the innate immune system relies on germ-line encoded, non-rearranged receptors held in common by the specific cell type, innate immunity is more rapidly responsive. It can initiate in minutes to hours and generally precedes development of a primary acquired immune response by at least several days.

Cells of the immune system

The major cellular constituents of both innate and acquired immunity originate in the bone marrow where they differentiate from multipotent hematopoietic stem cells along several pathways to become granulocytes, lymphocytes, and antigen-presenting cells (Chapter 2).

Table 1.1 Features of innate and acquired immune systems

Distinguishing features	
Innate immunity	**Acquired immunity**
Receptors fixed and based on pathogen molecular patterns	Receptors clonally variable and based on gene rearrangement
Does not require immunization	Consequence of B- and/or T-cell activation
Limited memory	Immunologic memory well developed
Includes physical barriers to pathogen	Antibody and cytotoxic T cells
Common features	
Cytokines and chemokines	
Complement cascade	
Phagocytic cells	
NK cells	
"Natural" autoantibodies	

Granulocytes

Polymorphonuclear leukocytes (granulocytes) are classified by light microscopy into three types. By far the most abundant in the peripheral circulation are neutrophils, which are principal defense-effector cells of antibody and complement-mediated immune responses (Chapter 21). They are phagocytic cells that ingest, kill and degrade microbes and other targets of an immune attack within specialized cytoplasmic vacuoles. The phagocytic activity of neutrophils is promoted by their surface display of receptors for antibody molecules (specifically the Fc portion of IgG molecules) (Chapter 14) and complement proteins (particularly the C3b component) (Chapter 20). Neutrophils are the predominant cell type in acute inflammatory infiltrates and are the primary effector cells in immune responses to pyogenic organisms (Chapter 24).

Eosinophils (Chapter 23) and basophils (Chapter 22) are the other circulating forms of granulocytes. A close relative of the basophil, but derived from distinct bone marrow precursors, is the tissue mast cell, which does not circulate in the blood. Eosinophils, basophils, and mast cells are important in defenses against multicellular pathogens, particularly helminths (Chapter 29). Their defensive functions are not based on phagocytic capabilities, but rather on their ability to discharge potent biological mediators into the cellular microenvironment. This process, termed degranulation, can be triggered by antigen-specific IgE molecules that bind to basophils and mast cells via high-affinity receptors for the Fc portion of IgE (FcεR) on their surfaces. In addition to providing a mechanism for helminthic host defenses, this is also the principal mechanism involved in acute (IgE-mediated) allergic reactions (Chapters 39–47).

Lymphocytes

Four broad categories of lymphocytes are identified based on display of particular surface molecules: B cells, T cells, NK cells, and natural killer T (NKT) cells. All lymphocytes differentiate from common lymphoid stem cells in the bone marrow. B cells create their immunoglobulin receptors in the bone marrow, and differentiate into antibody-producing cells in the periphery

(Chapter 7). T cells undergo further maturation and selection in the thymus for the rearrangement and expression of antigen receptors useful in self/nonself discrimination (Chapter 8).

T and B cells are the heart of specific immune recognition, a property reflecting their clonally-specific cell surface receptors for antigen (Chapter 4). The T-cell receptor (TCR) for antigen is a heterodimeric integral membrane molecule expressed exclusively by T lymphocytes. B-cell receptors for antigen (BCR) are membrane immunoglobulin (mIg) molecules of the same antigenic specificity that the cell and its terminally differentiated progeny, plasma cells, will secrete as soluble antibodies. Non-dividing, long-lived plasma cells, resident in bone marrow and solid lymphoid organs, may account substantially for persistence of antibody responses (including production of autoantibodies) over many years.[6]

Receptors for "antigen" on the third class of lymphocytes, NK cells, are not clonally expressed. Expressing receptors, however, for moieties that can be regarded as molecular signatures of pathogens, NK cells serve as major constituents of innate immunity. They also recognize target cells that might otherwise elude the immune system (Chapters 2, 17). Recognition of NK-cell targets is based largely on what their targets lack rather than on what they express. NK cells express receptors of several types for major histocompatibility complex (MHC) class I molecules via killer cell immunoglobulin-like receptors (KIR).[5,7] KIR can either inhibit or activate NK-cell activity utilizing receptors for MHC class I molecules or other immune adaptor molecules that express in their intracellular domain a tyrosine-based inhibitory-motif (ITIM) or tyrosine-based activation motif (ITAM), respectively. NK cells will kill target cells unless they receive an inhibitory signal transmitted by an ITIM receptor. Virus-infected cells and tumor cells that attempt to escape T-cell recognition by downregulating their expression of class I molecules become susceptible to NK-cell-mediated killing.

Although NK-cell-mediated innate immunity has been long considered to lack immunologic memory, recent studies suggest that NK cells may "remember" previous encounters with microbes or other antigens, the molecular basis of which is ill-defined.[5] NK cells can also participate in antigen-specific immune responses by virtue of their surface display of the activating ITAM receptor CD16, which binds the constant (Fc) region of IgG molecules. This enables them to function as effectors of a cytolytic mechanism termed antibody-dependent cellular cytotoxicity (ADCC), a mechanism exploited clinically with monoclonal antibody therapeutic agents.[8]

In general, pathways leading to differentiation of T cells, B cells, and NK cells are mutually exclusive, representing a permanent lineage commitment. No lymphocytes express both mIg and TCR. However, NKT cells exhibit both NK-like cytotoxicity and antigen-specific T-cell responsiveness, although with limited receptor diversity.

Antigen-presenting cells

● K E Y C O N C E P T S

Features of antigen-presenting cells

- Capacity for protein antigen uptake and partial degradation
- Expression of MHC molecules (class I and class II)
- Expression of accessory molecules for interaction with T cells
- Cytokine secretion

A morphologically and functionally diverse group of cells, all of which are derived from bone marrow precursors, is specialized for presentation of antigen to lymphocytes, particularly T cells (Chapter 6). Included among such cells are monocytes (present in the peripheral circulation); macrophages (solid tissue derivatives of monocytes); cells resident within the solid organs of the immune system such as dendritic cells; cutaneous Langerhans cells (Chapter 18) and constituents of the reticular endothelial system within other solid organs. B lymphocytes that specifically capture antigen by virtue of mIg receptors can also function efficiently in antigen presentation to T cells.

Cardinal features of antigen presenting cells (APCs) include their expression of both class I and class II MHC molecules (the latter either expressed constitutively or induced by cytokines) as well as requisite accessory molecules for T-cell activation (e.g., B7-1, B7-2/CD80, CD86).[9] Upon activation, APCs elaborate cytokines that induce specific responses in cells to which they are presenting antigen.

APCs differ substantially among themselves with respect to mechanisms of antigen uptake and effector functions. Monocytes and macrophages are actively phagocytic, particularly for antibody and/or complement-coated (opsonized) antigens that bind to their surface receptors for Fcγ and C3b. These cells are also important effectors of immune responses, especially in sites of chronic inflammation. Upon further activation by T-cell cytokines, they can kill ingested microorganisms by oxidative pathways similar to those employed by polymorphonuclear leukocytes. Moreover, they can kill adjacent target cells by a cytotoxic mechanism. Mature dendritic cells are especially efficient in antigen presentation and T-cell activation, but have little phagocytic function. Their maturation is induced in actively phagocytic immature dendritic cells by inflammatory stimuli, especially via cells of the innate immune system.[10]

The interaction between B cells acting as APCs and T lymphocytes is notable as the cells are involved in a mutually amplifying circuitry of antigen presentation and response. The process is initiated by antigen capture through B-cell mIg and ingestion by receptor-mediated endocytosis. This is followed by antigen degradation and then display to T cells as oligopeptides bound to MHC molecules. Like other APCs, B cells display CD80, thereby providing a requisite second signal to the antigen responsive T cell via its accessory molecule for activation, CD28 (Fig. 1.1).[9] As a result of T-cell activation, T-cell cytokines that regulate B-cell differentiation and antibody production are produced and T cells are stimulated to display the surface ligand CD40L (CD154), which can serve as the second signal for B-cell activation through its inducible surface molecule CD40.

Basis of acquired immunity

The essence of acquired immunity is molecular distinction between self constituents and potential pathogens (for simplicity, self/non-self discrimination, but perhaps more precisely discrimination between molecular species perceived as signaling potential "danger" and those that do not). This discrimination is predominantly a responsibility of T lymphocytes. It reflects the selection of thymocytes that have generated specific antigen receptors, and that upon later encounter can bind both self MHC molecules and non-self antigenic peptides. The consequence of this selection process is that foreign proteins are recognized as antigens whereas self proteins are tolerated (i.e., are not perceived as antigens).

T lymphocytes generally recognize antigens as a complex of short linear peptides bound to MHC molecules on the surfaces of APCs (Chapter 6). With the exception of superantigens (see below), T cells do not bind antigen in native conformation, nor do they recognize antigen in solution. The vast majority of antigens for T cells are oligopeptides. However, the antigen receptors of NKT cells can recognize lipid and glycolipid antigens that are presented to them by MHC-like CD1 molecules.[11]

Antigen recognition by T cells differs fundamentally from that by antibodies, which are produced by B lymphocytes and their derivatives. Antibodies, unlike T cells, can bind complex macromolecules and can bind them either at cell surfaces or in solution. Moreover, antibodies show less preference for recognition of proteins; antibodies against carbohydrates, nucleic acids, lipids, and simple chemical moieties can be readily produced. Although B cells can also be rendered unresponsive by exposure to self-antigens, particularly during differentiation in the bone marrow, this process does not define foreignness within the context of self-MHC recognition.

Clonal basis of immunological memory

An essential element of self/nonself discrimination is the clonal nature of antigen recognition. Although the immune system can recognize a vast array of distinct antigens, all of the receptors of a single T cell or B cell (and their clonal progeny) have identical antigen-binding sites and hence a particular specificity (Chapter 4). A direct consequence is the capacity for antigen-driven immunologic memory. This phenomenon derives from the fact that, after an initial encounter with antigen, clones of lymphocytes of appropriate specificity proliferate, resulting in

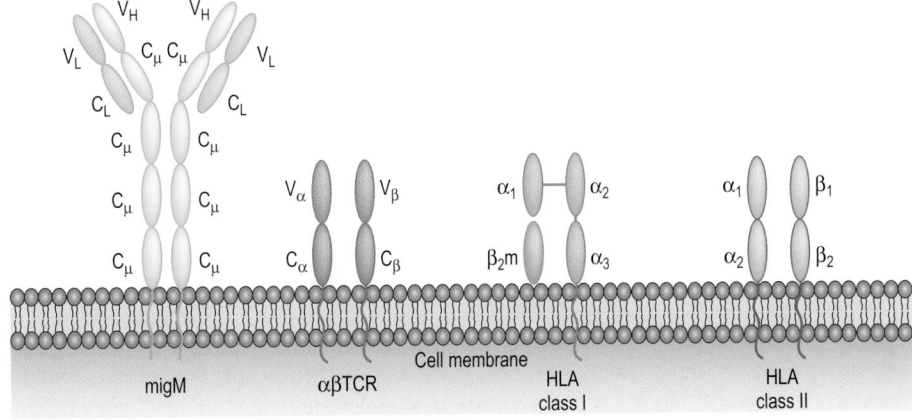

Fig 1.1 Antigen-binding molecules. Antigen-binding pockets of immunoglobulin (Ig) and T-cell receptor (TCR) are comprised of variable (V) segments of two chains translated from transcripts that represent V(D)J or VJ gene segment rearrangements. Antigen-binding pockets of Ig molecules are formed from contributions of V regions of both light (L) and heavy (H) chains. Antigen-binding grooves of MHC molecules are formed with contributions from α_1 and β_1 domains of class II molecules and from α_1 and α_2 domains of class I molecules. In contrast to Ig and TCR, MHC binding sites do not reflect genetic rearrangements. All of these molecules are members of the immunoglobulin superfamily. C, constant-region domain; β_2m, beta-2 microglobulin; mIgM, membrane immunoglobulin M; HLA, human leukocyte antigen.

a greater and more rapid response upon subsequent antigen encounter. These two hallmarks of the specific immune system, clonal specificity and immunological memory, provide a conceptual foundation for the use of vaccines in prevention of infectious diseases (Chapter 90). Immunologic memory involves not only the T cells charged with antigen recognition, but also the T cells and B cells that mediate the efferent limb of an inflammatory response. In its attack on foreign targets, the immune system can exhibit exquisite specificity for the inducing antigen, as is seen in the lysis of virus-infected target cells by cytolytic T cells. However, an immunologic attack *in vivo* also has important elements that are independent of antigen recognition, such as the response of phagocytes to inflammatory mediators.

Antigen-binding molecules

> ● KEY CONCEPTS
>
> **Features of the immunoglobulin superfamily**
>
> - Large family of ancestrally related genes (probably > 100 members)
> - Most products involved in immune system function or other cell–cell interactions
> - Proteins exhibit domain structure of ∼100 amino acids, usually translated from a single exon and characteristically with a single intra-domain disulfide bond
> - Tertiary structure of protein typified by anti-parallel strands forming a pair of β-pleated sheets

Three sets of molecules are responsible for the specificity of acquired immune responses by virtue of their capacity to bind foreign antigen. These molecules are immunoglobulins (Ig), TCRs and MHC molecules (Fig. 1.1) (Chapters 4, 5). All are products of a very large family of ancestrally-related genes, the immunoglobulin superfamily (IgSF).[12] Members of the IgSF family, which includes many other molecules essential to induction and regulation of immune responses, exhibit characteristic structural features. The most notable of these is organization into homologous domains of approximately 110 amino acids that are usually encoded by a single exon and characteristically have an intra-domain disulfide bond. Typically, each domain assumes a configuration of anti-parallel strands that form two opposing β-pleated sheets.

Immunoglobulins and T-cell receptors

The remarkable specificity of Ig and TCR molecules for antigen is achieved by a mechanism of genetic recombination that is unique to Ig and TCR genes (Chapter 4). The antigen-binding site of both types of molecules is comprised of a groove formed by contributions from each of two constituent polypeptides. In the case of immunoglobulins, these are a heavy (H) chain and one of two alternative types of light (L) chains, κ or λ. In the case of TCR, either of two alternative heterodimers can constitute the antigen-binding molecule, one comprised of α and β chains, and the other of γ and δ chains. The polypeptides contributing to both Ig and TCR can be divided into an antigen-binding amino-terminal variable (V) domain and one or more carboxy-terminal constant (i.e., non-variable) domains. Ig constant region domains generally include specific sites responsible for the biological effector functions and other activities of the antibody molecule (Chapter 14).

> ● KEY CONCEPTS
>
> **Comparison of T-cell and B-cell receptors for antigen**
>
> **Similarities**
>
> - Members of the Ig superfamily
> - Heterodimeric antigen-binding groove
> - Divided into variable and constant regions
> - Variable regions constructed by V(D)J rearrangements
> - Non-genomic N-nucleotide additions at V(D)J junctions
> - Exhibit allelic exclusion
> - Mature T cells and B cells display receptors of one and only one antigenic specificity
> - Negative selection for receptors with self-antigen specificity
> - Transmembrane signaling involving co-receptor molecules
>
> **Differences**
>
> - Ig can be secreted; TCR is not
> - Ig can bind antigen in solution; TCR binds antigen when presented by MHC molecule on APC
> - Somatic hypermutation of Ig genes
> - Isotype switching of Ig genes
> - Inflammatory effector functions by the Ig constant domains
> - Selection of TCR for self-MHC recognition

The most noteworthy feature of the vertebrate immune system is the process of genetic recombination that generates a virtually limitless array of specific antigen receptors from a rather limited genomic investment. This phenomenon is accomplished by the recombination of genomic segments that encode the variable portions of Ig and TCR polypeptides (Chapter 4).[13] The products of these rearranged genes provide a specific B or T cell with its unique antigen receptor. The mature receptor consists of the products of two or three such rearranged segments. These are designated V (variable) and J (joining), for IgL chains and TCR α and γ chains, and V, D (diversity), and J, for IgH and TCR β and δ chains. In addition to rearrangement, N-nucleotide addition also contributes substantially to potential receptor diversity. N-nucleotide addition results in the insertion at the time of rearrangement of one or more nongenomic nucleotides at the junctions between V, D, and J segments.[13] This permits receptor diversity to extend beyond germline constraints.

DNA rearrangement involved in generating T- and B-cell receptors is controlled by recombinases that are active in early thymocytes and in B precursor (p) cells in the bone marrow. The process is sequential and carefully regulated, generally leading to translation of one receptor of unique specificity for any given T or B lymphocyte. This result is achieved through a process termed allelic exclusion, wherein only one member of a pair of allelic genes potentially contributing to an Ig or TCR molecule is rearranged at a time.[14] The frequency of nonproductive rearrangements is high, two out of three. If a productive rearrangement is achieved, i.e., a full-length transcript that will encode the appropriate protein product, the other member of the allelic pair is permanently inactivated. If, on the other hand, the first effort at rearrangement is not productive, resulting in a truncated transcript, two alternatives are presented. The cell can attempt a second (or more) rearrangement at the same gene, depending upon the availability of unrearranged gene segment partners. Alternatively, the process can move to the second member of the pair on the homologous chromosome, which will similarly undergo rearrangement. This affords a cell several opportunities to construct a variable region sequence that encodes a full-length receptor transcript.

The process of allelic exclusion is not absolute, and a small number of lymphocytes will express dual in-frame Ig or TCR transcripts and in some cases surface receptors of dual specificity.[15] But B cells exclusively rearrange Ig genes, not TCR genes, and vice versa for T cells. Moreover, B cells sequentially rearrange L chain genes, typically κ before λ. Thus, B cells express either κ or λ chains, but not both. Similarly, thymocytes express α and β genes or γ and δ genes, and, with the caveat that some Vδ gene segments can rearrange with some Jα and vice versa, one never finds T cells with αδ or γβ receptors.

There is one feature of V region construction that is essentially reserved to B cells. This is somatic hypermutation (SHM), a process that can continue throughout the life of a mature B cell at the hypervariable sites of both the V_H and V_L genes.[13] The amino acid products of these sites, particularly at V, D, and J junctions, are the specific points of contact with antigen within the binding groove. As antigen is introduced into the system, mature B cells remain genetically responsive to the antigenic environment. As a consequence, through SHM of mIg, a few B cells increase their affinity for antigen. Such cells are preferentially activated, particularly at limiting doses of antigen. Thus, the average affinity of antibodies produced during the course of an immune response increases, a process termed affinity maturation. The process of SHM is not limited to V-region coding segments, but extends to 3′ and 5′ flanking sequences; indeed the start of the hypermutation domain lies within the V-gene promoter. SHM is driven by an enzyme, activation-induced cytidine deaminase (AID), that catalyzes mutation of deoxycytidine to deoxyuracil in single-stranded DNA.[16] Inactivation of AID is associated with development of hyper-IgM syndrome (Chapter 34). The process of SHM is also of pathogenetic importance in a variety of B-cell lymphomas and leukemias and in some nonlymphoid malignancies.[17]

T-cell receptors generally do not show evidence of SHM. This absence may be related to the focus on selection in the thymus involving co-recognition of a self-MHC molecule and self-peptides[18] (Chapter 8) rather than the continuous process of antigen-driven selection in the periphery by B cells after SHM. Thymic selection results in deletion by apoptosis of the vast majority of differentiating thymocytes by mechanisms that place stringent boundaries around the viability of a thymocyte with a newly expressed TCR specificity. Once a T cell is fully mature and ready for emigration from the thymus, its TCR is essentially fixed, thus reducing the likelihood of emergent autoimmune T-cell clones in the periphery.

Receptor selection

The receptor expressed by a developing thymocyte must be capable of binding with low level affinity to some particular MHC self-molecule, either class I or class II, expressed by a resident thymic APC. If it does not exhibit such binding affinity, the TCR can make further attempts to construct an appropriate receptor by additional Vα→Jα rearrangements. If it is not ultimately successful, the developing thymocyte dies. Because their receptors are generated by a process of semi-random selection of rearranging exon segments coupled with N-nucleotide additions, most thymocytes fail this test. They are consequently deleted as not being useful to an immune system that requires T cells to recognize self-MHC molecules. Thymocytes surviving this hurdle are said to have been "positively selected"[18] (Fig. 1.2A). Conversely, a small number of thymocytes bind with an unallowably high affinity for a combination of MHC molecule plus antigenic peptide expressed by a thymic APC. Because the peptides available for MHC binding at this site are derived almost entirely from self proteins, differentiating thymocytes with such receptors are intrinsically dangerous as potentially autoimmune. This deletion of thymocytes with

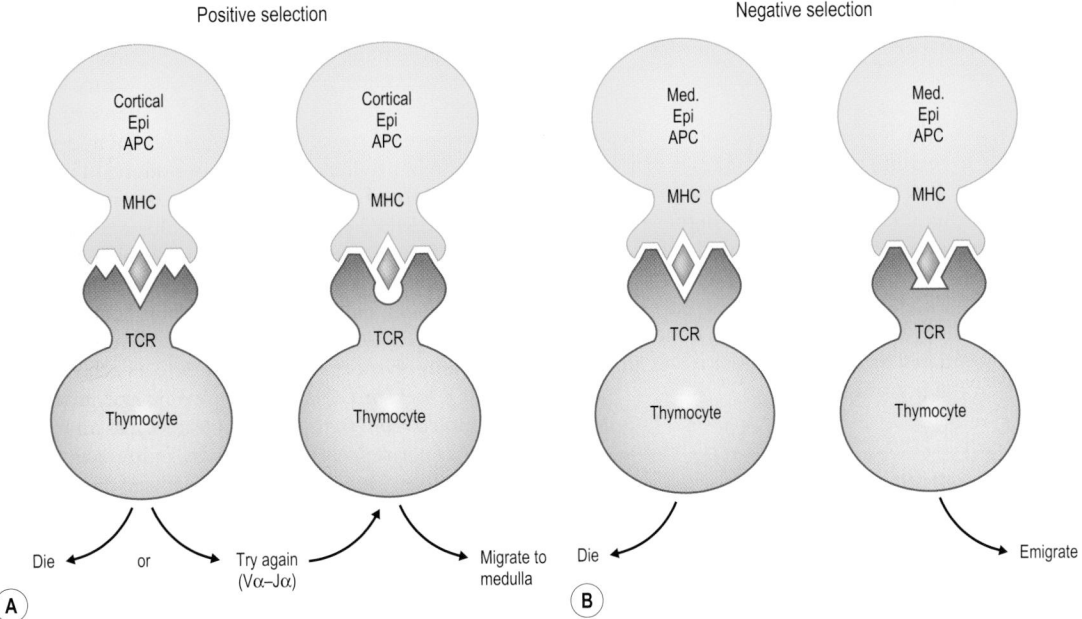

Positive selection   Negative selection

A   B

Fig 1.2 Two-stage selection of thymocytes based on binding characteristics of randomly generated TCR. (A) *Positive selection.* "Double-positive" (CD4+, CD8+) thymocytes with TCR capable of *low* avidity binding to some specific self-MHC molecule (either class I or class II) expressed by thymic cortical epithelial cells are positively selected. This process may involve sequential attempts at α gene rearrangement in order to express an αβ TCR of appropriate self-MHC specificity. If binding is to a class I molecule, the positively-selected thymocyte becomes CD8 single-positive; and if to a class II molecule, a CD4 single-positive. Thymocytes that are unsuccessful in achieving a receptor with avidity for either a class I or a class II self-MHC molecule die by apoptosis. The solid diamond represents a self-peptide derived from hydrolysis of an autologous protein present in the thymic microenvironment or synthesized within the thymic APC itself. **(B)** *Negative selection.* "Single-positive" (CD4+ *or* CD8+) thymocytes, positively selected in stage one, that display TCR with *high* avidity for the combination of self-MHC plus some self (autologous) peptide present in the thymus are negatively selected (i.e., die) as potentially "autoimmune." Those few thymocytes that have survived both positive and negative selection emigrate as mature T cells to the secondary lymphoid tissues.

high affinity receptors for self-MHC plus (presumptively) self-peptide is termed "negative selection" (Fig. 1.2B), a process that may also involve activity of regulatory T (Treg) cells.[19,20]

Although not selected for recognition of foreignness in the context of self, maturing pre-B cells in the bone marrow also are subject to negative selection upon encounter with "self" soluble or particulate antigen, and B cells in peripheral tissues can be rescued by ligand engagement in a process resembling positive selection.[21,22] Additionally, when an initial pre-B-cell mIg is cross-linked by encounter of relatively high affinity with self-antigen in the bone marrow, secondary rearrangements can occur. This process, termed receptor editing, can thus generate a new receptor lacking self reactivity (Chapter 7).[21]

Another feature that distinguishes B cells from T cells is that the cell surface antigen receptors of the former are secreted in large quantities as antibody molecules, the effector functions of which are carried out in solution or at the surfaces of other cells. Secretion is accomplished by alternative splicing of Ig transcripts to include or exclude a transmembrane segment of the Ig heavy chains.

Immunoglobulin class switching

In addition to synthesizing both membrane and secreted forms of immunoglobulins, B cells also undergo class switching. Antibody molecules are comprised of five major classes (isotypes). In order of abundance in the serum these are IgG, IgM, IgA, IgD, and IgE (Chapters 4 and 14). The IgG class is further subdivided into four subclasses and the IgA class into two subclasses. The class of immunoglobulin is determined by the sequence of the constant region of its heavy chain (C_H). The isotype-determining exons are located downstream (3') of the heavy chain variable (V_H) genes. Thus, an antibody-producing cell can change the class of antibody molecule that it synthesizes by utilization of different C_H genes without changing its unique antibody specificity. This process, termed class switch recombination, is regulated by cytokines and, like somatic hypermutation, is accomplished through the action of activation-induced cytidine deaminase.[23]

There is no process comparable to class switch recombination in T cells. The two types of TCR are products of four independent sets of V-region and C-region genes. A substantial majority of T cells express the αβ TCR; a small number express γδ TCR (usually 5% or less in peripheral blood). There is a higher representation of γδ T cells in certain tissues, particularly those lining mucous membranes, where they may be specialized for recognition of heavily glycosylated peptides or nonpeptide antigens. Thymocytes are committed to the expression of either αβ or γδ TCR and their differentiated progeny (T cells) never undergo secondary changes in the periphery.

Major histocompatibility complex

MHC molecules constitute a third class of antigen-binding molecules. When an MHC class I molecule was initially crystallized, an unknown peptide was found in a binding groove formed by the first two domains of the molecule ($α_1$ and $α_2$). This binding groove has since been established as a general feature of MHC molecules.[24,25] It is now known that the function of MHC molecules is to present antigen to T cells in the form of oligopeptides that reside within this antigen-binding groove (Chapter 6). The most important difference between the nature of the binding groove of MHC molecules and those of Ig and TCR is that the former does not represent a consequence of gene rearrangement.

Rather all the available MHC molecules in an individual are encoded in a linked array within the MHC, which in humans is located on chromosome 6 and designated HLA (Chapter 5).

MHC molecules are of two basic types, class I and class II. Class I molecules have a single heavy chain that is an integral membrane protein comprised of three external domains (Fig. 1.1). The heavy chain is noncovalently associated with $β_2$-microglobulin, a nonpolymorphic, non-membrane-bound, single-domain molecule that is not encoded within the MHC (although it is a member of the immunoglobulin superfamily). Class II MHC molecules, in contrast, are comprised of two polypeptide chains, α and β (or A and B), of approximately equal size, each of which consists of two external domains connected to a transmembrane region and cytoplasmic tail. Both chains of class II molecules are imbedded within the cell membrane, and both are encoded within the MHC. Class I and class II molecules have a high degree of structural homology and both fold to form a peptide-binding groove on their exterior face, with contribution from the $α_1$ and $α_2$ domains for class I molecules and from $α_1$ and $β_1$ domains for class II.[24]

There are three class I loci (HLA-A, -B, and -C) and three class II subregions (HLA-DR, -DQ, and -DP) that are principally involved in antigen presentation to T cells (Chapter 5). The functions of other class I and class II genes within this complex are less clear. Some at least, appear to be specialized for binding (presentation) of peptide antigens of restricted type or source (e.g., HLA-E),[26] and others are clearly involved in antigen processing (e.g., HLA-DM and HLA-DO) (Chapter 6).[27] Additionally, members of a family of "non-classical" class Ib molecules, $CD1_{a-d}$, which are encoded outside the MHC (on chromosome 1) are specialized for binding and presentation of lipid and lipid-conjugate antigens to T cells.[11,28]

The HLA complex represents an exceedingly polymorphic set of genes (Chapter 5). Consequently, most individuals are heterozygous at each major locus, having inherited one allele from the father and an alternative at each locus from the mother. In contrast to TCR and Ig, the genes of the MHC are co-dominantly expressed, i.e., allelic exclusion does not operate on MHC genes. Thus, at a minimum, an APC can express six class I molecules and six class II molecules (the products of the two alternative alleles of three class I and three class II loci). This number is, in fact, usually an underestimate for two reasons. First, as noted above, there may be products of other (non-classical) MHC genes with specialized functions. Second, the class II loci are somewhat more complex than just suggested. For example, the DRβ locus is duplicated so that most individuals express from each chromosome at least two different dimers, each comprised of a different β chain joined to an identical nonpolymorphic α chain. Additionally, because both the α and β loci for DQ are polymorphic and gene products can be assembled from *trans*-encoded transcripts, unique DQ αβ combinations, not represented in *cis* by either parental chromosome, are possible. Class I molecules are found on the surface of almost all somatic cells, whereas cell-surface expression of class II genes is restricted primarily to cells specialized for APC function.

Antigen presentation

Because MHC genes do not undergo recombination, the number of distinct antigen-binding grooves that they can form is many orders of magnitude less than that for either TCR or Ig. Oligopeptides that bind to MHC molecules are the products of self or foreign proteins. They are derived by hydrolytic cleavage within the APC and are loaded into MHC molecules before expression at the cell surface (Chapter 6). Indeed, stability of MHC molecules at the cell surface requires the presence of a peptide in the antigen-binding groove. Since most hydrolyzed proteins are of self origin, the binding groove of most MHC molecules contains a self peptide. Class I and class II molecules differ from one another in the length of peptides that they bind, usually 8–9 amino acids for class I and 14–22 amino acids for class II.[25] Although important exceptions are clearly demonstrable, they also generally differ with respect to the source of peptide. Those peptides binding to class I molecules usually derive from proteins synthesized intracellularly (e.g., autologous proteins, tumor antigens, viruses and other intracellular microbes), whereas class II molecules commonly bind peptides derived from proteins synthesized extracellularly (e.g., extracellular bacteria, non-replicating vaccines). Endogenous peptides are loaded into newly synthesized class I molecules in the endoplasmic reticulum following active transport from the cytosol. Loading of exogenous peptides into class II molecules, in contrast, occurs in acidic endosomal vacuoles.

In addition, to the recognition of lipids and lipid-conjugates presented by CD1 molecules, there are other exceptions to the generalization that MHC molecules only present (and T cells only recognize) oligopeptides. It has been known for many years that T cells can recognize haptens, presumably covalently or non-covalently complexed with peptides residing in the antigen-binding groove. This phenomenon is familiar to physicians as contact dermatitis to non-peptide antigens such as urushiol (from poison ivy) and nickel ion. Certain γδ T cells can recognize a variety of nonpeptide phosphoantigens, such as phosphorylated nucleotides, other phosphorylated small molecules and alkylamines, by a process that is not thought to require presentation by MHC molecules.[29]

Another exception to the generalization of T-cell recognition of oligopeptides is represented by a group of proteins termed superantigens (SAg).[30] SAg, of which the staphylococcal enterotoxin A (SEA) represents a prototype, are produced by a broad spectrum of microbes, ranging from retroviruses to bacteria. They differ from conventional peptide antigens in their mode of contact both with MHC class II molecules and TCR (Chapter 6). They do not undergo processing to oligopeptides, but rather bind to class II molecules and TCR as intact (~30 kDa) proteins outside the antigen-binding grooves. Their interaction with TCR is predominantly determined by polymorphic residues of the TCR Vβ region. Because SAg bind independently (more or less) of the TCR α chain and the other variable segments of the β chain, they are capable of activating much larger numbers of T cells than do conventional peptide antigens; hence the name. A secondary consequence of T-cell activation by SAg is death by apoptosis of appropriate Vβ-expressing cells. The initial response, however, is a wave of activation, proliferation and cytokine production that can have profound clinical consequences, leading to development of such diseases as toxic shock syndrome.[30] Interestingly, it is now apparent that certain bacterial products (e.g., protein A of *Staphylococcus aureus*) can similarly act on B cells, both to activate and then to delete B cells. Similarly to T-cell SAgs, B-cell SAgs interact with conserved sites in the variable regions of either Ig heavy or light chains outside the conventional antigen-binding region of an antibody.[31]

Lymphocyte adhesion and trafficking

The capacity to survey continuously the antigenic environment is an essential element of immune function. APCs and lymphocytes must be able to find antigen wherever it occurs in the body. Surveillance is accomplished through an elaborate interdigitated circulatory system of blood and lymphatic vessels that establish connections between the solid organs of the peripheral immune system (e.g., spleen and lymph nodes) in which the cellular interactions between immune cells predominantly occur (Chapter 2).

The trafficking and distribution of circulating cells of the immune system is largely regulated by interactions between molecules on the surfaces of such cells with ligands on vascular endothelial cells (Chapter 11). The leukocyte-specific cellular adhesion molecules can be expressed constitutively or can be induced by cytokines (e.g., as a consequence of an inflammatory process). Several families of molecules are involved in the regulation of lymphocyte trafficking. Particularly important are selectins and integrins, which regulate lymphocyte traffic and assure that mobile cells home to appropriate locations within lymphoid organs and other tissues.[32] Selectins are proteins characterized by a distal carbohydrate-binding (lectin) domain. They bind to a family of mucin-like molecules, the endothelial vascular addressins. Integrins are heterodimers essential for the emigration of leukocytes from blood vessels into tissues. Members of the selectin and integrin families are involved not only in lymphocyte circulation and homing, but are also important in interactions between APCs, T cells and B cells in induction and expression of immune responses. Certain endothelial adhesion molecules, mostly members of the Ig superfamily, are similarly involved in promoting interactions between T cells and APCs, as well as in leukocyte transmigration from the vasculature. Additionally, receptors for chemokines are important determinants of lymphocyte migration, particularly in guiding tissue-selective cell trafficking.[33]

Lymphocyte activation

For both B cells and T cells, initial activation is a two-signal event (Chapter 12).[34] This generalization is particularly true for cells that have not been previously exposed to antigen. The first signal is provided by antigen. Most commonly, antigens for B cells are proteins with distinct sites, termed epitopes, that bind to membrane Ig. Such epitopes can be defined by a contiguous amino acid sequence or (more frequently) can be conformationally defined by the 3-dimensional structure of the antigenic molecule. Epitopes can also be simple chemical moieties (haptens) that have been attached, usually covalently, to amino acid side-chains (Chapter 6). In addition to proteins, some B cells have receptors with specificity for carbohydrates, and less commonly lipids or nucleic acids. Antigens that stimulate B cells can be either in solution or fixed to a solid matrix (e.g., a cell membrane). As previously noted, the nature of antigens that stimulate T cells is more limited. T-cell receptors do not bind antigen in solution, but are usually stimulated only by small molecules, primarily oligopeptides, that reside within the antigen-binding cleft of a self-MHC molecule.

The second signal requisite for lymphocyte activation is provided by an accessory molecule expressed on the surface of the APC (e.g., B7/CD80) for stimulation of T cells or on the surface of a helper T cell (e.g., CD40L/CD154) for activation of B lymphocytes. The cell surface receptors for this particular second signal on T cells is CD28 and on B cells is CD40 (Fig. 1.3). Other cell surface ligand-receptor pairs may similarly provide the second signal (Chapters 8, 13). The growth and differentiation of both T cells and B cells additionally requires stimulation with one or more cytokines, which are peptide hormones secreted

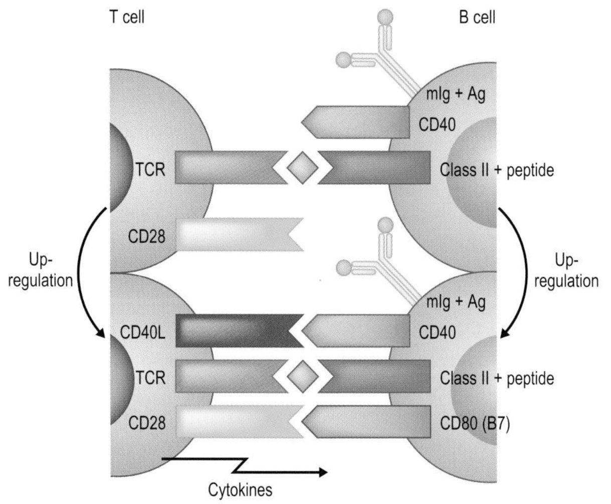

Fig. 1.3 Reciprocal activation events involved in mutual simulation of T cells and B cells. T cells constitutively express TCR and CD28. B cells constitutively express mIg and MHC class II. Antigen is endocytosed and processed to peptide constituents, binds to class II and is then presented to TCR. Activation of B cells by Ag upregulates expression of CD80 causing activation of T cells, which upregulates CD40L (CD154) and induces cytokine synthesis. Co-stimulation of B cells by antigen, CD40L and cytokines leads to Ig production.

in small quantities by activated leukocytes and APC for function in the cellular microenvironment.[35]

In the absence of a second signal, cells stimulated only by antigen become unresponsive to subsequent antigen stimulation (anergic) (Chapter 12).[36] T cells can also be "tolerized" by minor changes in the sequence of the stimulatory antigenic peptide that can convert an activating (agonist) signal into an inactivating (antagonist) signal.[37] This capacity to fundamentally alter the outcome of T-cell stimulation by means of minor changes in the antigen suggests exciting opportunities for development of future therapeutic agents.

Signal transduction through the antigen receptor is a complex process involving interactions between the specific receptor and a set of molecules co-expressed in the cell membrane.[38] For B cells, this set of molecules is a heterodimer, Igαβ; and for T cells it is a macromolecular complex, CD3, usually comprised of γ, δ, εε, and ς chains.

Within the cell membrane, antigen receptor stimulation induces phosphorylation of CD3 subunits and hydrolysis of phosphotidylinositol 4,5-bisphosphate by phospholipase C, leading to generation of diacylglycerol (DAG) and inositol 1,4,5-trisphosphate (IP$_3$). As a consequence of signal transduction and secondarily of DAG and IP$_3$ generation, tyrosine and serine/threonine protein kinases are activated. In turn, these kinases catalyze phosphorylation of a number of signal transducing proteins, leading to activation of cytoplasmic transcription factors NF-AT and NF-κB. These transcription factors then translocate to the nucleus, where they bind to 5′ regulatory regions of genes that are critical to generalized lymphocyte activation (Chapter 12).[38,39]

Cell-mediated immune responses

T-cell subsets

T lymphocytes expressing an αβ TCR can be divided into two major subpopulations based upon the class of MHC molecule that their TCR recognizes and the consequent expression of

one of a pair of TCR accessory molecules, CD4 or CD8 (Chapters 4, 8). By binding to MHC molecules on APCs, CD4 and CD8 contribute to the overall strength of intercellular molecular interactions. The ratio of CD4-to-CD8 cells in peripheral blood is usually about 2:1.

CD4 T cells, cytokines, and chemokines

The activities of CD4 T lymphocytes, commonly referred to as T helper (Th) cells, are mediated predominantly through the secretion of cytokines (Chapter 9). Cytokines are small ($\sim$12–30 kDa) protein hormones that control growth and differentiation of cells in the microenvironment. This activity can include autostimulation (autocrine function) if the cell producing the cytokine also expresses a surface receptor for it, or stimulation of other cells in the microenvironment (paracrine function) including B cells, APC, and other T cells. Although it is now recognized that their biological effects are broader than implied by their name, many of the principal cytokines active in the immune system are known as interleukins (ILs).

The specific profile of cytokines produced by CD4 T cells allows further functional subdivision (Chapters 15, 16).[35,40] CD4 T cells elaborating the "inflammatory" cytokines involved in effector functions of cell-mediated immunity, such as IL-2 and interferon (IFN)-γ, are designated Th1 cells. Other CD4 T cells synthesize cytokines such as IL-4 and IL-13 that control and regulate antibody responses, and are designated Th2 cells. Differentiation of Th1 versus Th2 subsets is a process substantially controlled by positive feedback loops, being promoted particularly by IL-12 in the case of Th1 cells and IL-4 in the case of Th2 cells. It is important to note that generalizations regarding cytokine activity are usually oversimplifications, reflecting a substantial overlap and multiplicity of functions (Chapter 9). For example, although IL-2 was initially identified as a T-cell growth factor, it also significantly affects B-cell differentiation. The prototypic inflammatory cytokine, IFN-γ, which promotes differentiation of effector function of CTL and macrophages, is also involved in regulation of Ig isotype switching. And IL-4, although known primarily as a B-cell growth and differentiation factor, can also stimulate proliferation of T cells.

A distinct subset of cytokines is a large group of highly conserved cytokine-like molecules, smaller than typical cytokines ($\sim$7–12 kDa), termed *chemo*tactic cyto*kines* or chemokines (Chapter 10).[41] Chemokines are classified based on the number and spacing of cysteine residues. They regulate and coordinate trafficking and activation of leukocytes, functioning importantly in host defenses, and also broadly in a variety of non-immunological processes including organ development and angiogenesis (Chapter 10).[35,41] They are characterized by binding to seven-transmembrane-domain G-protein-coupled receptors. Of particular interest to clinical immunologists, two chemokine receptors are utilized by HIV as co-receptors (together with CD4) to gain entry into target cells.[42]

Cytokines produced by activated T cells can downregulate as well as initiate or amplify immune responses.[43] Cytokines with such activity include IL-10 (produced by both T cells and B cells) and transforming growth factor β (TGF-β). The functions of IL-10 *in vivo* are thought to include both suppression of the production of pro-inflammatory cytokines and enhancement of IgM and IgA synthesis. TGF-β, produced by virtually all cells, expresses a broad array of biological activities, including the promotion of wound healing and the suppression of both humoral and cell-mediated immune responses.

In addition to their central role in initiation and regulation of immune responses, CD4 T cells are important effectors of cell-mediated immunity (Chapter 16). Through the elaboration of inflammatory cytokines, particularly IFN-γ, they are essential contributors to the generation of chronic inflammatory responses, characterized histologically by mononuclear cell infiltrates, where their principal role is thought to be the activation of macrophages. Additionally, CD4 T cells, at least in some circumstances, are capable of functioning as cytotoxic effectors, either directly as CTL (in which case the killing is "restricted" for recognition of antigen-bound self-MHC class II) or through the elaboration of cytotoxic cytokines such as lymphotoxin and tumor necrosis factor alpha (TNF-α).

A third subset of Th cells, designated Th17, has been recognized more recently. With differentiation driven particularly by TGF-β and IL-23 and characterized by the production of the pro-inflammatory cytokine IL-17, Th17 cells are important in the induction and exacerbation of autoimmunity in a variety of disease models, as well as in host defenses against a broad spectrum of pathogens.[44,45]

A further subset of CD4 T cells, Tregs, suppresses the functions of other lymphocytes. Tregs can differentiate either in the thymus (natural Tregs) or in the periphery (converted Tregs).[46] They are characterized by surface expression of CD4 and CD25 and by nuclear expression of the transcription factor FOXP3. Peripheral activation of CD25$^+$ Tregs is via the TCR; the cells are IL-2-dependent and apparently require cell–cell contact for suppressive function. They can suppress functions of both CD4 and CD8 T cells, as well as B cells, NK cells, and NKT cells. In contrast to activation, suppressor effects are independent of the antigen specificity of the target cells. Other Tregs, are noted for production of inhibitory cytokines, including IL-10 and TGF-β-secreting Th3 cells and IL-10-producing Tr1 cells.[47]

CD8 T cells

The best understood function of CD8 T cells is that of cytotoxic effectors (CTL).[48] Such cells are of particular importance in host defenses against virus-infected cells and cancer cells, where they are capable of direct killing of target cells expressing an appropriate viral peptide bound to a self-MHC class I molecule (Chapter 17). This process is highly specific and requires direct apposition of CTL and target cell membranes. Bystander cells, expressing noncognate MHC molecules (e.g., that might be presented in an *in vitro* culture system) or different antigenic peptides are not affected. The killing is unidirectional; the CTL itself is not harmed and after transmission of a "lethal hit" it can detach from one target to seek another. Killing occurs via two mechanisms: a death-receptor-induced apoptotic mechanism, resulting in fragmentation of target cell nuclear DNA and a mechanism involving insertion of perforins and granzyme from the CTL into the target cell. CTL activity is enhanced by IFN-γ. As CTL function is dependent upon cell surface display of MHC class I molecules, a principle mechanism of immune evasion by viruses and tumors is elaboration of factors that downregulate class I expression (Chapter 27). However, this increases susceptibility of such cells to cytolytic activity of NK cells.

Antibody-mediated immune responses

The structure of antibodies permits the possibility of a virtually limitless binding specificity of its antigen-binding groove. Antigen binding can then be translated into biological effector functions based on the properties of the larger nonvariable (constant) portions of its heavy chains (Fc fragment) (Chapter 14). Moreover, in response to cytokines in the cellular microenvironment, through the mechanism of isotype switching an antibody-producing cell can alter the biological effects of its secreted product without affecting its specificity. With functional heterogeneity determined by isotype, the antibody molecules provide an efficient defense system against extracellular microbes or foreign macromolecules (e.g., toxins and venoms) (Chapters 14, 24).

● KEY CONCEPTS

Biological properties of immunoglobulin classes

- IgM: Principal Ig of primary immune responses
  Generally restricted to vascular compartment
  B cell antigen receptor (monomer)
  Fixes complement
- IgG: Principal Ig of secondary immune responses
  Binds to Fcγ receptors on neutrophils, monocytes/macrophages, NK cells.
  Fixes complement (except IgG$_4$ subclass)
- IgA: Principal Ig of mucosal immunity
- IgD: Antigen receptor for mature B cells
  Typically co-expressed with membrane IgM
- IgE: Binds to Fcγ receptors on mast cells and basophils
  Antibody of immediate hypersensitivity
  Important in defenses against helminths

Each of the antibody classes contributes differently to an integrated defense system. IgM is the predominant class formed upon initial contact with antigen (primary immune response). As a monomeric structure comprised of two light (κ or λ) and two heavy (μ) chains, it is initially expressed as an antigen receptor on the surface of B lymphocytes. It is secreted, however, as a pentamer composed of five of the monomeric subunits held together by a joining (J) chain. IgM is essentially confined to the intravascular compartment. As a multivalent antigen binder that can efficiently activate complement, it is an important contributor to an early immune response. The synthesis of IgM is much less dependent than other isotypes upon the activity of T lymphocytes.

IgG is the most abundant immunoglobulin in serum and the principal antibody class of a secondary (anamnestic or memory) immune response. IgG molecules are heterodimeric monomers with two light (κ or λ) and two heavy (γ) chains joined by interchain disulfide bridges. Because of its abundance, its capacity to activate (fix) complement and the expression on phagocytes of Fcγ receptors, IgG is the most important antibody of secondary immune responses. IgG is the only isotype that is actively transported across the placenta. These transported maternal IgG antibodies provide the neonate with an important level of antibody protection during the early months, when its own antigen-driven antibody responses are first developing.

IgA is the principal antibody in the body's secretions (Chapter 19). It is found in serum in monomeric form of two light and two heavy (α) chains or as a dimer joined by J chain. In secretions, it is usually present as a dimer joined by J chain and is actively secreted across mucous membranes by attachment of a specialized secretory component (SC). It is found in high concentration in tears, saliva, and the secretions of the respiratory, gastrointestinal, and genitourinary systems, and is relatively resistant to enzymatic digestion. It is particularly abundant in colostrum, where its concentration may be greater than 50 times that in serum, providing passive immunity to the gastrointestinal system of a nursing neonate. IgA does not fix complement by the antibody-dependent pathway and hence does not promote phagocytosis. Its role in host defenses lies in preventing a breach of the mucous membrane surface by microbes or their toxic products.

IgD and IgE are present in serum at concentrations much lower than that of IgG. The biological role of secreted IgD, if any, is unknown. However, IgD is important as a membrane receptor for antigen on mature B cells. The molecular mechanisms that allow IgD production simultaneously permit continued production of IgM. These mechanisms do not require T-cell help.

Although IgE is the least abundant isotype in serum, it has dramatic biological effects because it is responsible for immediate-type hypersensitivity reactions including systemic anaphylaxis (Chapter 40). Such reactions are a consequence of the expression of high affinity receptors for Fcε on the surfaces of mast cells and basophils. Crosslinking of IgE molecules on such cells by antigen induces their degranulation, with the synthesis and/or release of the potent biological mediators of immediate hypersensitivity responses. The protective role of IgE is in host defenses against parasitic infestation, particularly helminths (Chapter 29).

Complement and immune complexes

As noted, the biological functions of IgG and IgM are largely reflections of their capacities to activate the complement system. Through a series of sequential substrate-enzyme interactions, the eleven principal components of the antibody-dependent complement cascade (C1q, C1r, C1s, and C2-9) effect many of the consequences of an antigen–antibody interaction (Chapter 20). These include the establishment of pores in a target membrane by the terminal components (C5-9) leading to osmotic lysis; opsonization by C3b, promoting phagocytosis; the production of factors with chemotactic activity (C5a); and the ability to induce degranulation of mast cells (C3a, C4a, and C5a). There are three distinct pathways to complement activation.[49] The pathway mediated by the binding of IgG or IgM to the first component (specifically C1q), has been termed the "classical" pathway. The lectin pathway is similar to the classical pathway but is activated by certain carbohydrate-binding proteins, the mannose (or mannan)-binding lectin (MBL) and ficolins, which recognize certain carbohydrate repeating structures on microorganisms. MBL and ficolins are plasma proteins homologous to C1q and contribute to innate immunity through their capacity to induce antibody- and C1q-independent activation of the classical pathway. Finally, a large number of substances, including certain bacterial, fungal and viral products, can directly activate the cascade through a distinct series of proteins also leading to activation of the central C3 component. Although bypassing C1, C4, and C2, this distinct pathway can achieve all the biological consequences of C3–9 activation. Non-antibody induced activation of C3 is referred to as the alternative or properdin pathway. Additionally, the central components of the cascade (e.g., C5a) can be directly produced by the action of serine proteases of the coagulation system.[49] Reflecting these separate pathways to activation, the complement system is a major contributor to the efferent limbs of both innate and acquired immune systems.

In addition to their roles in pathogen/antigen elimination, constituents of the complement system, together with antigen-antibody (immune) complexes, act at leukocyte surfaces to regulate immune functions. For example, interaction of immune complexes via FcγR on B cells decreases their responsiveness to stimulation. In contrast, complement activation on B-cell surfaces co-ligates their receptors with B-cell receptors for antigen; the cells are more readily activated and become relatively resistant to apoptosis.

Apoptosis and immune homeostasis

An immune response is commonly first viewed in a "positive" sense, i.e., lymphocytes are activated, proliferate and carry out effector functions. It is equally important, however, that this positive response be tightly regulated by mechanisms that operate to turn off the response and eliminate cells no longer required.[50] Under physiologic circumstances, once an immune response fades, commonly as a consequence of antigen depletion, two pathways to terminal lymphocyte differentiation become available: apoptosis or differentiation into memory cells. Memory cells are, of course, a key to the effectiveness of the adaptive immune system. Once seen effectively, a second encounter with antigen (e.g., pathogen) is both more rapid and more productive. IgG antibodies are rapidly produced and/or clones of CTL effector cells are expanded as a consequence of prior exposure and clonal expansion. But the majority of lymphocytes in an active response are not required for maintenance of immunologic memory, and for these larger populations a need for immune homeostasis leads to apoptosis.

Apoptosis is a unique process of cellular death, widely conserved phylogenetically, and distinguished from death by necrosis by cellular shrinking, DNA fragmentation and breakdown of cells into "apoptotic bodies" containing nuclear fragments and intact organelles (Chapter 13). The process depends upon the activation of cysteinyl proteases, termed caspases, that cleave proteins involved in DNA repair and cellular and organelle architecture at specific aspartyl residues. Absent such mechanisms, massive proliferation of lymphoid tissues is a consequence, seen clinically as the autoimmune lymphoproliferative syndrome (ALPS), which is characterized by lymphocytosis with lymphadenopathy and splenomegaly as well as autoimmunity and hypergammaglobulinemia (Chapter 35).[51]

Mechanisms of immunologic diseases

The pathogenic pathways that lead to diseases of the immune system are based on an understanding of it physiology and its perturbations in disease states (Table 1.2). First, immunologic disease can reflect a failure or deficiency of the immune system (Chapters 30–38). This pathway is similar to that accounting for most diseases of other organ systems, i.e., a consequence of failure of physiologic function. For the immune system such

Table 1.2 Pathways to immunologic diseases

1. Immune system deficiency or failure
   a. Congenital
   b. Acquired
2. Malignant transformation
3. Immunologic dysregulation
4. Autoimmunity
5. Untoward consequences of physiologic immune function

failures are usually identified by increased susceptibility to infection (Chapter 31). Failure can be congenital (e.g., X-linked agammaglobulinemia) or acquired (e.g., AIDS). It can be global (e.g., severe combined immunodeficiency) or quite specific, involving only a particular component of the immune system (e.g., selective IgA deficiency).

A second mechanism, malignant transformation (Chapters 76–80), is also common to virtually all organ systems. Malignancies of the hematopoietic system are familiar to all physicians. Manifestations of these diseases are protean, most commonly reflecting the secondary consequences of solid organ or bone marrow infiltration or replacement by tumor cells, with resulting anemia and immune system deficiency.

The third, fourth, and fifth pathways to immunopathogenesis are more specific to the immune system. Dysregulation of an essentially intact immune system constitutes the third general pathway. Features of an optimal immune response include antigen recognition and elimination with little adverse effect on the host. Both initiation and termination of the response, however, involve regulatory interactions that can go awry when challenged by antigens of a particular structure or in a particular mode of presentation. Diseases of immune dysregulation reflect genetic and environmental factors that act together to subvert a normal immune response to some pathological end. Examples include the acute allergic diseases (Chapters 39–47). A particularly intriguing disease of this type is thought to reflect an insufficiency of exposure to non-pathogenic microbes in early childhood, resulting in an increased susceptibility to atopy and asthma once the immune system has matured (the so-called "hygiene hypothesis"),[52] perhaps reflecting the effects of specific gut-colonizing organisms in the initial establishment of immune homeostatis.[53]

The fourth pathway, mechanistically quite similar to the third, lies at the heart of acquired immunity, i.e., the molecular discrimination between self and non-self. Ambiguity in this discrimination can lead to autoimmune tissue damage (Chapters 48–75). Although such damage can be mediated by either antibodies or T cells, the common association of specific autoimmune diseases with inheritance of particular HLA alleles (Chapter 5) suggests that the pathogenesis of autoimmune diseases usually represents a failure of self/non-self discrimination by T cells. This failure to discriminate can be general, leading to development of systemic autoimmune diseases such as systemic lupus erythematosus; or local, as in the organ-specific autoimmune diseases. In the latter instance, attack is directed against specific cells and usually particular cell surface molecules. In most cases, pathology is a consequence of target tissue destruction (e.g., multiple sclerosis, rheumatoid arthritis, or insulin-dependent diabetes mellitus). However, it can also reflect hormone receptor blockade (e.g., myasthenia gravis or insulin-resistant diabetes) or hormone receptor stimulation (e.g., Graves' disease). It is hypothesized that ambiguity in self/non-self discrimination is commonly triggered by an unresolved encounter with an infectious organism or other environmental agent, although this remains a subject of controversy (Chapter 48).[54]

A fifth pathogenetic pathway is disease development as a result of physiologic rather than pathologic function. Inflammatory lesions in such diseases are the result of the normal function of the immune system. A typical example is contact dermatitis to such potent skin sensitizers as urushiol, the causative agent of poison ivy dermatitis (Chapter 42). These diseases can also have an iatrogenic etiology that can range from benign (e.g., delayed hypersensitivity skin test reactions) to life-threatening (e.g., graft-vs-host disease, organ graft rejection).

Host immune defenses summarized

The first response upon initial contact with an invading pathogen depends upon components of the innate immune system (Chapter 3). This response begins with expression of pathogen-associated molecular patterns (PAMPs) by cells of the pathogen. These include lipoproteins, lipopolysaccharide, CpG-DNA, and bacterial flagellin, among others. PAMPs bind to pattern-recognition receptors (PRRs) on effector cells of the host's innate immune system including dendritic cells, granulocytes and lymphocytes.[55] The best characterized PRRs are the Toll-like receptors (TLRs), first recognized as determinants of embryonic patterning in *Drosophila* and subsequently appreciated as components of host defenses in both insects and vertebrates. TLR subfamilies can be distinguished by expression either on the cell surface or in intracellular compartments. Binding of TLRs by a PAMP ligand triggers intracellular signaling pathways via multiple "adapters" leading to a vigorous inflammatory response. Based on involvement of the myeloid differentiation primary response gene 88 (MyD88), two principal pathways are recognized. Most TLRs are MyD88-dependent, whereas TLR3 and -4 signal via a MyD88-independent IFNβ pathway.

The innate immune response also includes the capacity of NK lymphocytes to identify and destroy, by direct cytotoxic mechanisms, cells lacking surface expression of MHC class I molecules, which marks them as potentially pathogenic.[5] Additionally, an innate immune response involves elements of the humoral immune system that function independently of antibody, especially the activation of the complement cascade through the lectin and alternative pathways, with consequent opsonization to promote phagocytosis and destruction.

The defenses of the acquired immune system to any particular pathogenic agent are determined largely by the context in which it is encountered. Regardless, effectiveness depends upon the four principal properties of specific immunity: (1) a virtually unlimited capacity to bind macromolecules, particularly proteins, with exquisite specificity, reflecting generation of antigen-binding receptors by genetic recombination and, in the case of B cells, somatic hypermutation; (2) the capacity for self/non-self discrimination, consequences of a rigorous process involving positive and negative selection during thymocyte differentiation, as well as negative selection during B-cell differentiation; (3) the property of immunological memory, reflecting antigen-driven clonal proliferation of T cells and B cells that results in increasingly rapid and effective responses upon second and subsequent encounters with a particular antigen or pathogen; and (4) mechanisms for pathogen destruction including direct cellular cytotoxicity, release of inflammatory cytokines, opsonization with antibody and complement and neutralization in solution by antigen precipitation or conformational alteration.

Although most acquired immune responses involve a multiplicity of available defense mechanisms, several generalizations may be conceptually useful. T-cell (and NK-cell)-mediated effector functions are particularly important in defenses against pathogens encountered intracellularly such as viruses and intracellular bacteria. These responses involve the production of inflammatory cytokines by CD4 Th1 cells, as well as the direct cytolytic activity of CD8 CTL. In contrast, host defenses to most antigens encountered primarily in the extracellular milieu are largely dependent upon humoral mechanisms (antibody and complement) for antigen neutralization, precipitation, or opsonization and subsequent destruction by phagocytes. Targets of antibody-mediated immunity include extracellular bacteria and toxins (or other foreign proteins). It is worth reiterating, however, that induction of an effective antibody response (including isotype switching) and development of immunological memory (resulting from B-cell clonal expansion) require antigen activation not only of specific B cells, but also CD4 T cells, particularly of the Th2 type.

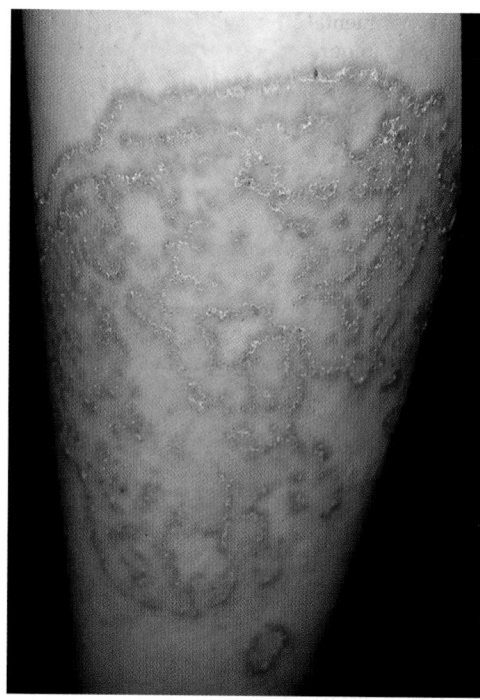

Fig 1.4 Leg of a 16-year-old patient with chronic mucocutaneous candidiasis as a consequence of congenital T-cell deficiency associated with hypoparathyroidism.

CLINICAL RELEVANCE

Characteristic infections associated with immune deficiency syndromes

- Deficiencies of T-cell-mediated immunity
  - Mucocutaneous fungal infections, especially *Candida albicans*
  - Systemic (deep) fungal infections
  - Systemic infection with attenuated viruses (e.g., live viral vaccines)
  - Infection with viruses of usually low pathogenicity (e.g., cytomegalovirus)
  - *Pneumocystis jiroveci* pneumonia
- Antibody deficiencies
  - Encapsulated bacterial infections (e.g., *Streptococcus* spp., *Haemophilus influenza*)
  - Recurrent pneumonia, bronchitis, sinusitis, otitis media
  - *Giardia lamblia* enteritis
- Phagocyte deficiencies
  - Gram-positive bacterial infection (e.g., staphylococci, streptococci)
  - Gram-negative sepsis
  - Systemic fungal infections (e.g., *Candida* spp., *Aspergillus* spp)
- Adhesion molecule deficiencies
  - Pyogenic bacterial infections (especially staphylococci)
  - Cutaneous and subcutaneous abscesses
- Complement component deficiencies
  - C3 deficiency—Infections with encapsulated bacteria
  - Deficiency of terminal components—Gram-negative bacteria, especially *Neisseria* spp.

Finally, clinical "experiments of nature" have proven particularly instructive in our efforts to understand the role of specific components of the immune system in overall host defenses (Chapter 31).[56] The importance of T cell-mediated immunity in host defenses to intracellular parasites, fungi (Fig. 1.4) and viruses is emphasized by the remarkable susceptibility of T cell-deficient patients to such organisms as *Pneumocystis jiroveci* and *Candida albicans,* and by the risks of utilizing attenuated live virus vaccines in such patients. Indeed, the relationship between susceptibility to particular potential pathogens and specific immunologic deficiencies is nicely illustrated by recent demonstrations that the pathogenesis of familial forms of chronic mucocutaneous candidiasis can reflect deficiency of IL-17-mediated immunity, either of the production of IL-17 F or in the IL-17 receptor A[57] or mutations affecting the coiled-coil domain of signal tranduceer and activator of transcription 1 (*STAT1*).[58]

On the other hand, patients with defects in antibody synthesis or phagocytic cell function are characteristically afflicted with recurrent infections with pyogenic bacteria, particularly Gram-positive organisms. And patients with inherited defects in synthesis of terminal complement components have increased susceptibility to infection with species of *Neisseria*.

In recent years immunology has entered the lay lexicon, largely as a result of the HIV pandemic. People throughout the world are now tragically aware of the consequences of immune deficiency. The remarkable progress in understanding this disease, however, depended substantially upon earlier studies of

relatively rare patients with primary immunodeficiency syndromes, more recently accelerated by progress in genomic definition of their molecular basis. Similarly, cure of patients with primary immunodeficiencies by cellular reconstitution, particularly bone marrow transplantation, presaged important recent progress in correction of such diseases by gene replacement therapy.[59] The "present" of clinical immunology is indeed bright. But its future potential to impact prevention and treatment of many challenging diseases through enhancement or suppression of global or antigen-specific immune responses is even more exciting to contemplate. A few approaches are broadly hinted at here, and it is hoped that readers will enjoy considering such opportunities "on the horizon" throughout the book. And given the nature of the immune system, will challenge themselves to transform a particular author's views to new and different clinical settings.

ON THE HORIZON

Enhancement of immune responses
- Gene replacement in monogenic immunodeficiency diseases with autologous induced pluripotent stem cells
- Cellular engineering to prevent T-cell infection by HIV

Suppression of immune responses
- Improvement in antigen-specific immunosuppression
- Specific suppression of long-lived antibody-producing cells
- Prevention of graft-versus-host disease in allogeneic bone marrow transplants
- Pharmacologic development of specific inhibitors of cytokines, chemokines, and their receptors

Immunodiagnostics
- Development of novel diagnostic tools based on nanotechnology arrays
- Clarification of role of exposure in childhood to specific bacteria and viruses in pathogenesis of allergy and asthma

Studies in experimental animal systems, especially the mouse, have been critical to our understanding of molecular aspects of immune system function and have contributed importantly to our appreciation of how aberrations of such functions are involved in the pathogenesis of disease. The new insights gained from use of transgenic mice (including murine expression of human genes) and constitutive or conditional gene-knockout mice are essential to a comprehensive view of the immune system at the advancing edge of its clinical application, implying that future progress in clinical immunology will equally depend upon detailed analysis in such systems. Nevertheless, the carefully studied patient will remain the ultimate crucible for understanding human immunity and the roles of the immune system in the pathogenesis of and protection from disease.

References

1. Flajnik MF, Kasahara M. Origin and evolution of the adaptive immune system: genetic events and selective pressures. Nat Rev Genet 2010;11:47–59.
2. Hancock RE, Brown KL, Mookherjee N. Host defence peptides from invertebrates—emerging antimicrobial strategies. Immunobiol 2006;211:315–22.
3. Lazzaro BP. Natural selection on the *Drosophilia* antimicrobial immune system. Curr Opin Microbiol 2008;11:284–9.
4. Mogensen TH. Pathogen recognition and inflammatory signaling in innate immune defenses. Clin Microbiol Rev 2009;22:240–73.
5. Vivier E, Raulet DH, Moretta A, et al. Innate or adaptive immunity? The example of natural killer cells. Science 2011;331:44–9.
6. Hiepe F, Dörmer T, Hauser AE, et al. Long-lived autoreactive plasma cells drive persistent autoimmune inflammation. Nat Rev Rheumatol 2011;7:170–8.
7. Marcenaro E, Carlomagno S, Pesce S, et al. Bridging innate NK cell functions with adaptive immunity. Adv Exp Med Biol 2011;780:45–55.
8. Alderson KL, Sondel PM. Clinical cancer therapy by NK cells via antibody-dependent cell-mediated cytotoxicity. J Biomed Biotechnol 2011;2011:379123.
9. Wang S, Chen L. T lymphocyte co-signaling pathways of the B7-CD28 family. Cell Mol Immunol 2004;1:37–42.
10. Münz C, Steinman RM, Fujii S. Dendritic cell maturation by innate lymphocytes: coordinated stimulation of innate and adaptive immunity. J Exp Med 2005;202:203–7.
11. Godfrey DI, Pellicci DG, Patel O, et al. Antigen recognition by CD1d-restricted NKT T cell receptors. Semin Immunol 2010;22:61–7.
12. Anderson MK, Rast JP. Evolution of antigen binding receptors. Annu Rev Immunol 1999;17:109–47.
13. Dudley DD, Chaudhuri J, Bassing CH, Alt FW. Mechanism and control of V(D)J recombination: similarities and differences. Adv Immunol 2005;86:43–112.
14. Corcoran AE. Immunoglobulin locus silencing and allelic exclusion. Semin Immunol 2005;17:141–54.
15. Brady BL, Steinel NC, Bassing CH. Antigen receptor allelic exclusion: an update and reappraisal. J Immunol 2010;185:3801–8.
16. Maul RW, Gearhart PJ. AID and somatic hypermutation. Adv Immunol 2010;105:159–91.
17. Okazaki IM, Kotani A, Honjo T. Role of AID in tumorigenesis. Adv Immunol 2007;94:245–73.
18. von Boehmer H. Selection of the T-cell repertoire: receptor controlled checkpoints in T-cell development. Adv Immunol 2004;84:201–38.
19. Wirnsberger G, Hinterberger M, Klein L. Regulatory T-cell differentiation versus clonal deletion of autoreactive thymocytes. Immunol Cell Biol 2011;89:45–53.
20. Simons DM, Picca CC, Oh S, et al. How specificity for self-peptides shapes the development and function of regulatory T cells. J Leukoc Biol 2010;88:1099–107.
21. Edry E, Melamed D. Receptor editing in positive and negative selection of B lymphopoeisis. J Immunol 2004;173:4265–71.
22. Goodnow CC, Vinuesa CG, Randall KL, et al. Control systems and decision making for antibody production. Nat Immunol 2010;11:681–8.
23. Goodman MF, Scharff MD, Romesberg FE. AID-initiated purposeful mutations in immunoglobulin genes. Adv Immunol 2007;94:127–55.
24. Madden DR. The three-dimensional structure of peptide-MHC complexes. Annu Rev Immunol 1995;13:587–622.
25. Yaneva R, Schneeweiss C, Zacharias M, Springer S. Peptide binding to MHC class I and II proteins: new avenues from new methods. Mol Immunol 2010;47:649–57.
26. Pietra G, Romagnani C, Manzini C, et al. The emerging role of HLA-E-restricted CD8 + T lymphocytes in the adaptive immune response to pathogens and tumors. J Biomed Biotechnol 2010;2010:907092.
27. Busch R, Rinderknecht CH, Roh S, et al. Achieving stability through editing and chaperoning: regulation of MHC class II peptide binding and expression. Immunol Rev 2005;207:242–60.
28. Cohen NR, Garg S, Brenner MB. Antigen presentation by CD1 lipids, T cells, and NKT cells in microbial immunity. Adv Immunol 2009;102:1–94.
29. Urban EM, Chapoval AI, Pauza CD. Repertoire development and the control of cytotoxic/effector function in human γδ T cells. Clin Dev Immunol 2010;2010:732893.
30. Fraser JD, Proft T. The bacterial superantigens and superantigen-like proteins. Immunol Rev 2008;225:226–43.
31. Silverman GJ, Goodyear CS. Confounding B-cell defences: lessons from a staphylococcal superantigen. Nat Rev Immunol 2006;6:465–75.
32. Smith CW. Adhesion molecules and receptors. J Allergy Clin Immunol 2008;121: S375–9.
33. Koelink PJ, Overbeek SA, Braber S, et al. Targeting chemokine receptors in chronic inflammatory diseases: an extensive review. Pharmacol Ther 2012;133:1–18.
34. Sharpe AH, Abbas AK. T-cell costimulation—biology, therapeutic potential and challenges. New Engl J Med 2006;355:973–5.
35. Commins SP, Borish L, Steinke JW. Immunologic messenger molecules: cytokines, interferons, and chemokines. J Allergy Clin Immunol 2010;125:S53–72.
36. Chappert P, Schwartz RH. Induction of T cell anergy: integration of environmental cues and infectious tolerance. Curr Opin Immunol 2010;22:552–9.
37. Madrenas J. Differential signaling by variant ligands of the T cell receptor and the kinetic model of T cell activation. Life Sci 1999;64:717–31.
38. Engels N, Wienands J. The signaling tool box for tyrosine-based costimulation of lymphocytes. Curr Opin Immunol 2011;23:324–9.
39. Schulze-Luehrmann J, Ghosh S. Antigen-receptor signaling to nuclear factor kappa B. Immunity 2006;25:701–15.
40. Zhu J, Paul WE. Peripheral CD4 + T-cell differentiation regulated by networks of cytokines and transcription factors. Immunol Rev 2010;238:247–62.
41. Rossi D, Zlotnik A. The biology of chemokines and their receptors. Ann Rev Immunol 2000;18:217–42.
42. Choi WT, An J. Biology and clinical relevance of chemokines and chemokine receptors CXCR4 and CCR5 in human diseases. Exp Biol Med 2011;236:637–47.
43. Taylor A, Verhagen J, Blaser K, et al. Mechanisms of immune suppression by interleukin-10 and transforming growth factor-beta: the role of T regulatory cells. Immunology 2006;117:433–42.
44. Korn T, Bettelli E, Oukka M, Kuchroo VK. IL-17 and Th17 cells. Annu Rev Immunol 2009;27:485–517.
45. O'Quinn DB, Palmer MT, Lee YK, Weaver CT. Emergence of the TH17 pathway and its role in host defense. Adv Immunol 2008;99:115–63.
46. Feuerer M, Hill JA, Mathis D, Benoist C. Foxp3 + regulatory T cells: differentiation, specification, subphenotypes. Nat Immunol 2009;10:689–95.
47. Peterson RA. Regulatory T-cells: diverse phenotypes integral to immune homeostasis and suppression. Toxicol Pathol 2012;40:186–204.
48. Chávez-Galán L, Arenas-Del Angel MC, Zenteno E, et al. Cell death mechanisms induced by cytotoxic lymphocytes. Cell Mol Immunol 2009;6:15–25.
49. Ehrnthaller C, Ignatius A, Gebhard F, Huber-Lang M. New insights of an old defense system: structure, function, and clinical relevance of the complement system. Mol Med 2011;17:317–29.
50. Boyman O, Létourneau S, Krieg C, Sprent J. Homeostatic proliferation and survival of naïve and memory T cells. Eur J Immunol 2009;39:2088–94.
51. Oliveira JB, Bleesing JJ, Dianzani U, et al. Revised diagnostic criteria and classification for the autoimmune lymphoproliferative syndrome (ALPS): report from the 2009 NIH international workshop. Blood 2010;116:e35–40.
52. Ege MJ, Mayer M, Normand AC, et al. Exposure to environmental microorganisms and childhood asthma. New Engl J Med 2011;364:701–9.
53. Atarashi K, Tanoue T, Shima T, et al. Induction of colonic regulatory T cells by indigenous *Clostridium* species. Science 2011;331:337–41.
54. Kivity S, Agmon-Levin N, Blank M, Shoenfeld Y. Infections and autoimmunity—friends or foes? Trends Immunol 2009;30:409–14.
55. Kumar H, Kawai T, Akira S. Pathogen recognition by the innate immune system. Int Rev Immunol 2011;30:16–34.
56. Notarangelo LD. Primary immunodeficiencies. J Allergy Clin Immunol 2010;125: S182–4.
57. Puel A, Cypowyi S, Busstamante J, et al. Chronic mucocutaneous candidiasis in humans with inborn errors of interleukin-17 immunity. Science 2011;332:65–8.
58. Van de Veerdonk FL, Plantinga TS, Hoischen A, et al. STAT1 mutations in autosomal dominant chronic mucocutaneous candidiasis. New Engl J Med 2011;365:54–61.
59. Qasim W, Gaspar HB, Thrasher AJ. Progress and prospects: gene therapy for inherited immunodeficiencies. Gene Ther 2009;16:1285–91.

2

Dorothy E. Lewis,
Gregory R.
Harriman, Sarah
E. Blutt

Organization of the immune system

The human immune system consists of organs, including the spleen, the thymus, and the lymph nodes; and movable cells, including cells from the bone marrow, blood and lymphatics. This design allows central locations for initial production and differentiation of committed cells from naïve precursors, as in the fetal liver, the bone marrow and the thymus; and more dispersed sites for selection and further differentiation of cells into mature effector cells, as in spleen, lymph nodes and intestinal Peyer's patches. This arrangement also allows the regulation of immune responses at locations peripheral to the primary lymphoid organs, and thus provides local control of infectious processes. The mechanisms responsible for the ability of nonspecific leukocytes and natural killer (NK) cells and antigen-specific T and B lymphocytes to respond rapidly are discussed in later chapters. This chapter is concerned with the basic features and ontogeny of cells involved in the immune response, as well as the essential structure of lymphoid organs.

Immune cell development

Ontogeny of the cells of the immune system

In the first month of embryogenesis in humans, stem cells capable of producing white blood cell progenitors are found in yolk sac erythropoietic islands physically attached to, but not inside, the embryo.[1] A specialized endothelial cell gives rise to the first progenitor cell.[2] An area adjacent to the liver, called the aorta–gonad–mesonephros (AGM), produces progenitor cells that develop into hematopoietic stem cells. In addition, the placenta has been identified as a separate possible source for fetal stem cells for both the AGM and the fetal liver. The properties of the HSC at different sites differ. For example, HSC in the fetal liver are in cycle, those in adult bone marrow are not. These progenitor stem cells first populate the embryonic liver and begin blood cell production in the sixth week of gestation, or just after the organ can be identified. By the eleventh week, the liver is the major source of hematopoiesis and remains so until the sixth month of gestation.

The first progenitor cells derived from hematopoietic stem cells (HSC) are colony-forming cells that can differentiate into granulocytes, erythrocytes, monocytes, megakaryocytes, and lymphocytes.[3] The elements of the skeleton are formed between the second and fourth months of gestation. After this process, white blood cell development shifts to the marrow of these bones. The transition from liver to bone marrow is completed in the sixth month of gestation. Cells that differentiate from early stem cells begin to populate the primary lymphoid organs, such

as the thymus, by 7–8 weeks' gestation.[4] At 8 weeks' gestation, T-cell precursors that have initiated T-cell receptor (TCR) rearrangement (Chapter 8) can be detected in thymic tissue. In the fetal liver, B-cell precursors initiate immunoglobulin (Ig) rearrangements by 7–8 weeks' gestation (Chapter 7). Late in the first trimester, B-cell development spreads to the bone marrow. In the bone marrow, B-cell progenitors congregate in the areas adjacent to the endosteum and differentiate in the direction of the central sinus. The association of B cells with stromal reticular cells is essential for eventual release of mature B cells into the central sinus. As in the case of T-cell development, a selection process causes many B-cell progenitors to die by apoptosis.

In adult humans the bone marrow is the chief source of stem cells. However, the peripheral blood can be induced to contain stem cells with different characteristics and limited self-renewal.[5]

Tools essential to an understanding of immune cell biology

Progress beyond morphologic categorization of hematopoietic cells was enhanced by monoclonal antibodies that identify stage-specific leukocyte cell surface antigens using flow cytometry. In the 1980s, the number of monoclonal antibodies raised against a multitude of human leukocyte antigens yielded a complicated nomenclature. In response, leukocyte differentiation antigen workshops were charged with the development of a more convenient naming system. The workshops grouped all the monoclonal antibodies that recognized a single molecule on leukocytes by the cluster pattern of cells with which they were identified, hence the term CD, or "cluster of differentiation" antigen (Table 2.1). As of 2010, 363 CD antigens had been officially recognized, with varying levels of characterization (see Appendix 1). Future human cell differentiation molecule workshops are planned to focus on markers of functional subsets of cells. A more extensive discussion of these markers can be found at http://www.hcdm.org

Hematopoiesis and lymphopoiesis

All mature cells of the hematopoietic and lymphoid lineages are derived from pluripotent stem cells.[6] These cells give rise to hematopoietic and lymphoid progenitors. The hematopoietic progenitors then mature into cells of the granulocytic, erythroid, monocytic–dendritic, and megakaryocytic lineages (GEMM colony-forming units, CFU-GEMM). Likewise, lymphoid progenitors mature into B lymphocytes, T lymphocytes, and NK cells (Fig. 2.1).

Table 2.1 Important cell surface antigens on hematopoietic cells

Cell type	Surface antigens	Predominant location
Hematopoietic stem cells		
Bone marrow	CD34⁻ or	Bone marrow
HSC	CD34⁺, Lin-, Thy1⁺	
Peripheral blood	CD34⁺, Lin-, CD38⁺, CD71⁺	Blood
HSC		
Myeloid cells		
Monocytes	CD14, CD35 (CR1), CD64 (FcRrγ1)	Blood
Macrophages	CD68, CD13, CD64, CD35	Tissues
Langerhans cells	CD1a, CD207 (Langerin), CD35, CD64	Skin
Follicular dendritic cells	CD80, CD56, Class II, CD83, CD40	B-cell areas, lymph nodes
Interdigitating dendritic cells	CD83, CD80, CD86, CD40	T-cell areas, lymph nodes
Dendritic cells	CD1a, CD11c	Mainly tissues
Myeloid dendritic cells	CD4, CCR5, CXCR4, CD123	
Plasmacytoid dendritic cells (IFN-α producing)		
Granulocytes		
Neutrophils	CD16 (FcγRIII), CD35 CD88 (C5aR)	Blood, tissues
Eosinophils	CD32 (FcγRII)	Blood, tissues
Basophils	CD23, (FcεRII), CD32	Tissues, blood
Mast cells	FcεRI αFcεRI α	Tissues, blood,
		Tissues
Lymphocytes		
T cells	CD7, CD3, CD4, CD8, CD28	Thymus, spleen, lymph nodes, MALT, blood
B cells	Surface Ig, class II,	Bone marrow, spleen, lymph nodes, MALT, blood
NK cells	CD19, CD20, CD22, CD40	Spleen, lymph nodes, mucosal tissues, blood
NKT cells	CD16, CD56, CD94	Blood, tissues
Tregs	CD3, CD56, Vα24 TCR	Thymus, blood, tissues
	CD4, CD25, Foxp3, GARP	

In the adult, hematopoiesis and lymphopoiesis occur in two distinct tissues. The development of hematopoietic lineage cells—that is, granulocytes, monocytes, dendritic cells, erythrocytes and platelets—occurs in the bone marrow (Table 2.2). B-lymphocyte development, through the stage of mature B cells, also occurs in the bone marrow (Chapter 7). On the other hand, T-cell progenitors leave the bone marrow, migrate to the thymus and differentiate into αβ and γδ T cells, as well as regulatory T cells (Chapter 8). Evidence also suggests that at least some NK cells develop from precursors in the thymus.[7] However, most NK-cell development occurs extrathymically, mainly in the bone marrow.

Characteristics of hematopoietic stem cells

The pluripotent stem cell gives rise to all red and white blood cell populations. Human hematopoietic stem cells (HSC) in the bone marrow are rare: 1 in 10 000 cells. They occupy a distant niche in the bone marrow closest to the bone and rely on osteoblasts for this localization. Several separation methods identify stem cells and their differentiative potential. Early observations showed that the HSC had characteristic flow cytometric light-scattering properties (low side scatter, medium forward scatter), no lineage (LIN)-specific markers (e.g., CD2, CD3, CD5, CD7, CD14, CD15, or CD16), and expressed CD34 on the cell surface.[8] However, hematopoietic reconstitution can occur with CD34⁻, noncycling LIN⁻ cells, suggesting that surface expression of CD34 is not a definitive marker of the most primitive precursors.[10] Indeed, characterization of the HSC based on cell surface/functional markers can be misleading.

A subpopulation of stem cells excludes nucleophilic dyes such as Hoechst dye and is called a "side population." This can give rise to a wide variety of cell types.[9] A key aspect of a long-term stem cell is its capacity for self-renewal via asynchronous division influenced by external factors, such as infection.[10] Hematopoietic stem cells circulate in the peripheral blood with 10–100 times less frequency. Mobilization of "stem cells" to the periphery can be induced with G-CSF. Of these, about 5–20% are true stem cells.[11] Enriched peripheral blood stem cells do not express lineage-associated antigens. A minor subpopulation expresses the B-cell antigens, CD19 and CD20, and there is variable expression of CD33 and CD13. Most peripheral blood stem cells express activation antigens, such as the transferrin receptor, CD71 and CD38. Peripheral blood HSC cells engraft 2–3 days faster than conventional bone marrow HSC, which is important for reduction of bone marrow transplantation morbidities. However, peripheral blood HSC are more differentiated than those obtained from the bone marrow and have only limited self renewal properties.[12]

Regulation of hematopoietic and lymphopoietic cell growth and differentiation

Regulation of stem cell differentiation occurs through interactions with a variety of microenvironmental factors in the bone marrow or thymus. Cell surface receptors recognize either soluble ligands (e.g., cytokines) released by other cells, or surface ligands (e.g., cell interaction molecules) expressed on adjacent cells. These receptors can facilitate differentiation. Stem cells can be exposed to spatially and temporally regulated ligands or factors. The differential expression of receptors on the stem cells allows control of proliferation and differentiation along one of the hematopoietic or lymphoid lineages.[11]

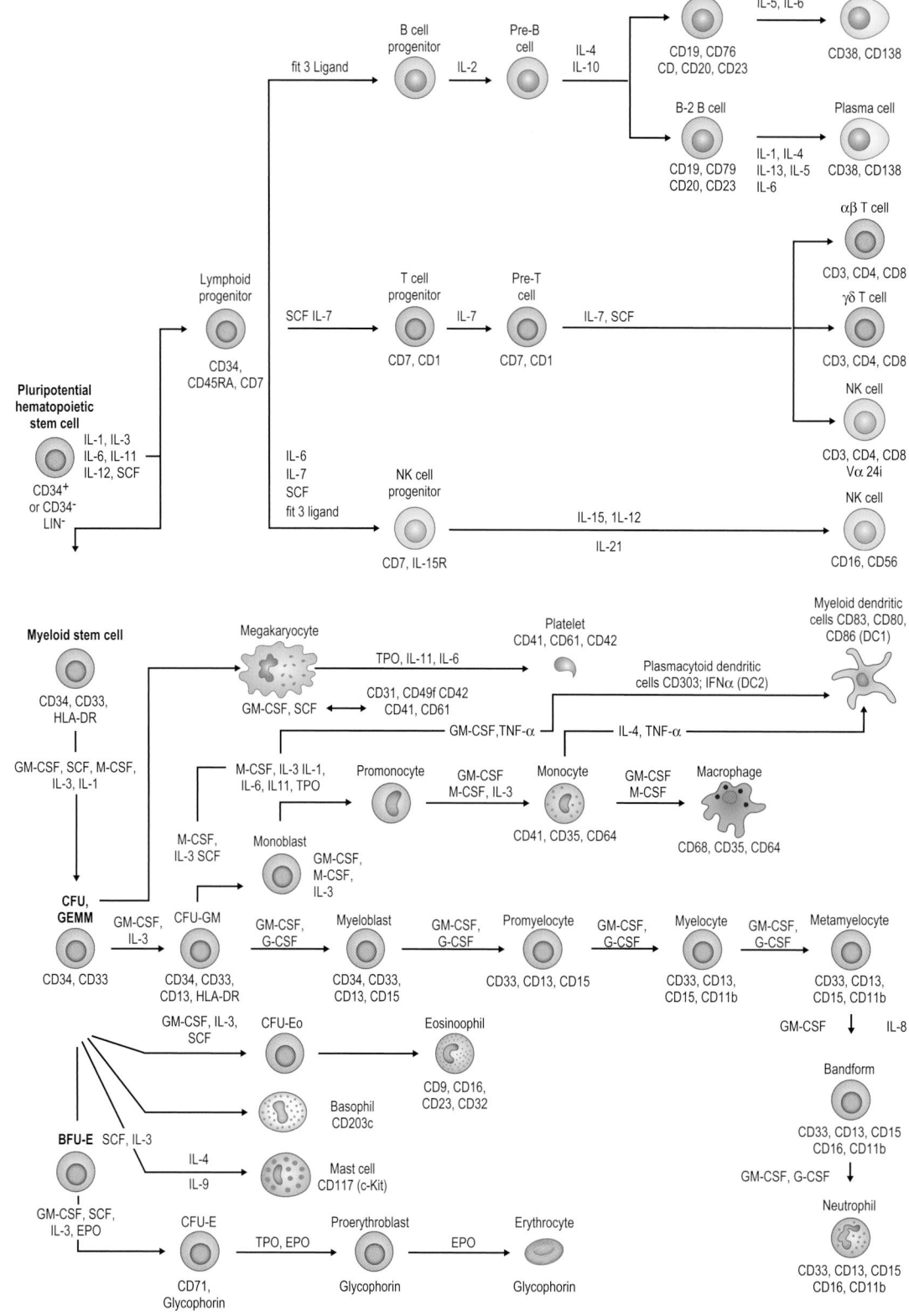

Fig. 2.1 The differentiation of hematopoietic cells.

Cytokines (Chapter 9) have pleiotropic effects on hematopoietic and lymphoid cell development. They affect both the growth and maintenance of pluripotent stem cells, as well as the development and differentiation of specific cell lineages. The effect of the cytokine often differs, depending on whether the cell has previously been or is concurrently being stimulated by other cytokines.

The stage of differentiation, as well as the presence or absence of the cytokine's receptor on the cell surface, also affects the cellular response. Although there are several cytokines, such as IL-6 and stem cell factor (SCF), that are considered to be classically involved in hematopoiesis, it has become clear in recent years that these cytokines can have non-hematopoietic functions, as well.

Table 2.2 Normal distribution of hematopoietic cells in the bone marrow

Cell type	Approximate proportion (%)
Stem cells	1
Megakaryocytes	1
Monocytes	2
Dendritic cells	2
Lymphocytes	15
Plasma cells	1
Myeloid precursors	4
Granulocytes	50–70
Red blood cell precursors	2
Immature and mature red blood cells	10–20

Stromal cells located within the bone marrow and thymus regulate hematopoietic and lymphoid cell growth and differentiation by releasing cytokines, such as the interleukins IL-4, -6, -7, and -11; leukemia inhibitory factor (LIF); granulocyte–macrophage colony-stimulating factor (GM-CSF); granulocyte colony-stimulating factor (G-CSF); and SCF.[13] Stromal cells also participate in cell–cell interactions with progenitors by means of the engagement of cell surface molecules that provide additional regulatory stimuli. In addition, stromal cells form the intercellular matrix (e.g., fibronectin and collagen) that binds to selectin and integrin receptors present on hematopoietic and lymphoid progenitors.[14]

Cytokines that affect the growth and maintenance of pluripotent and multipotent stem cells

Pluripotent stem cells are characterized by their ability to reconstitute cells of the hematopoietic and lymphoid lineages. Stem cells are resistant to 5-fluorouracil treatment, which indicates that they are dividing slowly at best. Maintenance of pluripotent capacity is mediated through differentiation antagonists, termed restrictins. Studies suggest that stromal cells maintain stem cell capacity by the release of factors such as restrictin-D or flt-3/flk-2 ligand, which either antagonize differentiation induced by other cytokines or facilitate stem cell self-renewal. Because the stem cell pool is depleted as their progeny differentiate, proliferation of the stem cells is required to avoid exhaustion. The entry of stem cells into the cell cycle and subsequent proliferation, as well as commitment to particular lineages, also appears to be controlled by cytokines. Recent studies have focused on discovery of in vitro conditions that maintain extended long-term cultures of stem cell populations. The data suggest that flt-3 ligand, c-kit ligand and megakaryocyte growth and development factor (MGDF) all promote long-term stem cell expansion. The combination of c-kit ligand, IL-3 and -6 causes more rapid expansion, but does not allow long-term extension of precursor cells.[15]

Several cytokines, either alone or in combination, have been shown to promote stem cell growth (Table 2.3).[16] In general, combinations of cytokines are more effective at inducing stem cell growth than are individual cytokines. For example, IL-1 promotes stem cell growth by inducing bone marrow stromal cells to release additional cytokines and by synergistically stimulating these cells in the presence of other cytokines. One of these other cytokines, IL-3, promotes the growth of hematopoietic progenitors. The effect is significantly enhanced by IL-6, IL-11, G-CSF, and SCF. IL-11, a stromal cell-derived cytokine, enhances IL-3-induced colony formation in 5-fluorouracil-resistant stem cells.

Similarly, other cytokines secreted by stromal cells, for example IL-6, G-CSF, and SCF, also exert their effects by shortening the G0 period in stem cells. In contrast, IL-3 acts on cells after they have left G0. IL-12 is unable to support the growth of primitive hematopoietic stem cells, either by itself or in conjunction with IL-11 or SCF. However, it does act in synergy with IL-3 and IL-11, or IL-3 and SCF, to enhance stem cell survival and growth. In some situations, cytokines can enhance the growth of hematopoietic and lymphoid cells, but in other circumstances the cytokine can inhibit cell growth or enhance differentiation. For example, the LIF cytokine can enhance the growth and development of bone marrow progenitor cells along multiple lineages in media containing IL-3, IL-6, and GM-CSF. However, in the absence of other cytokines or factors in serum, LIF has little effect on the growth and development of CD34$^+$ progenitor cells. Similarly, although transforming growth factor-β (TGF-β) and IL-4 are potent inhibitors of hematopoietic progenitor cell growth, they enhance granulocyte development. And, while tumor necrosis factor-α (TNF-α) inhibits the development of granulocytes, it can also potentiate the effects of IL-3 on hematopoietic progenitor cell proliferation.

Other cytokines have effects on the proliferation and differentiation of multipotent progenitors of hematopoietic and lymphoid cells. For example, GM-CSF and IL-3 promote the development of granulocytes, macrophages, dendritic cells and erythrocytes. IL-6 participates in the development of neutrophils, macrophages, platelets, T cells, and B cells. And thrombopoeitin signaling promotes stem cell self-renewal, which enhances transplantation success.[17]

Cytokines that inhibit hematopoietic stem cell growth

Cytokines produced by mature cells also downregulate hematopoietic stem cell growth. For example, macrophage inflammatory protein-1α (MIP-1α) is an inhibitor of hematopoietic progenitor cell proliferation. Other factors regulate stem cell growth through a variety of mechanisms, including the promotion of terminal differentiation (e.g., interferon-γ (IFN-γ) and TGF-β) or through the induction of apoptosis (e.g., TNF-α). When pathologic conditions exist, these cytokines can have adverse effects on hematopoietic and lymphoid cell development, resulting in various deficiency states.

● KEY CONCEPTS

Cells of the immune system

- Pluripotent stem cells in the bone marrow give rise to all the lineages of immune cells.
- The development and regulation of cells of the immune system is associated with the programmed appearance of specific cell surface molecules and responsiveness to selective cytokines.
- The mature cells of the immune system include the antigen-presenting cells of various types; other phagocytic cells, including neutrophils, eosinophils, basophils, and lymphocytes, which are T, B, or natural killer cells.
- Each lymphocyte lineage can be divided into discrete subpopulations which serve specialized functions. These include CD4 and CD8 T cells, T-helper (Th) subsets, CD16$^+$ and CD16$^-$ NK cells, and B-1 and conventional B-2 B cells.

Cytokines affecting development and differentiation of specific cell lineages

The initial event in differentiation involves the commitment of pluripotent stem cells to a specific lineage. Cytokines are important for this process and appear to have lineage-specific effects that act specifically at late stages of differentiation. For example, erythropoietin regulates the later stages of erythrocyte differentiation, whereas G-CSF induces granulocyte differentiation and macrophage colony-stimulating factor (M-CSF) is specific for macrophage maturation.[18] Cytokines that play an important role in the growth and development of specific cell lineages are described under each cell type.

Mature cells of the immune system

The mature cells of the immune system arise mainly from progenitor cells in the bone marrow. They include both nonspecific and antigen-specific effector cells. The central player in both lines of defense is the antigen-presenting cell (Chapter 6). In addition to their nonspecific effector functions, these cells are crucial for the development of specific immune responses. With maturation, these cells enter the blood (Table 2.4) where they circulate into the tissues and organs.

Antigen-presenting cells

Cells that act as antigen-presenting cells (APCs) include a diverse group of leukocytes such as monocytes, macrophages, dendritic cells (DCs), and B cells. In addition, endothelial or epithelial cells can acquire antigen-presenting abilities after upregulation of class II molecules of the major histocompatibility complex (MHC; Chapter 5) by various cytokines.

APC are found primarily in the solid lymphoid organs and skin (Chapter 18). The frequency of these cells varies between 0.1 and 1.0%. The specialized APC in B-cell areas of lymph nodes and spleen are termed follicular dendritic cells (FDCs). They trap antigen–antibody complexes and thus play a key role in the generation and maintenance of memory B cells. These cells do not express class II molecules, but do have receptors for IgG and complement component C3b, FcγR (CD64) and CR1 (CD35), respectively. DCs are also abundant in the thymic medulla and are involved in selection of thymocytes.

DCs residing in peripheral sites such as the skin, intestinal lamina propria, lung, genitourinary tract etc. are typically immature. These cells are more phagocytic and express fewer MHC class I, MHC class II, and co-stimulatory molecules. These immature dendritic cells take up antigens in tissues for subsequent presentation to T cells. During migration to the lymph nodes, dendritic cells undergo phenotypic and functional changes characterized by increased expression of MHC class I, MHC class II and co-stimulatory molecules (e.g., B7-1 [CD80] and B7-2 [CD86]) that react with ligands CD28 and CTLA-4 expressed by T cells.[19]

The predominant APCs of the skin are the Langerhans cells.[20] These are found in the epidermis and are characterized by rocket-shaped granules called Birbeck's granules. Upon migration from the skin, these cells deliver antigens entering the skin to the effector cells of the lymph nodes.

The immature tissue DCs in peripheral tissues also engulf and process antigens. They leave the tissues and home to T-cell areas

Table 2.3 Cytokines important for hematopoietic cell growth and differentiation

Cytokines	Stem cells	Thymocytes	B cells	NK cells
IL-1	Acts on stromal cells	Differentiation		
IL-2		Pleomorphic	Proliferation	Proliferation
IL-3	Proliferation			
IL-4		Pleomorphic	Promotes (low) Prevents (high)	Inhibits IL-2
IL-5			Proliferation/differentiation	
IL-6	Shortens G_0	Enhances stimulation	Maintains potential	Enhances IL-2
IL-7		Survival/proliferation	Proliferation of pro- and pre-B cells	Activation
IL-10			Survival	
IL-11 Oncostatin M	Shortens G_0		Maintains potential	
IL-12	Survival			Activation proliferation
IL-13			Activation/division of mature B cells	
IL-15			Proliferation	Development/survival
IL-21			Proliferation	Expansion
SCF/c-kit	Survival	Atrophy	Maintains potential	Expansion
G-CS	Shortens G_0		Maintains potential	
FLt3 ligand	Growth factor		Increases proliferation	Expansion
SDF1-α		Proliferation/Regeneration	Chemoattractant	
LIF	Proliferation	Atrophy		
Thrombopoietin	Expansion/regulates self-renewal			
TNF-α	Proliferation: inhibits granulocytes			
TGF-β	Inhibits growth enhanced granulocytes			
MIP-1α	Inhibits			
NGF			Proliferation/differentiation	Expansion

Table 2.4 Normal distribution of white blood cells in the peripheral blood of adults and children

Cell type	Approximate percentage		Range of absolute counts (no./μL)	
	Adults	**Children (0–2 yrs)**	**Adults**	**Children (0–2 yrs)**
Monocytes	4–13		400–1000	
Dendritic cells	0.5–1	ND[a]	30–170	ND
Granulocytes	35–73		2500–7500	1000–8500
Lymphocytes	15–52	34–75	1450–3600	3400–9000
As % of lymphocytes				
T cells	75–85	53–84	900–2500	2500–6200
CD4 cells	27–53	32–64	550–1500	1300–4300
CD8 cells	13–23	12–30	300–1000	500–2000
B cells	5–15	06–41	100–600	300–3000
NK cells	5–15	03–18	200–700	170–1100

[a]Not determined.
Child data adapted from Shearer W, Rosenblatt H, Gelman R, et al. Lymphocyte subsets in healthy children from birth through 18 years of age: The pediatric AIDS Clinical Trials Group P1009 study. J Allergy Clin Immunol 2003; 12: 973–980.

in the draining lymph nodes or spleen.[21] At these sites they can directly present processed antigens to resting T cells to induce their proliferation and differentiation. These effector cells then home to the site of the antigenic assault. The key distinction between mature DCs and macrophages in terms of antigen presentation is the ability of DCs to activate resting T cells directly. Modulation of DC maturation and viability are currently pursued strategies to improve vaccines for cancer and HIV.

Monocytes–macrophages

Cells of the monocyte–macrophage lineage exist in blood (~10% of white blood cells) primarily as monocytes, large 10- to 18-μm cells with peanut-shaped, pale purple nuclei as determined by Wright's staining (Table 2.4). The cytoplasm, which is 30–40% of the cell, is light blue and has azurophilic granules that resemble ground glass. There also are numerous intracytoplasmic lysosomes. The cells express MHC class II molecules, CD14 (the receptor for lipopolysaccharide), and distinct Fc receptors (FcR) for Ig. The latter include FcγRI (or CD64), which has a high affinity for IgG, and FcγRII (or CD32), which is of medium affinity and binds to aggregated IgG. FcγRIII (or CD16) has low affinity for IgG and is associated with antibody-dependent cellular cytotoxicity (ADCC); it is expressed on macrophages, but not on blood monocytes. Monocytes and macrophages also express CD89, the Fc receptor for IgA.

Macrophages are more differentiated monocytes that reside in various tissues, including lung, liver, and brain.[22] Most cells of the monocyte–macrophage lineage adhere strongly to glass or plastic surfaces, a property often used to deplete or purify them from mixed cell populations. Many cells of this lineage phagocytose organisms or tumor cells *in vitro*. Cell surface receptors, including CD14, Fcγ receptors and CR1 (CD35), are important in opsonization and phagocytosis. Cells of this lineage also express MHC class II molecules and some express the low-affinity receptor for IgE (CD23). Other cell surface molecules include myeloid antigens CD13 (aminopeptidase N) and CD15 (Gal (1–4) or [Fuc (1–3)] GlcNAc) and the adhesion molecules CD68 and CD29 or CD49d (VLA-4). In addition to phagocytic and cytotoxic functions, these cells have receptors for various cytokines such as IL-4 and IFN-γ that can regulate their function. Activated macrophages are also a major source of cytokines, including IFN, IL-1 and TNF, as well as complement proteins and prostaglandins.

Macrophages, along with DCs, are much more plastic in differentiation and function than previously realized. They can be alternatively activated and thereby become suppressive, developing anti-inflammatory properties that can be relevant in immune responses to cancer. Alternative activation is induced by T helper cell 2 (Th2) cytokines (Chapter 16) IL-4 and Il-13.[23]

Monocytes and macrophages arise from colony-forming unit granulocyte–monocyte (CFU-GM) progenitors that differentiate first into monoblasts, then promonocytes, and finally monocytes.[23] Mature monocytes leave the bone marrow and circulate in the bloodstream until they enter tissues, where they develop into tissue macrophages (alveolar macrophages, Kupffer cells, and microglial cells).

Several cytokines participate in the development of monocytes and granulocytes. For example, SCF, IL-3, IL-6, IL-11, and GM-CSF all promote the development of myeloid lineage cells from CD34[+] stem cells, especially those in the early stages of differentiation. Another cytokine, M-CSF, acts at the later stages of development and is lineage specific, inducing maturation into macrophages.[19]

Dendritic cells

Dendritic cells are accessory cells that express high levels of MHC class II molecules and are potent inducers of primary T-cell responses. Except for the bone marrow, they are found in virtually all primary and secondary lymphoid tissues, as well as in skin, mucosa, and blood. Dendritic cells are derived from CD34[+] MHC class II-negative precursors present in the bone marrow that also give rise to macrophages and granulocytes. GM-CSF and TNF-α are involved in the development of DCs from their precursors in bone marrow.[24] Langerhans cells are the immediate precursors of DCs in the skin. After encountering antigen, Langerhans cells migrate from the skin through afferent lymphatics and into draining lymph nodes, where they enter via the subcapsular sinus. Interdigitating DCs, which present peptide antigens bound to MHC class II molecules to T cells in the lymph nodes and spleen (Chapter 6), appear to derive from these Langerhans cell immigrants. TNF-α also maintains the viability of Langerhans cells in the skin and stimulates their migration. In Peyer's patches (Chapter 19), immature dendritic cells occur in the dome region underneath the follicle-associated epithelium (FAE), where they actively endocytose antigens taken up by M cells in the FAE. More mature interdigitating DCs are found in

T-cell regions, where they appear to be the major APC type. These cells, like their counterparts in the lungs, induce Th2 immune responses. There are at least two types of DC. DC1 are bone marrow derived and found in lymphoid tissues. They express CD1a and CD11c. Plasmacytoid DCs or DC2 are high producers of IFN-α. They express CD123 and not CD11c. Their derivation is debated, but they are derived from either myeloid or lymphoid lineages.[25,26]

Polymorphonuclear granulocytes

Polymorphonuclear (PMN) granulocytes arise from progenitors that mature in the bone marrow. They are released into the blood as short-lived (2–3 days), essentially end-stage, cells. They constitute 65–75% of the white blood cells in the peripheral blood, are 10–20 μm in diameter, and have features such as a multilobed pyknotic nucleus characteristic of cells undergoing apoptosis (Table 2.4).[27] PMNs are also found in tissues. They use diapedesis to gain access from the blood. Granulocytes act as early soldiers in the response to stress, tissue damage, or pathogen invasion. Because of their function in phagocytosis and killing, they possess granules whose unique staining characteristics are used to categorize the cells as neutrophils (Chapter 21), basophils (Chapter 22) or eosinophils (Chapter 23).

Neutrophils

Most circulating granulocytes are neutrophils (90%). Their granules are azurophilic and contain acid hydrolase, myeloperoxidase and lysozymes. These granules fuse with ingested organisms to form phagolysosomes, which eventually kill the invading organism. In some cases there is extracellular release of granules after activation via the Fc receptors. Neutrophils express a number of myeloid antigens, including CD13, CD15, CD16 (FcγRIII), and CD89 (FcαR). In response to bacterial infection, there is typically an increase in the number of circulating granulocytes. This often includes the release of immature granulocytes, called band or stab cells, from the bone marrow. In a mild infection, both the number and function of neutrophils are increased. This is associated with a delay in apoptosis. With a more severe infection there may actually be impairment of function owing to the release of immature cells.

Neutrophils derive from CFU-GM progenitor cells and differentiate within a 10- to 14-day period. These progenitors give rise to myeloblasts, which in turn differentiate into promyelocytes, myelocytes, and finally mature neutrophils. The cytokines SCF, IL-3, IL-6, IL-11, and GM-CSF promote the growth and development of neutrophil precursors, whereas certain cytokines are important for differentiation of CFU-GM progenitors into mature neutrophils.[28] For example, G-CSF induces maturation of neutrophil precursors into mature neutrophils. IL-4 enhances neutrophil differentiation induced by G-CSF, while at the same time inhibiting the development of macrophages induced by IL-3 and M-CSF.

Eosinophils

Eosinophils typically comprise 2–5% of the white cells in the blood. They exhibit a unique form of diurnal variation because the peak of production occurs at night, perhaps because glucocorticoid levels are lower at night. Eosinophils are capable of phagocytosis followed by killing, although this is not their main function. The granules in eosinophils are much larger than in neutrophils and are actually membrane-bound organelles. The crystalloid core of the granules contains a large amount of major basic protein (MBP), which can neutralize heparin and is toxic. During degranulation, the granules fuse to the plasma membrane and their contents are released into the extracellular space. Organisms that are too large to be phagocytosed, such as parasites, can be exposed to cell toxins by this mechanism. For example, MBP can damage schistosomes in vivo. However, tissue damage is kept to a minimum because the MBP is confined to a small area between the eosinophil and the schistosome. Eosinophils also release products that counteract the effects of mast cell mediators.

Eosinophils derive from a progenitor (CFU-Eo) that progresses through development stages similar to those of neutrophils.[29] These stages begin with an eosinophilic myeloblast, followed by an eosinophilic promyelocyte, a myelocyte, and finally a mature eosinophil. Three cytokines are important in the development of eosinophils: GM-CSF, IL-3 and IL-5. GM-CSF and IL-3 promote eosinophil growth and differentiation; SCF also has an effect on eosinophil function. IL-5 has more lineage-specific effects on eosinophil differentiation, although it also affects some subsets of T and B cells; it is also important for eosinophil survival and maturation.

Basophils and mast cells

Basophils represent less than 1% of the cells in the peripheral circulation, and have characteristic large, deep-purple granules. Mast cells are found in proximity to blood vessels and are much larger than peripheral blood basophils. The granules are less abundant and nucleus is more prominent. There are two different types of mast cell, designated mucosal or connective tissue depending on their location.[30] Mucosal mast cells require T cells for their proliferation, whereas connective tissue mast cells do not. Both types have granules that contain effector molecules. After degranulation, which is effected by cross-linkage of cell surface IgE bound to cells via the high-affinity receptor for IgE, the basophils–mast cells release heparin, histamine, and other effector substances to mediate an immediate allergic attack (Chapters 22 and 40).

Basophils and mast cells share a number of phenotypic and functional features that suggest derivation from a common precursor. They both contain basophilic-staining cytoplasmic granules; express the high-affinity IgE receptor (FcεRI); and release a number of similar chemical mediators that participate in immune and inflammatory responses, particularly anaphylaxis. However, basophils and mast cells have some distinct morphologic and functional characteristics that suggest they represent distinct lineages of cells, rather than cells at different stages within the same lineage. For example, in human transcription factor analysis seems to relate basophils closer to eosinophils than to mast cells.

Basophils mature from a progenitor (CFU-BM) into basophilic myeloblasts, then basophilic promyelocytes, myelocytes, and finally mature basophils. Less is known about the stages of mast cell development, although they are probably derived from the same CFU-BM progenitor as basophils.

In human, SCF induces the most consistent effects on the growth and differentiation of both basophils and mast cells. Both IL-3 and SCF are important for intestinal mast cell differentiation. Il-6 can also increase mast cell numbers. This probably explains why T cells are needed for their development.[31] In mice, both IL-4 and -9 stimulate mast cell development. However, in human only IL-9 acts in synergy with SCF to enhance mast cell growth. Additional cytokines that affect basophil growth include nerve growth factor and GM-CSF or TGF-β, and IL-5 for basophil differentiation.

Platelets and erythrocytes

Hematopoietic stem cells also give rise to platelets and erythrocytes. Platelets derive from CFU-GEMM progenitors, which in turn differentiate into burst-forming units for megakaryocytes (BFU-MEG). The BFU-MEG then differentiate into CFU-MEG, promegakaryoblasts, megakaryoblasts, megakaryocytes, and finally platelets.[32] Several cytokines, particularly thrombospondin, IL-1, IL-3, GM-CSF, IL-6, IL-11, and LIF, affect the growth and differentiation of platelets.

Erythrocytes also derive from CFU-GEMM progenitors, but their progenitors are burst-forming units for erythrocytes (BFU-E), which in turn differentiate into CFU-E, pronormoblasts, basophilic normoblasts, polychromatophilic normoblasts, orthochromic normoblasts, reticulocytes, and finally erythrocytes.[33] Again, several cytokines, notably GM-CSF, SCF, IL-9, thrombospondin, and erythropoietin, regulate erythrocyte development.

Lymphocytes

Lymphocytes, the central cell type of the specific immune system, represent about 25% of white cells in the blood (Table 2.4). Small lymphocytes range between 7 and 10 µm in diameter. They are characterized by a nucleus that stains dark purple with Wright's stain, and by a small cytoplasm. Large granular lymphocytes range between 10 and 12 µm in diameter and contain more cytoplasm and scattered granules. The three types of lymphocytes that circulate in the peripheral blood—T, B, and NK cells—constitute approximately 80, 10, and 10% of the total blood lymphocyte population, respectively (Chapters 7, 8, and 17). In the thymus most of the lymphocytes (90%) are T cells; however, in the spleen and lymph nodes only about 30–40% are T cells. The preponderant lymphocytes in these locations are B cells (60–70%).[34,35]

T lymphocytes

T lymphocytes arise from lymphocyte progenitors in the bone marrow that are committed to the T-cell lineage before homing to the thymus. In the early stages of embryogenesis, T-cell precursors migrate to the thymus in waves.[36,37] Associated with this migration is the developing ability of thymic education elements, epithelial cells, and DCs to select appropriate T cells.[38] In the thymus, T cells rearrange their specific antigen receptors (TCR) and then express CD3 along with the TCR on their surface (Chapter 8). Resting T cells in the blood typically range between 7 and 10 µm in diameter and are agranular, except for the presence of a structure termed a Gall body, which is not found in B cells (Table 2.4). The Gall body is a cluster of primary lysosomes associated with a lipid droplet. A minority of T cells in the blood (about 20%), are of the large granular type, meaning that they are 10–12 µm in diameter and contain primarily lysosomes that are dispersed in the cytoplasm. Golgi apparati also are found. The preponderant form of the TCR, found on about 95% of circulating T cells, consists of α and β chains (αβTCR+).[39] Some CD3+ cells do not express either CD4 or CD8 (double-negative or DN) and are characterized by having an alternative TCR composed of γ and δ chains (γδTCR+). Further differentiation in the thymus occurs from CD3+ cells that express both CD4 and CD8 (double-positive or DP) to cells expressing either CD4 or CD8 but not both (Chapter 8). These mature cells then circulate in the peripheral blood at a ratio of about 2:1 (CD4:CD8) and populate the lymph nodes, spleen and other secondary lymphoid tissues.

T-cell progenitors, which are CD7+, are believed to arise in the bone marrow from a multipotential lymphoid stem cell. After migration to the thymus, the CD7+ progenitors give rise to a population of CD34+, CD3-, CD4-, and CD8- T-cell precursors, which undergo further differentiation into mature T cells. Cytokines produced by thymic epithelial cells, e.g., IL-1 and soluble CD23, promote differentiation into CD2+, CD3+ thymocytes (Table 2.3). IL-7 induces the proliferation of CD3+ DN (CD4- CD8-) thymocytes, even in the absence of comitogenic stimulation. IL-7 is absolutely required for human T-cell development.[40] IL-2 and -4 demonstrate complex effects on thymocyte development. Both appear capable not only of promoting the development of prothymocytes, but also of antagonizing their development. IL-6 acts as a co-stimulator of IL-1- or -2-induced proliferation of DN thymocytes and can stimulate the proliferation of mature, cortisone-resistant thymocytes alone. Once T cells leave the thymus, a variety of cytokines affect their growth and differentiation.

Subpopulations of T cells

T cells can be divided into subsets based on surface expression of CD4 and CD8, as well as by function in the immune response. CD4 and CD8 T cells were originally characterized by expression of the respective antigen and association with functional ability. For example, human T cells expressing CD4 provide help for antibody synthesis, whereas cells expressing CD8 develop into cytotoxic T cells. These functional distinctions are not as definitive today. For example, there is ample evidence for cytotoxic cells that express CD4. Instead, the distinction involves which antigen-presenting molecule is used for TCR interaction. Thus, CD4 T cells recognize antigen in the context of MHC class II molecules, and CD8 T cells recognize antigen presented by class I molecules (Chapter 6).

T-helper (Th) cells mature in response to foreign antigens. Their function is dependent on the production of cytokine modules, which characterize them as Th type 1 (Th1), Th2 or Th17.[41] The precursor Th cell first differentiates into a Th0 cell producing interferon-γ (IFN-γ) and IL-4. The cytokine environment subsequently determines whether Th1 or Th2 cells predominate. Th1 cells produce primarily IFN-γ, IL-2, and TNF-α, and are important in cell-mediated immunity to intracellular pathogens, such as the tubercle bacillus. Th2 cells produce predominantly IL-4, -5, -6, -10, and -13, as well as IL-2, and predominate in immediate or allergic type 1 hypersensitivity. Other populations of CD4 T cells can develop and rely on IL-23 or -12 action upon the cells.[42] If T cells are exposed to IFN-γ, they upregulate both IL-12R and -23R, which then produce either conventional Th1 cells or another subset, Th17, which produces IL-17 and has been associated with autoimmunity. Conversely, IL-17-producing CD4 cells also result from the direct action of IL-23 without IL-12 involvement. It is likely that there are other epigenetically altered T cells that allow diversity of function during an immune response.

A minor subpopulation (<5%) of CD3+ cells in the peripheral blood express γδ TCR molecules. Most of these cells do not express CD4 or CD8. However, some intraepithelial lymphocytes that express γδ TCR also express CD8 αα homodimers in place of conventional CD8 αβ heterodimers. These cells, which are thymus independent, are involved in the initial response to bacterial antigens presented in mucosal epithelium. Another minor subpopulation of T cells, NKT cells, can be CD4+ or CD8+ and express a single Vα chain, Vα24, which recognizes glycolipids in the context of CD1a rather than a classical MHC molecule.[43,44] NKT cells express MIP-1 α and β, have a Th1 bias, but lack Il-10 production The final minor subset is regulatory T cells (Treg), which occur naturally and can be induced *in vitro*. They are CD4+

and express high levels of CD25 and the transcription factor Foxp3 and perhaps GARP.[45,46] These cells are important in regulatory immune responses. Treg are reduced in autoimmunity and increased in cancer.

B cells and plasma cells

B cells represent 5–10% of the lymphocytes in the blood (Table 2.4). They are typically 7–10 μm in diameter and lack Gall bodies and granules. The cytoplasm is characterized by scattered ribosomes and isolated rough endoplasmic reticulum (RER). The Golgi is not prominent, unless the cells are activated. B cells express cell membrane immunoglobulin (mIg), the majority expressing both IgM and IgD.[47] A small minority of B cells express either surface IgG or IgA. Plasma cells (10–15 μm) are not normally found in the blood. They display an eccentric nucleus and a basophilic cytoplasm with a well-developed Golgi. The plasma cell displays parallel arrays of expanded RER that contains Ig.

A number of other cell surface molecules are found on B cells (Chapter 7), including CD19, CD20, CD40, CD79, MHC class II, Fcγ RII receptors (CD32) and complement receptors C3b (CR1a; CD35) and C3d (CR2a; CD21). Similar to T cells, which surround the TCR with activation effector molecules termed CD3, the B-cell Ig also has a B-cell receptor complex consisting of CD19, CD21, and CD81 (Chapter 4). Upon activation and cross-linking of surface Ig by specific antigen, B cells undergo proliferation and differentiation to produce plasma cells. Plasma cells are nondividing, specialized cells terminally differentiated from B cells, the function of which is to secrete Ig. They lose expression of mIg and MHC class II molecules. B-cell proliferation and differentiation processes take place in the germinal centers of the lymph nodes.

Several cytokines influence the development of B lymphocytes. *In vitro* studies of cytokines involved in the development of early B-cell progenitors show that combinations of SCF (but not IL-3) with IL-6, IL-11 or G-CSF can maintain B-lymphoid potential.[47] Stromal cell-dependent differentiation of fetal pro-B cells occurs in conjunction with Flk-2/flt-3 ligand.

IL-4 has a variety of important effects on B-cell growth and differentiation. Low doses of IL-4 induce pre-B cells to differentiate into B cells expressing surface membrane IgM, whereas higher doses of IL-4 inhibit differentiation into B cells. In mature B cells, IL-4 increases expression of MHC class II, CD23 and CD40 molecules; promotes activation and progression to the G_1 stage of the cell cycle; enhances proliferation after stimulation through the Ig receptor; and induces immunoglobulin class switch in human to IgG_4 and IgE (IgG_1 and IgE in mouse). IL-13, which is closely related to IL-4, has many similar effects on B cells.

Other cytokines, such as IL-2, -5, -6, -11, and nerve growth factor (NGF), act on mature B cells and can either enhance their proliferation or promote their differentiation into immunoglobulin-secreting cells. In addition, IL-10 enhances the viability of B cells *in vitro*, increases MHC class II expression, and augments the proliferation and differentiation of B cells after stimulation through the Ig receptor or CD40. TGF-$β_1$ is a major switch factor for IgA. This cytokine induces human B cells triggered by mitogen to switch to both IgA_1 and IgA_2. SDF-1 (stromal cell-derived factor) attracts early-stage B-cell precursors and is a likely mechanism whereby B cells form islands in the bone marrow.[18] Best studied in mice, there are at least two major populations of B cells: B-1 cells that are found in the follicular mantle and the peritoneal cavity, and conventional B-2 cells, which are primarily found in lymphoid follicles. The B-1 lineage predominates early

in gestation and produces natural antibodies of the IgM isotype.[48]

There is good evidence for local expression of IgA plasma cell precursors in the ileum, which is important for bacterial containment.[49]

Natural killer cells

NK cells comprise the third major lymphocyte subset, i.e., 10–15% of circulating lymphocytes (Table 2.4). These cells are usually larger than typical lymphocytes (10–12 μm) and display less nuclear material and more cytoplasm than do small lymphocytes. They possess electron-dense peroxidase-negative granules and a well developed Golgi apparatus. Functional NK cells can be found in the fetal liver as early as 6 weeks' gestation. These fetal NK cells express cytoplasmic CD3 proteins, but exhibit no TCR rearrangements. Evidence suggests that an Fcγ receptor-positive cell that does not express lineage-specific markers (LIN⁻) exists in the fetal mouse thymus, where it normally gives rise to T cells. However, if removed from the thymus, the cells develop into CD3⁻ NK cells. Such CD3⁻ cells with variable CD16 expression exist in human thymocyte populations and can be induced to proliferate, express NK-associated antigens, and exhibit NK cell function *in vitro*. These cells also express substantial levels of CD3δ and CD3ε in the cytoplasm.[50]

Mature NK cells do not express conventional antigen receptors, such as TCR or Ig, and the genes for these receptors remain unrearranged. Some express FcγRIII (CD16) and others express CD56, an adhesion molecule. NK cells, like T cells, also express the CD2 molecule. NK cells express the β chain of the IL-2 receptor, CD122, which allows resting NK cells to respond directly to IL-2. The function of NK cells is to provide nonspecific cytotoxic activity towards virally infected cells and tumor cells (Chapter 17). NK cells also can kill specifically when they are provided an antibody. This death delivery mechanism, known as antibody-dependent cellular cytotoxicity (ADCC), occurs via binding of the antibody to the Fcγ receptor CD16. After activation, NK cells produce cytokines, such as IFN-γ, that can affect the proliferation and differentiation of other cell types, especially DCs. Some of the recognition molecules on human NK cells are activating, some are inhibiting, and some act as receptors for MHC class I molecules.

The ontogeny of NK cells is now better understood. Although they express a number of membrane antigens in common with T cells and share functional properties with some T-cell subsets, suggesting a common origin, NK cells are found in fetuses before the development of T cells or the thymus. In addition, NK cells appear to develop normally in nude, athymic mice. NK cells probably develop extrathymically, and recent data suggest that they can develop from stem cells in the lymph nodes. NK cells arise from triple-negative (CD3⁻CD4⁻CD8⁻) precursors that are CD56⁺, but do not express CD34 or CD5. T cells, on the other hand, develop from "triple-negative" precursors that are CD34⁺CD5⁺CD56⁺. It is likely that T and NK cells arise from a common "triple-negative" precursor with the phenotype CD7⁺CD34⁺CD5⁺CD56⁺.

The cytokine receptor that determines lineage specificity is the α chain of the IL-2 receptor, CD25. Once CD25 is upregulated, the cell is destined to become a T cell. The cytokines most important in the early development of NK cells are IL-15 and IL-7. Flt ligand and c-kit also facilitate NK cell expansion. Several cytokines promote the growth and differentiation of mature NK cells. IL-2, induces proliferation and activation of NK cells. This probably occurs via the IL-2 receptor β chain (CD122), as NK cells do not express CD25. IL-2 also induces the growth of NK cells from precursors in bone marrow cultures. Both IL-7 and IL-12 activate NK cells. Although IL-4 inhibits the effects of IL-2 or IL-7 on NK cells, it acts synergistically with IL-12 to induce proliferation of CD56$^+$ cells. IL-6, despite having no effect by itself, enhances NK cell activity in thymocytes cultured with IL-2. Finally, IL-15 is also involved in signalling NK cells for survival.[51]

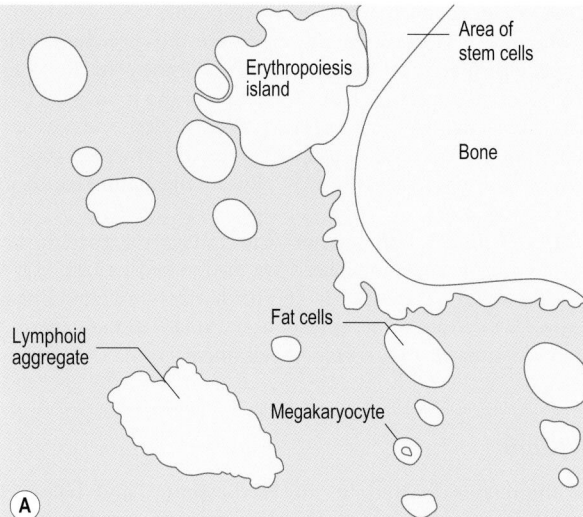

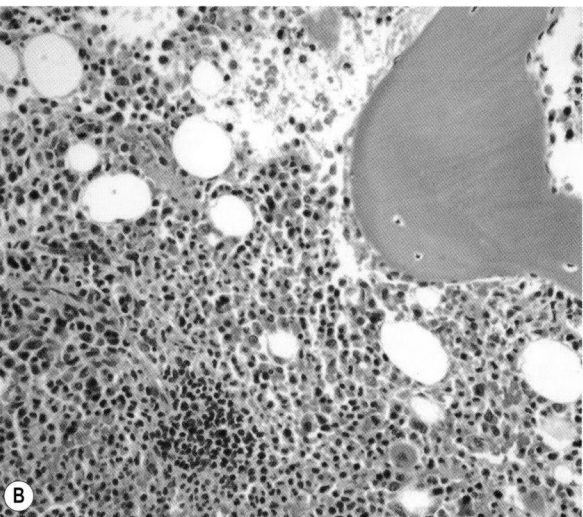

Fig. 2.2 Structure of the bone marrow, showing islands of erythropoiesis, granulopoiesis,and scattered lymphocytes.

● KEY CONCEPTS

Tissues of the immune system

- The immune system consists of central locations of immune cell production and differentiation, and dispersed organs, where encounter with and response to antigens occur.

- B cells and T cells develop in the bone marrow and thymus, respectively.

- The mucosal surfaces and skin provide the primary access for foreign antigens to cells of the immune system, where they first interact primarily with antigen-presenting cells.

- The secondary lymph organs, which include the spleen, lymph nodes, tonsils, and Peyer's patches, are where immune reactions occur.

Major lymphoid organs

The primary lymphoid organs are sites where lymphocytes differentiate from stem cells and proliferate and mature into effector cells. From birth to old age, these functions are carried out only in the bone marrow and the thymus.

Bone marrow

The bone marrow provides the environment necessary for the development of most of the white blood cells of the body (Fig. 2.2). At birth, most bone cavities are filled with actively dividing blood-forming elements known as "red" marrow. By 3–4 years, however, the tibia and femur become filled with fat cells, limiting their role in hematopoietic development. The ribs, sternum, iliac crest and vertebrae remain 30–50% cellular and produce hematopoietic cells throughout life.[1] Main components of the bone marrow include blood vessels, cells, and extracellular matrix. The production of cells from HSC occurs in areas separated by vascular sinuses. The walls of the surrounding sinus contain a layer of endothelial cells with endocytic and adhesive properties. These specialized endothelial cells of the sinuses probably produce type IV collagen and laminin for structural support. These cells also elaborate colony-stimulating factors and IL-6. The outer wall of the sinus is irregularly covered with reticular cells. These branch into areas where cells are developing and provide anchors for those cells by producing reticular fibers. Megakaryocytes lie against this wall, touching the endothelial cells. A functional unit of marrow, called a spheroid, contains adipocytes, stromal cell types and macrophages. These reticular cell networks compartmentalize the developing progenitor cells into separate microenvironments called *hematons*.

The distribution of stem and progenitor cells across the radial axis of the bone suggests that the HSC are next to the bone surface, whereas the more mature progenitor cells are nearer the central venous sinus. This distribution facilitates release of mature cells. The production of new progenitor cells from stem cells occurs as a result of interactions between stem cells and stromal cells. Given the right stimulus, most of the progeny proliferate and differentiate further, which may result in migration from the bone marrow. In migrating, the cells become detached from stromal elements and progress toward the central sinus. Control of hematopoiesis is regulated by both positive and negative cytokines and by up- and downregulation of various adhesion molecules in committed progenitor cells. The molecules involved include the fibronectin receptor, glycoproteins IIb and IIIa, ICAM-1 (CD54), LFA-1 (CD11, CD18), LFA-3 (CD58), CD2, and CD44. Adhesion molecules on stromal cell surfaces include fibronectin, laminin, ICAM-1 (CD54), types I, III and IV collagen, and N-CAM. The most clearly established role for adhesion molecules involves fibronectin, which allows erythroid precursors to bind to stromal cells and thus facilitates progression from erythroblast to reticulocyte.

The accessory cell populations in bone marrow regulate many aspects of hematopoiesis, both positively and negatively. The upregulation of growth of the earliest progenitor cells is mediated by cytokines. For example, macrophages produce IL-1, which then induces stromal cells to express growth factors such as GM-CSF, IL-6, and IL-11. However, downregulation can occur at any stage. For example, T cells regulate hematopoiesis by producing factors that act on early erythroid progenitor cells, BFU-E. Later progenitors, CFU-E, are then more fully differentiated by erythropoietin. By contrast, activated T cells produce factors that can suppress BFU-E and CFU-E *in vitro*.

Cells in the bone marrow were originally characterized by morphology. The predominant types are those of the myeloid lineage, which account for about 50–70% of the cells. Red blood cell precursors represent from 15 to 40% of the total cells. Other lineages exist in lower proportions (<5%). With the advent of cell surface antigen markers and flow cytometry, a more precise delineation could be made (Fig. 2.3). Thus, of the mature leukocytes in the bone marrow, approximately 70% are CD3$^+$, CD14$^+$, CD20$^+$, or CD11b$^+$. Both memory T and B cells return to the bone marrow after generation. These are designated as Lin$^+$. Of the Lin$^-$ cells, about 6% are CD33$^+$ and primarily of myeloid lineage. A Lin$^-$CD71$^+$ population represents about 18% of the total and is preponderantly of the red blood cell lineage.

Thymus

The thymus is located in the mediastinum and below the sternum. This bilobed organ develops from the third and fourth pharyngeal pouches and is endodermal in origin. It is organized into a loose lobular structure, with areas in each lobe consisting of a cortex of rapidly dividing cells and a medulla that contains fewer, but more mature, T cells (Figs 2.4, 2.5). This arrangement has long suggested a scenario for differentiation where cells progress from the cortex to the medulla. Non-lymphocyte cells play very important site-specific roles in the thymic development of T cells. Epithelial cells are scattered throughout the thymus. Depending on their location, they are known as nurse cells, cortical epithelial cells or medullary epithelial cells. Macrophage-type cells and interdigitating cells that are bone-marrow derived are located at the junction between cortex and medulla and are involved in T-cell selection.

Enlarged, activated T-cell precursors from the bone marrow begin by colonizing the subcapsular region of each lobe. These are actively proliferating and can self-renew. Selection begins when their progeny encounter MHC class II molecule-bearing cortical epithelial cells. A further education process probably occurs by interaction with macrophage-like cells found at the cortico-medullary junction and in the medulla.

Thymic nurse cells, found in the cortex, were originally thought to contribute to the thymic education of T cells. Because large numbers of thymic cells (50–200) can be found inside each nurse cell, it was believed that these structures provided an environment where selection and expansion could occur.

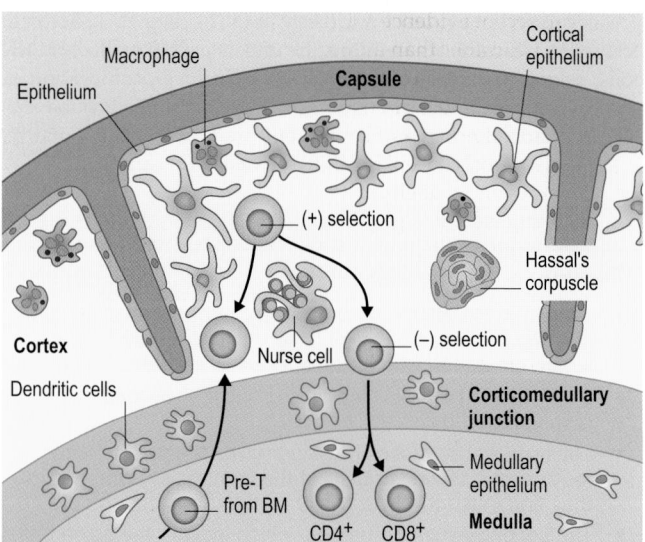

Fig. 2.4 Structure of the thymus, showing pre-T cells entering from the bone marrow (BM). Positive selection occurs on thymic epithelial cells; negative selection probably occurs during interactions with corticomedullary dendritic cells. This may explain why single-positive CD4 or CD8 cells are found primarily in the medulla. Nurse cells appear to remove negatively selected cells. Hassall's corpuscles are specialized cells producing thymic growth factors.

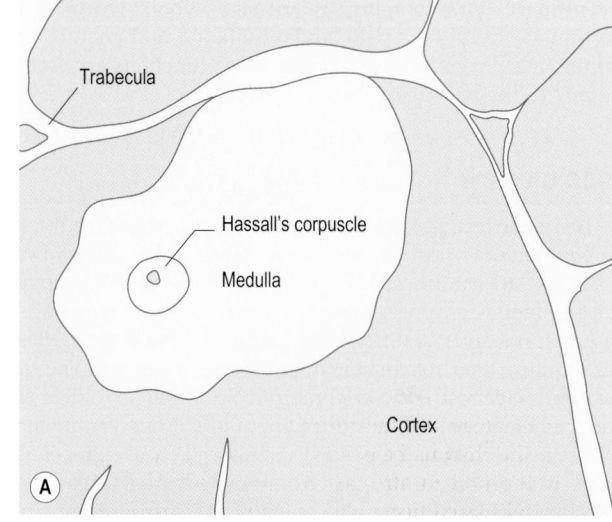

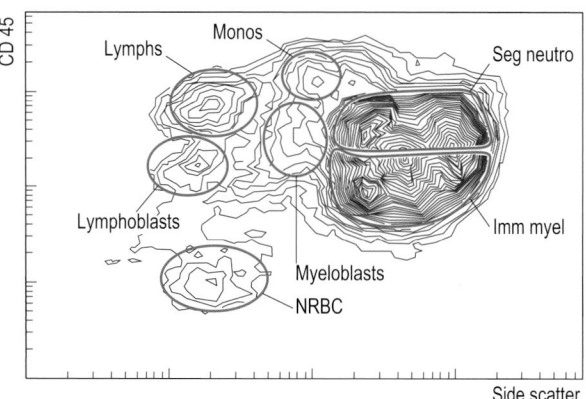

Fig. 2.3 Flow cytogram of normal human bone marrow based on CD45 expression and side scatter. Most of the major hematopoietic populations can be delineated. In this example 1.5% are red blood cell precursors (NRBC), 1.5% are lymphoblasts, 3.0% are mature lymphoytes (Lymphs), 3.0% are monocytes (Monos), 4.0% are myeloblasts, 45% are segmented neutrophils (Seg neutro),and 42% are immature myeloid cells (Imm myel).

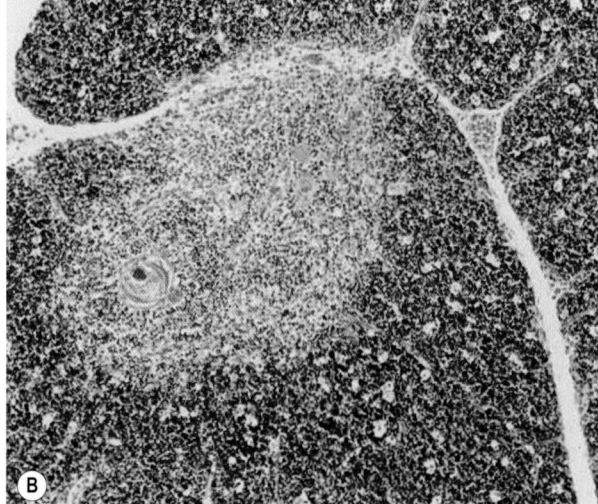

Fig. 2.5 Human thymus showing cortex and medullary areas. Cortical thymocytes are stained with an anti-CD1 antibody. Most medullary T cells do not express CD1.

However, recent evidence suggests that "nurse" may be a misnomer because, rather than aiding in their development, the nurse cells appear to dispose of developing T cells. Nurse cells are very busy, with about 90% of cortical T cells dying at this stage.

A structure known as Hassall's corpuscle, which consists of concentric whorls of epithelial cells, is found in the medulla, but its function is unclear. The Hassall's medullary epithelial cells contain secretory granules, and this network of cells may be active in the production of thymic hormones. In the fetus these bundles of cells are widely scattered, but become larger as the thymus matures. The center cells eventually become keratinized and die.

The thymic differentiation process (Chapter 8) involves rearrangement of functional TCR, surface expression of CD3, and both positive and negative selection that allows only a small percentage of T cells to survive. Pre-T cells in the thymus express CD2, CD5 and CD7, as well as activation antigens such as CD38 and the transferrin receptor (CD71). Pre-T cells express intracytoplasmic CD3 and exhibit rearrangements in the TCR-β chain. Successful rearrangement of TCR-α allows the cell to progress to the next stage of development, with functional TCR and CD3 on the cell surface.[38] Such later-stage cells represent most of the cells in the thymus (85%). These immature cells express both CD4 and CD8 on their surface, as well as CD1. CD69, an activation marker, is upregulated at this "double-positive" stage. CD69 continues to be expressed until the cell reaches the single-positive stage, where it expresses either CD4 or CD8, but not both. T cells are CD45RO$^+$ at the double-positive stage into the single-positive stage. Prior to leaving the thymus, CD45RO is downregulated and CD45RA appears. The most mature thymic cells lose CD1 expression and either CD4 or CD8 expression. Most of these mature cells are also negative for activation molecules (CD38 and CD71). However, they acquire an adhesion molecule called CD44, which is necessary for homing. Upon completion of this thymic selection and education process, mature CD4 or CD8 T cells leave the thymus and enter the peripheral circulation via the postcapillary venules at the corticomedullary junction.

After birth and during childhood, the thymus continues to grow and select and educate T cells. This process is probably necessary to develop a fully normal repertoire. Prior to puberty, however, the thymus begins to involute. The rapidly dividing cortex is the first to atrophy, leaving medullary areas intact. The sensitivity of cortical thymocytes to hormone-induced death probably accounts for the involution, although there is evidence that human thymocytes are less sensitive to glucocorticosteroids than are murine thymocytes. However, an increase in steroids reduces immature thymocyte numbers and enhances thymus involution. Recent evidence suggests that active TCR rearrangements, and hence T-cell development, continue in the adult thymus, albeit at a lower level than during childhood. There is an age-associated decline in new T-cell production, such that by age 75 the ability to make new T cells in humans is severely reduced.[52]

Development of hematopoietic and lymphoid cells

Although most of the key steps during the growth and development of hematopoietic and lymphoid cells occur in the bone marrow and thymus, additional maturation steps occur after the cells leave those tissues. For example, monocytes and dendritic cell precursors migrate from blood vessels into tissues where they mature into macrophages and dendritic cells, respectively. Likewise, mast cells and eosinophils undergo further differentiation

in resident tissues. After leaving the bone marrow and thymus, B and T cells undergo further maturation and memory cell development in secondary lymphoid organs. Some T cells, particularly γδ T cells residing in mucosal epithelium, may develop extrathymically.

Secondary lymphoid organs

Secondary lymphoid organs are sites where mature lymphocytes reside and where immune responses are generated. Secondary lymphoid organs belong to either the systemic or mucosal immune systems. The systemic immune system includes the spleen and lymph nodes and functions to protect the body from antigens in the lymphatic drainage and circulating in the bloodstream. The mucosal immune system responds to antigens that enter through mucosal epithelium and plays an important role in the inductive phase of the immune response. Unique features differentiate the mucosal immune system from the systemic immune system (Chapter 19). These include efferent but not afferent lymphatics, a specialized FAE involved in antigen sampling at the mucosal surface (Fig. 2.6), specialized dendritic cells that rapidly process and present antigens to initiate antigen-specific immune responses, unique distribution and subsets, and an environment that promotes class switching to IgA.

Systemic immune system
Spleen

The spleen is surrounded by a capsule of fibrous tissue with many trabeculae traversing from the capsule into the tissue of the spleen. These trabeculae branch and anastomose, forming a complex framework of lobules. Splenic blood vessels enter and exit through the hilum of the spleen and branch into smaller vessels within the trabeculae. Splenic tissue is supported by a fine network of reticular cells and fibers, called the reticulum, which connects and supports the trabeculae, blood vessels, and capsule. The lobules of the spleen can be functionally divided into two compartments, the red pulp and the white pulp. The largest compartment is the red pulp, which contains numerous venous sinuses situated between arteries and veins. Blood is filtered through these sinuses, which contain many macrophages that phagocytose senescent red and white blood cells, bacteria, and other particulate material. Other leukocytes are found in the red pulp, including neutrophils, eosinophils, and lymphocytes, particularly plasma cells.[53]

The white pulp consists of lymphoid tissue surrounding central arterioles, which are branches of trabecular arteries. This lymphoid tissue contains a T cell-predominant area immediately surrounding a central arteriole, the so-called periarteriolar lymphoid sheath (PALS), which contains both CD4 and CD8 T cells. It is punctuated at intervals by B-cell-predominant areas, follicles or so-called malpighian corpuscles. These B-cell-predominant areas contain primary and secondary follicles. Primary follicles consist of only a mantle zone, without germinal centers, whereas secondary follicles contain an inner germinal center in addition to the outer mantle zone (Fig. 2.7). Within the mantle zone are predominantly resting B cells, which express surface IgM/IgD and CD23 (FcεRII). It is within germinal centers that immunoglobulin class switch, affinity maturation through somatic mutation, and the development of memory B cells occurs. Germinal centers are more prevalent at younger ages and diminish with aging. CD4 T cells play a key role in B-cell responses through

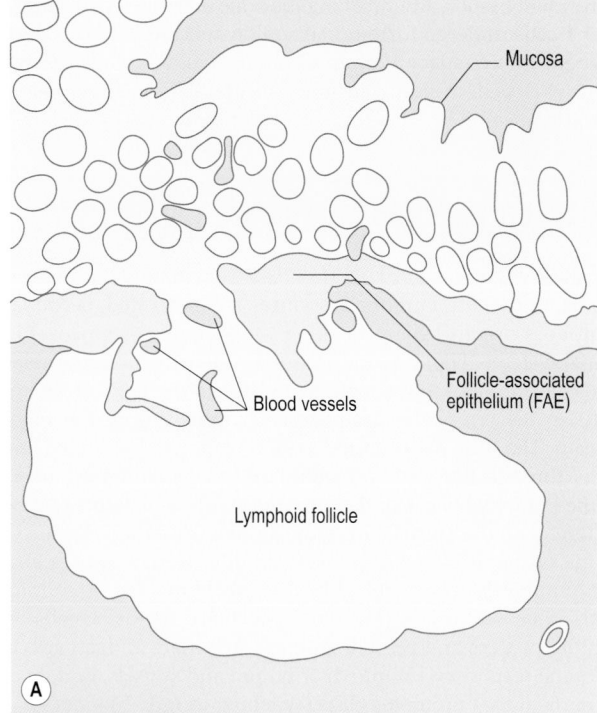

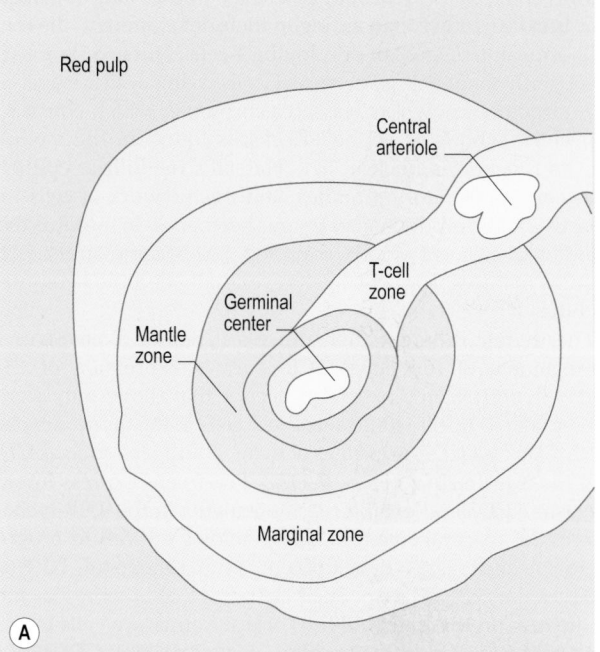

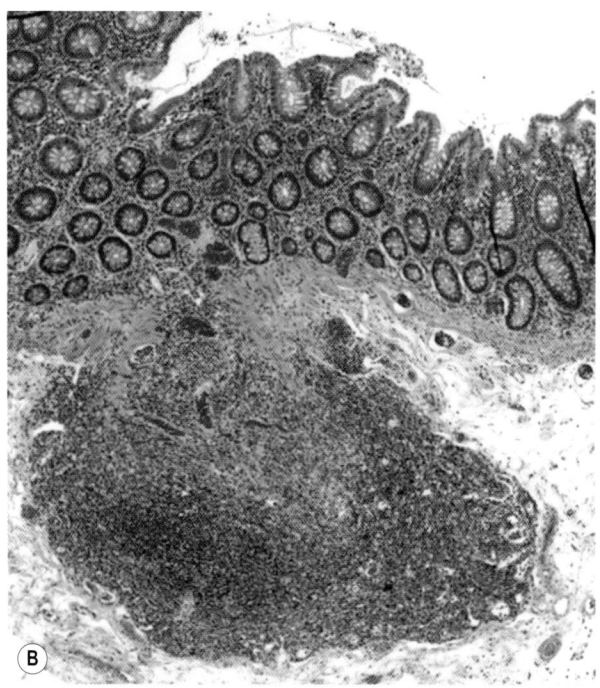

Fig. 2.6 **Lymphoid follicles in the human large intestine. FAE, follicule-associated epithelium.**

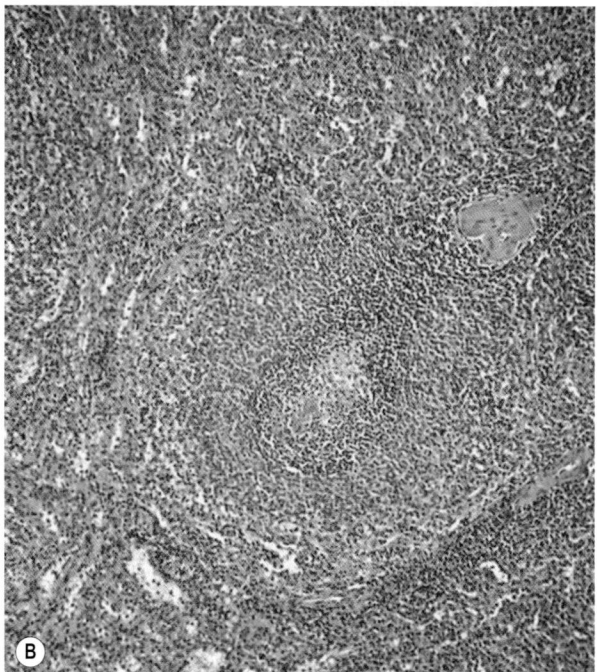

Fig. 2.7 **Human spleen showing a periarteriolar lymphoid sheath and germinal center.**

CD40L interactions. The signaling that occurs through this interaction is central to B-cell activation and class switching. In addition to activated B cells and CD4 T cells, the germinal center contains FDCs and macrophages.

At the interface between white pulp and red pulp is a region known as the marginal zone, which receives blood from branches of central arterioles opening into this region. It contains T cells, as well as subsets of macrophages and B cells. The marginal zone B cells (MZB), distinct from follicular B cells, express surface IgM, but only low levels of IgD and no CD23. The initial encounter of T cells and B cells with antigen occurs in the marginal zone after blood enters through branches of the central arteriole. Antigen presentation is enhanced by MZB cells, which are important in T cell-independent responses.

Lymph nodes and lymphatics

Lymph nodes occur as chains or groups located along lymphatic vessels. Lymph nodes exist in two major groups: those that drain the skin and superficial tissues (e.g., cervical, axillary, or inguinal lymph nodes), and those that drain the mucosal and deep tissues of the body (e.g., mesenteric, mediastinal, and periaortic lymph nodes). Lymph nodes are oval structures with an indentation at the region of a hilus, where blood vessels enter and leave the

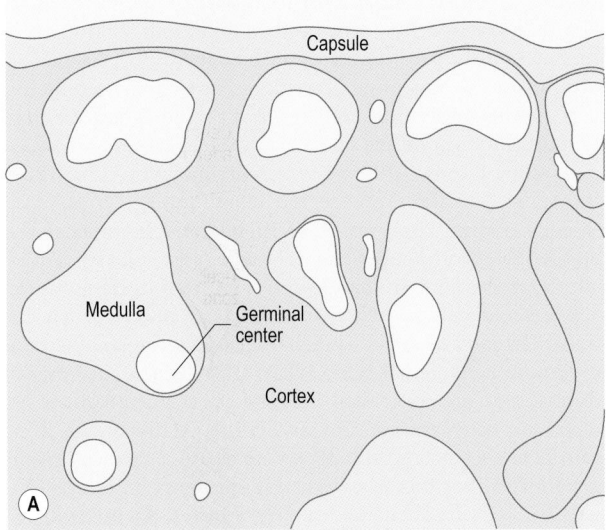

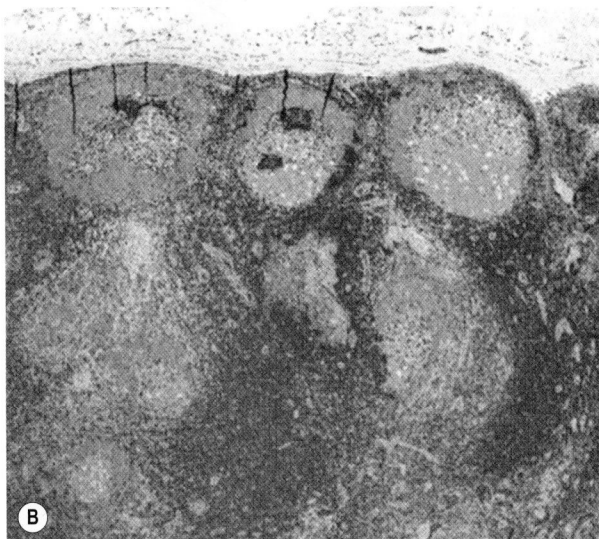

Fig. 2.8 Human lymph node showing cortex, medullary areas, and germinal centers.

node (Fig. 2.8). A lymph node is surrounded by a fibrous capsule contiguous with trabeculae traversing the node. Blood vessels and nerves, which enter through the hilus, branch through these trabeculae to the various parts of the node. Immediately beneath the capsule is a subcapsular (marginal) sinus. Afferent lymph vessels enter into this sinus opposite the hilus. Dendritic cells process antigen encountered in the skin and migrate into lymph nodes from afferent lymphatics through the subcapsular sinus and into the lymph node. Lymph nodes vary in size, from barely visible in an unstimulated state to several centimeters in size when undergoing an active immune response.

A lymph node is divided into two major regions, the cortex and the medulla. The cortex contains numerous primary and secondary lymphoid follicles, each approximately 0.5 mm in diameter, similar to those in the spleen. Surrounding the lymphoid follicles in the cortex is the paracortical region, which contains mostly T cells along with some macrophages and dendritic cells. Both CD4 and CD8 T cells are present, as are macrophages and B cells. The accessory cells, such as interdigitating dendritic cells, present peptide antigens in association with MHC molecules to the TCR on T cells to activate the T cells. Additional accessory

molecules (e.g., B7 [CD80] or LFA-3 [CD58]) on the accessory cell and their ligands (CD28 or CD2, respectively) on the T cell provide important co-stimulatory signals required for activation of the T cell. Other surface antigens, particularly adhesion molecules such as LFA-1 (CD18) and ICAM-1 (CD54), are involved in stabilizing cellular interactions, as well as providing additional signals between cells.

In the center of the lymph node, beneath the cortex, lies the medulla, which is divided into medullary cords. Surrounding the medullary cords are medullary sinuses that drain into the hilus. B and T cells migrate from the follicles and paracortical region to the medulla. Medullary cords contain T cells, B cells and macrophages, as well as a large number of plasma cells that produce immunoglobulin, which drains into medullary sinuses that empty into the hilus. Efferent lymphatic vessels leave the hilus carrying antibodies, together with mature B and T cells that migrate to other tissues and act as memory B and T cells. The lymphatic vessel system serves to carry lymphocytes derived from various tissue spaces through the network of lymph nodes eventually to the thoracic duct. This material is then drawn into the left subclavian vein and back into the circulation. By this mechanism, lymphocytes are circulated throughout the body. This system of transport develops early in gestation with both lymphatic muscle cells for propulsion and valves that regulate unidirectional lymph flow.[54]

Mucosal immune system

The mucosal immune system is located along the surfaces of mucosal tissues and has a unique organization (Chapter 19). Each mucosal immune system consists of organized secondary lymphoid structures, termed mucosa-associated lymphoreticular tissue (MALT), at which inductive immune responses occur, and more diffuse tissues such as the exocrine glands and lamina propria, where effector immune responses occur. Some mucosal sites, such as the intestine and lung, have well-developed MALT while others, like the vaginal-cervical mucosal surface, have minimally developed MALT. MALT resembles lymph nodes with B cell follicles, intervening T-cell zones and numerous antigen presenting cells such as DCs and macrophages.[55] In MALT, naïve T and B cells encounter antigen, become activated, exit the tissue via efferent lymphatics, and migrate to the mesenteric lymph nodes, then into the thoracic duct and finally to the bloodstream. The cells home to effector sites, particularly the lamina propria of various mucosal tissues. The intraepithelial lymphocytes contained within the epithelium of mucosa and the lamina propria located immediately beneath the epithelium are responsible for effector functions. They occur diffusely in mucosal tissues and lack the well-defined structure of the organized mucosal immune system.

The homing of activated lymphocytes from one inductive site to several mucosal surface effector sites has led to the concept of a common mucosal immune system (CMIS), although there is significant compartmentalization in humans.[56] Trafficking from MALT to the lamina propria is well regulated. Expression of cell surface molecules such as sphingosine 1 phospate (S1P), MAdCAM-1, VLA-1, LFA-1, VCAM-1, integrins such as $\alpha_4\beta_7$, and chemokines such as CCR9, CCL25, CCR10, and CCL28, are important in directing activated lymphocytes to the lamina propria surface.[57] At the mucosal surface, the environment is favorable for induction of IgA, a major effector of immunity. It is divided into two groups: low affinity, important for inhibition of commensal bacterial on mucosal surfaces and high affinity involved in neutralization of microbial pathogens.

Gastrointestinal tract

The organized MALT of the gastrointestinal system is termed the gut-associated lymphoreticular tissue (GALT). It is composed of Peyer's patches, cecal and rectal patches, and isolated lymphoid follicles. Isolated lymphoid follicles and cecal and rectal patches are found throughout the lamina propria and are similar to an individual follicle of a Peyer's patch. Peyer's patches consist of variably sized aggregates of closely associated lymphoid follicles located in the intestinal lamina propria, occurring predominantly in the ileum (Fig. 2.9).[58] Although these structures arise during fetal life, their full development, with follicles containing germinal centers, does not occur until several weeks after birth, presumably in response to antigenic stimulation. Their number and size increase until puberty and decline thereafter. Peyer's patches and lymphoid follicles have a structural organization that belies their function of presenting antigen from the intestinal lumen to T and B cells. The epithelium overlying lymphoid follicles and Peyer's patches — that is, the FAE (Fig. 2.6) — has a distinct structure. It lacks villi and contains very few goblet cells. Particulate antigen uptake via pinocytosis occurs in the FAE through specialized epithelial cells called M cells. The FAE expresses MHC class II molecules, with the exception of M cells. However, it does not express the polymeric immunoglobulin

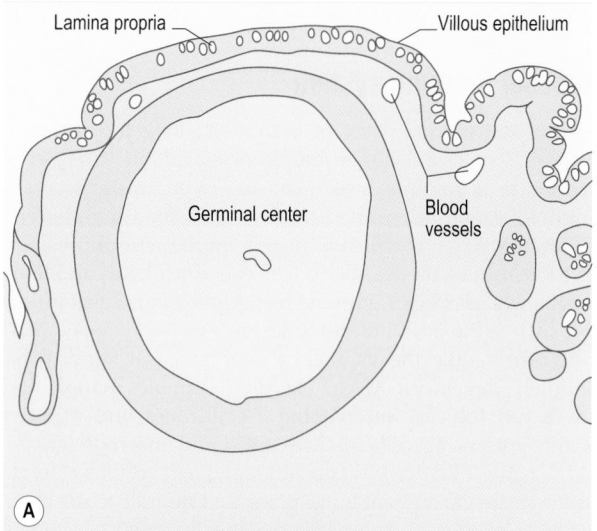

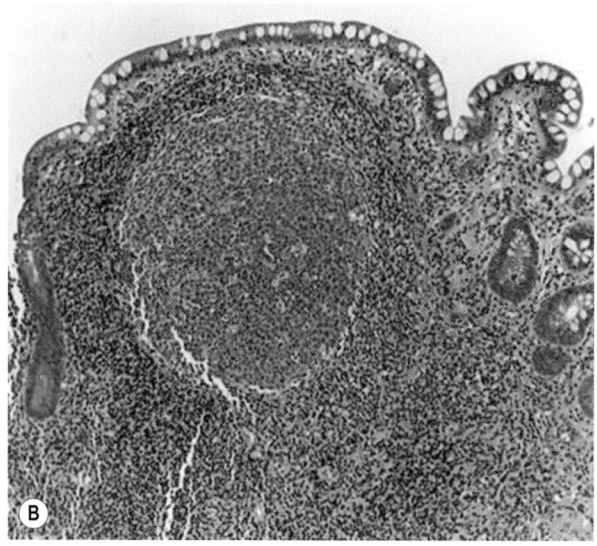

Fig. 2.9 Germinal center in terminal ilium.

receptor (secretory component) required for secretion of IgA, which is expressed by crypt epithelial cells in villous epithelium.[59] A substantial number of T cells, including CD4 T cells, are found in the subepithelial region. Beneath this epithelium, which overlies individual follicles, is a region called the dome. It contains large numbers of T cells, macrophages and DCs, as well as some B cells. Antigen, which is pinocytosed by M cells, is transported to the dome region where antigen presentation to T cells occurs. High levels of MHC class II molecules are expressed by macrophages and dendritic cells. Follicles lying beneath the dome contain mantle zones with predominantly resting B cells, most of which express IgM and IgD on their surface. Virtually all Peyer's patch follicles have germinal centers that contain activated B cells, FDCs, CD4 T cells, and tingible-body macrophages (so called because of their appearance after they have phagocytosed cellular debris). Many of the B cells within Peyer's patch germinal centers express surface IgA, and it is believed that this is where IgA class switch occurs. Very few CD8 T cells are located within the follicles. An interfollicular region contains predominantly CD4 and CD8 T cells, as well as dendritic cells, macrophages, and some B cells. CD4 T cells predominate over CD8 T cells in this region as well as in the dome.

The diffuse tissue of the gastrointestinal tract consists of two components: the lamina propria and intraepithelial lymphocytes (IEL). The lamina propria is located immediately beneath the epithelium. A key effector function of the lamina propria is the secretion of antibodies, primarily IgA. IgA is the major isotype produced by plasma cells in lamina propria regions. IgM represents 10–18% and IgG 3–5% of all Ig produced. Two IgA subclasses occur, IgA_1 and IgA_2, and the former represents >90% of IgA in the respiratory tract and >60% in the lamina propria of the small intestine.[60] Interestingly, IgA_2 increases in the lower ileum and becomes predominant in the colon and rectum. IgA is transported from the lamina propria into epithelial cells through polymeric immunoglobulin receptor-mediated uptake and subsequently secreted into the lumen. The lamina propria also contains large numbers of CD4 and CD8 T lymphocytes, CD4 T cells being about twice as prevalent as CD8 T cells. Almost all lamina propria T cells (>95%) express αβ TCR. The lamina propria also contains B lymphocytes, the majority of which express IgM. Normally, very few IgG B cells are in the lamina propria. However, under certain inflammatory conditions, such as inflammatory bowel disease, the number of IgG-producing B cells and plasma cells increases dramatically. Other cells, including macrophages, dendritic cells, eosinophils, mast cells, and a few neutrophils, are also found in the lamina propria and mediate effector functions. The gastrointestinal tract contains the largest number of resident macrophages in the body. These express CD68, lysozyme, ferritin, MHC II, and CD74.

Intraepithelial lymphocytes (IEL) are found at the basal surface of the epithelium as well as interdigitated with epithelial cells. The vast majority of IEL (>90%) are T cells, which are either $CD8^+$ or $CD4^-CD8^-$. Although the majority of IEL T cells express the αβ TCR, a substantial number express γδ TCR. The function of IEL remains incompletely understood, but they generate cytotoxic activity as well maintain oral tolerance. As part of their effector function, they produce several cytokines, including IL-5 and IFN-γ. Finally, epithelial cells in the small intestine express MHC class II molecules and likely present antigen to T cells.

Respiratory tract

Surrounding the entrance to the throat are the three tonsillar groups: palatine tonsil, lingual tonsil, and pharyngeal tonsil or adenoids.[61] They form a ring of lymphoid tissue surrounding the pharynx termed Waldeyer's ring. The tonsils reach full development in childhood and begin to involute by puberty. The palatine tonsils, one located on each side, lie at the entrance to the pharynx, each measuring approximately 2.5×1.25 cm. They are surrounded by a poorly organized capsule except at the pharyngeal surface, which is covered with stratified squamous epithelium. Trabeculae subdivide the tonsil into lobules. Blood vessels and nerves enter through the capsule and extend within trabeculae (Fig. 2.10). The surface of the tonsil is covered by pits, which are the openings of crypts. The crypts extend down into the tissue of the tonsil with branching, increasing surface area. There are abundant lymphoid follicles in each lobule that contain germinal centers that are predominantly B cells. By contrast, the lymphoid tissue surrounding the follicles contains T cells, macrophages, DCs, and some B cells. The lingual tonsils consist of 35–100 separate crypts surrounded by lymphoid tissue and are

located at the root of the tongue. The pharyngeal tonsils, or adenoids, are accumulations of lymphoid tissue, 2.5–4.0 cm long, located on the median dorsal wall of the nasopharynx. They contain a series of longitudinal folds but do not contain actual crypts. The lingual and pharyngeal tonsils also contain lymphoid nodules with germinal centers. The palatine tonsils and adenoids (nasopharyngeal tonsils) comprise the nasopharyngeal-associated lymphoreticular tissues (NALT).

Inductive immune responses to inhaled antigens within the respiratory tract occur mainly in the bronchus-associated lymphoid tissue (BALT). BALT consists of lymphoid aggregates located within the bronchial wall near bifurcations of the major bronchial branches (Fig. 2.11). These structures are analogous to the GALT present in the gastrointestinal tract and function to provide protection against inhaled microbes by induction of T- and B-cell responses. In human, BALT is

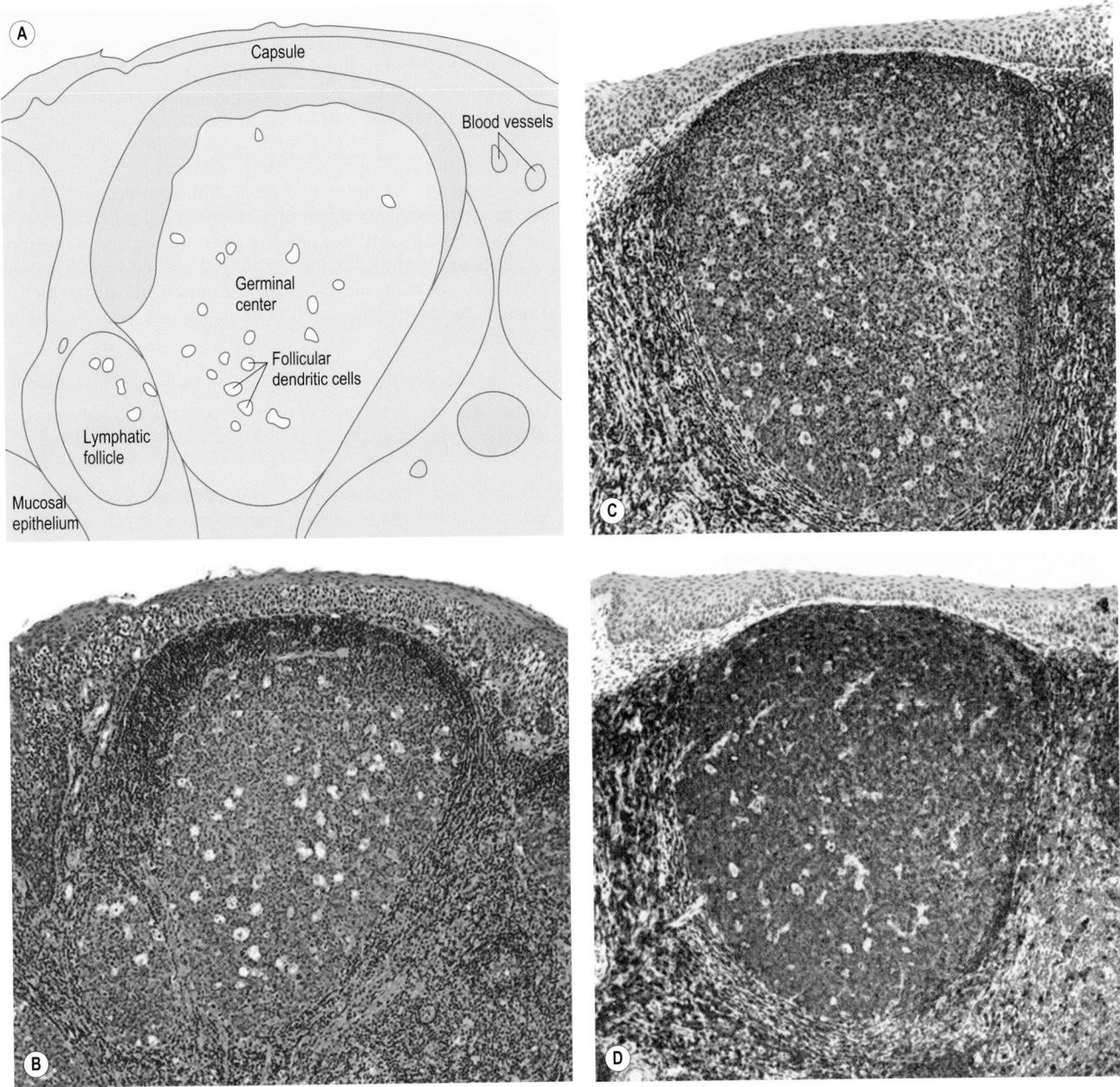

Fig. 2.10 Human tonsil. (A) Organization of lymphoid follicles and germinal centers. (B) Tonsillar tissue stained with hematoxylin and eosin. (C) Tonsillar tissue stained with anti-CD3 to demonstrate the distribution of T cells. (D) Tonsillar tissue stained with anti-CD19 to demonstrate the distribution of B cells.

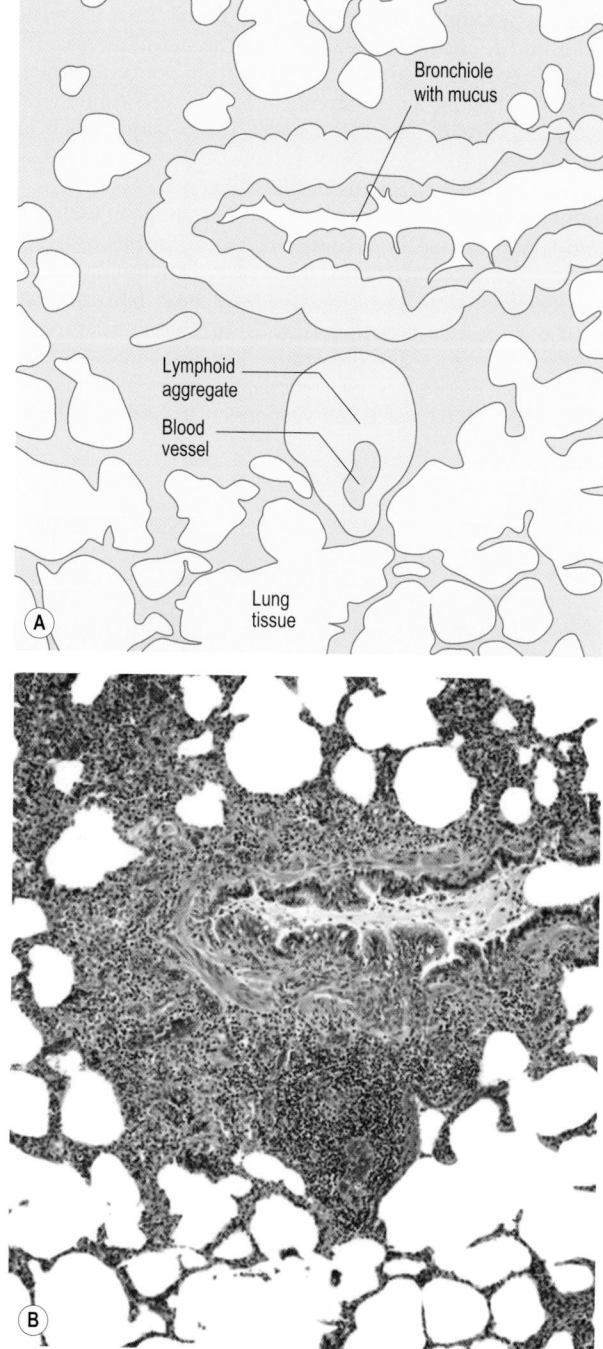

Fig. 2.11 **Lymphoid regions in the human lung.**

present at birth and rapidly expands when exposed to antigenic stimulation. The specialized epithelium overlying the lymphoid aggregates consists of M cells heavily infiltrated with lymphocytes and significant dendritic cell populations directly below the epithelium. As in the gastrointestinal tract, the main result of induction of immune responses in BALT is the production of secretory IgA.[62]

Although quite extensive in the gastrointestinal tract, the diffuse mucosal tissue of the respiratory tract is minimal. Pools of lymphocytes are present within the lung interstitium, made up of 10–20% T cells. Macrophages are present on both the air side

of the lung and airways as well as in the mucosa.[60] Minimal inflammation occurs in the bronchial mucosa owing to Tregs that inhibit T-cell activation and expansion. Instead, antigen is carried by local macrophages to the regional lymph nodes, where most respiratory effector immune responses originate.[61] Communication occurs between the gastrointestinal and respiratory mucosae through cell trafficking. Antigen-reactive T and B cells from the Peyer's patches can populate the bronchial mucosa. This common mucosal immune system feature has been exploited to develop oral vaccines against respiratory microbes.[63]

Genital tract

The male and female reproductive tracts are also components of the common mucosal system. The genital tract immune system must maintain a delicate balance between tolerance of germinal center cells, spermatozoa, and fetus, and the recognition of microbes. Most of what is known about the genital mucosal response has been learned from the female reproductive tract. Unlike the gastrointestinal and respiratory tracts, there is little induction of mucosal immune responses in the genital tract.[63] Most of the immune cells found in the mucosa derive from the induction of immune responses at other sites, predominately in the rectum and Peyer's patches, followed by homing of IgA cell precursors to the genital tract. Although secretory IgA is the predominant antibody found in the genital tract, monomeric IgA, IgM, and IgG are also present. The production and transport of antibody produced in the genital tract depends on hormonal and local factors, including IL-1b, IL-6, and IL-10, all of which influence the maturation of B cells to plasma cells within the mucosa.[64,65]

Skin

Although not a systemic or mucosal lymphoid organ per se, the skin is a specialized secondary immune organ involved in the induction of immune responses (Chapter 18). The skin consists of two layers, the epidermis and the dermis. The epidermis is the outermost layer and contains three distinct cell types: keratinocytes, melanocytes, and Langerhans cells (Fig. 2.12). Keratinocytes are squamous epithelial cells and are the principal cell type of the epidermis. Keratinocytes secrete a variety of cytokines, including IL-1, IL-6, IL-10, TGF-β, and TNF-α, which can profoundly influence immune responses. The second cellular constituent of the skin is the pigment-producing melanocyte. This cell is derived from the neural crest and resides in the basal layer of the epidermis. The third cellular component of the epidermis, and the one of particular importance for the immune system, is the Langerhans cell. Langerhans cells are found scattered throughout the epidermis within the malpighian layer, or prickle cell layer. Langerhans cells are important for both normal and pathologic cutaneous T-cell responses.. When they encounter antigen, in concert with exposure to cytokines provided by keratinocytes such as TNF-α and Il-6, Langerhans cells migrate from the epidermis to the dermis, then enter the afferent lymphatics and migrate to draining lymph nodes. There they participate in the generation of a primary immune response, presenting antigen to T cells.[66]

Under the epidermis is the dermis, which contains abundant fibroblasts producing collagen, a principal component of skin. The dermis also contains blood vessels and various epidermal

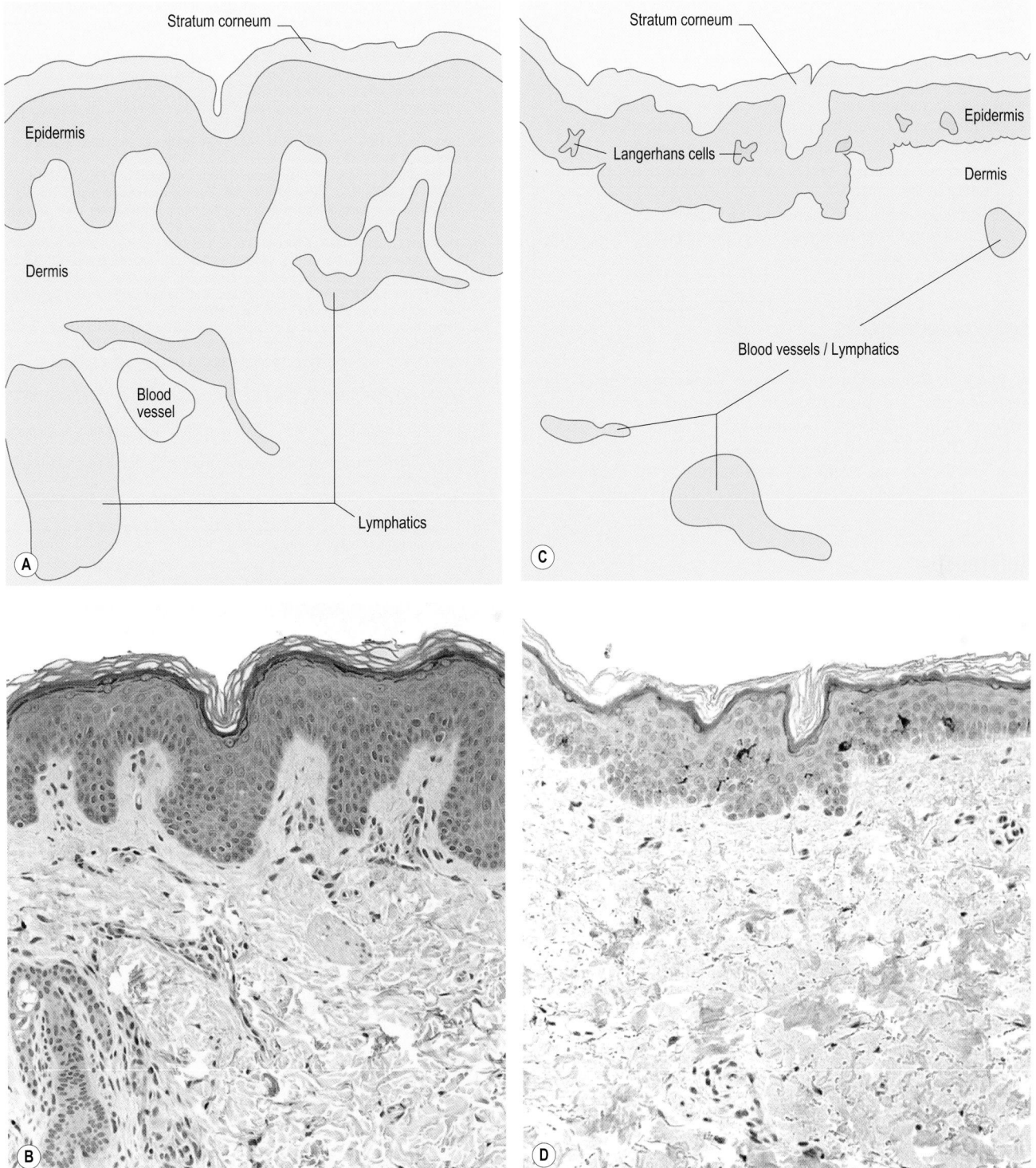

Fig. 2.12 Lymphoid regions in human skin. (A, C) Organization of the epithelial tissue. (B) Epithelial tissue stained with hematoxylin and eosin. (D) Epithelial tissue stained with anti-CD207 to demonstrate the distribution of Langerhans' cells (note brown cells).

adnexal structures, such as hair follicles, sweat glands, and sebaceous glands. The vasculature of the dermis consists of an extensive network of plexuses containing arterioles, capillaries, and venules. Dermal lymphatics are associated with the vascular plexuses. In normal skin, a small number of lymphocytes can be found in perivascular areas. These lymphocytes are mostly T cells with unique features, including expression of a memory phenotype (CD45RO+) and expression of a cutaneous lymphocyte-associated antigen that binds to the vascular addressing endothelial cell leukocyte adhesion molecule-1 (ELAM-1) (CD62E) present on the endothelium. This latter interaction plays an important role in homing of memory T cells to inflamed regions of the skin. The dermis also contains mast cells important for immediate hypersensitivity reactions.

Acknowledgments

We thank Dr Edwina Popek, Pathology Department, Texas Children's Hospital, Houston, Texas, for providing histopathological images of lymphoid tissues; Dr Gregory Stelzer and Wendy Schober for the flow cytometric display; Eleanor Chapman, Anna Wirt, Terry Saulsberry, and Yvette Wyckoff for typing the manuscript; and Dr Jerry McGhee for critical review of the first edition.

References

1. Rampon C, Huber P. Multilineage hematopoietic progenitor activity generated autonomously in the mouse yolk sac: analysis using angiogenesis-defective embryos. Int J Dev Biol 2003;47:273–80.
2. Gekas C, Dieterien-Lievre F, Orkin SH, Mikkola HK. The placenta is a niche for hematopoietic stem cells. Dev Cell 2005;8:297–8.
3. Orkin SH, Zon LI. Hematopoiesis: an evolving paradigm for stem cell biology. Cell 2008;132:631–44.
4. Haynes BF, Martin ME, Kay HH, et al. Early events in human T cell ontogeny: phenotypic characterization and immunohistological localization of T-cell precursors in early human fetal tissues. J Exp Med 1988;168:1061–80.
5. Drake AC, Khoury M, Leskov I, et al. Human CD34[+] CD133[+] hematopoietic stem cells cultured with growth factors including Angptl5 efficiently engraft adult NOD-SCID IL2rgamma -/- (NSG) mice. PLoS ONE 2011;6:18382–91.
6. Metcalf D. Hematopoietic cytokines. Blood 2008;111:485–91.
7. Raulet D. Development and tolerance of natural killer cells. Curr Opin Immunol 1999;11:129.
8. Moore KA, Lemischka IR. Stem cells and their niches. Science 2006;311:1880–5.
9. Bunting KD. ABC transporters as phenotypic markers and functional regulators of stem cells. Stem Cells 2002;20:11–20.
10. Wilson A, Laurenti E, Oser G, et al. Hematopoietic stem cells reversibly switch from dormancy to self-renewal during homeostasis and repair. Cell 2008;135:1118–29.
11. Wilson A, Trumpp A. Bone-marrow haematopoietic-stem-cell niches. Nature Immunol Rev 2006;6:93–107.
12. Lapidot T, Petit I. Current understanding of stem cell mobilization: The roles of chemokines, proteolytic enzymes, adhesion molecules, sytokines, and stromal cells. Exp Hematol 2002;30:973–87.
13. Bianco P, Riminucci M, Gronthos S, Robey PG. Bone marrow stromal stem cells: nature, biology, and potential applications. Stem Cells 2001;19:180–92.
14. Dorshkind K. Regulation of hemopoiesis by bone marrow stromal cells and their products. Annu Rev Immunol 1990;8:111–37.
15. Kondo M, Wagers MJ, Manz MG, et al. Biology of hematopoietic stem cells and progenitors: implications for clinical applications. Annu Rev Immunol 2003;21:759–806.
16. Zandstra PW, Conneally E, Petzer AL, et al. Cytokine manipulation of primitive human hematopoietic cell self-renewal. Proc Natl Acad Sci U S A 1997;94:4698–703.
17. Seita J, Ema H, Ooehara J, et al. Lnk negatively regulates self-renewal of hematopoietic stem cells by modifying thrombopoietin-mediated signal transduction. PNAS 2007;104:2349–54.
18. Barreda DR, Hanington PC, Belosevic M. Regulation of myeloid development and function by colony stimulating factors. Dev Comp Immunol 2004;25:509–54.
19. Shortman K, Liu YJ. Mouse and human dendritic cell subtypes. Nature Immunol Rev 2002;2:151–61.
20. Mende I, Karsunky H, Weissman IL, et al. Flk2[+] myeloid progenitors are the main source of Langerhans' cells. Blood 2006;107:1383–90.
21. Randolph GJ, Angeli V, Swartz MA. Dendritic-cell trafficking to lymph nodes through lymphatic vessels. Nature Immunol Rev 2005;5:617–28.
22. Takahashi K, Naito M, Takeya M. Development and heterogeneity of macrophages and their related cells through their differentiation pathways. Pathol Int 1996;46:473–85.
23. Bouhlel MA, Derudas B, Rigamonti E, et al. PPARgamma activation primes human monocytes into alternative M2 macrophages with anti-inflammatory properties. Cell Metab 2007;6:137–43.
24. Karsunky H, Merad M, Cozzio A, et al. Flt3 ligand regulates dendritic cell development from Flt3[+] lymphoid and myeloid commited progenitors to Flt3[+] dendritic cells in vivo. J Exp Med 2003;198:305–13.
25. Chicha L, Jarrossay D, Manz MG. Clonal type I interferon-producing and dendritic cell precursors are contained in both human lymphoid and myeloid progenitor populations. J Exp Med 2004;200:1519–24.
26. Onai N, Obata-Onai A, Tussiwand R, et al. Activation of the Flt3 signal transduction cascade rescues and enhances type I interferon-producing and dendritic cell development. J Exp Med 2006;203:227–38.
27. Friedman AD. Transcriptional regulation of granulocyte and monocyte development. Oncogene 2002;21:3377–90.
28. Lieber JG, Webb S, Suratt BT, et al. The in vitro production and characterization of neutrophils from embryonic stem cells. Blood 2004;103:852–9.
29. Rothenberg ME, Hogan SP. The eosinophil. Annu Rev Immunol 2006;24:147–74.
30. Kambe N, Hiramatsu H, Shimonaka M, et al. Development of both human connective tissue-type and mucosal-type mast cells in mice from hematopoietic stem cells with identical distribution pattern to human body. Blood 2004;103:860–7.
31. Matsuzawa S, Sakashita K, Kinoshita T, et al. IL-9 enhances the growth of human mast cell progenitors under stimulation with stem cell factor. Immunology 2003;170:3461–7.
32. Long MW. Megakaryocyte differentiation events. Semin Hematol 1998;35:192–9.
33. Malik P, Fisher TC, Barsky LL, et al. An in vitro model of human red blood cell production from hematopoietic progenitor cells. Blood 1998;91:2664–71.
34. Pelayo R, Welner R, Perry SS, et al. Lymphoid progenitors and primary routes to becoming cells of the immune system. Curr Opin Immunol 2005;17:100–7.
35. Blom B, Spits H. Development of human lymphoid cells. Annu Rev Immunol 2006;24:287–320.
36. Weerkamp F, Pike-Overzet K, Staal FJT. T-sing progenitors to commit. Trends Immunol 2006;27:125–31.
37. Haddad R, Guimiot F, Six E, et al. Dynamics of thymus colonizing cells during human development. Immunity 2006;24:217–30.
38. Spits H. Development of χβ T cells in the human thymus, thymic involution. Nature Immunol Rev 2002;2:760–72.
39. Gary DHD, Ueno T, Chidgey AP, et al. Controlling the thymic microenvironment. Curr Opin Immunol 2005;17:137–43.
40. Takhama Y. Journey through the thymus: stromal guides for T-cell development and selection. Nat Rev Immunol 2006;6:127–36.
41. Farrar JD, Asnagli H, Murphy KM. T helper subset development: roles of instruction, selection, and transcription. J Clin Invest 2002;109:431–5.
42. Bettelli E, Kuchroo VK. IL-12 and IL-23 induced T helper cell subsets: birds of the same feather flock together. J Exp Med 2005;201:169–71.
43. Kronenberg M. Towards an understanding of NKT cell biology: progress and paradoxes. Annu Rev Immunol 2005;26:877–900.
44. Synder-Cappione JE, Tincati C, Eccles-James IG, et al. A comprehensive Ex Vivo functional analysis of human NKT cells reveals production of MIP1 alpha and MIP-1 beta, a lack of IL17 and a Th1- bias in Males. PLoS ONE 2010;5:15412–20.
45. Jonuleit H, Schmitt E. The regulatory T cell family: distinct subsets and their interrelations. J Immunol 2003;171:6323–7.
46. Wang R, Kozhaya L, Mercer F, et al. Expression of GARP selectively identifies activated human FOXP3[+] regulatory T cells. PNAS 2009;106:13439–44.
47. Nagasawa T. Microenvironmental niches in the bone marrow required for B-cell development. Nature Immunol Rev 2006;6:107–16.
48. Herzenberg LA, Tung JW. B cell lineages: documented at last!. Nat Immunol 2006;7:225–6.
49. Barone F, Vossenkamper A, Boursier I, et al. IgA producing plasma cells originate from germinal centers that are induced by B cell receptor engagement in humans. Gastroenterology 2011;140:947–56.
50. Moretta L, Moretta A. Unravelling natural killer cell function: triggering and inhibitory human NK receptors. EMBO J 2004;23:255–9.
51. Farag SS, Caligiuri MA. Human natural killer cell development and biology. Blood 2006;20:123–37.
52. Naylor K, Guangjin LI, Vallejo AN, et al. The influence of age on T cell generation and TCR diversity. J Immunol 2005;174:7446–52.
53. Mebius RE, Kraal G. Structure and function of the spleen. Nature Immunol Rev 2005;5:606–16.
54. Petrenko VM, Gashev AA. Observations on the prenatal development of human lymphatic vessels with focus on basic structural elements of lymph flow. Lymphat Res Biol 2008;6:89–95.
55. Brandtzaeg P. Mucosal Immunity: Induction, Dissemination and Effector Functions. Scand J Immunol 2009;70:505–15.
56. Kunizawa J, Nochi T, Hiroshi K. Immunological commananlities and distinctions between airway and digestive immunity. Trends Immunol 2008;29:505–13.
57. Wright P. Inductive/effecor mechansims for humoral immunity at mucosal sites 2011;65:248–52.
58. Newberry RD, Lorenz RG. Organizing a mucosal defense. Immunol Rev 2005;206:6–21.
59. Woof JM, Mestecty J. Mucosal immunoglobulins. Immunol Rev 2005;206:64–82.
60. Bienenstock J, McDermott MRM. Bronchus- and nasal-associated lymphoid tissues. Immunol Rev 2005;206:22–31.
61. Lamm ME, Nedru JG, Kaetzel CS, Mazanec MB. IgA and mucosal defense. APMIS 1995;103:241–6.
62. Kyd JM, Foxwell AR, Cripps AW. Mucosal immunity in the lung and upper airway. Vaccine 2001;19:2527–33.
63. Boyaka PN, Tafaro A, Fischer R, et al. Therapeutic manipulation of the immune system; enhancement of innate and adaptive mucosal immunity. Curr Pharm Des 2003;9:1965–72.
64. Mestecky J, Moldoveanu Z, Russell MW. Immunologic uniqueness of the genital tract: challenge for vaccine development. Am J Reprod Immunol 2005;53:205–14.
65. Mestecky J, Rusell MW. Induction of mucosal immune responses in the human genital tract. FEMS Immunol Med Microbiol 2000;27:351–5.
66. Hayday A, Viney JL. The ins and outs of body surface immunology. Science 2000;290:97–100.

Innate immunity

Douglas R. McDonald, Ofer Levy

All living organisms are continually exposed to microbes within their environments. Therefore, an effective host defense against infectious agents is essential to survival. Innate immunity is the first line of host defense against infection. A defining characteristic of innate immunity is its existence prior to microbial exposure. Accordingly, upon microbial challenge, innate immune responses are initiated rapidly and precede the development of adaptive immune responses. The resulting adaptive immune response is characterized by remarkable diversity and specificity toward foreign antigens. In contrast, innate immune responses are directed towards essential and invariant structural components specific to microbes known as pathogen-associated molecular patterns, or PAMPs.[1] These PAMPs, which include microbial cell wall components and nucleic acids, are recognized by pattern recognition receptors (PRRs) and are highly potent and effective in initiating inflammatory responses.

● KEY CONCEPTS

The innate immune system

- The innate immune system provides the initial immune response to pathogens.
- The innate immune system is comprised of barriers to the environment (i.e., skin, mucosa), antimicrobial peptides and proteins, cells (i.e., neutrophils, macrophages, monocytes), and soluble factors (i.e., cytokines, chemokines, complement).
- Pathogen detection is mediated by a variety of germline-encoded pathogen recognition receptors (PRRs).
- PRRs recognize invariant microbial structures known as pathogen-associated molecular patterns (PAMPs).
- Activation of the innate immune system leads to subsequent activation of the adaptive immune system.
- Similar to the adaptive immune system, the innate immune system has a form of memory or "trained immunity" that allows a more robust innate immune response to a subsequent infection that occurs shortly after an initial infection.

Another classic characteristic that has differentiated adaptive from innate immunity is the concept of memory. The generation of memory B and T cells following infections allows a more rapid and robust immune response upon subsequent infections with the same organism. However, it is increasingly appreciated that microbial exposure can also be associated with enhanced subsequent innate immune responses, a phenomenon that has been referred to as "trained immunity."[2] Characteristics of enhanced or trained innate immunity are that it increases resistance of the host to re-infection, can provide "cross protection" against other infectious agents, but is less specific than adaptive immunity.

Macrophages and NK cells can mediate these enhanced responses through expansion and contraction of their cell populations. Additionally, they can upregulate expression of genes involved in pathogen recognition and presentation and secrete cytokines that augment the antimicrobial activity of bystander cells. Thus, there is a growing appreciation that the adaptive and innate immune systems may have many similar characteristics. The critical role of innate immunity in host defense is demonstrated by potentially life threatening infections that result from naturally occurring defects of the innate immune system, as reviewed in Chapter 36 of this book. This chapter reviews the principal components and functions of the innate immune system.

Barriers to infection

Skin and mucosa

Mechanical barriers to microbial entry, which include epithelial barriers such as skin and the linings of the gastrointestinal and respiratory tracts, play an essential role in host defense. Genetic disorders of the skin that compromise skin integrity, such as epidermolysis bullosa, can result in life threatening infections. More common are skin disorders that impair barrier function, such as eczema. Patients with eczematous skin have reduced expression of antimicrobial proteins and peptides (APPs) and are susceptible to cutaneous bacterial infections (e.g., *Staphylococcus* spp., *Streptococcus* spp.) and viral infections (e.g., herpes viruses).[3] Viral infections are the most common causes of respiratory tract infections. Influenza viruses and respiratory syncytial virus replicate in airway epithelial cells, leading to cell death and inflammation. The impaired barrier function of the airways can lead to increased susceptibility to secondary invasive bacterial infections by *Streptococcus pneumoniae* and other pyogenic bacteria. Inflammatory bowel diseases, such as Crohn's disease, also result in impaired barrier functions of the small and large intestines that can be associated with increased translocation of bacteria across gut mucosa, potentially leading to serious infection. Additionally, intestinal epithelial cells of some Crohn's disease patients produce reduced amounts of APPs, further increasing susceptibility to bacterial infection.[4]

Antimicrobial proteins and peptides

In addition to their function as a mechanical barrier, the epithelia of the skin and GI tract also produce APPs. These APPs include bactericidal/permeability-increasing protein (BPI), defensins (β-strand peptides connected by disulfide bonds) and catheliciдins (linear α-helical peptides) (Table 3.1).[5] Most APPs have a net positive charge, enhancing their affinity for the negatively charged microbial cell membrane. Binding of APPs to microbes can increase membrane permeability, and ultimately result in target cell death. Some APPs have enzymatic activity, such as lysozyme (Lz), which cleaves peptidoglycans found in cell walls of bacteria, especially Gram-positive bacteria. Other APPs bind to and compete for nutrients; for example, lactoferrin (Lf) binds iron.

BPI is a ~55-kDa cationic and hydrophobic protein with high affinity for the lipid A region of lipopolysaccharide (endotoxin). It is found in neutrophil primary (azurophilic) granules and is also inducible in epithelial cells. BPI inhibits Gram-negative bacteria by neutralizing endotoxin and through its microbicidal and opsonic properties.

Defensins are classified into different classes based upon the linking pattern of cysteines and their sizes. The α-defensins are expressed in neutrophils and Paneth cells of the small intestine; while β-defensins are expressed by mucosal surface epithelia, including cells found in skin, eye, oral mucosa, urogenital and respiratory tracts. Defensins have a broad specificity of antimicrobial activities against bacteria, mycobacteria, fungi, parasites, and viruses (Table 3.2). In addition to their anti-microbial functions, defensins have been shown to enhance antigen uptake and processing. They also stimulate the chemotaxis of monocytes, macrophages, and mast cells.[6,7] While the expression of

Table 3.1 Epithelial APPs

Antimicrobial peptide	Source	Target organism
Dermicidin	Eccrine sweat glands	Broad spectrum
Psoriasin	Keratinocytes, sebocytes	G-
RNase 7	Keratinocytes	Broad spectrum
RNase 5/ angiogenin	Keratinocytes	*C albicans*
Cathelicidin (LL-37)	Keratinocytes, sebocytes	G+, G-
BPI	Epithelia-oral, GI, urogenital tract	G-, (G+, fungi)
hBD-1	Keratinocytes, sebocytes	G-
hBD-2	Keratinocytes, sebocytes	G-
hBD-3	Keratinocytes	Broad spectrum
hBD-4	Keratinocytes	G+, G-
SLPI	Keratinocytes	Broad spectrum
Elafin	Keratinocytes	Broad spectrum
Adrenomedullin	Keratinocytes, hair follicles, eccrine/ apocrine sweat glands, sebocytes	G+, G-
MIP-3α/CCL20	Keratinocytes	Broad spectrum
Lysozyme	Keratinocytes, sebocytes, hair bulb cells	G+, G-
Lactoferrin	Milk, saliva, tears, nasal secretions, neutrophils	Broad spectrum

RNase, ribonuclease; BPI, bactericidal/permeability-increasing protein; hBD, human beta-defensin; SLPI, secretory leukocyte peptidase inhibitor; MIP, macrophage inflammatory protein; CCL, chemokine ligand

Table 3.2 Neutrophil-derived APPs

Neutrophil APP	Granule type	Target organism
Lysozyme	Azurophil, specific	G+, G-
Azurocidin	Azurophil, secretory	G+, G-, *C. albicans*
Elastase	Azurophil	G+, G-
Cathepsin G	Azurophil	G+, G-
Proteinase 3	Azurophil	G+, G-
BPI	Azurophil	G-, (G+, fungi)
α-defensins (HNP-1 to -4)	Azurophil	G+, G-, fungi, viruses
Cathelicidin (hCAP-18)	Specific	G+, G-, mycobacteria
Lactoferrin	Specific	G+, G-, fungi, viruses
SLPI	Specific	G+, G-, *A. fumigatus, C. albicans*
NGAL	Specific	G+, G-, fungi
Lysozyme	Azurophil, specific	G+, G-
Azurocidin	Azurophil, secretory	G+, G-, *C. albicans*
Elastase	Azurophil	G+, G-
Cathepsin G	Azurophil	G+, G-

BPI, bactericidal/permeability-increasing protein; HNP, human neutrophil peptide; hCAP, human cathelicidin antimicrobial protein; SLPI, secretory leukocyte peptidase inhibitor; NGAL, neutrophil gelatinase-associated lipocalin

several of the defensins is constitutive, inflammatory stimuli (bacterial products, pro-inflammatory cytokines) will increase the expression of defensins. Thus, in addition to their barrier function, epithelia elaborate APPs that can inhibit microbial colonization and modulate host defense.

Intraepithelial lymphocytes and B1 B cells

The intestinal mucosa and skin represent the largest surface areas of the body that are in contact with the external environment. Barrier epithelia of the skin and GI tract contain specific types of lymphocytes, e.g., intraepithelial T lymphocytes and B1 B cells, which respond to commonly encountered microbes. Within the epidermal layer, the main immune cell populations include keratinocytes, melanocytes, a type of dendritic cell (DC) known as the Langerhans cell, and intraepithelial T lymphocytes (Chapter 18).

Keratinocytes and melanocytes express a variety of PRRs that enable detection of microbes. Upon microbial detection, these cells then secrete cytokines (Chapter 9) that can contribute to innate immune responses through recruitment and activation of phagocytes.[8] Langerhans cells form an elaborate network of dendritic processes that allow them to capture antigens that gain access to skin. Following activation by microbes, Langerhans cells migrate to draining lymph nodes and express chemokine receptor-7 (CCR7) (Chapter 10), which allows them to migrate to the T-cell zones within the lymph node in response to chemokine ligand (CCL)-19 and CCL-21 and present antigen to T cells.[9]

Intraepidermal T lymphocytes constitute roughly 2% of lymphocytes within the skin. This special subset of lymphocytes expresses a more restricted set of αβ and γδ T-cell receptors than circulating T cells. This type of restriction is also seen in intraepithelial T lymphocytes found in the intestines. These specialized T cells appear to be committed to recognizing microbial peptide antigens commonly found at epithelial surfaces and thus function as components of the innate immune system.[10]

The B-1a and B-1b subsets of B lymphocytes are found mainly in the peritoneal and pleural cavities. In mice, they have been shown to also express an antigen receptor repertoire that differs from the more numerous conventional B-2 subset. B-1 cells can function as antigen presenting cells. However, unlike conventional B cells, upon antigen exposure B-1 cells do not develop into classic memory B cells and when they class switch they are more likely to switch into IgA than IgG. B-1 cells produce IgM antibodies that recognize polysaccharide and lipid antigens expressed on many types of bacteria. These antibodies provide protection against bacteria that have penetrated epithelial surfaces. Although antibodies produced by B-1 cells have low affinity for multiple antigens, the pentameric structure of IgM permits enhanced avidity.[11]

Mast cells are components of innate immunity that are also commonly found at the interface between host and environment. Mast cells are derived from progenitors in bone marrow and circulate as immature precursors to the periphery. They take up residence and mature in the skin, airways, and GI tract. As a result of their widespread distribution, mast cells are positioned to be the first responders to environmental stimuli, including infectious agents.[12] Stem cell factor (SCF, also known as c-kit ligand) is the main survival and developmental factor for mast cells. Mast cells express Toll-like receptor (TLRs, described below) 1 through 9 (Table 3.3), which allow them to respond to a wide variety of pathogens. TLR-induced mast cell activation leads to production of pro-inflammatory cytokines and chemokines that recruit and activate other inflammatory cells, including polymorphonuclear neutrophils (PMNs). Murine models of peritonitis, such as cecal ligation and puncture, have revealed that mast cells have the ability to enhance resistance to bacterial infection.[13] Mast cells are also well known for mediating allergic reactions through IgE-bound allergens that bind the high affinity IgE receptor, FcεRI, on the mast cell surface. Ligation of FcεRI leads to release of mast cell mediators, including tryptase, histamine, leukotrienes, prostaglandins, and cytokines, that mediate type 1 hypersensitivity reactions.

Humoral innate immunity

● KEY CONCEPTS

Humoral innate immunity

- Cytokines and chemokines are essential mediators of the innate immune response.
- Characteristics of cytokines include redundancy and pleotropism.
- Cytokine synthesis is a tightly controlled to allow effective immune responses and limit host tissue damage.
- Acute phase reactants (i.e., C-reactive protein (CRP)) are induced by cytokines (IL-6) and play roles in opsonization of microbes. CRP is measured from patient plasma clinically to monitor infections and inflammation.
- The complement system is an essential component of the innate immune system that destroys a wide variety of microbes.

The acute phase response

The innate immune response is initiated when cells of the innate immune system, including PMNs, monocytes, macrophages, and DCs encounter pathogens. Pathogen recognition occurs when PRRs expressed by a variety of cells recognize and bind to microbial molecules (e.g., lipopolysaccharide, DNA, RNA). These interactions activate signaling pathways that lead to the production of secreted factors, including cytokines and chemokines, involved in the inflammatory response. Characteristics of cytokines include pleotropism, e.g., the ability to act on multiple cell types, and redundancy. Cytokines can function locally, as well as distantly, and can affect the production of other cytokines. The effect of cytokines on target cells includes changes in gene expression that affect cell function (e.g., enhanced microbicidal activity, proliferation). The secretion of cytokines (IL-1β, IL-6, TNF-α) is a transient event, thereby limiting potential destruction of host tissue. However, severe infections with Gram-negative bacteria can lead to overproduction of TNF-α, IL-1β, and IFN-γ, which leads to vascular collapse, disseminated intravascular coagulation, and metabolic disturbances (septic shock) that can often be fatal. The synthesis of cytokines results from cytokine gene transcriptional activation. Cytokine synthesis is a transient process because the messenger RNA of most cytokines is unstable, thus limiting cytokine production. Production of certain cytokines is also regulated by a post-translational process. For example, TNF-α is a membrane-bound protein that is proteolytically cleaved by a membrane-associated metalloproteinase. IL-1β is a 33-kDa protein that is proteolytically processed by the IL-1β-converting enzyme caspase-1 to generate the biologically active 17-kDa mature IL-1β (described in more detail below).

Table 3.3 Classes of pattern recognition receptors

Pattern recognition receptor		Ligand
Toll-like receptors	TLR1/2	Triacyl lipopeptides
	TLR2	Zymosan
	TLR3	dsRNA
	TLR4	LPS, RSV glycoprotein, HSPs, pneumolysin
	TLR2/6	Diacyl lipopeptide
	TLR7	ssRNA
	TLR8	ssRNA
	TLR9	dsDNA, hemozoin
	TLR10	?
	TLR11	Profilin-like protein
NOD-like receptors (NLRs)	NOD1	DAP, MDP
	NOD2	MDP
	CIITA	?
	NAIP	*L. pneumophilia*, flagellin?
	IPAF	PAMPs
	NLRP1	PAMPs, MDP, microbial toxins
	NLRP2	?
	NLRP3	PAMPs, toxins, DAMPs
	NLRP4-14	?
RIG-like receptors (RLRs)	RIG-I	dsRNA, ssRNA
	MDA5	dsRNA, ssRNA
Scavenger receptors C-type lectin-like receptors	CD36, CD68, SRA, SRB	Oxidized lipoproteins, apoptotic cells,
	Mannose receptor	β-amyloid Bacterial carbohydrates
	Dectin-1	Fungal wall glucans

dsRNA, double stranded RNA; LPS, lipopolysaccharide; RSV, respiratory syncytial virus; ssRNA, single stranded RNA; CIITA, class II major histocompatibility complex transactivator; NAIP, neuronal apoptosis inhibitory protein; IPAF, IL-1 beta converting enzyme protease activating factor; NLRP, NOD-like receptor-related protein; SR, scavenger receptor; MDA-5, melanoma differentiation-associated gene-5

TNF-α and IL-1β can recruit PMNs and monocytes to sites of infection and enhance their ability to eliminate microbes. TNF-α and IL-1β induce expression of adhesion molecules, such as selectins (P-selectin, E-selectin) and the integrin ligands ICAM (intercellular adhesion molecule) and VCAM (vascular cell adhesion molecule) on vascular endothelial cells near the sites of infection. The expression of selectins on vascular endothelium induces leukocyte rolling on endothelium. Chemokines, like CXCL8, activate PMN and monocyte integrins and increase their affinity for ligands (ICAM, VCAM) on vascular endothelium, allowing migration of PMNs and monocytes to sites of infection. TNF-α and IL-1β both induce prostaglandin synthesis in the hypothalamus, which induces fever.

A variety of soluble proteins found in plasma play important roles in recognizing PAMPs and function as mediators of innate immunity. TNF-α and IL-1β induce production of acute phase reactants in hepatocytes, including members of the pentraxin family, such as serum amyloid A (SAA), serum amyloid P (SAP), and C-reactive protein (CRP), which bind to components of the bacterial cell wall.[14] TNF-α and IL-1β also induce production of IL-6 by a variety of cells, including mononuclear phagocytes, endothelial cells, and fibroblasts. IL-6 is another potent inducer of acute phase reactants, including CRP and fibrinogen. CRP, SAA, and SAP function as opsonins and can bind phosphorylcholine and phosphatidylethanolamine expressed on bacteria and apoptotic cells, enhancing phagocytosis of bacteria and apoptotic cells by macrophages. Lipopolysaccharide-binding protein (LBP) is an acute phase reactant synthesized by the liver in response to Gram-negative bacterial infections. LBP binds to LPS and subsequently forms a complex with CD14, TLR4, and MD-2, which functions as a high affinity receptor for LPS.[15] Mannose binding lectin (MBL) is a member of the calcium-dependent (C-type) lectins (collectins) produced by the liver in response to infection. MBL binds to carbohydrates with terminal mannose and fucose residues that are expressed on microbial cell surfaces.[16] MBL can bind to the C1q receptor on macrophages to enhance phagocytosis and can activate the complement system via the lectin pathway (discussed below). Surfactant protein-A and surfactant protein-D are collectins expressed in the lung that can bind a variety of microbes and inhibit their growth.[17] They also function as opsonins that promote ingestion by alveolar macrophages. Finally, ficolins are plasma proteins capable of binding to several types of bacteria and can activate complement.

The complement system

The complement system (Chapter 20) is an essential component of humoral innate immunity comprised of a collection of plasma proteins activated by microbes, which mediates microbial destruction and inflammation.[18] Complement activation can occur via three pathways: classical, alternative, and lectin. In the classical pathway the complement component C1 detects IgM, IgG1, or IgG3 bound to the surface of a microbe. C1 is composed of C1q, C1r, and C1s subunits that form multimeric complexes, which bind IgM or IgG bound to microbial surfaces. C1r and C1s are serine proteases. Activated C1s generates a C3 convertase (C4b2b) that is composed of C4b and C2b bound to the microbial surface. The C3 convertase cleaves C3, generating C3b, which covalently binds to C4b2b, generating the C5 convertase. The C5 convertase then activates the late steps of complement activation leading to assembly of the membrane attack complex (MAC) and subsequent cytolysis. The alternative pathway is initiated by small amounts of C3b, which are spontaneously generated in the plasma. C3b that remains unbound to a cell surface is rapidly hydrolyzed and inactivated. C3b bound to a microbe becomes a binding site for factor B. The bound factor B is then cleaved by factor D, generating factor Bb that covalently binds to C3b, forming the alternative pathway C3 convertase which activates the late steps of complement activation similar to the classical pathway. The lectin pathway is activated by MBL or ficolins binding to microbial surfaces. MBL then binds to MBL-associated serine proteases (MASPs)-1, -2, and -3. MASP-2 cleaves C4 and C2 to activate the complement cascade similar to the classical pathway (Fig. 3.1).

In addition to their role in microbial lysis, complement components also function as opsonins. Complement-coated microbes can be phagocytosed via complement receptors on phagocytes. Complement receptor type 1 (CR1) is a high affinity receptor for the C3b and C4b fragments of complement and mediates the internalization of C3b- and C4b-coated particles. CR1 on erythrocytes also mediates the clearance of immune complexes from the circulation. The complement type 2 receptor (CR2) is expressed on B cells and follicular dendritic cells and binds proteolytic fragments of C3, including C3d, C3dg, and iC3b. CR2 (also known as CD21) augments humoral immune responses by enhancing B cell activation by antigen and by promoting trapping of antigen-antibody complexes in germinal centers.[19]

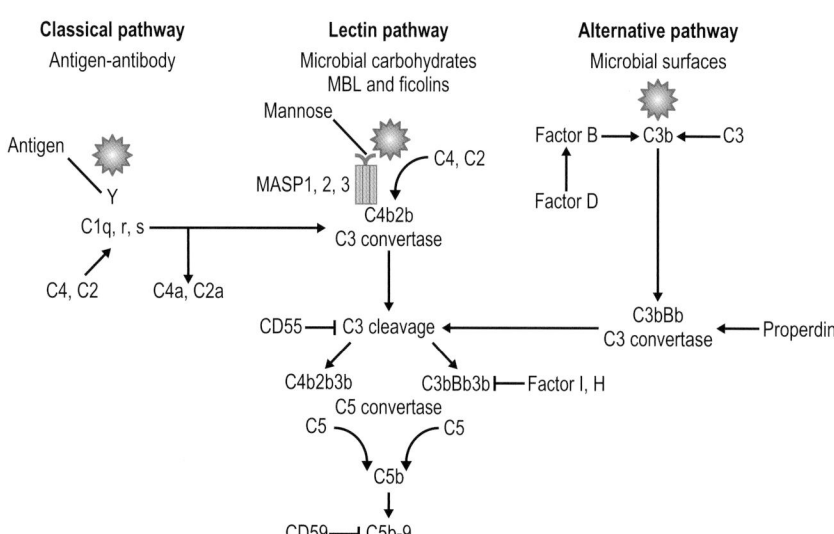

Fig. 3.1 Complement activation pathways. The classical complement cascade is activated by antibody bound to microbial surfaces, which is a binding site for the C1 complex. The alternative pathway is activated by the binding of spontaneously generated C3b to microbial surfaces. Microbial bound C3b binds factor B, which is converted to factor Bb, forming a C3 convertase. The lectin pathway is activated by the binding of MBL to mannose residues on microbial surfaces. MBL binds MBL-associated serine proteases, which bind and cleave C4 and C2, forming a C3 convertase.

Enhanced B cell activation through CR2 is another way in which the innate immune system influences subsequent adaptive immune responses. Additionally, CR2 is also the receptor for Epstein–Barr virus. Complement receptor 3 (CR3) is composed of CD18 and CD11b and is expressed in PMNs and mono-cytes/macrophages. CR3 binds to iC3b bound to the surface of microbes, leading to phagocytosis and destruction of the pathogen. The activation of complement via the alternative path-way can greatly enhance monocyte-generated TNF-α elicited by Gram-positive bacteria, such as group B streptococcus.[20]

There are multiple regulatory proteins within the complement pathways. C1-inhibitor (C1-INH) binds to and inhibits the enzy-matic functions of C1r and C1s within the classical pathway.[21] Properdin stabilizes the complex of C3b and Bb, increasing the lifespan of the alternative pathway C3 convertase. Conversely, factor H inhibits the formation of and degrades the C3bBb com-plex, whereas factor I inactivates C3b. CD55 (decay accelerating factor) and CD59 are cell surface, GPI-linked proteins that block complement-mediated cytolysis by inhibiting formation of the C3bBb complex and binding of C9 to the C5b678 complex, res-pectively. Absence of either CD55 or CD59 leads to paroxysmal nocturnal hemoglobinuria by complement-mediated intravascu-lar hemolysis.

Deficiencies of components of the complement system lead to a wide variety of diseases. Deficiencies of early components of the complement pathway are associated with invasive bacterial infections due to encapsulated organisms. Additionally, lack of early components of the complement pathway are associated with rheumatic disorders, including a lupus-like syndrome that may be due to impaired immune complex clearance, impaired clearance of apoptotic cells, and loss of complement-dependent B cell tolerance. Deficiency of Factor I is also associated with in-creased incidence of invasive infection with encapsulated bacte-ria, as well as glomerulonephritis and autoimmune disease. Deficiency of C1-INH protein and function, either hereditary or acquired, leads to angioedema. C1-INH inhibits C1, Factors XIa and XIIa, and kallikrein and, thus, dysregulation of these cas-cades leads to generation of vasoactive products that result in angioedema.[21,22] Deficiencies of late components of complement, including C5 through C9, as well as factors B, D, and properdin re-sult in susceptibility to meningococcal infections.[23] Deficiency of factor H function is associated with membranoproliferative glo-merulonephritis, hemolytic-uremic syndrome, and age-related macular degeneration.[24] Deficiency of MBL is associated with in-creased susceptibility to bacterial infections in infancy and in indi-viduals with other comorbid conditions, such as cystic fibrosis.[25]

Cellular innate immunity

Polymorphonuclear leukocytes

PMNs (Chapters 2, 21) are the most abundant leukocyte with ~10^9 PMNs produced per hour in the healthy adult, but have a short lifespan of ~5 days in circulation. PMNs are character-ized by segmented nuclei divided into 3 to 5 lobules and are thus readily identified by light microscopy. They are also referred to as neutrophils. The cytoplasm of PMN contains four types of granules, azurophilic (or primary), specific (or secondary), gelatinase, and secretory. PMN granules contain a wide variety of APPs with a broad spectrum of antimicrobial activities (Table 3.2). Azurophilic granules contain enzymes, such as pro-teinase 3, cathepsin G, and elastase, as well as α-defensins and BPI. Specific granules contain lactoferrin and the pro-forms of

cathelicidin peptides. Gelatinase granules are rich in gelatinase and are a marker of terminal neutrophil differentiation. Secre-tory granules contain a variety of receptors that are inserted into the cell membrane upon activation and exocytosis, converting the neutrophil into a cell responsive to many inflammatory stim-uli. PMNs are the earliest responders to infection. PMN that are not recruited to sites of infection undergo apoptosis and are cleared by the reticuloendothelial system.

Mononuclear phagocytes include monocytes and macrophages (Chapter 2). Monocytes originate in the bone marrow and migrate into the peripheral circulation. CD14$^+$ monocytes are effective at phagocytosis. They produce reactive oxygen interme-diates (ROIs) and pro-inflammatory cytokines in response to a wide variety of microbial stimuli. A recently characterized subset of monocytes that lacks CD14 expression (CD14^{dim}) but expresses CD16 is associated with vascular endothelia. This monocyte subset appears to be specialized for response to vi-ruses and nucleic acid-containing immune complexes and may also be involved in the pathogenesis of autoimmune disorders.[26] CD14$^+$ monocytes enter tissues where they mature into macro-phages. Macrophages in different tissues are given specific names, including the Kupffer cells of the liver, the alveolar mac-rophages of the lung, the osteoclasts in bone, and the microglia within the brain. Macrophages differ from PMNs in that they are not terminally differentiated and can proliferate at sites of infec-tion. Macrophages are longer lived than PMNs and are the pre-dominant innate immune cell several days after an infection.

Activated neutrophils and macrophages kill phagocytosed bacteria through production of microbicidal molecules within phagolysosomes. Microbes are detected by pattern recognition receptors, as well as by Fc and complement C3 receptors.[27] Bacteria are first internalized into phagosomes. Phagosomes fuse with lysosomes containing proteolytic enzymes (elastase, cathepsin G) to form phagolysosomes. Activated PMNs and macrophages also produce reactive oxygen intermediates (ROIs), which are toxic to microbes. ROI are produced by phagocyte-derived NADPH oxidase, an enzyme that consists of five subunits: p22^{phox}, p40^{phox}, p47^{phox}, p67^{phox}, and gp91^{phox}. The phagocyte oxidase is activated following engulfment of opsonized bacteria. A variety of stimuli lead to activation of the phagocyte oxidase complex, including the complement fragment C5a, formylated peptides like fMLP (N-formyl-methionine-leucine-phenylalanine), LTB4 (leukotriene B4), PAF (platelet activating factor), and pattern recognition receptors, like TLR4. Upon cellular activation, p40^{phox}, p47^{phox}, and p67^{phox} are phosphorylated and recruited to cellular membranes where they associate with membrane bound gp91^{phox} and p22^{phox} (also called flavocytochrome b$_{558}$) and GTP-bound Rac1 (monocytes) or Rac2 (neutrophils).[28] The function of the activated enzyme is to generate superoxide radicals. Superoxide radicals are converted to hydrogen peroxide by superoxide dismutase. Hydrogen peroxide is combined with halide ions by myeloperoxidase to generate hypohalous acids, which are toxic to bacteria. Another function of the phagocyte oxidase complex is to generate an environment within the phagolysosome required for activation of the proteolytic enzymes. The oxidase functions as an electron pump that generates an electrochemical gradient across the phagolysosomal membranes that is compensated by the movement of ions into the vacuole. This results in an increase in vacuolar pH and osmolarity, which is required for activation of elastase and cathepsin G.[29]

Macrophages produce reactive nitrogen intermediates in response to microbes. Nitric oxide (NO) is produced by inducible nitric oxide synthetase (iNOS). Expression of iNOS is induced by activation of TLRs and expression is augmented further by IFN-γ.[30] iNOS catalyzes the conversion of arginine to citrulline, releasing diffusible nitric oxide gas. Within phagolysosomes, NO can combine with hydrogen peroxide or superoxide to produce peroxynitrite radicals, which contribute to microbial killing. Although ROIs and NO are effective antimicrobial agents, they are non-specific. In the setting of strong and prolonged activation of PMNs and macrophages, ROIs and NO are capable of inducing damage to host tissues.

Dendritic cells (Chapter 2) are important in innate responses and for linking innate and adaptive immune responses.[31] DCs have long membranous extensions for surveying the local environment and are highly phagocytic. DCs are widely distributed throughout the body. They express a variety of PRRs that allow them to respond to microbes by increased antigen uptake and secretion of cytokines. Plasmacytoid dendritic cells (pDCs) are a subpopulation of DCs specialized for response to viral infection. pDCs secrete large amounts of type 1 interferons, which have potent antiviral activities. DCs link innate to adaptive immune responses after activation by microbes. Activated DCs rapidly uptake antigen and then home to draining lymph nodes where they localize to T-cell zones. During their migration to lymph nodes, DCs mature and become efficient antigen presenting cells (APCs). Once in the lymph node, DCs express high levels of costimulatory molecules, like B7 and IL-12p70, and present antigen to naïve T cells, inducing their differentiation into effector T cells (Th1 T cells).

Natural killer (NK) *cells* (Chapter 17) are derived from common lymphoid progenitor cells and constitute 5–20% of mononuclear cells in the periphery. NK cells were named based upon their ability to kill various target cells without the need for additional activation, in contrast to T lymphocytes that require activation prior to differentiation from naïve T cells into effector T cells. NK cells are a major source of IFN-γ, which augments the microbicidal functions of macrophages. Conversely, NK cells are primed by IL-15 derived from DCs and IL-12 or -18 derived from macrophages, demonstrating the regulatory interactions that occur between NK cells and other cells of the immune system. NK cells are distinct from B and T lymphocytes in that they do not express somatically rearranged antigen receptors, like immunoglobulin or T-cell receptor. Target cells are identified using germline DNA-encoded receptors.

NK cell function is regulated by a delicate balance between signals generated by inhibitory and activating receptors.[32] NK cells possess the ability to recognize and kill infected or malignantly transformed cells, while leaving healthy host cells unharmed. Inhibitory receptors on NK cells recognize class I major histocompatibility complex (MHC) molecules expressed on most healthy cells in the body. Examples of inhibitory receptors include three families of receptors: heterodimers composed of CD94 and NKG2A, the Ig-like transcripts (i.e., ILT-2), and the killer cell Ig-like receptor (KIR) family. Inhibitory receptors contain immunoreceptor tyrosine-based inhibition motifs (ITIMs) in their cytoplasmic tails. ITIMs recruit phosphatases [(SH2-containing protein phosphatase)-1, SHP-2, SHIP (SH2-containing inositol polyphosphate 5-phosphatase)] that oppose the effects of kinases induced by activating receptors. As a result, when NK cells encounter host cells expressing MHC class I molecules, protein tyrosine phosphatases are activated, reducing any signaling downstream of activating receptors and the NK cell is not activated (Fig. 3.2).

NK cells also possess activating receptors, including CD16, which mediates antibody-dependent cell cytotoxicity and natural cytotoxicity receptors (i.e., NKp46, NKp30, NKp44, NKG2D, CD94/NKG2C, 2B4). Activating receptors are linked to

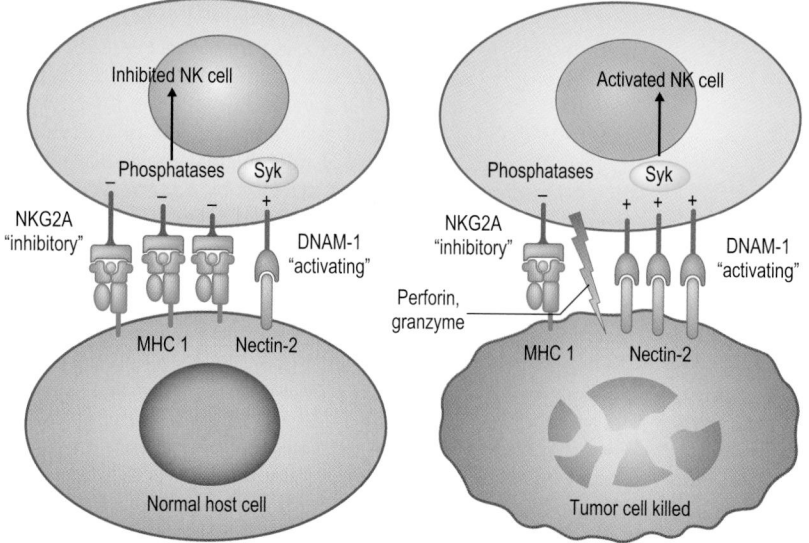

Fig. 3.2 Regulation of NK-cell function. Upon encountering normal host cells, inhibitory receptors on NK cells that contain ITIM motifs preferentially activate phosphatases (SHP-1/2, SHIP) that send inhibitory signals, inhibiting NK cell function. NK cells that encounter virally infected cells or tumor cells receive signals through activating receptors that contain ITAM motifs that activate tyrosine kinases, including SYK, which leads to NK cell activation, release of perforin and granzyme, and target cell death.

molecules (i.e., CD3ζ, FcRγ, or DAP12) that contain immunoreceptor tyrosine-based activation motifs (ITAMs). Upon ligand binding to activating receptors, tyrosine residues within ITAMs are phosphorylated by Src family kinases, and tyrosine phosphorylated ITAMs serve as binding sites for the activation of other protein tyrosine kinases, such as spleen tyrosine kinase (SYK) and zeta chain-associated protein kinase 70 (ZAP-70), which activate downstream effector molecules in a signaling cascade. Infection of host cells with some viruses can lead to reduced MHC class I expression as a way to reduce presentation of viral antigen to T cells. However, reduced MHC class I expression by infected cells results in reduced inhibitory signaling in the NK cell. Concomitantly, ligands for activating receptors are expressed by the infected cell, leading to NK cell activation and killing of the infected cell.

NK cells also play an important role in immunosurveillance against tumors.[33] In humans, the NK cell receptors that mediate tumor recognition include NKp46, NKp30, NKp44, DNAM-1 (DNAX accessory molecule-1), and NKG2D. The receptors used in NK-cell-mediated tumor lysis depend upon the ligands expressed by the target cells. Ligands expressed on target cells include MHC I-related chain (MIC)-A, MICB, unique long 16-binding proteins (ULBPs), poliovirus receptor (PVR), and nectin-2. DNAM-1 specific ligands include PVR and nectin-2, which are expressed in cell lines that include carcinomas, melanomas, and neuroblastomas. Nectin expression is not specific to tumors, since nectins are expressed on normal cells. DNAM-1-nectin interactions on normal cells do not result in NK cell lysis, however, because normal cells are protected by MHC class I expression. Conditions favoring NK-cell-mediated lysis include tumors in which nectins are overexpressed and/or MHC class expression is reduced, favoring NK-cell activation (Fig. 3.2).

Natural killer (NKT) *cells* are a small, but highly variable, population of thymus-derived T cells that express NK cell markers and a restricted repertoire of T-cell receptors (TCRs) (Chapter 4) that recognize lipids bound to the MHC-like molecule CD1d.[34] There appear to be unique phenotypic attributes among NKT cells. Type 1 NKT cells (also referred to as invariant NKT (iNKT) cells) express the invariant Vα24 and Jα28 TCR α chain, whereas type 2 NKT cells have a more diverse TCR repertoire. Current studies are attempting to further characterize subsets of NKT cells, suggesting that NKT cells are heterogeneous. Mature human NKT cells can be further divided into 3 groups, including CD4$^+$CD8$^-$, CD4$^-$CD8$^-$, and CD4$^-$CD8$^+$ subsets. The most completely characterized NKT antigen is the lipid α-galactosylceremide (αGalCer), which is often used to activate NKT cells experimentally. However, identification of natural NKT ligands has proven difficult. NKT cells express perforin and granulysin and are capable of cytotoxic activity. NKT cells are also able to influence innate and adaptive immune responses through release of large amounts of cytokines, including IFN-γ, TNF-α, IL-4, IL-13, IL-10, and GM-CSF. In general, NKTs found in blood can produce large amounts of cytokines, whereas NKTs in the thymus are poor cytokine producers.

The role of NKTs in human diseases is an area of active investigation. Some reports suggest that decreased NKT-cell frequency and/or function may increase susceptibility to some autoimmune diseases, including type 1 diabetes and multiple sclerosis. Mice with NKT defects are susceptible to tumors and adoptive transfer of normal NKTs can provide protection against the tumors, suggesting that NKT cells may play a role in tumor immunosurveillance. NKT cells may also contribute to the pathogenesis of the airway hyperresponsiveness (AHR) of asthma, which is dependent upon IL-4 and -13 production in the airways.

The iNKT cells are necessary for AHR in several murine models of asthma, since NKT deficient mice fail to develop AHR following allergen challenge, ozone challenge, or viral infection.[35] iNKT-cell deficiency was associated with severe varicella infection, demonstrating a role for iNKT cells in innate anti-viral immunity.[36]

Pattern recognition receptors

> ● **KEY CONCEPTS**
>
> **Pattern recognition receptors**
>
> - Toll-like receptors (TLRs) recognize endogenous and exogenous danger signals, consist of an extracellular domain containing leucine-rich repeats (LRRs) for ligand binding and a cytoplasmic Toll/IL-1 receptor domain that links to adapter proteins and complex signaling pathways.
> - Nucleotide oligomerization domain (NOD)-like receptors are a family of 22 proteins that contain LRRs for potential ligand binding, a NOD, and a caspase activation and recruitment domain (CARD), Pyrin domain, or a baculovirus inhibitor of apoptosis repeat (BIR) domain for initiation of signaling.
> - Retinoic acid-inducible gene (RIG)-like receptors consist of two N-terminal CARDs for signaling and an RNA helicase domain
> - C-type lectin receptors (CLRs) contain a C (Ca^{++})-type recognition domain and mediate diverse functions, depending upon the signaling pathways they activate.
> - Scavenger receptors (SRs) are a diverse group of receptors that recognize a variety of ligands, mediate uptake of oxidized lipoproteins, and may be involved in atherosclerotic plaque formation.

Our understanding of the mechanisms by which pathogens are detected has increased greatly over the past decade. Pathogen recognition by the innate immune system leads to engulfment, destruction, and often incomplete clearance of the invading pathogen. The subsequent adaptive immune response is required to completely clear the infection. The innate immune system expresses a wide variety of PRRs that mediate pathogen recognition, leading to production of pro-inflammatory cytokines, pathogen uptake and destruction, antigen processing and presentation, and initiation of adaptive immune responses that ultimately clear the host of pathogen. The detection of pathogens relies mainly upon PRRs that include the TLRs, nucleotide oligomerization domain (NOD)-like receptors (NLRs), and the retinoic acid-inducible gene-I (RIG-I)-like receptors (RLRs).[37] These receptors play an essential role in initiating the innate immune response. Unlike T- and B-cell antigen receptors, the PRRs are germline-encoded, do not undergo somatic recombination, and are expressed constitutively by immune and non-immune cells. PRRs recognize PAMPs, components of pathogens that are invariant and required for pathogen survival (Table 3.3). Although PRRs detect PAMPs expressed by microbes, they can also recognize self-molecules (i.e., host nucleic acids), which may play a role in the pathogenesis of some autoimmune diseases, such as lupus and rheumatoid arthritis.

Toll-like receptors

The *Toll* pathway was initially identified in *Drosophila melanogaster* as a receptor required for dorsal-ventral patterning. Subsequently, the *Toll* pathway was found to be an essential component of host defense against fungal infection, which led to cloning of mammalian homologues, the Toll-like receptors (TLRs). Mammalian TLRs consist of 11 members that can recognize a wide variety of PAMPs. The TLRs are type 1 integral membrane glycoproteins characterized by an extracellular domain with varying numbers of leucine-rich repeats (LRRs) and a cytoplasmic signaling domain homologous to the interleukin-1 receptor (IL-1R), referred to as the Toll/IL-1R (TIR) homology domain. The TIR domain links the receptor to adaptor proteins (like myeloid differentiation factor 88 (MyD88)) and downstream signaling molecules, leading to transcription of numerous genes that regulate inflammation (Fig. 3.3).

TLRs are widely expressed on or within cells of the immune system, as well as epithelial cells. TLRs detect a wide variety of pathogens, including bacteria, mycobacteria, viruses, fungi, and protozoa (Table 3.3). TLRs have been classified into subfamilies based upon their genetic tree. The subfamily of TLR1, TLR2, TLR6, and TLR10 recognize bacterial lipoproteins, whereas TLR3, TLR7, TLR8, and TLR9 recognize nucleic acids. TLR4, in conjunction with MD-2, recognizes lipopolysaccharide (LPS) and TLR5 binds bacterial flagellin. TLR11 has recently been found to recognize a profilin-like molecule of *Toxoplasma gondii*. However, ligand binding by TLRs can be promiscuous. For example, TLR4 can also bind respiratory syncytial virus F protein and pneumolysin of *S. pneumoniae*.[38,39] TLR9 binds malarial hemozoin, as well hypomethylated CpG-rich DNA. TLRs can also recognize endogenous danger signals, i.e., damage-associated molecular patterns (DAMPs), which include heat shock proteins.[40]

The cellular localization of TLRs varies. TLR1, TLR2, TLR4, TLR5, TLR6, TLR10, and TLR11 are localized to cell surfaces, whereas TLR3, TLR7, TLR8, and TLR9 are localized within endosomes. The cell surface expression of TLRs, such as TLR4, which recognizes LPS, is hypothesized to allow recognition of extracellular molecules released from pathogens. Endosomal expression of TLR3, 7, 8, and 9 allows recognition of microbial nucleic acids following their uptake and degradation in phagolysosomes. Additionally, endosomal expression of TLR3, 7, 8, and 9 is believed to prevent activation by host nucleic acids and the development

of autoimmunity. TLR expression is altered by exposure to pathogens, as well as by cytokines. The broad cellular expression of TLRs and their diverse and promiscuous agonist recognition allows detection of a wide variety of pathogens despite the existence of a limited number of TLRs.

The cellular responses that occur following TLR activation are essential to host defense. TLR activation stimulates a brief burst of macropinocytosis, which results in antigen uptake at sites of infection, allowing antigen presentation to T cells. TLR activation leads to production of pro-inflammatory cytokines, including TNF-α and IL-6, as well as chemokines, such as CXCL8. TLR pathway engagement induces transcription and translation of mRNA encoding pro-IL-1β. But production of mature IL-1β requires activation of the inflammasome, further described below. The production of pro-inflammatory cytokines recruits additional phagocytes to sites of infection and augments their antimicrobial functions. Production of IL-12p70 leads to activation of naïve T cells and their subsequent differentiation into effector T cells (Th1 T cells). Presentation of foreign peptides and increased expression of MHC molecules, along with expression of co-stimulatory molecules, like B7-1, B7-2, and IL-12p70, results in subsequent development of adaptive immune responses. IL-12p70 stimulates IFN-γ production by T cells, which further augments the microbicidal activities of phagocytes. Stimulation of TLR3, TLR7, TLR8, and TLR9 elicits the production of pro-inflammatory cytokines, as well as type 1 interferons, which play a crucial role in innate antiviral immunity and also influence adaptive immune responses.

Engagement of TLRs activates complex signaling pathways that have been characterized through biochemical analyses and through use of mice selectively deficient in these PRRs and downstream signaling proteins.[41-43] TLRs, IL-1R, and IL-18R share similar signaling pathways (Fig. 3.4). Upon ligand binding the cytoplasmic adaptor protein, MyD88, is recruited to the TIR domain of the receptor for all TLRs, except TLR3. Recruitment of MyD88 leads to recruitment of interleukin-1 receptor associated kinase-4 (IRAK-4), likely through death domain interactions. IRAK-4 activation leads to recruitment and activation of IRAK-1 and IRAK-2. In monocytes, IRAK-M is also recruited to this complex and functions as a negative regulator of signaling. Both IRAK-1 and IRAK-2 activation are required for full activation of NFκB and MAP kinases. IRAK activation leads to interaction with TNF-receptor-associated factor 6 (TRAF6), which is an E3 ubiquitin ligase. Along with the E2 conjugating complex of Ubc13 and Uev1a, TRAF6 is K-63 ubiquitinated, recruiting transforming growth factor β-activated protein kinase-1 (TAK-1). TAK-1 subsequently activates the inhibitor of NFκB (IκB) kinase complex (IKK), which consists of NFκB essential modifier (NEMO), IKKα and IKKβ, leading to phosphorylation of IκB (inhibitor of NFκB) proteins and their subsequent K-48 linked ubiquitination and degradation. NFκB is then released from inhibition, allowing translocation to the nucleus where it mediates transcriptional activation of numerous genes involved in inflammation. The transcription factor interferon regulatory factor-5 (IRF-5) is also activated downstream of TRAF6 and is required for production of pro-inflammatory cytokines. Additionally, TAK-1 activation leads to activation of p38 MAP kinase and c-Jun N terminal kinase (JNK), which, in turn, activates the AP1 transcriptional complex (Fig. 3.4).

TLR signaling demonstrates further complexity. TLR4 also interacts with the adaptors MAL (MyD88-like adaptor protein), TRAM (translocating chain-associating membrane protein), and TRIF (TIR domain containing adaptor inducing interferon β) (Fig. 3.4). TLR4 initially recruits MAL and MyD88 to trigger an "early phase" of NFκB and MAP kinase activation. TLR4 is

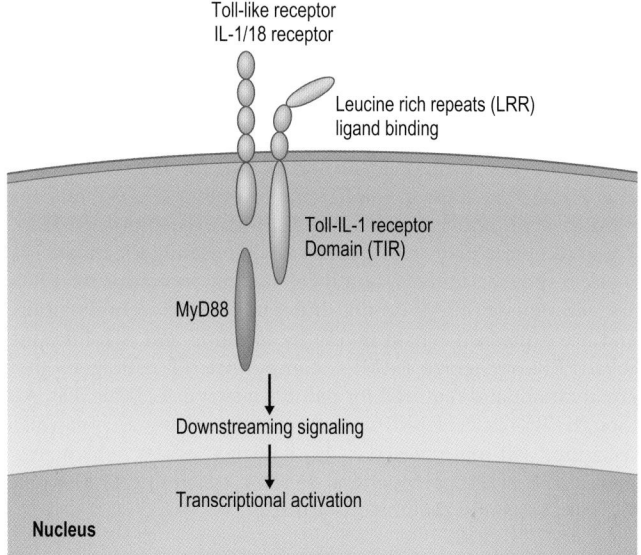

Fig. 3.3 TLRs and IL-1/18 receptors share a common signaling pathway. Upon ligand binding, signals are transduced intracellularly by the interaction of the adaptor protein, MyD88, with the TIR domain of receptor. MyD88 interacts with IRAK-4 through death domain interactions, leading to generation of a signaling cascade, which results in transcriptional activation of genes involved in inflammation.

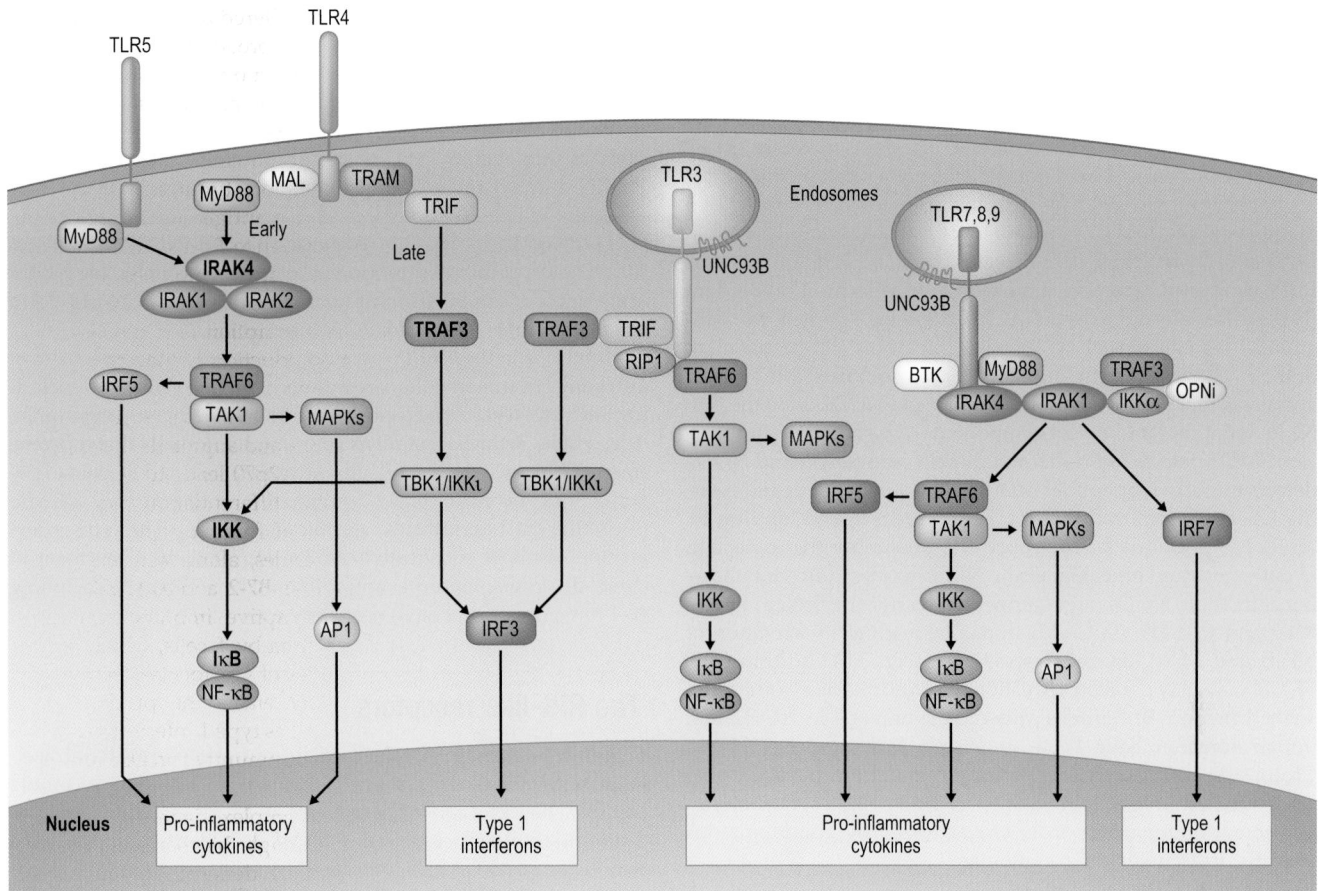

Fig. 3.4 MyD88 dependent and independent TLR signaling pathways. Activation of MyD88 dependent TLRs (TLR5) results in activation of IRAK4 and IRAK1, 2, leading activation of TRAF6 and TAK-1. Subsequently, activation of the IKK complex and MAP kinases lead to activation of NFκB and AP1 transcription factors, respectively. The transcription factor IRF5 is also activated downstream of TRAF6. The TLR4 signaling pathway utilizes four adaptor proteins. The adaptors MAL and MyD88 are activated upon ligand interaction at the cell surface, leading activation of an "early" signaling cascade through the IRAKs. Subsequently, TLR4 is internalized and a "late" signaling cascade dependent upon the adaptors TRAM and TRIF is activated. TLR3 activates a TRIF-dependent pathway that activates RIP1 and TBK1/IKKi, leading to production of pro-inflammatory cytokines and IFN-β. TLR7, 8, 9 are MyD88 dependent and activate the transcription factors NFκB, IRF5, AP1, and IRF7, resulting in production of pro-inflammatory cytokines and type 1 interferons.

subsequently endocytosed and trafficked to the endosome where it forms a signaling complex with TRAM and TRIF, which leads to activation of TANK-binding kinase-1 (TBK-1), IKKε, and IRF-3 and "late phase" activation of NFκB and MAP kinases. Activation of IRF3 induces IFN-β production.

The anti-viral TLRs are located in endosomes and interact with an endoplasmic reticulum membrane protein called UNC93B (Fig. 3.4).[44] Upon activation, TLR3 does not recruit MyD88, but rather TRIF, leading to recruitment of TRAF3 and activation of TBK1, IKKi, IRF-3, and IFN-β production. TRIF also recruits RIP1 and TRAF6, which leads to activation of NFκB. The other anti-viral TLRs (TLR7, TLR8, and TLR), are MyD88-dependent. However, they also activate a pathway utilizing IRAK-1, IKKα, TRAF3 and intracellular osteopontin (iOPN) that activates IRF7, leading to production of IFN-α. TLR7, TLR8, and TLR9 also utilize a TRAF6-dependent pathway that leads to NFκB/MAP kinase activation.[45] In addition, the tyrosine kinase, Bruton's tyrosine kinase (BTK), plays a critical role in TLR8- and TLR9-induced production of TNF-α and IL-6.[46] The signaling pathways activated by TLRs are complex and ongoing research continues to identify additional signaling components activated downstream of these receptors.

In natura, the innate immune system encounters intact pathogens that express multiple PAMPs, including bacterial cell wall components as well as microbial DNA and RNA, leading to activation of DCs and other phagocytes through multiple PRRs. The activation of DCs through combinations of TLRs, such as TLR4 and TLR8, results in synergistic production of Th1 T-cell-inducing cytokines, as well as the Th1-inducing ligand, Delta-4, leading to stronger Th1 differentiation of T cells than occurs following activation of single TLRs.[47] Interestingly, the use of combinations of TLR agonists on virus-sized nanoparticles containing antigen induce enhanced and better-sustained antibody responses in mice and non-human primates.[48] Thus, the use of combinations of TLR agonists as adjuvants in vaccines may result in enhanced efficacy of future vaccines, as well as in immunotherapy against tumors.

During an infection, multiple factors can mitigate TLR-induced inflammation. Adenosine, for example, is an endogenous purine metabolite whose levels rise during stress or hypoxia, Adenosine binds receptors expressed on leukocytes, leading to increased intracellular concentrations of cyclic adenosine monophosphate (cAMP), which in turn dampens TLR-mediated production of Th1-polarizing cytokines while preserving production of Th2 and anti-inflammatory cytokines. Resolvins and lipoxins are anti-inflammatory/pro-resolving lipid metabolites that can differentially regulate TLR4-mediated responses of macrophages, thereby inhibiting TNF response to pure LPS but enhancing uptake, killing, and TNF-α production of whole Gram-negative bacteria.[49]

NOD-like receptors

In addition to TLRs, other families of cytoplasmic PRRs have been identified, including NLRs and RLRs. NLRs mediate detection of intracytoplasmic bacterial products whereas RLRs detect the presence of viral nucleic acids generated by intracellular, replicating viruses. The currently known NLRs consist of 5 members of the NODs, 14 members of the NALP family, CIITA, IPAF and NAIP (Table 3.3). Proteins in the NLR family possess LRRs for ligand detection, a nucleotide oligomerization domain (NOD) also referred to as a NACHT domain, a domain for initiation of signaling, such as caspase activation and recruitment domain (CARD), pyrin domains, or baculovirus inhibitor of apoptosis repeat (BIR) domains. NOD1 and NOD2 were the first NLRs identified and detect components of bacterial peptidoglycan: NOD1 detects meso-diaminopimelic acid (DAP) and NOD2 detects muramyl dipeptide (MDP). Although direct ligand binding has been demonstrated for TLRs, direct ligand binding by NLRs has not, thus leaving open the possibility that detection of pathogens and other signals by NLRs may be indirect. Following activation, NODs oligomerize and recruit the protein kinase RIP2 and CARD9 via CARD domains, leading to activation of NFκB and MAP kinases, respectively (Fig. 3.5). Additionally, NOD2 may play a role in activation of some inflammasomes (described below). In humans, missense mutations in NOD2 that impair function have been associated with susceptibility to Crohn's disease. Conversely, missense mutations in NOD2 that lead to constitutive activation of NFκB lead to Blau syndrome, an autosomal dominant disorder characterized by granulomatous arthritis, iritis, and skin granulomas.

The inflammasomes

A variety of stimuli, including PAMPs, bacterial toxins, aluminum hydroxide (alum), UV light, as well as endogenous "danger signals" released by stressed or damaged host cells, referred to as damage-associated molecular patterns (DAMPs) (i.e., ATP, uric acid, hyaluronan), induce the processing of pro-IL-1β to mature IL-1β. The cytosolic cellular machinery responsible for IL-1β processing is termed the *inflammasome*. Prototypical inflammasomes include the NOD-like receptor-related protein-1 (NLRP1) inflammasome, the NLRP3 inflammasome, and the IL-1β-converting enzyme protease-activating factor (IPAF) inflammasome. NLRPs recruit ASC (apoptosis associated speck-like protein containing a CARD) via homotypic PYRIN domain interactions. ASC is an adaptor protein that contains a PYRIN domain and a CARD domain. Caspase-1 is subsequently recruited via CARD domains, leading to proteolytic processing of IL-1β and IL-18 (Fig. 3.5). Although NLRP1, NLRP3, and IPAF form prototypical inflammasomes, other NLRs, including NOD2 and neuronal apoptosis inhibitory protein (NAIP) can also form inflammasomes or modulate their activities.[50]

Mutations in the NLRP3 gene are associated with a spectrum of autosomal dominant inherited autoinflammatory diseases, including Muckle-Wells syndrome (sensineural deafness, urticaria, fevers, chills, arthritis), familial cold autoinflammatory syndrome (rash, conjunctivitis, fever, chills, arthralgias elicited by cold exposure), and neonatal onset multisystem inflammatory disease (NOMID) (rashes, arthritis, chronic meningitis). These disorders are the result of constitutive production of IL-1β. Treatment of these disorders involves anti-inflammatory therapy, including IL-1 antagonists that have been very effective.[51]

The RIG-like receptors

TLR-independent innate antiviral immune responses to intracellular replicating viruses are mediated by RIG-like receptors (RLRs). The RLRs consist of two receptors: RIG-I and (melanoma differentiation-associated gene-5) MDA-5. Both receptors have two N-terminal CARDs and an RNA helicase domain and appear to play important roles in virus-induced type 1 interferon expression in fibroblasts and conventional DCs. A third RLR, laboratory of genetics and physiology 2 (LGP2), lacks the N-terminal CARD domains and plays a role in repression of signaling. RIG-I and MDA-5 are activated by dsRNA generated during viral replication. RIG-I and MDA-5 have differing specificities for viral recognition. RIG-I detects orthomyxoviridae, rhabdoviridae, paramyxoviridae, and flaviviridae, whereas MDA-5 detects picornaviridae, caliciviridae, and coronaviridae. Poly inosine:cytosine (poly I:C) is a non-specific dsRNA analog used experimentally to activate TLR3 and RIG-I/MDA-5. Relatively short poly I:

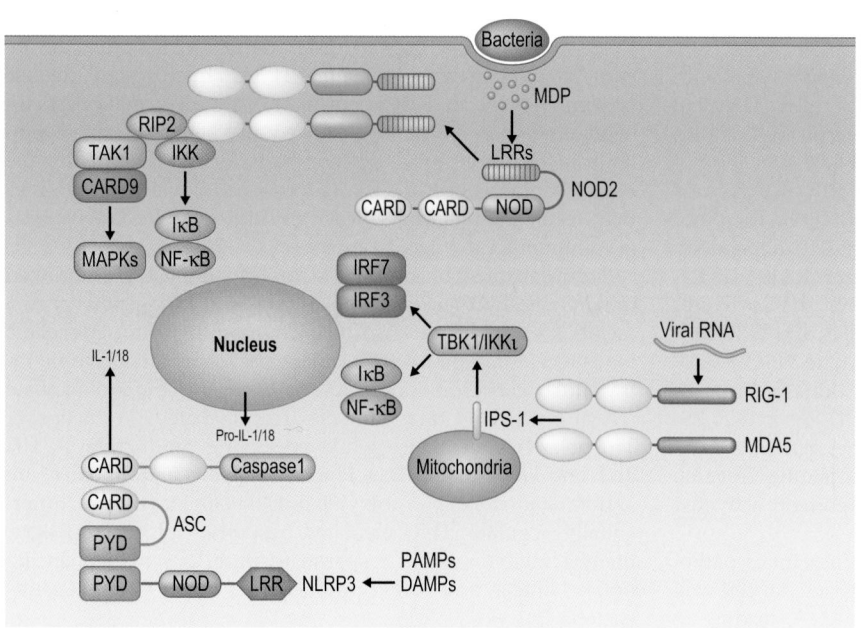

Fig. 3.5 NLR, RLR, and inflammasome signaling. NOD2 is activated following exposure to bacterial MDP, leading dimerization and activation of RIP2, TAK1, CARD9 and the IKK complex, leading to inflammatory gene transcription. RLRs, like RIG-I and MDA-5, are activated by double-stranded RNA generated by intracellular, replicating viruses, leading to activation of transcription factors, including NFκB, IRF3, and IRF7, leading to production of pro-inflammatory cytokines and type 1 interferons. Inflammasomes can be activated by microbial products (PAMPs), as well as endogenous products released by damaged host cells (DAMPs), leading to processing of pro-IL-1β to active IL-1β.

C (<1 kb) is recognized preferentially by RIG-I, whereas long poly I:C (>1 kb) is preferentially recognized by MDA-5.[38]

Activation of RIG-I and MDA-5 by dsRNA leads to their association with a mitochondria-associated adaptor known as interferon-β promoter stimulator-1 (IPS-1) or mitochondrial antiviral-signaling protein (MAVS) through CARD domain interactions. Downstream effectors include TBK-1 and IKKι, which activate IRF3 and IRF7, leading to production of type-1 interferons (Fig. 3.5). Of note, live bacteria are more effective inducers of STAT-1, type I IFN, and inflammasome pathways than killed organisms, a property that may reflect the importance of bacterial RNA to innate recognition of live infection.[52]

C-type lectin receptors

The C-type lectin receptors (CLRs) are a diverse group of receptors originally identified as Ca^{2+}-dependent carbohydrate binding proteins.[53] Currently, CLRs are defined as any protein that contains a C-type carbohydrate recognition domain (CRD), regardless of calcium or carbohydrate binding ability. CLRs include numerous members with diverse functions including cell adhesion, regulation of NK cell function, phagocytosis, endocytosis, platelet activation, complement activation, tissue remodeling, and innate immunity. In myeloid cells, CLRs can mediate internalization of microbes to allow for antigen processing and presentation. Some CLRs function analogously to TLRs, resulting in direct cellular activation and generation of inflammatory responses. Other CLRs are capable of binding PAMPs, but function to modulate cell activation (discussed below). The functions of myeloid CLRs are dictated by the signaling pathways they activate.

Dectin-1 is a CLR expressed on DCs and other myeloid cells that recognizes β-1, 3-linked glucans present in the cell wall of fungi, mycobacteria, and plants. Dectin-2 recognizes high mannose structures and α-mannans found in fungi, mycobacteria, and dust mites. Following ligand binding, Dectin-1 and Dectin-2 activate signaling pathways utilizing the tyrosine kinase SYK, CARD9, and RAF-1, leading to activation of the transcription factors NFκB, NFAT, and AP-1 and production of pro-inflammatory cytokines (Fig. 3.6). Activation of SYK

leads to generation of ROI, which can activate the NLRP3 inflammasome, leading to processing of pro-IL-1β to mature IL-1β. The importance of CLR function in anti-fungal immunity is demonstrated by inactivating mutations in Dectin-1 and CARD9 that lead to chronic mucocutaneous candidiasis, as well as invasive fungal infections in the case of CARD9 deficiency.[54]

Mincle (macrophage inducible C-type lectin) recognizes α-mannans and glycolipids and associates with the FcRγ chain. Upon ligand binding, SYK is recruited to the ITAM of FcRγ, leading to cellular activation. Mincle also binds the endogenous nucleoprotein SAP130, which is exposed by dead cells. The Mincle mediated response to dead cells leads to infiltration of PMNs into damaged tissue and is likely important for tissue repair.

Other CLRs, such as DCIR (DC-inhibitory receptor) possess an inhibitory ITIM motif. DCIR is expressed on myeloid cells, DCs, and B cells. DCIR inhibits TLR8-induced IL-12p70 and TNF-α production by myeloid DCs and TLR9-induced IFN-α production by pDCs. Inhibition of TLR responses is likely the result of inhibition of tyrosine kinases and/or PI3 kinase pathways.[53]

Pathogens express multiple PAMPs and CLRs and TLRs are known to cooperate in antimicrobial responses. Dectin-1 has been shown to assist TLR2 in the production of pro-inflammatory cytokines induced by zymosan, through activation of both Dectin-1-SYK and TLR2-MyD88 signaling pathways (Fig. 3.6). Additionally, DC-SIGN, which recognizes mycobacteria and viruses, can enhance TLR-induced NFκB activation through a RAF-1 dependent signaling pathway.[55]

Scavenger receptors

Scavenger receptors are a diverse group of receptors that include CD36, CD68, SR class A, and SR class B.[56] The receptors mediate the uptake of oxidized lipoproteins into cells. Scavenger receptors also mediate the uptake of microbes and contribute to the response of macrophages to mycobacteria. SR class A can also induce an inflammatory response to beta-amyloid fibrils, which may contribute to inflammation within senile plaques in the brains of Alzheimer's disease patients. (Table 3.3). Additionally, scavenger receptors

Fig. 3.6 C-type lectin signaling. CLRs, like Dectin-1, contain ITAM motifs that interact with the cytosolic tyrosine kinase, SYK, leading to activation of transcription factors including NFκB, NFAT, and AP1. Additionally, Dectin-1 activates the serine kinase, Raf1, which contributes to NFκB activation. TLRs, like TLR2, can cooperate with Dectin-1 signaling to activate NFκB, leading to an enhanced inflammatory response.

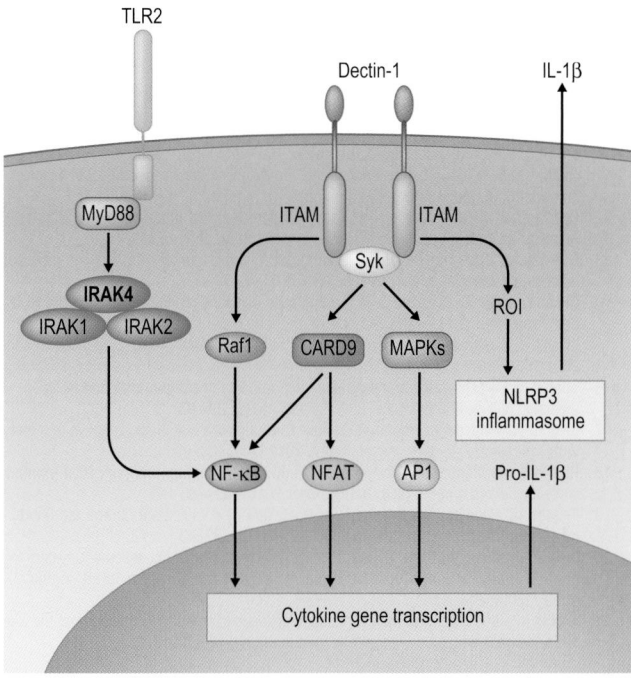

play a pathologic role in the generation of cholesterol-laden foam cells that comprise atherosclerotic plaques in blood vessels.

Summary

Our understanding of the complexity of innate immunity has advanced considerably over the past decade. The innate immune system consists of diverse populations of cells that include epithelia, which provide barrier functions and express PRRs and APPs that inhibit colonization by invading pathogens, as well as professional phagocytes that ingest and destroy pathogens and secrete cytokines and chemokines that recruit and activate other immune cells. Plasma factors, including acute phase proteins and complement proteins, are essential components of innate immunity and participate in optimal adaptive immune function. The innate immune system consists of a growing repertoire of PRRs, including TLRs, NLRs, RLRs, and CLRs which detect a broad spectrum of pathogens despite being germline encoded. Innate immune responses are responsible for initiating subsequent adaptive immune responses. The importance of the innate immune system to human health is underscored by single gene mutations, such as IRAK4 deficiency,[57] that result in immune deficiencies and infection, particularly in early life (to be described in Chapter 35. As innate immunity is expressed in an age-specific manner,[58] a better understanding of the ontogeny of the innate immune system, as well as the mechanisms by which innate and adaptive immunity interact, will guide development of adjuvants, resulting in more effective vaccines and tumor immunotherapy.[59,60]

References

1. Janeway Jr. CA, Bottomly K. Signals and signs for lymphocyte responses. Cell 1994;76(2):275–85.
2. Netea MG, Quintin J, van der Meer JW. Trained immunity: a memory for innate host defense. Cell Host Microbe 2011;9(5):355–61.
3. Ong PY, Ohtake T, Brandt C, et al. Endogenous antimicrobial peptides and skin infections in atopic dermatitis. N Engl J Med 2002;347(15):1151–60.
4. Nuding S, Fellermann K, Wehkamp J, Stange EF. Reduced mucosal antimicrobial activity in Crohn's disease of the colon. Gut 2007;56(9):1240–7.
5. Hazlett L, Wu M. Defensins in innate immunity. Cell Tissue Res 2011;343(1):175–88.
6. Schutte BC, McCray Jr PB. [beta]-defensins in lung host defense. Annu Rev Physiol 2002;64:709–48.
7. McDermott AM. Defensins and other antimicrobial peptides at the ocular surface. Ocul Surf 2004;2(4):229–47.
8. Miller LS. Toll-like receptors in skin. Adv Dermatol 2008;24:71–87.
9. Villablanca EJ, Mora JR. A two-step model for Langerhans cell migration to skin-draining LN. Eur J Immunol 2008;38(11):2975–80.
10. Hayday A, Theodoridis E, Ramsburg E, Shires J. Intraepithelial lymphocytes: exploring the Third Way in immunology. Nat Immunol 2001;2(11):997–1003.
11. Fagarasan S, Honjo T. T-Independent immune response: new aspects of B cell biology. Science 2000;290(5489):89–92.
12. Galli SJ, Tsai M. Mast cells in allergy and infection: versatile effector and regulatory cells in innate and adaptive immunity. Eur J Immunol 2010;40(7):1843–51.
13. Echtenacher B, Mannel DN, Hultner L. Critical protective role of mast cells in a model of acute septic peritonitis. Nature 1996;381(6577):75–7.
14. Deban L, Jaillon S, Garlanda C, et al. Pentraxins in innate immunity: lessons from PTX3. Cell Tissue Res 2011;343(1):237–49.
15. Miyake K. Endotoxin recognition molecules, Toll-like receptor 4-MD-2. Semin Immunol 2004;16(1):11–6.
16. Sharon N. Carbohydrates as recognition determinants in phagocytosis and in lectin-mediated killing of target cells. Biol Cell 1984;51(2):239–45.
17. Ledford JG, Pastva AM, Wright JR. Review: Collectins link innate and adaptive immunity in allergic airway disease. Innate Immun 2010;16(3):183–90.
18. Ricklin D, Hajishengallis G, Yang K, Lambris JD. Complement: a key system for immune surveillance and homeostasis. Nat Immunol 2010;11(9):785–97.
19. Rickert RC. Regulation of B lymphocyte activation by complement C3 and the B cell coreceptor complex. Curr Opin Immunol 2005;17(3):237–43.
20. Levy O, Jean-Jacques RM, Cywes C, et al. Critical role of the complement system in group B streptococcus-induced tumor necrosis factor alpha release. Infect Immun 2003;71(11):6344–53.
21. Kaplan AP. Enzymatic pathways in the pathogenesis of hereditary angioedema: the role of C1 inhibitor therapy. J Allergy Clin Immunol 2010;126(5):918–25.
22. Frank MM. Complement disorders and hereditary angioedema. J Allergy Clin Immunol 2010;125(2 Suppl. 2):S262–71.
23. Daha MR. Role of complement in innate immunity and infections. Crit Rev Immunol 2010;30(1):47–52.
24. Herbert AP, Deakin JA, Schmidt CQ, et al. Structure shows that a glycosaminoglycan and protein recognition site in factor H is perturbed by age-related macular degeneration-linked single nucleotide polymorphism. J Biol Chem 2007;282(26):18960–8.
25. Eisen DP. Mannose-binding lectin deficiency and respiratory tract infection. J Innate Immun 2010;2(2):114–22.
26. Cros J, Cagnard N, Woollard K, et al. Human CD14dim monocytes patrol and sense nucleic acids and viruses via TLR7 and TLR8 receptors. Immunity 2010;33(3):375–86.
27. Dale DC, Boxer L, Liles WC. The phagocytes: neutrophils and monocytes. Blood 2008;112(4):935–45.
28. Bokoch GM, Diebold B, Kim JS, Gianni D. Emerging evidence for the importance of phosphorylation in the regulation of NADPH oxidases. Antioxid Redox Signal 2009;11(10):2429–41.
29. Reeves EP, Lu H, Jacobs HL, et al. Killing activity of neutrophils is mediated through activation of proteases by K+ flux. Nature 2002;416(6878):291–7.
30. Kobayashi Y. The regulatory role of nitric oxide in proinflammatory cytokine expression during the induction and resolution of inflammation. J Leukoc Biol 2010;88(6): 1157–62.
31. Reis ESC. Harnessing dendritic cells. Semin Immunol 2011;23(1):1.
32. Bryceson YT, Chiang SC, Darmanin S, et al. Molecular mechanisms of natural killer cell activation. J Innate Immun 2011;3(3):216–26.
33. Stojanovic A, Cerwenka A. Natural killer cells and solid tumors. J Innate Immun 2011;3(4):355–64.
34. Berzins SP, Smyth MJ, Baxter AG. Presumed guilty: natural killer T cell defects and human disease. Nat Rev Immunol 2011;11(2):131–42.
35. Umetsu DT, Dekruyff RH. Natural killer T cells are important in the pathogenesis of asthma: the many pathways to asthma. J Allergy Clin Immunol 2010;125(5):975–9.
36. Levy O, Orange JS, Hibberd P, et al. Disseminated varicella infection due to the vaccine strain of varicella-zoster virus, in a patient with a novel deficiency in natural killer T cells. J Infect Dis 2003;188(7):948–53.
37. Kawai T, Akira S. Toll-like receptor and RIG-I-like receptor signaling. Ann N Y Acad Sci 2008;1143:1–20.
38. Kawai T, Akira S. The role of pattern-recognition receptors in innate immunity: update on Toll-like receptors. Nat Immunol 2010;11(5):373–84.
39. Malley R, Henneke P, Morse SC, et al. Recognition of pneumolysin by Toll-like receptor 4 confers resistance to pneumococcal infection. Proc Natl Acad Sci U S A 2003;100(4): 1966–71.
40. Vabulas RM, Wagner H, Schild H. Heat shock proteins as ligands of toll-like receptors. Curr Top Microbiol Immunol 2002;270:169–84.
41. Beutler B, Jiang Z, Georgel P, et al. Genetic analysis of host resistance: Toll-like receptor signaling and immunity at large. Annu Rev Immunol 2006;24:353–89.
42. O'Neill LA. The interleukin-1 receptor/Toll-like receptor superfamily: 10 years of progress. Immunol Rev 2008;226:10–8.
43. Kawai T, Akira S. Toll-like receptors and their crosstalk with other innate receptors in infection and immunity. Immunity 2011;34(5):637–50.
44. Tabeta K, Hoebe K, Janssen EM, et al. The Unc93b1 mutation 3d disrupts exogenous antigen presentation and signaling via Toll-like receptors 3, 7 and 9. Nat Immunol 2006;7(2):156–64.
45. Shinohara ML, Lu L, Bu J, et al. Osteopontin expression is essential for interferon-alpha production by plasmacytoid dendritic cells. Nat Immunol 2006;7(5):498–506.
46. Doyle SL, Jefferies CA, Feighery C, O'Neill LA. Signaling by Toll-like receptors 8 and 9 requires Bruton's tyrosine kinase. J Biol Chem 2007;282(51):36953–60.
47. Napolitani G, Rinaldi A, Bertoni F, et al. Selected Toll-like receptor agonist combinations synergistically trigger a T helper type 1-polarizing program in dendritic cells. Nat Immunol 2005;6(8):769–76.
48. Kasturi SP, Skountzou I, Albrecht RA, et al. Programming the magnitude and persistence of antibody responses with innate immunity. Nature 2011;470(7335):543–7.
49. Palmer CD, Mancuso CJ, Weiss JP, et al. 17(R)-Resolvin D1 differentially regulates TLR4-mediated responses of primary human macrophages to purified LPS and live E. coli. J Leukoc Biol 2011;90(3):459–70.
50. Schroder K, Tschopp J. The inflammasomes. Cell 2010;140(6):821–32.
51. Geyer M, Muller-Ladner U. Actual status of antiinterleukin-1 therapies in rheumatic diseases. Curr Opin Rheumatol 2010;22(3):246–51.
52. Sander LE, Davis MJ, Boekschoten MV, et al. Detection of prokaryotic mRNA signifies microbial viability and promotes immunity. Nature 2011;474(7351):385–9.
53. Osorio F, Reis ESC. Myeloid C-type lectin receptors in pathogen recognition and host defense. Immunity 2011;34(5):651–64.
54. Gross O, Gewies A, Finger K, et al. Card9 controls a non-TLR signalling pathway for innate anti-fungal immunity. Nature 2006;442(7103):651–6.
55. Gringhuis SI, den Dunnen J, Litjens M, et al. C-type lectin DC-SIGN modulates Toll-like receptor signaling via Raf-1 kinase-dependent acetylation of transcription factor NF-kappaB. Immunity 2007;26(5):605–16.
56. Greaves DR, Gordon S. The macrophage scavenger receptor at 30 years of age: current knowledge and future challenges. J Lipid Res 2009;50(Suppl):S282–86.
57. Picard C, von Bernuth H, Ghandil P, et al. Clinical features and outcome of patients with IRAK-4 and MyD88 deficiency. Medicine (Baltimore) 2010;89(6):403–25.
58. Levy O. Innate immunity of the newborn: basic mechanisms and clinical correlates. Nat Rev Immunol 2007;7(5):379–90.
59. Sanchez-Schmitz G, Levy O. Development of newborn and infant vaccines. Sci Transl Med 2011;3(90): 90 ps27.
60. Philbin VJ, Levy O. Developmental biology of the innate immune response: implications for neonatal and infant vaccine development. Pediatr Res 2009;65(5 Pt 2):98R–105R.

Antigen receptor genes, gene products, and co-receptors

Harry W. Schroeder, Jr., John B. Imboden, Raul M. Torres

In 1890, von Behring and Kitasato reported the existence of an agent in the blood that could neutralize diphtheria toxin. The following year, glancing references were made to "Antikörper" in studies describing the ability of the agent to discriminate between two immune substances, or bodies. The term antigen is a shortened form of "*Anti*somato*gen* + Immunkörperbildner," the substance that induces the production of an antibody. Thus, the definition of antibody and antigen represent a classic tautology.

In 1939, Tiselius and Kabat used electrophoresis to separate immunized serum into albumin, α-goblulin, β-globulin, and γ-globulin fractions. Absorption of the serum against the antigen depleted the γ-globulin fraction, yielding the terms gammaglobulin, immunoglobulin (Ig), and IgG. "Sizing" columns were then used to separate immunoglobulins into those that were "heavy" (IgM), "regular" (IgA, IgE, IgD, IgG), and "light" (light chain dimers), culminating with the discovery of the last major class of immunoglobulin, IgE, by Ishizaka and colleagues in 1966.

In 1949, Porter used papain to digest IgG molecules into two types of fragments, termed Fab and Fc. The constancy of the Fc fragment permitted its crystallization, and thus the elucidation of its sequence and structure. The variability of the Fab fragment precluded analysis until Bence-Jones myeloma proteins were identified as clonal, isolated light chains.

In 1976, Hozumi and Tonegawa demonstrated that the variable portion of κ chains was the product of the rearrangement of a variable (V) and joining (J) gene segment. In 1982, Alt and Baltimore reported that terminal deoxynucleotidyl transferase (TdT) could be used to introduce non-germline encoded sequence between rearranging V, D for diversity, and J gene segments, potentially freeing the heavy chain repertoire from germline constraints. In 1984, Weigert and colleagues determined that during affinity maturation variable domains could undergo mutation at rate of 10^{-3} per base pair, per generation. These discoveries clarified how lymphocytes could generate an astronomically diverse antigen receptor repertoire from a finite set of genes.

In 1982 Allison and colleagues raised antisera against a cell surface molecule that could uniquely identify individual T-cell clones. A year later, Kappler and a consortium of colleagues demonstrated that these surface molecules were heterodimers composed of variable and constant region domains, just like immunoglobulin. Subsequently, Davis and Mak independently cloned the β chain of the T-cell receptor (TCR). Initial confusion regarding the identity of the companion α chain led to the realization that there were two mutually exclusive forms of TCR, αβ and γδ.

Paratopes and epitopes

Immunoglobulins and T-cell receptors both belong to the eponymous immunoglobulin super-family (IgSF).[1] The study of antibodies precedes that of TCR by decades; hence much of what we know is based on knowledge first gleaned from the study of immunoglobulins.

Immunoglobulin-antigen interactions typically take place between the *paratope,* the site on the Ig at which the antigen binds, and the *epitope,* which is the site on the antigen that is bound. Thus lymphocyte antigen receptors do not recognize antigens, they recognize epitopes borne on those antigens. This makes it possible for the cell to discriminate between two closely related antigens, each of which can be viewed as a collection of epitopes. It also permits the same receptor to bind divergent antigens that share equivalent or similar epitopes, a phenomenon referred to as *cross-reactivity.*

Although both immunoglobulins and TCRs can recognize the same antigen, they do so in markedly different ways. Immunoglobulins tend to recognize intact antigens in soluble form, and thus preferentially identify surface epitopes that are often composed of conformational structures noncontiguous in the antigen's primary sequence. In contrast, TCRs recognize fragments of antigens, both surface and internal, that have been processed by a separate antigen presenting cell and then bound to an MHC class I or class II molecule (Chapters 5, 6).

The BCR and TCR antigen recognition complex

While the ability of the surface antigen receptor to recognize antigen was appreciated early on, the mechanism by which the membrane-bound receptor relayed this antigen recognition event into the cell interior was not understood since both BCR and TCR cytoplasmic domains are exceptionally short. This conundrum was solved when it was shown that BCR and TCR each associate non-covalently with signal transduction complexes: heterodimeric Igα:Igβ (also known as CD79a: CD79b, respectively) for B cells, and multimeric CD3 for T cells. Loss of function mutations in either of these complexes leads to cell death, which becomes clinically manifest as hypogammaglobulinemia in the case of B cells (Chapter 34), or severe combined immune deficiency (SCID) in the case of T cells (Chapter 35).

Immunoglobulins and TCR Structures

The Ig domain, the basic IgSF building block

Immunoglobulins consist of two heavy (H) and two light (L) chains (Fig. 4.1), where the L chain can consist of either a κ or a λ chain. T-cell receptors consist of either an αβ or a γδ heterodimer. Each component chain contains two or more IgSF domains, each of which consists of two sandwiched β pleated sheets "pinned" together by a disulfide bridge between two conserved cysteine residues.[1] Considerable variability is allowed to the amino acids that populate the external surface of the IgSF domain and the loops that link the β strands. These solvent exposed surfaces offer multiple targets for docking with other molecules.

Two types of IgSF domains, "constant" (C) and "variable" (V), are used in immunoglobulins and TCRs (Fig. 4.1). C-type domains, which are the most compact, have seven antiparallel strands distributed as three strands in the first sheet and four strands in the second. Side chains positioned to lie between the two strands tend to be nonpolar in nature, creating a hydrophobic core of considerable stability. Indeed, V domains engineered to replace the conserved cysteines with serine residues retain their ability to bind antigen. V-type domains add two additional anti-parallel strands to the first sheet, creating a five-strand–four-strand distribution. The two additional strands, which encode framework region 2 (FR2), are used to steady the interaction between

heterodimeric V domains, allowing them to create a stable antigen binding site.[2]

While each Ig and TCR chain contains only one NH2-terminal V Ig domain, the number of COOH-terminal C domains varies. Ig H chains contain between three and four C domains, and both Ig L chains and all four TCR chains contain only one C domain each. H chains with three C domains tend to include a spacer *hinge* region between the first (C_H1) and second (C_H2) domains. Each V or C domain consists of approximately 110–130 amino acids, averaging 12 000–13 000 kDa. A typical L or TCR chain will thus mass approximately 25 kDa, and a three C domain Cγ H chain with its hinge will mass approximately 55 kDa.

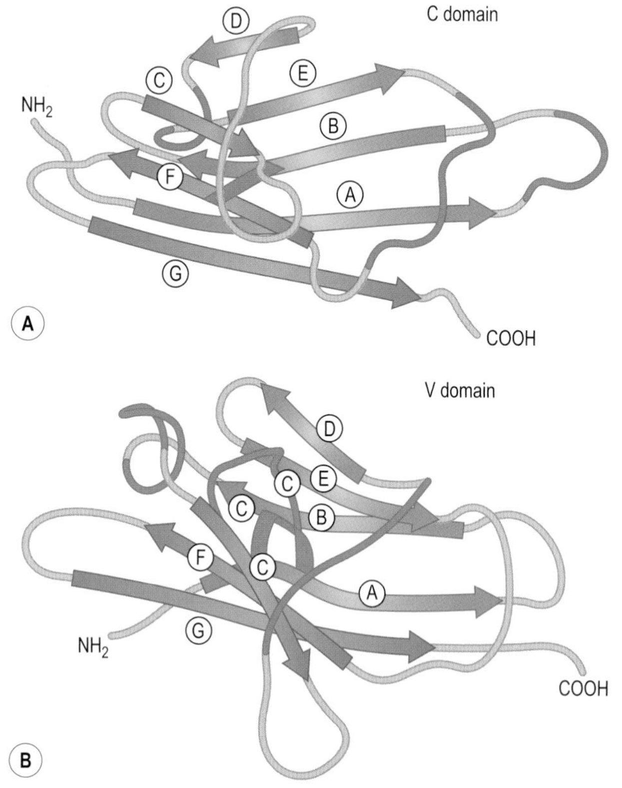

Idiotypes and isotypes

Immunization of heterologous species with monoclonal antibodies (or a restricted set of Igs) has shown that Igs and TCRs contain both common and individual antigenic determinants. Individual determinant(s), termed *idiotype(s)*, are contained within V domains. Common determinants, termed *isotypes*, are specific for the constant portion of the antibody and allow grouping of Ig's and TCRs into recognized classes, with each class defining an individual type of C domain. Determinants common to subsets of individuals within a species, yet differing between other members of that species, are termed *allotypes* and define inherited polymorphisms that result from allelic forms of the genes.[3]

The V domain

Early comparisons of the primary sequences of V domains identified three hypervariable intervals, termed complementarity determining regions or CDRs, situated between four framework regions of stable sequence (Fig. 4.2). The current definition of these regions integrates sequence diversity with three-dimensional structure.[4] The international ImMunoGeneTics information system, or IMGT, maintains an extremely useful website, http://www.imgt.org, which contains a large database of immunoglobulin and TCR sequences, as well as a multiplicity of software tools for their analysis.

Antigen recognition and the Fab

Studies of Ig structure were facilitated by the use of papain and pepsin to fragment IgG molecules. Papain digests IgG into two antigen-binding fragments (Fab) and a single crystallizable (or constant) fragment (Fc). Pepsin splits IgG into an Fc fragment and a single dimeric F(ab')$_2$ that can cross-link as well as bind antigens. The Fab contains one complete L chain in its entirety and the V and C_H1 portion of one H chain (Fig. 4.2). The Fab can be further divided into a variable fragment (Fv) composed of the V_H and V_L domains, and a constant fragment (Fb) composed of the C_L and C_H1 domains. Single Fv fragments can be genetically engineered to recapitulate the monovalent antigen binding characteristics of the original, parent antibody.[5] The extracellular domains of TCRαβ and TCRγδ correspond to Ig Fab.

Fig. 4.1 IgSF domain structures. (A) A typical compact C domain structure. The β strands are labeled A through G. The sequence at the core is conserved and nonpolar. The external surface and the β-loops are available for docking and often vary in sequence. (B) A typical V domain structure. Two additional strands, C' and C", have been added. Note the projection of the C-C' strands and loop away from the core.

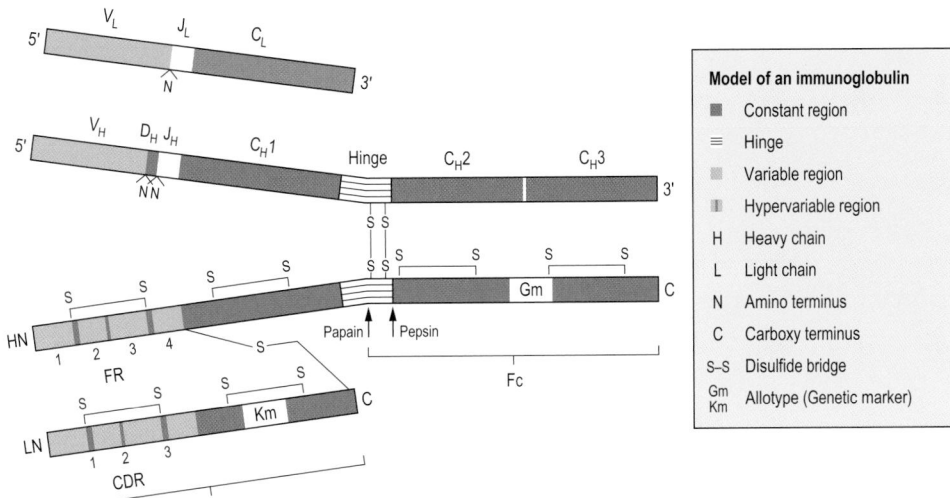

Fig. 4.2 A two-dimensional model of an IgG molecule. The top H and L chains illustrate the composition of these molecules at a nucleotide level. The bottom chains illustrate the nature of the protein sequence. See text for further details.

KEY CONCEPTS

Immunoglobulin and TCR structure

- Immunoglobulins and TCRs are heterodimeric proteins.
  - Immunoglobulins consist of two identical H and two L chains.
  - $\alpha\beta$ TCRs consist of one α and one β chain.
  - $\gamma\delta$ TCRs consist of one γ and one δ chain.
- Each Ig or TCR chain contains two or more domains with a characteristic beta barrel structure whose presence identifies a protein as a member of the immunoglobulin supergene family.
- Each Ig and TCR chain contains a V-type IgSF domain that will form one-half of the antigen binding site.
  - Each V domain contains three hypervariable intervals known as CDRs.
  - The CDRs of paired heterodimers chains are juxtaposed to form the antigen binding site.
- The C domains of Ig H chains define the immunoglobulin class or subclass.
- The two distal C IgH domains determine the effector function of the antibody.

Effector function and the Fc

The Fc portion (Fig. 4.2) encodes the effector functions of the immunoglobulin. These functions are generally inflammatory reactions that include fixation of complement, activation of complement,

and binding of antibody to Fc receptors on the surface of other cells. Each immunoglobulin class and subclass exhibits its own set of effector functions.[6] For example, the IgG C_H2 domain plays a key role in complement fixation and in binding to class-specific Fc receptors on the surface of effector cells. Both of these interactions are important in initiating the process of phagocytosis, in allowing certain subclasses to traverse the placenta, and in influencing the biologic functions of lymphocytes, platelets, and other cells.

Gm allotype system

A series of serologically defined genetic markers of the C domains of both H and L chains have been termed Gm for the gammaglobulin fraction of the serum in which they were first identified.[3] Different allelic forms have been defined for C domains of the γ_1, γ_2, γ_3, γ_4, α_2, and ε H chains and for the κ L chain. Associations between certain Gm allotypes and predisposition to develop certain diseases of immune function have been reported.

Immunoglobulin classes and subclasses

The constant domains of the H chain define the class and subclass of the antibody. Table 4.1 lists the five major classes of immunoglobulins in human and describes some of their physical and chemical features. Two of the five major H chain classes, α and γ, have

Table 4.1 Selected properties of immunoglobulin classes

	IgG	IgA	IgM	IgD	IgE
Molecular weight	160 000	170 000 or polymer	900 000	160 000	180 000
Approximate concentration in serum (mg/dL)	1000-1500	250-300	100-150	0.3-30	0.0015-0.2
Valence	2	2 (monomer)	10 (small antigen) 5 (large antigen)	2	2
Molecular formula	γ_2L_2	$(\alpha_2L_2)n$	$(\mu_2L_2)_5$	δ_2L_2	ε_2L_2
Half-life (days)	23	6	5	3	2.5
Special property	Placental passage	Secretory Ig	Primary response lymphocyte surface	Lymphocyte surface	Immediate hypersensitivity reactions

Table 4.2 Selected biologic properties of classes and subclasses of immunoglobulins

	IgG				IgA		IgM	IgD	IgE
	1	**2**	**3**	**4**	**1**	**2**			
Percentage of total (%)	65	20	10	5	90	10			
Complement fixation	++	+	++	-	-	-	++	-	-
Complement fixation (alternative)			+	+	+/-	+/-			
Placental passage	+	+	+	+	-	-	-	-	-
Fixing to mast cells or basophils	-	-	-	-	-	-	-	-	+
Binding to:									
Lymphocytes	+	+	+	+	-	-	+	-	-
Macrophages	+	+/-	+	+/-	-	-	-	-	-
Neutrophils	+	+	+	+	+	+	-	-	-
Platelets	+	+	+	+	-	-	-	-	-
Reaction with Staph. Protein A	+	+	-	+	-	-	-	-	-
Half-life (days)	23	23	8-9	23	6	6	5	3	2.5
Synthesis mg/kg/day	25	?	3.5	?	24	?	7	0.4	0.02

undergone duplication.[10] IgG1, IgG2, IgG3, and IgG4 all have the same basic structural design and differ only in the primary sequence of their constant regions and in the location of their interchain disulfide bonds. The H chain in each of these subclasses is referred to as γ_1, γ_2, etc. IgA consists of the two subclasses, α_1 and α_2. Table 4.2 compares the four subclasses of IgG, the two of IgA, and the classes of IgM, IgD, and IgE from the standpoint of their biologic functions. In human, two L chain classes exist, κ and λ. No specific effector function has been identified for either L chain class.

IgM

IgM exists in monomeric, pentameric, and hexameric forms. The 8 S monomeric 180 000-dalton IgM has the molecular formula $\mu_2 L_2$. It is a minor fraction in serum, but in its transmembrane form IgM plays a key role in B-cell development and function as the antigen recognition portion of the B-cell antigen receptor. The major form in serum is the 19 S, 900 000-dalton pentameric IgM, which contains five subunits [$(\mu_2 L_2)_5$] linked together by disulfide-bridges, and by one molecule of an additional polypeptide chain, the J chain, which joins two of the subunits by a disulfide bridge.[7]

IgM is the predominant immunoglobulin produced during the primary immune response. Occasionally, particularly in the case of carbohydrate Ags such as isohemagglutinins, it will remain the major or sole antibody class. IgM differs from most other immunoglobulins in having an extra C_H domain in place of a hinge.

IgM avidly fixes complement. This property is focused in C_H3, the homologue of IgG C_H2.[8] Although the valence of each $\mu_2 L_2$ subunit is 2, when binding to large protein antigens five of the 10 antigen binding sites in pentameric IgM appear blocked due to steric hindrance. As a consequence, the valence for large antigens is five.

IgG

IgG, the major immunoglobulin class, accounts for the bulk of serum antibody activity in response to most protein antigens. The four IgG subclasses are numbered in relation to their serum levels relative to each other, with IgG$_1$ predominant and IgG$_4$ the least common. IgG$_1$ and IgG$_3$ fix complement and bind phagocyte Fcγ receptors well, whereas IgG$_2$ fixes complement but binds Fcγ receptors more poorly. IgG$_4$ does not fix complement effectively in the native state, but has been reported to do so after proteolytic cleavage.[9] IgG$_1$ and IgG$_3$ are most frequently elicited by viral antigens,[10] IgG$_2$ by carbohydrates,[11] and IgG$_4$ by helminthic parasites.[12]

IgG4 has become a subject of intense study due to the recognition that the disulfide bonds of its hinge are easily reduced, thus allowing the heavy chains to separate and randomly re-associate to produce a mixed population of IgG$_4$ molecules with randomized heavy-chain and light-chain pairs.[13] This impairs the ability of IgG$_4$ to form immune complexes and thus has an anti-inflammatory effect, facilitating immunotherapy for allergic diseases (allergy shots). Overproduction of IgG$_4$ is seen in a disparate group of inflammatory diseases (including sclerosing forms of sialadenitis, pancreatitis, and cholangitis, as well as aortitis, thyroiditis, and retroperitoneal fibrosis). Together, these are referred to as IgG$_4$-related systemic disease (IgG$_4$-RSD). The role of IgG$_4$ in these diseases is unclear, but it appears to represent an important biomarker.

IgA

Although IgA generally exists in a monomeric form ($\alpha_2 L_2$) in the serum, it can interact with J chain to form a polymer ($\alpha_2 L_2)_{2/3}$-J. Second in concentration to IgG in serum, IgA functions as the predominant form of immunoglobulin in mucosal secretions.[14]

Secretory IgA is largely synthesized by plasma cells located in, or originating from, mucosal tissues. In the secretions, the molecule usually exists in an alternative polymeric form with two subunits in association with the 70 000-dalton secretory component ($\alpha_2 L_2)_2$-SC. SC is synthesized by the epithelial cells that line the lumen of the gut. The complete function of SC remains uncertain, but it appears to serve as a receptor for IgA and may play a role in attracting IgA-bearing lymphocytes to the gut and other organs of secretion. It also appears to render the secretory IgA complex more resistant to proteolytic digestion.

IgE

IgE is largely found in extravascular spaces. Its plasma turnover is rapid, with a half-life of about 2 days. IgE antibodies help protect the host from parasitic infections (Chapter 29). However, in Westernized, affluent societies, IgE is primarily associated with allergy. Through their interaction with Fcε receptors on mast cells and basophils, IgE antibodies, in the presence of antigens, induce the release of histamine and various other vasoactive substances, which are responsible for clinical manifestations of various allergic states.[15]

IgD

Although the H chain of IgD can undergo alternative splicing to a secretory form, IgD serum antibodies in human are uncommon and are absent in the serum of mice and primates. Instead, IgD typically is found in association with IgM on the surface of mature lymphocytes. The appearance of IgD is associated with the transition of a B lymphocyte from a cell that can be tolerized to antigen to a cell that will respond to antigen with the production of antibody (Chapter 7).

TCR $\alpha\beta$ and $\gamma\delta$

As members of the IgSF, TCR α, β γ, and δ chains share a number of structural similarities with immunoglobulin. Each chain contains a leader peptide, and extracellular, transmembrane, and intracytoplasmic components. The extracellular component can be divided into three domains: A polymorphic V domain encoded by VJ (α and γ chains) or VDJ (β and δ chains) gene segments, a C domain, and a hinge region.[16] The hinge region typically contains an extra cysteine (none in γ chains encoded by Cγ2) that forms a disulfide bond with the other partner of the heterodimer. The transmembrane domains all include a lysine and some contain an arginine residue that facilitate the association of the TCR heterodimer with components of the CD3 signal transduction complex, each of which has a matching negatively charged residue in their own transmembrane portions (see below). The intracytoplasmic components are tiny and play a minimal role in signal transduction.

TCR $\alpha\beta$

The TCR α and β chains are glycoproteins with molecular weights that vary from 42 to 45 kDa, depending upon the primary amino acid sequence and the degree of glycosylation. Deglycosylated forms have a molecular mass of 30 to 32 kDa. These chains share a number of invariant residues in common with immunoglobulin heavy and light chains, in particular residues that are thought to be important for interactions between heavy and light chains. The structures of several partial or full length TCRs have been solved by X-ray crystallography (Fig. 4.3).[17] In general, the structure of the TCR $\alpha\beta$ heterodimer is similar, but not identical, to that of an Ig Fab fragment.

TCR $\gamma\delta$

The TCR γ and δ chains are glycoproteins with a more complex molecular size pattern than α and β chains. TCRs that use the Cγ1 gene segment, which contains a cysteine-encoding exon are disulfide-linked (MW 36–42 kDa). TCRs that use Cγ2 exist in two non-disulfide-linked forms, one of 40–44 kDa and one of 55 kDa.[18,19] The differences in molecular size are due to variability of both N-linked glycosylation and primary amino acid sequence. The 55-kDa form uses a Cγ2 allele that contains three (rather than two) exons encoding the connecting piece, as well as more N-linked carbohydrate. The functional implication of three different TCR γ chain isoforms, if any, is unknown. The TCR δ chain is more straightforward, being 40–43 kDa in size

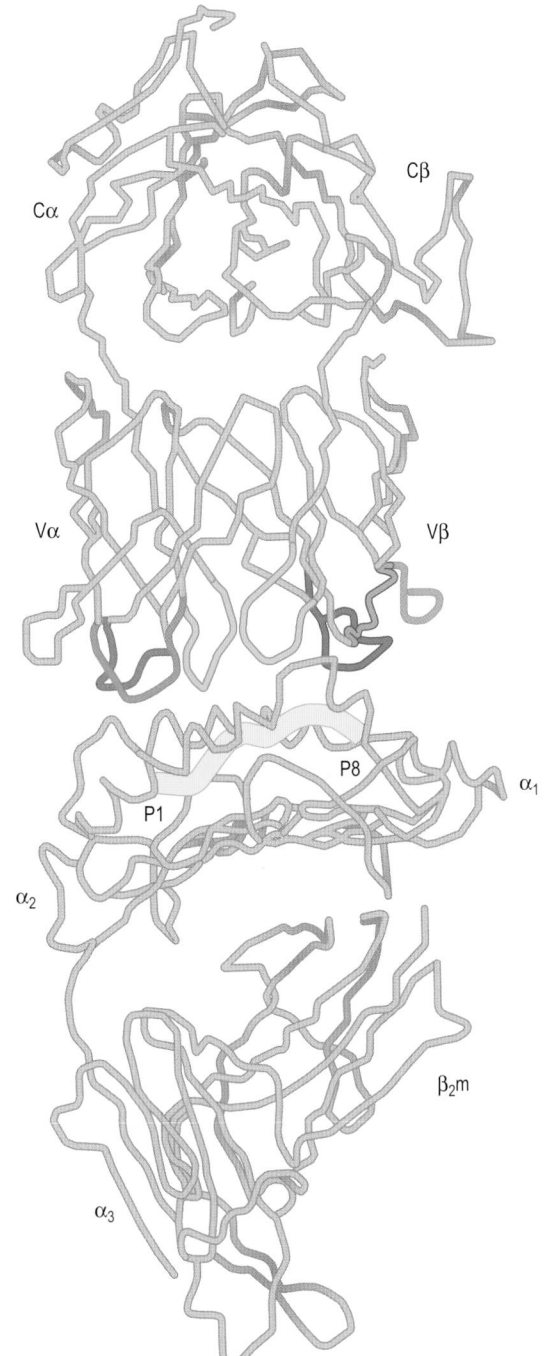

Fig. 4.3 Backbone representation of murine $\alpha\beta$ TCR bound to murine MHC class I and an octamer peptide. The TCR is above. The Vα CDR1 and CDR2 are magenta, Vβ CDR1 and CDR2 are blue, both CDR3s are green, and the Vβ HV4 is orange. β2M refers to β_2-microglobulin. The peptide is in yellow, and the NH$_2$-terminal and COOH-terminal residues are designated P1 and P8.
Reproduced with permission from Garcia et al.[23]

and containing two sites of N-linked glycosylation. The overall architecture of the $\gamma\delta$ TCR closely resembles that of $\alpha\beta$ TCRs and antibodies, although the angle between the V and C domains, known as the elbow angle, appears more acute.

Ligand recognition

Although TCR $\alpha\beta$ T cells primarily recognize peptide-MHC complexes (pMHC) (Fig. 4.3; Chapters 5, 6), other types of ligands exist. For example, some $\alpha\beta$ TCRs can bind nonpeptidic antigens (atypical antigens) that are bound to "non-classic" MHC Class Ib molecules. Many γδ T cells recognize atypical antigens that may or may not be associated with an antigen-presenting molecule, although some can bind peptides. Finally, many αβ TCRs bind superantigens (SAg) in a predominantly Vβ-dependent fashion (Chapter 6).

Binding to pMHC

TCRs recognize peptide antigens bound to the binding groove of MHC-encoded glycoproteins (Fig. 4.3). TCR recognition of pMHC requires a trimolecular complex in which all the components (antigen, MHC, and TCR) contact one another.[20-23] Thus, recognition is highly influenced by polymorphisms in the MHC molecule (Chapter 5). As in the case of Ig, TCR CDR1 and CDR2 are encoded in the germline V regions, whereas CDR3 is formed at the junction of the V gene with a J gene segment (TCR α and γ) or D and J gene segments (TCR β and δ chains).[24] Vβ also has a fourth region of variability near the other CDRs, hypervariable region 4 (HV4) or CDR4, which can participate in superantigen binding.

The co-crystallization of different combinations of soluble TCR αβ interacting with MHC class I bound to antigen peptide (pMHC) has made it possible to directly address the manner in which antigen recognition occurs (Fig. 4.3). The TCR αβ combining site is relatively flat, allowing it to interact with a rather broad surface at the point of contact with pMHC.

The TCR footprint on the pMHC complex tends to occur in a diagonal across the MHC antigen-binding groove, with TCR Vα positioned over the MHC α$_2$ helix and TCR Vβ overlying the MHC α$_1$ helix. This geometry would permit consistent access of the CD8 co-receptors to the MHC class I molecule. The CDR1 and CDR2 loops, which are entirely encoded by germline sequence, tend to interact more with the MHC molecule; whereas the CDR3 loops, which are composed of both germline and somatic (N region) sequence, appear to dominate the interaction with MHC bound peptide.

The binding of TCR to pMHC appears to be driven by enthalpy. That is, binding increases the stability of the CDR loops, especially CDR3. These results have led to the suggestion that initial binding focuses on the interaction between CDRs 1 and 2 and the MHC. After this initial recognition, the CDR3's change their shape to maximize the area of contact. Conformational flexibility, or "induced fit," would allow TCRs to rapidly sample many similar pMHC complexes, stopping only when their CDR3s are able to stabilize the interaction.

TCR binding affinity

The affinity with which the TCR ultimately binds its ligand is a critical determinant of T-cell activation. It is, however, only one factor in determining the overall *avidity* of the interaction, since other cell surface molecules of the T cell (e.g., CD4, CD8, CD2 and various integrins) bind to cell surface molecules on the antigen-bearing cell to stabilize cell–cell TCR–ligand interactions. Furthermore, since both the TCR and the pMHC ligand are surface membrane proteins, each T cell can provide multiple TCRs in the same plane that can bind multiple pMHC molecules on the surface of the antigen presenting cell. This makes binding of TCR to pMHC functionally multivalent, enhancing the apparent affinity of the interaction.

Atypical antigens

Some αβ T cells can recognize lipid antigens when they are complexed with members of the CD1 family.[25] The interaction of TCR αβ with CD1 resembles that of TCR αβ with MHC class I. Allelic polymorphism in CD1 is limited, which theoretically would restrict the range of lipid antigens that can be bound.

Rather than binding to a single groove on the MHC, lipids attach themselves to one of several hydrophobic pockets that can be found on the surface of CD1. Pocket volume can range from 1300 to 2200 Å^3. The number and length of the pockets differ between the various CD1 isoforms. For example, CD1b has three pockets that share a common portal of entry, as well as a fourth pocket that connects two of the three pockets to each other. This connecting pocket permits the insertion of lipids with a long alkyl chain, such as mycobacterial mycolic acid.

Antigen recognition by γδ TCRs resembles recognition of intact antigens by antibodies more closely than recognition of pMHC by αβ TCR.[26] γδ TCRs can recognize protein antigens, such as nonclassical MHC molecules and viral glycoproteins, as well as small, phosphate- or amine-containing compounds, such as pyrophosphomonoesters from mycobacteria and alkylamines.

Binding to non-peptide antigens plays an important role in the biology of γδ T cells. About 5% of peripheral blood T cells bear γδ TCRs, and most of these are encoded by Vγ9 JγP and Vδ2$^+$ gene segments. (In an alternative nomenclature, Vγ9 is known as Vγ2 and JγP as Jγ1.2. See the IMGT database at http://www.imgt.org.) These Vγ9 JγPVδ2$^+$ TCRs recognize non-peptide pyrophosphate- or amine-containing antigens, such as pyrophosphomonoesters from mycobacteria or isobutylamine from various sources.[26] Other common naturally-occurring small phosphorylated metabolites that stimulate γδ T cells include 2,3-diphosphoglyceric acid, glycerol-3-phosphoric acid, xylose-1-phosphate, and ribose-1-phosphate. In addition to mycobacteria, Vγ9 JγPVδ2$^+$ T-cell populations are seen to expand in response to listeriosis, ehrlichiosis, leishmaniasis, brucellosis, salmonellosis, mumps meningitis, malaria, and toxoplasmosis.

Recent work suggests that γδ T cells are easily activated by conserved stress-induced ligands, enabling them to rapidly produce cytokines that regulate pathogen clearance, inflammation and tissue homeostasis in response to tissue stress.[27]

Superantigens

Superantigens (SAgs) are a special class of TCR ligands that have the ability to activate large fractions (5–20%) of the T-cell population. Activation requires simultaneous interaction between the SAg, the TCR Vβ domain, and a major histocompatibility complex class II molecule on the surface of an antigen-presenting cell.[28]

Unlike conventional antigens, SAgs do not require processing to allow them to bind class II molecules or activate T cells. Instead of binding to the peptide antigen binding groove, SAgs interact with polymorphic residues on the periphery of the class II molecule. And, instead of binding to TCR β CDR3 residues, SAg interact with polymorphic residues in CDR1, CDR2, and HV4. Soluble TCR β chains can also bind the appropriate SAg in the absence of a TCR α chain. As a consequence, although SAg link the TCR to the MHC, the T-cell responses are not "MHC-restricted" in the conventional sense, since a T cell with the appropriate Vβ will respond to a SAg bound to a variety of polymorphic class II molecules.

Immunoglobulin gene organization

The component chains of immunoglobulins and T-cell receptors are each encoded by a separate multigene family.[29,30] The paradox of variability in the V region in conjunction with a nearly invariable constant region was resolved when it was shown that immunoglobulin V and C domains are encoded by independent elements, or gene segments, within each gene family. That is, more than one gene element is used to encode a single polypeptide chain. For example, while κ constant domains are encoded by a single Cκ exon in the κ locus on chromosome 2, κ variable domains represent the joined product of Vκ and Jκ gene segments (Fig. 4.4).

V_L gene segments typically contain their own promoter, a leader exon, an intervening intron of ~100 nucleotides, an exon that encodes the first three framework regions (FR 1, 2, and 3), the first two complementarity determining regions in their entirety, the amino terminal portion of CDR3, and a recombination signal sequence. A J_L (J for joining) gene segment begins with its own recombination signal, the remaining portion of CDR 3, and the complete FR 4 (Fig. 4.2).

(Use of the same abbreviation–V–for both the complete variable domain of an immunoglobulin peptide chain and for the gene segment that encodes only a portion of that same variable domain is the result of historic precedent. It is unfortunate that one must depend on the context of the surrounding text in order to determine which V region of the antibody is being discussed. The same holds true for the use of J to represent both the J gene segment and the J joining protein.)

The creation of a V domain is directed by the recombination signal sequences (RSS) that flank the rearranging gene segments.[31] Each RSS contains a strongly conserved seven base-pair, or heptamer, sequence (e.g., CACAGTG) that is separated from a less well-conserved nine base-pair, or nonamer, sequence (e.g., ACAAAACCC) by either a 12- or 23-base-pair (bp) spacer. For example, Vκ gene segments have a 12-bp spacer and Jκ elements have a 23-bp spacer. These spacers place the heptamer and nonamer sequences on the same side of the

Fig. 4.4 Rearrangement events in the human κ locus.
V = variable region; J = joining region; C = constant region of the κ light chain. See text for further description.
From Garcia KC, Degano M, Stanfield RL, et al. An alphabeta T cell receptor structure at 2.5 A and its orientation in the TCR-MHC complex. Science. 1996;274(5285):209-19.

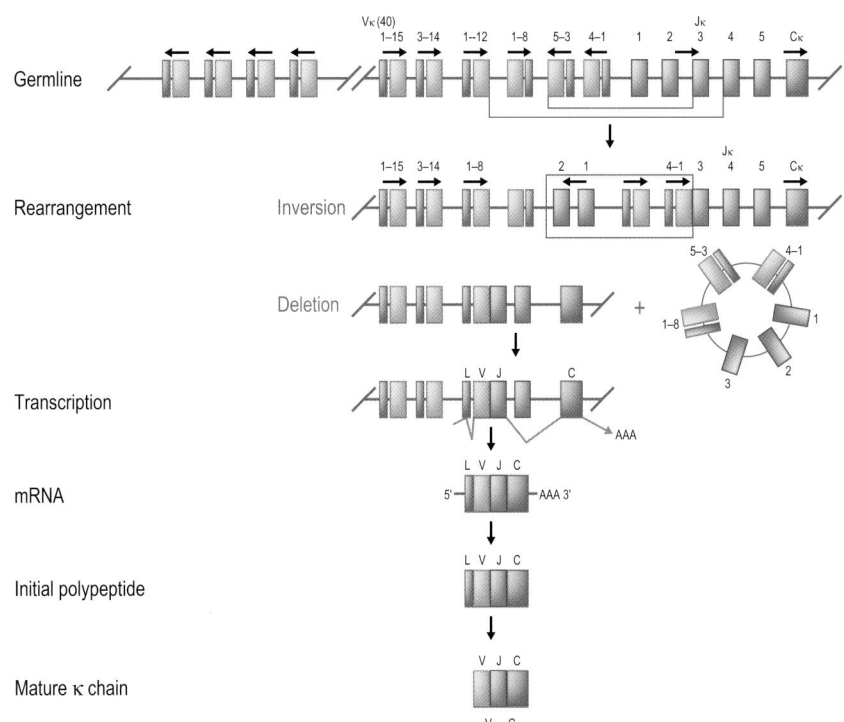

DNA molecule, separated by either one or two turns of the DNA helix. A one-turn recombination signal sequence (12-bp spacer) will preferentially recognize a two-turn signal sequence (23-bp spacer). This helps prevent wasteful V-V or J-J rearrangements.

Initiation of the V(D)J recombination reaction requires recombination activating genes 1 and 2 (*RAG1* and *RAG2*). These genes are expressed only in developing lymphocytes.[31] The gene products, RAG-1 and RAG-2, act by precisely introducing a DNA double-strand break (DSB) between the terminus of the rearranging gene segment and its adjacent recombination signal sequence (Fig. 4.5). These breaks are then repaired by ubiquitously expressed components of a DNA repair process that is known as nonhomologous end-joining (NHEJ). Lack-of-function mutations in NHEJ proteins yields susceptibility to DNA damage in all cells of the body.

The NHEJ process creates precise joins between the RSS ends, and imprecise joins of the coding ends. Terminal deoxynucleotidyl transferase (TdT), which is expressed only in lymphocytes, adds non-germline encoded nucleotides (N-nucleotides) to the coding ends of the recombination product.

Lymphoid-specific expression of RAG-1 and RAG-2 limits V(D)J recombination to B and T lymphocytes. However, to ensure that TCR genes are rearranged to completion only in T cells, and immunoglobulin genes are rearranged to completion only in

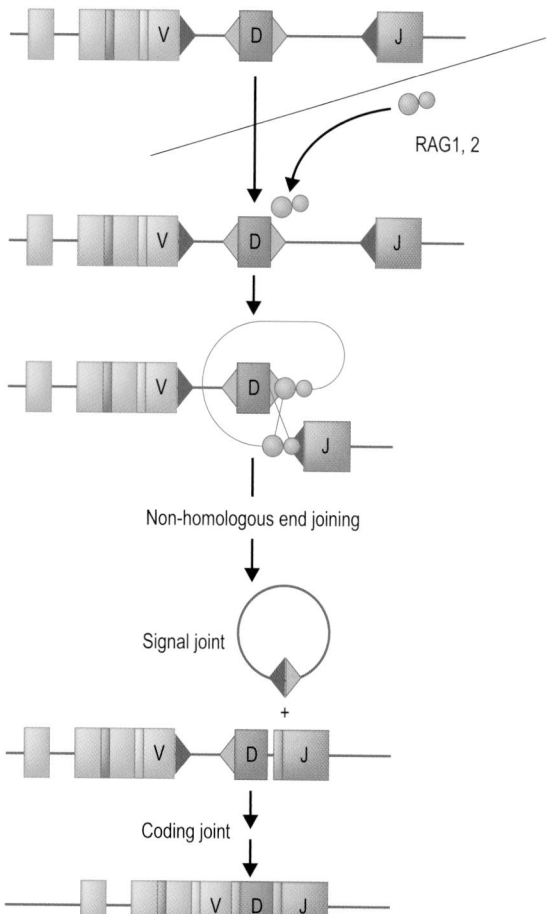

Non-homologous end joining

Signal joint

Coding joint

Fig. 4.5 VDJ Recombination. Lymphoid specific RAG-1 and RAG-2 bind to the recombination signal sequences (RSS) flanking V, D, or J gene segments, juxtapose the sequences, and introduce precise cuts adjacent to the RSS. Components of the non-homologous end joining repair pathway subsequently unite the cut RSS to form a signal joint, and the coding sequences of the rearranging gene segments to form a coding joint.

B cells. V(D)J recombination is further regulated by limiting the accessibility of the appropriate gene segments to the specific lineage as well as to the specific stage of development. For example, H chain genes are typically assembled before L chain genes.

The RAG-1 and RAG-2 recombinases cooperatively associate with 12- and 23-bp RSSs and their flanking coding gene segments to form a synaptic complex. Typically, the initial event will be recognition of the nonamer sequence of a 12-bp spacer RSS by RAG-1. RAG-1 binding to the heptamer provides specificity. RAG-2 does not bind DNA independently, but does make contact with the heptamer when in a synaptic complex with RAG-1. Binding of a second RAG-1 and RAG-2 complex to the 23-bp, two-turn RSS permits the interaction of the two synaptic complexes to form what is known as a paired complex. Creation of this paired complex is facilitated by the actions of the DNA-bending proteins HMG1 and HMG2.

After paired complex assembly, the RAG proteins single-strand cut the DNA at the heptamer sequence. The 3′ OH of the coding sequence ligates to 5′ phosphate and creates a hairpin loop. The clean cut ends of the signal sequences enable formation of precise signal joints. However, the hairpin junction created at the coding ends must be resolved by re-nicking the DNA, usually within four to five nucleotides from the end of the hairpin. This forms a 3′ overhang that is amenable to further diversification. It can be filled in via DNA polymerases, nibbled back, or serve as a substrate for TdT-catalyzed N-addition. DNA polymerase μ, which shares homology with TdT, appears to play a role in maintaining the integrity of the terminus of the coding sequence.

The cut ends of the coding sequence are then repaired by the non-homologous end joining proteins. NHEJ proteins involved in V(D)J recombination include Ku70, Ku80, DNA-PKcs, Artemis, XRCC4, XLF (Cernunnos), and ligase 4. Deficiency of any one of these proteins creates sensitivity to DNA breakage and can lead to a SCID phenotype (Chapter 35).

Ku70 and Ku80 form a heterodimer (Ku) that directly associates with DNA double-strand breaks to protect the DNA ends from degradation, permit juxtaposition of the ends to facilitate coding end ligation, and help recruit other members of the repair complex. The DNA protein kinase catalytic subunit (DNA-PKcs) phosphorylates Artemis, inducing an endonuclease activity that plays a role in the opening of the coding joint hairpin. Thus absence of DNA-PKcs or Artemis inhibits proper coding joint formation. Signal joint formation is normal in Artemis deficiency, but it is impaired in the absence of DNA-PKcs. This suggests an additional, as yet undefined, role for DNA-PKcs. Finally, XRCC4, XLF, and ligase 4 help rejoin the ends of the broken DNA.

Depending on the transcriptional orientation of the rearranging gene segments, recombination can result in either inversion or deletion of the intervening DNA (Fig. 4.3). The products of inversion remain in the DNA of the cell, whereas deletion leads to the loss of the intervening DNA. The increased proximity of the V promoter to the C domain enhancers promotes the subsequent transcription of the Ig gene product.

The κ locus

The κ locus is located on chromosome 2p11.2. It contains 5 Jκ and 75 Vκ gene segments upstream of Cκ (Fig. 4.6). The Vκ gene segments can be grouped into six different families of varying size.[32] Each family is comprised of gene segments that share extensive sequence and structural similarity.[33]

One-third of the Vκ gene segments contain frameshift mutations or stop codons that preclude them from forming functional protein, and of the remaining sequences less than 30 of the Vκ gene

Fig. 4.6 Chromosomal organization of the Ig H, κ, and λ gene clusters. The typical numbers of functional gene segments are shown. The κ gene cluster includes a κ deleting element that can rearrange to sequences upstream of Cκ in cells that express λ chains, reducing the likelihood of dual κ and λ light chain expression. These maps are not drawn to scale.

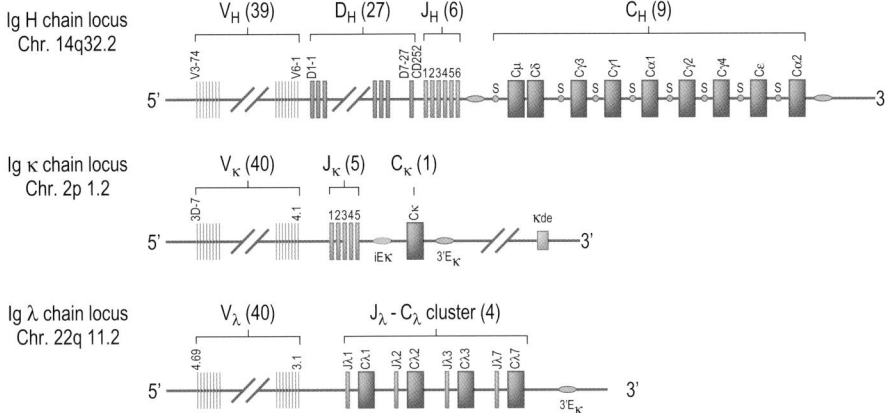

segments have actually been found in functional immunoglobulins. Each of these active Vκ gene segments has the potential to rearrange to any one of the 5 Jκ elements, generating a potential repertoire of more than 140 distinct VJ combinations. Even more diversity is created at the site of gene segment joining. The terminus of each rearranging gene segment can undergo a loss of 1 to 5 nucleotides during the recombination process. In human, but not mouse, N-addition can either replace some or all of the lost nucleotides or can be inserted in addition to the original germline sequence.[34] Each codon created by N-addition increases the potential diversity of the repertoire 20-fold. Thus, the initial diversification of the κ repertoire is focused at the VJ junction that defines CDR-L3.

The λ locus

The λ locus, on chromosome 22q11.2, contains four functional Cλ exons, each of which is associated with its own Jλ (Fig. 4.6). The Vλ genes are arranged in three distinct clusters, each containing members of different Vλ families.[35] Depending on the individual haplotype, there are approximately 30–36 potentially functional Vλ gene segments and an equal number of pseudogenes.

In addition to normal κ and λ peptides, H chains can also form a complex with unconventional λ light chains, known as surrogate or pseudo light chains (ΨLC). The genes encoding the ΨLC proteins, λ14.1 (λ5) and V_{preB}, are located within the λ light chain locus on chromosome 22 and are restricted in expression to discreet B-cell developmental stages.[36] Together, these two genes create a product with considerable homology to conventional λ light chains. The λ14.1 gene contains Jλ and Cλ-like sequences and the V_{preB} gene includes a Vλ-like sequence. A critical difference between these unconventional ΨLC genes and other L chains is that 14.1 and V_{preB} gene rearrangement is not required for ΨLC expression.

The H chain locus

The H chain locus, on chromosome 14q32.33, is considerably more complex than the κ and λ loci. There are ~80 V_H gene segments near the telomere of the long arm of chromosome 14.[37] Of these, approximately 39 are functional and can be grouped into seven different families of related gene segments. Adjacent to the most centromeric V_H, V6-1, are 27 D_H (D for diversity) gene segments (Fig. 4.6) and 6 J_H gene segments. Each V_H and J_H gene segment is associated with a two-turn recombination signal sequence, which prevents direct V → J joining. A pair of one-turn recombination signal sequences flanks each D_H. Recombination begins with the joining of a D_H to a J_H gene segment, followed by the joining of a

V_H element to the amino terminal end of the DJ intermediate. The V_H gene segment contains FR1, -2, and -3, CDR1 and -2, and the amino terminal portion of CDR3; the D_H gene segment forms the middle of CDR3; and the J_H element contains the carboxy terminus of CDR3 and FR4 in its entirety (Fig. 4.1). Random assortment of one of ~50 active V_H and one of 27 D_H with one of the 6 J_H gene segments can generate up to 10^4 different VDJ combinations (Fig. 4.7).

Although combinatorial joining of individual V, D, and J gene segments maximizes germline-encoded diversity, the major source of variation in the pre-immune repertoire is focused on the CDR-H3 interval which is created by VDJ joining (Fig. 4.7). First, D_H gene segments can rearrange by either inversion or deletion, and thus have the potential to be read backwards as well as forwards. Each D_H can be spliced and translated in each of the three potential reading frames. Thus, each D_H gene segment has the potential to encode six different peptide fragments. Second, the terminus of each rearranging gene segment can undergo a loss of one or more nucleotides during the recombination process. Third, the rearrangement process proceeds through a step that creates a hairpin ligation between the 5′ and 3′ termini of the rearranging gene segment. Nicking to resolve the hairpin structure leaves a 3′ overhang that creates a palindromic extension, termed a P junction. Fourth, non-germline-encoded nucleotides (N regions) can be used to replace or add to the original germline sequence. Every codon that is added by N-region addition increases the potential diversity of the repertoire 20-fold. N regions can be inserted both between the V and the D, and between the D and the J. Together, the imprecision of the joining process and variation in the extent of N addition permits generation of CDR-H3's of varying length and structure. As a result, more than 10^{10} different H chain VDJ junctions, or CDR-H3's, can be generated at the time of gene segment rearrangement. Together, somatic variation in CDR3, combinatorial rearrangement of individual gene segments, and combinatorial association between different L and H chains yields a potential pre-immune antibody repertoire of greater than 10^{16} different immunoglobulins.

Class switch recombination (CSR)

Located downstream of the VDJ loci are nine functional C_H gene segments (Fig. 4.7). Each C_H contains a series of exons, each encoding a separate domain, hinge, or terminus. All C_H genes can undergo alternative splicing to generate two different types of carboxy termini: either a membrane terminus that anchors immunoglobulin on the B lymphocyte surface, or a secreted terminus that occurs in the soluble form of the immunoglobulin. With the exception of $C_H1δ$, each C_H1 constant region is preceded by both an exon that cannot be translated (an I exon) and a region of

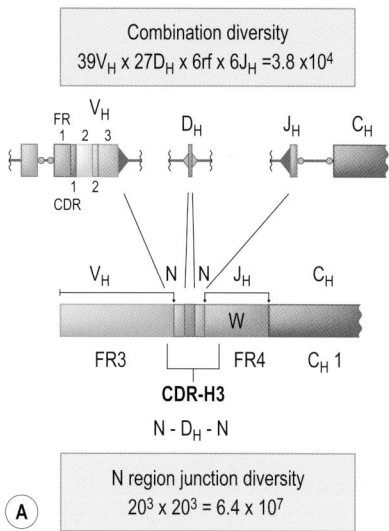

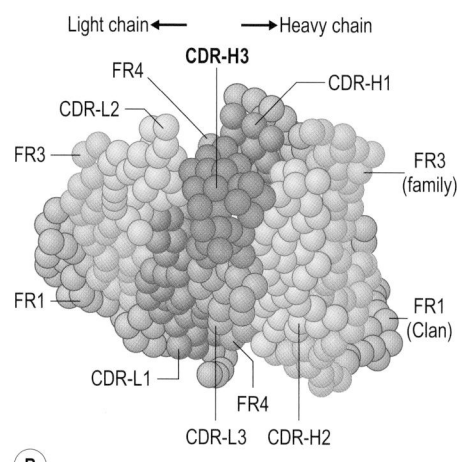

Fig. 4.7 The antigen binding site is the product of a nested gradient of diversity. (A) VDJ rearrangement yields 3.8 thousand different combinations. The CDR-H3 sequence contains both germline V, D, and J sequence and nongermline N nucleotides. The addition of nine N nucleotides on either side of the D gene segment yields 64 million different combinations. (B) The antigen binding site is created by the juxtaposition of the three complementarity determining regions (CDRs) of the H chain and the three CDRs of the light chain. The view is looking into the binding site as an antigen would see the CDRs. The V_H domain is on the right side. The central location of CDR-H3, which due to N addition is the focus for repertoire diversity, is readily apparent.

repetitive DNA termed the switch (S). Through recombination between the Cμ switch region and one of the switch regions of the seven other H chain constant regions (a process termed *class switching* or *class switch recombination (CSR)*), the same VDJ heavy chain variable domain can be juxtaposed to any of the H chain classes (Fig. 4.8).[38] Thus, the system can tailor both the receptor and the effector ends of the antibody molecule to meet a specific need.

Somatic hypermutation (SHM)

A final mechanism of immunoglobulin diversity is engaged only after exposure to antigen (39). With T-cell help, the variable domain genes of germinal center lymphocytes undergo *somatic hypermutation* (SHM) at a rate of up to 10^{-3} changes per base-pair per cell cycle. SHM is correlated with transcription of the locus and current studies suggest that at least two separate mechanisms are involved. The first mechanism targets mutation hot spots with the RGYW (purine/G/pyrimidine/A) motif and

the second mechanism incorporates an error-prone DNA synthesis that can lead to a nucleotide mismatch between the original template and the mutated DNA strand. SHM allows affinity maturation of the antibody repertoire in response to repeated immunization or exposure to antigen as B cells bearing receptors that have mutated to higher affinity for the cognate antigenic epitope are preferentially stimulated to proliferate, especially under conditions of limiting antigen concentration.

Activation-induced cytidine deaminase (AID)

AID plays a key role in both CSR and SHM.[39] AID is a single-strand DNA (ssDNA) cytidine deaminase that can be expressed in activated germinal center B cells. Transcription of an immunoglobulin V domain or of the switch region upstream of the C_H1 domain opens the DNA helix to generate ssDNA that can then be deaminated by AID to form mismatched dU/dG DNA base pairs. The base excision repair protein uracil DNA glycosylase (UNG) removes the mismatched dU base, creating an abasic site. Differential repair of this lesion leads to either SHM or CSR. The mismatch repair (MMR) proteins MSH2 and MSH6 can also bind and process the dU:dG mismatch. Deficiencies of AID, UNG underlie some forms of the hyper-IgM syndrome (Chapter 34).

Diversity and constraints on immunoglobulin sequence

In theory, combinatorial rearrangement of V(D)J gene segments, combinatorial association of H and L chains, flexibility in the site of gene segment joining, *N*-region addition, P junctions, hypermutation, and class switching can create an antibody repertoire the diversity of which is limited only by the total number of B cells in circulation at any one time. In practice, constraints and biases on both the structure and sequence of the antibody repertoire are apparent.

The representation of individual V gene elements is nonrandom. Among Vκ and V_H elements, half of the potentially functional V gene elements contribute minimally to the expressed repertoire. Among Vλ elements these restrictions are even greater, with three gene segments contributing to half of the expressed repertoire.

Particular patterns of amino acid composition in the sequences of the V domains create predictable canonical structures for several

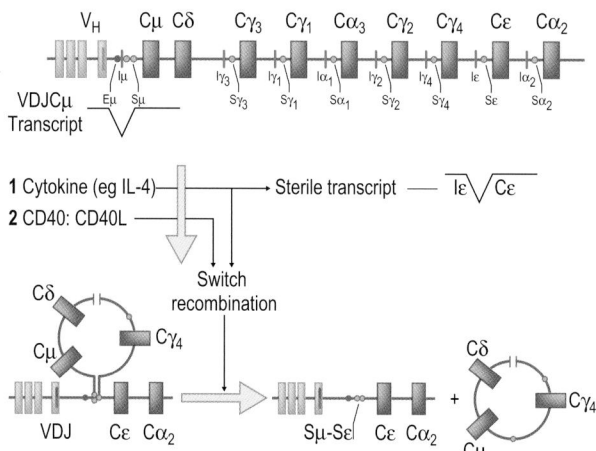

Fig. 4.8 Immunoglobulin H chain class switching. The molecular events involved in switching from expression of one class of immunoglobulin to another are depicted. At the top is the gene organization during μ chain synthesis. At the bottom a class switch recombination event has resulted in the deletion of the intervening DNA. Exposure to the appropriate cytokine or T-cell:B-cell interaction through the CD40: CD40L pathway results in activation of the I exon that yields a sterile epsilon transcript (Iε-Cε) (Chapter 7). The CD40:CD40L interaction is necessary for the subsequent replacement of Cμ by another constant gene (in this case, Cε). The S loci indicate switch-specific recombination signals.

of the hypervariable regions. In κ chains, CDR2 is found in a single canonical structure, whereas four structures are possible for CDR1.[40] In the H chain, most germline CDR1 and CDR2 elements encode one of three or one of five distinct canonical structures, respectively.[41] Preservation of these key amino acids during affinity maturation tends to maintain the canonical structure of CDR1 and CDR2 even while they are undergoing somatic hypermutation.[42]

The enhanced sequence diversity of the CDR3 region is mirrored by its structural diversity. Few canonical structures have been defined for the H chain CDR3, and even in κ chains 30% of the L chain CDR3 can be quite variable. However, at the sequence level there is a preference for tyrosine and glycine residues and a bias against the use of highly charged or hydrophobic amino acids in the H chain CDR3, which reflects preferential use of only one of the six potential D_H reading frames, natural selection of reading frame content, and selection during development.[43]

The TCR αδ-chain locus

The α and δ loci are located on chromosome 14q11-12. This region is unusual in that the gene segments encoding the two different TCR chains are actually intermixed (Fig. 4.9). There are 38–40 Vα, 5 Vα/Vδ, and 50 Jα functional gene segments, as well as one Cα gene.[44,45] Variation in numbers does occur between individuals. There are no Dα segments.

The δ locus lies between the Vα and Jα gene segments. There are 3 committed Vδ, 5 Vα/Vδ, 3 Dδ, and 3 Jδ gene segments, as well as one Cδ gene. Vδ3 lies 3′ of Cδ, and thus must rearrange by inversion. Although V region use by α and δ chains is largely independent of one another, this unusual gene organization is accompanied by sharing of 5 V gene segments. For example, Vδ1 can rearrange either to Dδ/Jδ or to Jα elements, and thus can serve as the V region for both γδ and αβ TCRs.

In the large majority of αβ⁺ T cells analyzed, the α chain on both chromosomes has rearranged. This occurs by the rearrangement of the 5′ recombination signal sequence δRec to a pseudo-J segment, ΨJα, at the beginning of the Jα cluster (Fig. 4.9) as well as by the subsequent rearrangement of Vα to Jα on both chromosomes. Both types of rearrangement delete all of the Dδ, Jδ, and Cδ genes, thus preventing co-expression of αβ and γδ TCRs.

The TCR β-chain locus

The β locus is positioned at chromosome 7q35.[44] It contains 40–48 functional Vβ genes, two Dβ, two Jβ clusters, each containing 6 or 7 gene segments, and two Cβ genes (Fig. 4.9). There is one Vβ immediately downstream of Cβ2, which rearranges by inversion. Each Cβ is preceded by its own Dβ–Jβ cluster. There is no apparent preference for Vβ gene rearrangement to either Dβ–Jβ cluster. Dβ1 can rearrange to the Jβ1 cluster or the Dβ2–Jβ2 cluster. Dβ2 can only rearrange to Jβ2 gene segments. The two Cβ segments differ by only six amino acids and are functionally indistinguishable from each other.

The TCR γ-chain locus

The γ locus is located at chromosome 7p14-15.[44] There are 4-6 functional Vγ region segments intermixed with pseudogenes and two J clusters with a total of 5 J segments. Each J cluster is 5′ to its C region (Fig. 4.9). The Vγ segments have been divided into 6 families, although only Vγ1 (9 members, 5 of them functional) and Vγ2 (one member) encode functional proteins. The number of Cγ gene exons varies: Cγ1 has three, while there are two alleles of Cγ2 that have 4 and 5, respectively. The first Cγ exon encodes most of the extracellular portion of this region. The last Cγ exon encodes the intracytoplasmic portion of the molecule. The middle exon(s) (one for Cγ1, two or three for Cγ2) encode the connecting piece, which does (Cγ1), or does not (Cγ2), include a cysteine. Since this cysteine can form a disulfide bond with another cysteine in the δ chain, TCRs using Cγ1 contain a covalently linked γ–δ pair, while TCRs using Cγ2 do not.

The nomenclature of the human γ locus differs between laboratories and reports, and is extensively cross-referenced on the IMGT website (http://www.imgt.org).

Allelic exclusion

Because of the inherently imprecise nature of coding joints, for both Ig and TCR only one in three V(D)J rearrangements will be in-frame and capable of creating a functional protein.[45]

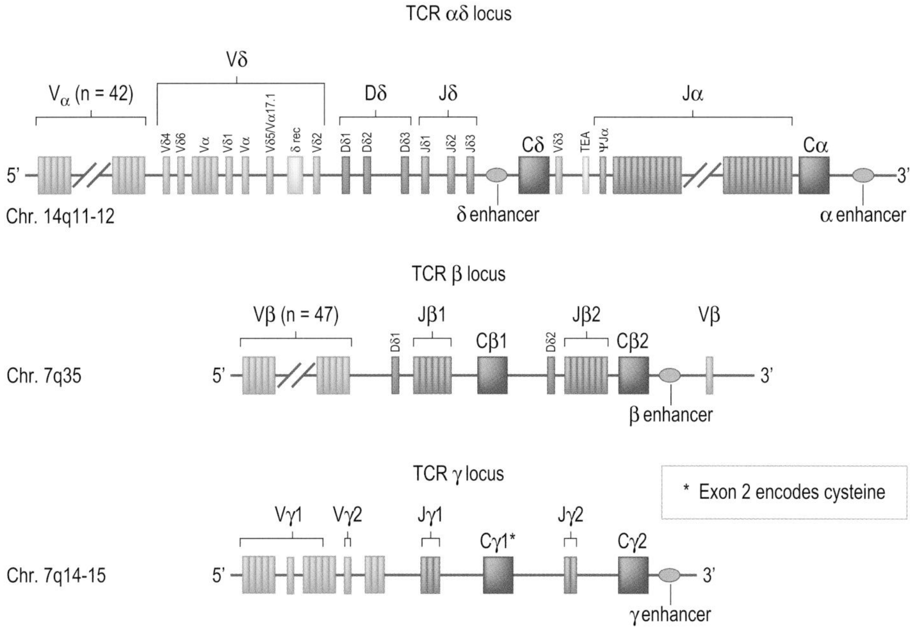

Fig. 4.9 Chromosomal organization of the TCR αδ, β, and γ gene clusters. Typical numbers of functional gene segments are shown. These maps are not drawn to scale.

TCR αδ locus

Vδ

Vα (n = 42)

Dδ   Jδ   Jα

Vβ4 Vβ6 Vα Vβ1 Vα Vβ5/Vα17.1 δ rec Vβ2   Dβ1 Dβ2 Dβ3 Jβ1 Jβ2 Jβ3   Cδ Vβ3 TEA ΨJα   Cα

5′ —   δ enhancer   α enhancer   —3′

Chr. 14q11-12

TCR β locus

Vβ (n = 47)   Jβ1   Jβ2   Vβ

Dβ1   Cβ1   Dβ2   Cβ2

5′ —   β enhancer   —3′

Chr. 7q35

TCR γ locus

Vγ1   Vγ2   Jγ1   Jγ2

Cγ1*   Cγ2

* Exon 2 encodes cysteine

5′ —   γ enhancer   —3′

Chr. 7q14-15

Theoretically, one in nine cells might be expected to express two different Ig or TCR chains. However, almost all B cells express the functional products of only one IgH allele and one IgL allele, and mature αβ T cells express only one functional TCRβ gene. The process of limiting the number of receptors expressed by an individual cell is known as *allelic exclusion*.[46]

Both stochastic and regulated models have been put forth to explain this process, but the precise mechanism remains unclear. The mechanism has been shown to be associated with the expression of a membrane-bound Ig or TCR product capable of transducing a signal. In pre-B cells, a functional μ H chain associates with the surrogate light chain to form the pre-B-cell receptor (pre-BCR). Similarly, in developing T-cell progenitors a productive TCR β chain associates with pre-Tα to form the pre-TCR. These preliminary antigen receptors signal to shut down RAG expression, promote cell division, and limit the accessibility of the IgH and TCRβ loci to further rearrangement while promoting the accessibility of the IgL and TCRα loci, respectively.

In pre-B cells, the κ locus is the first to rearrange, with λ rearrangement occurring in cells that have failed to produce a proper κ chain. Surface expression of an acceptable membrane-bound IgM B-cell receptor invokes the mechanism of allelic exclusion among the L chain loci, termed isotypic exclusion, and promotes further maturation of the B cell.

Productive TCRα rearrangement in CD4+CD8+ T-cell progenitors allows the expression of a functional TCR αβ heterodimer. Unlike IgH and TCRβ; TCRα does not undergo allelic exclusion at the level of gene rearrangement. Instead, in cells that express two functional TCRα alleles, one of the two alleles tends to preferentially pair with the one functional TCRβ chain. This is termed phenotypic allelic exclusion.

Allelic exclusion can be overcome by selection pressures. Cells that express self-reactive antigen receptors can downregulate IgH or TCR expression and reactivate gene rearrangement to replace one of the two offending chains. This process, termed *receptor editing*,[47] occurs most often in the IgL or TCRα loci, whose gene structures lend themselves to repeated rearrangement. Less commonly, the V_H in the H chain can be replaced by means of rearrangement to a cryptic RSS located at the terminus of the V_H gene segment.

KEY CONCEPTS

BCR and co-receptors

- The BCR–antigen complex consists of a membrane-bound Ig that is responsible for antigen recognition and an Ig-α/-β heterodimer that is responsible for transducing the recognition signal into the cell.
- BCR engagement leads to the phosphorylation of tyrosines in the Ig-α/-β ITAM motifs. This signal is then transmitted to one or more other intracellular signaling pathways.
- Recognition of antigen by B lymphocytes can also involve binding of antigen complexed with C3d and IgG to additional B-cell co-receptors.
- Binding of complexed antigen by individual coreceptors can lead to either positive or negative signals, each of which can influence the ultimate outcome of an antigen-B lymphocyte interaction.
- Deficiency of the components of the BCR antigen complex impairs B-cell development and can produce agammaglobulinemia.

B-cell receptor (BCR) complex: structure and function

Although the ability of surface immunoglobulin to recognize antigen was appreciated very early, the mechanism by which membrane-bound immunoglobulin (mIg) transmitted an antigen recognition event to the cell took longer to understand. Specifically, as the predominant isotypes expressed on the surface of mature B cells, mIgM and mIgD, contain only three amino acid residues exposed to the cytoplasm, it was thought unlikely that these Ig heavy chains could function as signal transduction molecules by themselves. This presumption was eventually proved correct when it was shown that all membrane immunoglobulin isotypes associated noncovalently with a heterodimeric complex consisting of two transmembrane proteins, Ig-α and Ig-β, each of which is capable of transducing signals into the cell (Table 4.3).

Membrane-bound immunoglobulin

Immunoglobulins mediate their effector functions as secreted products of plasma cells. However, as membrane-bound structures on mature B cells, immunoglobulins serve as the antigen recognition component of the B-cell receptor complex. Although all immunoglobulin classes can be expressed at the cell surface, the vast majority of circulating mature B cells co-express membrane-bound IgM and IgD. Appropriate activation of a naïve IgM and IgD expressing B cell leads to plasma cell differentiation and antibody secretion. The membrane-bound forms of IgM and IgD are the product of alternative splicing of the immunoglobulin transcript at the 3′, or carboxy terminus, of the heavy chain (Fig. 4.10). The two membrane exons encode the transmembrane hydrophobic stretch of amino acids and an evolutionarily conserved cytoplasmic tail encoding lysine, valine and lysine.

Table 4.3 The BCR and its co-receptor molecules

Molecule	M_r	Chromosome	Function
BCR			
mIgM (μ_2L_2)	180 000	14 (IgH; 14q.32) 2 (Igκ; 2p12) 22 (Igλ; 22q11.2)	Antigen recognition
Ig-α	47 000	19 (19q13.2)	Signal transducer
Ig-β	37 000	17 (17q23)	Signal transducer
Co-receptors			
CD21	140 000	1 (1q32)	Activating co-receptor Ligand for C3d, EBV, CD23
CD19	95 000	16 (16p11.2)	Activating co-receptor Signal transducer
FcγRIIB	40 000	1 (1q23-24)	Inhibitory co-receptor Low affinity receptor for IgG
CD22	140 000	19 (19q13.1)	Inhibitory co-receptor Adhesion molecule Signal transducer

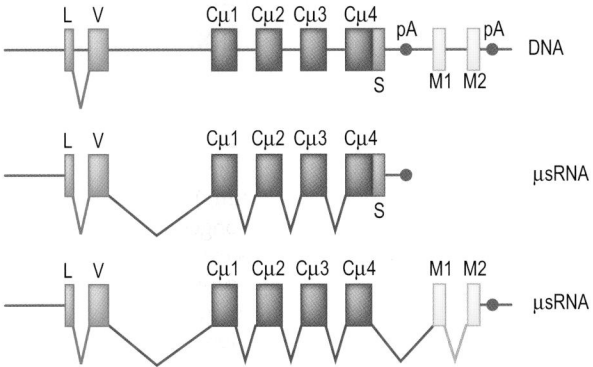

Fig. 4.10 Membrane and secretory IgM are created by alternative splicing. Alternative splicing of the Cm carboxy-terminal exons results in mRNA transcripts encoding either secreted IgM (μ_s RNA) or membrane-bound IgM (μ_m RNA).

Signal transduction and the Ig-α/β (CD79a/CD79b) heterodimer

The heterodimeric signal transduction component of the BCR complex that associates with membrane immunoglobulin has been designated CD79. It is composed of an Ig-α (CD79a) and Ig-β (CD79b) heterodimer. CD79 is responsible for transporting membrane-bound immunoglobulin (mIg) to the cell surface and for transducing BCR signals into the cell.[48,49]

CD79a/Ig-α is encoded by *CD79a/MB-1* (chromosome 19q13.2) as a 226 amino acid glycoprotein of approximately 47 kDa. The exact molecular weight depends on the extent of glycosylation. *CD79b/B29* (chromosome 17q23) encodes CD79b/Ig-β, which is a 229-amino acid glycoprotein of approximately 37 kDa. *CD79a* and *CD79b* share an exon–intron structure, which is similar to that of the genes that encode the CD3 TCR co-receptor molecules. These similarities suggest that both BCR and TCR co-receptors are the progeny of a common ancestral gene. Ig-α and Ig-β both contain a single IgSF Ig domain (111 residue C-type for Ig-α and 129 residue V-type for Ig-β). Each also contains a highly conserved transmembrane domain and a 61-(Ig-α) or 48- (Ig-β) amino acid cytoplasmic tail that also exhibits striking amino acid evolutionary conservation.

Ig-α and Ig-β are expressed by the earliest committed B-cell progenitors and before expression of Ig-μ heavy chain. The CD79 heterodimer has also been observed on the surface of early B-cell progenitors in the absence of μ heavy chain, although neither protein is required for progenitors to commit to the B-cell lineage.[50] Later in development, Ig-α and Ig-β are co-expressed together with Ig of all isotypes on the surface of B cells as a mature BCR complex.[48] The CD79 proteins are specific to the B lineage and are expressed throughout B lymphopoiesis. This has led to their use as markers for the identification of B-cell neoplasms.[51,52]

The signaling capacity of both Ig-α and Ig-β resides within an *immunoreceptor tyrosine-based activation motif* (*ITAM*) that has the consensus sequence of D/IxxYxxL(x)$_7$YxxL, where x is any amino acid. Similar ITAMs are also found within the cytoplasmic domain of the molecules that associate with, and signal for, the T-cell antigen receptor (CD3) and certain Fc receptors. The phosphorylation of both tyrosines in both Ig-α/β ITAMs is considered an obligate initial step in the propagation of antigen receptor engagement to the cell nucleus.[49,53] Tyrosine-phosphorylated ITAMs serve as efficient binding sites for Src homology 2 (SH-2) domains, which are present within a large number of cytosolic signaling molecules. Whether Ig-α

and Ig-β make qualitatively different contributions towards BCR signaling or are functionally redundant remains unclear, as evidence exists to support both views. Moreover, the high degree of evolutionary conservation within the non-ITAM portion of the cytoplasmic domains suggests additional, as yet uncharacterized, signaling roles for the cytoplasmic tails of these molecules over and above positive signaling via the ITAMs.

Ig-α and Ig-β are covalently associated by a disulfide bridge via cysteine residues that exist within the IgSF extracellular domains of both molecules. The association of the Ig-α/β heterodimer with membrane-bound Ig occurs though interaction within the transmembrane domains of these proteins.[48] The core BCR complex consists of a single Ig molecule associated with a single Ig-α/β heterodimer (H_2L_2/Ig-α/Ig-β) (Fig. 4.11).[54]

A current model for the initiation of signals originating from the BCR (Fig. 4.11) proposes that antigens induce the clustering of BCR complexes, increasing their local density. The increase in density leads to the transfer of phosphate groups to the tyrosine residues of the Ig-α/β ITAM motifs.[49,53] Src-family tyrosine kinases, of which LYN, FYN, and BLK are most often implicated, are believed to be responsible for ITAM phosphorylation upon aggregation of Ig-α/β. They have been shown to physically associate with the heterodimer. It has been suggested that a fraction of Src-family tyrosine kinases are associated with the Ig-α/β heterodimer and, upon aggregation, transphosphorylate juxtaposed heterodimers. However, the exact mechanism by which Ig-α/β undergoes initial tyrosine phosphorylation after antigen engagement remains uncertain. Regardless of mechanism, phosphorylated ITAMs subsequently serve as high-affinity docking sites for cytosolic effector molecules that harbor SH2 domains. The recruitment of the SYK tyrosine kinase, via its tandem SH2 domains, to doubly phosphorylated Ig-α/β ITAMs is thought to be a next step in propagating a BCR-mediated signal. Association of SYK with the BCR leads to its

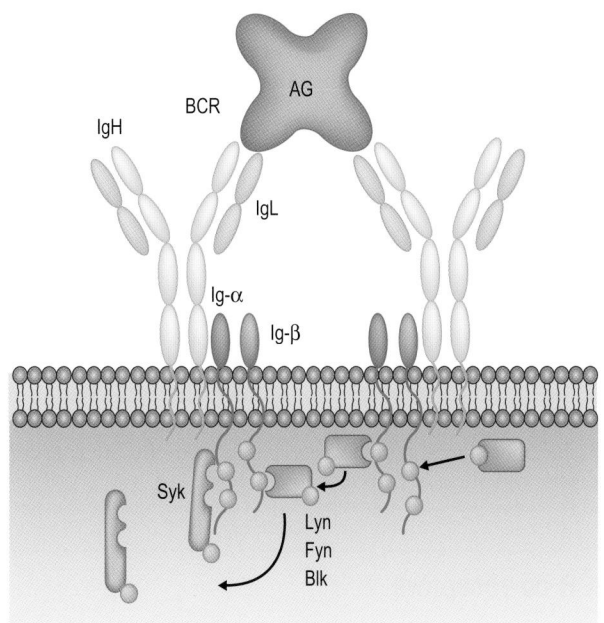

Fig. 4.11 The BCR core complex. The BCR core complex can be divided into an antigen recognition unit fulfilled by mIgM and a noncovalently associated signal transduction unit composed of the Ig-α/β (CD79) heterodimer. Antigen engagement of mIgM oligomerizes the BCR, allowing preassociated Src-family protein tyrosine kinases to phosphorylate neighboring Ig-α/β ITAM tyrosines. This promotes association of the SYK tyrosine kinase with the tyrosine phosphorylated ITAMs, allowing SYK to become a substrate for other Syk or Src-family tyrosine kinases and leading to its activation.

subsequent tyrosine phosphorylation by either Src-family or other Syk tyrosine kinases, further increasing kinase activity. Together, the concerted actions of the Syk and Src-family protein tyrosine kinases activate a variety of intracellular signaling pathways that can lead to the proliferation, differentiation, or death of the cell.[55]

Clinical consequences of disruptions in BCR signaling

Both the development of B lymphocytes and the maintenance of the mature antigen-responsive B-cell pool demand the presence of an intact BCR and its downstream signaling pathway(s). Disruption of these pathways can present clinically with hypogammaglobulinemia and an absence of B cells.

The most common such genetic lesions is BTK deficiency, which is an X-linked trait (Chapter 34).[56] BTK plays an important role in BCR signaling both during development and in response to antigen. Loss of function mutations in *BTK* results in the arrest of human B-cell development at the pre-B-cell stage.

BTK is intact in approximately 10 to 15% of patients with hypogammaglobulinemia and absence of B cells. Mouse models where BCR components or signaling pathways have been disrupted by targeted mutagenesis have provided insight into the basis of these atypical hypogammaglobulinemia disorders.[49] These studies have shown that an inability to express either a functional μ IgH chain, Ig-α, Ig-β, or the signaling adaptor molecule, BLNK, lead to an early, severe arrest in B lymphopoiesis, with subsequent agammaglobulinemia. Together, these experimental findings highlighted the central role of the BCR in the generation and function of B lymphocytes. They suggested that mutations in any component of the antigen receptor complex or immediate downstream effectors would have the potential to disrupt B-cell development and thus create an agammaglobulinemic state. These speculations were borne out when hypogammaglobulinemic individuals demonstrating an absence of B cells in the presence of normal BTK function were subsequently identified with mutations in Ig-μ heavy chain, Ig-α, or BLNK.[55]

Besides its important role in the maturation, differentiation and survival of B lymphocytes, the B-cell antigen receptor is responsible for initiating the humoral response to foreign antigen. Some of the variables that can influence the ultimate outcome of BCR–antigen interaction include the nature of the foreign antigen, the mode of activation, the developmental stage of the B cell, and the microenvironment in which antigen encounter occurs. Exactly how these variables ultimately result in the differential activation of diverse intracellular signaling pathways with fundamentally divergent outcomes is under study. Emerging from these studies is an appreciation of the role of BCR co-receptors, which have been shown to be capable of modulating antigen receptor signaling in response to antigen.

BCR co-receptors

The initiation of a humoral immune response results from antigen interaction with the antigen receptors on mature peripheral lymphocytes. However, the manner in which mature B and T lymphocytes recognize antigen is fundamentally different (Chapter 6). Surface Ig, as a component of the BCR on B lymphocytes, recognizes an antigenic epitope in its native three-dimensional configuration that, upon engagement with mIg, is capable of transmitting a signal to the cell interior. In contrast, the antigen receptor expressed by T lymphocytes recognizes an antigen-derived peptide associated with an appropriate MHC structure. Moreover, for a productive outcome of this T-cell recognition event, a CD4 or CD8 co-receptor must also bind to the MHC structure presenting the foreign antigen. Similarly, antigen recognition by the BCR on B lymphocytes is also influenced by co-receptors present on mature B cells (Table 4.3). In this case the co-receptors may also recognize antigen, but only in a form that has been modified by other components of the immune system, as described below. In general, these co-receptors and co-receptor complexes can be divided into those that regulate BCR signaling in a positive manner and those that regulate in a negative manner. Thus, the ultimate outcome of signaling via the BCR depends not only on the signals transduced via the Ig-α/β heterodimer, but also how these signals are perceived by the cell in association with the signals propagated by the various co-receptors that are concomitantly engaged.

Co-receptors that positively regulate BCR signaling
CD21

Mature B lymphocytes express two receptors for complement C3 components, CD35 (CR1) and CD21 (CR2) (Chapter 20). Of these, CD21 fulfills the requirements of a BCR co-receptor, as described below. The expression of CD21 is restricted to mature B cells and follicular dendritic cells, whereas CD35 is also found on erythrocytes, monocytes and granulocytes. CD21 is a 140-kDa surface glycoprotein encoded by the *CR2* locus on chromosome 1q32 (Table 4.3). Expression of CD21 begins at approximately the same time as IgD during B lymphopoiesis (Chapter 7). CD21 is subsequently expressed on all mature B cells until terminal differentiation. Within the mature population, marginal zone B cells express higher levels relative to follicular B cells. The extracellular domain of CD21 is composed of 15–16 short consensus regions (SCRs), each composed of 60–70 amino acids, and a relatively short 34-amino acid cytoplasmic tail. The two-amino terminal SCRs constitute the region that interacts with one of the third complement component (C3) cleavage products, iC3b, C3d, g, and C3d (Chapter 20).[57]

CD21 is a receptor for Epstein–Barr virus (EBV), which similarly binds the two *N*-terminal SCRs via its major envelope glycoprotein gp350/220. CD21, through its oligosaccharide chains, also binds CD23, the low-affinity IgE receptor (FcεRII). Whereas EBV utilization of CD21 for cell entry has clear physiological consequences in terms of infection, B-cell immortalization, and the potential for oncogenesis, the *in vivo* relevance of any CD21–CD23 interaction remains unclear.

CD19

CD19 is an IgSF surface glycoprotein of 95 kDa that is expressed from the earliest stages of B-cell development until plasma cell terminal differentiation, when its expression is lost.[58] Follicular dendritic cells also express CD19. *CD19* maps to chromosome 16p11.2, where it encodes a 540-amino acid protein with two extracellular C-type IgSF domains as well as a large, approximately 240-residue, cytoplasmic tail that exhibits extensive conservation between mouse and human. This relatively large cytoplasmic domain includes nine conserved tyrosine residues that, upon phosphorylation, serve as docking sites for other SH2-containing effector molecules. The signaling capacity of

CD19 has been shown to result from tyrosine phosphorylation, which occurs upon engagement of the BCR, CD19 or, optimally, by co-ligation of CD19 and IgM. Known signaling effector molecules that have been identified in association with tyrosine-phosphorylated CD19 include the LYN and FYN protein tyrosine kinases, the Rho-family guanine nucleotide exchange factor, VAV, and phosphatidyl inositol 3-kinase.[58] Although specific ligands for CD19 have been proposed, the physiological relevance of CD19 engagement by putative ligands has not been demonstrated.

In vitro studies using monoclonal antibodies (mAbs) directed against CD21 or CD19 provided initial evidence that these B-cell surface antigens could influence mIg-mediated signaling.[57,58] In the absence of identifying naturally occurring genetic deficiencies of CD21 or CD19, formal demonstration that these molecules played a physiological role in regulating B-cell responses has been provided by targeted mutagenesis in mouse models. CD21- and CD19-deficient mice demonstrate impaired antibody response to T-dependent antigens.[57–59] The paucity of CD5+ B cells in CD19-deficient mice also suggests a role for this molecule in the generation and maintenance of the B1 lineage of B cells (Chapter 7). CD19 is expressed from the earliest stages of B-cell ontogeny in both mice and humans and, accordingly, a signaling function for CD19 in B lymphopoiesis has been demonstrated.[60]

CD21–CD19 co-receptor complex

A mechanism by which these molecules could augment BCR-mediated signaling was provided by the identification of a CD21–CD19 co-receptor complex on mature B cells that also includes CD81 (Fig. 4.12). CD81, also known as TAPA-1, is a 26-kDa tetraspan molecule widely expressed on a number of cell types, including lymphocytes. The CD21–CD19 co-receptor model predicted that, as a result of complement activation, C3d would be deposited on an antigen, thereby providing a bridge by which a CD21–CD19 receptor complex could associate with mIgM and the B-cell receptor complex.[57–59] Clustering of

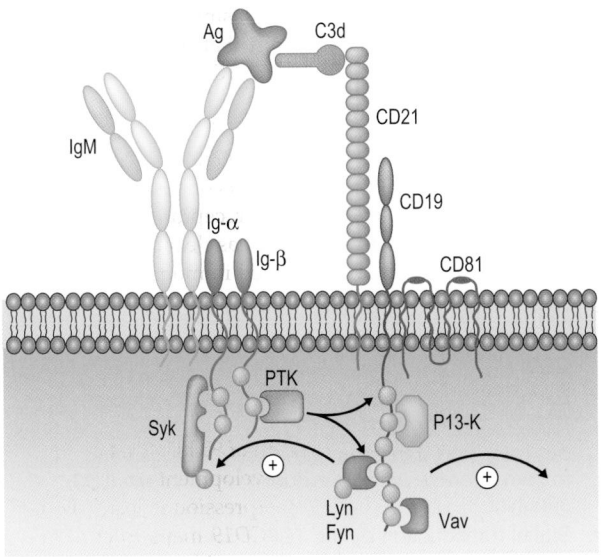

Fig. 4.12 Proposed mechanisms for the augmentation of BCR signaling by the CD21/19 co-receptor. Co-ligation of the BCR and CD21–CD19 complex by C3d–antigen complex allows a CD79-associated Src-family tyrosine kinase to phosphorylate tyrosine residues within the CD19 cytoplasmic domain. Subsequently, tyrosine-phosphorylated CD19 effectively recruits key SH2-containing signaling molecules to the BCR complex, allowing the initial BCR-mediated signal to quickly disseminate along different intracellular signaling pathways.

CD19 close to the BCR by the C3d–antigen complex would effectively recruit the signal transduction effector molecules associated with CD19 to the Ig-α/β heterodimer. As a consequence, the CD19-associated LYN and FYN tyrosine kinases, VAV, and PI3-kinase signaling effector molecules would be in a position to exert their activities on the Ig-α/β heterodimer-mediated signaling events initiated by antigen engagement of mIgM.

Strong support for CD21–CD19 co-receptor physiological function in BCR signaling was subsequently provided by experiments using a murine model of immune response. In these experiments, the immunization of mice with an antigen covalently attached to C3d dramatically reduced the signaling threshold necessary for antigen to elicit an immune response.[61] Antigen bearing either two or three copies of C3d was respectively 1 000 and 10 000 times more immunogenic than antigen alone. Thus, the CD21–CD19 co-receptor complex provides a link between the innate and adaptive immune responses. *In vivo*, CD19-deficient mice appear to have more severely affected T-dependent immune responses than do CD21-deficient animals, suggesting alternative roles for CD19 in regulating BCR signals beyond the CD21–CD19 co-receptor complex.

Co-receptors that negatively regulate BCR signaling

FcγRIIB

Among the several receptors for the Fc portion of immunoglobulin expressed by B cells, the Fc receptor for IgG, FcγRIIB (a member of the CD32 cluster), has an important role in negatively regulating BCR-mediated signal transduction.[62] FcγRIIB is a 40-kDa single-chain molecule that is encoded by single gene located on chromosome 1q23-24. Alternative splicing of different cytoplasmic exons permits expression of three isoforms. The extracellular domain of FcγRIIB is composed of two C-type IgSF domains that can bind with low affinity to IgG. All three FcγRIIB isoforms share a common cytoplasmic region that is important for negatively regulating activation signals delivered by associated surface receptors. The region within the cytoplasmic domain of FCγRIIB responsible for the inhibitory activity of this Fc receptor towards the BCR has been identified as a sequence that contains a tyrosine residue critical for its activity.[63] In analogy to the ITAM, which provides an activation signal, this inhibitory sequence has been referred to as an *i*mmunoreceptor *t*yrosine-based *i*nhibitory *m*otif, or *ITIM*. The ITIM is carried by the canonical sequence of I/L/VxYxxI/V/L (where x is any amino acid).[62] ITIMs are found in a number of other transmembrane structures, all of which share the ability to negatively regulate signaling by activating receptors.

The ability of passively administered soluble antibody to inhibit humoral responses has long been appreciated and was initially thought to occur by soluble antibody effectively masking all available antigen epitopes. The molecular mechanism accounting for this suppression is now known to be mediated by the binding of IgG to FcRγIIB and the subsequent recruitment of cytosolic phosphatases to the FcRγIIB ITIM upon tyrosine phosphorylation. Thus, the inhibitory effect of IgG on BCR-mediated B-cell activation is explained by the interaction of the FcγRIIB ITIM, and specifically associated phosphatases, with the BCR (Fig. 4.13). Co-ligation of the BCR and FcRγIIB by antigen–IgG complexes results in the tyrosine phosphorylation of the FcRγIIB ITIM, presumably by the BCR-associated tyrosine kinases. Phosphorylated FcRγIIB ITIMs then recruit two different SH2-containing phosphatases, SHIP and SHP-1, which

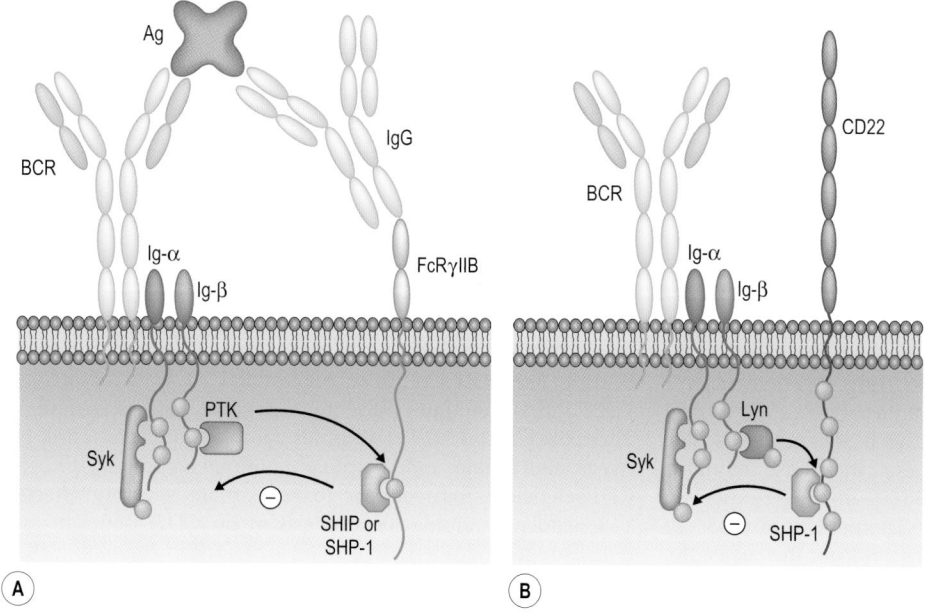

Fig. 4.13 Negative regulation of BCR signaling by Fcγ RIIB and CD22. (A) Soluble IgG–antigen immune complexes juxtapose the BCR with FcγRIIB. The BCR-associated LYN tyrosine kinase subsequently tyrosine phosphorylates the FcγRIIB ITIM. In turn, this leads to the recruitment of the SH2-containing inositol phosphatase SHIP and tyrosine phosphatase SHP-1 to the phosphorylated FcRγIIB ITIM. Both of these phosphatases have demonstrable inhibitory activity on BCR-mediated signaling. Although SHIP is believed to be the major effector in the FcRγIIB-mediated inhibition of BCR signaling,[64] the exact mechanism of its action in this context has not yet been elucidated. (B) CD22 associated with the BCR is tyrosine-phosphorylated upon antigen–BCR engagement. SH2-containing signaling molecules dock on tyrosine phosphorylated residues, including the SHP-1 tyrosine phosphatase that can subsequently dephosphorylate signaling molecules previously activated by a mIgM-mediated signal.

function to remove phosphate groups from inositol lipids or tyrosines, respectively. Although both phosphatases can negatively regulate BCR-mediated signaling events, SHIP appears to be the most relevant phosphatase in FcγRIIB inhibition of BCR signaling (Fig. 4.13).[64] Thus, once the majority of antigen exists in immune complexes together with antigen-specific IgG, attenuation of an ongoing immune response occurs by the juxtaposition of FcRγIIB with the BCR.

CD22

CD22 is a 135- to 140-kDa transmembrane glycoprotein that is restricted in its expression to the B lineage.[65] CD22 expression is limited to the cytoplasm of progenitor and pre-B cells in early B-cell development. Expression on the surface of the B cell occurs concomitant with the appearance of surface, or membrane, IgD. Upon B-cell activation, CD22 expression is initially transiently upregulated and subsequently down-modulated upon terminal differentiation to Ig-secreting plasma cells. Although the onset of CD22 expression follows a similar pattern during murine B lymphopoiesis, it is not restricted to the cytoplasm in early B lymphopoiesis but rather is expressed on the surface from the progenitor stage onward. The basis or function of CD22 intracellular retention in human B-cell development is not understood.

CD22 maps to chromosome 19q13.1 and encodes alternatively spliced forms of CD22, CD22α, and CD22β, of which the latter is the predominant species expressed by B cells. The CD22β isoform contains seven extracellular IgSF domains, of which all but one are of the C type. The single exception is the *N*-terminal domain, which is of the V type. CD22α lacks the IgSF third and fourth domains, although the significance of this minority alternatively spliced product remains unclear. The CD22 murine homolog has only been found as a full-length CD22β isoform. The extracellular domain of CD22 is homologous to the carcinoembryonic antigen subfamily of adhesion molecules, which includes the myelin-associated glycoprotein (MAG) and CD33. CD22 also functions as an adhesion molecule belonging to the Siglec subfamily of the Ig superfamily, whose members function as mammalian sialic acid-binding Ig-like lectins.[65] The two *N*-terminal IgSF domains have been shown to mediate adhesion to both B and T lymphocytes via the binding of structures carrying α2,6 sialic acids.

In addition to acting as an adhesion molecule, CD22 is also capable of modulating BCR signaling (Fig. 4.13). A fraction of CD22 associates with the BCR, and CD22 is rapidly tyrosine-phosphorylated upon mIgM engagement. Tyrosine-phosphorylated CD22 associates with several SH2-containing signaling molecules, including the LYN and SYK tyrosine kinases, PI3-kinase, phospholipase C-γ and SHP-1. The 140-amino acid cytoplasmic domain of CD22 includes six conserved tyrosine residues. Three of these tyrosines are located within conserved consensus ITIM sequences and possess a demonstrable capacity to bind the SH2 domain of the SHP-1 phosphatase. The presence of the multiple ITIMs and association with SHP-1 indicated that CD22 might impinge on BCR signaling in a negative manner. Physiological evidence that CD22 could act as a co-receptor to negatively regulate mIgM signaling was provided by the generation of CD22-deficient mice by targeted mutagenesis.[65] CD22-deficient B cells exhibited hyperactive B-cell responses upon BCR triggering, and an increased incidence of serum autoantibodies. This suggests that B-cell tolerance is altered and B cells are more readily activated in the absence of this negative regulator of BCR signaling.

● KEY CONCEPTS

TCR/CD3 complex

- Cell-surface expression of the TCR heterodimers requires association with a complex of invariant proteins designated CD3.

- Each TCR–CD3 complex contains 3 CD3 dimers.

- Assembly of the TCR–CD3 complex involves interactions between TCR transmembrane basic residues and transmembrane acidic residues in each of the CD3 subunits.

- Signal transduction by the TCR involves the phosphorylation of immunoreceptor tyrosine-based activation motifs (ITAMs) in the cytoplasmic domains of CD3 proteins.
  - Phosphorylated CD3 ITAMs recruit and activate the ZAP-70 protein tyrosine kinase.

- Deficiency of CD3 proteins impairs T-cell development and can produce SCID.

The T-cell receptor (TCR)–CD3 complex

The αβ and γδ TCR heterodimers, which are responsible for the recognition of specific antigen by T lymphocytes, associate with a complex of invariant proteins designated CD3. This association is necessary for TCR cell-surface expression and enables the TCR heterodimers, which have only short cytoplasmic domains, to couple to the intracellular signaling events that lead to the activation of T-cell effector function. There are four CD3 proteins: γ, δ, ε, and ζ (Fig. 4.14).[17,66]

CD3 proteins

CD3γ, CD3δ, and CD3ε are structurally similar, and the genes encoding them map to a locus in chromosome 11q23. The polypeptides range in size from 20 to 25 kDa. Each has an extracellular C-type IgSF domain, a transmembrane region that contains an acidic residue (aspartic acid in CD3δ and CD3ε, glutamic acid in CD3γ), and a cytoplasmic domain with a single immunoreceptor tyrosine-based activation motif (ITAM). The cytoplasmic domain of CD3ε (but not of CD3δ or CD3γ) has a net positive charge and can bind to the negatively charged inner leaflet of the plasma membrane with its ITAM inserted into the lipid bilayer. The CD3 chains are present in the TCR–CD3 complex in the form of noncovalently linked CD3γε and CD3δε heterodimers; interactions between the extracellular IgSF domains lead to the formation of these CD3 heterodimers.[17,66]

The 16-kDa CD3ζ differs substantially from the other CD3 proteins and is structurally homologous to the γ chain of the high affinity IgE receptor (FcRγ chain). The extracellular domain of CD3ζ is very short (only 9 amino acids) and is of unknown structure. As is the case with the other CD3 chains, the transmembrane region of CD3ζ contains an acidic residue (aspartic acid). The large cytoplasmic domain of CD3ζ has 3 ITAMs in tandem. and a net positive charge. Like the cytoplasmic domain of CD3ε, the transmembrane region of CD3ζ binds negatively charged lipids, suggesting that it also may associate with the inner leaflet of the plasma membrane.[17] CD3ζ is usually present in the TCR/CD3 complex in the form of disulfide-linked CD3ζζ homodimers.[17,22,66] The CD3ζζ homodimers form through interactions within the transmembrane domain. The NMR structure of the homodimer reveals helical transmembrane domains with co-localization of the two transmembrane aspartic acids at the interface of the two helices.[17]

Stoichiometry of the TCR–CD3 complex

The valency and stoichiometry of the TCR/CD3 complex remains a subject of considerable interest and of some uncertainty.[17,66,67] Although there is evidence that the complex may be bivalent (i.e., contains two TCR heterodimers), most studies conclude that the TCR/CD3 complex is univalent and that the αβTCR–CD3 complex consists of a single αβTCR heterodimer together with three CD3 dimers: CD3γε, CD3δε, and CD3ζζ (Fig. 4.14). The γδTCR–CD3 complex, in contrast, lacks CD3δ. On naïve T cells, this receptor complex contains two CD3εγ heterodimers and one CD3ζζ homodimer. Following activation of γδT cells, the TCR/CD3 complex incorporates the FcRγ chain, either as a homodimer or as heterodimer with CD3ζ.[17,22]

Assembly and cell-surface expression of the TCR-CD3 complex

Assembly begins with formation of the individual TCRαβ, CD3δε, and CD3γε heterodimers, processes that are driven by interactions between the extracellular domains of the pairing polypeptides. The subsequent higher order assembly of the TCRαβ with the CD3 dimers depends upon interactions between the potentially charged residues within their transmembrane regions. As noted above, each of the CD3 subunits has a transmembrane acidic residue while the transmembrane domains of the αβ and γδ TCRs contain basic residues. For example, the TCRα has an arginine and a lysine within its transmembrane domain while the transmembrane region of the TCRβ contains a lysine. Mutation of any of these transmembrane acidic or basic residues to neutral alanine impairs formation of the TCR/CD3 complex. TCRαβ appears to associate first with CD3δε and then with CD3γε. TCRα binds CD3δε, and TCRβ likely interacts with CD3γε. The incorporation of a CD3ζζ homodimer into the complex requires the prior formation of a TCRαβ–CD3εγ–CD3εδ hexamer and involves interactions between the arginine residue

Fig. 4.14 **Schematic representation of the human TCR and CD4 and CD8 co-receptors.** IgSF domains are represented by ovals. The four extracellular domains of CD4 are labeled D1-D4. Basic (+) and acidic (-) transmembrane charged residues are indicated, as are known and predicted sites of disulfide bonds. For schematic simplicity the cytoplasmic domains of the CD3 chains are shown as extending into the cytoplasm. The cytoplasmic domains of CD3ε and CD3ζ, however, are positively charged and likely are associated with the inner leaflet of the plasma membrane.

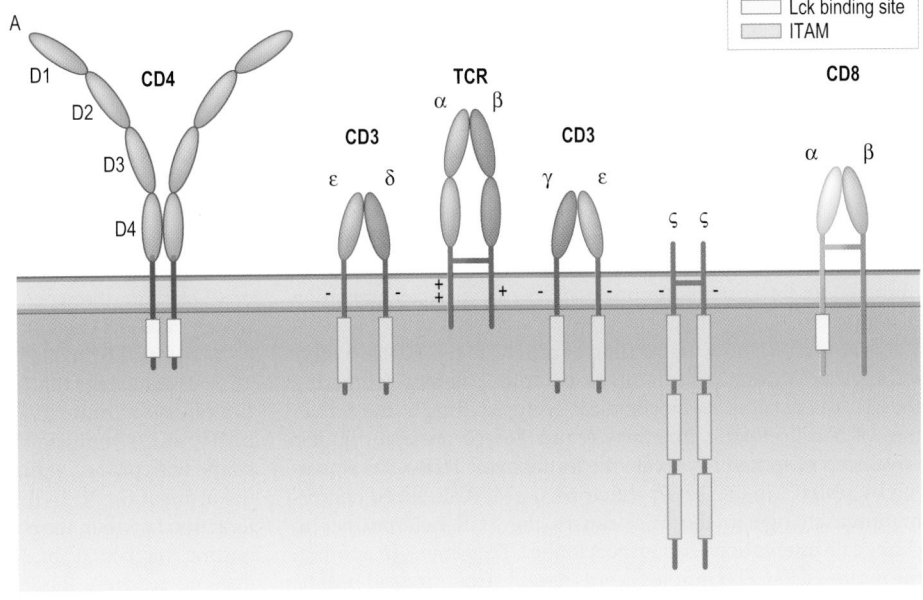

in the transmembrane domain of TCRα and the two co-localized aspartic acids in the transmembrane domains of the CD3ζζ homodimer.[17,66]

Formation of the TCR/CD3 complex is tightly regulated. For example, when there are deficiencies of CD3γ, CD3δ, or CD3ε, TCRα and β are retained in the endoplasmic reticulum and are rapidly degraded. In the absence of CD3ζ, the TCRαβ–CD3εγ–CD3εδ hexamer is exported to the Golgi but then is targeted to a lysosomal degradation pathway rather than the cell surface.[17,22,66]

Because the structures of most of the individual components of the TCR–CD3 complex are known, a model of the overall structure of the receptor has been proposed. This model envisions a compact TCR–CD3, with trimeric contacts occurring within the transmembrane regions of all components (i.e., TCRα–CD3ε–CD3δ, TCRβ–CD3ε–CD3γ, and TCRα–CD3ζ–CD3ζ) and with the TCRαβ extending further from the membrane than the CD3 chains.[17,66] The CD3 heterodimers localize to one side of TCRαβ, leaving the outer portion of the constant domain TCRα unobstructed and thus available to participate in TCR–CD3 dimerization during signal transduction.

Mutations in the *CD3D*, *CD3E*, *CD3G*, and *CD3Z* genes have been described in human.[68–70] The clinical consequences of these mutations underscore the importance of the CD3 proteins for the normal development and function of T cells. Homozygous mutations leading to complete deficiencies of either CD3δ, CD3ε, or CD3ζ protein produce a form of severe combined immunodeficiency (SCID) (Chapter 35) characterized by severe T-cell lymphopenia, but the presence of phenotypically normal B cells and NK cells (T⁻B⁺NK⁺SCID).[68,69] Interestingly, mutations in *CD3G* leading to deficiency of CD3γ produces considerable clinical heterogeneity ranging from severe immunodeficiency in infants to mild forms of autoimmunity in adulthood. Homozygous deficiency in CD3γ impaired, but did not abrogate, T-cell development, leading to mild T lymphopenia, reduction in cell-surface expression of TCR–CD3 complex on peripheral T cells by 75–80%, and impaired *in vitro* proliferative T-cell responses to lectins and to anti-CD3 monoclonal antibodies. In peripheral blood, there were differential effects on phenotypically defined T-cell subsets, with very few CD8⁺ T cells, a 10-fold reduction in CD4⁺CD45RA⁺ T cells ("naïve helper" subset), and normal numbers of CD4⁺CD45RO⁺ T cells ("memory" cells).[70]

Early events in TCR–CD3 signaling

Stimulation of the TCR–CD3 complex by pMHC, or by non-physiological agonists such as anti-CD3 monoclonal antibodies, leads to the phosphorylation of tyrosine residues of the CD3 ITAMs by the SRC-like protein tyrosine kinases, LCK and FYN.[71] The phosphorylated CD3 ITAMs in turn create high affinity binding sites for the SH2 domains of the ZAP-70 protein tyrosine kinase, leading to its recruitment to the TCR/CD3 complex and to its activation (Chapter 12).[71,72] The consequences of ZAP-70 deficiency (selective T-cell immunodeficiency in humans) underscore the centrality of its role in T-cell activation (Chapter 35).

It is not known how the binding of pMHC to the TCR transfers information through the receptor complex, thereby triggering the cascade of complex biochemical events leading to the activation of T-cell effector function. A number of possible models have been proposed to explain the initiation of TCR–CD3 signaling by pMHC. In one set of scenarios, a pMHC-induced conformational change in the TCR causes the TCR heterodimer to change its orientation with respect to the CD3 dimers. In another, the entire TCR–CD3 complex acts as a rigid structure, and pMHC

binding leads to displacement of the CD3 chains into the membrane or alters their orientation with respect to the membrane. Models for initiation of signaling also must accommodate recent findings that the ITAMs in the cytoplasmic domains of CD3ε and CD3ζ likely are inserted into the plasma membrane. Lipid binding appears to prevent phosphorylation of CD3ε and CD3ζ by Lck, indicating that these ITAMs must dissociate from the plasma membrane during the initiation of TCR–CD3 signaling. Following the initiation of signaling, sustained signaling appears to involve multimerization of TCR–CD3 complexes and engagement of co-receptors.[17,66]

T-cell co-receptors: CD4 and CD8

Expression of CD4 and CD8 divides mature T cells into two distinct subsets: CD4 T cells (Chapter 16), which recognize peptides in the context of class II MHC molecules, and CD8 T cells (Chapter 17), which recognize antigens presented by class I MHC molecules. Indeed, CD4 binds directly to class II MHC molecules, and CD8 interacts directly with class I MHC molecules (Fig. 4.15); in both cases binding involves non-polymorphic regions at the base of the MHC molecule. During antigen recognition, CD4 and CD8 are thought to bind the same pMHC complex as the TCR and thus are true co-receptors for the TCR. The cytoplasmic domains of CD4 and CD8 associate with LCK, and, in current models of TCR signaling, these co-receptors bring LCK into contact with the CD3 chains of the pMHC-engaged TCR–CD3 complexes and thus play an important role in the phosphorylation of CD3 ITAMs (Chapter 12). The CD4 and CD8 co-receptors are needed for full T-cell activation.[71,73,74]

The expression of the CD4 and CD8 co-receptors is highly regulated during T-cell development in the thymus (Chapter 8). Thymocytes initially express neither co-receptor ("double negative"). CD4⁻CD8⁻ thymocytes destined to become TCRαβ T cells progress through a CD4⁺CD8⁺ ("double-positive") stage to become mature CD4⁺CD8⁻ or CD4⁻CD8⁺ T cells. Positive and negative selection of thymocytes on the basis of their TCR specificities and commitment to the CD4 or CD8 lineages occur during the double-positive stage.

CD4: structure and binding to MHC class II molecules

A member of the immunoglobulin superfamily, CD4 is a 55-kDa glycoprotein that can be expressed either as a monomer or a dimer on the cell surface. Its relatively rigid extracellular region contains four IgSF domains (designated D1-4). The cytoplasmic domain of CD4 contains 2 cysteine residues that mediate its non-covalent interaction with LCK through a "zinc clasp"-like structure formed with a dicysteine motif in the *N*-terminal region of LCK.[71,73–75]

The crystal structure of the CD4 D1D2 fragment bound to pMHC class II demonstrates that the *N*-terminal domain (D1) of CD4 binds between the membrane-proximal α₂ and β₂ domains of MHC class II. Thus CD4 interacts with pMHC class II at a distance from the α-helices and peptide contacted by the TCR. This enables the TCR and CD4 to bind the same MHC class II molecule simultaneously. Models for the structure of TCRαβ–pMHC–CD4 indicate that this ternary complex assumes a V-shape with pMHC at the apex and with TCRαβ and CD4 forming the arms of the V. In this model, therefore, there is no direct interaction between the co-receptor and the TCR heterodimer, suggesting that pMHC brings the TCR and CD4 together. The model does not address the localization of the CD3 dimers, but raises

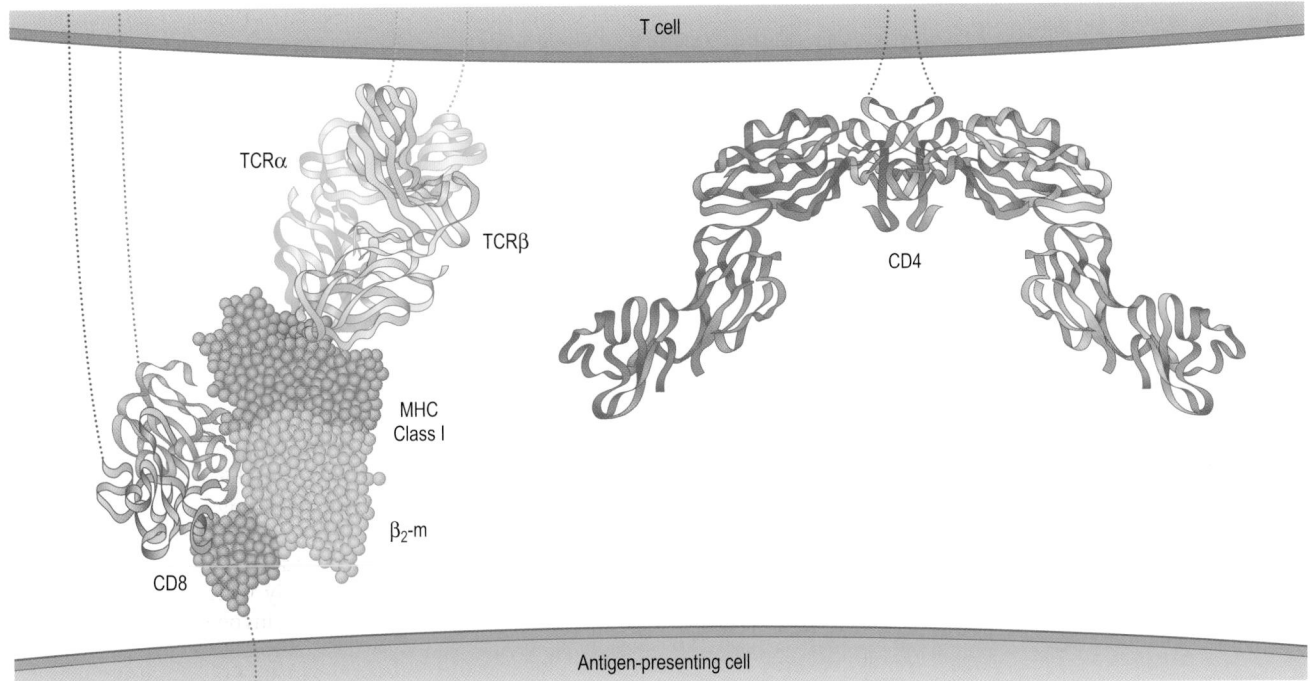

Fig. 4.15 Illustration of the interactions between the TCR, pMHC, and CD8. A composite illustration of the HLA-A*0201 structure in complex with a Tax peptide and its cognate T-cell receptor α and β chains (protein data bank (pdb) designation 1BD2) with the human CD8αα/HLA-A*0201 structure (pdb designation 1AKJ) was generated by superposition of the HLA moiety of the two structures. The HLA heavy chain is indicated as MHC, its light chain (β₂-microglobulin) as β₂-m, the CD8αα homodimer as CD8, the T-cell receptor α and β chains as TCRα and TCRβ. In addition, the CD4 homodimer (pdb file 1WIO) is shown to scale. Connecting peptides, transmembrane, and cytoplasmic domains are drawn by hand and indicated by dotted lines.

Figure courtesy of David H. Margulies, National Institute of Allergy and Infectious Diseases, National Institutes of Health.

the possibility that the CD3 chains lie within the open angle between TCRαβ and CD4, promoting interactions between CD3 chains and CD4-associated LCK.[71,73,74]

Experiments using soluble forms of CD4 and pMHC reveal that monomeric CD4 binds pMHC with very low affinity (Kd approximately 200 µM). The binding of CD4 to pMHC is of lower affinity than that TCRαβ to pMHC (Kd 1–10 µM) and displays a far more rapid off time. Because of the low affinity and the rapid off time, it is unlikely that interactions of CD4 with MHC class II molecules initiate the interaction between a T cell and an antigen-presenting cell. Rather, these binding characteristics are more compatible with a model in which the initial event is the interaction between the TCR and pMHC, followed by the recruitment of CD4, which acts primarily to promote signaling events through the delivery of LCK.[71,73,74]

CD8: structure and binding to MHC class I molecules

There are two CD8 polypeptides, α and β, and these are expressed on the cell-surface either as a disulfide-linked CD8αα homodimer or as a disulfide-linked CD8αβ heterodimer. On most αβ T cells, CD8αβ is the predominant form of CD8. However, natural killer (NK) cells (Chapter 17) and γδ T cells exclusively express CD8αα.[71,73–75]

CD8α, a 34- to 37-kDa protein, and CD8β, a 32-kDa protein, share about 20% amino acid sequence homology. Both are glycoproteins and IgSF members. Although CD8 subserves a co-receptor function similar to that CD4, in structure it differs substantially from CD4. The CD8 extracellular regions have single N-terminal IgSF V domains at the end of extended mucin-like stalk regions of 48 amino acids (CD8α) or 35–38 amino acids

(CD8β). A striking difference between the 2 forms of CD8 lies within the cytoplasmic domain. CD8α, like CD4, contains a cysteine-based motif that enables it to interact with LCK through a "zinc clasp"-like structure. In contrast, CD8β lacks this motif and does not associate with LCK. Interestingly, CD8αβ appears to be a more effective activator of TCR signaling than CD8αα. This may reflect the palmitoylation of the cytoplasmic domain of CD8β, which allows CD8αβ to associate with lipid rafts during T-cell activation.[71,73,74,76]

The structure of CD8αα–pMHC class I complexes demonstrates that CD8αα attaches primarily to the α3 domain of MHC class I (i.e., a non-polymorphic, membrane-proximal region of the molecule distinct from the peptide-binding groove engaged by the TCR) (Chapter 5). Compared to the interaction of CD4 and MHC class II, binding is more antibody-like, with a loop of the MHC α3 domain locked between the CDR-like loops of the two CD8α IgSF V domains. Models of the structure of the TCRαβ–pMHC–CD8 ternary complex propose a "V" shape similar to that of the model for TCRαβ–pMHC–CD4, with pMHC at the apex of the "V" and the TCR and CD8 forming the arms of the "V." CD8 binds to pMHC with lower affinity and with faster kinetics than the TCR. Thus, the binding properties of the CD8 co-receptor, like those of CD4, are consistent with a model in which the TCR initiates pMHC binding, followed by engagement of CD8 to the same pMHC.[71,73–76]

Co-stimulatory and inhibitory T-cell molecules: the CD28 family

Although the T-cell response to antigen requires the binding of the TCR and its co-receptors to pMHC, additional receptor-ligand interactions can affect the outcome by delivering signals

Table 4.4 CD28 superfamily

Receptor	Expression	Ligand	Function on T-cells
CD28	Most CD4 T cells 50% CD8 T cells	B7-1 (CD80) B7-2 (CD86)	Co-stimulation of IL-2 production and proliferation; Promotes T-cell survival
ICOS	Activated & memory T cells NK cells Not expressed by naïve T cells	ICOS ligand	Promotes T-cell differentiation and effector T-cell function
CTLA-4	Upregulated after T-cell activation	B7-1 (CD80) B7-2 (CD86)	Inhibits IL-2 production and proliferation; Promotes peripheral T-cell tolerance
PD-1	Upregulated after activation of T & B cells, myeloid cells	PD-L1 (B7-H1) PD-L2 (B7-DC)	Inhibits proliferations and cytokine production Promotes peripheral T-cell tolerance
BTLA	T & B cells, myeloid cells, dendritic cells	HVEM (herpesvirus-entry mediator)	Inhibits T-cell proliferation

CTLA-4 inhibits the response to TCR and CD28 signals and acts to terminate T-cell responses. T-cell activation induces CTLA-4, whose cell-surface expression is tightly regulated by the cytoplasmic motif YVKM. In the unphosphorylated state, this motif binds to AP-1 and AP-2 clathrin adaptor complexes that target CTLA-4 to intracellular compartments. Phosphorylation of the tyrosine releases the adaptor complexes and increases cell surface expression of CTLA-4.[77,79]

CD28 and CTLA-4 bind to the same ligands, B7.1 (CD80) and B7.2 (CD86), and interact with these B7 ligands through a conserved hydrophobic MYPPPYY motif in their extracellular domains. Nonetheless, CD28 and CTLA-4 differ in the valency of binding. CD28 is monovalent whereas CLTA-4 binds two B7 ligands. Moreover, the affinity of CTLA-4 for B7.1 and B7.2 is substantially greater than that of CD28.[78] Thus, the inhibitory complexes formed by CTLA-4, particularly those involving B7.1, are more stable that the co-stimulatory interactions involving CD28.

Inhibition of T-cell activation by CTLA-4 appears to involve competition for B7 ligands and the generation of intracellular signals. In addition, CTLA-4 can induce "reverse signaling" through B7.1 and B7.2 to the antigen-presenting cell, leading to the upregulation of the enzyme indoleamine 2,3-dioxygenase (IDO), which in turn breaks down tryptophan, a requirement for T-cell proliferation.[80]

The importance of CD28 co-stimulation has made it an attractive target for therapeutic intervention. Indeed, abatacept, a soluble fusion protein composed of the extracellular domain of human CTLA-4 and the constant regions of human IgG1, is an effective therapy for the treatment of rheumatoid arthritis (Chapter 51). Abatacept is thought to inhibit CD28 co-stimulation through blockade of its B7 ligands, but some of its immunosuppressive effects may be indirect through the induction of IDO and consequent local depletion of tryptophan.[81]

that promote activation (co-simulation) or that inhibit it (Table 4.4). Prominent among these are the interactions of members of the CD28 family with their cell-surface ligands on antigen-presenting cells. This family includes CD28, inducible co-stimulator (ICOS), cytotoxic T-lymphocyte-associated antigen-4 (CTLA-4), B- and T-lymphocyte attenuator (BTLA), and program death-1 (PD-1). CD28 and ICOS are co-stimulatory receptors; the major functions of CTLA-4, PD-1, and BTLA are inhibitory. CD28 and CTLA-4 are T-cell specific, whereas BTLA and PD-1 are also expressed by B cells and ICOS by NK cells.[77-79]

All members of the CD28 family have a single extracellular IgSF V domain and have, as their ligands, members of the B7 family of cell-surface molecules. CD28, CTLA-4, and ICOS are expressed on the cell-surface as disulfide-linked homodimers. Their cytoplasmic domains contain the SH2-binding motif YXXM. In contrast, PD-1 and BTLA are monomers whose cytoplasmic domains each contain an immunoreceptor tyrosine-based inhibitory motif (ITIM) and an immunoreceptor tyrosine-based switch motif (ITSM).

The best characterized members of the CD28 family are CD28 and CTLA-4. CD28 is the prototypic co-stimulatory receptor. Virtually all human CD4 T cells constitutively express CD28, as do half of the CD8 T cells. CD28 stimulation usually does not elicit a cellular response in the absence of TCR signaling. However, CD28 signals can act in concert with TCR signals to promote cytokine production, T-cell expansion, and T-cell survival. TCR signaling in the absence of CD28 co-stimulation can induce T-cell anergy (Chapter 12).

References

1. Williams AF, Barclay AN. The immunoglobulin superfamily–domains for cell surface recognition. Ann Rev Immunol 1988;6:381–405.
2. Padlan EA. Anatomy of the antibody molecule. Mol Immunol 1994;31(3):169–217.
3. Sanchez-Mazas A, Fernandez-Vina M, Middleton D, et al. Immunogenetics as a tool in anthropological studies. Immunology 2011;133(2):143–64.
4. Ehrenmann F, Kaas Q, Lefranc MP. IMGT/3Dstructure-DB and IMGT/DomainGapAlign: a database and a tool for immunoglobulins or antibodies, T cell receptors, MHC, IgSF and MhcSF. Nucleic Acids Res 2010;38(Database issue):D301–7.
5. Nelson AL. Antibody fragments: hope and hype. MAbs 2010;2(1):77–83.
6. Schroeder Jr. HW, Cavacini L. Structure and function of immunoglobulins. J Allergy Clin Immunol 2010;125(2 Suppl. 2):S41–52.
7. Johansen FE, Braathen R, Brandtzaeg P. Role of J chain in secretory immunoglobulin formation. Scand J Immunol 2000;52(3):240–8.
8. Chen FH, Arya SK, Rinfret A, et al. Domain-switched mouse IgM/IgG2b hybrids indicate individual roles for C mu 2, C mu 3, and C mu 4 domains in the regulation of the interaction of IgM with complement C1q. J Immunol 1997;159(7):3354–63.
9. Sensel MG, Kane LM, Morrison SL. Amino acid differences in the N-terminus of C(H)2 influence the relative abilities of IgG2 and IgG3 to activate complement. Mol Immunol 1997;34(14):1019–29.
10. Skvaril F, Schilt U. Characterization of the subclass and light chain types of IgG antibodies to rubella. Clin Exp Immunol 1984;55:671–6.
11. Barrett DJ, Ayoub EM. IgG2 subclass restriction of antibody to pneumococcal polysaccharides. Clin Exp Immunol 1986;63:127–34.
12. Otteson EA, Skvaril F, Tripathy SP, et al. Prominence of IgG4 in the IgG antibody response to human filiariasis. J Immunol 1985;134:2707–12.
13. Nirula A, Glaser SM, Kalled SL, Taylor FR. What is IgG4? A review of the biology of a unique immunoglobulin subtype. Curr Opin Rheum 2011;23(1):119–24.
14. Suzuki K, Ha SA, Tsuji M, Fagarasan S. Intestinal IgA synthesis: a primitive form of adaptive immunity that regulates microbial communities in the gut. Semin Immunol 2007;19(2):127–35.
15. Stone KD, Prussin C, Metcalfe DD. IgE, mast cells, basophils, and eosinophils. J Allergy Clin Immunol 2010;125(2 Suppl.):S73–80.
16. Davis MM, Bjorkman PJ. T-cell antigen receptor genes and T-cell recognition. Nature 1988;334:395–402.

17. Wucherpfennig KW, Gagnon E, Call MJ, et al. Structural biology of the T-cell receptor: insights into receptor assembly, ligand recognition, and initiation of signaling. Cold Spring Harb Perspect Biol 2010;2(4) a005140.

18. O'Brien RL, Roark CL, Jin N, et al. gammadelta T-cell receptors: functional correlations. Immunol Rev 2007;215:77–88.

19. Porcelli S, Brenner MB. Biology of the human gammadelta T-cell receptor. Immunol Rev 1991;120:137–83.

20. Marrack P, Rubtsova K, Scott-Browne J, Kappler JW. T cell receptor specificity for major histocompatibility complex proteins. Curr Opin Immunol 2008;20(2):203–7.

21. Krogsgaard M, Davis MM. How T cells "see" antigen. Nat Immunol 2005;6(3):239–45.

22. Rudolph MG, Stanfield RL, Wilson IA. How TCRs bind MHCs, peptides, and co-receptors. Annu Rev Immunol 2006;24:419–66.

23. Garcia KC, Degano M, Stanfield RL, et al. An alphabeta T cell receptor structure at 2.5 A and its orientation in the TCR-MHC complex. Science 1996;274(5285):209–19.

24. Davis MM. The evolutionary and structural "logic" of antigen receptor diversity. Semin Immunol 2004;16(4):239–43.

25. Cohen NR, Garg S, Brenner MB. Antigen presentation by CD1 lipids, T cells, and NKT cells in microbial immunity. Adv Immunol 2009;102:1–94.

26. Allison TJ, Garboczi DN. Structure of gammadelta T cell receptors and their recognition of non-peptide antigens. Mol Immunol 2002;39:1051–61.

27. Bonneville M, O'Brien RL, Born WK. Gammadelta T cell effector functions: a blend of innate programming and acquired plasticity. Nat Rev Immunol 2010;10(7):467–78.

28. Li H, Llera A, Malchiodi EL, Mariuzza RA. The structural basis of T cell activation by superantigens. Annu Rev Immunol 1999;17:435–66.

29. Tonegawa S. Somatic generation of antibody diversity. Nature 1983;302:575–81.

30. Krangel MS. Mechanics of T cell receptor gene rearrangement. Curr Opin Immunol 2009;21(2):133–9.

31. Schatz DG, Swanson PC. V(D)J recombination: mechanisms of initiation. Annu Rev Genet 2011;45:167–202.

32. Zachau HG. The immunoglobulin kappa gene families of human and mouse: a cottage industry approach. Biol Chem 2000;381(9–10):951–4.

33. Kirkham PM, Schroeder Jr. HW. Antibody structure and the evolution of immunoglobulin V gene segments. Semin Immunol 1994;6(6):347–60.

34. Lee SK, Bridges Jr. SL, Koopman WJ, Schroeder Jr. HW. The immunoglobulin kappa light chain repertoire expressed in the synovium of a patient with rheumatoid arthritis. Arthritis Rheum 1992;35:905–13.

35. Kawasaki K, Minoshima S, Nakato E, et al. One-megabase sequence analysis of the human immunoglobulin lambda gene locus. Genome Res 1997;7(3):250–61.

36. Vettermann C, Jack HM. The pre-B cell receptor: turning autoreactivity into self-defense. Trends Immunol 2010;31(5):176–83.

37. Matsuda F, Ishii K, Bourvagnet P, et al. The complete nucleotide sequence of the human immunoglobulin heavy chain variable region locus. J Exp Med 1998;188(11):2151–62.

38. Kracker S, Durandy A. Insights into the B cell specific process of immunoglobulin class switch recombination. Immunol Lett 2011;138(2):97–103.

39. Ganesh K, Neuberger MS. The relationship between hypothesis and experiment in unveiling the mechanisms of antibody gene diversification. Faseb J 2011;25(4):1123–32.

40. Tomlinson IM, Cox JP, Gherardi E, et al. The structural repertoire of the human V kappa domain. EMBO J 1995;14(18):4628–38.

41. Chothia C, Lesk AM, Gherardi E, et al. Structural repertoire of the human VH segments. J Mol Biol 1992;227:799–817.

42. Tomlinson IM, Walter G, Jones PT, et al. The imprint of somatic hypermutation on the repertoire of human germline V genes. J Mol Biol 1996;256(5):813–7.

43. Schroeder Jr. HW, Zemlin M, Khass M, et al. Genetic control of DH reading frame and its effect on B-cell development and antigen-specifc antibody production. Crit Rev Immunol 2010;30(4):327–44.

44. Arden B, Clark SP, Kabelitz D, Mak TW. Human T-cell receptor variable gene segment families. Immunogenetics 1995;42(6):455–500.

45. Jung D, Giallourakis C, Mostoslavsky R, Alt FW. Mechanism and control of V(D)J recombination at the immunoglobulin heavy chain locus. Annu Rev Immunol 2006;24:541–70.

46. Mostoslavsky R, Alt FW, Rajewsky K. The lingering enigma of the allelic exclusion mechanism. Cell 2004;118(5):539–44.

47. Nemazee D, Weigert M. Revising B cell receptors. J Exp Med 2000;191(11):1813–7.

48. Neuberger MS, Patel KJ, Dariavach P, et al. The mouse B-cell antigen receptor: definition and assembly of the core receptor of the five immunoglobulin isotypes. Immunol Rev 1993;132:147–61.

49. Wang LD, Clark MR. B-cell antigen-receptor signalling in lymphocyte development. Immunology 2003;110(4):411–20.

50. Pelanda R, Braun U, Hobeika E, et al. B cell progenitors are arrested in maturation but have intact VDJ recombination in the absence of Ig-alpha and Ig-beta. J Immunol 2002;169(2):865–72.

51. Mason DY, Cordell JL, Brown MH, et al. CD79a: a novel marker for B-cell neoplasms in routinely processed tissue samples. Blood 1995;86(4):1453–9.

52. Tsuganezawa K, Kiyokawa N, Matsuo Y, et al. Flow cytometric diagnosis of the cell lineage and developmental stage of acute lymphoblastic leukemia by novel monoclonal antibodies specific to human pre-B-cell receptor. Blood 1998;92(11):4317–24.

53. Gauld SB, Cambier JC. Src-family kinases in B-cell development and signaling. Oncogene 2004;23(48):8001–6.

54. Schamel WW, Reth M. Monomeric and oligomeric complexes of the B cell antigen receptor. Immunity 2000;13(1):5–14.

55. Niiro H, Clark EA. Regulation of B-cell fate by antigen-receptor signals. Nat Rev Immunol 2002;2(12):945–56.

56. Conley ME, Dobbs AK, Farmer DM, et al. Primary B cell immunodeficiencies: comparisons and contrasts. Annu Rev Immunol 2009;27:199–227.

57. Carroll MC. The role of complement and complement receptors in induction and regulation of immunity. Annu Rev Immunol 1998;16:545–68.

58. Fujimoto M, Poe JC, Inaoki M, Tedder TF. CD19 regulates B lymphocyte responses to transmembrane signals. Semin Immunol 1998;10(4):267–77.

59. Fearon DT, Carroll MC. Regulation of B lymphocyte responses to foreign and self-antigens by the CD19/CD21 complex. Annu Rev Immunol 2000;18:393–422.

60. Otero DC, Anzelon AN, Rickert RC. CD19 function in early and late B cell development: I. Maintenance of follicular and marginal zone B cells requires CD19-dependent survival signals. J Immunol 2003;170(1):73–83.

61. Dempsey PW, Allison ME, Akkaraju S, et al. C3d of complement as a molecular adjuvant: bridging innate and acquired immunity. Science 1996;271(5247):348–50.

62. Coggeshall KM. Positive and negative signalling in B lymphocytes. Curr Top Microbiol Immunol 2000;245:213–60.

63. Nimmerjahn F, Ravetch JV. Fcgamma receptors: old friends and new family members. Immunity 2006;24(1):19–28.

64. Ono M, Okada H, Bolland S, et al. Deletion of SHIP or SHP-1 reveals two distinct pathways for inhibitory signaling. Cell 1997;90(2):293–301.

65. Nitschke L. CD22 and Siglec-G: B-cell inhibitory receptors with distinct functions. Immunol Rev 2009;230(1):128–43.

66. Kuhns MS, Davis MM, Garcia KC. Deconstructing the form and function of the TCR/CD3 complex. Immunity 2006;24(2):133–9.

67. Schrum AG, Gil D, Turka LA, Palmer E. Physical and functional bivalency observed among TCR/CD3 complexes isolated from primary T cells. J Immunol 2011;187(2):870–8.

68. de Saint-Basile G, Geissmann F, Flori E, et al. Severe combined immunodeficiency caused by deficiency in either the delta or the epsilon subunit of CD3. J Clin Invest 2004;114(10):1512–7.

69. Roberts JL, Lauritsen JP, Cooney M, et al. T-B+NK+ severe combined immunodeficiency caused by complete deficiency of the CD3zeta subunit of the T-cell antigen receptor complex. Blood 2007;109(8):3198–206.

70. Recio MJ, Moreno-Pelayo MA, Kilic SS, et al. Differential biological role of CD3 chains revealed by human immunodeficiencies. J Immunol 2007;178(4):2556–64.

71. Gao GF, Rao Z, Bell JI. Molecular coordination of alphabeta T-cell receptors and coreceptors CD8 and CD4 in their recognition of peptide-MHC ligands. Trends Immunol 2002;23(8):408–13.

72. Palacios EH, Weiss A. Function of the Src-family kinases, Lck and Fyn, in T-cell development and activation. Oncogene 2004;23(48):7990–8000.

73. Wang JH, Reinherz EL. Structural basis of T cell recognition of peptides bound to MHC molecules. Mol Immunol 2002;38(14):1039–49.

74. van der Merwe PA, Davis SJ. Molecular interactions mediating T cell antigen recognition. Annu Rev Immunol 2003;21:659–84.

75. Artyomov MN, Lis M, Devadas S, et al. CD4 and CD8 binding to MHC molecules primarily acts to enhance Lck delivery. Proc Natl Acad Sci U S A 2010;107(39):16916–21.

76. Chang HC, Tan K, Ouyang J, et al. Structural and mutational analyses of a CD8alphabeta heterodimer and comparison with the CD8alphaalpha homodimer. Immunity 2005;23(6):661–71.

77. Riley JL, June CH. The CD28 family: a T-cell rheostat for therapeutic control of T-cell activation. Blood 2005;105(1):13–21.

78. Collins AV, Brodie DW, Gilbert RJ, et al. The interaction properties of costimulatory molecules revisited. Immunity 2007;17(2):201–10.

79. Bour-Jordan H, Esensten JH, Martinez-Llordella M, et al. Intrinsic and extrinsic control of peripheral T-cell tolerance by costimulatory molecules of the CD28/ B7 family. Immunol Rev 2011;241(1):180–205.

80. Grohmann U, Orabona C, Fallarino F, et al. CTLA-4-Ig regulates tryptophan catabolism in vivo. Nat Immunol 2002;3(11):1097–101.

81. Genovese MC, Becker JC, Schiff M, et al. Abatacept for rheumatoid arthritis refractory to tumor necrosis factor alpha inhibition. N Engl J Med 2005;353(11):1114–23.

Robert J.
Winchester

The major histocompatibility complex

The region of the genome that plays the central role in the regulation the adaptive immune response is termed the *major histocompatibility complex* (MHC). It is so designated because it was first identified as the site of numerous alternative genes, or *alleles*, that determined whether transplanted tissue would be compatible or rejected. Central among the well over one hundred genes now known to be situated in this region are a subgroup that encode what are termed *MHC molecules*. These are the *allotypic* molecules that were actually first recognized as markers of histocompatibility. In the human the genes encoding MHC molecules are alternatively termed *human leukocyte antigen* genes (HLA) and the MHC itself is sometimes termed the *HLA region*.

MHC molecules play a fundamental role in the adaptive immune system because they sample and bind small peptides derived from processed self-antigens, foreign antigens, and altered-self antigens and then present them on the cell surface where the MHC molecule bearing the peptide can then interact with a T-cell receptor (TCR) on the surface of the T cell. The interaction between MHC/peptide and the TCR plays a key role in the ability of the CD4 or CD8 T cell to recognize an infectious organism, or the products of such pathogens, as foreign. Conversely, major histocompatibility complex refers to the major role played by MHC molecules in determining the acceptability of transplanted cells or organs. Unexpectedly, however, the MHC molecules are also major determinants of susceptibility to autoimmune diseases.[1] This chapter explores the function of the various MHC genes and their polymorphisms in relation to these three quite different clinical features.

CLINICAL RELEVANCE

- MHC molecules regulate the recognition of particular pathogen peptides by CD4 and CD8 T cells in the adaptive immune response of immunity to infectious organisms.
- Certain MHC molecule allotypes are the major genetic determinants of susceptibility to many autoimmune diseases. This reflects the role of self-peptide and self-MHC in defining the recognition features of the T-cell arm of the adaptive immune system.
- MHC molecule allotypes play a key role in governing transplant rejection and appear to regulate placental development in pregnancy.

KEY CONCEPT

Perspective on the unique function of MHC molecules as a peptide binding and presenting structure

- The central role of the MHC is to function first as a receptor that binds a pathogen-derived peptide and then as ligand in the form of a p-MHC complex, which binds to the clonotypic T-cell receptor (TCR). There it triggers the activation and proliferation of the T cell in an adaptive immune response.
- As an evolutionary consequence of the plasticity of the TCR, which through thymic selection can adapt to a very large variety of p-MHC structures, the genes encoding the MHC are free to evolve a large number of genes encoding duplicated or alternative peptide presenting molecules with specificity to bind different peptides.
- This diversification of peptide presenting structures contrasts with the stereotyped structures of the innate immune system and fosters the development of different T-cell repertoires with completely different recognition properties. This thwarts the possibility that a pathogen will be able to evolve a way to bypass recognition.

Classical MHC molecules determine how T cells recognize processed antigen

Peptides derived from processed proteins of a pathogen or other antigen that are bound to classical MHC molecules average nine amino acids in length. Two or more of their amino acid side chains are used to anchor the peptide to pockets on the surface of the MHC. This complex ligand, which is composed of both the bound peptide and the presenting MHC molecule, or *p-MHC*, is the target of the TCR on the T-cell surface. Although the mode of TCR docking on MHC molecules is globally conserved, the shapes and chemical properties of the interacting surfaces found in these complexes are so diverse that no fixed pattern of contact has been recognized even between conserved TCR residues and conserved side chains of the MHC α-helices.[2] Indeed, of the amino acid side chains not bound to the MHC, only two or three are typically bound to the clonotypic TCR (Chapter 8). This limited contact yields considerable TCR plasticity, which has the important evolutionary implication of freeing the MHC molecule and the p-MHC complex from the strict stereochemical constraints that are usually imposed in receptor–ligand interactions. The consequence of TCR plasticity and this unusual receptor–ligand interaction has been the evolutionary development of a uniquely large number of different genes that encode various MHC structures, each of which is able to bind and present a different range of peptides to the same clonotypic TCR.

Peptides derived from external antigens, including pathogens, are typically absent during the formation of the T-cell repertoire in the thymus (Chapter 8). Thus self-peptide p-MHC complexes are used as surrogates for selecting, or training, individual T cells to recognize non-self-pathogen peptides.[3]

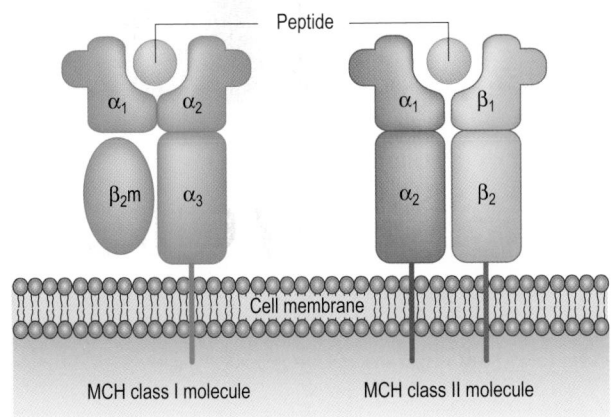

Fig. 5.1 MHC class I and II molecules have a homologous domain organization, but a different chain structure. Both class I and II molecules are expressed on the cell surface where they are accessible to T cells. The outermost domain contains a peptide-binding cleft that contains the peptide. In the case of class I molecules, a single alpha chain encodes the entire domain containing the peptide-binding cleft; while in class II molecules the domain is made up of an α- and a β-chain. These chains form supporting domains and anchor the molecule to the cell membrane. The class I molecule contains an extrinsic chain, β_2-microglobulin, that forms a separate domain.

For T cells, *immunologic self* is the set of self-peptides and self-MHC molecules that select the TCR repertoire. These self-peptides constitute the T-cell recognition component of an individual's adaptive immune system. This patterning of TCR recognition on self-peptides presented by self-MHC molecules is critical to the development of autoimmunity and allorecognition.

One basic task of the T cell is to protect the body from two major types of pathogens: viruses that would commandeer the replicative machinery of a cell, and bacteria that replicate autonomously and often extracellularly. These two types of pathogens present very different challenges to the immune system. To terminate viral infection, a cell harboring virus is killed by a cytotoxic CD8 T cell, whereas a bacterium can be eliminated by being phagocytized by a macrophage that has been selectively activated by a CD4 helper T cell that recognizes the peptides of this bacterium. The necessity of distinguishing between whether the presence of a pathogen peptide should elicit a killer or helper T-cell response is presumed to be the evolutionary drive that resulted in the creation of two specialized forms of MHC molecules, class I and class II (Fig. 5.1).[2,4]

The evolutionary consequence of the diversification of genes encoding MHC molecules is seen at two levels. The first is at the level of the *individual* and is characterized by the presence of different MHC class I and class II loci, each of which codes for one or more different peptide-presenting MHC molecules. The second is at the level of the *population* and is evidenced by the development of a very large number of alleles at each locus, with each allele coding for alternative polymorphic gene forms and thus for various peptide-presenting allotypes, each of which has the potential to bind a different set of peptides. Duplication of MHC genes involved in peptide presentation is a genetic strategy that increases the range of peptide-presenting structures available to the individual, thus enhancing the variety of presented peptides that can be recognized and bound.[5] There are three types of MHC class Ia (or classical class I) molecules, HLA-A, HLA-B, and HLA-C. These are encoded in three duplicated loci. HLA-B and HLA-C are quite near to each other in the primary sequence of the genome, whereas HLA-A is at some distance. Similarly, there are three types of class IIa (or classical class II) MHC molecules, HLA-DR, HLA-DQ, and HLA-DP. These are also encoded in three sets of duplicated loci (Fig. 5.2).[6] Each type

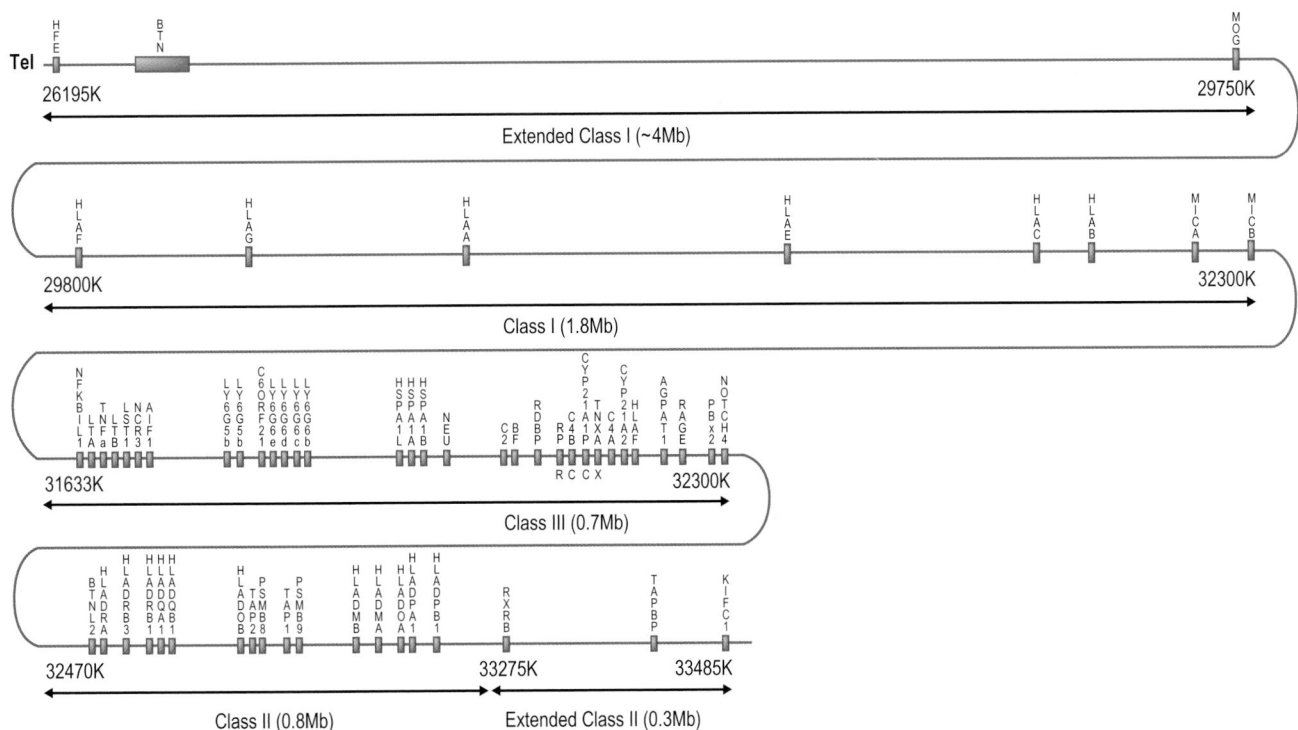

Fig. 5.2 Gene map of the extended HLA complex depicting the immune-related expressed genes, and certain reference genes. The HLA complex consists of five regions: extended class I, class I, class III, class II, and extended class II. Numbering of the sequence begins at the telomere. The approximate locations of genes near the start or end of the regions are indicated. The class III region is distinguished by genes for C2 and C4, TNF-α, and a cluster of genes in the LY6 family that were revealed in the sequencing of the genome. The genes of the RCCX region are indicated and the order of the principal duplicated genes shown. The expressed genes in the HLA-DR haplotypes encoding HLA-DR3, e.g., HLA-DRB1*03:01, are located within the class II region.
Modified from Beck S, Trowsdale J. The human major histocompatibility complex: lessons from the DNA sequence. Annu Rev Genomics Hum Genet 2000; 1: 117-137.

Table 5.1 Contrast of classical and non-classical MHC class I and II molecules

	MHC class			
	Ia	**Ib**	**IIa**	**IIb**
Polymorphism	High	Low	High	Low
Distribution	All nucleated cells	Restricted	Professional APCs	Restricted, endosome
Loci	HLA-A, B, C	HLA-E, G	HLA-DR, DQ, DP	HLA-DM, DO
Receptors	TCR αβ, γδ, KIR	CD94/NKG2A, C	TCR αβ	None, chaperone function
Presents	Many cytoplasmically self and non-self-derived peptides	Few peptides, e.g., class Ia leader	Peptides from ingested proteins and self-peptides	HLA-DR, DQ, DP

of MHC molecule in an individual selects its own repertoire of T cells that is restricted in its ability to react only to peptides presented in the context of the same type of MHC molecule. Because the genetic polymorphism of the MHC usually results in different maternal and paternal MHC genes, the range of MHC molecules can increase up to at least 12 separate types, each of which presents peptides to create 12 homologous TCR p-MHC-binding repertoires. The HLA region, located on the short arm of chromosome 6, also contains non-classical class Ib and class IIb genes, such as class Ib HLA-E and HLA-G and class IIb HLA-DM and HLA-DO (Fig. 5.2, Table 5.1).

The mechanism by which MHC class I and class II molecules present peptides became clear when the structures of these two molecules were determined. A simplified cartoon of the domain structure of MHC class I and class II proteins is depicted in Fig. 5.1. A more intricate ribbon structure of the actual class I molecule interacting with the TCR is presented in Chapter 4 (Fig. 4.3). For both class I and class II, the peptide-binding structure takes the shape of a beta-pleated floor with two alpha-helix walls. The peptide lies within the groove created by these structures (Figs. 5.3 and 5.4). Although the shapes of that portion of the class I and class II MHC molecules that interacts with the TCR are generally similar, the domain chain structures of the two types of molecule differ (Fig. 5.1). In the case of class I molecules, both halves of the peptide-binding domain of are encoded by the α-chain genes of the HLA-A, HLA-B, or HLA-C loci. β_2-Microglobulin, the partner chain for the class I heterodimer, has a purely structural role. For the class II molecules, however, one half of the peptide-binding domain is encoded by the α-chain and the other by the β-chain gene. The second domains of α- and β-chains create the pedestal upon which the peptide-binding domain rests. Thus, a genetic lesion of the β_2-microglobulin gene eliminates class I expression only. The class II α- and β-chains are both encoded within the MHC. The HLA-DRA, HLA-DQA, and HLA-DPA loci encode α-chains, while the HLA-DRB1, HLA-DQB1, and HLA-DPB1 (and often an additional DRB locus, commonly HLA-DRB3) loci code for the β-chains (Fig 5.2).

Among the evolutionary strategies used for viral survival, some virally encoded genes decrease the expression of the class I MHC surveillance system, which would otherwise alert the immune system to the presence of an infected cell (Chapters 17 and 27).[7] This attempt to escape surveillance by downregulation of class I MHC is countered by the extensive interaction of class I molecules with various NK receptors expressed on NK cells or T-cell subsets. These interactions provide a mechanism for detecting decreases in MHC class I expression, which is termed recognition of *missing self*.[8] There are two principal types of NK receptor used to detect missing self, members of the

immunoglobulin superfamily, such as killer immunoglobulin receptors (KIR), which bind directly to intact class I molecules, and members of the C type lectin family, such and CD94/NKG2C, which recognize the leader of class I molecules that selectively binds to HLA-E molecules (Table 5.1).

Biology and clinical consequences of the many MHC allotypes

Pathogens characterized by different proteins and peptides, either in different epidemics or endemic to regions, account for much of the evolutionary drive responsible for the large number of alternative gene forms and their regional diversity across the human race. An individual with an adaptive immune system based on MHC molecules that effectively bind peptides derived from common pathogens is much more likely to have an effective response against that common pathogen. This results in selection of individuals with a particular allotype, encoded by an allele.

● KEY CONCEPTS

Functional Biology of Classical MHC Genes

- T-cell recognition of processed peptides depends on the property of MHC molecules to bind small peptides through allotype-specific pockets that bind the amino acid side chains of the peptide.
- The *immunologic self* is the set of self-peptides and self-MHC molecules that select the TCR repertoire in the thymus and which constitute the T-cell recognition component of an individual's adaptive immune system.
- Non-self-peptide MHC complexes are recognized by T cells during an adaptive immune response.
- MHC class I and II MHC genes are extremely *polymorphic*. Each allele at each HLA locus encode molecules with different peptide-binding properties that influence the particular peptides recognized by the T cells and thereby determine the peptide recognition features of the adaptive immune response.
- MHC allotype polymorphisms are maintained by *frequency-dependent selection*, where the fitness of an individual bearing a common allele decreases because certain pathogens can adapt to the particular common structure and infect them more efficiently.

A *genetic polymorphism* implies that alleles of a gene are present at a frequency greater than expected from random mutation due to selection for diversity. In the case of the HLA genes, there

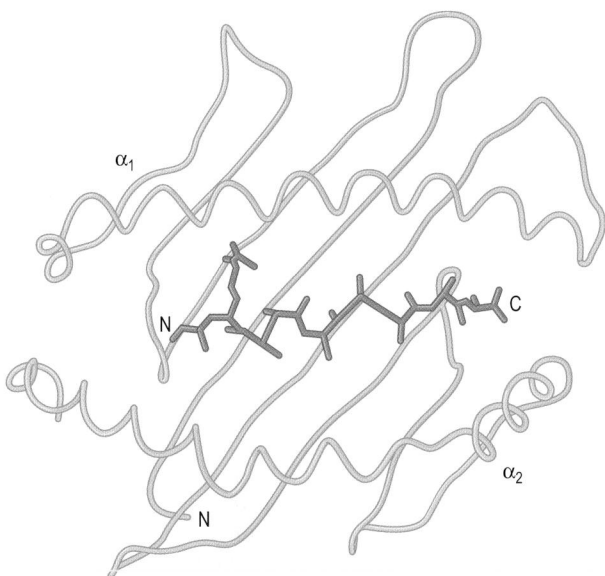

Fig. 5.3 The three-dimensional structure of HLA-B27. The α-helical margins of the peptide-binding cleft contain the bound peptide RRIKAITLK, which is oriented with its amino terminus to the left. There are extensive contacts at the ends of the cleft between peptide main-chain atoms and conserved MHC side chains, with the peptide amino and carboxyl termini tethered by H bonds and charge interactions. The peptide reciprocally stabilizes the three dimensional fold of HLA-B27. The side chain of arginine in the P2 position of the peptide inserts into the B pocket, which contains an oppositely charged glutamic acid at its base. The resulting salt bridge is the dominant anchor for the peptide. Side chains P4, P6, and P8 make minor contributions to the interaction of the peptide with the HLA-B27 molecule. The central region of the peptide is left free to interact with a TCR. Modified from Madden DR, Gorga JC, Strominger JL, Wiley DC. The three-dimensional structure of HLA-B27 at 2.1 A resolution suggests a general mechanism for tight peptide binding to MHC. Cell 1992; 70: 1035.

specific, but alternative, MHC molecules that differ in their binding pockets, present different peptides, and select different T-cell repertoires. This prevents the creation of antigen recognition structures shared by many individuals that a pathogen could readily counter by means of mutation. This illustrates *frequency-dependent selection*, where the fitness of an individual bearing a common allele decreases because certain pathogens can adapt to the particular common structure and more efficiently infect those bearing a common MHC peptide-binding structure. Moreover, selection also operates on the pathogen, encouraging peptide variation. Variation in peptides drawn from common pathogens, and the introduction of novel pathogens with novel peptides, results in pressure on the species to create variation in MHC molecules among individual members of that species. The remarkably different frequency of the HLA alleles in different ethnic subsets tells the history of the successful adaptation of our ancestors' adaptive immune systems to a new environment with different pathogens, as well as bottlenecks resulting from migration and perhaps survival during periods of massive epidemics.

MHC polymorphisms have clinical consequences. The large number of different HLA alleles greatly reduces the probability that two unrelated individuals will inherit an identical set of MHC genes, making the immunologic self close to unique for each unrelated individual. The phenomenon of near universal rejection of transplants between unrelated individuals is a reflection of this, because one person's T-cell repertoire will typically recognize another individual's self-peptide:MHC molecules as basically equivalent to a pathogen peptide:MHC complex. Thus, while it is the diversity of MHC allotypes that are recognized by the TCR repertoire of an individual, it is the TCR repertoire based on different MHC allotypes that is responsible for transplantation recognition.

Conversely, selection on self-peptide presented by self-MHC allotypes in the thymus can predispose to autoimmunity because the T-cell portion of the adaptive immune system is entirely selected on self-peptide. The inherent autoreactivity of the T-cell system can thus set the stage for the development of autoimmune

is no preponderant wild type allele, an example of *balancing selection*, and virtually all alleles qualify as genetically polymorphic. These reflect prior successful selection events. MHC polymorphisms provide a major evolutionary survival benefit, since they equip the species with a large number of very

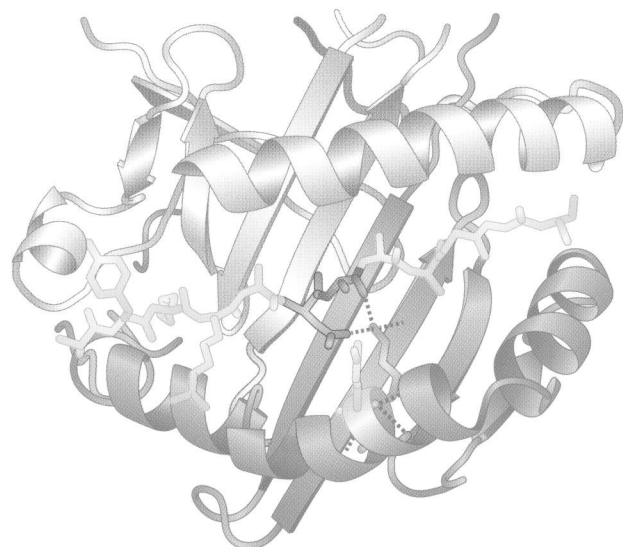

Fig. 5.4 Structure of a MHC class II molecule containing a peptide prepared using PyMol from published coordinates. The structure of the MHC molecule is largely shown as a ribbon diagram, while the peptide is a stick diagram. The peptide-binding groove is delimited by α-helices. The upper helix is encoded by the α-chain, and the lower helix by the β-chain. β-Pleated sheets form the saddle-like floor. Side chains are depicted on the β-chain at positions 70 and 71, a region involved in specifying the side chain pocket P4. This pocket binds the fourth side chain of the peptide contained within the MHC molecule. The side chains shown are respectively glutamine and lysine, which form part of the "shared epitope" structure associated with susceptibility to rheumatoid arthritis. The lysine is shown forming hydrogen bonds with the antigenic peptide.

diseases associated with the recognition of particular self-peptides, or peptides from external antigens that mimic these self-peptides and are ably presented by self-MHC.[9] The second key element is the important fact that certain alleles encode MHC molecules that bind peptides from molecules expressed in sites favoring autoimmune recognition by T cells. These target molecules become the focus of the adaptive immune response. Together, features specific to certain sets of self-peptides and to certain self-MHC molecules can contribute to the progressive development of autoimmunity, and ultimately autoimmune disease.

KEY CONCEPTS

Three features of the adaptive immune system set the stage for autoimmunity

- The first element is that the individual's adaptive immune system is determined by the set of self-peptides and self-MHC molecules that select the TCR repertoire. This contrasts with the pathogen-specific receptors of the innate immune system.
- The second element is the drive to genetic polymorphism that generates many different alternative forms of peptide-binding MHC molecules.
- The third element is that certain MHC allotypes bind particular self-peptides from critical target antigenic molecules. This can lead to the development of autoimmunity and autoimmune disease.

Principal genes of the MHC and their immunologic role

The MHC genes are organized into regions that perform different functions, but are inherited together in large blocks. The short arm of chromosome 6 (6p22.2-p21.3) contains the 3.6 million bases of the HLA complex, and this area is relatively enriched in genes interspersed among the HLA genes. Of the 128 expressed genes in the HLA complex, over 50 appear likely to have an immune function. According to the distribution of the HLA genes, it is subdivided into two principal regions (Fig. 5.2). The class I region is found at the telomeric end of the locus and is principally concerned with CD8 T-cell peptide recognition and NK cell recognition. The class II region is located at the centromeric end of the locus and is principally concerned with CD4 T-cell peptide recognition as well as the processing of peptides for class I molecules. The identification of additional genes of immunologic importance lying on either side of the classic MHC locus has extended these class I and class II regions, enlarging the MHC to a span of nearly 8 million bases. Interposed between the class I and II regions is the class III region, which also contains a number of genes that play different roles in the immune response, e.g., some complement components, TNF, etc.

peptide-binding portion of the molecule and the surface that interacts with the TCR or NKR (Fig. 5.1).

The ends of the class I peptide-binding cleft are closed and fix the peptide's orientation. The sides of the peptide-binding cleft are composed of α-helices and the floor is composed of symmetric strands of β-pleated sheet (Fig. 5.3). Two to three amino acid side chains of the peptide bind to pockets formed into the side and base of the groove. Consistent with their surveillance role for viral infections, classical class I molecules are expressed on nearly all nucleated cells. The expression of class I molecules is upregulated by α-, β-, and γ-interferons, GM-CSF and certain other cytokines. Expression is governed by the class I regulatory element (CRE) located ~160 nucleotides upstream from the initiation site that binds a number of regulatory factors, including those induced by interferons.

The MHC class Ia (classical) and Ib (non-classical) molecules have different functions and tissue distributions (Table 5.1). Class Ia genes are expressed on virtually all nucleated cells. Class Ib genes do not present non-self- peptide to the TCR of CD8 T cells and contain a very limited variety of self-peptides. These self-peptides include the leader peptide of the classical class Ia MHC molecules, and their binding to inhibitory receptors like CD94/NKG2A is an important part of the surveillance mechanism for missing self. Intact HLA-A, -B, or -C molecules are also ligands for a different group of NKR, the killer immunoglobulin receptors (KIR) (Chapter 17).[10,11]

HLA-G is highly expressed by placental trophoblast cells. HLA-F has a small binding cleft that does not contain peptide and its functions are not well understood. HFE, a member of the class I family, regulates iron absorption by controlling the interaction of the transferrin receptor with transferrin. HFE has a binding cleft that is too small to contain a peptide. HFE defects can lead to hereditary hemochromatosis or porphyria.

KEY CONCEPTS

Class I MHC genes

- The class I region contains the polymorphic *HLA-A*, *-B*, and *-C* genes and the less polymorphic, non-classical class Ib genes, *HLA-E*, *HLA-F*, and *HLA-G* genes.
- HLA-A, -B, and -C molecules are expressed on the surface of virtually all nucleated cells.
- HLA-A, -B, and -C are loaded with antigenic peptides derived from cytoplasmic proteins that are cleaved in the proteasome, and presented to clonal peptide-specific TCR of CD8 T cells.
- Each MHC allotype selects its own T-cell repertoire. Thus there are usually 6 different repertoires in a person's CD8 T cell population, each specialized for a maternal or paternally derived HLA-A, -B, and -C allotype.
- Class Ib molecules bind a very limited variety of self-peptides and engage lectin family natural killer receptors (NKR) in the recognition of *missing self*.

Class I MHC molecules

The genetically polymorphic 44-kDa α-chain of the, HLA-A, HLA-B or HLA-C, molecule is 362–366 amino acids long and consists of 5 domains. The ~30-amino-acid C-terminal cytoplasmic domain is connected to a ~25-amino-acid transmembrane domain (Fig. 5.1). The extracellular portion of the molecule consists of a ~90-amino-acid supporting stalk, the α_3 domain, and the similarly sized α_1 and α_2 domains that together form the

The class I region

The class I region also includes *MICA* and *MICB* (MHC class I polypeptide-related sequence A and B), the products of which are more distantly related members of the class I family that neither associate with β_2-microglobulin nor bind peptides.[5] These molecules are expressed as "danger signals" by virus-infected or otherwise stressed cells. MICA and MICB are ligands for the activating NKG2D molecule (*KLRK1*), another member of the killer cell lectin-like receptor complex[12] that appear on memory-effector T cells or NK cells, providing a signal to help activate their effector cytolytic response. Half of the expressed genes in the class I region have no apparent function in the immune system, including some ancient genes that antedate the development of the adaptive immune system.

HLA allele detection, nomenclature, and inheritance

The initial recognition of HLA molecules involved the use of human allosera that arose from alloimmunization during pregnancy or transplantation. The first nomenclature reflected the history of this discovery effort. Allosera were gradually supplanted by gel analysis and DNA-based methods. At the time this chapter was written, 6403 alleles of the class I and II HLA genes had been recognized. These include 1601 HLA-A, 2125 HLA-B, 1102 HLA-C, 10 HLA-E, 22 HLA-F, and 47 HLA-G named class I alleles, as well as 1027 HLA-DRB, 44 HLA-DQA1, 153 HLA-DQB1, 32 HLA-DPA1, and 149 HLA-DPB1 alleles. A modification of HLA terminology developed in 2010 has codified the allele designations in a manner that more directly corresponds with functional significance. The first element is the gene or locus name, e.g., HLA-B. This is followed by an asterisk separator mark and the usually two-digit allele group or allotype family, e.g., HLA-B*27. This in turn is followed by a colon field separator mark and the usually two- or three-digit designation of the allele subtype, which results in a distinct HLA protein due to a non-synonymous coding change, e.g., HLA-B*27:05. Additional colon field separator marks are used to separate additional features, such as noncoding changes that distinguish the nearly 100 HLA-B*27 alleles, e.g., HLA-B*27:05:02. Sequencing has also revealed null alleles that contain stop codons, e.g., HLA-B*27:59 N. Since there is no transcribed and expressed product, individuals with this null allele are not tolerized to determinants expressed by HLA-B*27 molecules and may make a strong alloimmune response to tissue expressing a non-null HLA-B*27 allotype. Different alleles occur at highly different frequencies among different ethnic and racial groups reflecting earlier success in surviving epidemics, founder effects, and more recent genetic admixture.

An important genetic principle of the MHC is that its many genes are not inherited separately. Large regions of the MHC are virtually devoid of crossing over, with certain alleles of different gene loci inherited together far more frequently than expected from the product of their frequencies, a phenomenon termed *linkage disequilibrium*.[13] The haplotype is the unit of inheritance of the MHC from either parent. For most haplotypes, linkage disequilibrium extends over the entire extended MHC, so that large groups of genes with distinct functions are inherited together. There is an evident strong selective pressure that has apparently maintained these ancestral haplotypes over millennia and suggests that particular alleles on a haplotype function cooperatively in the adaptive immune response. This linkage of many polymorphic alleles makes it difficult to identify the genes within the MHC that determine disease susceptibility or a particular immnophenotype.[1] The particular combinations of alleles in a haplotype and the frequency of the given haplotype vary among different populations, reflecting distant selection by pathogens, genetic bottlenecks, and ethnic admixture.

One should also be aware that there are two ways of counting the frequency of HLA alleles or haplotypes: allele (haplotype) or phenotype (genotype) frequency. The allele frequency counts the number of alleles per haploid chromosome, totaling 100% or 1.0. It is usually used in genetic literature. The phenotype frequency, which is identical to the genotype frequency in the case of HLA, enumerates the frequency of alleles in a population of diploid individual, considers both the maternal and paternal haplotypes, and totals up to 200%. The genotype frequency is the clinically relevant number for disease associations.

The genetic relationships among members of a family are important for disease inheritance and transplantation. Each parent shares one haplotype with each of their children and typically differs from a child by one haplotype. Two siblings may share two, one, or no haplotypes, and thus range from being HLA-identical, through haplo-identical, to HLA-disparate. A parent is usually only haploidentical with their child. Exceptions to this rule will occur most frequently in inbred populations, where both parents may share an identical MHC allele by descent.

Peptide-binding function

The peptide is a critical structural component of the classical class I and II MHC molecules. If a peptide is not loaded into a molecule or somehow escapes from the binding groove, the molecule becomes unstable and disassociates into its component chains.

Binding to MHC class I molecules follows several rules. Usually peptides are 9 amino acids in length and are always oriented with their NH_2 terminus to the "left" (Fig. 5.3). Allotypes are generally distinguished by different patterns of peptide binding, as illustrated for selected HLA-B molecules in Table 5.2.[14] In class I molecules, one or a few amino acid changes may alter considerably the functional consequences of a pocket and confer different binding properties. The table illustrates three motifs. In a healthy non-endocytosing cell, MHC molecules are filled with a variety of peptides from self-molecules, with the peptides selected according to the binding motif of the particular allotype. Even during viral infection or upon pathogen phagocytosis the number of non-self-peptides may not be high.

The biological consequences of the different patterns of peptide binding shown in Table 5.2 are significant. In the response to HIV-1 (Chapter 37), the presence of HLA-B*27 is associated with long-term non-progression to AIDS, while HLA-B*35 denotes rapid progressors.[15] Table 5.2 shows that 15 different peptides in a particular HIV envelope molecule can bind to the HLA-B*27 molecule, while no peptide contains motifs that preferentially bind to HLA-B*35. The HIV infection is controlled by a CD8 T-cell response in the long-term non-progressor for a period of years, and the length of this time is proportional to the number of viral peptides recognized.[16] Presumably one of the peptides bound by HLA-B*27 is in a part of a viral structure, such as an enzyme active site, or critical ligand, where a change in amino acid confers a selective disadvantage on the virus.

● ON THE HORIZON

Individualized MHC-based medicine

- Continued definition of the peptide-binding properties of individual MHC alleles.
- Continued definition of the epitopes expressed by pathogens and other antigens of interest.
- Use of genetic and sequencing technologies to identify individual MHC haplotypes and thus better predict immune responses to pathogens and vaccines.

Table 5.2 The peptide-binding motifs encoded by different HLA alleles influence the number of peptides in a protein that can be recognized by a MHC molecule (e.g., HIV envelope protein)

Allele designation:	HLA-B*27:05	HLA-B*35:01	HLA-B*07:02
Peptide binding motif	XRXXXXXX [KRYL]	XPXXXXXY	XPXXXXXL
Peptides from the HIV envelope protein able to bind to each allotype	IRGKVQKEY IRPVVSTQL TRPNNNTRK IRIQRGPGR SRAKWNNTL LREQFGNNK FRPGGGDMR WRSELYKYK KRRVVQREK ARILAVERY ERDRDRSIR LRSLCLFSY TRIVELLGR CRAIRHIPR IRQGLERIL	None	DPNPQEVVL KPCVKLTPL RPVVSTQLL SPLSFQTHL IPRRIRQGL
Number of peptides bound	15	0	5

Single-letter amino acid codes are used. X denotes any amino acid; R, arginine; K, lysine; Y, tyrosine; L, leucine; P, proline, etc.

Autoimmune disease

One of the more extraordinary observations in the MHC field was made in 1973 when the frequency of HLA specificity HLA-B27 was found to be 95% in those with the disease *ankylosing spondylitis* compared to around 5% in healthy controls. The odds of being HLA-B*27 positive if one has ankylosing spondylitis are thus $0.95/0.05 = 19$, and the odds of being HLA-B*27 positive if one is a control are $0.05/0.95 = 0.053$. Thus, the odds of developing ankylosing spondylitis if one is HLA-B*27 positive is $19/0.053 = 358:1$, an impressive observation that implicates HLA-B*27 in the pathogenesis of this disease. However, there are several points about this to emphasize. First, ankylosing spondylitis is a relatively rare disease with a prevalence of ~130 per 100 000, or 0.013%. Consequently, for every HLA-B27 patient with ankylosing spondylitis there are over 4 000 healthy HLA-B*27-positive persons without the disease $(5.0/(0.013 \times 0.95)$. Second, it is quite clear that the HLA-B*27 allele conferring susceptibility does not differ from the "wild-type" allele found in the healthy population and is also positively selected in the overall population. Third, there are over 90 alleles of HLA-B*27, of which HLA-B*27:05 is the most common; and most, but not all, of these alleles are associated with susceptibility to ankylosing spondylitis. The B27 molecules associated with susceptibility are often distinguished by the presence of a cysteine in the P2 pocket that potentially can dimerize to another HLA-B27 molecule. The dimeric B27 molecule is recognized by a particular KIR and can trigger an inflammatory response.[17] This allotype also has a tendency to fold slowly and somewhat unstably, as well as a peptide-binding motif that often recognizes a large proportion of peptides.

The class II region

The genes of the class II region are almost exclusively concerned either with recognition of peptide expressed by CD4 T cells or with processing of peptides for class I molecules. In the course of an immune response, non-self-proteins are endocytosed by "professional" phagocytes, processed and reduced to non-self-peptides, and presented by class II molecules expressed on these cells for recognition by the TCRs of CD4 T cells (Chapter 6).

Of the 18 expressed HLA genes in the class II region (Fig. 5.1, Table 5.1), eleven encode either the α-chains, HLA-DPA, HLA-DQA, and HLA-DRA; or the β chains, HLA-DPB, HLA-DQB, HLA-DRB1, HLA-DRB3 of the HLA-DP, HLA-DQ, and HLA-DR molecules; or the analogous α and β chains of HLA-DM and HLA-DO molecules.[5] With the exception of HLA-DRA, classical class II molecules are highly polymorphic. As with class I molecules, this polymorphism determines the particular peptides they present to CD4 T cells, thus regulating the CD4 T-cell immune response. The non-polymorphic non-classical class II molecules HLA-DM and HLA-DO are exclusively expressed in endosomes. They regulate peptide binding to the classical MHC class II molecules. HLA-DM, a peptide editor, plays a central role in peptide loading of MHC class II molecules.[18] HLA-DO interacts with HLA-DM, but its expression is more restricted.

The products of four genes in the class II region are involved with processing and loading peptides onto class I molecules (see Fig. 5.1 above). PSMB8 and PSMB9 are proteasome subunits and TAP1 and TAP2 transport the peptides from the cytoplasm to the endoplasmic reticulum.

KEY CONCEPTS

Class II MHC genes

- The class II region contains the genes encoding HLA-DR, DQ and DP molecules, which bind peptides recognized by CD4 T cells, and PSMB8, PSMB9, TAP1, and TAP2, which help process peptides for class I molecules.
- During the synthesis of MHC class II molecules, occupation of the peptide-binding groove by the N terminal part of the invariant chain prevents the binding of self-peptides. This structure also directs the class II molecule to the endosome.
- MHC class II molecules are constitutively expressed on B cells, professional antigen presenting cells (APC), thymic epithelial cells, and activated T cells.
- Interferon-γ induces the expression of MHC class II molecules on a wide variety of stromal, parenchymal, and vascular cells.

Class II molecules

Unlike class I molecules, which encode the peptide-binding pocket in a single protein chain, class II molecules are constructed from two structurally homologous α and β chains that each contributes half of the peptide-binding groove (Fig. 5.1). Both of these chains are encoded within the MHC. The α_2 domain of the α-chain contributes the left four strands of the β-pleated sheet floor and the upper α-helix, while the β_2 domain of the β chain contributes the right four strands of the β-pleated sheet floor and the lower α-helix (Fig. 5.4). The α_3 and β_3 domains, similar to the class I α_3 domain, form a supporting stalk and are each connected to trans-memebrane and intracytoplasmic domains (Fig. 5.1).

The peptide-binding region differs from that of the class I molecule in that the antigen-binding groove is open at both ends.

Thus, the MHC class II heterodimer does not interact with either the N or C terminus of the peptide. Accordingly, the MHC class II binding peptides may be of varying lengths, up to about 30 amino acids, and their N and C termini extend outwards from the peptide-binding groove (Fig. 6.2). Side chains in the middle of the peptide tether it to pockets in the center portion of the peptide-binding groove (Fig. 5.4).

In HLA-DP and HLA-DQ molecules, both the α- and β-chains are polymorphic and each contributes to overall peptide-binding characteristics of the molecule. The α- and β-chains in HLA-DP and HLA-DQ can come either from genes on the same haplotype, *cis*, or from the α- and β-chain genes on opposite haplotypes, *trans*. This complementation between genes encoded by different parental haplotypes generates novel MHC molecules with peptide-binding characteristics not found in either parent. These novel MHC molecules select additional T-cell repertoires that operate in parallel to the other T-cell repertoires. This mechanism is clinically relevant and is involved in the determination of *celiac disease* susceptibility, where the inheritance of the DQA1*05:01 allele and the DQB1*02:01 allele confers disease risk whether or not the genes are inherited on the same paternal or maternal haplotype, where they are encoded in *cis*, or through *trans* complementation.

The structure of the DR region between DRA and DRB1 is a complex polymorphic region that varies across different haplotypes.[5] While all MHC haplotypes have a single DRB1 locus, additional DRB genes are found in most, but not all haplotypes. These additional genes vary in number and position reflecting their origin by duplication and recombination events. The DRB3 locus is present in DRB1*03 and *11, *12, *13, and *14 haplotypes and encodes the HLA-DRw52 specificity. The DRB4 locus is present in evolutionarily more ancient DRB1*04, *07, and *09 haplotypes, and encodes the DRw53 specificity. The DRB5 locus is present in DRB1*15 and DRB1*16 haplotypes and encodes the DRw51 specificity.

The expression of MHC class II molecules is much more intricately regulated than that of class I MHC.[19] In addition to professional phagocytes, class II molecules are expressed on thymic epithelial cells and activated T cells. Interferon-γ expression occurring during tissue infiltration by activated T cells or NK cells also induces MHC class II molecule expression on a wide variety of stromal, parenchymal, and vascular cells. The MHC class II molecule expression is regulated within a lineage according to developmental stage. In the myeloid lineage, committed neutrophil progenitors express class II molecules through the myeloblast stage. Expression diminishes upon maturation of monocytes to macrophages, unless it is re-induced by interferon-γ. MHC class II is expressed on B cells but that expression is lost upon their differentiation into plasma cells.

Expression of class II molecules is regulated by a promoter located within 150 base pairs of the transcription initiation site in exon 1. A variety of cooperative *trans*-acting factors bind to the promoter. MHC2TA is a critical co-activator for MHC class II expression that binds to these subunits. Genetic defects in the expression of these factors results in the *bare lymphocyte syndrome*. MHC2TA is induced in activated T cells and by interferon-γ, resulting in upregulation of class II MHC expression. This upregulation is opposed by Th2 or anti-inflammatory cytokines such as TGF-β, IL-4, and IL-10.

Class II-associated autoimmune diseases

Susceptibility to a large number of autoimmune diseases, especially those characterized by autoantibodies, is influenced by a number of MHC class II alleles. The inheritance of *rheumatoid arthritis* is an interesting instance where susceptibility maps to a set of HLA-DRB1 alleles, all of which are intriguingly characterized by a similar amino acid motif involving neutral or positively charged amino acids around position 70–74 in the β-chain that has been designated the *shared epitope*.[20,21] In Fig. 5.4 the yellow-colored residue in the α-helical ribbon is glutamine and the magenta residue is positively charged lysine. It is seen hydrogen bonding to two side chains in the peptide. The region around position 70 is involved in the formation of a peptide side chain binding pocket that binds the fourth amino acid side chain contained within the MHC molecule. The presence of a negatively charged residue at position 71 or 74 removes susceptibility for rheumatoid arthritis. The presence of two alleles of this group increases susceptibility and favors development of more severe disease.[22] DRB1*01:01, *04:01, *04:04, *04:05, *04:08, *10:01, and *14:02 all encode a similar motif of neutral and positively charged residues in this region that confer susceptibility to rheumatoid arthritis.

The class III region

The MHC class III region is the shortest (0.7 Mb), most gene dense (58 genes; one every ∼15 kbp of DNA), and evolutionarily the most ancient and stable within the MHC since it contains highly conserved genes and the fewest pseudogenes.[5] It is delimited by the telomeric *BAT1* and the centromeric *NOTCH4*. Among the immune-related genes are three encoding complement components C2, fB, and C4; three members of the TNF family, TNF, LTA, and LTB; members of the Ly6 superfamily; three genes encoding heat shock protein; and the gene for the receptor for advanced glycation products, RAGE. Among non-immune genes is 21-hydroxylase (*CYP*).

With one major exception, there is little evidence of gene duplication in the class III region. The exception is the polymorphic subregion that contains the C4 and 21-hydroxylase loci. The duplicated C4 gene results in two functionally different forms, C4A (acidic) and C4B (basic) (Chapter 20). Some individuals may lack either the C4A or C4B gene and the variation in copy number of the C4 gene, mainly between 2 and 6 copies, contributes to the large range of stable normal C4 levels. Similarly the 21-hydroxylase gene is duplicated, as *CYP21A*, a pseudogene, and *CYP21B*.[23]

Extended class I and class II regions

The most telomeric member of the class I family, *HFE*, marks the beginning of the extended class I region that ends with *MOG*.[24] It also contains two clusters of olfactory receptor genes that have been considered to play a part in mating choice, and could influence selection of polymorphic HLA genes.[25] The presence of linkage disequilibrium also extends centromeric from the MHC to kinesin family member C1, *KIFC*. This region contains *TAPBP*, TAP binding protein (tapasin), a transmembrane glycoprotein that mediates interaction between newly assembled MHC class I molecules by binding to TAP1.

Future learning and resources:

This chapter provides only a limited sketch of this fascinating, but complex, topic. The reader is referred to the *HLA Facts Book* for a more detailed and very accessible presentation, though slightly out of date.[6] There are also a number of websites with extremely useful information. Four stand out in terms of their utility and the curated quality of the information. The IMGT/HLA Database contains all MHC sequences and has a variety of sequence alignments of different alleles as well as specialized sequence searches, http://www.ebi.ac.uk/imgt/hla/index.html. The NCBI maintains dbMHC, which includes several components of the international histocompatibility working group (IHWG) that are of interest. Among these are the anthropology database that contains HLA class I and class II allele and haplotype frequencies in various human populations: http://www.ncbi.nlm.nih.gov/projects/mhc/. Information about the genes and the genetic organization of the MHC is contained in several sites, but perhaps the most comprehensive and comprehensible is that using the Entrez search engine: http://www.ncbi.nlm.nih.gov. A comprehensive database of MHC ligands and peptide motifs is located at http://www.syfpeithi.de.

References

1. Trowsdale J. HLA genomics in the third millennium. Curr Opin Immunol 2005;17:498–504.
2. Housset D, Malissen B. What do TCR-pMHC crystal structures teach us about MHC restriction and alloreactivity? Trends Immunol 2003;24:429–37.
3. Stefanova I, Dorfman JR, Tsukamoto M, Germain RN. On the role of self-recognition in T cell responses to foreign antigen. Immunol Rev 2003;191:97–106.
4. Trowsdale J, Parham P. Mini-review: defense strategies and immunity-related genes. Eur J Immunol 2004;34:7–17.
5. Beck S, Trowsdale J. The human major histocompatibility complex: lessons from the DNA sequence. Annu Rev Genomics Hum Genet 2000;1:117–37.
6. Marsh SGE, Parham P, Barber LD. The HLA facts book. San Diego: Academic Press; 2000.
7. Lilley BN, Ploegh HL. Viral modulation of antigen presentation: manipulation of cellular targets in the ER and beyond. Immunol Rev 2005;207:126–44.
8. Raulet DH. Missing self recognition and self tolerance of natural killer (NK) cells. Semin Immunol 2006;18:145–50.
9. Winchester R. The genetics of autoimmune-mediated rheumatic diseases: clinical and biologic implications. Rheum Dis Clin North Am 2004;30:213–27, viii.
10. Kelley J, Walter L, Trowsdale J. Comparative genomics of natural killer cell receptor gene clusters. PLoS Genet 2005;1:129–39.
11. Parham P. Immunogenetics of killer cell immunoglobulin-like receptors. Mol Immunol 2005;42:459–62.
12. Lanier LL. On guard—activating NK cell receptors. Nat Immunol 2001;2:23–7.
13. Stewart CA, Horton R, Allcock RJ, et al. Complete MHC haplotype sequencing for common disease gene mapping. Genome Res 2004;14:1176–87.
14. Lund O, Nielsen M, Kesmir C, et al. Definition of supertypes for HLA molecules using clustering of specificity matrices. Immunogenetics 2004;55:797–810.
15. Winchester RJ, Charron D, Louie L, et al. The role of HLA in influencing the time of development of a particular outcome of HIV-1 infection, In: Charron D, editor. Proceedings of the Twelfth International Histocompatibility Workshop and Conference Sèvres, France EDK; 1997.
16. McMichael AJ, Ogg G, Wilson J, et al. Memory CD8+ T cells in HIV infection. Philos Trans R Soc Lond B Biol Sci 2000;355:363–7.
17. Bowness P, Ridley A, Shaw J, et al. Th17 cells expressing KIR3DL2+ and responsive to HLA-B27 homodimers are increased in ankylosing spondylitis. J Immunol 2011;186:2672–80.
18. Karlsson L. DM and DO shape the repertoire of peptide-MHC-class-II complexes. Curr Opin Immunol 2005;17:65–70.
19. Ting JP, Trowsdale J. Genetic control of MHC class II expression. Cell 2002;109(Suppl): S21–33.
20. Winchester R. The molecular basis of susceptibility to rheumatoid arthritis. In: Advances in Immunology, vol. 56. San Diego: Academic Press; 1994. p. 389–466.
21. Goronzy JJ, Weyand CM. Rheumatoid arthritis. Immunol Rev 2005;204:55–73.
22. Michou L, Croiseau P, Petit-Teixeira E, et al. Validation of the reshaped shared epitope HLA-DRB1 classification in rheumatoid arthritis. Arthritis Res Ther 2006;8:R79.
23. Gruen JR, Weissman SM. Human MHC class III and IV genes and disease associations. Front Biosci 2001;6:D960–72.
24. Horton R, Wilming L, Rand V, et al. Gene map of the extended human MHC. Nat Rev Genet 2004;5:889–99.
25. Ehlers A, Beck S, Forbes SA, et al. MHC-linked olfactory receptor loci exhibit polymorphism and contribute to extended HLA/OR-haplotypes. Genome Res 2000;10:1968–78.

Antigens and antigen presentation

John R. Rodgers,
Robert R. Rich

Antigens

By the late nineteenth century, "antibodies" were the hypothesized molecular entities that mediated specific immune memory, could neutralize toxins, and resulted in the formation of precipitates when mixed with the molecular species that induced their formation. In almost all cases, evidence for the presence of such antibodies required the prior exposure of responding animals to the very substances (or ones closely related, as in the case of toxoids) with which the antibodies reacted. This *specific* relationship of inducing agent and antibody led to the concept of an *antigen:* that molecular entity that could induce, in the blood of exposed animals, the formation of antibodies specific for it. By inventing the concept of the specific *receptor*, with a specificity analogous to the lock-and-key model of enzymes, Paul Ehrlich could explain the specificity of antibodies in molecular terms of a reciprocal interaction between receptor and its binding partner (*ligand*).[1] This explanation, though refined by methodological advances in biochemistry and molecular biology, has become a fact: an "antigen" is any molecule that binds specifically to the antigen-binding domain of an "antigen receptor" (antibody or T-cell receptor — TCR). This view of "antigen" is that of the investigator who uses antibodies as biochemical tools for detection or purification of some molecule of interest.

In contrast, Ehrlich proposed several tantalizing but unsatisfying explanations for the other critical property of antigens: that they *induce* the formation of their own antibodies. This view of "antigen" is that of the vaccinologist, who wants to induce effective immunity to an organism expressing that antigen, or of a clinician wondering why a patient does or does not respond to a particular allergen, self-antigen or tumor antigen. More than a century later, explaining the antigenicity of antigens remains an important and ongoing problem — why we fail to respond adequately to some pathogen or tumor antigens and how we can improve vaccines; why we respond to our own self-antigens (autoantigens) or antigens present in tissue grafts (alloantigens) and how we can prevent or treat autoimmune and tissue graft-related diseases (graft-versus-host disease (GVHD) and graft rejection). The cellular mechanisms governing how and when we respond to antigens remains at the cutting edges of both laboratory science and clinical medicine.

As a result of advances in the domain of *innate immunity*, it has become challenging, but all the more important, to distinguish between antigens and the many ligands for innate immune receptors (Chapter 3). Innate receptor ligands are often described as exhibiting patterns or motifs characteristic of a microbial class or physiological condition. To capture these notions Janeway[2] and Matzinger[3] coined the terms "pathogen-associated molecular patterns" (PAMP) and "danger signals," respectively. A prototypical innate ligand is lipopolysaccharide (endotoxin),

produced by many bacteria and a ligand for Toll-like receptor 4. Another is dsRNA, an obligatory intermediate in RNA virus replication and a ligand for TLR3. Both have features characteristic of a pathogen class. However, a variety of ligands that bind to TLR4 that have no obvious "motif" shared with LPS. Moreover, danger signals also do not exhibit an obvious "motif" but instead can be merely characteristic of a physiological state. For example, the receptor for advanced glycan intermediates, RAGE, is also a receptor for HMGB1, a nuclear transcription factor released to function as an inflammatory cytokine by macrophages. Thus, it is problematic to define innate receptor ligands in terms of intrinsic properties. Moreover, ligands for innate receptors can also be ligands for antigen receptors. Consequently, the conceptual difference between antigens and innate receptor ligands depends not on intrinsic properties of the ligands, but on the properties of the receptors to which they bind.

It has become a cottage industry to reveal "bridges" between innate and acquired immunity, blurring the formerly clear-cut distinctions between the two. Moreover, we see an a continual expansion of the function of innate receptors as registrars of states of internal stress (Matzinger's "danger") rather than as primarily monitors of external threats (Janeway's "stranger"). It is thus useful to see the categories of innate and acquired immune receptors as a continuum rather than as essentially distinct and in need of "bridges."

At one extreme, purely innate receptors are expressed constitutively among tissues and over time. They are present in the "ground state" of the organism and thus are innate. They function like most other receptors of the body to respond homeostatically to perturbations in the internal milieu of the organism, particularly to an experience of physiologic stress to immunologic homeostasis, but also to a molecular threat of stress as flagged by microbial products.

At the other extreme, acquired receptors are pleomorphic rather than unimorphic, inducible rather than constitutive. In the case of the two acquired immune receptors defined in mammals, antibodies and T-cell receptors, the induction is mediated by irreversible changes in the DNA sequence encoding them. The function of acquired immune receptors (antigen receptors) is to record exposure to an inciting antigen and thus mediate specific immune memory: the "faster, stronger" response of a secondary immune response. In particular, many T- and B-cell responses are accompanied by rapid proliferation of those cells expressing unique and specific antigen receptors (clonal selection and expansion).

In so-called "bridge" mechanisms, we see aspects of short-term memory (often called "priming") effected by innate mechanisms and acquired mechanisms that fail to exhibit memory. Thus, preexposure to activation of certain Toll-like receptors can lead to enhanced responses through the same or other innate receptors over a period of half a day, and some T- and B-cell responses exhibit a strong "primary" response to antigen without evidence of an enhanced memory responses. Likewise, priming through innate receptors is a critical mechanism for enhancing acquired immunity.

This chapter is organized around five themes: *antigen*, how antigens are manipulated by cellular and enzymatic machinery to permit recognition by antigen receptors (*antigen acquisition*, *processing*, and *presentation*), and, finally, the *antigen-presenting cells* (APC) themselves. A central function of APC is to present antigens to antigen-receptors on lymphocytes (signal 1) but also to provide co-stimulatory signals (signal 2) and regulatory signals (signal 3) to those lymphocytes.

Antigens in the sense of *ligand* are defined tautologically as the ligands for antigen receptors (Fig. 6.1). This definition includes the *acquired* antigen receptors found on B cells ((BCR), also known as membrane-bound immunoglobulin (mIg)) and T cells (TCR). Studies of natural killer cells in mice strongly suggest mammals have a third kind of acquired antigen receptor that recognize haptens and viruses.[4]

It is important to distinguish the antigen receptors just described from class I and class II major histocompatibility complex (MHC) *antigen-presenting molecules* (Chapter 5). MHC molecules bind short peptides (*oligopeptides*) and certain other molecules and present them to the TCR on T cells and, in some cases, to innate immune receptors on natural killer cells. MHC molecules themselves are innate receptors in that they are encoded in the germline and their expression is regulated homeostatically.

The antigen bound by a particular antigen receptor is sometimes called its *cognate antigen*. This makes sense because of

the allied concept that the great majority of lymphocytes express only a single antigen receptor due to the mechanism of allelic exclusion, with singular specificity for its own cognate antigen (Chapter 4). This concept is useful even if up to 5% of lymphocytes actually express more than one receptor. Because lymphocytes retain expression of that singular receptor when they divide, we can describe clones of lymphocytes that recognize the same cognate antigen, and distinct clones can recognize different aspects of the same cognate antigen.

Whether or not a particular molecule will serve as cognate antigen for any receptor depends on many factors. Because of the random mechanisms of forming antigen-receptors (albeit with selection bias in V region usage)[5] and the relatively short life span of most naïve lymphocytes there is a real possibility that many potential antigens, especially those present at low concentrations, never encounter a cognate receptor in the lifetime of the individual. Or the antigen might be sequestered within the cell or body in such a way as to escape detection by lymphocytes. Such antigens are sometimes called *cryptic antigens*. Many *self-antigens* are recognized briefly by T cells in the thymus or developing B cells in the bone marrow, causing the clonal deletion of responding lymphocytes. Only a few of these self-antigens escape this tolerance mechanism and threaten to become *auto-antigens*.

The term *immunogen* refers to "antigen" in the classic, second sense, of an antigen that, when used to immunize an animal, stimulates an immune response to itself. Likewise, an *allergen* is an antigen that stimulates an allergic response.

Special terms refer to facets of antigen as ligand for receptor and antigen as inducer of antibodies. Thus, "hapten," "epitope," and "determinant" refer to molecular structures that physically engage the antigen receptor (Fig. 6.1). Antigens that are not also immunogens are "incomplete antigens"; conversely, immunogens are also called "complete antigens."

Finally, we draw an important distinction between the terms "immunogen" and "adjuvant." Many immunogens are inactive unless mixed with adjuvant. Adjuvants, such as alum (a form of aluminum hydroxide), have two critical functions in vaccines (Chapter 90): a depot effect and an immunostimulatory effect. As a depot, the adjuvant allows retention of the antigen in the tissue to provide steady stimulation, as an immunostimulant it activates antigen-presenting cells to acquire, process, and present antigen.

Antigens for antibodies

Antibodies are classically defined as soluble molecules, immunoglobulins, in the blood and lymph fluids and permeating the tissues. When imbedded in the membrane of the producing B cells they are called B-cell receptors (Chapter 4). In addition, soluble forms can bind via their Fc domains to Fc receptors (FcR) or other moieties (e.g., complement receptors) on a variety of other molecules (Chapter 14). Antibodies bind antigens through their *antigen-binding domains* located at the *N*-termini of the heavy and light chains. Antibodies can signal the presence of antigen to the antibody-producing B cell or to cells expressing Fc or complement receptors. Antibodies can also mediate *antigen acquisition* by B cells or FcR-positive APC by receptor-mediated endocytosis (Fig. 6.2).

The *antigen-binding site* of the BCR is formed typically by the interface of the antigen-binding domains of the mIg light and heavy chains (Fig. 6.1). This site can be in the form of a shallow groove or a deep pocket, and can accommodate molecular structures as small as a single sugar molecule and as large as an oligosaccharide or oligopeptide of six or seven residues. These minimal structures are called *epitopes*. In contrast, antigens,

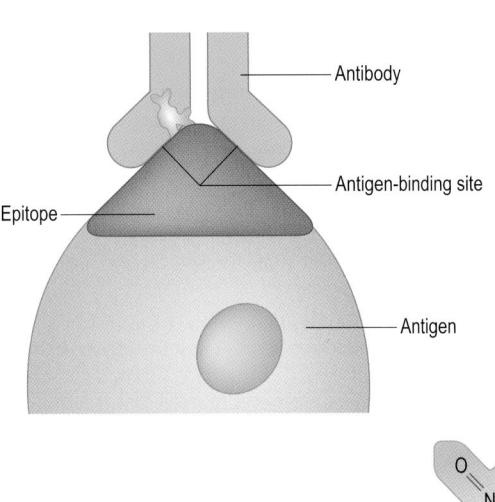

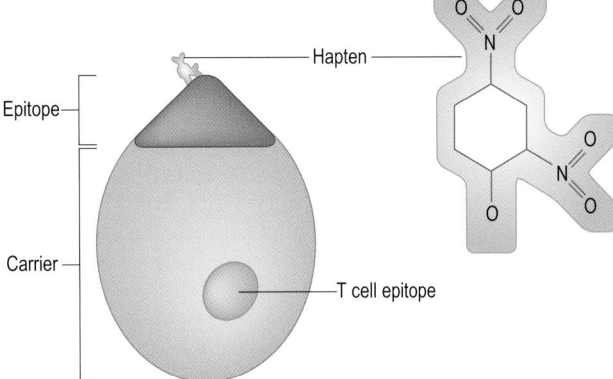

Fig. 6.1 Hapten, carriers, and two kinds of antigens. The antigen-binding site of an antibody binds an antigen through the latter's epitope: this is the biochemical sense of antigen used in ELISA, flow-cytometry, and Western blot analysis. Haptens are self-conjugating antigen moieties that can modify epitopes and provide new binding specificities. Haptens and many antigens by themselves are not immunogens, the second sense of "antigen." Immunogens (complete antigens) are processed by antigen-presenting cells to reveal T-cell epitopes presented by MHC molecules.

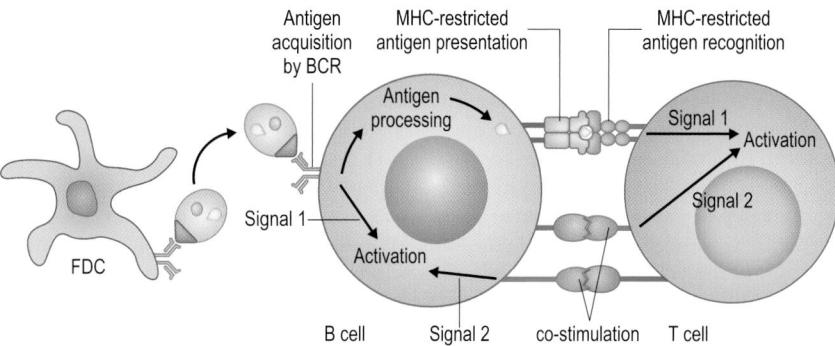

Fig. 6.2 **Antigen presentation.** Follicular dendritic cells (FDC) in germinal centers present antigens bound to local antibodies stored in their surface iccosomes. B cells acquire antigens through their BCR and present processed peptide epitopes via MHC molecules to T cells. T cells recognize antigens presented by MHC molecules on antigen-presenting cell. B and T cells receive signal 1 through the BCR and TCR, respectively.

Trinitrophenol
(Picric acid)

Urushiol
(poison ivy)
R= aliphatic chain

Penicillin

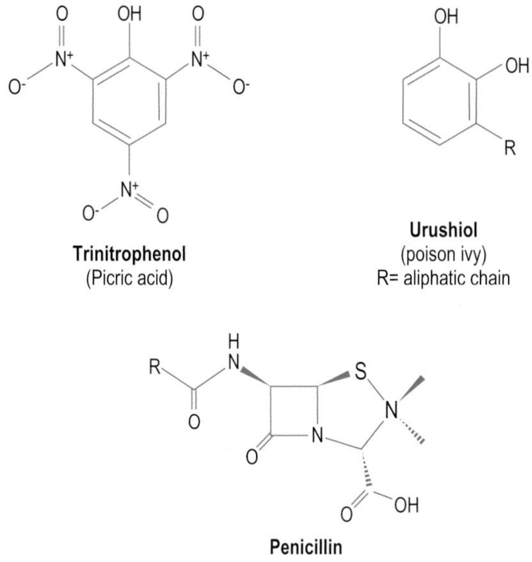

Fig. 6.3 **Some examples of haptens.**

which might contain many epitopes, can be much larger—e.g., as large as a protein, virus, or bacterium.

Epitopes can be formed by a string of contiguous residues of a protein or other polymer, or by a set of non-contiguous residues that folded together in the three-dimensional structure of the parent antigen. The latter epitopes are called *conformational* epitopes because they are present in the antigen only when it is properly folded, and are destroyed if the protein is denatured as, for example, on a Western blot. Conformational epitopes are typically found on the surface of native proteins and are often important for neutralizing antibodies, which must detect the epitope on a three-dimensional antigen surface. Linear epitopes for antibodies are usually available only when the protein is denatured or if they are present in external loops of a protein. It is important to realize that "conformational" is an empirical definition. Thus, binding of CD4 to the gp120 envelope protein of HIV induces conformational epitopes in gp120 representing a transition state of folding. Some CD4-induced epitopes are cryptic linear epitopes buried within the native conformation of gp120. Others, however, are chimeric epitopes formed by peptides from both CD4 and gp120 envelope.[6]

The term *hapten* comes from a Greek word meaning "hold" and is drawn from the dye industry where the word referred to the ability of dyes to *hold fast* to fabrics despite washing. A hapten is the smallest chemical moiety of an epitope that can bind effectively to the antigen-binding site of an antibody and is usually used in relationship to the "hapten-carrier" concept. In additional to highly reactive synthetic dyes, naturally occurring haptens include contact-sensitizing metals such as nickel and plant products such as urushiol, the toxin from poison ivy (Fig. 6.3).

Haptens, as exemplified by the small molecule dinitrophenol, are not immunogens for two reasons. First, by themselves they form few electrochemical contacts with the antibody and so their binding strength is usually very low. Second, they are so small that they cannot be subdivided to produce multiple epitopes, a feature critical to immunogenicity. In particular, haptens are typically monovalent and so do not themselves cross-link BCRs. When chemically conjugated to proteins they can become multivalent and by modifying self-peptides they can create epitopes for T cells.

KEY CONCEPTS

Antigens for B cells

- Immunogens contain
  - Epitopes that bind to the antigen-binding sites of antibodies
  - Class II epitopes for T helper cells
- Haptens can have almost any chemical nature.
- Epitopes on native proteins are usually discontinuous segments of amino acids at the cell surface.

Immunogens for B cells are either T-cell-dependent (TD) or T-independent (TI). TI antigens come in two flavors. Type 1 TI antigens can stimulate antibody production from even neonatal B cells in the absence of MHC-restricted T-cell help. The prototype of TI antigens is lipopolysaccharide (LPS), also known as *endotoxin*, derived from the cell wall of bacteria. LPS drives polyclonal responses of mouse B cells because it is an activating ligand for the Toll-like receptor TLR4 (Chapter 3) found on B cells in rodents; LPS also stimulates proliferation of B cells with LPS-specific antigen-receptors. Moreover, LPS can induce class-switching by B cells and thus generates IgG and IgA responses. Human B cells normally do not express TLR4 and are unresponsive to LPS. However, TLR4 and LPS responsiveness is inducible in human B cells by ligands for other TLR molecules and patients with Crohn's disease do express functional TLR4.[7]

Type 2 TI antigens stimulate antibody production from mature but not neonatal B cells. These antigens, which include the ABO blood group antigens, are typically polysaccharides or glycolipids with repeating epitopes. These can cross-link multiple BCR on a single B cell and thereby activate it. If Type 2 TI cannot stimulate a TLR, how do they activate B cells sufficiently to induce antibody production? It appears this is due to stimulation of other cells, perhaps through complement receptors, that provide sufficient co-stimulation. Thus, NK or even T cells contaminating a B-cell preparation might provide this function.[8]

However, B cells activated in this manner usually need help from T cells to undergo class-switching. Thus, antibodies against

ABO antigens and other type 2 TI antigens are of the IgM class. Since IgM cannot be transported across the placenta by the IgG transporter, FcRn, this explains why incompatible ABO blood groups rarely present a problem for the fetus or newborn.

On the other hand, T-dependent antigens contain epitopes recognized by T cells as well as by B cells (Fig. 6.1). B cells endocytose the parent antigen through the BCR, then process and present peptide epitopes to helper T cells within the germinal center. The T and B cells provide co-stimulation for each other, and CD40L on T cells induces class-switching and somatic hypermutation of immunoglobulin genes in the paired B cell. As a result, most antibody responses to B cells quickly switch from an initial IgM response to one dominated by one or more of the "downstream" Ig isotypes, IgG, IgA and IgE. For example, the food allergen ovalbumin, the major constituent of egg whites, contains peptides recognized by T cells. The simultaneous and cooperative responses of T and B cells in the *germinal center* reaction facilitate immune responses of both cell types.

T-dependent antigens can be modeled by the hapten-carrier concept, in which B-cell responses to the hapten require help from T cells responding to the epitopes within a carrier protein (Fig. 6.1). Experimentally, carrier proteins are typically foreign proteins. However, self-antigens can also serve as carriers in clinically relevant examples. For example, both urushiol, the active ingredient of poison ivy, and penicillin (Fig 6.3) readily form covalent adducts with cellular proteins (Fig. 6.4). These haptenated self-proteins constitute *neo-antigens,* which in this case elicit both T- and B-cell allergic responses.

Haptens are actually not the smallest moieties that can be recognized specifically by antibodies. *Determinants* are the molecular structures that actually *determine specificity*, and these can be as small as single side chain of an amino acid. For example,

antibodies can be generated that recognized the difference between a serine and a phosphoserine as part of a larger protein: the determinant here is the phosphate group. A single nitrate group is the determinant differentiating the two haptens dinitrophenol and trinitrophenol.

Using appropriate carriers and adjuvants, antibodies can be raised *in vivo* against almost any chemical moiety. Antigens as ligands include naturally occurring proteins, lipids, steroids, sugars, and nucleic acids, as well as synthetic compounds. From such studies there seem to be only two limitations to what can be an antigen in the sense of ligand: the antigen must be perceived as "foreign" in some sense to the responding animal, and it must provide a surface to which an antibody can form an electrochemical attachment. It is often possible to trick the immune system into generating autoreactive antibodies, and many of these arise in autoimmune reactions. Similarly, bacteriophage libraries of recombinant antibodies (*phage display libraries*) can be screened for almost any chemical specificity without regard for self/non-self discrimination.

The notion that "anything goes" is powerful theoretically but has its practical limitations. On the one hand, the powerful adjuvants and immunization protocols that can be used in experimental animals cannot be used in humans, so that vaccinologists are still frustrated by their inability reproducibly to stimulate effective immunity to many antigens. On the other, a variety of substances are effectively and fortunately hypoallergenic or hypoantigenic, permitting their use in cosmetic and implantable devices. These substances are non-proteinaceous and so lack T-cell epitopes, and are chemically inert, so unable to haptenate proteins. In addition, though sometimes polymeric, they seem to lack a suitable chemical surface for forming high affinity bonds with antibodies. For example, despite efforts to find contrary evidence, polysiloxane ("silicone") is immunologically inert even in experimental models.[9] This compound is used in contact lenses, breast implants, and other medical devices. These practical comments do not exclude the theoretical possibility that some individuals might generate antibodies reactive with some hypoantigenic substances.

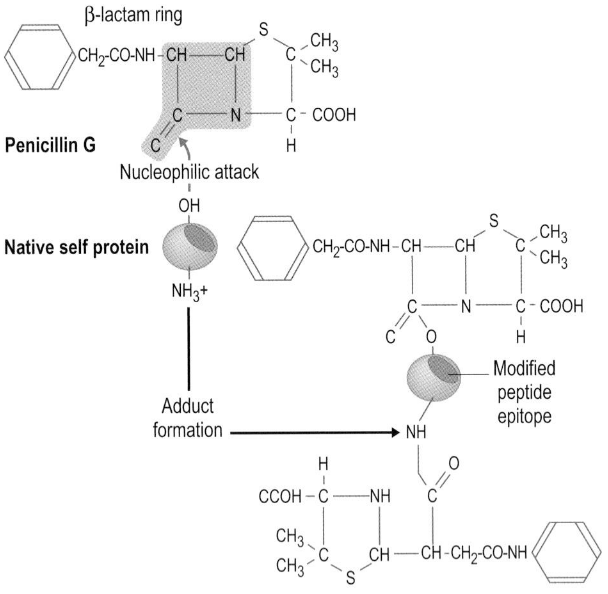

Fig. 6.4 Sensitizing agents create neoantigens by forming covalent adducts with self-proteins. Penicillin allergies involve both antibodies against penicillin and with T-cell responses to penicillin-modified self-proteins. The same chemical reaction that allows penicillin to inhibit peptidoglycan formation in bacteria leads to adduct formation of cellular proteins. Nucleophilic attack by penicillin G (upper left) on the β-lactam ring (shaded) opens the ring and creates an adduct (lower left) with a protein's serines (shown) and lysines. The lactam adducts can be presented to B cells as modified self-proteins or processed for presentation by MHC molecules to T cells as lactam-conjugated self-peptides.

Carbohydrate antigens

As already mentioned, polysaccharides tend to be type 2 TI antigens. Examples include the pneumococcal capsular polysaccharides targeted by pneumococcal vaccines and the human ABO blood group antigens. The latter are a "family" of related antigens expressed by most tissues and by many kinds of commensal bacteria. The polymorphic *ABO* locus encodes a glycosyltransferase that functions as a haptenating enzyme to modify the H antigen, a polysaccharide found on many different glycoproteins and glycolipids. The common *O* allele is functionally silent, so that only the H antigen is generated. Both active enzymes (alleles *A* and *B*) transfer a uridylate diphosphate (UDP)-charged sugar to glycoproteins and glycolipids. The *A* and *B* enzymes use UDP-*N*-acetyl-galactosamine and UDP-galactose, respectively, as sugar donors.

Individuals of genotypes *AA*, *BB*, or *AB* express enzyme A only, B only or both A and B antigens as self-antigens and are tolerant of them and of bacterial antigens with the same sugars (Chapters 30 and 95). In contrast, *O*-type individuals make neither *A* nor *B* antigens. As a result, both antigens appear foreign to *O* individuals and exposure to common bacteria induces both anti-*A* and anti-*B* antibodies. Similarly, *A*-type individuals (genotype *AO* or *AA*) make anti-B antibodies and B–type individuals (*BO* or *BB*) make anti-A antibodies. These systems are called "blood type" referring to the *type of antibodies the person does not make.* The antigens, however, are found in all tissues, including red blood cells. Infants are exposed to the type 2 TI A and B antigens through environmental exposure soon after birth. Anti-A and anti-B antibodies consequently begin to accumulate early in life (though use diagnostically isn't valid during the first year) and appear as "natural antibodies" of the IgM isotype.

Antigens as ligands for T-cell receptors

Most epitopes recognized by TCR are short peptides generated from proteins through *antigen processing.* Consequently, as peptides rather than native proteins, epitopes recognized by T cells are generally linear. The biochemical definition of antigen indicates that epitopes recognized by T-cell receptors should bind directly to them. However, although direct binding of epitope to TCR can be demonstrated in rare cases, usually the affinity of these interactions is too weak for measurement and probably too weak for biological effects. The weak affinity of TCR for its epitope is probably not an intrinsic property of TCR, but a result of thymic education, which has several mechanisms to select against T cells that recognize epitopes directly. Instead, epitopes for TCR first bind tightly to MHC molecules (class I for CD8 T cells and class II MHC for CD4 T cells) and it is the molecular complex of MHC plus peptide that is recognized by the TCR (Chapter 4).

Conventional oligopeptide epitopes can include modified amino acids such as phosphoserine or sugar residues. Hapten-modified self-peptides are major determinants of allergic responses to non-protein environmental agents, such as metals, cosmetics, and antibiotics. However, certain class Ib (or "nonclassical") MHC molecules (Chapter 5) seem to be specialized for recognizing non-peptide antigens. In particular, CD1 presents certain lipids, both endogenous and bacterial, to invariant natural killer (iNKT) cells; these are acquired through an endocytic pathway.[10] Similarly, MR1, recognized by mucosa-associated invariant TCR (MAIT) T cells, presents unidentified bacterial ligands acquired through an endocytic pathway.[11]

With rare exceptions, MHC molecules are not able to discriminate between self and foreign peptides and, indeed, the vast majority of epitopes bound by MHC molecules are self-epitopes.

The short length of peptide epitopes for MHC class I molecules is enforced by a closed-ended binding cleft that binds both amino and carboxyl termini (Fig. 6.5). In contrast, both ends of the binding cleft of class II MHC molecules are open, allowing longer peptides to bind. Because the ends of these peptides are usually degraded before presentation to T cells, most peptides presented by class II molecules are still short–on the order of 15 to 20 amino acids.

The binding site for peptides in both class I and class II molecules is a deep cleft that interacts with the peptide backbone and intimately with two or three of the side chains. The latter are considered *anchor* residues of the epitope and define the *binding motif* of the MHC molecule. The need for terminal anchoring severely limits the length of epitopes for class I MHC molecules to seven to ten amino acids, though longer peptides can sometimes bind by looping out central residues.

Three factors generally control whether a given peptide will be recognized by T cells as antigen: foreignness, binding affinity and antigen processing. Roughly half of all pathogen peptides are identical to self-peptides and, except for cases of autoimmunity, are tolerated by the immune system. The binding affinity of an epitope for most class I MHC molecules can be predicted fairly well. However, naturally occurring proteins must be processed proteolytically (see below) and many sequences that

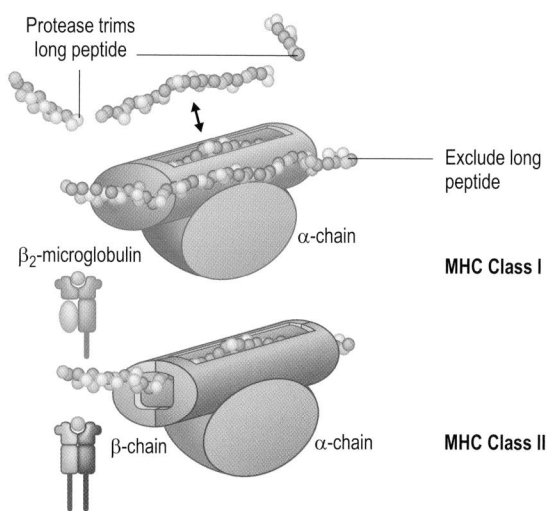

Fig. 6.5 Peptide binding by MHC class I and II molecules. Class I molecules are usually closed at both ends. The peptide termini must interact with terminal sockets. Peptides that are too long must be cleaved (arrows) prior to entry into the binding site. The clefts of class II molecules are open at the ends, permitting the binding of long peptides.

could be good epitopes are either not generated effectively or are destroyed proteolytically. For example, the chicken egg white protein ovalbumin contains three sequences that bind very tightly to class I MHC molecules in the C57BL/6 laboratory mouse and each of these is a potent antigen on its own. However, only one of these is produced naturally from the parent protein. Identifying the mechanisms and rules governing the proteolytic production of epitopes remains a major challenge.

The fact that any given allelic form of MHC molecule recognizes two or three anchor residues with high specificity severely limits the "universe" of peptides that it can present to T cells. Thus, a given class I allele can recognize only about 0.01% of all possible octamer peptides. Two different MHC alleles may recognize distinct anchors and thus see radically distinct antigenic universes. Nonetheless, most proteins have few potential T-cell epitopes and some proteins will not be antigenic in certain individuals simply because they do not produce a foreign peptide that binds with sufficient strength to any of the individual's MHC molecules. Consequently peptide modification to enhance MHC binding is an approach of interest in improving vaccine immunogenicity.[12,13]

Human populations have hundreds of allelic forms of class I and class II MHC molecules. The high polymorphism of MHC molecules has three important biological implications. First, most individuals from unrelated parents are heterozygous for each MHC locus, effectively doubling the size of their antigenic universe. Second, while many individuals may be unable to respond to certain pathogens, at least a few individuals are likely to be protected. This may account for the prevalence of certain MHC haplotypes in populations exposed to malaria, and for genetic vulnerabilities or resistance to HIV. Finally, epitopes detected by one individual may be invisible to the T cells of another person; subunit vaccines effective for some MHC haplotypes may be ineffective for others. For example, the hepatitis B surface antigen subunit vaccine is often ineffective in individuals homozygous for certain *HLA* haplotypes.

MHC restriction

Recognition of peptides by TCR is said to be "MHC-restricted." This has two meanings, molecular and genetic; in both, "restriction" is seen as a limitation or condition on the ability of T cells to recognize their antigens. In the newer, molecular, view, the ability of T cells to recognize their peptide epitopes is "restricted" by the MHC molecules that physically present the epitopes to them. Indeed, X-ray crystallography has shown that about 90% of the contacts made between TCR and the MHC:peptide complex are with the MHC molecule. However, the older, genetic meaning of "MHC-restricted" is more severe: T cells can recognize their cognate epitope *only* when it is presented by a particular allelic form of MHC molecule. This property was revealed long ago because of the extraordinary genetic diversity (polymorphism) of most class I and class II molecules in most species including humans. Most MHC alleles are very distinct from each other and most of the differences are concentrated in the portions of the MHC molecules that bind peptide and TCR. As a result, different allelic forms of MHC differ both in what peptide they can bind and how they will be seen by the TCR. Due to thymic selection (Chapter 8), TCRs have specificity for both the particular peptide and a particular MHC molecule and are unable to recognize other combinations of peptide and MHC. Thus, antigen-specific T cells from one individual are unable to recognize even the same peptide presented by antigen-presenting cells from other individuals, unless they happen to be MHC-matched.

How can we rationalize the operation of MHC-restriction? Why do T cells not recognize their antigens as do B cells—with no need for antigen-presentation? Because alloreactive T cells distinguish between self and non-self MHC molecules, it is tempting to think that MHC restriction mediates self-non-self discrimination. However, it is clear that allospecific antibodies also distinguish self from non-self MHC molecules.

Instead, MHC restriction may function in two opposing ways (Fig. 6.6). First, antigen-processing increases the complexity of pathogen antigens by exposing epitopes not available on the surface of pathogens. As discussed below, MHC molecules are "merely" the mechanism for acquiring peptides processed in inbtracellular compartments, transporting them to the cell surface and presenting them to T cells. In principal, a non-specific peptide binding protein, such as a heat shock protein, could carry out this function. The exquisite specificity of MHC molecules seems like a liability, because it reduces the universe of detectable foreign peptides. However, the same specificity reduces the universe of detectable self-proteins, reducing the risk of autoimmunity. Secondly, the requirement that T cells not respond unless activated by co-stimulation from the APC is enforced by anchoring MHC molecules on the APC. Thus, MHC restriction forces a T cell to be restricted by antigen-presenting cells.

Alloantigens

● KEY CONCEPTS

Properties of superantigens

Defining properties

- Presented and recognized as an unprocessed, native protein.
- Contact TCR and MHC molecules outside the traditional antigen-binding groove.

Specific properties

- Selectively stimulate T cells expressing certain TCR Vβ chains.
- TCR recognition is not MHC allele-restricted.
- Stimulate both CD4 and CD8 T cells in an MHC class II-dependent manner.

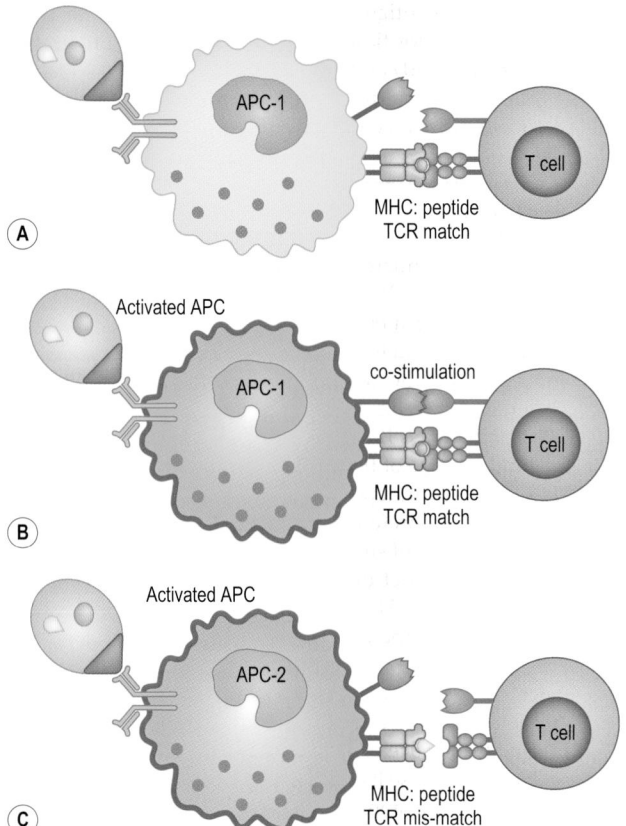

Fig. 6.6 MHC restriction carries out two critical functions. First, by presenting processed peptides derived from within proteins and pathogens, MHC molecules sample a broader antigenic landscape than antibodies, whose epitopes are surface oriented. Second, naive T cells respond to cognate epitopes only when presented by an activated APC (B) but not when the APC is resting (A). Experimentally observed MHC restriction results when an activated APC cannot present the proper MHC/peptide pair (C).

Thymic selection ensures that T cells recognize non-self peptides in the context of self-MHC molecules. A clinically important exception to this specificity manifests as "alloreactivity." If lymphocytes from imperfectly matched donors are mixed in a mixed-leukocyte reaction (MLR), about 5% of the T cells from one donor cross-react with some of the MHC:peptide complexes of the other. Thus, a T cell specific for a peptide from cytomegalovirus (CMV) and restricted by the class I molecule HLA-A2 might recognize some other peptide presented by HLA-B7 from the other donor. Disparities in the *major histocompatibility complex antigens* (MHC molecules, also known as *major transplantation antigens*) between an organ donor and recipient are very likely to stimulate graft rejection because of the high probability of cross-reactivity. But even if the donor is perfectly matched for MHC molecules (as happens in one-fourth of full-sibling pairs), minor histocompatibility differences can also cause tissue rejection. The *minor antigens* are proteins that are polymorphic or of limited expression in a species and thus in humans represent donor–recipient disparities in one or more of the roughly 30 000 different proteins encoded by the genome. A prominent example of a minor histocompatibility antigen is the H-Y antigen, encoded by the Y chromosome, which causes T-cell-mediated rejection of male donor tissue by female recipients. The MLR is extraordinarily sensitive to the presence of alloantigens and is a good predictor of whether organ transplants will be accepted.

The alloantigens just described are recognized by T cells, but alloantigens detected by antibodies are also important mediators of graft rejection. In this regard, the most important alloantigens are the blood group antigens; mismatch for ABO causes hyperacute rejection of donor tissues due to the presence in serum of pre-existing anti-A and/or anti-B antibodies (Chapter 81). Antibodies against HLA and minor histocompatibility antigens are important mediators of acute and chronic rejection.

Superantigens

"Superantigens" are microbial proteins that bind both class II MHC molecules and TCR, causing activation of the T cell. Superantigens include certain bacterial toxins, such as staphylococcal enterotoxin A (SEA) and toxic shock syndrome toxin (TSST), and viral proteins such as the mouse mammary tumor virus (MMTV) superantigen. Superantigens are not processed intracellularly. Instead, they bind class II MHC molecules as intact macromolecules and bind outside of the peptide–antigen binding groove.[14] Class II binding is independent of the specific MHC allele (though often with preference for one class II isotype — DR, DQ, or DP). Each type of superantigen also binds TCR belonging to a characteristic subset of Vβ families and in some case also makes contact with the TCR Vα chain. Recent evidence suggests that at least some superantigens also engage CD28.[15] Nonspecific T-cell activation appears to be a bacterial strategy to avoid microbe-specific recognition. However, by stimulating large numbers of clones of a specific Vβ family, bacterial superantigens can also induce an overwhelming T-cell response with massive cytokine release leading, for example, to food poisoning and toxic shock syndrome.

Antigen-presenting cells

Cells that present antigens to B cells: follicular dendritic cells (FDC)[16]

In many respects, B cells do not need antigen to be presented to them by any other cell: they express high-affinity antigen-receptors that have no contextual requirement for antigen-binding. However, it is clear that engaging B cells with soluble, especially monovalent, antigen can tie up the B-cell receptor in a non-signaling and even tolerogenic mode. Efficient B-cell activation requires either a polyvalent antigen, as with TI antigens, or some form of additional mechanism that effectively cross-links the BCR and induces signaling. Such cross-linking can be mediated by immune complexes (assemblies of antigens and antibodies), by antigens found on the surface of pathogens (thus rendered polyvalent), or by antigens fixed by complement. Two complement receptors on B cells (CR1 = CD35; CR2 = CD21) bind fragments of C3 and C4 attached to antigens.

Most B cells are activated in the limiting architecture of the germinal center; clonal activation leads to nearly monoclonal responses in each center. In this context, a unique cell, the *follicular dendritic cell* (FDC; Chapter 2) plays a special role in presenting antigens to B cells. FDC represent less than 1% of the cells within a germinal center and are tightly associated with B cells and associated macrophages. The bulk of published evidence suggests that FDC are stromal, not hematopoietic, in origin and are required for the formation of germinal centers. The presence and activity of FDC in germinal centers requires the presence of lymphotoxin, a member of the tumor necrosis family, apparently provided by lymphocytes. FDC play an organizing role by secreting the chemokine CXCL13, which binds to

CCR5 on lymphocytes, inducing the secretion of lymphotoxin. FDC trap and accumulate antigens through Fc receptors and complement receptors (especially CR1 and CR2 and C4bR) and store them in *iccosomes* (immune complex-coated bodies). Antigen in iccosomes is stable for months. The ability of FDC to accumulate antibodies secreted by local B cells gives them a high-affinity trapping mechanism with a specificity cognate with those B cells. FDC are thought to be critical for isotype switching, affinity maturation, and B-cell memory. Because C4b is a surrogate activator of CD40, FDC-presented antigen can drive these processes in the absence of CD40L, likely explaining the efficacy of many T-independent antigens. FDC are non-phagocytic, do not express MHC class II or T-cell activation molecules such as B7/CD80/CD86, and do not present antigens to T cells. However, by providing antigen to B cells or germinal center dendritic cells, FDC can activate germinal center T cells indirectly.

FDC are probably critical to the formation of tertiary lymphoid tissues in inflamed tissues and to resulting unwanted immune reactions, such as in chronic organ rejection and autoimmunity associated with vascular inflammation such as SLE. On the other hand, recent reports suggests that maternal lymph node FDC accumulate fetal antigens shed from trophoblasts and may be important in suppressing some T-cell responses to fetal antigens. These observations suggest that manipulating FDC may be therapeutically useful in controlling autoimmunity.

Cells that present antigens to T cells

Cells that present antigens to and activate *naïve* T cells are called *professional antigen-presenting cells* or, more commonly, just APC. Naïve T cells have a high threshold for activation and require co-stimulatory ligands found on professional APC. These are B cells, macrophages, mast cells and basophils, and both myeloid and plasmacytoid dendritic cells (DC).

In contrast, activated T cells have vastly reduced requirements for co-stimulation and their responses are proportional to the level of MHC expression. For typical class I molecules, this means almost all nucleated cells are potential targets for CD8 T cells. However, because most cells do not express co-stimulatory molecules, they do not stimulate naïve T cells. Unlike class I MHC molecules, class II molecules are expressed almost exclusively by professional APC. Among human cells, MHC class II and co-stimulatory molecules can also be expressed by activated T cells and inflamed endothelial cells. In addition, MHC class II is expressed by medullary and cortical epithelial cells in the thymus, where they play an important role during positive and negative selection.

The different types of professional APC have distinct but overlapping properties as APC. Conventional (myeloid) DC (cDC) are by far the most potent in terms of their ability to present a wide variety of antigens to naïve T cells. cDC in their immature form are constitutively tissue-resident phagocytes, actively engulfing and digesting any antigen in their vicinity. In this stage they express few co-stimulatory or class II MHC molecules. Once activated by a "danger" signal, cDC mature rapidly. They stop phagocytosis and begin to express recently digested antigens through upregulated MHC molecules. They become mobile, and follow a chemokine trail from the tissue to nearby draining lymphatics, through which they reach lymph nodes where they begin to present their antigens to T cells. Upregulated co-stimulatory molecules and cytokines allow the DC to activate naïve T cells and direct their differentiation.

cDC functions can be modulated. In the absence of full activation, they tend to be tolerogenic. Once activated by certain innate receptor ligands, cDC express IL-12 and drive a Th1 response (Chapter 16). However, if IL-10 is provided by some other cell type, cDC secrete little IL-12 and drive a predominantly IL-2 response. Other cytokine environments are able to skew cDC functions so that they drive Th-17 or Treg pathways. The rules governing these pathways are still poorly understood.

Although cDC are extremely potent on a per-cell basis, the activity of other professional APC types should not be underestimated, because they vastly outnumber the cDC. Macrophages are active phagocytes and can activate naïve T cells. B cells are not phagocytic but can internalize cognate antigens through their BCR. As a result they are several orders of magnitude more sensitive than cDC to limiting antigen concentrations. Dividing B cells asymmetrically partition endocytosed antigen and antigen-presentation into one of the two daughter cells, suggesting a mechanism for maintaining efficient engagement with T cells for a few clonal derivatives and antigen-free expansion for the majority.[17] Plasmacytoid DC, which seem to be produced by both myeloid and lymphoid progenitors, secrete very high levels of type I interferon but are not potent antigen-presenters. In contrast, mast cells are not phagocytic but may be specialized for presenting antigens acquired through Fc receptors.

Antigen acquisition

We have hinted that APC acquire antigens through multiple mechanisms. From a topological perspective, antigens are either exogenous or endogenous. Exogenous antigens (i.e., antigens synthesized external to the APC) are acquired by the cells and its associated antigen-processing apparatus chiefly through endocytosis. Endogenous antigens (i.e., antigens synthesized within the APC) are already "acquired" by the cell, but are often in the wrong cellular compartment. Viral capsid proteins synthesized by an infected cell and inserted into in the cell membrane can be internalized by endocytosis for antigen presentation. Autophagy is an important mechanism for digesting internal structures including invasive bacteria but also mitochondria and other organelles, and is part of cellular physiology of most cell types. In APC, autophagy mediates presentation of internal antigens. Finally, most peptides presented by class I MHC molecules are "acquired" through a non-phagocytic mechanism involving ubiquitin, specialized proteases, and both peptide and protein transporters located in the membrane of the endoplasmic reticulum.

Pinocytosis, essentially very small scale reversible endocytosis of the cell membrane, samples the fluid phase outside the cell. This takes place in many cells but is a property of the "ruffled" membrane edges found at the leading edge of mobile cells.

Receptor-mediated endocytosis through clathrin-coated pits internalizes many receptors and their cargo ligands. This is a property of most cell types, but is a major mechanism for acquiring antigens for APC. Here we find some exquisite specialization. Typical FcR for IgG, such as found on mast cells, macrophages, and dendritic cells, internalize readily upon cross-linking. These cells readily present antigens found in immune complexes. In contrast, B cells express an alternatively spliced form of this receptor that binds antibodies at the surface but does not internalize. As a group, B cells are not effective at presenting generic antigens acquired through FcR. However, the B-cell receptor itself readily internalizes after being cross-linked, and B cells are exquisitely adept at presenting their cognate antigen.

Phagocytosis is a mechanism for internalizing particles that may be as large as the cell itself. Initial engagement of multiple receptors causes a local deformation of the cell surface and a partial invagination of the cell membrane. This deformation coupled with the triggering of specific receptors leads to subcellular enzyme activity that changes the lipid composition of the membrane bilayer and remodels the cytoskeleton in the vicinity of the particle. This relaxes the membrane, allowing deeper invagination and creating the *phagocytic cup*. If the particle is small enough, the cup deepens until, when the particle is nearly engulfed, the outer edge of the cup closes like a purse-string, leading to membrane fusion and creating a new external surface and a subcellular vesicle. The endocytic vesicle undergoes successive fusion with other vesicles until fusion with the lysosome. Phagocytosis is a property of phagocytes, chiefly DC, macrophages, and neutrophils and in these cells is accompanied by further inflammatory activation of the phagocyte.

Many cell types in addition to professional phagocytes can phagocytose apoptotic cells using a specialized set of receptors that detect apoptotic cells; many cells can mediate this process, including those that do not possess large lysosomes. This accounts for the appearance of apoptotic bodies in otherwise normal cells in pathology sections. Phagocytosis of apoptotic cells by APC is often anti-inflammatory. In contrast, phagocytosis of microbes or necrotic cells, including cells undergoing secondary necrosis after apoptosis, is inflammatory.

Autophagy, found in even the simplest eukaryotes, is a major mechanism for mediating normal protein turnover, protection from intracellular pathogens, and resistance to starvation, as it allows a cell to recycle its own organelles. Perhaps 50% of the peptides presented by class II MHC molecules are endogenous peptides acquired through autophagy. In addition, autophagy mediates presentation by class I MHC molecules of exogenous and some endogenous peptides.[18]

Three broad categories of autophagic mechanisms have been described. Macroautophagy mediates engulfment of microbes or organelles through autophagosomes. Microautophagy closely resembles the vesicle fusion described for phagocytosis. Chaperone-induced autophagy allows vesicles including lysosomes to import proteins directly from the cytoplasm.

The three forms of autophagy are linked by their reliance on a set of *ATG* (autophagy) gene products. Through a cascade of activation events, ATG8 and ATG12, both ubiquitin-like proteins, nucleate a phagophore attached to an invading microbe or targeted organelle, followed by rapid recruitment of a lipid membrane to seal the object into an autophagosome. Macroautophagy can be induced by bacterial produces such as LPS but also by drugs, including rapamycin. Complicating the interpretation of many experiments, autophagy can control the activity of specific cellular proteins, including NFκB, so that the role of ATG proteins may be very indirect.

Cross-presentation refers to the idea that an APC can present antigens produced by some other cell. Since "cross-presentation by class II MHC molecules" is the norm, the term is used most often to describe cross-presentation by MHC class I, where it is critical for activation of CD8 T cells by APC. Cross-presentation can also inhibit immune responses. For example, antigen-specific B cells present epitopes from their cognate antigens and thereby become targets for CTL. In this way, CTL can suppress B-cell responses to some antigens.

Antigen processing

T cells recognize their cognate antigens in the form of short peptides embedded in MHC molecules—X-ray crystallography shows that roughly 90% of the molecular surface recognized by the TCR is the MHC molecule. *Antigen processing* excises these peptides from their parent protein antigens and loads them onto MHC molecules. The processing can take place in different cellular compartments, but loading takes place chiefly in specialized loading compartments. Class I MHC molecules load chiefly in the endoplasmic reticulum, though some loading might take place in endosomal compartments during *cross-presentation*. In contrast, specific mechanisms prevent class II loading in the ER but facilitate it in the specialized endosomal loading compartments.

Endogenous peptides presented by class I molecules derive from proteins made on the cell's own ribosomes. The chief mechanism for degrading large proteins into small peptides is the *proteasome*, a macromolecular tubular structure containing multiple protease activities that cleaves proteins into small fragments of 8 to 14 residues. There are at least four mechanisms that feed proteins into proteasomes. First, nascent cytoplasmic polypeptides that fail to fold properly are attacked by enzymes that attach chains of the protein *ubiquitin* to the protein targeted for destruction. Second, nascent proteins that are translocated into the endoplasmic reticulum endosome but do not fold properly can be exported back to the cytosol by a protein transporter called Sec61. This mechanism is called endoplasmic reticulum-associated protein degradation (ERAD). These two mechanisms are the most important and together represent the defective ribosome products (DRiP) model. Increasing evidence suggests the "DRiP" pathway is not simply an error-dependent pathway but rather represents a specialized mechanism of sampling open reading frames.[19] Third, properly folded mature proteins are ubiquitinated in the course of normal activity—part of the normal course of protein turnover. Finally, in autophagy and cross-presentation, proteins engulfed by phagocytes are partially degraded in lysosomes before transfer into the cytosol.

The DRiP mechanism provides a conceptual core for understanding how class I MHC molecules can sample internally generated antigens, a key requirement for targeting virus-infected or malignant cells. Degradation of mature proteins has a half-time of hours to months, but virus replication can take place on the order of hours. If MHC molecules were to sample antigens as they degrade through normal channels, surface representation would lag considerably behind internal processes. By sampling proteins during their synthesis, or if they fail to fold properly immediately after synthesis, DRiP mechanisms ensure that cytotoxic T cells receive a timely report of internal states.

All four class I MHC pathways make heavy use of the "UPS" (ubiquitin/proteasome) system for protein degradation found in all cells. UPS is initiated by heat shock chaperone proteins recognizing a malfolded protein and inducing covalent tagging of the protein with a single copy of ubiquitin, a 76-amino acid protein. This triggers polyubiquitination in which succeeding ubiquitins are attached to the preceding ubiquitin. Polyubiquitin tails are recognized by the regulatory subunit of the proteasome, a

multi-subunit cylindrical machine. Substrates are fed through the central channel and digested by proteolytic subunits, producing a residue of peptides roughly 8 to 14 amino acids long.

These products are substrates for the *transporter associated with antigen processing* (TAP), a member of the ATP-binding cassette (ABC) transporter family. Heterodimers of TAP1 and TAP2 subunits form peptide pumps that burn ATP to drive peptides from the cytosol into the lumen of the ER. Without a ready source of peptides in the ER, class I MHC molecules are extruded into the cytosol by Sec61 to be recognized by the UPS. TAP mutations are involved in many cases of type I bare lymphocyte syndrome (BLS) (Chapter 35) and many tumor cells lack class I expression due to mutations in their *TAP* genes (Chapter 5). There are several allelic forms in humans with modest differences in specificity. Cells not expressing TAP express low levels of certain MHC alleles and can be highly resistant to specific CTL. However, mice and humans lacking TAP are not profoundly immunodeficient and produce TAP-independent class I MHC-restricted CTL (Chapter 35). These findings suggest alternative mechanisms for loading class I MHC molecules are important even if not dominant in normal circumstances.

Interferon-γ induces an alternative set of proteolytic and regulatory subunits for the proteasome to create the "immunoproteasome." This has altered specificity and activity and may favor the production of peptides suitable for transport by TAP or alternative pathways.

A minor subset of peptides enters the ER independently of TAP through the protein secretory pathway. Nascent polypeptides bearing a *signal peptide* are recognized and transported into the lumen by the *signal recognition particle* (SRP). The signal peptide itself is cleaved by a *signal peptidase*. By inserting the sequence of a CTL epitope behind a signal peptide, this pathway can be used to deliver the epitope directly into the MHC class I loading compartment. Peptides that are too long to bind MHC class I molecules may be retained temporarily in the ER by additional peptide-binding proteins such as BiP, pumped back into the cytosol by an undefined non-TAP mechanism, or trimmed by cytosolic aminopeptidases.

The luminal proteases appear quite efficient, apparently reducing the steady-state concentration of free antigenic peptides in the ER to very low levels. As a result of differences in protease specificities and/or kinetic effects, different epitopes can be carved out of the same protein, depending on whether it follows the proteasome/TAP or the secretory pathway into the ER. Finally, different peptides within a single protein can be degraded or protected at different rates, leading to immunodominance of a subset of potential epitopes for a given MHC molecule.

The production of an immunodominant epitope from influenza A nucleoprotein (NP) illustrates how extra-epitope residues might affect non-proteasome, non-ubiquitin processing.[20] The optimal NP peptide in one mouse strain is the nonamer TYQRTRALV. The three *C*-terminal residues are efficiently removed from a related 12-mer peptide TYQRTRALVRTG. However, an 11-mer, TYQRTRALVTG, is impotent at producing the epitope. The terminal TG sequence represents a "block" to epitope production. All of these complexities in antigen processing make it difficult at present to predict which potential epitopes, identified on the basis of their ability to bind to class I molecules, will be immunodominant *in vivo*.

Class I MHC trafficking (Fig. 6.7)

Nascent Class I MHC molecules are inserted into the ER membrane via the protein secretory pathway. Nascent chains bind first to the membrane-bound chaperone calnexin until they begin

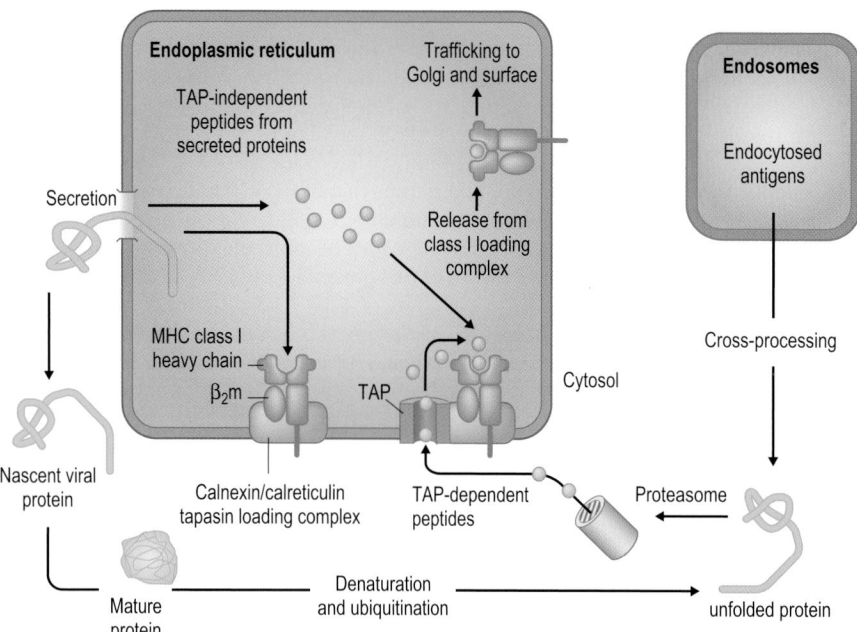

Fig. 6.7 Antigen processing for MHC class I. Two chief pathways for antigen processing intersect within the cytosol. Most endogenous antigens are synthesized on cytosolic ribosomes, processed by proteasomes, and enter the ER through the TAP transporter. A minor set of antigens are processed within the ER from proteins secreted into the ER. Professional antigen-presenting cells transfer endocytosed antigens into the cytosol for processing.

to fold into association with β₂-microglobulin light chains (β₂m). Heterodimers of β₂m and heavy chain are released by calnexin and bind the soluble chaperone, calreticulin. This assembly engages a *class I loading complex*, which includes a 60-kDa thiol reductase, the TAP heterodimer and another MHC-encoded protein, tapasin. Tapasin retains class I molecules in the complex until they bind peptide. MHC molecules failing to attract peptides misfold and are exported by Sec61 to the cytosol. Only those that bind peptide are released by tapasin from the loading complex, migrate to the Golgi where they undergo glycan maturation, and then traffic to the cell surface for recognition by CD8 T cells.

> ## KEY CONCEPTS
>
> ### Antigen processing for class II MHC
>
> - Class II MHC expressed constitutively only by professional APC (dendritic cells, macrophages, and B cells).
> - Epitopes presented by professional APC are acquired mostly through endocytosis and autophagocytosis.
> - Peptides (10–15 amino acids) often have terminal extensions, extending outside the antigen-binding groove.

Antigen processing for class II-restricted T cells

MHC class II molecules assemble in the ER where they associate with *invariant* chain, a 31-kDa protein that chaperones nascent dimers of class II molecules into endosomes. A segment of invariant chain, called CLIP, blocks class II molecules from binding peptides in the ER. CLIP may be removed along with the rest of invariant chain once in the endosomes Alternatively, a CLIP fragment may be left occupying the binding cleft; many class II MHC molecules traffic to the cell surface with CLIP embedded.

MHC class II molecules are loaded with peptides digested by lysosomes. Antigens acquired through endocytosis or autophagy are unfolded and partially degraded in endosomal and acidic lysosomal subcompartments by disulfide isomerase (which unlinks disulfide loops) and a variety of proteases. Most peptides presented by class II molecules are processed from parent proteins and loaded on to class II molecules within a specialized loading compartment of the endosomes. Within this general scheme there are at least two pathways for epitope production, distinguishable in part by their dependence on the function of DM molecules (Fig. 6.8). DM molecules (heterodimers of DMA and DMB subunits that are homologous to MHC class II proteins) catalyze the exchange of CLIP for processed epitopes. In the DM-independent pathway, peptides are loaded onto class II molecules recycling from the cell surface in the absence of CLIP.

The initial ligand for binding class II molecules is a large unfolded protein or protein fragment, rather than the oligopeptide ultimately displayed at the cell surface. This MHC-polypeptide complex is the substrate for trimming exopeptidases. Endosomal aminopeptidases cannot cleave at proline residues; prolines are found near the *N*-terminus of many mature epitopes. Trimming of the extra-cleft residues can continue even after the MHC–peptide complex has reached the surface through the activity of the membrane-bound surface enzyme aminopeptidase N.

As in the case of epitope formation for class I molecules, the initial conformation of the antigen can affect the production of specific linear epitopes. For example, vaccinating mice with synthetic peptides elicits class-II-restricted T cells specific for at least two HIV gp160 epitopes, of which only one is detected on infected cells. Similarly, prior denaturation or mutational destabilization of viral influenza hemagglutinin abolishes its ability to be processed for presentation to some Th clones.

Predicting epitopes for TCR

The critical role of antigens for T cells in driving both T- and B-cell responses to antigen has fueled attempts to use antigen sequence information to predict T-cell epitopes.

The characterization of *binding motifs* for a large number of class I and a smaller number of class II molecules has facilitated computer-based algorithms for predicting potential epitopes from a linear protein sequences. These motifs reflect the chemical affinity of the binding cleft for various amino acid side chains. In many cases it is possible to show that multiple alleles of class I or class II molecules recognize the same or very closely related

Fig. 6.8 Two pathways for loading antigens onto class II MHC molecules. Autophagy and endocytosis transfer cytosolic and external antigens, respectively, into the endosomes. Nascent class II molecules are chaperoned to the endosomes from the Golgi by the invariant chain. The DM molecules catalyze the exchange of antigenic peptides for invariant chain. Mature class II molecules recycling from the cell surface can acquire peptides in a DM-independent manner. Antigens binding initially as polypeptides are trimmed into oligopeptides in the endosomes and at the surface.

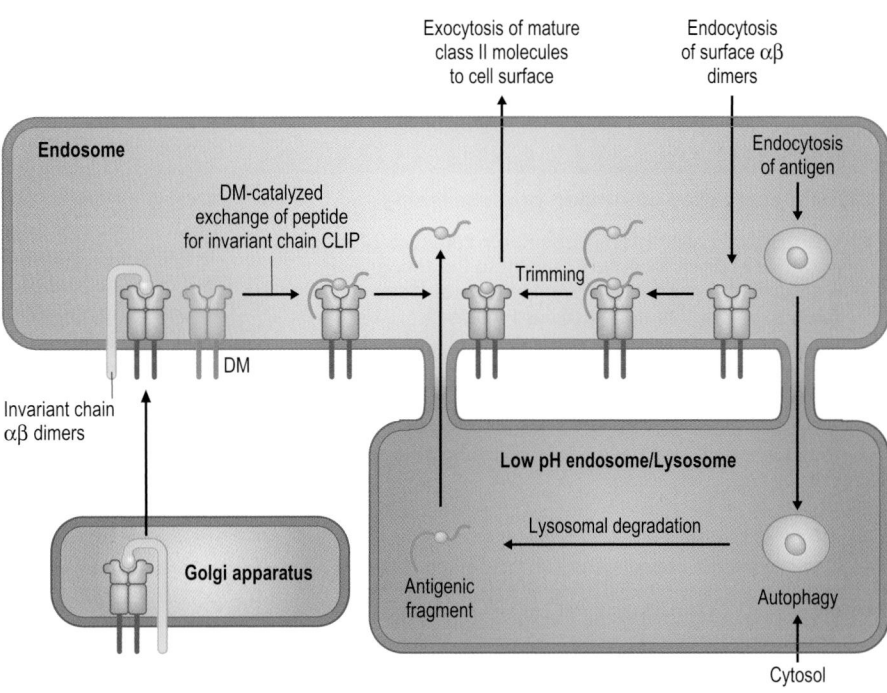

epitopes. These groups of MHC alleles are called "supertypes" and can facilitate the prediction of epitopes for a large number of alleles.[21] Because of the complexity of endoprotease and exoprotease cleavage during processing of epitopes for both class I and class II MHC molecules, it is difficult to predict whether a given epitope will actually be used *in vivo*.

Prediction algorithms have gotten quite sophisticated for predicting class I MHC binding properties but still fail to predict which peptides are produced by antigen processing. Prediction for class II peptides is still difficult.

Antigen presentation

Once loaded with peptide, MHC molecules move to the cell surface where they can be recognized by T cells. This is antigen presentation at the bare minimum and is sufficient for triggering effecter responses from pre-activated T cells. Presentation to naïve T cells requires additional factors and efficient activating of the TCR requires adhesion molecules. These additional processes are usually included under the rubric of "antigen processing." Antigen recognition/presentation of both naïve and activated T cells is mediated by the "immune synapse" although this structure might not be required in all cases.

The immune synapse represents a very close and tight association of APC and T cell resembling tight junctions and may even mediate trogocytosis, through which process peptide-loaded MHC molecules are transferred to the T cell itself.[22] The synapse is initiated when the leading edge of a T cell engaged in amoeboid motion through a tissue meets a potential APC or target cell. Initial low avidity interactions between the T-cell integrins CD11a and VLA-4 mediate a weak approximation of the two cellular surfaces. If MHC molecules on the APC present cognate antigen, the TCR will bind with maximum affinity. The co-receptors CD8 and CD4 bind to class I and class II MHC molecules, respectively. Their cytoplasmic tails, already loaded with the protein kinase Lck, are swept into proximity with the cytoplasmic domains of the T-cell receptor

chains, leading to phosphorylation of the latter and initiating downstream signaling events. An immediate effect is the thousand-fold upregulation of the integrin avidities. The costimulatory receptor CD28 migrates to the field, engaging its ligands on the APC. At the surface, the synapse matures as TCR and CD28 and their ligands concentrate at the center of the synapse, surrounded by a ring of integrins. Internally, the ongoing signaling events cause an arrest of cell migration, a re-organization of the microtubules to permit trafficking of vacuoles to the synapse. Vacuolar contents are delivered into the intercellular space of the synapse, where, if the T cell is a CTL, they will induce apoptosis in the opposite cell.

Microbial interference with antigen processing and presentation

Considering the importance of class I-mediated immune responses in antiviral immunity, it is not surprising to find pathogens using a variety of mechanisms for subverting antigen processing. Proteins from several serotypes of human adenovirus, as well as HIV-1 tat protein inhibit class I MHC transcription. Other viral factors inhibit class I MHC maturation in the endoplasmic reticulum. Proteins US2 and US11 from the human cytomegalovirus (CMV) target nascent class I molecules for destruction through ERAD. The CMV US6 and herpes simplex virus ICP47 proteins inhibit TAP function, indirectly starving MHC molecules of peptide. In contrast, the CMV US3 protein binds class I molecules that have already engaged peptides, but retains them in the ER. The HIV-1 protein nef binds the intracellular tails of mature class I MHC molecules, targeting them for increased endocytosis and degradation. Other pathways are also affected by pathogens. For example the protein ICP345 from herpes simplex virus inhibits ATG6, a critical autophagy-initiating protein. *Mycobacterium tuberculosis* suppresses acidification of lysosomes in macrophages to create for itself an environment conducive to its own replication inside lysosomes.

A clinical coda

If microbes can manipulate specific mechanisms of antigen processing and presentation, it should be obvious that human genetic variation in these pathways should be able to contribute to immune competency or, through deficiency, to immune dysfunctions. These may result in specific or global defects in antigen processing and recognition, such as the bare lymphocyte syndrome (BLS) (Chapter 35). Type I BLS involves general loss of class I surface expression, typically the result of mutations in the TAP peptide transporter. Type II BLS reflects loss of class II MHC expression; defects in any of at least four different transcription factors can cause this disease. In type III BLS, defects in the RFX transcription factor depress expression of both class II MHC molecules and the β_2-microglobulin light chain shared by all class I MHC proteins.

Growing evidence supports the notion that allergens are unusual antigens. It has been long known that allergens inducing delayed-type hypersensitivity are often drugs or environmental compounds able to form covalent adducts with self-proteins, thus generating neoantigens. Additional evidence supports the view that allergens inducing immediate hypersensitivity are (or are associated with) proteases.[23] Through a still-unknown mechanism, these proteases are thought to drive a Th2 response by T cells.

Self-antigens recognized by autoimmunity are so-far chemically unremarkable. The principles that govern pathological self-recognition appear to be the same as for healthy self-tolerance or recognition of foreign antigens: the availability of particular processed peptides at appropriate times for tolerance induction of T-cell activation.

Two nonexclusive models have emerged that may begin to account for why certain individuals are predisposed to autoimmunity and why certain self-antigens are likely to become autoantigens (Chapter 48). The first is the concept of *molecular mimicry*. According to this idea, exposure to sufficient doses of a pathogen-derived epitope that cross-reacts with a previously ignored or *cryptic* self-epitope can break self-tolerance to that epitope. A newer concept in autoantigenicity can explain why many autoantigens are proteins normally found intracellularly, where they are involved in nucleic acid and protein metabolism: small nuclear riboproteins, histones, and heat-shock proteins. This involves the observation (discussed earlier with regard to cross-presentation) that apoptotic bodies are efficiently recognized by dendritic cells, and that many intranuclear and intracellular antigens are exposed on the extraverted surfaces of apoptotic bodies. Thus it is possible that certain predisposing infections, by inducing apoptosis, can elicit autoimmune reactions to cryptic self-epitopes.

Finally, tumor-specific and tumor-associated antigens are typically self-proteins. In rare human cases, such as a peptide derived from papilloma virus type 16, they can be encoded by tumor viruses. Some tumor antigens, such as carcinoembryonic antigen (CEA), prostate-specific antigen (PSA), or the MAGE proteins of melanomas, are normal proteins that are merely overexpressed by tumor cells. These can serve as diagnostic markers or as a target for tumor-selective immunity. The antigenic products of mutated tumor suppressor genes and other oncogenes, such as *HER2*, the retinoblastoma protein RB, and the breast cancer-associated antigen BRAC, are also called *neoantigens* and are potentially more specific targets for immunotherapy. The neoantigens expressed by these tumors arise as chance mutations during the many steps of carcinogenesis. The immune system itself provides a unique category of neoantigens that can be targets of immunotherapy, the clonally distributed products of rearranged antigen receptor genes—idiotypes—expressed by malignancies such as myelomas.

Translational research in antigen processing and presentation

Several areas are ripe for new insights with probable application to clinical immunology. These include deeper understanding of peptide processing for presentation by class I MHC molecules, identification of antigenic ligands recognized by CD1- and MR1-restricted T cells, and identification of the putative antigen receptor expressed by NK cells. Although it now widely accepted that dendritic cells present endocytosed antigens for presentation by MHC class I, the mechanisms and rules governing this process remain unclear. Moreover, the rules governing production of CTL epitopes are uncertain. Better understanding of these pathways may make it easier to predict and identify relevant antigen targets for anti-tumor and anti-viral CTL.

Likewise, autophagy mediates processing of endogenous antigens in both MHC class I and class II pathways and is likely important in cross-presentation. Pathogens can both be cleared by autophagy but also can wrest control of autophagy for their own purposes, probably including redirection of antigen processing. Analysis of the role autophagy in antigen processing is still in its infancy and we expect progress in this direction to yield new tools for controlling infection and vaccine design.

The CD1 and MR1 class Ib MHC molecules present non-peptide ligands to specialized invariant NKT cells and these appear to have important regulatory functions in suppressing autoimmunity, especially in the gut. Ligands for MR1 are unknown and the endogenous ligands for CD1 are largely unknown. This is an area of growth in the next several years and will likely prove important for understanding and treating autoimmunity and some infectious diseases.

Finally, it now appears almost certain that some NK cells in mice and humans express novel species of antigen receptors in a clonal fashion. These receptors and their mechanism of clonal expression or clonal licensing will likely to be solved in the next few years, opening a new chapter in acquired immunity. These receptors are likely to be important for anti-microbial immunity.

References

1. Silverstein AM. Paul Ehrlich's receptor immunology: the magnificent obsession. New York: Academic Press; 2001.
2. Medzhitov R, Janeway Jr. CA. Decoding the patterns of self and nonself by the innate immune system. Science 2002;296:298–300.
3. Matzinger P. The danger model: a renewed sense of self. Science 2002;296:301–5.
4. Paust S, von Andrian UH. Natural killer cell memory. Nat Immunol 2011;12:500–8.
5. Schroeder Jr. HW, Zemlin M, Khass M, et al. Genetic control of DH reading frame and its effect on B-cell development and antigen-specific antibody production. Crit Rev Immunol 2010;30:327–44.
6. Lewis G, Fouts T, Ibrahim S, et al. Identification and characterization of an immunogenic hybrid epitope formed by both HIV Gp120 and human CD4 proteins. J Virol 2011;85(24):13097–104.
7. Ganley-Leal LM, Liang Y, Jagannathan-Bogdan M, et al. Differential regulation of TLR4 expression in human B cells and monocytes. Mol Immunol 2010;48:82–8.
8. Mond JJ, Lees A, Snapper CM. T cell-independent antigens type 2. Annu Rev Immunol 1995;13:655–92.
9. Tugwell P, Wells G, Peterson J, et al. Do silicone breast implants cause rheumatologic disorders? A systematic review for a court-appointed national science panel. Arthritis Rheum 2001;44:2477–84.
10. Brennan PJ, Tatituri RV, Brigl M, et al. Invariant natural killer T cells recognize lipid self antigen induced by microbial danger signals. Nat Immunol 2011;12:1202–11.
11. Le Bourhis L, Guerri L, Dusseaux M, et al. Mucosal-associated invariant T cells: unconventional development and function. Trends Immunol 2011;32:212–8.
12. Houghton CS, Engelhorn ME, Liu C, et al. Immunological validation of the EpitOptimizer program for streamlined design of heteroclitic epitopes. Vaccine 2007;25:5330–42.
13. Cole DK, Edwards ESJ, Wynn KK, et al. Modification of MHC anchor residues generates heteroclitic poptides that alter TCR binding and T-cell recognition. J Immunol 2010;185:2600–10.
14. Fraser JD, Proft T. The bacterial superantigens and superantigen-like proteins. Immunol Rev 2008;225:226–43.
15. Arad G, Levy R, Nasie I, et al. Binding of superantigen toxins into the CD28 homodimer interface is essential for induction of cytokine genes that mediate lethal shock. PLoS Biol 2011;9: e1001149.
16. Deshane J, Chaplin DD. Follicular dendritic cell makes environmental sense. Immunity 2010;33:2–4.
17. Thaunat O, Granja AG, Barral P, et al. Asymmetric segregation of polarized antigen on B cell division shapes presentation capacity. Science 2012;335:475–9.
18. Virgin HW, Levine B. Autophagy genes in immunity. Nat Immunol 2009;10:461–70.
19. Dolan BP, Bennink JR, Yewdell JW. Translating DRiPs: progress in understanding viral and cellular sources of MHC class I peptide ligands. Cell Mol Life Sci 2011;68:1481–9.
20. Yellen-Shaw AJ, Eisenlohr LC. Regulation of class I-restricted epitope processing by local or distal flanking sequence. J Immunol 1997;158:1727–33.
21. Greenbaum J, Sidney J, Chung J, et al. Functional classification of class II human leukocyte antigen (HLA) molecules reveals seven different supertypes and a surprising degree of repertoire sharing across supertypes. Immunogenetics 2009;63:325–35.
22. Dopfer EP, Minguet S, Schamel WW. A new vampire saga: the molecular mechanism of T cell trogocytosis. Immunity 2011;35:151–3.
23. Porter PC, Ongeri V, Luong A, et al. Seeking common pathophysiology in asthma, atopy and sinusitis. Trends Immunol 2011;32:43–9.

7

Harry W.
Schroeder, Jr.,
Andreas
Radbruch,
Claudia Berek

B-cell development and differentiation

B lymphocytes arise from multipotent hematopoietic stem cells that successively populate the embryonic para-aortic splanchnopleure, the fetal liver, and then the bone marrow. Stem cell daughter cells give rise to lymphoid primed multipotent progenitors (LMPPs), which in turn can give rise to either myeloid or lymphoid cells.[1,2] LMPPs then produce common lymphoid precursors (CLPs), which can generate T cells, B cells, NK cells, and dendritic cells. Final B-cell differentiation requires the exposure of CLP daughter cells to specialized microenvironments, such as those found in the fetal liver and the bone marrow. These two tissues are the primary B lymphoid organs. The shift from fetal liver to bone marrow begins in the middle of fetal life and ends just prior to birth. B cells continue to be produced in the bone marrow throughout the life of the individual, although the rate of production decreases with age.

An intact and functional B-cell antigen receptor (BCR) complex, which consists of membrane bound immunoglobulin (mIg), the Igα and Igβ co-receptors, and ancillary signal transduction components, must be present in order for the developing B cell to survive (Chapter 4). The composition of the BCR is subject to intense selection. In the primary organs, hazardous self-reactive BCRs, as well as non-functional ones, can be culled by altering the composition of the receptor (receptor editing), by cell anergy, or by apoptosis of the host cell. Survivors of this initial selection process are released into the blood and thence to the spleen, lymph nodes, and other secondary lymphoid tissues and organs where selection for specificity continues (Chapter 2).

B-cell differentiation (Fig. 7.1) is commonly presented as a linear process defined by the regulated expression of specific sets of transcription factors, immunoglobulin, and cell surface molecules. Given the central role of the BCR (Chapter 4), initial developmental steps are classically defined by the status of the rearranging immunoglobulin loci. With the development of monoclonal antibody technology, analysis of cell surface markers such as CD10, CD19, CD20, CD21, CD24, CD34, and CD38 (e.g., Fig. 7.2) has facilitated definition of both early and late stages of development,[3,4] especially in those cases where immunoglobulin cannot be used to distinguish between cell types. Of these, CD19, a signal transduction molecule expressed throughout B-cell development up to, but not including, the mature plasma cell stage[5] warrants special mention as the single best clinical marker for B-cell identity.

In practice, B-cell development is a more complex process than the simple, linear pathways depicted in Figs. 7.1 and 7.2. For example, pro-B cells typically derive from a common lymphoid progenitor, but they can also develop from a bipotent B/macrophage precursor. Thus, B lineage subsets identified by one fractionation scheme may consist of mixtures of subsets identified by others. It therefore behooves the practitioner to clarify the fractionation scheme used by the reference laboratory when comparing patient findings to the literature.

Initial commitment to the B-cell lineage requires activation of a series of transcriptional and signal transduction pathways. At the nuclear level, the transcription factors PU.1, Ikaros, ID-1, E2A, EBF, and PAX-5 play major roles in committing progenitor cells to the B-cell lineage.[6] However, after lineage commitment has been established, it is the composition of the BCR that controls further development.

Each B-cell progenitor has the potential to produce a large number of offspring. Some will develop into plasma or memory B cells, while others, the majority, will perish.[7] Most of the defined steps in this process of development represent population bottlenecks; developmental checkpoints wherein the developing B cell is tested to make sure that its BCR will be beneficial. In the periphery, exposure to antigen is associated with class switching and hypermutation of the variable domains of the antigen receptor. A few select survivors earn long lives as part of a cadre of memory B cells. These veterans are charged with the responsibility to rapidly engage antigen to which they have been previously exposed, providing experienced protection against repeated assault.

● KEY CONCEPTS

B-cell development in the primary lymphoid organs

- Commitment to the B-cell lineage reflects differential activation of transcription factors that progressively lock the cell into the B-cell pathway
- B-cell development is typically viewed as a linear, step-wise process that is focused on the assembly and testing of immunoglobulin function, first in the fetal liver and bone marrow, and then in the periphery:
  - Failure to assemble a functional receptor leads to cell death
  - Expression of a functional receptor subjects the B cell to antigen selection
  - B cells with inappropriate specificities tend to be eliminated.
  - B cells responding appropriately to external antigen can develop either into immunoglobulin-secreting plasma cells or into memory cells
- At the clinical level, B-cell development can be monitored by examining the pattern of expression of lymphoid-specific surface proteins

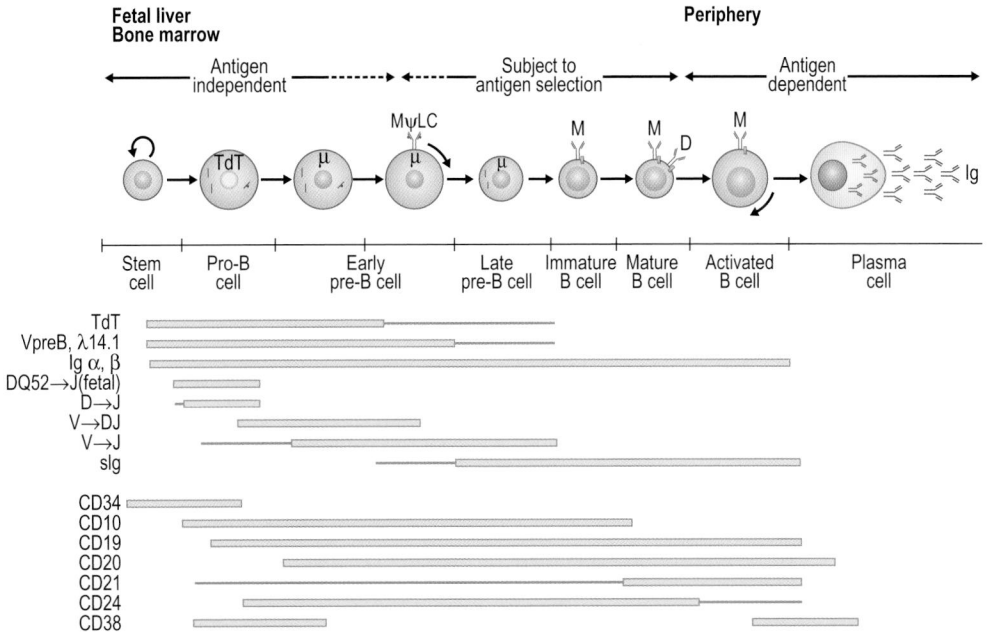

Fig. 7.1 Model of B-cell differentiation. B-cell development is typically viewed as a linear progression through different stages of differentiation. The various processes associated with the assembly of the B-cell antigen receptor complex and the expression pattern of surface molecules whose presence or absence are illustrated through use of bars. The various steps in immunoglobulin rearrangement and the pattern of expression of these surface molecules can be used to characterize stages in B-cell development.

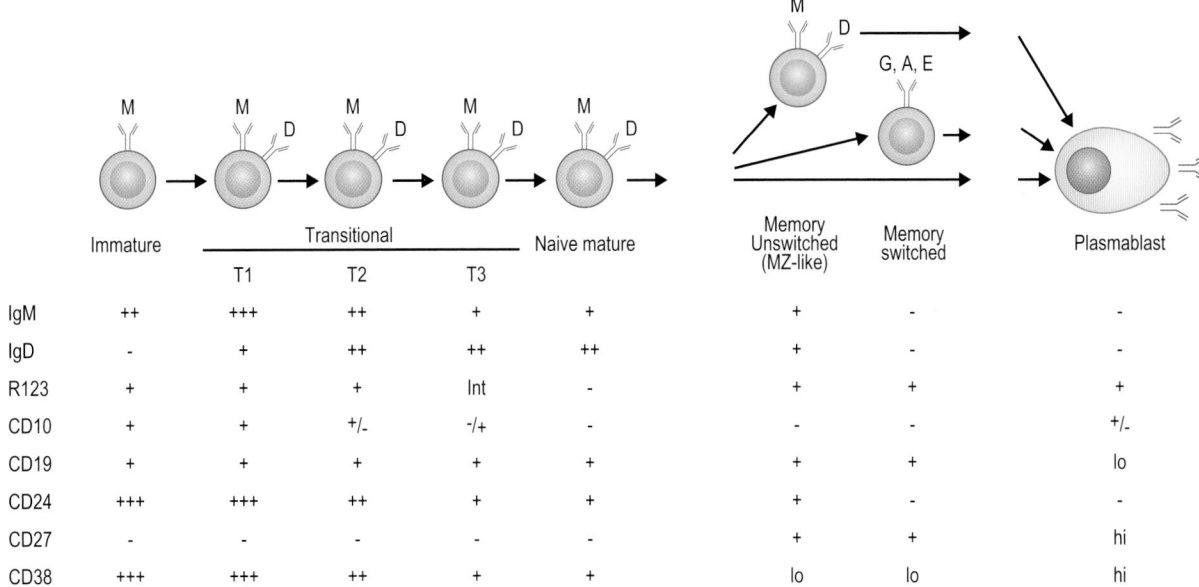

	Immature	T1	T2	T3	Naïve mature	Memory Unswitched (MZ-like)	Memory switched	Plasmablast
IgM	++	+++	++	+	+	+	-	-
IgD	-	+	++	++	++	+	-	-
R123	+	+	+	Int	-	+	+	+
CD10	+	+	+/-	-/+	-	-	-	+/-
CD19	+	+	+	+	+	+	+	lo
CD24	+++	+++	++	+	+	+	-	-
CD27	-	-	-	-	-	+	+	hi
CD38	+++	+++	++	+	+	lo	lo	hi

Fig. 7.2 B-cell subsets in the peripheral blood can be identified by differential staining for IgM, IgD, CD10, CD19, CD24, CD27, CD38, and use of the rhodamine dye R123, which is extruded by the ABCB1 transporter expressed in naïve, mature B cells and, to a lesser extent, T3 transitional B cells.[3] Currently B cells that are CD20$^+$CD27$^+$CD43$^+$CD70$^-$ are currently the best candidates for the human B-1-cell counterparts.[4] In addition to these subsets found in the blood, germinal center B cells found in the spleen and lymph nodes are characterized as IgD$^-$CD38^{++}CD10$^+$CD27$^{+/-}$; marginal zone B cells are typically CD27$^+$, CD21^{++}, CD23$^{+/-}$, CD1c$^+$, and IgD$^-$; and long-lived plasma cells found in the bone marrow, spleen, and tonsils are CD138$^+$CD38^{++}.

Specialized microenvironments also play a role in peripheral B-cell development (Chapter 2), each of which enables the B cell to properly engage different types of antigens or venues of attack. In the marginal zone, mature splenic B cells await bacterial pathogens. In the lymphoid follicles, B cells reactive with a given antigen collaborate with follicular T cells and dendritic cells in order to maximize the immune response. In the germinal centers, B cells use class switching and somatic mutation to modify and optimize the function and affinity of their immunoglobulins. And, underneath mucosal surfaces, B cells are primed to express IgA.

B-cell development begins in the primary lymphoid organs

Generation of a functioning antigen receptor is key to the viability of a B cell

Immunoglobulin rearrangement is hierarchical. In pro-B cells, $D_H \rightarrow J_H$ joining precedes $V_H \rightarrow DJ_H$ rearrangement (Chapter 4); followed by $V_L \rightarrow J_L$ joining in late stage pre-B cells.

Production of a properly functioning B-cell receptor is essential for development beyond the pre-B-cell stage. For example, function-loss mutations in RAG-1/2 and DNA dependent protein kinase (DNA-PKcs, Ku 70/80) preclude B-cell development. Each pro-B cell faces the probability that only one of three possible splices will place the V_H and J_H in the same reading frame. The opportunity to try rearrangement on the second chromosome gives failing pro-B cells a second opportunity. Together, this provides the cell with five chances out of nine for initial survival ($\frac{1}{3} + \frac{1}{3} \times \frac{2}{3}$). In-frame, functional VDJ_H rearrangement allows the pro-B cell to produce μ H chains, most of which are retained in the endoplasmic reticulum. The appearance of cytoplasmic μ H chains marks initiation of the pre-B-cell stage. These early pre-B cells tend to be large in size.

VpreB and λ14.1 [λ5], which together form the surrogate light chain (ψLC), and Igα and Igβ are constitutively expressed by pro-B cells. Pre-B cells whose μ H chains can associate with surrogate light chain form a pre-B-cell receptor. Its appearance signals the termination of further H chain rearrangement (allelic exclusion), which is followed by four to six cycles of cell division;[1] a process associated with a progressive decrease in cell size. Late pre-B daughter cells reactivate RAG1 and RAG2 and begin to undergo $V_L \rightarrow J_L$ rearrangement. Successful production of a complete κ or λ light chain permits expression of conventional IgM on the cell surface (sIgM), which identifies the *immature* B cell. Immature cells expressing self-reactive IgM antibodies may undergo repeated rounds of light chain rearrangement to lessen the self-specificity of the antibody, a process termed *receptor editing*.[8]

Immature B cells that have successfully produced an acceptable IgM B-cell receptor extend transcription of the H chain locus to include the Cδ exons downstream of Cμ. Alternative splicing permits co-production of IgM and IgD. These now newly *mature* IgM$^+$IgD$^+$ B cells enter the blood and migrate to the periphery where they form the majority of the B-cell pool in the spleen and the other secondary lymphoid organs. The IgM and IgD on each of these cells share the same variable domains.

Tyrosine kinases play key roles in B-cell development

Signaling through the BCR is required for continued development. Bruton tyrosine kinase is an important component of the phospholipase Cγ (PCLγ) pathway, which is used in BCR signaling. Deficiency of BTK function results in the arrest of human B-cell development at the pre-B-cell stage[9] and is the genetic basis of X-linked agammaglobulinemia (XLA) (Chapter 34).

BLNK is a SRC homology 2 (SH2) domain-containing signal transduction adaptor. When phosphorylated by SYK, BLNK serves as a scaffold for the assembly of cell activation targets that include GRB2, VAV, NCK, and phospholipase C-[γ] (PLCγ). An agammaglobulinemic patient lacking pre-B and mature B cells has been reported with a loss of function mutation in BLNK.

FLT3 (FLK2) is a receptor tyrosine kinase belonging to the same family as c-FMS, the receptor for colony stimulating factor-1 (CSF-1). FLT3 ligand, which has homology to CSF-1, is a potent co-stimulator of early pro-B cells. In mice, targeted disruption of *flt3* leads to a selective deficiency of primitive B-cell progenitors.

Cell surface antigens associated with B-cell development

B-cell development is associated with the expression of a cascade of surface proteins, each of which plays a key role in the fate of the cell (Fig. 7.1, Table 7.1). The timing of the appearance of each of these proteins can be used to further analyze the process of B-cell development.

CD34 is a highly glycosylated Type I transmembrane glycoprotein that binds to CD62L (L-selectin) and CD62E (E-selectin) and thus likely aids in cell trafficking (Chapter 12). It is expressed on a small population (1–4%) of bone marrow cells that includes hematopoietic stem cells. Minimal hematopoietic defects have been documented in mice deficient in CD34. However, such observations must be viewed with caution when extrapolated to human, because CD34 is not expressed on hematopoietic stem cells in the mouse.

CD10, also known as neprilysin, neutroendopeptidase, and the common acute lymphocytic leukemia antigen (CALLA), is a type II membrane glycoprotein metalloprotease. CD10 has a short N-terminal cytoplasmic tail, a signal peptide transmembrane domain, and an extracellular C-terminal domain that includes six N-linked glycosylation sites. The extracellular domain contains 12 cysteines whose disulfide bonds help stabilize its zinc-binding pentapeptide motif, which is involved in its zinc-dependent metalloprotease catalytic activity. By virtue of its protease activity, it is thought to downregulate cellular responses to peptide hormones and cytokines. Inhibition of CD10 activity on bone marrow stromal cells enhances B-cell maturation. CD10 (CALLA) is used as a marker for pre-B acute lymphocytic leukemias and for certain lymphomas.

CD19 is a cell-surface glycoprotein of the immunoglobulin superfamily that is exclusively expressed throughout B-cell development from the pro-B-cell stage up to, but not including, the plasma cell stage (Fig. 7.1).[5] CD19 exists in a complex with CD21 (complement receptor 2: CDR2), CD81 (TAPA-1) and Leu 13. With the help of CD21, CD19 can bind the complement C3 cleavage product C3d. The simultaneous binding of sIgM and CD19 to a C3d-antigen complex enables CD19 and the BCR to interact and thereby provides a link between innate and adaptive immune responses (Chapter 3). CD19-BCR interactions permit the cell to reduce the number of antigen receptors that need to be stimulated in order to activate the cell. Co-activation also reduces the threshold required for B-cell proliferation in response to a given antigen.

The cytoplasmic domain of CD19 contains nine conserved tyrosine residues which, when phosphorylated, allow CD19 to associate with PI-3 kinase and the tyrosine kinase VAV. Patients deficient in CD19 have normal numbers of CD20$^+$ B cells in the blood, but are pan-hypogammaglobulinemic and are susceptible to sinopulmonary infections.

CD20 contains four transmembrane domains and cytoplasmic C- and N– termini. It is a member of the CD20/FcεRIβ superfamily of leukocyte surface antigens. Differential phosphorylation yields three forms of CD20 (33, 35, and 37 kDa). Activated B cells have increased fractions of the 35- and 37-kDa forms of the antigen. CD20 appears to function as a B-cell Ca^{2+} channel subunit

Table 7.1 Cell surface proteins active in early B-cell development

Gene	Class or alternative name	Associated or targeted genes or molecules	B-cell developmental phenotype in human or *mouse* associated with disrupted function of the indicated gene
B-cell receptor complex			
μ chain	Immunoglobulin superfamily	κ,λ L chains, ΨL chain, CD79 a,b (Igα,β)	*Arrest at pre-B-cell stage*
λ14.1	Immunoglobulin superfamily	VpreB, μ H chain	*Arrest at pre-B-cell stage*
CD79a,b (Igα,β)	Immunoglobulin superfamily, cytoplasmic ITAM motifs	H chain, LYN, FYN, BLK, SYK	*Arrest at pro-B-cell stage*
Other cell surface proteins			
CD10	Type II metalloproteinase	Hydrolyzes peptide hormones, cytokines	*Not expressed in murine B-cell progenitors*
CD19	Immunoglobulin superfamily	mIgM, PI-3 kinase, VAV, LYN?,. FYN?	CVID3: panhypogammaglobulinemia, normal numbers of $CD20^+$ B cells in the blood
CD20	Four transmembrane domain surface molecule	B-cell Ca^{2+} channel subunit; indirectly interacts with LYN, FYN, LCK	CVID5: low IgG, normal IgM, variable IgA *20–30% reduction in B-cell numbers*
CD21	Complement control protein	iC3b, C3dg, C3d, CD19, CD81, Leu 13, CD23	*Diminished T-cell-dependent immune responses, decreased germinal center formation, reductions in affinity maturation*
CD24	GPI-linked sialoglycoprotein	Ligand for P-selectin (CD62P)	A57V polymorphism associated with increased risk of multiple sclerosis. *Deletion in mice leads to reductions in late pre-B and immature B-cell populations*
CD34	Type I transmembrane glycoprotein	Ligand for L-selectin (CD62L) and E-selectin (CD62E)	*Not expressed in murine B-cell progenitors*
CD38	Type II transmembrane glycoprotein ADP-ribosyl cyclase, Cyclic ADP-ribose hyroxylase	ADP Ribosylates proteins	*Diminished T-cell-dependent immune responses, augmented responses to T-cell-independent type 2 polysaccharide antigens*

and regulates cell cycle progression. It can interact directly with MHC class I and II molecules, as well as members of another family of four transmembrane domain proteins known as the TM4SF, e.g., CD43, CD81, and CD82. It also appears to interact indirectly with LYN, FYN, and LCK. In mice, loss of CD20 function leads to a 20–30% reduction in B-cell numbers. B-cell development, tissue localization, proliferation, T-cell-dependent antibody responses and affinity maturation are otherwise normal.

CD21 (complement receptor 2: CR2) is a cell surface protein that contains a small cytoplasmic domain and an extracellular domain consisting of a series of short consensus repeats termed complement control protein (CCP) domains. These extracellular domains can bind three different products of complement C3 cleavage, iC3b, C3dg, and C3d. When binding these products, CD21 acts as the ligand-binding subunit for the CD19/CD21/CD81 complex, tying the innate immune system to the adaptive immune response.[5] Mice that lack CD21 exhibit diminished T-dependent B-cell responses. However, serum IgM and IgG are in the normal range. A single 28-year-old male patient lacking CD21 has been described. He presented with mild clinical disease. *In vitro*, B cells showed reduced binding to C3d-containing immune complexes. CD40 function appeared intact and somatic hypermutation and class switching were present.

CD24 is a GPI-linked sialoprotein that serves as a ligand for P-selectin (CD62P). It is expressed on progenitor, immature, and mature B cells. Its expression decreases in activated B cells and is lost entirely in plasma cells. Monoclonal antibodies against CD24 inhibit human B-cell differentiation into plasma cells. In mice, CD24 is also known as HSA, or heat stable antigen.

Mice made deficient for CD24 show a leaky block in B-cell development with a reduction in late pre-B and immature B-cell populations. However, peripheral B-cell numbers are normal and no impairment of immune function has been demonstrated.

CD38 is a bifunctional enzyme that can synthesize cyclic ADP-ribose (cADPR) from nicotinamide adenine dinucleotide (NAD^+) and also hydrolyze cADPR to ADP-ribose. It is presumed that the enzyme exists to ADP-ribosylate target molecules. CD38 is expressed on pre-B cells, activated B cells, and early plasma cells; but not on immature or mature B cells or on mature plasma cells. Antibodies to CD38 can inhibit B lymphopoiesis, induce B-cell proliferation, and protect B cells from apoptosis. CD38 knockout mice exhibit marked deficiencies in antibody responses to T-cell-dependent protein antigens and augmented antibody responses to T-cell-independent type 2 polysaccharide antigens.

Transcription factors control early B-cell differentiation

Ultimately, B-cell development is a function of differential gene expression. Deficiencies in the function of the transcription factors that regulate lymphoid-specific gene expression can thus be expected to result in abnormal B-cell development (Fig. 7.3, Table 7.2).

PU.1 is an ETS family loop-helix-loop (winged helix) transcription factor. ETS proteins contain a structure that binds purine-rich DNA sequences. PU.1 regulates a number of lymphoid

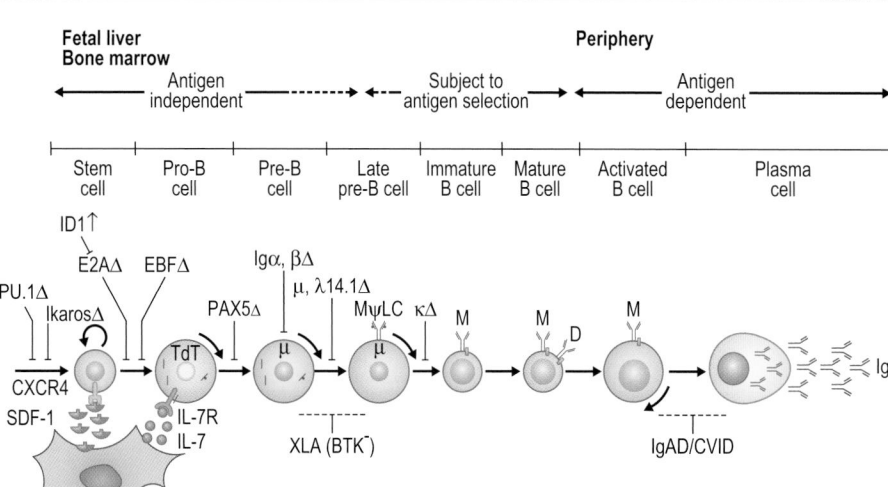

Fig. 7.3 Changes in the function of genes involved in early B-cell development can reduce or prevent the production of B cells and immunoglobulin. The stage of development at which abnormal function of selected set of transcription factors, cytokines, chemokines, and signal transduction elements can influence B-cell development is illustrated. A Greek delta (Δ) or a dash (−) indicates a loss of function of the gene in question. An upward arrow (↑) indicates an increase in the function of the gene in question.

Table 7.2 Nuclear and cytoplasmic factors active in early B-cell development

Gene	Class or alternative name	Associated or targeted genes or molecules	B-cell developmental phenotype in human or *mouse* associated with disrupted function of the indicated gene
Transcription factors			
PU.1	Loop-helix-loop (winged helix)	CD79a (Igα), μ H chain	*Arrest prior to the pro-B-cell stage*
Ikaros	Zinc finger	RAG1, TdT, IL2R, VpreB, LCK	*Arrest prior to the pro-B-cell stage*
Aiolos	Zinc finger	RAG1, TdT, IL2R	*Aging mice develop symptoms of systemic lupus erythematosus*
E2A	Basic helix-loop-helix (BHLH)	RAG1, IgH, Igκ, TdT, EBF, PAX5	*Arrest prior to the pro-B-cell stage*
EBF	EBF/Olf helix-loop-helix (HLH)-like	CD79a (Igα), λ14.1, VpreB, PAX5	*Arrest prior to the pro-B-cell stage*
PAX5	Paired-domain	CD19, λ14.1, VpreB, BLK kinase, J chain, V_H promoters, Vκ promoters	*Arrest at pro-B-cell stage*
The recombinase complex			
RAG1, RAG2	Recombinase	Recombination signal sequences of immunoglobulin gene segments	*Arrest at pro-B-cell stage*
TdT	Non-templated DNA polymerase	Coding ends of rearranging immunoglobulin gene segments	*Absence of N nucleotides, diminished production of pathogenic anti-DNA autoantibodies, loss of heterosubtypic immunity against influenza virus*
DNA-PK	DNA repair complex	Multimeric complex consisting of DNA-PKcs, Ku70, Ku80, which repairs double-stranded DNA breaks	*Arrest at pro-B-cell stage, original mouse SCID mutation identified as a loss of function mutation in DNA-PKcs*
Protein tyrosine kinases			
FLK2/FLT3	Class III receptor tyrosine kinase	GRB2, SHC	*Selective deficiency of primitive B-cell progenitors*
BLNK	SH2 adaptor protein	SYK, GRB2, VAV, NCK, Phospholipase Cγ (PLCγ)	*Arrest at pro-B-cell stage*
BTK	BTK/TEC protein tyrosine kinase	Phospolipase Cγ (PLCγ), SAB	*X-linked agammaglobulinemia - arrest at pre-B-cell stage*

specific genes, including CD79a (Igα), J chain, μ chain, κ chain, λ chain, RAG1, and TdT. ETS family members are relatively weak transcriptional activators and typically require the presence of other factors in order to activate or repress their target genes; PU.1 is no exception. PU.1 cooperates with PIP (LSIRF, IRF4), c-JUN, and c-FOS. PU.1 deficient mice demonstrate defective generation of progenitors for monocytes, and granulocytes as well as B and T lymphocytes, indicating a role in the generation of MPPs as well as LMPPs. PIP deficient mice lack germinal centers in peripheral lymphoid organs and exhibit defects in B-cell activation.

Ikaros and Aiolos belong to the same zinc finger transcription factor family. Both are expressed during lymphoid development, but Ikaros is expressed in stem cells and in mature lymphocytes, whereas Aiolos is only expressed after commitment to the B-cell lineage. Ikaros transcripts are subject to alternative splicing, generating several isoforms, each of which differ in their DNA binding patterns, tendency to dimerize, and their nuclear localization. Among the genes bound by Ikaros are TdT, λ14.1 (λ5), VpreB, and LCK. Ikaros deficient mice lack B cells. Aiolos deficient mice exhibit elevated levels of IgG and IgE. With age, these mice tend to develop autoantibodies and B-cell lymphomas.

The *E2A* locus encodes two basic helix-loop-helix transcription factors that represent two alternately spliced products, E12 and E47.[10] Targets for E2A include RAG-1 and terminal deoxynucleotidyl transferase (TdT), the enzyme responsible for *N* addition (Chapter 4). The functions of E12 and E47 overlap. However, E47 appears to play a greater role in driving TdT and RAG-1, whereas E12 is a better activator of EBF and PAX5, and thus helps commit developing cells to the B-cell lineage. In mice with disruptions in the *E2A* gene, B-cell development is arrested at an extremely early stage, prior to the first transcription of *RAG-1*.

ID-1 has a helix-loop-helix domain, but lacks a DNA binding domain. Thus, it can function as a dominant negative factor, inhibiting the function of helix-loop-helix transcription factors, such as E2A. ID-1 is expressed only in pro-B cells. *ID-1* transgenic mice have a phenotype similar to *E2A* knockout mice, suggesting that Id-1 can regulate E2A function.

EBF, or early B-cell factor, is a helix-loop-helix like transcription factor. EBF is expressed at all stages of differentiation except plasma cells and in mice has been shown to be critical in the progression of B cells past the early pro-B-cell stage. The developmental block in B-cell differentiation is similar to that seen in E2A mutants, suggesting that these transcription factors act co-operatively and regulate a common set of genes.

PAX5 is a paired-box, or domain, transcription factor that, among the progeny of hematopoietic stem cells, is expressed exclusively in cells of the B-cell lineage. PAX5 has both a positive and a negative effect on B-cell differentiation. In mice, B-cell precursors require Pax5 in order to progress beyond the pro-B-cell stage. The presence of Pax5 also prevents early B lineage progenitors from transiting into other hematopoietic pathways, including those leading to the development of granulocytes, dendritic cells, macrophages, osteoclasts, NK cells, and T cells.

MicroRNAs (miRNA) and B-cell development

MicroRNAs are a recently discovered class of small, noncoding RNAS that downregulate target genes at a post-transcriptional level.[11] These RNAs are process from longer transcripts by the sequential action of RNA polymerase II, the nuclear nuclease Drosha and the cytosolic nuclease Dicer. Mature miRNAs are incorporated into the multiprotein RNA induced silencing complex (RISC), which repress target mRNAs by either inducing mRNA cleavage or mRNA degradation, or by blocking mRNA translation. Critical miRNAs include miR-150, miR-155, and miR-17-92. Several of these miRNAs play a role in both early and late B-cell development. Abnormal function these miRNAs can contribute to oncogenesis and immune dysfunction.

Modulation of B-cell development by chemokines, cytokines, and hormones

Stromal cells can influence the microenvironment surrounding B-cell precursors through cytokines and chemokines, which exert local effects on B-cell development (Fig. 7.3). For example, CXCL12, also known as pre-B-cell growth-stimulating factor and as stromal cell-derived factor-1 (PBSF/SCF-1), promotes pro-B-cell proliferation. Mice with a targeted disruption of this gene exhibit impaired B lymphopoiesis in fetal liver and bone marrow, and fail to undergo bone marrow myelopoiesis.[12] The mechanism by which CXCL12 regulates early B-cell development remains unclear. However, disruption of its receptor CXCR4 leads to failure of in the homing of plasma cells to the bone marrow.

IL-7 has a minimal proliferative effect on human B-cell progenitors and, unlike mouse, is not essential for B lineage differentiation. Nevertheless, IL-7 enhances CD19 expression. IL-7 treatment of human pro-B cells also leads to a reduction in the expression of RAG-1, RAG-2, and TdT and thus can modulate the process of immunoglobulin gene segment rearrangement.

Interferons-α and -β (IFN-α/β) are potent inhibitors of IL-7-induced growth of B lineage cells in mice.[13] The inhibition is mediated by apoptotic cell death. One potential source of IFN-α/β is bone marrow macrophages. Another macrophage-derived cytokine, IL-1, can also act as a dose-dependent positive or negative modulator of B lymphopoiesis.

Systemic hormones also regulate lymphopoiesis.[14] A role for sex steroids is suggested by the reduction in pre-B cells during pregnancy. Estradiol can also alter later stages of B-cell development, promoting expansion of the marginal zone compartment. Prolactin appears to enhance production of both marginal zone and follicular B cells. Mice with a loss of function mutation in the *Pit-1* transcription factor gene do not produce growth hormone, prolactin, or thyroid-stimulating hormone. These dwarf mice exhibit a defect in B-cell development that is correctable by the thyroid hormone thyroxine.[15]

● KEY CONCEPTS

B-cell development in the periphery

- T-independent activation of naïve B cells results in terminal differentiation into short-lived plasma cells.
- T-dependent activation of B cells:
  - Leads to germinal center formation, permitting somatic hypermutation and class switch recombination
  - Results in differentiation into high affinity memory B cells (reactive memory) and plasma cells secreting high affinity antibodies (protective memory)
  - Generates long-term humoral immune protection
- The longevity of plasma cells is supported by highly specialized survival niches in the bone marrow
- Tfh cells control late B-cell differentiation by cell-bound ligands and secreted cytokines.
- Activated B cells control T-cell development by presentation of antigen and co-stimulation

B-cell development in the periphery: Differentiation and the response to antigen

The life span of mature B cells expressing surface IgM and IgD appears entirely dependent on antigen selection. After leaving the bone marrow, unstimulated cells live for only a few days.

Deletion of the transmembrane/intracellular domains of the B-cell antigen receptor of mature B cells disables their survival, which indicates that signaling through the BCR is essential for their survival. As originally postulated by Burnet´s "clonal selection" theory, B cells are rescued from apoptosis by their response to a cognate antigen.

The reaction to antigen leads to activation, which can then be followed by diversification. The nature of the activation process is critical. T-cell-independent stimulation of B cells induces differentiation into short-lived plasma cells with limited class switching. T-dependent stimulation adds additional layers of diversification, including somatic hypermutation of the variable domains, which permits affinity maturation, class switching to the entire array of classes available (Chapter 4), and differentiation into the long-lived memory B-cell pool or into the long-lived plasma cell population.

BAFF and APRIL can play key roles in the development of mature B cells

B cells leave the bone marrow while still undergoing initial maturation, demonstrating progressively higher levels of IgD expression with a commensurate lowering of IgM. They need the splenic environment in order to complete this maturation process. Immigrant splenic maturing B cells pass through two transitional stages, known as transitional stages 1 (T1) and 2 (T2). Only a minority of these cells successfully make the transition, as this differentiation step is a crucial checkpoint for controlling self reactivity. Passage through this checkpoint requires the interaction of soluble B-cell activating factor of the tumor necrosis family (BAFF), with its receptor, BAFF-R, which is expressed primarily on B cells.[16] Death signals triggered through interaction of the B-cell receptor with self-antigen can be counter balanced by stimulation of BAFF-R, which enhances expression of survival factors such as Bcl-2 and at the same time downregulates pro-apoptotic factors.

BAFF and a second TNF family member APRIL (a proliferation-inducing ligand) are essential factors for B-cell development and also for their long-term maintenance. With the development of plasma cells, BAFF-R is downregulated and instead the receptors TACI (transmembrane activator and calcium-modulator and cyclophilin ligand interactor) and BCMA (B-cell maturation antigen) are upregulated. In contrast to the BAFF-R these members of the TNF-R family can bind both BAFF and APRIL. APRIL can induce isotype switching in naïve human B cells; more importantly, it is a crucial survival factor supporting the longevity of plasma cells.[16,17]

T-independent responses

Unlike T cells, which require presentation of antigen by other cells, B cells can respond directly to an antigen as long as that antigen is able to cross-link the antibodies on the B-cell surface. Such antigens, especially those that by nature cannot be recognized by T cells (e.g., DNA or polysaccharides) can induce a B-cell response independent of T-cell help. Depending on the cytokine milieu, the B cells may even class switch, although the range of available classes appears to be restricted. B cells that are activated by antigen alone do not take part in a germinal center reaction (see below).

T-dependent responses

Activated B cells express both MHC class I and class II molecules (Chapter 5) on their cell surface. They can thus present both intracellular and extracellular antigens to CD4 T helper and CD8 T cytotoxic lymphocytes. Their role as antigen presenting cells is enhanced when they present peptides from the same antigen they have taken up with their antibodies (Chapter 7). Cognate recognition of the same antigen by both a B cell and a T cell permits each of these cells to reciprocally activate the other. In particular, T-cell-activated B cells express the co-stimulatory molecules CD80 and CD86, which are in turn required for activation of T cells via CD28, as well as their inactivation by CD152 (CTLA-4). Since B cells do not express IL-12, they do not induce expression of IFN-γ in the activated T cells, but rather favor the differentiation of activated T cells into IL-4, -5, -10, and −13 expressing Th2 cells and IL-21 secreting T follicular helper cells (Tfh). These cytokines can support the CD40 induced expansion of memory B cells (IL-4), CD40 induced class switch recombination (CSR) to IgG4 or IgE (IL-4) and differentiation of antigen activated B cells into high affinity plasma cells (IL-21).

Organization of the peripheral lymphoid organs

Compartmentalization in the immune system facilitates efficiency and regulation of the immune response. During development, the primary and secondary lymphoid organs are built up in an organized way.[18] The process involves multiple factors that play various roles in the development, maintenance, and function of the lymphoid organs.

B lymphocytes enter the secondary lymphoid organs through defined ways. Each organ exhibits a preferred route of entry.[19] For example, most lymphocytes enter the spleen through the bloodstream whereas lymphocytes enter lymph nodes and Peyer´s patches through high endothelial venules. In general, lymphocyte migration and the tissue specific homing is strictly controlled by chemokines (Chapter 13). Dendritic cells, macrophages, and other highly specialized cells transport antigens from peripheral sites of entry into the secondary lymphoid organs. Within these organs, circulating lymphocytes survey available antigens. Binding to a cognate antigen activates the cell. Contact between a T cell and a B cell that have been activated by the same antigen permits initiation of a T-cell-dependent immune response.

The spleen

In the secondary lymphoid organs, T cells and B cells are segregated into clearly defined areas (Chapter 2). Figure 7.4 illustrates the pattern observed in the white pulp of the spleen. It is in these areas where the antigen-dependent B-cell activation occurs and where the cells subsequently undergo further differentiation. The marginal sinuses, the site of entry for lymphocytes, macrophages, and dendritic cells, separate the white pulp from the red pulp. These sinuses are lined with a mucosal addressin cell adhesion molecule-1 (MAdCAM-1) expressing endothelium (Chapter 11). In the marginal sinuses, one finds a specialized layer of metallophilic macrophages that are thought to control the entry of antigen into the white pulp.

Follicular dendritic cells (FDC) are highly specialized cells that present antigen to B cells (Chapter 2). In contrast to other types of

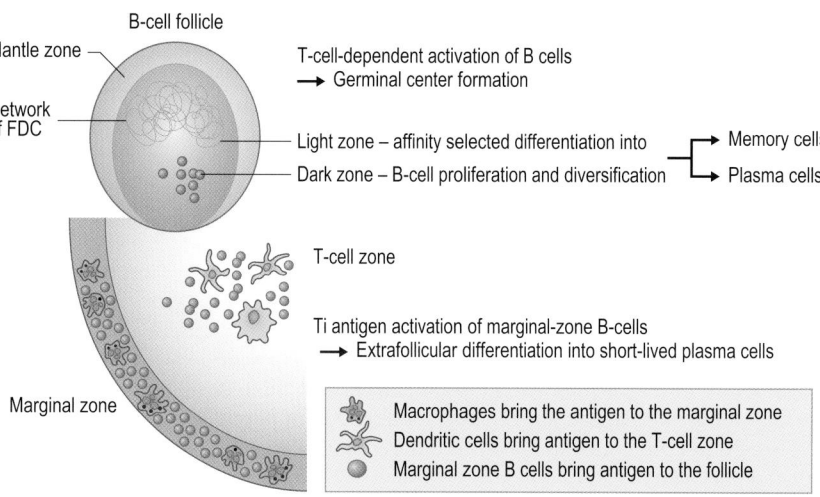

Fig. 7.4 T-cell and B-cell compartments within the white pulp of the spleen. Most splenic T cells can be found in a compartment that surrounds the central arterioles. This compartment is also referred to as the periarteriolar lymphocyte sheath (PALS). Most splenic B cells are found in two separate compartments, the marginal zone and the follicles. The marginal zone is located next to the marginal sinuses. The primary follicles are located within, but separate from, the T-cell zones. Within these primary follicles, B cells are embedded within a network of follicular dendritic cells (FDC).

dendritic cells, FDC do not process antigen. Instead, FDC have abundant complement receptors and Ig Fc receptors that allow accumulation of antigen in the form of immune complexes within the B follicle. FDC are crucial for B-cell maintenance as well as for their activation and differentiation (see below).

Chemokines (Chapter 10) and cytokines (Chapter 9) play a major role in the organized development of the secondary lymphoid organs.[20] For example, mice deficient for the B-cell chemokine receptor CXCR5 fail to develop primary B-cell follicles in the spleen. In these mice, B cells enter the spleen through the marginal sinuses just as they do in their wildtype littermates. However, B cells in these CXCR5 deficient mice fail to move into the areas where B-cell zones would normally develop. Instead, a broad ring of B cells surrounds the T-cell zone.

The proinflammatory cytokine tumor necrosis factor (TNF-α) and its receptor TNFR1 play an important role in the organogenesis of the spleen. In mice deficient for TNF-α, the marginal zones are expanded whereas the primary follicles are missing. The disruption of B-cell follicles in these mice is similar to that observed in CXCR5 deficient mice. However, in contrast to the CXCR5-deficient mouse, no network of FDC develops.

Deficiency of lymphotoxin (LTα) has even more profound effects. This can be explained by the fact that the LTα exists in two forms, a soluble homotrimer that is released from the cell membrane after cleavage and interacts with the TNFR1 molecule and a membrane bound heterotrimer LTα$_1$/LTβ$_2$ that interacts with the LTβ receptor (LTβR). Thus, in mice deficient for LTα, both interactions are interrupted. The expression of LTα$_1$/LTβ$_2$ on B cells is crucial for the organized development of lymphoid structures and hence the induction of memory humoral immune responses. LTα$_1$/LTβ$_2$-positive B cells by themselves are necessary and sufficient for the formation of the FDC network.[18]

The marginal zone provides a home for B-cell early responders

Mature B cells are not homogenous. Functionally and developmentally distinct subsets exist. In the spleen, follicular B cells have a key role in the adaptive immune response, whereas marginal zone (MZ) B cells are now seen as major players at the interface between the initial innate immune response and the delayed adaptive response.[21] The ability of MZ B cells to rapidly respond to encapsulated bacteria by differentiating into antigen

specific plasma cells helps keep such infections under control. MZ B cells take time to develop and are not present in young infants. The MZ becomes fully populated only after the age of two. In the physiologic absence of these MZ cells, a poor response to blood borne infections is commonly observed.[22]

Germinal centers

T-cell-dependent activation of follicular B cells can induce the formation of a germinal center (GC), which is the microenvironment where affinity maturation of the humoral immune response takes place. The interplay of hypermutation followed by antigen selection is the basis of affinity maturation. In the germinal center, B cells that express antibodies of high affinity are selected to develop into memory and long-living plasma cells.[23]

Germinal centers develop only after T-cell-dependent activation of B cells. Their full function is dependent on the interaction between CD40 expressed on B cells and CD40L (CD154) expressed on activated T cells. Patients with loss of function mutations in CD40L have high serum levels of IgM and suffer from recurrent infections (hyper-IgM syndrome, Chapter 34).[24]

In a primary immune response, it takes about a week for the complex GC structure to develop. In the spleen, a few days after activation of antigen specific B cells and T cells small clusters of proliferating B cells are observed at the border of the T-cell zone and the primary B-cell follicle.[25] The rapidly expanding B-cell clone seems to push the naïve B cells towards the edge of the primary follicle. The naïve B cells form a mantle zone around the newly developing GC and the primary follicle changes into a secondary follicle. Subsequently, the network of FDC becomes filled with proliferating, antigen-activated B cells. In addition, an influx of antigen activated Tfh is observed. These helper cells can enter the B-cell follicle as they express the chemokine receptor CXCR5, which is normally only expressed on B cells. Thus, during the GC reaction expression of the chemokine CXCL13 by the FDC attracts both antigen activated B and Tfh cells.

About the second week after immunization, the GC matures into a classical structure that contains a dark zone and a light zone. At this stage of GC development, proliferation is restricted to the dark zone. In the network of FDC, the B cells differentiate into plasma cells and memory cells. In the fully developed GC, dividing cells are termed centroblasts, whereas differentiating cells within the FDC network are termed centrocytes.

In the dark zone, proliferating B cells activate a mechanism of somatic hypermutation.[26] This is a highly specific process that is targeted towards the gene segments that encode the antigen-binding domain of the antibody molecule. Hypermutation introduces single nucleotide changes into the rearranged variable genes of the Ig molecules. Thus, within the dark zone, a clone of variants expressing antigen receptors with various affinities for the antigen is generated from a single B-cell progenitor. By chance a few of these mutations result in a receptor with higher affinity for antigen. B cells expressing such receptors are favored for activation and proliferation, particularly late in an immune response, when availability of antigen is limiting.

FDC present antigen to B cells, but only those with high affinity receptors are able to internalize the antigen via their BCR. Processing of the internalized antigen and presentation of peptides to Tfh cells are prerequisites for B-cell differentiation into memory and plasma cells. Thus, only the few B cells with high affinity receptors get adequate help.[27] IL-21 provided by the Tfh cells is crucial in this differentiation phase and, since it controls the fate of the GC B cell, it is essential for affinity maturation of the immune response.[28]

B-1 cells

In addition to the MZ and conventional (B-2) subsets, differential expression of the cell surface molecules IgD, CD5, CD11b/CD18, CD23, and CD45 have allowed the identification of two additional peripheral B-cell subsets, B-1a and B-1b.[21,22,29] "Conventional" B cells (B-2 cells) express high levels of IgM and IgD, whereas "CD5" B cells (B-1 cells) express minimal surface IgD. B-1 cells express little CD45 and virtually no CD23. They all express CD5 mRNA, although some display CD5 on their cell surface (B-1a) and some do not (B-1b).

B-1 cells seem to develop from distinct progenitors that represent a majority of B cells in fetal life.[30] Accordingly, in mouse fetal liver, all B cells, and in fetal spleen, 40 to 60% of B cells are B-1 cells. Later in development, B-1 cells comprise less than 10% of the splenic IgM$^+$ B cells. In the peritoneal cavity B-1 cells are abundant.

Natural antibodies are found in every serum. These IgM antibodies are produced by B-1 cells. They tend to have specificity for bacterial antigens as well as autoantigens. In general, they are of low affinity and polyreactivity, with self-reactivity appearing to play a role in tissue homeostasis. These antibodies also appear to provide an important and immediate defense against many infectious organisms.

The frequent presence of CD5 on chronic lymphocytic leukemia (CLL) B cells and their tendency to produce poly- and self-reactive antibodies led many to conclude that CLL was a leukemia of human B-1 cells. When it became clear that CD5 was not a definitive marker for B-1 cells in humans, considerable effort was expended searching for this elusive subset. Currently B cells that are CD20$^+$CD27$^+$CD43$^+$CD70$^-$ appear to be the best candidates.[4]

Regulatory B cells

Although incompletely understood, a number of observations point to the existence of B cells with antibody-independent, immunosuppressive functions.[31] These regulatory B (B$_{reg}$) cells appear to exert their immunosuppressive effects on Th1 cells via the release of IL-10 and cell-cell contact.

Molecular mechanism of somatic hypermutation (SHM) and class switch recombination (CSR)

Immunoglobulin SHM and CSR are essential mechanisms for the generation of a high affinity, adaptive humoral immune response. They allow the generation of effector plasma cells secreting high affinity IgG, IgA, and IgE antibodies.

Somatic hypermutation

Hypermutation occurs only during a narrow window in B-cell development. The mechanism is induced during B cell proliferation within the microenvironment of the GC.[32] With a high rate of about 10^{-3}/base pair/generation, single nucleotide exchanges are introduced in a stepwise manner into the rearranged V-region and its 3' and 5' flanking sequences. Mutations are randomly introduced, although there is a preference for transitions (cytidine $\rightarrow$ thymidine or adenosine $\rightarrow$ guanine) over transversions. Analysis of the pattern of somatic mutations has revealed that the sequence of the complementarity determining regions (CDRs; Chapter 4), the loops that form the antigen binding site, have been selected to form mutation hot spots.

Effective hypermutation requires the V-gene promoter and transcription enhancer sequences. Indeed, the position of the V-gene promoter defines the start of the hypermutation domain, which spans about 2000 nucleotides. Any heterologous sequence that is introduced into the V gene segment locus will become a target of the hypermutation machinery. Thus, somatic hypermutation can sometimes play a role in lymphomas and leukemias where oncogenes have been linked to Ig promoters and enhancers.

Class switch recombination

Upon transition from the immature to the mature state and leaving the bone marrow, the B cell starts to express IgD as well as IgM. Both IgM and IgD antibodies use the same V$_H$DJ$_H$-exon and promoter (Fig. 7.5). The molecular basis of co-expression of IgM and IgD by the same B cell is due to differential termination of transcription and splicing of the primary transcripts. Although sequences have been identified that are required for the control of termination and splicing of the Cμ and Cδ transcripts, none of the proteins involved are known. The role of IgD remains unclear. In mice, targeted inactivation of IgD has shown that it is not critical for B-cell activation and differentiation. IgD$^{-/-}$ B cells show a slightly reduced capability for affinity maturation, but no other defect has yet been described.

Unlike IgD, the other antibody classes are not stably expressed together with IgM. B cells can switch from expression of their V$_H$DJ$_H$-exon with Cμ to expression of the same V$_H$DJ$_H$-exon with any of the downstream C$_H$ genes (e.g., C$\alpha_{1,2}$, C$\gamma_{1,2,3,4}$, or Cϵ) (Chapter 4). Class switching, like somatic hypermutation, is a hallmark of B-cell activation. It can be induced by T-cell-independent signals (e.g., LPS) or by signals derived from T cells (e.g., CD40L). CD40L-deficient humans (X-linked hyper-IgM syndrome; Chapter 34) are severely impaired in the expression of Ig classes other than IgM.

TATA-less promotors located in front of the switch regions respond to signals from cytokines and B-cell activation-inducing ligands, like CD40L binding to CD40 on the B cell. Transcription starting from these promoters, which starts with a small I-exon

Fig. 7.5 Antibody class switch recombination.
Recombination between switch regions (Sμ and Sε) is preceded by transcription of these switch regions. Transcription is targeted by cytokines to distinct switch regions.

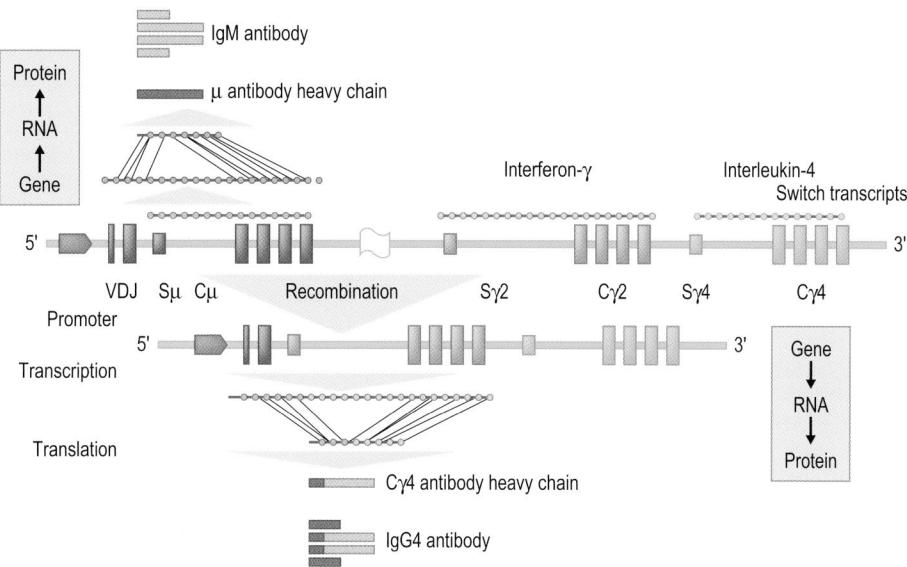

located between the promoter and the switch region, continues through the switch region itself, and finishes after including the entire C$_H$ gene sequence, is essential in targeting switch recombination to the transcribed switch region.

The choice of C$_H$ gene targeted for switch recombination in a particular B cell appears to be dependent on external cytokine signals. IFN-γ targets CSR to IgG2 in humans and IgG2a in mice, IL-4 to IgG4 and IgE in humans and IgG1 and IgE in mice, and transforming growth factor-β (TGF-β) to IgA in both humans and mice. Other switch targeting-cytokines have been described, although our knowledge is far from complete. It is evident however, that those cytokines central for the organization of cellular, humoral and mucosal immunity, respectively, recruit exactly those classes of antibodies that provide the most useful functions for their respective branches of the immune system.

Both SHM and CSR require activation-induced cytidine deaminase (AID)

Both molecular mechanisms, CSR and SHM are dependent on an activation-induced cytidine deaminase (AID).[33] Mice deficient for this enzyme express only IgM antibodies without somatic mutations, and patients with homozygous AID loss-of-function mutations present with hyper-IgM syndrome (Chapter 34). The mechanism of action remains controversial, in particular, the targeting of the DNA modifications to the rearranged V region gene that encodes the antigen–binding portion of the antibody molecule. Recently it was shown that DNA modifications are not limited to the rearranged V-region gene.[34] As AID is active on single-stranded DNA, it may target all genes that are transcribed during GC reaction. Subsequently all DNA modifications except the ones introduced into the rearranged V-region sequence undergo repairs. As a result, retained somatic mutations are concentrated on the V-regions of the BCR alone.

Hypermutation is proposed to occur in two steps.[26] The mechanism is induced by AID catalysed deamination of deoxycytydine (C) to deoxyuridine (U). The mispairing of U and deoxyguanosine (G) is than processed by uracil DNA glycosilase and targeted by repair pathways. As a consequence mutations at C–G pairs are observed. In the second step, mutations at A–T pairs are induced, probably during a mutagenic patch repair

of U–G mismatches introduced by AID. A number of proteins, such as MSH2 and MHS6 (homologues 2 and 6 of the *E. coli* MutS), polymerase η or exonuclease-1 seem to be involved, however, the mechanism is not clear.

In CSR AID is targeted to the switch regions located upstream (5′) of each C$_H$ gene. These switch regions are composed of 1 to 6 kilobase-long GC-rich repetitive sequence motifs. G–C pairs within these motifs are targeted by AID. Deamination of C and processing by uracil DNA glycosylase creates an abasic site that facilitates the introduction of double-strand DNA breaks. Joining and repair requires the presence of DNA-phosphokinases, Ku70, Ku80, and probably other members of the general double-strand repair mechanism (Chapter 4).

Both mechanisms, SHM and CSR, need to be tightly controlled, since the introduction of double-strand breaks into the DNA cannot only pose a risk to the longevity of the B cell, but also permit translocations involving and activating oncogenes.[35] For example, for Burkitt lymphoma cells and for plasma cell-derived myeloma cells the translocation and ectopic expression of the *c-MYC* gene is an apparent consequence of abnormal SHM and CSR.

B-cell memory

One of the key features of the immune system is immunological memory for antigens encountered in the past. In humoral immune responses there are two layers of memory, long-lived B memory cells and long-lived B effector cells (i.e., the plasma cells).

Plasma cell

Immunological memory of B lymphocytes is dependent on T helper lymphocytes. While primary B-cell responses start with secreted low affinity IgM antibodies after a lag-phase of 1–2 days and only gradually develop high affinity antibodies of other classes, secondary responses start faster and with high affinity antibodies of IgM and other classes. This protective humoral memory is provided by long-lived plasma cells.[35] These cells are generated in the secondary lymphoid organs and then

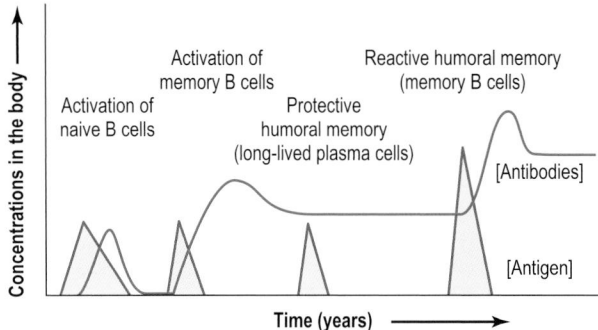

Fig. 7.6 The two types of B-cell memory, reactive memory of memory B cells and protective memory of long-lived plasma cells. The relative concentrations of antibody and antigen over time are indicated.

migrate to the bone marrow or to a site affected by inflammation. In the bone marrow, plasma cells survive in highly specialized niches provided by the underlying reticular stromal cells.[36] Here they can live on for long periods without further activation and proliferation, but their maintenance is dependent on survival factors such as APRIL and IL-6. Eosinophils were shown to be the main providers of these cytokines and, when they are depleted, plasma cells rapidly go into apoptosis.[37]

By continuously secreting antibodies, long-lived plasma cells provide the individual with long-term humoral protection. If the original antigen recurs at higher concentrations, free antigen can activate memory B cells and induce again differentiation into high affinity antibodies secreting effector plasma cells (Fig. 7.6).

Memory B cells

Memory B cells are derived from naïve B cells activated by antigen and T-cell help in extrafollicular or germinal center reactions. The differentiation to memory B cells is critically dependent on CD40 of the B cell and CD40L expressed by T cells. Inactivation of the CD40 or CD40L genes by targeted mutation in the murine germline or by accidental mutation in humans leads to a hyper-IgM syndrome and a general lack of B-cell memory (Chapter 34). Interestingly, using CD27 as a marker for B-cell memory cells, a small fraction of IgM memory B cells have been detected in the peripheral blood of some patients with hyper-IgM syndrome. The pattern of cell surface antigen expression suggested that these cells are MZ B cells. In human, hypermutation is a mechanism that occurs during a narrow window of B-cell development in the GC. However, it seems possible that under certain circumstances the mechanism of hypermutation might be induced when B cells are activated in a T-independent response, perhaps in the gut by signals delivered through Toll-like receptors. Recent results coming from a detailed V-gene repertoire analysis support the notion that IgM memory B cells can develop independently of the GC reaction.[38]

Although long-term protection of the organism is provided by both memory B and plasma cells, their contribution varies from individual to individual; some individuals are protected mainly by memory B cells whereas others are primarily protected by plasma cells. This can be of vital importance in special situations such as transplantation where activation of the immune system should be avoided. For example, treatment of recipients with rituximab, a monoclonal antibody specific for CD20, depletes memory B cells; but has no effect on long living plasma cells secreting transplant specific antibodies.

Abnormal B-cell development and diseases of immune function

- Failure to generate B cells or a normal repertoire of antibodies leads to humoral immune deficiency, which is commonly marked by recurrent sinopulmonary infections.
- Failure to prevent the formation of antibodies with high avidity or high affinity to self-antigens can lead to autoimmune diseases.
- The process of antibody repertoire diversification lends itself to the creation of mutations that can activate and modify oncogenes as well, leading to leukemia or lymphoma. Mechanisms include:
    - RAG1/2 catalyzed juxtaposition of an oncogene to an immunoglobulin promoter or enhancer, activating the oncogene.
    - AID-induced somatic hypermutation of the oncogene, altering its function.

Development of ectopic lymphoid tissue in autoimmune disease

In immune diseases such as myasthenia gravis, Sjögren syndrome, Hashimoto disease, or rheumatoid arthritis, ectopic lymphoid tissue can develop in the affected tissue or organ. Inflammatory cytokines and the presence of B cells can support the development of additional lymphoid tissue.

The growth of ectopic lymphoid tissue in rheumatoid synovium offers an excellent example of this disease-related phenomenon. In healthy individuals, the synovium is made up by a thin lining layer of synoviocytes. In contrast, in patients with rheumatoid arthritis the diseased joint is highly infiltrated with varying numbers of T cells, B cells, plasma cells, macrophages, and dendritic cells. In the majority of patients, these mononuclear cells are dispersed loosely throughout the synovium. However, in some patients well-organized, large lymphoid structures can develop that are similar in appearance to the lymphoid follicles seen in the secondary lymphoid organs.[39,40] At the center of these cell clusters one finds a network of FDC. Antigen presented by the FDC appears to activate B cells, which induces proliferation. A layer of T cells, which may support B-cell differentiation into plasma cells, surrounds the central B cells. The analysis of the V-gene repertoire expressed in synovial B cells has demonstrated that during proliferation hypermutation is activated in a pattern similar to that observed in normal secondary lymphoid organs. Thus, in rheumatoid arthritis a germinal center reaction can be induced within the synovial tissue. A central question is which antigens drive the immune response and select B cells to differentiate into memory and plasma cells. The ectopic lymphoid tissue may function as additional lymphoid tissue, in which case the immune response is no longer restricted to the peripheral lymphoid organs. Equally well, the ectopic lymphoid tissue may support a self-specific immune response. These questions remain active topics of investigation.

References

1. Matthias P, Rolink AG. Transcriptional networks in developing and mature B cells. Nat Rev Immunol 2005;5(6):497–508.
2. Nagasawa T. Microenvironmental niches in the bone marrow required for B-cell development. Nat Rev Immunol 2006;6(2):107–16.
3. Manjarrez-Orduno N, Quach TD, Sanz I. B cells and immunological tolerance. J Invest Dermatol 2009;129(2):278–88.

4. Griffin DO, Holodick NE, Rothstein TL. Human B1 cells in umbilical cord and adult peripheral blood express the novel phenotype CD20 + CD27 + CD43 + CD70. J Exp Med 2011;208(1):67–80.

5. Haas KM, Tedder TF. Role of the CD19 and CD21/35 receptor complex in innate immunity, host defense and autoimmunity. Adv Exp Med Biol 2005;560:125–39.

6. Santos PM, Borghesi L. Molecular resolution of the B cell landscape. Curr Opin Immunol 2011;23(2):163–70.

7. Rajewsky K. Clonal selection and learning in the antibody system. Nature 1996;381(6585):751–8.

8. Nemazee D, Weigert M. Revising B cell receptors. J Exp Med 2000;191(11):1813–7.

9. van der Burg M, van Zelm MC, Driessen GJ, van Dongen JJ. Dissection of B-cell development to unravel defects in patients with a primary antibody deficiency. Adv Exp Med Biol 2011;697:183–96.

10. Rothenberg EV, Telfer JC, Anderson MK. Transcriptional regulation of lymphocyte lineage commitment. Bioessays 1999;21(9):726–42.

11. Kotani A, Harnprasopwat R, Toyoshima T, et al. miRNAs in normal and malignant B cells. Int J Hematol 2010;92(2):255–61.

12. Nagasawa T, Hirota S, Tachibana K, et al. Defects of B-cell lymphopoiesis and bone-marrow myelopoiesis in mice lacking the CXC chemokine PBSF/SDF-1. Nature 1996;382(6592):635–8.

13. Wang J, Lin Q, Langston H, Cooper MD. Resident bone marrow macrophages produce type 1 interferons that can selectively inhibit interleukin-7-driven growth of B lineage cells. Immunity 1995;3(4):475–84.

14. Grimaldi CM, Hill L, Xu X, et al. Hormonal modulation of B cell development and repertoire selection. Mol Immunol 2005;42(7):811–20.

15. Foster M, Montecino-Rodriguez E, Clark R, Dorshkind K. Regulation of B and T cell development by anterior pituitary hormones. Cell Mol Life Sci 1998;54(10):1076–82.

16. Ng LG, Mackay CR, Mackay F. The BAFF/APRIL system: life beyond B lymphocytes. Mol Immunol 2005;42(7):763–72.

17. Castigli E, Geha RS. TACI, isotype switching, CVID and IgAD. Immunol Res 2007;38(1–3):102–11.

18. Fu YX, Chaplin DD. Development and maturation of secondary lymphoid tissues. Annu Rev Immunol 1999;17:399–433.

19. Butcher EC, Williams M, Youngman K, et al. Lymphocyte trafficking and regional immunity. Adv Immunol 1999;72:209–53.

20. Cyster JG. B cell follicles and antigen encounters of the third kind. Nat Immunol 2010;11(11):989–96.

21. Lopes-Carvalho T, Kearney JF. Marginal zone B cell physiology and disease. Curr Dir Autoimmun 2005;8:91–123.

22. Carsetti R, Rosado MM, Wardmann H. Peripheral development of B cells in mouse and man. Immunol Rev 2004;197:179–91.

23. Allen CD, Okada T, Cyster JG. Germinal-center organization and cellular dynamics. Immunity 2007;27(2):190–202.

24. Facchetti F, Appiani C, Salvi L, et al. Immunohistologic analysis of ineffective CD40-CD40 ligand interaction in lymphoid tissues from patients with X-linked immunodeficiency with hyper-IgM. Abortive germinal center cell reaction and severe depletion of follicular dendritic cells. J Immunol 1995;154(12):6624–33.

25. Camacho SA, Kosco-Vilbois MH, Berek C. The dynamic structure of the germinal center. Immunol Today 1998;19(11):511–4.

26. Di Noia JM, Neuberger MS. Molecular mechanisms of antibody somatic hypermutation. Annu Rev Biochem 2007;76:1–22.

27. Victora GD, Schwickert TA, Fooksman DR, et al. Germinal center dynamics revealed by multiphoton microscopy with a photoactivatable fluorescent reporter. Cell 2010;143(4):592–605.

28. Zotos D, Coquet JM, Zhang Y, et al. IL-21 regulates germinal center B cell differentiation and proliferation through a B cell-intrinsic mechanism. J Exp Med 2010;207(2):365–78.

29. Hayakawa K, Hardy RR. Development and function of B-1 cells. Curr Opin Immunol 2000;12(3):346–53.

30. Herzenberg LA, Tung JW. B cell lineages: documented at last! Nat Immunol 2006;7(3):225–6.

31. Mauri C, Blair PA. Regulatory B cells in autoimmunity: developments and controversies. Nat Rev Rheumatol 2010;6(11):636–43.

32. Wagner SD, Neuberger MS. Somatic hypermutation of immunoglobulin genes. Annu Rev Immunol 1996;14:441–57.

33. Honjo T, Muramatsu M, Fagarasan S. AID: how does it aid antibody diversity? Immunity 2004;20(6):659–68.

34. Liu M, Schatz DG. Balancing AID and DNA repair during somatic hypermutation. Trends Immunol 2009;30(4):173–81.

35. Manz RA, Hauser AE, Hiepe F, Radbruch A. Maintenance of serum antibody levels. Annu Rev Immunol 2005;23:367–86.

36. Radbruch A, Muehlinghaus G, Luger EO, et al. Competence and competition: the challenge of becoming a long-lived plasma cell. Nat Rev Immunol 2006;6(10):741–50.

37. Chu VT, Frohlich A, Steinhauser G, et al. Eosinophils are required for the maintenance of plasma cells in the bone marrow. Nat Immunol 2011;12(2):151–9.

38. Wu YC, Kipling D, Leong HS, et al. High-throughput immunoglobulin repertoire analysis distinguishes between human IgM memory and switched memory B-cell populations. Blood 2010;116(7):1070–8.

39. Weyand CM, Klimiuk PA, Goronzy JJ. Heterogeneity of rheumatoid arthritis: from phenotypes to genotypes. Springer Semin Immunopathol 1998;20(1–2):5–22.

40. Scheel T, Gursche A, Zacher J, et al. V-region gene analysis of locally defined synovial B and plasma cells reveals selected B cell expansion and accumulation of plasma cell clones in rheumatoid arthritis. Arthritis Rheum 2011;63(1):63–72.

Louise Swainson,
Stephanie C. De
Barros, Marco
Craveiro, Valérie
S. Zimmermann,
Naomi Taylor

T-cell development

T-cell development begins in the fetal liver during early embryogenesis and later continues within a specialized primary lymphoid organ, the thymus. The prominent role of the thymus in T-cell generation (thymopoiesis), which was first established in the mouse,[1] is made clear through the study of DiGeorge syndrome, a rare congenital disorder characterized by varying levels of thymic dysgenesis. The level of dysgenesis correlates with T-cell numbers, with a small subset of patients with minimal thymic tissue severely immunocompromised owing to a complete lack of T cells. A landmark study by Markert et al. showed that transplantation of allogeneic thymus tissue into these patients resulted in the appearance of mature T lymphocytes, thus rescuing the T-cell deficiency.[2] Similarly, in patients with FOXN1 deficiency, a primary immunodeficiency characterized by athymia, the same group has recently shown that thymus transplantation leads to T-cell reconstitution and function.[3] These results have conclusively demonstrated the essential role of the thymus in T-cell development in humans.

KEY CONCEPTS

The thymus

- T cells develop in the thymus.
- The thymus consists of three major regions: the cortex, the medulla, and the corticomedullary junction.
- Progenitor cells enter the thymus at the corticomedullary junction.
- Most immature T cells, termed thymocytes, are found in the cortex.
- The corticomedullary junction contains large numbers of macrophages and dendritic cells that arise from mesodermal tissue.
- As thymocytes mature, they migrate to the medulla, in a chemokine-dependent manner.
- Mature thymocytes express either CD4 or CD8 and are found exclusively in the medulla.

Following commitment of hematopoietic stem cell (HSC) precursors to the T-cell lineage, thymocytes pass through a series of stages that can be identified by phenotypic changes in the expression of selected cell surface markers. The four predominant thymocyte populations are characterized by expression of the TCR coreceptors CD4 and CD8; the earliest of these stages is represented by CD4$^-$CD8$^-$ double-negative (DN) cells, which can be further subdivided based on CD1A cell surface expression in humans, or CD25 and CD44 expression in mice. Co-expression

of CD4 and CD8 with an αβ TCR occurs at the CD4$^+$CD8$^+$ double-positive (DP) stage of development. The interaction of the TCR with self peptide–MHC complexes, under conditions where they are not self-reactive, leads to the development of CD8$^+$ single-positive (SP) or CD4$^+$ SP cells and is discussed in more detail below.[4] The fundamental stages of thymocyte development in humans and mice are shown in Figure 8.1.

Thymocyte differentiation is a strictly regulated process, highly dependent on cytokines and cell–cell interactions between thymic stroma and T-cell precursors. Numerous checkpoints must be overcome before developing T cells emigrate to the periphery to generate a diverse repertoire of mature, immunocompetent T lymphocytes.

T-cell commitment from HSC precursors

T-cell differentiation in the thymus begins in progenitor cells that are the daughters of bone marrow HSCs. It is, however, important to note that HSC themselves do not appear capable of seeding the thymus under physiological conditions and those cells that naturally migrate to the thymus are not capable of supporting long-term thymopoiesis but rather promote only a single wave of short-term thymopoiesis lasting 3–4 weeks.[5] Based on these experimental data, it had been concluded that long-term thymocyte differentiation requires an ongoing migration of donor progenitors from the BM to the thymus because under physiological conditions, the progenitor cells entering the thymus have a limited life span. However, under the right conditions, progenitor cells can sustain long-term T-cell production. For example, in the context of an immunodeficient mouse strain (ZAP-70-deficient) wherein there is available "space" for a precursor niche, forced intrathymic administration of hematopoietic progenitors can promote and sustain long-term thymopoiesis.[6] This potential for thymic reconstitution has led to many studies aimed at elucidating the characteristics of the T progenitor cells responsible for seeding the thymus in both mice and humans.[7]

In humans, the CD34$^+$ hematopoietic precursors that seed the thymus can differentiate into multiple lineages. They have the potential to give rise to T, B, and NK cells of the lymphoid compartment, and to myeloid cells such as dendritic cells (DCs) and erythrocytes.[4] T-cell commitment thus occurs after entry of precursors into the thymus. The long-standing model for hematopoiesis has placed the first step in hematopoietic development as the differentiation of HSCs into either myeloid or lymphoid lineage restricted precursors, the latter known as a common

Fig. 8.1 Species differences in thymocyte differentiation. Fundamental thymocyte developmental stages in humans and mice are indicated with respect to established phenotypic markers and selection checkpoints. The major differences between these species are different phenotypic markers used to define the DN stages, the site of β-selection, and the inverted expression of CD4 and CD8 within the ISP populations. The site of β-selection in humans is simplified for clarity.

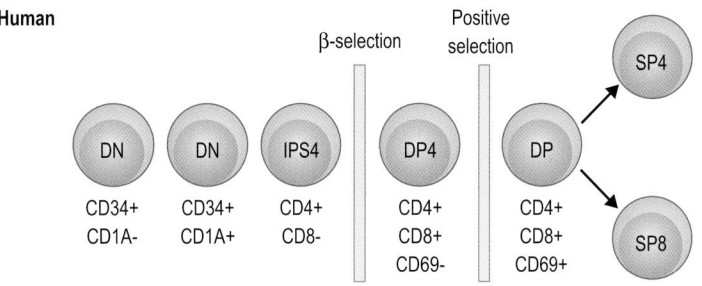

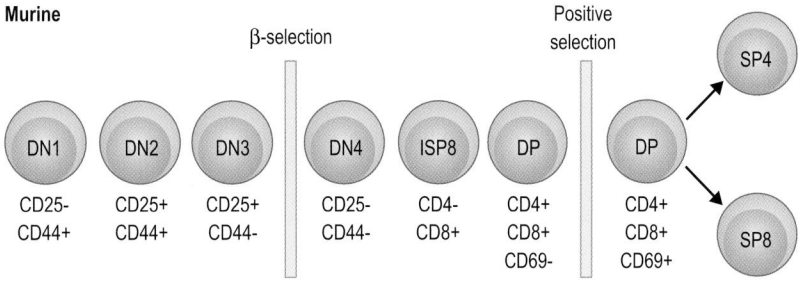

lymphoid precursor (CLP). This CLP then has the ability to generate T, B, and NK cells.[4] However, there is now some controversy regarding this issue as it has been reported by some investigators, and refuted by others, that progenitor cells in the murine thymus which have lost the potential to develop into B cells, but not T cells, can still give rise to myeloid cells.[8–10] In humans, a CD34$^+$ subset with a CD10$^+$CD24$^-$ phenotype (Chapter 7) has been shown to possess the characteristics of a CLP, retaining the ability to generate B, T, and NK lineages, but having lost myeloid potential.[11] These progenitors are present in cord blood and in the bone marrow, and can also be found in the blood throughout life. As such, they may constitute the proximal thymic precursor in man. Nonetheless, the question as to whether pro-T cells in the murine and human thymus retain a common T and myeloid potential will require further study.

At what developmental stage does a human precursor cell become destined to pursue a T lineage fate? Over the past few decades, the various transitional stages of T-cell development in the human thymus have been characterized as a function of phenotype, developmental potential, and status of T-cell receptor (TCR) gene rearrangements (Chapter 4). In the earliest stages of development, CD34$^+$ early thymic progenitors (ETP) lack CD1A, a member of the CD1 family of MHC-like glycoproteins. The acquisition of this marker is strongly associated with T-cell commitment. CD34$^+$CD1A$^+$ pre-T cells, in contrast to their upstream CD34$^+$CD1A$^-$ precursors, have rearrangements of TCRβ, γ, and δ loci, and appear unable to develop into non-T lineages.[4]

In the mouse thymus, the immature ETP expresses markers distinct from those expressed on human progenitor cells. These mouse progenitors are characterized as Lin$^-$CD44$^+$CD25$^-$Sca-1$^+$CD117c$^-$kit$^+$ (Lineage-negative, Sca-1$^+$, Kit$^+$; LSK) with only low CD127 (IL-7Rα) expression. Multipotent progenitors (MPP), retaining both myeloid and lymphoid potential, are generated from HSC and are characterized by the upregulation of the Fms-like tyrosine kinase receptor 3 (Flt3/CD135; resulting in LSK/CD135$^+$ cells). Subsets of MPP, characterized by expression of molecules such as RAG-1 and P-selectin, can also give rise to thymic precursors. This is also the case for the more committed CLP that lack myeloid potential. At least two major CLP subsets have been identified: CLP-1 (Lin$^-$Sca-1$^+$CD117$^{+/lo}$ CD127$^+$CD135$^+$B220$^-$)

and CLP-2 (Lin$^-$Sca-1$^+$CD117$^-$CD127$^+$ CD135$^+$B220$^+$), with the latter thought to be the most differentiated population with T-cell potential before commitment to the B-cell lineage. It is likely that MPP are capable of directly entering the thymus and it is notable that these cells are responsible for a more extended thymopoiesis than CLP (reviewed in Bhandoola et al.).[7]

Orchestrating thymocyte differentiation via an interplay of Notch and IL-7 signals

Notch1 is a member of a highly conserved family of transmembrane receptors that are involved in the regulation of cell fate choices in many lineages. Interaction of Notch1 with thymic stromal cells expressing its ligand Delta like-1 (DL-1) results in the proteolytical cleavage of its cytoplasmic portion, which translocates to the nucleus to mediate transcription of target genes.[12] The role of Notch1 in commitment to the T-cell lineage has been elegantly demonstrated by two ground-breaking studies. Retroviral-mediated overexpression of constitutively active Notch1 in hematopoietic precursors results in αβ T-cell development in the bone marrow, producing CD1A$^+$ DP cells normally only present in the thymus, while concomitantly blocking B lymphopoiesis.[13] Conversely, the conditional ablation of Notch1 expression causes an early block in T-cell development and results in the development of phenotypically normal immature B cells in the thymus.[14]

Signals mediated through Notch1,[15] IL-7R,[15] stem cell factor receptor (SCFR),[16] and CXCR4[17] are implicated in the survival and proliferation of early T-cell progenitors prior to the β-selection checkpoint. This early expansion results in an increase in the number of precursor cells upon which β-selection will act, enhancing the number of different productive TCRβ gene rearrangements that will be expressed in the developing thymocyte pool.

In addition to signals transmitted through the pre-TCR complex, it has become apparent that concomitant Notch1 signaling is also critical for driving developing thymocytes through the β-selection checkpoint. Notch1 ligation by DL-1 has previously been shown to regulate rearrangement of the TCRβ gene (Chapter 4)[18] and expression of pre-TCRα (pTα).[19] However, in mice bypassing pre-TCR receptor formation (see below) via expression of active downstream signaling mutants does not alleviate the requirement for Notch1 in progressing through β-selection to the DP stage.[20] The situation contrasts markedly in humans, where in the absence of Notch, human thymocyte precursors, including immature CD34[+] cells, can efficiently proceed to a mature DP stage, albeit with a significantly reduced proliferation.[21,22] The differentiation of these human thymocytes is dependent on IL-7, whereas in mice IL-7 signaling is not required.[15,23]

In the human thymus, high Notch activation appears to inhibit TCR-αβ differentiation, skewing human progenitors toward the γδ lineage. In order to rescue human αβ lineage differentiation, the level of Notch activation must be reduced.[24] This is intriguing as in mice, TCR-γδ-expressing cells can survive and expand in the absence of Notch, whereas high Notch levels are required for TCR-αβ differentiation as described above.[25]

The differential responsiveness of human and murine thymocytes to IL-7 likely reflects distinct expression profiles of the cytokine receptor (IL-7Rα) itself, as well as the stage at which β-selection occurs. IL-7Rα is not expressed on post-selection murine DP thymocytes,[26] but is easily detectable on the human DP subset at both the protein[27,28] and mRNA levels (our unpublished observations). In agreement with these data, murine DP thymocytes fail to phosphorylate Stat5 or upregulate Bcl-2[29,30] following IL-7 stimulation, while human DP thymocytes show an induction of STAT5 phosphorylation in response to this cytokine (our unpublished observations). In mice, an IL-7-insensitive stage between the β-selection and positive selection checkpoints is considered to be essential for the death of unsignaled thymocytes (death by neglect). While IL-7 stimulates STAT5 phosphorylation in human DP cells, it is important to note that the level of signaling is significantly lower than that detected in SP thymocytes, with an absence of blast formation, proliferation, and GLUT1 upregulation (our unpublished observations). Thus, these results suggest that even in the presence of an IL-7R complex, IL-7-mediated signals are dampened at the DP stage of human thymocyte differentiation. It will be important to determine the nature of the factors, such as SOCS family members, that inhibit IL-7 signaling in human DP thymocytes.

Beta selection

The first of two thymocyte proliferative phases occurs in DN thymocytes prior to recombinase activating gene (RAG) expression and TCR gene rearrangements (Chapter 4).[31] Importantly, CXCR4 signaling has recently been shown to play a key role in promoting the expansion of DN3 thymocytes, facilitating pre-TCR signals.[32,33] β-Selection allows the further differentiation of only those precursor T cells with productive, in-frame rearrangements of the TCRβ locus mediated by expression of RAG proteins. Extensive PCR and sequencing studies performed by Joachims et al. have demonstrated that, in humans, the TCRγ and TCRδ genes are rearranged first and lead to γδ T-cell development by default. Thymocytes unable to produce a functional γδ TCR are then diverted to the αβ lineage if they subsequently undergo an in-frame TCRβ rearrangement.[34] The formation of the pre-TCR constituting a nascent TCRβ chain in association with the pre-TCRα and CD3 molecules is necessary to pass the β-selection checkpoint. Indeed, failure to generate a functionally rearranged TCRβ chain at this stage of development results in thymocyte death by apoptosis. Signals derived from the pre-TCR complex trigger a maturation program within developing thymocytes that includes rescue from apoptosis, cessation of TCRβ gene rearrangement (allelic exclusion), initiation of TCRα

chain rearrangement, and a proliferative expansion that accounts for over 70% of total thymic cellularity.[35] Results from gene-deficient mouse models have illustrated that all components of the pre-TCR are essential for the cell to pass β-selection. In the absence of TCRβ rearrangement, due to RAG1 or RAG2 deficiency or deletion of the TCRβ loci, thymocyte development arrests at the β-selection checkpoint. The pTα, as well as the ε and γ signaling chains of the CD3 molecule, are also indispensable for differentiation beyond the pre-T stage (reviewed in Blom and Spits).[4] Analysis of a CD3δ-deficient human fetus indicates that absence of the δ chain also results in an inability of thymocytes to progress beyond β-selection.[36]

The phenotype of thymocytes at the stage where β-selection takes place in humans is somewhat controversial, with several lines of evidence indicating that β-selection can occur in distinct populations of cells differing in CD4 and CD8 expression. Intracytoplasmic (ic) TCRβ[−] populations have been found in CD4[+] ISP cells and in CD4[+]CD8α[+]β[−] early DP thymocytes, thus demonstrating that not all populations beyond the CD34[+]CD1A[+] stage are post β-selection cells. Blom and Spits have reported that β-selection can occur at the CD4[+] ISP stage, as TCRβ V-D-J recombination is present in a low level in CD4[+] ISP cells and 5% of CD4[+] ISP cells express TCRβ protein in their cytoplasm.[4] The group of Toribio, however, located the β-selection checkpoint at a later stage, namely, in CD4[+]CD8α[+]CD8β[+] cells that express a complex of TCRβ and pTα on the cell membrane.[37] Thus, it appears that expression of a TCRβ protein and subsequent β-selection occur within a developmental window that is not tightly coupled to regulation of CD4, CD8α, and CD8β expression. In contrast, in mice, β-selection occurs at a precise stage of differentiation, within DN3 (CD25[+]CD44[−]) thymocytes.

The timing of the rearrangement has functional consequences. In mice, it is those DN4 cells that have undergone a productive TCRβ rearrangement that show a proliferative burst,[38] whereas in humans, we have found that it is the CD4ISP and CD4[hi] DP immature thymocytes (characterized as TCRαβ[lo]) thymocytes that are proliferating and express high levels of the ubiquitous glucose transporter Glut1, as shown in Figure 8.2.[28] In mice, it is known that β-selection and subsequent proliferation correlate with a reversal in the polarity of thymocyte migration from the subcapsullar zone back into the cortex,[39] and this requires an adherence to the extracellular matrix. In humans, the data indicate that it is the GLUT1[+]CD4[hi]TCRαβ[lo] DP population that is associated with this critical phase of migration within the thymus.[28] It will therefore be important to study the functionality of murine and human thymocyte populations based on their differentiation stage rather than based solely on the presence of cell surface markers.

POSITIVE AND NEGATIVE SELECTION

The signals generated at β-selection through the emergent pre-TCR, Notch1, and CXCR4 signals lead to extensive proliferation prior to the rearrangement of TCRα, broadening the lymphocyte repertoire by allowing multiple TCRα chains to pair with the same β chain in a mature TCR αβ heterodimer. αβ Thymocytes subsequently die from neglect unless they are rescued by a low affinity interaction of the TCRαβ heterodimer with self peptides complexed with MHC antigens that are expressed on thymic epithelial cells (Chapters 5, 6). This process of positive selection thus avoids the production of non-functional T cells that are unable to recognize self-MHC. Positive selection is affected by the deletion of genes that encode MHC molecules; mice deficient in either class I or class II MHC genes exhibit markedly decreased numbers of CD8[+] and CD4[+] T cells, respectively (Chapter 35).

Fig. 8.2 Identification of the GLUT1-expressing human thymocyte population. The phenotype of human thymocytes expressing GLUT1 was monitored by flow cytometry. These cells could be characterized as a CD4^{hi} DP thymocyte population with significant proliferation potential (approximately 50% of these cells are in the S, G2, or M phases of the cell cycle). The cells represent an early stage following β-selection as demonstrated by low levels of TCRαβ and CD3 with expression of the CD8 β chain.

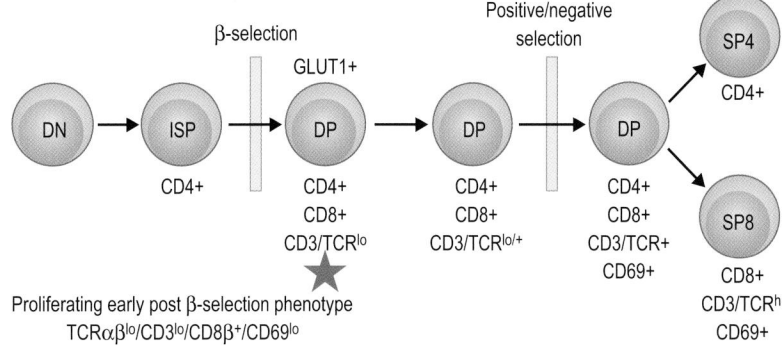

β-selection

Positive/negative
selection

GLUT1+

Proliferating early post β-selection phenotype
TCRαβ^{lo}/CD3^{lo}/CD8β^{+}/CD69^{lo}

DN → ISP → DP (CD4+ CD8+ CD3/TCR^{lo}) → DP (CD4+ CD8+ CD3/TCR$^{lo/+}$) → DP (CD4+ CD8+ CD3/TCR+ CD69+) → SP4 (CD4+) / SP8 (CD8+ CD3/TCR^{hi} CD69+)

ISP: CD4+

Thymocytes expressing high-affinity receptors for self-peptide–MHC are deleted in a process known as negative selection. The effect is to prevent the differentiation and export of potentially autoreactive cells into the periphery. It has long been questioned as to how T cells that are potentially autoreactive to antigens expressed solely in other tissues are culled by negative selection in the thymus. Much evidence has accumulated over the past decade showing that the autoimmune regulator gene (*AIRE*) plays a critical role in tolerizing thymocytes by inducing the expression of a battery of peripheral-tissue antigens in thymic medullary epithelial cells (reviewed in Gardner et al.).[40] *Aire*-deficient mice have reduced expression of peripheral antigens in thymic epithelial cells, and patients with mutations in the *AIRE* gene suffer from autoimmune polyendocrinopathy syndrome type-1 (APS-1), characterized by a spectrum of autoimmune diseases.[41]

There is considerable consensus that the fate of individual thymocytes is largely determined by the affinity and avidity (the product of affinity and the number of interactions) of their TCRs for the available self-peptide–MHC ligand; this process results in TCRs that are either included (positive selection) or excluded (negative selection) from the T-cell repertoire. It has been reported that the duration of TCR–ligand interactions helps to discriminate between low- and high-affinity ligands and a "zipper" mechanism initiates negative-selection signaling based on the interaction of the TCR and co-receptor molecules.[42]

This stringent developmental checkpoint allows less than 3% of thymocytes to pass αβ TCR selection. It is necessary for the elimination of self-reactive thymocytes, the maturation of which would result in autoimmunity. The resultant TCR signaling in CD3^{+}CD4^{+}CD8^{+} DP cells causes the termination of *RAG1* and *RAG2* gene expression, thereby fixing TCRα specificity. However, it is important to note that peripheral tolerance of self-reactive T cells that escape deletion is also required, and is largely facilitated by thymus-derived regulatory CD4^{+}FOXP3^{+} T cells (Treg) (Chapter 15).

Treg lineage commitment branches off from conventional CD4 T-cell (Tconv) development during thymocyte maturation. Current consensus favors the model that autoreactivity is a primary determinant of intrathymic Treg specification. This hypothesis is consistent with observations that Treg and Tconv TCR repertoires are largely distinct in mouse models (reviewed in Ohkura and Sakaguchi).[43] However, as TCR transgenic systems of self-antigen-driven intrathymic Treg development show that substantial negative selection of cells of the respective specificity also occur, other thymocyte intrinsic or extrinsic parameters are expected to influence the clonal deletion versus Treg cell fate decision (reviewed in Wirnsberger et al.).[44]

Strong evidence favors a "functional avidity" model according to which Treg specification occurs within an avidity window between positive selection and clonal deletion. Functional avidity incorporates determinants of the interaction between thymocyte and APC that extends beyond TCR affinity and number of peptide–MHC ligands, for example, co-stimulatory interactions or APC intrinsic properties, which may feed into signal integration by developing thymocytes.[44]

Lineage commitment

Following the successful rearrangement of an αβTCR, developing thymocytes undergo a lineage "choice" by differentiating into either CD4 helper or CD8 cytotoxic T cells. The cellular and molecular mechanisms regulating lineage fate have been arduously debated during the past 20 years. But it is important to note that almost all the proposed models have been based on experiments performed in mice.[45] This process is functionally important as the maintenance of the proper number and proportion of CD4^{+} and CD8^{+} T cells is essential for optimal host defense.

Early investigations led to the "instructive model" of lineage choice, which posits that co-engagement of the TCR and CD4 or CD8 initiates qualitatively or quantitatively distinct signals that direct downregulation of the inappropriate co-receptor and lineage choice. By expressing chimeric CD8/CD4 co-receptor transgenes in CD8α knockout mice, the Singer lab challenged the underpinnings of the instruction model, demonstrating that the identity of the co-receptor tail (CD4 or CD8) quantitatively influences the number of SP T cells generated, but does not alter the CD4/CD8 lineage decision. An alternative stochastic/selective model proposes that co-receptor downmodulation is a random process independent of TCR specificity, and thymocytes terminating the necessary co-receptor molecule for their TCR are subsequently eliminated as a result of inefficient TCR signaling. As a result, only thymocytes with correctly matching TCR and co-receptor molecules would survive to differentiate into mature T cells. This hypothesis no longer seems tenable as dead-end thymocytes expressing incorrect co-receptor–TCR combinations do not seem to occur in sufficient numbers to agree with the predictions of the model. Moreover, both the instructive and stochastic models are based on the premise that lineage commitment occurs in TCR signaled DP thymocytes simultaneously with positive selection, thus resulting in irreversible silencing of the opposite co-receptor gene. The discovery that signaled DP thymocytes initially terminate CD8 transcription even when differentiating into CD8^{+} T cells challenged this central paradigm and led to the now widely accepted "kinetic signaling" model of lineage commitment (reviewed in Singer et al.).[45]

The kinetic signaling model postulates that cell fate is determined by the duration of positive selection signaling. In this model, proposed by Alfred Singer and colleagues, DP thymocytes, regardless of their MHC specificity, respond to

TCR-mediated positive selecting signals by terminating *Cd8* gene expression and are thus converted into CD4$^+$CD8$^-$ intermediate thymocytes, making CD4 the initial choice of co-receptors. If positively selecting TCR signals are sustained, CD4$^+$CD8$^-$ intermediate thymocytes continue down the CD4$^+$SP T-cell differentiation pathway. For CD4$^+$CD8$^-$ cells interacting with MHC class I molecules, however, the downmodulation of CD8 at the CD4$^+$CD8$^-$ stage will lead to diminution, or loss, of TCR signaling. The resulting impairment of positively selecting TCR signals causes class I-restricted CD4$^+$CD8$^-$ cells to begin to transcribe *Cd8* again, and to terminate CD4 transcription (an event referred to as "co-receptor reversal"), thus switching them into the CD8$^+$SP T-cell differentiation pathway.

The cytokine IL-7 is crucial for mediating this co-receptor reversal and differentiation of mature CD8$^+$SP T cells.[46] The kinetic signaling model is strongly supported by experiments showing that when CD4 protein expression is placed under the control of CD8 transcriptional regulatory elements, class II-restricted cells undergo a complete shift in commitment to the CD8 lineage with expression of the Runx3 cytotoxic lineage factor, despite the MHC-II specificity and CD4 dependence of their TCRs.[47] Thus, T cells follow the CD4 differentiation pathway when TCR signaling persists, whereas IL-7 signaling promotes CD8 T-cell differentiation (Fig. 8.3).

Several of the mechanisms responsible for translating alternative TCR signals into alternative developmental programs of gene expression have been elucidated in the past few years. Transcription factors known to control the emergence of CD4 and CD8 lineages have been identified and include the zinc finger proteins ThPOK (T-helper inducing POZ-Kruppel factor) and Gata3 (for CD4), and the Runx factors Runx1 and Runx3 (for CD8). Constitutive expression of ThPok during thymic development restores normal development of class II-restricted T cells to the CD4 lineage in mice lacking this transcription factor and also causes a redirection of class I-restricted cells to the CD4 lineage. Furthermore, the binding of Runx3 to the ThPOK locus acts to repress ThPok expression and is required for development of CD8 T cells (reviewed in Naito and Taniuchi).[48]

Thymocyte migration and export

The thymus consists of many lobules, each of which has an inner medulla surrounded by an outer cortex. Studies in the mouse by Petrie and colleagues[49] have shown that an intricate movement through well-defined thymic regions occurs during thymocyte development, with lymphoid progenitors initially entering the thymus at the corticomedullary junction, then migrating to the subcapsular zone, which is located just under the outer border of the cortex. Here, thymocytes undergo β-selection-induced proliferation and differentiate into CD4$^+$CD8$^+$ DP cells, a phase that correlates with a reversal in the polarity of thymocyte migration from the subcapsular zone back into the medulla, where the final stages of T-cell development take place (reviewed in Blom and Spits).[4] Signals mediated via the CCR7 chemokine receptor are essential for the cortex-to-medulla migration of positively selected thymocytes in the thymus. The diverse nature of chemokines, adhesion molecules, and their receptors involved in thymocyte migration have been at least partially elucidated, and include the chemokines CXCL12, CCR19, and CCR21, P-selectins, recognition of VCAM1 and peptide-MHC on thymic epithelial cells, and signals mediated via the sphingosine

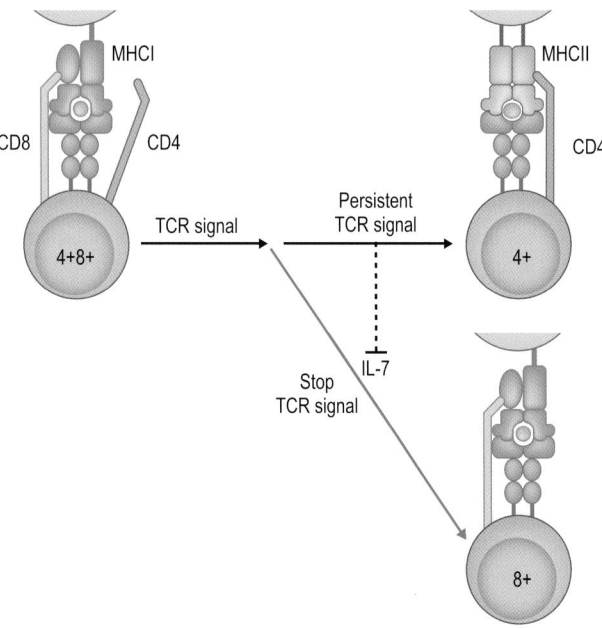

Fig. 8.3 The kinetic signaling model of lineage choice in mice. Positively selected DP thymocytes terminate *Cd8* gene expression and appear to be phenotypically CD4$^+$CD8^{low}. Under conditions where TCR signaling persists, due to an interaction with antigen presented by MCH–class II, IL-7 signaling is blocked and CD4 differentiation continues. However, under conditions wherein the selected TCR interacts with antigen presented by a MHC–class I complex, TCR signaling is disrupted, promoting IL-7 signaling and Runx3 expression. In mice, this cascade has been shown to result in the subsequent transcription of the *Cd8* gene, and the differentiation of CD8 cytotoxic cells.

(Adapted from A. Singer and colleagues.[45])

1-phosphate type 1 (S1P$_1$) receptor (reviewed in Takahama[50] and Love and Bhandoola).[51] The spatial journey of a thymocyte is thus, like all other processes and stages of thymopoiesis, dependent upon a multitude of interactions with other cells and soluble factors. Once mature CD4$^+$ SP and CD8$^+$ SP cells have completed their intrathymic differentiation, they undergo thymic export via blood vessels at the corticomedullary junction to the periphery, generating a diverse repertoire of mature, immunocompetent T lymphocytes.

● CLINICAL RELEVANCE

Abnormalities of T-cell development

- The importance of the thymus is underscored by the complete absence of T cells in patients in whom a thymus has failed to develop (e.g., complete DiGeorge syndrome, FOXN1 deficiency).

- T-cell development can be abrogated by the accumulation of toxic metabolites, such as seen in adenosine deaminase or purine nucleoside phosphorylase deficiencies.

- T-cell development requires expression of T-cell receptors (TCR); hence, loss-of-function mutations in RAG and associated genes typically results in the absence of T cells.

- T-cell survival and development require signal transduction through the TCR signaling complex and associated co-receptors; hence, loss-of-function mutations in TCR-CD3 components typically result in T-cell deficiency or dysfunction.

- The autoimmune regulator gene (AIRE) plays a critical role in tolerizing thymocytes; mutations in AIRE result in an autoimmune polyendocrinopathy (APS-1), characterized by a spectrum of autoimmune diseases.

References

1. Miller JF. Immunological function of the thymus. Lancet 1961;2:748–9.
2. Markert ML, Boeck A, Hale LP, et al. Transplantation of thymus tissue in complete DiGeorge syndrome. N Engl J Med 1999;341:1180–9.
3. Markert ML, Marques JG, Neven B, et al. First use of thymus transplantation therapy for FOXN1 deficiency (nude/SCID): a report of 2 cases. Blood 2011;117:688–96.
4. Blom B, Spits H. Development of human lymphoid cells. Annu Rev Immunol 2006;24:287–320.
5. Scollay R, Smith J, Stauffer V. Dynamics of early T cells: prothymocyte migration and proliferation in the adult mouse thymus. Immunol Rev 1986;91:129–57.
6. Vicente R, Adjali O, Jacquet C, et al. Intrathymic transplantation of bone marrow-derived progenitors provides long-term thymopoiesis. Blood 2010;115:1913–20.
7. Bhandoola A, von Boehmer H, Petrie HT, Zuniga-Pflucker JC. Commitment and developmental potential of extrathymic and intrathymic T cell precursors: plenty to choose from. Immunity 2007;26:678–89.
8. Wada H, Masuda K, Satoh R, et al. Adult T-cell progenitors retain myeloid potential. Nature 2008;452:768–72.
9. Bell JJ, Bhandoola A. The earliest thymic progenitors for T cells possess myeloid lineage potential. Nature 2008;452:764–7.
10. Schlenner SM, Madan V, Busch K, et al. Fate mapping reveals separate origins of T cells and myeloid lineages in the thymus. Immunity 2010;32:426–36.
11. Six EM, Bonhomme D, Monteiro M, et al. A human postnatal lymphoid progenitor capable of circulating and seeding the thymus. J Exp Med 2007;204:3085–93.
12. Allman D, Aster JC, Pear WS. Notch signaling in hematopoiesis and early lymphocyte development. Immunol Rev 2002;187:75–86.
13. Pui JC, Allman D, Xu L, et al. Notch1 expression in early lymphopoiesis influences B versus T lineage determination. Immunity 1999;11:299–308.
14. Radtke F, Wilson A, Stark G, et al. Deficient T cell fate specification in mice with an induced inactivation of Notch1. Immunity 1999;10:547–58.
15. Balciunaite G, Ceredig R, Fehling HJ, et al. The role of Notch and IL-7 signaling in early thymocyte proliferation and differentiation. Eur J Immunol 2005;35:1292–300.
16. Rodewald HR, Fehling HJ. Molecular and cellular events in early thymocyte development. Adv Immunol 1998;69:1–112.
17. Hernandez-Lopez C, Varas A, Sacedon R, et al. Stromal cell-derived factor 1/CXCR4 signaling is critical for early human T-cell development. Blood 2002;99:546–54.
18. Wolfer A, Wilson A, Nemir M, et al. Inactivation of Notch1 impairs VDJbeta rearrangement and allows pre-TCR-independent survival of early alpha beta Lineage Thymocytes. Immunity 2002;16:869–79.
19. Reizis B, Leder P. Direct induction of T lymphocyte-specific gene expression by the mammalian Notch signaling pathway. Genes Dev 2002;16:295–300.
20. Ciofani M, Schmitt TM, Ciofani A, et al. Obligatory role for cooperative signaling by pre-TCR and Notch during thymocyte differentiation. J Immunol 2004;172:5230–9.
21. Taghon T, Van de Walle I, De Smet G, et al. Notch signaling is required for proliferation but not for differentiation at a well-defined beta-selection checkpoint during human T-cell development. Blood 2009;113:3254–63.
22. Magri M, Yatim A, Benne C, et al. Notch ligands potentiate IL-7-driven proliferation and survival of human thymocyte precursors. Eur J Immunol 2009;39:1231–40.
23. Maillard I, Tu L, Sambandam A, et al. The requirement for Notch signalting at the beta-selection checkpoint in vivo is absolute and independent of the pre-T cell receptor. J Exp Med 2006;203:2239–45.
24. Van de Walle I, De Smet G, De Smedt M, et al. An early decrease in Notch activation is required for human TCR-alphabeta lineage differentiation at the expense of TCR-gammadelta T cells. Blood 2009;113:2988–98.
25. Garbe AI, Krueger A, Gounari F, et al. Differential synergy of Notch and T cell receptor signaling determines alphabeta versus gammadelta lineage fate. J Exp Med 2006;203:1579–90.
26. Sudo T, Nishikawa S, Ohno N, et al. Expression and function of the interleukin 7 receptor in murine lymphocytes. Proc Natl Acad Sci U S A 1993;90:9125–9.
27. Guillemard E, Nugeyre MT, Chene L, et al. Interleukin-7 and infection itself by human immunodeficiency virus 1 favor virus persistence in mature CD4(+)CD8(-)CD3(+) thymocytes through sustained induction of Bcl-2. Blood 2001;98:2166–74.
28. Swainson L, Kinet S, Manel N, et al. Glucose transporter 1 expression identifies a population of cycling CD4+ CD8+ human thymocytes with high CXCR4-induced chemotaxis. Proc Natl Acad Sci U S A 2005;102:12867–72.
29. Van De Wiele CJ, Marino JH, Murray BW, et al. Thymocytes between the beta-selection and positive selection checkpoints are nonresponsive to IL-7 as assessed by STAT-5 phosphorylation. J Immunol 2004;172:4235–44.
30. Yu Q, Park JH, Doan LL, et al. Cytokine signal transduction is suppressed in preselection doublepositive thymocytes and restored by positive selection. J Exp Med 2006;203:165–75.
31. Kawamoto H, Ohmura K, Fujimoto S, et al. Extensive proliferation of T cell lineage-restricted progenitors in the thymus: an essential process for clonal expression of diverse T cell receptor beta chains. Eur J Immunol 2003;33:606–15.
32. Janas ML, Varano G, Gudmundsson K, et al. Thymic development beyond {beta}-selection requires phosphatidylinositol 3-kinase activation by CXCR4. J Exp Med 2010;207(1):247–61.
33. Trampont PC, Tosello-Trampont AC, Shen Y, et al. CXCR4 acts as a costimulator during thymic beta-selection. Nat Immunol 2010;11(2):162–70.
34. Joachims ML, Chain JL, Hooker SW, et al. Human alpha beta and gamma delta thymocyte development: TCR gene rearrangements, intracellular TCR beta expression, and gamma delta developmental potential—differences between men and mice. J Immunol 2006;176:1543–52.
35. von Boehmer H, Fehling HJ. Structure and function of the pre-T cell receptor. Annu Rev Immunol 1997;15:433–52.
36. de Saint Basile G, Geissmann F, Flori E. Severe combined immunodeficiency caused by deficiency in either the delta or the epsilon subunit of CD3. J Clin Invest 2004;114:1512–7.
37. Carrasco YR, Trigueros C, Ramiro AR, et al. Beta-selection is associated with the onset of CD8beta chain expression on CD4(+)CD8alphaalpha(+) pre-T cells during human intrathymic development. Blood 1999;94:3491–8.
38. Hoffman ES, Passoni L, Crompton T, et al. Productive T-cell receptor beta-chain gene rearrangement: coincident regulation of cell cycle and clonality during development in vivo. Genes Dev 1996;10:948–62.
39. Takahama Y. Journey through the thymus: stromal guides for T-cell development and selection. Nat Rev Immunol 2006;6:127–35.
40. Gardner JM, Fletcher AL, Anderson MS, Turley SJ. AIRE in the thymus and beyond. Curr Opin Immunol 2009;21:582–9.
41. Nagamine K, Peterson P, Scott HS, et al. Positional cloning of the APECED gene. Nat Genet 1997;17:393–8.
42. Palmer E, Naeher D. Affinity threshold for thymic selection through a T-cell receptor-co-receptor zipper. Nat Rev Immunol 2009;9:207–13.
43. Ohkura N, Sakaguchi S. Regulatory T cells: roles of T cell receptor for their development and function. Semin Immunopathol 2010;32:95–106.
44. Wirnsberger G, Hinterberger M, Klein L. Regulatory T-cell differentiation versus clonal deletion of autoreactive thymocytes. Immunol Cell Biol 2011;89:45–53.
45. Singer A, Adoro S, Park JH. Lineage fate and intense debate: myths, models and mechanisms of CD4- versus CD8-lineage choice. Nat Rev Immunol 2008;8:788–801.
46. Park JH, Adoro S, Guinter T, et al. Signaling by intrathymic cytokines, not T cell antigen receptors, specifies CD8 lineage choice and promotes the differentiation of cytotoxic-lineage T cells. Nat Immunol 2010;11:257–64.
47. Sarafova SD, Erman B, Yu Q, et al. Modulation of coreceptor transcription during positive selection dictates lineage fate independently of TCR/coreceptor specificity. Immunity 2005;23:75–87.
48. Naito T, Taniuchi I. The network of transcription factors that underlie the CD4 versus CD8 lineage decision. Int Immunol 2010;22:791–6.
49. Prockop SE, Palencia S, Ryan CM, et al. Stromal cells provide the matrix for migration of early lymphoid progenitors through the thymic cortex. J Immunol 2002;169:4354–61.
50. Takahama Y. Journey through the thymus: stromal guides for T-cell development and selection. Nat Rev Immunol 2006;6:127–35.
51. Love PE, Bhandoola A. Signal integration and crosstalk during thymocyte migration and emigration. Nat Rev Immunol 2011;11:469–77.

9

John J. O'Shea,
Massimo Gadina,
Richard Siegel

Cytokines and cytokine receptors

● KEY CONCEPT

Cytokine characteristics

- Cytokines have pleotropic effects: they may have more than one receptor.
- Cytokines can be redundant—their receptors often share subunits.
- Cytokines can have specific and unique functions—their receptors typically have ligand-specific subunits as well.

Cytokines play pivotal roles in controlling the development and functions of a variety of immune and non-immune cells. They are of particular interest to immunologists because of their importance in immune regulation, their role in disease pathogenesis, and, increasingly, treatment. One of the barriers to learning about cytokines is the complicated nomenclature and system of classification. In part, this reflects the nonspecificity of the term cytokine. It does not encompass a class of factors that are structurally or functionally related: rather, it includes a number of different factors produced by lymphoid and non-lymphoid cells that mediate intercellular communication. The confusion in terminology arises partly from the history of the field. The various cytokines were discovered by researchers in several disciplines and many marked their cytokine with their original set of interests.

The term lymphokine was originally used to denote products of lymphocytes,[1] but Cohen et al.[2] coined the word cytokine to emphasize the point that these factors need not be made by one specific cell source. This was an important insight, because many immunologically relevant cytokines are made by nonlymphoid cells. Later, the term interleukin was introduced to emphasize the importance of these factors in communication between leukocytes.[3] Although this designation has remained in use, it is similarly inaccurate.

Cytokines can be defined operationally as polypeptides secreted by leukocytes and other cells that act principally on hematopoietic cells, the effects of which include modulation of immune and inflammatory responses. However, there are clear exceptions to even this broad definition. Some definitions distinguish cytokines from hormones and growth factors, which act on non-hematopoietic cells. Thus, cytokines are typically characterized as factors made by more than one cell type and act locally, whereas hormones are secreted by specialized cells and act at a distance on a restricted set of target cells. Although many cytokines act locally in an autocrine or paracrine fashion, some do enter the bloodstream and can act in a typical endocrine fashion. Consequently, the boundary between cytokines and hormones is rather indistinct. In fact, classic hormones such as growth hormone (GH), prolactin (PRL) and erythropoietin (EPO) are clearly cytokines, as is one of the newest hormones, leptin, as evidenced by the type of receptor they bind and their modes of signaling. Clear functional similarities and evolutionary relationships exist among these families of molecules that act on the immune, hematopoietic, endocrine and nervous systems.

A major challenge in discussing cytokines is their classification. One way is to group the factors by function. However, an important characteristic of cytokines is that they are often pleiotropic in their effects. They can have multiple target cells and consequently multiple actions. Second, structurally dissimilar cytokines can have overlapping but typically non-identical actions, a given effect often being mediated by several different cytokines. This is termed cytokine redundancy. Finally, a single cytokine frequently induces or influences the action of other cytokines, and can function synergistically. Thus understanding the exact properties of a given cytokine is a challenge. However, this complexity of cytokine action has been simplified to an extent by the generation of cytokine gene targeted mice.

The complexity in terms of action provides a strong rationale for an alternative nosology, and that is to group cytokines according to the type of receptor that they bind rather than by their function. This classification is also useful because it reflects the evolutionary relatedness of cytokines, growth factors, and hormones, and emphasizes similarities in modes of signal transduction. The classification used in this chapter is adapted from Vilcek[4] and includes the following receptors: the so-called type I (hematopoietin family) and type II (interferon family) cytokine receptors, tumor necrosis factor (TNF) family receptors, interleukin (IL)-1 receptor and the related Toll-like receptors (TLRs), IL-17 receptors, receptor tyrosine kinases, and the TGF-β family receptor serine kinases (Table 9.1, Fig. 9.1). A sixth group of cytokines, better known as chemokines, are considered to form a separate family in view of the structure of their seven transmembrane domain receptors (Chapter 10). This chapter reviews in detail only a selected set of cytokines with important immunological functions.

Type I and II cytokine receptors (hematopoietin family and interferon receptors)

Ligand and receptor structure

Cytokines (Table 9.1) that bind the class of receptors termed the type I or hematopoietic cytokine receptor superfamily include hormones such as EPO, thrombopoietin (TPO), PRL, GH, and leptin; colony-stimulating factors (CSF) such as granulocyte

Table 9.1 Cytokines classified by receptor families

Receptor family	Cytokine	Signaling	Source	Target	Action	Knockout phenotype
Type 1 (hemato-poietin)	GH	JAK2, STAT5b	Two GH genes, pituitary, placental	Diverse tissues	Growth, adipocyte differentiation	Dwarfism
	Prl	JAK2, STATa	Two Prl genes pituitary, uterus	Mammary epithelium	Growth, differentiation	Infertility, lactation defects
	Epo	JAK2, STAT5	Kidney, Liver	Erythroid precursors	Erythroid differentiation	Embryonic lethal, severe anemia
	Tpo	JAK2, STAT5	Liver, Kidney	Committed stem cells and megakaryocytes	Platelet	Severe thrombocytopenia
	Leptin	JAK2/STAT3	Adipocytes	Hypothalamus, thyroid	Satiety, controls metabolic rate	Obesity
	G-CSF	JAK2, STAT3	Many tissues, macrophages, endothelium, fibroblasts	Committed progenitors	Differentiation, activates mature granulocytes	Neutropenia
	IL-6	JAK1, STAT3	Macrophage, fibroblasts, endothelium, epithelium, T cells, other	Liver, B cell, T cell, thymocytes myeloid cells, osteoclasts	Acute-phase reactants proliferation, differentiation co-stimulation	Reduced Ig, esp. IgA, T lymphopenia, impaired acute-phase response, and Th17 cells
	IL-11	JAK1, STAT3	Stromal cells, Sinoviocytes, osteoblasts	Hematopoietic stem cells, hepatocytes, macrophages, neurons	Proliferation	Female infertility
	IL-27	JAK1, STAT1, STAT3, STAT4. STAT5	Activated DC, macrophages, epithelial cells	T and NK cells, other cells	Enhancement of Th1 responses, and IL-10; inhibition of Th1, Th2, and Th17 responses	Fatal inflammatory disease with infection
	IL-31	JAK1, STAT3, STAT5	Th2 cells CD8 T cells	Monocytes, epithelial cells Keratinocytes, eosinophils basophils	Induces chemokines, PMN recruitment	
	CNTF[a]	JAK1, STAT3	Schwann cells	Neuronal	Survival	Progressive atrophy and loss of motor neurons
	LIF[a]	JAK1, STAT3	Uterus, macrophage, fibroblasts, endothelium, epithelium, T cells	Embryonic stem cells, neurons hematopoietic	Survival	Decreased hematopoietic progenitors, defective blastocyst implantation
	Osm	JAK1, STAT3	Macrophage, fibroblasts, endothelium, epithelium	T cells, Myeloid cells, liver, embryonic stem cells	Differentiation, acute-phase induction	
	CT-1	JAK1, STAT3	T cells, others, Myocardial	Myocardium	Growth	
	GM-CSF	JAK1, STAT3	T cells, macrophages, endothelium, fibroblasts	Immature and committed myelomonocytic progenitors macrophages and granulocytes, DC	Growth, differentiation survival, activation	Pulmonary alveolar proteinosis
	IL-3	JAK2, STAT5	T cells Macrophages, mast cells, NKT cells Eosinophils	Immature hematopoietic progenitors of multiple lineages	Growth, differentiation survival	No defects in basal hematopoiesis

Table 9.1 Cytokines classified by receptor families—cont'd

Receptor family	Cytokine	Signaling	Source	Target	Action	Knockout phenotype
	IL-5	JAK2, STAT5	Th2 T cells, Activated eosinophils NK, NKT cells	Eosinophil, B cells, basophils, mast cells	Proliferation, activation	Decreased oesinophilla, defective CD5, B1-cell development
	IL-2	JAK1, JAK3, STAT5	T cells, NK cells, NKT cells	T, B, NK cells, macrophages	Proliferation, cytoxicity IFN-γ secretion, antibody production	Lymphoproliferation[a]
	IL-4[b]	JAK1, JAK3, STAT6	Th2 cells, cells mast cells, NKT cells, γ/δ T cells	T cell, B cell, macrophage	Proliferation, Th2 differentiation IgG^1 and IgE production Inhibition of cell-mediated immunity	Defective Th2 differentiation and IgE production, decreased allergic responses
	IL-7	JAK1, JAK3, STAT5	Bone marrow, thymic stromal cells, spleen DC, keratinocytes, Monocytes, macrophages	Thymocytes, T cells, B cells	Growth, differentiation, survival	SCID[a]
	IL-9	JAK1, JAK3, STAT5	Th2 and Th9 T cells, mast cells, eosinophils	T cells, B cells, mast cell precursors	Proliferation, Th1 inhibition	Not essential for Th2 pathology
	IL-15[b]	JAK1, JAK3, STAT5	Many cells	T-cells, especially memory cells, NK and NKT cells	Proliferation, survival and activation	Absence of NK and memory cells
	IL-21	JAK1, JAK3, STAT3	T cells, Th17 cells, Tfh cells	T, B, and NK cells, DC, macrophages, keratinocytes	Isotype switching, plasma cell differentiation, enhances CD8+ and NK cell responses, promotes Th17 cell differentiation	Acts in concert with IL-4 Decreased Th17 cells
	IL-13	JAK1, TYK2, STAT6	Activated T cells, NKT, mast cells, basophils	B cells, mast cells, macrophages, epithelial cells, smooth muscle cells	Co-stimulator of proliferation, IgE increased CD23 and Class II, Inhibits cytokine secretion and cell-mediated immunity	Defective Th2 responses and IgE production, decreased allergic responses
	IL-12	JAK2, TYK2, STAT4	Macrophages, DC, B cells	T cell, NK cell	Th1 differentiation, proliferation, cytotoxicity	Defective Th1 differentiation, susceptibility to bacterial infections*
	IL-23	JAK2, TYK2, STAT3, STAT5	Macrophages, DC	T cells, macrophages	IL-17 production	Reduced arthritis, inflammation,
	IL-35	?	Treg	T cells	Treg proliferation Suppresses proliferation and functions of Th17	Reduced Treg activity
	TSLP	JAK1, JAK2, STAT1 STAT3, STAT5	Epithelial cells, keratinocytes	DC (human) B cells (mouse)	TH2 differentiation (human)	Shared receptor usage with IL-7R
Type II (interferon)	IFN-α/β	JAK1, TYK2, STAT1, STAT2	Plasmacytoid DC, Macrophages, fibroblasts, other	All, NK cell	Antiviral, anti-proliferative increased MHC Class I activation	Susceptibility to viral infections[a]
	IFN-γ	JAK1, JAK2, STAT1	Th1 T cells NK cells	Macrophages, endothelium NK cells	Activation, increased MHC Class II expression, increased antigen presentation	Susceptibility to bacterial infections[a]
	IL-10	JAK1, TYK2, STAT3	Th2 T cells, other cells	Macrophages	Decreased MHC class II expression, decreased antigen presentation	Exaggerated inflammatory response and autoimmune disease

Table 9.1 Cytokines classified by receptor families—cont'd

Receptor family	Cytokine	Signaling	Source	Target	Action	Knockout phenotype
	IL-19, 20, 22, 24, 26	STAT1, STAT3	T cells, monocytes, melanocytes, NKT cells	T cells, keratinocytes, Epithelial cells	Induces production of inflammatory cytokines, Th2 responses, activation of epithelial cells	
	IL-28, 29, 30	STAT1, STAT2, STAT3, STAT4, STAT5	DC, Many cells	Many cells	Antiviral	
IL-1/TLR	IL-1α/β	IRAK, MyD88, TRAF6, NF-kB	Many cells, esp. macrophages	CNS, endothelial cell liver, thymocyte, macrophage , T cells	Fever, anorexia, activation acute-phase reactants co-stimulation, activation, cytokine secretion, differentiation of Th17 cells	Reduced inflammation, cooperates with TNF in host defense
	IL-1 F, G					
	IL-18	IRAK, MyD88, TRAF6, NF-kB	Many cells, esp. macrophages, keratinocytes, osteoblast	T cells, NK cells, Macrophages, epithelial cells cells		Increased susceptibility to infection, Reduced arthritis
	IL-33			T cells, nuocytes	Enhanced Th2 responses	
	IL-37					
IL-17	IL-17A		Th17 cells, CD8 T cells, γ/δ T cells	Endothelium, many cells	Inflammation	Susceptibility to extracellular bacteria
	IL-17B,C,D		Many cells	Monocytes, epithelial cells	Inflammation, chondrogenesis	
	IL-17E (IL-25)	TRAF2	mast cells Th2 cells	Th2 cells	Enhanced Th2 responses	Increased susceptibility to helminths
	IL-17 F		Th17 cells, CD8 T cells γ/δ T cells	Endothelium, many cells	Inflammation	
TGF-β receptor serine kinase family	TGF-β 1,2, 3		T cells, macrophages other	T cells, macrophages other	Inhibits growth and activation, promotes Th17	
Receptor tyrosine kinases	Stem cell factor	Ras/Raf/ MAPK Stromal cell	Bone marrow	Pluripotent stem cell	Activation, growth	Defective hematopoietic stem cell proliferation, melanocyte production and development
	CSF-1 (M-CSF)	Ras/Raf/ MAPK	Macrophage, endothelium, fibroblast, other	Committed myelomonocytic progenitors	Differentiation proliferation, survival	Monocytopenia, osteopetrosis, female infertility
	Flt-3 ligand	Ras/Raf/ MAPK	Diverse tissue	Myeloid cells, especially DC	Proliferation, differentiation	Reduced repopulating hematopoietic stem cells; reduced B-cell precursors
	IL-32	NF-κB, p38 MAPK	T, NK cells, monocytes, epithelia	Monocytes	Induces TNF, IL-1, IL-6, IL-8	
	IL-16		T and B cells, mast cells, eosinophils	CD4 T cells		
	IL-3	ERK	Many cells	Monocytes	Proliferation binds CSF-1 receptors	

[a]A LIFR is shared by these cytokines.
[b]Note that two forms of the IL-4 and perhaps IL-15 receptor exist.
In cases where STAT5a or STAT5b are designated, the cytokines appear to use either interchangeably.

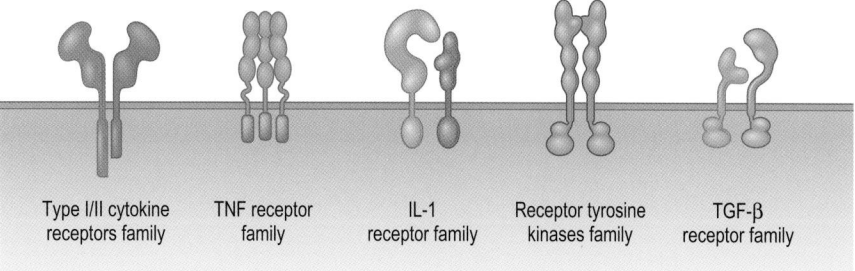

Fig. 9.1 Schematic representation of prototypical receptors from five of the major cytokine receptor superfamilies.

Labels under figure:
Type I/II cytokine receptors family — TNF receptor family — IL-1 receptor family — Receptor tyrosine kinases family — TGF-β receptor family

(G)-CSF, granulocyte–macrophage (GM)-CSF; and interleukins (IL)-2–IL-7, IL-9, IL-11–IL-13, IL-15, IL-21, IL-23, IL-27, IL-31, and IL-35. Also included in this family are ciliary neurotrophic factor (CNTF), leukemia inhibitory factor (LIF), oncostatin M (OSM), and cardiotropin 1 (CT-1). Closely related are the interferons (IFN-α, -β, -τ, -ω, limitin) and IL-10-related cytokines, IL-19, IL-20, IL-22, IL-24, IL-26, and the interferon-related cytokines IL-28A (IFN-γ2), IL-28B (IFN-γ3), IL-29 (IFN-γ1), which bind type II receptors. The ligands and receptors in this superfamily are structurally similar and utilize related molecules for signal transduction.[5]

A central feature of type I cytokines is a similarity in their basic structure. Each contains four anti-parallel α helices with two long and one short loop connections arranged in an up–up–down–down configuration. Because of this structure, these cytokines have also been referred to as the α-helical bundle cytokine family.

Structurally, the receptors in the type I family have conserved cysteine residues, a conserved Trp–Ser–X–Trp–Ser motif (where X indicates any amino acid), and fibronectin-like repeats in their extracellular domains. These receptors have a single transmembrane domain and divergent cytoplasmic domains. Within the cytoplasmic portion of these receptors two segments of homology can be discerned, termed the Box 1 and Box 2 motifs. The membrane proximal domain binds Janus kinases (JAKs; see below). Some of the cytokine receptors are homodimers, such as the receptors for EPO, TPO, PRL, and possibly leptin; whereas other receptors for type I cytokines are heterodimers, containing two distinct receptor subunits. Based on this characteristic, the type I family of receptors can be divided into subfamilies. Each member of the subfamily uses a shared receptor subunit in conjunction with a ligand-specific subunit. For example, the receptors for IL-2, IL-4, IL-7, IL-9, IL-15, and IL-21 all use a common cytokine γ chain, γc (Table 9.1), whereas a common β chain, βc, is shared by IL-3, IL-5, and GM-CSF. Similarly, gp130 is a shared subunit for IL-6 family cytokines (IL-6, IL-11, IL-27, CNTF, LIF, OSM and CT-1). IL-12 and IL-23 also share a receptor subunit, as do members of the IL-10 family.

Other levels of shared receptor usage also exist. For example, the receptors for LIF, CNTF, OSM, and CT-1 all share the LIF receptor subunit, IL-31 and OSM also share one receptor chain; whereas IL-2 and IL-15 utilize the same β and γc chains. Conversely, IL-4 can bind two different receptor complexes. The classic IL-4 receptor is composed of the IL-4Rα chain and the γc chain. Additionally, IL-4 can also bind the IL-13 receptor, which comprises a heterodimer of the IL-4Rα chain and the IL-13Rα chain. IL-13 only utilizes the IL-13 receptor complex for signaling.

The utilization of common receptor subunits explains the phenomenon of shared biological activities (cytokine redundancy) between cytokines that belong to the same subfamily. Within a subfamily, actions distinct for each cytokine can be attributed, at least in part, to the ligand-specific subunits. The pleiotropic effects of a single cytokine can be accounted for by the existence of more than one receptor for that cytokine.

Family members and their actions

Homodimeric receptors

Many of the cytokines that use homodimeric receptors are classic hormones. These include the factors GH, PRL and leptin. Several hormones that regulate hematopoiesis also exist as homodimers. EPO, for example, is required for erythrocyte growth and development and is widely used to treat anemia. Similarly, TPO is required for megakaryocyte development and may have a use in the treatment of thrombocytopenia. G-CSF regulates the production of neutrophils through its action on committed progenitor cells, but also supports the survival of mature neutrophils, enhancing their functional capacity. G-CSF is widely used clinically to treat patients with granulocytopenia. As one would predict, G-CSF-deficient mice have marked neutropenia, and mutations of the G-CSFR result in severe congenital neutropenia in humans.

Cytokine receptors utilizing gp130

gp130 is a receptor component for IL-6, IL-11, IL-27, and IL-31, as well as for several cytokines that are important in development.[6] Targeted disruptions of the gp130 gene are lethal in early embryogenesis. The mice exhibit defects in myocardial, hematologic, and placental development. LIF binds to a receptor that comprises gp130 in association with the LIF receptor (LIFR), as do the cytokines OSM, CNTF, and CT-1. Targeted disruptions of the LIFR gene are also embryonically lethal, creating defects in placental architecture and developmental abnormalities in neural tissue and bone. Targeted disruptions of LIF lead to failure of blastocyst implantation. Another critical role of LIF is the maintenance of stem cell pluripotency in culture.

Interleukin-6

The IL-6 receptor (IL-6R) consists of an 80-kDa IL-6 binding protein (α chain) (CD126) and gp130. IL-6 has a wide array of biological actions on both lymphoid and non-lymphoid cells. It is important in host defense and in inflammatory responses. Accordingly, IL-6-deficient mice are highly susceptible to infection by Candida and Listeria. IL-6 is an important growth and differentiation factor for B cells, inducing the production of immunoglobulin, including IgE. IL-6$^{-/-}$ mice have normal numbers of B cells, but have a reduced immunoglobulin response to neoantigen and a marked reduction in IgA production. IL-6 also promotes T-cell growth and differentiation. Consequently, IL-6$^{-/-}$ mice have reduced numbers of thymocytes and peripheral T cells. IL-6 is important for Th17 differentiation, and the cytotoxic T-cell response to viruses. IL-6 functions synergistically with IL-3 in hematopoiesis, and IL-6-deficient mice have reduced numbers of progenitor cells.

IL-6 serves as a major inducer of fever and the synthesis of acute-phase proteins (fibrinogen, serum amyloid A, haptoglobin, C-reactive protein, etc.) in the liver. The elevation of the erythrocyte sedimentation rate (ESR) in inflammatory disease largely reflects the accelerated synthesis of these proteins, and IL-6-deficient mice are defective in this response. Following exposure to IL-6, the liver reduces synthesis of albumin and transferrin and initiates hepatocyte regeneration. IL-6 induces adrenocorticotrophic hormone and anterior pituitary hormones such PRL, GH and luteinizing hormone. IL-6 also plays a role in osteoporosis by affecting osteoclast function. For example, IL-6-deficient mice are protected from bone loss following estrogen depletion.

Unlike many cytokines, IL-6 can be detected in the serum, although baseline levels are low in the absence of inflammation. However, IL-6 is rapidly produced in response to bacterial and viral infections, inflammation, or trauma. Patients with rheumatoid arthritis, cardiac myxoma, Castleman's disease, and other autoimmune diseases have high serum levels of IL-6. This cytokine may also contribute to malignancies such as multiple myeloma.

IL-6 is produced by a range of cell types, but its expression in mononuclear phagocytes has been well documented. Stimulation of monocytes with IL-1, TNF, or LPS stimulates the expression of IL-6, whereas IL-4 and IL-13 inhibit its production. The promoter of the IL-6 gene contains a number of binding sites for the following transcription factors: nuclear factor-κB (NF-κB), nuclear factor for IL-6 (NF-IL-6, or CCAAT element-binding protein), activator protein-1 (AP-1), cAMP response element-binding protein (CREB), and the glucocorticoid receptor.

Interleukin-11

IL-11 and its receptor are widely expressed. It stimulates stem cells, megakaryocytes, myeloid precursors and erythroid precursors, as well as promoting B-cell differentiation. It also acts on non-hematopoietic cells, including bone and liver. IL-11 is induced by pro-inflammatory cytokines (IL-1, TNF) and by TGF-β.

Interleukin-27

IL-27, like IL-12, is composed of two subunits designated EBI3 and p28. It signals through a receptor comprising gp130 and WSX-1/TCCR (T-cell cytokine receptor), which is expressed on naïve CD4 T cells. IL-27 promotes Th1 differentiation, but also has essential anti-inflammatory properties.[7] It inhibits Th17 differentiation and enhances IL-10 production.

Cytokine receptors utilizing the β$_c$ chain

The cytokines IL-3, IL-5 and GM-CSF all bind to receptors that share a common βc receptor subunit (common β subunit). Each of the individual receptors for these cytokines has a ligand-specific α subunit. Mice, but not humans, have a second β chain, βIL3. This species-specific redundancy may explain why gene targeting of βc in the mouse did not result in loss of IL-3 responses, although βc-null mice did have reduced GM-CSF and IL-5 responses.

Interleukin-3

IL-3 binds to a receptor composed of a unique IL-3Rα subunit and the common βc subunit. IL-3 synergizes with other cytokines to stimulate the growth of immature progenitor cells of all lineages, and is therefore a multi-lineage colony-stimulating factor

(CSF). It prevents cell death and promotes the survival of macrophages, mast cells, and megakaryocytes. IL-3 is produced mainly by lymphoid cells, but also by mast cells and eosinophils. IL-3-deficient mice have no obvious defect in hematopoiesis, suggesting that the major role of IL-3 *in vivo* may be in the response to stress.

Interleukin-5

IL-5 is unusual among cytokines in that it is a disulfide-linked homodimer, with each component containing three α-helical bundles. Its major action is to promote the growth, differentiation, and activation of eosinophils. As such, it is very important in pathogenesis of allergic disease. IL-5$^{-/-}$ mice fail to develop eosinophilia in response to parasitic or aeroallergen challenge. Remarkably, these mice exhibit minimal signs of inflammation and damage to the lungs. IL-5 deficiency does not affect the worm burden of infected mice, indicating that eosinophilia per se may not play an essential role in the host defense against helminths. Both IL-5 and IL-5R knockout mice have decreased numbers of CD5$^+$ B cells (B-1 cells), concomitant with low serum concentrations of IgM and IgG3. IL-5 is produced by activated helper T cells of the Th2 phenotype (see below), mast cells, and eosinophils in an autocrine manner.

Granulocyte–Macrophage-CSF

GM-CSF acts on hematopoietic precursors to support myelomonocytic differentiation. It activates mature neutrophils and macrophages, increasing their microbicidal activity and inducing the production of pro-inflammatory cytokines. Along with IL-4 and IL-13, GM-CSF is a major stimulatory cytokine for the *in vitro* production of dendritic cells (DCs). GM-CSF induces proliferation and activation of eosinophils and upregulates adhesion molecules on fibroblasts and endothelial cells. Homozygous inactivation of the GM-CSF gene in mice, however, does not affect steady-state hematopoiesis. Instead, these animals develop alveolar proteinosis and lymphoid hyperplasia, which is not due to a detectable infectious agent. βc$^{-/-}$ mice also develop alveolar proteinosis, characterized by the accumulation of surfactant in the lungs. A similar defect may be responsible for disease in a subset of humans with this abnormality.

The production of GM-CSF can be induced by pro-inflammatory cytokines and LPS. Unsurprisingly, GM-CSF is made by activated lymphocytes and other stimulated cells. GM-CSF is not ordinarily detectable in blood except under pathologic conditions such as asthma. GM-CSF has been used clinically to treat chemotherapy-induced neutropenia, especially in the context of certain infections (e.g., fungal). It has also been tested in myelodysplastic syndrome and aplastic anemia.

Cytokine receptors utilizing the γ$_c$ chain

The cytokines IL-2, IL-4, IL-7, IL-9, IL-15, and IL-21 all bind to receptors that share a common γc receptor subunit. The γc subunit and the ligand-specific subunits are expressed predominantly on lymphocytes, although they can be found on other hematopoietic cells as well. Proof of their importance was provided when it was shown that mutation of the γc gene was responsible for X-linked severe combined immunodeficiency (SCID), which is characterized by a lack of T cells and NK cells, and poorly functioning B cells (Chapter 35).[8] This disorder, which has proved to be the most common form of SCID in humans, is thus designated as a T$^-$B$^+$ SCID. γc knockout mice were found to also have a SCID phenotype, although one that, unlike human, lacked B cells. The lack of γc abrogates signaling by all of the cytokines that utilize this subunit (IL-2, IL-4, IL-7, IL-9, IL-15, and IL-21), but the lack of IL-7 signaling is predominantly responsible for the SCID phenotype. Thus, the lesser importance of IL-7 signaling in human B-cell development probably explains the less severe block on B-cell function seen in patients with X-linked SCID.

Interleukin-2

The IL-2 receptor consists of three subunits, α, β, and γc. The latter two are members of the type I cytokine receptor family. NK cells constitutively express these latter two subunits and respond to high doses of IL-2, whereas in T cells the IL-2Rα subunit is induced upon activation, where it creates a high-affinity receptor for IL-2. IL-2Rα is also inducible in activated monocytes and B cells. IL-2Rα, however, is not a member of the type I cytokine receptor family. Rather, it resembles members of the complement family and IL-15R (see below). Thymocytes express high levels of IL-2Rα, but a role of IL-2 in thymic development is not evident with IL-2 and IL-2Rα-deficient mice exhibiting normal thymocyte development.

IL-2, one of the first cytokines to be intensively studied, is produced principally by activated T cells and is a prototypical autocrine T-cell growth factor that is required for progression from the G1 to the S phase of the cell cycle in T cells activated *in vitro*. It is an important factor in determining the magnitude of T-cell and NK-cell responses, augmenting the cytolytic activity of T and NK cells and inducing IFN-γ secretion. IL-2 is also important in programming CD8 memory T cells, which undergo secondary expansion in viral infections.[9] IL-2 is a growth factor for B cells and induces class switching. It also activates macrophages. Targeted deletion of the genes encoding IL-2, IL-2Rα, and IL-2Rβ yielded surprising phenotypes. T-cell development in these mice appears normal, but they succumb to autoimmune and lymphoproliferative disease, pointing to the existence of a separate, *in vivo* role of IL-2 whose function is to maintain lymphoid homeostasis and thus help prevent autoimmune disease.[10] IL-2-deficient mice develop massive enlargement of peripheral lymphoid organs, hemolytic anemia, inflammatory bowel disease, and infiltrative granulopoiesis. In addition, they have high levels of IgG1 and IgE. Paradoxically, their T cells proliferate poorly *in vitro* in response to either polyclonal activators or antigen-specific signals. A similar phenotype is seen in humans with IL-2Rα mutations.

Whereas the T-cell hyperplasia and tissue infiltration observed in IL-2 or IL-2Rα chain-deficient individuals was originally thought to be due to a defect in the re-stimulation-induced cell death of activated T cells, abnormal regulatory T (Treg) cell function may provide an alternative mechanism (Chapter 15). Naturally arising Treg cells in both mice and humans express high levels of IL-2Rα, and maintenance of peripheral Treg cell numbers has been shown to be dependent on IL-2.[11] In addition, IL-2 inhibits Th17 differentiation.

IL-2 is produced almost exclusively by activated T cells. It is rapidly induced upon recognition of foreign antigen. Indeed, IL-2 production is one of the key indicators of T-cell activation. The IL-2 promoter has been extensively characterized and contains binding sites for nuclear factor of activated T-cells (NFAT), AP-1, and NF-κB. IL-2 production is also regulated by stabilization of its mRNA.

IL-2 has been used in a number of clinical circumstances, both to treat malignancies and to boost CD4 T-cell counts in HIV. The clinical utility of IL-2 therapy is limited by its toxicity, two important manifestations being hepatic dysfunction and the so-called capillary or vascular leak syndrome. On the other hand, anti-IL-2Rα monoclonal antibodies, daclizumab and basiliximab, are used to prevent rejection of allotransplants. Polymorphisms of IL-2Rα are associated with multiple sclerosis.

Interleukin-4

Two classes of IL-4R appear to exist.[12] One consists of the IL-4Rα subunit in conjunction with γc and is expressed on hematopoietic cells. The other, a "type II" receptor, appears to consist of the IL-4Rα subunit in association with the α chain of IL-13R. This latter receptor appears to be widely expressed. However, two IL-13R subunits have been cloned, so the exact composition of the type II IL-4R remains uncertain. The existence of two receptors helps explain why IL-4 has diverse actions on both hematopoietic and non-hematopoietic cells. The loss of IL-4Rα would be predicted to block the actions of both IL-4 and IL-13, which could explain why gene targeting of IL-4Rα leads to a more severe phenotype than that observed in IL-4-deficient mice. Polymorphisms of IL-4Rα have been reported to be associated with a propensity towards atopy.[13]

In general, IL-4 serves to promote allergic response and to inhibit cell-mediated immune responses. Among the most important roles of IL-4 is its ability to promote differentiation of naïve CD4 T cells into a subset that produces IL-4 and IL-5.[14,15] These cells are denoted the so-called T-helper 2 (Th2) subset, as opposed to T-helper 1 (Th1) cells, which produce lymphotoxin-α and IFN-γ (Chapter 16). In conjunction with CD40 activation, IL-4 also promotes B-cell proliferation and class switching, particularly to IgG1 and IgE in mice and to IgG4 and IgE in humans. Mice deficient in IL-4 have normal B lymphopoiesis, but marked reductions in IgG1 and IgE production in response to parasites. However, these mice have residual Th2 responses, because IL-13, which also binds IL-4Rα, can partially compensate for the defect.

IL-4 also upregulates the expression of surface IgM, MHC class II, and CD23 on B cells. In conjunction with GM-CSF, it is also a growth factor for mast cells and basophils, as well as a potent inducer of DC differentiation. IL-4 inhibits macrophage activation and the production of pro-inflammatory cytokines. It antagonizes the effects of IFN-γ, blocks cytokine-induced proliferation of synoviocytes, downregulates the expression of adhesion molecules, and antagonizes the induction of some acute-phase reactants in hepatocytes by IL-6.

IL-4 is made by the Th2 subset of CD4 T cells, basophils and mast cells. A minor population of NK1.1$^+$ CD4 T cells also produces large amounts of IL-4. Based on the tight regulation of IL-4 production, the IL-4 promoter has received considerable attention. A number of transcription factors appear to be important in regulating IL-4 production, including NFAT, NF-IL6, C/EBP, c-MAF, and GATA-3. The IL-4 promoter has a Stat6 binding site, which is consistent with the fact that IL-4 regulates its own expression. Epigenetic control and chromatin remodelling are also important aspects.[16]

Clinically, IL-4 has been tested in the treatment of malignancies and some autoimmune disorders. The ability of IL-4 to generate DCs is being exploited in the use of tumor vaccines. Conceivably, soluble IL-4R might also be useful in the treatment of allergic disease.

Interleukin-7

The IL-7 receptor consists of the IL-7Rα chain (CD127) in association with γc. It is expressed on both immature and mature thymocytes. Humans with loss-of-function mutations of IL-7Rα have T$^-$B$^+$ SCID but, unlike individuals with γc mutations, display normal NK-cell development (Chapter 35).[8] Gain-of-function mutations of the IL-7Rα chain result in constitutive

JAK1 signaling and cell transformation, and give rise to T cell acute lymphoblastic leukemia.[17]

IL-7Rα expression is tightly regulated during thymocyte development (Chapter 8). IL-7 plays an important role in both developing thymocytes and mature T cells. It is expressed in double-negative thymocytes, downregulated in double-positive cells, and then re-expressed in single-positive thymocytes. It is also expressed in mature peripheral T cells. This may be a reflection of its anti-apoptotic effects, which are attributable to the induction of Bcl-2 family members. IL-7 promotes the growth of thymocytes, as well as the expression and rearrangement of TCR genes and the expression of RAG1 and RAG2 (Chapter 4). IL-7Rα is expressed on cutaneous T-cell lymphomas, which also produce this cytokine; thus the autocrine response to IL-7 may contribute to the growth of these tumors.

IL-7- and IL-7R-deficient mice exhibit impairments in both T- and B-cell development. Postnatal B-cell development in IL-7$^{-/-}$ mice is blocked at the transition to pre-B cells and is arrested even earlier in IL-7Rα$^{-/-}$ mice. This suggests that IL-7Rα binds a cytokine other than IL-7, perhaps the thymic stroma-derived lymphopoietin. Why these abnormalities do not occur in humans with IL-7Rα mutations is not clear; presumably a factor that does not bind IL-7R regulates this step in human B-cell development.

IL-7 is produced by a wide variety of cells, including marrow and perhaps thymic stromal cells, as well as in the kidney, spleen, epithelial cells, and keratinocytes. This is consistent with its role in the maintenance of function in both immature and mature lymphocytes.

Clinically, IL-7 may be useful to restore immune function in some congenital immunodeficiencies, after bone marrow transplantation, or in HIV infection. Polymorphisms of the IL-7R are associated with multiple sclerosis.

Interleukin-9

IL-9 has some of the same properties as IL-4. It strongly synergizes with stem cell factor to promote the growth and differentiation of mast cells and is a potent regulator of mast cell function. IL-9 also potentiates IgE production induced by IL-4 in B cells. Although it was first identified as a T-cell growth factor, a physiologic role in T-cell development has not been established. IL-9 is produced by activated Th2 cells, mast cells and eosinophils. Recently, a new subset of Th cells termed Th9 has been proposed.[18] These cells have been shown to also secrete IL-10, but to enhance inflammatory responses. Interestingly, IL-9 inhibits Th1 cytokine production. Some lymphoid tumors also produce IL-9, where it may serve as an autocrine growth factor.

Interleukin-15

The IL-15 receptor consists of the IL-2Rβ and γc subunits in association with a unique ligand-specific subunit, IL-15Rα, which is homologous to IL-2Rα.[19] These receptor proteins contain protein-binding motifs termed "sushi domains". In both human and mouse these receptors and their cognate ligands are physically linked in the genome. Given their shared receptor usage, there are many similarities in the actions of IL-2 and IL-15, particularly in terms of the effects on lymphoid cells. Like IL-2, IL-15 induces proliferation and cytokine production in T and NK cells. However, despite the similarities between these two ligands/receptors there are a number of important differences. IL-15Rα is more widely expressed than IL-2Rα, IL-2Rβ, and γc. In addition to lymphoid cells, IL-15Rα is expressed in fibroblasts, epithelial, liver, intestine, and other cells. IL-15 and IL-15Rα knockout mice are defective in NK-cell production and in the generation of

memory T cells, explaining the absence of NK development in patients with γc mutations.

The production of IL-15 is very different from that of IL-2. IL-15 mRNA is expressed broadly in hematopoietic and non-hematopoietic cells, although it is not typically produced by T cells. (HTLV-I-transformed T cells are an exception in that they produce abundant IL-15.) Following the pattern seen in IL-7 and IL-9, there are multiple upstream AUGs in the 5′ untranslated portion of the IL-15 message that interfere with translation. Thus, IL-15 is controlled by translational regulation. IL-15 protein is also controlled at the level of secretion of the protein, but this is incompletely understood. High levels of IL-15 protein have been reported in synovial fluids from patients with rheumatoid arthritis, alveolar macrophages from patients with sarcoidosis, and peripheral blood mononuclear cells from patients with ulcerative colitis. A monoclonal anti-IL-15 antibody is being tested in rheumatoid arthritis.

Interleukin-21

IL-21 is a T-cell-derived cytokine that works in concert with other γc cytokines. It synergizes with IL-7 and IL-15 to expand and activate CD8 T cells. IL-21 also augments the activity of NK cells. Recently, it has been shown that IL-21, along with IL-6 drive differentiation of follicular helper T cells (Tfh). Cells of this subset of Th cells are found preferentially in B-cell follicles where, under control of the transcription factor BCL6, they regulate B-cell development, activation and class switching. Tfh are also a source of IL-21. IL-21 appears to have some anti-cancer properties and it has been tested in the treatment of melanoma.[20]

Other heterodimeric receptors

Interleukin-12. IL-12 is a heterodimer composed of two disulfide-linked polypeptide chains, p35 and p40, derived from two distinct genes.[21,22] IL-12 p35 shares homology with other cytokines, such as IL-6, whereas p40 resembles the IL-6 receptor. Thus, IL-12 can be viewed as being synthesized as a ligand–receptor complex. Two chains of IL-12R have been identified. Because the ligand already comprises the α subunit, the two chains of the IL-12R are denoted IL-12Rβ1 and β2. Expression of high-affinity IL-12R is very restricted, being found predominantly on T and NK cells. IL-12R expression is also notable in that it is regulated by the activation state of the cell. IL-12Rβ1 and β2 are highly inducible upon T-cell activation, and IL-4 inhibits IL-12Rβ2 expression. This is important because IL-12Rβ2 is required for IL-12 signaling and the activation of the transcription factor STAT4. NK cells constitutively express IL-12Rβ1 and IL-12Rβ2.

IL-12 plays a pivotal role in promoting cell-mediated immune responses. Humans with IL-12R mutations, as well as mice with IL-12 and IL-12R deficiency, have very blunted immune responses and are highly susceptible to infections by intracellular pathogens.[23] An important function of IL-12 is that it promotes the differentiation of uncommitted helper T cells to the Th1 subset, i.e., T cells that produce LT-α and INF-γ. Th1 differentiation is markedly impaired in IL-12- and IL-12R-deficient mice. A major action of IL-12 is its ability to induce the production of IFN-γ, doing so synergistically in combination with IL-2 or IL-18. Consequently, many of the actions of IL-12 are blocked in IFN-γ or IFN-γR knockout mice. IL-12 also induces proliferation and cytolytic activity of T and NK cells.

DCs and macrophages are the major producers of IL-12 in response to various pathogens, occupancy of Toll-like receptors and CD40. The IL-12p40 promoter is complex and contains NF-κB sites, interferon response elements (IREs), and ETS binding sites. As with other cytokine genes, nucleosome remodelling is important in the regulation of IL-12.[24]

Because of its profound effects on cell-mediated immunity, IL-12 has been used in the treatment of malignancies and infectious diseases, but its utility has been limited due to significant toxicity. IL-12 may also have use in vaccines as an adjuvant. Conversely, antagonizing the actions of IL-12 has been found to be useful in Th1-mediated diseases, including inflammatory bowel disease (Chapter 74).

Interleukin-23. IL-23 is another heterodimeric type I cytokine. It is composed of two disulfide-linked polypeptide chains, p19 and IL-12 p40. The IL-23 receptor also shares the IL-12Rβ1 chain paired to the IL-23R.[25] The IL-23R complex is expressed on activated T cells. Its function relates to a third T lineage of differentiated helper cells, which produce high levels of the cytokine IL-17 (Th17, see below). IL-23 is thought to be important in the maintenance of Th17 cells. As such, IL-23 is thought to be important in host defense against extracellular bacteria and the pathogenesis of autoimmune and autoinflammatory disorders. It is notable in this regard that therapies that target IL-12p40 antagonize both IL-12 and IL-23. IL-23 is produced primarily by DCs in response to TLR agonists. IL-23R polymorphisms are associated with inflammatory bowel disease, ankylosing spondylitis and other autoimmune diseases.

Interleukin-35. IL-35 is a newly described cytokine that is a dimer consisting of IL-12 p35 and EB13. This cytokine appears to be preferentially produced by Treg cells, as the expression of EBI3 is directly regulated by the Treg-specific transcription factor FoxP3. Tregs are also the main cellular target of IL-35, where it induces proliferation and production of IL-10. A synthetic form of IL-35, obtained by covalently linking EBI3 to IL-12p35, can reduce the incidence of arthritis in mouse models.[26]

Interleukin-13. IL-13 has many of the same effects as IL-4 and shares a receptor subunit(s) with IL-4. IL-13-deficient mice have reduced levels of IL-4, IL-5, and IL-10. They also have lower IgE levels and eosinophilia. In mice deficient for both IL-4 and IL-13, these Th2 responses are abolished and the ability to clear parasites is severely impaired. These double-knockout mice default to Th1 responses, with concomitant production of INF-γ, IgG2a and IgG2b. It appears that IL-4 and IL-13 cooperate in promoting Th2 responses, having both overlapping and additive roles.

Interleukin-31. IL-31 signals through the heterodimeric receptor IL-31RA and oncostatin M receptor (OSMR). It is produced by activated Th2 cells. Overexpression of IL-31 results in atopic dermatitis but, surprisingly, IL-31RA-deficient mice showed an increased Th2 response.[27,28]

Thymic stromal lymphopoietin (TSLP)

TSLP is an IL-7-like cytokine expressed by epithelial cells and keratinocytes. Its receptor comprises TSLPR and IL-7Rα, which is expressed primarily on monocytes and myeloid-derived DCs, as well as on B cells. Signaling events downstream of this heterodimeric receptor includes activation of JAK1 and JAK2 and STAT1, 3, and 5 phosphorylation.[29] This cytokine appears to have different effects in mouse and human cells. TSLP-treated human DCs promote Th2 differentiation.[30] A major means by which TSLP exerts its effect is through promotion of basophil hematopoiesis.[31] Elevated TSLP levels have been found in humans and animal models of airway inflammatory disease and atopic dermatitis. In the mouse, TSLP contributes to prenatal B-cell development.

Interferons

Type I interferons

The type I interferons include IFN-α, IFN-ω, and IFN-β. IFN-β and IFN-ω are encoded by single genes, whereas IFN-α includes at least 14 separate genes, each encoding structurally distinct forms. These intronless genes are all clustered on the short arm of chromosome 9 and appear to have diverged from a common ancestor more than 100 million years ago. Each of these molecules binds to the same IFN-α/β receptor and their actions are similar. The receptor is a heterodimer composed of two subunits termed IFNAR1 and IFNAR2. These subunits have limited similarity to type I cytokine receptors, although they lack the WSXWS motif.

A major effect of type I interferons is their antiviral action.[32] Discovered in 1957, they act on all cells to inhibit viral replication as well as cellular proliferation. It is unclear why there are so many type I genes. Given that their relative potencies differ; it is possible that these genes evolved in response to various viral pathogens. Alternatively, IFN gene duplication may affect the magnitude of antiviral responses. A major mechanism is the inhibition of protein translation. They also upregulate MHC class I and downregulate MHC class II expression. IFN-α/β increase the cytolytic activity of NK cells. Predictably, IFNARI knockout mice are extremely susceptible to infections, even though lymphoid development is normal.

Interferons are produced ubiquitously, viral infection being a major inducer of their transcriptional regulation. Type I IFN is also induced by intracellular bacterial pathogens and LPS. Immunoregulatory effects of IFN-α/β are being increasingly recognized, and it is notable that a subset of DCs produces very high levels.[33,34] The promoter for IFN-β has been intensively analyzed. It binds a variety of transcription factors, including NF-κB and interferon regulatory factor 1 (IRF-1). IRF-2 also binds to this promoter and functions as a repressor.

Type I IFN is used clinically in the treatment of certain infections, e.g., viral hepatitis. Owing to its antiproliferative action, it is also used in the treatment of certain malignancies, particularly hairy cell leukemia. IFN-β is used in the treatment of multiple sclerosis.

Newer interferon-like cytokines including IL-28A, IL-28B, and IL-29 (also designated IFN-λ1, -λ2, and -λ3) have been identified. They bind to a receptor designated IL-28R. The exact *in vivo* functions of these interferon-like cytokines are poorly understood, although they probably contribute to antiviral responses.

Interferon-γ

IFN-γ is a major activator of macrophages, enhancing their ability to kill microorganisms by augmenting their cytolytic machinery. IFN-γ exerts this effect by causing the cell to increase its production of reactive oxygen intermediates, including hydrogen peroxide, nitric oxide, and indoleamine dioxygenase. It also upregulates MHC class II expression. IFN-γ also acts on CD4 T cells to promote Th1 differentiation while inhibiting the generation of Th2 cells. It promotes the maturation of CD8 T cells to cytotoxic cells. In mice, IFN-γ augments NK cytolytic activity, promotes switching to IgG2a and IgG3, and inhibits switching to IgG1 and IgE. Endothelial cells and neutrophils are also activated by IFN-γ. Like IFN-α/β, IFN-γ also contributes to antiviral defenses.

The IFN-γ receptor is a heterodimer composed of IFN-γRα and IFN-γRβ subunits. When one IFN-γ homodimer binds, a complex of two α and two β receptors is created.[35] Mice with a disrupted

IFN-γR develop normally and have normal lymphoid development, but are highly susceptible to viral and bacterial infections, especially intracellular microbes. They have diminished macrophage MHC class II expression, decreased NK function, and reduced serum IgG_{2a} concentrations. Humans with mutations of IFN-γR subunits are also susceptible to mycobacterial and Salmonella infections.

The control of IFN-γ production is tightly regulated, T cells of the Th1 subset and NK cells being the major producers. Transcription factors, including STAT4, T-BET, and EOMES, play an important roles in IFN-γ gene regulation.[16] IFN-γ has been used to treat patients with immunodeficiencies (e.g., chronic granulomatous disease) and in certain patients with disseminated mycobacterial infections.[36] A monoclonal anti-IFN-γ antibody, fontolizumab, is being studied in the treatment of autoimmune disease.

Interleukin-10 and related cytokines

The major function of IL-10 is to serve as an anti-inflammatory and immunosuppressive cytokine. Unlike other cytokines in this family, it is a disulfide-linked dimer. A single IL-10R has been cloned, but the receptor may have additional components. IL-10R is expressed on macrophages, mast cells, and most other hematopoietic cells. It is also inducible in non-hematopoietic cells by stimuli such as LPS.

IL-10 strongly inhibits the production of IL-1, IL-6, IL-8, IL-12, TNF, and other immune and inflammatory cytokines. It inhibits macrophage antigen presentation and decreases expression of MHC class II, adhesion molecules, and the co-stimulatory molecules CD80 (B7.1) and CD86 (B7.2). The importance of IL-10 as an endogenous inhibitor of cell-mediated immunity is emphasized by the finding that IL-10-deficient mice develop autoimmune disease, which manifests with severe inflammatory bowel disease and exaggerated inflammatory responses. Delayed-type hypersensitivity and contact hypersensitivity responses are also prolonged and amplified.

IL-10 is made by Th1 and Th2 cells, although a subset of T cells that preferentially produces IL-10 and TGF-β is sometimes denoted Th3. IL-10 is also produced by activated B cells, macrophages, keratinocytes and bronchial epithelial cells. LPS and TNF are inducers of IL-10. IL-10 is readily detected in the blood of patients with septic shock and other inflammatory and immune disorders. Owing to its anti-inflammatory properties, IL-10 has been used experimentally in the treatment of some Th1-mediated autoimmune diseases. Paradoxically, IL-10 is elevated in patients with systemic lupus erythematosus, and there is a correlation between levels of IL-10 and autoantibody production.

There are viral homologues of IL-10 that may blunt the immune response to these pathogens. IL-10 also contributes to the immunosuppression seen in lepromatous leprosy or parasitic infestations. Other IL-10-related cytokines include IL-19, IL-20, IL-22, IL-24, and IL-26, but their biological actions are incompletely understood.[37]

Cytokines and the differentiation of T cells to helpers and effectors

Classically, precursor CD4 T-cell differentiation was viewed as polarization into one of two phenotypes: Th1 or Th2 (Fig. 9.2, Chapter 16). Th1 cells drive the immune response towards cell-mediated immune responses, whereas Th2 cells promote a humoral or allergic response. The latter is protective against helminthic and other parasitic infestations. Th1 cells produce IL-2, LT-α, and IFN-γ, whereas Th2 cells produce IL-4, IL-5, and IL-10.

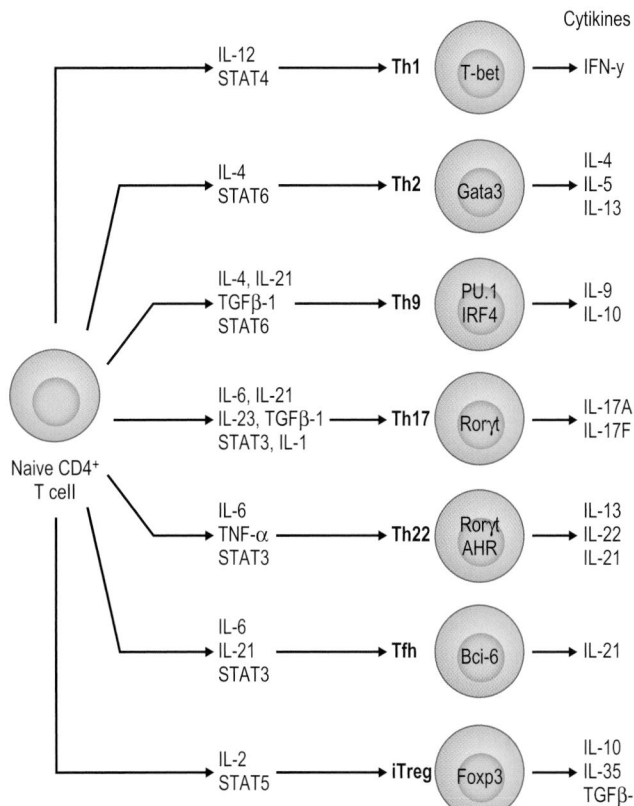

Fig. 9.2 Differentiation of T-helper cell subtypes.

Both subsets produce IL-3. More recently, other T-cell subsets have been identified, e.g., Th17 and Treg.

The differentiation of helper T cells has important implications for host defense. In mouse models of parasitic disease, the failure of some strains to mount a Th1 response results in the majority of the animals succumbing to the infection. Conversely, in other disease models the production of a Th2 response results in enhanced survival, whereas a Th1 response causes more damage to the host.

Although the mechanisms by which Th1 and Th2 development is governed are not fully understood, differentiation into each of these subsets is regulated by different cytokines. For example, IL-4 promotes Th2 differentiation and antagonizes Th1 responses. Conversely, IL-12 and IFN-γ promote Th1 differentiation and antagonize Th2 development. A number of transcription factors have been reported to regulate this response. GATA-3, c-MAF, and NFATp regulate IL-4 production and Th2 differentiation, whereas STAT4 and T-BET promote Th1 differentiation.[15,22]

The immunopathogenesis of autoimmune disease does not fit quite so neatly into the standard Th1/Th2 dichotomy. CD4 T cells can differentiate into cells that produce IL-10 and transforming growth factor-β (TGF-β) — so-called Th3 cells — and they can also become "adaptive" Treg cells; with both types appearing to protect against autoimmunity.[38] As discussed above, IL-2 and TGF-β are important for Treg cell differentiation. Models of autoimmunity have pointed to the importance of yet another subset of Th cells that produces IL-17 and are now termed Th17 cells. TGF-β and IL-6 are thought to promote Th17 differentiation from naïve progenitors, whereas IL-23 is important for the maintenance of these cells. In addition to a role in autoimmunity, IL-17 is important in host defense against extracellular bacteria.[39] New, recently described subsets of Th cells include Th9; Th22, which infiltrate the epidermis in inflammatory diseases and secrete IL-22 and TNF-α and angiogenetic and chemotactic factors; and Tfh, whose main role is to regulate the evolution of effector and memory B-cell responses by secreting cytokines such as IL-17 and IL-21.

Signaling

Neither type I nor type II receptors exhibit intrinsic enzymatic activity. However, the conserved membrane proximal segment of each of these receptors serves as the site at which these receptors bind Janus kinases (JAKs) (Table 9.1). These JAKs play a pivotal role in signaling via this family of cytokine receptors .

Janus kinases

Four mammalian Janus kinases, JAK1, JAK2, JAK3, and TYK2, have been identified. JAKs are structurally unique, consisting of a C-terminal catalytically active kinase domain that is preceded by a segment termed the pseudokinase domain. The latter gives JAKs their name and has regulatory functions. A key feature of the JAKs is their association with cytokine receptors, which appears to be mediated by the N terminus.

Ligand binding to type I and II receptors induces the aggregation of receptor subunits, which brings JAKs in close proximity and allows them to phosphorylate and activate each other. After activation, the JAKs phosphorylate receptor subunits on tyrosine residues, which allow the recruitment of proteins with SRC homology-2 (SH2) or phosphotyrosine-binding (PTB) domains. These proteins can also be phosphorylated by JAKs. Phosphorylation results in the activation of a number of biochemical pathways. Importantly, phosphorylation of cytokine receptors generates docking sites for a class of SH2-containing transcription factors termed the STATs (see below) (Fig. 9.3).

The pivotal function of the JAKs is vividly illustrated by mice or humans that are deficient in these kinases. The association of JAK3 with the common gamma chain, γc, suggested that JAK3 mutations might also cause SCID, and indeed it was found that mutation of JAK3 results in autosomal recessive T^-B^+ SCID (Chapter 35).[40] JAK3 knockout mice also proved to exhibit SCID. Indeed, mutation of either γc or JAK3 leads to the same

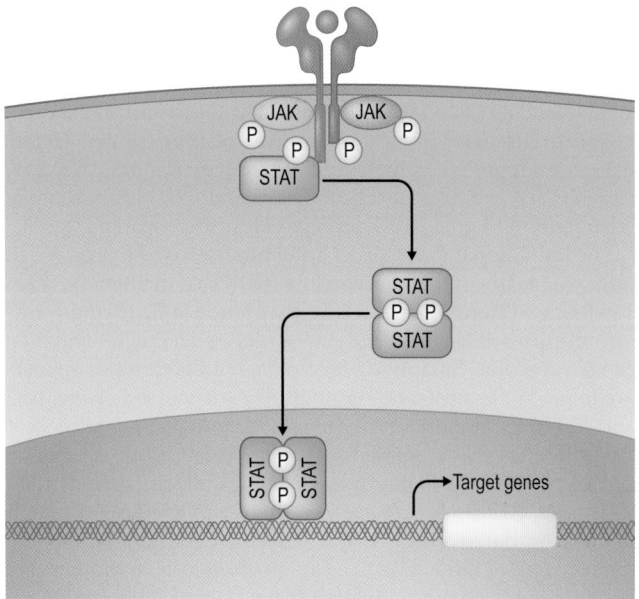

Fig. 9.3 The roles of JAKs and STATs in signal transduction by type I and II cytokine receptors.

functional defects. These findings led to the notion that a JAK3 inhibitor might represent a new class of immunosuppressant drug. One such inhibitor, CP 690,550, was effective in preclinical studies.[41] This drug is currently being tested in humans.

In contrast to JAK3-deficient mice and humans, gene targeting of jak1 and jak2 results in more diverse abnormalities. Jak1$^{-/-}$ mice die perinatally from neurologic defects, but also have a SCID phenotype similar to jak3$^{-/-}$ mice. This is explained by the fact that γc-containing cytokine receptors utilize JAK1 in association with their ligand-specific receptor subunit. Other cytokines that are dependent on JAK1 include those that use gp130 cytokine receptors (IL-6, LIF, OSM, CNTF, and IL-11) and type II receptors (IL-10, IFN-γ, and IFN-α/β). Gene-targeting of jak2 was embryonically lethal, principally because JAK2 is essential for EPO function and the mice fail to form blood. In addition, JAK2 is necessary for signaling of other cytokines, including IL-3.

The importance of the JAKs has been substantiated by the identification of chromosomal translocations in various leukemias resulting in TEL (a transcription factor)/JAK fusion proteins, which have constitutive kinase activity and uncontrolled signaling. For example, a mutation in the pseudokinase domain of JAK2 underlies most cases of polycythemia vera. Gain-of-function mutations of JAK3 can contribute to leukemia. And, mutations of TYK2 are associated with hyper-IgE syndrome.

STATs

Members of the signal transducer and activator of transcription (STAT) family of DNA-binding proteins serve a key role in transducing signals from cytokine receptors on the cell surface to the nucleus, where they regulate gene transcription. STATs are latent, cytosolic transcription factors that have SH2 domains (phosphotyrosine-binding modules) that allow them to be recruited to phosphorylated cytokine receptors (Fig. 9.3). Different STATs bind to specific cytokine receptors (Table 9.1). STATs are themselves tyrosine phosphorylated by JAKs, and this promotes their dimerization. STATs translocate to the nucleus, bind DNA, and regulate transcription.

There are seven mammalian STATs: STAT1, STAT2, STAT3, STAT4, STAT5a, STAT5b, and STAT6. Stat knockout mice document the essential and specific functions of these transcription factors in transmitting cytokine signals. Stat1$^{-/-}$ mice develop normally, but have extreme susceptibility to viral and some bacterial infections, consistent with the defects seen in IFNγ$^{-/-}$ and IFNγR$^{-/-}$ mice, and in IFNβR-deficient humans. STAT1 also appears to be important in regulating apoptosis. Its absence is associated with tumorigenesis in mice. Humans with mutations of STAT1, which is activated by IFNs, present with increased susceptibility to *Salmonella* and mycobacterial infections as well as autosomal dominant chronic mucocutaneous candidiasis.[42] Gene targeting of stat3 leads to early embryonic lethality, the lethality being related in part to interference with Lif function. Conditional knockouts of stat3 in myeloid cells display exaggerated inflammatory responses, evidently due to a failure of IL-10 signaling. STAT3 is also essential for Th17 cells. Mutations of Stat3 underlie the primary immunodeficiency known as hyper-IgE syndrome or Job's syndrome. An important aspect of the susceptibility of these patients to infection is the failure to generate Th17 cells. Conversely, polymorphisms of Stat3 are associated with inflammatory bowel disease (Chapter 74). As might be expected from the fact that STAT4 is activated by IL-12; stat4$^{-/-}$ mice develop normally but have defective cell-mediated immune responses and Th1 differentiation combined with augmented Th2 development. This phenotype is consistent with the abnormalities seen in IL-12$^{-/-}$ mice, IL-12R$^{-/-}$ mice, and IL-12R-deficient humans.

STAT6 is activated by IL-4. Stat6$^{-/-}$ mice have defective Th2 development with defective IgE responses following infection with parasites. Lack of STAT6 dramatically attenuates allergic and asthmatic disease in animal models of these diseases. IL-13 also activates STAT6, and its responses are abrogated in stat6$^{-/-}$ mice.

STAT5a and STAT5b are highly homologous, but nonetheless have different functions. Stat5a$^{-/-}$ mice have impaired mammary gland development and failure of lactation, whereas stat5b$^{-/-}$ mice have defective sexually dimorphic growth and growth hormone-dependent regulation of liver gene expression. Stat5a/5b doubly-deficient mice manifest increased perinatal lethality, decreased size, female infertility, and impaired lymphocyte development. Stat5$^{-/-}$ mice develop lymphoproliferative disease reminiscent of IL-2- and IL-2R-deficient mice, presumably related to loss of Treg cells. A single patient with STAT5b mutations has been identified and she manifests impaired responses to GH and immune dysregulation.

CLINICAL RELEVANCE

Types I and II cytokine receptors

- IL-7R, γc, and JAK3 mutations cause SCID
- TYK2 and STAT3 mutations cause hyper-IgE syndrome.
- IL-12, IL-12R, and IFNγR mutations are associated with susceptibility to intracellular infections.
- Polymorphisms of IL-2R and IL-7R are associated with multiple sclerosis.
- Polymorphisms of IL-23R are associated with inflammatory bowel disease.
- Polymorphisms of STAT4 are associated with RA and SLE.
- EPO, G-CSF, and TPO are used to treat cytopenias.
- Anti-IL-2R mAb is used to prevent transplant rejection.
- Anti-IL-12p40 is used to treat inflammatory bowel disease.

Attenuation of type-I and type-II cytokine signaling

Perhaps as important as the triggers that initiate signal transduction are the mechanisms for extinguishing the response.[43] There are several families of proteins involved in downregulating cytokine signaling. Among these are phosphatases, cytokine-inducible inhibitor molecules, and transcriptional repressors. The phosphatase SHP-1 interacts with cytokine receptors and downregulates signaling. Moth-eaten mice lack a functional SHP-1 protein and die at an early age from autoimmune disease.

Another family of proteins that attenuate cytokine signaling is the suppressors of cytokine signaling (SOCS), which are alternatively termed JAB, SSI, and CIS. These are SH2-containing proteins that bind to either cytokine receptors or to JAKs and inhibit signaling. There are at least eight members of this family. Largely due to systemic hyperresponsiveness to IFN-γ, Socs-1$^{-/-}$ mice die within a few weeks of birth. SOCS-2 has been recently shown to regulate Th2 differentiaion and allergic responses. Another family member, SOCS-3, is important in controlling Th17 differentiation.[39,44,45]

KEY CONCEPT

Properties of the TNF receptor superfamily

- Activation of a TNF receptor can lead to a wide range of effects, from proliferation to apoptosis.
- Transduction of signals through TRAFs leads to the enhancement of survival.
- Signaling through death domains leads to the induction of apoptosis.

TNF receptor and ligand superfamilies

This large family of structurally related ligands, receptors, and inhibitory decoy receptors has various roles both within and without the immune system. The first two members of this family to be discovered were TNF and lymphotoxin-α (LTα; sometimes formerly referred to as TNF-β). These molecules are secreted principally by activated myeloid and T cells. They have similar pro-inflammatory functions and belong to a large family of related molecules that includes CD30 ligand, CD40 ligand, FAS ligand, and TRAIL. Indeed, the TNF cytokine family now contains more than 2018 members, each of which exhibits marked differences in tissue expression, ligand specificity, receptor binding and biological function (Fig. 9.4; Tables 9.2 and 9.3). This section describes general aspects of TNF and TNFR biology, with examples from three of the best-studied TNF-family members: TNF, lymphotoxin, and FAS ligand.

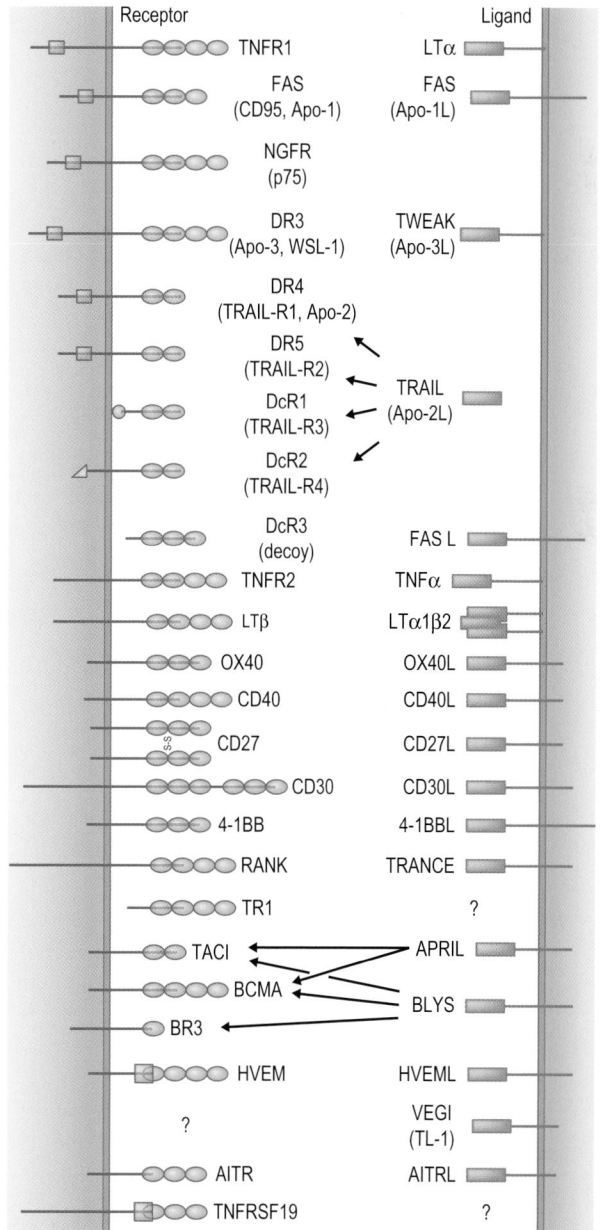

Fig. 9.4 Schematic representation of members of the TNF ligand and receptor superfamily.

Table 9.2 TNF superfamily cytokines

Symbol	Common name	Aliases	Binds to receptor(s)	OMIM ID	Key functions	Phenotype associated with over expression	Phenotype associated with deficiency	Human genetic disease associations
TNFSF1	Lymphotoxin alpha (Lα)	LT, TNFB, TNFSF1	TNFR2 (1B), TNFR1 (1A), HVEM (14)	153440	Lymphoid organ formation		Absence of LN and PP, defective GC formation	
TNFSF2	Tumor necrosis factor (TNF)	DIF, TNFA, TNFSF2, CACHECTIN	TNFR2 (1B), TNFR1 (1A)	191160	Inflammation	Wasting syndrome, arthritis	Defective GC formation, resistance to endotoxic shock and experimental arthritis	TNF2 (G-308A) promotor polymorphism associated with increased susceptability to septic shock, asthma and RA severity
TNFSF3	Lymphotoxin beta (LTβ)	p33, TNFC, TNFSF3	As a $β_2-α_1$ heterotrimer with LTα binds to LTβ receptor (3)	600978	Lymphoid organ formation	Ectopic lymphoid organ formation		
TNFSF4	OX40 Ligand	GP34, OX4OL, TXGP1, CD134L, OX-40 L	OX40 (4)	603594	CD4 T-cell expansion, survival, and Th2 development	Increased Th2 responses	Th2 deficiency, blockade improves EAE	Associated with SLE in GWAS
TNFSF5	CD40 Ligand	IGM, IMD3, TRAP, gp39, CD154, CD40L, HIGM1, T-BAM,	CD40 (5)	300386	Co-stimulation and differentiation of B cells and APC	Constitutive expression in B cells or keratinocytes leads to SLE-like syndrome	Immunodeficiency due to Defective Ig class switching and germinal center formation	X-linked hyper-IGM syndrome associated with CD40L loss of function mutations
TNFSF6	Fas Ligand	FASL, CD178, CD95L, APT1LG1	Fas (6), DcR3 (6B)	134638	Mediator of CD4(+) T-cell apoptosis due to restimulation and apoptosis in other cell types		Lymphadenopathy and Systemic Autoimmunity	Autoimmune Lymphoproliferative Syndrome (ALPS) type Ib
TNFSF7	CD27 Ligand	CD70, CD27L, CD27LG	CD27 (7)	602840	T-cell co-stimulation	T-cell hyperactivation eventually leading to immunodeficiency (HIV-like)		
TNFSF8	CD30 Ligand	CD153, CD30L, CD30LG	CD30 (8)	603875	T-cell co-stimulation			
TNFSF9	4-1-BB Ligand	4-1BB-L	4-1BB (9)	606182	T-cell co-stimulation			
TNFSF10	(TNF-like apoptosis inducing ligand) TRAIL	TL2, APO2L, TRAIL, Apo-2 L	DR4 (10A), DR5 (10B), DcR1 (10 C), DcR2 (10D)	603598	Dendritic cell apoptosis, NK-cell mediated tumor cell killing		defective NK-mediated tumor eradication	

Symbol	Common names	Receptor (TNFRSF)	OMIM	Function	Phenotype	Disease / additional
TNFSF11	RANK-L	ODF, OPGL, sOdf, RANKL, TRANCE, hRANKL2	RANK (11A)	602642	Mediates osteoclast formation and bone remodeling. Stimulation of APC		
TNFSF12	TWEAK	APO3L, DR3LG, TWEAK, MGC20669	TWEAK-R (12A)	602695	Potential role in inflammation and lymphocyte function		
TNFSF13	APRIL	APRIL, TALL2, TWE-PRIL	TACI (13B), BCMA (17)	604472	Promotes T-independent type-2 responses through interactions with TACI	overexpression in T cells produces prolonged T-cell survival and enhanced TI-2 responses	
TNFSF13B	BlyS, BAFF	BAFF, BLYS, TALL1, THANK, ZTNF4	TACI (3B), BAFF-R (13 C), BCMA(17)	603969	Promotes B-cell maturation, plasmablast survival	SLE-like systemic autoimmunity and arthritis	
TNFSF14	LIGHT	LTg, TR2, HVEML, LIGHT	HVEM (14), LT-βR (3), DcR3 (6B)	604520	CD8 T-cell and APC co-stimulation	inflammation, T-cell hyperactivation Th1 bias	Defective CD8 T-cell co-stimulation
TNFSF15	TL1A	TL1, TL1A, VEGI	DR3 (25)	604052	Ligand for DR3 (TNFRSF25) on lymphocytes	T-cell activation, IL-13 dependent small interstinal hyperplasia and inflammation.	Common variant associated with Inflammatory Bowel Disease through GWAS
TNFSF18	GITR Ligand	TL6, AITRL, GITRL, hGITRL	GITR (18)	603898	T-cell co-stimulation (+) CD25(+) regulatory T cells		Reduced immunopathology in T-cell-dependent autoimmune diseases
ED1	ectodermal dysplasia 1, anhidrotic (EDA1)	EDA, HED, EDA1, XHED, XLHED	EDAR	305100	Tooth, hair and sweat gland formation		X-linked ectodermal dysplasia

Table 9.3 TNF superfamily receptors (receptors in italics have a C-terminal death domain)

Symbol	Common name(s)	Aliases	Binds to ligand(s)	OMIM ID	Key functions	Phenotype associated with deficiency	Human genetic diseases
TNFRSF1A	Tumor necrosis factor receptor 1 (TNF-R1)	FPF, p55, p60, TBP1, TNF-R, TNFAR, TNFR1, p55-R, CD120a, TNFR55, TNFR60, TNF-R-I, TNF-R55, MGC19588	TNF-α (2), Ltα (1)	191190	Mediates TNF-induced inflammation (and apoptosis in some cells)	resistance to TNF-induced arthritis models, resistant to endotoxic shock, Increased sensitivity to bacterial pathogens	Periodic fever syndrome (TRAPS) associated with heterozygous extracellular mutaions. Locus associated with primary biliary cirrhosis and multiple sclerosis in GWAS
TNFRSF1B	Tumor necrosis factor receptor 2 (TNF-R2)	p75, TBPII, TNFBR, TNFR2, CD120b, TNFR80, TNF-R75, p75TNFR, TNF-R-II	TNF-α (2), Ltα (1)	191191	May enhance pro-apoptotic effect of TNFR1	still susceptible to TNF-induced arthritis models, defective CD8(+) T-cell apoptosis after restimulation, increased sensitivity to bacterial pathogens	
TNFRSF3	Lymphotoxin β receptor	LTBR, CD18, TNFCR, TNFR-RP, TNFRSF3, TNFR2-RP, LT-BETA-R, TNF-R-III	LIGHT (14), LTβ (3)	600979	lymphoid organ formation	No LN, PP, defective GC formation	
TNFRSF4	OX40	OX40, ACT35, CD134, TXGP1L	OX40L (4)	600315	T-cell co-stimulation	Defective CD4 T-cell responses	
TNFRSF5	CD40	p50, Bp50, CD40, CDW40, MGC9013	CD40L (5)	109535	Co-stimulation and differentiation of B cells and APC	Defective Ig class switching and germinal center formation	Autosomal hyper-IgM syndrome associated with loss-of function mutations. Locus associated with rheumatoid arthritis through GWAS.
TNFRSF6	*Fas, CD95*	FAS, APT1, CD95, APO-1	FasL (6)	134637	Apoptosis of restimulated CD4 T cells, B cells, ? others	Defective apoptosis of restimulated CD4(+) T cells	Autoimmune Lymphoproliferative Syndrome (ALPS) associated with heterozygous dominant-interfering mutations
TNFRSF6B	Decoy receptor 3	M68, TR6, DCR3, DJ583P15.1.1	FasL (6), TL1A (15), LIGHT (14)	603361	Soluble decoy receptor for FasL, LIGHT, and TL1A. May have a role in tumor immune evasion		Associated with Inflammmatory bowel disease in GWAS
TNFRSF7	CD27	T14, CD27, S152, Tp55, MGC20393	CD27L (7)	186711	T-cell co-stimulation	Defective T-cell responses	
TNFRSF8	CD30	CD30, KI-1, D1S166E	CD30L (8)	153243	?Inhibition of CD8 T-cell effector function		
TNFRSF9	4-1BB, CD137	ILA, 4-1BB, CD137, CDw137, MGC2172	4-1BBL (9)	602250	T-cell co-stimulation	Defective CD8 T-cell responses	Locus associated with ulcerative colitis in GWAS
TNFRSF10A	*Death Receptor 4 (DR4)*	DR4, APO2, MGC9365, TRAILR1, TRAILR-1	TRAIL (10)	603611	Mediator of dendritic cell and tumor cell apoptosis		
TNFRFRSF10B	*Death Receptor 5 (DR5)*	DR5, KILLER, TRICK2, TRICKB, ZINFR9, TRAILR2, TRICK2A, TRICK2B, TRAIL-R2, KILLER/DR5	TRAIL (10)	603612	Mediator of dendritic cell and tumor cell apoptosis		
TNFRSF10C	Decoy receptor 1	LIT, DCR1, TRID, TRAILR3	TRAIL (10)	603613	GPI-linked decoy receptor, interferes with TRAIL function		

Gene symbol	Name	Other names	Ligand	OMIM ID	Function	Phenotype	Disease association
TNFRSF10D	Decoy receptor 2	DCR2, TRUNDD, TRAILR4	TRAIL (10)	603614	Transmembrane decoy receptor, interferes with TRAIL function		
TNFRSF11A	(Receptor activator of NF-κB) RANK	OFE, ODFR, PDB2, RANK, TRANCER	RANKL (11)	603499	Mediates DC co-stimulation and osteoclast maturation and activation	Osteopetrosis due to osteoclast deficiency, no lymph nodes, impaired B-cell development	
TNFRSF11B	Osteoprotegerin (OPG)	OPG, TR1, OCIF, MGC29565	TRAIL (10), RANKL (11)	602643	Soluble decoy receptor for RANK	osteoporosis, arterial calcification	
TNFRSF12A	TWEAK-receptor	FN14, TWEAKR	TWEAK (12)	605914			
TNFRSF13B	TACI	TACI	APRIL (13), BAFF (13B)	604907	May inhibit some of the pro-survival effects of BAFF-R	Decreased TI-2 B-cell responses, but B-cell hyperplasia and autoimmunity	Loss of function mutations associated with familial CVID.
TNFRSF13C	BAFF receptor (BAFF-R)	BAFF/BLyS receptor 3	BAFF (13B)	606269		Impaired survival of immature transitional B cells	
TNFRSF14	Herpes virus entry mediator (HVEM)	TR2, ATAR, HVEA, HVEM, LIGHTR	LIGHT (14), herpes viruses	602746			Locus associated with rheumatoid arthritis and ulcerative colitis in GWAS
TNFRSF16	NGF-R	TNFRSF16, p75(NTR)	NGF (not a TNF family member)	162010	NGF receptor - evolutionary outlier as NGF not classic TNF family molecule	Defective sensory neuron innervation; impaired heat sensitivity	
TNFRSF17	B-cell maturation antigen (BCMA)	BCM	APRIL (13), BAFF (13B)	109545		Apparently no B-cell phenotype	
TNFRSF18	Glucocorticoid-induced TNF receptor (GITR)	AITR, GITR, GITR-D	GITRL (18)	603905	T-cell co-stimulation, marker for CD4(+)CD25(+) Treg cells, modulates Treg function	T-cell hyperactivation	
TNFRSF19	Toxicity and JNK inducer (TAJ)	TROY, TRADE, TAJ-alpha		606122	Similar to EDAR, expressed in skin and brain		
TNFRSF19L	RELT	RELT, FLJ14993			Possible T-cell co-stimulator		
TNFRSF21	Death Receptor 6 (DR6)	DR6, BM-018		605732	Negative regulator B- and T-cell responses	Enhanced T and B-cell activation	
TNFRSF25	Death Receptor 3 (DR3)	DR3, TR3, DDR3, LARD, APO-3, TRAMP, WSL-1, WSL-LR, TNFRSF12	TL1A (15)	603366		Impaired thymic negative selection. Reduced immunopathology and T-cell accumulation at site of autoimmune disease	
EDAR	Ectodysplasin 1, anhidrotic receptor	DL, ED3, ED5, ED1R, EDA3, EDA-A1R	E1	604095	Tooth, hair, sweat gland formation	abnormal tooth, hair, and sweat gland formation	Ectodermal Dysplasia
XEDAR	XEDAR; ectodysplasin A2 isoform receptor	EDAA2R, EDA-A2R	EDA-A2	300276			

Locuslink ID: Gene 'homepage' curated by NCBI. Go To and type the locuslink ID in the search window.
OMIM: ID in the Online Mendelian Inheritance in Man Database. Go to and type in the OMIM ID in the search window.
LN, lymph node; PP, Peyer's patch; GC, germinal center.

Ligand and receptor structure

Much of our understanding of the structural and functional characteristics of the TNF ligand and receptor superfamilies has been learned from analysis of TNF (TNFSF2), LTα (TNFSF1), FASL (TNFSF6), and their receptors. TNF and LTα are closely related homotrimeric proteins (32% identity). Human TNF is synthesized as a 233-amino acid glycoprotein. It contains a long (76 residue) amino-terminal sequence that anchors it to the cell membrane as a 25-kDa type II membrane protein. A secreted 17-kDa form of TNF is generated through the enzymatic cleavage of membrane-bound TNF by a metalloproteinase termed TNF-α-converting enzyme (TACE). Both soluble and membrane forms of TNF are thought to be noncovalent homotrimers held together by a trimerization domain in the secreted molecule. When bound, both forms of TNF are biologically active. They have different affinities for the two TNF receptors and thus can exhibit different biological properties (see below).

LTα differs from TNF in that it is synthesized as a secreted glycoprotein. Human LTα is synthesized as a 205-amino acid glycoprotein that in native form exists as a 25-kDa homotrimer. It can bind both TNF receptors with affinities comparable to those of TNF, and has similar biological effects. A membrane-bound form of LT has been identified that consists of a heterotrimeric complex containing one LTα subunit noncovalently linked to two molecules of an LTα-related type II membrane protein termed LTβ. The LTα1β2 heterotrimer, also known as mLT, is not cleaved by TACE and is thought to exist exclusively as a membrane-bound complex. mLT does not bind either of the two TNF receptors, but rather exerts its effects on another member of the TNF receptor superfamily, the lymphotoxin β receptor (LTβR). TNF and the two LT subunits are encoded by closely linked single-copy genes situated in the class III major histocompatibility locus, at chromosome 6p21.3 in humans (Chapter 5).

The two receptors for TNF (and LTα) are type-I transmembrane glycoproteins. They are designated TNFR1 (also termed p60 in humans, p55 in mice, official designation TNFRSF1A) and TNFR2 (also known as p80 in humans, p75 in mice, TNFRSF1B). These receptors are characterized by cysteine-rich repeats of about 40 amino acids in their amino-terminal extracellular domains. Each extracellular domain consists of three or four cysteine-rich regions containing four to six cysteines involved in intrachain disulfide bonds. The cytoplasmic domains of these receptors have no obvious similarity to any known kinase and are thought to lack intrinsic enzymatic activity. Signal transduction is therefore achieved by the recruitment and activation of adaptor proteins that recognize specific sequences in the cytoplasmic domains of these receptors. Recruitment of adaptor molecules activates a number of characteristic signaling pathways that can lead to a remarkably diverse set of cellular responses, including differentiation, activation, release of inflammatory mediators and apoptosis.

Family members and their actions

Tumor necrosis factor (TNF), lymphotoxin-α (LTα), and receptors

TNF is a major physiologic mediator of inflammation.[46] It initiates the response to Gram-negative bacteria that produce lipopolysaccharide (LPS). IFN-γ also induces TNF and augments its effects. TNF has been shown to induce fever, activate the coagulation system, induce hypoglycemia, depress cardiac contractility, reduce vascular resistance, induce cachexia and activate the acute-phase response in the liver. Thus, TNF is the major mediator of septic shock. TNF also upregulates MHC class I and class II expression, activates phagocytes, and induces mononuclear phagocytes to produce cytokines such as IL-1, IL-6, chemokines, and TNF itself. Activation by TNF causes increased adhesion of cells to endothelium and can be cytotoxic, particularly to tumor cells. TNF-deficient mice are resistant to septic shock induced by high doses of LPS, but have increased susceptibility to bacterial infection. The dual role of TNF in controlling bacterial replication and in septic shock emphasizes the point that although the goal of an immune response is to eliminate invading microorganisms, the response itself can be injurious to normal host tissues. Septic shock is an extreme example of this. Although the primary source of TNF is the mononuclear phagocyte, it is also produced by T cells, NK cells, and mast cells. LTα shares many of the same biological effects as TNF, owing mainly to its ability to bind the same receptors. However, LTβR plays a unique role in the development of secondary lymph nodes.

Fas ligand (FasL) and its receptor, Fas/APO-1/CD95

FAS (Apo-1/CD95/TNFRSF6) is a type I integral membrane protein that is structurally related to TNFR1. FAS is thought to trimerize and transduce pro-apoptotic signals upon binding of its ligand, FASL. Similar to TNF, the physiologic ligand for FAS (CD95L or FASL) is synthesized as a type II membrane protein and is expressed on activated B cells, T cells, and NK cells. FAS-induced apoptosis is thought to play an essential role in the termination of T-cell responses, particularly in the peripheral immune system. FAS also plays a key role in the induction of cell death by cytotoxic T cells (CTLs) and natural killer (NK) cells, where it functions in conjunction with perforin.

CD40 Ligand and CD40

CD40 is expressed by a variety of cell types, including B cells, DCs, monocytes, macrophages and endothelial cells. It plays a major co-stimulatory role in B-cell differentiation and recombination, and promotes survival through the induction of BCL-2 family members. Studies of both CD40-deficient mice and patients with hyper-IgM syndrome (Chapter 34) reveal that its function extends beyond the humoral immune response, with CD40 signaling also playing a role in cell-mediated immunity. CD40 ligand (CD154) is a 39-kDa protein expressed by activated CD4 T cells that can bind to and activate CD40 by cell–cell contact.

Other members

Other members of the TNFR family play various roles in the development and function of the immune system. CD40, OX-40, CD27, CD30, and 4-1BB can mediate co-stimulation of T-cell activation, albeit through different mechanisms. CD154 on T cells triggers antigen-presenting cell (APC) activation, including upregulation of the CD28 ligands B7-1 and B7-2. This indirectly boosts co-stimulation of the T-cell response. OX-40, CD27, CD30, and 4-1BB more likely act as direct co-stimulators of T-cell activation. The TNF family ligand BAFF (BlyS/TALL1/TNFSF13B) has a special role in B-cell maturation and can bind three distinct receptors, TACI (TNFRSF13B), BADD-R (TNFRSF13C), and BCMA (TNFRSF17).

Signaling

The TNF receptor superfamily can be divided into three subfamilies on the basis of the types of intracellular signaling molecules recruited, e.g., FADD, TRADD or TRAF (Fig. 9.5).[47]

Fig. 9.5 The role of the death domain- and death effector domain-containing molecules in signaling by TNFR1 and TNFR2.

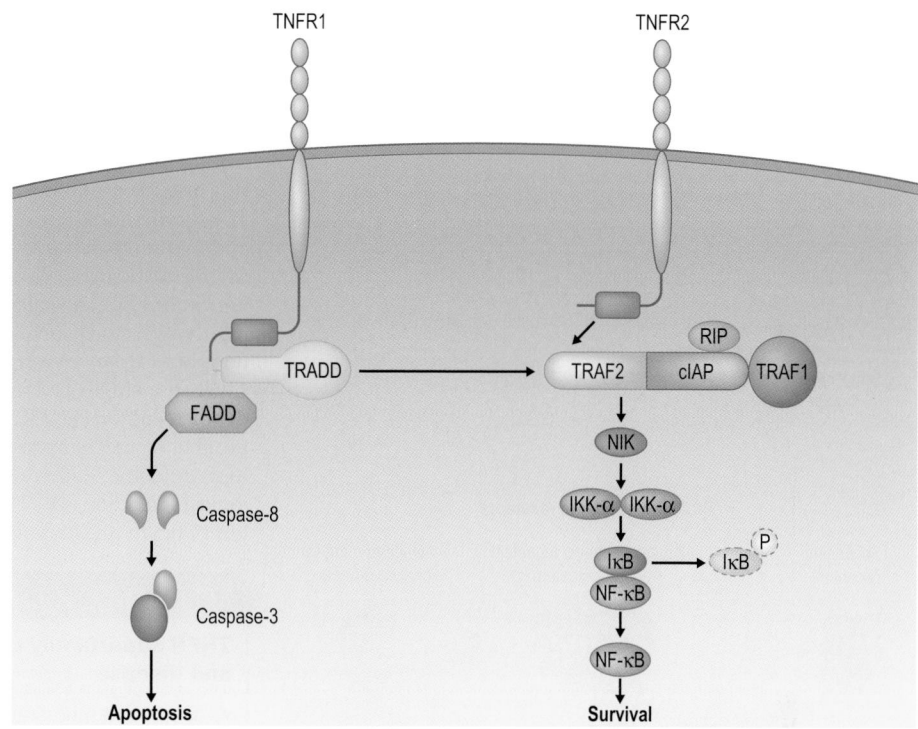

The cytoplasmic domains of several receptors, including TNFR1, FAS, DR3, DR4, and DR5, contain a conserved ~80-amino acid motif termed the death domain (DD). This element is required for recruitment of DD-containing adaptor molecules that are involved in the initiation of apoptotic cell death (see below). For this reason, these receptors have been termed "death receptors." The function of a number of death receptors can be regulated by decoy receptors, cell surface molecules that bind ligand, but lack functional intracellular domains. Other TNF receptor superfamily receptors that lack death domains (e.g., CD27, CD30, CD40, HVEM, TNFR2, LT-βR, OX-40, and 4-1BB) associate with different types of adapter molecules, most importantly members of the TRAF (TNFR-associated factor) family, as described below.

Death domains: TRADD and FADD

The primary molecule transducing signals in TNFR1 is TNF receptor-associated death domain (TRADD), which is directly recruited to TNFR1 after activation by TNF. The death domain mediates the interaction between TNFR1 and TRADD. This death domain motif is found in both adaptor molecules such as TRADD and the cytoplasmic domains of the receptor itself (Fig. 9.6). The binding of TRADD to TNFR1 leads to the recruitment and activation of numerous associated signaling molecules. TNF-induced apoptosis is generally thought to be achieved by the interaction of TRADD with FADD (FAS-associated death domain; also known as MORT1), a ~27-kDa protein that oligomerizes with TRADD through the death domains contained in both molecules. In turn, recruitment of FADD coordinately activates several members of the caspase family.[48] Caspase-8, which is generally considered to be the apical caspase in the TNF and FAS pathways, is recruited to FADD in the activated complex. It is thought to be activated by a self-cleavage reaction. Cleaved caspase-8 can subsequently activate downstream caspases, notably caspase-3, which play a more proximal role in apoptosis. In addition to FADD, TRADD also has a TRAF-binding motif that leads to the recruitment of TRAF1 and 2 and

the subsequent TRAF-dependent activation of pro-inflammatory signaling mediated by activation of NF-κB and MAP-kinase pathways. Although cell death in tumor cells can be induced by TNF, the most common result of TNFR1 ligation in primary immune cells is inflammation and sometimes protection from TNF-induced apoptosis. Recent evidence suggests that activation of pro-apoptotic and pro-inflammatory signaling by TNFR1 is not simultaneous, but proceeds by sequential steps.

Unlike TNFR1, FAS can directly recruit FADD to its cytoplasmic death domain, leading to the rapid formation of a death-inducing signaling complex (DISC), which contains FADD/MORT1 and caspase-8, thereby permitting activation of downstream caspases. The FADD death domain is recruited through interactions between charged residues in the death domains of FAS and FADD. Caspase-8 recruitment is accomplished through a structurally related domain termed the death-effector domain (DED). FADD DED contains two hydrophobic patches not present in the DD that are vital for binding to the death-effector domains in the pro-domain of caspase-8 and for apoptotic activity.[48]

The cytoplasmic domains of many receptors in the TNFR superfamily, including TNFR2, CD30, and CD40, do not contain death domains. Instead, the cytoplasmic domains contain short peptide consensus sequences that enable recruitment of TRAF proteins, which are a different family of adaptor proteins. A separate consensus sequence has been identified for TRAF6 versus other TRAF proteins, and other mechanisms probably operate to maintain the specificity of TRAF recruitment. Structural studies have revealed a mushroom-like structure for the TRAF proteins, with a trimer of the three TRAF subunits stabilized by a stalk-like coiled-coil domain.

TRAF proteins activate NF-κB and MAP-kinase pathways through recruitment and activation of protein complexes that activate these signaling cascades. The exact mechanisms by which this occurs are not yet clear, but recent studies have called attention to the ability of TRAF proteins to catalyze ubiquitination of target signaling complexes, which can function as an

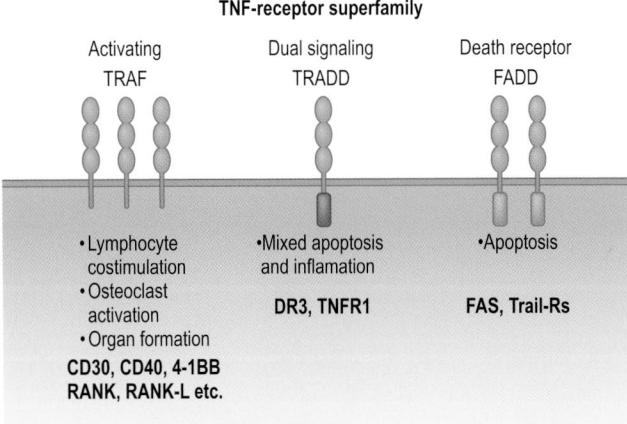

translocate to the nucleus, where they regulate the expression of a wide variety of genes involved in the inflammatory response.

Some TNF-family receptors use other mechanisms to activate NF-κB. For example, LTβ receptor activates the IKK complex via the serine–threonine kinase NIK, which was initially identified through its ability to associate with TRAF2. A naturally occurring mouse mutation termed alymphoplasia (aly) is the result of a point mutation of NIK. Aly/aly mice lack lymph nodes and Peyer's patches, and also exhibit disorganized splenic and thymic structures. This mutation, and the phenotype of LTβR knockout mice, revealed the critical role of this receptor in normal lymph node development and the formation of "tertiary" lymphoid tissue in inflammation.

When a single TNF-family ligand, such as TNF, binds both a death receptor (TNFR1) and a non-death receptor (TNFR2), a number of mechanisms regulate receptor signaling and the cellular outcome. Rather than functioning in cell death, the physiological function of TNFR2 may be as a co-stimulator of lymphocyte proliferation.[50]

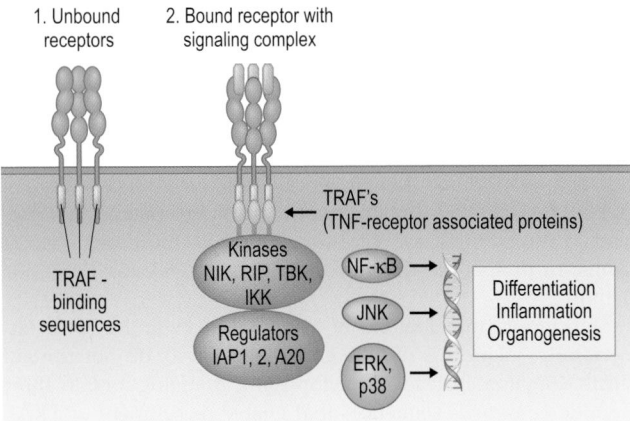

Fig. 9.6 Signaling by TNF family cytokines and their receptors

CLINICAL RELEVANCE

TNFR superfamily cytokines and receptors and disease

- Dominant mutations of TNFRI are associated with autosomal dominant periodic fever syndromes known as TNFR1-associated periodic syndromes (TRAPS).
- Mutations in CD40L are associated with X-linked hyper-IgM syndrome (X-HIM).
- Dominant mutations in FAS are associated with autoimmune lymphoproliferative syndrome (ALPS).
- Rheumatoid arthritis often responds to therapeutic use of TNF antagonists.

Clinical relevance

Mutations of TNFR1 are associated with autosomal dominant periodic fever syndromes (Chapter 59).[51] These patients have missense mutations in exons encoding the extracellular regions of *TNFR1* that are thought to affect normal *TNFR1* function, prompting the designation *TNFR1*-associated periodic syndromes, or TRAPS. Although the precise role of *TNFR1* has yet to be elucidated, patients with TRAPS typically have low serum levels of soluble TNF receptors that might normally serve to neutralize and control serum TNF levels. Recent work has shown mutated TNFR1 accumulates intracellularly and may signal in a TNF-independent fashion to amplify inflammatory responses.[52] Clinical studies are in progress to test the potential efficacy of TNF blockade with etanercept in controling fevers in TRAPS patients.

The *in vivo* role of FAS signaling in the regulation of the immune system was confirmed when the naturally arising lpr and gld mouse strains were found to harbor homozygous mutations of Fas and Fas ligand, respectively. Both of these mouse strains are characterized by lymphadenopathy and splenomegaly due to the accumulation of unusual CD4⁻CD8⁻ T cells, as well as the production of autoantibodies. Subsequently, humans with heterozygous FAS receptor were identified with similar symptoms and autoantibodies.[53] In this disease, the autoimmune lymphoproliferative syndrome or ALPS, FAS mutants act as dominant negative inhibitors of intracellular signaling, causing defective apoptosis in all carriers of *FAS* mutations and overt disease in a variable percentage of family members (Chapter 35).

activating step. TRAF6, which mediates NF-κB activation by a number of TNF-family receptors, associates with a protein complex that mediates K63-linked ubiquitination and activation of the inhibitor of κB kinase (IKK) complex, which consists of two catalytic subunits, IKKα and IKKβ and a regulatory protein IKKγ or NEMO.[49] Rather than causing degradation of IKK, K-63 linked ubiquitination activates kinase activity, leading to phosphorylation and degradation of IκB (inhibitor of NF-κB) and the release of active NF-κB subunits. Active NF-κB subunits

The gene encoding CD40 ligand is defective in X-linked hyper-IgM syndrome (X-HIM), a rare inherited disorder in which affected male children generate only IgM antibodies, many of which are autoantibodies (Chapter 34). Patients with X-HIM frequently suffer opportunistic infections, usually bacterial, and have an increased susceptibility to cancer. The physiologic role of the BAFF receptor in mouse B-cell development is illustrated by BAFF-R mutations in the A/WySnJ mouse, which lacks peripheral B cells. TACI knockout mice have hyperactive B cells, but in humans, dominant negative TACI mutations have been found in patients with common variable immunodeficiency affecting B-cell numbers and function (Chapter 34), arguing that in humans TACI serves as a positive modulator of B cells.[54]

Interleukin-1/Toll-like receptor family

Ligand and receptor structure

The IL-1/Toll-like family of receptors comprises at least 11 members, including the IL-1RI, IL-1RII, IL-1R-associated protein (IL-1RAcP), IL-18R, IL-18RAcP, IL-1Rrp2, IL-1RAPL, IL-33R(T1/ST2), TIGGIR, SIGGIR, and the mammalian Toll-like receptors (TLR1–10).[55,56] The ligands for these receptors include IL-1, IL-18 and IL-1 F5–10, IL-33 and IL-37.[56,57]

Family members and their actions

Interleukin-1

There are two cell surface receptors for IL-1, type I (IL-1RI) and type II (IL-1RII). Both of these bind ligand (Fig. 9.4), but only IL-1RI transduces signals. The extracellular domain of IL-1RI has three immunoglobulin-like domains and a 200-amino acid cytoplasmic domain. Upon ligand binding, IL-1RI associates with IL-1R accessory protein (IL-1RAcP), which is critical for the initiation of signaling. The IL-1RII cytoplasmic domain is extremely short and has been suggested to be a "decoy" receptor, competing with IL-1RI for ligand binding and attenuating signaling. Both IL-1Rs are susceptible to proteolytic cleavage near the membrane surface. Therefore, they can be found as soluble proteins, functioning as another mechanism to "buffer" IL-1 signaling. These soluble receptors are readily detectable in the circulation. IL-1R also associates with a second subunit, termed the IL-1R associated protein (IL-1Rap).

There are three members of the IL-1 gene family: two agonists, IL-1α and IL-1β, and one antagonist, IL-1 receptor antagonist (IL-1Ra). IL-1α and IL-1β are structurally similar and have similar actions, but they are regulated differently. IL-1β is regulated at the levels of mRNA stabilization and translation. Both IL-1α and IL-1β are synthesized as precursor proteins. The pro-form of IL-1α has biological activity, whereas that of IL-1β does not. Pro-IL-1β remains in the cytoplasm until it is cleaved by caspase-1, otherwise known as IL-1β-converting enzyme (ICE).

It is then transported out of the cell. IL-1α is thought to be processed by a calpain-like converting enzyme.

The cleavage occurs in a multi-protein complex called the inflammasome. There are two key components of the inflammasome: caspase-1 and a recognition/assembly component which is a so-called NOD-like receptor (NLR). Often another protein called ASC (a simple adapter protein containing both pyrin and CARD domains) is required to facilitate assembly. NLR proteins are intracellular pattern-recognition receptors that contain 3 domains: a segment with multiple leucine-rich repeats whose role is to recognize the trigger for activation (whether directly or indirectly remains unclear); a portion called a NACHT domain that leads to ATP-dependent dimerization of the NLR after trigger recognition; and a protein-protein interaction domain, most commonly either a pyrin or a CARD domain, that recruits caspase-1.

The best-studied inflammasome is the so-called NLRP3 inflammasome. Recognition of the trigger by NLRP3 causes its dimerization, recruitment of ASC via interaction of the pyrin domains of NLRP3 and ASC, and subsequent recruitment of caspase-1 via the CARD domains present in both ASC and caspase-1. The dimerization of caspase-1 upon inflammasome assembly allows it to auto-activate by cleavage of the pro-form to generate active enzyme. The NLRP3 inflammasome can be activated by *ATP*; components of Gram-positive *bacterial cell walls*, such as muramyl dipeptide; *intracytoplasmic DNA*, such as occurs during viral infection; *molecules resulting from tissue damage*, such as hyaluronin fragments; *crystals*, including those of uric acid (released from necrotic cells), *alum* (a commonly-used adjuvant), *silica and asbestos* (environmental contaminants that lead to lung disease; and *amyloid-β*, a key protein in Alzheimer's disease. Cigarette smoke as well as uric acid and cholesterol crystals also leads to activation of caspase-1.[58]

Principal functions of IL-1 include the induction of acute-phase protein synthesis, cachexia and fever. In fact, it was the first endogenous pyrogen to be identified. It induces the production of IL-6 and chemokines, promotes hematopoiesis, stimulates adhesion of vascular leukocytes to endothelium, and has procoagulant effects. Importantly, IL-1 is a critical differentiation factor for Th17 cells, which underscores the role of this cytokine in inflammation and inflammatory diseases. Unlike TNF, however, it does not induce cell death. The major source of IL-1 is mononuclear phagocytes. However, other cells also produce it. IL-1RI$^{-/-}$ and IL-1β$^{-/-}$ mice have blunted fever responses to some (but not all) stimuli. This indicates that despite the impressive actions of IL-1, it is evidently redundant to some extent in febrile responses.

Interleukin-18

IL-18R was first designated IL-1Rrp (IL-1R related protein) before being recognized as the receptor for IL-18. The receptor is expressed predominantly on T cells, B cells, and NK cells. It associates with an accessory protein, IL-18RAcP. A major action of IL-18 is the induction of IFN-γ, a function it typically performs synergistically with IL-12. IL-18-null mice have deficiencies in IFN-γ production, NK cell activity, and Th1 responses. IL-18 can also induce IL-4 and IL-13 production, indicating a somewhat broader range of action. IL-18-binding protein interacts with IL-18 and prevents association with IL-18R.

Interleukin-33

IL-33 (previously known as IL-1 F11) appears to be a cytokine that acts by binding to a specific extracellular receptor, namely the IL-1 receptor-related protein ST2, also known as IL-33R.

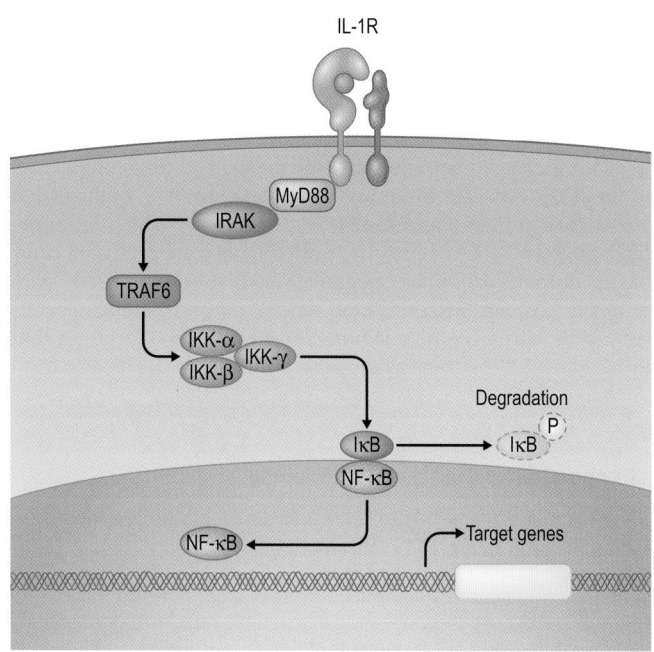

It also acts as a transcriptional regulator intracellularly. Because of this dual effect and because of the expression of ST2 on different cell types, IL-33 acts on both immune and non-immune cells. It acts on T and B cells promoting Th2-associated cytokines, including IL-4, IL-5 and IL-13.[59] And, it acts on mast cells, promoting degranulation, an effect also shown on basophils and granulocytes in general, but also enhancing cell survival. Interestingly, IL-33-treated basophils have been shown to suppress arthritic inflammation. Among IL-33 non-hematopoietic targets, this cytokine showed activity on endothelial and epithelial cells where it induces angiogenesis and production of other cytokines and chemokines.

Other IL-1 family members

IL-37 (also known as IL-1 F7) exists in several splice variants of which IL-1F 7b has been the most studied. IL-37 binds to IL-18Rα chain, although with a lower affinity than IL-18. Despite binding to the same receptor and its capacity to complex with IL-18Acp, IL-37 does not seem to act as a receptor antagonist for IL-18. IL-37 also translocates to the nucleus and binds Smad3, enabling it to regulate gene transcription. The biologic function of IL-37 is to negatively regulate excessive inflammatory response. Macrophages expressing IL-37 no longer secrete pro-inflammatory cytokines and IL-37 transgenic mice are resistant to LPS-induced shock.[60]

IL-1 F5, F6, and F9 act via a receptor complex formed from the IL-1R homolog IL-1Rrp2 (HUGO nomenclature IL-1RL2) and AcP.[55,56] IL-1 F5, also known as IL-36 receptor antagonist (IL-36RA), acts as an antagonist for IL-36α, IL-36β, and IL-36γ (respectively IL-1 F6, IL-1 F8, and IL-1 F9). Mutations in this gene have been associated with generalized pustular psoriasis. Keratinocytes from patients with deficiency of IL-36 receptor antagonist (DITRA) have elevated levels of multiple inflammatory cytokines in lesional skin.[59] They are highly expressed in skin and airway, and may be involved in skin diseases such as psoriasis. IL-1 F5 serves to antagonize these three ligands, in a manner similar to IL-1Ra antagonism of IL-1α and IL-1β.

The remaining members of the IL-1 and IL-1R families are the receptor homologues APL and TIGIRR. Both of these have limited tissue distribution, with TIGIRR found almost exclusively in brain and APL in brain and a small number of other tissues.[61] Little is known of about the function of TIGIRR, or about APL in any organ other than the brain. Most insight into APL has come from the finding that deletions or mutations of this gene cause mental retardation.

Signaling

Ligand binding to IL-1R, IL-18R, and TLRs results in NF-κB activation (Fig. 9.7). These receptors all associate with the adapter protein MyD88. MyD88 has a C-terminal TIR domain and an N-terminal death domain. MyD88 allows the recruitment of IL-1 receptor-associated kinase (IRAK), which also has an N-terminal death domain. IRAK, in turn, permits the recruitment and activation of a member of the TNF receptor-associated factor (TRAF) family, TRAF6. This leads to the activation of the serine kinases TAB2, TAK1 and inhibitor of κB kinases, IKKα and IKKβ. With IKKγ or NEMO, these kinases phosphorylate IκB, which leads to its degradation within proteasomes, freeing bound NF-κB for nuclear translocation. Mice deficient in MyD88, IRAK, and TRAF6 have diminished responses to IL-1R/TLR family ligands. Other adapter molecules, including Mal and TRIF, are involved in TLR signaling.

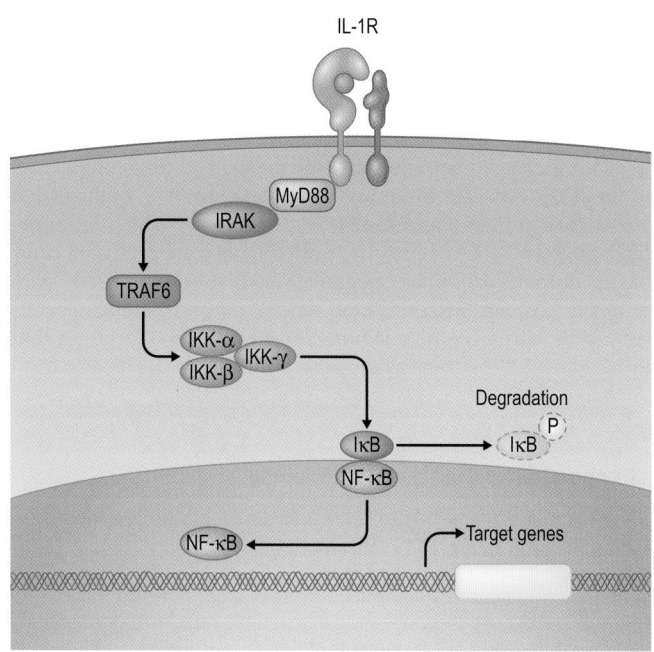

Fig. 9.7 Mechanism of signal transduction by IL-1R and related receptors.

Clinical relevance

The actions of IL-1 are tempered by the actions of a critical natural cytokine antagonist, IL-1 receptor antagonist (IL-1Ra), which is encoded by the *IL1RN* gene. Mutations in *IL1RN* can cause a systemic autoinflammatory disease denoted Deficiency of IL-1Ra or DIRA.[62] Mutations in *NLRP3* contribute to several hereditary periodic fever syndromes, including Familial Cold Autoinflammatory Syndrome (FCAS), Muckle-Wells syndrome, and neonatal onset multi-organ inflammatory disease (NOMID; in Europe called chronic infantile, neurological, cutaneous, articular syndrome or CINCA). NLRP3 is also called cryopyrin, thus these disorders have been collectively referred to as cryopyrinopathies.[49]

Interleukin-17 receptors

Although their precise functions are incompletely understood, IL-17 and related cytokines are major inducers of inflammation and serve to recruit inflammatory cells.

Ligand and receptor structure

The IL-17 receptor family is incompletely understood, but comprises at least five receptors, IL-17AR and IL-17BR (IL-17RH1), IL-17RL (receptor like), IL-17RD and IL-17RE, which are ubiquitously expressed.[25,63] These receptors have a single transmembrane domain and exceptionally large cytoplasmic tails. The ligands in the IL-17 family include IL-17A-F, but the precise interactions between ligands and receptors have not been defined. A viral IL-17 homolog, designated HVS-13, is present in the herpesvirus saimiri genome. Structurally, this family of cytokines forms cystine knots. In this respect, these cytokines are related to other, better-known cytokines such as nerve growth factor. IL-17 (IL-17A) is located on human chromosome 6 (mouse chromosome 1) and is produced by activated CD4, γ/δ and CD8 T cells. Recent findings have suggested that CD4 T cells that preferentially produce IL-17 (Th17 cells) represent a distinct lineage of effector Th cells.[64] These cells can be differentiated via a varied sets of stimuli that include IL-1β, IL-6, IL-21, and TGF-β. IL-23 appears to have a critical role in regulating the biological activity of these cells. IL-17 F is located adjacent to IL-17. Although it seems to be regulated in a similar manner, it may be more widely expressed than IL-17. Less well studied are IL-17 B, IL-17 C, and IL-17 D. All of these are thought to be expressed in a variety of non-hematopoietic tissues, although IL-17 D is reported to be produced by CD4 T cells.

With respect to their biological actions, IL-17 A and IL-17 F are most intensively studied. These cytokines evoke inflammation largely by inducing the production of chemokines, G-CSF, and GM-CSF, with the subsequent recruitment of polymorphonuclear leukocytes. IL-17 also induces production of matrix metalloproteinase by epithelial cells, which may be an important aspect of the pro-inflammatory effects. IL-17 family cytokines appear to be important in host defense against *Klebsiella pneumoniae* and *Mycobacterium tuberculosis*. Abundant data also point to pathogenic roles of IL-17A in models of immune-mediated disease and in human autoimmune disorders.

IL-17 E, which is also known as IL-25, is produced by Th2 cells and mast cells. It evokes an inflammatory response characterized by overproduction of Th2 cytokines, mucus production, epithelial cell hyperplasia, and eosinophilia. This cytokine is essential for the elimination of helminthic parasites.[65,66]

Signaling

Engagement of the IL-17 receptor activates MAP kinases, the PI3 kinase pathway and NF-κB. Signaling via IL-25 is reported to be dependent upon the adapter molecule TRAF6. IL-17 acts synergistically with TNF.[67] The IL-17R associates with an adapter molecule called Act through the SEFIR domains which are part of both the receptor and the adaptor.

Clinical relevance

Many human diseases and animal models of autoimmune disease have been associated with increased levels of IL-17. The inflammatory effects of IL-23 and IL-17 also appear to be associated with malignant transformation. Because of this, targeting IL-17 ligands and receptors could be a useful strategy. Importantly though, IL-17A and IL-17 F are essential for mucocutaneous immunity against *Candida albicans*. Deficiency in this pathway or high titres of neutralizing autoantibodies (auto-Abs) against IL-17A and IL-17 F results in chronic mucocutaneous candidiasis.[68,69]

Receptor tyrosine kinases

Ligand and receptor structure

Many growth factors, such as insulin and epidermal growth factor, utilize receptor tyrosine kinases (RTKs). Some, but not all, of these factors can be classified as cytokines. These include CSF-1 (colony-stimulating factor-1 or M-CSF), stem cell factor (SCF, c-KIT ligand, or steel factor), platelet-derived growth factor (PDGF), and FLT3 ligand (FMS-like tyrosine kinase 3 ligand, FLT3-L). All of these have important hematologic effects and tend to be included in discussions of cytokines. The structure of SCF and CSF-1 is similar to that of the cytokines that bind type I receptors, as they too form four α-helical bundles, even though

their receptors are entirely distinct. The similarities in their three-dimensional structures point to a common evolutionary ancestor. The receptors in this subfamily typically have five immunoglobulin-like loops in their ligand-binding extracellular domains. The cytoplasmic domain contains a tyrosine kinase catalytic domain interrupted by an "insert region" that does not share homology with other tyrosine kinases. This segment is used to recruit various signaling molecules.

Family members and their actions

Bone marrow stromal cells can synthesize stem cell factor (SCF, c-KIT ligand, or Steel factor) as either a secreted or a transmembrane protein. SCF is required to make stem cells responsive to other CSFs. SCF is widely expressed during embryogenesis and is also detectable in the circulation of normal adults. It has effects on germ cells, melanocytes, and hematopoietic precursors; as well as important effects on the differentiation of mast cells. Naturally occurring mouse mutations of SCF (Steel) or its receptor (W) have been recognized for many years. These mice have defects in hematopoiesis and fertility, lack mast cells, and have absent coat pigmentation.

CSF-1, also known as monocyte–macrophage-CSF or macrophage-CSF (M-CSF), is a hematopoietic growth factor that supports the survival and differentiation of monocytic cells. It is produced by a wide variety of cells, including monocytes, smooth muscle cells, endothelial cells, and fibroblasts. M-CSF-deficient mice manifest monocytopenia and osteopetrosis. IL-34 is a new cytokine that binds to the CSF-1 receptor. FLT3-L synergizes with other cytokines, including SCF, in inducing proliferation of hematopoietic precursors. FLT3-L is also an important regulator of DCs.

Signaling

The first step in signaling by the RTKs is ligand-induced receptor dimerization (Fig. 9.8). Dimerization brings the two kinase domains into proximity and results in the activation of

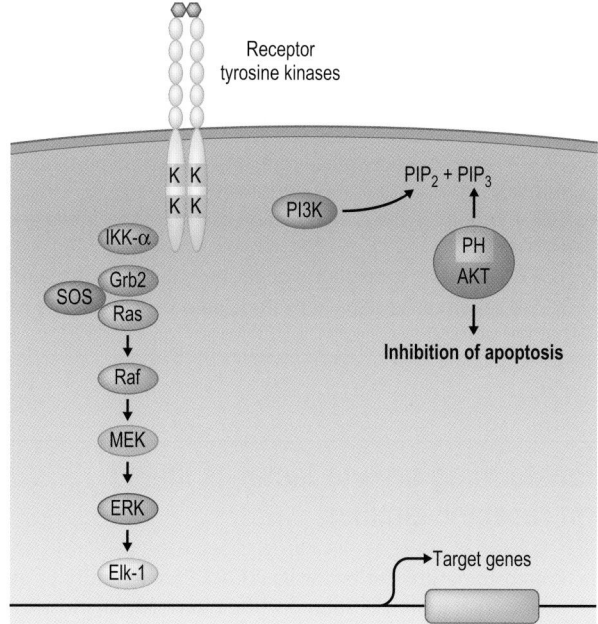

Fig. 9.8 Mechanism of signal transduction by receptor tyrosine kinases.

phosphotransferase activity. This leads to autophosphorylation of the receptor subunits on the tyrosine residues, which are then bound by a variety of signaling molecules, initiating signal transduction.[70] During this important step, the signaling and adapter molecules recognize phosphotyrosine residues on the RTKs by virtue of either their SH2 (src homology 2) domains or their phosphotyrosine binding (PTB) domains.

A major pathway activated by RTKs is the RAS/RAF/ERK pathway. RAS is a small G protein with intrinsic low GDP/GTP exchange activity. In RTK signal transduction, two adapter proteins, GRB2 and SHC, have important functions in RAS activation. In some cases, GRB2 binds directly to phosphotyrosine residues on the cytoplasmic tail of the receptor via its SH2 domain. Alternatively, SHC can bind first and then recruit GRB2. In addition to an SH2 domain, GRB2 has two SH3 domains that bind proline-rich segments of the guanine nucleotide exchange factor son of sevenless protein (SOS), recruiting it to the membrane and allowing it to activate RAS. Activated RAS binds and activates the serine/threonine kinase RAF, which in turn phosphorylates the dual-specificity kinase MEK. Activated MEK phosphorylates and activates ERK (extracellular signal-regulated kinase), which then translocates to the nucleus, where it phosphorylates and modulates the activity of various transcription factors, including ELK-1. Accordingly, mutations of RAS that lead to the constitutive activation of the ERK pathway have been found in a wide variety of human cancers.

Another important pathway activated by RTKs is the phosphatidylinositol 3'-OH kinase (PI3-kinase) pathway.[71] PI3-kinase catalyzes the formation of phosphatidylinositol-3,4,5-trisphosphate (PtdIns(3,4,5)P3) and PtdIns(3,4)P2. These phospholipids are recognized by proteins with pleckstrin homology (PH) domains. One such protein is protein kinase B (PKB or AKT), which has been implicated in the regulation of apoptosis. The PI3-kinase pathway is inhibited by the lipid phosphatase PTEN, which dephosphorylates PI3-kinase-generated phosphatidylinositides. Deletion of PTEN has been found in numerous tumor types, demonstrating a role for this protein as a tumor suppressor.

Gain-of-function mutations of c-kit result in a disorder termed systemic mastocytosis. Mutations resulting in a fusion between the PDGFRA and FIP1L1 genes underlie hypereosinophilic syndrome.[72,73]

● **KEY CONCEPT**

Properties of the TGF-β receptor family

- TGF-β receptors play a key role in lymphoid homeostasis, with pro- and anti-inflammatory actions.
- TGF-β promotes the differentiation of regulatory T cells and Th17 cells.
- TGF-β receptors transduce signals through SMAD proteins.
- TGF-β receptor function is dysregulated in many forms of human cancer.

Transforming growth factor-β ligand and receptor families

The transforming growth factor-βs (TGF-β) are a family of over 40 cytokines that inhibit cellular proliferation and can induce apoptosis of a variety of cell types. TGF-βs are involved in a number of biological processes, including tissue remodelling, wound repair, development, and hematopoiesis. Mutations of the elements in this pathway also contribute to malignant transformation. The mammalian ligands that belong to this family include TGF-β1, -β2, and -β3, bone morphogenic proteins (BMPs), activins, inhibins, and müllerian-inhibiting substance. Despite the name, TGF-βs inhibit the growth of many other cells, and, in combination with other cytokines and growth factors, may induce growth instead. TGF-βs also induce collagen and fibronectin production by fibroblasts, which is thought to be responsible, at least in part, for diseases characterized by fibrosis (e.g., systemic sclerosis and pulmonary fibrosis). Functionally, TGF-β inhibits many aspects of lymphocyte function, including T-cell proliferation and CTL maturation. Transgenic mouse studies have been performed using dominant negative forms of the TGF-β receptor. These mice exhibit massive expansion of lymphoid organs and develop T-cell lymphoproliferative disorders, suggesting a critical role for TGF-β in T-cell homeostasis.[39]

Ligand and receptor structure

The TGF-βs are expressed as biologically inactive disulphide-linked dimers that are cleaved to form active dimers. On translocation into the endoplasmic reticulum, the N-terminal leader peptide is cleaved and the mature protein is subsequently generated by a second cleavage event that releases an N-terminal pro-region. The pro-region can remain associated with the biologically active C-terminal region, inhibiting its activity.

The biological effects of the TGF-βs and their related ligands are mediated by two classes of receptor, designated type I (RI) and type II (RII).[74] A third group of receptors, denoted type III, also exists (e.g., TGF-βRIII in the case of TGF-β). This latter group does not actively participate in signal transduction, but is thought to function to present ligands to the functional receptors. Similar to the RTKs described previously, the cytoplasmic domains of TGF-β receptors possess intrinsic kinase activity. However, TGF-βRI and TGF-βRII encode serine/threonine kinases. The signaling cascade appears to be initiated by the binding of TGF-β to the type II receptor, inducing the assembly of a ternary complex containing TGF-β, TGF-βRII, and TGF-βRI.

Family members and their actions

The three known human TGF-βs—TGF-β1, TGF-β2, and TGF-β3—all have expressed molecular weights of 25 kDa. These three isoforms of TGF-β are closely related and have very similar biological functions. TGF-β_1, the most abundant form, is the only isoform found in platelets. T cells and monocytes mainly synthesize TGF-β_1, a critical function of which is to antagonize lymphocyte responses.

Approximately half of TGF-$\beta 1^{-/-}$ mice survive until birth, and 3–4 weeks later they typically succumb to an overwhelming autoimmune state characterized by lymphoid and mononuclear infiltration of the heart, lung, and other tissues, and by autoantibody production. These studies, along with selective inhibition of TGF-β function in T cells, indicate that TGF-β plays a crucial role in T-cell homeostasis and the prevention of spontaneous T-cell differentiation. TGF-β_1 clearly has very complex actions. It induces FoxP3, promotes adaptive Treg cell differentiation, and inhibits IFN-γ production. Conversely, TGF-β_1 with IL-6 induces IL-17, a pro-inflammatory cytokine. Thus, TGF-β_1 has both pro-inflammatory and anti-inflammatory activities.

TGF-β_2 is the most abundant TGF-β isoform in body fluids, whereas TGF-β_3 is the least abundant of the three. TGF-β_2 and TGF-β_3-null mice exhibit defects distinct from those observed in TGF-β_1 knockouts, particularly in bone and internal organ formation. Their deficiency is embryonically lethal, demonstrating that although the three isoforms functional similarly *in vitro*, they play distinct roles *in vivo*.

The human type II receptor is an 80-kDa glycoprotein which, as mentioned above, is the principal receptor for TGF-β. Upon binding of its ligand to RII, the type I receptor is recruited into the complex and activated through phosphorylation of its GS domain. The principal type I receptor in the TGF-β pathway is the ~55-kDa activin-like kinase-5 (ALK-5). ALK-1 can also be recruited into the complex and can transduce TGF-β-mediated signals.

Signaling

Ligand binding to the type II receptor allows the recruitment of the type I receptor (Fig. 9.9).[75] Although the receptor subunits have some affinity for one another, the complex of the receptor subunits bound to ligand is more stable. The type II receptor is thought to be a constitutively active kinase. Upon ligand binding, the type II receptor phosphorylates the type I receptor. The type I receptor is structurally distinct from the type II receptor in having a juxtamembrane domain that precedes the kinase domain, which is referred to as the GS domain. It is this site that is phosphorylated by the type II receptor. In turn, the type I receptor is responsible for phosphorylating key signaling intermediates. It is not clear whether activation of the type I receptor is due to enhancement of its kinase activity, to the appearance of substrate-binding sites, or to a combination of the two.

SMADs

The primary substrates activated by the type I receptors are SMADs, a group of related proteins that have been highly conserved throughout evolution and play a critical role in TGF-β signal transduction.[76] Eight mammalian SMADs have been identified. All exhibit a high degree of specificity for conserved motifs in the cytoplasmic tail of type I receptors. These proteins do not contain any previously known structural or enzymatic motifs. However, they have two homology domains, termed the MH1 and MH2 domains, at the *N*- and *C*-termini, respectively, which are separated by a central linker domain. The extreme *C*-terminus of some SMADs is a critical site of phosphorylation, as described below.

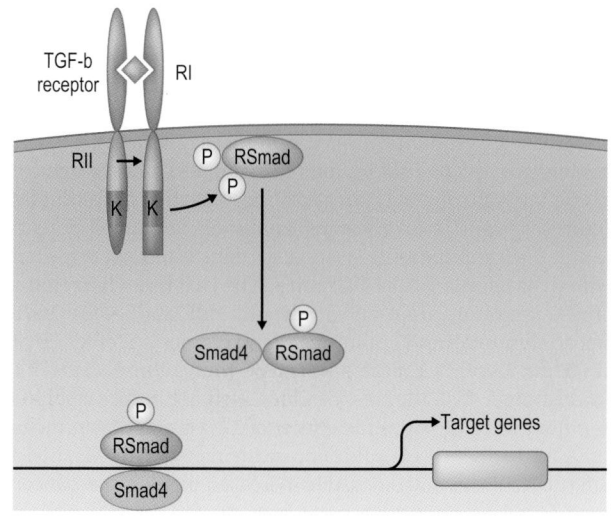

TGF-b receptor   RI

RII   K K   P RSmad   P

P Smad4 RSmad

P RSmad   Smad4   →Target genes

Fig. 9.9 SMADs and signaling by TGF-β superfamily receptor serine kinases.

SMADs have been subdivided into three classes based on functional distinctions. The receptor-regulated SMADs (R-Smads) directly interact with, and are phosphorylated by, the type I receptor. These include SMAD1, -2, -3, -5, and -8. Smad2 and Smad3 are phosphorylated in response to TGF-β, whereas Smad1, -5, and -8 are primarily activated in response to BMP activation. R-SMADs bind to the GS domain of type I receptor and are phosphorylated at a conserved SSXS motif in their C terminus. The interaction of R-SMADs with TGF-β receptors can also be regulated by another molecule termed SARA (SMAD anchor for receptor activation). SARA binds unphosphorylated SMAD2 and SMAD3. By virtue of its FYVE domain, SARA can bind phospholipids and localize SMADs to the plasma membrane, facilitating receptor binding. Phosphorylation of SMADs also permits dissociation from SARA.

Upon recruitment to their cognate activated type I receptor, R-SMADs are phosphorylated on *C*-terminal serine residues, triggering homodimerization of R-SMADs or heterodimerization with another class of SMAD, the common SMAD or C-SMAD. SMAD4 is the only known C-SMAD in vertebrates. It is thought to function as the central and essential downstream mediator of other SMADs in all TGF-β/BMP pathways. The SMAD MH2 domain is important for both receptor interaction and SMAD dimerization. However, SMAD4 lacks the SSXS element conserved in the R-SMADs and thus is not phosphorylated, rendering it unable to bind type I receptors directly.

The third subfamily of SMADs is the inhibitory SMADs, or I-SMADs. In mammals, SMAD6 and SMAD7 are the I-SMADs. I-SMADs may have different modes of function. For example, SMAD7 is induced by TGF-β and binds to TGF-β receptors inhibiting the phosphorylation of R-SMADs, thus serving as a classic feedback inhibitor. SMAD6 utilizes an alternative mechanism, and is thought to function by competing with SMAD4 for binding to an R-SMAD.

Consistent with their key functions in development, gene targeting of SMAD molecules has been shown to produce severe phenotypic abnormalities. SMAD2 null mice lack anterior/posterior specification and fail to develop mesoderm. SMAD3-deficient mice have limb malformations and defective immune function. SMAD3 null mice exhibit defective TGF-β responses. However, these mice also display accelerated wound healing compared to normal mice, which seems to contradict the role of SMAD3 as a positive regulator of TGF-β in enhancing wound healing. SMAD4-deficient mice die early in embryogenesis and exhibit severe defects in gastrulation. Of the I-SMADs, studies with SMAD6-deficient mice indicate a role in the development and homeostasis of the cardiovascular system.

Once phosphorylated, R-SMADs dissociate from the activated type I receptor and associate with SMAD4 in the cytoplasm. This is followed by nuclear translocation of the heteromeric SMAD complex, the binding to cognate DNA motifs in the promoters of TGF-β-responsive genes, and the concomitant induction of transcription. The SMAD MH1 motif mediates sequence-specific DNA binding, whereas the MH2 domain contains the transcriptional activation domain.

Other TGF-β-activated pathways

Although a canonical SMAD DNA-binding element (SBE) has been described (AGAC), comparison of the TGF-β responsiveness of synthetic promoters to natural promoters has revealed that SMADs can only partially account for the gene-regulatory effects of TGF-β signaling. SMADs also interact with a variety of other transcription factors, transcriptional co-activators, and transcriptional co-repressors to coordinately regulate transcription of a select subset of complex promoters. For example, FAST-1 (forkhead activin signal transducer), a winged helix forkhead transcription factor, associates with the SMAD2/ SMAD4 complex. Moreover, SMADs also bind to c-JUN/ c-FOS, and AP-1 sites frequently overlap with SBE sites in the naturally occurring promoters of TGF-β-responsive genes. SMADs can also bind ATF2, the vitamin D receptor, and other transcription factors, and can recruit the co-activators CBP/ p300. Additionally, the SKI and SNON co-repressors can interact with SMADs and antagonize TGF-β signaling.

Other signaling pathways are known to mediate TGF-β signals. In particular, a number of members of the mitogen-activated protein kinase (MAPK) family are activated in response to TGF-β. TGF-β induces ERK, JNK and p38 MAPK activity. Inhibition of several of these pathways inhibits TGF-β-mediated transcriptional activation. In addition, a mitogen-activated protein kinase family member, TAK1 (TGF-β-associated kinase-1), has been implicated in TGF-β signaling. TAK1 is activated in response to ligand binding and has been shown to associate with another molecule, TAB1 (TAK1-asociated binding protein), that activates TAK1 kinase activity. Together, they have been reported to activate the MAPK pathway(s), leading to activation of p38/MPK2 and c-JUN N-terminal kinase (JNK), with evidence that this may take place via MKK6 and MKK4, respectively.

Clinical relevance

Although the relevance of TGF-β to clinical immunology remains unclear, defects in the TGF-β pathway have been identified in a range of human cancers. SMAD4 is deleted in half of all human pancreatic carcinomas. Mutations in SMAD2 have been identified in patients with colon cancer, and somatic mutations in TGF-β receptors have been identified in colon and gastric cancers. Loss of SMAD3 is associated with leukemia. In addition, oncogenic RAS has been shown to repress SMAD signaling by negatively regulating SMAD2 and SMAD3.

Other cytokines

Interleukin-14

Several new cytokines have been identified, but their functions are less clear than those discussed above. IL-14 was identified as a high molecular weight B-cell growth factor produced by T cells and some B-cell tumors. The precise nature of this putative cytokine is still uncertain.

Interleukin-16

IL-16 was formerly termed lymphocyte chemoattractant factor, because of its ability to recruit CD4 T cells.[76] It is unrelated to other cytokines and its only known receptor is the CD4 molecule. It was originally identified as a product of CD8 T cells, but its message is widely expressed. CD4 T cells, eosinophils and mast cells can all secrete IL-16. It is present in bronchoalveolar lavage fluids from asthmatics and sarcoid patients. It has also been detected in blister fluid from bullous pemphigoid lesions. The physiologic function of IL-16 has yet to be clarified.

Interleukin-32

IL-32 is one of the newest cytokines and it too is structurally distinct.[77] It is inducible by the combination of IL-12 and IL-18. IL-32 induces the expression of various cytokines, including TNF, IL-1, IL-6, and chemokines, and can synergize with muramyl dipeptides. IL-32 signals via NF-κB and p38. IL-32 is present in rheumatoid synovium, and injection of IL-32 induces inflammation and recruitment of inflammatory cells.

Therapeutic targeting of cytokines and cytokine receptors

Because of all the important activities in numerous diseases outlined in this chapter cytokines and their receptors have been actively studied as therapeutic targets or as therapeutic agents (Table 9.4; Chapter 92). Interferons were the first cytokines to be considered as antiviral agents. Currently, Type I IFN are used to treat a wide array of disease from viral hepatitis C infection (IFN-α and IFN-λ) to multiple sclerosis (IFN-β). IL-2 is currently marketed (as aldesleukin) for the treatment of renal cancer and melanoma. TNF was investigated after its discovery as an anti-tumor agent, but its inflammatory properties made it a highly successful target for autoimmune and inflammatory diseases.

With the advent of molecular biology techniques and monoclonal antibody engineering, targeting of these molecules has become a highly successful strategy to modulate the immune response. IL-2 is not only a therapeutic protein but also a target. Daclizumab and basiliximab are monoclonal antibodies directed against the IL-2Rα chain and have been approved for use in transplantation, multiple sclerosis, uveitis and ulcerative colitis.

IL-6, one of the most important pro-inflammatory cytokines, has also been targeted and several anti-IL-6 antibodies are now under development. Tocilizumab, which targets the IL-6R, has been approved for several autoimmune diseases ranging from RA to ankylosing spondilytis.

The effective targeting of the p40 subunit of IL-12/IL-23 with the human monoclonal antibody ustekinumab has resulted in effective treatment of some forms of psoriasis, psoriatic arthritis, and Crohn's disease. However, ustekinumab is not effective in multiple sclerosis.

Many studies have implicated TNF in the pathogenesis of the chronic inflammatory diseases such as RA and Crohn's disease. Levels of TNF are highly elevated in the synovial fluid and the serum of patients with RA, as well as in the gastrointestinal mucosa of patients with Crohn's disease. This suggests that the pro-inflammatory effects of TNF might underpin the severe inflammatory symptoms observed in these diseases. Of particular relevance to RA, TNF inhibits the synthesis of cartilage components such as proteoglycan and bone formation and stimulates bone resorption. These findings prompted the development of specific TNF inhibitors that have demonstrated great promise in the treatment of RA and Crohn's. The two best-characterized of these inhibitors are monoclonal anti-TNF antibodies (infliximab, adalimumab and golimumab) and chimeric TNFR2-Fc protein (etanercept). Clinical studies of these compounds have demonstrated that they can induce striking improvement in RA patients (Table 9.4). Side effects of TNF-antagonism include increased incidence of infection, particularly with Mycobacterium tuberculosis, and a possible increased incidence of cancer.[78] Other TNF-like molecules have been targeted for therapeutic purposes. Targeting of RANKL with denosumab has been used

Table 9.4 Recombinant cytokines and biologic agents currently in clinical use or being tested for clinical application

NName	Commercial name	Target	Type	Phase	Indications
Daclizumab	Zenapax	IL-2Rα	Humanized MAb	FDA approved	Transplantation, Multiple Sclerosis
Basiliximab	Simulect	IL-2Rα	Chimeric (mouse/human) MAb	In clinic	Transplantation uveitis, ulcerative colitis,
REGN-688		IL-4R	Human MAb	II	Asthma, atopic eczema
Benralizumab		IL-5R	Humanized MAb	II	Asthma, COPD
Reslizumab	Cinquil	IL-5R	Humanized MAb (from rat)	II/III	Asthma, inflammation of skin and gastrointestinal tract
Mepolizumab	Bosatria (proposed)	IL-5	Humanized MAb	III	Asthma, nasal polyp
Tocilizumab	Actemra	IL-6R	Humanized Mab	FDA approved	RA, JIA, Castleman's disease, Ankylosing spondylitis
ALD518		IL-6	Humanized MAb	II	RA, cancer
SA-237		IL-6	Humanized MAb	I	RA
Siltuximab		IL-6	Chimeric Mab (mouse/human)	II	Cancer, leukemia
SirukMab		IL-6	Human MAb	II	Lupus erithematosus, Lupus nephritis, RA
CYT 99 007		IL-7R	rHuman IL-7	II	Immunodeficiency
Eenokizumab		IL-9	Humanized Mab	II	Asthma
Oprelvekin	Neumega	IL-11R	rHuman IL-11	II	Thrombocytopenia, Von Willebrand Disease
Ustekinumab	Stelara	IL-12/23 p40	Human Mab	FDA approved	Psoriasis, psoriatic arthritis, Crohn's disease, sarcoidiosis, palmoplantar pustulosis
Briakinumab		IL-12/23 p40	Human Mab	III	Psoriasis, Crohn's disease
Lebrikizumab		IL-13	Humanized MAb	II	Asthma
Tralokimumab		IL-13	Human MAb	II	Athma, COPD
Anrukinzumab		IL-13	Humanized MAb	II	Ulcerative colitis
TNX-650		IL-13	Humanized Mab	I/II	Hodgkin Lymphoma
LY2439821		IL-17	Humanized Mab	II	RA, psoriasis
RG-4934		IL-17	Human MAb	I	RA, psoriatic arthritis
Secukinumab		IL-17	Human MAb	III	Psoriasis, psoriatic arthritis, ankylosing spndylitis, RA, Crohn's disease, multiple sclerosis, xerophtalmia
GSK-1070806		IL-18	Humanized Mab	I	Inflammatory bowel disease
NNC-114-0005		Il-21	Human MAb	I	RA
Denenicokin		IL-21R	rHuman IL-21	II	Cancer
Fezakinumab		IL-22	Human Mab	II	RA, Psoriasis
SCH-900222		IL-23		II	Plaque psoriasis
Anakinra	Kineret	IL-1	Human recombinant IL-1RA	FDA approved	Autoinflammatory syndromes, RA
IL-Trap/Rilonacpet	Arcalyst	IL-1	Human IL-1R-Fc (IgG1) fusion protein	FDA approved	Autoinflammatory syndromes, RA, gout, JIA
Canakinumab	Ilaris	IL-1β	Human MAb	FDA approved	Autoinflammatory syndromes, RA
MABp1		IL-1α	Human Mab	I/II	Cancer, atherosclerosis, RA
Gevokizumab		IL-1β	Humanized MAb	II	RA, typeI and type II diabetes, Behcet's disease, uveitis,
LY-2189102		IL-1β	Human MAb	I	Atherosclerosis
Sifalimumab		IFNα	Human MAb	II	Lupus, Dermatomyositis, Polymyositis
Rontalizumab		IFNα	Humanized MAb	II	Lupus
Etanercept	Enbrel	TNFα	TNFR2-Fc (IgG1) fusion protein	FDA approved	RA, JRA, psoriatic arthritis, plaque psoriasis, ankylosing spondylitis

Continued

Table 9.4 Recombinant cytokines and biologic agents currently in clinical use or being tested for clinical application—cont'd

NName	Commercial name	Target	Type	Phase	Indications
Infliximab	Remicade	TNFα	Chimeric MAb	FDA approved	RA, Psoriasis, Crohn's disease, ankylosing spondylitis, psoriatic arthritis, ulcerative colitis
Adalimumab	Humira	TNFα	Human MAb	FDA approved	RA, plaque psoriasis, Crohn's disease, ankylosing spondylitis, psoriatic arthritis, ulcerative colitis, JIA
Golimumab	Simponi	TNFα	Human MAb	FDA approved	RA, ankylosing spondylitis, psoriatic arthritis
Pegsunercept		TNFα	PEGylated TNFR2-Fc (IgG1) fusion protein	FDA approved	RA, JRA, psoriatic arthritis, plaque psoriasis, ankylosing spondylitis
Certolizumab	Cimzia	TNFα	PEGylated Fab' fragment of humanized MAb	FDA approved	RA, JRA, psoriatic arthritis, plaque psoriasis, ankylosing spondylitis
Belimumab	Benlysta	BAFF/BLyS	Human MAb	FDA approved	Lupus erythematosus
Brentuximab vedotin	Acderis (proposed)	TNFRSF8 (CD30)	Chimeric MAb	I/II	Lymphoma
Denosumab	Prolia or Xgeva	RANKL	Human MAb	FDA approved	Osteoporosis, RA, hypercalcemia of malignancy, cancer
Fresolimumab		TFGβ 1,2 and 3	Human MAb	II	Systemic sclerosis, renal sclerosis, pulmonary fibrosis, cancer, renal fibrosis, liver fibrosis

Source: Pipeline (Drug pipeline information database by Citeline, Inc.)

for the treatment of osteoporosis as well as the hypercalcemia that results from some forms of cancer.

Because of the importance of IL-1 in the pathogenesis of fever, it would be expected that agents that inhibit IL-1 would be therapeutically useful. Indeed, IL-1Ra, the naturally produced antagonist, has been studied in a variety of settings. It has been found to be somewhat efficacious in the treatment of rheumatoid arthritis. The drug anakinra is also effective in other autoinflammatory disorders, including Muckle–Wells disease, neonatal multisystem inflammatory disease, and Still's disease as well as in the treatment of gout and type II diabetes.[79] Rilonacept is a fusion protein containing the extracellular portions of the two IL-1 receptor components IL-1R and AcP and it has been approved by the FDA for the treatment of cryopyrinopathies. Similarly, the human monoclonal canakinumab has entered the clinical arena with overlapping applications while other are in various stages of clinical development.

Finally, one of the latest, and most exciting, new anti-receptor antibodies is belimumab which targets BAFF, a B-cell stimulatory TNF family member. Belimumab is the first licensed drug for the treatment for lupus erythematosus in more than 50 years and its mechanism of action is believed to be interference with B-cell survival, differentiation and autoantibody formation.[80] Beyond their beneficial effects to patients, the clinical effect of specific cytokine blockade with these agents is the ultimate test of the pathogenic role of the targeted cytokine. Bringing cytokine blockade into the clinics has helped to unravel the complex web of interactions between cytokines in human autoimmune and inflammatory conditions.

Conclusions and summary

Cytokines encompass a wide range of molecules that are essential for communication between cells of the immune system and other non-immune cells. Although the number of cytokines already seems vast, it is likely that more will be discovered in the future. Considerable progress has been made in defining the *in vivo* functions of various cytokines. Equally impressive have been advances in our understanding how dysregulation of cytokines and cytokine signaling contribute to human disease. Cytokine and anti-cytokine therapies are being successfully used in the clinic. It is likely that their use will increase with advances in the understanding of the immunobiology of these cytokines.

References

1. Dumonde DEA. "Lymphokines": non-antibody mediators of cellular immunity generated by lymphocyte activation. Nature 1969;224:38.
2. Cohen S, Bigazzi PE, Yoshida T. Similarities of T cell function in cell-mediated immunity and antibody production. Cell Immunol 1974;12:150.
3. Thompson AW, Lotze MT. The cytokine handbook. San Diego, CA: Academic Press; 2003.
4. Vilcek J. The cytokines: an overview. In: Lotte M, Thompson AW, editors. The cytokine hand book, vol. I, 4th ed. Amsterdam: Academic Press; 2003. p. 3–18.
5. Boulay JL, O'Shea JJ, Paul WE. Molecular phylogeny within type I cytokines and their cognate receptors. Immunity 2003;19:159–63.
6. Taga T, Kishimoto T. Gp130 and the interleukin-6 family of cytokines. Annu Rev Immunol 1997;15:797–819.
7. Hunter CA. New IL-12-family members: IL-23 and IL-27, cytokines with divergent functions. Nat Rev Immunol 2005;5:521–31.
8. Kovanen PE, Leonard WJ. Cytokines and immunodeficiency diseases: critical roles of the gamma(c)-dependent cytokines interleukins 2, 4, 7, 9, 15, and 21, and their signaling pathways. Immunol Rev 2004;202:67–83.
9. Williams MA, Tyznik AJ, Bevan MJ. Interleukin-2 signals during priming are required for secondary expansion of CD8+ memory T cells. Nature 2006;441:890–3.
10. Malek TR, Bayer AL. Tolerance, not immunity, crucially depends on IL-2. Nat Rev Immunol 2004;4:665–74.
11. Sakaguchi S, Sakaguchi N. Regulatory T cells in immunologic self-tolerance and autoimmune disease. Int Rev Immunol 2005;24:211–26.
12. Nelms K, Keegan AD, Zamorano J, et al. The IL-4 receptor: signaling mechanisms and biologic functions. Annu Rev Immunol 1999;17:701–38.
13. Risma KA, Wang N, Andrews RP, et al. V75R576 IL-4 receptor alpha is associated with allergic asthma and enhanced IL-4 receptor function. J Immunol 2002;169:1604–10.
14. Mosmann TR, Coffman RL. TH1 and TH2 cells: different patterns of lymphokine secretion lead to different functional properties. Annu Rev Immunol 1989;7:145–73.
15. Murphy KM, Reiner SL. The lineage decisions of helper T cells. Nature Rev Immunol 2002;2:933–44.

16. Lee GR, Kim ST, Spilianakis CG, et al. T helper cell differentiation: regulation by cis elements and epigenetics. Immunity 2006;24:369–79.

17. Zenatti PP, Ribeiro D, Li W, et al. Oncogenic IL7R gain-of-function mutations in childhood T-cell acute lymphoblastic leukemia. Nat Genet 2011;43(10):932–9.

18. Li H, Rostami A. IL-9: basic biology, signaling pathways in CD4 + T cells and implications for autoimmunity. J Neuroimmune Pharmacol 2010;5:198–209.

19. Tagaya Y, Bamford RN, DeFilippis AP, Waldmann TA. IL-15: a pleiotropic cytokine with diverse receptor/signaling pathways whose expression is controlled at multiple levels. Immunity 1996;4:329–36.

20. Crotty S. Follicular helper CD4 T cells (TFH). Annu Rev Immunol 2011;29:621–63.

21. Trinchieri G, Pflanz S, Kastelein RA. The IL-12 family of heterodimeric cytokines: new players in the regulation of T cell responses. Immunity 2003;19:641–4.

22. Watford WT, Hissong BD, Bream JH, et al. Signaling by IL-12 and IL-23 and the immunoregulatory roles of STAT4. Immunol Rev 2004;202:139–56.

23. Picard C, Fieschi C, Altare F, et al. Inherited interleukin-12 deficiency: IL12B genotype and clinical phenotype of 13 patients from six kindreds. Am J Hum Genet 2002;70:336–48.

24. Smale ST, Fisher AG. Chromatin structure and gene regulation in the immune system. Annu Rev Immunol 2002;20:427–62.

25. McKenzie BS, Kastelein RA, Cua DJ. Understanding the IL-23-IL-17 immune pathway. Trends Immunol 2006;27:17–23.

26. Collison LW, Workman CJ, Kuo TT, et al. The I hibitory cytokine IL-35 contributes to regulatory T-cell function. Nature 2007;450:566–9.

27. Dillon SR, Sprecher C, Hammond A, et al. Interleukin 31, a cytokine produced by activated T cells, induces dermatitis in mice. Nat Immunol 2004;5:752–60.

28. Perrigoue JG, Zaph C, Guild K, et al. IL-31-IL-31R interactions limit the magnitude of Th2 cytokine-dependent immunity and inflammation following intestinal helminth infection. J Immunol 2009;182:6088–94.

29. Rochman Y, Kasyap M, Sakamoto K, et al. Thymic stromal lymphopoietin-mediated STAT5 phosphorylation via kinases JAK1 and JAK2 reveals a key difference from IL-7-induced signaling. Proc Natl Acad Sci U S A 2010;107:19455–60.

30. Watanabe N, Hanabuchi S, Soumelis V, et al. Human thymic stromal lymphopoietin promotes dendritic cell-mediated CD4 + T cell homeostatic expansion. Nat Immunol 2004;5:426–34.

31. Siracusa MC, Saenz SA, Hill DA, et al. TSLP promotes interleukin-3-independent basophil hematopoiesis and type 2 inflammation. Nature 2011;477:229–33.

32. Garcia-Sastre A, Biron CA. Type I interferons and the virus-host relationship: a lesson in detente. Science 2006;312:879–82.

33. Siegal FP, Kadowaki N, Shodell M, et al. The nature of the principal type 1 interferon-producing cells in human blood. Science 1999;284:1835–7.

34. Asselin-Paturel C, Boonstra A, Dalod M, et al. Mouse type I IFN-producing cells are immature APCs with plasmacytoid morphology. Nat Immunol 2001;2:1144–50.

35. Bach EA, Aguet M, Schreiber RD. The IFN gamma receptor: a paradigm for cytokine receptor signaling. Annu Rev Immunol 1997;15:563–91.

36. Rosenzweig SD, Holland SM. Defects in the interferon-gamma and interleukin-12 pathways. Immunol Rev 2005;203:38–47.

37. Donnelly RP, Sheikh F, Kotenko SV, Dickensheets H. The expanded family of class II cytokines that share the IL-10 receptor-2 (IL-10R2) chain. J Leukoc Biol 2004;76:314–21.

38. Li MO, Wan YY, Sanjabi S, et al. Transforming growth factor-beta regulation of immune responses. Annu Rev Immunol 2006;24:99–146.

39. Ghoreschi K, Laurence A, Yang XP, et al. Transforming growth factor-beta induces development of the T(H)17 lineageT cell heterogeneity and pathogenicity in autoimmune disease. Trends Immunol 2011;32:395–401.

40. Pesu M, Candotti F, Husa M, et al. Jak3, severe combined immunodeficiency, and a new class of immunosuppressive drugs. Immunol Rev 2005;203:127–42.

41. Changelian PS, Flanagan ME, Ball DJ, et al. Prevention of organ allograft rejection by a specific Janus kinase 3 inhibitor. Science 2003;302:875–8.

42. Liu L, Okada S, Kong XF, et al. Gain-of-function human STAT1 mutations impair IL-17 immunity and underlie chronic mucocutaneous candidiasis. J Exp Med 2011;208:1635–48.

43. Wormald S, Hilton DJ. Inhibitors of cytokine signal transduction. J Biol Chem 2004;279:821–4.

44. Chen Z, Laurence A, Kanno Y, et al. Selective regulatory function of Socs3 in the formation of IL-17-sweeting T cells. Proc Natl Acad Sci USA 2006;103:8137–42.

45. Knosp CA, Carroll HP, Elliott J, et al. SOCS2 regulates T helper type 2 differentiation and the generation of type 2 allergic responses. J Exp Med 2011;208:1523–31.

46. Beutler BA. The role of tumor necrosis factor in health and disease. J Rheumatol 1999;57:16–21.

47. Siegel RM, Muppidi J, Roberts M, et al. Death receptor signaling and autoimmunity. Immunol Res 2003;27:499–512.

48. Siegel RM. Caspases at the crossroads of immune-cell life and death. Nat Rev Immunol 2006;6:308–17.

49. Deng L, Wang C, Spencer E, et al. Activation of the IkappaB kinase complex by TRAF6 requires a dimeric ubiquitin-conjugating enzyme complex and a unique polyubiquitin chain. Cell 2000;103:351–61.

50. Kim EY, Priatel JJ, Teh SJ, Teh HS. TNF receptor type 2 (p75) functions as a costimulator for antigen-driven T cell responses in vivo. J Immunol 2006;176:1026–35.

51. Kastner DL, Aksentijevich I, Goldbach-Mansky R. Rapid autoinflammatory disease reloaded: a clinical perspective. Cell 1999;140:784–90.

52. Simon A, Park H, Maddipati R, et al. Concerted action of wild-type and mutant TNF receptors enhances inflammation in TNF receptor 1-associated periodic fever syndrome. Proc Natl Acad Sci U S A 2006;107:9801–6.

53. Straus SE, Sneller M, Lenardo MJ, et al. An inherited disorder of lymphocyte apoptosis: the autoimmune lymphoproliferative syndrome. Ann Intern Med 1999;130:591–601.

54. Wood PM. Primary antibody deficiency syndromes. Curr Opin Hematol 2010;17:356–3661.

55. Dunne A, O'Neill LA. The interleukin-1 receptor/Toll-like receptor superfamily: signal transduction during inflammation and host defense. Sci STKE 2003;25 Febuary, re3.

56. Dinarello C, Arend W, Sims J, et al. IL-1 family nomenclature. Nature Immunol 2011;1:973.

57. Nold MF, Nold-Petry CA, Zepp JA, et al. IL-37 is a fundamental inhibitor of innate immunity. Nature Immunol 2010;11:1014–42.

58. Martinon F, Mayor A, Tschopp J. The inflammasomes: guardians of the body. Annu Rev Immunol 2009;27:229–65.

59. Schmitz J, Owyang A, Oldham E, et al. IL-33, an interleukin-1-like cytokine that signals via the IL-1 receptor-related protein ST2 and induces T helper type 2-associated cytokines. Immunity 2005;23:479–90.

60. Sims J, Towne J, Blumberg H. 11 IL-1 family members in inflammatory skin disease. Ernst Schering Res Found Workshop 2006;56:187–91.

61. Carrie A, Jun L, Bienvenu T, et al. A new member of the IL-1 receptor family highly expressed in hippocampus and involved in X-linked mental retardation. Nat Genet 1999;23(1):25–31.

62. Aksentijevich I, Masters SL, Ferguson PJ, et al. An autoinflammatory disease with deficiency of the interleukin-1-receptor antagonist. N Engl J Med 2009;360:2426–37.

63. Kawaguchi M, Adachi M, Oda N, et al. IL-17 cytokine family. J Allergy Clin Immunol 2004;114:1265–73.

64. Dong C. Diversification of T-helper-cell lineages: finding the family root of IL-17-producing cells. Nat Rev Immunol 2006;6:329–33.

65. Fort MM, Cheung J, Yen D, et al. IL-25 induces IL-4, IL-5, and IL-13 and Th2-associated pathologies in vivo. Immunity 2001;15:985–95.

66. O'Shea JJ, Paul WE. Mechanisms underlying lineage commitment and plasticity of helper CD4 + T cells. Science 2010;327:1098–102.

67. Maezawa Y, Nakajima H, Suzuki K, et al. Involvement of TNF receptor-associated factor 6 in IL-25 receptor signaling. J Immunol 2006;176:1013–8.

68. Puel A, Picard C, Cypowyj S, et al. Inborn errors of mucocutaneous immunity to Candida albicans in humans: a role for IL-17 cytokines? Curr Opin Immunol 2010;22:467–74.

69. Puel A, Cypowyj S, Bustamante J, et al. Chronic mucocutaneous candidiasis in humans with inborn errors of interleukin-17 immunity. Science 2011;332:65–8.

70. Pawson T, Scott JD. Signaling through scaffold, anchoring, and adaptor proteins. Science 1997;278:2075–80.

71. Cantley LC. The phosphoinositide 3-kinase pathway. Science 2002;296:1655–7.

72. Longley BJ, Reguera MJ, Ma Y. Classes of c-KIT activating mutations: proposed mechanisms of action and implications for disease classification and therapy. Leuk Res 2001;25:571–6.

73. Cools J, DeAngelo DJ, Gotlib J, et al. A tyrosine kinase created by fusion of the PDGFRA and FIP1L1 genes as a therapeutic target of imatinib in idiopathic hypereosinophilic syndrome. N Engl J Med 2003;348:1201–14.

74. Heldin CH, Miyazono K, ten Dijke P. TGF-beta signalling from cell membrane to nucleus through SMAD proteins. Nature 1997;390:465–71.

75. Massague J, Gomis RR. The logic of TGFbeta signaling. FEBS Lett 2006;580:2811–20.

76. Wilson KC, Center DM, Cruikshank WW. The effect of interleukin-16 and its precursor on T lymphocyte activation and growth. Growth Factors 2004;22:97–104.

77. Felaco P, Castellani ML, De Lutiis MA, et al. Interleukin-32: a newly-discovered proinflammatory cytokine. J Biol Regul Homeost Agents 2009;23:141–7.

78. Bongartz T, Sutton AJ, Sweeting MJ, et al. Anti-TNF antibody therapy in rheumatoid arthritis and the risk of serious infections and malignancies: systematic review and meta-analysis of rare harmful effects in randomized controlled trials. JAMA 2006;295:2275–85.

79. Goldbach-Mansky R. Current status of understanding the pathogenesis and management of patients with NOMID/CINCA. Curr Rheumatol Rep 2011;13:123–31.

80. Pipeline (Drug pipeline information database by Citeline, Inc.).

Philip M. Murphy

Chemokines and chemokine receptors

Chemokines form a large family of small secreted proteins whose main immunologic function is to coordinate leukocyte trafficking by activating G protein-coupled receptors. The immunologic functions of chemokines may be beneficial, for example in support of host defense and tissue repair, or harmful, for example in support of chronic inflammation and autoimmunity. The chemokine system is also a major target for immune system evasion or exploitation by pathogens (e.g., in HIV/AIDS and *Plasmodium vivax* malaria). Increasingly, non-immunologic chemokine functions are being recognized, and these may also be beneficial (e.g., organ development and angiogenesis), or harmful (e.g., cancer metastasis). This chapter focuses on the basic principles and clinical correlates of chemokine regulation of the immune system, including novel chemokine-targeted therapeutics.

KEY CONCEPTS

Chemokine and chemokine receptors at a glance

- *Definition:* Chemokines are defined by a common structure, the chemokine fold; chemokine receptors are defined by a common biochemical function: chemokine binding-dependent cell signaling. Most chemokine receptors catalyze guanine nucleotide-exchange on Gi-type G proteins.

- *Classification:* Chemokines form four main structural subclasses (C, CC, CXC, and CX3C) and two main immunological subclasses (inflammatory and homeostatic).

- *Evolution:* Chemokines and chemokine receptors arose in vertebrates and have been copied or mimicked by many viruses. Chemokines and chemokine receptors are rapidly evolving; the repertoires can differ among species and among individuals of the same species.

- *Ligand–receptor promiscuity:* Most chemokine receptors pair promiscuously with chemokine ligands, but are restricted to a single chemokine subclass.

- *Cell biology:* Chemokines coordinate leukocyte trafficking, but can have prominent non-trafficking functions (e.g., lymphocyte proliferation/apoptosis/differentiation/activation, granulocyte degranulation/superoxide production, direct antimicrobial activity), as well as effects on other cell types in non-immunologic contexts (e.g., development, cancer, angiogenesis).

- *Biology:* Chemokines act redundantly or non-redundantly *in vivo*, depending on the context. Host chemokine receptors mediate antimicrobial defense, but certain pathogens (e.g., HIV and *Plasmodium vivax*) can exploit chemokine receptors to infect the host. Moreover, excessive or inappropriate chemokine expression may pathologically amplify immunologically mediated disease.

Molecular organization of the chemokine system

Chemokines

Chemokines are defined by structure, not function.[1] The tertiary folded structure is highly conserved, in part because of uniformly spaced, disulfide-bonded cysteines (Fig. 10.1), which provide a logical approach to subclassification of the family. All chemokines have at least two cysteines, and all but two have at least four. In the four cysteine group, the first two are either adjacent (CC motif, $n=24$) or separated by either one amino acid (CXC motif, $n=16$) or three amino acids (CX3C motif, $n=1$). C chemokines ($n=2$) have only two cysteines, corresponding to C-2 and C-4 in the other groups. Disulfide bonds link C-1 to C-3 and C-2 to C-4. Chemokines contain 3 β-sheets arranged in the shape of a Greek key, overlaid by a C-terminal α-helical domain and flanked by an N-terminal domain that lacks order. Sequence identity is less than 30% for any two chemokines from different groups, but ranges between 30 and 99% for any two chemokines from the same group. The group names are used as roots followed by the letter "L" and a number (e.g., CXCL1) in a systematic nomenclature that was established to resolve competing aliases.[2]

CC and CXC chemokines can be subclassified by additional motifs. The 7 CXC chemokines with glu-leu-arg (ELR) N-terminal to C-1 share greater than 40% sequence identity, attract neutrophils, bind the same CXCR2 receptor, and are angiogenic (Table 10.1). Among CXC chemokines lacking ELR, CXCL12 is angiogenic and attracts neutrophils; CXCL9-11 are also greater than 40% identical and share a receptor (CXCR3), but are angiostatic.

There are two CC subgroups that have two additional cysteines, one in the C-terminal domain. They are distinguished by the location of the sixth cysteine, which can be found either in the C-terminal domain or between C-2 and C-3 (Table 10.2). CXCL16 and CX3CL1 cross classes to form a unique multimodular subgroup. Each has a classic chemokine domain, a mucin-like stalk, a transmembrane domain, and a C-terminal cytoplasmic module, and each can exist as either a membrane-bound form or shed form, enabling either direct cell–cell adhesion or chemotaxis, respectively. Chemokine monomer, dimer and tetramer structures can occur. Complex quaternary structures bound to glycosaminoglycans (GAGs) on the surface of cells can also be important for function *in vivo*.[1] A native heterodimer composed of CCL3 and CCL4 subunits has been purified from activated human monocytes and peripheral blood lymphocytes.

Fig. 10.1 Chemokine classification and nomenclature. Chemokine classes are defined by the number and arrangement of conserved cysteines, as shown. Brackets link cysteines that form disulfide bonds. ELR refers to the amino acids glu-leu-arg. X refers to an amino acid other than cysteine. The underscore is a spacer used to optimize the alignment. The N- and C-termini can vary considerably in length (not illustrated). For molecules with four cysteines, there are approximately 24 amino acids between Cys-2 and Cys-3, and 15 amino acids between Cys-3 and Cys-4. At right are listed the nomenclature system and the number of human chemokines known in each class (N).

Class					Names	N
CX3C:		CXXXC	C	C	CX3CL1	1
Non-ELR CXC:		CX_C	C	C	CXCL#	9
ELR CXC:	ELR	CX_C	C	C	CXCL#	7
4C CC:		C_C	C	C	CCL#	19
6C CC:		C_C C	C	C C	CCL#	5
C:			C	C	XCL#	2

Table 10.1 The human CXC, CX3C, and C chemokine families

ELR motif	Chemokine	Common aliases	Main source	Main immunologic roles
ELR+	CXCL1 CXCL2 CXCL3	GROα MGSA GROβ GROγ	Inducible in most hematopoietic and tissue cells Many tumors	Neutrophil trafficking
ELR-	CXCL4	PF-4	Preformed in platelets	Procoagulant
ELR+	CXCL5 CXCL6 CXCL7 CXCL8	ENA-78 GCP-2 NAP-2 IL-8	Induced in epithelial cells of gut & lung; N, Mo, Plts, EC Induced in lung microvascular EC; Mo; alveolar epithelial cells, mesothelial cells, EC & MΦ Preformed in platelets Induced in most cell types	Neutrophil trafficking
ELR-	CXCL9 CXCL10 CXCL11 CXCL12 CXCL13 CXCL14	Mig IP-10 I-TAC SDF-1, PBSF BCA-1 BRAK	Induced in PMN, MΦ, T cells, astrocytes, microglial cells, hepatocytes, EC, fibroblasts, keratinocytes, thymic stromal cells Induced in ECs, Mo, keratinocytes, respiratory & intestinal epithelial cells, astrocytes, microglia, mesangial cells, smooth muscle cells ECs, Mo, Constitutive in bone marrow stromal cells; most tissues Constitutive in follicular HEV of secondary lymphoid tissue Constitutive in most tissues, breast and kidney tumors	Th1 response Myelopoiesis HPC, neutrophil homing to BM B lymphopoiesis Naïve B- & T-cell homing to follicles B$_1$-cell homing to peritoneum Natural Ab production Macrophage migration
ELR+	(CXCL15)	(mouse only)	Constitutive in lung epithelial cells	Neutrophil trafficking
ELR-	CXCL16 CXCL17	Sexckine	Constitutive in spleen; DCs of the T zone Lung, heart, tumor cells	T-cell and DC homing to spleen Immature myeloid DC trafficking
NA	CX3CL1 XCL1 XCL2	Fractalkine Lymphotactin α Lymphotactin β	EC, neurons, Mo, DC γδ epidermal T cells, NK, NK-T, activated CD8 and Th1 CD4 T cells	NK, monocyte, MΦ, and Th1-cell migration CD62L^{lo} T effector cell migration

NA, not applicable. Mo, monocyte; PMN, neutrophil; DC, dendritic cell; EC, endothelial cell; HEV, high endothelial venule; MPC, myeloid progenitor cell; plt, platelet; MΦ, macrophage; GRO, growth-related oncogene; PF-4, platelet factor-4; GCP, granulocyte chemoattactant protein; ENA-78, 78 amino acid epithelial cell-derived neutrophil activator; NAP, neutrophil activating protein; IL-8, interleukin-8; Mig, monokine induced by IFN-γ; I-TAC; interferon-inducible T-cell alpha chemoattractant; SDF, stromal cell-derived factor; BCA, B-cell-activating chemokine; BRAK, breast and kidney-associated chemokine.

Chemokine receptors

Chemokine receptors are defined as mediators that activate cellular responses upon binding chemokines. All 19 known human subtypes are members of the 7-transmembrane (7TM) domain superfamily of G protein-coupled receptors.[3] Chemokine binding, membrane anchoring and signaling domains come from a single polypeptide chain. Homo- and heterodimers have been reported, but the physiologic form has not been clearly delineated.

Table 10.2 The human CC chemokine family

Chromosomal location	Chemokine	Common aliases	Sources	Main immunologic roles
17q11-12	CCL1	I-309	Inducible in Mo & CD4$^+$ and CD8$^+$ $\alpha\beta$ and CD4$^-$CD8$^-$ $\gamma\delta$ T cells	Th2 response
	CCL2	MCP-1	Inducible in Mo, fibroblasts, keratinocytes, EC, PMN, synoviocytes, mesangial cells, astrocytes, lung epithelial cells & MΦ. Constitutively made in splenic arteriolar lymphatic sheath and medullary region of lymph node, many tumors, & arterial plaque EC.	Innate immunity Th2 response CD4$^+$ T-cell differentiation
	CCL3	MIP-1α LD78α MIP-1αS	Inducible in Mo/MΦ, CD8 T cells, B cells, plts, PMN, Eo, Ba, DC, NK, mast cells, keratinocytes, fibroblasts, mesangial cells, astrocytes, microglial cells, epith cells	Innate immunity Th1 response CD4 T-cell differentiation
	CCL3L1	LD78β MIP-1αP	Similar to CCL3	Probably similar to CCL3
	CCL4	MIP-1β	Similar to CCL3	Innate immunity Th1 response
	CCL5	RANTES	Inducible in EC, T cells, epithelial cells, Mo, fibroblasts, mesangial cells, NK cells Constitutively expressed and stored in plt and Eo granules	Innate immunity Th1 and Th2 response
NA	(CCL6)	Mouse only	Inducible in bone marrow and peritoneal-derived MΦ	ND
17q11-12	CCL7	MCP-3	Inducible in Mo, plts, fibroblasts, EC, skin, bronchial epithelial cells, astrocytes	Th2 response
	CCL8	MCP-2	Inducible in fibroblasts, PMN, astrocytes Constitutively expressed in colon, small intestine, heart, lung, thymus, pancreas, spinal cord, ovary, placenta	Th2 response
NA	(CCL9/10)	Mouse only	Constitutively expressed in all mouse organs except brain; highest in lung, liver and thymus Induced in heart and lung	ND
17q11	CCL11	Eotaxin	Epithelial cells, EC, smooth muscle, cardiac muscle, Eo, dermal fibroblasts, mast cells, MΦ, Reed–Sternberg cells	Th2 response Eosinophil trafficking Mast cell trafficking Basophil trafficking, degranulation
NA	(CCL12)	Mouse only	Inducible in lung alveolar MΦ & smooth muscle cells; spinal cord. Constitutive expression in Lymph node and thymic stromal cells	Allergic inflammation
17q11-12	CCL13	MCP-4	Inducible in nasal and bronchial epithelial cells; dermal fibroblasts; PBMCs; atherosclerotic plaque EC and MΦ Constitutively expressed in small intestine, colon, thymus, heart and placenta	Th2 response
	CCL14a	HCC-1	Constitutively expressed in most organs; high plasma levels	ND
	CCL14b	HCC-3	Same as CCL14b except absent from skeletal muscle and pancreas	ND
	CCL15	HCC-2; Lkn-1	Inducible in Mo and DC Constitutive RNA expression in liver, gut, heart and skeletal muscle, adrenal gland and lung leukocytes.	ND
	CCL16	HCC-4; LEC	Constitutively expressed in liver, possibly many other organs. Also, Mo, T cells and NK cells express mRNA.	ND
16q13	CCL17	TARC	Constitutive in normal DC and Reed-Sternberg cells of Hodgkin's disease	Th2 response
17q11.2	CCL18	DC-CK1, PARC	Constitutive in Mo/MΦ, germinal center DC	DC attraction of naïve T cells
9p13.3	CCL19	ELC, MIP-3β	Constitutive on interdigitating DC in secondary lymphoid tissue	Naïve and memory T-cell & DC homing to lymph node
2q36.3	CCL20	LARC MIP-3α	Constitutive in lymph nodes, peripheral blood leukocytes, thymus, and appendix Inducible in PBMC, HUVEC	DC homing to Peyer's patch Humoral response
9p13.3	CCL21	SLC, 6Ckine	Constitutive in lymphatic EC, HEV & interdigitating DC in T areas of 2° lymphoid tissue, thymic medullary epith cells & EC	Naïve and memory T-cell & DC homing to lymph node

Table 10.2 The human CC chemokine family—cont'd

Chromosomal location	Chemokine	Common aliases	Sources	Main immunologic roles
16q13	CCL22	MDC	Constitutive in DC and MΦ Inducible in Mo, T and B cells	Th2 response
17q12	CCL23	MPIF-1	Constitutive in pancreas & skeletal muscle	ND
7q11.23	CCL24	Eotaxin-2	Inducible in Mo	Eosinophil migration
19p13.3	CCL25	TECK	Constitutive in thymic stromal cells & small intest	Thymocyte migration Homing of memory T cells to gut
7q11.23	CCL26	Eotaxin-3	Constitutive in heart & ovary Inducible on dermal fibroblasts & EC	Th2 response
9p13.3	CCL27	CTACK, Eskine	Constitutive in placenta, keratinocytes, testis and brain	Homing of memory and effector T cells to skin
5p12	CCL28	MEC	Constitutive in epith cells of gut, airway	Homing of T cells to mucosal surfaces

NA, not applicable; Mo, monocyte; PMN, neutrophil; DC, dendritic cell; EC, endothelial cell; HEV, high endothelial venule; MPC, myeloid progenitor cell; plt, platelet; MΦ, macrophage MCP, monocyte chemoattractant protein; MIP, macrophage inflammatory protein; RANTES, regulated upon activation normal T cell expressed and secreted; MRP, MIP-related protein; HCC, hemofiltrate CC chemokine; TARC, thymus and activation-related chemokine; PARC, pulmonary and activation-related chemokine; ELC, Epstein–Barr virus-induced receptor ligand chemokine; LARC, liver and activation-related chemokine; SLC, secondary lymphoid tissue chemokine; MDC, macrophage-derived chemokine; MPIF, myeloid progenitor inhibitory factor; TECK, thymus-expressed chemokine; CTACK, cutaneous T-cell-associated chemokine; MEC, mucosa-associated epithelial cell chemokine.

Some chemokine receptors pair monogamously with their chemokine ligand. However, most are promiscuous, but restricted to one chemokine group (Fig. 10.2). The receptors are named based on the ligand group specificity. Each chemokine has a unique receptor specificity profile, and vice versa. Almost all chemokines are chemotactic agonists, and a few may be agonists at one receptor and antagonists at another. Differential receptor usage and differential regulation of expression may account for non-redundant function *in vivo* observed for chemokines acting at the same receptor.

Atypical chemokine system components

There are three classes of atypical chemokine system components. First, three human 7TM chemokine binding proteins have been identified (DARC (Duffy antigen receptor for chemokines), D6, and CCX CKR) that are able to bind chemokines promiscuously without signaling or with atypical signaling. These proteins are thought to function as chemokine scavengers.[4] Second, there are an increasing number of endogenous non-chemokine agonists recognized that act at chemokine receptors (e.g., β-defensin-2 at CCR6). Third, many viruses encode chemokines, structurally related 7TM chemokine receptors, structurally unique chemokine binding proteins (scavengers), and non-chemokine chemokine receptor ligands (agonists or antagonists).[5] For example, the HIV-encoded proteins gp120 and tat are chemokine mimics with agonist and antagonist activity, respectively. Viral chemokine elements can function to evade the immune system, recruit new target cells, reprogram gene expression for cell proliferation and angiogenesis, or target cell entry (e.g., HIV gp120).[6] Secreted chemokine-binding proteins have even been identified in tick saliva, which could explain the lack of inflammation associated with tick bites.[7]

● KEY CONCEPTS

Immunologic classification of the chemokine system

- *Homeostatic system*: Constitutively expressed ligands and receptors. Important in hematopoiesis and immune surveillance. Key receptors: CXCR4 on all leukocytes, especially hematopoietic progenitor cells; CXCR5 on naïve B cells; CCR7 on mature dendritic cells and naïve T cells; and gut and skin-specific T-cell homing receptors CCR9 and CCR10, respectively).

- *Inflammatory system*: In innate immunity, inducible ligands, and constitutively expressed receptors (e.g. neutrophil CXCR2, monocyte/macrophage CCR2 and CX3CR1, eosinophil CCR3, and NK cell CX3CR1). In adaptive immunity, inducible ligands and inducible receptors (e.g., CXCR3, CCR4, and CCR6 on Th1, Th2, and Th17 subsets of CD4 T cells, respectively).

- *Decoy receptors*: Some 7TM proteins that bind chemokines do not signal and act instead as scavengers/"decoy receptors" to limit chemokine action.

Immunologic classification

All leukocyte subtypes respond to chemokines via chemokine receptors, and each subtype expresses a characteristic subset of receptors. The chemokine system can be subclassified into two main subsystems, *homeostatic* and *inflammatory* based on receptor expression patterns. Homeostatic chemokines are differentially and constitutively expressed in specific microenvironments of primary and secondary immune organs. They recruit hematopoietic precursor cells, dendritic cells (DC), neutrophils and naïve and memory lymphocyte subsets via constitutively expressed receptors. Noxious stimuli induce inflammatory chemokines in diverse tissue cells and leukocytes. Inflammatory chemokine receptors are constitutively expressed on myeloid and NK cells, but must be induced on activated effector

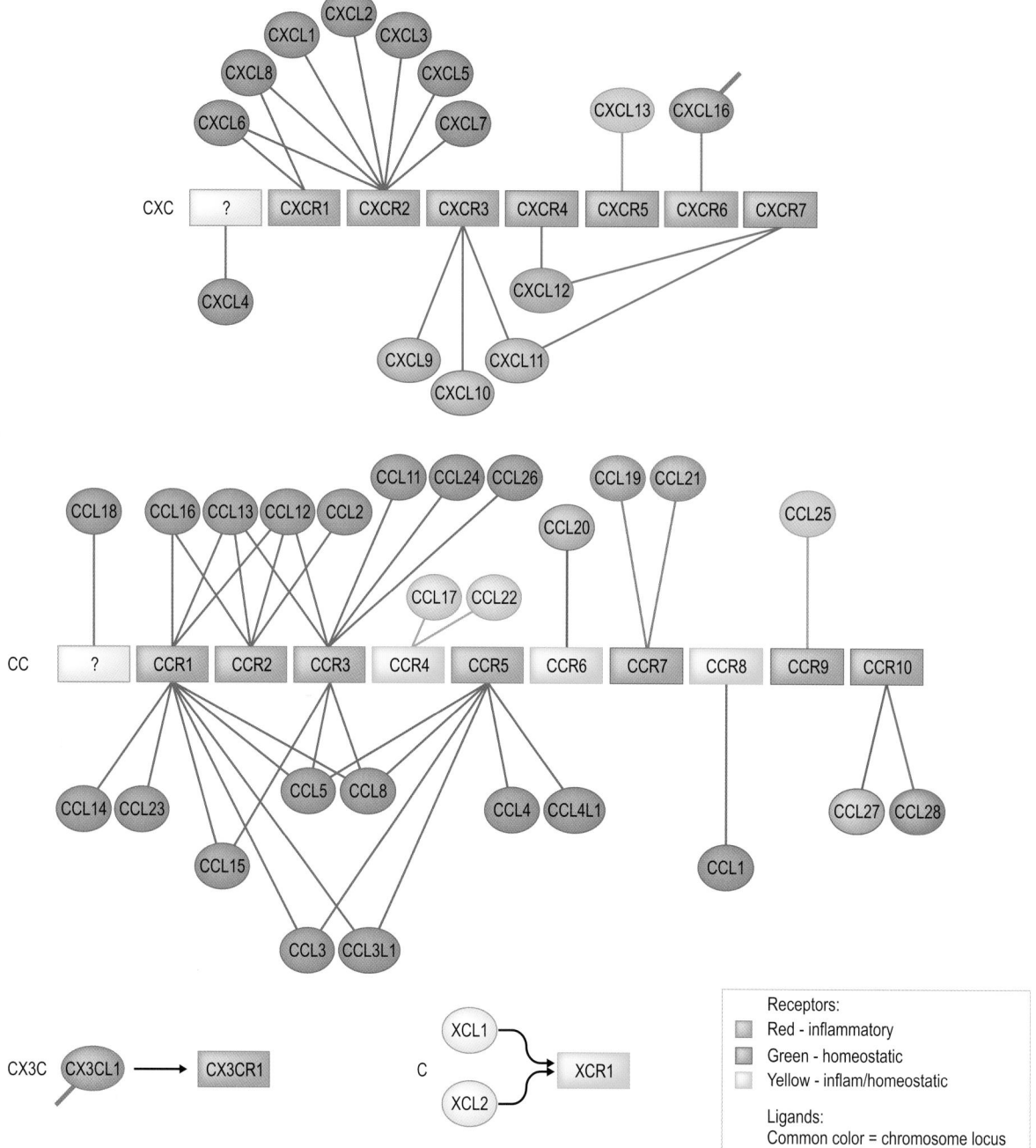

Fig. 10.2 Human chemokine agonist specificities for chemokine receptors. See box inset for color code. Note that chemokines encoded by clustered genes tend to bind to the same or similar receptors. ?, receptor not yet determined at the molecular level; handle, mucin-like stalk found in CXCL16 and CX3CL1. This arrangement is a modification of a previously published concept, first developed by M. Baggiolini and co-workers.

lymphocytes. Dynamic shifts in receptor expression occur during DC and NK cell maturation and during lymphocyte maturation, activation and differentiation.

Inflammatory CXC and CC chemokine genes are found in two main clusters on human chromosomes 4q12-q21 and 17q11-q21, respectively. However, homeostatic chemokine gene distribution is a diaspora involving small clusters on multiple chromosomes. Thirteen of the 19 human chemokine receptor genes are clustered at 3p21-23, and *CXCR1* and *CXCR2* are adjacent at 2q34-q35. The chemokine and chemokine receptor repertoire may vary even among closely related species. Gene copy number (e.g., for CCL3) and sequence can vary among individuals of a species, and this variation can affect the risk of acquiring certain diseases.

Chemokine presentation mechanisms

Chemokines act locally. They are probably presented tethered to matrix or to endothelial cells via glycosaminoglycans or, in two cases (CX3CL1 and CXCL16), by transmembrane domains.[1] The tethering cell may have produced the chemokine or else imported it by transcytosis from neighbors. The ligand binding site includes the receptor N-terminus and one or more extracellular loops, which allow docking of the chemokine N-loop domain; and 7TM domains, which accept the chemokine's N-terminus and are critical for triggering.

Leukocyte responses to chemokines

Whereas all leukocyte subtypes migrate in response to chemokines, each subtype can also respond in additional stereotypical ways. For example, lymphocytes can proliferate, undergo apoptosis, or release immunoregulatory and cytotoxic factors; and granulocytes can release antimicrobial and inflammatory mediators (e.g., superoxide, defensins, proteases, histamine, eicosanoids). The mechanism of leukocyte migration can vary depending on the leukocyte and the environment.[8] It is best understood for transendothelial migration (Chapter 11).[9] In an initial chemokine-independent step, leukocytes roll on inflamed endothelium in a selectin-dependent manner. Next, chemokines posted on endothelium stimulate rolling leukocytes to express activated β_2 integrins, which mediate firm adhesion via endothelial ICAMs. Leukocytes sense chemokine gradients, polarize and become poised to crawl. Motion involves shear-dependent coordinated cytoskeletal remodeling, involving expansion of the leading edge (lamellipodium), myosin-based contraction at the trailing edge (uropod), release of the uropod from substrate, and membrane lipid movement.[10] Navigation through tissue may require relays of chemokines and adhesion molecules.

Chemokine signaling pathways

Chemokines trigger chemokine receptors to act as guanine nucleotide exchange factors (GEF) mainly for heterotrimeric Gi-type G proteins, releasing GDP from and binding GTP to the Gi alpha subunit.[11] This results in G protein dissociation into α and $\beta\gamma$ subunits, which in turn activates diverse G protein-dependent effectors, including phospholipases A2, C (subtypes β_2 and β_3) and D, phosphatidylinositol-3-kinase γ (PI3Kγ), protein tyrosine kinases (PTK) and phosphatases, low molecular weight GTPases, and mitogen-activated protein kinases (Fig. 10.3).

Cytosolic and calcium-independent PLA2 catalyze formation of arachidonic acid from membrane phospholipids and enhance chemokine activation of human monocyte chemotaxis. PLC hydrolyzes PI bisphosphate (PIP$_2$) to form 1,2-diacylglycerol (DAG) and inositol-1,4,5-trisphosphate (IP$_3$). IP$_3$ induces Ca^{2+} release from intracellular stores, which acts with DAG to activate protein kinase C (PKC). PI3Kγ phosphorylates PIP$_2$ to form PIP$_3$, which recruits proteins containing pleckstrin homology (PH) or PHOX (PX) domains to lamellipodium, thereby converting shallow extracellular chemokine gradients to steep intracellular effector gradients. Four PH domain-containing targets—Akt, and GEFs for Rac, Rho, and Cdc42—modulate distinct phases of cell movement in various model systems. Rho regulates cell adhesion and chemotaxis, and myosin contraction. Rac and Cdc42 control lamellipodia and filipodia formation, respectively. Downstream targets of Rac include Pak1, which also regulates myosin contraction.

Regulation of chemokine action

Chemokine and chemokine receptor expression can be positively or negatively regulated at the transcriptional level by diverse factors, including pro-inflammatory cytokines, oxidant stress, viruses, bacterial products such as LPS and *N*-formylpeptides, cell adhesion, antigen uptake, T-cell co-stimulation, and diverse transcription factors (e.g., NF-κB). In innate immunity, pro-inflammatory cytokines such as IL-1, TNF, and IL-15 induce expression of inflammatory chemokines important for recruitment of myeloid and NK cells. In adaptive immunity, signature cytokines of polarized helper T cells establish positive feedback loops for production of signature chemokines able to specifically recruit these cells. For example, Th1 cells produce IFN-γ, which induces expression of CXCL9, 10, and 11, the chemokine agonists specific for the signature Th1 cell chemokine receptor CXCR3, thereby amplifying Th1 cell recruitment. Similar loops may exist for Th2 cells involving CCL17/CCR4 and IL-4, as well as for Th17 cells involving CCL20/CCR6 and IL-17. Interferons, glucocorticoids and anti-inflammatory cytokines (e.g., IL-10, TGF-β)

Fig. 10.3 Chemokine signal transduction in chemotaxis. Depicted are key steps in two of the main pathways induced by most chemokines. The PI3Kγ pathway is particularly important for cell migration. Chemokines are able to activate other pathways as well, including non-Gi-type G proteins, protein tyrosine kinases, and MAP kinases. These pathways influence cell proliferation and activation. The model is modified from the Alliance for Cell Signaling (http://www.signaling-gateway.org). PLC, phospholipase C; PI3K, phosphatidylinositol-3-kinase; RGS, regulator of G protein signaling; DAG, diacylglycerol; IP3, inositol trisphosphate; PIP, phosphatidylinsol phosphate; GAG, glycosaminoglycan; CK, chemokine; PKC, protein kinase C; GRK, G protein-coupled receptor kinase; GEF, guanine nucleotide exchange factor.

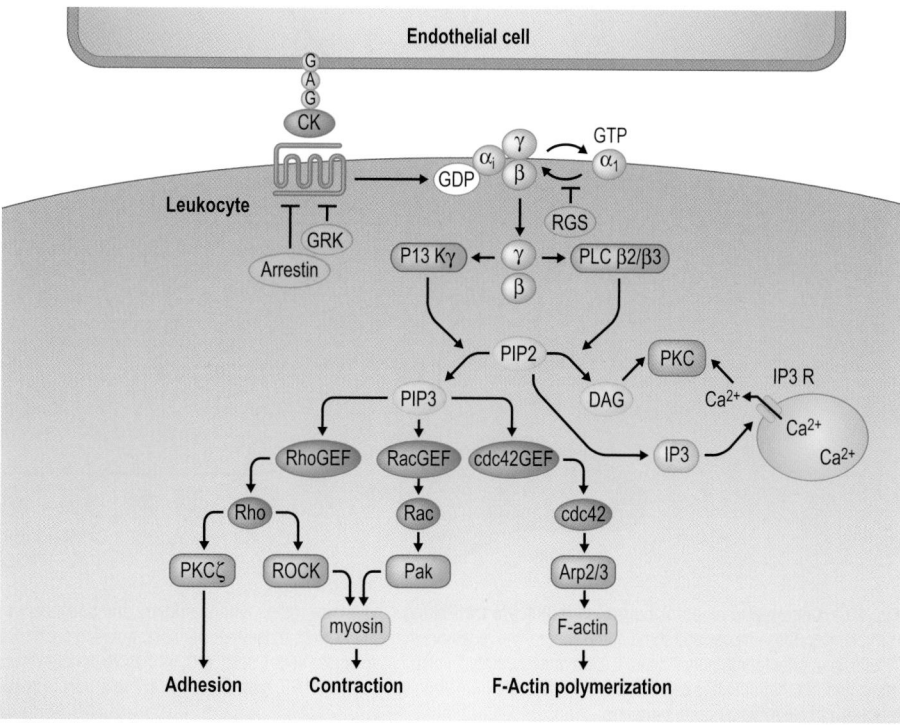

can inhibit inflammatory chemokine gene expression. Chemokines can also be regulated at the level of mRNA stability.

A chemokine gene can generate families of proteins varying in activity and potency by alternative splicing and post-translational modification, especially N- and C-terminal proteolytic trimming.[12] Proteases can target many chemokines (e.g., CD26 [dipeptidyl peptidase IV] and matrix metalloproteinases (MMP)), or few or only one (e.g., TACE (the TNF-α converting enzyme), plasmin, urokinase plasminogen activator and cathepsin G). Chemokine action can be blocked by chemokine-binding proteins (e.g., Duffy), endogenous receptor antagonists, receptor decoys and autoantibodies. In addition, cytokines may convert a signaling receptor into a decoy (e.g., IL-10 inactivates CCR2 on monocytes).

Chemokine regulation of hematopoiesis

Most chemokines that modulate hematopoietic progenitor cell (HPC) proliferation *ex vivo* act early during hematopoiesis and are inhibitory. CXCL12, the most abundant chemokine in bone marrow, is an important exception. CXCL12 signaling through its receptor CXCR4 is critical for bone marrow myelopoiesis and B-cell lymphopoiesis. CXCR2 and CXCR4 both regulate neutrophil egress from bone marrow, and CXCR4 is also critical for mobilization of HPCs from bone marrow.[13] A second CXCL12 receptor, CXCR7, does not regulate hematopoiesis, but interestingly also binds CXCL11 and is an essential factor responsible for cardiac valve development and marginal zone B-cell positioning in spleen. CCR2 is important for monocyte release from bone marrow.

During development T cells must migrate from the thymic cortex to the medulla. Chemokines and chemokine receptors are differentially expressed in thymus and could coordinate migration.[14] However, their precise roles remain unclear.

CCR9 and its ligand, CCL25, may be important since competitive transplantation of CCR9$^{-/-}$ bone marrow is less efficient than normal marrow at repopulating the thymus of lethally irradiated Rag-1$^{-/-}$ mice. CCL25 is expressed by medullary dendritic cells and both cortical and medullary epithelial cells. CCR9 is expressed on the majority of immature CD4$^+$CD8$^+$ thymocytes, but is downregulated during transition to the CD4$^+$ or CD8$^+$ single-positive stage (Fig. 10.4). Just before thymic egress, thymocytes become CCR9 negative and upregulate L-selectin. Transition from CD4$^+$CD8$^+$ thymocytes in the cortex to CD4$^+$ or CD8$^+$ single positive thymocytes in the medulla is associated with upregulation of CCR4 and CCR7, receptors for CCL22, and CCL19 and CCL21, respectively, which are expressed in the medullary stroma. Accordingly, these chemokines attract thymocytes between the late cortical and medullary stages of development *in vitro*. Neutralization studies suggest that egress of newly formed T cells from fetal thymus to the circulation is mediated by CCL19, which is selectively localized on endothelial cells of medullary venules and acts at CCR7 on mature thymocytes.

Once myeloid cells are released from the bone marrow, they undergo specific trafficking itineraries and in some cases become resident in tissue. This is regulated, in part, by specific chemokines. For example, CXCL14 is important for macrophage positioning in lung, and CCL11 and its receptor CCR3 for eosinophils in spleen and the gastrointestinal tract. CCR6 regulates positioning of immature myeloid CD11c$^+$CD11b$^+$ DC in the subepithelial dome of Peyer's patches. This may partly explain why humoral immune responses within the gut mucosa are abnormal in CCR6$^{-/-}$ mice. CX3CR1 regulates localization of myeloid DCs in Peyer's patches and may be important for antigen sampling from the intestine.

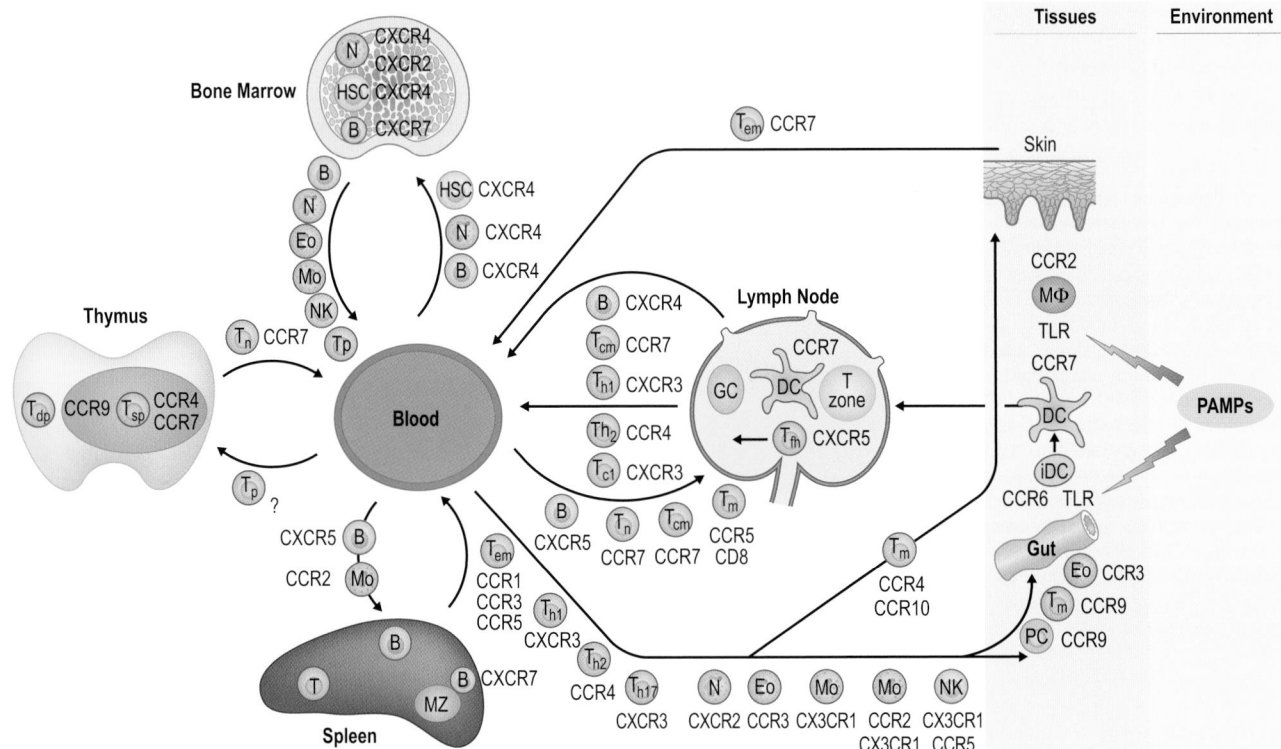

Fig. 10.4 Chemokine receptor control of leukocyte trafficking. Shown are routes among primary and secondary immune organs and the periphery, leukocyte subtypes trafficking on those routes and some of the chemokine receptors that appear to be most important in regulating each route. Tn, naïve T cells; Tp, precursor T cells; Tm, memory T cells; T$_{EM}$, effector memory T cells; T$_{CM}$, central memory T cells; T$_{FH}$, follicular help T cells; iDC, immature dendritic cells; N, neutrophil; Eo, eosinophil; Mφ, macrophage; Mo, monocyte; NK, natural killer cell; PC, plasma cell; HSC, hematopoietic stem cell; GC, germinal center. The model is based primarily on studies of mice where the relevant gene has been inactivated by gene targeting.

Chemokine regulation of the immune response

The innate and adaptive immune systems are deployed separately, but assembled, in part, by specific sets of chemokines and chemokine receptors (Fig. 10.4).[15]

Innate immunity

Platelet-derived chemokines

Made primarily during platelet development, stored in platelet α granules, and rapidly released during platelet degranulation; CXCL4 and CXCL7 are among the first chemokines to appear at sites of tissue injury and infection, particularly when there is hemorrhage and vascular damage, and can reach high concentrations.[16] CXCL7 can function as an immediate-early mediator of neutrophil recruitment released from platelets at sites of inflammation. Although it is not a prominent leukocyte chemoattractant and does not induce degranulation of neutrophil lysosomal enzymes, CXCL4 is able to induce neutrophil secondary granule exocytosis and release of matrix-degrading enzymes, which may facilitate neutrophil penetration of infected or injured tissues.

CXCL8 and CXCR2

All 7 ELR$^+$ CXC chemokines preferentially recruit neutrophils *in vitro* by binding to CXCR2. Two of these, CXCL6 and CXCL8, are also potent agonists at CXCR1, which is coexpressed at similar levels on neutrophils.[17] These 7 chemokines are rapidly inducible, but may differ biologically due to temporal and spatial differences in expression, which provide a mechanism for graded navigation of neutrophils through tissue. Blocking studies in multiple animal models have demonstrated the importance of CXCL8 and CXCR2 in neutrophil accumulation in response to infectious and non-infectious stimuli. Intradermal injection of CXCL8 in man causes rapid ($<$30 min) and selective accumulation of large numbers of neutrophils in perivascular regions of the skin without causing edema. Moreover, tissue-specific transgenic overexpression of mouse CXCL8 paralogues KC and MIP-2 suggests that *in vivo* these factors may recruit cells, but not independently activate cytotoxic mechanisms. In a human blister model, endogenous CXCL8 peaks at ~24 hours, whereas C5a and leukotriene B4, which also recruit neutrophils, appear earlier. Thus the primary role of CXCL8 may be to amplify early inflammatory responses initiated by immediate early chemoattractants such as leukotriene B4.[18] CXCL1, 2, 3, 7 and 8 have also been reported to induce basophil chemotaxis and histamine release *in vitro*, which together with other factors such as complement-derived anaphylatoxins promote vasodilatation during early stages of the innate immune response.

Monocyte recruitment typically follows neutrophil accumulation with delayed kinetics and can be mediated by multiple inflammatory CC receptors and CX3CR1. CCR2 and CX3CR1 are particularly important and define two monocyte subsets, CX3CR1^{hi}CCR2$^-$ and CX3CR1^{lo}CCR2$^+$, which are referred to as "resident" and "inflammatory" monocytes because of their distinct trafficking characteristics.[19]

NK cells

Human NK cell subsets express unique repertoires of chemokine receptors.[20] The CD56^{dim}CD16$^+$ subset, which is associated with high cytotoxic capacity and low cytokine production, expresses primarily CXCR1 and CX3CR1. The minor subset of CD56^{bright}CD16^{dim} cells, which produce large amounts of cytokines but have low killing capacity, preferentially express CCR7. The exact profile of chemokine receptor expression can be modulated by adherence and stimulation *ex vivo* with IL-2. Cognate chemokines chemoattract NK cells and promote degranulation and killing.

The importance of chemokines in NK cell function *in vivo* is illustrated well by mouse cytomegalovirus (MCMV) infection, a cause of hepatitis. MCMV induces CCL3 production in the liver, which is required for recruitment of NK cells. NK cells are the major source of IFN-γ in this model, and IFN-γ induces CXCL9, which is required for protection. Thus a cytokine to chemokine to cytokine cascade is required for NK cell-mediated host defense against this pathogen.

Dendritic cells and transition to the adaptive immune response

Transition from innate to adaptive phases of the immune response involves antigen uptake by antigen-presenting cells, especially dendritic cells, mediated by Fc and complement phagocytic receptors; as well as pattern recognition receptors (PRRs), including DC-SIGN and Toll-like receptors (TLRs). Both TLR2 and TLR4 signaling induces expression of CCL3, CCL4 and CCL5. However, TLR2 selectively induces CXCL8, whereas TLR4 selectively induces CXCL10. CXCL8 increases neutrophil migration to the site, whereas CXCL10 enhances NK cell or Th1 effector T-cell trafficking. Pathogens can skew the nature and magnitude of the immune response in a specific direction by means of specific PRR ligands.

The chemokine receptors expressed on DCs vary depending on the nature of the inflammatory stimulus and type. For example, blood-derived plasmacytoid and myeloid DCs express a similar repertoire of inflammatory chemoattractant receptors, but they are functional only on myeloid DCs. CCL3, CCL4 and CCL5 may be particularly important for recruiting additional mononuclear phagocytes and DCs to sites of infection. This can amplify the late stage of the innate immune response. In the extreme, this can devolve into endotoxic shock. Consistent with this idea, genetic disruption of the CCL3/CCL4/CCL5 receptor CCR5 renders mice relatively resistant to LPS-induced endotoxemia.

Adaptive immunity

Afferent trafficking to secondary lymphoid tissue

The homeostatic receptors CXCR5 and CCR7 and their ligands are major regulators of the immune response, acting at the level of B and T lymphocyte and DC trafficking to and within secondary lymphoid tissue.[21,22] DC maturation in peripheral tissues is associated with downregulation of inflammatory receptors, which is important for recruitment, migration and retention in the periphery; and reciprocal upregulation of CCR7, which mediates mature DC migration to draining lymph nodes. Inflammatory receptors also contribute to afferent trafficking, as demonstrated for CCR2 on Langerhans cells in a mouse model of *Leishmania* infection. CCR7 is also a major lymph node trafficking receptor for naïve T cells and can mediate activated T-cell exit from inflamed tissue.

The CCR7 ligand CCL21 is constitutively expressed on afferent lymphatic endothelium, high endothelial venules (HEV), stromal cells and interdigitating dendritic cells in T zones of lymph node, Peyer's patch, mucosa-associated lymphoid tissue and spleen.[8] It is not expressed in B-cell zones or sinuses. CCL19, another CCR7 ligand, is also restricted to the T zone and is expressed on interdigitating DCs.

CCR7[-/-] mice and the *plt* mouse, which is naturally deficient in CCL19 and a CCL21 isoform expressed in secondary lymphoid organs, have similar phenotypes: atrophic T-cell zones populated by a paucity of naïve T cells. This and the failure of activated DC to migrate to lymph node from the skin of these mice explain why contact sensitivity, delayed type hypersensitivity and antibody production are severely impaired.

CXCR5 is expressed on all peripheral blood and tonsillar B cells, but only on a fraction of bone marrow B cells. Its ligand CXCL13 is expressed constitutively on follicular high endothelial venules (HEV) and controls trafficking of CXCR5 positive B and T cells from the blood into follicles. In *CXCR5*[-/-] mice, B cells do not migrate to lymph node, Peyer's patches are abnormal, and inguinal lymph nodes are absent. CXCL13 is also required for B1 cell homing, natural antibody production, and body cavity immunity. *CXCR5*[-/-] mice still can produce antibody, perhaps in part because B cells and follicular DC, by an unknown mechanism, are able to form ectopic germinal centers within T-cell zones of the periarteriolar lymphocyte sheath of spleen.

Migration within lymph node microenvironments

CXCR5 is expressed on a majority of memory CD4 T cells in the follicles of inflamed tonsils. Follicular helper T cells (T_{FH}), a CD57[+] subset of CXCR5[+] T cells, lack CCR7, which licenses them to move from the T zone following activation to the follicles where they provide help for B-cell maturation and antibody production. Reciprocally, B cells activated by antigen in the follicles upregulate CCR7 and move towards the T-cell zone. Thus B-T interaction can be facilitated by reciprocal movement of these cells, which may be influenced by the balance of chemokines made in adjacent lymphoid zones.[23] CXCR4 signaling is also important in naïve and memory B-cell trafficking to germinal centers, and CCR5 ligands can guide naïve CD8 T cells to sites of CD4 T cell–dendritic cell interaction in lymph nodes.

Efferent trafficking

Naïve lymphocytes that do not encounter antigen continue to recirculate between the blood and secondary lymphoid tissue without acquiring any tissue-specific homing properties. Most antigen-stimulated T cells die by apoptosis. The survivors can be divided into functionally distinct subsets marked by characteristic patterns of chemokine receptor expression. In general, the trafficking properties of these cells are not well-understood. Among CD4 T cells, three memory subsets and two main effector subsets have been proposed. The memory subsets include follicular helper (T_{FH}) cells; effector memory (T_{EM}); and central memory cells (T_{CM}). T_{EM} do not express L-selectin or CCR7. They traffic through peripheral tissues as immune surveillance cells, rapidly releasing cytokines in response to activation by recall antigens. T_{CM} express CCR7 and lymph node homing receptors. They traffic between the blood and secondary lymphoid organs, but are not polarized and lack immediate effector function. Instead, they efficiently interact with DCs in lymph node and differentiate into effector cells upon secondary stimulation. Highly heterogeneous, multifunctional human T_{EM} cells are produced early in differentiation and may become stable resting cells.[24]

Upon antigen activation, the classic effector CD4 T-cell subsets, Th1, Th2, and Th17, downregulate CCR7 and upregulate inflammatory chemokine receptors. Exit from lymph node via efferent lymphatics is mediated by S1P receptor signaling. *In vivo*, Th1 cells more frequently express CXCR3, CXCR6, CCR2, CCR5, and CX3CR1 than Th2 cells, and the pattern of receptor expression is a function of maturation and age.[25] In contrast, Th2 cells more frequently express CCR3, CCR4, and CCR8 than Th1 cells. CXCR3 expression has been most consistently associated with Th1 immune responses and Th1-associated diseases. Consistent with this, its agonists CXCL9-11 are highly induced by IFN-γ but not IL-4. "Th1 chemokines" also help maintain Th1 dominance through their ability to block CCR3. Similarly, in Th2 immunity IL-4 and IL-13 made at inflamed sites in the periphery induce production of CCL7, CCL11 and other CCR3 ligands, the CCR4 ligands CCL17 and CCL22, and the CCR8 ligand CCL1. CCR3 is expressed on a subset of Th2 T lymphocytes as well as on eosinophils and basophils, the three major cell types associated with Th2-type allergic inflammation. Th2 cells are also associated with CCR4 expression. Arrival of Th2 cells amplifies a positive feedback loop through secretion of additional IL-4. CCL7 and CCL11 can block Th1 responses by antagonizing CCR2, CXCR3 and CCR5. Th17 cells are all found within the CCR6[+] subset of CD4 T cells.[26] There may also be a positive feedback loop for IL-17 induction of the CCR6 ligand CCL20 as a mechanism to recruit additional Th17 cells to inflamed sites.

Tissue-specific lymphocyte homing

Cutaneous lymphocyte-associated antigen (CLA[+]) T lymphocytes, which home to skin, preferentially express CCR4 and CCR10.[24] The CCR4 ligand CCL22 is made by resident dermal macrophages and DCs, whereas the CCR10 ligand CCL27 is made by keratinocytes. Blocking both of these pathways, but not either one alone, has been reported to inhibit lymphocyte recruitment to the skin in a delayed-type hypersensitivity model. This implies that these two molecules act redundantly as well as independently of inflammatory chemokines.

Homing to small intestine is determined in part by T lymphocyte expression of the integrin $\alpha_4\beta_7$ and CCR9.[27] The $\alpha_4\beta_7$ ligand MAdCAM-1 and the CCR9 ligand CCL25 colocalize on normal and inflamed small intestine endothelium. Most T cells in the intraepithelial and lamina propria zones of the small intestine express CCR9. These cells, which are mainly TCRγδ[+] or TCRαβ[+]CD8αβ[+], are reduced in small intestine from CCR9[-/-] mice.

As B cells differentiate into plasma cells, they downregulate CXCR5 and CCR7 and exit the lymph node. B immunoblasts expressing IgG coordinately upregulate CXCR4, which promotes homing to the bone marrow, whereas B immunoblasts expressing IgA specifically migrate to mucosal sites. Like gut-homing T cells, B immunoblasts that home to small intestine express $\alpha_4\beta_7$ integrin and CCR9 and respond to CCL25.

Chemokines and disease

There is a vast literature correlating the presence of chemokines with diverse human diseases, but strong evidence that they are actually involved in pathogenesis is available for only a small subset, which constitutes the focus of this section.

Examples of chemokine and chemokine receptor determinants of human disease

- *WHIM syndrome*: Caused by truncating gain-of-function mutations in *CXCR4*
- Plasmodium vivax *malaria*: Protection conferred by a non-functional promoter variant in Duffy
- *HIV infection*: Protection conferred by homozygous *CCR5Δ32*
- *AIDS disease progression rate*: Slowed by heterozygous *CCR5Δ32*
- *West Nile virus disease*: Increased risk with homozygous *CCR5Δ32*
- *Kaposi's sarcoma*: Human herpesvirus 8 vGPCR
- *Age-related macular degeneration*: Increased risk with *CX3CR1 M280* allele
- *Cardiovascular disease*: Decreased risk with *CX3CR1 M280* allele
- *Autoimmune heparin-induced thrombocytopenia*: Caused by CXCL4 autoantibodies
- *Chronic renal allograft rejection*: Reduced risk with homozygous *CCR5Δ32*
- *Rheumatoid arthritis*: Reduced risk with *CCR5Δ32*
- *Eosinophilic esophagitis*: Associated with CCL26 variant

Opposite effects of CCR5 in HIV and West Nile virus infection

HIV envelope glycoprotein gp120 mediates fusion of viral envelope with the target cell membrane by binding to CD4 and a chemokine receptor.[6] Both CCR5 and CXCR4 physically associate with CD4 and gp120, and are therefore referred to as "HIV coreceptors" (Chapter 37). HIV strains are functionally classified and named according to their specificity for CXCR4 (X4 strains), CCR5 (R5 strains), or both (R5X4 strains).

The importance of CCR5 in clinical HIV/AIDS is revealed most clearly by *CCR5Δ32*, a non-functional allele that occurs in ~20% of North American Caucasians. Homozygotes are highly resistant to R5 HIV, the main transmitting strain; and HIV-infected heterozygotes have slower disease progression. Homozygotes appear healthy, as do unstressed CCR5 knockout mice. This has led to FDA approval of the specific CCR5 antagonist maraviroc for treatment of patients with HIV/AIDS.[28] An HIV+ patient from Germany with leukemia who fortuitously received a bone marrow transplant from a *CCR5Δ32* homozygote after cytoreductive therapy for the leukemia has remained well off antiretroviral therapy with undetectable viral load.[29] This has fortified efforts to develop zinc finger nuclease and other genetic methods to block CCR5 in patients.

FDA-approved drugs targeting the chemokine system

- Maraviroc: CCR5 antagonist for HIV/AIDS that works by blocking HIV target cell entry
- Plerixafor: CXCR4 antagonist indicated together with G-CSF for HPC mobilization in autologous stem cell transplantation of patients with multiple myeloma and non-Hodgkin lymphoma receiving cytoreductive therapy

CCR5 is also important in the pathogenesis of West Nile virus (WNV) infection in both mouse and man, but in this case it plays a protective role.[30] The mechanism appears to be decreased antiviral defense by diminishing recruitment of CCR5+ leukocytes into brain. Theoretically, therefore, CCR5 blocking agents could increase the risk of WNV disease in infected individuals, particularly in the setting of HIV/AIDS where the immune system is already compromised.

Malaria

Plasmodium vivax also uses a chemokine receptor for target cell entry.[31] The parasite ligand, named the *Plasmodium vivax* Duffy Binding Protein (PvDBP), is expressed in micronemes of merozoites and binds to the *N*-terminal domain of DARC (Duffy Antigen Receptor for Chemokines) on erythrocytes via a cysteine-rich domain. This interaction is required for junction formation during invasion, but not for initial binding or parasite orientation. *P. vivax*-malaria is rare in sub-Saharan Africa due to genetic deficiency in Duffy caused by a single nucleotide substitution in the Duffy promoter (–46 C) affecting an erythroid-specific GATA-1 site. Fixation of the mutation in Africa presumably occurred because of positive selective pressure from malaria. Duffy deficiency in man and in Duffy knockout mice is not associated with any known health problems. Duffy is an obvious drug target, but to date no candidates have been reported.

WHIM syndrome

Truncating mutations in the *C*-tail of CXCR4 that increase receptor signaling are the cause of WHIM syndrome, a rare disease characterized by *w*arts, *h*ypogammaglobulinemia, *i*nfection, and *m*yelokathexis (neutropenia without maturation arrest).[32] Myelokathexis and infection can be explained by exaggeration of the normal bone marrow retention action of CXCR4 for myeloid cells, inhibiting their egress to blood. The exact mechanism underlying the selective predisposition to human papillomavirus infection is unknown. Dialing down the pathologically increased CXCR4 activity with a specific CXCR4 antagonist is a direct and rational strategy for treatment of patients with WHIM syndrome. In this regard, clinical trials are in progress to repurpose plerixafor (Mozobil, AMD3100), a CXCR4 antagonist approved by the FDA for use with G-CSF to mobilize HSCs for autologous transplantation in patients with multiple myeloma or lymphoma undergoing cytoreductive therapy.[33,34]

Atherosclerosis

Macrophages are the dominant leukocyte present in atherosclerotic lesions and are associated with the presence of macrophage-targeted chemokines such as CCL2, CCL5 and CX3CL1.[35] *CCL2-/-*, *CCR2-/-*, *CX3CL1-/-*, and *CX3CR1-/-* mice on the atherogenic *ApoE-/-* genetic background demonstrate smaller lesions and reduced accumulation of macrophages in the vessel wall. Adoptive transfer studies with bone marrow from *CXCR2-/-* mice have also revealed a role for CXCR2 in promoting atherosclerosis in mouse models, apparently by promoting monocyte adhesion to early atherosclerotic endothelium through interaction with its mouse ligand KC and activation of the VLA-4/VCAM-1 adhesion system.

The CX3CR1 genetic variant CX3CR1-M280, which lacks normal CX3CL1-dependent adhesive function under conditions of physiologic flow, has been associated with reduced risk of atherosclerotic vascular disease in human. Mechanistic studies suggest that CX3CL1 on coronary artery smooth muscle cells anchors macrophages via CX3CR1.

The viral chemokine system

Studies of the viral chemokine system can yield insight into the role of chemokines in immunoregulation. Viral chemokine elements may also have applications as therapeutic agents.

Structural classification

- Chemokines (e.g., HHV8 vMIP-I, II, and III)
- 7TM chemokine receptors (e.g., HCMV US28, HHV8 vGPCR)
- Chemokine-binding proteins (e.g., γHV68 vCKBP-III)
- Chemokine mimics (e.g., HIV gp120)

Functional classification

- Cell entry factors (e.g., HIV gp120)
- Leukocyte chemoattractants (e.g., HHV8 vMIP-II)
- Immune evasion
  - Chemokine scavengers (e.g., γHV68 vCKBP-III)
  - Chemokine receptor antagonists (e.g., MCV MC148-R)
- Angiogenic factors (e.g., HHV8 vGPCR)
- Growth factors (e.g., HHV8 vGPCR)
  - In mice, overexpression of this viral chemokine receptor induces KS-like lesions.

Kaposi's sarcoma

HHV8 is an example of a virus laden with genes encoding pirated chemokines and chemokine receptors. It encodes three CC chemokines, vMIP-I, II, and III, as well as a constitutively active CC/CXC chemokine receptor named vGPCR, encoded by ORF74. All of these factors are angiogenic and may contribute to the pathogenesis of Kaposi's sarcoma (KS), a highly vascular multicentric non-clonal tumor caused by HHV8, typically in the setting of immunosuppression such as in HIV/AIDS. Consistent with this, vGPCR induces KS-like tumors when expressed in transgenic mice. The mechanism may involve activation of NF-κB and induction of angiogenic factors and pro-inflammatory cytokines. This virus appears to have converted a hijacked receptor, probably CXCR2, into a regulator of gene expression.[36]

Autoimmunity

Two human diseases have been identified in which chemokines act as autoantigens for autoantibodies. The first, heparin-induced thrombocytopenia (HIT), is the only human autoimmune disease directly linked mechanistically to chemokines.[37] An established risk factor for thromboembolic complications of heparin therapy, HIT occurs in 1–5% of patients treated with heparin and is the result of autoantibodies that bind specifically to CXCL4-heparin complexes in plasma. The second, autoimmune myositis, is associated with autoantibodies to histidyl tRNA synthetase, a protein synthesis factor that is also able to induce DC chemotaxis, apparently by acting as an agonist at CCR5. Its exact importance in promoting inflammation in myositis has not been established.

In general, T-cell-dependent autoimmune diseases in human, such as psoriasis, multiple sclerosis (MS), rheumatoid arthritis (RA), and Type I diabetes mellitus, are associated with inflammatory chemokines and tissue infiltration by T lymphocytes and monocytes expressing inflammatory chemokine receptors. The relative importance of these is not fully known. Patients homozygous for the CCR5 null allele CCR5Δ32 have been reported who have MS, indicating that this receptor is not required for disease. An association of this allele with outcome

in MS has not been firmly established. CCL2 and CCR2 and to a lesser extent CCL3 and CCR1 knockout mice have reduced disease in experimental allergic encephalomyelitis (EAE), a model of MS. Moreover, neutralization of CCL3 and CCL2 markedly reduced the early and relapsing phases of EAE, respectively.

A dominant negative antagonist of CCL2 inhibits arthritis in the MRL-*lpr* mouse model of RA, suggesting a potential role for CCL2 and CCR2. Met-RANTES, a chemically modified variant of CCL5 that blocks CCR1, CCR3 and CCR5, was beneficial in a collagen-induced arthritis model in DBA/I mice. A meta-analysis has shown a protective effect for CCR5Δ32 in RA. However, in clinical trials the CCR5 antagonist maraviroc was ineffective. In the NOD mouse model of diabetes, insulitis and hyperglycemia were reduced in CCL3 knockout mice.

Paradoxically, in some cases blocking chemokine receptors can lead to increased inflammation as shown for CCR1 and CCR2 in nephrotoxic nephritis and glomerulonephritis mouse models. This is associated with increased renal recruitment of CD4 and CD8 T cells, macrophages, and enhanced Th1 immune responses. The mechanism remains unclear.

Acute neutrophil-mediated inflammatory disorders

Many neutrophil-mediated human diseases have been associated with the presence of CXCL8, including psoriasis, gout, acute glomerulonephritis, ARDS, rheumatoid arthritis and ischemia-reperfusion injury. Systemic administration of neutralizing anti-CXCL8 antibodies is protective in diverse models of neutrophil-mediated acute inflammation in the rabbit (skin, airway, pleura, glomeruli), providing proof-of-concept that CXCL8 is a non-redundant mediator of innate immunity and acute pathologic inflammation in these settings. CXCR2 knockout mice are less susceptible to acute urate crystal-induced gouty synovitis. And, SB-265610, a nonpeptide small molecule antagonist with exquisite selectivity for CXCR2, prevents neutrophil accumulation in the lungs of hyperoxia-exposed newborn rats. Together these results identify CXCL8 and its receptors as candidate drug targets for diseases mediated by acute neutrophilic inflammation. CXCR2 knockout mice also have delayed wound healing.

Transplant rejection

An advantage of transplant rejection over other animal models of human disease is that in both the human and animal situation the time of antigenic challenge is precisely known. The most extensive analysis of the role of chemokines in transplant rejection has been carried out in an MHC class I/II-mismatched cardiac allograft rejection model in the mouse, which is mediated by a Th1 immune response.[36] Similar sets of inflammatory chemokines are found in the mouse model as in the human disease and appear in a strict temporal sequence.

Analysis of knockout mice has demonstrated that while multiple chemokine receptors contribute to rejection in this model, there is a marked rank order: CXCR3 > > CCR5 > CCR1 = CX3CR1 = CCR2. Most impressively, rejection and graft arteriosclerosis do not occur if the recipient mouse, treated with a brief, subtherapeutic course of cyclosporine, is *CXCR3-/-* or if the donor heart is *CXCL10-/-*. This identifies the CXCR3/CXCL10 axis as a potential drug target. Neutralization of CXCL9, a CXCR3 ligand which appears later than CXCL10, can also prolong cardiac allograft survival.

In man, CCR5 may be important in chronic kidney allograft rejection, since individuals homozygous for *CCR5Δ32* are under-represented among patients with this outcome in a large German kidney transplantation cohort.

Allergic airway and intestinal disease

Chemokine receptors associated with asthma include CXCR2, CCR3, CCR4 and CCR8.[38] CCR3 is present on eosinophils, basophils, mast cells and some Th2 T cells. CCR4 and CCR8 identify airway T cells of allergen-challenged atopic asthmatics. CCR8 knockout mice have reduced allergic airway inflammation in response to three different Th2-polarizing antigens: *Schistosoma mansoni* soluble egg antigen, ovalbumin and cockroach antigen. A role for the CCR3 axis in asthma has been supported by CCL11 neutralization in guinea pig, and CCR3 gene knockout in mouse. The effect of CCR3 knockout depends dramatically on the specific method of sensitization and challenge due to complex and opposite effects on eosinophil and mast cell trafficking. Thus *CCR3-/-* mice sensitized intra-peritoneally have reduced eosinophil extravasation into the lung, but an increase in mast cell homing to the trachea. The net result is a paradoxical increase in airway responsiveness to cholinergic stimulation. Mast cell mobilization is not seen after epicutaneous sensitization, and these animals have reduced airway eosinophilia on challenge and no increase in airway hyperresponsiveness. *CCR6-/-* mice have decreased allergic airway inflammation in response to sensitization and challenge with cockroach antigen, which is consistent with the induction of its ligand CCL20 in this model. *CCR6-/-* mice are also protected from a mouse model of psoriasis, although the mechanism does not involve CCR6 expression on Th17 cells. Eosinophilic esophagitis has been associated with a CCL26 variant. Although there is no CCL26 homologue in mouse, other mouse CCR3 ligands have been implicated in a mouse model of this disease. CCR9 is an attractive drug target in Crohn's disease due its important role in T-cell homing to gut. Preclinical studies have provided proof of principle for this and clinical trials using a small molecule antagonist are underway.

Cancer

Many chemokines have been detected *in situ* in tumors, and cancer cells have been shown to produce chemokines and express chemokine receptors. However, the role played by endogenous tumor-associated chemokines in recruiting tumor-infiltrating lymphocytes and tumor-associated macrophages and in promoting an anti-tumor immune response has not been delineated. On the contrary, there are data from mouse models suggesting that the overall effect may be to promote tumorigenesis through additional effects on cell growth, angiogenesis, apoptosis, immune evasion and metastasis.[39,40] Controlling the balance of angiogenic and angiostatic chemokines may be particularly important. Chemokine receptors on tumor cells have been shown to directly mediate chemokine-dependent proliferation.

Therapeutic applications

Chemokines and chemokine receptors as targets for drug development

Efforts to develop chemokine blocking agents over the past 20 years have recently led to FDA approval of two drugs, maraviroc targeting CCR5 as a viral entry factor in HIV/AIDS

and plerixafor targeting CXCR4 in HSC mobilization from bone marrow for transplantation of cancer patients (see above).[28,33] Chemokine receptors are the first cytokine receptors for which potent, selective non-peptide small molecule antagonists have been identified that work *in vivo*. Targeting host determinants, as in the case of CCR5 in HIV/AIDS, is a new approach in the development of antimicrobial agents. Other candidate disease indications are Duffy in *P. vivax* malaria; CXCR4 in WHIM syndrome; CXCR2 in acute neutrophil-mediated inflammation; CXCR3 and CCR2 in Th1-driven disease; CCR2 and CX3CR1 in atherosclerosis; CCR3 and possibly CCR4 and CCR8 in Th2 diseases such as asthma; CCR9 in inflammatory bowel disease; and CCR6 in Th17 diseases such as psoriasis.

Potent and selective non-peptide small molecule antagonists of chemokine receptors, including CXCR2, CXCR3, CXCR4, CCR1, CCR2, CCR3, CCR5 and CCR9 have been reported. These molecules share a nitrogen-rich core and appear to block ligand binding by acting at a conserved allosteric site analogous to the retinal-binding site in the transmembrane region of rhodopsin. Although small molecules taken as pills are the main goal, other blocking strategies are also under consideration, such as (1) ribozymes, (2) modified chemokines (e.g., amino-terminally-modified versions of CCL5), (3) intrakines, which are modified forms of chemokines delivered by gene therapy that remain in the endoplasmic reticulum and block surface expression of newly synthesized receptors, (4) monoclonal antibodies, and (5) zing finger nuclease-mediated homologous gene therapy.

The fact that viral anti-chemokines typically block multiple chemokines acting at multiple receptors hints that the most clinically effective chemokine-targeted anti-inflammatory strategy will need to provide broad-spectrum coverage. In this regard, the viral anti-chemokines themselves may have a place therapeutically, although issues of antigenicity may be limiting for chronic inflammatory diseases.

Chemokines as biological response modifiers

Both inflammatory and homeostatic chemokines are being evaluated for therapeutic potential as biological response modifiers, acting mainly as immunomodulators or as regulators of angiogenesis. Studies to date have not revealed major problems with toxicity, and efficacy has been noted in models of cancer, inflammation and infection. Clinical trials in cancer and stem cell protection have been disappointing. Chemokines are also being developed as vaccine adjuvants. Chemokine gene administration has also been shown to induce neutralizing antibody against the encoded chemokine, which is able to block immune responses and to ameliorate EAE and arthritis in rodent models.

Many chemokines, when delivered pharmacologically as recombinant proteins or by plasmid DNA or in transfected tumor cells, are able to induce immunologically-mediated anti-tumor effects in mouse models and could be clinically useful. Mechanisms may differ depending on the model, but may involve recruitment of monocytes, NK cells and cytotoxic CD8 T cells to tumor. Chemokines may also function as adjuvants in tumor antigen vaccines. Chemokine-tumor antigen fusion proteins represent a novel twist on this approach that facilitates uptake of tumor antigens by APCs via the normal process of ligand–receptor internalization. Non-ELR CXC chemokines such as CXCL4 also exert anti-tumor effects through angiostatic mechanisms.

Conclusion

The chemokine system occupies a central place in immunoregulation and is an attractive source of potential drug targets for any disease with an innate or adaptive immune component. A basic outline for how the system works has been established using mouse models, and there has now been tangible progress translating this knowledge to the clinic. Two major successes, CCR5 inhibition in HIV/AIDS and CXCR4 inhibition for HPC mobilization, are pioneers demonstrating the feasibility of targeting the chemokine system therapeutically in humans. However, both are eccentric indications that address unusual, niche roles of chemokine receptors. Chronic immune-mediated diseases remain a major unmet medical need, where the chemokine system offers many targets and challenges for the future.

Acknowledgments

This review was supported with funding from the Division of Intramural Research, National Institute of Allergy and Infectious Diseases, NIH.

References

1. Allen SJ, Crown SE, Handel TM. Chemokine: receptor structure, interactions, and antagonism. Annu Rev Immunol 2007;25:787–820.
2. Zlotnik A, Yoshie O, Nomiyama H. The chemokine and chemokine receptor superfamilies and their molecular evolution. Genome Biol 2006;7:243.
3. Murphy PM, Baggiolini M, Charo IF, et al. International union of pharmacology. XXII. Nomenclature for chemokine receptors. Pharmacol Rev 2000;52:145–76.
4. Ulvmar MH, Hub E, Rot A. Atypical chemokine receptors. Exp Cell Res 2011;317:556–68.
5. Slinger E, Langemeijer E, Siderius M, et al. Herpesvirus-encoded GPCRs rewire cellular signaling. Mol Cell Endocrinol 2011;331:179–84.
6. Berger EA, Murphy PM, Farber JM. Chemokine receptors as HIV-1 coreceptors: roles in viral entry, tropism, and disease. Annu Rev Immunol 1999;17:657–700.
7. Deruaz M, Frauenschuh A, Alessandri AL, et al. Ticks produce highly selective chemokine binding proteins with antiinflammatory activity. J Exp Med 2008;205:2019–31.
8. Schumann K, Lammermann T, Bruckner M, et al. Immobilized chemokine fields and soluble chemokine gradients cooperatively shape migration patterns of dendritic cells. Immunity 2010;32:703–13.
9. Butcher EC. Leukocyte-endothelial cell recognition: three (or more) steps to specificity and diversity. Cell 1991;67:1033–6.
10. Alon R, Shulman Z. Chemokine triggered integrin activation and actin remodeling events guiding lymphocyte migration across vascular barriers. Exp Cell Res 2011;317:632–41.
11. Thelen M, Stein JV. How chemokines invite leukocytes to dance. Nat Immunol 2008;9:953–9.
12. Mortier A, Gouwy M, Van Damme J, Proost P. Effect of posttranslational processing on the in vitro and in vivo activity of chemokines. Exp Cell Res 2011;317:642–54.
13. Martin C, Burdon PC, Bridger G, et al. Chemokines acting via CXCR2 and CXCR4 control the release of neutrophils from the bone marrow and their return following senescence. Immunity 2003;19:583–93.
14. Bunting MD, Comerford I, McColl SR. Finding their niche: chemokines directing cell migration in the thymus. Immunol Cell Biol 2011;89:185–96.
15. Charo IF, Ransohoff RM. The many roles of chemokines and chemokine receptors in inflammation. N Engl J Med 2006;354:610–21.
16. Vandercappellen J, Van Damme J, Struyf S. The role of the CXC chemokines platelet factor-4 (CXCL4/PF-4) and its variant (CXCL4L1/PF-4var) in inflammation, angiogenesis and cancer. Cytokine Growth Factor Rev 2011;22:1–18.
17. Stillie R, Farooq SM, Gordon JR, Stadnyk AW. The functional significance behind expressing two IL-8 receptor types on PMN. J Leukoc Biol 2009;86:529–43.
18. Chou RC, Kim ND, Sadik CD, et al. Lipid-cytokine-chemokine cascade drives neutrophil recruitment in a murine model of inflammatory arthritis. Immunity 2010;33:266–78.
19. Geissmann F, Jung S, Littman DR. Blood monocytes consist of two principal subsets with distinct migratory properties. Immunity 2003;19:71–82.
20. Morris MA, Ley K. Trafficking of natural killer cells. Curr Mol Med 2004;4:431–8.
21. Forster R, Davalos-Misslitz AC, Rot A. CCR7 and its ligands: balancing immunity and tolerance. Nat Rev Immunol 2008;8:362–71.
22. Muller G, Hopken UE, Lipp M. The impact of CCR7 and CXCR5 on lymphoid organ development and systemic immunity. Immunol Rev 2003;195:117–35.
23. Cyster JG. Chemokines, sphingosine-1-phosphate, and cell migration in secondary lymphoid organs. Annu Rev Immunol 2005;23:127–59.
24. Tubo NJ, McLachlan JB, Campbell JJ. Chemokine receptor requirements for epidermal T-cell trafficking. Am J Pathol 2011;178:2496–503.
25. Zhang HH, Song K, Rabin RL, et al. CCR2 identifies a stable population of human effector memory CD4 + T cells equipped for rapid recall response. J Immunol 2010;185:6646–63.
26. Singh SP, Zhang HH, Foley JF, et al. Human T cells that are able to produce IL-17 express the chemokine receptor CCR6. J Immunol 2008;180:214–21.
27. Koenecke C, Forster R. CCR9 and inflammatory bowel disease. Expert Opin Ther Targets 2009;13:297–306.
28. Singh IP, Chauthe SK. Small molecule HIV entry inhibitors: Part I. Chemokine receptor antagonists: 2004–2010. Expert Opin Ther Pat 2011;21:227–69.
29. Hutter G, Nowak D, Mossner M, et al. Long-term control of HIV by CCR5 Delta32/Delta32 stem-cell transplantation. N Engl J Med 2009;360:692–8.
30. Lim JK, Murphy PM. Chemokine control of West Nile virus infection. Exp Cell Res 2011;317:569–74.
31. Gaur D, Mayer DC, Miller LH. Parasite ligand-host receptor interactions during invasion of erythrocytes by Plasmodium merozoites. Int J Parasitol 2004;34:1413–29.
32. Kawai T, Malech HL. WHIM syndrome: congenital immune deficiency disease. Curr Opin Hematol 2009;16:20–6.
33. Pusic I, DiPersio JF. Update on clinical experience with AMD3100, an SDF-1/CXCL12-CXCR4 inhibitor, in mobilization of hematopoietic stem and progenitor cells. Curr Opin Hematol 2010;17:319–26.
34. Dale DC, Bolyard AA, Kelley ML, et al. The CXCR4 antagonist plerixafor is a potential therapy for myelokathexis, WHIM syndrome. Blood 2011;118:4963–6.
35. Barlic J, Murphy PM. Chemokine regulation of atherosclerosis. J Leukoc Biol 2007;82:226–36.
36. Grisotto MG, Garin A, Martin AP, et al. The human herpesvirus 8 chemokine receptor vGPCR triggers autonomous proliferation of endothelial cells. J Clin Invest 2006;116:1264–73.
37. Cuker A. Recent advances in heparin-induced thrombocytopenia. Curr Opin Hematol 2011;18:315–22.
38. Medoff BD, Thomas SY, Luster AD. T cell trafficking in allergic asthma: the ins and outs. Annu Rev Immunol 2008;26:205–32.
39. Wu X, Lee VC, Chevalier E, Hwang ST. Chemokine receptors as targets for cancer therapy. Curr Pharm Des 2009;15:742–57.
40. Strieter RM. Chemokines: not just leukocyte chemoattractants in the promotion of cancer. Nat Immunol 2001;2:285–6.

Lymphocyte adhesion and trafficking
Sirpa Jalkanen,
Marko Salmi

Proper control of the movement of lymphocytes through the body is a prerequisite for mounting an effective immune response. Lymphocyte trafficking provides the means by which the few lymphocytes that carry a specific antigen receptor have the opportunity to encounter their counter-antigen. Antigens can be introduced into the body via practically any surface that is exposed to the environment. Not only is the area to be protected vast (about 500 m^2 of epithelial surfaces in the skin, gut and lungs), but also the huge numbers of recirculating lymphocytes (about 10^{11}), the total length of the vascular tree (>100 000 km) and the velocity of the blood-borne lymphocytes in the vessels provide formidable challenges. An elaborate process termed lymphocyte trafficking has evolved to overcome these physical constraints.[1–4] The process relies on the basic concept of compartmentalizing specific functions into discrete anatomical organs and then connecting them by means of continuous lymphocyte recirculation. Both lymphoid and nonlymphoid organs and tissues are connected by two different types of vessels. The blood vessels transport lymphocytes into the various organs, where they have a chance to leave the blood and enter the tissue stroma. Vessels of the lymphatic system then collect the extravasated lymphocytes from these various organs and return them to the circulation (Fig. 11.1).

Early lymphocyte precursor trafficking to the primary lymphoid organs

Lymphocyte trafficking begins at an early stage of human ontogeny, when lymphocyte precursor cells first appear and migrate into the primary lymphoid organs.[5] The multipotent hematopoietic stem cells from the yolk sac and from the aorta–gonad–mesonephros migrate via the circulation to the liver and spleen, which are important organs supporting B-lymphocyte production in the embryo (Chapter 7), and then into the bone marrow. Thereafter, the developmental maturation of B cells takes place solely in the bone marrow. T cells, on the other hand, require an additional migratory event, which involves the entry of marrow-derived T-cell progenitors into the thymus (Chapter 8). These early T-cell progenitors enter the thymus via the vessels in the cortical region. Concomitant with their differentiation and maturation via positive and negative selection, they pass from the cortex into the medulla.

Migration of naïve mature lymphocytes from the blood to the secondary lymphoid organs

After completing their initial course of development, newly arisen naïve B and T cells exit the primary lymphoid organs and travel through the blood into the secondary lymphoid organs. These include the peripheral lymph nodes, the organized lymphoid tissues of the gut (e.g., Peyer's patches and the appendix) and the spleen (Chapter 2). In the lymph nodes most lymphocyte trafficking from the blood to the tissues takes place in specialized postcapillary venules. The venule endothelial cells exhibit a characteristic high cuboidal morphology that has given them their name: high endothelial venules (HEV).[6] The protrusion of the surface of these endothelial cells into the vascular lumen promotes the interaction of leukocytes in the relatively low-shear venular part of the circulatory system with the endothelial surface membrane (Fig. 11.2). HEV carry many unique adhesion molecules that enable the capture of passing lymphocytes. They also have special intercellular connections that facilitate the penetration of the vessel walls by these emigrating lymphocytes. It has been estimated that more than 50% of incoming lymphocytes make transient contacts with the vascular lining in the lymph nodes, and that as many as one passing cell in four adheres to the endothelium and then extravasates into the tissue.[7]

● KEY CONCEPTS

Lymphocytes recirculate

- Lymphocytes recirculate continuously between blood and lymphoid organs.
- 80% of lymphocytes enter the lymph nodes via specialized vessels called high endothelial venules (HEV).
- The remaining lymphocytes enter the lymph nodes together with dendritic cells and antigens via afferent lymphatics.
- Lymphocytes leave the lymph nodes via efferent lymphatics.
- Lymphocyte recirculation allows the lymphocytes to meet their cognate antigens and other leukocyte subsets to evoke an efficient immune response.

Antigens are gathered into these secondary lymphoid organs by a different route. Most antigens in the periphery can be taken up by dendritic cells (Chapter 6), which subsequently migrate into the secondary lymphoid organs via the afferent lymphatics.[8]

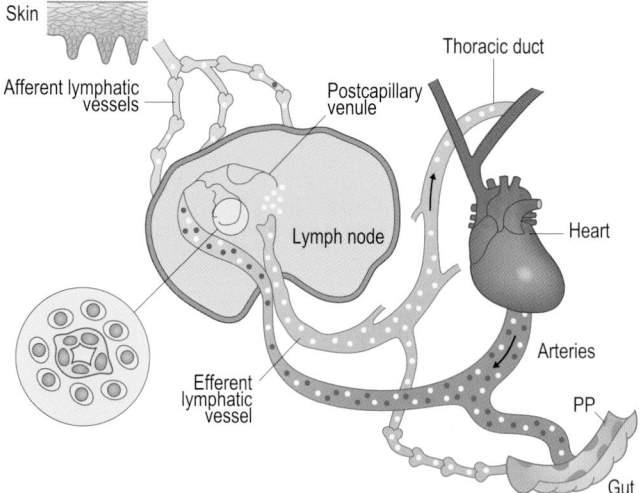

Fig. 11.1 Lymphocyte recirculation routes under physiologic conditions.
A low level of continuous antigenic transport into lymphoid organs takes place via afferent lymphatics draining the skin and the epithelium of the gut. Blood borne lymphocytes enter the organized lymphatic tissues (lymph nodes and Peyer's patches—PP) from the circulation via the arterial tree, flow through the capillary bed, and then extravasate in the postcapillary high endothelial venules (HEV). The extravasated lymphocytes percolate through the tissue parenchyma, enter the lymphatic vessels, and are then carried via the efferent lymphatics back to the systemic circulation. Most of the venous circulation has been omitted from the figure. Inset: an HEV.
From Salmi M, Jalkanen S. How do lymphocytes know where to go: current concepts and enigmas of lymphocyte homing. Adv Immunol 1997; 64: 139, with permission from Elsevier.

These afferent lymph channels open into the subcapsular sinus of the lymph node. Individual dendritic cells subsequently penetrate the lymphatic endothelium and emigrate into the stroma. Unbound, or free, antigens that diffuse by chance into these secondary lymphoid organs can also be captured by the professional antigen-presenting cells of the lymph nodes. Lymph nodes thus serve as traps for the immune system, collecting lymphocytes from the blood and antigens from the lymph (see Fig. 11.1). In these organs, lymphocytes percolate through the tissue in search of their cognate antigens. If a given lymphocyte does not find its antigen, it will leave the organ by entering the efferent lymphatics that drain the medullary sinuses. The frustrated cell is then transported via a major lymphatic trunk, such as the thoracic duct, back into the large systemic veins. After re-entering the circulation, the cell can then randomly gain access to another lymph node, where it has another chance to extravasate into the tissue and find its cognate antigen. One round of recirculation from the blood to the lymph node stroma, to a lymphatic vessel and then back to the blood takes about 1 day. Naïve lymphocytes continue circulating in the blood until they either find their cognate antigen or die.[3,6]

Activated lymphocytes display selective tissue homing patterns

In a secondary lymphoid organ a successful encounter between a lymphocyte and its cognate antigen leads to the proliferation of the cell within the organ and the maturation of its progeny.[3,6] Simultaneously, a process called imprinting leads to a profound change in the subsequent pattern of migration of the antigen-responsive cell. During the imprinting local dendritic cells give educational clues, such as vitamin A and D metabolites, to the

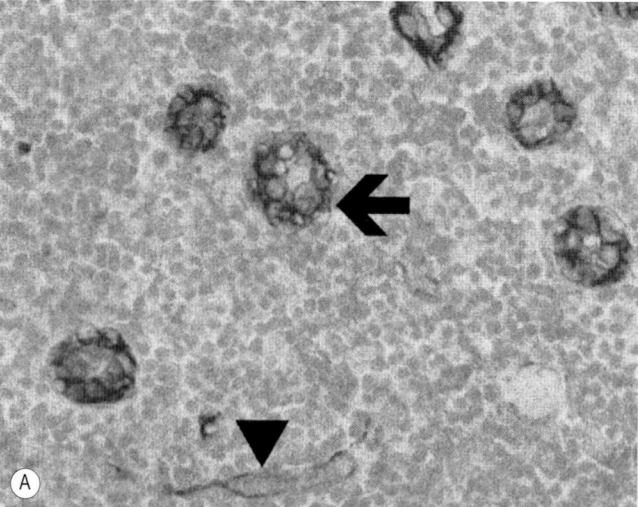

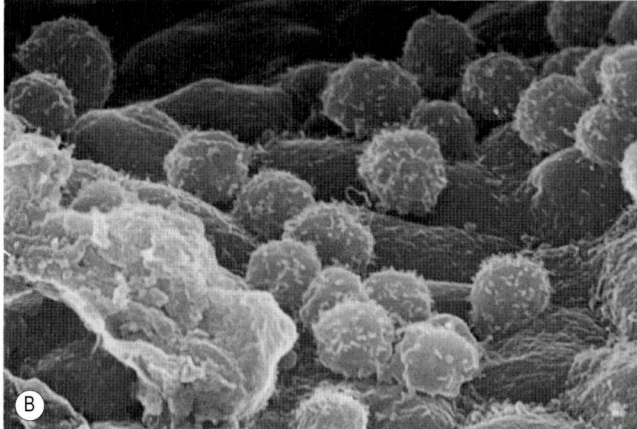

Fig. 11.2 Characteristic features of HEV. (A) In this immunoperoxidase staining with anti-CD31 antibody, six HEV are seen with typical plump endothelial cells. One HEV is identified by an arrow; a vessel with flat endothelium is also seen in this figure (arrowhead). (B) In this scanning electron micrograph lymphocytes are adhering to HEV.

lymphocytes, which lead to changes in the chemoattractant and adhesion receptor repertoire of the lymphocytes.[9,10] Although these responding cells leave the node via the lymphatics and are carried back to the systemic circulation, unlike naïve cells they no longer migrate randomly to any lymphoid tissue. Instead, imprinting primes the cells to preferentially seek the peripheral tissues in which the inciting antigen was originally ingested by the dendritic cell. In this way, selective homing of lymphocytes according to their previous history allows the organism to focus the immune response to the tissues where the effector cells can do the most good.

Among T cells, distinct pools of central and effector memory cells can be distinguished. The different profile of adhesion molecule and chemokine receptor expression allows central memory cells to continue migration through lymph nodes, whereas effector memory cells are dispersed to patrol peripheral tissues.[11]

Under normal conditions, two distinct routes of lymphocyte recirculation can be discerned.[3,4,6] One targets lymphoid cells to the peripheral lymph nodes, and the second targets them to gut-associated lymphoid tissues (GALT; Chapter 19). Although the common gut-associated lymphoid system has long been considered to include both the respiratory and the genitourinary tracts, differences in the fine specificity of lymphocyte homing between these targets do exist.

Distinct recirculation routes in spleen

The spleen holds a unique place in the panoply of secondary lymphoid tissues.[12] It contains more lymphocytes than all the peripheral lymph nodes put together, and the number of lymphocytes recirculating through it daily is the equivalent of the total pool of circulating lymphocytes. In the spleen, which lacks HEV, lymphocytes enter the tissue through the marginal zone sinuses, where macrophage-like cells may play an important role. Once in the splenic parenchyma, T cells accumulate in the regions surrounding the central arteriole in white pulp, a location known as the periarteriolar sheath. B cells are scattered in the corona that surrounds these T-cell areas. Most splenic lymphocytes leave the spleen via the splenic vein. The mechanisms that control the entry and exit of lymphocytes from the spleen remain incompletely understood. However, they appear to be quite distinct from those that operate in the peripheral lymph nodes and GALT.

● KEY CONCEPTS

Adhesion molecules in inflammation

- Adhesion molecules are important in directing leukocyte traffic to sites of inflammation.
- Numerous inflammatory mediators upregulate and/or induce expression of several endothelial-cell adhesion molecules.
- Harmful inflammation can be prevented and cured by blocking the function of adhesion molecules.

Inflammation-induced changes in leukocyte trafficking

During an acute inflammatory response to an antigenic insult, leukocytes can migrate into all nonlymphoid tissues, which are normally virtually devoid of lymphocytes. The inflammation-induced leukocyte immigration takes place in characteristic waves.[4,13] First, the polymorphonuclear leukocytes rapidly (typically within 1–4 hours) infiltrate into the inflammatory focus. They are followed by mononuclear cells (monocytes and

lymphocytes). In a primary challenge it may take 3 days or more before antigen-specific immunoblasts are seen at the peripheral scene of inflammation. However, a secondary response by memory lymphocytes typically has a much shorter lag period. Different CD4 T-helper subpopulations, including Th1, Th2, Th17, and T regulatory cells (Chapters 8, 15, and 16), and CD8 T-cytotoxic cells (Chapter 17) can all enter the inflamed tissue using basically the same mechanisms, although the ratio of these populations and the individual molecules employed may vary. Successful resolution of an inflammatory reaction appears to also be dependent on a coordinated program involving lipoxins, resolvins and protectins, all of which serve to halt cell recruitment and initiate apoptosis.[14,15]

The normal vascular endothelium in nonlymphoid tissues has a flat, inactive morphology. With inflammation, a series of events renders postcapillary venules in these tissues capable of binding lymphocytes. The most important changes are due to the proadhesive effects of a multitude of proinflammatory cytokines that are released by a variety of cell types after being subjected to inflammatory stimuli.[4,13]

If inflammation becomes chronic, marked histological manifestations become apparent in affected nonlymphoid tissues.[16] Most notably, the venules in these chronically inflamed tissues acquire many of the characteristics of HEV. Also, immigrating lymphocytes can form lymphoid follicles that resemble those seen in lymph nodes. These alterations have consequences for lymphocyte recirculation pathways. For example, the inflamed skin display characteristics of lymphocyte homing that are clearly distinct from those of either mucosal or peripheral lymph node systems.[9,10,17]

Molecular mechanisms involved in leukocyte extravasation from the blood into the tissues

The adhesion cascade

Dynamic interactions between leukocytes and endothelial cells can be observed both *in vitro* and *in vivo*. By means of intravital microscopy, for example, leukocyte adhesion can be followed *in vivo* in experimental animals and even in human tissues (Fig. 11.3). Leukocyte–endothelial-cell interaction during the

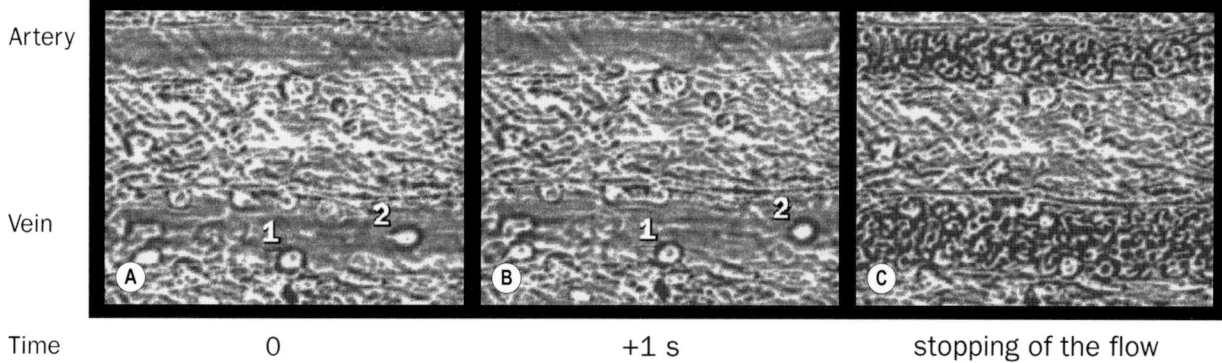

Artery

Vein

Time   0   +1 s   stopping of the flow

Fig. 11.3 Intravital microscopy of mesenteric vessels. In these video frames taken at indicated intervals from the same field, a vein, an artery, leukocytes and the transparent mesenteric membrane are seen. Within the vein rolling and adherent leukocytes are visible, whereas no such cells are seen in the artery. Leukocyte 1 is attached to the vessel wall and leukocyte 2 is slowly rolling. Compare the locations of these cells in A and B to stationary leukocytes outside the vessels. Leukocyte 1 is at the same location in both panels, whereas leukocyte 2 has moved a distance corresponding to roughly the length of its diameter. Under normal conditions, freely flowing cells move so fast that they cannot be visualized. However, in panel C the flow has been transiently stopped. Under this static condition, the large number of hematopoietic cells (mainly erythrocytes) traveling within the bloodstream can be seen.
Courtesy of S. Tohka, University of Turku, Finland.

extravasation cascade can be divided into a series of phases, or steps, that all leukocyte subtypes are thought to follow (Fig. 11.4).[2,3] First, the leukocytes marginate out of the main bloodstream and begin to tether and roll on the endothelial cell surface. This step is mediated primarily by selectin adhesion molecules and their mucin-like counter-receptors. This slow-velocity movement culminates in an activation phase, during which the leukocyte chemokine receptors transmit activation signals by recognizing their chemokine ligands presented on the endothelial-cell surface. This leads to avidity and/or affinity changes in leukocyte integrins that bind the leukocytes firmly to their immunoglobulin superfamily ligands on the endothelial cells. The lymphocytes then begin to transmigrate through the endothelium, a process that also involves leukocyte integrins and other molecules. Leukocytes diapedese between the endothelial cells through the endothelial cell junction, which opens transiently and subsequently closes.[18] This process requires proteinases, such as matrix metalloproteinase-2 (MMP-2), which is induced in T cells upon adhesion to endothelial cells, as well as other, as yet to be defined, repair mechanisms that subsequently close the path of transmigration. However, leukocytes can also migrate through the endothelial cells in a subtype-specific fashion. For example, polymorphonuclear leukocytes prefer entering via the inter-endothelial junctions, whereas non-activated lymphocytes may choose the transcellular route.[19]

● KEY CONCEPTS

Leukocyte-endothelial interactions

- Leukocytes interact with the vessel wall in a multistep fashion, using several leukocyte surface molecules that recognize their counter-receptors on endothelial cells.
- The rolling and tethering of leukocytes on the vessel wall is mediated by selectins.
- Chemokines and their receptors are needed to activate leukocyte integrins.
- Only activated integrins are able to mediate firm adhesion between leukocytes and endothelium.
- The transmigration of leukocytes into the tissues requires proteinases and repair mechanisms.

An additional complexity to the extravasation system is created by the fact that certain endothelial molecules involved in the adhesion cascade show organ-specific expression patterns. Analogously, leukocyte-associated homing molecules display subtype-specific expression profiles. Therefore, only those leukocytes that have the proper set of molecules on their surface can enter a particular tissue, because the entering leukocyte has to find a correct endothelial partner molecule at each step of the adhesion cascade. Thus, leukocyte–endothelial-cell interaction takes place in a well-coordinated multistep fashion, in which every step must be properly executed in order before the leukocyte can be guided into the tissue. The multistep nature of the leukocyte adhesion cascade is thus reminiscent of the cascades involved in blood clotting and complement-mediated killing.

Receptors and their ligands in leukocyte–endothelial-cell interaction

A variety of molecules belonging to several molecular families are expressed on both leukocyte and endothelial-cell surfaces and participate in the complex extravasation process.[6] Most of these molecules exert their function in successive, but overlapping, phases of the adhesion cascade. In addition, proper functioning of multiple intracellular signaling molecules is needed for execution of a successful extravasation.[4,20] In the following section, only the best-known surface molecules in this process are discussed (Fig. 11.5). A summary of the phenotypes exhibited by mice that are deficient for these molecules is presented in Table 11.1.

Selectins and their ligands

Three members of the selectin family mediate leukocyte trafficking. L-selectin is expressed on several leukocyte subpopulations. E-selectin is expressed on endothelium, and P-selectin is expressed on both platelets and endothelium. An important structural feature of selectins is the presence of a terminal lectin domain that is used to bind to their counter-receptors. The counter-receptor is typically decorated by a sialyl Lewis X (sLeX) carbohydrate, which is a prototype recognition domain for selectins in general.[21] The interaction between selectins and their counter-receptors is transient and weak, which allows leukocytes effectively to form and break contacts with endothelium during tethering and rolling under shear stress.

L-selectin preferentially mediates lymphocyte migration to peripheral lymph nodes. However, it also participates in the homing of lymphocytes to organized MALT, e.g., Peyer's patches (Chapter 19). L-selectin is also an important contributor

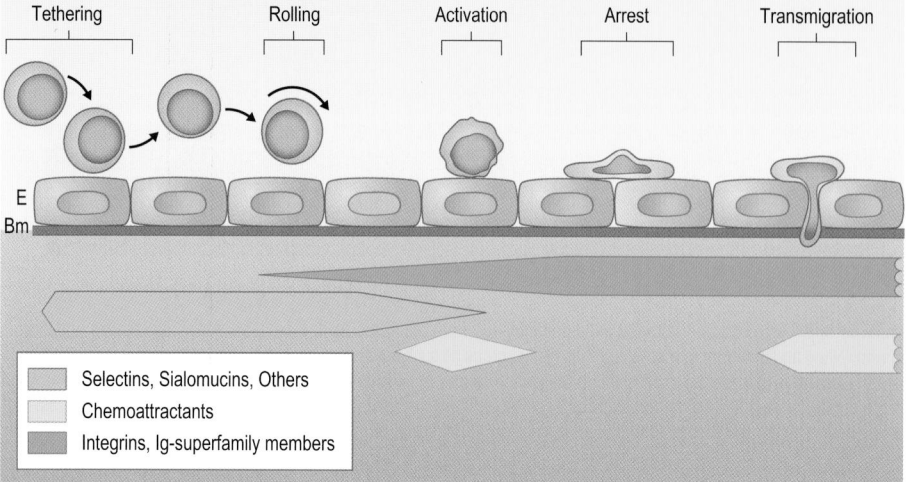

Fig. 11.4 **The multistep cascade of lymphocyte extravasation.** The blood-borne cell makes transient initial contacts with endothelial cells, which leads to the cell rolling along the vascular lining. If the cell becomes activated, it can subsequently adhere firmly to the endothelial cells, seek for an interendothelial junction, and then migrate through the basement membrane into the tissue. The contribution of major superfamilies of adhesion-associated molecules at each step is depicted below. E, endothelial layer; Bm, basement membrane.

Tethering | Rolling | Activation | Arrest | Transmigration

E
Bm

☐ Selectins, Sialomucins, Others
☐ Chemoattractants
☐ Integrins, Ig-superfamily members

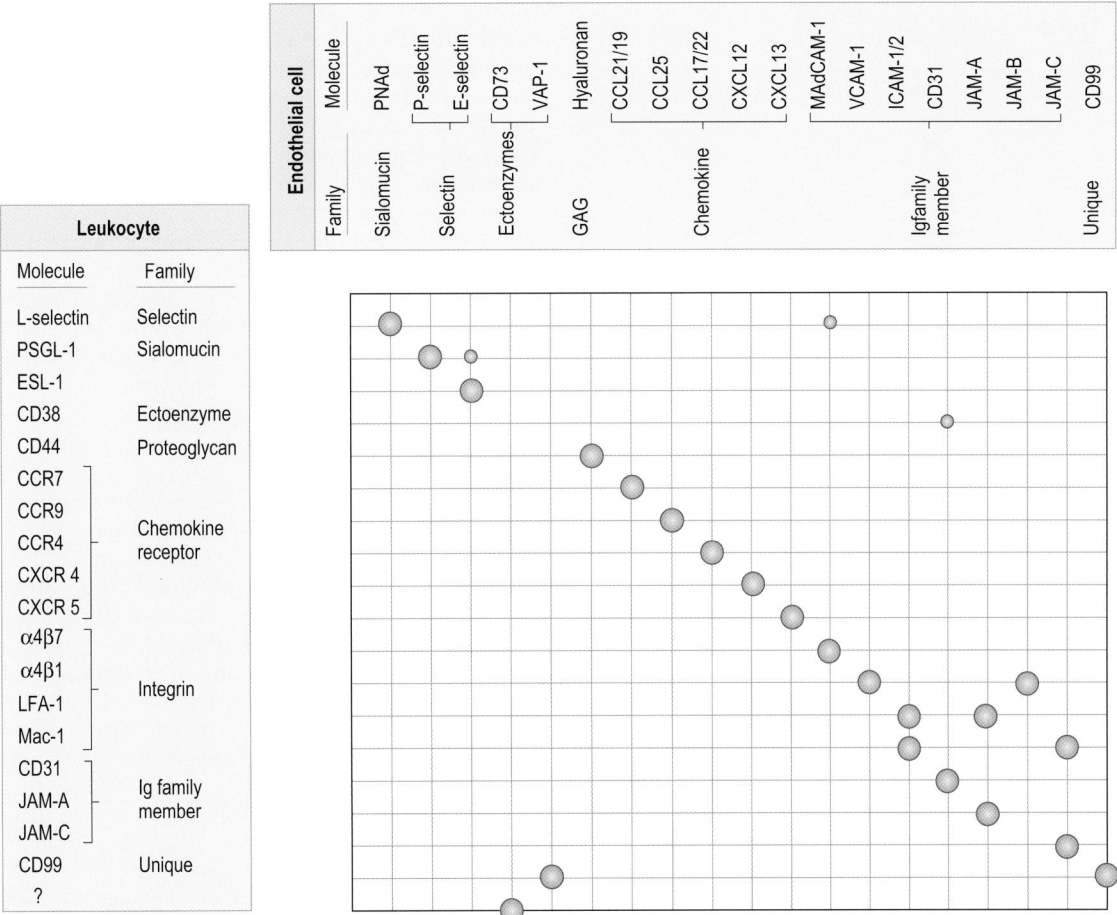

Fig. 11.5 Adhesion molecules mediating leukocyte traffic. The most relevant proteins involved in leukocyte–endothelial-cell interactions are shown as receptor–ligand pairs. GAG, glycosaminoglycan.

to the process of leukocyte trafficking to sites of inflammation. Peripheral lymph node addressins (PNAd) are the best-characterized counter-receptors for L-selectin. This group consists of at least six different molecules that are decorated with a sulfated and fucosylated sLeX that serves as a recognition motif for L-selectin. PNAds include glycosylation-dependent cell adhesion molecule-1 (GlyCAM-1), CD34, podocalyxin, endomucin, nepmucin, and mucosal addressin cell adhesion molecule-1 (MAdCAM-1). MAdCAM-1 is decorated with recognition epitopes for L-selectin on HEV in the organized lymphoid areas of the gut, but not on the flat-walled vessels in lamina propria. The importance of post-translational carbohydrate modifications for the function of selectin ligands has been well demonstrated in knockout mice deficient for fucosyl, glucosaminyl, galactosyl, sialyl or sulfotransferases. For example, mice with a targeted disruption of fucosyltransferase VII (Fuc-TVII) are unable to glycosylate L-selectin ligands appropriately. These mice exhibit severe defects in lymphocyte homing and in the extravasation of leukocytes to sites of inflammation. In contrast, core 2 β 1,6-N-acetylglucosaminyltransferase (C2 β GlcNAcT) knockout mice that have deficient glycosylation of their P- and E-selectin ligands demonstrate normal lymphocyte homing to lymph nodes, but impaired leukocyte trafficking to sites of inflammation.[21] Interestingly, L-selectin also facilitates entry of leukocytes into the tissues by mediating leukocyte tethering and rolling of endothelium-bound leukocytes by binding to P-selectin glycoprotein ligand-1 (PSGL-1).

E-selectin and P-selectin are inflammation-inducible molecules. Within minutes, P-selectin can be translocated from intracellular storage granules onto the endothelial cell surface, where it binds to its leukocyte receptor, PSGL-1 (Fig. 11.5). P-selectin and PSGL-1 mediate rolling at early time points during inflammation. Platelet P-selectin can facilitate lymphocyte entry into the tissues, because it can simultaneously bind to PNAd on endothelium and PSGL-1 on lymphocytes. E-selectin upregulation requires new protein synthesis. It is maximally expressed about 4 hours after the induction of inflammation. E-selectin is needed for slow rolling of leukocytes. It also has an affinity towards PSGL-1, as well as a specific glycoform of PSGL-1, cutaneous lymphocyte antigen (CLA). CLA specifically directs lymphocyte trafficking to inflamed skin. In addition to PSGL-1, E-selectin has a more private leukocyte receptor called E-selectin ligand-1 (ESL-1) (Fig. 11.5).[22] Mice deficient for both E- and P-selectin have more drastic defects in their rolling and leukocyte migration to sites of inflammation than could have been anticipated from the mice deficient in only one of the two selectins. This suggests that E- and P-selectins have overlapping functions and can compensate for each other.

Chemokines and their receptors

Chemotactic cytokines and their receptors (Chapter 10) are grouped into four different families based on their primary protein structure. The families are defined by a cysteine signature motif—CXC, CC, C, and CX3C—where C is a cysteine and X any amino acid residue.[23] Most chemokines are small, soluble heparin-binding chemoattractants. The relevant chemokines for leukocyte extravasation are presented to bloodborne

Table 11.1 Phenotypes of mice deficient in homing-associated molecules

Molecule	Main abnormalities in leukocyte trafficking
L-selectin	Impaired lymphocyte homing to peripheral lymph nodes
E-selectin	Increased velocity of rolling leukocytes
P-selectin	Decreased leukocyte rolling at early stages of inflammation
PSGL-1	Decreased leukocyte rolling at early stages of inflammation
ICAM-1	Impaired neutrophil migration to sites of inflammation
ICAM-2	Delayed eosinophil accumulation in the airway lumen in allergy, impaired neutrophil transmigration
VCAM-1	Embryonic lethal
CD31	Deficient migration through basement membrane
JAM-A	Increased dendritic cell homing to lymph nodes and reduced transendothelial migration
$S1P_1$	Embryonic lethal
CD11a	Reduced lymphocyte trafficking to peripheral lymph nodes and to Peyer's patches
CD11b	Decreased leukocyte trafficking to sites of inflammation; Decreased neutrophil emigration in ischemia/reperfusion injury
β_2-integrin	No neutrophil emigration into the skin, normal emigration into inflamed peritoneum and increased migration into inflamed lung
α_4-integrin	Embryonic lethal, chimeric mice have reduced lymphocyte homing into Peyer's patches
β_7-integrin	Impaired lymphocyte migration into Peyer's patches
CD44	Decreased lymphocyte migration to peripheral lymph nodes and thymus
VAP-1	Faster rolling, decreased firm adhesion and transmigration and diminished leukocyte infiltration to sites of inflammation
CD73	Increased leukocyte traffic to sites of inflammation in ischemia
CD38	Defective chemotaxis of granulocytes and dendritic cells in severe inflammations
CCR9	Reduced number of intraepithelial T cells and IgA-positive plasma cells in lamina propria
CCR7	Defective lymphocyte entry to lymph nodes and formation of T-cell areas
CCL19/CCL21	Impaired homing of lymphocytes (especially T cells) to lymph nodes
CXCR5/CXCL13	Defect in the formation of follicles in the lymph nodes
CXCR4	Aberrant B-cell follicles
CCR4	Prolonged graft survival due to reduced T-cell trafficking

lymphocytes by proteoglycan molecules present on endothelial cell surfaces. During the adhesion cascade they activate integrins by signaling via serpentine receptors, which are pertussis-toxin sensitive and G-protein linked.[24]

Different leukocyte subsets bear their own distinct sets of receptors, which enable them to respond to chemokines presented on the vascular endothelium as well as within the tissues.

For example, CCL21 and CCL19 are preferentially expressed by HEV that are found in interfollicular areas within a lymph node. They preferentially attract T cells bearing the CCR7 receptor, and thus draw T lymphocytes from the blood and into these areas. Fractalkine, a CX3C chemokine, can be produced in either a soluble or a membrane-anchored form. It can be found on HEV in peripheral lymph nodes and has potent chemoattractant activity for T cells. The major attractants for B cells are CXCL12 and CXCL13. Although many chemokines are present in different organs in the body, some selectivity in their expression can guide tissue-selective leukocyte trafficking. For example, CCL25 attracts CCR9 positive lymphocytes to the small intestine, and CCL17/CCL22 attract CCR4-bearing lymphocytes to the skin.

Integrins and their immunoglobulin superfamily ligands

Integrins are a large family of heterodimeric molecules consisting of an α and a β chain.[25] Traditionally they are thought to mediate firm adhesion between leukocytes and endothelial cells; although in specific low-shear conditions they can also participate in rolling. The most important integrins with regard to leukocyte trafficking are $\alpha_4\beta_7$, $\alpha_4\beta_1$ and LFA-1. $\alpha_4\beta_7$ is a principal homing receptor for lymphocyte trafficking to mucosa-associated lymphatic tissues. It binds to MAdCAM-1 on HEV in organized mucosal lymphatic tissues, such as Peyer's patches and appendix, and to flat-walled venules in the lamina propria.

α_4-Integrin can also pair with a β_1 chain to form an $\alpha_4\beta_1$ dimer, which lymphocytes utilize primarily in inflammatory conditions. It binds to endothelial vascular cell adhesion molecule-1 (VCAM-1) on endothelium.

Lymphocyte function-associated antigen-1 (LFA-1/CD11a/CD18) is a member of the group of leukocyte integrins that contain a unique α chain (CD11 a, b, c and d), but share a common β chain (β_2/CD18). LFA-1 is present on practically all leukocyte subsets. LFA-1 interacts with its counter-receptors, intercellular adhesion molecules (ICAM-1 and ICAM-2) on the endothelial cell surface (Fig. 11.5). ICAM-1 is upregulated at sites of inflammation, whereas ICAM-2 is constitutively present on vascular endothelium. LFA-1 must be activated to be functional. Activation of LFA-1 is thought to be primarily a product of chemokine signaling, although alternative activation pathways exist. These include triggering through glycosyl-phosphatidylinositol (GPI)-linked molecules, CD44, as well as other costimulatory lymphocyte surface molecules.[20] LFA-1-dependent pathways display no significant organ specificity in their function. Mac-1 (CD11b/CD18) is also involved in leukocyte migration, although its contribution is overshadowed by LFA-1. Like LFA-1, Mac-1 uses ICAM-1 and ICAM-2 as its ligands (Fig. 11.5).

Other homing-associated molecules

Several other molecules belonging to various molecular families also participate in the adhesion cascade. CD44 is a multifunctional proteoglycan that is found on a large variety of different cell types.[26] Using endothelial hyaluronan as its ligand, it mediates lymphocyte rolling. It can form bimolecular complexes with $\alpha_4\beta_1$ that strengthens leukocyte–endothelial-cell interaction. In vivo inhibition studies using function-blocking antibodies indicate that CD44 plays an important role in directing lymphocyte trafficking to sites of inflammation, e.g., skin and joints.

CD31, a member of the immunoglobulin superfamily, is found on many subsets of lymphocytes and in the continuous endothelium of all vessel types. It is expressed primarily at the intercellular junctions and is involved in a stimulus-specific manner in transmigration, especially through the endothelial basement membrane. Other molecules involved in the transmigration process are CD99 and junctional adhesion molecules (JAM) A, B, and C, which are expressed both on leukocytes and endothelial cells. These molecules interact sequentially in a homotypic fashion during diapedesis. In addition, endothelial JAM-A can use LFA-1 as leukocyte ligands. JAM-B uses $\alpha_4\beta_1$ and JAM-C may utilize Mac-1.

The role of ectoenzymes in the adhesion cascade has been recently recognized.[27,28] Vascular adhesion protein-1 (VAP-1), CD73, and CD38 have well established roles in leukocyte trafficking. Owing to their enzymatic properties, they can rapidly modify adhesive interactions and modulate the microenvironment. VAP-1 is a homodimeric sialoglycoprotein that, under conditions of inflammation, is rapidly translocated on to the endothelial cell surface. It mediates early phases of leukocyte interaction with endothelium, as well as transmigration. Besides its adhesive function, it also possesses an amine oxidase activity that can produce potent immunomodulators such as H_2O_2 and aldehyde as end products. CD73 is present both on a subpopulation of lymphocytes and on endothelium. It is an ectonucleotidase. The main product of its enzymatic activity in dephosphorylation of AMP is adenosine, which is highly anti-inflammatory in nature. Endothelial CD73 may also have a counter-receptor on the lymphocyte surface, because lymphocyte binding to endothelium inhibits the enzymatic activity of CD73. This facilitates the extravasation process of the lymphocyte. CD38, an ADP-ribosyl cyclase, is expressed on most lymphoid cells and can use CD31 as its endothelial cell ligand. Via its enzymatic activity it regulates calcium fluxes and the sensitivity of leukocytes to chemokine signals.

Intraorgan lymphocyte localization

Following its extravasation from the blood vessels, a lymphocyte needs to interact with several matrix molecules, such as fibronectin, laminin and collagens. Adhesive interactions between a lymphocyte and the extracellular matrix molecules are largely mediated by β_1-integrins, although lymphocytes can also use CD44 to interact with fibronectin and collagens. The directional movement and the final localization of a lymphocyte within the tissues are controlled by chemokines.[13,23,29] Modern two-photon imaging has provided detailed information about the kinetics and directionality of lymphocyte movement in living tissues.[30]

Besides directing the entry of T cells into the tissues, CCL21 and CCL19 also determine the final destination of the T lymphocyte within lymph nodes, spleen and Peyer's patches. CCL19 and CCL21 produced by stromal cells in the T-cell areas within the lymphoid tissues guide the T lymphocyte into the interfollicular space. In an analogous manner, B-cell-attracting chemokine-1 CXCL13 is produced by a subset of follicular dendritic cells found in secondary lymphoid organs. It attracts B cells possessing CXCR5 to the light zone of the follicles. CXCL12, on the other hand, guides CXCR4 positive B cells to the dark zone (Fig. 11.6).

Correct localization of a lymphocyte and an antigen-presenting cell within the lymph node is a prerequisite for an optimal immune response. Dendritic cells that carry antigens from the peripheral tissues into the lymph node enter the node via afferent lymphatic vessels (Fig. 11.6). An interaction between the dendritic cell and the T cell in the T-cell area is then crucial for T-cell activation. B-cell collaboration with T cells is ensured by upregulation of CXCR5 expression on a subpopulation of T cells, and of CCR7 on certain B cells that allow the movement

Fig. 11.6 Role of chemokines in the entry and localization of lymphocytes within lymphoid organs. CCL19 and CCL21 are involved in the entry of T lymphocytes into the lymph node via HEV. They also guide T cells to the interfollicular areas within the node. In contrast, CXCL12 and CXCL13 attract B lymphocytes on the vessel wall and direct their localization within the follicles.

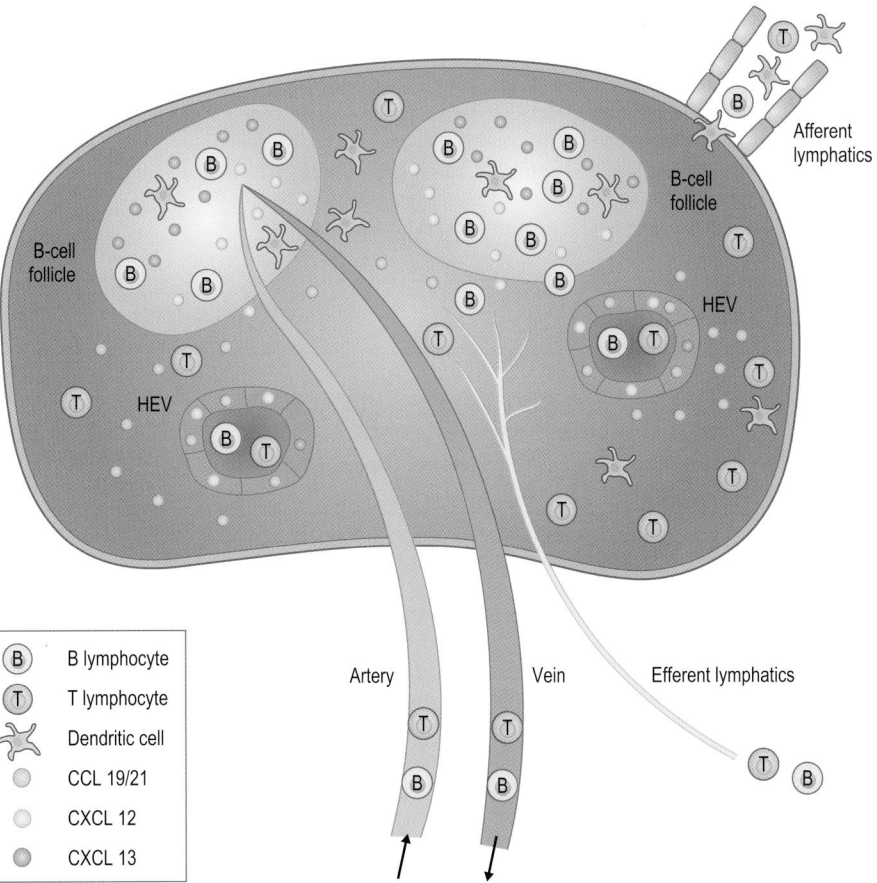

of these cells to the boundary of the B- and T-cell zones. The importance of CCL21 and CCL19 in lymphocyte trafficking is demonstrated by a spontaneous mutant mouse strain, *plt*, which has reduced expression of these chemokines. In these mice, both lymphocyte entry via HEV and the organization of T-cell areas within lymph nodes are defective. This phenotype is recapitulated in CCR7 knockout mice. CCL21/CCL19 and CXCL12/CXCL13 are currently the best-known determinants of lymphocyte localization within lymphoid tissues, although several other chemokines are also needed for optimal encounters between various cell populations in order to create a crisp immune response.

Cell trafficking within lymphatics

Although leukocyte trafficking within the lymphatics is an essential part of the recirculation process and the immune response in general, very little is known about the molecular mechanisms that regulate this tightly controlled and cell type-selective migration. CCL21 on lymphatic endothelium attracts CCR7-positive dendritic cells and lymphocytes into the afferent lymphatics and hence to the draining lymph nodes. JAM-A may also control the traffic of dendritic cells, as dendritic cells defective for JAM-A show increased motility and enhanced trafficking via the afferent lymphatics into the draining lymph nodes. Other adhesion molecules, such as macrophage mannose receptor and common lymphatic endothelial and vascular endothelial receptor-1 (CLEVER-1), mediate lymphocyte migration into the lymphatics. Lymphocytes adhere to lymphatic vessels via these molecules in *in vitro* assays and inhibition and/or lack of these molecules impair lymphocyte trafficking within lymphatics *in vivo*.[31,32] Sphingosine 1 phosphate receptor 1 (S1P$_1$), which is expressed in many different cell types, also participates in lymphocyte entrance into the afferent lymphatics and lymphocyte exit from the lymph nodes into the efferent lymphatics. Although its absence leads to defects in vascular development and embryonic lethality, studies of conditional knockout mice have shown that lymphocytes lacking S1P$_1$ can enter the lymph nodes normally. However, they are not able to exit from the lymph nodes into the efferent lymphatics. Additional studies indicate that S1P$_1$ may control lymphocyte trafficking by regulating endothelial permeability and/or suppressing lymphocyte chemotaxis in S1P$_1$ gradients.[29,33]

Clinical implications

Leukocyte trafficking plays a pivotal role in the pathogenesis of all infectious and inflammatory diseases.[13] It is essential for mounting a proper immune response against an invading microbe. However, in many other cases inappropriate leukocyte migration also causes tissue destruction. Here we have chosen a few representative examples to illustrate some of the general principles.

Immunodeficiencies

Various defects in leukocyte trafficking have been identified during the past two decades.[34] Leukocytes from patients with Wiskott–Aldrich syndrome, for example, show reduced migration to chemokines CCL2, CCL3, and CXCL12 owing to a mutation in the gene encoding an intracellular WAS protein responsible for proper cytoskeletal organization of the hematopoietic cells. Mutations of CXCR4 in WHIM (warts, hypogammaglobulinemia, infections and myelokathexis) patients lead to an enhanced chemotactic response to CXCL12 expressed on bone marrow endothelium and leukocyte accumulation in the bone marrow. A single case of inherited dysfunction of E-selectin has also been reported. The patient had recurrent infections but did not demonstrate neutrophilia. She could not synthesize E-selectin on endothelium, although her serum level of soluble E-selectin was increased.[35]

Three different forms of adhesion defect in integrins lead to poor or total lack of homing of certain leukocyte populations.[36,37] Their typical features are listed in Table 11.2. These diseases are extremely rare, but they recapitulate in humans the basic principles of leukocyte trafficking first deciphered in animal models.

LAD I

Patients with leukocyte adhesion defect-1 (LAD-1) have defects in the synthesis, pairing or expression of β$_2$-integrins.[37] The severe form leads to the total or almost total absence of CD11a/CD18 (LFA-1), CD11b/CD18 (Mac-1), CD11c/CD18, and CD11d/CD18. Although these patients exhibit neutrophilia, they suffer from severe recurrent bacterial infections owing to defects in leukocyte extravasation into sites of inflammation. They usually die young. Patients suffering from a milder form of LAD-1 (<10% of normal β$_2$-integrins) demonstrate impairment in leukocyte migration and suffer from frequent infections as well, but usually survive until adulthood. In these patients

Table 11.2 Clinical features of immunodeficient patients with abnormalities in homing-associated molecules

	LADI	LADII	LADIII
Clinical manifestation			
Recurrent bacterial infections	+++	+	+++
Neutrophilia	yes	yes	yes
Developmental abnormalities	no	yes	no
Laboratory findings			
CD18 expression	Marked decrease or absence	Normal	Normal
sLex expression	Normal	Absent	Normal
Neutrophil rolling	Normal	Markedly decreased	Normal
Neutrophil firm adherence	Markedly decreased	Mild decrease	Markedly decreased
Likely gene affected	CD18	FUCT1	KINDLIN3

lymphocyte migration to inflammatory sites is close to normal, probably because lymphocytes can utilize the VLA-4-VCAM-1 pathway to compensate for the lack of β_2-integrins. LAD-1 variants with modestly reduced β_2-integrin expression have been associated with mutations which create heterodimers that do not bind ligands. In all types of LAD I, granulocytes typically show normal rolling, but failure to arrest on endothelial cells.

LAD II

LAD II patients suffer from several abnormalities, including recurrent infections, neutrophilia, impaired pus formation, mental retardation, growth defects, and deficiency in H blood group antigen.[37] The cause of the disease is impaired transport of GDP-fucose from the cytoplasm to the Golgi lumen as a result of mutations in a GDP-fucose transporter. The defect leads to impaired modification of selectin ligands, notably that of PSGL-1, with fucose. Consequently, they demonstrate a marked decrease in leukocyte rolling under flow conditions. Interestingly, some patients respond to treatment with oral fucose.

LAD III

The third LAD syndrome involves defective inside-out signaling of β_1, β_2, and β_3 integrins.[37] In the leukocytes of these patients, activation of multiple leukocyte integrins, including LFA-1 and VLA-4, by chemokine-triggered G-protein-coupled signals is genetically defective. Concurrent defects in platelet integrins lead to a bleeding diathesis. LAD III is caused by mutated Kindlin3, which is a major cytoplasmic activator of integrins.

Diseases of autoimmunity

Multiple sclerosis

Migration of lymphocytes through the blood–brain barrier into the central nervous system is a key pathogenetic event that occurs during the development of multiple sclerosis (MS) and its widely used animal model, experimental allergic encephalomyelitis (EAE).[38] *In vivo* animal studies have shown that the disease course can be dramatically altered by blocking the function of leukocyte α_4-integrin. This treatment is able to prevent the disease and even reverse the paralytic disease and lymphocytic infiltrations in the brain. Antibodies against $\alpha_4\beta_1$ show this remarkable efficacy even if started a month after the onset of the clinical disease. Certain EAE models can also be blocked by targeting the α_4-integrin ligand VCAM-1, or by blocking the function of CD44. In contrast, lack of many other adhesion molecules, such as L-selectin, PSGL-1, E- and P-selectin, fail to yield a consistent effect on EAE. It should also be noted that although $\alpha_4\beta_1$-integrin is very important for lymphocyte homing to brain, it is not a brain-specific zip code as it is also involved in leukocyte trafficking to other organs, such as pancreas and gut.

Transplant rejection

In all forms of rejection, activation of vascular endothelium of the graft with the ensuing lymphocyte infiltration is a critical parameter. In heart transplantation, for example, multiple endothelial adhesion molecules (such as P-selectin, ICAM-1, and PNAd) normally absent from the organ are rapidly induced in a rejected organ. *In vivo* studies have shown that blocking the function of these molecules prevents the unwanted binding of lymphocytes to the graft.[39] For example, in rodent allograft models rejection is significantly reduced if lymphocyte LFA-1 and endothelial

ICAM-1 are rendered nonfunctional by monoclonal antibodies or by disruption of these molecules through gene deletion. The chemoattractant system has also been extensively targeted for inhibiting lymphocyte influx into transplants. For instance, FTY720, a small molecule that inhibits S1P$_1$ receptor, promotes long-term graft survival in murine models.

Ischemia–reperfusion injury

When blood flow is restored to an ischemic organ a massive influx of granulocytes into the hypoxic tissue can be seen. This ischemia–reperfusion injury is due to the activation of the endothelial cells in the insulted organ. In many cases it has been shown that depletion of circulating neutrophils, or blockage of their entry into the ischemic tissue through anti-adhesive therapy, can reduce tissue necrosis by up to 50% and prevent the death of cells in the zone of reversibly damaged tissue.[40] Myocardial ischemia–reperfusion injury, for example, is alleviated in CD18, ICAM-1, P- and E-selectin-deficient mice. In many cases similar results have been obtained by using antibodies to block the function of these adhesion proteins, which are induced in the ischemic tissue.

Cancer

Lymphocyte trafficking can be harnessed to improve the outcome of cellular immunotherapy against cancer.[41] Infusion of activated or genetically modified effector T cells would benefit from a more effective targeting of the cells into the tumor. On the other hand, anti-adhesive therapies targeting inappropriate accumulation of regulatory T cells in the tumor would also enhance anti-cancer immune responses.

● THERAPEUTIC PRINCIPLES

- Pro-adhesive strategies are mainly developed using gene therapy.
- Inappropriate inflammation associated with many diseases can be dampened by anti-adhesive therapeutics.
- Humanized, function-blocking monoclonal antibodies are effective anti-adhesive molecules.
- Cell migration can also be blocked by ligand and receptor analogs, small molecule inhibitors and genetic means (e.g., RNA interference).

Adhesion molecules as diagnostic targets

Immunodeficiency disorders

In classic LAD I deficiency, a definitive diagnosis can be established by flow-cytometric analysis of immunofluorescent-stained CD18 integrin on blood leukocytes.[37] In normal individuals, practically all peripheral blood lymphocytes are CD18 positive. In severe cases of LAD I deficiency there is a complete absence of this adhesion molecule, whereas in moderate deficiency about 1–10% of control levels is seen. LAD II can be diagnosed with commercially available antibodies by documenting a lack of fucosylated adhesion molecules, e.g., abnormal expression of sLeX on blood leukocytes. Diagnosis of LAD III requires activation of the cells, the use of mAbs that recognize specific activation epitopes or functional assays.

Soluble adhesion molecules

Most adhesion molecules are found in soluble forms in body fluids. They can be produced by alternative splicing of the mRNA leading to the lack of transmembrane anchors, by proteolytic cleavage of cell bound proteins by various sheddases (proteases), or by cleavage of the GPI linkage. The soluble forms can either function as molecular sinks, competing for their specific ligand(s) with the membrane-bound forms, or trigger biological responses by interacting with their ligand-bearing cells.

The availability of commercial kits for measuring the levels of soluble adhesion molecules has led to numerous reports describing an increase or a decrease of certain adhesion molecules in different diseases. In most cases there appears to be little or no additional diagnostic or predictive value derived from the use of these tests compared to more traditional parameters of inflammation activity. At present, therefore, the indications for measurements of soluble adhesion molecules, or chemokines, in inflammatory and cancerous diseases remain to be defined.

Imaging

The use of neutrophil scans or radioactively labeled nonspecific molecules to localize inflammatory foci is not satisfactory in terms of timing, expense, biohazards, specificity or sensitivity. Hence, there have been trials to radioactively or nonradioactively label monoclonal antibodies that recognize endothelial adhesion molecules, infuse them intravenously, and follow their accumulation by appropriate imaging devices.[42] Inflammation-inducible molecules such as E-selectin and MAdCAM-1 have been used as target antigens. The utility of this approach in the case of radioactively labeled E-selectin antibodies has been verified in patients.

> ### CLINICAL PEARLS
> - Blocking of α_4-integrin with natalizumab ameliorates disease activity in multiple sclerosis.

Therapeutic application of adhesion modulating therapies

Pro- and anti-adhesive therapies have long been an obvious pharmaceutical goal in the field of leukocyte trafficking. Inflammation-promoting strategies would be beneficial in diseases such as immune deficiencies, persistent infections and cancer. Moreover, pro-adhesive control of lymphocyte traffic would benefit areas such as vaccine development and bone-marrow cell transplantation. In fact, lymphocyte recirculation routes have been already empirically exploited by choosing optimal primary and secondary vaccination regimens at different anatomical locations. Anti-adhesive therapy, on the other hand, can be seen as a form of treatment applicable to all disease categories involving an inflammatory component. In addition, it could provide novel precision drugs individually tailored for organ-specific inflammatory disorders, which would be predicted to diminish the problems of generalized immunosuppression.

From antibodies to small molecular drugs

A number of specific antagonists of adhesion molecules have been developed.[43] Function-blocking monoclonal antibodies have often been the drug candidates used for proof-of-principle experiments. These include both chimeric and fully humanized antibodies against important adhesion molecules and chemokines. In parallel, recombinant ligand or receptor analogs have been developed. Knowledge of the structure of the adhesion molecules has allowed the design of rational, small molecular drugs such as those affecting the conformational state of leukocyte integrins.[44] Recently, the ability to modulate mRNA expression of adhesion molecules through RNAi has added another potential tool to the pharmaceutical armamentarium.

Although all these forms of therapy have been enormously successful in a panoply of different animal models, transfer to the clinic has been difficult. However, a small number of very potent drugs targeting adhesion molecules have been introduced.

Adhesion-modulating drugs in clinical use

The first two selective adhesion molecule inhibitors (SAM) developed were natalizumab and efalizumab. The efficacy of α_4 blocking in EAE (see above) paved the way for natalizumab, a humanized anti-α_4-integrin antibody. Monthly intravenous injection of natalizumab in patients with relapsing multiple sclerosis led to more than 90% fewer lesions than with placebo.[45] Moreover, the risk of sustained progression of disability was reduced by more than 40% and the rate of clinical relapses declined by almost 70%. Even in patients who relapsed in the presence of β-interferon treatment, the addition of natalizumab to the treatment regimen reduced the formation of new or enlarging lesions by more than 80% and diminished the number of clinical relapses by about 50%. These data indicate that natalizumab may be more effective in the treatment of multiple sclerosis than any of the currently employed therapies. Because α_4 can also pair with β_7, natalizumab has also been tested in patients with Crohn's disease. A subpopulation of these patients has responded favorably to long-term treatment.

Efalizumab is a humanized, function-blocking antibody directed against CD11a. It has been used in patients with plaque psoriasis. Weekly subcutaneous injections of the antibody have improved the disease score by more than 75% in 22–39% of patients, compared to a similar response in 5% of placebo-treated patients.[46] In addition, in more than 30% of patients other clinical endpoints, including physician-assessed disease activity, have improved significantly.

At the time this chapter was written, approximately almost 10 000 patients had been treated natalizumab. Compared to placebo groups, one type of serious adverse reaction was associated with therapy.[47] During natalizumab treatment, reactivation of a polyoma JC virus caused progressive multifocal leukoencephalopathy in 124 patients, which turned fatal in approximately 20% of cases. Early reports of potentially deadly complications led to the temporary withdrawal of natalizumab from the market, but the benefits of the therapy were thought to outweigh the potential risks, and the drug was returned to the market. Apart from the incidence of leukoencephalopathy, only fatigue and allergic reactions have been more common in natalizumab-treated patients than in controls. Progressive multifocal leukoencephalopathy has also occurred among efalizumab-tretaed patients, and this led to withdrawal of the drug from the market in 2009. Other potential problems with SAM therapy include a rebound type of exacerbation of the disease after discontinuation of the drugs, and the induction of an immune response against the antibodies, which blunts the efficacy of the therapy. Finally, it should be emphasized that natalizumab and efalizumab may have anti-inflammatory properties, such as an ability to block T-cell activation, that are not related to their central role in leukocyte recirculation. In any case natalizumab is the first evidence that the understanding of lymphocyte trafficking can be successfully harnessed in clinical medicine.

Lymphocyte migration can also be targeted therapeutically by modulating lymphocyte exit from the lymph nodes. Fingolimod/FTY720 causes S1P$_1$ receptor internalization and degradation. Consequently, it inhibits lymphocyte egress from lymphoid organs. It may selectively retain the CCR7-positive T cells, including central memory T cells, which may be particularly important for the pathogenesis of brain inflammation, while sparing CCR7-negative effector memory cells. It has been approved by FDA as a first-line treatment for relapsing multiple sclerosis, and it is the first orally active disease modifying drug for the this immunological disease.[48]

References

1. Gowans JL, Knight EJ. The route of re-circulation of lymphocytes in rat. Proc R Soc Lond B Biol Sci 1964;159:257–82.
2. Springer TA. Traffic signals for lymphocyte recirculation and leukocyte emigration: the multistep paradigm. Cell 1994;76:301–14.
3. Butcher EC, Picker LJ. Lymphocyte homing and homeostasis. Science 1996;272(5258):60–6.
4. Ley K, Laudanna C, Cybulsky MI, et al. Getting to the site of inflammation: the leukocyte adhesion cascade updated. Nat Rev Immunol 2007;7(9):678–89.
5. Moore MA. Commentary: the role of cell migration in the ontogeny of the lymphoid system. Stem Cells Dev 2004;13(1):1–21.
6. von Andrian UH, Mempel TR. Homing and cellular traffic in lymph nodes. Nat Rev Immunol 2003;3(11):867–78.
7. Hay JB, Hobbs BB. The flow of blood to lymph nodes and its relation to lymphocyte traffic and the immune response. J Exp Med 1977;145(1):31–44.
8. Randolph GJ, Angeli V, Swartz MA. Dendritic-cell trafficking to lymph nodes through lymphatic vessels. Nat Rev Immunol 2005;5(8):617–28.
9. Mora JR, Iwata M, von Andrian UH. Vitamin effects on the immune system: vitamins A and D take centre stage. Nat Rev Immunol 2008;8(9):685–98.
10. Sigmundsdottir H, Butcher EC. Environmental cues, dendritic cells and the programming of tissue-selective lymphocyte trafficking. Nat Immunol 2008;9(9):981–7.
11. Sallusto F, Lanzavecchia A. Heterogeneity of CD4 + memory T cells: functional modules for tailored immunity. Eur J Immunol 2009;39(8):2076–82.
12. Mebius RE, Kraal G. Structure and function of the spleen. Nat Rev Immunol 2005;5(8):606–16.
13. Luster AD, Alon R, von Andrian UH. Immune cell migration in inflammation: present and future therapeutic targets. Nat Immunol 2005;6(12):1182–90.
14. Serhan CN, Chiang N, Van Dyke TE. Resolving inflammation: dual anti-inflammatory and pro-resolution lipid mediators. Nat Rev Immunol 2008;8(5):349–61.
15. Nathan C, Ding A. Nonresolving inflammation. Cell 2010;140(6):871–82.
16. Aloisi F, Pujol-Borrell R. Lymphoid neogenesis in chronic inflammatory diseases. Nat Rev Immunol 2006;6(3):205–17.
17. Kupper TS, Fuhlbrigge RC. Immune surveillance in the skin: mechanisms and clinical consequences. Nat Rev Immunol 2004;4(3):211–22.
18. Muller WA. Mechanisms of leukocyte transendothelial migration. Annu Rev Pathol 2011;6:323–44.
19. Salmi M, Jalkanen S. Lymphocyte homing to the gut: attraction, adhesion, and commitment. Immunol Rev 2005;206:100–13.
20. Kinashi T. Intracellular signalling controlling integrin activation in lymphocytes. Nat Rev Immunol 2005;5(7):546–59.
21. Rosen SD. Ligands for L-selectin: homing, inflammation, and beyond. Annu Rev Immunol 2004;22:129–56.
22. Ley K, Kansas GS. Selectins in T-cell recruitment to non-lymphoid tissues and sites of inflammation. Nat Rev Immunol 2004;4(5):325–35.
23. Moser B, Wolf M, Walz A, et al. Chemokines: multiple levels of leukocyte migration control. Trends Immunol 2004;25(2):75–84.
24. Sallusto F, Baggiolini M. Chemokines and leukocyte traffic. Nat Immunol 2008;9(9):949–52.
25. Carman CV, Springer TA. Integrin avidity regulation: are changes in affinity and conformation underemphasized? Curr Opin Cell Biol 2003;15(5):547–56.
26. Steeber DA, Venturi GM, Tedder TF. A new twist to the leukocyte adhesion cascade: intimate cooperation is key. Trends Immunol 2005;26(1):9–12.
27. Salmi M, Jalkanen S. Cell-surface enzymes in control of leukocyte trafficking. Nat Rev Immunol 2005;5(10):760–71.
28. Salmi M, Jalkanen S. Homing-associated molecules CD73 and VAP-1 as targets to prevent harmful inflammations and cancer spread. FEBS Lett 2011;585(11):1543–50.
29. Cyster JG. Chemokines, sphingosine-1-phosphate, and cell migration in secondary lymphoid organs. Annu Rev Immunol 2005;23:127–59.
30. Germain RN, Miller MJ, Dustin ML, et al. Dynamic imaging of the immune system: progress, pitfalls and promise. Nat Rev Immunol 2006;6(7):497–507.
31. Marttila-Ichihara F, Turja R, Miiluniemi M, et al. Macrophage mannose receptor on lymphatics controls cell trafficking. Blood 2008;112(1):64–72.
32. Karikoski M, Irjala H, Maksimow M, et al. Clever-1/Stabilin-1 regulates lymphocyte migration within lymphatics and leukocyte entrance to sites of inflammation. Eur J Immunol 2009;39(12):3477–87.
33. Rosen H, Goetzl EJ. Sphingosine 1-phosphate and its receptors: an autocrine and paracrine network. Nat Rev Immunol 2005;5(7):560–70.
34. Notarangelo LD, Badolato R. Leukocyte trafficking in primary immunodeficiencies. J Leukoc Biol 2009;85(3):335–43.
35. DeLisser HM, Christofidou-Solomidou M, Sun J, et al. Loss of endothelial surface expression of E-selectin in a patient with recurrent infections. Blood 1999;94(3):884–94.
36. Badolato R. Leukocyte circulation: one-way or round-trip? Lessons from primary immunodeficiency patients. J Leukoc Biol 2004;76(1):1–6.
37. Etzioni A. Defects in the leukocyte adhesion cascade. Clin Rev Allergy Immunol 2010;38(1):54–60.
38. Greenwood J, Heasman SJ, Alvarez JI, et al. Review: leucocyte-endothelial cell crosstalk at the blood-brain barrier: a prerequisite for successful immune cell entry to the brain. Neuropathol Appl Neurobiol 2011;37(1):24–39.
39. Yopp AC, Krieger NR, Ochando JC, et al. Therapeutic manipulation of T cell chemotaxis in transplantation. Curr Opin Immunol 2004;16(5):571–7.
40. Kakkar AK, Lefer DJ. Leukocyte and endothelial adhesion molecule studies in knockout mice. Curr Opin Pharmacol 2004;4(2):154–8.
41. Ruffell B, DeNardo DG, Affara NI, et al. Lymphocytes in cancer development: polarization towards pro-tumor immunity. Cytokine Growth Factor Rev 2010;21(1):3–10.
42. Marshall D, Haskard DO. Clinical overview of leukocyte adhesion and migration: where are we now? Semin Immunol 2002;14(2):133–40.
43. Mackay CR. Moving targets: cell migration inhibitors as new anti-inflammatory therapies. Nat Immunol 2008;9(9):988–98.
44. Shimaoka M, Springer TA. Therapeutic antagonists and conformational regulation of integrin function. Nat Rev Drug Discov 2003;2(9):703–16.
45. Ropper AH. Selective treatment of multiple sclerosis. N Engl J Med 2006;354(9):965–7.
46. Kupper TS. Immunologic targets in psoriasis. N Engl J Med 2003;349(21):1987–90.
47. Major EO. Reemergence of PML in natalizumab-treated patients–new cases, same concerns. N Engl J Med 2009;361(11):1041–3.
48. Brinkmann V, Billich A, Baumruker T, et al. Fingolimod (FTY720): discovery and development of an oral drug to treat multiple sclerosis. Nat Rev Drug Discov 2010;9(11):883–97.

Erik J. Peterson,
Jonathan S.
Maltzman, Gary A.
Koretzky

T-cell activation and tolerance

Activation of T lymphocytes during an immune response triggers a series of programmed gene regulation, proliferation, differentiation, and effector functions. These programs are designed to allow the immune system to react against foreign antigens without initiating self-reactivity or autoimmunity. Each of these functions is fully dependent on environmental cues that are recognized by cell surface receptors and then translated by means of a series of biochemical alterations within the cell. This chapter discusses signal transduction through one of the most studied of these receptors, the antigen-specific T-cell receptor (TCR) complex. It addresses the mechanisms whereby signals propagated through the TCR combine with those from co-stimulatory receptors to produce either productive activation or immune tolerance. It also discusses how abnormal signaling can contribute to T-cell dysfunction and disease (Table 12.1).

● CLINICAL RELEVANCE

Dysfunction or deficiency of T-cell signaling proteins (induced or spontaneous) has been causally linked to several disease states in animal or human models.

Molecules wherein mutations may lead to immune deficiency:

- CD45
- LCK
- ZAP-70
- SLP-76
- LAT
- IL-2R γ chain

Molecules wherein mutations may lead to lymphocyte hyperproliferation:

- CTLA-4
- SHP-1
- CD95/CD95 ligand
- SAP
- CBL/CBL-b
- ZAP-70
- LYP
- DGK

The T-cell antigen receptor complex

The TCR complex consists of a ligand-binding α/β or γ/δ heterodimer in association with the CD3/ζ chain complex, which provides transmembrane signal transduction capability.[1] Specificity of the TCR for antigen resides exclusively within the highly polymorphic clonotypic ligand-binding α/β or γ/δ chains. Although many of the biochemical events leading to α/β and γ/δ T-cell activation are similar, there are differences between these cell types in regard to their development, their spectrum of antigen reactivity, and their role in specific immune responses. This chapter focuses on α/β T cells.

The α/β TCR specifically recognizes short peptide ligands bound to major histocompatibility complex (MHC) antigens (Chapter 5) on the surface of antigen-presenting cells (APCs) (Chapter 6). Co-receptor molecules expressed on subsets of α/β T cells determine whether the TCR recognizes class I or class II MHC. CD4 T cells are stimulated by processed exogenous antigen presented by class II MHC molecules on the surface of professional APCs. CD8 T cells respond to peptides synthesized by the presenting cells and presented by class I molecules. CD4 and CD8 associate with MHC class II and class I molecules, respectively, to stabilize the tripartite interaction between the TCR, antigen, and MHC, which increases the effectiveness of TCR engagement.

Although the α/β chains of the TCR contain all of the information necessary for antigen/MHC binding, these proteins cannot initiate the intracellular biochemical events that signal antigen recognition. Instead, signal transduction is accomplished by the noncovalently associated CD3 and TCRζ polypeptides, which include several pairs of transmembrane hetero- or homo-dimers (Fig. 12.1) (Chapter 4). Each CD3 and ζ chain derives signaling capacity from the presence of one or more cytoplasmic regions known as an immunoreceptor tyrosine-based activation motifs (ITAMs).[2]

● KEY CONCEPTS

Protein tyrosine kinase activation

The earliest detectable biochemical event following T-cell receptor engagement is activation of protein tyrosine kinases:

- Src family: LCK, FYN
- Syk family: ZAP-70
- Tec family: ITK, RLK

Activation of protein tyrosine kinases by the TCR and the role of the ITAMs

The first biochemical event known to occur following engagement of the TCR is the activation of LCK and FYN, two members of the SRC family of protein tyrosine kinases (PTKs).[3] Similar to all SRC PTKs, LCK and FYN possess a number of features critical for their function (Fig. 12.2). These include an amino-terminal

Table 12.1 Phenotypes associated with deficient function of selected T-cell signaling molecules

Molecule	Affected signaling event	Phenotype Mouse	Human
TCR signaling			
CD3 γ	TCR expression	B⁺T⁺NK⁺ SCID	B⁺T⁺NK⁺ SCID
CD3 ε	TCR expression	B⁺T⁻NK⁺ SCID	B⁺T⁺/⁻NK⁺ SCID
CD3 δ	TCR expression	B⁺T⁻NK⁺ SCID	B⁺T⁻NK⁺ SCID
CD3 ζ	TCR expression, TCR-mediated PTK activation	B⁺T⁺NK⁺ SCID	B⁺T⁺NK⁺ SCID
ZAP-70	TCR-mediated PTK activation	B⁺T⁺/⁻NK⁺ SCID. TCRαβ T cells are absent, but TCRγδ T cells survive. Arthritis occurs in some inbred strains	B⁺T⁺/⁻NK⁺ SCID. CD8 T-cell lymphopenia. Overexpressed in some hematologic malignancies
LCK	TCR-mediated PTK activation	B⁺T⁺/⁻NK⁺ SCID. Impaired thymopoiesis and proliferation	B⁺T⁺NK⁺ SCID. CD4 lymphopenia, absent CD28 expression on CD8 T cells, and hypogammaglobulinemia
CD45	Maintenance of SRC family PTK in "open" conformation	B⁺T⁺/⁻NK⁺ SCID. Impaired thymopoiesis	B⁺T⁺/⁻NK⁺ SCID. Impaired thymopoiesis, decreased cytotoxic T-cell responses, progressive hypogammaglobulinemia, genetic polymorphisms may correlate with increased prevalence of autoimmune disease
SAP	SHP-2 binding to SLAM	Increased susceptibility to lymphocytic choriomeningitis virus, reduced IgE production, NKT-cell deficiency	X-linked lymphoproliferative disease (XLP) with B-cell hyper-responsiveness, NKT-cell deficiency
WASP	Actin polymerization	Decreased T-cell proliferation and IL-2 production	Wiscott–Aldrich syndrome (immunodeficiency, atopic dermatitis, thrombocytopenia, bloody diarrhea)
CBL/CBL-b[a]	E3 ubiquitin ligase. Recruitment of CrKL/C3G inhibitory complex	Hyperproliferative T cells[a]	Proto-oncogene for leukaemia
LAT	Coupling PTK activation to downstream signals	B⁺T⁻NK⁺ SCID. Absolute block in thymopoiesis	
SLP-76	Coupling PTK activation to downstream signals	B⁺T⁻NK⁺ SCID. Absolute block in thymopoiesis. Defect in vascular/lymphatic development	
ITK/RLK	Amplification of proximal PTK signals. Activation of PLC-γ1	Defective Th2 immune responses	
CTLA-4	Inhibition of CD28-mediated co-stimulation	Fatal lymphoproliferative disease with myocarditis, pancreatitis	Allelic variants associated with autoimmunity, including Hashimoto's thyroiditis, Graves' disease, and systemic lupus erythematosus
SHP-1	Downregulation of PTK activity	Autoimmunity, inflammatory lung disease. "Motheaten" mice	
LYP (Lymphoid phosphatase; *PTPn22* gene product)	Attenuation of lck activity	Augmented TCR-stimulated IL-2 production and proliferation	Allelic variants are associated with increased risk of rheumatoid arthritis, systemic lupus, type I diabetes mellitus.
DGKζ	Downregulation of DAG-dependent Ras activation	Impaired T-cell anergy induction	
IL-2R signaling			
γc	Coupling IL-2 binding to JAK activation	B⁺T⁻NK⁻ SCID	B⁺T⁻NK⁻ SCID, X-linked SCID
JAK3	Phosphorylation of STAT proteins	B⁺T⁻NK⁻ SCID	B⁺T⁻NK⁻ SCID

[a]CBL and CBL-b are closely-related; CBL-b-deficient mice develop autoimmune features and more severe lymphoproliferative disease than mice lacking CBL. γc, common γ-chain (IL2Rγ); IgE, immunoglobulin E; NK, natural killer; SCID, severe combined immunodeficiency; TCR, T-cell receptor.

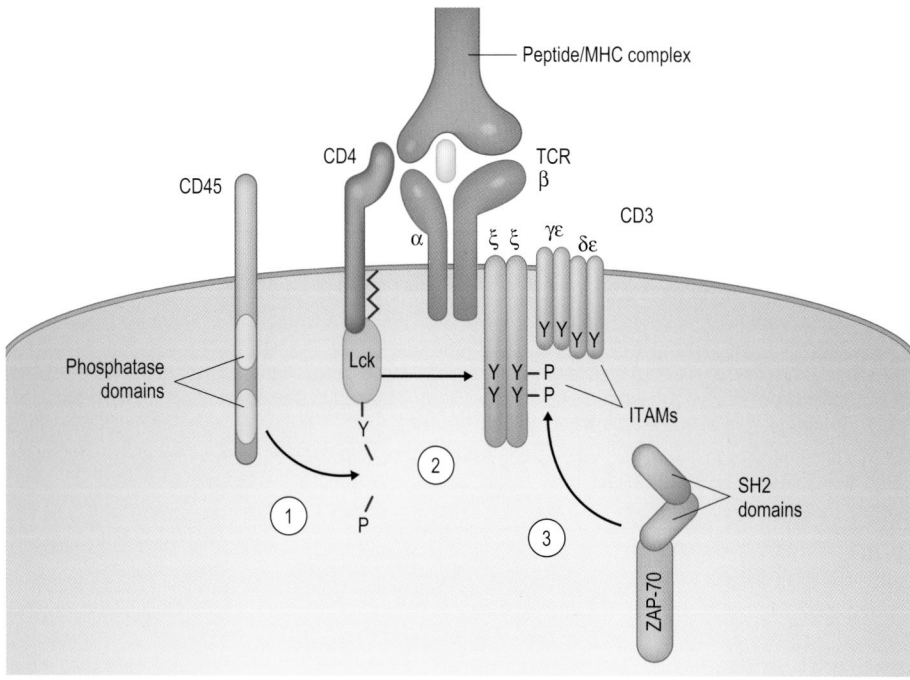

Fig. 12.1 **Biochemical events in early T-cell receptor (TCR) signaling.** The tyrosine phosphatase CD45 dephosphorylates the negative regulatory tyrosine residue on the CD4-associated protein tyrosine kinase (PTK) LCK, maintaining LCK in an activatable conformation (1). Engagement of the TCR α/β heterodimer and the CD4 (or CD8) co-receptors by MHC-bound peptide antigen brings activated LCK into proximity with immunoreceptor tyrosine-based activation motif (ITAM)-bearing CD3 chains. LCK phosphorylates the CD3ζ chain within ITAMs (2). The phosphorylated CD3ζ-chain ITAMs interact with the tandem SH2 domains of the cytoplasmic PTK ZAP-70 (3), permitting activation of ZAP-70 and phosphorylation of downstream substrates.

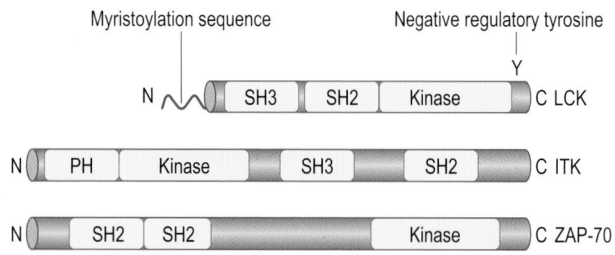

Fig. 12.2 **Domain organization of T-cell receptor (TCR)-stimulated protein tyrosine kinases (PTKs).** Comparative schematic representation of members of three families of PTKs required for T-cell-activating signals. In addition to catalytic domains, LCK (SRC family), ITK (TEC family), and ZAP-70 (SYK family) each contain regions responsible for mediating protein–protein interactions, including SH3 and SH2 domains. SH3, Src homology 3; SH2, Src homology 2; PH, pleckstrin homology.

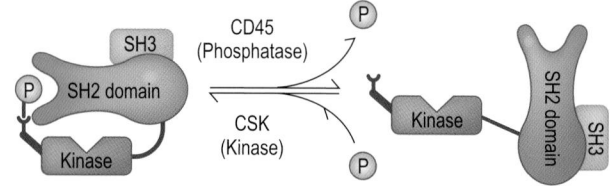

Fig. 12.3 **Model for dynamic regulation of LCK by intramolecular interaction between an SH2 domain and phosphotyrosine.** The transmembrane phosphatase CD45 dephosphorylates tyrosine 505 in the carboxyl-terminus of the SRC family protein tyrosine kinase (PTK) LCK. CD45 activity maintains LCK in an "open" conformation, permitting LCK kinase domain access to intracellular substrates. CSK activity opposes that of CD45; phosphorylation of tyrosine 505 results in an intramolecular interaction between the SH2 domain and phosphotyrosine. Inhibition of LCK kinase activity correlates with the "closed" conformation (left).

myristoylation sequence that directs membrane localization, a SRC homology 3 (SH3) domain that permits associations with other proteins containing regions rich in proline residues, a SRC homology 2 (SH2) domain that dictates interactions with proteins phosphorylated on tyrosine residues, a catalytic region, and a carboxyl-terminal tyrosine residue. The precise mechanism whereby LCK and FYN are stimulated by the TCR is not clear, but both have been shown to associate physically with TCR CD3 components and/or CD4 and CD8. SRC family PTK enzymatic function is regulated, in part, by the state of tyrosine phosphorylation of the kinase. When the conserved carboxyl-terminal tyrosine residue is phosphorylated, the SRC family PTKs adopt a closed conformation that is the product of an intramolecular interaction between that phosphotyrosine and the SH2 domain (Fig. 12.3). This intramolecular interaction inhibits the enzymatic activity of the PTK, limiting subsequent tyrosine phosphorylation-dependent signaling events. Phosphorylation of the carboxyl-terminal tyrosine (Y505 in LCK and Y527 in FYN) is dynamically regulated.[4] Phosphate is transferred to this residue by the cytoplasmic PTK CSK and is removed by the transmembrane protein tyrosine phosphatase CD45.

The phenotypes of CD45-deficient cells, mice, and humans highlight the critical regulatory importance of the carboxyl-terminal tyrosine in SRC family PTKs.[5] TCR signal transduction in cell lines lacking CD45 is blocked at the most proximal step, and mice that have been genetically modified to lack CD45 expression exhibit profound defects in thymocyte development and subsequent T-cell activation. CD45 deficiency in humans creates a T^-, B^+, NK^+ severe combined immunodeficiency (SCID) (Chapter 35). These outcomes correlate with markedly impaired LCK enzymatic activity and hyperphosphorylation on the regulatory tyrosine.

Following TCR engagement and PTK activation, numerous cellular substrates become tyrosine-phosphorylated, including the CD3 and ζ ITAMs (Fig. 12.1). In resting T cells, key tyrosine residues within the ITAMs are embedded within the hydrophobic core of the plasma membrane lipid bilayer. Upon TCR triggering, conformational changes induced within the CD3 cytoplasmic tails result in enhanced tyrosine accessibility to the action of SRC family kinases.[2] ITAM phosphorylation creates a docking site for another cytosolic PTK, ζ-associated phosphoprotein of 70 kDa (ZAP-70). ZAP-70, a member of the

SYK family PTKs, contains a catalytic domain that is located carboxyl-terminal to two tandem SH2 domains (Fig. 12.2). The ZAP-70 SH2 domains have affinity for phosphotyrosine present within ITAMs. Thus, inducible phosphorylation of the CD3 and ζ ITAMs results in the recruitment of ZAP-70 to these components of the TCR. Upon TCR recruitment, ZAP-70 enzymatic activity is increased owing to phosphorylation by LCK as well as autophosphorylation. The net result of these phosphorylations is conversion of the TCR from an enzymatically inactive complex to a potent PTK.

The critical importance of LCK, FYN, and ZAP-70 for both thymocyte development and mature T-cell activation has been established by studies in mutant cell lines, mice, and humans. Jurkat T cells (a human leukemic cell line commonly employed as a model for mature T-cell activation) deficient in expression of either LCK or ZAP-70 cannot be activated via the TCR.[6] Mice deficient in Zap-70 or Lck, but not in Fyn, exhibit a significant yet incomplete block in early T-cell development. This phenotype suggests that the pre-TCR (a complex present on immature thymocytes that includes signaling components thought to be similar to the TCR on mature T cells) also requires Src and Syk family PTKs to transduce signals. ZAP-70 deficiency and abnormal LCK function in humans create a T$^-$, B$^+$, NK$^+$ SCID (Chapter 35).[7]

In addition to SRC and SYK family PTKs, TCR engagement results in the activation of a third family of cytosolic PTKs, the Tec family.[8] Members of this family in T cells include TEC, ITK, and RLK. TEC PTKs contain SH2, SH3, and catalytic domains, as well as pleckstrin homology (PH) domains that mediate interactions with membrane-localized phospholipids (Fig. 12.2). PH domains permit the recruitment of TEC family kinases to the plasma membrane, where they can phosphorylate important substrates. Activation of Tec family members is dependent upon the prior activation of SRC and SYK family PTKs. ITK positively regulates antigen receptor signaling through recruitment and activation of the lipid modulator PLCγ to a "signalosome" nucleated by the cytoplasmic adaptor protein SLP-76 (see below). The importance of normal ITK signaling was recently shown in humans where homozygous mutation led to immunodeficiency resulting in death from Epstein–Barr virus (EBV)-associated lymphoproliferation.[9]

Tec family kinases are thought to act as modulators of TCR signal strength. Mice deficient in Tec kinases display variable partial defects in thymocyte development and peripheral T-cell maturation. T cells deficient in Tec PTKs display alterations in actin polymerization and cytoskeletal polarization that promote recruitment of adhesion-related proteins including β2 integrins and signaling mediators such as Vav to membrane regions important for propagating activation signals.

● KEY CONCEPTS

TCR signaling pathways

T-cell receptor engagement leads to the initiation of signaling cascades, including:

- PLCγ1 activation
  - Calcium flux
  - DAG formation
- RAS/MAPK
- NF-κb

Second-messenger cascades downstream of the TCR-stimulated PTKs

All of the well-established signaling pathways initiated by TCR engagement are dependent upon the activation of ZAP-70 and its association with the CD3 and ζ chain ITAMs. One consequence of effective TCR stimulation is activation of the membrane-associated enzyme phospholipase Cγ1 (PLCγ1) (Fig. 12.4).[10] PLCγ1 is phosphorylated by multiple TCR-dependent PTKs, including both ZAP-70 and members of the Tec family. TCR-stimulated tyrosine phosphorylation alone is not sufficient to activate PLCγ1; relocalization of the enzyme into adaptor-protein nucleated complexes probably plays a critical role.

Activated PLCγ1 catalyzes the hydrolysis of phosphatidylinositol-4,5-bisphosphate (PIP$_2$), a minor plasma membrane phospholipid. PIP$_2$ hydrolysis gives rise to two biochemical second

Fig. 12.4 Signaling pathways activated by T-cell receptor (TCR) engagement. TCR ligation results in activation of protein tyrosine kinases (PTKs) such as LCK and ZAP-70. Phospholipase Cγ1 (PLCγ1) becomes phosphorylated and activated by ITK and PI3K. Hydrolysis of phosphatidyl inositol bisphosphate (PIP$_2$) by PLCγ1 releases diacylglycerol (DAG) and inositol trisphosphate (IP$_3$). IP$_3$ stimulates an increase in intracellular calcium concentration, which activates the phosphatase calcineurin. Calcineurin dephosphorylates NFAT, thereby signaling NFAT translocation to the nucleus. The formation of DAG leads to activation of RAS-GRP1 GEF activity and RAS activation. Active RAS binds and stimulates the kinase RAF1, initiating a cascade of serine/threonine kinases (MAPK cascade) leading to phosphorylation and nuclear translocation of the ERK kinases. DAG formation also results in activation of the CARMA/BCL-1/MALT1 complex leading to phosphorylation of IκB kinase (IKK). Active IKK phosphorylates IκB-α, leading to IκB-α degradation and release of NF-κB to the nucleus. Transcription factors NFAT, NFκB, and those activated by the MAPK pathway cooperate to upregulate transcription of genes such as IL-2 critical for T-cell activation.

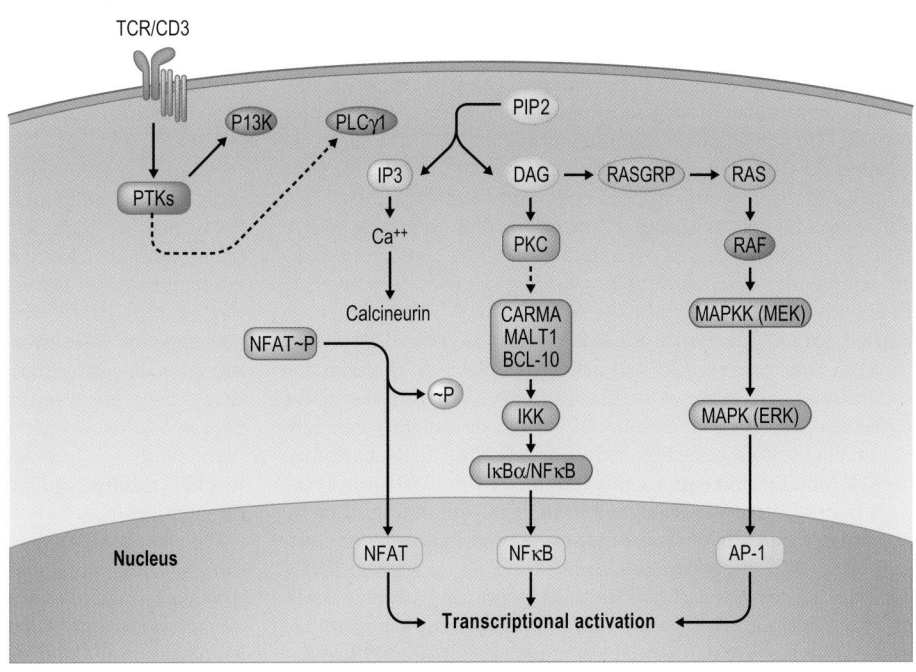

messengers, the soluble sugar inositol-1,4,5-trisphosphate (IP_3) and the lipid diacylglycerol (DAG). IP_3 binding to a cognate receptor on endoplasmic reticulum (ER) results in the release of calcium from this organelle. The IP_3-mediated reductions in calcium ER concentrations are sensed by STIM1, an EF-hand domain-containing protein localized in the ER membrane.[11] STIM1 aggregation induces clustering and augmented function of store-operated calcium entry (SOCE) channels, including the transmembrane protein ORAI. Marked calcium influx from the extracellular milieu attends channel activation. TCR-triggered calcium flux results in the activation of calcineurin, a serine/threonine phosphatase. Substrates of calcineurin include members of the nuclear factor of activated T cells (NFAT) family. In resting T cells, NFAT proteins are phosphorylated and reside in the cytosol. Activated calcineurin dephosphorylates NFAT, allowing it to translocate to the nucleus and bind response elements in the promoters of genes important for T-cell activation.

Knowledge of the calcineurin pathway has been exploited clinically. The compounds cyclosporine and tacrolimus both inhibit calcineurin-dependent T-cell activation, but via distinct mechanisms. These drugs are mainstays in the prevention of human solid-organ transplant rejection (Chapter 80) and can also be used to treat T-cell driven autoimmune diseases such as systemic lupus erythematosus and rheumatoid arthritis, although they are not first-line therapy for these disorders (Chapter 51).

The second major product of PIP_2 hydrolysis, DAG, functions as a physiological activator of TCR signaling intermediates, including protein kinase D (PKD), Ras guanyl nucleotide releasing proteins (RASGRP), and members of the protein kinase C (PKC) family of serine/threonine kinases.[12] PKD cooperates with PKC-dependent signals to activate high-affinity binding capacity and clustering of integrins, a family of molecules that mediate TCR signal-augmented cell binding to adhesion molecules on APCs.[13] RasGRP mediates activation of the Ras cascade. The importance of the RasGRP pathway in TCR-mediated signaling is highlighted by the finding that deletion of RasGRP1 leads to severe defects in thymocyte development in mice. PKC is essential for full activation of the TCR-stimulated Ras/ERK and NF-κB cascades (see below) that are required to mount an activating gene transcriptional program.

In T lymphocytes, exchange of guanosine triphosphate (GTP) for guanosine diphosphate (GDP)-bound RAS can occur through one of two distinct molecular mechanisms involving the guanine exchange factors (GEFs) son of sevenless (SOS) or RasGRP1.[14] Following TCR activation, SOS is recruited to the plasma membrane through its interaction with the GRB2 adaptor protein. This mechanism is similar to events leading to RAS activation downstream of growth receptors with intrinsic tyrosine kinase activity in nonlymphoid cells. Activation via the GRB2-SOS pathway acts as a digital "on–off" switch, whereas activation RASGRP-mediated activation can be envisioned as an analog rheostat, leading to varying degrees of activation depending on the strength of signal.[15] RAS activity may be curbed through the hydrolysis of RAS-bound GTP to GDP, either through the intrinsic GTPase activity of RAS or through the recruitment of GTPase-activating proteins (GAPs) to the active RAS molecule. Thus, the ability of RAS to modulate T-cell activation events is governed by both signals leading to the exchange of GTP for GDP and signals affecting the rate of GTP hydrolysis.

Active RAS recruits RAF to the plasma membrane, thereby activating a cascade of serine-threonine protein kinases, including MEK, and the extracellular signal-regulated kinase (ERK). This kinase cascade culminates with the nuclear translocation of ERK. Upon entry into the nucleus, ERK can phosphorylate and activate several transcription factors that are critical for TCR-induced transactivation of cytokines and other activation genes. Evidence for the central importance of RAS activation for T-cell function has come from studies in cell lines and in genetically altered mice. Jurkat T cells expressing inhibitory mutant forms of RAS fail to produce IL-2 following TCR engagement. In contrast, Jurkat cells expressing an activated form of RAS produce IL-2 much more readily than do wild-type cells. Similarly, mice transgenic for activating Ras mutants show alterations in thymocyte development and demonstrate a partially stimulated state in the absence of antigen binding.

Stimulation of T cells also involves activation of the lipid kinase phosphatidylinositol 3'-hydroxyl kinase (PI3K) (Fig. 12.4).[16] PI3K phosphorylates phosphoinositides, which play an important role in the regulation of several downstream serine/threonine kinases. The activation of PI3K requires phosphorylation of a regulatory subunit that controls catalytic activity conferred by a 110-kDa subunit. Although TCR engagement alone can stimulate some degree of PI3K function, full activity of the lipid kinase appears to require co-stimulation of the T cell through receptors such as CD28 (see below).

Cross-linking of the TCR also leads to activation and nuclear translocation of members of the nuclear factor-κB (NFκB) family of transcription factors (Fig. 12.4).[17] Normally, NFκB family members are sequestered in the cytoplasm through interaction with inhibitors of NFκB (IκBs). TCR stimulation results in the formation of a multimolecular complex composed of CARMA1, BCL-10, and MALT1 (CBM). Assembly of the complex is dependent upon activation of PKC-θ. CBM complex formation lies upstream of signals leading to activation of IκB kinases (IKKs), phosphorylation and degradation of IκB, and subsequent release and translocation to the nucleus of NFκB. Defects in T-cell activation and survival result from deficiencies in CBM proteins.

Integration of second-messenger pathways by adaptor proteins

Considerable insight into how intracellular signaling pathways initiated by TCR cross-linking can be integrated has come from the characterization of adaptor proteins.[18,19] Adaptors lack enzymatic or transcriptional regulatory activity. Instead, they possess modular domains responsible for subcellular relocalization and intermolecular interactions. Both constitutive and induced intermolecular interactions mediated by adaptor molecules can provide the necessary scaffold to promote signal transduction events.

Adaptor proteins commonly contain modular domains that exhibit affinity for phosphorylated tyrosine residues (Fig. 12.5A). Such regions include the SH2 and phosphotyrosine-binding (PTB) domains. Each of these domains recognizes phosphorylated tyrosine residues within a specific sequence context. For example, PTB domains obtain their specificity based on residues amino-terminal to the phosphotyrosine, whereas SH2 domains recognize particular sequence motifs carboxyl-terminal to the key phosphotyrosine. Other adaptor domains include SH3 modules, which bind proline-rich regions, WW regions responsible for interactions with proline/tyrosine or proline/leucine motifs, and PH domains that have specificity for phospholipids.

It is clear that many ubiquitously expressed adaptors as well as others with more restricted tissue distribution function in diverse cellular processes. Several hematopoietic-specific adaptors are now known to play essential roles in T-cell development, in coordinating the signals necessary for mature T-cell activation,

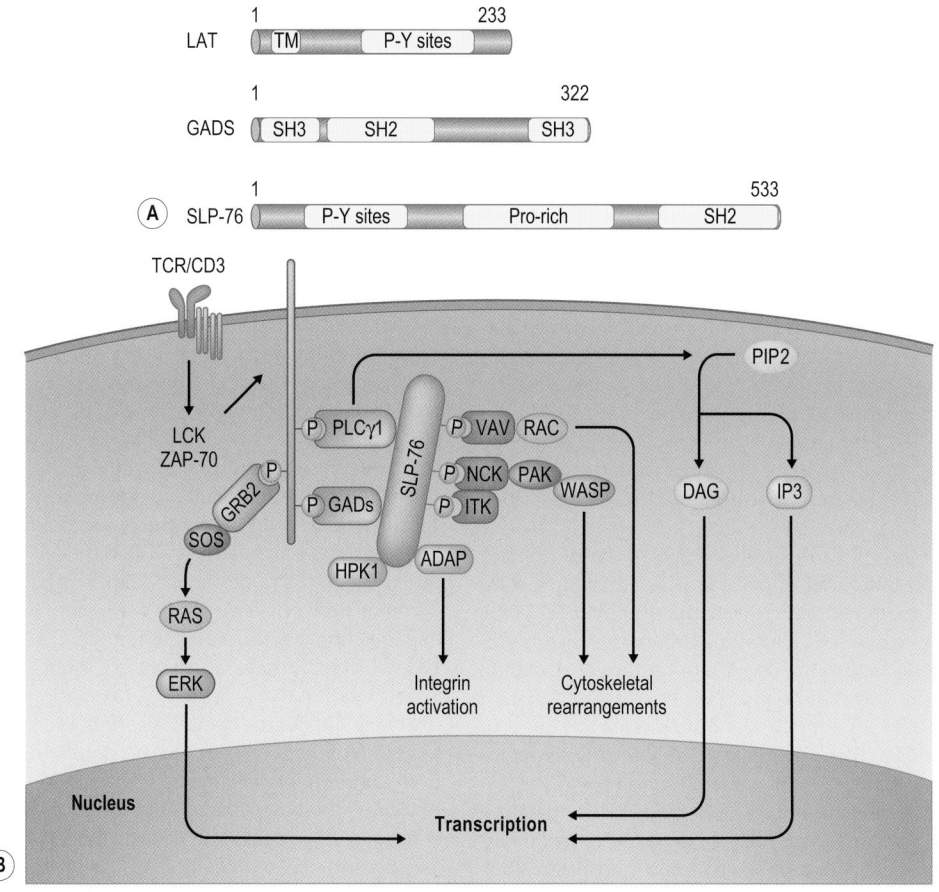

Fig. 12.5 Model for adaptor protein-mediated coupling of the T-cell receptor (TCR) to phospholipase Cγ1 (PLCγ1) activation. (A) Structural schematics of three adaptors implicated in plasma membrane proximal biochemical events. SH3 domains mediate association with proline-rich regions; SH2 domains associate with phosphorylated tyrosine residues. (B) LAT and SLP-76 are among the substrates of the TCR-activated protein tyrosine kinases (PTKs). When tyrosine residues within the LAT cytoplasmic tail are phosphorylated, GADS binds to LAT through the GADS SH2 domain. Recruitment of GADS results in relocalization of SLP-76, as the proline-rich region of SLP-76 mediates constitutive association with the SH3 domain of GADS. Tyrosine-phosphorylated SLP-76, in turn, becomes associated with ITK via the ITK SH2 domain. ITK is thus brought into proximity with membrane-localized substrates, including PLCγ1. Activation of PLCγ1 leads to hydrolysis of phosphatidylinositol 4,5-bisphosphate (PIP2) and activation of transcription factors such as nuclear factor-κB (NFκB), activating protein 1 (AP-1), and nuclear factor of activated T cells (NFAT). SH2 domain containing leukocyte phosphoprotein of 76 kDa (SLP-76) also recruits several other signaling molecules, such as VAV, NCK, HPK1, and ADAP, thereby regulating changes in the actin cytoskeleton and adhesion. Phosphorylation of linker of activated T cells (LAT) also leads to recruitment of Grb2/SOS and an additional pathway for RAS activation. TM, transmembrane domain; P-Y, sites for phosphorylation of tyrosine; pro-rich, proline-rich regions.

and in the process of terminating T-cell responses. Two adaptors critical for T-cell activation, linker of activated T cells (LAT) and SH2 domain-containing leukocyte phosphoprotein of 76 kDa (SLP-76), are described in this section.

Both LAT and SLP-76 were identified in efforts to characterize substrates of the PTKs stimulated by TCR engagement. LAT is a 36-kDa integral membrane protein that contains numerous tyrosine residues within its cytoplasmic tail (Fig. 12.5A). The tyrosines exist within the correct sequence motifs needed to bind the SH2 domains of other T-cell signaling molecules. In stimulated T cells, LAT inducibly associates with the SH2 domains of GRB2, GADS (another Grb2 family member), PLCγ1, and the p85 subunit of PI3K. It is likely that these induced intermolecular interactions are critical for communicating TCR engagement to downstream second-messenger cascades. The importance of LAT for T-cell activation was suggested by the signaling phenotype of LAT-deficient variants of the Jurkat T-cell leukemic line. Engagement of the TCR on these cells fails to result in signaling events downstream of ZAP-70 activation. Furthermore, examination of Lat-deficient mice revealed an

essential role for Lat in T-cell development. The Lat[−/−] mice have significantly decreased numbers of thymocytes, which are arrested at an early stage during development. Arrested thymocyte development leads to the complete lack of T cells in Lat[−/−] peripheral lymphoid organs. In recent *in vivo* studies, a knockin of a PLCγ1-binding mutant of Lat partially restored thymocyte development but also resulted in a lymphoproliferative phenotype in adult animals.

Using similar approaches, it was shown that SLP-76 is absolutely required for both T-cell development and signaling via the mature TCR.[10] Thus, mice deficient in SLP-76 show a complete block in thymocyte development. In mutant T-cell lines lacking SLP-76, the PLCγ1 and RAS/MAPK signaling cascades are not activated by TCR ligation, despite normal TCR-stimulated activation of Zap-70. SLP-76 contains an amino-terminal region with tyrosine phosphorylation sites, a central proline-rich domain, and a carboxyl-terminal SH2 domain. Unlike LAT, SLP-76 does not possess a transmembrane domain. By means of its proline-rich region, SLP-76 constitutively associates with the adaptor GADS, and through the SLP-76 SH2 domain can inducibly interact with other tyrosine-phosphorylated adaptors such as HPK-1 and ADAP. Following tyrosine phosphorylation, SLP-76 inducibly binds other SH2-domain-containing proteins (e.g., VAV, an exchange factor for the RAC GTP-binding protein, NCK, an adaptor protein, and ITK). Each of the SLP-76 domains appears critical for its function, as the overexpression of mutant variants of SLP-76 is unable to restore TCR signaling efficiency fully in either Jurkat T cells or SLP-76-deficient mice. In contrast, overexpression of wild-type SLP-76 dramatically augments TCR-stimulated second-messenger production.

One model of how SLP-76 and LAT functionally interact is as follows.[20] Following TCR engagement, the two adaptors associate with each other, bridged by GADS and PLCγ1. These interactions anchor a multimolecular "signalosome" at the plasma membrane (Fig. 12.5B). Formation of this complex brings Itk into proximity of PLCγ1, resulting in its phosphorylation and activation and leading to the generation of IP$_3$ and DAG, as described above.

Along with LAT and SLP-76, T cells express a large number of other adaptor proteins that appear to play important roles in promoting TCR-mediated signal transduction events. Many of these are widely expressed, and some are expressed only in hematopoietic cells. Adaptors are important for the coordination of both positive and negative aspects of TCR activation. For example, in the absence of antigen, the transmembrane adaptor PAG binds to the PTK CSK, bringing it to the plasma membrane.[21] Membrane-localized CSK phosphorylates the regulatory tyrosine of LCK, thus keeping LCK inactive. Delineating the positive and negative aspects of signal transduction mediated by subcellular localization of kinases and phosphatases is an ongoing area of active research by multiple laboratories worldwide.

Co-receptors transduce signals that are integrated with TCR signals

T-cell proliferation and the initiation of effector function require that the T cell must receive signals in addition to the TCR via other cell surface receptors.[22] This requirement for multiple signals allows the T cell to be extremely sensitive to TCR binding while protecting against the inappropriate activation of potentially dangerous effector cells. Because T cells respond to antigens presented on APCs, stimulation under physiological conditions involves the potential engagement of multiple ligand co-receptors on the T cell by various ligands on the APC. Many of these co-receptors have been characterized, and progress has been made in our understanding of how these molecules promote T-cell activation. One obvious way in which co-receptors may function is to increase the avidity of the interaction between the T cell and the APC. Interestingly, however, many co-receptors are also capable of transducing signals themselves, some independent of and others synergistic with the TCR. Additionally, co-receptors are often important as recruiters of the cytoplasmic signaling molecules and the adaptor proteins described above.

The most intensively studied co-receptors are CD4 and CD8 (Chapter 4). CD4 and CD8 expression defines subsets of T cells responding to class II or class I-bound peptide antigen, respectively (Chapter 8). Either molecule can contribute to enhanced TCR signal strength, because they each associate with LCK.[23] This constitutive interaction, which occurs via specific residues within the CD4 and CD8 cytoplasmic domains, localizes a key effector enzyme to the TCR complex.

Co-stimulatory molecules are required for optimal T-cell activation

As stated earlier, T-cell stimulation is a composite of TCR crosslinking and co-stimulatory signals. In contrast to the CD4 and CD8 co-receptors that bind to MHC molecules, other ligands on APCs interact with T-cell surface proteins termed co-stimulatory molecules. The importance of co-stimulatory molecules is implied by the large number of proteins expressed on the cell surface of T cells and the number of ligands expressed on APCs. Initially, it was thought that there is redundancy in co-stimulation, with numerous T-cell proteins capable of transducing co-stimulatory signals, each sufficient to attain an activation threshold. However, it is now clear that co-stimulatory receptor–ligand pairs differ in their expression patterns and confer diverse phenotypic responses.

The best-characterized co-stimulatory molecule present on T cells is CD28, a constitutively expressed homodimeric transmembrane glycoprotein.[24] CD28 binds to two ligands expressed on APCs, B7.1 (CD80) and B7.2 (CD86). Ligation of CD28 on its own has little effect on T-cell activation; however, when CD28 is engaged along with the TCR, many TCR signals are augmented. Indeed, concomitant CD28 and TCR engagement is required for activation of naïve T cells. Co-stimulation of the TCR plus CD28 dramatically augments IL-2 production, both by increasing transcription of the IL-2 gene and by stabilizing its mRNA. If the TCR is engaged in the absence of CD28 co-stimulation, such a stimulus leads not to activation but either to T-cell death by apoptosis (Chapter 13) or to a state of unresponsiveness known as anergy (see below).

CD28 ligation engages several signal transduction pathways implicated in T-cell activation.[25] CD28 contains no intrinsic enzymatic activity, but it is inducibly phosphorylated on tyrosine residues during T-cell activation. These phosphorylated tyrosines recruit several signal-transducing molecules possessing SH2 domains, including GRB2 and the 85-kDa subunit of PI3K. TCR- and CD28-dependent co-activation of PI3K leads to transactivation of the pro-survival genes *BCL-2* and *BCL-XL*. GRB2 association with CD28 may be important for efficient activation of the GEF VAV1. Active VAV1 can potentiate activation of PKCθ, which lies upstream of an NF-κB-dependent survival program. VAV1 may also mediate CD28-driven activation of the GTP-binding protein RAS-related C3 botulinum toxin substrate 1 (RAC1). RAC1 function is crucial for TCR-dependent activation of c-JUN N-terminal kinase (JNK), which plays an important role in CD28-dependent T-cell cytokine production and apoptosis resistance.

CD28 is the prototype member of a receptor family characterized by the presence of extracellular immunoglobulin-like domains.[24] Other family members include CTLA-4 (cytotoxic T lymphocyte-associated antigen 4), ICOS (inducible co-stimulator), PD-1 (programmed death 1), and BTLA (B- and T-lymphocyte attenuator). Cellular expression patterns and signaling functions vary drastically for molecules in this group. While CD28–B7 interactions are co-stimulatory, ligation of CTLA-4 by B7 is inhibitory (see T-cell anergy section below).

As its name implies, ICOS is not expressed on naïve cells but is induced following combined TCR and CD28 stimulation in an ERK and MAPK-dependent manner.[26] ICOS–ICOS-L interaction is required for IL-21-dependent development of T follicular helper (Tfh) cells, a subset of CD4 cells required for germinal center formation and B-cell antibody class switching. In animals treated with ICOS blocking antibodies, reduced Tfh and germinal center formation correlates with suppression of autoimmune responses in murine models of rheumatoid arthritis and multiple sclerosis. ICOS deficiency is also associated with human common variable immune deficiency (CVID) (Chapter 34).

PD-1 serves as a negative regulator of T-cell activation.[27] PD-1 antagonizes T-cell activation through attenuation of PI3K and Akt activation. Advanced live cell imaging studies suggest that PD-1 enforces T-cell tolerance (see below) by inhibiting TCR-mediated "stop signals" that promote stable, prolonged physical association between T cells and APCs in lymphoid tissue. Disruption of the PD-1 gene in mice results in autoantibody formation and glomerulonephritis. In chronic viral infections, CD8 T cells display a hyporesponsive "exhausted" phenotype associated with elevated surface expression of PD-1. Antibody blockade of PD-1/PDL-1 interactions results in restoration of effector functions in exhausted T cells. Together, these observations suggest that PD-1 may be a therapeutic target for autoimmune and/or infectious disease management.

A second large class of co-stimulatory molecules includes members of the tumor necrosis factor receptor (TNFR) family.[24] Co-stimulatory TNFR family members include OX40 (CD134), 4-1BB (CD137), herpesvirus entry mediator (HVEM), CD30, and glucocorticoid induced TNF receptor (GITR). Cytoplasmic domains within these type I transmembrane proteins contain sequences that recruit a family of adaptor molecules known as TNF receptor-associated factors (TRAFs). Antigen receptor co-stimulation functions for both CD4 and CD8 T cells have been described for each member of this family. With regard to positive regulation of T-cell signaling, the best-studied member of this group is OX40.[28] Compared with the IL-2 receptor, OX40 is upregulated on activated CD4 T cells with delayed kinetics, as peak OX40 levels occur 48 hours after CD3/CD28 stimulation. Trimerization of OX40 induced by engagement of APC-expressed OX40L leads to recruitment of TRAF2, TRAF3, and TRAF5. TRAF complexes control activation of a survival-enhancing NF-κB pathway. OX40 deficiency leads to defects in CD4 T-cell proliferation, reduced survival of effector memory T cells, and impaired formation of effective responses to secondary T-cell stimulation with antigen. Antibody-mediated blockade of OX40-OX40L results in reduced induction of experimental autoimmune responses (EAE) and collagen-induced arthritis.[28]

Spatial and temporal distribution of TCR signaling proteins

Recent methodological advances in live cell imaging and engineering of lipid bilayers that mimic physiological antigen-presenting surfaces have permitted exciting insights into the temporal-spatial relationships between signaling molecules. A highly organized interface forms between the T cell and the APC, and this interface has been termed the immunological synapse (IS). Following TCR engagement, several transmembrane and cytoplasmic proteins are coordinately polarized toward the IS and form a structure called the supramolecular activation cluster (SMAC).[29] The SMAC is composed of concentric rings with a central region (cSMAC) enriched in TCR and CD3/ζ. The more peripheral ring (pSMAC) is enriched for the integrin leukocyte function-associated antigen-1 (LFA1). Inhibitory signaling molecules such as the transmembrane phosphatase CD45 are excluded from the SMAC. These observations initially suggested that formation of the SMAC is required for signal initiation. The subsequent finding of a paucity of active signaling molecules located in the SMAC has led to alternative models in which the SMAC is involved in directed cytokine secretion or in signal termination.

Complexes composed of TCR, active kinases, and adaptor molecules termed microclusters form at the immune synapse within seconds following TCR engagement.[30] TCR microclusters are dynamically regulated in space and time. Within 2–3 minutes of formation, microclusters migrate along polymerized actin from the periphery to the center of the IS, where dephosphorylation and dissociation of the components occurs. Sustained TCR signaling depends upon constant reformation of microclusters containing SLP-76 and ZAP-70 at the periphery of the central zone. Co-stimulatory signals generated by CD28 or the integrin very late antigen-4 (VLA4) can alter the dynamics of microcluster formation and movement and enhance T-cell activation. The functions of either the SMAC or the microclusters in TCR signal initiation and termination remain incompletely understood.

> ● KEY CONCEPTS
>
> Mechanisms of tolerance can be divided into central and peripheral:
>
> **Central**
> - Clonal deletion/AIRE
>
> **Peripheral**
> - Immune privilege
> - Anergy
> - Regulation

Tolerance

Tolerance is an inherent property of the immune system that governs the ability to respond against foreign antigens (nonself) without attacking the host (self). A lack of self-tolerance leads to autoimmune disease. The immune system in any individual must therefore be able to distinguish subtle differences between self and nonself. Multiple complementary mechanisms of immune system tolerance have developed to calibrate immune responsiveness to maintain maximum protective activation capacity. The remainder of this chapter discusses tolerance in the T-cell compartment.

The concept of immune tolerance pre-dated understanding of the cellular and molecular bases for the phenomenon. Owen's experiments in cattle showed that a shared blood supply during development led to lifelong immune tolerance.[31] Billingham, Brent, and Medawar expanded upon the experiments in 1953 by showing that *in utero* inoculation with foreign tissue resulted in tolerance to foreign skin grafts later in life.[32]

Establishment of immune tolerance to self may occur either during T-lymphocyte development or after maturation in the tissues.[33] Central tolerance refers to tolerance that is induced during development of T cells in the thymus (Chapter 8). Despite the presence of mechanisms that promote expression of a full repertoire of self-peptides (see below) in the thymus, establishment of central tolerance alone is inadequate to prevent tissue damaging autoimmune responses. Some self-reactive T cells normally develop and emigrate from the thymus to the peripheral lymphoid compartment. Control of such "escaped" autoreactive cells is achieved through a series of non-thymus dependent processes; these are referred to in aggregate as peripheral tolerance.

Central tolerance/clonal deletion

The recent development of techniques and reagents capable of tracking the fate of clonal T-cell populations has allowed progress on the elucidation of molecular mechanisms of clonal deletion.[34,35] Monoclonal antibodies specific for Vβ17 TCR variable regions were used to establish the developmental timing of clonal deletion in early studies. Endogenous retrovirus-derived "self" peptides form the dominant antigens for Vβ17-bearing thymocytes. In normal murine thymus, Vβ17-expressing CD4+CD8+ [double-positive (DP)] thymocytes are present, but more mature CD4+ single-positive (CD4SP) or CD8SP are not. Absence of Vβ17-expressing mature thymocytes suggests that clonal deletion occurs at the DP to SP transition.

TCR transgenic mice expressing a single specificity TCR potentiated additional investigation into central tolerance. The majority of developing T cells in H-Y mice, the first TCR-transgenic model of clonal deletion, is reactive against a Y-chromosome-encoded antigen, H-Y. Massive deletion of these cells results in small thymi in self-antigen-expressing (male) mice with only a small number of DP thymocytes able to survive the antigen-induced cell death. In contrast, transgenic T cells develop normally in mice lacking the H-Y antigen (female). Later studies of animals engineered to express autoreactive TCR at more physiologic developmental stages have shown that clonal deletion can occur prior to, during, or after the DP stage.

Deletion for self-reactivity implies that the extent of autoreactivity of the developing thymocytes is systematically calibrated. A currently favored model is one that employs strength of signal as determined by a combination of TCR affinity and co-stimulation to assess the extent of self-reactivity.[36] Signals that go beyond a threshold of acceptability lead to clonal deletion. This model is supported by experiments in which the TCR signaling machinery has been genetically altered to increase or decrease signal intensity from each TCR. For example, an increase in the number of ITAMs (presumably leading to increases in downstream signals) enhances clonal deletion in a TCR transgenic system.[2]

For clonal deletion to establish comprehensive self-tolerance, T cells must come into contact with all potential self-antigens during thymocyte maturation. It is easy to recognize how deletion of cells reactive to MHC and other widely expressed protein products can occur in the thymus. However, there are also self-antigens whose expression is restricted to a specific tissue or developmental time point.

The complex mechanisms whereby clonal deletion of developing thymocytes reactive with tissue-restricted antigens (TRAs)— expressed only in the pancreas or testes, for example—is achieved are beginning to be unraveled. Some evidence supports the possibility that all TRAs are transported to the thymus by APCs such as migratory dendritic cells.[37] Another, non-mutually exclusive model holds that subsets of thymus-resident APCs may "ectopically" express TRAs. The leading candidate for controlling TRA expression within medullary thymic epithelial cells (mTECs) is the transcription factor AIRE (autoimmune regulator).[38] AIRE expression ectopically drives mTECs to express peptides from open reading frames. Self-reactive developing T cells are thus exposed to tissue-specific self-peptides in the thymus and are deleted. AIRE-deficient humans and mice develop autoimmune polyendocrinopathy-candidiasis-ectodermal dystrophy (APS-1 or APECED in humans; Chapter 35), emphasizing the role of central tolerance in preventing T-cell-mediated autoimmune disease.

Isolated TRA presentation by mTECs is unlikely to fully account for successful clonal deletion, given the relative rarity of mTECs in thymic stroma and the abundance of autoreactive thymocytes. One potential mechanism for enhancing exposure of autoreactive cells to deleting TRA-driven signals is antigen presentation by additional thymic stroma resident cells. In support of this model is the recent observation that intercellular transfer of TRAs between mTECs and thymic-resident or immigrant dendritic cells readily occurs.[36]

Peripheral mechanisms of tolerance

Clonal deletion, like all biological processes, is not perfect. Given the potential for autoimmune tissue damage should clonal deletion fail (as exemplified in those humans and mice carrying AIRE mutations), there must be "backup" mechanisms to control autoreactivity for those few cells that manage to escape the thymus. These mechanisms include immune privilege, anergy, and regulation.

Immune privilege

Medawar first described the concept of "immune privilege" more than 50 years ago. Typically described areas of immune privilege include the anterior chamber of the eye, the brain, and the fetus in pregnant females.[39] Both the eye and the brain have a limited capacity for regeneration, and thus uncontrolled destructive immune responses in these organs could have permanent devastating effects on individual survival fitness. As a fetus expresses MHC derived from both parents, peripheral tolerance of the mother to the fetus is required for fetal survival.

Immune privileged tissues evade or suppress immune effector functions through multiple mechanisms. Cells of the eye, brain, and the fetal villous trophoblast display low level or absent surface expression of classical MHC class Ia protein. This feature likely protects them from CTL-mediated lysis (Chapter 17). Ocular cells express pro-apoptotic cell surface molecules such as FAS ligand (FASL) and TRAIL (Chapter 13). These TNF family members may contribute to apoptosis of infiltrating T and other inflammatory cells bearing "death receptors." In mice, the presence of FasL on ocular cells is critical in the acceptance of corneal allografts. Soluble factors elaborated by ocular dendritic cells likely contribute to immune privilege. These include the cytokines TGFβ and IL-10, which may lead to induction and or recruitment of T regulatory cells (Tregs), and migration inhibitory factor (MIF) that suppresses NK-cell-dependent cytolytic capacity. In addition, ocular dendritic cells may produce high levels of indoleamine oxidase, an enzyme that supports Treg differentiation.

T-cell anergy

Cellular proliferation and/or potentiation of T-cell effector function are not inevitable consequences of TCR engagement. In fact, under some conditions TCR ligation results in anergy, a cellular fate characterized by reduced proliferation and cytokine production in response to subsequent TCR engagement.[40] T-cell anergy can ensue either when the TCR is engaged without concomitant co-stimulation or when the ligand for the TCR is not of sufficient affinity to initiate the full spectrum of biochemical second messengers. This phenomenon was first noted by stimulating T cells in the presence of metabolically inactivated APCs. Subsequently, it was shown that CD28 co-stimulation could prevent the induction of anergy. Interestingly, supplementation of cultures with IL-2 can overcome the anergic state *in vitro*. In addition to TCR and co-stimulatory signals, recent work has shown that environmental cues such as nutrient and energy store availability and the products of regulatory T cells (described below) also control the anergy/activation fate choice.

T-cell anergy can be induced by activation of the calcineurin/NFAT pathway without concomitant increases in the RAS/ERK pathway-dependent activating protein 1 (AP-1) transcription factor activity (Fig. 12.6A). Relatively unopposed NFAT activity can be induced experimentally either by treatment with calcium ionophore or stimulation through the TCR while blocking CD28 co-stimulation. Concurrent treatment of TCR-stimulated cells with protein synthesis inhibitors or with NFAT pathway inhibitors, such as cyclosporine, abrogates the development of later unresponsiveness, supporting the notion that anergy induction

and maintenance depends upon transcription and translation of anergy-associated factors.[41]

Numerous biochemical and gene regulatory events correlate with observed inhibition of Ras pathway function in anergized versus fully activated T cells (Fig. 12.6B).[42] First, preferential FYN kinase-dependent activation of c-CBL within anergized cells leads to recruitment of the RAF kinase to the nucleotide exchange factor RAP1. The RAF-RAP1 association prevents RAF recruitment to RAS, and thus engenders reduced ERK pathway activation. Second, upregulation of NFAT-dependent transcription factors EGR2 and EGR3 results in transactivation of proteins implicated in the restraint of T-cell activation, including GRAIL, CBL-b, and ITCH.[41] E3 ubiquitin

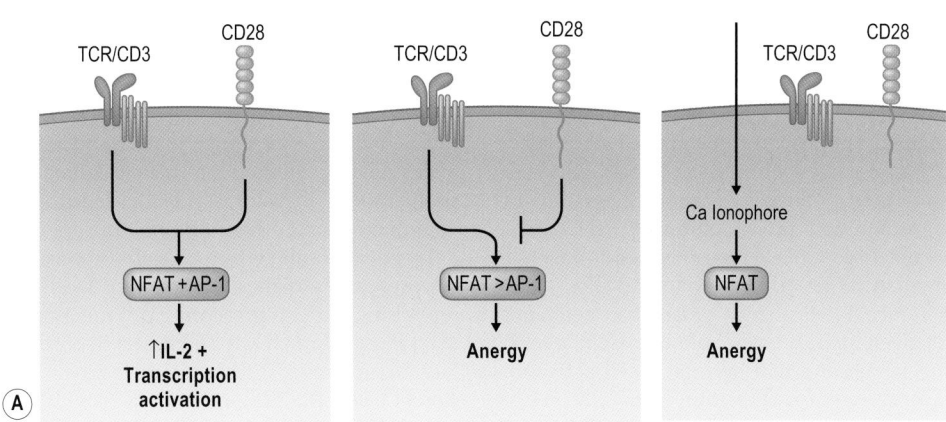

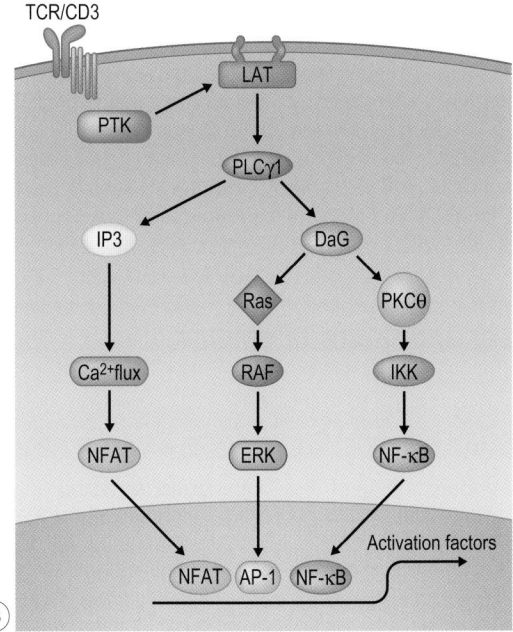

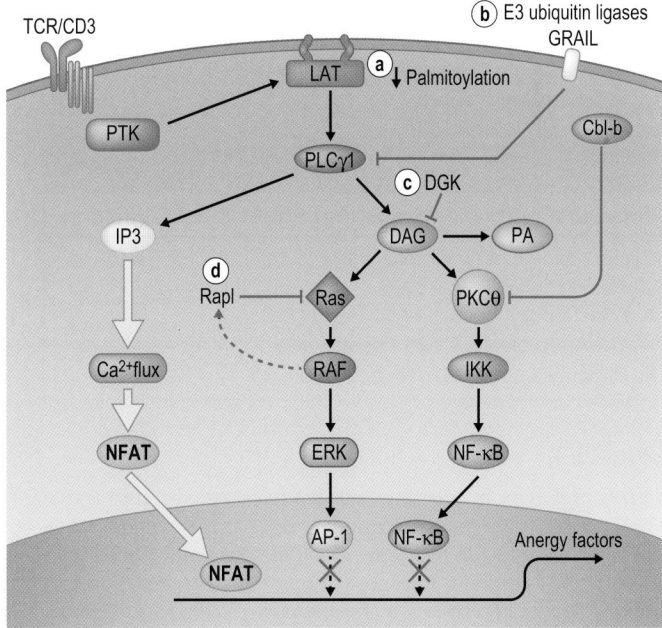

Fig. 12.6 T-cell anergy induction and maintenance correlates with differential activation of TCR-dependent second-messenger signaling cascades. (A) Stimulation of T cells by cross-linking of both T-cell receptor (TCR)/CD3 and CD28 lead to upregulation of both the nuclear factor of activated T cells (NFAT) and activating protein 1 (AP-1) transcription factors, leading to increased transcription of the interleukin-2 (IL-2) gene and activation. An imbalance of activated NFAT and AP-1 by blockade of CD28 signals (middle) or calcium ionophore (right panel) leads to an anergic phenotype. (B) TCR signaling required for full T cell activation features Calcium flux-, Ras-, and PKC-dependent biochemical events leading to cooperative transcriptional regulation by NFAT, AP-1, and NF-κb transcription factors (left panel). In anergized cells, TCR-dependent signaling is differentially impaired (DAG-dependent events more so than Calcium-dependent events) through multiple mechanisms: a) decreased palmitoylation of LAT results in diminished recruitment to the immunological synapse, b) upregulated GRAIL and CBL-b degrade positive signaling regulators PLCγ1 and PKCθ, c) Diacylglyerol kinases (DGK) convert DAG (PKC and RAS activator) to phosphatidic acid (PA); d) active RAP1 recruits RAF, thus preventing RAS-mediated signaling to ERK. Anergy mechanisms and mediators are highlighted in red.

ligase activity associated with a number of these factors is responsible for ubiquitin-mediated proteolysis of TCR signal-promoting molecules such as PKCθ and RAS-GRP. Third, post-translational modification of the positive TCR signaling mediator LAT is also observed in anergy.[43] As described above, LAT is normally palmitoylated and its membrane localization restricted to detergent-insoluble lipid rafts. In previously anergized T cells, however, LAT palmitoylation and phosphorylation are both decreased. Fourth, anergy-associated increased expression of members of the diacylglycerol kinase family (DGKα and DGKζ) represents augmented capacity for phosphorylation-dependent conversion of DAG, the key lipid mediator upstream of RAS and NF-κB signaling, into phosphatidic acid (PA), an inactive compound with respect to ERK pathway activation.[12]

Cellular sensing of adequate nutrient and energy stores required for optimal differentiation and proliferation regulates the anergy/activation T-cell fate decision. The importance of amino acid- and energy-sensing pathways was suggested by observations that anergy is induced in T cells activated in the presence of antagonists to leucine or glucose, despite the presence of robust combined antigen receptor and co-stimulatory pathway signaling.[40] Several lines of evidence suggest that establishment of "metabolic anergy" after integration of signaling inputs from antigen recognition (TCR), immune (CD28, IL-2 receptor), and metabolic (e.g., GLUT1) receptors and sensors is governed by mammalian target of rapamycin (mTOR).[44] TCR and CD28 ligation induce T-cell anergy rather than activation when the stimuli are given in the presence of rapamycin, a selective mTOR inhibitor, suggesting that optimal T-cell activation and avoidance of anergy requires activation of mTOR. mTOR is activated by signals that communicate abundant nutrients (e.g., leucine-stimulated RAG proteins). Conversely, mTOR is inhibited by activated AMPK, an enzyme that responds to low energy stores reflected by increased AMP:ATP ratios. Through mediators such as AKT, mTOR activation functions to promote cell cycle entry and prevent transcriptional activation of anergy factors GRAIL and CBL-b.

KEY CONCEPTS

Immunosuppressive drugs that affect T-cell signaling

Cyclosporine and tacrolimus inhibit T-cell receptor (TCR)-generated signals:
- Anti-TCR antibodies block TCR signals
- CTLA-4Ig blocks CD28 signals
- Rapamycin inhibits mTor activation

Regulation

Subsets of T lymphocytes can enforce tolerance through active regulation of autoreactive immune responses. So-called Tregs can suppress effector functions of other immune cells of both myeloid and lymphoid lineages (Chapter 15). Proliferation and cytokine production by naïve and memory T cells constitute the most extensively studied immune functions that are susceptible to Tregs, which inhibit these processes through both cell contact-dependent and soluble molecule secretion mechanisms.[45] By regulating the activation and proliferation of antigen-specific effectors, Tregs promote tolerance to self and suppress autoimmunity *in vivo*.

Identification of Tregs was initially described based on correlation between potent suppressive activity and the co-expression of CD4 and high levels of CD25. Most Tregs also express GITR,

CD103, CTLA-4, lymphocyte activation gene 3 (LAG-3), and low levels of CD45RB. However, there remains no single surface marker that is entirely specific for Tregs. That Treg suppressive capacity does reflect a unique CD4 T-cell differentiation pathway is strongly suggested by findings that expression of the transcription factor Foxp3 correlates tightly with regulatory capacity in mice.[46] The absence of Foxp3 either through spontaneous mutation (exemplified by the *scurfy* mouse) or through targeted disruption of the gene leads to the complete loss of T cells with regulatory activity. Conditional deletion of Foxp3 in peripheral T cells results in loss of the suppressive phenotype. Conversely, overexpression of Foxp3 by transgenesis or retroviral methods leads to an excess of T cells with regulatory activity, strongly suggesting that FoxP3 is both necessary and sufficient for Treg suppressive functions. Inducible Foxp3 expression and development of suppressive capacity can be observed in naïve CD4 T cells after exposure to TGFβ or retinoic acid, but the physiologic relevance of inducible Treg *in vivo* remains unclear.[47]

In humans, mutations in *FOXP3* account for a majority of cases of immune dysfunction/polyendocrinopathy/enteropathy/X-linked (IPEX) syndrome. The signs and symptoms of FOXP3-deficient disease are similar in mice and humans. Affected human males develop an autoimmune syndrome consisting of lymphoproliferation, thyroiditis, insulin-dependent diabetes mellitus, enteropathy, and other immune disorders.

Tregs can inhibit effector T-cell responses through secretion of suppressive cytokines, induction of T-cell apoptosis, or through repressing antigen presenting cell function.[45] Key Treg-secreted cytokines include IL-10, TGFβ, and IL-35; each of these molecules has the capacity to induce cell cycle arrest. Tregs, via high expression of CD25 (IL-2Rα), may compete with neighboring T effector cells for limited supplies of IL-2. The resulting growth factor deprivation can kill proliferating T cells in a BIM-dependent manner. Tregs preferentially express Galectin-1, a β-galactoside binding protein that ligates CD45 and other lymphocyte surface molecules and that may suppress lymphocyte activation through induction of cell cycle arrest. Treg surface proteins that work to effectively decrease efficiency of antigen presentation by dendritic cells include CTLA-4, which interferes with CD28-dependent T-cell costimulation, LAG3, which binds to MHC class II molecules and prevents dendritic cell maturation, and Nrp1, which mediates prolonged Treg/DC interactions that may restrict access of effector T cells to the DC.

Summary and future directions

ON THE HORIZON

- Better understanding of T-cell intracellular signaling pathways should lead to improved, immunomodulatory therapies.
- Promising targets of current investigation include:
  - Positive and negative aspects of signal transduction mediated by subcellular localization of kinases and phosphatases.
  - Modulation of the negative regulator of T-cell activation PD-1 in management of autoimmunity and infectious diseases.

Antigen receptor signaling controls key T cell developmental checkpoints as well as mature T cell fate and behavior decisions. Membrane-proximal TCR signaling depends upon tyrosine phosphorylation events that are coupled to "second messenger" cascades through adaptor proteins. TCR affinity for ligand is the major determinant for life or death decisions by immature thymocytes that result in establishment of a broadly self-tolerant mature T cell repertoire. In peripheral T cells, auxiliary signals from co-stimulatory molecules, co-receptors, growth factor receptors, and metabolic sensors each shape the transcriptional regulation programs that govern cell function. T cells proliferate and produce cytokines when members of the CD28 or TNFR families of receptors signal in tandem with the TCR. Immunoreceptor and costimulatory signals are also critical in maintaining immune tolerance through clonal deletion, anergy, and peripheral suppression by regulatory T cells. Better understanding of T cell intracellular signaling pathways will lead to improved, targeted immunomodulatory therapies.

References

1. Weiss A, Littman DR. Signal transduction by lymphocyte antigen receptors. Cell 1994;76(2):263–74.
2. Guy CS, Vignali DA. Organization of proximal signal initiation at the TCR:CD3 complex. Immunol Rev 2009;232(1):7–21.
3. Salmond RJ, Filby A, Qureshi I, et al. T-cell receptor proximal signaling via the Src-family kinases, Lck and Fyn, influences T-cell activation, differentiation, and tolerance. Immunol Rev 2009;228(1):9–22.
4. Mustelin T, Vang T, Bottini N. Protein tyrosine phosphatases and the immune response. Nat Rev Immunol 2005;5(1):43–57.
5. Hermiston ML, Xu Z, Weiss A. CD45: a critical regulator of signaling thresholds in immune cells. Annu Rev Immunol 2003;21:107–37.
6. Abraham RT, Weiss A. Jurkat T cells and development of the T-cell receptor signalling paradigm. Nat Rev Immunol 2004;4(4):301–8.
7. Buckley RH. Primary immunodeficiency diseases due to defects in lymphocytes. N Engl J Med 2000;343(18):1313–24.
8. Readinger JA, Mueller KL, Venegas AM, et al. Tec kinases regulate T-lymphocyte development and function: new insights into the roles of Itk and Rlk/Txk. Immunol Rev 2009;228(1):93–114.
9. Huck K, Feyen O, Niehues T, et al. Girls homozygous for an IL-2-inducible T cell kinase mutation that leads to protein deficiency develop fatal EBV-associated lymphoproliferation. J Clin Invest 2009;119(5):1350–8.
10. Smith-Garvin JE, Koretzky GA, Jordan MS. T cell activation. Annu Rev Immunol 2009;27:591–619.
11. Oh-hora M, Rao A. Calcium signaling in lymphocytes. Curr Opin Immunol 2008;20(3):250–8.
12. Zhong XP, Guo R, Zhou H, et al. Diacylglycerol kinases in immune cell function and self-tolerance. Immunol Rev 2008;224:249–64.
13. Burbach BJ, Medeiros RB, Mueller KL, Shimizu Y. T-cell receptor signaling to integrins. Immunol Rev 2007;218:65–81.
14. Roose JP, Mollenauer M, Gupta VA, et al. A diacylglycerol-protein kinase C-RasGRP1 pathway directs Ras activation upon antigen receptor stimulation of T cells. Mol Cell Biol 2005;25(11):4426–41.
15. Das J, Ho M, Zikherman J, et al. Digital signaling and hysteresis characterize ras activation in lymphoid cells. Cell 2009;136(2):337–51.
16. Deane JA, Fruman DA. Phosphoinositide 3-kinase: diverse roles in immune cell activation. Annu Rev Immunol 2004;22:563–98.
17. Thome M, Charton JE, Pelzer C, Hailfinger S. Antigen receptor signaling to NF-kappaB via CARMA1, BCL10, and MALT1. Cold Spring Harb Perspect Biol 2010;2(9):a003004.
18. Jordan MS, Singer AL, Koretzky GA. Adaptors as central mediators of signal transduction in immune cells. Nat Immunol 2003;4(2):110–6.
19. Balagopalan L, Coussens NP, Sherman E, et al. The LAT story: a tale of cooperativity, coordination, and choreography. Cold Spring Harb Perspect Biol 2010;2(8): a005512.
20. Koretzky GA, Abtahian F, Silverman MA. SLP76 and SLP65: complex regulation of signalling in lymphocytes and beyond. Nat Rev Immunol 2006;6(1):67–78.
21. Simeoni L, Lindquist JA, Smida M, et al. Control of lymphocyte development and activation by negative regulatory transmembrane adapter proteins. Immunol Rev 2008;224:215–28.
22. Nurieva RI, Liu X, Dong C. Yin-Yang of costimulation: crucial controls of immune tolerance and function. Immunol Rev 2009;229(1):88–100.
23. Artyomov MN, Lis M, Devadas S, et al. CD4 and CD8 binding to MHC molecules primarily acts to enhance Lck delivery. Proc Natl Acad Sci USA 2010;107(39):16916–21.
24. Sharpe AH. Mechanisms of costimulation. Immunol Rev 2009;229(1):5–11.
25. Rudd CE, Taylor A, Schneider H. CD28 and CTLA-4 coreceptor expression and signal transduction. Immunol Rev 2009;229(1):12–26.
26. Simpson TR, Quezada SA, Allison JP. Regulation of CD4 T cell activation and effector function by inducible costimulator (ICOS). Curr Opin Immunol 2010;22(3):326–32.
27. Fife BT, Pauken KE. The role of the PD-1 pathway in autoimmunity and peripheral tolerance. Ann N Y Acad Sci 2011;1217:45–59.
28. Croft M. Control of immunity by the TNFR-related molecule OX40 (CD134). Annu Rev Immunol 2010;28:57–78.
29. Dustin ML, Chakraborty AK, Shaw AS. Understanding the structure and function of the immunological synapse. Cold Spring Harb Perspect Biol 2010;2(10): a002311.
30. Yokosuka T, Saito T. Dynamic regulation of T-cell costimulation through TCR-CD28 microclusters. Immunol Rev 2009;229(1):27–40.
31. Owen RD. Immunogenetic consequences of vascular anastomoses between bovine twins. Science 1945;102(2651):400–1.
32. Billingham RE, Brent L, Medawar PB. Actively acquired tolerance of foreign cells. Nature 1953;172(4379):603–6.
33. Singh NJ, Schwartz RH. Primer: mechanisms of immunologic tolerance. Nat Clin Pract Rheumatol 2006;2(1):44–52.
34. von Boehmer H, Kisielow P. Negative selection of the T-cell repertoire: where and when does it occur? Immunol Rev 2006;209:284–9.
35. Gallegos AM, Bevan MJ. Central tolerance: good but imperfect. Immunol Rev 2006;209:290–6.
36. Klein L, Hinterberger M, Wirnsberger G, Kyewski B. Antigen presentation in the thymus for positive selection and central tolerance induction. Nat Rev Immunol 2009;9(12):833–44.
37. Bonasio R, Scimone ML, Schaerli P, et al. Clonal deletion of thymocytes by circulating dendritic cells homing to the thymus. Nat Immunol 2006;7(10):1092–100.
38. Taniguchi RT, Anderson MS. The role of Aire in clonal selection. Immunol Cell Biol 2011;89(1):40–4.
39. Forrester JV, Xu H, Lambe T, Cornall R. Immune privilege or privileged immunity? Mucosal Immunol 2008;1(5):372–81.
40. Chappert P, Schwartz RH. Induction of T cell anergy: integration of environmental cues and infectious tolerance. Curr Opin Immunol 2010;22(5):552–9.
41. Mueller DL. Mechanisms maintaining peripheral tolerance. Nat Immunol 2010;11(1):21–7.
42. Saibil SD, Deenick EK, Ohashi PS. The sound of silence: modulating anergy in T lymphocytes. Curr Opin Immunol 2007;19(6):658–64.
43. Hundt M, Tabata H, Jeon MS, et al. Impaired activation and localization of LAT in anergic T cells as a consequence of a selective palmitoylation defect. Immunity 2006;24(5):513–22.
44. Powell JD, Delgoffe GM. The mammalian target of rapamycin: linking T cell differentiation, function, and metabolism. Immunity 2010;33(3):301–11.
45. Shevach EM. Mechanisms of foxp3 + T regulatory cell-mediated suppression. Immunity 2009;30(5):636–45.
46. Littman DR, Rudensky AY. Th17 and regulatory T cells in mediating and restraining inflammation. Cell 2010;140(6):845–58.
47. Sakaguchi S, Miyara M, Costantino CM, Hafler DA. FOXP3 + regulatory T cells in the human immune system. Nat Rev Immunol 2010;10(7):490–500.

Helen C. Su,
Andrew L. Snow,
Michael J.
Lenardo

Programmed cell death in lymphocytes and associated disorders

Normal immune cell homeostasis reflects a dynamic balance between cell proliferation and cell death.[1] During the first week following an immune response to pathogen, antigen-specific lymphocyte cell numbers will increase 100- to 5000-fold. As the infection resolves, the majority of these expanded clones will die with up to a twenty-fold decrease in the first month.

Mechanisms of programmed cell death have evolved to counterbalance cell proliferation because immunological space is limited. For example, during antigen encounter individual clones must compete with other lymphocytes for access to the antigen on antigen presenting cells, to co-stimulatory signals and to cytokines. The presence of previously expanded lymphocytes could thus potentially hinder efficient immune responses to new antigens. A failure to remove senescent, damaged, or autoreactive cells can also predispose to autoimmunity or neoplasia.

Genetic programs of cell death are highly conserved and contribute to the proper development of both immune and non-immune organ systems.[2] These mechanisms of programmed cell death are necessary for the development and function of both T cells and B cells.[3,4] This chapter focuses on mechanisms of programmed cell death that operate in mature lymphocytes as revealed by studies of humans with rare genetic disorders. For further details, we refer readers to several recent reviews.[5-7]

Forms of programmed cell death

Forms of programmed cell death include necrosis, apoptosis and autophagy. Necrosis, which induces a local inflammatory reaction, is characterized by cell swelling, an apparent disorganized breakdown of organelles, and plasma membrane rupture and leakage (Fig. 13.1).[8] It can be induced by many stimuli, including hypoxia, mechanical damage, and chemicals.

Autophagy is a catabolic process. It features characteristic double-membrane vacuoles. Autophagy normally occurs as a survival response during cellular starvation.

Apoptosis literally means "falling off," as of leaves or petals. Morphologically, apoptotic cells exhibit shrinkage, rounding, vacuolar and vesicular formation, nuclear condensation with fragmentation, membrane blebbing, and a breakdown into apoptotic bodies containing nuclear fragments and intact organelles (Fig. 13.1).[8] *In vivo*, apoptotic bodies are rapidly engulfed by phagocytes, thus preventing an inflammatory response. Apoptotic cells can also undergo secondary necrosis, especially when death outpaces phagocytosis. Although usually thought to be an "accidental" form of death, necrosis can be a form of programmed cell death initiated when apoptosis is blocked. Programmed necrosis may promote innate immunity during infections with certain pathogens.

KEY CONCEPTS

Apoptosis

- Programmed cell death is a normal physiologic process of mature peripheral lymphocytes.
  - The best characterized form of programmed cell death is apoptosis.
- The signaling pathway for apoptosis is conserved among worms, mice, and humans.
- Apoptosis can proceed through an extrinsic pathway involving death receptors, or an intrinsic pathway involving mitochondria (Fig. 13.2).
  - Both pathways activate caspases in an intracellular enzymatic cascade that leads to the morphological features of cell death.
- Actively cycling lymphocytes are most susceptible to death.
  - Excess antigen can induce apoptosis via death receptors.
  - Limited antigen levels can lead to cytokine withdrawal, which can in turn induce apoptosis.
- Lymphocyte and dendritic cell apoptosis serves to maintain tolerance and prevent autoimmunity.

Apoptosis signaling pathways

Basic components of a conserved signaling pathway for apoptosis were first identified genetically in the nematode *Caenorhabditis elegans*.[2] During *C. elegans* development, 131 of the 1090 cells generated disappear in the adult animal. Several key genes—*ced-3*, *ced-4*, *ced-9*, and *egl-1*—control the death of these cells. These genes have mammalian homologs: caspases, APAF-1, BCL-2, and BH3-only proteins of the BCL-2 family, respectively. Both the worm proteins, and their human homologs, link to form a signaling pathway in which CED-3 kills, CED-4 promotes CED-3 killing, CED-9 blocks CED-4, and EGL-1 in turn blocks CED-9.

The outcome—apoptosis—hinges critically upon its last step, activation of caspases. These key enzymes are cysteinyl proteases that cleave after specific aspartyl residues. Although certain caspases participate in pro-inflammatory cytokine maturation, the rest participate in apoptosis induction. Caspases exist in the cytoplasm as inactive zymogens. The key to their regulation is proteolytic processing and rearrangement of their conformation into a highly active form. Various stimuli can trigger the formation of signaling platforms that are anchored by either mitochondria-derived proteins or death receptors. Oligomerization into these stoichiometric activation complexes activates initiator caspases, which then cleave and activate effector caspases.

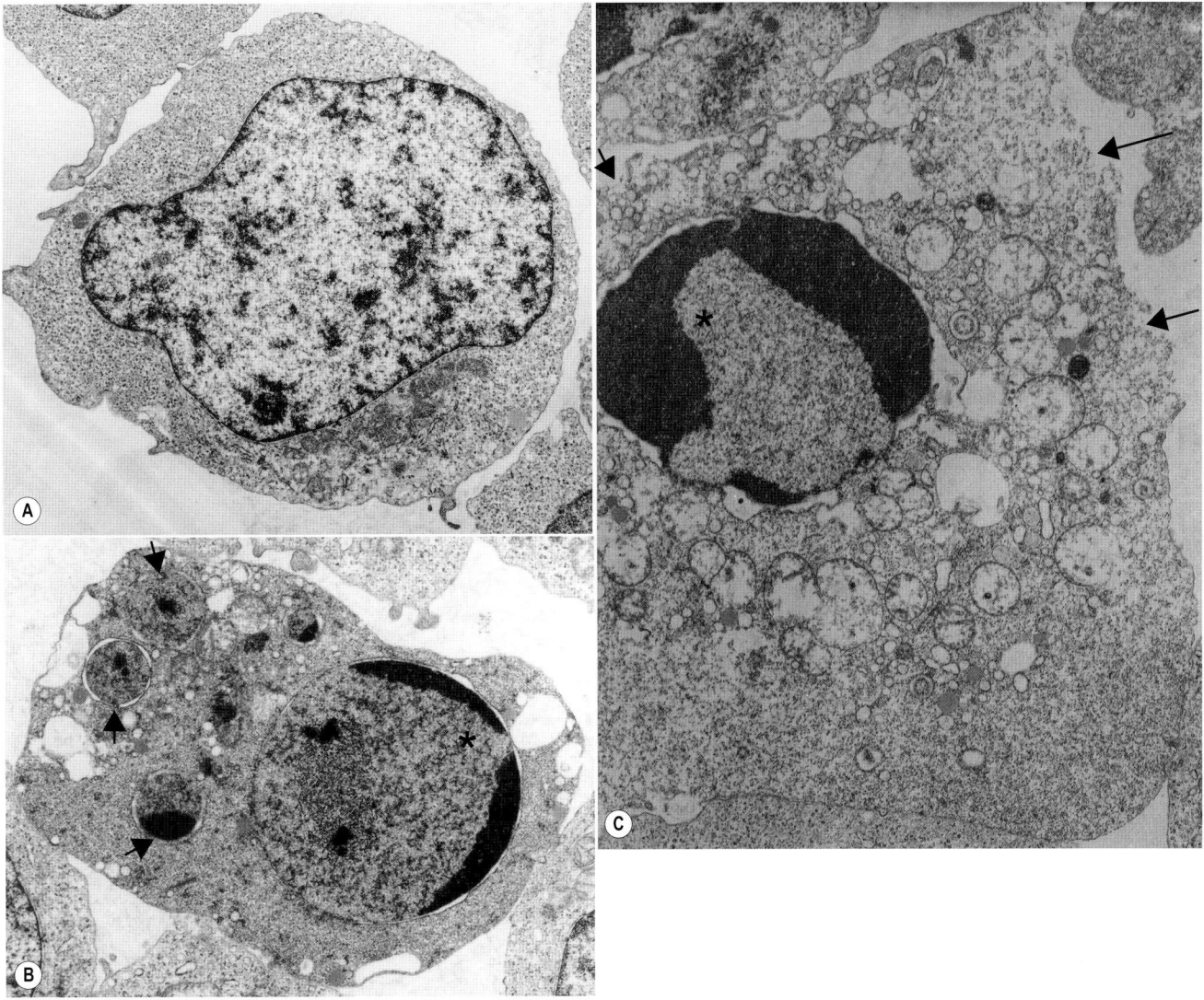

Fig. 13.1 Transmission electron micrographs showing morphologic features of dying Jurkat T cells. (A) A normal cell is shown for comparison. The apoptotic cell in (B) is shrunken and displays chromatin condensation (asterisk at electron dense crescent) and many apoptotic bodies (arrows). Membrane blebbing is not seen in this image. The necrotic cell in (C) is swollen and displays numerous disintegrated organelles and disruption of its plasma membrane (arrows). The chromatin condensation (asterisk) is consistent with secondary necrosis occurring during late apoptosis.
Courtesy of Dr. Lixin Zheng, NIAID, NIH.

Effector caspases cleave protein substrates that help to repair DNA, maintain the integrity of plasma membrane and subcellular organelle compartments, and form part of the architecture of the nucleus and the cytoskeleton. Proteolysis of these substrates presumably leads to the morphologic changes seen in apoptosis.

In mammals, two principal pathways initiate apoptosis (Fig. 13.2). The intrinsic (mitochondrial) pathway mirrors the core signaling pathway elucidated in nematodes. The extrinsic (death receptor) pathway proceeds separately and is not found in simple invertebrates. Both pathways lead to caspase activation.

Intrinsic (mitochondrial) pathway

Many physiologically important stimuli trigger the intrinsic pathway of apoptosis. These include negative selection of T cells during thymic education, growth factor or cytokine deprivation, DNA damage, and treatment with cytotoxic drugs such as chemotherapeutic agents. Proteins of the B-cell lymphoma 2 (BCL-2)

family control the intrinsic pathway.[9] The fine balance between the levels and activation status of the pro- and anti-apoptotic members of this family determines the cell's fate. Structurally, all members of the BCL-2 family share one or more of the four known BCL-2 homology regions (BH). The pro-survival members share three or four BH regions and include BCL-2, BCL-X$_L$, and MCL-1. The pro-apoptotic members, which have two or three BH regions, structurally resemble their prosurvival relatives, and include BAX and BAK. Finally, a subgroup of pro-apoptotic members named "BH3-only" proteins contain only one BH region. This subgroup includes BAD, BID, BIM, NOXA, and PUMA/BBC3.

The most accepted current model of how these proteins control the intrinsic apoptosis pathway is illustrated in Fig. 13.2. The BH3-only proteins seem to act as sensors for different apoptotic stimuli. For example, BIM serves as a sensor for growth factor withdrawal, whereas PUMA senses DNA damage. Activated BH3-only proteins bind and sequester anti-apoptotic BCL-2 members, and then induce the translocation of the pro-apoptotic protein BAX from the cytosol to the mitochondria where it clusters

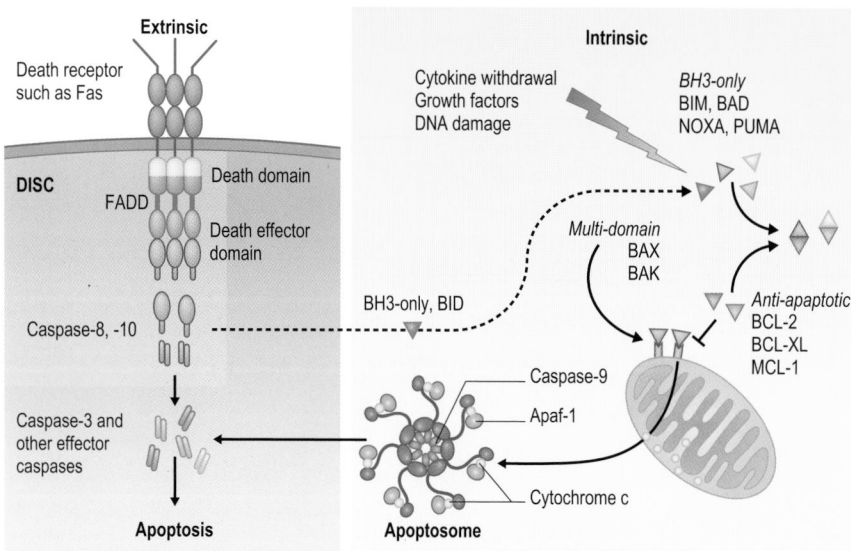

Fig. 13.2 Extrinsic and intrinsic signaling pathways for apoptosis. Two pathways exist for activating the effector caspases for lymphocyte apoptosis induction and propriocidal regulation. The extrinsic pathway activates initiator caspases-8 and -10 in death-inducing signaling complexes (DISC) anchored by death receptors. The intrinsic pathway activates initiator caspase-9 within the apoptosome. This structure is assembled when mitochondria are permeabilized. BCL-2 family members either facilitate or antagonize mitochondrial permeability and can link the intrinsic to the extrinsic pathway. See text for more details.

with BAK. This leads to pore formation in the outer mitochondrial membrane, loss of inner mitochondrial transmembrane potential, and the release of several apoptotic proteins such as SMAC/DIABLO, apoptosis inducing factor (AIF), and cytochrome c. Released cytochrome c oligomerizes in the cytosol with APAF-1 and procaspase-9 to form a Ca^{2+}- and ATP-dependent caspase-9-activating complex called the apoptosome. Once activated within this complex, the initiator caspase-9 cleaves and activates downstream effector caspases such as caspase-3, leading to cell death. Anti-apoptotic BCL-2 members may promote survival by binding BAX and inducing its retro-translocation from the mitochondria back to the cytosol, preserving mitochondrial integrity and cell survival.

Extrinsic (death receptor) pathway

Apoptosis can be triggered by extracellular signals that activate cell surface death receptors of the tumor necrosis factor (TNF) receptor superfamily.[7,10] Members of this superfamily exist as pre-assembled trimers and include the prototypical death receptor Fas (CD95, or Apo1) and TNFR1. Death receptors have cytoplasmic death domains (DD), which bind to DD-containing adaptor molecules through homotypic interactions (Fig. 13.2). The adaptor molecule FADD is crucial for signal transduction because it also possesses a death effector domain (DED). This domain enables FADD to bind homotypically to the initiator caspases-8/10, which also contain DED. Upon receptor-ligand binding, recruitment of caspases-8/10 into the large death-inducing signaling complex (DISC) causes their oligomerization and enzymatic activation. Clusters of DISC form higher order signaling protein oligomerization transduction structures (SPOTS), which promote further caspase activation leading to cell death.

The extrinsic pathway can feed into the intrinsic pathway to amplify signals for death.[11] Activated caspase-8 can cleave BID, a pro-apoptotic BH3-only BCL-2 family member analogous to the *C. elegans egl-1* gene. Truncated BID improves the binding of the pro-apoptotic multi-domain BAX and BAK proteins to mitochondrial membranes, increasing mitochondrial permeability. Cells that depend upon this mitochondrial amplification for death-receptor mediated death include peripheral blood lymphocytes. By contrast, other cell types that exhibit more efficient

DISC formation for caspase-8 and downstream caspase-3 activation die independently of mitochondrial involvement.

Engagement of death receptors can trigger cellular responses other than death. For example, Fas stimulation also activates the transcription factor NF-κB and mitogen-activated protein kinases (MAPK) p38 and ERK1/2. Activation of these signaling pathways can counterbalance signals for death. However, Fas mutations generally impair death signals more readily than growth-promoting signals.

Lymphocyte death during an immune response

Mature peripheral lymphocytes vary in their susceptibility to apoptosis. Resting cells and cells undergoing initial activation are typically refractory to death, allowing them to respond to antigenic challenge. However, once cells proliferate and enter the late G1/S phase of the cell cycle, their sensitivity to death increases. The acquisition of death sensitivity occurs at the height of an ongoing immune response and at its conclusion. Thus, lymphocytes possess a built-in rheostat that can regulate cell death as a function of the rapidity by which the cells are progressing through the cell cycle.[4]

The sensitivity of lymphocytes to antigen-driven cell death during an immune response, termed propriocidal regulation, is a major negative feedback mechanism that can be used to control the intensity of immune responses.[4,6] Two events contribute to antigen receptor restimulation-induced propriocidal death (Fig. 13.3). First, high levels of antigen stimulate the production of high levels of interleukin (IL)-2, which drives lymphocytes into cell cycle. Cells respond by undergoing molecular changes that render them susceptible to the extrinsic pathway or "active" apoptosis. This process may involve increased Fas expression and downregulation of anti-apoptotic molecules such as c-FLIP, but once the Fas receptor is engaged the process is independent of new protein or mRNA synthesis. As a consequence, T and B lymphocytes are triggered to die when their Fas receptors interact with membrane-bound, but not soluble, FasL.[12] CD8 cells also die when triggered through their TNF receptors. In addition, the antigen receptor appears to directly connect to the pro-apoptotic molecule BIM. This mechanism helps limit the magnitude of the immune response, protecting the host in the presence of continuous or repeated antigenic stimulation.

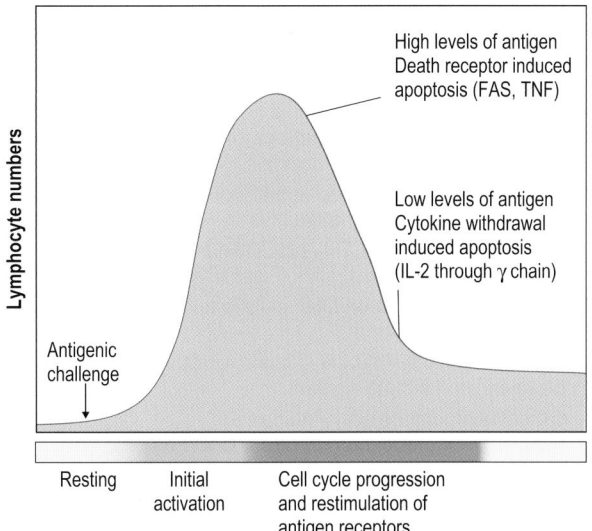

Fig. 13.3 Propriocidal regulation of actively cycling lymphocytes involves apoptosis induced primarily through (1) death receptors at the height of the immune response, and (2) upon cytokine withdrawal at the end of the response.

The second mechanism contributing to death of lymphocytes occurs when an immune response wanes (Fig. 13.3). A falling level of antigen markedly decreases the amount of IL-2 produced. This in turn decreases CD25—a component of the high affinity IL-2 receptor complex the expression of which is IL-2-dependent—and renders the cells increasingly non-responsive to IL-2. Cytokine withdrawal drives the intrinsic pathway of apoptosis in a process that requires new protein and mRNA synthesis. Death can be blocked by addition of common γ chain receptor cytokines besides IL-2, such as IL-4, -7, and -15, or by overexpressing anti-apoptotic BCL-2/BCL-X$_L$ proteins that restrain apoptosis at the mitochondria. This mechanism facilitates contraction of the immune response following pathogen elimination.

Thus, actively cycling lymphocytes die by means of mechanisms that involve antigen receptor-induced death. These mechanisms, mediated partly by death receptors Fas and TNF, and partly by cytokine withdrawal, act to limit the magnitude and duration of an immune response by eliminating activated cells.

In vivo importance of apoptosis

Apoptosis is a normal physiological process that maintains immunologic tolerance and prevents development of autoimmunity.[7,13] *Lpr* (lymphoproliferation) is an immune phenotype first noted in mice with a loss of function mutation in *Fas*. Homozygous mutant *lpr* mice develop splenomegaly and lymphadenopathy. Depending upon the genetic background, they also develop hypergammaglobulinemia, autoantibodies, glomerulonephritis, polyarteritis, sialoadenitis, arthritis, or primary biliary cirrhosis. Similar disease features are seen in mice with the *gld* (generalized lymphoproliferative disease) phenotype, which results from a homozygous loss of function mutation in Fas ligand (*FasL*). Furthermore, when the Fas death receptor pathway is selectively blocked in dendritic cells, dendritic cell numbers and antigen presenting cell (APC) function are enhanced, and disease is surprisingly severe. The death of

dendritic cells, acting in concert with propriocidal death of lymphocytes, may thus enforce tolerance and prevent autoimmunity *in vivo*.

● CLINICAL RELEVANCE

- Genetic impairment of lymphocyte apoptosis is the cause of the autoimmune lymphoproliferative syndrome (ALPS).
- Mutations in *TNFRSF6* *(FAS)* underlie most cases of ALPS.
  - A proportion of ALPS is caused by somatic *FAS* mutations affecting DNT cells, sometimes in addition to germline *FAS* mutations.
  - A minority of ALPS is caused by mutations in *TNFSF6* (Fas ligand) or *CASP10* (caspase 10).
  - These mutations all impair the Fas-mediated extrinsic pathway of apoptosis.
  - Most are dominant interfering because they prevent formation of an effective death-inducing signaling complex (DISC).
- ALPS predisposes to autoimmunity and lymphomas.
  - The most typical autoimmune findings are autoantibodies, Coombs positive hemolytic anemia, or chronic idiopathic thrombocytopenic purpura.
  - Hodgkin and non-Hodgkin lymphomas both occur.
- Mutations in other components of the Fas death receptor signaling complex give rise to immunodeficiency states superimposed upon ALPS-like features.
  - Caspase-8 deficiency state reflects the loss of participation of caspase-8 in two different signaling complexes—one for death induction, and another for NF-κB activation.
  - FADD deficiency may reflect the loss of participation of FADD in antiviral innate immunity mediated by type I interferon, as well as in apoptosis induction.
- RALD results from a defect in the cytokine withdrawal-induced intrinsic pathway of apoptosis.
  - A somatic *NRAS* or *KRAS* gain-of-function mutation that prevents BIM induction is responsible.
  - Due to effects on generalized leukocyte homeostasis, disease resembles juvenile myelomonocytic leukemia as well as ALPS.
- X-linked lymphoproliferative disease (XLP) due to loss of SAP expression impairs T-cell receptor restimulation-induced apoptosis and leads to the overaccumulation of CD8 T cells.

The autoimmune lymphoproliferative syndrome (ALPS)

Clinical features

In 1992, Sneller and colleagues described a childhood syndrome of immune cell dysregulation including autoimmunity, hypergammaglobulinemia, lymphadenopathy, and lymphocytosis. The lymphocytosis reflected expansion of an unusual T-cell population bearing rearranged TCR-α/β but lacking CD4 or CD8 co-receptor expression (double-negative T cells or DNT). Like *lpr* mice, these patients had *FAS* mutations leading to the defective lymphocyte apoptosis that was critical for disease pathogenesis. The human disease was therefore termed auto-immune lymphoproliferative syndrome (ALPS).

Diagnostic criteria for ALPS

- Required criteria
  - Chronic non-malignant lymphadenopathy and/or splenomegaly
  - Increased peripheral CD4⁻CD8⁻TCRα/β (DNT) cells
- Supporting criteria (primary)
  - Lymphocyte apoptosis defect
  - Mutations in *FAS*, *FASLG*, or *CASP10*
- Supporting criteria (secondary)
  - Elevated biomarkers (sFASL, IL-10, B$_{12}$, or IL-18)
  - Characteristic histopathology
  - Autoimmune manifestations
  - Family history of ALPS

For a definitive diagnosis of ALPS, both required criteria plus at least one primary supporting criterion are needed. For a probable diagnosis of ALPS, both required criteria plus at least one secondary supporting criterion are needed.

● CLINICAL PEARLS

- Classification is based upon findings that may be present or have resolved.
- Despite its moniker, at least one-fifth of patients with ALPS lack evidence of autoimmunity.
- Variable penetrance means that not all individuals with mutations manifest disease.
- TCRγ/δ cells lacking CD4 and CD8 co-receptors may falsely elevate the double negative T-cell (DNT) count.
- Expression of B220 on DNT cells is a finding specific to ALPS.
- Elevated soluble FasL, B$_{12}$ levels, or other biomarkers can be used as a simple screen.
- Other helpful laboratory findings are hypergammaglobulinemia, direct Coombs test, or anti-cardiolipin antibodies.
- Patients without known mutations should be directly analyzed for somatic mutations in sorted DNT cells.
- Apoptosis assays may be normal in the case of *FASLG* or somatic *FAS* mutations, but is no longer required for establishing a definitive diagnosis.
- RALD, previously classified as a form of ALPS, is a non-malignant condition that can be confused with juvenile myelomonocytic leukemia.

ALPS is a rare condition with variable disease penetrance that affects an estimated 500 persons worldwide.[5] Diagnostic criteria, which were revised in 2009, reflect deranged lymphocyte homeostasis.[14] Patients present with a chronic non-malignant accumulation of lymphocytes with lymphadenopathy and/or splenomegaly, and with elevated DNT numbers in peripheral blood. Autoimmunity is often seen, or more rarely lymphoma, but these are not required for diagnosis.

Signs and symptoms of ALPS usually emerge in infancy or early childhood when patients typically first undergo medical investigation for unexplained splenomegaly, lymphadenopathy, or autoimmune destruction of blood cells. Often there is painless enlargement of peripheral lymphoid organs, but no fever or weight loss unless complicated by lymphoma. The thymus or liver can also be enlarged. Although lymphoid hyperplasia can fluctuate, even without treatment it tends to gradually improve with age. Up to 80% of ALPS patients have circulating autoantibodies, although only half have actual autoimmune disease. Coombs positive hemolytic anemia and chronic immune thrombocytopenic purpura are the most common autoimmune diseases. These manifestations tend to be severe, but often follow a variable course. When seen at initial presentation, ALPS can be mistaken for Evans syndrome.[12,15] Neutropenia due to hypersplenism or autoimmunity can occur, but is usually mild. The high incidence of anti-cardiolipin or anti-neutrophil antibodies has no correlation with the clinical manifestations of thrombosis or neutropenia. Rare autoimmune manifestations include antinuclear antibodies, rheumatoid factor, glomerulo-nephritis, optic neuritis or uveitis, Guillain–Barré syndrome, primary biliary cirrhosis, anti-factor VIII antibodies with coagulopathy, autoimmune hepatitis, vasculitis, and linear IgA dermopathy.

DNT expansion is peculiar to, and required for, the diagnosis of ALPS. Normally, DNT comprise 1.5% or less of lymphocytes in the peripheral blood or in lymphoid tissues. However, they can reach up to 40% in ALPS patients. These cells are distinct from the immature DNT cells developing in the thymus that have not yet rearranged their TCR genes or expressed TCR on their cell surface. They are thought to represent aging mature T cells that have lost CD8 co-receptor expression, but the details

of their origin are obscure. In ALPS patients the expanded DNT produce high levels of IL-10. As elevations in IL-4 and -5 are also seen, the resulting T helper type 2 (Th2) cytokine profile probably contributes to the observed polyclonal hyperglobulinemia and autoantibodies. The demonstration that some ALPS patients are mosaics—with *FAS* mutations in DNT but not all T cells—implicates these double-negative T cells in the pathogenesis of the disease.

Lymphoproliferation in ALPS is not limited to DNT. Patients have increased numbers of total T cells, with contributions from CD8 cells expressing CD57 as well as TCRγ/δ⁺ cells that lack CD4 and CD8 expression. Both total B cells and CD5⁺ B cells are increased. By contrast, CD4⁺CD25⁺ T cells are low, resulting in no overall change in CD4 cell numbers. NK cell numbers are also unchanged. Lymph node biopsy reveals a characteristic histopathology showing follicular hyperplasia with polyclonal plasmacytosis, and paracortical expansion with infiltrating DNT.

Because apoptosis assays often yield apparent normal results for patients who have somatic *FAS* mutations or *FASLG* mutations, abnormal apoptosis is now considered an adjunct for diagnosing ALPS. Alternatively, certain biomarkers can be measured to help diagnose ALPS. For example, the presence of high levels of circulating soluble FASL or cobalamin (vitamin B$_{12}$) is predictive of ALPS, especially those due to either germline or somatic *FAS* mutations.[14,16,17]

Although initially non-malignant, the lymphoproliferation in ALPS predisposes to lymphoid malignancy, which develops in 10% of ALPS patients. In rare instances, ALPS patients are diagnosed when they initially present with lymphoma. Compared to the general population, ALPS patients with *FAS* mutations have a 51-fold and 14-fold elevated incidence of Hodgkin and non-Hodgkin lymphoma, respectively. Median age of diagnosis was 11 years for Hodgkin lymphoma and 21 for non-Hodgkin lymphoma; however, lymphomas were identified anywhere between 2 to 50 years of age. Lymphomas are primarily of B-cell origin but of diverse histological type, thus betraying a general anti-neoplastic role for propriocidal death of lymphocytes. The lymphomas display neither loss of heterozygosity for the *FAS* mutation nor increased resistance to apoptosis. Most patients who develop malignancy have mutations in the DD region, with severe impairment in FAS-mediated lymphocyte apoptosis but continued FAS-mediated activation of NF-κB and MAPK for growth promotion.

Defective apoptosis in ALPS also affects antigen presenting cells.[12] The ensuing accumulation of dendritic cells and histiocytes can lead to a clinical presentation that resembles sinus histiocytosis with massive lymphadenopathy or Rosai-Dorfman disease. The subsequent development of histiocytic sarcomas suggests that this accumulation not only exacerbates lymphocyte function, but can also predispose to myeloid malignancy.

Molecular etiology and classification

The current ALPS classification based on underlying genetic defects is presented in Table 13.1.[14] Most ALPS patients bear heterozygous mutations in the *FAS (TNFRSF6)* gene located on chromosome 10q24.1. Mutations can be found throughout the gene, either in coding regions or in splice sites, with the majority (~2/3) affecting the intracellular death domain (DD) encoded by exon 9. (A description of all mutations can be found in the ALPS database at http://www.niaid.nih.gov/topics/ALPS/research/Pages/mutationDatabase.aspx.) Autosomal dominant disease transmission occurs because most mutations exert a dominant interfering effect. This effect is explained by understanding that the association of six normal FAS with five (to seven) normal FADD molecules in a complex is required for receptor death signaling function (Fig. 13.2).[18] In heterozygous patients, while only half of FAS proteins are abnormal, the majority of FAS complexes will contain at least one mutant protein, which inhibits complex function. Severity is greatest for DD mutations, which disrupt the homotypic interactions required for FADD and initiator caspase recruitment into the death-inducing signaling complex (DISC). Those that do not affect DISC formation can impair downstream formation of higher order signaling protein oligomerization transduction structures (SPOTS), which are necessary for efficient caspase activation. In a proportion of ALPS patients, *FAS* somatic mutations have been found in purified DNT cells and a fraction of peripheral lymphocytes, monocytes and hematopoietic precursors. Notably, their (non-DNT) T cells lacked *FAS* mutations and apoptosis defects when expanded *in vitro*. Additional somatic *FAS* mutations have recently been found in several patients who have "milder" germline *FAS* mutations that affect the extracellular domain.[19] While only a few ALPS patients have compound heterozygous loss-of-function mutations that cause haploinsufficiency, individuals with complete loss of function due to homozygous mutations often manifest more severe symptoms.

A minority of ALPS patients harbor mutations in other components of the Fas pathway. Heterozygous mutations in Fas ligand (*FASLG*, *TNFSF6*) have been reported for a systemic lupus erythematosus (SLE) patient with lymphadenopathy, splenomegaly, and defective lymphocyte apoptosis after TCR restimulation, but no apparent DNT expansion, as well as a patient with a more classic ALPS phenotype.[20] Although caspase-10 functional polymorphisms may influence disease, at least two heterozygous caspase-10 mutations in three ALPS patients have been identified that cause defective apoptosis in lymphocytes and dendritic cells.[21] Finally, a subgroup of ALPS patients fulfills diagnostic criteria including increased DNT but lacks known mutations in the Fas pathway.

The relationship between genotype and phenotype is complex. In large kindreds, family members with the same mutation and degree of defective *in vitro* FAS-mediated apoptosis had very different clinical manifestations. In-depth analysis revealed that penetrance was greatest with intracellular DD mutations and least with extracellular mutations. For several small families who had "milder" germline *FAS* mutations that affect the extracellular domain, disease occurred only in those individuals who had also accumulated somatic *FAS* mutations.[19] It is not known whether a similar mechanism explains the variable disease penetrance in large kindreds, or whether other as yet identified factors, genetic and/or environmental, influence the clinical phenotype.

ALPS-like diseases

Some patients have features that overlap with, but do not fulfill, diagnostic criteria for ALPS. Understanding the molecular etiology of these conditions has led to their classification as separate clinical entitites. These can be grouped into ALPS-like diseases that target other components central to the extrinsic (death receptor) pathway, or that involve the intrinsic (mitochondrial) pathway.

ALPS-like diseases that target other components central to the extrinsic (death receptor) pathway

ALPS-like diseases can reflect not only defective apoptosis, but also abnormalities in non-apoptotic pathways that regulate lymphocyte growth and activation. One such molecule is caspase-8. Its deficiency, found in two siblings with homozygous mutations, led to an immune dysregulation syndrome we term caspase-8 deficiency state (CEDS).[5,22] Consistent with the known role of caspase-8 as an initiator caspase in the DISC, these patients had mild lymphadenopathy and splenomegaly, as well as lymphocyte apoptotic defects, but marginal elevations in DNT. More importantly, unlike classical ALPS patients, the CEDS patients had recurrent sinopulmonary infections and mucocutaneous herpesvirus infections. They had low serum immunoglobulin levels and poor humoral responses to polysaccharide antigens, as well as impaired activation of T cells, B cells, and natural killer (NK) cells. The impaired lymphocyte activation resulted from a defect in the kinetics of activation of the critical transcription factor NF-κB in response to stimulation through antigen receptors, TLR-4, and FcγRIII. This defect occurred because caspase-8 participates in a signaling complex that includes other proteins such as Bcl-10, MALT-1, and IKK in an NF-κB activating signalosome. This complex differs from the DISC and is not affected in classical ALPS patients.

Table 13.1 Revised ALPS classification by molecular defect

Classification	Genetic defect
ALPS-FAS	*FAS (TNFRSF6)*
ALPS-FAS/sFAS*	Germline plus somatic *FAS* mutations
ALPS-sFAS	Somatic *FAS* mutations
ALPS-FASLG	*FASLG (TNFSF6)*
ALPS-CASP10	*CASP10*
ALPS-U	Unknown mutation
*Provisional	

FADD is the other instance of a molecule that participates in apoptosis but has other important functions in lymphocytes. Recently, four related patients were identified who had homozygous mutations that resulted in FADD deficiency.[23] FADD is well-known as an adapter molecule that brings caspase-8 into the DISC to activate it. Nevertheless, although defective lymphocyte apoptosis, increased DNT, elevated serum biomarkers, and autoantibodies were seen in one patient, none of the patients had lymphadenopathy or splenomegaly, which is a required criterion for a diagnosis of ALPS. Furthermore, unlike classic ALPS, the patients all had recurrent episodes of fever with encephalopathy and liver dysfunction, which were usually associated with viral infections. In the one tested patient, antiviral innate immunity mediated by type I interferon was impaired, which was consistent with a previously identified role for FADD in other experimental systems. Several patients also had invasive pneumococcal disease, functional asplenia, cardiovascular malformations, and cerebral atrophy.

Interestingly, both caspase-8 and FADD participate in apoptosis; but they also have been implicated in regulating programmed necrosis, especially in mice. The signaling pathway for programmed necrosis is still being worked out, but seems to require RIP1 and RIP3 kinases in a complex called the necrosome. The necrosome is antagonized by caspase-8, FADD, and c-FLIP within the DISC, which explains why programmed necrosis occurs when apoptosis is blocked. Finally, autophagic cell death has also been observed in monocytes, where it is antagonized by caspase-8. Whether programmed necrosis or autophagic death contributes to CEDS or FADD deficiency disease phenotypes in humans remains unclear. Identifying other patients with CEDS or FADD deficiency will help to address this important question.

RAS-associated autoimmune leukoproliferative disease (RALD)

No human disease involving mutations in signaling components of the intrinsic apoptosis pathway has yet been identified. However, an ALPS-like disease has been defined whose signaling pathway feeds into and affects the intrinsic apoptosis pathway. The disease, RAS-associated autoimmune leukoproliferative disease (RALD), is characterized by defective lymphocyte apoptosis upon cytokine withdrawal.[14,24,25] This discovery was initially made in a patient who fulfilled other diagnostic criteria for ALPS (lymphadenopathy, splenomegaly, mild DNT elevation, and autoantibodies). However, he had less typical features including monocytosis, lymph nodes that showed follicular hyperplasia with sinus histiocytosis, and a history of what had been termed childhood leukemia but was apparently cured by oral therapy alone. The patient had a gain-of-function somatic mutation in the gene NRAS, which caused MEK (MAPK kinase)/ERK hyperactivation leading to diminished expression of the pro-apoptotic molecule BIM. This loss of BIM induction thus accounted for failure to induce apoptosis upon cytokine withdrawal. Additional patients having gain-of-function somatic mutations in NRAS or its homolog KRAS were subsequently identified. Overall, the disease is characterized by hepatosplenomegaly, lymphadenopathy, autoimmune cytopenias, monocytosis, either normal or marginally increased DNT levels, and defective lymphocyte apoptosis upon cytokine withdrawal. This disease, which is strongly reminiscent of juvenile myelomonocytic leukemia, is now considered to be distinct from classic ALPS.

Apoptosis in other immunodeficiencies

X-linked lymphoproliferative disease (XLP) due to *SH2D1A* mutations is another ALPS-like disease that features impaired lymphocyte apoptosis.[6,26] XLP patients may present with dysgammaglobulinemia or lymphoma, but more commonly with fulminant mononucleosis and lymphoproliferation. The acute lymphoproliferative disease in XLP presents with lymphadenopathy, splenomegaly, interstitial lung disease, and/or hemophagocytic lymphohistiocytosis/macrophage activation syndrome. Cytotoxic T lymphocytes (CTL) from XLP patients are defective in killing EBV-infected cells, and the T cells vigorously expand during infection. Their accumulation is exacerbated by an intrinsic defect in the T cells to undergo TCR restimulation-induced apoptosis. Without the *SH2D1A*-encoded SAP protein, TCR signal strength is insufficient for optimal expression of pro-apoptotic molecules such as FasL and BIM. The mechanism by which SAP normally increases TCR signal strength involves its recruitment to NTB-A with displacement of SHP-1 and simultaneous colocalization of NTB-A with the CD3 complex. Thus, study of XLP has shed new light on how the TCR sigaling pathway normally links to downstream cell death pathways to maintain lymphocyte homeostasis.

⬤THERAPEUTIC PRINCIPLES

ALPS

- Disease can improve with age.
- Corticosteroids are useful for rapidly bringing autoimmune disease under control.
- If unable to discontinue medications, low-dose corticosteroids given every other day, mycophenolate mofetil, or rapamycin may be useful in preventing recurrence of autoimmune disease.
- Rapamycin is the only medication that treats lymphoproliferation as well as autoimmune disease.
- Rituximab has resulted in persistent hypogammaglobulinemia when given to ALPS patients.
- Splenectomy should be considered only when hypersplenism contributes to severe refractory cytopenias.
- The risk of post-splenectomy sepsis necessitates lifelong antibiotic prophylaxis.
- Cytotoxic agents or matched unrelated donor allogeneic bone marrow transplantation can be considered for worst case scenarios.
- Patients should undergo periodic monitoring for development of lymphoma.
- When they develop, ALPS lymphomas tend to respond to conventional therapies.

Therapies for ALPS

Although symptoms can remit with age, some ALPS patients require continued treatment to control autoimmune disease.[27] Treatment for autoimmune cytopenias is similar to that used in patients without ALPS. A high-dose pulse of corticosteroid (5-30 mg/kg methylprednisolone i.v.) is useful in bringing autoimmune cytopenias rapidly under control. This is followed by a low-dose course (1-2 mg/kg prednisone orally) that can be tapered and eventually discontinued after several weeks to months. Adjuncts to corticosteroids include intravenous immunoglobulin for autoimmune thrombocytopenia or hemolytic anemia, and granulocyte-colony stimulating factor (G-CSF, 1-2 µg/kg from three times a week to once daily) for autoimmune neutropenia. In some patients, autoimmune disease promptly recurs after discontinuing corticosteroids. These patients may need to be maintained on a minimal dose every other day. Such patients may benefit by switching to the immunosuppressant mycophenolate mofetil ($\sim$600 mg/M^2/dose orally, twice daily) for long-term maintenance therapy. The long-term corticosteroid- and splenectomy-sparing effects of this agent are particularly advantageous in children. Alternatively, rapamycin (steady-state serum trough of 4-15 ng/mL) is highly efficacious. For patients who fail these approaches, cytotoxic agents can be tried. Success has been anecdotally reported using azathioprine, vincristine, or rituximab (anti-CD20 monoclonal antibody, 375 mg/M^2/week I.V. ×4). However, in several ALPS patients rituximab has been associated with development of persistent hypogammaglobulinemia after use.[28] Allogeneic bone marrow transplantation has been curative when undertaken in the rare instances of severely and intractably affected patients who have homozygous *FAS* mutations and complete absence of FAS. However, given the associated high risks of complications and death, use of matched unrelated donor allogeneic bone marrow—which is likely to be required to avoid repopulating with lymphocytes from family members having the same mutation—should be considered a therapy of last resort.

Although lymphadenopathy and splenomegaly may be unsightly, these disease manifestations are usually not treated unless medically indicated. Hypersplenism can contribute to low blood cell counts when splenic pooling exacerbates autoimmune-mediated destruction. Notably, except for rapamycin, none of the current agents used to treat ALPS improves lymph node or spleen size, including sulphadoxine-pyrimethamine (Fansidar) or pyrimethamine alone. Splenectomy may be required if immunosuppressant agents fail to improve cytopenias. Due to an increased risk for post-splenectomy pneumococcal sepsis, splenectomy should be undertaken with caution. Patients should be immunized against *Streptococcus pneumoniae*, *Haemophilus influenzae*, and *Neisseria meningitides* before splenectomy. Following splenectomy, patients should be re-immunized with conjugate plus polysaccharide pneumococcal vaccines when titers wane. Lifelong antibiotic prophylaxis with penicillin or fluoroquinolones is essential. Splenectomized patients should be instructed to seek immediate medical attention to rule out bacteremia during febrile illnesses.

Distinguishing between a newly developing or relapsed lymphoma and a benign lymphadenopathy requires careful periodic examinations and surveillance by serial computed tomography (CT) scans. Suspiciously enlarging lymph nodes may necessitate biopsy to assess for clonality and chromosomal abnormalities. Positron emission tomography (PET) scans, which detect areas of high cellular glucose uptake, are useful for identifying and following suspicious lesions.[24] Fortunately, lymphomas in ALPS patients tend to respond to conventional therapies.

Future directions

Over the coming years, high-throughput genomics should continue to yield insights into the etiology and molecular pathogenesis of aberrant lymphocyte homeostasis. In particular, whole exome sequencing makes it possible to screen all coding regions of every gene for novel mutations in atypical cases of ALPS, XLP, and related disorders. Similarly, RNA-Seq technology allows for simultaneous quantification and deep sequencing of every mRNA transcript expressed in a given cell type, providing a powerful tool for uncovering somatic mutations in specific cell populations (e.g., DNTs) or lymphomas and assessing relative RNA expression patterns. High-throughput genomics may also pinpoint genetic variations that modify disease penetrance in large kindreds in diseases such as ALPS. Over time, integration of these technologies into clinical laboratories should revolutionize screening and diagnosis of lymphoproliferative disorders linked to impaired apoptosis. Earlier genetic diagnoses of pediatric ALPS-related disorders, combined with gene expression and biomarker profiling, should pave the way for tailored patient-specific therapies.

Conclusion

Programmed cell death is an essential regulatory mechanism to establish equipoise with growth, differentiation, and proliferation of lymphocytes. Studies in humans with the rare genetic disorder autoimmune lymphoproliferative syndrome (ALPS) have demonstrated that apoptosis is physiologically important for maintaining lymphocyte homeostasis, preventing autoimmunity, and suppressing lymphomagenesis. Patients with caspase-8 deficiency state (CEDS) or FADD deficiency have revealed that molecules responsible for death can also participate in other intracellular signaling pathways for normal lymphocyte function. Other ALPS-like disorders, such as RAS-associated autoimmune leukoproliferative disease (RALD) or X-linked lymphoproliferative disease (XLP), have also shed light into the role of programmed cell death for leukocyte homeostasis and how TCR restimulation-induced lymphocyte apoptosis is regulated during viral infections. Defining the genetic abnormalities responsible for ALPS and related disorders should continue to provide insights into the mechanisms that regulate immune cell homeostasis *in vivo*.

● ON THE HORIZON

- Next-generation sequencing technology will streamline the discovery of novel genetic variants linked to lymphoproliferative disease and other immune system disorders.
- Integration of genomics-based tools in the clinic will provide more rapid genetic diagnosis and augment patient-specific therapeutic interventions.

Acknowledgments

We thank Koneti Rao, Thomas Fleisher, and João Bosco de Oliveira for helpful discussions. We also thank João Bosco de Oliveira for his contributions to an earlier edition of this chapter. This manuscript was supported by the Intramural Research Program of the National Institute of Allergy and Infectious Diseases, NIH.

References

1. Ahmed R, Gray D. Immunological memory and protective immunity: understanding their relation. Science 1996;272(5258):54–60.
2. Horvitz HR. Nobel lecture. Worms, life and death. Biosci Rep 2003;23(5–6):239–303.
3. Ranger AM, Malynn BA, Korsmeyer SJ. Mouse models of cell death. Nat Genet 2001;28(2):113–8.
4. Lenardo M, Chan KM, Hornung F, et al. Mature T lymphocyte apoptosis – immune regulation in a dynamic and unpredictable antigenic environment. Annu Rev Immunol 1999;17:221–53.
5. Su HC, Lenardo MJ. Genetic defects of apoptosis and primary immunodeficiency. Immunol Allergy Clin North Am 2008;28(2):329–51, ix.
6. Snow AL, Pandiyan P, Zheng L, et al. The power and the promise of restimulation-induced cell death in human immune diseases. Immunol Rev 2010;236:68–82.
7. Bidere N, Su HC, Lenardo MJ. Genetic disorders of programmed cell death in the immune system. Annu Rev Immunol 2006;24:321–52.
8. Edinger AL, Thompson CB. Death by design: apoptosis, necrosis and autophagy. Curr Opin Cell Biol 2004;16(6):663–9.
9. Youle RJ, Strasser A. The BCL-2 protein family: opposing activities that mediate cell death. Nat Rev Mol Cell Biol 2008;9(1):47–59.
10. Ashkenazi A, Dixit VM. Death receptors: signaling and modulation. Science 1998;281(5381):1305–1308.
11. Kantari C, Walczak H. Caspase-8 and Bid: Caught in the act between death receptors and mitochondria. Biochim Biophys Acta 2011;1813(4):558–63.
12. Lenardo MJ, Oliveira JB, Zheng L, et al. ALPS – ten lessons from an international workshop on a genetic disease of apoptosis. Immunity 2010;32(3):291–5.
13. Siegel RM, Chan FK, Chun HJ, et al. The multifaceted role of Fas signaling in immune cell homeostasis and autoimmunity. Nat Immunol 2000;1(6):469–74.
14. Oliveira JB, Bleesing JJ, Dianzani U, et al. Revised diagnostic criteria and classification for the autoimmune lymphoproliferative syndrome: report from the 2009 NIH International Workshop. Blood 2010;116(14):e35–e40.
15. Seif AE, Manno CS, Sheen C, et al. Identifying autoimmune lymphoproliferative syndrome in children with Evans syndrome: a multi-institutional study. Blood 2010;115(11):2142–5.
16. Caminha I, Fleisher TA, Hornung RL, et al. Using biomarkers to predict the presence of FAS mutations in patients with features of the autoimmune lymphoproliferative syndrome. J Allergy Clin Immunol 2010;125(4):946–949. e6.
17. Magerus-Chatinet A, Stolzenberg MC, Loffredo MS, et al. FAS-L, IL-10, and double-negative CD4- CD8- TCR alpha/beta+ T cells are reliable markers of autoimmune lymphoproliferative syndrome (ALPS) associated with FAS loss of function. Blood 2009;113(13):3027–30.
18. Wang L, Yang JK, Kabaleeswaran V, et al. The Fas-FADD death domain complex structure reveals the basis of DISC assembly and disease mutations. Nat Struct Mol Biol 2010;17(11):1324–9.
19. Magerus-Chatinet A, Neven B, Stolzenberg MC, et al. Onset of autoimmune lymphoproliferative syndrome (ALPS) in humans as a consequence of genetic defect accumulation. J Clin Invest 2011;121(1):106–12.
20. Bi LL, Pan G, Atkinson TP, et al. Dominant inhibition of Fas ligand-mediated apoptosis due to a heterozygous mutation associated with autoimmune lymphoproliferative syndrome (ALPS) Type Ib. BMC Med Genet 2007;8:41–55.
21. Zhu S, Hsu AP, Vacek MM, et al. Genetic alterations in caspase-10 may be causative or protective in autoimmune lymphoproliferative syndrome. Hum Genet 2006;119(3):284–94. Epub 2006 Jan 31.
22. Su H, Bidere N, Zheng L, et al. Requirement for caspase-8 in NF-kappaB activation by antigen receptor. Science 2005;307(5714):1465–8.
23. Bolze A, Byun M, McDonald D, et al. Whole-exome-sequencing-based discovery of human FADD deficiency. Am J Hum Genet 2010;87(6):873–81.
24. Niemela JE, Lu L, Fleisher TA, et al. Somatic KRAS mutations associated with a human nonmalignant syndrome of autoimmunity and abnormal leukocyte homeostasis. Blood 2011;117(10):2883–6.
25. Takagi M, Shinoda K, Piao J, et al. Autoimmune lymphoproliferative syndrome-like disease with somatic KRAS mutation. Blood 2011;117(10):2887–90.
26. Snow AL, Marsh RA, Krummey SM, et al. Restimulation-induced apoptosis of T cells is impaired in patients with X-linked lymphoproliferative disease caused by SAP deficiency. J Clin Invest 2009;119(10):2976–89.
27. Teachey DT. Autoimmune lymphoproliferative syndrome: new approaches to diagnosis and management. Clin Adv Hematol Oncol 2011;9(3):233–5.
28. Rao VK, Price S, Perkins K, et al. Use of rituximab for refractory cytopenias associated with autoimmune lymphoproliferative syndrome (ALPS). Pediatr Blood Cancer 2009;52(7):847–52.

Immunoglobulin function

Neil S. Greenspan, Lisa A. Cavacini

Antibody-mediated immunity generally requires noncovalent contact between an antibody and the antigen. The ability of an antigen to bind noncovalently to an antibody, termed *antigenicity*, is a physical-chemical property evaluated with respect to a given antibody population. In contrast, *immunogenicity*, the ability to induce the biosynthesis and secretion of soluble antibody molecules, is a biological property. Thus its measurement requires *in vivo* studies. While antigenicity is necessary for immunogenicity (as defined by the production of antibodies), it is not sufficient. Moreover, the immunogenicity of a given molecule or molecular complex is influenced by host genetic variation. When an antibody binds to a macromolecular antigen, it directly contacts only a portion of the molecular surface of that antigen. Similarly, only a portion of the antibody molecule makes direct contact with the antigen. By convention, the portion of an antibody or T-cell receptor that makes physical contact with an antigen is referred to as the *paratope* or combining site. Conversely, the region of the antigen in physical contact with the paratope, the antigenic determinant, is termed the *epitope*. Most of the amino acids in an antibody variable domain that contact a given antigen are located in the hypervariable regions (also termed complementarity determining regions or CDRs). However, X-ray crystallographic analyses of antibody–protein antigen complexes have shown that contact residues can reside in the framework regions,[1] as well.

Although an epitope (paratope, etc.) is usually defined in terms of intermolecular contact, the region of a molecule involved in physical contact with another molecule may not correspond exactly to the structural correlates for energetics and specificity.[2]

Antigen binding and molecular Identity

Physical aspects of binding

Antibody–antigen interactions are, with rare exceptions, *noncovalent*. This fact is significant in that these interactions are, in principle, spontaneously reversible under the conditions of temperature, pressure, pH, and ionic strength that generally prevail in living organisms.

Several types of noncovalent bonds have been shown to contribute to antibody–antigen binding. These include van der Waals forces, hydrogen bonds, ionic bonds, and hydrophobic interactions. Individually the strength of these bonds is in the range of one to a few kcal/mole, versus 50–100 kcal/mole for covalent bonds. Since the potential to engage in these types of bonds is shared by many of the components of biological macromolecules, individual weak bonds do not usually confer a high degree of specificity. For example, any two atoms can interact through van der Waals forces. It is only through the simultaneous action of many such bonds that molecular specificity arises. Hence, the importance of a close fit, often referred to as *complementarity*, between the epitope and the paratope.

Complementarity can be maximized by matching the physical-chemical properties of the epitope and paratope. For example, binding can be facilitated when one molecule is concave and the other is convex, when one molecule is positively charged and the other is negatively charged, or when one molecule is a hydrogen bond donor whereas the other offers a hydrogen bond acceptor. It is expected that the greater the complementarity between receptor and ligand the stronger the interaction (greater affinity) between the two molecules. Specificity (see below) is also expected to be influenced by complementarity.[3]

In rationalizing the strength of interactions between antibodies and antigens, it is important to remember that the antibody competes with solvent for binding to antigen. Therefore, the thermodynamics of the interaction between these two structures reflects the influence of the interaction on the solvent and other solutes. Furthermore, bound water molecules may make important, even crucial, contributions to an interaction between two biomolecules.

Antibody recognition of antigen serves as a paradigm for understanding molecular recognition in the immune system and in biology in general. As will be discussed below, this fact, coupled with the inducibility of antibodies, permits antibodies to be used as surrogate ligands for almost any receptor (or vice versa).

Affinity is the concept used to convey how strongly two molecules bind to each other. In Table 14.1, antibody–antigen interactions are categorized with respect to the numbers of different kinds of paratope-epitope bonds and the absolute number of such bonds of each kind. Reflecting the different types of antibody–antigen interaction, two categories of affinity merit consideration: *intrinsic affinity* and *functional affinity*. It should be noted that some immunologists use the term "avidity" in place of "functional affinity."

Intrinsic affinity is a measure of the strength of the *monovalent* interaction between a particular paratope and a particular epitope under defined conditions of temperature, pressure, ionic strength, and pH (Fig. 14.1). By convention, the intrinsic affinity is taken to be the equilibrium association constant characterizing the paratope–epitope pair. It is the reciprocal of the concentration of monovalent antigen at which half of the paratopes will be occupied. It is not an intrinsic property of either the paratope or the epitope but rather, intrinsic affinity characterizes the relationship between two molecules under defined conditions.

Table 14.1 Antigens and valence

Number of types of epitope	Epitope copy number	Examples
Monodeterminant	Monovalent	Hapten: DNP, digoxin
Monodeterminant	Multivalent	Polysaccharide: dextran[a]
Multideterminant[b]	Monovalent	Monomeric protein: myoglobin
Multideterminant	Multivalent	Virion: influenza virus

[a]Even a polysaccharide composed of one type of hexasaccharide can have two or more different kinds of epitope: terminal versus internal residues, for instance. However, a given antiserum may preferentially contain antibodies specific for only one such epitope.
[b]Typically, multideterminance can only occur with respect to a polyclonal antibody.
Adapted from Benjamini E, Leskowitz S. Immunology: a short course, 2nd edn. New York: Wiley-Liss, 1991, with permission from Wiley-Liss, Inc., a subsidiary of John Wiley & Sons, Inc.

The intrinsic affinity of an antibody for a small molecule, such as a drug (e.g., digoxin) or a hormone (e.g., insulin), can be clinically important both *in vivo* and *in vitro*.[4] For example, the *in vivo* effectiveness of antibody F(ab) fragments in removing toxic levels of the drug, digoxin, from patients being treated for congestive heart failure likely depends on the intrinsic affinity of the F(ab) fragments for the drug. Alternatively, antibody intrinsic affinity can limit the analytical sensitivity of an *in vitro* immunoassay designed to determine the concentration of an analyte, such as a hormone (e.g., insulin, parathyroid hormone), or a drug (e.g., digoxin).

In contrast, functional affinity is defined as the equilibrium association constant characterizing the interaction between an intact antibody and an *intact* antigen. For a monovalent IgG antibody–antigen interaction, the intrinsic affinity and the functional affinity will be the same. However, if two paratopes interact simultaneously with two epitopes on the same antigen, referred to as *monogamous bivalency* (Fig. 14.2), the functional affinity of the antibody for the *multivalent* antigen may be substantially greater (as much as 10 000-fold for IgG) than the intrinsic affinity of that antibody for the relevant epitope on that same antigen.[5] Functional affinity is also influenced by the degree to which the geometric relationships among the epitopes are optimal for the paratopes, which will depend on the quaternary structure and segmental flexibility of the antibody molecule. In the presence of non-optimal geometry, the average number of engaged sites may be less than maximal, and energy may be expended in achieving some epitope–paratope contacts. Therefore, the functional affinity for a multivalent interaction does not necessarily increase in direct relationship to the maximal number of binding sites that can be engaged simultaneously by an antibody molecule. For example, the effective valency of pentameric IgM with 10 paratopes is typically half that.

Intrinsic affinity provides information, qualified as above, on the degree of complementarity between epitope and paratope. Functional affinity accounts for properties influenced by structural features outside of the epitope and paratope, as normally conceived. Both concepts of affinity are valuable. Maximization of intrinsic affinity may be of prime importance for antibody-mediated inactivation of toxins or enzymes, which frequently involve monovalent interactions. However, in cases where antibodies bind to repeated epitopes on the surfaces of bacteria, viruses, fungi, parasites, or mammalian cells, the functional affinity may play a much larger role influencing the biological consequences of the interaction.

Bivalent (IgG, IgE) or multivalent (IgA, IgM) antibodies carry with them the potential to bind simultaneously to two or more epitopes on different antigenic particles, crosslinking them

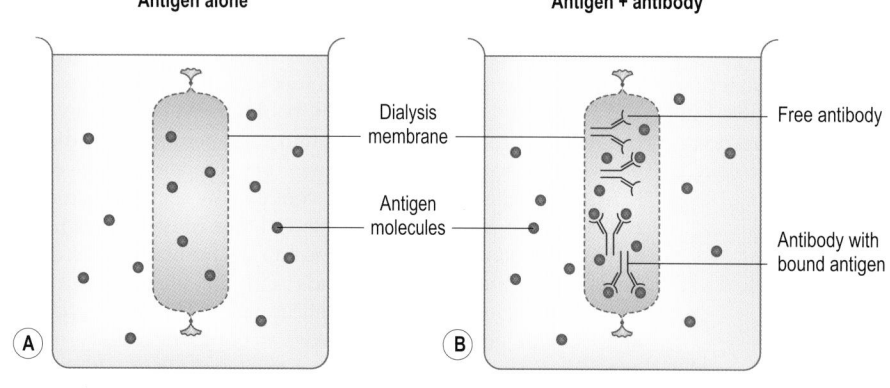

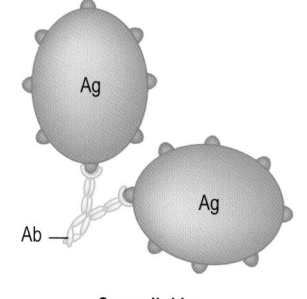

Antigen alone   **Antigen + antibody**

Dialysis membrane

Antigen molecules

Free antibody

Antibody with bound antigen

Fig. 14.1 Measurement of the intrinsic affinity characterizing an interaction between antibody and antigen (hapten) by equilibrium dialysis. At equilibrium (A), the amount of diffusible free hapten inside the dialysis bag will be equal to the amount of free hapten outside of the dialysis bag. However, in the presence of hapten-specific antibody (B) the total hapten concentration will be greater inside of the dialysis bag (free + antibody-bound) than outside of the bag (free). The extent of this difference can be used to determine the intrinsic affinity of the antibody for the hapten.
With permission from Abbas AK, Lichtman AH, Pober JS, Cellular and Molecular Immunology, 1991, W. B. Saunders Company.

Fig. 14.2 Interaction of a bivalent antibody, such as IgG, with multivalent antigens can result in monogamous bivalent binding (B) or crosslinking (C). The complexes in (B) are referred to as cyclic antibody–antigen complexes.
With permission from Eisen HN, General Immunology, 1990, J. B. Lippincott Company.

(A) **Monovalent binding**   (B) **Monogamous bivalent binding**   (C) **Cross-linking (bivalent) binding** rather than engaging in monogamous bivalency or monogamous multivalency (Fig. 14.2). This phenomenon has played an important historical role in immunology. It is the basis for the clinical method for typing erythrocyte antigens (e.g., ABO and Rh antigens), which still rely on agglutination of red cells by antibodies (or lectins). Such antibodies may also participate in the inactivation of complex antigens such as are found on the surface of HIV. Many neutralizing epitopes of HIV are normally not well exposed on native virus; however, conformational changes following antibody binding may expose these epitopes for neutralization by other antibodies.

KEY CONCEPTS

Binding of antibody to antigen

- Paratopes interact with epitopes through multiple noncovalent (weak) bonds, each of which is reversible at room temperature.
- For the clinician, immunological specificity needs to be viewed in its biologic rather than physical context.
- Intrinsic affinity and functional affinity both refer to the strength of antigen–antibody interactions, but often play separate roles in the biology of that interaction.
- Intrinsic affinity measures the strength of the interaction between a monovalent epitope and the paratope on the antibody. This can be determined by the equilibrium association constant. Intrinsic affinity is influenced both by the degree of complementarity between epitope and paratope and by ambient conditions, including the temperature, pressure, ionic strength, and pH.
- Functional affinity is a measure of the average strength of the interaction between a multivalent antigen and an intact antibody. It is influenced by the spatial relationships characterizing the epitopes that are being recognized as well as the physical properties of the underlying substrate.

Immunological specificity

The concept of specificity is fundamental to an understanding of the nature and consequences of interactions between immunological receptors and antigens. However, in the immunologic context, the term specificity encompasses several different aspects.[6] Several of these aspects are discussed below.

One aspect of specificity focuses on the goodness of fit between the paratope and the epitope. Intrinsic affinity is regarded as a reasonable measure of this goodness of fit. However, substantial conformational adjustments of either the paratope or the epitope may be necessary for formation of the complex.[7] Such conformational changes will generally incur energetic costs. Consequently, intrinsic affinity and final complementarity may not be perfectly correlated.

A second aspect of specificity focuses on the ability of a paratope to distinguish among different epitopes. Such specificity is most readily studied when the epitope is in monovalent form and evaluated relative to a specified set of ligands. Thus, one should be cautious about extrapolating claims that one antibody is more or less specific than another antibody without any reference to the relevant universe of ligands. However, there are practical cases where it is justifiable to speak globally of more- or less-specific antibodies. Polyspecific antibodies have been described in the neonatal primary repertoire.[8] These antibodies appear to be globally less discriminating than antibodies typical of the immune repertoire (secondary or later response) when tested on large panels of antigens.

Nevertheless, it is important to note that even antibodies derived from secondary (or later) responses are not,[9] and cannot be, absolutely specific.[10,11] The impossibility of perfect recognition or discrimination can be understood in both thermodynamic and structural terms. First, perfect fit and absolute discrimination would imply infinite intrinsic affinity (negative free energy change of complex formation), which is not physically plausible.[10] Second, the convexity of atoms prevents perfect shape complementarity between antibody (receptor) and antigen (ligand).[11] Recent results also indicate that at least some antibodies can adopt two or more different unbound conformations, each of which exhibits a different ligand-binding profile. Such paratopes may undergo further structural adjustment in the process of binding to an epitope.[12] This property can be advantageous to the function of an antibody. Antibodies that react with multiple conformations of a viral surface antigen may be much more likely to interfere with viral infection because they can bind more rapidly to the virus than the virus can bind to its receptor, as demonstrated for HIV.[13]

Whereas the first two aspects of specificity focused on the epitope, a third relates to the ability of an antibody to discriminate among antigens that display multiple copies of one or more distinct epitopes. An antigen expressing many copies of one epitope is termed *multivalent*, and an antigen that expresses two or more structurally distinguishable epitopes is referred to as *multideterminant* (Table 14.1). Because two different cells, bacteria, viruses, etc., may both express multiple copies of the same or nearly the same epitope, an antibody that is highly specific (in the first aspect above) for such a shared epitope may be a poor discriminator between such multivalent particles.[6] Yet, an antibody with a relatively poor degree of complementarity and intrinsic affinity for an epitope found on only one of two or more multivalent targets may be superior at discriminating among these antigens. Furthermore, antibodies (or other molecules) expressing two or more binding sites of identical structure may not discriminate identically among antigens displaying the same epitope in different two- or three-dimensional distributions.[6]

We offer some final points regarding specificity. First, the interactions between molecules such as CD4 and MHC class II, which are not clonally distributed, are often described as non-specific, meaning not specific for an antigen under consideration. The contrast being drawn is with the antigen-specific receptors, Ig or TCR. However, from the point of view of the first or second category of specificity described above (goodness of fit, discrimination between ligands), the interaction between molecules like CD4 and MHC class II may be as biochemically specific as that between an antibody and a class II molecule. Ideally, this sense of "non-specific" should be modified by the preceding term "antigen." If not, the meaning must be inferred from the context. Second, for many purposes immunological specificity has an ultimately biological, not a physical, definition. If the endpoint of analysis is the triggering of a complex response, such as cell activation or initiation of the complement cascade, then the presence, absence, or the extent of that response, and not the extent of receptor-antigen interaction, will be the ultimate criterion for evaluating specificity. Such biological specificity is not always directly correlated with specificity as determined by the analysis of binding.[6] Third, the enormous utility of antibodies is crucially dependent on the discriminatory abilities of these molecules with respect to other molecules or molecular aggregates. However, given that the discrimination mediated by antibodies is not absolute, the usefulness of a particular antibody may depend on the context. For example, which antigens or potential antigens in addition to the preferred target are available for binding to the antibody. Fourth, apparent antibody specificity may vary with the methods used for analysis, as these methods may differ in sensitivity and the conditions (pH, ionic strength, temperature) of application such that the relevant intrinsic affinities may vary among the different assays.

Protein epitopes

Based on the proximity of the relevant amino acids in the primary structure of the protein, several categories of epitopes have been defined for protein antigens (Fig. 14.3). The simplest is the *linear* epitope, where all of the relevant amino acids are derived from a contiguous stretch of the polypeptide chain. However, many, perhaps most, epitopes on globular proteins involve amino acids from two or more stretches of polypeptide that are distant from one another in the primary structure. Such an epitope is referred to as a *conformational*, or *discontinuous*, epitope. In some cases, such as with the capsids of non-enveloped viruses, a conformational epitope may contain amino acids that are derived from separate polypeptide chains, but that are next to each other in the final capsid structure. Another category of protein epitope, the *neo-epitope*, is reserved for those antigenic sites that become recognizable only after a post-translational event, such as proteolytic cleavage. For example, several neo-epitopes have been defined on cleavage products of human C1q, C3, and C9, components of the complement pathway.[14] Antibodies recognizing such neo-epitopes can be used to monitor the extent of activation of the complement pathway.[14]

Studies in the 1970s on the sizes of epitopes associated with synthetic peptide antigens yielded results suggesting that protein epitopes would maximally involve six or seven amino acids. However, the first structure of an antibody variable module in complex with a globular protein antigen, determined by X-ray crystallography,[1] indicated that protein epitopes, defined on the basis of intermolecular contact, could be as large as 15–20 amino acids. A similar number of amino acids in the antibody V domains constituted the paratope. And, even peptide antigen–antibody interaction can involve at least twelve peptide amino acids in contact with the antibody. Still, it is possible that there are smaller epitopes on globular proteins, particularly for regions of proteins that protrude or have a high radius of curvature.

Antibodies specific for both linear and conformational epitopes have important practical applications. For example, a synthetic peptide corresponding in amino acid sequence to a segment of the polypeptide chain predicted from the nucleotide sequence can be used to elicit antibodies.[15] Antibodies with the potential to recognize a linear epitope available in a denatured form of the gene product can be used to identify the protein following expression, electrophoresis, and blotting under denaturing conditions. Some antibodies raised by challenge with synthetic peptides that bind to linear epitopes can recognize a protein in denatured form but will not bind to or alter the function of the native protein.

Antibodies with the ability to neutralize protein function generally recognize conformations accessible to the native protein, usually at discontinuous epitopes. Thus antibodies specific for peptides (that correspond in amino acid sequence to a portion of a native protein) or denatured protein that can cross-react with the protein in a native (folded, functional) state can be extremely valuable. Such cross-reactivity is more likely to occur when the region being recognized is relatively disordered in the native structure.[16]

Carbohydrate epitopes

The classical studies of Kabat on the binding of antibodies to dextran led to the concept that epitopes on carbohydrate antigens could be as large as six or seven monosaccharides.[17] However, minimal carbohydrate epitopes can probably be as small as one or two monosaccharides. Even in the case of larger epitopes, it is typical for the terminal groups to play a dominant role in determining antibody specificity for carbohydrate antigens. Recent studies suggest that polysaccharide epitopes can sometimes also result from conformational properties of polysaccharides.

Interactions between antibodies and polysaccharides are typically characterized by relatively low intrinsic affinities in comparison to antibody–protein interactions.[5] Relatively weak antibody–carbohydrate binding can result from biological constraints related to protection against self-recognition and consequent tissue damage or from physical-chemical constraints related to the conformational freedom and high degree of solvation of unbound carbohydrates.

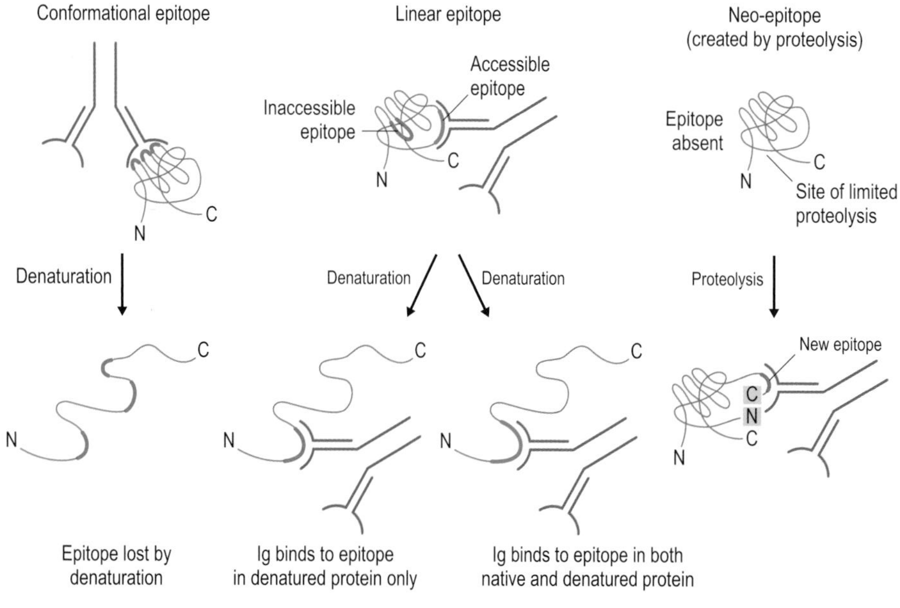

Fig. 14.3 Types of protein epitopes. Some antibodies recognize structural features of proteins that arise from the folding of the polypeptide backbone (conformational epitope). Other antibodies recognize groups of amino acid residues that are contiguous, or nearly so, in the primary (covalent) structure of the protein (linear epitope). If such a linear determinant is inaccessible in the native structure of the protein, the corresponding antibodies may only be elicited by the denatured form of the protein. Neo-epitopes are created by covalent post-translational modifications, such as proteolytic cleavage. With permission from Abbas AK, Lichtman AH, and Pober JS, Cellular and molecular immunology, 3rd edition, 1997, W. B. Saunders Company.

Conformational epitope | Linear epitope | Neo-epitope (created by proteolysis)

Accessible epitope

Inaccessible epitope

Epitope absent — Site of limited proteolysis

Denaturation

Denaturation / Denaturation

Proteolysis

New epitope

Epitope lost by denaturation | Ig binds to epitope in denatured protein only | Ig binds to epitope in both native and denatured protein

Another important feature of polysaccharide antigens is that they are generally multivalent. Bacterial polysaccharide epitope densities can approach values in the millions per square micrometer, which is probably one to several orders of magnitude greater than the epitope densities for protein determinants on mammalian cells. Therefore, multipoint attachment and functional affinity are likely to be critical factors in the mediation of immunity by anti-polysaccharide antibodies or other carbohydrate-specific proteins.

Immune complexes *in vivo*

● KEY CONCEPTS

Immune complexes

- Immune complexes are aggregates of antibody and antigen.
- Immune complexes can form in tissues, or they can form in the circulation and subsequently deposit in tissues.
- Immune complexes can activate complement or Fc receptor-bearing cells, leading to tissue damage.
- The composition, size, charge, and antibody isotypes characterizing a given population of immune complexes will influence the pathogenic potential of the complexes.

Interactions between antibodies and antigens *in vivo* can result in the formation of molecular aggregates, referred to as *immune complexes*. Deposition of immune complexes in tissues, such as blood vessels, renal glomeruli, renal tubules, the thyroid gland, and the choroid plexus, can result in pathological conditions.[18] Immune complexes can form in the circulation prior to deposition in a given tissue or they can form directly in the affected tissue. Variables such as concentration, composition, size, charge, and antibody isotype will influence the magnitude and sites of tissue deposition for these complexes. The magnitude of complement activation and the extent of interaction with Fc and complement receptors, in conjunction with the sites and extent of tissue deposition, determine the biological properties of the complexes. Antigen–antibody lattice size is determined by antigen valence, epitope geometry, antibody valence, the intrinsic affinity of paratope for epitope, antibody and antigen flexibility, the ratio of antibody to antigen, and the absolute concentrations of antibody and antigen. The potential diversity of immune complex morphologies is illustrated in Fig. 14.4. These complexes, between a monoclonal antibody specific for a bacterial polysaccharide and various anti-idiotypic or anti-isotypic monoclonal antibodies, are visualized by electron microscopy.

Immune complexes have also been found to have immunoregulatory effects,[19] particularly with respect to antibody responses. Immune complexes can bind simultaneously to B cell surfaces through antigen (to B cell surface immunoglobulin), antibody (to Fc receptors), and associated complement components (to complement receptors). The interaction with FcγRIIB, on the B lymphocyte membrane, has the effect of diminishing the B-cell response (Chapter 4). The molecular events underlying these immunoregulatory effects are being intensively studied, and they have been exploited clinically for many years. Antibody to the erythrocyte Rh antigens is used to prevent immunization of an Rh⁻ mother by an Rh⁺ fetus, thereby avoiding *hemolytic disease of the newborn* in a subsequent Rh⁺ fetus (Chapter 61).

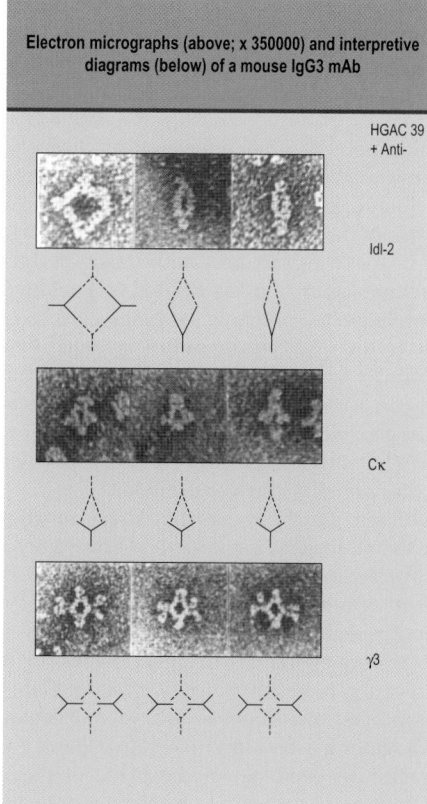

Electron micrographs (above; × 350000) and interpretive diagrams (below) of a mouse IgG3 mAb

HGAC 39 + Anti-

Idl-2

Cκ

γ3

Fig. 14.4 Electron micrographs (above; × 350 000) and interpretive diagrams (below) of a mouse IgG3 mAb (HGAC 39; specific for a bacterial polysaccharide) in complex with mAbs specific for, respectively, an idiotope (Idl-2; top), a light chain isotypic determinant (Cκ; middle), and a heavy chain isotypic determinant (γ₃; bottom). The different antibodies are not intrinsically distinguishable in the electron micrographs, but the interpretations take into account information in addition to that provided directly by the electron microscopic images. In the top series of micrographs, the choice of which molecules to represent as solid or dotted figures is arbitrary.

With permission from Greenspan NS, Analyzing immunoglobulin functional anatomy with monoclonal anti-immunoglobulin antibodies, BioTechniques 1989; 7: 1086.

Correlations between C_H region structure and antibody function

● KEY CONCEPTS

Structure–function relationships of C_H domains

- Immunoglobulin function is influenced by differences in quaternary structure and segmental flexibility.
- The hinge region helps control segmental flexibility in IgG molecules.
- When interacting with multivalent antigens, IgM molecules can adopt a dislocated configuration (staple configuration) in which the Fab arms are bent out of the plane of the Fc regions.

Antibodies are heterodimeric proteins that can be functionally divided into variable domains, which bind antigen, and constant domains, which define the effector function of the immunoglobulin. This dual function allows an antibody to physically link a specific antigen to a separate antigen-non-specific effector molecule, such as a component of complement or a cell-bound

Fc receptor. Many features of C_H domain structure exhibited by the immunoglobulin isotypes can be understood in the context of this requirement for linkage between antigens and an antigen-non-specific effector molecules.

One property of prime significance for antibody function is intramolecular mobility, often referred to as *segmental flexibility.* Hydrodynamic methods, electron microscopy, X-ray crystallography, and fluorescence polarization have all been used to evaluate the degree of flexibility exhibited by IgG, IgM, IgA, and IgE molecules.[20] In the case of the best studied isotype, IgG, it is clear that the structural feature most associated with relative motion of one subunit relative to another is the hinge, which connects the C_H1 domain to the C_H2 domain and is encoded by a separate exon. The human IgG3 subclass has an extended hinge region that can impart increased flexibility. In the case of IgA, the IgA1 hinge is flexible such that the F(ab) arms can range from the typical "Y" configuration to a "T" configuration whereas IgA2 molecules are relatively constrained.[21]

Immunoglobulin flexibility has important functional consequences for the antibody. First, inter-F(ab) movements can play an important role in permitting antibodies to bind in monogamous bivalent (or multivalent) fashion to antigenic surfaces that display repetitive epitopes. Second, efficiency in precipitation of multivalent antigen molecules or agglutination of multivalent antigen particles can be correlated with inter-F(ab) flexibility. And third, optimal interactions of effector molecules with IgG antibody Fc regions has been postulated to depend on the ability of the Fc region to bend out of the plane of the F(ab) arms (*dislocation*) (but see discussion on complement activation below).

Functions mediated by antibody alone

While it is clear that in many *in vivo* situations antibodies mediate their effects with the aid of other molecules and, in selected cases, cells (see next section), there are circumstances where the antibody can influence antigenic targets directly, at least *in vitro.* The very name "antibody" implies the negation of some activity, and antibodies were first defined as factors that could inactivate or neutralize toxins. Subsequent studies have shown inactivation of viruses, parasites, and enzymes, as well.

Virus neutralization

> ### ● KEY CONCEPTS
>
> **Virus neutralization**
>
> - Antibodies can neutralize (decrease the replication of) viruses by several mechanisms, including blocking attachment to the host cell, preventing penetration of the host cell membrane, or interfering with uncoating of the virus within the cell.
> - Neutralizing antibodies typically recognize proteins or glycoproteins on the virion surface.
> - Some antibodies that bind to virion surface proteins or glycoproteins are not neutralizing. In some cases such antibodies may contribute to immunity, whereas in others they may actually enhance infection.
> - The magnitude of neutralization mediated by a given antibody may vary with the host cell used for the measurement.
> - Neutralization *in vitro* is usually related to protection *in vivo*, but these two properties are not always perfectly correlated.

A phenomenon of fundamental medical and biological importance is the *neutralization* of viruses by antibodies.[22] Although neutralization is defined as the elimination or reduction of the virus's ability to replicate, it does not imply a particular mechanism of interference with the process of replication. Moreover, the measurement of neutralization can depend on the choice of host cell. Thus, the neutralizing activity of a given antibody for a given virus is not an intrinsic property of the antibody, but is a property of the relationship between antibody and virus, under defined conditions. Consequently, neutralization titers in serum do not always correlate perfectly with protection from infection or disease *in vivo.*

There are several mechanisms by which antibodies can inactivate viruses. The process by which a virus infects a cell involves multiple steps. These include attachment to one or more membrane components, penetration of or fusion with the membrane, uncoating, and genome expression. Although the most obvious mechanism of neutralization is prevention of viral attachment to the host cell surface, some antibodies can block other steps. For example, neutralizing antibodies for enveloped viruses, such as influenza virus, have been shown to prevent fusion between the virion and cell membranes, and neutralizing antibodies for polio virus have been shown to interfere with viral uncoating in the host cell.

Different isotypes of antibodies may employ different neutralization mechanisms to varying degrees, although this statement should not be interpreted to mean that there is a one-to-one correspondence between isotypes and neutralization mechanisms. For example, in the blood IgG or IgM antibodies can mediate protection against a virus either directly, in some cases, or with the assistance of complement components in others. However, IgA, the dominant isotype in mucosal secretions, operates under conditions where complement is less plentiful than in the blood. Thus virus-specific IgA is more likely to utilize virus-inactivating mechanisms that do not require complement, such as prevention of attachment.

Traditional thinking maintains that antibody mediates any protective effects extracellularly. However, it has been reported that IgA antibodies, being transported by the polymeric immunoglobulin receptor, can mediate protection against intracellular influenza virus.[23] Similar phenomena have been reported for rotavirus and HIV.

There are several other notable features of antibody–virus interactions. Not all antibodies that bind to molecules on the virion surface will neutralize the virus in all conditions. For a given virus-encoded gene product, such as the influenza virus hemagglutinin, binding of antibodies to some sites, but not others, will effect neutralization. Some gene products on the virion surface may fail to routinely support viral neutralization (e.g., influenza neuraminidase). However, antibody to influenza neuraminidase, while non-neutralizing, is thought to slow the spread of infection by interfering with the escape of progeny virions from an infected cell. Non-neutralizing antibodies, or neutralizing antibodies at suboptimal concentrations, have been found in some instances to enhance the infection of host cells by virus (e.g., HIV-1 or dengue virus). It should be noted however, that the clinical relevance of this enhancement, at least in regards to HIV, remains to be determined. Finally, some non-neutralizing antibodies, or those antibodies that fail to directly neutralize virus in an *in vitro* assay, can mediate protective effects *in vivo*, presumably by engaging antigen-non-specific effector mechanisms (i.e., complement or Fc receptor-bearing cells) or perhaps through cellular signal transduction.[24]

Neutralization of toxins and enzymes

In many bacterial infections, the clinical consequences of infection result from toxic molecules liberated by the bacterial cells rather than from the presence of the microorganisms themselves. Antibodies to such toxins can provide life-saving protection from disease, while not directly eliminating the bacteria producing the toxins. The classical example of this situation is infection with *Corynebacterium diphtheriae*, which secretes a potentially lethal exotoxin. Bacteria can also produce additional virulence factors, such as enzymes that facilitate spreading of the pathogen through tissues. Host antibodies that inactivate such enzymes can have a beneficial influence on the clinical course. Inactivation of toxins or enzymes is presumed to result from direct competition between antibody and the target molecule or substrate of the toxin or enzyme or from the stabilization or induction of conformations incompatible, to some degree, with the normal function(s) of the toxin or enzyme. However, recent evidence in mice suggests that the protection afforded by exotoxin-neutralizing antibodies can depend on the presence of Fcγ receptors.[25]

Functions mediated by antibody and additional molecules or cells

Complement activation

Regardless of whether binding of antibody to antigen directly mediates protective effects, antibody bound *in vivo* will activate antigen-nonspecific effector mechanisms. The exact mechanisms will depend on the isotype of the antibody as well as on other factors. One critical set of these effector mechanisms is encompassed by the classical pathway of complement activation. The human antibody isotypes vary considerably in their intrinsic ability to activate this pathway. The consensus view is that IgM, IgG1, and IgG3 isotypes are effective activators. While some sources state that IgG2, IgG4, and IgA are weak or non-activators of the classical complement pathway, evidence suggests that when epitope density is high, IgG2 can also activate the classical pathway effectively.[26] Instead of attempting to decide which subclass is absolutely superior, it is more useful to recognize that complement-fixing ability may not be determined solely by the subclass of an IgG antibody.

One obvious source for the isotype-related variation in complement activating ability is variation in affinity for C1q (IgG3>IgG1>IgG2>IgG4), the portion of the first component in the classical pathway that physically contacts the C_H2 domains of antibodies. The intrinsic affinity of the C1q globular heads for Fc regions of any isotype is relatively low, which may account in part for the observation that two or more IgG molecules in proximity are required for activation of the classical pathway beginning with C1. Thus, in the activation of the classical pathway, the functional affinity of C1q for antibody Fc regions is a crucial parameter.

IgG subclass-associated differences in some measures of complement activation have been found, under some experimental conditions, to depend on quantitative differences in steps of the cascade subsequent to the binding of C1q to antibody. While there have been speculations regarding the role of segmental flexibility in complement activation, there is no simple correlation between this physical property and activity in fixing the classical complement pathway.[27]

While it is generally agreed that IgA does not activate the classical pathway, its ability to activate the alternative complement pathway has been controversial. Studies with recombinant IgA molecules have suggested that neither IgA1 nor IgA2 activates either complement pathway.[28] However, aberrantly glycosylated IgA and polymeric IgA may activate the lectin/and or alternative pathway, and this activation has been postulated to be associated with IgA nephropathy.[29]

Antibody-mediated activation of the classical complement pathway has a variety of potential consequences, including creation of additional sites on a foreign particle to which phagocytic cells can attach and ingest the particle (opsonization), elaboration of substances that mediate leukocyte chemotaxis, additional metabolic changes involved in the destruction of pathogens by leukocytes, and changes in vascular permeability (Chapter 20). In this process, it is the antibody that provides the specificity whereas the other molecules function without specificity for the epitopes involved.

Receptors for Fc regions

> **● KEY CONCEPTS**
>
> **Antibody effector systems**
>
> - Multivalence of Fc regions is often important in activating antibody effector functions.
> - The occurrence and magnitude of effector function activation varies with antibody isotype.
> - Effector mechanisms are inherently non-specific with respect to antigen.
> - Antibody Fc regions provide the mechanistic link between antigen-specific V domains and antigen non-specific effector mechanisms.

The other major system by which antibodies mediate effector functions is cellular. The specific molecules with which cells recognize antibodies are called Fc receptors (FcR).[30] In humans, there are several Fc receptors for IgG (FcγRI, FcγRII, FcγRIII), as well as other Fc receptors for IgA, IgE, and IgM (Fig. 14.5). We describe selected features of Fc receptors that help to illuminate the principles by which they function.

Some receptors (FcγRI, FcεRI) have relatively high intrinsic affinities for antibody molecules, and can therefore bind significant fractions of monomeric Ig at physiological concentrations. For example, the high-affinity receptor for IgE (FcεRI) binds IgE with an intrinsic affinity of approximately 1×10^{10} M^{-1}. Therefore, single IgE molecules can bind to mast cells or basophils through cell surface FcεRI prior to interacting with allergen (antigen). In contrast, FcγRII and FcγRIII have relatively weak intrinsic affinities for IgG Fc regions. Consequently, multivalent forms of IgG, such as are found in complexes of antibody and multivalent antigens (immune complexes), are much more readily bound to these FcR. Thus, for both the complement-dependent and the FcR-dependent effector function pathways, multivalency of Fc regions (functional affinity) plays a critical role.

Several types of functional consequences can follow ligation of FcR by antibody–antigen complexes. These include activation

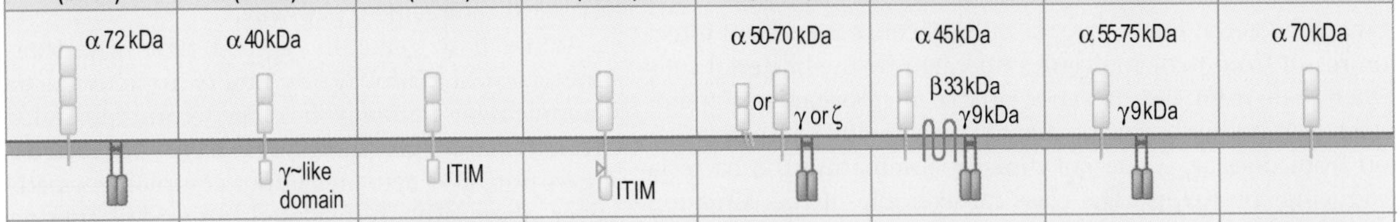

Receptor	FcγRI (CD64)	FcγRII-A (CD32)	FcγRII-B2 (CD32)	FcγRII-B3 (CD32)	FcγRIII (CD16)	FcεRI	FcαRI (CD89)	Fcα/μR
Structure	α 72 kDa	α 40 kDa			α 50-70 kDa or γ or ζ	α 45 kDa β 33 kDa γ 9 kDa	α 55-75 kDa γ 9 kDa	α 70 kDa
		γ~like domain	ITIM	ITIM				
Binding Order of affinity	IgG1 10^8 M^{-1} 1) IgG1=IgG3 2) IgG4 3) IgG2	IgG1 2×10^6 M^{-1} 1) IgG1 2) IgG3=IgG2* 3) IgG2	IgG1 2×10^6 M^{-1} 1) IgG1=IgG3 2) IgG4 3) IgG2	IgG1 2×10^6 M^{-1} 1) IgG1=IgG3 2) IgG4 3) IgG2	IgG1 5×10^5 M^{-1} IgG1=IgG3	IgE 10^{10} M^{-1}	IgA1, IgA2 10^7 M^{-1} IgA1=IgA2	IgA, IgM 3×10^9 M^{-1} 1) IgM 2) IgA
Cell type	Macrophages Neutrophils† Eosinophils† Dendritic cells	Macrophages Neutrophils Eosinophils Platelets Langerhans' cells	Macrophages Neutrophils Eosinophils	B cells Mast cells	NK cells Eosinophils Macrophages Neutrophils Mast cells	Mast cells Eosinophils† Basophils	Macrophages Neutrophils Eosinophils‡	Macrophages B cells
Effect of ligation	Uptake Stimulation Activation of respiratory burst Induction of killing	Uptake Granule release (eosinophils)	Uptake Inhibition of stimulation	No uptake Inhibition of stimulation	Induction of killing (NK cells)	Secretion of granules	Uptake Induction of killing	Uptake

Fig. 14.5 Domain structures, binding properties, cellular expression patterns, and functional effects of human Fc receptors. A given FcR may exhibit differences in composition depending on the cell type expressing it. For example, FcγRIII is expressed on neutrophil plasma membranes bearing a glycosylphosphotidylinositol anchor, without FcR γ chains, while it is expressed on NK-cell plasma membranes as a conventional transmembrane protein in association with FcR γ chains. Similarly, FcγRII-B1 contains an additional stretch of polypeptide encoded by an exon whose product is not represented in the intracellular domain of FcγRII-B2. This additional portion of the polypeptide is believed to prevent the internalization of FcγRII-B1 subsequent to crosslinking.

*A subset of FcγRII-A allotypes bind to human IgG2. †For these cells, FcR expression is inducible, not constitutive. ‡The molecular weight of CD89α chain is 70–100 kDa in eosinophils. With permission from Janeway CA Jr, Travers P, Walport M, Shlomchik M. Immunobiology: the immune system in health and disease, 6th edition. New York: Garland Science; 2004.

and metabolic alteration of the FcR$^+$ cells, phagocytosis of antibody-coated particulate antigens, antibody-dependent cellular cytotoxicity (ADCC), and release of mediators that promote inflammation. The end result of Fc binding depends not only on the receptor, but on the cell on which it is expressed and on co-stimulation, if any, of additional receptors on that cell. As an example, the most studied FcR are those that bind IgG and these receptors are expressed on many hematopoietic and even non-hematopoietic cells. In humans, there are three classes of receptors (I, II, and III). The latter two FcR each exist in two isoforms (A and B). Of interest to the regulation of the immune response, the B isoform for FcγRII transmits an inhibitory signal while the A isoform transmits an activating signal.

CD89 has been identified in humans as a receptor for IgA and it is expressed on myeloid cells including PMN, monocytes, and a population of dendritic cells.[31] Signaling through CD89 involves an ancillary chain that transmits an activating signal. However, not all CD89 molecules associate with this chain in which case bound IgA is endocytosed and recycled back to the surface of the cell.[31] Interestingly, Fc binding to CD89 may be more potent at mediating antibody-dependent cellular cytotoxicity than binding to one of the FcγR. Recent data suggest another possible function that depends on the interaction between antibody (IgA) and a cell surface receptor able to bind to polymeric immunoglobulins (pIgR). Transport of IgA-antigen complexes across epithelial surfaces by pIgR may represent a form of antibody-facilitated antigen excretion.[32]

Antibodies as surrogate ligands

The notion that one molecule can mimic a second molecule, in one respect or another, is of extraordinarily broad applicability and profound biological significance. At least three types of mimicry can be distinguished, and each type can be regarded as a continuous (as opposed to discrete) variable.[33] First, one can conceive of limited structural mimicry of one molecule by another. By chance, two otherwise different molecules could have regions that happen to contain the same or similar (in key respects), atoms in the same, or almost the same, three-dimensional arrangement. Second, there is mimicry at the level of noncovalent interaction. In this case, the question of interest is whether the model (object of mimicry) and the mimic bind the same receptor sites and with the same affinities. Third, there is mimicry of more complex biological functions, such as cellular or enzymatic inactivation. It is important to make these distinctions because the extent of mimicry of one type is not a perfect predictor of the extent of mimicry of another type. We have already noted that slight changes in structure sometimes have slight effects on binding affinity or specificity, yet in other cases they have dramatic effects on binding affinity or specificity. Thus, structural similarity (mimicry), as we perceive it, is not perfectly correlated with mimicry at the level of binding or the level of elicitation of higher biological function.

There are two aspects of receptor-ligand interaction that antibodies can potentially mimic. First, as noted earlier, the inducibility of a vast repertoire of antibody specificities suggests the potential for identifying, through screening or selection, antibodies that can bind any given target molecule at (near) a given site. Thus, there should be a reasonable probability of obtaining antibodies that bind to a particular receptor at a site bound by some other, perhaps physiological, ligand or co-receptor. Evidence that antibodies can mimic the functional effects of other molecules is provided by many investigations of anti-idiotypic antibodies and conventional anti-receptor antibodies.[33]

Second, as noted earlier, the triggering event for many cellular and effector processes in the immune system is the aggregation of receptor molecules by clustered ligands. Therefore, the ability of antibodies, which naturally have a maximal valence of two or greater, to crosslink cell surface molecules and initiate signal transduction contributes to the abilities of antibodies to serve as surrogate co-receptors for cell surface molecules. This property of antibodies has greatly facilitated the identification and functional characterization of many of these molecules and is also being exploited for therapeutic uses.[34]

Functional properties of engineered antibody molecules

Monoclonal antibodies

Many modern applications of antibodies in research, medicine, veterinary medicine, and other fields rely heavily, although not exclusively, on monoclonal antibodies. By definition, a monoclonal antibody population is derived from a clonal population of B lineage cells. Therefore, all of the molecules express identical variable domains and identical antigen specificities. It is the homogeneity of V domain structure associated with monoclonal antibodies that most crucially distinguishes them from polyclonal antibodies, such as those conventionally derived from the serum. Homogeneous antibodies give more reproducible and more easily interpreted results for many kinds of assays.

● KEY CONCEPTS

Monoclonal antibodies from hybridomas

- Hybridomas are created by fusing normal lymphocytes, typically from animals immunized with an antigen of choice, and transformed cells of B lymphocyte lineage (myeloma cells).
- Monoclonal antibodies produced by a hybridoma are homogeneous, expressing a single amino acid sequence.
- Hybridomas can be grown indefinitely in tissue culture or in the peritoneal cavities of syngeneic mice (for murine hybridomas).
- Hybridomas can be selected on the basis of the antigenic specificity or functional properties of the monoclonal antibody secreted by the hybridoma.

Monoclonal antibodies of selected specificity were first produced by cells referred to as hybridomas.[35] In contrast, a myeloma protein would be an example of a monoclonal antibody of unselected specificity. Hybridomas are hybrid transformed cells that are created by the fusion of two types of cells, with each parental cell endowing the hybridoma with desirable properties. One parent of a hybridoma (the fusion partner) is a transformed cell, usually a myeloma cell line, which contributes a metabolism that supports unlimited growth in tissue culture and high rates of immunoglobulin synthesis and secretion. Myeloma cell lines currently used as hybridoma fusion partners have been genetically manipulated such that they no longer synthesize an immunoglobulin molecule and they can be selected against in special culture media. The second parental cell is a B lymphocyte which provides the genetic information for the production of a particular antibody. Note that the choice of specificity on the part of the investigator is influenced at two stages in the process, including the choice of immunogen and the nature of the screening assay. By screening a population of hybridomas, most of which will secrete different antibodies, with an appropriately designed assay it is possible to identify the minority of cells that secrete a monoclonal antibody of desired specificity.

Monoclonal antibodies are useful for the identification and quantitation of diverse molecules of biological or synthetic origin, including human immunoglobulins (e.g., paraproteins), antigens from infectious agents (e.g., HIV p24), hormones, drugs, and toxins. They have also been exploited for therapeutic purposes, such as reversing allograft rejection, killing tumor cells, or preventing cytokine activity contributing to autoimmune disease (Chapter 92).

Recombinant antibodies

● ON THE HORIZON

Recombinant antibodies–antibody engineering

- Increase potency by changes in Fc
  - Activate effector functions
  - Increase half-life
  - Reduce or eliminate bystander effects
- Expand repertoire/targeting
  - Nanobodies
  - Drug or toxin conjugation
  - Multispecific/meric constructs
- Vaccine design
  - Role of isotype in protection
  - Glycosylation effects

The ability to manipulate the genes that encode antibodies, and thereby manipulate the structures of antibodies, has opened a new era in the study and application of antibodies (Fig. 14.6). Progress includes expression of recombinant intact IgG molecules,[36] expression of Ig fragments (F(ab), Fv) in eukaryotic and prokaryotic host cells,[37] expression of combinatorial libraries of antibody fragments displayed on the surfaces of filamentous phage particles,[37] and bispecific antibodies.[38] Recombinant antibodies are also being designed to improve distribution and half-life of administered antibodies (Chapter 92). Not only does antibody engineering contribute to the design of potential therapeutics, but important basic science information has been gained using recombinant antibodies.[39] For example, advances in understanding the role of specific effector functions in tumor cell destruction have been possible using mutant and engineered recombinant antibodies, with rituximab being an illustrative example.

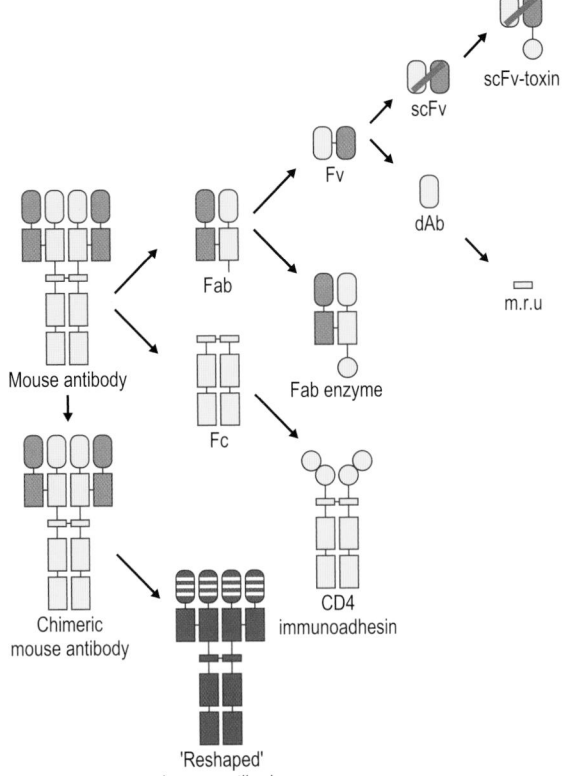

Fig. 14.6 Examples of engineered antibodies and antibody-derived fragments that can be created through the manipulation of antibody genes. Each closed rectangular (constant) or rounded (variable) box represents a domain. The molecule at the bottom of the figure represents a humanized antibody, where the constant domains and variable domain framework regions correspond to human amino acid sequences. Only the hypervariable regions, and in some cases a small number of framework residues, correspond to mouse or rat antibody amino acid sequences. Other structures depicted include an Fab fragment; an Fv fragment; a single-chain Fv fragment (scFv) in which the C-terminus of the V_H domain is linked covalently by a linker peptide to the N-terminus of the V_L domain; an Fab-enzyme fusion protein; an scFv-toxin fusion protein; an immunoadhesin in which extracellular domains from CD4 have been covalently attached to human heavy chain constant domains; a single V_H domain (dAb); and a peptide derived from a hypervariable region (minimal recognition unit, or mru).

With permission from Winter G, Milstein C, Man-made antibodies, Nature 1991: 349: 293.

References

1. Amit AG, Mariuzza RA, Phillips SEV, et al. Three-dimensional structure of an antigen-antibody complex at 2.8 Å resolution. Science 1986;233:747–53.
2. Greenspan NS, Di Cera E. Defining epitopes: it's not as easy as it seems. Nat Biotechnol 1999;17:936–7.
3. Pauling L. Molecular structure and intermolecular forces. In: Landsteiner K, editor. The specificity of serological reactions. New York: Dover; 1962. p. 275–93.
4. Steward MW. The biological significance of antibody affinity. Immunol Today 1981;2:134–9.
5. Karush F. The affinity of antibody: range, variability, and the role of multivalence. In: Litman GW, Good RA, editors. Immunoglobulins. New York: Plenum; 1978. p. 85–116.
6. Greenspan NS, Cooper LJN. Complementarity, specificity, and the nature of epitopes and paratopes in multivalent interactions. Immunol Today 1995;16:226–30.
7. Rini JM, Schulze-Gahmen U, Wilson IA. Structural evidence for induced fit as a mechanism for antibody–antigen recognition. Science 1992;255:959–65.
8. Holmberg D, Forsgren S, Forni L, et al. Reactions among IgM antibodies derived from neonatal mice. Eur J Immunol 1984;14:435–41.
9. Kramer A, Keitel T, Winkler K, et al. Molecular basis for the binding promiscuity of an anti-p24 (HIV-1) monoclonal antibody. Cell 1997;91:799–809.
10. Alberts B, Bray D, Lewis J, et al. Molecular biology of the cell. 2nd ed. New York/London: Garland; 1989. p. 94.
11. Náray-Szabó G. Analysis of molecular recognition: steric electrostatic and hydrophobic complementarity. J Mol Recognit 1993;6:205–10.
12. James LC, Roversi P, Tawfik DS. Antibody multispecificity mediated by conformational diversity. Science 2003;299:1362–7.
13. Kwong P, Doyle M, Casper D, et al. HIV-1 evades antibody-mediated neutralization through conformational masking of receptor-binding sites. Nature 2002;420:678–82.
14. Mollnes TE, Harboe M. Neoepitope expression during complement activation—a model for detecting antigenic changes in proteins and activation of cascades. The Immunologist 1993;1:43–9.
15. Walter G, Scheidtmann K-H, Carbone A, et al. Antibodies specific for the carboxy- and amino-terminal regions of simian virus 40 large tumor antigen. Proc Natl Acad Sci USA 1980;77:5197–200.
16. Berzofsky JA. Intrinsic and extrinsic factors in protein antigenic structure. Science 1985;229:932–40.
17. Kabat EA. The upper limit for the site of the human antidextran combining site. J Immunol 1960;84:82–5.
18. Mannik M. Physicochemical and functional relationships of immune complexes. J Immunol 1980;74:333–8.
19. Heyman B. The immune complex: possible ways of regulating the antibody response. Immunol Today 1990;11:310–3.
20. Nezlin R. Internal movements in immunoglobulin molecules. Adv Immunol 1990;48:1–40.
21. Boehm MK, Woof JM, Kerr MA, Perkins SJ. The Fab and Fc fragments of IgA1 exhibit a different arrangement from that in IgG: a study by X-ray and neutron solution scattering and homology modelling. J Mol Biol 1999;86(5):1421–47.
22. Dimmock NJ. Neutralization of animal viruses. Curr Top Microbiol Immunol 1993;183:1–146.
23. Mazanec MB, Kaetzel CS, Lamm ME, et al. Intracellular neutralization of virus by immunoglobulin A antibodies. Proc Natl Acad Sci USA 1992;89:6901–5.
24. Binder GK, Griffin DE. Immune-mediated clearance of virus from the central nervous system. Microbes Infect 2003;5(5):439–48.
25. Abboud N, Chow SK, Saylor C, et al. A requirement for FcγR in antibody-mediated bacterial toxin neutralization. J Exp Med 2010;207(11):2395–405.
26. Garred P, Michaelsen TE, Aase A. The IgG subclass pattern of complement activation depends on epitope density and antibody and complement concentration. Scand J Immunol 1989;30:379–82.
27. Tan LK, Shopes RJ, Oi VT, et al. Influence of the hinge region on complement activation, C1q binding, and segmental flexibility in chimeric human immunoglobulins. Proc Natl Acad Sci USA 1990;87:162–6.
28. Chintalacharuvu KR, Morrison SL. Production and characterization of recombinant IgA. Immunotechnology 1999;4(3–4):165–74.
29. Oortwijn BD, Eijgenraam JW, Rastaldi MP, et al. The role of secretory IgA and complement in IgA nephropathy. Semin Nephrol 2008;28:58–65.
30. Nimmerjahn F, Ravetch JV. Fcgamma receptors as regulators of immune responses. Nat Rev Immunol 2008;8(1):34–47.
31. Monteiro RC. Role of IgA and IgA fc receptors in inflammation. J Clin Immunol 2010;30(1):1–9.
32. Kaetzel CS, Robinson JK, Chintalacharuvu KR, et al. The polymeric immunoglobulin receptor (secretory component) mediates transport of immune complexes across epithelial cells: a local defense function for IgA. Proc Natl Acad Sci USA 1991;88:8796–800.
33. Greenspan NS. Relections on internal images. Nat Biotechnol 1997;15:123–4.
34. Cragg MS, French RR, Glennie MJ. Signaling antibodies in cancer therapy. Curr Opin Immunol 1999;11:541–7.
35. Kohler G, Milstein C. Continuous cultures of fused cells secreting antibody of predefined specificity. Nature 1975;256:495–7.
36. Morrison SL. In vitro antibodies: strategies for production and application. Annu Rev Immunol 1992;10:239–65.
37. Hudson PJ. Recombinant antibody constructs in cancer therapy. Curr Opin Immunol 1999;11:548–57.
38. Fanger MW, Morganelli PM, Guyre PM. Bispecific antibodies. Crit Rev Immunol 1992;12:101–24.
39. Deckert PM. Current constructs and targets in clinical development for antibody-based cancer therapy. Curr Drug Targets 2009;10:158–75.

Regulatory T cells

Shimon Sakaguchi, Kajsa Wing, Makoto Miyara

The normal mammalian immune system protects the individual from a myriad of potentially pathogenic micro-organisms while simultaneously avoiding harmful reactions against the normal constituents of the body, i.e., maintaining immunological self-tolerance. The mechanisms that control this fundamental property of the system are of interest to both basic and clinical immunologists, as the failure of protective immunity can lead to an enhanced susceptibility to infectious diseases, and loss of self-tolerance may trigger an autoimmune disorder. Furthermore, it is often clinically desirable to enhance an immune response to certain self (or quasi-self) antigens, such as tumor antigens, or to induce immune suppression for the purpose of facilitating organ transplant acceptance. Elucidation of the mechanisms responsible for immune regulation and maintenance of self-tolerance is, therefore, one of the primary goals of current medical immunology.

One key feature of the adaptive immune response is that, once triggered, it shows essentially the same effector activity whether the target antigen is a microbe or a self-antigen, leading to elimination of the microbe or destruction of self-tissue. To prevent self-destructive immune responses while allowing protective immune responses to non-self-antigens, the mammalian immune system has evolved various regulatory contrivances that either inhibit the generation of potentially harmful self-reactive T and B lymphocytes—termed central tolerance—or, after lymphocyte generation, downregulate cellular activation and expansion upon encounter with self-antigens, termed peripheral tolerance. For T cells, central tolerance is established in the thymus where many of the potentially dangerous lymphocytes that carry high-affinity T-cell receptors (TCR) for self-antigens are deleted via negative selection during development. This results in the generation of a peripheral T-cell repertoire that is largely self-tolerant. However, there is abundant evidence that some auto-reactive T cells escape thymic deletion, and potentially pathogenic self-reactive T cells are indeed present in most individuals. Nevertheless, autoimmune diseases only occur infrequently, thus indicating that auto-reactive T cells are somehow controlled in the periphery. Such peripheral mechanisms of self-tolerance include further deletion of self-reactive T cells, the seclusion of self-antigen from T lymphocytes, low TCR affinity, or lack of co-stimulation in antigen recognition (clonal ignorance), inactivation of auto-reactive T lymphocytes upon encounter with antigen without co-stimulation (clonal anergy), or active suppression of self-reactive lymphocytes by other T cells (dominant suppression).[1,2]

Among various mechanisms of peripheral self-tolerance, this chapter deals with dominant suppression mediated by regulatory T cells (Tregs). Several types of T cells with regulatory activity have been described, including subpopulations of γδ T cells, NKT cells, CD8[+] and CD4[+] T cells (Table 15.1, Fig. 15.1).[3] Some of these Tregs are naturally produced in the immune system, while others are induced from naïve T cells as a product of a particular mode of antigen stimulation in a particular cytokine milieu. Although it remains to be determined how each cell population is functionally stable and physiologically important, this abundance and apparent redundancy of Treg populations may not be surprising when one considers how essential it is to maintain immune homeostasis and self-tolerance.

This chapter focuses on CD4 Tregs, in particular naturally occurring CD25[+]CD4[+] Tregs that specifically express the transcription factor Foxp3. Foxp3[+]CD25[+]CD4[+] Tregs have been the subject of the majority of recent Treg studies, and may have the broadest implication to our understanding of the mechanism of various immunological disorders. There is evidence that an anomaly in Foxp3[+] natural Treg function or number can be a primary cause of autoimmune disease, allergy, and inflammatory disorders such as inflammatory bowel disease (IBD) in humans. Because of their natural presence in the immune system, they also pose as a good target for the treatment and prevention of immunological diseases.[4]

CD4 regulatory T cells

CD4 Tregs can be divided into two categories: naturally occurring and induced. The naturally occurring Foxp3[+] Tregs, also referred to as CD25[+] Tregs because of their constitutive expression of CD25, are primarily generated in the thymus in a functionally mature form but can also arise *de novo* in the periphery from naïve CD4 T cells. Induced CD4 Tregs, such as IL-10-secreting Type 1 regulatory T cells (Tr1) and TGF-β-secreting T helper 3 cells (Th3) also differentiate from naïve

Table 15.1 Subsets of natural and induced Treg

	Natural FOXP3+ Treg	Induced Tr1 and Th3	Qa-1-restricted CD8+ Treg	CD8+CD28- Treg	NKT cell	gdT cell
Site of generation	Thymus	Periphery/ *in vitro*	Periphery	Periphery/ *in vitro*	Periphery	Periphery
Marker	Foxp3, CD25, CTLA-4, GITR	IL-10 TGF-β	Non-classical MHC Ib Qa-1	Not specified	invariant TCR chain Va14 (mouse), Va24 (human)	Various subsets Vg5+ (mouse) Vg1+ (human)
Specificity	Peptide plus MHC class II	Peptide plus MHC class II	Peptide plus MHC class Ib	Peptide plus MHC class I	Glycolipids plus CD1d	Glycolipids plus CD1, Peptide plus MHC class Ib
Target cell	T cells, B cells, APC, NK cells NKT cells	T cell	T cell	DC/APC	T cells, APC	T cell, APC, epithelial cells
Suppressive mechanisms	Cell-contact Co-stimulation modification Cytokine production	IL-10 TGF-β	CD94-NKG2	Induction of ILT3/ILT4 in DC	IL-10, Th2 cytokines	Lysis, CD95-CD95 ligand pathway, thymosin-b4
Reported suppressive function	Autoimmunity Transplantation Allergy Infection Cancer	Autoimmunity Transplantation Allergy	Autoimmunity	Autoimmunity Transplantation	Autoimmunity Transplantation Cancer	Autoimmunity Allergy (dermatitis) Infection

APC, antigen presenting cell; DC, dendritic cell; ILT, immunoglobulin transcript; Tr1, regulatory type 1 cell; Th3, T helper 3 cell; Treg, regulatory T cell; MHC, major histocompatibility complex.

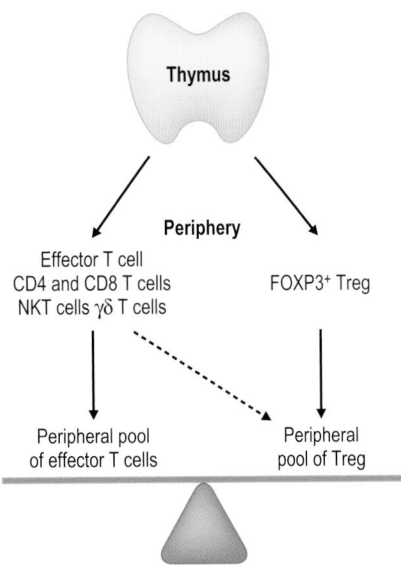

Fig. 15.1 Developmental pathways of regulatory T cells. Treg cells can develop either in the thymus or the periphery and are vital for maintaining tolerance as a counter-balance to effector T cells. Thymically generated Tregs, also known as naturally occurring Tregs or CD4+CD25+ Tregs, express Foxp3 and develop within the thymus according to a specialized combination of TCR and co-stimulatory signals. Extra-thymic development of CD4+ Tregs and CD8+ Tregs can ensue from a host of different conditions, such as high concentrations of TGF-β, IL-10, or other particular circumstances surrounding antigen priming. The signals that control differentiation of γδ T cells and NKT cells to cells with regulatory properties are less well defined.

T cells following antigen stimulation in conjunction with specific conditions in the periphery but do not express Foxp3. Although both natural Foxp3+ Tregs and induced Foxp3- Tregs are suppressive, they differ in their development, phenotype, and function and they are thus considered to be of separate lineages (Table 15.1, Fig. 15.1).[5]

Thymically derived CD4+ regulatory T cells

The first report of autoimmune-preventive thymically derived T cells in the normal immune system occurred about 40 years ago when thymectomy on day 3 of life (d3Tx) was said to inflict organ-specific autoimmune diseases, such as oophoritis, in otherwise healthy mice.[6] Subsequent studies showed that the development of autoimmune disease could be inhibited if the thymectomized animals were reconstituted with CD4+CD8- thymocytes or CD4+ splenocytes from histocompatible immune-uncompromised animals. In order to pinpoint a specific phenotype for CD4 T cells with regulatory function, surface markers with more restricted expression patterns have been explored, and among these CD5high, CD45RBlow, CD38low, and CD62Lhigh expression have been shown to characterize naturally occurring CD4+ Tregs in mice.[6] To date the functionally most useful and specific surface marker of natural Tregs is their high and stable expression of the interleukin-2 (IL-2) receptor α-chain, CD25. Between 5 and 10% of CD4+ T cells express CD25 constitutively in the thymus and periphery of mice. Importantly, transfer of CD4 lymphocytes depleted of CD25+ cells induces autoimmunity in athymic nude mice, while co-transfer of CD4+CD25+ cells protects the mice from disease induction (Fig. 15.2). Other markers shown to be associated with CD25+ Tregs are cytotoxic T lymphocyte antigen 4 (CTLA-4; CD152) and glucocorticoid-induced tumor necrosis factor receptor protein (GITR). However, neither these nor CD25 can be considered specific markers of natural Tregs since conventional T cells upregulate GITR, as well as CTLA-4 and CD25, after activation.[4,7] This dilemma is especially apparent when investigating naturally occurring Tregs in humans where up to 30% of CD4+ T cells in peripheral blood express CD25, yet only 2-4% of CD4+ T cells, enriched among cells with the highest expression level of CD25 (CD25high), have suppressive properties (Fig. 15.3).[8] The fact that CD25+ Tregs is not a discrete population in humans poses a problem both when obtaining cells for experimental purposes and when evaluating

Fig. 15.2 Dominant self-tolerance in rodents and humans. Transfer of T-cell suspensions depleted of Foxp3⁺CD4⁺ Tregs induces autoimmune disease and IBD, and heightens immune responses to non-self-antigens in athymic nude or SCID mice (left). Male children are afflicted with IPEX. Their mothers with hemizygous defects of the *FOXP3* gene bear defective and normal Tregs as a mosaic because of random inactivation of the X chromosome in each Treg cell. They are completely normal because normal Tregs dominantly control the activation and expansion of effector T (Teff) cells that mediate autoimmune disease, IBD, and allergy (right). Open circles represent intact Treg or Teff cells; closed circles represent defective Tregs.

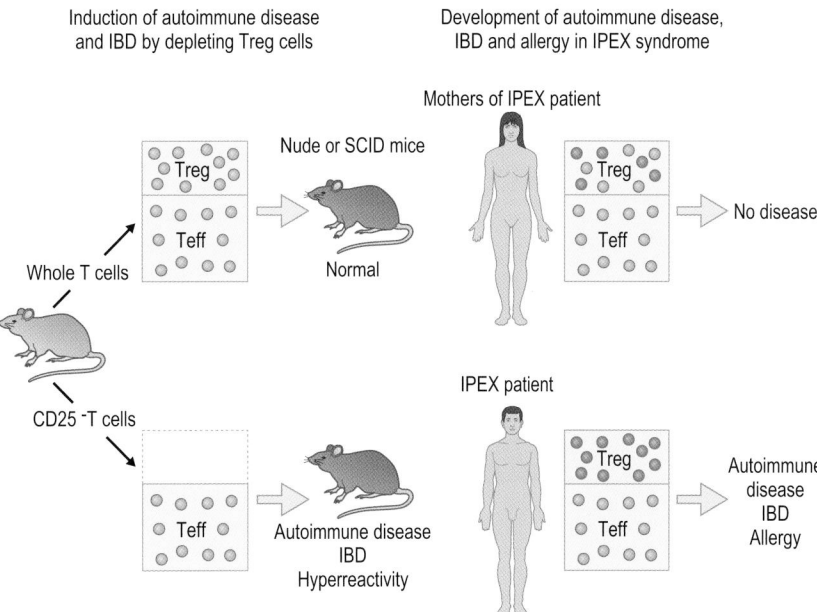

their role in a clinical setting. Therefore, finding more specific cell surface markers of CD4⁺ natural Tregs remains an important future goal.

Thymically derived CD25⁺ Tregs express the transcription factor Foxp3

A major breakthrough was achieved when natural CD25⁺ Tregs were found to specifically express the transcription factor Foxp3 that is closely linked with their development and function.[9] The first hint as to the significance of Foxp3 was given by studies of the Scurfy mutant mouse. This mouse strain suffers from a spontaneous X-linked mutation of the *Foxp3* gene, which leads to fatal lymphoproliferative disease associated with multiorgan infiltrates and early death by 3-4 weeks of age in hemizygous males. Similarly, mutations in the human orthologue *FOXP3* are linked to immune dysregulation, polyendocrinopathy, enteropathy, X-linked (IPEX) syndrome, which is an X-linked immunodeficiency syndrome associated with organ-specific autoimmune diseases such as type 1 diabetes, inflammatory bowel disease, allergic dermatitis, food allergy, hyperimmunoglobulinemia E, hematological disorders, and severe infections (Fig. 15.2).[7] Common features of the human IPEX syndrome and scurfy mice are deficient levels of CD25⁺ Tregs. CD25⁺CD4⁺ T cells and CD25⁺CD4⁺CD8⁻ thymocytes specifically express *Foxp3* mRNA in contrast to the cell surface markers used to date. In addition, other thymocytes/T cells, T helper 1 (Th1) or T helper 2 (Th2) cells scarcely express *Foxp3* even after stimulation.[9] Intranuclear staining of the Foxp3 protein shows that while the majority of Foxp3⁺ cells in mice reside in the CD4⁺CD25⁺ T-cell population, some can also be found in the CD4⁺CD25⁻ population (Fig. 15.3). Importantly, retroviral transduction of *Foxp3* in naïve CD25⁻ T cells can convert them to regulatory cells with similar function and phenotype as natural Tregs. Basically, the same pattern of FOXP3 expression can be observed in humans, with most FOXP3⁺ cells among CD4⁺CD25^high T cells, with a few being CD25⁻ or CD25^low (Fig. 15.3). One difference between mice and humans is that human CD8 T cells with suppressive function can, in some cases, express FOXP3. Another disparity is that low levels of FOXP3 can be transiently induced by TCR stimulation in non-regulatory T cells. These T cells can be

detected directly in blood as CD4⁺ T cells with a memory phenotype and a weak expression of FOXP3, but with no suppressive function.[8] Human FOXP3⁺ Tregs with suppressive function can be divided into two subsets: CD45RA⁺FOXP3^low naïve Tregs (nTregs) and CD45RA⁻FOXP3^high effector Tregs (eTregs) (Fig. 15.3). Naïve Tregs that express CD31, a marker for recent thymic emigrants, correspond to murine naturally occurring Treg cells that arise from the thymus. They differentiate *in vitro* upon activation and *in vivo*, probably in response to various self- or non-self antigens, into FOXP3^high effector Treg cells.

● CLINICAL RELEVANCE

IPEX is a result of FOXP3⁺ Treg deficiency

When the *Foxp3/FOXP3* gene has a loss-of-function mutation FOXP3⁺ Tregs fail to develop or Foxp3 protein is dysfunctional, and a fatal autoimmune/autoinflammatory disease develops. This monogenic X-linked disease directly demonstrates how crucial natural FOXP3⁺ Tregs are for maintaining self-tolerance and immune homeostasis.

Cardinal features of IPEX are:

- Autoimmune diseases (type 1 diabetes, thyroiditis, hemolytic anemia)
- Allergy (dermatitis, hyperimmunoglobulinemia E, food allergy)
- Inflammatory bowel disease

It is likely that Foxp3 can specify the Tregs cell lineage, regardless of whether the Tregs are CD4⁺ or CD8⁺, or are major histocompatibility complex (MHC) class II- or class I-restricted. Collectively, natural CD4⁺ Tregs are best recognized by their expression of Foxp3. However, since the Foxp3 protein is expressed in the nucleus, it is not useful for the isolation of live cells and, for that purpose, CD25 remains the most commonly used marker.

Development and maintenance of Foxp3⁺ Tregs

Several findings point to the thymus as central in the generation of Foxp3⁺ Tregs. First, CD25⁺Foxp3⁺ T cells are found in both periphery and thymus. Second, both peripheral and thymic CD25⁺Foxp3⁺ T cells suppress the proliferation and cytokine

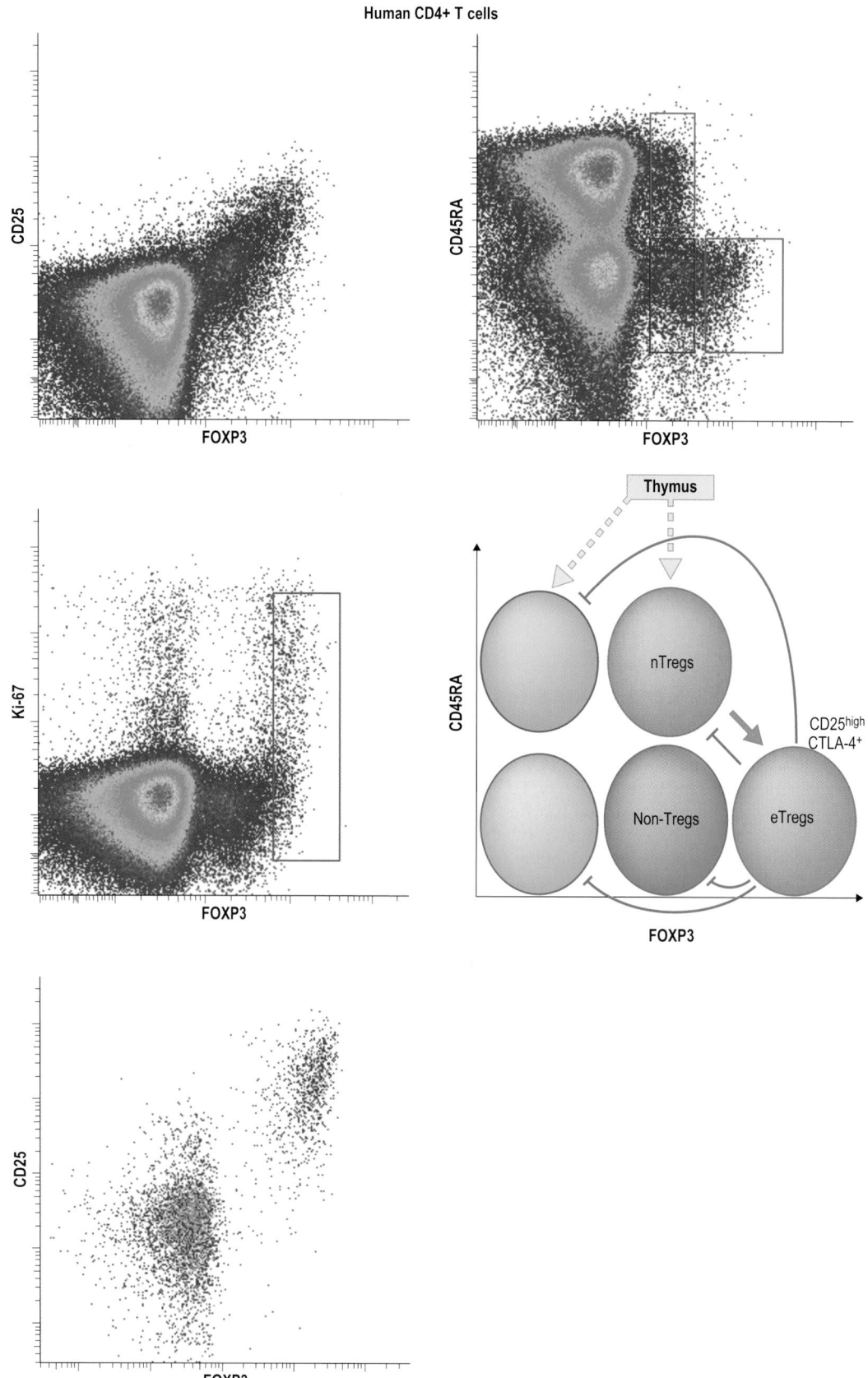

Fig. 15.3 Expression of CD25 and Foxp3 denotes natural Tregs in mice and in humans. In mice, between 5 and 10% of CD4$^+$ T cells express CD25 and, among these, almost all are Foxp3$^+$. In addition, a few Foxp3-expressing cells reside among CD4$^+$CD25$^-$ T cells. In the peripheral blood of humans, expression of surface marker CD25 is well correlated with intracellular FOXP3, especially when the levels of CD25 and FOXP3 are high (top left). CD45RA and intracellular expression of FOXP3 enables the definition of 3 distinct subsets within FOXP3$^+$CD4$^+$ T cells: CD45RA$^-$ effector Treg cells with high expression of FOXP3 (blue box), CD45RA$^+$ naïve Treg cells with low expression of FOXP3 (red box) and CD45RA$^-$ non-Treg cells with low expression of FOXP3 (purple box) (top right). Effector FOXP3^{high} Treg cells correspond to actively proliferating Treg cells *in vivo* as they express Ki-67 (bottom left, purple box). Thymus produces CD45RA$^+$FOXP3^{low} nTregs as well as naïve CD45RA$^+$ non-Treg cells. Upon antigenic stimulation, nTregs differentiate to CD45RA$^+$FOXP3^{high} eTregs, which are potently suppressive and capable of suppressing the proliferation of other Tregs as well as non-Tregs *in vitro* (bottom right).

production of conventional CD4 or CD8 T cells *in vitro*. Third, athymic mice transferred with CD25⁻ T cells or thymocytes spontaneously develop organ-specific autoimmune diseases, which can be reversed by co-transfer of either CD25⁺CD4⁺ thymocytes or CD25⁺CD4⁺ splenocytes from normal adult mice.[4] Therefore, the thymus not only contributes to self-tolerance by deleting auto-reactive T cells but also by producing Foxp3⁺ Tregs. Foxp3⁺ Tregs are thought to arise from T-cell clones with relatively high reactivity to self-antigens presented in the thymus. It is yet unclear how these cells are spared from negative selection and how the Tregs developmental pathway is initiated.[7] It is nevertheless likely that a higher responsiveness to self-antigen is a benefit when suppressing hazardous auto-reactive T cells since Foxp3⁺ Tregs would be more easily and strongly activated when presented with self-antigens in the context of tissue damage. In addition to TCR interaction, it seems that accessory signals, such as co-stimulation through CD28-B7 or CD40-CD40L, play an important role in the production of Foxp3⁺ Tregs in the thymus, since animals that lack CD28 or CD40 expression generate only minute numbers of Foxp3⁺ T cells in the thymus (Table 15.2).[7]

In the periphery, the maintenance of Foxp3⁺ Tregs requires antigenic priming and cytokines. It is vital that Foxp3⁺ Tregs encounter specific antigens to remain in the Tregs pool. For example, cell transfer experiments in d3Tx models have demonstrated that Tregs from donors of the same sex are better at protecting against orchitis or oophoritis than Tregs from donors of the opposite sex, and that Tregs from ovariectomized mice are less competent in preventing oophoritis than those from normal females. In general, Foxp3⁺ Tregs behave similarly to conventional T cells as they have been shown to recirculate between the blood and lymph and then home to organ-draining lymph nodes where they effectively expand in response to their specific antigen.[10]

IL-2 is vital for the maintenance of natural Tregs and CD25 is accordingly not a mere marker but also a functionally indispensable molecule for Tregs as a key component of the high affinity IL-2 receptor. Mice genetically deficient in IL-2 or IL-2 receptor α-chain (CD25) or β-chain (CD122) develop a severe lymphoproliferative disease with lymphocyte infiltration in multiple organs, resulting in early death.[4] Moreover, genetic deficiencies of CD25 in humans generate a comparable clinical and pathological pattern. It is now known that IL-2 deficient animals have substantially reduced, although not completely depleted, numbers of

Foxp3⁺ T cells, and that disease can be prevented by adoptive transfer of normal Foxp3⁺ Tregs (Table 15.2). TGF-β is another cytokine that is important for the maintenance of Foxp3⁺ Tregs as it is shown to enhance expression of *Foxp3* and also induce *de novo* Foxp3 expression in naïve T cells, thus making them suppressive.[5]

In addition to antigen recognition and cytokines, Foxp3⁺ Tregs require appropriate interactions with antigen-presenting cells (APC) for their function and survival. Several molecules of cell adhesion and co-stimulation are important for function and homeostasis of Tregs, including CD18/CD11a, GITR, CD28, CTLA-4, and Toll-like receptors (TLR).[4] Although Foxp3⁺ Tregs express these markers and direct signalling takes place through these molecules, indirect effects on Tregs via effector T cells also likely exist and must be taken into account. For example, CD28 provides naïve T cells with a co-stimulatory signal for promoting IL-2 secretion and preventing cell death and since Foxp3⁺ Tregs likely survive on exogenously produced IL-2 this may result in significant reduction of Foxp3⁺ Tregs. APCs, in particular dendritic cells (DCs), express TLRs, which recognize pathogen-associated molecular patterns shared among microbes or certain self-molecules (e.g., heat-chock proteins) released during inflammation. Strong activation of APCs via TLRs instigates DCs to mature and strongly activate and expand not only naïve T cells but also natural Foxp3⁺ Tregs. Furthermore, CD25⁺ Tregs express TLR 2, 5, and 8, and stimulation of Tregs through these TLRs may suppress excessive anti-microbial immune responses that could incur immunopathological tissue damage (Table 15.2).[4]

Suppressive function of Foxp3⁺ Tregs

The standard assay to analyze the suppressive function of CD25⁺ Tregs is to co-culture purified cell fractions of T cells with Tregs and then measure the proliferative response upon antigenic stimulation in the presence of APC. Such assays show that freshly isolated Foxp3⁺CD25⁺ Tregs are not able to suppress T-cell responses *in vitro* unless they are first stimulated via the TCR with a specific antigen. However, once activated, they suppress other CD4 and CD8 T cells irrespective of their antigen specificities.[11] Foxp3⁺ Tregs can inhibit proliferation and cytokine production of naïve T cells. They can also suppress the

Table 15.2 Signals with impact on FOXP3⁺ Treg induction, maintenance, and suppression

	Development	**Maintenance/survival**	**Suppressive function**
Peptide MHC II interaction	Yes (high affinity)	Yes	Yes at least initially
CD28	Yes (crucial)	Yes (indirectly by induction of IL-2 production in effector T cells)	Not crucial for induction of suppression but high expression on APC breaks suppression
CD40	Yes	No	No
CTLA-4	No	Unclear	Yes
GITR	No	Modest positive effect	Breaks suppression
TLR ligands	No	Yes	TLR ligands initially break suppression but this is followed by induction of enhanced suppression
IL-2	Yes (but not crucial)	Yes (crucial)	High levels break suppression
TGF-β	Not required for thymic differentiation but may be involved in peripheral induction	Yes	Yes (not crucial)

MHC II, major histocompatibility complex II; IL-2, interleukin 2; APC, antigen presenting cell; TGF-β, transforming growth factor β; CTLA-4, cytotoxic T lymphocyte antigen 4; GITR, glucocorticoid-induced tumor necrosis factor receptor protein; TLR, toll-like receptor.

function of already differentiated Th1 and Th2 cells *in vitro* and have been shown to reverse ongoing immunopathology like colitis *in vivo*.[12] Furthermore, in addition to suppressing T-cell function, Foxp3[+] Tregs are also able to suppress B cells, NK cells, and NKT cells.[13]

Foxp3[+] Tregs likely suppress by multiple mechanisms including both soluble and cell surface-bound mediators (Fig. 15.4). *In vitro* studies have shown that Foxp3[+] Tregs need direct cell-to-cell contact with responder cells, and that suppression does not occur if Tregs are separated from effector T cells by a semi-permeable membrane even if this allows for the passage of soluble factors.[11] Moreover, Foxp3[+]CD25[+] Tregs are not prominent producers of either IL-10 or TGF-β *in vitro*. These features are quite different from Tr1 or Th3 cells, which solely rely on soluble immunosuppressive cytokines, such as IL-10 and TGF-β, for their inhibitory function.

Although Foxp3[+] Tregs have been shown to suppress effector T cells under APC-free conditions *in vitro*, presumably by absorbing IL-2, it is reasonable that Foxp3[+] Tregs *in vivo* control immune responses also by regulating APC. Indeed, by using two-photon laser-scanning microscopy, it has been shown *in vivo* that while there are limited contacts between Foxp3[+] Tregs and effector T cells, stable interactions exist between Foxp3[+] Tregs and DC during ongoing suppression in lymph nodes.[10] One way that Foxp3[+] Tregs regulate immune responses may be through competition with effector T cells for access to APC.[7] Foxp3[+] Tregs have, relative to conventional T cells, a more activated phenotype (e.g., high expression of adhesion molecules such as LFA-1) in normal healthy individuals, which gives an advantage when engaging with APC and results in the prevention of naïve T-cell priming. Interestingly, Foxp3[+] Tregs have been

shown to modify the function of the APC. APCs cultured with Foxp3[+] Tregs downregulate CD80 and CD86 by a CTLA-4 dependant mechanism and become impaired in their ability to stimulate T cells. Additionally, CTLA-4 expressing Tregs can induce production of the enzyme indoleamine dioxygenase (IDO), which catalyzes the amino acid tryptophan to the metabolite kynurenine that represses T-cell responses. Importantly, CTLA-4 expression by Foxp3[+] Tregs has been shown to be critical for tolerance *in vivo* since mice with deletion of this co-inhibitory molecule only in Foxp3-expressing cells develop lethal autoimmunity. Other proposed suppressive mechanisms that involve close contact between Foxp3[+] Tregs and target cells include surface-bound TGF-β, which is inhibitory at a close range, and perforin/granzyme B, which kills target cells (Fig. 15.4).[14]

Despite the fact that immunosuppressive cytokines are redundant for suppression *in vitro*, the *in vivo* situation seems somewhat different. Recently, the immune suppressive cytokine IL-35 has been implicated in Treg-mediated suppression and both TGF-β and IL-10 expressed by Foxp3[+] Treg are important in prevention of IBD in mice.[15] Curiously, adoptive transfer of IL-10-deficient CD25[+] Tregs failed to protect against colitis, although it could inhibit the development of gastritis. Furthermore while perforin- or granzyme-expressing Foxp3[+] Tregs are rare in the spleen they are abundant in a tumor environment.[7] Taken together, Foxp3[+] Tregs can use several different mechanisms of suppression and one or another seems to play more prominent roles than others depending on the local cytokine milieu, the strength, and type of immune response.

Peripherally induced CD4 regulatory T cells

In addition to thymus-derived natural CD25[+]CD4[+] Tregs, there is abundant evidence in mice that supporting the peripheral development of T cells with suppressive properties and an anergic phenotype. For example, Foxp3-expressing CD25[+]CD4[+] Tregs, functionally and phenotypically similar to natural Tregs, can be induced from naïve T cells by *in vitro* antigenic stimulation in the presence of TGF-β and IL-2 or by specific ways of *in vivo* antigenic stimulation, e.g., targeting of antigen to immature DC or chronic low-dose antigen administration.[16] Recent findings indicate that both murine and human natural Treg cells express Helios, an Icaros family transcription factor, while induced FoxP3-expressing CD4 T cells do not, which indicates that some differences exists between thymically derived and peripherally induced Foxp3[+] Tregs.[17] Other induced Tregs include TGF-β-secreting Th3 cells and IL-10-secreting Tr1 cells, which have been shown to be present and functional in humans following bone marrow transplantation and in response to allergens (Table 15.1).

Tr1 cells were initially generated *in vitro* from CD4 T cells rendered anergic by chronic stimulation in the presence of IL-10, which is a potent negative regulator of inflammation and lymphoproliferation.[18] T cells obtained in such a fashion produce a unique pattern of cytokines distinct from Th1 or Th2 cells, with IL-10 as the signature cytokine. In addition Tr1 cells secrete some TGF-β, IFN-γ, and IL-5 but no IL-4 or IL-2. Tr1 cells are anergic but can proliferate in the presence of IL-2. Currently there is no specific surface marker for Tr1 cells and their identification relies on the IL-10 they produce, which, together with TGF-β, forms the basis for their suppressive function. Notably, Tr1 cells do not express high constitutive levels of CD25 nor do they express Foxp3, which clearly separates them from Foxp3[+] natural Tregs. In addition, antigenic stimulation with immature DCs (i.e., low levels of co-stimulatory molecules), or DCs pre-treated with

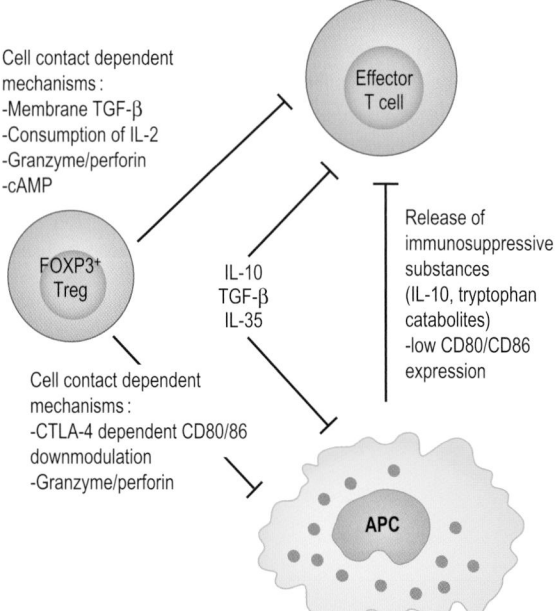

Fig. 15.4 Proposed suppressive mechanisms of FoxP3[+] Tregs. Foxp3[+]CD25[+] Tregs can inhibit many different types of effector cells and can also suppress immune responses at multiple stages, including the initial priming in the lymph node and effector actions at the site of inflammation. The precise mechanism is not known, but numerous theories have been proposed and it is likely that Foxp3[+]CD25[+] Tregs suppress by several different mechanisms. *In vivo* Tregs can act in a cell contact-dependent manner by competing directly for stimulatory ligands on the APC, by absorbing essential growth factors such as IL-2, or by directly transmitting an as-yet uncharacterized negative signal to either the T cell or APC. Alternatively, Tregs can use long-range suppressive mechanisms by means of the cytokines IL-10, IL-35, and TGF-β.

IL-10/TGF-β, confers naïve CD4 T cells with an anergic and suppressive phenotype both *in vitro* and *in vivo*.[18]

Several investigations show that Tr1 cells take part in the tolerance process in humans. For example, the presence of Tr1 cells can be correlated with lack of graft-versus-host disease in bone marrow transplantation and Tr1 cells are also induced following specific immunotherapy in allergic patients. Experimental data from a murine model shows that Tr1 cells can prevent IBD. Interestingly, Tr1 cells specific for *Escherichia coli* proteins can be isolated from the intestinal mucosa of healthy donors. In pemphigus vulgaris, which is an autoimmune disorder with circulating autoantibodies against desmoglein-3 (Chapter 62), Tr1 cells specific for desmoglein-3 can be isolated from pemphigus vulgaris-prone but apparently healthy individuals, while pemphigus patients rarely have such cells. Collectively, Tr1 cells can be induced to auto-antigens as well as foreign antigens as a component of the mechanisms that maintain tolerance to both self and non-self.[18]

Th3 cells were identified in mice during investigations of the mechanisms of oral tolerance. Oral tolerance has presumably evolved to prevent hypersensitivity reactions to food and microbial antigens present in the mucosal flora. It was found that mice fed with myelin basic protein, a neuronal auto-antigen, developed T cells that preferentially produced TGF-β together with varying amounts of IL-4 and IL-10. These T cells had suppressive properties, mediated by TGF-β, and could prevent the induction of experimental autoimmune encephalomyelitis (EAE), the murine equivalent of multiple sclerosis (MS) (Chapter 65). Th3 cells can be identified by their surface expression of latency-associated peptide (LAP), which binds inactive TGF-β. Recently, LAP+ Tregs have been shown to be induced after oral or nasal administration of tolerogenic CD3 monoclonal antibodies. Th3 cells can also be generated *in vitro* if grown in the presence of TGF-β, IL-4, and IL-10. Since the intestinal mucosa has high basal levels of all these cytokines, which are upregulated after antigen administration, it is conceivable that this particular environment drives the formation of Th3 cells while a different setting may produce Tregs of another phenotype.[16]

Other subsets of regulatory T cells

In addition to CD4+ Tregs, other types of T cells with immunosuppressive properties are also found, and these can recognize antigens different from those typically presented to CD4 T cells via MHC class II and may therefore serve to induce tolerance in other settings (Table 15.1). One example is CD8 T cells with TCRs that recognize antigen presented by the mouse MHC class lb Qa-1 molecule (HLA-E in humans). Qa-1 has limited polymorphisms, is expressed solely by activated T cells, and can present both foreign and self-peptides. Since Qa-1 peptide complexes on, for example, CD4 T cells can bind the inhibitory CD94-NKG2 receptor complex on CD8 T cells, this is believed to be one way that Qa-1-restricted CD8 T cells regulate T-cell responses.[19] Another subset of regulatory CD8 T cells are CD8+CD28- Tregs, which can suppress immune responses by direct interaction with APCs. These cells are generated by multiple rounds of *in vitro* stimulation with allo-antigen and can downregulate co-stimulatory molecules or upregulate the inhibitory immunoglobulin-like transcript 3 (ILT3) and ILT4 receptors on DCs, thus leading to the impaired activation of effector T cells.[19]

γδ T cells with a regulatory phenotype exist as a subset of the epithelial γδ T cells, which can be found in mice. Mice deficient in γδ T cells do not appropriately regulate responses to various pathogens. This inappropriate regulation manifests as immunopathology in conjunction with the robust development of

immunity. γδ T cell-deficient mice also show accelerated autoimmune responses in models of systemic lupus erythematosus (SLE) and spontaneously develop dermatitis when bred on certain genetic backgrounds. Commonly, these conditions are driven by αβ T cells and the γδ T cells will inhibit αβ T cells predominantly in the local environment. In humans, which lack an equivalent population of intraepithelial γδ cells, it is plausible that this immune regulation is provided by other types of suppressive cells.[20]

NKT cells respond to the non-classical class I antigen presenting molecule CD1d, which binds glycolipids rather than peptides. NKT cells can induce either pro-inflammatory (IFN-γ) or anti-inflammatory (IL-4, IL-10, IL-13) immune responses, but the prerequisites for this choice are ill defined. Nevertheless, under appropriate conditions, NKT cells clearly promote tolerance, which is illustrated in studies of transplantation and oral tolerance (Table 15.1).[21]

Clinical relevance of regulatory T cells

Abundant evidence strongly supports natural Tregs as key controllers of self-tolerance, and Tregs of various subsets take an active part in the control of almost all types of physiological and pathological immune responses, which also makes them suitable targets for immunotherapy (Table 15.1, Table 15.3).

⬤ THERAPEUTIC PRINCIPLES

Adjustment of the immune response by FOXP3+ Treg

Reduction of FOXP3+ Treg suppression or reducing Treg numbers
- Enhancement of tumor immunity
- Clearance of infections
- Improvement of responses to vaccines

Boost of FOXP3+ Treg function or increasing Treg numbers
- Treatment of autoimmunity
- Treatment of allergic responses
- Induction of transplantation tolerance
- Control of excessive immunopathology to foreign antigens (i.e. pathogens)
- Maintenance of feto-maternal tolerance in pregnancy

Autoimmunity

As discussed above, natural Foxp3+CD4+ Tregs are engaged in active suppression of autoimmune disease since their depletion results in spontaneous development of autoimmune disease in rodents. Furthermore, genetic anomaly of Tregs development or function can be a direct cause of autoimmune disease in humans, as exemplified in IPEX.[7] A reduction of Foxp3+ Tregs in number or function has been reported in systemic autoimmune diseases such as SLE, Sjögren syndrome, ANCA-associated vasculitis, Kawasaki disease, systemic sclerosis, psoriasis, autoimmune hepatitis, myasthenia gravis, and IBD.[17] Of note, type II autoimmune polyglandular syndrome, which resembles the systemic disease induced in nude mice reconstituted with splenocytes devoid of CD4+CD25+ T cells, is also characterized by Treg functional deficiency. On the other hand, studies of multiple sclerosis (MS) and type 1 diabetes did not detect any

Table 15.3 Potential therapeutic approaches for Treg-based therapy

Increase of Treg numbers or function	Reduction of Treg numbers or function
Ex vivo expansion of pure natural FOXP3$^+$ Treg with allo- or auto-antigens plus growth factors such as IL-2 and chemicals such as rapamycin *Ex vivo* induction of Treg from conventional T cells by cytokines (IL-10, TGF-β), pharmacological agents or modified DC *In vivo* promotion of Tregs rather than effector T cells using monoclonal Ab treatment or pharmacological agents (anti-CD3 Ab, anti-CD40L Ab, etc)	Transient reduction of FOXP3$^+$ Treg and/or perturbation of suppression *in vivo* (anti-CD25 Ab, anti-CTLA-4 Ab, or anti-IL-2 Ab) Render effector T cells resistant to suppression (GITR signalling)

Treg, regulatory T cell; IL-2, interleukin-2; IL-10, interleukin-10; TGF-β, transforming growth factor β; DC, dendritic cell; CTLA-4, cytotoxic T lymphocyte antigen 4; GITR, glucocorticoid induced tumor necrosis factor receptor protein.

differences between patients and controls and conflicting data have been reported in rheumatoid arthritis (RA) with regard to both function and numbers of CD25^{high} Tregs. A general observation is that FOXP3$^+$ Tregs increase in number at the site of inflammation.[17] In the case of RA, synovial fluid from patients with ongoing RA was found to contain increased numbers of Foxp3$^+$CD25$^+$ Tregs as compared to the levels in peripheral blood. CD25$^+$ Tregs from synovial fluid from patients with RA are largely functional, although their numbers or suppressive function is apparently not enough to halt the inflammatory process. In contrast, CD25$^+$ Tregs obtained from the blood of MS patients have reportedly decreased abilities to suppress proliferation of effector T cells. In summary, reduced levels of FOXP3$^+$CD25$^+$ Tregs in peripheral blood are not a general finding in autoimmune disease and may not necessarily reflect the actual conditions at the site of inflammation. It remains to be determined whether an imbalance between natural Tregs and self-reactive T cells somehow plays a causative role in common autoimmune diseases.[22]

Allergic disease

CD25$^+$ natural Tregs play an important role in suppressing the development of allergic reactions to innocuous environmental substances. This is best illustrated by IPEX, which is accompanied not only by organ-specific autoimmune diseases but also by severe eczematous dermatitis, high levels of serum IgE and sometimes eosinophila.[4] Indeed, FOXP3$^+$CD25$^+$ Tregs from the blood of healthy non-allergic donors suppress both proliferation and production of Th2 cytokines when challenged with specific allergens *in vitro*. If the same experiment is performed with Tregs from allergic individuals a marked difference is seen, as they fail to downregulate Th2-related responses to allergens. Since the suppressive ability for polyclonal stimuli is retained in allergic patients this deficiency is directly related to the allergen the individual is sensitized to, and thus probably does not reflect a general Tregs deficiency. The inability to suppress Th2 responses induced by birch or grass pollen is more aggravated when the allergic reaction is ongoing and effector cells are fully activated, as during spring and summer compared to wintertime. Addition of IL-4 can attenuate the CD25$^+$ Tregs-mediated suppression of Th2 clones *in vitro* in the same way as IL-2, which may provide an explanation for the insufficient control of ongoing allergic responses by Tregs.[13] Both non-allergic and allergic individuals harbor allergen-specific IL-4-producing effector T cells, IL-10-producing Tr1 cells, and CD25$^+$ Tregs, but in different proportions. The balance between Th2 and certain Tregs populations may therefore dictate whether clinical allergy will develop. Indeed, in the setting of curative specific allergy immunotherapy (SIT), allergen-specific IL-10-producing T cells can be induced. Furthermore, children who "grow out" of their cow milk allergy have higher numbers of CD4$^+$CD25$^+$ T cells specific for β-lactoglobulin than children with clinically active allergy. This suggests that certain allergies can be cured by the induction/expansion of antigen-specific Tregs and that the balance of Tregs versus effector T cells is of importance to prevent allergy.[23]

Transplantation

The ultimate goal of organ transplantation is to establish tolerance to allogeneic organ grafts as effectively and stably as to self-tissues, but without the need for continuous general immunosuppression (Chapter 81).[24] Needless to say, Tregs have sparked a lot of attention in this area of research. CD25$^+$ Tregs were first shown to suppress graft versus host disease (GVHD) in murine models of allogeneic bone marrow transplantation. Similarly, nude mice transplanted with allogeneic skin rejected the graft when reconstituted with CD4$^+$CD25$^-$ T cells alone but retained the graft when large enough numbers of CD25$^+$ Tregs were co-transferred. In humans, attempts have been made to prevent GVHD in bone marrow transplantation and induce graft tolerance in organ transplantation by the use of purified CD25$^+$ Tregs.[25] Efforts have also been made to expand donor-specific Tregs *ex vivo* to enhance suppression and lower the number of Tregs needed for tolerance induction. Other means to establish tolerance to grafts include administration of monoclonal antibodies (mAb) to various cell surface molecules such as CD4, CD8, and CD40L on T cells and CD40, CD80/86 on APC or CD11a and CD54 expressed by both T cells and APC.[24] These treatments may more potently suppress the activation and expansion of effector T cells than that of CD25$^+$ natural Tregs, and thus allow the latter to expand in a graft-specific fashion and tip the scale in favor of dominant tolerance. In addition, such mAb treatments can also induce Tregs of extra-thymic origin. Indeed, several types of inducible Tregs including CD8$^+$ Tregs and Tr1 are shown to contribute to graft tolerance.[18,19] A third potential way to promote the induction of Tregs in organ transplantation is to evaluate the effects of various immunosuppressants in terms of altering the balance between Tregs and effector T cells. Different immunosuppressants target different pathways in cell metabolism and can therefore have different effects on cell populations that behave in dissimilar ways, such as effector T cells and Tregs. Dosage and timing of administration, as well as specific drug combinations, seem to be a promising angle of transplantation immunotherapy with the purpose of inducing graft tolerance and preventing graft rejection. Tregs have been shown to home to, and reside within, the graft, which is stably accepted once a dominance of Tregs has become established. Treg-mediated transplantation tolerance is not a systemic phenomenon, but rather localized to the graft, and as such it would not incur the dangers that accompany general immunosuppression.[24]

Tumor immunity

It is now well known that many of the tumor-associated antigens recognized by a patient's T cells are normal self-constituents, indicating that anti-tumor immune responses are within the range of Foxp3[+] Treg control. Therefore, the presence of natural Tregs in the normal immune system may not only prevent autoimmunity but also hamper immune surveillance of cancer.[26] In fact, Foxp3[+] Tregs are shown to reside in the tumor mass where they likely block any immune response targeting malignant cells. Studies performed on human malignancies show that the frequency of Foxp3[+] Tregs is increased in tumors of, for example, metastatic melanoma or cancers in the pancreas and lung. Moreover, high levels of Foxp3[+] Tregs in the tumor are correlated with a poor prognosis and survival. Treg cells are not only involved in solid tumors but also in hematologic malignancies.[27] For example, the architectural pattern of Treg cells in follicular lymphomas is associated with the prognosis of the disease. Whether the elevated levels are due to migration of Tregs into the tumor or to an expansion on the site is not clear, but evidence exists in support of both events. For example, ovarian tumor cells and infiltrating macrophages secrete the Treg-recruiting chemokine CCL22, which binds to CCR4 expressed by Tregs, and, in addition, many tumors produce TGF-β, which contributes to the maintenance of Foxp3[+] Tregs and may also induce Foxp3 expression in non-Treg cells within the tumor microenvironment. It is now evident that both effector T cells and Tregs must be assessed in monitoring the efficacy of anti-cancer immunotherapy.[26]

Involvement of Tregs in tumor immunity indicates that anti-tumor immune responses can be provoked or enhanced by depleting Tregs in a host that is otherwise responding poorly. Experimental mouse models have indeed demonstrated that simple depletion of CD25[+] Tregs with anti-CD25 Ab results in tumor eradication, and similar effects can be achieved with *in vivo* administration of agonistic anti-GITR or anti-CTLA-4 blocking Abs.[28] Depletion of CD25[+] T cells also enhances the effect of vaccination with tumor antigens. Pharmacological agents are another possible way of altering the effector T cell/Tregs ratio. For example, fludarabine was shown to selectively decrease the frequency of CD25[+] Tregs in patients receiving chemotherapy. Conversely, previously used regimens, such as administration of exogenous IL-2, are now being re-evaluated since IL-2 may expand Tregs. As expected from the role of Tregs in self-tolerance, a caveat of Treg-based therapies of cancer is the possible development of autoimmunity that may depend on the degree and period of *in vivo* systemic Tregs depletion as well as the genetic make-up of the host.[26]

Infectious disease

Immune responses to infectious agents, such as bacteria and viruses, often result in tissue damage, which might be more severe if it were not for the involvement of Tregs. On the downside, in many cases Tregs can contribute to the development of chronic infections. As previously discussed, Foxp3[+]CD25[+] Tregs have the potential to directly respond to microbial products and are believed to be engaged in suppressing responses to infectious agents. A number of studies show that the outcome of an infection partly hinges on the proper balance between effector T cells and Tregs.[29] For example, in the murine model of colitis effector T cells, in the absence of Treg, are triggered by the commensal bacteria to cause intestinal inflammation in immunodeficient hosts, while co-transfer of CD25[+] Tregs protects the animals

through an IL-10-dependent mechanism.[15] Adoptive transfer of CD25[+] Tregs prevents lethal pneumonia in T-cell-deficient mice infected with *Pneumocystis jiroveci*, but at the expense of a deficient protective response and microbial clearance. Similarly, CD25[+] Tregs suppress Th1 responses in mice infected with *Helicobacter pylori*, thereby limiting the mucosal inflammation, but resulting in a higher bacterial load. Human studies show that CD25[+] Tregs from carriers of *H. pylori* suppress responses to *H. pylori* antigens *in vitro* and have increased frequencies of CD25[high] T cells in both the stomach and the duodenal mucosa compared with healthy controls. Taken together, modulation of the infectious response by Foxp3[+] Tregs can limit tissue damage, but may enhance pathogen survival. This sort of compromise may not always be adverse to the host. For example, in murine *Leishmania major* infection, CD25[+] Tregs prevent complete eradication of the parasites, which results in the persistence of low numbers of microbes that have proven to be essential for the development of T-cell memory and prevention of re-infection. However, this delicate balance can be tipped in favor of the pathogen, which can be seen in the case of malaria and various viral infections, such as human immunodeficiency virus (HIV). For example, HIV-specific CD4 and CD8 T-cell responses are substantially suppressed by Foxp3[+]CD25[+] Tregs *in vitro* in most HIV-infected individuals. Taken together, future treatments, and also vaccine design, will need to take Tregs into account and, depending on the pathogen in question, it might be necessary to reduce or enhance the activity of Tregs to achieve a favorable outcome (Table 15.3).[29]

Translational research

Manipulations of Foxp3[+] Tregs in animal models of, for example, autoimmune disease, cancer, transplantation, and infection have shown a great potential for modulation of immunological diseases by this subset. The findings in animals have already started to make their way into clinical practice and more is likely to come within the next 5-10 years. In cases when immunity needs to be boosted, such as in cancer and during infection, the approach is to identify molecules that inhibit function and differentiation of Tregs as well as molecules that locally deplete them. Such examples in current therapy are CTLA4-specific blocking antibody (Ipilimumab (MDX-010; Bristol-Myers Squibb)) to dampen Treg function and enhance effector T-cell activity and DAB389-IL-2 (denileukin difitox (Ontak; Eisai)) to deplete Tregs. In cases when tolerance should be reinforced (autoimmunity, transplantation, allergy, feto-maternal tolerance) molecules that either mimic or enhance Tregs function and survival is under investigation. In the former case CTLA4-Ig (Abatacept (Orencia; Bristol-Myers Squibb)) that in part mimics the effect of Tregs on antigen-presenting cells is currently being used for the treatment of, for example, rheumatoid arthritis. In addition, cellular therapy by infusion of *ex vivo* expanded Tregs is in small-scale use in patients with GVHD after hematopoetic stem cell transplantation. Cell-based therapies are indeed a promising strategy for managing various immunological diseases and immune responses, but require further improvement in the purity and functional stability of *ex vivo* expanded or induced Foxp3[+] Tregs. This is attainable by determining specific Treg markers for isolation of a pure Treg population and by generating a suitable mix of cytokines and chemicals that favor survival and expansion of Tregs over conventional T cells, while at the same time stabilizing FOXP3 expression. The development of such a "cocktail" will be a major endeavor for the years to come.

ON THE HORIZON

■ Treg-based therapeutics consisting of small chemical compounds as well as biologicals that can either reinstate tolerance when needed in the case of autoimmunity, transplantation, allergy, feto-maternal tolerance or locally downregulate Tregs in cancer and infection.

■ *Ex vivo* expansion and/or induction protocols that generate pure and stable FOXP3⁺ Tregs that can be used in a wide variety of immunological disorders.

References

1. Palmer E. Negative selection—clearing out the bad apples from the T-cell repertoire. Nat Rev Immunol 2003;3(5):383–91.

2. Van Parijs L, Abbas AK. Homeostasis and self-tolerance in the immune system: turning lymphocytes off. Science 1998;280(536156):243–8.

3. Bach JF. Regulatory T cells under scrutiny. Nat Rev Immunol 2003;3(3):189–98.

4. Sakaguchi S. Naturally arising Foxp3-expressing CD25+CD4+ regulatory T cells in immunological tolerance to self and non-self. Nat Immunol 2005;6(4):345–52.

5. Curotto de Lafaille MA, Lafaille JJ. Natural and adaptive foxp3+ regulatory T cells: more of the same or a division of labor? Immunity 2009;30(5):626–35.

6. Sakaguchi S, Wing K, Miyara M. Regulatory T cells—a brief history and perspective. Eur J Immunol 2007;37(Suppl. 1):S116–23.

7. Wing K, Sakaguchi S. Regulatory T cells exert checks and balances on self tolerance and autoimmunity. Nat Immunol 2010;11(1):7–13.

8. Sakaguchi S, Miyara M, Costantino CM, Hafler DA. FOXP3+ regulatory T cells in the human immune system. Nat Rev Immunol 2010;10(7):490–500.

9. Zheng Y, Rudensky AY. Foxp3 in control of the regulatory T cell lineage. Nat Immunol 2007;8(5):457–62.

10. Bluestone JA, Tang Q. How do CD4+CD25+ regulatory T cells control autoimmunity? Curr Opin Immunol 2005;17(6):638–42.

11. Piccirillo CA, Thornton AM. Cornerstone of peripheral tolerance: naturally occurring CD4+CD25+ regulatory T cells. Trends Immunol 2004;25(7):374–80.

12. Duchmann R, Zeitz M. T regulatory cell suppression of colitis: the role of TGF-beta. Gut 2006;55(5):604–6.

13. Wing K, Suri-Payer E, Rudin A. CD4+CD25+-regulatory T cells from mouse to man. Scand J Immunol 2005;62(1):1–15.

14. Tang Q, Bluestone JA. The Foxp3+ regulatory T cell: a jack of all trades, master of regulation. Nat Immunol 2008;9(3):239–44.

15. Izcue A, Coombes JL, Powrie F. Regulatory T cells suppress systemic and mucosal immune activation to control intestinal inflammation. Immunol Rev 2006;212:256–71.

16. Weiner HL, da Cunha AP, Quintana F, Wu H. Oral tolerance. Immunol Rev 2011;241(1):241–59.

17. Miyara M, Gorochov G, Ehrenstein M, et al. Human FoxP3(+) regulatory T cells in systemic autoimmune diseases, Autoimmun Rev [Internet] 2011 May 18 [cited 2011 Jul 26]; available from: http://www.ncbi.nlm.nih.gov/pubmed/21621000.

18. Battaglia M, Gregori S, Bacchetta R, Roncarolo M-G. Tr1 cells: from discovery to their clinical application. Semin Immunol 2006;18(2):120–7.

19. Smith TRF, Kumar V. Revival of CD8 + Treg-mediated suppression. Trends Immunol 2008;29(7):337–42.

20. Hayday A, Tigelaar R. Immunoregulation in the tissues by gammadelta T cells. Nat Rev Immunol 2003;3(3):233–42.

21. Godfrey DI, Kronenberg M. Going both ways: immune regulation via CD1d-dependent NKT cells. J Clin Invest 2004;114(10):1379–88.

22. Dejaco C, Duftner C, Grubeck-Loebenstein B, Schirmer M. Imbalance of regulatory T cells in human autoimmune diseases. Immunology 2006;117(3):289–300.

23. Akdis M, Blaser K, Akdis CA. T regulatory cells in allergy: novel concepts in the pathogenesis, prevention, and treatment of allergic diseases. J Allergy Clin Immunol 2005;116(5):961–8; quiz 969.

24. Wood KJ, Sakaguchi S. Regulatory T cells in transplantation tolerance. Nat Rev Immunol 2003;3(3):199–210.

25. Randolph DA, Fathman CG. CD4+CD25+ regulatory T cells and their therapeutic potential. Annu Rev Med 2006;57:381–402.

26. Baecher-Allan C, Anderson DE. Immune regulation in tumor-bearing hosts. Curr Opin Immunol 2006;18(2):214–9.

27. Nishikawa H, Sakaguchi S. Regulatory T cells in tumor immunity. Int J Cancer 2010;127(4):759–67.

28. Yamaguchi T, Sakaguchi S. Regulatory T cells in immune surveillance and treatment of cancer. Semin Cancer Biol 2006;16(2):115–23.

29. Belkaid Y, Rouse BT. Natural regulatory T cells in infectious disease. Nat Immunol 2005;6(4):353–60.

Helper T-cell subsets and control of the inflammatory response

Todd N. Eagar,
Stephen D. Miller

T cells are a critical component of the immune system and are key regulators of inflammation. T cells provide three distinct elements to the response against pathogens. First, through the use of the T-cell antigen receptor (TCR), T cells promote immune responses against discrete protein antigens. Second, T cells differentiate to the specific effector phenotypes required to remove the foreign antigen. Finally, at the resolution of the initial immune response T cells provide long-term memory. The contributions of T cells to host protection are highlighted by the clinical presentation of individuals lacking a functional T-cell compartment. For instance, patients with severe combined immunodeficiency (e.g., T⁻B⁺ SCID) or acquired immunodeficiency (e.g., AIDS) experience recurrent bacterial, fungal, and viral infections and if untreated have a dramatically shortened life expectancy. On the opposite side of the spectrum, rampant inflammation and autoimmunity are associated with conditions such as autoimmune lymphoproliferative syndrome (ALPS), autoimmune polyendocrine syndrome type 1 (APS-1), and immune dysregulation, polyendocrinopathy, enteropathy, X-linked syndrome (IPEX) in which T-cell responses are dysregulated. This chapter examines the role of CD4 T cells as regulators of inflammation. The discussion addresses the processes required to generate functional T-cell immunity, the pathways regulating established immune responses, and the heterogeneity within the T-cell compartment.

Initiating a functional T-cell response

Naïve T cells

As discussed in Chapter 8, T cells are generated in the thymus from lymphocyte precursor cells. Following emigration from the thymus, mature $CD4^+$ and $CD8^+$ T cells enter the peripheral immune system. Prior to exposure to cognate antigen and appropriate co-stimulation, T cells are considered to be in a naïve state. Phenotypically, naïve T cells are small cells with little cytoplasm; they express surface markers such as CD45RA, CCR7, CD62L, CD127, and CD132. They lack expression of markers of previous activation such as CD25, CD44, CD69, CD45RO, and HLA-DR. In their naïve state, T cells have a low level of metabolism and lack the ability to produce pro-inflammatory cytokines.[1] Their survival is dependent on their close proximity to dendritic cells (DCs) and stromal cells within the lymph nodes where they receive low levels of TCR signals and IL-7.[2] Functionally, naïve T cells are not capable of participating in immune responses; they must first go through the processes of activation, proliferation, differentiation, and migration.

KEY CONCEPTS

T-cell-mediated inflammation requires activated or memory T cells

Naïve T cells
- Low frequency
- Traffic through circulatory and lymphatic systems
- Require professional APCs for activation
- Require strong costimulation
- Delayed expansion
- Delayed cytokine production
- Dependent on IL-7

Activated T cells
- Traffic through most tissues
- Respond to antigen presented by nonprofessional APCs
- Require less costimulation
- Rapidly expand following antigen encounter
- Rapidly produce effector cytokines
- Dependent on IL-2

Memory T cells
- Traffic through most tissues
- Dependent on IL-7 and IL-15
- Respond to antigen presented by nonprofessional APCs
- Require less co-stimulation
- Rapidly expand following antigen encounter

T-cell activation

T-cell function is intimately tied to the activation process. Activation is required for the naïve T cell to acquire an effector or memory phenotype. A second round of activation is required to elicit effector cytokine production from the effector or memory T cell. Full activation of a T cell requires the cell to receive and integrate signals from a minimum of three diverse types of receptors: the T-cell receptor (TCR, signal 1), co-stimulatory receptors (signal 2), and cytokines (signal 3).[3] Each of these signals elicits biochemical signaling cascades and provides information to the T cell to help shape the generation of effector T cells. These signals are in large part generated by the innate immune system and allow the T cell to sense the environmental context of the activation process. As discussed later, this requirement for multiple signals in T-cell activation is itself a method for limiting immune-mediated damage to the host that might result from inappropriate T-cell activation.

The most critical signals required for T-cell activation are delivered through the TCR. Each T cell expresses a TCR that is generated through the process of somatic recombination (Chapter 4).

Through the processes of thymic selection, TCR gene products are selected for their recognition of self-major histocompatibility complex (MHC) proteins (Chapter 6). The absolute requirement for self-MHC in TCR signaling enforces a need for close interactions between the T cell and an antigen presenting cell (APC) and allows for the APC to provide additional signals to help shape the T-cell response. The primary APC type involved in activating naïve T cells is the DC.[4] DCs are widely distributed in tissues throughout the body where they function as phagocytes. Exposure to pathogens via Toll-like receptor (TLR) signals, tissue damage, or other stimuli induce DC maturation. As DCs mature, they reduce the rate of phagocytosis, increase the levels of surface MHC and co-stimulatory molecule expression, and migrate from the tissue into the regional lymph nodes where they enter the T-cell-rich areas.[5]

Upon entering the lymph node through the high endothelial venules (HEV), T cells interact with numerous DCs as they scan for cognate antigen. In the absence of TCR signaling these interactions are of short duration. Successful TCR engagement elicits the T cell to adhere to the DC in an interaction that may last up to 20 hours.[6] Firm adhesion to an APC is required to facilitate the long-term interactions required for full activation. The affinity and avidity of TCR and MHC/peptide is insufficient to stably maintain contact with an APC. When the T cell initially scans the APC for the presence of cognate peptide, weak adhesion bonds are formed. Engagement of TCR promotes signals that activate tight adhesion using molecules such as the integrin LFA-1 (CD11a) binding to ICAM (CD54) to maintain contact between the T cells and APCs. A key step in T-cell activation is the development of a structured signaling complex known as an immunological synapse. The immunological synapse is formed as the T-cell receptor and its signaling components are actively brought together with accessory or co-stimulatory molecules.[7] Co-stimulatory receptors help to provide additional information to the T cell and allow the APC to provide information regarding the environment from which the antigen was derived. For example, the expression of many co-stimulatory ligands, including the B7 molecules CD80 and CD86, which are ligands for the co-stimulatory receptor CD28, are upregulated in dendritic cells following TLR signaling and therefore serve as a method for the T cell to sense the presence of microbial activity. Ligation of co-stimulatory molecules such as CD28 provides activating stimuli to the T cell and can decrease the amount of TCR engagement required for full activation. Co-stimulatory molecules possess structured domains that interact with components of several intracellular signaling pathways. When properly engaged, the combination of TCR, adhesion, and co-stimulatory signals can lead to the induction of biochemical signaling pathways leading to T-cell activation (Chapter 12). In the presence of incomplete stimulation, i.e., if co-stimulation is lacking, T cells are prevented from participating in inflammation and may become unresponsive to further stimulation (anergic) or undergo apoptosis (Chapter 13). This is an important safety mechanism used to prevent inappropriate T-cell activation. This is one of the key processes by which peripheral self-tolerance is maintained in T cells.

T-cell activation is critically tied to the activation state of the dendritic cell. Immature dendritic cells are incapable of stimulating functional T-cell responses and may in fact induce tolerance or anergy. DC maturation is dependent on external stimuli and in effect allows the DC to integrate tissue and inflammatory factors. For instance, TLR stimulation induces elevated expression of MHC class II, B7-1, B7-2, CD40, and inflammatory cytokines, thereby making the mature DC able to fully elicit T-cell activation. Mature DCs provide information to the T cell through the expression of co-stimulatory molecules and cytokines. Factors such as vitamin D, TGF-β, and IL-10, which are present in the tissue from which the DC migrated, can greatly impact the ability of the DC to activate T cells by altering the extent of co-stimulatory ligands and the type of cytokines expressed by the T cell. In this manner, DCs from immune-privileged sites such as the eye may suppress potentially damaging T-cell responses.[8]

The T-cell activation process is an important target for immunosuppression. Therapies targeting key biochemical pathways leading to activation are in current use to prevent rejection in solid organ transplantation, to treat graft-versus-host disease in bone marrow transplantation, and to reduce the severity of autoimmune diseases or other immune-mediated disorders. Inhibitors such as cyclosporine and tacrolimus block the enzyme calcineurin that is induced following TCR engagement. These inhibitors prevent effective signals mediated through the **n**uclear **f**actor of **a**ctivated **T** cells (NFAT) and block the full activation of the T cell as indicated by a reduction of IL-2 synthesis and entry of the T cells into the cell cycle. Another commonly used immunosuppressant, rapamycin, targets a distinct biochemical signal. Rapamycin specifically inhibits the function of the kinase **m**ammalian **t**arget **o**f **r**apamycin (mTOR) that is induced by TCR and CD28 engagement or by IL-2 receptor signaling. By disrupting mTOR signaling, rapamycin reduces the ability of T cells to enter the cell cycle. Rapamycin therapy is also thought to favor the generation of T cells with regulatory ability.[9] Several monoclonal antibodies and fusion proteins are in clinical use for the treatment of autoimmune disease and the prevention of graft rejection. A chimeric fusion of the extracellular domain of cytotoxic lymphocyte antigen 4 (CTLA-4; CD152) with the Fc portion of IgG (CTLA-4 Ig) is used to prevent T-cell activation by blocking the interactions between CD28 and its ligands CD80 and CD86. Antibodies against the alpha chain of the IL-2R function to block the IL-2-driven activation of T cells and reduce the numbers of activated T cells. On the opposite side of the spectrum, antibodies that block the inhibitory receptor CTLA-4 are currently being employed to enhance anti-tumor T-cell responses and promote tumor rejection.[10]

Clonal expansion of T cells

T-cell activation can be detected within 8 hours of antigen exposure; however, days are required until T-cell responses can be detected from a naïve host. This delay is partially due to the need for generating sufficient numbers of T cells to produce a detectable and effective response. It has been estimated that the frequency of T cells specific for any given antigen is approximately one per 1×10^6 total CD4 T cells.[11] Considering the total number of CD4 T cells present in an individual, the total number of T cells recognizing a single peptide epitope could be estimated at around 100 cells per mouse or 10^5 per human. These estimates are supported by experimental evidence in which 20-200 CD4 T cells reactive against a single epitope were sorted from unimmunized mice.[12] Given the low initial numbers of T cells specific for a given epitope, T cells must go through several rounds of division to achieve sufficient numbers to mount an effective response. Following antigen exposure, cellular proliferation is initially slow, taking 2 days for the first divisions to occur in the lymph nodes and spleen. Cell numbers increase rapidly between day 2 and day 7 post-antigen exposure when peak expansion has occurred. By this point in time many T cells have undergone as many as 8 rounds of division. This process is known as clonal expansion (Fig. 16.1). For instance, a single precursor T cell following 8 rounds of division can yield 256 daughter cells, each possessing the same TCR. Through the combined proliferative responses of

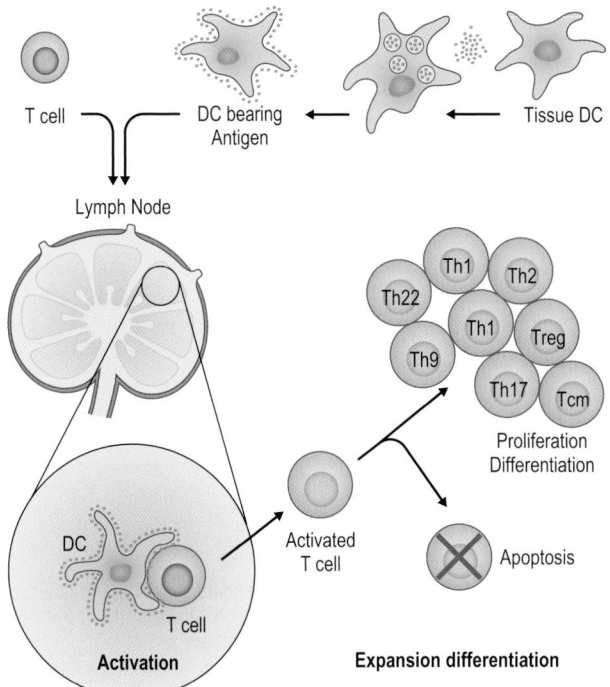

Fig. 16.1 T-cell expansion and differentiation. Following emigration from the thymus, CD4 T cells travel through the lymph nodes. Inflammation results in the recruitment of tissue dendritic cells (DCs) into the draining lymph nodes. In the lymph nodes, DCs present antigen to naïve T cells. Effective antigen presentation stimulates the activation, proliferation and differentiation of T cells into Th1, Th2, Th9, Th17, Th22, or uncommitted T central memory cells.

multiple T-cell clones responding to different epitopes of the same antigen or multiple antigens produced by the same pathogen, a rapid net increase in pathogen-reactive T cells will occur within the draining lymph node.

In the clinical setting, T-cell proliferation is targeted by four major immunosuppressants: azathioprine, cyclophosphamide, methotrexate, and mycophenolate mofetil. Azathioprine, methotrexate, and mycophenolate mofetil suppress proliferation by inhibiting nucleotide synthesis. Cyclophosphamide, on the other hand, is an alkylating agent that suppresses DNA replication. These agents are used in the treatment of autoimmune diseases and for the prevention of graft loss in transplantation (Chapter 88).

T-cell trafficking

There are several key differences between naïve (resting) and activated T cells that influence their ability to participate in inflammatory processes. Among these differences is the ability to migrate to tissue sites and carry out effector functions. As discussed in Chapter 11, T-cell migration relies upon three basic types of interactions between the T cell and the vascular endothelium. The first step is a rolling process mediated by the interaction of selectin molecules (L, E, or P) with their ligands. Selectins slow the T cell and allow close contact with the endothelial cell glycocalyx. The second step is mediated by chemokines. Binding of chemokines to their receptors on the T cell leads to rapid G-protein-coupled receptor signaling, calcium flux, and activation of integrins. Integrins mediate the last stages by stimulating strong adhesion to the endothelial cell, thereby arresting the T-cell movement on the luminal side of the blood vessel and allowing the subsequent transmigration of the T cell across the vessel wall and entry to the tissue site of inflammation.[13]

Naïve T cells and effector T cells traffic through different tissues. This differential trafficking is due to varied expression of selectins, chemokine receptors, and integrins by the T cells and endothelial cells. Naïve T cells circulate almost exclusively through the secondary lymphatic organs. Following thymic maturation and export from the thymus to peripheral lymphoid tissue, naïve T cells recirculate from the blood into lymph nodes and then travel through the lymphatic ducts back into the circulation. This pattern of movement relies upon the expression of CCR7, L-selectin or (CD62L), and LFA-1 ($\alpha_L\beta_2$, integrin, CD11a, CD18). T cells expressing CCR7 follow gradients of CCL21 (SLC) as they migrate through the HEV and into T-cell-rich areas of the lymph nodes, Peyer's patches, and spleen. L-selectin expression allows adherence to the HEV found in the cortex of lymph nodes. LFA-1 interacts with ICAM-1 (CD54) and ICAM-2 (CD102). Interactions with LFA-1 and ICAM-1 are essential for T-cell extravasation into the lymph nodes. Migration to Peyer's patches requires $\alpha_4\beta_7$ integrin in addition to LFA-1. T cells are also subject to control by their ability to leave lymph nodes. Following entry from the blood, the release of T cells from the lymph nodes is regulated by sphingosine-1-phosphate (S1P), a secreted phospholipid. Sensitivity to S1P is mediated by sphingosine-1-phosphate receptor 1 (S1P1), a G protein-coupled receptor. While circulating in the blood where S1P levels are high, T cells become insensitive to S1P by downregulating the expression of S1P1. Due to the low S1P levels found within the lymph nodes, S1P1 is re-expressed and T cells regain the ability to respond to S1P and exit the lymph nodes in 12-18 hours after entry.[14]

Through the process of activation, T cells alter the pattern of homing receptor expression, reducing their ability to migrate within the secondary lymphatic system and gaining receptors needed for trafficking in the peripheral tissues. Very rapidly following TCR engagement, T cells downregulate S1P1 and express CD69, which suppresses chemotactic migration in response to S1P. Another early consequence of T-cell activation is the shedding of L-selectin from the T-cell surface and the expression of ligands for E and P selectin. The change in selectin/ligand expression allows the activated T cells to interact with endothelium at sites distal from the lymph node. Specificity for tissue entry can be at the level of selectins. For example, while entry into the lymph nodes is mediated by L-selectin, entry into skin or lung requires ligands for E or P selectin, respectively.[13] Upon activation, T cells also express a new set of chemokine receptors. Activated T cells respond to chemokines such as CCL3 (MIP-1α). Recent research has shown that damage within specific tissues relates with the attraction of T cells using different chemokine gradients. For example, expression of CCR4 appears to assist in the homing of T cells to the skin, while other chemokine receptors are used by activated T cells trafficking to other areas. There also appears to be a temporal regulation of chemokine expression during ongoing inflammation. In a murine model of CNS autoimmunity, relapsing experimental autoimmune encephalomyelitis (R-EAE), different chemokines are expressed in the spinal cord at different stages of the immune response. This suggests a model for recruitment of T cells of different specificities, as well as monocytes, which are intimately involved in the tissue damage.[15] Another level of control of tissue migration is exerted by the integrins. Following activation, LFA-1 expression is markedly increased as is the expression of other integrins. The importance of differential integrin expression is manifest as more is learned about their role in migration into specific tissues. For instance, VLA-4 (CD49d) is important for T-cell migration into a variety of sites including the CNS, lungs, and intestines.[15]

Taken together, the differences in homing receptor expression between naïve and activated T cells reflect their diverse roles in immune response. Naïve T cells are restricted to the lymph nodes and circulatory system in order to be in close proximity to a concentrated collection of dendritic cells while the homing receptor expression pattern expressed by activated T cells permits their migration into diverse tissues as they participate in immune surveillance. Due to the multistep process of migration and the tissue selective expression patterns of selectins and integrins, a number of therapies targeting T-cell migration have been developed. Antibodies targeting CD62L and LFA-1 have been developed to prevent the entry of T cells into lymph nodes. In addition, the S1P1 inhibitor drug fingolimod is a recently approved therapy for the treatment of multiple sclerosis. Fingolimod is thought to prevent the egress of recently activated T cells from the lymph nodes. Natalizumab, a monoclonal antibody against the α4 integrin, is utilized in multiple sclerosis and Crohn's disease to prevent the migration of T cells into the CNS and intestines, respectively.

Differentiation of CD4 Th subsets

The idea that T helper cell subpopulations can possess distinct phenotypes with relation to the cytokines that they produce was first demonstrated by experiments using long-term murine CD4 T helper cell clones and cell lines.[16] It was observed that after repeated, long-term stimulation T-cell clones would produce two distinct patterns of cytokines. Based on the cytokine expression phenotype of the cells, they were designated T helper 1 (Th1) and T helper 2 (Th2). It is now appreciated that CD4 T cells can differentiate into a plethora of phenotypes (Fig. 16.1). For convenience, these can be grouped into four general categories of cell types based on function: (1) those possessing pro-inflammatory effector characteristics; (2) those possessing regulatory or anti-inflammatory activities; (3) those that function to promote B-cell follicle development; and (4) those functioning as memory cells. The pathways leading to the T cell developing a stable phenotype are initiated at the time of T-cell activation.[17] Signals through the TCR induce the expression of receptors and signaling intermediates that allow the T cell to become sensitive to cytokines produced by the dendritic cell or other cell types in the environment. Signals through cytokine receptors lead to the expression of lineage-specific transcription factors that promote the adoption of an individual cell's effector phenotype. In addition, during the proliferative stages of activation changes in chromatin structure and accessibility function to reinforce the phenotype of the T cell. The end result of this differentiation process ultimately dictates what type of immune response will be produced.

Effector cell phenotypes

T effector cells are those that promote inflammatory processes through the release of cytokines (Fig. 16.2). These cells function by modifying or promoting the activity of accessory cells that ultimately mediate the inflammatory processes required for clearance of the antigen. Based on the profiles of cytokine production and ultimately the types of inflammation that they promote (Table 16.1), effector T cells are divided into five basic groups, Th1, Th2, Th9, Th17, and Th22. Table 16.2 summarizes responses to selective pathogens in which Th1 and Th2 effector responses have been implicated.

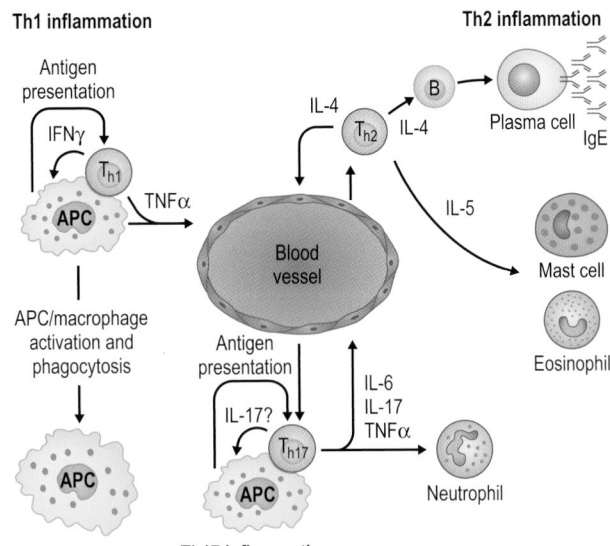

Fig. 16.2 Generalized model for Th-mediated inflammation. *Top left*: Introduction of an infectious agent stimulates the release of chemokines and TNF-α from tissue macrophages, stimulating the recruitment (upward arrows) of T cells and monocytes through the local vasculature. Antigen recognition by T cells stimulates the local production of Th1 cytokines. IFN-γ activates macrophages enhancing the clearance of infectious agents. *Top right*: Trafficking to sites of Th2 responses is stimulated by local chemokine expression, leading to T-cell recruitment. Antigen recognition leads to IL-4 production by Th2 cells, which stimulates B cell IgE class switching. Production of IL-5 activates eosinophils. Cross-linking of FcεR1 molecules bound to IgE leads to the degranulation of mast cells and eosinophils. *Bottom*: Recruitment of Th17 cells and restimulation by antigen results in the release of IL-6, IL-17, and TNF-α, which promotes the recruitment, activation, and function of many cells, particularly neutrophils.

Table 16.1 T-helper cell effector function through cytokine secretion

Th1	
IL-2	T-cell growth and potentiation of Fas-mediated apoptosis NK-cell growth and cytolytic activity B-cell growth and antibody production
IFN-γ	Increases class I and class II MHC molecule expression on numerous cell types Promotes Th1 differentiation Macrophage activation, stimulates phagocytic killing and oxidative bursts Induces IgG2α and IgG3 class switching Inhibits IgG1 and IgE class switching Inhibits Th2 proliferation Activates neutrophils Activates endothelium to promote CD4 T-cell adhesion Stimulates NK-cell cytolytic activity Required for the activation of CD8 CTLs
TNF-α	Activates vascular endothelial cells, enhancing leukocyte recruitment Activates neutrophils, eosinophils, and macrophages Stimulates IL-1, IL-6, TNF, and chemokine expression by macrophages Protects against viral infections, similar to IFNs Increases class I MHC molecule expression Induces fever Activates coagulation
LT (TNF-β)	Activates neutrophils and osteoclasts Activates vascular endothelial cells, enhancing leukocyte recruitment Cytotoxic activity against tumor cells Stimulates adhesion molecule expression Increases class I MHC molecule expression
Th2	
IL-4	Growth and differentiation of Th2 cells B-cell growth and class II MHC molecule upregulation Induces IgG4 class switching (IgG1 in mice) and IgE Inhibits IgG2a and IgG3 class switching Mast cell growth Inhibits macrophage activation Induces VCAM expression on endothelium—recruits eosinophils/monocytes
IL-5	B-cell growth and activation Eosinophil differentiation, activation, and survival
IL-10	Inhibits cytokine and chemokine production in monocytes, especially TNF, IL-1, and IL-12 Inhibits macrophage activation and function Inhibits T-cell-mediated inflammation Induces IgG4 class switching (IgG1 in mice)
IL-13	Upregulates class MHC molecule expression on monocytes and B cells Inhibits pro-inflammatory cytokine production by monocytes B-cell co-stimulation Induces IgG4 class switching (IgG1 in mice) and IgE Increases class I MHC molecule expression
Th9	
IL-9	Mast cell expansion and recruitment T-cell growth factor
IL-21	Promotes Th17 differentiation B-cell survival, antibody class switching Enhances NK-cell proliferation, promotes killer function
Th17	
IL-6	Activation of acute phase response inducing fever and antibacterial responses Stimulation of CRA and SAA production in liver Promotes Th2 and Th17 differentiation Activation and elicitation of NK responses Promotes plasma cell differentiation and Ig production
IL-17	Increases T-cell proliferation Promotes neutrophil recruitment and activity Promotes cytokine production including IL-6 and TNF-α Induces chemokine production
IL-21	See above
TNF-α	See above
Th22	
IL-22	Activation of acute phase response inducing fever and antibacterial responses
IL-13	See above
TNF-α	See above

Table 16.2 T-cell effector responses to selected pathogens

Organism	Nature of the immune response
Bacteria	
Borrelia burgdorferi	Th1 responses associated with protection and joint pathology
Chlamydia trachomatis	Th1 responses protective and source of pathology
Helicobacter pylori	Th1 responses involved in ulcer formation
Legionella pneumophila	Th1 responses associated with immunity
Listeria monocytogenes	Th1 responses are protective: IFN-γ from γδ and CD8 T cells is important
Mycobacterium leprae	Severity and phenotype of disease depends on Th1 and Th2 predominance
Mycobacterium tuberculosis	Th1 responses control infection
Treponema pallidum	Th1 resolves infection, Th2 chronic
Yersinia pestis	Th1 responses associated with immunity
Fungi	
Aspergillus fumigatus	Th2 production predominate: does Th1 offer protection?
Blastomyces dermatitidis	Th1 and Th17 cells protect: Th2 switch in progressive disease
Candida albicans	Th1 and Th17 responses are protective
Cryptococcus neoformans	Susceptibility associated with Th2 response, Th1 response associated with protection
Paracoccidioides brasiliensis	Infection stimulates Th2 response, but Th1 and Th17 responses protect
Parasites	
Leishmania spp.	Th1 responses are protective, Th2 responses allow chronic infection
Filaria	Initiates Th2 production, Th1 response appears protective
Schistosoma mansoni	Th1 and humoral responses protect, typically Th2 responses directed against eggs
Trypanosoma cruzi	Th1 responses inhibit parasite replication, but protection is not completely CD4 dependent
Giardia lamblia	Th1 and Th2 responses protect
Viruses	
Measles	Th1 responses are protective
Hepatitis B	Th1 responses seen in spontaneous recovering patients
Human immunodeficiency virus	Shift from Th1 to a Th0 (Th2?) response late in disease correlates with susceptibility to pathogens
Respiratory syncytial virus	Th1 response protects, Th2 response kills

Th1

Th1 cells are classically defined by their production of the cytokines IFN-γ, GM-CSF, IL-2, and lymphotoxin (LT, TNF-β). The critical decision to produce Th1 cells is dependent upon the innate immune response to infection by intracellular bacteria, fungi, and viruses. Infection with these pathogens leads to the activation of TLR signaling and the subsequent production of

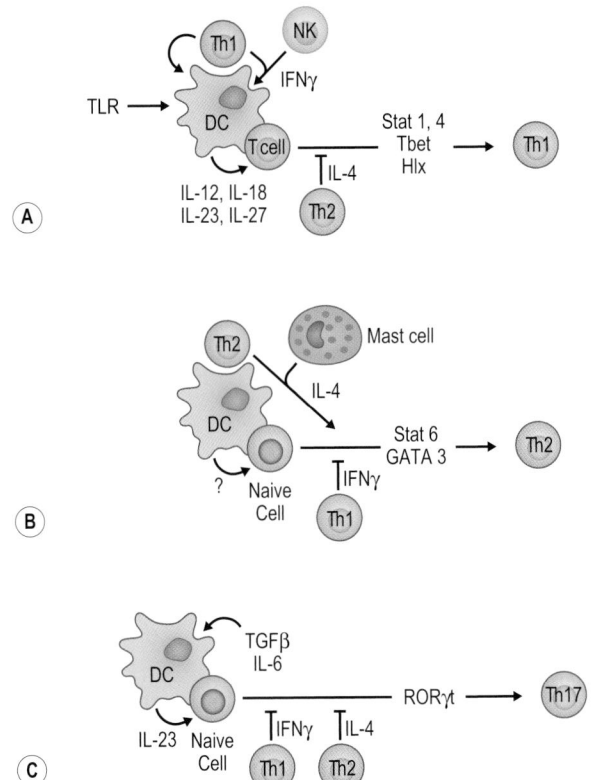

Fig. 16.3 Factors influencing T effector differentiation. Cytokine exposure during the activation stage of naïve T cells strongly influences T effector differentiation. Depicted here are the factors promoting and inhibiting Th1 (A), Th2 (B), and Th17 (C) following functional activation of undifferentiated T cells.

cytokines critical for Th1 development by dendritic cells and NK cells. Th1 differentiation is promoted by IL-12, IL-18, IFN-γ, and type 1 interferons while being inhibited by IL-4, IL-10, and TGF-β (Fig. 16.3). Th1 differentiation is enhanced by exposure to IFN-γ. A variety of cells such as NK cells and previously committed Th1 cells are thought to be important early sources of IFN-γ. The function of IFN-γ in Th1 differentiation is through STAT1 signaling downstream of the IFN-γ receptor. IFN-γR/STAT1 signaling stimulates the production of the Th1 restricted transcription factor Tbet. IL-12 produced by mature dendritic cells is thought to be the critical factor associated with Th1 commitment. T-cell activation and STAT1 signals lead to the expression of IL-12Rβ, which upon binding of IL-12 signals through Jak-2 and Tyk-2 to activate STAT 4. STAT4 enters the nucleus where it elicits the expression of Th1-lineage-specific transcription factors such as Tbet. Tbet serves to reinforce the Th1 phenotype by promoting IFN-γ and IL-12Rβ2 expression.[17] IL-18 plays a dual role in Th1 function by promoting Th1 commitment and eliciting IFN-γ production by fully differentiated Th1 cells.

Th1 cells promote cell-mediated inflammatory responses through inducing the activation of macrophages, NK cells, B cells, and CD8 T cells. Th1 cells regulate macrophage function at several levels. GM-CSF promotes the production of monocyte lineage cells from the bone marrow, thereby increasing the pool of macrophage precursors. IFN-γ is a potent macrophage activator, enhancing microbiocidal activity by initiating nitric oxide (NO) production from iNOS, upregulating production of oxygen radicals, increasing phagocytic function. IFN-γ also promotes antigen presentation by upregulating MHC class I, MHC class II, and co-stimulatory molecule expression by macrophages (Fig. 16.2). IFN-γ can activate NK cells and also promote humoral responses in B cells to mediate antibody class switching to an IgG1 isotype (IgG2a in mice).[18] IgG1 activates the classical complement pathway and can bind Fcγ receptors expressed on phagocytic cells, thereby promoting opsonization. Lastly, IFN-γ acts in conjunction with another Th1 cytokine, IL-2, to promote differentiation of CD8 T cells into cytotoxic effector cells. Macrophage-dependent Th1-mediated inflammatory responses are known as delayed-type hypersensitivity responses (DTH). *In vivo*, DTH responses are critical for protection from intracellular pathogens including bacteria, fungi, and viruses. Additionally, Th1 cells have been implicated in the pathogenesis of many autoimmune diseases including multiple sclerosis, type 1 diabetes mellitus, rheumatoid arthritis, and Crohn's disease.

Th2

Th2 cells are defined by their production of IL-4, IL-5, IL-9, IL-10, and IL-13. *In vitro*, the critical step in Th2 cell differentiation is the presence of exogenous IL-4 and the absence of IFN-γ during T-cell activation. *In vivo* Th2 differentiation is thought to require IL-4 produced by basophils, eosinophils, mast cells, NKT cells, or even previously differentiated Th2 cells. Naïve T cells express the IL-4R, and the combination of TCR (NFAT), co-stimulatory (CD28 and ICOS), and IL-4R/STAT6 signaling promotes IL-4 transcription and the production of the transcription factors c-Maf and GATA3. c-Maf functions to promote IL-4 production and suppress IFN-γ, thereby helping to establish Th2 polarity. GATA3 also appears to inhibit IFN-γ production, but additionally plays a critical role in establishing Th2 cells by promoting IL-5 and IL-13 production (Fig. 16.3).[19]

Th2 cells release IL-4 and IL-5, which attract and activate the function of eosinophils and mast cells. Th2-type cytokines also enhance the class switching of B cells to induce the production of IgG1, IgE, and sIgA. High levels of IgE in Th2 reactions, combined with antigen exposure and FcεR1 receptor expression by eosinophils or mast cells, results in triggering and release of inflammatory factors such as histamine, platelet activating factor, prostaglandins, and leukotrienes (Fig. 16.2). These factors act on the local environment, producing vascular dilation and leakage, bronchial constriction and intestinal hypermotility. On a more systemic level anaphylaxis may be produced. These eosinophil and mast cell-dependent reactions are known as immediate-type hypersensitivity (ITH). ITH responses are important for ridding the body of intestinal helminths (Chapter 29); in fact components of helminth eggs strongly promote Th2 differentiation. Th2 responses are also associated with atopy and hyper-responsive airway conditions such as asthma and allergies.

Th17

CD4 T cells possessing a Th17 phenotype are characterized by the production of IL-17a/f, IL-21, IL-22, IL-26, GM-CSF, and TNF-α. Th17 differentiation has been described to require the presence of IL-1β, IL-6, IL-23, and TGF-β and the absence of type 1 interferons, IFN-γ and IL-4 (Fig. 16.3). Much of the Th17 cell potency can be attributed to the production of IL-17. Other sources of IL-17 are neutrophils, CD8 T cells, and γδ T cells. IL-17 is a potent promoter of inflammation particularly with regard to cellular recruitment. IL-17 induces the expression of adhesion molecules and the production of the pro-inflammatory mediators IL-6, GM-CSF, G-CSF, a wide variety of chemokines, prostaglandin E2, and matrix metalloproteinases (Fig. 16.2). The effect of Th17 cells on recruitment is further enhanced by the

production of TNF-α. IL-21 regulates B-, T-, and NK-cell functions.[20] In B cells, IL-21 has been found to regulate plasma cell differentiation and promote IgM and IgG1 antibody production. IL-21 is a T-cell growth factor; in the presence of TCR signals, it promotes T-cell activation, proliferation, and survival. It therefore appears that Th17 cells are important for the recruitment of effector cells including neutrophils and monocytes.

In many ways, Th17 cells appear to be potent cell-mediated effectors with similarities to Th1 cells. Th17 responses are thought to be elicited in response to infection with extracellular bacteria and fungi. In addition, Th17 cells have been implicated in the pathogenesis of a broad spectrum of autoimmune diseases, including systemic lupus erythematosus, atopic dermatitis, psoriasis, rheumatoid arthritis, multiple sclerosis, and inflammatory bowel disease.[21]

Th9

Although Th2 cells have long been known to produce IL-9, the proposition that an IL-9-producing T-cell subset is a separate lineage has only been described recently. Human Th9 cells have been shown to produce IL-9 and IL-21. IL-9 is an important growth factor for T cells, mast cell, and hematopoietic stem cells. IL-9 functions by preventing apoptosis. The differentiation of naïve T cells into a Th9 phenotype is thought to be dependent on the presence of IL-4 and TGF-β.[22] Th9 cells express the transcription factor PU.1, which is necessary and sufficient for the Th9 phenotype (and lack Gata3 and RORγt expression). Similar to Th2 cells, Th9 cells are thought to play a role in protection from helminths. In addition, Th9 cells play a role in asthma where they promote airway restriction and mucus secretion. Experimental models also suggest that Th9 cells may contribute to the pathogenesis of autoimmune disease.

CLINICAL RELEVANCE

Diseases associated with CD4 T effector responses

Th1
- Multiple sclerosis
- Psoriasis
- Type 1 diabetes melitus
- Tuberculoid leprosy

Th2
- Allergy and asthma
- Helminthic infections
- Lepromatous leprosy

Th9
- Asthma
- Helminthic infections

Th17
- Asthma
- Multiple sclerosis
- Psoriasis
- Rheumatoid arthritis
- Transplant rejection

Th22
- Psoriasis
- Wound healing

Th22

A population of IL-22, IL-13, and TNF-α-secreting CD4 T cells was identified from the skin of patients with inflammatory skin disorders.[3] The IL-22 expressing cell population was found to express the skin-homing receptor CCR10. These cells, labeled Th22 cells, have been subsequently found to differentiate in the presence of IL-6 and TNF-α.[23] Phenotypically, Th22 cells express a gene profile different from other Th cell types. They also produce fibroblast growth factors that promote epidermal repair. The hallmark cytokine IL-22 is a member of the IL-10 family with important functions in regulating skin homeostasis and protection from infection. Much remains to be learned about the function of this effector T-cell subset.

Regulatory T cells

Regulatory T cells (Tregs) possess the ability to suppress or otherwise downregulate the function of other pro-inflammatory T cells. Although multiple T-cell subsets may possess regulatory T-cell activity, our understanding of regulatory function was greatly enhanced by the discovery of CD25 and FoxP3 as markers for a regulatory subpopulation of CD4 T cells. Regulatory cell function is described in much greater detail in Chapter 15. This discussion focuses on the involvement of two populations of peripherally derived regulatory cell phenotypes: adaptive Tregs and Tr1 cells.

Adaptive Tregs

In mice, the majority of CD4$^+$ CD25$^+$ FoxP3$^+$ Treg cells (natural Treg) are thought to develop regulatory ability in the thymus. A separate population, known as adaptive Treg cells, has been found to develop in the periphery. Once differentiated, the adaptive Treg cells are similar in phenotype to natural Tregs in that they express CD4, CD25, CD38, CD62L, CD103, and FoxP3. Although not fully characterized, adaptive Tregs are thought to be generated in response to a widely expressed antigen, through prolonged exposure to antigen or polyclonal stimuli. Differentiation to become adaptive Tregs may therefore result from antigen presentation by poor APCs such as immature DC or other non-professional APC. Some experiments suggest that stimulation in the presence of inhibitory cytokines such as IL-10 and TGF-β also favors adaptive Treg differentiation. Similar to natural Tregs, adaptive Treg cells are capable of suppressing CD4 and CD8 T-cell responses *in vitro* and *in vivo*. Unlike natural Tregs, which function in a cell-contact-dependent manner, adaptive Tregs appear to function at least in part through the secretion of IL-10 and TGF-β. These cytokines may directly regulate effector T cells or may inhibit dendritic cell activity. The generation of adaptive Tregs is of great interest as a cell-based therapy for inflammatory diseases including autoimmunity.[24]

Tr1 cells

Tr1 cells have been defined as a population of CD4 T cells that produce IL-10 in response to stimulation. Unlike adaptive Tregs, Tr1 cells do not express FoxP3 and do not necessarily express CD25. Tr1 cells are described to be produced *in vivo* following antigen delivery to or infection of the respiratory system. It is thought that antigen exposure in the presence of IL-10 and TGF-β normally found in the lungs is important for Tr1 differentiation. Experimentally, Tr1 cells can be induced by repeated intranasal antigen delivery.[25] In fact, it has also been reported that Tr1 cells are induced during the course of infection by *Bordetella pertussis*.[26] Tr1 cells function by producing IL-10 to block proliferation of naïve T cells, to prevent Th1 differentiation by blocking IL-12 production, and to enhance differentiation of T cells toward a Tr1 phenotype.

Follicular helper T cells (Tfh)

One of the earliest described roles of CD4 T cells is their ability to promote or "help" generate effective antibody production by B cells. Th1 and Th2 cells are well known for their ability to promote specific B-cell effector responses. Evidence supports the role of a distinct subpopulation of T cells, known as T follicular helper (Tfh) cells, as playing a key role in regulating T-cell-dependent B-cell responses.

Tfh cells are identified by their surface expression of CXCR5, ICOS, PD-1, CD200, BTLA, OX40, and SAP while lacking the expression of CD127 and CCR7.[27] Tfh differentiation is promoted by signals through ICOS and the presence of IL-6 and IL-21. The presence of CXCR5 and lack of CCR7 are particularly important because these chemokine receptors control homing to the B-cell follicle and T-cell areas, respectively. Considering that B cells are an important source of IL-6 and ICOSL expression, it is likely that Tfh differentiation occurs in concert with the generation and expansion of antigen-specific B cells. Tfh also express the transcription factor BCL6, which is absolutely required for their differentiation and function. BCL6 antagonizes T-cell differentiation into different helper phenotypes by altering of the effector-specific functions of Tbet, Gata3, and RORγt. Unlike Th1, Th2, or Th17 effector T cells, however, dual expression of BCL6 with other Th lineage-specific markers is common. The fact that there is not a complete separation between Tfh and other T effector lineages might suggest that the Tfh phenotype is generated in parallel with T-effector-cell differentiation and in response to inflammatory cues present in the lymph nodes.

Memory T cells

A critical contribution of adaptive immune cells to the host defense is the generation of immunological memory. Following an immune response, small numbers of T cells persist long term and are called memory T cells. Memory T cells function to protect the host from reinfection by the same micro-organisms and protection correlates with the number of specific memory cells present in the host. This is also a critical process in T cell-dependent vaccination strategies (Chapter 90). Memory cells are uniquely capable of accelerating responses against repeat antigen for several reasons. First, memory cells are maintained at higher frequencies than naïve cells. Second, memory T cells proliferate and produce cytokines in response to stimulation with lower doses of antigen, less co-stimulation, and much faster kinetics than do naïve cells. Third, memory cells can promote APC function and secrete polarizing cytokines such as IFNγ or IL-4 and accelerate activation and differentiation of naïve T cells.

Memory T cells can be divided into two general subgroups based on their patterns of migration. Central memory cells are T cells that have re-expressed secondary lymphoid homing receptors CCR7 and L-selectin following activation.[28] This allows the central memory T cells to recirculate through the secondary lymphatic organs similar to naïve T cells. Lymph node circulation is beneficial because dendritic cells from diverse tissue sites continuously bring antigen to the draining lymph nodes, thereby increasing the effective area of memory cell surveillance. Effector memory T cells express homing receptors similar to those of activated T cells. This prevents effector memory cells from trafficking through the lymph nodes but allows the effector memory T cells to migrate through the peripheral tissues either through uninflamed tissues or in response to localized inflammatory stimuli. Thus memory cell responses are bolstered through the process of immune surveillance at distinct sites. Differentiation to become central or effector memory cells might be through distinct mechanisms. Central memory cells develop from T cells that have failed to fully proliferate or differentiate to a specific Th phenotype.[29] These central memory cells can differentiate during subsequent antigen encounters. On the other hand, effector memory cells are thought to differentiate from previously committed T cells and retain their effector characteristics allowing for rapid tissue responses.

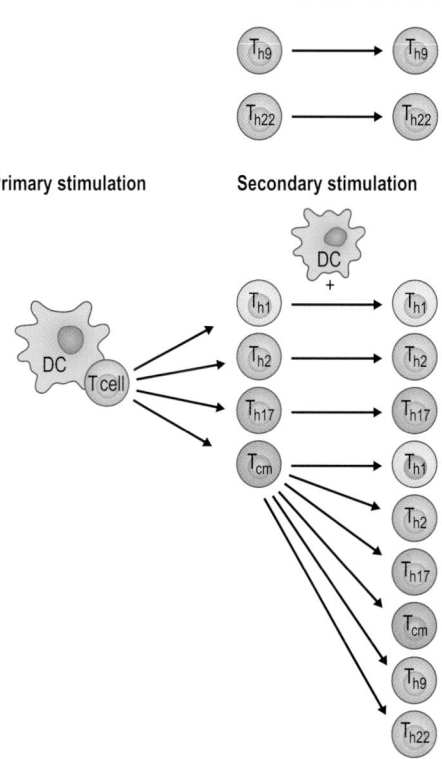

Fig. 16.4 Mechanism of Th phenotype shift. Under appropriate conditions, T-cell activation may result in daughter cells adopting one of several T effector phenotypes. Within a polarized population of Th cells, there may exist a subset of undifferentiated T lymphocytes (here referred to in the general category as Tcm). Fully committed Th1, Th2, or Th17 cells upon restimulation will produce; Th1, Th2, or Th17, respectively. Tcm or other uncommitted cell types retain the potential to differentiate into T effectors of any phenotype, depending on the context of the secondary stimulation.

General considerations in effector T-cell differentiation

Several key concepts of T helper maturation should be discussed with regards to the cellular differentiation of CD4 T cells. First and foremost, all T effector, T regulatory, and memory T cells are thought to arise from a naïve thymic emigrant precursor. This is evident considering that T cells from TCR transgenic mice can differentiate to many different effector, regulatory, and memory phenotypes while possessing the same TCR.

Second, differentiation to a specific phenotype is self-promoting and inhibitory to other phenotypes through production of effector cytokines (Fig. 16.3). IFN-γ production early in Th1 differentiation promotes signaling through the IFNγR, leading to STAT1 signals, which has the dual function of promoting IL-12R expression and inhibits IL-4R expression. Similarly, IL-4 expression promotes Th2 differentiation while also suppressing responsiveness to IL-12 and IFN-γ. Additionally, expression of critical transcription factors Tbet (Th1) or gata3 (Th2) results in reinforced expression of factors that promote only one phenotype and downregulation of other phenotypes; this is due to the establishment of specific patterns of gene expression and chromatin remodeling.

Third, polarization is incomplete. Following exposure to antigen, responding T cells may possess multiple phenotypes. Heterogeneity of Th phenotypes is a common feature of diseases such as asthma where Th2, Th9, and Th17 responses are thought to contribute to disease; in psoriasis where Th1, Th17, and Th22 cell types are detectable; and in multiple sclerosis where Th1, Th17, and Th22 cells are thought to mediate inflammation. A portion of the T cells may persist as undifferentiated (Th0) cells or uncommitted central memory cells.

Fourth, Th phenotypes are for the most part stable. As part of the differentiation process, T cells express phenotype-reinforcing transcription factors and go through epigenetic changes that make the phenotype of fully committed T cells difficult to change (Fig. 16.4). For example, Th1 cells do not express Th2 cytokines despite extended culture under Th2-skewing conditions. There is, however, growing evidence of plasticity and interconversion between T helper subsets.[30] For instance, experiments tracing T-cell lineage commitment have shown that T cells that once expressed FoxP3 could become Th17 effector cells if stimulated in the presence of IL-6. It remains to be determined what portion of this plasticity reflects incomplete differentiation or whether our previous models of complete lineage commitment were based on non-physiological stimuli. Lastly, *in vitro* or *in vivo*, differentiation can be incomplete. The presence of undifferentiated precursor cells or central memory cells can adopt different Th phenotypes upon subsequent antigen stimulation (Fig. 16.4).

Termination of T-cell responses

● KEY CONCEPTS

Regulation of T-cell responses

- Cell death pathways
  - TNF family receptors: Fas/FasL, TRAIL and TNFR1
- Inhibitory receptor activity
  - CTLA-4 and PD1
  - Inhibition of TCR signaling
- Cytokine mediated regulation
  - Anti-inflammatory cytokine production (IL-10, TGF-β)
  - Cytokines that promote and inhibit inflammation at different stages of a response (IFNγ, IL-2, IL-27)
  - Regulation of apoptosis (LT, TNF-α)
  - Growth factor withdrawal (IL-2, IL-7, IL-15)

During inflammation there is an enormous expansion of T-cell numbers and activity. Termination of an immune response and return to homeostasis requires a sharp decrease in both T-cell numbers and activity.

Three possible outcomes may result from not returning to pre-inflammation T-cell numbers and activity. First, with each succeeding infection, the body would be increasingly burdened by the energy requirements of maintaining larger T-cell numbers. Second, there would be a loss of TCR diversity resulting from the overrepresentation of clonally expanded T cells. Third, there is an increased risk of damage to self by the presence of large numbers of activated effector T cells that are easily retriggered. The termination of T-cell responses and restoration of homeostasis does not only result from the loss of the original stimulus but relies upon the active control processes including the induction of cell death, activation of inhibitory signaling pathways, and cytokine function. These processes function to eliminate large numbers of effector T cells and down-modulate their function.

Cell death pathways active in T-cell homeostasis

Several cell death pathways are important in regulating the process of activation-induced cell death (AICD) and restoring homeostasis. Deletion of peripheral T cells following an immune response has been attributed primarily to the interactions of Fas (CD95) and Fas ligand (FasL; CD95L), which promote apoptosis (Chapter 13). Following activation T cells upregulate the surface expression of Fas and FasL. T cells are sensitive to Fas-mediated apoptosis either by stimulation from another cell (death signal) or also as stimulated by molecules on the same cell (suicide signal). This process is known as AICD. Mutations in Fas and FasL result in the accumulation of activated lymphocytes in the periphery. Another TNF-family member, TRAIL, has also been associated with AICD. Mice genetically deficient in TRAIL showed enhanced susceptibility to autoimmune disease. Some evidence suggests that TRAIL regulates AICD primarily in Th2 cells.[31]

Action of inhibitory receptors

T cells express several Ig-family transmembrane proteins containing immune tyrosine inhibitory motifs (ITIMs). Two of these, CTLA-4 and PD-1, are expressed following activation and play an important role in terminating T-cell responses *in vivo*. The first, CTLA-4, is expressed on peripheral T cells following activation. CTLA-4 binds to B7-1 and B7-2, thereby sharing ligands with the positive co-stimulatory molecule CD28. CTLA-4 engagement inhibits T-cell function by competing with CD28 for available ligand and inhibiting proximal TCR signaling through its association with the phosphatases SHP-2 and PP2A. Underscoring the importance of CTLA-4 in T-cell homeostasis, mice that are genetically deficient in CTLA-4 develop a severe CD28-dependent lymphoproliferative disease, tissue infiltration, and early death.[32] PD-1 interacts with two ligands, PD-L1 and PD-L2, which possess different expression patterns throughout the immune system and peripheral tissues. Like CTLA-4, engagement of PD-1 limits T-cell cytokine production and proliferation. PD1 signals may also enhance T-cell apoptosis. Loss of PD-1 has been associated with autoimmune cardiomyopathy, arthritis, and a lupus-like glomerulonephritis disease.[33]

Cytokine-mediated inhibition

Another method of controlling T-cell activity is through cytokine signaling. Cytokines function to terminate immune responses in three basic methods: by loss or withdrawal of growth factors; by promoting cell death; and by direct anti-inflammatory properties. IL-2 functions in the early stages of an immune response as a growth factor by promoting T-cell survival and expansion. IL-2 and its receptors are rapidly expressed by CD4 T cells upon activation. Loss of IL-2 signals through decreased production or loss of receptor expression deprives the cell of survival signals, resulting in AICD. IL-7 is another growth factor important for the survival of naïve and memory T cells. Similar to IL-2, loss of IL-7 or IL-7 receptor results in increased apoptosis among activated and memory populations.[34] As discussed in Chapter 13, cell death by growth factor withdrawal results from activation of the mitochondrial pathway of apoptosis.

Cytokines may function to limit T-cell responses directly. Apart from its role in Th1 inflammation and macrophage activation, IFN-γ functions to downregulate CD4 T-cell responses. Mice deficient in IFN-γ or the IFNγR show heightened T-cell responses and the accumulation of activated T cells. Another cytokine, IL-10, plays an important role in suppressing inflammation by inhibiting macrophage activation, downregulating chemokine production, and diminishing T-cell responses by suppressing co-stimulatory molecule expression by APCs. IL-10 is produced by Th2, adaptive Tregs, and Tr1 cells, as well as monocytes and macrophages. IL-10-deficient mice develop inflammatory bowel disease due to dysregulated Th1 responses. A role for IL-27 in downregulating T-cell responses has recently been described. Mice genetically deficient for the IL-27 receptor develop exaggerated CD4 T-cell responses and inflammatory diseases. These effects of IL-27 can be attributed to its role in suppressing Th1 responses and CD4 T-cell proliferation.[35] TGF-β$_1$ is another anti-inflammatory cytokine that is produced by subsets of regulatory T cells and a variety of other cell types throughout the body. Unlike IL-10, which targets APCs, TGF-β$_1$ directly inhibits T-cell proliferation and Th1 differentiation.[36] Mice deficient in TGF-β$_1$ have multi-tissue infiltration of activated lymphocytes and macrophages. Interestingly, IL-2 signaling has also been identified to play a positive role in the termination of T-cell responses by promoting the activity of regulatory T cells. Tregs express high levels of IL-2R and require constant IL-2 signals for survival. The third method by which cytokines can quell T-cell responses is through promoting apoptosis of the T cell. TNF-α is well characterized as possessing pro-apoptotic function. TNFR1 possesses a death domain and binding of TNF-α results in the activation of the caspase pathway and apoptosis.

Therapeutic regulation of T-cell responses for treatment of immune-mediated diseases

It is critically important clinically to be able to control inflammation to treat immune-mediated disease, including autoimmune diseases and allergy. As discussed above, some of the most effective techniques to control inflammation are aimed directly at T cells, especially at the various steps involved in T-cell activation, differentiation, trafficking, or effector functions (Fig. 16.5). The following are included among the many potential approaches currently being employed or in development for therapeutic regulation of inflammatory diseases: (a) blockading appropriate

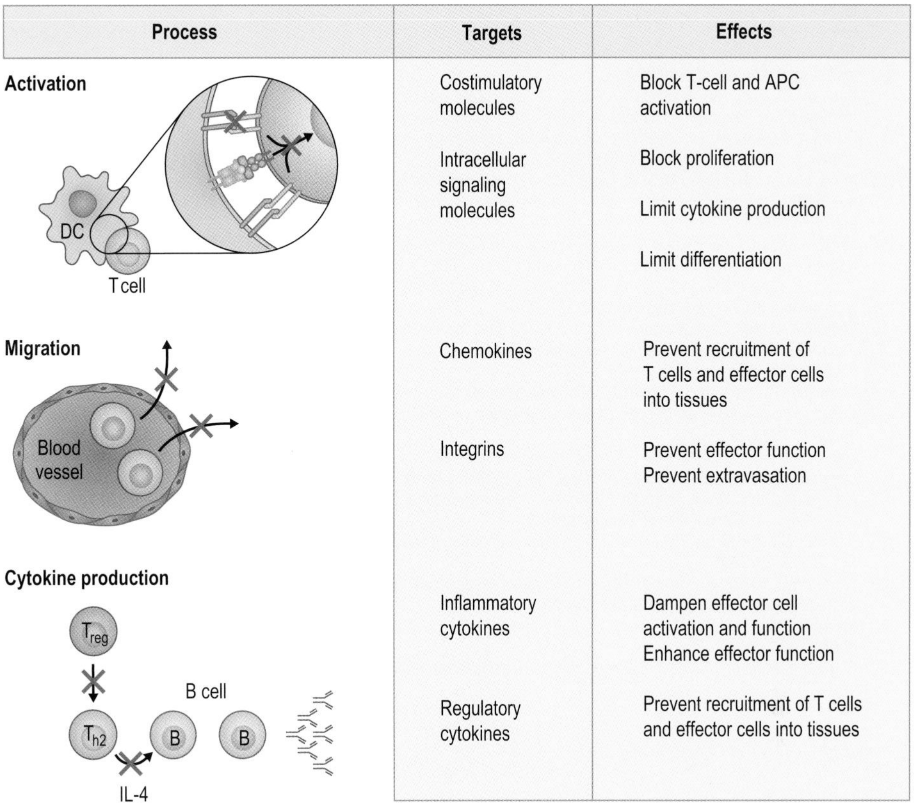

Fig. 16.5 Therapeutic regulation of inflammation Several techniques have been employed to reduce T-cell responses in cases of inflammation. Among these are inhibiting T-cell activation and differentiation by blocking co-stimulatory interactions with APC (top), inhibiting T-cell and effector cell trafficking by blocking molecules required for chemotaxis (middle), and limiting the effect of T helper responses by decreasing the availability of inflammatory cytokines (bottom).

Process	Targets	Effects
Activation	Costimulatory molecules	Block T-cell and APC activation
	Intracellular signaling molecules	Block proliferation
		Limit cytokine production
		Limit differentiation
Migration	Chemokines	Prevent recruitment of T cells and effector cells into tissues
	Integrins	Prevent effector function Prevent extravasation
Cytokine production	Inflammatory cytokines	Dampen effector cell activation and function Enhance effector function
	Regulatory cytokines	Prevent recruitment of T cells and effector cells into tissues

co-stimulatory signals or intracellular signaling molecules to prevent T-cell activation or to control ongoing effector inflammatory responses; (b) preventing recruitment of effector T cells into inflammatory sites by targeting various selectins, integrins, and/or chemokine receptors by blocking the binding of these molecules to their ligands or blocking their downstream signaling pathways; (c) neutralizing the pro-inflammatory cytokines (e.g., IFN-γ, IL-17, or TNF-α) and other effector molecules (e.g., iNOS, reactive oxygen intermediates, etc.) involved in the effector limb of destructive inflammatory processes; and (d) using regulatory cytokines such as TGF-β, IL-4, or IL-10 to regulate pro-inflammatory responses.

Opportunities for translational research

● ON THE HORIZON

- Development of effective techniques to identify antigens targeted in organ-specific autoimmune and allergic diseases, and in transplant rejection.
- Development and implementation of an effective tolerance inducing strategy capable of regulating T-cell responses in an antigen-specific manner.
- Identification of tolerance-specific biomarkers/assays to clearly delineate successful therapy of inflammatory diseases.

A major challenge in the next 5-10 years is to develop safe and effective immunoregulatory strategies in which pathogenic inflammatory T cells are suppressed in an antigen-specific manner leaving the remainder of the immune system undisturbed. The gold standard for treatment of immune-mediated inflammatory conditions—including autoimmune disease, allergy and asthma, prevention of rejection of allogeneic organ and tissue transplants, and prevention of immune response to replacement proteins in patients with enzyme deficiency diseases—involves the induction of antigen-specific immune tolerance only against the targeted proteins. This strategy avoids the serious side effects, including increased rates of infection with opportunistic pathogens and increased rates of development of neoplastic disease, which can accompany the use of immunosuppressive agents and immune subset depleting antibodies. There are a number of tolerance-inducing strategies both in pre-clinical development and currently undergoing initial clinical trials that hold great promise for specific therapy of immune-mediated diseases. Broadly, these strategies are attempting to target the activation of naïve pathogenic T cells and/or the pro-inflammatory functions of effector T cells either directly (via the induction T-cell intrinsic anergy) and/or indirectly via the activity of antigen-specific regulatory T cells.

References

1. Takada K, Jameson SC. Naive T-cell homeostasis: from awareness of space to a sense of place. Nature Rev 2009;9:823–32.
2. Tan JT, Dudl E, LeRoy E, et al. IL-7 is critical for homeostatic proliferation and survival of naive T cells. Proc Natl Acad Sci USA 2001;98:8732–7.
3. Smith-Garvin JE, Koretzky GA, Jordan MS. T cell activation. Annu Rev Immunol 2009;27:591–619.
4. Watts C, West MA, Zaru R. TLR signalling regulated antigen presentation in dendritic cells. Curr Opin Immunol 2010;22:124–30.
5. Randolph GJ, Angeli V, Swartz MA. Dendritic-cell trafficking to lymph nodes through lymphatic vessels. Nat Rev Immunol 2005;5:617–28.
6. Mempel TR, Henrickson SE, Von Andrian UH. T-cell priming by dendritic cells in lymph nodes occurs in three distinct phases. Nature 2004;427:154–9.
7. Friedl P, den Boer AT, Gunzer M. Tuning immune responses: diversity and adaptation of the immunological synapse. Nat Rev Immunol 2005;5:532–45.

8. Manicassamy S, Pulendran B. Dendritic cell control of tolerogenic responses. Immunol Rev 2011;241:206–27.
9. Thomson AW, Turnquist HR, Raimondi G. Immunoregulatory functions of mTOR inhibition. Nature Rev 2009;9:324–37.
10. Quezada SA, Peggs KS, Simpson TR, Allison JP. Shifting the equilibrium in cancer immunoediting: from tumor tolerance to eradication. Immunol Rev 2011;241:104–18.
11. Blattman JN, Antia R, Sourdive DJ, et al. Estimating the precursor frequency of naive antigen-specific CD8 T cells. J Exp Med 2002;195:657–64.
12. Moon JJ, Chu HH, Pepper M, et al. Naive CD4(+) T cell frequency varies for different epitopes and predicts repertoire diversity and response magnitude. Immunity 2007;27:203–13.
13. Ley K, Kansas GS. Selectins in T-cell recruitment to non-lymphoid tissues and sites of inflammation. Nat Rev Immunol 2004;4:325–35.
14. Cyster JG. Chemokines, sphingosine-1-phosphate, and cell migration in secondary lymphoid organs. Ann Rev Immunol 2005;23:127–59.
15. Rebenko-Moll NM, Liu L, Cardona A, Ransohoff RM. Chemokines, mononuclear cells and the nervous system: heaven (or hell) is in the details. Curr Opin Immunol 2006;18:683–9.
16. Mosmann TR, Cherwinski H, Bond MW, et al. Two types of murine helper T cell clone. I. Definition according to profiles of lymphokine activities and secreted proteins. J Immunol 1986;136:2348–57.
17. Zhu J, Paul WE. Peripheral CD4+ T-cell differentiation regulated by networks of cytokines and transcription factors. Immunol Rev 2010;238:247–62.
18. Coffman RL, Lebman DA, Rothman P. Mechanism and regulation of immunoglobulin isotype switching. Adv Immunol 1993;54:229–70.
19. Paul WE, Zhu J. How are T(H)2-type immune responses initiated and amplified? Nature Rev 2010;10:225–35.
20. Leonard WJ, Spolski R. Interleukin-21: a modulator of lymphoid proliferation, apoptosis and differentiation. Nature Rev 2005;5:688–98.
21. Korn T, Bettelli E, Oukka M, Kuchroo VK. IL-17 and Th17 cells. Annu Rev Immunol 2009;27:485–517.
22. Soroosh P, Doherty TA. Th9 and allergic disease. Immunol 2009;127:450–8.
23. Eyerich S, Eyerich K, Pennino D, et al. Th22 cells represent a distinct human T cell subset involved in epidermal immunity and remodeling. J Clin Invest 2009;119:3573–85.
24. Masteller EL, Tang Q, Bluestone JA. Antigen-specific regulatory T cells—ex vivo expansion and therapeutic potential. Semin Immunol 2006;18:103–10.
25. Roncarolo MG, Gregori S, Battaglia M, et al. Interleukin-10-secreting type 1 regulatory T cells in rodents and humans. Immunol Rev 2006;212:28–50.
26. Byrne P, McGuirk P, Todryk S, Mills KH. Depletion of NK cells results in disseminating lethal infection with Bordetella pertussis associated with a reduction of antigen-specific Th1 and enhancement of Th2, but not Tr1 cells. Eur J Immunol 2004;34:2579–88.
27. Nutt SL, Tarlinton DM. Germinal center B and follicular helper T cells: siblings, cousins or just good friends? Nat Immunol 2011;12:472–7.
28. Lanzavecchia A, Sallusto F. Understanding the generation and function of memory T cell subsets. Curr Opin Immunol 2005;17:326–32.
29. Catron DM, Rusch LK, Hataye J, et al. CD4+ T cells that enter the draining lymph nodes after antigen injection participate in the primary response and become central-memory cells. J Exp Med 2006;203:1045–54.
30. O'Shea JJ, Paul WE. Mechanisms underlying lineage commitment and plasticity of helper CD4+ T cells. Science 2010;327:1098–102.
31. Roberts AI, Devadas S, Zhang X, et al. The role of activation-induced cell death in the differentiation of T-helper-cell subsets. Immunol Res 2003;28:285–93.
32. Chikuma S, Bluestone JA. CTLA-4 and tolerance: the biochemical point of view. Immunol Res 2003;28:241–53.
33. Okazaki T, Honjo T. The PD-1-PD-L pathway in immunological tolerance. Trends Immunol 2006;27:195–201.
34. Rochman Y, Spolski R, Leonard WJ. New insights into the regulation of T cells by gamma (c) family cytokines. Nature Rev 2009;9:480–90.
35. Hunter CA. New IL-12-family members: IL-23 and IL-27, cytokines with divergent functions. Nat Rev Immunol 2005;5:521–31.
36. Li MO, Wan YY, Sanjabi S, et al. Transforming growth factor-beta regulation of immune responses. Annu Rev Immunol 2006;24:99–146.

17

Cytotoxic T lymphocytes and natural killer cells

Stephen L. Nutt,
Sebastian
Carotta, Axel
Kallies, Gabrielle
T. Belz

Cytotoxic T lymphocytes (CTL) and natural killer (NK) cells represent two distinct but related lineages that are important for the control of viral, bacterial, and parasitic infections. These cells also play a prominent and complementary role in the sensing and elimination of malignant cells. Although the approaches by which CTL and NK cells kill their target cells and produce immunomodulatory cytokines are quite similar, the mechanisms by which they recognize their targets are distinctly different. CTL are CD8 T cells (Chapter 8) that recognize targets via the interaction of a diverse repertoire of polyclonally rearranged T-cell receptors (TCR) (Chapter 4) with a peptide-MHC class I complex (Chapter 6) and are a component of the adaptive immune response. MHC class I molecules are expressed on virtually all cells in the body and allow the CTL to scan the tissues for cells expressing foreign or cancer-associated peptides (Chapter 5). In contrast, NK cells are members of the innate immune system (Chapter 3) that use an array of invariant activating and inhibitory receptors to control their activity and specificity.[1] These fundamentally distinct approaches to the recognition of antigen allow for complementary functions, with CTL being specialized in detecting cells infected with intracellular pathogens such as viruses, whereas a prominent function of NK cells is to eliminate those cells where the pathogen or oncogene has blocked display of MHC class I molecules on the surface of the affected cell. As one of the principal immune-evasion mechanisms of viruses and tumors is to suppress MHC class I expression, NK cells provide a key line of defense against this strategy.

The importance of the lytic function of CTL and NK cells has been demonstrated in animal models as well as in patients with defective cytotoxicity. A number of recessive genetic syndromes that affect cytotoxic function have been reported, including familial hemophagocytic lymphohistiocytosis (FHL), which results from mutations in the perforin gene.[2] FHL patients present with severe immunodeficiency often associated with uncontrolled viral infections, including cytomegalovirus (CMV), herpes simplex virus (HSV) and Epstein–Barr virus (EBV). Similarly, mice genetically deficient or depleted for CTL and NK cells are overtly susceptible to viral pathogens as well as displaying impaired tumor rejection capabilities.[2]

With this potent ability to control pathogen-infected and malignant cells, it is not surprising that the modulation of cytolytic activity is an aim of many immune therapies (see Section 10). These strategies involve either the dampening of CTL function in situations such as transplantation or autoimmunity, or enhancing CTL and NK-cell function via vaccination or cytokine therapy. However, tight controls need to be maintained over these effector cells, as deregulated CTL activity plays a direct role in a variety of immunopathological settings, including autoimmune diseases, hypersensitivity reactions, graft-versus-host disease and transplant rejection. To maintain the discrimination between killing unwanted or infected cells while not killing healthy neighboring cells, numerous layers of regulation operate to control cytotoxic functions.

CLINICAL RELEVANCE

Functions of CTL and/or NK cells

Protective functions include

Host defense against:

- Viruses, including HIV, EBV, pox virus and CMV
- Bacteria, including *Listeria monocytogenes*
- Parasites, including *Plasmodium falciparum* and *Toxoplasma gondii*
- Primary and metastatic tumors

Positive regulation of:

- Graft versus leukemia effect
- Placental vascularization by uterine NK cells

Uncontrolled cytotoxicity contributes to

- Some autoimmune disease, including diabetes and rheumatoid arthritis
- Hypersensitivity reactions
- Graft-versus-host disease
- Transplant rejection

Effector Functions/Mechanisms

KEY CONCEPTS

CTL and NK cell effector mechanisms

Cytotoxicity

- Killing by the perforin/granzyme pathway
- Death receptor mediated apoptosis, including Fas and TRAIL

Immune modulation

- Inflammatory cytokine production, including IFN-γ and TNF
- Chemokine secretion
- Immunomodulatory cytokines, including IL-10 and GM-CSF

Cytotoxicity

Cytotoxic cells kill their targets via two major pathways, perforin/granzyme-mediated lysis and death receptor-induced

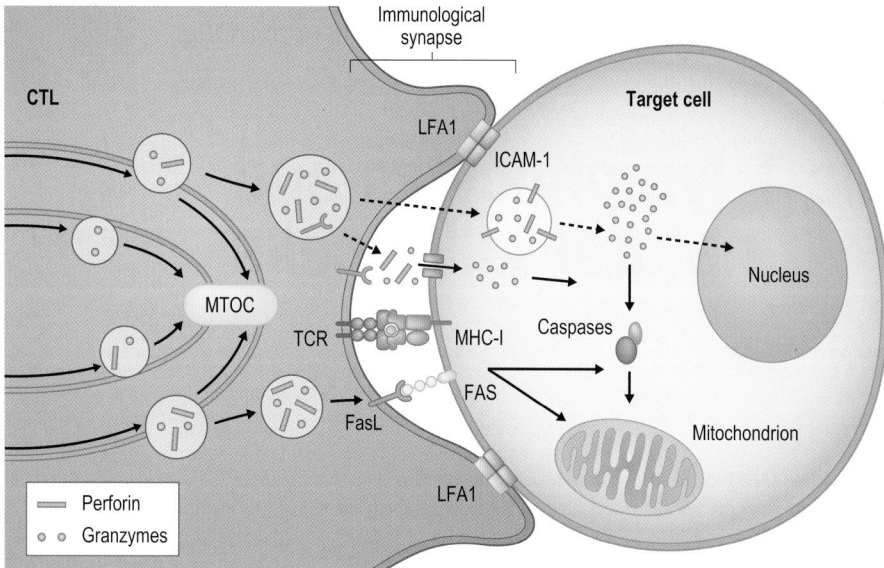

Fig. 17.1 Mechanisms of CTL-induced cell death. The CTL recognizes its target via the interaction of the TCR and the peptide–MHC class I complex on the target cell. TCR signaling induces the formation of an immunological synapse that is stabilized by the binding of LFA1 to ICAM on the target cell. Lytic granules containing perforin, granzymes, and FasL are polarized along microtubules and move toward the microtubule-organizing center (MTOC). Lytic granules are then either endocytosed intact into the target cell, or their contents are secreted into the synapse by a process that requires perforin. Both mechanisms permit granzymes to gain entry into the target cell and induce apoptosis by caspase-dependent and independent pathways that result in DNA cleavage and mitochondrial damage. Membrane bound FasL can bind to its receptor on target cells and induce apoptosis independently of the perforin/granzyme pathway.

apoptosis. Both require intimate contact between the lytic cell and its target (Fig. 17.1).[3] Although the processes are similar for CTL and NK cells, CTL lytic activity is acquired only after activation and differentiation, whereas NK cells have a "natural killing" capacity that does not require pre-stimulation. Despite this, NK-cell killing is significantly increased by prior activation by cytokines or inflammatory signals. Both cell types also produce cytokines, most notably IFN-γ, that further enhance the immune response.

Perforin/granzyme pathway

Perforin is a membrane-disrupting protein that, together with a family of serine proteases (granzymes), forms the bulk of lytic granules. The process of lysis has been most extensively studied in CTL, where, upon interaction between the TCR and an appropriate MHC class I peptide, a synaptic complex forms between the CTL and its target.[3] Lytic granules can then be observed moving along a microtubule network toward the microtubule-organizing center that localizes at the synapse (Fig. 17.1). This process allows the polarized secretion of lytic granules precisely at the CTL–target cell interface. Perforin functions to disrupt the target cell membrane, including either the plasma membrane or the lysosomal membrane. Once the lytic lysosome is internalized into the target cell, it is granzymes that are the initiators of cell death. Granzymes function directly by cleaving substrates, or indirectly via initiating a protease cascade. One important substrate of granzyme B is the pro-apoptotic protein BID (BH3-interacting domain death agonist), which induces cell death via mitochondrial mediators such as cytochrome c. Granzyme A, in contrast, kills via cleavage of nuclear proteins and facilitates double-stranded DNA breaks. Other granzymes must also play an important role in cytotoxicity, as mice deficient for both granzyme A and B are capable of tumor rejection and target cell lysis.

Death receptor-induced apoptosis

Cytotoxic cells also have a receptor-based system to induce apoptosis of target cells (Chapter 13). This pathway uses members of the tumor necrosis factor receptor (TNFR) superfamily that are expressed on the target cells. These receptors have an intracellular signaling motif, called the death domain, which recruits molecules such as FADD (Fas-associated death domain) that transduce the death signal. The two most prominent apoptosis-inducing TNFR family members are Fas (CD95)[4] and TRAIL (TNF-related apoptosis inducing ligand).[5] Whereas Fas is expressed on a wide variety of tissues, Fas ligand (FasL) expression is restricted to activated CTL and NK cells, where it is stored in lytic granules and, upon activation, released to the effector cell membrane. The Fas/FasL pathway is important in controlling T-cell numbers through activation-induced cell death (AICD), as well as in the rejection of some tumors. Cytotoxic cells also express TRAIL, which upon binding to TRAIL receptors induces apoptosis in a wider selection of targets.[5] Of particular therapeutic interest is the fact that tumor cells are often exquisitely sensitive to TRAIL.

Cytokines

Antigen-stimulated CTL and activated NK cells modulate the immune response by their ability to produce a variety of cytokines, most notably IFN-γ and TNF. These potent inflammatory cytokines activate macrophages and lymphocytes at the site of infection. IFN-γ helps establish a Th1 response (Chapter 16) and further stimulates differentiated CTL. NK cells are also a potent source of a diverse range of cytokines, including GM-CSF, IL-5, IL-10, and IL-13 (Chapter 10). The capacity to secrete a broad spectrum of cytokines provides NK cells with a wide range of regulatory capabilities. CTL and NK cells are capable of secreting a number of chemokines (Chapter 11), including CCL3, CCL4, and CCL5. These chemokines help recruit additional lymphocytes into the immune reaction.

Cytotoxic T cells

The development and tissue distribution of CTL

CD8 T lymphocytes develop in the thymus, where they are selected for their ability to recognize nonself-peptides in the context of MHC class I molecules (Chapter 8). Upon thymic export these cells acquire a quiescent state and are termed

Table 17.1 Properties of CTL populations

Marker	Naïve CD8 T cell	Effector CTL	Effector memory (T$_{EM}$)	Central memory (T$_{CM}$)
CD25	−	+++	++	−
CD62L	++	−	−	++
CD44	+	+++	+++	+++
CCR7	+	−	−	+
IL7R (CD127)	++	+	+	++
IL2Rβ (CD122)	+	+	++	+++
Main tissue distribution	Lymph nodes, spleen, blood	Lymph nodes, spleen, blood, nonlymphoid tissue (lung, liver)	Nonlymphoid tissue (lung, liver), spleen	Lymph nodes, spleen, blood
Cytotoxic function	−	+++	++	−
IFN-γ	−	+++	+++	+
Self-renewal capacity	+++	+	++	+++

"naïve." Naïve CD8 T cells circulate between the peripheral lymphoid organs such as the spleen and lymph nodes via the arterial and lymphatic systems. The tissue distribution of lymphocytes is determined by targeting proteins, which can be divided into three categories: selectins, chemokine receptors, and integrins.[6,7] Naïve and activated CD8 T cells display distinct sets of these targeting proteins, allowing for the differential homing abilities of these cells (Chapter 11). Naïve CD8 T cells express high levels of the lymph node homing receptor L-selectin (CD62L) and CCR7, a chemokine receptor that recognizes the chemokines CCL19 and CCL21, which are produced in the T-cell areas of secondary lymphoid organs (Table 17.1, Chapter 10).[6,7] Here naïve T cells interact with antigen-presenting cells (APC), in particular dendritic cells (DC). If a naïve CD8 T cell does not encounter its specific antigen, it leaves the lymph node. This "egress" is regulated by the sphingosine-1-phosphate receptor-1 (S1P1).[6,7] If, however, a CD8 Tcell encounters the correctly presented peptide–MHC-I complex, a dramatic change in its localization and homing properties ensues. These cells shut down their egress program, and undergo multiple rounds of proliferation to become activated CTL. After the proliferative phase, the CTL then re-acquire egress capacity by downregulating the molecules that recruited them to the lymph node in the first place, CD62L and CCR7.[6,7] Egress also requires the re-expression of S1P1 and the downregulation of CD69, an early activation marker of T cells.

Activated CTL travel via the circulation to nonlymphoid sites where they tether to endothelial cells and extravasate into tissue. This transmigration occurs in both inflamed and noninflamed sites, such as the skin, gut, or lung. Many of the effector memory CTL are retained in nonlymphoid tissues, where they are poised to respond rapidly should the antigen be encountered again. A smaller number of memory cells reacquire CD62L and CCR7 expression and circulate through the blood and lymphoid organs and provide long-term memory.

The CTL response

The CTL response to an acute infection consists of three phases: first, the initial activation and proliferation of the CTL; second, the contraction of effector populations; and third, the long-term maintenance of memory cells.

Initial activation of the CTL response

Naïve T cells constantly circulate through the secondary lymphoid organs, where antigen encounter occurs. For a CTL response, antigen is brought to the lymph node via the lymphatic system by APC (Fig. 17.2). These APC are typically DC that mature after antigen acquisition in the nonlymphoid tissues and migrate to the lymph node. Although DC appear to be the most important "professional" APC, macrophages and B cells are also able to present antigens in a similar manner. These antigens are not recognized in isolation but only when complexed to MHC molecules. APC efficiently degrade self or foreign (pathogen-derived) proteins into shorter fragments (generally 8-10 amino acids in length) by the action of proteases in the cytosol. They are then transported into the lumen of the endoplasmic reticulum where they are loaded onto newly synthesized MHC class I molecules for presentation at the cell surface (Chapter 6). This then enables the APC to communicate with the antigen-specific CD8 T cells via interactions between the T-cell receptor and MHC molecules.

In the lymph node, naïve CD8 T lymphocytes scan the APC for the presence of antigenic peptides complexed with the MHC class I molecules, a process termed "immune surveillance." The scanning process is not completely random. In the case of an infection, inflammatory signals in the lymph node induce the chemokine receptor CCR5 expression on naïve CD8 T cells, which allows individual cells to be attracted to sites of antigen-specific DC-CD4 T-cell interactions as signaled by a gradient of the chemokines CCL3 and CCL4.[8] In the absence of a specific recognition by the TCR, the encounter is only transient and the T cell continues on to another APC to repeat the process. If the MHC class I–peptide complex is bound by the TCR and initiates signaling, a more lasting interaction occurs.

TCR activation promotes the polarization of the T cell and the formation of the "immunological synapse."[9] The immunological synapse is a highly structured body that functions to concentrate TCR signaling in a defined area. It is associated with the selective recruitment of signaling molecules and exclusion of negative regulators. The synapse is stabilized by a ring of adhesion molecules, including, for example, LFA1, which binds to ICAM1 on the APC (Fig. 17.1). For a T cell to become fully active, co-stimulation through a second signaling pathway is required. Many co-stimulators have been identified that share

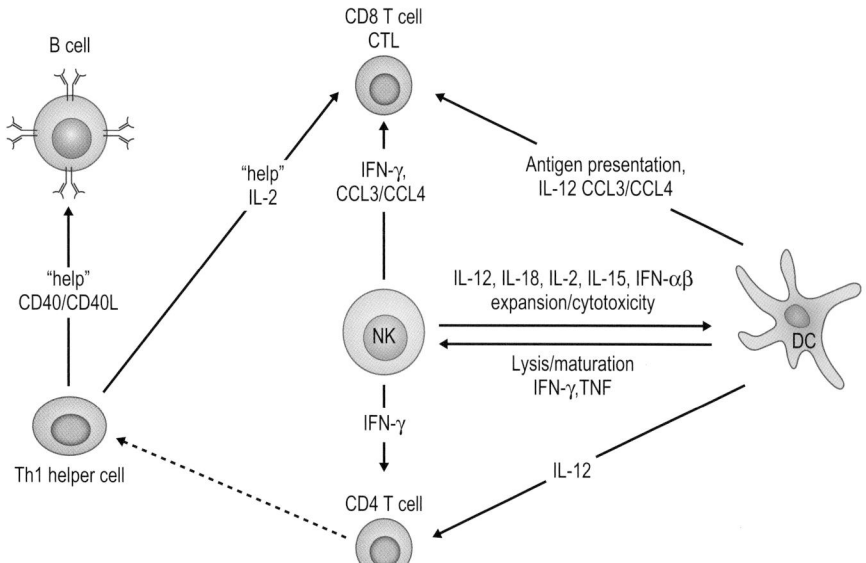

Fig. 17.2 Cellular interactions during an immune response in the lymph node. After their encounter with antigen DC move to the draining lymph node, where they initiate an antigen-specific immune response. In the very early stages, NK cells are recruited to the lymph node and modulate various aspects of this response. NK cells provide cytokines that induce the maturation of DC, which enables these cells to efficiently present the antigen to T cells in the context of co-stimulatory signals. NK cells also have the ability to eliminate immature DC and to provide "early" IFN-γ for the initiation of a Th1-type CD4 T-cell response. Finally, NK cells produce a range of chemokines, most notably CCL3 (MIP-1α) and CCL4 (MIP-1β), which are crucial for the recruitment of CD8 T cells into the immune response.

the common characteristic of being transmembrane receptors, often of the TNFR superfamily, that bind transmembrane ligands on the APC. The most important co-stimulator, CD28, binds the ligands CD80 (B7.1) and CD86 (B7.2), both of which are expressed on activated APC. Co-stimulation results in the clonal expansion of CTL with the selected antigen specificity. The expression of CD80/86 is tightly regulated. High-level expression occurs only after an APC receives activation signals, such as inflammatory cytokines, or components of the pathogens such as lipopolysaccharide. Co-stimulation via CD28 is most critical during the initiation of the immune response, as it promotes IL-2 production that, in turn, supports the development of effector T cells.[10] Naïve T cells that receive TCR stimulation in the absence of co-stimulatory signals can become nonresponsive to antigen, a state termed "anergy."

Cross-presentation and priming

After it was established that only direct interaction with an APC and appropriate co-stimulation led to full CTL activity, a problem arose in explaining the mechanism by which antigens in non-APC were recognized by CTL. This dilemma was resolved by the discovery that there are two distinct mechanisms by which CTL encounter peptide–MHC class I complexes.[11] If the APC expresses the antigen, for example if it is infected by a virus, then the APC can process the antigen via the endogenous MHC class I pathway for presentation. The more intriguing situation arises when the APC does not express the antigen. In this case the APC acquire and process the antigen via a process termed "cross-presentation" (Chapter 6).[11] Cross-presentation is initiated by the capture of foreign or exogenous antigens by phagosomes. The antigens are then processed by an unusual mechanism that directs the peptides to the MHC class I pathway and presentation on the cell surface. An encounter of a CTL with an antigen processed in this pathway is termed "cross-priming."[11] This strategy assists the CTL in viral control in two ways. First, cross-priming alleviates the need for the DC to be infected for detection, and therefore prevents viruses escaping immune detection by avoiding infection of DC. Second, viruses often attempt to evade CTL by downregulating the MHC class I pathway. "Cross-dressing" is a process related to cross-priming but involves the direct exchange of preformed peptide–MHC

complexes to uninfected cells. This mechanism acts to significantly amplify the magnitude of priming of T cells, and like cross-presentation, potentially circumvents immune evasion strategies used by pathogens.[12]

The contraction of effector populations

After activation of the CTL in the secondary lymphoid organs, an immune response is characterized by the rapid proliferation of antigen-specific cells and their acquisition of effector functions. CTL proliferate at one of the fastest rates known for mammalian cells, with a cell cycle time of approximately 6 hours in both humans and rodents. Infection leads to a dramatic increase in the numbers of pathogen-specific CTL, from almost undetectable initial levels to several million cells in the course of a single week. The magnitude of this response is dependent on the kind of infection and the dose of the antigen. It is controlled by the number of precursors recruited into the response.[10,13] The expansion phase is followed by a contraction of the CTL population that is independent of both the magnitude of the response and clearance of the antigen. This phase is essential to prevent nonspecific tissue damage through uncontrolled cytokine release and cytolytic activity. Contraction also preserves the flexibility of the T-cell response to new infections while memory of previously encountered antigens is maintained. Typically, 5% of the expanded antigen-specific population survives in the long-lived memory pool.

The long-term maintenance of memory cells

The production of long-lasting antigen-independent memory cells is essential for a rapid response should re-infection occur. CTL memory provides a more vigorous response than the primary challenge for both quantitative and qualitative reasons.[10,13] Quantitatively, owing to the substantial clonal expansion during a primary infection, the precursor frequency of antigen-specific CTL is vastly higher in immune individuals than in naïve subjects, thus allowing for a stronger response. Qualitatively, memory CTL exhibit a striking efficiency in elaborating effector functions associated with the rapid production of IFN-γ. This enhanced response is the result of reprogramming of gene expression profiles by epigenetic changes in DNA methylation or chromatin structure. The CTL memory compartment is composed of two cell types, effector memory (T_{EM}) and central memory (T_{CM}). These subsets differ in their surface molecule expression and in their ability to exhibit effector functions (Table 17.1).[12] Like their naïve counterparts, T_{CM} express high levels of CD62L and CCR7 and reside primarily in the secondary lymphoid organs. T_{CM} are capable of prolonged homeostatic self-renewal in the absence of antigen. T_{EM}, on the other hand, are characterized by low expression of CD62L and CCR7 and are distributed throughout the body, including peripheral tissues such as lung and gut, where they can immediately confront invading pathogens. The development of these distinct memory cell types is not fully understood. The conventional linear model of memory formation proposes that memory cells are derived directly from the remaining effector cells after the contraction phase.[10,13] An alternative model proposes that pathways exist that allow the differentiation of memory cells without passing through an effector stage. CD4 T-cell help and cytokines, including IL-15 and IL-7 and their receptors, have been identified as crucial for the survival and maintenance of the memory T-cell pool.[10,13,14]

CD4 T-cell help

The final player in the initial activation of CTL is the "help" provided by CD4 T cells specific for an antigen linked to the CTL epitope (Chapter 16). The discovery of cross-priming by DC led to a model whereby both CD4 and CD8 T cells recognize antigen on the same APC via MHC classes II and I, respectively.[11] Subsequent studies demonstrated that the function of the CD4 T cells in the process is to activate the DC. The requirement for CD4 help to generate a CTL response in the absence of an inflammatory stimulus contrasts with the fact that CD4 T cells are not required for a strong primary CTL response to many model infectious agents, such as lymphocytic choriomeningitis virus (LCMV) and *Listeria monocytogenes*.[10] This CD4 independence is explained by direct activation of the APC by the pathogen through activation of the Toll-like receptors that induce pro-inflammatory cytokines, thereby bypassing the need for CD4 help. It is likely that a role for help in primary responses depends on a number of variables, such as the degree of APC activation, inflammatory cytokine production, mode of infection or immunization, and the sensitivity of the assays employed to detect primary and memory CTL responses.

The processes by which help is provided are poorly understood. It is likely that cytokines such as IL-2 and IL-21 are involved.[10,15] These cytokines, provided by the CD4 T cells, promote the survival, proliferation and programming of the memory CTL. CD4 T-cell-deficient mice have been developed to study these CTL responses. Interestingly, "helpless" CD8 T cells strongly resemble CTL in chronic infections in which pathogens are not cleared despite a robust CTL response. In these studies two molecules have been found that mediate the defects in helpless CTL responses. Firstly, re-stimulation of helpless CTL leads to an abortive response due to activation-induced cell death, which is mediated by TRAIL.[16] IL-21 produced by CD4 T cells acts to enhance proliferation of virus-specific CD8 T cells and reduce TRAIL expression.[17] Secondly, PD-1 (programmed *death* 1), an inhibitory member of the TNFR family, is expressed on both helpless CTL and on CTL cells during chronic infections. Blocking the interaction of PD-1 with its ligands greatly enhances the numbers and functions of the impaired CTL.[18]

Detection and analysis of CTL function

Much progress in our understanding of the generation of CTL in an immune response has resulted from the development of several accurate and sensitive assays for CTL function. Traditional CTL assays were performed on bulk populations of effector cells and included chromium (^{51}Cr) release assays. In these assays, target cells are labeled with ^{51}Cr and then pulsed with peptide-antigen. Peptide-specific CTL are incubated with the target cells. Lytic activity is then measured by the release of ^{51}Cr into the culture supernatant. Although the release of ^{51}Cr represents a powerful quantitative assay for CTL activity, it has the distinct disadvantage of requiring pre-stimulation of the CTL population for 1–2 weeks to expand the numbers of antigen-specific CTL to detectable levels. In mice this limitation was overcome by the development of animals that were monoclonal for the TCR. These mouse strains express transgenic TCR that recognize either MHC class I (CD8) or MHC class II (CD4) specific epitopes. Such T cells, which are specific for a single peptide, have proved extremely useful in the study of CTL responses, as antigen-specific cells can be easily detected.

Although they are powerful tools, TCR transgenic mouse models have some limitations, as they do not recapitulate the diversity of the normal immune response and represent an approach that cannot be used in human studies. The development of labeled tetramers of MHC class I–peptide complexes that bind to the endogenous TCR has made a major contribution to alleviating these previous limitations, as they allow the detection of antigen-specific CTL within a polyclonal population.[19] This technique is simple and broadly applicable. It can accurately detect rare antigen-specific populations from patient material or animal tissue (Fig. 17.3). The ability to prospectively identify antigen-specific CTL has been combined with single-cell functional assays such as ELISpot or intracellular cytokine assays. These techniques enable the identification of individual cytokine or chemokine-secreting CTL in a population by either flow-cytometric or colormetric (ELISpot) assays (Fig. 17.3). The finding that the lysosomal compartment proteins LAMP1/2 (CD107a/b) can be detected on the cell surface of degranulating CTL provides another powerful flow cytometry-based single-cell assay to investigate CTL lytic function.[20]

Natural killer cells

Properties of NK cells

NK cells are a lymphoid lineage that, owing to the absence of antigen–receptor rearrangements, belongs to the innate immune response. Compared to CTL, NK cells are relatively large, granular, and do not require pre-activation in order to recognize and lyse malignant or aberrant cells. NK cells also produce copious amounts of cytokines and chemokines, which enable them to modulate the immune system. Whereas the development of B and T lymphocytes has been extensively studied and anatomical sites and major mediators are well characterized, NK cells have proven more elusive. Part of the problem lies in their relative scarcity, amounting to less than 2% of cells in bone marrow or spleen and to ~15% of the lymphocytes in blood. The lack of appropriate markers to distinguish NK cells, coupled with phenotypic heterogeneity between species and within mouse strains, has also complicated their analysis.

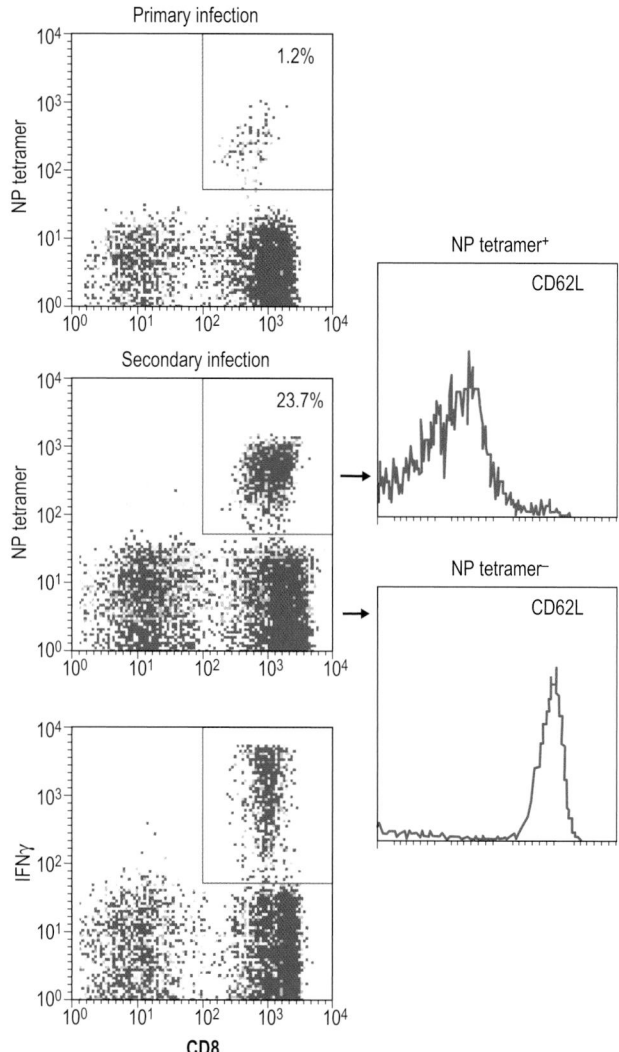

Fig. 17.3 Monitoring a virus-specific CTL response. A fluorescent-labeled tetramer complex comprising an MHC class I molecule and a virus-specific nucleoprotein (NP) antigen peptide is used to detect NP-specific CD8 T cells in the spleens of mice infected with influenza virus. During the primary response, virus-specific CTL expand in the draining lymph node of the lung and later exit to the lung and spleen (upper left). After the infection is resolved, a small population of virus-specific memory CTL reside in the spleen. A second infection with influenza results in very high numbers of virus-specific CTL in the spleen (middle left) and lung. Specific CTL can be re-stimulated with the NP peptide *in vitro*, inducing IFN-γ secretion that is detected by intracellular staining with a labeled anti-IFN-γ antibody (lower left). Staining with an antibody to CD62L shows the typical profile of effector CD8 T cells in the NP-tetramer positive CTL (upper right) and of naïve CD8 T cells in the tetramer negative population (lower right).

In recent years it has become apparent that NK cells develop in the bone marrow from a lymphoid progenitor.[21] IL-15 is essential throughout NK-cell development *in vivo*, but can be substituted for *in vitro* by high concentrations of IL-2. The IL-15R consists of three components, the IL-2/15β chain (CD122), a unique IL-15Rα chain, and the common γ chain, which contains the intracellular signaling component of the receptor.[22] The importance of this receptor complex is emphasized by the lack of NK cells in X-linked SCID patients, and in dogs and mice that have mutations in the common γ-chain gene. In contrast to the B- and T-cell lineages, where the requirement for cytokines changes throughout their development and activation state, NK cells appear to constantly require IL-15 for

their survival.[21] However, the IL-15/IL-15R complex does not function in a manner similar to other cytokines that are produced as soluble ligands and bind to their receptor in a paracrine or autocrine manner. Surprisingly, IL-15 is virtually undetectable in body fluids or cell culture supernatants, despite the ubiquitous distribution of the mRNA. The solution to this paradoxical observation is that IL-15 function requires the presence of the IL-15Rα in the same cell. The IL-15/IL-15Rα complex is then presented on the cell surface in *trans* to the NK cell expressing the IL-15Rαβγ complex.[22] In this manner IL-15 is thought to maintain the homeostatic levels of NK cells in the body. Once NK cells have acquired IL-15 responsiveness, they proceed through an ordered differentiation process that results in an expansion phase and the acquisition of a panel of activating and inhibitory receptors (Table 17.2).[1,21] It was previously assumed that these bone marrow derived NK cells were fully functional, but recent data suggest that NK-cell maturation entails multiple steps and activation states.[1,23]

Table 17.2 Human and mouse NK cell receptors (partial list)

Gene	Function	Ligands
Human		
LILRB1	Inhibitory	HLA-class I
KIR2DL1, 2, 3	Inhibitory	HLA-C
KIR2DL4	Activating	HLA-G
KIR2DL5	Inhibitory	?
KIR3DL1	Inhibitory	HLA-B, HLA-A
KIR3DL2	Inhibitory	HLA-A, CpG-ODN
KIR3DL3	Inhibitory	?
KIR2DS1, 2, 3, 4, 5	Activating	HLA-class I
KIR3DS1, 3	Activating	?
CD94/NKG2A	Inhibitory	HLA-E
CD94/NKG2C, E	Activating	HLA-E
NKG2D	Activating	MICA/B, ULBP1-6, H60, MULT1
CD16 (FcγRIII)	Activating	Immune complexes
CD27	Activating	CD70
CD244 (2B4)	Activating	CD48
NKR-P1A	Inhibitory	LLT1 (CLEC2D)
Mouse		
Ly49A-C, E-G, I-O	Inhibitory	MHC-class I
Ly49D	Activating	H-2D^d
Ly49H, P	Activating	MCMV m157
CD94/NKG2A	Inhibitory	Qa-1b
CD94/NKG2C, E	Activating	Qa-1b (mouse poxvirus)
NKG2D	Activating	RAE-1
KLRG1	Inhibitory	E-, R-, N-cadherins
CD16 (FcγRIII)	Activating	Immune complexes
CD27	Activating	CD70
CD244 (2B4)	Inhibitory	CD48
NKR-P1A, F	Activating	Clr-g
NKR-P1B, D	Inhibitory	Clr-b
PILRα/PILRβ	Inhibitory	O-glycosylated CD99
NKp46	Activating	hemagglutinin
DNAM-1 (CD226)	Activating	CD112, CD155

Fig. 17.4 Schematic representation of human NK cells. The human NK-cell subsets show distinct receptor expression and effector functions. CD56^bright NK cells produce high levels of cytokines and have patterns of chemokine and homing receptor expression that distinguish them from CD56^dim NK cells. CD56^dim NK cells express high levels of KIR and cytotoxic activity. The relative level of receptors and effector molecules is indicated on an arbitrary scale, with $+/-$ being weak and $+++$ being strong expression.

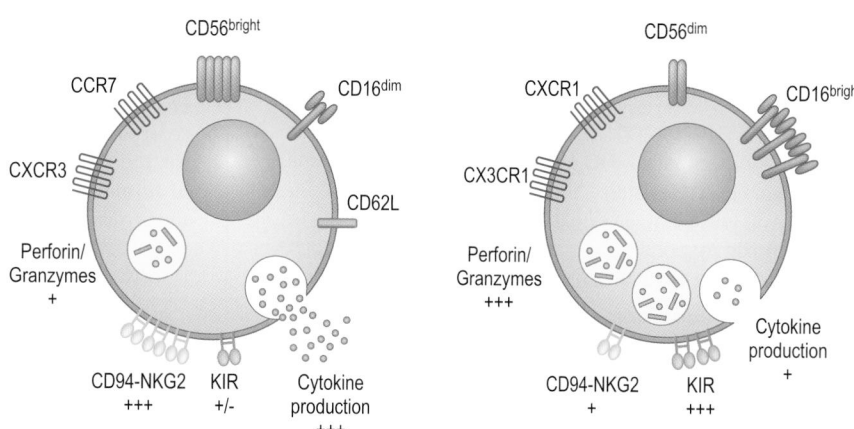

Tissue distribution and diversity of NK cells

In line with their surveillance function, NK cells are found at many sites in the body. In mice, where the tissue distribution has been thoroughly studied, NK cells are found in bone marrow, peripheral blood, thymus and spleen, with the thymic NK cells potentially representing a distinct cell lineage.[21] NK cells also represent one of the predominant hematopoietic cell types in organs such as liver and lung, and the decidual lining of the uterus. Few are present in nonimmunologically activated lymph nodes.

The broad range of tissue distribution suggests that there is diversity in the function of mature NK cells. Indeed, human NK cells can be divided into two subsets based on the expression of CD16 (FcγRIII) and the adhesion molecule CD56 (Fig. 17.4). CD56^dim NK cells represent >90% of the peripheral blood NK cells, are CD16+KIR+, and display greater cytotoxicity. By contrast, CD56^bright NK cells show greater proliferative potential, greater cytokine production, and are the principal NK-cell population in secondary lymphoid organs.[24] NK-cell progenitors in the lymph node that are CD56^bright develop through a series of intermediaries into CD56^dim cells.[24] It is not clear whether the CD56^dim cells in the blood represent an even more immature cell stage or a separate population.

One important limitation in understanding the functional role played by the NK-cell subsets has been the inability to identify populations corresponding to the CD56^bright and CD56^dim populations in rodents, as this molecule is not expressed in mouse NK cells. NK-cell heterogeneity, based on the differential expression of CD11b (integrin αM) and CD27, has been dissected in mice. Whereas developing NK cells in the bone marrow are CD27+CD11b^dim, these cells differentiate into CD27+CD11b^bright and CD27−CD11b^bright stages in the spleen.[23] Interestingly, CD27+ cells are found in lymph nodes, whereas the CD27− NK cells are localized predominantly in the peripheral blood and lung. Comparative studies showed that human CD56^dim NK cells are CD27−, while CD56^bright cells are CD27++ suggesting that the CD27 marker now enables the direct comparisons of NK-cell subsets in mouse and human.[23]

Cytokine regulation of NK-cell activation, function, and homeostasis

NK cells rely on IL-15 for their development and homeostatic maintenance in the peripheral organs. However, cultured NK cells also respond to other cytokines, including IL-2, -4, -12, -18, and -21.[25] Surprisingly, NK-cell numbers are relatively normal in mice deficient for these other cytokines, suggesting that they may be more important for function than for development.[21] The IL-2R shares its β and γ subunits with the constitutively expressed IL-15R (Chapter 9). The dimeric IL-2Rβγ is able to respond to the high levels of IL-2 supplied *in vitro* to induce proliferation of NK cells that were historically called lymphokine-activated-killer or LAK cells. IL-2 activation will also induce the IL-2Rα chain to complete the high-affinity trimeric receptor. IL-4 activates human NK cells, and promotes the proliferation of a fraction of NK cells characterized by their ability to produce IL-13.

The cytokines IL-12 and -18 have profound effects on NK-cell function. IL-12 and -18 are produced by macrophages and DC during inflammatory immune activation, such as viral infection.[26] While NK cells are present in IL-12- or -18-deficient mice and only marginally reduced in double mutant animals, cytotoxic activity and the ability to respond to infections such as mouse CMV (MCMV) is impaired.[26] Cultivation of NK cells in IL-12 and/or IL-18 induces short-term activation, cytotoxicity and IFN-γ production, whereas longer cultures produce more specialized cytokine-producing cells.[25]

Another NK cell-activating cytokine is IL-21.[27] IL-21 is a member of the common γ chain family of cytokines produced by CD4 T cells and, in contrast to IL-2 or -15, does not promote proliferation. Instead, it enhances maturation and effector function. Mouse NK cells treated with IL-21 display a broad-spectrum increase in cytotoxic function and produce cytokines including IFN-γ and IL-10.[27] Importantly, mice treated with IL-21 show a marked increase in NK-cell-mediated tumor rejection, highlighting the potential for use of this cytokine in anti-cancer therapeutics.[28] Human NK cells respond similarly to IL-21, but there is also a role for IL-21 in early NK development that is not present in the mouse.

NK-cell receptors

NK cells differ from CTL in that they do not require the expression of MHC class I to recognize target cells. In fact, the re-introduction of MHC class I molecules into previously susceptible cell lines confers resistance to NK cell-mediated killing. These observations led to the missing-self hypothesis, which proposes that NK cells survey tissues for the usually ubiquitous MHC class I expression.[1] Encounter with MHC class I sends an inhibitory signal to the NK cell, which then moves on in search of other targets. However, if a cell downregulates MHC class I to avoid CTL activity, these cells are killed by NK cells. The

● KEY CONCEPTS

NK-cell receptors

Inhibitory receptors:

- Recognize mostly MHC class I ligands with high affinity
- Signal via ITIM motifs
- Recruit phosphatases (SHP and SHIP) to prevent a cytotoxic response
- Required for NK-cell licensing

Activating receptors:

- Do not bind MHC class I molecules with high affinity
- Ligands include viral molecules and stress induced proteins
- Signal via ITAM motifs.
- Use several signaling adaptors, including DAP12

missing-self hypothesis, although altered over time to encompass other observations, has been extremely useful in providing a predictive framework by which to investigate NK-cell receptors and the recognition of target cells (Fig. 17.5).

In the past two decades a large number of NK-cell receptors have been identified, (Table 17.2)[1] the ligands for many of which are known. Although a number of these NK-cell receptor ligands are the MHC class I molecules themselves, as predicted by the missing-self hypothesis, there are many other classes of ligands. NK-cell receptors are classified into either activating or inhibitory types. This distinction was initially based on the *in vitro* properties of antibodies against these receptors, but is increasingly regarded as the expression of the biochemical signal-transduction pathways activated by the receptor.[1] Interestingly, although this conceptual strategy of target recognition is conserved in all mammals tested, rodents and humans have evolved their receptors from two independent gene families, the killer immunoglobulin-like receptors (KIR) in humans and the Ly49 family in mice (Table 17.2).

NK-cell receptor signaling

The signals derived from NK receptors are defined as inhibitory or activating in terms of their effect on NK-cell function. All extensively characterized inhibitory receptors carry an immunoreceptor tyrosine-based inhibitory motif (ITIM) in their intracellular domain. Ligation of ITIM-containing receptors causes tyrosine phosphorylation and the recruitment of a variety of phosphatases, including SHP and SHIP, that act to damp downstream signaling pathways and NK-cell effector functions.[1] In contrast, activating receptors use immunoreceptor tyrosine-based

activation motifs (ITAM) to transduce stimulatory signals. Engagement of an ITAM-containing receptor results in tyrosine phosphorylation and recruitment of adaptor molecules, including FcεR1γ, CD3ζ, or DAP12. The best-characterized activating receptor is CD16, an Fc receptor that binds IgG and is responsible for the antibody-dependent cell-mediated cytotoxicity (ADCC) of human NK cells. CD16 recruits FcεR1γ and CD3ζ, which in their turn attract the tyrosine kinases syk and ZAP70.[1] These pathways then promote effector functions via multiple signal transduction pathways.

NK receptors that recognize MHC-I molecules

NK cells recognize a wide variety of MHC class I molecules of both classic and nonclassic types. The receptors providing this recognition fit broadly into the immunoglobulin-like and lectin-like superfamilies. They show significant differences between mice and humans.

Killer cell immunoglobulin-like receptors (KIR) in humans

The KIR genes represent a family of 15 genes that are physically linked on chromosome 19.[29] The locus shows a high degree of variation in humans with both the number of KIR genes varying between individuals and extensive allelic polymorphisms. The KIR family was originally called killer inhibitory receptors, but subsequent studies have demonstrated that activating receptors are also encoded by the KIR locus. As expected, the inhibitory KIR contain ITIM, whereas all activating KIR utilize DAP12 to transduce signals from an ITAM.[1] Individual KIR genes are expressed by only a subset of NK cells. This expression pattern is stably maintained in a clonal manner. Similarly to most other NK-cell receptors, KIR can also be expressed by some T cells after activation.

KIR recognize the human MHC class I molecules HLA-A, -B, and -C (Table 17.2). The specificity of the inhibitory KIR has been extensively characterized, with, for example, the different isoforms of KIR2D recognizing all known alleles of HLA-C.[1,29] The ligands of the activating KIR are less clear; however, they do not bind with high affinity to HLA molecules. KIR2DL4 is the most evolutionarily distinct member of the family and appears to be expressed in all activated NK cells in culture and on the CD56[bright] subset in peripheral blood. KIR2DL4 also has some distinct structural features and may act as an unconventional activating receptor binding HLA-G.[1,29]

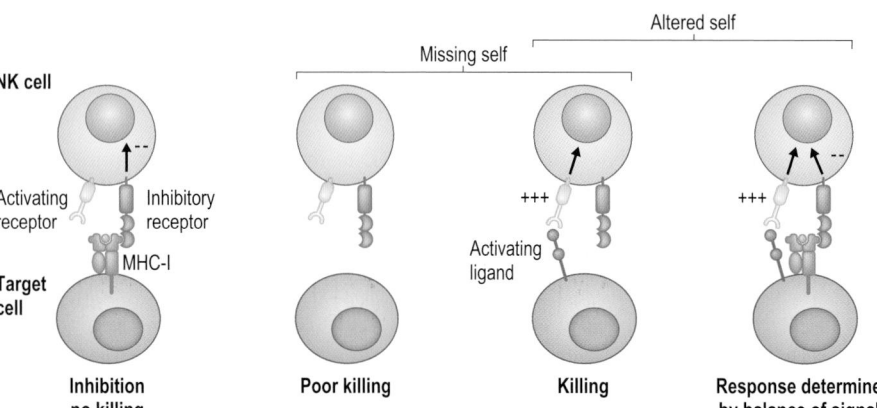

Fig. 17.5 NK-cell recognition of target cells. NK cells express inhibitory receptors for MHC class I and activating receptors for a variety of cellular, viral, and stress-induced ligands that alter the outcome of encounter with a target cell. The missing-self hypothesis initially predicted that NK cells would be activated to kill in the absence of MHC class I inhibition. However, an activating signal is also required. This activating signal can be provided by cellular ligands, or by viral or stress-induced proteins, termed "altered self." In the presence of both inhibitory and activating signals the outcome is determined by quantitative differences in signal strength between the two.

There are epidemiological data implicating particular KIR in a variety of autoimmune pathologies and viral responses.[30] For example, individuals with KIR2DS2 and some HLA-C alleles are predisposed to rheumatoid arthritis with vascular complications. Conversely, HIV-infected individuals who are homozygous for HLA-Bw4 progress to AIDS more slowly than those with other haplotypes, especially when they have the *KIR3DS1* gene. The mechanism by which this occurs is unknown, but the activity suggests that KIR recognize an HIV-associated peptide in the context of HLA-Bw4 (Chapter 37).[31]

The Ly49 family in rodents

In a remarkable example of the power of selection to shape the evolution of the immune system, a multigenic locus with functional properties almost identical to those of the KIR genes has evolved independently in rodents. Mice, which have only two Kir genes of unknown function, have an analogous cluster of type II transmembrane spanning lectin-like genes called the Ly49 family on chromosome 6.[1] This family consists of more than 20 members and is highly polymorphic between mouse strains. Like KIR molecules, Ly49 receptors are also highly variegated in their expression in NK cells. Ly49 genes encode activating and inhibitory receptors that bind to MHC class I molecules and signal via ITAM and ITIM motifs, respectively (Table 17.2). Ligand-binding studies have revealed that the inhibitory Ly49 receptors such as A, C, and I function to prevent autoaggression by NK cells by binding to MHC class I molecules. The function of the activating receptors has proved more difficult to elucidate. Ly49D is known to have high affinity for the MHC class I H-2D^d allele and is involved in rejecting bone marrow allografts expressing H-2D^d, whereas the function of Ly49D in the normal immune response is unclear. For one activating receptor, Ly49H, the physiological function is known, as it recognizes the m157 molecule of MCMV and is important in viral control.[1,32]

CD94 and NKG2 family

Unlike the KIR or Ly49s, the CD94/NKG2 complex is present both in rodents and humans. CD94/NKG2 receptors recognize nonclassic MHC class I ligands, such as HLA-E in humans and Qa1^b in mice. A single CD94 gene is physically linked to four NKG2 (A, C, E, and a truncated F) genes in humans. CD94 is found on the cell surface either alone or with the NKG2 proteins. The NKG2 family also consists of activating (C, E) and inhibitory forms (A). Interestingly, both the activating and the inhibitory complexes recognize HLA-E that present predominantly the leader peptides of other HLA molecules, but not HLA-E itself. This system may provide a mechanism for NK cells to monitor the expression of multiple MHC class I proteins using HLA-E as a surrogate, with a prominent example being the requirement of CD94 for the control of mouse ectromelia virus.[33]

NKG2D

NKG2D, which is only distantly related to the NKG2 family, is a single, nonpolymorphic gene that is expressed on all NK cells from an early stage. In the mouse NKG2D signals through both DAP12 and another adaptor, DAP10, whereas human NK cells use only DAP10.[1] Activation of NKG2D using a specific antibody results in enhanced cytotoxicity and cytokine secretion.[34] The ligands of NKG2D are a family of molecules with structural similarity to MHC class I proteins, including MICA/B in

humans and RAE-1 in mice. These ligands represent a diverse array of sequences, yet all bind with high affinity to NKG2D.[34] Interestingly, the MIC family in humans is highly polymorphic, suggesting that in this receptor–ligand interaction the diversity comes from the ligands rather than the receptors. Transfection of otherwise resistant tumor cells with NKG2D ligands restores the susceptibility of these cells to NK-cell cytotoxic function. The key to understanding NKG2D function lies in the fact that the ligands are inducible and provide a mechanism for NK cells to detect stressed tissue, such as virally infected or malignant cells,[34] a phenomenon that has been termed "altered self" (Fig. 17.5).

NK receptors that recognize non-MHC I molecules

Beyond the multiple systems of activating and inhibitory receptors that NK cells have evolved to recognize MHC class I molecules and their structural variants, they also have several other receptor families that bind non-MHC class I ligands. These include the NKR-P1 family, which is a polymorphic multigene family in rodents consisting of activating (A, C, F) and inhibitory forms (D), but consists of only a single member in humans, whose activity is inhibitory. The ligands for some family members have been recently reported and are themselves lectin family receptors, including clr-b and clr-g in mice and LLT1 in humans. Another NK receptor that is conserved between species is CD244 (2B4), a pan-NK-cell-expressed molecule whose ligand is CD48. Based on antibody cross-linking studies, human CD244 is designated an activating receptor. However, analysis of CD244-deficient mice suggests that the mouse homolog is inhibitory. A number of additional activating receptors exist, including the natural cytotoxicity receptors NKp30, NKp44, and NKp46. NKp30 and NKp46 are broadly expressed on human NK cells, and NKp46 is expressed on all mouse NK cells. NKp44 is specifically expressed on activated human NK cells. These receptors can be activated by antibody cross-linking and, although their ligands are unknown, there is evidence that NKp46 binds hemagglutinin on influenza virus-infected cells, and mice deficient for NKp46 have impaired response to influenza infection.[34] Therefore, the natural cytotoxicity receptors are likely to play a critical role in some aspects of NK-cell function.

NK-cell licensing and self-tolerance

The plethora of MHC class I-binding inhibitory receptors, as proposed by the missing-self hypothesis, explains the influence of MHC class I on NK-cell lytic function against tumors. However, how self-tolerance is achieved has been less clear. The initial theory to explain self-tolerance was the "at least one receptor" model, which proposed that NK cells must express at least one self-MHC class I inhibitory receptor. A second model suggested that the receptor repertoire is shaped by selection by the specific MHC haplotype and the presence of self-ligands. The observation that NK cells are not autoreactive in the absence of any inhibitory ligands (MHC class I-deficient mice) and are actually poor killers suggests that the situation is more complex than these models would allow for.[1] A concept termed "licensing" was proposed to account for these observations.[1] Under this model, NK cells are initially unresponsive or "unlicensed" and acquire functional competency through binding of at least one inhibitory receptor before they can be activated and display cytotoxic function. An alternative "disarming" model proposes that all NK cells are initially responsive, but that chronic stimulation by normal cells renders these cells unresponsive, or "anergic" unless the stimulation is opposed by MHC class I-specific inhibitory receptors. More recently a third "rheostat" model has also been proposed whereby the number and affinity of inhibitory receptors it expresses tune NK-cell reactivity in a quantitative manner.[1] Regardless of the exact tolerance mechanism it is interesting, that unlike T cells there is no evidence for clonal deletion of autoreactive NK cells. Unlicensed NK cells can still have a function as inflammatory signals and viral infection can, at least partially, overcome the defects in unlicensed cells.[1]

Specific NK-cell functions

The increasing ability to separate NK cells from T cells both phenotypically and genetically has greatly enhanced the understanding of NK-cell functions. Although some cytotoxic and immunomodulatory capacities overlap with those of T cells, it is also apparent that some functions of NK cells are unique. Specific examples of NK-cell functions are discussed below.

Control of viral infections

NK-cell activity rises early in the course of viral infection, partly driven by the release of IL-12, IL-18, and IFN-α/β, which stimulates activation (Chapter 27). The evidence that NK cells are essential for host defense against viruses comes directly from patients and mice lacking NK-cell function and indirectly from viral strategies to avoid NK-cell recognition. Human patients with selective deficiencies in NK cells show a pronounced susceptibility to recurrent severe infections, especially with HSV and CMV.

A powerful example of the role of NK-cell-activating receptors in viral control is NK-cell-mediated resistance to mouse cytomegalovirus (MCMV). Mouse strains that lack Ly49H are highly susceptible to MCMV, leading to uncontrolled viral replication and death.[32] Importantly, this protection is mediated by the recognition of the m157 protein of MCMV by Ly49H. As a consequence, whereas in the early stages of MCMV infection the NK-cell response is nonspecific, subsequent control of the virus depends on the proliferation and effector function of the Ly49H$^+$ NK-cell subset in the presence of the activating ligand. The rapid accumulation of Ly49H$^+$ NK cells during MCMV infection is the first example of clonal expansion of NK cells in a manner similar to that of B and T cells.[32] Surprisingly these studies also found compelling evidence for the maintenance of a long-lived NK-cell "memory"-like population, blurring the line between innate (NK cells) and adaptive (B and T cells) immune cells.[32]

As mentioned earlier, there is also evidence that NK cells have direct effects on the progression of HIV infection (Chapter 37).[31] NK cells are able to lyse HIV-infected target cells either directly or by ADCC. Despite this ability, NK-cell responses are impaired in HIV-infected patients as infected T-cell blasts selectively downregulate some HLA genes to avoid CTL activity but remain resistant to NK-cell cytotoxicity. NK cells also secrete large quantities of the chemokines CCL3, CCL4, and CCL5, which are the ligands for CCR5 and inhibit CCR5-dependent entry of HIV into target cells. These findings are supported by studies that show that high-risk, but uninfected, individuals appear to have increased NK-cell activity, and that the combination of the expression of HLA-Bw4 and the *KIR3DS1* gene is associated with

delayed progression to AIDS.[31] Finally, HIV viremia induces several functional abnormalities on NK cells, suggesting that this complex virus and NK cells interact at multiple levels.

Control of malignant cells

A function for NK cells in protective tumor immune surveillance, although hypothesized many years ago, is still uncertain. One limitation in testing this hypothesis has been the lack of a mouse model that is NK-cell-deficient but has an otherwise competent immune system. There is good evidence that NK cells can reject tumor cells in animal models, and that the administration of cytokines that enhance NK-cell function, including IL-2, -12, and -21, or those that induce IFN-α production, are protective against metastasis.[28,35] In light of this, there have been many clinical trials to assess either cytokine treatment or the injection of *ex vivo* treated NK cells (Chapter 77). Unfortunately, the high doses of IL-2 required for efficacy are relatively toxic, and transferred NK cells have proved difficult to target to tumors.[35,36] Despite this, some successes have been demonstrated for melanoma, leukemia, lung, and hepatic cancers. Current trials are now testing combination therapies such as low dose IL-2 and -12 or IFN-α as well as more targeted NK-cell transfer.

Role of NK cells in hematopoietic stem cell transplantation

⬤ CLINICAL PEARLS

Exploiting NK cells in leukemia therapy

- Hematopoietic stem cell transplantation requires donor and recipient HLA matching to reduce graft-versus-host disease (GvHD) mediated by transplanted CTL.
- Haploidentical donors and recipients (those that share only one HLA haplotype) represent 50% of unrelated transplants and undergo a stronger conditioning regimen to avoid GvHD.
- Alloreactive NK cells are present after haploidentical transplant and provide a potent graft-versus-leukemia (GvL) effect in animal models.
- Transplantation from NK-cell-alloreactive donors controls leukemia relapse and improves engraftment without causing GvHD.

NK cells in an F1 offspring of two mouse strains can reject parental bone marrow, a process termed "hybrid resistance." This is in contrast to organ grafts from the same mice that are tolerated by CTL owing to their expression of MHC class I molecules from each parent. This phenomenon is mediated by the interaction of host NKG2D and its ligands, RAE-1, on the repopulating bone marrow cells, as treatment with a neutralizing antibody to NKG2D prevented hybrid resistance.[37] This raises the possibility that stem cells or tissues upregulate the expression of NKG2D ligands after transplantation, and that NKG2D may contribute to some graft rejection in immunocompetent hosts.

In humans, allogeneic bone marrow transplantation can cure leukemia through the reaction of donor CTL in the graft against the residual leukemic cells. These transferred T cells also mediate graft-versus-host disease (GvHD). The need to prevent GvHD by strong immunosuppression is the major cause of transplantation failure, due to infection and cancer relapse. It has been proposed that transplantation with a haploidentical donor (identical at one HLA haplotype and fully mismatched on the other, for example a parent) provides allogeneic NK cells with an HLA haplotype that supplies more KIR ligand than a matched recipient would provide. Hence it would yield a stronger graft-versus-leukemia effect.[36] Indeed, mice treated with alloreactive NK cells tolerate 30 times the lethal dose of mismatched bone marrow cells without developing GvHD, and alloreactive NK cells eradicated human acute myeloid leukemia (AML) transplanted into NOD/SCID mice.[36] Retrospective studies on acute myelogenous leukemia (AML) and acute lymphoblastic leukemia (ALL) patients that received haploidentical grafts revealed that transplants with alloreactive NK cells showed better engraftment and GvHD protection, and less relapse.[38]

These studies suggest that therapeutic treatment with alloreactive NK cells will be effective in eliminating residual cancer cells following front line treatments or in preventing cancer relapse. Feasibility studies have shown that the production of clinical grade cultured human NK cells is possible and that the transferred cells persist for some time in the patient. An alternative strategy is the use of monoclonal antibodies directed against particular inhibitory KIR. Pre-clinical studies suggest that blockade of the inhibitory KIR enhances anti-tumor activities of the endogenous NK cells, providing a rationale for initiating clinical trials to test this approach.[32,36]

● ON THE HORIZON

Clinical trials of transferred alloreactive NK cells

- Adoptive transfer of cultured clinical grade NK cells has proven feasible and well tolerated by patients and is a promising therapy to limit relapse in patients with cancer.

- A treatment regimen comprising pre-conditioning with chemotherapeutic reagents followed by alloreactive NK cells and IL-2 administration is in clinical trials.

- Therapeutic blockade of inhibitory NK-cell receptors using anti-KIR monoclonal antibodies is also undergoing clinical trials for their efficacy in boosting NK cell mediated killing of cancer cells.

NK cells and pregnancy

During pregnancy, maternal (self) and paternal (non-self) antigens are expressed in the embryo and placenta. The reasons why the maternal immune system temporarily tolerates the fetus remain poorly understood. Interestingly, the majority of leukocytes present at the site of implantation are a distinct subset of NK cells known as uterine NK (uNK) cells. Mice deficient in uNK cells show some changes in decidual blood vessels and reduced fertility, supporting a role for these cells, but how they function is unclear.[39,40] uNK cells have low cytotoxic activity and, in addition to IFN-γ and TNF, secrete angiogenic factors such as vascular endothelial growth factor (VEGF-C) and angiopoietin-2. This suggests that uNK cells can influence maternal arterial integrity and trophoblast invasion.[39]

uNK cells can recognize HLA-C/E/G on paternal trophoblasts. Recently, it has been found that KIR expression on maternal uNK cells is a key factor in the development of pre-eclampsia (a serious complication of pregnancy in which the fetus receives an inadequate supply of blood due to failure of trophoblast invasion). Mothers lacking most activating KIR when the fetus possessed HLA-C2 were at a greatly increased risk of pre-eclampsia. Thus, the maternal KIR and trophoblast interaction

appears to play a positive physiological role related to placental development, suggesting that too great an inhibition of uNK cells is detrimental to the process. This has clearly been selected against, as human populations have a reciprocal relationship between certain KIR haplotypes and HLA-C2 frequency.[40]

Interactions of CTL and NK cells in the immune response

Although studies of CTL and NK cells in isolation have greatly advanced our understanding of their functions, it is obvious that these immune cells function in a system that depends on numerous interactions between the various cell types at multiple levels. In the case of cytotoxic cells, these immunomodulatory interactions are becoming increasingly appreciated (Fig. 17.2). In particular, it has become apparent that NK cells and DC interact specifically to promote outcomes such as the maturation of NK cells.[26] CTL activation by mature DC is influenced directly by NK cell-derived IFN-γ, and indirectly through the role of NK cells in promoting a Th1 response in CD4 T cells (Chapter 16).

Increasing evidence has emerged to implicate DC-NK-cell cross-talk in various aspects of the immune response. DC produce a variety of cytokines that modulate NK-cell behavior, including IL-12, IL-15, IL-18, and IFN-α.[26] Interestingly, the outcome of these interactions for the DC depends on its maturity; with immature DC being killed by NK cells, whereas mature DC are resistant to lysis. The interactions of mature DC and NK cells would be expected to occur at the site of infection, where DC provide inflammatory stimuli for NK cells. The other site of encounter is the lymph node, where, during an immune reaction, NK cells are recruited by chemokines and interact with mature DC and CD4 T cells to induce a Th1 response. This process requires IFN-γ production from NK cells (Fig. 17.2).

NK cell and CTL interactions are also important in generating an immune response to tumors that are, in general, poorly immunogenic. DC that are matured *in vitro* by NK cells show strongly enhanced ability to induce Th1 and CTL responses, including cytokine secretion. IFN-γ in particular is very important in the rejection of primary tumors and the formation of CTL memory to tumors. It is also likely that killing by NK cells and CTL provides DC with increased access to tumor antigens and promotes further adaptive immunity. Using DC to harness the helper function of NK cells as well as the cytotoxic functions of both CTL and NK cells offers therapeutic promise and is currently being tested in a variety of cancers.[26]

Evasion of the cytotoxic response

Viruses

As one principal function of CTL and NK cells is the control of viral infections, it is not surprising that viruses have strategies to interfere with the host response (Chapter 27). The multiplicity of these evasion strategies indicates that this is an essential step for long-term viral persistence.[41]

These strategies include:

1. *Latency.* This involves minimizing viral gene expression and thereby avoiding detection. Examples include HSV in neurons, HIV in T cells, and EBV in B cells.
2. *Antigenic variation.* The virus possesses the ability to rapidly mutate its genome and produce escape variants that are no

longer visible to CTL. Such mutations were shown for LCMV in mouse and HIV infection in humans.

3. *Infection of immune nonaccessible sites.* Such inaccessible sites include infection of the CNS by HSV or rubella.

4. *Production of viral defense molecules (immunoevasins).* Many viruses, including adenovirus and EBV, interfere with cytotoxic activity by producing proteins that either hinder Fas or TNF-mediated killing or inhibit the function of antiviral cytokines such as IFN-α/β. A number of viruses, including EBV, produce homologs of anti-apoptotic molecules, such as Bcl2, to inhibit killing by CTL. Various members of the poxvirus family have evolved homologs of the naturally occurring IL-18-binding protein that inhibits IL-18 activity and NK-cell function.[42]

5. *Modulation of molecules involved in recognition.* A widely utilized viral strategy to evade the cytotoxic response is to interfere with antigen processing, presentation, or the expression of other molecules required for CTL recognition (Chapter 6). Several viruses, including adenovirus, downregulate MHC class I expression on the cell surface. This can be achieved by a number of mechanisms. For example, adenovirus type 2 E3 protein forms a complex with MHC class I to prevent antigens from being processed; MCMV gpm152 protein causes retention of the MHC class I molecules in the Golgi compartment; and CMV proteins US2 and US11 promote the rapid degradation of newly synthesized MHC class I complexes. An alternative approach is to interfere with antigen processing, either inhibiting the expression of the TAP protein, as is the case for HSV, or producing proteins that are resistant to antigen digestion by the proteasome, such as the EBNA-1 protein of EBV.[43] This inhibition strategy is not restricted to MHC class I, as human and mouse CMV express proteins that inhibit the cell surface expression of NKG2D ligands.

Tumor cells

Part of the evidence that CTL and NK cells function to control malignant cells comes from the effort tumor cells will go to avoid cytotoxic activity (Chapter 76). Conversely, promoting the cytotoxic response either through specific tumor antigens or through polyclonal stimulation remains one of the most actively pursued strategies in cancer therapy.

Tumors evade cytotoxic function in a number of ways:

6. *Downregulation or loss of MHC class I expression.* This strategy is common in solid tumors, including metastatic melanoma and breast cancer, where MHC class I downregulation accounts for up to 50% of samples.[44] MHC class I loss is also induced by mutations in the gene encoding β2-microglobulin or transcription factors that regulate its expression. MHC class I downregulation is associated with changes in the regulatory mechanisms controlling antigen presentation, and can often be corrected by treatment with cytokines such as IFN-γ.

7. *Antigenic mutation.* Tumors can also avoid CTL activity by antigenic loss. This strategy takes the form of silencing or mutating epitopes that are particularly immunogenic to CTL. This phenomenon has been shown most clearly for the loss of immunogenicity of serially transferred tumor cell lines in the mouse. In human malignancies, tumor antigens such as MART-1 are lost in metastatic melanoma independent of treatment.[45]

8. *Immune modulation by tumor-produced factors.* Tumors express a variety of factors that can modulate the immune response, including FasL, which protects the tumor by inducing apoptosis in activated Fas-expressing CTL. This model is not universally accepted and a role for FasL in inducing the expression of inflammatory cytokines is also possible. Tumors are also known to express TGF-β, which acts on CTL and NK cells to inhibit the expression of effector molecules such as perforin and granzymes. TGF-β also acts on NK cells to downregulate the expression of NKG2D. In addition, tumors can produce soluble decoy ligands such as MIC, which suppresses NKG2D function.

References

1. Orr MT, Lanier LL. Natural killer cell education and tolerance. Cell 2010;142:847–56.
2. Voskoboinik I, Dunstone MA, Baran K, et al. Perforin: structure, function, and role in human immunopathology. Immunol Rev 2010;235:35–54.
3. Jenkins MR, Griffiths GM. The synapse and cytolytic machinery of cytotoxic T cells. Curr Opin Immunol 2010;22:308–13.
4. Strasser A, Jost PJ, Nagata S. The many roles of FAS receptor signaling in the immune system. Immunity 2009;30:180–92.
5. Johnstone RW, Frew AJ, Smyth MJ. The TRAIL apoptotic pathway in cancer onset, progression and therapy. Nat Rev Cancer 2008;8:782–98.
6. Cyster JG. Chemokines, sphingosine-1-phosphate, and cell migration in secondary lymphoid organs. Annu Rev Immunol 2005;23:127–59.
7. Ley K, Kansas GS. Selectins in T-cell recruitment to non-lymphoid tissues and sites of inflammation. Nat Rev Immunol 2004;4:325–35.
8. Castellino F, Huang AY, Altan-Bonnet G, et al. Chemokines enhance immunity by guiding naive CD8+ T cells to sites of CD4+ T cell-dendritic cell interaction. Nature 2006;440:890–5.
9. Fooksman DR, Vardhana S, Vasiliver-Shamis G, et al. Functional anatomy of T cell activation and synapse formation. Annu Rev Immunol 2010;28:79–105.
10. Ahmed R, Bevan MJ, Reiner SL, et al. The precursors of memory: models and controversies. Nat Rev Immunol 2009;9:662–8.
11. Heath WR, Belz GT, Behrens GM, et al. Cross-presentation, dendritic cell subsets, and the generation of immunity to cellular antigens. Immunol Rev 2004;199:9–26.
12. Wakim LM, Bevan MJ. Cross-dressed dendritic cells drive memory CD8+ T-cell activation after viral infection. Nature 2011;471:629–32.
13. Parish IA, Kaech SM. Diversity in CD8(+) T cell differentiation. Curr Opin Immunol 2009;21:291–7.
14. Pellegrini M, Calzascia T, Toe JG, et al. IL-7 engages multiple mechanisms to overcome chronic viral infection and limit organ pathology. Cell 2011;144:601–13.
15. Cox MA, Harrington LE, Zajac AJ. Cytokines and the inception of CD8 T cell responses. Trends Immunol 2011;32:180–6.
16. Janssen EM, Droin NM, Lemmens EE, et al. CD4+ T-cell help controls CD8+ T-cell memory via TRAIL-mediated activation-induced cell death. Nature 2005;434:88–93.
17. Barker BR, Gladstone MN, Gillard GO, et al. Critical role for IL-21 in both primary and memory anti-viral CD8+ T-cell responses. Eur J Immunol 2010;40:3085–96.
18. Barber DL, Wherry EJ, Masopust D, et al. Restoring function in exhausted CD8 T cells during chronic viral infection. Nature 2006;439:682–7.
19. Altman JD, Moss PA, Goulder PJ, et al. Phenotypic analysis of antigen-specific T lymphocytes. Science 1996;274:94–6.
20. Betts MR, Brenchley JM, Price DA, et al. Sensitive and viable identification of antigen-specific CD8+ T cells by a flow cytometric assay for degranulation. J Immunol Methods 2003;281:65–78.
21. Huntington ND, Vosshenrich CA, Di Santo JP. Developmental pathways that generate natural-killer-cell diversity in mice and humans. Nat Rev Immunol 2007;7:703–14.
22. Bulfone-Paus S, Bulanova E, Budagian V, et al. The interleukin-15/interleukin-15 receptor system as a model for juxtacrine and reverse signaling. Bioessays 2006;28:362–77.
23. Hayakawa Y, Huntington ND, Nutt SL, et al. Functional subsets of mouse natural killer cells. Immunol Rev 2006;214:47–55.
24. Caligiuri MA. Human natural killer cells. Blood 2008;112:461–9.
25. Brady J, Carotta S, Thong RP, et al. The interactions of multiple cytokines control NK cell maturation. J Immunol 2010;185:6679–88.
26. Ferlazzo G, Munz C. Dendritic cell interactions with NK cells from different tissues. J Clin Immunol 2009;29:265–73.
27. Zwirner NW, Domaica CI. Cytokine regulation of natural killer cell effector functions. Biofactors 2010;36:274–88.
28. Skak K, Kragh M, Hausman D, et al. Interleukin 21: combination strategies for cancer therapy. Nat Rev Drug Discov 2008;7:231–40.
29. Parham P. MHC class I molecules and KIRs in human history, health and survival. Nat Rev Immunol 2005;5:201–14.
30. Khakoo SI, Carrington M. KIR and disease: a model system or system of models? Immunol Rev 2006;214:186–201.
31. Fauci AS, Mavilio D, Kottilil S. NK cells in HIV infection: paradigm for protection or targets for ambush. Nat Rev Immunol 2005;5:835–43.
32. Vivier E, Raulet DH, Moretta A, et al. Innate or adaptive immunity? The example of natural killer cells. Science 2011;331:44–9.
33. Fang M, Orr MT, Spee P, et al. CD94 is essential for NK cell-mediated resistance to a lethal viral disease. Immunity 2011;34:579–89.

34. Stern-Ginossar N, Mandelboim O. An integrated view of the regulation of NKG2D ligands. Immunology 2009;128:1–6.
35. Smyth MJ, Cretney E, Kershaw MH, et al. Cytokines in cancer immunity and immunotherapy. Immunol Rev 2004;202:275–93.
36. Moretta L, Locatelli F, Pende D, et al. Killer Ig-like receptor-mediated control of natural killer cell alloreactivity in haploidentical hematopoietic stem cell transplantation. Blood 2011;117:764–71.
37. Ogasawara K, Benjamin J, Takaki R, et al. Function of NKG2D in natural killer cell-mediated rejection of mouse bone marrow grafts. Nat Immunol 2005;6:938–45.
38. Velardi A, Ruggeri L, Mancusi A, et al. Natural killer cell allorecognition of missing self in allogeneic hematopoietic transplantation: a tool for immunotherapy of leukemia. Curr Opin Immunol 2009;21:525–30.
39. Parham P. NK cells and trophoblasts: partners in pregnancy. J Exp Med 2004;200:951–5.
40. Trowsdale J, Moffett A. NK receptor interactions with MHC class I molecules in pregnancy. Semin Immunol 2008;20:317–20.
41. Horst D, Verweij MC, Davison AJ, et al. Viral evasion of T cell immunity: ancient mechanisms offering new applications. Curr Opin Immunol 2011;23:96–103.
42. Alzhanova D, Fruh K. Modulation of the host immune response by cowpox virus. Microbes Infect 2010;12:900–9.
43. Lilley BN, Ploegh HL. Viral modulation of antigen presentation: manipulation of cellular targets in the ER and beyond. Immunol Rev 2005;207:126–44.
44. Chang CC, Campoli M, Ferrone S. HLA class I antigen expression in malignant cells: why does it not always correlate with CTL-mediated lysis? Curr Opin Immunol 2004;16:644–50.
45. Jager D, Jager E, Knuth A. Immune responses to tumour antigens: implications for antigen specific immunotherapy of cancer. J Clin Pathol 2001;54:669–74.

Hui Xu, Laura Timares, Craig A. Elmets

Host defenses in the skin

The skin, which includes the hair and nails, is the largest organ in the body and is the major interface between an individual and his/her environment.[1] It comprises 12-15% of the body's weight and serves several different functions. It plays an important role in temperature, water and electrolyte regulation; it is a major source of vitamin D for the body; and it serves as a protective barrier against invading pathogens, exogenous chemicals, mechanical insults and the destructive effects of physical agents such as sun, wind, and heat. To perform these various activities, the skin is comprised of multiple different cell types in three self-regenerating compartments layered one on top of the other (Fig. 18.1). Adnexal tissues, which include the sebaceous glands and eccrine and apocrine sweat glands, are embedded within these tissues and have specialized functions.

The *epidermis* is the outermost layer. It does not contain any blood or lymphatic vessels and relies on the dermal microvasculature for oxygen and nutrients.

Keratinocytes, which comprise ~95% of the cells within the epidermis, form a self-renewing stratified squamous epithelium that differentiates from cuboidal shaped cells in the basal layer to flat, anucleate cells of the most superficial part of the epidermis called the stratum corneum. Keratins are the major proteins produced by keratinocytes. These intermediate keratin

KEY CONCEPTS

The primary functions of skin

- The body's largest organ, which represents 12–15% of body weight and spans a surface area of $\sim 2\ m^2$.

- A homeostatic organ that, due to the skin's large surface area, regulates fluid retention/evaporation and functions as the principal organ for thermoregulation.

- A tactile interface with the world by virtue of an array of specialized sensory cells that may be distributed at very high densities in skin at critical points of the body (e.g., finger tips may have 2500 sensory cells/cm²).

- A photosynthetic organ that transforms 7-dehydrocholesterol to vitamin D_3 after exposure to UV radiation, an essential step in the biosynthetic pathway of vitamin D.

- A strong physical barrier that withstands physical stresses endured by exposure to the forces of nature. These include shear forces, extreme temperatures, wind and water. Granular layer keratinocytes are bound together through tight junctions, providing an effective seal that blocks entry of small molecules and microbes.

- A pharmacological barrier provided by the production of enzymes that detoxify or repair damage caused by chemicals and other carcinogens, such as ultraviolet and ionizing radiation.

- A regenerative organ that can eliminate damaged skin cells, especially those that have received excessive amounts of ultraviolet radiation, in which the damage cannot be sufficiently repaired to restore normal function.

- An immunological barrier provided by a complex integration of innate and adaptive immune mechanisms that serve to protect against entry by microbial pathogens and to neutralize or eliminate potentially harmful exogenous antigens and endogenous neoplastic cells.

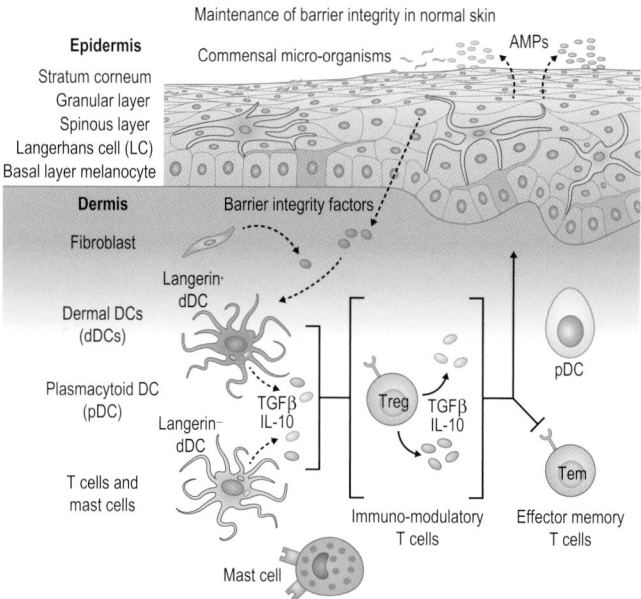

Fig. 18.1 Histological features of normal skin. The epidermis is made up of keratinocytes organized into stratified layers. The most superficial layer is the stratum corneum (light pink). The granular layer cells are connected through tight junctions. Granular layer cells also secrete anti-microbial peptides (AMPs). The basal layer (tan) contains the proliferative cells that give rise to all the differentiated suprabasal keratinocytes. Basal cells are bound to the basement membrane and share that scaffold with interspersed melanocytes (brown). Langerhans cells (LCs) (blue) are epidermal antigen presenting cells that reside in the spinous layer of the epidermis (tan). The dermis contains a number of DC subsets that, under resting conditions, are conditioned by barrier integrity factors. Two of the myeloid dermal DC (dDC) subsets have been described are langerin⁺ and langerin⁻ DCs. Plasmacytoid DCs (pDCs) are also present in the dermis and secrete type I interferons (yellow). Resident memory T cells (T_{EM}) (yellow) represent previously primed T cells in many lineages (Th1, CTL, Th17, Tc17, Treg) poised to respond when their specific antigens are presented locally, but remain quiescent in uninfected skin. Mast cells (green) reside near endothelial venules (not shown). Normal skin produces immunomodulatory factors, such as IL-10 and TGF-beta, which inhibit immune activation of resident cells and act on skin to maintain barrier integrity.

cytoskeletal filaments attach to desmosomal proteins at the plasma membrane. These desmosomal proteins help form the adherens junctions that attach keratinocytes with each other. During the differentiation process, the composition of the keratin and desmosomal proteins changes. Basal layer keratinocytes synthesize keratins 5 and 14, and desmoglein 3 is more abundant than desmoglein 1. Keratins 1 and 10 predominate in the stratum corneum. In the superficial epidermis desmoglein 1 predominates and desmoglein 3 is not expressed. These differences in keratins and desmogleins have immunologic consequences.[2] For example, pemphigus vulgaris, with anti-desmoglein 1 and anti-desmoglein 3 antibodies, presents with blisters that originate in the suprabasal layer of the epidermis, whereas pemphigus foliaceus, with anti-desmoglein 1 only, results in blisters located in the upper epidermis.

The remainder of cells within the epidermis are pigment-producing melanocytes; Merkel cells, which are neuroendocrine cells important for mechanoreception; and Langerhans cells, antigen presenting cells (APCs) within the epidermis.

The *dermis,* which lies beneath the epidermis, contains fibroblasts that synthesize collagen, elastic fibers and a variety of glycoproteins, proteoglycans and glycosaminoglycans. These provide elasticity and tensile strength to the skin. Collagen

production is a dynamic process of continual remodeling with ongoing synthesis and degradation.[1] Matrix metalloproteinases, which degrade collagen, are synthesized by dermal fibroblasts. Scleroderma and morphea (localized scleroderma) are autoimmune diseases characterized by overproduction of collagen in the dermis (Chapter 54). Other dermis cell types include mast cells and diverse sets of tissue macrophages and dendritic cells (DCs).[1]

The microvasculature of the skin is found within the dermis. Dermal endothelial cells are the main components of the arterioles, capillaries and post-capillary venules of the dermal microvasculature. They both produce and respond to cytokines and chemokines. The endothelial cells express E-selectin and P-selectin to which lymphocytes expressing cutaneous lymphocyte-associated antigen (CLA) and P-selectin glycoprotein ligand (PSGL), respectively, can attach.[3] This allows for a specific subset of lymphocytes to selectively recirculate back and forth to the skin and allows for recruitment of leukocytes to the skin during the process of inflammation (Table 18.1). The egress of leukocytes from the blood occurs primarily through the post-capillary venules.

The dermis is separated from the epidermis by the *basement membrane zone,* an elaborate complex of molecules that serves as a scaffold to which keratinocytes attach and that functions as a diffusion barrier for cells and macromolecules.[4] Antigen–antibody complexes concentrate at the basement membrane zone in the involved and uninvolved skin of systemic lupus erythematosus patients (Chapter 50). Molecules present at the dermal–epidermal junction are also targets in autoimmune blistering diseases, including bullous pemphigoid and epidermolysis bullosa acquisita (Chapter 62).

Beneath the dermis is the *subcutaneous tissue,* which is enriched for adipose cells. Adipose cells produce leptin, which has been implicated in a variety of inflammatory diseases including psoriasis.

In toto the skin functions as a protective barrier, and this task is achieved by a variety of means.[1]

(1) The hair and the stratum corneum serve as a physical barrier. The stratum corneum is an impermeable cover that hinders the entry of invading microorganisms and prevents access to potentially toxic chemicals. It reflects and absorbs ultraviolet radiation, preventing damage to the deeper layers of skin.

(2) Enzymes synthesized by the skin function as a pharmacological barrier. Some metabolize chemicals and others repair DNA damage that has occurred from ultraviolet radiation and xenobiotics that have evaded the physical barrier.

(3) It provides a complex immunological barrier with components, both cells and molecules, unique to the skin. This immunological barrier protects against potentially harmful chemicals, microorganisms and neoplastic cells.

The skin has been recognized as a target for immunological assault for many years. It possesses a distinct set of resident immunocompetent cells, lymphocytes and macrophages that preferentially recirculate to the skin, as well as cytokines and other immunological mediators that influence immune responses. This "skin associated lymphoid tissue"[5] contains components necessary for both innate and acquired immunity that act locally to enhance the protective functions of the skin and systemically to serve notice to the rest of the body to augment host defenses. Disturbances in these protective activities can result in an increase in infections and malignancies when deficient, or in immunologically mediated skin diseases when excessive (Table 18.2).

● KEY CONCEPTS

Immunological defenses of the skin

- The innate defenses of the skin provide the first line of defense against exogenous antigens and invading pathogens.

- Granular layer keratinocytes are the main producers of cutaneous microbicidal peptides β-defensin and cathelecidin, which are generated in response to pathogen-associated molecular patterns (PAMPs) and danger-associated molecular patterns (DAMPs). In addition, they, like all keratinocytes, produce pro-inflammatory mediators such as IL-1α & β, IL-6, and TNFα.

- Tricellulin molecules are specialized tight junction proteins that regulate sampling of the external microbial environment by protruding dendrites of Langerhans cells (LC) residing in the suprabasal layer of the epidermis.

- LCs internalize microbes and, in response, produce IL-1β, IL-6, and other cytokines.

- Mediators derived from a variety of cells within the epidermis and dermis activate neighboring keratinocytes and LCs, thereby perpetuating a pro-inflammatory signal cascade throughout the epidermal layers.

- LCs become activated in response to a combination of signals (TLRs, NLRs, IL-1β, and TNFα) and migrate from skin to reach regional lymph nodes where they mature into potent antigen presenting cells, which can instruct both T cells and lymph node resident dendritic cells (DCs), through delivery of cutaneous antigens and other information.

- Keratinocyte-derived pro-inflammatory mediators and chemokines (CXCL8/IL-8) act on post endothelial venules to promote extravasation of inflammatory cells from the circulation into the dermis. Recruited inflammatory cells include neutrophils, monocytes/macrophages, plasmacytoid DCs, NK cells, and memory T cells.

- Inflammatory leukocytes enter the epidermis and attach to keratinocytes through interactions with CD54 (ICAM-1) proteins on activated keratinocytes, to clear invading pathogens and cellular debris.

- Immune cells that are resident in healthy skin are epidermal LCs, dermal leukocytes, mast cells, macrophages, and dermal dendritic cells.

Table 18.1 T-cell subsets and trafficking in skin

T-cell subset	Homing-R[a]	Chemokine-R	From	Homing to	Ligands for homing and chemokine receptors
Naïve T cells	L-selectin (CD62L) LN homing receptor	CCR7+	Blood	LN	L-selectin ligand: GlyCAM-1 integrin on LN HEV[b]
Central memory T cells (T_{CM}) CD45RA+	L-selectin	CCR7+	LN	LN & the circulation	CCR7 ligand: LN-derived chemokine CCL21 (aka 6Ckine, secondary lymphoid-tissue chemokine (SLC))
Effector memory T cells (T_{EM}) CD45RO+	CLA+ (PSGL-1) Skin homing receptor	CCR4+	LN	Blood/dermis	CLA ligand: E-selectin on activated post-capillary venules CCR4 ligand: skin-derived inflammatory chemokines: MCP-1, MIP-1, RANTES, TARC, CCL22

T_{EM} subsets resident in dermis	Homing-R	Chemokine-R	Function	Cytokines produced	Notes
Treg	CLA+	CCR5+	Regulatory; resolution phase; inhibit auto reactivity	IL-10, TGFβ	• T regs are 5–10% of CLA+ dermal T cells • Tregs two-way trafficking–migration from dermis to LN, then recirculate to dermis • CCR5 binds RANTES, MIP-1
Th1, Tc1	CLA+	CCR4+	Type I anti-viral	IFNγ, TNFα, IL-2	• Promotes cellular immunity • Development of cytotoxic T cells (CTL)
Th2, Tc2	CLA+	CCR4+	Type II Parasites cleared	IL-4, IL-5, IL-10, and IL-13	• Promotes humoral immunity • Recruitment of eosinophils
Th17, Tc17	CLA+	CCR4+	Inflammatory; anti-fungal; anti-bacterial	IL-17A, IL-17 F, TNF-α, IL-21 and IL-22	• Activation is dependent on IL-23 derived from keratinocytes/LCs/DCs

Twenty billion T cells are resident in healthy dermal tissue, representing twice the number of circulating T cells present in the entire circulation. (T-cell distribution density in skin ~1 million T cells/cm^2)

[a]Homing-R—an adhesion molecule on leukocytes that recognizes and binds site-specific adhesion molecules expressed on high endothelial venules in the LN and activated post capillary venules in the dermis and other organs. L-selectin is the lymph node homing receptor while CLA is the skin homing receptor.

[b]HEV—high endothelial venules are post-capillary venous swelling in LNs and most secondary lymphoid organs

Innate immunity and the skin

Pattern recognition receptors

Epidermal keratinocytes are among the first responders deployed as sentinels in the rapid response to microbial pathogens and environmental toxins. These cells have been programmed to recognize highly conserved sequence patterns in macromolecules expressed primarily by microbial pathogens and host derived danger signals (Chapter 3). This responsibility for identification of pathogen-associated molecular patterns (PAMP) and danger-associated molecular patterns (DAMP) is undertaken in part by pattern-recognition receptors (PRRs), which include the plasma membrane and intra-vesicular membrane-bound Toll-like receptors (TLRs) and cytosolic nucleotide-binding domain, leucine-rich repeat containing receptors (NLRs) (formerly termed NOD-like receptors).[6,7] An array of TLRs and NLRs is expressed by cells at epithelial interfaces, including skin keratinocytes, dendritic cells (DCs), macrophages, natural killer cells, mast cells and granulocytes. Of the greater than 10 TLRs that have been identified, eight (TLR1–7 and 9) are found on keratinocytes.[7] Myeloid DC subsets, known for their potent antigen presenting capabilities, express combinations of TLRs 1–5 and 8, while plasmacytoid DCs, which secrete type I interferons, express TLRs7 and 9.[8]

Human keratinocytes express NOD1 and mRNA transcripts for 11 of 14 pyrin domain containing NLR genes.[9] NLRs act independently, but in synergy with TLR signals to trigger potent innate immune responses in the skin against microbes by either promoting NFκB activation or forming inflammasomes—specialized protein complexes that activate caspase-1 or caspase-5 enzymes and precursor forms of the pro-inflammatory cytokines IL-1β, -18, and -33 to produce active mediators.

The value of cutaneous TLR activation in the skin for host defense responses is exemplified by the use of imiquimod as a therapeutic agent. This imidazoquinolone is a known TLR7 ligand agonist and is applied topically to treat human papilloma virus-induced genital warts and nonmelanoma skin malignancies and premalignancies.[10]

Keratinocytes, dendritic cells and monocytes also express the PRR dectin-1. Dectin-1 is a membrane associated glycoprotein that serves as the receptor for β-glucan, a polysaccharide found in several species of fungi. Once ligand binding has occurred, dectin-1 initiates a signaling pathway that includes the intracellular adapter molecule caspase recruitment domain-containing protein 9 (Card9). This signal transduction pathway results in production of the cytokines IL-1β, -6, and -23 and the development of Th17 cells, which are essential for antifungal immunity. The clinical relevance of dectin-1 and its associated pathway to antifungal immunity has been demonstrated. People with early stop codon mutations in dectin-1 have been noted to have

Table 18.2 Immunodermatological disorders that affect the skin

Papulosquamous disorders
Psoriasis
Lichen planus
Cutaneous graft vs host disease
Acute, subacute and discoid lupus erythematosus
Eczematous disorders
Atopic dermatitis
Allergic contact dermatitis
Urticarial disorders
Urticaria and angioedema
Erythema multiforme
Stevens Johnson syndrome
Toxic epidermal necrolysis
Cryopyrin-associated periodic syndromes
    Muckle Wells syndrome
    Familial cold urticaria
Neonatal onset multisystem inflammatory disease (NOMID)
Deficiency of the interleukin-1–receptor antagonist (DIRA)
TNF receptor associated periodic syndrome (TRAPS)
Purpuric disorders
Leukocytoclastic vasculitis
Medium vessel vasculitides (polyarteritis nodosa, Wegener's granulomatosis, Churg-Strauss vasculitis)
Vesiculobullous diseases
Pemphigus
Bullous pemphigoid
Paraneoplastic pemphigus
Epidermolysis bullosa acquisita
Dermatitis herpetiformis
Linear IgA bullous dermatoses
Pemphigus gestationis
	Pigmentary disorders
	Vitiligo
	Hair disorders
	Alopecia areata
	Autoimmune disorders
	Dermatomyositis
	Mixed connective tissue disease
	Scleroderma and morphea
	Photodermatoses
	Polymorphous light eruption
	Solar urticaria
	Chronic actinic dermatitis
	Photoallergic contact dermatitis
	Allergic drug eruptions
	Disorders of the subcutaneous tissues
	Erythema nodosum
	Erythema induratum
	Immunodeficiencies
	Ataxia telangiectasia
	Chronic mucocutaneous candidiasis
	Chronic granulomatous disease
	Hyper-Immunoglobulin E syndrome
	Leukocyte adhesion molecule deficiency
	Severe combined immunodeficiency
	Warts–hypogammaglobulinemia–infections–myelokathexis syndrome (WHIM syndrome)
	Wiskott–Aldrich syndrome
	Organ transplant recipients on immunosuppressive medications

deficiencies in Th17 cells and recurrent vulvovaginal *Candida albicans* infections and onychomycosis.[11,12] Mutations in Card9 also lead to a Th17 deficiency that is associated with chronic mucocutaneous candidiasis.

Cutaneous production of cytokines and chemokines

Types of cytokines and chemokines

The skin is a rich source of cytokines and chemokines (Chapters 9, 10)[9,13] which play a major role in both the local and systemic responses to injury and contribute to non-immunological processes such as wound healing, carcinogenesis and pigmentation. Cytokine and chemokine production in the skin involves several different cell types including keratinocytes, melanocytes, DCs, fibroblasts and mast cells. Keratinocytes, for example, produce multifunctional pro-inflammatory cytokines IL-1, -6, -33, and TNF-α; immunosuppressive and anti-inflammatory cytokines IL-10, TGF-β, and IL-1 receptor antagonist (IL-1RA); colony stimulating factors GM-CSF, G-CSF, and M-CSF; immunomodulatory cytokines IL-7, -12, -15, -18, -19, -20, and -23; and the chemokines CXCL8/IL-8, CCL2/MCP-1, CCL20/MIP3α, and CCL5/RANTES. IL-1β, -12, and -23, CCL3/MIP1α, CCL4/MIP1β, and CCL5/RANTES are among the cytokines and chemokines produced by Langerhans cells.[9] Cytokines can have unique effects on skin cells, e.g., the ability of IL-1 to remodel the dermis by stimulating matrix metalloproteinase synthesis, while at the same time augmenting collagen production. Mutant forms of cytokines can result in diseases with cutaneous manifestations. For example, loss of function mutations of IL-1–receptor antagonist can present with the autoinflammatory syndrome, called deficiency of IL-1–receptor antagonist (DIRA) which is characterized by severe pustulosis, ichthyosiform lesions, psoriasis-like changes, and nail abnormalities.[14]

Phases of active cutaneous cytokine secretion

In response to immunologic and inflammatory stimuli, three phases of keratinocyte activated secretion have been described.

Initiation

In healthy skin, keratinocytes constitutively produce inactive pro-IL-1α, -1β, and -18. In response to the presence of DAMPs from cell-derived components following infection, photodamage by UV radiation, or application of haptens, keratinocytes rapidly form inflammasomes and quickly secrete pro-inflammatory molecules including IL-1, IL-6, TNFα, and many others.[9] IL-1β is a potent stimulator of endothelial cell activation, resulting in rapid infiltration of inflammatory leukocytes and circulating T cells into the dermis. TNFα contributes to the inflammatory process by causing dermal microvascular endothelial activation and proliferation, recruitment of neutrophils, macrophages and lymphocytes to the inflammatory site, and augmentation of intercellular adhesion molecule-1 (ICAM-1, CD54) expression on keratinocytes and endothelial cells. IL-6 plays an important role in the development of Th-17 cells, which produce IL-17 and more IL-6. Thus, IL-6 can perpetuate chronic inflammation. In later phases of the cutaneous response, IL-6 mediates inhibitory effects on TNFα and IL-1 through the activation of IL-1R antagonist and induction of IL-10 synthesis by keratinocytes.

Amplification

A second wave of secretion during the amplification phase produces another set of cytokines and chemokines (e.g. GM-CSF, TNFα, and IL-8). These mediators amplify pro-inflammatory signals through activation of surrounding keratinocytes. In addition, they set the stage for the generation of adaptive immune responses by stimulating cutaneous LCs and DCs to mature into potent APCs that can either migrate to draining lymph nodes to activate T cells, or activate memory antigen-specific T cells present in the skin, resulting in local amplification of effector T-cell subpopulations. Keratinocyte-derived CXCL8/IL-8 is a potent chemoattractant for neutrophils. Activated keratinocytes and dermal fibroblasts express ICAM-1, which is the ligand for the β_2 integrin molecule Leukocyte Function Antigen (LFA-1) present on migratory T cells. This permits infiltration into the affected dermal and epidermal layers. While in the steady state some macrophages and inflammatory cells are resident in the dermis; in the presence of inflammatory signals, more are recruited along with granulocytes, which are activated to scavenge pathogens and tissue debris.

As part of the innate immune response, small numbers of resident dermal plasmacytoid DCs can be activated through TLRs 7 and 9 by virus infection to produce abundant amounts of type I interferons.[15] They can produce inducible nitric oxide synthase (iNOS) and arginase, which can act to destroy invading organisms.

Resolution

Once clearance of invading pathogens and infected cells is complete, the resolution phase begins. Keratinocytes produce immunomodulatory factors such as IL-10 and -1 receptor antagonist (IL-1RA). IL-10 can also be produced by recruited leukocytes during this phase. IL-10 potently inhibits adaptive and inflammatory cellular responses, while IL-1RA effectively blocks the activity of IL-1β. Both are thus important mediators that help to return the skin to its pre-inflammatory state. Macrophages and selected DC subsets also inhibit ongoing adaptive immune responses through expression of indoleamine 2,3 dioxygenase (IDO), an enzyme that alters tryptophan metabolism in T cells.

Antimicrobial peptides

The skin is a production site for antimicrobial peptides that play an important role in the innate immune response.[16] These agents, of which over 20 have been described, were originally thought to operate as a barrier to microorganisms that were able to breach the stratum corneum. Their antimicrobial effect was achieved by disrupting bacterial and fungal cell membranes and viral envelopes. This class of compounds has broad effects on innate and adaptive immune responses. The two best characterized antimicrobial peptides in the skin are the cathelicidins and β-defensins. They are made by keratinocytes, cells of the sebaceous and eccrine glands, and mast cells. Cathelicidins are secreted as a precursor protein, hCAP18, which is then processed to the active form of the molecule, LL-37. Following infection or disruption of the epidermal barrier, levels of cathelicidins are strongly increased.

Cathelicidins interact with a variety of cell surface receptors including Toll-like, G-protein coupled and EGF receptors to initiate host immune and inflammatory responses. Cathelicidins increase leukocyte migration, stimulate the secretion of chemokines and cytokines and promote angiogenesis. Among the cytokines and chemokines stimulated are IL-6, -10, -18, CCL2/MCP-1, CCL20/MIP3α, and CCL5/RANTES. Interestingly, vitamin D$_3$, the synthesis of which is initiated in the skin by ultraviolet radiation, plays an important role in regulating cathelicidin expression through epigenetic mechanisms.

Abnormalities in antimicrobial peptides have been implicated in a variety of immunological and non-immunological skin diseases, including atopic dermatitis, psoriasis and rosacea.[16] In atopic dermatitis deficiencies in antimicrobial peptide levels have been found. This may help to explain why individuals with this disease are at increased risk for viral (herpes simplex, human papilloma virus-induced warts and poxvirus-induced molluscum contagiosum) and bacterial (*Staphylococcus aureus*) skin infections.

Disruption of the skin barrier caused by physical stresses, such as shear forces, chemical, thermal, or UV damage, can compromise barrier integrity and stimulates production of pro-inflammatory mediators, including antimicrobial peptides to protect vulnerable sites during wound healing.

Adaptive immunity and the skin

While the innate immune response forms the first line of host defense against pathogenic stimuli in the skin, the adaptive immune response amplifies innate immunity by providing antigen-specific protection against intracellular and extracellular pathogens. In contrast to innate immunity, adaptive immunity is able to distinguish self from non-self and eliminate non-self microbial and mutated cancer cells without damaging normal self tissues and cells. The adaptive immune response in the skin is carried out primarily by T cells and IgE antibodies. The T cells that mediate cutaneous host immune defenses preferentially recirculate between the skin and regional lymph nodes (Table 18.1). T-cell-mediated adaptive immunity is dependent on APCs that can process antigens and provide the necessary secondary signals for T-cell activation (Chapter 6). The skin contains unique subpopulations of myeloid DCs that perform this antigen presenting function. Analyses of the phenotype of skin resident DC have thus far identified multiple distinct types of DCs in the skin. Major specialized functions have been ascribed to each.

Dendritic cells

Dendritic cells (DCs) are a heterogeneous group of cells that are distinguished by a typical morphology (Fig. 18.2) that allows for a large surface area to cell volume ratio. These cells are commonly divided into two types—myeloid and plasmacytoid. Myeloid DCs are the most powerful APCs for the induction of adaptive immune responses. They express a wide array of antigen capture receptors that are responsible for internalizing and processing antigens from invading organisms and coupling them into peptide–MHC complexes that are presented to naïve and memory T cells (Chapter 6). Through integration of environmental signals (via TLR, NLR, and antigen capture receptors) myeloid DCs are able to engage T cells and program their differentiation into subsets of skin homing effector cells capable of eliminating an invading pathogen.

Epidermal Langerhans cells

In normal skin, Langerhans cells (LCs) reside in the suprabasal layer of the epidermis and in that location form a network that is poised to sense and respond to microbial and non-microbial environmental stimuli (Fig. 18.2). LCs are identified by their expression of the C-type lectin langerin (CD207) protein and the conventional DC marker CD11c. Langerin is an antigen capture receptor that internalizes to form a Langerhans cell specific organelle called the Birbeck granule, believed to be a specialized

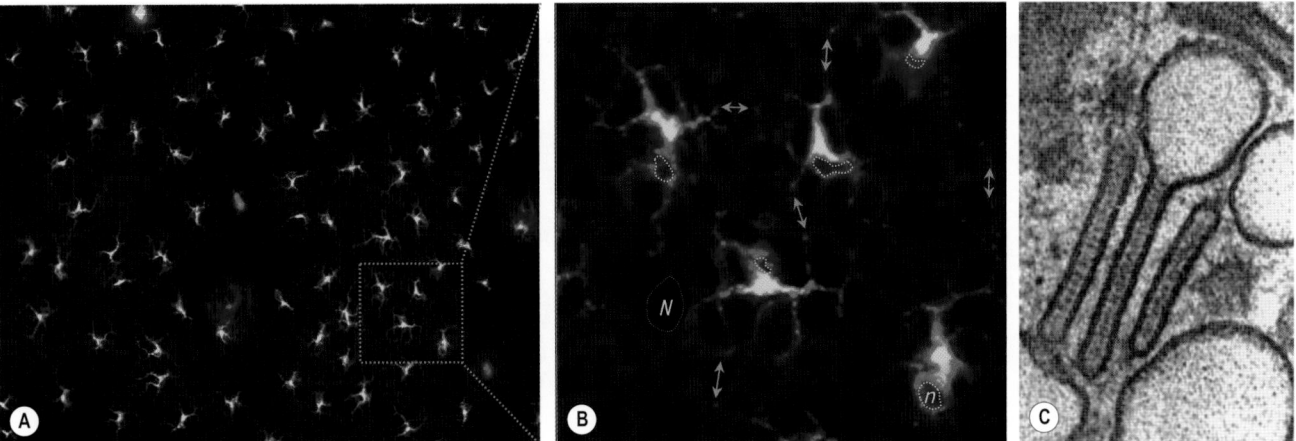

Fig. 18.2 (A) Langerhans cells (LCs). A horizontal view of epidermis (murine) stained with an antibody to MHC class II molecules, of which only LCs are positive. Dendritic shaped LCs are spaced throughout the epidermis with dendrites stretching out to meet and communicate with neighboring LCs. (B) High power view of LCs. Note the short distance between dendrites of adjacent LCs. (C) Transmission electron microscopy of Birbeck granules in Langerhans cells from human epidermis. The Birbeck granule has a "tennis racket" morphology and is formed by internalized langerin molecules.
From Romani N, Clausen BE, Stoitzner P. Langerhans cells and more: langerin-expressing dendritic cell subsets in the skin. Immunol Rev 2010; 234: 120–141.

antigen-processing compartment. Human LCs are also identified by their expression of CD1a, a protein structurally similar to MHC class I molecules that presents lipid antigens, rather than peptide epitopes, to T cells. Recent studies in mice have revealed that LCs can respond to danger signals by extruding their dendritic processes through a specialized tight junction pore called tricellulin, which is present at tricellular contacts in the granular layer.[17] To capture external pathogens, LCs redistribute their langerin receptors and concentrate them at the tips of the extruded dendrites, then internalize the receptors to form Birbeck granules.

LCs have long been considered responsible for inducing cutaneous effector T-cell responses. However, recent *in vivo* studies using animal models have called this into question and have suggested that they may be more effective at activating suppressive Treg cells and thus may prevent pathogenic overreactions to environmental stimuli[18,19] Other *in vivo* studies indicate mouse LCs are potent inducers of Th17 cells.[20] While human and mouse LCs demonstrate a breadth of potent antigen presenting functions *in vitro*, the T-cell subpopulations that they activate *in vivo* and the conditions under which they are activated still need to be definitively established.

Dermal dendritic cells

Dermal DCs efficiently present antigens that have reached the dermis. In the dermis of normal skin, there are multiple subpopulations of resident DCs.[21,22] In mice, dermal DCs are langerin+ and langerin−, and are developmentally distinct from LCs. Notably, human dermal DCs do not express langerin. In mouse skin, langerin+ dermal DCs represent <5% of identifiable skin DCs.[21] These cells specialize in cross-presentation of antigen, which permits presentation of intracellular bacterial or viral antigens without being directly infected by the pathogen. This subset is able to acquire intracellular antigens from keratinocytes and present them to CD8 T cells. The function of this dermal DC subset is of importance in the induction of CD8 T-cell responses to intracellular microbially infected cells and cancer cells in the skin.[22] Other studies have shown that they are required for induction of IgG2a/c and IgG2b isotype antibodies.[21] It is

important to note that resting DCs and LCs have a low level of T-cell stimulating activity, and that antigen presentation by resting DCs induces unresponsiveness of T cells under normal conditions. This is a key mechanism for maintaining immune tolerance, which is needed to prevent the immune system from attacking self tissues.

T cells and immune responses in the skin

Phases of the cell-mediated immune response in the skin

A consequence of antigen exposure via the skin is triggering of the adaptive immune response (Fig. 18.3). This has been divided into two phases. The first exposure of naïve T cells to antigens is called the *sensitization* or *immunization* phase. Re-exposure to the same antigen is called the *elicitation*, or *effector*, phase.

Immunization/sensitization phase of cutaneous immune responses

Cutaneous APCs "take up" and process the antigens, then migrate from the skin to the draining lymph nodes where they present processed antigens to T cells. During the migratory process, LCs and DCs undergo maturational changes that allow them to effectively present the antigens to T cells once they arrive in the lymph nodes. They increase their expression of MHC class I and II, the co-stimulatory molecules CD80 and CD86, and the adhesion molecule ICAM-1. At the same time, expression of the adhesion molecule E-cadherin, which allows Langerhans cells to remain in the epidermis by attaching to adjacent keratinocytes, is lost and the capacity to internalize exogenous antigens is diminished. The naïve T cells in the lymph nodes that are activated by these APCs express T-cell receptors specific for the antigen presented to them. As a result of this interaction, they become effector or memory T cells. Naïve T cells in skin draining lymph nodes express high levels of the lymph node homing receptors chemokine receptor CCR7 and the adhesion molecule L-selectin. When they are activated by cutaneous DCs, they downregulate CCR7 and L-selectin, and upregulate

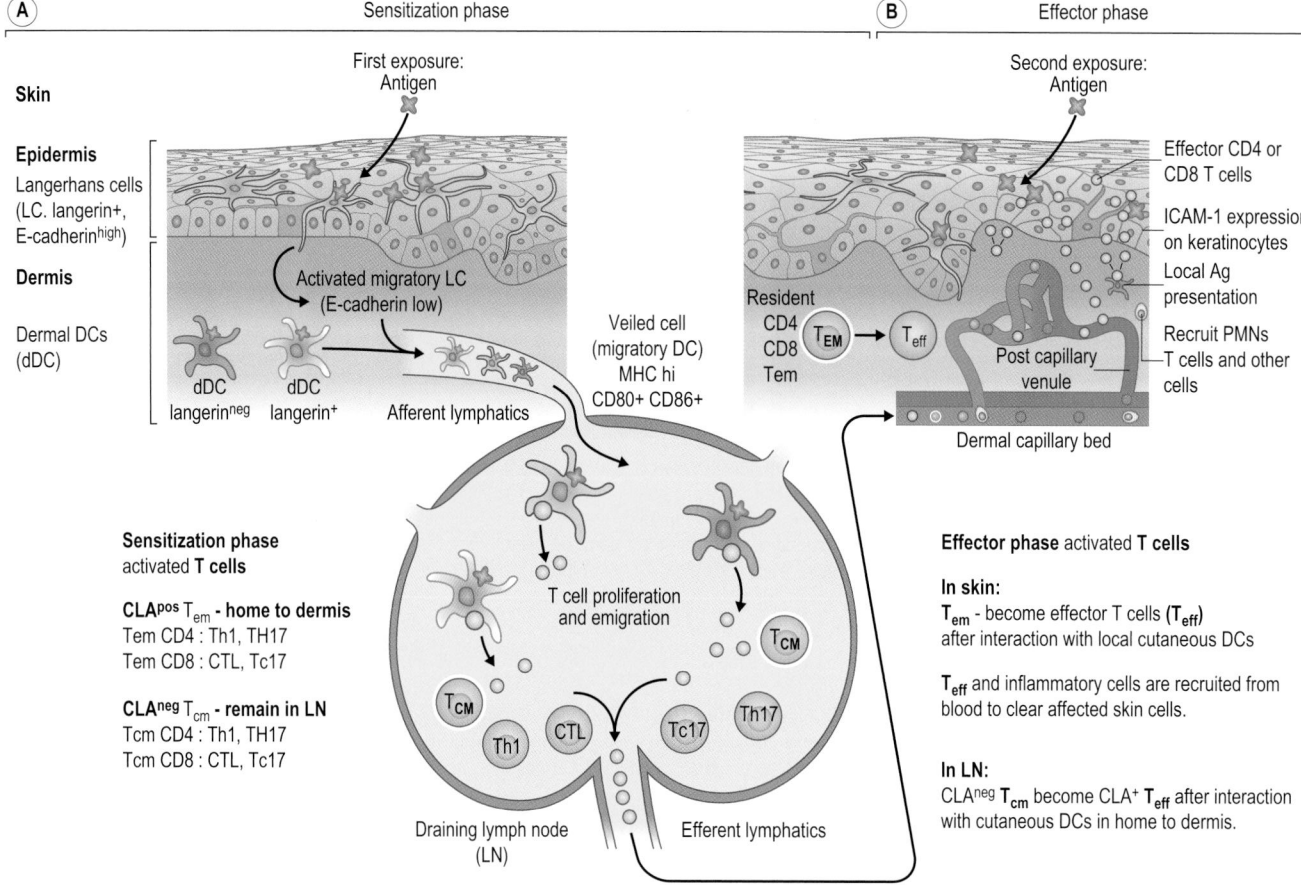

Fig. 18.3 Phases for the development of immune responses in the skin. During the sensitization phase, dendritic cells capture pathogens in the skin and migrate through afferent lymphatics to the skin draining lymph nodes (LN) where they present the antigens to naïve T cells. T-cell differentiation is induced by activated cutaneous DCs and they develop into T_{EM} cells and T_{CM} cells representing different lineages (Th1, CTL, Th17, Tc17), depending on DC programming. T_{EM} migrate to the dermis and become skin resident T_{EM}, while T_{CM} stay in lymph nodes. The effector phase occurs in response to a second exposure to antigen, which activates DCs that in turn activates local T_{EM} to become effector cells *in situ*. Activated cutaneous DCs that reach the draining LN can activate T_{CM} to become skin homing T effector cells, in concert with recruited cells, will enter into the epidermal layer by binding ICAM-1 molecules present on activated keratinocytes, to clear infection, eliminate pathogen-infected cells, remove debris, and repair the skin barrier.

the skin-specific homing receptor cutaneous leukocyte antigen (CLA) and chemokine receptors CCR4 and CCR10.[23] This allows activated T cells to migrate out of lymph nodes and to recirculate to the skin.[23] Unless antigen is present for an extended period of time, immunization/sensitization of cutaneous immune responses (the first exposure to antigen) does not cause an inflammatory reaction, and therefore often goes unnoticed.

Elicitation/effector phase of cutaneous cell-mediated immune responses

In resting, normal skin, a large number of memory T cells, previously activated during the sensitization phase, reside in the dermis.[23] These resident cutaneous CD8 and CD4 T cells are effector memory T cells (T_{EM}). Their strategic location allows them to quickly develop into effector cells for rapid responses to clear infected or damaged skin. They differ from their counterpart, central memory T cells (T_{CM}), which are present in lymph nodes, because Tem express the skin homing receptors CLA and CCR4 and have different response patterns to antigen re-stimulation.[23] Following re-exposure to antigen presenting LCs and dermal DCs, T_{EM} are able to rapidly respond locally, leading to full secondary immune responses *in situ*. T_{CM} present in draining lymph nodes or spleen can also be activated to

develop into effector cells that can then migrate into the sites where antigen is present to elicit an immune response.[23] These cells switch to become circulating effector T cells following their interaction with cutaneous DCs that have migrated from the area of skin where antigen is present. The T cells migrate out of the draining lymph nodes and attach to activated post-capillary venules in the dermis, where they migrate into the affected skin site. Once antigen-specific memory CD4 and CD8 T_{EM} and T_{CM} become activated effector cells, they can directly recognize and eliminate pathogens, interact with cutaneous LCs or DCs to further amplify the response, and produce cytokines and chemokines that recruit and stimulate antigen non-specific inflammatory leukocytes.

T-cell subpopulations and immune responses in the skin

In response to antigen presented by cutaneous DCs, activated T cells expand and develop into different T-cell subsets, each mediating subset-specific functions for protecting against an array of pathogens. Currently, the main CD4 subsets are designated as Th1, Th2, Th17, and Treg cells (Table 18.1) (Chapter 8). Recently, a Th22 subset has been described. It is induced by LCs and has been implicated in human inflammatory skin diseases.[24] Although the primary function of CD8 T cells is cytotoxic activity, Tc1, Tc2, and Tc17 subsets have also been identified.[25] These cells have many of the same functions as their Th counterparts.

T-cell subpopulations and the skin

Th1 cells

Th1 cells preferentially produce IFN-γ and IL-2 and are the principal regulators of type 1 immunity against intracellular pathogens, such as viral infections and tumors. IFN-γ stimulates macrophages to phagocytose and induce oxidative bursts, aiding in intracellular killing of microbes. IFN-γ also upregulates expression of class I and class II MHC molecules and ICAM-1 on keratinocytes, dermal microvascular endothelial cells and fibroblasts and induces them to secrete proinflammatory cytokines and chemokines such as IL-12, CXCL10/IP-10, CXCL9/Mig, and CCL5/RANTES.[26] In animal models, deficiencies in IFN-γ render them more susceptible to microbial infections in the skin and cutaneous tumors. Th1 cells have been shown to be important for cutaneous delayed type hypersensitivity responses such as the tuberculosis skin test reaction, nickel allergic contact dermatitis, and most likely allergic contact dermatitis to other haptens such as those in poison ivy.

Th2 cells

Th2 cells produce IL-4, -5, -10, and -13 and help regulate humoral immune responses to extracellular parasites and bacterial infections. Th2 cell-mediated inflammation is characterized by the presence of eosinophils and basophils, and by mast cell degranulation due to cross-linking of surface-bound IgE.[27] IL-4 and -13 activate B-cell proliferation, antibody production, and class-switching to IgE. IL-5 is a potent hematopoietic cytokine that stimulates bone marrow production of eosinophils, as well as activation and chemotaxis of eosinophils and basophils to affected tissue. In animal models, a deficiency of Th2 cells profoundly increases susceptibility to *Leishmania* infection in the skin. In humans, Th2 cells appear to play a critical role in the pathogenesis of atopic dermatitis (Chapter 42).

Th17 cells

Th17 cells produce IL-17A, -17 F, -21, and -22.[28] (IL-17A is commonly called IL-17.) Th17 cells have protective effects against extracellular bacterial and fungal infections in the skin. Both IL-17A and -17 F enhance protective immune responses by inducing the production of CXC chemokines, G-CSF, and antimicrobial peptides by keratinocytes and other organ system epithelial cells. Mice that are deficient in IL-17A are highly susceptible to *S. aureus* infections in the skin. IL-22 is required for the early host responses against *Citrobacter rodentium* in mice. The Th17 cytokines IL-17 and -22 are important mediators for psoriasis responses and other skin autoimmune disorders.[28] In clinical trials, a majority of patients with psoriasis treated with a neutralizing anti-IL-17 antibody showed improvement.[28] Animal models also suggest that IL-17 promotes tumor development in the skin.

Regulatory T cells (Treg)

Regulatory T cells (Tregs) help establish a balance between defense against pathogens and avoidance of autoimmune disease. Tregs are either naturally occurring or induced by antigens (Chapter 15). Treg cells are commonly characterized as CD4+/CD25+/Foxp3+ cells. Treg cells inhibit immune responses through production of the immunosuppressive cytokines IL-10 and TGF-β and by expression of immunoregulatory surface molecules such as CTLA-4 and LAG-3. Treg cells can directly inhibit the activation and function of T cells and they can suppress the activity of antigen presenting DCs. A defect in Treg function can result in autoimmune and inflammatory diseases. About 5-10% of the T cells resident in normal human skin are Treg.[23, 29–31] In allergic contact dermatitis, Treg cells have important functions in dampening immune and inflammatory responses, thus limiting tissue damage.[31] In contrast, increased Treg activities enhance immunosuppression, impairing host immune defenses against tumors.[23] In ultraviolet (UV) irradiation-induced skin tumors, UV induced immunosuppression is considered a critical mechanism for tumor development and this is, to a great extent, mediated by UV-induced Treg cells (see below).[32,33]

CD8 T-cell immunity

CD8 T cells produce large amounts of IFN-γ and express killer molecules Fas-L, perforin, and granzyme B, which eliminate virally infected cells and tumor cells.[34] The presence of CD8 T cells in tumor tissues is a good prognostic factor for certain types of cancer.[35] and in animal models a deficiency in CD8 T cells diminishes anti-tumor immunity and increases the susceptibility to tumor development. This has also been shown for both squamous cell and basal cell carcinomas of the skin in humans and in animal models.[36–38] CD8 Tc1 and Tc17 cells, which produce IFN-γ and IL-17, respectively, have been reported to take part in the development of allergic contact dermatitis.[39] The cytotoxic activity of CD8 T cells, which is mediated by Fas-L and perforin, also contributes to allergic contact dermatitis.[40]

γδT cells

γδT cells, also known in mouse skin as dendritic epidermal T cells, express T-cell receptor gamma and delta chains in place of conventional expressing alpha and beta TCR. γδT cells reside in epithelial tissues such as skin, gut, lung, and reproductive tract where they provide a first line of defense against pathogenic attacks.[41] In humans, γδT cells account for at least 10% of the T cells in the epithelium. Epithelium-resident γδT cells differ from circulating peripheral γδT cells in their development, selection, TCR diversity, and effector functions. γδT cells in murine epidermis express CCR10 and migrate to the skin in response to the specific ligand CCL27 produced by keratinocytes. Additionally, CCR4, E- and P-selectins also play roles in support of their localization in the skin.

Unlike conventional αβT cells, epithelial γδT cell activation is not restricted by MHC class I and class II molecules. Moreover, alternate sets of co-stimulatory molecule interactions, such as the junctional adhesion molecule like protein (JAML) and its ligand, the coxsackie and adenovirus receptor (CAR), have recently been shown to regulate γδT-cell activation. γδT cells in skin recognize microbial and stress- or damage-induced tissue antigens which are presented by non-classical MHC molecules such as CD1 molecules. Epithelial γδT cells are believed to be partially activated under static conditions, and can therefore rapidly mount responses to pathogenic stimuli.

γδT cells can function as effector cells in protection against microbial and environmental pathogens and elimination of cancer cells. They also have an important role in wound repair by stimulating keratinocyte proliferation. γδT cells can interact with monocytes, granulocytes and DC to regulate their functions in innate immune responses. Crosstalk between γδT cells and DC not only stimulates γδT cell functions, but also has important effects on αβT-cell-mediated adaptive immune responses by affecting DC activation and function. Activated γδT cells can also act as antigen presenting cells to directly present antigens to and activate αβT cells.

Cytokines and chemokines and the adaptive immune response in the skin

Although pro-inflammatory mediators are intimately involved in the innate immune response, they are also known to influence adaptive immunity. IL-1 activates LC and dermal DC migration and maturation that include upregulation of the expression of co-stimulatory molecules, such as CD80 and CD86. It also stimulates T-cell differentiation factors, such as IL-12. IL-12 plays a pivotal role in Th1 T-cell differentiation, thereby biasing the immune response toward Th1 cells at the expense of Th2 and Th17 cells. In contrast, IL-23, which is also produced by keratinocytes and Langerhans cells, leads to preferential development of Th17 cells. IL-6 and TGF-β also help promote a Th17 response.

Chemokines are primary facilitators for the regulation of leukocyte migration and play important roles in the development of inflammation in the skin (Chapter 10). In addition to facilitating cell migration, chemokines can induce integrin activation during leukocyte-endothelial interactions, leukocyte degranulation and mediator release, and angiogenesis. Specific chemokines are produced upon pathogenic stimulation and regulate the migration of DCs and T cells in and out of the skin, which is mediated by specific chemokine receptors expressed by DCs and T cells. Once DCs in the skin have encountered antigen, CCL21 and CXCL12 facilitate their migration out of the skin into draining lymph nodes. CCL21 and CCL19 enable homing of naïve T cells to lymph nodes where they are able to interact with and become activated by antigen presenting DCs. Following T-cell activation, effector T cells express chemokine receptors CCR4 and CCR10 and migrate to the skin in response to chemokines CCL17 and CCL27, which are produced by keratinocytes and mesenchymal cells in cutaneous tissues.[42] Human skin resident T cells express a specific chemokine receptor CCR8, which is rarely detected on T cells in other organs. CCL1, the selective ligand for CCR8, is produced in cutaneous tissues and regulates the migration of the skin homing T cells.[43] Additionally, CXCL1 and CXCL8/IL-8 facilitate the infiltration of granulocytes and monocytes into the skin during inflammation.[44]

Mast cells and the skin

The skin is a rich source of mast cells.[45] These cells derive from CD34+ progenitors in the bone marrow and migrate into many different tissues in the body, especially at environmental interfaces. In the skin, they are found in the dermis and are concentrated around the dermal microvasculature, appendages and nerves. Their density in the skin has been estimated to be 7 000–20 000/mm². At least two types of tissue mast cells have been identified—connective tissue and mucosal. Those that are present in the skin resemble mucosal mast cells and possess the neutral proteases tryptase and chymase. Mast cells are difficult to recognize histologically on hematoxylin and eosin stained skin sections, but can be identified by using metachromatic stains such as toluidine blue and Giemsa, which stain mast cells a purple color.

The distinguishing feature of mast cells is their collection of cytoplasmic granules (Chapter 22). These granules contain preformed mediators that are released when stimulated to degranulate. The mediators include histamine, heparin, the proteases tryptase, chymase, carboxypeptidase, arylsulfatase A, β-hexosaminodase and β-glucuronidase, and the cytokines TNF-α, GM-CSF, IL-3, -4, -5, -6, -8, and -13. In addition, mast cells, upon stimulation, synthesize platelet activating factor and the eicosanoids prostaglandin D_2 and the leukotrienes C_4, D_4, and E_4. These mediators have pro-inflammatory effects on the skin, causing vasodilatation and edema, stimulating the immigration of leukocytes, including eosinophils into the skin, and causing pruritus.

Mast cells have a number of receptors on their cell surface. They express the high affinity surface receptor for the Fc portion of the IgE molecule (FcεRI). Antigen-specific binding allows for cross-linking of IgE molecules that have bound to FcεRI on the mast cell surface. This initiates a sequence of calcium and energy dependent events that culminate in fusion of granules to the plasma membrane, eventuating in release of the granule contents. The degranulation and release of potent prostinoids, histamines, and inflammatory cytokines can rapidly recruit inflammatory cells. Mast cells also express opioid, adenosine and β-adrenergic receptors, and, as a result, mast cell stimulation can proceed through actions independent of FcεRI. Non-antigenic stimuli include opiates, C5a anaphylatoxin, stem cell factor and substance P.

Mast cells participate in the host response to parasitic infections and tumors, and have been implicated in bullous pemphigoid, leukocytoclastic vasculitis, atopic dermatitis, allergic contact dermatitis and mastocytosis (urticaria pigmentosa). They also play a prominent role in the pathogenesis of urticaria and angioedema.

Antibodies and the skin

Much less is known about B cells in the skin, although the antibodies that they produce play a key role in the pathogenesis of several different dermatological diseases. Although not specifically made in the skin, IgE plays a critical role in a number of skin diseases. IgE antibodies have been postulated to be one of the major defenses against parasitic infections. It has also been suggested that they play an important role in immune surveillance, either for the early recognition of immunogenic moieties or to augment the immune response by facilitating the presentation of antigen.[46] In the skin, IgE is considered an essential element of several skin diseases including urticaria and angioedema, atopic dermatitis, hyper-immunoglobulin E syndrome and bullous pemphigoid. As its name implies, it also plays an essential role in hyper-IgE syndrome. Patients with this autosomal dominant disease develop cutaneous manifestations of severe dermatitis, recurrent staphylococcal abscesses and, in some individuals, recurrent cutaneous candidiasis. Hyper-IgE syndrome is associated with dominant negative mutations in the signal transducer and activator of transcription 3 (STAT3) gene. Among the known activities of STAT3 is stimulation of the production of β-defensins in the skin, possibly explaining the clinical manifestations of the disease.[47]

The role of IgG in normal immune homeostasis in the skin is less certain. However, IgG is intimately involved in a number of blistering disorders including pemphigus, bullous pemphigoid, epidermolysis bullosa acquisita and paraneoplastic pemphigus as well as in antigen-antibody complex disorders such as leukocytoclastic vasculitis. The role of IgA under normal conditions is also unknown. It plays a critical role in the pathogenesis of dermatitis herpetiformis, linear IgA bullous dermatosis and IgA-mediated cutaneous vasculitis.

Ultraviolet radiation and cutaneous immunity

Sunlight is the major environmental agent to which the skin is exposed. While its presence is essential for life, injudicious exposure to wavelengths in the ultraviolet spectrum can lead to sunburn, aging of the skin, skin cancer and a variety of photosensitivity diseases, many of which have an immunologic pathogenesis. There has been great interest in defining the effects of this form of radiant energy on cutaneous immunological processes because of the belief that UV-induced alterations in immunological function contribute in a fundamental way to the pathogenesis of skin cancer and to some immunologically mediated skin diseases. Although much of the investigation into the immunological effects of ultraviolet radiation has been conducted in animal models, many of the observations have been corroborated in humans.

In mice, as in humans, chronic UV exposure results in the development of highly antigenic skin cancers capable of stimulating a vigorous anti-tumor response. Despite the antigenic nature of the tumors and thus the potential for inducing a robust host immune response to eradicate them, these tumors grow progressively in the original host.[48] This apparent paradox was resolved in studies that showed that UV, in addition to producing mutant cells, also impairs host cell-mediated immune responses that have evolved to identify and eradicate the mutant cells before they develop into clinically apparent malignancies.[32,33,48] Only when there are mutant cells in an environment of immune suppression will tumors occur. For example, organ transplant recipients who are treated with immunosuppressive medications have a greatly increased risk of UV-induced skin cancers and the tumors that do develop behave more aggressively.[49]

Ultraviolet radiation, which penetrates no further than the superficial dermis, mediates its effects by perturbing the function of APCs in the skin.[50] Specifically, UV-irradiated DCs are ineffective at activating Th1 cells but are unimpaired at activating specific populations of T cells that suppress the response, thereby shifting the balance from one of immune activity towards one of antigen-specific immunological tolerance. The immunosuppressive effect is mediated at least in part through UV-induced augmentation in the production of the immunosuppressive cytokine IL-10 and inhibition of the synthesis of the Th1-stimulating cytokine IL-12. It may seem surprising that an environmental carcinogen such as UV radiation suppresses immunological function in the skin. One proposed explanation is that an alteration of epithelial proteins by continuous environmental stresses such as UV radiation necessitates induction of immune tolerance mechanisms to preserve the integrity of the skin barrier.

The immunosuppressive effect of UV radiation has been exploited for therapeutic purposes. Ultraviolet radiation phototherapy is used as a modality for the management of immunologically mediated skin diseases such as psoriasis and atopic dermatitis.

ON THE HORIZON

- Inhibitors of TNF-α and IL-12/IL-23 are being employed in the management of psoriasis, providing an opportunity to broaden the spectrum of skin diseases for which these agents can be used. TNF-α inhibitors, for example, are being evaluated for the management of pemphigus and bullous pemphigoid.

- The identification of a unique phenotypic profile for T cells that preferentially recirculate to the skin should provide the impetus for development of agents that specifically inhibit the activity of those cells, while leaving the functions of those T cells that circulate to other parts of the body intact.

- Knowledge of several types of dendritic cells in the skin that are specialized in the type of T cells they activate provides the basis for their utilization to improve vaccination procedures. It is likely that cutaneous dendritic cells will be employed for vaccination against tumors such as melanoma and selected infectious agents.

- Continued clarification of the role of cytokines in cutaneous diseases will be employed in treatment of immunologically mediated skin diseases. For example, the identification of Th17 cells in the inflammatory infiltrate of psoriasis has stimulated interest in the evaluation of biologic inhibitors of IL-17 as a therapy for the disease.

CLINICAL RELEVANCE

- Knowledge of involvement of the immune system in psoriasis has led to introduction of drugs that target various aspects of the immune response in this disease. These include biologic response modifiers that target T cells (alefacept), TNF-α (etanercept, infliximab, adalimumab), and the p40 peptide common to both IL-12 and -23 (ustekinumab).

- Understanding of suppressive effects of ultraviolet radiation on the immune system has been exploited by using it as a treatment for such immunologically mediated skin diseases as psoriasis, atopic dermatitis, and cutaneous graft versus host disease.

- Identification of antigens targeted in several autoimmune blistering diseases (pemphigus, bullous pemphigoid) has resulted in greater precision in the categorization of these diseases and in better diagnostic methods. In cases in which the diagnosis of a particular bullous disease is uncertain, immunoblotting procedures can be helpful.

References

1. Chu DH, et al. The structure and development of skin. In: Freedberg IM, et al., editors. Fitzpatrick's dermatology in general medicine. New York: McGraw-Hill; 2003.
2. Amagai M. Pemphigus. In: Bolognia J, Jorizzo JL, Rapini RP, editors. Dermatology. St. Louis: Mosby/Elsevier; 2008. p. 417–29.
3. Kupper TS, Fuhlbrigge RC. Immune surveillance in the skin: mechanisms and clinical consequences. Nat Rev Immunol 2004;4(3):211–22.
4. Yancey KB, Allen DM. The biology of the basement membrane zone. In: Bolognia J, Jorizzo JL, Rapini RP, editors. Dermatology. St. Louis: Mosby/Elsevier; 2008. p. 403–15.
5. Streilein JW. Lymphocyte traffic, T-cell malignancies and the skin. J Invest Dermatol 1978;71(3):167–71.
6. McInturff JE, Modlin RL, Kim J. The role of toll-like receptors in the pathogenesis and treatment of dermatological disease. J Invest Dermatol 2005;125(1):1–8.
7. Nestle FO, Di Meglio P, Qin JZ, Nickoloff BJ. Skin immune sentinels in health and disease. Nat Rev Immunol 2009;9(10):679–91.
8. Kadowaki N, Ho S, Antonenko S, et al. Subsets of human dendritic cell precursors express different toll-like receptors and respond to different microbial antigens. J Exp Med 2001;194(6):863–9.
9. Watanabe H, Gaide O, Pétrilli V, et al. Activation of the IL-1beta-processing inflammasome is involved in contact hypersensitivity. J Invest Dermatol 2007;127(8):1956–63.
10. Grossberg AL, Gaspari AA. Topical antineoplastic agents in the treatment of mucocutaneous diseases. Curr Probl Dermatol 2011;40:71–82.
11. Ferwerda B, Ferwerda G, Plantinga TS, et al. Human dectin-1 deficiency and mucocutaneous fungal infections. N Engl J Med 2009;361(18):1760–7.
12. Glocker EO, Hennigs A, Nabavi M, et al. A homozygous CARD9 mutation in a family with susceptibility to fungal infections. N Engl J Med 2009;361(18):1727–35.
13. Steinhoff M, Brzoska T, Luger TA. Keratinocytes in epidermal immune responses. Curr Opin Allergy Clin Immunol 2001;1:469–87.
14. Aksentijevich I, Masters SL, Ferguson PJ, et al. An autoinflammatory disease with deficiency of the interleukin-1-receptor antagonist. N Engl J Med 2009;360(23):2426–37.
15. Zaba LC, Krueger JG, Lowes MA. Resident and "inflammatory" dendritic cells in human skin. J Invest Dermatol 2009;129(2):302–8.

16. Schauber J, Gallo RL. Antimicrobial peptides and the skin immune defense system. J Allergy Clin Immunol 2008;122(2):261–6.

17. Kubo A, Nagao K, Yokouchi M, et al. External antigen uptake by Langerhans cells with reorganization of epidermal tight junction barriers. J Exp Med 2009;206(13):2937–46.

18. Allan RS, Smith CM, Belz GT, et al. Epidermal viral immunity induced by CD8alpha+ dendritic cells but not by Langerhans cells. Science 2003;301(5641):1925–8.

19. Loser K, Mehling A, Loeser S, et al. Epidermal RANKL controls regulatory T-cell numbers via activation of dendritic cells. Nat Med 2006;12(12):1372–9.

20. Igyarto BZ, Haley K, Ortner D, et al. Skin-resident murine dendritic cell subsets promote distinct and opposing antigen-specific T helper cell responses. Immunity 2011;35(2):260–72.

21. Nagao K, Ginhoux F, Leitner WW, et al. Murine epidermal Langerhans cells and langerin-expressing dermal dendritic cells are unrelated and exhibit distinct functions. Proc Natl Acad Sci U S A 2009;106(9):3312–7.

22. Henri S, Guilliams M, Poulin LF, et al. Disentangling the complexity of the skin dendritic cell network. Immunol Cell Biol 2010;88(4):366–75.

23. Clark RA. Skin-resident T cells: the ups and downs of on site immunity. J Invest Dermatol 2010;130(2):362–70.

24. Fujita H, Nograles KE, Kikuchi T, et al. Human Langerhans cells induce distinct IL-22-producing CD4+ T cells lacking IL-17 production. Proc Natl Acad Sci U S A 2009;106(51):21795–800.

25. He D, Wu L, Kim HK, et al. CD8+ IL-17-producing T cells are important in effector functions for the elicitation of contact hypersensitivity responses. J Immunol 2006;177(10):6852–8.

26. Schroder K, Hertzog PJ, Ravasi T, Hume DA. Interferon-gamma: an overview of signals, mechanisms and functions. J Leukoc Biol 2004;75(2):163–89.

27. Leung DY, Boguniewicz M. Advances in allergic skin diseases. J Allergy Clin Immunol 2003;111(Suppl. 3):S805–12.

28. Iwakura Y, et al. Functional specialization of interleukin-17 family members. Immunity 2011;34(2):149–62.

29. Sakaguchi S, Yamaguchi T, Nomura T, Ono M. Regulatory T cells and immune tolerance. Cell 2008;133(5):775–87.

30. Dudda JC, Perdue N, Bachtanian E, Campbell DJ. Foxp3+ regulatory T cells maintain immune homeostasis in the skin. J Exp Med 2008;205(7):1559–65.

31. Dubois B, Chapat L, Goubier A, et al. Innate CD4+CD25+ regulatory T cells are required for oral tolerance and inhibition of CD8+ T cells mediating skin inflammation. Blood 2003;102(9):3295–301.

32. Krutmann J, Elmets CA. Photoimmunology. Oxford/Cambridge, MA: Blackwell Science; 1995. p. xii, 303.

33. Elmets CA, Bergstresser PR, Tigelaar RE, et al. Analysis of the mechanism of unresponsiveness produced by haptens painted on skin exposed to low dose ultraviolet radiation. J Exp Med 1983;158(3):781–94.

34. Yusuf N, Nasti TH, Katiyar SK, et al. Antagonistic roles of CD4+ and CD8+ T-cells in 7,12-dimethylbenz(a)anthracene cutaneous carcinogenesis. Cancer Res 2008;68(10):3924–30.

35. Finn OJ. Cancer immunology. N Engl J Med 2008;358(25):2704–15.

36. Kaporis HG, Guttman-Yassky E, Lowes MA, et al. Human basal cell carcinoma is associated with Foxp3+ T cells in a Th2 dominant microenvironment. J Invest Dermatol 2007;127(10):2391–8.

37. Clark RA, Huang SJ, Murphy GF, et al. Human squamous cell carcinomas evade the immune response by down-regulation of vascular E-selectin and recruitment of regulatory T cells. J Exp Med 2008;205(10):2221–34.

38. He D, Li H, Yusef N, et al. IL-17 promotes tumor development through the induction of tumor promoting microenvironments at tumor sites and myeloid-derived suppressor cells. J Immunol 2010;184(5):2281–8.

39. He D, Wu L, Kim HK, et al. IL-17 and IFN-gamma mediate the elicitation of contact hypersensitivity responses by different mechanisms and both are required for optimal responses. J Immunol 2009;183(2):1463–70.

40. Kehren J, Desvignes C, Krasteva M, et al. Cytotoxicity is mandatory for CD8(+) T cell-mediated contact hypersensitivity. J Exp Med 1999;189(5):779–86.

41. Witherden DA, Havran WL. Molecular aspects of epithelial γδT cell regulation. Trends Immunol 2011;32(6):265–71.

42. Homey B, Alenius H, Müller A, et al. CCL27-CCR10 interactions regulate T cell-mediated skin inflammation. Nat Med 2002;8(2):157–65.

43. Schaerli P, Ebert L, Willimann K, et al. A skin-selective homing mechanism for human immune surveillance T cells. J Exp Med 2004;199(9):1265–75.

44. Kunkel EJ, Butcher EC. Chemokines and the tissue-specific migration of lymphocytes. Immunity 2002;16(1):1–4.

45. Longley J, Duffy TP, Kohn S. The mast cell and mast cell disease. J Am Acad Dermatol 1995;32(4):545–61; quiz 562–564.

46. Wang B, Rieger A, Kilgus O, et al. Epidermal Langerhans cells from normal human skin bind monomeric IgE via Fc epsilon RI. J Exp Med 1992;175(5):1353–65.

47. Minegishi Y, Saito M, Nagasawa M, et al. Molecular explanation for the contradiction between systemic Th17 defect and localized bacterial infection in hyper-IgE syndrome. J Exp Med 2009;206(6):1291–301.

48. Kripke ML. Antigenicity of murine skin tumors induced by ultraviolet light. J Natl Cancer Inst 1974;53(6):1333–6.

49. Boyle J, Mackie RM, Briggs JD, et al. Cancer, warts, and sunshine in renal transplant patients. A case-control study. Lancet 1984;1(8379):702–5.

50. Toews GB, Bergstresser PR, Streilein JW. Epidermal Langerhans cell density determines whether contact hypersensitivity or unresponsiveness follows skin painting with DNFB. J Immunol 1980;124(1):445–53.

Host defenses at mucosal surfaces

Kohtaro Fujihashi, Prosper N. Boyaka, Jerry R. McGhee

Mammals have evolved a sophisticated network of molecules and cells that serves to maintain homeostasis on exposed mucosal surfaces. This system is anatomically and functionally distinct from its blood-borne counterpart and is strategically located at the portals by which most microorganisms enter the body. This specific branch of the immune system may have developed in response to the size of the mucosal surfaces, which cover an area of ~400 m² in the adult human, and the large number of exogenous antigens to which these surfaces are exposed.

The innate mucosal defense system

The innate defense of the mucosa includes the physical barrier provided by epithelial cells, the movement of the epithelial cilia, the production of mucus by goblet cells, the secretion of molecules with innate antibacterial activity, and the cytolytic activity of NK cells (Fig. 19.1). These innate mechanisms provide a first line of defense against exogenous antigens and invading pathogens.

KEY CONCEPTS

Innate defenses of the mucosal immune system

The innate defenses of the mucosal immune system provide a first line of defense against exogenous antigens and invading pathogens. These defenses include:

- Physical barriers: the epithelium, the epithelial cilia, goblet cell mucus production;
- Mucosal antibacterial molecules: Paneth cell production of α-defensins in the small intestine; epithelial cell production of β-defensins in the oral mucosa, trachea, bronchi, mammary glands and salivary glands; lactoferrin, lysozyme, lactoperoxidase, and secretory leukocyte protease inhibitor (SLPI);
- Cellular innate immunity: mucosal natural killer (NK) cells, dendritic cells and PMNs.

Physical barrier provided by epithelial cells

Mucosal surfaces are covered by a layer of epithelial cells that prevent the entry of exogenous antigens into the host while permitting the absorption of nutrients.[1] In the GI tract, the barrier effect of tightly joined epithelial cells, termed enterocytes, is facilitated by the mucus blanket that covers these cells. Mucus is secreted by goblet cells and consists of glycoproteins of various molecular sizes that tend to interfere with the attachment of microorganisms.

Damaged or infected enterocytes are replaced by crypt epithelial cells, which differentiate into enterocytes as they migrate toward the desquamation zone at the villus tip. Multilayered squamous epithelial cells cover the epithelia of other mucosal surfaces, including the oral cavity, the pharynx, the tonsils, the urethra, and the vagina. These epithelia, which lack tight junctions, secrete a glycoprotein mucus that coats the intercellular space between the lower stratified layers. Additional barrier effects are provided by polymeric IgA (pIgA), and by the renewal of exposed epithelial cell layers by cells from subjacent layers.

Defensins and other mucosal antimicrobial peptides

Cells of the epithelium produce antimicrobial β-sheet proteins that range between 30 and 40 amino acids in length termed defensins. These cells exhibit antimicrobial effects similar to those of antibiotics, as well as anti-viral activity. Defensins can be grouped into two distinct structural categories, α and β. α-Defensins, which contain two contiguous cysteine residues, are smaller than β-defensins, whose cysteine residues are separated by six amino acids. α-Defensins are secreted by tracheal epithelial cells and by Paneth cells in the crypt regions of villi. This allows them to be secreted into the lumen of the small intestine. α-Defensins are homologous to peptides that function as mediators of nonoxidative microbial cell killing in neutrophils (termed human neutrophil peptides, or HNPs).[2] β-Defensins, such as human β-defensin 1 (HBD-1), are expressed in the epithelial cells of the oral mucosa, trachea, bronchi, mammary glands, and salivary glands. Inflammatory cytokines such as interleukin-1 (IL-1), tumor necrosis factor-α (TNF-α) and bacterial lipopolysaccharide (LPS) play a role in their induction.

Other potent antimicrobial products of the epithelium include lactoferrin, lysozyme, the peroxidases, secretory phospholipase A2, and cathelin-associated peptides. Some are secreted by intestinal Paneth cells, but all are produced by polymorphonuclear neutrophils (PMNs). Lactoferrin, a member of the transferrin family, is found in exocrine secretions such as milk. High concentrations of lysozyme (1209–1325 μg/mL) are found in tears and other secretions, such as saliva, colostrum, serum and urine. Human milk contains lysozyme in concentrations ranging from 20 to 245 μg/mL, depending on the lactation period. It also contains at least two peroxidases. Milk leukocytes produce myeloperoxidase (MPO) and mammary gland cells produce human lactoperoxidase (hLPO). Both peroxidases display properties similar to those of human salivary peroxidases (hSPO). Secretory

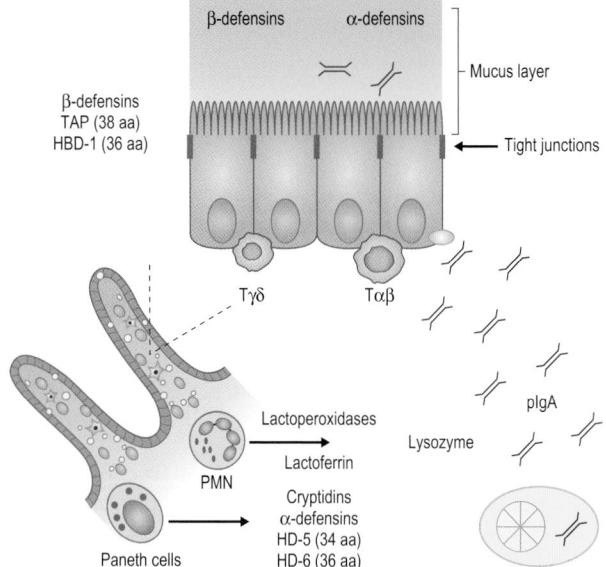

Fig. 19.1 Innate mucosal host defense factors. A thick coat of mucus prevents penetration of macromolecules and potential pathogens. The epithelial cell barrier is connected via tight junctions and contains both αβ and γδ intraepithelial T lymphocytes (IELs). The crypt regions contain Paneth cells, which produce cryptins (α-defensins). The β-defensins are products of epithelial cells and form a defensin network. Other innate factors, such as lysozyme, lactoperoxidase, lactoferrin, and phospholipases, also serve in antimicrobial defense.

phospholipase A2 (S-PLA2) is released by Paneth cells upon exposure to cholinergic agonists, bacteria or LPS. Secretory leukocyte protease inhibitor (SLPI) is found in human saliva, nasal secretions, tears, cervical mucus and seminal fluid. It is believed to be responsible for the anti-HIV properties of external secretions.

Mucosal natural killer cells

Natural killer (NK) cells are found in the lamina propria and the intraepithelial compartment, where they appear as large granular lymphocytes. Nonspecific recruitment of cytotoxic effector cells into the intestinal mucosa occurs in either antigen-primed or virus-infected mice. As NK cells secrete IFN-γ and IL-4 after infection, they can influence the development of effector T cells, as well (Chapter 17).

A common adaptive mucosal immune system

Higher mammals have developed an organized secondary lymphoid tissue system in the gastrointestinal (GI) and upper respiratory tracts. The gut-associated lymphoreticular tissues (GALT) include Peyer's patches (PPs), the appendix, and solitary lymphoid nodules in the GI tract. The tonsils and adenoids comprise the nasal-associated lymphoreticular tissues (NALT). Experimental animals such as rabbits, rats and guinea pigs exhibit organized bronchus-associated lymphoreticular tissues (BALT) that rarely occur in human airway branches.[1] Together, GALT and NALT in humans and GALT, BALT and NALT in experimental species are termed mucosa-associated lymphoreticular tissue, or MALT.

The vast areas of the mucosal immune system characterized by diffuse collections of lymphoid cells are termed the effector tissues. These include the interstitial tissues of the mammary, lacrimal, salivary, sweat and all other exocrine glands; as well as the lamina propria and the epithelium of the GI tract. The

lamina propria areas of the upper respiratory and genitourinary tracts are also lymphoid effector sites. MALT is connected with effector sites through the migratory patterns of lymphoid cells.

KEY CONCEPTS

The common mucosal immune system

The mucosa-associated lymphoreticular tissues (MALT) comprise discrete and diffuse collections of lymphoid tissues that share distinctive features, including a unique type of epithelium, a distinct architecture, a unique set of antigen-presenting cells (APCs), and B cells, where switching to IgA predominates. The involved tissues include:

- The gut-associated lymphoreticular tissues (GALT): Peyer's patches, the appendix, and solitary lymphoid nodules in the GI tract;
- The nasal-associated lymphoreticular tissues (NALT): the tonsils and adenoids;
- The effector tissues: the interstitial tissues of the mammary, lacrimal, salivary, sweat and all other exocrine glands; the lamina propria and the epithelium of the GI tract; and the lamina propria areas of the upper respiratory and genitourinary tracts.

MALT as an inductive site

MALT has a unique type of epithelium for antigen uptake. Its features include a characteristic architecture; antigen-presenting cells (APCs), such as dendritic cells that differ from APCs in spleen; and B-cell areas with germinal centers where switches to IgA predominate. The columnar epithelium that covers MALT is infiltrated with lymphocytes and APCs, leading to the term follicle-associated epithelium (FAE). Lacking goblet cells, the FAE is covered with far less mucus than normal enterocytes. Soluble and particulate luminal antigens are taken up by microfold (M) cells and are delivered to adjacent APCs. M cells have been described in Peyer's patches, the appendix and tonsils, and represent 10–15% of cells within the FAE.[3] M cells are also found in isolated lymphoid follicles (ILFs), and at the tips of the villus where they are termed villous M cells.[4] The microvilli of these cells, which are less dense than those of adjacent enterocytes (Fig. 19.2), offer a portal of entry into the MALT. The M cell is often identified by an invagination of the basolateral membrane into a 'pocket' normally occupied by lymphocytes and APCs (Fig. 19.3).

M cells appear ideal for antigen uptake owing to a well developed microvesicle system that contains endosomes. However, it remains unclear whether M cells act as classic APCs. M cells also provide a portal of entry for some invasive pathogens, such as invasive strains of *Salmonella typhimurium*; but not for noninvasive strains of *S. typhimurium* and reoviruses.

Gut-associated lymphoreticular tissues (GALT)

Each Peyer's patch contains a dome region that is positioned under the FAE. This dome region is populated by T cells, B cells, macrophages (MØ), and dendritic cells (DC). It includes follicles that contain germinal centers. The presence of all three major APC types in the dome, i.e., memory B cells, MØ, and DCs, makes it likely that antigen uptake occurs immediately following release from M cells (Fig. 19.4A). M-cell pockets in Peyer's patches contain approximately equal numbers of T and B cells, but fewer MØ. Approximately 75% of the T cells are T helper (Th) cells.

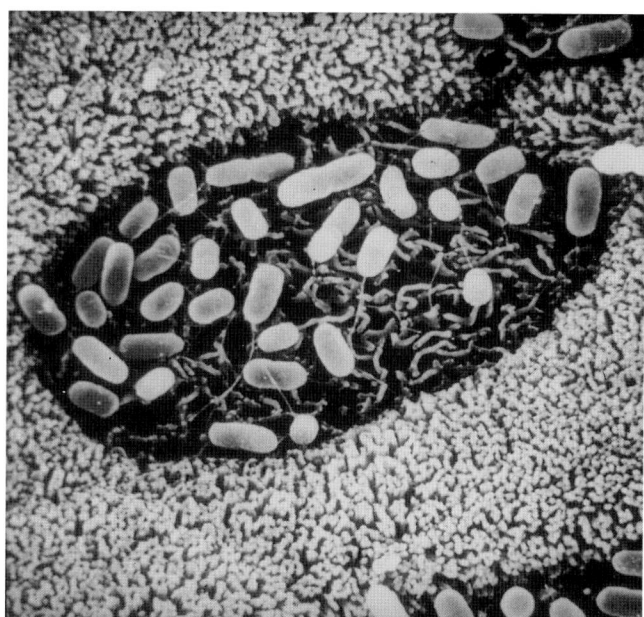

Fig. 19.2 The microfold (M) cell. A scanning electron micrograph of an M cell with adjacent enterocytes. The M cell has selectively bound *E. coli* 0157. Note that a thick brush border is lacking, facilitating the binding and uptake of microparticles.
Courtesy of Dr. Tatsuo Yamamoto, Niigata University.

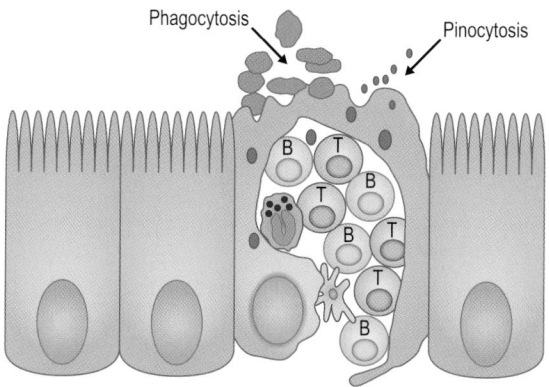

Fig. 19.3 Microanatomical features of M cells. The M cell forms a "pocket" containing memory lymphocytes. It actively pinocytoses soluble antigens and phagocytoses particulates such as viruses, bacteria, and microspheres.
Courtesy of Dr. Svein Steinsvoll, University of Oslo.

GALT B-cell follicles are enriched for IgA-bearing B cells.[1] Thus, germinal centers in MALT are thought to be the major sites for B-cell μ to α switching (Chapters 4 and 7). The interfollicular regions of Peyer's patches contain the high endothelial venules (HEVs), which represent the major point of entry for T and B cells, as well as an interdigitating network of dendritic cells and mature T cells. Both CD4 and CD8 TCRαβ T cells are found in these interfollicular regions, with CD4 cells representing the predominant phenotype. Both naïve and memory T cells are present in Peyer's patches with one-third in cell cycle (Fig. 19.4, Table 19.1).

The structurally and functionally related cytokines, lymphotoxin-α (LT-α), lymphotoxin-β (LT-β), and TNF-α (Chapter 9), are critical for lymphoid organogenesis. LT-α$^{-/-}$ mice are markedly deficient in secondary lymph nodes,[5] whereas LT-β$^{-/-}$ mice have mesenteric and cervical lymph nodes, but lack peripheral lymph nodes and Peyer's patches. TNF-RI$^{-/-}$ mice are characterized by an absent or abnormal

Peyer's patch structure, whereas TNF-α$^{-/-}$ mice exhibit normal patches. In humans, PPs develop during prenatal life, a situation also seen in sheep, pigs, dogs, and horses. ILF formation occurs postnatally in response to lumenal stimuli, including the normal bacterial flora.[6] Mature ILFs contain mostly conventional B cells and small numbers of CD4 T cells.[6]

Nasal-associated lymphoreticular tissues (NALT)

Strategically positioned at the entry of the respiratory, as well as the digestive, tracts are the accumulations of lymphoid tissues that comprise the palatine, lingual and nasopharyngeal tonsils, which collectively form Waldeyer's ring. These tissues resemble both lymph nodes and Peyer's patches, including an FAE with M cells in the tonsillar crypts that is essential for selective antigen uptake (Fig. 19.3). Germinal centers containing B and T cells, plasma cells and professional APCs are also present. Tonsillar tissues can serve as a source of precursors of IgA plasma cells found in the upper aerodigestive tracts, as well as an inductive site for more generalized mucosal and systemic immune responses.[7] Induction through the nasal cavity may well exceed that induced by oral immunization. When viral and bacterial antigens are introduced into the nasal cavity, usually along with mucosal adjuvants such as cholera toxin (CT) and/or its B subunit (CT-B), optimal immune responses are induced in external secretions, such as saliva and, surprisingly, in secretions of the female genital tract.[1]

NALT develops postnatally. The LTα$_1$β$_2$ signaling pathway appears to be essential for the maintenance, but not the initiation, of NALT organogenesis.[4] Signaling via the IL-7/IL-7R and the L-selectin/PNAd adhesion molecules both play important roles in the organization of NALT.[4] Thus cytokine signaling cascades, and in particular the LTα$_1$β$_2$-LTβR signaling pathway, are essential for the maintenance of NALT architecture.

Other potential sites for mucosal induction of an immune response

The follicular structures analogous to PPs found in the large intestine and especially in the rectum, which are known as rectal-associated lymphoreticular tissues (RALT), are another IgA-inductive site and a source of IgA plasma cell precursors. Unlike most other mucosal tissues, the lamina propria of the large intestine is characterized by a predominance of IgA2 versus IgA1 producing cells.[1] It has been shown that the eye drop administration of antigen elicits secretory immunoglobulin A (S-IgA) responses in ocular and nasal mucosa. Thus, both tear-duct associated lymphoreticular tissue (TALT) and conjunctiva-associated lymphoreticular tissue (CALT) are able to uptake antigens for the initiation of mucosal immune responses as the parts of MALTs.[8,9]

Lymphocyte homing into mucosal compartments

There is a direct route for B-cell migration between PPs and GI lamina propria (Fig. 19.4B). Indeed, the mesenteric lymph nodes of orally immunized animals can repopulate the lamina propria of gut, mammary glands, lacrimal glands, and salivary glands with antigen specific IgA plasma cells (Fig. 19.4B),[1] pointing to the existence of a 'common' mucosal immune system. This concept has undergone further refinement, as studies now show that

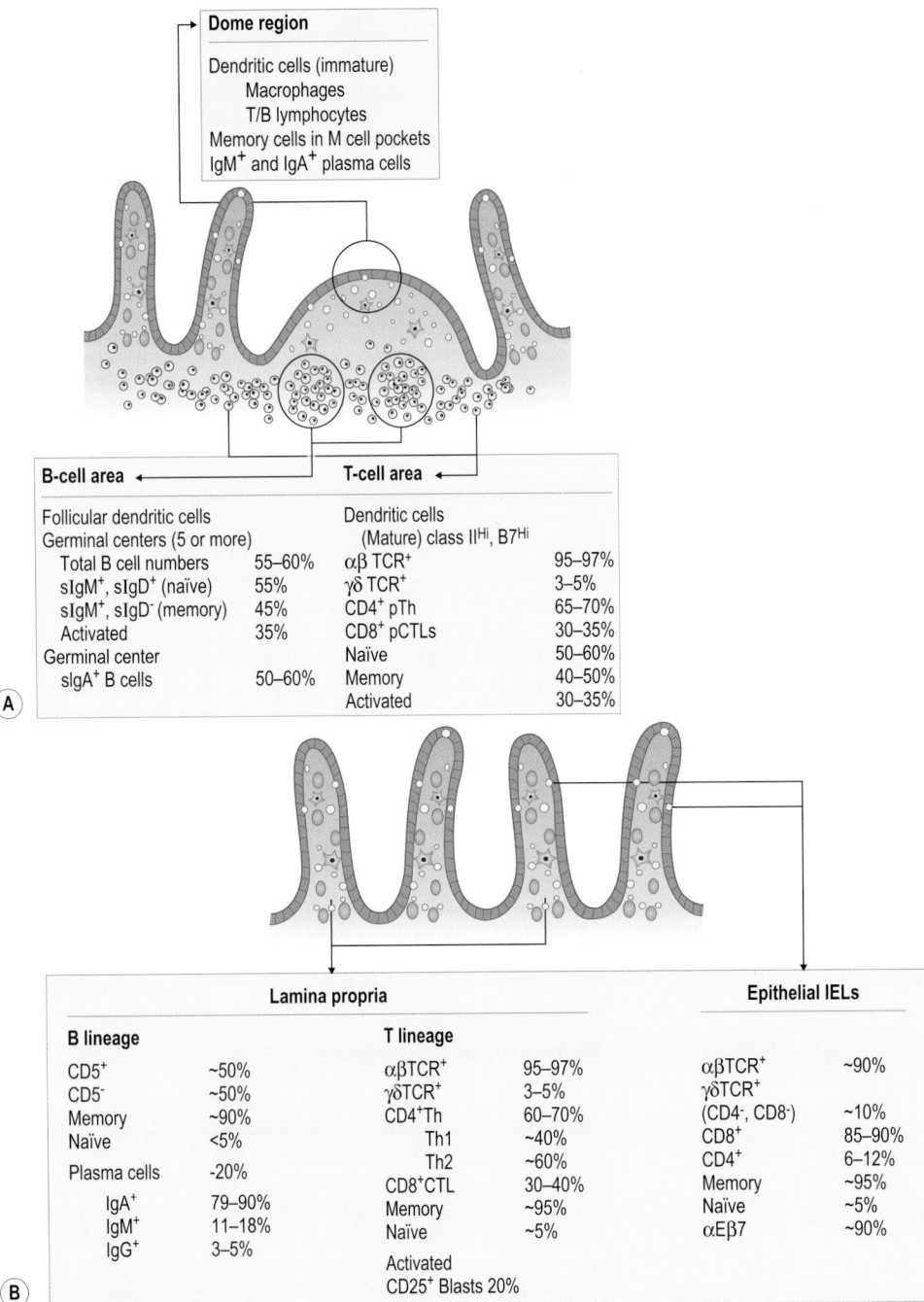

Dome region

Dendritic cells (immature)
　Macrophages
　T/B lymphocytes
Memory cells in M cell pockets
IgM$^+$ and IgA$^+$ plasma cells

B-cell area			T-cell area	
Follicular dendritic cells			Dendritic cells	
Germinal centers (5 or more)			(Mature) class II^{Hi}, B7^{Hi}	
Total B cell numbers	55–60%		αβ TCR$^+$	95–97%
sIgM$^+$, sIgD$^+$ (naïve)	55%		γδ TCR$^+$	3–5%
sIgM$^+$, sIgD$^-$ (memory)	45%		CD4$^+$ pTh	65–70%
Activated	35%		CD8$^+$ pCTLs	30–35%
Germinal center			Naïve	50–60%
sIgA$^+$ B cells	50–60%		Memory	40–50%
			Activated	30–35%

Ⓐ

Lamina propria					Epithelial IELs	
B lineage			**T lineage**			
CD5$^+$	~50%		αβTCR$^+$	95–97%	αβTCR$^+$	~90%
CD5$^-$	~50%		γδTCR$^+$	3–5%	γδTCR$^+$	
Memory	~90%		CD4$^+$Th	60–70%	(CD4$^-$, CD8$^-$)	~10%
Naïve	<5%		Th1	~40%	CD8$^+$	85–90%
Plasma cells	~20%		Th2	~60%	CD4$^+$	6–12%
			CD8$^+$CTL	30–40%	Memory	~95%
IgA$^+$	79–90%		Memory	~95%	Naïve	~5%
IgM$^+$	11–18%		Naïve	~5%	αEβ7	~90%
IgG$^+$	3–5%		Activated			
			CD25$^+$ Blasts 20%			

Ⓑ

Fig. 19.4 Structural features and cellular components of gut-associated lymphoreticular tissues (GALT). (A) The dome region is covered by the follicle-associated epithelium (FAE) with its characteristic microfold or M cells. Major features of the dome include M cells with lymphocyte pockets, scattered plasma cells, and immature dendritic cells (DCs). The B-cell area contains five or more germinal centers with high frequencies of surface IgA$^+$ B cells. The adjacent T-cell area contains mature interdigitating DCs and precursors of CD4 Th and CD8 CTLs. (B) Structural features and cellular characteristics of mucosal effector sites. The lamina propria is equally populated by B$_1$ and B$_2$ cells, both of which differentiate into IgA$^+$ plasma cells. Note that memory B and T lymphocytes are also both present in this compartment. Although intraepithelial lymphocytes (IELs) in human are mainly TCRαβ$^+$, significant numbers of TCRγδ$^+$ T cells are also found in this compartment.

the migration of cells into and from NALT adheres to rules different from those for cell migration into and from GALT and the GI tract.

Lymphocyte homing in the GI tract

Naïve lymphocytes enter mucosal or systemic lymphoid tissues from the blood through specialized high endothelial venules (HEV), which consist of cuboidal endothelial cells (Fig. 19.5A). In GALT, HEV are present in the interfollicular zones, which are rich in T cells.[10] In effector sites such as the lamina propria of the GI tract, the endothelial venules are less pronounced and tend to occur near villus crypt regions (Fig. 19.5B). Mucosal addressin cell adhesion molecule-1 (MAdCAM-1) is the most important addressin expressed by Peyer's patch HEV or lamina

propria venules (LPV) (Chapter 11). Peripheral lymph node addressin (PNAd) and vascular cell adhesion molecule (VCAM-1) are the principal addressins expressed by peripheral lymph node and skin HEV, respectively.

The major homing receptors expressed by lymphocytes are the integrins, a large class of molecules characterized by a heterodimeric structure of α and β chains (Chapter 11). In general, the type of homing receptor is determined by the integrin expressed with the α$_4$ chain; the β$_1$-integrin characterizes the homing receptor for the skin, whereas the β$_7$-integrin characterizes the receptor for the gut. The pairing of α$_4$ with β$_7$ is thus responsible for lymphocyte binding to the MAdCAM-1 that is expressed on HEVs in PPs and GI tract LPVs (Fig. 19.5).[11]

The C-type lectins L-, E-, and P-selectins (Chapter 11) also serve as homing receptors. L-selectin has a high affinity for carbohydrate-decorated PNAd, which is of central importance

Table 19.1 Major T-cell subpopulations associated with Peyer's patches

T-cell phenotype	Percentage of total T cells
CD3$^+$αβ TCR$^+$	95–97
CD3$^+$γδ TCR$^+$	3–5
CD3$^+$, CD4$^+$ (precursors of Th)	65–70
CD3$^+$, CD8$^+$ (precursors of CTLs)	30–35
Naïve (CD45RB^{Hi})	50–60
Memory (CD45RB^{Lo}, CD45RO^{Hi})	40–50
Blasts (in cell cycle)	30–35

in peripheral lymph node homing of B and T cells. L-selectin can also bind to carbohydrate-decorated MAdCAM-1 and is an important initial receptor for homing into GALT HEVs.

Chemokines are also involved in lymphocyte homing, with different chemokine-receptor pairs controling migration into different lymphoid tissues (Chapter 10). For example, loss of secondary lymphoid tissue chemokine (SLC) results in lack of naïve T cell or dendritic cell migration into spleen or Peyer's patches. CCR4, which responds to the thymus activation-regulated chemokine (TARC) and macrophage-derived chemokine (MDC), mediates the arrest of skin-homing T cells, but does not affect $\alpha_4\beta_7{}^{hi}$ T-cell migration in the GI tract. Conversely, memory $\alpha_4\beta_7{}^{hi}$ T cells that express the receptor for thymus-expressed chemokine (TECK), CC9, migrate into the lamina propria of the GI tract. Both human $\alpha_E\beta_7{}^+$ and $\alpha_4\beta_7{}^{hi}$ CD8 T cells

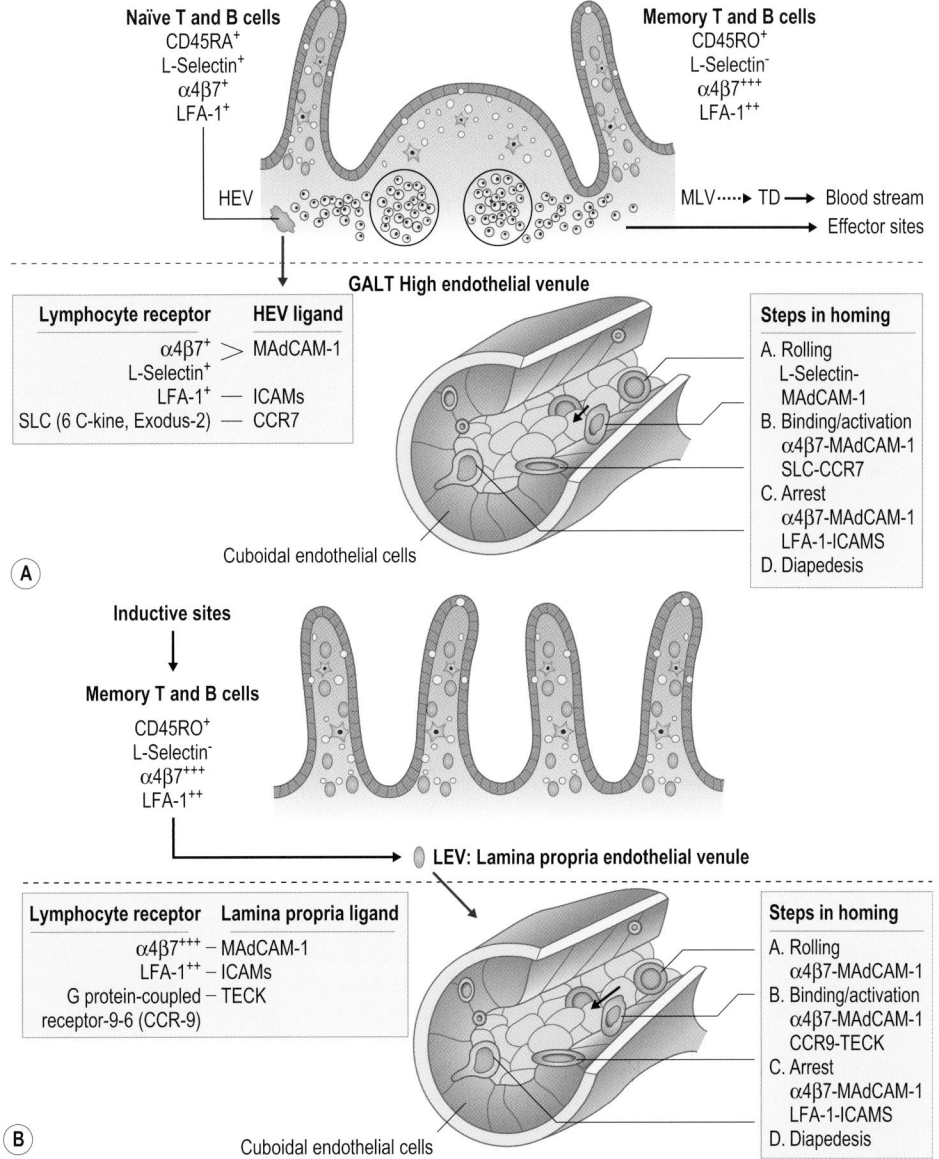

Fig. 19.5 Structural features and lymphocyte homing into GALT. (A) High endothelial venules (HEV) occur in T-cell areas and express the ligands MAdCAM-1, ICAM-1, and CCR7. Naïve T and B cells, which are L-selectin$^+$, $\alpha_4\beta_7{}^+$ and LFA-1$^+$, all participate in rolling, binding activation, arrest and diapedesis in the HEV. Memory B and T cells express $\alpha_4\beta_7$ and LFA-1 at a higher level. (B) Lymphocyte receptors and addressin ligands involved in homing into mucosal effector sites of the GI tract. The majority of B and T cells exhibit a memory phenotype with coexpression of high levels of $\alpha_4\beta_7$ and LFA-1. The expression of the G-protein-coupled receptor CCR9 allows the homing steps that occur on lamina propria venules.

express CCR9, suggesting that TECK-CCR9 is also involved in lymphocyte homing and the arrest of IELs in the GI tract epithelium (Fig. 19.4).

Peyer's patches and GALT contain both naïve and memory T- and B-cell subsets, whereas lamina propria consists of memory T and B cells and terminally differentiated plasma cells (Table 19.1, Fig. 19.4). Naïve B cells and T cells destined for GALT express L-selectin, moderate levels of $\alpha_4\beta_7(\alpha_4\beta_7{}^+)$ and LFA-1. Memory lymphocytes destined for lamina propria express higher levels of $\alpha_4\beta_7$ $(\alpha_4\beta_7{}^{hi})$ and lack L-selectin. Initial rolling is dependent upon $\alpha_4\beta_7$ interaction with LPV MAdCAM-1. Activation-dependent binding and extravasation require LFA-1–ICAM binding. $\alpha_4\beta_7$ also mediates binding to E-cadherin, and CCR9 expression can result in activation-dependent entry into the epithelial cell compartment.

Migration out of the lymph nodes similarly appears to depend on addressins. Cryosections of human tissues have revealed naïve T and B cells in HEV that express both L-selectin and $\alpha_4\beta_7$, whereas memory T and B cells in efferent lymphatics express $\alpha_4\beta_7$ but not L-selectin. The majority of cells in mesenteric lymph nodes, including B-cell blasts, tend to be of the memory phenotype and are $\alpha_4\beta_7{}^{hi}$, L-selectin^{lo}. Ig-containing B-cell blasts also express high levels of $\alpha_4\beta_7$.

The separation of naïve and memory T and B cells for entry into GALT HEV or LPV has important implications in vaccine development (Chapter 90). Recent studies offer strong evidence that peripheral blood mononuclear cells, which are assumed to home to systemic lymphoid tissues, are also destined for mucosal effector sites in the GI tract. For example, an oral cholera vaccine elicited transient IgA antibody-forming cells (AFC) in blood and subsequent IgA anticholera toxin AFC in duodenal tissues.[12] In a separate study, most peripheral blood AFC induced after parenteral immunization were L-selectin$^+$, whereas those induced after oral and rectal immunization were predominantly $\alpha_4\beta_7{}^+$ AFCs.[13] In this latter study most of the AFCs produced IgA, but some also expressed IgG. Interestingly, AFC after nasal immunization expressed both L-selectin and $\alpha_4\beta_7$ homing receptors. These results suggest that enteric immunization of GALT can trigger the appearance of $\alpha_4\beta_7{}^+$ memory IgA and IgG B cells, which can then migrate into the bloodstream.

Lymphocyte homing in NALT and lung-associated tissues

Unlike Peyer's patch HEVs, which are found in T-cell zones, murine NALT HEV are found in B-cell zones and express PNAd either alone or associated with MAdCAM-1. Moreover, anti-L-selectin Abs — but not anti-MAdCAM-1 Abs — block the binding of naïve lymphocytes to NALT HEV, suggesting a predominant role for L-selectin and PNAd in the binding of naïve lymphocytes to these HEV.[14]

During pulmonary immune responses, induction of VCAM-1, E-selectin and P-selectin in the pulmonary vasculature is matched by increased expression of P-selectin ligand on peripheral blood CD4 and CD8 T cells.[15] As the cells accumulate in the bronchoalveolar fluid, the number of cells that express P-selectin ligand in the blood declines. Very late antigen (VLA-4) appears to be involved, as migration of VLA-4$^+$ T cells into bronchoalveolar fluid is impaired following treatment with anti-α_4 Ab. Antigen-specific L-selectin^{low} cytotoxic T-lymphocyte (CTL) effectors also accumulate in the lung.

Following systemic immunization, most NALT effector B cells express L-selectin, with only a few cells expressing $\alpha_4\beta_7$. In contrast, after enteric (oral or rectal) immunization the opposite holds true.[16] Effector B cells induced by nasal immunization display a more promiscuous pattern of adhesion molecules, with a large majority expressing both L-selectin and $\alpha_4\beta_7$.

The common mucosal immune system revisited

The existence of a common muscosal immune system has become almost a matter of dogma, and so the homing pattern that has been elucidated in the GI tract after immunization of GALT has been taken to be the model for all mucosal immune sites. However, the more recent studies summarized above suggest instead that the specific set of homing receptors and ligand addressins expressed in the GI tract are absent in NALT or associated lymph nodes. The failure of tonsillar cells to demonstrate selective $\alpha_4\beta_7$ expression, and the lack of MAdCAM-1 expression on tonsil HEVs, makes it likely that gut-homing does not extend to human NALT and associated lymph nodes. It remains possible, and even likely, that memory T and B cells from the gut may enter NALT for additional priming and reprogramming of homing receptors. Likewise, memory T and B cells induced in NALT may traffic to lung and genitourinary tract tissues, as well as to the GI tract. Thus, the rules for the homing of naïve T- and B-cell precursors into NALT need to be more clearly defined.

Induction of mucosal immunity

Immune responses expressed in mucosal tissues are typified by S-IgA Abs, which constitute the predominant Ig isotype in external secretions. The resistance of S-IgA to endogenous proteases makes Abs of this isotype uniquely suited to protect mucosal surfaces. The development of mucosal immunity requires T cells, including CD4 T helper (Th) cell subsets, CD8 CTLs, and other T-cell subsets. B-cell commitment (Cμ to Cα switching) and B-/T-cell interactions are of central importance, resulting in the induction of plasma cells producing pIgA. Cytokines produced by CD4 and CD8 T-cell subsets; by DCs, MØs, and B cells; and by nonclassic APCs (e.g., epithelial cells) all contribute to induction of normal mucosal immune responses.

Mucosal antigen-presenting cells

Large macromolecules are taken up by M cells in the GI tract. N418$^+$, 2A1$^+$, NLDC-145$^-$, M342$^-$ DCs form a dense layer of cells in the subepithelial dome (SED) just beneath the follicle epithelium where CD4, but not CD8, T cells can be found.[17] Another subset of DCs, N418$^+$, 2A1$^+$, NLDC-145$^+$ and M342$^+$, populates the interfollicular T-cell regions where both CD4 and CD8 T cells reside. DCs in the dome region are immature, highly endocytic, and express low levels of MHC and B7 molecules. DCs in the T-cell area are mature, with low endocytic activity and high levels of MHC class I and II molecules and B7 molecule expression. Antigen taken up by M cells appears to be first endocytosed in the dome region by immature DCs, which then migrate to T-cell interfollicular areas where maturation occurs (Fig. 19.4A). DCs are also found in NALT such as human tonsils and lung, where they play the same role as in the GALT.

Intestinal epithelial cells (IECs) express MHC class II and class I molecules and present peptides to primed CD4 and CD8 T cells. However, it is still unclear whether IECs can process antigen or if the MHC class II molecules on these cells only serve as receptors for predigested peptides that result from enzymatic lysis in the stomach. Human and murine IECs also express CD1d, a non-classical MHC class I molecule that is also found on DCs and MØ and that appears to be involved in the presentation of lipid and glycolipid antigens (Chapter 6).

CD4 T-helper cell subsets in mucosal immunity

Th cell subsets are classified as either Th1, Th2 or Th17 according to the pattern of cytokines produced (Chapter 16). Th1 cells selectively produce IL-2, IFN-γ, LT-α, LT-β and TNF-α, whereas Th2 cells produce IL-4, IL-5, IL-6, IL-9, IL-10 and IL-13 (Fig. 19.6). Both Th1 and Th2 cells develop from naïve CD4 T cells through the same T-cell precursor (Th0) phase (Chapter 8). IL-2 is produced by Th0 cells upon antigen exposure and serves as an important growth factor. IL-12 induces NK cells to produce IFN-γ that, together with IL-12, triggers Th0 cells to differentiate along the Th1 pathway.

In mouse, Th1-type responses are associated with the development of cell-mediated immunity, as manifested by delayed-type hypersensitivity (DTH) and by B-cell responses with a characteristic IgG Ab subclass (IgG2a) pattern. Th2 cells support the production of IgA, as well as IgG1, IgG2b and IgE. IFN-γ produced by Th1 cells inhibits both Th2 cell proliferation and B-cell isotype switching stimulated by IL-4. Likewise, Th2 cells regulate Th1 cell effects by secreting IL-10, which inhibits IFN-γ secretion by Th1 cells. This decreased IFN-γ production allows the development of Th2-type cells.

In human, Th1 and Th2 cells also reciprocally regulate the development of the opposite subset through IFN-γ and IL-4 secretion, respectively (Fig. 19.6). Antigen-specific IgG subclass responses in patients with Lyme borreliosis, a pathology known to induce Th1 cells and strong IFN-γ responses, consisted of IgG1 and IgG3 C-fixing Abs with low IgG2 and undetectable IgG4 Ab levels,[18] suggesting that in human IL-4 promotes switching to IgG4 and IFN-γ promotes switching to IgG1 (Fig. 19.6).

In addition to these Th1 and Th2 cells, regulatory T cells (Treg) and Th17 cells are known to be involved in mucosal homeostasis and inflammatory responses (Chapter 15). Further, human tonsil CD4 T cells expressing B-cell follicle homing receptor CXCR5 are identified as follicular Th (Tfh) cells to help B-cell differentiation.[19,20] Foxp3+ Treg cells in Peyer's patches can apparetnly differentiate into Tfh cells, which express the chemokine CXCR5, the transcription factor Bcl-6, and the cytokine IL-21 to promote germinal center formation and IgA synthesis in the gut.[21]

Cytokines in mucosal immunity

B-cell isotype switching and IgA plasma cell differentiation

Isotype switching is preceded by transcriptional activation of the isotype in question (Chapter 4). Two major cytokines, IL-4 and TGF-β, induce surface IgM-positive (sIgM+) B cells to switch to downstream isotypes, including IgE and IgA. The addition of TGF-β1 to LPS-triggered mouse B-cell cultures can lead to increased IgA synthesis, an effect that can be enhanced by IL-2 or IL-5. TGF-β1 can also induce sIgM+ to sIgA+ B-cell switches. In human, anti-CD40 stimulation of tonsillar B cells, together with TGF-β1 in the presence of IL-10, stimulates IgA synthesis.[1] Cα1 transcripts can also be induced by B-cell mitogen plus TGF-β, and Cα2 transcripts can be induced by TGF-β together with IL-10, suggesting that switches to IgA2 are more T cell- and Th2-cytokine dependent.

DCs can also induce the S-IgA Ab response through novel CD40-independent mechanisms . DCs can directly interact with B cells through the B-cell activation factor of the TNF family (BAFF), also called lymphocyte stimulator protein (BLyS), and a proliferation-inducing ligand (APRIL) in order to induce

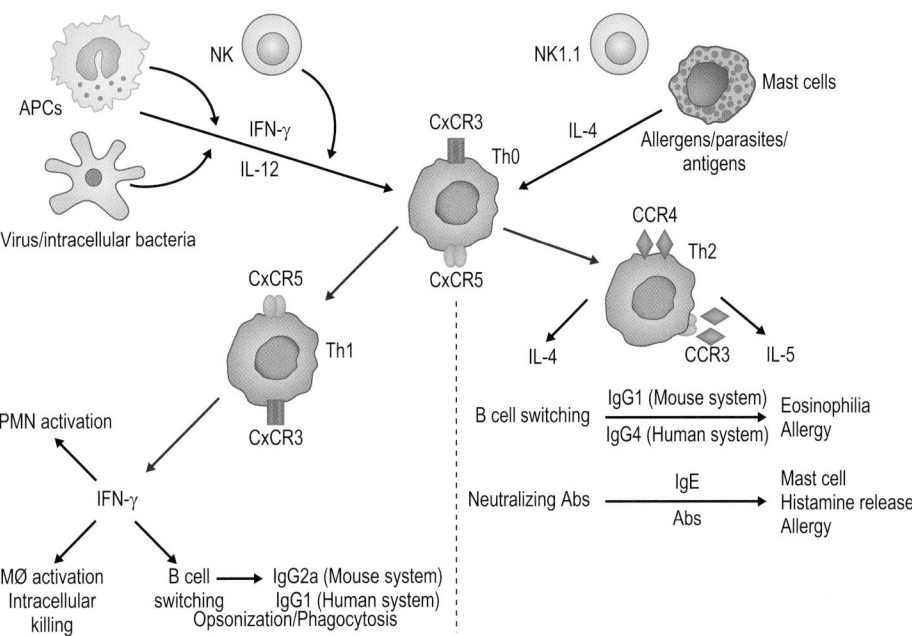

Fig. 19.6 T-helper cell subset development. The cellular and cytokine environment induces Th0 cells to develop into either Th1 or Th2 subsets. APCs produce IL-12 in response to microbial assault and, together with IFN-γ produced by NK cells, induce mature Th1 cells. Th1 cells express select chemokine receptors and, through IFN-γ synthesis, activate MØ and induce B cells to produce opsonizing Abs. Other cells, such as NK1.1 and mast cells, respond to antigen/allergen with IL-4, which induces Th0 to Th2 switching. Th2 cells produce IL-4, -5, -6, -10, -9, and IL-13, which help regulate mucosal S-IgA Ab responses.

surface IgA$^+$ B cells (or post-switched IgA committed B cells).[22] APRIL-transmembrane activator and CAML interactor (TACI) signal transduction has been shown to play a key role in the induction of CD40-independent IgA class switching in mice.[23] Altered function mutations in TACI can also result in IgA deficiency in human (Chapter 34). Differentiation of sIgA$^+$ B cells into IgA-producing plasma cells is particularly dependent on the Th1 cytokines IL-5 and IL-6.[24]

Vaccine development and mucosal immune responses

Mucosal immune responses include a major B-cell component that is characterized by secretory IgA (S-IgA) Ab, as well as T-helper cell and CTL responses. These responses can be induced by pathogens triggering the organized mucosal inductive sites. Effective protection against strong mucosal pathogens requires prophylactic immune responses that can be achieved by mucosal vaccines. In contrast to systemic challenge, vaccines administered via mucosal routes can trigger both mucosal immune responses as a first line of defense at the portal of pathogen entry and systemic immune responses that neutralize pathogens that have penetrated that barrier.

Because it is now well accepted that Th1-type responses result in B- and T-cell responses distinct from those induced by Th2-type cells, mucosal adjuvants, vectors and delivery systems are being developed for vaccines that can specifically induce Th1- or Th2-type responses (Chapter 90). For example, in mice the mucosal adjuvant cholera toxin (CT) has been shown to promote mucosal S-IgA as well as serum anti-vaccine and anti-CT-B subunit (CT-B) Ab (IgG1 and IgE) responses associated with CD4 Th2 cells (see below).[25] Conversely, recombinant *Salmonella typhimurium* BRD 847 (*aroA$^-$*, *aroD$^-$*) expressing the C fragment of tetanus toxin has been shown to be an excellent oral vaccine vector for the induction of Th1-type responses with brisk mucosal S-IgA as well as serum Ab (IgG2a) responses.[25]

New mucosal adjuvants and delivery systems for the induction of targeted immunity

Bacterial enterotoxins and their nontoxic derivatives

Two bacterial enterotoxins (i.e., cholera toxin (CT) and heat-labile toxin (LT) from *Escherichia coli*) are now established as effective for the induction of both mucosal and systemic immunity to coadministered protein antigens. Cholera toxin consists of two structurally and functionally separate A and B subunits (Fig. 19.7). The B subunit of CT (CT-B) binds to GM1 gangliosides, which on epithelia allows the A subunit to reach the cytosol of target cells, where it acts to elevate cAMP thereby promoting secretion of water and chloride ions into the intestinal lumen. The labile toxin (LT) from *E. coli* is closely related to CT and binds to GM1 and GM2 gangliosides as well. Thus, LT also

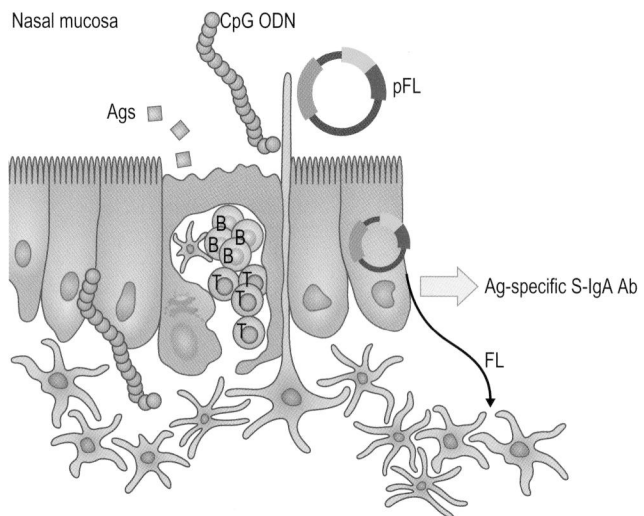

Fig. 19.7 Dendritic cell-targeting nasal adjuvant. Nasal administration of CpG oligodeoxynucleotide (ODN) and plasmid expressing Flt3 lignd cDNA (pFL) specifically target dendritic cells in NALT. These nasal dendritic cell-targeting vaccines successfully elicit protective Ag-specific S-IgA Ab responses in the elderly.

binds GM2 and asialo-GM1 gangliosides. In order to circumvent toxicity, mutant CT (mCT) and LT (mLT) molecules have been generated by site-directed mutagenesis wherein single amino acid substitutions have been made in the active site of the A subunit of CT or LT, or in the protease sensitive loop of LT. The levels of antigen-specific serum IgG and secretory IgA Abs induced by these mutants are comparable to those induced by wild-type CT, and significantly higher than those induced by recombinant CT-B.[26] One of the mutants also induces Th2-type responses through a preferential inhibition of Th1-type CD4 T cells.

Mutant LT molecules, whether possessing a residual ADP-ribosyltransferase activity (e.g., LT-72R) or totally devoid of it (e.g., LT-7 K and LT-6 K3), can also function as mucosal adjuvants when administered intranasally to mice together with unrelated antigens.[27] As LT induces a mixed CD4 Th1- (i.e., IFN-γ) and Th2-type (i.e., IL-4, IL-5, IL-6 and IL-10) response,[25] one might envisage the use of LT mutants when both Th1- and Th2-type responses are desired.

Safety of mucosal adjuvants and delivery systems

The olfactory neuroepithelium in the nasopharynx constitutes approximately 50% of the nasal surface and has direct neuronal connection to the olfactory bulbs (OBs) in the central nervous system (CNS). While diarrhea is the primary limiting factor for the use of oral enterotoxin as an adjuvant in humans, major safety concerns with mucosal adjuvants and delivery systems for nasal vaccination are also important since they can enter and/or target olfactory neurons, and therefore gain access to OBs and deeper structures in the brain parenchyma. These adverse effects appear in large part to be mediated by the ADP-ribosyl transferase activity and the nature of the cellular receptors targeted. Both CT and LT mutants bind to GM1 on epithelial cells and require endocytosis followed by transport across the epithelial cell to reach the basolateral membrane. GM1 gangliosides are also abundantly expressed by cells of the CNS and their concentration on neuronal and microglial cells varies during the development of various cell types and different regions of the brain.[28]

CT or CT-B, when given nasally to mice, enter the olfactory nerves and epithelium (ON/E) and OBs by mechanisms that are selectively dependent upon GM1.[29] nCT as adjuvant also promotes the uptake of nasally co-administered, unrelated proteins into the ON/E. The targeting of CNS tissues by nasally administered bacterial enterotoxins is clearly related to a higher incidence of Bell's Palsy (facial paresis) among volunteers of a nasal vaccination trial given nLTh-1 as mucosal adjuvant. Bell's Palsy among study subjects that in 2000 received nonliving nasal influenza vaccine (Nasalflu® led to its withdrawal from the market (www.niaid.nih.gov/dmid/enteric/intranasal.htm).

The use of GM1-receptor binding holotoxins as nasal mucosal adjuvants is currently inadvisable due to the risk for their accumulation in the CNS. However, development of nontoxic mCTs could overcome these potential problems. To this end, a model adjuvant has been developed by combining the ADP-ribosylating ability of nCT with a dimer of an Ig-binding fragment, D, of *Staphylococcus aureus* protein A.[30] This CTA1-DD molecule directly binds to B cells of all isotypes, but not to MØ or DCs. Despite the lack of a mucosal binding element, the B cell-targeted CTA1-DD molecule is as strong an adjuvant as nCT. Notably, CTA1-DD promoted a balanced Th1/Th2 response with little effect on IgE Ab production. CTA1-DD did not induce inflammatory changes in the nasal mucosa, and most importantly did not bind to or accumulate in the OBs or the CNS.[31] CTA1-DD is an example of the use of non-ganglioside

targeting adjuvants and delivery systems as new tools for the development of safe and effective nasal vaccines.

Immunostimulatory DNA sequences

Plasmid DNA for gene vaccination can be functionally divided into two distinct units: a transcription unit and an adjuvant/mitogen unit.[32] The latter contains immunostimulatory sequences consisting of short palindromic nucleotides centered around a CpG dinucleotide core, as for example 5′-purine-purine-CG-pyrimidine-pyrimidine-3′. The adjuvant effect of these sequences is mediated by bacterial but not by eukaryotic DNA, owing to its high frequency of CpG motifs and to the absence of cytosine methylation. CpG motifs can induce B-cell proliferation and Ig synthesis as well as cytokine secretion (i.e., IL-6, IFN-α, IFN-β, IFN-γ, IL-12, and IL-18) by a variety of immune cells.

Because CpG motifs create a cytokine microenvironment favoring Th1-type responses, they can be used as adjuvants to stimulate antigen-specific Th1-type responses or to redirect harmful allergic or Th2-dominated autoimmune responses. Indeed, coinjection of bacterial DNA or CpG motifs with a DNA vaccine or with a protein antigen promotes Th1-type responses even in mice with a pre-existing Th2-type immunity. CpG motifs can enhance both systemic and mucosal immune responses when given nasally to mice.[33]

Mucosal cytokines and innate factors as adjuvants

Mucosal delivery of cytokines offers a means to prevent the adverse effects associated with the large and repeated parenteral doses often required for the effective targeting of tissues and organs. For example, nasal delivery permits acquisition of significant serum levels of IL-12 at one-tenth the dose required for inhibition of serum IFN-γ by parenteral administration.[1] A nasal vaccine of tetanus toxoid (TT), given with either IL-6 or IL-12, induced serum TT-specific IgG Ab responses that protected mice against lethal challenge with tetanus toxin.[34] Also, nasal administration of TT with IL-12 as adjuvant induced high titers of S-IgA Ab responses in the GI tract, vaginal washes and saliva.[34] Similar results were reported when mice were nasally immunized with soluble influenza H1 and N1 proteins and IL-12. In related studies, IL-12 was shown to redirect CT-induced antigen-specific Th2-type responses toward the Th1 type when given by oral or intranasal routes.[1] And, IL-12 was shown to promote both Th1- and Th2-type responses when administered by a separate mucosal route.[1] These observations document the power of IL-12 for the induction of targeted immunity.

Innate molecules secreted in the epithelium provide another mechanism by which the adaptive mucosal immune system might be activated. To test this concept, protein antigens were given with either IL-1, α-defensins (i.e., human neutrophil peptides, HNPs) or lymphotactin.[1] Lymphotactin, a C chemokine (Chapter 10) produced by NK and CD8 T cells such as TCRγδ IELs, is chemotactic for T and NK cells and induces the migration of memory T cells across endothelial cells. IL-1 is produced by a number of cells, including macrophages and epithelial cells, whereas α-defensins are produced by Paneth cells. Nasal administration of protein antigens with these innate molecules enhanced systemic immune responses to coadministered antigens. However, whereas both IL-1 and lymphotactin produced mucosal S-IgA Ab responses, the defensins failed to do so.[1] Thus, some, but not all, inflammatory cytokines and molecules of the innate immune system can be effectively administered by mucosal routes to regulate both systemic and mucosal immune responses.

Flt3 ligand (FL) binds to the *fms*-like tyrosine kinase receptor Flt3/Flk2. FL mobilizes and stimulates myeloid and lymphoid progenitor cells, DCs, and NK cells. Although FL dramatically augments numbers of DCs *in vivo*, it fails to induce their activation. Treatment of mice by systemic FL injection can induce marked increases in the numbers of DCs in both systemic (i.e., spleen) and mucosal lymphoid tissues (i.e., iLP, PPs and mesenteric lymph nodes [MLN]). This increase in mucosal DCs can, in some cases, initially enhance induction of oral tolerance.[35] In others it can favor the induction of immune responses by mucosal, systemic or cutaneous routes. It was reported that nasal administration of plasmid or adenovirus encoding FL cDNA (pFL or Ad-FL) with protein Ags resulted in the induction of Ag-specific S-IgA as the protective immunity.[36-38] These studies confirm the adjuvant activity of FL for both Ab- and CMI-responses and suggest that the costly treatment of using FL protein may now be replaced by use of FL cDNA.

Transgenic plants

Plants can be engineered to synthesize and assemble one or more Ags that retain both T- and B-cell epitopes, thereby inducing systemic and mucosal immune responses in both mice and humans.[39,40] In order to circumvent potential denaturation of antigen during cooking, recombinant bananas have been developed that can accumulate up to 1 milligram of vaccine Ag per 10 grams of banana. Most recently, CT-B subunit has been expressed under the control of the rice seed storage protein glutelin promoter (MucoRice-CT-B). Oral feeding of powdered MucoRice-CT-B to mice and non-human primates resulted in the induction of both systemic and mucosal Ab responses for the protection against CT.[41-43]

> ● ON THE HORIZON
>
> **Development of transgenic plants as vehicle for vaccine administration**
>
> - MucoRice system is potent and ideal strategy for vaccine development.
> - MucoRice system may also be used as a passive neutralizing antibody delivery system.

Synthesis and functions of secretory antibodies

Mucosal S-IgA differs from bone marrow-derived serum IgA in both molecular composition and specific Ab activity. Humans possess two Cα gene segments, Cα1 and Cα2 (Chapter 4), the use of which defines the two IgA subclasses, IgA1 and IgA2.[44] These IgA subtypes differ primarily in their hinge regions. IgA1 Abs contain an additional set of 13 amino acid residues in the hinge region that renders them more flexible and susceptible to IgA1 specific proteases produced by certain bacteria. IgA1 secreting plasma cells are prevalent in most human mucosal tissues, especially the small intestine and the respiratory tract, whereas the human colon and genital tract are enriched for IgA2 secreting cells. Although S-IgA at mucosal surfaces has often been viewed as a barrier to prevent adhesion and colonization of pathogens, as well as an effective means to neutralize viruses and toxins, these antibodies confer the additional advantage of providing anti-inflammatory properties.[8]

In external secretions, adult levels of S-IgA are reached considerably earlier (1 month to 2 years) than in the serum (adolescence)

(Chapter 32). Approximately 98% of S-IgA antibodies are produced locally in mucosal tissues, with only a minor fraction deriving from the circulation.

> ● KEY CONCEPTS
>
> **Secretory IgA**
>
> - Unlike serum IgA, mucosal secretion of IgA reaches adult levels early in life (1 month to 2 years).
> - The polymeric Ig receptor (pIgR) is expressed on the basolateral surface of epithelial cells and facilitates the active transport of secretory IgA, as well as pentameric IgM, into the mucosal secretions.
> - Secretory IgA protects the host by inhibiting microbial adherence; neutralizing viruses, enzymes, and toxins; and engaging in anti-inflammatory activities by means of inhibiting IgM and IgG complement activation.
> - Clinically, selective IgA deficiency, which is the most common primary immune deficiency, is characterized by recurrent mucosal infections, including sinusitis, otitis media, bronchitis, and pneumonias of viral or bacterial origin, as well as acute diarrhea caused by viruses, bacteria, or parasites such as *Giardia lamblia*.

Polymeric Ig receptor and pIgA transport

The polymeric Ig receptor (pIgR) is synthesized as a transmembrane protein by epithelial cells and is found on the basolateral surface of epithelial cells. It acts as a receptor for the endocytosis of polymeric IgA (pIgA) and pentameric IgM, both of which typically contain a J chain. pIgR is produced by bronchial epithelial cells, renal tubules, glands and the epithelium of the small and large intestine.[1] pIgR is not expressed by the FAE (including M cells) of Peyer's patches, but only by the adjacent columnar epithelial cells. It is expressed mainly in the upper respiratory tract, which includes the nasal cavity, tonsils, trachea, bronchi and tracheobronchial glands. Expression in the lower tract is restricted to the pulmonary alveolar cells.

In the female reproductive tissues, the expression of pIgR is influenced by sex hormones. It is low in the vagina, absent in the ovary and myometrium, and very high in the fallopian tubes and uterus. Normal kidneys do not express pIgR, whereas epithelial cells in the lower urinary tract may normally express pIgR and transport pIgA into urine. The expression of pIgR can be upregulated by cytokines such as IFN-γ, TNF-α, IL-1α, IL-1β, and TGF-β.

IgA-mediated inhibition of microbial adherence

The inhibition of microbial adherence plays a critical initial role in the protection of the host. This inhibition is mediated by both specific and nonspecific mechanisms. Secretory and polymeric IgA are more effective at agglutinating microorganisms than is membrane-bound IgA, and the agglutinating ability of S-IgA specific for capsular polysaccharides of *Haemophilus influenzae* appears to be crucial in order to prevent colonization by *H. influenzae*.[45] When a microorganism interacts with S-IgA molecules, its surface becomes less hydrophobic and thus less likely to interact with the mucosal epithelium, but at the same time more likely to be entrapped in the mucus. Carbohydrate chains on the S-IgA molecule bind to bacteria and other antigens, and so represent another nonspecific mechanism that inhibits microbial adherence.

Neutralization by S-IgA of viruses, enzymes and toxins

S-IgA Abs have been shown to be effective at neutralizing viruses in several experimental systems (e.g., influenza, Epstein–Barr virus, HIV, etc.) and at different steps in the infectious process. S-IgA specific to influenza hemagglutinin can interfere with the initial binding of influenza virus to target cells or with the internalization and the intracellular replication of the virus. Indeed, *in vitro* experiments employing polarized murine epithelial cells have demonstrated that Abs specific to rotavirus and hepatitis virus can neutralize the viruses inside epithelial cells. Finally, S-IgA can neutralize the catalytic activity of many enzymes of microbial origin.

Anti-inflammatory actions mediated by S-IgA Abs

IgA Abs are unable to activate complement by either the classic or the alternative pathway (Chapter 20). Nevertheless, they can interfere with IgM- and IgG-mediated complement activation.[37] S-IgA can inhibit phagocytosis, bactericidal activity and chemotaxis by neutrophils, monocytes and macrophages. IgA can downregulate the synthesis of TNF-α and IL-6, as well as enhancing the production of IL-1R antagonists by LPS-activated human monocytes. Thus, the antiflogistic properties of IgA are of significant importance for the integrity of the mucosa in that IgA can limit bystander tissue damage that may result from the continuous interactions of the mucosa with myriad dietary and environmental antigens. Systemically, circulating IgA also appears to help limit inflammatory reactions that result from complement fixation and phagocyte activation, and it contributes to the inhibition of IgE-dependent anaphylactic responses.

IgA deficiency

After AIDS, selective IgA deficiency (IgAD) is the most primary immune deficiency in individuals of European descent (Chapter 34). The clinical diagnosis of IgA deficiency depends on the relative absence of IgA in the serum. However, the most important manifestations of the disorder primarily reflect the absence of both S-IgA1 and S-IgA2 in the external secretions. Thus, IgA deficiency affects both the mucosal and systemic immune compartments, with only rare individuals exhibiting a superselective loss of either IgA1 or IgA2 alone.[46]

Mucosal cytotoxic T lymphocytes

M cells have specific receptors for mucosal virus that allow certain viruses, such as the reovirus, to enter the cells in both NALT and GALT. It is likely that enteric viruses such as rotavirus, and respiratory pathogens such as influenza and respiratory syncytial virus (RSV), also enter the mucosal inductive pathway via M cells.[47] After enteric infection or immunization, antigen-stimulated CTLs are disseminated from Peyer's patches into mesenteric lymph nodes via the lymphatic drainage. Oral immunization with live virus can thus induce antigen-specific CTLs in both mucosal tissues for mucosal and systemic lymphoid tissues.

Mucosal cytotoxic T cells

- After enteric infection or immunization, antigen-stimulated CTLs are disseminated from Peyer's patches into mesenteric lymph nodes via the lymphatic drainage.
- Oral immunization with live virus can induce antigen-specific CTLs in both mucosal inductive and effector tissues for mucosal responses, as well as in systemic lymphoid tissues.

Enteric viruses and mucosal cytotoxic T lymphocytes

CD8 CTLs (Chapter 17) play a central role in rotavirus and reovirus immunity.[48,49] Reovirus-induced CTL precursors (pCTLs) in GALT migrate to the systemic compartment. Reovirus-specific CD8 CTLs associated with the αβ T-cell population are also observed in the IELs. Oral delivery of rotavirus increases pCTLs in GALT and results in their dissemination throughout the murine lymphoid system within 3 weeks. Moreover, adoptively transferred CD8 T cells mediate the clearance of rotavirus infection in SCID mice.

Respiratory viruses and mucosal CTLs

Studies of immune responses after intranasal infection with influenza virus in CD4-coreceptor knockouts or other mice in which this subset had been depleted have shown that CD4 T cells do not affect the induction of pCTLs or significantly alter clearance of infection.[50] Clearance of influenza is unaltered by the use of β₂-microglobulin knockout mice, which lack CD8 T cells, or of mice that have been treated with monoclonal anti-CD8. γδ T cells with several Vδ chain specificities increase in the infected site as clearance occurs, which suggests a regulatory role for γδ T cells in antiviral immunity.[51]

Mucosal AIDS models for CTL responses

Approximately 80% of new HIV-1 infections result from sexual transmission (Chapter 37). Thus, significant efforts have been focused on the development of mucosal immunity in the genital tract. Studies using the Rhesus macaque and the simian immunodeficiency virus (SIV) vaginal infection model have provided direct evidence that pCTLs occur in female macaque reproductive tissues, and that infection with SIV induces CTL responses. This important finding was recently extended to vaginal infection with an SIV/HIV-1 chimeric virus (SHIV) containing HIV-1 89.6 *env* gene.[52] Recent work has shown that intranasal immunization with SIV/HIV components induces antibody responses in vaginal secretions. Intranasal immunization of mice with HIV-1 T-cell epitopes and the mucosal adjuvant CT has been shown to induce functional CTLs.

Other mucosal CTL systems

Salmonella can elicit CD8 T-cell responses, including CTLs, to expressed proteins; and CD8 T cells induced to the parasite *Toxoplasma gondii* have been shown to be protective. Thus, mucosal CD8 CTLs can also be induced in nonviral situations. Significant questions remain as to the mechanism by which naïve CD8 T cells can be triggered to expand into pCTLs and to the rules for expression of effector CTLs and memory in the actual mucosal compartment that manifests the infection. It has been shown that pCTLs accumulate in immunologically privileged sites but do not develop a cytotoxic function until they encounter infected class I MHC-presenting target cells. It is possible that this mechanism protects the common mucosal immune system network from inadvertent cytotoxic inflammatory events.

Mucosal immune responses in aging

Immune functions are known to deteriorate with age in several species. The risk and severity of infections are higher, and the susceptibility to certain types of autoimmune diseases and cancer are greater in the elderly,[53] while responses to vaccination are diminished. These studies provide evidence of dysregulation and of an overall decline in host immunity with increasing age. In systemic immune compartments, the age-associated alterations have been studied extensively. Dysfunctions occur in both B and T cells, though the latter are considered to be more susceptible to immunosenescence.

In humans, it has been shown that elderly subjects have significantly higher concentrations of salivary S-IgA Abs than younger subjects, whereas whole gut lavages of aged and young subjects contain similar amounts of Abs.[54] Analogous results have also been obtained for total IgA Ab responses in serum of aged animals and humans. These results indicate an absence of aged-associated impairment in total IgA Ab levels in external secretions.

Ag-specific IgA B-cell responses play a central role in the induction of mucosal immunity to infectious diseases.[1] The GI tract in the elderly is particularly susceptible to infectious diseases. Ag-specific mucosal IgA Ab responses are diminished in aged animals, especially those in the GALT.[54]

In elderly humans, pathogens that invade through mucosal surfaces such as the influenza virus and the bacterial pathogen *Streptococcus pneumoniae* cause more severe and more frequently lethal infections. The development of effective vaccines for the elderly remains a largely unmet goal. In order to provide effective protection against influenza and *S. pneumoniae* in the elderly, one should strongly consider developing a new generation of vaccines that could induce pathogen-specific immunity in the respiratory tract. Although it has been shown that effective protection can be provided by pathogen-specific systemic IgG without mucosal IgA responses, pathogen-specific S-IgA responses are a necessary component for providing a first line of effective immunity against these respiratory pathogens at their entry site.

● KEY CONCEPTS

Mucosal immunosenescence

- Early mucosal aging is evident in the GI immune system.
- Nasal immunization is an effective route for the induction of mucosal and systemic immune responses in aging mice.
- Dendritic cell-targeting mucosal adjuvants are able to elicit protective pathogen-specific S-IgA Ab responses in aged mice.

References

1. Mestecky J, Blumberg RS, Kiyono H, McGhee JR. The Mucosal Immune System. In: Paul WE, editor. Fundamental immunology. Philadelphia, PA: Lippincott Williams & Wilkins; 2003. p. 965.
2. Porter EM, Liu L, Oren A, et al. Localization of human intestinal defensin 5 in Paneth cell granules. Infect Immun 1997;65:2389.
3. Kato T, Owen R. Structure and function of intestinal mucosal epithelium. In: Mestecky J, Lamm ME, Strober W, et al., editors. Mucosal immunology, vol. 1, 3rd edn. Burlington, VT: Elsevier Academic Press; 2005: p. 131.
4. Kiyono H, Fukuyama S. NALT- versus Peyer's-patch-mediated mucosal immunity. Nat Rev Immunol 2004;4:699.
5. Fu YX, Chaplin DD. Development and maturation of secondary lymphoid tissues. Annu Rev Immunol 1999;17:399.
6. Lorenz RG, Chaplin DD, McDonald KG, et al. Isolated lymphoid follicle formation is inducible and dependent upon lymphotoxin-sufficient B lymphocytes, lymphotoxin beta receptor, and TNF receptor I function. J Immunol 2003;170:5475.
7. Quiding-Jarbrink M, Granstrom G, Nordstrom I, et al. Induction of compartmentalized B-cell responses in human tonsils. Infect Immun 1995;63:853.
8. Knop N, Knop E. Conjunctiva-associated lymphoid tissue in the human eye. Invest Ophthalmol Vis Sci 2000;41:1270.
9. Nagatake T, Fukuyama S, Kim DY, et al. Id2-, RORγt-, and LTβR-independent initiation of lymphoid organogenesis in ocular immunity. J Exp Med 2009;206:235.
10. Youngman KR, Lazarus NH, Butcher E. Lymphocyte homing: Chemokines and adhesion molecules in T cell and IgA plasma cell localization in the mucosal immune system. In: Mestecky J, Lamm ME, Strober W, et al., editors. Mucosal immunology, vol. 1, 3rd edn. Burlington, VT: Elsevier Academic Press; 2005: p. 667.
11. Holzmann B, McIntyre BW, Weissman IL. Identification of a murine Peyer's patch-specific lymphocyte homing receptor as an integrin molecule with an α chain homologous to human VLA-4 alpha. Cell 1989;56:37.
12. Quiding M, Nordstrom I, Kilander A, et al. Intestinal immune responses in humans. Oral cholera vaccination induces strong intestinal antibody responses and interferon-gamma production and evokes local immunological memory. J Clin Invest 1991;88:143.
13. Quiding-Jarbrink M, Lakew M, Nordstrom I, et al. Human circulating specific antibody-forming cells after systemic and mucosal immunizations: differential homing commitments and cell surface differentiation markers. Eur J Immunol 1995;25:322.
14. Csencsits KL, Jutila MA, Pascual DW. Nasal-associated lymphoid tissue: phenotypic and functional evidence for the primary role of peripheral node addressin in naive lymphocyte adhesion to high endothelial venules in a mucosal site. J Immunol 1999;163:1382.
15. Wolber FM, Curtis JL, Milik AM, et al. Lymphocyte recruitment and the kinetics of adhesion receptor expression during the pulmonary immune response to particulate antigen. Am J Pathol 1997;151:1715.
16. Quiding-Jarbrink M, Nordstrom I, Granstrom G, et al. Differential expression of tissue-specific adhesion molecules on human circulating antibody-forming cells after systemic, enteric, and nasal immunizations. A molecular basis for the compartmentalization of effector B cell responses. J Clin Invest 1997;99:1281.
17. Kelsall BL, Strober W. Distinct populations of dendritic cells are present in the subepithelial dome and T cell regions of the murine Peyer's patch. J Exp Med 1996;183:237.
18. Widhe M, Ekerfelt C, Forsberg P, et al. IgG subclasses in Lyme borreliosis: a study of specific IgG subclass distribution in an interferon-gamma-predominated disease. Scand J Immunol 1998;47:575.
19. Breitfeld D, Ohl L, Kremmer E, et al. Follicular B helper T cells express CXC chemokine receptor 5, localize to B cell follicles, and support immunoglobulin production. J Exp Med 2000;192:1545.
20. Schaerli P, Willimann K, Lang AB, et al. CXC chemokine receptor 5 expression defines follicular homing T cells with B cell helper function. J Exp Med 2000;192:1553.
21. Tsuji M, Komatsu N, Kawamoto S, et al. Preferential generation of follicular B helper T cells from Foxp3+ T cells in gut Peyer's patches. Science 2009;323:1488.
22. Litinskiy MB, Nardelli B, Hilbert DM, et al. DCs induce CD40-independent immunoglobulin class switching through BLyS and APRIL. Nat Immunol 2002;3:822.
23. Castigli E, Scott S, Dedeoglu F, et al. Impaired IgA class switching in APRIL-deficient mice. Proc Natl Acad Sci (USA) 2004;101:3903.
24. Fujihashi K, McGhee JR, Lue C, et al. Human appendix B cells naturally express receptors for and respond to interleukin 6 with selective IgA1 and IgA2 synthesis. J Clin Invest 1991;88:248.
25. Fujihashi K, McGhee JR. Th1/Th2/Th3 cells for regulation of mucosal immunity, tolerance and inflammation. In: Mestecky J, Lamm ME, Strober W, et al., eds. Mucosal immunology, vol. 1, 3rd edn. Burlington, VT: Elsevier Academic Press 2005. p. 539.
26. Yamamoto S, Kiyono H, Yamamoto M, et al. A nontoxic mutant of cholera toxin elicits Th2-type responses for enhanced mucosal immunity. Proc Natl Acad Sci (USA) 1997;94:5267.
27. Rappuoli R, Pizza M, Douce G, Dougan G. Structure and mucosal adjuvanticity of cholera and *Escherichia coli* heat-labile enterotoxins. Immunol Today 1999;20:493.
28. Mancini P, Santi PA. Localization of the GM1 ganglioside in the vestibular system using cholera toxin. Hear Res 1993;64:151.
29. van Ginkel FW, Jackson RJ, Yuki Y, McGhee JR. The mucosal adjuvant cholera toxin redirects vaccine proteins into olfactory tissues. J Immunol 2000;165:4778.
30. Agren L, Lowenadler B, Lycke N. A novel concept in mucosal adjuvanticity: the CTA1-DD adjuvant is a B cell-targeted fusion protein that incorporates the enzymatically active cholera toxin A1 subunit. Immunol Cell Biol 1998;76:280.
31. Eriksson AM, Schon KM, Lycke NY. The cholera toxin-derived CTA1-DD vaccine adjuvant administered intranasally does not cause inflammation or accumulate in the nervous tissues. J Immunol 2004;173:3310.
32. Tighe H, Corr M, Roman M, Raz E. Gene vaccination: plasmid DNA is more than just a blueprint. Immunol Today 1998;19:89.
33. Moldoveanu Z, Love-Homan L, Huang WQ, Krieg AM. CpG DNA, a novel immune enhancer for systemic and mucosal immunization with influenza virusd. Vaccine 1998;16:1216.
34. Boyaka PN, Marinaro M, Jackson RJ, et al. IL-12 is an effective adjuvant for induction of mucosal immunity. J Immunol 1999;162:122.
35. Williamson E, Westrich GM, Viney JL. Modulating dendritic cells to optimize mucosal immunization protocols. J Immunol 1999;163:3668.

36. Kataoka K, McGhee JR, Kobayashi R, et al. Nasal Flt3 ligand cDNA elicits CD11c⁺ CD8⁺ dendritic cells for enhanced mucosal immunity. J Immunol 2004;172:3612.

37. Sekine S, Kataoka K, Fukuyama Y, et al. A novel adenovirus expressing Flt3 ligand enhances mucosal immunity by inducing mature nasopharyngeal-associated lymphoreticular tissue dendritic cell migration. J Immunol 2008;180:8126.

38. Fukuyama Y, King JD, Kataoka K, et al. Secretory-IgA antibodies play an important role in the immunity to *Streptococcus pneumoniae*. J Immunol 2010;185:1755.

39. Haq TA, Mason HS, Clements JD, Arntzen CJ. Oral immunization with a recombinant bacterial antigen produced in transgenic plants. Science 1995;268:714.

40. Tacket CO, Mason HS, Losonsky G, et al. Immunogenicity in humans of a recombinant bacterial antigen delivered in a transgenic potato. Nat Med 1998;4:607.

41. Nochi T, Takagi H, Yuki Y, et al. Rice-based mucosal vaccine as a global strategy for cold-chain- and needle-free vaccination. Proc Natl Acad Sci (USA) 2007;104:10986.

42. Nochi T, Yuki Y, Katakai Y, et al. A rice-based oral cholera vaccine induces macaque-specific systemic neutralizing antibodies but does not influence pre-existing intestinal immunity. J Immunol 2009;183:6538.

43. Tokuhara D, Yuki Y, Nochi T, et al. Secretory IgA-mediated protection against *V. cholerae* and heat-labile enterotoxin-producing enterotoxigenic *Escherichia coli* by rice-based vaccine. Proc Natl Acad Sci (USA) 2010;107:8794.

44. Mestecky J, Moro I, Kerr MA, Woof JM. Mucosal immunoglobulins. In: Mestecky J, Lamm ME, Strober W, et al., editors. Mucosal immunology, vol. 1, 3rd edn. Burlington, VT: Elsevier Academic Press; 2005. p. 153.

45. Kauppi-Korkeila M, van Alphen L, Madore D, et al. Mechanism of antibody-mediated reduction of nasopharyngeal colonization by *Haemophilus influenzae* type b studied in an infant rat model. J Infect Dis 1996;174:1337.

46. Burrows PD, Cooper MD. IgA deficiency. Adv Immunol 1997;65:245.

47. Neutra MR, Kreahenbuhl JP. Cellular and molecular basis for antigen transport accross epithelial barriers. In: Mestecky J, Lamm ME, Strober W, et al., editors. Mucosal immunology, vol. 1, 3rd edn. Burlington, VT: Elsevier Academic Press: 2005, p. 111.

48. Burns JW, Siadat-Pajouh M, Krishnaney AA, Greenberg HB. Protective effect of rotavirus VP6-specific IgA monoclonal antibodies that lack neutralizing activity. Science 1996;272:104.

49. Cuff CF, Cebra CK, Rubin DH, Cebra JJ. Developmental relationship between cytotoxic α/β T cell receptor-positive raepithelial lymphocytes and Peyer's patch lymphocytes. Eur J Immunol 1993;23:1333.

50. Allan W, Tabi Z, Cleary A, Doherty PC. Cellular events in the lymph node and lung of mice with influenza. Consequences of depleting CD4⁺ T cells. J Immunol 1990;144:3980.

51. Carding SR, Allan W, Kyes S, et al. Late dominance of the inflammatory process in murine influenza by γ/δ⁺ T cells. J Exp Med 1990;172:1225.

52. Miller CJ, McChesney MB, Lu X, et al. Rhesus macaques previously infected with simian/human immunodeficiency virus are protected from vaginal challenge with pathogenic SIVmac239. J Virol 1997;71:1911.

53. Miller RA. The aging immune system: primer and prospectus. Science 1996;273:70.

54. Fujihashi K, Kiyono H. Mucosal immunosenescence: new developments and vaccines to control infectious diseases. Trends Immunol 2009;30:334.

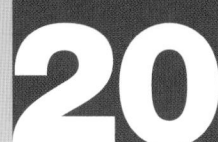

Terry W. Du Clos,
Carolyn Mold

Complement in host deficiencies and diseases

The complement system is an important part of the innate immune system and a major effector mechanism of humoral immunity.[1] It is comprised of a group of serum proteins that are activated through sequential protease-based steps similar to the coagulation, fibrinolytic, and contact pathways. Complement activation is linked to cellular responses by the recognition of cleaved complement proteins by receptors on leukocytes and vascular cells. The components of the complement system, including complement regulatory proteins and receptors, are shown in Table 20.1. The three primary roles of complement in host defense against infection are: (1) to activate an inflammatory response; (2) to opsonize microbial pathogens for phagocytosis and killing; and (3) to lyse susceptible organisms. The complement system also provides a bridge between the innate and adaptive immune responses through receptors on lymphocytes and antigen-presenting cells (APC). Three pathways have been described that share these functions. These pathways differ in their initiation steps and thus are activated in response to different threats. Activation of the complement cascade is amplified at several key steps so that it has the potential to induce a rapid, massive inflammatory response. Complement activation is normally targeted and highly regulated to focus this response. However, complement activation also contributes to tissue injury in infectious, autoimmune, and inflammatory diseases where it is an essential component of the response to immune complex deposition and tissue damage. This chapter gives an overview of the complement system, a review of complement deficiency screening and clinical effects, and a brief discussion of the role of complement in diseases of inflammation and autoimmunity.

Complement pathways

Three pathways of complement activation have been described: the classical, alternative, and lectin pathways (Fig. 20.1). The classical pathway is the complement pathway that is initiated by immunoglobulin M (IgM) and IgG antibody binding to antigen. The classical pathway may also be activated by innate pattern recognition molecules such as the pentraxins, C-reactive protein (CRP) and serum amyloid P (SAP) component,[2] and the membrane-bound lectin, SIGN-R1.[3] It participates with natural IgM in early host defense,[4,5] and provides a mechanism for immune complex and apoptotic cell clearance.[1] The lectin pathway uses most of the classical-pathway components, but is activated by mannan-binding lectin (MBL) and the ficolins, which are lectins that recognize repeating carbohydrate patterns on micro organisms.[6] The alternative pathway is believed to be the most ancient pathway in an evolutionary sense, and also has the broadest recognition ability. The alternative pathway is

activated by surface components of all types of microorganisms, including bacteria, fungi, parasites, viruses, and virus-infected cells. The alternative pathway differs from the classical and lectin pathways in its ability to autoactivate when tightly regulated inhibitory signals are absent. Activation of the alternative pathway is also initiated by properdin, a molecule that binds to pathogens and apoptotic cells.[7] This mechanism promotes its function as an innate and rapid response to infection. The alternative pathway is an important amplification mechanism for classical or lectin-pathway activation, resulting in greater opsonization and generation of the terminal lytic pathway.[8]

The cleavage of C3 to C3a and C3b is central to all three pathways of complement activation. This enzymatic step exposes a highly reactive thioester bond through which C3b covalently attaches to nearby molecules (Fig. 20.2). Activation of C3 to C3b also exposes sites for interactions with other complement proteins and receptors, as discussed below. Recent results have shed new light on the structural basis for C3 activation. In 2006 three papers reported the first X-ray structure of C3b, the activated product C3.[9–11] The results revealed a major conformational change in C3 upon cleavage to C3b that exposes the reactive thioester group as well as cryptic binding sites for complement receptors and regulatory proteins.

Classical pathway

● KEY CONCEPTS

Structural and functional homologies in complement pathways

- Recognition: C1q, MBL, Ficolins
- Initiating enzymes: C1r, C1s, MASP-1, MASP-2, fD
- C3 convertases: C4b2b, C3bBb
- C5 convertases: C4b2b3b, C3bBb3b
- Enzyme subunits of convertases: C2b, Bb
- Assembly subunits: C3b, C4b, C5b
- Anaphylatoxins: C3a, C5a
- MAC subunits: C6, C7, C8, C9
- Regulatory proteins: C4BP, fH, CR1, CR2, MCP, DAF

The classical pathway is usually focused by antibody (or pentraxin) binding to a target antigen. In general, the ability of antibodies to activate complement is: IgM > IgG3 > IgG1 > IgG2 > IgG4. Binding of these antibodies exposes sites in the Fc region for attachment of the first subcomponent of complement, C1q. C1 is a large calcium-dependent complex composed of C1q, and two molecules each of

Table 20.1 Proteins of the complement system

Component	Function
Classical pathway (CP)	
C1q	Part of C1. Binds to surface-bound IgM, IgG, pentraxins, ligands on apoptotic cells to initiate CP activation.
C1r	Part of C1. After auto-activation cleaves C1s.
C1s	Part of C1. After activation by C1r cleaves C4 and C2.
C4	Cleaved by C1s to form C4b, part of the CP and LP C3 and C5 convertases.
C2	Binds to C4b, cleaved by C1s to form C2b, the enzymatic component of the CP and LP C3 and C5 convertases.
Lectin pathway (LP)	
MBL	Recognition component for LP activation. Binds to mannose-rich glycans through C-type lectin domains.
MASP-1	Associated with MBL and ficolins. Cleaves C2, but not C4. Cleaves pro-factor D into factor D.
MASP-2 Ficolins 1-3	Associated with MBL and ficolins. Cleaves C2 and C4. Recognition components for LP activation. Bind to glycans through fibrinogen-like recognition domains.
Alternative pathway (AP)	
C3	Cleaved by C3 convertases to form C3b and C3a. C3b is opsonic, part of the AP C3 convertase, part of all C5 convertases. C3b is further cleaved to opsonic iC3b and CR2 ligands C3dg and C3d. C3a is an anaphylatoxin.
Factor B	Binds to C3b, cleaved by factor D to form Bb, the enzymatic component of the AP C3 and C5 convertases.
Factor D	Cleaves factor B bound to C3b to form AP convertases.
Properdin	Stabilizes AP convertases. Binds to microbial ligands to initiate AP activation.
Membrane attack complex (MAC)	
C5	Cleaved by C5 convertases to form C5b and C5a. C5b initiates MAC formation. C5a is an anaphylatoxin.
C6	Part of the MAC. Binds membranes
C7	Part of the MAC. Binds membranes
C8	Part of the MAC. Initiates pore formation.
C9	Part of the MAC. Polymerizes to form lytic pores.
Soluble regulatory proteins	
C1-INH	Serine protease inhibitor of C1r, C1s, MASP-1, MASP-2, kallikrein, factor XII.
C4BP	Binds C4b. Decay accelerating and cofactor activities for C4b-containing convertases.
Factor H	Binds C3b and polyanions. Has decay-accelerating and cofactor activities for C3b-containing convertases.
Factor I	Cleaves C3b or C4b bound to a cofactor.
Vitronectin	Binds C5b-7, prevents membrane insertion and lysis.
Clusterin	Binds C8 and C9, prevents MAC assembly and lysis.
Membrane regulatory proteins	
CD55 (DAF)	Accelerates decay of C3 and C5 convertases.
CD46 (MCP)	Cofactor for factor I cleavage of C3b and C4b.
CD59	Binds to C8 and C9, prevents MAC assembly and lysis.
Receptors	
CD35 (CR1)	Opsonic receptor for C3b and iC3b. Has decay accelerating and cofactor activity for C3b-containing convertases.
CD21 (CR2)	Receptor for C3dg and C3d. Enhances B cell activation.
CD11b/CD18 (CR3)	Opsonic receptor for iC3b. Leukocyte adhesion integrin.
CD11c/CD18 (CR4)	Opsonic receptor for iC3b. Leukocyte adhesion integrin.
CRIg	Opsonic receptor for iC3b and C3c. Inhibits C5 convertases.
C5aR (CD88)	Proinflammatory and chemotactic receptor for C5a and C5a$_{desarg}$
C5L2	Receptor for C5a and C5a$_{desarg}$. Function not fully defined.
C3aR	Proinflammatory and chemotactic receptor for C3a.

the proenzymes, C1r and C1s. C1q is a 410-kDa protein with six globular heads connected by a collagen-like tail. For IgM, which is pentameric, binding to antigen creates a conformational change that exposes the C1q binding site in the Cμ3 domain. For IgG, at least two closely bound molecules are required to provide multiple attachment points for C1q binding to the Cγ2 domain. Similarly, CRP or SAP molecules bound to ligand provide multiple C1q binding sites resulting in classical pathway activation. IgM, IgG, and CRP bind C1q through its globular head groups.[12] Membrane lipids exposed on apoptotic cells or mitochondrial membranes,

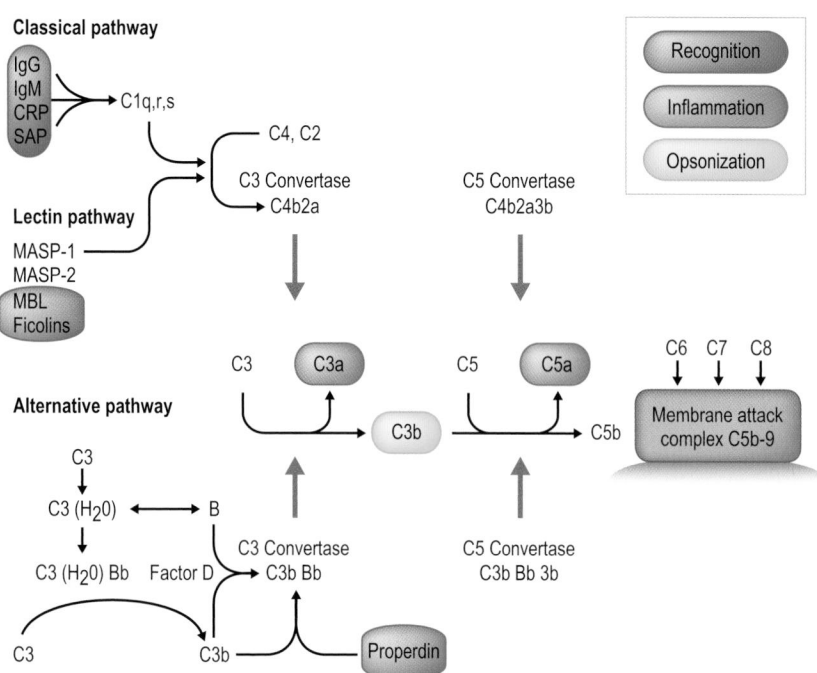

Fig. 20.1 **Overview of the complement pathways indicating components required for recognition, enzymatically active components and complexes, major opsonic, inflammatory and membranolytic products.**

polyanions, nucleic acids, retroviruses, and endotoxins can also activate the classical pathway.

Once C1q binds to an activator through several globular heads, C1r is cleaved and activated by an autocatalytic process.[13] Activated C1r then cleaves and activates C1s, which cleaves circulating C4. C4 and C3 are highly homologous proteins that share an unusual internal thioester bond (see Fig. 20.2).[14] Cleavage of C4 releases the C4a fragment, and exposes the reactive thioester bond in the larger C4b fragment. This allows C4b to attach covalently to nearby target structures, through either amide or ester bonds, to amino or carboxyl groups on proteins, glycoproteins, or polysaccharides on cell surfaces, antibodies, and antigens. The exposed thioester bond is reactive, but susceptible to rapid hydrolysis, and only about 5% of the C4 typically becomes attached to the target. Bound

C4b provides an anchor site for C2 attachment, which is then cleaved by C1s, releasing the smaller fragment, C2a. (A nomenclature change for the C2 fragments designating the smaller fragment C2a and the larger fragment C2b has been agreed upon by the field, and is used here.)

The complex of C4b2b is termed the classical-pathway C3 convertase, because it has the capacity to cleave C3, releasing C3a. The C2b component of the complex contains the active enzymatic site. C3 cleavage is similar to C4 cleavage in that the larger fragment, C3b, contains a thioester site (Fig. 20.2) that can mediate covalent attachment to nearby surface structures, including the antigen, antibody, and the attached C4b. C3 is found at higher concentration in serum than C4, and its cleavage is amplified by the alternative pathway. Thus, efficient complement activation will result in a cluster of multiple bound C3b molecules that can be recognized by cellular receptors. C3b that attaches to C4b within the C3 convertase produces the trimolecular complex C4b2b3b, which is a C5 convertase. Cleavage of C5 produces C5a, which has potent inflammatory activity and C5b, which initiates the formation of the membrane attack complex (MAC)), also known as the terminal complement complex (TCC) (Fig. 20.3).

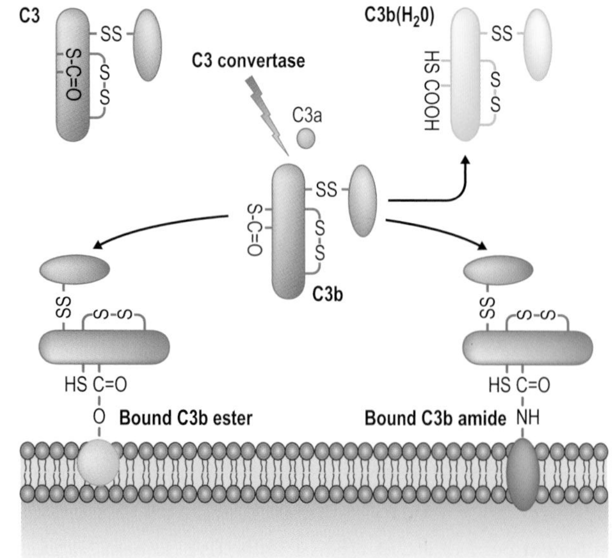

Fig. 20.2 **Exposure and reactivity of the C3 thioester bond.** C3 cleavage by a C3 convertase generates metastable C3b with a reactive thioester. Metastable C3b may be hydrolyzed to form C3b(H$_2$O) or may react with hydroxyl or amino groups to become covalently bound to a surface.

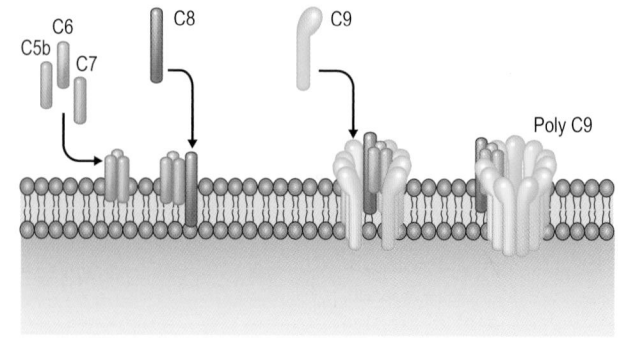

Fig. 20.3 **Sequence of protein interactions in the assembly of the membrane attack complex (MAC).** C5b, generated by C5 convertase cleavage of C5, combines with C6 and C7 to form a hydrophobic complex capable of membrane interaction. Binding of C8 allows the complex to insert further into the membrane and forms a site for C9 polymerization. C9 polymers form the transmembrane pore-associated complement-mediated lysis of membranes.

Lectin pathway

The lectin pathway is similar to the classical pathway, except that it uses pattern recognition molecules, MBL, ficolins-1, 2, and 3, instead of antibody to target activation.[6,15] MBL is structurally similar to C1q, with a collagen-like region and globular heads. The globular heads of MBL are C-type lectin domains specific for repeating carbohydrate structures found on microorganisms. Like C1q, MBL and ficolins are found in complex with serine proteases, MASPs (MBL-associated serum protease), which are structurally and functionally similar to C1r and C1s. MASP-1 and -2 are active proteases, but only MASP-2 cleaves both C4 and C2 to generate C4b2b, the same C3 convertase as the classical pathway. MASP-1 can supplement activation by cleaving C2, but not C4. Two non-proteolytic splice products of the *MASP2* and *MASP1/3* genes, sMAP and MAP-1, compete with MASP-1 and -2 for binding to MBL to regulate the lectin pathway. Subsequent steps in the lectin pathway are identical to the classical pathway. MASP-1 may also contribute to the alternative pathway by cleaving pro-factor D to active factor D.[16]

Alternative pathway

The alternative pathway uses proteins that are structurally and functionally homologous to those of the classical pathway, but this pathway has unique features that play three important roles in the complement cascade. The surveillance role of the alternative pathway is mediated by a low level of spontaneous activation that results from the hydrolysis of the C3 thioester bond.[1] Hydrolyzed C3, $C3(H_2O)$, assumes a conformation similar to that of C3b and can bind factor B (homologous to C2), which is cleaved by factor D (homologous to C1s) to form a fluid-phase C3 convertase. This convertase cleaves C3 to generate C3b, which can covalently bind to nearby structures and provide the basis for a bound C3 convertase (C3bBb). Because C3b is both a part of this enzyme and a product of the reaction, a positive feedback loop is formed that rapidly deposits more C3b. This low level of activation is tightly regulated on host cells and tissues by plasma and membrane bound complement regulatory proteins, and it is the lack of regulation that restricts alternative-pathway activation to microbial targets. The plasma protein factor H (fH) is particularly important in controlling alternative-pathway activation both in the fluid phase and on "non-activating" surfaces, which recruit fH through its binding sites for polyanions including sialic acid and glycosaminoglycans. "Activating" surfaces, such as microbial polysaccharides, lipopolysaccharides, and glycoproteins, provide C3b attachment sites that are protected from regulatory proteins. Similar to the classical pathway, the alternative-pathway C5 convertase (C3bBb3b) is formed when C3b attaches to the C3 convertase. The alternative-pathway C3 and C5 convertases are stabilized by properdin (factor P), for which this pathway was originally named.

More recently, an additional role for properdin in initiating alternative-pathway activation was rediscovered. Properdin is a pattern recognition molecule with specificity for microbes and damaged cells. Once bound, properdin can recruit fluid-phase C3b, independent of covalent binding, and thereby provide a platform for the assembly of the alternative-pathway convertase.[7] Thus, properdin binding can direct alternative-pathway activation, similar to MBL in the lectin pathway. Properdin binding to certain *Neisseria* species potently activates the alternative pathway and this may account for the susceptibility of properdin-deficient individuals to infection with *Neisseria meningitidis*.

The third important role of the alternative pathway is the amplification of C3b deposition and C5 convertase generation that is initiated by the classical or lectin pathways.[8] This function of the alternative pathway is critical in complement-mediated pathology, as it increases the generation of C5a and the MAC, the most inflammatory components of the system. It is the amplification role of the alternative pathway that makes it a therapeutic target.

Membrane attack complex

All three complement pathways merge with the cleavage of C5 into C5a and C5b. Although C5 is structurally homologous to C3 and C4, it lacks the internal thioester bond that allows covalent attachment to surfaces. C3a and C5a are also structurally homologous and as described below are the most potent proinflammatory mediators of the complement system. C5b initiates the formation of the MAC (Fig. 20.3), a complex of C5b, C6, C7, C8, and multiple C9 molecules. This complex, as indicated by its name, penetrates membrane bilayers to form pores that disrupt the osmotic barrier, leading to swelling and lysis of susceptible cells. Lysis of antibody-sensitized erythrocytes by the MAC is the basis of the hemolytic complement assay or CH_{50}. C5b initiates the formation of the MAC without further proteolytic steps. C5b binds to C6, and this complex binds to C7. The C5b67 complex is lipophilic and associates with cell membranes, if available, or with serum lipoproteins. Once bound to a membrane, C5b67 recruits C8 and the complex penetrates more deeply into the membrane. However, complete lysis requires C9, a pore-forming molecule with homology to perforin, a protein used by cytotoxic T cells and natural killer cells for killing virus-infected targets. The complex of C5b678 forms a nidus for C9 binding and polymerization. Although complement-dependent lysis of bacteria can be observed *in vitro*, most pathogens have evolved mechanisms to circumvent this activity of complement.[17] Sublytic MAC contributes to the deleterious effects of complement activation in inflammatory diseases.[18]

Regulation of complement activation

The complement cascade is rapidly activated and highly amplified by the generation of C3 and C5 convertases. There are three main levels of control that serve to limit the potential harm that uncontrolled complement activation might cause. These three levels are: (1) the initiation step in the classical and lectin pathways; (2) the C3 and C5 convertases of all three pathways; and (3) the assembly of the MAC. Both soluble and membrane-bound regulatory proteins serve these functions, which help terminate complement activation as well as direct it to appropriate targets.[19]

C1 esterase inhibitor

C1 esterase inhibitor (C1-INH) is a serum glycoprotein and a serine proteinase inhibitor (serpin). C1-INH covalently binds to activated C1r and C1s, irreversibly inhibiting their activity and thereby limiting classical-pathway activation. C1-INH inactivation of C1r and C1s also removes them from the C1 complex, exposing sites on the collagen-like region of C1q. C1-INH also inhibits MASP-1 and -2, kallikrein, factor XIa, XIIa and plasmin of the lectin pathway and the contact, coagulation, and fibrinolytic systems. Inherited deficiency of C1-INH is the basis of hereditary angioedema, a disease characterized by recurrent attacks of subcutaneous or submucosal edema (Chapter 42).[20]

Regulators of the C3 and C5 convertases

The C3 and C5 convertases are central to the generation of the inflammatory and opsonic products of complement activation and are highly regulated by fluid-phase and membrane-bound regulatory proteins. The convertases themselves are complexes of two or three components and one mechanism of regulation is the dissociation of these complexes. This type of regulation is termed "decay acceleration." A second mechanism of regulation is the enzymatic inactivation of the C4b and C3b components of the convertases (Fig. 20.4). This is accomplished by the plasma enzyme factor I, which however only acts on C4b or C3b in complex with one of several regulatory proteins. The binding of regulatory proteins to C4b or C3b to enable factor I cleavage is termed "cofactor activity."

Factor I

Factor I (C3b inactivator, C3bINA) cleaves C4b and C3b into products that are recognized by specific cellular receptors, as discussed below. The sequential cleavages of C3b by factor I to iC3b and C3dg is depicted in Fig. 20.4. C4b is cleaved in an analogous manner to C4d. (The iC4b intermediate is found only transiently.) The regulatory proteins that facilitate this cleavage by cofactor activity and those that inactivate C3 and C5 convertases by decay-accelerating activity are not enzymes, but are members of a family of structurally related proteins encoded within the regulators of complement activation (RCA) genetic locus. This family is characterized by a repeating structure that consists of subunits, termed complement control protein repeats (CCP) of about 50 amino acids with a conserved pattern of disulfide bonds.

Soluble regulatory proteins, C4b-binding protein and factor H

C4b-binding protein (C4bp) and factor H(fH) are fluid-phase regulatory proteins with both decay-accelerating and cofactor activities. C4bp is multimeric, being composed of seven identical subunits, each containing eight CCPs. fH is a single-chain protein composed entirely of 20 CCPs. C4bp is specific for C4b and the C4b-containing convertases of the classical pathway (C4b2b, C4b2b3b), whereas fH regulates C3b and C3b-containing convertases (C3bBb, C3bBb3b, C4b2b3b). fH is essential for regulation of C3 "tickover," and fH deficiency results in

acquired deficiency of C3. Additional binding sites on fH that recognize polyanions such as sialic acid and glycosaminoglycans provide targeted regulation of alternative-pathway activation on surfaces.[21-23]

Membrane regulatory proteins, CD55 (DAF), CD46 (MCP), CD35 (CR1), and CRIT

The RCA family also includes the membrane regulatory proteins decay-accelerating factor (CD55, DAF), membrane cofactor protein (CD46, MCP), and complement receptors CR1 (CD35) and CR2 (CD21).[24] CD55 (DAF) and CD46 (MCP), as their names imply, have decay-accelerating and cofactor activities that prevent complement activation on cell membranes. Each has an extracellular domain composed exclusively of four CCPs. CD55, a glycophosphatidylinositol (GPI)-anchored protein, and CD46, a transmembrane protein, are widely distributed on cells in contact with the blood, with the exception that erythrocytes lack CD46. Soluble CD55 is also found in most biological fluids. Both protect cells from complement-mediated lysis. CD35 (CR1) has decay-accelerating and cofactor activity and is a receptor for bound C3b. The function of CD35 as a complement receptor is discussed later in the chapter.

Complement C2 receptor inhibitor trispanning (CRIT), is a non-RCA membrane regulator of the classical pathway. CRIT was originally identified on Schistosoma and Trypanasoma parasites and later found to be widely expressed on human tissues and blood cells, except for neutrophils and erythrocytes.[25] CRIT competes with C2 for binding to C4b, blocking the formation of the classical-pathway C3 convertase.

Properdin

In contrast to the regulatory proteins discussed above, properdin (factor P) stabilizes C3 and C5 convertases of the alternative pathway, increasing their activity. Properdin is found as noncovalently linked dimers, trimers, tetramers, and larger species composed of identical 56-kDa chains. The majority of the protein consists of a series of six thrombospondin type 1 modules. Properdin binds to C3b and to Bb, preventing the spontaneous or induced decay of the alternative-pathway C3 and C5 convertases. Its multimeric structure promotes interaction with clustered C3b. As discussed above, bound properdin can recruit C3b to provide a site of assembly for the alternative-pathway C3 convertase.[7]

Regulators of the MAC

The MAC is also regulated by both fluid-phase and membrane regulatory proteins.[1,24]

Soluble MAC inhibitors, vitronectin, and clusterin

Soluble hydrophobic proteins can block the incorporation of MAC into membranes. Two well-characterized proteins with this activity are vitronectin (S protein), and clusterin (SP-40,40, apolipoprotein J). Vitronectin is found in the serum and extracellular matrix and binds to C5b-7. C8 and C9 can still bind to the complex, but membrane insertion and C9 polymerization are prevented. Soluble complexes of vitronectin and C5b-9 are found in the serum during complement activation and an enzyme-linked immunosorbent assay (ELISA) specific for this complex has been used to monitor activation of the MAC. Clusterin is found in the serum, in the male reproductive tract, and on

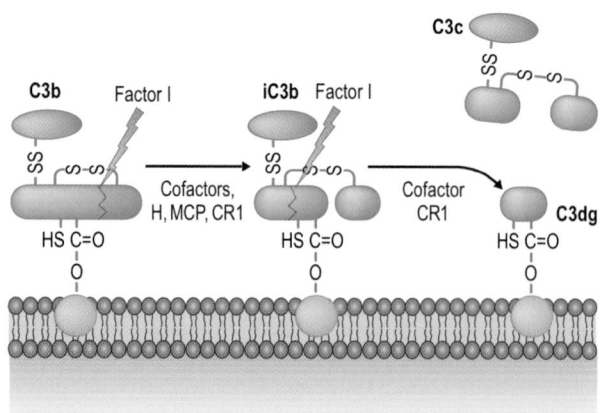

Fig. 20.4 Factor I-dependent cleavage of C3 showing the structures of the products and the required cofactors.

endothelial cells of normal arteries. It is also associated with amyloid deposits, including β amyloid in Alzheimer's disease. Clusterin forms an inactive complex with C5b-9, preventing membrane insertion.

Membrane MAC inhibitor, CD59

The primary membrane-bound inhibitor of MAC is CD59.[24] CD59 is a GPI-anchored protein found on most cells. CD59 binds to C8 and C9, preventing the incorporation and polymerization of C9.

Complement receptors

Many of the biological effects of complement activation are mediated by cellular receptors for fragments of complement proteins. These include receptors for the small soluble complement fragments, C5a and C3a, and receptors for bound complement fragments, C1q and cleaved forms of C4b and C3b. Receptors for bound C3 are specific for not only C3b, but further breakdown products generated by the enzymatic processing by factor I in conjunction with the cofactor proteins mentioned above. The breakdown of C3 and intermediate products are shown in Fig. 20.4 and the receptors for these components in Fig. 20.5.

C1q receptors

C1q shares the same general structure with a family of proteins termed 'soluble defense collagens' that includes the "collectins" (MBL, surfactant proteins A and D, conglutinin), and the ficolins. These proteins have collagen-like regions associated with globular recognition domains. The collectins have C-type lectin

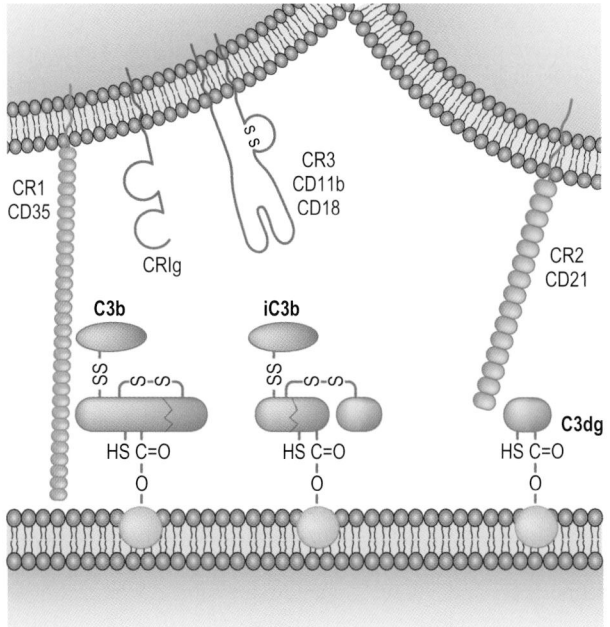

Fig. 20.5 Receptors for bound C3b and its cleavage products. Receptors shown are CD35 and CD21 composed of CCP (SCR) subunits, CD11b/CD18 (CR3), a β2 integrin, and CRIg with 1 or 2 Ig domains. The specificities of the receptors are: CD35 for C3b, C4b > C3b; CRIg for iC3b > 3b; CD11b/CD18 for iC3b; CD21 for C3dg, C3d > C3b. CD11c/CD18 (CR4) is similar to CD11b/CD18 and is not shown. Receptors are not drawn to scale. Their molecular weights are listed in Table 20.1.

carbohydrate recognition domains. Ficolins also recognize acetyl groups on carbohydrates and other molecules using fibrinogen-like recognition domains. The globular head groups of C1q are not lectins, but rather bind to amino acid motifs on IgG, IgM, and pentraxins. In general, this group of proteins broadly recognizes pathogen-associated carbohydrate patterns and damaged or apoptotic cells. Reported direct effects of C1q and other defense collagens on leukocytes include enhanced phagocytosis, respiratory burst, and regulation of cytokine responses. Several cell surface proteins that are important for these activities of C1q or other soluble defense collagens have been proposed, including CD93 (C1qRp), CD35 (CR1), α2β1 integrin, calreticulin in complex with CD91, gC1qbp, and SIPRα. However, none of these have been definitively established as receptors in the classical sense.[26]

Complement receptor 1 (CD35, CR1)

There are five identified receptors for bound fragments of C3 and/or C4. CD35 (CR1) is a large protein composed of a linear string of CCPs, a transmembrane region, and a short intracytoplasmic domain. Different allelic forms of CD35 are found, the most common being composed of 30 CCPs with a molecular weight of 190 kDa. These CCPs are organized into groups of seven, creating structures termed long homologous repeats (LHRs), each of which contains a single binding site. The predominant allele of CD35 contains two binding sites for C3b, one for C4b and one for C1q. CR1 is found on human erythrocytes, monocytes and macrophages, neutrophils, B lymphocytes, a small percentage of T lymphocytes, eosinophils, follicular dendritic cells (FDC), and glomerular podocytes.

CD35 on primate erythrocytes provides a noninflammatory mechanism for clearing soluble immune complexes from the circulation. Although the number of receptors on each erythrocyte is low, the large number of erythrocytes provides the major pool of CR1 in the circulation. Soluble immune complexes that fix complement attach quickly to erythrocytes in the circulation, bypassing monocytes and neutrophils. These erythrocyte-bound complexes are taken to the liver where they are transferred to Kupffer cells expressing Fc and complement receptors and destroyed. The erythrocytes exit into the circulation to pick up more immune complexes. This clearance pathway is impaired in patients with systemic lupus erythematosus (SLE) due to decreased complement in the circulation, decreased CD35 on erythrocytes, and saturated Fc receptors in the liver and spleen.

CD35 on monocytes and neutrophils promotes binding of microbes with bound C3b and C4b, facilitating their phagocytosis through Fc receptors. CD35 can directly mediate uptake of microbes when phagocytic cells have been activated by chemokines or integrin interactions with matrix proteins. CD35 is a member of the RCA family and has decay-accelerating and cofactor activity in addition to its function as a receptor. It differs from the membrane regulatory proteins DAF (CD55) and MCP (CD46) in its ability to bind to C3b and C4b extrinsically (on targets other than the cell expressing it), and in its cofactor activity for C3b processing. CD35 is the most effective cofactor for factor I(fI) cleavage of C3b and iC3b to the smallest covalently bound fragment, C3dg. C3dg is the major ligand for CR2 on B lymphocytes, described below. The cofactor activity of CD35 on B lymphocytes can process bound C3b to C3dg, facilitating binding to CR2 and lowering the threshold for B-cell activation.[27]

Complement receptor 2 (CD21, CR2)

CD21 (CR2) is also an RCA family protein composed of 15–16 CCPs. CD21 has a limited range of expression that includes B lymphocytes, FDC, and some epithelial cells. CD21 is specific for the smallest covalently bound C3 fragments, C3dg and C3d, and has weaker binding to iC3b. CD21 is also the Epstein–Barr virus receptor on B lymphocytes and nasopharyngeal epithelial cells and binds to CD23, a low-affinity IgE receptor.

CD21 on B lymphocytes serves a co-stimulatory role. It is expressed on mature B cells as a complex with CD19 and CD81 (TAPA-1). Co-ligation of CD21 and the B-cell antigen receptor induces the phosphorylation of CD19, activating several signaling pathways and strongly amplifying B-cell responses to antigen. This role of CD21 is believed to contribute to the strong adjuvant effect produced by attaching C3d to antigen.[27]

Complement receptors 3 and 4

CR3 and CR4 are the β2-integrins commonly known as CD11b/CD18 (Mac-1) and CD11c/CD18. β2-integrins are large heterodimers found on neutrophils and monocytes with multiple roles in adhesion to endothelium and matrix molecules as well as direct recognition of microbial pathogens. The binding activities of β2-integrins are regulated by cellular activation often through chemokine receptors. Both CD11b/CD18 and CD11c/CD18 are expressed primarily on neutrophils, monocytes, and natural killer cells and bind to iC3b and, to a lesser extent, C3b. CD11b/CD18 has been studied more extensively than CD11c/CD18. CD11b/CD18 expression, clustering, and conformation are all rapidly upregulated by chemokine activation of neutrophils, leading to increased responses to ligand. CR3 plays an essential role in neutrophil attachment to and migration through activated endothelium to sites in inflammation and in the regulation of neutrophil apoptosis. Deficiency of the β2-chain (CD18) results in leukocyte adhesion deficiency, characterized by recurrent pyogenic infections and defects in inflammatory and phagocytic responses. Complement receptors CD11b/CD18 and CD11c/CD18 provide an essential function for the removal of microbial pathogens following complement activation, since C3b processing often occurs rapidly following deposition.[28]

Complement receptor of the immunoglobulin superfamily (CRIg)

CRIg is a receptor for iC3b and C3b found on Kupffer cells in the liver as well as other tissue macrophages, but absent from splenic macrophages, peripheral blood cells, bone marrow-derived macrophages, and monocyte/macrophage cell lines.[29] Two alternative-spliced forms of human CRIg were identified with one and two Ig domains. The mouse receptor has a single Ig domain. CRIg is thought to function in the removal of C3b or iC3b-opsonized particles from the circulation by the liver.

C5a and C3a receptors

During complement activation, the homologous proteins C3 and C5 are each cleaved near the amino-terminus of the α–chains to release a soluble peptide fragment of approximately 8 kDa. These fragments are designated C3a and C5a. C5a may also be generated locally by direct cleavage of C5 by thrombin or leukocyte proteases.[30] C3a and C5a are termed "anaphylatoxins"

Table 20.2 Cellular targets and effects of complement anaphylatoxins

	Target	Effects
C3a, C5a	Mast cells, basophils	Degranulation, release of vasoactive amines: contraction of smooth muscle, increased vascular permeability
C3a	Eosinophils	Chemotaxis, degranulation
C5a	Endothelium	Increased adhesion of leukocytes, chemokine and cytokine synthesis
C5a	Neutrophils, monocytes/macrophages, eosinophils, basophils, astrocytes	Chemotaxis
C5a	Neutrophils, monocytes/macrophages	Priming: activation of receptors, assembly of NADPH oxidase; activation: degranulation, respiratory burst
C5a	Resident macrophages	Regulation of FcγR expression (↑activating, ↓ inhibitory)
C5a	Hepatocyte	Acute phase protein synthesis
C3a, C5a	Lymphocytes, antigen-presenting cells	Regulation of T cell responses to antigen

because of their ability to increase vascular permeability, contract smooth muscle, and trigger the release of vasoactive amines from mast cells and basophils. C5a is 10- to 100-fold more active than C3a. These peptides are also chemotactic: C5a is specific for neutrophils, monocytes, and macrophages, whereas C3a is specific for mast cells and eosinophils. Other biological activities of complement anaphylatoxins are summarized in Table 20.2.[1,31]

Structurally the anaphylatoxins are compact structures consisting of multiple helices cross-linked by disulfide bonds with more flexible carboxy-terminal regions. The C-terminal peptide of C3a interacts with the C3aR and can reproduce C3a agonist activity. In contrast, C5a interacts with the C5aR at multiple sites. Serum carboxypeptidases cleave the C-terminal arginine from C3a and C5a producing the des Arg forms. This inactivates C3a; however, C5a$_{desarg}$ retains much of its biological activity. The C5aR (CD88 and C5L2) and the C3aR are rhodopsin-type receptors with seven transmembrane-spanning domains coupled to G-protein signaling pathways.[32] C5aR is expressed at high levels on neutrophils and is also found on macrophages, mast cells, basophils, smooth muscle cells, and endothelial cells. When C5a is generated locally, for example in an extravascular site of infection, it helps induce an acute local inflammatory response including vasodilation, edema, neutrophil chemotaxis, and activation of neutrophils and macrophages for enhanced phagocytosis and killing.[32] The inflammatory activities of C5a may also contribute to complement-mediated pathology in conditions such as sepsis, acute respiratory distress syndrome, and ischemia–reperfusion injury, making the C5a–C5aR interaction an attractive therapeutic target.

The C5L2 receptor binds to both C5a and C5a$_{desarg}$. C5L2 was initially believed to be a default or decoy receptor for C5a, because it is uncoupled from G proteins. Genetic deletion of C5L2 (Gpr77-/-) in mice resulted in enhanced neutrophil infiltration and cytokine production in the pulmonary Arthus reaction, supporting an anti-inflammatory role for C5L2 in immune complex disease where genetic deletion of C5aR is fully protective.[33] However, studies in a cecal ligation and puncture (CLP) model of sepsis found increased survival in mice lacking either C5aR or C5L2.[34] The results suggest an active pro-inflammatory role for C5L2 that requires C5a and results in the release of the inflammatory signal, high-mobility group box-1 protein (HMGB1) from phagocytic cells. Thus, both C5aR and C5L2 may contribute synergistically to harmful inflammatory events during sepsis.

Complement in host defense and immunity

Complement in host defense

Complement activation provides a coordinated response to infection that results in the opsonization of microbial pathogens and the attraction and activation of phagocytic cells to kill them. Complement-dependent opsonization is of greatest importance in infections with encapsulated extracellular bacteria, and individuals with deficiencies in antibody production, neutrophil function, or C3 share increased susceptibility to these organisms, including *Streptococcus pneumoniae* and *Haemophilus influenzae*. MBL deficiency is also associated with recurrent pyogenic infections in young children. In general, activation of complement by natural antibody or MBL results in C3b and iC3b deposition on these pathogens, overcoming the anti-phagocytic effects of the capsule. Phagocytic cells ingest and kill the organisms using CD35, CD11b/CD18, and CD11c/CD18 receptors in conjunction with other innate and Fc receptors. C5aR signaling activates these receptors, leading to increased phagocytosis. Gram-negative bacteria are susceptible to complement-dependent lysis. This is evident in the increased incidence of disseminated neisserial infection in individuals deficient in C3, any of the MAC components, or properdin, as discussed below.

Complement in inflammation

An essential function of complement in host defense is the coordination of the local inflammatory response. C5a is the most potent complement product in this activity.[32] Sublytic deposition of MAC on endothelial cells and platelets and C3a interaction with the C3aR also contribute to the proinflammatory effects of complement activation. As discussed below, these potent inflammatory fragments of complement, when generated in high amounts or targeted inappropriately, result in many of the disease-related deleterious effects of complement. Local production of C5a at a site of infection occurs either through local complement activation or through direct cleavage of C5 by tissue macrophages or thrombin.[30] This C5a is released and sets up a chemotactic gradient for neutrophils and macrophages. In addition, C5a activates endothelial cells to express P-selectin and synthesize chemokines, including IL-8. Interaction of C5a with mast cells releases vasoactive amines, increasing endothelial permeability. Neutrophils and macrophages are "primed" by interaction of C5a with its receptor. Priming includes enhancement of chemotaxis, activation of complement receptors for phagocytosis,[28]

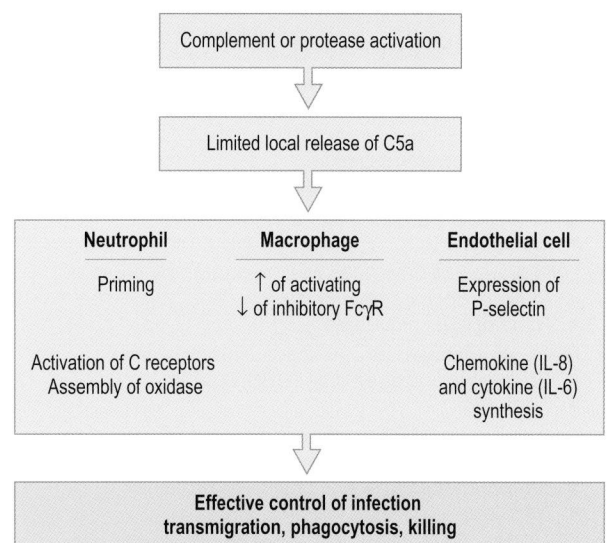

Fig. 20.6 **C5a in local host defense.**

increased expression of activating FcγR,[35] and assembly of the NADPH-oxidase that is required for effective killing of microbes after phagocytosis. C5a also prevents neutrophil apoptosis, prolonging survival and contributing to local accumulation. Together these actions result in the attraction and activation of potent anti-microbial cells and resolution of infection (Fig. 20.6).

Pathogen evasion of complement

Further evidence of the host defense function of complement is the association of complement evasion strategies with virulence. Pathogenic Gram-negative bacteria, such as Salmonella, have lipopolysaccharides with long O-polysaccharide side chains that promote rapid shedding of the MAC and prevent its insertion into the cell membrane. *Neisseria* species have several factor H-binding components that help restrict alternative-pathway activation and protect against lysis. Group A and B streptococci and *S. pneumoniae* have cell surface components (M protein, Bac or beta, PspC, Hic) that bind to factor H and/or C4bp, restricting complement activation. Other organisms, including type 3 group B streptococci, elaborate sialic acid-containing capsules or cell walls to limit alternative-pathway activation.

Although complement deficiencies are not generally associated with viral infections, the importance of complement in host defense against viruses is suggested by the multiple strategies used by viruses to evade complement. Several viruses produce complement regulatory proteins, including vaccinia virus complement control protein, and herpes virus glycoprotein C, which facilitate breakdown of C3b and C4b. Some viruses, such as human immunodeficiency virus (HIV), incorporate complement regulatory proteins into the viral envelope, a strategy that is also used by other pathogens, such as Schistosoma.

There are also many examples of complement receptors and membrane regulatory proteins being exploited as receptors for pathogens to invade cells. Examples of these include strategies of direct pathogen binding to receptors as well as deposition of C3 fragments followed by invasion through host C3 receptors.[17]

Role of complement in adaptive immunity

Over the past 10 years there has been renewed interest in the role of the innate immune system in adaptive immune responses.[1] The importance of complement in humoral immunity has been recognized since the observation that complement depletion of mice prior to immunization decreased antibody responses to thymus-dependent antigens. Further studies have shown that complement receptors CR1 (CD35) and CR2 (CD21) are also required. In humans these receptors are found together on B lymphocytes and FDC. CD35 is also expressed on a number of other cell types (described above), including erythrocytes and phagocytic cells.

Effects of complement on the humoral immune response

Results obtained by experimental manipulation of C3, C4 and their receptors in mouse models indicate roles for these complement components at multiple levels in the humoral immune

response.[27] One caveat regarding these studies is that in the mouse CD35 and CD21 are alternative splice products of the same gene, and genetically deficient animals lack both receptors. In humans CD35 and CD21 are encoded by separate genes. The first role of CD35/CD21 is in B-cell development, indicated by a pronounced defect in B-1 cell development in CD35/CD21-deficient mice. B-1 cells are generally found outside lymphoid follicles, have a restricted repertoire, and are essential in the production of natural antibodies to pathogens, such as *S. pneumoniae*, and to self antigens exposed on damaged cells, such as phosphatidylcholine and DNA. Although the mechanism of this defect in CD35/CD21-deficient mice is not fully understood, these mice have an altered repertoire of natural antibody and B-1 cells.[36] Decreased natural antibody may contribute to susceptibility to infection and autoimmune disease in hereditary complement deficiency (discussed below).

A second role for complement in the antibody response is the well-described function of CD21 as a co-receptor for the mature B-cell response to antigen.[27] As described above, CD21 is associated with the signaling complex of CD19 and CD81 (TAPA-1) in the B-cell membrane. Co-ligation of CD21 with the B-cell antigen receptor occurs naturally when the antigen activates complement and covalently binds C3dg. This co-ligation of the B-cell receptor with CD21 greatly decreases the threshold for B-cell activation and blocks Fas-initiated apoptosis of B cells. B cells activated by complement-opsonized antigen have increased ability to present antigen as well as survival and proliferation during encounters with T-dependent antigens.

The expression of CD35 and CD21 on FDC is also important in the antibody response. FDC trap antigen in the germinal centers and provide selection of somatically mutated high-affinity B-cell clones. Antigen trapped on FDC also provides a source of long-term stimulation for maintenance of memory B cells. FDC use complement receptors (CD35 and CD21) and FcγR to trap and retain antigen for these functions. Expression of CD21 on both FDC and B cells is required for effective affinity maturation of the antibody response and for the development and maintenance of memory B cells.

Complement and T-cell activation

Recent studies in primary pulmonary infection with influenza indicate that C3-deficient mice have a defect in influenza-specific CD4 and CD8 T-cell priming.[37] CR1/2 deficiency had no effect. The mechanism is unknown, but may be more efficient uptake and presentation of C3-opsonized virus by APC through CR3 and CR4 or stimulation of T-cell responses through the C3aR.

Co-stimulation of human T cells *in vitro* through CD3 and CD46 leads to the development of T cells with a regulatory phenotype characterized by synthesis of IL-10 in the absence of other Th2 cytokines (IL-2, -4) (Chapter 10).[38] The induction of regulatory T cells was seen in response to both anti-CD46 cross-linking and natural ligands (C3b dimers, streptococcal M protein).

CD55-deficient mice showed enhanced T-cell responses to immunization and increased T-cell-dependent autoimmune disease. These effects were complement-dependent and apparently involve the loss of CD55 regulation of local complement synthesis by APC during cognate interactions with T cells. One postulated mechanism is that CD55 inhibits the generation of C3a and C5a by APC, preventing their interactions with C3aR and C5aR on T cells.[39] Complement anaphylatoxins, C3a and C5a, have many important effects in inflammatory diseases that include attraction and activation of inflammatory cells, as well as regulation of APC and T-cell responses. Examples of these will be discussed in the sections below.

Role of complement in clearance of apoptotic cells

Damaged tissue and dead and dying cells activate complement through several pathways. This may increase local inflammation and injury, as in ischemia/reperfusion injury and hemolytic–uremic syndrome (HUS) (discussed below). Complement activation by apoptotic cells contributes to their opsonization and clearance, and may prevent the development of autoimmunity. The deleterious consequences of complement activation following tissue damage are mainly attributable to alternative-pathway-dependent generation of C5a and the MAC,[8,40] whereas the beneficial effects are dependent on early classical-pathway components and innate recognition molecules.[41]

Necrosis, as occurs following ischemic tissue injury, exposes phospholipids and mitochondrial proteins that activate complement directly or indirectly. The pathways are different depending on the tissue involved.[40] For example, renal reperfusion injury appears to be initiated by the alternative pathway, possibly secondary to the loss of regulatory proteins on tubular epithelial cells. Intestinal ischemia–reperfusion injury is initiated by natural IgM antibodies and requires both the classical pathway for initiation, and the alternative pathway for injury. MBL and CRP-initiated complement activation have been proposed to contribute to myocardial reperfusion injury after coronary artery ligation.

Apoptotic cells are recognized by multiple receptors and opsonins.[41,42] The association between early classical-pathway deficiencies and systemic lupus erythematosus (SLE) (see below and Chapter 50) has been attributed to a failure of complement-dependent opsonization, resulting in accumulation of apoptotic cells and released autoantigens. Support for this hypothesis is provided by studies of mice deficient in C1q, IgM, or SAP, all of which develop autoantibodies against phospholipid and nuclear antigens characteristic of SLE, and by the therapeutic effect of CRP in mouse models of SLE.[2] The role of complement in apoptotic cell recognition and uptake by macrophages is depicted in Fig. 20.7. MBL, C1q, and SP-D bind to apoptotic cells and facilitate clearance through direct binding to cellular receptors as well as complement activation.[42] Natural IgM antibodies, CRP, and SAP bind to phospholipids exposed on late apoptotic cells. All three proteins can also activate the classical pathway generating C1q, C4b, C3b, and iC3b ligands for complement receptors. CRP and SAP also directly opsonize apoptotic cells for uptake through Fcγ receptors.[43] Phagocytosis of apoptotic cells generally induces anti-inflammatory cytokines, transforming growth factor-β (TGF-β) and IL-10.[44,45]

Targeted activation of complement for opsonization

Interestingly, CRP and SAP also bind complement regulatory proteins, factor H and C4bp, which helps to limit complement activation to the deposition of opsonic components with little or no lysis or generation of C5a.[45,46] This type of complement activation was also observed on acrosome-activated spermatozoa. In this case the classical pathway was activated by CRP from follicular fluid, resulting in bound C3b and iC3b that are proposed to bind complement receptors on the egg and facilitate fertilization. Riley-Vargas, et al. have proposed the acronym TRACS (targeted and restricted activation of the complement system) for this type of limited complement activation that occurs as part of normal processes such as the acrosome reaction, and the recognition and removal of ischemic tissue and apoptotic cells.[47]

Complement deficiencies

Genetics and incidence

Complete genetic deficiencies of complement proteins are rare, with an estimated combined prevalence of 0.03% for any inherited complete deficiency (excluding MBL deficiency) in the general population.[48,49] For most components, inheritance is autosomal and expression is codominant, so complete deficiency is homozygous recessive and heterozygotes express half levels. There are two C4 genes (C4A and C4B), so a range of partial deficiencies may be observed. All cases of C1-INH deficiency have been heterozygous, and properdin deficiency is X-linked. MBL is found in multiple allelic forms with different levels of expression ranging from 5 ng/mL to more than 5 μg/mL in plasma. Deficiencies specific to the lectin pathway are not detected by the screening assays described below, but may be determined by specific assays.[6] A 10% incidence of MBL deficiency and a single case of MASP-2 deficiency have been described.

The most common clinical presentations of patients with complement deficiencies are recurrent infections with encapsulated bacteria, recurrent neisserial infections, and systemic autoimmune disease (Table 20.3). Populations with these disease manifestations have a much higher incidence of complement deficiency. For example, in white patients with SLE, the incidence of C2 deficiency is nearly 1%, 100-fold higher than in the general population. Screening of patients with autoimmune disease for complement deficiencies is useful, as these individuals are at higher risk for certain disease manifestations and may be at greater risk for infectious complications. Complement deficiency is found in as many as 20% of patients with recurrent disseminated neisserial infections. Evaluation of complement function is highly recommended in patients

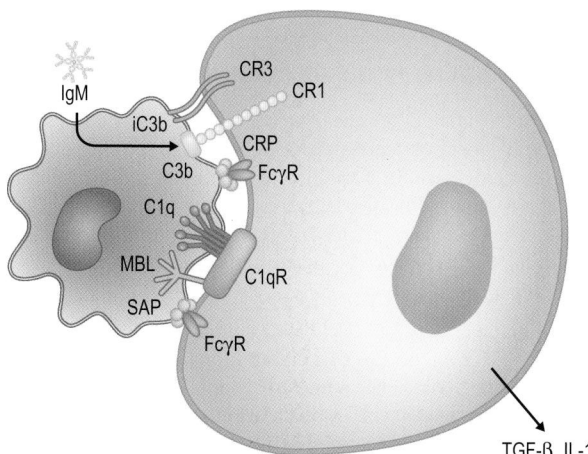

Fig. 20.7 Pathways of opsonization of apoptotic cells by complement. Innate recognition of apoptotic cells by natural immunoglobulin M (IgM), C-reactive protein (CRP), serum amyloid P (SAP), C1q, and mannose-binding lectin (MBL) is shown. Each reaction activates complement leading to opsonization by C3b and iC3b. In addition, C1q and MBL bind to collectin receptors, and CRP and SAP bind to FcγR on macrophages. Cytokine responses to apoptotic cells opsonized by complement include the anti-inflammatory cytokines, transforming growth factor-β (TGF-β) and interleukin-10 (IL-10).

Table 20.3 Clinical effects of genetic complement deficiency

Deficient component	Resulting defect	Clinical associations
C1q, C1r, C1s, C4, C2	Inability to activate the classical pathway	Systemic lupus erythematosus
Factor D, properdin	Inability to activate the alternative pathway	Infection, *Neisseria meningitidis*
MBL, MASP-2	Decreased or absent ability to activate the lectin pathway	Recurrent childhood infection, pyogenic bacteria
C3	Lack of opsonization inability to generate C5a and form the MAC	Recurrent childhood infection *N. meningitidis*, *Streptococcus pneumoniae*, other encapsulated bacteria, autoimmune disease
Factor H, factor I, NeF	Lack of regulation of fluid-phase C3 convertases, severe acquired C3 deficiency	Infection, membranoproliferative glomerulonephritis
C5, C6, C7, C8, C9	Inability to form the MAC	Recurrent, disseminated neisserial infection
Serum carboxy-peptidase N	Failure to control C3a, C5a, bradykinin	Recurrent angioedema
C1 INH	Loss of regulation of C1 and bradykinin	Recurrent angioedema
Factor H, factor I, CD46	Lack of regulation of membrane C3 convertases	Atypical hemolytic-uremic syndrome, age-related macular degeneration
DAF, CD59	Failure to regulate complement activation on autologous cells	Paroxysmal nocturnal hemoglobinuria

C1 INH, C1 esterase inhibitor; DAF, decay-accelerating factor; MAC, membrane attack complex; MASP, MBL-associated serine protease; MBL, mannan-binding lectin; NeF, nephritic factor.

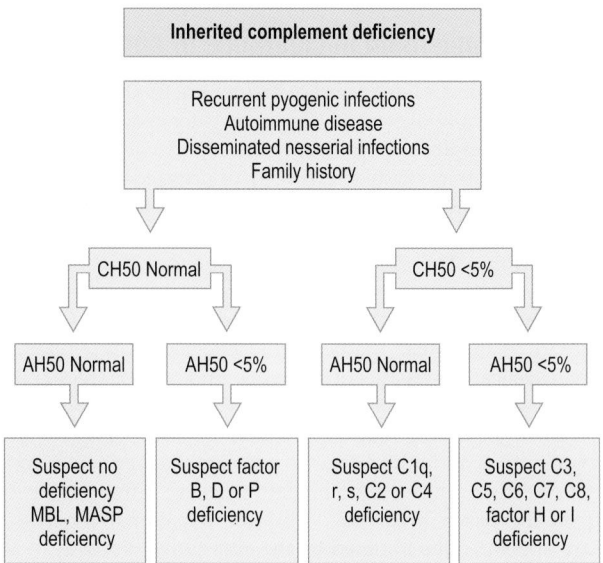

C9 deficiency may have up to 30% normal CH50 with low AH50

Fig. 20.8 Flow chart for the evaluation of inherited complement deficiencies using hemolytic screening assays for the classical (CH_{50}) and alternative pathways (AH_{50}). For each assay, the entire activation pathway including the membrane attack complex (MAC) is required for lysis.

CLINICAL RELEVANCE

Value of screening for complement deficiencies

- Patients with infection and complement deficiency are much more likely to have recurrent infection.
- Prophylactic antibiotics and immunization should be considered in complement-deficient individuals.
- Complement deficiency in patients with autoimmune disease may indicate increased risk for infectious complications. Prophylactic antibiotics and immunization should be used where appropriate.
- Patients with recurrent or disseminated neisserial infection should be evaluated for deficiency of C3–C9 by CH_{50}.

with recurrent or disseminated neisserial infections so that appropriate immunization and antibiotic prophylaxis can be instigated.

Complement deficiencies are most readily detected by hemolytic screening assays[49] – the CH_{50} and AH_{50}, which determine the dilution of patient's serum needed to lyse 50% of erythrocytes sensitive to the classical (CH_{50}) or alternative pathway (AH_{50}). Deficiency of any C1 subcomponent, or any of the other classical-pathway components (C2–C8) will result in little or no lysis in the CH_{50} (CH_{50} values less than 5%). C9-deficient patients may have residual activity in this assay (CH_{50} values less than 30%). Little or no lysis is observed in the AH_{50} assay if factor D, properdin, or any of the components C3–C9 are deficient. Deficiency of factor B has not been described. By comparing the results in the two assays it is possible to narrow the search for the deficient component (Fig. 20.8). Hemolytic and antigenic assays may be done for each individual component to confirm the deficiency.

Classical-pathway deficiencies

Patients with deficiencies of early classical-pathway components (C1, C4, C2) are most commonly identified as having systemic autoimmune disease, but are also at increased risk of infection. The primary infectious agents in these patients are encapsulated bacteria, *S. pneumoniae*, *H. influenzae*, *N. meningitidis*, and *Streptococcus agalactiae*, which rely on antibody and classical-pathway opsonization for clearance.

C1 deficiency

C1-deficient patients most commonly lack C1q, but C1r or C1s deficiency also results in nonfunctional C1 and no classical-pathway activity. Absence of C1q is highly associated with the development of SLE, with an incidence of 90%. It has been proposed that this association is related to defective clearance of apoptotic cells.[60] Apoptotic cells may be opsonized by IgM, or pentraxins leading to activation of the classical pathway, which may be initiated by IgM or pentraxin (CRP and SAP). Cells may also be cleared by direct C1q binding, leading to attachment and uptake through other phagocytic receptors, e.g., the phosphatidylserine receptor.[44] Other proposed mechanisms to account for the strong association between C1 and C4 deficiency (see below) and SLE include defective immune complex clearance and defective development and maintenance of B-cell tolerance.

C4 deficiency

There are two C4 genes, C4A and C4B, located within the major histocompatibility complex (MHC) on chromosome 5. The two forms of C4 have similar function, but different substrate preferences for the covalent binding reaction that occurs on activation to C4b. C4A is more efficient in attaching to amino groups on proteins, such as immune complexes, whereas C4B is more efficient in attaching to carbohydrates. Complete C4 deficiency requires four null alleles and is rarely found, but is highly associated with SLE (75% incidence). Partial C4 deficiencies with one to three null alleles, however, are relatively common, found in up to 25% of individuals. Complete C4A deficiency is greatly over-represented in the SLE population. C4A deficiencies are found in about 1% of the general population and 10–15% of patients with SLE. Complete C4B deficiencies are more commonly associated with bacterial infections, suggesting that the functionally different C4 genes contribute differently to host defense and autoimmunity.

C2 deficiency

The gene for C2 is also located within the MHC. C2 deficiency is the most common complete complement deficiency, with about 0.01% incidence in the population. About half of C2-deficient individuals are clinically normal. The remaining individuals have recurrent pyogenic infections and/or rheumatologic diseases. The most common infectious agents are *S. pneumoniae*, *H. influenzae*, *N. meningitidis*, and *S. agalactiae*. Infections are invasive and mainly found in childhood, suggesting that the immune defect may be overcome by development of acquired immune defenses.[50] The rheumatologic diseases include SLE (15%) vasculitis, polymyositis, and Henoch–Schönlein purpura. The SLE associated with C2 deficiency has some features that distinguish it from other SLE, including equal expression in males and females, early onset, increased photosensitivity, decreased renal disease, lower frequency of anti-dsDNA antibodies, and higher frequency of anti-SSA/Ro and anti-C1q antibodies.[48]

Lectin-pathway deficiencies

MBL deficiency was originally found as a serum defect in opsonization of yeast in pediatric patients with recurrent infections. There are multiple MBL polymorphisms in the population both in the promoter and coding regions, and MBL deficiency is common (estimated to be 14% in the normal Swedish population).[48] In addition to the association of MBL deficiency in children with recurrent infections, there is a two- to threefold increased frequency of MBL deficiency in SLE and these individuals have more frequent and more severe infections during the course of their disease. Serious infectious complications are also more frequent in the subgroups of cystic fibrosis and rheumatoid arthritis (RA) patients that have MBL deficiency.[49]

A single homozygous MASP-2 deficiency has been reported.[6] The patient was asymptomatic until the age of 13, when he was diagnosed with ulcerative colitis. Additional autoimmune manifestations developed along with recurrent severe infections with *S. pneumoniae*.

Alternative-pathway deficiencies

Individuals with complete deficiencies of factor D or properdin have been reported. Factor D-deficient patients have presented with recurrent infections due to *Neisseria* and other organisms. Properdin deficiency is X-linked and patients most commonly have severe childhood infections with *N. meningitidis*.

C3 deficiencies

C3 is central to all three complement activation pathways. Nineteen families have been reported with primary inherited deficiency of C3.[50] The most common presentation is with recurrent life-threatening infections in early childhood (before the age of 2), sometimes followed by immune complex disease. The infections observed are primarily respiratory tract infections (48%) and meningitis (34%) with a variety of pathogens, especially encapsulated bacteria. The organisms most often involved are *N. meningitidis* and *S. pneumoniae*, but other encapsulated Gram-negative and -positive bacteria have also been observed. Recurrent infections are seen in more than half of C3-deficient patients. This clinical presentation is similar to that seen in hypogammaglobulinemia. C3-deficient individuals may develop renal disease (26%), including membranoproliferative and mesangiocapillary glomerulonephritis and autoimmune disease (26%), most commonly SLE.

Acquired C3 deficiency: genetic deficiencies of factor H and I, C3 and C4 nephritic factors

Factors H and I are required to control the fluid-phase alternative-pathway C3 convertase. Complete deficiency of either protein results in C3 cleavage and depletion to very low levels. C5, factor B, and properdin levels may also be reduced. The clinical presentation of patients with factor H or factor I deficiency resembles that of primary C3 deficiency.[50] The highest disease association is recurrent infection with *N. meningitidis* and *S. pneumoniae*, and there is also an increased incidence of SLE. Factor H deficiency is more commonly associated with renal disease than C3 or factor I deficiency (73% of factor H-deficient individuals compared to 13% of factor I-deficient and 26% of C3-deficient individuals).

Nephritic factors (NeF) are autoantibodies specific to classical and alternative-pathway C3 convertases (C4b2a or C3bBb) or the alternative-pathway C5 convertase that stabilize these enzyme complexes and prevent normal regulatory control. The alternative-pathway C3Nef induces unregulated complement activation, resulting in acquired C3 deficiency. NeF are often associated with membranoproliferative glomerulonephritis (MPGN) type II. C3NeF is also associated with partial lipodystrophy, a condition in which fat is lost from the waist upward.

Deficiencies of complement receptors
Deficiencies of CR1 (CD35) and CR2 (CD21)

Complete genetic deficiencies of CR1 or CR2 have not been reported. However, partial deficiencies of CR1 on erythrocytes, B lymphocytes, and polymorphonuclear leukocytes and of CR2 on B lymphocytes have been reported in SLE patients. Decreased CR1 on erythrocytes may be acquired as a result of immune complex clearance.

Leukocyte adhesion deficiency (LAD): CR3 and CR4 deficiency

Leukocyte adhesion deficiency (LAD; Chapter 21) is a syndrome caused by mutations of the common β2-integrin chain, CD18, found in LFA-1, CR3, and CR4. Defects are related to adhesion and activation of phagocytic cells and the clinical presentation includes childhood infections with pyogenic bacteria.

Deficiencies of regulatory proteins

Hereditary angioedema: C1 INH deficiency

Hereditary angioedema (HAE) is found in individuals with heterozygous deficiency of C1-INH. Complete genetic deficiency of C1-INH has never been reported, and HAE is the only complement deficiency with an autosomal dominant pattern of inheritance. C1-INH is a serine protease inhibitor (serpin) with regulatory activity for C1r, C1s, MASP-1 and MASP-2 of the complement system, factor XII (Hageman factor), and kallikrein of the contact system, factor XI and thrombin of the coagulation system, and plasmin and tissue plasminogen activator (tPA) of the fibrinolytic system. Although previous studies implicated a C2 product (C2 kinin) as a mediator, more recent information, including studies in a C1-INH deficient mouse model, indicate that bradykinin is the primary biological mediator of angioedema in HAE.[20] In the more common form of HAE (type I, 85% of patients), reduced synthesis of C1-INH is found (5–30% of normal), along with decreased serum C4 and C2. In type II HAE, an abnormal C1-INH is synthesized making antigenic levels normal or elevated with reduced functional activity and decreased C4 and C2. Clinically, type I and type II HAE are indistinguishable.

Clinically, HAE presents in childhood or adolescence as recurrent episodes of swelling that are subcutaneous and/or submucosal, nonpainful, nonpruritic and nonpitting. Urticaria is not present. Episodes are self-limited, usually peaking at 24 hours and resolving over 2–5 days. Attacks are variable in frequency, severity, duration, and location, and initiating factors are poorly understood. The most common areas involved are the extremities, face, genitals, respiratory tract, and gastrointestinal tract. Intestinal attacks are often associated with vomiting and diarrhea and are extremely painful. Laryngeal attacks may result in life-threatening respiratory obstruction. Recurrent attacks continue throughout the life of the patient and may involve multiple sites or progress from one site to another. Diagnosis of HAE is suggested by family history and clinical findings. Confirmation is based on decreased C1-INH functional activity (< 10–35% of normal). It is important to note that, although C1-INH protein is decreased in type I HAE, it can be normal or even elevated in type II HAE. C4 levels are below normal in 95% of HAE patients. Acquired forms of C1-INH deficiency have been described, usually in elderly patients with lymphoproliferative diseases. These may be caused by autoantibodies to C1-INH and are distinguished from HAE by a lack of family history and decreased C1q, as well as C4. The management and treatment of HAE are discussed in Chapter 42.

Paroxysmal nocturnal hemoglobinuria: DAF and CD59 deficiency

Paroxysmal nocturnal hemoglobinuria (PNH) is a rare acquired disorder in which a somatic mutation in the Pig-A gene in a clone of bone marrow stem cell results in defective synthesis of GPI-anchored proteins.[51] PNH is characterized clinically by intravascular hemolysis with periodic hemoglobinuria and venous thrombosis. DAF and CD59 are GPI-anchored complement regulatory proteins expressed on erythrocytes, and PNH erythrocytes are highly susceptible to lysis. Studies of individuals with isolated DAF and CD59 deficiencies indicate that hemolysis is more highly associated with CD59 deficiency. The basis for thrombosis in PNH is poorly understood.

Control of localized complement activation: atypical hemolytic–uremic syndrome, age-related macular degeneration

Hemolytic-uremic syndrome (HUS) is a rare disease characterized by microangiopathic hemolytic anemia, thrombocytopenia, and acute renal failure. "Typical" HUS is found in children and is caused by E. coli, mainly 0157:H7, producing a shiga-like toxin. Atypical HUS affects older children and adults and is not associated with infection. Recently, mutations in complement regulatory proteins, factor H, factor I, or CD46 have been identified in approximately 50% of patients with atypical HUS.[52,53] The factor H mutations associated with HUS are clustered in the C-terminal end of the molecule in CCP20, a region that is required for factor H binding to polyanions and endothelial cells. The ability of factor H to regulate fluid-phase alternative-pathway activation is not affected and C3 levels are normal. These findings have led to the hypothesis that local complement regulation is essential for preventing renal disease following endothelial cell injury, and that factor H acts locally after binding to exposed matrix or damaged endothelium. Factor H and the membrane protein CD46 are both cofactors for factor I-mediated cleavage of C3b.

An additional factor H polymorphism (Tyr/His402) identified by genetic screening has been shown to be associated with the development of age-related macular degeneration (AMD), a major cause of blindness in the elderly.[54] This polymorphism is located in CCP7 in a region of factor H that binds heparin and CRP.[55] As is the case for the mutations associated with HUS, this region of factor H is not required for regulation of the fluid-phase alternative-pathway convertase. AMD develops when abnormal deposits of protein, termed drusen, form in the retina. Recent findings support the view that the local inflammatory response, including complement activation with MAC deposition, damages the retina leading to vision loss. Additional genetic analyses identified protective factor H variants as well as protective and high-risk polymorphisms in the factor B gene. Although complement factors are not the only genes linked to AMD, they are estimated to account for more than 50% of cases. These findings may lead to the development of new complement based therapeutics that could provide protection from a very common form of age-related visual loss.

Complement in disease

Measurement of complement in a clinical setting

Laboratory tests for complement include functional assays for the classical pathway (CH_{50}), the alternative pathway (AH_{50}), and the lectin pathway.[49,56] Functional and antigenic assays for each of the individual components are available in specialty laboratories. The CH_{50} is a hemolytic assay in which sheep erythrocytes sensitized with rabbit antibody are incubated with dilutions of the patient's serum. The titer is the dilution at which 50%

of the sheep erythrocytes are lysed. The CH_{50} requires all of the classical-pathway and terminal components (C1–C9). A comparable assay for the alternative pathway uses a buffer that blocks classical-pathway activation and rabbit erythrocytes in place of sensitized sheep erythrocytes. Rabbit erythrocytes spontaneously activate the human alternative pathway and are lysed in the assay. The AH_{50} requires all of the alternative-pathway and terminal components (factor B, D, P, C3–C9). The combined use of the CH_{50} and AH_{50} is the most effective screening method for genetic deficiencies of complement components. Complete deficiency will generally result in titers of $<5\%$ in one or both assays. Because C3–C9 are common to both pathways, the combined results of the two assays can rapidly determine whether the deficiency is one of these shared components, one of the unique classical-pathway components (C1, C2, C4) or one of the alternative-pathway components (factor B, D, properdin) (Fig. 20.8). Properdin deficiency results in low, but not absent, lysis in the AH_{50}, and C9-deficient patients may have values up to 30% of normal in the CH_{50}. Deficiencies of factor H and I and nephritic factors often result in very low C3 levels leading to reduced titers in both assays.

Lectin-pathway function (and MBL deficiency) is determined using an ELISA in which the patient's serum is placed into wells coated with mannan. Binding MBL and activation of the lectin pathway results in the deposition of C4b and C4d that are detected with monoclonal antibodies. MBL levels may also be determined antigenically.

Heterozygous C1-INH deficiency as described above is associated with the clinical syndrome HAE.[20] The diagnosis may be made based on clinical findings and family history. C1 INH activity is reduced in these patients and C4 protein is also low in 95% of patients, especially during attacks of edema. In type I HAE (85% of cases), C1 INH protein levels are low, but in type II HAE (15% of cases), an abnormal C1 INH protein is made and antigenic levels are normal or elevated. There is an acquired form of C1 INH deficiency associated with lymphoma in which low C1 INH is accompanied by decreased C1q as well as C4 and C2.

Complement levels may also be decreased in diseases or conditions in which complement is activated, leading to consumption.[49,56] In contrast to genetic deficiencies, complement consumption characteristically results in low, but not absent, functional activity. In addition, multiple components of one or more pathways are expected to be low, and these decreased levels of complement are often correlated with disease activity. The most commonly used and most readily available complement tests are C3 and C4 protein and the CH_{50}. Diseases accompanied by classical-pathway activation result in decreased CH_{50}, C4, and C3 levels. The alternative pathway is spared. These are primarily immune complex-associated diseases, both autoimmune and infectious, and are listed in Table 20.4. In addition 20% of cases of acute renal allograft rejection are associated with decreased CH_{50} and C2. Another cause of selective classical-pathway activation is essentially a laboratory artifact in which clotting of the blood sample is associated with consumption of the early classical pathway. Plasma CH_{50}, C3, and C4 levels are all normal, but serum CH_{50} values are markedly decreased.

The alternative pathway is activated in gram-negative sepsis, post-streptococcal glomerulonephritis, MPGN, IgA nephropathy, factor H or factor I deficiency, and PNH. Laboratory values may show decreased C3 with decreased or normal CH_{50}, and normal C4 levels (Table 20.4). Alternative-pathway activation is not always reflected in decreased C3, because C3 is found at the highest concentration of all complement components and is an acute-phase reactant with elevated synthesis during disease states.

Table 20.4 Complement test interpretation

Pathway	CH_{50}	C4	C3	Related diseases
Classical	↓	↓	↓	SLE, serum sickness, vasculitis, hepatitis C vasculitis, subacute bacterial endocarditis, type I MPGN
Alternative	↓	N	↓	Post-streptococcal GN, gram negative bacteremia, pancreatitis, type II MPGN
Fluid-phase activation of classical pathway	↓	↓	N	C4NeF, HAE, cryoglobulinemia, hypergammaglobulinemia
Fluid-phase activation of alternative pathway	↓	N	↓	Factor H or factor I deficiency, C3NeF, type II MPGN
Acute phase response	↑	↑	↑	Chronic inflammation in the absence of immune complexes
Sample mishandling; coagulation-associated activation	↓	N	N	
Biosynthetic defects in complement proteins	↓	N	↓	Severe liver disease, decreased C3, C6, C9

N, normal; SLE, systemic lupus erythematosus; MPGN, membranoproliferative glomerulonephritis; NeF, nephritic factor.

In clinical practice evaluation of complement levels may be useful in a variety of circumstances. Initial consideration of complement deficiency may be appropriate in patients presenting with autoimmune or infectious diseases (Table 20.3). The complement profile may also be helpful in differential diagnoses (Table 20.4). Monitoring complement levels is frequently used to follow disease activity in SLE patients. Complement levels may predict renal disease activity and may reflect a response to therapy in SLE. However, complement levels are rarely useful in isolation and should be taken in the context of clinical assessment and other laboratory values as reflected in disease activity index scores (e.g., the Systemic Lupus Erythematosus Disease Activity Index 2000).

Role of complement in specific immunological diseases

The following sections briefly describe contributions of complement activation to the pathogenesis of immunological diseases. Emphasis is given to conditions in which animal models have helped to define the relative roles of different pathways and activities of complement. A general concept emerging from current research in this area is that most of the pathogenic effects of complement depend on generation of C5a and MAC. Further, it is becoming recognized that, regardless of the initial activation mechanism, alternative-pathway amplification is needed to produce sufficient quantities of these mediators to cause disease.

Systemic lupus erythematosus (Chapter 50)

Complement plays a dual role in SLE. There is a strong association of genetic deficiencies of C1, C4, C2, and C3 with SLE, indicating a protective role. Three complement-dependent mechanisms have been proposed: (1) complement-dependent clearance of immune complexes; (2) an essential role for complement in the development and maintenance of self-tolerance in B lymphocytes; and (3) a requirement for complement in the clearance of apoptotic cells and potential autoantigens released from such cells. On the other hand, complement activation is believed to play a pathogenic role in tissue damage induced by autoantibodies in SLE. There is evidence for complement activation in SLE skin and renal lesions, as well as in autoantibody-mediated hemolytic anemia and thrombocytopenia. In mouse models of SLE genetic deficiency or blockade of alternative-pathway activation is protective, whereas deficiency of C4 exacerbates autoimmunity and disease.[8,40]

The pathogenesis of SLE is due in large part to the inflammatory response to immune complexes formed by autoantibody binding to antigens from dead and dying cells. The Arthus reaction is often used to study the inflammatory response to passively administered IgG antibody and antigen (usually ovalbumin) independent of autoimmune disease. The response is FcγR-dependent and includes increased vascular permeability with edema and rapid influx of neutrophils into the site. Depending on the route of injection, the Arthus reaction can be elicited in the skin, lungs, or peritoneum, with some differences in cells and effector pathways. Recent findings have shed new light on a long-standing controversy regarding the roles of complement and FcγR in the Arthus reaction. In the current model C5a has an essential role, not as a neutrophil chemoattractant, but as a modulator of FcγR expression on resident macrophages.[57] C5a may be generated through immune complex-initiated complement activation or directly from C5 by proteolytic cleavage. C5a binding to the C5aR makes resident macrophages responsive to immune complexes by increasing expression of stimulatory FcγR and decreasing expression of inhibitory FcγRIIb. This pathway is likely to apply to lupus nephritis where pathogenesis requires stimulatory FcγR, is increased in the absence of FcγRIIb, and can be treated by blocking C5 cleavage.

Anti-phospholipid syndrome (Chapter 60)

The anti-phospholipid syndrome is characterized by anti-phospholipid antibodies, recurrent fetal loss, vascular thrombosis, and thrombocytopenia. Anti-phospholipid antibodies are found in 50% of lupus patients and thrombotic events occur in about half of these patients. Anti-phospholipid antibodies found in patients without SLE have similar clinical consequences. Disease pathogenesis has been attributed to procoagulant effects of anti-phospholipid antibodies. A mouse model was recently described in which injection of pregnant mice with human IgG anti-phospholipid antibodies resulted in fetal loss and wasting.[58] In this model complement is required for pathogenesis and treatment with complement inhibitors is protective. Studies in the mouse model are consistent with initial complement activation by anti-phospholipid antibodies bound to the decidua, followed by C5a generation and recruitment of neutrophils. The alternative as well as the classical pathway was required for pathology. Interestingly, C3 deposition in the decidua was decreased if neutrophils were depleted, suggesting an amplification pathway mediated either by tissue damage or by neutrophil release of complement components.

Rheumatoid arthritis (Chapter 51)

Patients with RA generally have normal or elevated complement values systemically. There is, however, evidence for local complement activation in joint fluid, in synovia, and in rheumatoid nodules. Complement activation products in the joint are not specific to RA, but are also found in patients with osteoarthritis, SLE, Reiter's syndrome, and gout. Concentrations of C3a and C5a in joint fluid are higher in RA than in other types of arthritis. An important role for complement activation in the pathogenesis of RA is suggested by studies in two animal models – collagen-induced arthritis and the K/BxN-derived antibody transfer model. In the first model, inflammatory joint disease was ameliorated by treatment with an antibody to C5 that blocks its cleavage, preventing generation of C5a and the MAC. In the second model, disease was prevented by genetic deficiency of factor B, but not C4, indicating an essential involvement of the alternative pathway.

Vasculitis (Chapters 57, 58)

Human vasculitides encompass a spectrum of disease mechanisms and clinical manifestations. Some, such as giant-cell arteritis and the anti-neutrophil cytoplasmic antibody (ANCA)-associated vasculitides, Wegener's granulomatosis, microscopic polyangiitis, and Churg–Strauss syndrome, are not associated with local complement deposition or evidence of systemic complement depletion. In others, particularly those with circulating immune complexes, C3b, MAC and/or alternative-pathway components are deposited in lesions and complement profiles consistent with activation are found (Table 20.4). Classical-pathway activation is found in polyarteritis nodosa, hypersensitivity vasculitis, rheumatoid vasculitis, SLE vasculitis, and mixed cryoglobulinemia. The vasculitis of Henoch–Schönlein purpura has features of alternative-pathway activation.

Immunologic renal diseases (Chapter 67)

Complement activation is evident in most types of glomerulonephritis, with the site and pathway of activation dependent on the site of immune complex or autoantibody deposition.[59] Alternative-pathway activation is associated with IgA nephropathy, post-streptococcal glomerulonephritis, and membranoproliferative glomerulonephritis (MPGN) type II. In IgA nephropathy, C3, properdin and the MAC co-localize with IgA in glomerular mesangium. Earlier studies demonstrated activation of the alternative pathway by aggregated IgA. More recent results have implicated activation of the lectin pathway in IgA nephropathy.[60] In a recent analysis of 60 renal biopsies from patients with IgA nephropathy, 25% showed deposition of MBL, along with L-ficolin, MASP, and C4d, indicating activation of the lectin pathway.[61] Glomerular deposition of MBL was associated with greater histological damage and higher proteinuria.

MPGN is a chronic progressive form of glomerulonephritis characterized by endocapillary proliferation and thickening of glomerular capillaries producing enlarged glomerular tufts. MPGN is divided into three histological groups, designated type I, II, and III based on electron microscopy of the glomerular lesion. Complement activation is present in all forms of MPGN with decreases in circulating levels and the presence of C3 on biopsy. MPGN type II differs from the other two forms in that serum levels of C4 are not decreased and renal biopsies do not usually demonstrate IgG or C4 deposition. MPGN type II is associated with three conditions that lead to unregulated alternative-pathway activation, factor H deficiency, inhibitory antibodies to factor H, and C3NeF.[50] Complete factor H deficiency is rare, but strongly associated with renal disease (73% of cases), suggesting that unregulated alternative-pathway activation can damage the kidney. Factor H-deficient pigs and mice also develop MPGN that in mice could be alleviated by combined deletion of factor B.[50] C3NeF is an autoantibody that binds to the alternative-pathway C3 convertase (C3bBb), preventing its decay and regulation by factor H and I. C3NeF is found in as many as 80% of patients with MPGN type II.

In glomerulonephritis secondary to immune complex disease, such as SLE and MPGN type I, complement activation is primarily by the classical pathway and C4 is found deposited along with C3 and IgG in glomerular deposits. Complement activation contributes to disease by attracting and activating inflammatory cells through C5a and by direct damage to cells through MAC. Pathology due to inflammatory cell infiltration is predominant when subendothelial immune complex deposition and complement activation occur. Subepithelial deposits are associated with membranous disease characterized by minimal inflammation but also by direct damage to podocytes by MAC. In the Heymann nephritis model of human membranous nephropathy, there is strong experimental evidence that MAC insertion into glomerular epithelial cells is responsible for proteinuria, and beneficial effects can be seen with complement activation antagonists and anti-C5 antibody.

Asthma (Chapter 39)

Asthma is a chronic inflammatory disease of the lung in which Th2 responses to environmental allergens frequently play a critical role. The development of mice deficient in receptors for C3a and C5a has led to a new understanding of the roles of the complement anaphylatoxins in asthma. Several studies demonstrated a correlation between C3a and C5a release in asthmatic lungs and the influx of eosinophils and neutrophils. C3-deficient and C3aR-deficient mice were protected from development of acute bronchoconstriction, airway inflammation, and airway hyper-responsiveness. C5a inhibition had similar effects on the response to challenge in an established allergic environment. However, in contradiction to these findings, C5 deficiency was genetically linked to susceptibility to experimental allergic asthma. Further studies found that C5a signaling (most likely through the C5aR on pulmonary dendritic cells) during initial pulmonary exposure to allergen decreased Th2 cytokine and IgE production, thereby preventing the initiating of the allergic response.[62]

Ischemia/reperfusion injury

Ischemia/reperfusion (I/R) injury refers to injury induced by inflammatory mediators, such as reactive oxygen intermediates produced by activated neutrophils, following the reperfusion of hypoxic tissue. Different pathways of complement activation may be important in different sites of injury, possibly due to differences in expression of complement regulatory proteins. The complement mediators of tissue injury are C5a and MAC acting locally, and in some cases C5a acting systemically. In experimental renal I/R injury and in human tubular necrosis, the alternative pathway appears to be directly activated and neither antibody nor the classical pathway is required. However, in intestinal I/R injury, the classical pathway as well as the alternative pathway is required and a natural IgM antibody to a newly exposed antigen on damaged endothelium initiates complement activation. In coronary artery ligation/reperfusion models, innate recognition of epitopes on ischemic tissue by MBL and CRP leads to lectin and classical pathway activation.

Neurological disease

Complement is found in the central and peripheral nervous system. In the central nervous system complement enters from the blood when the blood–brain barrier is impaired. Low levels of hemolytic complement (0.25% of serum levels) can be measured in the cerebrospinal fluid if care is taken to stabilize it with gelatin during storage. Complement proteins and regulatory proteins are synthesized by glial cells and astrocytes and synthesis is enhanced by inflammatory cytokines. There is evidence both from human multiple sclerosis (Chapter 65) and the animal model, experimental allergic encephalitis (EAE), that complement activation with the generation of the MAC contributes to the demyelination in these diseases. Generation of the MAC can lead to oligodendrocyte death, generation of inflammatory mediators, or a repair process in which myelin synthesis is decreased. Complement activation on myelin and oligodendrocytes is initiated by anti-myelin antibodies or directly by myelin through the classical pathway. There is evidence of MAC formation in the cerebrospinal fluid of patients with multiple sclerosis, and complement depletion, inhibition, and genetic deficiency are protective in rat and mouse models of EAE.

There is evidence of complement activation in degenerative neurological conditions such as Alzheimer's disease.[63,64] In Alzheimer's disease neurofibrillary tangles and senile plaques composed of β-amyloid and other proteins develop, resulting in neuronal loss and dementia with progressive loss of cognitive function. Complement activation products C1q, C4, C3, and MAC components, as well as clusterin and vironectin, are found deposited in areas of amyloid, suggesting classical-pathway activation. Peptides derived from β-amyloid were shown to activate C1 directly by binding to the collagen-like domain. SAP, a component of all types of amyloid, including β-amyloid, activates the classical pathway as well. There are limited data on the role of complement in Alzheimer's disease pathogenesis, with some studies reporting enhanced disease following complement inhibition and another finding decreased inflammatory changes and neuronal degeneration in C1q deficiency.

Future directions in complement research

- Functional analysis of polymorphisms in complement proteins and receptors identified in genome wide association studies (GWAS) of inflammatory and autoimmune diseases will be functionally characterized to provide insight into pathogenesis and treatment.

- Genetic sequencing of entire complement pathways in patients with inflammatory and autoimmune diseases will reveal novel pathogenic mechanisms and approaches to diagnosis and therapy.

- Structural analysis of complement protein complexes will lead to targeted small molecules to inhibit or enhance complement activation.

- Therapeutic trials of existing agents and those in development will refine therapy of complement-mediated diseases.

- Proteome studies in patients with infectious, inflammatory and autoimmune diseases will reveal patterns of complement activation and biomarkers for diagnosis, disease activity, and monitoring responses to therapy.

Complement-based therapeutics

The multiple roles of complement in inflammatory and autoimmune diseases make it an attractive target for therapeutic intervention. Recombinant complement inhibitors, inhibitory monoclonal antibodies and peptide-based receptor inhibitors have been developed to block complement effects.[65] As described above, complement has many beneficial effects in host defense and the adaptive immune response. The detrimental effects of complement activation are for the most part associated with C5a and the MAC.[40] Thus targeting either the generation of C5a or the C5aR might be expected to control inflammation while maintaining other important functions such as opsonization. An anti-C5 monoclonal antibody (eculizumab) that prevents C5 cleavage was effective in murine lupus and Heymann nephritis. In human trials, eculizumab was of benefit in patients with PNH and is now approved for human use in this condition and is being evaluated for treatment of SLE and atypical hemolytic-uremic syndrome. Peptides and monoclonal antibodies directed at the C5aR are effective in a number of inflammatory models in animals and have potential in the treatment of sepsis, reperfusion injury, and asthma. Other approaches that are being developed will target complement regulatory proteins to specific cell or tissue targets. As complement has been the object of increasing importance in a variety of inflammatory diseases, it is likely that further research will establish new complement-based therapeutic agents for additional applications.

Translational research

The distance traveled over the past 50 years in phagocyte defects has been remarkable, spanning initial identification, phenotyping, and molecular characterization. Just the last 10 years have seen the advent of oral antifungals, potent oral antibiotics, oral antivirals, and reduced intensity conditioning for bone marrow transplantation. These advances have transformed the quality of life and longevity of all patients with immune deficiencies. We now need further in depth study of mechanisms to drive

novel insights into disease pathophysiology. The advent of therapeutic cytokines, small molecule inhibitors and agonists, RNA inhibitors, and effective means of gene transfer should make directed approaches to disease modification a reality. However, we must be sure we know exactly what functions need addressing. The downstream effects of genetic defects are surprisingly complex, and not always as straightforward as was anticipated. More detailed clinical and functional phenotyping, careful examination of developmental and gene expression effects, and continued longitudinal studies of large cohorts will convert these severe diseases punctuated by acute, life-threatening infections, into chronic conditions that are successfully treated medically, or successfully managed until successful bone marrow transplantation is available.

References

1. Ricklin D, Hajishengallis G, Yang K, et al. Complement: a key system for immune surveillance and homeostasis. Nat Immunol 2010;11:785–97.
2. Marnell L, Mold C, Du Clos TW. C-reactive protein: ligands, receptors and role in inflammation. Clin Immunol 2005;117:104–11.
3. Kang YS, Do Y, Lee HK, et al. A dominant complement fixation pathway for pneumococcal polysaccharides initiated by SIGN-R1 interacting with C1q. Cell 2006;125:47–58.
4. Ravetch JV, Clynes RA. Divergent roles for Fc receptors and complement in vivo. Annu Rev Immunol 1998;16:421–32.
5. Brown JS, Hussell T, Gilliland SM, et al. The classical pathway is the dominant complement pathway required for innate immunity to *Streptococcus pneumoniae* infection in mice. Proc Natl Acad Sci U S A 2002;99:16969–74.
6. Sorensen R, Thiel S, Jensenius JC. Mannan-binding-lectin-associated serine proteases, characteristics and disease associations. Springer Semin Immunopathol 2005;27:299–319.
7. Spitzer D, Mitchell LM, Atkinson JP, et al. Properdin can initiate complement activation by binding specific target surfaces and providing a platform for de novo convertase assembly. J Immunol 2007;179:2600–8.
8. Lachmann PJ. The amplification loop of the complement pathways. Adv Immunol 2009;104:115–49.
9. Janssen BJ, Christodoulidou A, McCarthy A, et al. Structure of C3b reveals conformational changes that underlie complement activity. Nature 2006;444:213–6.
10. Abdul Ajees A, Gunasekaran K, Volanakis JE, et al. The structure of complement C3b provides insights into complement activation and regulation. Nature 2006;444:221–5.
11. Wiesmann C, Katschke KJ, Yin J, et al. Structure of C3b in complex with CRIg gives insights into regulation of complement activation. Nature 2006;444:217–20.
12. Gaboriaud C, Juanhuix J, Gruez A, et al. The crystal structure of the globular head of complement protein C1q provides a basis for its versatile recognition properties. J Biol Chem 2003;278:46974–82.
13. Gaboriaud C, Thielens NM, Gregory LA, et al. Structure and activation of the C1 complex of complement: unraveling the puzzle. Trends Immunol 2004;25:368–73.
14. Dodds AW, Ren XD, Willis AC, et al. The reaction mechanism of the internal thioester in the human complement component C4. Nature 1996;379:177–9.
15. Matsushita M. Ficolins: complement-activating lectins involved in innate immunity. J Innate Immun 2010;2:24–32.
16. Takahashi M, Ishida Y, Iwaki D, et al. Essential role of mannose-binding lectin-associated serine protease-1 in activation of the complement factor D. J Exp Med 2010;207:29–37.
17. Lambris JD, Ricklin D, Geisbrecht BV. Complement evasion by human pathogens. Nat Rev Microbiol 2008;6:132–42.
18. Cole DS, Morgan BP. Beyond lysis: how complement influences cell fate. Clin Sci (London) 2003;104:455–66.
19. Zipfel PF, Skerka C. Complement regulators and inhibitory proteins. Nat Rev Immunol 2009;9:729–40.
20. Zuraw BL. Clinical practice. Hereditary angioedema. N Engl J Med 2008;359:1027–36.
21. Giannakis E, Jokiranta TS, Male DA, et al. A common site within factor H SCR 7 responsible for binding heparin, C-reactive protein and streptococcal M protein. Eur J Immunol 2003;33:962–9.
22. Manuelian T. Mutations in factor H reduce binding affinity to C3b and heparin and surface attachment to endothelial cells in hemolytic uremic syndrome. J Clin Invest 2003;111:1181–90.
23. Morgan HP, Schmidt CQ, Guariento M, et al. Structural basis for engagement by complement factor H of C3b on a self surface. Nat Struct Mol Biol 2011;18:463–70.
24. Kim D, Song W. Membrane complement regulatory proteins. Clin Immunol 2006;118:127–36.
25. Inal JM, Hui KM, Miot S, et al. Complement C2 receptor inhibitor trispanning: a novel human complement inhibitory receptor. J Immunol 2005;174:356–66.
26. Bohlson SS, Fraser DA, Tenner AJ. Complement proteins C1q and MBL are pattern recognition molecules that signal immediate and long-term protective immune functions. Mol Immunol 2007;44:33–43.
27. Roozendaal R, Carroll MC. Complement receptors CD21 and CD35 in humoral immunity. Immunol Rev 2007;219:157–66.
28. van Lookeren Campagne M, Wiesmann C, Brown EJ. Macrophage complement receptors and pathogen clearance. Cell Microbiol 2007;9:2095–102.
29. Helmy KY, Katschke Jr KJ, Gorgani NN, et al. CRIg: a macrophage complement receptor required for phagocytosis of circulating pathogens. Cell 2006;124:915–27.

30. Huber-Lang M, Sarma JV, Zetoune FS, et al. Generation of C5a in the absence of C3: a new complement activation pathway. Nat Med 2006;12:682–7.
31. Klos A, Tenner AJ, Johswich K-O, et al. The role of the anaphylatoxins in health and disease. Mol Immunol 2009;46:2753–66.
32. Ward PA. Functions of C5a receptors. J Mol Med 2009;87:375–8.
33. Gerard NP, Lu B, Liu P, et al. An anti-inflammatory function for the complement anaphylatoxin C5a-binding protein, C5L2. J Biol Chem 2005;280:39677–80.
34. Rittirsch D, Flierl MA, Nadeau BA, et al. Functional roles for C5a receptors in sepsis. Nat Med 2008;14:551–7.
35. Kumar V, Ali SR, Konrad S, et al. Cell-derived anaphylatoxins as key mediators of antibody-dependent type II autoimmunity in mice. J Clin Invest 2006;116:512–20.
36. Holers VM, Kulik L. Complement receptor 2, natural antibodies and innate immunity: Inter-relationships in B cell selection and activation. Mol Immunol 2007;44:64–72.
37. Kopf M, Abel B, Gallimore A, et al. Complement component C3 promotes T-cell priming and lung migration to control acute influenza virus infection. Nat Med 2002;8:373–8.
38. Kemper C, Chan AC, Green JM, et al. Activation of human CD4 + cells with CD3 and CD46 induces a T-regulatory cell 1 phenotype. Nature 2003;421:388–92.
39. Hawlisch H, Kohl J. Complement and Toll-like receptors: key regulators of adaptive immune responses. Mol Immunol 2006;43:13–21.
40. Thurman JM, Holers VM. The central role of the alternative complement pathway in human disease. J Immunol 2006;176:1305–10.
41. Taylor PR, Carugati A, Fadok VA, et al. A hierarchical role for classical pathway complement proteins in the clearance of apoptotic cells in vivo. J Exp Med 2000;192:359–66.
42. Poon IK, Hulett MD, Parish CR. Molecular mechanisms of late apoptotic/necrotic cell clearance. Cell Death Differ 2010;17:381–97.
43. Du Clos TW, Mold C. Pentraxins (CRP, SAP) in the process of complement activation and clearance of apoptotic bodies through Fcgamma receptors. Curr Opin Organ Transplant 2010; Dec 9 [Epub ahead of print].
44. Fadok VA, Bratton DL, Henson PM. Phagocyte receptors for apoptotic cells: recognition, uptake, and consequences. J Clin Invest 2001;108:957–62.
45. Gershov D, Kim S, Brot N, et al. C-Reactive protein binds to apoptotic cells, protects the cells from assembly of the terminal complement components, and sustains an antiinflammatory innate immune response: implications for systemic autoimmunity. J Exp Med 2000;192:1353–64.
46. Mold C, Gewurz H, Du Clos TW. Regulation of complement activation by C-reactive protein. Immunopharmacology 1999;42:23–30.
47. Riley-Vargas RC, Lanzendorf S, Atkinson JP. Targeted and restricted complement activation on acrosome-reacted spermatozoa. J Clin Invest 2005;115:1241–9.
48. Sjoholm AG, Jonsson G, Braconier JH, et al. Complement deficiency and disease: an update. Mol Immunol 2006;43:78–85.
49. Wen L, Atkinson JP, Giclas PC. Clinical and laboratory evaluation of complement deficiency. J Allergy Clin Immunol 2004;113:585–93; quiz 594.
50. Reis ES, Falcao DA, Isaac L. Clinical aspects and molecular basis of primary deficiencies of complement component C3 and its regulatory proteins factor I and factor H. Scand J Immunol 2006;63:155–68.
51. Parker C, Omine M, Richards S, et al. Diagnosis and management of paroxysmal nocturnal hemoglobinuria. Blood 2005;106:3699–709.
52. Kavanagh D, Richards A, Atkinson J. Complement regulatory genes and hemolytic uremic syndromes. Annu Rev Med 2008;59:293–309.
53. Noris M, Remuzzi G. Atypical hemolytic uremic syndrome. N Engl J Med 2009;361:1676–87.
54. Hecker LA, Edwards AO, Ryu E, et al. Genetic control of the alternative pathway of complement in humans and age-related macular degeneration. Hum Mol Genet 2009;19:209–15.
55. Okemefuna AI, Nan R, Miller A, et al. Complement factor H binds at two independent sites to C-reactive protein in acute phase concentrations. J Biol Chem 2010;285:1053–65.
56. Glovsky MM, Ward PA, Johnson KJ. Complement determinations in human disease. Ann Allergy Asthma Immunol 2004;93:513–22; quiz 523–515, 605.
57. Shushakova N, Skokowa J, Schulman J, et al. C5a anaphylatoxin is a major regulator of activating versus inhibitory FcgammaRs in immune complex-induced lung disease. J Clin Invest 2002;110:1823–30.
58. Holers VM, Girardi G, Mo L, et al. Complement C3 activation is required for antiphospholipid antibody-induced fetal loss. J Exp Med 2002;195:211–20.
59. Lesher AM, Song W-C. Review: Complement and its regulatory proteins in kidney diseases. Nephrology 2010;15:663–75.
60. Seelen MA, Roos A, Daha MR. Role of complement in innate and autoimmunity. J Nephrol 2005;18:642–53.
61. Roos A, Rastaldi MP, Calvaresi N, et al. Glomerular activation of the lectin pathway of complement in IgA nephropathy is associated with more severe renal disease. J Am Soc Nephrol 2006;17:1724–34.
62. Hawlisch H, Wills-Karp M, Karp CL, et al. The anaphylatoxins bridge innate and adaptive immune responses in allergic asthma. Mol Immunol 2004;41:123–31.
63. Kolev MV, Ruseva MM, Harris CL, et al. Implication of complement system and its regulators in Alzheimer's disease. Curr Neuropharmacol 2009;7:1–8.
64. Fonseca MI, Chu S-H, Berci AM, et al. Contribution of complement activation pathways to neuropathology differs among mouse models of Alzheimer's disease. J Neuroinflammation 2011;8:4.
65. Ehrnthaller C, Ignatius A, Gebhard F, et al. New insights of an old defense system: structure, function, and clinical relevance of the complement system. Mol Med 2011;17:317–29.

Gülbû Uzel,
Steven
M. Holland

Phagocyte deficiencies

We have learned a great deal about phagocytes since their discovery by Metchnikoff in 1905: neutrophils, monocytes, macrophages, and eosinophils traffic to the site of infection or inflammation and engulf micro-organisms and apoptotic cells as the lead players in the innate immune response.

Neutrophils

Neutrophils, also known as granulocytes because of their numerous cytoplasmic granules, are crucial for the host defense against bacteria and fungi. They are bone marrow-derived, terminally differentiated cells incapable of further cellular division. They have a short lifespan in the circulation ($t_{1/2} \sim 7$ hours), but survive an additional 1–2 days in the tissue. In the peripheral blood, they are normally maintained at 3000–6000 cells/mm^3 and represent 30–50% of the circulating leukocytes. There are four pools of neutrophils *in vivo*: (1) the bone marrow pool ($\sim 90\%$ of the total); (2) the circulating pool ($\sim 3\%$ of the total); (3) the marginated pool (adherent to the endothelium, $\sim 4\%$ of the total); and (4) those located in the tissues as extravasated or exudative neutrophils. About 55–60% of the bone marrow is dedicated to the production of neutrophils.

Myeloid cell differentiation is a complex step-wise process that typically extends over two weeks in the bone marrow. The pluripotent stem cell, the precursor for all hematopoiesis, develops into lineage-committed progenitors proceeding to terminally differentiated distinct cells, all the while preserving and regenerating more pluripotent stem cells.[1]

Production of macrophages and granulocytes

The pluripotent stem cell gives rise to the myeloid stem cell from which the colony-forming unit granulocyte/erythrocyte/macrophage/megakaryocyte (CFU-GEMM) is derived. Among the growth factors that are influential at this step are stem cell factor (SCF), interleukin-3 (IL-3), and granulocyte/macrophage colony-stimulating factor (GM-CSF).[2] The CFU-GEMM further differentiates into the colony-forming unit–granulocyte/macrophage (CFU-GM) under the continuing influence of these growth factors. The colony-forming unit–granulocyte (CFU-G), a neutrophil lineage committed precursor, is derived from CFU-GM under the control of IL-3, GM-CSF, and granulocyte colony-stimulating factor (G-CSF). The myeloblast is formed from the CFU-G under the influence of GM-CSF and G-CSF and is the first morphologically distinct cell of the neutrophil lineage. Promyelocyte, myelocyte, metamyelocyte, band form and mature neutrophil formation follow consecutively under the ongoing control of G- and GM-CSF.

The maturation process from stem cell to the myelocyte stage takes 4–6 days and an additional 5–7 days for the myelocyte to form the mature neutrophil, all in the bone marrow. The half-life of neutrophils in the circulation is only 7 hours, and an astounding 10^{11} neutrophils are generated daily, a number that can be further expanded in the setting of infection.

Macrophage differentiation is similar to granulocyte differentiation in many respects. The CFU-GM differentiates into the colony-forming unit-macrophage (CFU-M) followed by the formation of the monoblast, promonocyte and monocyte under the influence of macrophage colony-stimulating factor (M-CSF).[3] After monocytes are released into blood, they circulate for 1–4 days before entering tissues where they further differentiate into macrophages.

Evolution of neutrophil granules

During myelopoiesis in the bone marrow, the first granules form at about the promyelocyte stage, stain blue with a Wright or Romanowsky stain, and are called primary or azurophilic granules. Their formation ceases at the myelocyte stage and they are distributed among the daughter cells. These primary granules contain microbicidal enzymes including defensins, hydrolases and proteases (Table 21.1). As the granulocyte precursors mature and divide, the number of primary granules per cell decreases. After the promyelocyte stage, secondary or specific granules form. In the mature neutrophil they comprise about two thirds of the granules. The secondary granules are less dense and contain cytochrome b558, lysozyme, lactoferrin, and collagenase. The gelatinase-containing tertiary granule probably forms after the metamyelocyte stage and can be detected in the band form and mature granulocyte.

Disorders of neutrophil production

Chronic neutropenia refers to conditions with absolute neutrophil counts (ANC) of less than 500/μL lasting more than 6 months. Chronic neutropenia can have many etiologies, as listed in Table 21.2

Severe congenital neutropenia (SCN) and cyclic neutropenia (CN)

While Kostmann originally described an extensive northern Swedish kindred with both recessive and dominant neutropenia, subsequently sporadic cases were added, making this a confusing melange of neutropenia syndromes.[4] Severe congenital

Table 21.1 Neutrophil granule components

Granule	Contents	Properties
Primary (azurophilic) granules	*Lysosomal hydrolases* Myeloperoxidase Defensins Lysozyme Elastase Cathepsin G Azurocidin Proteinase 3 Bacterial—permeability increasing protein (BPI) *Acid hydrolases* Cathepsin B Cathepsin D β-Glycerophosphatase granulocyte β-Glucuronidase N-acetyl-β-glucosaminidase α-Mannosidase *Other* Collagenase	• First formed during myelopoiesis at promyelocye stage • Appear blue when stained with Wright's stain • Least mobilizable granule • Measure ~0.8 μm • Defensins constitute 30–50% of granule contents • Augment the microbial damage initiated by reactive oxidants • Help digest dead microbes and host cells • BPI neutralizes Gram-negatives
Secondary (specific) granules	*Lysosomal hydrolases* Lysozyme *Other* Collagenase Gelatinase Lactoferrin Vitamin B_{12} binding proteins Cytochrome b_{558} Histaminidase FMLP receptors C3bi receptors	• Synthesis begins at the myelocyte stage • These granules are specific to phagocytes • Measure ~0.5 μm • Binding proteins deprive microorganisms of nutrients • Most are positively charged, enhancing cell surface
Tertiary (smaller) granules	*Acid hydrolases* Cathepsin B Cathepsin D β-Glycerophosphatase granulocyte β-Glucuronidase N-acetyl-β-glucosaminidase α-Mannosidase *Other* Gelatinase	• Heterogeneous population of organelles including C-particles and secretory vesicles • Detected in the band form and mature neutrophils

Table 21.2 Causes of neutropenia

Classification	Etiology
Hematological	Kostmann syndrome Severe congenital neutropenia Cyclic neutropenia Myelodysplastic syndrome Aplastic anemia Leukemia
Immunological/inflammatory disorders	SCID Hyper-IgM syndrome (CD40L) Chediak–Higashi syndrome Cartilage–hair hypoplasia Reticular dysgenesis Dyskeratosis congenita Autoimmune neutropenia Isoimmune neutropenia
Infections	HIV Parvovirus Epstein–Barr virus Malaria Cytomegalovirus
Inborn errors of metabolism/ nutritional disorders	Gaucher's disease Glycogen storage disease, type Ib Transcobalamin deficiency Vitamin B12, folate deficiency
Other	Schwachman-Bodian-Diamond syndrome Idiopathic neutropenia Chemotherapy Radiation therapy Drugs (e.g., vancomycin, chloramphenicol, sulfamethoxazole, clozapine) Toxins (e.g., benzene) Dialysis Reticuloendothelial sequestration

neutropenia is now known to be a heterogeneous group of disorders that present similarly. The genes involved are neutrophil elastase (*ELANE* or *ELA2*), *HAX1*, *G6PC3*, *GFI1*, and activating mutations in the Wiskott–Aldrich syndrome (*WAS*) gene.

SCN is usually diagnosed in the neonatal period or early infancy due to life-threatening pyogenic infections, cellulitis, stomatitis, peritonitis, perirectal abscess or meningitis. The most common bacteria isolated are *Staphylococcus aureus, Escherichia coli,* and *Pseudomonas aeruginosa*. Patients usually have an ANC below 200/μL, mild anemia and hypergammaglobulinemia, sometimes with eosinophilia and monocytosis. SCN represents an impairment of myeloid differentiation due to maturational arrest of neutrophil precursors at the level of promyelocytes or myelocytes in the bone marrow. A subset of patients with SCN (7.5–10%) subsequently develops a myelodysplastic syndrome (MDS) or acute myeloid leukemia (AML), which has been associated with acquired truncation mutations of the G-CSF receptor (G-CSFR).

The majority of patients with SCN have heterozygous mutations in the neutrophil elastase (*ELANE*, formerly *ELA2*).[4] The clinically fascinating cyclic form of this disorder has oscillating neutrophil counts with 21-day cycles, hence the name cyclic neutropenia (CN). These mutations are transmitted as autosomal dominants but also occur spontaneously. There is no clear genotype-phenotype correlation between which specific *ELANE* mutations lead to cyclic as opposed to severe congenital neutropenia. These typically missense mutations lead to intracellular accumulation of mutant proteins that are inappropriately trafficked into azurophil granules.[5] This mutated, aberrantly folded protein is thought to contribute to neutrophil precursor apoptosis and the clinical phenotype of neutropenia, but the mechanisms by which this occurs are still somewhat obscure. Treatment with subcutaneous G-CSF can typically increase the ANC above 1000/μL with a decrease in the frequency of infections and significant clinical improvement overall.[6] SCN patients who have received long term G-CSF are at an increased risk of developing AML or MDS, which correlates with overall G-CSF responsiveness.

Homozygous loss-of-function mutations in *HAX1* account for the majority of recessive cases of SCN,[7] some of which were in original pedigree described by Kostmann. Patients may have isolated SCN or associated neurological problems (cognitive impairment, developmental delay or epilepsy) depending on which isoform of *HAX1* is mutated. Patients with mutations affecting isoform A have only SCN, as opposed to patients with mutations affecting both isoforms (A and B), who develop neurological problems in addition to SCN.[8]

Dominant zinc finger mutations disabling transcriptional repressor activity of *growth factor independent 1 (GFI1)* have been described in a few patients with SCN.[4] GFI1 is a transcriptional repressor pro-oncogene controlling normal hematopoietic cell differentiation, which also regulates *ELANE* as well as several of the CAAT enhancer binding proteins (C/EBP). Mutations in *GFI1* are also associated with aberrations in lymphoid and myeloid cells, leading to a circulating population of immature myeloid cells. *Gfi1* knockout mice have impaired Th2 regulation and B cell, Th17 and dendritic cell differentiation.

Mutations in the *glucose-6-phosphatase catalytic subunit 3 (G6PC3)* gene complex cause another form of SCN along with developmental and somatic problems.[9] G6PC3 encodes glucose-6-phosphatase-β, which hydrolyzes glucose-6-phosphate in the final step of gluconeogenesis and glycogenolysis. It is coupled to a glucose transporter (G6PT) that facilitates glucose-6-phosphate transport from the cytoplasm to the endoplasmic reticulum. Mutations in *G6PT* lead to glycogen storage disease type Ib, which has variable neutropenia and infections and other complications such as liver adenomas, growth retardation, osteoporosis, polycystic ovaries, and inflammatory bowel disease. These children have increased susceptibility to bacterial infections and cardiovascular abnormalities, including prominent ectatic superficial veins.

Shwachman–Bodian–Diamond syndrome (SBDS)

Shwachman–Bodian–Diamond syndrome was first described in 1964 as a disorder with pancreatic exocrine insufficiency and bone marrow dysfunction. Today it is recognized as the second most common cause of inherited exocrine pancreatic insufficiency after cystic fibrosis. It is autosomal recessive (located at 7q11) with an estimated incidence of 0.5–1:100000.[10] The SDBS protein belongs to a highly conserved protein family involved in RNA metabolism. Mutations cause defects in the development of the exocrine pancreas, hematopoiesis and chrondrogenesis. Recurring mutations result from gene conversion due to recombination with a pseudogene in 89% of unrelated patients; 60% carry two converted alleles. (Pseudogene conversion is also the cause of the majority of cases of p47^{phox}-deficient chronic granulomatous disease [CGD].)

Patients present with recurrent infections, failure to thrive, hematopoietic dysfunction, metaphyseal dysostosis, growth retardation, and fatty replacement of the pancreas. The majority of the patients have mild neutropenia, while a minority have neutrophil counts below 500/μL, which can be intermittent or chronic.[11] Anemia and thrombocytopenia are associated with neutropenia. Congenital aplastic anemia is an unusual presentation. Upper and lower respiratory tract pyogenic infections are common and related to neutropenia. Short ribs with broadened anterior ends are common radiologic findings, along with metaphyseal dyschondroplasia of the femoral head. The diagnosis is suggested by neutropenia, radiological findings, and abnormal pancreatic exocrine function. It is confirmed by gene sequencing.

Autoimmune neutropenia

Autoimmune neutropenia (AIN) is caused by peripheral destruction of neutrophils due to granulocyte-specific autoantibodies.[12]

Primary autoimmune neutropenia

Primary AIN is seen in infancy unassociated with other systemic immune-mediated disorders and is the most common form of neutropenia, equally affecting boys and girls at around 1/100000.[12] The average age at diagnosis is 8 months. The majority present with mild skin and upper respiratory tract infections; some patients remain asymptomatic despite low neutrophil counts. The majority of patients have a neutrophil count greater than 500/μL at the time of diagnosis, but the ANC may transiently increase two- to threefold during severe infection. Bone marrow shows normal to increased cellularity. Myeloid precursors typically reach the myelocyte/metamyelocyte stage. Phagocytosed granulocytes in the bone marrow may indicate removal of sensitized granulocytes there. Granulocyte-specific antibodies are detected by direct granulocyte immunofluorescence testing (D-GIFT); the vast majority of which are IgG against glycoproteins of the granulocyte membrane designated neutrophil antigens (NA). The NA are located on IgG receptor IIA or IIIB (FcγRIIa and FcγRIIIb).

AIN is generally self-limited. Disappearance of the antibodies from the circulation precedes normalization of neutrophil counts. Prophylactic antibiotic treatment should be reserved for those with recurrent infections. Alternative treatment strategies for severe infections and in the setting of emergency surgical interventions include high-dose intravenous immunoglobulin (IVIG), corticosteroids, and G-CSF, with the latter being the most effective at increasing the ANC.

Secondary autoimmune neutropenia

Secondary AIN can be seen at any age and has a more variable clinical course. Hepatitis, systemic lupus erythematosus or Hodgkin disease may underlie it, as well as cause other autoimmune problems, as well. The antineutrophil antibodies have pan-FcγRIII specificity. CD18/CD11b antibodies have been detected in a subset of patients with secondary AIN. This neutropenia responds poorly to most therapies.

Alloimmune neonatal neutropenia (ANN)

First described by Lalezari in 1966, ANN is caused by the transplacental transfer of maternal antibodies against the fetal neutrophil antigens NA1, NA2, and NB1 leading to immune destruction of neonatal neutrophils.[13] These complement-activating antineutrophil IgG antibodies can be detected in about 1/500 live births. Antibody coated neutrophils in ANN are phagocytosed by the reticuloendothelial system and removed from circulation, leaving the neutropenic neonate at risk for infections. Omphalitis, cellulitis, and pneumonia typically occur within the first two weeks of life in association with neutropenia. The diagnosis can be made by detection of neutrophil-specific alloantibodies in the maternal serum. ANN responds to G-CSF or high-dose IVIG, but most patients improve without specific treatment in a few weeks to 6 months with the waning of maternal antibody.

Defects of leukocyte adhesion

Migration of circulating leukocytes from the bloodstream into the tissues depends on complex bidirectional interactions between leukocytes and endothelial cells (Chapter 11). The initial steps involve the activation of circulating leukocytes by signal molecules released from inflamed tissues or from bacteria themselves. After activation by chemotactic factors such as the complement fragment C5a, IL-8, leukotriene B4 (LTB4) or the bacterial product fMetLeuPhe, leukocytes rapidly become adhesive to the endothelium, other leukocytes or laboratory surfaces. The activation process involves translocation of subcellular granules containing adhesion molecules (CD18/CD11b) to the polymorphonuclear leukocyte (PMN) surface and qualitative alterations in the adhesion molecules constitutively expressed on the plasma membrane. Adhesion and transmigration of leukocytes occur as a result of interactions between three groups of molecules: leukocyte integrins, endothelial intercellular adhesion molecules (ICAMs, members of the immunoglobulin supergene family) and glycosaminoglycans or selectins (Fig. 21.1). The first step in targeting PMNs to inflamed tissues is the rolling or tethering of PMNs on the endothelium of postcapillary venules.[14] This is due to the interactions between CD15s (sialyl Lewis^X or SLe^X) expressed on the leukocyte surface and P-selectin or E-selectin—members of the selectin family of adhesion molecules—expressed on the vascular endothelium. In addition, L-selectin on the leukocyte surface interacts with its counterligands P-selectin, CD34, glyCAM-1 and other glycoproteins located on the endothelial surface. Rolling, a relatively low affinity interaction mediated by selectins, is followed by firm adhesion, which is a high affinity interaction between integrins on the neutrophil and ICAMs on the endothelium. Adhesion is followed by the transmigration of neutrophils between endothelial cells out to the extracellular matrix.

Leukocyte adhesion deficiency I (LAD I)

In the 1970s infants and children were recognized with severe, recurrent life-threatening bacterial infections affecting the skin, gingiva and lung. A common clinical feature was delayed separation of the umbilical stump with severe omphalitis. These patients were shown to have defects in membrane expression of the leukocyte adhesion glycoproteins of the integrin superfamily.[15,16]

Integrins are noncovalently-associated, heterodimeric cell surface receptors, comprised of one α subunit (CD11a, CD11b, or CD11c) and a common β-chain (CD18), which is required for surface expression of the CD11 chains. These proteins mediate leukocyte adhesion to the endothelium and other leukocytes. LAD I results from mutations in CD18 (*ITGB2*), located on chromosome 21q22. Patients with LAD I have defective polymorphonuclear cell adherence, leading to defective chemotaxis and trafficking, as well as low natural killer (NK) and cytotoxic T lymphocyte (CTL) activity. The absence of CR3 leads to loss of complement-mediated phagocytosis and bacterial killing. LAD-1 is often manifested by delayed umbilical cord separation, omphalitis, persistent leukocytosis, destructive periodontitis and recurrent infections with *S. aureus*, *Pseudomonas aeruginosa*, and *Klebsiella* sp. Patients with some residual CD18 expression and function (i.e., hypomorphic mutations), live beyond childhood with less frequent or severe infections and do not typically have delayed umbilical cord separation. Persistent neutrophil leukocytosis (usually > 15 000/μL) in the absence of infection is common in all patients, driven by both low level ongoing infection and impaired exit of neutrophils from the circulation. Oral ulcers, severe periodontitis, gingivitis with apical bone loss (Fig. 21.2), and eventual loss of permanent teeth are major problems in LAD I. Necrotizing cutaneous ulcers with delayed wound healing and lingering eschar formation are common (Fig. 21.3). Defective chemotaxis and adhesion mean that leukocytes fail to migrate to sites

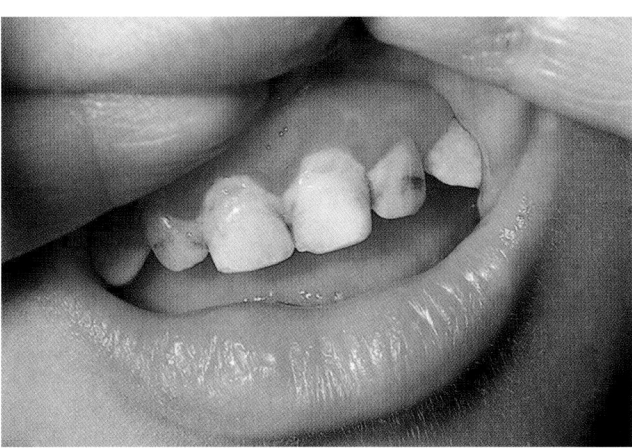

Fig. 21.2 Oral pathology in a patient with leukocyte adhesion deficiency type I (LAD I). Gingivitis and severe periodontitis are hallmarks of LAD I.

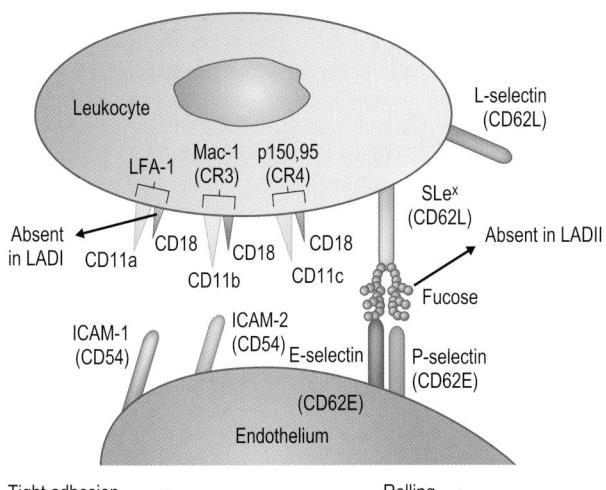

Fig. 21.1 Leukocyte adhesion to nonlymphoid endothelium. Selectins (L-selectin/CD62L, P-selectin/CD62P, and E-selectin/CD62E), integrins (CD18/CD11a or LFA-1, CD18/CD11b or Mac-1, and CD18/CD11c or p150,95), and intercellular adhesion molecules (ICAMs) are involved in leukocyte adhesion to the nonlymphoid endothelium. Rolling, the initial step of leukocyte adhesion, is mediated by the interactions of E-selectin and P-selectin on endothelial surfaces with the sialyl Lewis^X (SLe^X or CD15s) of leukocytes as well as L-selectin on the leukocyte surfaces with its counter-ligands CD34 or glyCAM-1. This low-affinity tethering or rolling facilitates tight adhesion as a result of the interactions of LFA-1 with ICAM-1 or ICAM-2 and Mac-1 with ICAM-2. CD18 is the molecule that is missing or dysfunctional in LAD I; SLe^X is the missing molecule in LAD II.

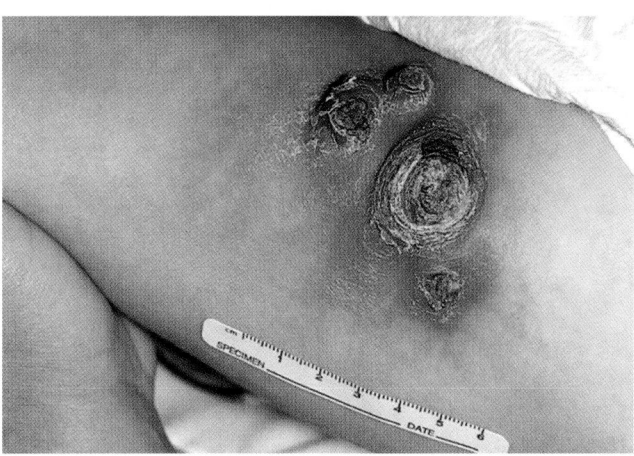

Fig. 21.3 Skin infection of a patient with leukocyte adhesion deficiency type I (LAD) I). Failure to form pus, inability to demarcate the fibrotic skin debris, and limited inflammation. *Enterococcus gallinarium* was cultured from the wound.

of infection, accounting for the inability to form pus and erythema at the site of infection. Biopsies of the ulcers characteristically show poorly formed granulation tissue and scant fibrinous exudate without neutrophils. Ulcerative gastrointestinal disorders resembling idiopathic inflammatory bowel disease are also recognized in LAD-1, especially as patients age.

Although most cases of CD18 deficiency are homozygous, compound heterozygotes also occur.[17] The diagnosis is usually made by flow cytometric analysis of neutrophils showing decreased or absent CD18 and its associated heterodimers: CD11a, CD11b, and CD11c, and confirmed by mutational analysis of *ITGB2*. More subtle phenotypes can be detected by testing for mobilization of CD18 complexes, such as CD18/CD11b from neutrophils upon cellular stimulation. Definitive therapy of LAD I is bone marrow transplantation. Infections must be managed aggressively since inflammatory responses and clinical signs are unreliable in these patients with profoundly impaired innate responses. Surgery is often essential for debridement of nonhealing ulcers, which frequently need tissue grafts.

KEY CONCEPTS

Leukocyte adhesion deficiency

- Three types of adhesion defect are known: LAD 1, II, and III. There are two phenotypes for LAD I: moderate and severe.
- LAD I results from mutations in CD18; LAD II is due to mutations in sialyl Lewis^X (CD15s); LAD III is due to mutations in *FERMT3*
- High white cell count, delayed umbilical cord separation, recurrent bacterial infections, skin ulcers, defective wound healing, gingivitis, and periodontitis are the hallmarks of LAD I.

Leukocyte adhesion deficiency II (LAD II)

A distinct defect of leukocyte adhesion with susceptibility to infection was described by Etzioni et al. in 1992 and named LAD II.[15,18] It is characterized by growth and mental retardation, hypotonia, seizures, dysmorphic features, strabismus and persistent periodontitis. In contrast to LAD I, wound healing is not impaired, nor is the susceptibility to bacterial infections as severe as in LAD I. Hypofucosylation of the protein CD15s (sialyl Lewis^X, SLe^X) on neutrophils impairs the rolling step of neutrophil adhesion. The underlying defect is in GDP-fucose biosynthesis, due to mutation in GDP-fucose transporter-1 (*FUCT1* or *SLC35C1*), hence the designation of this disease as a congenital disorder of glycosylation IIc (CDGIIc). In addition to severe impairment in neutrophil migration to the skin similar to LAD I, lymphocyte homing to the skin is also defective in LAD II. Patients with LAD II have had relatively mild courses of infections with several pneumonias and superinfection of varicella lesions,[18] and some have reportedly improved with fucose supplementation. In addition to SLe^X, fucosylated blood group antigens are also affected, leading to the Bombay blood group phenotype (lack of the H antigen) and Lewis a$^-$b$^-$ in these patients. Absence of CD15s on patient neutrophils can be detected by flow cytometry. Effective and prompt treatment of infections is central to the management of LAD II.

Leukocyte adhesion deficiency III (LAD III)

Following the elucidation of LADI and LADII, another leukocyte adhesion deficiency was recognized, initially named LAD1/variant (LAD1v), then LADIII. It had a distinct infantile

bleeding diathesis similar to Glanzmann-type thrombasthenia along with defective leukocyte adhesion.[19] While CD18/CD11a (LFA-1 or $\alpha_1\beta_2$) is the main integrin on leukocytes, $\alpha_{IIb}\beta_3$ (also called GPIIb-IIIa), allows platelets to bind fibrinogen to promote clotting. This was initially described in Turkish patients and ascribed to *FERMT3*, which encodes KINDLIN3, an adaptor protein expressed in hematopoietic cells that regulates integrin activation.[20,21] KINDLIN3 activates integrins through binding to distinct motifs on the short tails of the integrin β subunits. Phenotypically, leukocytes and platelets in LADIII have defective β_3, β_2, and β_1 integrin activation due to loss of "inside-out" or chemokine-mediated LFA-1 activation and intrinsic LFA-1/$\alpha_1\beta_2$ adhesiveness. In addition, these cells have decreased adherence to endothelial cells and reduced expression of the Rap-1 guanine nucleotide exchange factor, CalDAG-GEFI (CDGI). Based on the location and severity of mutation, LADIII leukocytes may also display loss of adhesion to VCAM-1. LADIII platelets have decreased binding to soluble fibrinogen, do not respond properly to thrombin via thrombin receptors (PARs) and therefore have poor platelet granule secretion through integrin activation. Bone marrow transplantation is curative.

Chronic granulomatous disease (CGD)

Chronic granulomatous disease (CGD) was first described in 1954 as a disorder with recurrent infections and hypergammaglobulinemia (in contrast to Bruton's agammaglobulinemia described in 1952). CGD is due to defective phagocyte superoxide production leading to impaired microbial killing. It is comprised of a group of five genotypes with a common phenotype (Table 21.3), characterized by recurrent severe bacterial and fungal infections and tissue granuloma formation.[22] CGD occurs with a frequency of around 0.5–1/100 000. It is inherited in X-linked and autosomal recessive patterns, with the relative frequencies of recessive disease depending on the rates of consanguinity in different countries. In the United States the X-linked form accounts for about 65% of cases and p47^{phox} deficiency for about 25%.

Patients with CGD often present with pneumonia, liver abscess, skin infections, lymphadenitis, or osteomyelitis; bacteremia is relatively uncommon. Initial presentation with inflammatory bowel disease is not unusual. Exuberant tissue granuloma formation at the sites of infection, at surgical wounds and in hollow viscera are frequent problems seen more often in patients with the X-linked form of CGD.

Table 21.3 Notation used to describe different phenotypes of X-linked CGD

	X91^0	X91$^-$	X91$^+$
gp91^{phox} protein as determined by immunoblot or spectral analysis	Undetectable	Diminished	Normal
Cytochrome b$_{558}$ spectrum	Absent	Low	Absent or normal
Type of mutations in CYBB	Deletions, insertions, splice site mutations, missense mutations, nonsense mutations	Missense mutation	Missense mutations

The NADPH oxidase and its activity

The NADPH oxidase is a multicomponent system that transfers an electron to molecular oxygen by way of FAD and heme to form O_2^- (Fig. 21.4). Cytochrome b_{558} is a membrane-bound heterodimer lodged in the wall of the secondary granules; the large glycosylated β subunit is gp91^{phox} (*p*hagocyte *ox*idase) and the small nonglycosylated α subunit is p22^{phox}. The cytoplasmic tail of gp91^{phox} binds FAD, heme, and NADPH which are required for electron transfer to O_2. Neutrophil stimulation leads to aggregation and phosphorylation of of p47^{phox}, p67^{phox}, p40^{phox}, and the small GTP binding proteins p21rac1/p21rac2. These dock with the cytochrome at the membrane through binding of p47^{phox} and p22^{phox}.

Segal et al. showed that much of the killing effect of neutrophils is actually carried out by proteases, enhanced by NADPH oxidase activity.[23] Charge created by electron flux across the membrane is compensated mostly by K^+ flux, which enhances microbial killing. Zychlinksy et al. have identified neutrophil extracellular traps (NETs; extruded DNA with attached antimicrobial peptides), which depend on superoxide generation and are deficient in CGD.[24]

Mutations leading to CGD

X-linked CGD

The most common form of CGD is caused by mutations in *CYBB*, which encodes gp91^{phox} (located at Xp21.1) (Table 21.3). Mutations include deletions (22.2%), insertions (7%), deletion/ insertions (1.5%), nonsense (29.8%), missense (19.4%), splice sites (19.5%), and promoters (0.6%).[25] The spontaneous mutation rate is approximately 11%. With large interstitial deletions adjacent genes are deleted as well, leading to complex phenotypes. Telomeric deletions cause McLeod syndrome (*KX* or Kell antigen deletion), Duchenne's muscular dystrophy (*DMD*), and X-linked retinitis pigmentosa (*RPGR*) along with CGD.[26] The phenotype of McLeod syndrome includes absent erythrocyte Kx protein and diminished levels of Kell blood group antigens. Patients may eventually develop progressive neurodegenerative symptoms such as areflexia, dystonia and choreiform movements. McLeod syndrome patients form anti-Kx and anti-Km antibodies when transfused, making future transfusions extremely difficult. Deletions centromeric from *CYBB* may cause ornithine decarboxylase deficiency along with CGD.[27]

Autosomal recessive CGD

Mutations in p47^{phox} (*NCF1*, located at 7q11.23) cause the majority of the recessive cases of CGD, around 25%, usually due to homozygous deletions of the canonical GT splice site at the start of exon. 2[28] p22^{phox} (*CYBA*, located at 16q24), and p67^{phox} (*NCF2*, located at 1q25) are responsible for less than 5% of CGD cases, each. p40^{phox} (*NCF4*, located at 22q13.1) deficiency has been reported in a single boy with early onset severe granulomatous fistulizing colitis without a significant infectious phenotype.[29] No autosomal dominant cases of CGD have been identified.

Clinical manifestations of CGD

The first severe infection is usually in infancy or childhood, but can occur in adulthood. Later diagnoses usually occur in patients with residual superoxide production, either hypomorphic gp91^{phox} or p47^{phox} deficiency.[22,30] The constellation of signs and symptoms that suggest CGD range from failure to thrive, to inflammatory bowel disease, to visceral abscesses, to recurrent sinopulmonary infections, to characteristic infections. Infections are most commonly pneumonia, lymphadenitis, liver abscess, skin abscess, perianal abscess, and osteomyelitis. As in other neutrophil defects, the most common pathogen is *S. aureus*. Characteristic infections are due to catalase-positive organisms such as *S. aureus*, *Burkholderia cepacia* complex, *Serratia marcescens*, *Nocardia* sp., and *Aspergillus* sp. (Fig. 21.5).

Staphylococcal liver abscesses in CGD are dense and necrotic and cause significant morbidity. Their fibrocaseous consistency means that percutaneous drainage is rarely successful and open surgery is required.[31] The inflammatory liver involvement is the likely cause of the splenomegaly commonly seen in CGD. Further, liver involvement is closely tied to mortality.[32]

Fig. 21.4 Schematic representation of the NADPH oxidase system. Chemoattractants interact with their receptors on the neutrophil surface, leading to an increase in intracellular calcium concentration. This activation results in the assembly of the NADPH oxidase complex following phosphorylation of cytosolic factors. This in turn leads to superoxide production. DAG = diacylglycerol; PIP_2 = phosphatidylinositol bisphosphate; IP_3 = inositol triphosphate; α, β, γ = subunits of the GTP-coupled receptors.

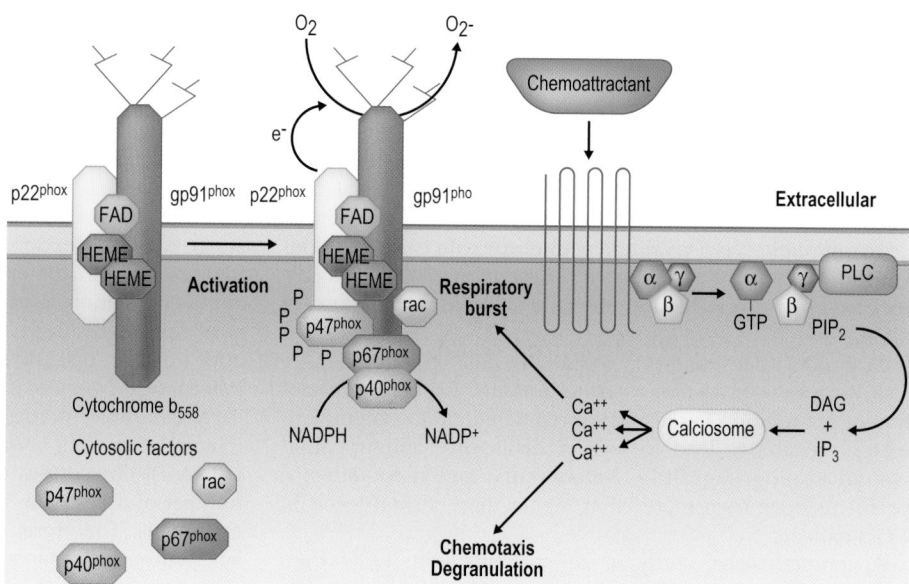

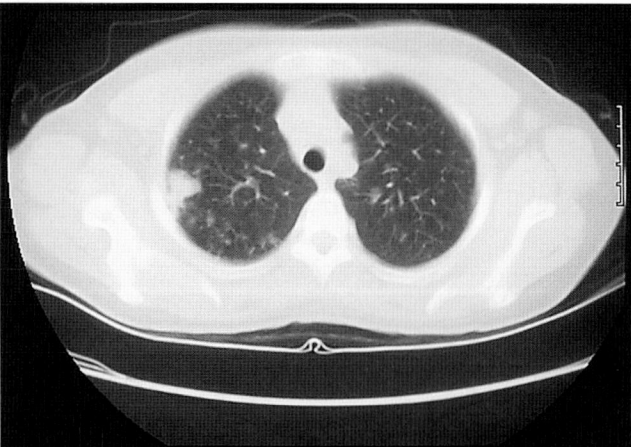

Fig. 21.5 CT scan of the lungs of a patient with CGD and *Aspergillus* pneumonia. *Aspergillus* pneumonia is detected as a peripheral consolidation in the lung parenchyma.

Pulmonary aspergillosis was previously the primary cause of death in CGD.[22] *A. fumigatus* is the most commonly isolated fungus, but it is now easily and successfully treated with azole antifungals. In contrast, *A. nidulans* and *A. viridinutans*, species with low pathogenicity in the normal host, cause severe disease in CGD.[33,34] Thoracic wall invasion may occur, leading to osteomyelitis of the ribs, perforation of the diaphragm or cutaneous abscesses. Surgical resection of these infections is often required. *Aspergillus* infections in CGD are often unaccompanied by systemic symptoms or signs of infection (e.g., fever, leukocytosis) and therefore should be suspected in any case of an asymptomatic pulmonary infiltrate.[33] A characteristic presentation of acute fungal infectoin in CGD is referred to as mulch pneumonitis, a syndrome of fever, hypoxia, and diffuse pulmonary infiltrates caused by inhalation of fungi, typically during mulching, leaf raking, or gardening.[35] This syndrome can be the initial presentation of CGD in older children and adults and is important to recognize since it best responds to a combination of antifungals and steroids.

Septicemia is relatively uncommon, but may occur with *B. cepacia* complex and *Chromobacterium violaceum*. *Granulobacter bethesdensis* is a novel Gram-negative rod that causes chronic necrotic lymph node and spleen involvement in CGD.[36]

Inflammatory granuloma formation is one of the hallmarks of CGD. Pyloric outlet obstruction, bladder outlet obstruction and ureteral obstruction are common. Crohn's-like inflammatory bowel disease affects between 30-50% of patients, predominantly X-linked, and may involve the esophagus (Fig. 21.6), jejunum, ileum, cecum, rectum, and perirectal area.[37] Gastrointestinal manifestations can include diarrhea, malabsorption, abdominal pain, growth delay, and hypoalbuminemia. The median age of initial GI manifestations is 5 years and abdominal pain is common. Interestingly, GI involvement has no effect on mortality, is not associated with liver disease and is unaffected by the use of interferon-γ.[30,32,37]

Granulomata respond very well to steroids, and often require a slow taper over several weeks to months. Exuberant formation of granulation tissue and dysregulated cutaneous inflammatory responses lead to wound dehiscence and impaired wound healing (Fig. 21.7). Autoimmune and rheumatologic problems have been reported at higher than normal levels in CGD patients.[38]

A comprehensive study of 287 patients with CGD from 244 kindreds correlated the production of reactive oxygen

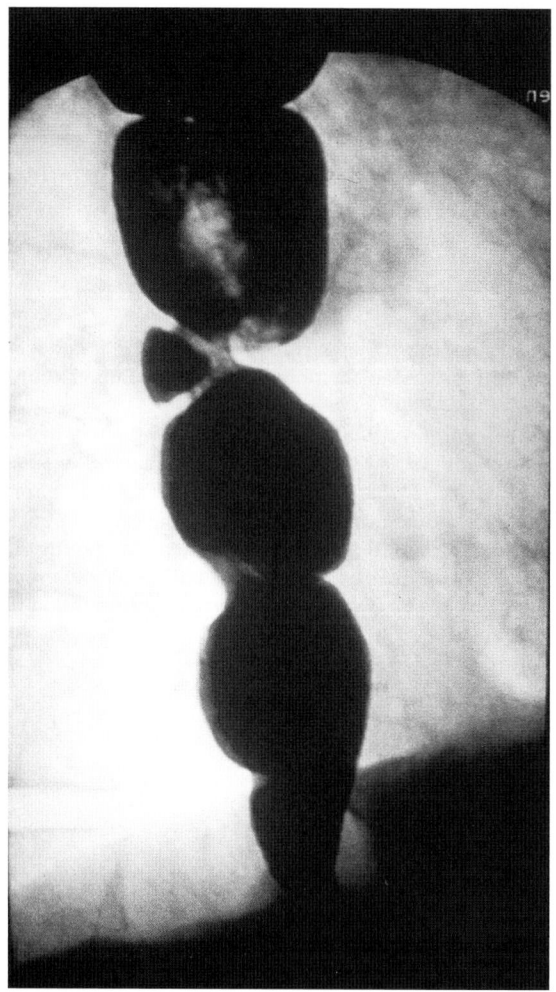

Fig. 21.6 Esophageal involvement in CGD. Esophageal strictures caused by granuloma formation as seen by barium swallow.

intermediates with survival.[30] Patients with residual superoxide production had significantly better long-term survival than patients without residual superoxide production. Confirming the importance of this association, there was a direct correlation between the degree of superoxide and survival. Consistent with their previously recognized milder disease and better survival, patients with mutations in p47[phox] had significant residual superoxide production. For those with gp91[phox] mutations, the findings were more surprising. X-linked CGD patients with residual superoxide production were those with missense or splice mutations in the first 309 amino acids of gp91[phox]. Those with missense mutations from amino acids 310-587 had no residual superoxide production, regardless of protein levels. Therefore, identification of the specific molecular subtype of CGD and specific mutation has important implications for severity and survival. Interestingly, mortality curves did not diverge until after age 20, suggesting that residual superoxide production determines later toxicities, such as liver dysfunction, not early childhood mortality from infection. It is critical to keep in mind that this comprehensive study included data from patients followed for up to 30 years, meaning that a significant number of cases were born before the advent of modern antimicrobials. Therefore, survival of a child born in the current age with ideal management may well exceed that in the reported population.

nitroblue tetrazolium reduction (NBT) and dichlorofluorescein (DCF), but these are somewhat more complicated to perform or more prone to reader effects (Fig. 21.8). One important false-positive to keep in mind in DHR testing is myeloperoxidase (MPO) deficiency. MPO deficiency gives a DHR result consistent with CGD, but when superoxide production is measured by NBT or the more specific ferricytochrome c reduction, it is normal to increased.

Treatment of CGD

Prophylactic trimethoprim–sulfamethoxazole (TMP–SMX) significantly reduces the frequency of bacterial infections in CGD, especially those caused by *S. aureus*. TMP–SMX prophylaxis is ineffective against fungal infections but does not encourage them. Prophylactic itraconazole prevents fungal infections. IFN-γ is beneficial as a prophylactic treatment in CGD. In a multicenter placebo-controlled trial of IFN-γ, the number and severity of infections were significantly reduced by IFN-γ. The exact mechanism of action of IFN-γ is not known but it has multiple effects, including stimulation of components of NADPH oxidase in partial deficiencies, increased bactericidal activity through neutrophil granule components, and Fc receptor expression. Subcutaneous administration of recombinant IFN-γ three times a week at a dose of 50 µg/m^2 (for those with body surface area greater than 0.5 m^2) is recommended. The adverse effects of recombinant IFN-γ in patients with CGD have been limited to fever, chills, headache, flu-like illness and diarrhea. Leukocyte transfusions are sometimes used during severe infections in addition to antibiotics, although the benefits are unproven and neutrophils for transfusion are difficult to obtain.

Because CGD is predominantly a hematopoietic disorder, bone marrow transplantation can cure CGD, even in the setting of active infection.[39] The type of transplant that is used in CGD patients varies with the center, but both fully myeloablative and partially myeloablative transplants (reduced intensity conditioning) have been effective. Although active infection is a relative contraindication for bone marrow transplantation overall, there are certain infections in CGD, especially those due to atypical *Aspergillus* species infections, that are not curable with standard antifungal therapy. The role of bone marrow transplantation early after the diagnosis of CGD is emerging, since it often prevents not only recurrent life-threatening infections, but also gastrointestinal disease and growth retardation.

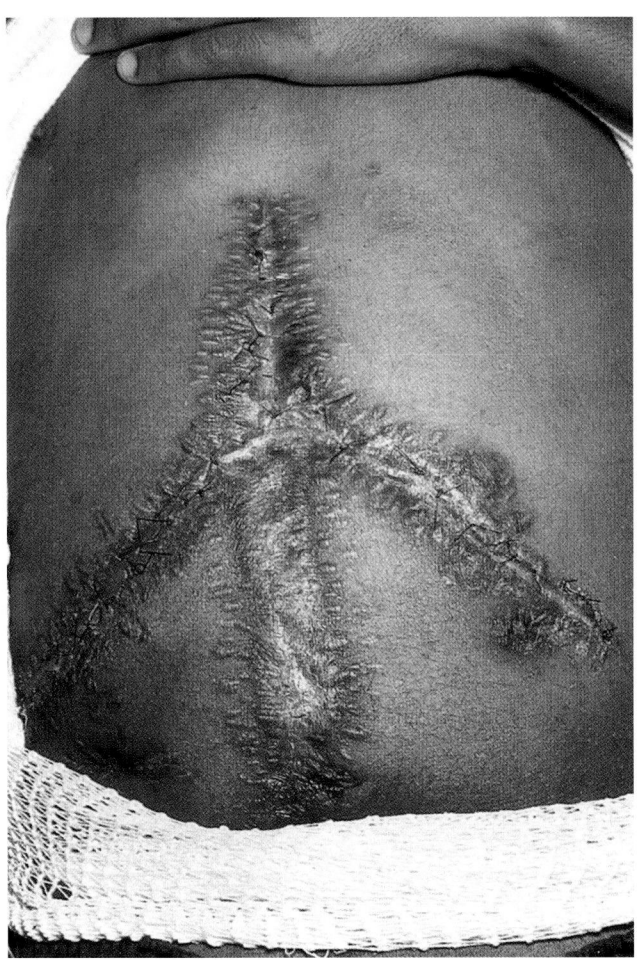

Fig. 21.7 Exuberant granuloma formation in CGD. Wound dehiscence and impaired wound healing at surgical incision sites due to dysregulated inflammatory responses in an X-linked CGD patient.

● CLINICAL PEARLS

Chronic granulomatous disease (CGD)

- CGD comprises a group of five inherited disorders with a common phenotype.
- Infections with catalase-positive bacteria and fungi, and granuloma formation in the gastrointestinal and urinary tract are the major problems in CGD.
- Oral prophylactic antibiotics and subcutaneous IFN-γ injections three times a week are currently recommended for CGD.
- Diagnosis can be made via NBT test or DHR assay, the latter being a more sensitive diagnostic tool.

Diagnosis of CGD

The diagnosis of CGD is most easily established by the dihydrorhodamine (DHR) assay, which measures the hydrogen peroxide dependent conversion of dihydrorhodamine 123 to rhodamine 123, which is accompanied by fluorescence. This test is relatively reproducible and can be quantized on a flow cytometer allowing the determination of a DHR index, which correlates with residual superoxide production capacity. Other assays include

Myeloperoxidase (MPO) deficiency

MPO is a heme-containing enzyme necessary for the conversion of H_2O_2 to HOCl. MPO is expressed early in myeloid differentiation and resides in the azurophilic granules of neutrophils and the lysosomes of monocytes.[40] The resulting mature protein is a symmetric molecule of four peptides with each half consisting of a heavy–light chain heterodimer. Neutrophils of MPO-deficient individuals fail to produce HOCl upon stimulation, while the NADPH oxidase system remains unaffected. Prolonged supranormal levels of superoxide and H_2O_2 production follow stimulation in MPO-deficient neutrophils. This may be due to the lack of negative feedback regulation of HOCl on the NADPH oxidase, although the exact mechanism is unknown. MPO deficiency can be primary (congenital) or secondary (acquired).

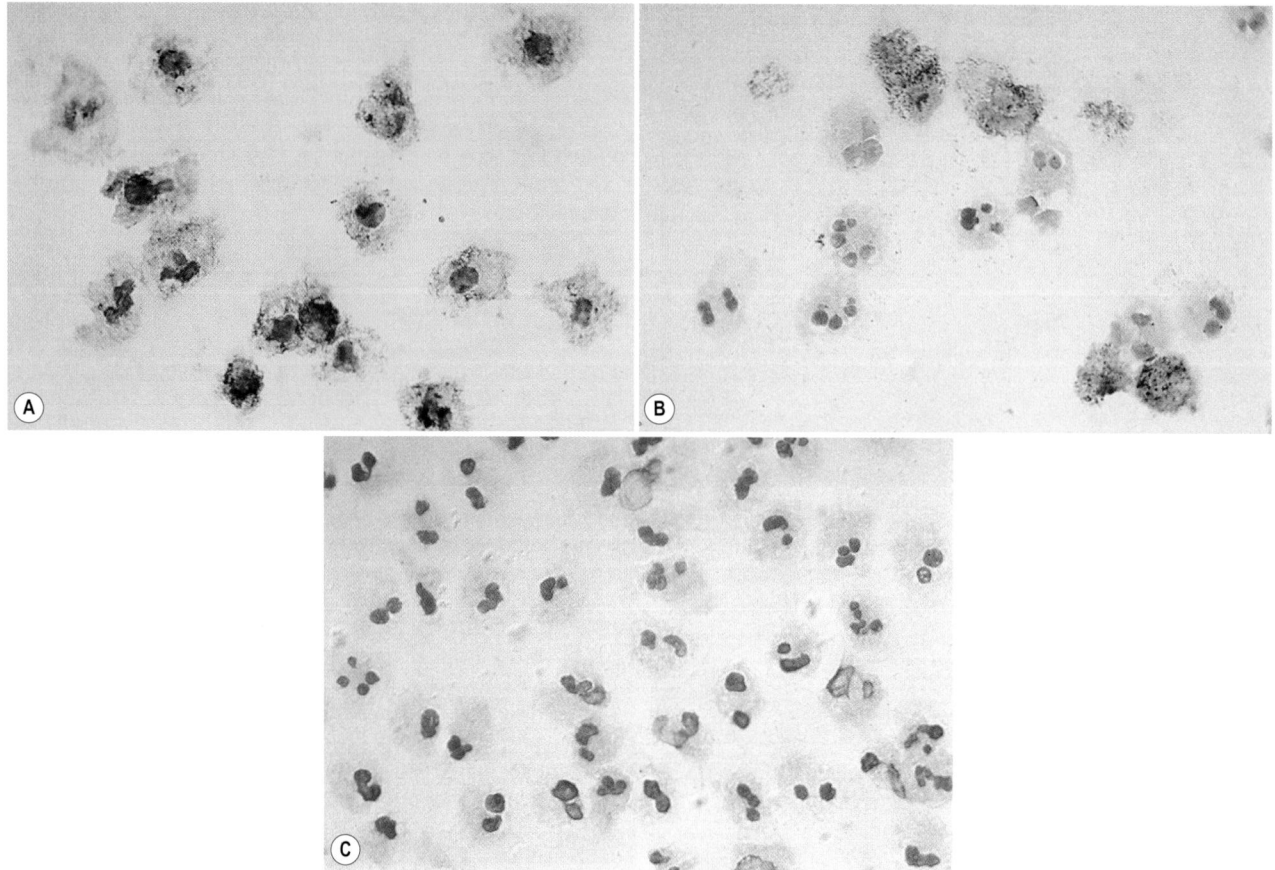

Fig. 21.8 Laboratory diagnosis of CGD with the nitroblue tetrazolium test (NBT). (A) NBT reduction by purified normal neutrophils following stimulation with phorbol esters and calcium ionophore. NBT is reduced by all neutrophils, showing a blue/purple deposit. (B) NBT reduction by purified neutrophils from an X-linked CGD carrier; two different populations of cells are seen. Normal (unaffected cells) reduce the NBT dye and stain blue/purple, whereas affected cells fail to reduce the NBT dye and appear clear. (C) Neutrophils from a patient with CGD fail to reduce the NBT dye and appear clear.
Courtesy of Dr. Douglas B. Kuhns, SAIC, Frederick, MD.

Primary MPO deficiency

Primary MPO deficiency is the most common phagocyte defect with a frequency of 1:4000. There is heterogeneity among patients in the degree of MPO deficiency; both total and partial deficiencies have been described. Patients with primary MPO deficiency do not usually have an increased incidence of infections, probably because MPO-independent mechanisms compensate for the lack of MPO-dependent microbicidal activity. In some patients visceral candidiasis has occurred in the setting of concurrent diabetes. However, the frequency of such cases is very low. Affected patients may develop nonfungal infections, malignancies and certain skin disorders. In several cohorts of complete MPO-deficient patients, an increased incidence of solid or hematologic tumors has been observed.[39] MPO deficient neutrophils have no apparent defect in phagocytosis of bacteria or fungi, but microbicidal activity is slower than normal. MPO-deficient neutrophils are severely impaired in killing *Candida* spp. or *Aspergillus* spp. *in vitro*, despite the fact that MPO-deficient patients do not develop significant fungal infections. This suggests that the mucosal barrier to fungal infection is independent of MPO activity and is able to prevent invasive infection.

The most common mutation is a missense replacement of arginine 569 with tryptophan (R569W), causing maturational arrest of the MPO precursor and preventing heme incorporation. Most patients are compound heterozygotes. The diagnosis of MPO deficiency is made using anti-MPO monoclonal antibodies in flow cytometric analysis of neutrophils. No MPO expression is seen in the congenital deficiency, whereas near-normal antigenic reactivity may be seen with the acquired form.[40] Maintenance antibiotic or antifungal therapy is not routinely recommended. In patients with diabetes mellitus and congenital MPO deficiency, who may develop localized or systemic infections, prompt and prolonged therapy is advised.

Secondary or acquired MPO deficiency

In the majority of patients, MPO deficiency is partial and transient. Secondary MPO deficiency occurs under certain clinical conditions, such as some hematologic malignancies or disseminated cancers, exposure to cytotoxic agents or anti-inflammatory medications, iron deficiency, lead intoxication, thrombotic diseases, renal transplants, and pregnancy. MPO activity in the bone marrow myeloid precursors as well as peripheral blood cells may vary from cell to cell. Treatment of the underlying condition typically corrects the defect. This deficiency is most likely linked to somatic mutations in the case of malignancy or toxic-metabolic effects on MPO activity.[40]

Specific granule deficiency

Neutrophil-specific granule deficiency (SGD) is a rare disorder of leukocyte maturation in which neutrophil secondary granules and some primary granule proteins are absent due to mutations in CCAAT/enhancer binding protein epsilon (C/EBPε, located at 14q11.2), a member of the leucine zipper family of transcription factors.[41] SGD is characterized by frequent, severe pyogenic infections, a paucity or absence of neutrophil-specific granule proteins and defensins, and atypical neutrophil nuclear structure with mostly bi-lobed nuclei. *In vitro*, these patients' cells show diminished neutrophil migration, reduced staphylococcal killing, reduced phagocytosis and increased cell surface/volume ratio. Eosinophils and platelets are also affected in SGD. Platelets lack high-molecular-weight (HMW) von Willebrand factor multimers, and have reduced platelet fibrinogen and fibronectin due to diminished platelet α granules. Bleeding diatheses and neutrophil phagocytosis of platelets are seen in SGD. In addition, SGD eosinophils are deficient in the eosinophil-specific granule proteins eosinophil cationic protein (ECP), eosinophil-derived neurotoxin (EDN) and major basic protein (MBP), despite the presence of mRNA transcripts for these proteins. Few patients have been reported to have survived beyond adolescence except for a milder dominant form. Bone marrow transplantation should be considered early in the disease.

●KEY CONCEPTS

Specific granule deficiency (SGD)

- SGD is caused by promyelocyte–myelocyte transition block due to a mutation in the *C/EBPε* gene.
- Absence of secondary granule proteins, and a selective loss of the primary granule defensins are the pathologic findings in SGD granulocytes.
- The prognosis is very poor in recessive forms of SGD.

Chediak–Higashi syndrome

Chediak–Higashi syndrome (CHS) is a rare, autosomal recessive disorder characterized by partial oculocutaneous albinism, increased susceptibility to infections, deficient natural killer cell (NK) activity and abnormal giant primary granules in neutrophils.[42] This immunodeficiency was first reported by Beguez-Cesar in 1943 and then further described by Chediak and Higashi a decade later. The hallmark of CHS is giant abnormal granules in all granule-containing cells including melanocytes (melanosomes are members of the lysosomal lineage of organelles), neutrophils, central and peripheral nerve tissue, fibroblasts, and hair. The problem is the inability to form appropriate lysosomes and cytoplasmic granules. CHS granulocytes lack cathepsin G and elastase, but the defensin content is normal. The giant granules of CHS are derived predominantly from the azurophilic granules. CHS is classically described as a biphasic immunodeficiency, in which susceptibility to infection marks the first phase and an accelerated lymphoproliferative syndrome with histiocytic infiltration of various tissues marks the second. Rarely, the accelerated phase may be the initial presentation. The giant organelles are derived from the late compartments of the endocytic pathway, affecting specifically late endosomes and lysosomes with minimal or no effect on early endosomes. *CHS1* encodes a 3801 amino acid

peptide (Lyst, lysosomal transporter) that has a vital role in lysosomal trafficking. Lysosomal exocytosis triggered by membrane wounding is impaired in Chediak-Higashi fibroblasts. The reduced survival of fibroblasts after wounding indicates that impaired lysosomal exocytosis inhibits membrane resealing. Inability of cells to repair plasma membrane lesions may contribute to the pathology of CHS. The degree of albinism may vary from a slightly diluted skin pigment to hypopigmented skin and hair, photophobia, nystagmus, strabismus, macular hypoplasia and reduced visual acuity. Skin biopsies show large irregular melanin granules in melanocytes. Microscopic analysis of hair also shows poor distribution of melanin. Pancytopenia, neutropenia, and lack of NK-cell activity result in frequent pyogenic infections, usually due to staphylococci or streptococci. Hepatosplenomegaly and lymphadenopathy are common. A mild bleeding diathesis is due to platelet storage pool deficiency. Neurologic dysfunction has been noted in CHS, including mental retardation, seizures, cranial nerve palsies and progressive peripheral neuropathy.

The lymphoma-like lymphohistiocytic accelerated phase is characterized by increased hepatosplenomegaly, lymphadenopathy and worsened pancytopenia, which may resemble the virus-associated hemophagocytic syndromes or familial erythrophagocytic lymphohistiocytosis. Although chemotherapy can induce transient remissions, relapses are common. Bone marrow transplantation prevents the accelerated phase and restores NK-cell function, but it does not resolve the central or peripheral nervous abnormalities. Demonstration of giant azurophilic cytoplasmic inclusions on peripheral blood smear is very suggestive of the diagnosis of CHS; mutation analysis confirms the diagnosis.

Hyper-IgE recurrent infection (HIES or Job) syndrome

Davis et al. first described hypoinflammatory recurrent infections with severe eczema in 1966. This was further refined and expanded by Buckley et al. in 1972, who recognized the characteristic IgE elevation. We now consider this to be a multisystem autosomal dominant disorder caused by heterozygous mutations in signal transducer and activator of transcription 3 (STAT3, located at 17q21).[43] Mutations in STAT3 are mostly missense and clustered in either the DNA-binding domain or Src homology 2 (SH2) domains. The disease is characterized by recurrent infections of the lower respiratory system and skin, chronic eczema, arterial anomalies, including coronary arterial tortuosity and aneurysms, extremely elevated IgE levels and eosinophilia (Table 21.4). HIES occurs in all racial and ethnic groups.

Facial, skeletal, and dental abnormalities

Facial abnormalities seen in the majority of the patients are a protruding, prominent mandible and forehead, apparent ocular hypertelorism, a broad nasal bridge and a wide, fleshy nasal tip with increased interalar distance (Fig. 21.9). Midline anomalies common in this disorder are high-arched palate and midline sagittal clefts of the tongue.

Skeletal abnormalities are common. Grimbacher, et al. noted pathologic fractures in 57% and scoliosis in 76% (Fig. 21.10). Low bone density and cortical bone loss are also common, but not clearly correlated with the fracture rate. Other infrequent skeletal abnormalities reported in HIES are craniosynostosis, spina

Table 21.4 Clinical and laboratory findings in patients with the hyper-IgE syndrome

Findings	Incidence (%)
Eczema	100
High IgE levels (> 2000 IU/mL)	97
Eosinophilia (> 2 sd above the mean for normals)	93
Boils	87
Pneumonia	87
Mucocutaneous candidiasis	83
Characteristic facies (in those ≥ 16 years)	83
Lung cysts	77
Scoliosis (for those ≥ 16 years)	76
Hyperextensible joints	68
Delayed shedding of primary teeth	72
Bone fractures	57

Adapted from Grimbacher B, Holland SM, Gallin JI, et al. Hyper-IgE syndrome disorder. N Engl J Med 1999; 340: 692.

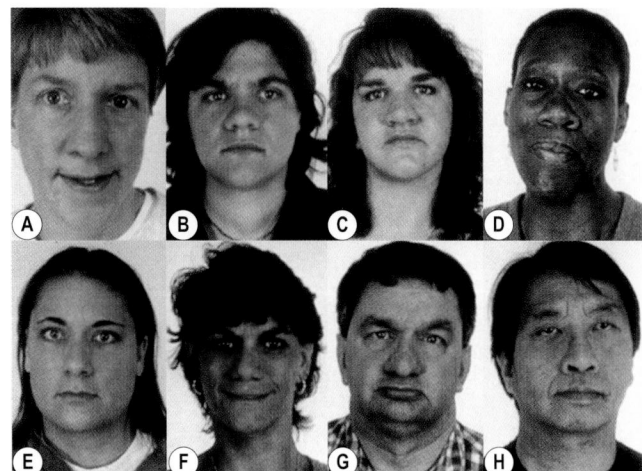

Fig. 21.9 Facial abnormalities seen in patients with hyper-IgE recurrent infection syndrome (HIES). Protruding prominent mandible and forehead, hypertelorism, broad nasal bridge with a wide nasal tip, and increased interalar distance are commonly seen facial features of HIES.

With permission from Grimbacher B, Holland SM, Gallin JI, et al. Hyper-IgE syndrome with recurrent infections–an autosomal dominant multisystem disorder. N Engl J Med 1999; 340:692.

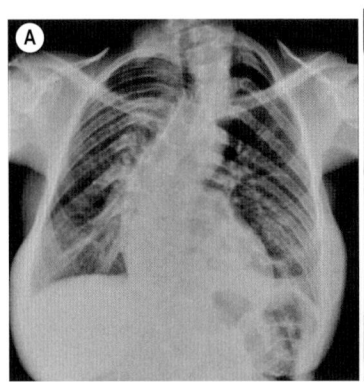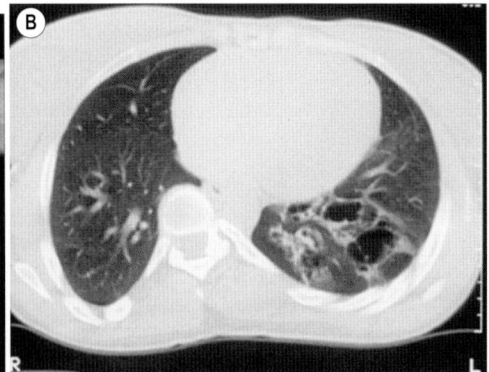

Fig. 21.10 Thoracic pathology in hyper-IgE recurrent infection syndrome (HIES). (A) Chest X-ray of a patient with scoliosis. (B) CT scan of the lungs in the same patient demonstrates multiple pneumatoceles due to prior infections.

bifida, bifid rib, wedge-shaped lumbar vertebra, hemivertebra and pseudoarthritis of the hip. Hyperextensibility of joints is common. A unique dental abnormality seen in this syndrome is retained primary teeth causing delayed eruption of the permanent teeth.

KEY CONCEPTS

Hyper-IgE recurrent infection syndrome (HIES) or Job syndrome

- Recurrent infections of the lower respiratory system and skin, chronic eczema, extremely elevated IgE levels, and eosinophilia are the hallmarks of the syndrome.
- Facial, skeletal and dental abnormalities are very common.
- Lung abscesses and pneumatoceles following pneumonias caused by *Staphylococcus aureus* and *Haemophilus influenzae* are the major factors for morbidity.

Infections and immunologic characteristics

Moderate to severe eczema presenting within the first hours to weeks of life is almost universal in HIES. Mucocutaneous candidiasis involving finger and toenails, mouth, vagina and intertriginous areas is seen in most patients. Primary pulmonary infections are caused by *S. aureus, Haemophilus influenzae*, and *Streptococcus pneumoniae*. These pneumonias are often associated with abscess formation and usually lead to the development of pneumatoceles (see Fig. 21.10). Once lung cavities are formed, they provide an attractive environment for superinfection with *Pseudomonas* or *Aspergillus* spp. The clinical morphotype suggests abnormal tissue remodeling, and associated with abnormal matrix metalloproteinase (MMP) 3, 8, and 9 levels. *Pneumocystis jiroveci* pneumonia, *Cryptococcus neoformans* esophageal infection and intestinal histoplasmosis have been reported. IgE levels are usually above 2000 IU/mL, but substantial fluctuations in IgE levels have been recorded over time and the IgE levels do not correlate with disease activity or eosinophilia. Total serum IgG levels are usually within the normal range. Eosinophilia is common; the white blood cell count is usually normal to low.

Mutations in *STAT3* lead to disruption of cytokine signaling, inlcuding IL-6, IL-10, IL-11, and IL-17. STAT3 deficiency leads to a proinflammatory state with elevated TNF-α and IFN-γ, but also results in inability to form IL-17 producing T cells (Th17 cells), which may explain the predisposition to mucocutaneous candidiasis.[44] Memory B and T cells are low. Shingles eruptions are increased in Job syndrome, despite the fact that primary varicella zoster virus infections are normally handled. Lymphomas, but not epithelial malignancies, are increased in STAT3 deficiency.

DOCK8 deficiency (autosomal recessive hyper-IgE syndrome)

During the phenotyping of Job syndrome, it became clear that there was a partially overlapping syndrome with an autosomal recessive pattern of transmission. This disease overlaps with Job syndrome in its elevated IgE, eczema, and eosinophilia. However, dedicator of cytokinesis 8 (DOCK8, located at 9p24) deficiency also includes food allergies, asthma, herpesvirus infections, human papilloma virus and molluscum contagiosum virus infections, which are not part of STAT3 deficiency. In addition to the infection susceptibility, DOCK8-deficient patients are predisposed to cutaneous and lymphoid malignancies.[45] While Th17 cells are markedly diminished in STAT3-deficient patients, they are less severely reduced in DOCK8-deficient patients (the HIES-like patients in ref 44). The specific contributions of these relatively IL-17-deficient states are areas of active investigation.

GATA2 deficiency (MonoMAC syndrome)

GATA2 (located at 3q21.3) is an early hematopoietic transcription factor most active in myeloid development. Human haploinsufficiency of GATA2 leads to this unusual syndrome.[46] The syndrome of monocytopenia and mycobacterial disease (monoMAC) is characterized by late childhood or adult-onset disseminated nontuberculous mycobacterial disease or disseminated fungal disease. These patients' hemograms are remarkable for absolute circulating monocytopenia, NK cell cytopenia, and B cell lymphopenia. Despite these circulating cytopenias, there are tissue macrophages and plasma cells, and immunoglobulin levels are normal to elevated. Neutrophils are variably affected. Other infections in this syndrome include human papilloma virus, molluscum contagiosum, histoplasmosis, and aspergillosis. Progressive pulmonary alveolar proteinosis is common, as are cytogenetic abnormalities in bone marrow such as trisomy 8 and monosomy 7. Diagnosis is suspected based on the infections and the abnormal hemogram. Since most routine hematologic laboratory studies allow normal monocyte percentages to range quite low, it is necessary to look at absolute monocyte numbers. Other presentations of this syndrome include aplastic anemia, acute myelogenous leukemia, and chronic myelomonocytic leukemia. Sequencing of GATA2 is the preferred diagnostic approach.

● ON THE HORIZON

- Early recognition and molecular diagnosis of all phagocyte defects, leading to prophylactic antimicrobial treatment, where indicated.
- Improvement in bone marrow transplantation technology to allow early, safe, successful, fertility-preserving transplantation in all cases.
- Understanding the mechanisms of the hepatic complications of CGD that correlate with mortality.
- Characterizing the pathways that converge on STAT3 signaling causing the complex somatic and immune disorder, hyper-IgE recurrent infection syndrome.

Assessment of neutrophil function

Discrete abnormalities in neutrophil function lead to recurrent bacterial or fungal infections. Assays have been developed to interrogate those functions. However, since neutrophils cannot be viably stored or frozen, samples are usually examined fresh with simultaneous normal volunteer controls. The techniques discussed here are reviewed in detail in reference[47] and Chapter 96.

Isolation of neutrophils

Most assays require neutrophils to be purified away from other leukocytes and blood components. Blood is usually anticoagulated using either citrate or heparin (10 units/mL) tubes and maintained at 20–25°C (room temperature) in polypropylene containers. Most protocols use differences in the cell density as the basis for the separation by sedimentation or centrifugation, or both. Typically, $1–2 \times 10^6$ neutrophils can be isolated per milliliter of whole blood.

Neutrophil adherence

The adhesive function of phagocytes is commonly assessed by passage of 1 mL of whole blood through a column filled with nylon wool. Adherence is measured as the difference in the absolute neutrophil count of the pre-column sample and of the sample after passage through the nylon wool column. Alternatively, isolated neutrophils can be induced to bind to plastic using a 96-well plate either uncoated, or coated with fetal bovine serum, a ligand like ICAM-1, or a specific extracellular matrix protein such as fibrinogen or fibronectin. Endothelial cell monolayers harvested from human umbilical veins may serve as a more physiological substrate for the measurement of cell adhesion. Isolated neutrophils are pre-loaded with the cell permeant, acetoxymethyl ester derivative of the fluorescent dye, calcein (calcein-AM). Nonspecific esterases in the cytosol cleave the ester linkage, trapping the fluorescent probe in the cytosol. The labeled neutrophils are added to each well and incubated in the absence or presence of phorbol myristate acetate (PMA) to promote adherence through activated integrins. At the end of the incubation, the wells are washed to remove nonadherent cells. The fluorescence of each well is determined with a fluorescent microplate reader and compared to the fluorescence of a control well with a fixed number of fluorescent cells. Under control conditions, fewer than 10% of the neutrophils adhere to plastic or to plastic coated with fetal bovine serum. Slightly more neutrophil adherence is observed on wells coated with fibrinogen. Treatment of normal neutrophils with PMA for 30 minutes results in the adherence of 100% of the neutrophils under all conditions. This adherence is abnormal in patients with leukocyte adhesion deficiency. Neutrophils isolated from patients with typical LAD-1 generally exhibit markedly reduced adherence under both unstimulated and PMA conditions.

Neutrophil chemotaxis

Neutrophil chemotaxis *in vivo* can be evaluated using skin windows. Skin blisters are gently raised on the volar surface of the forearm using a vacuum pump and an 8-well blister device, with little hemorrhage or vascular damage. The roof of the blister is removed and the exposed skin lesion is bathed with autologous serum using a skin window chamber. In 24 hours, exudative neutrophils accumulate in the autologous serum bathing the skin lesion. The skin chamber provides a mechanism for characterizing the immune cells, as well as soluble immune mediators, that accumulate in the autologous serum during the evolution of the inflammatory response. Chemotaxis *in vitro* is generally measured using a Boyden chamber. The Boyden chamber includes three components: a lower (chemoattractant) chamber, a nitrocellulose or polycarbonate filter layer, and an upper cell chamber. The lower compartments of the Boyden chamber are filled with a chemoattractant such as fMLF (10^{-8} M) or IL-8 (10 ng/mL). Recently, an improved rapid fluorescence-based measure of neutrophil chemotaxis has been developed that uses a new 96-well disposable chemotaxis chamber that can be read in a fluorescence microplate reader.

Expression of surface antigens

The expression of cell surface antigens on neutrophils relies on labeled monoclonal antibodies analyzed by flow cytometry. The panel may include the β_2 integrins (CD11a, CD11b, CD11c, and CD18), selectins (CD62L), Fcγ receptors I, II, and III (CD64, CD32 and CD16), leukosialin (CD43), the common leukocyte antigen (CD45), and markers for the specific granules (CD67) and azurophilic granules (CD63). The expression of surface antigens can be used to assess the responsiveness of neutrophils to particular ligands such as fMLF and LPS.

Neutrophil degranulation

The proteases, acid hydrolases, and inflammatory mediators released from storage granules in neutrophils can mediate bacterial killing, tissue damage, healing, and immune regulation. Lactoferrin from specific granules can chelate iron, resulting in a bactericidal or bacteriostatic effect. Stimulation of neutrophils with various secretagogues can release granular enzymes into the extracellular fluid. Treatment of the neutrophils with cytochalasin b (5 μg/mL) disrupts microfilament assembly and facilitates the release of both specific and azurophilic enzymes. To differentiate degranulation from cell lysis, release of the cytosolic enzyme lactate dehydrogenase should be monitored simultaneously. The release of azurophilic granules can be assessed by determination of β-glucuronidase activity. Supernatant fluids or cell extracts obtained from stimulated neutrophils are incubated with 4-methylumbelliferyl-β-D-glucuronide. Alternatively, myeloperoxidase can be determined using commercially available enzyme-linked immunoassays. CD63 is also found in the membrane of azurophilic granules and migrates to the neutrophil surface after stimulation with fMLF in the presence of cytochalasin b. The release of specific granules can be assessed by determination of lactoferrin levels using an enzyme-linked immunoassay. The carcinoembryonic antigen CD66b (formerly CD67) is found on the neutrophil surface and in the specific granules, and its expression on the surface of the neutrophils is increased after stimulation with fMLF or lipopolysaccharide. Detection of the constituents of secretory granules can be assessed by flow cytometric analysis of the change in expression of surface proteins such as adhesion molecules, and cytochrome b$_{558}$ of the NADPH oxidase.

Generation of reactive oxygen species

The release of reactive oxygen intermediates such as O_2^- and H_2O_2 is an important component of the neutrophil bactericidal machinery. Neutrophils isolated from patients with CGD are unable to generate superoxide, leading to their oxygen-dependent bactericidal defect. The production of superoxide (O_2^-) can be detected using the reduction of cytochrome c. Because O_2^- causes a one-to-one stoichiometric reduction of ferricytochrome c to ferrocytochrome c, the resultant increase in the absorption spectrum at 550 nM can be used to quantitate the production of O_2^-. Superoxide dismutase is added to an identical tube to control for the nonspecific reduction of cytochrome c. However, since cytochrome is not permeable to the cells, the detection of O_2^- is limited to that released into the extracellular milieu. Neutrophils isolated from patients with CGD fail to produce O_2^- in response to phorbol myristate acetate (PMA) in 10 minutes. However, some patients with forms of CGD associated with residual superoxide production have low, but detectable O_2^- production in 60 minutes. Neutrophils isolated from X-linked heterozygous carriers of CGD can yield a full spectrum of O_2^- production, while neutrophils from autosomal recessive carriers of CGD generally yield a normal response. Although the detection of O_2^- by reduction of cytochrome c is useful in the diagnosis of patients with CGD, it cannot be used in the diagnosis of carriers because of the wide spectrum of responses that result from the degree of X chromosome lyonization.

The extracellular release of H_2O_2 can be measured using horseradish peroxidase-induced oxidation of either phenol red or Amplex red. Polymorphonuclear neutrophil suspensions in the presence of horseradish peroxidase and one of the chromophores are exposed to either PMA or buffer alone. Changes in optical density of phenol red at 600 nm can be determined with a standard microplate reader. Amplex red is a much more sensitive fluorescent chromophore and H_2O_2-dependent changes in fluorescence can be determined with a fluorescence microplate reader.

The nitroblue tetrazolium (NBT) test is a qualitative assay of O_2^- production. Either whole blood or isolated neutrophils are mixed with NBT in a chamber slide and stimulated with PMA for 15–30 minutes at 37 °C. The slide is counterstained with 0.1% safranin, and examined under a microscope. The NBT test yields a visual record of the reduction of NBT dye to the insoluble, blue-black deposits of formazan. Normal neutrophils, but not neutrophils from CGD patients, reduce the yellow dye to black-brown-blue aggregates in the cells. The NBT can be used to diagnose X-linked carriers of CGD but cannot differentiate autosomal carriers from normal subjects.

An alternative to the NBT test is a flow cytometric assay using the dye, dihydrorhodamine-1,2,3. Neutrophils are loaded with the nonfluorescent dye, and then stimulated with PMA for 15 minutes at 37 °C. The H_2O_2 produced oxidizes the dye and results in increased fluorescence, detectable with a flow cytometer. Catalase is added to prevent cell-to-cell diffusion of H_2O_2. Since dye is localized to the cytoplasm, and catalase is present in the extracellular fluid, the dihydrorhodamine-1,2,3 assay detects the intracellular production of reactive oxygen metabolites. Stimulation of normal neutrophils with PMA results in a two-log shift in the fluorescence intensity. Neutrophils from an X-linked carrier of CGD exhibit mosaicism with a negatively-stained (abnormal) population and a brightly-stained positive population. Neutrophils from a patient with X-linked CGD that lack gp91^{phox} express little increase in fluorescence while neutrophils from a patient with a deficiency in p47^{phox} exhibit a slight increase in fluorescence. The major advantages of the dihydrorhodamine-1,2,3 assay are the sensitivity, the signal-to-noise ratio, and the ease of counting a large number of cells.

Western blot for determination of NADPH oxidase defect

Determination of the specific protein defect in CGD by western blot analysis also provides direction for the genetic defect. A validated normal control and a typical gp91^{phox} CGD are included on each blot to insure adequate development of p22^{phox}. Patients with p47^{phox} CGD are Western blot-negative. Patients with p67^{phox} CGD are generally Western blot-negative. Because p22^{phox} and gp91^{phox} exist as a membrane complex, patients with a defect are p22^{phox}, in general, are Western blot-negative for both p22^{phox} and gp91^{phox}. In contrast, defects in gp91^{phox} yield more variable results. In general, patients with nonsense defects in gp91^{phox} exhibit low but detectable levels of p22^{phox}. Patients with missense mutations in gp91^{phox} that yield detectable gp91^{phox} protein exhibit proportionately higher levels of p22^{phox}.

Translational research

The distance traveled over the past 50 years in phagocyte defects has been remarkable, spanning initial identification, phenotyping, and molecular characterization. Just the last 10 years have seen the advent of oral antifungals, potent oral antibiotics, oral antivirals, and reduced intensity conditioning for bone marrow transplantation. These advances have transformed the quality of life and longevity of all patients with immune deficiencies. We now need further in depth study of mechanism to drive novel insights into disease pathophysiology. The advent of therapeutic cytokines, small molecule inhibitors and agonists, RNA inhibitors, and effective means of gene transfer should make directed approaches to disease modification a reality. However, we must be sure we know exactly what functions need addressing. The downstream effect of genetic defects are surprisingly complex, and not always as straightforward as was anticipated. More detailed clinical and functional phenotyping, careful examination of developmental and gene expression effects, and continued longitudinal studies of large cohorts will convert these severe diseases punctuated by acute, life-threatening infections, into chronic conditions that are successfully treated medically, or successfully managed until successful bone marrow transplantation is available.

Acknowledgment

This work was supported by the intramural program of the National Institute of Allergy and Infectious Diseases. Neither author has any conflicts to disclose.

References

1. Kaushansky K. Lineage-specific hematopoietic growth factors. N Engl J Med 2006;354:2034–45.
2. Berliner N. Lessons from congenital neutropenia: 50 years of progress in understanding myelopoiesis. Blood 2008;111(12):5427–32.
3. Geissmann F, Manz MG, Jung S, et al. Development of monocytes, macrophages, and dendritic cells. Science 2010;327(5966):656–61.
4. Bouma G, Ancliff PJ, Thrasher AJ, Burns SO. Recent advances in the understanding of genetic defects of neutrophil number and function. Br J Haematol 2010;151(4):312–26.
5. Kollner I, Sodeik B, Schreek S, et al. Mutations in neutrophil elastase causing congenital neutropenia lead to cytoplasmic protein accumulation and induction of the unfolded protein response. Blood 2006;108(2):493–500.
6. Dale DC, Welte K. Cyclic and chronic neutropenia. Cancer Treat Res 2011;157:97–108.
7. Klein C, Grudzien M, Appaswamy G, et al. HAX1 deficiency causes autosomal recessive severe congenital neutropenia (Kostmann disease). Nat Genet 2007;39(1):86–92.
8. Germeshausen M, Grudzien M, Zeidler C, et al. Novel HAX1 mutations in patients with severe congenital neutropenia reveal isoform-dependent genotype-phenotype associations. Blood 2008;111(10):4954–7.
9. Boztug K, Appaswamy G, Ashikov A, et al. A syndrome with congenital neutropenia and mutations in G6PC3. N Engl J Med 2009;360(1):32–43.
10. Boocock GR, Marit MR, Rommens JM. Phylogeny, sequence conservation, and functional complementation of the SBDS protein family. Genomics 2006;87(6):758–71.
11. Huang JN, Shimamura A. Clinical spectrum and molecular pathophysiology of Shwachman-Diamond syndrome. Curr Opin Hematol 2010; Nov 30 [Epub ahead of print].
12. Capsoni F, Sarzi-Puttini P, Zanella A. Primary and secondary autoimmune neutropenia. Arthritis Res Ther 2005;7(5):208–14.
13. Maheshwari A, Christensen RD, Calhoun DA. Immune neutropenia in the neonate. Adv Pediatr 2002;49:317–39.
14. Borregaard N. Neutrophils, from marrow to microbes. Immunity 2010;33(5):657–70.
15. Etzioni A. Genetic etiologies of leukocyte adhesion defects. Curr Opin Immunol 2009;21(5):481–6.
16. Kishimoto TK, Hollander N, Roberts TM, et al. Heterogeneous mutations in the beta subunit common to the LFA-1, Mac-1, and p150,95 glycoproteins cause leukocyte adhesion deficiency. Cell 1987;50(2):193–202.
17. Roos D, Meischl C, de Boer M, et al. Genetic analysis of patients with leukocyte adhesion deficiency: genomic sequencing reveals otherwise undetectable mutations. Exp Hematol 2002;30(3):252–61.
18. Etzioni A, Gershoni-Baruch R, Pollack S, Shehadeh N. Leukocyte adhesion deficiency type II: long-term follow-up. J Allergy Clin Immunol 1998;102(2):323–4.
19. Alon R, Etzioni A. LAD-III, a novel group of leukocyte integrin activation deficiencies. Trends Immunol 2003;24(10):561–6.
20. Malinin NL, Zhang L, Choi J, et al. A point mutation in KINDLIN3 ablates activation of three integrin subfamilies in humans. Nat Med 2009;15(3):313–8.
21. Svensson L, Howarth K, McDowall A, et al. Leukocyte adhesion deficiency-III is caused by mutations in KINDLIN3 affecting integrin activation. Nat Med 2009;15(3):306–12.
22. Winkelstein JA, Marino MC, Richard Johnston J, et al. Chronic Granulomatous Disease: Report on a National Registry of 368 Patients. Medicine 2000;79:155–69.
23. Segal AW. How neutrophils kill microbes. Annu Rev Immunol 2005;23:197–223.
24. Papayannopoulos V, Zychlinsky A. NETs: a new strategy for using old weapons. Trends Immunol 2009;30(11):513–21.
25. Roos D, Kuhns DB, Maddalena A, et al. Hematologically important mutations: X-linked chronic granulomatous disease (third update). Blood Cells Mol Dis 2010;45(3):246–65.
26. Royer-Pokora B, Kunkel LM, Monaco AP, et al. Cloning the gene for an inherited human disorder–chronic granulomatous disease—on the basis of its chromosomal location. Nature 1986;322(6074):32–8.
27. Deardorff MA, Gaddipati H, Kaplan P, et al. Complex management of a patient with a contiguous Xp11.4 gene deletion involving ornithine transcarbamylase: a role for detailed molecular analysis in complex presentations of classical diseases. Mol Genet Metab 2008;94(4):498–502.
28. Roos D, Kuhns DB, Maddalena A, et al. Hematologically important mutations: the autosomal recessive forms of chronic granulomatous disease (second update). Blood Cells Mol Dis 2010;44(4):291–9.
29. Matute JD, Arias AA, Wright NA, et al. A new genetic subgroup of chronic granulomatous disease with autosomal recessive mutations in p40 phox and selective defects in neutrophil NADPH oxidase activity. Blood 2009;114(15):3309–15.
30. Kuhns DB, Alvord WG, Heller T, et al. Residual NADPH oxidase and survival in chronic granulomatous disease. N Engl J Med 2010;363(27):2600–10.
31. Lublin M, Bartlett DL, Danforth DN, et al. Hepatic abscess in patients with chronic granulomatous disease. Ann Surg 2002;235(3):383–91.
32. Feld JJ, Hussain N, Wright EC, et al. Hepatic involvement and portal hypertension predict mortality in chronic granulomatous disease. Gastroenterology 2008;134(7):1917–26.
33. Segal BH, DeCarlo ES, Kwon-Chung KJ, et al. Aspergillus nidulans infection in chronic granulomatous disease. Medicine 1998;77(5):345–54.
34. Vinh DC, Shea YR, Jones PA, et al. Chronic invasive aspergillosis caused by Aspergillus viridinutans. Emerg Infect Dis 2009;15(8):1292–4.
35. Siddiqui S, Anderson VL, Hilligoss DM, et al. Fulminant mulch pneumonitis: an emergency presentation of chronic granulomatous disease. Clin Infect Dis 2007;45(6):673–81.
36. Greenberg DE, Shoffner AR, Zelazny AM, et al. Recurrent Granulibacter bethesdensis infections and chronic granulomatous disease. Emerg Infect Dis 2010;16(9):1341–8.
37. Marciano BE, Rosenzweig SD, Kleiner DE, et al. Gastrointestinal involvement in chronic granulomatous disease. Pediatrics 2004;114(2):462–8.
38. De Ravin SS, Naumann N, Cowen EW, et al. Chronic granulomatous disease as a risk factor for autoimmune disease. J Allergy Clin Immunol 2008;122(6):1097–103.
39. Kang EM, Marciano BE, DeRavin S, et al. Chronic granulomatous disease: overview and hematopoietic stem cell transplantation. J Allergy Clin Immunol 2011;127(6):1319–26.
40. Lanza F. Clinical manifestation of myeloperoxidase deficiency. J Mol Med 1998;76(10):676–81.
41. Gombart AF, Koeffler HP. Neutrophil specific granule deficiency and mutations in the gene encoding transcription factor C/EBP(epsilon). Curr Opin Hematol 2002;9(1):36–42.
42. Kaplan J, De Domenico I, Ward DM. Chediak–Higashi syndrome. Curr Opin Hematol 2008;15(1):22–9.
43. Freeman AF, Holland SM. Clinical manifestations, etiology, and pathogenesis of the hyper-IgE syndromes. Pediatr Res 2009;65:32R–7R.
44. Milner JD, Sandler NG, Douek DC. Th17 cells, Job's syndrome and HIV: opportunities for bacterial and fungal infections. Curr Opin HIV AIDS 2010;5:179–83.
45. Zhang Q, Davis JC, Lamborn IT, et al. Combined immunodeficiency associated with DOCK8 mutations. N Engl J Med 2009;361(21):2046–55.
46. Hsu AP, Sampaio EP, Khan J, et al. Mutations in GATA2 are associated with the autosomal dominant and sporadic monocytopenia and mycobacterial infection (MonoMAC) syndrome. Blood 2011;118:2653–5.
47. Elloumi HZ, Holland SM. Diagnostic assays for chronic granulomatous disease and other neutrophil disorders. Methods Mol Biol 2007;412:505–523.

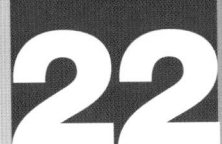
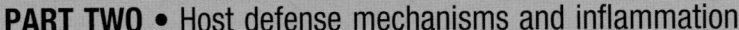
Martin Metz, Knut
Brockow, Dean
D. Metcalfe,
Stephen J. Galli

Mast cells, basophils, and mastocytosis

Mast cells and basophils are critical effector cells in IgE-associated allergic diseases, in host responses to parasites, and in many other processes.[1–3] Mast cells and basophils share several features in addition to the metachromatic staining properties of their prominent cytoplasmic granules (Table 22.1). Both are derived from bone marrow progenitors, express high-affinity IgE Fc receptors (FcεRI) on their surface, are major sources of histamine and other potent inflammatory mediators, and can be activated to release a wide array of mediators after sensitization with IgE and subsequent exposure to specific multivalent antigen.[1–4] However, mast cells and basophils differ in their responsiveness to other potential activators of secretion and in the specific pattern of mediators released by the activated cells.[1–3] Moreover, basophils and mast cells exhibit several differences in morphology, particularly by transmission electron microscopy (Table 22.2 and Fig. 22.1).

● **KEY CONCEPTS**

Origins of basophils and mast cells

- Mast cells and basophils represent distinct hematopoietic lineages.
- Basophils are granulocytes that mature in the bone marrow, circulate in the blood, and can be recruited into peripheral tissues at sites of immunologic or pathologic responses.
- Mast cell progenitors also arise in the bone marrow, but mast cells mature in peripheral tissues.
- Mast cells are present throughout virtually all normal connective tissues, and are particularly abundant near epithelial surfaces exposed to the environment.
- The KIT ligand stem cell factor (SCF) is critical for mast cell development and survival and can influence mast cell function.
- IL-3 is not required for normal basophil development in mice, but is critical for the basophilia associated with certain Th2 responses.

Development and distribution of mast cells

Distribution and heterogeneity

Unlike mature basophils, mature mast cells do not normally circulate in the blood but are ordinarily distributed throughout the connective tissues, where they often lie adjacent to blood and lymphatic vessels, near or within nerves, and beneath epithelial surfaces that are exposed to the external environment (e.g., lung, gut, and skin).[1,2]

The numbers of mast cells in normal tissues vary considerably by anatomic site, and their distribution can change during perturbations of homeostasis.[1–3] For example, in certain inflammatory or immunologic reactions mast cells can appear within the respiratory or gastrointestinal epithelium and in their associated secretions.[1–3] Mast cell numbers at sites of chronic inflammation may be many times higher than in the corresponding normal tissues.[1–3] The extent to which such changes reflect proliferation of resident mast cell populations, as opposed to the recruitment and differentiation of mast cell precursors, remains unclear.

The phenotype of different populations of mast cells, including morphology, histochemistry, mediator content and response to drugs and stimuli of activation, can also vary.[1–3] It is possible that mast cells of different phenotypes have different roles in health and disease, and may respond differently to drugs used in clinical settings. In mice and rats, connective tissue mast cells (CTMCs) and mucosal mast cells (MMCs) exhibit significant differences in multiple aspects of phenotype.[1–3] In humans, some mast cells express immunoreactivity for both tryptase and chymase (MC_{TC}), whereas others are immunoreactive for tryptase (MC_T) but lack detectable chymase (<0.04 pg/cell).[1,2,5] MC_T predominate in lung and small intestinal mucosa and MC_{TC} predominate in skin and small intestinal submucosa. A few mast cells that apparently express chymase (MC_C) but no detectable tryptase have also been reported.

Mast cell phenotypic variation could reflect any one or more of the following mechanisms: distinct mast cell lineages; the process of cellular maturation and differentiation; the functional status of the cell; and the influence of microenvironmental factors.[2]

Mast cell development in mice and rats

An essentially homogeneous population of growth factor-dependent immature mast cells develops when mouse hematopoietic cells are cultured in media containing interleukin (IL)-3.[2] Although such IL-3-induced bone marrow-derived cultured mast cells (BMCMCs) share some phenotypic characteristics with mouse MMCs, both *in vivo* and *in vitro* studies indicate that these cells acquire phenotypic features more similar to those of CTMCs when placed in an appropriate environment.[1,2] In vitro, fibroblasts provide factors, particularly stem cell factor (SCF), that promote IL-3-induced BMCMCs to develop features of CTMCs.[1,2] Indeed, studies in both mice and humans indicate that many aspects of mast cell development and survival

Table 22.1 Natural history, major mediators and surface membrane structures of human mast cells and basophils

Characteristic	Basophils	Mast cells
Natural history		
Origin of precursor cells	Bone marrow	Bone marrow
Site of maturation	Bone marrow	Connective tissues (a few in the bone marrow)
Mature cells in the circulation	Yes (usually <1% of blood leukocytes)	No
Mature cells recruited into tissues from circulation	Yes (during immunologic, inflammatory responses)	No
Mature cells normally residing in connective tissues	No (not detectable by microscopy)	Yes
Proliferative ability of morphologically mature cells	None reported	Yes (in certain circumstances)
Life span	Days (like other granulocytes)	Weeks to months (based on studies in rodents)
Mediators		
Major mediators stored preformed in cytoplasm	Histamine, chondroitin sulfates, neutral protease with bradykinin-generating activity, β-glucuronidase, elastase, cathepsin G-like enzyme, major basic protein, Charcot–Leyden crystal protein, tryptase[a], chymase[a], carboxypeptidase A[a]	Histamine, heparin and/or chondroitin sulfates, neutral proteases (chymase and/or tryptase), many acid hydrolases, cathepsin G, carboxypeptidase A
Major lipid mediators produced upon appropriate activation	Leukotriene C_4 (LTC_4)	Prostaglandin D_2, LTC_4, platelet-activating factor
Cytokines, chemokines and growth factors released upon appropriate activation	IL-4, IL-13	Tumor necrosis factor, IL-1, IL-3, IL-4, IL-5, IL-6, IL-10, IL-13, IL-16, VPF/VEGF, GM-CSF, MIP-1α, MCP-1
Surface structures[b]		
Ig receptors	FcεRI, FcγRII (CDw32), FcγRIIB	FcεRI, FcγRI, FcγRII, FcγRIIB
Cytokine/growth factor receptors	IL-1RIIb (CD121b), IL-2R (CD25), IL-3Rα, IL-4Rα, IL-5Rα, GM-CSFRα, TrK-A, CCR-2, CCR-3, CXCR1, CXCR4, KIT (some basophils express low numbers of KIT receptors)	KIT (SCF receptor), CCR-3, CCR-5, CXCR1, CXCR2, CXCR3, CXCR4, IL-4Rα, IL5Rα, IL-6R, IFN-γRα, TrkA, T1/ST2/IL-1R4
Cell adhesion structures	LFA-1 α chain (CD11a), C3bi receptor (CD11b), CR4 (CD11c), sLe^x(CD15s), LFA-1 β chain (CD18), $β_1$integrin (CD29), leukosialin (CD43), PECAM-1 (CD31), CD44, ICAM-3 (CD50), ICAM-1 (CD54), LFA-3 (CD58), L-selectin (CD62L), CD102, $β_7$-integrin, neurothelin (CD147), PETA-3 (CD151), BST-1 (CD157), PSGL-1 (CD162)	CD11a, CD11b, CD11c, CD18, CD29, CD43, CD44, CD49a, CD49b, CD49c, CD49d, CD49e, CD50, CD51, CD54, CD58, CD61, CD81, CD102, CD147, CD151, CD157

IL, interleukin; SCF, stem cell factor; LFA, lymphocyte function-associated antigen; CR, complement receptor; ICAM, intercellular adhesion molecule; sLe^x sialyl Lewis^x, PECAM-1, platelet-endothelial cell adhesion molecule-1; PETA-3, platelet-endothelial cell tetra-span antigen; BST-1, bone marrow stromal cell antigen-1; PSGL-1, P-selectin glycoprotein ligand-1.
[a]Expressed in peripheral blood basophils of asthma, allergy, and drug-reactive patients (Li L, Li Y, Reddel SW, et al. Identification of basophilic cells that express mast cell granule proteases in the peripheral blood of asthma, allergy, and drug-reactive patients. J Immunol 1998; 161: 5079–5086).
[b]Some mast cell surface structures have been detected in either mast cells cultured from human umbilical cord blood (expression varies during differentiation), skin mast cells or lung mast cells (Valent P. Immunophentypic characterization of human basophils and mast cells. Chem Immunol 1995; 61: 34–48). Basophils and various populations of mast cells also can express several TLRs. [8,9,15].

are critically regulated by SCF, the ligand for the KIT tyrosine growth factor receptor, which is expressed on the mast cell surface.[1,2]

Several other cytokines also promote mast cell development and/or proliferation *in vitro*, including IL-4, IL-9, and IL-10.[1,2] In contrast, granulocyte–macrophage colony-stimulating factor (GM-CSF) and transforming growth factor (TGF)-β1 can inhibit mouse BMCMC proliferation in response to IL-3.[2]

Mast cell development in humans

Human mast cell progenitors are present in umbilical cord blood, as well as in the bone marrow and the peripheral blood, and highly enriched populations of mast cells develop from these and other sources of human hematopoietic cells when they are maintained *in vitro* in media containing recombinant human

SCF (rhSCF).[1,2,6] rhSCF also promotes the development of human mast cells *in vivo*.[7]

Development and distribution of basophils

Basophils differentiate and mature in the bone marrow and then circulate in the blood. In the blood, the basophil is the least common blood granulocyte, with a prevalence of approximately 0.5% of total leukocytes and approximately 0.3% of nucleated marrow cells.[2] Basophils are not ordinarily found in connective tissues. Because the normal frequency of blood and bone marrow basophils is so low, accurate determinations ordinarily require absolute counting methods. The basophil's prominent metachromatic cytoplasmic granules permit it to be identified easily in Wright–Giemsa-stained preparations of peripheral blood or bone marrow cells. Both cytogenetic evidence and

Table 22.2 Morphologic features of mature basophils and mast cells

Characteristic	Basophils	Mast cells
Size	5–7 μm	6–12 μm
Surface	Irregular, short, thick processes	Numerous, uniformly distributed, elongated thin processes
Nucleus	Segmented (usually; occasionally nonsegmented)	Nonsegmented (usually round to oval in electron micrographs)[a]
Nuclear chromatin condensation	Marked	Moderate
Cytoplasmic granules	Fewer and larger than in mast cells; contain predominantly electron-dense particulate material with occasional membranous whorls	Smaller, more numerous, and generally more variable than in basophils; contain scroll-like structures, particles, or crystals, alone or in combination
Aggregates of cytoplasmic glycogen	Present	Absent
Cytoplasmic lipid bodies	Rare	Common but not present in all cells
Granule–granule fusion during anaphylactic degranulation	Rare (granule membranes usually fuse individually with plasma membrane)	Common

[a]Human mast cells generated *in vitro* can exhibit multilobulated nuclei. From Galli SJ, Lichtenstein LM. In: Middleton E Jr, Reed CE, Ellis EF, et al., eds. Allergy: principles and practice, 3rd edn. St Louis: Mosby, 1988; with permission from Elsevier.

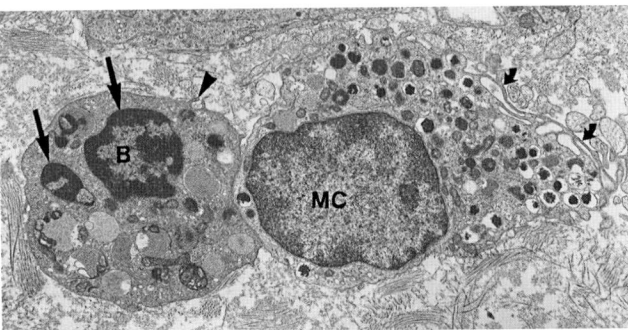

Fig. 22.1 Mast cell and basophil ultrastructure. A basophil (B) adjacent to a mast cell (MC) in the ileal submucosa of a patient with Crohn disease. The basophil exhibits a bilobed nucleus (solid arrows) whose chromatin is strikingly condensed beneath the nuclear membrane. The basophil surface is relatively smooth with a few blunt processes (arrowhead). The mast cell nucleus is larger and its chromatin less condensed than that of the basophil. The mast cell's granules are smaller, more numerous and more variable in shape and content than those of the basophil. The mast cell surface has numerous elongated, thin folds (curved arrows). (Original magnification ∼ ×9000). From Dvorak AM, Monahan RA, Osage JE, Dickersin GR. Crohn's disease: transmission electron microscopic studies. Hum Pathol 1980; 11: 606–619, with permission from Ann M. Dvorak.

in vitro studies indicate that basophils share a precursor with other granulocytes and monocytes.[1,2] The ultrastructural features of human basophils are summarized in Table 22.2 and illustrated in Fig. 22.1. The extent of the biochemical similarities between basophils and mast cells continues to be explored.[8,9]

Under physiological conditions basophils have a lifespan of days. IL-3 promotes the production and survival of basophils *in vitro* and can induce basophilia *in vivo*. Findings in IL-3$^{-/-}$ mice indicate that IL-3 is not necessary for the development of normal numbers of bone marrow or blood basophils, but is essential for the bone marrow and blood basophilia associated with certain Th2 cell-associated immunologic responses.[2,9]

Biologic mediators produced by mast cells and basophils

Basophils and mast cells contain, or elaborate on appropriate stimulation, a diverse array of potent biologically active mediators.[1–3,5,6,8–13] These agents mediate a wide array of effects in inflammation, immunity and tissue remodeling, and can also influence the clotting, fibrinolytic, complement and kinin systems. Some of these products are stored pre-formed in cytoplasmic granules (e.g., proteoglycans, proteases, histamine, certain cytokines), and others are synthesized upon activation of the cell by IgE and antigen or other stimuli (e.g., products of arachidonic acid oxidation through the cyclo-oxygenase or lipoxygenase pathways and, in some cells, platelet-activating factor (PAF), as well as cytokines, chemokines, and growth factors).[1–3,5,6,8–13]

● KEY CONCEPTS

Mast cell and basophil mediators

- Mast cells and basophils are sources of distinct, but overlapping, panels of mediators with diverse biologic effects.
- Some mast cell and basophil mediators are preformed and stored in cytoplasmic granules (e.g., histamine, heparin and other proteoglycans, proteases). They can be released rapidly upon degranulation induced by cellular activation.
- Mast cells and basophils also produce lipid mediators (e.g., PGD$_2$, LTC$_4$), which are derived from arachadonic acid and are newly synthesized upon appropriate activation of the cell.
- Mast cells can transcribe and secrete many cytokines/chemokines/growth factors, including (in mouse and/or human mast cells) IL-1, IL-2, IL-3, IL-4, IL-5, IL-6, IL-8, IL-10, IL-13, IL-16, GM-CSF, TNF, IFN-γ, TGF-β, bFGF, VPF/VEGF, NGF, and many C-C chemokines.
- In response to cellular activation (e.g., through the FcεRI), mast cells can release at least two cytokines, TNF and VPF/VEGF, from both stored and newly synthesized pools.
- Induction of cytokine mRNA in mast cells is not always accompanied by the release of detectable cytokine bioactivity.
- In some circumstances, induction and/or release of mast cell cytokines can occur in response to stimuli that do not induce a detectable release of histamine.
- Release of some cytokines (e.g., TNF) can continue for hours after initial FcεRI-dependent mast cell activation.
- Mast cell cytokine mRNA expression and/or cytokine release can be inhibited by cyclosporine or dexamethasone.
- Basophils appear to produce a more restricted spectrum of cytokines than do mast cells, but these include IL-4 and IL-13.

Mediators that are pre-formed

Mediators stored pre-formed in the cytoplasmic granules include histamine, proteoglycans, serine proteases, carboxypeptidase A, and small amounts of sulfatases and exoglycosidases. Studies in mice indicate that mast cells account for nearly all of the histamine stored in normal tissues, with the exception of the glandular stomach and the CNS.[2] Basophils are the source of most of the histamine in normal human blood.[2] Mouse and rat mast cells (and some human mast cells), but not human basophils, contain serotonin.[1,2]

Human mast cells contain variable mixtures of heparin (about 60 kDa) and chondroitin sulfate proteoglycans.[1,2] Although the sulfated glycosaminoglycans of normal human blood basophils have not been characterized, chondroitin sulfates account for the majority of the proteoglycans in the basophils of patients with myelogenous leukemia.[2]

Neutral proteases are the major protein component of mast cell secretory granules. The three major families of proteases found in mast cell granules are represented by the serine proteases chymase and tryptase and the metalloprotease carboxypeptidase A. In mice, five different chymases (mouse mast cell protease [mMCP]-1, -2, -4, -5, and -9) and four different tryptases (mMCP-6, -7 and -11 and mouse transmembrane tryptase [mTMT]) have been described;[12,13] in humans, it appears that there is only one chymase and four different tryptases (α, β, γ, and δ, encoded by several genes and alleles).[5,11,12] Mast cell protease content varies depending on the microenvironment, and can therefore contribute significantly to mast cell heterogeneity. Several potential functions have been associated with various mast cell proteases (e.g., effects that promote bronchomotor tone and degradation of fibrinogen, extracellular matrix proteins and endogeneous or exogenous peptides, including components of animal venoms),[1-3,5,11-14] and it is likely that additional biological roles will be identified.

Mediators that are newly synthesized

Activated mast cells initiate the *de novo* synthesis of several lipid-derived substances. Of particular importance are the cyclo-oxygenase and lipoxygenase metabolites of arachidonic acid, which have potent inflammatory activities and which may also play a role in modulating the release process itself.[10] The major cyclo-oxygenase product of mast cells is prostaglandin D_2 (PGD_2), and the major lipoxygenase products derived from mast cells and basophils are the sulfidopeptide leukotriene LTC_4 and its peptidolytic derivatives LTD_4 and LTE_4.[1,2,8,10] Mast cells isolated from a variety of tissues release both LTC_4 and PGD_2, whereas peripheral blood basophils release LTC_4 but not PGD_2. Mast cells also produce LTB_4, although in much smaller quantities than PGD_2 or LTC_4, and some mast cell populations represent a potential source of PAF.[1,2,8,10]

Cytokines, chemokines and growth factors

The ability of mast cells and basophils to produce cytokines, chemokines and growth factors greatly expands the list of possible mechanisms by which these cells may contribute to the pathophysiology of allergic and immunologic diseases, host defense or homeostasis.[1-3,6,8,15] Mast cells are a source for IL-1, -2, -3, -4, -5, -6, -8, -10, -13, -16, GM-CSF, TNF, NGF, bFGF, TGF-β1, and VPF/VEGF, as well as several C-C chemokines (Chapters 9 and 10). These products are released when the cells are activated via IgE-dependent mechanisms, and are also produced under other circumstances (e.g., in response to stimulation by bacterial products).[1-3,6,8,15]

The first cytokine bioactivity to be clearly associated with normal mast cells was TNF.[1] Some of the TNF released from mouse mast cells upon appropriate stimulation (e.g., via IgE-dependent activation) reflects cytokine that is rapidly released from pre-formed stores, and even larger amounts of newly synthesized TNF are released over a period of hours after cell activation.

The first cytokine bioactivity to be associated with normal basophils was IL-4, and mature human basophils isolated from peripheral blood can release IL-4 (and IL-13) in response to FcϵRI-dependent activation.[2,7,8] Basophils and mast cells express CD40 ligand (CD40L, CD154), and thus may also contribute to IgE production by promoting immunoglobulin class switching.[2,16]

Mechanisms of activation of mast cells and basophils

● KEY CONCEPTS

Mechanisms of mast cell and basophil activation

- Mast cells and basophils have cell-surface high-affinity IgE receptors (FcϵRI) that confer on these cells the ability to express specific immunological functions.

- Mast cells and basophils can be activated *in vivo* either by signaling through the FcϵRI or by a variety of nonimmunologic signals (e.g., certain neuropeptides, anaphylatoxins, f-Met-Leu-Phe, bacterial products/TLR ligands, animal venom components).

- The responses of basophils and/or different subpopulations of mast cells to stimuli other than IgE and antigen vary: some populations respond weakly or not at all to some stimuli.

- Some stimuli activate cells to release a panel of mediators quantitatively or qualitatively more limited than that induced by IgE and antigen.

- The susceptibility of mast cells or basophils to activation by IgE and specific antigen or other stimuli can be regulated by cytokines (e.g., SCF, IL-3), as well as by other microenvironmental factors.

- Certain mast cell populations can exhibit downregulation of FcϵRI-dependent activation via signaling by FcγRIIB or other receptors (such as members of the KIR family).

FcϵRI-mediated activation

Mast cells and basophils express FcϵRI, the high-affinity receptor for IgE.[1-4] Whereas high "constitutive" levels of FcϵRI expression apparently are restricted to mast cells and basophils, in humans low levels of expression are detected in Langerhans' cells, peripheral blood dendritic cells, and monocytes.[1-4] In mast cells and basophils, FcϵRI has a tetrameric structure composed of a single IgE-binding α chain, a single β chain and two identical disulfide-linked γ chains. All three subunits must be present for efficient cell surface expression in rodents, but human cells can express FcϵRI in the absence of the β chain. In humans, the FcϵRI expressed by hematopoietic cells other than mast cells and basophils consists of only the $\alpha\gamma\gamma$ form.[4] The aggregation of FcϵRI that is occupied by IgE is sufficient for initiating downstream signal transduction events that activate the mast cells or basophils to degranulate and to secrete lipid mediators

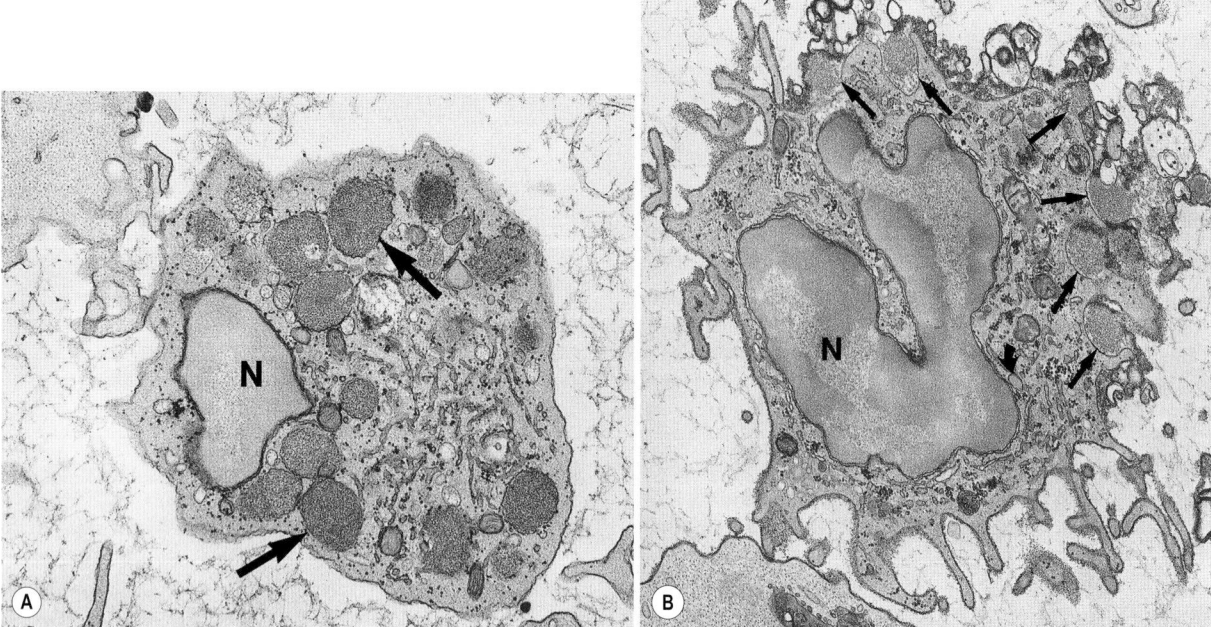

Fig. 22.2 (A) Transmission electron micrograph of a human basophil in a preparation of peripheral blood leukocytes obtained by separation over Ficoll-Hypaque. All of the cytoplasmic granules (some indicated by solid arrows) contain particulate electron-dense material. N, nucleus. (Original magnification ~ ×19 800). (B) A human basophil 2 minutes after exposure to antigen *in vitro*. The cell exhibits extrusion of granules from six separate sites on the plasma membrane (small arrows). At this time after cell stimulation, particle-filled granules retain their shape and characteristic structure even after exposure to extracellular milieu. Cationized ferritin coats the cell surface and enters culs-de-sac that contain exteriorized granules. The cell exhibits no fully intracytoplasmic typical basophilic granules, but one of the smaller kind of granules (curved arrow) can be observed in the perinuclear region. N, nucleus. (Original magnification ~ ×19 200).
From Dvorak AM, Newball HH, Dvorak HF, Lichtenstein LM. Antigen-induced IgE-mediated degranulation of human basophils. Lab Invest 1980; 43: 126-139, with permission from Nature Publishing Group Ltd.

and cytokines.[1-4] The FcεRI β chain functions as an amplifier of signaling through FcεRI, which can markedly upregulate the magnitude of the mediator release response to FcεRI aggregation.[4] Certain mutations that result in amino acid substitutions in the human β chain may be linked to atopic disease.[4]

At the ultrastructural level, stimulation of appropriately sensitized human basophils with specific antigen provokes fusion of the membranes enveloping individual cytoplasmic granules with the plasma membrane (Fig. 22.2).[2] As a result, the granules' contents, including stored mediators, are released via multiple narrow communications between single granules and the cell surface. IgE-dependent degranulation of human lung mast cells also results in the fusion of granule membranes with the plasma membrane (Fig. 22.3).[2] However, in this cell type the first ultrastructural changes detectable in the stimulated cells are granule swelling, followed by fusion of individual granule membranes forming interconnecting chains of swollen granules; histamine release is initiated by the opening of these channels to the exterior through multiple narrow points of fusion with the plasma membrane.[2]

Both *in vitro* and *in vivo*, levels of FcεRI surface expression on mast cells and basophils correlates positively with the concentration of IgE.[1] IgE-dependent upregulation of FcεRI expression *in vitro*, which reflects stabilization of expression of FcεRI on the cell surface, permits mast cells to secrete strikingly increased amounts of mediators after anti-IgE challenge, and to exhibit IgE-dependent mediator release at lower concentrations of specific antigen. Furthermore, mast cells that have undergone IgE-dependent upregulation of surface FcεRI expression may, upon subsequent FcεRI-dependent activation, secrete cytokines and growth factors that are released at very low levels (or not at

all) by mast cells with low levels of FcεRI expression.[2] These findings strongly suggest that basophils and mast cells in subjects with high levels of IgE (as typically characterizes patients with allergic disorders or parasitic infections) may be significantly enhanced in their ability to express IgE-dependent effector functions or, via cytokine production, potential immunoregulatory functions.[2] *In vitro* data from studies with mouse or human mast cells indicates that, under some circumstances, the binding of certain IgE antibodies to FcεRI can promote mast cell survival and/or mediator secretion, even in the absence of known specific antigen.[1] The clinical significance of these findings is not yet clear.

In addition to the high-affinity IgE receptor, mouse mast cells and human basophils express the low-affinity IgG receptor FcγRIIB. Co-aggregation of FcγRIIB and FcεRI has been shown to diminish IgE-dependent activation of mouse mast cells, RBL cells and human basophils *in vitro* and to diminish the expression of IgE- and mast cell-dependent allergic reactions *in vivo*.[17]

Activation by nonimmunologic means

In addition to IgE and specific antigen, a variety of biologic substances, including products of complement activation and neuropeptides, as well as certain bacterial products, cytokines, animal venom components, chemical agents and physical stimuli, elicit the release of basophil or mast cell mediators.[1-3,8,14,15] Morphine and other narcotics are among the pharmacological agents that can induce the release of mast cell mediators, especially from skin mast cells, and intravenous infusion of large

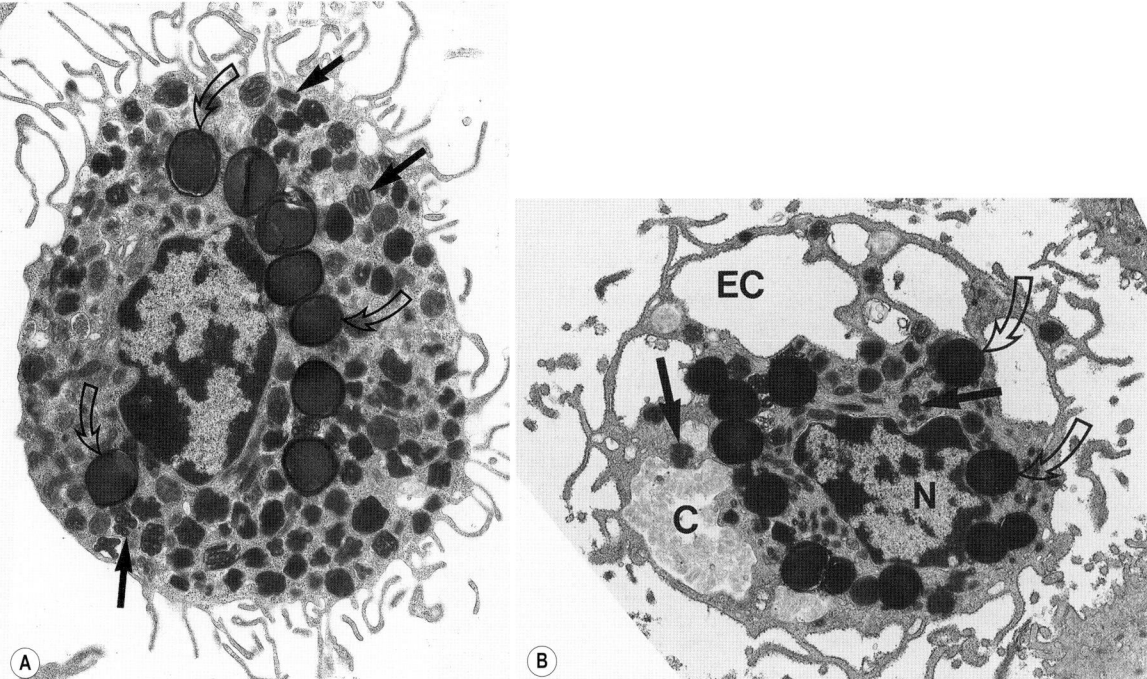

Fig. 22.3 (A) Mast cell purified from human lung. The cell contains many cytoplasmic granules with scroll-like substructural elements (solid arrows) and eight large nonmembrane-bound lipid bodies (open arrows). The plasma membrane has prominent folds. N, nucleus. (Original magnification ~ × 12 900). (B) An isolated human lung mast cell 10 minutes after exposure to anti-IgE *in vitro*. Some degranulation channels (C), formed by fusion of membranes surrounding individual cytoplasmic granules, contain altered granule matrix; others (EC) are empty. Cationized ferritin stains the plasma membrane and the membranes of some empty degranulation channels (EC). The membranes lining other channels (C) are unstained. A few unaltered scroll-containing granules (solid arrows) remain. Numerous lipid bodies are also present (open arrows). The cytoplasm contains prominent filaments. N, nucleus. (Original magnification ~ × 9 100).
From Galli SJ, Dvorak AM, Dvorak HF. Prog Allergy 1984; 34: 1, with permission from Ann M. Dvorak.

doses of morphine regularly causes an increase in plasma histamine levels and often results in shock.[1,2]

HIV glycoprotein 120, as well as protein Fv (pFv), which is released into the intestinal tract in patients with viral hepatitis, can interact with the heavy-chain variable domain of IgE antibodies that use VH3 gene segments (Chapter 4) and thereby induce the release of histamine, IL-4 and IL-13 from human basophils and mast cells.[8] Basophils also respond to stimulation with immobilized secretory IgA (sIgA) by releasing both histamine and LTC[4], but only if the cells have first been primed by pretreatment with IL-3, IL-5, or GM-CSF.[18] Furthermore, certain bacterial products — including lipopolysaccharide (LPS) and other ligands of TLRs — directly induce the release of some mast cell products; pathogens can also activate mast cells indirectly via activation of the complement system.[2,15]

It should be emphasized that the responsiveness of basophils and different populations of mast cells to individual stimuli varies; e.g., cutaneous mast cells appear to be much more sensitive to stimulation by neuropeptides than are pulmonary mast cells.[1,2] Moreover, some stimuli induce a pattern of mediator release that differs from the one associated with IgE-dependent mast cell activation. For example, LPS induces mast cells to release certain cytokines preferentially over pre-formed mediators.[15]

Mast cells, basophils, and allergic inflammation

The immediate hypersensitivity reaction is the pathophysiologic hallmark of allergic rhinitis, allergic asthma, and anaphylaxis, and the central role of the mast cell in the pathogenesis of the

acute manifestations of these disorders is widely accepted. To avoid confusion between immunologic mechanisms and clinical syndromes in the discussion of these disorders, it is essential to begin by defining some key terms.

Type I hypersensitivity reaction

Also known as the allergic or immediate hypersensitivity reaction, a type I hypersensitivity reaction, as originally described by Gell and Coombs, is now understood to be a pathologic immune response initiated in appropriately sensitized subjects by the interaction of antigen-specific IgE molecules on the surface of mast cells and/or basophils with the relevant multivalent antigen.[1-4] The physiologic effects are due to the biologic responses of target cells (vascular endothelial cells, smooth muscle, glands, leukocytes, etc.) to mediators released by activated mast cells and/or basophils. The term refers to an immunopathologic mechanism: it conveys no information about the severity or distribution of the reaction.

Immediate- or early-phase responses

The signs and symptoms that develop at the site of antigen exposure within the first few minutes of a type I reaction reflect the biologic activities of the mast cell- and/or (especially in systemic reactions) basophil-derived mediators that are released immediately after the activation of these cells. In sites that do not contain basophils, such as normal skin, these mediators are derived largely — perhaps exclusively — from mast cells. Thus, in most allergic patients, intradermal challenge with specific antigen or anti-IgE induces an immediate wheal and flare reaction, accompanied by intense pruritus, which reaches a maximum 15–30 minutes later.[1,2] Such immediate allergic reactions are usually accompanied by an increase in local levels of LTC_4 and PGD_2, and by the liberation of histamine and tryptase.

Studies in wild-type and c-*KIT* mutant genetically mast cell-deficient mice, and c-*KIT* mutant mice that have been selectively engrafted with mast cell populations (i.e., mast cell knock-in mice), have shown that essentially all of the augmented vascular permeability, tissue swelling and deposition of cross-linked fibrin associated with IgE-dependent passive cutaneous anaphylaxis reactions or with IgE-dependent reactions in the stomach wall were mast cell dependent.[2] In humans, studies of nasal secretions or skin blister fluids induced by exposure to allergen demonstrate the release of both histamine and tryptase, with a strong correlation between levels of these two mediators, implicating mast cells in these reactions.[2]

CLINICAL RELEVANCE

Mast cells and basophils in health and disease

- Mast cells and basophils are primary effector cells in atopic disorders (allergic rhinitis, allergic asthma, anaphylaxis).
- Antigen-specific mast cell activation results in an immediate reaction, and in many cases contributes to a late-phase response in the involved tissues.
- The late consequences of mast cell activation reflect the actions of cytokines, chemokines, growth factors, and other mediators derived from mast cells and from other cells resident at or recruited to these sites whose recruitment, phenotype, or function can be influenced by mast cell-derived products.
- Mast cells and basophils may also contribute to host defense against certain parasites and have been implicated in a wide variety of other diseases and host responses, including innate immunity to microbial infection.

Anaphylaxis

Traditionally, this term has been used to describe an antigen-specific IgE-mediated reaction that is both life-threatening and systemic, with several organ systems involved (Chapter 40). In this context anaphylaxis can be considered a severe, systemic type I immediate hypersensitivity reaction. However, because degranulation of mast cells and/or basophils can occur via non-IgE-dependent mechanisms, and because the biologic effects of the liberated mast cell and/or basophil mediators are the same regardless of the mechanism by which they are released, the term anaphylaxis sometimes also is used to describe a clinical syndrome that is severe, abrupt, and manifested by cutaneous (urticaria, angioedema), respiratory (asthma, laryngeal edema), cardiovascular (hypotension, cardiovascular collapse), and/or gastrointestinal (nausea, vomiting, diarrhea, cramping) signs and symptoms that occur either singly or in combination, whether or not the underlying mechanism is dependent on IgE. When used in this fashion, the term does not imply any particular pathologic mechanism. Several lines of evidence indicate that systemic anaphylaxis in humans is associated with extensive mast cell activation. Increased levels of mast cell tryptase have been detected in the serum after the onset of anaphylactic symptoms, but little or no tryptase can be detected in serum from normal controls.[2,3,5] The histamine detected in the plasma of patients with anaphylaxis can be derived from both mast cells and basophils.[2,3,5]

Late-phase responses

In many allergic patients the immediate reaction to cutaneous antigenic challenge is followed 4–8 hours later by persistent swelling and leukocyte infiltration, which is termed the late-phase response (LPR).[1–3] LPRs can develop following IgE-dependent reactions in the respiratory tract, the nose and the skin, and in other anatomic locations. Many of the clinically significant consequences of IgE-dependent reactions, both in the respiratory tract and in the skin, are thought to reflect the actions of the leukocytes recruited to these sites, rather than the direct effects of the mediators released by mast cells at early intervals after antigen challenge.

Both clinical and animal studies suggest that mast cell activation contributes to the leukocyte infiltration that is associated with LPRs, via effects of mast cell products on adhesion molecule expression by vascular endothelial cells and other cells at the reaction site, as well as by the production of chemokines and other chemoattractants.[1–3,8] However, in actively sensitized hosts, LPRs can be induced by peptides that can activate T cells but which cannot induce IgE-dependent mast cell activation.[19] Such evidence indicates that both IgE- and T-cell-dependent mechanisms can contribute to the elicitation of LPRs in actively immunized subjects.

The leukocytes recruited to sites of experimentally induced LPRs include basophils, eosinophils, neutrophils, lymphocytes, and macrophages. Thus, the expression of features of LPRs reflects the contributions of mast cells, T cells, and many other cell types; the relative importance of these potential effector cells probably varies depending on the individual circumstances.

Chronic allergic inflammation

In patients with chronic atopic diseases, including allergic asthma, allergic rhinitis and atopic dermatitis, the sites of pathology contain complex inflammatory infiltrates, including monocytes, macrophages, eosinophils, neutrophils, mast cells, basophils, and T cells, especially those that produce the Th2-type pattern of cytokines that can promote allergic responses. It is likely that all of these participants significantly influence the course of these allergic disorders and, in the aggregate, contribute to the development of the pathology associated with these conditions. Although the recruitment and function of some of these leukocytes can be regulated by mechanisms that are largely independent of the activity of mast cells and basophils, recent findings suggest that mast cell and basophil products may play a larger role in the chronic manifestations of allergic inflammation than was previously supposed.

IgE-dependent activation induces mast cells to release TNF and a broad panel of other cytokines, chemokines and growth factors.[1–3] Upon appropriate activation, basophils produce IL-4 and IL-13.[2,8,9] Such cytokines have the potential to influence many aspects of the pathophysiology at sites of allergic diseases, including some of the chronic changes (e.g., fibrosis, enhanced mucus production) associated with these disorders.[2,3,8,9,16] Given that mast cell degranulation results in the local release of proteoglycans that are able to bind a variety of growth factors, FcεRI-mediated mast cell activation may also regulate the function, concentration, and spatial distribution of cytokines and growth factors, whether derived from mast cells or other sources, within the tissue microenvironment. In other words, the traditional concept of the self-limited allergic reaction, which was thought to reflect the release of mast cell mediators whose biologic half-lives were measured in minutes or hours, must now be recognized as incomplete. Indeed, the complex and prolonged consequences of cytokine expression, together with the potential long-term effects of some of the cells' other mediators, suggest that mast cell activation can contribute importantly to many of the chronic features of allergic diseases and other disorders associated with mast cell activation.[2,3,8,9,16] Many other factors probably also contribute to the chronicity of allergic inflammation. These include prolonged or repeated exposure to relevant allergens, basophil functions that can increase the magnitude and duration of the inflammation associated with certain IgE and allergen specific immune responses[9] and perhaps the diminished threshold for mast cell activation observed *in vivo* after even a single antigenic challenge.

Mast cells and basophils in disease and host defense

Mast cells and basophils are thought of primarily as proinflammatory effector cells, but some of their products can have anti-inflammatory or immunosuppressive actions.[1–3,8,9,16] Studies in mast cell knock-in or mast cell-associated-protease-deficient mice have identified examples of innate or acquired immune responses in which mast cells can significantly reduce the intensity and/or duration of the response.[2,3,14,16] Such findings support the hypothesis that mast cells, and perhaps basophils, can both help to initiate and amplify and downregulate or resolve biological responses that contribute to health or disease.

Asthma

Approximately 80–90% of individuals who develop asthma before the age of 30 have an allergic component to the disease. Several lines of evidence indicate that mast cells contribute significantly to the initiation and maintenance of the pathology of allergic asthma.[1–3,8,10] In patients with allergic asthma, evidence of mast cell degranulation is provided by elevated levels of histamine and tryptase in the bronchoalveolar lavage fluid of those with moderately symptomatic asthma, and in bronchoalveolar lavage fluids after endobronchial allergen challenge.[8]

There is growing agreement that the local elaboration of multiple cytokines, chemokines, and growth factors, by mast cells and many other cell types, contributes importantly to the pathophysiology of asthma. Evidence includes the extended time course of release observed for some of these mast cell-derived products, the potent biological activities of such molecules, and the amplification and prolongation of the response achieved by the recruitment of additional effector cell types, each capable of contributing additional mediators to the inflammatory response. Mast cells have been proven to contribute to multiple features of asthma in certain mouse "models" of the disorder, including allergen-induced bronchial constriction and hyperreactivity to methacholine, eosinophil and T-cell infiltration, lung collagen deposition, and increased numbers of epithelial goblet cells and proliferating cells in the airway epithelium.[2,3] TNF may be especially important in these reactions, as this cytokine can be produced by both mast cells and eosinophils and can augment T-cell proliferation and cytokine production and enhance nonspecific bronchial hyperresponsiveness, as well as mediating many other proinflammatory effects.[1,16] However, many cells other than mast cells, such as eosinophils and lymphocytes, as well as structural cells in the lungs such as epithelial cells, fibroblasts

and smooth muscle cells, also represent a potentially important source of cytokines, chemokines, and growth factors in the chronic allergic inflammation of allergic asthma.[2,8,16] Moreover, mast cell and basophil mediators other than cytokines can also significantly influence disease pathophysiology. Clinical and *in vitro* studies indicate that LTC_4 and its peptidolytic derivatives LTD_4 and LTE_4, derived from mast cells, basophils, and other sources, can contribute importantly to disease manifestations in many subjects with atopic asthma.[8,10]

Parasitic diseases

IgE-associated allergic disorders are not thought to confer any benefit to the host, and may cause significant pathology or death. What then is the selective advantage of IgE-associated immune responses? Several lines of evidence suggest that mast cells and basophils represent important components of host defense against parasites (Chapter 29).

Parasitic infections often induce strong primary and secondary IgE responses, with some of the IgE being specific for parasite antigens. Parasite infections are also associated with increased levels of circulating basophils and eosinophils, and markedly increased serum levels of IgE. This leads to enhanced expression of FcεRI on basophils and mast cells. There are also increased numbers of mast cells at sites of parasitic infection. However, it has been difficult to prove that individual components of this IgE-associated immune response to helminths are truly essential for the expression of protective host immunity to the parasite.

Studies of infection with the nematode *Strongyloides venezuelensis* (Sv) in $Kit^{W/W-v}$ and congenic normal mice have documented increased numbers of mast cells at sites of parasite infection in the wild-type mice, and a delayed clearance of the parasite in $Kit^{W/W-v}$ mice that lack mast cells.[2] However, expulsion of the parasite did eventually occur even in the absence of mast cells. $Kit^{W/W-v}$ mast cell-deficient mice which were also devoid of IL-3 exhibited a striking impairment in their ability to expel a primary infection with Sv.[2,3] In guinea pigs, basophils appear to be required for the expression of immune resistance to cutaneous feeding by larval *Amblyomma americanum* ticks,[2] whereas the expression of IgE-dependent immune resistance to the cutaneous feeding by larval *Haemaphysalis longicornis* ticks in mice is dependent on mast cells and basophils.[9] These data, as well as many other lines of evidence, suggest that mast cells and basophils may provide similar or overlapping effector functions in parasite immunity, with the relative contributions of one or the other cell type varying according to such factors as the species of the parasite, the specific host and the site of infection. Given the importance of maintaining effective immune resistance to helminth parasites, it is perhaps not surprising that the responses remain largely intact despite the loss of a single effector component, such as IgE or mast cells.

Mast cells in innate immunity

Mast cells may contribute significantly to several aspects of host defense during innate immune responses to bacterial infection. Mast cell knock-in mice and mice lacking mMCP-6 were used to show that mast cells can represent a central component of host defense against certain bacterial infections, and that the recruitment of circulating leukocytes with bactericidal properties is dependent on mast cells.[2,3,16] Certain bacterial or viral products—including LPS and other ligands of TLRs—also directly induce the release of some mast cell products.[2,3,15]

Pathogens can also activate mast cells indirectly via activation of the complement system.[2,3,15] Mast cell function in such settings can reflect the interaction between products of complement activation and complement receptors on mast cells and/or the response of mast cells to products of other cells that have been activated by complement-dependent mechanisms.[1,2] Clearly, a lack of mast cells can impair the effectiveness of some innate immune responses, at least in mice. However, in two mouse models of severe bacterial infections, evidence in mast cell knock-in mice indicates that mast cell-derived TNF can increase mortality.[3]

Many animal venoms can activate mast cells and, in mice, mast cells can enhance resistance to the toxicity of the venoms of some reptiles and the honeybee, at least in part by secreting carboxypeptidase A and other proteases that can degrade components of these venoms.[2,3,14]

Other diseases

Mast cells or basophils or their products have been implicated in a bewildering variety of diseases not thought to be associated with an IgE response (e.g., scleroderma, pulmonary fibrosis of diverse origins, inflammatory bowel disease, and peptic ulcer disease), as well as in angiogenesis, adaptive immune responses, protective responses to toxic agents, and reparative responses such as wound healing.[1–3, 8,9,15,16] Mast cells have been implicated in the pathogenesis of experimental allergic encephalomyelitis (an animal model of multiple sclerosis) and rheumatoid arthritis.[2] Recently, IgE and basophils have been implicated in the pathology of lupus erythematosus.[20] However, many of the roles proposed for mast cells or basophils in nonimmunological diseases, adaptive responses or tissue remodeling have not been evaluated using mast cell knock-in mice, basophil-deficient mice, or other genetic approaches. Accordingly, the actual importance of the mast cell or the basophil in many of these settings remains to be determined.

Mastocytosis

Mastocytosis is a heterogeneous disorder that is associated with mast cell accumulation in the skin, bone marrow, gastrointestinal tract, liver, spleen, and lymph nodes. The true prevalence is unknown. The incidence has been estimated between 3 and 7 new patients per million people.[21] Mastocytosis may present at any age, but has a typical onset either in infancy or in early to mid-adulthood. Most cases are sporadic, and only a few cases of familial mastocytosis have been described.

Description and natural history

The clinical signs and symptoms of disease observed in patients with mastocytosis are in large part explained by tissue mast cell hyperplasia and an excess production of mast cell mediators (Fig. 22.4). The skin is involved in most cases, but mastocytosis can occur without visible skin manifestations. The term "systemic mastocytosis" (SM) has been used to categorize patients in whom increased numbers of mast cells are found in organ systems other than the skin.[22]

Adult and pediatric populations exhibit important differences in clinical presentation, pathogenesis, and prognosis. Whereas mastocytosis in childhood tends to be self-limited and to involve only the skin, the course in patients with adult-onset disease is usually prolonged and includes systemic involvement. Associated hematologic disorders exist or develop in up to 10% of adult patients.[22]

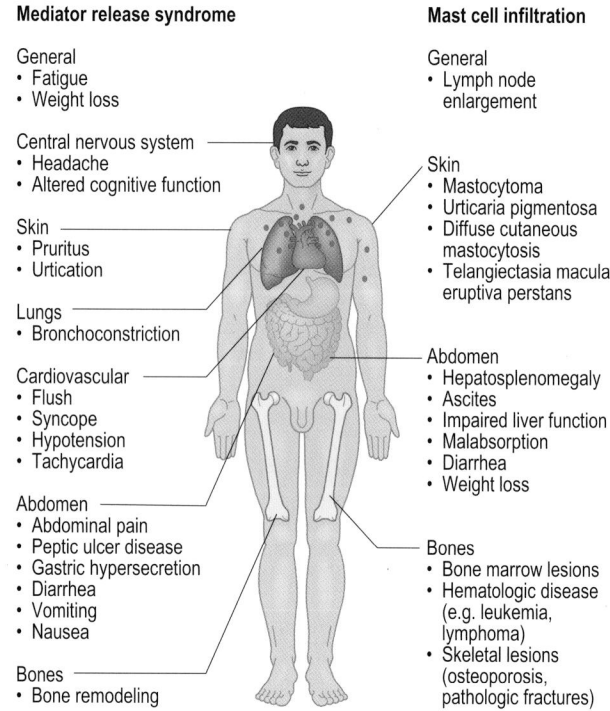

Mediator release syndrome

General
• Fatigue
• Weight loss

Central nervous system
• Headache
• Altered cognitive function

Skin
• Pruritus
• Urtication

Lungs
• Bronchoconstriction

Cardiovascular
• Flush
• Syncope
• Hypotension
• Tachycardia

Abdomen
• Abdominal pain
• Peptic ulcer disease
• Gastric hypersecretion
• Diarrhea
• Vomiting
• Nausea

Bones
• Bone remodeling

Mast cell infiltration

General
• Lymph node enlargement

Skin
• Mastocytoma
• Urticaria pigmentosa
• Diffuse cutaneous mastocytosis
• Telangiectasia macularis eruptiva perstans

Abdomen
• Hepatosplenomegaly
• Ascites
• Impaired liver function
• Malabsorption
• Diarrhea
• Weight loss

Bones
• Bone marrow lesions
• Hematologic disease (e.g. leukemia, lymphoma)
• Skeletal lesions (osteoporosis, pathologic fractures)

Fig. 22.4 Clinical manifestations of mastocytosis.

Cutaneous lesions

More than 90% of all patients with mastocytosis initially present with hyperpigmented skin lesions (maculopapular cutaneous mastocytosis [MPCM] or urticaria pigmentosa). These skin lesions are disseminated brownish-red macules or slightly elevated papules that may urticate spontaneously or after trauma. This reaction elicited in lesional skin after stroking or rubbing is referred to as Darier's sign. In children, the lesions tend to be well demarcated and may form raised nodules or plaques, whereas in adults, they may become confluent (Figs. 22.5A, B).[23] Although lesions may involve all sites of the integument including mucous membranes, the trunk and proximal extremities typically have the highest density of lesions.

Mastocytosis has two additional cutaneous manifestations: solitary mastocytoma, a flat or mildly elevated, and well demarcated, solitary yellowish red-brown lesion, typically 2–5 cm in diameter, that occurs in infants and children, and diffuse cutaneous mastocytosis (DCM). DCM is a rare disorder that presents in infants in the first year of life. It may involve the entire integument (erythrodermic mastocytosis). DCM presents with edema and doughy thickening of the skin. Serious systemic complications may occur, including hypotension and gastrointestinal hemorrhage.

Infants and young children with mastocytosis in the skin sometimes exhibit blister formation. A biopsy from a mastocytosis skin lesion typically shows increased numbers of normal-looking mast cells in the papillary dermis (Fig. 22.5C).

Bone marrow and hematologic involvement

Eighty percent or more of adults with SM show focal to diffuse collections of spindle-shaped mast cells in the bone marrow (Fig. 22.5D). Fibrotic lesions may develop. Patients also may have a definable hematologic disorder such as a myelodysplastic

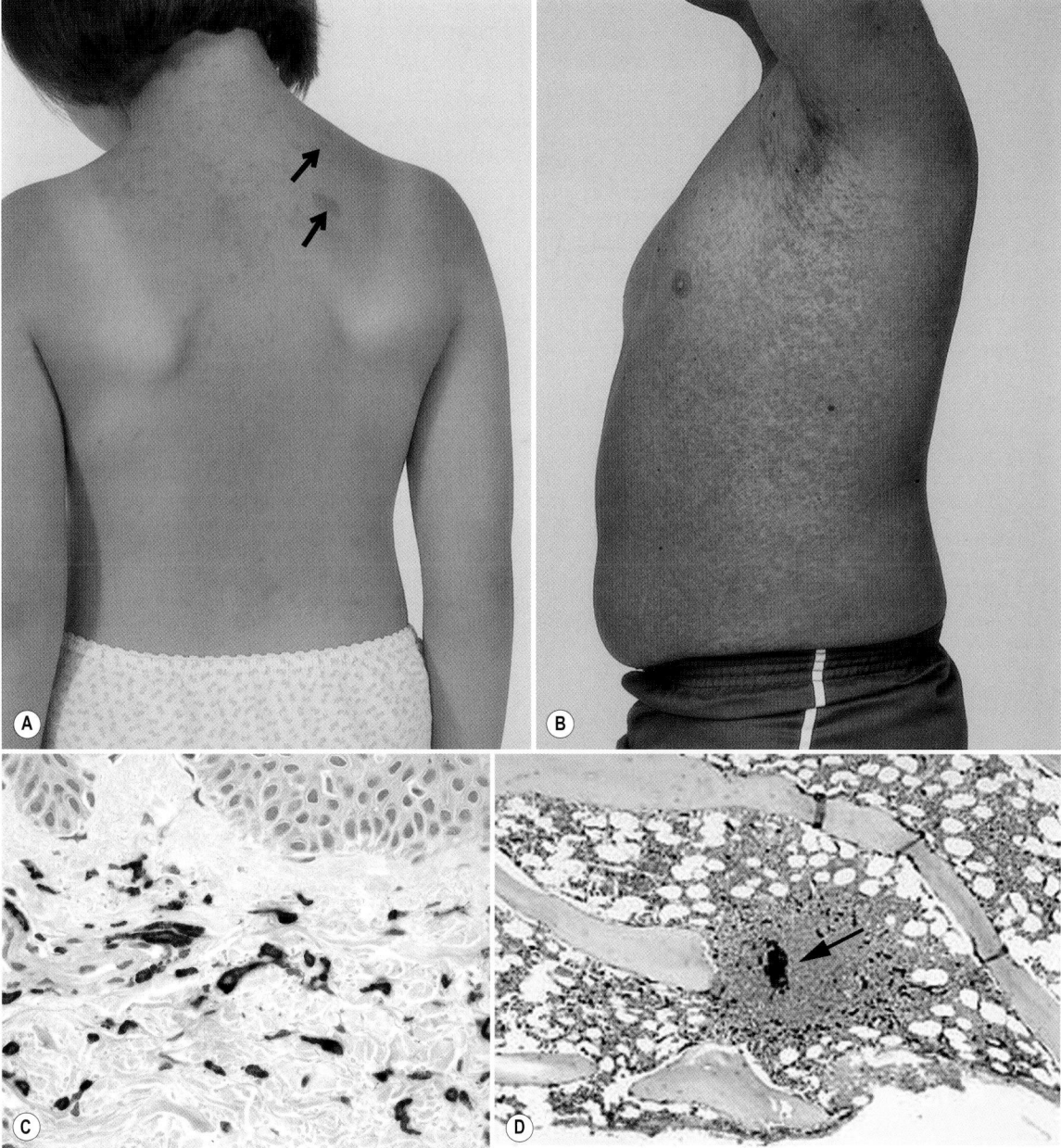

Fig. 22.5 Cutaneous mastocytosis and histopathology. Urticaria pigmentosa is the most common form of cutaneous mastocytosis. In childhood, lesions are disseminated and consist of well-demarcated hyperpigmented macules (e.g., arrows) (A). In adults, lesions may be numerous with less well-demarcated brownish-red macules and papules (B). Histopathology of cutaneous mastocytosis shows many mast cells containing abundant tryptase immunoreactive cytoplasmic granules in the papillary dermis (antitryptase, AA1 clone, Dako; original magnification ∼ × 400) (C). Bone marrow pathology of indolent mastocytosis is characterized by paratrabecular lymphoid nodule containing small, well-differentiated lymphoid cells around substantial numbers of fusiform cells with prominent granules in the tryptase stain (arrow) (antitryptase, AA1 clone, Dako; original magnification ∼ × 250) (D).
Courtesy of Cem Akin.

syndrome, myeloproliferative disorder, acute leukemia, or a malignant lymphoma.[22] Anemia, thrombocytopenia, and eosinophilia may occur, predominantly in patients with more aggressive disease.

Osteoporosis, osteopenia, sclerosis, or cystic lesions of bone are present in approximately one third of patients with SM. In severe disease, pathologic fractures may occur. The long bones, pelvis, ribs, skull, and vertebrae are the most common sites of skeletal involvement. Some patients report associated musculoskeletal or fibromyalgia-like pain.

Mast cell mediator-induced symptoms

Flushing, shortness of breath, palpitations, nausea and diarrhea, hypotension and occasionally syncope are sometimes experienced by patients with mastocytosis and are believed to result from an excess release of mast cell mediators.[24] Patients may describe recurrent episodes with a combination of these symptoms. Such episodes typically last for 30 minutes. Lethargy and fatigue lasting several hours may follow. Systemic episodes occur spontaneously, or they may be provoked in some individuals by stimuli such as hymenoptera insect stings, aspirin and other NSAIDs, opiates (including morphine and morphine-derivatives), muscle relaxants, ethanol, allergies to inhalants or foods, contrast media, surgery or endoscopy, infection (bacteria, viruses, others), and certain physical stimuli such as friction, heat or exercise.

The cumulative prevalence of anaphylaxis in the history of adults with mastocytosis has been reported to be between 22 and 49%, depending on the population and the definition.[25,26] Severe or protracted anaphylaxis may occur and fatal reactions have been described. For example, in addition to spontaneous episodes, patients with mastocytosis may develop life-threatening anaphylaxis after hymenoptera stings, during the course of insect venom hyposensitization, or after receiving iodinated contrast materials. SM is diagnosed with greater frequency in patients with a history of hymenoptera sting anaphylaxis and who are found to have an elevated serum tryptase level.[27]

Involvement of the gastrointestinal tract is common in patients with SM.[28] Abdominal pain or discomfort, diarrhea and nausea are typical symptoms sometimes associated with food intake, but not necessarily with specific foods. Diarrhea is not generally related to gastric hypersecretion; and has been attributed to altered intestinal secretion, structural mucosal abnormalities and hypermotility. Associated malabsorption is usually mild and not clinically important.

A number of patients present with a constellation of signs and symptoms that variably include pruritus, flushing, urticaria, nasal pruritus or congestion, wheezing, throat swelling, headache, hypotension, or diarrhea and in whom an allergic etiology and mastocytosis have been excluded as diagnoses.[29] Because mast cell activation occurs in such clinical scenarios, it has been proposed that such individuals may either have a mast cell population that is abnormally sensitive to activation by unknown stimuli or have mast cells themselves that are susceptible to spontaneous degranulation.[29,30] The associated clinical syndrome has been termed "mast cell activation syndrome," or MCAS. Diagnostic criteria have been proposed for MCAS which require that the signs and symptoms recorded are those seen with mast cell mediated allergic reactions, that there is documentation of release of mast cell mediators during episodes, and that there is some response to anti-mediator therapy. To date, insufficient clinical evidence exists to firmly establish this syndrome.

Other manifestations

Mast cell infiltrates are commonly found in liver and spleen biopsies of patients with SM.[25] In one series of 41 patients, hepatomegaly has been reported in 24% and elevated levels of liver enzymes in 54%. However, severe liver disease was unusual, except for those with aggressive disease. In these patients, fibrosis, cirrhosis, ascites, and portal hypertension were reported to be more frequent. Splenomegaly and lymphadenopathy may also occur and are more pronounced in patients with associated hematologic disorders and more aggressive disease.

Patients with mastocytosis sometimes report neuropsychiatric problems. Altered cognitive or emotional function, such as poor attention, irritability, impaired memory, personality change, and depression, have been observed in association with mastocytosis. Fatigue is often present, especially in those with more aggressive disease.

Prognosis and classification

The clinical course varies from asymptomatic with normal life expectancy to highly aggressive. Prognosis depends on the variant of disease and the presence of the D816V *c-KIT* mutation within hematopoietic cell lineages. The WHO classification defines 7 variants of mastocytosis (Table 22.3).[31] SM is defined in the WHO classification by major and minor criteria (Table 22.4). Criteria defining the mast cell burden, involvement of non-mast cell-lineages and aggressiveness of disease are applied to subclassify SM in subvariants.[31]

In children, mastocytosis of the skin, or cutaneous mastocytosis (CM), may be the only manifestation of disease; and resolves in the majority of patients by adulthood. In one study, the disease resolved in 67% and a major or partial regression occurred in 33% of the cases.[32] SM was a predictor of persistent disease in three children. Most adults fall within the indolent SM category and the disease tends to remain relatively stable over many years.[33] Evolution of disease into more aggressive categories is uncommon and particularly occurs in those carrying high numbers of neoplastic mast cells with an immature phenotype and with a c-KIT mutation detectable not only in mast cells, but also in other hematological myeloid or lymphomatoid lineages.

Table 22.3 WHO classification of mastocytosis

Cutaneous mastocytosis
Indolent systemic mastocytosis
Systemic mastocytosis with an associated clonal hematologic non-mast-cell lineage disease
Aggressive systemic mastocytosis
Mast cell leukemia
Mast cell sarcoma
Extracutaneous mastocytoma

Table 22.4 Diagnosis of systemic mastocytosis based on WHO criteria[a]

Major criterion:
Multifocal, dense infiltrates of mast cells ($>/= 15$ mast cells in aggregates) detected in sections of bone marrow and/or other extracutaneous organ(s)

Minor criteria:
1. More than 25% of mast cells in biopsy sections of bone marrow or other extracutaneous organs are spindle shaped or display atypical morphology, or, of all mast cells in bone marrow aspirate smears, >25 % are immature or atypical
2. Detection of an activating point mutation at codon 816 of *c-KIT* in blood, bone marrow, or another extracutaneous organ
3. Mast cells in the bone marrow, blood, or other extracutaneous organs express CD2 and/or CD25 in addition to normal mast cell markers
4. Serum total tryptase persistently exceeds 20 ng/ml

[a]One major and one minor, or three minor, criteria are needed for the diagnosis of systemic mastocytosis.
Data from Horny HP, Metcalfe DD, Bennett JM, et al. Mastocytosis In: WHO Classification of Tumors of Hematopoietic and Lymphoid Tissues. Swerdlow SH, Campo E, Harris NL, Jaffe ES, Pileri SA, Stein H, Thiele J, Vardiman JW, editors. World Health Organization classification of tumors Lyon: IARC Press 2008: 54-63.

Patients classified as having a non-indolent variant generally have a less favorable prognosis and some may experience a rapid progression.[22] Patients in these categories are less likely to exhibit involvement of the skin. Factors influencing the clinical course are the associated hematologic abnormalities and the rapidity of the increase in mast cell numbers, especially in aggressive mastocytosis and mast cell leukemia.

Mast cell leukemia is the rarest form and has the most fulminant behavior. Survival of those with mast cell leukemia is generally less than one year.

Etiology and pathogenesis

The most important survival/growth factor for mast cells is the KIT ligand, stem cell factor (SCF). At least in adults, it is thought that one initial event which can facilitate the development of mastocytosis is an activating mutation in c-KIT, the gene for KIT.[34] KIT, a transmembrane thyrosine kinase receptor encoded by the prooncogene c-KIT, is expressed on mast cells, melanocytes, hematopoietic stem cells, interstitial cells of Cajal, and germ cell lineages. Ligation of KIT by SCF promotes dimerization of the receptor and subsequently induces intrinsic tyrosine kinase activation. The resulting phosphorylated tyrosine residues serve as docking sites for intracellular downstream signaling pathways leading to cell proliferation and activation. The most commonly detected mutation is Asp816Val, which has been identified not only in bone marrow mast cells, but also in other hematopoietic cell lineages, and in the skin and spleen in some patients. These findings support the conclusion that the disease is clonal. The reason(s) for the different behavior of indolent versus aggressive variants of mastocytosis, however, remain(s) unknown, although mutations in other signalling molecules including NRAS have now been reported. Patients with hypereosinophilia and high numbers of mast cells on the basis of a FIP1L1-PDGFRA fusion have been described.[35]

The Asp816Val c-KIT mutation in exon 17 and additional c-KIT mutations outside exon 17 have been detected in some children in biopsies of lesional skin. However, a clear genotype-phenotype correlation could not be demonstrated. These findings raise the possibility that mastocytosis in many children has a different basis from that in most adults. This could provide an explanation for the generally more benign course of some cases of childhood CM.

Diagnosis

Most patients with mastocytosis present with characteristic cutaneous lesions that support the diagnosis. Clinical examination of the entire skin should be performed at initial presentation and a biopsy may be taken. Mast cells within skin biopsies are identified using toluidine blue or Giemsa stains, or by immunohistochemistry using antibodies to mast cell tryptase. A 10- to 20-fold increase in mast cell numbers has been reported in lesions of urticaria pigmentosa, but the increase may be less pronounced. However, a 2- to 4-fold increase in mast cell numbers has been observed in unrelated conditions including idiopathic anaphylaxis, flushing, chronic urticaria, and eczema.

Biochemical demonstration of elevated serum levels of mast cell tryptase (>20 ng/mL) supports the diagnosis of SM, whereas in CM tryptase levels may be normal.[36] In addition, elevation in urinary histamine and its metabolites may be observed in SM. However, mast cell tryptase and histamine can also be elevated in association with acute exacerbations of allergic diseases, including anaphylaxis, and therefore such elevations, in isolation, are not diagnostic of mastocytosis.

A bone marrow biopsy and aspiration should be considered in patients with elevated basal serum tryptase levels, particularly in adults, if there are accompanying signs or symptoms of disease and if heterophilic anti-mouse antibodies have been excluded, which may interfere with the tryptase assay. In patients with anaphylaxis and elevated tryptase levels, clonal mast cells carrying the Asp816Val c-KIT mutation and expressing an abnormal CD25$^+$ phenotype have been described.[37] Some of these patients do not fulfill all criteria for systemic mastocytosis and the diagnosis in such situations is thus monoclonal mast cell activation syndrome (MMAS) to reflect the clonal nature of the findings.[22,29,37] Especially in males with insect sting anaphylaxis, elevated basal tryptase levels and hypotensive episodes, but without urticaria, appear to identify those with a high risk for clonal mast cell disease.[38] A bone marrow biopsy is also useful for staging the disease by excluding associated hematologic abnormalities. In patients with an associated hematologic disorder, identification of mast cells in the bone marrow may be difficult if the mast cells are dysplastic and when mast cell granules are more coarse than normal, or are even absent.[39] The most accurate stain for the detection of mast cells in mastocytosis is an immunohistochemical stain with antibody to mast cell tryptase. Identifying the coexpression of CD2 and/or CD25 in CD117 (KIT)-positive mast cells by flow cytometry of bone marrow aspirates, or by immunohistochemical analysis of bone marrow biopsies, has been considered to be the most sensitive and specific method to diagnose SM in the bone marrow.[40]

Analysis of c-KIT mutations, especially the Asp816Val mutation, in bone marrow or skin specimens should be performed in patients in whom the diagnosis is uncertain, presentation is untypical, or therapy with tyrosine kinase inhibitors is being considerd.

In patients with SM, the size of the liver and spleen should be measured by ultrasound or CT and osteodensitometry should be done by the DXA method to evaluate for osteoporosis. SM is classified into one of the more aggressive variants of disease when bone marrow involvement of non-mast cell-lineages, organ dysfunction and/or a high mast cell burden are present.

Further studies, such as gastrointestinal endoscopy or biopsy to obtain tissue specimens from the liver, spleen, gastrointestinal tract, or lymph nodes are usually considered only when these organs are suspected to be involved and the biopsy would yield clinically useful information.

Physical examination, serum tryptase determination, and a complete blood count should be done at yearly intervals in patients with MMAS or with indolent SM.

Therapy

There currently is no cure for mastocytosis. Treatment is symptomatic and is tailored to the symptoms of the individual patient.[22] Prominent mast cell mediator-induced symptoms include hypotension, gastric hypersecretion, abdominal pain, and pruritus. Aggressive forms of therapy are not indicated in patients with indolent mastocytosis, as this disorder has a favorable prognosis. In patients with aggressive disease or associated hematologic disorders, treatment is a therapeutic challenge.

Therapy of cutaneous and indolent disease

In patients with indolent disease, management includes reassurance of the patients, avoidance of exacerbating factors, and treatment that offers symptomatic relief. Information about the nature of the disease, an explanation of expected symptoms, and discussion of prognosis will address the most common concerns of patients with mastocytosis. Factors known to provoke episodes of flushing and hypotension should be reviewed with the patient and avoided. Patients with mastocytosis and hymenoptera venom exposure are at risk for anaphylaxis. Epinephrine is the drug of choice for anaphylaxis and should be kept available by patients at risk at all times. Immediate self-administration during anaphylaxis may be life-saving. Insect venom immunotherapy when appropriate, and premedication with antihistamines and corticosteroids prior to general anesthesia, should be seriously considered.

Nonsedating H_1-antihistamines are the drugs of choice for pruritus and urtication. For prophylaxis of recurrent episodes, antihistamines should be administered daily. For some patients, classical sedating H_1-blockers, such as hydroxyzine or diphenhydramine, seem to be more effective. The addition of an H_2-receptor antagonist is also an option. Gastric acid hypersecretion, peptic ulcer disease, and reflux esophagitis are managed with H_2-receptor blockers and proton pump inhibitors. Cromolyn sodium may be used, particularly for gastrointestinal symptoms. Anticholinergics are an option for control of diarrhea. Systemic corticosteroids are used in cases of malabsorption or ascites. Calcium, vitamin D, and biphosphonates are the drugs of choice for osteoporosis.

Application of topical corticosteroids under occlusion or topical PUVA (psoralen plus UVA radiation) treatment may be considered in patients with CM. Oral PUVA (psoralen plus UVA radiation) and UVA_1 radiation are effective in reducing pruritus and urtication. However, relapse typically occurs a few months after therapy is discontinued, as is the case with topical application of corticosteroids. The benefits of these forms of therapy have to be weighed against the potential of inducing atrophy associated with glucocorticosteriod applicaction and cutaneous malignancies associated with long-term UV exposure.

Therapy of aggressive disease and associated hematologic disorders

Patients with mastocytosis and an associated hematologic disorder should be managed using appropriate therapy for the associated disorder.[22] Chemotherapy has not been shown to produce remission, or to prolong survival, in mast cell leukemia. Chemotherapy is not indicated in indolent mastocytosis, as it may lead to bone marrow suppression without improving the symptoms of mastocytosis. A partial response to interferon-α2b has been reported in patients with aggressive mast cell disease. Cladribine (2-cholorodeoxyadenosine) has also been reported to reduce mast cell burden and may be considered in aggressive mastocytosis.

New therapeutic approaches should target neoplastic mast cells. The tyrosine kinase inhibitor imatinib is not generally considered to be indicated in patients with Asp816Val mutations in KIT, as sterical conformations of the receptor interfere with the action of the drug in this setting. However, the drug has been reported to reduce mast cell load and symptoms in patients with mutations in other c-*KIT* exons. Other tyrosine kinase inhibitors have been developed which may also inhibit KIT with mutations in codon 816, and some of these are currently in clinical trials. Bone marrow transplantation may evolve as an option, although results to date have been disappointing.

Translational research

The challenges in the next 5-10 years include improving our understanding of the molecular abnormalities underlying mastocytosis and contributing to the pathology in various clinical subgroups of patients with such disorders, and continuing to seek better agents to treat such disorders. We also need better approaches to detect and monitor the involvement of mast cells and basophils in allergic disorders and other diseases involving these cell types.

Acknowledgments

Some of the work reviewed in this chapter was supported by the Division of Intramural Research, NIAID/NIH, United States Public Health Service grants AI 23990, CA72074 and A170813, by Deutsche Forschungsgemeinschaft grant ME2668/1-1 and/or by AMGEN Inc.; Dr Galli has consulted for Genentech Inc. and AMGEN Inc. under terms that are in accord with Stanford University conflict-of-interest guidelines.

References

1. Metcalfe DD. Mast cells and mastocytosis. Blood 2008;112:946–56.
2. Galli SJ, Metcalfe DD, Arber DA, Dvorak AM. Basophils and mast cells and their disorders. In: Kaushansky KLM, Beutler E, Kipps TJ, Seligsohn U, Prchal JT, editors. Williams Hematology. 8th ed. New York: McGraw-Hill Medical; 2010. p. 915–32.
3. Galli SJ, Tsai M. Mast cells in allergy and infection: versatile effector and regulatory cells in innate and adaptive immunity. Eur J Immunol 2010;40:1843–51.
4. Kraft S, Kinet JP. New developments in FcepsilonRI regulation, function and inhibition. Nat Rev Immunol 2007;7:365–78.
5. Schwartz LB. Effector cells of anaphylaxis: mast cells and basophils. Novartis Found Symp 2004;257:276–85.
6. Inomata N, Tomita H, Ikezawa Z, et al. Differential gene expression profile between cord blood progenitor-derived and adult progenitor-derived human mast cells. Immunol Lett 2005;98:265–71.
7. Costa JJ, Demetri GD, Harrist TJ, et al. Recombinant human stem cell factor (kit ligand) promotes human mast cell and melanocyte hyperplasia and functional activation in vivo. J Exp Med 1996;183:2681–6.
8. Marone G, Triggiani M, Genovese A, et al. Role of human mast cells and basophils in bronchial asthma. Adv Immunol 2005;88:97–160.
9. Karasuyama H, Mukai K, Obata K, et al. Nonredundant roles of basophils in immunity. Annu Rev Immunol 2011;29:45–69.
10. Boyce JA. Mast cells and eicosanoid mediators: a system of reciprocal paracrine and autocrine regulation. Immunol Rev 2007;217:168–85.
11. Caughey GH. Mast cell tryptases and chymases in inflammation and host defense. Immunol Rev 2007;217:141–54.
12. Pejler G, Abrink M, Ringvall M, et al. Mast cell proteases. Adv Immunol 2007;95:167–255.
13. Stevens RL, Adachi R. Protease-proteoglycan complexes of mouse and human mast cells and importance of their beta-tryptase-heparin complexes in inflammation and innate immunity. Immunol Rev 2007;217:155–67.
14. Metz M, Piliponsky AM, Chen CC, et al. Mast cells can enhance resistance to snake and honeybee venoms. Science 2006;313:526–30.
15. Hofmann AM, Abraham SN. New roles for mast cells in modulating allergic reactions and immunity against pathogens. Curr Opin Immunol 2009;21:679–86.
16. Galli SJ, Grimbaldeston M, Tsai M. Immunomodulatory mast cells: negative, as well as positive, regulators of immunity. Nat Rev Immunol 2008;8:478–86.
17. Zhu D, Kepley CL, Zhang K, et al. A chimeric human-cat fusion protein blocks cat-induced allergy. Nat Med 2005;11:446–9.
18. Iikura M, Yamaguchi M, Fujisawa T, et al. Secretory IgA induces degranulation of IL-3-primed basophils. J Immunol 1998;161:1510–5.
19. Ali FR, Oldfield WL, Higashi N, et al. Late asthmatic reactions induced by inhalation of allergen-derived T cell peptides. Am J Respir Crit Care Med 2004;169:20–6.
20. Charles N, Hardwick D, Daugas E, et al. Basophils and the T helper 2 environment can promote the development of lupus nephritis. Nat Med 2010;16:701–707.
21. Rosbotham JL, Malik NM, Syrris P, et al. Lack of c-kit mutation in familial urticaria pigmentosa. Br J Dermatol 1999;140:849–52.
22. Valent P, Akin C, Escribano L, et al. Standards and standardization in mastocytosis: consensus statements on diagnostics, treatment recommendations and response criteria. Eur J Clin Invest 2007;37:435–53.
23. Brockow K, Akin C, Huber M, et al. Assessment of the extent of cutaneous involvement in children and adults with mastocytosis: relationship to symptomatology, tryptase levels, and bone marrow pathology. J Am Acad Dermatol 2003;48:508–16.
24. Brockow K. Urticaria pigmentosa. Immunol Allergy Clin North Am 2004;24:287–316, vii.
25. Gonzalez de Olano D, de la Hoz Caballer B, Nunez Lopez R, et al. Prevalence of allergy and anaphylactic symptoms in 210 adult and pediatric patients with mastocytosis in Spain: a study of the Spanish network on mastocytosis (REMA). Clin Exp Allergy 2007;37:1547–55.
26. Brockow K, Jofer C, Behrendt H, et al. Anaphylaxis in patients with mastocytosis: a study on history, clinical features and risk factors in 120 patients. Allergy 2008;63:226–32.
27. Bonadonna P, Perbellini O, Passalacqua G, et al. Clonal mast cell disorders in patients with systemic reactions to Hymenoptera stings and increased serum tryptase levels. J Allergy Clin Immunol 2009;123:680–6.
28. Jensen RT. Gastrointestinal abnormalities and involvement in systemic mastocytosis. Hematol Oncol Clin North Am 2000;14:579–623.
29. Akin C, Valent P, Metcalfe DD. Mast cell activation syndrome: Proposed diagnostic criteria. J Allergy Clin Immunol 2010;126:1099–1104 e4.
30. Valent P, Akin C, Arock M, et al. Definitions, criteria, and global classification of mast cell disorders with special reference to mast cell activation syndromes: A consensus proposal. Int Arch Allergy Immunol 2011;157:215–25.
31. Horny HP, Metcalfe DD, Bennett JM, et al. Mastocytosis. In: Swerdlow SH, Campo E, Harris NL, et al., editors. WHO Classification of Tumors of Hematopoietic and Lymphoid Tissues. World Health Organization classification of tumors. Lyon: IARC Press; 2008. p. 54–63.
32. Uzzaman A, Maric I, Noel P, et al. Pediatric-onset mastocytosis: a long term clinical follow-up and correlation with bone marrow histopathology. Pediatr Blood Cancer 2009;53:629–34.
33. Brockow K, Scott LM, Worobec AS, et al. Regression of urticaria pigmentosa in adult patients with systemic mastocytosis: correlation with clinical patterns of disease. Arch Dermatol 2002;138:785–90.
34. Akin C, Metcalfe DD. The biology of Kit in disease and the application of pharmacogenetics. J Allergy Clin Immunol 2004;114:13–9; quiz 20.
35. Pardanani A, Ketterling RP, Brockman SR, et al. CHIC2 deletion, a surrogate for FIP1L1-PDGFRA fusion, occurs in systemic mastocytosis associated with eosinophilia and predicts response to imatinib mesylate therapy. Blood 2003;102:3093–6.
36. Schwartz LB, Irani AM. Serum tryptase and the laboratory diagnosis of systemic mastocytosis. Hematol Oncol Clin North Am 2000;14:641–57.
37. Akin C, Scott LM, Kocabas CN, et al. Demonstration of an aberrant mast-cell population with clonal markers in a subset of patients with "idiopathic" anaphylaxis. Blood 2007;110:2331–3.
38. Alvarez-Twose I, Gonzalez de Olano D, Sanchez-Munoz L, et al. Clinical, biological, and molecular characteristics of clonal mast cell disorders presenting with systemic mast cell activation symptoms. J Allergy Clin Immunol 2010;125:1269–78 e2.
39. Horny HP, Valent P. Histopathological and immunohistochemical aspects of mastocytosis. Int Arch Allergy Immunol 2002;127:115–7.
40. Escribano L, Orfao A, Diaz-Agustin B, et al. Indolent systemic mast cell disease in adults: immunophenotypic characterization of bone marrow mast cells and its diagnostic implications. Blood 1998;91:2731–6.

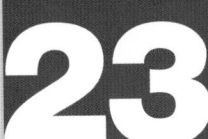

Anna Kovalszki,
Javed Sheikh,
Peter F. Weller

Eosinophils and eosinophilia

Eosinophils are terminally differentiated, bone marrow-derived granulocytes that normally circulate in the blood in low numbers and tend to localize in those tissues with mucosal epithelial surfaces. Increased blood or tissue eosinophils occur with helminth parasite infections as well as with allergic diseases and a variety of other, often idiopathic conditions. Conventionally the major focus on eosinophils has been delineating the "effector" functions of these end-stage granulocytes, including what roles these cells play as helminthotoxic effector cells and the contribution they make to the immunopathogenesis of allergic diseases. More recent findings indicate that eosinophil functions are considerably more extensive.[1-4] Eosinophils contain stores of multiple pre-formed cytokines, engage in cognate cell–cell interactions with other cell types, including lymphocytes, and have roles in varied host immune and inflammatory responses not conventionally marked by quantitatively extensive eosinophil infiltration.[4]

Production and distribution of eosinophils

Eosinophilopoiesis

The development of eosinophils in the bone marrow can be elicited by three cytokines. Granulocyte–macrophage colony-stimulating factor (GM-CSF), interleukin (IL)-3 and IL-5 each promote eosinophilopoiesis. In contrast to IL-3 and GM-CSF, which also promote the development of other lineages, IL-5 uniquely promotes the development and terminal differentiation of eosinophils. Although IL-5 is produced by CD8 T cells, NK cells, and other leukocytes, including eosinophils themselves, IL-5 is a defining cytokine product of Th2 CD4 T cells. The production of IL-5 by Th2 lymphocytes accounts for the eosinophilia accompanying Th2 cell-mediated immune responses characteristic of helminth infections and allergic diseases.

Eosinophilopoiesis develops over about a week. Retained in the marrow is a pool of mature eosinophils. IL-5, alone and in concert with the chemokine eotaxin-1 (CCLII), rapidly releases this pool of mature eosinophils into the circulation to acutely increase blood eosinophilia and facilitate recruitment of eosinophils to sites of inflammation.[1] Blood eosinophils circulate with a half-life of about 8–18 hours. Eosinophils leave the circulation and localize in tissues, especially those with mucosal interfaces with the outside world, such as the gastrointestinal, and lower genitourinary tracts. Although the mechanisms governing this homing of eosinophils to mucosal tissues are not

fully known, the chemokine eotaxin-1 is involved in the homing of eosinophils to the gastrointestinal, but not the respiratory, tract.[2] Eosinophils live longer than neutrophils and probably persist in tissues for several weeks. They are principally tissue-dwelling cells: as demonstrated in rodents, for every eosinophil present in the circulation there are 300–500 in the tissues.

Eosinophil adherence mechanisms

The transit of eosinophils from the marrow, through the circulation and into tissues is governed in part by multiple adherence molecules expressed on eosinophils (Fig. 23.1).[5] As for other leukocytes, recruitment of eosinophils into tissue sites of inflammation utilizes combinatorial interactions involving specific adhesion molecules (via their expression and altered affinity states) that mediate cellular interactions with the vascular endothelium and actions of chemoattractant molecules. Eosinophils express several adhesion molecules broadly shared with other leukocytes that mediate their initial rolling and subsequent adherence to endothelial cells. Similar to neutrophils, eosinophils can adhere via CD11/CD18 heterodimeric β_2-integrins to the intercellular adhesion molecules ICAM-1 and ICAM-2. Likewise, specific sialoglycoproteins mediate adherence between eosinophils and endothelial E- and P-selectins. Unlike neutrophils, but similar to lymphocytes, eosinophils are able to bind to vascular cell adhesion molecule-1 (VCAM-1). Eosinophils express two α_4-integrins, very late activation antigen-4 (VLA-4, $\alpha_4\beta_1$) and $\alpha_4\beta_7$, that bind to VCAM-1. Moreover, $\alpha_4\beta_7$ binds to the mucosal addressin cell adhesion molecule (MadCAM). The β_2-integrin, $\alpha d\beta_2$, which binds ICAM-3 and is expressed on other leukocytes, is an additional integrin that mediates eosinophil adhesion to VCAM-1. Enhanced expression of VCAM-1 on the vascular endothelium, as elicitable by IL-4 or IL-13 stimulation, may contribute to the localization of eosinophils in some tissue sites of inflammation.

In addition to mediating interactions with the endothelium, eosinophil adherence molecules, by their interactions with extracellular matrix components, modulate the activity of eosinophils that have exited the bloodstream. Eosinophil VLA-6, $\alpha_6\beta_1$, binds laminin. Both $\alpha_4\beta_1$ and $\alpha_4\beta_7$ interact with specific domains of tissue fibronectin, and these interactions can enhance eosinophil functional responses. Eosinophils express CD44 (PGP-1), which binds hyaluronic acid. Siglec-8, a sialic acid-binding immunoglobulin-like lectin, is expressed on eosinophils and binds sialoglycoconjugates.[6]

Fig. 23.1 Adherence mechanisms utilized by human eosinophils to bind to vascular endothelial cells and the extracellular matrix molecules. ICAM, intercellular adhesion molecule; VCAM, vascular cell adhesion molecule; MadCAM, mucosal addressin cell adhesion molecule; VLA, very late activation antigen.

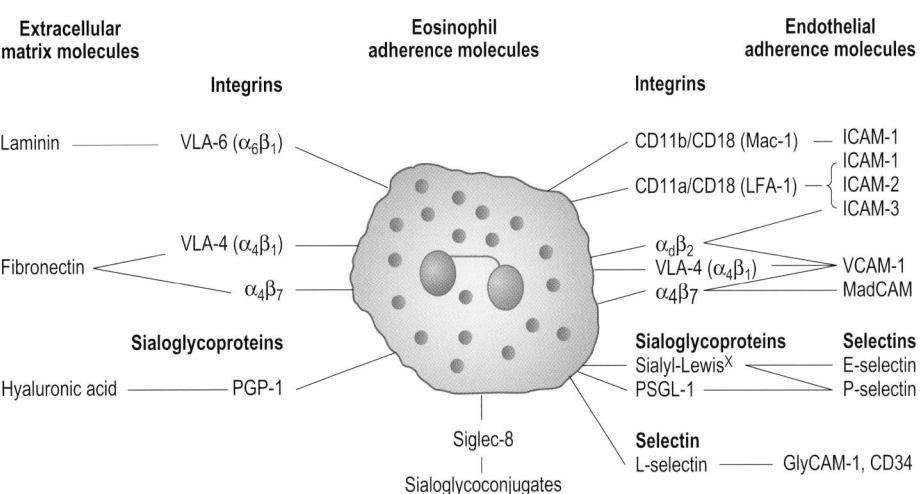

KEY CONCEPTS

Actions of eosinophilopoietic cytokines IL-3, GM-CSF, IL-5

- Promote eosinophil development and maturation in the marrow (IL-5).
- Release a pool of matured eosinophils from the marrow (IL-5).
- Sustain the viability and antagonize apoptosis of mature eosinophils, enhance multiple effector responses of mature eosinophils.

Eosinophil chemoattractants

Mobilization of eosinophils into tissues is governed by receptor-mediated chemoattractant stimuli. Chemoattractants promote the directed migration of eosinophils and may enhance the adhesion of eosinophils to vascular endothelium and their subsequent migration through the endothelium. Many compounds have been identified as eosinophil chemoattractants, including humoral immune mediators, such as platelet-activating factor (PAF) and the complement anaphylatoxins C5a and C3a; certain cytokines; and several chemokines, most notably the eotaxins. None of these is specific solely for eosinophils, but eotaxin-1, eotaxin-2, and eotaxin-3 exhibit the most restricted specificity.[1] Eotaxins signal through CCR3 chemokine receptors that are expressed on eosinophils as well as basophils, some Th2 cells and some mast cells. Thus, recruitment of eosinophils to sites of immunologic reactions is governed by their response to chemoattractants that facilitate intravascular emigration and direct migration of extravascular eosinophils, as well as by the functional states of eosinophil adherence molecules and the differential expression of endothelial cell adherence ligands.

Structure of eosinophils

Human eosinophils, unlike neutrophils, usually have a bilobed nucleus (Fig. 23.2). Defining attributes of eosinophils are their large, cytoplasmic "specific" granules that are morphologically distinct because of their unique content of crystalloid cores. Crystalloid cores are recognizable by transmission electron microscopy and usually appear electron dense (Fig. 23.2). The cores

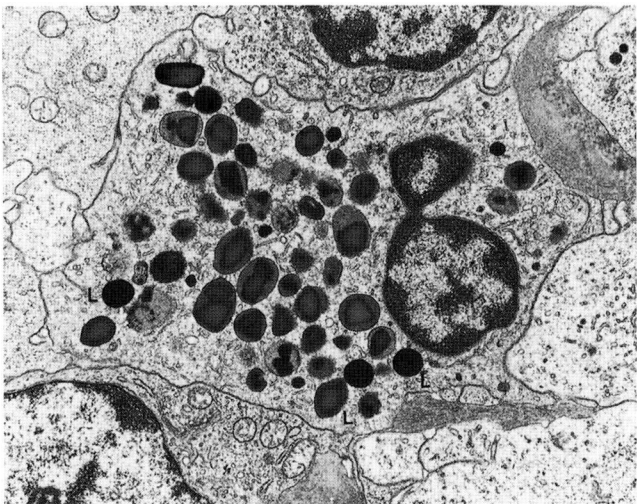

Fig. 23.2 Transmission electron micrograph of a human eosinophil. The numerous cytoplasmic specific granules contain the electron-dense crystalline cores that are unique to eosinophils. In addition, lipid bodies are visible as globular, uniformly dark structures. (Original magnification × 11,180.)
Courtesy of Dr Ann M. Dvorak, Israel Deaconess Medical Center, Harvard Medical School, Boston.

and surrounding matrices of specific granules contain cationic proteins that account for the tinctorial staining of granules with eosin. Eosinophils at sites of inflammation can exhibit morphologic changes in their specific granules, including loss of either matrix or core components from within intact granules, compatible with the extracellular release of granule constituents.

Lipid bodies, cytoplasmic structures distinct from granules (Fig. 23.2), are roughly globular in shape and range in size from minute to the size of specific granules. Lipid bodies are dissolved by common alcohol-based hematologic stains, but with osmium fixation are preserved and stain darkly. Lipid bodies lack a delimiting membrane, but contain internal membranes that are often obscured by overlying lipid. Lipid bodies are found in neutrophils and other cells, especially in association with inflammation; but eosinophils typically contain more lipid bodies than neutrophils. Lipid body formation in eosinophils is rapidly inducible within minutes. In eosinophils, key enzymes involved in eicosanoid formation, including prostaglandin H synthase, the 5- and 15-lipoxygenases and leukotriene (LT) C_4 synthase, localize at lipid bodies; and lipid bodies are sites of eicosanoid synthesis.[7]

Cell surface receptors and proteins

Eosinophil receptors for immunoglobulins include those for IgG, IgE, and IgA. The receptor for IgG on eosinophils is principally the low-affinity FcγRII (CD32), whereas neutrophils have FcγRII and FcγRIII (CD16). Exposure of eosinophils to interferon (IFN)-γ elicits expression of a phosphatidylinositol-linked form of CD16 on eosinophils, and CD16 may be expressed on eosinophils from some patients with eosinophilic disorders.

Eosinophil IgE receptors include the high-affinity IgE receptor FcεRI, typically found on basophils and mast cells, as well as FcεRII, the low-affinity IgE receptor, like CD23 found on lymphocytes, monocytes, and antigen-presenting cells. Although FcεRI α chain protein is present within eosinophils, its surface expression can be low or undetectable. Engagement of eosinophil FcεRI does not elicit exocytotic degranulation, as it does on basophils and mast cells. FcεRI may participate in IgE-mediated antigen uptake by antigen-presenting eosinophils. Eosinophil expression of IgE receptors is notable because IgE levels and eosinophil numbers frequently increase concomitantly in helminth parasitic infections as well as allergic diseases.

Eosinophils express FcαRI (CD89), which binds secretory IgA more potently than other forms of IgA. Engagement of FcαRI triggers eosinophil release of granule proteins. With the characteristic localization of eosinophils to mucosal surfaces of the respiratory, gastrointestinal, and genitourinary tracts, this IgA receptor enables eosinophils to engage secretory IgA present at these mucosal sites.

Eosinophils have receptors for complement components including C1q (CR1), C3b/C4b (CR1), iC3b (CR3), C3a, and C5a. Both C3a and C5a are eosinophil chemoattractants and stimulate the production of oxygen radicals by eosinophils. Eosinophils express several receptors for chemokines. CCR1 is a receptor for MIP-1α, MCP-3 and RANTES, whereas CCR3 is a receptor for eotaxin-1, eotaxin-2, eotaxin-3, MCP-3, and RANTES. Eosinophils express CXCR4 and respond to the ligand for this receptor, stromal cell-derived factor-1α.

Mature eosinophils, like their immature precursors, express receptors for the three cytokines, GM-CSF, IL-3, and IL-5, that promote eosinophilopoiesis and stimulate the functioning of mature eosinophils. In addition, eosinophils have receptors for a broad range of other cytokines, including IL-1α, IL-2, IL-4, IFN-α and IFN-γ, TNF-α, stem cell factor (c-KIT), and IL-16 (which signals via CD4 on eosinophils). Thus, eosinophils are subject to stimulation by many cytokines, although little is understood about how many of them affect eosinophil functioning *in vivo*.

Of pertinence to interactions between eosinophils and B and T lymphocytes, eosinophils can express several relevant plasma membrane proteins. Class II MHC proteins, generally absent on blood eosinophils, are induced for expression on eosinophils in sites of inflammation. In addition, eosinophils can express CD40, CD154 (CD40 ligand), CD153 (CD30 ligand), CD28 (B7-2), and CD86.[4]

Eosinophils express receptors for several lipid mediators, including platelet-activating factor (PAF) and leukotriene B_4 (LTB$_4$), which are chemoattractants for eosinophils and stimulate eosinophil degranulation and respiratory burst activity. Eosinophils also have receptors for prostaglandins D_2, and E_2 and for cysteinyl leukotrienes.

Constituents of eosinophils

Eosinophil specific granules contain pre-formed proteins that include both specific cationic proteins and stores of diverse cytokines and chemokines.

Cationic granule proteins

Eosinophil granule cationic proteins have been extensively studied because of their abundance in the granules and their capacity to exert multiple effects on host cells and microbial targets. Major basic protein (MBP), named for its quantitative predominance within the granule and its markedly cationic (basic) isoelectric point of about 11, is a 13.8- to 14-kDa protein. A homolog of MBP that is somewhat smaller (13.4 kDa) and less basic (pI 8.7) has been identified. MBP lacks enzymatic activity and probably exerts its varied effects via its markedly cationic nature. MBP was found to be toxic to both airway epithelium and helminths, and to have antibacterial effects.[8]

A second granule protein is eosinophil peroxidase (EPO), an enzyme distinct from neutrophil myeloperoxidase. Cationic EPO (pI 10.8) uses hydrogen peroxide and halide ions to form hypohalous acids, which are toxic for parasites, bacteria, and tumor and host cells. EPO utilizes bromide in preference to chloride and is even more active with a pseudohalide, thiocyanate, to generate oxidant products, including hypobromous and hypothiocyanous acids.

Two additional granule proteins are eosinophil cationic protein (ECP) (18 kDa, pI 10.8) and eosinophil-derived neurotoxin (EDN) (18–19 kDa, pI 8.9). EDN, never demonstrated to be neurotoxic for humans, is so named because, after it is injected intracerebrally into test rabbits, it elicits a characteristic neuropathologic response. Both ECP and EDN are ribonucleases (RNases). EDN expresses 100 times more RNase activity than does ECP, although their toxic effects on bacterial, parasitic and mammalian target cells are not simply due to their RNase catalytic activities.

Within the specific granule, MBP is localized to the crystalloid core, whereas ECP, EDN, and EPO are localized in the matrix of the granule around the core (Fig. 23.2). MBP is also found in low amounts (~3% of eosinophil levels) in basophils, but whether this reflects endocytosis or endogenous synthesis is not known. Uptake of MBP and EPO into mast cells is known to occur via endocytosis. Small amounts of EDN and ECP are present in neutrophils, and as neutrophils contain mRNA transcripts for these, EDN and ECP are likely synthesized by neutrophils. Nevertheless, eosinophils are the dominant source of these four cationic proteins. The properties of these proteins and their numerous biologic effects have been reviewed,[8] as these proteins have major effects not only in the potential role of eosinophils in host defense against helminthic parasites, but also in contributing to tissue dysfunction and damage in eosinophil-related allergic and other diseases.

Cytokines and chemokines

Eosinophils are capable of elaborating at least four dozen diverse cytokines and chemokines, and studies continue to identify more cytokines released by eosinophils. The potential activities of eosinophil-derived cytokines are extensive. Eosinophil-derived cytokines include those with autocrine growth factor activities for eosinophils and those with potential roles in acute and chronic inflammatory responses. A notable feature of eosinophils as a source of cytokines is that they contain stores of these cytokines pre-formed within eosinophil granules and secretory vesicles.[9] Thus, in contrast to most lymphocytes, which must be induced to synthesize de novo cytokines destined for release, eosinophils can immediately release pre-formed cytokine and chemokine proteins into the surrounding milieu. Although levels of pre-formed cytokines in eosinophils may be lower than those of specifically stimulated lymphocytes, local and rapid release of eosinophil-derived cytokines in tissues could readily induce a response in various adjoining cell types.

Eosinophils synthesize the three growth factor cytokines GM-CSF, IL-3 and IL-5, which promote eosinophil survival, antagonize eosinophil apoptosis, and enhance eosinophil effector responses. Other cytokines elaborated by human eosinophils that may have activities in acute and chronic inflammatory responses include IL-1α, IL-6, IL-8, IFN-γ, TNF-α, and MIP-1α. Human eosinophils can elaborate other various "growth" factors, including transforming growth factor (TGF)-α, TGF-β$_1$, vascular endothelial growth factor, platelet-derived growth factor (PDGF)-β, and heparin-binding epidermal growth factor. These cytokines may have a role in contributing to epithelial hyperplasia and fibrosis, as well as other activities. In addition, eosinophils are recognized as sources of specific cytokines and chemokines capable of stimulating or inhibiting lymphocyte responses, including IL-2, IL-4, IL-10, IL-12, IL-16, RANTES, and TGF-β$_1$. Of note, eosinophil cytokines include those associated with Th2 (IL-4, IL-5, IL-13), Th1 (IL-12, IFN-γ), and T-regulatory (IL-10, TGF-β) responses, emphasizing the diverse immunoregulatory potentials for eosinophil-secreted cytokines.[9]

Activated eosinophils

A well-recognized attribute of eosinophils is that, in conjunction with eosinophilic diseases, some blood and tissue eosinophils may exhibit various alterations indicative that these cells have been "activated." These changes include increased metabolic activity, diminished density ("hypodense"), enhanced LTC$_4$ formation, and morphologic alterations, including cytoplasmic vacuolization, alterations in granule numbers and size, and losses within specific granules of MBP-containing cores or matrices. Activated eosinophils may exhibit enhanced plasma membrane expression of some proteins, including CD69, HLA-DR, and CD25.

Features associated with in vivo "activated" eosinophils can be elicited in part by exposing eosinophils to specific stimuli, including GM-CSF, IL-3, and IL-5. In addition, interactions with extracellular matrix components can further contribute to eosinophil activation. Eosinophil "activation," however, is not a singularly binary process, and some attributes of activation can be elicited without other attributes by mediators and mechanisms that remain to be delineated.

Mechanisms of eosinophil degranulation

As eosinophil granules contain four major cationic proteins and a multitude of pre-formed cytokines and chemokines, the processes by which eosinophils mobilize these granule constituents for their extracellular release are important in understanding the regulated functioning of eosinophils. Unlike mast cells or basophils that undergo acute exocytotic degranulation in response to cross-linking of their high-affinity Fcε receptors, an analogous mechanism to elicit comparable exocytotic degranulation of

fluid-phase eosinophils has not been identified. Cross-linking of eosinophil IgG or IgA Fc receptors can stimulate release of eosinophil cationic proteins, but this rapid FcR-mediated acute "degranulation" process is cytolytic for eosinophils. In contrast, observations of eosinophils on the surfaces of large non-phagocytosable multicellular helminth parasites do provide evidence that eosinophils can degranulate by exocytosis to release granule contents on the surfaces of target parasites.

An alternative mechanism of mobilizing granule contents for secretion that eosinophils utilize is a process of vesicular transport-mediated "piecemeal" degranulation. Electron microscopic observations of lesional eosinophils provided evidence that eosinophil granule contents were mobilized in vivo by selective incorporation into small vesicles that traffic to the cell surface and release these granule contents. By this process, there may be agonist-elicited selective secretion of certain eosinophil-derived cytokines.[10] Ultrastructural studies have demonstrated that secretory vesicles arise from granules and transport cytokines, such as IL-4.[10] Insights into the selectivity and mechanisms of differential cytokine secretion have been indicated by finding, at least for IL-4, that a receptor for IL-4 mediates the transport of IL-4 from granules and within secretory vesicles.[11] How this process of vesicular transport is regulated and functions to selectively mobilize specific eosinophil granule-derived cytokines or cationic proteins remains under investigation.

In addition to regulated release of granule contents from viable eosinophils, a common, but often overlooked, occurrence is the apparent lysis of eosinophils. Both cutaneous and pulmonary biopsies of eosinophil-associated diseases contain free, extracellular, but still membrane-bound eosinophil granules. These free extracellular granules express cytokine, chemokine, and cysteinyl leukotriene receptors and are secretion competent even outside of intact eosinophils.[12,13] The mechanism of cytolysis in such reactions is undefined, but may represent eosinophil apoptosis and occur more commonly than heretofore recognized. Eosinophils can release mitochondrial DNA-containing "traps," that also contain cytotoxic granule-derived proteins, into the extracellular space.[14]

Functions of eosinophils

Conventional considerations of the roles that eosinophils may play have been guided by quantitative considerations, so that those diseases characteristically marked by more prominent eosinophilia have occasioned the most interest. Thus, studies have focused on the "effector" roles eosinophils play in host defense against helminth infections and in the immunopathogenesis of allergic and other eosinophilic diseases. Additional roles for eosinophils must be considered in immune or inflammatory responses not conventionally recognized to contain abundant eosinophils.[4]

Roles in host defense

Because the host response to infections with multicellular helminth parasites is characteristically associated with eosinophilia, it is often believed that eosinophils evolved to have a role in killing helminths, especially during their larval stages. Indeed, in vitro eosinophils can kill numerous helminths, organisms too large to be phagocytosed. Eosinophils adhere to the parasite and deposit eosinophil granule contents onto its surface. Cell products that can contribute to parasite death include MBP, ECP, EDN, and EPO.

As reviewed,[15] the helminthotoxic roles of eosinophils *in vivo* are less certain in humans and rodents. In eosinophil-depleted mice, the intensities of primary and secondary infections with some helminths have not been greater than in eosinophilic mice, nor have IL-5 transgenic mice exhibited increased resistance to infection with some helminth species. Moreover, schistosome infections in two lines of eosinophil-ablated mice have shown no differences in measures of infection compared to normal mice.[16] Nevertheless, murine studies need to be interpreted with caution. Some helminth infections elicit Th1-biased responses in mice, which differ from Th2-biased responses in humans or rats. Many experimental infections involve introducing helminth infections that are often host species-restricted into unnatural host mice, in which innate immune responses may be prominent. Natural human infections are usually a consequence of repeated exposures, during which acquired, rather than innate, immunity becomes prominent. Thus, eosinophil functions as helminthotoxic cells *in vivo* remain unclear. Eosinophils might have alternative functions in host responses to helminths, including functioning as antigen-presenting cells and even favoring the survival of *Trichinella* larvae in muscles.[17,18]

Roles in disease pathogenesis

The ability of eosinophils to release biologically active lipids as paracrine mediators of inflammation and to release pre-formed cationic and cytokine granule constituents enables them to contribute to the immunopathogenesis of various diseases, including asthma.[1] Eosinophils form several classes of biologically active lipids. Eosinophils may liberate PAF, whose diverse activities can be mediated either directly or by stimulating other cells to release leukotrienes, prostaglandins, and complement peptides. Stimulated eosinophils release LTC_4. LTD_4 and LTE_4 are formed from LTC_4 by the sequential enzymatic removal of glutamic acid and glycine from its tripeptide glutathione side chain. LTC_4 and especially LTD_4 have bronchoconstrictor activities, constrict terminal arterioles, dilate venules, and stimulate airway mucus secretion. Thus, eosinophils are a potential source of two major types of mediator lipids, the sulfidopeptide leukotrienes and PAF.

Oxidants released by eosinophils, including superoxide anion, hydroxyl radical, and singlet oxygen, and EPO-catalyzed hypothiocyanous acid and other hypohalous acids have the potential to damage host tissues.

Released eosinophil granule proteins are immunochemically detectable in fluids, including blood, sputum, and synovial fluids, and in tissues, including the respiratory and gastrointestinal tracts, skin, and heart, in association with various eosinophil-related diseases. The eosinophil cationic proteins, including MBP, ECP, and EPO, can damage various cell types. Thus, extracellular release of eosinophil granule proteins, by degranulation or cytolysis of eosinophils, could contribute to local tissue damage by causing dysfunction and damage to adjacent cells.

Other eosinophil functions

Other potential functions for the eosinophil are not fully defined. In addition to the acute release of lipid, peptide, and cytokine mediators of inflammation, eosinophils probably contribute to chronic inflammation, including the development of fibrosis. Eosinophils can be a major source of the fibrosis-promoting cytokine TGF-β. Additional roles of eosinophils in modulating extracellular matrix deposition and remodeling are suggested by studies of normal wound healing. During dermal wound healing, eosinophils infiltrate into wound sites and sequentially express TGF-α early and TGF-$β_1$ later during wound healing. These findings suggest that eosinophils may contribute to the more chronic subepithelial airway fibrosis characteristic of chronic asthma.

Additional functions for eosinophils are indicated by the findings that they may be induced to express class II MHC proteins and can function as antigen-presenting cells.[19] Blood eosinophils lack HLA-DR expression, but eosinophils recovered from the airways 48 hours after segmental antigen challenge have been shown to express HLA-DR. Cytokines, including GM-CSF, IL-3, IL-4, and IFN-γ, induce eosinophil HLA-DR expression. Both murine and human eosinophils can function as HLA-DR-dependent MHC-restricted antigen-presenting cells in stimulating proliferation of T cells. *In vivo*, murine eosinophils can process exogenous antigens in the airways, traffic to regional lymph nodes, and function as antigen-specific antigen-presenting cells to stimulate responses of CD4 T cells.[20]

Because eosinophils normally become resident in submucosal tissues, they undoubtedly participate in ongoing homeostatic immune responses at these sites. Eosinophils are even found in the thymus. Further investigations will help delineate their functional roles and interactions with other cells, including lymphocytes, so that the scope of eosinophil function will probably extend beyond its currently more defined role as an effector cell contributing to allergic inflammation.

Eosinophilia and eosinophilic disorders

Diverse infectious, allergic, neoplastic and idiopathic disease processes can be associated with increased blood and/or tissue eosinophil numbers. Blood eosinophilia, present when eosinophil numbers are in excess of their usual level of $<450/\mu L$ of blood, may be intermittently, modestly or less frequently markedly increased. Blood eosinophil numbers are not necessarily indicative of the extent of eosinophil involvement in affected tissues.

Some patients with sustained blood eosinophilia can develop organ damage, especially cardiac. This cardiac involvement can include the formation of intraventricular thrombi and endomyocardial fibrosis with secondary mitral or tricuspid regurgitation (Fig. 23.3). Such damage can complicate the sustained eosinophilia of hypereosinophilic syndromes and has been noted with eosinophilias accompanying other diseases, including eosinophilia with carcinomas, lymphomas, GM-CSF, or IL-2 administration, drug reactions, and parasitic infections. Most patients with eosinophilia, however, develop no evidence of endomyocardial damage. Conversely, cardiac disease can rarely present in patients without known eosinophilia. The pathogenesis of eosinophil-mediated cardiac damage involves both usually heightened numbers of eosinophils and some activating events, as yet ill-defined, that promote eosinophil-mediated tissue damage.

Cardiac damage progresses through three stages. In the first, there is damage to the endocardium and infiltration of the myocardium with eosinophils and lymphocytes, with eosinophil degranulation and myocardial necrosis. Elevated plasma levels of troponin can be a sensitive assay of early eosinophil-mediated cardiac damage. A similar acute eosinophilic myocarditis can develop with drug hypersensitivity reactions and may be more fulminant. The first stage is frequently clinically occult, although subungual splinter hemorrhages may be prominent. Elevations of serum troponins as a measure of myocardial injury should be evaluated. Echocardiography usually detects no abnormalities at this stage, although cardiac magnetic resonance imaging

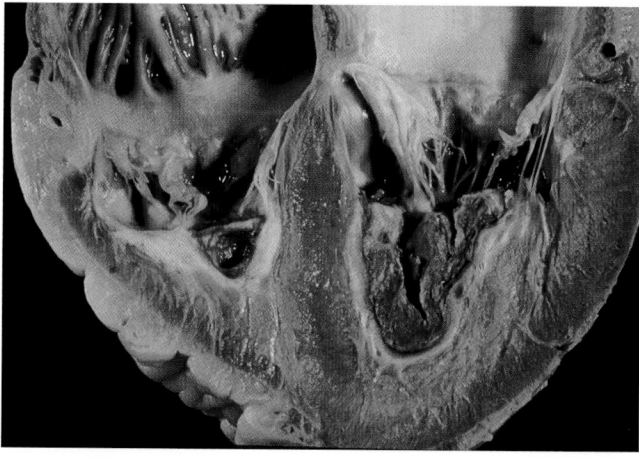

Fig. 23.3 Eosinophil endomyocardial disease. A large thrombus is present in the apex of the left ventricle and the chordae tendineae are entrapped, leading to severe mitral valve regurgitation.

(MRI) is evolving as a technique to potentially detect cardiac involvement at an earlier stage. Uncommonly, death due to acute progressive cardiac disease can occur. Corticosteroid therapy during the acute stage may help control and prevent the evolution of myocardial fibrosis.

The second stage of heart disease, the formation of thrombi along the damaged endocardium, affects either or both ventricles and occasionally the atrium. Outflow tracts near the aortic and pulmonic valves are usually spared. These thrombi can embolize to the brain and elsewhere. Finally, in the fibrotic stage, progressive scarring leads to entrapment of chordae tendineae with the development of mitral and/or tricuspid valve regurgitation and to endomyocardial fibrosis, producing a restrictive cardiomyopathy. Echocardiography and MRI are valuable in detecting intracardiac thrombi and the manifestations of fibrosis. Patients with sustained eosinophilia should be monitored by echocardiography and serum troponin assays for evidence of cardiac disease. In an older series of patients referred to the NIH, much of the mortality in these patients with hypereosinophilia was attributable to end-stage congestive heart failure. In contemporary times, earlier recognition of cardiac involvement, mitral valve replacement with bioprostheses and additional therapeutic options for hypereosinophilic syndromes (see below) have largely minimized the morbidity and mortality attributable to end-stage eosinophilic endomyocardial disease.

Infectious diseases associated with eosinophilia

Eosinophilia is encountered only with specific infectious diseases. With active bacterial or viral infections, eosinopenia is characteristic. This suppression of blood eosinophils is due in part to heightened endogenous corticosteroid production as well as to inflammatory mediators released during these infections. This suppression of eosinophilia, with either serious bacterial infections or marked inflammation, accounts for the absence of otherwise expected eosinophilia in some patients with helminth infections, including those with hyperinfection strongyloidiasis.[21] As a general clinical guideline, patients with a febrile illness and an increased or even normal blood eosinophilia are not likely to have common bacterial or viral infections, unless they have adrenal insufficiency or a confounding medication-elicited eosinophilia.

Helminth parasites

Helminth parasites are multicellular metazoan organisms—the "worm" parasites. Infections with diverse helminths elicit eosinophilia (Chapter 29).[21] Although eosinophilia may provide a hematologic clue to the presence of helminth infection, the absence of blood eosinophilia does not exclude such infections. The eosinophilic response to helminths is determined both by the host's immune response and by the parasite, including its distribution, migration and development within the infected host. The level of eosinophilia tends to parallel the magnitude and extent of tissue invasion by helminth larvae or adults. For several helminth infections the migration of infecting larvae or subsequent developmental stages through tissues is greatest early in infection, and hence the magnitude of the elicited eosinophilia will be the greatest in these early phases. For established infections, local eosinophil infiltration will often be present around helminths within tissues, without a significant blood eosinophilia. Eosinophilia may be absent in those helminth infections that are well contained within tissues (e.g., intact echinococcal cysts) or are solely intraluminal within the intestinal tract (e.g., Ascaris, tapeworms). For some established infections, increases in blood eosinophilia may be episodic. Intermittent leakage of cyst fluids from echinococcal cysts can transiently stimulate increases in blood eosinophilia and also cause symptoms attributable to allergic or anaphylactic reactions (urticaria, bronchospasm). For tissue-dwelling helminths, increases in eosinophilia may occur principally in association with migration of adult parasites, as in loiasis and gnathostomiasis.

Helminth infections more likely to elicit prolonged hypereosinophilia in adults include filarial and hookworm infections and strongyloidiasis (Table 23.1).[21] Trichinellosis can elicit an acute hypereosinophilia. *Strongyloides stercoralis* infection, difficult to diagnose solely by stool examinations, is especially important to exclude, not only because it elicits modest to even marked eosinophilia, but also because, unlike other helminths, it can develop into a disseminated, often fatal, disease (hyperinfection syndrome) in patients given immunosuppressive corticosteroids.[21] An ELISA serology has proved valuable in detecting strongyloidiasis and should be obtained for eosinophilic patients likely to receive corticosteroids. Some tissue- or blood-dwelling helminths that are not diagnosable by stool examinations but that can cause marked eosinophilia require diagnostic examination of blood or biopsied tissues or specific serologic tests.[21] Infections with these organisms include filarial infections, trichinellosis, and visceral larva migrans. In children, owing to their propensity for geophagous pica and ingestion of dirt contaminated by dog ascarid eggs, visceral larva migrans due to *Toxocara canis* is a potential etiology for sustained eosinophilia. ELISA serologic testing can evaluate this possibility.

Other infections: protozoa and fungi

Infections with single-celled protozoan parasites do not characteristically elicit eosinophilia. This is true of all intestinal, blood- and tissue-infecting protozoa, with two exceptions. Two intestinal protozoans, *Dientamoeba fragilis* and *Isospora belli*, can at times be associated with low-grade eosinophilia. Hence, in patients with symptoms of enteric infection and eosinophilia, diagnostic trophozoites of *D. fragilis* or oocysts of *I. belli* should be sought in stool examinations. Fecal examinations for *I. belli* oocysts must be specifically requested, as they are not usually detected in routine stool ova and parasite examinations. Other enteric protozoa do not elicit eosinophilia and, if detected in stool examinations, should not be accepted as causes of eosinophilia.

Table 23.1 Parasitic diseases capable of causing marked (>3000/μL) or long-standing eosinophilia

Helminth infection	Hypereosinophilia	Chronic eosinophilia
Angiostrongyliasis costaricensis		
Ascariasis	+ during early lung migration	
Hookworm infection	+ during early lung migration	+ common cause of low-grade eosinophilia
Strongyloidiasis	uncommonly	+ self-perpetuating, may last >50 years
Trichinosis	+ with heavy infections	
Visceral larva migrans	+ principally in children	
Gnathostomiasis		
Cysticercosis		
Echinococcosis		+ may be episodic with cyst fluid leakage
Filariases:		
Tropical pulmonary eosinophilia	+	+
Loiasis	+ especially in expatriates	+
Onchocerciasis	+	+
Flukes:		
Schistosomiasis	+ during early infection in nonimmunes	+
Fascioliasis	+ during early infection	+
Clonorchiasis	+ during early infection	+
Paragonimiasis	+ during early infection	+
Fasciolopsiasis	+ during early infection	+

Adapted from Wilson ME, Weller PF. Eosinophilia. In: Guerrant RL, Walker DH, Weller PF, eds. Tropical infectious diseases: principles, pathogens and practice, 3rd edn. Philadelphia: Churchill Livingstone, 2011; p. 943.

Three fungal diseases may be associated with eosinophilia. Aspergillosis is accompanied by eosinophilia only in the form of allergic bronchopulmonary aspergillosis, not when it is an invasive pathogen. Coccidioidomycosis, following primary infection, especially in conjunction with erythema nodosum, and at times with progressive disseminated disease, may elicit blood eosinophilia and may cause an eosinophilic meningitis. Basidiobolomycosisis may also be associated with eosinophilia.[21]

HIV and retroviral infections

Eosinophilia may uncommonly accompany HIV infections for several reasons. First, leukopenia may increase eosinophil percentages without reflecting true eosinophilia. Second, adverse reactions to medications may elicit eosinophilia. Third, patients with AIDS who develop adrenal insufficiency due to cytomegalovirus and other infections may exhibit eosinophilia as a consequence. In addition, usually modest, and uncommonly marked eosinophilia, is observed in some HIV-infected patients.[21] Eosinophilia more commonly develops with HTLV-1 infections.[21]

Allergic diseases associated with eosinophilia

Among the noninfectious diseases associated with eosinophilia (Table 23.2) are allergic diseases, notably those mediated by IgE-dependent mechanisms. In these diseases, including allergic rhinitis, conjunctivitis, and asthma, eosinophils are present in involved tissues as well as often being increased in the blood.

Myeloproliferative and neoplastic disease

Eosinophilia may occur with specific neoplastic diseases, as well as in some disorders of uncertain etiology, including some hypereosinophilic syndromes.

Hypereosinophilic syndromes

A syndrome previously termed the idiopathic hypereosinophilic syndrome is not a single entity but rather a constellation of leukoproliferative disorders characterized by sustained overproduction of eosinophils. The three original diagnostic criteria for this syndrome are: eosinophilia in excess of 1500/μL of blood persisting for longer than 6 months; lack of an identifiable parasitic, allergic or other etiology for eosinophilia and an absence of other eosinophilic syndromes clinically distinct from the hypereosinophilic syndrome; and signs and symptoms of organ involvement. In contemporary practice, one can no longer wait for 6 months before diagnostic and therapeutic interventions are needed for a hypereosinophilic patient with organ involvement. If the other criteria are reliably met prior to the 6-month time frame, a diagnosis can be made and treatment promptly initiated. Moreover, in recent years there has been increasing recognition that hypereosinophilic syndromes (HES) encompass a spectrum of disorders, and notable progress has been made in identifying the underlying defects in some of these (Fig. 23.4).[22,23]

> ● KEY CONCEPTS
>
> **Hypereosinophilic syndromes**
>
> - Eosinophilia sustained in excess of 1500/μL.
> - Absence of allergic, parasitic, or other etiologies for eosinophilia.
> - Evidence of organ involvement.

Some patients with HESs exhibit features common to myeloproliferative disorders, including elevated vitamin B_{12} and LDH levels, splenomegaly, cytogenetic abnormalities, myelofibrosis, anemia, and myeloid dysplasia. This is termed the myeloproliferative variant of HES, and patients often also have an elevated serum level of tryptase. In many patients with myeloproliferative HESs, the molecular defect has been identified as a chromosome 4 deletion that yields a fusion gene encoding a FIP1LI/PDGFRA (platelet-derived growth factor-α receptor) (F/P) protein that constitutively expresses receptor kinase activity. This fusion gene can be diagnostically evaluated by RT-PCR or FISH (fluorescence in situ hybridization) (Chapter 98). Importantly, the majority of patients with this fusion mutation respond to therapy with imatinib, which is considered the first line of

Table 23.2 Eosinophil-associated diseases and disorders

Allergic or atopic diseases

Asthma
Allergic rhinitis
Eosinophilic esophagitis
Atopic dermatitis
Allergic urticaria
Nasal polyps

Myeloproliferative and neoplastic disorders

Hypereosinophilic syndromes: myeloproliferative, lymphoproliferative
  and others
Leukemia
Lymphoma- and tumor-associated
Mastocytosis

Pulmonary syndromes

Parasite-induced eosinophilic lung diseases:
Loeffler syndrome: patchy migratory infiltrates, resolving over weeks,
  seen with transpulmonary migration of helminth parasites, especially
  Ascaris
Tropical pulmonary eosinophilia: miliary lesions and
  fibrosis; heightened immune response causing one form of
  lymphatic filariasis; increased IgE and antifilarial antibodies
Pulmonary parenchymal invasion: paragonimiasis
Heavy hematogenous seeding with helminths: trichinellosis,
  schistosomiasis, larva migrans
Allergic bronchopulmonary aspergillosis
Chronic eosinophilic pneumonia: dense peripheral infiltrates,
  fever; progressive; blood eosinophilia may be absent; steroid
  responsive
Acute eosinophilic pneumonia: acute presentation diagnosed
  by bronchoalveolar lavage or biopsy
Churg–Strauss vasculitis: small and medium sized arteries; granulomas,
  necrosis; asthma often antecedent; extrapulmonary (e.g., neurologic,
  cutaneous, cardiac, or gastrointestinal) involvement likely
Drug- and toxin-induced eosinophilic lung diseases
Other: hypereosinophilic syndromes, neoplasia, bronchocentric
  granulomatosis

Skin and subcutaneous diseases

Skin diseases: atopic dermatitis, blistering diseases, including bullous
  pemphigoid, urticarias, drug reactions
Diseases of pregnancy: pruritic urticarial papules and plaques
  syndrome, herpes gestationis
Eosinophilic pustular folliculitis
Eosinophilic cellulitis (Wells syndrome)
Kimura's disease and angiolymphoid hyperplasia with
  eosinophilia
Shulman's syndrome (eosinophilic fasciitis)
Episodic angioedema with eosinophilia: recurrent
  periodic episodes with fever, angioedema, and secondary
  weight gain; may be long-standing without untoward cardiac
  dysfunction

Gastrointestinal disorders

Eosinophilic gastroenteritides
Inflammatory bowel disease: eosinophils in lesions; occasionally blood
  eosinophilia with ulcerative colitis

Rheumatologic diseases

Vasculitis: Churg–Strauss and cutaneous necrotizing eosinophilic
  vasculitis

Immunologic reactions

Medication-related eosinophilias
Immunodeficiency diseases: Job's syndrome and Omenn's syndrome
Transplant rejections

Endocrine

Hypoadrenalism: Addison's disease, adrenal hemorrhage,
  hypopituitarism

Other causes of eosinophilia

Atheromatous cholesterol embolization
Hereditary
Serosal surface irritation, including peritoneal dialysis and pleural
  eosinophilia

Adapted from Weller PF. Eosinophilia and eosinophil-related disorders.
In: Adkinson NF Jr, Yunginger JW, Busse WW, et al, eds. Allergy: principles
and practice, 6th edn. Philadelphia: Mosby, 2003; p. 1105.

therapy for FIP1LI/PDGFRA-positive myeloproliferative HES.[24,25] For patients with any evidence of cardiac involvement, including elevated troponin levels, it is recommended to administer glucocorticoids along with the initiation of imatinib. Other eosinophilic patients without F/P mutations have also responded to imatinib, indicating that other receptor tyrosine kinase mutations can underlie some of these myeloproliferative forms of HES.[26] In addition, clonal abnormalities in the eosinophil lineage have been reported in a few patients (Fig. 23.4).

Another variant form of HES is a lymphoproliferative form due to clonal expansions of lymphocytes, often CD4+CD3− Th2-like lymphocytes, that elaborate IL-5.[27] These aberrant T cells can be sought by flow cytometry or T-cell receptor analysis. These patients, who may have elevated IgE levels, usually do not develop eosinophilic cardiac disease, but are at risk for developing T-cell lymphomas.[27]

In addition to these recognized variants, there are yet a substantial number of HES patients for whom the etiologies of the eosinophilia remain unknown. Some such patients develop no signs or symptoms of disease and can be followed without therapy. For those who require therapy, including those with lymphoproliferative variants, glucocorticosteroids are the mainstay of treatment.[27] With glucocorticoid therapy, partial or complete remission of eosinophilia within one month has been reported to occur in 85% of patients.[25] Second-line agents include hydroxyurea and IFN-α.[28] A neutralizing anti-IL-5 monoclonal antibody (mepolizumab) has been evaluated and shown to have steroid-sparing effects in those affected with FIP1L1-PDGFRA negative hypereosinophilic syndrome, but it is not FDA approved.[29] Anti-CD52 monoclonal antibody (alemtuzumab) and allogenic hematopoietic cell transplantation have been used for particularly severe and refractory HES.

Historically, initial reports and case series suggested a high rate of morbidity and mortality from HES, but with earlier diagnosis and therapy, and with more varied drug options, morbidity, and particularly mortality, have been reduced.

Eosinophilia with tumors or leukemias

The F/P-positive myeloproliferative variant of HES can be considered a form of chronic eosinophilic leukemia.[30] Eosinophilia is a characteristic of the M4Eo subtype of acute myeloid leukemia, having the common M4 characteristic of chromosomal 16 abnormalities. Other forms of eosinophilic leukemia, often with specific cytogenetic and molecular genetic abnormalities, have been recognized.[30] Eosinophilia may accompany chronic myelogenous leukemia (often with basophilia), but is uncommon with acute lymphoblastic leukemia. Eosinophilia may be observed in some lymphoma patients, including Hodgkin's disease, especially the nodular sclerosing form, T-cell lymphoblastic lymphoma, and adult T-cell leukemia/lymphoma. A small proportion of patients with carcinomas, especially of mucin-producing epithelial cell origin, have associated blood and tissue eosinophilia. Eosinophilia

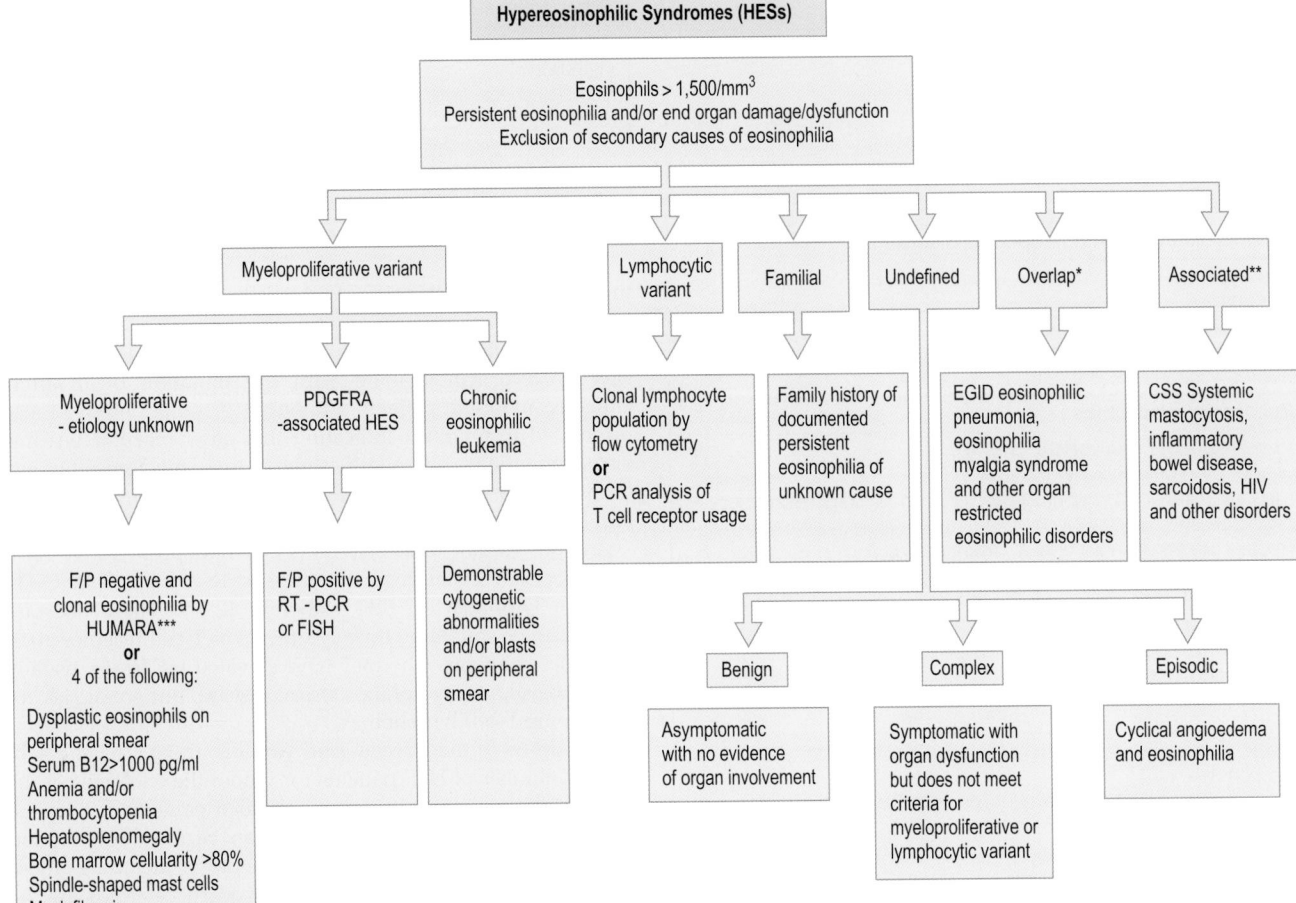

Fig. 23.4 Classification of hypereosinophilic syndromes based on a Workshop Summary report. Specific syndromes discussed at the workshop are indicated in bold. *Incomplete criteria, apparent restriction to specific tissues/organs. **Peripheral eosinophilia, > 1500/mm³ in association with a defined diagnosis. †Presence of the FLPL1/PDGFRA (F/P) mutation. *** Clonality analysis based on the digestion of genomic DNA with methylation-sensitive restriction enzymes followed by PCR amplification of the CAG repeat at the human androgen receptor gene (HUMARA) locus at the X chromosome. CSS, Churg-Strauss Syndrome; EGID, eosinophil gastrointestinal diseases; FISH, fluorescence *in situ* hybridization.
From Klion AD et al. Approaches to the treatment of hypereosinophilic syndromes: A workshop summary report. J Allergy Clin Immunol 2006; 117: 1294, with permission from the American Academy of Allergy, Asthma and Immunology.

may accompany angioimmunoblastic lymphadenopathy, mycosis fungoides, Sézary syndrome and lymphomatoid papulosis. Eosinophilia occurs in about 20% of patients with systemic mastocytosis and may be the presenting finding in the absence of cutaneous manifestations.

Organ system involvement and eosinophilia

Eosinophilic syndromes limited to specific organs, such as eosinophilic pneumonias or eosinophilic gastroenteritides (EGID) (Chapter 44), characteristically do not extend beyond their own target organ, and hence lack the multiplicity of organ involvement often found with nonorgan-specific hypereosinophilic syndromes. They also do not have the predilection to develop secondary eosinophil-mediated cardiac damage, for reasons that are not known.

Pulmonary eosinophilias

Blood eosinophilia can infrequently accompany pleural fluid eosinophilia, which is a nonspecific response seen with various disorders, including trauma and repeated thoracenteses. In addition, several pulmonary parenchymal disorders may be associated with eosinophilia (Table 23.2).

Helminth parasites are responsible for four forms of eosinophilic lung disease.[21] The first of these is Loeffler's syndrome, which is marked by blood eosinophilia, eosinophilic patchy pulmonary infiltrates that appear and resolve over weeks and, at times, bronchospasm. This syndrome is typically caused by those helminth parasites (*Ascaris lumbricoides*, and less commonly hookworm and *Strongyloides*) that migrate through the lungs early in their developmental lifecycle.[21] Stool examinations are not helpful, as the pulmonary response is elicited by infecting larval forms months before productive egg-laying from later adult stages begins in the intestines. In some cases, such as suspected strongyloidiasis, serology may be helpful in the early stage of disease. Diagnosis is made on epidemiologic grounds.[21]

The second form of helminth-induced lung disease is the syndrome of tropical pulmonary eosinophilia, which develops in a minority of patients infected with lymphatic-dwelling filarial species.[21] This syndrome is characterized by marked blood eosinophilia, a paroxysmal nonproductive cough, wheezing, and occasional weight loss, lymphadenopathy and low-grade fevers. On chest X-rays increased bronchovesicular markings, diffuse interstitial lesions 1–3 mm in diameter or mottled opacities, usually more prominent in lower lung fields, are common. Patients have markedly increased numbers of blood and alveolar eosinophils, and elevations in both total serum IgE and anti-filarial antibodies.

A third form of helminth-induced lung disease is caused by helminths that invade the pulmonary parenchyma, notably lung flukes that cause paragonimiasis. The fourth form of lung disease is caused by larger than usual numbers of helminth organisms that are carried hematogenously into the lungs. Examples include schistosomiasis, trichinellosis, and larva migrans.

Bronchopulmonary aspergillosis constitutes another type of eosinophil-associated pulmonary disease. Two forms of idiopathic eosinophilic pneumonia are recognized. In chronic eosinophilic pneumonia patients may exhibit peripheral pulmonary infiltrates that may extend across lobar fissures. Uncommonly, chronic eosinophilic pneumonia is antecedent to Churg–Strauss syndrome vasculitis. Blood eosinophilia is present in most patients, but not all. Chronic eosinophilic pneumonia is of unknown etiology and is responsive to corticosteroids, but prone to relapse. An acute form of eosinophilic pneumonia, manifest by fever, pulmonary infiltrates and respiratory insufficiency, is diagnosable by finding eosinophils in bronchoalveolar lavage fluids or on lung biopsy. Acute eosinophilic pneumonia, which often follows new exposures to smoke or dusts, responds to corticosteroid treatment and does not relapse.

The major vasculitis associated with eosinophilia is the Churg–Strauss syndrome (Chapter 58). Late-onset asthma, eosinophilia, and at times transient pulmonary infiltrates, antedate the development of systemic vasculitis in about half of cases. Pulmonary involvement is seen in almost all patients, and pulmonary infiltrates occur in three-quarters. Nasal and sinus involvement is common. Corticosteroids, anti-IgE monoclonal antibody or anti-cysteinyl leukotriene agent therapies for asthma may mask the evolution of Churg–Strauss syndrome. Neurologic, cutaneous, cardiac and gastrointestinal organ involvement is common (Chapter 57).[31] Cardiac involvement includes pericarditis and small vessel cardiac vasculitis, and much less commonly endomyocardial thrombosis and fibrosis.

Diverse medications and other drugs are capable of eliciting pulmonary eosinophilia. More commonly implicated medications include nonsteroidal anti-inflammatory drugs (NSAIDs) and antimicrobial medications. Likewise, toxic agents, including from occupational exposure, can be responsible for pulmonary eosinophilia. Each of these reactions has a defined etiologic stimulus and hence differs from idiopathic and other eosinophilic diseases, but the clinical presentation of drug- and toxin-elicited pulmonary eosinophilias can resemble other forms of pulmonary eosinophilia, including acute or chronic eosinophilic pneumonia.

Skin and subcutaneous diseases

A number of cutaneous diseases can be associated with heightened blood eosinophils, including atopic dermatitis, blistering disorders including bullous pemphigoid, drug reactions, and two diseases associated with pregnancy, herpes gestationis and the syndrome of pruritic urticarial papules and plaques of pregnancy. Eosinophilic pustular folliculitis is seen mostly in patients with HIV infections and in those treated for hematologic malignancies or after bone marrow transplantation. For patients with cutaneous involvement and eosinophilia, angiolymphoid hyperplasia with eosinophilia and Kimura's disease, eosinophilic cellulitis (Wells syndrome), eosinophilic fasciitis, and eosinophilic pustular folliculitis can be differentiated based on the histopathology of biopsied lesions. Another syndrome, episodic angioedema with eosinophilia, is characterized by recurring episodes of angioedema, urticaria, fever, and marked blood eosinophilia. This syndrome responds to glucocorticosteroid therapy.

Gastrointestinal diseases

The eosinophilic gastrointestinal disorders (EGIDs), including eosinophilic esophagitis, eosinophilic gastroenteritis and eosinophilic colitis, represent a heterogeneous collection of disorders in which there may be eosinophilic infiltration of the mucosa, the muscle layer or the serosa, the last of which can lead to eosinophilic ascites (Chapter 44).[32,33] Peripheral blood eosinophilia may occur in the EGIDs, although with eosinophilic esophagitis, peripheral blood eosinophil counts are often normal. Eosinophils are present in the lesions of collagenous colitis and ulcerative colitis, but blood eosinophilia is usually absent. Gastrointestinal eosinophilia elicited by intestinal helminths and eosinophilic enterocolitis due to hypersensitivity reactions to medications must be excluded in patients with these diseases who have tissue eosinophilia.

Rheumatologic disorders

Of the various forms of vasculitis, only two are commonly associated with eosinophilia. The principal eosinophil-related vasculitis is the Churg–Strauss syndrome (as discussed above; and in Chapter 57). Cutaneous necrotizing eosinophilic vasculitis with hypocomplementemia and eosinophilia is a distinct vasculitis of small dermal vessels that are extensively infiltrated with eosinophils. This form of vasculitis may occur in patients with connective tissue diseases. In addition, eosinophilia may uncommonly accompany rheumatoid arthritis itself, but is more commonly due to adverse reactions to treatment medications (including NSAIDs, gold and tetracyclines) or due to concomitant vasculitis. An uncommon disorder, characterized by the association of *n*odules, *e*osinophilia, *r*heumatism, *d*ermatitis, and *s*welling (NERDS), includes prominent para-articular nodules, recurrent urticaria with angioedema, and tissue and blood eosinophilia.

Immunologic disorders

Adverse reactions to medications are a common cause of eosinophilia (Chapter 46 and Clinical Pearls box on page 11). Although often considered as hypersensitivity reactions, in most instances of drug-associated eosinophilia the mechanism leading to eosinophilia is not understood. Eosinophilia may develop without other manifestations of adverse drug reactions, such as rashes or drug fevers. In addition, drug-induced eosinophilia may be associated with distinct clinicopathologic patterns in which eosinophilia accompanies drug-induced diseases that are characteristically limited to specific organs with or without associated blood eosinophilia. When organ dysfunction develops, cessation of drug administration is necessary. Drug-induced interstitial nephritis may be accompanied by blood eosinophilia, and eosinophils may be detectable in urine.[34] Unlike G-CSF therapy, therapy with GM-CSF can lead to prominent blood and tissue eosinophilia. Administration of IL-2 or of IL-2-stimulated lymphocytes can be followed by the development of eosinophilia, most likely due to stimulated production of IL-5. Reactions to medications, often anticonvulsants, minocycline and allopurinol, can elicit DRESS, *d*rug *r*eaction with *e*osinophilia and *s*ystemic *s*ymptoms.[35] In addition to cutaneous eruptions, fever, lymphadenopathy, hepatitis, nephritis, atypical lymphocytosis, GI tract involvement, eosinophilia are common but variable elements of this drug-induced syndrome, which can be fatal. The triggering medication must be stopped, and corticosteroids are often administered.

Some primary immunodeficiency syndromes are associated with eosinophilia. The hyper-IgE syndrome is characterized by recurrent staphylococcal abscesses of the skin, lungs and other sites, pruritic dermatitis, hyperimmunoglobulinemia E, and eosinophilia of the blood, sputum and tissues. Eosinophilia is characteristic of Omenn's syndrome, combined immunodeficiency with hypereosinophilia (Chapter 35).

Infiltration of eosinophils accompanies rejection of lung, kidney, and liver allografts. Tissue and blood eosinophilia occur early in the rejection process, and eosinophil counts and eosinophil granule protein levels (in urine, bronchoalveolar lavage fluids, and involved allograft tissues) have correlated with prognosis, severity, and response to rejection therapy.

CLINICAL PEARLS

Eosinophilia and drug reactions

Drug reactions	Examples
Interstitial nephritis	Semisynthetic penicillins, cephalosporins
Pulmonary infiltrates	Nitrofurantoin, sulfas, NSAIDs
Pleuropulmonary	Dantrolene
Hepatitis	Semisynthetic penicillins, tetracyclines
Hypersensitivity vasculitis	Allopurinol, phenytoin
Asthma, nasal polyps	Aspirin
Eosinophilia–myalgia	L-Tryptophan contaminant syndrome
Asymptomatic	Ampicillin, penicillins, cephalosporins
Cytokine-mediated	GM-CSF, IL-2
DRESS (drug reaction with eosinophilia and systemic symptoms)	Minocycline, allopurinol, anticonvulsants

Adapted from Weller PF. Eosinophilia and eosinophil-related disorders. In: Adkinson NF Jr, Yuninger JW, Busse WW, et al, eds. Allergy: principles and practice, 6th edn. Philadelphia: Mosby, 2003; p. 1105.

Endocrine diseases

The loss of endogenous adrenoglucocorticosteroid production in Addison's disease, adrenal hemorrhage or hypopituitarism can cause increased blood eosinophilia, although usually not more than mild to moderate.

Other causes of eosinophilia

The syndrome of atheromatous cholesterol embolization is at times associated with hypocomplementemia, eosinophilia, and eosinophiluria. Uncommonly, kindreds with hereditary eosinophilia have been recognized. Irritation of serosal surfaces can be associated with eosinophilia, and related diseases can include Dressler's syndrome; eosinophilic pleural effusions; peritoneal, and at times blood, eosinophilia developing during chronic peritoneal dialysis; and perhaps the eosinophilia that follows abdominal irradiation.

Evaluation of eosinophilia

Because a diversity of disorders may be accompanied by eosinophilia, evaluation of the patient with eosinophilia requires a consideration of features based on the patient's history, physical examination, and other laboratory, radiographic or diagnostic testing.[28,36] An initial approach can focus on identifying eosinophilic diseases that have a defined treatable etiology. These include infections with helminth parasites, and for these the approach should be guided by information obtained from the history regarding potential exposures; from the history and physical examinations regarding signs and symptoms of any clinically apparent associated illness; from standard biochemical and radiographic testing for evidence of organ involvement; and from specific parasitologic tests, including potentially stool, urine, blood, sputum, or tissue examinations, as well as serologic tests.[21] The duration and magnitude of the eosinophilia may help suggest some entities, especially if it is prolonged or markedly elevated (Table 23.1). Other causes of eosinophilia that are amenable to treatment include eosinophilia secondary to medications, for which cessation of the offending drug may be indicated if the eosinophilia is accompanied by organ damage. Likewise, if eosinophilia is secondary to glucocorticosteroid deficiency, diagnostic testing can corroborate this deficiency and lead to the administration of replacement corticosteroids and consequent resolution of the eosinophilia.

Because allergic diseases usually are associated with at least some degree of eosinophilia, clinical and laboratory evidence of such disease should be sought. If the eosinophilia is not attributable to allergic diseases, parasitic infections, medications or steroid deficiency, further evaluation will be guided by whether the patient has evidence of organ disease and, if so, which organs are involved (Table 23.2). This is germane, for instance, in defining whether the patient has a distinct eosinophilic pulmonary, gastrointestinal, or cutaneous syndrome. Bone marrow examinations in most patients with eosinophilia are not usually informative, revealing only evidence of enhanced eosinophilopoiesis; but marrow should be examined if there is concern for a hematologic malignancy or myeloproliferative disorder. For patients with sustained eosinophilia who meet the criteria for HES, diagnostic testing should aim to identify which variant form of HES the patient may have, in which case, bone marrow examination is often needed (Fig. 23.4).

THERAPEUTIC PRINCIPLES

Therapy of specific eosinophilic diseases

Eosinophil-associated diseases with identifiable etiologies

Parasitic infections	Treat causative parasite
Drug-reaction related eosinophilias	Terminate eliciting medication
Adrenal insufficiency	Corticosteroid replacement therapy
Allergic/atopic diseases	Varied, may include topical or inhaled corticosteroids

Distinct eosinophilic syndromes involving specific organs

Eosinophilic pulmonary diseases:

Acute eosinophilic pneumonia	Corticosteroids
Chronic eosinophilic pneumonia	Corticosteroids, interferon-α
Churg–Strauss vasculitis	Corticosteroids, interferon-α

Hypereosinophilic syndromes

F/P-positive myeloproliferative	Imatinib
Lymphoproliferative and other	Corticosteroids, interferon-α, hydroxyurea, anti-IL-5 monoclonal antibody, other

References

1. Blanchard C, Rothenberg ME. Biology of the eosinophil. Adv Immunol 2009;101:81–121.
2. Akuthota P, Xenakis JJ, Weller PF. Eosinophils: offenders or general bystanders in allergic airway disease and pulmonary immunity? J Innate Immun 2011;3:113–9.
3. Spencer LA, Weller PF. Eosinophils and Th2 immunity: contemporary insights. Immunol Cell Biol 2010;88:250–6.
4. Shamri R, Xenakis JJ, Spencer LA. Eosinophils in innate immunity: an evolving story. Cell Tissue Res 2011;343:57–83.
5. Gonlugur U, Efeoglu T. Vascular adhesion and transendothelial migration of eosinophil leukocytes. Cell Tissue Res 2004;318:473–82.
6. Bochner BS. Siglec-8 on human eosinophils and mast cells, and Siglec-F on murine eosinophils, are functionally related inhibitory receptors. Clin Exp Allergy 2009;39:317–24.
7. Bozza PT, Magalhaes KG, Weller PF. Leukocyte lipid bodies—biogenesis and functions in inflammation. Biochim Biophys Acta 2009;1791:540–51.
8. Hogan SP, Rosenberg HF, Moqbel R, et al. Eosinophils: biological properties and role in health and disease. Clin Exp Allergy 2008;38:709–50.
9. Spencer LA, Szela CT, Perez SA, et al. Human eosinophils constitutively express multiple Th1, Th2, and immunoregulatory cytokines that are secreted rapidly and differentially. J Leukoc Biol 2009;85:117–23.
10. Melo RC, Weller PF. Piecemeal degranulation in human eosinophils: a distinct secretion mechanism underlying inflammatory responses. Histol Histopathol 2010;25:1341–54.
11. Spencer LA, Melo RCN, Perez SAC, et al. Cytokine receptor-mediated trafficking of preformed IL-4 in eosinophils identifies an innate immune mechanism of cytokine secretion. Proc Natl Acad Sci U S A 2006;103:3333–8.
12. Neves JS, Perez SA, Spencer LA, et al. Eosinophil granules function extracellularly as receptor-mediated secretory organelles. Proc Natl Acad Sci U S A 2008;105:18478–83.
13. Neves JS, Weller PF. Functional extracellular eosinophil granules: novel implications in eosinophil immunobiology. Curr Opin Immunol 2009;21:694–9.
14. Yousefi S, Gold JA, Andina N, et al. Catapult-like release of mitochondrial DNA by eosinophils contributes to antibacterial defense. Nat Med 2008;14:949–53.
15. Klion AD, Nutman TB. The role of eosinophils in host defense against helminth parasites. J Allergy Clin Immunol 2004;113:30–7.
16. Swartz JM, Dyer KD, Cheever AW, et al. Schistosoma mansoni infection in eosinophil lineage-ablated mice. Blood 2006;108:2420–7.
17. Padigel UM, Hess JA, Lee JJ, et al. Eosinophils act as antigen presenting cells to induce immunity to Strongyloides stercoralis in mice. J Infect Dis 2007;196:1844–51.
18. Fabre V, Beiting DP, Bliss SK, et al. Eosinophil deficiency compromises parasite survival in chronic nematode infection. J Immunol 2009;182:1577–83.
19. Akuthota P, Wang HB, Spencer LA, et al. Immunoregulatory roles of eosinophils: a new look at a familiar cell. Clin Exp Allergy 2008;38:1254–63.
20. Wang HB, Ghiran I, Matthaei K, et al. Airway eosinophils: allergic inflammation recruited professional antigen-presenting cells. J Immunol 2007;179:7585–92.
21. Wilson ME, Weller PF. Eosinophilia. In: Guerrant RL, Walker DH, Weller PF, editors. Tropical Infectious Diseases: Principles, Pathogens and Practice. 3rd ed. Philadelphia: Elsevier; 2011. p. 939–49.
22. Klion AD, Bochner BS, Gleich GJ, et al. Approaches to the treatment of hypereosinophilic syndromes: a workshop summary report. J Allergy Clin Immunol 2006;117:1292–302.
23. Simon HU, Rothenberg ME, Bochner BS, et al. Refining the definition of hypereosinophilic syndrome. J Allergy Clin Immunol 2010;126:45–9.
24. Baccarani M, Cilloni D, Rondoni M, et al. The efficacy of imatinib mesylate in patients with FIP1L1-PDGFRalpha-positive hypereosinophilic syndrome. Results of a multicenter prospective study. Haematologica 2007;92:1173–9.
25. Ogbogu PU, Bochner BS, Butterfield JH, et al. Hypereosinophilic syndrome: a multicenter, retrospective analysis of clinical characteristics and response to therapy. J Allergy Clin Immunol 2009;124:1319–25.
26. Eling T, Tainer B, Ally A, et al. Separation of arachidonic acid metabolites by high-pressure liquid chromatography. Methods Enzymol 1982;86:511–7.
27. Roufosse F, Cogan E, Goldman M. Lymphocytic variant hypereosinophilic syndromes. Immunol Allergy Clin North Am 2007;27:389–413.
28. Roufosse F. Hypereosinophilic syndrome variants: diagnostic and therapeutic considerations. Haematologica 2009;94:1188–93.
29. Rothenberg ME, Klion AD, Roufosse FE, et al. Treatment of patients with the hypereosinophilic syndrome with mepolizumab. N Engl J Med 2008;358:1215–28.
30. Bain BJ, Fletcher SH. Chronic eosinophilic leukemias and the myeloproliferative variant of the hypereosinophilic syndrome. Immunol Allergy Clin North Am 2007;27:377–88.
31. Pagnoux C, Guilpain P, Guillevin L. Churg-Strauss syndrome. Curr Opin Rheumatol 2007;19:25–32.
32. Straumann A. Idiopathic eosinophilic gastrointestinal diseases in adults. Best Pract Res Clin Gastroenterol 2008;22:481–96.
33. DeBrosse CW, Rothenberg ME. Allergy and eosinophil-associated gastrointestinal disorders (EGID). Curr Opin Immunol 2008;20:703–8.
34. Wang YC, Lin YF, Chao TK, et al. Acute interstitial nephritis with prominent eosinophil infiltration. Clin Nephrol 2009;71:187–91.
35. Ben m'rad M, Leclerc-Mercier S, Blanche P, et al. Drug-induced hypersensitivity syndrome: clinical and biologic disease patterns in 24 patients. Medicine (Baltimore) 2009;88:131–40.
36. Klion A. Hypereosinophilic syndrome: current approach to diagnosis and treatment. Annu Rev Med 2009;60:293–306.

PART THREE
Host defenses to infectious agents

24.

Host defenses to extracellular bacteria

David S. Stephens, William M. Shafer

The human host has evolved protective mechanisms to deal with the multitude of bacterial species encountered in nature. These host defenses include nonspecific mechanisms of clearance, and innate as well as specific adaptive immune responses. Partly because of these mechanisms, the vast majority of bacterial species (e.g., ~10 000 different species of bacteria per gram of soil) do not cause human disease. A smaller number of bacterial species (~10^3) have established symbiotic or commensal relationships with the human host and colonize skin and mucosal surfaces.[1] These commensals are generally of low virulence except in individuals whose host defenses are compromised. A few (~10^2) pathogenic bacterial species or subpopulations of those species have evolved virulence factors or strategies that can overcome or circumvent human host defense mechanisms and cause local or invasive clinical disease. In fact, defects in host defenses are often suggested by the infecting bacteria (Table 24.1). Many of these bacterial pathogens reside mostly extracellularly. Examples are pathogens such as *Neisseria meningitidis*, *Neisseria gonorrhoeae*, *Haemophilus influenzae*, group A streptococci, *Bordetella pertussis*, and *Streptococcus pneumoniae*, which are transmitted from one individual to another by close contact. Other "extracellular" bacterial pathogens, such as *Vibrio cholerae*, *Shigella dysenteriae*, enteropathogenic *Escherichia coli*, *Bacillus anthracis*, and *Clostridium tetani*, are acquired through food, water, animal, or other environmental contact. *Staphylococcus aureus* is an important extracellular pathogen for humans and can be acquired from other humans, animals, or through environmental contacts.

"Extracellular" bacterial pathogens usually produce acute inflammatory and purulent infectious diseases such as meningitis, septicemia, pneumonia, urethritis, pharyngitis, inflammatory diarrhea, cellulitis, and abscesses, and/or produce disease by the release of toxins. Disease associated with some extracellular bacteria (e.g., *Helicobacter pylori*) results from chronic colonization. Susceptibility to extracellular bacterial pathogens is enhanced by hereditary, acquired or age-related defects in epithelial, humoral, and phagocytic host defenses. Enhanced resistance to extracellular bacterial pathogens or their toxins can be accentuated by chemoprophylaxis, by vaccines, and by other immune modulation processes (e.g., passive immune globulin administration). Caution is urged in the interpretation of the term "extracellular," as some of these pathogenic bacterial species invade host cells as a part of their normal lifecycle and during steps in the disease process.

Host defenses and immune responses at epithelial surfaces

Clearance and nonspecific host defenses at epithelial surfaces

Intact skin and mucosal surfaces provide a formidable barrier to most bacterial species.[2] Damage to epithelial barriers by trauma, co-infections, drugs such as those used in chemotherapy, environmental factors such as smoking, allergies or low humidity, catheterization and intubation circumvent these barriers and allow bacteria access to subcutaneous tissues, blood vessels, and other normally sterile sites (Table 24.2). Skin is a relatively dry, acidic (pH 5–6) barrier that contains growth-inhibiting fatty acids and antimicrobial peptides (see below),[2] characteristics that are detrimental to many bacteria. The stratified desquamatory epithelial surface of the skin also helps in the removal of micro-organisms. Repeated trauma to skin (e.g., dialysis and IV drug use) enhances skin colonization with pathogens such as *S. aureus*.

Mucosal surfaces have additional nonspecific antibacterial defenses. Lysozyme is found in most mucosal secretions and lyzes bacterial cell walls by splitting muramic acid β(1–4)-N-acetyl-glucosamine linkages. The mucociliary blanket of the respiratory tract (Fig. 24.1) and the female urogenital tract (fallopian tube) moves bacteria away from epithelial surfaces, as does the flushing of the urinary tract with urine and the bathing of the conjunctiva with tears. Phospholipase A2, particularly in tears, has

Table 24.1 Host defense defects suggested by infecting bacteria

Bacteria	Defective system
Staphylococci, aerobic Gram-negative bacilli	Skin and mucous membrane barriers, phagocyte dysfunction
Haemophilus influenzae, pneumococci	Antibody, mucous membrane barriers
Neisseria meningitidis and *Neisseria gonorrhoeae*	Complement pathways, antibody
Mycobacterium, Salmonella	Cell-mediated immunity

Table 24.2 Bacterial infections associated with impaired skin and mucous membrane barriers

Compromised physical barriers
Cystic fibrosis (mucoid *P. aeruginosa*)
Immotile cilia syndromes (recurrent sinopulmonary infections with pyogenic bacteria)
Tracheostomy and tracheal intubation (aerobic Gram-negative bacteria)
Urinary tract obstructive lesions and bladder catheters (Gram-negative bacilli)
IV catheters, other mucosal disruption (tumor, ulceration, etc.) (*S. aureus* and Gram-negative bacilli, mixed aerobic and anaerobic infections in diabetics)
Surgical procedures and skin trauma (*S. aureus*)
Burns (aerobic Gram-negative bacilli, *S. aureus*)
Smoking (*H. influenzae*, pneumococci, meningococci)
Achlorhydria (*Salmonella*, tuberculosis)
Slowing peristalsis with opium alkaloids (prolongs symptomatic shigellosis)

Alteration of normal flora
Antibiotics: *Candida* overgrowth, *C. difficile* colitis
Alcoholism: *Klebsiella* pharyngeal colonization, tuberculosis
Severe illness: colonization of oropharynx by Gram-negative bacilli and nosocomial pneumonias
Alteration of the normal microbial flora by antibiotics, alcoholism, and severe illness may lead to colonization or production of disease by extracellular bacteria. For example, colonization of the respiratory tract with aerobic Gram-negative bacilli may follow treatment with broad-spectrum antibiotics that eradicate the normal upper respiratory tract flora. Serious Gram-negative bacilli pneumonia may occur, especially if other host abnormalities are also present

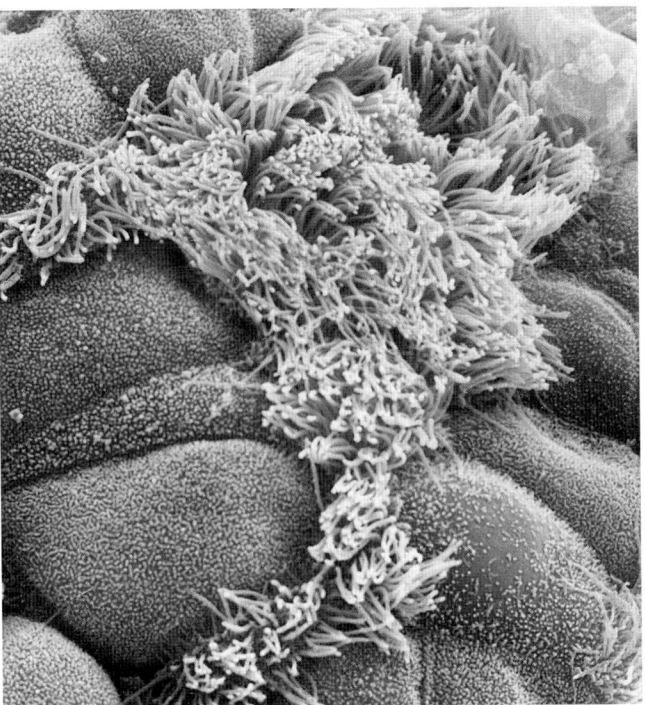

Fig. 24.1 Mucociliary host defense. Scanning electron micrograph of human upper respiratory mucosa showing the ciliated and nonciliated epithelial surface (×16000).[27]

Table 24.3 Immune microbial pattern recognition molecules

Toll-like receptors (TLR)
NOD, Caterpillar proteins, PGRPs
RNA helicases/PkR
Complement proteins: C1q, C1 inhibitor
Antimicrobial peptides
Collectins and surfactants
C- and S-lectins: mannose-binding lectin, L-ficolin

received attention as an antibacterial agent. The acid pH of the stomach, intestinal peristalsis, and the antibacterial effect of proteolytic enzymes present in intestinal secretions are important gastrointestinal tract host defenses against bacteria.

The normal flora of the skin, upper respiratory and gastrointestinal tracts, and the genital tract of females is also a major barrier to colonization by newly acquired pathogens.[1,3] Altering normal flora or protective barriers, for example by creating pharmacologic or surgical gastric achlorhydria or by the use of broad-spectrum antibiotics, can lead to the acquisition and overgrowth of pathogenic bacteria such as *Salmonella typhimurium*, *Clostridium difficile*, or antibiotic-resistant Gram-negative bacilli. Normal flora also facilitate a high level of priming of the immune system by maintaining high levels of MHC class II molecule expression on macrophages and other antigen-presenting cells.[2]

Bacterial attachment and colonization of mucosal surfaces can be inhibited by bacterial binding to human cellular antigens present in secretions, such as ABO blood group antigens. Cell adhesion and extracellular matrix molecules such as fibronectin and proteoglycans can also inhibit or enhance bacterial binding to epithelial surfaces. The Tamm–Horsfall glycoprotein, found in urine, can bind avidly to a variety of bacteria and facilitate clearance. Proteins such as lactoferrin (LF), present at mucosal surfaces, bind iron, an important requirement for bacterial growth. This action may reduce microbial proliferation, but some mucosal pathogens bind LF and remove iron for growth.

Innate and acquired immune defenses at mucosal surfaces

Immune pattern recognition molecules (Table 24.3) are a major arm of the innate immune system and are released or expressed by a range of host cells, including lymphocytes, macrophages or tissue histiocytes, dendritic cells, polymorphonuclear leukocytes (PMNs), and epithelial cells (Chapter 3). These cells also protect mucosal surfaces from microbial invasion. In acquired immunity, mucosal immunoglobulins are a major protection against extracellular bacteria.

Pattern recognition molecules

The discovery and characterization of specific pattern recognition molecules has revolutionized our understanding of the initial specific events occurring between microbes and human cells. The identification and function of these molecules is rapidly expanding and include Toll-like receptors, NOD and caterpillar proteins, RNA helicases, complement proteins, antimicrobial peptides, collectin and surfactants, C- and S-lectins such as mannose-binding lectin and L-ficolin.[4–7] A family of major importance are the Toll-like receptors[4–7] (TLR1–10) (Table 24.4) found on macrophages, neutrophils, and other host cells. These receptors recognize a variety of microbial ligands or pathogen-associated molecular patterns (PAMPs), including lipoproteins, LPS, flagellin, and nucleic acids produced by Gram-negative and/or -positive bacteria. Alterations (polymorphisms) in TLRs (e.g., TLR4) and other pattern recognition molecules is associated with susceptibility or severity of specific infections (e.g., sepsis).[6] TLR expression can be regulated by type I interferons and by microRNAs (miRNAs) and the dysregulation of TLRs can be involved in acute and chronic inflammatory diseases and cancer.[7]

Table 24.4 Human Toll-like receptors and microbial ligands

TLR1-lipopeptide PAMPs (pathogen-associated molecular patterns)
TLR2-lipopeptiode PAMPs
TLR3-dsRNA
TLR4-LPS
TLR5-flagellin
TLR6-lipopeptide PAMPs
TLR7-nucleic acid PAMPs
TLR8-nucleic acid PAMPs
TLR9-nucleic acid PAMPs, CpG DNA
TLR10-lipopeptide PAMPs

Dendritic cells

Discovered in the early 1970s by Steinman and Cohen,[8] dendritic cells (DCs) are now recognized as important and potent antigen-processing and -presenting cells that are crucial for the induction of T- and B-cell responses (Chapter 6). They present peptides and proteins to both T and B cells. DCs have been thought of as the pacemaker of the immune response[9] and are widely distributed in tissues, especially those that interface with the environment. They are a heterogeneous group of antigen-processing cells that arise from three pathways that are lymphoid or myeloid related in their origin. They employ pattern recognition receptors (e.g., TLRs) to detect pathogens (viruses and bacteria) in their environment. In most tissues, DCs are at low levels and are immature, but upon activation they take up and process antigen. DC activation has a number of important consequences in immunity, including activation of naïve T cells. DCs are an important source of IL-23, which can activate macrophages and Th17 CD4 T cells, and as a consequence, DCs perform a key role in host defense against viral, fungal, and bacterial pathogens. The recently described but rare condition of monocytopenia with B and NK lymphoid deficiency also includes a significant reduction in DCs and is associated with disseminated nontuberculosis mycobacterial infection as well as papilloma virus infection.[10] Skin contains a major supply of tissue DCs (Langerhans' cells) and their involvement in combating skin and soft tissue infection must be considered along with their function and contribution to stimulating immunity during vaccination. Limited information is available regarding their role in host resistance to extracellular bacteria, but studies have been performed that examine the interaction of bacteria with DCs. For instance, Unkmeir et al.[11] studied the interaction of serogroup B meningococci with DCs. Infection of DCs by meningococci resulted in a significant and rapid production of pro-inflammatory cytokines and chemokines, including TNF-α, IL-6, and IL-8 through a lipo-oligosaccharide (LOS)-dependent mechanism.

Lymphocytes

Mucosa-associated lymphocyte tissue (MALT) is comprised of intraepithelial lymphocytes (IELs), lamina propria lymphocytes and lymphoid follicles (e.g., Peyer's patches), and is sometimes divided into the gut-associated (GALT), bronchial-associated (respiratory tract) (BALT), and genitourinary tract lymphoid tissues (Chapter 19).[12] These cells are important for homeostatic regulation and the maintenance of immune response against microbes at mucosal surfaces, including "extracellular" bacteria. One in five cells in the intestinal epithelium is a lymphocyte. These cells express pattern recognition receptors (e.g., TLRs), have constitutive cytotoxic activity, secrete chemokines and cytokines important in regulation and host defense, and act in concert with mucosal epithelial cells and exocrine glands. For example, depression of IEL response (e.g., the production of IL-2/IFN-γ), is observed in experimental sepsis and following IEL exposure to lysates of enteropathogenic *E. coli* and other intestinal pathogens. *H. pylori*-associated gastritis is characterized by cytokine release and increased IEL infiltration, and can result in gastric MALT lymphomas. Eradication of *H. pylori* causes a reduction in IEL infiltrates.

Macrophages

Phagocytic cells, macrophages and PMNs are also present at mucosal surfaces (Fig. 24.2). These cells express pattern recognition receptors and migrate to mucosal surfaces by chemotaxis and diapedesis between epithelial cells. Macrophages are also encountered after crossing the epithelial barrier. Specialized epithelial M cells of mucosal surfaces are key sites for antigen sampling, including viruses, and bacteria and macrophages surround these sites.[13] However, enteroinvasive pathogens such as *Shigella* can resist macrophages. *Shigella* induce macrophage apoptotic death by direct interaction of the bacterial protein IpaB with interleukin-1β-converting enzyme. Viral co-infections may prime macrophages for LPS-induced apoptosis.[14]

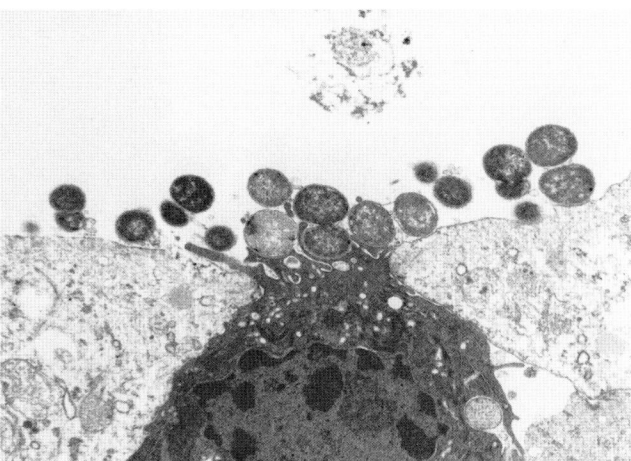

Fig. 24.2 Bacterial phagocytosis at mucosal surfaces. Transmission electron micrograph of phagocyte engulfing *N. meningitidis* at a human respiratory epithelial mucosal surface (×19 000).[27]

Polymorphonuclear leukocytes

In areas of epithelial inflammation, polymorphonuclear leuko-cytes (PMNs) or neutrophils can be recruited to mucosal and skin surfaces. PMNs are more effective in the presence of specific immune defenses, such as antibody and complement components. PMNs express pattern recognition receptors and have both oxygen-dependent and -independent mechanisms of killing (Chapter 21). Extracellular bacteria typically evade these bactericidal processes by resisting phagocytosis (Fig. 24.3). Resistance to phagocytosis can be due to the action of carbohydrate capsules, which impede the engulfment of phagocyte-associated bacteria. Other microbial surface structures, such as the pili of the gono-coccus, can "stiff-arm" neutrophils, keeping them at a distance.[15] A number of pyogenic bacteria (e.g., *S. aureus*) secrete leukoci-dins, which lyse phagocytes. Other pathogens (e.g., group A streptococci) inhibit chemotaxis of neutrophils through the elaboration of enzymes (e.g., C5a peptidase) that proteolytically cleave chemotactic signals. Regardless of the mechanism by which bacteria resist phagocytes, opsonic antibody can often overcome these forces and promote killing. The importance of PMNs in host defense against extracellular pathogens can best be highlighted by the increased frequency of bacteremias and other life-threatening infections in neutropenic patients or those individuals with neutrophil deficits (e.g., chronic granulomatous disease, Chediak–Higashi syndrome or specific granule deficiency, to name but a few) (Chapter 21).

Antimicrobial peptides (AMPS) and antimicrobial proteins

Extracellular pathogens are likely to be confronted with both myeloid-derived AMPs (e.g., the α-defensins stored within neutrophil granules) and nonmyeloid antibacterial peptides and proteins.[16] AMPs, which are typically cationic, amphipathic molecules, represent an integral part of the innate host defense system for humans and other vertebrates, invertebrates and plants.[17] Many of these AMPs from evolutionary diverse sources share structural similarities, suggesting their importance in host defense throughout evolution. In general terms, these AMPs (often effective at micromolar concentrations *in vitro*) can either be constitutively synthesized (e.g., the α-defensins of neutrophils) or their production can be induced in a variety of epithelial cells (e.g., Paneth cells of the small intestine) by a variety of stimuli, including infection. Cationic and anionic dermicidin-derived AMPs are produced by eccrine sweat glands and have antibacterial action against pathogens that cause skin and soft tissue infections. Humans produce two main classes of AMPs: defensins[16] and cathelicidins. Defensins (3–4 kDa) are cysteine-rich peptides with intramolecular disulphide bonds and are classified as α- and β-defensins. α-Defensins are major components of neutrophil granules capable of reaching mg/mL concentrations in phagolysosomes and small intestinal Paneth cells. β-Defensins are produced by a large variety of epithelial cells, mucosal surfaces, skin, and organs. The circular θ-defensins of rhesus macaques are produced by a unique ligation reaction of two peptides, but owing to a premature stop mutation are not produced by humans; θ-defensins can have potent antiviral effects. Unlike many other vertebrates, humans produce only one cathelicidin, designated LL-37, which is synthesized by both PMNs and epithelial cells. The "cathelin" domain of the precursor protein resembles inhibitors of cysteine proteases and is removed by proteolytic cleavage to liberate the LL-37 AMP, an α-helical, linear peptide of 37 amino acids. Larger neutrophil proteins[15] derived from granules can have direct antibacterial and anti-endotoxin activities and these include bactericidal permeability-increasing protein (BPI), cathepsin G, azurocidin, and lysozyme. BPI is a tenacious binder of lipopoly-saccharide (LPS) and has functional as well as structural characteristics similar to LPS-binding protein (LBP), which is critically involved in delivering lipopolysaccharides to host cells (see below).

AMPs probably exert their lethal effect at the bacterial inner membrane, causing rapid depolarization and loss of membrane potential,[17] although some evidence exists that certain peptides have cytosolic targets. Bacteria have evolved multiple ways of circumventing or expressing decreased susceptibility to AMPs.[17] Bacteria can avoid AMPs to some extent by reducing the electro-negativity of their microbial cell surface, which reduces electrostatic interactions with cationic regions of the peptide. Bacterial surface modifications that impede AMP binding due to masking or reduction of negatively charged groups include the presence of capsule, decoration of lipid A by modification of phosphates with 4' phosphoethanolamine or 4'-amino-arabinose, the presence of phosphorylcholine attached to oligosaccharides of LPS, and, in Gram-positive pathogens, incorporation of D-alanine to teichoic acid. Other mechanisms used by bacteria to subvert the lethal action of AMPs include energy-dependent efflux to the extracellular fluid, transporter-dependent influx to the bacterial cytosol where they are degraded by proteases, extracellular proteolytic degradation, L-lysinylation of membrane phosphotidylglycerol, production of AMP-binding proteins, reduction of cytoplasmic membrane potential, and biofilm production. The regulation of genes encoding products involved in such resistance has been extensively studied and certain two-component regulatory systems (e.g., *pmrAB* and *phoPQ* in *Salmonella* and *misRS* in meningococci and gonococci) or transcriptional regulators can be involved in determining levels of bacterial susceptibility to AMPs.

AMPs probably contribute to host defense through their antibiotic-like action and by virtue of their immunomodulatory properties. In this respect, they should be viewed more broadly as host defense peptides.[18] They can effectively bind and neutralize endotoxin and capsular polysaccharides, act as chemokines,

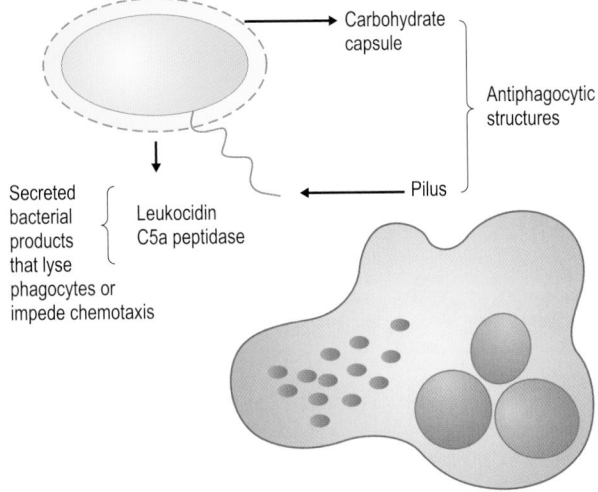

Fig. 24.3 Bacterial resistance to PMNs in the extracellular environment. The two principal mechanisms of bacterial resistance to PMN killing. These consist of resistance to phagocytosis as a result of bacterial surface components (e.g., capsule or pili) and the action of extracellular proteins that can lyse PMNs (e.g., leukocidins) or decrease chemotaxis (e.g., C5a peptidase). Bacteria growing in biofilms may be more protected from PMNs than bacteria growing in the planktonic state.

and induce chemokine synthesis, which results in recruitment and accumulation of phagocytes at sites of infection. AMPs can also promote wound healing, and have been proposed to link innate and adaptive immune responses.[19] Mice expressing human defensin-5 are more resistant to lethal *Salmonella* infection, providing evidence that human AMPs are important in host defense.[20] AMPs present at the human vaginal and cervical mucosal surfaces may also be important in host defense against sexually transmitted infections or in reducing the incidence of vaginosis. LL-37 and β-defensins are probably important in the antimicrobial defense of human skin (Chapter 18). Mice deficient in the murine version of LL-37 (CRAMP) are more susceptible to group A streptococcal skin and soft tissue infections and invasive disease. Patients with psoriasis or atopic dermatitis provide an example of where AMP levels are altered. Thus, keratinocytes of inflamed psoriatic lesions produce increased levels of certain AMPs, and such patients rarely have secondary bacterial infections.[19] In contrast, keratinocytes from patients with atopic dermatitis do not overproduce AMPs and often have skin infections caused by *S. aureus*. Human synthesis of β-defensin 2 is significantly decreased in patients with acute burns, which may partly explain their increased susceptibility to *Pseudomonas aeruginosa* infections. The rare patients with PMN-specific granule deficiency are deficient in defensins and other neutrophil components, and these individuals have life-threatening infections.[16] The severe congenital neutrophil deficiency termed morbus Kostmann disease can be treated with G-CSF to restore neutrophil levels, but such phagocytes fail to produce LL-37 and such patients often have frequent and life-threatening infections as well as periodontal disease. As a final example, individuals with single nucleotide polymorphisms in the promoter for transcription of the human β-defensin 1 (hBD-1) gene are at increased risk for dental caries, periodontal disease, and Crohn's disease. hBD-1 has important antimicrobial action against anaerobic Gram-positive commensal bacteria, which may help to prevent their unwanted overgrowth, and the opportunistic fungus *Candida albicans*, but only after intramolecular disulphide bonds are reduced to produce a linear peptide; *in vivo*, this reduction occurs by the thioredoxin system.[21] Thus, taken together, there is increasing evidence that AMPs are important in the overall integrity of the human host defense scheme, and a combination of their antimicrobial and immunomodulatory activities is involved in protection against extracellular pathogens.

Immunoglobulins

Immunoglobulins, principally secretory IgA and IgG, are present at mucosal surfaces and in mucosal secretions. Important in the generation of these immunoglobulins at mucosal surfaces is the dissemination of IgA and IgG class-committed B- and T-helper cells with specificity to an antigen encountered and processed at one mucosal site to local and distant mucosal sites. Protective mucosal antibodies against bacteria may be derived from prior colonization, vaccines, or shared cross-reactive antigens on normal flora. Mucosal immunoglobulins may neutralize bacterial toxins, facilitate phagocytosis or bactericidal activity, inhibit bacterial adherence ligands, or sterically hinder other events necessary for bacterial colonization and invasion. Many extracellular bacterial pathogens (*N. meningitidis*, *N. gonorrhoeae*, *H. influenzae*, certain streptococci) colonize and/or infect mucosal surfaces where protective IgA1 antibodies could become available.[22] These pathogens secrete an IgA1 protease that cleaves IgA1, thereby inactivating it. IgA1 protease can also recognize other substrates, notably LAMP-1, that are important in host defense. Bacterial infections associated with abnormal immunoglobulin production or function are summarized in Table 24.5 and Chapter 34.

Bacterial pathogens at epithelial surfaces

"Extracellular" bacteria that cause disease in humans are transferred from person to person by direct contact, contact with feces, respiratory droplets or other secretions, or from contaminated food or water. Acquisition of these pathogenic bacteria may be transient, or lead to colonization or local and invasive disease. To colonize human epithelial barriers and mucosal surfaces, bacteria overcome the nonspecific clearance (e.g., mucus, ciliary activity) and other local immune defense mechanisms (e.g., mucosal cellular defenses, immunoglobulins, fatty acids, lactoferrin). For example, bacteria can transverse mucus by expressing motility factors (e.g., pili, flagella) or mucinases (e.g., *V. cholerae*),

---

⬤ THERAPEUTIC PRINCIPLES

Managing defects in host defenses

- Impaired skin and mucous membrane barriers—protect skin from maceration and injury, frequent change of IV catheters. Antibiotic prophylaxis, such as use of trimethoprim-sulfamethoxazole, remains controversial.

- Defects or polymorphisms in innate immune mechanisms—may lead to select cytokine use or other adjuvant therapy such as activated protein C in sepsis.

- Abnormal humoral immunity—intravenous immune serum globulin.

- Complement system abnormalities—fresh plasma or, if available, individual complement components to replace deficient factor.

- Defective cell-mediated immunity reversal of malnutrition—reduction in dosage of immunosuppressive drugs (corticosteroids); other therapy in selected patients (transfer factor, bone marrow transplantation, replacement of missing enzymes).

- Phagocyte dysfunction—GM-CSF or G-CSF to increase neutrophil numbers.

- Immunization with pneumococcal, meningococcal, *H. influenzae*, and influenza vaccines in selected patients.

Table 24.5 Bacterial and other infections associated with abnormal humoral immunity

Primary deficiency
Congenital or X-linked agammaglobulinemia (Bruton's agammaglobulinemia) is manifested by recurrent bacterial infections of the middle ear and sinopulmonary tract, often with complicating bacteremias. Infections with enteroviruses also occur.
Selective immunoglobulin deficiency: IgA—variable course, often free of infection; IgG, IgG subclass deficiency, IgM—recurrent pyogenic bacterial infections.
Common variable immunodeficiency ("acquired" hypogammaglobulinemia) is associated with various bacterial sinopulmonary infections, giardiasis, increased risk of lymphomas, and gastric carcinomas.

Secondary deficiency
Multiple myeloma and chronic lymphocytic leukemia (CLL) are associated with infections caused by encapsulated bacteria, Gram-negative bacilli, *S. aureus*, and giardiasis.
Splenectomy—severe infections with pneumococci, other streptococci, *H. influenzae*, and meningococci.

and induce ciliostasis or decrease motility by direct contact or by the release of toxins.

Initial attachment of bacteria to human epithelial cells is, in part, mediated by pili, fimbriae, or other bacteria ligands, and close adherence involves the cell wall, outer membrane proteins, lipopolysaccharide, and other bacterial surface structures. The attachment of bacteria to human epithelial cells prevents loss from the host. Attachment can also induce cytoskeletal rearrangements, such as elongation and branching of the microvilli, the accumulation of actin, and calcium efflux, which facilitates close adherence and invasion of epithelial cells by normally "extracellular" bacteria, especially at sites with rapidly moving fluid. The entry of bacteria into epithelial cells provides access to nutrients and protection from host defenses, allows protected multiplication, and leads to shedding of organisms back to the mucosal surface, to facilitate transmission and further spread of the infection on the epithelium. Attachment can also initiate epithelial cell apoptosis or toxin-mediated cell death and lead to the breakdown of the epithelial barrier.

N. meningitidis (the meningococcus), for example, is transmitted from person to person by large respiratory droplets or close contact with secretions. During the process of colonization of human upper respiratory mucosal surfaces (e.g., the nasopharynx) meningococci utilize phase-variable meningococcal surface ligands and multiple human epithelial cell surface receptors.[23,24] Meningococci that are acapsulate, piliated, express high levels of the outer membrane protein, Opc (formerly class 5C protein) and the nonsialylated LOS structure containing a terminal Galβ1–4Glu group (L8 immunotype) attach to and interact with human epithelial cells most effectively (Fig. 24.4). These characteristics correspond to the predominant phenotype of meningococci retrieved from the nasopharynx of human carriers. Pili facilitate twitching motility and microcolony formation, which allows the penetration of mucus and provides initial attachment. Post-translational modification of pili by addition of phosphoglycerol to the Ser-93 residue of pilin by the action of a phosphotransferase (PptB), which is interestingly increased in levels when meningococci attach to epithelial cells, helps to release bacteria and promotes their migration across the mucosal epithelia. This process has been advanced as a mechanism to allow meningococci to colonize new sites, migrate and disseminate, leading to invasive disease.[25] The outer membrane adhesin, Opc, mediates meningococcal attachment and invasion by binding vitronectin, which attaches to and is internalized by the vitronectin receptor αvβ3 found on epithelial cell surfaces.[23] Class V (opacity) meningococcal proteins interact directly with members of the carcinoembryonic (CD66) antigen family.[23] The expression of a sialic acid capsule and sialylatable LOS structures, such as the L3,7,9 immunotype, interfere with Opc-mediated attachment and invasion and facilitate spread and transmission.[26] Other surface proteins such as NadA and factor H-binding protein (fHbp) also play a role in pathogenesis and are included in new serogroup B vaccines. Meningococci at mucosal surfaces bind and utilize lactoferrin as an iron source and secrete a protease that cleaves IgA1. Meningococcal colonization of the human upper respiratory (nasopharyngeal) epithelium is also associated with ciliostasis and sloughing of ciliated cells, which occur at a distance from the sites of bacterial attachment.[26,27] Ciliostasis may be caused by a diffusible toxin, such as LPS, which may directly or indirectly cause cytotoxicity by the induction of inflammatory cytokines. Other co-factors, such as smoking or viral infections, facilitate meningococcal invasion at nasopharyngeal mucosal surfaces.

Immune responses during local and systemic invasion by extracellular bacterial pathogens

Bacteria that breach mucosal and skin barriers and reach submucosal tissues and/or the bloodstream induce immune responses, including cytokine release, phagocytosis, complement activation, antibody release or production, and other local or systemic induction of the inflammatory cascade. The survival of bacteria following colonization of the epithelium and access to the bloodstream depends on the integrity of the host immune response (including variability due to genetic polymorphism) and on the ability of the bacteria to resist this response. Host factors that increase the risk for the development of systemic disease due to extracellular bacteria include polymorphisms in innate immune mechanisms, the absence of bactericidal or opsonizing antibodies, deficiencies in the complement pathways,[28] and an absence of or reduction in neutrophil function or levels.

As noted above, immune pattern recognition molecules[4] expressed or released by a variety of host cells, especially PMNs, monocytes, macrophages and dendritic cells, are important initiators of the immune response to extracellular bacteria. Interaction with microbial ligands (LPS, lipoproteins) leads to release of chemokines and cytokines (Chapters 9 and 10) that mediate the local and systemic inflammatory response to extracellular bacteria. Phagocytes can ingest bacteria by opsonin-independent (less efficient) or -dependent mechanisms. Mononuclear phagocytes in the blood, liver, spleen, and lung remove particles, including bacteria. Complement components, fibronectin, or other extracellular matrix proteins that bind to bacteria facilitate recognition. Bacteria ingested by phagocytes are killed by toxic O_2 radicals and/or H_2O_2 through myeloperoxidase-dependent or -independent mechanisms. The elaboration

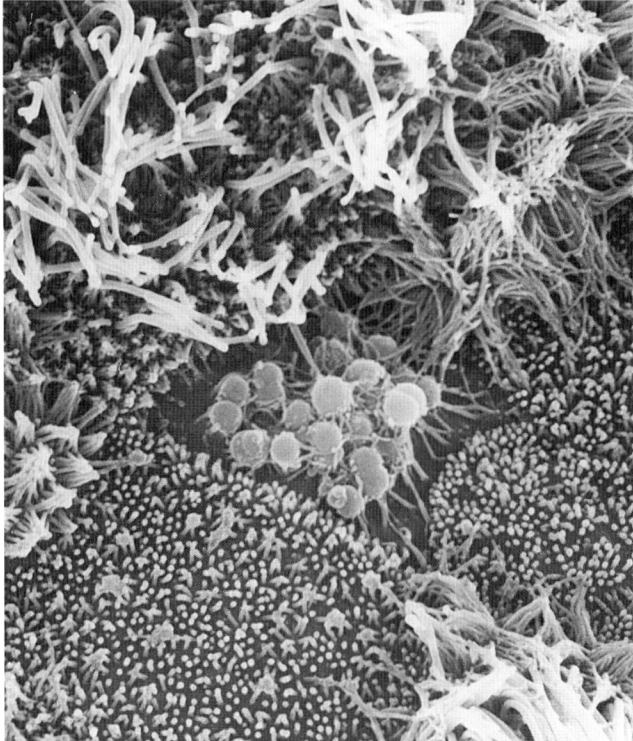

Fig. 24.4 Colonization and adherence of extracellular bacteria at mucosal surfaces. Scanning electron micrograph of *N. meningitidis* adherence and microcolony formation of a human upper respiratory mucosa ($\times 16\,250$).[27]

of superoxide dismutase and catalase can reduce the efficacy of O_2-dependent killing of bacteria, but the high levels of O_2 radicals that accumulate in PMNs probably overcome these bacterial enzymes, as evidenced by the susceptibility of *S. aureus* to intraleukocytic killing. Oxygen-independent systems caused by the action of AMPs (see above) also contribute significantly to phagocytic killing. Bacterial infections associated with phagocytic dysfunction are described in Chapters 21 and 31. Activated neutrophils can release granule proteins with direct antibacterial action (e.g., BPI) or degradative activity (e.g., elastase) and chromatin containing the antibacterial histone H2A.[29] These released compounds work together to form extracellular fibers, termed neutrophil extracellular traps (NETs), that can trap and kill Gram-positive and -negative bacteria as well as degrade their virulence factors. NETs have been observed in instances of acute inflammation (experimental dysentery and spontaneous appendicitis) and provide a mechanism for reducing bacterial spread at sites of acute infection. Complement, a series of more than 20 proteins, is activated by microbial surfaces (alternative complement cascade) or via antibody or by the mannose-binding lectin system (Chapter 20). Complement activation leads to microbial lysis and the release of opsonins and chemoattractant molecules for phagocytic cells. Complement activity is mediated by the classic complement pathway, which can be initiated either by antibody binding to cell surface epitopes or by antibody-independent autocatalytic activation of C1 to form C1q. Initiation of the alternative pathways by bacterial products or mannose-binding protein leads to the direct deposition of the C3b complex on the bacterial surface. Complement activation results in the activation of the late components of the complement pathway, which results in the formation of a membrane attack complex (MAC), insertion in the bacterial cell, and bactericidal activity. Gram-positive extracellular pathogens resist the bacteriolytic action of MAC as a result of their thick peptidoglycan layer, which impedes the insertion of MAC C5b-9 complex. Gram-negative bacteria can resist MAC through structural alterations in their LPS (the possession of O antigen keeps MAC at a distance from the bacterial surface) or by masking or deleting the epitope(s) responsible for binding bactericidal antibody. The initiation of the complement cascade is also an essential step in opsonization and the eventual phagocytosis and ingestion of invading bacteria.

In infants, antibacterial activity wanes as levels of passively transferred maternal antibody fall. This waning of antibody is correlated with the highest incidence of several "extracellular" pyogenic bacterial diseases (*S. pneumoniae*, *N. meningitidis*, *H. influenzae* type b) in young children. During childhood and adolescence, levels of bactericidal antibodies rise and rates of these diseases decline. Specific antibodies are acquired through carriage and through cross-reacting epitopes on other commensal species. For example, cross-reactive antibodies to *N. meningitidis* are acquired by colonization with commensal *Neisseria* spp. (e.g., *Neisseria lactamica*) and unrelated bacteria (e.g., *Enterococcus faecium*, *Bacillus pumilus*, and *E. coli*). The lack of bactericidal antibodies against a strain acquired in the upper respiratory tract is an important risk factor for invasive meningococcal disease.

Complement deficiencies, either congenital or acquired, also increase the risk for invasive bacterial diseases (Chapter 20). Because C3 plays a critical role in the complement cascade, congenital C3 deficiency or conditions that reduce C3 (e.g., systemic lupus erythematosus, cirrhosis, nephritis, C3 nephritic factor) increase the risk for invasive disease due to pyogenic bacteria such as *S. pneumoniae* and *N. meningitidis*. Mannose-binding lectin (MBL) is a plasma opsonin that initiates complement activation.

MBL gene polymorphisms are found in children with meningococcal and pneumococcal sepsis. Properdin deficiency, leading to defective alternative pathway killing, is also associated with severe and recurrent meningococcal infections. Terminal complement deficiencies (C5–C8) are also associated with recurrent invasive bloodstream meningococcal and gonococcal infections, indicating an important role for insertion of the complement membrane attack complex in the bactericidal activity of human serum against pathogenic *Neisseria*.[30] In adults, 10–20% of invasive meningococcal disease is associated with a defect in the complement system.[30] Enteric colonization by bacteria that have similar antigenic epitopes has been proposed to induce these blocking antibodies. Screening tests useful for the evaluation of humoral, complement, and other immune defects are discussed in Chapter 30.

In addition to defects in innate immunity, immunoglobulins and complement deficiencies, human genetic polymorphisms are associated with an increased risk or severity of bacterial diseases. For example, FcγIIa (CD32) receptor polymorphisms, Fcγ-receptor III (CD16), MBL, TLR4, TNF promoter region polymorphisms, plasminogen activator and inhibitor expression, and hereditary differences in cytokine induction influence susceptibility to meningococcemia.[30] Each of these polymorphisms can influence the course of invasive bacterial infection by influencing the response of the inflammatory cascade.

Induction of the inflammatory cascade, acute-phase reaction or response, augments humoral defense components, increases the number and function of phagocytic cells, and facilitates the delivery of humoral cellular molecules to sites of bacterial invasion.[2] Components of this reaction include cytokines, mannose-binding protein, fibronectin, haptoglobin, transferrin, C-reactive protein, platelet-activating factor, prostaglandins, lipopolysaccharide-binding protein (LBP), α1-antitrypsin and α2-macroglobulin. Acute-phase reaction components induce fever and the catabolism of muscle protein, decrease available iron, increase phagocyte activity, increase vascular permeability, and induce the release of hormones and neurotransmitters.

Pyogenic extracellular bacteria have evolved strategies to avoid or overcome immune responses. For example, meningococci isolated from the bloodstream or cerebrospinal fluid are characteristically encapsulated and express the sialylatable lacto-N-neotetraose-containing L3,7,9 LPS immunotype. The co-expression of both of these structures is necessary for meningococcal systemic disease in the infant rat model, influences neutrophil activation and endothelial injury in cell monolayer models, and is required for resistance to complement-mediated killing. The similarity of capsules such as the serogroup B (α2→8)-linked polysialic acid and of lacto-N-neotetraose and other α-chain LPS structures with complex human sugars, glycosphingolipids, makes these structures infrequent targets for bactericidal antibody recognition.[31] Encapsulation of *N. meningitidis* downregulates the activation of the alternative pathway and is protective against phagocytosis by human macrophages and monocytes. Sialylation of LOS in meningococci has been shown to increase resistance to classic and alternative complement-mediated killing by decreasing the deposition of C3b and IgM on the cell surface, irrespective of capsular phenotype. Bacterial surface proteins can also influence activation of complement pathways. Thus, the factor H-binding protein on the surface of meningococci serves to downregulate activation of the alternative pathway of complement. Phase-variable expression of the length of the gonococcal LOS or the presence of certain forms of the major outer membrane protein (Por1A) can alter levels of gonococcal susceptibility to complement killing. The complement regulatory protein C4BP, which dampens activation of the classical pathway, can interact with most gonococcal Por1A serovars (and some select Por1B serovars) and this provides a mechanism by which gonococci can evade killing by human serum.

Sepsis

Septicemia remains a leading cause of death in the United States.[32] It also accounts for several billion dollars of the USA's annual healthcare expenditure. Both Gram-negative and -positive bacteria can trigger sepsis and septic shock (Table 24.6). Septic shock is a result of initial and widespread overstimulation of the pro-inflammatory response in the systemic vasculature followed by anti-inflammatory cytokine activation, and may be characterized by a number of clinical findings, including hypotension, organ failure, and death. The severity of sepsis can also be influenced by polymorphic alleles of genes involved in the inflammatory cascade.[28, 30, 33] A related syndrome (systemic immune response syndrome, or SIRS) may be seen with the release of bacterial toxins or products from sites of colonization or local infections.

Peptidoglycan, DNA CpG motifs or LPS released by bacterial lysis or growth and toxins or superantigens are major initiators of the hypotension and shock of septicemia or SIRS, either directly through interaction with host cell membranes or indirectly through the release of host inflammatory mediators or T-cell proliferation (Fig. 24.5). The morbidity and mortality of bacteremia have been directly correlated with increased levels of pro-inflammatory cytokines and the amount of circulating bacterial components. Indeed, the severity of Gram-negative sepsis has been equated with high levels of endotoxin, increased levels of cytokines, and excessive activation of the alternative complement pathway. Disseminated intravascular coagulation, which often accompanies Gram-negative sepsis, is due to excessive activation of the coagulation cascade and downregulation of the fibrinolytic system associated with high levels of LPS. Levels of natural anticoagulants in the vasculature, such as antithrombin and protein C, are often low in Gram-negative sepsis. The onset and severity of disseminated intravascular coagulation may be influenced by genetic polymorphisms in plasminogen activation or inhibition. The altered vascular endothelial lining facilitates thrombosis and thrombocytosis. Although much remains to be learned about the mechanisms by which Gram-negative and -positive bacteria and their products trigger sepsis, significant advances have been recently made, particularly with LPS. Advances during the past decade include the identification of certain LPS–host protein interactions that result in delivery

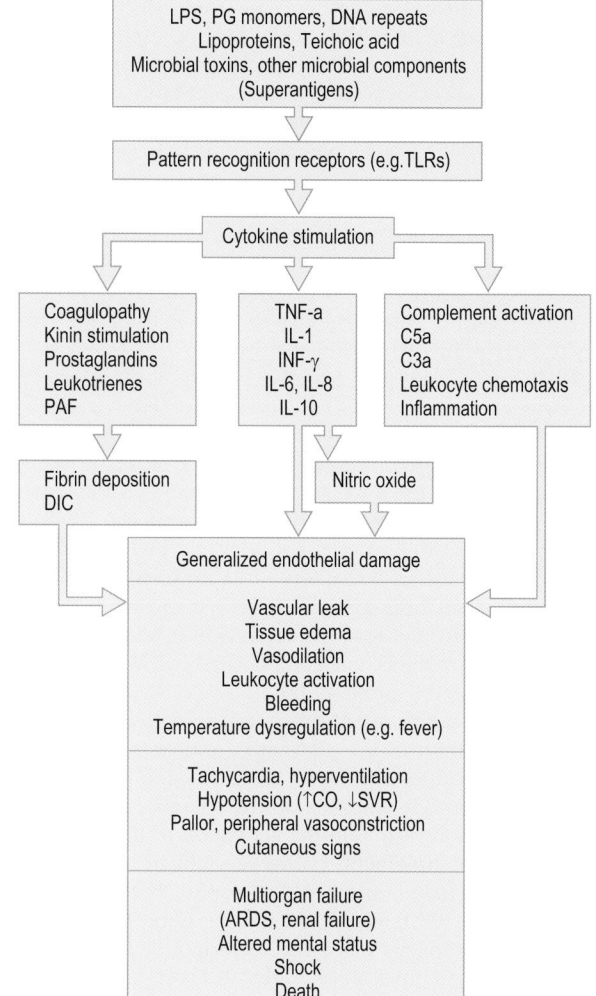

Fig. 24.5 Inflammatory cascade initiated during sepsis.

of LPS to host cell receptors and gene activation events that result in elevated expression of a diverse array of pro-inflammatory mediators.

KEY CONCEPTS

Definitions of septicemia and sepsis syndrome

- *Septicemia*—Life-threatening bacterial infection of the bloodstream caused by Gram-positive or -negative bacteria.
- *Sepsis syndrome*—Clinical evidence of infection, plus evidence of systemic response to infection and altered organ perfusion, but may not have documented bacterial infection in bloodstream. May be due to toxin, microbial product release into bloodstream.
- *SIRS (systemic inflammatory response syndrome) or MODS (multiple organ dysfunction syndrome)*—Response to a wide variety of clinical insults, both infectious and noninfectious (pancreatitis, burns); similar pathophysiology to septicemia and sepsis syndrome.

A general scheme (summarized in Fig. 24.6) for the development of endotoxic shock is as follows:

1. LPS becomes available in host fluids through rapid bacterial multiplication, release of outer membrane vesicles or the bacteriolytic action of antibiotics or antimicrobial systems (e.g., complement) in the host.

Table 24.6 Major agents of septicemia

Staphylococcus aureus
Enterococci
Streptococcus pneumonia
Haemophilus influenzae
Streptococcus pyogenes
Streptococcus agalactiae

Gram-negative aerobic bacilli

E. coli	*Enterobacter* spp.
Pseudomonas aeruginosa	*Morganella morganii*
Serratia marcescens	*Proteus mirabilis*
Klebsiella pneumoniae	*Providencia stuartii*
Citrobacter spp.	*Acinetobacter* spp.
Neisseria meningitidis	*Pasteurella* spp.

Fig. 24.6 LPS triggering of cytokine production by macrophages. Steps known or presumed to be necessary for LPS triggering of pro-inflammatory cytokines.

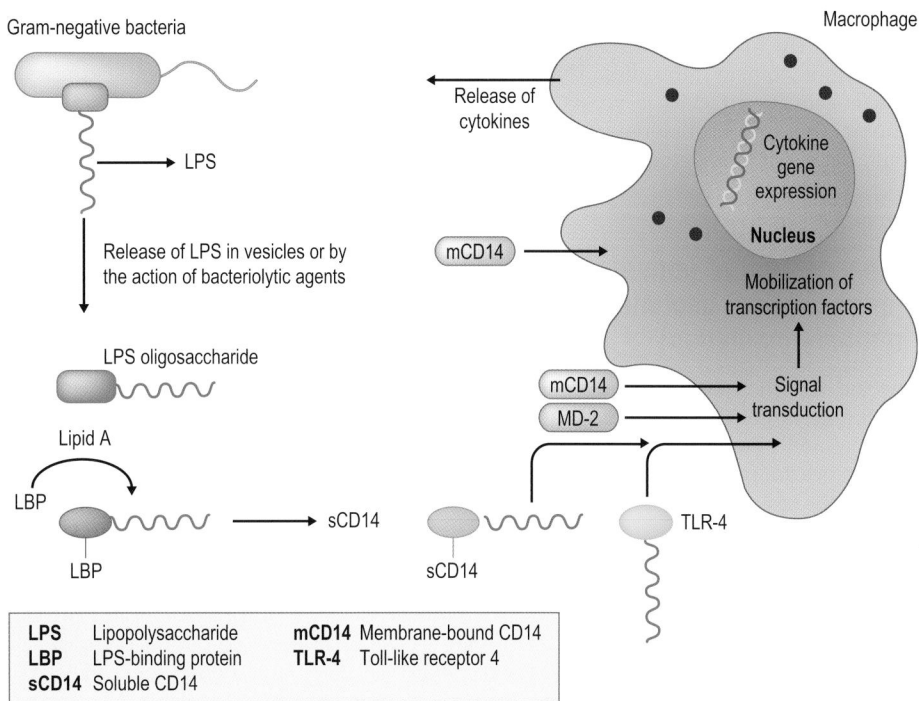

LPS   Lipopolysaccharide   **mCD14** Membrane-bound CD14
LBP LPS-binding protein   **TLR-4** Toll-like receptor 4
sCD14 Soluble CD14

2. During the acute-phase response the production of a serum glycoprotein of 60 kDa, termed lipopolysaccharide-binding protein (LBP), is increased; although structurally similar to bactericidal permeability increasing protein (BPI), LBP lacks bactericidal activity. LBP binds lipid A, the toxic domain of LPS, with high affinity.

3. The LBP–LPS complex is then transferred to CD14, which exists in both soluble and membrane states. The primary role of LBP is to accelerate this transfer reaction.[33] CD14 is clearly important in the development of endotoxic shock, as CD14-deficient mice are resistant to lethal challenge with LPS.[34] However, membrane CD14 does not have "signaling" ability. Soluble CD14 can accept LPS from the LBP complex and transfer it to an LPS receptor on the macrophage surface, which does have signaling ability.

4. The nature of this LPS receptor has been defined. Poltorak et al.[35] ascribed the relevant genetic defect in endotoxin-resistant C3H/HeJ mice to a missense mutation in the Toll-like receptor-4 gene (*Tlr4*).

TLR4 belongs to a family of transmembrane receptors originally identified in *Drosophila* as being important in controlling dorso-ventral patterning and antifungal responses (Chapter 3). TLR4 signaling requires an accessory protein, myeloid differentiation protein-2 (MD-2),[36] that binds directly to endotoxin. The key point, however, is that the LPS engagement of MD-2/TLR4 on host cells, particularly macrophages, triggers intracellular signaling events that ultimately, through NF-κB and other pathways, result in cytokine gene activation and the overproduction of pro-inflammatory cytokines (TNF-α, IL-1, IL-6, IL-8, interferons). Different TLRs (e.g., TLR2) play a critical role in the recognition of lipoproteins and the recognition of these components is a likely key determinant in the development of septic shock seen with Gram-positive infections. TLR5 recognizes bacterial flagella, and such recognition is of likely importance in the host response to motile bacteria; some human pathogens (e.g., *H. pylori*) produce flagellin molecules that do not engage TLR5.[37] Another TLR (TLR9) has been shown to recognize

bacterial DNA CpG dinucleotides.[38] Taken together, the clinical syndrome of septic shock represents a series of interactions of bacterial products with pattern recognition molecules on serum proteins (LBP and soluble CD14), and with host cell receptors (MD-2/TLR4 and TLR2, other TLR receptors) that recognize and bind bacterial products, leading to signaling events and transcriptional factors that modulate cytokine gene expression. These events trigger further events in the inflammatory cascade, leading to massive activation of the coagulation, complement, and kinin pathways.

Early and effective antimicrobial therapy is the primary goal in the treatment of sepsis. Adjuvant therapy is reviewed elsewhere.[39] For example, recombinant protein C is approved for use in patients with sepsis, but is associated with an increased risk of cerebral hemorrhage.[39] In contrast to the initial phase of sepsis characterized by the release of TNF-α, IL-1, IL-6, and interferon-γ,

CLINICAL RELEVANCE

Signs of septicemia

- Shaking chills, spiking fevers or hypothermia (< 36 °C)
- Tachycardia, hyperventilation
- Pallor (peripheral vasoconstriction) and acrocyanosis, but 10–20% are flushed "warm shock"
- Nausea/vomiting, diarrhea
- Hypotension < 90 mmHg or > 40 mmHg decrease from baseline, in 20–35% of cases
- Cardiac output, decreased systemic vascular resistance (SVR)
- Cutaneous signs: purpura fulminans, petechiae, palpable purpura, echthyma gangrenosum
- Change in mental status
- Signs may be more subtle in elderly and uremic (renal failure) patients
- WBC count > 12 000/mm³ or < 4000 cells/mm³ with > 10% immature (band) forms
- Oliguria (< 20 mL/h of urine)

during the latter phase an anti-inflammatory response may predominate. The failure of anti-inflammatory therapeutic mediators (anti-endotoxin antibodies, TNF-α, antagonists of IL-1 or platelet-activating factor) in sepsis suggests that this hypoinflammatory state encountered in many patients at presentation could be an additional target of immune modulation.

Enhancement of immune responses to "extracellular" bacteria (vaccines and immunomodulation)

Vaccines are the most affordable and cost-effective health intervention for enhancing the immune response to extracellular bacterial and other microbial pathogens (Chapter 90). The use of vaccines to prevent diphtheria, pertussis, tetanus, certain serogroups of N. meningitidis, H. influenzae b (Hib), and S. pneumoniae is a major public health success. The efficacy of vaccines to extracellular bacteria is most often correlated with enhanced bactericidal antibodies, opsonic antibodies and/or neutralizing antibodies, both systemically and at mucosal surfaces. Enhancement of these immune mechanisms can provide protection even in immunocompromised individuals. For example, vaccination with meningococcal capsular polysaccharide vaccines protects patients with hereditary complement deficiencies by enhancing opsonophagocytic activity. However, some older vaccines had limitations in terms of long-lived immune responses, safety issues, and poor responses in certain populations (extremes of age) when infections with extracellular bacteria are most common.

Advances in genetic engineering, immunology, molecular pathogenesis, vaccine adjuvants and delivery systems are leading to the development of new vaccines and vaccine approaches that enhance the immune response to extracellular bacterial pathogens. The introduction of acellular pertussis vaccines and pneumococcal and meningococcal conjugate vaccines are recent examples.

The conjugation of bacterial polysaccharides to carrier proteins such as diphtheria or tetanus toxins has been a major advance in stimulating immune responses to saccharide bacterial antigens. Polysaccharide capsules, for example, when used alone, are "T-independent" antigens; they do not require the presence of T cells to induce an immune response, and generate IgM as the dominant antibody produced (Chapter 6). There is also a failure to induce memory and failure of affinity maturation following polysaccharide immunization. Thus, polysaccharides are poorly immunogenic in infants, the elderly, and those with impaired antibody production—groups most susceptible to encapsulated bacterial pathogens. Covalent linkage of the polysaccharide to a carrier protein converts the polysaccharide to a thymus-dependent antigen generating IgG anticapsular antibodies and memory B cells. Because these vaccines induce vigorous mucosal immune responses they also protect by herd immunity. A major (and unanticipated) result of vaccination with the H. influenzae (Hib), meningococcal and pneumococcal conjugate vaccines was the interruption of mucosal carriage, decreased transmission and herd immunity. They are now used as part of the routine childhood and adolescent immunization series.

The presentation to CD4 T cells of an antigen by MHC class II molecules is critical for an immune response and influences the amount of antibody, the affinity of that antibody and the duration of response. The two major subsets of CD4 T cells (i.e., Th1 and Th2) influence the qualitative and quantitative features of an immune response to vaccines and bacterial antigens (Chapters 15-17). Th1 responses are characterized by complement-fixing antibody and are associated with the release of IFN-γ, IL-2, and IL-12. Th2 responses result in high circulating and secreting antibody levels and the induction of cytokines IL-4, IL-5, and IL-10.

Considerable progress is being made in the development of new vaccine adjuvants and immune modulators (see Chapter 90 for update information). Aluminum salts, used since the 1930s in many vaccines against bacteria, induce a >90% Th2 response. As noted above, bacterial toxins as conjugates can be used to enhance immunogenicity. In addition, saponin adjuvants, liposomes, CpG DNA repeats, and immunostimulating complexes are under development as adjuvants. Monophosphoryl lipid A, long known to be an effective adjuvant in animal models, has recently been approved by the FDA for human use and may significantly improve immunogenicity of new vaccines. Cytokines such as IL-1, IL-2, IL-12, IL-18, and GM-CSF also modify and enhance immune responses to vaccines IL-12, for example, induces strong Th1 shifts, and GM-CSF is a co-migrating signal for dendritic cells and stimulates antigen processing and presentation. Antigen recognition and processing in macrophages is critical to determining Th1 and Th2 responses and can be manipulated by selected adjuvants. Immune modulation is being evaluated not only for the enhancement of bacterial vaccines, but also as adjunct therapy for serious bacterial infections such as sepsis. Vaccines and specific immunotherapeutic approaches such as cytokines may also find use against chronic tissue-damaging inflammatory reactions created by persistent extracellular bacteria (e.g., Helicobacter) and autoimmune reactions that may be induced by cross-reactive bacterial antigens (e.g., Campylobacter jejuni and Guillain–Barré syndrome).[40]

Translational research opportunities

● ON THE HORIZON

- Tailored vaccine design based upon assessment of innate immune molecular signatures.
- Discovery of small molecule inhibitors or enhancers specifically targeting innate immune pathways.
- Identification of immune responses that prevent or eliminate mucosal bacterial pathogen colonization.
- Development of new therapies modulating immune response in sepsis.

An important challenge for the next 5-10 years will be to take the rapidly expanding basic discoveries in innate immunity and response to bacterial antigens into clinical applications. The design and use of bacterial vaccines through the assessment of innate immune molecular signatures after vaccination, both for general use and for subpopulations of non-responders, is one example. A second is the continued development of small molecule inhibitors or enhancers that specifically target innate immune pathways in order to modulate bacterial immune responses. A third is the control of mucosal immune responses to prevent or eliminate bacterial pathogen colonization. Finally, the development of new therapies for acute bacterial sepsis will be based upon improved understanding and control of the immune responses in sepsis.

References

1. Gill SR, Pop M, Deboy RT, et al. Metagenomic analysis of the human distal gut microbiome. Science 2006;312:1355–9.
2. Dieffenbach CW, Tramont EC. Innate (general or nonspecific) host defense mechanisms. In: Mandell GL, Bennett JE, Dolin R, editors. Principles and practice of infectious diseases, vol. 1. 6th ed. Philadelphia: Elsevier; 2005. p. 34.
3. Mackowiak PA. The normal microbial flora. N Engl J Med 1982;307:83.
4. Pasare C, Medzhitov R. Toll-like receptors: linking innate and adaptive immunity. Adv Exp Med Biol 2005;560:11–8.
5. Akira S, Uematsu S, Takeuchi O. Pathogen recognition and innate immunity. Cell 2006;124:783.
6. Beutler B, Jiang Z, Georgel P, et al. Genetic analysis of host resistance: Toll-like receptor signaling and immunity at large. Annu Rev Immunol 2006;24:353–89.
7. Quinn SR, O'Neill LA. A trio of microRNAs that control Toll-like receptor signalling. Int Immunol 2011;7:421–5.
8. Steinman R, Cohn Z. Identification of a novel cell type in peripheral lymphoid organs of mice. J Exp Med 1973;137:1142–62.
9. Banchereau J, Steinman RM. Dendritic cells and the control of immunity. Nature 1998;392:245–52.
10. Bigley V, Haniffa M, Doulatov S, et al. The human syndrome of dendritic cell, monocyte, B and NK lymphoid deficiency. J Exp Med 2011;208:227–34.
11. Unkmeir A, Kammerer U, Stade A, et al. Lipopolysaccharide and polysaccharide capsule: virulence factors of Neisseria meningitidis that determine meningococcal interaction with human dendritic cells. Infect Immun 2002;70:2454.
12. Yoshikai Y. The interaction of intestinal epithelial cells and intraepithelial lymphocytes in host defense. Immunol Res 1999;20:219.
13. Sansonetti PJ, Phalipon A. M cells as ports of entry for enteroinvasive pathogens: mechanisms of interaction, consequences for the disease process. Semin Immunol 1999;11:193.
14. Jungi TW, Schweizer M, Perler L, Peterhans E. Supernatants of virus-infected macrophages prime uninfected macrophages for lipopolysaccharide-induced apoptosis by both an interferon-dependent and an independent mechanism. Pathobiology 1999;67:294.
15. Shafer WM, Rest RF. Interactions of gonococci with phagocytic cells. Annu Rev Microbiol 1989;43:121.
16. Ganz T. Defensins: antimicrobial peptides of innate immunity. Nat Rev Immunol 2003;3:710.
17. Peschel A, Sahl H-G. The co-evolution of host cationic antimicrobial peptides and microbial resistance. Nat Microbiol Rev 2006;4:529.
18. Bowdish OME, Davidson DJ, Hancock REW. Immunomodulatory properties of defensins and cathelicidins. In: Shafer WM, editor. Antimicrobial peptides and human disease. Heidelberg: Springer Verlag; 2006. p. 27.
19. Braff MH, Gallo RL. Antimicrobial peptides: an essential component of the skin defensive barrier. In: Shafer WM, editor. Antimicrobial peptides and human disease. Heidelberg: Springer Verlag; 2006. p. 91.
20. Salzman NH, Ghosh D, Huttner KM, et al. Protection against enteric salmonellosis in transgenic mice expressing a human intestinal defensin. Nature 2003;422:522.
21. Schroeder BO, Wu Z, Nuding S, et al. Reduction of disulphide bonds unmasks potent antimicrobial activity of human β-defensin 1. Nature 2011;469:419–23.
22. Mulks MH, Plaut AG. IgA protease production as a characteristic distinguishing pathogenic from harmless neisseriaceae. N Engl J Med 1978;299:973.
23. Virji M, Makepeace K, Ferguson DP, Watt SM. Carcinoembryonic antigens (CD66) on epithelial cells and neutrophils are receptors for Opa proteins of pathogenic neisseriae. Mol Microbiol 1996;22:941.
24. Merz AJ, So M. Interactions of pathogenic Neisseriae with epithelial cell membranes. Annu Rev Cell Dev Biol 2000;16:423–57.
25. Chamot-Rooke J, Mikaty G, Malosse C, et al. Posttranslational modification of pili upon cell contact triggers N. meningitidis dissemination. Science 2011;331:778–82.
26. Stephens DS, Spellman PA, Swartley JS. Effect of the (α2→8)-linked polysialic acid capsule on adherence of Neisseria meningitidis to human mucosal cells. J Infect Dis 1993;167:475.
27. Stephens DS, Hoffman LH, McGee ZA. Interaction of Neisseria meningitidis with human nasophrayngeal mucosa: attachment and entry into columnar epithelial cells. J Infect Dis 1983;148:369.
28. Ellison RTD, Kohler PF, Curd JG, et al. Prevalence of congenital or acquired complement deficiency in patients with sporadic meningococcal disease. N Engl J Med 1983;308:913.
29. Brinkman V, Reichard U, Goosmann C, et al. Neutrophil extracellular traps kill bacteria. Science 2004;303:1532–5.
30. Emonts M, Hazelzet JA, de Groot R, Hermans PW. Host genetic determinants of Neisseria meningitidis infections. Lancet Infect Dis 2003;3:565–77.
31. Kahler CM, Stephens DS. Genetic basis for biosynthesis, structure, and function of meningococcal lipooligosaccharide (endotoxin). Crit Rev Microbiol 1998;24:281–334.
32. Martin GS, Mannino DM, Eaton S, Moss M. The epidemiology of sepsis in the United States from 1979 through 2000. N Engl J Med 2003;348:1546.
33. Hyakushima N, Mitsazawa H, Nishitani C, et al. Interaction of soluble form of recombinant extracellular TLR4 domain with MD-2 enables lipopolysaccharide binding and attenuates TLR4-mediated signaling. J Immunol 2004;173:6949–54.
34. Jiang Z, Georgel P, Du X, et al. CD14 is required for MyD88-independent LPS signaling. Nat Immunol 2005;6:565–70.
35. Poltorak A, He X, Smirnova I, et al. Defective LPS signaling in C3H/HeJ and C57BL/10ScCr mice: mutations in Tlr4 gene. Science 1998;2085:282.
36. Zughaier SM, Tzeng YL, Zimmer SM, et al. Neisseria meningitidis lipooligosaccharide structure-dependent activation of the macrophage CD14/Toll-like receptor 4 pathway. Infect Immun 2004;72:371–80.
37. Andersen-Nissen E, Smith KD, Strobe KL, et al. Evasion of Toll-like receptor 5 by flagellated bacteria. Proc Natl Acad Sci U S A 2005;102:9247.
38. Hemni H, Takenchi O, Kawai T, et al. A Toll-like Receptor recognizes bacterial DNA. Nature 2000;408:740.
39. Gischer M, Hilinski J, Stephens DS. Adjuvant therapy for meningococcal sepsis. Pediatr Infect Dis J 2005;24:177–8.
40. Hughes RA, Hadden RD, Gregson NA, Smith KJ. Pathogenesis of Guillain–Barré syndrome. J Neuroimmunol 1999;100:74.

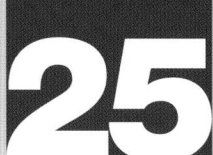

Host defenses to intracellular bacteria

Stephen T. Reece, Stefan H.E. Kaufmann

The evolutionary relationship between humans and bacteria is so intimate that it is impossible to imagine the development of one without the other.[1] While this coexistence is generally mutually beneficial, clear boundaries exist between the two that are intensely defended. We tend to think of the human host as the defender and bacteria as transgressors of these boundaries. However, evolution of human immunity has been accompanied by evolution of ingenious bacterial mechanisms to not only survive its onslaught, but also to manipulate it to enhance survival. This idea is instructively mirrored in the lifestyle of intracellular bacteria. These bacteria actively seek out an environment inside human cells in which to flourish; this is not an easy environment to survive in. Human cells have developed an ability to differentiate bacterial from host components and direct host cells to clear the invader. In some instances this works well, for example, during listeriosis. This is, however, a rare exception. In most cases intracellular bacteria are long-lived in the human body, sometimes for the entire human lifetime. This chapter dissects the current interpretation of this fascinating interaction between human and microbe, sheds light on how our immune system functions and describes how it helps drive novel approaches to vaccination.

● CLINICAL PEARLS

Distinguishing clinical characteristics of infections with intracellular bacteria

- Nonsterilizing immunity
- Persistent bacteria, sometimes latent infection
- Formation of long-lasting tissue granulomas containing low numbers of viable bacteria
- Critical role of T cells in protection, role of antibodies less well established but could be important
- Critical role of immune response in pathology
- Lack of effective available vaccines

Balance of protection and pathology defines the chronic nature of intracellular bacterial infection

Only a few intracellular bacteria, such as *Listera monocytogenes*, are eradicated once the immune response has reached its height. More often, the intracellular habitat provides a protective niche that promotes persistent infection in the face of an ongoing immune response. In this case the bacteria can persist for long periods of time without causing clinical signs of illness,

and are reactivated to cause disease only after the immune response has become compromised. This occurs in *Mycobacterium tuberculosis* infection, resulting in disease years or decades after primary contact. In fact, disease need not arise from infection at all: in many regions, for example, the majority of adults harbor *M. tuberculosis* without suffering from clinical disease. Alternatively, disease can develop directly after primary infection, during maturation of the immune response, or with regression once the immune response is sufficiently strong. Yet sterile eradication of the pathogen is rarely achieved: bacteria persist latently and illness may re-emerge at a later time. For example, *Rickettsia prowazekii* may persist for decades after convalescence from typhus, to later cause Brill–Zinsser disease.

Several intracellular bacteria possess components that profoundly influence the course of disease, for example, the lipopolysaccharides (LPSs) of brucellae and salmonellae. Chronic persistence inside host cells, however, depends on the target cell remaining intact and physiologically active. Accordingly, many intracellular bacteria are of low toxicity and do not have dramatic direct effects on their host. Instead, pathogenesis is largely determined by the immune response. Classic examples of this concept include granuloma liquefaction in acute tuberculosis (TB), which severely affects lung function, and eye scarring as a consequence of chronic or recurring *Chlamydia trachomatis* infection that ultimately leads to trachoma.

The survival of intracellular bacteria has major consequences for pathology. Although many intracellular bacteria show some organ tropism, dissemination to other organs frequently occurs, resulting in different disease forms. For example, TB is generally manifested in the lung, yet any other organ can be affected. In contrast to other *Salmonella enterica* serovars, the serovars *Typhi* and *Paratyphi* are not restricted to the gastrointestinal tract but are disseminated to internal organs, primarily the liver and spleen. In these cases the type of clinical disease depends markedly on the infected tissue type.

● KEY CONCEPTS

Characteristic features of intracellular bacterial infections

- Persistence of bacteria inside mononuclear phagocytes (i.e., macrophages)
- Low to absent bacterial-mediated toxicity to the host
- Protection requires cytokine-mediated activation of infected phagocytes
- IFN-γ and TNF-α produced by antigen-specific T cells are key cytokines for protection

Intracellular bacterial infections of clinical relevance (Table 25.1)

Granulomatous infections

Tuberculosis

Tubercle bacilli are typically inhaled in microdroplets ranging from 1 to 3 μm in diameter and then engulfed by alveolar macrophages, which transport the pathogens to the lung interstitia. There, as well as in the draining lymph nodes, primary lesions develop that rarely cause disease directly.[2] The combination of both types of lesions is called a Ghon complex. The infection remains dormant under the control of the immune system. Once the immune response becomes debilitated, however, dormant bacteria are reactivated and pulmonary TB develops. Bacteria disseminate to other sites in the lung and occasionally to other organs, including the kidneys, liver and central nervous system. Infection of immunocompromised patients, notably those with AIDS, or newborns results in the rapid development of disease (miliary TB). TB represents a major health problem worldwide, including an increasing incidence in many industrialized countries. In 2007, up to 10 million active TB cases were diagnosed worldwide, and close to 2 million people died of the disease. The much larger estimated number of 2 billion individuals infected with *M. tuberculosis* well illustrates the dissociation of infection from disease. The emergence of multidrug-resistant strains has further complicated the situation, and a recent study has conclusively demonstrated that, following successful treatment, reinfection can occur later in life. The currently available vaccine Bacille Calmette–Guérin (BCG), an attenuated strain derived from the etiological agent of bovine TB, *M. bovis*, shows only low and variable protection against pulmonary TB in adults.

Leprosy

M. leprae is most likely transmitted by contact with patients who shed microorganisms in nasal secretions and lesion exudates. It primarily affects the nerves and the skin, frequently leading to stigmatizing deformities. Leprosy is a spectral disease. At the tuberculoid pole, rigorous T-cell responses succeed

Table 25.1 Major infectious diseases caused by intracellular bacteria

Disease	Pathogen	Prevalence	Incubation time	Route of infection	Target cell
Granulomatous intracellular bacteria					
Tuberculosis	*Mycobacterium tuberculosis*	Worldwide	Years (latency after primary infection and disease reactivation) Weeks (miliary TB)	Inhalation of bacteria-containing micro-droplets	Macrophage
Leprosy	*M. leprae*	South America Africa India Southeast Asia	Years	Unknown	Macrophage Schwann cell
Typhoid fever	*Salmonella enterica* serovars *Typhi* and *Paratyphi*	Worldwide	7–10 days	Fecal-oral	Macrophage
Brucellosis	*Brucella* spp.	Worldwide	Weeks to months	Zoonosis; cows, goats, pigs Inhalation, gut, skin abrasion	Macrophage
Listeriosis	*Listeria monocytogenes*	Worldwide	Days to months	Fecal-oral	Macrophage Hepatocyte
Nongranulomatous intracellular bacteria					
Legionnaires' disease	*Legionella pneumophila*	Worldwide	2–10 days	Inhalation	Macrophage
Rocky Mountain spotted fever	*Rickettsia rickettsia*	Western hemisphere	1 week	Tick bite	Vascular endothelial cell Smooth muscle cell
Urogenital infection	*Chlamydia trachomatis* serovars D-K	Worldwide	1–3 weeks	Sexual intercourse	Epithelial cell
Conjunctivitis, trachoma	*Chlamydia trachomatis* serovars D-K	Africa	Conjunctivitis: 1–3 weeks Trachoma: years	Eye	Epithelial cell
Cat scratch disease	*Bartonella henselae* *B. quintana* *B. bacilliformis*	Worldwide	Bacillary angiomatosis Peliosis hepatis Endocarditis Bacteremia with fever Neuroretinitis: 1–3 weeks	Flea, sandfly or mosquito bite Animal scratch or bite	Erythrocyte Endothelial cell

in restricting microbial growth in well-defined lesions containing few bacilli. In contrast, at the lepromatous pole bacterial growth is unrestricted and lesions contain abundant bacilli within macrophages lacking signs of activation. Regulatory T (Treg) cells and other types of immunosuppression have been implicated in this latter type of disease. Throughout the spectrum Schwann cells are affected, promoting nerve damage and anesthesia. This results in injuries and secondary infections that significantly exaggerate the disease. Despite the success of multidrug therapy in reducing the number of registered leprosy cases worldwide, the annual rate of new case detection remains unchanged, at approximately 700 000 cases per year, with children representing 15% of new cases. This suggests that active transmission of M. leprae is still occurring, but the route and mechanism of this transmission remains unclear.[3]

Atypical mycobacterial infections

These environmental microbes are unable to persist within activated macrophages and thus rarely cause disease in individuals with competent immune status.[4] M. scrofulaceum occasionally causes lymphadenitis in children, and M. kansasii primarily causes infections in elderly men with pre-existing lung disease. As a consequence of HIV infection, however, nontuberculous mycobacteria (NTM), primarily M. avium / M. intracellulare, have gained clinical importance, and these infections are recognized as one of the most common complications of AIDS in industrialized nations.

Typhoid or enteric fever

Typhoid is a foodborne disease caused by Salmonella enterica serovars Typhi and Paratyphi in humans. The pathogens are disseminated within mononuclear phagocytes (MPs) from the gastrointestinal tract to macrophage-rich organs, particularly the liver, spleen, and lymph nodes. Accordingly, typhoid is characterized by systemic symptoms such as prolonged fever and malaise with sustained bacteremia, although diarrhea or constipation may also be present. In some cases an asymptomatic carrier state can persist as a result of chronic infection of the gallbladder, which maintains the environmental reservoir of infection in endemic areas. Typhoid fever remains a major cause of morbidity and mortality, with approximately 16 million cases and 220 000 deaths annually worldwide.[5]

Gastroenteritis

S. enterica serovars Typhimurium and Enteritidis are the major causes of salmonella gastroenteritis in humans, which occurs mainly as a result of the ingestion of contaminated food or water. The bacteria rapidly cross the intestinal epithelia and replicate in the lamina propria, inducing an influx of polymorphonuclear neutrophils (PMNs), which is generally sufficient to resolve the infection within 7 days. In rare cases the bacteria enter the bloodstream and cause systemic bacteremia, most notably in AIDS patients, where death can occur as a result of septic shock.[5]

Listeriosis

Although epidemic outbreaks of this food-borne disease have been observed, disease manifestations are most severe in patients with a compromised immune system where the central nervous system becomes involved and fatal bacteremia can

result.[6] Additionally, as these bacteria are able to cross the placenta, listeriosis is a major cause of perinatal and neonatal disease, typically resulting in abortion. Between 2004 and 2005 an incidence rate of 2.5–3.0 cases per million population was reported in the USA with 30% of cases affecting pregnant women.

Brucellosis

This globally distributed zoonosis afflicts various domestic animals but is rare in humans. It is caused by Brucella abortus, B. melitensis or B. suis, which primarily infect cows, goats and pigs, respectively.[7] The bacteria are transmitted to humans via inhalation, through abraded skin or the gastrointestinal tract. Lesions are primarily found within macrophage-rich tissues, especially the spleen and bone marrow. Human brucellosis is characterized by systemic symptoms, particularly undulant fever. Although the disease often remains subclinical, in some patients it becomes chronic, and relapses and remissions may occur.

Lymphogranuloma venerum

Lymphogranuloma venerum, a sexually transmitted disease, is highly prevalent in Africa, Southeast Asia, and South America. It is caused by the L1, L2, and L3 serotypes of C. trachomatis, which are disseminated from the urogenital tract to local lymph nodes and then to the skin. Accordingly, lymphogranuloma venerum is characterized by lymph node swelling and skin lesions that are accompanied by systemic complications.[8]

Melioidosis

Burkholderia pseudomallei is a Gram-negative bacillus and the causative agent of meliodiosis, endemic in Southeast Asia and northern Australia. The disease can be acquired through inhalation, ingestion or through cuts in the skin. Susceptible hosts can suffer abscess formation in multiple organs and in some cases disseminated infection resulting in septic shock accompanied by pneumonia.[9]

Tularemia

This rare zoonosis in humans caused by Francisella tularensis is mainly found in rabbits and has recently gained wider recognition due to its potential for dual use.[10] This Gram-negative bacterium survives in macrophages and primarily causes acute pneumonia as well as sores of the skin, with subsequent involvement of the lymph nodes.

Nongranulomatous infections
Legionnaires' disease or legionellosis

Legionnaires' disease is caused by Legionella pneumophila, an environmental bacterium that persists within amoeba living in water reservoirs (e.g., air-cooling systems), from where it is spread aerogenically.[11] Infection is exacerbated by a compromised immune status. Characteristically, Legionnaires' disease presents as atypical pneumonia associated with general symptoms and is complicated by extrapulmonary infection, renal failure, and lung abscesses.

Chlamydial urethritis, cervicitis, and conjunctivitis

Chlamydia trachomatis serovars D–K remain in epithelial cells of the urogenital tract, causing cervicitis and urethritis. In women, infertility may develop as a result of chronic or recurrent infection. In neonates, congenital infection during birth may result in conjunctivitis and pneumonia. Urogenital infections by chlamydiae occur worldwide and are now considered to be the most common bacterial sexually transmitted disease, with an estimated 100 million new infections occurring annually.

Trachoma

Smear infections of the eye with *C. trachomatis* serovars A, B, and C cause inclusion conjunctivitis. As a consequence of multiple chronic infections and of the resulting immune response, scars develop that eventually injure the cornea, leading to trachoma. Approximately 84 million people are infected with *C. trachomatis* worldwide, 7.6 million of whom suffer visual impairment.[12]

Chlamydia pneumoniae

C. pneumoniae (formerly known as *C. trachomatis* TWAR strain) is the cause of mild respiratory disease in young adults and may cause serious infections in older, more debilitated patients. Atypical pneumonia may also be caused as a result of infection with *C. psittaci*, although this zoonosis, transmitted by birds, is relatively rare.

Typhus

Rickettsia prowazeckii, R. typhi, and *R. tsutsugamushi* cause diseases of varying severity.[13] They are transmitted by arthropods and infect vascular endothelial cells at the site of an insect bite or scratch, causing skin reactions. Subsequently, pathogens are disseminated to the central organs and more general symptoms develop. Globally, typhus is of minor importance.

Rocky Mountain spotted fever, Ehrlichiosis

Rocky Mountain spotted fever is caused by *R. rickettsii*. Infection of the vascular endothelium leads to systemic symptoms and skin manifestations that may be followed by shock and neurological complications.[13] Worldwide, this disease, as well as Mediterranean spotted fever caused by *R. conorii*, is of minor importance; as is probably Ehrlichiosis, a newly emerging zoonosis transmitted by ticks and caused by various *Ehrlichia* spp., mainly *E. chaffeensis*.[14] Disease manifestations include generalized symptoms such as fever and muscle pain.

Bartonella

Bartonella spp. represent Gram-negative faculative intracellular pathogens transmitted by insect vectors such as fleas, sandflies and mosquitoes.[15] The most clinically relevant species are *B. henselae, B. quintana,* and *B. bacilliformis*. *B. henselae* causes cat scratch disease (CSD) resulting in local lymphadenopathy in the lymph node draining the scratch site accompanied by fever, headache and splenomegaly. Oculoglandular involvement (Parinaud's syndrome), encephalopathy, neuroretinitis, or osteomyelitis can occur, although in rare cases. In immunosuppressed patients bacillary angiomatosis and peliosis can occur, characterized by pseudotumoral proliferation of endothelial cells.

Granuloma pathology as hallmark of intracellular bacterial infection

● KEY CONCEPTS

Balance of protection and host pathology in granulomas

- Macrophage activation results in bacterial death (protective)
- Intracellular bacterial killing by "killer molecules" from T cells (protective)
- Lysis of infected macrophages by T cells results in release of bacteria and killing by more effective effector cells (protective) or bacterial dissemination (pathogenic)
- Development of central necrosis in granulomas results in death of tissue and bacteria (protective/pathogenic)
- Fibrotic encapsulation of granuloma results in containment of infection (protective)
- Over-exuberant tissue fibrosis and necrosis (pathogenic)
- Liquefication of central necrotic tissue in granulomas results in bacterial replication, cavity formation, and transmission of bacteria (pathogenic and contagious)

A characteristic feature of many infections caused by intracellular bacteria is the need for tissue remodeling by the host at the site of infection. This produces structures called granulomas, which are the result of an inability to rapidly clear the tissue of intracellular bacteria (Fig. 25.1). The longevity of the granuloma depends directly on the continuous presence of the microbial pathogen, and the lesion generally disappears after its sterile eradication. Granulomas form the focus of the coordinated cross talk between different types of T cells, B cells, and infected and uninfected mononuclear phagocytes (MPs) and dendritic cells (DCs). Even if the immune system fails to completely eliminate bacteria inside the granuloma, the latter performs a protective function by containing microbes within distinct foci and preventing their dissemination. At the same time, the granuloma can be detrimental to the host because it can interfere with physiologic organ functions.[16]

Granulomatous lesions are generally initiated by nonspecific inflammatory signals mediated by bacterial products, chemokines and pro-inflammatory cytokines that are produced by endothelial cells and MPs at the site of infection. Inflammatory phagocytes are attracted to the site of microbial replication and an infiltrative, sometimes exudative, lesion develops. Following the accumulation and activation of increasing numbers of MPs and DCs, this lesion takes a more granulomatous form. A significant number of B cells is also found, which seem to influence granuloma morphology. Once specific T and B cells have been attracted to the lesion, it transforms into a productive granuloma that provides the most appropriate tissue site for antibacterial protection. Here, activation of macrophages by interferon-gamma (IFN-γ) and tumor necrosis factor-alpha (TNF-α) inhibits microbial growth. Cytolytic T cells are able to target bacteria within cells that are not able to efficiently kill bacteria themselves. At the same time, IL-10 produced by Treg cells prevents exacerbated immunopathology associated with this mechanism. Eventually, the granuloma is encapsulated by a fibrotic wall and its center becomes necrotic.[17] Both tissue reactions are primarily protective, the former by promoting bacterial containment and the latter by reducing the nutrient and oxygen supply to the pathogen. The combined effects of chronic macrophage activation, persistence of intracellular bacteria and hypoxia likely lead to enhanced cell death in the center of granulomas resulting

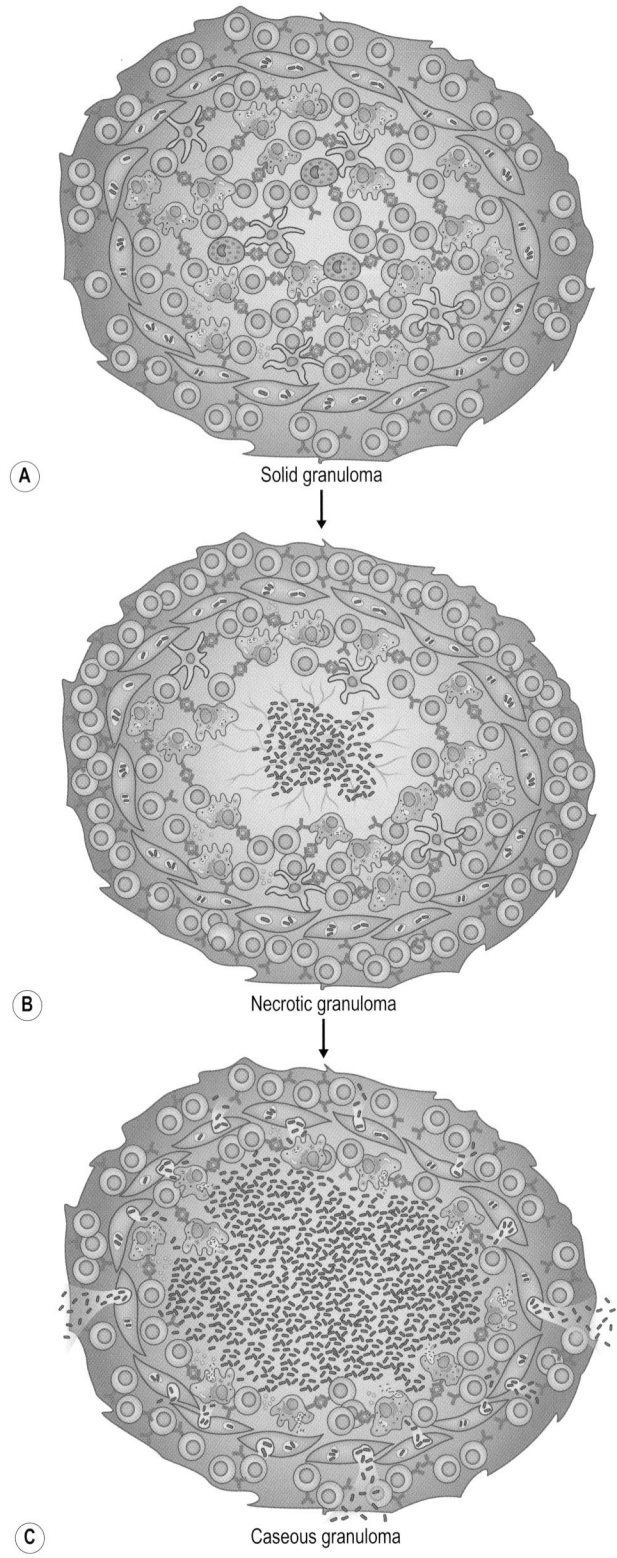

(A) Solid granuloma

(B) Necrotic granuloma

(C) Caseous granuloma

Fig. 25.1 Development of granuloma pathology and implications for TB. This figure depicts three distinct yet continuous stages of granuloma pathology in the lung due to *M. tuberculosis* intracellular infection. (A) Solid granuloma: Composed largely of T cells and infected and uninfected MPs. These granulomas are defined by a lack of central necrosis and likely are representative of an ability to control *M. tuberculosis* replication. (B) Caseous/necrotic granulomas: These structures contain a central region of demarcated necrotic cell death. Bacteria are often detected within the caseous necrotic region and in proximal cells, notably MPs. Since calcified caseous granulomas containing few bacteria have been observed, development of central necrosis may be a consequence of antibacterial mechanisms resulting in sacrifice of host cells to contain infection. (C) Cavity formation: These structures result from inability of caseous granulomas to contain bacterial proliferation. The acellular necrotic region, containing a large number of extracellular bacteria, increases in size and can liquefy and empty into the lung airways, resulting in transmission of viable bacteria via cough. Therefore granuloma formation is central to human-to-human spread of TB. Dissemination of bacteria through the blood stream results in disease manifestation in other organs, such as meninges and urinary bladder.

The interdependence of innate and adaptive immunity in protection against intracellular bacteria

Innate immune mechanisms as first-line defenses

The interaction between host cell and pathogen that defines the intracellular lifestyle consists of a number of different layers. Each layer of interaction mediates a facet of host protection that attempts at eliminating the invading bacterial pathogen. Bacteria are first engulfed, normally by professional phagocytes including tissue macrophages, DCs and PMNs. Binding of a bacterium to certain host receptors leads to the active internalization by professional phagocytes. This process is enhanced by complement components and immunoglobulin, which bind to complement receptors (CRs) and Fc receptors, respectively, on professional phagocytes. In some cases intracellular bacteria can exploit nonprofessional phagocytes, which provide a less hostile environment owing to their inability to mobilize antibacterial effector mechanisms. *Bartonella* spp., uniquely among intracellular bacteria, are also able to enter red blood cells allowing transmission via blood-sucking insect vectors. This represents a particularly advantageous niche as red blood cells lack the machinery to drive the adaptive immune responses required for protection. Vascular endothelial cells, epithelial cells, Schwann cells and hepatocytes are the preferred habitats for *Rickettsia* spp., *C. trachomatis*, *M. leprae*, and *L. monocytogenes*, respectively. These host cells express minimal phagocytic activity, thereby requiring that the bacteria induce their own internalization. The invasion process necessitates tight adhesion to specific cellular receptors that are capable of mediating the uptake process, including members of the integrin and growth factor receptor families. The tight binding of bacteria to these receptors activates the intracellular cytoskeleton to cause macropinocytosis, that is, membrane ruffling, invagination, and finally phagosome formation.[18]

At this juncture the host exploits an ability to discriminate between host and bacterial molecules. This occurs via recognition of conserved molecular motifs by host receptors broadly defined as pattern recognition receptors (PRRs, Table 25.2; Chapter 3). The best-characterized group of PRRs is the so-called Toll-like receptors (TLRs). The TLR system constitutes an innate scanning mechanism for microbial patterns to recognize and distinguish between a wide array of microbes, notably bacteria and viruses. TLRs are present as homo- or hetero-dimers on the plasma membrane or within endosomes/phagosomes.[19] TLR ligands of

in the formation of caseum. Development of caseum may also favor the local replication of facultative intracellular bacteria in the cellular detritus, as well as microbial dissemination to distant tissue sites and to the environment to transmit infection.

Table 25.2 Pattern recognition receptors (PRRs) involved in detection of intracellular bacteria

PRR	Location	Ligand
Toll-like receptors		
TLR1	Plasma membrane	Triacyl lipoprotein
TLR2	Plasma membrane	PGA, porins, LAM
TLR4	Plasma membrane	LPS
TLR5	Plasma membrane	Flagellin
TLR6	Plasma membrane	Diacyl lipoprotein
TLR7(human TLR8)	Endosome	ssRNA
TLR9	Endosome	CpG DNA
Scavenger receptors		
SR-A	Plasma membrane	LPS, LTA, CpG DNA, proteins
MARCO	Plasma membrane	LPS, proteins
CD36	Plasma membrane	Diacyl lipoprotein
LOX-1	Plasma membrane	Protein
SREC	Plasma membrane	Protein
C-type lectins		
DC-SIGN	Plasma membrane	LPS, ManLAM, capsular polysaccharide
MINCLE	Plasma membrane	Mycobacterial cord factor: TDM
NOD-like receptors		
NOD1	Cytoplasm	D-glutamyl-meso-diaminopimelic acid
NOD2	Cytoplasm	MDP
NLRP1	Cytoplasm	MDP
NLRP3	Cytoplasm	RNA, LPS, LTA, MDP
NLRC4	Cytoplasm	Flagellin
Naip5	Cytoplasm	Flagellin

We omit PRRs (i.e., TLR3, which binds viral-produced double-stranded RNA) not classically associated with intracellular bacteria. Toll-like receptors (TLR); peptidoglycans (PGA); lipoarabinomannan (LAM); mannose lipoarabinomannan (ManLAM); lipopolysaccharide (LPS); scavenger receptors (SR); lipteichoic acid (LTA); trehalose dimycolate (TDM); dendritic cell-specific intercellular adhesion molecule-3-grabbing nonintegrin (DC-SIGN); macrophage-inducible C-type lectin (MINCLE); muramyl dipeptide (MDP); nucleotide-binding domain (NOD); NOD-like receptors (NLR); single stranded RNA (ssRNA); cytosine-phosphatidyl-guanine DNA (CpGDNA); macrophage receptor with collagenous structure (MARCO); cluster of differentiation 36 (CD36); lipoxygenase1 (LOX-1); scavenger receptor expressed by endothelial cell-l (SREC).

bacterial origin comprise di- and tri-acylic lipoproteins, LPSs, and flagellin, which are recognized by TLR-2/6, TLR-2/1, TLR-4/4, or TLR-5/5, respectively. The vast array of mycobacterial cell wall lipids such as lipoarabinomannan (LAM), trehalose dimycolate (TDM), and phosphatidyl inositol mannosides (PIMs) bind either TLR-2 or TLR-4. Lipoteichoic acid (LTA) of Gram-positive bacteria is recognized by TLR-2. TLR-9 binds low methylated bacterial DNA containing CpG motifs within endosomes.

Scavenger receptors and C-type lectins are also considered PRRs and function at the cell membrane.[20] Scavenger receptors were first defined by their ability to transport modified forms of low density lipoproteins inside cells indicating their ability to also interact with host molecules. However, receptors such as SR-A, MARCO, CD36, LOX-1, and SREC can bind a wide array of bacterial molecules such as lipids, CpG DNA and protein (see Table 25.2 for binding specificities). SR-A is important for clearance of extracellular bacteria from the spleen and liver. MARCO expressed on alveolar macrophages is implicated in clearance of pneumococcal bacteria preventing pneumonia. C-type lectins are similarly membrane-expressed and include DC-specific intercellular adhesion molecule-3-grabbing nonintegrin (DC-SIGN), mannose receptor, dectin-1, dectin-2, which chiefly recognize fungal components and MINCLE, which recognizes trehalose dimycolate (TDM), the cord factor of *M. tuberculosis*.

The cellular cyoplasm is monitored for presence of molecules of bacterial origin by a further group of PRRs, the nucleotide oligomerization domain protein-like receptors (NLRs). These molecules are characterized by presence of a nucelotide-binding domain and leucine-rich repeat motifs. Molecules from this group recognizing bacterial components are nucleotide-binding oligomerization domain (NOD)-containing proteins NOD1 and NOD2, NOD-like receptors (NLR)P1, NLRP3, and Naip5 (see Table 25.2).[21]

It has been suggested that, whereas scavenger receptors and C-type lectins are required to bind and internalize the bacillus, it is the TLRs that discriminate between the pathogens and initiate the necessary intracellular signaling events. It should, however, be noted that intracellular signaling events can also be triggered by other interactions such as ligand binding to macrophage mannose receptor (MMR), dectin 1, or DC-SIGN.[21] Far from a one-ligand, one-receptor binary mechanism of sensing and signaling, PRRs often collaborate to produce multiprotein complexes. CD14, MD2 and TLR4 collaborate for LPS sensing and signaling. Similarly, MARCO and TLR2 synergize to recognize TDM. To allow signaling these complexes interact with adaptor proteins containing immunoreceptor tyrosine-based activation motif (ITAM)-like or Toll/interleukin-1 receptor (TIR) domain motifs. TLR signaling occurs via the adaptor proteins MyD88, TIRAP/Mal and Trif. These molecules then orchestrate a downstream signaling cascade culminating in induced patterns of gene transcription. The cytoplasmic NLRs lead to activation of the multiprotein complex called the inflammasome leading to cleavage of pro-IL-1ß and pro-IL-18 to their active forms. Activation of other members of this group, NOD1 and NOD2 results in inflammatory cytokine secretion. This could indicate that presence of bacterial molecules in the cytoplasm may require a specific cytokine-mediated response. PRRs are also receptive to certain endogenous "danger" signals produced by tissues undergoing stress, damage or abundant cell death. These include endogenous heat shock proteins, host nucleotides and the chromatin component HMGB1. Therefore, PRRs mediate signals not only emanating from intracellular bacteria but also the cellular detritus resulting from infection. Understanding how these two inputs mesh to produce a coherent disease-specific output remains an exciting challenge for future research.

Ultimately, the culmination of PRR collaborative sensing and signaling is the induction of inflammatory genes that results in mobilization of the adaptive immune response. These include cytokines that act both locally and systemically and are important mediators of protection against intracellular bacteria via specific signaling through engagement of host cell surface receptors. Such engagement both mobilizes critical mechanisms of host protection and orchestrates the mobilization of adaptive immune responses.

Cytokines as mediators of defense against intracellular bacteria

We have already mentioned the range of cytokines produced by the signaling mechanisms that result from engagement of PRRs. These serve by both enhancing intracellular mechanisms of bacterial killing and mobilizing adaptive immune mechanisms, representing the next layer of host defense. Because these responses allow an amplification of the potency of the initial innate immune responses they must be carefully regulated by the host to prevent extensive tissue pathology. In fact, we might view the development of a granuloma as the sequela of a balance between bacterial killing mechanisms orchestrated by adaptive immunity and the need to control tissue pathology. On initiation of signaling cascades by PRRs, such cytokines are ultimately produced by multiple cell types including adaptive T cells, B cells, innate T cells, MPs, DCs, PMNs and even epithelial cells. These small molecules can act locally and systemically to directly signal cells, to produce antibacterial molecules, to combat intracellular infection and both to increase numbers of immune cells and to direct the composition of the cellular infiltrate. We will first consider the hierarchy by which these cytokines act in the controlling of intracellular bacterial infection and the antibacterial mechanisms they augment. We will then return to the generation and regulation of the cells that produce them.

●KEY CONCEPTS

T-cell-mediated mechanisms underlying protection

- IFN-γ- and TNF-α-mediated activation of ability of phagocytes to kill bacteria by means of:
  - ROI and RNI
  - Delivery of lysosomal hydrolytic enzymes and antimicrobial peptides to the bacteria-containing phagosome
  - Autophagy
  - Formation and maintenance of granulomas
- T-cell-mediated response controls but does not eradicate the pathogen

---

IFN-γ, TNF-α, IL-12, and IL-18

By far, the cytokine with the clearest demonstrable potency against intracellular bacteria is IFN-γ. Extensive studies on the activation of antibacterial effector functions in macrophages have revealed a central role for IFN-γ.[22] Accordingly, IFN-γ neutralization with antibodies, or deletion of the IFN-γ gene by homologous recombination, markedly exacerbates infectious diseases such as listeriosis, TB, or typhoid in experimental animals. Similarly, the action of TNF-α appears to augment IFN-γ and is also important in control of intracellular infection. This has been demonstrated in humans through use of blocking of TNF-α by antibodies as antiinflammatory therapy. Such treatments can activate clinical TB in individuals harboring a latent infection. A central antimicrobial mechanism stimulated by IFN-γ and TNF-α is production of reactive nitrogen intermediates (RNIs) via the induction of NOS2 and reactive oxygen intermediates (ROIs) via activation of NADPH-dependent oxidative burst. They also synergize to augment autophagy, a mechanism that plays an increasingly appreciated role in host cell defense. It

is now clear that the production of IFN-γ depends on prior activation by IL-12 and/or -18. IL-12 in concert with TNF-α induces a cytokine loop resulting in the production of IFN-γ, which sustains the production of IL-12 and -18. The importance of these cytokines in host defense against intracellular pathogens has been demonstrated using gene knockout mice. These mice exhibit overwhelming susceptibility to infections with mycobacteria, salmonellae, and listeriae as a direct result of the lack of macrophage activation mediated by IFN-γ. Recently these observations have been extended to humans. Patients with mutations in genes for the IFN-γ receptor or IL-12 and its receptor are highly susceptible to infections with salmonellae and mycobacteria, including BCG.[23]

Many nonprofessional phagocytes also respond to IFN-γ causing some microbial growth inhibition. IFN-γ also induces two families of guanidine triphosphatases, which appear to confer resistance against intracellular bacteria. These two groups are p47 immunity-related GTPases (p47 IRGs) and p65 guanylate-binding proteins (p65 GBPs). Mice deficient in p47 IRG, LRG-47, are highly susceptible to *M. tuberculosis*.[24] p65 GBPs contribute to elimination of mycobacteria and listeriae by potentiating intraphagosomal oxidative mechanisms, antimicrobial peptides and autophagy effectors (see below).[25]

Pro-inflammatory cytokines and phagocyte attraction

The recruitment of more phagocytes to the site of infection represents a vital process in the resolution of infection. Phagocyte recruitment is achieved via the secretion by macrophages and endothelial cells of cytokines of the IL-1 family, TNF-α, IL-6, and chemokines. Signaling via members of the IL-1 family is considered closely related to that of the TLRs due to close homology of the cytoplasmic domains of TLRs and IL-1 family receptors. The most studied member of the family is IL-1β, which in synergy with chemokines and TNF-α increases the expression of adhesion molecules on the vascular epithelium and which promotes the extravasation of the inflammatory infiltrate into infected tissues. Chemokines are a family of structurally-related proteins (Chapter 10). The positions of the first two cysteine residues in the protein sequence have been used to divide chemokines into four subfamilies: CC (MIP-1β, MCP-1, -2, -3), CXC (MIP-2, IL-8), C (lymphotactin) and CX3C chemokines (fractalkine), where C represents cysteine and X represents any amino acid other than cysteine. These molecules are critical in controlling the migration of PMNs (IL-8) and monocytes (MCP-1) from the bloodstream to infected tissue.[26] Recently the role of chemokines in intracellular infections has been increasingly appreciated, e.g., with mice lacking the receptor for MCP-1 being deficient in their ability to clear listeria infection.

Cytokine-induced host-protective cellular mechanisms

RNIs and ROIs

Activation of a membrane-bound NADPH oxidase by stimulation with IFN-γ or IgG initiates an oxidative burst that generates the ROI, O^-_2, H_2O_2, OH^-, $^1O_2$, and •OH radical (Table 25.3).[27] In human PMNs and blood monocytes that possess myeloperoxidase, ROI activity is further augmented by the formation of hypochlorous acid. Oxidation and/or chlorination of bacterial lipids and proteins results in bacterial killing. The importance of ROIs in antibacterial defense is underlined by recurrent infections in patients whose phagocytes fail to generate an oxidative burst (Chapter 21). NOS2 is an inducible cytosolic enzyme in

Table 25.3 Antibacterial effector mechanisms of activated macrophages and corresponding microbial evasion strategies

Macrophage effector mechanism	Microbial evasion strategy
Production of reactive oxygen intermediates (ROI)	Uptake via complement receptors; Production of ROI detoxifying molecules (superoxide dismutase, catalase); Bacterial ROI scavengers (phenolic glycolipids, sulfatides, lipoarabinomannans)
Production of reactive nitrogen intermediates	Inhibition of phagosome maturation via blockage of H^+ ATP pump, indirect effect of ROI detoxifying molecules
Autophagy, intraphagolysosomal killing	Egression into cytoplasm; Resistant cell wall
Phagosomal acidification, phagosome–lysosome fusion	Inhibition of phagosome maturation
Defensins	Modification of cell wall lipid A to resist action of defensins
Reduced iron supply (transferrin receptor downregulation, lipocalins)	Expression of microbial siderophores to increase iron uptake
Tryptophan degradation	Upregulation of bacterial tryptophan synthesis

professional phagocytes that delivers NO to the phagolysosome harboring bacteria while consuming O_2 and L-arginine. NO is further oxidized to NO^-_2 and NO^-_3. Nitrification and/or oxidation then functions by inactivating bacterial molecules needed for bacterial growth.[28] The formation of •NO is catalyzed by NOS2, which is promoted by both immunological stimuli such as IFN-γ and TNF, and microbial products such as LPSs, lipoteichoic acid, and mycobacterial lipids. RNIs exert their bactericidal activity by destroying iron-/sulfur-containing reactive centers of bacterial enzymes, and by synergizing with ROIs to form highly reactive peroxynitrite ($ONOO^-$). A central role for NOS2 in protection against intracellular bacteria is well established in murine models of infection. Whether NOS2 plays such a similarly central role in humans is still unclear.

Apoptosis and autophagy

Apoptosis is a highly regulated form of cell death that plays a central role in control of cell turnover, a vital process for tissue homeostasis.[29,30] Macrophage apoptosis also constitutes a defense mechanism, allowing removal of phagocytes containing intracellular bacteria without the need to generate significant inflammation. Apoptosis, in contrast to cellular necrosis, results in cell death without permeabilization of the host cell membrane. The process can be triggered by TNF-α signaling and augmented by IFN-γ, resulting in activation of cellular caspases, mitochondrial membrane permeability and cytochrome c release. These processes result in cellular disintegration and production of apoptotic bodies that are engulfed and digested by neighboring phagocytic cells. An indication of the key importance of apoptosis in control of intracellular infection comes from the fact that *M. tuberculosis* inhibits apoptosis, allowing protection of the intracellular niche for bacterial proliferation.

Autophagy, a process common to all cells, delivers cytoplasmic biomass to lysosomal structures for degradation. Until recently, autophagy was considered a mechanism for removal of dysfunctional or damaged cellular organelles. However, it is becoming appreciated as a mechanism critical for defense against intracellular bacteria. This is underlined by the fact that IFN-γ and engagement of PRRs enhance autophagy. Increased autophagy allows sequestration of intracellular bacteria in a specialized double-membraned autophagosome to which lysosomal contents are delivered. The resulting autolysosome focuses antimicrobial mechanisms to kill and digest the bacteria. Autophagy has been shown to occur after infection of macrophages with *M. tuberculosis* and defects in autophagic mechanisms are consistent with TB susceptibility in humans.

Nutrient deprivation

Deprivation of required nutrients appears to be an obvious strategy for microbial killing, yet it seems to be employed rarely, with restricted tryptophan supply being the best-known example. Tryptophan degradation is achieved by the enzyme indolamine 2,3-deoxygenase (IDO), which degrades tryptophan to kynurenine (Table 25.3). This reaction is induced by IFN-γ in both MPs and IFN-γ-responsive nonprofessional phagocytes and inhibits the growth of *C. psittaci* and *C. trachomatis* inside human macrophages and epithelial cells.[31]

Production and regulation of antimicrobial peptides

Defensins are small lysosomal polypeptides that are microbicidal at basic pH and are particularly abundant in phagocytes.[32] Many of these compounds have microbicidal activity against intracellular bacteria, particularly granulysin, which is present in the granules of human natural killer (NK) cells and cytolytic T cells. This molecule kills a number of pathogens *in vitro*, including *L. monocytogenes*, *S. enteric* serovar Typhimurium, and *M. tuberculosis*.[33] Another antimicrobial peptide, cathelicidin, is regulated by vitamin D in a TLR-2-dependent manner. This mechanism operates uniquely in human cells where IL-15 signaling of *M. tuberculosis*-infected macrophages upregulates vitamin D receptor expression resulting in increased cathelicidin expression.[34] Cathelicidin is cleaved to produce an antimicrobial peptide, which controls intracellular *M. tuberculosis*. The exact mechanism that leads to intracellular microbial killing by antimicrobial peptides remains to be established.

Lysis, tissue damage, and bacterial killing

Cytolytic phenomena generally accompany infections with intracellular bacteria. Cells with cytolytic potential that are activated during such infections include PMNs, blood monocytes, NK cells, and T cells.[35-37] PMNs and blood monocytes that are attracted to foci of bacterial growth nonspecifically destroy the surrounding tissue, primarily by secreting hydrolytic enzymes, including elastase, collagenase, and gelatinase. These enzymes affect the integrity of both cells and extracellular matrix. They are at least partially responsible for the exudative character of early lesions. NK cells and T cells express nonspecific or specific cytolytic activity, respectively, further contributing to tissue damage. Tissue damage is generally localized to the site of microbial implantation or persistence, for example, the granuloma. Cytolytic T cells probably act at advanced stages of infection and contribute to the liquefaction that follows the reactivation of dormant bacteria. Without doubt, the tissue damage caused by cytolytic mechanisms significantly determines the pathology of an infectious disease. Furthermore, the release of bacteria contained within distinct foci may promote the dissemination of pathogens to distant sites. However, cytolytic mechanisms are required for protection against microbes living in protective niches, such as deactivated macrophages or epithelial cells. Transmission of bacteria from an incapacitated cell to a highly activated professional phagocyte could significantly improve bacterial elimination. Finally, cytolytic T cells may also attack intracellular microbes. Once the target cells have been lysed by perforin, bacteria can be killed by means of a specific molecule, granulysin, which is contained within the granules of the cytotoxic T cell.

Evasion from, interference with, and resistance to microbial killing

Strategies against toxic effector molecules

Many intracellular bacteria have exploited successful strategies against macrophage effector molecules (Table 25.3). One mechanism of evasion is determined by the receptor that is used for pathogen entry into the host cell. Internalization via CRs inhibits the production of IL-12, a cytokine critical in facilitating macrophage activation.[38] Engulfment by this receptor also bypasses activation of the oxidative burst, thereby avoiding ROI production. Similarly, engaging MMR and DC-SIGN for uptake triggers secretion of the suppressive cytokines IL-10 and TGF-β. Several intracellular bacteria also produce ROI detoxifiers, including superoxide dismutase and catalase, which nullify O_2 and H_2O_2, respectively. Finally, a number of small bacterial products, such as the phenolic glycolipid and LAM of mycobacteria, scavenge ROIs. Many of the strategies used to counteract the effects of ROIs also overlap in their effects on RNI. A modification of lipid A renders Gram-negative bacteria, including salmonellae, resistant to the effects of host antimicrobial peptides.[32]

Intraphagosomal survival

Inhibition of phagolysosome fusion represents a major intracellular survival strategy for a number of intracellular bacteria, including *M. tuberculosis*, *Francisella* spp., *Brucella* spp., and *L. monocytogenes* (Fig. 25.2). After engulfment, these pathogens manipulate the endocytic fate of the phagosome that contains them. This is achieved in part by manipulation of Rab GTPases, proteins required for normal endocytic trafficking, positioned in the phagosome membrane.[39] The mycobacteria-containing phagosome acquires Rab5 but not the late endosomal markers Lamp-1, -2 and Rab7, enabling arrest of maturation of this compartment at an early endosomal stage. This compartment does not acidify, due in part to a paucity of vacuolar H^+ ATPase; at the same time, it exchanges molecules with the plasma membrane such as the transferrin receptor to access iron.[40] Activation of macrophages with IFN-γ restores maturation of the mycobacterial phagosome, resulting in a drop in mycobacterial viability. Francisella and brucella are engulfed by phagosomes that acquire the early endosomal markers EEA1 and Rab5.[41] The franciscella-containing vacuole acquires late endosomal markers but escapes into the cytosol by perforating the late endosomal membrane. After a transient phagosomal stage, brucellae enter compartments enclosed by endoplasmic reticulum (ER) membranes to escape delivery to phagolysosomes.

Escape into cytoplasm

A successful strategy for survival inside activated macrophages is egression from the phagosome into the cytoplasm, which has been exploited by *L. monocytogenes* and the various pathogenic *Rickettsia* spp. (Fig. 25.2).[42,43] This has the advantage of both avoiding the cellular defense mechanisms within the phagosome and providing the bacteria with a nutrient-rich environment. *L. monocytogenes* possesses several virulence factors to facilitate its escape from the phagolysosome, a pore-forming hemolysin (listeriolysin, LLO) that acts together with

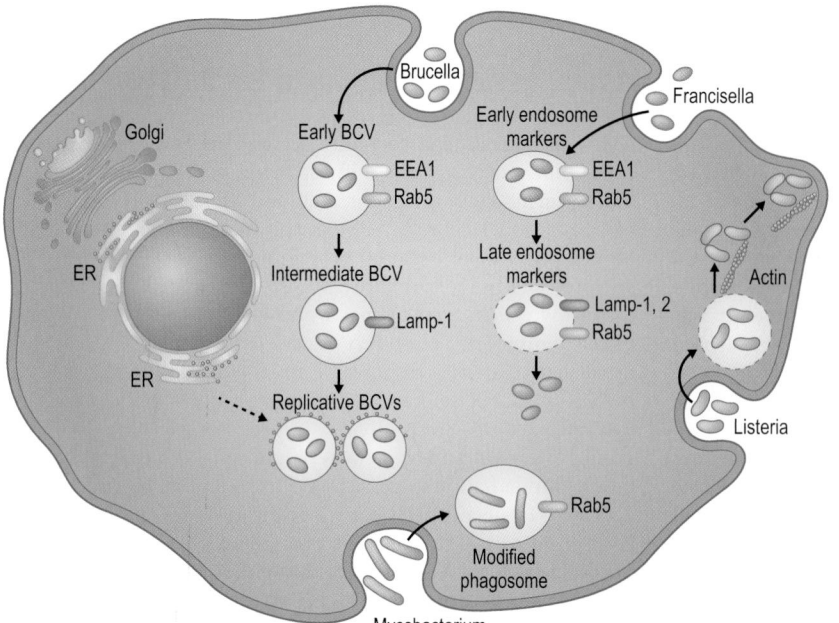

Fig. 25.2 Inhibition of phagolysosome fusion represents a major survival strategy for a number of intracellular bacteria, including *M. tuberculosis*, *Francisella* spp., *Brucella* spp., and *L. monocytogenes*. The mycobacteria-containing phagosome acquires Rab5 but not the late endosomal markers Lamp-1 and 2, enabling arrest of maturation of this compartment at an early endosomal stage. *Francisella* spp. and *Brucella* spp. are engulfed by phagosomes that acquire the early endosomal markers EEA1 and Rab5. The francisella-containing vacuole acquires late endosomal markers but escapes into the cytosol by perforating the late endosomal membrane. A similar strategy is adopted by *L. monocytogenes*. After a transient phagosomal stage, brucellae enter compartments enclosed by endoplasmic reticulum (ER) membranes to escape delivery to phagolysosomes. Brucella-containing vacuole (BCV).

a metalloproteinase, a lecithinase, and two phospholipases to efficiently promote the rupture of the phagosomal membrane, as well as spreading to other cells. Recent data indicate that *M. tuberculosis* and *M. leprae* can also egress from the phagosome into the cytoplasm of macrophages and DCs.[44] This behavior is dependent on secreted bacterial virulence factors and may contribute to increased levels of cell death. These bacterial virulence factors are not expressed by BCG, which hence does not show this phenotype.

Cell-to-cell spreading

For a bacterial pathogen that is very well adapted to the intracellular milieu and vulnerable to extracellular defense mechanisms, it is highly desirable to remain within host cells.[42] Yet once a sufficiently large number of bacteria have proliferated, the original cell dies and bacteria are released into the extracellular space. To avoid this fate some intracellular bacteria have developed mechanisms that allow their direct spreading to other cells. *L. monocytogenes* induces polar actin polymerization by means of a surface protein ActA. A polymerized actin tail is formed that pushes the bacteria through the cell, forcing the host cell membrane to protrude into a neighboring cell. This cell engulfs this protrusion, and eventually both the new membrane and the host membrane are dissolved by phospholipases.

T lymphocytes as specific mediators of acquired resistance

Whereas activated macrophages act as the nonspecific executors, T lymphocytes are the specific mediators of acquired resistance against intracellular bacteria. The dramatic increase in the incidence of TB and other intracellular bacterial infections in AIDS patients illustrates the central role of T lymphocytes. For instance, at least 0.5 million individuals are co-infected with HIV and *M. tuberculosis* and HIV increases the risk of developing TB by several orders of magnitude. At the site of microbial growth, T lymphocytes not only initiate the most potent defense mechanisms available, they also focus this response to the site of encounter, thus minimizing collateral damage to the host. Although protective T-cell responses are multifactorial, they can be reduced to a few principal mechanisms (Fig. 25.3).

T cells inevitably also produce pathology, and the pathogenesis of infections with intracellular bacteria is significantly determined by T cells. It is therefore important that the T-cell response be tightly controlled and downregulated when necessary. Regulatory mechanisms, including Treg cells, are in place to limit immunopathology.[16]

Protective immunity involves conventionally defined T-cell sets, CD4 αβ T cells, and CD8 αβ T cells, as well as unconventional T cells, such as γδ T cells, CD1-restricted αβ T cells, and T cells that recognize antigen in the context of other nonclassical MHC class I molecules (Fig. 25.3). Although these T-cell sets perform different tasks, substantial redundancy exists. Furthermore, these T-cell populations act in a coordinated way in close interaction with other leukocytes, such as NK cells. Depending on the etiologic agent and the stage of disease, the relative contribution of the different T-cell subsets to acquired resistance may vary. The conventional αβ T cells make up more than 90% and γδ T cells less than 10% of all lymphocytes in the blood and peripheral organs of humans and mice. However, γδ T cells represent a significant proportion of the intraepithelial lymphocytes in mucosal tissues, suggesting a particular role at this important port of microbial entry (Chapter 19). Implication of T-cell populations is primarily derived from studies with experimental animals and immunohistological *in-situ* hybridization studies of lesions.

CD4 T cells

Overwhelming evidence, including experimental animal studies, their abundance in "protective" granulomas of patients suffering from bacterial infections, and the high prevalence of disease caused by intracellular bacteria in CD4 T-cell-deficient AIDS patients, supports the important role of CD4 T cells in immune defense against intracellular bacteria. Such T cells recognize antigenic peptides in the context of MHC class II molecules. MHC II molecules pick up antigenic peptides within the endosomal system (Fig. 25.3). Thus, antigens from all intracellular bacteria, even those that evade the phagosome at later stages, are accessible to processing and presentation through the MHC class II pathway. A potential problem with CD4 T cell-mediated defense mechanisms relates to their failure to recognize infected cells that are constitutively MHC class II negative. These include endothelial cells, epithelial cells, hepatocytes, and Schwann cells, the potential targets of *Rickettsia* spp., *C. trachomatis*, *L. monocytogenes*, and *M. leprae*, respectively.

The CD4 T-cell population can be further subdivided into distinct subsets, according to their pattern of cytokine production (Chapter 16). The first two subsets were discovered over 20 years ago and are identified in both mouse and humans; Th1 cells which overwhelmingly produce IFN-γ and IL-2, and Th2 cells which produce IL-4, -5, and -13. The Th1 subset can also be defined on the basis of the Tbet transcription factor, while Th2 classification is consistent with expression of the transcription factor GATA-3.[45] It is tempting to assume that different T-cell subsets have emerged to combat different pathogens. IL-2 and IFN-γ from Th1 cells promote cell-mediated immunity, characterized by macrophage activation, stimulation of cytolytic CD8 T cells, and the production of opsonizing IgG antibodies. In contrast, Th2 cells control the differentiation of B cells into plasma cells and promote Ig class switching. NK T cells that arise rapidly after infection to secrete both IFN-γ and IL-4 could be instrumental in determining the emergent T-cell subset during an infection.[43]

More recently, a further distinct Th-cell population, termed Th17, was identified that produces IL-17, IL-22, and GM-CSF. Th17 cells are also characterized by expression of the transcription factor RORγt. Cytokines of the IL-17 family are strong inducers of granulopoiesis, of pro-inflammatory mediators such as IL-6, and of the chemokines CXCL1, CXCL8, and CXCL6, which attract neutrophilic and eosinophilic granulocytes and prolong their survival.[46] Th17 cells, too, have limited importance for protection in murine models against primary infection with mycobacteria, salmonellae and listeriae. However, Th17 cells can drive more rapid Th1 responses against pulmonary TB in mice after vaccination, resulting in enhanced protection. And recent work demonstrated IL-17 was required for optimally protective Th1 responses during murine *F. tularensis* infection.[47]

Despite the convenience of defining T-cell populations in terms of subsets, recent evidence suggests considerable plasticity in cytokine production by T cells. This was first suggested by demonstration that all subsets could produce the T-cell regulator cytokine IL-10, which regulates potency of T-cell responses

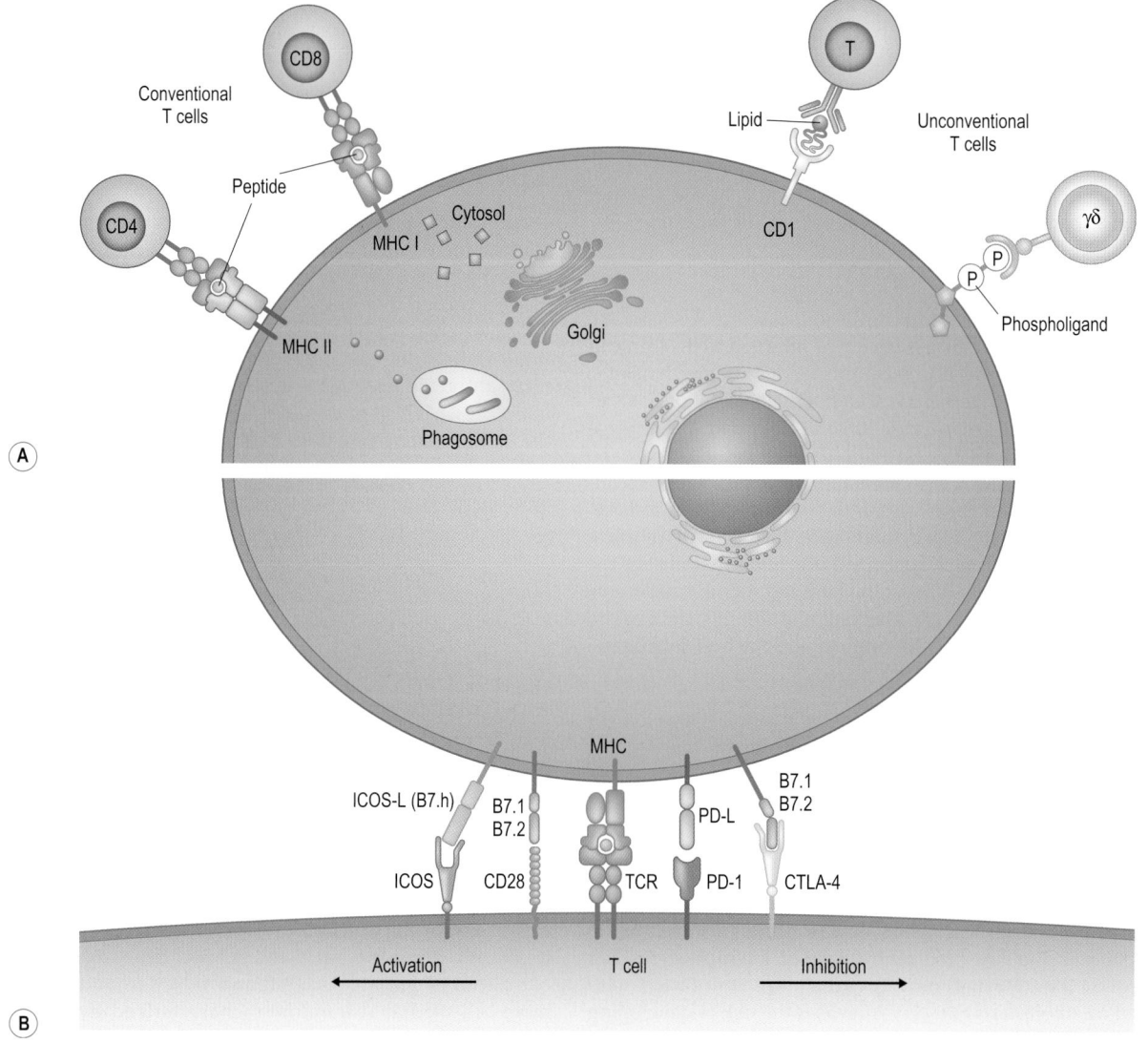

Fig. 25.3 T-cell stimulation during intracellular infection. Recognition of bacterial antigen by T cells (A). Antigen originating from intracellular bacteria is presented to CD4 and CD8 T cells. Unconventional T cells comprising γδ T cells and CD1-restricted T cells are also activated. Human γδ T cells recognize small molecules containing pyrophosphate residues; CD1-restricted T cells recognize glycolipids in the context of CD1 molecules. (B) CD4 T cells can be subdivided into different T helper (Th) cells according to their cytokine expression pattern. Th1 cells are critical for protection against intracellular bacteria. They typically produce interferon-gamma (IFN-γ), tumor necrosis factor-alpha (TNF-α), lymphotoxin (LT), interleukin (IL)-2, and granulocyte-macrophage colony-stimulating factor (GM-CSF). Th2 cells stimulate humoral immune responses via secretion of IL-4 and -5. Other cytokines produced by Th2 cells include IL-13 and -25. Th17 cells produce IL-6, -17, -21, and -22, which probably contribute to early protection. Regulatory T cells (Treg) produce tumor growth factor beta (TGF-β) and IL-10, which suppress immune responses. See Chapters 9 and 12 for details.
Modified from Kaufmann SHE, Parida SK, Tuberculosis in Africa: Learning from Pathogenesis for Biomarker Identification, Cell Host & Microbe, 2008: (4)3, 219-228, with permission of Elsevier.

to limit host collateral damage during immune responses. IL-10 expression might be an intrinsic control mechanism common to all T cells. However, reduction in T-cell potency also favors chronic intracellular bacterial infection. T-cell subsets may acquire the ability to produce additional cytokines by expression of additional transcription factors or by remodeling chromatin structure.[48] Future research will surely redefine T-cell behavior during intracellular bacterial infection.

CD8 T cells

Infection of mice deficient in specific T-cell subsets has conclusively demonstrated a role for CD8 T cells during listeriosis and TB.[49] Furthermore, CD8 effector T cells have been identified in granulomas of tuberculoid leprosy patients that contain

minute numbers of bacteria. The cytolytic potential of these T cells can serve two roles in infection of intracellular bacteria, namely target cell killing or the lysis of cells that are unable to control the infection, thus releasing the bacteria for phagocytosis by more activated cells. In humans CD8-mediated killing is cell contact-dependent and based on production of perforin, granzymes, and granulysin (Chapter 17).[37] Finally, CD8 T cells are also a potent source of IFN-γ and TNF-α, thus contributing to direct activation of infected macrophages to enhance protective mechanisms (Fig. 25.3).

CD8 T cells recognize antigenic peptides in the context of MHC class I gene products, which are responsible for presentation of antigens residing in the cytosol (Chapter 6). Initially, therefore, it was mysterious how CD8 T cells were stimulated by intracellular bacteria, which were thought to have a uniquely restricted phagosomal residence. However, with the knowledge that many intracellular bacteria egress into the cytoplasm, one major mechanism for MHC class I processing became obvious: proteins secreted by bacteria in the cytoplasm undergo antigen processing and presentation similarly to newly synthesized host proteins.[50] Yet, alternative contact points for MHC class I molecules and bacterial peptides should exist. Cross-presentation by noninfected APCs of antigens engulfed within apoptotic blebs from infected cells represents a critical pathway to induce CD8 T cells by phagosomal bacteria (see below). One major advantage of CD8 T cells over CD4 T cells is their recognition of antigen bound by MHC class I gene products, which are expressed by almost all host cells. Thus, CD8 T cells recognize professional and nonprofessional phagocytes equally well.

Cross-presentation

Many intracellular bacteria such as chlamydiae and rickettsiae dwell within nonprofessional APCs, which do not express MHC class II constitutively at high levels and lack the expression of co-stimulatory molecules.[51] Those living inside professional APCs, such as salmonellae and mycobacteria, interfere with expression of antigen-presenting molecules in general, thereby inhibiting T-cell activation. Those intracellular bacteria that do not egress from the phagosome are secluded from the classical cytoplasmic MHC class I processing pathway. Despite this, all intracellular bacteria are able to activate CD4 and CD8 T cells, suggesting that alternative mechanisms of T-cell priming must be associated with the intracellular lifestyle. Cross-presentation by noninfected APCs, at least in TB and salmonellosis, could represent one such mechanism.[52] Noninfected cells engulf bacterial antigens associated with vesicles produced by apoptotic cells. Apoptosis as a prerequisite for this pathway is induced by many intracellular bacteria including salmonellae, mycobacteria, and listeriae. This cross-presentation pathway in infections with intracellular bacteria adds an essential function to the physiological role of apoptosis in maintenance of tissue integrity and growth.

γδ T cells

The relevance of the γδ T-cell set to bacterial immunity is incompletely understood. γδ T cells produce cytokines and are cytolytic; hence they cover a functional spectrum similar to that of their αβ T-cell counterparts. Although the genetic restriction of antigen recognition by γδ T cells remains elusive, it is clear that they are less fastidious than αβ T cells in this respect. Hence, in principle, all infected host cells are potential targets for γδ T cells. Experimental mouse studies revealed the early accumulation of γδ T cells at sites of bacterial deposition. γδ T cells have also been identified in certain forms of disease, including tuberculous lymphadenitis and leprosy lesions during reactional stages. Because of their less demanding activation and antigen recognition requirements, γδ T cells may fill a gap between nonspecific resistance and the more specific αβ T-cell response. Furthermore, transient participation of γδ T cells in protection and a unique requirement for γδ T cells in granuloma formation have been described for experimental listeriosis and TB in mice. In mice, antigens recognized by γδ T cells appear to comprise heat shock protein-derived peptides presented by nonpolymorphic MHC class I-like molecules. In contrast, human γδ T cells respond to nonpeptidic phosphorylated metabolites of the isoprenoid pathway of bacterial and host origin.[53] In addition, γδ T cells

constitute a major source of IL-17 early in primary *M. tuberculosis* infection of mice, perhaps until Th1 cells can take over after generation of T-cell immunity.

T cells controlled by CD1 molecules

CD1 comprise a group of nonpolymorphic MHC-related molecules that can present glycolipid antigens to unconventional T cells. They are divided into two groups. In humans, T cells that respond to group I CD1 molecules, that is, CD1a, b and c, are either CD4−/CD8− or CD8+ and express the αβ TCR. These cells can respond to a variety of microbial glycolipids, including LAM, PIMs, mycolic acids, sulfatides, sulfoglycolipids, and lipopeptides.[54] Group I CD1 molecules are absent in mice. Upon antigen stimulation respective T cells can proliferate and secrete IFN-γ, and lyse macrophages infected with mycobacteria. The group II CD1 molecule CD1d is present in both humans and mice and controls development of NKT cells that express both the NK cell marker NK1.1 and an invariant evolutionarily conserved TCR. Upon antigen activation these T cells rapidly produce cytokines and are capable of producing both IL-4 and IFN-γ. As bacterial antigens recognized by NKT cells, PIMs from mycobacteria and glycosphingolipids from *Ehrlichia* and *Sphingomonas* species have been identified. Recent data also suggest that NKT cells can respond to host endogenous lysosomal lipids loaded onto CD1d.[55] These lipids accumulate due to a temporary downregulation of the enzyme α-galactosidase A, mediated through TLR signaling, during intracellular infection. The α-galactosidase A processes these lipids during homeostatic metabolism.

B cells

Although B cells and antibodies appear to have a minor biological role in infections with intracellular bacteria, IgG and IgA probably play a role at the epithelial port of entry.[56] Furthermore, some facultative intracellular bacteria spend some time outside their host cells, where they are accessible for antibodies. Therefore it is not surprising that antibodies are protective against salmonellae and listeriae. B cells are also potent APCs for soluble antigens including lipids presented by CD1c, and secrete many cytokines otherwise associated with T cells, DCs, and macrophages. B-cell signaling via MyD88 during *S. typhimurium* infection has been associated with B-cell production of IL-10 and mice with B-cell-specific deficiency in MyD88 were more resistant to infection demonstrating that, like T cells, B cells can perform regulatory functions.[57]

T-cell memory and regulation of immune responses

Memory T cells

Similar to other infectious agents, protective immunity against intracellular bacteria relies on immune memory. In fact, memory induction forms the basis of the success of all vaccines (Chapter 90). Protective immunity in humans can last for decades after infections with various viruses or bacteria. For vaccine development against intracellular bacteria, it is essential to identify conditions leading to long-lasting T-cell immunity.

It is thought that during an ongoing immune response, most T cells become effector T cells and eventually die of exhaustion.

A small proportion that receive stimulatory signals of intermediate strength change their phenotype and become long-lived memory T cells. To become a memory T cell, anti-apoptotic molecules are produced and responsiveness to the homeostatic cytokines IL-7 and -15 is increased through expression of the respective cytokine receptors.[58] Two types of memory T cells, central memory T cells (T_{CM}) and effector memory T cells (T_{EM}), have been defined based on differential surface molecules and functions.[58] T_{EM} lose their lymph node homing properties (CCR7, CD62L) but rather migrate to peripheral tissues where they express effector functions, namely, cytokine secretion and cytotoxicity. Their daily proliferation rate in humans has been estimated at 4.7% compared to 1.5% for T_{CM}. T_{CM} persist in lymph nodes and express the IL-2 receptor, which enables them to quickly propagate upon IL-2 stimulation. Although it is generally accepted that memory T cells can survive in the absence of antigen and MHC molecules, the situation may be different during chronic infections with intracellular bacteria, and little is known about the induction and maintenance of long-lasting T-cell immunity in this scenario.[59] In experimental listeriosis of mice, induction of T memory cells depends on the duration of infection. Further studies on this issue are required for rational design of novel vaccines to achieve long-lasting T-cell immunity against intracellular bacteria.

● KEY CONCEPTS

How might a vaccine work?

- Activation of innate immunity for instruction of appropriate acquired immune response (PRRs)
- Activation of a broad array of T-cell populations
- T-cell secretion of appropriate cytokine combination
- Efficient development of T-cell memory
- Efficient activation of antibacterial effector mechanisms
- Best case scenario: sterile pathogen eradication
- Second best case scenario: driving the infection "deeper" into latency, thus efficiently preventing reactivation of disease

Regulatory T cells

Similar to most infectious agents, intracellular bacteria can cause detrimental inflammation and tissue damage due to IFN-γ-mediated Th1 responses and ultimately exacerbated pathology by TNF-α. Under normal circumstances, control mechanisms are in place to limit immunopathology. Such countermeasures are elicited as part of the ongoing immune response during infection. The main cytokines, which limit inflammation and control IFN-γ production, are IL-10 and TGF-β. Although macrophages and DCs produce these cytokines, their main producers are Treg cells, which are the prime cells involved in immune regulation. Natural Treg cells are responsive to IL-2 due to constitutive CD25 expression and are characterized by expression of the transcription factor FOXP3 (Chapter 15).[60] Expansion of Treg cells appears to be both antigen-dependent and -independent. In addition, Treg cells selectively express TLRs and can be activated, for example, by LPSs and possibly other TLR ligands. This makes their immediate activation during bacterial infection a probable scenario. Although Treg cells limit CD8 T-cell responses in experimental listeriosis, their general role in infections by intracellular bacteria has not been fully elucidated. However, their regulatory function in other infections is better established. Suppression of T-cell responses and anergy have been frequently clinically documented for TB and leprosy. Although

Treg functions can limit detrimental T-cell responses and immunopathology, they can also prevent elimination of bacteria, and hence are likely a key factor in promoting the persistent chronic state of infection with intracellular bacteria.

Concluding remarks

● ON THE HORIZON

- Development and refinement of diagnostics based on light emitting diode (LED) microscopy and DNA amplification tests for more sensitive and more specific point-of-care tests for TB.
- Design of biomarkers to discriminate latent infection from active TB.
- Development and clinical testing of new drugs for MDR/XDR-TB and dormant *M. tuberculosis*.
- Development and clinical testing of new vaccines that protect against pulmonary TB in adults.
- Reduction of the unequal burden of TB in developing and industrialized countries by public health measures, education, and socioeconomic advances.

The intracellular pathogen *M. tuberculosis* remains the single most lethal pathogen for humankind. The current vaccine, BCG, protects against newborn TB but not against the most prevalent pulmonary TB in adults. TB can be cured by chemotherapy. However, the increasing incidence of multidrug-resistant (MDR)- and extensively drug-resistant (XDR)-TB call for new drugs. These drugs should act on novel molecular targets in order to be active against MDR- and XDR-TB, should not antagonize antiretroviral therapy (ART) in HIV-co-infected individuals and should act on dormant *M. tuberculosis* to reduce treatment time. Finally, new diagnostic measures are needed to improve on the high proportion of false-negative TB cases diagnosed. Novel diagnostic techniques should not only include detection of the pathogen by microscopy, culture and DNA amplification but also through biomarkers of the host response. New biomarkers are currently being defined that not only distinguish between latent infection and active TB disease, but in the future may predict the risk of latently infected individuals developing active TB during lifetime. Development of novel intervention measures for TB is laborious and time-consuming and in addition suffers from the unequal distribution of the disease in developing and industrialized countries. Yet, with numerous new candidate vaccines and drugs in clinical trials and several novel diagnostics in testing, chances are good that new measures will become available within 5–10 years. Combined, these intervention measures could reduce—by more than half—morbidity and mortality of this disease. Development of new intervention measures against the major scourge amongst intracellular bacteria will provide guidelines for specific intervention measures for other intracellular bacterial pathogens.

It is being increasingly recognized that the interaction between intracellular bacteria and the immune system is not of the "all or nothing" type but is instead a "continuous struggle." This realization has far-reaching implications for preventive and therapeutic strategies against intracellular bacterial infections. First, vaccination against intracellular bacteria has not yet been effected satisfactorily because of the involvement of several distinct T-cell subsets with different modes of stimulation and activity profiles. Second, chemotherapy has frequently proved suboptimal for the sterile eradication of bacteria hidden in cellular niches. A better understanding of the complex cross talk between cytokines, T lymphocytes, macrophages, and infected host cells will no doubt directly promote the development of improved control measures. It is interesting in conclusion to recall that the discovery of several fundamental principles of immunology was stimulated by early attempts to treat and prevent infections with intracellular bacteria. These include the characterization of macrophages and their contribution to antibacterial defense by Elias Metchnikoff, and the description of granulomatous lesions in TB by Robert Koch.

Acknowledgments

We are grateful to Mary Louise Grossman for excellent assistance and Diane Schad for the figures.

References

1. Kaufmann SHE, Rouse B, Sacks D, editors. The immune response to infection. Washington, DC: ASM Press; 2011.
2. Kaufmann SHE, van Helden PD, editors. Handbook of tuberculosis, vol. 3: Clinics, diagnostics, therapy and epidemiology. Weinheim: Wiley-VCH; 2008.
3. Britton WJ, Lockwood DN. Leprosy. Lancet 2004;363:1209–19.
4. Cosma CL, Sherman DR, Ramakrishnan L. The secret lives of the pathogenic mycobacteria. Annu Rev Microbiol 2003;57:641–76.
5. Crump JA, Mintz ED. Global trends in typhoid and paratyphoid fever. Clin Infect Dis 2010;50:241–6.
6. Pamer EG. Immune responses to Listeria monocytogenes. Nat Rev Immunol 2004;4:812–23.
7. Roop 2nd RM, Bellaire BH, Valderas MW, Cardelli JA. Adaptation of the Brucellae to their intracellular niche. Mol Microbiol 2004;52:621–30.
8. Pathela P, Blank S, Schillinger JA. Lymphogranuloma venereum: old pathogen, new story. Curr Infect Dis Rep 2007;9:143–50.
9. Cheng AC. Melioidosis: advances in diagnosis and treatment. Curr Opin Infect Dis 2010;23:554–9.
10. Sjostedt A. Intracellular survival mechanisms of Francisella tularensis, a stealth pathogen. Microbes Infect 2006;8:561–7.
11. Neild AL, Roy CR. Immunity to vacuolar pathogens: what can we learn from Legionella? Cell Microbiol 2004;6:1011–8.
12. Wright HR, Turner A, Taylor HR. Trachoma. Lancet 2008;371:1945–54.
13. Parola P, Paddock CD, Raoult D. Tick-borne rickettsioses around the world: emerging diseases challenging old concepts. Clin Microbiol Rev 2005;18:719–56.
14. Winslow GM, Bitsaktsis C. Immunity to the ehrlichiae: new tools and recent developments. Curr Opin Infect Dis 2005;18:217–21.
15. Biswas S, Rolain JM. Bartonella infection: treatment and drug resistance. Future Microbiol 2010;5:1719–31.
16. Dorhoi A, Reece ST, Kaufmann SH. For better or for worse: the immune response against Mycobacterium tuberculosis balances pathology and protection. Immunol Rev 2011;240:235–51.
17. Ulrichs T, Kaufmann SH. New insights into the function of granulomas in human tuberculosis. J Pathol 2006;208:261–9.
18. Abrahams GL, Hensel M. Manipulating cellular transport and immune responses: dynamic interactions between intracellular Salmonella enterica and its host cells. Cell Microbiol 2006;8:728–37.
19. O'Neill LA. How Toll-like receptors signal: what we know and what we don't know. Curr Opin Immunol 2006;18:3–9.
20. Taylor PR, Martinez-Pomares L, Stacey M, et al. Macrophage receptors and immune recognition. Annu Rev Immunol 2005;23:901–44.
21. Strober W, Murray PJ, Kitani A, Watanabe T. Signalling pathways and molecular interactions of NOD1 and NOD2. Nat Rev Immunol 2006;6:9–20.
22. Schroder K, Hertzog PJ, Ravasi T, Hume DA. Interferon-gamma: an overview of signals, mechanisms and functions. J Leukoc Biol 2004;75:163–89.
23. Ottenhoff TH, Verreck FA, Lichtenauer-Kaligis EG, et al. Genetics, cytokines and human infectious disease: lessons from weakly pathogenic mycobacteria and salmonellae. Nat Genet 2002;32:97–105.
24. MacMicking JD, Taylor GA, McKinney JD. Immune control of tuberculosis by IFN-gamma-inducible LRG-47. Science 2003;302:654–9.
25. Kim BH, Shenoy AR, Kumar P, et al. A family of IFN-gamma-inducible 65-kD GTPases protects against bacterial infection. Science 2011;332:717–21.
26. Le Y, Zhou Y, Iribarren P, Wang J. Chemokines and chemokine receptors: their manifold roles in homeostasis and disease. Cell Mol Immunol 2004;1:95–104.
27. Werner E. GTPases and reactive oxygen species: switches for killing and signaling. J Cell Sci 2004;117:143–53.
28. Bogdan C. Nitric oxide and the immune response. Nat Immunol 2001;2:907–16.
29. Rudel T, Kepp O, Kozjak-Pavlovic V. Interactions between bacterial pathogens and mitochondrial cell death pathways. Nat Rev Microbiol 2010;8:693–705.
30. Deretic V. Autophagy in immunity and cell-autonomous defense against intracellular microbes. Immunol Rev 2011;240:92–104.
31. Rottenberg ME, Gigliotti-Rothfuchs A, Wigzell H. The role of IFN-gamma in the outcome of chlamydial infection. Curr Opin Immunol 2002;14:444–51.
32. Lehrer RI. Primate defensins. Nat Rev Microbiol 2004;2:727–38.
33. Lieberman J. The ABCs of granule-mediated cytotoxicity: new weapons in the arsenal. Nat Rev Immunol 2003;3:361–70.
34. Jo EK. Innate immunity to mycobacteria: vitamin D and autophagy. Cell Microbiol 2010;12:1026–35.
35. Orange JS, Ballas ZK. Natural killer cells in human health and disease. Clin Immunol 2006;118:1–10.
36. Segal AW. How neutrophils kill microbes. Annu Rev Immunol 2005;23:197–223.
37. Stenger S, Rosat JP, Bloom BR, et al. Granulysin: a lethal weapon of cytolytic T cells. Immunol Today 1999;20:390–4.
38. Stuart LM, Ezekowitz RA. Phagocytosis: elegant complexity. Immunity 2005;22:539–50.
39. Brumell JH, Scidmore MA. Manipulation of rab GTPase function by intracellular bacterial pathogens. Microbiol Mol Biol Rev 2007;71:636–52.
40. Russell DG. Mycobacterium tuberculosis: here today, and here tomorrow. Nat Rev Mol Cell Biol 2001;2:569–77.
41. Salcedo SP, Holden DW. Bacterial interactions with the eukaryotic secretory pathway. Curr Opin Microbiol 2005;8:92–8.
42. Stavru F, Archambaud C, Cossart P. Cell biology and immunology of Listeria monocytogenes infections: novel insights. Immunol Rev 2011;240:160–84.
43. Cooper AM. Cell-mediated immune responses in tuberculosis. Annu Rev Immunol 2009;27:393–422.
44. van der Wel N, Hava D, Houben D, et al. M. tuberculosis and M. leprae translocate from the phagolysosome to the cytosol in myeloid cells. Cell 2007;129:1287–98.
45. Yagi R, Junttila IS, Wei G, et al. The transcription factor GATA3 actively represses RUNX3 protein-regulated production of interferon-gamma. Immunity 2010;32:507–17.
46. Iwakura Y, Ishigame H, Saijo S, Nakae S. Functional specialization of interleukin-17 family members. Immunity 2011;34:149–62.
47. Lin Y, Ritchea S, Logar A, et al. Interleukin-17 is required for T helper 1 cell immunity and host resistance to the intracellular pathogen Francisella tularensis. Immunity 2009;31:799–810.
48. O'Shea JJ, Paul WE. Mechanisms underlying lineage commitment and plasticity of helper CD4+ T cells. Science 2010;327:1098–102.
49. Cox MA, Harrington LE, Zajac AJ. Cytokines and the inception of CD8 T cell responses. Trends Immunol 2011;32:180–6.
50. Dussurget O, Pizarro-Cerda J, Cossart P. Molecular determinants of Listeria monocytogenes virulence. Annu Rev Microbiol 2004;58:587–610.
51. den Haan JM, Bevan MJ. Antigen presentation to CD8+ T cells: cross-priming in infectious diseases. Curr Opin Immunol 2001;13:437–41.
52. Winau F, Hegasy G, Kaufmann SH, Schaible UE. No life without death—apoptosis as prerequisite for T cell activation. Apoptosis 2005;10:707–15.
53. Bonneville M, O'Brien RL, Born WK. Gammadelta T cell effector functions: a blend of innate programming and acquired plasticity. Nat Rev Immunol 2010;10:467–78.
54. Brigl M, Brenner MB. CD1: antigen presentation and T cell function. Annu Rev Immunol 2004;22:817–90.
55. Darmoise A, Teneberg S, Bouzonville L, et al. Lysosomal alpha-galactosidase controls the generation of self lipid antigens for natural killer T cells. Immunity 2010;33:216–28.
56. Joller N, Weber SS, Oxenius A. Antibody-Fc receptor interactions in protection against intracellular pathogens. Eur J Immunol 2011;41:889–97.
57. Neves P, Lampropoulou V, Calderon-Gomez E, et al. Signaling via the MyD88 adaptor protein in B cells suppresses protective immunity during Salmonella typhimurium infection. Immunity 2010;33:777–90.
58. Lanzavecchia A, Sallusto F. Understanding the generation and function of memory T cell subsets. Curr Opin Immunol 2005;17:326–32.
59. Scott P. Immunologic memory in cutaneous leishmaniasis. Cell Microbiol 2005;7:1707–13.
60. Belkaid Y, Rouse BT. Natural regulatory T cells in infectious disease. Nat Immunol 2005;6:353–60.

Chris M. Olson, Jr.,
Erol Fikrig, Juan
Anguita

Host defenses to spirochetes

Characteristics of spirochetes

Spirochetes constitute a unique and diverse group of bacteria that inhabit many different environments such as soil, deep marine sediments, arthropods and mammals. These microorganisms cause numerous human illnesses, including syphilis and Lyme disease. Spirochetes share a typical spiral shape with distinctive flat-wave morphology. Cellular dimensions vary over a wide range, with a diameter between 0.09 to 0.75 µm, and lengths that range from 3 to 500 µm. They are motile organisms with a multilayered outer membrane that encapsulates a peptidoglycan layer surrounding their inner membrane. Motility is due to the presence of endoflagella located in the periplasmic space. These axial filaments are arranged in a bipolar fashion and extend toward the opposite end of the cell (Fig. 26.1). The viability of the organism is dependent on an intact outer membrane, which can be damaged by variations in osmolarity, antibodies or complement resulting in the loss of intracellular components and ultimately death of the bacterium.

Several spirochetal species are able to induce disease in mammals (Table 26.1). Lyme disease was first discovered in 1976 as an illness affecting a cluster of children in Lyme, Connecticut. Several manifestations of the disease, however, had been known for over a century in parts of Europe. In 1982 the agent of Lyme disease was identified as *Borrelia burgdorferi*.[1]

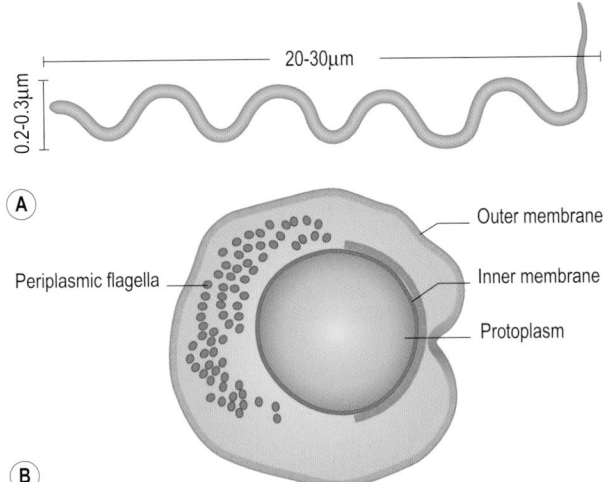

Fig. 26.1 *B. burgdorferi* structure is characterized by a distinctive flat-wave morphology consisting of approximately 18 bends and a length of 20-30 µm (A). A cross-section of this spirochete reveals the endo-flagella, which are responsible for the unique morphology and motility of this organism (B).

Labels (A): 20-30µm; 0.2-0.3µm

Labels (B): Periplasmic flagella; Outer membrane; Inner membrane; Protoplasm

In contrast, *Treponema pallidum* subspecies *pallidum* is the causative agent of venereal syphilis, a disease that has been recognized for over 5 centuries, although its agent was not determined until 1905.[2]

The genomes of *B. burgdorferi* and *T. pallidum* have been sequenced.[3,4] Despite similar ancestry and morphological features, these spirochetes have striking differences at the genetic level that may account for the differences in their life cycles, environmental adaptations and the diseases they cause. Both *B. burgdorferi* and *T. pallidum* have relatively small genomes when compared to other microorganisms. *B. burgdorferi*, however, has one of the most complex genomes known among prokaryotes. This spirochete has a single linear chromosome and 21 plasmids, the largest number of plasmids of any characterized prokaryote. Of the 21 plasmids, nine are circular and 12 are linear. Furthermore, less than 10% of *B. burgdorferi* plasmid-coding regions are found in other microorganisms, including spirochetes, which underscores the uniqueness of this spirochete amongst microorganisms. Unlike *B. burgdorferi*, *T. pallidum* contains a single circular chromosome with no plasmids. Yet, 476 open reading frames (ORFs) in *T. pallidum* have orthologous genes in *B. burgdorferi*. Almost 60 of these orthologous genes encode proteins of unknown biological functions that are specific to spirochetes and may be involved in the pathology associated with infection.

In contrast to other spirochetes, *B. burgdorferi* and *T. pallidum* do not contain lipopolysaccharide (LPS). Lipoproteins are the major immunogens of *B. burgdorferi* and most likely *T. pallidum*, and thus they are their dominant pro-inflammatory agonists. Five percent of the chromosomal ORFs of *B. burgdorferi* encode putative lipoproteins, whereas 14.5 to 17% of the functionally complete ORFs contained in these plasmids encode lipoproteins. Interestingly, only 2.1% of the *T. pallidum* ORFs encode putative lipoproteins. The abundant lipoprotein coding potential of *B. burgdorferi* suggests that they may be important for the survival of the spirochete. In fact, as a result of increased temperature and nutrient availability, as well as reduced pH, expression of several *B. burgdorferi* lipoproteins is augmented upon tick feeding and transmission into the mammalian host.[5] For instance, the lipoprotein outer surface protein (Osp) A is expressed at high levels in the gut of the unfed tick, but upon feeding OspA expression is downregulated, and the expression of OspC increases 90-fold.[5] It is thought that many Osps have adhesive functions, and it has been shown that OspA is involved in the attachment of *B. burgdorferi* to the gut of the tick through an interaction with the tick receptor TROSPA.[6] Furthermore, OspC may be necessary for the migration of *B. burgdorferi* from the gut of the tick to the salivary glands, where it is transmitted into the mammalian host during tick engorgement. OspC may also be required for survival in the mammalian host.

Clinical manifestations

Lyme disease

B. burgdorferi sensu stricto (*B. burgdorferi*) is the etiologic agent of Lyme disease in the United States and other parts of the world, while *B. afzelii* and *B. garinii* are agents of Lyme disease that are restricted to Europe and Asia.[1] Infection with Lyme disease-causing spirochetes has also been observed in Japan, Russia, and China. In the United States, transmission of the spirochete is by hard-bodied ticks of the *Ixodes* complex, mainly *I. scapularis* and *I. pacificus*. According to the Centers for Disease Control and Prevention, Lyme disease is the most common tick-borne disease in the United States.[7]

An early hallmark of infection is the appearance of a skin rash known as *erythema migrans* (Fig. 26.2), which appears at the inoculation site, often during the first week of infection (Stage I, Lyme disease), as a result of local inflammatory responses. Other symptoms secondary to the local inflammatory responses

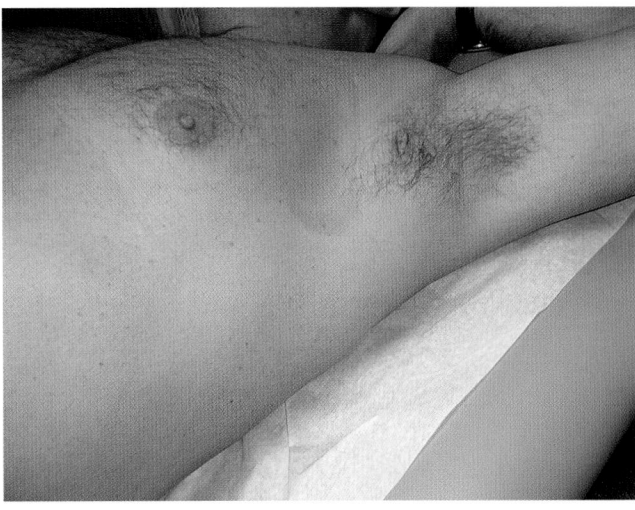

Fig. 26.2 Erythema migrans due to infection with *Borrelia burgdorferi*, the Lyme disease agent.
Courtesy of Gary Wormser, M.D.

Table 26.1 Spirochetes are the causative agents of many diseases, which can have social as well as lasting health-related consequences

Major diseases caused by spirochetal infection				
Disease	**Agents**	**Distribution**	**Transmission**	**Symptoms**
Lyme disease	*Borrelia burgdorferi*	North America, Europe	Tick engorgement	Development of a skin rash known as *erythema migrans*, accompanied by other symptoms such as malaise, myalgia, and/or arthralgia. Symptoms can progress to include carditis and arthritis. Persistent infection can result in chronic arthritis, neuroborreliosis, or cutaneous symptoms (acrodermatitis chronica atrophicans)
	B. garinii	Asia, Europe		
	B. afzelii	Asia, Europe		
	B. andersoni	North America		
	B. japonica	Japan		
	B. lusitaniae	Southern Europe		
	B. valaisiana	Europe, Ireland, UK		
Relapsing fever	*B. hermsii*	Western USA	Tick engorgement	Clinical manifestations of infection include high-density spirochetemia, high fever, myalgias, and arthralgias, and can even include cerebral hemorrhage and fatality
	B. turicatae	Southwestern USA, Mexico		
	B. parkeri	Western USA		
	B. mazzotti	Central America		
	B. venezuelensis	Central America		
	B. duttoni	Sub-Saharan Africa		
	B. crocidurae	North Africa, Middle East		
	B. persica	Middle East, Central Asia		
	B. hispanica	Iberian peninsula, North Africa		
	B. latyschewii	Iran, Iraq, Eastern Europe		
	B. caucasia	Iraq, Eastern Europe		
Venereal syphilis	*Treponema pallidum pallidum*	Worldwide	Sexual contact	Disease progresses from a primary lesion (chancre) to a secondary eruption and then a latent period, and if left untreated tertiary symptoms may appear.
Endemic syphilis or Bejel syphilis	*T. pallidum endemicum*	Eastern Mediterranean region, West Africa	Nonsexual skin contact	Symptoms begin with a slimy patch on the inside of the mouth followed by blisters on the trunk and limbs. Bone infection in the legs soon develops, and, in the later stages, lumps may appear in the nose and on the soft palate of the mouth
Yaws	*T. pertenue*	Humid equatorial countries	Nonsexual skin contact	Destructive lesions of the skin and bones, which is rarely fatal but can be debilitating
Pinta	*T. carateum*	Mexico, Central America,, South America	Nonsexual skin contact	Dark skin lesions found on those areas of the body that are exposed to sunlight. Eventually, the skin lesions become discolored
Leptospirosis	*L. interrogans*	Worldwide	Urine from an infected animal	Symptoms include fever, headache, chills, nausea, and vomiting, eye inflammation, and muscle aches. In more severe cases, the illness can result in liver damage and kidney failure

occurring during Stage I can affect more distal sites and may include fever, headache, malaise, myalgia and/or arthralgia. Hematogenous dissemination of the spirochete is Stage II, Lyme disease and results in colonization of different tissues and/or organs and presentation of a range of symptoms such as conduction system abnormalities, meningitis, and acute arthritis. Joint inflammation appears in 60% of untreated individuals in the USA and predominately affects large joints, especially the synovium of the knee. Some untreated individuals develop stage III Lyme disease, which is generally characterized by prolonged infection with the spirochete. Late stage symptoms may include chronic arthritis, neuroborreliosis, or cutaneous lesions such as *acrodermatitis chronica atrophicans*.

Diagnosis

A detailed clinical history and comprehensive physical examination are critical for the accurate diagnosis of Lyme disease. Appropriate laboratory testing, however, is a valuable diagnostic aid. A two-tiered approach for the serodiagnosis of Lyme disease is standard. Using this approach, serum is first tested for the presence of *B. burgdorferi*-specific antibodies by a sensitive method, such as enzyme-linked immunosorbent assay (ELISA) or an immunofluorescent assay (IFA) (Chapter 93). Sera testing negative for antibodies generally need not be tested further; however, those found to be positive or equivocal are further evaluated by the more specific immunoblotting for IgM and IgG antibodies. The detection of at least two of three specific bands in IgM or 5 of 10 specific bands in IgG is considered positive. Patients with early Lyme disease often report to a physician during the first few days of infection, at which time a detectable humoral response may not have developed. Consequently, the two-tiered approach is considered highly sensitive during the later stages of the disease (>90%), and less sensitive during very early infection. Furthermore, a positive serologic test, particularly IgG, is evidence of exposure to *B. burgdorferi*, but it does not necessarily indicate active infection. All serologic tests must then be evaluated in conjunction with the clinical assessment by the attending physician. Other diagnostic methods, such as culture and PCR (Chapter 98)-detection of *B. burgdorferi*, may be very useful to detect active infection, particularly of the skin, joints and central nervous system. Culture, however, is generally limited to research labs, and the sensitivity and specificity of PCR can vary greatly among testing centers.

Treatment

During early stages of Lyme disease, such as that during which *erythema migrans* is present, oral administration of doxycycline (100 mg twice daily) or amoxicillin (500 mg 3 times a day) for approximately 2 weeks is recommended.[8] Doxycycline has the advantage of being effective against *Anaplasma phagcytophilum*, which may also be transmitted by ticks. In areas where *B. burgdorferi* infection is prevalent, some experts recommend antibiotic therapy for individuals who served as hosts to *I. scapularis* ticks that were attached longer than 40–48 hours—the time required for transmission of the spirochete. It is extremely difficult, however, to consistently make accurate determinations of the species of tick and the degree of engorgement. Furthermore, randomized double-blind clinical trials involving individuals who were bitten by *I. scapularis* ticks led to the conclusion that treating all individuals who remove vector ticks with antibiotics is probably not warranted.[8]

Venereal syphilis

Infection with the agent of syphilis, *T. pallidum* subspecies *pallidum*, occurs worldwide. *T. pallidum* is an obligate human parasite that is almost exclusively transmitted when contact with infectious exudates from lesions of the skin and mucous membranes of infected individuals occurs. Clinically, this treponemal infection is first characterized by the formation of a hardened and painless ulcer at the initial site of infection. This primary lesion, called a chancre, forms after invasion of the bloodstream by the spirochete. Four to 6 weeks following infection, the edges of the chancre roll inwards and upwards and, in most cases, a secondary eruption appears, often accompanied by a rash on the palms of the hands and the soles of the feet. The secondary manifestations resolve within weeks to a year following the development of a vigorous cell-mediated immune response. Long periods of latency, and late lesions of the skin, bone, viscera, cardiovascular and central nervous systems can follow despite the clearance of the majority of the treponemes, which coincides with the resolution of the primary syphilitic lesion.

Diagnosis

Much like Lyme disease, the diagnosis for syphilis is based on the clinical presentations of the disease and serologic tests. In addition, dark-field microscopy may be used for the identification of *T. pallidum* in the serous exudates of the chancre. This approach, however, is limited by the number of live treponemes in the exudates and by the presence of non-pathologic treponemes in oral and anal lesions; as such, negative examinations on three independent days are required before a lesion is considered negative for *T. pallidum*.

Infection with *T. pallidum* leads to the production of non-specific antibodies, which is the basis for other diagnostic tests, such as the traditional non-treponemal serologic tests including the VDRL (Venereal Disease Research Laboratory) and RPR (rapid plasma regain) tests. Because these tests are non-specific, false-positive reactions may occur as a result of pregnancy, auto-immune disorders, or infections. Therefore, treponemal-specific tests, which detect antibodies to various antigens of *T. pallidum* are often used to confirm the results of a non-specific test. Interestingly, treponemal-specific tests are just as sensitive as non-treponemal tests; however, they are much more difficult and expensive to perform, which limits their use. These tests include, but are not limited to, the enzyme immunoassay test for *T. pallidum*-specific IgG (EIA), *T. pallidum* hemagglutination test (TPHA), fluorescent treponemal antibody-absorbtion test (FTA-abs) and ELISA.

Treatment

Susceptibility to infection with *T. pallidum* is universal, although only 30% of exposures with lesions teeming with the spirochete result in infection. Infection results in gradual development of immunity against *T. pallidum* and often against heterologous treponemes as well. However, treatment with long-acting penicillin subverts the development of immunity against *T. pallidum*. 2.4 million units in a single intramuscular dose the day that the primary, secondary or latent syphilis is diagnosed is effective at killing the spirochetes. For people who are allergic to penicillin, there are alternative treatments such as doxycycline.

Host defenses to *B. burgdorferi*

● KEY CONCEPTS

Protective versus pathological responses to *Borrelia burgdorferi*

- The early immune response to *B. burgdorferi* is necessary to control spirochetal burden; however, alone it is not sufficient to resolve infection.
- The T-cell-mediated response appears to be involved in pathology arising from infection.
- A T-cell-independent B-cell response is sufficient to resolve infection with *B. burgdorferi*.

Since its discovery, the Lyme disease spirochete has been the subject of intensive investigation in order to elucidate the mechanisms that contribute to its ability to cause persistent infection and multi-systemic disease, despite the development of strong immune responses. *B. burgdorferi* virulence is owed, in part, to the evolution of sophisticated tactics to evade killing mechanisms during all stages of the immune response; the first stage beginning with transmission into the host via tick engorgement, at which time the spirochete is exposed to serum complement and cellular immunity, and the second and third stages being homogenous dissemination to and colonization of peripheral sites, at which points the host is producing specific antibodies. Both the innate and adaptive immune responses elicited by *B. burgdorferi* are discussed, with the supposition that these responses are required for efficient bacterial clearance while acknowledging that unnecessarily prolonged or intense responses may contribute to pathology arising from infection. Indeed, predisposition to infection could be the result of one or more monogenic traits that confer primary immunodeficiencies; whether or not this is the case waits to be determined, but human studies have shown that responses to *B. burgdorferi* are diminished in individuals with specific mutations in or diminished expression of innate immune cell receptors (NOD-2 and TLR-1). Much of the knowledge we have regarding host defenses to *B. burgdorferi* has been elucidated from murine models of infection.

Innate immune responses

The initial recognition of pathogens with cells of the host relies on a complex interplay between pathogen recognition receptors (PRRs) and bacterial constituents, which initiates a cascade of responses leading to the upregulation of chemokines and cytokines, adhesion molecules and a vast array of other effector molecules (Chapter 3). This response is often initiated by endothelial and/or epithelial cells, and is aimed at the recruitment of different types of innate immune cells, their activation and ultimately pathogen clearance. Each PRR recognizes a specific structure that is present in a group or groups of microorganisms and that distinguishes them from the more specific recognition of antigens by the T- and B-cell receptors. The recognition of patterns instead of specific antigens provides the innate immune system with a rapid way to respond to infecting organisms until the more specific response mediated by T and B cells develops.

A distinct innate cellular infiltration profile has been observed in *B. burgdorferi*-infected tissues. Based on studies using mice, the inflamed heart appears to be predominately comprised of macrophages, with smaller amounts of T and invariant natural killer

T cells (iNKT cells). However, neutrophils are the primary innate immune cell found in the joints. This tissue-specific tropism complicates our understanding of the host defense against the spirochete, but might suggest that macrophages are more efficient at preventing successful colonization of *B. burgdorferi*, because carditis is a less frequent manifestation of Lyme disease. Importantly, these early defense responses also have a role in determining the type, strength and duration of the more specific adaptive immune response, beyond their direct bacterial-killing capability.

Early pathogen recognition

The most extensively studied *B. burgdorferi* molecular pattern recognized by innate immune receptors is the large (over 150) group of surface lipoproteins. The interaction of *B. burgdorferi* lipoproteins with complexes formed by Toll-like receptors (TLRs) 1 and 2 initiates a series of signaling cascades that results in the production of proinflammatory cytokines (IL-1β, TNF, IL-12, and IL-18, among others), chemokines (IL-8, MCP-1, KC), metalloproteinases, adhesion molecules (E-selectin, VCAM-1 and ICAM-1)[9] and type I interferons. These interactions are critical for generating an effective spirochete-clearing inflammatory response, as demonstrated by experiments using mice deficient for TLR1, TLR2 or their adaptor molecule, MyD88. These mice had significant increases in *B. burgdorferi* burdens following infection. Moreover, humans with decreased TLR1 expression are hyporesponsive to the original OspA-based Lyme disease vaccine, and macrophages from these subjects also have diminished inflammatory responses to the lipoprotein. Importantly, the development of inflammatory arthritis in the absence of TLRs or MyD88 was the first suggestion that alternative pathways exist that trigger the inflammatory response to the spirochete.

The interaction of several cell types with the spirochetes also involves receptors other than TLRs, including several integrins belonging to the β$_1$, β$_2$, and β$_3$ groups. Integrins are heterodimers composed of α and β subunits that are classified according to the β chain they contain. Integrins are involved in the adhesion of cells to a variety of ligands and mediate essential cellular processes, including attachment and cell migration (Chapter 11). Some integrins have also been associated with the phagocytosis of microorganisms. For the most part, the study of the interaction between the spirochete and integrins has focused on their role as molecules aiding the adhesion of *B. burgdorferi* to cells and the colonization of tissues, and as receptors that contribute to signals that induce the production of pro-inflammatory factors (Fig. 26.3).

Phagocytic cell recruitment and spirochetal clearance

The recruitment of phagocytic cells and other cell types into sites of infection is mediated by the production of chemokines, increased vascular permeability, and upregulated expression of cell adhesion molecules in endothelial cells. *B. bugdorferi* induces the upregulation of these factors in different cell types. Chemokine production at sites of pathology in disease-susceptible C3H/HeJ mice and -resistant C57BL/6 J mice show that inflammation is related to increased production of neutrophil and monocyte-macrophage chemokines, KC and MCP-1, respectively. In patients, the production of chemokines, especially IL-8, during the initial response to *B. burgdorferi* correlates well with the onset of symptoms known to occur during the early stages of infection, suggesting that their production is increased during

Professional antigen presenting cell

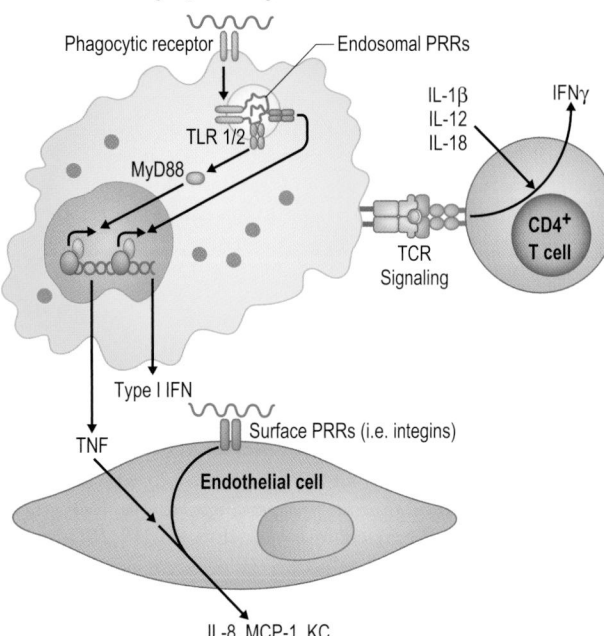

Fig. 26.3 The interaction of *B. burgdorferi* with PRRs in innate immune cells and endothelial cells mediates the inflammatory response to the spirochete. Phagocytosis induces TLR-driven pro-inflammatory cytokine production as well as antigen presentation by professional APCs that leads to the activation of CD4 effector T cells, which is marked by the production of IFN-γ. Likewise, PRR- and TNF receptor signaling lead to the upregulation of chemokines by endothelial cells. Overall, these responses lead to increased activation and recruitment of innate immune cells in sites of infection.

the beginning of the infection to recruit phagocytic cells, which are involved in the initial clearance of the spirochete.

Phagocytosis plays a major role in the pathogenesis of Lyme disease through the control of bacterial numbers, and the modulation of the potency and quality of pro-inflammatory cytokine induction. Indeed, studies using the murine model of Lyme borreliosis have shown that the protective role of the cytokine IFNγ in cardiac inflammation occurs at least partly, through increased phagocytosis of the spirochete. However, despite the importance of this cardinal mechanism of pathogen clearance, little is known about the molecular events or receptors that mediate *B. burgdorferi* phagocytosis. MyD88-mediated signals substantially mediate the phagocytosis of *B. burgdorferi*. However, MyD88-mediated phagocytosis occurs independently of any known *B. burgdorferi*-recognizing TLRs. The mechanism of MyD88-mediated phagocytic uptake is therefore unclear and the subject of intensive investigation. Furthermore, the analysis of MyD88-deficient macrophages shows that although reduced, phagocytosis is not absent in these cells. The uptake of *B. burgdorferi* by phagocytic cells seems to be therefore mediated by more than one receptor with MyD88-dependent and independent components.

Complement

The complement system is a key component of the innate immune system (Chapter 3). It is comprised of a collection of serum proteins and cell surface receptors that are involved in the early response to pathogens, including *B. burgdorferi*.[10] Destruction of micro-organisms via complement involves the formation of a pore in the microbial cell membrane by the membrane attack complex (MAC), which results in the lysis of the organism. Three

different pathways elicit complement activation: the classical (antigen/antibody-mediated), lectin and alternative (pathogen surface) pathway. These pathways converge at the level of C3 convertase, a protease that cleaves complement component C3 into C3a and C3b. As a result, C3b can (1) bind to the surface of the bacteria and facilitate internalization of the spirochete via opsonization or (2) bind C3 convertase and facilitate the deposition of downstream components onto the surface of the spirochete resulting in the formation of MAC and lysis of the cell.

B. burgdorferi activates the classical and alternative pathways of the complement cascade.[11] Moreover, the activation of complement has been associated with dramatic decreases in spirochetal numbers in different tissues of infected mice, indicating the importance of the complement system early in *B. burgdorferi* infection. However, complement-independent, antibody-mediated killing of spirochetes has been extensively reported, although the relative contribution of the two mechanisms *in vivo* remains uncertain.

The members of the *B. burgdorferi* sensu lato group, which includes *B. burgdorferi* sensu stricto, *B. garinii*, and *B. afzelii*, have evolved a variety of mechanisms enabling them to escape complement-mediated lysis, including the expression of complement regulator-acquiring surface proteins (CRASPs). Of these CRASPs, the ERP (OspEF-related protein) family of outer membrane proteins serve as binding sites for the complement inhibitor factor H and factor H-like protein 1 (FHL-1).[9] The interaction of factor H with these proteins recruits a protease (factor I) that cleaves and inactivates the complement serum proteins, C3b and C4b. Cleavage of these two complement proteins prevents the deposition of downstream components onto the surface of the spirochete; thereby, halting the formation of the membrane attack complex. *B. burgdorferi* also express a CD59-like molecule on the outer membrane that can inactivate MAC and prevent complement-mediated lysis.[12] It has been speculated that most borreliae are able to evade complement-mediated lysis, and recently a novel protein expressed by *B. hermsii* (a relapsing fever spirochete) has been discovered that affords protection to spirochete by inactivating C3b.[13]

Adaptive immune responses

T-cell-mediated responses

Upon antigen presentation by macrophages, dendritic cells or B cells, naïve CD4 T cells are activated and differentiate into effector T cells. Effector CD4 T cells are classified based on their cytokine production profile, which determines their mode of action and downstream effects (Chapter 16). The characterization of effector CD4 T-cell subsets keeps evolving, from the original Th1 (IFNγ-producing)/Th2 (IL-4, IL5, IL-13) dichotomy, to the more recent inclusion of novel subsets, such as Th17 (IL-17), Th9 (IL-9), and Tregs (IL-10). The most powerful inducer of differentiation of naïve CD4 T cells is the local cytokine environment. Interaction of *B. burgdorferi* antigen with TLRs induces the production of IL-12, which drives the differentiation of CD4 T cells into Th1 effector cells. Thus, TLRs are important to bridge the innate and adaptive immune responses. Through their production of IFNγ and TNFβ, Th1 cells are regulators of the cell-mediated inflammatory reaction, which is characterized by macrophage activation, including phagocytosis, stimulation of CD8 T cells, and production of opsonizing IgG antibodies. While IFNγ and Th1 CD4+ T cells have been shown to be protective during cardiac inflammation with *B. burgdorferi*, joint inflammation is independent of this effector cell type. However, in patients with

Lyme disease, Th1 cells dominate in the synovial fluid, and the severity of arthritis directly correlates with increased levels of Th1 cells in the synovium.[14] Whether neutrophilic infiltration during joint infection with the spirochete is influenced by Th effector cells that more directly affect this cell type, such as Th17 cells (through the production of IL-17) remains to be elucidated. Overall, the studies performed in the murine model of infection underscore the complexity of the nature of a "protective" response that may be highly dependent on the local composition of inflammatory cells.

B-cell-mediated responses

Antibodies are specific and powerful effector molecules of the adaptive immune response. Once antibodies bind to their specific foreign antigen, they confer protection to the host using a variety of effector mechanisms: antibodies contribute to adaptive immunity by neutralizing microbes or their products, activation of complement, and opsonization, which leads to phagocytosis of microorganisms. The activation of B cells and their differentiation into antibody secreting plasma cells often requires an interaction with helper T cells, which controls isotype switching as well as somatic hypermutation. However, in response to *B. burgdorferi*, T-cell-independent humoral responses also confer protection to the host. Thus, T-cell-, CD40L-, and MHC class II-deficient mice infected with *B. burgdorferi* mount a protective antibody response, which upon passive serum transfer affords protection to severe combined immune deficient (SCID) mice from homologous challenge. However, mice that lack both B and T cells developed severe arthritis and carditis in response to infection with *B. burgdorferi*.

The role of antibodies in controlling *B. burgdorferi* infection may be more important during the hematogenous dissemination phase, where they are easily accessible, than once the spirochetes have colonized tissues. *B. burgdorferi* is able to evade the humoral response by interacting with the extracellular matrix of the mammalian host via attachment to decorin, a major component of the extracellular matrix. *B. burgdorferi* attaches to decorin with a ligand-binding lipoprotein known as decorin-binding protein A (DbpA). A deficiency in decorin reduces the incidence of Lyme arthritis in mice, suggesting that the interaction of DbpA with the extracellular matrix provides a protective niche for *B. burgdorferi*, and thus prevents humoral-mediated bacterial killing. Once in the joints and heart, clearance of the spirochete may be more dependent on cellular responses (such as macrophages in the heart), than antibodies. In fact, the lack of IFNγ-mediated activation of macrophages has profound consequences on murine cardiac inflammation, even in the presence of strong antibody responses. Furthermore, the bacterial clearance potential of infected mouse sera administered in newly infected mice is lost when administered 4-8 days after infection. Although interpreted as proof of bacterial adaptation to the murine host, bacterial clearance can also be the result of the colonization of tissues into which antibodies are less able to penetrate.

B. burgdorferi can also avoid clearance by antibodies through antigenic diversity. *B. burgdorferi* differentially expresses outer membrane antigens under pressure from the immune response, which might contribute to the spirochetes' ability to persist in the host. A mechanism that is potentially essential for spirochetal immune escape is the recombination that takes place at the *vls* locus,[15] which consists on a *vls* expression site (*vlsE*) located near the right telomere of the linear plasmid lp28-1 and 15 silent cassettes upstream. *vlsE* encodes a surface-exposed, immunogenic protein of 34 kDa.

B. burgdorferi is also able to evade antibody responses during transmission from the tick by attachment to the tick salivary protein, Salp15. Adherence of Salp15 to *B. burgdorferi* through an interaction with OspC protects the spirochete from antibody-mediated killing,[16] increasing the pathogen's capacity to infect and colonize the mammalian host upon tick feeding.

Host defenses to *T. pallidum*

● KEY CONCEPTS

Protective versus pathological responses to *Treponema pallidum*

- The role of the early innate response to *T. pallidum* is still poorly understood because immunogenic cell surface proteins able to activate pattern recognition receptors remain to be found.
- It is likely that the cell-mediated immune response to *T. pallidum* is involved in the development of pathology following infection with the spirochete. Likewise, this response seems to be involved in the resolution of infection with *T. pallidum*.
- The protection that the humoral response affords to the host is unclear. Furthermore, no definite antigens have been isolated from the spirochete, due to the inability to cultivate this organism *in vitro*.

Treponema pallidum is known colloquially as "The Stealth Pathogen" because of its denuded outer membrane, which is comprised of mostly non-immunogenic transmembrane proteins, while highly immunogenic lipoproteins are contained within the periplasmic space.[17] This molecular architecture, coupled with the ability to generate antigenic variants, is responsible for the treponemes remarkable ability to cause persistent infection with relatively few organisms.[18,19]

For more than 500 years, syphilis has been a recognized disease; however, we have yet to elucidate many of the specific immunologic phenomena that occur as a result of infection with the treponeme and that are inherent to the clinical manifestations of the disease. Our limited understanding of immunological phenomena during infection is mainly due to our inability to culture these organisms *in vitro* and to reproducibly infect an animal model. Consequently, our understanding of the immune responses to this pathogen is not nearly as detailed as our knowledge of those elicited in response to infection with *B. burgdorferi*.

Innate immune responses

Only recently has the contribution of innate immune responses to syphilis pathology and disease resolution been addressed. Similar to *B. burgdorferi* lipopoproteins, treponemal lipoproteins appear to be the major pro-inflammatory agonists during treponeme infection through engagement with their cognate receptors, TLR1/2 and CD14. The inflammatory milieu established by treponemal lipoproteins is a principal driving force for immune cell recruitment to *T. pallidum*-infected tissues. The importance of this immune system compartment during the response to *T. pallidum* is further supported by the systemic upregulation of innate immune cells during treponemal dissemination and by demonstration that macrophages are principal effectors of treponemal clearance during infection.[20]

Early pathogen recognition

Dendritic cells are among the most potent antigen-presenting cells of the immune system and are critical for the initiation of T-cell responses against bacterial invaders. Because of their location in the skin (i.e., Langerhans cells), they likely mediate the initial responses to treponemes at the primary syphilitic lesion. Due to the denuded outer membrane of *T. pallidum*, extremely high treponeme to dendritic cell ratios (500:1 and higher) are required for observable levels of phagocytosis *in vitro*. Thus, unhindered replication of spirochetes at the initial site of infection probably underlies the vigorous cell-mediated immune response, and chancre appearance, that ensues following antigen presentation to and differentiation and activation of CD4 T cells.

Phagocytic cell recruitment and spirochetal clearance

It is not until after the recruitment of macrophages and their activation via CD4 T-cell-derived IFN-γ, that the majority of spirochetes are killed and resolution of syphilitic lesions occurs. Activated macrophages readily phagocytose antibody-opsonized treponemes through Fc receptor-mediated uptake. However, as with DCs, uptake via a direct PAMP:PRR interaction does not occur readily, and because of treponemal antigenic variation, not all spirochetes will be eliminated via opsonophagocytosis despite the vigorous inflammatory response. The relatively few remaining spirochetes are able to cause persistent infection.

Complement

The immunoprotection afforded by human syphilitic serum is in large part due to the activation of the complement cascade by bactericidal antibodies and spontaneous hydrolysis of C3. Thus, like *B. burgdorferi*, *T. pallidum* activates the classical and alternative pathways of the complement cascade, and there is a considerable amount of evidence for an important role of these pathways in syphilitic lesion resolution during experimental and human infection with treponemes. Unlike *B. burgdorferi*, there is no evidence indicating that *T. pallidum* has evolved mechanisms to evade complement-dependent killing, suggesting that these complement pathways have a larger role in controlling treponemal infection than *B. burgdorferi*.

During experimental syphilis, immunization with purified outer membrane vesicles (OMV) isolated from *T. pallidum* results in complement-dependent bactericidal activity.[21] More recently, immunization with OMVs led to the isolation of a bactericidal monoclonal antibody, called M131, that provides partial protection to experimental syphilis. M131 binds to a phosphorylcholine surface epitope of *T. pallidum* and is the first demonstration of such an antigen on the surface of the spirochete.[22]

Adaptive immune responses

T -cell-mediated responses

The infiltration of T cells (CD4 and CD8) and macrophages into the primary and secondary syphilitic lesion facilitates local clearance of the majority of treponemes and lesion resolution via a vigorous cell-mediated immune response characteristic of a delayed-type hypersensitivity or Th1 response.[23,24] CD4 T cells are the principal T-cell subset found in the lesions and are believed to promote macrophage activation and subsequent treponeme clearance through IFN-γ secretion. The role of

CD8+ cells is not clear, but throughout the course of primary lesion development during experimental syphilis, their proportion related to CD4 T cells increases. Once the treponemes are cleared and the lesion heals, a latency stage ensues, which is characterized by long-lasting, protective T-cell memory to *T. pallidum* antigens. Importantly, the clearance of treponemes from syphilitic lesions and the development of T-cell memory require cooperation between the cellular and humoral arms of the immune system.

B-cell-mediated responses

There are many functional activities of human syphilitic serum originating from B-cell responses to *T. pallidum*. Infection with *T. pallidum* invokes a humoral immune response early in the course of infection, which strengthens as the number of recognizable antigens increases during the progression of infection. A polymorphic gene family of *T. pallidum*, called *T. pallidum* repeat (*tpr*), has been recently identified and shown to be related to the major surface protein (Msp) genes of *T. denticola*.[25] A single member of the *tpr* family, *tpr*K, serves as an antigen for opsonizing antibodies, suggesting that this protein is a surface antigen of *T. pallidum*. However, there are only inferential indications that surface antigens of *T. pallidum* exist. So, although candidate *T. pallidum* surface proteins have been advanced on the basis of porin activity or homology with a surface protein of *T. denticola*, there is no direct evidence identifying specific surface antigens on *T. pallidum*. Furthermore, like most pathogenic organisms, *T. pallidum* has evolved various mechanisms to escape host killing. TprK is an immunogen with seven discrete variable regions differing among isolates of the spirochete.[25] In fact, the antibody response to *T. pallidum* is directed against these variable regions, which leads to immune selection of new TprK variants because of macrophage-mediated opsonophagocytosis; thus, antigenic variation is involved in the reinfection of hosts despite robust immune responses.[25,26]

Translational research

ON THE HORIZON

- Efficient diagnostic methods are required to rapidly identify infection and procure antimicrobial treatments.
- Development of new generation vaccines for Lyme disease.
- Attention to communities at risk for contracting syphilis with investments in prophylaxis and efficient treatments.

The challenge in the next 5-10 years is to develop effective diagnostic methods for both Lyme disease and syphilis as well as devise new preventative measures. For Lyme disease, advances in genetic manipulation as well as other means to study structure/function of key components of the spirochete would allow the development of single or combination vaccines. Further, the identification of host factors that mediate a protective response as well as those that contribute to inflammation could lead to a better understanding of the disease. Overall, the identification of the elements that mediate specific tissue tropisms for the bacterium and their interaction with local/infiltrating cellular components can permit the design of targeted therapies in conjunction with antimicrobial treatments.

For syphilis, the study of the micro-organism is hampered by the difficulties associated with its culture and manipulation.

This creates a significant challenge. Although advances have been made in our understanding of the pathology associated with infection, a significant challenge in the near future is to fully understand this pathogen. An area in which advances can be made in the next decade consists on the better education of populations that are at risk of acquiring the infection. Because these populations are usually associated with poor communities, a significant investment needs to be made in order to allow persons at risk to better evade the transmission of the pathogen, through education, better diagnostics and rapid antimicrobial treatment.

Conclusion

Spirochetes are a phylogenetically ancient and distinct group of microorganisms. Because of their propensity to cause diseases in humans, *B. burgdorferi* and *T. pallidum* are the two most well-studied spirochetes. However, the inability to culture *T. pallidum in vitro* has made researching this spirochete very difficult, and as a consequence our understanding of the immune response following infection with this spirochete is more limited.

The etiologic agents of Lyme disease and syphilis are similar in having relatively small genomes, surviving only in association with a host and eliciting inflammatory disease, but genomic comparison clearly shows that *T. pallidum* and *B. burgdorferi* are not closely related. It seems likely that, despite some similarities, these spirochetes evolved independently from a more complex ancestor, resulting in differences in their life cycles, environmental adaptations and the pathology associated with their infection. Therefore, it is not surprising to learn of differences in the host immune response to *B. burgdorferi* and *T. pallidum*. Both the host response to these spirochetes and the infectivity of the bacterium determine the extent of pathology following infection.

References

1. Burgdorfer W, Barbour AG, Hayes SF, et al. Lyme disease—a tick-borne spirochetosis? Science 1982;216:1317–9.
2. Krause RM. Metchnikoff and syphilis research during a decade of discovery, 1900-1910. Development of an animal model and a preventive treatment set the stage for progress. ASM News 1996;62:307–10.
3. Fraser CM, Norris SJ, Weinstock GM, et al. Complete genome sequence of *Treponema pallidum*, the syphilis spirochete. Science 1998;281:375–88.
4. Fraser CM, Casjens S, Huang WM, et al. Genomic sequence of a Lyme disease spirochaete, *Borrelia burgdorferi*. Nature 1997;390:580–6.
5. Anguita J, Hedrick MN, Fikrig E. Adaptation of *Borrelia burgdorferi* in the tick and the mammalian host. FEMS Microbiol Rev 2003;27:493–504.
6. Pal U, Li X, Wang T, et al. TROSPA, an *Ixodes scapularis* receptor for *Borrelia burgdorferi*. Cell 2004;119:457–68.
7. Lyme Disease—United States, 2001-2002. MMWR 2004;53:365–9.
8. Wormser GP, Nadelman RB, Dattwyler RJ, et al. Practice guidelines for the treatment of Lyme disease. The Infectious Diseases Society of America. Clin Infect Dis 2000;31(Suppl. 1):1–14.
9. Guerau-de-Arellano M, Huber BT. Chemokines and Toll-like receptors in Lyme disease pathogenesis. Trends Mol Med 2005;11:114–20.
10. Lawrenz MB, Wooten RM, Zachary JF, et al. Effect of complement component C3 deficiency on experimental Lyme borreliosis in mice. Infect Immun 2003;71:4432–40.
11. Kochi SK, Johnson RC. Role of immunoglobulin G in killing of *Borrelia burgdorferi* by the classical complement pathway. Infect Immun 1988;56:314–21.
12. Pausa M, Pellis V, Cinco M, et al. Serum-resistant strains of *Borrelia burgdorferi* evade complement-mediated killing by expressing a CD59-like complement inhibitory molecule. J Immunol 2003;170:3214–22.
13. Hovis KM, McDowell JV, Griffin L, Marconi RT. Identification and characterization of a linear-plasmid-encoded factor H-binding protein (FhbA) of the relapsing fever spirochete *Borrelia hermsii*. J Bacteriol 2004;186:2612–8.
14. Gross DM, Steere AC, Huber BT. T helper 1 response is dominant and localized to the synovial fluid in patients with Lyme arthritis. J Immunol 1998;160:1022–8.
15. Zhang JR, Hardham JM, Barbour AG, Norris SJ. Antigenic variation in Lyme disease borreliae by promiscuous recombination of VMP-like sequence cassettes. Cell 1997;89:275–85.
16. Ramamoorthi N, Narasimhan S, Pal U, et al. The Lyme disease agent exploits a tick protein to infect the mammalian host. Nature 2005;436:573–7.
17. Cox DL, Chang P, McDowall AW, Radolf JD. The outer membrane, not a coat of host proteins, limits antigenicity of virulent *Treponema pallidum*. Infect Immun 1992;60:1076–83.
18. Salazar JC, Hazlett KR, Radolf JD. The immune response to infection with *Treponema pallidum*, the stealth pathogen. Microbes Infect 2002;4:1133–40.
19. Sellati TJ, Bouis DA, Caimano MJ, et al. Activation of human monocytic cells by *Borrelia burgdorferi* and *Treponema pallidum* is facilitated by CD14 and correlates with surface exposure of spirochetal lipoproteins. J Immunol 1999;163:2049–56.
20. Salazar JC, Cruz AR, Pope CD, et al. *Treponema pallidum* elicits innate and adaptive cellular immune responses in skin and blood during secondary syphilis: a flow-cytometric analysis. J Infect Dis 2007;195:879–87.
21. Blanco DR, Champion CI, Lewinski MA. Immunization with *Treponema pallidum* outer membrane vesicles induces high-titer complement-dependent treponemicidal activity and aggregation of *T. pallidum* rare outer membrane proteins (TROMPs). J Immunol 1999;163:2741–6.
22. Blanco DR, Champion CI, Dooley A, et al. A monoclonal antibody that conveys in vitro killing and partial protection in experimental syphilis binds a phosphorylcholine surface epitope of *Treponema pallidum*. Infect Immun 2005;73:3083–95.
23. McBroom RL, Styles AR, Chiu MJ, et al. Secondary syphilis in persons infected with and not infected with HIV-1: a comparative immunohistologic study. Am J Dermatopathol 1999;21:432–41.
24. Van Voorhis WC, Barrett LK, Koelle DM, et al. Primary and secondary syphilis lesions contain mRNA for Th1 cytokines. J Infect Dis 1996;173:491–5.
25. Centurion-Lara A, Castro C, Barrett L, et al. *Treponema pallidum* major sheath protein homologue Tpr K is a target of opsonic antibody and the protective immune response. J Exp Med 1999;189:647–56.
26. Giacani L, Molini BJ, Kim EY, et al. Antigenic variation in *Treponema pallidum*: TprK sequence diversity accumulates in response to immune pressure during experimental syphilis. J Immunol 2010;184:3822–9.

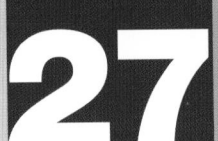

Scott N. Mueller,
Barry T. Rouse

Host defenses to viruses

Viruses as obligate intracellular parasites require their host to replicate them and to facilitate their spread to others. In humans, viral infections are rarely lethal, even if they are highly cytolytic to individual cells. Mortality commonly occurs when viruses jump species (such as Ebola or human immunodeficiency virus (HIV)), when the virus undergoes a major antigenic change (i.e., influenza viruses), or when host immunity is compromised. HIV represents one of the most dramatic human examples of an exotic virus that kills its host. However, HIV kills slowly, providing ample time to spread to new hosts and an effective strategy for persistence in the species. Death or dire consequences following virus infection in mammals with inadequate immunity are well illustrated by observations that fetuses or neonates, especially if deprived of passive immunity, succumb to many agents well tolerated by normal adults. The increasing wealth of immunological tools, such as transgenic animal models and major histocompatibility complex (MHC) tetramers, have provided sensitive methods for defining the relevance of immune mechanisms for antiviral defense. In most situations, defense against viruses involves multiple immune components, and the impact of a single mechanism varies greatly according to the method by which individual viruses enter, replicate, and spread within the host. In this chapter, we highlight the principal means by which the host achieves immunity following infection by viruses. Table 27.1 presents an overview.

Viral entry and infection

Access to target tissues presents numerous obstacles for entry and infection by most human viruses. Most effective of these are the mechanical barriers provided by the skin and mucosal surfaces, as well as the chemically hostile environment of the gut (Fig. 27.1). A number of common human viral pathogens enter through the gastrointestinal tract, including rotavirus, enteric adenoviruses, and hepatitis A virus (HAV). These are usually spread via person-to-person contact or contaminated food and water. Respiratory infections caused by influenza viruses, rhinoviruses, coronaviruses, measles virus, varicella-zoster virus (VZV), and respiratory syncytial virus (RSV) are often spread by aerosol transmission, as well as person-to-person contact. Many of the herpes viruses target the skin or the mucosae, such as herpes simplex virus (HSV) and VZV. HSV in particular can infect oral and genital mucosa, the eye, and the skin through small cuts and abrasions. Other herpes viruses, such as Epstein–Barr virus (EBV) and cytomegalovirus (CMV), target the mucosa. CMV can also spread vertically from mother to baby or rarely via blood transfusions. Human papillomavirus (HPV) targets skin and mucosa and causes warts and may transform cells, inducing cancers such as cervical cancer. Viruses such as West Nile virus, Dengue virus and Semliki forest virus may also enter through the skin via insect vectors. HIV and hepatitis B virus (HBV) are commonly spread via sexual contact. HIV, HBV, and hepatitis C virus (HCV) can also infect humans via direct entry into the bloodstream via transfusions or contaminated needles.

Most human viruses replicate only in certain target tissues, this being mainly the consequence of viral receptor distribution. Many viruses use two receptors, such as the use of the CD4 co-receptor and the chemokine receptor CCR5 by HIV. After attachment to a cellular receptor, viruses may fuse with the cell membrane or be endocytosed and then gain entry into the cytoplasm or nucleus by fusing with the vesicular membrane (enveloped viruses such as HSV and HIV), or translocate across the cell membrane or induce lysis of the endocytic vesicle once in the cytoplasm (nonenveloped viruses such as Norwalk virus and poliovirus).[1] Viruses then utilize host cell machinery and specialized virally encoded proteins to replicate rapidly within the cell. Once they have multiplied within the cell, many viruses induce cytolysis in order to facilitate release of new infectious virions (the poxviruses, poliovirus, and herpes viruses, for example). Other viruses are released from infected cells by budding through the cell membrane in the absence of cell death (e.g., HIV and influenza virus). Having entered the body, however, viruses encounter numerous innate defenses and activate the components of adaptive immunity. The latter usually assures that clinical disease, if not infection, will not become evident. Successful exploitation of these defenses through the use of vaccines remains a central challenge for many human viruses, particularly those that cause chronic infections such as HIV and HCV.[2]

Innate immunity to viruses

Viral infection induces an extensive array of defense mechanisms in the host. Innate defenses come into play to block or inhibit initial infection, to protect cells from infection, or to eliminate virus-infected cells; these occur well before the effectors of adaptive immunity become active (Chapter 3). The innate immune defenses are initiated via pathogen recognition receptors (PRRs), which recognize pathogen-associated molecular patterns (PAMPs). These include transmembrane receptors of the Toll-like receptor (TLR) family, two families of intracellular receptors including the NOD-like receptors (NLRs) and the RIG-I-like helicases (RLHs), as well as the sensor molecule absent in melanoma 2 (AIM2) (Table 27.2). These cellular sensors promote the expression of interleukin-1 (IL-1) and IL-18, type I (α/β) interferons (IFN-I) and a variety of IFN-stimulated genes and inflammatory cytokines. TLRs are cell surface or endosomal

Table 27.1 Viral infections and immunity

Viral event	Obstacles	Time course
Transmission	Mechanical and chemical barriers	0
Infection and replication	Innate immunity	0 →
Infection stopped or spreads	Viral antigens transported to lymphoid tissues	Within 24 hours
Infection controlled	Specific antibodies and cell-mediated immunity	4–10 days
Sterile immunity	Immune memory	14 days to years
Viral persistence if infection not controlled	Immune disruption or evasion	Weeks to years

Table 27.2 Sensors of viral infection

Toll-like receptors (TLRs)		
TLR3	dsRNA, MCMV, VSV, LCMV, HSV, EBV	
TLR7 and TLR8	ssRNA, Influenza virus, HIV, VSV	
TLR9	dsDNA, HSV, MCMV	
TLR2	MV hemagglutinin protein, HSV, HCMV	
TLR4	MMTV envelope protein, RSV	
RIG-I-like helicases (RLHs)		
RIG-I	Influenza virus, VSV, HCV, JEV, MV, RSV, Sendai virus, EBV	
MDA-5	Poly(I:C), MV, Sendai virus, VSV, MCMV, Picornaviruses	
NOD-like receptors (NLRs)		
NLRP3	Influenza virus, Sendai virus, Adenovirus, Vaccinia virus	
NOD2	Influenza virus, VSV, RSV	
AIM2	Vaccinia virus, MCMV	
DAI	Cytosolic dsDNA, HSV	

AIM2, absent in melanoma 2; DAI, DNA-dependent activator of IFN; dsRNA, double-strand RNA; EBV, Epstein-Barr virus; HCMV, human cytomegalovirus; HCV, hepatitis C virus; HIV, human immunodeficiency virus; HSV, herpes simplex virus 1/2; JEV, Japanese encephalitis virus; LCMV, lymphocytic choriomeningitis virus; MCMV, murine cytomegalovirus; MDA-5, melanoma differentiation-associated gene; MMTV, mouse mammary tumor virus; MV, measles virus; NLR, NOD-like receptor; RLH, RIG-I-like helicase; RSV, respiratory syncytial virus; ssRNA, single-strand RNA; TLR, Toll-like receptor; VSV, vesicular stomatis virus.

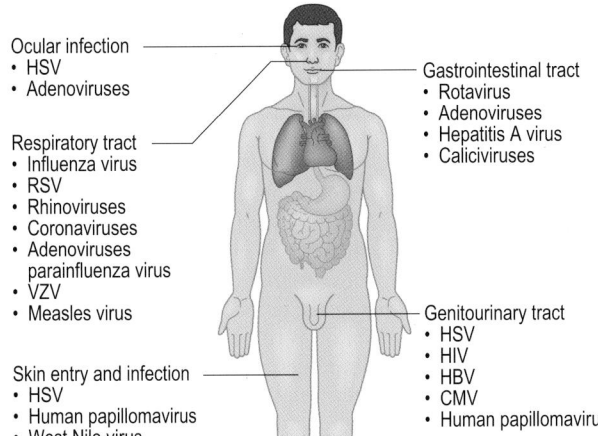

Fig. 27.1 Common routes of entry and infection for human viral pathogens. CMV, cytomegalovirus; HBV, hepatitis B virus; HIV, human immunodeficiency virus; HSV, herpes simplex virus; RSV, respiratory syncytial virus; VZV, varicella-zoster virus.

Ocular infection
• HSV
• Adenoviruses

Respiratory tract
• Influenza virus
• RSV
• Rhinoviruses
• Coronaviruses
• Adenoviruses parainfluenza virus
• VZV
• Measles virus

Skin entry and infection
• HSV
• Human papillomavirus
• West Nile virus

Gastrointestinal tract
• Rotavirus
• Adenoviruses
• Hepatitis A virus
• Caliciviruses

Genitourinary tract
• HSV
• HIV
• HBV
• CMV
• Human papillomavirus

immunity: the NLRP3 inflammasome, the RIG-I inflammasome, and the AIM2 inflammasome. Other cytoplasmic sensors of viruses, such as the more recently discovered cytosolic dsDNA sensor DAI (**D**NA-dependent **a**ctivator of **I**FN), may also play important roles in sensing viral pathogens.

membrane-bound proteins expressed by numerous cells including dendritic cells (DC), macrophages, lymphocytes, and parenchymal cells. Expression of TLRs is largely inducible in most cell types, though some (TLR7/8/9) are constitutively expressed at high levels by specialized plasmacytoid DC for rapid IFN production. Different TLR molecules recognize specific viral products such as single- and double-stranded RNA (TLR 3 and TLR7/8, respectively) or double-stranded DNA (TLR9). Much of our understanding of the roles of TLRs to antiviral defense have been discovered in mice, yet our understanding of the similarities and differences in the functions of human TLRs is rapidly improving.[3]

The more recently discovered RLHs, retinoic acid-inducible gene I (RIG-I) and melanoma differentiation-associated gene (MDA-5), mediate cytoplasmic recognition of viral nucleic acids.[4] These activate mitochondrial antiviral signaling proteins (MAVS) to stimulate IFN-I production and activate the inflammasome, a molecular complex that facilitates the activation of caspases and induces the production of proinflammatory IL-1β and IL-18.[5] NLRs are a second class of cytosolic sensors of PAMPS that activate the inflammasone.[6] These include the NLRP (or NALP), NOD, and IPAF/NAIP receptors. Three major inflammasomes have been shown to be involved in antiviral

KEY CONCEPTS

Major antiviral innate defense mechanisms

Acting to block infection:
- Natural antibodies
- Complement components
- Some cytokines and chemokines

Acting to protect cells from infection:
- Interferon-α/β
- Interferon-γ
- IL-1, IL-18

Acting to destroy or inhibit virus-infected cells:
- Natural killer cells
- NKT cells
- Macrophages
- Neutrophils
- γδ T cells
- Nitric oxide

Involved in regulating antiviral inflammatory response:
- Interleukins-1, 6, 10, 12, 18, 23, 33
- Transforming growth factor-β
- Chemokines (CCL2, 3, 4, 5)

The innate defense system consists of multiple cellular components and many specialized proteins. The longest known and best studied antiviral proteins are the α/β IFNs, which act by binding to the type I IFN receptor and result in the transcription of more than 100 IFN-stimulated genes. One consequence of this "antiviral state" is the inhibition of cell protein synthesis and the prevention of viral replication.[7] Type I IFNs also activate natural killer (NK) cells and induce other cytokines such as IFN-γ and IL-12 that promote NK responses (Chapter 17). NK cells produce pro-inflammatory cytokines, they can kill infected cells and interact with DC, and are an important component of innate defense against viruses. NK cells are regulated by an array of activating and inhibitory receptors whose expression and function are just beginning to be understood. Uninfected cells are usually protected from NK cell cytolysis as they deliver negative signals such as high expression of MHC molecules. In contrast, virus-infected cells are killed either because they deliver positive signals or because they lack adequate MHC-negative signals. The NK defense system appears important against some herpes viruses, which downregulate MHC expression in the cells they infect. NK cells are also important in resistance to mouse and human cytomegalovirus, and possibly to HIV, influenza virus, and Ebola viruses.[8] A distinct NK cell population, NKT cells, may provide some antigen-specific innate immune protection against certain viruses.[9] Many other leukocytes are involved in innate defense, including macrophages, DC, neutrophils, and perhaps T cells expressing $\gamma\delta$ T-cell receptors for antigen. Furthermore, tissue cells including fibroblasts, epithelial and endothelial cells express PRRs and can respond to viral infection via the production of innate cytokines, including IFN-I and IL-1.

Several classes of innate host proteins function in antiviral defense. These include natural antibody, which may play a role in defense against some virus infections, as well as the pentraxins and complement proteins.[10] Some viruses may be directly inactivated by complement activation or be destroyed by phagocytic cells that bind and ingest complement-bound virions. Several pro-inflammatory cytokines and chemokines induced by virus infection also play key roles in defense. Foremost among these is IL-1 and other members of the IL-1 family, including IL-18 and IL-33.[11] These cytokines influence both innate and adaptive immune cells and play critical roles in antiviral defense. Other anti-viral cytokines are produced early following infection, such as TNF-α, IFN-γ, IL-12, IL-6, and chemokines such as MIP-1α. In particular, IL-12 is a potent inducer of IFN-γ from NK cells. Inflammatory chemokines may also play an important role in innate antiviral defense by orchestrating macrophage, neutrophil, DC, and NK responses at the site of infection (Chapter 10). Not only are these components of innate immunity involved in mediating initial protection against viruses; several components (such as the PRRs, the cytokines IFN-I, IL-I, and IL-12, and phagocytes including macrophages, monocytes, and DC) serve to shape the nature and effectiveness of the subsequent adaptive response to viral pathogens.

Adaptive immunity to viruses

Innate immunity generally serves to slow, rather than stop, viral infection, allowing time for the adaptive immune response to begin. The two major divisions of adaptive immunity, antibody and T-cell-mediated, are mainly directed at different targets. Antibodies usually function by binding to free viral particles, and in so doing block infection of the host cell. In contrast, T cells act principally by recognizing and destroying virus-infected cells, or by orchestrating an inflammatory response that includes several antiviral components. As all viruses replicate within cells and many can spread directly between cells without re-entering the extracellular environment, resolution of infection is reliant more on T-cell function than on antibody. Antiviral antibody, however, does assume considerably more importance as an additional immunoprotective barrier against reinfection. It is the presence of antibody at portals of entry—most often mucosal surfaces—that is of particular relevance to influenza, HSV, and HIV infections.[12] Accordingly, vaccinologists try to design vaccines that optimally induce mucosal antibody.

Initiation of adaptive immunity is closely dependent upon early innate mechanisms that activate antigen-presenting cells (APC), principally subsets of DC. APC and lymphocytes are drawn into lymphoid tissues by chemokine and cytokine signals and retained there for a few days in order to facilitate effective interactions between these cells. The architecture of the secondary lymphoid tissues supports the coordinated interactions between cells of the adaptive immune system through a network of supportive stromal cells and local chemokine gradients.[13] The induction events occur in lymph nodes draining the infection site, or in the spleen if virus enters the bloodstream. The passage of viral antigens to lymph nodes usually occurs in DCs.[14] Some viruses are able to compromise the function of APC, such as HSV and measles virus, which can inhibit DC maturation.

B-cell activation occurs following antigen encounter in the B-cell follicles, and possibly the T-cell zones, in the spleen or lymph nodes.[15] Some activated B cells become short-lived plasma cells while others move to the edges of the B-cell follicles and interact with antigen-specific helper CD4 T cells via presentation of antigenic peptides on B-cell MHC class II molecules. These activated B cells initiate germinal center (GC) reactions, which ensure somatic hypermutation and affinity maturation for the selection of high-affinity, antibody-producing long-lived plasma cells, as well as memory B cells (Chapter 7). Recent advances have greatly improved our understanding of the signals that control the generation of these important B-cell subsets, particularly at the molecular level.[16] We now know that upregulation of the transcription factors Blimp-1, XBP-1, and IRF-4 dictates plasma cell formation, whereas Pax-5 expression delineates B cells destined for GC reactions and the memory B-cell lineage.

Antibody binding to epitopes expressed by native proteins at the surface of free virions usually blocks viral attachment or penetration of target cells. Sometimes the consequence is viral lysis (with complement proteins also involved), opsonization, or sensitization for destruction by Fc receptor-bearing cells that mediate antibody-dependent cellular cytotoxicity (ADCC). Occasionally, however, Fc receptor binding of antibody-bound virus may facilitate infection and result in more severe tissue damage. This occurs in dengue fever and may happen in some instances in HIV infection.

As indicated previously, antibody may function most effectively to prevent reinfection, especially at mucosal surfaces. The antibody involved in humans is predominantly secretory immunoglobulin A (IgA), but serum-derived IgG may also be protective, particularly in sites such as the vaginal mucosa. Both antibody isotypes act mainly to block infection of epithelial cells, although in some instances the antibody may transport antigen from within the body across epithelial cells to the outside. Mucosal antibody persists for a much shorter period than does serum antibody, which explains in part why immunity to mucosal pathogens is usually of much shorter duration than is immunity to systemic virus infections.

Antiviral T- and B-cell immunity

Effector systems	Recognized molecules	Control mechanisms
Antibody	Surface proteins or virions	Neutralization of virus, opsonization, or destruction of infected cells by ADCC
Antibody + complement	Surface proteins expressed on infected cells	Infected cell destruction by ADCC or complement-mediated lysis
Mucosal antibody (IgA)	Surface proteins or virions	Viral neutralization, opsonization, and transcytosis
CD4 T cells	Viral peptides (10–20 mers) presented on MHC class II – surface, internal or nonstructural proteins presented by APC	Antiviral cytokine and chemokine production; help for CD8 T-cell and B-cell responses; killing infected cells; regulatory functions to reduce immunopathology
CD8 T cells	Viral peptides (8–10 mers) presented on MHC class I – surface, internal or nonstructural proteins presented on infected cells or by cross-presentation	Killing infected cells or purging virus without cell death; antiviral cytokine and chemokine production

ADCC, antibody-dependent cellular cytotoxicity; APC, antigen-presenting cell; IgA, immunoglobulin A; MHC, major histocompatibility complex.

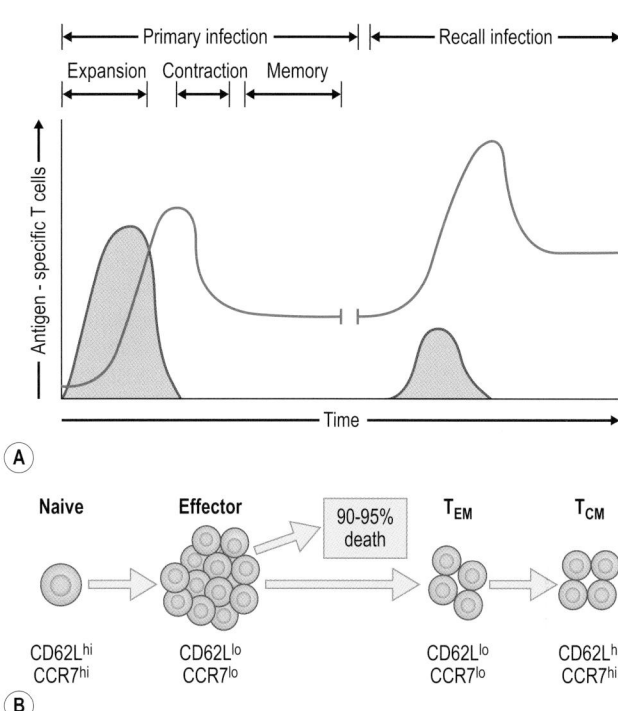

Fig. 27.2 Expansion/contraction/memory phases of adaptive immunity and memory cell subsets. (A) Dynamics of primary and secondary (recall) T-cell responses to viral infection. Both primary and recall T-cell responses undergo expansion and contraction phases, followed by stable immune memory. Recall responses induce a larger effector pool and reduced contraction further boosting the memory pool. (B) Effector and memory T-cell differentiation. Antigen stimulation expands effector cells, most of which die during the contraction phase. T_{EM} cells that are formed gradually convert to T_{CM} cells over time, with corresponding changes in surface marker expression.

Like B-cell responses, T-cell responses to viral infections also begin within the lymphoid tissues. Specific CD8 cytotoxic T lymphocyte (CTL) precursors recognize antigen in the context of MHC class I–peptide antigen complexes on professional APC, such as DC. The CD8 T cells become activated, proliferate, and differentiate into effectors. Expansion of these naïve antigen-specific precursors is considerable, often exceeding 10,000-fold, and results in an effector population that can account for 40% or more of a host's total CD8 T-cell population (Fig. 27.2). Various factors, including antigen and APC, co-stimulatory molecules (such as CD28 and 4-1BB), and inflammatory cytokines (such as IFN-I and IL-12) are required to program the development of functional effector lymphocytes.[17] The CTL effectors enter the efferent lymph and bloodstream and access almost all body locations, including both primary and subsequent sites of infection. However, effectors do not stay activated for long once the virus is cleared, and approximately 95% die by a process termed activation-induced cell death. Following this contraction phase, the remaining cells differentiate into memory cells, which remain as a more or less stable population in the host for many years. They represent an expanded pool of CTL precursors that can be activated upon secondary encounter with antigen, and provide enhanced protection upon reinfection with the same virus (see next section). Though much of our knowledge of T-cell responses to viruses have been obtained using mice, recent work has demonstrated that most of the fundamental principles (described below) are the same or similar in humans.[18]

T-cell immunity against a particular virus commonly involves both CD4 and CD8 T-cell subsets. Both CD4 and CD8 T cells recognize peptides derived from viral antigens bound to surface MHC proteins (class II and class I, respectively). Complexes of viral peptides bound to MHC class II proteins are generated by APC from scavenged and processed virus-infected cells or viral particles. Antigen–MHC class I complexes are expressed on the surface of infected cells, and antigen can also be transferred to APC from infected cells by a process known as cross-presentation.[19] Recent experiments in mice have also demonstrated a role for transfer of antigen between DC[20] as they migrate from infected tissues to the lymphoid tissues. Curiously, although many peptides derived from viral proteins have an appropriate motif that permits MHC binding, the majority of CD8 T cells, and possibly CD4 T cells, are often specific for a few immunodominant epitopes. Use of MHC class I and class II tetramers to directly visualize antigen-specific CD8 and CD4 T-cell responses, respectively, has demonstrated the significant size of T-cell responses to viruses and that the majority of the activated T cells seen at the peak of the response are virus-specific.

CTL function by recognizing virus-infected cells and killing them (Chapter 17). This often involves perforins and cytotoxic granules containing granzymes. Effector CTL can also induce death in target cells following engagement of Fas ligand on the CTL with Fas on target cells. Both pathways lead to apoptosis of the target cell, involving the degradation of nucleic acids, including those of the virus. Alternatively, CD8 T cells also mediate defense through the release of various cytokines following antigen recognition. Some of the cytokines and chemokines most highly produced by CTL include IFN-γ, TNF-α, lymphotoxin-α, and RANTES (Chapters 9 and 10). These cytokines can have multiple antiviral effects on infected cells and the cells around them, including purging of virus from infected cells without killing the cell. This is particularly important for viruses like HSV, which infects non-rejuvenating cells such as nerve cells.

CD4 T cells are also involved in antiviral defense. They are important for controlling infections such as HSV, influenza virus, HIV, and many others. CD4 T cells participate in antiviral immunity in several ways. First, the subset acts as helper cells for the induction of both antiviral antibodies and CD8 T-cell responses to most virus antigens.[21] CD4 T cells also function as antiviral effector cells, and generate stable memory cell populations similar to those of CD8 T cells. The differentiation of CD4 T cells into effectors occurs in a manner very similar to that with CD8 T cells. At present less is known about the size and specificity of CD4 T-cell responses, but effector CD4 T-cell populations appear to consist of a broader epitope specificity than CD8 T cells responding to a given virus. CD4 T cells are activated by recognizing viral peptides associated with class II MHC molecules, which are present on more specialized cells such as APC. Thus, CD4 T cells rarely recognize viral epitopes present on cells as a consequence of viral gene expression within that cell, dictating their function as helper cells for B cells and CD8 T cells, and as producers of cytokines for help and viral clearance.

In some instances CD4 T cells can perform cytotoxic functions, though not as effectively as CD8 CTL. More commonly, however, effector CD4 T cells act by synthesizing and releasing numerous cytokines following their reaction with antigen (Chapter 9). Subsets of CD4 T effectors produce different groups of cytokines. The type most often involved in antiviral defense are designated T-helper 1 (Th1) cells, and primarily produce IFN-γ, LTα, TNF-α, and IL-2 to help orchestrate the inflammatory response and act directly or indirectly in antiviral defense. Conversely, Th2 effectors produce an array of cytokines that may downregulate the protective function of Th1 cells, such as IL-4, IL-5, and two anti-inflammatory cytokines, IL-10 and transforming growth factor-β (TGF-β). Th2 T cells play a protective function against some parasite infections (Chapter 29), though in some virus infections an exuberant Th2 response may be associated with immunopathology or impaired immunity. Indeed, blocking the Th2 cytokine IL-10 was recently shown to assist in the clearance of chronic viral infection. Th17 cells that produce IL-17, and also IL-22, are generated under certain inflammatory conditions, though it is unclear whether these cells play a vital role during viral infections.[22] Lastly, CD4 T cells can differentiate into T follicular helper (Tfh) cells following interactions with antigen-specific B cells, which are important for germinal center formation and antibody responses to viruses.[23]

Immunological memory

Immunological memory is a cardinal feature of adaptive immunity. The goal of vaccinology is to induce long-lived immunological memory to protect against reinfection. Following infection with certain viruses, memory can be exceptionally long-lived, potentially for the life of the host (e.g., yellow fever and smallpox viruses).[18,24] Memory is defined by the persistence of specific lymphocytes and antibody-producing plasma cells, rather than that of antigen to induce continuous lymphocyte activation. Humoral memory to viruses involves long-lived plasma cells in the bone marrow that provide a continuous low-level source of serum antibody. This maintenance of humoral immunity also involves a population of homeostatically maintained memory B cells, which may be required to maintain stable numbers of

long-lived plasma cells over time. The pool of memory T cells is regulated by low-level homeostatic division controlled by the cytokines IL-7 and -15. For memory CD8 T cells, IL-7 is primarily important for survival while IL-15 is crucial for low-level proliferation to maintain the size of the memory T-cell pool.[25]

● KEY CONCEPTS

Principles of antiviral immunity

- Many human viral infections are successfully controlled by the immune system
- Certain emerging viruses may overwhelm the immune system and cause severe morbidity and mortality
- Other viruses have developed mechanisms to overwhelm or evade the immune system and persist
- Individuals with defects in innate or adaptive immunity demonstrate more severe viral infections
- T-cell immunity is more important for control than antibody with many viral infections
- Antibody is important to minimize reinfection, particularly at mucosal sites
- Immune memory is often sufficient to prevent secondary disease, though not in all viral infections
- Tissue-specific immune memory may be important to rapidly protect against reinfection at peripheral sites (such as the skin and mucosae)

Immunological memory is defined by a pool of antigen-specific cells whose increased frequency enables rapid control of viral reinfection (Fig. 27.2). A population of IL-7Rα-expressing effector cells are the precursors of this memory pool.[26] This population of cells, which constitutes about 5–10% of the effector pool, preferentially survives the contraction phase, and gradually differentiates into a stable memory population. Upon reinfection, these memory cells can be rapidly activated, and by virtue of their increased frequency mediate more rapid clearance of the viral pathogen. Moreover, repeated stimulation of memory cells via multiple infections with the same virus, or prime-boost vaccine regimes, further increases the size of the antigen-specific memory T-cell pool.[27] Re-stimulation also affects the activation status and tissue distribution of memory T cells, which may enhance protection from viral infection in mucosal, and other, tissues.

Experiments in humans and mice have demonstrated that memory T cells are heterogeneous.[27] Memory T cells have been divided into effector memory (T_{EM}) and central memory (T_{CM}) subsets, defined by expression of two surface molecules involved in T-cell migration: CD62L and CCR7. The CD62L^{lo}CCR7^{lo} T_{EM} subset is found primarily in non-lymphoid tissues and spleen, whereas the CD62L^{hi}CCR7^{hi} T_{CM} subset is largely present in the lymph nodes and spleen. The current model predicts that effector T cells form the T_{EM} subset and these cells gradually convert to a T_{CM} phenotype over time. Though the conditions that control the rate of this conversion are unknown, it is likely that the amount of antigen and inflammatory signals received during the effector phase greatly influences this. It has also been shown that CD4 T-cell help is required for the generation of long-lived memory CD8 T cells, via interactions with DC.[21]

Studies suggest that T_{CM} are capable of mounting stronger proliferative responses following reinfection. However, the tissue-specific homing of T_{EM} cells permits them to reside in sites of potential viral infection, such as the skin and mucosae. Indeed, the hallmark of a recently described subset of memory CD8 T cells involves long-term residence within tissues at sites of previous viral infection.[28–30] This includes the skin, intestine, and brain.

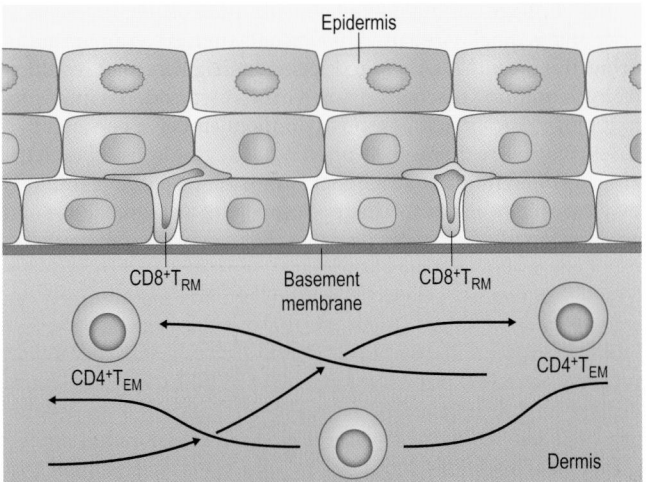

Fig. 27.3 Unique subsets of memory CD8 and CD4 T cells reside within peripheral tissues, at sites of previous viral infection, and provide rapid protection against reinfection. Resident memory CD8 T cells (T_{RM}) remain localized in the epidermis in skin after HSV infection. CD4 T_{EM} continue to migrate through the dermal layers of skin, with access to the blood and the lymphoid tissues.

These resident memory T cells (T_{RM}) are sequestered from the circulation and provide rapid protection against viruses such as HSV in skin, where they localize with a unique dendritic morphology and undergo slow surveillance of the tissue (Fig. 27.3).[44] This is in contrast to CD4 T_{EM}, which continue to migrate through the non-lymphoid tissues rather than being sequestered in the peripheral tissues, and also differs from the CD8 and CD4 T_{CM}, which migrate largely through the lymphoid organs (spleen and lymph nodes). These differences may define the physiological *raison d'être* for these memory T-cell subsets. However, memory in certain peripheral tissues, such as the lungs, may be less effective or wane over time.[31] This may explain in part why vaccines against respiratory viruses have a poor record.

Immune evasion and immunity to chronic viral infections

Many, if not all, viruses employ immune blunting or delay tactics to circumvent aspects of the immune system, allowing them time to replicate further or escape detection (Table 27.3).[32] One such mechanism may involve killing or infecting APC. Viruses may also delay or prevent apoptosis induced by CTL within infected cells. Other viral evasion measures aimed at the CD8 T-cell-mediated antiviral defense system serve to inhibit antigen processing, thereby minimizing effector CTL induction. Many viruses also downregulate MHC molecules on the surface of infected cells to escape CTL killing. In addition, viruses may produce various mimics or modulators/inhibitors of cytokines, chemokines, or other components of the immune system or their receptors. Viruses also resort to antigenic hypervariability to escape antibody or T-cell recognition. This can occur during transmission from host to host (e.g., influenza virus), or within hosts during chronic infection through the generation of viral escape mutants. The latter is particularly important for HIV and HCV infections.

The success of many viral pathogens rests in their ability to subvert the host immune response. The most successful human viruses can escape the immune system and persist for the life of the host.[33] Two well-studied examples of this are CMV and EBV. T-cell responses to these viruses are prominent and readily

Table 27.3 Mechanisms and examples of viral immune evasion

Mechanism	Example
Interference with viral antigen processing and presentation	HSV (ICP47), EBV (EBNA-1), HIV (Nef, Tat), HPV (E5), CMV (UL6)
Evasion of NK cell function	HIV (Nef), EBV (EBNA-1), CMV (UL40, UL18)
Inhibition of cell apoptosis	Adenovirus (RID complex and E1B), HIV (Nef), EBV (BHRF-1)
Destruction of T cells	HIV
Interference with antiviral cytokines and chemokines	EBV (IL-10 homologue), CMV (US28 chemokine receptor homologue), vaccinia virus (IL-18-binding protein), HIV (Tat chemokine activity)
Inhibition of complement action	HSV, pox viruses
Inhibition of DC maturation	HSV, vaccinia virus
Frequent antigenic variation	Influenza virus, HIV
Infection of immune privileged site	Measles virus, VZV and HSV (neurons)
Immune exhaustion	HIV, HCV, HBV

CMV, cytomegalovirus; DC, dendritic cell; EBV, Epstein–Barr virus; HBV, hepatitis B virus; HCV, hepatitis C virus; HIV, human immunodeficiency virus; HPV, human papillomavirus; HSV, herpes simplex virus; IL-18, interleukin-18; NK, natural killer; RID, receptor internalization and degradation; VZV, varicella-zoster virus.

detectable in people, yet the immune system is unable to clear either pathogen completely. However, these viruses generally remain undetectable in immunocompetent individuals. Other viral infections, such as those caused by the herpes viruses HSV and VZV, are marked by periods of latency, where no virus can be detected. Yet periods of viral reactivation, often triggered by stress, can lead to episodes of disease. These are controlled by the immune response, which plays a central role in controlling herpes virus latency.[34]

Many of the most medically important human viruses are associated with persistent viremia. These include chronic infections such as HIV, HCV, HBV, and human T-lymphotropic virus (HTLV), among others. Such viral infections are marked by high levels of persisting antigen and can result in skewed T-cell immunodominance hierarchies, altered tissue localization of immune cells, and severely impaired T-cell function.[33] This altered T-cell function is hierarchical and results in functional T-cell defects ranging from reduced cytokine production and altered proliferative capacity (exhaustion) to death (deletion) of the responding T cells (Fig. 27.4). Recent work has shown that viral antigen levels are responsible for this immune dysfunction.[35] This is in stark

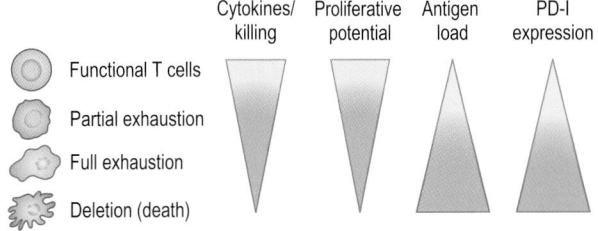

Fig. 27.4 Hierarchical model of T-cell exhaustion during persistent viral infection. T-cell function (cytokine production, killing, and proliferative potential) is negatively influenced by increasing levels of antigen. Low levels of persistent antigen may lead to partial loss of function and intermediate levels of programmed death (PD)-1 expression. High, sustained levels of antigen over time can lead to full loss of function, high levels of PD-1, and eventually cell death (deletion).

contrast to normal memory T-cell development, which occurs in the absence of persisting antigen (see previous section). Recent studies have demonstrated that signaling through the cell-surface receptor programmed death (PD)-1 on effector CTL causes exhaustion during chronic infections.[36] This pathway may be essential for preventing excessive immunopathology by effector T cells, yet appears to contribute directly to failed immunity to HIV infection, and other chronic human viral infections. These studies implicate this pathway as a potential therapeutic target.

Outcomes of virus infection: immunity or immunopathology

Typically, individual humans respond to a virus infection in different ways. When the common cold or even pandemic influenza infection occurs, only a small percentage of exposed persons may develop overt clinical disease. In the pre-vaccine days, poliomyelitis was a much-feared consequence of poliovirus infection, but only a very small percentage of infected persons developed the paralyzing complications. Similarly, only an unfortunate few develop life-threatening meningoencephalitis following infection with the insect–transmitted West Nile fever virus. It is particularly characteristic of chronic viral infections that clinical expression is highly variable. With hepatitis C, for example, 70-80% of patients develop some form of chronic liver disease and fail to clear infection. However, up to 30% do control the infection, clear virus, and can be immune to reinfection. The latter group of individuals make a type of immune response that includes protective antibodies along with an appropriate pattern of T-cell responsiveness.[37]

We do not fully understand the reasons for the varying outcome of virus infections in different persons and almost certainly multiple factors are involved. Many of these factors impact the response pattern made by the innate immune system that in turn affects the magnitude and type of adaptive immune response that occurs. Some of the circumstances that do influence the outcome of infection include genetic susceptibility of the host, the age of the host when infected, the dose and route of infection, the variable induction in the host of anti-inflammatory cells and proteins, and the presence of concurrent infections and past exposure to cross-reactive antigens.[37]

Immunopathology and autoimmunity

Immune responses against virus-infected cells often result in tissue damage, especially if cell killing is involved or there is extensive recruitment and activation of inflammatory cell types such as macrophages and sometimes neutrophils. If the response is brief and is quickly repaired, it is usually judged as an immunoprotective event. A prolonged tissue-damaging effect resulting from an immune reaction against viruses is considered immunopathology. Such situations most commonly involve persistent viruses, which are themselves often mildly cyto-destructive in the absence of an immune reaction. Chronic tissue damage initiated by viruses may also result in development of an autoreactive and an occasionally oncogenic response. For example, some autoimmune diseases (AID) may be initiated or exacerbated by virus infections, but no named virus has been regularly incriminated as a cause of human AID.[38] Circumstantial evidence exists for a virus link in multiple sclerosis (MS), insulin-dependent diabetes, and possibly systemic lupus erythematosus (SLE). In MS, many viruses have been isolated from patients, although no specific one has been tied to the disease etiology. The current hypothesis is that viral infections set up an inflammatory environment that may exacerbate or tip the balance towards disease in genetically susceptible individuals.[38]

Immunopathological reactions involving viruses have several mechanisms, but T cells are usually involved as orchestrators of the inflammatory events (Table 27.4). The clearest example of immunopathology involving a virus is lymphocytic choriomeningitis virus (LCMV) in the mouse. This model has dominated ideas and has set several paradigms in viral immunology in general. The first virus-induced immunopathological lesion recognized was glomerulonephritis and arteritis, noted in mice persistently infected with LCMV. The lesions were assumed to represent inflammatory reactions to tissue-entrapped immune complexes that activate complement. Similar immune complex-mediated lesions occur in other infections, which include lung lesions found in severe influenza and respiratory syncytial virus, as well as viral hepatitis and arthritis.[39] However, only rarely have viral antigens been shown to contribute to the antigen component of the complex. An example where the inclusion of viral antigen in immune complexes has been demonstrated is chronic hepatitis B virus infection of humans. Autoimmune disease such as SLE also results from immune complex-mediated tissue damage. However, evidence linking viruses to the etiology or pathogenesis of SLE is scarce, since the immune complexes in SLE do not appear at any stage to include viral antigens.

Thanks largely to the LCMV model, it is clear that CD8 T-cell recognition of viral antigens can result in tissue damage. In LCMV damage occurs in the leptomeninges of immunocompetent mice infected intracerebrally. Hepatitis can also occur in mice infected intravenously. Neither lesion becomes evident if the CD8 T-cell response is suppressed. CD8 T-cell-mediated immunopathology is a causative mechanism of chronic hepatitis associated with hepatitis C and B infection as well as with some lesions that occur

Table 27.4 Lesions resulting from immunopathology

Primarily involving CD8 T cells acting as cytotoxic T lymphocytes or sources of pro-inflammatory cytokines:	Murine lymphocytic choriomeningitis virus; Hepatitis B virus-induced chronic hepatitis; Coxsackie B virus-induced diabetes; Coxsackie B virus-induced myocarditis; Demyelination caused by some strains of mouse coronavirus and Theiler's virus
Primarily involving CD4 T cells that produce Th1 cytokines:	Demyelination caused by some strains of mouse coronavirus and Theiler's virus; Herpes simplex virus-induced stromal keratitis
Involvement of CD4 T cells that produce Th2 cytokines:	Respiratory syncytial virus-induced pulmonary lesions
Involvement of antibody:	Glomerulonephritis in chronic hepatitis B; Dengue hemorrhagic fever

during HIV infection.[40] The immunopathological mechanisms involved in hepatitis B infection have been carefully analyzed in a mouse model in which the whole HBV was expressed as a transgene. In this model, CD8 T cells orchestrated the immunopathology, but the process was complex. Initially, CTL-mediated killing events occurred, but since hepatocytes die by apoptosis it was not clear how this related to subsequent inflammatory events. However, the CD8 T cells also released numerous cytokines and chemokines that recruited inflammatory cells, primarily macrophages. Interestingly, liver-infiltrating CTL have been shown to be inhibited by PD-1–PD-L1 interactions, which may greatly reduce the severity of local immunopathology. Additional viral immunopathology models where lesions result primarily from CD8 T-cell involvement include myocarditis and insulin-dependent diabetes associated with coxsackie B virus infection. In both instances, CD8 T cells mainly orchestrate events, but tissue damage may result from the bystander effects of cytokines and other molecules such as lipid mediators, metalloproteinases, and components of the oxygen burst. Although coxsackie virus can be a cause of diabetes in the mouse, attempts to relate viral infection directly to the etiology of human diabetes have so far failed.[38]

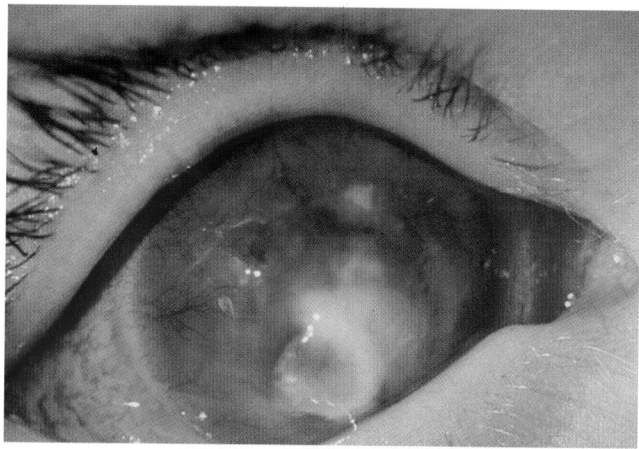

Fig. 27.5 Example of herpetic stromal keratitis (HSK) in the human eye after herpes simplex virus-1 (HSV-1) infection. Inflammation of the eye and eyelid can be observed, as well as neovascularization, and substantial necrosis, ulceration, and opacity of the cornea.

CLINICAL RELEVANCE

Hypothesized role of viruses in autoimmunity

- Molecular mimicry: similar epitopes shared by virus and host
- Bystander activation: chronic release of cytokines and host antigens activates local autoreactive lymphocytes
- Viral persistence: chronic viral antigen presentation on host cells leads to prolonged immunopathology

---

Immunopathological reactions against viruses can also involve subsets of CD4 T cells. Most commonly Th1 cells are responsible for such reactions, but Th17 and occasionally Th4 subsets may also play the main role. One well-studied example involves persistent infection with Theiler's virus in mice.[41] This infection causes a demyelinating syndrome that resembles the AID experimental allergic encephalomyelitis. In both situations, CD4 T cells that produce Th1 cytokines appear to serve as the pathologic mediators. Furthermore, in both models an increase in the involvement of myelin-derived autoantigens occurs as the disease progresses. Once again, such observations indicate the possible role of a virus in an autoimmune disease. With the Theiler's virus model the virus persists in the nervous system and chronically stimulates CD4 T cells to secrete an array of cytokines. The demyelinating events appear to result from cytokine action on oligodendrocytes. Myelin components such as myelin basic protein, proteolipid protein, and myelin oligodendroglial glycoprotein may be released and participate as additional antigens in immunoinflammatory events. This scenario is referred to as epitope spreading.

Another model of virus-induced immunopathology that mainly involves the Th1 subset of CD4 T cells is stromal keratitis caused by herpes simplex virus infection (Fig. 27.5).[42] The pathogenesis of this immunopathological lesion is unusual in that it occurs and progresses when viral antigens can no longer be demonstrated. The chronic immunoinflammatory lesions are mainly orchestrated by CD4 T cells, but multiple early events occur that induce the subsequent pathology. Viral replication, the production of certain cytokines and chemokines (IL-1,

IL-6, IL-12, and CXCL8), recruitment of inflammatory cells (such as neutrophils), and neovascularization of the avascular cornea all precede immunopathology.[42] Recently, it has become evident that Th17 T cells participate in stromal keratitis lesions. The role of Th17 T cells as orchestrators of inflammatory reactions has been a major research focus especially in lesions of AID.[22] When Th17 T cells are the principal mediators of tissue damage, there is an abundance of neutrophils recruited to the inflammatory sites, with such cells mainly responsible for the tissue damage.

A further mechanism of viral-induced immunopathology and autoimmunity is molecular mimicry.[38] Molecular mimicry represents shared antigenic epitopes, either B- or T-cell antigens, between the host and virus (Chapter 48). The idea began for streptococci and their association with rheumatic fever. With human autoimmune disease, there is little direct support for viral molecular mimicry; however, some animal models have been used to prove the theoretical case, using a model where a viral antigen is expressed as a self-protein in the islet cells of the pancreas. In this model subsequent infection with the virus induces diabetes. However, this is not true mimicry and may be more closely related to viral antigen persistence in a model such as Theiler's disease.

Recently it has become apparent that immunopathology can result from an imbalance in the types of functional effector T cells induced.[37] Tissue damage can be the bystander consequences of a dysregulated immune response to infection. The magnitude of the response can be influenced by the activity of one or more types of regulatory T cells (Tregs) (Chapter 15). Recent research has emphasized the role of natural CD4$^+$CD25$^+$FoxP3$^+$ Tregs, which are considered important for controlling the onset of autoimmune disease. These Tregs can also influence that magnitude of the protective immune response to viruses.[43] Natural FoxP3$^+$ Tregs, or other types of regulatory T cells that produce an abundance of anti-inflammatory cytokines IL-10 and TGF-β, are known to be involved in limiting excessive immunopathology associated with ongoing immune responses to persistent viral infection. Evidence for this has been reported in several viral infections, including HCV, HIV, and influenza virus.[43] It is interesting to note that Treg function may be both beneficial to the host, by limiting immunopathology, and detrimental, due to reduced local T-cell responses and thus prolonged viral persistence.

Phases of immunity affected by regulatory T cells (Tregs)

- Interference with antigen presentation by dendritic cells
- Inhibition of T-cell proliferation
- Inhibition of molecules involved in tissue-specific migration of effector cells
- Inhibition of T-cell effector functions in lymphoid and nonlymphoid tissues

Translational research opportunities

Reversing T-cell exhaustion in patients suffering from chronic infections or cancer will be a key clinical target in the near future. The discovery of multiple inhibitory receptors on exhausted T cells (including PD-1, LAG-3, 2B4, TIM-3, etc.) provides the opportunity to selectively improve T-cell function through blockade of these inhibitory receptors. This may be combined with blockade of immunosuppressive cytokines (such as IL-10), or enhancement of signals stimulatory to the response (such as IL-7 therapy), as well as with more traditional anti-viral therapies and vaccination. The challenge that lies ahead will be in determining which combination of inhibitory and stimulatory signals will need to be manipulated in different diseases and in different groups of patients.

The design of new generation vaccines to target diseases such as HIV and influenza virus may require tailor-made solutions for patients who respond poorly to vaccination, or respond improperly through adverse effects such as autoimmune reactions. High throughput approaches now allow for the generation of a molecular signature of vaccination or infection. Such systems biology approaches are expected to result in novel screening for immune protection parameters after vaccination. In the near future this should also assist in the formulation of new vaccines containing key immune activators, such as those that stimulate certain subsets of T cells, or induce appropriate homing molecule expression on these cells to direct them to tissues where they are required to mediate protection (such as mucosal sites, or the skin).

Clinically needed research opportunities

- Overcoming immune dysfunction during chronic viral infections essential for successful viral clearance.
- Improving the efficacy of vaccines to viruses using systems biology approaches.
- Therapies for reducing immunopathology during viral infections.

In some individuals viral infections cause mild, or sometimes debilitating, tissue damage. Factors that influence whether a viral infection results in immunopathology varies from individual to individual. These factors include age, the route of infection, pre-existing immunity, host genetics and the host's viral burden or virome. Our knowledge of the influence of these factors on the outcome of viral infection is expected to improve rapidly in the coming decade. Recent advances have shed considerable light on the various pro-inflammatory and anti-inflammatory mediators produced during viral infections. These represent key targets for novel therapies in the near future via the use of small-molecule inhibitors or treatment with endogenous chemical mediators such as resolvins or protectins.

Conclusions

Humans are infected by many pathogenic viruses. In most cases, these infections are controlled by the immune system with limited damage to the host. However, certain viruses, particularly in cases where the host's immune system is impaired, can cause significant damage to the host's tissues. As our understanding of the mechanisms underlying innate immune defenses, antigen presentation, T- and B-cell responses, and Tregs continues to improve, so too does the ability to design better vaccines and therapies to boost the immune control of viral infections. Although this remains a challenging goal, particularly for many human viruses such as HIV, HCV, and HSV, these rapid advances continue to provide many avenues for further investigation.

Acknowledgments

Barry T. Rouse is supported by grants from the National Institutes of Health and Scott N. Mueller by the Australian Research Council.

References

1. Marsh M, Helenius A. Virus entry: open sesame. Cell 2006;124(4):729–40.
2. Bachmann MF, Jennings GT. Vaccine delivery: a matter of size, geometry, kinetics and molecular patterns. Nat Rev Immunol 2010;10(11):787–96.
3. Casanova JL, Abel L, Quintana-Murci L. Human TLRs and IL-1Rs in host defense: natural insights from evolutionary, epidemiological, and clinical genetics. Annu Rev Immunol 2011;29:447–91.
4. Kawai T, Akira S. Innate immune recognition of viral infection. Nat Immunol 2006;7(2):131–7.
5. Kanneganti TD. Central roles of NLRs and inflammasomes in viral infection. Nat Rev Immunol 2010;10(10):688–98.
6. Martinon F, Mayor A, Tschopp J. The inflammasomes: guardians of the body. Annu Rev Immunol 2009;27:229–65.
7. Garcia-Sastre A, Biron CA. Type 1 interferons and the virus-host relationship: a lesson in detente. Science 2006;312(5775):879–82.
8. Lodoen MB, Lanier LL. Natural killer cells as an initial defense against pathogens. Curr Opin Immunol 2006;18(4):391–8.
9. Godfrey DI, Stankovic S, Baxter AG. Raising the NKT cell family. Nat Immunol 2010;11(3):197–206.
10. Bottazzi B, Doni A, Garlanda C, et al. An integrated view of humoral innate immunity: pentraxins as a paradigm. Annu Rev Immunol 2010;28:157–83.
11. Sims JE, Smith DE. The IL-1 family: regulators of immunity. Nat Rev Immunol 2010;10(2):89–102.
12. Iwasaki A. Antiviral immune responses in the genital tract: clues for vaccines. Nat Rev Immunol 2010;10(10):699–711.
13. Mueller SN, Germain RN. Stromal cell contributions to the homeostasis and functionality of the immune system. Nat Rev Immunol 2009;9(9):618–29.
14. Randolph GJ, Ochando J, Partida-Sanchez S. Migration of dendritic cell subsets and their precursors. Annu Rev Immunol 2008;26:293–316.
15. Okada T, Cyster JG. B cell migration and interactions in the early phase of antibody responses. Curr Opin Immunol 2006;18(3):278–85.
16. Martins G, Calame K. Regulation and functions of Blimp-1 in T and B lymphocytes. Annu Rev Immunol 2008;26:133–69.
17. Mescher MF, Curtsinger JM, Agarwal P, et al. Signals required for programming effector and memory development by CD8 + T cells. Immunol Rev 2006;211:81–92.
18. Ahmed R, Akondy RS. Insights into human CD8(+) T cell memory using the yellow fever and smallpox vaccines. Immunol Cell Biol 2011;89(3):340–5.
19. Heath WR, Belz GT, Behrens GM, et al. Cross-presentation, dendritic cell subsets, and the generation of immunity to cellular antigens. Immunol Rev 2004;199:9–26.
20. Heath WR, Carbone FR. Dendritic cell subsets in primary and secondary T cell responses at body surfaces. Nat Immunol 2009;10(12):1237–44.
21. Castellino F, Germain RN. Cooperation between CD4 + and CD8 + T cells: when, where, and how. Annu Rev Immunol 2006;24:519–40.
22. Korn T, Bettelli E, Oukka M, et al. IL-17 and Th17 Cells. Annu Rev Immunol 2009;27:485–517.
23. Crotty S. Follicular helper CD4 T cells (T(FH)). Annu Rev Immunol 2011;29:621–63.

24. Amanna IJ, Slifka MK, Crotty S. Immunity and immunological memory following smallpox vaccination. Immunol Rev 2006;211:320–37.
25. Surh CD, Boyman O, Purton JF, et al. Homeostasis of memory T cells. Immunol Rev 2006;211:154–63.
26. Williams MA, Bevan MJ. Effector and memory CTL differentiation. Annu Rev Immunol 2007;25:171–92.
27. Jameson SC, Masopust D. Diversity in T cell memory: an embarrassment of riches. Immunity 2009;31(6):859–71.
28. Bevan MJ. Memory T cells as an occupying force. Eur J Immunol 2011;41(5):1192–5.
29. Gebhardt T, Wakim LM, Eidsmo L, et al. Memory T cells in nonlymphoid tissue that provide enhanced local immunity during infection with herpes simplex virus. Nat Immunol 2009;10(5):524–30.
30. Masopust D, Choo D, Vezys V, et al. Dynamic T cell migration program provides resident memory within intestinal epithelium. J Exp Med 2010;207(3):553–64.
31. Woodland DL, Kohlmeier JE. Migration, maintenance and recall of memory T cells in peripheral tissues. Nat Rev Immunol 2009;9(3):153–61.
32. Finlay BB, McFadden G. Anti-immunology: evasion of the host immune system by bacterial and viral pathogens. Cell 2006;124(4):767–82.
33. Virgin HW, Wherry EJ, Ahmed R. Redefining chronic viral infection. Cell 2009;138(1):30–50.
34. Rouse BT, Kaistha SD. A tale of 2 alpha-herpesviruses: lessons for vaccinologists. Clin Infect Dis 2006;42(6):810–7.
35. Mueller SN, Ahmed R. High antigen levels are the cause of T cell exhaustion during chronic viral infection. Proc Natl Acad Sci U S A 2009;106(21):8623–8.
36. Keir ME, Butte MJ, Freeman GJ, et al. PD-1 and its ligands in tolerance and immunity. Annu Rev Immunol 2008;26:677–704.
37. Rouse BT, Sehrawat S. Immunity and immunopathology to viruses: what decides the outcome? Nat Rev Immunol 2010;10(7):514–26.
38. Fujinami RS, von Herrath MG, Christen U, et al. Molecular mimicry, bystander activation, or viral persistence: infections and autoimmune disease. Clin Microbiol Rev 2006;19(1):80–94.
39. Polack FP, Teng MN, Collins PL, et al. A role for immune complexes in enhanced respiratory syncytial virus disease. J Exp Med 2002;196(6):859–65.
40. Rehermann B. Hepatitis C virus versus innate and adaptive immune responses: a tale of coevolution and coexistence. J Clin Invest 2009;119(7):1745–54.
41. Olson JK, Ercolini AM, Miller SD. A virus-induced molecular mimicry model of multiple sclerosis. Curr Top Microbiol Immunol 2005;296:39–53.
42. Biswas PS, Rouse BT. Early events in HSV keratitis—setting the stage for a blinding disease. Microbes Infect 2005;7(4):799–810.
43. Belkaid Y, Tarbell K. Regulatory T cells in the control of host-microorganism interactions (*). Annu Rev Immunol 2009;27:551–89.
44. Gebhardt T, Whitney PG, Zaid A, et al. Different patterns of peripheral migration by memory CD4+ and CD8+ T cells. Nature 2011;477(7363):216–19.

Peter C. Melby,
Gregory M.
Anstead

Host defenses to protozoa

Protozoal infections are an important cause of morbidity and mortality worldwide (Table 28.1). Protozoan pathogens exact their major toll in the tropics, but infection with these parasites remains a significant problem in developed countries, owing to travel to and emigration from developing countries, the susceptibility of AIDS patients to opportunistic protozoans, and episodic transmission within communities.

> ● KEY CONCEPTS
>
> ### Host defense against protozoa
>
> - Interaction of the parasite with host cells induces an array of cytokines that stimulate the innate and adaptive immune responses to eliminate the pathogen, and/or cytokines that inhibit or downregulate the antiparasitic responses to enable the initiation of tissue parasitism.
> - The outcome of infection is determined by the balance between the infection-promoting and the host-protective cytokines and effector cells. Often there is a mixed response, resulting in a persistent subclinical infection.
> - A persistently infected host may develop clinical disease if there is a waning of the immune mechanisms (e.g., in AIDS) that are critical to the control of infection.

Protozoan pathogens make up a group of highly diverse organisms that utilize a wide array of mechanisms of pathogenesis and evasion of the host immune response. There are numerous host targets for the intracellular protozoan parasites, including erythrocytes (*Babesia* and *Plasmodium*), macrophages (*Leishmania* and *Toxoplasma gondii*), or multiple cell types (*Trypanosoma cruzi*). The luminal parasitic protozoan may be extracellular, such as the amebae and the flagellates (*Giardia* and *Trichomonas*), or primarily intracellular, such as the coccidian parasite *Cryptosporidium*.

The innate and acquired immune systems respond to the blood and tissue and intestinal protozoan pathogens with a diverse array of weapons.[1,2] Neutrophils and macrophages are the effector cells that mediate the innate response against the extracellular protozoan parasites. The natural killer (NK)-cell-activated macrophage system is central to the innate response to the intracellular parasites (Fig. 28.1) (Chapters 3, 17). The innate cytokine response also plays a critical role in the generation of the adaptive immune response. For the intracellular pathogens (e.g., *Leishmania* spp., *T. cruzi*, *T. gondii*), the early production of IL-12 and IFN-γ drives the differentiation of T cells to a protective Th1 phenotype. In most cases CD4 T cells play a primary role in acquired cellular immunity, but CD8 T cells can play a critical role through cytokine production (e.g., *Plasmodium* spp., *T. cruzi*, *T. gondii*) or direct cytotoxic activity (e.g., *Cryptosporidium*). For the

parasites that have an extracellular stage (e.g., *Plasmodium* spp., the trypanosomes, *Giardia* and *Trichomonas*), specific antibodies play a role in the acquired immune response.

Intensive effort has been dedicated to the development of effective vaccines for protozoal diseases, but to date none has reached the stage of clinical use. A review of all the potential vaccine candidates is beyond the scope of this chapter and the reader is referred to a number of excellent reviews.[3–6] A discussion of the immune responses to some of the individual protozoal pathogens follows.

Plasmodium spp.

Pathogenesis

Soon after *Plasmodium* spp. sporozoites are injected into the bloodstream by the *Anopheles* mosquito they invade hepatocytes and undergo schizogony (asexual reproduction). A dormant form of *P. vivax* and *P. ovale* (hypnozoites) can reside within hepatocytes for months and then cause a clinical bloodstream infection. Following schizogony, merozoites are released from ruptured hepatocytes into the bloodstream, where they invade red blood cells to produce ring-stage parasites. These parasites mature into trophozoites, which again undergo schizogony leading to rupture of the erythrocyte and the release of merozoites. The merozoites then invade fresh RBCs, or develop into male or female gametocytes that can then be picked up by another feeding mosquito to continue the transmission cycle.

The clinicopathological features of malaria are caused by the intraerythrocytic stage. Schizogony and rupture of RBCs is associated with fever. Much of the tissue damage is mediated by the adherence of *P. falciparum*-infected RBCs to endothelial cells through multiple ligand–receptor interactions and plugging of microcapillary beds. Several *P. falciparum* trophozoite proteins, most notably belonging to the erythrocyte membrane protein 1 (EMP-1) family, interact either directly or indirectly with the RBC membrane resulting in abnormalities that promote cytoadherence.[7] A number of endothelial adhesion molecules including intercellular adhesion molecule-1, vascular cell adhesion molecule-1, thrombospondin, E-selectin, CD31, CD36, hyaluronic acid, and chondroitin sulphate A mediate cytoadherence. Sequestration of parasitized RBCs in the capillary beds offers a survival advantage to the parasites by removing them from splenic circulation. Along with the sequestered RBCs there is accumulation of intravascular macrophages, neutrophils and platelets.

Table 28.1 Worldwide significance of the major protozoal infections

Parasite	Estimated worldwide cases (annual mortality)	Clinical manifestations
Plasmodium spp.	400–490 million (*P. falciparum*: > 2 million deaths/year, primarily children)	Fever with potential complications of severe hemolysis, renal failure, pulmonary edema, cerebral involvement
Leishmania spp.	10–50 million people infected, 1.2 million new cases per year	Asymptomatic infection; skin ulcers or nodules; destructive oropharyngeal lesions; visceral disease with fever, hepatosplenomegaly, cachexia, pancytopenia
Trypanosoma cruzi	24 million (60 000 deaths)	Asymptomatic infection; dysrhythmias or chronic heart failure; hypertrophy and dilation of the esophagus, colon
Toxoplasma gondii	Several hundred million people infected worldwide. 5–70% of healthy US adults are seropositive	Self-limited fever, hepatosplenomegaly; lymphadenopathy and encephalitis (reactivation in AIDS patients); congenital infection, with fetal death, chorioretinitis, meningoencephalitis
Entamoeba histolytica	50 million (100 000 deaths)	Asymptomatic infection, diarrhea, dysentery, or liver abscess
Giardia lamblia	200 million (most common in young children and immunocompromised persons)	Asymptomatic infection, chronic diarrhea
Cryptosporidium parvum and *C. hominis*	Prevalence 3–10% in patients with diarrhea in developing countries	Self-limited diarrhea in immunocompetent persons, severe intestinal and biliary disease in AIDS patients
Trichomonas vaginalis	170 million/year	Asymptomatic infection, vaginal discharge, urethritis

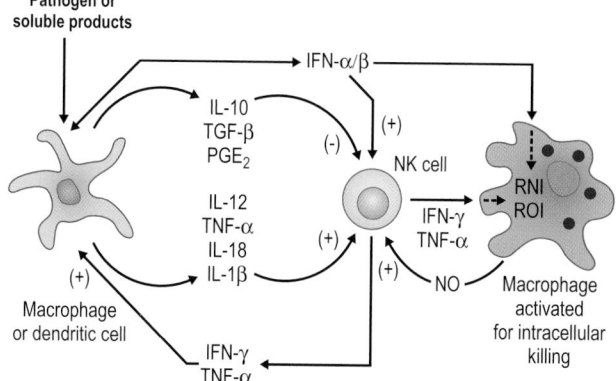

Fig. 28.1 Macrophage, NK cell, and cytokine interactions in the innate immune response to intracellular protozoa. Exposure of macrophages or dendritic cells to a pathogen or microbial product can result in the relase of cytokines and inflammatory mediators that may stimulate (+) or suppress (-) NK cell activation. Activated NK cells produce cytokines that can then activate macrophages for intracellular killing. It must be recognized that this diagram is oversimplified and that these cytokines, most notably IFN-α/β, IL-10, TGF-β, and IL-12, may be produced by other types of cells, such as epithelial cells or enterocytes. NO, nitric oxide; RNI, reactive nitrogen intermediates; ROI, reactive oxygen intermediates.

and cerebral malaria, acts to limit the inflammatory response. The induction of nitric oxide (NO) synthesis by endothelial cells may also contribute to inflammatory lesions in the brain.

KEY CONCEPTS

Immunopathogenesis of severe *Plasmodium falciparum* malaria

- Release of malarial antigens stimulates TNF-α production.
- TNF-α induces expression of endothelial adhesion molecules (e.g., intercellular adhesion molecule-1, vascular cell adhesion molecule-1, thrombospondin, E-selectin, and chondroitin sulphate A).
- *P. falciparum* trophozoite proteins interact with the plasma membrane of the infected RBC to form knob-like protrusions and other membrane abnormalities.
- Infected RBCs with altered membrane surface adhere to upregulated endothelial adhesion molecules.
- Trapped infected RBCs are sequestered away from the splenic defense and cause microcapillary plugging, leading to inflammatory pathology and possible tissue ischemia.

The induction of a proinflammatory cytokine cascade and counter-regulatory responses play a central role in the pathogenesis of *P. falciparum* malaria and its complications. Parasite antigens, particularly those having glycophosphatidyl inositol (GPI) membrane anchors, released during the rupture and reinvasion of RBCs, activate the innate immune response. The production of proinflammatory cytokines (IL-1, TNF-α, IL-12, and IFN-γ), that leads to fever, expression of endothelial adhesion molecules, and cytoadherence is mediated in part by TLR-2 and is MyD88-dependent.[7] T cells primed by previous exposure to either malaria or cross-reacting antigens also produce IFN-γ, which contributes to the production of a pathologically high level of TNF-α. IL-10-mediated downregulation of the Th1 immune response and TNF-α production, which has a role in severe

Innate immunity

Complement-mediated lysis can occur at the sporozoite and merozoite stages. Although sporozoites rapidly transit to the liver, some can activate dendritic cells at the site of inoculation or in the regional lymph node.[8] An IL-12 and IFN-γ-dependent pathway of innate resistance to exoerythrocytic stages of murine malaria has been identified. NK cells are probably the source of the IFN-γ. Although high levels of TNF-α are associated with severe malaria, physiological levels are protective through the activation of macrophages that can clear pre-erythrocytic-stage parasites.

The role of T cells in innate immunity to *Plasmodium* spp. is unclear. Malaria-reactive CD4 T cells, which express the αβ TCR and are MHC Class II restricted, have been identified in nonexposed individuals. Additionally, γδ TCR$^+$ T cells that respond to phosphorylated nonpeptide antigens on live parasites have been demonstrated. Both of these cell populations can secrete IFN-γ, and could therefore lead to phagocyte activation and killing of parasites.

Acquired immunity

Partial immunity to *Plasmodium* spp. infection is acquired slowly following repeated exposure in endemic areas.[9] In areas of intense perennial *P. falciparum* transmission the density of parasitemia, the morbidity and the incidence of cerebral malaria and malaria-related deaths is highest in the early childhood years, declining thereafter. The onset of puberty is associated with enhanced naturally acquired immunity, but pregnancy leads to reduced immune-mediated protection.

Acquired immune mechanisms active at the pre-erythrocytic stage have largely been identified through studies in which mice were vaccinated with large numbers of irradiated sporozoites and challenged with murine *Plasmodium* spp. For reasons that are not clear, vaccination with sporozoites in experimental systems induces much stronger immunity compared to that induced by natural infection. Antisporozoite antibody-mediated immunity requires the presence of high antibody titers to prevent sporozoite invasion of the hepatocyte, which occurs within minutes of inoculation. Acquired immunity to the pre-erythrocytic stage is primarily mediated through Class I-restricted parasite-specific CD8 T cells, and to a lesser extent CD4 T cells, via secreted IFN-γ, which induces nitric oxide-dependent killing of the intrahepatocyte parasites.[10]

Both antibody-dependent and cell-mediated (antibody-independent) immune mechanisms are active against the erythrocytic stage of infection.[11] Immunity develops following drug-cured blood-stage infection in laboratory animals, and the immunity is stronger after repeated episodes of infection/cure. Adoptive transfer of antibodies from drug-cured mice confers protection to naïve mice. Similarly, adoptive transfer of immune human serum is protective for naïve individuals. Antibodies directed against merozoite surface proteins can inhibit invasion. The IgG1 and IgG3 isotypes play a role in naturally acquired immunity by opsonizing schizont- and trophozoite-infected RBCs (recognizing parasite antigens on the surface of the RBC) so that they can be cleared by phagocytic cells, especially in the spleen.

CD4 T cells are also able to confer immunity to blood-stage infection when adoptively transferred from immune mice. The mechanism(s) of CD4 T cell-mediated immunity is unclear, but MHC Class II-restricted antigen presentation and T-cell co-stimulation is required and the generation of cytokines and nitric oxide has been implicated. Protective cellular immune responses (CD4 and CD8 T-cell proliferation, IFN-γ production and NO synthesis) in the absence of detectable antibody responses were identified in naïve volunteers who were repeatedly exposed to low doses of blood stage parasites. T cells expressing the γδ receptor have recently been shown to play a role in the control of chronic parasitemia in mice. The T-cell effector mechanisms that are active in acquired immunity to human malaria have not been defined. Regulatory T cells maintain homeostasis by controlling the intensity of the immune response.

Evasion of host immunity

The malaria parasite uses several different mechanisms to evade the host immune response.[12] Sporozoites and merozoites evade circulating antibody by rapidly entering hepatocyte or RBCs,

respectively. Some sporozoite proteins enter the hepatocyte nucleus and influence the expression of a number of host genes, thereby favoring parasite survival. Mature RBCs do not express MHC molecules on their surface, and so avoid recognition by T cells. The few parasite proteins that are expressed on the erythrocyte surface exist in multiple allelic forms that have variable B-cell epitopes that induce only variant-specific antibody responses. Many of the immunodominant antigens in *Plasmodium* spp. are proteins having extensive repeat sequences that vary from strain to strain and tend to function as T-independent antigens that induce short-lived, low-affinity antibodies. The population of CD4+CD25+ regulatory T cells is expanded during malaria infection, and these cells suppress anti-malarial T-cell immunity in mice, possibly through production of IL-10 and TGF-β. Both TGF-β and IL-10 may suppress host effector mechanisms, but the absence of these counter-regulatory cytokines leads to enhanced inflamatory pathology and mortality in rodent malaria models.

Leishmania spp.

Pathogenesis

The intracellular *Leishmania* amastigote replicates within macrophages in the vertebrate host, and the extracellular promastigote develops within the insect vector. The female phlebotomine sand fly becomes infected by ingesting amastigotes during a blood meal. In the sand fly gut the amastigotes differentiate into infectious metacyclic promastigotes that infect the vertebrate host during the next blood meal. The surface lipophosphoglycan (LPG) plays a central role in the parasite's entry and survival in host cells. Immunomodulatory factors present in the sand fly saliva may enhance the infectivity of the parasite. Once introduced into the skin the promastigotes are phagocytosed (through complement–complement receptor-mediated coiling phagocytosis) by neutrophils, dendritic cells, and macrophages, where they transform to amastigotes and replicate within the acidic and hostile environment of the phagolysosome. Eventually the phagocytes rupture and release amastigotes to infect other macrophages or a sand fly.

Innate immunity

Much of what we know of immunity in leishmaniasis comes from studies of inbred mouse strains, which demonstrate a genetically-determined spectrum of innate and adaptive immune responses that determine the outcome of infection. The innate immune response to *Leishmania* is mediated by NK cells, cytokines and phagocytes.[13] The production of IL-12 early in the course of infection by dendritic cells leads to the early activation of NK cells and the production of IFN-γ. Chemokines (IP-10, MCP-1 and lymphotactin), as well as LPG-TLR4 interaction can also promote the early NK cell activation. Activated NK cells have been shown to be cytolytic for *Leishmania*-infected macrophages, but NK cell-derived IFN-γ plays a more prominent role in host defense by activating macrophages to kill the intracellular parasite through the generation of reactive oxygen intermediates (ROI) or reactive nitrogen intermediates (RNI). Parasite-induced MyD88-dependent signaling through TLR2, TLR3, and TLR4 contributes to macrophage activation and NO production. Activated polymorphonuclear leukocytes can kill parasites through oxidative mechanisms, but there are conflicting data concerning the role of neutrophils *in vivo*. An important study demonstrated that infiltrating neutrophils promote sand fly-transmitted infection, probably through modulation of macrophage function by apoptotic neutrophils.[14] Type 1 interferons participate in the early induction of NO and control of parasite replication early in infection.

Acquired immunity

Within an endemic area there is acquisition of immunity in the population over time. Retrospective epidemiological studies indicate that most individuals with prior (primary) infection (subclinical or healed) are immune to a subsequent clinical infection. Following primary infection parasites persist for the life of the host and maintain long-term immunity.

There is extensive evidence from experimental models that cellular immune mechanisms mediate acquired resistance to *Leishmania* infection, and human studies have generally confirmed this. Antileishmanial antibodies, which are produced at a low level in localized cutaneous leishmaniasis (LCL) and at a very high level in visceral leishmaniasis (VL), play no role in protection. The general mechanisms of cellular immunity in leishmaniasis can be summarized (Fig. 28.2). Following infection in the skin, migratory dermal dendritic cells phagocytose *Leishmania* and presumably transport the intracellular parasite to the regional lymph node, where they induce a T-cell response. Acquired immunity is mediated by parasite-induced

production of IFN-γ by CD4 T cells (Th1 subset). CD4 T cells are absolutely required, but immunity to cutaneous disease can develop in the absence of CD8 T cells. Both CD4 and CD8 T cells are required for an effective defense against murine visceral *L. donovani* infection, but the precise role of CD8 T cells is unclear. The generation of the Th1 response is critically dependent on CD40-CD40L-mediated IL-12 production and driven by NK-cell-derived IFN-γ. IL-12 and STAT4 are required for the maintenance of immunity. Tumor necrosis factor-α (TNF-α) contributes to protective immunity by synergizing with IFN-γ to activate macrophages. Recently, nuclear factor-kappa B (NF-κB) family members have been shown to regulate T-cell responses and immunity to *L. major* infection in mice.

Two sub-populations of CD4 T cells mediate immunity induced by primary infection.[15] Effector memory cells, which are short-lived and dependent on the persistence of antigen, rapidly respond to secondary infection by migrating to the infected tissue and generating effector cytokines. Central memory T cells, which can be maintained in the absence of persistent antigen, circulate throughout the lymphatic system and upon secondary challenge migrate to and proliferate in the draining lymph node, gain the capacity to produce IFN-γ, and then migrate to the site of infection. Thus, central memory T cells act as a reserve of antigen-reactive T cells that can expand and become effector T cells in response to secondary antigenic challenge.

The generation of RNI by activated macrophages is the primary mechanism of parasite killing in the murine model.[16] Although IFN-γ-induced production of NO may not be detectable in human macrophages, inhibition of nitric oxide synthase 2 (NOS2) was shown to impair killing of intracellular *Leishmania*.

Several adaptive immune mechanisms promote parasite replication and disease.[17] The progression of murine *L. major* infection has been correlated with the expansion of Th2 cells and the production of IL-4, IL-5, and IL-10. In susceptible mice, IL-4 production within the first day of infection was shown to downregulate IL-12 receptor β-chain expression and drive the response to a Th2 phenotype. However, other non-susceptible mouse strains appear to be able to overcome an early IL-4 response and develop a resistant phenotype, and susceptibility to some *L. major* strains is not strictly mediated by IL-4 (IL-13 and/or IL-10 may have a prominent role). The production of transforming growth factor beta (TGF-β) or prostaglandin E$_2$ (PGE$_2$) may also contribute to susceptibility.[15]

Peripheral blood mononuclear cells (PBMCs) isolated from patients with localized cutaneous leishmaniasis demonstrate a Th1 response to *Leishmania* antigens, and in the cutaneous lesion there is an exuberant Th1 and granulomatous response that mediates parasite killing and localized tissue damage, which usually leads to a scar. Patients with mucosal leishmaniasis (ML) exhibit vigorous cellular immune responses characterized by high levels of TNF-α and Th1 and Th17 cytokines; it is postulated that this hyperresponsive state contributes to the prominent tissue destruction of ML. Patients with diffuse cutaneous leishmaniasis (DCL) resemble the progressive infection caused by *L. major* in BALB/c mice in that there is minimal or absent *Leishmania*-specific lymphoproliferative responses, and predominant Th2 cytokine expression. During active VL in humans there is a marked depression of *Leishmania*-specific lymphoproliferative and IFN-γ responses, as well as an absence of delayed-type hypersensitivity (DTH) response to parasite antigens. This anergy appears to be mediated, at least in part, by a suppressive effect of IL-10 and low levels of IL-12. Successful treatment of active disease restores an antigen-specific Th1 response.

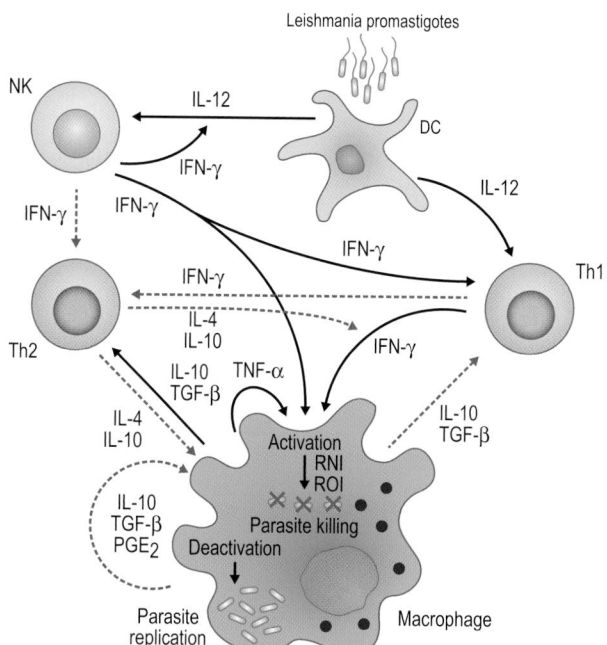

Fig. 28.2 Immunity in leishmaniasis. Exposure of dendritic cells to parasites or parasite antigens leads to the release of IL-12, which induces NK cells to produce IFN-γ and drives the acquired immune response toward a protective Th1 phenotype. IL-12 production by dendritic cells and IFN-γ production by NK and Th1 cells negatively regulates the Th2 response. IFN-γ activates macrophages to kill the intracellular pathogen. In genetically susceptible individuals a counter-regulatory Th2 cytokine response can suppress the Th1 response and impair classical macrophage activation, leading to parasite replication and uncontrolled infection. Counterprotective macrophage-derived cytokines can also inhibit the Th1 response, stimulate the Th2 response, and impair classical activation through an autocrine loop. Activating stimuli are shown by solid arrows, and deactivating stimuli are shown by dashed arrows.

Evasion of host immunity

The *Leishmania* parasite has numerous ways in which it adapts to and survives within the vertebrate host.[16,17] In the skin the promastigotes may be phagocytosed by neutrophils and macrophages, which, unlike dendritic cells, do not actively participate in T-cell priming. Furthermore, the clearance of apoptotic neutrophils is likely to make macrophages more permissive to infection. The parasite's surface LPG (and to a lesser extent the surface protein gp63) plays an important role in the entry and survival of *Leishmania* in the mammalian host by conferring complement resistance, and by facilitating the entry of complement-opsonized parasites into the macrophage without triggering a respiratory burst. Macrophage phagosome–endosome fusion and phagolysosomal biogenesis are also inhibited by the parasite LPG.

Leishmania-infected macrophages have a diminished capacity to initiate and respond to a T-cell response, and the impaired antimicrobial effector activity provides a safe haven for the intracellular parasite.[16] Infected macrophages have decreased synthesis of IL-1 and IL-12, and blunted IFN-γ-mediated activation through the disruption of signal transduction pathways involving JAK/STAT, protein kinase C, p38 MAPK, ERK, AP-1, and NF-κB. Signaling mediated by tyrosine phosphorylation is decreased by the rapid induction of the host phosphotyrosine phosphatase SHP-1. Conversely, there is increased synthesis of the immunosuppressive molecules IL-10, TGF-β and PGE$_2$. The IL-4/IL-13-enhanced expression of arginase by infected macrophages (termed alternatively activated macrophages) contributes to depletion of L-arginine and reduced NO production. IL-10 produced by CD4$^+$CD25$^+$ T regulatory (Treg) cells has an essential role in parasite persistence. Recently it was shown that metastasizing parasites that cause mucosal disease harbor a high burden of *Leishmania* RNA virus, which subverts the host immune response and promotes parasite persistence through activation of TLR3.[18]

Trypanosoma cruzi

Pathogenesis

T. cruzi is transmitted to the mamalian host when the infectious metacyclic trypomastigote, which is deposited on the skin in the feces of the reduvid insect vector while it takes a blood meal, is scratched into the wound or transferred to a mucous membrane (e.g., the eyes). The trypomastigotes can infect almost any cell type, and replicate as amastigotes in the cytoplasm. Eventually the amastigotes transform back into trypomastigotes and rupture the cell to enter the bloodstream, whence they invade other cells or are picked up by another insect vector.

Following primary infection the parasites replicate locally and then disseminate through the bloodstream to a variety of tissues. Muscle and glial cells are the most frequently infected cells, and acute myocarditis or meningoencephalitis can develop. In most cases, however, primary infection occurs without clinical symptoms and the infected individual may enter an indeterminate phase of asymptomatic seropositivity. Only 10–30% of chronically infected individuals will ultimately develop symptomatic Chagas' disease, usually involving the heart or gastrointestinal tract. Pathologically there are few parasites observed in cardiac tissue, but an intense chronic inflammatory infiltrate with fibrosis and loss of muscle fibers is evident.

In the digestive tract there is lymphohistiocytic infiltration of the myenteric plexuses, with a dramatic reduction in the number of ganglion cells.

The tissue damage of acute *T. cruzi* infection is the result of a direct effect of the parasite and the acute host inflammatory response. In chronic infection the balance between immune-mediated parasite containment and host-damaging inflamation determines the course of disease. The pathological mechanisms related to chronic Chagas' disease are controversial, but whether tissue damage is caused directly by parasites or indirectly through parasite-directed inflammatory or autoimmune mechanisms, it is clear that parasite persistence is required for disease (Table 28.2).[19] Autoimmunity could arise from molecular mimicry of self by parasite antigens, or by the release of self molecules from damaged or dying host cells within the environment of an activated innate immune response. The production of IL-10 by *T. cruzi*-infected cells may downregulate the pathologic cellular immune response.

Innate immunity

The early innate immune response to *T. cruzi* infection is mediated primarily by NK cells, dendritic cells and macrophages.[20,21] Macrophages and DCs exposed to *T. cruzi* trypomastigote antigens produce proinflammatory cytokines including IL-12 and TNF-α, through a MyD88-dependent mechanism.

Table 28.2 Evidence for autoimmune and parasite-induced inflammatory mechanisms in chronic Chagas' disease

Evidence for autoimmune-mediated disease	Evidence for parasite-induced inflammatory disease
Inflammatory disease presents in tissues with few or no parasites on routine histopathology studies.	Sensitive parasite detection techniques (PCR, immunohistochemistry) strongly correlate presence of parasites (or parasite material) and severity of inflammatory disease.
Peculiar pattern of organ involvement (heart and gastrointestinal tract) in patients with chronic disease.	Organs free of parasites (by sensitive parasite detection techniques) are also free of disease.
Long delay in the onset of chronic disease following infection; only a minority of infected persons develops disease.	Absence of effective cellular immune response (in mice or humans) almost invariably exacerbates rather than reduces the parasite burden and disease.
Wide variability in the expression of disease among infected people.	In chronically infected mice the destruction of a transplanted heart is dependent on parasite infiltrating the transplanted tissue.
Self-reactive antibodies and T cells demonstrable in infected people and in experimental animals. Level of antibodies to the ribosomal P protein (R13 peptide) and cardiac myosin (B13 antigen) correlate with cardiac disease.	Degree of disease in hearts transplanted into chronically infected mice correlates with level of parasite burden in transplanted tissue.
Transient or limited disease reported in experimental models following lymphocyte transfer.	Reduction of parasite burden by chemotherapy leads to decreased tissue inflammation and disease.

MyD88-deficient mice had impaired inflammatory responses and host defense against *T. cruzi*. Signaling through another protein involved in TLR2 signaling, the Toll/IL1R domain-containing adapter protein inducing interferon beta (TRIF) promotes resistance through production of IFN-β and downstream expression of IFN-β inducible genes such as the p47 GTPase *IRG47*.[22] IL-12 activates NK cells to secrete IFN-γ, which synergizes with TNF-α to activate macrophages to control parasite replication. The generation of NO is the primary trypanocidal mechanism in murine macrophages. A number of trypomastigote antigens, including free glycosyl-phosphatidylinositol (GPI) anchors, glycoinositol phospho-lipids (GIPLs), GPI-linked glycoproteins, and GPI-mucins activate the innate immune response, at least in part through TLR-2 and possibly TLR4. CpG motifs in the *T. cruzi* genome have also been shown to activate TLR9. Several other TLR-independent mechanisms of innate immunity, including the activation of NOD-like receptors, have been identified.[21]

Acquired immunity

The innate immune response, through production of IL-12, type I interferons, and other proinflammatory mediators, is critically linked to the generation of an effective adaptive immune response.[20] In infected mice the parasitemia (trypomastigotes) increases until 3–4 weeks after infection, when either the mice die or the infection is controlled by the acquired immune response. Antibodies contribute to immunity through opsonization, complement activation and antibody-dependent cellular cytotoxicity.

Several lines of evidence establish the importance of T cells in acquired immunity to *T. cruzi* infection. Parasite-specific CD4 and CD8 T cells are activated in response to infection, and mice lacking CD4 or CD8 T cells have impaired ability to control the infection. CD8 T cells with cytotoxic activity against *T. cruzi*-infected cells have been identified in infected mice, and these cells confer protection against challenge when passively transferred to naïve mice. In the early stage of infection CD4 T cells are the predominant subset recruited to the myocardium, but activated CD8 T cells soon dominate the inflammatory process in cardiac tissue. Cytokine production (IFN-γ and TNF-α) by parasite-specific CD8 T cells is more important than cytolytic activity in the control of infection.[23]

T. cruzi infection leads to a mixed Th1/Th2 cytokine response and in general the Th1/Th2 balance determines resistance or susceptibility. As noted earlier, IL-12/STAT4-dependent IFN-γ production by NK cells in early infection and later by T cells, clearly has an important protective function. IL-4 does not appear to play a major role in susceptibility to *T. cruzi* infection, but IL-10 promotes parasite replication by inhibiting macrophage trypanocidal activity. IL-10 also plays a critical role in minimizing inflammation-mediated tissue pathology by regulating the Th1 and proinflammatory cytokine (predominantly TNF) responses. Polymorphisms in the IL-10 gene that lead to reduced IL-10 production are associated with increased severity of cardiomyopathy in patients with Chagas' disease. Similarly, TGF-β has been shown to inhibit macrophage trypanocidal activity and increase parasitemia and mortality. In addition to the production of these regulatory cytokines, the secretion of prostaglandins and NO, the induction of apoptosis of T and B cells, and the expansion of a myeloid suppressor cell population serve to control the intensity of the immune response.

Evasion of host immunity

A significant part of the pathogenesis following *T. cruzi* infection is its dissemination through the bloodstream to many tissues. *T. cruzi* bloodstream trypomastigotes resist complement lysis because the parasite has a complement regulatory protein (GP-160), which is functionally similar to mammalian decay-accelerating factor in that it inhibits C3 convertase formation and activation of the alternate complement pathway.

The establishment of chronic infection by *T. cruzi* is favored by a generalized depression of T-cell responses. A number of different mechanisms may contribute to this, including low IL-2 production or IL-2 receptor expression; downregulation of components of the T-cell–receptor complex; T-cell receptor dysfunction; apoptosis of T cells; defects in the processing and presenting of antigens in the Class II (but not the Class I) pathway; T-cell or macrophage suppressor activity; and PGE$_2$ production. Within foci of myocarditis, apoptosis of both parasites and host cells occurs; the phagocytosis of these apoptotic cells by macrophages leads to their deactivation or acquisition of an alternatively activated phenotype, which enables parasite replication and persistence. The rapid escape of the parasite from the phagosome into the cytoplasm through the action of acid-activated porins enables the organism to avoid enzymatic destruction.

Toxoplasma gondii

Pathogenesis

Transmission occurs via the ingestion of oocysts, which are shed in the feces of felines or present in undercooked meat. Following the oral ingestion of cysts, intestinal epithelial cells are infected by trophozoites that enter via the laminin receptor. The parasite transforms into intracellular tachyzoites, which replicate within a parasitophorous vacuole (PV) and ultimately rupture the cell. The released tachyzoites can disseminate to invade virtually any nucleated cell type, but mononuclear phagocytes are the preferred host cell. The toxoplasma transmembrane adhesin MIC2 has a major role in the process of host cell invasion. Under pressure from exogenous stressors, including the host immune response, tachyzoite replication is controlled and tissue cysts, which are a modified parasitophorous vacuole containing slowly replicating bradyzoites, are formed. The tissue cysts persist as a chronic latent infection as long as the host immune function is intact. If the latently infected person is immunosuppressed reactivation occurs and tachyzoites are released to infect more cells. Because tissue cysts (bradyzoites) are found in proportionately larger numbers in the brain, reactivation of latent infection in the immunocompromised host is most commonly manifest as encephalitis.

Innate immunity

IL-12, IFN-γ, TNF-α and NK cells contribute to the control of the early stages of *T. gondii* infection. CD8α$^+$ dendritic cells are the primary producers of IL-12, which is essential to host resistance. IL-12 is produced through a MyD88-dependent mechanism, at least in part through the interaction of parasite-derived proteins and TLR2 and TLR11.[24] and activation of CCR5. IL-12-dependent activation of NK cells leads to IFN-γ, production, which in turn activates macrophages to limit parasite replication. T cells expressing the $\gamma\delta$ receptor are also an early source of IFN-γ and TNF-α. Recruitment of inflammatory macrophages, but not neutrophils, to the site of infection is crucial to control of parasite replication and dissemination.

The mechanism(s) of IFN-γ-mediated macrophage activation for the control of early parasite replication in humans is unclear. In murine macrophages the primary mechanism of acute control is the IFN-γ-induced immunity-related GTPases. The production of nitric oxide and generation of reactive oxygen intermediates by activated macrophages are important in control of chronic infection.

Acquired immunity

The systemic antibody response does not play a role in acquired immunity to *T. gondii*. Mucosal IgA, however, does play a role in resistance to oral infection with *T. gondii* cysts. *T. gondii* is a potent activator of CD4 and CD8 T cells, which are required for acquired immunity to *T. gondii*. As such, patients with defects in T-cell-mediated immune responses (e.g., patients with AIDS) are at risk for reactivation of latent infection.

NK-cell-derived IFN-γ drives the differentiation of T cells into type 1 CD4 and CD8 T cells that are essential to acquired immunity. The route by which peptides enter the Class I and Class II antigen-processing pathways have not been fully defined, but evidence supports that cross-presentation of exogenous soluble antigens by CD8α^+ dendritic cells, perhaps derived from dead or dying parasites, as an important requirement for generation of CD8 T-cell responses. Parasite-specific cytolytic T cells have been demonstrated but CD8 T cells mediate protection primarily through the generation of IFN-γ. The dominant fully mature CD8 effector T cells, which express the killer cell lectin-like receptor G1 (KLRG1) marker and high levels of granzyme B and IFN-γ, are driven by IL-12.[25] However, the combination of IL-7 and IL-15, but not IL-12, appears to be required for central memory T-cell differentiation. CD4 and CD8 T cells act synergistically to prevent cyst reactivation during chronic infection.

IFN-γ-induced macrophage activation is the key effector mechanism in acquired immunity to *T. gondii*. In mice, the induction of immunity-related GTPases, which damage the parasitophorous vacuole membrane and kill *T. gondii* within the cytosol, is the primary macrophage effector mechanism.[26] The generation of reactive nitrogen and oxygen intermediates, degradation of tryptophan, and the production of leukotrienes have also been implicated in the control of *T. gondii* in human macrophages. Anti-inflammatory molecules, particularly IL-10 and IL-27, play an important role in modulating the adaptive immune response and restricting host tissue damage.[27]

Evasion of host immunity

T. gondii escapes early macrophage killing in a number of ways.[27] Virulent parasites are protected by localization to the parasitophorous vacuole, which does not fuse with host cell lysosomes (probably because the PV membrane proteins are of parasite rather than host origin) and the vacuole is not acidified. The infected macrophage is also a suboptimal target for T-cell-induced immunity because of reduced expression of MHC Class II and costimulatory molecules. Infection also induces the production of counter-regulatory molecules such as IL-10, TGF-β, lipoxin A4, or members of the suppressor of cytokine synthesis (SOCS) family. These protect the host by downregulating a potentially pathologic inflammatory response, but also inhibit

Th1 cytokine synthesis and macrophage antimicrobial activity. Some clonal populations of *T. gondii* secrete ROP16, a parasite kinase that activates host STAT6 and leads to a M2 macrophage phenotype that is permissive to infection.

Entamoeba histolytica

Pathogenesis

E. histolytica causes asymptomatic intestinal colonization, acute diarrhea, dysentery, colitis, liver abscess, and, rarely, disseminated disease.[28] Susceptibility to amebiasis is determined by the host's nutritional status, intestinal microflora, genetics, and gender. *E. histolytica* cysts are ingested through consumption of food or water contaminated by feces. After excystation, the motile trophozoites penetrate the colonic mucus barrier by mechanical disruption. The trophozoites adhere to the colonic epithelial cells by a galactose/*N*-acetylgalactosamine-inhibitable adhesin (Gal/GalNAc lectin). Epithelial cells with adherent amebae undergo microvilli shortening and apical separation, and the trophozoites penetrate between the epithelial cells. This invasion is facilitated by cysteine proteases and a surface metallocollagenase, which attack the components of connective tissue ground substance causing ulceration of the colonic mucosa and submucosa (Fig. 28.3). The trophozoites of *E. histolytica* can lyse multiple cell types, including neutrophils, which release enzymes that further damage the tissue. The cytotoxic effects of amebae are mediated by a secreted cysteine protease, the Gal/GalNAc lectin, phospholipase A, and contact-dependent cytolysis, in which an ion channel (amebapore) is inserted into the membrane of target cells. *E. histolytica* can induce apoptosis in mammalian cells by caspase-dependent, TNF-α/Fas-independent process. Amebic liver abscesses develop when trophozoites erode through the intestinal submucosa, enter the portal circulation and are deposited in the liver.[28,29] Transcriptional profiling comparing virulent and nonvirulent *Entamoeba* species has identified novel virulence factors in *E. histolytica*.[30]

Innate immunity

Trophozoites bind to the intestinal epithelial cells, stimulating the release of IL-1α, IL-1β, IL-6, IL-8, and GM-CSF, which act as neutrophil chemoattractants and activators. The trophozoite cysteine proteinase 5 (*Eh*CP5) promotes inflammation by cleaving pre-IL-1β and by binding to integrin on the intestinal epithelial cells, causing NF-κB activation. Neutrophils release reactive oxygen species that are amebicidal, but also cause damage to host tissue. However, the amebae can also destroy neutrophils and express several enzymes that disarm the oxidative burst. The ability of neutrophils to tip the balance toward resolution of infection depends on appropriate activation by IFN-γ and TNF-α. Host IL-10, derived from CD4 lymphocytes and acting on intestinal epithelial cells, is essential to maintain the integrity of the intestinal mucosa during amebiasis. IL-10 has multiple activities: it decreases pro-inflammatory NF-κB signaling, increases mucin production, suppresses activation of antigen-presenting cells, promotes induction of CD4 T regulatory cells, affects B-cell class switching to IgA, and has anti-apoptotic effects on the epithelium.[29]

Invariant natural killer T (iNKT) cells, which comprise about 30% of the hepatic lymphocytes, play a central role in host defense against *E. histolytica* in the liver. The binding of amebic

Fig. 28.3 Immunopathogenesis of intestinal protozoal pathogens. After adherence (*Giardia* and *Entamoeba*) or epithelial invasion (*Entamoeba* and *Cryptosporidium*), there is release of various inflammatory mediators from macrophages and neutrophils. This causes the activation of resident phagocytes and recruitment of phagocytes into the lamina propria. Enterocyte death can be due to direct action of the parasites or to immune-mediated damage from complement, cytotoxic lymphocytes, proteases, and reactive oxygen and nitrogen intermediates (ROI and RNI, respectively). The inflammatory mediators also act on enterocytes and the enteric nervous system, inducing the secretion of water and chloride. In response to enterocyte damage, under the influence of activated T lymphocytes, the crypts undergo hyperplasia and the villi become shorter (villous atrophy). The immature hyperplastic cells have poor absorptive ability, but retain secretory ability. Damage to the epithelium can cause leakage (exudation) from lymphatics and capillaries. Similar mechanisms are probably responsible for the diarrhea that occurs in infection with *Cyclospora* and *Isospora*. *Isospora* is unique in causing an eosinophilic infiltrate.

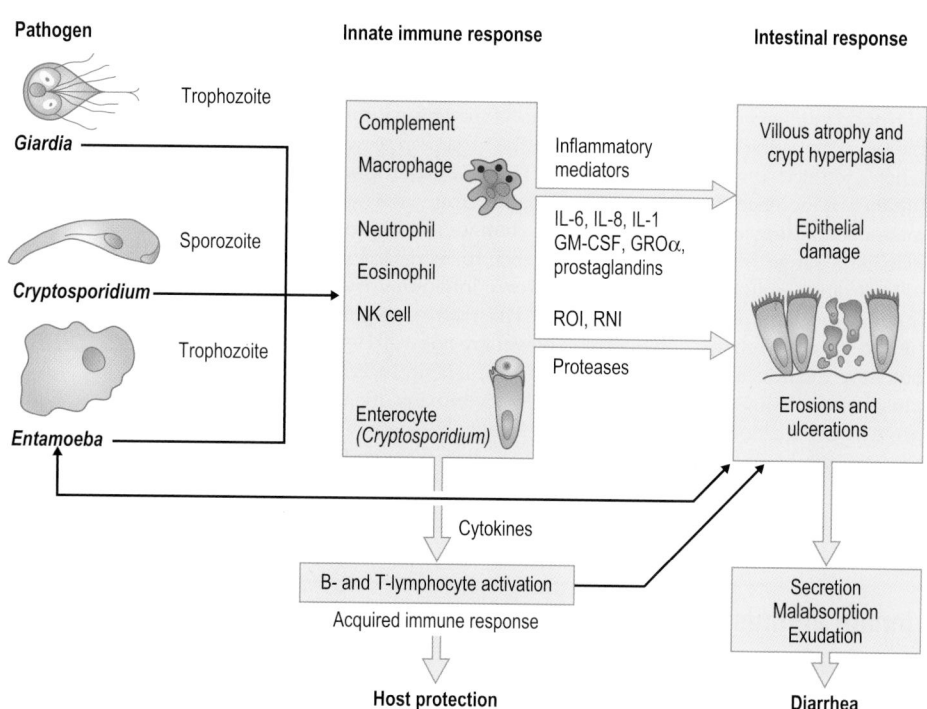

lipopeptidephosphoglycan (LPPG) to iNKT cells stimulates IFN-γ release. Neutrophils also flood into the liver in the initial phases of abscess formation.[29]

Acquired immunity

E. histolytica infection elicits an intestinal IgA response to the parasite surface adhesin, Gal/GalNAc lectin, which is important for resistance to colonization and invasion. In addition to preventing trophozoite adherence, *E. histolytica*-specific sIgA acts to prevent invasion and maintain a commensal relationship between host and parasite by decreasing the host inflammatory response. Engagement of Gal/GalNAc lectin by sIgA can also modulate the virulence of the ameba.[29]

Dendritic cells are activated by both the amebic Gal/GalNAc lectin and LPPG to produce IL-12 and TNF-α, thereby driving a protective Th1 immune response.[30] IFN-γ produced by CD4 cells activates macrophages to release NO, which is amebicidal. By contrast, IL-4, IL-5, and IL-13 production by Th2 cells leads to chronic, non-healing granulomatous lesions. The Th2 cytokines upregulate macrophage arginase-1, which depletes the arginine required for NO production, and generates ornithine, which promotes fibroblast proliferation and collagen deposition. Trophozoites can erode through the granuloma walls, and disseminate within the liver. The conditions that generate a Th2 response are not clearly known, but host genetics probably plays a role.[29] Dissemination of infection may occur when cell-mediated immunity is impaired, and HIV-infected patients have higher rates of seroconversion, invasive amebiasis, and liver abscesses.[30]

Evasion of host immunity

E. histolytica utilizes a number of strategies to circumvent the immune defenses of the host. It resists complement-mediated lysis during hematogenous spread by proteolytic degradation of C3a and C3b. In addition, the Gal/GalNac lectin binds to C8 and C9, preventing assembly of the C5b-9 membrane attack complex.[31]

The cytolytic capability of *E. histolytica* affords protection from neutrophils, macrophages, and eosinophils, unless these cells are activated.[29] Cytolysis by *E. histolytica* can occur via necrosis and apoptosis. Trophozoites also inhibit the macrophage respiratory burst and the production of IL-1 and TNF-α. A protective antibody response is subverted by the degradation of IgA and IgG by amebic cysteine proteases, and by capping, ingesting or shedding ameba-specific antibodies.[29] These proteases can also cleave the Fc region so that interaction with host cell surface receptors is avoided. Another secreted product of *E. histolytica*, monocyte locomotion inhibition factor (MLIF), inhibits monocyte locomotion and the monocyte and neutrophil respiratory burst and NO production; enhances anti-inflammatory cytokine and chemokine release from host cells; and alters adhesion molecule expression on macrophages. The suppression of host macrophage NO production by an array of trophozoite secretory products, including parasite-derived PGE$_2$, is a major factor in the persistence of amebic liver abscesses.[29] In chronic infection, *E. histolytica* promotes the development of Treg cells that suppress the proliferation of responder T cells by releasing IL-10, TGF-β, and IL-35.[29]

Giardia lamblia

Pathogenesis

Recent studies of *Giardia lamblia* have identified eight genotypes, two of which infect humans (assemblages A and B).[32] The severity of giardiasis ranges from asymptomatic carriage to chronic watery diarrhea, epigastric pain, nausea, vomiting, and weight loss, depending on host factors and the virulence of the *Giardia* strain.[32,33] Younger age, malnutrition, and immunodeficiency increase the severity of infection.[33] After ingestion of the *Giardia* cyst in fecally contaminated food or water, the cyst survives its trip through the acidic stomach, and excystation and multiplication of trophozoites occurs in the small bowel. As they transit through the lower intestine they encyst, allowing the organism to survive when excreted into the environment. The *Giardia* trophozoite initiates adherence to the intestinal epithelium via a surface mannose-binding lectin. Histopathologic changes in symptomatic giardiasis range from a normal appearance to increased crypt-villous ratios, epithelial damage, and chronic inflammatory infil-trate in the lamina propria (Fig. 28.3). The factors responsible for the structural changes in the small bowel are not well defined, but may include injury from adherence, parasite-induced apo-ptosis of epithelial cells, and the release of cytotoxins, including proteases. Additional epithelial damage may be mediated by the host cellular immune response. Diarrhea arises from epithelial barrier dysfunction, reduction in microvillous surface area, chlo-ride hypersecretion, and glucose and sodium malabsorption.[33]

Innate immunity

Giardia lacks catalase, superoxide dismutase, and glutathione reductase, so it has limited capacity to neutralize reactive oxygen species produced by intestinal epithelial cells. Nitric oxide, pro-duced by both epithelial cells and macrophages, has giardicidal effects; however, *Giardia* may circumvent this defense by com-peting with these host cells for arginine uptake.[34] The antimicro-bial peptide defensin is produced by Paneth cells and thus can also participate in host defense against *Giardia*. Few macro-phages are found in the intestinal mucosa during giardiasis, which suggests they do not play an important role in the innate immune response. The infection is rare in breast-fed infants because breast milk contains free fatty acids lethal to *Giardia* cysts and, in endemic areas, anti-*Giardia* antibodies.

Acquired immunity

Several lines of evidence suggest the importance of the humoral immune response in the control of giardiasis. Infection with *Giar-dia* results in the production of anti-*Giardia* antibodies in the se-rum and mucosal secretions. Human immunodeficiency syndromes that affect antibody production are associated with chronic giardiasis. Mast cells of the intestinal mucosa play a piv-otal role in parasite elimination, perhaps by promoting IgA production by B cells.[32]

There is also evidence for a role of T-cell-dependent immunity in the control of giardiasis, but the mechanisms have not been fully defined. T-cell-deficient mice and mice treated with anti-CD4 antibody are unable to control *Giardia* infection. CD8 T lymphocytes are not important in protective immunity. Epide-miologic studies indicate that partial immunity is acquired from *Giardia* infection, which leads to reduced risk and severity of subsequent infections.[32]

Evasion of host immunity

Giardia evades the host humoral immune response by under-going surface antigenic variation by altering a group of variant-specific surface proteins (VSPs). Selection occurs by an immune-mediated process because switching occurs when intestinal anti-VSP IgA responses are first detected.[33] *Giardia lam-blia* also produces a protease that cleaves IgA. Although *Giardia* activates dendritic cells for antigen presentation, it also inhibits IL-12 production, in part by enhancing IL-10 release; the net re-sult is the mollification of a local anti-parasitic inflammatory re-sponse.[32] The trophozoite also releases arginine deiminase, which degrades arginine, making it less available for host NO production.[34]

Cryptosporidium parvum and *Cryptosporidium hominis*

In humans, there are four intestinal coccidians that are intra-cellular parasites of enterocytes: *Isospora belli*, *Cyclospora caye-tanensis*, and two species of *Cryptosporidium*, *Cr. parvum*, and *Cr. hominis*. *Cryptosporidium* has the greatest epidemiologic sig-nificance: in 1993 a huge outbreak involving 403,000 persons occurred in Milwaukee, Wisconsin.[35] Because of their similar-ity, only the immunology of cryptosporidiosis will be discussed.

Pathogenesis

Cryptosporidium typically causes self-limited (but often pro-longed) diarrhea in the immunocompetent host. However, in patients with the acquired immunodeficiency syndrome (AIDS), *Cryptosporidium* can cause severe diarrhea, with malabsorption and wasting, and cholangiopathy.[36] Infection with *Cryptosporid-ium* occurs when sporulated oocysts are ingested and excyst in the proximal small bowel, invade the intestinal epithelial cells (facilitated by a cysteine protease), develop into trophozoites and undergo schizogony, with a resultant merozoite-containing schizont. The merozoites are extruded and invade other epithelial cells. The merozoites may continue an asexual cycle or develop into macro- or microgametes that fuse to form oocysts. Histolog-ically, in the infected small bowel there is villous atrophy and blunting, and crypt hyperplasia with increased infiltration of lym-phocytes, macrophages and plasma cells. Intraepithelial lympho-cytes are uncommon; neutrophils and occasional eosinophils are present between the epithelium and the lamina propria. Disorga-nized cells undergoing necrosis replace normal enterocyte archi-tecture (Fig. 28.3). There is an association between the degree of intestinal injury and malabsorption and the intensity of infection, as measured by oocyst excretion.

The neuropeptide substance P, which is produced by endothe-lial cells, lymphocytes and monocytes of the lamina propria, con-tributes to diarrhea by increasing intestinal chloride secretion and glucose malabsorption. Increased expression of substance P is observed in AIDS patients with cryptosporidiosis and severe diarrhea.[37]

Innate immunity

The type I and type II interferons play a key role in the innate protective response against cryptosporidium.[38] Because of the parasite's intracellular location near the luminal surface of the enterocyte, the macrophages of the lamina propria are spa-tially isolated from the parasite. Thus, the intestinal epithelium mounts its own assault on the invading microbe through TLR2/TLR4-dependent activation of NF-κB and release of the microbiocidal peptide β-defensin-2, TNF-α, and the chemokines IL-8, RANTES, and GRO-α, which act as chemoattractants and activators of neutrophils. In patients with AIDS and cryptosporidiosis, the HIV Tat protein may sabotage host defense against *Cryptosporidium* by inhibiting cholangiocyte TLR-4 expression.[36]

IL-15, produced by activated monocytes, stimulates NK cell proliferation, cytotoxicity, and cytokine production, including IFN-γ. There is significant IL-15 expression in the jejunal mucosa in immunocompetent patients with cryptosporidiosis, and IL-15 levels inversely correlate with parasite burden. However, in AIDS patients with chronic uncontrolled cryptosporidiosis IL-15 is undetectable.[36]

Mannose-binding lectin (MBL) is a serum protein that binds to various pathogens, including *Cryptosporidium*. Upon binding, MBL activates complement, thereby promoting opsonization and phagocytosis. Low serum levels of MBL, which may result from malnutrition or polymorphisms in the MBL gene, increase susceptibility to cryptosporidiosis.[36] Infected intestinal cells also release TGF-β, which decreases necrosis and stimulates the synthesis of extracellular matrix proteins, which limit epithelial damage.

Prostaglandins E_2 and $F_{2\alpha}$, released by infected enterocytes, promote secretory diarrhea, but also upregulate mucin production, which may hinder parasite attachment. In addition, these prostaglandins stimulate the release of β-defensin-2, which has direct anti-cryptosporidial activity and is chemotactic for T cells and dendritic cells.[36]

Acquired immunity

Specific IgG and IgA production occurs in patients infected with *Cryptosporidium* but the antibody response does not influence the symptoms of infection. CD4 T cells play a central role in the control of cryptosporidiosis in adult mice, although they are not essential in neonates, in which innate immune mechanisms are sufficient to control the infection. In immunocompetent mice CD4 intraepithelial lymphocytes (IELs) initiate early control of infection, whereas cytotoxic CD8 IELs appear later and function in parasite elimination. Resolution of infection depends on a balance of Th1 cytokines (IFN-γ, IL-18) needed to control the infection and Th2 cytokines (IL-4, IL-10, and IL-13) that limit immunopathologic damage. In mice, γδ T cells are rapidly recruited to control cryptosporidial infection, but their role in human infection is unknown. Severe intestinal disease or biliary involvement is usually seen in AIDS patients whose CD4 count is <50/μL. HIV-infected patients with CD4 counts >200/μL usually experience self-limited disease.

Evasion of host immunity

Cryptosporidium evades host defense primarily by exerting control over infected enterocyte apoptosis.[39] One of the upregulated genes is osteoprotegerin, which inhibits apoptosis by acting as a decoy receptor for TNF-related apoptosis-inducing ligand (TRAIL).[37] Control of host apoptosis is complex; early inhibition of apoptosis by NF-κB activation allows the parasite to complete its life cycle, whereas the late promotion of apoptosis facilitates merozoite release. Nevertheless, the infected cells secrete FasL, which promotes apoptosis in uninfected bystander cells. In this way, the host counters the anti-apoptotic activity of the parasite by surrounding the parasitized cells by a zone of apoptotic cells.[39]

Trichomonas vaginalis

Pathogenesis

Trichomonas vaginalis is a flagellated protozoan parasite of the human urogenital tract that exists only as a trophozoite. It causes vaginitis, cervicitis, and urethritis. Its adherence to the vaginal squamous epithelium is facilitated by a number of adhesins. *Trichomonas* causes tissue damage by contact-dependent cytolysis due to pore-forming proteins and proteases, and secretion of a glycoprotein cell-detaching factor that causes sloughing of the vaginal epithelium. Levels of the cell-detaching factor correlate with the severity of the disease, and vaginal antibodies directed against this factor modulate its effects. Inflammation in the genital mucosa and submucosa leads to copious secretions, and the surface epithelium may slough, causing focal erosions and hemorrhage.

The increased risk of HIV transmission in women with trichomoniasis may be due to increased recruitment of inflammatory cells, mucosal erosion, or degradation of secretory leukocyte protease inhibitor (SLPI) by trichomonal proteases. Lower levels of SLPI are found in the vaginal fluid of women with trichomoniasis, which can lead to increased tissue damage and HIV transmission.[40] The lipophosphoglycan of *Trichomonas* induces production of the chemokines IL-8 and CCL20, which, which can also facilitate HIV infection by promoting dendritic cell recruitment.[40]

Innate immunity

Although trichomoniasis has recently received increased attention as a risk factor for HIV transmission and obstetric complications, there is little known about the protective immune response against this organism. *Trichomonas* secretes a factor that promotes neutrophil chemotaxis, causing profuse leukorrhea, but the oxidative microbicidal mechanisms of the neutrophils have decreased efficacy in the anaerobic vaginal environment. Activated macrophages can destroy trichomonads in a T and B cell-independent manner, and release IL-lβ and TNF-α, which are chemotactic for neutrophils.[41] *Trichomonas* induces neutrophil apoptosis, and macrophage clearance of these apoptotic cells causes release of IL-10, which may contribute to resolution of the inflammatory response.[42]

Acquired immunity

Repeated infections with *T. vaginalis* do not induce immunity; however, the infection is self-limited in most cases, so there are effective mechanisms of host defense. *T. vaginalis* induces the production of antibodies in both the serum and vaginal secretions. The serum antibody response correlates with active infection, and serum, but not vaginal, IgG from infected patients displays complement-mediated lytic activity against trichomonads in culture.[43]

Evasion of host immunity

Although *T. vaginalis* activates the alternative pathway of complement, the cervical mucus and menstrual blood are low in complement. Menstrual blood also supplies iron, which upregulates trichomonal adhesins and cysteine proteases, causing the degradation of complement component C3 bound to the surface of the parasite. Parasite virulence is thus enhanced, and the symptoms are exacerbated during menses. Cysteine proteases secreted by *T. vaginalis* also degrade immunoglobulins, sabotaging the antibody response. The parasite also secretes soluble antigens that act as decoys for neutralizing antibodies or cytotoxic T cells, and disguises itself by binding to host plasma proteins. Phenotypic variation of surface markers is also a means of antibody evasion.[43]

References

1. Lavelle EC, Murphy C, O'Neill LA, Creagh EM. The role of TLRs, NLRs, and RLRs in mucosal innate immunity and homeostasis. Mucosal Immunol 2010;3(1):17–28.
2. Rasmussen SB, Reinert LS, Paludan SR. Innate recognition of intracellular pathogens: detection and activation of the first line of defense. APMIS 2009;117(5–6):323–37.
3. Bethony JM, Cole RN, Guo X, et al. Vaccines to combat the neglected tropical diseases. Immunol Rev 2011;239(1):237–70.
4. Crompton PD, Pierce SK, Miller LH. Advances and challenges in malaria vaccine development. J Clin Invest 2010;120(12):4168–78.
5. Magez S, Caljon G, Tran T, et al. Current status of vaccination against African trypanosomiasis. Parasitology 2010;137(14):2017–27.
6. Coler RN, Reed SG. Second-generation vaccines against leishmaniasis. Trends Parasitol 2005;21(5):244–9.
7. Schofield L, Grau GE. Immunological processes in malaria pathogenesis. Nat Rev Immunol 2005;5(9):722–35.
8. Good MF, Doolan DL. Malaria's journey through the lymph node. Nat Med 2007;13(9):1023–4.
9. Doolan DL, Dobano C, Baird JK. Acquired immunity to malaria. Clin Microbiol Rev 2009;22(1):13–36.
10. Doolan DL, Martinez-Alier N. Immune response to pre-erythrocytic stages of malaria parasites. Curr Mol Med 2006;6(2):169–85.
11. Marsh K, Kinyanjui S. Immune effector mechanisms in malaria. Parasite Immunol 2006;28(1–2):51–60.
12. Casares S, Richie TL. Immune evasion by malaria parasites: a challenge for vaccine development. Curr Opin Immunol 2009;21(3):321–30.
13. Liese J, Schleicher U, Bogdan C. The innate immune response against *Leishmania* parasites. Immunobiology 2008;213(3–4):377–87.
14. Peters NC, Egen JG, Secundino N, et al. In vivo imaging reveals an essential role for neutrophils in leishmaniasis transmitted by sand flies. Science 2008;321(5891):970–4.
15. Scott P, Artis D, Uzonna J, Zaph C. The development of effector and memory T cells in cutaneous leishmaniasis: the implications for vaccine development. Immunol Rev 2004;201:318–38.
16. Olivier M, Gregory DJ, Forget G. Subversion mechanisms by which *Leishmania* parasites can escape the host immune response: a signaling point of view. Clin Microbiol Rev 2005;18(2):293–305.
17. Sacks D, Anderson C. Re-examination of the immunosuppressive mechanisms mediating non-cure of *Leishmania* infection in mice. Immunol Rev 2004;201:225–38.
18. Ives A, Ronet C, Prevel F, et al. Leishmania RNA virus controls the severity of mucocutaneous leishmaniasis. Science 2011;331(6018):775–8.
19. Golgher D, Gazzinelli RT. Innate and acquired immunity in the pathogenesis of Chagas disease. Autoimmunity 2004;37(5):399–409.
20. Junqueira C, Caetano B, Bartholomeu DC, et al. The endless race between *Trypanosoma cruzi* and host immunity: lessons for and beyond Chagas disease. Expert Rev Mol Med 2010;12:e29.
21. Kayama H, Takeda K. The innate immune response to *Trypanosoma cruzi* infection. Microbes Infect 2010;12(7):511–7.
22. Koga R, Hamano S, Kuwata H, et al. TLR-dependent induction of IFN-beta mediates host defense against *Trypanosoma cruzi*. J Immunol 2006;177(10):7059–66.
23. Martin D, Tarleton R. Generation, specificity, and function of CD8+ T cells in *Trypanosoma cruzi* infection. Immunol Rev 2004;201:304–17.
24. Yarovinsky F, Zhang D, Andersen JF, et al. TLR11 activation of dendritic cells by a protozoan profilin-like protein. Science 2005;308(5728):1626–9.
25. Wilson DC, Grotenbreg GM, Liu K, et al. Differential regulation of effector- and central-memory responses to *Toxoplasma gondii* Infection by IL-12 revealed by tracking of Tgd057-specific CD8+ T cells. PLoS Pathog 2010;6(3):e1000815.
26. Zhao YO, Khaminets A, Hunn JP, Howard JC. Disruption of the *Toxoplasma gondii* parasitophorous vacuole by IFNgamma-inducible immunity-related GTPases (IRG proteins) triggers necrotic cell death. PLoS Pathog 2009;5(2):e1000288.
27. Aliberti J. Host persistence: exploitation of anti-inflammatory pathways by *Toxoplasma gondii*. Nat Rev Immunol 2005;5(2):162–70.
28. Ralston KS, Petri Jr WA. Tissue destruction and invasion by *Entamoeba histolytica*. Trends Parasitol 2011;27(6):254–63.
29. Mortimer L, Chadee K. The immunopathogenesis of *Entamoeba histolytica*. Exp Parasitol 2010;126(3):366–80.
30. Baxt LA, Singh U. New insights into *Entamoeba histolytica* pathogenesis. Curr Opin Infect Dis 2008;21(5):489–94.
31. Santi-Rocca J, Rigothier MC, Guillen N. Host-microbe interactions and defense mechanisms in the development of amoebic liver abscesses. Clin Microbiol Rev 2009;22(1):65–75.
32. Solaymani-Mohammadi S, Singer SM. *Giardia duodenalis*: the double-edged sword of immune responses in giardiasis. Exp Parasitol 2010;126(3):292–7.
33. Ankarklev J, Jerlstrom-Hultqvist J, Ringqvist E, et al. Behind the smile: cell biology and disease mechanisms of *Giardia* species. Nat Rev Microbiol 2010;8(6):413–22.
34. Pavanelli WR, Gutierrez FR, Silva JJ, et al. The effects of nitric oxide on the immune response during giardiasis. Braz J Infect Dis 2010;14(6):606–12.
35. Mac Kenzie WR, Hoxie NJ, Proctor ME, et al. A massive outbreak in Milwaukee of *Cryptosporidium* infection transmitted through the public water supply. N Engl J Med 1994;331(3):161–7.
36. Kothavade RJ. Challenges in understanding the immunopathogenesis of *Cryptosporidium* infections in humans. Eur J Clin Microbiol Infect Dis 2011;30(12):1461–72.
37. Pantenburg B, Dann SM, Wang HC, et al. Intestinal immune response to human *Cryptosporidium* sp. infection. Infect Immun 2008;76(1):23–9.
38. Barakat FM, McDonald V, Foster GR, et al. *Cryptosporidium parvum* infection rapidly induces a protective innate immune response involving type I interferon. J Infect Dis 2009;200(10):1548–55.
39. Liu J, Deng M, Lancto CA, et al. Biphasic modulation of apoptotic pathways in *Cryptosporidium parvum*-infected human intestinal epithelial cells. Infect Immun 2009;77(2):837–49.
40. Thurman AR, Doncel GF. Innate immunity and inflammatory response to *Trichomonas vaginalis* and bacterial vaginosis: relationship to HIV acquisition. Am J Reprod Immunol 2011;65(2):89–98.
41. Han IH, Goo SY, Park SJ, et al. Proinflammatory cytokine and nitric oxide production by human macrophages stimulated with *Trichomonas vaginalis*. Korean J Parasitol 2009;47(3):205–12.
42. Ahn MH, Song HO, Ryu JS. *Trichomonas vaginalis*-induced neutrophil apoptosis causes anti-inflammatory cytokine production by human monocyte-derived macrophages. Parasite Immunol 2008;30(8):410–6.
43. Petrin D, Delgaty K, Bhatt R, Garber G. Clinical and microbiological aspects of *Trichomonas vaginalis*. Clin Microbiol Rev 1998;11(2):300–17.

Host defenses to helminths

Subash Babu,
Thomas B.
Nutman

Parasitic helminths are complex eukaryotic organisms, characterized by their ability to maintain long-standing, chronic infections in human hosts, sometimes lasting decades. Hence, parasitic helminths are a major health care problem worldwide, infecting more than two billion people, mostly in developing countries (Fig. 29.1). Common helminth infections, such as intestinal helminths, filarial and schistosome infections, are a major medical, social and economic burden to the countries in which these infections are endemic. Chemotherapy, while highly successful in some areas, still suffers from the disadvantages of the length of treatment, the logistics involved in the distribution of drugs and in some cases, the emergence of drug resistance. Vector control measures are at best an adjunct measure in the control of helminth infections but also suffer from the same social, logistic and economic obstacles as mass chemotherapy. Therefore, the study of the immune responses to helminth infections attains great importance both in terms of understanding the parasite strategies involved in establishing chronic infection and in the delineation of a successful host immune response to develop protective vaccines against infection.

Spectrum of host–parasite interactions

While both protozoa and helminths can cause parasitic infections, the biology and the host response to each are extremely different. Protozoa are small, unicellular organisms that multiply intracellularly and pose an extreme immediate hazard to the host immune system. Helminths, in contrast, are large (often centimeters to meters in length), extracellular (the exception being *Trichinella spiralis*), and typically do not multiply in their vertebrate host and therefore do not present an immediate threat during initial infection.

Helminths have characteristically complex life cycles with many developmental stages.[1] Thus, the host is exposed during the course of a single infection to multiple life cycle stages of the parasites, each stage with both a shared and a unique antigenic repertoire. Thus, in *Schistosoma mansoni*, infection begins with penetration of the skin of humans exposed to infested waters by the free swimming cercariae, which then develop into tissue dwelling schistosomula. In the liver and mesenteric veins, schistosomula differentiate into sexually dimorphic adult worms, which mate and the resultant eggs produced migrate through tissues into the lumen of the intestine or bladder for environmental release. Similarly, in lymphatic filarial infection, the host is exposed to the infective stage larvae in the skin, lymph nodes and lymphatics, to the adult worms in the lymph nodes and lymphatics and finally to the microfilariae in the peripheral circulation. Hence, the host–helminth interaction is complex not only due to the multiple life cycle stages of the parasite but also because of the tissue tropism of the different stages.

Antigenic differences between the life cycle stages can lead to distinct immune responses that evolve differentially over the course of a helminth infection. In addition, depending on the location of the parasite, the responses are compartmentalized (intestinal mucosa and draining lymph nodes in intestinal nematode infection or skin/subcutaneous tissue and draining lymph nodes in onchocerciasis) or systemic (lymphatic filariasis or schistosomiasis). Moreover, the migration patterns of the parasite might elicit varied cutaneous, pulmonary and intestinal inflammatory pathologies as seen, for example, in *Ascaris* or *Stronglyloides* infection during their migratory phase. This is further complicated by the fact that human hosts are often exposed to multiple life cycle stages of the parasite at the same time. Thus, a chronically infected patient with lymphatic filariasis harboring adult worms and microfilariae might be exposed to insect bites transmitting the infective stage parasite. The immune response that ensues will not only be a reaction to the invading organism but will also bear an imprint of the previous exposures and the concurrent infection.

> ## ● KEY CONCEPTS
>
> ### Helminth infection
>
> - Divided into nematodes, trematodes, and cestodes.
> - Produce chronic infections that can persist for decades.
> - Characteristically cause morbidity rather than mortality.
> - Multicellular parasites that do not multiply in the definitive host but can reproduce sexually to produce larval stages that ensure continued transmission.

Helminth infections can elicit a spectrum of clinical manifestations mirroring diversity in host immune responses. For example, in lymphatic filariasis, most infected individuals remain clinically asymptomatic despite harboring significant worm burdens felt to reflect the induction of parasite-specific tolerance in the immune system. Others exhibit acute manifestations including fever and lymphadenopathy that is felt to reflect inflammatory processes induced by incoming larvae, dying worms or superadded infections. Individuals who mount a strong but inappropriate immune response end up with lymphatic damage and subsequent immune-mediated pathology — hydrocele and elephantiasis. Finally, a group of infected individuals mount exuberant immune responses often resulting in unusual pathology such as tropical pulmonary eosinophilia. Thus, the clinical manifestations of lymphatic filariasis exemplify the spectrum of host–parasite interactions that occur during helminth infections (Fig. 29.2).

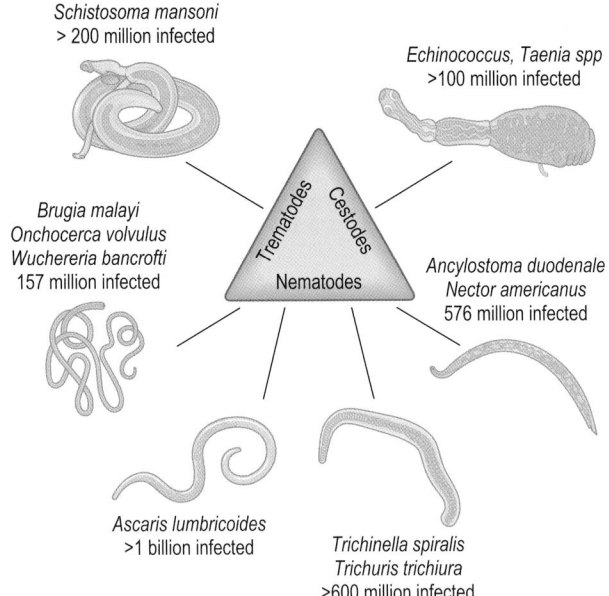

Schistosoma mansoni
> 200 million infected

Echinococcus, Taenia spp
>100 million infected

Brugia malayi
Onchocerca volvulus
Wuchereria bancrofti
157 million infected

Ancylostoma duodenale
Nector americanus
576 million infected

Trematodes

Cestodes

Nematodes

Ascaris lumbricoides
>1 billion infected

Trichinella spiralis
Trichuris trichiura
>600 million infected

Fig. 29.1 Common and medically relevant helminth infections and their global prevalence.

Another hallmark of all helminth infections is their chronic nature, with many helminths surviving in the host for decades. For example, adult schistosomes and filariae can survive in host tissues for as long as 30 years, producing eggs and larval stages all the time. Similarly, *Strongyloides stercoralis*, due to their ability to "auto-infect," can maintain their life cycle for decades. Chronic infections certainly reflect an adaptation that leads to "parasitism" in that causing mortality would prevent parasite

transmission, if the host were to die before larval release or egg production could occur. In addition to the long-lived nature of the infection, helminths frequently live within a balanced host–parasite interface so that relatively asymptomatic carriers are available as reservoirs for ongoing transmission. When this balanced co-existence is interrupted, pathology—exemplified by cirrhosis and portal hypertension in schistosomiasis and elephantiasis associated with lymphatic filariasis—can ensue.

Prototypical host responses to helminths

The canonical host immune response to all helminths is of the Th2 type and involves the production of cytokines—IL-4, -5, -9, -10, and -13, the antibody isotypes—IgG1, IgG4 and IgE, and expanded populations of eosinophils, basophils, mast cells and alternatively activated (M2) macrophages.[2] While the Th2 response induced by helminth parasites is a stereotypical response of the host, its initiation requires interaction with many different cells, most notably: (1) stromal cells; (2) dendritic cells and macrophages; (3) eosinophils; (4) mast cells; (5) basophils; and (6) epithelial and innate helper cells.[2] These in turn can induce and culminate in type-2 responses. Over time, with chronic infection, these prototypical type-2 responses are modulated by both adaptive and natural regulatory T cells, alternatively activated macrophages, eosinophils, and likely other, heretofore unidentified, cell populations (Fig. 29.3).

Helminths and dendritic cells

Dendritic cells (DC) are professional antigen-presenting cells that play an essential role in presenting antigen to T cells to initiate immune responses (Chapter 6). For Th1 responses,

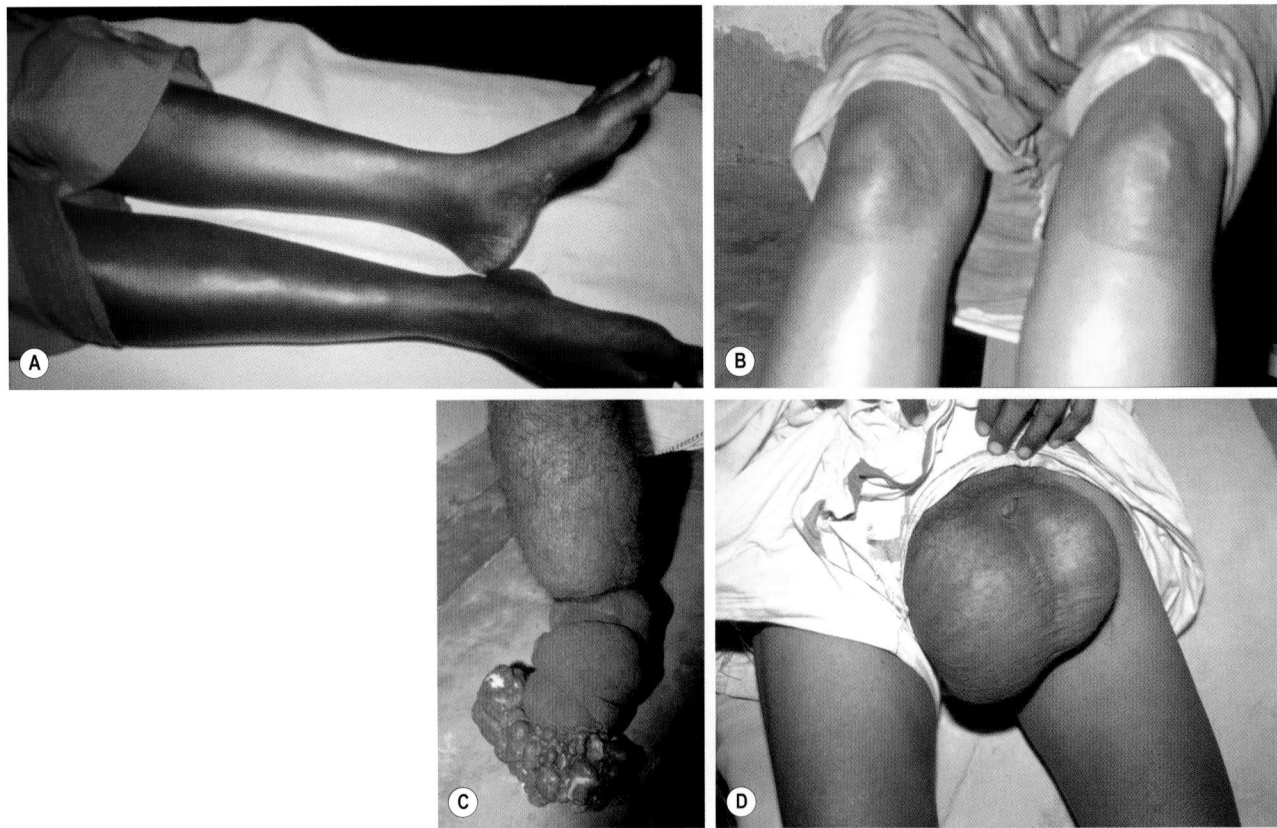

Fig. 29.2 The clinical manifestations of lymphatic filariasis including (A) mild lymphedema, (B) severe lymphedema, and (C) elephantiasis and (D) hydrocele.

Fig. 29.3 Regulation of the T-cell response in helminth infection. IL, interleukin; Th0, precursor T helper cell; Th2, T helper 2 cell; Treg, regulatory T cell; Tfh, T follicular helper cell. TSLP, thymic stromal lymphopoietin; RELMα, resistin-like molecule-alpha.

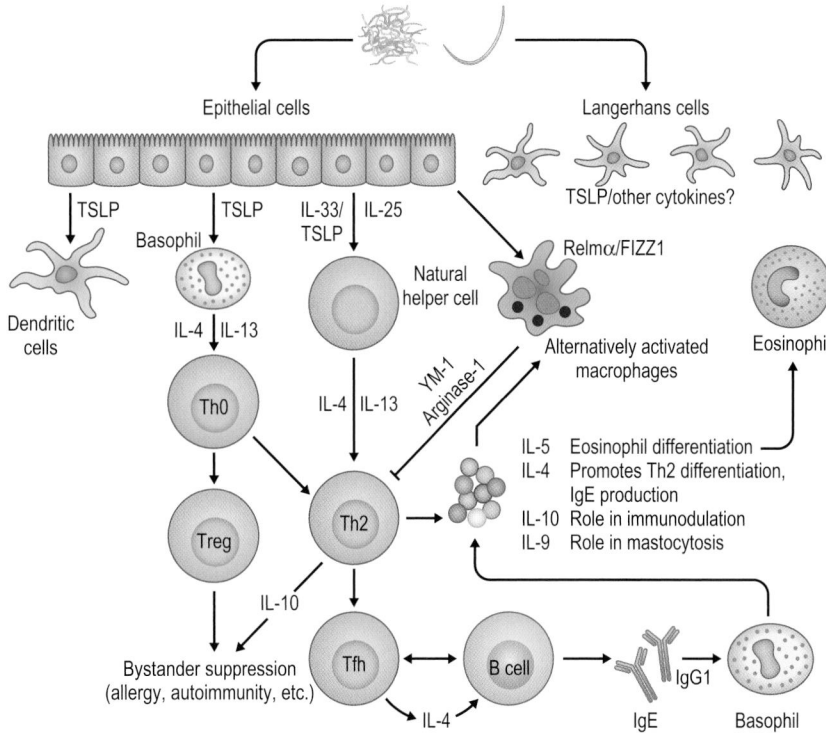

dendritic cells present bacterial or protozoal antigens in the context of upregulated co-stimulatory molecules—CD80 and CD86; Th1-biasing pattern recognition receptors, e.g., Toll-like receptors (TLRs); and a cytokine milieu of IL-12.[3] In terms of Th2 responses, *in vivo* depletion of dendritic cells has been shown to inhibit the induction of Th2 responses to *S. mansoni*. Helminth products can prime DC for the induction of Th2 responses by interaction with pattern recognition receptors such as TLRs and C-type lectin receptors (CLRs). This interaction, which depends on TLR and CLR signaling, can promote Th2 responses by suppressing antigen-presentation, co-stimulation, and/or expression of Th1 promoting cytokines by directly interfering with these pathways. This has been demonstrated in various helminth systems including schistosomes, hookworm, and filarial parasites.[4] Moreover, helminth modulation of DC function can also occur in a pattern recognition receptor-independent fashion—this is mainly dependent on the enzymatic activity of helminth derived products. For instance, omega-1, a glycosylated RNAse secreted by schistosome eggs, can drive Th2 responses via functional modulation of DC directly. While the exact mechanism behind DC-driven Th2 induction is still not clearly understood, various molecules and pathways including thymic stromal lymphopoietin (TSLP), CD40-CD40L, OX-40-OX-40 L, the Notch ligands, delta-4 and jagged-2, and suboptimal TCR triggering are thought to play important roles. The modulation of DC function by helminth antigens appears to be generalizable and impairs their ability to respond to other infectious stimuli (e.g., *Mycobacterium tuberculosis*).[5]

Helminths and macrophages

Macrophages are the other important class of antigen-presenting cells that can serve as protective effector cells in bacterial and protozoal infections by their production of nitric oxide and other mediators. Helminth interaction with macrophages induces a population of macrophages preferentially expressing arginase

instead of nitric oxide due to increased activation of arginase-1 by IL-4 and IL-13.[6] These macrophages, termed alternatively activated (or M2) macrophages, are characterized by their ability to upregulate arginase-1, chitinase 3-like proteins 3 and 4 (also known as YM1 and YM2, respectively), and resistin-like molecule-α (RELMα). These alternatively activated macrophages are known to be important in wound healing and have been postulated to play a potential role in repairing wound damage that occurs during tissue migration of helminth parasites. By virtue of expressing regulatory molecules such as IL-10, TGF-β, and programmed cell death 1 ligand 2 (PDL2), these macrophages may have a predominantly regulatory role in helminth infections. These anti-inflammatory macrophages can suppress T-cell responses through arginase-1 production and PDL2 expression and inhibit classical macrophage inflammation and recruitment through arginase-1, RELMα, triggering receptor expressed on myeloid cells 2 (TREM2), and other molecules. Interestingly, these helminth-induced macrophages exhibit a unique feature of proliferation *in situ* at the site of infection as an alternative mechanism of inflammation, which allows macrophages to accumulate in sufficient numbers to perform critical anti-helminth functions without cell recruitment from the periphery. While helminth infection does induce expression of these cells in humans, early interaction of parasites or parasite antigens leads to a predominantly pro-inflammatory response with expression of genes involved in inflammation and adhesion, including TNF-α, IL-6, IL-1-β, MIP-1-β, MIP-3-β, IL-8 as well as CD44 and ICAM-1.[7]

Helminths and T cells

Typically, infections with tissue invasive helminths induce a robust Th2 response manifested by enhanced expression of IL-4, -5, -9, -10, and -13 in response to live parasites, parasite antigens or mitogens.[2,4] The central player in Th2 immunity is the CD4 Th2 cell, which expresses all or most of the cytokines listed above as well as certain key chemokines such as CC chemokine ligand–11 (CCL-11, also known as eotaxin-1). It is clear that IL-4Rα, which is a component of both the IL-4 and -13 receptors, is at the epicenter of Th2 immunity, since IL-4 and/or -13 are critical for resistance to most helminth parasites.[8,9] Indeed, mice lacking IL-4Rα, signal transducer and activator of transcription 6 (STAT6), or the transcription factor GATA-binding protein 3 (GATA3) exhibit severely compromised anti-helminth immunity. Interestingly, in terms of the initiation of Th2 responses, most of these factors appear dispensable—thus neither IL-4 nor STAT6 is necessary for initiation of Th2 responses. In addition to the early expression of IL-4, other factors including expression of co-stimulatory molecules on naïve T cells play an important role in Th2 differentiation. Thus, CD80, CD86 interaction with CD28 and ICOS-ICOSL as well as OX40–OX40L interaction are involved in initiation or maintenance of the Th2 response. Finally, induction of GATA-3 and downregulation of the transcription factor T-bet in T cells are important steps in T-cell differentiation to the Th2 phenotype in helminth infections. Interestingly, chronic helminth infections are associated with a down-modulation of parasite antigen specific proliferative responses as well as IFN-γ and IL-2 production, but with intact IL-4 responses to parasite antigens and global downregulation of both Th1 and Th2 responses to live parasites.[2,4]

Recently, a new subset of T cells expressing IL-9 and -10, but not IL-4 (and therefore different from Th2), has been described in allergic inflammation and in response to intestinal parasites.[10] These cells appear to be under the control of TGF-β and IL-4 and dependent on the molecular factors STAT6, GATA-3, interferon regulatory factor 4 (IRF-4), and PU.1. While these cells might not represent a distinct phenotype from Th2 cells, the effector functions suggest that they might be part of a continuum of phenotypes that respond to helminth infections.

T follicular helper cells (Tfh) are a subset of CD4 T cells that migrate to B-cell follicles after activation and promote germinal center formation and B-cell isotype switching.[11] These cells, which form an independent lineage of CD4 T cells, have been recently identified to be the predominant IL-4-producing T cells early in helminth infection. In addition, Tfh are major producers of IL-21, a cytokine that plays a crucial role in supporting polarized Th2 responses *in vivo*.

In mouse models of filariasis and schistosomiasis, parasite survival is linked to the activity of regulatory T cells (Treg; Chapter 15) and immunity to infection can be boosted by the depletion of these cells. Tregs of both innate and adaptive origins can be induced in helminth infections—the former can arise directly from developing T cells in the thymus and the latter can be induced in the periphery by conversion from naïve T cells (for example, by TGF-β). In *Heligmosomoides polygyrus* infections, forkhead box P3 (FOXP3)-expressing Tregs are induced in greater numbers, express higher levels of CD103, and mediate more potent suppression than Tregs from uninfected mice. Similarly, in the periphery, FOXP3[-] cells are converted to FOXP3[+] Tregs by both helminth products and host-induced TGF-β.[2]

Helminths and B cells

Helminth interactions with B cells occur both at the B-cell cytokine level and at the level of antibody production. Interactions at the cellular level primarily result in B-cell activation and cytokine production, most notably IL-10.[12] B cells are important for the Th2 responses to certain helminths, possibly through expression of co-stimulatory molecules and/or production of IL-10. Immune regulation by B cells has also been recognized

in schistosome infection, where B-cell deficiency leads to enhanced Th2-dependent immunopathology. However, it is at the level of antibody production that B cells play a profound role in helminth infections. One of the most consistent findings in helminth infections, in both mice and humans, is the elevated level of IgE observed following exposure to helminths. Most of the IgE produced is not antigen specific, perhaps representing nonspecific potentiation of IgE producing B cells or deregulation of a normally well-controlled immune response. Interestingly, these IgE antibodies persist many years after the infection has been treated, indicating the presence of long-lived memory B cells or plasma cells in helminth infections. IgE production both in mice and humans is dependent on IL-4 or -13. Other isotypes commonly elevated in chronically helminth-infected humans are IgG4 and IgG1, the former being more dependent on both IL-4 and -10.

Helminths and eosinophils

Blood and tissue eosinophilia is characteristic of helminth infection and is mediated by IL-5 (probably in concert with IL-3 and GM-CSF). Recruitment of eosinophils to the site of infection occurs very early in experimental helminth infection—as early as 24 hours following exposure. Kinetics in humans is harder to determine but is postulated to occur as early as 2-3 weeks following infection, as demonstrated in experimental infections of volunteers. Apart from the rapid kinetics of recruitment, eosinophils in the blood and tissue also exhibit morphological and functional changes attributable to eosinophil activation. These include decreased density, upregulation of surface activation molecules such as CD25, CD69, CD44, and HLA-DR, enhanced cellular cytotoxicity, and release of granular proteins, cytokines, leukotrienes, and other mediators of inflammation.[13] Activation of eosinophils requires T cells since in the absence of T cells, eosinophils accumulate at the site of infection but do not degranulate or become cytotoxic. In addition, eosinophils have recently been shown to be important in metabolic homeostasis through maintenance of alternatively activated macrophages in adipose tissue.

Helminths and basophils/mast cells

Basophils are an important component of the immune response to helminth infections.[14] Basophils have gained prominence recently due to their possible role in Th2 cell differentiation as sources of IL-4 and even as antigen-presenting cells (APCs).[15] Basophils in humans and mice readily generate large quantities of IL-4, in IgE-dependent and -independent manners, in response to various stimuli, including FcεR1 crosslinking with IgE and allergens, IL-3, micro-organism- and parasite-derived antigens, and some proteases. Basophils have been reported to critically contribute to Th2 cell differentiation *in vivo* in certain models such as papain-elicited Th2 responses through their production of IL-4 in lymph nodes. In addition, basophils have also been reported to be critical APCs for driving Th2 cell differentiation in different models of helminth infection. However, other studies have failed to corroborate a role for basophils in mediating Th2 priming *in vivo*.

Mast cells may also contribute to inflammatory reactions directed against invasive helminth parasites. These cells express high-affinity Fcε receptors that are sensitized with parasite-antigen specific IgE and that can be triggered by parasite antigens. It has been postulated that cytokines and other mediators released by sensitized mast cells contribute to (1) the recruitment and activation of effector eosinophils; (2) increased local concentrations of antibody and complement; and (3) mucus hypersecretion and increased peristalsis of the gastrointestinal tract, which plays an important role in resistance to certain gastrointestinal nematode infections.[16]

Helminths and epithelial/innate lymphoid cells

Epithelial cells are the first barrier layer exposed to or breached by most helminths, and the capacity of these cells to respond by initiating an "alarm" response has recently been recognized.[17] Epithelial cells are capable of interacting with helminth parasites through pattern recognition receptors (for example, Toll-like receptors (TLRs) and NOD-like receptors (NLRs)) and producing cytokines such as IL-25, IL-33, and TSLP, which are considered to be Th2 cell-inducing "alarmins." TSLP also promotes IL-3 independent basophil hematopoiesis and type-2 inflammation in helminth infections. In addition, epithelial cells in the intestine are in constant contact with beneficial and pathogenic bacteria and hence ideally located for immunological surveillance of the intestinal lumen. This recognition of signals by intestinal epithelial cells is essential to mucosal homeostasis, implicating these cells as central modulators of inflammatory responses. Indeed, microRNAs expressed by epithelial cells have been shown to mediate mucosal-immune system cross-talk, resulting in protective Th2 responses to intestinal helminths. Finally, epithelial cells can directly deliver inhibitory or tolerogenic signals to T and B cells (including control of B-cell class switching to IgA producing cells).

Innate lymphoid cells (ILCs) represent a novel family of hematopoietic effectors that serve protective roles in innate immune responses to infectious microorganisms, in lymphoid tissue formation and in homeostasis of tissue stromal cells.[18] One of the novel subsets of ILCs recently discovered is the "natural helper" (NH) cells or "nuocytes," which produce IL-5 and -13 associated with Th2 responses. These cells lack known lineage markers, are dependent on the gamma-c family of cytokines, and are present in adipose tissues, lymph nodes, and spleen. Another cell type identified as important in Th2 immunity are the multi-potent progenitor type-2 cells, which might represent precursors of Th2 cytokine-producing innate leukocytes, including basophils, mast cells, and IL-13-producing ILCs.[19,20]

Protective immunity against helminths

Susceptibility to helminth infection

Multiple factors play a role in susceptibility to helminth infection including age, gender, and genetics. Most helminth infections are acquired relatively early in life and resistance to infection or re-infection develops with increasing age and exposure.[21] Interestingly, gender also plays an important role in susceptibility, with males—both humans and mice—being more susceptible to some but not all helminth infections. In addition to prevalence, the intensity of infection is also higher in males. This trend might be the result of either innate male susceptibility or behavior-related increases in exposure to parasites. However, animals housed under controlled conditions also exhibit this gender dichotomy, implicating host male physiology as a contributing factor to this phenomenon. Several studies link gender differences in immunological function to circulating hormones, such as testosterone, estradiol, and progesterone as well as glucocorticoids. Finally, a genetic predisposition to innate resistance to parasitic helminths is considered a factor with major histocompatibility complex (MHC) genes playing an important role in susceptibility to infection.

Evidence for protective immunity in humans

Although acquired immunity is difficult to demonstrate definitively in many helminth infections, three important lines of evidence for the presence of acquired, immunologically mediated resistance exist. First, epidemiologic studies (flattening of age prevalence curves) suggest that in schistosomiasis and in all the filarial infections, resistance occurs and is acquired with increasing age. Second, a phenomenon known as concomitant immunity, i.e., resistance to re-infection in the presence of ongoing infection, has also been demonstrated to exist in helminth infections.[22] Finally, a genetic predisposition to mounting an effective immune response has been suggested and linkage mapping techniques are now being utilized to map quantitative trait loci (QTL) associated with resistance to helminths using microsatellite markers.[23] Study of candidate gene polymorphisms, as well as whole genome scans in resistant and susceptible populations, would help shed more light on the genetics of host resistance to helminths.

Protective immunity to helminths

The mechanism of protective immunity to helminths is dependent on the location of the helminth infection.[24] Clearly, T cells are central to resistance against helminths. For example, T cells are essential in mediating the expulsion of gastrointestinal nematodes.[8] Mice lacking T cells are defective in their ability to expel *Trichuris muris* but resistance can be reconstituted by transfer of T cells from normal mice. Also, CD4 T cells from infected mice could transfer protective immunity to SCID mice (lacking both B and T cells), the data suggesting that CD4 T cells, but not CD8 T cells, are important for protective immunity. Similarly, T cells are required for expulsion in *Nippostrongylus brasiliensis* infection. Both nude mice and SCID mice are susceptible to infection with Brugian parasites, whereas mice that lack either CD4 or CD8 T cells are not. In schistosome-infected mice, T cells are essential in forming host-protective granulomas around the eggs deposited in the liver. Indeed, SCID mice infected with *S. mansoni* die because of the exacerbated egg-induced inflammation related to their inability to form granulomas to sequester the eggs in the tissues.

The role of cytokines in protective immunity has been extensively studied in murine models of both gastrointestinal helminths and tissue-invasive helminths.[8] Pathways of immune clearance mediated by Th2 cells are more clearly defined in the intestinal setting than in the tissues, but in both instances, multiple mechanisms are in play. The cytokines involved in both responses are IL-4, -5, -9, and -13. Most of the studies examining resistance to intestinal helminths involve four parasitic gastrointestinal nematode infections of rodent models—*T. spiralis*, *H. polygyrus*, *N. brasiliensis*, and *T. muris*. These studies show that: (1) CD4 T cells are crucial for host protection; (2) IL-4 is required for host protection and limits host pathology; (3) IL-13 can substitute for IL-4 in some but not all infections; (4) IL-2 and IFN-γ inhibit protective immunity; and (5) IL-4 and -13 have multiple effects on the immune system and gut physiology leading to protection. Th2 responses are initiated and sustained by innate populations (including epithelial cells) through IL-25 and -33.

This in turn is amplified by a network involving innate lymphoid cells that constitutively express IL-13 and promote Th2 immunity. IL-4 and -13 can act through a common receptor—IL-4Rα that signals through Stat6, both of which are required for host protection (either IL-4Rα- or Stat6-deficient mice fail to clear infection). Type-2 cytokines mobilize a broad range of downstream effector mechanisms.[24,25] Epithelial cells in the gut promote goblet cell differentiation, enhancement of mucus secretion, and the production of resistin-like molecule-β (RELMβ), which is an innate effector molecule with direct anti-helminth activity. Goblet cells can also secrete gel-forming mucins, which are major macromolecular components of the mucus barrier—two of which, Muc2 and Muc5ac, are critical in resistance to intestinal nematode infection. IL-4Rα activation also leads to increased intestinal smooth muscle hypercontractility and accelerated epithelial turnover to promote an effector response akin to an "epithelial escalator," which together with epithelial secretions helps expel intestinal helminths. Mucosal mast cells release mast cell proteases that can degrade epithelial tight junctions, thereby increasing fluid flow as part of the "weep and sweep" response. Alternatively activated macrophages in the gut can also entrap intestinal worms and cause death by compromising worm vitality.

While the role of Th2 cytokines in immunity to gastrointestinal helminth infection is well defined, their role in protective immunity to tissue-invasive helminths is not as clear.[24] In murine models of schistomiasis, protective immune responses can be generated by vaccination with irradiated cercariae. This resistance is dependent upon a Th1-mediated immune response consisting of macrophages and endothelial cells activated by IFN-γ and TNF-α producing nitric oxide and Th1-associated antibodies—IgG2a and IgG2b. In contrast, studies in rats and epidemiological studies in humans suggest Th2-mediated effector mechanisms involving IgA and IgE antibodies, as well as eosinophils, as central to protective immunity. In addition, control of a primary infection in a naïve mouse is dependent on the presence of IL-4 and -10, in the absence of which exacerbated pathology results. Protective immunity to filarial infections in mice is dependent primarily on Th2 responses in mice. Thus, mice lacking IL-4, IL-4R, or Stat6 are all susceptible to infection with *Brugia* parasites. Interestingly, IFN-γ also has a protective role since mice lacking IFN-γ exhibit impairment in the elimination of the parasite. Therefore, protective immunity to tissue-invasive helminths requires coordination of both Th1 and Th2 responses.

In tissue-invasive helminth infections, effector mechanisms involve multiple innate immune cells,[2] with antibodies acting as initiators of immunity by activating Fc receptor expressing cells. Basophils, by their ability to produce high levels of IL-4, act as effectors to promote helminth killing in secondary or challenge infections. However, they do not appear to be essential for the clearance of primary infections. Although eosinophils are crucial players in producing early IL-4, they are also amplifiers of immune responses rather than critical mediators of primary immunity since depletion of eosinophils did not alter the course of several helminth infections. The mechanism of protection mediated by eosinophils is thought to be antibody-dependent cell-mediated cytotoxicity as observed in *S. mansoni* studies *in vitro* or through release of eosinophil granule contents. Purified eosinophil granule contents have been demonstrated to effectively kill *Brugia malayi* microfilariae, schistosomula, and *T. spiralis* newborn larvae *in vitro*. Similarly, neutrophils can attack helminth larvae in response to IL-4 and -5, but their importance in resistance to primary helminth infections is not known.

Antibodies play a major role in mediating protection to some but not all helminth infections.[24] In human studies on schistosome-infected individuals, it is clear that elevated parasite-specific IgE correlates with resistance to reinfection and acquisition of primary resistance. IgE has been implicated in the expulsion of nematodes from the gut and respiratory tract, in part by enhancement of eosinophil cytotoxic responses in an antibody-dependent cell-mediated cytotoxicity mechanism, and indeed this has been demonstrated *in vitro* for *S. mansoni*. In addition, *in vivo* data from mice deficient in IgE showed increased worm burdens with *S. mansoni* and *B. malayi*, indicating an important role for IgE in host defense. Again using genetically manipulated mice models, IgM has been shown to be crucial for host protection against *B. malayi* and to *S. stercoralis*. B₁ B cells, a subset of B cells that secrete IgM, appear to be an important component of this protective axis.

> ### ● KEY CONCEPTS
>
> **Helminth-induced immune responses**
>
> - Characterized by IgE antibody production, tissue and peripheral blood eosinophilia, mast cell involvement, and type-2 cytokines
> - Implicated both in pathogenesis of helminth infections and in mediating immunologic protection
> - In mucosal immunity to helminths, Th2 responses are initiated and sustained by innate populations (including innate lymphoid cells) through IL-25 and -33
> - In tissues, helminths are acted upon by host innate effectors, including macrophages, neutrophils, eosinophils, and basophils
> - Regulated by T cells and other cells producing IL-4, -5, -9, -10, and/or -13
> - Characterized by the induction of regulatory T cells that mediate down-modulation of immune responses to helminth infections and impact bystander phenomena such as allergy and autoimmunity

Finally, a major mechanism of protection appears to be the formation of multicellular, immune cell aggregates called granulomas around incoming infectious larvae or eggs.[24] In murine models of schistomiasis and filariasis, granulomas are primarily composed of T cells (which help in the recruitment of other cell types as well as mediating alternative activation of macrophages), B cells (particularly the B₁ subset), and macrophages and eosinophils. While the exact mechanism by which granulomas mediate killing of the parasite remains unknown, it is clear that formation of these structures is an important host defense mechanism. One cell type that can mediate effector functions within the granuloma is the alternatively activated macrophage, for example, by targeting the glycan chitin frequently expressed by helminths but not by the host. The chitinase and fizz family proteins (ChaFFs), which include chitinase and chitinase-like secreted proteins, are prime candidates for mediating host resistance. These proteins include acidic mammalian chitinase (AMCase) and the RELM family proteins and are capable of enzymatic activities that potentially damage certain helminths.

Pathology associated with immune responses in parasitic helminth infection

Typically, characteristic pathological findings are associated with each parasitic infection and relate to the presence of the parasites in host tissues. But there are also pathologic reactions that stem directly from the host response.

necessary and sufficient to reconstitute granuloma formation in SCID mice.

Lymphatic filariasis is associated with similar fibrotic reactions, wherein adult parasites residing in the afferent lymphatic channels and lymph nodes induce "scarring," thought to be partially responsible for the lymphedema and chyluria found in this condition.

Fibrosis

Fibrosis is commonly associated with chronic helminth infections that result in chronic inflammation and dysregulated wound healing.[29] These infections activate macrophages and fibroblasts resulting in the production of TGF-β, PDGF, IL-1β, and other factors. Macrophages also promote inflammation by recruiting and activating monocytes and neutrophils, as well as activating CD4 T cells. CD4 T cells coordinate the immune response with the production of various cytokines—enhancing neutrophil recruitment with IL-17, activating macrophages with IL-4 and -13 or IFN-γ, and inducing collagen production by fibroblasts through IL-4, IL-13, and possibly TGF-β. In addition, fibroblasts are stimulated to synthesize matrix metalloproteinases (MMPs) and tissue-inhibitors of metalloproteinases (TIMPs), leading to extracellular matrix remodeling and fibrosis.

Toll-like receptors

Immunopathology in lymphatic filariasis is associated with the presence of an endosymbiotic *Rickettsia*-like bacterial organism *Wolbachia*. *Wolbachia* stimulate immune cells through TLR2 and TLR4 and release pro-inflammatory cytokines, as well as vascular endothelial growth factors (VEGF) that might contribute to lymphatic pathology.[30] In addition, *Wolbachia*–TLR4 interaction is the major mechanism of corneal inflammation in onchocerciasis.

Immediate hypersensitivity responses

Immediate hypersensitivity responses are associated with the early and/or acute phase of infections with invasive helminth parasites—such as *Ascaris*, hookworm, schistosomes, or filariae. Patients manifest symptoms suggestive of allergic reactivity, such as wheezing or urticaria. Furthermore, in clinical syndromes associated with *Loa loa* infection (with its angioedematous Calabar swellings; Fig. 29.4), with tropical pulmonary

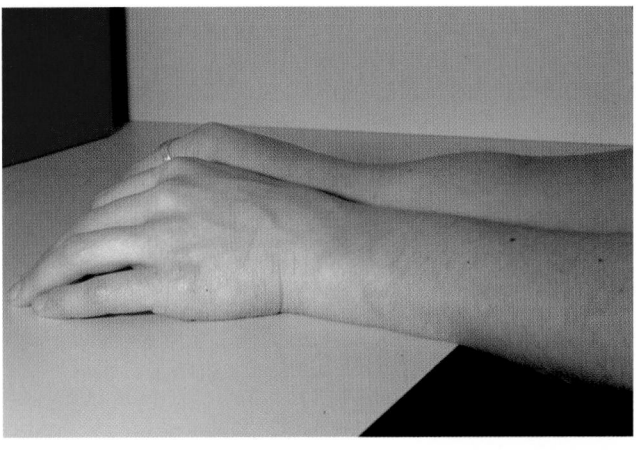

Fig. 29.4 Angioedema (Calabar swelling) of the forearm in a patient with *Loa loa* infection.

Immune complexes

Immune complexes are potent mediators of localized inflammatory processes that occur in many parasitic infections, presumably due to the chronic low-dose antigen release seen in these infections. Circulating immune complexes have been identified in both experimental and human filarial and schistosomal infections. They induce lymphatic inflammation and vasculitis in a filarial infection as a result of their deposition. In addition, immune complex glomerulonephritis (ICGN), a common manifestation of immune complex-mediated pathology, has been documented by renal biopsy in patients with schistosomiasis and filarial infections. Although the incidence of helminth-induced ICGN is unknown, proteinuria and/or hematuria have been reported in up to 50% of patients with loiasis or lymphatic filariasis, and may be exacerbated by chemotherapy. Other manifestations of immune complex mediated damage, such as reactive arthritis and dermatitis, have also been described in patients with helminth infections.

Autoantibodies

Autoantibodies have been implicated in disease pathogenesis in a variety of helminth infections, including filarial infections, schistosomiasis, and hookworm infection, and are thought to reflect a polyclonal B-cell expansion that often accompanies these infections.[26] Autoantibodies against nuclear material have been found in a vast majority of patients with chronic schistosomiasis. In addition, antibodies to calreticulin and the neutrophil granule protein defensin are common in individuals with a hyperresponsive form of onchocerciasis (sowda) characterized by severe skin pathology. Anti-retinal antibodies in serum and ocular fluids are found in onchocerciasis and are postulated to play a role in the pathogenesis of retinal degeneration and optic atrophy occurring in the infection.

Granulomatous reactions

While granuloma formation is the mainstay of the protective immune response to certain helminths, it can also lead to deleterious effects in the form of pathology. Although granulomatous reactions occur in many helminth infections (e.g., toxocariasis, *Angiostrongylus* infections, and lymphatic filariasis), parasitic granulomata have been best studied in *S. mansoni* infections, where granulomatous and fibrosing reactions against tissue-trapped eggs are orchestrated by CD4 T cells, and the fibrosis that results from the cellular response is the principal cause of morbidity in infected patients. The severity of the inflammatory process markedly varies both in humans and in experimental animal models, with severe pathology associated with Th1 and Th17 responses and milder pathology with Th2-dominant responses.[27]

Studies in murine models of granuloma formation have demonstrated the important roles of IL-13 and TNF-α.[28] IL-13 is a key mediator of chronic infection-induced liver pathology. However, IL-13 can also bind to a decoy receptor composed of IL-13Rα-2, which acts to inhibit the actions of IL-13. IL-13Rα-2 appears to play an important role in preventing pathology since mice lacking IL-13Rα-2 fail to limit granuloma formation in the chronic phase of *S. mansoni* infection. In addition, IL-13Rα-2-deficient mice develop severe IL-13-dependent fibrosis and portal hypertension, and succumb to infection. Finally, TNF-α is required for egg-laying and excretion of eggs from the host and in addition, TNF-α is eosinophilia, and with larva currens in strongyloidiasis, IgE-mediated reactions are thought to underlie these signs and symptoms.[31] Eosinophil-associated pathology, on the other hand, is found even more frequently in response to helminth infection. Evidence has been accumulating in parasitic diseases associated with profound or extreme hypereosinophilia, as in endomyocardial fibrosis associated with loiasis, or in the tropical pulmonary eosinophilia syndrome, that the major cause of tissue destruction appears to be the eosinophil and its toxic-granule associated molecules.[13]

Mechanisms of evasion and immune regulation by helminth parasites

Helminths exert profound immunoregulatory effects on the host immune system, with both parasite-antigen-specific and more generalized levels of immune suppression. Patients with schistosomiasis or filariasis have markedly diminished responses to parasite antigens and in addition, some measurable attenuation in responses to bystander antigens and routine vaccinations. Thus, while host immunosuppression is usually antigen-specific, chronic infection can be associated with some spill-over effects.[4,5] The long lifespan of helminth parasites is major evidence of successful immune evasion strategies of these parasites. Among the mechanisms utilized by parasites to avoid immune-mediated elimination are those of evasion — the use of sequestration, camouflage, and antigenic variation — and suppression, regulation, or blockade of immune effector pathways.[32]

Mechanisms of evasion

Sequestration

Pathogens become sequestered when they enter into intra- or extracellular compartments, such as the central nervous system, that are not accessible to all components of the immune response. Encystation, as occurs in infections with the metacestodes, *Echinoccous* spp., and *Taenia solium* or *T. spiralis*, is considered a mechanism of protection against immune attack. Similarly, in *Onchocerca volvulus* infection, the parasites are surrounded by a relatively avascular, acellular fibrotic capsule that serves as a barrier to the host response. Tropism for environments that are immunologically relatively protected (e.g., the eye in *O. volvulus* infection and the intestinal lumen for intestinal nematodes) contributes to sequestering the parasite from the host effector systems.

Camouflage and shedding of surface antigen and bound antibodies

Schistosomes adsorb host molecules on to their tegument, including MHC antigens, the Fc portion of immunoglobulin, and blood group antigens. They probably serve to disguise the parasite from host immune attack. Shedding of antigen upon recognition by host antibody may also enhance parasite survival; this phenomenon has been described for *S. mansoni*. Tissue- and intestinal-dwelling nematodes also periodically release portions of their outer glycocalyx coat and finally discarded or secreted antigens might serve as soluble decoys to divert the immune system. The activation of complement is inhibited in *Echinococcus granulosus* infection by the uptake of host inhibitory factor H onto the hydatid cyst wall.

Parasite-derived factors

Parasite-derived products play a very important role in host immune evasion.[33,34] Parasite products such as the schistosome-secreted proteins, alpha-1 and omega-1, promote Th2 differentiation. Alpha-1 (also known as IL-4-inducing principle of schistosome eggs or IPSE), released by schistosome eggs, induces IL-4 release and degranulation by human and mouse basophils by cross-linking surface IgE. Omega-1 is a ribonuclease abundantly secreted by eggs, which conditions dendritic cells to drive Th2 polarization.

Phosphorylcholine (PC) is a small hapten-like moiety present in the excretory/secretory products of many helminths, and one particular PC–containing molecule, ES-62, from filarial worms has a wide variety of immunomodulatory properties. Thus, ES-62 can inhibit the proliferation of CD4 T cells and conventional B cells, decrease IL-4 and IFN-γ production, promote proliferation and IL-10 production by B_1 B cells, and condition APCs to drive Th2 differentiation with concomitant inhibition of Th1 responses. ES-62 also exhibits bystander anti-inflammatory activity in collagen-induced arthritis, chemical contact sensitivity, and airway hyper-reactivity. Helminths utilize glycans (including antigens Le(X) (Galβ1-4[Fcα1-3]GlcNac-), LDNF (GalNAcβ1-4[Fucα1-3]GlcNac-), LDN (GalNAcβ1-4GlcNAc-), and Tn (GalNacα1-O-Thr/Ser)) within glycoproteins and glycolipids, which mimic host glycans, to regulate host immune responses. In addition, these host-like helminth glycans can directly interact with host glycan-binding proteins such as C-type lectin receptors and galectins to shape innate and adaptive immune responses. Helminth lipids have also been implicated in immune modulation; schistosome phosphatidylserine induces dendritic cells to polarize IL-4-producing T cells, whereas schistosome lyso-phosphatidyl serine induces dendritic cells to activate IL-10 secreting Tregs.

Helminth parasites also utilize mechanisms involving cytokine mimicry and interference to establish chronic infection. Thus parasites produce cytokine- and chemokine-like molecules to interfere with the function of host innate immune products. The first helminth cytokines were found to be homologs of TGF-β expressed by *B. malayi*; both schistosomes and filarial parasites express members of the TGF-β receptor family. Similarly, *E. granulosus* expresses a TGF-β ligand, and thus all helminth groups might have the potential to exploit TGF-β–mediated immune suppression. Various helminths including *B. malayi* produce homologs of macrophage migration inhibitory factors (MIF), which activate an anti-inflammatory pathway through SOCS-1, a molecule involved in cytokine signaling. *T. muris* expresses a homolog of IFN that binds to the IFN-γ receptor *in vitro* and induces signaling. As *T. muris* is expelled by IL-4, secretion of an IFN-γ-like protein can prolong its survival.

Similarly, helminth parasites utilize chemokine- or chemokine receptor-like proteins to evade protective immunity. *Ascaris suum* expresses a neutrophil chemoattractant with chemokine-binding properties. *S. mansoni* eggs secrete a protein (*S. mansoni* chemokine-binding protein, smCKBP) that binds the chemokines CXCL8 and CCL3 and inhibits their interaction with host chemokine receptors and their biological activity, resulting in suppression of inflammation.[35] Cells of the innate immune system utilize C-type lectin receptors such as DC-SIGN, L-SIGN, the mannose receptor, macrophage galactose-binding lectin, and other lectins to recognize particular glycan antigens from helminth parasites. Interestingly, parasites like *S. mansoni* and *Toxocara canis* express their own glycan and lectin antigens that act as molecular mimics of host antigens, thereby interrupting or misdirecting host inflammatory responses. Similarly, *B. malayi* expresses galectins that can bind host immune cells in a carbohydrate-dependent manner.

Helminths secrete two major classes of protease inhibitors called the cystatins and serpins, each with proposed immunomodulatory roles. Cystatins inhibit cysteine proteases (cathepsins and aspartyl endopeptidases) required for antigen processing and presentation, thereby inhibiting T-cell activation. They also elicit the regulatory cytokine IL-10, leading to direct impairment of T-cell proliferation. The serpins are serine protease inhibitors, which can cause specific inhibition of neutrophil proteinases, cathepsin G, and neutrophil elastase. Aspartic proteases from *Ascaris lumbricoides* block efficient antigen processing dependent on proteolytic lysosomal enzymes.

Other parasite products mediate their effect by blocking effector functions including recruitment and activation of inflammatory cells and limiting the destructive potential of activated granulocytes or macrophages in the local extracellular milieu. For example, the host chemoattractant platelet activating factor (PAF) is inactivated by a complementary enzyme PAF hydrolase secreted by *N. brasiliensis*. Eotaxin-1, a potent eosinophil chemoattractant, is degraded by metalloproteases from hookworms. *Ancylostoma caninum* secretes a protein, neutrophil inhibitory factor, that binds the integrins CD11b/CD18 and blocks adhesion of activated neutrophils to vascular endothelial cells and also the release of H_2O_2 from activated neutrophils. *Necator americanus* ES products also bind to host NK cells and augment the secretion of IFN-γ, which might cross-regulate deleterious Th2 responses.[36] Other modulators, such as prostaglandins and other arachidonic acid family members, such as PGE2 and PGD2, inhibit IL-12 production by dendritic cells.

Finally, helminths susceptible to oxidant-mediated killing express both secreted and membrane-associated enzymes, such as superoxide dismutase, glutathione-S-transferase, and glutathione peroxidase, molecules thought to play a significant role in assisting parasite survival in inflamed tissues. Recently, a family of helminth defense molecules, secreted by parasitic helminths, has been shown to exhibit biochemical and functional characteristics similar to human anti-microbial peptides such as LL-37. These molecules can modulate innate cell activation by classical TLR ligands such as LPS.

Host-related factors

Regulatory T cells

Natural regulatory T (Treg) cells play an important role in down-modulation of immune responses in infectious diseases, tumor immunology, and auto-immunity (Chapter 15).[37,38] They are characterized by the expression of surface markers, CD25 and to a lesser extent GITR, and by the transcription factor FOXP3. Natural Tregs can turn off effector T-cell responses, primarily by a direct contact-mediated mechanism, but can also act via suppressive cytokines. Adaptive Tregs, which also express CD25, act through immunosuppressive mechanisms including IL-10 and TGF-β. Evidence for the involvement of Tregs in helminth-mediated down-modulation of the immune response has been accumulating in recent years.[39] IL-10 and TGF-β, both factors associated with Tregs, are elicited in response to helminth infections, and *in vitro* neutralization of IL-10 and TGF-β at least partially restores T-cell proliferation and cytokine production in lymphatic filariasis. Similar reversals of immunosuppression are observed in onchocerciasis and schistosomiasis, with IL-10 producing natural Tregs from egg-induced granulomas being important for host survival. In addition, T-cell clones secreting IL-10 and TGF-β have

been isolated in onchocerciasis. Evidence from humans and mouse models argues for a major role of $CD25^+Foxp3^+$ Tregs in controlling pathology and immunity during helminth infections. For example, in *H. polygyrus*-infected mice, natural Tregs are present in greater frequencies and also express higher levels of CD103 and are more potent immune suppressors than Tregs from naïve mice. In murine filarial infections, parasite survival is linked to Treg activity and immunity to infection can be restored by Treg depletion. Similarly, Tregs are instrumental in controlling Th2 responses in chronic *S. mansoni* infection.

Hyporesponsive T cells

Effector T-cell responses can be turned off or modulated through a variety of mechanisms including through CTLA-4 and PD-1.[40] Interestingly, increased expression of CTLA-4 and PD-1 has been demonstrated in filarial infections, and blocking of CTLA-4 can restore partially a degree of immunological responsiveness in cells from infected individuals. Moreover, T cells have decreased induction of T-bet, the Th1 master regulatory transcription factor, indicating a failure at the transcriptional level to differentiate into Th1 cells. Finally, T cells from filarial infected individuals exhibit classical signs of anergy, including diminished T-cell proliferation to parasite antigens, lack of IL-2 production, and increased expression of E3 ubiquitin ligases. Similarly, anergic T cells are found in both humans and mice with schistosomiasis and, in the latter case, these T cells express high levels of the anergy molecule GRAIL (gene related to anergy in lymphocytes).

Modulation of APC function

Dendritic cells are the first antigen-presenting cells usually to encounter parasites and helminth modulation of DC function has been well characterized.[41] Filarial parasites induce down-regulation of MHC class I and class II as well as cytokines and other genes involved in antigen presentation, thereby rendering DCs suboptimal in activation of CD4 T cells. Schistosomes induce similar effects on DCs with subsequent Th2 polarization and inhibited responses to Th1-inducing TLR ligands. In addition, schistosomes also modulate the activation of Nlrp3 (NLR family, pyrin domain containing 3) inflammasome and thus IL-1β production. The role of helminth infections in modulating the activation status of macrophages is discussed above. Alternatively activated macrophages are able to markedly suppress target cell proliferation, as well as mediating repair of tissue damaged by parasites. Helminth infections can also elicit a population of regulatory B cells that can inhibit immune responses through both IL-10-dependent and -independent mechanisms. Helminth antigens can also modulate MHC class II and CD80/86 expression on "antigen-presenting" basophils to induce the development of Th2 cells. Finally, a heterogeneous population of immature myeloid cells that share the common property of suppressing immune responses are termed myeloid-derived suppressor cells (MDSC). Although these MDSC have been well characterized in cancer immunology, their role in helminth infections is still being explored. But it is known that several helminth parasites are adept at increasing the rate of medullary or extramedullary myelopoiesis and inducing the expansion and accumulation of MDSC.

Apoptosis

Another mechanism of immune evasion is the ability of some helminths to induce host cell apoptosis.[32] In schistosomes, a molecule termed "Schistosome apoptosis factor" induced apoptosis of CD4 T cells through a Fas-FasL-dependent mechanism. Apoptosis of CD4 T cells has also been demonstrated *in vivo* in the spleens of *Brugia*-infected mice. Finally, *Brugia* microfilariae can interact with dendritic cells and NK cells and induce their apoptosis.

Regulation of allergy and autoimmunity in helminth infection

The hygiene hypothesis postulates that the stimulation of the immune system by microbes or microbial products protects from the development of inflammatory and atopic disorders.[42] Human studies have demonstrated that people living in areas endemic for helminth infections have a decreased reactivity to skin tests for allergens and milder forms of asthma.[43] Experimental animal models also reveal the protective effect of helminth infections against atopy and asthma. Several mechanisms have been proposed for the helminth-induced protection, the chief of which are the induction of regulatory T-cell activity, regulatory B-cell activity, and immuno-suppressive cytokines including IL-10 and TGF-β. Similarly, exposure to helminth parasites has been reported to prevent the onset of Th1-mediated diseases such as multiple sclerosis, diabetes mellitus, and Crohn's disease in experimental animal models.[43] Finally, helminth infection may prove useful as a therapeutic tool for autoimmune disease, as evidenced by the promising preliminary data relating to the ingestion of *Trichuris suis* eggs and the improvement of disease symptoms in individuals suffering from inflammatory bowel disease.[44]

Vaccines against helminth parasites

Vaccines against helminth infections are a necessary tool for their elimination and eradication for several reasons.[45] First, reinfection after chemotherapy is common and occurs rapidly in a majority of intestinal helminths and in some of the tissue-invasive ones as well. Hence, with sustained, continued community-based treatment, high rates of community transmission occur. In addition, there is evidence for the emergence of drug resistance, albeit rare. Second, control of the vectors involved in transmission (e.g., mosquitoes in lymphatic filarial parasites) or intermediate hosts (e.g., snails in schistosomiasis) has been difficult to achieve for both logistical and economic reasons; the emergence of pesticide resistance is also problematic. Third, although much of the geohelminth burden could be reduced by improvements in sanitation, water management, and housing, for the areas most intensely endemic for helminth parasites this has not been achieved. Thus, vaccination may ultimately provide the most efficacious way to both prevent parasitic disease and interrupt transmission.

Very few helminth vaccine candidates have reached human clinical trials.[46] One of the most promising vaccine candidates is the 28-kDa glutathione-S-transferase protein from *S. mansoni* and its homolog in *Schistosoma hematobium* (Sh28-GST). This vaccine (in alum) has been shown to elicit antibody responses characteristic of Th2 immunity in human trials. This vaccine is primarily aimed at reducing morbidity by affecting female worm fecundity, thereby improving the efficacy of chemotherapy. Similarly, *Ancylostoma*-secreted protein-2, a secreted protein from *N. americanus*, was selected for evaluation as a recombinant vaccine candidate based on human epidemiological and experimental animal model studies. The vaccine has completed Phase II trials but

unfortunately, because of IgE-mediated allergic reactions in previously hookworm-infected individuals, this vaccine candidate has been shelved in favor of potential new candidates [e.g., glutathione-S-transferase-1 (GST1) and aspartic protease-1 (APR1)].

With rapid advances in parasite genomics and proteomics, as well as newer and better vaccine delivery systems offering better and more rapid assessment, prospects for new anti-helminth vaccines are excellent, although the potential lack of commercial markets imposes a significant impediment to their development.

● ON THE HORIZON

Anticipated approaches to improved control and treatment of helminthic diseases

- Point of care species-specific diagnostics
- Vaccines for several soil-transmitted and tissue-invasive helminths
- Decoding genomes and proteomes of each of the major pathogenic helminths for humans
- Understanding the role of infection chronicity on the regulation of the immune response to parasitic helminths
- Gaining insight into the regulation by pre-existing helminth infection on the outcome of co-incident non-helminth infections, allergic and autoimmune diseases

Translational research opportunities and challenges

An important challenge in the next 5-10 years will be to use the discoveries made in the genomics and proteomics of the pathogenic helminth parasites into useful diagnostics, therapeutics, and preventative vaccines. But because so many of these helminth parasites result in diseases that have traditionally been "neglected" (the so-called Neglected Tropical Diseases [NTDs]) by both commercial entities and funding agencies, a further major need will be to translate fundamental insights from parasite biology into low cost deliverables to individuals and populations in resource-limited areas of the world.

References

1. Keusch GT. Immune responses in parasitic diseases. Part A: general concepts. Rev Infect Dis 1982;4:751–5.
2. Allen JE, Maizels RM. Diversity and dialogue in immunity to helminths. Nat Rev Immunol 2011;11:375–88.
3. Sher A, Pearce E, Kaye P. Shaping the immune response to parasites: role of dendritic cells. Curr Opin Immunol 2003;15:421–9.
4. Maizels RM, Yazdanbakhsh M. Immune regulation by helminth parasites: cellular and molecular mechanisms. Nat Rev Immunol 2003;3:733–44.
5. van Riet E, Hartgers FC, Yazdanbakhsh M. Chronic helminth infections induce immunomodulation: consequences and mechanisms. Immunobiology 2007;212:475–90.
6. Kreider T, Anthony RM, Urban Jr JF, Gause WC. Alternatively activated macrophages in helminth infections. Curr Opin Immunol 2007;19:448–53.
7. Semnani RT, Nutman TB. Toward an understanding of the interaction between filarial parasites and host antigen-presenting cells. Immunol Rev 2004;201:127–38.
8. Finkelman FD, Shea-Donohue T, Goldhill J, et al. Cytokine regulation of host defense against parasitic gastrointestinal nematodes: lessons from studies with rodent models. Annu Rev Immunol 1997;15:505–33.
9. Wynn TA. IL-13 effector functions. Annu Rev Immunol 2003;21:425–56.
10. Noelle RJ, Nowak EC. Cellular sources and immune functions of interleukin-9. Nat Rev Immunol 2010;10:683–7.
11. Crotty S. Follicular helper CD4 T cells (TFH). Annu Rev Immunol 2011;29:621–63.
12. Harris N, Gause WC. To B or not to B: B cells and the Th2-type immune response to helminths. Trends Immunol 2011;32:80–8.

13. Klion AD, Nutman TB. The role of eosinophils in host defense against helminth parasites. J Allergy Clin Immunol 2004;113:30–7.
14. Karasuyama H, Mukai K, Obata K, et al. Nonredundant roles of basophils in immunity. Annu Rev Immunol 2011;29:45–69.
15. Siracusa MC, Comeau MR, Artis D. New insights into basophil biology: initiators, regulators, and effectors of type 2 inflammation. Ann N Y Acad Sci 2011;1217:166–177.
16. Galli SJ, Tsai M. Mast cells in allergy and infection: versatile effector and regulatory cells in innate and adaptive immunity. Eur J Immunol 2010;40:1843–51.
17. Artis D, Grencis RK. The intestinal epithelium: sensors to effectors in nematode infection. Mucosal Immunol 2008;1:252–64.
18. Spits H, Di Santo JP. The expanding family of innate lymphoid cells: regulators and effectors of immunity and tissue remodeling. Nat Immunol 2011;12:21–7.
19. Neill DR, McKenzie AN. Nuocytes and beyond: new insights into helminth expulsion. Trends Parasitol 2011;27:214–21.
20. Saenz SA, Noti M, Artis D. Innate immune cell populations function as initiators and effectors in Th2 cytokine responses. Trends Immunol 2010;31:407–13.
21. Anderson RM, May RM. Helminth infections of humans: mathematical models, population dynamics, and control. Adv Parasitol 1985;24:1–101.
22. Maizels RM, Bundy DA, Selkirk ME, et al. Immunological modulation and evasion by helminth parasites in human populations. Nature 1993;365:797–805.
23. Quinnell RJ. Genetics of susceptibility to human helminth infection. Int J Parasitol 2003;33:1219–31.
24. Anthony RM, Rutitzky LI, Urban Jr JF, et al. Protective immune mechanisms in helminth infection. Nat Rev Immunol 2007;7:975–87.
25. Maizels RM, Pearce EJ, Artis D, et al. Regulation of pathogenesis and immunity in helminth infections. J Exp Med 2009;206:2059–66.
26. Zandman-Goddard G, Shoenfeld Y. Parasitic infection and autoimmunity. Lupus 2009;18:1144–8.
27. Wynn TA, Thompson RW, Cheever AW, Mentink-Kane MM. Immunopathogenesis of schistosomiasis. Immunol Rev 2004;201:156–67.
28. Wynn TA. Common and unique mechanisms regulate fibrosis in various fibroproliferative diseases. J Clin Invest 2007;117:524–9.
29. Allen JE, Wynn TA. Evolution of Th2 immunity: a rapid repair response to tissue destructive pathogens. PLoS Pathog 2011;7:e1002003.
30. Pfarr KM, Debrah AY, Specht S, Hoerauf A. Filariasis and lymphoedema. Parasite Immunol 2009;31:664–72.
31. Pritchard DI. The pro-allergic influences of helminth parasites. Mem Inst Oswaldo Cruz 1997;92(Suppl. 2):15–8.
32. Maizels RM, Balic A, Gomez-Escobar N, et al. Helminth parasites—masters of regulation. Immunol Rev 2004;201:89–116.
33. Harnett W, Harnett MM. Helminth-derived immunomodulators: can understanding the worm produce the pill? Nat Rev Immunol 2010;10:278–84.
34. Hewitson JP, Grainger JR, Maizels RM. Helminth immunoregulation: the role of parasite secreted proteins in modulating host immunity. Mol Biochem Parasitol 2009;167:1–11.
35. Smith P, Fallon RE, Mangan NE, et al. *Schistosoma mansoni* secretes a chemokine binding protein with antiinflammatory activity. J Exp Med 2005;202:1319–25.
36. Loukas A, Constant SL, Bethony JM. Immunobiology of hookworm infection. FEMS Immunol Med Microbiol 2005;43:115–24.
37. Belkaid Y, Rouse BT. Natural regulatory T cells in infectious disease. Nat Immunol 2005;6:353–60.
38. Shevach EM. Mechanisms of foxp3 + T regulatory cell-mediated suppression. Immunity 2009;30:636–45.
39. Belkaid Y, Tarbell K. Regulatory T cells in the control of host-microorganism interactions (*). Annu Rev Immunol 2009;27:551–89.
40. Fife BT, Bluestone JA. Control of peripheral T-cell tolerance and autoimmunity via the CTLA-4 and PD-1 pathways. Immunol Rev 2008;224:166–82.
41. Everts B, Smits HH, Hokke CH, Yazdanbakhsh M. Helminths and dendritic cells: sensing and regulating via pattern recognition receptors, Th2 and Treg responses. Eur J Immunol 2010;40:1525–37.
42. Yazdanbakhsh M, Kremsner PG, van Ree R. Allergy, parasites, and the hygiene hypothesis. Science 2002;296:490–4.
43. Wilson MS, Maizels RM. Regulation of allergy and autoimmunity in helminth infection. Clin Rev Allergy Immunol 2004;26:35–50.
44. Elliott DE, Weinstock JV. Helminthic therapy: using worms to treat immune-mediated disease. Adv Exp Med Biol 2009;666:157–66.
45. Bethony JM, Cole RN, Guo X, et al. Vaccines to combat the neglected tropical diseases. Immunol Rev 2011;239:237–70.
46. Hotez PJ, Bethony JM, Diemert DJ, et al. Developing vaccines to combat hookworm infection and intestinal schistosomiasis. Nat Rev Microbiol 2010;8:814–26.

PART FOUR
Immunologic deficiencies

Approach to the evaluation of the immunodeficient patient

Javier Chinen,
Mary E. Paul,
William T.
Shearer

Immunodeficiency diseases often present with increased susceptibility to infection but may also include conditions that reflect dysregulation of the immune response, such as allergies, autoimmunity or lymphoproliferation. Primary immunodeficiencies (PID) are inherited diseases that can affect any aspect of the immune response, and are usually manifested in childhood. In contrast to PIDs, secondary immunodeficiencies (discussed in detail in Chapters 37 and 38) can present at any age, in that they are acquired disruptions of the immune function caused by environmental, metabolic disease, anatomical abnormalities or infectious agents. Examples of PIDs include severe combined immune deficiencies (SCID), complete DiGeorge syndrome, and chronic granulomatous disease. The best known and most significant secondary immunodeficiency is caused by the human immunodeficiency virus (HIV) (Chapter 37). This chapter presents an approach to the evaluation of the immunodeficient patient.

KEY CONCEPTS

Features of congenital antibody deficiencies

- Free of infections until 6–9 months of age, when maternal antibodies that passed through the placenta to infant are below protective levels.
- Severe infections with bacterial organisms, especially sinusitis, otitis media, and pneumonias caused by encapsulated bacteria such as *Streptococcus pneumoniae*.
- Growth failure is generally not seen, except in the patient who has been chronically ill with severe infection.

Frequency and differential diagnosis

Estimates of the incidence of PIDs or congenital immunodeficiencies varies from selective IgA deficiency, a relatively common condition, (1:223–1:1000 people)[1] to the rare severe combined immunodeficiency (estimated 1:50,000–1:100,000 live births).[2] With universal newborn screening for T-cell deficiencies established in a few states of the USA the true incidence of SCID will soon be available. Chronic granulomatous disease (CGD) is estimated to occur with an incidence of 1:200,000 live births.[3] A household-based telephone survey suggested that 1 in 1200 persons in the USA is diagnosed with a primary immunodeficiency.[4] HIV infection continues to be prevalent locally and worldwide: in 2009, 6 in 1000 adults in the USA were infected with HIV, with other countries having up to 25 times this incidence.[5] The hallmark of immunodeficiency is recurrent serious infection with repeated antibiotic treatment failures and unusual severity of disease. Acquired and non-immunological causes for recurrent infections should be first considered in the differential diagnosis of the patient with frequent infections. Examples of extrinsic factors that can affect the immune system include disorders that disrupt usual mucosal clearance mechanisms, such as posterior urethral valves or urethral stenosis in patients with recurrent urinary tract infection; or cystic fibrosis in individuals who have recurrent sinusitis or pneumonia and/or diarrhea. Disruption of natural barriers can similarly lead to increased risk of infection in patients with skin lesions due to eczema or burns. Patients with low immunoglobulin levels may be able to produce antibodies normally, and have loss of antibodies due to a protein-losing enteropathy, nephropathy, or massive protein loss through the skin. Secondary immunodeficiency can result from other conditions affecting cell metabolism, for example, malnutrition, diabetes mellitus, and sickle cell anemia; or could be secondary to predictable or idiopathic adverse effects of drugs. Optimal management of these conditions often results in improved immunity.

Evaluation of the patient with suspected immunodeficiency

The evaluation of patients for immunodeficiency is based on a careful evaluation of the history and physical examination, accompanied by limited initial laboratory testing. With this information, the clinician can often tell patients (or parents) whether their (or their child's) immune system is significantly compromised (Fig. 30.1). Often the medical history and initial laboratory testing provide clues suggesting a specific immune disorder, and studies of specific components of the immune response and diagnostic tests for specific immunodeficiencies might be indicated. For example, an increased frequency of infections affecting only the respiratory tract and caused by encapsulated bacteria direct the diagnostic work-up to defects in humoral immunity and complement; in contrast, a history of *Aspergillus* pneumonia would suggest neutropenia and chronic granulomatous disease. According to the severity of the illness, clinical immunologists may recommend an initial exploration of the major components of the immune system: lymphocyte subset distribution, antibody responses, T-cell function, phagocyte oxidative burst, and the complement system.

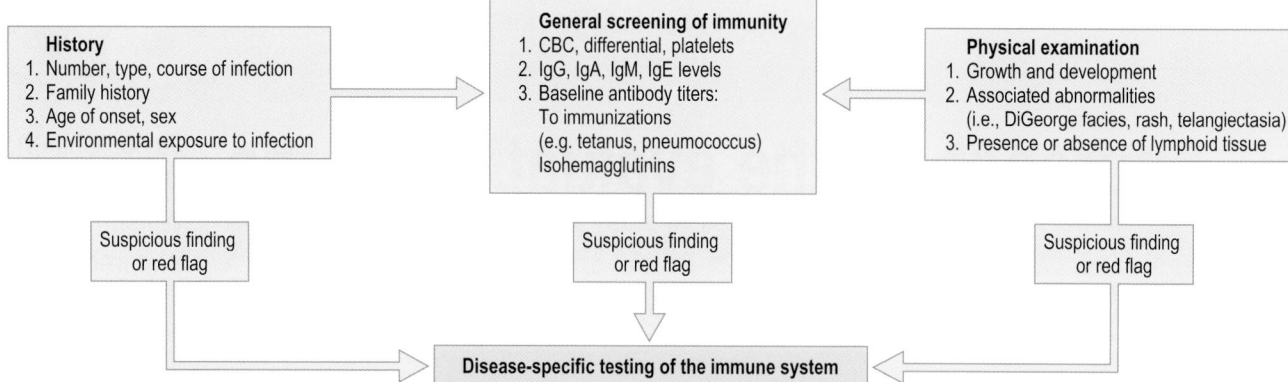

Fig. 30.1 Evaluation of immunity in a patient for immunodeficiency starts with a careful history and physical examination. Clues in the history for further evaluation include: an excess of respiratory tract infections of unusual severity; life-threatening infections; infections with unusual organisms; a family history of immunodeficiency. The outlined laboratory tests provide an adequate screen of immunity in a patient with no specific findings.

KEY CONCEPTS

Features of congenital T-cell immunodeficiency

- Onset of thrush, diarrhea, and failure to thrive in the first months of life.
- Severe infections with opportunistic microorganisms such as *Pneumocystis jiroveci*, *Candida albicans*, adenovirus, cytomegalovirus, Epstein–Barr virus (EBV).
- "BCGitis" in areas where BCG immunization is mandatory.
- Absolute and relative lymphopenia.

Medical history

Age and environment

The differential diagnosis of immunodeficiency varies with the age of onset of symptoms. Infants from birth to 3 months of age are likely to have maternal immunoglobulins present unless they were born prematurely. Therefore, deficiencies in the immune system at this age presenting with frequent infections are most likely due to severe deficiencies in other immune components, such as neutrophils, complement components, or T cells. Older patients might present with increased risk of infections secondary to comorbid conditions, such as diabetes mellitus, or to a normal decline of immune responses, a process known as immunosenescence.[6]

Environmental conditions may influence the risk of infection. Infants frequently exposed to other infants with infections, such as in the setting of a daycare facility, have more infectious illnesses than those who are not exposed. Passive cigarette smoke inhalation also predisposes to infections, including otitis media, pneumonia, and bronchitis, by inducing an inflammatory response of the respiratory mucosa.[7] The hygienic practices of the patient, caretakers and family members have an impact on the frequency of infections such as impetigo and furunculosis.

History of immunization and previous infections

The immunization history provides significant clues since the efficacy of vaccines depends on intact immunity. Incomplete schedule of immunizations easily explains the incidence of preventable diseases. A history of an adverse reaction to a live viral vaccine is suspicious for immunodeficiency, as infants with T-cell defects, B-cell defects, and combined T- and B-cell defects are susceptible to severe or even fatal infections from live attenuated vaccines. These infections include measles and chicken pox pneumonitis, rotavirus vaccine-induced diarrhea,[8] and lymphadenitis caused by BCG.

Historical information regarding the frequency, type and severity of illness and infections should be sought. Individuals with immunodeficiency may have infections with unusually prolonged courses, unusual severity, or can present as unexpected complications (Fig. 30.2). Recurrent infections that involve more than one site are more suspicious for immune deficiency than those involving a single site. Also suggestive of immune compromise are severe and invasive infections such as recurrent pneumonia, meningitis, sepsis, septic arthritis, osteomyelitis, or abscess and infections with organisms usually of low pathogenicity, such as *Candida albicans* or *Pneumocystis jiroveci* (Table 30.1). Patients with antibody deficiency disorders tend to present with infections caused by extracellular pyogenic organisms such as *Haemophilus* spp., *Pneumococcus* spp., and *Streptococcus* spp. In contrast, patients with defects in cell-mediated immunity are more likely to present with recurrent viral, fungal, protozoan, and mycobacterial infections. Furthermore, infections with catalase-positive bacteria

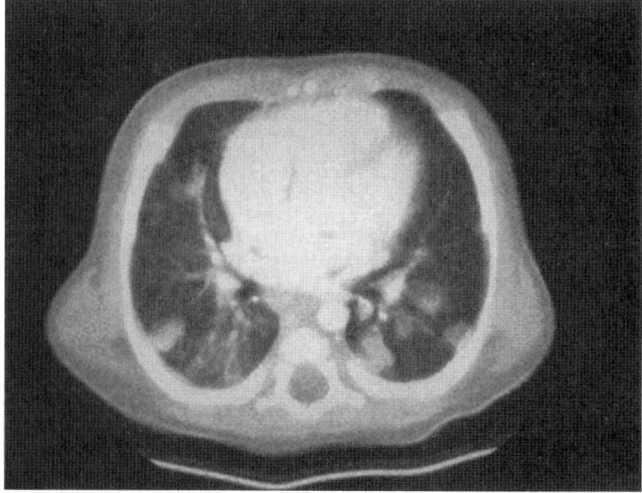

Fig. 30.2 CT scan in an infant with CGD. Multiple nodular opacities are seen throughout both lung fields due to fungal pneumonia in an infant with CGD.

From Seeborg et al. A five-week-old HIV-1-exposed girl with failure to thrive and diffuse nodular pulmonary infiltrates. J Allergy Clin Immunol 2004; 113: 629, with permission from Elsevier.

Table 30.1 Clinical clues of significance for the diagnosis of immunodeficiencies

	T-cell function-defect	Antibody defect	Granulocyte defects	Complement defect	IFN-γ/IL-12 defect
Recurrent or severe common bacterial infections	X	X	X (Catalase positive)	X (Encapsulated bacteria)	
Systemic mycobacterial infections	X				X
Recurrent or severe viral infections	X	X	X		X
Invasive fungal infections	X		X		
Opportunistic infections	X				X
Failure to thrive	X	X	X		
Autoimmunity	X	X	X	X	
Lymphoma	X	X (CVID)			

such as *Serratia marcescens* may indicate a possible neutrophil oxidative burst defect. Recurrent neisserial infections can be found in individuals deficient in the terminal complement components.

A relatively normal incidence of infections followed by a sudden occurrence of repeated infections in an adult or adolescent suggests a secondary immunodeficiency, including HIV infection.

Comorbid conditions

Apart from frequent infection, other important aspects of the history and physical exam can suggest congenital syndromes associated with immune defects (Table 30.2). Neutrophil adhesion defects lead to delayed (beyond 2 weeks of age) umbilical cord separation because of omphalitis and poor wound healing. DiGeorge syndrome patients usually present very early with hypocalcemic seizures associated with hypoparathyroidism, velopalatal insufficiency or with cardiovascular malformations rather than with recurrent infections. Infants with Wiskott–Aldrich syndrome—immunodeficiency, thrombocytopenia and eczema—present with petechiae and bruises in the neonatal period.

Obtaining a history of atopic disease is helpful. Mucosal inflammation due to allergic rhinitis predisposes to sinusitis and otitis media.[9] For most patients, once the allergic rhinitis is well managed the frequency of upper respiratory tract infection

Table 30.2 Non-immune clinical findings present in immunodeficiency syndromes

Non-immune clinical finding	Immunodeficiency
Small platelets, thrombocytopenia, eczema	Wiskott–Aldrich syndrome
Conical teeth, ectodermal dysplasia	NEMO defect
Delayed shedding of primary teeth, frequent fractures, hyperextensibility	Autosomal dominant hyper-IgE syndrome
Cerebellar ataxia, telangiectasia	Ataxia-telangiectasia
Hypoparathyroidism, conotruncal heart defect, velopalatal insufficiency	DiGeorge syndrome
Short limbs	Cartilage-hair hypoplasia
Microcephaly	DNAse IV-deficient SCID, Nijmegen syndrome
Silvery hair, albinism	Pigment dilution disorders
Pectum carinatum, skeletal dysostosis, pancreatic insufficiency	Shwachman–Diamond syndrome

diminishes. Also, it is important to elicit a history of recurrent wheezing. At times, an initial history of recurrent pneumonia is actually associated with radiological findings of perihilar cuffing and atelectasis secondary to reactive airways disease or asthma. Other significant conditions include renal disease causing proteinuria, or enteropathies, which result in protein losses and secondary hypogammaglobulinemia.

Use of medications

Use of particular drugs might also cause immunodeficiency, which could be *predictable*, such as the use of Rituximab (anti-CD20 antibody) resulting in B-cell depletion and potential antibody deficiency, or *idiopathic*, such as hypogammaglobulinemia that might develop with the use of anticonvulsants.[10]

Family and social history

Family history is essential in the evaluation of suspected immunodeficiency. A history of early infant deaths and possible consanguinity should be sought. A clear pattern of inheritance may define an X-linked, autosomal dominant or autosomal recessive genetic syndrome. Family members of immunodeficient patients might also have a history of autoimmune disease or of connective tissue disease. Many of the most common primary immunodeficiency disorders have X-linked inheritance patterns. Familial cases of selective IgA deficiency and common variable immunodeficiency have been reported, and a susceptibility trait can sometimes be traced through many generations. Socieconomical factors often determine malnutrition, known to be of a significant impact on immune function.[11]

Physical examination

Attention to detail in the physical exam can supply important clues that suggest immune dysfunction. In a normal child, a paucity of lymphoid tissue such as tonsils and lymph nodes might reflect impaired development in patients with X-linked agammaglobulinemia. Certain physical findings are characteristic of specific immunodeficiency syndromes, such as telangiectasias over the bulbar conjunctivae and face with or without ataxia in ataxia-telangiectasia; chronic eczema and delayed shedding of primary teeth in hyper-IgE syndrome; severe eczema in immunodeficiency, polyendocrinopathy and enteropathy, X-linked (IPEX) syndrome and Wiskott–Aldrich syndrome; chronic periodontitis in chemotactic defects of the neutrophils; and silvery hair, pale skin, and photophobia in Chediak–Higashi syndrome. Investigation for Shwachman–Diamond syndrome should be considered in neutropenic patients; especially if also presenting with *skeletal dysplasia*, DiGeorge syndrome and NEMO deficiency patients present with a characteristic facies.

Patients with immunodeficiencies most often present with clinical findings secondary to the excess of infections. Some children are small for their age with growth delay secondary to recurrent infections. Hepatosplenomegaly and diffuse lymphadenopathy can suggest HIV infection or a disorder of immune dysregulation. Children with leukocyte adhesion deficiency (LAD) can present with severe gingivostomatitis and dental erosion as a consequence of abnormal leukocyte function (Fig. 30.3). Multiple scars from skin abscesses might suggest neutrophil defects, and scarred tympani with reduced hearing can indicate a history of recurrent otitis media that can be associated with antibody deficiency.

Many patients with increased frequency of infections may not have abnormal results in clinically available immunological testing and may not give clear evidence of a secondary etiology in the medical evaluation. In these difficult cases, referral to tertiary care and research centers for investigation of rare diseases is recommended.

> ● KEY CONCEPTS
>
> **Screening tests for suspected immunodeficiency**
>
> - Evaluate for neutropenia, lymphopenia, thrombocytopenia, and/or small platelets
> - Immunoglobulin levels and specific antibodies to childhood immunizations
> - Lateral chest radiograph in infants for thymus shadow
> - Delayed hypersensitivity skin tests (Candida, tetanus antigens; PPD if received BCG)
> - Consider flow cytometry to quantify T cells, T-cell subsets, B cells, and NK cells (especially in infants)
> - Measurement of CH50 activity
> - Test for oxidative burst in phagocytes

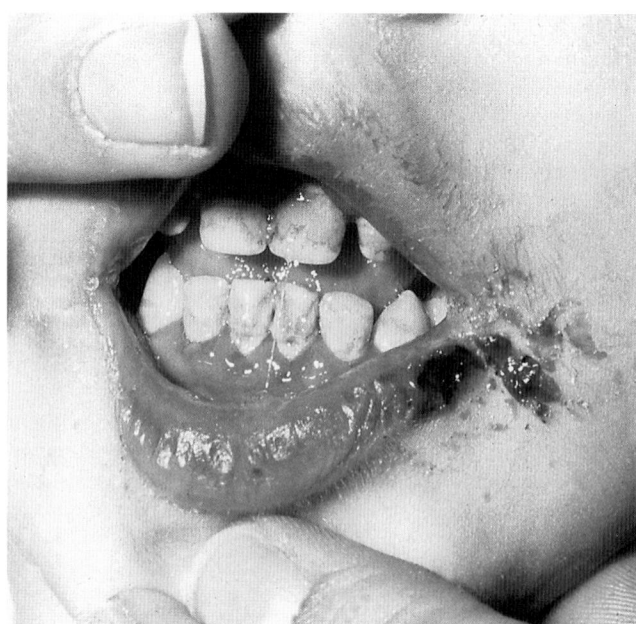

Fig. 30.3 Severe gingivostomatitis and dental erosion in a 2-year-old child with LAD.
Courtesy of Dr DC Anderson.

Laboratory investigations

Common screening tests

Practitioners suspecting immunodeficiency can learn a great deal from commonly ordered tests. The complete blood count (CBC) with differential and platelet determination is ordered to evaluate the total white blood cell count and total numbers of neutrophils, lymphocytes, eosinophils, and platelets. Abnormal counts should be determined using age-specific ranges. Leukocytosis, neutropenia, lymphopenia, and abnormalities in white blood cell morphology can be detected from this test. Anemia may be present in children with chronic disease. Platelet counts may be abnormally low in children with poor bone marrow function or autoimmune disease, and platelets will be reduced in number and will be morphologically small in children with Wiskott–Aldrich syndrome. Abnormal results on chemistry panels, including serum liver enzymes levels, can suggest organ compromise as a result of infections or autoimmunity associated with immunodeficiency. Low protein levels suggest malnutrition and conditions associated with protein losses, which may cause hypogammaglobulinemia. A chest radiograph can reveal absence of the thymus shadow, suggesting impaired T-cell development.

HIV infection can be ruled-out by screening by measuring anti-HIV antibodies, by ELISA or by rapid HIV test. In those individuals with a suspected defect in humoral immunity and in children younger than 18 months of age, a polymerase chain reaction (PCR)-based test to detect HIV viremia should be performed to avoid false negatives and confounding maternal anti-HIV antibodies, respectively.

Immunology testing

Specific immunological testing is guided by clues obtained from the history and physical exam, and results of the common screening laboratory tests.

Immunoglobulin levels

The immunoglobulins IgG, IgA, IgE, and IgM levels can be measured. The IgA level is especially helpful in that it is low in all permanent types of agammaglobulinemia and in selective IgA deficiency. IgE level measurement is of significance for the diagnosis of hyperimmunoglobulin E syndrome. Serum IgG subclass levels can be determined; however, rather than using as a screen for immunodeficiency, measurement of IgG subclass levels is best utilized when patients have clinical conditions associated with specific antibody deficiencies but normal total IgG levels. In some of these patients, IgG subclass deficiency, particularly IgG_2 and IgG_3 deficiencies, might be present. IgG_2 deficiency has been linked with selective IgA deficiency and deficiency of antipolysaccharide antibodies. IgA subclass levels IgA_1 and IgA_2 are not associated with a specific immune defect and there is no clinical indication for these measurements. The variation of normal ranges of human serum immunoglobulins with age is an important consideration in children, since IgA and IgG subclass levels may not reach normal adult reference ranges until 6 years of age.[1,12]

B-cell function: specific antibody production

To properly assess B-cell function, specific antibody production must be measured. Patients with recurrent infections may warrant this test even if immunoglobulin levels are normal; cases of antibody deficiency have been documented in patients with normal immunoglobulin and immunoglobulin subclass levels. An initial screen of antibody production may involve the quantification of isohemagglutinins. Isohemagglutinins occur in all individuals except those with blood type AB; they are natural IgM antibodies to polysaccharide blood group antigens A and/or B, which are not expressed on the red blood cells of the patient tested. Children less than one year of age do not reliably have measurable serum isohemagglutinins because of the limited exposure. These antibodies should normally be present in titers greater than 1:10. Specific IgG antibody production can be measured as a challenge following immunization with protein antigens (Chapter 95), such as toxins derived from tetanus and diphtheria organisms, and polysaccharide antigens, such as those produced by pneumococci and *Haemophilus influenzae*. For pneumococcal immunization, there are two vaccines that need to be differentiated. The conjugated vaccine containing 13 pneumococcal seroptypes (PCV13, Wyeth) is currently included in the universal schedule of immunizations for infants and toddlers, and induces a robust, T cell-dependent immune response. The unconjugated 23-valent pneumococcal polysaccharide vaccine (Pneumovax, Merck) is available for immunization of adults and children aged 2 years and older. The immune response for this vaccine is considered to be less dependent on T cells and is also not as long-lived as the conjugated vaccine. The pneumococcal antigen challenge using the unconjugated vaccine is not recommended for children under 2 years of age because normal children are not thought to reliably respond to the unconjugated antigen at this age. However, this view has been challenged by newer information showing that one-year-old children produce normal antibody responses to this unconjugated vaccine.[13,14] Normal antibody responses are usually demonstrated with a rise greater than twofold in specific antibody levels within 2 weeks for protein antigens and within 4–6 weeks for polysaccharide antigens. Patients with agammaglobulinemia have difficulty with all antibody production, whereas those with IgG_2 subclass deficiency or specific antibody deficiency with normal levels of immunoglobulin may only have difficulty with antibody production following immunization with polysaccharide antigens. By definition, patients with selective IgA deficiency alone or with transient hypogammaglobulinemia of infancy have normal specific IgG antibody production. The pneumococcal seroptypes included in the current conjugated anti-pneumococcal vaccine, serotypes 1, 3, 4, 5, 6A, 6B, 7 F, 9 V, 14, 18 C, 19A, 19 F, and 23 F, were estimated to be responsible for approximately 90% of invasive pneumococcal disease in children less than 5 years of age worldwide.[15] Previous immunization with the conjugate vaccine does not preclude use of the unconjugated pneumococcal polysaccharide vaccine. The 23-valent polysaccharide vaccine provides the potential for stimulation and measurement of a protective immune response to 11 serotypes (2, 8, 9 N, 10A, 11A, 12 F, 15B, 17 F, 20, 22 F, 33 F) not included in the conjugated vaccine. Testing for antibodies against serotypes not included in the two vaccines and comparing the antibody titers in the pre- and post-immunization blood samples helps with the assessment of specific increase of specific anti-serotype antibody titers as a response to the vaccine administration.

Evaluation of cellular immunity

Screening tests: chest radiography and delayed-type hypersensitivity (DTH) skin tests

Examination of the posteroanterior and lateral chest radiographs to look for a thymic shadow can be helpful. This is especially appropriate in infants. However, the thymus can shrink in response to such stresses as surgery and infection, or with high-dose corticosteroid treatment. Cellular immune function can be screened with the use of the DTH skin test. Delayed-type hypersensitivity reactions occur 48-72 hours after antigen exposure, although antigens used to test DTH can occasionally produce immediate hypersensitivity reactions.

Delayed-type hypersensitivity reactions involve the production of local edema and vasodilation as a result of inflammatory cytokines secreted by antigen-specific T cells, followed by lymphocyte infiltration and maximal induration 48 hours after antigen exposure. Generally, DTH skin tests are performed using vaccine antigens or microbial agents to which the patient has been previously exposed. Commonly used antigens include tetanus toxoid, mumps, and extracts from *Candida albicans* and *Trichophyton* spp. The purified protein derivative (PPD) or tuberculin, can serve as a negative control in most patients in developed countries with a low incidence of tuberculosis. The antigens are injected intradermally using a volume of 0.1 mL with a 25- to 27-gauge needle. Standard dilutions generally used are 1:100 for *Candida albicans* and tetanus toxoid, 1:10,000 for PPD, and 1:30 for trichophyton antigen. Reactions are measured at 24, 48, and 72 hours. Patients should be cautioned that rarely, a local severe Arthus reaction (Gel and Coombs type III hypersensitivity) due to circulating IgG and IgM complement-fixing antibodies, might occur ~24 hours after injection; this reaction can be manifest by warmth, erythema, edema, petechiae, and ulceration. A positive DTH reaction is determined if there is ≥ 5 mm of induration at 48 hours for antigens other than PPD, where an induration of ≥ 10 mm is considered a positive reaction specific for *M. tuberculosis*. To avoid false negatives, a history of adequate previous exposure to antigen is important. Virtually all children and adults with previous exposure should respond to at least one antigen in a panel of tetanus toxoid, mumps and *C. albicans*. Anergy, or nonresponse to the antigen following previous exposure, can indicate a cellular defect. A nonresponder should be retested with more concentrated antigens, or may require an *in vitro* lymphocyte evaluation in the absence of a secondary cause for anergy, such as the use of immunosuppressive therapy.

Lymphocyte subset enumeration

Quantitation of B- and T-cell subsets narrows the differential diagnosis and provides evidence for the diagnosis of combined, cellular, or antibody immunodeficiency (Chapters 34, 35, 94, 95, and 96). Both T and B cells can be identified and labeled using flow cytometry and fluorescent monoclonal antibodies. T-cell enumeration involves the use of a pan-T-cell monoclonal antibody specific for CD3. The CD4 marker serves as identification for T-helper (Th) cells. B cells can be identified by using monoclonal antibodies against the cell surface markers CD19 or CD20. Natural killer (NK) cells can be identified using monoclonal antibodies against CD16 and CD56. Specialized clinical laboratories are available to measure lymphocyte markers of importance to particular diseases; for instance, the proportion of αβTCR and γδTCR double-negative $CD3^+$ T cells is of relevance in the diagnosis of autoimmune lymphoproliferative syndrome (ALPS). Also, the proportion of class-switched B cells has a predictive value for autoimmune and granulomatous complications in common variable immunodeficiency (CVID). Using flow cytometry, the fluorescence intensity corresponding to cells labeled with each specific antibody is obtained (Fig. 30.4) and the percentage of the specific lymphocyte subset can be estimated. A reference range is available for each subset defining normal values as those whose values fall between the fifth and 95th

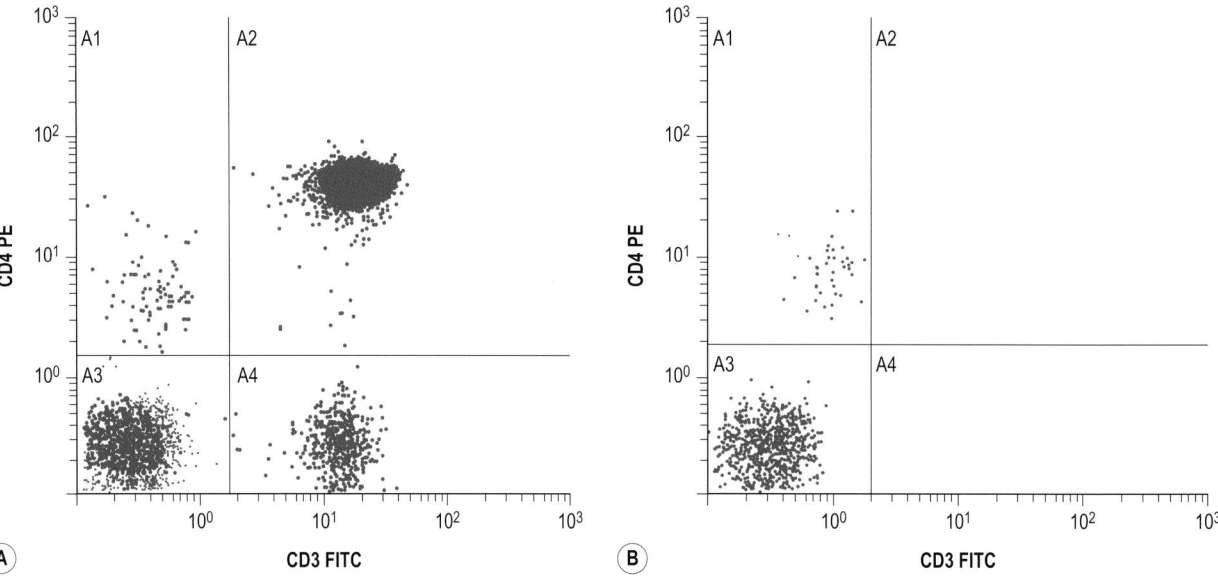

Fig. 30.4 Histograms of fluorescently-stained lymphocytes. The quadrant of interest, A2, shows lymphocytes that are positive for labeling with both fluorescein isothiocyanate (FITC)-tagged monoclonal antibodies specific for CD3 and phycoerythrin (PE)-tagged monoclonal antibodies specific for CD4. The histogram on the left (A) shows normal fluorescence due to CD4$^+$ T lymphocytes in quadrant A2. The histogram on the right (B) shows absence of CD4$^+$ T lymphocytes in an infant with SCID.

percentages for this population. Separate ranges should be used for children because infants and children generally have higher absolute numbers of T-cell subsets and higher percentages of CD4 cells (Fig. 30.5). Non-immune factors, such as age, gender, and adrenocorticoid levels, influence the expression of blood lymphocyte subset populations. Therefore, interpretation of lymphocyte phenotyping should take into consideration the clinical status of the patient. For example, transient moderate lymphopenia with predominance of T cells and NK cells might be seen in patients admitted to intensive care units. HIV infection causes progressive depletion of CD4 T cells.

Lymphocyte functional analysis

To test lymphocyte function in the laboratory, mitogen- and antigen-induced lymphocyte proliferation or transformation studies are performed (Chapter 95). For these studies, lymphocytes are stimulated to proliferate involving new DNA synthesis and cell division. This response *in vitro* correlates with the *in vivo*

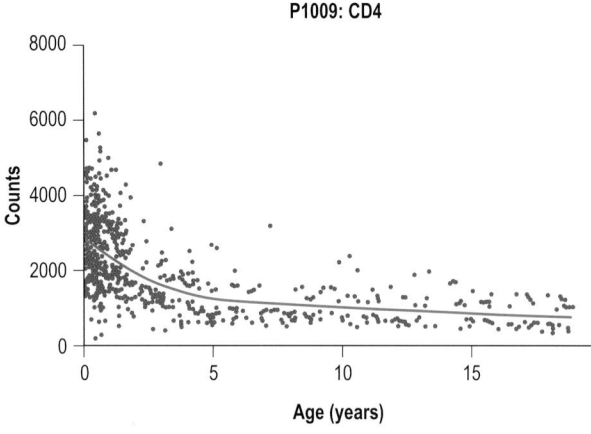

Fig. 30.5 Change in distribution of peripheral blood CD4 T-cell subsets with age in healthy children. Scatter plot indicates peripheral blood CD4$^+$ T-cell counts (cells/μL) by age, with lowest curves in healthy children from birth to 18 years of age. From Shearer et al. Lymphocyte subsets in healthy children from birth through 18 years of age: The Pediatric AIDS Clinical Trials Group P1009 study. J Allergy Clin Immunol 2003; 112: 973, with permission from Elsevier.

DTH response. Mitogens such as concanavalin A, phytohemagglutinin, and pokeweed stimulate proliferation of normal T cells, as can allogeneic histocompatibility antigens when leukocytes from two donors are mixed in culture. Proliferation of lymphocytes can be evaluated by the demonstration of cell division, or by increased DNA synthesis. Increased DNA synthesis is monitored by the incorporation of radiolabeled nucleotides, usually tritiated thymidine, in culture media. Other assays to assess mitogen-induced cell proliferation measure either deoxybromouridine incorporation, the change in the pH or the ATP concentration of the culture media. These assays are being increasingly used as surrogate markers of cellular immunity. However a comparison with the traditional assay based on radiolabeled nucleotide is not available.

Of note, a flow cytometry assay that measures cell division using carboxyfluorescein succinimidyl ester (CFSE), a fluorescent compound that distributes evenly in cells and is increasingly used in clinical immunology laboratories.[16] CFSE is distributed equally in dividing cells, and each progeny cell has half the fluorescence intensity of CFSE than the parent cell. After mitogen or antigen stimulation, mononuclear cells can be stained with specific labeled antibodies, allowing the identification of cell subsets that proliferate.

Phagocytes

The laboratory evaluation of a patient with a suspected phagocyte deficiency should begin with a complete blood count. Neutropenia is the most frequently encountered disorder of the phagocyte system.[17] Neutrophilia, at values exceeding those associated with acute infection, is a common finding in leukocyte adhesion deficiency type I.

Abnormalities of white blood cell function involve difficulty with adherence, locomotion, deformability, recognition, attachment, engulfment, phagosome formation, phagocytosis, degranulation, microbial killing, and elimination of engulfed material (Chapter 21). The number of clinical assays to evaluate neutrophil function is limited. Chronic granulomatous disease is diagnosed by demonstrating absent or markedly reduced oxidase activity in neutrophils in response to stimulation. Oxidase activity can be detected by a flow cytometry assay measuring the oxidation of dihydrorhodamine (DHR) 123 in phagocytes, resulting in fluorescent rhodamine-123.[18] For patients with suspected LAD I deficiency, neutrophils are labeled with monoclonal antibody directed against the adhesion molecule CD11/CD18 heterodimer. Absence of fluorescence indicates lack of expression of the adhesion molecule. In addition, an increase of fluorescence intensity after stimulation can be documented in normal individuals, indicating the normal upregulation of this molecule after cell activation.[19]

Other laboratory techniques used to identify phagocytic defects include assays for chemotaxis and bactericidal activity. A major pitfall for neutrophil studies is the spontaneous cell activation that might occur *in vitro* when cells are not tested within a few hours of sample procurement, resulting in artifactual values.

Complement

Laboratory tests for complement components include tests for functional activity of the classic pathway with a CH50 assay and the alternative pathway with an AH50 assay, and immunochemical methods to measure complement component levels.[20] The CH50 evaluation tests the ability of fresh serum from the patient to lyse antibody-coated sheep erythrocytes. This reflects the activity of all numbered components of the classic complement pathway, C1–C9, and terminal components of the alternative complement pathway. A total deficiency of one of the classic complement pathway components will result in a CH50 assay approaching zero (Chapter 20). Patients with complement deficiency are rare, and complement test abnormalities are often transient due to increased consumption or activation. It is recommended to repeat abnormal complement tests if the sample was taken when the patient had an acute illness. Quantitative tests for components C3 and C4 are utilized in testing for complement deficiencies and for evaluation of complement activation (Chapter 20).

Innate immunity: INF-γ levels, Toll-like receptor assay

The importance of the many components of innate immunity are increasingly recognized, as single gene defects in this immune compartment have been found to cause susceptibility to specific infections (Chapter 36).[21] For example, patients with defects in the proteins constituting the interferon gamma (INF-γ) receptor may have elevated serum INF-γ levels, even when there is no infection. The IFN-induced response associated kinase 4 (IRAK4) defect, observed with susceptibility to pneumococcal infection, can be associated with abnormal Toll-like receptor assay responses. It should be noted that the clinical value of most of these innate immunity tests as screening or diagnostic tools for immune defects has not been clearly established.

Testing for specific primary immune defects

Molecular testing for specific primary immunodeficiency disorders is available through commercial and research laboratories.[22] Specialized functional tests for immune deficiency are available in reference centers, for instance the testing of lymphocyte apoptosis in a patient who may have ALPS, the evaluation of NK cell function for suspected familial hemophagocytic lymphohistiocytosis, or the evaluation of each component of the complement cascade. If autosomal recessive SCID is suspected, the ADA and PNP enzyme activities in the red blood cells should be determined. White blood cells must be used to measure the activity of these enzymes in recently transfused individuals, since donor red blood cells will elevate the enzyme activity in deficient patients. Ataxia–telangiectasia (AT) has the consistent laboratory finding of elevated α-fetoprotein levels along with variable abnormalities in B- and T-cell function.

Genetic testing in primary immunodeficiencies

Although there are congenital immunodeficiency syndromes without known etiology, defective genes and gene products have been identified in over 170 PIDs.[23] For a rapidly growing number of immune deficiency disorders, an abnormal gene has been located and/or the specific gene product and its function are known. In these cases, the diagnosis can be confirmed by molecular genetic analysis (Chapter 98). For example, gene mutations in *BTK* leading to the absence of Bruton's tyrosine kinase results in arrest of B-cell development at the pre-B-cell stage in congenital X-linked agammaglobulinemia. Similarly, abnormal T-cell development leading to SCID results from mutations in at least 15 genes, including *IL2RG* and *JAK3*. Patients with gene mutations that have not been shown to be causative factors in a disease need to be carefully evaluated to demonstrate the pathogenic nature of the genetic change.

Recently, universal newborn screening for T-cell deficiencies has been developed in Wisconsin, Massachusetts, California and New York, by detecting T-cell receptor excision circles (TRECs, DNA recombination byproducts) in blood spots from Guthrie cards.[24–28] Newborns presenting with SCID and other T-cell deficiencies were identified.[2] In June 2010, the US Department of Health and Human Services approved the addition of SCID to the universal newborn screening panel. As it is adopted in more states, this program is likely to diagnose many more children with severe immunodeficiency before fatal infections occur, leading to significantly improved treatment outcomes.

● CLINICAL PEARLS

- Lymphopenia is a hallmark of T-cell immunodeficiency in infancy. Unexplained lymphopenia should be recognized and evaluated.
- Normal range for immunoglobulin levels and lymphocyte counts varies with age; age-matched controls should be used for interpretation.
- Survival and morbidity outcomes of hematopoietic stem cell transplantation for SCID are best when performed in the first 3.5 months of age.
- Delays in treatment of immunodeficiency leads to infections that cause permanent damage to organ systems such as the lungs, where bronchiectasis or bronchiolitis obliterans may develop secondary to recurrent pneumonias.

● ON THE HORIZON

- Early diagnosis of SCID and non-SCID is the key to successful hematopoietic stem cell transplantation.
- Implementation of universal screening of newborn infants by DNA analysis of dried blood spots on Guthrie cards (T-cell receptor excision circle, TREC) will detect almost all severe T-cell deficiencies.
- Development of DNA sequence analysis for >170 types of primary immunodeficiency performed in one test.
- Improving outcomes through a network of centers of excellence for diagnosis and definitive treatment of primary immunodeficiencies.

Translational research

A challenge in the next 5-10 years is to take laboratory discoveries into the clinical diagnosis and management of severe primary immunodeficiencies. No child with T-cell primary immunodeficiency should go undiagnosed and suffer the ravages of debilitating opportunistic infections that reduce the success rate of immunoreconstitution with hematopoietic stem cells. The TREC (T-cell receptor excision circle) assay makes it possible to detect T-cell deficient infants shortly after birth. This information should find the way into medical practice much like early detection of metabolic diseases has with the dried blood spot (Guthrie cards). However, while the TREC assay is a means to detect insufficient T-cell numbers, development of gene-specific DNA probes that could take advantage of the same blood spot collection system are needed in order to identify the molecular defect, not only of T-cell deficiencies, but those of B cells, monocytes/macrophages, natural killer cells, complement factors, and Toll-like receptors. Highly trained specialists in primary immunodeficiencies at centers of excellence need these tools of early diagnosis of newborn immunodeficiencies to speed the definitive therapies of these children.

Conclusions

The approach to the patient with suspected immune deficiency requires knowledge of developmental pathways and function of the different compartments of the immune system, as well as the clinical presentation of these uncommon disorders. The medical history, particularly the frequency, severity, and etiology of infections, is most helpful to orient the diagnostic workup. Commonly ordered tests in primary care, such as a complete blood cell count and serum immunoglobulin levels, are helpful to support possible diagnosis and referral to a clinical immunologist. Immunological testing according to clues obtained from the medical history helps to narrow the differential diagnosis to specific immunodeficiencies, which are confirmed by molecular methods.

Description of new T-cell subsets, e.g., Th17 and regulatory T cells, has helped to explain the immunopathogenesis of certain clinical manifestations, such as the occurrence of autoimmunity in patients with combined immunodeficiency, and "cold abscesses" in the autosomal dominant hyper-IgE syndrome. Testing for these lymphocyte phenotypes is now being integrated into the clinical evaluation.

Illustrative cases

Case 1

A 6-month-old Caucasian female presented with a history of rash and otitis media that had been recurrent since 2 weeks of age. She had poor weight gain, frequent spitting up, coughing spells, and persistent diarrhea. Maternal HIV testing was negative. The physical examination showed an emaciated infant without palpable lymphoid tissue and with severe oral thrush. Cystic fibrosis was ruled out by genetic studies. Stool viral cultures were persistently positive for rotavirus.

Humoral immunity showed immunoglobulin levels below or just above the lower limit of normal (Table 30.3). Isohemagglutinins were not tested as the patient was less than one year old. As she had not been immunized, specific antibody titers to vaccines

were not tested. Stool α1-antitrypsin levels were normal, suggesting that protein was not being lost in the stool, and urinalysis did not show protein loss. The complete blood count revealed profound lymphopenia and absolute neutropenia. The neutropenia resolved on subsequent evaluations but the lymphopenia persisted. The thymic shadow was not present on chest radiograph. Delayed hypersensitivity skin tests were not placed as the patient would not have been expected to have a reliable response at this age. Evaluation of lymphocytes subsets by flow cytometry revealed that the CD4$^+$ and CD8$^+$ T- and B-cell numbers were all markedly low. The patient's lymphocytes had no proliferative response when stimulated with phytohemagglutinin. The history and physical examination, along with the laboratory values, including low immunoglobulin levels and markedly low lymphocyte numbers with poor proliferative response to mitogen stimulation, strongly suggested the diagnosis of SCID. The patient had low levels of adenosine deaminase (ADA) and increased levels of the toxic nucleotide metabolites. SCID due to ADA deficiency was diagnosed.

Following ADA enzyme replacement therapy and immunoglobulin infusions the patient thrived and had fewer infections. Lymphocyte numbers and function improved.

Case 2

A 4-year-old female presented with history of frequent upper and lower respiratory infections and short stature. Family history was not contributory. Physical examination was remarkable for height and weight less than fifth percentile for age and a significant chest deformity (Fig. 30.6). Radiological examination demonstrated metaphyseal dysplasia and *pectum carinatum*, with significant bilateral lung atelectasis. A hematology evaluation showed severe neutropenia (570 cells/μL [1500-8000]), normal lymphocyte count and mild thrombocytopenia (Table 30.3). Examination of bone marrow resulted mild dysplasia with presence of three lineages, and no evidence of chronic viral infections. Evaluation for failure to thrive was significant for low levels of pancreatic enzymes. A sweat test was done to screen for cystic fibrosis and was reported normal.

Immunological evaluation showed normal serum levels of Ig G, A, and M, with mildly increased IgE levels. Specific antibody responses to childhood vaccines were protective to tetanus, diphtheria and *H. influenzae* antigens, and to only two of 14 pneumococcal serotypes measured, despite being fully immunized. Lymphocyte phenotyping revealed low B cells and NK cells. A diagnosis of Shwachman–Diamond syndrome (SDS) was made based on the patient's unique clinical manifestations.[24] Genetic sequencing analysis of the SDS gene identified one mutated allele that had not been previously reported while molecular investigations for chromosomal breakage defects, other skeletal genetic syndromes and mitochondrial defects were negative. The patient was treated with pancreatic enzyme replacement, antibiotic prophylaxis and close hematological management.

Case 3

A 12-year-old Caucasian male presented at 8 months of age with diarrhea for one month, nuchal rigidity, left facial weakness, and a left sixth cranial nerve palsy. He had been well for the first 6 months of life. The family history was negative for immunodeficiency. The patient had received his childhood immunizations, including the live polio virus vaccine. Physical examination revealed an absence of tonsillar tissue, and the patient had no

Table 30.3 Results of screening tests and special evaluations of illustrative cases.

Test	Case number			
	1	2	3	4
Antibody function				
Serum immunoglobulin (mg/dL)				
IgG	235 (208–686)	Normal	41 (256–1067)	748 (520–1340)
IgA	<8 (10–62)	Normal	7 (12–103)	40 (25–81)
IgM	<7 (43–183)	Normal	14 (47–173)	78 (64–275)
Isohemagglutinins	ND	ND	Negative	Normal
Functional antibody tests				
Antitetanus	ND	Normal	Undetectable	0.28
Antidiphtheria	ND	Normal	Undetectable	0.12
Antipneumococcus	ND	2 of 14 protective	ND	Normal
Lymphocyte function				
Lymphocyte count (x10e3 cell/μL)	0.217 (2.5–16.5)	2.8 (2.3–5.4)	2.56 (4.0–13.5)	10.60 (3.0–9.5)
CD4 number (x10e3 cell/μL)	0.009 (1.6–4.0)	1.27 (0.9–2.4)	1.72 (1.4–4.3)	ND
CD8 number (x10e3 cell/μL)	0.008 (0.5–1.7)	1.5 (0.5–1.5)	0.73 (0.5–1.7)	ND
CD19 number (x10e3 cell/μL)	0.010 (0.3–2.0)	0.023 (0.4–1.4)	0.107 (0.6–2.6)	ND
Functional antibody				
Proliferation (counts/min)				
PHA	546 (55494)	Normal	210973 (177195)	ND
ConA	ND	Normal	124680 (143591)	ND
PWM	ND	Normal	162646 (138684)	ND
Complement function				
Total hemolytic complement (U/ml)	ND	ND	618 (300–500)	<100 (300–500)
Phagocyte function				
Neutrophil count (x10e3 cell/μL)	0.109 (1.0–9.0)	0.570 (1.5–8.5)	3.3 (1.0–8.5)	4.2 (1.5–8.5)
Monocyte count (x10e3 cell/μL)	0.546 (mean 0.7)	Normal	0.11 (mean 0.6)	0.65 (mean 0.5)
Oxidative activity (DHR)	ND	Normal	Normal	ND

Normal values are reported in parentheses. Normal values may vary from laboratory to laboratory due to technique and may vary owing to age.

palpable lymph nodes. The presenting neurologic symptoms resolved, but the patient subsequently developed a lower-extremity flaccid paralysis that had persisted.

Immunodeficiency was suspected because of the chronicity of the illness, the lack of lymphoid tissue on physical examination, and the finding of an unusual infectious agent causing severe sequelae to infection. The age at presentation was typical for patients with a defect in humoral immunity. Immune system evaluation (Table 30.3) showed a normal absolute neutrophil count and a low absolute lymphocyte count. The CH50 was mildly elevated; ruling-out a complement component deficiency. Immunoglobulin levels were low. Antibody levels to diphtheria and

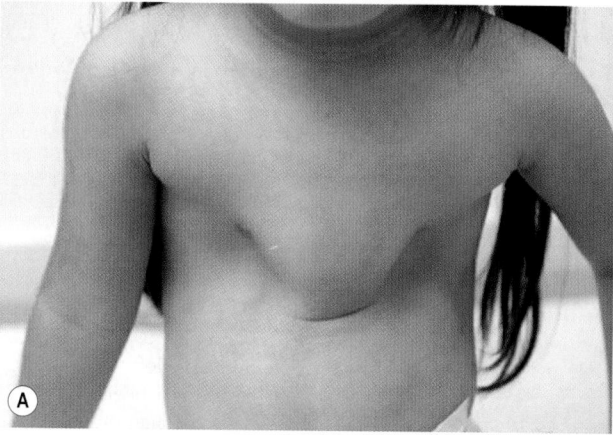
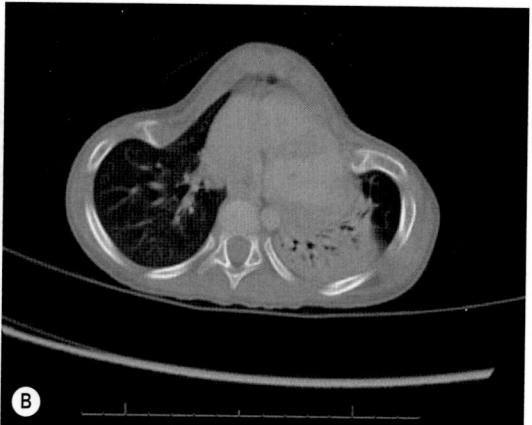

Fig. 30.6 A 4 year old girl presenting with congenital neutropenia, small stature and pancreatic insufficiency. Genetic sequencing analysis confirmed diagnosis of Shwachman–Diamond syndrome. A, *Pectus carinatum*; B, chest CT (computed tomograph) scan;

(Continued)

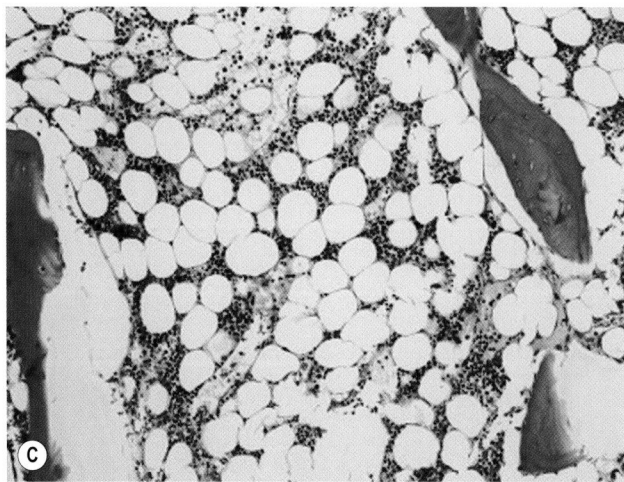

Fig. 30.6—cont'd C, bone marrow biopsy (H&E stain, 100×).
From Shah SS, et al. Diagnosis of primary immunodeficiency: let your eyes do the talking. J Allergy Clin Immunol 2009; 124: 1363–4, with permission from Elsevier.[29]

tetanus were very low. The thymus was present on the chest radiograph. Lymphocyte evaluation showed normal numbers and percentages of T cells and absent numbers and percentages of B cells. Proliferative responses of lymphocytes to mitogens were normal. Molecular testing showed a mutation in the gene encoding Bruton's tyrosine kinase (BTK). The cerebrospinal fluid was remarkable for a lymphocytic pleocytosis with normal protein and glucose levels. Stool and throat cultures grew vaccine strain poliovirus. The patient was diagnosed with vaccine acquired polio virus infection and X-linked agammaglobulinemia.

The patient receives monthly immunoglobulin replacement therapy and is otherwise well.

Case 4

The patient was a 3 year old girl hospitalized for pneumonia. The past medical history was significant for recurrent otitis media and bronchitis. Two siblings had had a history of recurrent otitis media and bronchitis. The physical examination revealed normal tonsillar tissue and the presence of small lymph nodes in the cervical region.

Laboratory values (Table 30.3) were normal except that the CH50 level was below the lowest measurable level. C3 and C4 levels were normal, but the level of C2 was 0. The patient's father, mother, and brother had levels of C2 which were half of the normal value, consistent with being heterozygous for an abnormal C2 allele. C2 deficiency was diagnosed. The patient has had chronic sinusitis and bronchitis despite antibiotic prophylaxis. C2 deficiency is most frequently associated with autoimmune disease; this patient has not had autoimmune disease and undergoes yearly surveillance examinations.

References

1. Yel L. Selective IgA deficiency. J Clin Immunol 2010;30:10–6.
2. Chase NM, Verbsky JW, Routes JM. Newborn screening for T-cell deficiency. Curr Opin Allergy Clin Immunol 2010;10:521–5.
3. Stasia MJ, Li XJ. Genetics and immunopathology of chronic granulomatous disease. Semin Immunopathol 2008;30:209–35.
4. Boyle JM, Buckley RH. Population prevalence of diagnosed primary immunodeficiency diseases in the United States. J Clin Immunol 2007;27:497–502.
5. UNAIDS. AIDS epidemic update: November 2009. Copyright Joint United Nations Programme on HIV/AIDS (UNAIDS) and World Health Organization (WHO); 2009.
6. Agarwal S, Busse PJ. Innate and adaptive immunosenescence. Ann Allergy Asthma Immunol 2010;104:183–90.
7. Jones LL, Hashim A, McKeever T, et al. Parental and household smoking and the increased risk of bronchitis, bronchiolitis and other lower respiratory infections in infancy: systematic review and meta-analysis. Respir Res 2011;12:5.
8. Werther RL, Crawford NW, Boniface K, et al. Rotavirus vaccine-induced diarrhea in a child with severe combined immunodeficiency. J Allergy Clin Immunol 2009;124:600.
9. Skoner AR, Skoner KR, Skoner DP. Allergic rhinitis, histamine, and otitis media. Allergy Asthma Proc 2009;30:470–81.
10. Guerra IC, Fawcett WA, Redmon AH, et al. Permanent intrinsic B cell immunodeficiency caused by phenytoin hypersensitivity. J Allergy Clin Immunol 1986;77:603–7.
11. Jones KD, Berkley JA, Warner JO. Perinatal nutrition and immunity to infection. Pediatr Allergy Immunol 2010;21(4 Pt 1):564–76.
12. Ozen A, Baris S, Karakoc-Aydiner E, et al. Outcome of hypogammaglobulinemia in children: immunoglobulin levels as predictors. Clin Immunol 2010;137:374–83.
13. Fried AJ, Bonilla FA. Pathogenesis, diagnosis, and management of primary antibody deficiencies and infections. Clin Microbiol Rev 2009;22:396–414.
14. Balloch A, Licciardi PV, Russell FM, et al. Infants aged 12 months can mount adequate serotype-specific IgG responses to pneumococcal polysaccharide vaccine. J Allergy Clin Immunol 2010;126(2):395–7.
15. Johnson HL, Deloria-Knoll M, Levine OS, et al. Systematic evaluation of serotypes causing invasive pneumococcal disease among children under five: the pneumococcal global serotype project. PLoS Med 2010;7(10):pii: e1000348.
16. Kurata Y, Kato M, Kuzuya T, et al. Pretransplant pharmacodynamic analysis of immunosuppressive agents using CFSE-based T-cell proliferation assay. Clin Pharmacol Ther 2009;86:285–9.
17. Segel GB, Halterman JS. Neutropenia in pediatric practice. Pediatr Rev 2008;29:12–23.
18. Kuhns DB, Alvord WG, Heller T, et al. Residual NADPH oxidase and survival in chronic granulomatous disease. N Engl J Med 2010;363:2600–10.
19. Etzioni A. Defects in the leukocyte adhesion cascade. Clin Rev Allergy Immunol 2010;38(1):54–60.
20. Frank MM. Complement disorders and hereditary angioedema. J Allergy Clin Immunol 2010;125(2 Suppl.):S262–S271.
21. Notarangelo LD. Primary immunodeficiencies. J Allergy Clin Immunol 2010;125(2 Suppl. 2):S182–S194.
22. Waggoner DJ, Pagon RA. Internet resources in medical genetics. Curr Protoc Hum Genet 2009 [chapter 9]. Unit 9.12.
23. International Union of Immunological Societies Expert Committee on Primary Immunodeficiencies, Notarangelo LD, Fischer A, Geha RS, Wedgwood J, et al. Primary immunodeficiencies: 2009 update. J Allergy Clin Immunol 2009;124:1161–78.
24. Puck JM. Laboratory technology for population-based screening for severe combined immunodeficiency in neonates: the winner is T-cell receptor excision circles. J Allergy Clin Immunol 2012;129(3):607–16.
25. Buckley RH. The long quest for neonatal screening for severe combined immunodeficiency. J Allergy Clin Immunol 2012;129:597–604.
26. Verbsky J, Thakar M, Routes J. The Wisconsin approach to newborn screening for severe combined immunodeficiency. J Allergy Clin Immunol 2012;129:622–7.
27. Hanson IC, Shearer WT. Ruling out HIV infection when testing for severe combined immunodeficiency and other T-cell deficiencies. J Allergy Clin Immunol 2012;129:875–6.
28. Shearer WT. Screening for severe combined immunodeficiency in newborns. J Allergy Clin Immunol 2012;129:619–21.
29. Shah SS, Bacino CA, Sheehan AM, et al. Diagnosis of primary immunodeficiency: let your eyes do the talking. J Allergy Clin Immunol 2009;124:1363–4.

Infections in the immunocompromised host

Jennifer Cuellar-Rodriguez, Alexandra F. Freeman

Due to improved antimicrobials and immunosuppressant agents, there are increasing numbers of hosts with immune deficiencies, either acquired primarily through genetic defects or acquired secondarily, for example, through treatment for malignancy and autoimmune disease, or after solid or hematopoietic stem cell transplantation. Understanding both the genetic defects as well as the immunologic targets of immunosuppressant agents will help further the knowledge of host control of infection. In this chapter, we review the infection spectrum of some of the major classes of primary immunodeficiencies, as well as acquired immunodeficiency.

Primary immunodeficiencies

Phagocyte defects (Chapter 21)

The phagocytic neutrophils and monocytes are key members of the primary immune response. Neutrophils are essential in the initial host defense against microbes. Antimicrobial peptides, cytokines, and chemokines released at the site of microbial entry cause neutrophils to migrate to the site of inflammation (chemotaxis), ingest, and then kill the microbe through oxygen-dependent or -independent mechanisms. Defects in quantity or quality of neutrophils can predispose to infection, which is primarily with fungi and bacteria (Table 31.1). Defects in monocytes are less frequent, and contribute to control of intracellular bacteria, mycobacteria, and fungi.

Chronic granulomatous disease

Chronic granulomatous disease (CGD) causes the most common qualitative neutrophil immunodeficiency. Defects in the NADPH oxidase cause an abnormal neutrophil respiratory burst leading to recurrent bacterial and fungal infections. However, it is interesting that the spectrum of infections is fairly limited with the most common pathogens being: *Staphylococcus aureus*, *Burkholderia cepacia*, *Serratia marcescens*, *Nocardia* species, and *Aspergillus* species.[1-3] Other infecting organisms occur less frequently, but are rare outside of CGD including *Chromobacteria violaceum*, *Aspergillus nidulans*, and the newly identified bacteria *Granulibacter bethesdensis*.[4]

Infections in CGD are typically of the lung, lymph nodes, liver and bone (Fig. 31.1). Identification of the infecting organism is essential in CGD to guide antimicrobial therapy. CGD is characterized by exuberant granulomatous inflammation, both in areas without clear infection, such as in the gastrointestinal and genitourinary tract, but also in response to infection.[1,2] Therefore, although necrotic and purulent centers may form in liver and lymph node infections, the yield with drainage may be poor due to the thicker consistency of granulomatous inflammation. At times, the infected lymph nodes may need resection to cure infections. Likewise, in lung infections, fine needle aspirate frequently provides a higher yield than bronchoscopy due to the nature of inflammation.

The granulomatous inflammation may be intense enough to impede successful treatment of infection solely with antimicrobials and necessitate corticosteroid addition to appropriate antimicrobials. For instance, "mulch pneumonitis" occurs in CGD with large inhalations of decaying organic matter, as occurs with mulching.[5] A diffuse pneumonitis associated with *Aspergillus* results, and can be quite fulminant with a high mortality if the inflammatory response is not treated (such as with corticosteroids) in addition to antifungals. There is suggestion that the addition of corticosteroids may help with other infections in CGD such as *Nocardia* pneumonia.[6]

CGD is one of the few primary immunodeficiencies in which prophylactic antimicrobials have been systemically studied in a randomized, controlled manner. Trimethoprim-sulfamethoxasole has activity against the majority of bacterial pathogens in CGD, and thus is an ideal prophylactic antibiotic and has been shown to significantly decrease bacterial infections.[7] Itraconazole was shown to be effective in preventing some of the fungal infections.[8] The newer triazoles, including voriconazole and posaconazole, have not been studied as prophylactic antimicrobials in this setting, but have extended spectrum and would likely be effective as well.

Leukocyte adhesion deficiencies

Leukocyte adhesion deficiencies (LAD) result from the inability of neutrophils to migrate to the site of infection.[2] LAD-1 is most frequent, resulting from a defect in β-2 integrin, and presenting typically with failure of umbilical cord separation and omphalitis. The spectrum of infection is not as specific as with CGD, but limited typically to bacterial infections. Gingivitis and periodontitis lead to frequent oral bacterial infections. Necrotizing, ulcerative skin infections and respiratory tract infections are also common, typically with *S. aureus* or Gram-negative bacteria. Although primarily a defect of neutrophils resulting in bacterial infections, viral warts are not infrequent. Fungal infections are unusual. Little is known about antimicrobial prophylaxis for LAD-1, but typically prophylaxis with some coverage for oral flora, *S. aureus*, and Gram-negative organisms is provided, such as with amoxicillin/clavulanate.[9] Other rare neutrophil defects, including Chediak–Higashi and Griscelli syndromes, also are characterized by recurrent pyogenic infections.

Table 31.1 Infection susceptibility of select primary immunodeficiencies

Immunodeficiency	Genetic defect	Functional defect	Infection susceptibility
Chronic granulomatous disease	Gp91^{phox}, p22^{phox}, p40^{phox}, p47^{phox}, p67^{phox}	Defect in NADPH oxidase leading to abnormal superoxide production	Catalase positive bacteria (e.g., *Staphylococcus aureus*, *Burkholderia*, *Serratia*, *Nocardia*) and filamentous molds
Leukocyte adhesion disorder-1	Beta-2-integrin	Neutrophil migration	Bacteria, typically *S. aureus*, Gram negatives
Severe congenital neutropenia	*HAX1*, *ELANE*	Neutropenia	Bacteria, typically streptococci, *S. aureus*, Gram negatives
X-linked agammaglobulinemia	Bruton tyrosine kinase (BTK)	Absence of B cells, antibody production	Encapsulated bacteria, Enterovirus, *Helicobacter* and related species
CD40 ligand deficiency	CD40 ligand	Impaired B-cell class switching	Encapsulated bacteria, *Pneumocystis jiroveci*, *Cryptosporidium*
Severe combined immunodeficiency (SCID)	Multiple genes such as IL2RG, RAG1/2, ADA, JAK3, etc.	T-cell lymphopenia, variable B and NK expression	Bacteria, virus, *P. jiroveci*, *Candida*, BCG
DiGeorge syndrome	Deletion of chromosome 22q11 in majority	Thymic hypoplasia or aplasia	Viruses, opportunists infrequent
AD-HIES	STAT3	Impaired Th17 cell differentiation	*S. aureus*, *Candida*, dimorphic fungi; secondary infection of pneumatocoeles with molds, Gram-negative bacteria and nontuberculous mycobacteria
DOCK8 deficiency	DOCK8	T-cell lymphopenia, defect still being delineated	*S. aureus*, *Candida*, *Molluscum contagiosum*, human papilloma virus (HPV), herpes viruses
IL-12/IFN-γ axis defects	IFN-γR1, IFN-γR2, IL-12, IL-12R, NEMO	Failure of STAT1 activation, intracellular killing	*Mycobacteria*, *Salmonella*, dimorphic fungi
Complement C5-9 defects	Specific complements	Impaired membrane attack complex killing	*Neisseria* species

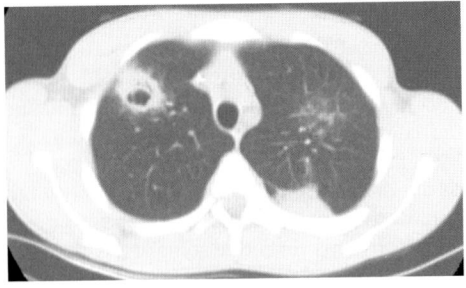

Fig. 31.1 Chest CT of a *Nocardia* pneumonia in a 17-year-old man with chronic granulomatous disease.

● KEY CONCEPTS

Infection risks in primary immunodeficiencies

- Neutrophil defects present primarily with bacterial and fungal infections.
- Humoral immunodeficiencies present with impaired antibody formation and primarily sinopulmonary infections with encapsulated organisms.
- Severe primarily T-cell defects usually present with opportunists such as *Pneumocystis*.
- Abnormalities of the IL-12/interferon-γ axis commonly present with nontuberculous mycobacteria infections.
- Cytokine autoantibody syndromes are being increasingly recognized with infection susceptibility dependent on the involved cytokine.

Quantitative phagocyte defects

Neutropenia is the most common quantitative defect of phagocytes and typically results from cytotoxic agents as discussed later in this chapter. However, there are also genetic and acquired defects not associated with pharmaceuticals that result in neutropenia. Autosomal recessive defects in *HAX1* cause Kostmann's syndrome, a type of severe congenital neutropenia, which typically presents in infancy with recurrent bacterial infections.[10,11] Autosomal dominant defects in the neutrophil elastase gene *ELANE* cause severe congenital neutropenia and cyclic neutropenia. Benign ethnic neutropenia is seen primarily in individuals of African descent and it is usually asymptomatic. Secondary causes of neutropenia include antineutrophil antibodies and hypersplenism with sequestration.

Infections associated with neutropenia relate to the etiology as well as the degree and duration of neutropenia. Cyclic neutropenia may be largely asymptomatic, with self-limited fevers and oral ulcers or cervical lymphadenopathy as opposed to the severe chronic neutropenia of infancy that has more serious infections. Neutropenia is most frequently associated with bacterial infections, often localized to the mouth, cervical lymph nodes, lungs, and perianal area. Gram-positive bacteria, such as streptococci and staphylococci, and enteric Gram-negative bacteria are frequent. Fungal infections are more frequent in the prolonged and severe neutropenias associated with hematologic malignancies and hematopoietic transplantation. Fever in the setting of neutropenia requires rapid assessment, with particular focus on physical examination to areas with high bacterial colonization such as the oral cavity and perianal region as well as sites of indwelling intravenous catheters. Empiric broad-spectrum antibiotics after obtaining appropriate cultures are often prudent.

Two recently described genetic defects are associated with monocytopenia and with disseminated mycobacterial disease. One is an autosomal dominant disorder associated with *GATA2* mutations and characterized by opportunistic infections with mycobacteria, fungi, disseminated warts, pulmonary alveolar proteinosis, and myelodysplasia.[12,13] Onset is typically in adulthood, and in addition to monocytopenia, lymphocytopenia may also be present. A second disorder with monocytopenia and disseminated BCG has been described with mutations in interferon regulatory factor 8 (*IRF8*).[14]

Humoral immunodeficiencies (Chapter 34)

Humoral immunodeficiencies are characterized by absent or defective B cells with resultant lack of specific antibody responses leading predominantly to infections with encapsulated bacteria. There is a spectrum of severity with X-linked agammaglobulinemia (XLA) characterized by a total absence of B cells and presentation in the first years of life and the later presentations of common variable immunodeficiency (CVID).[15]

XLA presents typically with recurrent ear, sinus and lung infections in late infancy as maternally derived IgG is depleted. Typical bacterial etiologies are *Streptococcus pneumoniae* and *Haemophilus influenzae*. Despite immunoglobulin replacement, bronchiectasis may occur, and with it the spectrum of pulmonary infections may broaden requiring careful microbiologic monitoring.[16] Neutropenia may occur, frequently when replacement immunoglobulin is not provided, and may be associated with a broader spectrum of infection with more severe *S. aureus* and *Pseudomonas* infections. Persistent *Helicobacter*, *Flexispira*, and *Campylobacter* species infections are infrequent, and are characterized by ulcerative skin lesions.[17,18] Bacteremia, even without significant systemic symptoms, may be present. These infections require a high suspicion to identify as special microbiology media with longer lengths of incubation may be required. Eradication of infection, even with a combination of intravenous antibiotics is often difficult. Chronic *Mycoplasma* and *Ureaplasma* species infections can occur leading to lung disease and arthritis. *Giardia* can be a source of gastrointestinal disease. Severe meningoencephalitis with enteroviral infections may occur and can be quite devastating and difficult to treat. Replacement immunoglobulin therapy given intravenously or subcutaneously is used to minimize the recurrent encapsulated bacterial infections and diminish the risk of enterovirus infection. The role of prophylactic antibiotics is not well studied, and varies between centers.

CD40 ligand deficiency (X-linked hyper-IgM) is the most common of the immunoglobulin class switch defects.[15] Sinopulmonary infections similar to XLA typically arise in early childhood. However, as opposed to XLA, *Pneumocystis jiroveci* pneumonia (PCP) occurs and may be the initial infection. Other infections indicative of T-cell defects occur as well including cytomegalovirus (CMV), toxoplasmosis and cryptosporidiosis. Cryptosporidial infection can be a chronic and severe problem and may lead to sclerosing cholangitis.

Primary cellular and combined immunodeficiencies (Chapter 35)

Severe combined immunodeficiency

Severe combined immunodeficiency (SCID) results from a severe deficiency in the number or function of T cells. Depending on the genetic defect, B and/or NK cells are affected as well. Presentation is typically very early in life, with significant compromise within the first few months of life. In recent years, there has been more recognition of "leaky" forms of SCID in which the defects are not complete and presentation can be later and more variable.[19,20]

SCID is associated with recurrent and persistent viral, bacterial and fungal infections. PCP frequently occurs in early infancy, and prophylaxis should be provided. Mucocutaneous candidiasis is frequent, and may require antifungal suppressive therapy. Diarrhea from viral and other etiologies frequently leads to failure to thrive. Severe respiratory viral infections and CMV occur as well. In countries where BCG vaccine is given, disseminated infection may result; with transplantation, an immune reconstitution syndrome may be seen in which sites of BCG infection become inflamed and abscesses may form.

DiGeorge syndrome

Immune deficiency in DiGeorge syndrome results from varying degrees of thymic hypoplasia or aplasia.[21] Other manifestations include congenital heart disease, characteristic facies and palate anomalies, hypocalcemia and learning disabilities. With the exception of severe cases in which there is thymic aplasia and severe T-cell lymphopenia, opportunistic infections are infrequent. Upper respiratory tract infections predominate, and prophylactic antibiotics may not be necessary. With the more mild defects, live viral vaccination may be considered safe.[22]

Autosomal dominant hyper-IgE syndrome (Job's syndrome)

Autosomal dominant hyper-IgE syndrome (Job's syndrome; HIES), resulting from *STAT3* mutations, has been frequently characterized as a phagocytic defect. However, in recent years it has been recognized that the immune defects center around the failure of Th17 cell differentiation and a decrease in memory T and B cells.[23–25] A lack of Th17 cells resulting in impaired IL-17 and -22 signaling, and diminished antimicrobial peptide upregulation appears to at least explain some of the infection susceptibility.

AD-HIES is characterized by recurrent skin and lung bacterial infections, mucocutaneous candidiasis, eczema and a variety of connective tissue, skeletal and vascular abnormalities.[26] *S. aureus* skin abscesses start early in life and *S. aureus* colonization appears to drive the eczema. *Staphylococcus aureus*, *Streptococcus pneumonia*, and *Haemophilus influenzae* pneumonias typically start in the first few years of life, and prophylactic antimicrobials such as trimethoprim-sulfamethoxazole may be useful in diminishing the frequency. Healing of pneumonias appears aberrant, and bronchiectasis and pneumatoceles frequently result. The lung with these parenchymal abnormalities is then predisposed to mold infections (most frequently *Aspergillus* and *Scedosporium*

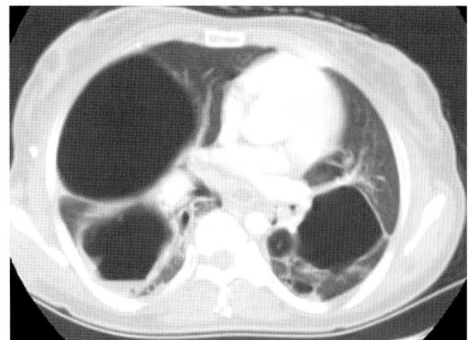

Fig. 31.2 **Chest CT of a pneumatocele with secondary *M. abscessus* and *Pseudomonas aeruginosa* infection in a 25-year-old woman with AD-HIES.**

species), Gram-negative infections such as *Pseudomonas aeruginosa* and nontuberculous mycobacteria (Fig. 31.2).[27,28] These secondary infections can be quite difficult to eradicate. Mucocutaneous candidiasis is the most frequent fungal infection. PCP is much less frequent, typically occurring in infancy, potentially as the first pneumonia.[29] Disseminated cryptococcal infection has been described causing meningitis or gastrointestinal infection. *Histoplasma* and *Coccidioides* infections have also been described, typically localized to a region of the gastrointestinal tract.

DOCK8 deficiency

DOCK8 deficiency is a combined defect that is one cause of an autosomal recessive hyper-IgE syndrome.[30,31] Compared to AD-HIES, DOCK8 deficiency is characterized by severe cutaneous viral infections in addition to sinopulmonary infections. Recurrent cutaneous herpes simplex virus (HSV) and varicella-zoster virus (VZV) occur, as well as severe, disfiguring warts and *Molluscum contagiosum* infection. Mucocutaneous candidiasis occurs, but less frequently than with AD-HIES. DOCK8 deficiency has an overall worse prognosis than AD-HIES, with frequent occurrence of malignancies, typically squamous cell carcinoma and lymphomas.

Defects of the IL-12/interferon-γ axis

Defects of the IL-12/interferon-γ axis are characterized by mycobacterial infections. Monocyte-derived macrophages ingest intracellular bacteria such as *Mycobacteria* and *Salmonella*, leading to IL-12 secretion. IL-12 binds to its receptor on T lymphocytes and NK cells leading to IFN-γ secretion, which then binds to its heterodimeric receptor on macrophages, activating microbial killing through STAT1. Many defects along this pathway have been described, including mutations in IL-12, IL-12 receptor, IFN-γ receptor, STAT1, and NFκB essential modulator operon (NEMO).[31–33] Defects along this pathway show varying susceptibility to nontuberculous mycobacteria (NTM), *Salmonella*, and endemic dimorphic fungal infection (Fig. 31.3).[34–36] For example, individuals with dominant IFN-γ receptor defects retain some IFN-γ signaling and tend to have localized NTM infections, often presenting with osteomyelitis, and infrequently other opportunistic infections, such as disseminated histoplasmosis.[36] Treatment of the dominant IFN-γ receptor defects is typically successful with combination anti-mycobacterial agents with or without exogenous IFN-γ. On the other hand, autosomal recessive IFN-γ receptor defects, in which there is typically no residual IFN-γ signaling, have much more severe disease, with earlier onset of disseminated NTM or BCG disease, poor response to

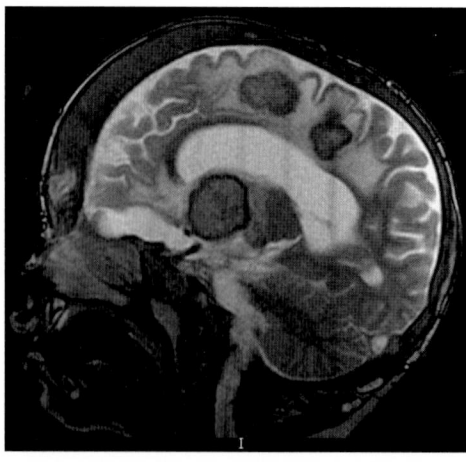

Fig. 31.3 **Brain MRI showing BCG abscesses in a 3-year-old boy with an IFN-γ receptor defect.**

therapy with frequent relapse and a greater susceptibility to infection including some viral susceptibility. Death in childhood is frequent and hematopoietic stem cell transplantation is typically considered.

Complement deficiencies (Chapter 20)

Infections with encapsulated organisms are the typical manifestations of complement defects.[37] C3 deficiency is associated with recurrent and severe infections with *Streptococcus pneumoniae*, *Haemophilus influenzae*, and *Neisseria meningitidis*, whereas deficiencies of the components of the terminal pathway composing the membrane attack complex, C5-9, result in *N. gonorrhoeae* and *N. meningitidis* infections.

Asplenia

The spleen acts as both a source for antibody production as well as a filter to remove pathogens through phagocytic cells. Spleens can be physically absent, either congenitally or through surgical resection (such as with intractable hemolytic anemia or thrombocytopenia, malignancy, trauma), or functionally absent as is seen with increased age in sickle cell disease. Infection associated with asplenia includes sepsis with encapsulated bacteria, namely *Streptococcus pneumoniae* and *Haemophilus influenzae*, and *Babesia*, a protozoa that infects erythrocytes and causes fever and hemolysis with asplenia.[37] Similar to babesia, malaria infection can be more severe in patients without a spleen. The risk of infection differs with the etiology of asplenia, with splenectomy associated with trauma having the lowest risk as typically small amounts of splenic tissue remain. In addition, infection with encapsulated organisms appears to be more common in children with asplenia than in asplenic adults.

Secondary non-medication-associated immunodeficiency

Cytokine autoantibodies

In recent years, there has been greater recognition of infection susceptibility associated with anti-cytokine autoantibodies.[38] Autoimmune polyendocrinopathy with candidiasis and ectodermal dysplasia (APOCED) is a disorder caused by mutations in the autoimmune regulator gene (AIRE). Many autoimmune manifestations are seen in APOCED including hypoparathyroidism, diabetes and adrenal failure as a result of persistent autoreactive T cells due to failure of thymic deletion. The main infectious complication is severe chronic mucocutaneous candidiasis (CMCC). Neutralizing autoantibodies to IL-17 and -22 have been detected, and are thought to be the cause of the CMCC, similar to other defects along the Th17/IL-17/IL-22 pathway such as AD-HIES.[39,40] Neutralizing autoantibodies IFN-γ have been described, leading to disseminated NTM infections.[41] This disorder typically presents in adulthood, and has an increased prevalence in Asians. Although the primary manifestation of autoantibodies against GM-CSF antibodies is pulmonary alveolar proteinosis (PAP), an increased frequency of opportunistic infections such as *Nocardia* and nontuberculous mycobacteria has been described.[42]

HIV

Infection with human immunodeficiency virus (HIV) leads to progressive CD4 lymphocyte destruction with resultant increase in opportunistic infection (Chapter 37). In addition to the T lymphocyte abnormalities, B-cell dysfunction leading to abnormal antibody formation is frequent. Infection susceptibility is tied closely to the CD4 lymphocyte count.[43,44] At any CD4 count, encapsulated sinopulmonary bacterial infections may occur, in addition to recurrent mucosal candidiasis and herpes simplex infection. Hepatitis B, C, and D may lead to chronic hepatitis, and HPV infection may lead to condyloma acuminata. With CD4 counts of less than 500/μL in adults, an increase in infection-related malignancy is seen including Kaposi sarcoma from HHV-8, lymphoma, and oral hairy leukoplakia from EBV infection, and cervical or anorectal dysplasia from HPV infection. An increase in pulmonary tuberculosis is also seen. With a CD4 count of less than 200/μL there is an increase in opportunists causing infection such as *Pneumocysis jiroveci*, *Toxoplasmosis gondii*, microsporidia, and protozans such as *Cryptosporidium* and *Isospora* species. There is an increase in dissemination of tuberculosis and syphilis, and etiologic agents of bacterial dysentery, such as *Salmonella* and *Campylobacter* species, may lead to bacteremia. At CD4 counts of less than 100/μL, disseminated fungal and nontuberculous mycobacterial infections including *Histoplasma*, *Cryptococcus*, *Penicillium marneffei*, and *Mycobacterium avium* complex are seen. CMV can cause severe disease such as retinitis, and JC virus causes progressive multifocal leukoencephalopathy. Herpes simplex and herpes zoster infections become disseminated as well.

● T H E R A P E U T I C   P R I N C I P L E S

Prevention of infection in patients with a defect in host defenses

- Use of prophylactic antibiotics in patients at high risk for a specific type of infection.
- Immunization to prevent specific bacterial and viral infections:
  - Active immunization, especially in patients who should be capable of mounting an effective response (e.g., before elective splenectomy or before elective initiation of immunosuppressive therapy)
  - Passive immunization through administration of high-titer pooled immunoglobulin to patients exposed to or at high risk of specific viral infections.

Infections in patients receiving immunosuppressive medications

Immunosuppressive drugs have been used for over 60 years,[45] and have been essential for the management of autoimmune and inflammatory diseases, hematologic and oncologic malignancies, and in transplant recipients. Early immunosuppressive agents lacked specificity, and therefore led to serious and numerous adverse effects. As understanding of the immune system has evolved, more specific and sometimes more potent agents that target particular components of the immune response have been developed.

Newer immunosuppressive agents have revolutionized the treatment of multiple diseases, and have markedly improved the outcomes of solid organ and hematopoietic stem cell transplant (Chapter 81). However the improvement gained could be jeopardized by a potential increase in infectious complications, and monitoring of infectious complications has not always been extensive in clinical trails.[46] Notably, immunosuppressive agents are used most of the time in combination with other agents, and therefore establishing an association of a specific type of infection with a particular drug is challenging.

Described below are the most common classes of immunosuppressive drugs that have been linked to infectious complications.

Cytotoxic agents (e.g., cyclophosphamide, methotrexate, azathioprine)

Initially developed to control neoplastic growth in oncologic and hematologic malignancies, cytotoxic drugs have also found their niche as an essential component of the conditioning regimen for hematopoietic stem cell transplant (HSCT) and solid organ transplant (SOT), and as immunomodulators in autoimmune, inflammatory disorders, and graft-versus-host disease (GVHD). In general, these drugs interfere with DNA synthesis by blocking different steps in the cell cycle and inducing apoptosis. They inhibit B- and T-cell proliferation, and hinder cellular and humoral immune responses in a dose-dependent fashion.[47] One of the main side effects of these agents is toxicity on hematopoietic cells; they can induce neutropenia to varying degrees. Fever occurs during chemotherapeutic-induced neutropenia in 10–50% of patients with solid tumors, and in >80% of those with hematologic malignancies.[48] Common sites of infection include the intestinal tract, lung and skin; bacteremia occurs in up to 25% of patients. Probably due to the high incidence of indwelling catheters and the widespread use of prophylactic antibiotics, currently coagulase-negative staphylococci are the most common blood isolates, followed by Enterobacteriaceae and non-fermenting Gram-negative rods (e.g., *Pseudomonas aeruginosa*).[48] Invasive mold infections (e.g., *Aspergillus* spp.) typically occur after prolonged neutropenia (>2 weeks). Invasive yeast (usually *Candida* spp.) infections are more commonly seen in patients with severe mucositis and neutropenia. Detailed guidelines for the use of antimicrobial agents in the setting of chemotherapy-induced neutropenic fever have been published.[48] Although bacterial infections are the most common infections associated with the use of cytotoxic drugs, when used as immunomodulators a higher frequency of opportunistic infections, such as *Pneumocystis*, *Listeria* spp., nontuberculous mycobacteria (NTM), *Cryptococcus* spp., and varicella zoster virus (VZV) has been described.

Glucocorticoids

Depending on the dose and duration, glucocorticoids can induce a vast range of immune defects. Glucocorticoids bind a cytosolic receptor which then translocates to the nucleus to act as a transcription factor affecting the expression of multiple genes.[47] They target transcription factors such as activator protein 1 and NFκB.[49] The overall results are decreased cytokine production (IL-1, IL-6, and TNF-α), and impaired leukocyte chemotaxis, cell adhesion, phagocytosis and lymphocyte function. Neutrophils increase in the peripheral circulation, primarily because of demargination; however, trafficking and bacterial killing appear to be impaired. In contrast, monocytes and lymphocytes decrease in the peripheral blood. Lymphopenia, particularly T-cell lymphopenia, results from increased apoptosis and inhibition of IL-2-mediated proliferative responses. At large doses, antibody responses (B cells) are also impaired.[47]

Infections are a frequent complication of corticosteroid use, and differences in the type and frequency of infections are dependent on dose and duration of treatment.[50] Bacterial infections are the most common infectious complications of corticosteroid use.[51] However, opportunistic fungal, viral, and mycobacterial infections are also seen, particularly with high doses and long durations of systemic glucocorticoid therapy. Some of the infections that have been associated with their use are: Gram-positive and Gram-negative bacteria, superficial and invasive *Candida* spp. infections, invasive and pulmonary aspergillosis and nocardiosis, *Cryptococcus* spp., *P. jiroveci* pneumonia (PCP), *Listeria monocytogenes*, endemic mycosis, *M. tuberculosis*, NTM, and VZV, among others. Outside of the setting of SOT and HSCT, routine use of antimicrobials for patients receiving corticosteroids is not recommended except for antituberculous treatment (e.g., isoniazid) for those with a positive tuberculin skin test (PPD) or a positive IFN-γ release assay, and trimethoprim-sulfamethoxazole in patients receiving high-dose steroid for extended periods.[52] Alternate-day use of corticosteroids has been associated with a lower risk of severe infection, therefore whenever possible this dosing schedule should be used.[51]

Calcineurin inhibitors

Cyclosporine and tacrolimus have been cornerstones in improving the outcome of transplant recipients by preventing allograft rejection in SOT, and GVHD in HSCT. Cyclosporine is a small cyclic polypeptide of fungal origin that interacts with cylophilin to create a complex that inhibits calcineurin, leading to the inhibition of IL-2 production and other cytokines, and therefore diminished T-cell activation. Tacrolimus, a macrolide antibiotic also of fungal origin, exhibits a similar mechanism of action; it binds to FK-binding protein (FKBP) and inhibits calcineurin.[49] Although there has been a lower rate of infection in solid organ transplant recipients since the introduction of cyclosporine and tacrolimus, a significant infection risk remains, and infection remained the most common cause of death in a trial that compared cyclosporine to tacrolimus based regimens in kidney transplant recipients.[53] Infectious complications seem to be dose-dependent and, as it is usually the case, seen more often when these drugs are used in combination with other immunosuppressive drugs.

Mammalian target of rapamycin (mTOR) inhibitors

Sirolimus and everolimus interfere with cell cycle proliferation, and exert an effect on signal transduction pathways that mediate specific cytokine responses. They specifically bind to FKBP, which in turn inhibits the mTOR. mTOR inhibitors have been associated with a lower incidence of CMV infection, when compared to other immunosuppressive regimens used in transplantation.[46] Impaired wound healing has been seen. However, this has not correlated with an increased incidence of bacterial or fungal infections.

Mycophenolate mofetil (MMF)

MMF is a prodrug of mycophenolic acid, which inhibits inosine monophosphate dehydrogenase, a key enzyme in purine synthesis. It is a cytotoxic drug with antiproliferative effect on T and B lymphocytes.[49] In addition to its potential myelosuppressive effect, it has been associated in some studies of SOT to a higher risk of CMV infection.[46]

Antithymocyte globulin (ATG)

ATG is a polyclonal immunoglobulin prepared by immunizing horses or rabbits with human thymocytes, and harvesting the IgG. These antibodies produce a profound lymphopenia that can last well beyond one year. Although differences exist between the half-life of horse and rabbit ATG, their functional half-life is not well established, but rabbit ATG is more potent than horse ATG.[49] Used for induction or rejection therapy in transplant recipients, their use has been associated consistently with a greater risk of CMV disease and post-transplant lymphoproliferative disease (PTLD).[54] Because these are foreign proteins, serum sickness can develop between 1 and 2 weeks after treatment.

Monoclonal antibodies

Monoclonal antibodies, as well as small molecules that target similar specific cellular steps or factors, have made it possible to manipulate disease pathways in such a way that has led to astonishing clinical responses for previously untreatable or intractable illnesses.[55] However, many of these biologic agents interfere with natural immunity, and have therefore increased rates of both common and uncommon infections.[56] As with many other immunosuppressive drugs, establishing causality is a challenge; only those associated with a probable increase in the risk of infection are described below (Table 31.2).

Tumor necrosis factor-α (TNF-α) inhibitors

TNF-α is a cytokine that plays a central role in macrophage and phagosome activation, differentiation of monocytes into macrophages, recruitment of neutrophils and macrophages, and granuloma formation and maintenance. Blockade results in increased risk of infection, and although granulomatous infections such as tuberculosis have received the most attention, clinical trials suggest that there is also an increased risk of bacterial, viral, fungal and parasitic infections.[56,57] TNF-α infliximab, adalimumab and golimumab are monoclonal antibodies directed against TNF-α; certolizumab pegol is a pegylated Fab fragment of a humanized anti-TNF-α monoclonal antibody, and etanercept is a soluble

Table 31.2 Selected monoclonal antibodies and small molecules and their risk of infection

Drug name	Target	Serious infections
Adalimumab Certolizumab pegol Etanercept Golimumab Infliximab	TNF-α*	TB, NTM, endemic mycoses, listeriosis, candidiasis, invasive mold infections, nocardiosis, bacterial infections, VZV and HBV reactivation, severe malaria and leishmaniasis
Rituximab	CD20	HBV reactivation, PML, PCP, enteroviral meningoencephalitis, CMV disease, VZV, babesiosis, parvovirus, nocardiosis
Anakinra Rilonacept	IL-1	Bacterial infections (cellulitis and pneumonia)
Alentuzumab	CD52	Herpes viruses reactivation (EBV, VZV, CMV, HHV-6), severe respiratory viral infections (adenovirus, RSV, parainfluenza, influenza), PCP, invasive mold infections, histoplasmosis, cryptococcosis, PTLD, bacterial meningitis, toxoplasmosis, PML, parvovirus, nocardiosis, TB, NTM, acanthamebiasis and *Balamuthia mandrillaris*
Muromonab	CD3	Bacterial infections, listeriosis, nocardiosis, aspergillosis, candidiasis, cryptococcosis, toxoplasmosis, CMV, HSV, VZV, adenovirus, RSV, PCP and enteroviruses
Basiliximab Daclizumab	CD25	Bacterial infections, CMV, HSV, EBV-associated PTLD, RSV, adenovirus, influenza, BK virus, invasive mold infections, candidiasis, nocardiosis, TB, NTM, toxoplasmosis
Natalizumab	α-4 Integrin	PML, respiratory viral and bacterial infections, UTI, viral meningitis and encephalitis, CMV, IA, PCP, VZV, NTM, cryptyosporidiasis
Abatacept Belatacept	T-cell co-stimulation blockade	Bacterial infections, ?EBV-associated PTLD
Alefacept	Inhibits T-cell activation	1 case of MAI bursitis, 1 case of nocardiosis when co-administered with infliximab
Gemtuzumab	CD33	Bacteremia, bacterial pneumonia, and HSV reactivation.

*TNF-α: tumor necrosis factor-α; IL-1: interleukin 1; TB: tuberculosis; NTM: non-tuberculous mycobacteria; VZV: varicella zoster virus; HBV: hepatitis B virus; PML: progressive multifocal leukoencephalopathy; PCP: *Pneumocystis jiroveci* pneumonia; CMV: cytomegalovirus; EBV: Epstein–Barr virus; HHV-6: human herpes virus 6; RSV: respiratory syncytial virus; PTLD: post-transplant lymphoproliferative disease; HSV: herpes simplex virus; UTI: urinary tract infection; IA: invasive aspergillosis.

including granulomatous infections, appears to be lower with the use of etanercept than with the other TNF-α blockers, probably due to differences in mechanism of action and pharmacokinetics.[55]

The association between tuberculosis and anti-TNF-α therapy was noted shortly after the initial approval of infliximab, and has been noted for all the anti-TNF-α therapies.[57] NTM infections have also been associated with anti-TNF-α therapy. Most reported cases have been MAI infections, but many other NTM, as well as other rare mycobacterial pathogens (e.g., *M. szulgai*) and *M. leprae* have been reported. Risk of disseminated fungal infections, particularly histoplasmosis, but also coccidiodomycosis, is significantly increased in patients treated with TNF-α blockers. Other notable infections that have been described in the setting of anti-TNF-α blockers are *Listeria* spp., *Legionella*, salmonellosis, recurrent or relapsing leishmaniasis, overwhelming *Plasmodium falciparum* infection, and invasive mold infections (i.e., aspergillosis and mucormycosis). Risk of certain viral infection also appears to be increased, particularly herpes zoster. Several cases of severe hepatitis B virus (HBV) reactivation in patients with positive surface antigen at the start of treatment have been reported. Patients receiving anti-TNF-α therapy should be screened for TB (latent or active), HBV and HCV before starting treatment.[58]

Rituximab

Rituximab is a chimeric murine-human monoclonal antibody that targets CD20 on mature B lymphocytes. It results in rapid and profound depletion of B cells that can last up to several months.[59] In most adults, serum immunoglobulin levels remain largely stable, since plasma cells do not express CD20. Initial trials suggested that rituximab had minimal effect on the occurrence of infections, however more recent meta-analyses have reported a higher relative risk of infections. The increase in the risk of infection seems to be more prominent in the setting of repeated administration and in patients with underlying immune defects or concomitant significant immunosuppression.[59] HBV reactivation occurs with rituximab treatment. There have been reports of fulminant hepatitis and even death in patients who experienced hepatitis B flare after rituximab treatment, particularly when used in combination therapy (e.g., R-CHOP). Also a reverse seroconversion phenomenon has been described, with loss of protective HBV surface antibodies and reactivation. Most cases of reactivation have occurred within 6 months of therapy, but there are case reports of reactivation occurring as late as a year after treatment.[58] Assessment of HBV status before starting rituximab is recommended. To reduce the risk of reactivation, HBV suppression with lamivudine or lamivudine and tenofovir (in HIV-infected individuals) should be considered.

Since the initial approval of rituximab, there have been approximately 80 cases of progressive multifocal leukoencephalopathy (PML) associated with its use. Most cases have been reported in patients with hematologic malignancies. However, some have been reported in patients with systemic lupus erythematosus, rheumatoid arthritis and idiopathic thrombocytopenic purpura, who have had other immunusuppressants as well, and therefore causality is still not well understood. There have been many reports of PCP following rituximab, and although the evidence is far from conclusive because most patients also received other immunosuppressive therapies, it is well known that B cells are necessary for clearance of *Pneumocystis* in mouse models. The need for PCP prophylaxis

receptor for TNF-α.[55,58] There is substantial discrepancy between studies on the overall incidence of serious infections associated with the use of anti-TNF-α therapy and although most studies have concluded that there is an increased risk of serious infections, particularly in the first few months after treatment, the true relative risk is still unknown.[57,58] The risk of serious infections, in patients receiving rituximab remains to be determined. Other rare infections that have been described in the setting of rituximab use are enteroviral meningoencephalitis, CMV disease, disseminated VZV, refractory babesiosis, parvovirus B19, and nocardiosis.[54,55]

IL-1 antagonists: anakinra and rilonacept

IL-1 is a cytokine secreted by numerous cell types in response to inflammatory antigens; it mediates the febrile response to infection and inflammation, B-cell activation, stimulation of T-cell maturation by inducing IL-2. It also induces IL-6, TNF-γ, and IL-8. Anakinra is a recombinant IL-1 receptor antagonist that competitively inhibits the binding of IL-1 to IL-1 type-I receptor.[58] Rilonacept is a human dimeric fusion protein, made up of the extracellular component of the IL-1 receptor and the Fc portion of IgG1; it binds with very high affinity to circulating IL-1α and -1β, thereby inhibiting IL-1.[55] Their use has been associated with a small increase in the risk of serious bacterial infections, mostly pneumonia and cellulitis.

Alentuzumab

Alentuzumab is a humanized IgG1 that targets CD52 on B and T lymphocytes, monocytes, macrophages, and NK cells. It lyses these cell populations, and results in profound and sustained deficits in cellular and humoral immunity that lasts for several months; CD4 and CD8 cell count reach their nadir approximately 4 weeks after treatment, but median counts remain at less than 25% of baseline for approximately 9 months.[58] Opportunistic and non-opportunistic infections have been associated with its use, particularly reactivation of herpes virus (e.g., Epstein–Barr virus (EBV), CMV, disseminated VZV) and fungal infections (e.g., PCP, invasive molds and dimorphic fungi). Also several cases of TB and NTM have been reported. The incidence of these opportunistic infections (OIs) varies with the administered dose, and whether it is used as a single agent or in combination with other immunosuppressants (e.g., induction therapy (4.5%) versus treatment for rejection (21%) in SOT).[56,58] When used for T-cell depletion in allogeneic HSCT it has been associated with a very high risk of CMV reactivation (50–85%) and disease, severe adenovirus infection, human herpes virus 6 encephalitis, respiratory viral infections that frequently progress to pneumonia (e.g., influenza, parainfluenza, RSV) and PTLD. Other infections that have occurred are overwhelming bacteremia, bacterial meningitis, toxoplasmosis, PML, disseminated amoebiasis, parvovirus, and nocardiosis. All patients receiving alentuzumab should receive PCP and herpesvirus prophylaxis for a minimun of 2 months after therapy or until CD4 counts are ≥ 200 cells/μL (Campath package insert). Given the high incidence of CMV reactivation and disease, prophylaxis or preemptive therapy is warranted.[59]

Muromonab (OKT3)

OKT3 is a murine IgG2 monoclonal antibody that binds the CD3 molecule on T lymphocytes. Binding of OKT3 to T cells results in an early nonspecific T-cell activation with cytokine release, followed by a transient and profound lymphocyte depletion.[56] T-cell function returns to normal within a week after therapy. Bacterial infections are the most common reported infections, although not significantly different from

non-monoclonal antibody containing regimens. Other reported infections include listeriosis, nocardiosis, aspergillosis, candidiasis, cryptococcosis, toxoplasmosis, CMV, HSV, VZV, adenovirus, RSV, PCP, and enteroviruses.

Daclizumab and basiliximab

Daclizumab and basiliximab are humanized and chimeric monoclonal antibodies, respectively, that target CD25, the α chain of the IL-2 receptor complex expressed on activated alloantigen-reactive T lymphocytes. It competitively inhibits IL-2 binding and prevents IL-2 mediated activation of lymphocytes and cytokine release. They are mainly used in transplantation to prevent rejection or steroid-refractory GVHD.[55] When used as prophylaxis for rejection in solid organ transplantation, their use does not seem to be associated with an increased risk in infections. In allogeneic HSCT recipients a high rate of mortality and of opportunistic infections (95%) has been reported in patients receiving daclizumab for steroid-refractory GVHD; however, given the high risk for OIs in this population in general, the actual role of daclizumab is unclear. Infections described in this setting are common bacterial infections, viral reactivations (CMV, BK virus, adenovirus, HSV, RSV, influenza), EBV-associated PTLD, invasive fungal infections (*Aspergillus, Scedosporium, Cunninghamela,* and *Candida*), as well as *Legionella, Nocardia,* NTM, TB, and toxoplasmosis.[58]

Natalizumab

Natalizumab is a humanized IgG4 that targets the α_4 subunit of $\alpha_4\beta_1$ and $\alpha_4\beta_7$ integrins, found in lymphocytes; it inhibits their binding to cellular adhesion molecules (vascular cell adhesion molecule 1(VCAM-1) and mucosal addressin-cell adhesion molecule 1) in the central nervous system and gastrointestinal tract, thereby attenuating inflammation in these tissues.[60] It is associated with a profound decrease in CD4, CD8, and CD19 lymphocytes in the cerebrospinal fluid, and it is used in the treatment of multiple sclerosis and Crohn's disease. Natalizumab was temporarily withdrawn from the market in 2005 after 3 cases of PML were reported in patients with prolonged exposure. It has now been reintroduced with a black box warning about the risk of PML. Other infections reported with natalizumab include upper and lower respiratory tract viral and bacterial infections, urinary tract infections, viral meningitis and encephalitis, CMV infection, pulmonary invasive aspergillosis, PCP, VZV pneumonia, MAI, and *Cryptosporidium parvum* infection; however, most patients with these infections were receiving concurrent immunosuppression.

Abatacept and belatacept

Abatacept and belatacept are fusion proteins that prevent the interaction of CD80/CD86 on antigen-presenting cells and CD28 on T lymphocytes, preventing T-lymphocyte activation. An increased risk of serious infections, mainly bacterial, was reported in a randomized trial of rheumatoid arthritis (RA) when abatacept was compared to placebo, particularly in patients receiving other biologic therapies.[56] A recent metanalysis of trials in RA did not show a statistically significant increase in the risk of infections. Most of the infections reported associated with abatacept use were pneumonias and other bacterial infections.[58] The experience with belatacept is limited, and when compared to cyclosporine in kidney transplant recipients, there was no significant increase in infections; however, 3 cases of EBV-associated PTLD occurred in the belatacept arm.[56]

Infections in solid organ transplant recipients

● KEY CONCEPTS

Determinants of the risk for infections in transplant recipients

- Epidemiologic exposures (e.g., residing in a histoplasma endemic area)
- Immunosuppressive drugs
- Antimicrobial prophylaxis
- Type of transplant (e.g., cord transplant vs matched related donor transplant)
- Time after transplant

Despite significant improvement in the survival of solid organ transplant recipients, infectious complications remain a major cause of morbidity and mortality. The risk of infection is determined by the interaction of various factors, such as age of the recipient, type of transplant, invasive procedures, dose and duration of immunosuppressive drugs, epidemiologic exposures of the donor and the recipient, use of antimicrobial prophylaxis, donor-recipient serostatus to certain infections (e.g., CMV, EBV, toxoplasmosis), and ongoing viral replication (so-called indirect effects).[61] Assessment of a recipient's risk for infection should help tailor specific prophylactic strategies and infectious work-up when an infection is suspected.

Age is an important determinant of susceptibility to infections; it impacts the likelihood of prior exposures to microbial pathogens, either by primary infection or vaccination. History of exposure to different pathogens can have either positive or negative effects. Older patients are more likely to have encountered pathogens that can remain latent and reactivate at the time of transplant (e.g., CMV, *T. cruzi*, toxoplasmosis); younger patients have a higher risk of acquiring primary infections after transplant, which tend to be more severe than disease secondary to reactivation of a latent infection. In addition, younger patients may lack pre-existing immunity that can have a protective effect against clinical disease (e.g., EBV-associated PTLD).[62]

The type of allograft affects the specific infectious risk, usually as a result of technical factors associated with the transplant procedure, but also inherent to the transplanted organ. These are important determinants of both the location and type of infections. For example urinary tract infections are most common after kidney transplant, usually as a result of catheter placement or ureteric stenting. BK virus is ubiquitous, but disease with associated nephropathy (BKVAN) is most common after kidney transplant, and it is an important cause of allograft loss. Infection after liver transplant frequently is from leaks from biliary, pancreatic and gastrointestinal anastomoses. Cardiac assist devices in heart transplant recipients are a frequent source of infection. Tracheal anastomotic infections, particularly due to yeast, are a significant complication of lung transplantation. In single lung transplants, recurrent infections of the native lung, such as Gram-negative bacteria or fungi, can extend to the transplanted lung. Small intestine transplant recipients are at particularly high risk of opportunistic and non-opportunistic viral infections of the gastrointestinal tract that can be severe and even life threatening, such as norovirus and EBV.[63,64]

Despite all the differences in individual risk of infection, the general patterns of infection in the absence of antimicrobial intervention are similar among solid organ transplant recipients. This predictable temporal pattern (timeline of infection after organ transplantation) has enabled the institution of specific prophylactic strategies that have been extremely successful in lowering the incidence of certain infections, and in developing a differential diagnosis in transplant recipients in whom an infection is suspected.[65]

● CLINICAL PEARLS

Infections in solid-organ transplant recipients

- Most infections occur in the first 6 months following transplantation.
- In the first month, most infections are nosocomial or are related to surgical procedures or pre-existing infection in the donor or recipient.
- Infections between 1 and 6 months following transplantation are commonly secondary to the use of immunosuppressive drugs, with a predominance of cytomegalovirus infection.
- Infections after 6 months are usually due either to chronic viral infection, acquired earlier, or to chronic allograft dysfunction, necessitating repeated courses of high-dose immunosuppression.

Infections in the first month after transplant

Infections in this period are generally associated with technical complications of the surgery (e.g., infected hematoma in the surgical bed), nosocomial (e.g., catheter-related infections, *C. difficile*), donor-transmitted infections (e.g., lymphocytic choriomeningitis virus, HIV, TB, histoplasmosis) or recipient's prior infections (e.g., colonization and infection with MDR bacteria, HSV reactivation).[61,66]

Infections 1 to 6 months after transplant

Before routine antimicrobial prophylaxis, this period was typically characterized by the presence of opportunistic infections, such as PCP and CMV.[65] However, the incidence of disease secondary to these pathogens has been significantly reduced or delayed since the routine use of TMP-SMX prophylaxis and anti-CMV prophylactic or preemptive therapy. Reactivation of latent infections such as TB, Chagas disease, endemic fungal infections, and cryptococcosis; viral infections such as BK virus, adenovirus, RSV, HBV, and EBV are also common (Fig. 31.4). Invasive fungal infections, specifically *Aspergillus* and non-*Aspergillus* mold infections, can also be problematic during this period of heightened immune suppression.[61]

Infections 6 months after transplant

This period is less well defined; patients with satisfactory allograft function develop more severe manifestations of community acquired infections, but the risk of opportunistic infections is generally lower. Patients with poor allograft function, and therefore increased immunosuppression, or those with ongoing chronic

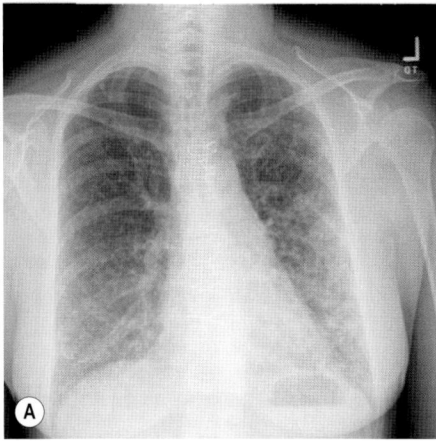
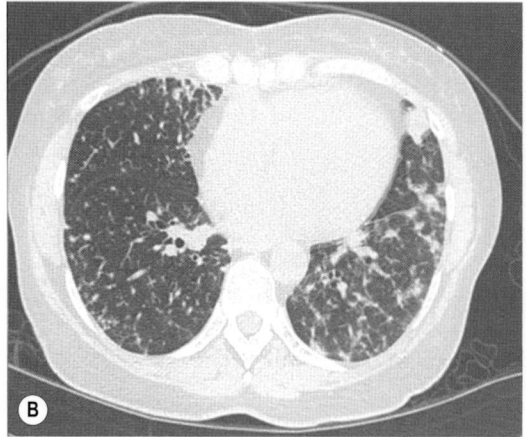
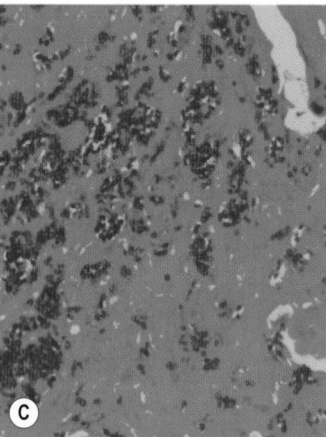

Fig. 31.4 Disseminated histoplasmosis in a patient from an endemic area 3 months after a heart transplant. (A) Chest X-ray with bilateral reticulonodular infiltrates. (B) Computed tomography of the chest with bilateral patchy and nodular infiltrates. (C) Lung biopsy. Gomori methanine silver (GMS) stain shows yeast forms compatible with *Histoplasma capsulatum*.

viral infections, are considered at high risk for opportunistic infections such as invasive fungal infections, late-onset CMV disease, nocardiosis, PCP, listeriosis, and EBV-associated PTLD. In addition, lung transplant recipients with chronic graft dysfunction develop bronchiolitis obliterans, which predisposes them to recurrent bacterial pneumonia. Similarly liver transplant recipients with chronic graft dysfunction frequently develop biliary strictures and recurrent cholangitis.[61]

Infections in hematopoietic stem cell transplant

● CLINICAL PEARLS

Infections in bone marrow transplant recipients

- Infections 2–4 weeks post-transplantation are usually due to profound neutropenia and damage to mucosal surfaces.
- Between the period of engraftment and weeks 15–20 post-transplant, opportunistic infections predominate and are commonly associated with the development of acute graft-versus-host disease and its treatment.
- Serious infections occurring 4–6 months following transplantation are seen predominantly in patients with chronic graft-versus-host disease.

Survival after hematopoietic stem cell transplant has significantly improved during the last decade. Factors contributing to the increase in survival are the use of less toxic, non-myeloablative conditioning regimens, use of peripheral blood stem cells (PBSC) that has led to faster neutrophil recovery, use of antimicrobial prophylaxis or preemptive therapy, and use of ursodiol to prevent cholestasis.[67] Despite these advances, infectious complications are still a frequent cause of morbidity and mortality.

The risk for infection is influenced by several factors, and varies significantly between type of transplant (autologous vs allogeneic), stem cell source (bone marrow, peripheral blood stem cells and cord blood), degree of HLA matching, hematopoietic potential of the graft (number of infused CD34 cells), T-cell depletion, type of conditioning (myeloablative vs reduced intensity vs non-myeloablative), presence of graft rejection or GVHD,

donor-recipient serostatus to certain infections (e.g., CMV), and use of antimicrobial prophylaxis.[68,69]

Autologous stem cell transplantation refers to the patient serving as his or her own donor to allow administration of myeloablative chemotherapy. The patient's cells are harvested before the procedure, cryopreserved, and then infused into the recipient after receiving a pre-transplant conditioning regimen. Because there is no risk of rejection or GVHD, and because after engraftment there is an early and progressive recovery of cell-mediated immunity, the risk for infection in autologous SCT is much higher before engraftment. The major compromises in host defenses during this period are neutropenia and mucosal injury, which last between 10 and 14 days. After engraftment the incidence of infections decreases dramatically, and most infections are secondary to use of central venous catheters.[68]

In allogeneic SCT, the risk for infection can be divided into three time intervals: pre-engraftment, early post-engraftment, and late post-engraftment.

Pre-engraftment period

As with autologous SCT, the major impairments in host defenses before engraftment are neutropenia and mucosal injury. The pre-engraftment period varies widely between the different types of conditioning regimens and the stem cell source. In general terms when ablative regimens are used, engraftment occurs anywhere between 15 to 45 days after transplant, and can be as short as 5 to 7 days when non-ablative regimens are used.[68] Peripheral blood stem cell (PBSC) grafts are associated with faster neutrophil engraftment compared to cord blood units and therefore lower rates of infection during this period.[70] Bacterial infections are most common. However, when neutropenia is prolonged, the risk of fungal infection, such as *Candida*, *Aspergillus* and other invasive molds, increases significantly. Without acyclovir prophylaxis, severe HSV reactivation is frequent. The approach to neutropenic patients in whom an infection is suspected or identified is discussed in detail elsewhere.[48]

Early post-engraftment period

The resolution of neutropenia marks the beginning of the second period of risk for infection, and usually lasts 2 to 3 months (Fig. 31.5). This period is characterized by a progressive recovery

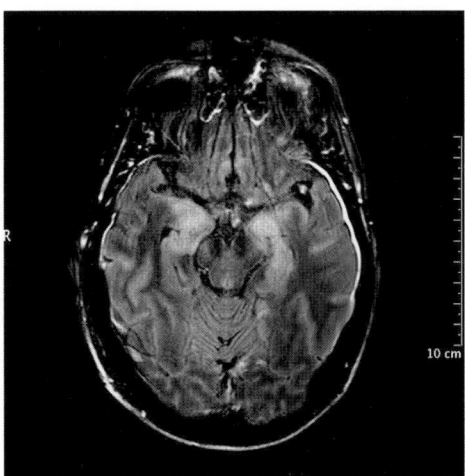

Fig. 31.5 MRI of the brain of a patient with HHV-6 encephalitis 36 days after a matched unrelated donor hematopoietic stem cell transplant for diffuse large B-cell lymphoma. Flair axial image shows bilateral medial temporal lobe edema compatible with limbic encephalitis.

of B- and T-lymphocyte function. However, this is a slow process; thus opportunistic viral and fungal infections are frequent during this period. The risk of infection is higher in patients who develop acute GVHD, and therefore require high dose steroids. Bacterial infections can still occur, and are usually related to use of indwelling catheters or GVHD of the gut. CMV viremia is common during this period. However, routine use of preemptive or prophylactic therapy has been effective in preventing life-threatening CMV disease. The risk of PCP has also decreased significantly since the introduction of PCP prophylaxis.[68,69]

Late post-engraftment period

This period is the period of late immune recovery and ends when the patient regains normal immunity. In the absence of chronic GVHD, this period can last up to 2 years. The development of chronic GVHD delays immune restoration, and can extend this period for many years (as long as immunosuppressive drugs are required). Viral and bacterial infections of the respiratory tract are common during this period. Infections with encapsulated bacteria are common in patients with chronic GVHD, as well as opportunistic viral and fungal infections such as VZV, CMV, invasive aspergillosis and non-*Aspergillus* mold infections, and PCP, among others.[68]

Infections of particular importance in transplant recipients

CMV

CMV is one of the most important pathogens affecting transplant recipients. It is widely distributed in the general population; seropositivity for CMV varies in different geographic regions, and it ranges from 30–97%.[71] Before widespread use of interventions aimed at reducing the incidence of CMV disease and infection, CMV disease (i.e., pneumonitis, gastroenteritis, hepatitis, encephalitis, etc.) occurred frequently during the first 3 months after transplantation. In SOT the highest risk for CMV disease is in patients in whom the donor is seropositive and the recipient is seronegative for CMV (D+/R-). CMV has a predilection to invade the allograft, possibly due to an aberrant immune response within the graft. The risk of infection varies also with the type of transplant; lung, small intestine and pancreas transplant recipients have a higher risk for CMV, while liver and kidney recipients are at lower risk. In SOT, CMV infection has been found consistently to be an independent risk factor for other infectious complications, as well as graft rejection.[71] In HSCT, infection is usually the result of reactivation of endogenous virus; hence the highest risk is in seropositive recipients. Without prophylaxis, up to 80% of seropositive recipients will experience CMV infection after HSCT. Seronegative individuals have a 30–40% chance of becoming infected when receiving unscreened blood products or stem cells from a seropositive donor. Risk factors for CMV disease are acute and chronic GVHD, use of high-dose corticosteroids, use of cord blood, T-cell depletion and use of mismatched or unrelated donors.[72]

Typically, CMV viremia precedes CMV disease by 1 to 2 weeks; therefore close monitoring of CMV reactivation by PCR assays or pp65 antigenemia allows the detection of early CMV replication, and therefore institution of appropriate antiviral therapy (ganciclovir, valganciclovir, or foscarnet) before the development of end-organ disease. This approach, termed pre-emptive therapy, has the advantage of effectively decreasing the incidence of early CMV disease, and limiting the drug-related toxicity. In addition, a limited amount of viral replication may allow for the development of CMV-specific immune reconstitution. Pre-emptive therapy is the preferred method for preventing CMV disease in HSCT[72] and is widely used in SOT in patients with intermediate risk for CMV disease. In solid organ high-risk recipients (D+/R-), although pre-emptive therapy is an accepted alternative, universal prophylaxis is preferred. It has the theoretical advantage of preventing reactivation of other herpes viruses, and may be more likely to prevent the indirect effects of CMV. CMV prophylaxis, as opposed to preemptive therapy, is effective in preventing CMV disease early after the transplant, but is associated with an increased risk of late-onset CMV viremia and disease.[71]

Other herpes viruses

HSV infection is common in both SOT and HSCT recipients, particularly during the first month after transplant. Routine use of antiviral prophylaxis has successfully decreased the incidence of severe HSV reactivation. However, breakthrough mucocutaneous HSV infection and even disseminated disease can still occur. VZV reactivation is also a common complication of transplant recipients. Routine use of acyclovir prophylaxis has decreased the incidence of disseminated VZV significantly. As with HSV, severe VZV disease is typically treated with IV acyclovir.[63]

Although EBV can cause a wide spectrum of disease, EBV-associated post-transplant lymphoproliferative disorder (PTLD) is the most feared complication of EBV infection after SOT and HSCT. The term EBV-associated PTLD is generally used to describe a heterogeneous group of clinical syndromes associated with uncontrolled lymphoproliferation, which can result in true malignancies containing clonal chromosomal abnormalities. Early diagnosis requires a high index of suspicion. EBV viral load monitoring and radiological evaluation can assist in early diagnosis. Reduction of immunosuppression should be the initial strategy in managing the disease. Timing of additional therapies such as antivirals, rituximab and chemotherapy remain controversial.[63,68,69]

HHV-6 has been associated with disease after transplant, and although a variety of clinical manifestations have been described in transplant recipients, the more convincing association is with encephalitis. The initial presentation may be subtle with memory loss or disorientation. However, it may progress to severe mental status abnormalities and seizures. The diagnosis is established with a positive PCR in the CSF, and absence of other infectious agents. Treatment is with ganciclovir or foscarnet.[69]

Invasive filamentous fungal infections

Invasive *Aspergillus fumigatus* is the most common species of *Aspergillus* causing clinical disease in transplant recipients. However, other species of *Aspergillus* have been implicated in significant disease, mainly *A. terreus*, *A. nidulans*, *A. flavus*, and *A. ustus*. Invasive pulmonary aspergillosis is the most common presentation,[73] with subsequent dissemination such as to the sinuses and brain. Risk factors are prolonged neutropenia, high-dose corticosteroids, cord blood transplantation, CMV disease, GVHD, rejection and lung transplantation. Manifestations of filamentous fungi that are almost exclusively seen in lung transplant recipients are tracheobronchitis, characterized by ulceration and cartilage invasion, and bronchial anastomotic infections, which frequently lead to stenosis or fistulas.[74]

Voriconazole is considered the drug of choice for invasive aspergillosis. However, drug–drug interaction can be problematic in transplant patients, limiting its use. The alternative treatments are less efficacious. Monitoring serum *Aspergillus* galactomannan in high-risk patients, such as those with prolonged neutropenia, as well as CT imaging, can assist in the early diagnosis of invasive aspergillosis.[74] Despite early diagnosis and treatment, the mortality associated with invasive aspergillosis, in particular in HSCT recipients, is still high (60–85%).[75] Therefore, anti-aspergillus prophylaxis should be considered in patients in whom prolonged neutropenia is expected, in patients with chronic GVHD receiving high-dose corticosteroids and in lung transplant recipients.

Fusarium spp., *Scedosporium* spp., mucormycosis, and dematiaceous molds are increasingly recognized as significant pathogens in transplant recipients. Clinical disease can be very similar to the infection caused by *Aspergillus* spp.; invasive pulmonary infection and sinusitis remain the most common sites of infection. *Fusarium* spp. frequently disseminates hematogenously and can be isolated in blood cultures. Many of these infections are resistant to most antifungal drugs, and remain an important cause of transplant-related mortality.[73,76]

Invasive candidiasis

Before routine use of antifungal prophylaxis, invasive candidiasis was the most common invasive fungal infection in transplant recipients. In SOT, most *Candida* infections occur during the first month after transplant, usually related to the surgical procedure. Liver, pancreas and small bowel transplant recipients are at particularly high risk for invasive candidiasis; also lung transplant recipients can develop bronchial anastomotic infections.[74] In HSCT, most *Candida* infections occur in the pre-engraftment period, and are associated with the mucosal injury that results from the conditioning regimen, and with the widespread use of antibiotics for the treatment or prevention of fever and neutropenia. Fluconazole-resistant *Candida* species are now increasingly isolated, requiring alternative therapies such as echinocandins. Antifungal prophylaxis has been proven

to reduce the incidence of invasive fungal infections after HSCT, and to reduce the infection-related mortality and overall mortality.[75] In SOT, antifungal prophylaxis is recommended for high-risk liver transplant recipients, and in small bowel and lung transplant recipients.

Translational research

● ON THE HORIZON

- CMV, EBV, and adenovirus remain problematic infections in both hematopoietic stem cell and solid organ transplant recipients, and medications currently available to treat these infections have significant associated toxicities, or lack efficacy.
- Adoptive immunotherapy, in which virus specific donor-derived T cells are expanded and infused into the transplant recipient, will likely become more widespread in treating these infections.

Viral reactivation and disease are still a major cause of morbidity and mortality among transplant recipients. CMV, EBV and adenovirus are particularly problematic once disease develops. Preemptive strategies have substantially decreased the incidence of invasive CMV disease; nevertheless a significant number of patients still go on to develop invasive disease. Preemptive therapy and treatment is limited by the toxicity associated with the available antivirals, and the lack of efficacy against EBV and adenovirus. In addition, development of resistance can complicate therapy. Development of new effective antivirals has been slow. Cidofovir has a good activity against DNA viruses *in vivo* and *in vitro*. However, it lacks oral bioavailability (there is only an IV formulation), and it has dose-associated limiting toxicity. Hexadecyloxypropyl-cidofovir (CMX001) is an ether lipid ester analog of cidofovir that has been reported to be 1000-fold more potent than cidofovir against DNA viruses such as CMV and adenovirus. It is available in an oral formulation that is said to lack the nephrotoxic effects of cidofovir. There are ongoing clinical trials to determine the efficacy and safety of CMX001 for the treatment of DNA viruses. There are other antivirals in the pipeline, but they are at much earlier stages of development. Because of the scarcity of effective, non-toxic antivirals and because uncontrolled viral infections correlate with a lack of cellular immunity against viruses, several groups are working on the development of adoptive immunotherapy, which is the artificial reconstitution of virus-specific T cells with *in vitro* expanded T cells. A number of small studies have now shown that virus-specific T cells are effective in controlling CMV and EBV infections in transplant recipients. The translation of adoptive immunotherapy into the clinic has been limited by technical difficulties associated with the generation of viral-specific cells that are not alloreactive, that can be produced from naïve T cells, and that can be developed rapidly and cost-effectively. However significant advances continue to be seen in the field of cellular therapy, and these could become part of the armamentarium against viruses in the next decade.

Conclusions

Immunocompromised hosts are surviving longer as antimicrobials improve and as immunosuppressant agents become less toxic. Both monogenetic primary immunodeficiencies and the increasingly specific immunosuppressant agents allow insight into host control of specific microbes. With this knowledge, new types of immunodeficiencies are being recognized, such as the autoantibody cytokine disorders described above. In addition, the knowledge of specific host immunity will help in developing therapies to boost host responses in the increasing challenges of treatment-resistant microbes.

References

1. Holland SM. Chronic granulomatous disease. Clin Rev Allergy Immunol 2010;38:3–10.
2. Rosenzweig SD, Holland SM. Phagocyte immunodeficiencies and their infections. J Allergy Clin Immunol 2004;113:620–6.
3. Winklestein JA, Marino MC, Johnston Jr RB, et al. Chronic granulomatous disease. Report on a national registry of 368 patients. Medicine (Baltimore) 79:155–69.
4. Greenberg DE, Ding L, Zelazny AM, et al. A novel bacterium associated with lymphadenitis in a patient with chronic granulomatous disease. PLoS Pathog 2006;2:e28.
5. Siddiqui S, Anderson VL, Hilligoss DM, et al. Fulminant mulch pneumonitis: an emergency presentation of chronic granulomatous disease. Clin Infect Dis 2007;45:673–81.
6. Freeman AF, Marciano BE, Anderson VL, et al. Corticosteroids in the treatment of severe Nocardia pneumonia in chronic granulomatous disease. Pediatr Infect Dis J 2011;30:806–8.
7. Margolis DM, Melnick DA, Alling DW, Gallin JI. Trimethoprim-sulfamethoxasole prophylaxis in the management of chronic granulomatous disease. J Infect Dis 1990;162:723–6.
8. Gallin JI, Alling DW, Malech HL, et al. Itraconazole to prevent fungal infections in chronic granulomatous disease. N Engl J Med 2003;348:2416–22.
9. Freeman AF, Holland SM. Antimicrobial prophylaxis for primary immunodeficiencies. Curr Opin Clin Immunol 2009;9:525–30.
10. Palmblad J, Papadaki HA. Chronic idiopathic neutropenias and severe congenital neutropenia. Curr Opin Hematol 2008;15:8–14.
11. Boztug K, Klein C. Genetic etiologies of severe congenital neutropenia. Curr Opin Pediatr 2011;23:21–6.
12. Hsu AP, Sampaio EP, Khan J, et al. Mutations in GATA2 are associated with the autosomal dominant and sporadic monocytopenia and mycobacterial infection (MonoMac) syndrome. Blood 2011;118:2653–5.
13. Vinh DC, Patel SY, Uzel G. Autosomal dominant and sporadic monocytopenia and susceptibility to mycobacteria, fungi, papillomaviruses and myelodysplasia. Blood 2010;115:1519–29.
14. Hambleton S, Salem S, Bustamante J, et al. IRF8 mutations and human dendritic-cell immunodeficiency. N Engl J Med 2011;365:127–38.
15. Conley ME, Dobbs AK, Farmer DM, et al. Primary B cell immunodeficeincies: comparisons and contrasts. Ann Rev Immunol 2009;27:199–227.
16. Tarzi MD, Gringoriadou S, Carr SM, et al. Clinical immunology review series: an approach to the management of pulmonary disease in primary antibody deficiency. Clin Exp Immunol 2008;155:147–55.
17. Cuccherini B, Chua K, Gill V, et al. Bacteremia and skin/bone infections in two patients with X-linked agammaglobulinemia caused by an unusual organism related to *Flexispira/Helicobacter* species. Clin Immunol 2000;97:121–9.
18. Murray PR, Jain A, Uzel G, et al. Pyoderma gangrenosum-like ulcer in a patient with X-linked agammaglobulinemia: identification of *Helicobacter bilis* by mass spectrometry analysis. Arch Dermatol 2010;146:523–6.
19. Van der Burg M, Gennery AR. Educational paper: the expanding clinical and immunological spectrum of severe combined immunodeficiency. Eur J Pediatr 2011;170:561–71.
20. Puck JM. Severe combined immunodeficiency: new advances in diagnosis and treatment. Immunol Res 2007;38:64–7.
21. Kobrynski LI, Sullivan KE. Velocardiofacial syndrome, diGeorge syndrome: the chromosome 22q11.2 deletion syndromes. Lancet 2007;1443–52.
22. Perez EE, Bokszczanin A, McDonald-McGinn D. Safety of the live viral vaccines in patients with chromosome 22q11.2 deletion syndrome (diGeorge/velocardiofacial syndrome). Pediatrics 2003;112:e325.
23. Ma CS, Chew GY, Simpson N, et al. Deficiency of Th17 cells in hyper IgE syndrome due to mutations in STAT3. J Exp Med 2008;65:1551–7.
24. Milner JD, Brenchley JM, Laurence A, et al. Impaired T(H) 17 cell differentiation in subjects with autosomal dominant hyper-IgE syndrome. Nature 2008;452:773–6.
25. Renner ED, Rylaarsdam S, Anover-Sombke S, et al. Novel signal transducer and activator of transcription 3 (STAT3) mutations, reduced T(H) 17 cell numbers, and variably defective STAT3 phosphorylation in hyper-IgE syndrome. J Allergy Clin Immunol 2008;122:181–7.
26. Freeman AF, Holland SM. Clinical manifestations, etiology, and pathogenesis of the hyper-IgE syndromes. Pediatr Res 2009;65:32R–37R.
27. Melia E, Freeman AF, Shea YR, et al. Pulmonary nontuberculous mycobacterial infections in hyper-IgE syndrome. J Allergy Clin Immunol 2009;124:617–8.
28. Vinh DC, Sugui JA, Hsu AP, et al. Invasive fungal disease in autosomal-dominant hyper-IgE syndrome. J Allergy Clin Immunol 2010;125:1389–90.
29. Freeman AF, Davis J, Anderson VL, et al. Pneumocystis jiroveci infection in patients with hyper-immunoglobulin E syndrome. Pediatrics 2006;118:e1271.
30. Engelhardt KR, McGhee S, Winkler S, et al. Large deletions and point mutations involving the dedicator of cytokinesis 8 (DOCK8) in the autosomal-recessive form of hyper-IgE syndrome. J Allergy Clin Immunol 2009;124:1289–302.
31. Zhang Q, Davis J, Lamborn IT, et al. Combined immunodeficiency associated with DOCK8 mutations. N Engl J Med 2009;361:2046–55.
32. Al-Muhsen S, Casanova JL. The genetic heterogeneity of mendelian susceptibility to mycobacterial diseases. J Allergy Clin Immunol 2008;122:1043–51.
33. Holland SM. Interferon gamma, IL-12, IL-12R and STAT1 immunodeficiency diseases: disorders of the interface of innate and adaptive immunity. Immunol Res 2007;38:342–6.
34. Averbuch D, Chapgier A, Boisson-Dupuis S, et al. The clinical spectrum of patients with deficiency of signal transducer and activator of transcription 1. Pediatr Infect Dis J 2011;30:352–5.
35. Vinh DC, Masannat F, Dzioba RB, et al. Refractory disseminated coccidioidomycosis and mycobacteria in interferon-gamma receptor 1 deficiency. Clin Infect Dis 2009;49:e62–e65.
36. Zerbe CS, Holland SM. Disseminated histoplasmosis in persons with interferon-gamma receptor 1 deficiency. Clin Infect Dis 2005;41:e38–41.
37. Ram S, Lewis LA, Rice PA. Infections of people with complement deficiencies and patients who have undergone splenectomy. Clin Microbiol Rev 2010;23:740–80.
38. Browne SK, Holland SM. Anticytokine autoantibodies in infectious diseases: pathogenesis and mechanisms. Lancet Infect Dis 2010;10:875–85.
39. Kisand K, Boe Wolff AS, Podkrajsek KT. Chronic mucocutaneous candidiasis in APECED or thymoma patients correlate with autoimmunity to Th17 associated cytokines. J Exp Med 2010;207:299–308.
40. Puel A, Doffinger R, Natividad A, et al. Autoantibodies against IL-17A, IL-17F, and II-22 in patients with chronic mucocutaneous candidiasis and autoimmune polyendocrine syndrome type 1. J Exp Med 2010;207:291–7.
41. Patel SY, Ding L, Brown MR, et al. Anti-IFN-gamma autoantibodies in disseminated nontuberculous mycobacterial infections. J Immunol 2005;175:4769–76.
42. Trapnell BC, Uchida K, Suzuki T. Pulmonary alveolar proteinosis, a primary immunodeficiency of impaired GM-CSF stimulation of macrophages. Curr Opin Immunol 2009;21:514–21.
43. Aberg JA, Gallant JE, Anderson J. Primary care guidelines for the management of persons infected with human immunodeficiency virus: recommendations of the HIV Medicine Association of the Infectious Diseases Society of America. Clin Infect Dis 2004;39:609–29.
44. Kaplan JE, Masur H, Holmes KK. Preventing opportunistic infections among HIV-infected persons-2002. MMWR Recomm Rep 2002;51(RR-8):1–52.
45. Allison AC. Immunosuppressive drugs: the first 50 years and a glance forward. Immunopharmacology 2000;47:63–83.
46. Mueller NJ. New immunosuppressive strategies and the risk of infection. Transpl Infect Dis 2008;10:379–84.
47. Chinen J, Shearer WT. Secondary immunodeficiencies, including HIV infection. J Allergy Clin Immunol 2010;125:S195–203.
48. Freifeld AG, Bow EJ, Sepkowitz KA, et al. Clinical practice guideline for the use of antimicrobial agents in neutropenic patients with cancer: 2010 update by the Infectious Diseases Society of America. Clin Infect Dis 2011;52:e56–93.
49. Halloran PF. Immunosuppressive drugs for kidney transplantation. N Engl J Med 2004;351:2715–29.
50. Lionakis MS, Kontoyiannis DP. Glucocorticoids and invasive fungal infections. Lancet 2003;362:1828–38.
51. Gea-Banacloche JC, Opal SM, Jorgensen J, et al. Sepsis associated with immunosuppressive medications: an evidence-based review. Crit Care Med 2004;32:S578–590.
52. Kang I, Park SH. Infectious complications in SLE after immunosuppressive therapies. Curr Opin Rheumatol 2003;15:528–34.
53. Marcen R. Immunosuppressive drugs in kidney transplantation: impact on patient survival, and incidence of cardiovascular disease, malignancy and infection. Drugs 2009;69:2227–43.
54. Gaber AO, Knight RJ, Patel S, Gaber LW. A review of the evidence for use of thymoglobulin induction in renal transplantation. Transplant Proc 2010;42:1395–400.
55. Salvana EM, Salata RA. Infectious complications associated with monoclonal antibodies and related small molecules. Clin Microbiol Rev 2009;22:274–90.
56. Gea-Banacloche JC, Weinberg GA. Monoclonal antibody therapeutics and risk for infection. Pediatr Infect Dis J 2007;26:1049–52.
57. Martin-Mola E, Balsa A. Infectious complications of biologic agents. Rheum Dis Clin North Am 2009;35:183–99.
58. Koo S, Marty FM, Baden LR. Infectious complications associated with immunomodulating biologic agents. Infect Dis Clin North Am 2010;24:285–306.
59. Gea-Banacloche JC. Rituximab-associated infections. Semin Hematol 2010;47:187–98.
60. Polman CH, O'Connor PW, Havrdova E, et al. A randomized, placebo-controlled trial of natalizumab for relapsing multiple sclerosis. N Engl J Med 2006;354:899–910.
61. Fishman JA, Issa NC. Infection in organ transplantation: risk factors and evolving patterns of infection. Infect Dis Clin North Am 2010;24:273–83.
62. Michaels MG, Green M. Infections in pediatric transplant recipients: not just small adults. Hematol Oncol Clin North Am 2011;25:139–50.
63. Fonseca-Aten M, Michaels MG. Infections in pediatric solid organ transplant recipients. Semin Pediatr Surg 2006;15:153–61.
64. Fishman JA. Introduction: infection in solid organ transplant recipients. Am J Transplant 2009;9(Suppl. 4):S3–6.
65. Fishman JA, Rubin RH. Infection in organ-transplant recipients. N Engl J Med 1998;338:1741–51.
66. Fisher RA. Cytomegalovirus infection and disease in the new era of immunosuppression following solid organ transplantation. Transpl Infect Dis 2009;11:195–202.
67. Gooley TA, Chien JW, Pergam SA, et al. Reduced mortality after allogeneic hematopoietic-cell transplantation. N Engl J Med 2010;363:2091–101.

68. Wingard JR, Hsu J, Hiemenz JW. Hematopoietic stem cell transplantation: an overview of infection risks and epidemiology. Infect Dis Clin North Am 2010;24:257–72.

69. Hiemenz JW. Management of infections complicating allogeneic hematopoietic stem cell transplantation. Semin Hematol 2009;46:289–312.

70. Szabolcs P, Cairo MS. Unrelated umbilical cord blood transplantation and immune reconstitution. Semin Hematol 2010;47:22–36.

71. Humar A, Snydman D. Cytomegalovirus in solid organ transplant recipients. Am J Transplant 2009;9(Suppl. 4):S78–86.

72. Ljungman P, Hakki M, Boeckh M. Cytomegalovirus in hematopoietic stem cell transplant recipients. Infect Dis Clin North Am 2010;24:319–37.

73. Person AK, Kontoyiannis DP, Alexander BD. Fungal infections in transplant and oncology patients. Infect Dis Clin North Am 2010;24:439–59.

74. Nucci M, Anaissie E. Fungal infections in hematopoietic stem cell transplantation and solid-organ transplantation—focus on aspergillosis. Clin Chest Med 2009;30:295–306 vii.

75. Wirk B, Wingard JR. Current approaches in antifungal prophylaxis in high risk hematologic malignancy and hematopoietic stem cell transplant patients. Mycopathologia 2009;168:299–311.

76. Maschmeyer G, Calandra T, Singh N, et al. Invasive mould infections: a multi-disciplinary update. Med Mycol 2009;47:571–83.

Maturing of the fetal and neonatal immune system

David B. Lewis

The fetus and neonate are more vulnerable than older children and adults to severe infection with a variety of pathogens, including pyogenic bacteria, fungi, viruses, and intracellular protozoa,[1] indicating substantial limitations in innate and adaptive immunity in prenatal and early postnatal life. The results of hematopoietic stem-cell transplantation using cord blood also suggest impairment of neonatal cellular immunity, e.g., the significantly lower risk of acute graft-versus-host disease compared to bone marrow and peripheral blood transplants containing adult T cells.[2] These clinical observations have made defining the physiologic immaturity of the human fetal and neonatal immune system of great interest.

CLINICAL RELEVANCE

Examples of infections more frequent or severe in the fetus and neonate than in older children and adults

- Bacteremia and meningitis due to pyogenic bacteria, e.g., group B streptococcus—higher rate in neonatal period than any other age group.
- Primary herpes simplex virus infection—approximately 20% mortality in the neonate even with current antiviral therapy, e.g., acyclovir.
- Enteroviral infection—severe infection, e.g., hepatic necrosis with disseminated intravascular coagulation, which is unusual outside the neonatal period except in cases of severe T-cell immunodeficiency such as severe combined immunodeficiency (SCID).
- Toxoplasmosis—congenital infection typically disseminates to the retina; disseminated infection is unusual in postnatally acquired infection.
- *Mycobacterium tuberculosis* acquired congenitally or perinatally has a high risk of progressing to miliary disease and meningitis.
- Mucocutaneous candidiasis is more frequent in the otherwise healthy neonate than in older children and adults.

Dendritic cells and antigen presentation

Activated CD11c$^+$ dendritic cells (DCs) are myeloid derived cells that participate in antigen presentation to T and B cells and produce critical cytokines, e.g., interleukin (IL)-12 p70 (a heterodimer of the IL-12/IL-23 p40 subunit and IL-12 p35) and IL-15, which provide early innate immune protection and influence later adaptive immunity (Fig. 32.1). Plasmacytoid dendritic cells (pDCs) are a distinct DC population that at rest lack the characteristic dendrite-like protrusions of CD11c$^+$ DCs. pDCs are found in lymphoid tissue, circulation, and certain sites of tissue inflammation,

e.g., the skin in herpes simplex virus (HSV) infection. Activated pDCs are an important source of type I interferon (IFN), which provides early innate antiviral immunity and enhance the differentiation of Th1 lymphocytes from naïve CD4 T-cell precursors. DCs are activated by a variety of stimuli, including following recognition of conserved structures of microbial pathogens by Toll-like receptors (TLRs), C-lectin type receptors, RIG-I-like receptors, and NOD- and LRR-receptors (NLRs) (Chapter 3).[3]

DCs in tissues

The colonization of CD11c$^+$ DCs in extra-lymphoid and lymphoid tissues is developmentally regulated and independent of exposure to inflammatory mediators. Immature CD11c$^+$ DC lineage cells are found in the interstitial regions of solid organs, including the kidney, heart, pancreas, and lung by 12 weeks of gestation, and progressively increase until 21 weeks.[3] Epidermal HLA-DR$^+$ DC-like cells are found in the skin even earlier (7 weeks gestation) and are probably derived from CD45$^+$ HLA-DR$^+$ cells that enter the epidermis, extensively proliferate, and then acquire CD1c, langerin, and CD1a in a stepwise manner.[4]

Circulating and monocyte-derived DCs

Circulating CD11c$^+$ DCs are typically CD11c^{high} and major histocompatibility complex (MHC) class IIhigh but lineage-negative (Lin$^-$), i.e., lacking markers for other cell lineages, such as T cells, monocytes, B cells, NK cells, granulocytes, and erythroid cells. Human pDCs are CD11c^{low}Lin$^-$ and express high levels of CD123 (IL-3 receptor α-chain) and BDCA-2 (CD303 or CLEC4C), a type II transmembrane C-type lectin. The concentrations and surface phenotype of CD11c$^+$ DCs in cord blood and adult peripheral blood are similar.[3] An exception is CD86 (B7-2) T-cell co-stimulatory protein, which is lower on cord blood CD11c$^+$ DCs. The concentration of pDCs in cord blood is significantly higher than in adult peripheral blood, and gradually declines after birth.[3]

Circulating neonatal DCs have selective limitations in the TLR-mediated upregulation of expression of molecules involved in T-cell co-stimulation by engagement of CD28 (CD80 and CD86) and other DC–T-cell interactions (MHC class II and CD40) compared to those of the adult.[3] For example, cord blood CD11c$^+$ DCs have reduced expression of CD40 in response to ligands for TLR-2/6 (*Mycoplasma fermentans*), TLR-3 (poly I:C), TLR-4 (lipopolysaccharide (LPS)), and TLR-7 (imiquimod), and reduced CD80 in response to TLR-3 or -4 ligands. In contrast, CD11c$^+$ DC upregulation of CD40 in response to GU-rich single-stranded RNA, a TLR-8 ligand, is similar, as is MHC class II and CD86

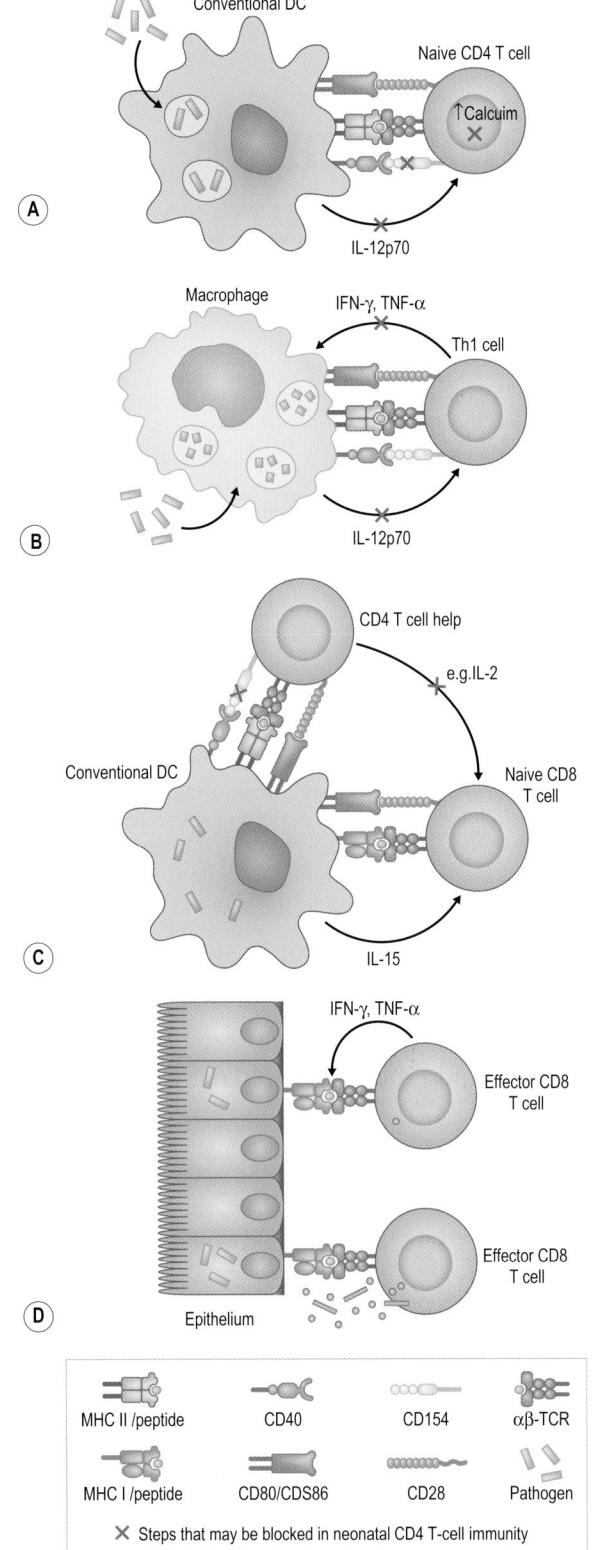

upregulation after stimulation with TLR-3 and -4 ligands. Cord blood and adult peripheral blood pDCs also similarly upregulate HLA-DR, CD80, and CD86 after stimulation with TLR-9 ligands, i.e., synthetic DNA oligonucleotides lacking methylated CpG residues (CpG DNA).[3]

Th1 immunity may be particularly limited in the neonate and young infant compared to older individuals because of decreased IL-12 p70 production by CD11c$^+$ DCs, e.g., in response to LPS plus IFN-γ.[1] However, this limitation may be pathogen-dependent, as decreased IL-12 production by cord blood CD11c$^+$ DCs is probably comparable to adult CD11c$^+$ DCs after stimulation with certain Gram-positive and -negative bacteria or meningococcal outer-membrane proteins.[1] Circulating DCs from cord blood can also allogeneically stimulate cord blood T cells *in vitro*,[1] but it is unclear if they are as effective as adult DCs in promoting Th1 differentiation in an allogeneic context.

The production of type I IFN by circulating CD11c$^+$ DCs and pDCs is also reduced in cord blood, and may limit the control in the neonate of pathogens such as herpes simplex virus (HSV) (see below). For example, IFN-α production by cord blood CD11c$^+$ DCs in response to a TLR-3 ligand and by cord blood pDCs in response to TLR-9 ligands—such as live or inactivated HSV, or CpG DNA is reduced compared to adult DCs.[3] This decreased TLR9-mediated production of type I IFN by neonatal DCs appears to be due to reduced nuclear translocation of interferon regulatory factor 7 (IRF7), a transcription factor that is essential for the induction of type I IFN.[3]

Monocyte-derived dendritic cells (MDDCs) are produced by culturing cord blood or adult peripheral blood monocytes *in vitro* with cytokines, such as granulocyte–macrophage colony-stimulating factor, IL-4, and tumor necrosis factor (TNF)-α. In general, cord blood MDDCs have reduced levels of IL-12 p70 expression after stimulation, but it remains unclear if these and other functional and phenotypic differences apply to neonatal and adult DCs of the tissues. Gene expression profiling suggests that MDDCs may best model inflammatory DCs, which are generated from monocytes *in vivo* at sites of marked tissue inflammation, such as during Th1-driven reversal reactions of leprosy,[3] but it is unclear to what extent inflammatory DCs are generated in the fetus and neonate.

Postnatal DC maturation

HLA-DR expression and CD80 expression induced by LPS, which is significantly reduced in cord blood CD11c$^+$ DCs, reaches adult DC levels by 3 months of age.[5] In a longitudinal study of Gambian infants, TNF-α, IL-6, and IL-12/IL-23p40 expression by CD11c$^+$ DCs in response to LPS (TLR-4) at 1 year and 2 years of age was significantly greater than at birth or compared to those of adult cells.[6] In contrast, CD11c$^+$ DCs from newborns and infants at 1 and 2 years of age all had higher levels of production of these cytokines in response to PAM (a TLR-2 agonist) or

Fig. 32.1 T-cell activation and differentiation in response to antigen. Steps that may be blocked in neonatal CD4 T cells are indicated as red Xs. (A) Th1 generation from naïve CD4 T cells requires that CD11c$^+$ dendritic cells (DCs) present antigenic peptides bound to major histocompatibility complex (MHC) class II and co-stimulatory molecules, such as CD80 and CD86. T-cell activation results in calcium-dependent increases in CD154 on the CD4 T-cell surface. The CD154–CD40 interaction enhances CD11c$^+$ DC production of interleukin (IL)-12p70, which promotes Th1 differentiation. (B) Differentiated Th1 cells help kill intracellular pathogens, such as *Mycobacterium tuberculosis*, that hide in the intracellular microvesicular compartments of macrophages. Pathogen-derived peptides bound to

MHC class II displayed on the infected cell surface engage the $\alpha\beta$-T-cell receptor (TCR) of the Th1 cell, triggering its secretion of interferon (IFN)-γ and tumor necrosis factor (TNF)-α. These cytokines bind to specific surface receptors on the infected cell and increase its microbicidal activity. (C) The generation of CD8 T-cell effectors from naïve CD8 T cells requires $\alpha\beta$-TCR engagement by cognate peptide/MHC class I complexes on the CD11c$^+$ DC, CD80/CD86-CD28 co-stimulation, CD11c$^+$ DC-derived IL-15, and, possibly, cytokines from CD4 T cells. (D) CD8 T-cell effectors secrete perforin and granzymes, which kill target cells displaying viral peptide/MHC class I, and IFN-γ and TNF-α, which have antiviral activity and enhance antigen presentation.

3 M-003 (a TLR-7/8 agonist). For pDCs, adult levels of HLA-DR and CD80 expression induced by CpG (a TLR-9 ligand) were not achieved until 6–9 months of age.[6] The pDC production of TNF-α, IL-6, and in response to either TLR-7/8 or TLR-9 agonists at 1 year of age was similar to those of adult pDCs.

T cells

Ontogeny of thymic development

Initial colonization of the fetal thymus by prothymocytes occurs at 8.5 weeks of gestation, with dramatic increases in thymic cellularity during the second and third trimesters. Transient thymic involution, particularly of cortical double-positive (CD4^{high} CD8^{high}) thymocytes, may occur at the end of the third trimester due to a prenatal surge in the circulating levels of glucocorticoids.[1] This involution is followed by thymic recovery at 1 month of age, with peak thymic cellularity in relation to body size and, presumably, output of recent thymic emigrants (RTEs), between 6 and 12 months of age.[1,7]

Repertoire of Alpha/Beta T-cell receptors

The usage of T-cell receptor (TCR) D and J gene segments in the thymus is initially less diverse than subsequently. The complementarity determinant region 3 (CDR3) region of the TCR chain transcripts is also reduced in length and sequence diversity between 8 and 15 weeks of gestation. This is most likely due to decreased activity of terminal deoxynucleotidyl transferase (TdT), which performs N-nucleotide addition during V(D)J recombination. The impact of limitations in αβ-TCR diversity on the ability of the fetus to respond to congenital infection is likely to be most pronounced in the first trimester of pregnancy, as intrathymic TdT activity, CDR3 length, and V segment diversity during the second trimester are similar to that of postnatal thymic tissue.[1] A low-resolution analysis of the TCR repertoire expressed on cord blood T cells indicates that the diversity of TCR usage and CDR3 length are similar to that of antigenically naïve T cells in adults and infants, suggesting that the functional pre-immune repertoire is well formed by birth.

TCR excision circles (TREC) are generated during TCR gene rearrangement of thymocytes, and may persist for long periods in T-lineage cells that do not proliferate. TREC levels in cord blood are relatively high compared to adult peripheral blood, as would be expected given the predominance of naïve (CD45RA^{high}CD45R0^{low}) T cells and recent thymic emigrants (RTEs) in cord blood (see below). In addition, the cord blood T cells are likely enriched in RTEs,[8] which also have a higher TREC content than more mature circulating naïve T cells.[1,8]

Fetal T-cell development and phenotype

By 14 weeks of gestation, CD4 and CD8 T cells are found in the fetal circulation, liver, and spleen, and CD4 T cells are detectable in lymph nodes. The percentage of circulating T cells gradually increases during the second and third trimesters of pregnancy through about 6 months of age, followed by a gradual decline to adult levels. The ratio of CD4 to CD8 T cells in the circulation is relatively high during fetal life (about 3.5) and gradually declines with age.

Most circulating CD4 T cells in the term and preterm neonate and in the second and third trimester fetus express a CD45RA^{high}CD45R0^{low}CCR7$^+$CD25$^-$CD95$^-$ surface phenotype characteristic of antigenically naïve CD4 T cells found in adults. However, second trimester naïve CD4 T cells have higher basal levels of Foxp3, and, upon allogeneic stimulation, are highly skewed toward regulatory T-cell (Treg) phenotype and function compared to adult peripheral blood naïve CD4 T cells, which preferentially differentiate into effector cells.[9] Tregs are also more abundant in peripheral lymphoid tissue in the fetus compared to that in the adult.[10] This Treg skewing appears to be a characteristic of CD4 T cells derived from fetal hematopoietic stem cells (HSCs) rather than adult HSCs, and is likely an important mechanism for fetal–maternal tolerance.[9]

Protein tyrosine kinase 7 (PTK7) identifies RTEs among adult naïve CD4 T cells and is also expressed at high levels by cord blood T cells and post-natal thymocytes.[8] These observations are consistent with the fetal and neonatal peripheral T-cell compartment being enriched in RTEs, which is also supported by the high degree of thymic cellularity in the newborn and young infant.[7] Cord blood T cells may be more prone than adult naïve T cells to undergo homeostatic proliferation because of a greater sensitivity to the mitogenic effects of IL-7, and this may also be a reflection of RTE enrichment.[1,8]

CD4 T-cell responses

Herpes virus infections

One of the most striking limitations in neonatal T-cell immunity is the reduced and delayed HSV-specific CD4 T-cell proliferation and cytokine (IL-2, IFN-γ, and TNF-α) production in neonates compared to adults after primary HSV infection.[11] Older infants and young children also have reduced CD4 T-cell immunity (IL-2, IFN-γ, and CD40-ligand (CD154) expression) after primary infection with cytomegalovirus (CMV) compared to adults,[12] which is associated with persistent CMV shedding in the urine and saliva. These reduced responses after primary CMV infection likely also applies to the neonate and young infant with congenital, perinatal, or postnatally acquired CMV infection, resulting in persistent shedding of CMV for years following its acquisition.

Vaccines

Vaccination with bacille Calmette-Guérin (BCG) at birth versus 2 or 4 months of age is equally effective in inducing CD4 T-cell proliferative and IFN-γ responses to mycobacterial antigens, and does not result in increased Th2 skewing, i.e., production of IL-4, -5, and -13 and reduced levels of IFN-γ.[1] However, the Th1 responses of infant vaccine recipients have not been directly compared with those of older children and adults. In contrast, the CD4 T-cell response to oral poliovirus vaccine (OPV) may be reduced in the neonate and young infant: Newborns given OPV at birth, 1, 2, and 3 months of age have lower OPV-specific CD4 T-cell proliferation and IFN-γ production compared to adults immunized in childhood.[1] In contrast, the neonate's and infant's antibody titres are higher than those of adults, suggesting that CD4 follicular T-cell help for B cells is not impaired. In contrast to BCG, the administration of pertussis vaccine in the neonatal period may result in a subsequent skewing of pertussis antigen-specific T cells toward a Th2 phenotype.[13]

Mechanisms for reduced immunity

● KEY CONCEPTS

Mechanisms that may account for delayed CD4 T-cell immunity to infection and vaccination in the fetus and neonate

- Decreased CD154 (CD40-ligand) expression by naïve CD4 T cells after activation by antigen
- Decreased production by conventional dendritic cells of IL-12 p70, a key cytokine for Th1 differentiation
- Increased methylation of the interferon-γ gene resulting in decreased gene transcription in response to T-cell activation
- Decreased expression of STAT4 protein and IL-12-induced STAT4 tyrosine phosphorylation in neonatal CD4 T cells
- Reduced expression by neonatal CD4 T cells of NFAT family transcription factors required for CD154 and cytokine gene transcription

Normal CD4 T-cell activation by engagement of the αβ-TCR and CD28 (Fig. 32.1) results in the activation of NFAT-, AP-1-, and NF-κB-dependent transcription of genes such as IL-2 and CD154. IL-2 promotes CD4 T-cell proliferation in an autocrine and paracrine fashion, and CD154 engages CD40 on the CD11c$^+$ DC to increase its expression of CD80, CD86, and IL-12 p70. In addition to limitations in DC function discussed above, multiple potential mechanisms intrinsic to the neonatal CD4 T cell that may limit its ability to expand into memory/effector Th1 cells have been revealed by *in vitro* studies (Fig. 32.1).[1] These impairments include reduction in neonatal CD4 T-cell NFAT proteins, which is mediated by microRNA-184,[14] IL-2 and CD154 expression,[15] and IL-12-induced STAT4 activation.[15] The IFN-γ gene may also be more highly methylated in neonatal than adult naïve CD4 T cells,[1] limiting its accessibility to transcription factors. Reduced CD154 expression may decrease CD40 engagement of CD11c$^+$ DCs and their production of IL-12 p70.[1] Finally, decreased STAT4 signaling, which normally enhances IFN-γ gene transcription, may also impair Th1 differentiation.[1]

CD8 T-cell AND γδ-T-CELL responses

CD8 T-cell responses to herpes viruses, such as CMV, acquired congenitally are similar to those of adults or the responses to infection acquired in infancy or early childhood.[1] Congenital CMV infection also elicits a robust fetal γδ-T-cell response, including IFN-γ production and the expression of cytotoxins.[16] Neonates with congenital Chagas disease also have a readily detectable CD8 T-cell responses to this pathogen,[1] which appears to influence the subsequent quality of immune responses to vaccination with unrelated antigens. These apparently robust responses do not rule out a brief, but potentially important, lag in the onset of CD8 or γδ-T-cell immunity that might compromise the early control of these pathogens. CD8 T-cell responses to HIV-1 in perinatally or *in utero*-infected infants suggest that CD8 T cells capable of mediating cytotoxicity are also typically generated *in vivo* in the fetus.[1,17] Interestingly, the suppressive effects of HIV-1 on CD8 T-cell responses appear to be relatively specific, as HIV-1-infected infants with poor HIV-1-specific CD8 T-cell responses maintain CD8 T cells to herpes viruses.[1]

B cells

Ontogeny of B cells

Pre-B cells are first detected in the human fetal liver and omentum by 8 weeks of gestation and in the fetal bone marrow by 13 weeks of gestation. By mid-gestation the bone marrow is the predominant site of pre-B-cell development, and by 30 weeks of gestation it is the sole site.

By 16 weeks of gestation, all heavy-chain isotypes are detectable in fetal bone marrow B cells. The stimulus for this fetal isotype switching remains unclear. The frequency of B cells in tissues rapidly increases so that by 22 weeks' gestation the proportion of B cells in the spleen, blood, and bone marrow is similar to that in the adult. Cord blood B cells expressing surface IgG or IgA are typically very rare (i.e., < 1% of circulating B cells). True germinal centers in the spleen and lymph nodes are absent during fetal life, but appear during the first months after postnatal antigenic stimulation.

A distinct feature of fetal and cord blood B cells is their high frequency of markers, e.g., CD5, CD9, CD10, and CD38, that are found on transitional and pre-naïve B cells in healthy adults, and that predominate during early immune reconstitution of B-lineage cells following hematopoietic stem cell transplantation.[18] This finding is consistent with the rapid expansion of the B-cell compartment during late fetal and early post-natal ontogeny. Cord blood B cells, particularly from those prematurely born, have significantly reduced expression of CD40, CD80, CD86, and BAFF-receptor and a reduced ability to proliferate in response to BAFF and a BCR signal or to produce IgM, IgG, and IgA in response to CD154 and IL-10.[19] It is unclear how long after birth this reduction in surface expression and function of naïve B cells in the preterm infant persists, but the similar level of antibody responses to for most T-dependent antigens in vaccines in 2-month-old preterm versus term infants suggests that this functional impairment is largely resolved by this chronological age (see below).

Immunoglobulin repertoire

The preimmune immunoglobulin repertoire consists of antibodies that can be expressed prior to encounter with antigen and is determined by the number of different B-cell clones with distinct antigen specificity.[20] During early to mid-gestation this repertoire is limited by less diverse usage of V segments, but by the third trimester is as diverse as that of the adult. There is over- or under-representation of a V(D)J segments in the neonate, but their importance in limiting the neonatal humoral immune response remains unclear. The length of the CDR3 region of the immunoglobulin heavy chain, which is located at the center of the antigen-combining site, is shorter in the mid-gestation fetus than at birth or in adulthood; this is most likely due to decreased TdT activity. As the CDR3 region is the most hypervariable portion of immunoglobulins, a short CDR3 region significantly reduces the diversity of the fetal immunoglobulin repertoire[20] and may compromise the antibody response of the fetus, e.g., following congenital infection. CDR3 length of the immunoglobulin heavy chain progressively increases during the third trimester and reaches the length of adult B cells (12–13 amino acids) by 2 months after birth.[20] Somatic hypermutation is limited or absent for neonatal B-cell responses to protein antigens, e.g., encoded by respiratory syncytial virus (RSV), but is similar to adult levels by 3 months of age.[21]

B1 B cells

B1 B cells constitute 4% of cord blood B cells and have a CD20$^+$CD27$^+$CD43$^+$ surface phenotype.[22] They exhibit tonic intracellular signaling, are highly effective at stimulating allogeneic CD4 T cells, and spontaneously secrete IgM that is encoded by heavy chain immunoglobulin genes with minimal somatic hypermutation but a substantial amount of N-region additions.[22] Like murine B1 B cells, those of adult peripheral blood are enriched for certain specificities, such as phosphorylcholine. Thus, human B1 B cells may be considered a part of the innate immune system in providing protection against pathogens, such as certain encapsulated bacteria.

Ontogeny of responsiveness to T-dependent and -independent antigens

The chronology of the antibody response to different antigens differs depending on the need for cognate CD4 T-cell help (Table 32.1). Antigens that depend on cognate help (direct CD4 T-cell–B-cell interactions) include most proteins and polysaccharide–protein conjugates (T-dependent (TD) antigens). The response to TD antigens is characterized by the generation of memory B cells with somatically mutated, high-affinity immunoglobulin and the potential for isotype switching. Antigens that are partially or completely independent of CD4 T-cell help (T-independent antigens) can be divided into T-independent type 1 (TI-1) and type 2 (TI-2) antigens (Chapter 6). TI-1 antigens directly bind to B cells and fully activate them to produce antibodies, e.g., fixed *Brucella abortus* bacteria and CpG DNA. TI-2 antigens include bacterial capsular polysaccharides and require additional signals for optimal antibody production, such as TLR ligands that are directly recognized by B cells or cytokines produced by non-B cells (e.g., NK cells, NK T cells, γδ-T cells, or DCs). The response to TI-2 antigens is characterized by a lack of B-cell memory or somatic hypermutation and isotype expression that is largely restricted to IgM and IgG2.

The capacity of the neonate and young infant to respond to TD antigens is well established at birth, as reflected in the immune response to most protein and polysaccharide conjugate vaccines (Table 32.2). Nevertheless, there are clear differences between

Table 32.1 Postnatal ontogeny of competence for antibody responses to T-cell-dependent (TD) and T-cell independent type 1 (TI-1) and type 2 (TI-2) antigens

Antigen type	Nature of antigen	Age for competent response
TD	Proteins and protein-conjugated polysaccharides	Birth
TI-1	Certain microbial-derived products that directly activate B cells, e.g., *Brucella abortus*, CpG DNA	Birth
TI-2	Unconjugated polysaccharides, such as those from bacterial capsules	Delayed (6–24 months of age)

Table 32.2 Postnatal antibody responses of infants 6 month of age or younger to selected vaccines

Vaccine	Antigen type	Antibody response in neonate and young infant
Diphtheria toxoids	TD	Immunogenic at birth, but response superior when vaccination series delayed until 1 month of age
Haemophilus influenzae type b polysaccharide-conjugate vaccine	TD	Immunogenic at birth, but response superior when vaccination series delayed until 2 months of age
Haemophilus influenzae type b polysaccharide unconjugated vaccine	TI-2	Not reliably immunogenic until 18–24 months of age
Hepatitis B surface antigen	TD	Moderately decreased with vaccination at birth compared to 1 month of age; decreased response in premature compared to term neonate; delay of vaccination series recommended for premature infants of HbsAg mothers
Meningococcal polysaccharide-conjugated vaccine (types A, C, Y, W-135)	TD	Increased antibody titers in response to vaccination beginning at 2 months of age, with evidence of priming—efficacy?
Meningococcal polysaccharide vaccine—unconjugated (types A, C, Y, W-135)	TI-2	Serotype A immunogenic as early as 3 months of age; other serotypes not reliably immunogenic until 24 months of age; vaccination with type C induces tolerance to subsequent immunization in adults and presumably all age groups
Pertussis vaccine—acellular	TD	Immunogenic when series begun at 2 months of age; Th2 skewing when given at birth
Pertussis vaccine—whole cellular	TD	Tolerance to pertussis toxin after vaccination at birth but not at 1 month of age; mechanism?
Pneumococcal polysaccharide-conjugate vaccine—7, 11, or 13 valent	TD	Protective to majority of serotypes after three doses when series is begun at 2 months of age.
Pneumococcal polysaccharide unconjugated vaccine—23 valent	TI-2	Reliably immunogenic down to 12 months of age for most serotypes
Tetanus toxoids	TD	Protective in vaccinated neonates but relatively delayed response compared to 2-month-old infants

neonates and older infants in the magnitude of the antibody response to protein neoantigens. For example, in the case of hepatitis B surface antigen (HBsAg), the initial antibody response in term neonates immunized shortly after birth is substantially lower than if primary immunization is begun at 1 month of age.[1] The neonate's ultimate anti-HBsAg titres achieved after secondary and tertiary immunizations are similar to those of older children, indicating that neonatal immunization does not result in tolerance. Together, these results indicate that the developmental limitations responsible for reduced antibody responses are transient, although the precise mechanisms remain undefined.

Antibody production by human neonatal B cells to a TI-1 antigen *in vitro* (*B. abortus*) is only modestly reduced (Table 32.1) and may reflect a decreased ability of antigen-activated B cells to proliferate rather than a decreased precursor frequency of antigen-specific clones.

The response to TI-2 antigen is the last to appear chronologically, and accounts for the neonate's poor antibody response to infection with encapsulated bacteria, e.g., group B streptococci (GBS) and/or vaccination with unconjugated polysaccharide antigens, such as for *Hemophilus influenzae* and *Streptococcus pneumoniae* (Table 32.2). The response to some unconjugated polysaccharide antigens can be demonstrated by 6 months of age, but the response to vaccination with *H. influenzae* type b capsule or *Neisseriae meningitidis* type C is poor until approximately 18–24 months. Responses to pneumococcal polysaccharide have been proven adequate at 12 months of age.[29,30] This poor response in children less than 2 years of age is associated with a lack of circulating memory (CD27[high]) B cells that express IgM and have not undergone isotype switching. These IgM memory B cells are also absent in adults after splenectomy, suggesting that they depend on the spleen microenvironment for their generation and/or long-term survival. It is unclear whether decreased TI-2 antigen responses in early childhood are due to an intrinsic immaturity in B cells or APCs or both of the spleen, or to other limitations in the spleen microenvironment.

Antibody responses of the premature infant

There is a limited antibody response of premature infants to immunization with protein antigens during the first month of life but not by 2 months of age (Table 32.2). Thus, postnatal age is more of a determinant of antibody responses to TD antigens than is gestational age.[1] This may be of particular clinical relevance for HBsAg vaccine, which in term neonates is effective when given immediately after birth. As in term infants, the antibody responses to TI-2 antigens in premature infants are delayed until 6–24 months of age, depending on the particular antigen.

Maternal–fetal transfer of IgG

IgG is transported from the mother to the fetus by transcytosis and is detectable in the fetus by 17 weeks of gestation. Circulating concentrations of IgG in the fetus rise steadily and may exceed those of the mother after 34 weeks of gestation, consistent with the transfer being an active transport mechanism. The fetus synthesizes little IgG so that the concentration *in utero* is almost entirely maternally derived (Fig. 32.2). Accordingly, the degree of prematurity is reflected in proportionately lower neonatal IgG concentrations.

Fetal and postnatal immunoglobulin synthesis

IgG is the predominant immunoglobulin isotype at all ages (Fig. 32.2). The IgG plasma half-life is about 21 days, and maternally derived IgG levels fall rapidly after birth. IgG synthesized by the neonate and that passively derived from the mother are approximately equal when the neonate reaches 2 months of age; by 10–12 months of age the IgG is nearly all infant-derived. Values reach a nadir of ~400 mg/dL in term infants at 3–4 months of age and rise thereafter (Fig. 32.2). The premature

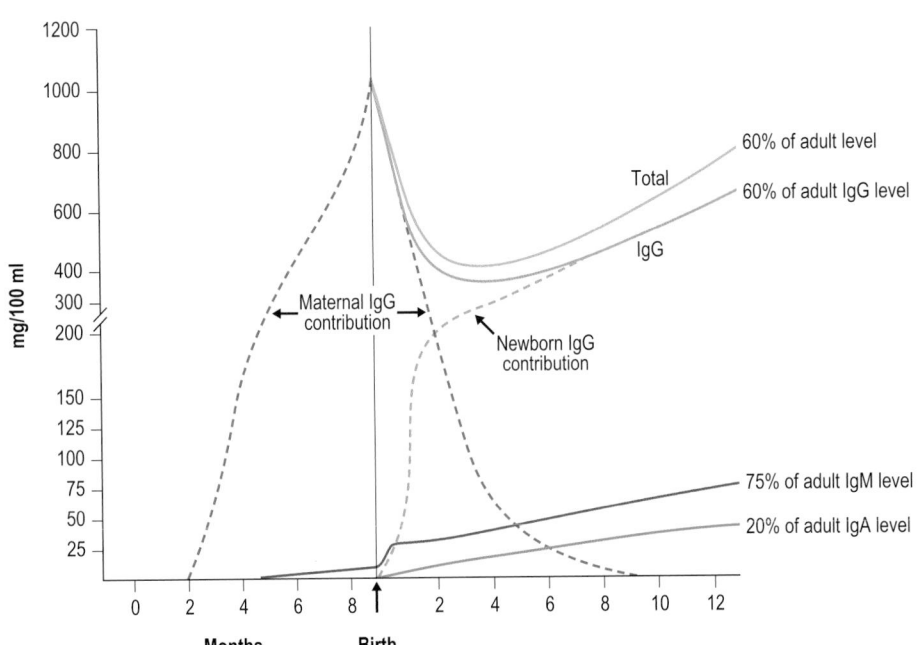

Fig. 32.2 IgG, IgM, and IgA levels in the fetus and in the infant in the first year of life. IgG of the fetus and newborn are solely of maternal origin. Maternal IgG disappears by 9 months of age, by which time endogenous synthesis is well established. IgM and IgA of the neonate are due solely to endogenous synthesis because these immunoglobulin isotypes do not cross the placenta.
From Remington JS, Klein JO, Wilson CB, et al. (eds) Infectious Diseases of the Fetus and Newborn Infant, 7th edn. Philadelphia: Elsevier; 2006: Fig. 4-16.

infant has a lower IgG concentration at birth, and reaches a nadir at 3 months of age. The slow onset of IgG synthesis in the neonate is predominantly an intrinsic limitation of the neonate rather than inhibitory effect of maternal antibody, as a similar pattern of IgG development is observed in neonates born to mothers with untreated agammaglobulinemia.

IgM does not cross the placenta. It increases from a mean of 6 mg/dL in premature infants less than 28 weeks of gestation to 11 mg/dL at term, which is approximately 8% of the maternal IgM level. This IgM, which is likely to be pre-immune or "natural," is enriched for polyreactive antibodies produced by B1 cells, and may play a role in the innate defense against infection. Postnatal IgM concentrations rise rapidly in premature and term infants in the first month and then more gradually thereafter, presumably in response to antigenic stimulation (Fig. 32.2). Elevated (> 20 mg/dL) IgM concentrations in cord blood suggest possible intrauterine infections, but this is not a sensitive screen for congenital infections.

IgA also does not cross the placenta and has a concentration in cord blood of about 0.1–5.0 mg/dL, approximately 0.5% of the levels in maternal sera. Concentrations are similar in term and premature neonates, and increase to 20% of those in adults by 1 year of age (Fig. 32.2). Increased cord blood IgA concentrations are observed in some infants with congenital infection, and elevated IgA is common in young infants infected by vertical transmission with HIV. IgA has a relatively short half-life in plasma of approximately 5 days. Secretory IgA is present in substantial amounts in the saliva by 10 days after birth.

The concentration of IgE in cord blood is typically only about 0.5% of those of maternal levels. The rate of postnatal increase varies, and is greater in infants predisposed to allergic disease or greater environmental exposure to allergens. Although the level of cord blood IgE has been reported to also predict the risk of the subsequent development of atopy, elevated serum IgE levels at birth may also reflect maternally derived IgE in a substantial number of cases, which may obscure the predictive value of this measurement.[23] The mechanisms by which maternal IgE can be transferred to the fetus remain unclear.

NK cells

The human fetal liver produces NK cells as early as 6 weeks of gestation, but the bone marrow is the major site for NK-cell production from late gestation onward. NK cells are present in greatest numbers in the circulation during the second trimester of fetal development, and comprise ~15% of total lymphocytes in the neonatal circulation, which is typically equal to or greater than in adults. IL-15 appears to play a central role in NK-cell development, suggesting that NK lineage cells in fetus and neonate have normal IL-15 responsiveness.

NK cells can be divided into CD56[bright] and CD56[dim] populations that are, respectively, specialized for cytokine production and cell-mediated cytotoxicity (Chapter 17).[1] Cord blood CD56[dim] NK cells have markedly higher levels of expression of the CD94/NKG2A inhibitory receptor and significantly lower expression of several types of killer inhibitory receptors (multiple KIRs and LIR-1/ILT2), and the NKG2D activating receptor than adult peripheral blood NK cells.[24] The functional consequence of these differences in receptor expression remains unclear. Cord blood NK cells overall have a markedly reduced capacity for cytotoxic granule release and natural cytotoxicity against K562 erythroleukemia cells and for antibody-dependent cellular cytotoxicity against anti-CD20 mAb-coated Raji cells compared to adult NK cells.[24] Full cytotoxic function is not

probably achieved until at least 9–12 months of age.[1] NK cells from the premature infant also have more pronounced reductions in cytotoxic function than those of the term neonate. In contrast, IL-2-stimulated killing of K562 cells by cord blood NK cells is comparable to that by adult NK cells, suggesting a potential cytokine immunotherapeutic strategy, and CD56[dim] cord blood NK cells have a markedly greater capacity to produce IFN-γ in response to IL-12 p70 and IL-18 stimulation compared to their adult NK cell counterparts.[24] Thus, neonatal NK cells do not have generalized immaturity in function, but rather have a functional capacity that is distinct from that of adult NK cells.

Phagocytes

Neutrophils

Mature neutrophils are first detected by 14–16 weeks of gestation. At mid-gestation, postmitotic neutrophils constitute only 10% of circulating leukocytes and are also in markedly lower numbers in the bone marrow compared to term newborns and adults. Sepsis and other perinatal complications can cause neutropenia, and severe or fatal sepsis is often associated with persistent neutropenia, particularly in preterm neonates. Neutropenia may be associated with increased margination of circulating neutrophils, which occurs early in response to infection. Sustained neutropenia often reflects depletion of the neonate's limited postmitotic neutrophil storage pool. Importantly, septic neutropenic neonates in whom the neutrophil storage pool is depleted are more likely to die than are those with normal neutrophil storage pools. Reduced G-CSF production can also be a factor in neutropenia, although this does not appear to be a major mechanism in most cases of neutropenia associated with sepsis.

Neonatal phagocytic function is also limited by reduction or delays in neutrophil migration from the blood to sites of infection and inflammation.[1] This may explain why the early inflammatory response in neonatal skin often contains a larger number of eosinophils than in adult skin and why the transition from a neutrophilic to a mononuclear cell-dominated response is delayed in the newborn. The combination of a deficiency in the abundance of L-selectin and ability to shed this protein from the surface of neonatal neutrophils, and decreased binding of these cells to P-selectin may contribute to defective cell adhesion to activated endothelium. Neonatal neutrophil chemotaxis leukotrienes, IL-8, and other stimuli may also be impaired. In contrast, phagocytosis and killing by neonatal neutrophils, including by NADPH oxidative and nonoxidative mechanisms, are largely intact, but can be compromised when opsonins are limiting or the bacterial density is high. These deficits in uptake and killing are greater in preterm neonates. The NADPH oxidative pathway of signaling is also involved in the generation of neutrophil extracellular traps (NETs), which are lattices of extracellular DNA, chromatin, and antibacterial proteins. Cord blood neutrophils from both preterm and term deliveries have impaired NET formation compared to adult peripheral blood neutrophils, and this may compromise the antibacterial defenses of neonates.[25]

Mononuclear phagocytes

Blood monocytes of neonates and adults are similar in number and phagocytic and microbicidal activity. By contrast, migration of neonatal monocytes into sites of inflammation, such as delayed-type hypersensitivity reactions, is reduced.[1] The capacity of mononuclear phagocytes to produce pro-inflammatory cytokines, e.g., IL-1β, -6, -8, and -12/-23 p40 is substantially reduced in premature neonates[1,26] and is associated with decreased expression of signaling molecules, such as MyD88.[26] These limitations in mononuclear cell function may be compounded by a concomitant deficiency in production of IFN-γ by neonatal T cells and NK cells, and by impaired responsiveness of neonatal mononuclear phagocytes to IFN-γ.[1] However, cord blood monocytes of term newborns have a significantly greater capacity than adult peripheral monocytes to express IL-12/-23 p40 and a reduced capacity for TNF-α production in response to TLR ligands.[1]

Humoral mediators of inflammation and opsonization

Compared with adults, neonates have moderately diminished alternative complement pathway activity and slightly diminished classic complement pathway activity (Chapter 20). Fibronectin and mannan-binding lectin concentrations are also slightly lower. Consistent with these findings, neonatal sera are less effective than adult sera in opsonization either in the absence of antibody or at low titers of antibody. Generation of complement-derived chemotactic activity is also moderately diminished. These differences are greater in preterm than in term neonates. Preterm neonates may also have compromised lung defenses as a result of reduced abundance of surfactant apoprotein A. These deficiencies, in concert with phagocyte deficits described above, may contribute to delayed inflammatory responses and impaired bacterial and fungal clearance in neonates.

Host defense mechanisms against specific pathogens

Herpes simplex virus

> #### ● KEY CONCEPTS
>
> **Potential mechanisms contributing to the severity of primary herpes simplex virus (HSV) infection of the neonate**
>
> - Reduced type I interferon production by plasmacytoid dendritic cells
> - Decreased production of IL-12 p70 by CD11c+ dendritic cells
> - Decreased natural killer cell-mediated and antibody-dependent cellular cytotoxicity against HSV-infected target cells
> - Diminished and delayed HSV-specific CD4 T-cell responses, including Th1 cells

HSV infection is severe in term infants infected at the time of parturition or postnatally up to 4 weeks of age, and characteristically spreads rapidly to produce disseminated disease, in which liver involvement and disseminated intravascular coagulation and/or central nervous system disease in is frequent.[11] Deficiencies in the function of neonatal NK cells, CD11c+ DCs, and pDCs are probably important contributors to the poor early control

of infection by the mechanisms of innate immunity. Reduced pDC function, including type I IFN secretion, and based on murine studies, the activation by pDCs of CD4 T cells in the tissues may be particularly important in the severity of neonatal HSV infection.[3] Fetal and neonatal NK cells have reduced natural and antibody-dependent cytotoxicity against HSV-infected target cells. These decreased NK-cell responses are likely to be relevant, as rare patients with selective NK-cell deficiency are also highly susceptible to severe and early disseminated infection with HSV and other herpes viruses.

Following primary HSV infection neonates do not achieve HSV-specific CD4 T-cell responses until 3–6 weeks after clinical presentation, whereas adults develop robust responses within 1 week.[11] Since CD4 T cells provide multiple effector functions that may be critical for the resolution of HSV infection, this marked lag could be an important contributor to the tendency for dissemination and severe organ damage. The basis for the delayed development of HSV antigen-specific CD4 T cells in neonates is not known, nor is it clear if this applies to CD8 T-cell responses. Neonates also have a reduced HSV-specific antibody response following infection compared to adults with primary infection,[11] and passively acquired maternal antibody could play a role in decreasing transmission or ameliorating disease severity in neonatal HSV.

Group B streptococci

> #### ● KEY CONCEPTS
>
> **Potential mechanisms that may contribute to the high frequency and severity of group B streptococcal (GBS) infections in the neonate**
>
> - Reduced surfactant apoprotein A in the lungs of preterm neonates
> - Decreased numbers of alveolar lung macrophages, particularly in the preterm neonate, that can effectively phagocytose and kill GBS in the lung
> - Limitations in the local generation of chemotactic factors and/or deficits in the chemotactic responses of neonatal neutrophils
> - Decreased neutrophil killing at sites of infection because of limited amounts of opsonins and, in some individuals, neutrophil microbicidal activity
> - Decreased killing due to engagement of Siglec-5 on neutrophils and mononuclear phagocytes by GBS proteins
> - Limited neutrophil storage pool in bone marrow compartment—important cause of neutropenia in overwhelming infection.

In the absence of maternally derived type-specific antibodies, the neonate is at risk for GBS infection. There are subtle but cumulative limitations in a number of other host defense mechanisms that account for the marked susceptibility of the neonate to GBS infection.[1] For example, neonates lack secretory IgA and have reduced amounts of fibronectin in their secretions compared to older individuals. Reduced amounts of surfactant apoprotein A in the lungs of preterm neonates, a paucity of alveolar macrophages in the lungs, particularly in preterm infants, and diminished phagocytosis and killing of GBS by these cells may facilitate invasion through the respiratory tract. Limitations in the generation of chemotactic factors and/or deficits in the chemotactic responses of neonatal neutrophils may delay recruitment of neutrophils to sites of infection. Neonatal neutrophils that reach sites of infection may kill bacteria less efficiently because of limited amounts of opsonins available for a high local density of GBS, or because the microbicidal activity of neutrophils from certain neonates is decreased. Rapidly progressive infection can deplete the limited marrow neutrophil reserve compounding this problem. GBS may compound these developmental limitations in phagocyte function by its β protein engaging Siglec-5 on neutrophils and mononuclear phagocytes, which impairs phagocytosis, the oxidative burst, and extracellular trap production.[27]

Once GBS infection is established, the adequacy of neutrophil production may be critical for preventing morbidity and mortality. Severe or fatal sepsis from GBS is often associated with persistent neutropenia, particularly in preterm neonates, and most likely reflects the depletion of the postmitotic neutrophil storage pool in the bone marrow.

Although the use of intravenous immunoglobulin in the prevention or treatment of neonatal GBS and other pyogenic infections is theoretically attractive, multiple clinical trials suggests that this approach does not consistently reduce mortality.[1] However, monoclonal antibody therapy for neonatal sepsis holds promise based on the results from a study using an anti-lipotechoic humanized monoclonal antibody to prevent staphylococcal sepsis in prematurely born neonates.[28]

Summary

The human fetus and neonate have both quantitative and qualitative deficiencies of innate and acquired immunity as well as skewing of innate immune response toward particular effector functions compared to the adult. Increased bacterial infections of the neonate, as seen in neonatal nurseries and intensive care units in major medical centers, result from impaired production or function of soluble factors that serve as opsonins and defective mobility and chemotaxis of phagocytes, as well as their inability to be produced at high levels under stress. Increased viral infections in neonates obtains from functional deficiencies of NK cells, CD11c+ DCs, and pDCs as well as diminished and delayed CD4 T-cell responses that stimulate cytolytic CD8 T cells. Thus, the very beginning of life is marked by a period of high risk for infection. Better countermeasures are needed for the protection of infants during this time, which may include specific immunotherapy.

References

1. Lewis DB, Wilson CB. Developmental immunology and role of host defenses in the fetal and neonatal susceptibility to infection. In: Remington JS, Klein JO, Wilson CB, et al., editors. Infectious Diseases of the Fetus and Newborn Infant. 7th ed Philadelphia: Elsevier; 2010. p. 80–191.
2. Merindol N, Charrier E, Duval M, Doudeyns H. Complimentary and contrasting roles of NK cells and T cells in pediatric umbilical cord blood transplantation. J Leukoc Biol 2011;90:49–60.
3. Lewis DB. Neonatal T-cell immunity and its regulation by innate immunity and dendritic cells. In: Ohls R, Yoder MC, editors. Hematology, Immunology, and Infectious Diseases: Neonatology, Questions and Controversies. Philadelphia: Elsevier; 2011; in press.
4. Schuster C, Vaculik C, Fiala C, et al. HLA-DR+ leukocytes acquire CD1 antigens in embryonic and fetal human skin and contain functional antigen-presenting cells. J Exp Med 2009;206:169–81.
5. Nguyen M, Leuridan E, Zhang T, et al. Acquisition of adult-like TLR4 and TLR9 responses during the first year of life. PLoS One 2010;5:e10407.
6. Corbett NP, Blimkie D, Ho KC, et al. Ontogeny of Toll-like receptor mediated cytokine responses of human blood mononuclear cells. PLoS One 2010;5:e15041.
7. Weerkamp F, de Haas E, Naber B, et al. Age-related changes in the cellular comparison of the thymus in children. J Allergy Clin Immunol 2005;115:834–40.
8. Haines CJ, Giffon TD, Lu LS, et al. Human CD4+ T cell recent thymic emigrants are identified by protein tyrosine kinase 7 and have reduced immune function. J Exp Med 2009;206:275–85.
9. Mold JE, Venkatasubrahmanyam S, Burt TD, et al. Fetal and adult hematopoietic stem cells give rise to distinct T cell lineages in humans. Science 2010;330:1695–9.
10. Michaelsson J, Mold JE, McCune JM, Nixon DF. Regulation of T cell response in the developing fetus. J Immunol 2006;176:5741–8.
11. Muller WJ, Jones CA, Koelle DM. Immunobiology of herpes simplex virus and cytomegalovirus infections of the fetus and newborn. Curr Immunol Rev 2010;6:38–55.
12. Tu W, Chen S, Sharp M, et al. Persistent and selective deficiency of CD4+ T cell immunity to cytomegalovirus in immunocompetent young children. J Immunol 2004;172:3260–7.
13. White OJ, Rowe J, Richmond P, et al. Th2-polarisation of cellular immune memory to neonatal pertussis vaccination. Vaccine 2010;28:2648–52.
14. Weitzel RP, Lesniewski ML, Havernik P, et al. microRNA 184 regulates expression of NFAT1 in umbilical cord blood CD4+ T cells. Blood 2009;94:6648–57.
15. Chen L, Cohen AC, Lewis DB. Impaired allogeneic activation and T-helper 1 differentiation of human cord blood naïve CD4 T cells. Biol Blood Marrow Transplant 2006;12:160–71.
16. Vermijlen D, Brouwer M, Donner C, et al. Human cytomegalovirus elicits fetal γδ T cell responses in utero. J Exp Med 2010;207:807–21.
17. Thobakgale CF, Ramduth D, Reddy S, et al. Human immunodeficiency virus-specific CD8+ T-cell activity is detectable from birth in the majority of in utero-infected infants. J Virol 2007;81:12775–84.
18. Suryani S, Tangye SG. Therapeutic implications of advances in our understanding of transitional B-cell development in humans. Exp Rev Clin Immunol 2010;6:765–75.
19. Kaur K, Chowdhury S, Greespan NS, et al. Decreased expression of tumor necrosis factor family receptors involved in humoral immune responses in preterm neonates. Blood 2007;110:2948–54.
20. Schroeder Jr HW. Similarity and divergence in the development and expression of the mouse and human antibody repertoires. Dev Comp Immunol 2006;30:118–35.
21. Williams JV, Weitkamp J-H, Blum DL, et al. The human neonatal B cell response to respiratory syncytial virus uses a biased antibody variable gene repertoire that lacks somatic mutations. Mol Immunol 2009;47:407–14.
22. Griffin DO, Holodick NE, Rothstein TL. Human B1 cells in umbilical cord and adult peripheral blood express the novel phenotype CD20+CD27+CD43+CD70-. J Exp Med 2011;208:67–80.
23. Bennelykke K, Pipper CB, Bisgaard H. Transfer of maternal IgE can be a common cause of increased IgE levels in cord blood. J Allergy Clin Immunol 2010;126:657–63.
24. Le Garff-Tavernier M, Veziat V, Decocq J, et al. Human NK cells display major phenotypic and functional changes over the life span. Aging Cell 2010;9:527–35.
25. Yost CC, Cody MJ, Harris ES, et al. Impaired neutrophil extracellular trap (NET) formation: a novel innate immune deficiency of human neonates. Blood 2009;113:6419–27.
26. Lavoie PM, Huang Q, Jolette E, et al. Profound lack of interleukin (IL)-12/IL-23-40 in neonates born early in gestation is associated with an increased risk of sepsis. J Infect Dis 2010;202:1754–63.
27. Carlin AF, Chang Y-C, Areschoug T, et al. Group B Streptococcus suppression of phagocyte functions by protein-mediated engagement of human Siglec-5. J Exp Med 2009;206:1691–9.
28. Weisman LE, Thrackray HM, Steinhorn RH, et al. A randomized study of a monoclonal antibody (pagibaximab) to prevent staphylococcal sepsis. Pediatrics 2011;128:271–9.
29. Balloch A, Licciardi PV, Russell FM, et al. Infants aged 12 months can mount adequate serotype-specific IgG responses to pneumococcal polysaccharide vaccine. J Allergy Clin Immunol 2010;126:395–7.
30. Licciardi PV, Balloch A, Russell FM, et al. Pneumococcal polysaccharide vaccine at 12 months of age produces functional immune responses. J Allergy Clin Immunol 2012;129:794–800.

Jörg J. Goronzy,
Cornelia M.
Weyand

Aging and the immune system

It is not surprising that the quality and quantity of an immune response is primarily determined by age. This age dependency is apparent throughout life. Many infectious childhood diseases take a different course when the infection is first encountered during adulthood. More strikingly, morbidity and mortality from infections increase in the elderly population. As early as at age 40, vaccine responses to selected vaccines, e.g., hepatitis B, start to decline. Incidence of herpes zoster, a reactivation of latent varicella zoster virus (VZV), starts to increase at the age of 50 years, as does morbidity and mortality from influenza infection. The decline in immune competence is not linear; in particular, a more abrupt transition appears to occur in the eighth decade of life.

The mechanisms underlying the immune dysfunction in the elderly are broadly termed immunosenescence.[1] In terms of public health, immunosenescence is of increasing importance because of the changing population demographics, with increases in the percentage of individuals older than 65 years in both industrialized and developing countries (although to a lesser extent in the latter). Infections are a major cause for morbidity in the elderly. Vaccinations that have changed the infectious landscape in children and young adults have only been partially successful in the elderly. Moreover, a functional immune system is important for tissue repair, of increasing importance with age in degenerative diseases, and in cancer surveillance.

● KEY CONCEPTS

Immune aging is associated with:
- Declined ability to fight infection and cancer
- Reduced vaccine responses
- Increased propensity for autoimmunity
- Constitutive production of inflammatory mediators

The term immunosenescence is reminiscent of cellular senescence, which was originally defined as the inability of somatic cells to proliferate. Senescent cells not only have a cell cycle arrest, but also a change in morphology and metabolic behavior.[2] A convenient marker of a senescent cell is the increased activity of the lysosomal enzyme β-galactosidase (senescence-associated β-galactosidase or SAβ-gal). Functionally more important are changes in gene expression in senescent cells, in particular, of inflammatory cytokines in various cell types, including cells not derived from hematopoietic precursor cells (HPCs). As the immune system is a highly dynamic and proliferative system, with kinetics and growth-stimulating and control mechanisms vastly distinct for different cellular constituents, it is under constant stress to maintain homeostasis and at risk to develop an imbalance between subpopulations with age.

Age and immune cell generation

The immune system is in constant demand for cellular replenishment to compensate for peripheral losses and cell death. For neutrophils, which have a short half-life, the body needs to produce $\sim 10^{10}$ cells/kg per day. Even for lymphocytes, which are more long-lived but are also more frequent due to their settling in lymphoid tissues, the daily need is on the order of several billion cells. The principal precursor cell for all myeloid and lymphoid lineages is the hematopoietic stem cell (HSC). Studies in the 1960s showed that the hematopoietic tissue in bone marrow decreases with age. A similar decline is seen when the frequencies of peripheral $CD34^+CD45^+$ HSC are determined (Fig. 33.1). Primitive HSC appear to be spared from this decline; in fact, Rossi, Weissmann, and colleagues found an age-related increase in the frequencies of lineage $CD34^+CD38^-CD90^+$ HSC.[3] Functionally, aged HSC are compromised. Telomerase expression in the peripheral HPC is not fully protective and a shortening in telomeric length is seen with age in humans, similar to more differentiated peripheral mononuclear cells. Reconstitution potential is reduced, possibly driven by accumulated DNA damage. Interestingly, gene expression in HSC does not only exhibit quantitative, but also qualitative changes. The activation and repression of lineage-specific gene programs is age-dependent.[4] As a consequence, lineage potential shifts from the lymphoid to the myeloid line. This shift may contribute to the clinical observation that HSC-derived leukemia preferentially has a lymphoid phenotype in the young and a myeloid one in the elderly. Epigenetic dysregulation of differentiation programs in clonal HSC populations can give rise to

● KEY CONCEPTS

Influences of age on immune cell generation
- Hematopoietic stem cells are reduced in frequency and biased towards the myeloid and against the lymphoid lineages
- Myeloid cell generation is largely intact
- B-cell generation declines and B-cell repertoire selection is disturbed
- Thymic involution causes a decline and eventual demise of T-cell generation
- Homeostatic proliferation of peripheral T cells takes over as the major source of T-cell production
- Ability to rebuild a T-cell repertoire after lymphocyte-depleting interventions is severely compromised after mid-adulthood

myelodysplastic syndromes. Moreover, in the healthy elderly individual myeloid cells do not decrease, and may even increase, with age. And peripheral neutrophil numbers do not decline and are able to recover after therapy-induced depletion (e.g., chemotherapy). Furthermore, there is no loss in the ability to generate robust neutrophilia in response to infection or other stressors (Fig. 33.1).

In contrast to myeloid cells, generation of naïve B cells declines with age (Fig. 33.1). In addition to HSC-intrinsic lineage commitments, defects in blood-borne factors and bone marrow niches contribute.[5] The majority of investigators describe a decline in the absolute and relative numbers of memory CD27[+] B cells with not all memory B-cell subsets being equally affected.[6] Reduced B-cell generation and expansion of antigen-specific B cells with age should result in a contraction of the aging repertoire. Preliminary studies have shown that this is indeed the case, in particular in frail elderly.[7] Also, monoclonal gammopathies of undetermined significance representing clonal benign expansion of plasma cells are observed in more than 5% of individuals older than 70 years. Purging of autoreactive cells during B-cell selection may be compromised in an attempt to compensate for the reduced B-cell generation that would explain that autoantibodies are a common phenomenon with increasing age.[8] B-cell responses may primarily rely on the adaptation of existing memory sequences per hypermutation rather than recruitment of new naïve B cells. Moreover, in clinical settings where B cells are specifically depleted in the treatment of B-cell malignancies or autoimmune diseases or are killed as a side effect of chemotherapy, recovery in the elderly host will be incomplete and delayed.[9]

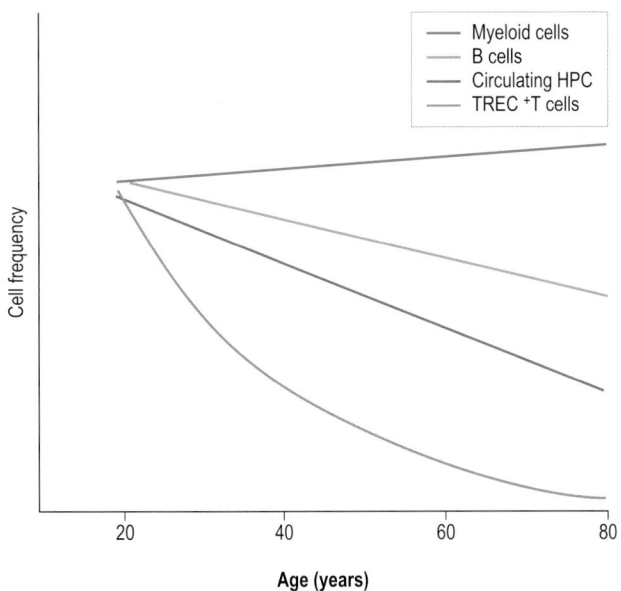

Fig. 33.1 Influence of age on the regeneration of hematopoietic lineages. The schematic diagram illustrates the effect of age on the generation of hematopoietic cell lineages. Frequencies of CD45RA[+]CD38[+] hematopoietic precursor cells, myeloid cells, T-cell receptor excision circle (TREC)-containing T cells and naïve B cells in the blood are arbitrarily set at 100% at age of 20 years. Because of their short half-life and lack of peripheral proliferation, frequencies of myeloid cells reflect their generation. T-cell receptor excision circles are a marker of recent thymic emigrants, although they tend to overestimate thymic production, in particular in later age. In most individuals, thymic production is irrelevant after the age of 50 years. Hematopoietic precursor cells do not only show a decline with age, but also a qualitative switch towards production of myeloid instead of lymphoid cells. T-cell generation is additionally impacted by thymic involution.

T-cell generation is more affected by aging than any other myeloid or lymphoid systems due to the involution of the thymus. The thymus undergoes dramatic structural changes that begin during childhood and puberty. Thymopoietic niches disappear and the frequency of thymic epithelial cells and thymocytes declines. In parallel, the thymic perivascular space increases.[10] One major structural change is the accumulation and infiltration of adipocytes in the perivascular space that does not appear to be a compensatory response, but rather an active and regulated developmental step in thymic organ transformation.[11,12] However, thymic activity during adult life has a crucial role as thymic resection in children undergoing cardiac surgery can reproduce many of the T-cell repertoire changes in a 20-year-old individual that are usually seen in elderly 70 to 80 year-olds.[13] Single joint T-cell receptor excision circles, taken as an indicator of thymic output, exhibit a log linear decline with age (Fig. 33.1). The low frequencies in the elderly cannot be taken as evidence for ongoing production, but may indicate the survival of long-lived naïve T cells. Intervention studies, mostly in bone marrow transplantation patients or patients undergoing chemotherapy, but also after treatment with T-cell-depleting antibodies, have suggested that after the age of 40 to 50 years the regenerative capacity is too miuscule to rebuild a naïve T-cell repertoire in the vast majority of individuals.

Throughout adulthood, homeostatic proliferation of naïve T cells accounts for the bulk and eventually for all of T-cell generation. Homeostatic cytokines such as IL-7 and recognition of self major histocompatibility complex (MHC) molecules regulate proliferation and survival. For human CD4 T cells, this process is relatively robust under steady state conditions (Fig. 33.2); frequencies of naïve CD4 T cells only moderately decline with age.[14] Only after the age of 70 to 75 years, contraction in diversity is seen, possibly as a consequence of accelerated cell death.[15] In general, homeostatic proliferation in a lymphopenic host, e.g., after cytotoxic medical interventions, cannot restore a functional naïve T-cell system. Accelerated homeostatic proliferation is associated with transition into a memory-like or even an effector cell type.[16] The CD8 T-cell compartment is less stable with age (Fig. 33.2); it is unclear whether this is due to defective T-cell generation or a consequence of chronic immune stimulation (see below).

Cumulative antigenic stimulation with age and T-cell population homeostasis

The adaptive system responds to antigenic challenges with clonal expansion and differentiation into effector cells followed by clonal downsizing and persistence of long-lived memory T cells. Infections therefore leave a permanent imprint on the immune system, on which vaccinations capitalize. However, the pathogen-induced clonal expansion also represents a challenge to homeostatic mechanisms that are supposed to maintain a balance among naïve, memory, and effector cells. This is particularly evident in persisting infections where the offending pathogen cannot be cleared. Most of the current understanding is based on T-cell homeostasis in chronic viral infections, although B cells are certainly also affected. Persistent infections represent a continuum from latent infections with no or infrequent reactivation such as seen with herpes viruses to continuous viral replication at different rates such as with hepatitis C and human immunodeficiency virus. Chronic infection with replicating viruses leads to clonal exhaustion, an actively induced program that limits immune responses through the expression

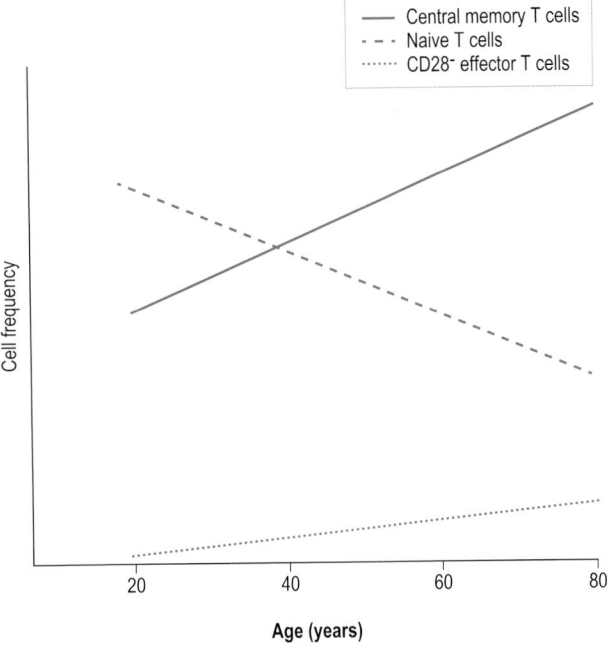

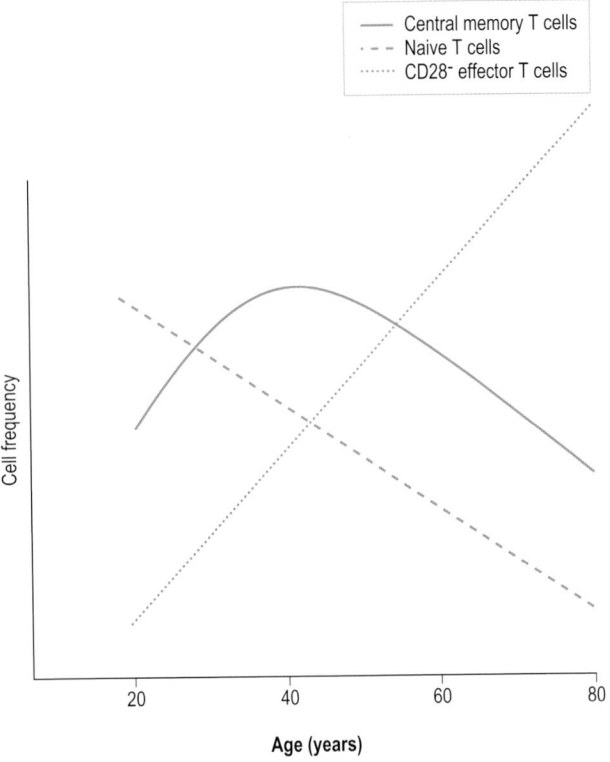

Fig. 33.2 Influence of age on T-cell subset distribution. CD4 and CD8 memory and effector T-cell frequencies increase with age at the expense of naïve T cells. Most remarkable is an increase in end-differentiated effector CD8 T cells, in part driven by chronic cytomegalovirus infection. In general, subset homeostasis is more robust for CD4 than CD8 T cells.

of inhibitory receptors PD1, TIM3, and LAG3 and additional functional defects.[17] T-cell exhaustion is typical for these diseases, but is not a general feature of immune aging. In contrast, herpes virus infections are highly prevalent in apparently healthy population without causing an active disease, as they establish latency in specific cell types. Classical examples are varicella zoster virus (VZV), Epstein-Barr virus (EBV), and cytomegalovirus (CMV). The effects of these herpes viruses with immune aging differ largely; the mechanisms for these differences are unknown. VZV tends to relapse with age, and episodes of reactivation present as shingles. A decrease in the frequency of VZV-specific CD4 memory T cells has been postulated to explain this lack in viral control mechanisms.[18] In contrast, EBV and CMV infections only relapse in severely immunocompromised individuals, but not during normal immune aging. Chronic CMV infection is particularly instructive from an immune aging perspective. The virus can be acquired throughout a lifetime, with about 30% of all individuals infected by the age of 20 and nearly 90-100% in the elderly. The CD8 T-cell response to CMV is extraordinarily large, suggesting a lack in clonal downsizing. CD8 T cells to one single CMV epitope can encompass between 1 and 20% of the entire T-cell compartment; the entire CMV response can entail more than 50% of all CD8 cells in an elderly individual. Many of these cells have the phenotype of end-differentiated effector T cells that lack the expression of CD28 and CD27 and re-express CD45RA.[19] The expansion of these end-differentiated cells compromises the size of naïve and central memory CD8 cell compartments (Fig. 33.2). This memory inflation appears to have broad implication for overall immune health.[20] The size of the CD8+CD28− T-cell compartment is predictive of defective vaccine responses to influenza and has been associated with a shorter lifespan in octogenarians. The mechanism of how expanded CMV-specific cells affect the overall immune system are unknown; possibly memory inflation has a negative impact due to space competition or expanded highly differentiated T cells have a direct regulatory effect and suppress activation of unrelated T cells. Memory inflation is seen much less frequently for EBV and certainly not for VZV, raising the question why CMV has such an unusual role. Memory inflation to CMV also occurs for CD4 cells, however, without causing an imbalance between different memory cell subpopulations; expansion of end-differentiated CD28−CD4+ effector T cells in healthy elderly is much less frequent than for the CD8 compartment. The expansion of the CD8+CD28−CD45RA+ compartment, including but not limited to CMV-specific cells, is likely the major component of the immune-risk phenotype, originally defined as an inverted ratio of CD4 to CD8 T cells that has been associated with increased mortality and immune dysfunction. CD8+CD28−CD45RA+ T cells differ substantially from exhausted CD8 T cells seen with chronic highly replicating viruses. CD45RA+CD28− end-differentiated effector cells do not express the inhibitory receptors PD1, TIM, or LAG3, or the pro-apoptotic molecule Bim, nor are they defective in cytotoxic activity or production of IFN-γ or TNF-α, all characteristic features of exhausted cells. However, they express MHC class I recognizing inhibitory receptors of the killer cell lectin-like, killer immunoglobulin-like receptors, and immunoglobulin-like transcript families.[21] These inhibitory receptors do not appear to affect effector functions *in vivo*, but their expression may be beneficial by constraining otherwise unopposed expansion of these cells.

KEY CONCEPTS

Depending on virus and host, chronic viral infection with increasing age is associated with:

- T-cell exhaustion and accumulation of dysfunctional T cells (e.g., hepatitis C)
- Memory inflation and accumulation of terminally differentiated, fully functional CD8 effector T cells (e.g., CMV)
- Loss of antigen-specific T cells (e.g., VZV)

Inflamm-aging and the aging host environment

The aging host environment is characterized by the continuous presence of inflammatory mediators independent of acute or chronic disease (Fig. 33.3).[22] Even for the healthy elderly, IL-6 and tumor necrosis factor levels are two- to fourfold higher than in the serum of young adults. Indisputably, low-level systemic inflammation plays an important role in the progression of several age-related diseases including Alzheimer's disease, atherosclerosis, and cancer. Moreover, inflammatory markers are associated with several conditions that are characteristic of the elderly. IL-6 serum concentrations have been correlated with loss of mobility and disability; increased mortality among older individuals has been shown for those who have higher levels of TNF-α. Increased IL-6 and C-reactive protein serum levels and increased white blood cell counts, presumably due to increased numbers of neutrophils, predispose for, and are associated with, frailty. A causative relationship may also exist between the increased production of IL-6 and TNF-α and the age-associated loss in muscle mass eventually presenting as sarcopenia. Long-lived individuals, such as centenarians, tend to have lower levels of pro-inflammatory cytokines and increased levels of anti-inflammatory mediators such as cortisone and IL-10, supporting the concept that low-level inflammation is detrimental for healthy aging.

Production of inflammatory cytokines is driven by several mechanisms with contributions differing in individuals. The immune system itself, in particular the innate immune system, is certainly a major source. Senescence of the adaptive immune system leads to a less effective control of chronic viral infections as well as incomplete response to exogenous challenges, thereby leading to increased and prolonged innate immune activation. The gastrointestinal system plays a unique role. Defective epithelial barrier function, as well as decline in the mucosa-associated lymphoid tissue, results in a lack of containment of bacterial growth. The relevance of this mechanism has been shown for HIV-infected patients in whom the mucosa-associated lymphoid tissue is destroyed and who have increased systemic levels of lipopolysaccharides. In addition to innate immune activation, remodeling of the adaptive immune system also favors an inflammatory response. As delineated above, aging is associated

with the expansion of effector cell populations, in part driven by chronic viral infections. Such CD8 effector cells acquire many features of NK cells, are cytotoxic, and produce IFN-γ and TNF-α, both in response to antigen and after nonspecific stimulation.

> ● **KEY CONCEPTS**
>
> Increased constitutive production of inflammatory mediators with age (inflamm-aging) is caused by:
> - Activation of the innate immune system due to defective epithelial barrier function and defective adaptive immunity
> - Accumulation of adipocytes producing inflammatory mediators
> - Accumulation and activation of T-effector-cell populations
> - DNA damage-induced gene activation in senescent cells

The immune system, however, is not the only source of inflammatory cytokines. Cell senescence has been associated with the production of cytokines. Persistent DNA damage response signaling will not only develop an irreversible cell cycle block characteristic of cellular senescence, but will also initiate a transcriptional program to secrete numerous growth factors, proteases, and cytokines, also termed the senescence-associated secretory phenotype (SASP). SASP has been shown to provide a pro-inflammatory environment that is locally conducive to cancer cell transformation and growth, but also that systemically contributes to the chronic inflammation characteristic of the elderly.

Cellular defects and senescence

Depending on the cell type and the pathway, the cytokine milieu in the elderly conditions activates as well as attenuates signaling pathways. Low responsiveness to cytokine stimuli is frequently seen in those cells that have increased baseline activation of a signaling pathway (e.g., cells that constitutively have increased STAT3 or STAT1 phosphorylation respond less to IL-6/GM-CSF or type I/II interferons, cytokines that activate these STATs). Attenuation of signaling pathways by induction of negative feedback loops in part explains the reduced responsiveness

Fig. 33.3 Inflamm-aging. The schematic diagram depicts possible mechanisms that account for the increased production of inflammatory mediators with age. These mediators contribute to many of the age-associated diseases.

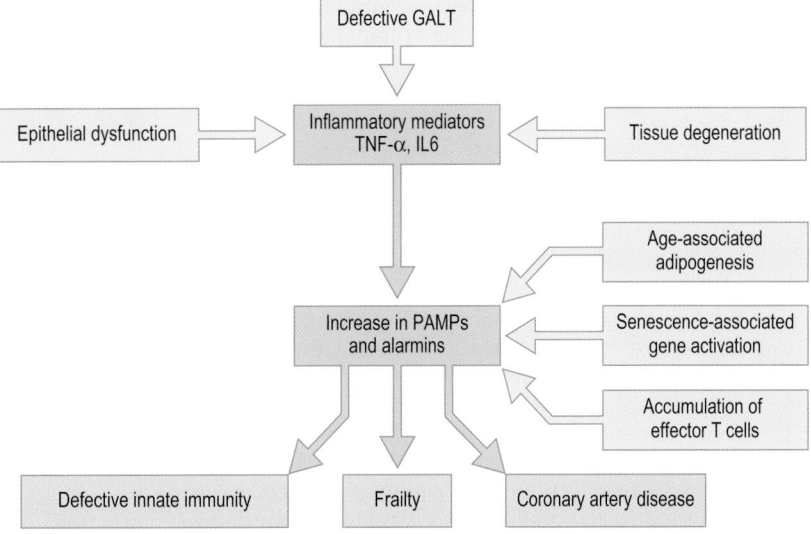

and functionality of cells of the innate immune system. Obviously, it is important to know whether cellular defects are intrinsic or conferred by the host environment, because therapeutic approaches are different.

KEY CONCEPTS

Influences of age on cells of the immune system
- Telomeric erosion impairs proliferative competence and restraints clonal expansion
- End-differentiation reduces functional plasticity
- Activation of specific gene programs modifies cell function

  - Genes associated with T-cell exhaustion (e.g., PD1)
  - Loss of CD28 on T cells
  - Gain in NK cell-associated regulatory receptors on T cells (e.g., KIR, KLR, ILT)
  - Senescence-associated gene activation (e.g. inflammatory mediators)
  - Global epigenetic changes

While neutrophil and monocyte/macrophage numbers are normal in old age, many of their functions decline with age.[23,24] Decreased chemotaxis in neutrophils delays tissue infiltration; reduced phagocytosis and respiratory burst compromise the ability to control bacterial infections; TLR-induced monocyte/macrophage activation is reduced in the elderly. In a recent study, the delayed hypersensitivity reaction to *Candida albicans* antigen in the skin of elderly individuals was attributed to decreased activation and cytokine production of macrophages *in situ* that hampered recruitment of T cells to the antigenic challenge.[25] When stimulated *ex vivo*, macrophage dysfunction was not apparent. A similar dichotomy has been shown for dendritic cells. Plasmacytoid and myeloid dendritic cells studied directly *ex vivo* exhibited declines in Toll-like receptor responses, which correlated with the ability to respond to flu vaccination. In contrast, dendritic cells established from monocytes of elderly individuals by *in vitro* cultures with growth factors had increased production of inflammatory cytokines.

Adaptive immune cells are also directly affected by the proinflammatory environment in the aging host, but age-related activation of genetic response programs are of at least equal relevance.[26,27] The program most obviously influenced by age is the induction of cellular senescence. In all hematopoietic cell lineages including stem cells, telomeric lengths decline with age.[28] This is of particular importance for T cells because much of their response depends on their ability to proliferate and clonally expand. Telomeric erosion is due to cumulative replicative history and DNA damage, but also because the ability to express telomerase and repair telomeric ends declines with cell differentiation and aging.

Lymphocytes in the elderly are always more differentiated than those in the young. While most obvious for CD8 T cells, increasing differentiation can also be noted for B cells and CD4 T cells. Differentiation into memory and effector cells is generally driven by antigen recognition, but may also occur in the absence of exogenous antigen under the influence of cytokines. A classical example is that under lymphopenic conditions, increased T-cell homeostatic proliferation is associated with the acquisition of memory-like and effector phenotypes.[16] Most striking in the elderly is the accumulation of a terminally differentiated CD8 effector T-cell population, phenotypically defined by the expression of CD45RA and eventually CD57 and the loss of CD27 and CD28.[19] These cells are highly equipped to exert effector functions including the production of cytokines and cytotoxic

activity, but can no longer differentiate into memory cells. One of their hallmarks is the expression of MHC class I recognizing receptors including killer lectin-like receptors (KLRG) and killer immunoglobulin-like receptors (KIRs), as well as NKG2D and ILT2. With the exception of NKG2D and a few KIR isoforms, most of these receptors are inhibitory; they express an ITIM motif in their cytoplasmic domain and suppress activation signals delivered through stimulatory receptors by recruiting a phosphatase. Some of these receptors, such as NKG2D, KIR2DL4, and the KIR2DS isoforms have stimulatory or co-stimulatory function. Because the combination of regulatory receptors on individual cells is stochastic, T cells with predominantly stimulatory or inhibitory receptors can be found. In general, inhibitory receptors prevail and proliferation and clonal expansion is inhibited, but only to a lesser degree T-cell effector function.

Terminal T-cell differentiation is different from the T-cell exhaustion program, which is not a feature of healthy aging but occurs in response to chronic infections with high rate of viral replication.[29] Elderly T cells display additional changes in gene expression, which cannot all be summoned under the mechanisms described above (inflammatory cytokine-induced, senescence-associated, differentiation, and exhaustion).

Clinical consequences of immune aging—immunodeficiency, autoimmunity, and accelerated degenerative diseases

The most profound and most noted consequence of human senescence is the increased susceptibility to infections. Upper respiratory bacterial infections (e.g., by *Streptococcus pneumoniae*) and urinary tract infections are frequent in an elderly population and less well contained by the innate immune system and pre-existing adaptive immunity. Not surprisingly, the elderly immune system is not able to induce a protective response to new mostly viral challenges to which the individual has not been exposed to in the past. Clinically important examples are the recent SARS epidemic and infections with the West Nile fever virus. First-time vaccinations with live viruses, for example yellow fever virus, are associated with increased morbidity and even mortality in the elderly. Despite annual vaccination, influenza infections remain a major threat in the elderly population associated with high morbidity and mortality. Pneumonia due to respiratory syncytial virus, usually infecting young children, is not uncommon. Immune competence to chronic infections is also compromised with age. The best example here is the reactivation of the VZV that presents as chickenpox in

---

CLINICAL RELEVANCE

Immune aging accounts for:
- Increased morbidity and mortality from bacterial infections (e.g., pneumococci)
- Increased morbidity and mortality from viral infection (e.g., influenza, West Nile fever)
- Reactivation of latent virus (e.g., VZV)
- Ineffective primary and booster vaccinations
- Acceleration of degenerative diseases due to the production of inflammatory mediators (e.g., atherosclerotic disease, Alzheimer disease, osteoarthritis)
- Increased incidence of autoimmune disease (e.g., polymyalgia rheumatica, giant cell arteritis, rheumatoid arthritis)

---

the young and relapses as shingles in the elderly. The one exception of a chronic persisting infection is CMV for which even in the very elderly reactivation with clinical complications is rarely observed. Vaccinations against pneumococcal antigens, influenza strains, and VZV are recommended in the elderly; however, vaccine efficacy is limited and unsatisfactory.[30]

The degenerative process associated with immune aging also predisposes for autoimmune manifestations and a breakdown in self-tolerance (Fig. 33.4). Autoantibodies are a common finding in healthy elderly; many of these autoantibodies are specific for common autoantigens such as antibodies to IgG Fc or to nuclear components. The risk for several autoimmune diseases increases with age. This is most strikingly the case for polymyalgia rheumatica and giant cell arteritis.[31] While polymyalgia rheumatica predominantly presents as an activation of the innate immune system, giant cell arteritis is clearly a disease of the adaptive immune system with T-cell-dependent granulomatous inflammation in the vascular wall of mid-sized and large arteries. Incidence of many other autoimmune diseases that can occur in middle-aged adults continues to rise with increasing age including rheumatoid arthritis and many other less frequent diseases.[32]

The low-grade inflammatory process in the aging host has direct clinical consequences (Fig. 33.3). Inflammation promotes frailty and sarcopenia; it accelerates numerous degenerative diseases including coronary artery disease, osteopenia, and degenerative diseases of the nervous system including Alzheimer's disease. Accelerated immune aging may be one of the reasons that autoimmune diseases, such as rheumatoid arthritis, are associated with a shorter lifespan and increased risk for cardiovascular morbidity. Inflammation as a cause of accelerated aging has been also implicated to explain the increased morbidity and mortality of HIV-infected patients on higly active antiretroviral therapy (HAART).[33]

Strategies and interventions on the horizon

Vaccinations hold the promise to reduce the increased infectious susceptibility in the elderly, but improving vaccine responses has proven to be a challenge.[34] Deficiency in the antigen-presenting system and in the co-stimulatory signals may be overcome by identifying new adjuvants instead to the currently employed aluminum salts.. Stimulation of Toll-like receptors is one promising approach to improve activation of antigen presenting cells in the elderly. In trials, so far TLR9 agonists improved the vaccine response to hepatitis B, which starts to decline after the age of 40. Increasing the vaccine dose is another promising approach. The VZV vaccine used to boost the immune response in the elderly to prevent herpes zoster flares is about 14-fold higher than in the vaccine used to immunize children. Also live vaccines or self-replicating constructs that also accomplish higher antigen loads may not have a sufficient safety profile in the elderly.

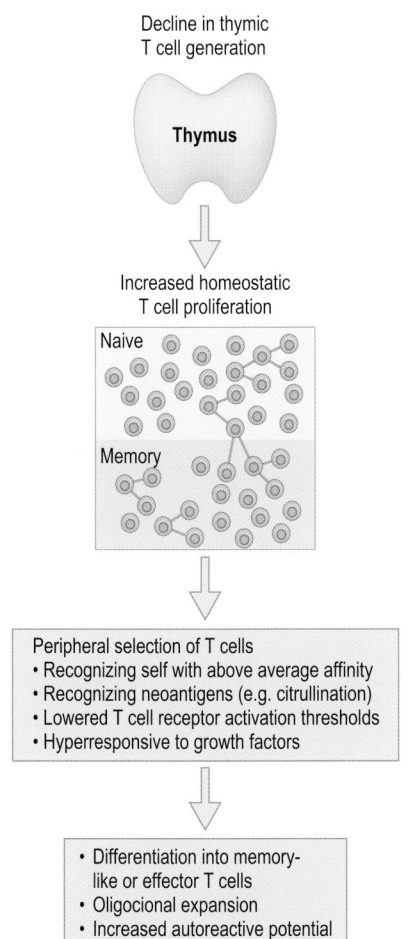

Decline in thymic
T cell generation

Thymus

Increased homeostatic
T cell proliferation

Naive

Memory

Peripheral selection of T cells
• Recognizing self with above average affinity
• Recognizing neoantigens (e.g. citrullination)
• Lowered T cell receptor activation thresholds
• Hyperresponsive to growth factors

• Differentiation into memory-
  like or effector T cells
• Oligoclonal expansion
• Increased autoreactive potential

Fig. 33.4 Influence of age on T-cell tolerance. Age is associated with a defect in tolerance mechanisms that range from harmless autoantibody production to increased risk for several autoimmune diseases. Regulatory T cells do not appear to be reduced or defective with age. The diagram shows a model where T-cell homeostatic mechanisms in the absence of thymic production generate a repertoire that is prone to autoimmunity. A similar model has been proposed for B-cell selection.

ON THE HORIZON

- Thymic rejuvenation (e.g., with KGF, IL-7, and other mediators)
- Prevention of chronic infection that accelerate immune aging (e.g., immunization for CMV)
- Improved vaccination strategies and technologies (e.g., novel adjuvants, novel vaccine delivery systems, pharmacological approaches to improve T- and B-cell activation, clonal expansion and differentiation)

Obviously, a proper T-cell response to infectious organisms or to vaccines depends on the availability of a T-cell repertoire that includes specificities to respond. Thymic involution and memory inflation due to chronic infections are currently implicated in compromising the T-cell repertoire. The true impact of memory inflation and the underlying mechanisms are currently under investigation and may eventually lead to preventive interventions to prevent infections or to limit expansion and survival of disproportionately expanded T cells. Thymic rejuvenation is being explored in individuals who have a depleted T-cell repertoire, such as patients recovering from HIV infection or patients treated for cancer with chemotherapy and/or bone marrow transplantation. Approaches include manipulation of the concentration of various cytokines and hormones.[35,36] Beyond finding an effective way to restore thymic activity, future studies also need to keep in mind that thymic activity in the adult and in the elderly may have unwanted side effects as thymic involution is not a typical age degenerative process, but appears to be developmentally regulated.[12]

As it is unclear what drives increased inflammation in the elderly and the likely mechanisms are multifactorial, such interventions at present need to be nonspecific. Such immunomodulatory therapy is obviously standard practice in patients with autoimmune disease who exhibit accelerated aging and increased all-cause mortality, such as rheumatoid arthritis, Calorie restriction to slow immune aging is not well accepted by humans to an extent that it is effective. Statins and aspirin have been routinely used to prevent cardiovascular disease; their effect may be mostly anti-inflammatory. Treatment with hydroxychloroquine is explored in HIV patients under HAART treatment to reduce the increased incidence of cardiovascular disease and age-related degenerative disease of vital organ systems. If this concept proves to be effective, future applications will require the development of mild and low-toxicity medications to reduce low-grade inflammation.

References

1. Dicarlo AL, Fuldner R, Kaminski J, et al. Aging in the context of immunological architecture, function and disease outcomes. Trends Immunol 2009;30:293–4.
2. Rodier F, Campisi J. Four faces of cellular senescence. J Cell Biol 2011;192:547–56.
3. Beerman I, Maloney WJ, Weissmann IL, Rossi DJ. Stem cells and the aging hematopoietic system. Curr Opin Immunol 2010;22:500–6.
4. Geiger H, Rudolph KL. Aging in the lympho-hematopoietic stem cell compartment. Trends Immunol 2009;30:360–5.
5. Cancro MP, Hao Y, Scholz JL, et al. B cells and aging: molecules and mechanisms. Trends Immunol 2009;30:313–8.
6. Ademokun A, Wu YC, Dunn-Walters D. The ageing B cell population: composition and function. Biogerontology 2010;11:125–37.
7. Dunn-Walters DK, Ademokun AA. B cell repertoire and ageing. Curr Opin Immunol 2010;22:514–20.
8. Quinn 3rd WJ, Scholz JL, Cancro MP. Dwindling competition with constant demand: can homeostatic adjustments explain age-associated changes in peripheral B cell selection? Semin Immunol 2005;17:362–9.
9. Townsend MJ, Monroe JG, Chan AC. B-cell targeted therapies in human autoimmune diseases: an updated perspective. Immunol Rev 2010;237:264–83.
10. Lynch HE, Goldberg GL, Chidgey A, et al. Thymic involution and immune reconstitution. Trends Immunol 2009;30:366–73.
11. Dixit VD. Thymic fatness and approaches to enhance thymopoietic fitness in aging. Curr Opin Immunol 2010;22:521–8.
12. Dowling MR, Hodgkin PD. Why does the thymus involute? A selection-based hypothesis. Trends Immunol 2009;30:295–300.
13. Sauce D, Larsen M, Fastenackels S, et al. Evidence of premature immune aging in patients thymectomized during early childhood. J Clin Invest 2009;119:3070–8.
14. Goronzy JJ, Lee WW, Weyand CM. Aging and T-cell diversity. Exp Gerontol 2007;42:400–6.
15. Goronzy JJ, Weyand CM. T cell development and receptor diversity during aging. Curr Opin Immunol 2005;17:468–75.
16. Surh CD, Sprent J. Homeostasis of naive and memory T cells. Immunity 2008;9(29):848–62.
17. Kim PS, Ahmed R. Features of responding T cells in cancer and chronic infection. Curr Opin Immunol 2010;22:223–30.
18. Arvin A. Aging, immunity, and the varicella-zoster virus. N Engl J Med 2005;352:2266–7.
19. Akbar AN, Fletcher JM. Memory T cell homeostasis and senescence during aging. Curr Opin Immunol 2005;17:480–5.
20. Derhovanessian E, Larbi A, Pawelec G. Biomarkers of human immunosenescence: impact of Cytomegalovirus infection. Curr Opin Immunol 2009;21:440–5.
21. Weng NP, Akbar AN, Goronzy J. CD28(-) T cells: their role in the age-associated decline of immune function. Trends Immunol 2009;30:306–12.
22. Kanapuru B, Ershler WB. Inflammation, coagulation, and the pathway to frailty. Am J Med 2009;122:605–13.
23. Kovacs EJ, Palmer JL, Fortin CF, et al. Aging and innate immunity in the mouse: impact of intrinsic and extrinsic factors. Trends Immunol 2009;30:319–24.
24. Panda A, Arjona A, Sapey E, et al. Human innate immunosenescence: causes and consequences for immunity in old age. Trends Immunol 2009;30:325–33.
25. Agius E, Lacy KE, Vukmanovic-Stejic M, et al. Decreased TNF-alpha synthesis by macrophages restricts cutaneous immunosurveillance by memory CD4 + T cells during aging. J Exp Med 2009;206:1929–40.
26. Maue AC, Yager EJ, Swain SL, et al. T-cell immunosenescence: lessons learned from mouse models of aging. Trends Immunol 2009;30:301–5.
27. Nikolich-Zugich J, Rudd BD. Immune memory and aging: an infinite or finite resource? Curr Opin Immunol 2010;22:535–40.
28. Hodes RJ, Hathcock KS, Weng NP. Telomeres in T and B cells. Nat Rev Immunol 2002;2:699–706.
29. Akbar AN, Henson SM. Are senescence and exhaustion intertwined or unrelated processes that compromise immunity? Nat Rev Immunol 2011;11:289–95.
30. Chen WH, Kozlovsky BF, Effros RB, et al. Vaccination in the elderly: an immunological perspective. Trends Immunol 2009;30:351–9.
31. Weyand CM, Goronzy JJ. Medium- and large-vessel vasculitis. N Engl J Med 2003;349:160–9.
32. Goronzy JJ, Shao L, Weyand CM. Immune aging and rheumatoid arthritis. Rheum Dis Clin North Am 2010;36:297–310.
33. Deeks SG. HIV infection, inflammation, immunosenescence, and aging. Annu Rev Med 2011;62:141–55.
34. Aspinall R, Del Giudice G, Effros RB, et al. Challenges for vaccination in the elderly. Immun Ageing 2007;4:9.
35. Taub DD, Murphy WJ, Longo DL. Rejuvenation of the aging thymus: growth hormone-mediated and ghrelin-mediated signaling pathways. Curr Opin Pharmacol 2010;10:408–24.
36. Dorshkind K, Montecino-Rodriguez E, Signer RA. The ageing immune system: is it ever too old to become young again? Nat Rev Immunol 2009;9:57–62.

34.

Primary antibody deficiencies

Harry W. Schroeder, Jr., Ewa Szymanska-Mroczek

Primary antibody deficiency diseases are characterized by an inability of the humoral immune system to produce sufficient quantities of protective antibodies to properly protect the host from hazardous antigens.[1] This inability may be evident from birth or it may manifest at a later age. In some cases, the deficiency may either resolve or worsen with time.[2] Many of these diseases are caused by mutations that alter the function of genes that regulate B-cell development or homeostasis. Others reflect mutations in the immunoglobulin genes themselves. In some of the most common conditions, a genetic predisposition has been well documented, but the underlying defect remains unclear. The typical patient will present with a history of recurrent upper or lower respiratory infections and reduced serum concentrations of one or more classes of immunoglobulin (IgM, IgG, or IgA). However, patients with normal serum immunoglobulin levels may exhibit specific deficits in their ability to mount a protective response against certain antigens, and some virtually agammaglobulinemic patients can be remarkably asymptomatic. A classification of primary antibody deficiency diseases can be found in Table 34.1.

Primary immune deficiency disorders are the consequence of specific defects in B-cell development (Chapter 7). B-cell production begins in the fetal liver, and shifts to the bone marrow in the latter stages of fetal life (Fig. 34.1). As B cells mature, they leave the liver and the bone marrow and migrate via the blood into secondary lymphoid organs, primarily the spleen but also the lymph nodes, as well as other peripheral and mucosal tissues. Contact with a polymeric cognate antigen, such as a polysaccharide, activates the B cell and allows it to differentiate into an antibody producing plasma cell. The response to protein antigens, including toxins and viral proteins, requires T-cell help. In the germinal centers, B cells can replace an upstream heavy (H) chain constant domain with a downstream one, e.g., IgM to IgG_1, altering effector function. They can also introduce mutations at a high level into the variable domains, tailoring the antibody to the antigen, a process termed affinity maturation.

Clinical manifestations

Patients with antibody deficiencies most commonly present with a history of recurrent sinusitis, bronchitis and pneumonia. Patients may also present with recurrent cellulitis, boils, gastrointestinal discomfort, myalgias, arthralgias, fatigue and depression. The respiratory infections typically involve encapsulated bacterial pathogens such as *Streptococcus pneumoniae* and *Haemophilus influenzae*. Protection against these bacteria requires production of anti-polysaccharide antibodies, which does not require T-cell help. Because a similar susceptibility for infection is seen among patients who are deficient in neutrophil function or in the pivotal third component of complement (C3), all three of these arms of the host defense system should be evaluated in patients who suffer with recurrent bacterial infections.

The clinical course of uncomplicated primary infections with viruses such as varicella zoster or mumps does not differ significantly from that of the normal host. However, antibody-deficient patients have difficulty generating long-lasting immunity, thus chickenpox may repeatedly recur as shingles. This suggests that while T cells are sufficient to control established viral infections, antibodies best function to limit the initial dissemination of virus and prevent re-infection. There are exceptions to this general rule. Hypogammaglobulinemic patients can have difficulty clearing hepatitis B virus from the circulation, poliovirus from the gut, and enterovirus from the brain, leading to progressive and sometimes fatal outcomes.

Because sinopulmonary infections are also commonly seen in normal infants and children, in allergic individuals, in smokers, and in patients with other diseases such as cystic fibrosis, the threshold for an extensive evaluation for immunodeficiency can be a matter of clinical judgment. However, two or more episodes of bacterial pneumonia within a five-year period, unexplained bronchiectasis, *H. influenzae* meningitis in an older child

---

⬤ CLINICAL PEARLS

Clinical manifestations of antibody deficiency

- Recurrent bacterial infections
  - Early in untreated disease, infections are primarily due to encapsulated pyogenic bacteria (e.g., *Streptococcus pneumoniae* and *Haemophilus influenzae* type b).
  - Later in untreated disease, damage to mucosal surfaces engenders susceptibility to staphylococci, nontypable *H. influenzae*, and Gram-negative rods, as well.
- Recurrent viral infections
  - In most cases, viral infections are cleared normally, but protective immunity does not develop. For example, recurrent shingles can be a common symptom in untreated patients.
  - In some cases, patients may continue to excrete virus after resolution of their clinical symptoms.
- Increased prevalence of other immunologic disorders
  - Paradoxic increased risk of antibody-mediated autoimmune disorders, such as idiopathic thrombocytopenia, autoimmune thyroiditis, systemic lupus erythematosus, and celiac disease
  - Lymphoid hypertrophy.
  - Increased risk of allergic disorders, especially among patients with IgA deficiency.

Table 34.1 Primary antibody deficiencies

Disorder	Gene or locus	Chromosome
IgA deficiency/Common variable immunodeficiency		
IgA deficiency/Common variable immunodeficiency	MHC	6p21.3
TACI deficiency (AD/AR)	*TNFRSF13B* (IgAD2, CVID2)	17p11.2
ICOS deficiency (AR)	*ICOS* (CVID1)	2q33
BAFF-R (AR)	*TNFRSF13C* (CVID4)	22q13.1-q13.31
CD19 deficiency (AR)	*CD19* (CVID3)	16p11.2
CD20 deficiency (AR)	*CD20* (CVID5)	11q13
CD81 deficiency (AR)	*CD81* (CVID6)	11p
Transient hypogammaglobulinemia of infancy (THI)	Unknown	Unknown
X-linked agammaglobulinemia (XL)	*BTK*	Xq21.3-q22
X-linked agammaglobulinemia with growth hormone deficiency (XL)	*BTK*	Xq21.3-q22
Hyper-IgM syndrome		
X-linked hyper-IgM syndrome (XHM)(XL)	*CD154 or CD40L* (HIGM1)	Xq26
Activation-induced cytidine deaminase deficiency (AR/AD)	*AID* (HIGM2)	12p13
CD40 deficiency (AR)	*CD40* (HIGM3)	20q12-q13.2
Uracil-DNA glycosylase (UNG) deficiency (AR)	*UNG* (HIGM5)	12q23-q24.1
XHM with ectodermal dysplasia (XHM-ED) (XL)	*NEMO* (HIGM6)	Xq28
Autosomal agammaglobulinemia (AGM)		
Ig-associated Igα deficiency (AR)	*CD79A* (AGM3)	19q13.2
Ig-associated Igβ deficiency (AR)	*CD79B* (AGM6)	17q23
Ig μ H chain deficiency (AR)	*IGHG1* (AGM1)	14q32.33
BLNK deficiency (AR)	*BLNK* (AGM4)	10q23.2
Surrogate light chain deficiency (AR)	*IGLL1* (AGM2)	22q11.21
LRRC8 truncation (AD)	*LRRC8* (AGM5)	9q34.13
Selective IgG subclass deficiencies		
Immunoglobulin γ H chain deficiencies (AR)	*IGHG1*	14q32.33
Selective κ light chain deficiency (AR)	*IGKC*	2p12
Selective λ light chain deficiency (AR)	*IGLC*	22q11.2
Antibody deficiency with normal serum immunoglobulin levels		
Vκ A2 deficiency (AR)	*IGKV2D-29*	2p12

Autosomal dominant (AD), autosomal recessive (AR), X-linked (XL).

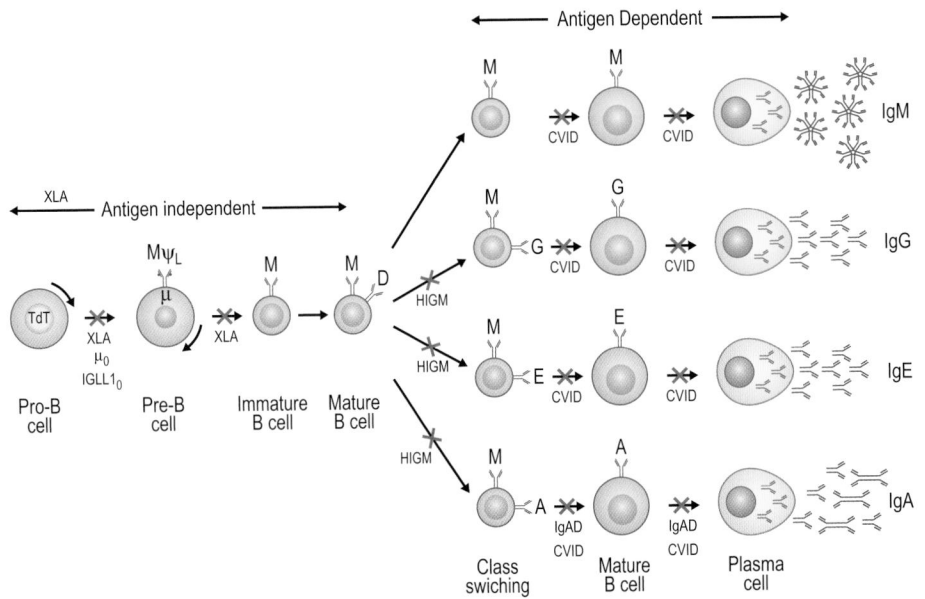

Fig. 34.1 Defects in B-cell development can lead to humoral immune deficiency. X-linked agammaglobulinemia (XLA) and autosomal agammaglobulinemias (AGM) result from either a failure to generate a functional antibody receptor signaling complex or a failure to transmit signals from this complex. These failures obstruct production of immature B cells. Hyper-IgM syndromes (HIGM) result from either a failure to engage in proper cognate interactions with T cells or disruptions in the genes that permit class switch recombination or somatic hypermutation. These failures inhibit class switching to IgG, IgA, and IgE, as well as limiting affinity maturation. Common variable immune deficiency (CVID), IgG subclass deficiencies (IgSD), selective IgA deficiency (IgAD), and transient hypogammaglobulinemia of infancy (THI) reflect a selective or generalized failure to progress from the immature B-cell stage to the plasma cell stage. This failure can occur as a consequence of an abnormal BCR co-receptor complex (CD19, CD81), of limitations in factors controlling B-cell homeostasis (TACI, BAFFR) or from difficulty receiving late stage T-cell help (ICOS).

or adult, chronic otitis media in an adult, recurrent intestinal infections and diarrhea due to *Giardia lamblia*, or a family history of immunodeficiency all warrant evaluation.

The purest forms of antibody deficiency result from mutations that allow VDJ rearrangement but prevent the expression or function of the pre-B-cell receptor. For example, a function-loss mutation of the μ heavy chain or components of the surrogate light chain (VpreB, λ14.1(λ5)) will affect only the B-cell lineage. However, these rare immune deficiencies are the exception, because most of the diseases associated with primary antibody deficiency involve more than one cell lineage. For example, *X-linked agammaglobulinemia* (XLA) is the product of loss-of-function mutations in Bruton tyrosine kinase *(BTK),* a key component of the BCR signal transduction pathway. BTK is also expressed in neutrophils, and under stressful conditions XLA patients have developed recurrent neutropenia. Patients with *X-linked hyper-IgM syndrome* (HIGM1) may also exhibit T-cell dysfunction, placing them at risk for infection with *Pneumocystis jiroveci.* Immune deficiency also appears to place patients at risk for autoimmunity, which is increased among patients with *IgA deficiency* (IgAD), *common variable immunodeficiency* (CVID), and hyper-IgM syndrome.[3]

Clinical manifestations of the primary immunodeficiency will also be heavily influenced by the patient's medical history. Patients with a delayed diagnosis or in situations wherein their infections have not been treated aggressively may suffer permanent damage to the respiratory or gastrointestinal mucosa, creating susceptibility to nontypable *H. influenzae,* staphylococci, *Pseudomonas* spp., and enteric bacteria as well.

Principles of diagnosis and treatment

Diagnostic tests and their interpretation

Testing for immune deficiency should be performed when the patient has a history of repeated infections that exceeds expectations for normal individuals, when an opportunistic pathogen or one of a low virulence is responsible for an infection, when a diagnosis of a disorder frequently associated with immunodeficiency has been made, or when there is a family history of

Table 34.2 Laboratory diagnosis of primary antibody deficiency

Level	Test	Application(s)
I	CBC with differential	Primary screening tests
	Complement (CH$_{50}$, C3, C4) ESR Quantitative serum IgM, IgG, and IgA levels	
Ia	Urinalysis, 24-hour urine for protein Stool for α-1-antitrypsin	Symptoms suggest protein loss through kidneys or GI tract
II	B-cell functional evaluation	Level I normal but history suggests antibody deficiency
	Quantitative IgG subclasses, IgE Natural or commonly acquired antibodies (isohemagglutinins, rubella, rubeola, tetanus) Response to immunization T-cell-dependent antigens (tetanus) T-cell-independent antigens (unconjugated pneumococcal vaccine, unconjugated *H. influenzae* B vaccine)	Better definition of a Level I defect
III	Quantification of blood T- and B-cell subpopulations by immunofluoresence assays using monoclonal antibody markers T cells: CD3, CD4, CD8 B cells: CD19, CD20, CD21, Ig (μ, δ, κ, λ),	Panhypogammaglo-bulinemia or severely low IgM and IgA
IV	Disease-specific analysis Gene expression Gene sequencing	Gene-specific diagnosis Genetic counseling

primary immunodeficiency. Table 34.2 illustrates four levels of testing complexity and when such testing might commonly be undertaken.

Level I testing is both revealing and cost effective. It includes measuring serum immunoglobulin (IgM, IgG, and IgA), complement (50% hemolytic power of serum (CH$_{50}$) and complement components C3, and C4, a complete blood count with differential (CBC/diff), and an erythrocyte sedimentation rate (ESR). Lymphopenia is found most often in disorders that affect the production or function of T cells (Chapter 35), but can also occur in patients with CVID. Congenital absence of an individual complement component will result in total absence of measurable complement-mediated hemolysis (Chapter 20). The ESR is often, although not always, elevated in individuals with inflammatory disorders and can be useful in the evaluation of patients with a questionable or unclear history of recurrent or chronic infection.

Interpretation of the significance of the quantitative immunoglobulin determinations requires appreciation of age-related changes in immunoglobulin concentrations (Fig. 34.2).[4,5] At the end of the second trimester of pregnancy, there is active transport of IgG across the placental barrier. At birth the infant's serum IgG concentration is typically 20–25% higher than that of the mother. Catabolism of maternal IgG coupled with the slow development of endogenous antibody function leads to a physiologic nadir of serum IgG in infants of 4–6 months of age. In normal infants, this loss of maternal protection is often associated with the first appearance of otitis media or bronchitis. Thus, the onset of sinopulmonary infections within the first three months of age should also raise the index of suspicion for immunodeficiency in the mother. After age 6 months, maternally derived IgG has largely been lost and IgG antibodies specific for diphtheria or tetanus become useful functional measures.

CLINICAL PEARLS

Interpreting quantitative immunoglobulins

- Normal ranges of serum immunoglobulin levels vary with age; hence, evaluation should take the age of the patient into account.
  - As the mother's transplacental contribution of IgG is catabolized, total serum IgG concentrations reach a nadir at 4 to 6 months of age.
  - IgG$_2$ and IgG$_4$ subclass levels rise more slowly than IgG$_1$ and IgG$_3$; hence, reference to adult controls can lead to the false diagnosis of IgG subclass deficiency in young children.
  - Serum IgA concentrations typically do not achieve adult values until puberty. They are often the first to decline in many primary immunodeficiencies.

IgM is the first isotype to reach young adult levels, followed by total IgG and then IgA. This physiologic delay in the production of serum IgA can complicate the diagnosis of IgA deficiency in infants and young children. Serum immunoglobulin concentrations in healthy adults tend to remain remarkably constant, but can increase dramatically in response to infection as well as suffer a decline in response to immunosuppressive agents, such as corticosteroid administration. With increasing age, serum immunoglobulin may continue to rise.[5] The physiologic significance of this increase in the elderly is unclear, although in some cases it reflects an accumulation of expanded B-cell clones or monoclonal gammopathies (Chapter 80).

KEY CONCEPTS

Functional Tests of Specific Antibody Production

- IgM T-independent responses may be assessed by measurement of serum isohemagglutinins (anti-A and anti-B titers) in patients who are not blood type AB.
- IgG T-independent responses may be assessed by measurement of antibodies produced in response to immunization with unconjugated purified pneumococcal polysaccharide vaccine.
- IgG T-dependent recall responses may be assessed by measurement of a fourfold or greater rise in titer of antibodies to diphtheria or tetanus toxoid alter booster immunization.

The common laboratory practice of defining the lower range of normal for serum immunoglobulin levels as two standard deviations below the age-adjusted mean carries with it the risk of falsely labeling otherwise normal patients immunodeficient. Immunoglobulin levels vary widely with environmental exposure and normal biologic variation is much broader than that defined by the mean of the population. Symptomatic patients with IgA deficiency may demonstrate normal total IgG levels, but have a high IgG$_1$ level that masks deficiencies of IgG$_2$ and IgG$_4$. Patients with a combined deficiency of IgA and an IgG subclass may benefit from more aggressive therapy; thus quantitative measurements of all four IgG subclasses IgG$_1$, IgG$_2$, IgG$_3$, and IgG$_4$ can be useful in fully defining the extent of humoral immune deficiency. Among patients with borderline serum IgG levels, tests to evaluate the host's ability to produce functional specific antibody should be performed prior to making a

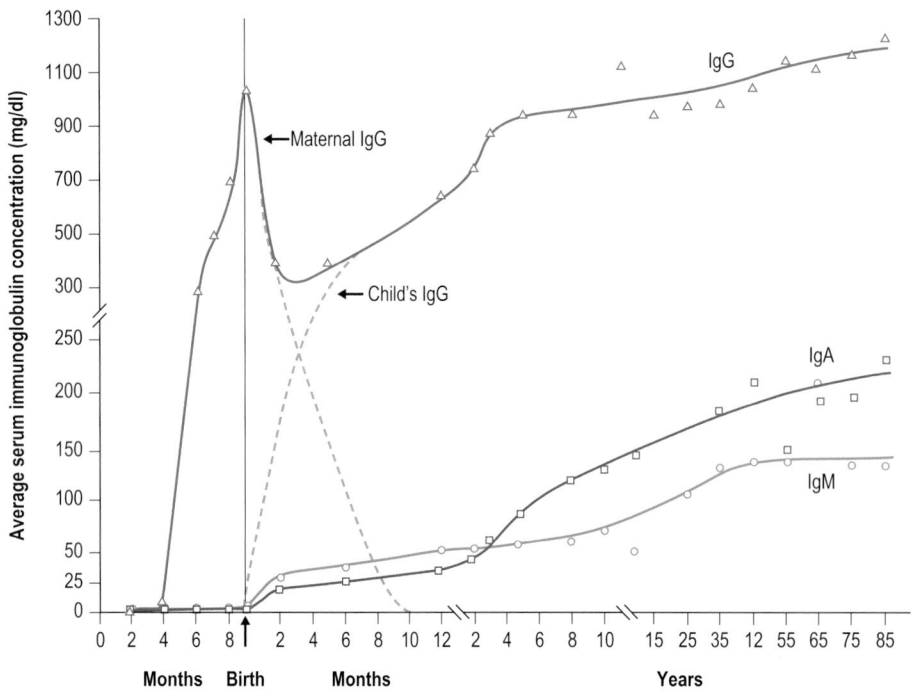

Fig. 34.2 Age-related changes in the serum concentration of immunoglobulins. Average serum immunoglobulin concentrations of the major isotypes are shown as a function of age.[5,6]

decision to institute a more aggressive therapy, especially among patients receiving corticosteroids, which can lower total serum IgG while preserving function. The most commonly employed tests include measurement of isohemagglutinins (naturally occurring IgM antibodies to the polysaccharide antigens that define the ABO blood type system on red blood cells) and post-immunization responses to polysaccharide antigens (e.g., pneumovax or unconjugated *H. influenzae* B vaccine) and protein antigens (e.g., tetanus or diphtheria toxoids) (Chapter 95). IgM is made by the newborn, and most infants can generate isohemagglutinins, making determination of anti-A and anti-B titers a useful measurement of B-cell function even in infants. (In older children and adults, isohemagglutinin titers of less than 1:8 are considered significant.[6]) Serum for specific antibody titers should be obtained before and 3 to 4 weeks after immunization. Optimally, the paired sera should be assayed simultaneously to avoid confusion that may result from single-tube dilution differences at the time the assay is performed. As a general rule, a high baseline titer or a fourfold or greater rise in a specific titer in individuals with a low baseline titer confirms that a specific humoral response is intact. Measurement of anti-pneumococcal polysaccharide titers can be complicated by the physiologic unreliability of responses to unconjugated polysaccharides prior to the age of 2 (although this belief has been challenged).[7] The development of conjugated polysaccharide vaccines further complicates analysis for children and young adults who have received such a vaccine, although information can still be gleaned from study of responses to polysaccharide antigens present only in multi-valent unconjugated vaccines.

Because of its relatively low molecular weight and slow turnover compared with other isotypes, protein loss through the kidneys or gastrointestinal tract can result in the selective loss of IgG. Should symptoms warrant, 24-hour urine for protein or a stool sample for α-1-antitrypsin level can document protein loss.

An elevated IgE level can support a suspicion of allergy as an underlying explanation of sino-pulmonary symptoms. Serum IgE concentrations are often elevated in patients with IgA deficiency. Extreme elevations of IgE suggest the *hyper-IgE syndrome*.

Enumeration of B and T cells should be performed for any individual who has severe panhypogammaglobulinemia. The most widely used method of demonstrating B cells relies on immunofluorescent labeling of surface CD19, which is restricted in expression to mature B cells. Because an infant may have serum IgG of maternal origin for the first several months of life, the determination of the number of circulating B cells is the single most useful test in making the presumptive diagnosis of XLA, a disorder in which pre-B cells in the bone marrow fail to develop to cells of mature phenotype. Absence of circulating B cells also characterizes the *immunodeficiency associated with thymoma* in adults, whereas adults with *chronic lymphocytic leukemia* may have hypogammaglobulinemia with an overabundance of circulating B cells that typically express CD5.

X-linked hyper-IgM syndrome (HIGM1) represents the product of a loss-of-function mutation of the *CD154* (*CD40L*) gene. CD154, a surface antigen found on activated T cells, binds CD40 on B cells to facilitate class switching, survival, and proliferation (Chapter 12). A fluorescent-labeled CD40 fusion protein can be used to evaluate the expression of functional CD154 on T cells by flow cytometry. X-linked agammaglobulinemia (XLA) reflects a loss-of-function mutation of *BTK*. As typical for previously lethal X-linked disorders, a high percentage of cases represent new mutations. Confirmation of the diagnosis, carrier detection, and prenatal diagnosis often depend on a molecular or sequence analysis of the gene in question.

Replacement therapy with human immunoglobulin

There are a number of commercial preparations of human immunoglobulin that are FDA approved and available in the USA (Chapter 85). No commercial preparations are available in the USA to supplement IgM or IgA. All commercial human immunoglobulin preparations are effective in treating patients with immunodeficiency disorders. Clinically relevant differences relate to the route of administration, which can be by intravenous or subcutaneous means, to the method of stabilization and storage, and to quantities of contaminating serum IgA in the preparations. Low IgA content is a concern for those rare individuals with immunodeficiency and absent IgA who manufacture IgG or IgE antibodies directed against IgA and have a history of anaphylactic reactions upon infusion of IgA-containing blood products.[8]

Immunoglobulin replacement therapy is not indicated for patients whose immune deficiency is limited to the selective absence of IgA. Indeed, selective IgA deficiency has long been viewed as a relative contraindication for immunoglobulin replacement because of the risk of anaphylaxis upon receipt of IgA-containing products, even though such reactions are extremely rare. However, immunoglobulin replacement therapy has been found to be beneficial in patients with a combined deficit of IgA and IgG subclasses who exhibit impaired antibody responses to carbohydrate antigens.

The goal of immunoglobulin replacement is to provide sufficient concentrations of functional antibodies to prevent disease, not to achieve a target IgG level in the serum. Specific approaches to and protocols for immunoglobulin replacement therapy[9] are described in detail in Chapter 85. The only indication for immunoglobulin replacement in a patient with immunodeficiency is severe impairment of the ability to produce functional antibody. Such impairment exists in primary immunodeficiency diseases associated with low levels of all five isotypes of immunoglobulin, such as XLA, CVID, HIGM, and *severe combined immunodeficiency* (SCID). Patients with a documented inability to produce specific antibodies after immunization with a history of significant morbidity from infections are also candidates for intravenous immunoglobulin (IVIG) therapy even though they present with normal or near-normal levels of IgG. This includes certain cases of IgG subclass deficiency such as those associated with compound IgA, IgG_2, and IgG_4 deficiency, boys with Wiskott–Aldrich syndrome, and patients with ataxia-telangiectasia. Since most patients with transient hypogammaglobulinemia of infancy can produce normal amounts of specific antibodies after immunization despite having a low total serum IgG, they usually are not candidates for immunoglobulin replacement, although again patients with a history of significant infections may benefit.[10] IVIG is unlikely to be beneficial in selective IgA deficiency or selective IgG_4 deficiency.

X-linked agammaglobulinemia

Diagnosis

XLA, also known as Bruton agammaglobulinemia, is the prototypic humoral immunodeficiency.[11] Function-loss mutations in *BTK* lead to a block in B-cell maturation, a near total absence of B cells in the periphery, and pan-hypogammaglobulinemia. Due to the transplacental transfer of maternal immunoglobulin, affected boys typically do not begin to suffer recurrent pyogenic infections until after age 6 months. The normal delay in endogenous immunoglobulin production and the presence of maternal IgG requires that testing of infants known or suspected to have XLA should begin with examination of the number of B cells in the blood. Deficient expression of BTK protein can be detected by flow cytometry, a technique that can also be used for carrier detection. For those cases where protein is present but the phenotype suggests XLA, analysis of the *BTK* gene at the nucleotide level remains the definitive diagnostic procedure. A large number of different mutations have been found and collected into a disease-specific database known as BTKbase (http://bioinf.uta.fi/BTKbase). As with most X-linked lethal diseases, approximately one-third of sporadic cases are due to *de novo* mutations and diagnosis may require individual mutation analysis. There can be significant variation in the manifestations of the disease in any given family member, thus a paucity of symptoms should not prevent diagnostic evaluation even in adults.[12]

Clinical manifestations

Although patients begin to suffer recurrent infections by age 1 year, with antibiotics and good hygiene it is not uncommon to delay suspicion of the diagnosis until well into mid-childhood. Indeed, diagnoses have been made in older adults, including aged male relatives of affected probands.[12] Recurrent upper and lower respiratory tract infections, including otitis media, sinusitis, bronchitis, and pneumonia, are common. Untreated, these infections can lead to bronchiectasis (Fig. 34.3), pulmonary failure, and death at an early age. The infections are typically due to pyogenic encapsulated bacteria including *S. pneumoniae*, *H. influenzae*, *Staphylococcus aureus*, and *Pseudomonas* spp. Diarrhea due to *G. lamblia* is also common, although less so than in CVID. Systemic infections include bacterial sepsis, meningitis,

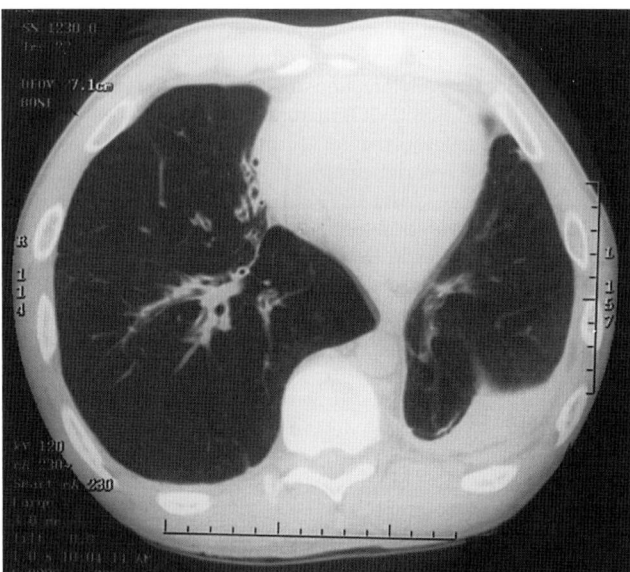

Fig. 34.3 A CT scan, with contrast, demonstrates bronchiectasis, bronchitis, and emphysema in the lungs of a 36-year-old man with XLA. Due to a left lower lobe lobectomy, the mediastium has shifted to the left. As a result of bronchiectatic scarring, the diameter of the bronchi in the right lung is greater than the diameter of the corresponding blood vessels, and the bronchi remain dilated in the periphery. Bronchial plugs can be seen filling some of the bronchi on the right. Finally, due to emphysema, the right upper lobe demonstrates greater radiolucency. In addition to suffering from XLA, this patient has a thirty pack-year history of smoking, which has exacerbated his clinical condition.

osteomyelitis, and septic arthritis. *Mycoplasma* and *Chlamydia* infections of the urogenital tract can lead to epididymitis, prostatitis, and urethral strictures. Skin infections include cellulitis, boils, and impetigo.

Although patients with XLA can resolve most viral infections, they are unusually sensitive to infections with enteroviruses, including echovirus, coxsackievirus, and poliovirus. Patients with XLA can develop paralytic poliomyelitis after vaccination with live virus. Echovirus and coxsackie virus infections can involve multiple organs with patients going on to develop chronic meningoencephalitis, dermatomyositis, and/or hepatitis.

Untreated patients often complain of arthritis affecting the large joints. This appears to have an infectious etiology, because the arthritis typically resolves with immunoglobulin replacement therapy. Enterovirus and *Mycoplasma* have been identified in the affected joints of these patients.

Infections with opportunistic organisms, such as tuberculosis, histoplasmosis and *P. jiroveci*, and malignancies are rare, likely reflecting intact cell-mediated immunity.

Origin and pathogenesis

BTK belongs to a subfamily of the Src cytoplasmic protein-tyrosine kinases. BTK is phosphorylated following activation of the B-cell receptor (BCR). It plays a critical role in the proliferation, development, differentiation, survival, and apoptosis of B lineage cells. Individuals with XLA begin with normal numbers of early B-lineage progenitors in their bone marrow. These B-cell progenitors express the expected markers of B differentiation, including terminal deoxyribonucleotide transferase (TdT), CD19 and CD10. There is, however, a relative deficiency of cells containing cytoplasmic μ heavy chains in the bone marrow. Development of cells beyond the pre-B stage is even more severely impaired. Those cells that make it through the gauntlet can produce antigen-specific antibodies. Although in low numbers, the presence of these B cells in lymphoid tissues enables XLA patients to express endogenous immunoglobulin, class switch, and even suffer allergic or autoantibody-mediated reactions.

Patients have been described with an X-linked recessive form of agammaglobulinemia that is associated with growth hormone deficiency. Genetic analysis of the *BTK* gene in one such patient identified a frameshift mutation leading to a premature stop codon and the loss of carboxy terminal amino acids.

Treatment and prognosis

The primary goal of therapy is to prevent damage to the lungs. Human immunoglobulin replacement therapy should be started as soon as the diagnosis is made (Chapter 85). Patients treated with sufficient quantities (0.4–0.6 g/kg every 3 to 4 weeks for IVIG or 100–150 mg/kg every week for subcutaneous immunoglobulin (SQIG) suffer few lower respiratory tract infections. However, these patients remain at risk for viral infections, including enteroviral meningoencephalitis. Since mucosal immunoglobulin cannot be replaced, the patients also remain at risk for recurrent upper respiratory infections, which may require prophylactic antibiotic therapy. Immunoglobulin-treated patients can lead normal lives without concern about exposure to infectious agents in childcare settings or classrooms.[13] Immunizations designed to elicit protective antibodies are unnecessary because the monthly replacement therapy will provide passive protection. Since patients are unable to mount antibody responses and vaccines, especially live vaccines, carry some risk of untoward side effects, they are relatively contraindicated.

An XLA patient who develops symptoms of enteroviral central nervous system or neuromuscular infection should have appropriate culture of the involved organ system. CSF culture and analysis for cells and protein should be performed and a muscle biopsy for culture should be considered if virus is not recoverable from stool or CSF. Although there are no clear guidelines for managing patients with chronic enteroviral infections, immunoglobulin therapy should be accelerated for at least several weeks and higher doses maintained until symptoms cease and the virus can no longer be detected.

Autosomal agammaglobulinemia

Origin and pathogenesis

The pre-B-cell receptor and signal transduction axis

Expression of the pre-B-cell receptor is a key step in the maturation of the pre-B cell (Chapter 7).[14] Function-loss mutations in any one of the genes that code for components of the pre-BCR and its associated signaling complex can inhibit pre-B-cell development, leading to an absence of mature B cells. This phenotype is seen in patients with biallelic function-loss mutations of the μ heavy chain region (μ$_0$, AGM1), the λ-like surrogate light chain (IGLL1, AGM2), the immunoglobulin-associated α (Igα, CD79A, AGM3) and β (Igβ, CD79B, AGM6) chains and the adaptor B-cell linker protein (BLNK, AGM4), which is a key cytoplasmic component of the pre-BCR signaling pathway.

LRRC8

An absence of B cells has also been reported in a patient with a truncation of *LRRC8* (AGM5), a gene of unknown function that is expressed in progenitor B cells. In this case, the patient was heterozygous for the molecular defect.

Diagnosis and Treatment

Diagnosis in each of these cases requires gene mutation analysis. Treatment follows the same guidelines given for XLA.

Hyper-IgM syndrome

Diagnosis

Patients with the hyper-IgM syndrome exhibit markedly reduced serum concentrations of IgG, IgA, and IgE with normal to elevated levels of IgM and normal numbers of circulating B cells.[15] The altered distribution of immunoglobulin isotypes reflects a block in the ability of B lymphocytes to switch from IgM to the other isotypes. Increased IgM reflects polyclonal expansion of IgM synthesis in response to infection. HIGM patients suffer the same infections with encapsulated bacteria common to all patients with antibody deficiency. The HIGM phenotype can be inherited as an X-linked, autosomal recessive or autosomal dominant trait. The phenotype can also be acquired in association with neoplasia or congenital rubella.

Hyper-IgM syndrome type 1 (HIGM1): CD40L (CD154) deficiency

Class switch recombination is a multi-step process that requires exquisite coordination between the B cell and its cognate helper T cell. A key step in the initiation of the process is the binding of constitutively expressed CD40 on the B cell to its ligand, CD40L (CD154), which is expressed on activated T cells. The most common X form of the disease, X-linked hyper-IgM syndrome (HIGM1) results from loss-of-function mutations in *CD154* (Xq26).

Hyper-IgM syndrome type 2 (HIGM2): AID dysfunction

Activation-induced cytidine deaminase (AID, 12p13), a member of the cytidine deaminase family, is required for class switch recombination between immunoglobulin H chain constant domains and for somatic hypermutation of the immunoglobulin V domains (Chapter 4). AID is expressed only in activated B cells. The hyper-IgM phenotype can result from either biallelic *AID* function-loss mutations or from a dominant negative mutation on only one of the *AID* alleles.

Hyper-IgM syndrome type 3 (HIGM3): CD40 deficiency

The cognate partner for CD40L (CD154) is CD40, the gene for which is located on an autosome (20q12-q13.2). HIGM3 patients with function-loss mutations on both alleles of the *CD40* gene present with a phenotype indistinguishable from HIGM1, with the exception that as an autosomal recessive condition females and males are equivalently affected.

Hyper-IgM syndrome type 4 (HIGM4): as yet unknown causes

Patients presenting with an HIGM-like phenotype, but lacking demonstrable mutations in genes previously associated with HIGM, such as *CD40*, *CD154*, *NEMO*, *AID*, and *UNG*, have been grouped by some immunologists into a category termed HIGM4. B cells from HIGM4 patients demonstrate defective class switch recombination, but normal somatic hypermutation. A genetic cause has yet to be identified and spontaneous recovery has been reported.[16]

Hyper-IgM syndrome type 5 (HIGM5): UNG deficiency

AID acts by deaminating cytidine nucleotides in DNA, leaving a uracil nucleotide in its place. Uracil-DNA glycosylase (*UNG*, 12q23-24.1) can remove the uracil, permitting normal or error-prone repair. Patients with function-loss mutations on both alleles of the *UNG* gene have presented with a history of bacterial infections, hyperplasia, increased serum IgM levels, and low IgG and IgA.

Hyper-IgM Syndrome type 6 (HIGM6): X-Linked hyper IgM with hypohydrotic ectodermal dysplasia (XHM-ED)

The nuclear factor kappa B (NF-κB) essential modulator (NEMO) plays a key role in the CD40 signal transduction pathway. *NEMO* is located on the X-chromosome (Xq28) and its protein product also influences ectodermal development. In addition to hypogammaglobulinemia, XHM-ED patients with mutations in *NEMO* can also present with conical teeth, an absence of eccrine sweat glands, and a paucity of hair follicles.

Clinical manifestations

CD40-CD154 axis (HIGM1, HIGM3, and HIGM6/XHM-ED)

The majority of patients with HIGM have inherited disruptions in the CD40-CD154 axis. The spectrum of disease in these patients has been well-characterized. Recurrent upper and lower respiratory tract infections are the most common clinical complaint. Patients may also exhibit recurrent neutropenia with oral ulcers and perirectal abscesses and opportunistic infections with *P. jiroveci*, *Toxoplasma gondii*, or *Cryptosporidium* cholangitis. Autoimmunity is observed in approximately 20% of patients, and lymph nodes and spleen are deprived of germinal centers. These features signal a compromise in cell-mediated immunity as well as the characteristic flaw in antibody production.

Without prophylaxis, one third of patients develop *P. jiroveci* pneumonia which can be the presenting complaint in affected infants. These patients are also at risk for serious infections with cytomegalovirus (CMV), adenovirus, *Cryptococcus neoformans*, or mycobacteria.

Chronic diarrhea occurs in more than half of the patients. Organisms include *Cryptosporidium*, *G. lamblia*, *Salmonella*, and *Entamoeba histolytica*. One quarter may require total parenteral nutrition due to diarrhea or to perirectal abscesses. Oral ulcers, gingivitis, and perirectal ulcers are associated with neutropenia, which may occur chronically or intermittently in up to two-thirds of the patients. One-fifth of the patients develop sclerosing cholangitis that can lead to hepatic failure. Cryptosporidiosis is present in half of these patients. Infections with hepatitis B and C are associated with exposure to blood products.

Although originally distinguished by the high level of serum IgM, IgM levels are often normal in affected individuals. IgG is low in all patients. IgA and IgE are usually low, but can be normal or even elevated in one-tenth of the patient population. B- and T-cell counts are within the normal range in more than 90% of the patients, and depressed in the rest.

Lymphoid hyperplasia is a common finding in CD40–CD154 axis patients with active infections. Individual nodes may become extremely large and some patients develop splenomegaly. Hilar adenopathy causes a diagnostic dilemma, as the risk of lymphoma is increased in HIGM. Although the lymphoid tissue is usually histologically abnormal, reactive processes are far more common than malignancy. Plasma cells may be abundant or sparse. Primary follicles are poorly developed. The most characteristic abnormality is the absence of germinal centers. Nodular lymphoid hyperplasia of the intestine is frequent and can be accompanied by malabsorption and protein-losing enteropathy. Diffuse lymphoid infiltration of various organs and tissues can also occur.

AID-UNG axis (HIGM2 and HIGM5)

Infected AID-UNG-deficient patients can present with giant germinal centers filled with highly proliferating B cells, presumably due to intense antigen stimulation. Approximately 25% of HIGM2 patients, but not HIGM5, present with evidence of autoimmunity. Manifestations include hemolytic anemia, thrombocytopenia and autoimmune hepatitis. Autoantibodies in these patients are of the IgM isotype. Unlike deficiencies of the CD40–CD154 axis, cell-mediated immunity is unaffected.

Origin and pathogenesis

CD40-CD154 axis (HIGM1, HIGM3, and HIGM XHM-ED)

CD154, a member of the tumor necrosis factor (TNF) family, is a type II transmembrane protein that is predominantly expressed on mature, activated CD4 T cells. Its expression peaks at 6–8 hours post-activation and then falls to resting levels by 24 to 48 hours. CD154 is also expressed on CD4 thymocytes, activated CD8 T cells, NK cells, monocytes, basophils, mast cells, activated eosinophils, and activated platelets. Newborn T cells are deficient in CD154 expression, although they can be induced to express the antigen if strongly stimulated.

CD40 is a member of the TNF receptor superfamily. It is constitutively expressed on pro-B, pre-B, and mature B cells, as well as on interdigitating cells, follicular dendritic cells, thymic epithelial cells, monocytes, platelets, and some carcinomas.

Engagement of B cell CD40 with CD154 on an activated T cell that also expresses Fas ligand (FasL or CD95L) leads to the upregulation of Fas (CD95) on the B cell (Chapter 12). NEMO is a part of the signaling pathway. If the B cell has concomitantly bound its cognate antigen and engaged the B-cell receptor-signaling pathway, it becomes resistant to Fas-mediated apoptosis and expresses CD80/CD86 on the cell surface. The activated B cell can then engage CD28 on the T-cell surface and trigger the T cell to secrete its cytokines. If the B cell fails to engage its BCR, the Fas pathway predominates and the B cell is eliminated. With proper activation of the CD40-CD154 pathway, exposure to IL-2 and -10 induces production of IgM, IgG_1, and IgA; and exposure to IL-4 induces production of IgG_4 and IgE. This change in immunoglobulin isotype reflects both induction of switching and the enhanced survival and proliferation of the B cell. In the absence of CD154, B cells can express IgM, but have difficulty switching and are likely to undergo apoptosis rather than proliferate in response to antigen.

CD40-CD154 interactions between CD154$^+$ T cells and CD40$^+$ macrophages lead to enhanced production of IL-12, which then stimulates T cells to release interferon-γ. Activation of this pathway appears necessary for the defense against *P. jiroveci* and other opportunistic organisms. Its absence likely contributes to cell-mediated immune deficiency.

Treatment and prognosis

The availability of human immunoglobulin replacement therapy has greatly improved the quality of life in HIGM. Adequate replacement can result in the reduction of serum IgM concentrations, prevention of infections with encapsulated bacteria, resumption of growth, and the gradual resolution of splenomegaly and lymphoid hyperplasia. Neutropenia persists but may be clinically silent. Autoimmune and lymphoproliferative complications may respond to anti-CD20 therapy (rituximab).[17]

However, despite the improvement granted by immunoglobulin replacement, the prognosis of patients with defects in the CD40–CD154 axis remains guarded. Among patients in a European Registry,[18] one-quarter of HIGM1 patients died before the age of 25. These deaths were primarily the result of opportunistic infections, including pneumocystis pneumonia (*PCP*), cholangitis, CMV, mycobacterial infections, and cirrhosis secondary to hepatitis. Prophylaxis with trimethoprim-sulfamethoxazole can significantly reduce the risk of PCP. There is also an increased incidence of carcinomas of the liver, pancreas and biliary tree, and perirectal abscesses can prove difficult to manage. Regular monitoring of gastrointestinal manifestations and management of neutropenia are mandatory. Bone marrow transplantation is a viable option for patients who fail to respond to supportive therapy.

IgA deficiency

Selective IgAD, selective IgG subclass deficiencies, CVID, and a syndrome of recurrent sinopulmonary infections (RESPI) with normal serum immunoglobulin levels appear to share an overlapping set of gene defects.[19] Clinically, these disorders are marked by an increased susceptibility to upper and lower respiratory infections with encapsulated bacteria. IgAD and CVID feature similar B-cell differentiation arrests, but differ in the extent of immunoglobulin deficits. The correlation between serum immunoglobulin levels and severity of infection is not absolute. Virtually agammaglobulinemic patients may suffer with only occasional sinusitis, whereas patients with near normal serum immunoglobulin levels may present with recurrent pneumonia and bronchiectasis.[20]

Diagnosis

Approximately 1 in 600 individuals of European ancestry are unable to produce detectable quantities IgA_1 and IgA_2, making selective IgAD the most frequently recognized primary immunodeficiency in the Americas, Australia, and Europe. The diagnosis is dependent on the sensitivity of the laboratory measurement. The clinical laboratory typically reports serum IgA levels of less than 7 mg/dL, the concentration below which nephelometry becomes unreliable.

Uncomplicated patients with IgAD have normal serum levels of IgM, normal or elevated levels of IgG, and demonstrate normal cell-mediated immunity. A minority of patients demonstrate additional evidence of immune dysfunction, with inability to generate appropriate IgG_2 anti-carbohydrate antibodies, frank IgG subclass deficiencies, or evidence of impairment of T-cell function. Patients with IgA serum levels that fall more than two standard deviations below the mean serum level for their age are considered to have partial IgA deficiency. These patients can also suffer from recurrent infections.

Clinical manifestations

The likelihood that an IgA-deficient individual who was identified serendipitously will require medical attention is difficult to assess because most studies in the literature reflect patients who were ascertained as a result of clinical symptoms. Among IgAD patients referred to immunology clinics, more than 85% present with recurrent infections, typically with encapsulated bacteria such as *H. influenzae* and *S. pneumoniae*. Among affected children, symptoms can begin in the first year of life, although the physiologic lag in serum IgA can delay the diagnosis until after the age of 2. In some patients, respiratory infections disappear with maturity. In others, infections may persist throughout adult life. Rarely, IgAD patients experience recurrent bronchitis, pneumonia and even bronchiectasis. These more severely afflicted patients often exhibit IgG_2 and IgG_4 subclass deficiencies, as well. Chronic intermittent diarrhea due to *G. lamblia* is a common complaint although there are indications that this may track more closely with related deficits in IgG function. Systemic infections such as viral hepatitis, meningoencephalitis, and

septicemia can also occur. Some symptomatic patients have elevated IgE levels, which can introduce an allergic or asthmatic component to respiratory dysfunction. The rise in IgE has been explained as a compensatory response to the absence of IgA. This appears to be a double-edged sword, because up to 20% of patients complain of allergic rhinitis, conjunctivitis, urticaria, and atopic eczema. Allergic reactions may be enhanced due to the lack of IgA blocking antibodies in the serum, and unusually severe asthma has also been associated with IgAD.

Among those less common IgA-deficient patients who are truly devoid of IgA, as many as three-fifths produce IgG or IgE anti-IgA antibodies.[21] These uncommon patients are at an uncertain risk for adverse reactions following transfusion with blood products as mentioned previously, plasma from normal donors, or from some preparations of immunoglobulin replacement therapy, which, of course, contain IgA. Patients with high anti-IgA levels (greater than 1:1000) typically have potent antibodies directed against all IgAs. These patients are at risk for severe anaphylaxis. Patients with low anti-IgA antibody titers (less than 1:256) are often multiparous or multi-transfused patients. These patients rarely demonstrate severe anaphylaxis after infusion with plasma or blood products, but do present with hives and rashes. Serum complement typically falls as a result of this type of reaction.

IgAD patients often develop autoimmune diseases. These include juvenile rheumatoid arthritis, systemic lupus erythematosus, Addison's disease, chronic nephritis, dermatomyositis, Evans syndrome, isolated hemolytic anemia, isolated idiopathic thrombocytopenic purpura, insulin-dependent diabetes mellitus, pulmonary hemosiderosis, sarcoidosis, Sjögren's syndrome, Henoch-Schönlein syndrome or hemorrhagic purpura, and thyroiditis. Gastrointestinal disorders include pernicious anemia, inflammatory bowel disease, intestinal disaccharidase deficiency, lactase deficiency, pancreatic insufficiency, and celiac disease. The latter in particular can be difficult to diagnose without biopsy since serologic diagnosis often relies on detection of anti-tissue transglutaminase, anti-endomysial or anti-gliadin IgA antibodies.[22] Hepatobiliary disorders include chronic active hepatitis, cholelithiasis, lupoid hepatitis, and primary biliary cirrhosis. Skin disorders include pyoderma gangrenosum, perinychia, and vitiligo. It is unclear whether this autoimmune diathesis is the end result of recurrent infections, the product of recurrent insult by antigens that would otherwise be cleared by IgA, or whether the underlying deficit that leads to IgAD also increases the risk of developing an autoimmune disorder. For example, autoimmune disorders such as insulin-dependent diabetes mellitus and celiac disease are associated with the same MHC haplotypes (Chapter 5) as IgAD and CVID.

IgAD is associated with an increased risk for the development of malignancies[23,24] epithelial tumors such as gastric and colonic adenocarcinoma, Hodgkin's disease, and acute lymphoblastic leukemia. Hepatoma, lymphosarcoma, melanoma, multiple myeloma, ovarian carcinoma, squamous cell carcinoma, and malignant thymoma have also been reported. Cervical and bronchial lymphadenopathy can be found in IgAD patients who suffer from recurrent sinopulmonary infections. Patients with chronic gastrointestinal infections may demonstrate a nodular lymphoid hyperplasia of the small intestine that can lead to intestinal obstruction. Histologic evaluation reveals active B lymphocyte proliferation in the germinal centers of the Peyer's patches. These enlarged lymph nodes have been mistaken for lymphoma. In some cases, it is possible to attribute the increased risk of malignancy to the lack of protection against ingested carcinogens. In others, the simultaneous presence of IgAD and malignancy may simply reflect the high prevalence of IgAD in the Caucasian population.

Origin and pathogenesis

IgAD, selective IgG subclass deficiencies, and CVID are diseases that are defined by a quantitative phenotype, a paucity of serum immunoglobulins of a given isotype despite the presence in the blood of B-lymphocytes bearing the missing isotypes. By definition, the fundamental defect involves the failure of B-lymphocytes bearing a given isotype to differentiate into plasma cells. These diseases appear to represent a common endpoint for multiple pathogenic processes. All three phenotypes may be acquired and many of the recognized precipitating causes, such as phenytoin, are the same (see Table 34.3).

IgA deficiency (IgAD1) is associated with MHC haplotypes (6p21.3) that are more common in European populations than in the peoples of sub-Saharan Africa and east Asia. In the United States, the prevalence of IgAD among African Americans is one-twentieth of that observed among Americans of European descent and in Japan the incidence is approximately 1 in 18,500. IgA deficiency (IgAD2) has also been observed in family members of CVID patients with altered function of the transmembrane activator and CAML interactor (*TACI*, 17p11.2), which is a receptor for B-cell-activating factor (BAFF).

Table 34.3 Other conditions associated with humoral immunodeficiency

Genetic disorders	
Monogenic diseases	Ataxia-telangiectasia
	Autosomal forms of SCID
	Transcobalamin II deficiency and hypogammaglobulinemia
	Wiskott–Aldrich syndrome
	X-linked lymphoproliferative disorder (EBV associated)
	X-linked SCID
Chromosomal anomalies	Chromosome 18q- Syndrome
	Monosomy 22
	Trisomy 8
	Trisomy 21
Systemic disorders	
Malignancy	Chronic lymphocytic leukemia
	Immunodeficiency with thymoma
	T-cell lymphoma
Metabolic or physical loss	Immunodeficiency caused by hypercatabolism of immunoglobulin
	Immunodeficiency caused by excessive loss of immunoglobulins and lymphocytes
Environmental exposures	
Drug-induced	Antimalarial agents
	Captopril
	Carbamazepine
	Glucocorticoids
	Fenclofenac
	Gold salts
	Imatinib
	Penicillamine
	Phenytoin
	Sulphasalazine
Infectious diseases	Congenital rubella
	Congenital infection with CMV
	Congenital infection with Toxoplasma gondii
	Epstein–Barr virus
	Human immunodeficiency virus

Treatment and prognosis

Most individuals with IgAD suffer respiratory infections no more frequently than the average individual and thus require no special treatment. All individuals with IgA deficiency should be warned of the risk of serious transfusion reactions caused by antibodies to IgA. Wearing a medical alert bracelet is recommended. Should transfusion be necessary, the ideal donors are other individuals with IgAD. Washed erythrocytes are safer than whole blood.

Patients with selective IgA deficiency who suffer from clinically significant, recurrent upper respiratory infections often respond to prophylactic antibiotics with potency against encapsulated bacteria. Treatment of allergy in those patients with a compensatory increase in IgE is helpful. Patients who present with combined IgA and IgG subclass deficiencies may require subcutaneous or intravenous immunoglobulin replacement therapy.

Common variable immunodeficiency

Diagnosis

The diagnostic category of CVID includes a heterogeneous group of patients, mostly adults, who exhibit deficient production of more than one different major class of antibodies. These patients tend to have normal numbers of B cells in their blood that are clonally diverse. B cells in CVID patients can recognize antigens and respond with proliferation, but they appear quantitatively impaired in their ability to become memory B cells and mature plasma cells. In infected patients, abortive differentiation can lead to massive B lymphocyte hyperplasia, splenomegaly, and intestinal lymphoid hyperplasia.

With an estimated prevalence of 1 in 25 000; CVID is the most prevalent human primary immunodeficiency requiring medical attention.[25] Men and women are equally affected. As with IgAD, the prevalence among African Americans is one-twentieth that of Americans of European descent. Some patients present during childhood, but most are diagnosed after the third decade of life. The typical patient reports a normal pattern of recurrent otitis media as an infant and toddler that resolved in childhood. During adolescence, respiratory infections appear and steadily increase in frequency and duration. Recurrent pneumonia as a young or middle-aged adult is often the precipitating complaint that brings the patient to the attention of the clinical immunologist. Although CVID thus appears to be an acquired disorder, family studies have clearly documented that susceptibility for the disease can be inherited and the manifestations of the disorder can change with time. Transitions within the spectrum of normal serum immunoglobulin concentrations to IgA deficiency to IgA deficiency with IgG subclass deficits to frank CVID have been documented in both sporadic and familial cases.[2]

Common variable immunodeficiency is a diagnostic category of primary immunodeficiencies that includes a number of immune disorders. Most CVID patients of Northern European descent exhibit a distinctive phenotype characterized by a broad deficiency of immunoglobulin isotypes despite the presence of normal numbers of surface immunoglobulin bearing B-cell precursors in the peripheral blood. Almost all of these patients are IgA deficient and, by definition, demonstrate total serum IgG levels of less than 500 mg/dL. Some IgG subclasses are more affected than others, with the sequential order of involvement being $IgG_4 > IgG_2 > IgG_1 > IgG_3$. Most patients are also deficient in IgM and IgE. This pattern is common to patients with specific MHC susceptibility haplotypes as well as to those who have inherited function-loss mutations in the genes for ICOS (CVID1), an immune co-stimulator molecule used by T cells to activate B cells in germinal centers, BAFFR (CVID4) and TACI (CVID2), the receptors for B-cell-activating factor (BAFF), CD19 (CVID3) and CD81 (CVID6), components of the B-cell co-stimulatory receptor, and CD20 (CVID5). TLR7 and TLR9 activation can be deficient in these patients, although the genes are intact.[26]

Uncomplicated patients demonstrate normal cell-mediated immunity, although a minority of patients may have evidence of T-cell dysfunction as well as other hematopoietic cell types. In some cases, B-cell numbers are reduced, although not to the extent exhibited by disorders of pre-BCR formation or signaling as discussed in the sections on XLA and autosomal agammaglobulinemia or in the agammaglobulinemia associated with thymoma with pure red cell aplasia.

IgAD and CVID have been associated with congenital infection with rubella virus, cytomegalovirus, and *T. gondii*. The administration of certain drugs has also been linked to a depression in serum immunoglobulin levels. Up to 20% of patients treated with phenytoin for idiopathic epilepsy suffer a mild decrease in serum IgA levels, and a minority may progress to a CVID-like phenotype. Medications used for the treatment of rheumatoid arthritis, inflammatory bowel disease, and chronic myelogenous leukemia can also decrease production of antibody. Persistence of antibody deficiency usually requires continued administration of the drug or continued infection with the virus or parasite. Recovery of immunoglobulin production may take months or years.

Clinical manifestations

Although some CVID patients have reduced numbers of circulating B cells, the majority have normal quantities of IgA, IgG, and IgM-bearing B-cell precursors in the blood. Defects in B-cell survival, number of circulating $CD27^+$ memory B cells (including IgM^+CD27^+ B cells), B-cell activation after antigen receptor cross-linking, T-cell signaling, and cytokine expression have been observed. A decrease in the relative numbers of CD4 to CD8 T cells is common and cutaneous anergy is a frequent finding. Alteration of the CD4/CD8 ratio can reflect expansion of the CD8 natural killer cell population or an increase in the subset of $CD8^+$, $CD57^+$ T cells and NK cells. In some patients inversion of the ratio reflects a true decline in the absolute number of CD4 helper T cells.

The clinical manifestations of CVID are similar but more severe than the ones seen in IgAD. Respiratory symptoms often begin with recurrent sinusitis, otitis media, and mild bronchitis, which are typically due to, encapsulated bacteria such as *H. influenzae* and *S. pneumoniae*. The frequency and severity of the upper respiratory infections worsen in the young adult and lower respiratory infections such as pneumonia become common. Apparently asymptomatic, untreated patients may suffer recurrent subclinical pulmonary infections that can lead to irreversible chronic lung damage with bronchiecstasis, unilateral hyperlucent lung, emphysema, and cor pulmonale. With damage to pulmonary mucosa, the spectrum of bacterial pathogens broadens to include *S. aureus* and *Pseudomonas aeruginosa*. Recurrent cellulitis, boils, folliculitis, impetigo or erythroderma can be presenting complaints.

Intermittent or chronic diarrhea due to *G. lamblia* is a common complaint. Some unfortunate patients develop a malabsorption syndrome that resembles celiac sprue but is unresponsive to the avoidance of gluten (Fig. 34.4). Although allergic disorders are rare in CVID, antigen-specific IgE can be produced in sufficient quantities to enable anaphylactic reactions. Untreated patients often complain of asymmetrical, oligoarticular arthralgias or frank arthritis, which in some cases reflect infections with encapsulated organisms or with *Mycoplasma* spp. and thus require antibiotic therapy. These arthritic complaints typically respond to immunoglobulin replacement therapy.

CVID patients are often anergic, but only a minority suffer infections characteristic of cell-mediated immune dysfunction, such as mycobacteria, *P. jiroveci*, and fungi. CD8 T-cell numbers may be depressed in such patients. Most viral infections are cleared normally. Exceptions include enteroviral infections, including meningoencephalitis, as well as hepatitis B and C, which can progress to a fatal chronic active hepatitis. Lack of humoral immunity enhances susceptibility to viral reactivation. Untreated patients often complain of recurrent herpes zoster (shingles).

Autoimmune diseases are common in CVID and include pernicious anemia, autoimmune neutropenia, Graves disease, hypothyroidism, rheumatoid arthritis, systemic lupus erythematosus, and Sjögren syndrome. Coombs positive hemolytic anemia with idiopathic thrombocytopenic purpura, a combination known as Evans syndrome, may predate the diagnosis of CVID.

Non-caseating granulomas in the lung, lymph nodes, skin, bone marrow and liver reminiscent or indistinguishable from sarcoid-like syndrome, is more common in patients of African descent, but can be seen in up to one-fifth of all patients. Occasionally the granulomas result from mycobacterial and fungal infections. In the majority of cases, the cause remains unclear and the granulomas resolve spontaneously.

There is an increased risk for the development of gastrointestinal and lymphoid malignancies, especially non-Hodgkin's lymphomas. Confounding the diagnosis of malignancy is the propensity of patients to develop benign lymphoproliferative

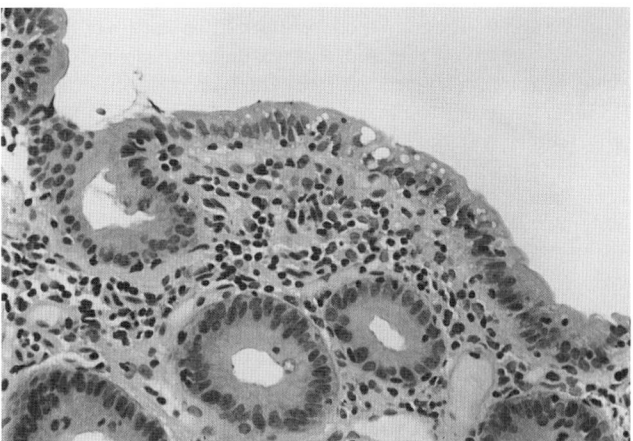

Fig. 34.4 Hypogammaglobulinemic sprue in a 41-year-old white male with CVID and insulin-dependent diabetes mellitus. The patient suffered from intractable diarrhea. A hematoxylin and eosin stain of a duodenal biopsy obtained by endoscopy is shown. The villi are blunted and there is a marked increase in intraepithelial lymphocytes. However, unlike typical celiac disease, the villi are not completely blunted and few plasma cells are seen. The patient is homozygous for the HLA-B8,-DR3 haplotype. Although the patient failed to respond to a gluten-free diet, the diarrhea resolved with corticosteroid therapy.

disorders. Lymphadenopathy, splenomegaly, or both are common in untreated patients. The lymph node architecture is usually preserved, but in some patients the lymph node architecture is disrupted by a polymorphic lymphocytic infiltrate. Lymphoid aggregates with an abnormal architecture can also develop in the skin, bone marrow, or other tissues. This atypical lymphoid hyperplasia can be difficult to differentiate from a malignant lymphoma.

Origin and pathogenesis

The typical presenting manifestation of CVID is hypogammaglobulinemia, not agammaglobulinemia; suggesting a partial or varying block in B-cell maturation. Careful analysis of B cells in patients has also revealed a spectrum of immune deficiency ranging from the nearly complete absence of memory B cells to a less severe disorder. All of these findings serve to underline the complex etiology for the disorder, and many details remain to be elucidated. As with IgAD1, the MHC represents the most common genetic susceptibility locus for CVID. Due to linkage disequilibrium, the gene, or genes, within this locus that create susceptibility have yet to be identified with certainty. For example, *MSH5*, a gene in the class III region of the MHC is variously identified as a causative agent and as a marker for an associated extended haplotype. Non-MHC associated single gene defects have been identified, although they represent only a minority of patients with CVID. These defects influence BCR signal transduction in mature B cells (CD19, CD81), B-cell homeostasis (BAFFR, TACI), late stage B-cell differentiation (CD20), and late stage B-cell–T-cell interactions (ICOS).

The major histocompatibility complex (MHC)

A large array of genes that play important roles in the control of the immune response are located in the HLA major histocompatibility complex on chromosome 6 (Chapter 5). Studies at the University of Alabama at Birmingham have shown that in the Southeastern United States the majority of IgAD and CVID patients share parts or all of one of three extended HLA haplotypes marked by either HLA-DR3,-B8, HLA-DR7,-B44 and HLA-DR4,-B44. The combined results of three studies of patients from Alabama, New England, and Australia indicate a 13% prevalence of immunodeficiency in individuals homozygous for HLA-DR3,-B8. These HLA alleles are also more common in patients who suffer with diabetes mellitus, pernicious anemia, celiac disease, autoimmune thyroid disease and myasthenia gravis. Remarkably, several individuals with TACI mutations had also inherited MHC haplotypes associated with the disease,[27] suggesting the possibility of epistatic interactions between MHC and TACI (CVID2) alleles.

The CD19 (CVID3), CD81 (CVID6), CD21 B-cell co-receptor complex

CD21 (complement component C3d/Epstein–Barr virus receptor 2) binds to membrane- IgM-bound antigen when complement C3d is also attached to that antigen (Chapter 20). In association with CD81 and CD19, this co-receptor complex enhances the antigen-binding signal, promoting B-cell activation. Patients with mutations in CD19 and CD81 have been reported. It is likely that mutations in CD21 will yield a similar phenotype.

The BAFF, BAFFR (CVID4), and TACI (CVID2) axis

The TNF family members B-cell activating factor of the TNF family (BAFF) and a proliferation-inducing ligand (APRIL) bind to two receptors, B-cell maturation antigen (BCMA) and transmembrane activator and calcium-modulator and cyclophilin ligand interactor (TACI), both of which are members of the TNF-R family. BCMA is exclusively expressed on B cells, whereas TACI is expressed on B cells and activated T cells. A third receptor, BAFF-R, which is unique for BAFF, is expressed mainly on B cells but is also expressed on a subset of T cells. This BAFF/APRIL system plays a key role in mature B-cell homeostasis and development. BAFF and APRIL also can induce isotype switching in naïve human B cells. Loss-of-function (autosomal recessive) or altered-function (autosomal dominant) TACI alleles have been found in approximately 10% of CVID patients in many series.[28] Two polymorphic alleles, A181E and C104R, are present in the majority of CVID patients with TACI alterations. These alleles are also present in approximately 2% of the normal population, suggesting that the presence of these altered alleles functions as a susceptibility factor for the development of the disease. Family members may have IgA deficiency or may have no evidence of immune dysfunction. However, CVID patients with these altered alleles have a higher prevalence of complications from CVID, including lymphoproliferation, splenomegaly and autoimmune phenomena.[29]

CD20 (CVID5)

CD20 encodes a B-cell membrane-spanning molecule that plays an as yet unidentified role in the development and differentiation of B cells into plasma cells. One inbred patient with a CD20 mutation and CVID has been reported.

ICOS (CVID1)

Function-loss mutations in the genes for ICOS, an immune co-stimulator molecule used by T cells to activate B cells in germinal centers, BAFFR, and CD19, the B-cell co-stimulatory receptor have also been reported in isolated CVID patients. All of these genes play key roles in the maturation, proliferation, and longevity of mature B cells.

Treatment and prognosis

Therapy in CVID begins with the aggressive treatment of ongoing infections and the institution of prophylactic measures to prevent or ameliorate future infection. Patients suffering from moderate upper respiratory tract infections and bronchitis will likely benefit from empiric therapy with agents effective against encapsulated organisms such as *H. influenzae* and *S. pneumoniae*. Patients with recurrent pneumonia and evidence of bronchiectasis may be infected with *Pseudomonas* spp., *S. aureus*, or other aggressive organisms; thus every effort should be made to identify the inciting agent. The course of treatment for immunodeficient patients is often prolonged and intravenous administration of antibiotics may be required.

The most effective therapy for hypogammaglobulinemic patients is replacement therapy with human immunoglobulin (Chapter 85). A number of studies have demonstrated a steadily decreasing incidence of infection with increasing frequency of immunoglobulin administration. At higher doses, even patients with bronchiectasis may experience improvement in pulmonary function. Each patient may demonstrate his or her own individual response to therapy, exhibiting dramatic differences in the frequency and severity of infections with moderate changes in the replacement dose. Patients suffering from a serious acute infection often benefit from one-time booster doses of immunoglobulin. Ultimately, replacement dosage must be individualized based upon the response of the patient. Adverse reactions occur most frequently at the time of the first administration of immunoglobulin, likely because of concurrent infection increasing the potential for generation of immune complexes. If the patient demonstrates no evidence of adverse reactions, administration of intravenous or subcutaneous immunoglobulin can be performed at home.

Some patients with CVID sustain severe anaphylaxis when given IVIG or other blood products that contain serum or plasma. These patients may possess anti-IgA antibodies, including IgE anti-A antibodies.[30] For patients with a history of severe adverse reactions, it is advisable to try lots of IVIG with the lowest IgA possible and to test the patient with the different lots in an intensive care unit. Once having identified a lot that can be tolerated, the patient may receive therapy under more relaxed conditions.

Serum immunoglobulin concentrations in patients with CVID can change over time,[2] with rare patients regaining normal serum IgG levels and no longer requiring immunoglobulin therapy. Careful review of the clinical history of these patients may reveal evidence of exposure to pharmacologic agents associated with the development of hypogammaglobulinemia (e.g., phenytoin). However, the overwhelming majority of patients require replacement therapy for life.

Although IgG can be replaced, at present IgM and IgA cannot be provided to the patient. The absence of these multimeric proteins may help explain why even patients on high dose replacement therapy can continue to suffer from recurrent sinusitis or gastrointestinal discomfort.[31] Recurrent sinusitis can be ameliorated with continued prophylactic therapy with antibiotics effective against encapsulated bacteria. Patients with CVID also are at risk from *G. lamblia*, as well as other enteric pathogens. Patients with chronic diarrhea often respond to treatment with empiric antibiotic therapy. Gastroesophageal reflux disease (GERD) is a common complaint, best treated symptomatically. Some patients develop lactose intolerance or gluten-sensitive enteropathy. Gluten avoidance ameliorates symptoms in only a minority of cases. A majority responds to corticosteroids or anti-TNF agents. The use of these agents can be a double-edged sword, however, since resistance to infection will decrease in a patient who is already immune-deficient. Other patients develop a malabsorption syndrome that can lead to hypoalbuminemia and hypocalcemia (due to malabsorption of vitamin D), and decreased levels of vitamin A and carotene.[32] The cause of diarrhea and malabsorption in this latter patient subset remains unclear, and treatment is limited to supportive measures, with vitamin and mineral replacement as indicated.

Patients with bronchiectasis should be treated aggressively with replacement therapy. In severe cases, aggressive pulmonary toilet will benefit the patient, including bronchodilator therapy, position and postural drainage, or other physical therapies. The use of corticosteroids should be avoided.

IgA-deficient mothers fail to secrete IgA in their colostrum. Although colostral IgM levels may be elevated in an attempt to compensate for the lack of maternal IgA, the newborn remains relatively unprotected against intestinal pathogens. Of greater concern are the children of mothers with untreated CVID who are born in a state of humoral immunodeficiency and are at great risk for life-threatening sinopulmonary infection. In order to compensate for the loss of IgG across the placenta and to provide the infant with the passive immunity it will require, IVIG therapy should be initiated in untreated patients; in patients on immunoglobulin replacement the dose of IVIG should be increased by 50% during the third trimester of pregnancy.

Splenomegaly is common in untreated patients. Hypersplenism in most patients responds to aggressive therapy with antibiotics and IVIG. The presumption is that the hypersplenism is secondary to reactive hyperplasia of lymphoid follicles within the spleen, reflecting a response to infection. Development of esophageal varices or other hematologic manifestations of hypersplenism (refractory thrombocytopenia, anemia, neutropenia, and lymphopenia) may require splenectomy as the therapy of last resort. The outcome for most such patients has been good, with resolution of symptoms; although patients with altered TACI alleles tend to do less well. For those patients who undergo splenectomy, the risk of infection from encapsulated organisms increases, and they should be placed on penicillin prophylaxis (or an equivalent).

The development of constellation of pulmonary abnormalities that include granulomatous and lymphoproliferative (lymphocytic interstitial pneumonia (LIP), follicular bronchiolitis, and lymphoid hyperplasia) histopathologic patterns, termed granulomatous-lymphocytic interstitial lung disease (GLILD), can be an ominous sign. These patients appear more likely to develop granulomatous liver disease, autoimmune hemolytic anemia, lymphoproliferative disease, and progressive pulmonary disease. In one study,[33] median survival was reduced by more than 50%.

● THERAPEUTIC PRINCIPLES

- The primary goal of treatment is to keep the patient infection free.
- In patients whose respiratory mucosa is intact, intravenous or subcutaneous replacement IgG therapy is generally effective in protecting the patient from pulmonary infections.
- For those patients who have developed bronchiectasis or who continue to subject themselves to environmental toxins (e.g., smoking), replacement IgG will ameliorate but may not prevent all such infections.
- Because mucosal immunoglobulin cannot be replaced, even patients on adequate IgG replacement therapy remain at risk for sinus or gastrointestinal infections.
- Prophylactic antibiotics that are effective against encapsulated organisms can significantly reduce the frequency of upper respiratory tract infections in patients who continue to suffer despite replacement therapy with IVIG.
- Prolonged diarrhea in hypogammaglobulinemic patients is often caused by *Giardia lamblia* and responds well to metronidazole therapy.
- Patients with primary antibody deficiencies should not receive live vaccines.

Selective IgG subclass deficiencies

Diagnosis

A diagnosis of clinical immunodeficiency should be supported by clear evidence of functional impairment. Most individuals with modest reductions in serum IgG subclass levels are functionally normal. Indeed, individuals with deletions of the heavy chain immunoglobulin gene locus, some of whom completely lack IgG_1, IgG_2, IgG_4, and IgA_1,[34] have been reported to be asymptomatic. This experiment of nature is a further reminder of the fact that absence of serum immunoglobulin is not necessarily synonymous with clinical immune deficiency.

The diagnosis of a functional IgG subclass deficiency can thus be made with confidence only when there is both a significant decrease in the serum concentration of a specific isotype and there is clear evidence of abnormal specific antibody production. Up to 10% of normal males and 1% of normal females are IgG_4 deficient, which makes a diagnosis of immunodeficiency as a result of an isolated IgG_4 subclass deficiency problematic. Thus, among patients with a deficiency of IgG_1 or IgG_3, documentation of the ability to produce protective titers of anti-tetanus toxin and anti-diphtheria toxin antibodies following standard tetanus toxoid and diphtheria immunizations is a strong indication that replacement immunoglobulin therapy is likely unwarranted. Similarly, documentation of a strong anti-pneumococcal polysaccharide response in patients with an apparent IgG_2 deficiency would suggest immunoglobulin replacement is likely not required. IgG_2 levels normally begin to rise in childhood later than other subclasses, and a low value in a child may be a temporary finding. Conversely, the lack of a response to vaccination calls for appropriate prophylactic therapy.

Clinical manifestations

The clinical spectrum of isolated IgG subclass deficiency is quite variable and deficiencies of each of the four IgG subclasses have been described. Some individuals are referred to the clinical immunologist with only a mild reduction of total IgG, but most symptomatic patients have marked deficiencies of one or more IgG subclasses despite normal total IgG concentrations. Since IgG_1 makes up the majority of serum IgG in most patients, a deficiency of IgG tends to correlate with depressed serum levels of total IgG.

Determination of IgG subclasses is rarely performed on asymptomatic individuals, thus most patients with an isolated IgG_2 deficiency come to medical attention as a result of recurrent sinusitis, otitis media, or pulmonary infections. Individuals may have few residual symptoms between infections, but some have severe chronic inflammation with refractory sinusitis, pulmonary fibrosis, or bronchiectasis. Because protective antibodies directed against carbohydrate antigens are usually of the IgG_2 subclass, many affected patients exhibit an impairment of their ability to mount specific protective responses to encapsulated pathogens. However, normal responses have also been described.[35] The response to polysaccharides is typically tested by challenge with a pneumococcal polysaccharide vaccine. Diagnosis is complicated by the fact that interpretation of pneumococcal polysaccharide vaccine responses remains controversial. Many clinicians would agree, however, that IgG_2-deficient patients who suffer with recurrent sinopulmonary infections and who respond to less than half of the polysaccharide antigens with which they have been challenged meet the standard for functional immune deficiency and thus, should the infections be severe, warrant aggressive prophylactic therapy up to and including immunoglobulin replacement.

IgG_3 deficiency can occur alone or in association with IgG_1 deficiency. Recurrent infection of the respiratory tract with chronic lung disease has been reported. With a serum half-life only two weeks, IgG_3 levels can be consumed rapidly during the course of an active infection in an otherwise normal individual.[36] Consequently, before making the diagnosis of IgG_3 deficiency, serum levels of IgG_3 should be re-checked when the individual is asymptomatic.

When compared with the serum, IgG_4 is over-represented in secretions, and IgG_4-committed B cells are present at mucosal sites, suggesting a role in mucosal immunity. Since IgG_4 is normally present in the serum in very low concentrations, the significance of a low serum level in a patient with recurrent infection remains unclear.

Origin and pathogenesis

The origin of IgG subclass deficiency is unknown. Homozygous deletions of portions of the immunoglobulin heavy chain constant locus associated with total absence of IgG_2, IgG_3, and IgG_4 or combinations of these isotypes have been described in healthy individuals. IgG_2 deficiency is often found in association with selective IgA deficiency with or without IgG_4 deficiency, and patients with selective IgG subclass deficiencies have been shown to have inherited the same MHC haplotypes as those who suffer with IgAD and CVID. These observations suggest that patients with recurrent infections have a more complex defect than the mere elimination of one or more IgG isotype. In some instances, subclass deficiency is associated with a T-cell defect, as in chronic mucocutaneous candidiasis and ataxia-telangiectasia. IgG subclass deficiency can also be acquired. Acute infections, medications, chemotherapy, irradiation, surgery, and HIV infection have all been temporally linked to the development of a deficiency in one or more IgG subclass.[37]

Treatment and prognosis

The natural history of IgG subclass deficiency plus or minus IgA deficiency, especially in children, is not constant.[38] Some children improve, whereas for others subclass deficiency can progress into frank CVID. Associated allergic rhino-sinusitis and asthma must be aggressively treated with conventional therapy for these disorders, as these conditions increase the risk of purulent sinusitis and pneumonia. Causes of anatomic obstruction should be sought when persistent infection of a sinus or pulmonary segment is the presenting complaint; the role of surgical therapy for anatomic obstruction should not be overlooked.

Many patients with IgG subclass deficiency do well on prophylactic antibiotics and will never need immunoglobulin supplementation. However, immunoglobulin replacement therapy can be beneficial in patients with severe, recurrent infections. Patients who begin therapy should improve within the first 2 months, but to avoid misinterpretation of a placebo effect, a full 6-month trial is recommended. A reduction in frequency of viral respiratory infections is likely to occur in any individual receiving IVIG because of the broad spectrum of antibodies present, thus relative freedom from trivial infections should not be taken as evidence of need for permanent replacement therapy.

Antibody deficiency with normal serum immunoglobulin levels

Occasional patients may present with normal serum immunoglobulin concentrations and a selective inability to respond to infections with pyogenic organisms. Diagnosis requires documentation of an inability to respond to antigenic challenge. These patients may respond to replacement immunoglobulin therapy. The antibody response to specific polysaccharide antigens can be very selective. In human, most protective anti-*H. influenzae* type b (anti-Hib) antibodies utilize the rare Vκ A2 gene.[39] The Navajo population in the southwestern United States suffers a five- to tenfold increased incidence of Hib disease. This population also exhibits a high prevalence of an A2 allele with a defective recombination signal sequence, preventing use of germline-encoded antibodies that can generate protective antigen binding sites. With the development of high throughput sequencing technologies, it is likely that many more such subtle defects that underlie susceptibility to infectious diseases will be identified in the coming years.

A recent analysis of a group of well-characterized patients, mostly female, with a history of recurrent sinopulmonary infections (RESPI) and normal serum immunoglobulin levels revealed a high prevalence of the same MHC haplotypes observed in IgAD, selective IgG subclass deficits, and CVID.[20] This is further evidence that the presence of serum immunoglobulin is not necessarily synonymous with clinical immune sufficiency. These patients tend to respond to aggressive antibiotic therapy, including prophylaxis.

Selective light chain deficiency

Selective deficiencies of either κ or λ light chains have been reported.[40–42] In one such case, the patient was the offspring of a consanguineous (uncle-niece) union; and in the second, a molecular analysis demonstrated different loss of function mutations in the patient's Cκ alleles. The parents of these children had no health difficulties, but each of the patients required medical attention for recurrent sinopulmonary infections and diarrhea. Two of the κ-deficient patients exhibited IgA deficiency and the remaining κ- and the λ-deficient patients were panhypogammaglobulinemic.

Transient hypogammaglobulinemia of infancy

Diagnosis

As infants make the transition from dependence on maternal immunoglobulin to reliance on endogenously produced antibodies, they suffer a physiologic nadir of serum immunoglobulin at 4 to 6 months of age, a period associated with susceptibility to mild upper respiratory infections and otitis media (see Fig. 34.2). Children, both male and female, who (a) exhibit serum concentrations of one or more of the three major immunoglobulin classes that fall below the 95% confidence interval for age on two or more occasions during infancy, (b) demonstrate a rise in these values to or toward normal over time, and (c) lack features consistent with other forms of primary immunodeficiency fall within the catch-all diagnosis of transient hypogammaglobulinemia of infancy (THI).[43,44] By definition, the diagnosis of THI can be made with certainty only in retrospect.

Clinical manifestations

Immunoglobulin concentrations are rarely measured in infants unless there is some reason to suspect an immunodeficiency. Most patients with this diagnosis come to medical attention due to either recurrent infections or to routine screening studies of relatives of other immunodeficient patients. Yet bearing in mind that 2.5% of normal infants will fall below the 95%

confidence range at any one time, the diagnosis of THI is remarkably rare. Among two major centers, one in the USA and one in Germany, the diagnosis was given to only 16 of 18 000 children in whom the index of suspicion warranted immunoglobulin determinations.[45,46]

Patients with THI typically are able to synthesize specific antibodies in response to immunization with T dependent antigens (e.g., tetanus and diphtheria toxoids).[45] They may have difficulty, however, responding to polysaccharide antigens (e.g., isohemagglutinins and pneumococcal vaccine). Some will fail to sustain protective antibody responses to antigen. Most patients with THI, especially those ascertained as a result of family studies or mild upper respiratory infections alone, exhibit fewer infections over time. The great majority of infants with THI will normalize their serum immunoglobulin levels within 24 months of age. However, a minority fails to normalize IgG, continues to suffer with recurrent infections and may develop evidence of autoimmune disease. IgM levels may be reduced and laboratory studies may demonstrate a reduced frequency of switched memory B cells. These patients often become part of the hypogammaglobulinemia syndrome complex that includes CVID and may ultimately require long-term therapy with immunoglobulin, prophylactic antibiotics, or both.

Treatment and prognosis

Children with suspected THI should be monitored with serial determination of serum immunoglobulins and isohemaglutinin titers in order to confirm acquisition of normal immune function. Some children will not achieve normal levels of IgG for several years, and some will remain IgG subclass or IgA deficient. Treatment of transient hypogammaglobulinemia with IVIG is generally not warranted unless the child suffers from persistent, recurrent, invasive infections including pneumonia.

● ON THE HORIZON

- Elucidation of the molecular basis of selective defects in humoral responses to pathogens, in part through the use of high throughput sequencing to characterize the precise molecular composition of antibody responses in immune deficiencies.
- Further elucidation of the molecular basis of common variable immune deficiency, hypogammaglobulinemia, and IgA deficiency.

Frontiers in research

Bruton reported the first case of agammaglobulinemia in 1952, as well as the first successful therapy for this classic primary antibody deficiency. There has been remarkable progress in the identification of single gene disorders since that time. However, the underlying pathogenesis of the most common manifestation of primary antibody deficiency in our population, hypogammaglobulinemia in the adult, remains unclear. It seems likely that this disorder is multifactorial in nature, dependent on the inheritance of certain susceptibility loci in association with either environmental influences or random chance. In rare cases, patients with hypogammaglobulinemia have shown resolution of their symptoms, suggesting that a better understanding of pathogenesis might yield therapies of remission. The molecular basis of selective deficiencies in the response to pathogens in the presence of normal serum immunoglobulin levels also remains unclear. It is likely that a more exhaustive evaluation of the antibody repertoire in these patients, which is now possible through high throughput sequencing, may yield new insights into antibody deficiency syndromes and offer new potential therapies.

References

1. Notarangelo LD. Primary immunodeficiencies. J Allergy Clin Immunol 2010;125: S182–94.

2. Johnson ML, Keeton LG, Zhu ZB, et al. Age-related changes in serum immunoglobulins in patients with familial IgA deficiency and common variable immunodeficiency (CVID). Clin Exp Immunol 1997;108:477–83.

3. Cunningham-Rundles C. Autoimmunity in primary immune deficiency: taking lessons from our patients. Clin Exp Immunol 2011;164(Suppl. 2):6–11.

4. Stiehm ER, Fudenberg HH. Serum levels of immune globulins in health and disease. A survey. Pediatrics 1966;37:715–27.

5. De Greef GE, Van Tol MJ, Van Den Berg JW, et al. Serum immunoglobulin class and IgG subclass levels and the occurrence of homogeneous immunoglobulins during the course of ageing in humans. Mech Ageing Dev 1992;66(1):29–44.

6. Soothill JF, Hayward AR, Wood CB. Pediatric immunology. Oxford: Blackwell Scientific; 1983.

7. Balloch A, Licciardi PV, Russell FM, et al. Infants aged 12 months can mount adequate serotype-specific IgG responses to pneumococcal polysaccharide vaccine. J Allergy Clin Immunol 2010;126:395–7.

8. Buckley RH, Schiff RI. The use of intravenous immune globulin in immunodeficiency disease. N Engl J Med 1991;325:110–7.

9. Ballow M. Safety of IGIV therapy and infusion-related adverse events. Immunol Res 2007;38(1–3):122–32.

10. Duse M, Iacobini M, Leonardi L, et al. Transient hypogammaglobulinemia of infancy: intravenous immunoglobulin as first line therapy. Int J Immunopathol Pharmacol 2010;23(1):349–53.

11. Lindvall JM, Blomberg KE, Valiaho J, et al. Bruton's tyrosine kinase: cell biology, sequence conservation, mutation spectrum, siRNA modifications, and expression profiling. Immunol Rev 2005;203:200–15.

12. Nelson KS, Lewis DB. Adult-onset presentations of genetic immunodeficiencies: genes can throw slow curves. Curr Opin Infect Dis 2010;23(4):359–64.

13. Winkelstein JA, Conley ME, James C, et al. Adults with X-linked agammaglobulinemia: impact of disease on daily lives, quality of life, educational and socioeconomic status, knowledge of inheritance, and reproductive attitudes. Medicine 2008;87(5):253–8.

14. Conley ME, Dobbs AK, Farmer DM, et al. Primary B cell immunodeficiencies: comparisons and contrasts. Annu Rev Immunol 2009;27:199–227.

15. Durandy A, Taubenheim N, Peron S, et al. Pathophysiology of B-cell intrinsic immunoglobulin class switch recombination deficiencies. Adv Immunol 2007;94:275–306.

16. Karaca NE, Durandy A, Gulez N, et al. Study of patients with Hyper-IgM type IV phenotype who recovered spontaneously during late childhood and review of the literature. Eur J Pediatr 2011;170(8):1039–47.

17. Hennig C, Baumann U, Ilginus C, et al. Successful treatment of autoimmune and lymphoproliferative complications of patients with intrinsic B-cell immunodeficiencies with Rituximab. Br J Haematol 2010;148(3):445–8.

18. Levy J, Espanol-Boren T, Thomas C, et al. Clinical spectrum of X-linked hyper-IgM syndrome. J Pediatr 1997;131(1 Pt 1):47–54.

19. Schroeder Jr HW, Schroeder III HW, Sheikh SM. The complex genetics of common variable immunodeficiency. J Investig Med 2004;52(2):90–103.

20. Johnston DT, Mehaffey G, Thomas J, et al. Increased Frequency of HLA -B44 in Recurrent Sino-Pulmonary Infections (RESPI). Clin Immunol 2006;119:346–50.

21. Nielsen LK, Dziegiel MH. Recombinant human immunoglobulin (Ig)A1 and IgA2 anti-D used for detection of IgA deficiency and anti-IgA. Transfusion 2008;48(9):1892–7.

22. Borrelli M, Maglio M, Agnese M, et al. High density of intraepithelial gammadelta lymphocytes and deposits of immunoglobulin (Ig)M anti-tissue transglutaminase

23. antibodies in the jejunum of coeliac patients with IgA deficiency. Clin Exp Immunol 2010;160(2):199–206.

24. Cunningham-Rundles C, Bodian C. Common variable immunodeficiency: clinical and immunological features of 248 patients. Clin Immunol 1999;92(1):34–48.

25. Salavoura K, Kolialexi A, Tsangaris G, et al. Development of cancer in patients with primary immunodeficiencies. Anticancer Res 2008;28(2B):1263–9.

26. Castigli E, Geha RS. Molecular basis of common variable immunodeficiency. J Allergy Clin Immunol 2006;117(4):740–7.

27. Yu JE, Knight AK, Radigan L, et al. Toll-like receptor 7 and 9 defects in common variable immunodeficiency. J Allergy Clin Immunol 2009;124(2):349–56.

28. Salzer U, Chapel HM, Webster AD, et al. Mutations in TNFRSF13B encoding TACI are associated with common variable immunodeficiency in humans. Nat Genet 2005;37(8):820–8.

29. Salzer U, Bacchelli C, Buckridge S, et al. Relevance of biallelic versus monoallelic TNFRSF13B mutations in distinguishing disease-causing from risk-increasing TNFRSF13B variants in antibody deficiency syndromes. Blood 2009;113(9):1967–76.

30. Zhang L, Radigan L, Salzer U, et al. Transmembrane activator and calcium-modulating cyclophilin ligand interactor mutations in common variable immunodeficiency: clinical and immunologic outcomes in heterozygotes. J Allergy Clin Immunol 2007;120(5):1178–85.

31. Burks AW, Sampson HA, Buckley RH. Anaphylactic reactions after gamma globulin administration in patients with hypogammaglobulinemia. Detection of IgE antibodies to IgA. N Engl J Med 1986;314:560–4.

32. Malamut G, Verkarre V, Suarez F, et al. The enteropathy associated with common variable immunodeficiency: the delineated frontiers with celiac disease. Am J Gastroenterol 2010;105(10):2262–75.

33. Sneller MC, Strober W, Eisenstein E, et al. New insights into common variable immunodeficiency. Ann Int Med 1993;118:720–30.

34. Bates CA, Ellison MC, Lynch DA, et al. Granulomatous-lymphocytic lung disease shortens survival in common variable immunodeficiency. J Allergy Clin Immunol 2006;114(2):415–21.

35. Lefranc MP, Hammarström L, Smith CI, Lefranc G. Gene deletions in the human immunoglobulin heavy chain constant region locus: molecular and immunological analysis. Immunodefic Rev 1991;2(4):265–81.

36. Shackelford PG, Granoff DM, Madassery JV, et al. Clinical and immunologic characteristics of healthy children with subnormal serum concentrations of IgG2. Pediatr Res 1990;27(1):16–21.

37. Tabata N, Azuma E, Masuda S, et al. Transient low level of IgG3 induced by sepsis. Acta Paediatr Jpn 1995;37(2):201–2.

38. Morell A. IgG subclass deficiency: a personal viewpoint. Pediatr Infect Dis J 1990;9: S4–S8.

39. Kutukculer N, Karaca NE, Demircioglu O, et al. Increases in serum immunoglobulins to age-related normal levels in children with IgA and/or IgG subclass deficiency. Pediatr Allergy Immunol 2007;18(2):167–73.

40. Feeney AJ, Atkinson MJ, Cowan MJ, et al. A defective Vkappa A2 allele in Navajos which may play a role in increased susceptibility to *Haemophilus influenzae* type b disease. J Clin Invest 1996;97(10):2277–82.

41. Bernier GM, Gunderman JR, Ruymann FB. Kappa-chain deficiency. Blood 1972;40(6):795–805.

42. Barandun S, Morell A, Skvaril F, et al. Deficiency of kappa- or lambda-type immunoglobulins. Blood 1976;47:79–89.

43. Stavnezer-Nordgren J, Kekish O, Zegers BJ. Molecular defects in a human immunoglobulin kappa chain deficiency. Science 1985;230(4724):458–61.

44. Stiehm RE. The four most common pediatric immunodeficiencies. Adv Exp Med Biol 2007;601:15–26.

45. Moschese V, Graziani S, Avanzini MA, et al. A prospective study on children with initial diagnosis of transient hypogammaglobulinemia of infancy: results from the Italian Primary Immunodeficiency Network. Int J Immunopathol Pharmacol 2008;21(2):343–52.

46. Tiller Jr TL, Buckley RH. Transient hypogammaglobulinemia of infancy: review of the literature, clinical and immunologic features of 11 new cases, and long-term follow-up. J Pediatr 1978;92:347–53.

47. Dressler F, Peter HH, Muller W, et al. Transient hypogammaglobulinemia of infancy: Five new cases, review of the literature and redefinition. Acta Paediatr Scand 1989;78:767–74.

Primary T-cell immunodeficiencies

Chaim M. Roifman, Eyal Grunebaum

This chapter is dedicated to the diagnosis and management of inherited immune defects associated with predominantly T-cell dysfunction. One of the central roles of T cells is coordinating the activity of other arms of the immune system; therefore T-cell deficiencies are often accompanied with dysfunction of other cell types such as B and NK cells. Patients with profound T-cell deficiency (TD) typically present with repeated respiratory and gastrointestinal infections, oral thrush and failure to thrive. Such patients are classified as having severe combined immune deficiency (SCID) if their lymphocyte numbers are extremely low. Other patients with TD may have sizeable numbers of autologous circulating T cells and either a clinical presentation identical to SCID or somewhat delayed and atypical features. The latter patients are traditionally referred to as having combined immunodeficiency or T-cell deficiency with autologous T cells (TDA).

In recent years, studying the pathogeneses of human TD diseases has led to major advances in understanding T-cell development and function. Therefore, prior to describing the clinical and laboratory features as well as the etiology and management of each TD, the maturation, selection, activation and death of T cells are briefly reviewed, with emphasis on genes and pathways involved in the TD described below.

T-cell development and function

T-cell maturation

In humans, lymphoid progenitor cells originating from the bone marrow reach the thymus and mature into functional T cells. Various defects in this process can cause profound T-cell deficiencies (Fig. 35.1). Thymocyte maturation consists of sequential well-defined stages that can be followed by gene expression and by the presence of cell surface receptors (Chapter 8).[1] During the first major stage of thymocyte differentiation there is no expression of CD4 or CD8, therefore the cells are often referred to as double-negative (DN) cells. Successful re-arrangement of the β chain of the T-cell receptor for antigen (TCR) and pairing of the β chain with the pre-Tα chain allows progression of the DN cells into the second major stage of differentiation. In this second stage thymocytes express both CD4 and CD8, hence they are termed double-positive (DP) cells. Rearrangement of the TCR α chain allows expression of the combined TCRαβ on the surface of DP thymocytes. At the DP stage, positive and negative selection of thymocytes (also known as central selection) occurs, which is described in more detail below. Thymocytes that survive this selection mature into the third major stage of differentiation where they downregulate the expression of either CD4 or

CD8, resulting in CD4⁻CD8⁺ or CD4⁺CD8⁻ cells, respectively, which are also known as single-positive (SP) cells. SP cells can emigrate from the thymus to the blood and secondary lymphatic organs, where they encounter antigens and exert their biological functions.

T-cell selection

Ensuring T-cell reactivity against foreign antigens and not against self-antigens is crucial for survival. Two major mechanisms of selecting T cells have been identified, the first occurs in the thymus and is known as central selection, while the other occurs outside of the thymus and is known as peripheral selection.[2] Central selection is thought to depend on the affinity and avidity between the TCR and the major histocompatibility complex (MHC)–peptide complex presented by the thymic epithelial cells. According to this model, more than 80% of thymocytes express TCR that do not recognize any complex or have only low affinity, leading to apoptosis of these cells "by neglect." On the opposite side of the spectrum, thymocytes expressing TCR with high avidity (and that hence may become self-reactive), receive a signal to undergo deletion or inactivation. Only a small fraction of thymocytes, possibly in the order of 5%, which express TCR with intermediate affinity, are positively selected by a survival signal. Recent studies have identified the important roles of medullary thymus epithelial cells (mTEC) and the transcription factor *auto*immune *reg*ulator (AIRE) within these cells for central selection and prevention of autoimmunity. The thymus is also the site for generating natural regulatory T cells (Treg), characterized by the expression of CD4, CD25 and the transcription factor FoxP3. Together with induced regulatory T cells, produced in the periphery from conventional T cells, Treg are essential for the maintenance of peripheral immune tolerance.

T-cell activation

T-cell signaling is often initiated by TCR binding to peptide-MHC complexes expressed on the surface of antigen presenting cells. This engagement leads to a series of intracellular signaling cascades that culminate in the generation of a T-cell response (Fig. 35.2) (Chapter 12). The protein tyrosine kinase LCK is first activated with resultant phosphorylation of CD3 co-receptor cytoplasmic domain, specifically at tyrosine-based activation motifs (ITAMs) of immune receptors. These phosphorylated ITAMs on CD3ζ serve as binding sites for the ζ chain-associated protein kinase 70 (ZAP-70). Activated ZAP-70 phosphorylates a variety of downstream linker and adapter proteins including LAT and SLP-76. Other signaling proteins are subsequently recruited, resulting in calcium mobilization, actin cytoskeleton rearrangement and activation of Ras GTPase. These events result in activation of transcription factors, such as nuclear factor of activated

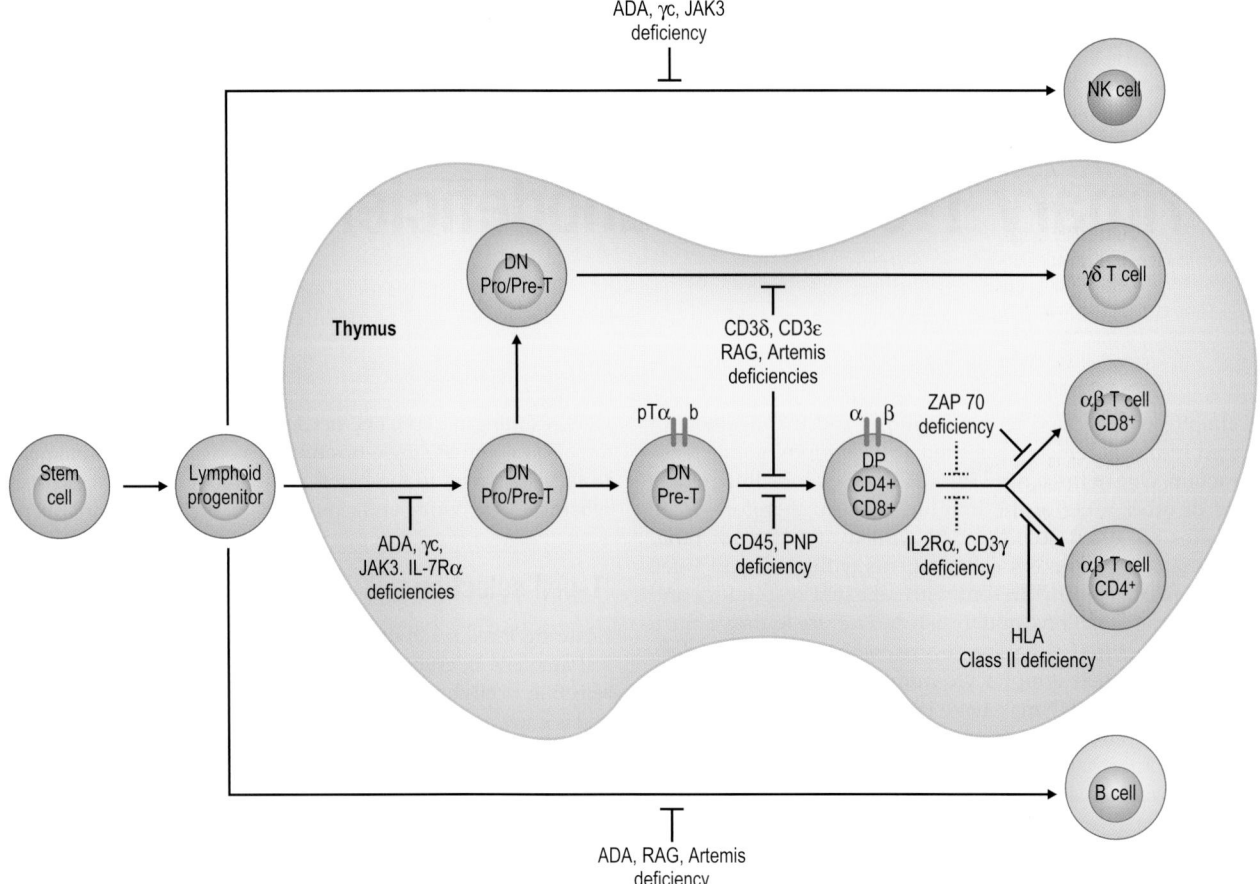

Fig. 35.1 Impaired maturation of T lineage cells in the thymus can lead to profound T-cell deficiency. Lymphoid progenitor cells that reach the thymus mature through consecutive steps into functional T cells. Blocked lines indicate specific stages impaired by known genetic abnormalities. Some defects can also interfere with maturation of B and natural killer (NK) cells. Abbreviations: ADA, adenosine deaminase deficiency; γc, gamma common chain of the interleukin (IL)-2 receptor; JAK3, Janus activated kinase 3; IL7Rα, alpha chain of the IL7 receptor; DN, double negative; RAG, recombination activating genes; PNP, purine nucleoside phosphorylase; ZAP 70, ζ-chain-associated protein kinase 70; IL2Rα, alpha chain of the IL2 receptor; MHC, major histocompatibility complex.

T cells (NF-AT), activator protein (AP-1) and nuclear factor kappa-light-chain-enhancer of activated B cells (NF-κB), which trigger changes in the pattern of T-cell gene expression, secretion of cytokines such as interleukin (IL)-2 and receptor expression, such as IL-2 receptor (IL2R). IL-2 is one of the key factors for differentiation of thymocytes as well as activation and proliferation of T lymphocytes. IL-2 binds the IL2R, which is composed of the α (CD25), β (CD122) and γ (CD132) chains. IL2Rα plays a critical role in sensitizing target cells to physiological levels of IL-2; however, because of the short cytoplasmic tail, the α chain does not contribute directly to signaling, which is performed by the β and γ chains through JAK1 and JAK3 respectively. Both JAK1 and JAK3 can activate Signal transducer and activator of transcription (STAT) 5. The γ chain also participates in signaling through other receptors including IL-4, -7, -9, -15, and -21; therefore it is often referred to as the γ common chain (γc). In addition to the role in T-cell activation, the IL-2 receptor has a critical role in maintaining self-tolerance[3] as well as promoting the survival and function of NK cells.[4] The IL7R, although it also shares the γc chain, has been shown to be primarily important for early stages of T-cell development, but not NK cells, as well as for maintaining of T-cell homeostasis in the periphery.

T-cell death

The tremendous capacity of T cells to undergo proliferation and activation carries also an inherent risk of over-expansion. Hence appropriate and timely induction of apoptosis of T cells at

various stages of development is crucial (Chapter 13). Some of the mechanisms leading to T-cell apoptosis in the thymus, particularly during the negative selection of DP thymocytes, were described above. These mechanisms often involve down-regulation of anti-apoptosis molecules such as BCL-2 and upregulation of pro-apoptotic molecules such as BIM and BAX. In peripheral T lymphocytes, ligation of the FAS receptor initiates apoptosis through the adaptor molecule FAS-associated protein with death domain (FADD), caspase 8, and other members of the caspase cascade pathways culminating in cell death. In addition, improper DNA maintenance, as well as malfunction of several DNA-damage repair molecules also induces apoptosis of T cells.[5] Importantly, decreased apoptosis can cause autoimmunity and malignancy, while exaggerated apoptosis can cause reduced thymic output and TD.

Profound T-cell immune deficiencies

TD can be divided into three groups including (A) presentation with absent or very low CD3[+] T cells (<500 cell/μL), commonly referred to as classical SCID; (B) T-cell immunodeficiency with autologous T cells (TDA) with CD3[+] T cells ≥500/μL caused either by hypomorphic mutations in genes associated with SCID or by genetic abnormalities presenting predominantly with TDA; and

Fig. 35.2 T-cell signaling cascade. Activation of T cells following specific peptide by major histocompatibility complex (MHC) to the T-cell receptor (TCR) involves signaling through IL receptors, co-receptors, and calcium tunnels. Recruitment of additional intracellular molecules triggers changes in gene expression, cytokine secretion, and receptor expression. Abbreviations: TAP, transporter associated with antigen presentation; TAPBP, TAP binding protein; MHC, major histocompatibility complex; CIITA, class II MHC transactivator; IL-7, interleukin-7; IL7Rα, alpha chain of the IL7 receptor; CD40L, CD40 ligand; ZAP-70, ζ-chain-associated protein kinase 70; JAK, Janus activated kinase; γc, gamma common chain of the IL-2 receptor; LCK, lymphocyte-specific protein tyrosine kinase; STAT, signal-transducer and activator of transcription; CBL, Casitas B-lineage lymphoma; WASP, Wiskott–Aldrich syndrome protein; SLP76, SH2 domain containing leukocyte protein of 76 kDa; LAT, linker for activation of T cells; PLC1, Phospholipase C 1; GRB2, growth factor receptor-bound protein 2; DAG, diacylglycerol; RAS, rat sarcoma; MAPK, mitogen-activated protein kinase; PKC, Protein kinase C; NF-κB, nuclear factor kappa-light-chain-enhancer of activated B cells; NFAT, nuclear factor of activated T cells; RAG, recombination activating genes; LIG4, DNA ligase 4; ATM, ataxia telangiectasia mutated; DCLRE1C, DNA cross-link repair 1 C; MRE11A, MRE11 meiotic recombination 11 homolog A; RMRP, RNA component of mitochondrial RNA processing endoribonuclease.

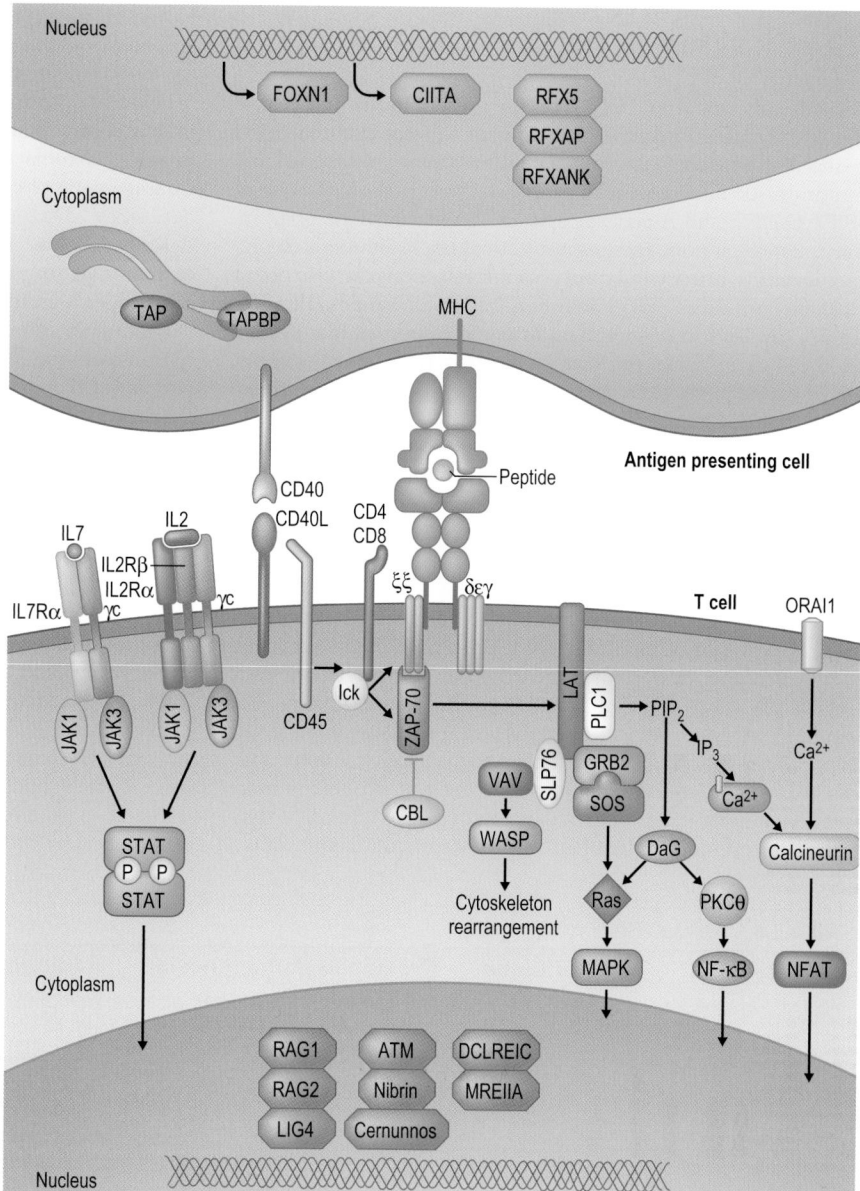

(C) well-defined syndromes with prominent multi-system involvement including TDA. However, this classification should not be used dogmatically, as there is a wide clinical and immunological spectrum, reflecting effects of different mutations within TD-causing genes, as well as genetic, epigenetic, and environmental factors. For example, although adenosine deaminase (ADA) deficiency typically causes SCID with absent or very low circulating T cells, few ADA-deficient patients develop Omenn syndrome (OS), while others may present later in life with features of TDA. Conversely, while most patients with cartilage hair hypoplasia (CHH) have only mild to moderate immune abnormalities, few have also been identified with SCID or OS.

Importantly, the diagnosis of TD should be considered after excluding secondary non-hereditary causes of severe immune deficiency, such as infections, medications, malignancies, nutritional deficiencies and others (Chapter 38). In the past, the frequency of TD was estimated at 1:50 000–1:100 000 live births. However, increased awareness and improved diagnosis, as well as preliminary data from neonatal screening programs, now suggest a frequency of 25 000–30 000, particularly among populations with increased parental consanguinity or founder effects.

● **KEY CONCEPTS**

Profound T-cell immunodeficiency: clinical and laboratory features

- Patients with profound T-cell immunodeficiency typically present in infancy with repeated, invasive, difficult-to-treat infections caused by routine or opportunistic pathogens.
- Patients with profound T-cell immunodeficiency typically have small/absent lymphatic tissue and thymus.
- Profound T-cell immunodeficiency can also present with autoimmunity/Omenn's syndrome, granulomatous disease or malignancy, in infancy or later in life.
- Profound T-cell immunodeficiency can be associated with well-defined multi-system disorders with known genetic defects.
- Profound T-cell immunodeficiency can be associated with markedly reduced/absent or non-functional B and NK cells.
- Absence or presence of T, B, and NK cells help identify the molecular causes of profound T-cell immunodeficiency.
- T cells can be present in patients with profound T-cell immunodeficiency; however, their diversity and ability to respond appropriately to stimulations are severely impaired.

TD with absent or very low T cells (SCID)

Patients suffering from SCID typically present in the first year of life with repeated invasive and difficult to treat bacterial, viral (particularly cytomegalovirus, parainfluenza and rotavirus) and opportunistic infections such as *Pneumocystis jiroveci pneumoniae* (PJP), *Candida* and *Aspergillus* species. These infections often involve the respiratory and gastrointestinal track, although meningitis, arthritis, urinary tract and systemic infections can also occur. Epstein–Barr virus (EBV) infection, although rare in this age group, can lead to uncontrolled immune responses manifesting as B-cell lymphoma or hemophagocytic lymphohistiocytosis. Diarrhea and increased resting energy expenditure also contribute to the frequent failure to thrive observed in these patients.[6]

Family history is extremely important in the diagnosis and evaluation of TD. Early death of a family member from infection and parental or ancestral consanguinity are vital clues to the putative diagnosis of TD. Moreover, the presence of a male sibling or a maternal uncle with TD suggests an X-linked recessive mode of inheritance. However, lionization of X chromosome in females, mosaic expression, partial and variable penetration as well as presence of modifying genes can pose diagnostic challenges. Another important clue is the family's origin, as some defects are more common among specific ethnic groups. For example, Artemis gene mutations are prevalent among the Athabascan-speaking Navajo and Apache Native Americans;[7] mutations in the recombination activating gene *RAG2* are more frequent among Palestinian patients with TD,[8] while CD3δ deficiency is commonly identified in the Mennonite community.[9]

However, in most patients with TD such indicators are absent, emphasizing the crucial role of universal neonatal screening for the early diagnosis of TD.

Physical examination of patients with typical TD reveals lack of lymphatic tissue including absence of tonsils while chest imaging is remarkable for the absence of a thymus shadow. Characteristic physical features can aid in identifying immunodeficiency diseases associated with defined syndromes, as described below. In a few patients with TD, allogeneic T cells of maternal origin or transmitted through blood transfusion can trigger a graft versus host (GvH)-like disorder.

Laboratory investigations in patients with SCID reveal severe lymphopenia stemming from marked reduction in the number of circulating T lymphocytes, which are typically < 500 cell/μL.[10] Expansion of other lymphocyte lineages such as B cells in patients with γc mutations or NK lymphocytes in patients with RAG mutations can lead to normal or increased lymphocyte counts. Therefore, enumeration of lymphocyte populations should be done by flow cytometry using fluorescent antibodies to antigens expressed on the cell surface (Chapter 94). This analysis should include CD2, CD3, CD4, and CD8 for T cells, CD19 or CD20 for B cells, and CD16 or CD56 for NK cells. The absence or presence of the various lymphocyte lineages also allows grouping of SCID as absent (or low) T, B, and NK cells (T⁻B⁻NK⁻ SCID, Table 35.1), absent (or low) T and NK cells with normal B cells (T⁻B⁺NK⁻ SCID, Table 35.2), absent (or low) T and B cells with normal NK cells (T⁻B⁻NK⁺ SCID, Table 35.3), or absent (or low) T cells with normal B and NK cells (T⁻B⁺NK⁺ SCID, Table 35.4). In addition, *in vitro* response of T cells to mitogen stimulation with PHA or anti-CD3 antibody, which can be

Table 35.1 T⁻B⁻NK⁻ SCID

Disease	Inheritance	Presumed pathogenesis	Additional features	Treatment
Reticular dysgenesis	AR	Impaired mitochondrial energy metabolism and leukocyte differentiation	Severe neutropenia, deafness. Mutations in adenylate kinase 2	gCSG HSCT
Adenosine deaminase deficiency	AR	Accumulation of toxic purine nucleosides	Neurological, hepatic, renal, lung, and skeletal and bone marrow abnormalities	HSCT, PEG-ADA, gene therapy

Table 35.2 T⁻B⁺NK⁻ SCID

Disease	Inheritance	Presumed pathogenesis	Additional features	Treatment
IL2Rγ deficiency	X-linked	Abnormal signaling through by IL-2 receptor and other receptors containing γc (IL-4, -7, -9, -15, -21)	None	HSCT
JAK3 deficiency	AR	Abnormal signaling downstream of γc	None	HSCT

Table 35.3 T⁻B⁻NK⁺ SCID

Disease	Inheritance	Presumed pathogenesis	Additional features	Treatment
RAG1 and 2 deficiency	AR	Defective V(D)J recombination	None	HSCT
Artemis deficiency	AR	Defective V(D)J recombination, radiation sensitivity	*DCLERE1C* gene defects	HSCT
DNA-PK deficiency	AR	Defective V(D)J recombination	None	HSCT
DNA ligase IV deficiency	AR	Defective V(D)J recombination, radiation sensitivity	Growth delay, microcephaly, bone marrow abnormalities, lymphoid malignancies	HSCT
Cernunnos-XLF	AR	Defective V(D)J recombination, radiation sensitivity	Growth delay, microcephaly, bird-like facies, bone defects	HSCT

Table 35.4 T⁻B⁺NK⁺ SCID

Disease	Inheritance	Presumed pathogenesis	Additional features	Treatment
CD3δ deficiency	AR	Arrest of thymocytes differentiation at the CD4⁻CD8⁻ stage	Thymus size may be normal	HSCT
CD3ε deficiency	AR	Arrest of thymocytes differentiation at the CD4⁻CD8⁻ stage	γ/δ T cells absent	HSCT
CD3ζ deficiency	AR	Abnormal signaling	None	HSCT
IL7Rα deficiency	AR	Abnormal IL7R signaling	Thymus absent	HSCT
CD45 deficiency	AR		None	HSCT
Coronin 1A deficiency	AR	Abnormal T-cell egress from thymus and lymph nodes	Normal thymus size. Attention deficit disorder.	HSCT

quantified by measuring [³H]thymidine incorporation into the DNA of replicating cells, should be assessed. Typically, T cells from patients with profound TD have <50% of the response observed in healthy controls. Alternative methods to assess T-cell responses have been introduced in recent years, including measurement of cell proliferation by dilution of carboxyfluorescein diacetate (CFDA) or incorporation of non-radioactive bromo-deoxyuridine (BrDU) and ethynyl-2'-deoxyuridine (EdU) into DNA, which are detected by fluorescence-activated cell sorting.[11] Other methods to assess T cells *in vitro* include measuring cytokine secretion by the cells or determining the cells' cytotoxic activity in "mixed lymphocyte reaction" (Chapter 95).

Analysis of thymopoiesis can also help in the diagnosis of TD. T-cell receptor excision circles (TREC), which are fragments of genomic DNA formed during V(D)J recombination in thymocytes, have been shown to reflect thymus activity (Chapter 101). In our lab, TREC levels in patients with TD are typically below 400/μg DNA. The stability of genomic DNA, which can be accurately quantified by PCR, even from Guthrie cards, has become the mainstay of TD neonatal screening programs. Indeed, combining T-cell enumeration, measurement of T-cell responses to mitogens and TREC are sufficient to establish the diagnosis of TD, which can often be confirmed by identification of a molecular defect. Generation of naïve T cells by the thymus can also be assessed by the percentage of T cells expressing CD45RA relative to the memory T cells expressing CD45RO.

SCID is a medical emergency, as patients are extremely susceptible to developing additional severe and debilitating infections. A team experienced in the management of SCID should provide care for these patients. Patients should be placed in protective isolation and receive aggressive treatment and prophylaxis for infections. Many patients cannot produce appropriate antibodies; therefore intravenous immunoglobulin replacement therapy should be initiated. Patients should not receive any live vaccines, such as BCG, oral polio, VZV, MMR, or rotavirus, as these attenuated pathogens can cause fatal infections. In addition, patients should only receive irradiated blood products, T-cell depleted and from CMV-negative donors. Appropriate nutrition should also be planned once the patient is stabilized.[6] Correction of the immune deficiency can often be accomplished by hematopoietic stem cells transplantation (HSCT), which should be done as quickly as possible (Chapter 82). Best results are achieved when a family related HLA-identical donor is used, with long-term survival approaching 90%.[12] However, such donors are available for less than 20% of patients. Alternatively, we have shown that the use of HLA-matched unrelated donors (MUD) provides excellent survival (>80%) and long-term immune reconstitution.[12] In the absence of MUD, stem cells from a haplo-identical family donor can be used. Unfortunately, in many large and experienced centers, HSCT with haplo-identical

donors are associated with up to 30% graft loss, increased frequency of lung complications, delayed and impaired immune reconstitution and <60% survival.[12,13] Indeed, in the absence of a related HLA-identical donor, the current European EBMT/ ESID guidelines indicate that MUD transplantations are preferable to the use of a haplo-identical family donor. Gene therapy using the patient's own hematopoietic stem cells has also been attempted in patients with SCID (Chapter 86). Unfortunately, 25% of patients developed leukemia after gene therapy for IL2Rγ deficiency.[14] Gene therapy for ADA deficiency has been more successful as most patients have been free of infections, growing well, and so far have not developed leukemia;[15] however, long-term efficacy and safety of ADA gene therapy are still not known.

● KEY CONCEPTS

Profound T-cell immunodeficiency: classification

- Absent or very low CD3⁺ T cells (<500 cell/μL), commonly referred to as classical severe combined immunodeficiency.
- T-cell immunodeficiency with autologous CD3⁺ T cells (≥500 /μL) caused by hypomorphic mutations in SCID-associated genes or by genetic abnormalities, which predominantly present as T-cell immunodeficiency with autologous T cells.
- Well-defined syndromes with prominent multi-system involvement as well as T-cell immunodeficiency with autologous T cells.

With the availability of flow cytometry analysis in most pediatric centers, categorization of profound T-cell deficiency in accordance to the affected lymphocyte lineages has become a resourceful tool for many clinicians, as detailed in the following sections. It should, however, be remembered that different mutations within TD-causing genes, as well as genetic, epigenetic, and environmental factors, may result in variation of the phenotype.

TD with absent (or low) T, B, and NK cells (T⁻B⁻NK⁻SCID)

Reticular dysgenesis

Absence of all lymphocyte lineages is a very rare form of TD that has been reported commonly among patients with reticular dysgenesis. Typically, patients with reticular dysgenesis suffer from a block in myeloid differentiation, resulting in severe neutropenia that leads to disseminated fungal infections very early in life. Deafness has also been reported in these patients. Recently, mutations in the gene encoding the mitochondrial energy metabolism adenylate kinase 2 (AK2), an enzyme important for leukocyte differentiation, were found in patients with autosomal recessive reticular dysgenesis.[16,17] The neutropenia is often unresponsive to gCSF treatment and the only cure for these patients is HSCT.

Adenosine deaminase deficiency

ADA is a central enzyme in the degradation and salvage of adenosine and deoxyadenosine, which are important for many biological processes, including energy transfer, extra and intracellular signaling and DNA formation (Fig. 35.3). In 1972, inherited ADA defects were recognized as causing autosomal recessive SCID with no or low T cells. ADA deficiency is estimated to account for 15–25% of SCID. All lymphocyte lineages might be affected by accumulation of toxic metabolites, resulting in absent or low T, B, and NK cells. However, as purine metabolite accumulation can occur over a period of time and because different lymphocyte lineages display diverse sensitivity to this intoxication, the immunological phenotype of patients can vary over time. Thus, ADA deficient patients can present with $T^-B^+NK^+$, $T^-B^-NK^+$, or $T^-B^-NK^-$ phenotype. In addition, leaky and hypomorphic mutations in ADA can result in OS,[18] while "partial" ADA deficiency can cause autoimmunity[19] as well as milder and delayed presentation, even in adulthood.[20] While TD remains the dominant phenotype of this metabolic disease, other organs and tissues can also be affected, including the brain, skeleton, liver, kidneys, lung, and bone marrow.[21–23] The diagnosis of ADA deficiency is often established by demonstrating lack of ADA enzyme activity in patients' erythrocytes (if the patient did not receive recent red blood cell transfusions) and supported by demonstrating significant increase of deoxyadenosine nucleotides (dAXP) in the patient's cells. To prevent the progressive toxicity, correction of the metabolic defect should be attempted as quickly as possible. Previously, frequent transfusions of red blood cells, which contain high concentrations of ADA enzyme, were given to ADA-deficient patients. Subsequently, bovine ADA enzyme, which was coupled with polyethylene glycol in order to reduce immunogenicity and extend biological activity (PEG-ADA), was shown to improve the immune and non-immune abnormalities in more than 80% of ADA-deficient patients.[24] However, the benefits of PEG-ADA

are often partial and temporary, resulting in increased susceptibility to infections, autoimmunity, and malignancy at an older age.[25,26] Gene therapy has also been attempted in ADA deficiency. In recent years, the addition of mild myeloablative medications and discontinuation of PEG-ADA prior to the infusion of the gene-corrected cells improved immune reconstitution of ADA-deficient patients.[15] However, long-term engraftment and benefits of ADA gene therapy await further studies. Until better protein or gene therapy becomes available, HSCT remains the only corrective treatment offered to most ADA-deficient patients. However, the success rate of such procedures is significantly lower than that observed in non-ADA deficient SCID. The disappointing outcome of HSCT in ADA deficiency might be related to pre-existing non-reversible damage to immune and non-immune organs, increased sensitivity of the patient's organs to chemotherapy or delayed donor immune reconstitution in the toxic purine-rich environment. Best results are achieved when an HLA-matched sibling donor is available, and often such transplants are performed without any myeloablative conditioning. Particularly disappointing are the results of HSCT when haplo-identical donors, are used.[27] Therefore, the recent European guidelines suggest that in the absence of an HLA-matched family donor, an HLA-matched unrelated donor should be sought.

TD with absent (or low) T and NK cells but normal B cells (T⁻B⁺NK⁻SCID)

IL-2R (γc) deficiency

Defects in the γ chain of the IL2R are the most common cause of SCID, and patients are frequently referred to as X-linked SCID because the γ chain maps to Xq12-13. IL2Rγ-deficient patients often present in infancy with typical SCID features. While T and NK cells are absent, there is often significant increase in the number of B lymphocytes; therefore the absolute number of lymphocytes in these patients may be misleading. The few T cells that might be detected in the peripheral blood do not respond to stimulation with mitogens and TREC levels are undetected. HSCT either from an HLA-matched sibling donor, which can often be done without myeloablation, or from an HLA-matched unrelated donor result in excellent survival rates and long-term immune reconstitution. Gene therapy has also been attempted

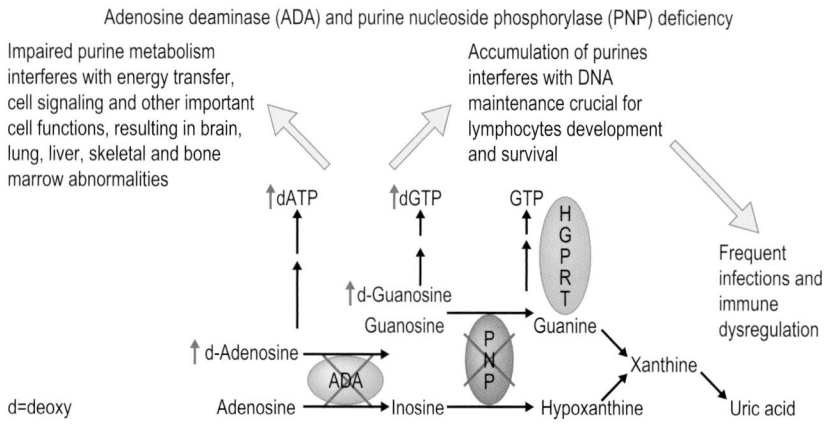

Adenosine deaminase (ADA) and purine nucleoside phosphorylase (PNP) deficiency

Impaired purine metabolism interferes with energy transfer, cell signaling and other important cell functions, resulting in brain, lung, liver, skeletal and bone marrow abnormalities

Accumulation of purines interferes with DNA maintenance crucial for lymphocytes development and survival

Frequent infections and immune dysregulation

↑dATP   ↑dGTP   GTP

↑d-Guanosine

Guanosine

↑d-Adenosine

Adenosine → Inosine → Hypoxanthine

Guanine

Xanthine

Uric acid

d=deoxy

ADA   PNP   HGPRT

Fig. 35.3 Adenosine deaminase and purine nucleoside phosphorylase deficiency. Adenosine deaminase and purine nucleoside phosphorylase are ubiquitous enzymes important for the degradation and salvage of purine metabolites. Inherited ADA or PNP defects cause accumulation of the enzyme's substrates, leading to increased concentrations of dATP or dGTP, respectively. The latter interfere with DNA maintenance, energy transfer, and cell signaling. Abbreviations: d, deoxy; HGPRT, hypoxanthine-guanine phosphoribosyltransferase.

in more than 30 patients; however, the high rate of fatal leukemia in addition to uncertainty of long-term correction of this defect has resulted in suspension of the procedure until gene delivery and safety are improved.

JAK3 deficiency

The IL2Rγ uses the JAK3 tyrosine kinase to transmit intracellular signaling; therefore it was not surprising that inherited defects in JAK3 also result in a T⁻B⁺NK⁻ SCID phenotype, practically indistinguishable from IL2Rγ deficiency.[29] JAK3 maps to chromosome 19; therefore, its inheritance follows an autosomal recessive pattern. Hence, in males with T⁻B⁺NK⁻ SCID and normal IL2Rγ as well as female patients with T⁻B⁺NK⁻ SCID, sequencing of JAK3 is needed to establish a molecular diagnosis. Currently the only definitive treatment for JAK3 deficiency is allogeneic HSCT, preferably from HLA-matched related or unrelated donors.[12]

TD with absent (or low) T and B cells but normal NK cells (T⁻B⁻NK⁺ SCID)

An inability to properly recombine the V(D)J gene segments interferes with T- and B-cell receptor formation, which severely impairs maturation and function of T and B cells. In contrast, NK cells, which do not require V(D)J gene rearrangement remain unaffected, resulting in a T⁻B⁻NK⁺ phenotype. Moreover, in some patients the number of NK cells is significantly elevated. Abnormalities in several genes important for V(D)J recombination have already been recognized as causing SCID with absent (or low) T and B cells but normal NK cells. Laboratory evaluations in these patients reveal practically absent T cells and no TREC. B cells are also very low and patients are unable to produce antibodies. If T cells are detectable, these cells are unable to respond to stimulation. There are several methods to measure the effects of *RAG1* and *RAG2* mutations on V(D)J recombination activity.[29,30] However, the clinical relevance of this analysis is not clear yet.

Patients with T⁻B⁻NK⁺ SCID can only be cured by HSCT. Initially, the outcome of such patients was reported to be lower than that of other forms of SCID.[31] However, recently we showed that with early diagnosis, proper myeloablative conditioning prior to HSCT and careful donor selection, patients with T⁻B⁻NK⁺ SCID have long-term survival rates and immune reconstitution similar to other forms of SCID.[12] Gene therapy by *ex vivo* insertion of wild-type gene copies, targeted *in situ* gene correction, directing genes into "safe harbors"[32] or compounds that can induce readthrough of nonsense mutations may become alternative treatment options for some of these patients.

RAG1 and RAG2 deficiency

Defects in recombination activating genes *RAG1* and *RAG2* were the first to be identified in patients T⁻B⁻NK⁺ SCID and they account for the majority of these patients. Patients typically have no T or B cells, while NK cells are normal or even elevated. RAG1 and 2 deficiencies are autosomal recessive diseases, which only affect the immune system, in contrast to some of the other T⁻B⁻NK⁺ SCID that are associated with non-immune consequences.

Artemis deficiency

Defects in Artemis, which is encoded by the *DCLRE1C* (DNA cross-link repair 1 C) gene, also causes autosomal recessive T⁻B⁻NK⁺ SCID secondary to abnormal V(D)J recombination.

In addition, patients' bone marrow cells and fibroblasts demonstrate increased sensitivity to irradiation. Because of a founder effect, Artemis deficiency is particularly common among the Athabascan speaking indigenous North American natives, although mutations in RAG and IL2Rγ are also found in this population.[7]

DNA-PK deficiency

Recently mutations in the DNA-dependent protein kinase (DNA-PK), an enzyme important for approximation of the hairpin extremities of the V(D)J coding sequences, together with Ku70/80, were identified in a 5-month-old female with autosomal recessive SCID and virtually absent T and B cells but normal NK cells.[33]

DNA ligase IV deficiency

Inherited defects in DNA ligase IV and Cernunnos-XLF deficiency can also cause SCID with absent (or low) T and B cells but normal NK cells. However, mutations in these genes are associated with typical non-immune abnormalities; therefore they will be described below in the section of "well-defined syndromes with prominent multi-system involvement including SCID."

TD with absent (or low) T with normal B and NK cells (T⁻B⁺NK⁺ SCID)

The TCR initiates signaling through activation of the invariant CD3 chains; hence mutations in the CD3 complex or its downstream signaling cascade often cause TD. B and NK cells are not dependent on this pathway; therefore patients typically present with absent or low T cells while B and NK cells are normal.

CD3δ deficiency

Mutations in the CD3δ gene were the first among the CD3 chains to be identified as a cause of autosomal recessive T⁻B⁺NK⁺ SCID.[9] In a kindred of Mennonite descent, we described patients who developed typical SCID features before 3 months of age. The patients had no circulating CD4⁺ or CD8⁺ T cells, but preserved B and NK cells, resulting in a T⁻B⁺NK⁺ phenotype. Interestingly, in contrast to most other forms of SCID, the size of the thymus in these patients was nearly normal. Analysis of thymus sections revealed preserved lobular structures with moderate populations of T-cell precursors; however, Hassall corpuscles were absent and there was no typical intra-lobar corticomedulla distinction. Microarray analysis of gene expression in the thymus of the patients revealed reduction in the transcripts of CD3δ and sequencing the patients CD3δ genes identified homozygous mutations that led to a premature stop in the CD3δ. The CD3δ defect causes arrest of thymocyte differentiation at the DN (CD4⁻CD8⁻) stage with accumulation of early thymocyte precursors. The presence of increased thymocyte precursors in the thymus of CD3δ patients is likely responsible for the increased frequency of engraftment failure following allogeneic HSCT performed without myeloablative conditioning.[34]

CD3ε deficiency

Mutations in CD3ε can also cause complete deficiencies in peripheral T cells, including γ/δ T cells.[35] Patients with this autosomal recessive T⁻B⁺NK⁺ SCID present before 2 months of age with cytomegalovirus pneumonitis, diarrhea and candidiasis.

CD3ζ deficiency

Defects in the CD3ζ chain were reported in a single patient with autosomal recessive T⁻B⁺NK⁺ SCID.[36] The female patient suffered from pneumonia at 4 months of age, followed by persistent cough, recurrent otitis media, failure to thrive, chronic mild rash, *Salmonella* gastroenteritis, thrombocytopenia, and CMV infection. T-cell numbers were initially very low, although subsequent studies demonstrated a large population of T cells with low expression of TCRε. These T cells did not respond to *in vitro* stimulation with PHA or anti-CD3 antibody. The patient received allogeneic HSCT at 12 months of age.

IL-7Rα deficiency

The IL7R, formed by the common γc chain and the IL7Rα chain, is crucial for the development of early thymocytes. Hence it was not surprising that null mutations in the IL7Rα were identified as a cause for autosomal recessive T⁻B⁺NK⁺ SCID.[37] Even missense mutations, which preserve production and expression of the IL7R, can cause T⁻B⁺NK⁺ SCID.[38] Importantly, early identification followed by allogeneic HSCT is curative for these patients.

CD45 deficiency

CD45 deficiency was reported in only 2 patients who presented in the first months of life with SCID features including disseminated CMV. Laboratory evaluations demonstrated lymphopenia with practically no CD4⁺ T cells and no *in vitro* response of T cells to mitogens.[39,40] In contrast, γδ T cells were not affected. The proportion of NK cells, defined by CD3⁻/CD16⁺/CD56⁺ expression, was below the normal level in one patient, leading some authors to categorize this autosomal recessive defect as T⁻B⁺NK⁻ SCID, although most consider CD45 deficiency as T⁻B⁺NK⁺ SCID.

Coronin 1A deficiency

The single patient described so far with coronin-1A deficiency, suffered from respiratory tract infections and oral thrush since infancy. She then developed extensive mucocutaneous chickenpox following vaccination with live attenuated varicella vaccine. Immune evaluation revealed very low T cells, with normal B and NK cell numbers. Responses of T cells to mitogens were initially normal but subsequently became severely depressed. Interestingly, the thymus was of normal size. It is thought that coronin is required for proper actin-cytoskeletal mediated egress of T cells from thymus and lymph nodes.[41]

⬤ T H E R A P E U T I C   P R I N C I P L E S

Profound T-cell immunodeficiency: management principles

- Profound T-cell immunodeficiency is a medical emergency.
- Profound T-cell immunodeficiency evaluation and treatment should be coordinated by a pediatric immunologist experienced in the management of such patients.
- Patients with profound T-cell immunodeficiency should be maintained in an isolated environment, receive prophylactic antibiotics and intravenous immunoglobulin, and appropriate nutrition.
- Patients with profound T-cell immunodeficiency should only receive CMV-negative, irradiated blood products and irradiated breast milk.
- Patients with profound T-cell immunodeficiency should not receive live vaccines.

T-cell deficiency with autologous T cells

T-cell immunodeficiency diseases with autologous T cells (TDA), also known as combined immunodeficiency, have been recognized at increasing frequency over the past two decades. Many of the affected patients present in infancy with features identical to SCID despite the presence of residual circulating T cells. Some patients with TDA present in infancy with a well-defined clinical phenotype, such as OS, while others have a delayed presentation with less frequent infections. Additionally, patients with TDA can present beyond the first year of life, or with recurrent infections, autoimmunity and hematological malignancy. Respiratory infections often lead to bronchiectasis, while gastrointestinal infections can result in failure to thrive and short stature. Cutaneous and mucosal candida infections, as well as herpes and papilloma virus infections can cause significant morbidity. In recent years, among patients with TDA there has been a surge in recognition of additional opportunistic infections including JC virus, herpes simplex virus 8 and others. Allergic manifestations such as eczema, asthma, urticaria and food allergy are also common. Autoimmunity develops in more than half of these patients, often resulting in difficult-to-treat hematopoietic cytopenias, hepatitis, and brain and kidney vasculitis.

Immunological assessment in patients with TDA reveals the presence of substantial numbers of circulating T cells (CD3⁺ cells ≥ 500/μL). Frequently, these cells represent mono- or oligoclonal T-cell expansion that lack the typical diversity of a normal T-cell repertoire. T-cell diversity can be analyzed by flow cytometry using fluorescent antibodies against Vβ families or by spectrotype determination of PCR-amplified CDR3 species. The flow cytometry analysis is relatively easy to perform using fresh samples, provides rapid results and allows separate assessment of CD4⁺ and CD8⁺ T cells, while spectroscopy provides more detailed analysis and can be performed on stored DNA samples. These T cells often have an increased percentage of memory cells (CD45RO⁻) and reduced levels of naïve cells (CD45RA⁺). In many cases, but not all, TREC levels are significantly reduced compared to normal age-matched controls. Regulatory T cells, characterized as CD4⁺CD25⁺Foxp3⁺, are often decreased. *In vitro*, responses to mitogens may be low, but not uniformly abnormal. Diagnosis of some TDA can be challenging as in some instances full immune evaluation does not decisively establish the diagnosis of TD. In these rare cases analysis of thymus morphology can be very helpful. Although normal thymus morphology does not exclude the possibility of TD, abnormal thymus morphology, including lack of Hassall corpuscles and/or loss of cortico-medulla demarcation, is consistently found in TD. Our evaluation strategy has been proven safe and beneficial for patients with TDA. It also allowed for earlier introduction of curative treatment such as HSCT, which is associated with improved outcome. Two striking examples of the benefit of this strategy have been the identification of an abnormal thymus in patients with ZAP-70 and CD25 deficiency, which led to successful HSCT many years prior to discovering the molecular diagnosis of these conditions.[42]

Management of patients with TDA includes prophylactic antibiotics, antifungal treatment, and immunoglobulin replacement. Patients should not receive live vaccines, and should be treated promptly once exposed to infections. Nutritional supplements and physiotherapy as well as psychological support to the patient and family are important. Historically, the outcome of patients with TDA was generally poor, as many died early in life from uncontrolled infections, organ failure, autoimmunity or malignancy. This could mostly be attributed to the lack or delay in recognizing and diagnosing these patients. Hence, curative HSCT should be considered as early as possible, taking into consideration multiple factors, including the age of the patient, the type of donor available, the severity and reversibility of existing non-immune organ damage, etc. For instance, cartilage-hair hypoplasia (CHH) could be an indication for HSCT, but not ataxia telangiectasia.

The circulating autologous T lymphocytes may have variable functions that can interfere with engraftment of donor cells; therefore patients suffering from TDA often need myeloablative conditioning prior to HSCT. Indeed, survival rate following HSCT of patients with TDA who did not receive conditioning has been traditionally low, while myeloablative regimens have resulted in far superior results.[43] Myeloablative doses of busulphan and cyclophosphamide have been used with excellent results with practically no short or long-term toxicity. Best outcomes following HSCT for patients with TDA remain with the use of a family related HLA-identical sibling donor. In the absence of HLA-identical siblings, some centers had opted for the use of HLA haplo-identical family members. However, compiled European experience has shown disappointing survival rate with frequent engraftment failure. In contrast, we chose more than 20 years ago to use MUD transplantations for these patients, resulting in outstanding survival rates (>85%) and long-term immune reconstitution.[44] In our experience, the most common complication following MUD HSCT in TDA was GvH disease, which often could be controlled with a pulse of methylprednisolone.[45] Nevertheless, GVH disease remains the direct culprit of mortality in most patients. Importantly, following MUD HSCT, and in contrast to haplo-HSCT, life-threatening infections were extremely rare, with an average of only 1 major infection following MUD HSCT.[46]

THERAPEUTIC PRINCIPLES

Profound T-cell immunodeficiency: transplantations

- Profound T-cell immunodeficiency can often be corrected by allogeneic hematopoietic stem cell transplantation.
- Transplantations should be performed as quickly as possible, while considering the patient's clinical status and donor availability.
- Best transplantations results are achieved when HLA-identical family donors are used.
- Transplantations using an HLA-matched unrelated donor are often associated with excellent long-term survival and immune reconstitution.
- Patients with profound T-cell immunodeficiency and autologous T cells often need myeloablative conditioning prior to transplantations.
- Patients with profound T-cell immunodeficiency caused by defects in adenosine deaminase can also benefit from enzyme replacement therapy or gene therapy.

TDA caused by hypomorphic mutations in genes associated with SCID

Omenn syndrome

OS was first described as familial reticuloendotheliosis with eosinophilia. The combination of fatal TD with generalized severe erythroderma and lymphadenopathy was initially thought to be

Table 35.5 T-cell immunodeficiency with autologous T cells associated with Omenn syndrome

Gene defect	Immune phenotype	Additional features
RAG1 deficiency	T$^{-/+}$B$^-$NK$^+$	None
RAG2 deficiency	T$^{-/+}$B$^-$NK$^+$	None
Artemis	T$^{-/+}$B$^-$NK$^+$	Irradiation sensitivity
DNA ligase IV deficiency	T$^{-/+}$B$^-$NK$^+$	Irradiation sensitivity, microcephaly
Adenosine deaminase deficiency	T$^{-/+}$B$^{-/+}$NK$^{-/+}$	Multi-system involvement
RMRP deficiency	T$^{-/+}$B$^+$NK$^-$	Cartilage hair hypoplasia
IL2Rγ deficiency	T$^{-/+}$B$^+$NK$^-$	X-linked
IL7Rα deficiency	T$^{-/+}$B$^+$NK$^+$	Autosomal recessive
CHD7	T$^{-/+}$B$^+$NK$^+$	CHARGE syndrome
22q11.2 microdeletion	T$^{-/+}$B$^+$NK$^+$	DiGeorge syndrome

caused only by hypomorphic mutations in RAG1 or RAG2; however, recent studies have shown that practically all TD that allow for some T-cell propagation can be associated with OS (Table 35.5). Patients with OS, similar to SCID, frequently present during the first year of life with chronic diarrhea, pneumonitis, and failure to thrive. However, in contrast to the typical paucity or absence of lymph nodes in SCID, patients with OS have enlarged lymph nodes, spleen and liver. In addition, they suffer from generalized erythroderma, which may be accompanied with alopecia and loss of eyebrows and eyelashes. Significant protein loss through the skin and the gut can lead to generalized edema and metabolic disturbances as well as failure to thrive. Importantly, signs and symptoms of OS can evolve with time, and might be triggered following exposure to food antigens or infections.

CLINICAL PEARLS

Guidelines for the diagnosis of T-cell immunodeficiency with autologous T cells

- Presentation with typical infections such as *Pneumocystis jiroveci* pneumonia, CMV pneumonitis, oral thrush, or recurrent invasive infections.
- Disseminated or atypical disease after exposure to live vaccines or common pathogens.
- Presentation with severe gastrointestinal manifestations, autoimmunity, granuloma formation, or lymphoid malignancy in early age.
- Family history of profound T-cell immunodeficiency.
- CD3$^+$ T cells usually ≥500 cell/μL.
- Restricted diversity of T-cell repertoire.
- Low CD45RA$^+$ T cells or TREC.
- Decreased or deteriorating function of circulating T cells.
- Dysplastic thymus morphology.
- Identification of defect in a gene/protein involved in T-cell development or function.
- Signs and symptoms relevant to the syndrome such as short stature (cartilage-hair hypoplasia), microcephaly (DNA ligase IV deficiency), or facial features (DiGeorge syndrome).

Immune evaluations in patients with OS pose a diagnostic challenge because they often reveal normal or high lymphocyte counts, unlike typical SCID.[47] The assessment of lymphocyte markers by flow cytometry is helpful in most cases, but could be misleading as the number of circulating CD3[+], CD4[+], and CD8[+] T cells may be normal. Importantly, and in contrast with observations in healthy infants, a substantial portion of T lymphocytes from patients with OS co-express activation markers including CD45RO and HLA-DR. Similar clinical and laboratory features can also be observed among SCID patients with maternal T-cell engraftment. Despite the normal or increased number of circulating T cells, the responses of T cells from patients with OS to stimulation with mitogens and antigens *in vitro* are often severely reduced. Another hallmark of OS is the abnormal mono- or oligoclonal T-cell expansion in peripheral blood and tissues. Quantitative assessment of the T-cell repertoire in these patients may reveal overrepresentation of a few T-cell clones and under-representation or complete absence of most other Vβ families.[48] The expansion of T cells in the periphery also causes dilution of TRECs; hence patients with OS typically have markedly reduced or absent TREC levels. The number of B and NK cells varies in accordance to the molecular defects, as described above for patients with SCID. Humoral immunity is invariably depressed, similar to most other types of SCID, while IgE levels are frequently elevated. Skin biopsies may be helpful in guiding to the diagnosis of OS.[47] Typically, staining with hematoxylin and eosin shows acanthosis and parakeratosis. Dyskeratosis and spongiosis are seen in the Malpighian layer and vacuolation is often observed in the basal layer. Inflammatory cells can be present in the epidermis but are typically more prominent in the dermis and to a lesser degree at the dermal–epidermal junction. Inflammatory infiltrates consist predominantly of mononuclear cells and eosinophils. Immunohistochemistry in the skin of patients with OS often demonstrates CD3[+] T cells (mostly of the CD4[+] subset) and a small number of macrophages.

The clonal T-cell expansion in OS is attributed in part to hypomorphic mutations that hamper but do not completely abolish thymocyte maturation, resulting in a "leaky" defect. Interestingly, although there is extensive variability in the representation of T-cell clones among patients with OS, few Vβ families appear dominant (Vβ 17, Vβ 14, Vβ 13, and Vβ 3), even across different genotypes, suggesting possibly a common (auto)antigen-driven mechanism for the T-cell expansion.[47] Recently we provided evidence for an additional mechanism to generate autoreactive T cells. We showed reduced AIRE expression by medullary thymic epithelial cells in thymuses of patients with OS that could lead to impaired negative selection.[49] Regardless of the cause for dysregulated T-cell development, these cells may infiltrate target tissues such as the skin, gut, and liver, and secrete cytokines inducing local damage. The T-cell clones in the peripheral blood of patients with OS are predominantly of the Th2 phenotype, hence they secrete IL-4 and -13, -9, and -5, which promote IgE production as well as expansion of eosinophil and mast cell populations. Together with the impaired production of Treg in the dysfunctional thymus of OS patients, these processes can lead to uncontrolled allergy, inflammation and autoimmunity.

We and others have identified OS in association with hypomorphic mutations in many SCID-causing genes (Table 35.5), including Artemis, DNA ligase IV, RMRP, ZAP-70, γc, IL7Rα, CD3δ, ADA, RAG1, and RAG2.[34] Interestingly, hypomorphic mutations in some of these genes, such as RAG and IL7Rα, can in some siblings cause OS, while other siblings may present as typical SCID with no or very low T cells.[50] Moreover, changes over time in the same patient suggest the immune phenotype is influenced by epigenetic or modifier genes.[51] Regardless of the molecular cause of OS, patients require systemic corticosteroids and/or cyclosporine to suppress the uncontrolled inflammation. Ultimately, patients with OS can only be cured with allogeneic HSCT. Initial results of HSCT for OS were disappointing, possibly because of late diagnosis, inadequate control of the severe inflammation, selection of less favorable (haplo-identical) donors or avoidance of proper myeloablative regimens. We have recently reported excellent survival and long-term immune function following busulphan and cyclophosphamide conditioning and HLA-matched related or unrelated HSCT in OS.[46]

Hypomorphic mutations in γc

We identified several unrelated male infants who grew normally until the age of 6 to 9 months, when oral thrush, PJP and recurrent skin infections developed.[52] Patients had normal-sized tonsils and cervical lymph nodes, as well as normal thymus size. Peripheral lymphocyte markers, including CD3[+], CD4[+] and CD8[+], CD19[+], and CD56[+] cells as well as T-cell repertoire and *in vitro* T-lymphocyte responses to PHA and anti-CD3 were comparable to control samples. Thymic biopsy demonstrated the presence of Hassall corpuscles and clear corticomedulla demarcation. Sequencing of the patient's DNA revealed a single amino acid change (R222C) in the γc gene. Allogeneic HSCT in these patients provided long-term immune reconstitution.

Table 35.6 T-cell immunodeficiency diseases associated with growth and skeletal defects

Disease	Gene(s) affected	Inheritance	Immunological characteristics	Additional features
Cartilage hair hypoplasia	RMRP	AR	SCID, Omenn syndrome, susceptibility to VZV, impaired antibody production, autoimmunity	Short-limbed dwarfism, fine light-colored hair, bone marrow dysplasia, abnormal intestinal plexus neurons, impaired spermatogenesis, malignancy
Adenosine deaminases deficiency	ADA	AR	SCID, Omenn syndrome, partial and delayed TDA, autoimmunity	Chondro-osseous, neurological, hepatic, renal, lung, and bone marrow abnormalities
DiGeorge syndrome	22q11.2	AD	SCID, Omenn syndrome, TDA, autoimmunity	Cardiac defects, hypocalcemia, dysmorphism, cleft palate, short stature, neuropsychiatric problems
Dyskeratosis congenita	Dyskerin TERT bNOP10 NHP2 TERC TINF2	X-linked, AD, AR	SCID, TDA	Growth delay, nail and skin defects, non-infectious enteropathy, developmental delay, microcephaly, and cerebellar hypoplasia

Hypomorphic mutations in JAK3

Brugnoni, et al. described an infant with JAK3 mutations that affected but did not abolish JAK3 protein expression and function. By 3 months of age, the patient had circulating autologous $CD3^+CD4^+$ T cells, which climbed beyond 3000 cells/μL.[53] These cells showed a primed-activated phenotype, defective secretion of T-helper 1 and 2 cytokines, reduced proliferation to mitogens and a high *in vitro* susceptibility to spontaneous and activation-induced cell death. A restricted T-cell receptor repertoire was observed, with oligoclonal expansion within each of the dominant segments. Milder phenotypes were also described in association with hypomorphic JAK3 mutations, including a thriving female baby who presented at 19 months of age with recurrent mild respiratory tract infections and persistent candidiasis.[54] Another patient was diagnosed at 6 years of age when searching for a bone marrow donor for her younger brother. The sister remained clinically well for many years without transplant, complaining primarily of disseminated warts. In another family with JAK3 mutations, an 8-year-old patient suffered from lymphoproliferative disease while an 18-year-old sibling carrying the same mutations was practically healthy.[55] Thus screening for *JAK3* gene mutations should be considered in patients with ill-defined T-cell deficiencies.

Hypomorphic mutations in RAG1 and 2

RAG1 and *RAG2* hypomorphic mutations, in addition to causing OS, can lead to autosomal recessive TDA with various phenotypes. These phenotypes include:

(a) non-infectious granulomas of the skin, bones, lymph nodes, spleen, sinus or cartilaginous laryngeal structures, which may appear before the development of opportunistic infections.[30,56] The granulomas are often extensive, and persist despite treatment with topical steroids, tacrolimus and broad-spectrum antibiotics. The granulomas do resolve after HSCT, suggesting that they are caused by immune dysregulation. Similar granulomas were also reported recently among patients with hypomorphic mitochondrial RNA-processing endoribonuclease (*RMRP*) and Artemis mutations.[57,58]

(b) autoimmune blood cell cytopenia and disseminated CMV infection.[59]

(c) $CD4^+$ lymphocytopenia, as reported recently in an adolescent female who suffered from extensive chickenpox and recurrent pneumonia. The latter patient had reduced naïve T and B cells with intact proliferative capacity and normal antibody production. T-cell receptor-Vβ repertoire was polyclonal but TREC levels were markedly reduced.[60]

Hypomorphic mutations in ADA

In addition to classical SCID, patients with *ADA* gene mutations that permit some enzyme activity can have an attenuated phenotype or present beyond infancy and into adulthood.[20,61] These late-onset ADA deficient patients suffer predominantly from recurrent sinopulmonary bacterial infections, autoimmune hypothyroidism, diabetes mellitus, hemolytic anemia, and idiopathic thrombocytopenia. Some patients also develop recalcitrant warts, severe lung disease and bronchiectasis. In addition to lymphopenia, laboratory evaluations in these patients often show eosinophilia and markedly elevated IgE levels. The optimal management of these patients is not yet clear. While ADA replacement therapy with PEG-ADA may provide temporary benefit, long-term immune function and survival with this treatment has not been established.

Genetic aberrations presenting predominantly with TDA

Several genetic abnormalities can present predominantly with TDA. They frequently predispose to autoimmunity and malignancy, in addition to susceptibility to infections and failure to thrive.

ζ-Associated protein (ZAP-70) deficiency

ZAP-70 deficiency is an autosomal recessive TDA that often results in a distinct phenotype. The essential role of ZAP-70 in TCR-mediated signal transduction was first uncovered by this human T-cell deficiency. Moreover, ZAP-70 deficiency was the first *in vivo* demonstration that a protein tyrosine kinase is absolutely required for T-cell activation and proliferation. ZAP-70 deficiency was originally described among patients who presented with *Pneumocystis jiroveci* pneumonitis and normal numbers of CD4 circulating T cells, but low to absent CD8 T cells. The circulating CD4 T cells failed to respond to *in vitro* stimulation with PHA or anti-CD3 antibody; however, incubation of these cells with TPA and ionomycin rescued the proliferative response. The thymus of patients with ZAP-70 deficiency reveals the presence of Hassall corpuscles, normal architecture and normal numbers of $CD4^+CD8^+$ thymocytes in the cortex but reduced numbers of $CD8^+$ cells in the medulla.[42] Surprisingly, TREC levels are reduced in these patients despite the relatively preserved thymus, indicating that thymopoiesis is depressed.[43,44] In addition, analysis of sequential recombination events involving the TCR genes indicates that T-cell differentiation is impaired before the δREC-ψJα rearrangement, a late TCR delta-deleting rearrangement. Allogeneic HSCT can completely correct the immunodeficiency. Clinical presentations of ZAP-70 deficiency also include OS, ulcerative colitis and thrombocytopenia, lymphoma, unusual pustular skin lesions, or a delayed moderate course of recurrent infections beyond infancy.[62-64]

CD25 (IL2Rα) deficiency

IL2Rα deficiency was the first single gene defect shown to directly cause autoimmunity. We identified a male patient that suffered from cytomegalovirus pneumonitis, persistent oral thrush and candida esophagitis from 6 months of age, followed by adenovirus gastroenteritis, chronic diarrhea and failure to thrive.[3] From 8 months of age, lymphadenopathy and hepatosplenomegaly became increasingly apparent with chronic inflammation of his mandible and chronic lung disease. The absolute number of peripheral $CD3^+$ T lymphocytes was relatively low with significant reduction in $CD4^+$ cells. The response of T cells to stimulation by PHA and anti-CD3 was reduced and could not be corrected by addition of exogenous IL-2. Analysis of the patient's thymus revealed a normal sized thymus with minimal Hassall corpuscles and a lack of distinct cortico-medulla demarcation. There was also dense lymphocytic infiltration into the lung, liver, gut, soft tissue, and bone, accompanied by tissue atrophy and chronic inflammation. Immunohistochemical analysis of the thymus revealed absence of CD25 expression. In addition, the patient had multiple autoantibodies, including anti-mitochondrial and anti-nuclear antibodies, as well as antibodies to recombinant human PDC-E2, sp100, F-actin, and chromatin. These autoantibodies may have contributed to the patient's primary biliary cirrhosis. Allogeneic HSCT after myeloablative conditioning corrected the susceptibility to infections and completely reversed the autoimmunity associated with this autosomal recessive disorder. Other cases of CD25 deficiency were subsequently reported with endocrinopathy, severe eczema and cytopenia.[65]

Orai1 and Stim1 deficiencies

Orai1 and Stim1 are important for calcium influx and their deficiency can cause autosomal recessive TDA.[66] Patients often suffer from recurrent and severe bacterial, viral and opportunistic infections in the first few months of life, although one patient survived until 9 years of age. Laboratory evaluations in these patients show normal numbers of lymphocytes, total T lymphocytes as well as CD4$^+$ and CD8$^+$ T cells. In contrast, *in vitro* T-cell activation through TCR dependent or independent pathways is impaired. Some, but not all, of the patients, have normal T-cell stimulation with PMA and ionomycin. T-cell repertoire is preserved, suggesting normal T-cell development. B-cell numbers and immunoglobulin levels are also normal, although patients often fail to mount an adequate antibody response following vaccinations. A few patients also suffer from autoimmunity, particularly hematopoietic cytopenia, as well as lymphoproliferation. In addition to the immune defects, patients display congenital non-progressive myopathy (that may manifest as moderate to severe hypotonia), anhydrotic ectodermal dysplasia (associated with mutations in Orai1) and dental enamel defects. Allogeneic HSCT can correct the immune deficiency but not the myopathy.

FOXP3 deficiency

Mutations in the FOXP3 transcription factor cause an X-linked recessive disorder known as IPEX (Immune dysregulation, polyendocrinopathy, enteropathy X-linked) syndrome.[67] Similar to CD25 deficiency, affected male patients suffer from severe autoimmunity in infancy. Watery, difficult to control, or bloody diarrhea is often the predominant symptom. Neonatal-onset insulin-dependent diabetes mellitus and thyroid disease are reported in 30% of patients. Eczema is also a prominent manifestation. In addition, lymphadenopathy, hepatosplenomegaly, cholestatic hepatitis, nephropathy, hemolytic anemia, thrombocytopenia, neutropenia, seizures, sarcoidosis, vasculitis, arthralgia and arthritis have been reported. The immune abnormalities, as well as the decreased barrier function of the skin and the gut, likely contribute to the increased frequency of infections, including sepsis, meningitis, pneumonia and osteomyelitis. Histological examination of affected organs frequently reveals infiltration of CD3$^+$ T cells, eosinophils, and plasma cells as well as severe tissue destruction. Circulating CD4 and CD8 T cells are present in normal numbers and they respond appropriately to mitogen stimulation. TREC levels are also normal. However, the number and function of CD4$^+$CD25$^+$FOXP3$^+$ regulatory T cells is reduced. B and NK cells numbers are often normal and patients are able to produce protective antibodies; however, they also generate a variety of autoantibodies against the small intestine, pancreatic islet cells, thyroid, kidney, and hematopoietic cells. Immunosuppressive drugs such as steroids, cyclosporine, tacrolimus, sirolimus and others can transiently control the autoimmune phenomena, but allogeneic HSCT offers the best option for cure, particularly if performed early, before development of irreversible organ damage. Until now only few patients have received HSCT, with mixed results. Some centers have elected reduced-intensity conditioning, yet long-term correction of the immune defect was not always accomplished.

IL-10, IL-10 receptor α and β deficiencies

IL-10, produced mainly by T cells and macrophages, is an important anti-inflammatory cytokine. The role of IL-10 and its receptor IL10R, composed of α and β chains, in modulating immune responses was further emphasized by the discovery of autosomal recessive mutations in these genes among patients with early onset inflammatory bowel disease.[68] Peripheral-blood mononuclear cells from these patients secrete increased amounts of TNF-α and other proinflammatory cytokines. Some patients develop enteric fistulas as well as perianal abscesses and fistulas, often requiring partial bowel resections and ileostomy. Moreover, because IL-10 signaling is crucial for activation of regulatory T cells (Treg), cells that are central in preventing autoimmunity, some patients with IL-10/IL10R deficiency also develop autoimmune manifestations such as rheumatoid arthritis. Corticosteroids, methotrexate, thalidomide and anti-TNF-α monoclonal antibodies provide only partial and temporary remission. Reversal of the inflammation occurred in several patients following allogeneic HSCT.

CD40 ligand deficiency

Mutations in the gene encoding CD40 ligand cause X-linked hyper-IgM syndrome. These male patients typically present in infancy with bacterial or opportunistic sinopulmonary infections.[69] Some suffer from chronic *Cryptosporidium* infection, which may contribute to the increased frequency of sclerosing cholangitis and liver failure observed in these patients. Patients are also prone to develop autoimmunity and malignancy. The numbers of circulating T, B, and NK cells are normal, as is the response of T cells to stimulation. IgM levels are elevated in most, but not all, patients while IgG and IgA are markedly reduced. The diagnosis is supported by flow cytometric analysis, demonstrating inability of T cells to upregulate CD40 ligand expression following over-night stimulation. However, because patients may have missense mutations that allow some CD40L expression, the diagnosis is often established by gene sequencing. Allogeneic HSCT, particularly if performed at an early age with an HLA-matched sibling donor, can correct the immune deficiency, although the long-term benefits of such procedures need to be established. A similar phenotype was also described in a few patients with autosomal recessive hyper-IgM syndrome, which is caused by defects in CD40. In these patients the diagnosis is supported by reduced or absent expression of CD40 on B lymphocytes and is confirmed by gene sequencing. Hyper-IgM syndrome with an autosomal inheritance pattern can also be caused by mutations in activation-induced cytidine deaminase and uracil N-glycosylase; however, while these patients suffer from bacterial infections and lymphadenopathy they do not develop opportunistic infections, reflecting the sparing of T cells in these primarily B-cell lineage immune abnormalities.

MHC class II deficiency

MHC class II deficiency (also known as bare lymphocyte syndrome, type II) is caused by inherited defects in at least one of the four transacting regulatory genes *CIITA*, *RFXANK*, *RFX5* and *RFXAP* that are required for transcription of MHC class II genes.[70] Patients with this autosomal recessive TD may present in infancy with typical features of SCID, although some are diagnosed later in life. MHC class II deficiency is common in North African and Mediterranean descendants, although patients from other ethnic groups have been described. Typically, circulating CD4 T cells are reduced, but the response of T cells to mitogens is usually preserved. In contrast, the responses of T cells to antigens or in the "mixed leukocyte reaction" are compromised. The diagnosis can be readily established by flow cytometric analysis demonstrating absent MHC class II expression on B and T cells. Unfortunately, HSCT for MHC class II deficiency has been less successful than for other forms of TD, with frequent graft rejection and reduced survival.

MHC class I deficiency

MHC class I deficiency (or bare lymphocyte syndrome, type I) is often associated with skin and nasopharyngeal destructive granulomatous disease and vasculitis.[47] This deficiency consists of a group of autosomal recessive diseases caused by mutations in TAP-1, TAP-2, and TAP-binding protein, which are important for intracellular loading of antigens into MHC class I molecules and stabilizing the complex (Chapter 6). MHC class I deficient patients often suffer chronic lung infections in the first or second decade of life, which are frequently complicated by bronchiectasis. The numbers of circulating CD8 T cells are often, although not universally, reduced while CD4 T- and B-cell numbers are normal. The diagnosis of MHC class I deficiency can be suspected by observing markedly reduced cell surface expression of class I molecules by flow cytometric analysis, with occasional increase in TCRγ/δ bearing T cells or reduced circulating NK cells.

Purine nucleoside phosphorylase (PNP) deficiency

PNP deficiency is an uncommon cause of autosomal recessive TD. PNP-deficient patients typically suffer from progressive cellular immunodeficiency. While they can often tolerate BCG vaccine at birth,[71,72] they might develop fatal infections following live viral vaccines or common wild-type viruses such as varicella, parainfluenza and JC in the first years of life.[73,74] In up to one-third of PNP-deficient patients, the TD also results in autoimmunity, particularly autoimmune cytopenia, as well as hematological malignancies.[75,76] Similar to ADA deficiency, immune evaluation shortly after birth in PNP-deficient patients might be normal, as the damage to immune cells is caused by gradual accumulation of purine metabolites. Over time, T cell numbers, particularly CD4 T cells, decrease and their response to in vitro stimulation diminishes.[77] Although B and NK cells are typically spared, some PNP-deficient patients have low immunoglobulin levels and poor antibody responses to immunizations.[77] PNP is a ubiquitous enzyme and tight purine homeostasis is crucial for function of all cells (Fig. 35.3); hence, it is not surprising that non-immune abnormalities are also common in PNP-deficient patients. Indeed >50% of the patients suffer from neurological defects consisting of developmental delay, mental retardation, hyper- or hypotonia and ataxia, which often precede the immune abnormalities.[71,78,79] A few patients have associated bone marrow dysplasia,[80] as well as sclerosing cholangitis.[81] PNP deficiency interferes with the production of uric acid, which provides a readily available test, although with low sensitivity and specificity. The diagnosis of PNP deficiency is often established by demonstrating markedly reduced (<5% of normal) enzyme activity in red blood cells or even in dried blood spots from Guthrie cards[72] and by demonstrating increased concentrations of the PNP substrate deoxyguanosine and dGTP. Definitive diagnosis can be established by demonstrating a deleterious mutation in the PNP gene.[82] Management of PNP-deficient patients has been challenging. Currently the only definitive treatment option is allogeneic HSCT. Unfortunately, HSCT for PNP deficiency is often associated with engraftment failure, GvH disease and persistence of the neurological deficits.[83] As an alternative, we are developing PNP gene and protein replacement therapies, which have shown promise in a relevant animal model.[84,85]

CD3γ deficiency

Mutations in the CD3γ chain can cause autosomal recessive TDA. Affected patients show partial TCR/CD3 expression, mild to moderate T-cell lymphocytopenia, poor in vitro T-cell responses to mitogens as well as very low TREC and CD45RA$^+$ T cells.[86] Some of the patients develop severe enteropathy early in life and die in infancy. Other family members that carry the same mutations have reached adulthood, possibly reflecting the involvement of either environmental or additional genetic factors in determining the phenotype.

Wiskott–Aldrich syndrome

Wiskott–Aldrich syndrome is a rare X-linked recessive condition, typically diagnosed in infancy and characterized by thrombocytopenia, skin eczema and recurrent infections.[87] The platelets are smaller than normal and appear to be rapidly cleared from the circulation. The abnormal coagulation in these patients is associated with bloody stools and life threatening intracranial bleeding. Patients suffering from Wiskott–Aldrich syndrome may have increased susceptibility to bacterial, viral and opportunistic organisms including PJP. Autoimmunity and malignancy, particularly lymphoma, have been frequently reported in these patients. T-cell numbers tend to decrease over time, resulting in mild-to-moderate lymphopenia. Typically, IgM is low, IgG is normal, while IgA and IgE are elevated. Furthermore, antibody production to polysaccharide antigens is markedly depressed. Patients with WAS should be given prophylaxis against PJP, as well as platelet support, until they receive HSCT from HLA-matched related or unrelated donors. Splenectomy should be avoided in patients with Wiskott–Aldrich syndrome unless they develop uncontrolled bleeds. Gene therapy for WAS is also being currently studied in a few centers.

X-linked lymphoproliferative syndromes (XLP)

Patients suffering from XLP typically present with extreme susceptibility to EBV infection, which frequently leads to uncontrolled lymphoid proliferation. XLP may be caused by hemizygous mutations in the genes SH2D1A or BIRC4 (both on the X-chromosome) resulting in XLP-1 or XLP-2, respectively.[88] Following EBV infection, but also without EBV, patients may develop severe infectious mononucleosis, which can progress into hepatic necrosis, aplastic anemia, lymphomatoid granulomatosis or malignant lymphoma. Patients may also present with bone marrow hypoplasia and splenomegaly as part of a hemophagocytic lymphohistiocytosis-like picture, hypogammaglobulinemia or dysgammaglobulinemia, lymphocytic vasculitis or chronic colitis. Circulating T, B, and NK cells and proliferation of T cells in vitro are typically normal, although NK cell activity has been shown to be impaired in some patients. A comparison between patients with XLP-1 and XLP-2 suggests that the former leads more frequently to lymphoma while the latter is associated with colitis. Sequencing of both genes or determining their expression should be completed in suspected cases. Moreover, following the diagnosis of XLP, other male family members, even if asymptomatic, should be screened. Patients who are unable to produce antibodies should receive immunoglobulin replacement. Allogeneic HSCT can cure the susceptibility to EBV, and should be attempted particularly for patients diagnosed at an early age who have a healthy HLA-matched sibling donor that is XLP-gene mutation negative.

EBV-induced lymphoid proliferation can also be inherited in an autosomal recessive pattern. Female patients from a consanguineous family were found to have mutations in the IL-2 inducible T-cell Kinase (*ITK*) gene.[89] The clinical and immunological phenotypes are identical to the X-linked disease. Therefore, *ITK* gene sequencing should be done for EBV-associated lymphoid proliferation in females or males with normal *SH2D1A* and *BIRC4* genes.

Well-defined syndromes with prominent multisystem involvement including TDA

Many well-defined multisystem disorders with known genetic defects have been shown to cause TDA.

Cartilage hair hypoplasia

Cartilage hair hypoplasia (CHH) is caused by autosomal recessive mutations in the ribonuclease mitochondrial RNA processing (*RMRP*) gene. The immune deficiency of patients with CHH is variable.[90] Some present in infancy with SCID or OS and require HSCT. In others, T-cell numbers, responses of T cells to mitogens and TREC levels may be depressed with restricted T-cell receptor repertoire. Some patients have autoimmunity, increased susceptibility to varicella zoster infections, inability to produce antibodies following vaccinations or even normal immunity. Patients are often identified early in life because of spondylometaphyseal chondrodysplasia that results in short-limbed dwarfism, although normal skeletal development and height have been reported. Typically the patient's hair is fine, sparse and light-colored, with an abnormally small caliber. Patients may also suffer from bone marrow dysplasia, abnormal intestinal plexus neurons, impaired spermatogenesis, and predisposition to malignancy.

Dyskeratosis congenita

Dyskeratosis congenita (DKC) is a heterogeneous group of disorders that may be associated with varying degrees of TD.[91] A few patients, particularly those with the X-linked form caused by mutations in the gene for dyskerin, can present in infancy with a SCID phenotype, including markedly reduced numbers of T and/or B cells and increased susceptibility to opportunistic infections. These patients often suffer from somatic abnormalities including significant intrauterine growth retardation, short stature, severe, chronic, non-infectious enteropathy, microcephaly, developmental delay, and cerebellar hypoplasia, a constellation of features also known as Hoyeraal-Hreidarsson syndrome. Most patients present in adolescence or later in life with nail dystrophy, skin abnormalities and oral leukoplakia. Many also suffer from growth delay, which may aid in the diagnosis

(Table 35.6). Bone marrow failure, pulmonary fibrosis and malignancy are often the cause of death. DKC is caused by defects in telomerase maintenance proteins such as dyskerin, which is inherited as an X-linked disease and is the most common cause of DKC. Mutations in telomerase reverse transcriptase (*TERT*), *NOP10*, *NHP2*, and *C16ORF57* have been shown to cause autosomal recessive DKC, while mutations in telomerase RNA component (*TERC*), *TERT* and *TINF2* can cause autosomal dominant DKC.[92] Allogeneic HSCT has been attempted in patients with DKC, primarily for the bone marrow failure or malignancy, with disappointing results, in part because of the associated somatic abnormalities.

DNA ligase IV and Cernunnos-XLF deficiencies

Increased sensitivity to irradiation is a feature of several immunodeficiency disorders. Mutations in Artemis, DNA ligase IV and Cernunnos-XLF can cause autosomal recessive SCID with absent or very low T and B cells , while sparing NK cells as well as TDA. DNA ligase IV deficient patients also demonstrate increased sensitivity to irradiation, genome instability and bone marrow abnormalities. Microcephaly, unusual facial features, growth delay and varying degrees of developmental delay are commonly seen. Patients might also be at increased risk for lymphoid malignancy. Allogeneic HSCT can correct the immune abnormalities, although it remains unclear whether this procedure might prevent malignancy. A similar TD phenotype has been reported in patients with inherited Cernunnos-XLF defects.[93] The patients suffer from bacterial and opportunistic infections; however, the infections are not fatal in the first decade of life. Immune evaluations demonstrate lymphopenia with decreased numbers of T cells, which are mostly memory T cells (CD45RO+), although the *in vitro* responses of T cells to mitogen stimulation are preserved in some patients. In contrast, B-cell number and immunoglobulin production are markedly reduced. NK cells are not affected. In addition, patients display severe pre- and post-natal growth retardation, microcephaly, bird-like facies and bony malformations, as well as increased sensitivity of skin fibroblasts to ionizing radiation. Correction of the immune deficiency can be achieved by allogeneic HSCT.[94]

Ataxia telangiectasia (AT), AT-like disease, and Nijmegen breakage syndrome

AT, AT-like disease, and Nijmegen breakage syndrome (NBS) are also TD associated with increased sensitivity of cells to irradiation. AT is an autosomal recessive multisystem disorder characterized by progressive cerebellar ataxia, telangiectasia and increased susceptibility to malignancies, particularly lymphomas and leukemia. Although many patients may have TD, systemic bacterial as well as severe viral and opportunistic infections are uncommon. Laboratory immune investigations typically show decreased peripheral T cells, particularly of naïve T cells, with abnormal *in vitro* response to mitogens. The thymus is hypoplastic and TREC levels are markedly reduced.[95] In addition, most AT patients have decreased serum IgA and IgG concentrations with normal or raised IgM levels, a phenotype reminiscent of hyper-IgM syndrome, which may be associated with more severe infections. Many patients are unable to produce polysaccharide antibodies. Truncal ataxia develops early and within several years there are additional peripheral coordination abnormalities, resulting in frequent aspirations and recurrent lung infections. Neurological disturbances also include extrapyramidal symptoms. From about 10 years of age, most children become wheelchair-bound. The telangiectasia, which involves the conjunctiva and skin, usually appears at about 4 to 6 years of age. Diagnosis of AT, suggested by elevated α-feto-protein and increased sensitivity of patients' cells to irradiation, can be confirmed by identifying a mutation in the *ATM* gene. Treatment is mostly supportive, with antibiotic and immunoglobulin replacement, if needed, as well as intensive physiotherapy. Patients should be followed closely for the development of malignancies. Unfortunately, HSCT is not beneficial for these patients. Hence, alternative approaches, including small molecules that can correct aberrant gene splicing, are being explored.

An autosomal recessive AT-like disease, with reduced T-cell numbers and function as well as increased sensitivity of cells to irradiation, can also be caused by hypomorphic mutations in MRE11, a molecule involved in cell cycling and double strand DNA repair.[96]

Reduced, albeit not absent, T-cell numbers and mitogen responses together with impaired antibody production are often found in patients suffering from Nijmegen breakage syndrome (NBS), an autosomal recessive disorder. Granulomas have also been reported in some patients. Notably, patients have impaired DNA repair resulting in increased frequency of malignancy. In addition, NBS is characterized by extremely small head circumference, bird like facial features and growth retardation. Diagnosis is usually established by sequencing of the *NBS* gene. Among NBS patients of eastern European descent, a founder homozygous mutation g.657_671delACAAA is commonly present. Management is primarily supportive, although recently a few reported patients received allogeneic HSCT following non-myeloablative conditioning.[97]

DiGeorge syndrome

DiGeorge syndrome (DGS) is the most common TD in humans, with an estimated incidence of 1:4000 live births.[98] DGS is inherited in an autosomal dominant fashion, with hemizygous chromosome 22q11.2 microdeletion identified in >90% of patients, although most cases arise from de novo mutations. More than 75% of the patients have variable degrees of T-cell defects, most commonly reduced numbers of T cells, attributed to impaired T-cell generation by the underdeveloped thymus. However, the ability of these T cells to respond to stimulation *in vitro* and *in vivo* is often preserved. Hence, while these patients have an increased frequency of infections, it is often by anatomical rather than T-cell abnormalities. Nevertheless, 0.5–1% of patients with DGS present as SCID with no or very low T cells, a condition known as complete DGS, which has been treated with allogeneic thymus transplantation (Chapter 84) or HSCT with variable long-term outcome. DGS patients can also suffer from OS and autoimmunity. Because of the immune deficiency, administration of live vaccines to these patients has been controversial. We have recently shown safe administration of the measles-mumps-rubella vaccine in a large group of patients with a 22q11.2 microdeletion who had >500 circulating CD4 T cells/μL and adequate *in vitro* mitogenic responses. Interestingly, patients were often unable to maintain protective antibodies to the vaccines.[99] The 22 chromosome haploinsufficiency and disturbance in formations of the third and fourth pharyngeal pouches cause many additional features that often aid in the diagnosis. These include cardiac defects, hypoparathyroidism, dysmorphic facial features, cleft palate, feeding difficulties, renal abnormalities, short stature, and neuropsychiatric problems.

FOXN1 deficiency

Patients with FOXN1 deficiency typically suffer from alopecia totalis, nail dystrophy and abnormal thymus development. T cells, particularly CD4 T cells, are reduced, with impaired responses to mitogenic stimulation. TREC and naïve T cells are absent while flow cytometry and spectrotyping demonstrate oligoclonal expansion of T cells, which is in part due to expansion of $CD4^-CD8^-$ DN cells. Similar to patients with severe DGS, few patients with FOXN1 deficiency have been treated by either allogeneic HSCT or thymus transplantations, with variable results.[100]

Translational research

● ON THE HORIZON

New T-cell disorders

- T-cell deficiencies of the future will reveal the more complex nature and many will be associated with unexpected autoimmune conditions and lymphoid malignancies.
- Delineation of aberrant pathways of T-cell activation are critical for developing appropriate therapeutic approaches, which may include selective immune suppressant therapy.
- Expansion of primary immunodeficiency into areas of autoimmunity, inflammatory diseases, and lymphoid malignancies will broaden the spectrum of responsibilities for the clinical immunologist.

The traditional clinical as well as laboratory definitions of profound T-cell deficiencies, although still helpful in many cases, may no longer be sufficient for newer forms of immunodeficiency. An example of this apparent discord is the FOXP3 deficiency in which *in vitro* responses to mitogens as well as TREC levels can be normal. There is a growing awareness of the two-sided nature of primary immunodeficiency and autoimmune disease. We therefore need to broaden our definitions to include severe autoimmune/inflammatory conditions, as main or prominent clinical features of profound T-cell deficiency, in addition to recurrent opportunistic infections. Other clinical features, such as granulomata and lymphoma have also been reported recently as sole manifestations of T-cell immunodeficiencies.

There is no doubt that with the increased recognition of the genetic aberrations linked to these diseases, we are likely to see a great expansion of novel phenotypes associated with known genotypes. This new area of T-cell deficiencies will require careful evaluation. It will be necessary to possibly consider selective immunosuppression in these new forms of primary immunodeficiency associated with autoimmune disease and lymphoid malignancies, a concept unthinkable but a few years ago.

Prospective trials should help in the future to determine the validity of transplantation as compared with immunosuppressive therapy in these patients.

References

1. Sebzda E, Mariathasan S, Ohteki T, et al. Selection of the T cell repertoire. Annu Rev Immunol 1999;17:829–74.
2. Hogquist KA, Baldwin TA, Jameson SC, et al. Central tolerance: learning self-control in the thymus. Nat Rev Immunol 2005;5:772–82.
3. Sharfe N, Dadi HK, Shahar M, et al. Human immune disorder arising from mutation of the alpha chain of the interleukin-2 receptor. Proc Natl Acad Sci U S A 1997;94: 3168–71.
4. Huang Y, Lei Y, Zhang H, et al. Role of interleukin-18 in human natural killer cell is associated with interleukin-2. Mol Immunol 2010;47:2604–10.
5. Strasser A, Puthalakath H, O'Reilly LA, et al. What do we know about the mechanisms of elimination of auto reactive T and B cells and what challenges remain? Immunol Cell Biol 2008;86:57–66.
6. Barron MA, Makhija M, Hagen LE, et al. Increased resting energy expenditure is associated with failure to thrive in infants with severe combined immunodeficiency. J Pediatr 2011;159:628–632.e1.
7. Xiao Z, Yannone SM, Dunn E, et al. A novel missense RAG-1 mutation results in T-B-NK + SCID in Athabascan-speaking Dine Indians from the Canadian Northwest Territories. Eur J Hum Genet 2009;17:205–12.
8. Dalal I, Tasher D, Somech R, et al. Novel mutations in RAG1/2 and ADA genes in Israeli patients presenting with T-B- SCID or Omenn syndrome. Clin Immunol 2011;140:284–90.
9. Dadi HK, Simon AJ, Roifman CM, et al. Effect of CD3delta deficiency on maturation of alpha/beta and gamma/delta T-cell lineages in severe combined immunodeficiency. N Engl J Med 2003;349:1821–8.
10. Buckley RH, Schiff RI, Schiff SE, et al. Human severe combined immunodeficiency: genetic, phenotypic, and functional diversity in one hundred eight infants. J Pediatr 1997;130:378–87.
11. Yu Y, Arora A, Min W, et al. EdU incorporation is an alternative non-radioactive assay to [(3)H]thymidine uptake for in vitro measurement of mice T-cell proliferations. J Immunol Methods 2009;350:29–35.
12. Grunebaum E, Mazzolari E, Porta F, et al. Bone marrow transplantation for severe combined immune deficiency. JAMA 2006;295:508.
13. Gennery AR, Slatter MA, Grandin L, et al. Inborn errors working party of the european group for blood and marrow transplantation; European Society for Immunodeficiency. Transplantation of hematopoietic stem cells and long-term survival for primary immunodeficiencies in Europe: entering a new century, do we do better? J Allergy Clin Immunol 2010;126:602–10.
14. Hacein-Bey-Abina S, Hauer J, Lim A, et al. Efficacy of gene therapy for X-linked severe combined immunodeficiency. N Engl J Med 2010;363:355–64.
15. Aiuti A, Cattaneo F, Galimberti S, et al. Gene therapy for immunodeficiency due to adenosine deaminase deficiency. N Engl J Med 2009;360:447–58.
16. Lagresle-Peyrou C, Six EM, Picard C, et al. Human adenylate kinase 2 deficiency causes a profound hematopoietic defect associated with sensorineural deafness. Nat Genet 2009;41:106–11.
17. Pannicke U, Hönig M, Hess I, et al. Reticular dysgenesis (aleukocytosis) is caused by mutations in the gene encoding mitochondrial adenylate kinase 2. Nat Genet 2009;41:101–105.
18. Roifman CM, Zhang J, Atkinson A, et al. Adenosine deaminase deficiency can present with features of Omenn syndrome. J Allergy Clin Immunol 2008;121:1056–8.
19. Somech R, Lai YH, Grunebaum E, et al. Polyethylene glycol-modified adenosine deaminase improved lung disease but not liver disease in partial adenosine deaminase deficiency. J Allergy Clin Immunol 2009;124:848–50.
20. Ozsahin H, Arredondo-Vega FX, Santisteban I, et al. Adenosine deaminase deficiency in adults. Blood 1997;89:2849–55.
21. Nofech-Mozes Y, Blaser SI, Kobayashi J, et al. Neurologic abnormalities in patients with adenosine deaminase deficiency. Pediatr Neurol 2007;37:218–21.
22. Sauer AV, Mrak E, Hernandez RJ, et al. ADA-deficient SCID is associated with a specific microenvironment and bone phenotype characterized by RANKL/OPG imbalance and osteoblast insufficiency. Blood 2009;114:3216–26.
23. Sokolic R, Maric I, Kesserwan C, et al. Myeloid dysplasia and bone marrow hypocellularity in adenosine deaminase-deficient severe combined immune deficiency. Blood 2011;118:2688–94.
24. Booth C, Hershfield M, Notarangelo L, et al. Management options for adenosine deaminase deficiency; proceedings of the EBMT satellite workshop (Hamburg, March 2006). Clin Immunol 2007;123:139–47.
25. Chan K, Puck JM. Development of population-based newborn screening for severe combined immunodeficiency. J Allergy Clin Immunol 2005;115:391–8.
26. Husain M, Grunebaum E, Naqvi A, et al. Burkitt's lymphoma in a patient with adenosine deaminase deficiency-severe combined immunodeficiency treated with polyethylene glycol-adenosine deaminase. J Pediatr 2007;151:93–5.
27. Antoine C, Müller S, Cant A, et al. European Group for Blood and Marrow Transplantation; European Society for Immunodeficiency. Long-term survival and transplantation of haemopoietic stem cells for immunodeficiencies: report of the European experience 1968–99. Lancet 2003;361:553–60.
28. Roberts JL, Lengi A, Brown SM, et al. Janus kinase 3 (JAK3) deficiency: clinical, immunologic, and molecular analyses of 10 patients and outcomes of stem cell transplantation. Blood 2004;103:2009–18.
29. Villa A, Santagata S, Bozzi F, et al. Partial V(D)J recombination activity leads to Omenn syndrome. Cell 1998;93:885–96.
30. De Ravin SS, Cowen EW, Zaremba KA, et al. Hypomorphic Rag mutations can cause destructive midline granulomatous disease. Blood 2010;116:1263–71.
31. Bertrand Y, Landais P, Friedrich W, et al. Influence of severe combined immunodeficiency phenotype on the outcome of HLA non-identical, T-cell-depleted bone marrow transplantation: a retrospective European survey from the European group for bone marrow transplantation and the European Society for Immunodeficiency. J Pediatr 1999;134:740–8.
32. Pessach IM, Notarangelo LD. Gene therapy for primary immunodeficiencies: looking ahead, toward gene correction. J Allergy Clin Immunol 2011;127:1344–50.
33. van der Burg M, Ijspeert H, Verkaik NS, et al. A DNA-PKcs mutation in a radiosensitive T-B- SCID patient inhibits Artemis activation and no homologous end-joining. J Clin Invest 2009;119:91–8.
34. Marcus N, Takada H, Law J, et al. Hematopoietic stem cell transplantation for CD3δ deficiency. J Allergy Clin Immunol 2011;128(5):1050–7.
35. De Saint Basile G, Geissmann F, Flori E, et al. Severe combined immunodeficiency caused by deficiency in either the delta or the epsilon subunit of CD3. J Clin Invest 2004;114:1512–47.
36. Roberts JL, Lauritsen JP, Cooney M, et al. T⁻B⁺NK⁺ severe combined immunodeficiency caused by complete deficiency of the CD3zeta subunit of the T-cell antigen receptor complex. Blood 2007;109:3198–206.
37. Puel A, Ziegler SF, Buckley RH, et al. Defective IL7R expression in T(-)B(+)NK(+) severe combined immunodeficiency. Nat Genet 1998;20:394–7.
38. Roifman CM, Zhang J, Chitayat D, et al. A partial deficiency of interleukin-7R alpha is sufficient to abrogate T-cell development and cause severe combined immunodeficiency. Blood 2000;96:2803–7.
39. Kung C, Pingel JT, Heikinheimo M, et al. Mutations in the tyrosine phosphatase CD45 gene in a child with severe combined immunodeficiency disease. Nat Med 2000;6:343–5.
40. Tchilian EZ, Wallace DL, Wells RS, et al. A deletion in the gene encoding the CD45 antigen in a patient with SCID. J Immunol 2001;166:1308–13.
41. Shiow LR, Paris K, Akana MC, et al. Severe combined immunodeficiency (SCID) and attention deficit hyperactivity disorder (ADHD) associated with a Coronin-1A mutation and a chromosome 16p11.2 deletion. Clin Immunol 2009;131:24–30.
42. Roifman CM. Studies of patients' thymi aid in the discovery and characterization of immunodeficiency in humans. Immunol Rev 2005;203:143–55.
43. Roifman CM, Somech R, Grunebaum E. Matched unrelated bone marrow transplant for T+ combined immunodeficiency. Bone Marrow Transplant 2008;41:947–52.
44. Roifman CM. Hematopoietic stem cell transplantation for profound T-cell deficiency (combined immunodeficiency). Immunol Allergy Clin North Am 2010;30:209–19.
45. Somech R, Kavadas FD, Atkinson A, et al. High-dose methylprednisolone is effective in the management of acute graft-versus-host disease in severe combined immune deficiency. J Allergy Clin Immunol 2008;122:1215–6.
46. Nahum A, Reid B, Grunebaum E, et al. Matched unrelated bone marrow transplant for Omenn syndrome. Immunol Res 2009;44:25–34.
47. Villa-Forte A, de la Salle H, Fricker D, et al. HLA class I deficiency syndrome mimicking Wegener's granulomatosis. Arthritis Rheum 2008;58:2579–82.
48. Zhang J, Quintal L, Atkinson A, et al. Novel RAG1 mutation in a case of severe combined immunodeficiency. Pediatrics 2005;116:e445–9.
49. Poliani PL, Facchetti F, Ravanini M, et al. Early defects in human T-cell development severely affect distribution and maturation of thymic stromal cells: possible implications for the pathophysiology of Omenn syndrome. Blood 2009;114:105.
50. Giliani S, Bonfim C, de Saint Basile G, et al. Omenn syndrome in an infant with IL7RA gene mutation. J Pediatr 2006;148:272–4.
51. Dalal I, Tabori U, Bielorai B, et al. Evolution of a T-B- SCID into an Omenn syndrome phenotype following parainfluenza 3 virus infection. Clin Immunol 2005;115:70–3.
52. Somech R, Roifman CM. Mutation analysis should be performed to rule out gammac deficiency in children with functional severe combined immune deficiency despite apparently normal immunological tests. J Pediatr 2005;147:555–7.
53. Brugnoni D, Notarangelo LD, Sottini A, et al. Development of autologous, oligoclonal, poorly functioning T lymphocytes in a patient with autosomal recessive severe combined immunodeficiency caused by defects of the Jak3 tyrosine kinase. Blood 1998;91(3):949–55.
54. Mella P, Schumacher RF, Cranston T, et al. Eleven novel JAK3 mutations in patients with severe combined immunodeficiency-including the first patients with mutations in the kinase domain. Hum Mutat 2001;18:355–6.
55. Frucht DM, Gadina M, Jagadeesh GJ, et al. Unexpected and variable phenotypes in a family with JAK3 deficiency. Genes Immun 2001;2:422–32.
56. Schuetz C, Huck K, Gudowius S, et al. An immunodeficiency disease with RAG mutations and granulomas. N Engl J Med 2008;358:2030–8.
57. Moshous D, Meyts I, Fraitag S, et al. Granulomatous inflammation in cartilage-hair hypoplasia: Risks and benefits of anti-TNF-α mAbs. J Allergy Clin Immunol 2011;128:847–53.
58. Ijspeert H, Lankester AC, van den Berg JM, et al. Artemis splice defects cause atypical SCID and can be restored in vitro by an antisense oligonucleotide. Genes Immun 2011;12:434–44.
59. de Villartay JP, Lim A, Al-Mousa H, et al. A novel immunodeficiency associated with hypomorphic RAG1 mutations and CMV infection. J Clin Invest 2005;115:3291–9.
60. Kuijpers TW, Ijspeert H, van Leeuwen, et al. Idiopathic CD4+ T lymphopenia without autoimmunity or granulomatous disease in the slipstream of RAG mutations. Blood 2011;117:5892–6.
61. Hershfield MS. Adenosine deaminase deficiency: clinical expression, molecular basis, and therapy. Semin Hematol 1998;35:291–8.
62. Roifman CM, Dadi H, Somech R, et al. Characterization of ζ-associated protein, 70 kd (ZAP70)-deficient human lymphocytes. J Allergy Clin Immunol 2010;126(6):1226.
63. Picard C, Dogniaux S, Chemin K, et al. Hypomorphic mutation of ZAP70 in human results in a late onset immunodeficiency and no autoimmunity. Eur J Immunol 2009;39:1966–76.
64. Turul T, Tezcan I, Artac H, et al. Clinical heterogeneity can hamper the diagnosis of patients with ZAP70 deficiency. Eur J Pediatr 2009;168:87–93.
65. Newell A, Dadi H, Goldberg R, et al. Diffuse large B-cell lymphoma as presenting feature of Zap-70 deficiency. J Allergy Clin Immunol 2011;127:517–20.

66. Caudy AA, Reddy ST, Chatila T, et al. CD25 deficiency causes an immune dysregulation, polyendocrinopathy, enteropathy, X-linked-like syndrome, and defective IL-10 expression from CD4 lymphocytes. J Allergy Clin Immunol 2007;119:482–7.

67. Feske S, Picard C, Fischer A. Immunodeficiency due to mutations in ORAI1 and STIM1. Clin Immunol 2010;135:169–82.

68. Torgerson TR, Ochs HD. Immune dysregulation, polyendocrinopathy, enteropathy, X-linked: forkhead box protein 3 mutations and lack of regulatory T cells. J Allergy Clin Immunol 2007;120:744–50.

69. Glocker EO, Kotlarz D, Boztug K, et al. Inflammatory bowel disease and mutations affecting the interleukin-10 receptor. N Engl J Med 2009;361:2033–45.

70. Davies EG, Thrasher AJ. Update on the hyper immunoglobulin M syndromes. Br J Haematol 2010;149:167–80.

71. Picard C, Fischer A. Hematopoietic stem cell transplantation and other management strategies for MHC class II deficiency. Immunol Allergy Clin North Am 2010;30:173–8.

72. Markert ML. Purine nucleoside phosphorylase deficiency. Immunodefic Rev 1991;3:45–81.

73. Iangari A, Al-Harbi A, Al-Ghonaium A, et al. Purine nucleoside phosphorylase deficiency in two unrelated Saudi patients. Ann Saudi Med 2009;29:309–12.

74. Banzhoff A, Schauer U, Riedel F, et al. Fatal varicella in a 5-year-old boy. Eur J Pediatr 1997;156:333–4.

75. Parvaneh N, Teimourian S, Jacomelli G, et al. Novel mutations of NP in two patients with purine nucleoside phosphorylase deficiency. Clin Biochem 2008;41:350–2.

76. Watson AR, Evans DI, Marsden HB, et al. Purine nucleoside phosphorylase deficiency associated with a fatal lymphoproliferative disorder. Arch Dis Child 1981;56:563–5.

77. Grunebaum E, Roifman CM. Gene abnormalities in patients with hemophagocytic lymphohistiocytosis. Isr Med Assoc J 2002;4:366–9.

78. Myers LA, Hershfield MS, Neale WT, et al. Purine nucleoside phosphorylase deficiency (PNP-def) presenting with lymphopenia and developmental delay: successful correction with umbilical cord blood transplantation. J Pediatr 2004;145:710–2.

79. Ozkinay F, Pehlivan S, Onay H, et al. Purine nucleoside phosphorylase deficiency in a patient with spastic paraplegia and recurrent infections. J Child Neurol 2007;22:741–3.

80. Moallem HJ, Taningo G, Jiang CK, et al. Purine nucleoside phosphorylase deficiency: a new case report and identification of two novel mutations (Gly156A1a and Val217Ile), only one of which (Gly156A1a) is deleterious. Clin Immunol 2002;105:75–80.

81. Dror Y, Grunebaum E, Hitzler J, et al. Purine nucleoside phosphorylase deficiency associated with a dysplastic marrow morphology. Pediatr Res 2004;55:472–7.

82. Aytekin C, Dogu F, Tanir G, et al. Purine nucleoside phosphorylase deficiency with fatal course in two sisters. Eur J Pediatr 2010;169:311–4.

83. Grunebaum E, Zhang J, Roifman CM. Novel mutations and hot-spots in patients with purine nucleoside phosphorylase deficiency. Nucleosides Nucleotides Nucleic Acids 2004;23:1411.

84. Baguette C, Vermylen C, Brichard B, et al. Persistent developmental delay despite successful bone marrow transplantation for purine nucleoside phosphorylase deficiency. J Pediatr Hematol Oncol 2002;24(1):69–71.

85. Toro A, Grunebaum E. TAT-mediated intracellular delivery of purine nucleoside phosphorylase corrects its deficiency in mice. J Clin Invest 2006;116:2717–26.

86. Liao P, Toro A, Min W, et al. Lentivirus gene therapy for purine nucleoside phosphorylase deficiency. J Gene Med 2008;10:1282–93.

87. Recio MJ, Moreno-Pelayo MA, Kiliç SS, et al. Differential biological role of CD3 chains revealed by human immunodeficiencies. J Immunol 2007;178:2556–64.

88. Notarangelo LD, Miao CH, Ochs HD. Wiskott-Aldrich syndrome. Curr Opin Hematol 2008;15:30–6.

89. Pachlopnik Schmid J, Canioni D, Moshous D, et al. Clinical similarities and differences of patients with X-linked lymphoproliferative syndrome type 1 (XLP-1/SAP deficiency) versus type 2 (XLP-2/XIAP deficiency). Blood 2011;117:1522–9.

90. Huck K, Feyen O, Niehues T, et al. Girls homozygous for an IL-2-inducible T cell kinase mutation that leads to protein deficiency develop fatal EBV-associated lymphoproliferation. J Clin Invest 2009;119:1350–8.

91. Kavadas FD, Giliani S, Gu Y, et al. Variability of clinical and laboratory features among patients with ribonuclease mitochondrial RNA processing endoribonuclease gene mutations. J Allergy Clin Immunol 2008;122:1178–84.

92. Jyonouchi S, Forbes L, Ruchelli E, et al. Dyskeratosis congenita: a combined immunodeficiency with broad clinical spectrum—a single-center pediatric experience. Pediatr Allergy Immunol 2011;22(3):313–9.

93. Savage SA, Bertuch AA. The genetics and clinical manifestations of telomere biology disorders. Genet Med 2010;12(12):753–64.

94. Buck D, Malivert L, de Chasseval R, et al. Cernunnos, a novel nonhomologous end-joining factor, is mutated in human immunodeficiency with microcephaly. Cell 2006;124:287–99.

95. Cağdaş D, Ozgür TT, Asal GT, et al. Two SCID cases with Cernunnos-XLF deficiency successfully treated by hematopoietic stem cell transplantation. Pediatr Transplant 2011 Apr 27. doi:10.1111/j.1399-3046.2011.01491.x. [Epub ahead of print].

96. Giovannetti A, Mazzetta F, Caprini E, et al. Skewed T-cell receptor repertoire, decreased thymic output, and predominance of terminally differentiated T cells in ataxia telangiectasia. Blood 2002;100:4082–9.

97. Taylor AM, Groom A, Byrd PJ. Ataxia-telangiectasia-like disorder (ATLD)—its clinical presentation and molecular basis. DNA Repair (Amst) 2004;3:1219–25.

98. Albert MH, Gennery AR, Greil J, et al. Successful SCT for Nijmegen breakage syndrome. Bone Marrow Transplant 2010;45:622–6.

99. McDonald-McGinn DM, Sullivan KE. Chromosome 22q11.2 deletion syndrome (DiGeorge syndrome/velocardiofacial syndrome). Medicine (Baltimore) 2011;90:1–18.

100. Al-Sukaiti N, Reid B, Lavi S, et al. Safety and efficacy of measles, mumps, and rubella vaccine in patients with DiGeorge syndrome. J Allergy Clin Immunol 2010;126:868–9.

101. Markert ML, Marques JG, Neven B, et al. First use of thymus transplantation therapy for FOXN1 deficiency (nude/SCID): a report of 2 cases. Blood 2011;117:688–696.

Capucine Picard,
Anne Puel,
Jacinta
Bustamante,
Emmanuelle
Jouanguy, Shen-
Ying Zhang,
Stéphanie
Dupuis-Boisson,
Jean-Laurent
Casanova

Inherited disorders of IFN-γ-, IFN-α/β/λ-, and NF-κB-mediated immunity

In the past 15 years, new primary immunodeficiencies (PIDs) affecting interferon (IFN)-γ-mediated immunity, IFN-α/β-λ-mediated immunity, Toll and interleukin-1 receptor (TIR) domain, and nuclear factor (NF)-κB-mediated immunity have been identified. Some of these genetic defects are "conventional" PIDs, associated with a broad range of infections, but others provide a molecular explanation for severe pediatric infectious diseases previously thought to be idiopathic (Table 36.1). These "nonconventional" PIDs may be associated with severe and/or recurrent infections caused by a single family of micro-organisms, a situation strongly contrasting with that for "conventional" PIDs.[1] Standard immunologic explorations are generally normal in these patients, whether they are susceptible to one or many infectious agents. Despite the lack of a clear immunological abnormality, infections in these patients are typically severe and often fatal. In this chapter, we describe these PIDs. They include disorders of the interleukin (IL)-12/23–IFN-γ circuit and phagocytic burst (CYBB gene) associated with the syndrome of Mendelian susceptibility to mycobacterial disease (MSMD). Combined disorders of IFN-γ- and IFN-α/β-λ-mediated immunity are associated with mycobacterial and viral diseases. We also describe three genetic defects affecting primarily the Toll-like receptor (TLR)-3 pathway.[2–4] The predominant infectious phenotype of patients with any of these three defects is herpes simplex virus (HSV)-1 encephalitis (HSE) in childhood. Finally, we describe four PIDs associated with impaired signaling downstream from or via the TLR-IL-1R (TIR) canonical pathway, with mutations in IRAK4, MYD88, NEMO, and IKBA.[5–10] Mutations in NEMO and IKBA also impair the alternative, TRIF-dependent pathway. The principal infectious phenotype

of patients with any of these four defects is the occurrence of pyogenic bacterial infections. Collectively, all these disorders were initially thought to be rare, but they have since been diagnosed in about 500 patients around the world (Table 36.1).

Mendelian susceptibility to mycobacterial disease: inherited disorders of the IL-12/23–IFN-γ circuit and the respiratory burst pathway

Inherited disorders of the IL-12/23-IFN-γ circuit are associated with a selective susceptibility to weakly pathogenic mycobacteria and *Salmonella* (MSMD, OMIM: 209950) (Fig. 36.1).[11] These PIDs are caused by mutations in seven genes involved in IFN-γ-mediated immunity: *IFNGR1* and *IFNGR2*, encoding the two chains of the receptor for IFN-γ, a pleiotropic cytokine secreted by NK and T cells; *STAT1*, encoding a transcription factor essential to the IFN-γR signaling pathway; *IL12B*, encoding the p40 subunit of IL-12 and -23, IFN-γ-induced cytokines secreted by macrophages and dendritic cells (DCs); *IL12RB1*, encoding the β1 chain of the receptor for IL-12 and -23, which is expressed on NK and T cells;[12] *NEMO*, encoding NF-κB essential modulator (NEMO), which is involved in the CD40-dependent induction of IL-12; and *IRF8*, encoding an interferon regulatory factor inducible by IFN-γ.[13] Some mutations in *STAT1* and most mutations in *NEMO* are associated with a much broader range of infectious diseases (see below), and complete interferon regulatory factor 8 (IRF8) deficiency is associated with a lack of circulating monocytes and DCs, and severe clinical disease, mimicking combined immunodeficiency (CID). The molecular and clinical features of MSMD have been reviewed elsewhere.[14] Most of the identified mutations in MSMD patients concern genes of the IL-12/23-IFN-γ circuit, but two different mutations in a single gene, *CYBB*, encoding the gp91^{phox} subunit of the nicotinamide adenine dinucleotide phosphatase (NADPH) oxidase involved in the respiratory burst pathway, have recently been described. The MSMD-causing mutations in *CYBB* affect the respiratory burst selectively in macrophages.

● **KEY CONCEPTS**

- New PIDs should be sought in patients with unexplained infectious diseases.
- Children with severe infectious diseases should be repeatedly investigated for known and unknown immunodeficiency conditions.
- The exploration of idiopathic infections leads to the discovery of new PIDs and to a better understanding of immunity to pathogens.

Table 36.1 New inherited disorders

Gene	Form	Inheritance	Infections						EDA	Inflammatory signs
			Mycobacteria	Salmonella	Viruses	HSE	Pyogenic bacteria	Fungi		
IFNGR1	Complete	AR	++	+	+[1]	-	+/-[2]	-	-	N
	Partial	AR	++	+	-	-	+	-	-	N
	Partial	AD	++	+	-	-	-	+/-[3]	-	N
IFNGR2	Complete	AR	++	-	+	-	-	-	-	N
	Partial	AR	++	-	-	-	-	-	-	N
IRF8	Complete	AR	++	-	-	-	-	-	-	N
	Partial	AD	++	-	-	-	-	-	-	N
IL12RB1	Complete	AR	++	++	-	-	-	+	-	N
IL12B	Complete	AR	++	++	-	-	-	+	-	N
STAT1	Partial	AD	++	-	-	-	-	-	-	N
	Partial	AR	++	-	++	-	-	-	-	N
	Complete	AR	++	-	++	+	-	-	-	N
CYBB	Partial	XR	++	-	-	-	-	-	-	N
TLR3	Hypomorphic	AD	-	-	HSV-1	++	-	-	-	N
UNC93B1	Amorphic	AR	-	-	HSV-1	++	-	-	-	N
TRAF3	Hypomorphic	AD	-	-	HSV-1	++	-	-	-	N
NEMO	Hypomorphic	XR	+	+	+	+	++	+	+/-	Weak
IKBA	Hypermorphic	AD	-	+	+	+	++	+	+	Weak
IRAK4	Amorphic	AR	-	-	-	-	++	-	-	Weak
MyD88	Amorphic	AR	-	-	-	-	++	-	-	Weak

AR: autosomal recessive, AD: autosomal dominant, XR: X-recessive, HSE: herpes simplex encephalitis, EDA: ectodermal anhidrotic dysplasia, N: normal.
[1]One complet IFNGR1-defient patient presented a Kaposi Sarcoma.
[2]One complet IFNGR1-defient patient had Listeria monocytogenes meningitis.
[3]One PD IFNGR1-deficient patient presented one episode of Histoplasma capsulatum infection; another patient presented coccidiodomycosis.

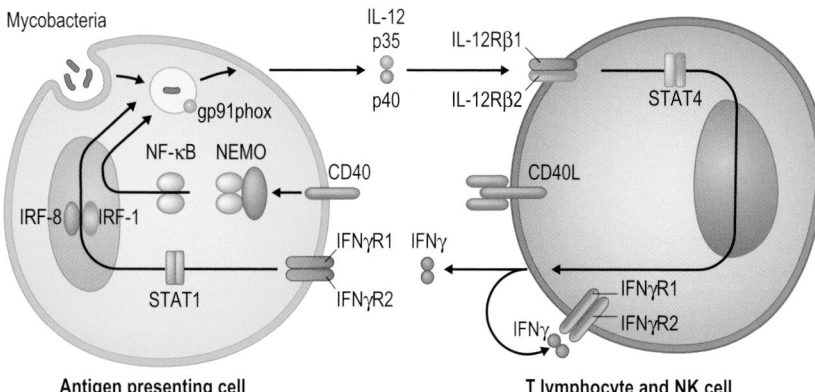

Fig. 36.1 Genetic etiologies of Mendelian susceptibility to mycobacterial infection. IL-12 is secreted principally by the phagocytes and DCs and binds to a heterodimeric receptor consisting of β1 and β2 chains, which is expressed specifically on NK and T lymphocytes. IFN-γ is secreted by NK and T lymphocytes and binds to a ubiquitous receptor made of two chains, a ligand-binding (IFN-γR1) and a signaling-associated chain (IFN-γR2). STAT-1 is phosphorylated in response to IFN-γ and is translocated to the nucleus as a homodimer. NEMO is a regulatory protein in the NF-κB pathway. The engagement of CD40 signaling via the NF-κB pathway is important for IL-12 production and for protective immunity against mycobacterial infection. IRF8 is an IFN-γ-inducible transcription factor required for the induction of various target genes, including IL-12. Gp91^{phox} is a key component of the phagocyte NADPH oxidase. The eight molecules shown in red have been found to be mutated in certain patients with severe mycobacterial infection.

Complete autosomal recessive IFN-γ receptor 1 deficiency

Complete IFN-γ receptor 1 (IFN-γR1) deficiency (OMIM 107470) is caused by recessive null *IFNGR1* mutations precluding the expression of IFN-γR1 on the cell surface[15,16] or recognition of the ligand, IFN-γ, by surface-expressed receptors.[17,18] Therefore, affected patients fail to respond to IFN-γ and have high serum concentrations of IFN-γ after infection.[14] More than 30 such patients have been reported and all have suffered from disseminated infections caused by environmental mycobacteria (EM) and/or bacille Calmette–Guérin (BCG) vaccines, with impaired granuloma formation (Fig. 36.2A).[14,19–23] Infections usually began early in life, often before the age of 3 years. A few of these patients have presented with nontyphoid salmonellosis and one presented with recurrent invasive infection caused by *Listeria monocytogenes*.[19] Three patients had respiratory viral infections and one had a fatal human herpes virus-8-driven Kaposi's sarcoma.[19,24] Multiple antibiotics against mycobacteria should be administered without interruption and vaccination with live BCG is contraindicated. The prognosis is very poor, with only 25% of patients surviving to the age of 15 years in the absence of haematopoietic stem cell transplantation (HSCT).[19,25] HSCT is best carried out once mycobacterial disease has been controlled, is the only curative treatment, but has proven to be associated with an unusually high rate of graft rejection, making transplantation particularly difficult.

THERAPEUTIC PRINCIPLES

For MSMD Patients

- Vaccination with live BCG is contraindicated.
- Multiple antibiotics against mycobacteria should be administered without interruption in patients with complete IFN-γR1 or IFN-γR2 deficiency.
- Antimycobacterial antibiotics may be associated with IFN-γ injections in selected patients with partial IFN-γR1 or IFN-γR2 deficiency, complete IL-12p40 or IL-12Rb1 deficiency.
- HSCT should be considered in selected patients with complete IFN-γR1 or IFN-γR2 deficiency.

Complete autosomal recessive IFN-γ receptor 2 deficiency

Seven children with complete IFN-γR2 signaling chain deficiency (OMIM 147569) have also been reported.[14,26,27] Mutations

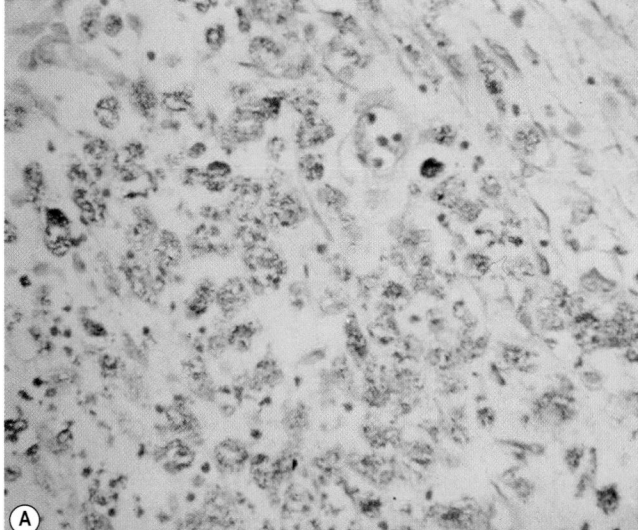

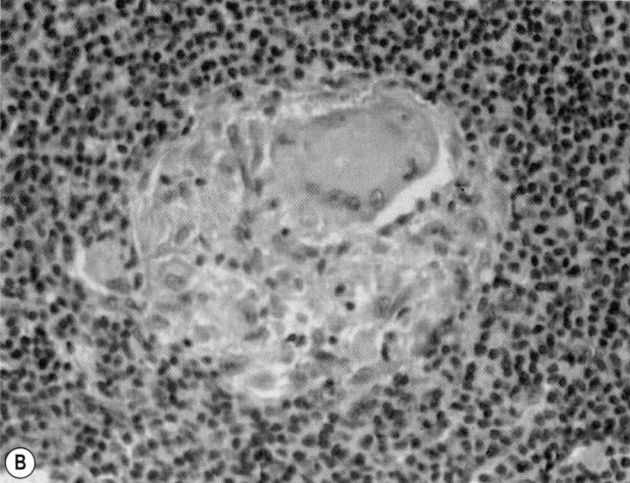

Fig. 36.2 Two types of granuloma. (A) The lepromatous-like type consisted of poorly defined, poorly differentiated granulomas, with few, if any giant cells and lymphocytes, but widespread macrophages loaded with acid-fast bacilli. (B) The tuberculoid type consisted of well-circumscribed and differentiated granulomas, with epithelioid and multinucleated giant cells containing very few acid-fast rods, surrounded by lymphocytes and fibrosis, occasionally with central caseous necrosis.

in the *IFNGR2* gene encoding IFN-γR2 lead to a complete loss of cellular responsiveness to IFN-γ, whether due to a lack of receptor expression or to the surface expression of nonfunctional receptors. All children with complete IFN-γR2 deficiency had severe, early-onset infections due to EM and/or BCG, all requiring continuous multidrug therapy. Three of these patients also had cytomegalovirus infection. Two patients underwent HSCT, which was successful in one case. Three of the other five patients died of disseminated mycobacterial infection at the age of 5 years and the two remaining patients are currently on antibiotic treatment at the ages of 3 and 9 years, respectively. Multiple antibiotics against mycobacteria should be administered without interruption and vaccination with live BCG is contraindicated. These patients should also be considered candidates for HSCT. Overall, the immunological features of IFN-γR2-deficient patients are essentially indistinguishable from those with complete IFN-γR1 deficiency with early-onset, recurrent, multiple, and life-threatening mycobacterial infections with impaired granuloma formation (Fig. 36.2A).

Partial autosomal recessive IFN-γR1 and IFN-γR2 deficiencies

Fourteen patients from 11 unrelated kindreds with autosomal recessive (AR) partial IFN-γR1 deficiency (OMIM 107470) have been identified.[18,28] A founder effect had been described for the two mutations, that affect the extracellular domain of IFNGR1: V63G and I87T. Patients with partial IFN-γR1 deficiency have a less severe clinical phenotype than patients with complete deficiency. Disseminated BCG was observed in five patients. One patient, who had not been vaccinated with BCG, had curable symptomatic primary tuberculosis. *Mycobacterium abscessus* caused a disseminated infection in one patient. Other non-mycobacterial infections were reported caused by nontyphoid systemic *Salmonella*, *Shigella sonnei*, *Haemophilus influenzae*, *Legionella* spp., *Mycoplasma pneumoniae*, and *Klebsiella* spp. These patients had well-circumscribed and differentiated tuberculoid granulomas (Fig. 36.2B). Ten patients are currently free of infection with no prophylaxis. One patient with recessive partial IFN-γR2 deficiency (OMIM 147569) has also been reported.[14] A homozygous nucleotide substitution was found in *IFNGR2*, resulting in a single amino-acid substitution in the extracellular domain. The young adult patient concerned has had BCG and *M. abscessus* infections and is now well at 25 years of age. Thus, a diagnosis of partial recessive IFN-γR1 or IFN-γR2 deficiency should be considered in children and adults with mycobacterial and *Salmonella* infections with a mild clinical and histological phenotype. For these patients, antimycobacterial treatment can eventually be stopped, but not within the first year after control of the infection is achieved after which the patients should be closely monitored.

Partial autosomal dominant IFN-γR1 deficiency

Patients from more than 40 unrelated kindreds were found to have a autosomal dominant (AD) form of partial IFN-γR1 deficiency (OMIM 107470).[14,19,29] These patients have a heterozygous small frameshift deletion in *IFNGR1*, downstream from the segment encoding the transmembrane domain, but upstream from the recycling motif and JAK-1 and STAT-1 docking sites. This heterozygous mutation is therefore dominant negative and decreases cellular responses to IFN-γ. More than 60 patients with this condition have been identified, most bearing the same 818del4 heterozygous mutation (or another mutation in the same region), defining the first hotspot for small deletions.[19, 30–34] The clinical phenotype is characterized by EM and BCG

infections, often affecting the bones.[19] A diagnosis of mycobacterial osteomyelitis is highly suggestive of dominant IFN-γR1 deficiency.[19] Only two of the patients in the largest cohort of patients with heterozygous 818del4 (of 35 patients) have presented with nontyphoid salmonellosis, one presented with a single episode of infection with *Histoplasma capsulatum*, eight are asymptomatic, and two died of disseminated mycobacterial infection at the ages of 17 and 27 years, respectively. Antimycobacterial treatment could be combined with IFN-γ therapy in cases of disseminated infection. Antibiotics can be stopped, but not within the first year after the infection is brought under control and vaccination with live BCG is contraindicated. The clinical outcome of patients with partial dominant IFN-γR1 deficiency, like that of patients with partial recessive IFN-γR1 and IFN-γR2 deficiencies, is much better than that of children with complete IFN-γR deficiency, because there is some residual IFN-γ signaling defining a strong correlation between *IFNGR1* genotype, cellular and clinical phenotype.[19]

IL-12 p40 deficiency

Twenty-two patients with complete recessive IL-12p40 deficiency (OMIM 161561) have been reported.[14,35–37] These patients have mutations in *IL12B*, either small insertions or large deletions. Two founder mutational events have been identified in four kindreds from Saudi Arabia and in two kindreds from the Indian subcontinent. Children with this deficiency produce abnormally low levels of IFN-γ, due to a lack of stimulation by IL-12. This defect can be partially corrected, in a dose-dependent manner, with exogenous recombinant IL-12.[35] All children inoculated with live BCG vaccine developed clinical infection, two children had infection caused by EM, and one had an infection caused by *Mycobacterium tuberculosis*. Five patients presented nontyphoid salmonellosis and one presented with a single episode of infection caused by *Nocardia asteroides*, an acid-fast agent closely related to *Mycobacterium*. One of these patients is asymptomatic, but six died of infection between the ages of 1 and 11 years. The survivors are currently well between 2 and 23 years of age and most are not receiving prophylactic treatment.

Complete AR IL-12Rβ1 deficiency

More than 140 patients with recessive complete IL-12 receptor β1 (IL-12Rβ1) deficiency (OMIN 601604), with no cellular expression or with expression of the mutated form (in only one patient) have been identified.[38] The cellular phenotype of IL-12Rβ1-deficient patients is a lack of response of NK and T lymphocytes to IL-12 and IL-23, resulting in low levels of IFN-γ production. The clinical phenotype is characterized by EM/BCG infections, with half the patients also presenting with nontyphoid salmonellosis.[38] Most of the children inoculated with live BCG vaccine developed clinical infection: 13% had infections caused by EM (alone or associated with other infections), and four had infections caused by *M. tuberculosis*. The low penetrance for the case-definition phenotype of BCG/EM disease led to the discovery of tuberculosis as the sole infectious phenotype in several patients, providing the first cases of Mendelian predisposition to tuberculosis.[39] Half the patients presented nontyphoid salmonellosis and one presented a single episode of infection caused by *Paracoccidioides brasiliensis*. Eight of these patients are asymptomatic, but more than 27% have died from mycobacterial or *Salmonella* infection. A substantial fraction of IL-12Rβ1-deficient patients also presented with mild forms of chronic mucocutaneous candidiasis (CMC),[38,40] an observation probably related to the impairment of the IL-23-IL-17 circuit in these patients.[41] The survivors are currently well between 1 and 46 years of age.

For IL-12p40 and IL-12Rβ1 deficiencies, antimycobacterial treatment can be combined with IFN-γ therapy in cases of disseminated infection. Antibiotics can be stopped, but not within the first year after the infection is brought under control. Granuloma formation is preserved, but may be multibacillary in these patients. Thus, a diagnosis of IL-12p40 or IL12-Rβ deficiency should be considered in children and adults with mycobacterial and *Salmonella* infections that have a milder clinical and histological phenotype. Vaccination of these patients with live BCG is contraindicated. The prognosis is nevertheless good, partly owing to the incomplete clinical penetrance of primary mycobacterial infection, the favorable response of infections to treatment and the rarity of recurrent or multiple mycobacterial infections. Indeed, children with primary mycobacterial disease can mount a fully protective immune response against a secondary mycobacterial disease. However, the high incidence of recurrent salmonellosis in these patients suggests that IL-12 is required for both primary and secondary immunity to *Salmonella*.

Partial AD STAT-1 deficiency

Four kindreds with heterozygous mutations in *STAT1* causing an AD partial deficiency of the signal transducer and activator of transcription (STAT)-1 (OMIM 600555) have been described.[42–44] STAT-1 is a critical transducer of IFN-mediated signals, either as STAT-1 homodimers—γ-activating factor (GAF)—or as STAT-1/STAT-2/IRF-9 trimers, known as interferon-stimulated gene factor 3 (ISGF3) (Fig. 36.3). These heterozygous *STAT1* mutations reduce the cellular response to IFN-γ, but not to IFN-α. Two patients suffered from disseminated BCG infection with tuberculoid granulomas, one suffered from local BCG infection and two others had disseminated *Mycobacterium avium* infection. The other four patients are asymptomatic. All patients are currently well between 10 and 43 years of age. Antimycobacterial treatment can be stopped, but not during the first year after the infection is brought under control and vaccination with live BCG is contraindicated. Observations of affected patients suggest that STAT-1 and GAF are required for human IFN-γ-mediated mycobacterial immunity. In conclusion, patients with partial dominant STAT-1 deficiency have clinical and cellular phenotypes (i.e., susceptibility to mycobacterial disease and impaired GAF activation) similar to those of patients with partial IFN-γR deficiency and should be treated in a similar manner.

Complete AR and partial AD IRF8 deficiency

Two types of IRF8 deficiency have recently been reported (OMIM 601565).[13] In a child born to consanguineous parents, disseminated BCG disease led to the discovery of a lack of circulating monocytes and dendritic cells (DCs). The severity of the disease, mimicking CID, made HSCT necessary. Candidate gene studies showed that the child had AR complete IRF8 deficiency. The IL-12-IFN-γ circuit was therefore profoundly disrupted. Other mechanisms may account for BCG disease and vulnerability to other infectious agents. In two other adult patients with a history of pure MSMD, the same heterozygous mutation was found in *IRF8*, defining an AD, partial IRF8 deficiency. The mutation was severely hypomorphic and dominant-negative. Interestingly, the IL-12-IFN-γ circuit did not appear to be disrupted in tests on whole blood. Nevertheless, the two unrelated patients with AD IRF8 deficiency lacked circulating CD1c$^+$ CD11c$^+$

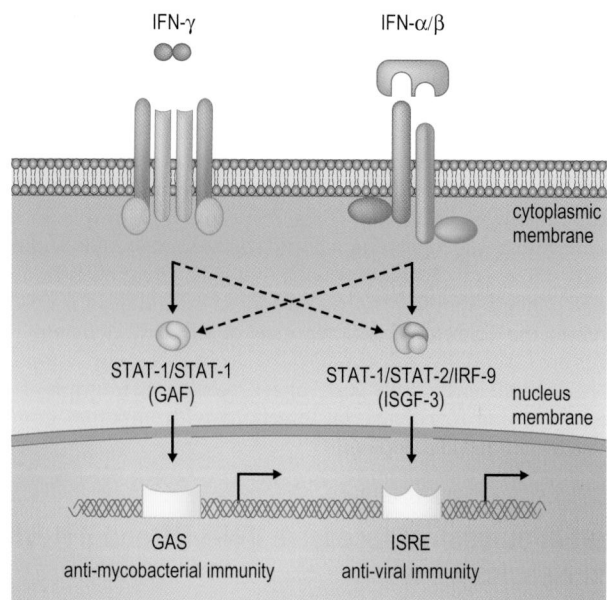

Fig. 36.3 STAT-1 pathway. The binding of homodimeric IFN-γ to its tetrameric receptor leads to activation of the constitutively associated JAK kinases JAK-1 and JAK-2, which then phosphorylate tyrosine residues in the intracellular part of IFN-γR1. Upon IFN-γ stimulation, unphosphorylated STAT-1 molecules are directly recruited to IFN-γR1 docking sites. They are then phosphorylated and released into the cytosol as phosphorylated STAT-1 homodimers, which form γ-activating factors (GAF) that are translocated to the nucleus. GAF binds γ-activating sequences (GAS) present in the promoters of target genes. Following monomeric IFN-α/β stimulation, STAT-2 is recruited to the phosphorylated IFN-αR1 chain of the heterodimeric IFN-αR, which is in turn phosphorylated by JAK-1 and TYK-2. This leads to the phosphorylated STAT-2-mediated recruitment of STAT-1, which is then phosphorylated. Active phosphorylated STAT-1/STAT-2 heterodimers are released into the cytosol and translocated to the nucleus with IRF-9, to form interferon-stimulated gene factor-3 (ISGF-3) heterotrimers. ISGF-3 binds IFN-α/β sequence response elements (ISRE) in the promoters of target genes via the DNA-binding domains of STAT-1 and IRF-9. In humans, recessive complete STAT-1 deficiency results in impaired responses to both IFN-γ and -α/β. It is associated with a specific syndrome, different from MSMD, of susceptibility to both mycobacteria (impaired IFN-γ-mediated immunity) and viruses (impaired IFN-α/β-mediated immunity).

DCs. This population of cells produces large amounts of IL-12 in normal individuals, and its absence therefore probably contributed to the MSMD phenotype.

Partial X-recessif CYBB deficiency

A X-linked recessive MSMD has recently been reported (OMIM 300645).[45] The seven patients from two unrelated French families were identified as suffering from mycobacterial disease. The *CYBB* or gp91^{phox} (NOX2) mutations identified in these seven patients had not been previously described and affect the transmembrane domain as well as an extracellular loop. *CYBB* encodes the major component of the NADPH oxidase complex.[45] Mutations in any of the genes encoding molecules from this complex generally result in chronic granulomatous disease (CGD).[46] However, unlike the cells of CGD patients, neutrophils and monocytes from these seven patients with XR-MSMD displayed a perfectly functional respiratory burst.[45] These patients produce only small amounts of neutrophil and monocyte gp91^{phox} protein, but normal amounts of cytochrome b558 (association of gp91phox and p22phox). However, differentiated macrophages and Epstein-Barr virus (EBV)-transformed B cells display a much more profound defect of gp91^{phox} expression, resulting in impaired cytochrome b558 assembly and impaired superoxide production and hydroxide peroxide release.[45] Thus, the respiratory burst in human macrophages is a crucial effector mechanism for protective immunity to tuberculous mycobacteria. None of the seven patients suffered from any other infectious diseases and they are all currently well between 37 and 61 years of age without prophylactic antibiotics. Vaccination with live BCG is contraindicated. Infections can be successfully treated with multiple antibiotics.

Inherited disorders of IFN-γ- and IFN-α/β-mediated immunity

Complete AR and partial AD STAT-1 deficiency

Five children from three unrelated kindreds with complete recessive STAT-1 deficiency (OMIM 600555) have also been identified (unpublished data).[47,48] These patients carried homozygous mutations that completely abolished the STAT-1-dependent cellular responses to IFN-g and IL-27, but also to IFN-a/b and IFN-l which may explain their susceptibility to mycobacteria and viruses, respectively. All patients had disseminated BCG disease. One patient died of recurrent encephalitis caused by HSV, a second died of an undocumented illness thought to be of viral origin, and a third died 3 months after HSCT, from EBV lymphoproliferative disorder. Recent data indicate that the two remaining children with complete STAT-1 deficiency died of unknown viral diseases, (unpublished data).[48] The mortality associated with viral illnesses in children with complete STAT-1 deficiency suggests that the STAT-1-dependent response to human IFN-α/β is necessary for effective anti-viral immunity. The patients with complete STAT-1 deficiency had multiple, severe, early-onset viral infections. Multiple antibiotics against mycobacteria, and possibly antiviral treatment directed against herpes viruses, should be administered without interruption and these patients should be considered for HSCT. Vaccination with live BCG is contraindicated. AR partial, as opposed to complete, STAT1 deficiency has recently been described in three unrelated kindreds. [49–51] These patients suffered from mild mycobacterial and viral disease. They displayed an impaired, but not abolished, response to IFN-γ and IFN-α in terms of GAF- and ISGF3-mediated immunity. Complete and partial recessive STAT-1 deficiency define an innate immunodeficiency ranging from lethal to moderate clinical disease that should be considered in infants and children with infectious diseases, notably (but not exclusively) mycobacterial and viral in nature.

Inborn errors of the TLR3-IFN-α, IFN-β, and IFN-λ pathway

This group of inherited disorders leads to impaired TLR3 signaling and susceptibility to HSE in childhood. The affected patients bear mutations in *TLR3*, *UNC93B1*, or *TRAF3* (Fig. 36.4). The

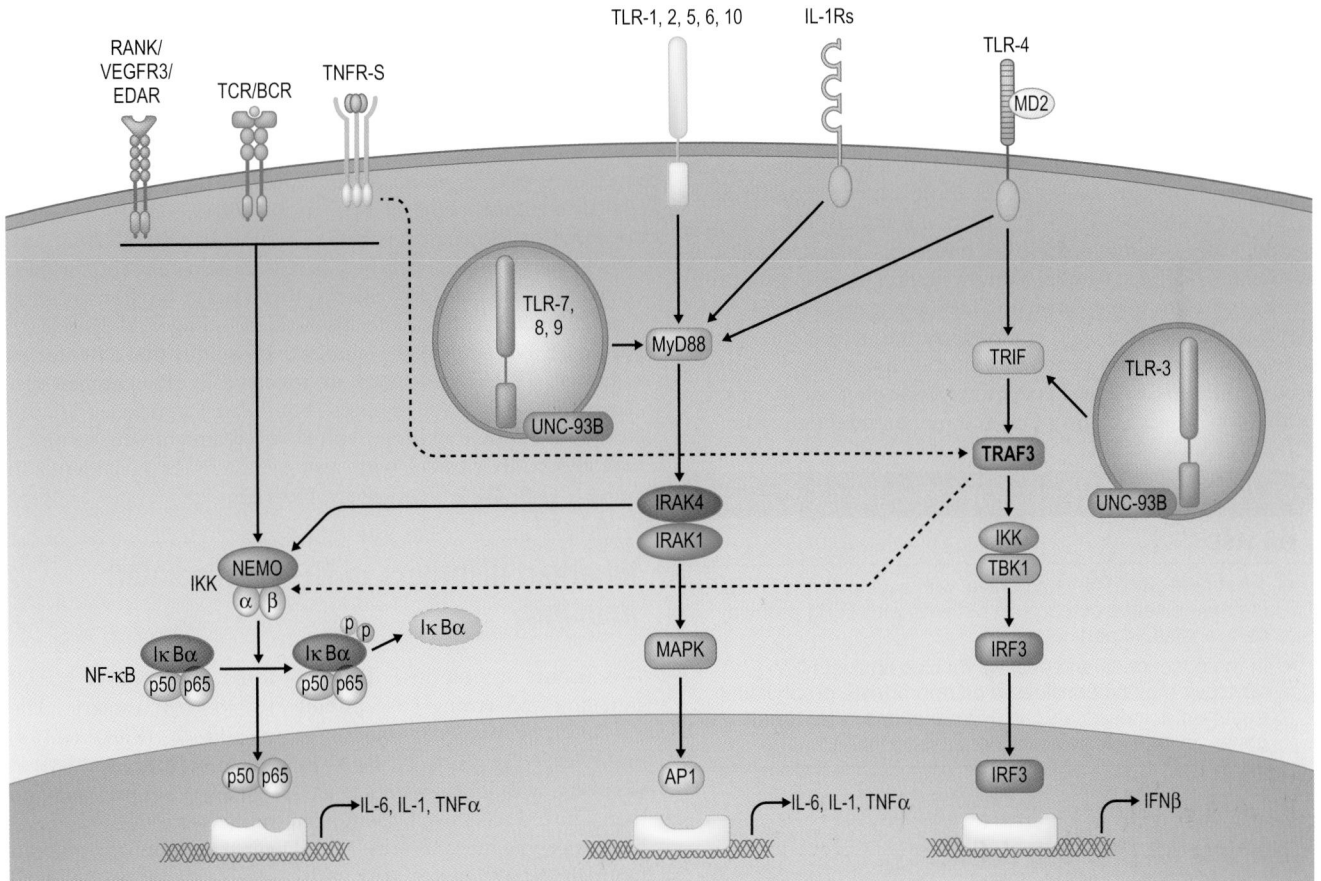

Fig. 36.4 Human defects involving IFN-α/-β, IFN-λ, and NF-κB pathways. Immune receptor signaling pathways leading to NF-κB activation can be grouped into four categories on the basis of the surface receptors involved: developmental receptors RANK, VEGFR3, and EDAR; antigen receptors (TCR and BCR); members of the TNF receptor superfamily (TNF-Rs) and members of the TIR superfamily (IL-1Rs/TLRs). The two proteins of the TIR signaling pathway (MyD88, IRAK-4) and the two proteins of the NF-κB signaling pathway (NEMO and IκBα) responsible for PIDs are shown in red. The defect in UNC-93B abolishes cellular responses to TLR3 and 7-9 agonists. The defect in TRAF3 impairs cellular responses to TLR3 and other pathways. The three proteins of the TLR3 signaling pathway (TLR3, UNC-93B, and TRAF3) responsible for PIDs are shown in red.

signaling pathway controlled by TRIF, which is mediated by TLR3 and TLR4, leads to activation of the transcription factors IRF3 and NF-κB (Fig. 36.4).[52] TRIF recruits TRAF6 and activates TAK1 for NF-κB activation. TRIF also recruits a signaling complex involving TBK1 and IKKε via TRAF3 for IRF3 activation.[52] This signaling pathway induces the production of type I and type III IFNs and inflammatory cytokines, and is important in antiviral immunity.[52] UNC-93B is a 12-transmembrane domain protein present in the ER and delivers the nucleotide-sensing receptors TLR3, 7, 8, and 9 from the ER to endolysosomes.[53] TRAF-3 has functions downstream from multiple TNF receptors and the receptors inducing IFN-α, -β, and -λ production, including TLR3. *UNC93B1* and *TRAF3* defects also impair the TLR7-9 pathway, but with no known clinical consequences.

Partial AD TLR3 deficiency

An AD form of TLR3 deficiency due to a heterozygous dominant-negative mutation of *TLR3* was identified in 2007 (OMIM 613002).[3] Seven patients from two unrelated kindreds with the same missense mutation in *TLR3* have been reported. Monocyte-derived DCs, NK, and CD8 T cells from TLR3-deficient patients have an impaired response to stimulation with a TLR3 agonist. The fibroblasts of the patients produce low levels of the antiviral molecules IFN-β/-λ in response to a TLR3 agonist and HSV-1, leading to higher levels of viral replication and virus-induced cell death than for healthy control cells. Only one child from each kindred identified developed HSE. The first patient developed HSE at 5 years of age, during primary infection with HSV-1. Nineteen months later, HSE recurred. The second patient presented an episode of meningo-encephalitis at the age of 5 months. Both patients have been exposed to other viruses during 8 and 20 years of follow-up, respectively, as shown by the positive serological results obtained for other herpes viruses with no subsequent acute events. None of the other five individuals with the dominant *TLR3* mutation developed HSE, despite serologically documented HSV-1 infection. Treatment with recombinant IFN-α, in parallel with acyclovir, may help to improve disease outcome in patients with TLR3 deficiency and HSE. TLR3 deficiency thus displayed complete penetrance at the cellular level, but incomplete penetrance at the clinical level. Multiple factors may affect clinical penetrance, including age at infection with HSV-1, the viral inoculum and human modifier genes.

THERAPEUTIC PRINCIPLES

For HSE

- Treatment with IFN-α, in parallel with acyclovir, may help to improve disease outcome in patients with TLR3 pathway deficiencies, in particular.
- In the absence of an effective vaccine against HSV-1, acyclovir may be considered an appropriate prophylactic treatment in individuals carrying mutations in TLR3 pathway genes, even if serologically negative for HSV-1.

Complete AR UNC-93B deficiency

AR UNC-93B deficiency was identified in 2006 as the first genetic etiology of isolated HSE (OMIM 610551).[2] Three individuals from two consanguineous kindreds were found to carry homozygous mutations in *UNC93B1*. UNC-93B deficient fibroblasts and leukocytes did not respond to TLR3, or to TLR7-9

agonists, respectively, in terms of IFN-α, -β, and -λ production. The fibroblasts from UNC-93B-deficient patients displayed abnormally high levels of viral replication and cell death after infection with HSV-1. Two of the three UNC-93B-deficient individuals developed HSE. The first patient presented recurrent episodes of HSE at the age of 11 months, 14 months, and 3 and a half years. During 14 years of follow-up, this patient has experienced no subsequent acute events. The second patient presented recurrent episodes of HSE at the ages of 5 and 17 years. She is now 21 years old and her clinical status has not worsened since the second episode of HSE. One sibling of the second patient, who carries the same homozygous mutation in *UNC93B1*, is now 30 years old and has not developed HSE, despite serologically documented HSV-1 infection. The two patients with UNC-93B deficiency and HSE have been exposed to other viruses with no evident clinical manifestations.[2] Treatment with recombinant IFN-α may also be considered, in parallel with acyclovir, in patients with UNC-93B deficiency and HSE.

Partial AD TRAF3 deficiency

A French patient with AD tumor necrosis factor (TNF) receptor-associated factor 3 (TRAF3) deficiency and HSE has recently been identified.[4] The *de novo* germline heterozygous missense mutation in this patient is loss-of-expression, loss-of-function, and dominant-negative. Fibroblasts from the patient displayed impaired responses to TLR3 agonist stimulation, in terms of IFN-β and -λ production. Various TRAF3-dependent pathways were impaired in the patient's cells, including the IFN-α/-β- and -λ-inducing and TNF-R-responsive pathways. However, there was sufficient residual TRAF3-dependent signaling for most other pathways to remain clinically silent. By contrast, the impaired TLR3 response was symptomatic and caused HSE, implying that the TLR3 pathway is critically dependent on TRAF3 and essential for immunity to HSV-1 in the CNS. The first clinical signs of HSE in the TRAF3-deficient patient appeared at the age of 4 years. The patient with TRAF3 deficiency and HSE described here is now 18 years old and has otherwise remained healthy with no prophylaxis. She shows normal resistance to other infectious diseases, including viral diseases in particular. We cannot yet exclude the possibility that other forms of human TRAF3 deficiency are involved in other human diseases, including viral diseases, but TRAF3 deficiency should be sought in other children with HSE. Treatment with recombinant IFN-α, in parallel with acyclovir, may be considered in patients with TRAF3 deficiency and HSE.

Inherited disorders of NF-κB-mediated immunity

This group of inherited disorders leads to impaired NF-κB signaling and strong susceptibility to pyogenic bacteria. The affected patients bear mutations in *NEMO*, *IKBA*, *IRAK4*, or *MyD88* (Fig. 36.4).[7,54] Patients with anhidrotic ectodermal dysplasia with immunodeficiency (EDA-ID) syndrome carry either X-linked recessive hypomorphic mutations in *NEMO* or AD hypermorphic mutations in *IKBA*. Diverse mutations have been found in *NEMO*, associated with various cellular and clinical phenotypes (see above and below).[9] Patients with AR amorphic mutations in *IRAK4* or in *MyD88* present a more restricted, purely immunological defect, with specific impairment of the TIR-interleukin receptor-associated kinase (IRAK) signaling pathway.[7] Patients with NEMO or IκBα deficiencies are susceptible to multiple infectious agents, including pyogenic bacteria, mycobacteria, and viruses. By contrast, patients with IRAK-4 and MyD88 deficiencies seem to be specifically prone to pyogenic bacterial diseases.

X-linked recessive hypomorphic NEMO deficiency

X-linked anhidrotic ectodermal dysplasia with immunodeficiency (XL-EDA-ID) is a rare PID associated with a developmental disorder (OMIM 300291). Patients with XL-EDA-ID carry hypomorphic mutations in the gene encoding IKK-γ/NEMO, a protein essential for activation of the ubiquitous transcription factor NF-κB. To date, up to 100 patients with NEMO deficiency have been reported.[9,55] The most consistent immunological abnormality in NEMO-deficient patients is an absence of serum antibodies against carbohydrates. Some patients have hypogammaglobulinemia, more rarely hyper-IgM syndrome and a few have NK-cell abnormalities.[9] Most NEMO-deficient patients fail to produce IL-10 in response to activation with TNF-α in whole-blood assays.[9]

An X-linked recessive form of MSMD (XR-MSMD) was discovered in three unrelated kindreds caused by two neighboring mutations (E315A and R319Q) in *NEMO*.[64] These two missense mutations, which affect two neighboring residues in the leucine zipper domain that normally form a salt bridge, are responsible solely for impairing the CD40-triggered induction of IL-12 production by monocyte-derived cells upon stimulation with CD40L-expressing T cells. Four maternally related male family members in two successive generations presented only *M. avium* infection and the other two, unrelated, patients suffered from only mycobacterial disease. These patients had a purely mycobacterial infectious phenotype, with no sign of EDA with the exception of conical decidual incisor teeth in one patient.

The infectious phenotype for the other NEMO-deficient patients is characterized mostly by infections due to encapsulated pyogenic bacteria, such as *H. influenzae* and *Streptococcus pneumoniae*. Infections caused by weakly pathogenic microorganisms, such as *M. avium* and *Mycobacterium kansasii*, have also been diagnosed in patients.[55] Other infectious diseases, including salmonellosis, pneumocystosis, and viral illnesses caused by HSV and cytomegalovirus, have been reported. Infectious episodes were marked by a poor clinical and biological inflammatory response.[9] One third of the NEMO-deficient patients died from invasive infection, demonstrating the severity of this disorder.[9] About 80% of the reported NEMO deficient patients to date have had EDA-ID, which is characterized by hypohidrosis, widely spaced cone- or peg-shaped teeth, and hypotrichosis (Fig. 36.5).[9,54] These features result from defective signaling via the ectodysplasin receptor signaling pathway. In some other NEMO-deficient patients, osteopetrosis (O) and lymphoedema (L) have been found associated with the EDA phenotype.[8,9,59] Some patients also have dysmorphia with mild frontal bossing.[60,61] However, about 10 % of NEMO-deficient patients do not display any of the classical features of the EDA phenotype.[9,62,63]

Prophylactic trimethoprim-sulfamethazole and/or penicillin V treatment should also be considered and IgG substitution should be carried out in patients with NEMO deficiency presenting with an impairment of B-cell immunity. NEMO-deficient patients with functional B-cell immunity should be immunized with *S. pneumoniae* conjugated and nonconjugated vaccines, *H. influenzae* conjugated vaccine and *Neisseria meningitidis* conjugated and nonconjugated vaccines. Vaccination with live BCG is contraindicated. The families and physicians of NEMO-deficient patients should note that it is important to initiate empiric

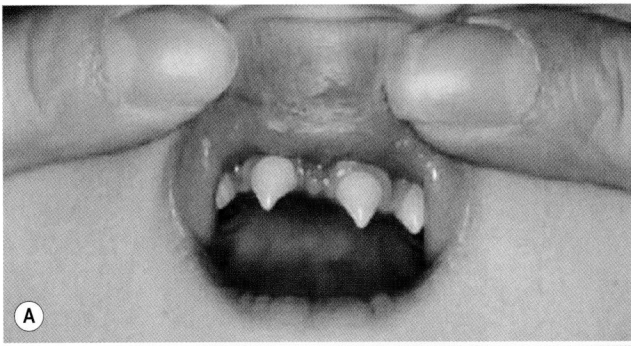

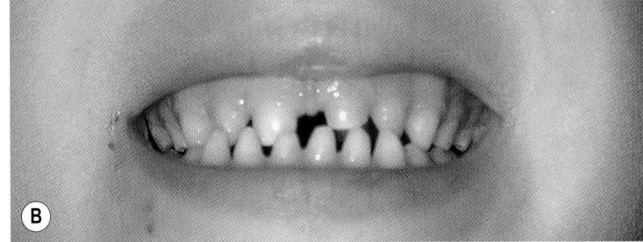

Fig. 36.5 Two patients with EDA-ID, one of whom presented widely spaced cone- or peg-shaped teeth, the other having conical incisors.

parenteral antibiotic treatment against *S. pneumoniae, Staphylococcus aureus, Pseudomonas aeruginosa*, and *H. influenzae* as soon as infection is suspected or the patient develops a moderate fever as patients may die from rapid invasive bacterial infection despite appropriate prophylaxis. Patients with a severe infectious phenotype should be considered for HSCT (unpublished data).[60,65–69] The NEMO–NF-κB signaling pathway includes a large number of receptors involved in the development of ectodermal-derived structures (EDAR, RANK, and VEGFR) and in immunity (antigen receptors (TCR and BCR), members of the TNF receptor superfamily (such as CD40 or TFNR), and members of the TIR superfamily). Clinical variability therefore probably results from differences in the impact of the various hypomorphic mutations in this pathway downstream from these receptors.

⬤ THERAPEUTIC PRINCIPLES

For inherited disorders of TIR-mediated immunity

- Patients should receive conjugated and nonconjugated vaccines against encapsulated bacteria (pneumococcus, *H. influenzae*, meningococcus).
- A preventive treatment, including antibiotic prophylaxis with cotrimoxazole and/or penicillin V, should be administered throughout the life of the patient.
- Monthly prophylactic administrations of intravenous or subcutaneous immunoglobulins should be considered in selected patients.
- Empiric parenteral antibiotic treatment against *S. pneumoniae, S. aureus*, and *P. aeruginosa* should be initiated as soon as an infection is suspected or if the patient develops a moderate fever, without taking inflammatory parameters into account.
- HSCT should be considered in selected patients with NEMO and IκBα deficiency.

AD IκBα deficiency

Five patients with three different hypermorphic mutations of *IKBA*, which encodes an inhibitor of NF-κB (OMIM 164008), have been identified since 2003, one of whom displays complex partial mosaicism.[10,56–58] IκBα deficiency leads to a severe impairment of TCR signaling.[10] IκBα-deficient patients have hypogammaglobulinemia and do not produce specific antibodies. Some also have low proportions of memory CD4[+] and CD8[+] T cells, no TCRγ/δ T cells, and severe impairment of T-cell proliferation in response to anti-CD3. All IκBα-deficient patients without mosaicism described to date have EDA.[9,54] One IκBα-deficient patient with complex mosaicism has no features of EDA.[56] All five IκBα-deficient patients have developed recurrent bacterial infections: pneumonia in five cases, sepsis or meningitis in three cases, and arthritis in one case.[56–58,70] They are also prone to opportunistic infections, three of these patients having had pulmonary pneumocystosis and CMC. Finally, four of these patients have presented recurrent diarrhea and/or colitis. Thus, a diagnosis of IκBα deficiency should be considered in children with EDA and CID with impaired T-cell immunity. Antibiotic prophylaxis with cotrimoxazole and/or penicillin V should be proposed and IgG substitution should be carried out in patients with IκBα deficiency. The recommendations for NEMO-deficient patients with fever should also be applied to IκBα-deficient patients. HSCT has been reported in two patients with severe IκBα deficiency causing CID.[65,70] One of these patients is alive and well, with no treatment, 8 years after haploidentical HSCT, whereas the other patient died of bacterial sepsis during the period of aplasia.[65,70]

AR IRAK4 deficiency

Inherited interleukin-1 receptor-associated kinase-4 (IRAK-4) deficiency (OMIM 607676) is an AR disorder first described in 2003.[5] In total, 52 patients have since been identified, from 33 kindreds.[7,55] The blood cells of these patients fail to produce pro-inflammatory cytokines upon stimulation with all known TLR agonists (with exception of TLR3 agonists), IL-1β, and IL-18. IRAK-4-deficient patients seem to have normal antigen-specific T- and B-cell responses, as shown in routine immunological investigations, with two notable exceptions.[70] First, the glycan-specific immunoglobulin (Ig)G and IgM antibody responses to pneumococcal and AB glycans (allohemagglutinins of the ABO system) are impaired in up to one-third of the patients explored.[7] Second, serum IgE and IgG4 concentrations are high in up to two-thirds and one-third, respectively, of patients tested.[7]

IRAK-4-deficient patients suffer from recurrent infections caused by pyogenic bacteria, mostly *S. pneumoniae, S. aureus,* and *P. aeruginosa,* with little or no fever or inflammatory response.[7] The leading pathogen responsible for infections in these patients is *S. pneumoniae,* which was found in half the cases of documented invasive infection (septicemia, meningitis, abscesses, or arthritis), whereas *S. aureus* and *P. aeruginosa* were found in 14 and 19% of such episodes, respectively. IRAK-4-deficient patients also suffer from noninvasive pyogenic bacterial infections, mostly affecting the skin and upper respiratory tract, with necrotizing infections particularly common. The principal bacterial strains isolated during noninvasive infections in IRAK-4-deficient patients were *S. aureus* in 43% of episodes, *P. aeruginosa* in 22% of episodes, and *S. pneumoniae* in 16% of episodes. All sudden invasive infections occurred before the age of 14 years. IRAK-4 deficiency is a life-threatening disease, resulting in the deaths of 20 of the 52 known patients, all of whom died before the age of 8 years. Eleven of these patients died of invasive pneumococcal disease. There is an overall trend towards improvement with age, as shown by the seven adult patients doing well with no treatment at 18 to 37 years of age.

Patients with IRAK-4 deficiency should also be immunized with *S. pneumoniae* conjugated and nonconjugated vaccine, *H. influenzae* conjugated vaccine, and *N. meningitidis* conjugated and nonconjugated vaccine. A preventive treatment, including antibiotic prophylaxis with cotrimoxazole plus penicillin V, should be administered throughout the life of the patient. Given the severity of bacterial infection during childhood and the defective antibody production found in some IRAK-4-deficient patients, we also recommend the administration of empiric IgG injections until the patient is at least 10 years old. This prophylaxis seems to decrease the incidence of invasive bacterial infections.[7] The families and physicians of IRAK-4-deficient patients should note that it is important to initiate empiric parenteral antibiotic treatment against *S. pneumoniae, S. aureus,* and *P. aeruginosa* as soon as an infection is suspected or if the patient develops a moderate fever, because patients may die from rapid invasive bacterial infection despite appropriate prophylaxis. A diagnosis of IRAK-4 deficiency should be considered in children presenting with recurrent invasive pyogenic infection and poor inflammatory responses.

AR MyD88 deficiency

MyD88 deficiency is an AR disorder recently described in 22 patients (OMIM 612260).[6,7,55,72] MyD88-deficient patients display a lack of production of pro-inflammatory cytokines by whole blood and no CD62L shedding from granulocytes following activation with most of the TLR and IL-1R agonists tested, with the exception of TLR3, which uses a MyD88-independent pathway.[3,6,73] Thus, there seems to be no overt defect of leukocyte development in MyD88-deficient patients, and antigen-specific T- and B-cell responses appear to be normal, as shown by routine immunological analyses, in most cases.[6,71] Some of the modest, subclinical abnormalities of B-cell responses, such as the production of low levels of antibodies against carbohydrates in some patients, may thus reflect impaired TACI responses, rather than impaired TLR and IL-1R responses.[74] MyD88 deficiency, like IRAK-4 deficiency, confers a predisposition to severe bacterial infection, with impairment of the ability to increase plasma CRP concentrations and to mount fever at the beginning of infection. However, pus formation has been observed at various sites of infection.

Patients with MyD88 deficiency present a narrow susceptibility to invasive pyogenic bacterial infections.[7,55,72] *S. pneumoniae* was involved in 41% of the documented invasive episodes in MyD88-deficient patients, whereas *S. aureus* and *P. aeruginosa* were found in 20 and 16 % of such episodes, respectively. Most MyD88-deficient patients suffered from their first bacterial infection before the age of 2 years. Nine patients died from invasive bacterial infections, all before the age of 4 years, and most before the age of 1 year.[7,55,72] Seven of these patients died from invasive pneumococcal disease. However, MyD88 deficiency seems to improve with age, and none of the patients has presented invasive bacterial infection after adolescence.[7] MyD88 deficiency also confers a predisposition to noninvasive pyogenic bacterial infections, mostly affecting the skin and upper respiratory tract. The principal bacterial strains found during noninvasive infections were *S. aureus* in 53% of patients, *S. pneumoniae* in 20% of patients, and *P. aeruginosa* in 13% of patients. Most MyD88-deficient patients have had noninvasive bacterial infections, with half the patients suffering from their first noninvasive bacterial infection before the age of 2 years. MyD88-deficient patients continue to suffer from skin infections, sinusitis, or pneumonia, even after reaching adolescence. The therapeutic recommendations in

MyD88-deficient patients are the same as those for IRAK-4-deficient patients (see above). A diagnosis of MyD88 deficiency should be considered in children presenting with recurrent pyogenic infection with poor inflammatory responses.

Conclusion

An understanding of the molecular basis of these PIDs affecting the innate immune responses mediated by IFN-γ, IFN-α/β/λ, TIRs, or NF-κB has provided detailed insight into the pathogenesis of infections in affected patients, paving the way for genetic counseling and rational treatment design.[75] These PIDs should be sought in patients with unexplained infectious diseases, whether caused by a single or multiple infectious agents, even if all standard immunological explorations are normal.[76-78] Interestingly, even common infectious diseases, such as tuberculosis, invasive pneumococcal disease, and herpes encephalitis, may be favored by Mendelian immune disorders. The discovery of many new PIDs is an exciting perspective, not only increasing our understanding of immunity to pathogens, but also benefiting patients. It is thought that most children with severe infectious diseases probably suffer from an underlying PID, and they should therefore be repeatedly investigated for known and unknown immunodeficiency conditions.

Acknowledgments

We thank our laboratory colleagues, our collaborators at Hospital Necker-Enfants Malades and elsewhere, and our patients and families for their assistance in making possible the studies contained in this chapter. We thank all the members of the Human Genetics of Infectious Diseases Laboratory for helpful discussions, including, in particular, Laurent Abel, Pegah Ghandil, and Maya Chrabieh. JLC was an International Scholar of the Howard Hughes Medical Institute. The Laboratory of Human Genetics of Infectious Diseases is supported by grants from the Rockefeller University Center for Clinical and Translational Science grant 5UL1RR024143-03 and the Rockefeller University. The Laboratory of Human Genetics of Infectious Diseases was supported by the March of Dimes, the Dana Foundation, the ANR, the INSERM, the FRM, and the PHRC.

References

1. Notarangelo LD, Fischer A, Geha RS, et al. Primary immunodeficiencies: 2009 update. J Allergy Clin Immunol 2009;124(6):1161–78.
2. Casrouge A, Zhang SY, Eidenschenk C, et al. Herpes simplex virus encephalitis in human UNC-93B deficiency. Science 2006;314(5797):308–12.
3. Zhang SY, Jouanguy E, Ugolini S, et al. TLR3 deficiency in patients with herpes simplex encephalitis. Science 2007;317(5844):1522–7.
4. Perez de Diego R, Sancho-Shimizu V, Lorenzo L, et al. Human TRAF3 adaptor molecule deficiency leads to impaired Toll-like receptor 3 response and susceptibility to herpes simplex encephalitis. Immunity 2010;33(3):400–11.
5. Picard C, Puel A, Bonnet M, et al. Pyogenic bacterial infections in humans with IRAK-4 deficiency. Science 2003;299(5615):2076–9.
6. von Bernuth H, Picard C, Jin Z, et al. Pyogenic bacterial infections in humans with MyD88 deficiency. Science 2008;321(5889):691–6.
7. Picard C, von Bernuth H, Ghandil P, et al. Clinical features and outcome of patients with IRAK-4 and MyD88 deficiency. Medicine (Baltimore) 2010;89(6):403–25.
8. Doffinger R, Smahi A, Bessia C, et al. X-linked anhidrotic ectodermal dysplasia with immunodeficiency is caused by impaired NF-kappaB signaling. Nat Genet 2001;27(3):277–85.
9. Hanson EP, Monaco-Shawver L, Solt LA, et al. Hypomorphic nuclear factor-kappaB essential modulator mutation database and reconstitution system identifies phenotypic and immunologic diversity. J Allergy Clin Immunol 2008;122(6):1169–77.
10. Courtois G, Smahi A, Reichenbach J, et al. A hypermorphic IkappaBAlpha mutation is associated with autosomal dominant anhidrotic ectodermal dysplasia and T cell immunodeficiency. J Clin Invest 2003;112(7):1108–15.
11. Casanova JL, Abel L. Genetic dissection of immunity to mycobacteria: the human model. Annu Rev Immunol 2002;20:581–620.
12. Picard C, Casanova JL. Inherited disorders of cytokines. Curr Opin Pediatr 2004;16(6):648–58.
13. Hambleton S, Salem S, Bustamante J, et al. IRF8 mutations and human dendritic-cell immunodeficiency. N Engl J Med 2011;365(2):127–38.
14. Filipe-Santos O, Bustamante J, Chapgier A, et al. Inborn errors of IL-12- and IFN-gamma-mediated immunity: molecular, cellular, and clinical features. Semin Immunol 2006;18(6):347–61.
15. Newport MJ, Huxley CM, Huston S, et al. A mutation in the interferon-gamma-receptor gene and susceptibility to mycobacterial infection. N Engl J Med 1996;335(26):1941–9.
16. Jouanguy E, Altare F, Lamhamedi S, et al. Interferon-gamma-receptor deficiency in an infant with fatal bacille Calmette-Guerin infection. N Engl J Med 1996;335(26):1956–61.
17. Jouanguy E, Dupuis S, Pallier A, et al. In a novel form of IFN-gamma receptor 1 deficiency, cell surface receptors fail to bind IFN-gamma. J Clin Invest 2000;105(10):1429–36.
18. Sologuren I, Boisson-Dupuis S, Pestano J, et al. Partial recessive IFN-γR1 deficiency: genetic, immunological and clinical features of 14 patients from 11 kindreds. Hum Mol Genet 2011;20(8):1509–23.
19. Dorman SE, Picard C, Lammas D, et al. Clinical features of dominant and recessive interferon gamma receptor 1 deficiencies. Lancet 2004;364(9451):2113–21.
20. Al-Muhsen S, Casanova JL. The genetic heterogeneity of mendelian susceptibility to mycobacterial diseases. J Allergy Clin Immunol 2008;122(6):1043–51; quiz 1052–1053.
21. Marazzi MG, Chapgier A, Defilippi AC, et al. Disseminated *Mycobacterium scrofulaceum* infection in a child with interferon-gamma receptor 1 deficiency. Int J Infect Dis 2010;14(2):e167–e170.
22. Prando C, Boisson-Dupuis S, Grant AV, et al. Paternal uniparental isodisomy of chromosome 6 causing a complex syndrome including complete IFN-gamma receptor 1 deficiency. Am J Med Genet A 2010;152A(3):622–9.
23. Kong XF, Vogt G, Chapgier A, et al. A novel form of cell type-specific partial IFN-gammaR1 deficiency caused by a germ line mutation of the IFNGR1 initiation codon. Hum Mol Genet 2010;19(3):434–44.
24. Camcioglu Y, Picard C, Lacoste V, et al. HHV-8-associated Kaposi sarcoma in a child with IFNgammaR1 deficiency. J Pediatr 2004;144(4):519–23.
25. Roesler J, Horwitz ME, Picard C, et al. Hematopoietic stem cell transplantation for complete IFN-gamma receptor 1 deficiency: a multi-institutional survey. J Pediatr 2004;145(6):806–12.
26. Rosenzweig SD, Dorman SE, Uzel G, et al. A novel mutation in IFN-gamma receptor 2 with dominant negative activity: biological consequences of homozygous and heterozygous states. J Immunol 2004;173(6):4000–8.
27. Vogt G, Chapgier A, Yang K, et al. Gains of glycosylation comprise an unexpectedly large group of pathogenic mutations. Nat Genet 2005;37(7):692–700.
28. Jouanguy E, Lamhamedi-Cherradi S, Altare F, et al. Partial interferon-gamma receptor 1 deficiency in a child with tuberculoid bacillus Calmette-Guerin infection and a sibling with clinical tuberculosis. J Clin Invest 1997;100(11):2658–64.
29. Jouanguy E, Lamhamedi-Cherradi S, Lammas D, et al. A human IFNGR1 small deletion hotspot associated with dominant susceptibility to mycobacterial infection. Nat Genet 1999;21(4):370–8.
30. Okada S, Ishikawa N, Shirao K, et al. The novel IFNGR1 mutation 774del4 produces a truncated form of interferon-gamma receptor 1 and has a dominant-negative effect on interferon-gamma signal transduction. J Med Genet 2007;44(8):485–91.
31. Storgaard M, Varming K, Herlin T, Obel N. Novel mutation in the interferon-gamma-receptor gene and susceptibility to mycobacterial infections. Scand J Immunol 2006;64(2):137–9.
32. Lee WI, Huang JL, Lin TY, et al. Chinese patients with defective IL-12/23-interferon-gamma circuit in Taiwan: partial dominant interferon-gamma receptor 1 mutation presenting as cutaneous granuloma and IL-12 receptor beta1 mutation as pneumatocele. J Clin Immunol 2009;29(2):238–45.
33. van de Vosse E, van Dissel JT, Ottenhoff TH. Genetic deficiencies of innate immune signalling in human infectious disease. Lancet Infect Dis 2009;9(11):688–98.
34. Vinh DC, Masannat F, Dzioba RB, et al. Refractory disseminated coccidioidomycosis and mycobacteriosis in interferon-gamma receptor 1 deficiency. Clin Infect Dis 2009;49(6):e62–e65.
35. Picard C, Fieschi C, Altare F, et al. Inherited interleukin-12 deficiency: IL12B genotype and clinical phenotype of 13 patients from six kindreds. Am J Hum Genet 2002;70(2):336–48.
36. Pulickal AS, Hambleton S, Callaghan MJ, et al. Biliary cirrhosis in a child with inherited interleukin-12 deficiency. J Trop Pediatr 2008;54(4):269–71.
37. Elloumi-Zghal H, Barbouche MR, Chemli J, et al. Clinical and genetic heterogeneity of inherited autosomal recessive susceptibility to disseminated Mycobacterium bovis bacille calmette-guerin infection. J Infect Dis 2002;185(10):1468–75.
38. de Beaucoudrey L, Samarina A, Bustamante J, et al. Revisiting human IL-12Rbeta1 deficiency: a survey of 141 patients from 30 countries. Medicine (Baltimore) 2010;89(6):381–402.
39. Boisson-Dupuis S, El Baghdadi J, Parvaneh N, et al. IL-12Rbeta1 deficiency in two of fifty children with severe tuberculosis from Iran, Morocco, and Turkey. PLoS One 2011;6(4):e18524.
40. de Beaucoudrey L, Puel A, Filipe-Santos O, et al. Mutations in STAT3 and IL12RB1 impair the development of human IL-17-producing T cells. J Exp Med 2008;205(7):1543–50.
41. Puel A, Picard C, Cypowyj S, et al. Inborn errors of mucocutaneous immunity to Candida albicans in humans: a role for IL-17 cytokines? Curr Opin Immunol 2010;22(4):467–74.
42. Dupuis S, Dargemont C, Fieschi C, et al. Impairment of mycobacterial but not viral immunity by a germline human STAT1 mutation. Science 2001;293(5528):300–3.
43. Averbuch D, Chapgier A, Boisson-Dupuis S, et al. The clinical spectrum of patients with deficiency of signal transducer and activator of transcription-1. Pediatr Infect Dis J 2011;30(4):352–5.

44. Chapgier A, Boisson-Dupuis S, Jouanguy E, et al. Novel STAT1 alleles in otherwise healthy patients with mycobacterial disease. PLoS Genet 2006;2(8):e131.

45. Bustamante J, Arias AA, Vogt G, et al. Germline CYBB mutations that selectively affect macrophages in kindreds with X-linked predisposition to tuberculous mycobacterial disease. Nat Immunol 2011;12(3):213–21.

46. Segal BH, Leto TL, Gallin JI, et al. Genetic, biochemical, and clinical features of chronic granulomatous disease. Medicine (Baltimore) 2000;79(3):170–200.

47. Dupuis S, Jouanguy E, Al-Hajjar S, et al. Impaired response to interferon-alpha/beta and lethal viral disease in human STAT1 deficiency. Nat Genet 2003;33(3):388–91.

48. Chapgier A, Wynn RF, Jouanguy E, et al. Human complete Stat-1 deficiency is associated with defective type I and II IFN responses in vitro but immunity to some low virulence viruses in vivo. J Immunol 2006;176(8):5078–83.

49. Chapgier A, Kong XF, Boisson-Dupuis S, et al. A partial form of recessive STAT1 deficiency in humans. J Clin Invest 2009;119(6):1502–14.

50. Kong XF, Ciancanelli M, Al-Hajjar S, et al. A novel form of human STAT1 deficiency impairing early but not late responses to interferons. Blood 2010;116(26): 5895–906.

51. Kristensen IA, Veirum JE, Moller BK, Christiansen M. Novel STAT1 alleles in a patient with impaired resistance to mycobacteria. J Clin Immunol 2011;31(2):265–71.

52. Kawai T, Akira S. The role of pattern-recognition receptors in innate immunity: update on Toll-like receptors. Nat Immunol 2010;11(5):373–84.

53. Kim YM, Brinkmann MM, Paquet ME, Ploegh HL. UNC93B1 delivers nucleotide-sensing toll-like receptors to endolysosomes. Nature 2008;452(7184):234–8.

54. Puel A, Picard C, Ku CL, et al. Inherited disorders of NF-kappaB-mediated immunity in man. Curr Opin Immunol 2004;16(1):34–41.

55. Picard C, Casanova J-L, Puel A. Infectious diseases in patients with IRAK-4, MyD88, NEMO, or I(kappa)B(alpha) deficiency. Clin Microbiol Rev 2011;24(3):490–7.

56. Janssen R, van Wengen A, Hoeve MA, et al. The same IkappaBalpha mutation in two related individuals leads to completely different clinical syndromes. J Exp Med 2004;200(5):559–68.

57. McDonald DR, Mooster JL, Reddy M, et al. Heterozygous N-terminal deletion of IkappaBalpha results in functional nuclear factor kappaB haploinsufficiency, ectodermal dysplasia, and immune deficiency. J Allergy Clin Immunol 2007;120(4):900–7.

58. Lopez-Granados E, Keenan JE, Kinney MC, et al. A novel mutation in NFKBIA/IKBA results in a degradation-resistant N-truncated protein and is associated with ectodermal dysplasia with immunodeficiency. Hum Mutat 2008;29(6):861–8.

59. Roberts CM, Angus JE, Leach IH, et al. A novel NEMO gene mutation causing osteopetrosis, lymphoedema, hypohidrotic ectodermal dysplasia and immunodeficiency (OL-HED-ID). Eur J Pediatr 2010;169(11):1403–7.

60. Dupuis-Girod S, Corradini N, Hadj-Rabia S, et al. Osteopetrosis, lymphedema, anhidrotic ectodermal dysplasia, and immunodeficiency in a boy and incontinentia pigmenti in his mother. Pediatrics 2002;109(6):e97.

61. Mancini AJ, Lawley LP, Uzel G. X-linked ectodermal dysplasia with immunodeficiency caused by NEMO mutation: early recognition and diagnosis. Arch Dermatol 2008;144(3):342–6.

62. Mooster JL, Cancrini C, Simonetti A, et al. Immune deficiency caused by impaired expression of nuclear factor-kappaB essential modifier (NEMO) because of a mutation in the 5' untranslated region of the NEMO gene. J Allergy Clin Immunol 2010;126(1): 127–32.

63. Puel A, Reichenbach J, Bustamante J, et al. The NEMO mutation creating the most-upstream premature stop codon is hypomorphic because of a reinitiation of translation. Am J Hum Genet 2006;78(4):691–701.

64. Filipe-Santos O, Bustamante J, Haverkamp MH, et al. X-linked susceptibility to mycobacteria is caused by mutations in NEMO impairing CD40-dependent IL-12 production. J Exp Med 2006;203(7):1745–59.

65. Fish JD, Duerst RE, Gelfand EW, et al. Challenges in the use of allogeneic hematopoietic SCT for ectodermal dysplasia with immune deficiency. Bone Marrow Transplant 2009;43(3):217–21.

66. Permaul P, Narla A, Hornick JL, Pai SY. Allogeneic hematopoietic stem cell transplantation for X-linked ectodermal dysplasia and immunodeficiency: case report and review of outcomes. Immunol Res 2009;44(1–3):89–98.

67. Tono C, Takahashi Y, Terui K, et al. Correction of immunodeficiency associated with NEMO mutation by umbilical cord blood transplantation using a reduced-intensity conditioning regimen. Bone Marrow Transplant 2007;39(12):801–4.

68. Pai SY, Levy O, Jabara HH, et al. Allogeneic transplantation successfully corrects immune defects, but not susceptibility to colitis, in a patient with nuclear factor-kappaB essential modulator deficiency. J Allergy Clin Immunol 2008;122(6): 1113–1118 e1.

69. Minakawa S, Takeda H, Nakano H, et al. Successful umbilical cord blood transplantation for intractable eczematous eruption in hypohidrotic ectodermal dysplasia with immunodeficiency. Clin Exp Dermatol 2009;34(7):e441–e442.

70. Dupuis-Girod S, Cancrini C, Le Deist F, et al. Successful allogeneic hemopoietic stem cell transplantation in a child who had anhidrotic ectodermal dysplasia with immunodeficiency. Pediatrics 2006;118(1):e205–e211.

71. Ku CL, von Bernuth H, Picard C, et al. Selective predisposition to bacterial infections in IRAK-4-deficient children: IRAK-4-dependent TLRs are otherwise redundant in protective immunity. J Exp Med 2007;204(10):2407–22.

72. Conway DH, Dara J, Bagashev A, Sullivan KE. Myeloid differentiation primary response gene 88 (MyD88) deficiency in a large kindred. J Allergy Clin Immunol 2010;126(1):172–5.

73. von Bernuth H, Ku CL, Rodriguez-Gallego C, et al. A fast procedure for the detection of defects in Toll-like receptor signaling. Pediatrics 2006;118(6):2498–503.

74. He B, Santamaria R, Xu W, et al. The transmembrane activator TACI triggers immunoglobulin class switching by activating B cells through the adaptor MyD88. Nat Immunol 2010;11(9):836–45.

75. Casanova JL, Abel L, Quintana-Murci L. Human TLRs and IL-1Rs in host defense: natural insights from evolutionary, epidemiological, and clinical genetics. Annu Rev Immunol 2011;29:447–91.

76. Alcais A, Abel L, Casanova JL. Human genetics of infectious diseases: between proof of principle and paradigm. J Clin Invest 2009;119(9):2506–14.

77. Alcais A, Quintana-Murci L, Thaler DS, et al. Life-threatening infectious diseases of childhood: single-gene inborn errors of immunity? Ann NY Acad Sci 2010;1214(1):18–33.

78. Casanova JL, Abel L. Inborn errors of immunity to infection: the rule rather than the exception. J Exp Med 2005;202(2):197–201.

HIV infection and acquired immunodeficiency syndrome

Susan L. Gillespie, Mary E. Paul, Javier Chinen, William T. Shearer

In the past 3 decades remarkable progress has been made in both the prevention and treatment of HIV infection. The infection has gone from a cause of widespread certain death to a chronic disease manageable with appropriate care and treatment. Certain preventive measures have shown remarkable ability to cut the spread of HIV infection from HIV-infected to HIV-uninfected persons. Yet, a vaccine is still critically needed and there is some positive news in that regard at long last. This chapter on HIV infection and AIDS records a perceptible pulse of progress throughout: epidemiology; virology; routes of infection; immunopathogenesis; clinical features; diagnostic tests; treatment; immune reconstitution; and prevention.

Epidemiology of HIV

Global perspective

Over the past few years, there has been stabilization of the overall growth of the global AIDS epidemic. The number of new infections has steadily declined since the late 1990s and there are fewer AIDS-related deaths due to the scale up of antiretroviral therapy since 2004.

According to the Joint United Nations Programme on HIV/ AIDS (UNAIDS) 33 million people worldwide were estimated to be living with HIV or AIDS at the end of 2009 (Fig. 37.1).[1] New HIV infections are declining in most countries. The annual number of incident HIV infections peaked at >3 million in the late 1990s and has steadily declined thereafter. In 2009, 2.6 million people were newly infected, with approximately 1% of these infections (370 000 cases) occurring in children younger than 15 years of age. The decline in new HIV infections is most clearly reflected in the fact that HIV incidence has fallen by more than 25% in 33 countries between 2001 and 2009. It is imperative, however, that prevention and treatment efforts continue with a global emphasis because HIV incidence increased by more than 25% in seven other countries in that same period.

There has been slow but continued reduction in the number of people dying from AIDS-related conditions worldwide. AIDS mortality peaked at 2.1 million in 2004 and settled at 1.8 million in 2009. The decline reflects increased access to antiretroviral therapy for, and improvements in care and support of, infected individuals. Mortality of children younger than 15 years of age has also declined, due to the expansion of services to prevent mother-to-child transmission (PMTCT) of HIV to infants

and an increase in access to care and treatment for children. Although access to care and treatment services for HIV-infected children in resource-limited settings is expanding, it is estimated that only 28% of children in need received life-saving antiretroviral therapy and an estimated 260 000 children died of AIDS-related illnesses in 2009.

● KEY CONCEPTS

Trends in HIV infection

- Global rates of HIV infection have stabilized but there is great heterogeneity in disease incidence between countries and regions.
- Although most countries had a reduction in disease incidence between 2001 and 2009, seven countries had increases in disease incidence by more than 25% over that period.
- The age demographic most affected in the developing world, i.e., those aged 25–44 years, includes men and women who are economically productive and women of childbearing potential.
- Worldwide, most infections are acquired through heterosexual contact.
- In the USA, African Americans and men who have sex with men (MSM) are disproportionately infected.
- The numbers of infections transmitted from mother to child are declining as access to prophylactic medications to prevent infection improves.

Sub-Saharan Africa bears the greatest share of the global HIV burden. In 2009, the number of people living with HIV in sub-Saharan Africa reached 22.5 million or 68% of the global total. Furthermore, an estimated 130 000 children became perinatally HIV-infected in 2009 at a time when mother-to-child transmission is virtually preventable. The estimated 1.3 million people who died of HIV-related illnesses in sub-Saharan Africa represented 72% of the global total deaths attributed to the epidemic in 2009.[1]

US perspective

The Centers for Disease Control and Prevention (CDC) estimate that almost 1.2 million adults and adolescents were living with HIV in the USA at the end of 2008, including 236 400 (20%) whose infection was undiagnosed. This represents an increase of approximately 6% from the previous estimate in 2006.[2] Despite

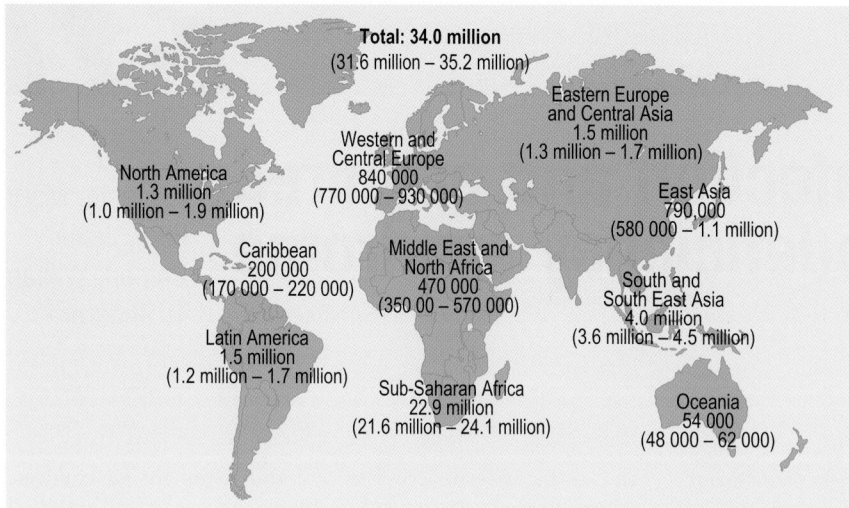

Fig. 37.1 Global prevalence of HIV infection: 33.3 million.
(Modified from UNAIDS, 2010).

ongoing prevention efforts designed to reduce the number of new cases of HIV infection, the number of newly diagnosed infections in the USA has remained unchanged from 2006 to 2009, approximately 40 000 to 50 000 per year. Within the USA there is great variability in both the geographic and demographic distribution of the disease with certain segments of the American population being disproportionately affected, specifically men who have sex with men (MSM) and ethnic and racial minorities including African Americans and Latino Americans (Fig. 37.2).[3] In the USA and other developed countries, in contrast to more resource-limited parts of the world, the number of children newly infected with HIV has decreased dramatically as a consequence of successful PMTCT interventions.[3] The CDC estimates that the number of infants born annually with HIV in the USA dropped from 1 650 in 1991 to fewer than 200 in 2004. At the same time, new pediatric AIDS cases and AIDS deaths also have plummeted, in large part due to powerful combinations of antiretroviral drugs.

Virology

Classification

HIV is an enveloped, positive-sense RNA virus with icosahedral symmetry and two copies of its genome. It belongs to the lentivirinae group of retroviruses (Fig. 37.3). As with all retroviruses, it contains the enzyme reverse transcriptase capable of turning its RNA genome into DNA, which is integrated into the host cell genome and can then be translated to produce viral proteins and new virions. Like other lentiviruses, HIV has a long latency period before causing clinical disease.

There are two distinct types of HIV, HIV-1 and HIV-2. Both cause human immunodeficiency, but HIV-2 is mostly found in West Africa, is less pathogenic than HIV-1 and may have a longer latency period. Phylogenetic studies have found that HIV-2 is

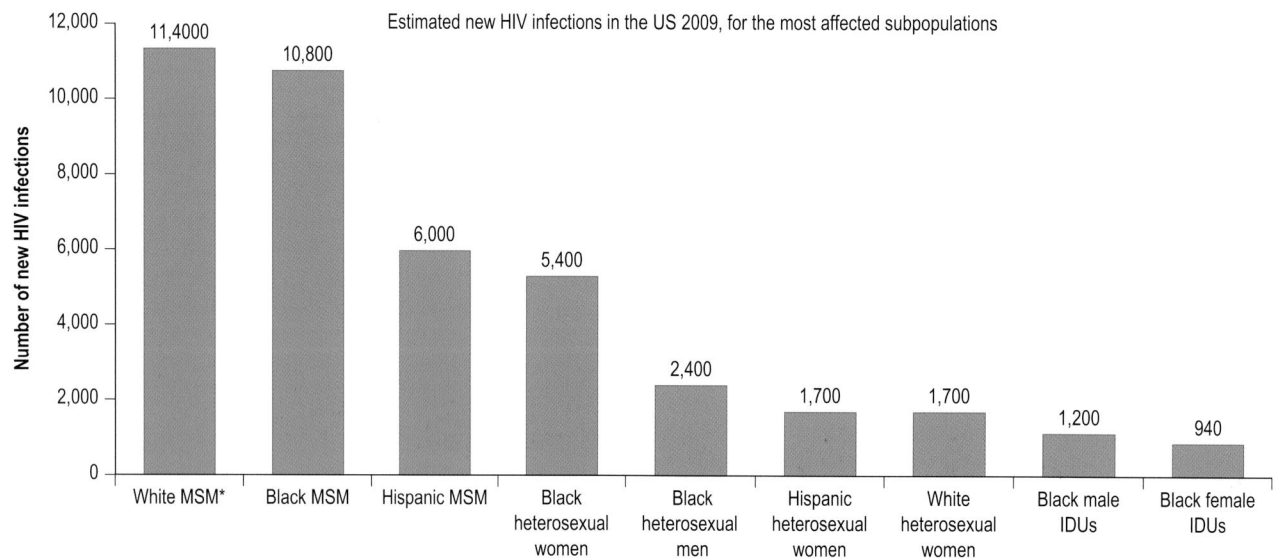

Estimated new HIV infections in the US 2009, for the most affected subpopulations

Fig. 37.2 US trends in HIV infection by race and mode of transmission.
From Centers for Disease Control and Prevention. HIV surveillance—United States, 1981-2008. MMWR Morb Mortal Wkly Rep 2011; 60: 689-693. Atlanta: US Department of Health and Human Services, Centers for Disease Control and Prevention, 2011. Also available at http://www.cdc.gov/hiv/topics/surveillance/resources/reports.gov

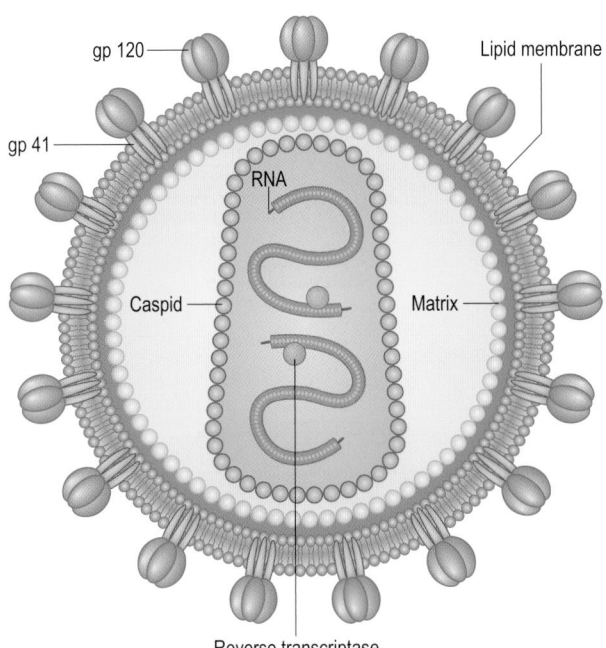

Fig. 37.3 Structure of HIV virion.
From Baliga CS, Shearer WT. HIV/AIDS. In: Fireman P, ed. Atlas of allergy. Philadelphia: Elsevier Science (USA), 3 rd edn, 2005: pp. 351-367.

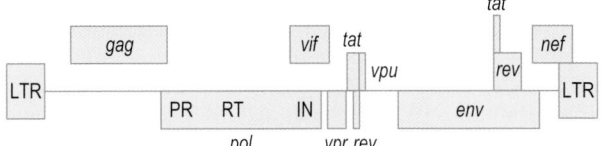

Fig. 37.4 HIV genome. LTR = long terminal repeat; the products of *pol*: PR = protease; RT = reverse transcriptase; IN = integrase.

Table 37.1 HIV proteins and their major functions

Structural proteins	Gag	Cleavage gives rise to capsid, matrix, nucleocapsid and p6
	Pol	Cleavage gives rise to protease, integrase, RNAse H, reverse transcriptase
	Env	gp120 and gp41
Regulatory proteins	Tat	Stabilizes transcription complex on the LTR and increases processivity of the complex
	Rev	Allows export of the viral RNA out of the nucleus
Accessory proteins	Nef	Downregulates MHC class I expression
	Vif	Ubiquitination and subsequent degradation of APOBEC3G
	Vpr	Arrests cell in G2/M phase of cell cycle
	Vpu/Vpx	Ubiquitinates CD4 in the endoplasmic reticulum

more closely related to Simian Immunodeficiency Virus (SIV), found in certain species of monkeys, whereas HIV-1 is more closely related to SIV_{cpz} (SIV from chimpanzees) supporting the presumed origin theory of HIV-1 evolving from infected chimpanzees in approximately 1930.

HIV-1 can be further subdivided based on the genetic divergence in the *env* gene.[4] With divergences of 30–50%, HIV-1 has been divided into three groups, M (major or most), O (outlier), and N (new or non-M, non-O). The M group is further subdivided into clades (A–H, J, K, and O), each of which differs from each other by 20–30%. Clade B is most common in the industrialized world, including the USA. C is the most common clade worldwide, being present in Africa and South Asia.

Structural genes: *gag, pol*, and *env*

The HIV genome is 9.8 kb in length and can be divided into three groups of genes: structural, regulatory, and accessory (Fig. 37.4 and Table 37.1).

● KEY CONCEPTS

HIV as a Zoonosis

- The natural reservoir of HIV prior to widespread human infection seems to have been chimpanzees for HIV-1, and sooty mangabeys for HIV-2.
- Each of the three groups of HIV-1, M, N, O, are thought to represent separate transmission events from chimpanzees to humans.
- The natural hosts of the SIV have a less robust immune response than humans, have poorer viral control, but only rarely show CD4 T-cell loss or progress to immunodeficiency.
- The ability of SIV to replicate in some non-human primates without causing overt disease may hold important knowledge needed for the management of the pandemics in humans.

The 55-kDa Gag polyprotein (p55) is encoded by the HIV *gag* gene. After translation, the N-terminal is myristolated causing it to localize to the cell membrane where it recruits two copies of viral RNA and other viral and cellular proteins, culminating in the budding and release of intact HIV particles.

The *pol* gene encodes protease (PR, p10), integrase (IN, p50), RNAse H (p15), and reverse transcriptase (RT, p31). Pol is translated in a complex with Gag (Gag-Pol, p160) by a ribosomal frame-shifting event toward the distal end of *gag*. PR cleaves the Gag-Pol complex into Gag and Pol. It further cleaves Pol into the above components. Functional PR exists as a dimer and is an aspartyl protease. The IN protein has three functional activities: an exonuclease, endonuclease, and a ligase. It first removes the terminal two nucleotides from the linear double-stranded viral DNA through its exonuclease function. Finally, utilizing its ligase function, it covalently joins the viral DNA with the host's. RNAse H is capable of cleaving RNA if it is part of an RNA-DNA duplex. This is important in removing the RNA template from the negative-strand DNA and allowing the positive strand of DNA to be synthesized by RT p31.

The protein Env, or gp160, is the product of the gene *env*. After translation, Env is glycosylated in the Golgi bodies. A cellular protease cleaves gp160 into gp120 and gp41. The transmembrane domain of Env is gp41. This is also the fusion domain involved in HIV infection. Glycoprotein 120 acts as the ligand for HIV, binding to CD4 and the chemokine receptors CXCR4 and CCR5.

Regulatory proteins: Tat and Rev

The regulatory proteins Tat and Rev are essential for HIV replication. Tat stands for trans-activating factor.[5] Although the HIV viral promoter LTR (long terminal repeat) is efficient in initiating DNA translation, without Tat the processivity is poor, and only 10% of the RNA products are complete. Tat binds to the transactivation response element (TAR) and facilitates the binding of several accessory proteins to the transcription complex, notably the Tat-associated kinase (Tak). HIV encodes 11 proteins from a single RNA transcript, which is then multiply spliced. To perform this task, HIV's Rev binds to the Rev responsive element (RRE) in the *env* sequence as well as to a nuclear export signal known as CRM1, which directs the RNA to an accessory pathway in the nucleus. This pathway is permissive to the passage of RNA messages containing both introns and exons into the cytoplasm. Without Rev, only Tat and Nef would be synthesized by HIV.[6]

Accessory proteins: Nef, Vif, Vpr, and Vpu/Vpx

The accessory proteins, Nef, Vif, Vpr, and Vpu (or Vpx in HIV-2) are not required for viral replication, but they help the efficiency of this process. Nef has numerous effects (Fig. 37.5).[7] It downregulates CD4 by promoting its endocytosis and lysosomal degradation. This helps the virus budding by removing the Env receptor from the cell surface. Nef also reduces the expression of major histocompatibility complex (MHC) class I on the cell's surface, thus limiting the ability of infected cells to be cleared by the immune system. It also activates T cells by binding to the T-cell receptor and several down-stream effectors. Activated T cells translocate transcription factors NFAT and NF-κB to the nucleus where they are thought to prime the viral promoter leading to greater HIV transcription.

Vif stands for virion infectivity factor. Vif can at least partially overcome the inhibitory action that a cellular factor, APOBEC3G, can have on HIV replication. Retroviruses have genomes containing many adenines. APOBEC3G is a cytosine deaminase that mutates cytosines to uracils on the first strand of HIV DNA synthesized during viral replication (Fig. 37.6), resulting in the second strand containing an adenine instead of a guanine as the retroviral reverse transcriptase recognizes uracil as a thymidine. APOBEC3G is part of a family of APOBEC proteins (apolipoprotein B (APOB) mRNA-editing, catalytic polypeptide), which work by deaminating cytosine and inducing mutations, either to generate genetic diversity or inactivate viruses such as HIV or hepatitis B. Vif acts along with several other cellular cofactors like elongin B, elongin C, cullin-5 (CUL5), to form an ubiquitin-ligase complex, which leads to the polyubiquitination of APOBEC3G and to a proteosomal degradation pathway.[8]

The viral protein R (Vpr) has several functions assigned to it.[7] It is best known for its ability to arrest the cell cycle in the G2/M

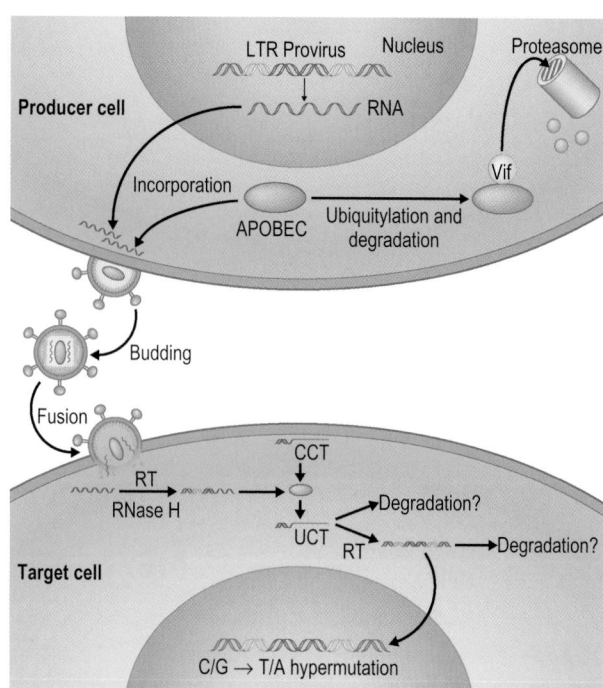

Fig. 37.6 Vif and APOBEC3G. APOBEC3G acts on the first strand of synthesized viral DNA to deaminate cytosine, thus converting it to uracil. The uracil leads to the incorporation of an adenine into the complementary DNA strand instead of a guanine, thus affecting a C/G → T/A mutation on the viral genome. The presence of uracils in single-stranded DNA can directly lead to the degradation of that DNA strand. Vif and other proteins bind to APOBEC and ubiquitinate it, leading to proteasomal degradation.
From Harris RS, Liddament NT. Retroviral restriction by APOBEC proteins. Nat Rev Immunol 2004; 4: 868-877.

phase through phosphorylation of Cdc2 and inhibition of the phosphorylase Cdc25C, as well as for its part in helping the pre-integration complex navigate through the cytosol into the nucleus. It recognizes various nuclear localization signals and disrupts the nuclear membrane in non-dividing cells. Vpr has been implicated in the induction of apoptosis. While low levels of expression seem to have an anti-apoptotic effect, higher levels promote apoptosis through caspase-dependent mechanisms.

Viral protein U (Vpu) is found in HIV-1 and SIV_{CPZ}.[9] Vpu binds to CD4 in the ER and leads to the ubiquitylation of CD4 to allow free Env migration to the cell surface and into nascent HIV particles.

Routes of infection

HIV is transmitted through three routes of infection: sexual, parenteral, and perinatal (Table 37.2). In general, higher viral loads, lower CD4 T-cell count, and larger viral inoculum size are all associated with a greater risk of transmission.

Sexual HIV transmission

Sexual transmission is the most common mode of infection, responsible for 70–80% of worldwide infections. Besides the factors mentioned above, recipients of penetrative intercourse are more likely to become infected. Anal intercourse carries the greatest risk, followed by vaginal intercourse, with oral

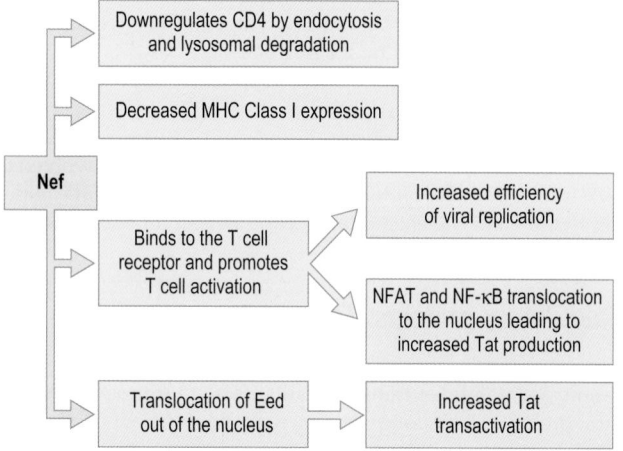

Fig. 37.5 The many functions of Nef.

Table 37.2 Routes of HIV infection

Mode of transmission worldwide	Percentage of cases
Sexual	70–80
Vaginal intercourse	60–70
Anal intercourse	5–10
Perinatal	5–10
In utero and intrapartum	2.5–5.0
Postpartum	2.5–5.0
Parenteral	8–15
Injecting drug abuse	5–10
Blood transfusions	3–5

From Baliga CS, Shearer WT. HIV/AIDS. In: Fireman P, ed. Atlas of allergy. Philadelphia: Elsevier Science (USA), 3rd edn, 2005: pp. 351-367.

intercourse the least likely to spread the virus. The presence of other sexually transmitted diseases, especially ulcerative lesions such as those seen in herpes simplex or syphilis infection, increases the risk of transmission.

Parenteral HIV transmission

Parenteral transmission is the second most common route of HIV infection, accounting for 8 to 15% of all HIV infections. Examples include contaminated needles among injection drug users (IDU), accidental needle sticks among health care workers, improperly sterilized hospital equipment, and contaminated blood products. Use of contaminated needles by IDUs is the largest risk factor for parenteral transmission. Infection control efforts have greatly reduced the risk but HIV transmission by transfusion of contaminated blood products remains significant, particularly in resource limited settings where there is a dependence upon family/replacement and paid blood donors, and where the infrastructure for routine blood screening is suboptimal.[1,10]

Perinatal HIV transmission

Perinatal transmission accounts for the majority of pediatric HIV cases and for 5–10% of HIV infections in patients of all ages. The virus is capable of infecting the child in utero, during labor, and after delivery through breastfeeding. Without preventive therapy, the risk of a child contracting HIV from the mother during gestation or during labor is about 25%. The majority of transmission events occur during the passage of the fetus through the birth canal, by exposure of the baby to infected maternal blood, amniotic fluid, and/or cervical and vaginal secretions. Although breastfeeding confers an additional 15–29% increased risk of transmission of the virus from mother to child, to prevent morbidity and mortality related to diarrheal diseases, breastfeeding is still recommended in settings where access to replacement feeding is limited.

Immunopathogenesis

The mechanisms of immunodeficiency induced by HIV are not limited to depletion of its main target cell, the CD4 T cell; HIV infection ultimately leads directly or indirectly to the impairment of every arm of the immune system.[10] The time of progression from infection to the development of AIDS is not the same for all infected individuals, and several explanations have been proposed including genetic resistance genes and presence of low virulence mutant viral particles. The study of long-term non-progressor individuals has helped to define T-cell and antibody features associated with anti-HIV immunity in the search for the optimal vaccine design, focusing on minimizing escape variants and inducing persistent specific viral neutralization or inhibition of replication.[11] HIV researchers have also explored the role of chronic immune activation processes that are associated with progression to AIDS, which also helps to explain the diverse clinical impact of this viral infection in different individuals.[12]

Mucosal dendritic cells: myeloid vs plasmacytoid

Following a mucosal inoculation of HIV, CD4 T cells are generally infected by CCR5-tropic virus, also called R5 or M-tropic virus.[13] After approximately one week, the virus becomes detectable in draining regional lymph nodes. *Myeloid dendritic cells are not infected with HIV*; rather HIV gp120 binds to dendritic cell-specific intercellular adhesion molecule-grabbing nonintegrin (DC-SIGN) in the cell membrane. The resulting complex is internalized as a phagosome and then presented on the cell surface. As there is no fusion of the HIV Env with the dendritic cell membrane, infection does not occur. *Plasmacytoid dendritic cells, on the other hand, express CD4 and the co-receptors CXCR4 and CCR5 and thus become infected by the virus.* Infection leads to expression of CCR7, which acts as a homing signal for the lymph nodes; it is in lymph nodes where the virus infects CD4 T cells, and significant viral replication occurs, resulting in detectable viremia and dissemination through lymphoid tissues. Of interest, the target cells for HIV infection, CD4 T cells and monocyte/macrophage cells, are also reservoirs for the virus. HIV infected cells carry a stable provirus integrated in the cell genome and transcriptionally silent until the cell is activated. These cells can reestablish HIV viremia even after prolonged anti-viral treatment, since viral reservoirs are unlikely to be eradicated within a life time.[14]

Gastrointestinal system: early target

Within days of infection, 20% of CD4 T cells found in gut-associated lymphoid tissue (GALT) are infected. Of these, up to 80% are killed, by both lytic infection and Fas mediated apoptosis of both infected and non-infected cells, mainly $CD4^+CCR5^+$ memory T cells.[15] By the time of peak viremia, 60% of the mucosal memory CD4 T cells are infected. Because their destruction is less drastic, circulating CD4 T-cell counts do not reflect the magnitude of CD4 T-cell death taking place in the GALT. Following acute HIV infection, a massive activation of the immune system occurs. Inadequate memory T-cell responses can lead to infection and inflammation of the entire bowel. The presence of immune activators over the massive surface area of the bowel has been hypothesized to result in the profound immune activation seen in HIV. Mucosal Th17 cells are a preferential target for HIV, further weakening mucosal immunity and favoring microbial infection. The viremia decreases spontaneously from as high as 10 million copies of HIV RNA/mL during the acute illness to a stable level many orders of magnitude lower called the viral setpoint. It is known that higher setpoints of viral load and lower T-cell counts are loosely predictive of shorter periods of clinical latency.[16] Eventually, a prolonged period of homeostasis between the virus and the immune system collapses and AIDS ensues.

Chronic immune activation and progression to AIDS

After the acute stage, HIV infection induces a high degree of proliferation and turnover of CD4 and CD8 T cells. The massive immune activation can be explained by the circulation of many soluble factors, including Toll-like receptor (TLR) ligands. HIV infection appears to activate plasmacytoid dendritic cells by stimulation of TLR7 to secrete IFN-α and proinflammatory cytokines,[17] and use both TLR8 and DC-SIGN to infect these cells.[18] In turn, stimulated dendritic cells activate T cells, which are also being directly activated through TLR ligands. Bacterial products from the mucosa[19] and HIV protein products like Nef, Env, Vif, etc., are mediators of this immune activation. Other microbial infections, viral, bacterial or fungal, can stimulate the different TLRs and result in CD4 and CD8 T-cell activation and apoptosis.[20] This rampant immune activation is thought to lead to the eventual collapse of the immune system.

Anti-HIV cellular immunity

Studies in macaque primates have shown that when CD8 T cells are depleted, animals experience increased viral loads and rapid clinical progression toward SAIDS.[21] In HIV-infected humans, the initial control of viremia occurs with the initial expansion of HIV-specific CD8 T cells.[11] The importance of anti-HIV cytotoxic T cells is suggested by the development of viral escape mutations that are driven by immune selection pressure and evade the immunological response.[22,23] In addition to their cytotoxicity, CD8 T cells secrete chemokines such as RANTES and MIP-1β that inhibit viral entry via CCR5, and IFN-γ, that activates immune cells and increases HLA expression. Recent reports suggest that non-cytotoxic mechanisms are perhaps the major anti-HIV activity of CD8 T cells.[24,25] Though severely reduced in number, IFN-γ-secreting HIV-specific CD4 T cells are present in HIV-infected individuals.[26] The role of adaptive cellular immunity in protection against natural infection is currently challenged, since about 40–60% of non-infected but exposed individuals do not present with detectable anti-HIV responses.[27]

Mechanisms of T-cell depletion

Three major mechanisms of T-cell depletion have been reported: direct lytic infection, apoptosis and autophagy.

Apoptosis

Increased apoptosis of T cells in HIV infection was described early in the epidemic. Several explanations have been offered:

(1) HIV-induced apoptosis of infected cells (viral cytopathic effect);
(2) A bystander effect from HIV-infected neighbor cells releasing viral proteins;
(3) Death of HIV-specific effectors following their migration to infected sites;
(4) Perturbation of proapoptotic signaling molecules on immune cells secondary to the chronic immune activation; and
(5) Destruction of HIV-infected cells by immune effectors.[28]

Late HIV infection is associated with the dominance of a syncytia-inducing form of the virus. Syncytia formation (clustering of CD4 T cells and membrane fusion) occurs through the interaction of HIV Env and CD4/CXCR4 on neighboring cells.

These cells are more prone to undergo apoptosis through a Fas-dependent pathway. Most of the HIV proteins have been implicated at one time or another in HIV-induced apoptosis.

Autophagy

Autophagy is a process by which cytoplasm and organelles are sequestered and directed toward lysosomal pathways. This process has been implicated in both preventing and inducing apoptosis, reflecting common regulating factors shared by both, e.g., TNF-related apoptosis-inducing-ligand (TRAIL), FADD, DAPk, ceramide, and Bcl-2.[29] HIV Env has been shown to be a stimulus for autophagy in uninfected CD4 T cells via its interaction with CXCR4.[30] Inhibition of the autophagic pathway prevented Env-induced cell death in uninfected cells *in vitro* and demonstrates that this mechanism contributes to the loss of uninfected cells.

Anti-HIV humoral immunity

After establishment of HIV infection, neutralizing antibodies are produced; however, the virus quickly mutates to avoid them, such that the host continues to respond to evolving viral mutants. The fact that antibodies can be effective in protecting hosts from HIV infection has been demonstrated in macaques and in a humanized mouse model of HIV infection.

Innate immunity

Innate immunity mechanisms are characterized by their lack of antigen specificity and include epithelial barriers, the complement system, phagocytes and antigen presenting cells. Their role in HIV pathogenesis is complex as their function is of most importance during acute infection, but their contribution to immune activation may be deleterious in the chronic stage. Studies including individuals exposed to HIV who do not develop infection suggest that an increased innate immune response generated in the mucosal microenvironment may explain the failure to develop a specific anti-HIV response.[31]

NK cells in HIV infection

NK cells are dramatically altered in HIV infection.[32] A small subset of NK cells has been found to express both CD4 and CCR5 or CXCR4. These NK cells can be infected by HIV and may serve as one of the sites of latent infection or can be activated and contribute with the state of immune chronic activation. CCR5 and inhibitory receptor expression are higher on NK cells in HIV-infected patients than in HIV seronegative subjects. In contrast, there is reduced expression of surface receptors on NK cells, that induce cytotoxic activity, such as NK-cell protein 30 (NKp30), NKp44, and NKp46. Antibody-dependent cell-mediated cytotoxicity (ADCC) is reduced in HIV-infected patients, as well as the NK-cell responsiveness to IL-2. The expression of HLA-C-specific inhibitory NK-cell receptors has been found to be increased in HIV patients. Interestingly, studies of Vietnamese seronegative but HIV-exposed intravenous drug users (IDUs) showed that their NK cells not only secreted greater quantities of chemokines than controls, but they also had greater direct cytotoxicity. Genetic studies suggest that inheritance of particular killer inhibitor receptor (KIR) alleles with their HLA ligands delays disease progression.[33] The two subsets of dendritic cells, myeloid and plasmacytoid, play an additional role in HIV infection by stimulating innate immune responses such as the type-I interferons against HIV via plasmacytoid dendritic cells. Dendritic cells may have opposing roles, with myeloid dendritic cells acting as reservoirs and favoring HIV dissemination while plasmacytoid dendritic cells inhibit HIV replication by cytokine secretion. In fact, low levels of plasmacytoid dendritic cells correlate with high viral loads, low CD4 T-cell counts, opportunistic infections, and disease progression.

Cytokines in HIV infection

The dysregulation of the immune system produced by HIV infection includes significant perturbation in the balance of T-cell helper 1 (Th1) and Th2 cytokine levels. The Th1 cytokines IL-2, TNF-α, IFN-γ, and IL-12 decrease during HIV infection, while the Th2 cytokines, IL-10 and -4, increase or remain normal. In addition, levels of proinflammatory cytokines such as IL-1, -6, and -8 also increase.[34] Viral replication in HIV-infected T cells and monocytes is induced by IL-2, -7, and -15, and by pro-inflammatory cytokines. These cytokines appear to induce viral replication by activating the host cell, a requirement for HIV productive replication. Some cytokines, such as IL-10, decrease HIV production, likely by inhibiting the synthesis of the activating cytokines, and by decreasing the expression of CCR5 and other chemokine receptors. In addition, the HIV LTR promoter contains sequences that bind cellular factors that are activated as a response to cytokine binding, such as NF-κB and AP1. IFN-α and -β have activity against HIV, although their role of these cytokines *in vivo* is not well established and may have only an adjuvant effect.[35] Their activity might favor HIV infection, as shown by the upregulation of CCR5 by IFN-α, which can facilitate viral entry.[36] Chemokines inhibit HIV infection by competing viral binding sites. The α-chemokine SDF-1 competes with lymphotropic HIV strains for binding to CXCR4, while the β-chemokines MIP1-α, MIP1-β, and RANTES compete with macrophage-tropic strains for binding to CCR5.

Clinical features

Acute HIV infection

Untreated, the natural history of HIV infection involves the progression through four clinical phases: acute retroviral syndrome, asymptomatic or latent infection, symptomatic HIV infection and finally AIDS. Each clinical phase correlates with specific events in the interaction between HIV and the host immune system. A small percentage of patients become long-term non-progressors, and an even smaller percentage become elite controllers (see below).

Soon after infection, unopposed by effective host immune responses, HIV rapidly replicates and disseminates to lymphoid tissues (see Immunopathogenesis: Gastrointestinal system) and to the systemic circulation with viremia reaching as high as 10 million copies per milliliter. Plasma viremia typically peaks three to four weeks after transmission then, due to the depletion of susceptible CD4 T cells and HIV-specific immune responses, the virus load precipitously declines, followed by more gradual decline for several weeks before reaching the set point.

Clinically the acute phase of HIV infection is manifested by a flu-like illness, the acute retroviral syndrome.[37] Two to 4 weeks after transmission, coinciding with the period of high plasma viremia and dissemination of virus to lymphoid organs, the majority of infected individuals experience a nonspecific infectious mononucleosis-like illness that lasts from a few days to several weeks. As the host develops HIV-specific immunity, the virus load decreases, CD4 and CD8 T cells recover, and the symptoms of the acute infection resolve. Although up to 90% of patients seek medical care for this illness, the nonspecific nature of the symptoms makes diagnosis of acute infection difficult and most newly infected individuals are not diagnosed until much later. The public health implications of the acute HIV infection are enormous because the risk of transmission from individuals with acute infection appears to be much higher than from those with established infection, in part because of the high viral load.

● CLINICAL PEARLS

Acute infection as an opportunity for early HIV diagnosis

- Acute HIV infection is a non-specific viral syndrome, often described as being similar to infectious mononucleosis.
- Many patients present to a clinician at this stage, but most are not recognized as HIV infection.
- Irreparable damage to the host immune system occurs during this stage of HIV infection resulting in chronic immune activation and the eventual collapse of the immune system.
- HIV viral latency is established during the acute infection as HIV DNA integrates with the host genome resulting. Integrated viral genetic material makes cure of HIV impossible even after prolonged viral suppression with highly active antiretroviral therapy (HAART).
- HAART initiated during the acute infection can halt the destruction of the body's memory T cells in the GALT and lead to better long-term outcomes for the patient.
- The practical importance of early therapy of acute infection remains in question because patients who are able to achieve and maintain undetectable viral loads on antiretroviral therapy do well, despite having commenced treatment long after their acute infection.

Asymptomatic HIV infection

The acute infection is followed by a prolonged asymptomatic or latent period that may last 8–10 years in adults, but is much shorter in children. During this time, the HIV viral load fluctuates around a relatively stable setpoint. The viral setpoint is a major determinant of infectivity and risk of disease progression with higher viral loads being more likely associated with viral transmission, more rapid disease progression and greater risk of death. The host immune response is insufficient to eradicate the infection but is enough to contain viral replication for many years. While commonly thought to represent a stalemate between viral replication and CD4 T-cell production, this period is actually characterized by a steady and inexorable decline of CD4 T cells (50–75 cells per year).

Symptomatic HIV infection (pre-AIDS syndrome)

As the infection progresses, most individuals develop clinical symptoms. The ability of the immune system to contain viral replication is overcome and the viral load begins to increase. There is usually an inflection point in the CD4 T-cell curve marking the start of a period of more rapid decline in CD4 T-cell counts. As these counts fall, immunodeficiency, symptomatic disease and AIDS eventually occur (Fig. 37.7).

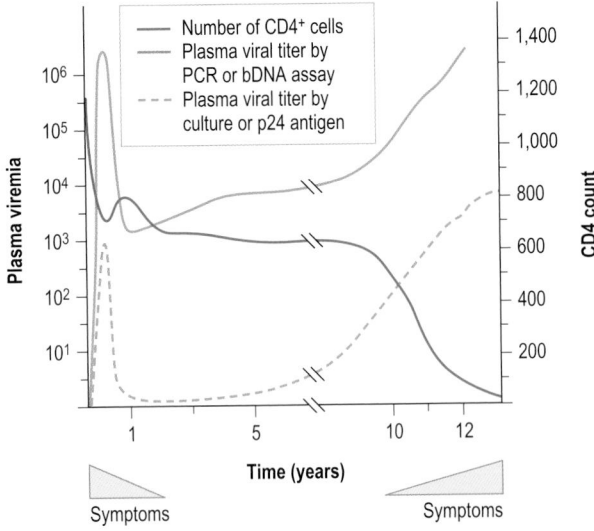

Fig. 37.7 Natural course of HIV infection. The relationship between CD4 T-cell counts and viral loads over the course of infection in the absence of treatment. From Baliga CS, Shearer WT. HIV/AIDS. In: Fireman P, ed. Atlas of allergy. Philadelphia: Elsevier Science (USA), 3rd edn, 2005: pp. 351-367.

End-stage HIV infection: AIDS

As the CD4 T-cell count drops below 200 cells/μL, the immune system's ability to fight infection is sufficiently compromised that AIDS-defining illnesses appear. Based upon the CD4 T-cell count, prophylaxis for opportunistic infections is administered (Table 37.3). Without treatment, most patients will succumb to opportunistic infections within 2 years of developing AIDS.

Long-term non-progressors/elite controllers

Some HIV-infected patients are called long-term non-progressors (LTNP) because they do not progress to AIDS after a defined period of time. One explanation for this phenomenon is the deletion of 32 nucleotides in the *CCR5* gene (*CCR5-δ32*). This deletion, postulated to have originated from selective pressure exerted by the bubonic plague, is found in people of European Caucasian ancestry. The deletion renders the CCR5 receptor non-functional, and offers protection against viral infection. Other mutations have been identified, such as the *CCR2-64I* mutation, the *SDF1-3'A* mutation, and the *RANTES-28 G* mutation, however, these mutations are found in only a minority of LTNPs.

APOBEC3G mRNA levels have been found elevated in LTNPs compared to non-infected controls and most HIV-infected patients. An explanation for the APOBEC3G findings in LTNPs is that they are infected with a defective or less fit virus. More conventional mechanisms have been proposed for LTNPs, such as strong and broad neutralizing antibody and/or cytotoxic T-cell responses. HLA-B27 and -B57 have also been correlated with LTNPs. In children, CD8 HLA-DR T-cell percentages <5% at 1–2 months of age have been implicated in predicting LTNPs.[39]

In a subset of LTNPs, circulating auto-antibodies to a conformational epitope in the extra membrane loop of CCR5 have been found that induce downregulation of the coreceptor. Interestingly, if the levels of those antibodies waned, the LTNPs were more likely to progress to symptomatic disease.[40]

A rare group of HIV infected individuals are able to control the viral load at very low levels without antiretroviral therapy. These elite controllers display high expression of the T-bet transcription factor perforin, and granzyme B.[38] Table 37.4 summarizes factors that can affect HIV progression.

Table 37.3 Opportunistic infection prophylaxis and treatment in adolescents and adults*

Risk factor	Agent	Prophylactic medication
CD4 cell count <200 cells/μL	*Pneumocystis jiroveci*	Trimethoprim sulfamethoxazole (TMP-SMX) or dapsone plus or minus pyrimethamine and leucovorin or aerosolized pentamidine or atovaquone
	Coccidioidomycosis	In endemic areas: fluconazole or Itraconazole
CD4 T cell count <100 cells/μL	*Toxoplasma gondii*	TMP-SMX or dapsone plus pyrimethamine plus leucovorin or atovaquone plus pyrimethamine plus leucovorin
	Histoplasmosis	In endemic areas: Itraconazole
CD4 T cell count <50 cells/μL	*Mycobacterium avium* complex (MAC)	Macrolide (clarithromycin or azithromycin) or rifabutin
	Cryptococcosis	In endemic areas: fluconazole or itraconazole
PPD >5 mm induration or recent TB contact but no active TB and no history of treatment for active or latent TB	*Mycobacterium tuberculosis*	INH + pyridoxine for 9 months; if unlikely to complete 9 month course and on HAART: rifabutin plus pyrizinamide for 2 months
Contact with chickenpox or shingles in varicella zoster sero-negative individuals	Varicella zoster	Varicella zoster immunoglobulins (VZIG)
HIV-infected	*Streptococcus pneumoniae* Meningococcus— for youth attending the military or college and consider For unvaccinated adults	Pneumovax Menactra
Negative anti-HBc and previously unimmunized or underimmunized to hepatitis B	Hepatitis B	Recombivax-HB or Energerix-B
Negative anti-hepatitis A serology	Hepatitis A	Havrix

*For additional information see the current US guidelines at http://AIDSinfo.nih.gov.

Table 37.4 Factors affecting HIV disease progression

Inoculum size	Higher the inoculum the faster the disease progression
Age	Infected infants have a higher risk of rapidly developing AIDS at any given CD4 percentage. This is less common in adults
Viral setpoint	The higher the viral setpoint the faster the disease progression
Broad and robust cellular and humoral immune responses	These correlate with lower setpoints, but what parts of these and which one is more important are unknown
Coreceptor mutations: δ32 CCR5, CCR2-64 I, SDF 1-3' A	Homozygotes for the δ32 CCR5 mutation fail to develop disease; heterozygotes have a much longer period of clinical latency
Th1 responses: IL-2 and IFN-γ levels Autoantibodies to CCR5 HLA-B27, -B57, -DLR	Found in subsets of LTNPs
APOBEC3G levels	Higher levels are associated with slower progression
Viral fitness	Less fit viruses are associated with slower disease progression

Diagnosis and monitoring of HIV infection

Diagnostic tests

The diagnosis of HIV infection depends upon the detection of biological markers, produced either by the virus or by the infected host, that appear in a chronology that is typically consistent between individuals. The earliest virologic markers, HIV RNA and HIV p24, can be measured 9–12 days and 14–19 days after infection respectively. The period of time between infection and detection of HIV RNA is called the "eclipse period".[42]

Enzyme immunoassays

Various generations of screening enzyme immunoassays (EIAs) are able to detect anti-HIV antibody 2–6 weeks after HIV RNA is detected. Traditionally, the period between infection and detection of HIV antibody by a particular test is referred to as the "window period" for that assay. The window period for new generation combination EIAs has been shortened to about 2 weeks because in addition to detecting antibody to both HIV-1 and -2 they also detect p24 antigen.[41]

Rapid HIV EIA tests

Rapid enzyme immunoassays are the most commonly used HIV screening tests. Rapid HIV tests are self-contained EIAs that detect HIV in whole blood or oral fluid specimens and can be used at the point of care yielding results within 30 minutes. Because results of rapid tests are available quickly, individuals can learn their results within the same encounter. In health care facilities, rapid tests have been useful when immediate results are needed to direct decisions about treatment. In labor and delivery, for example, rapid tests are performed on pregnant women with unknown serostatus to determine the need for antiretroviral (ARV) treatment to prevent mother-to-child transmission.

For both EIAs and rapid tests, a negative result is conclusive and generally requires no follow up testing. In individuals with possible recent exposure, antibody tests may be negative in the window period before seroconversion so testing should be repeated within 2–3 months. A reactive EIA or rapid test requires further testing to confirm the diagnosis. The Western blot assay identifies specific HIV antigens to which IgG antibodies in the patient's serum react and historically has been used to confirm positive screening tests results. However, because Western blots do not become diagnostically reactive until approximately 5–6 weeks after infection, nucleic acid amplification tests are now commonly used to confirm infection because they detect HIV infection well before the Western blot is positive.

Nucleic acid amplification tests

Nucleic acid amplification tests (NAAT) are used to detect HIV RNA or DNA in biological samples in order to diagnose and/or monitor HIV infection. *HIV RNA PCR is used to quantify the virus load or the extracellular viral RNA in plasma.* HIV RNA detection plays a valuable role in identifying early infection prior to seroconversion and in confirming reactive screening tests. Quantification of HIV RNA is also used to monitor the effectiveness of antiretroviral therapy in suppressing viral replication. *HIV DNA PCR is a qualitative assay used to detect HIV viral DNA in peripheral blood mononuclear cells.* Detecting HIV DNA has allowed the early diagnosis of HIV in perinatally exposed infants.

Monitoring tests

Once infection is confirmed, specific laboratory tests are performed at baseline and then periodically to monitor disease status and progression, to inform treatment decisions, and to identify end organ toxicity. The CD4 T-cell count is used to assess immune function and is the most important factor in deciding whether to initiate ARV therapy and/or prophylactic medications for opportunistic infections. Once a patient is on ARV therapy, an increasing CD4 T-cell count also helps to confirm the efficacy of antiretroviral therapy.[43] In children younger than 5 years of age, CD4 percentage is preferred because it typically remains stable in the setting of age-related changes in absolute CD4 count in this age group.[44]

HIV viral load

Particularly for patients on ARV therapy, plasma HIV RNA (viral load) is the most important indicator of response to therapy. Optimal viral suppression is generally defined as a viral load persistently below the level of detection (<20–75 copies/mL, depending on the assay used) and is usually achieved in 12–24 weeks of effective ARV treatment.[43] Failure to achieve maximal viral suppression or detectable virus after a period of maximal suppression may indicate virologic failure attributable to drug resistance.

Drug resistance: HIV genotype vs phenotype

Viral resistance to antiretroviral agents can be assessed by either HIV genotype or phenotype assays. Genotype assays, based on PCR and genomic sequencing, identify the presence of key mutations that confer anti-HIV drug resistance. Phenotype assays assess the ability of HIV to replicate *in vitro* in the presence of antiretroviral agents. The assay is performed by isolating certain key regulatory genes from HIV, usually protease and reverse transcriptase, inserting them into standardized viral constructs containing an indicator cassette, and infecting cell lines in the presence of antiretroviral agents. The results are compared against control viral isolates and expressed as a fold-change in viral susceptibility. Phenotyping assays remain very expensive and large studies have failed to conclusively prove a clinical advantage of phenotypes over genotypes. The phenotype assay quantifies susceptibility and is typically used by experts evaluating individuals who have accumulated resistence and failed multiple regimens.

Testing for viral tropism and abacavir hypersensitivity

Additional assays should be performed prior to the initiation of specific antiretroviral medications. A viral tropism assay should be performed prior to initiation of a CCR5 antagonist and HLA-B*5701 testing before initiation of abacavir (ABC).

Treatment

Antiretroviral therapy: attacking HIV's life cycle

Combinations of ARV medications are used to maximally inhibit HIV replication to reduce HIV-associated morbidity and mortality. Highly-active combination ARV therapy (HAART) refers specifically to a combination of at least three ARVs inhibiting the HIV lifecycle (Fig. 37.8). Current US guidelines recommend initiation of antiretroviral-naïve persons with a combination of two nucleoside reverse transcriptase inhibitors (NRTI) plus either a non-nucleoside reverse transcriptase inhibitor (NNRTI), a ritonavir-boosted protease inhibitor (PI), or an integrase inhibitor. In treatment-experienced patients, modification of ARV regimens and use of other classes of ARVs is guided in part by consideration of a number of factors including viral resistance patterns, potential side effects, available medication formulations, pill burden, frequency of dosing, tolerability, short and long-term adverse event profiles, desire for pregnancy and desire to preserve subsequent treatment options.[43]

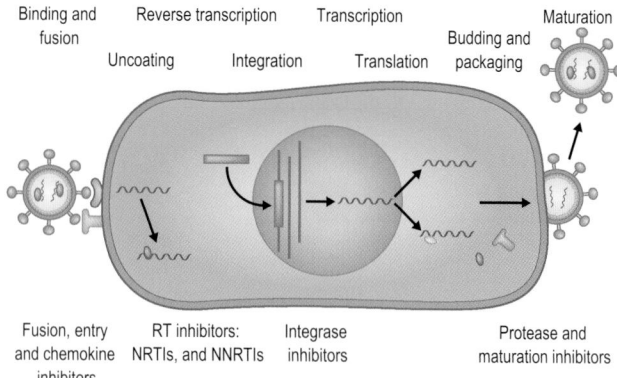

Fig. 37.8 Life cycle of HIV and the sites of action of antiretroviral agents. HIV binds to CD4 and its chemokine coreceptor (CCR5 and CXCR4). The viral particle is then uncoated and reverse transcription takes place. The viral DNA is then transported to the nucleus where it integrates with the host DNA. Through transcription and translation, the viral genome is copied for either packaging into new virions or for production of viral proteins. The genome and proteins are transported to the cell membrane where they are incorporated into budding viral particles. Following release, maturation occurs to create an infectious virion. Classes of antiretroviral agents are listed below the steps where they act.

Early vs delayed therapy: importance of CD4 T-cell count

There is still significant controversy regarding whether to initiate treatment for HIV-infected adolescents and adults early while the individual is still asymptomatic or later after there has been clinical or immunologic deterioration. US treatment guidelines[43] recommend initiating ARV therapy in all adult patients with (1) symptomatic infection, including AIDS-defining illness; (2) CD4 count <350 cell/μL; and/or (3) certain medical conditions, regardless of CD4 T-cell count, such as pregnancy, HIV-associated nephropathy, or hepatitis B or hepatitis C co-infection.

For asymptomatic adults with CD4 T-cell counts between 350 and 500 cells/μL, observational cohort studies have demonstrated benefit of treatment so ARV therapy is now recommended by many experts for individuals with CD4 cell counts ≤500 cells/μL. Decisions to start ARV therapy should be based on comorbidities, risk of disease progression, and patient willingness and ability to adhere to long-term treatment. Initiation of ARV therapy in patients with CD4 T-cell counts >500 cells/μL is optional, to be considered on a case by case basis. Earlier initiation of ARV therapy, at CD4 counts >500 cells/μL, may be associated with a survival benefit and may prevent the development of HIV-associated non-AIDS-defining illness, including malignancies and cardiovascular, renal or hepatic diseases. These advantages should be weighed against such factors as cost, drug-related complications, nonadherence to lifelong therapy in asymptomatic patients and the potential for developing drug resistance.[43]

Stratification of treatment by age of patients

Recommendations for initiating therapy have been relatively more aggressive in children when compared to adolescents and adults because most infected children were infected perinatally, and experience rapid disease progression.[45] As for adults, the risk of disease progression in children is inversely related to CD4 count or percentage; however, the risk of disease progression associated with a specific CD4 count varies with the age of the child. Infants <12 months of age experience higher risks of progression or death than older children for any given CD4 count, whereas those risks in children age 5 years or older are more similar to those of adolescents and adults. Thus, current pediatric treatment guidelines distinguish between infants less than 12 months of age, children between 1 and 5 years, and older children. ARV therapy is recommended for all infants <12 months of age regardless of clinical status, CD4 percentage or viral load. Early initiation of children perinatally infected with HIV has been shown to be most beneficial with initiation of ARV therapy in children before rather than after the age of 3 months being associated with a 75% reduction in mortality.[45]

In children one year of age or older, ARV therapy is recommended for any child with clinical signs or symptoms of advanced HIV disease regardless of CD4 absolute count or percentage or virus load. For children with no or mild symptoms, ARV therapy is initiated when they meet age-related CD4 thresholds, have high HIV viral loads and/or are affected by specific clinical conditions.[46]

Antiretroviral agents

There are more than twenty approved antiretroviral drugs that are classified into six classes based upon their chemical structure or the viral lifecycle step that they inhibit. The classes of antiretroviral agents currently available include NRTIs, NNRTIs, protease inhibitors (PIs), fusion inhibitors, integrase inhibitors and CCR5 antagonists (Table 37.5).

Reverse transcriptase inhibitors, protease inhibitors and integrase inhibitors

Modified versions of cellular nucleosides, NRTIs, once triphosphorylated *in vivo*, are incorporated into the proviral DNA by HIV reverse transcriptase and induce premature chain termination, thereby inhibiting successful conversion of the viral RNA to DNA. NNRTIs bind to RT and induce a conformational change such that RT is unable to bind with nucleotides. PIs act on viral protease, preventing the cleaving of the posttranslational viral polyproteins necessary for maturation and infectivity of viral particles. Integrase inhibitors prevent strand transfer of viral DNA and thus block the incorporation of the completed HIV DNA copy into the host cell DNA.

Fusion inhibitors, CCR5 blockers, and small molecular weight inhibitors

Fusion inhibitors and CCR5 antagonists inhibit HIV entry into host cells. Fusion inhibitors bind to viral gp41 and block the conformational changes necessary to induce fusion of the viral particle with the host cell. CCR5 antagonists bind to the CCR5 chemokine coreceptor on host cells, induce a conformational

Table 37.5 FDA-approved antiretroviral agents*

Generic name	Abbreviation	Brand name	Generic name	Abbreviation	Brand name
Nucleoside reverse transcriptase inhibitors (NRTIs)			**Non-nucleoside reverse transcriptase inhibitors (NNRTIs)**		
Zidovudine	AZT, ZDV	Retrovir	Nevirapine	NVP	Viramune
Didanosine	ddl	Videx	Delavirdine	DLV	Rescriptor
Stavudine	d4T	Zerit	Efavirenz	EFV	Sustiva
Lamivudine	3TC	Epivir	Etravarine	ETR	Intelence
Abacavir	ABC	Ziagen	Rilpivirine	RPV	Edurant
Tenofovir DF	TDF	Viread	**Protease inhibitors (PIs)**		
Emtricitabine	FTC	Emtriva	Saquinavir	SQV, hgc SQV, sgc	Invirase Fortovase
Integrase inhibitor			Ritonavir	RTV	Norvir
Raltegravir	RAL	Isentress	Indinavir	IDV	Crixivan
CCR5 antagonist			Nelfinavir	NFV	Viracept
Maraviroc	MVC	Selzentry			
Fusion inhibitor			Amprenavir	APV	Agenerase
Enfuvirtide	T-20	Fuzeon	Atazanavir	ATV	Reyataz
Combination pills			Tipranavir	TPV	Aptivus
Efavirenz tenofovir DF and emtricitabine		Atripla	Darunavir	DRV	Prezista
Zidovudine and lamivudine		Combivir	Fosamprenavir	FPV	Lexiva
Abacavir and lamivudine Zidovudine, lamivudine and abacavir Tenofovir DF and Emtricitabine Efavirenz Tenofovir DF Rilpivirine		Epzicom Trizivir Truvada Complera	Lopinavir and ritonavir	LPV/r	Kaletra

*For additional information see the current US guidelines at http://AIDSinfo.nih.gov.

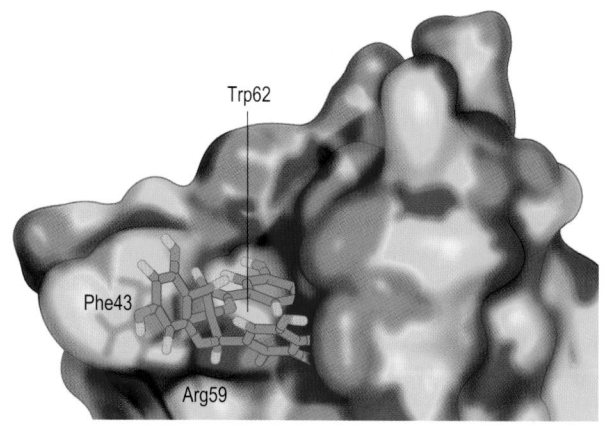

Fig. 37.9 Epigallocatechin gallate (EGCG) binding to CD4. Recent studies indicate that polyphenolic EGCG, a component of green tea, can bind to the HIV binding site of CD4 (KD = 10nM as measured by nuclear magnetic spectroscopy) and potentially interfere with viral infection by interaction with 3 key amino acids in the D1 domain of the CD4 molecule (tryptophane 62, phenylalanine 43 , and arginine 59).
From Williamson MP, McCormick TG, Nance CL, et al. Epigallocatechin gallate, the main polyphenol in green tea, binds to the T-cell receptor, CD4: Potential for HIV-1 therapy. J Allergy Clin Immunol 2006; 118: 1369-1374.

change that impedes CCR5 interaction with HIV gp120, thereby preventing HIV entry into host cells.

Small molecular weight inhibitors of HIV binding to the CD4 molecule are a new approach. Epigallocatechin gallate (EGCG), by blocking gp120 binding to the CD4 molecule, has been shown to inhibit the infections of CD4 T cells in culture by wild type viruses, setting the stage for a Phase I/II study in humans (Fig. 37.9).[47]

Immunoreconstitution after therapy

Return of T cells: memory then naïve

To varying degrees, the immune system is able to recover following initiation of therapy, a process called immunoreconstitution.[45] Upon starting HAART in patients who are compliant and able to tolerate the regimen, the initial CD4 T-cell count is the best predictor of a successful outcome. Rapid reduction in the viral load, often to undetectable, is one of the earliest changes following initiation of HAART, reflecting the ability of combination ARV therapy to rapidly suppress viral replication. Lagging behind the drop in viral load is the rise in CD4 T-cell values. An initial increase in circulating cells occurs in 3–6 months as a result of a decrease in immune activation and subsequent migration of memory T cells (CD4[+], CD45RO[+]) out of the lymphoid compartment. A more gradual rise in total CD4 T cells occurs over the course of three to five years with the appearance of new naïve (CD4[+], CD45RA[+], CD62L[+]) and memory T cells. Interestingly, a substantial minority of patients never reach a normal level of CD4 T cells, but instead reach a plateau at lower levels. Primary and some secondary drug prophylaxis for opportunistic infections may be discontinued in patients once the CD4 T-cell count is >200 cells/mm[3] for more than 3–6 months. Cellular and humoral responses to most pathogens also recover with rising CD4 T-cell counts. Of interest, a low CD4 T-cell count at the time of initiating HAART predicts a poor response to bacterial vaccines even after recovery of CD4 T-cell levels, suggesting a lag in the return of naïve CD4 T cells.

Immunoreconstitution inflammatory syndrome (IRIS)

- IRIS is typically found 2 to 3 weeks after initiating HAART.
- Patients often become profoundly ill and require hospitalization.
- Steroids are sometimes useful in the treatment.
- Clinicians may prevent IRIS by initiating HAART only after treating opportunistic infections.

Immune reconstitution inflammatory syndrome

Immune reconstitution inflammatory syndrome (IRIS) is a well known, if incompletely understood, response in AIDS patients after initiating antiretroviral therapy. IRIS is characterized by an acute paradoxical worsening of inflammatory symptoms of treated opportunistic infections or the unmasking of previously subclinical, untreated infections related to the recovery of immune responses to opportunistic pathogens. IRIS occurs within weeks of ART initiation as the memory and effector antigen-activated CD4 T-cell population recovers. A recent systematic review found that IRIS developed in 13% of patients initiating ART.[48] The most predictive risk factor for the development of IRIS was a low CD4 T-cell count at the start of ART, with the incidence of IRIS increasing exponentially as the CD4 T-cell count declined. IRIS develops more commonly in patients with cytomegalovirus retinitis, cryptococcal meningitis, progressive multifocal leukoencephalopathy and tuberculosis. As many as 4% of patients with IRIS died, but the proportion was much higher if the syndrome was associated with cryptococcal meningitis.[49]

Hyperallergenic state associated with immunoreconstitution

Another complication possibly associated with IRIS is the appearance of asthma and atopic dermatitis in perinatally HIV infected children, who received combination anti-retroviral therapies since infancy.[50] This condition may be mediated by CD4 T-cell activation, release of Th2-type cytokines, and loss of T regulatory cells and tolerance. In support of this concept, Gingo et al.[51] recorded at least a 20% prevalence of asthma in HIV-infected adults as compared to that of 8.8% in the general population.

Prevention

Prevention of mother-to-child transmission

More than 90% of children living with HIV worldwide were infected through mother-to-child transmission during pregnancy, around the time of birth or through breastfeeding. Efforts to PMTCT hold the most promise in reducing the number of children infected with HIV. These interventions include:

(1) Early identification of HIV infection in pregnant women through routine antenatal testing;
(2) Provision of antiretroviral medications to both the pregnant woman and her infant;
(3) Delivery by elective cesarean section when indicated;

(4) The complete avoidance of breastfeeding when safe and sustainable alternatives exist;

(5) The widespread availability of educational programs addressing HIV infection;

(6) Prevention of HIV perinatal transmission; and

(7) HIV counseling and testing services.[52]

Prevention of sexual transmission

Several biomedical interventions have the potential for radically changing the patterns and rates of HIV transmission. These include male circumcision, and expanded use of ART in infected individuals to prevent ongoing infection (treatment as prevention) or prophylactically in uninfected individuals either before or after potential exposure to HIV to prevent acquisition of infection (pre- and post-exposure prophylaxis).

Male medical circumcision

The penile foreskin contains HIV-susceptible cells and is a potential portal of viral entry. Randomized controlled trials in several African countries indicate that male medical circumcision reduces the risk in men of heterosexually acquiring HIV infection by 50–60%.[53] The World Health Organization recommends male circumcision as part of a comprehensive HIV prevention package; however, condom use and other prevention modalities remain important in HIV prevention. There was only a modest benefit for the female partners of the circumcised men.[54] In fact in some circumstances the risk of transmission to women by HIV infected men undergoing circumcision may be increased, perhaps through exposure to infected blood attributed to resumption of sexual activity before the circumcision site had fully healed.[55]

Pre-exposure prophylaxis

Recently, two different modalities of antiretroviral treatment have been found to decrease acquisition of HIV when used by uninfected individuals prior to their exposure to the virus as pre-exposure prophylaxis (PrEP): topically applied ARV medications and systemic ARV therapy. Topically applied ARVs have been shown to block the acquisition of HIV in women from their HIV infected partners by 35–54%. The Centre for the AIDS Program of Research in South Africa (CAPRISA 004) trial was the first double-blind, randomized controlled trial demonstrating efficacy of vaginally inserted gel containing the antiretroviral medication tenofovir disoproxil fumarate, when compared to a placebo gel in preventing HIV transmission from HIV-infected men to their uninfected partners.[56] Vaginal pre-exposure prophylaxis represents a promising intervention for preventing heterosexual transmission of HIV to women. This method may be particularly effective because women are able to initiate and control its use to protect themselves from infection.

Prophylactic ARV therapy

ARVs taken prophylactically have also been shown to be effective in reducing the transmission of HIV both in MSM and in heterosexual individuals and couples. The multinational Preexposure Prophylaxis Initiative (iPrEx) trial demonstrated that daily oral combination therapy emtricitabine and tenofovir disoproxil fumarate (FTC-TDF) reduced the incidence of HIV among MSM by 44% when compared to placebo.[57] Daily oral FTC-TDF was also shown to reduce HIV incidence among heterosexual individuals by 63–78%; and by 73% among heterosexual discordant couples. Despite these successful trials, preliminary results of one PrEP trial have failed to show similar efficacy for preventing HIV acquisition among heterosexual women.[58]

Expanded treatment with ARV therapy

The expanded use of ARV therapy in infected individuals has been shown to reduce HIV transmission to uninfected partners. Both "Treatment as Prevention" and "Test and Treat" strategies involve the use of ARV therapy in individuals who do not otherwise meet criteria for ARV therapy initiation with the express purpose of reducing transmission to others. In both approaches HAART is initiated regardless of CD4 count or viral load, in order to reduce the viral load in the genital secretions of the infected partner to thereby reduce HIV transmission to uninfected partners. The efficacy of the Treatment as Prevention model is demonstrated in the multinational HIV Prevention Trials Network (HPTN) 052 clinical trial that examined the effectiveness of ART to prevent the sexual transmission of HIV in serodiscordant couples. Serodiscordant couples (1763 in number) were randomly assigned to have the infected partner either start ART immediately upon enrollment or to defer ART until immunologic or clinical criteria were met. Of 28 genetically linked infections that occurred during the trial, only 1 infection occurred in couples assigned to receive immediate treatment, representing a 96% reduction in the risk of HIV transmission. There were also fewer morbidity and mortality events in the early treatment group suggesting a therapeutic benefit from early treatment as well.[59]

The fundamental paradigm for Test and Treat programs is the same as that in Treatment as Prevention. Test and Treat, however, emphasizes the need for universal voluntary routine HIV testing and initiating ART immediately in those found to be positive regardless of CD4 count or viral load. Although the approach remains controversial, with concerns regarding drug resistance, increased sexual risk taking in treated individuals, and societal cost-effectiveness, this approach may over time prove to be an effective prevention modality.

Preventive vaccines

A highly preventive vaccine that induces sterilizing antibody at all routes of entry of HIV (i.e., mucosal, blood) has been a 30-year quest of researchers the world over (Chapter 90).[60] The production of an effective HIV vaccine has been thwarted by the extreme rate of mutation in the virion and the sequestration of the virus in impenetrable reservoirs, predominantly the non-replicating CD4 T cell. More than 30 HIV vaccines have been tested in human trials, including those with recombinant env gp120 proteins with adjuvants, HIV DNA plasmids, viral vectors, and prime-boost designs.[61] These vaccines have for the most part yielded disappointing results. Phase III trials of VAX003 in Thailand (AIDSVAX B/E plus alum) and VAX004 in North America and Europe (AIDSVAX B/E plus alum) showed no protection against HIV infection. Naked HIV DNA with cytokines IL-15, IL-12, and chemokine receptor 005 with and without electroporation has not been effective. Pox virus HIV vaccines in the step trial of North and South American and the Phambili trial in South Africa (Ad5-HIV trivalent vaccine) were ineffective in stopping HIV entry or post-infection viremia.[62,63] However, the phase III trial RV144 in Thailand (ALVAC-HIV vCP1521+AIDSVAX gp120 B/E) showed possible protection against HIV infection in heterosexual men and women.[64]

In addition to the goal of developing an HIV vaccine that elicits neutralizing antibodies, the search for a vaccine that stimulates a protective CD8 cytotoxic T-cell response continues. Animal model studies with SIV demonstrate that the cytotoxic T cell has an essential role in limiting the concentrations of virus during acute infection and creates viral escape variants with reduced viral fitness.[65] Association of certain MHC molecules with HIV disease progression is clearly linked to the cytotoxic T-cell responses. Unfortunately the HIV vaccine-induced cytotoxic CD8 T-cell response is insufficient to halt acute or chronic HIV disease progression. This was clearly indicated in the STEP clinical trial in which the CD8 T-cell effects were the same between HIV-infected vaccinees and sham HIV-infected vaccinee controls.[63] Qualities of effector and central memory CD8 T cells that would be protective include: (1) production of cytotoxic cytokines (e.g., IFN-γ and IL-2), (2) rapidly replicating capacity, (3) cytotoxic potential, (4) high affinity for HIV antigens, (5) inhibition of HIV replication, (6) recognition of specific HIV epitopes restricted by protective HLA-B antigens, (7) central memory cells with long life spans, and (8) rapid attack memory cells at mucosal HIV entry sites.

Therapeutic vaccines

A therapeutic vaccine is one in which the vaccine is used after infection occurs, aiming to induce anti-viral immunity to alter the course of disease. This would be accomplished by controlling viremia or reducing the viral setpoint in infected patients. Primate models suggest that just such a result is possible, especially with cellular immunity-inducing vaccines. To date, however, data from human studies show no conclusive benefit from using therapeutic vaccines alone. Using a therapeutic vaccine in combination with HAART is another approach currently under investigation.

A small study of a therapeutic vaccine in 25 HIV-infected individuals produced a 1 $\log_{10}$ reduction in viral load as compared to placebo-treated HIV-infected individuals.[66] However, HIV disease progression was not seen with this therapeutic vaccine in limited follow-up, indicating the need for longer follow-up and larger clinical trials before any measure of success can be claimed.

Future for HIV vaccines

The general pessimism that prevailed in the scientific community after the failure of the STEP vaccine trial is gradually being replaced by a cautious optimism with limited success of the RV144 clinical trial in Thailand. Also, there is general belief that more basic research exploring vaccine design and trials in animals will lead to important clues for human study. Understanding the immune correlates of vaccine efficacy is an absolute requirement judging the success of an HIV vaccine.

● ON THE HORIZON

- Production of newer antiretroviral drugs, including those used for post-exposure prophylaxis with greater specificity for interrupting events in the viral lifecycle and with fewer side effects for patients.
- Investigation of new microbicidal drugs that can be safely applied prior to exposure for protection against HIV virus transfer.
- Development of preventive and therapeutic vaccines for HIV/AIDS that induce strong viral neutralizing antibody power and strong CD8 T cell cytotoxic responses.
- Testing of gene construct-modified autologous hematopoietic stem cells capable of halting HIV replication.

Translational research needs and conclusions

The quest for better ARV therapeutic agents continues, with the goal of greater selectivity and fewer side effects. However, the eradication of HIV/AIDS can only practically be approached with a preventive vaccine that elicits strong HIV-neutralizing ability and generates a strong cytotoxic CD8 T-cell response specific for HIV antigens. The approach to cure with gene therapy is perhaps the most sophisticated translational research venture. Using viral vectors to place gene constructs within nuclear DNA that prevent HIV replication is the goal of such research. Arguably, the most advanced form of this genetic engineering to halt HIV replication is the zinc finger endonuclease approach to disrupt specific genes necessary for the life cycle of HIV.[67] Adoptive transfer of antologous zinc finger-treated stem cells with infinite replication capacity may be an attractive future for patients already infected with HIV. The extraordinary experiment of HLA-matched and CCR5-δ35 deletion of hematopoietic stem cell immunoreconstitution of an HIV-infected patient (Berlin Man) is a proof of concept of molecular and genetic engineering to cure HIV infection, a technique totally impractical to the millions of HIV-infected patients worldwide.[68] Nevertheless, this "once in a million" chance experiment has demonstrated survival advantage of lymphocytes that cannot become infected with HIV.[64]

The human immunodeficiency retrovirus Type-1 contains but 9 genes, but those 9 genes have so far thwarted all scientific efforts for a cure of its infection in man. Optimism is warranted, however, because of the enormous knowledge base the study of HIV has produced in understanding the many arms of innate and adaptive immunity that protects humans and the promise of a curative treatment or vaccine for HIV. The HIV/AIDS pandemic has also brought the sobering realization that other new and potentially deadly pathogens may yet emerge to strike at man. Perhaps in no other disease has so much been learned so fast. In the developed world, HIV causes chronic infection rather than certain death, thanks in large part to the use of antiviral drugs. More novel drugs are in development due to newfound understanding of the molecular biology behind HIV. For virologists and immunologists, HIV continues to perplex and fascinate; for clinicians it continues to teach humility.

Acknowledgments

Supported in part by NIH Grants AI06944, HD052102, AI007456 AI36211, AI082978, and RR0188 and the Pediatric AIDS Fund of Texas Children's Hospital.

References

1. Joint United Nations Programme on HIV/AIDS (UNAIDS) . Global report: UNAIDS report on the global AIDS epidemic 2010.
2. Centers for Disease Control and Prevention. HIV surveillance—United States, 1981–2008. MMWR Morb Mortal Wkly Rep 2011;60:689–93.
3. Centers for Disease Control and Prevention. HIV surveillance report 2011;21.
4. Hemelaar J, Gouws E, Ghys P, Osmanov S. WHO-UNAIDS. Network for HIV Isolation and Characterisation. Global trends in molecular epidemiology of HIV during 2000–2007. AIDS 2011;25:679–89.
5. Narayan V, Ravindra KC, Chiaro C, et al. Celastrol inhibits Tat-mediated human immunodeficiency virus (HIV) transcription and replication. J Mol Biol 2011;410:972–83.
6. Grewe B, Überla K. The human immunodeficiency virus type 1 Rev protein: ménage à trois during the early phase of the lentiviral replication cycle. J Gen Virol 2010;91:1893–7.
7. Poropatich K, Sullivan Jr DJ. Human immunodeficiency virus type 1 long-term non-progressors: the viral, genetic and immunological basis for disease non-progression. J Gen Virol 2011;92:247–68.

8. Chiu Y-L, Greene WC. The APOBEC3 cytidine deaminases: An innate defensive network opposing exogenous retroviruses and endogenous retroelements. Annu Rev Immunol 2008;26:317–53.
9. Binette J, Cohen E. Recent advances in the understanding of HIV-1 Vpu accessory protein functions. Curr Drug Targets Immune Endocr Metabol Disord 2004;4:297–307.
10. McMichael AJ, Borrow P, Tamaras GD, et al. The immune response during acute HIV-1 infection: clues for vaccine development. Nat Rev Immunol 2010;10:11–23.
11. Koup RA, Safrit JT, Cao Y, et al. Temporal association of cellular immune responses with the initial control of viremia in primary human immunodeficiency virus type 1 syndrome. J Virol 1994;68:4650–5.
12. Cadogan M, Dalgleish AG. HIV immunopathogenesis and strategies for intervention. Lancet Infect Dis 2008;8:675–84.
13. Salazar-Gonzalez JF, Salazar MG, Keele BF, et al. Genetic identity, biological phenotype and evolutionary pathways of transmitted/founder viruses in acute and early HIV-1 infection. J Exp Med 2009;206:1273–89.
14. Dinosco JB, Kim SY, Wiegand AM, et al. Treatment intensification does not reduce residual HIV-1 viremia in patients on highly active antiretroviral therapy. Proc Natl Acad Sci U S A 2009;106:9403–8.
15. Brenchley JM, Price DA, Douek DC. HIV disease: fallout from a mucosal catastrophe? Nat Immunol 2006;7:235–9.
16. Ganesan A, Chattopadhyay P, Brodie T, et al. Immunologic and virologic events in early HIV infection predict subsequent rate of progression. J Infect Dis 2010;201:271–84.
17. Meier A, Alter G, Frahm N, et al. MyD88-dependent immune activation mediated by human immunodefieciency virus type 1-encoded toll-like receptor ligands. J Virol 2007;81:8180–91.
18. Gringhius SI, van der Vlist M, van den Berg LM, et al. HIV-1 exploits innate signaling by TLR8 and DC-SIGN for productive infection of dentritic cells. Nat Immunol 2010; II:419–28.
19. Funderburg N, Luciano AA, Jiang W, et al. Toll-like receptor ligands induce human T cell activation and death, a model for HIV pathogenesis. PLoS ONE 2008;3:e1915.
20. Jiang W, Lederman MM, Hunt P, et al. Plasma levels of bacterial DNA correlate with immune activation and the magnitude of immune restoration in persons with antiretroviral-treated hiv infection. J Infect Dis 2009;199:1177–85.
21. Matano T, Shibata R, Siemon C, et al. Administration of an anti-CD8 monoclonal antibody interferes with the clearance of chimeric simian/human immunodeficiency virus during primary infections of rhesus macaques. J Virol 1998;72:164–9.
22. Borrow P, Lewicki H, Wei X, et al. Antiviral pressure exerted by HIV-1-specific cytotoxic T lymphocytes (CTLs) during primary infection demonstrated by rapid selection of CTL escape virus. Nat Med 1997;3:205–11.
23. Goulder PJR, Phillips RE, Colbert RA, et al. Late escape from an immunodominant cytotoxic T-lymphocyte response associated with progression to AIDS. Nat Med 1997;3:212–7.
24. Killian MS, Johnson C, Teque F, et al. Natural suppression of human immunodeficiency virus Type 1 replication is mediated by transitional memory CD8+ T Cells. J Virol 2011;85:1696–705.
25. Wong JK, Strain MC, Porrata R, et al. In vivo CD8+ T-Cell suppression of SIV viremia is not mediated by CTL clearance of productively infected cells. PLoS Pathog 2010;6:1–12.
26. Pantaleo G, Koup RA. Correlates of immune protection in HIV-1 infection: what we know, what we don't know, what we should know. Nat Med 2004;10:806–10.
27. Lederman MM, Alter G, Daskalakis DC, et al. Determinants of protection among HIV-exposed seronegative persons: An overview. J Infect Dis 2010;202:S333–S338.
28. Gougeon M-L. Apoptosis as an HIV strategy to escape immune attack. Nat Rev Immunol 2003;3:392–404.
29. Levine B. HIV and CXCR4 in a kiss of autophagic death. J Clin Invest 2006;116:2078–80.
30. Espert L, Denizot M, Grimaldi M, et al. Autophagy is involved in T Cell death after binding of HIV-1 envelope proteins to CXCR4. J Clin Invest 2006;116:2161–72.
31. Tomescu C, Abdulhaqq S, Montaner LJ. Evidence for the innate immune response as a correlate of protection in human immunodeficiency virus (HIV)-1 highly exposed seronegative subjects (HESN). Clin Exp Immunol 2011;164:158–69.
32. Vieillard V, Fausther-Bovendo H, Samri A, et al. Specific phenotypic and functional features of natural killer cells from HIV-Infected long-term nonprogressors and HIV controllers. J Acquir Immune Defic Syndr 2010;53:564–73.
33. Martin MP, Qi Y, Gao X, et al. Innate partnership of HLA-B and KIR3DL1 subtypes against HIV-1. Nat Genet 2007;39:733–40.
34. Clerici M, Galli M, Bosis S, et al. Immunoendrocrinologic abnormalities in human immunodeficiency virus infection. Ann N Y Acad Sci 2000;917:956–61.
35. Vendrame D, Sourisseau M, Perrin V, et al. Partial inhibition of human immunodeficiency virus replication by type I interferons: Impact of cell-to-cell viral transfer. J Virol 2009;83:10527–37.
36. Stoddart CA, Keir ME, McCune JM. IFN-α-induced upregulation of CCR5 leads to expanded hiv tropism in vivo. PLoS Pathog 2010;6:1–10.
37. Cohen MS, Shaw GM, McMichael AJ, et al. Acute HIV-1 infection. N Engl J Med 2011;364:1943–54.

38. Hersperger AR, Martin JN, Shin LY, et al. Increased HIV-specific CD8+ T-cell cytotoxic potential in HIV elite controllers is associated with T-bet expression. Blood 2011;117:3799–808.
39. Paul M, Mao C, Charurat M, et al. Predictors of immunologic long-term nonprogression in HIV-infected children: implications for initiating therapy. JAllergy Clin Immunol 2005;115:848–55.
40. Pastori C, Weiser B, Barassi C, et al. Long-lasting CCR5 internalization by antibodies in a subset of long-term nonprogressors: a possible protective effect against disease progression. Blood 2006;107:4825–33.
41. Branson BM. The future of HIV testing. J Acquir Immune Defic Syndr 2010;55:S102–S105.
42. Fiebig EW, Wright DJ, Rawal BD, et al. Dynamics of HIV viremia and antibody seroconversion in plasma donors: implications for diagnosis and staging of primary HIV infection. AIDS 2003;17:1871–9.
43. Panel on Antiretroviral Guidelines for Adults and Adolescents. Guidelines for the use of antiretroviral agents in HIV-1-infected adults and adolescents. 2011.
44. Panel on Antiretroviral Therapy and Medical Management of HIV-Infected Children. Guidelines for the use of antiretroviral agents in pediatric HIV infection. 2010.
45. Violari A, Cotton M, Gibb D, et al. Early antiretroviral therapy and mortality among HIV-infected infants. N Engl J Med 2008;359:2233–44.
46. Panel on Antiretroviral Therapy and Medical Management of HIV-Infected Children. Guidelines for the use of antiretroviral agents in pediatric HIV infection. 2011.
47. Nance CL, Siwak EB, Shearer WT. Preclinical development of the green tea catechin, epigallocatechin gallate, as an HIV-1 therapy. J Allergy Clin Immunol 2009;123:459–65.
48. Muller M, Wandel S, Colebunders R, et al. Immune reconstitution inflammatory syndrome in patients starting antiretroviral therapy for HIV infection: a systematic review and meta-analysis. Lancet Infect Dis 2010;10:251–61.
49. Murdoch DM, Venter WD, Feldman C, et al. Incidence and risk factors for the immune reconstitution inflammatory syndrome in HIV patients in South Africa: a prospective study. AIDS 2008;33:601–10.
50. Siberry GK, Leister E, Jacobson D, et al. Increased risk of asthma and atopic dermatitis in perinatally HIV-infected children and adolescents. Clin Immunol 2012;142:201–8.
51. Gingo MR, Wenzel SE, Steele C, et al. Asthma diagnosis and airway bronchodilator response in HIV-infected individuals. J Allergy Clin Immunol 2012;129:708–14.
52. Panel on Treatment of HIV-Infected Pregnant Women and Prevention of Perinatal Transmission. Recommendations for use of antiretroviral drugs in pregnant HIV-1-infected women for maternal health and interventions to reduce perinatal HIV transmission in the United States. 2010.
53. Siegfried N, Muller M, Deeks JJ, et al. Male circumcision for prevention of heterosexual acquisition of HIV in men. Cochrane Database Syst Rev 2009; CD003362.
54. Baeten JM, Donnell D, Kapiga SH, et al. Male circumcision and risk of male-to-female HIV-1 transmission: a multinational prospective study in African HIV-1-serodiscordant couples. AIDS 2010;24:737–44.
55. Wawer M, Makumbi F, Kigozi G, et al. Circumcision in HIV-infected men and its effect on HIV transmission to female partners in Rakai, Uganda: a randomised controlled trial. Lancet 2009;374:229–37.
56. Abdool KQ, Abdool KS, Frohlich JA, et al. Effectiveness and safety of tenofovir gel, an antiretroviral microbicide, for the prevention of HIV infection in women. Science 2010;329:1168–74.
57. Grant RM, Lama JR, Anderson PL, et al. Preexposure chemoprophylaxis for HIV prevention in men who have sex with men. N Engl J Med 2010;363:2597–9.
58. FHI to initiate orderly closure of FEM-PrEP 2011. Accessed at http://www.fhi.org/en/Research/Projects/FEM-PrEP.htm.
59. Cohen MS, Chen YQ, McCauley M, et al. Prevention of HIV-1 infection with early antiretroviral therapy. N Engl J Med 2011;365:493–505.
60. McElrath M, Haynes B. Induction of immunity to human immunodeficiency virus type-1 by vaccination. Immunity 2010;33:542–54.
61. Ross A, Bråve A, Scarlatti G, et al. Progress towards development of an HIV vaccine: report of the AIDS Vaccine 2009 Conference. Lancet Infect Dis 2010;10:305–16.
62. Buchbinder S, Mehrotra D, Duerr A, et al. Efficacy assessment of a cell-mediated immunity HIV-1 vaccine (the Step Study): a double-blind, randomised, placebo-controlled, test-of-concept trial. Lancet 2008;372:1881–93.
63. Gray G, Buchbinder S, Duerr A. Overview of STEP and Phambili trial results: two phase IIb test-of-concept studies investigating the efficacy of MRK adenovirus type 5 gag/pol/nef subtype B HIV vaccine. Curr Opin HIV AIDS 2010;5:357–61.
64. Rerks-Ngarm S, Pitisuttithum P, Nitayaphan S, et al. Vaccination with ALVAC and AIDSVAX to prevent HIV-1 infection in Thailand. N Engl J Med 2009;361:2209–20.
65. Goulder P, Watkins D. Impact of MHC class I diversity on immune control of immunodeficiency virus replication. Nat Rev Immunol 2008;8:619–30.
66. Johnston M, Fauci A. HIV vaccine development—improving on natural immunity. N Engl J Med 2011;365:873–5.
67. Perez EE, Wang J, Miller JC, et al. Establishment of HIV-1 resistance in CD4+ T cells by genome editing using zinc-finger nucleases. Nat Biotechnol 2008;26:808–16.
68. Hutter G, Nowak D, Mossner M, et al. Long-term control by CCR5 Delta 32/Delta 32 stem-cell transplantation. N Engl J Med 2009;360:692–8.

Javier Chinen,
William T.
Shearer

External factors inducing immune deficiency

Clinicians often care for patients with an unusually high susceptibility to infections, who are characterized by either recurrent
infectious episodes or decreased response to antimicrobial treatment. The variability of clinical presentation of infectious diseases in different patients has been largely attributed to factors
specific to the infectious agent, such as virulence of different
strains. In the past few decades, in part due to the human immunodeficiency virus (HIV) epidemics, the role of the immune system on the course of infections has been recognized. Impaired
immunity function can adversely affect the outcomes of infectious diseases and significantly increase the morbidity and
mortality. HIV is likely the most well-known cause of secondary
immunodeficiency; however, many other factors extrinsic to the
immune system, such as malnutrition, immunosuppressive
agents, surgery, and trauma are more commonly encountered
compromising the immune system (Table 38.1). These factors
also include age extremes (i.e., prematurity and old age), adverse
environments (e.g., high altitude, space travel), and genetic
anomalies. This chapter reviews common conditions of genetic
(other than primary immune deficiencies), metabolic, and environmental etiology known to impair the immune function. The
immune defects caused by these conditions are usually heterogeneous in presentation, affecting humoral and cellular immunity
with variable degrees of severity. The understanding of the
mechanisms of disease helps in the assessment and management
of patients, because correction of the primary disorder or removal
of the immunosuppressive agents, when it is feasible, often leads
to prevention or reversal of the related immune defects.

KEY CONCEPTS

- Immunodeficiency commonly occurs as the result of
  diseases or conditions extrinsic to the immune system, such
  as malnutrition.
- Correction of the primary disorder leads to prevention or
  reversal of the associated immune defects.
- Environmental conditions, when severe, may induce
  immunodeficiency by acting as stressors or by suppression
  of the production and function of immune cells.

Immunological defects associated with genetic diseases other than primary immunodeficiencies

Genetic diseases include a number of rare conditions caused by
inherited or sporadic changes in the genetic information of individuals, which range from deleterious mutations in a single gene

to deletions or duplications of several genes, including entire
chromosomes. There are several genetic syndromes that may
be associated with mild to moderate degrees of immune compromise. The pathogenesis of the immune defects in these syndromes include deficiency of proteins such as cytokines and
adhesion molecules, weakening of natural epithelial barriers
and subtle defects in cell division and DNA repair affecting lymphocyte proliferation. The management of increased susceptibility to infections in patients with genetic diseases relies on
prevention, such as promoting hygiene measures and using
antibiotic prophylaxis when necessary.

Down syndrome

Down syndrome (DS) or trisomy of chromosome 21 is a relatively common congenital defect with an incidence of 1:600 to
1:800 live births. DS patients present with hypotonia, characteristic facies, heart and gastrointestinal defects and mental retardation. Infections are common, but usually not severe, such as
periodontitis and upper respiratory tract infections. Although
the risk of frequent infections can be attributed to poor hygiene
and institutionalization, immunological abnormalities have been
reported, including absolute lymphopenia with a decreased
number of naïve T cells,[1-3] possibly secondary to premature thymus involution. Also, an impaired antibody response has been
demonstrated, which could be associated with IgG subclass deficiency in some cases. Phagocytic cells from DS patients show
decreased chemotaxis, phagocytosis and bacterial killing. Autoimmune disease occurs at a higher frequency in DS, with its most
frequent manifestation, thyroiditis, developing before 8 years of
age in about half of DS children. Mononuclear cells from DS patients have increased expression of DSCAM (Down syndrome
cellular adhesion molecule), SOD1 (superoxide dismutase 1)
and Down syndrome critical region 1 (DSCR1) proteins encoded
in genes located in chromosome 21, which could explain
impaired pathogen clearance.[4] Decreased institutionalization
and better access to medical care have reduced the risk of infection and improved the life expectancy of DS patients.

Turner syndrome

Turner syndrome (TS) results from the presence of only one
X chromosome, with the other X chromosome missing or abnormally repressed. TS patients have short stature, do not develop
into puberty, and are infertile. They present with frequent respiratory infections and develop bronchiectasis at early age. There
are no consistent immune defects in all patients. It has been

Table 38.1 Common conditions associated with secondary immunodeficiencies

	Cellular immunity	Humoral immunity
Congenital		
Down syndrome	T-cell cytopenia, decreased LPR to mitogens, thymus hypotrophy, decreased naïve T cells, defective NK-cell activity, decreased phagocytosis and chemotaxis	Decreased antibody responses to vaccines, increased autoimmune antibodies
Turner syndrome	T-cell cytopenia, anergy, decreased LPR to mitogens	Decreased serum levels of IgG and IgM
Metabolic		
Protein-calorie malnutrition	T-cell cytopenia, thymus hypotrophy, impaired cytokine secretion, decreased phagocytosis, and chemotaxis	Decreased antibody responses to vaccines, decreased serum IgG levels
Diabetes mellitus	T-cell cytopenia, decreased LPR to mitogens, decreased phagocytosis and chemotaxis	Decreased antibody responses to vaccines
Uremia	Increased T-cell apoptosis, decreased LPR to mitogens, decreased phagocytosis and chemotaxis, decreased oxidative responses.	Decreased antibody responses to vaccines, decreased serum IgG levels
Infectious diseases		
HIV infection	CD4 T-cell cytopenia, decreased LPR to mitogens and antigens, thymus hypotrophy, decreased NK-cell and phagocytic activity	Decreased antibody responses to vaccines, nonspecific increased serum IgG levels
Viral infections—measles	Impaired cell antigen presentation and cellular anergy	Decreased antibody responses to vaccines, decreased serum IgG levels
Stress		
Trauma	Lymphopenia, decreased cellular responses, decreased chemotaxis	Decreased complement activity
Surgery—splenectomy	Not reported	Decreased antibody responses, negligible to polysaccharides
Environmental conditions		
Radiation and UV light	T-cell anergy, deficient antigen presentation, immunosuppression at high doses	Defective antibody response secondary to impaired T-cell function
High altitude and chronic hypoxia	T-cell cytopenia	Decreased antibody responses to vaccines, decreased serum IgG levels
Space flight conditions	Variable lymphopenia, decreased LPR to mitogens and antigens	Variable impairment of antibody responses

LPR, lymphoproliferative response.

shown that some patients have low immunoglobulin levels[5] and decreased T-cell proliferative responses to mitogens.[6]

Sickle cell disease and cystic fibrosis

◉ CLINICAL PEARLS

- Sickle cell disease (SCD) patients present with increased susceptibility to infections by encapsulated organisms, such as S. *pneumoniae*.
- Autosplenectomy occurs in most SCD patients by 2 years of age, and is associated with decreased or absent antibody responses to polysaccharide antigens, and inefficient complement activity.
- Prevention of infections in SCD patients should include completion of routine immunizations and anti-pneumococcal antibiotic prophylaxis.

Two genetic diseases with significant prevalence in general population and with increased susceptibility to infections are sickle cell disease (SCD) and cystic fibrosis (CF). SCD is an autosomal recessive disease that affects the expression of the beta-hemoglobin protein and causes anemia. Its prevalence is highest in individuals of African background at 1/500. SCD patients have an increased susceptibility for infections from encapsulated

organisms; for example, *Streptococcus pneumoniae*-related sepsis and meningitis occurs 30-300 times more often than in normal children. Autosplenectomy occurs in most SCD patients by the second year of life as a result of microinfarcts, becoming the major reason for the increased risk of infections. Absence of the spleen is associated with impaired antibody production to polysaccharides and with impaired complement alternative pathway in SCD patients.[7] SCD patients also present with an increased frequency of osteomyelitis caused by *Salmonella* spp.; however, it is not well understood why susceptibility to this pathogen is increased. Prevention of infections in SCD patients should include anti-pneumococcal prophylaxis and routine immunizations to encapsulated organisms. Penicillin-based prophylaxis regimens reduce the incidence of pneumococcal infections by 84%.[7]

CF is an autosomal recessive disorder caused by mutations in the cystic fibrosis transmembrane conductance regulator (*CFTR*) gene. It decreases the fluidity of secretions, causing blockade of secretory tubules and affecting organs such as the pancreas, salivary glands, genital tubules, and liver canaliculi. Most significantly, the mucociliary clearance of bacteria in the lungs is impaired. CF patients present with lungs colonized with *Pseudomonas aeruginosa*, and often present with pneumonia by this pathogen and other bacteria. Several lung bactericidal factors are decreased, such as lysozymes, defensins and cathelicidins.[8] This results in the inability to clear bacterial colonization, and eventual progression to pneumonia. Adaptive immunity is intact, demonstrated by the normal production of antibodies against *P. aeruginosa,* and increasing evidence of defects in mechanisms of innate immunity.[9] CF patients experiencing recurrent pneumonias benefit from respiratory therapy to clear secretions and from antibiotic prophylaxis.

Immunological defects secondary to metabolic diseases: malnutrition, diabetes mellitus and uremia

Taking into consideration that an immune response is mediated by lymphocyte proliferation, it is not surprising that metabolic disturbances and nutrient limitations affect this response and might result in increased morbidity and mortality from infections. Severe malnutrition and other conditions affecting the adequate absorption and metabolism of nutrients such as diabetes mellitus and protein-losing enteropathy may impair the functioning of all organs, including the immune system.

Malnutrition

Malnutrition is one of the most frequent causes of secondary immunodeficiency worldwide, affecting individuals of all ages (Fig. 38.1).[10] Protein-caloric malnutrition may result from poor intake, malabsorption or excessive loss of nutrients. Individuals with protein-caloric malnutrition progressively lose their T-cell production and T-cell function, resulting in immunodeficiency with increased incidence of diarrhea and respiratory infections. These conditions are complicated with concomitant deficit of micronutrients (e.g., zinc) that augment the susceptibility to infections by inducing defects in the barrier mucosae.[11] Serum immunoglobulin levels appear to remain normal for a relative prolonged period of time, as well as the effectiveness of vaccination to elicit antibodies. Nutritional replenishment of malnourished children results in reversal of deficiencies of lymphocyte proliferation and phagocytosis, and significant recovery of thymus size as measured by ultrasonography.

Micronutrient deficiencies are more prevalent in protein-caloric malnutrition, but may also present alone, and are usually subclinical in a healthy looking child. Feeding only half the recommended intake of iron, zinc, or vitamins B, C, and E cause oxidative damage and DNA breaks, with decreased NK cell cytotoxicity and monocyte phagocytic activity (Table 38.2).[12]

Vitamin A deficiency is manifested by night blindness, dry and scaly skin, apathy, anemia, retarded growth, elevated intracranial pressure and increased infections. Deficiency of vitamin

Table 38.2 Immune defects associated with micronutrient deficiencies

Vitamin A deficiency	T-cell cytopenia, decreased DTH, decreased phagocytic and NK-cell function. Decreased antibody responses to vaccines
Vitamin C deficiency	Decreased phagocytosis and decreased intracellular oxidative responses
Vitamin E deficiency	Decreased intracellular oxidative responses, increased PGE2 secretion (inhibitor of cell immunity)
Copper deficiency	Lymphopenia, neutropenia
Iron deficiency	Lymphopenia, decreased phagocytosis
Selenium deficiency	Decreased intracellular oxidative responses
Zinc deficiency	Lymphopenia, decreased DTH, impaired mucosal barrier, decreased T-cell-dependent antibody responses
DTH, delayed-type hypersensitivity.	

A and other micronutrients leads to impaired function of mucous membranes[13] and decreased interferon (IFN)-α production. Higher immunization rates are seen when vitamin A is given with measles vaccine in malnourished children. In the past few years, the essential role of vitamin D in the modulation of the immune response has been demonstrated, with most relevance to the development of Th1-cell mediated inflammatory (cytotoxic) responses and immunity to intracellular microbes such as *Mycobacterium tuberculosis*.[14]

In contrast to protein-caloric deficiency due to other causes, malnutrition resulting from eating disorders, such as anorexia nervosa and bulimia, does not result in increased frequency of infections.[15] However, patients with these disorders show leukopenia and lymphopenia with abnormal DTH (delayed-type hypersensitivity) skin test responses to antigens. Paradoxically, infections may occur during nutritional treatment, possibly because of reactivation of latent infections.

Protein-losing enteropathy with consequent hypogammaglobulinemia can be present in most patients with intestinal inflammatory diseases; however, the ability to produce antibodies is usually preserved. Thus, the need for treatment with intravenous immunoglobulin should be carefully assessed, because correction of the primary defect may reduce the predisposition to infection without a requirement for any other intervention. A similar disorder, intestinal lymphangiectasis, is characterized by congenital intestinal lymphatic obstruction and loss of lymph, with hypogammaglobulinemia and moderate to severe lymphopenia. Treatment with a diet enriched with medium-chain triglycerides reverses the symptoms and pathological findings.[16]

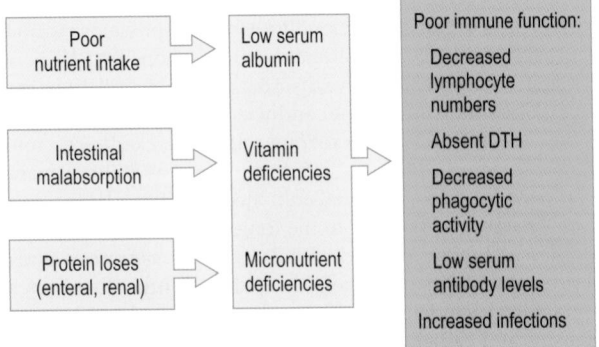

Fig. 38.1 Malnutrition results from decreased food intake, decreased gastrointestinal absorption of nutrients or protein losses due to inflammatory enteropathies or renal disease. Protein deficiency causes decreased production of immune cells and immunoglobulins, increasing susceptibility to infections.

Diabetes mellitus

Diabetes mellitus (DM) is characterized by insufficient production of insulin by the pancreas, which results in poor glucose cell metabolism. DM can result from autoimmune damage (type I, insulin dependent), or a decrease in the cell response to insulin (type II, non-insulin dependent). Both types of DM present with increased susceptibility to infections due to immune defects, poor glucose metabolism, poor blood supply and local tissue denervation. Altered immune defects that have been reported include lymphopenia, cutaneous anergy and impaired *in vitro* lymphocyte proliferation.[17] The humoral response usually remains intact, with normal antibody responses to routine immunizations. Diabetics can exhibit abnormal phagocytic adherence, chemotaxis phagocytosis and bactericidal activity. Maintenance of blood glucose levels in normal ranges results in improvement of phagocyte function and lower risk of infections.

Uremia

Treatment of uremia often requires either hemodialysis (HD) or peritoneal dialysis (PD). Unfortunately, both uremia and dialysis can impair the immune system, and thereby predispose patients to serious infections. Even when disparities in age, sex, race, and diabetes mellitus were taken into account, mortality rates in dialysis patients attributed to sepsis were higher by a factor of 100 to 300.[18] Sepsis secondary to vascular device infections or respiratory infections are common in dialysis patients. Their immune system dysregulation is characterized by immunodeficiency with a state of cellular activation, leading to a chronic inflammatory state and increased oxidative stress.[19] Several toxins targeting phagocytes have been identified in plasma and peritoneal fluid of uremic patients, including angiogenin, p-cresol, a form of ubiquitin, degranulatory inhibitory protein and a protein with homology to immunoglobulin light chains. Phagocytic cell dysfunction is the most common and consistent immune defect found in uremics. Diminished chemotaxis, phagocytosis, intracellular killing and oxygen radical production have been documented.[20] The molecular mechanisms of these are not clear. It has been suggested that increased intracellular calcium seen in end-stage renal diseases could impair phagocytosis. Iron overload in HD patients is associated with decreased phagocytic bacterial killing and increased risk of infection. Improvement of such immune defects is seen after iron chelation. Patients in hemodialyis often have an increased frequency of infections. Naïve T cells are decreased proportionally with increased apoptosis of these cells, and uremia. When dendritic cells were exposed to uremic sera from hemodialysis patients, endocytosis was reduced, but their ability to induce allogeneic T-cell proliferation was stimulated. Decreased lymphocyte counts, depressed lymphoproliferative response to mitogens and antigens and cutaneous anergy can also be seen in uremic patients. Most uremic patients show adequate antibody response to vaccines; however, antibody titers decline rapidly within 6 months, regardless of vaccination.

Immunological defects secondary to infectious diseases

During the encounter between a microbial pathogen and its host, a variety of complex biological processes occur, in which microbes attempt to proliferate and the host fights to eliminate them. Pathogens may interfere with a variety of immunological defenses in order to decrease their clearance and establish an infection. In some cases, this action also favors infection by other pathogens. For example, during influenza infection, the inflammatory response in the lung paradoxically increases the patient's susceptibility to bacterial pneumonias.[21] One infectious agent in particular, human immunodeficiency virus, targets the immune system itself by infecting CD4 T lymphocytes and causing severe immunodeficiency (Chapter 37). However, most immunological disturbances caused by microbial infections are transient and usually reflect a normal immune response rather than a weakening of the immune defenses. In some cases of chronic infections such as tuberculosis and parasites, immune suppression may be secondary to the state of wasting that is induced by these diseases. The following examples describe selected individual pathogens that characteristically induce immune suppression.

Viral pathogens
Measles virus

In the early 1900s, it was noted that the tuberculin DTH skin test response was blunted during acute measles infection. Measles infects lymphoid tissues through the CD46 molecule, a complement receptor present in monocytes and lymphocytes, affecting antigen presentation, cell-mediated killing and immunoglobin synthesis.[22,23] The period of immunosuppression lasts only a few weeks until the virus is cleared, but may linger in some hosts. In rare cases, persistent measles infection develops and causes subacute sclerosing panencephalitis, a progressive degeneration of the central nervous system, mediated by an inflammatory reaction triggered by persistent measles antigen, despite the presence of high-titer anti-measles antibodies.

Epstein–Barr virus (EBV)

EBV infection is present in almost 90% of the world's adult population, and usually occurs subclinically. It may occasionally manifest as a self-limiting lymphoproliferative disease known as acute infectious mononucleosis. EBV targets B cells using the CD21 surface antigen for entry and transforms these cells to establish a chronic infection. EBV-infected B cells fail to undergo apoptosis. Activated (also called "atypical", because of their morphology) T cells eliminate EBV-infected B cells, developing a massive expansion of a selected oligoclonal population with limited TCR (T-cell receptor) Vβ gene usage. As a result, there is a relative T-cell anergy, which can be demonstrated in in vitro experiments. There is also a concurrent polyclonal expansion of B cells with enhanced immunoglobulin production.[24] These changes last for only a few weeks.

The X-linked recessive lymphoproliferative syndrome (XLP) develops in individuals with mutations in the SHD1A gene, resulting in affected males unable to control EBV–infected cell proliferation. Impaired immune response, splenomegaly and lymphoproliferative disease are usually fatal to affected individuals.[25]

Cytomegalovirus (CMV)

Infection with CMV also leads to a mononucleosis illness. CMV-infected monocytes have a decreased ability to present antigens because of reduced MHC protein expression and function, using viral molecules that resemble MHC proteins. In addition CMV encodes a human IL-10 homolog, with demonstrated inhibitory activity of the activation of human lymphocytes.[26]

Influenza virus

Acute infection with influenza virus causes transient lymphopenia, primarily within the T-cell population. Other immunological alterations are reduced lymphocyte proliferation, increased NK cell activity and generation of regulatory T cells, as well as impairment of mucus clearance that enhances bacterial adherence and increases the susceptibility to secondary bacterial infections.[27] Bacterial pneumonias are the most common cause of mortality during influenza epidemics.[28]

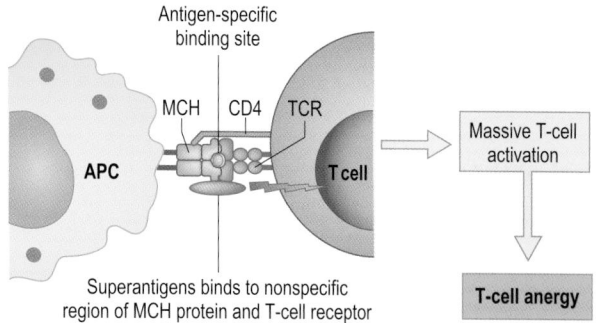

Fig. 38.2 **Superantigens are microbial proteins that bind nonspecific regions of MHC molecules expressed by antigen-presenting cells, and to one of over 20 subfamilies of T-cell receptor.** This results in activation of a large number of T cells, with release of cytokines and subsequent anergy.

Bacterial pathogens

Severe bacterial infections have been associated with alterations of innate immunity, such as decreased leukocyte chemotaxis and reduced reticuloendothelial function. However, these are not seen consistently and vary with bacterial invasiveness, production of bacterial toxic products and the host capacity to contain the dissemination of infection. For example, *Streptococcus* spp. and *Staphylococcus* spp. produce a family of toxins called superantigens, which induce nonspecific activation of T cells, massive cytokine release, and cell apoptosis. (Fig. 38.2) Superantigens also induce T-cell anergy. Several systemic illnesses result from superantigen effects, including toxic shock syndrome and scarlet fever. Over 40 bacterial superantigens have been described.[29] Early antibiotic therapy may reduce the incidence of immunological disturbances due to bacterial infections.

Immunological defects induced by surgery or trauma

Stress induced by surgery or trauma results in a metabolic and inflammatory response to control the injury and repair the damage. Local inflammation is necessary for wound healing and defense against microbial pathogens. The reaction to injury also initiates a systemic response with release of several inflammatory cytokines, which may affect the ability of the host to respond to immunological challenges and also predispose the patient to infection.[30] These responses may lead to adult respiratory distress syndrome (ARDS) if affecting the lungs and to multiorgan failure or systemic inflammatory response syndrome (SIRS). The term "sepsis" is reserved to SIRS of infectious etiology.

The series of events leading to the inflammatory response to trauma, whether accidental or operative, can be summarized into five steps: loss of epithelial barriers, vasodilation, increased vascular permeability, cellular activation and adhesion, and neuroendocrine cytokine release (Fig. 38.3).

CLINICAL PEARLS

- Surgery and severe trauma cause increased susceptibility to infections.
- In addition to physical loss of mucosal barriers, the inflammatory reaction after injury is followed by up to ten days of immunological anergy.
- Removal of dead tissue and foreign bodies, and prompt restoration of enteral feeding reduce the time period of increased risk of infections.

Mechanical or chemical injury during trauma can cause epithelial damage and allow vast quantities of microbial pathogens access to the host. In addition, postoperative changes such as decreased motility may also affect the mucosal barrier. The release of inflammatory mediators in response to tissue damage and microbial products induce the next steps of vasodilation, increased permeability and cell activation. Chemotaxis of polymorphonuclear cells is decreased following acute depletion of complement proteins and production of other acute plasma proteins. T-cell counts decrease between the second and fourth day after injury and correlate with the injury severity, although they may not correlate with clinical outcome.[31] Release of late phase cytokines is directed at control of the inflammatory response and may consequently impair the immune response.[32] Delayed-type hypersensitivity responses are depressed following major injury, with up to 90% of severely injured patients being anergic, as measured both by DTH skin testing and *in vitro* lymphocyte proliferation to mitogens and antigens. B-cell activation and antibody production are also impaired following trauma or major burns.

Stress, originated from trauma or other causes, stimulates the neuroendocrine axis to produce hormones such as vasopressin, aldosterone, catecholamines, and cortisol.[33] Elevated levels of cortisol increase the release of neutrophils to peripheral blood and produce lymphopenia. In addition, the regulated secretion of prostaglandins, thromboxanes, and leukotrienes are disturbed and may contribute to immunosuppression of the injured patient. Prostaglandin E2 inhibits lymphocyte proliferation, decreases IL-2 release and inhibits natural killer cells up to 7–10 days following major injury.

Control of tissue damage, pain relief, nutritional support and avoidance of ischemia decrease the release of inflammatory mediators and therefore reduce the immune abnormalities induced by surgical injury. Neutrophils from a well-perfused wound

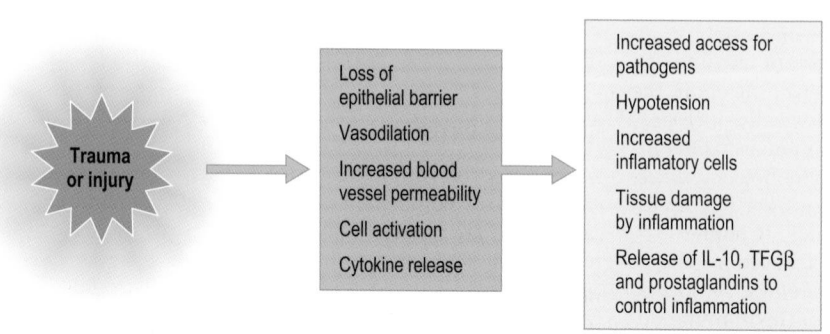

Fig. 38.3 **After trauma or injury, inflammation processes develop to promote tissue healing.** However, significant inflammation also contributes to tissue damage (e.g., systemic inflammatory response syndrome, SIRS, and acute respiratory distress syndrome, ARDS). Late phase immune regulatory mechanisms in response to inflammation may induce a transient immunosuppressive state, mediated by soluble mediators such as IL-10.

have better phagocytic and bactericidal activity than neutrophils from an ischemic wound.

The management of an injured patient should include prompt removal of all dead tissue to decrease the release of tissue degradation products and nonspecific immune activation. Although necessary in early time post injury, parenteral feeding leads to mucosal atrophy and increased risk of sepsis, and should be replaced or supplemented with enteral feedings when possible.

Splenectomy

Surgical removal of the spleen is indicated following trauma or in cytopenias induced by certain medical conditions involving excessive removal of red blood cells or platelets by the reticuloendothelial system. However, risks and benefits of splenectomy should be carefully assessed, because it may result in barely detectable immunological changes that, however, significantly increase the risk of bacterial sepsis. Splenectomized patients are particularly susceptible to infections by encapsulated organisms such as *S. pneumoniae* and *H. influenzae*. The mortality for sepsis in splenectomized patients is between 50% and 70%, emphasizing the need to avoid splenectomy when possible. Patients who are scheduled for splenectomy, should receive anti-penumococcal, anti-*H. influenzae* and anti-meningococcal immunizations at least two weeks prior to surgery.[34] Revaccination after splenectomy is not effective. In addition, splenectomized patients should receive life-long anti-pneumococcal antibiotic prophylaxis to reduce their risk of severe pneumonia and sepsis by S. *pneumoniae*.

Environmental conditions causing immunodeficiency

Ultraviolet (UV) light

UV light is a form of radiant energy, transmitted as electromagnetic waves with wavelengths ranging from 230 to 450 nm. It is classified as UVA if the wavelength is between 320 and 450 nm, as UVB if it is between 280 and 320 nm, and UVC if it is less than 280 nm. The effects of UVB are known to be mutagenic, by creating crosslinks between thymidines in DNA. The most common source of UV light affecting humans is exposure to sun, being most intense where the ozone layer is thinner, such as places close to the North Pole. Immunosuppression by UV light was first suspected because the incidence of malignant skin disorders increases upon exposure to sunlight. Photoimmunosuppression occurs even with low doses of UVB, possibly to prevent an inflammatory reaction that could damage sun-exposed skin. Delayed-type hypersensitivity skin test responses to antigens were compared in individuals using sunscreens with different levels of sun-protection factor (SPF) and UVA protection. DTH responses were reduced in participants without protection for UVA, regardless of the protection for UVB.[35] UV light induces the activation of NFκB, a second-signal molecule involved in T-cell activation and apoptosis (Fig. 38.4). It also affects the activation of antigen-presenting cells, the release of cytokines, and the expression of surface markers. The immunosuppressive effect of UV light may be regulated by soluble mediators released from epidermal cells, including melanocyte stimulating hormone, which induces hapten-specific tolerance in addition to its major role of activating melanocytes to protect the skin from sunlight. This modulation of the immune system by UV light has

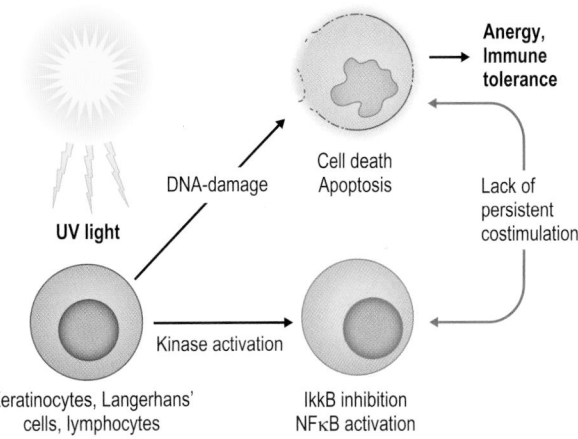

Fig. 38.4 UV light causes immunosuppression by two mechanisms: apoptosis of skin lymphocytes and dendritic cells by directly altering their DNA; and activating lymphocyte kinases that lead to cell apoptosis mediated by NFκB pathways.

been used to treat autoimmune skin disorders. UVB light and psoralen plus UVA light are the treatments of choice for severe psoriasis.[36] The most effective wavelength of UVB is approximately 313 nm. UVA light treatment may be combined with coal tar or an occlusive ointment for increased efficacy, and remission occurs in 80% of patients.

Ionizing radiation

Humans have been exposed to radiation in nuclear power plant accidents and in explosions of atomic bombs.[37] The immunosuppressive effect of ionizing radiation in the survivors of these exposures has been clinically evident by the increased susceptibility to infections and tumors. It has also been evident when used therapeutically against neoplastic diseases in humans, and experimentally in animal models. Irradiation significantly impairs cell-mediated immunity. The production of lymphocytes and neutrophils, as well as other blood lineages, is affected according to the radiation dose. Radiation causes apoptosis of hematopoietic cells in the bone marrow. When radiation is used at therapeutic doses for myeloablation in bone marrow transplants, neutrophil counts typically recover one month after exposure, and lymphocyte counts recover within 3 months. The immunosuppression by different radiotherapy regimens is usually measured by graft survival. All immunological components, including total, CD4 and CD8 T-cells, serum immunoglobulin levels, and the proliferative response to mitogens, decrease after radiotherapy. Specific immune responses are compromised primarily because of the lymphopenia. The number of cells of nonspecific immunity, such as macrophages and granulocytes, may also be decreased. Phagocytosis is relatively radioresistant, whereas antigen processing by macrophages is easily impaired by low-dose radiation. The radiation effect on humoral immunity also depends on the radiation dose, frequency of administration, rate and temporal relationship to antigen administration. When given in fractions, lymphocyte counts are reduced even more: in one study when administered in five fractions, mean lymphocyte counts were 1840 cells/μL, in 12 fractions were 1120 cells/μL, and in 20 fractions, 640 cells/μL.[38] The antibody response may be shortened or lengthened, although it is generally not affected. Children with cancer who are treated with craniospinal irradiation sustain lymphopenia and impaired *in vitro* lymphoproliferative responses to mitogens for more than a year after treatment.

High altitude and chronic hypoxia

Environmental extreme conditions, such as cold, heat or hypoxia, induce changes in the immune system, mostly due to acute stress. Exposure to these adverse conditions occurs during expeditions or with demanding outdoor activities, such as skiing and hiking. Acute stress temporarily increases immune function, as shown by increased mitogen proliferation. However, chronic stress causes immunosuppression, with decreases of T-cell and NK-cell counts, cytokine secretion and immunoglobulin levels.[39]

Populations living at high altitude, who are affected by both high altitude and hypoxia, have more infections than people living at sea level. However, poor living conditions, minimal access to medical care and low socio-economical levels are confounding factors that may contribute to their susceptibility to infection. There are few studies of the effect of high altitude on the immune function, and their results are equivocal. In decompression chamber studies, mitogen-induced T-cell proliferation is reduced, but T- and B-cells, and NK-cell activity are unchanged. Both men and mice develop good immune responses to meningococcal vaccine, at an altitude of 4930 m.[40] Changes induced by chronic hypoxia and high altitude quickly reverse when subjects return to sea level.

Space flights

Little is known about the effects of long-duration space flights on the immune system. Immune function may be affected by stress associated with sleep cycle alterations, confinement and isolation; and other factors, such as microgravity and space radiation. During space flight missions both increases and decreases in the numbers of total lymphocytes, both T and B cells have been reported.[41] Levels of immunoglobulins G, A, and M remain stable. However, inhibition of mitogen proliferation of both human and rat T cells *in vitro*, with a reduction of IL-2 receptor expression, was observed after exposure to microgravity and rotation, possibly as a result of decreased cell to cell contact. Lymphocytes stimulated with mitogens or antigens in microgravity, modeled or in a space, do not proliferate.[42] If the cells were stimulated before exposure to modeled microgravity, they retained their ability to proliferate. Other abnormalities were decreased NK-cell cytotoxic activity and decreased secretion of interleukins: IL-1, IL-2, and TNF-α. Studies of how space travel conditions may affect the immune system have included simulated isolation and sleep deprivation. A significant increase in plasma levels of soluble TNF-α receptor I and IL-6 occurred after four days of total sleep deprivation. There is also evidence of reactivation of chronic latent viruses after a simulated space flight.[43] More studies are being developed to define the effects of space travel upon the immune system.

Summary

Several clinical conditions of diverse pathogenesis are associated with immunological defects. These defects may be severe and of clinical significance, resulting in increased susceptibility to infections. The mechanisms of disease that secondarily lead to impaired immunity are many, involving metabolic abnormalities, such as lack of specific nutrients, and the insufficiency or excess of certain soluble factors, such as cortisol and prostaglandins. Physicians should be aware of the associations of these diseases with increased susceptibility of infections, because

appropriate management of the primary disorders often can prevent and reverse the associated immune dysfunction. Surgical stress, whether accidental or in the operating room, triggers a cascade of events to help tissue healing. However, it also releases inflammatory mediators that may result in immunosuppression of lymphocytes monocytes and neutrophils. Secondary immunodeficiency in trauma can be reduced by minimizing tissue damage, removing nonviable tissue, avoiding ischemia, and providing adequate nutritional support, particularly using an enteral route preferentially. Environmental conditions, in particular, UV and ionizing radiation, high altitude and chronic hypoxia, have a measurable effect in the immune system, which justifies their consideration in the approach of the patient presenting with immunodeficiency.

Translational research

● ON THE HORIZON

- Research opportunities for amelioration of secondary immunodeficiencies.
- Evaluation of micronutrients deficiency included in the diagnostic work up for immune deficiencies.
- Immunomodulation approaches to minimize the time of T-cell anergy following severe trauma or surgery.
- Development of immunization protocols in preparation of manned space flights.

Significant advances in the past decade have started to characterize the spectrum of immune disorders caused by factors extrinsic to the immune system. Deficiencies of many vitamins have been shown to modulate different intracellular pathways of the immune response, underscoring their role in the susceptibility to infections. Inflammatory mechanisms in response to injury are being characterized, with identification of cytokines and other mediators responsible for the different stages of healing, which secondarily affect systemic immunity. The role of gravity and other space flights factors in the immunological synapse is being established, prompting awareness of the impairment of the immune system for future human space expeditions.

References

1. Ram G, Chinen J. Infections and immunodeficiency in Down syndrome. Clin Exp Immunol 2011;164:9–16.
2. Kusters MAA, Vesterjegen RHJ, Gemen EFA, DeVries E. Intrinsic defect of the immune system in children with Down syndrome: a review. Clin Exp Immunol 2011;256:189–93.
3. Fisher BA, Charles P, Lundberg K, et al. Organ-specific autoantibodies but not anti-cyclic citrullinated peptides are a feature of autoimmunity in Down's syndrome. Ann Rheum Dis 2010;69:939–40.
4. De Vita S, Canzonetta C, Mulligan C, et al. Trisomic dose of several chromosome 21 genes perturbs haematopoietic stem and progenitor cell differentiation in Down's syndrome. Oncogene 2010;29:6102–14.
5. Cruz NV, Mahmoud SA, Chen H, et al. Follow-up study of immune defects in patients with dysmorphic disorders. Ann Allergy Asthma Immunol 2009;102:426–31.
6. Battersby AJ, Knox-Macaulay HH, Carrol ED. Susceptibility to invasive bacterial infections in children with sickle cell disease. Pediatr Blood Cancer 2010;55:401–6.
7. Adamkiewicz TV, Silk BJ, Howgate J, et al. Effectiveness of the 7-valent pneumococcal conjugate vaccine in children with sickle cell disease in the first decade of life. Pediatrics 2008;121:562–9.
8. Campodónico VL, Gadjeva M, Paradis-Bleau C, et al. Airway epithelial control of *Pseudomonas aeruginosa* infection in cystic fibrosis. Trends Mol Med 2008;14:120–33.
9. Brennan S. Innate immune activation and cystic fibrosis. Paediatr Respir Rev 2008;9:271–9.
10. Black RE, Allen LH, Bhutta ZA, et al. Maternal and Child Undernutrition Study Group. Maternal and child undernutrition: global and regional exposures and health consequences. Lancet 2008;371:243–60.

11. Cunningham-Rundles S, McNeeley DF, Moon A. Mechanisms of nutrient modulation of the immunoresponse. J Allergy Clin Immunol 2005;115:1119–28.

12. Prasad AS. Zinc: role in immunity, oxidative stress and chronic inflammation. Curr Opin Clin Nutr Metab Care 2009;12(6):646–52.

13. Huang J, Vieira A. Evidence for a specific cell membrane retinol-binding protein transport mechanism in a human keratinocyte line. Int J Mol Med 2006;17:62.

14. Adams JS, Liu PT, Chun R, et al. Vitamin D in defense of the human immune response. Ann N Y Acad Sci 2007;1117:94–105.

15. Nova E, Marcos A. Immunocompetence to assess nutritional status in eating disorders. Expert Rev Clin Immunol 2006;2:433–44.

16. Vignes S, Bellanger J. Primary intestinal lymphangiectasia (Waldmann's disease). Orphanet J Rare Dis 2008;3:5.

17. Daoud AK, Tayyar MA, Fouda IM, Harfeil NA. Effects of diabetes mellitus vs. in vitro hyperglycemia on select immune cell functions. J Immunotoxicol 2009;6:36–41.

18. Foley RN. Infectious complications in chronic dialysis patients. Perit Dial Int 2008;28 (Suppl. 3):S167–S171.

19. Raff AC, Meyer TW, Hostetter TH. New insights into uremic toxicity. Curr Opin Nephrol Hypertens 2008;17:560–5.

20. Lim WH, Kireta S, Leedham E, et al. Uremia impairs monocyte and monocyte-derived dendritic cell function in hemodialysis patients. Kidney Int 2007;72:1138–48.

21. Mills EL. Viral infections predisposing to bacterial infections. Ann Rev Med 1984; 35:469.

22. Kerdiles YM, Sellin CI, Druelle J, Horvat B. Immunosuppression caused by measles virus: role of viral proteins. Rev Med Virol 2006;16:49.

23. Griffin DE. Measles virus-induced suppression of immune responses. Immunol Rev 2010;236:176–89.

24. Williams H, Crawford DH. Epstein-Barr virus: the impact of scientific advances on clinical practice. Blood 2006;107:862.

25. Nichols KE, Ma CS, Cannons JL, et al. Molecular and cellular pathogenesis of X-linked lymphoproliferative disease. Immunol Rev 2005;203:180.

26. Loewendorf A, Benedict CA. Modulation of host innate and adaptive immune defenses by cytomegalovirus: timing is everything. J Intern Med 2010;267:483–501.

27. Bhatia A, Kast RE. How influenza's neuraminidase promotes virulence and creates localized lung mucosa immunodeficiency. Cell Mol Biol Lett 2007;12:111–9.

28. Cate TR. Impact of influenza and other community-acquired viruses. Semin Respir Infect 1998;13(1):17.

29. Fraser JD, Proft T. The bacterial superantigen and superantigen-like proteins. Immunol Rev 2008;225:226–43.

30. Ni Choileain N, Redmond HP. Cell response to surgery. Arch Surg 2006;141:1132–40.

31. Reikerås O. Immune depression in musculoskeletal trauma. Inflamm Res 2010;59:409–14.

32. Flohé SB, Flohé S, Schade FU. Deterioration of the immune system after trauma: signals and cellular mechanisms. Innate Immun 2008;14:333–44.

33. Godbout JP, Glaser R. Stress-induced immune dysregulation: implications for wound healing, infectious disease and cancer. J Neuroimmune Pharmacol 2006;1:421–7.

34. American Academy of Pediatrics . Pneumococcal infections. In: Pickering LK, editor. RedBook. 2009 Report of the Committee of Infections Diseases. 28th ed. Elk Grove Village, IL; 2009. p. 534–5.

35. Moyal DD, Fourtanier AM. Broad-spectrum sunscreens provide better protection from solar ultraviolet-simulated radiation and natural sunlight-induced immunosuppression in human beings. J Am Acad Dermatol 2008;58(5 Suppl. 2):S149–S154.

36. Patel RV, Clark LN, Lebwohl M, et al. Treatments for psoriasis and the risk of malignancy. J Am Acad Dermatol 2009;60:1001–17.

37. Kusunoki Y, Hayashi T. Long-lasting alterations of the immune system by ionizing radiation exposure: implications for disease development among atomic bomb survivors. Int J Radiat Biol 2008;84:1–14.

38. MacLennan IC, Kay HE. Analysis of treatment in childhood leukemia. IV. The critical association between dose fractionation and immunosuppression induced by cranial irradiation. Cancer 1978;41:108–11.

39. Mishra KP, Ganju L. Influence of high altitude exposure on the immune system: a review. Immunol Invest 2010;39:219–34.

40. Biselli R, Le Moli S, Matricardi PM, et al. The effects of hypobaric hypoxia on specific B cell responses following immunization in mice and humans. Aviat Space Environ Med 1991;62(9 Pt 1):870–4.

41. Gridley DS, Slater JM, Luo-Owen X, et al. Spaceflight effects on T lymphocyte distribution, function and gene expression. J Appl Physiol 2009;106:194–202.

42. Fitzgerald W, Chen S, Walz C, et al. Immune suppression of human lymphoid tissues and cells in rotating suspension culture and onboard the International Space Station. In Vitro Cell Dev Biol Anim 2009;45:622–32.

43. Shearer WT, Ochs HD, Lee BN, et al. Immune responses in adult female volunteers during the bed-rest model of spaceflight: antibodies and cytokines. J Allergy Clin Immunol 2009;123:900–5.

PART FIVE

Allergic diseases

Immunological mechanisms of airway diseases and pathways to therapy

David B. Corry,
Farrah Kheradmand,
Amber Luong,
Lavannya Pandit

The immunological airway diseases compose a large and disparate group of respiratory disorders that are characterized by airway and parenchymal inflammation that impairs sinus and lung function. The physiological importance of the airways combined with the need to respond immunologically to an extremely broad range of particulate and gaseous aerosols explains much of the diverse nature of airway immune disorders and their disproportionately large effect on human health. The allergic respiratory tract immune disorders covered in this chapter are extremely common conditions.

Allergic disorders have a common immune phenotype comprising highly characteristic cellular, humoral, biochemical, and molecular components, although individual variability means that not all these immunological features are equally expressed. The most studied and visually characteristic allergic immune cells are eosinophils and tissue mast cells, which are easily seen on conventional hematoxylin and eosin staining of pathological specimens. Eosinophils may far outnumber all other inflammatory cells. Less obvious on histochemical staining, but equally important to allergic diseases, are B cells that secrete the antibody isotypes IgE and IgG$_4$ and Th2 cells, which secrete a restricted repertoire of cytokines including IL-4, -5, -9, -10, and -13 that coordinate and activate other allergic effector cells (Chapter 16).

The allergic airway diseases are typically chronic and occasionally fatal, and although spontaneous remissions are not uncommon, none are curable. Recent insights have, however, vastly improved prospects for improved therapy.

Clinical presentation of allergic airway disease

Although the diverse effector cells and molecules that characterize allergic inflammatory exudates may be seen at any point along the respiratory tract, the functional impact of allergic disease is quite different in the upper and lower airways.

Chronic rhinitis and rhinosinusitis

Epidemiology and clinical presentation

The major allergic upper airway disorders are chronic rhinitis and rhinosinusitis. Allergic rhinitis (AR) involves allergic inflammation of the nasal mucosa and is the commonest type of chronic rhinitis, especially when symptoms are seasonal. Non-allergic rhinitis accounts for 30–70% of chronic perennial rhinitis. Typical symptoms of AR include clear rhinorrhea, sneezing, post-nasal drip, and nasal pruritus and congestion often in association with ocular symptoms such as conjunctivitis and tearing. Based on symptom

duration, AR is now classified as "intermittent" or "persistent" with severity of symptoms noted as "mild" or "moderate-severe."[1] Consequently, AR can be categorized into four groups based on the combination of the above two categories of frequency and severity of symptoms. Patients with persistent AR typically have daily symptoms year-round, but can also manifest seasonal fluctuations in the severity of their symptoms. The severity of symptoms on the impact of quality-of-life and productivity is reflected in the "mild" and "moderate-severe" categorization.

> ### KEY CONCEPTS
>
> **Classification of allergic rhinitis**
>
> | Frequency of symptoms | Severity of symptoms |
> |---|---|
> | **Intermittent**
 ■ Symptoms present for less than 4 days a week
 ■ Or for less than 4 weeks | **Mild**
 ■ No presence of sleep disturbance
 ■ Or impairment of daily activities, leisure and/or sport
 ■ Or impairment of school or work
 ■ Or troublesome symptoms |
> | **Persistent**
 ■ Symptoms present for more than 4 days a week
 ■ Or for more than 4 weeks | **Moderate-Severe**
 ■ Presence of sleep disturbance
 ■ And/or impairment of daily activities, leisure and/or sport
 ■ And/or impairment of school or work
 ■ And/or troublesome symptoms |

In contrast to rhinitis, which involves inflammation and symptoms confined to the nasal passages and mucosa, rhinosinusitis affects both the sinuses (maxillary, ethmoid, sphenoid, and frontal) and nasal mucosa. Rhinosinusitis is subdivided into four clinical categories including acute and chronic rhinosinusitis (ARS and CRS, respectively) with three recognized subgroups of CRS including CRS without nasal polyps (CRSsNP), CRS with nasal polyps (CRSwNP), and allergic fungal rhinosinusitis (AFRS).[2] ARS is defined as a disease process persisting for 3 weeks or less, while symptoms persisting for longer than 12 weeks are categorized as CRS. Another small subset of CRS patients are those with aspirin-exacerbated respiratory disease (AERD). These patients have the triad of CRSwNP, asthma, and history of nasal congestion and bronchospasm occurring within 2–3 hours after consumption of aspirin or other non-steroidal anti-inflammatory drugs that inhibit cyclooxygenase 1 (COX-1).

Signs and symptoms associated with rhinosinusitis in adults include facial pain and pressure, headaches, nasal congestion with or without obstruction, frontal or post nasal drainage, generalized malaise, and cough. Of these, nasal obstruction is the most common (81–95%), followed by facial pain and pressure (70–85%), discolored nasal drainage (51–83%), and hyposmia (61–69%).[3] In contrast, symptoms in children are age-related and require the caretaker to recognize them. Young children often present with a chronic cough, and irritability rather than facial pain.[4] Parents often also report halitosis and purulent nasal discharge. Although it is more difficult to determine the prevalence of rhinosinusitis in children because of shared symptoms with allergic rhinitis and viral upper respiratory tract infections, it appears to be inversely related to age. After childhood, rhinosinusitis can present at any age while AFRS more commonly presents in young adults.

Diagnosis

The diagnosis of allergic rhinitis is based on a history of typical symptoms and either *in vitro* or *in vivo* testing for elevated serum allergen-specific IgE antibodies. Common symptoms include post-nasal drainage, sneezing, itchy nose and eyes, and clear rhinorrhea. The frequency and effect of symptoms on sleep and productivity should be assessed in order to classify patients as intermittent or persistent and mild or moderate-severe.

Patients suffering from allergic rhinitis can present with "allergic shiner," a darkening of the infraorbital skin resulting from chronic venous pooling. In some children, wiping the front of the nose with the back of the hand in an upward motion (the allergic salute) creates a persistent horizontal crease across the nasal bridge that is a hallmark of chronic anterior rhinorrhea. Bilateral conjunctivitis may be present in patients with ocular involvement. On anterior rhinoscopy with a hand-held otoscope, engorged, boggy, and pale inferior turbinates also suggest allergic rhinitis. In addition, there is often a clear discharge coating the nasal cavity. Examination of the oropharynx often reveals cobblestoning of the mucosa, a sign of chronic post-nasal drainage.

The two tests used most commonly to demonstrate IgE-mediated allergic reactions are immediate-hypersensitivity skin testing and measurement of serum allergen-specific IgE levels. Skin prick tests correlate well with the symptoms of allergic rhinitis and with airway responsiveness to allergens.[1,5] Measuring serum allergen-specific IgE levels provides an *in vitro* means of supporting a diagnosis of allergic rhinitis. Compared to skin prick testing, the *in vitro* test is more specific, but less sensitive,[6] and more expensive. However, serum tests may be the only practical way of detecting allergen-specific IgE in some patients, especially those with urticaria and eczema.

The diagnosis of CRS requires the presence of two or more clinical symptoms persisting for longer than 12 weeks and objective evidence of inflammation within the sinus cavity; ARS is the same symptom complex, but present for a shorter duration. The symptoms of ARS/CRS can vary in severity and prevalence. The most specific symptom for rhinosinusitis is the presence of purulent rhinorrhea.[7] Since most symptoms of rhinosinusitis are non-specific, evidence of inflammation on nasal endoscopy or imaging is also necessary to make a diagnosis of CRS. On nasal endoscopy, inflammation is suggested by edema and/or drainage from the middle meatus; a diagnosis of CRSwNP is made when nasal polyps are visualized (Fig. 39.1). Inflammation

within the sinuses may not be apparent on nasal endoscopy and in patients with a strong history of CRS, computed tomographic (CT) scanning of the sinuses is necessary to detect mucosal thickening and fluid within the sinuses (Fig. 39.2).

● KEY CONCEPTS

Diagnosis of chronic rhinosinusitis

Chronic rhinosinusitis

- Presence of at least two of the following symptoms
  - Facial pressure or pain
  - Nasal obstruction or congestion
  - Anterior or posterior nasal drainage
  - Hyposmia or anosmia
- Edema or discolored drainage within the sinus cavity or middle meatus
- *Or* CT sinus showing fluid or mucosal thickening within sinus cavities

CRS without nasal polyps	CRS with nasal polyps
■ No evidence of nasal polyps within the middle meatus as noted on nasal endoscopy in a patient with no history of previous sinus surgery	■ Presence of nasal polyps within the middle meatus as noted on nasal endoscopy ■ History of nasal polyps within sinus cavity in a previously operated patient with CRS diagnosis

---

The most widely accepted diagnostic criteria for allergic fungal rhinosinusitis (AFRS) include five characteristics: nasal polyps; type I (immediate) hypersensitivity to fungi; radiographic imaging consistent with AFRS; eosinophilic mucin with evidence of fungi; and a lack of evidence of fungal invasion into the surrounding sinus tissue.[8] A diagnosis of AFRS may still be entertained in patients whose nasal polyps have been removed at surgery, but who manifest the other criteria. Type I hypersensitivity to fungi can be detected by positive skin testing to fungal antigens or assessed

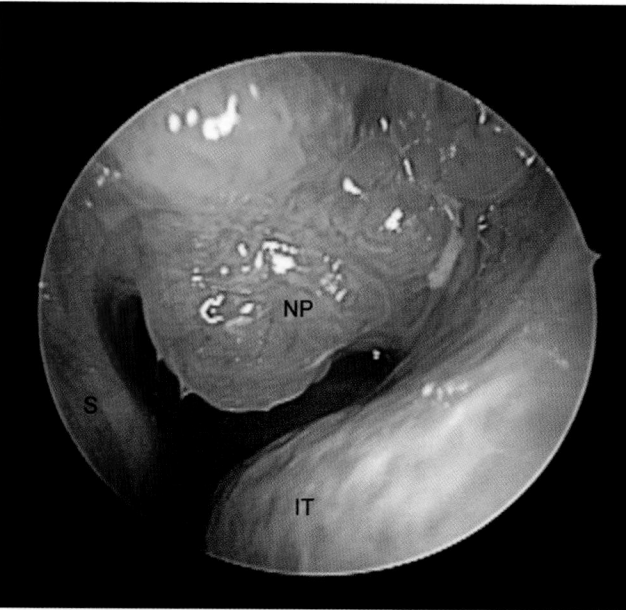

Fig. 39.1 Nasal polyposis. Seen on this nasal endoscopy are nasal polyps (NP) emanating from the sinus cavity into the nasal cavity between the septum (S) and the inferior turbinate (IT) of a patient with chronic rhinosinusitis.

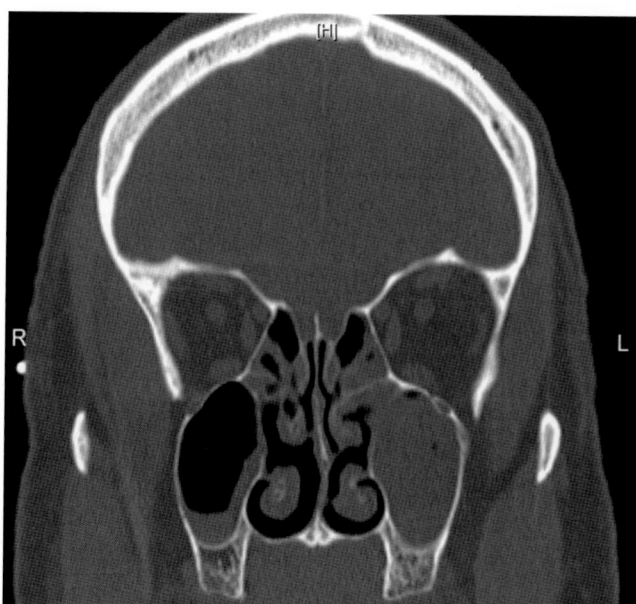

Fig. 39.2 Coronal sinus CT image from a patient with chronic rhinosinusitis. The maxillary sinuses (lateral to the nasal cavity) and ethmoid sinuses (medial to the orbital cavities) exhibit mucosal thickening and accumulation of obstructed secretions consistent with inflammatory changes within the paranasal sinuses.

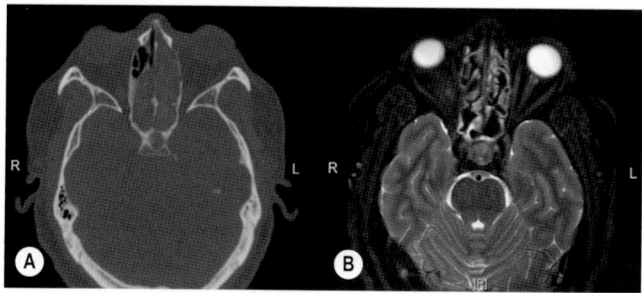

Fig. 39.3 CT and MRI images of ethmoid sinusitis from a patient with allergic fungal rhinosinusitis. The CT image (A) demonstrates inspissated mucus giving a hyperintense signal centrally within the ethmoid sinuses between the orbits. These same regions appear black (no signal) on the corresponding MRI image (B).

by elevated serum fungal-specific IgE titers. Imaging consistent with AFRS is based on the CT and magnetic resonance imaging (MRI) characteristics of eosinophilic mucin, which contains heavy metals such as iron, manganese, and calcium.[9] The presence of these metals along with inspissated secretions results in a heterogeneous signal with hyperintensity arising within the mucin on CT-based imaging. As assessed by MRI, involved sinuses have a drop signal as a result of the absence of freely mobile protons (Fig. 39.3).[9] Fulfilling the remaining criteria for AFRS requires histologic examination and microbiology for fungi within the mucin and tissue obtained at the time of surgery.

To make a diagnosis of aspirin-exacerbated respiratory disease requires meeting diagnostic criteria for CRS with nasal polyps, and either a history of respiratory symptoms exacerbated by oral intake of aspirin or other COX-1 inhibitors on at least two occasions, or a positive reaction on aspirin challenge.[10] Such patients should also be evaluated for asthma, if not already diagnosed.

Therapy

The most effective and widely used pharmaceutical approaches to control nasal and ocular symptoms of AR are intranasal glucocorticoids and anti-histamines. Intranasal glucocorticosteroids

(steroids) are the most efficacious medication class available for the management of allergic rhinitis symptoms, particularly nasal congestion, and are now considered first-line medical therapy.[1] They may also improve eye symptoms. Of the numerous formulations available, mometasone furoate demonstrates the highest anti-inflammatory potency and lowest systemic absorption as compared to other commonly used intranasal steroids.[11] However, no studies have shown any differences in clinical efficacy among the currently available intranasal steroids.

Antihistamines are also highly effective against the histamine-driven symptoms of sneezing, pruritus, and rhinorrhea. Second generation antihistamines are recommended over first generation formulations for their non-sedating effects and equivalent ability to reduce AR symptoms.[12] Intranasal antihistamines can be as effective as oral antihistamines for control of allergic and non-allergic rhinitis, but neither is as effective as intranasal steroids for nasal congestion. Other pharmacologic agents potentially useful in the management of rhinitis include oral steroids, oral leukotriene receptor antagonists, intranasal chromones, and intranasal ipratropium bromide.

In addition to pharmaceutical approaches, allergen immunotherapy has long been available as a means of providing long-term relief from rhinitis. Two types of immunotherapy are available: subcutaneous immunotherapy (SCIT) and sublingual immunotherapy (SLIT) (Chapter 91). An important concern with the use of SCIT is the risk of triggering anaphylaxis. Both SCIT and SLIT are widely available in Europe, while SCIT is preferred in the United States.[13]

Finally, although allergen avoidance seems a sensible tactic, multiple studies evaluating the effectiveness of single method avoidance measures have shown no clinically significant reduction in symptoms. On the other hand, use of multiple methods to control allergen exposure have suggested some potential clinical benefit.[14] The treatment of chronic rhinosinusitis is more controversial than that of allergic rhinitis. As the etiology and pathophysiology of CRS is unclear and data from controlled studies are limited, many of the treatment guidelines for CRS are highly dependent on expert opinion. Recent guidelines have followed similar protocols for the establishment of grades of evidence for clinical recommendations. These are generally based on the Grades of Recommendation, Assessment, Development, and Evaluation (GRADE) grading system of assessing studies and integrating their results with the risks and benefits of therapy. In general, CRS should first be treated maximally with medical therapy, followed by surgery in those who fail medical management. However, criteria defining maximal medical therapy have yet to be established.[10]

The cornerstone of medical therapy in CRS remains the use of anti-inflammatory agents, especially steroids delivered systemically or topically. Systemic steroid therapy significantly reduces nasal polyp size and should be included in the first-line management of CRSwNP. Although fewer clinical studies are available, steroids are also recommended in the treatment of CRSsNP. Long-term antibiotic therapy (>12 weeks using macrolides) has demonstrated symptomatic and objective improvements as compared to sinus surgery, although usage guidelines vary between countries.[15,16]

Of particular interest is the use of anti-fungal antibiotics in CRS given the strong association between CRS and filamentous fungi. However, oral anti-fungals have only proved effective in AFRS patients.[17,18] Topical anti-fungal preparations have not been found useful in the management of CRS. Although relatively understudied, an important adjunctive measure in the management of both rhinitis and CRS is to perform saline irrigation of the nasal passages, which improves disease symptoms and is virtually risk-free.

Patients with persistent symptoms despite medical therapy are candidates for functional endoscopic sinus surgery. Outcomes of medical versus sinus surgery combined with intranasal steroids showed similar improvements, but CRSwNP patients achieved improved asthma control with medical therapy.[15] For AFRS patients in which the sinuses are impacted with copious dried mucus requiring manual extraction and patients presenting with serious complications of CRS such as vision loss or intracranial extension of disease, endoscopic sinus surgery is mandatory.

Asthma

Epidemiology and clinical presentation

After several decades of rising incidence, asthma is now the most common chronic disease of childhood and one of the most common disorders of adults in the United States. Although most frequently initially diagnosed in childhood, asthma can be first diagnosed at any age. The widely prevalent and incurable nature of asthma will continue to assure its position as one of the most expensive of medical afflictions both in terms of total medical expenditure and in time lost from work and school. Asthma is a lower respiratory tract disease that is characterized by dyspnea and other symptoms including cough, chest tightness, chest pain, and wheezing. Persons with mild disease can often present only with a mild, chronic cough. In contrast to other obstructive lung diseases, asthma symptoms are present intermittently and are characteristically relieved by bronchodilator and anti-inflammatory therapy.[19]

Asthma patients are classified into distinct clinical subtypes according to characteristic environmental or occupational exposures that elicit disease symptoms, the presence or absence of concomitant atopy, temporal expression of symptoms, and responsiveness to anti-inflammatory therapy (Table 39.1). Respiratory viruses are the most frequently implicated causes of asthma attacks, especially in children, while tobacco smoke and air pollution are other major inciting agents. The majority of asthma patients are atopic, a term that reflects the production of IgE and both the genetic predisposition toward immediate-type immune reactions and exposure to causative environmental agents such as pollens, dust mites, fungi, and many insects.[20] If evidence for atopy is present, patients are referred to as extrinsic, atopic, or allergic asthmatics, whereas those who lack atopy are referred to as having intrinsic or non-allergic asthma. In general, airway constriction occurs and symptoms of asthma are provoked when triggering agents are inhaled from the environment, representing the clinical expression of airway hyper-reactivity,

which represents the exaggerated tendency of the asthmatic airway to constrict in response to exposure to a wide variety of provocative agents. Some of these agents, such as viruses and pollens, are only intermittently present, causing seasonal asthma, while other agents are encountered continuously (e.g., fungi), and cause persistent (or perennial) asthma. Occupational asthma is defined as asthma acquired in the workplace, where dozens of potentially toxic agents have been identified. Numerous additional clinical asthma subsets can be defined according to the factor or factors that most often elicit attacks of dyspnea. A final category of asthma, steroid resistant, refers to patients who are relatively unresponsive to anti-inflammatory steroid therapy (Table 39.1).[21]

Diagnosis

Asthma is often recognized on clinical grounds alone, with acute attacks marked by obvious dyspnea, wheezing, cough, and use of accessory muscles of respiration. Such attacks typically resolve with bronchodilator therapy. Spirometry can provide more objective evidence of airway obstruction as assessed by decrements in the forced expiratory volume in 1 second (FEV_1) and other measures of air flow. Nonetheless, a uniformly acceptable disease definition has remained elusive, at least partly because of the nonspecific nature of symptoms and a clinical spectrum that blends with many other disease processes. When the clinical presentation is uncertain, bronchial provocation tests can be used to determine the presence of airway hyper-responsiveness and thereby establish the diagnosis.[21] Additional laboratory data that support a diagnosis of allergic asthma include peripheral blood eosinophilia, elevated serum total and antigen-specific IgE levels, and positive skin prick test results against one or more allergens.

Therapy

As with rhinitis and rhinosinusitis, the therapy of asthma is generally non-specific and directed at improving airflow through bronchodilation and reducing inflammation. Immediate relief of bronchoconstriction and dyspnea is achieved with bronchodilating agents that activate the β_2 adrenergic receptor on airway smooth muscle (beta agonists). For long-term control of asthma, the most effective agent class is steroids, which reduce inflammation and suppress airway constriction and dyspnea. For mild to moderate disease, bronchodilating agents and steroids are typically administered by inhalation, which reduces but does not eliminate systemic side effects. A secondary agent class used for controlling bronchospasm is the anti-cholinergics, which are antagonists of the muscarinic acetylcholine receptor. Severe disease may also require treatment with steroids, which are given orally for relatively brief periods to minimize the often severe side effects that can follow systemic administration. Severe disease exacerbations, especially when life-threatening, are treated by intravenous administration of steroids and high-dose inhaled beta agonists (given by nebulizer).

Additional anti-inflammatory agents available for the treatment of asthma include leukotriene receptor antagonists, chromones, theophylline, and omalizumab, a monoclonal antibody that reduces circulating and mast cell-bound IgE. While beneficial in some patients, these latter agents are not as effective as inhaled steroids. Finally, as with rhinitis and rhinosinusitis, avoidance of exposures that typically elicit symptoms is an important adjunctive treatment measure. To be effective, allergen avoidance measures need to be very intensive, but can be effective in preventing disease exacerbations and reducing asthma symptoms.[22] However, it can be difficult to achieve this in a normal domestic setting.

Table 39.1 Clinical subsets of human asthma

Viral induced
Allergic
Non-allergic
Intrinsic
Extrinsic
Occupational
Persistent
Seasonal
Exercise induced
Nocturnal
Steroid resistant

Other airway allergic disease syndromes

In addition to the common allergic disorders discussed above, several other allergic airway diseases have been described and although not as common, these often cause profound morbidity. As with asthma, these disorders are clinically heterogeneous, but are believed to share a similar pathophysiology related to the inhalation of antigens that provoke airway eosinophil and Th2 responses. No single clinical, pathologic, or radiographic feature is pathognomonic for these diseases; and diagnosis relies on a constellation of findings, especially antigen exposures, radiographic details, and histopathology. Nonetheless, all of these disorders are prominently linked by the presence of eosinophils in peripheral blood and airway tissues.

Under the trophic influence of IL-5, eosinophils develop from precursor cells present largely in the bone marrow (Chapter 23). Early mature eosinophils are then released into the blood where they circulate for a brief period prior to entering the interstitium of airway tissues where they can reside for long periods. Chemotactic factors that enhance the extravasation of eosinophils include complement components, eosinophil chemotactic factor-A, leukotrienes, tumor-associated factors, and chemokines. Putative functions of tissue resident eosinophils range from host defense against parasites such as nematode helminths in diseases such as tropical pulmonary eosinophilia to mediators of end-stage tissue destruction and irreversible lung damage and fibrosis in other disorders such as acute and chronic eosinophilic pneumonia.

The eosinophilic disorders discussed below are organized according to whether there is an *extrinsic* or *intrinsic* cause of the eosinophilia (Table 39.2). Inhaled or ingested extrinsic factors, including medications and infectious agents (e.g., parasites, fungi, mycobacteria), can trigger an eosinophilic immune response. This may be mild and self-limited, as in Loeffler syndrome. Intrinsic pulmonary eosinophilic syndromes are, by definition, idiopathic and represent a varied group of diseases, often systemic in nature.

Extrinsic eosinophilic syndromes

Tropical eosinophilic pneumonias

The tropical eosinophilic syndromes are a group of clinically similar eosinophil-predominant inflammatory disorders characterized by chest pain, wheezing, cough, and airway hyper-responsiveness, often in the setting of a debilitating, but transient, febrile illness. Fleeting lung infiltrates may be seen on chest radiographs and laboratory studies often demonstrate strikingly high peripheral blood, lung and airway eosinophilia, and elevated serum IgE levels. Migrating parasites traversing the lungs are thought to be responsible for most cases of tropical eosinophilic pneumonia. Embolization of microfilariae (e.g., *Dirofilaria* spp.) or helminth eggs within the pulmonary microvasculature leads to antigen release and induction of a typically granulomatous allergic immune reaction. Persistent or chronic, recurrent infection with etiological organisms (e.g., *Strongyloides* spp. *Wucheria bancrofti*, *Brugia malayi*) leads to chronic inflammation that may cause parenchymal necrosis and irreversible fibrosis. In the United States, *Strongyloides* spp. are the most common cause of parasitic infection and tropical eosinophilic pneumonia. Patients who are immunocompromised, including those recently prescribed systemic steroids, may develop *Strongyloides* hyperinfection syndrome, in which large numbers of recently released larvae burrow through the intestine and migrate to the lungs,

Table 39.2 Eosinophilic lung disorders

Disease	Causative agent	Proposed immune mechanism
Loeffler syndrome	Inhaled food, infection, or medication	T-cell-mediated hypersensitivity reaction
Drug rash with eosinophilia and systemic symptoms (DRESS) syndrome	Drugs: sulfonamides, phenobarbital, sulfasalazine, carbamazepine, and phenytoin	Hypersensitivity reaction to drug
Parasitic infections	*Strongyloides* spp., *Wucheria bancrofti*, *Brugi malayi*	T-cell and B-cell clonal activation in response to parasite antigens and adjuvant factors.
Allergic bronchopulmonary aspergillosis	*Aspergillus*	IgE and immune complex deposition
Acute eosinophilic pneumonia	Fungal infections, cigarette smoking, post-stem cell transplant	Hypersensitivity response to inhaled antigen (infectious or otherwise)
Chronic eosinophilic pneumonia	Unknown systemic-mediated process	Unknown, but chronic nature evident with T-cell-mediated granuloma production
Idiopathic hypereosinophilic syndrome	Infections, systemic diseases and drugs that drive peripheral eosinophilia	Systemic responses caused in part due to excess IL-5 production from clonal expansion of Th2-cells as well as fusion gene *FIP1L1–PDGFR*
Churg-Strauss syndrome	Autoimmune vasculitis to unknown antigen, associated with asthma.	Decreased T-regulatory cell function with diminished IL-10 production

causing a severe and potentially fatal lung disease that is frequently complicated by sepsis (Fig. 39.4). A very similar disease, termed Loeffler syndrome, was originally reported to be caused by the larvae of *Ascaris* spp., but other helminths and hypersensitivity responses to medications have since been etiologically implicated. Therapy of parasite-related pulmonary eosinophilia syndromes is directed at relieving symptoms and eliminating the parasites.

DRESS syndrome

The drug rash with eosinophilia and systemic symptoms (DRESS) syndrome is a severe drug hypersensitivity reaction that has a constellation of systemic signs and symptoms including skin rash, fever, lymphadenopathy, and inflammation of the liver, lung, and heart. Numerous drugs have been reported to cause DRESS syndrome including sulfonamides, phenobarbital, sulfasalazine, and anti-seizure medications such as carbamazepine

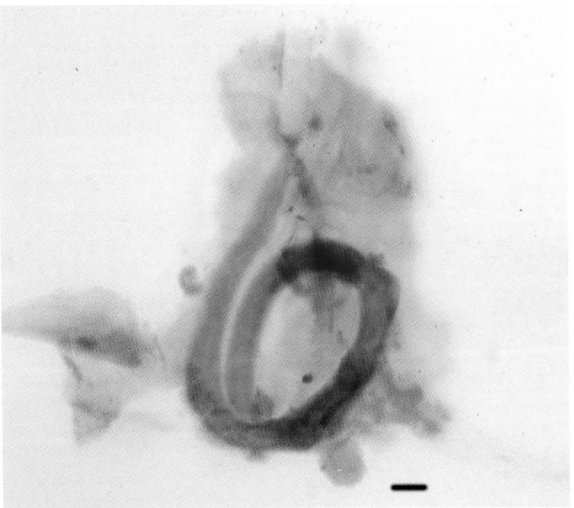

Fig. 39.4 Strongyloidiasis. The coiled larva of *Strongyloides stercoralis* is seen on this Papanicolau stain of a bronchoalveolar lavage sample from a patient with *Strongyloides* hyperinfection. Original magnification 400×; bar = 10 μm.

and phenytoin. Importantly, symptom onset may be delayed long after initiation of the drug.[23] The therapy of DRESS syndrome involves discontinuing the offending medication and providing supportive care in the setting of severe organ involvement.

Allergic bronchopulmonary aspergillosis (ABPA)

ABPA is a severe pulmonary allergic reaction to *Aspergillus* antigens that is seen almost exclusively in the setting of pre-existing asthma or cystic fibrosis.[24] Diagnostic criteria include asthma with wheezing, peripheral blood eosinophilia, detection of precipitating anti-*Aspergillus* antibodies, elevated serum total IgE levels, and radiographic evidence of fleeting pulmonary infiltrates often accompanied by central bronchiectasis. *Aspergillus* spp. and other filamentous fungal species can frequently be isolated from airway secretions of ABPA patients, suggesting that active and relatively unopposed fungal growth within the airways is responsible for the disease. Complications of chronic ABPA include severe airway hyperresponsiveness, bronchiectasis, eosinophilic pneumonia, pulmonary fibrosis, and invasive fungal disease. Treatment of ABPA aims to suppress the inflammatory response to the fungus and to control bronchospasm with glucocorticoid therapy, the duration of which may be shortened by concomitant use of oral anti-fungal agents such as itraconazole.[25]

Acute eosinophilic pneumonia (AEP)

AEP is an acute, often debilitating eosinophilic inflammatory syndrome that exclusively involves the lungs and is marked by pulmonary infiltrates, dyspnea progressing to frank respiratory failure, and fever. The diagnosis is dependent on eosinophils exceeding 25% of all inflammatory cells within the bronchoalveolar lavage fluid. Increasing evidence suggests an association between AEP and respiratory infections and new-onset cigarette smoking.[26,27] AEP has also been reported following allogeneic hematopoietic stem cell transplantation in the setting of graft versus host disease.[28] Prompt recognition of the disease and initiation of treatment with glucocorticoids usually results in rapid radiographic and clinical improvement.

Intrinsic eosinophilic syndromes

Chronic eosinophilic pneumonia (CEP)

This disorder presents similarly to AEP, but in a more chronic manner (greater than 6 weeks' duration). CEP can occur in isolation and/or in association with polyarteritis nodosa, rheumatoid arthritis, scleroderma, ulcerative colitis, breast carcinoma, and histiocytic lymphoma.[29] Most patients have evidence of asthma and atopy. Like AEP, CEP can present with striking eosinophilic inflammation of the lung (Fig. 39.5). Granulomas are occasionally seen on biopsy specimens, suggesting that an antigen-driven, T-cell-mediated process is involved in the chronicity of the disease. Treatment, as for AEP, is centered on steroid therapy, but unlike AEP, clinical relapse occurs frequently after discontinuation of treatment.

Idiopathic hypereosinophilic syndrome (IHES)

This multisystem disease is marked by the massive accumulation of eosinophils in many tissues and almost universally involves the lungs. Expansion of Th2 cells and local and systemic release of IL-4 and -5 is also frequently seen.[30] The clonal expansion of Th2 cells in the absence of known antigen exposures and the association of IHES with a variety of chromosomal aberrations strongly support the concept that IHES is a myeloproliferative disorder involving Th2 cells, although aberrant secretion of IL-5 by both solid and liquid tumors can produce very similar syndromes.[30] Many organs can be affected, resulting in dysfunction or failure of the gastrointestinal tract, skeletal muscles (leading potentially to respiratory failure), endomyocardial fibrosis, myocarditis, and congestive heart failure.[31] Pulmonary involvement manifests as obstructive airway disease, pulmonary edema, or pulmonary emboli due to a hypercoagulable state. In addition to hypereosinophilia, IHES patients may also have evidence of polyclonal hypergammaglobulinemia. Diagnosis is based on the discovery of elevated peripheral blood eosinophilia in the setting of a multisystem disorder, with evidence of aberrant Th2 responses or elevated IL-5 secretion. Interferon alpha can be administered in IHES to reduce IL-5 production by the abnormal Th2 cells.[30]

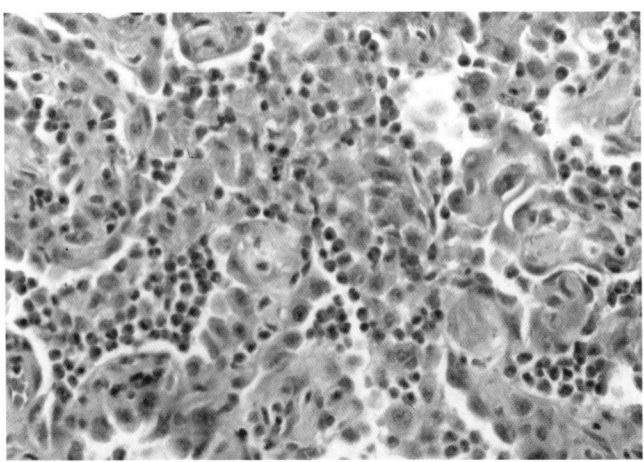

Fig. 39.5 Histology of chronic eosinophilic pneumonia. Lung biopsy specimen from a patient with chronic eosinophilic pneumonia demonstrates a confluent infiltrate with eosinophils filling alveoli together with large, multinucleate macrophages. Original magnification, 200×, hematoxylin and eosin stain.

Churg-Strauss syndrome (CSS)

Churg-Strauss syndrome, a necrotizing vasculitis of medium and small caliber vessels, is characterized by airway obstruction and eosinophilia and is virtually always seen in the setting of pre-existing asthma. The disease has an autoimmune nature given the presence of circulating anti-myeloperoxidase and anti-neutrophil cytoplasmic antibodies (p-ANCA). Because CSS is seen in patients with a history of asthma and allergies and the prominent pathologic feature is necrotizing vascular and tissue granulomas, the term "allergic granulomatosis and angiitis" is used synonymously. Inhaled or ingested antigens have been proposed as causative agents in susceptible individuals. Reports linking the syndrome with the leukotriene inhibitors zafirlukast and montelukast in the setting of steroid withdrawal suggest that these agents unmask pre-existing CSS rather than directly cause the disorder. Similar observations have been made with omalizumab treatment. The vasculitis of CSS can affect the sinuses, central and peripheral nervous systems, gastrointestinal tract, kidneys, and heart. Treatment of Churg-Strauss syndrome is based on reinstituting systemic steroids, which leads to disease resolution in the majority of patients. In severe steroid-resistant disease, cyclophosphamide and other immunosuppressants may be required.[32,33]

Immunological mechanisms of allergic airway disease

All major allergic airway disease syndromes include substantial patient subsets that unequivocally demonstrate evidence of allergic inflammation including elevated blood and airway eosinophilia, elevated serum total and antigen-specific IgE levels, and positive RAST skin testing. Specialized testing may also reveal predominant Th2 cytokine responses generated from peripheral blood mononuclear cells when challenged against common allergens *in vitro* and the presence of Th2 cells, eosinophils, IgE-secreting B cells, and secreted products of these cells within affected sinus and airway tissues. As well as the conventional causes of Th2-mediated airway inflammatory responses, fungal and bacterial infections also serve as distinct causes of inflammation.

The major effector immune mechanisms of disease proposed by Gell and Coombs in the 1960s remain essential to understanding the pathogenesis of allergic airway diseases.[34] While such mechanisms probably operate to some degree in all allergic diseases, their relative importance appears to vary, depending on whether the disease process predominantly affects the upper or lower respiratory tract (Fig. 39.6).

● KEY CONCEPTS

Immunopathogenesis of allergic airway disease

- Gell and Coombs' type 1 and type 4 hypersensitivity mechanisms contribute to disease expression, especially airway obstruction.
- Innate immune pathways involving TSLP, IL-25, and complement proteins critically contribute to the development of allergic airway inflammation.
- Environmental agents that are emerging as potentially important initiation factors for allergic airway inflammation include proteases, chitin, and endotoxin as derived from fungi, insects, and bacteria.
- Fungi and bacteria are further emerging as potentially important infectious causes of allergic disease of the upper and lower airways.

Type I (immediate) hypersensitivity

This form of hypersensitivity involves the activation of absophils and mast cells that release histamine and other inflammatory mediators that drive the clinical features of the response. Antigen recognition is via IgE antibodies, which bind through their Fc portion to high affinity receptors (FcεRI) and arm the effector cells. Th2 cells coordinate both the production of IgE antibodies

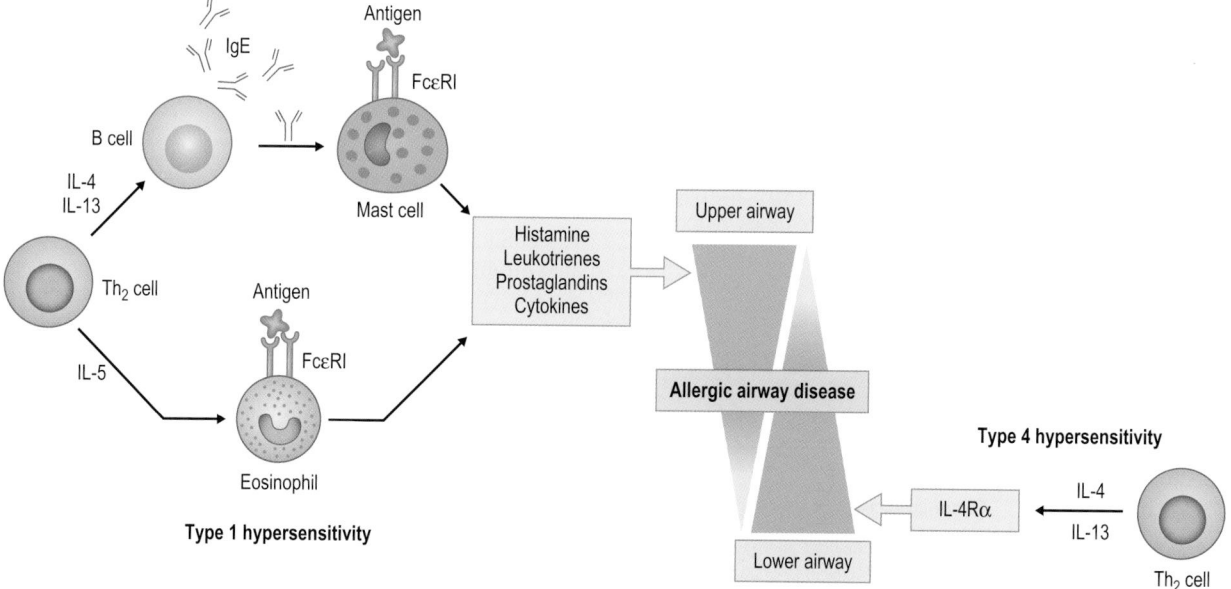

Fig. 39.6 Differential importance of allergic immune mechanisms according to airway level. Type I hypersensitivity (left), mediated by IgE-primed mast cells and eosinophils, is ultimately driven indirectly by the cytokines secreted by Th2 cells. In contrast, type IV hypersensitivity (right) is mediated directly by Th2 cytokines, especially IL-4 and -13, acting through a similar receptor that includes IL-4Rα. Both immune mechanisms are important to the expression of allergic disease at all airway levels, but type I hypersensitivity predominates in the upper airway, whereas type IV hypersensitivity likely assumes a more important role in the lower airway.

and the activation and recruitment of allergic effector cells to the airway. Antigen-specific IgE bound to the surface of mast cells and basophils is cross-linked upon exposure to relevant antigens, causing cellular activation and release of preformed mediators of inflammation such as histamine, proteases, leukotrienes, numerous cytokines, and other substances. Based on the study of human cells and rodents with experimental allergic disease, IL-4 and -13 released primarily by Th2 cells are especially important regulators of type I hypersensitivity reactions. IL-4 is required for B-cell maturation and IgE secretion, while IL-13 also contributes to IgE responses.

There is evidence that IL-4 and -13 can mediate distinct effector phenotypes in airway and tissue macrophages and dendritic cells. Two effector macrophage subtypes are currently recognized, including conventionally activated (M1) macrophages that arise under the predominant influence of type I cytokines, especially IFN-γ, and alternatively activated macrophages (M2) that arise under the influence of IL-4 and -13 in the relative absence of IFN-γ. M2 macrophages express a distinct gene profile that includes high-level expression of arginase 1, Ym1, Fizz1 (RELM), and PD-L2. While the specific functional roles of M2 cells in allergic disease remain to be determined, arginase 1, Fizz1, and PD-L2 are all regulatory molecules that suppress ongoing Th2 responses, suggesting that M2 cells prevent overly exuberant allergic responses.[35]

The effect of mediator release in immediate hypersensitivity reactions is most dramatically illustrated by the clinical syndrome of anaphylaxis, in which patients often exhibit profound bronchoconstriction and dyspnea accompanied by the extravasation of vascular solutes and fluid into the interstitium that produces diffuse edema and hypotension (Chapter 40). Type I hypersensitivity against inhaled allergens more commonly presents with symptoms of acute rhinitis. Rhinitis is the airway disease that is most responsive to agents that specifically interrupt type I hypersensitivity mechanisms, such as anti-histamines.[36,37]

Cell-mediated features of immediate hypersensitivity

Airway obstruction in allergen-sensitized asthma evolves over several hours after allergen exposure and is seen in two distinct phases. The early phase response is marked by airway constriction that becomes maximal ~30 minutes after allergen exposure and is fully relieved after approximately 2 hours (Fig. 39.7). Approximately 50% of asthmatic subjects tested will also develop a late phase airway response in which airway obstruction again develops 4–6 hours after allergen exposure. Late phase reactions

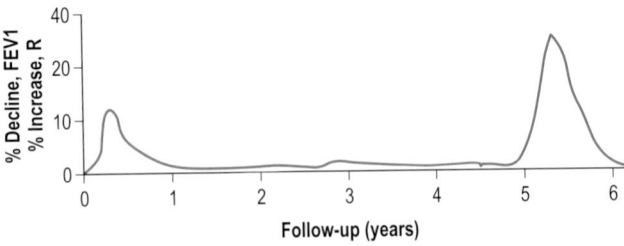

Fig. 39.7 Early and late phase airway changes following allergen challenge. This schematic diagram depicts the two phases of bronchoconstriction typically seen after allergen inhalation in sensitized, asthmatic subjects. Within 20–30 minutes after allergen inhalation, the first (early) phase of bronchoconstriction as assessed by either a decline in FEV$_1$ or increase in airway resistance (R) is seen. After quickly subsiding, approximately 4–6 hours (h) later, a second (late) phase of bronchoconstriction occurs.

are linked to the infiltration of the airways with Th2 cells and eosinophils and the accompanying bronchoconstriction is reversible with bronchodilating agents.[36]

Airway hyper-responsiveness is neurologically mediated through parasympathetic nerves such as the vagus and is fully reversible with bronchodilating agents that either interrupt muscarinic parasympathetic signaling directly (e.g., ipratropium bromide) or activate receptors (e.g., beta adrenergic) that antagonize muscarinic bronchoconstrictive pathways. Aside from its formal demonstration in the clinical laboratory through bronchial provocation testing, airway hyper-responsiveness is recognized clinically as episodic bronchoconstriction that is reversed with bronchodilating agents. Late phase responses after antigen challenge therefore represent a form of airway hyper-responsiveness and in part reveal the immunological nature of this ultimately neurological phenomenon.

More detailed analysis of the immunological mechanisms underlying airway hyper-responsiveness has been derived from experimental models of asthma, all of which manifest allergic airway disease, antigen-specific IgE responses, and airway hyper-responsiveness that resemble allergic asthma. Studies from many species have demonstrated that airway hyper-responsiveness in the setting of allergic inflammation is critically dependent on Th2 cells that have specifically been recruited to the lung. Moreover, it is now clear that IL-13 is the major Th2 cytokine that mediates airway hyper-responsiveness by acting directly on constitutive airway cells such as airway smooth muscle cells that express the IL-13 receptor. IL-13 administered directly to the airway is sufficient on its own to elicit airway hyper-responsiveness, independent of antibodies and even T cells. Mice completely deficient in B cells, IgE, and all other antibody isotypes, but with a full complement of T cells, develop airway hyper-responsiveness following allergen challenge to the same degree as wild type animals. Thus, experimental studies suggest that airway hyper-responsiveness is a cell-mediated hypersensitivity response mediated by Th2 cells and IL-13.[21]

It should be emphasized that IL-13 does not directly induce bronchoconstriction. Moreover, bronchoconstriction in asthmatic subjects, expressed as episodic bouts of dyspnea, is triggered by very diverse exogenous factors in addition to allergens (e.g., altered temperature and humidity, pungent odors, irritating aerosols) and endogenous stimuli (e.g., extreme emotional states) with little apparent connection to immunological mechanisms. Thus, rather than directly mediating airway obstruction, IL-13 instead establishes the basis for responding broadly to diverse agents with neurologically mediated bronchoconstriction. How IL-13 mediates these neurological changes is currently unknown.

A second and more insidious form of airway obstruction mediated through cell-mediated hypersensitivity and IL-13 is physical obstruction of the airways due to mucus that can accumulate in the airways as tenacious plugs, thereby obstructing airflow. IL-13, together with IL-9, is a trophic and differentiation factor for airway goblet cells and submucosal glands that enables the massive secretion of mucus by these cells, but again the final specific triggers of secretion are likely to be diverse and in part act through neurological pathways. Airway obstruction due to mucus is not immediately reversible with bronchodilators or other pharmacologic agents and is consequently the major cause of death, due to asphyxiation, in asthma.[38]

Finally, IL-4 and -13 further coordinate the recruitment and retention of allergic effector cells to airway epithelium and submucosa, an arrangement that facilitates rapid responses to inhaled allergens. Acting through a similar receptor that includes the alpha chain of the IL-4 receptor (IL-4Rα), IL-4 and IL-13 signal on

Table 39.3 Chemoattractants linked to the recruitment of allergic inflammatory cells

Chemokine	Receptor
CCL1	CCR8
CCL11	CCR3
CCL17, CCL22	CCR4
CX_3CL1	CX_3CR1
Prostaglandin D2	CRTh2
Leukotriene B4	BLT1

constitutive airway cells such as airway epithelial cells to induce secretion of a restricted repertoire of chemoattractants or chemotactic factors that promote the immigration of allergic cells expressing specific cognate receptors from the lung and airway microcirculation (Table 39.3).[39]

Contributing immune mechanisms in allergic airway disease

In addition to its critical role in promoting epsilon class switching and IgE secretion, IL-4 potentially contributes to airway hyper-reactivity and airway mucus secretion by signaling through the same or a very similar receptor used by IL-13 that includes IL4Rα and the $α_1$ chain of the IL-13 receptor (IL-13Rα1). More importantly, however, IL-4 is a critically important growth and differentiation factor for Th2 cells. Both IL-13 and -4 activate the transcription factor signal transducer and activator of transcription 6 (STAT6). In addition to these closely related cytokines, all components of the IL-4/-13 signaling pathway are required for expression of experimental allergic airway disease, especially airway hyper-responsiveness.[40]

IL-5 also contributes to both immediate and cell-mediated hypersensitivity reactions through its role in promoting the growth and differentiation of eosinophils. The degree to which eosinophils contribute numerically to airway inflammation varies widely based on diagnosis and prior use of glucocorticoids, which rapidly induce eosinophil apoptosis. Typically, however, eosinophils constitute 5–20% of airway inflammatory cells in asthma, but can massively outnumber all other airway cells in AFRS and eosinophilic pneumonia. Eosinophils potentially contribute to airway obstruction and disease through a variety of mechanisms. If sufficiently numerous, eosinophils can impair gas exchange based simply on their physical bulk within the small airways and alveolar walls. Eosinophils also secrete a variety of toxic granule products including major basic protein, eosinophil-derived neurotoxin, and eosinophil peroxidase, in addition to leukotrienes, cytokines, and many other mediators. Many eosinophil proteins are highly cationic and possess ribonuclease and antimicrobial activities, but the importance of these functions to the expression of allergic disease is largely unknown. Purified eosinophil proteins are highly toxic to cultured airway cells and damage the airways of experimental animals; on this basis the eosinophil has been presumed to be a major cause of airway dysfunction and remodeling in asthma, rhinosinusitis, and the eosinophilic pneumonias.[41] However, attempts to define the importance of eosinophils through experimental models and clinical trials using anti-IL-5 antibodies and other approaches have produced conflicting or inconclusive results and so the true relevance of eosinophils in allergic disease is unresolved.

In addition to Th2 cells, mast cells, and eosinophils, there are other pro-allergic cytokine producing cells within the airway mucosa with the potential to contribute to allergic reactions. These include γδ T cells and NK T cells. These cells behave in an innate immune manner in terms of their ability to rapidly secrete Th2 (and other) cytokines in response to provocative challenge, but NK T cells and γδ T cells also possess antigen receptors characteristic of adaptive immune cells. Despite their pro-inflammatory potential, direct analysis of NK T cells suggests that they contribute little to airway allergic reactions.[42] There is yet insufficient study of γδ T cells to determine their role in allergic airway disease.

In addition to the principal Th2 cytokines, numerous additional soluble mediators contribute to the expression of allergic disease. The complement system is especially important, and complement proteins C3a and C5a, the major anaphylatoxins, are both essential for the expression and regulation of asthma in experimental systems. C3a signaling through the C3a receptor C3aR is required for robust Th2 responses, allergic inflammation, and airway hyper-responsiveness in response to airway allergen challenge. In contrast, C5a, which can signal through two receptors, C5aR and C5L2, appears to inhibit Th2 responses, perhaps acting as a physiological antagonist of the allergic disease-promoting activity of C3a.[43]

Lipid mediators of inflammation of importance to allergic airway disease include the leukotrienes (LTs), prostaglandins (PGs), and others. The cysteinyl leukotrienes (CysLTC4, -D4, and -E4) signal through at least two major receptors to mediate some of the same allergic disease features as IL-13, including airway inflammation and airway hyper-reactivity. Full expression of experimental allergic disease in fact appears to require the concomitant expression of both IL-13 and the CysLTs.[44,45] IL-13 appears to be the dominant allergic mediator, however, perhaps accounting in part for why LT antagonism alone is not as effective as inhaled steroids in asthma.[46] Non-cysteinyl leukotrienes such as LTB4 also contribute to the expression of allergic airway inflammation by controlling the recruitment of allergic effector cells including Th2 cells.[47]

Similarly, PGD_2 is an important mediator of Th2 cell recruitment and allergic airway inflammation in rodents, most likely acting cooperatively with LTB4 and chemokines.[47] Most other prostaglandins are thought to promote allergic airway disease, especially in aspirin-sensitive rhinitis and asthma.[48] An important exception to this is PGE_2, which exhibits potent anti-allergic activity by signaling through one of its five known receptors, EP3.[49]

Other lipid mediators likely contributing to the expression of allergic inflammation and airway obstruction are the thromboxanes and lipoxins. Whereas thromboxane A_2 is a potent pro-inflammatory lipid derived from platelets, lipoxins have the opposite effect and are anti-inflammatory.[50]

Environmental factors and allergic disease initiation

The earliest immunological events that initiate Th2 responses and the environmental factors that trigger them are incompletely understood. Currently, asthma and to a large extent rhinosinusitis and rhinitis are believed to represent aberrant immunological responses to innocuous inhaled antigens. The very strong association between asthma and atopy supports this concept, with many allergens being relatively innocuous proteins derived from organisms such as dust mites, cats, dogs, and plants that are not otherwise harmful or infectious. Atopy is further thought to represent a fundamental underlying condition that leads in some cases to overt allergic disease, but whether atopy represents primarily a genetically or environmentally controlled condition remains unclear. Extensive analysis of allergens has revealed no consistent structural features suggesting that physical properties are highly relevant to atopy and allergic disease expression.[51]

A major exception to the intrinsically innocuous nature of allergens are, however, the filamentous fungi such as *Aspergillus* spp. and other potentially infectious causes of allergic disease. Atopy to filamentous fungi in distinct allergic disease populations varies widely, ranging from 100% in AFRS, up to 66% of children with asthma or allergies in Kuwait, and to as few as 32% of asthmatic adults in Greece. Fungal sensitization is viewed as being no different from sensitization to any other allergen ubiquitously present in human environments. However, fungi differ from all other allergen sources in that they are ubiquitous and able to actively infect and grow within the respiratory tract.[52]

Fungal respiratory tract infection has been linked to a variety of disease syndromes, most dramatically highly lethal invasive and disseminated disease that is seen almost exclusively in the setting of severe neutropenia, but that is not allergic in nature. However, a fungal infectious basis for non-invasive allergic disease is also suggested by (1) the high rate of isolation of filamentous fungi from the airways in CRS, especially AFRS, and ABPA; (2) the universal presence of fungus-specific immunity in AFRS and ABPA subjects; (3) the efficacy of anti-fungal antibiotics when given to fungus-sensitized asthmatic patients; and (4) experimental validation that filamentous fungi are infectious for the mouse airway and readily produce allergic airway disease that is comparable to asthma. However, not all patients with allergic airway disease demonstrate fungus-specific immunity, nor are anti-fungal antibiotics effective in all such patients, especially those with CRS, and hence fungal airway infections may be etiologically relevant to only a subset of allergic disease patients.[52]

Other infectious agents also potentially contribute to allergic airway diseases. CRS with polyposis is associated with the presence of bacteria in the nasal passages and sinuses, especially *Staphylococcus aureus*. Superantigens secreted by *S. aureus* both stimulate release of Th2 cytokines and *in situ* IgE production. Moreover, asthmatic patients are more likely than non-asthmatic patients to have serum specific IgE to *S. aureus* enterotoxins.[53] Atypical bacteria (*Mycoplasma* and *Chlamydia* spp.) can also contribute to allergic disease by inducing vascular remodeling that promotes airway obstruction.[54] However, the most prominent link between infectious agents and allergic airway disease involves respiratory viruses, especially human rhinovirus (HRV). Approximately 70–80% of children and adults test positive for HRV during acute disease exacerbations. Other respiratory viruses are likely to contribute to allergic disease pathogenesis, although the mechanisms remain obscure.[55]

Non-infectious particulate and gaseous matter can also contribute to the expression of allergic disease. Of particular interest are the potentially critical roles played by tobacco smoke, diesel exhaust particles, and other forms of smoke. Enhanced exposure to such air pollution, especially proximity to major roadways, is strongly linked to asthma exacerbation and enhanced atopy. Diesel exhaust particles further enhance allergic airway responses in allergen-challenged rodents. In addition to carbon-predominant aerosols, ozone also enhances allergic airway responses. A common link tying these various forms of air pollution to allergic disease may be the induction of oxidative stress, which ultimately leads to enhanced activation of nuclear factor kappa B (NF-κB), enhanced Th2 cytokine release, and increased allergic inflammation.[56,57]

When considering the etiological role of any agent in allergic disease, it is important to distinguish initiating from exacerbating factors. Staphylococci and other bacteria and viruses generally fail to produce overt allergic disease when administered to the airways of experimental animals, and allergic inflammation is typically not observed with these agents during acute, symptomatic airway infections in human subjects. Similarly, diesel exhaust particles, tobacco smoke extract, and ozone do not induce allergic disease if inhaled in the absence of other pro-allergic factors. These agents elicit enhanced allergic responses only when administered concomitantly with an allergen. Thus, bacteria, viruses, and common air pollutants are unlikely to be initiators of allergic airway disease, but can serve as important co-factors, especially in disease exacerbations. In contrast, fungi have been clearly shown as single agents to initiate allergic disease, at least experimentally. Moreover, fungal airway infection is sufficient to induce atopy to innocuous bystander antigens, suggesting that fungal infection may underlie both atopy and respiratory tract allergic disease.[52]

Research from experimental systems has shed additional light on how allergens initiate allergic inflammation and disease. Although structural features of allergens are not linked to their allergic character, a common biochemical feature is protease activity. Where used industrially, proteases derived from bacteria, fungi, and plants have also been linked to occupational asthma. Moreover, proteases as single molecules are as effective as any complex allergen or fungal infection in inducing allergic airway inflammation and airway hyper-reactivity when administered to rodents. It is possible, but unlikely, that there exists sufficient protease activity in some household aerosols to induce asthma; typical household dust protease levels are probably far too low to actually induce disease. However, many household proteases are derived from fungi, suggesting again that airway infection due to these organisms, which would result in *in situ* protease production, may be an important mechanism underlying allergic disease induction. Some viruses, especially HRV, also produce proteases that are highly allergenic.

Other substances produced by fungi, especially chitin, induce allergic cytokine production by eosinophils and basophils and most likely contribute to allergic disease initiation. Lipopolysaccharide (LPS; endotoxin) derived from the cell walls of Gram-negative bacteria has been associated with allergic disease, particularly when complexed with allergens derived from dust mites. Thus, diverse substances secreted or shed by common environmental microbes are capable of acting as adjuvant factors for initiating or promoting allergic inflammation and airway disease.[58–60]

The critical molecular pathways activated by proteases, chitin, and LPS that elicit Th2 responses and allergic disease are incompletely defined. Analyses of diverse allergenic proteases suggest that they initiate a complex, airway epithelial-centered mechanism in which the epithelial cytokines thymic stromal lymphopoietin (TSLP) and IL-25 are induced and lead to robust Th2 cell commitment and allergic responses. Fungal proteases also induce expression of airway matrix metalloproteinase (MMP) 7, which is required for the biological activity of IL-25, and promote secretion of allergy-promoting airway chemokines (e.g., CCL17 and CCL11). Additional cellular targets of allergenic proteases potentially include airway dendritic cells and perhaps macrophages, although the molecular targets and effector pathways resulting from protease activation of these cells are unknown (Fig. 39.8).[61]

Proteolytically active allergens such as Der p 1 promote permeabilization of the respiratory epithelium by disrupting tight junction proteins, an effect that potentially enhances antigen detection and allergic immune responses. Proteases also have broad potential to disrupt normal airway immune homeostasis by cleaving airway immune molecules such as CD25, CD23, and numerous cytokines, ultimately leading to a pro-allergic immune environment (Fig. 39.8). The LPS receptor Toll-like receptor 4 (TLR4) has been linked to allergic lung disease in some

Fig. 39.8 Mechanisms of allergenic proteinase-dependent induction of allergic airway disease. Inhaled proteinases or proteinase sources (e.g., fungal spores) initiate a series of molecular events in discrete lung compartments and involving distinct cell types that induce predominant airway Th2 responses that coordinate both the allergic inflammation and physiological changes that typify allergic respiratory tract disease. Initial innate immune responses induced by proteinases include induction of airway chemokines that favor recruitment of allergic effector cells including Th2 cells (1). Likely airway cellular targets of proteinases include basophils, airway epithelial cells, and possibly airway smooth muscle cells (2). Activation of these cells by cleavage of cell surface receptors such as PAR2 and CD23 potentially leads to activation of these cells to produce pro-allergic cytokines such as TSLP and IL-25, the latter of which is activated by MMP7, an endogenous proteinase also induced by allergenic proteinases. Allergenic proteinases also likely act on soluble substrates such as complement, especially C3 to generate C3a, the ligand for the C3aR. CD25 is another immune receptor present on T cells that can be cleaved by proteinases, potentially to favor Th2 cytokine secretion. Finally, proteinases act directly on antigen presenting cells such as dendritic cells through an unknown mechanism in secondary lymphoid organs such as lymph nodes to promote their maturation in a manner that favors Th2 cell differentiation from naïve precursor (ThP) T cells (3).
Modified from: Porter PC, Yang T, Luong A, et al. Proteinases as molecular adjuvants in allergic airway disease. Biochim Biophys Acta 2011; 1810(11): 1059–1065.

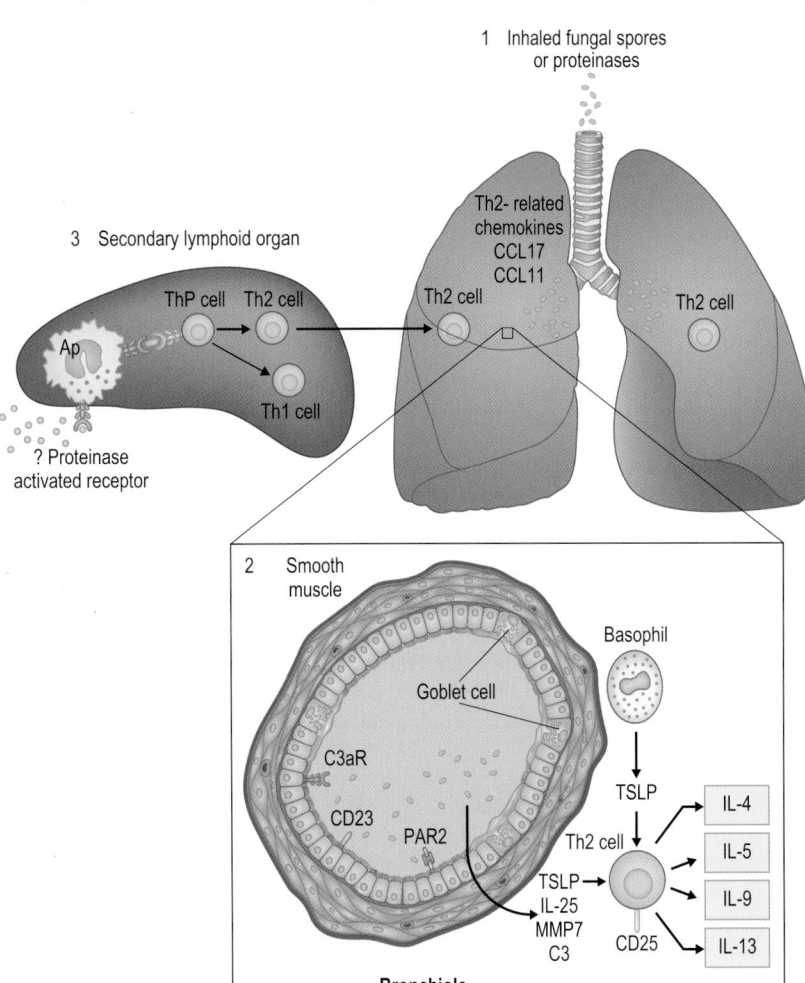

Non-allergic respiratory tract inflammatory syndromes

Although the majority of respiratory tract inflammatory disease is allergic, additional pulmonary immune-related disorders that are non-allergic exist and are responsible for considerable morbidity. The immunological mechanisms, etiologic environmental factors, and therapies for these diseases are distinct from common allergic disorders and hence warrant consideration in the differential diagnosis of airway inflammatory disorders. Two of the most important non-allergic airway obstructive immune disorders are hypersensitivity pneumonitis and chronic obstructive pulmonary disease.

Hypersensitivity pneumonitis (HP)

HP is a non-IgE-mediated inflammatory lung disease that results from recurrent exposure to any of a wide variety of inhaled antigenic aerosols containing organic and possibly infectious

contexts, but promotes an anti-allergic effect in others and thus plays an uncertain role in allergic disease. Activation of protease activated receptor 2 (PAR-2) and C3 may be important additional pathways by which allergenic proteases contribute directly to allergic disease initiation. Little is understood about possible chitin receptors in allergic disease.[61]

matter. Pulmonary involvement is typically diffuse and includes predominantly mononuclear inflammation of the terminal bronchioles, interstitium, and alveoli, with little involvement of the larger airways. Despite the term "extrinsic allergic alveolitis," another commonly used term for this disorder, low-grade eosinophilia is only seen in 1–3% of bronchoalveolar lavage specimens and is not a consistent or characteristic feature of disease. Over time, this pattern of inflammation leads to destruction of alveoli and to irreversible pulmonary fibrosis that may be fatal.

The etiology of HP is frequently idiopathic, but many cases can be traced to exposure to organic aerosols that contain thermophilic bacteria (e.g., *Saccharopolyspora rectivirgula*) commonly found in heated water reservoirs such as room humidifiers and hay; filamentous fungi (e.g., *Aspergillus* spp.); animal proteins and fecal matter (e.g., pigeon breeder's disease); and industrial chemicals such as isocyanates. Symptoms including chest tightness, chest pain, dyspnea, and fever appear 4 to 6 hours after exposure. Removal of the offending antigen may prevent the progression to chronic, irreversible disease. Other than oxygen therapy in the setting of profound hypoxemia, there is no defined medical therapy for HP; specifically, there is no role for glucocorticoids.

The immunopathogenesis of HP is complex and not well understood. During the acute presentation, the histological picture is that of an immune-complex mediated interstitial injury with a predominant neutrophilic infiltrate. Subsequent disease stages evolve into predominant mononuclear inflammatory infiltrates consisting of lymphocytes, plasma cells, and foamy macrophages, followed by granulomas. In advanced disease, fibrosis replaces the inflammatory infiltrates.

Acutely, HP is thought to be initiated by an immune-complex mediated hypersensitivity (type III) with *in situ* immune complex deposition in the lung interstitium that occurs as a result of the interaction of the inhaled antigen and pre-existing IgG antibodies in the alveolar spaces. Complement activation occurs and most likely contributes to the alveolitis and neutrophilia. However, many people with precipitating antibodies to putative HP antigens (precipitins) do not develop actual parenchymal or symptomatic disease.[62] Therefore, type IV or delayed type hypersensitivity reactions involving Th1 and possibly Th17 cells are also thought to play a role in disease expression.

Chronic obstructive pulmonary disease (COPD)

The disorder most frequently confused with asthma is COPD, which encompasses chronic bronchitis with or without emphysema. Chronic bronchitis is defined clinically by the presence of a daily cough productive of sputum for 3 months of a year for 2 consecutive years, while emphysema is an anatomical description of the enlargement and destruction of alveoli. COPD is currently the fourth leading cause of death in the world but is expected to reach third place by 2020. The most common cause of COPD is tobacco smoking, but chronic exposure to toxins such as coal dust, biomass fuels, and chronic respiratory infections have been linked to COPD in non-smokers. Because not all smokers develop COPD, disease initiation is thought to reflect the interaction of genetic susceptibility and environmental factors. To date, the only known gene linked to increased risk of early onset emphysema is mutations in the α_1-antitrypsin (*A1AT*) gene. Allelic variance in the *A1AT* gene accounts for only a small fraction of all cases of COPD, suggesting that many additional genes, as yet undiscovered, influence the expression of COPD.[63]

People who smoke often have low level respiratory symptoms and they only present to medical attention once these become disabling. In addition to cough and sputum production, COPD often presents clinically with an insidious onset of dyspnea and progressive and persistent exercise limitation, with minimal reversibility of airway obstruction. This contrasts with asthma, which is marked by paroxysms of dyspnea that usually resolve completely with therapy. Smokers with chronic bronchitis-predominant COPD with little emphysema often maintain normal body weight, but severe emphysema involving >25% of the lung is often associated with profound weight loss, cachexia, and airflow obstruction. Further, epidemiological studies have shown that lung cancer risk is strongly related to radiographic emphysema, independent of airflow obstruction. In contrast, non-smoking asthmatics carry no greater risk for lung cancer than the general non-smoking population.

The American Thoracic Society (ATS) and European Respiratory Society (ERS) have advocated the use of the lower limit of normal (LLN) based on the National Health and Nutrition Examination Survey (NHANES) data on lung function in a healthy population to diagnose COPD. Alternatively, the Global Initiative for Chronic Obstructive Lung Disease (GOLD) has in the past decade promoted the use of a fixed FEV_1/FVC ratio of less than 70% to diagnose COPD. This latter guideline is now widely used to classify smokers with and without COPD, but this stratification will exclude up to 20% of smokers with emphysema who have normal lung function.[64] Based on lung function and symptoms, smokers are categorized into one of four GOLD stages: mild, moderate, severe, and very severe. Radiographically, emphysema is characterized by hyperexpansion and hyperlucency of lung in the absence of pulmonary infiltrates and significant lung fibrosis. Computed tomography may also reveal generalized airway thickening and the abnormal enlargement of airspaces in a focal (centrilobular) or diffuse (panlobular) distribution, which despite its radiographic appearance, contains organized areas of inflammatory cell infiltrates (Fig. 39.9).

Macroscopically, the lungs of smokers with COPD are strikingly abnormal, virtually always assuming a diffuse dark brown or black appearance. Normal alveoli, which are typically of the order of 1 mm in size, are frequently replaced by much larger airspaces including blebs and bullae. Thickened airways with increased mucus content may also be seen grossly. Microscopically, the alveoli are often enlarged and contain increased numbers of macrophages containing black pigment. The alveolar walls and the peribronchiolar interstitium may contain a mixed inflammatory infiltrate consisting of neutrophils,

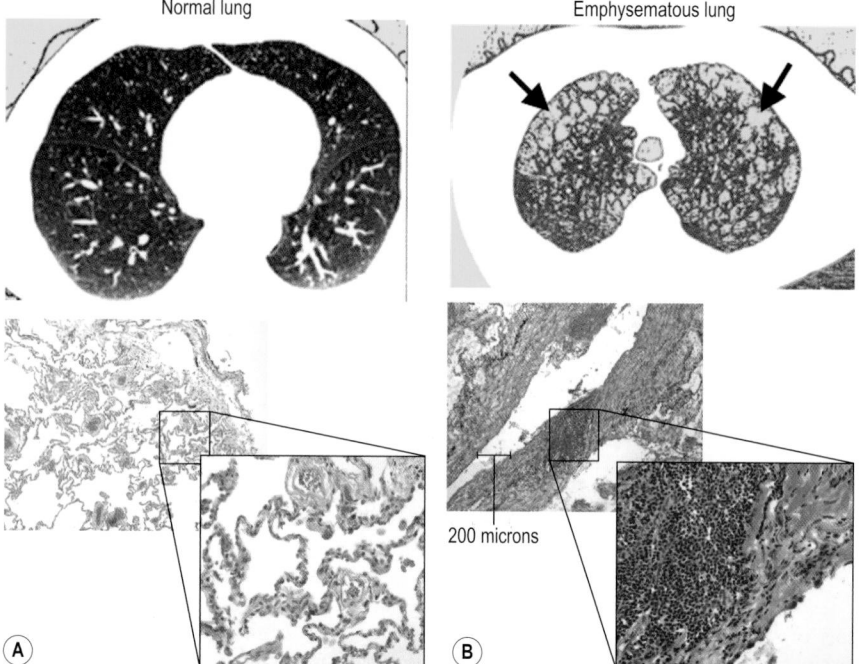

Normal lung

Emphysematous lung

200 microns

(A)   (B)

Fig. 39.9 Lung parenchymal destruction in smokers with COPD and emphysema. Representative computed tomography images show lungs of a smoker without (A) and with (B) emphysema; arrows point to low attenuation dark black areas devoid of lung tissue (emphysematous regions) within the diseased lung. Lower panels show representative low- and high-magnification histology images from human lung in each case; note the focal collection of mononuclear cells in emphysematous lung.

macrophages, and lymphocytes including plasma cells. Especially in chronic bronchitis, the smaller airways may be critically narrowed due to a combination of pathological changes that include squamous and goblet cell metaplasia of the airway epithelium, peribronchiolar inflammation, and mucus hypersecretion and impaction.

In contrast to asthma, airway obstruction, when present, is typically minimally or non-reversible in COPD even with use of bronchodilators. Moreover, lung destruction and airway obstruction often worsen irretrievably over time in emphysema despite smoking cessation, whereas acute episodes of airway obstruction in asthma are typically reversible. Loss of alveoli and permanent lung destruction are also not generally seen in asthma. Eosinophils are further distinctly absent in COPD that is not complicated by concomitant atopy and asthma. Thus, asthma and COPD are both common lung diseases marked by airway obstruction, but the environmental associations, natural histories, and radiographic and pathological manifestations that characterize the two disorders differ substantially.

The immunological basis of COPD differs markedly from asthma, but inflammation increasingly appears to be the fundamental underlying cause of both airway obstruction and lung destruction. In contrast to Th2 cells and other allergic effector cells that likely underlie disease in asthma, the major immune effector cells in COPD are Th1 and Th17 cells. Over the past five decades, macrophages and neutrophils were thought to drive the main pathophysiologic changes in human emphysema. Only after the discovery that adaptive immune cells are prominently recruited to the lungs of former smokers with emphysema did it become clear that T cells might be responsible for perpetuating inflammatory responses in the lungs even after cessation of tobacco smoke exposure.

Ultimately, lung destruction in COPD is due to enhanced production of matrix metalloproteinases and other enzymes that degrade elastin (elastases), including MMP2, MMP9, MMP12, and neutrophil elastase (NE). The activity of most of these enzymes is controlled by endogenous inhibitors such as tissue inhibitors of metalloproteinases (TIMPs) and A1AT, the principal antagonist of elastases. Cigarette smoke exposure is sufficient to both enhance elastase secretion from macrophages and neutrophils and reduce the activity of elastase inhibitors: in addition to elastin, MMP12 specifically inhibits A1AT, leading to unopposed NE activity. These biochemical events are critically important to the expression specifically of emphysema because elastin is an important matrix protein that is in part responsible for both the structural integrity of the lung and its elastance (ability to stretch). Emphysema, therefore, is the clinical expression of the immune-based loss of lung integrity due to enhanced expression of elastases.[65]

A highly characteristic feature of emphysema is its chronic and progressive nature despite smoking cessation, which suggests the involvement of adaptive immune mechanisms in addition to purely innate processes. Recent studies have confirmed the presence of activated T cells in lung interstitium in COPD that express characteristic markers of Th1 cells, including CXCR3. Further analysis of T cells extracted from the peripheral lung of smokers with stable, uncomplicated emphysema confirmed that these cells secrete IFN-γ and IL-17A in the absence of IL-4 and -13; T regulatory cells are also reduced in the lung periphery of these patients.

The discovery of Th1 and Th17 cytokines in emphysematous lung provides further insight into the immunological basis of lung destruction due to smoking. IL-17A promotes secretion of neutrophil chemokines, in part accounting for the chronic neutrophilia of COPD. IL-17A and IFN-γ further act coordinately to promote a pro-elastolytic lung environment. Chemokines induced by IFN-γ such as CXCL10 and IL-17A act directly to stimulate MMP12 secretion by macrophages. IL-17A further stimulates macrophage MMP12 secretion by promoting production of the chemokine CCL20, which simulates macrophage MMP12 release. Thus, tobacco smoke acutely elicits elastase secretion from innate immune cells, but ultimately induces a Th1/Th17-predominant adaptive immune response that underlies chronic inflammation and progressive emphysema even in persons who have stopped smoking.

The chronic, progressive, and incurable nature of emphysema further suggests an autoimmune basis to the underlying Th1 and Th17-predominant inflammation. Additional studies have confirmed that Th1 and Th17 cells from peripheral blood in severe emphysema are responsive to human elastin peptides, although other autoantigens likely exist. Thus, emphysema appears to be a Th1/Th17-driven lung inflammatory process that is initiated by cigarette smoke and involves both innate and autoimmune components that promote elastolysis, loss of lung integrity, and impaired lung function.[65] In addition to the lack of a prominent Th1/Th17 immune component, with the possible exception of severe disease exacerbation, no convincing evidence exists to suggest that asthma is an autoimmune disease.

Despite the marked pathophysiological differences between COPD and asthma, the treatment of COPD is, like asthma, aimed at reducing airway obstruction and other acute and chronic symptoms, including cough and mucus production. The most commonly used medications therefore include inhaled bronchodilators (beta agonists) and muscarinic antagonists such as ipratropium and tiotropium bromide supplemented with inhaled corticosteroids. The otherwise stable deterioration in lung function that characterizes COPD is punctuated in many patients by bouts of disease exacerbation marked by sudden, but transient worsening of lung function in the setting of an acute and febrile pneumonic or bronchitic syndrome. These episodes are thought to represent bouts of airway infection with viruses, especially HRV, or bacteria such as *Haemophilus influenzae*. Patients usually respond to anti-inflammatory therapy with glucocorticoids and antibiotics, but may not return to baseline lung function and often require mechanical ventilatory support.

Novel pathways to therapy in allergic airway disease

The long-standing perception that allergic airway disease is mediated primarily by IgE and immediate-hypersensitivity mechanisms has now yielded to the more nuanced view that allergic disease is immunologically quite complex and likely to involve multiple hypersensitivity mechanisms operating in parallel, likely with different mechanisms predominating at distinct levels of the airway (Fig. 39.6). Recent studies also suggest that factors other than allergens themselves likely critically influence the airway immune response to inhaled antigens. Such adjuvant factors potentially include cell wall products of bacteria and fungi such as LPS and chitin and secreted factors such as proteases. Evidence further increasingly suggests that asthma and rhinosinusitis may be linked to respiratory tract infections involving viruses, especially HRV, bacteria, especially *S. aureus*, and many filamentous fungi. Defining through additional studies how these factors contribute to allergic airway disease, if at all, has critically important implications for future therapy.

Current pharmacological therapy for asthma, rhinosinusitis, and rhinitis is non-specific and directed largely at the amelioration of inflammation and symptoms. Although surgical therapy for rhinosinusitis offers the possibility of substantial symptomatic relief, neither medical nor surgical therapies are sufficient to resolve disease. Moreover, the side effect burden of medical therapy for allergic disease is becoming increasingly apparent. In addition to the untoward effects of chronic glucocorticoid usage, involving weight gain and disorders of the gastrointestinal, cardiovascular, neurological, immune, and endocrine systems that may be fatal, long-acting beta agonists are now known to lead to worsening of asthma control and excess mortality when used as monotherapy.[66] Recently acquired insights into the pathophysiology of allergic airway disease, however, suggest that newer therapeutic approaches may be both more effective and safer than current approaches.

It will be essential as part of future studies to clarify the role of chronic infections due to bacteria and fungi in asthma and rhinosinusitis. Demonstration that fungal airway infection, for example, underlies disease in some patients would suggest that allergic airway inflammation is not an aberrant response to innocuous antigenic aerosols as currently believed, but may actually be beneficial in infection clearance.

Discovery that chronic airway infections cause or contribute to allergic disease expression would further support consideration of antimicrobial agents as the cornerstone of therapy. However, a major drawback to the use of antimicrobials for superficial, chronic mucosal infections is that it is not known if such agents, other than fluoroquinolones, concentrate in the respiratory tract lining fluid in microbicidal concentrations. The potential inhibitory effect of microbial biofilms and respiratory tract mucus and other secretions on antibiotic activity at the airway epithelial surface is further not well understood. Moreover, the frequency with which antibiotic resistance develops during chronic therapy of respiratory tract infections, especially with regard to fungi, is not known and, aside from monitoring symptoms, procedures for assessing antibiotic efficacy have not been established. Thus, much additional research is required to determine optimal medical therapy and monitoring of disease due to potential infectious agents. Protocols defining the optimal combinatorial use of surgery and antibiotics for chronic rhinosinusitis must also be established.

A major advantage to the therapy of respiratory tract disease of any kind is having the options for both aerosol delivery and topical therapy. Major agents used to treat asthma, rhinitis, and rhinosinusitis such as bronchodilators and glucocorticoids are available for aerosol delivery by metered dose inhalers or as additives to saline irrigations in addition to oral and parenteral formulations. Although potentially more costly on a weight basis when formulated for aerosol or topical delivery, less drug need be delivered for equivalent efficacy compared to other delivery routes. However, the greatest advantage of aerosol and topical delivery is the ability to direct drug only to where it is needed, thereby avoiding potentially serious side effects involving off-target organs. Due to technical difficulties in formulating for metered dose inhalers, which are commonly used devices for generating precisely dosed medication aerosols for inhalation, and the frequent denaturing of biologicals such as monoclonal antibodies during aerosolization through nebulization, future aerosolized medications for allergic airway disease are likely to be restricted to small molecules.

Regardless of the potential contribution of airway infections in asthma and rhinosinusitis, anti-inflammatory therapy will remain essential for disease control, but applied such that host defense is minimally compromised. Inhibition of type I hypersensitivity mechanisms with anti-IgE antibody (omalizumab), while modestly effective in asthma, has also shown modest benefit in rhinosinusitis. As established in experimental systems, inhibition of the IL-4/-13 signaling pathway with monoclonal antibodies is a potentially effective approach for asthma and initial clinical trials appear promising. However, the utility of this approach in upper respiratory tract allergic disease remains uncertain. Further approaches targeting other Th2 cytokines and effector cells such as IL-5, IL-9, and eosinophils are ongoing and may ultimately demonstrate effectiveness.

Perhaps more promising than targeting terminal allergic effector cells and cytokines is neutralization of early immune mediators of Th2 cell differentiation and recruitment, including IL-25, TSLP, MMP7, and airway chemokines, all of which are induced by proteases and participate critically in experimental allergic airway disease. Inhibition of C3a/C3aR signaling may also effectively preclude ongoing Th2 responses, but this complement anaphylatoxin pathway may be too generally important in host defense to represent a practical therapeutic target in allergic disease. Ultimately, the most specific, and likely most powerful, means of inhibiting allergic inflammation will be to block the immune receptors that initially respond to fungi, helminths, and other highly allergenic moieties. However, much further work is required to define such receptors and the critical signaling pathways that initiate robust and durable allergic responses required for allergic disease expression. Fundamental insight into the pathophysiology of airway inflammation has markedly advanced over the past decade of focused research and will increasingly influence how translational research on allergic and other airway disorders is conducted. Such research is already influencing the next generation of clinical trials in allergic disease. In addition to elucidating the molecular logic of how allergic inflammation mediates airway obstruction and other disease features, the critical role that environmental exposures play in initiating allergic inflammation has increasingly been recognized. Over the next decade, investigators must prioritize clarifying the importance of specific environmental factors, especially infectious agents such as fungi, bacteria, and viruses, and adjuvant substances such as proteases, chitin, and air pollutants, in the initiation and perpetuation of allergic inflammation and disease. Knowledge gained in these areas will subsequently drive creation of the next generation of diagnostic and therapeutic approaches critically needed to combat these most common of human immunological diseases.

References

1. Bousquet J, Khaltaev N, Cruz AA, et al. Allergic Rhinitis and its Impact on Asthma (ARIA) 2008 update. Allergy 2008;63(Suppl. 86):8–160.
2. Meltzer EO, Hamilos DL, Hadley JA, et al. Rhinosinusitis: developing guidance for clinical trials. J Allergy Clin Immunol 2006;118(5 Suppl.):S17–61.
3. Rosenfeld RM, Andes D, Bhattacharyya N, et al. Clinical practice guideline: adult sinusitis. Otolaryngol Head Neck Surg 2007;137(3 Suppl.):S1–31.
4. Wu AW, Shapiro NL, Bhattacharyya N. Chronic rhinosinusitis in children: what are the treatment options? Immunol Allergy Clin North Am 2009;29(4):705–17.
5. Cockcroft DW, Davis BE, Boulet LP, et al. The links between allergen skin test sensitivity, airway responsiveness and airway response to allergen. Allergy 2005;60(1):56–9.
6. Calabria CW, Dietrich J, Hagan L. Comparison of serum-specific IgE (ImmunoCAP) and skin-prick test results for 53 inhalant allergens in patients with chronic rhinitis. Allergy Asthma Proc 2009;30(4):386–96.
7. Pynnonen M, Fowler K, Terrell JE. Clinical predictors of chronic rhinosinusitis. Am J Rhinol 2007;21(2):159–63.
8. Bent 3rd JP, Kuhn FA. Diagnosis of allergic fungal sinusitis. Otolaryngol Head Neck Surg 1994;111(5):580–8.
9. Mukherji SK, Figueroa RE, Ginsberg LE, et al. Allergic fungal sinusitis: CT findings. Radiology 1998;207(2):417–22.
10. Scadding GK, Durham SR, Mirakian R, et al. BSACI guidelines for the management of rhinosinusitis and nasal polyposis. Clin Exp Allergy 2008;38(2):260–75.
11. Lumry WR. A review of the preclinical and clinical data of newer intranasal steroids used in the treatment of allergic rhinitis. J Allergy Clin Immunol 1999;104(4 Pt 1):S150–8.
12. Brozek JL, Bousquet J, Baena-Cagnani CE, et al. Allergic Rhinitis and its Impact on Asthma (ARIA) guidelines: 2010 revision. J Allergy Clin Immunol 2010;126(3):466–76.
13. Niggemann B, Jacobsen L, Dreborg S, et al. Five-year follow-up on the PAT study: specific immunotherapy and long-term prevention of asthma in children. Allergy 2006;61:855–9.
14. Bjornsdottir US, Jakobinudottir S, Runarsdottir V, Juliusson S. The effect of reducing levels of cat allergen (Fel d 1) on clinical symptoms in patients with cat allergy. Ann Allergy Asthma Immunol 2003;91(2):189–94.
15. Ragab SM, Lund VJ, Scadding G. Evaluation of the medical and surgical treatment of chronic rhinosinusitis: a prospective, randomised, controlled trial. Laryngoscope 2004;114(5):923–30.
16. Joe SA, Thambi R, Huang J. A systematic review of the use of intranasal steroids in the treatment of chronic rhinosinusitis. Otolaryngol Head Neck Surg 2008;139(3):340–7.
17. Seiberling K, Wormald PJ. The role of itraconazole in recalcitrant fungal sinusitis. Am J Rhinol Allergy 2009;23(3):303–6.
18. Chan KO, Genoway KA, Javer AR. Effectiveness of itraconazole in the management of refractory allergic fungal rhinosinusitis. J Otolaryngol Head Neck Surg 2008;37(6):870–4.
19. Anandan C, Nurmatov U, van Schayck OC, Sheikh A. Is the prevalence of asthma declining? Systematic review of epidemiological studies. Allergy 2010;65(2):152–67.
20. Peat JK, Salome CM, Woolcock AJ. Factors associated with bronchial hyperresponsiveness in Australian adults and children. Eur Respir J 1992;5(8):921–9.
21. Corry DB, Irvin CG. Promise and pitfalls in animal-based asthma research: Building a better mousetrap. Immunol Res 2006;35(3):279–94.
22. Kelly HW. Non-corticosteroid therapy for the long-term control of asthma. Expert Opin Pharmacother 2007;8(13):2077–87.
23. Lee JH, Park HK, Heo J, et al. Drug rash with eosinophilia and systemic symptoms (DRESS) syndrome induced by celecoxib and anti-tuberculosis drugs. J Korean Med Sci 2008;23(3):521–5.
24. Hartl D, Latzin P, Zissel G, et al. Chemokines indicate allergic bronchopulmonary aspergillosis in patients with cystic fibrosis. Am J Respir Crit Care Med 2006;173(12):1370–6.
25. Wark PA, Gibson PG, Wilson AJ. Azoles for allergic bronchopulmonary aspergillosis associated with asthma. Cochrane Database Syst Rev 2003;3:CD001108.
26. Swartz J, Stoller JK. Acute eosinophilic pneumonia complicating Coccidioides immitis pneumonia: a case report and literature review. Respiration 2009;77(1):102–6.
27. Uchiyama H, Suda T, Nakamura Y, et al. Alterations in smoking habits are associated with acute eosinophilic pneumonia. Chest 2008;133(5):1174–80.
28. Yoshimi M, Nannya Y, Watanabe T, et al. Acute eosinophilic pneumonia is a non-infectious lung complication after allogeneic hematopoietic stem cell transplantation. Int J Hematol 2009;89(2):244–8.
29. Cottin V, Frognier R, Monnot H, et al. Chronic eosinophilic pneumonia after radiation therapy for breast cancer. Eur Respir J 2004;23(1):9–13.
30. Bain B. The idiopathic hypereosinophilic syndrome and eosinophilic leukemias. Haematologica 2004;89(2):133–7.
31. Fauci AS, Harley JB, Roberts WC, et al. NIH conference. The idiopathic hypereosinophilic syndrome. Clinical, pathophysiologic, and therapeutic considerations. Ann Int Med 1982;97(1):78–92.
32. Wechsler ME, Finn D, Gunawardena D, et al. Churg-Strauss syndrome in patients receiving montelukast as treatment for asthma. Chest 2000;117(3):708–13.
33. Wechsler ME, Wong DA, Miller MK, Lawrence-Miyasaki L. Churg-Strauss syndrome in patients treated with omalizumab. Chest 2009;136(2):507–18.
34. Gell PGH, Coombs RRA. Clinical Aspects of Immunology. Oxford, England: Blackwell; 1963.
35. Huber S, Hoffmann R, Muskens F, Voehringer D. Alternatively activated macrophages inhibit T-cell proliferation by Stat6-dependent expression of PD-L2. Blood 2010;116(17):3311–20.
36. Fireman P. Understanding asthma pathophysiology. Allergy Asthma Proc 2003;24(2):79–83.
37. Rosenwasser LJ. Mechanisms of IgE inflammation. Curr Allergy Asthma Rep 2011;11(2):178–83.
38. Molfino NA, Nannini LJ, Martelli AN, Slutsky AS. Respiratory arrest in near-fatal asthma. N Engl J Med 1991;324(5):285–8.
39. Corry DB. Emerging immune targets for the therapy of allergic asthma. Nature Rev Drug Discov 2002;1:55–64.
40. Wills-Karp M. Immunologic basis of antigen-induced airway hyperresponsiveness. Annu Rev Immunol 1999;17:255–81.
41. Rothenberg ME, Hogan SP. The eosinophil. Ann Rev Immunol 2006;24:147–74.
42. Afshar R, Medoff BD, Luster AD. Allergic asthma: a tale of many T cells. Clin Exp Allergy 2008;38(12):1847–57.
43. Zhang X, Kohl J. A complex role for complement in allergic asthma. Exp Rev Clin Immunol 2010;6(2):269–77.
44. Vargaftig BB, Singer M. Leukotrienes mediate murine bronchopulmonary hyperreactivity, inflammation, and part of mucosal metaplasia and tissue injury induced by recombinant murine interleukin-13. Am J Respir Cell Mol Biol 2003;28(4):410–9.
45. Chavez J, Young HWJ, Corry DB, Lieberman MW. Interactions between leukotriene C4 and interleukin 13 signaling pathways in a mouse model of airway disease. Arch Pathol Lab Med 2006;130(4):440–6.
46. Montuschi P, Peters-Golden ML. Leukotriene modifiers for asthma treatment. Clin Exp Allergy 2010;40(12):1732–41.
47. Luster AD, Tager AM. T-cell trafficking in asthma: lipid mediators grease the way. Nat Rev Immunol 2004;4(9):711–24.
48. Guilemany JM, Roca-Ferrer J, Mullol J. Cyclooxygenases and the pathogenesis of chronic rhinosinusitis and nasal polyposis. Curr Allergy Asthma Rep 2008;8(3):219–26.
49. Corry DB. Resolving a case of split personality. Nat Immunol 2005;6(5):432–4.
50. Bonnans C, Levy BD. Lipid mediators as agonists for the resolution of acute lung inflammation and injury. Am J Respir Cell Mol Biol 2007;36(2):201–205.
51. Aalberse RC. Structural biology of allergens. J Allergy Clin Immunol 2000;106(2):228–38.
52. Porter P, Polikepahad S, Qian Y, et al. Respiratory tract allergic disease and atopy: experimental evidence for a fungal infectious etiology. Med Mycol 2011;49(1):S158–63.
53. Pastacaldi C, Lewis P, Howarth P. Staphylococci and staphylococcal superantigens in asthma and rhinitis: a systematic review and meta-analysis. Allergy 2011;66(4):549–55.
54. Metz G, Kraft M. Effects of atypical infections with Mycoplasma and Chlamydia on asthma. Immunol Allergy Clin North Am 2010;30(4):575–85.
55. Newcomb DC, Peebles Jr. RS. Bugs and asthma: a different disease? Proc Am Thorac Soc 2009;6(3):266–71.
56. Dozor AJ. The role of oxidative stress in the pathogenesis and treatment of asthma. Ann N Y Acad Sci 2010;1203:133–7.
57. Riedl M, Diaz-Sanchez D. Biology of diesel exhaust effects on respiratory function. J Allergy Clin Immunol 2005;115(2):221–8.
58. Reese TA, Liang H-E, Tager AM, et al. Chitin induces accumulation in tissue of innate immune cells associated with allergy. Nature 2007;447(7140):92–6.
59. Trompette A, Divanovic S, Visintin A, et al. Allergenicity resulting from functional mimicry of a Toll-like receptor complex protein. Nature 2009;457(7229):585–8.
60. Singh M, Lee SH, Porter P, et al. Human rhinovirus proteinase 2A induces TH1 and TH2 immunity in patients with chronic obstructive pulmonary disease. J Allergy Clin Immunol 2010;125(6):1369–78.
61. Porter PC, Yang T, Luong A, et al. Proteinases as molecular adjuvants in allergic airway disease. Biochim Biophys Acta 2011;1810(11):1059–65.
62. Richerson HB, Bernstein IL, Fink JN, et al. Guidelines for the clinical evaluation of hypersensitivity pneumonitis. Report of the Subcommittee on Hypersensitivity Pneumonitis. J Allergy Clin Immunol 1989;84(5 Pt 2):839–44.
63. Castaldi PJ, Cho MH, Cohn M, et al. The COPD genetic association compendium: a comprehensive online database of COPD genetic associations. Hum Mol Genet 2010;19(3):526–34.
64. Hesselbacher S, Ross R, Schabath M, et al. Cross-sectional analysis of the utility of pulmonary function tests in predicting emphysema in ever-smokers. Int J Environ Research Public Health 2011;8(5):1324–40.
65. Gadgil A, Duncan SR. Role of T-lymphocytes and pro-inflammatory mediators in the pathogenesis of chronic obstructive pulmonary disease. Int J Copd 2008;3(4):531–41.
66. Rodrigo GJ, Moral VP, Marcos LG, Castro-Rodriguez JA. Safety of regular use of long-acting beta agonists as monotherapy or added to inhaled corticosteroids in asthma. A systematic review. Pulm Pharmacol Ther 2009;22(1):9–19.

Elena Borzova,
Clive E.H. Grattan

Urticaria, angioedema, and anaphylaxis

Urticaria is a common skin disorder that can lead to severe impairment of quality of life. Recently, there has been substantial progress in our knowledge and understanding of the pathophysiology of the condition, offering new diagnostic and treatment approaches for at least some patients. However, in many cases, urticaria is still a disease of unknown etiology that is difficult to manage effectively.

Definition

Urticaria is a heterogeneous group of disorders that share a distinct skin reaction pattern, i.e., the development of urticarial skin lesions.[1] Urticarial lesions resulting from localized edema of the upper dermis are called wheals (Fig. 40.1), whereas pronounced swelling of deeper dermal layers, subcutis, and submucosal tissues is known as angioedema (Fig. 40.2).

KEY CONCEPTS

Definition of urticaria

- Urticaria is characterized by superficial and deep swellings.
- Wheals are superficial swellings of the dermis of skin: they are pale and itchy with surrounding redness when they appear and then become pink before fading.
- Angioedema is a deep swelling below the skin or mucosa that usually lasts longer than wheals and may be painful rather than itchy.
- Wheals may occur alone or together with angioedema in urticaria.
- Acute urticaria lasts less than 6 weeks. It is common and often caused by viral infections. Urticaria due to drugs and foods falls in this category, but the diagnosis is usually clear from the history.
- Chronic urticaria lasts 6 weeks or more with continuous disease activity. A cause may not be found. Urticaria occurring intermittently over a period of more than 6 weeks can be defined as episodic.
- When angioedema occurs without wheals, C1 esterase inhibitor deficiency should be excluded.

Epidemiology

Urticaria is common: up to 25% of the general population experience some form of urticaria at least once over their lifetime, whereas the lifetime prevalence of chronic urticaria (CU) is between 0.1 and 3% of the general population.[2,3] Acute urticaria affects mainly young adults with an obvious female preponderance,[3] whereas CU is more common in adults, affecting mainly middle-aged women, and is rare in children and adolescents.[2–4] By definition, acute urticaria resolves within 6 weeks, whereas CU may last for years. Rarely, CU may last for >10 years. However, CU is almost always a self-limiting disorder, resolving spontaneously in 50% patients within 6 months of onset.[4]

Genetics

With the exception of hereditary angioedema and the hereditary auto-inflammatory periodic syndromes, urticaria does not show mendelian inheritance. Nevertheless, there is some evidence of genetic predisposition and human leukocyte antigen (HLA) associations in CU.[5–8]

Although earlier studies found no association between HLA class I antigens and CU, a recent study suggested an increased frequency of HLA-Bw4 in CU.[5] Several associations have been reported for class II HLA antigens in CU in different ethnic populations. A link between CU and HLA-DRB1*04 (DR4) and its associated allele, DQB1*0302 (DQ8), was found in British CU patients with evidence of functional autoantibodies compared with a control population. This link with the HLA-DR4 haplotype was also confirmed in Turkish CU patients,[7] while strong associations with HLA-DRB1*1302 and DQB1*0609 alleles were found for aspirin-induced urticaria in Korean patients.[8]

Clinical patterns

Urticaria is often classified by the duration of continuous activity into acute (less than 6 weeks), chronic (6 weeks of more), or episodic, where short episodes occur repeatedly over a period of time. This classification has the merit of simplicity but takes no account of etiology or clinical features that may help clinical management or research. Classification of urticaria by etiology is satisfying academically but of little value in the clinic, where the etiology is often unknown and management decisions have to be based solely on the clinical assessment.[9]

Etiopathogenesis and etiological classification

Although many aspects of the pathophysiology of urticaria remain unclear, our understanding has advanced considerably over the last two decades, allowing an etiological classification (Table 40.1).

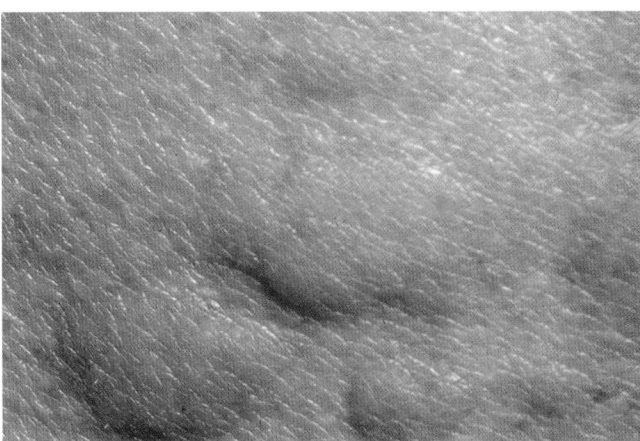

Fig. 40.1 Spontaneous wheals in severe ordinary urticaria showing superficial pink swellings with pale edematous centers.

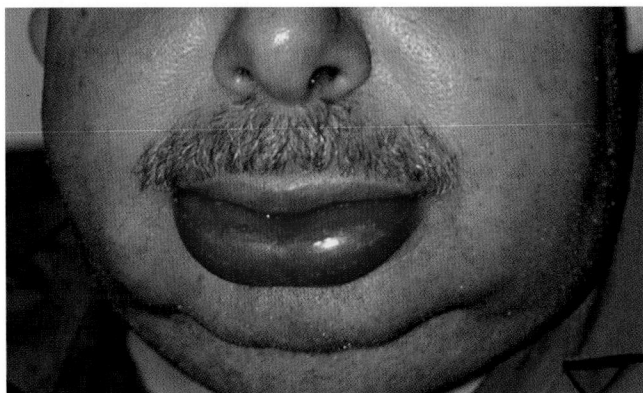

Fig. 40.2 Angioedema of the mouth in acquired C1 esterase inhibitor deficiency.

Table 40.1 Clinical patterns of urticaria
Spontaneous (ordinary) urticarial
Acute
Chronic
Episodic
Inducible urticaria
Mechanical: dermographism, delayed-pressure urticaria, vibratory angioedema
Thermal: cold-induced urticaria, localized heat-induced urticaria
Cholinergic urticaria and pruritus
Aquagenic urticaria and pruritus
Solar urticaria
Exercise (and food) induced anaphylaxis
Contact urticaria
Angioedema without wheals
Angioedema, due to C1 inhibitor deficiency
Angioedema with normal C1 inhibitor
Urticarial vasculitis
Normocomplementemic urticarial vasculitis
Hypocomplementemic urticarial vasculitis
Autoinflammatory syndromes (presenting with urticaria)
Hereditary (cryopyrin-associated) periodic syndromes
Familial cold autoinflammatory syndrome
Muckle–Wells syndrome
Chronic infantile neurological cutaneous and articular syndrome
Acquired
Schnitzler's syndrome

Mast cell-dependent mechanisms

Skin mast cells are key players in the pathogenesis of urticaria. They are predominantly located around the small blood and lymphatic vessels as well as around or within peripheral nerves.[3] Mast cell population density is greatest at distal body areas, including the face, hands, and feet.[10] There is conflicting evidence as to whether the number of cutaneous mast cells in urticaria patients is increased but there is general agreement that they release mediators more readily than normal.

Human skin mast cells contain preformed mediators in their granules, including histamine, proteases (tryptase, chymase), and heparin. They express many membrane receptors, including high-affinity immunoglobulin E (IgE) and low-affinity IgG receptors. Unlike mast cells elsewhere (pulmonary and intestinal), skin mast cells possess complement C5a receptors and activation sites for neuropeptides and basic secretagogues.[4]

Skin mast cell activation is central to the pathophysiology of CU. Mast cells can be activated by a variety of immunological and nonimmunological triggers (Fig. 40.3).[11] Immunological and nonimmunological pathways of mast cell activation are characterized by distinct patterns of mediator release. Immunological activation of mast cells requires prior sensitization and is triggered by cross-linking of high-affinity IgE receptors (FcεRI) by antigen bound to antigen-specific IgE, by anti-FcεRIa, or by anti-IgE antibodies. Histamine release peaks at 5–10 minutes, followed by *de novo* synthesis of lipid-derived mediators (leukotriene C4 and prostaglandin D2) and cytokines.[12] In contrast, nonimmunological stimulation of mast cells by neuropeptides, opiates, compound 48/80, or C5a leads to rapid histamine release within 15–20 seconds, without generation of eicosanoids and cytokines.[12] Moreover, prolonged and subthreshold immunological stimulation may result in a state of receptor desensitization. For example, desensitization of FcεRI may lead to basophil hyporesponsiveness to anti-IgE in autoimmune CU.[13] However, the desensitization of receptors by immunological stimulation does not affect nonimmunological release. Interestingly, enhanced responsiveness of skin mast cells to some nonimmunological stimuli has been observed in patients with CU.

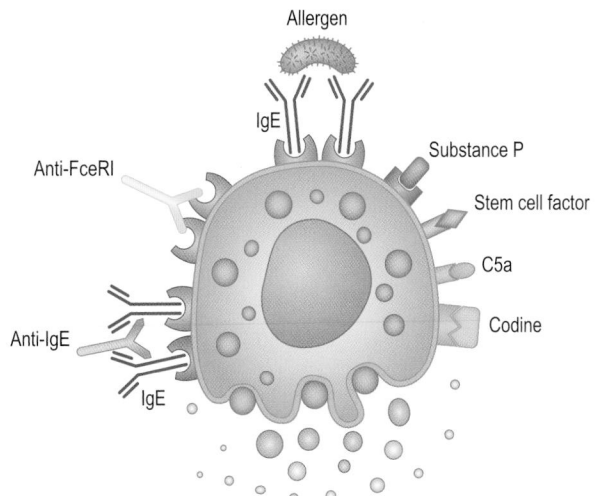

Fig. 40.3 Schematic representation of a mast cell or basophil illustrating activation of the immunoglobulin E (IgE) receptor by cross-linking with immunological stimuli (allergen/specific IgE binding, anti-IgE, or anti-FceRI autoantibodies) or independent activation by nonimmunological stimuli (substance P, stem cell factor, codeine, or C5a) leading to degranulation.

Allergic urticaria

Immunological triggers of mast cell activation play an important role in different types of urticaria.[3,11] The classical example of immunological mast cell activation via high-affinity IgE receptors is IgE-mediated urticaria (often termed allergic urticaria). In allergic urticaria, the cross-linking of receptor-bound IgE leads to the release of diverse preformed mediators and newly synthesized lipid mediators and cytokines, resulting in the early and late-phase IgE-mediated allergic inflammatory responses.

IgE-mediated mast cell activation usually presents as acute allergic urticaria in sensitized individuals and is very rarely, if ever, responsible for chronic whealing. Examples include some food- and drug-induced urticarias and latex-induced contact urticaria. Allergic urticaria to inhaled allergens (e.g., latex, animal epithelia) is often accompanied by respiratory symptoms. Generalized allergic urticaria may progress to anaphylaxis. Allergic urticaria resolves rapidly on withdrawal of allergen exposure and recurs with each re-exposure to the allergen or cross-reactive agents.

Autoimmune urticaria

Autoimmune urticaria is mediated by histamine-releasing auto-antibodies directed against the extracellular α-chain of FcεRI on dermal mast cells or basophils or, less frequently, against receptor-bound IgE. These functional autoantibodies have been demonstrated by several independent research groups in 25–50% of adult and pediatric patients with the ordinary presentation of CU.[13,14] The pathophysiology of autoimmune CU involves cross-linking of high-affinity IgE receptors by autoantibodies leading to degranulation of mast cells and basophils. There is good evidence that activation of cutaneous mast cells by IgG derived from CU sera *in vitro* is dependent on C5a but not all histamine-releasing IgG derived from CU sera are complement-dependent on basophil assays. Most functional autoantibodies are IgG1 or IgG3,[14] which are known to fix complement. By contrast, nonfunctional anti-FcεRI autoantibodies demonstrated by Western blot or enzyme-linked immunosorbent assay (ELISA) in other autoimmune diseases (including systemic lupus erythematosus and bullous pemphigoid) are generally from the noncomplement-fixing subclasses IgG2 and IgG4.[14]

Recently, anti-CD23 antibodies have also been detected in CU patients.[15] The low-affinity IgE receptor FcεRII/CD23 expressed on B lymphocytes and eosinophils may therefore be another target antigen for an autoimmune response in CU. The interaction between anti-CD23 antibodies and CD23 on eosinophils may induce release of major basic protein 1 (MBP-1), a potent IgE-independent histamine-releasing agent, resulting in activation of mast cells and basophils. The clinical relevance of anti-CD23 antibodies in CU remains to be elucidated but they may play a role in CU patients without autoantibodies against FcεRI or IgE.

Immune complex-mediated urticaria

Mast cell activation can result from binding of circulating immune complexes to FcγRIII, expressed on mast cells.[3,11] In addition, circulating immune complexes can activate complement, leading to C3a and C5a anaphylatoxin formation. Urticaria caused by immune complexes can occur in serum sickness-like reactions, transfusion reactions, some drug-induced urticarias, and urticaria associated with infectious or autoimmune diseases. Immune complex-mediated urticaria usually develops 1–3 weeks after initial exposure to the antigen and disappears several weeks after antigen discontinuation. Chronic immune complex-mediated urticaria is known as urticarial vasculitis (UV: see below). In this condition, urticaria can be associated with systemic symptoms, such as fever, arthritis, or nephritis. Damage to post-capillary venules results from the deposition of immune complexes in the vessel wall. Immune complexes are formed on exposure to external (drug or infections) or internal (collagen-like region of C1q) antigens. Complement activation via the classical pathway leads to neutrophil chemotaxis through cytokine expression and adhesion molecule activation (Fig. 40.4). Proteolytic enzymes released from neutrophils damage vessel walls, leading to wheal formation and red blood cell extravasation.

Nonimmunological mast cell activation

Skin mast cells can be activated nonimmunologically by many agents, including neuropeptides (substance P, neuropeptide Y, vasoactive intestinal peptide, or somatostatin), calcitonin gene-related protein, compound 48/80, and natural polyamines.[3,11,12] Drugs (e.g., opiates, muscle relaxants, radiocontrast media, polymyxin B) can also cause dose-dependent nonimmunological urticaria by activating membrane-associated G-coupled proteins. A classical clinical example is codeine-induced acute urticaria.

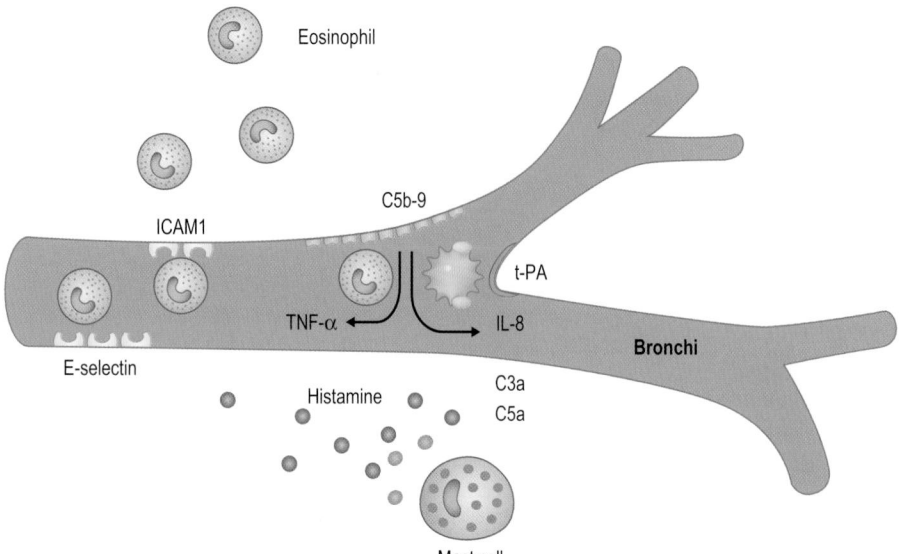

Fig. 40.4 Immune complex-mediated urticaria initiated by lodging of antigenic complexes in small blood vessels followed by C3a and C5a generation. This results in mast cell degranulation and cytokine upregulation of adhesion molecules (ICAM-1, E-selectin) by tumor necrosis factor-α (TNF-α) and interleukin-8 (IL-8), which leads to tissue recruitment of neutrophils and esoinophils and activation of tissue plasminogen activator (t-PA).

Mast cell and basophil releasability in urticaria

Besides the nature of the stimulus, the clinical signs of urticaria also depend on the releasability of effector mast cells in urticaria. In CU patients, dermal mast cells show a decreased activation threshold. Although CU basophils are hyporesponsive to immunological stimuli such as anti-IgE, they are paradoxically hyperresponsive to an as-yet unidentified factor in normal human serum.[14]

Skin response to mast cell activation in chronic urticaria

Despite there being different pathways for mast cell activation, the end result is degranulation with release or secretion of mediators. Histamine is crucial for the development of cutaneous manifestations of urticaria and is found in high concentrations in tissue fluid of wheals. It causes localized redness due to vasodilatation, wheal formation resulting from increased vascular permeability and edema, and a surrounding axon reflex-mediated flare. Histamine is also the main, if not the only, mediator of pruritus in urticaria. However, wheals caused by histamine alone are short-lived whereas urticarial lesions may persist up to 24 hours, implying that other pro-inflammatory mediators must also contribute.

Mast cell-independent mechanisms of urticaria

Pseudoallergy

Pseudoallergy or nonallergic hypersensitivity clinically mimics immediate-type allergic reactions without any evidence of underlying immunological mechanisms.[16] The most common triggers of pseudoallergic reactions are aspirin and other nonsteroidal anti-inflammatory drugs (NSAIDs) as well as some food ingredients and additives such as salicylates, benzoates, and tartrazine.[16] These reactions do not involve sensitization and can, therefore, occur on first exposure to the culprit agent. Pseudoallergic reactions are dose-dependent and usually occur with chemically nonrelated substances. The diagnosis is difficult because skin tests and serology are irrelevant. Diagnosis of nonallergic hypersensitivity is based on a distinctive clinical pattern, time course, clinical signs, and response on elimination of the cause. In the appropriate clinical context, pseudoallergy can be confirmed with oral challenge tests.

NSAIDs

Aspirin and other NSAIDs inhibit constitutive cyclooxygenase (COX-1) and inducible cyclooxygenase (COX-2), thereby diverting arachidonic acid metabolism towards the 5-lipoxygenase pathway in some cell types, notably eosinophils. This modulation of arachidonic acid metabolism results in overproduction of cysteinyl-leukotrienes LTC4, D4, and E4, leading to vasodilatation and edema. Furthermore, reduction of prostaglandin E2 formation by COX inhibition has two further effects that promote urticaria: first, by reducing inhibition of cysteinyl leukotriene production and second, by reducing an inhibitory effect on immunologically mediated mast cell degranulation (Fig. 40.5). Cross-sensitivity occurs with other nonselective NSAIDs in susceptible individuals, depending on their pharmacological potency for COX inhibition but not their chemical structure. Although coxibs, which are relatively selective inhibitors of the COX-2 isoenzyme, do not precipitate symptoms in most NSAID-sensitive patients, skin reactions have been reported.

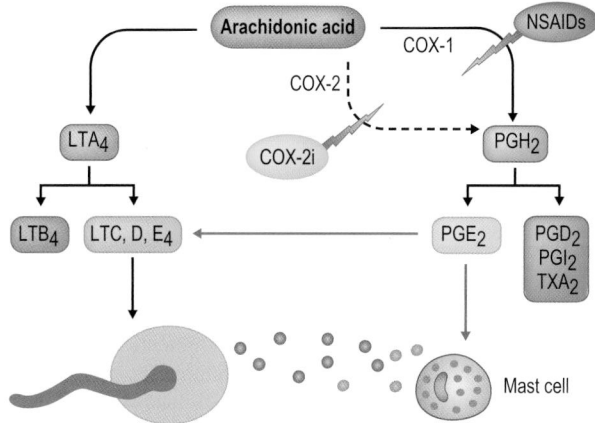

Fig. 40.5 Arachidonic acid pathways illustrating potential diversion from prostaglandin synthesis to cysteinyl leukotrienes (LTC4, D4, E4) by blocking cyclooxygenase (COX), leading to increased vasopermeability. Reduction of prostaglandin E2 also reduces its direct inhibitory effect on leukotriene production and on immunological mast cell degranulation.

Aspirin and NSAIDs can trigger acute urticaria as well as causing flare-ups of pre-existing chronic ordinary (but not physical) urticaria. Aspirin-induced exacerbations have been reported in 20–40% of patients with CU.[3,17] Moreover, acute aspirin-induced urticaria appears to be a risk factor for the development of CU.[17] In some patients aspirin can act as a co-factor in food- or exercise-induced anaphylaxis.

Urticaria can develop from a few minutes to 24 hours after aspirin ingestion but usually starts within 1–2 hours. Angioedema of the lips and tongue, impaired swallowing, and laryngeal edema develop occasionally. Aspirin-induced skin symptoms usually subside 24–48 hours after discontinuing the drug. However, severe exacerbations of CU caused by aspirin and other NSAIDs can last from several days to several weeks after aspirin intake.[17]

There are no skin tests or reliable *in vitro* diagnostic techniques for patients with aspirin-induced urticaria, and the diagnosis can only be established by challenge tests. Patients should avoid aspirin and other NSAIDs, but COX-2 inhibitors (coxibs) are usually well tolerated and can probably be used safely. Leukotriene receptor antagonists and 5-lipoxygenase inhibitors can be beneficial in the management of aspirin- and NSAID-evoked urticaria, but their efficacy still needs to be confirmed in well-designed studies.[18]

Food-induced pseudoallergic reactions in chronic urticaria

Pseudoallergic food reactions appear to be important in some CU patients. Pseudoallergic food triggers include natural salicylates and artificial food additives, such as benzoates and tartrazine. Low-molecular-weight aromatic compounds in tomatoes, white wine, and herbs have also been implicated.[16] Clinically, exacerbations of CU due to dietary pseudoallergens gradually subside within 10–14 days on an exclusion diet; in contrast, in 1–3 days in allergic urticaria. One study showed increased gastroduodenal and intestinal permeability in CU patients. Those who responded to elimination of pseudoallergens in their diet demonstrated normalization of mucosal permeability and skin symptoms. Although the underlying mechanisms for pseudoallergic reactions in CU remain unproven, an impaired gastroduodenal barrier function is likely to be a contributory factor.[19]

Kinin-mediated angioedema

Angioedema due to hereditary and acquired C1 esterase inhibitor (C1inh) deficiency and ACEI-induced angioedema involves kinins rather than histamine or leukotriene release. There is currently no evidence that kinins are involved in other types of urticaria or angioedema.

Clinical classification

History-taking and examination define distinctive patterns of urticaria that can indicate the likely pathogenesis, best management, and prognosis for each patient. Six clinical patterns of disease can be recognized.[3,9] These patterns are not completely distinct and can overlap in some patients.

Spontaneous urticaria

Spontaneous urticaria is the commonest presentation. The term "spontaneous" makes no assumption about etiology, which may include autoimmunity, allergy, pseudoallergy, or infection. Those cases for which a cause cannot be ascertained with reasonable confidence are called idiopathic. In practice, this may be the majority of patients. Spontaneous urticaria can be further classified by duration and frequency of attacks into acute, chronic, and episodic urticaria.

Acute urticaria

Acute urticaria is defined as continuous disease lasting less than 6 weeks. People with an atopic predisposition are at higher risk of acute urticaria; atopic diseases are found in about half of acute urticaria patients.[3] Most acute urticaria resolves spontaneously within 3 weeks but in 10% patients may progress to CU.

Foods, drugs, and infections are the commonest identifiable causes of acute urticaria, although many cases remain unexplained. Viral upper respiratory tract infections precede the onset of acute urticaria by a few days in 40% of patients.[3] Acute urticaria can also be seen in pre-icteric viral hepatitis A, B, and C. However, a specific cause of acute urticaria will not be found in about 50% of patients. Foods are the commonest cause of acute urticaria in children but are rarely responsible for acute urticaria in adults. In infancy, cow's milk allergy is a frequent cause of acute allergic urticaria. Drug-induced urticaria is the commonest presentation of drug hypersensitivity, accounting for a quarter of all adverse drug reactions, with penicillin and NSAIDs the commonest causes of allergic and nonallergic drug-induced urticaria, respectively. Drug-induced urticaria is more likely in the elderly, perhaps reflecting polypharmacy and age-related pharmacokinetic changes, and in patients with human immunodeficiency virus (HIV) infection, renal or liver diseases. Acute NSAID-induced urticaria may be a risk factor for CU.[17]

Chronic urticaria

Chronic urticaria is characterized by daily or almost daily itchy wheals on the skin with or without angioedema for 6 weeks or more. Chronic urticaria is thought to be mediated by functional autoantibodies against the alpha chain of the high-affinity IgE receptor or against IgE itself in 30–50% of patients.[9] Functional abnormalities of basophils have been described. However, in 50% patients the etiopathophysiology of the disease remains unknown.

Chronic urticaria affects women twice as often as men. There is a common link between chronic urticaria and thyroid autoimmunity (in about 14–25% of CU cases) as well as other autoimmune diseases including Graves disease, vitiligo, etc. Chronic urticaria is often associated with physical urticaria (e.g., delayed pressure urticaria is found in ~40% of patients with CU). Chronic urticaria can be aggravated by viral infections, stress, intake of aspirin and other NSAIDs, and it can worsen in women in the premenstrual period. More than 50% patients present with both wheals and angioedema. Chronic urticaria may have a continuous or a relapsing course. Chronic urticaria can cause serious disability for patients, including loss of sleep and energy, social isolation, altered emotional reactions and difficulties in aspects of daily living similar in degree to patients with severe ischemic heart disease.

Episodic urticaria

The cause of episodic urticaria often remains unknown but the possibility of an allergic or pseudoallergic cause needs to be considered.

Physical urticaria

Physically induced urticarias are common, accounting for 25% of all cases of CU. These include dermographism, cold contact urticaria, delayed-pressure urticaria (DPU), vibratory angioedema, localized heat urticaria, cholinergic, adrenergic, and aquagenic urticarias. Physical urticarias can coexist with chronic spontaneous urticaria, and more than one physical urticaria can occur in the same patient (e.g., dermographic and cholinergic urticarias), which may lead to difficulty in diagnosis. With the exception of DPU, physical urticarias develop rapidly after exposure to the relevant trigger and fade within an hour.[2,3]

The pathogenesis of physical urticarias is unclear. Physical stimuli lead to nonimmune activation of mast cells resulting in clinical manifestations that relate to the intensity, area, and duration of exposure. A diagnosis of physical urticaria is confirmed if the symptoms can be reproduced by challenge testing with the suspected stimulus. Challenge tests can also be used for monitoring threshold changes during treatment. In general, treatment of physical urticarias includes avoidance of known physical triggers and taking antihistamines. Sometimes tolerance can be induced for cold and solar urticarias.

Mechanical urticaria
Sympathetic dermographism

Dermographism is the commonest physical urticaria, mainly affecting young people. Typical red, itchy, linear wheals are evoked within minutes of stroking, friction, rubbing, or scratching the skin (Fig. 40.6). Overheating, stress, and anxiety usually aggravate symptoms. Transient dermographism may occur after some bacterial and fungal infections, in scabies, parasitosis, and after treatment with penicillin. The diagnosis of dermographism is confirmed by stroking the skin with a blunt firm object, usually on the upper back. Antihistamines are the mainstay of therapy. Ultraviolet B radiation may be effective for patients unresponsive to antihistamines.

Delayed pressure urticaria (DPU)

Isolated DPU occurs in just 2% of all urticaria patients but DPU coexists with CU in up to 40% of patients. DPU is the most debilitating of the physical urticarias, and is triggered by sustained local pressure, e.g., wearing tight shoes, carrying heavy bags, long

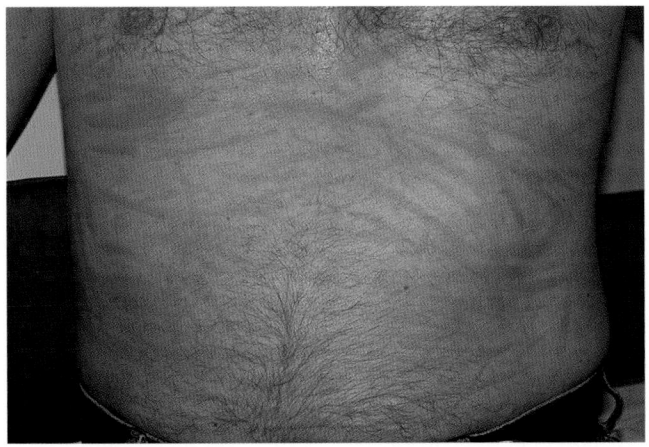

Fig. 40.6 Extensive induced dermographic whealing on the chest of a patient due to scratching.

walks, sitting or leaning against firm objects, climbing ladders, jogging, driving, or hand clapping. Deep and painful swellings, clinically resembling angioedema, develop 30 minutes–12 hours after sustained pressure, and may be associated with flu-like symptoms, fever, arthralgia, and fatigue. The most frequently affected sites are hands, soles, buttocks, shoulders, and areas under straps and belts. DPU lesions last 12–48 hours and are usually painful rather than itchy, especially on the hands and feet. Laboratory investigation reveals transitory leukocytosis and elevated erythrocyte sedimentation rate (ESR). Hanging a heavy weight suspended on a narrow band over the forearm or thigh for 15 minutes may be used as a challenge test, but more reliable results can be obtained with a dermographometer applied at $100 \, g/mm^2$ for 70 seconds. The reaction should be assessed after 6 hours. DPU is difficult to treat because it responds poorly to antihistamines. High doses of steroids may be required for control in severe cases.

Vibratory angioedema

Vibratory angioedema is very rare. Familial cases have been described. Local swelling develops several minutes to 6 hours after exposure to vibrating machinery, lawn mowing, after applauding and jogging, for instance. Systemic symptoms can occur (headache, tightness in chest, diffuse flare). Placing the hand on a laboratory vortex for 5–15 minutes is a useful challenge test. Avoidance of the trigger is the only helpful treatment strategy.

Thermal
Cold urticaria

Cold urticaria accounts for about 3% of physical urticarias.[20] It occurs in both children and adults, and is commoner in cold climates, in women, and in atopic patients. The majority of cases are primary with no identifiable cause but some cases are secondary to internal disease. Clinical manifestations can be local or generalized. Mucosal involvement may develop after drinking cold beverages. Systemic symptoms can be respiratory (laryngeal angioedema, tongue or pharyngeal swelling, wheezing), vascular (hypotension, tachycardia), gastrointestinal (hyperacidity, nausea, diarrhea), or neurological (disorientation, headache). Cold-induced urticaria can be evoked by low ambient temperature, contact with cold objects, food or beverages, and immersion in cold water. Wheals develop during the cold exposure or, more commonly, on warming up. The severity of cold urticaria

depends on the intensity and duration of the cold stimulus. Cold urticaria is potentially life-threatening with a risk of anaphylaxis and death on exposure of large areas to cold, for example jumping into cold water, hypothermia in neurosurgical and cardiothoracic operations. Familial cold urticaria is due to mutations in the cold-induced autoinflammatory syndrome 1 (NLRP-3) gene and is described below.

In 1–5% of patients, cold urticaria is secondary to cryoproteins (cryoglobulins, cryoagglutinins, cryofibrinogen, cryohemolysin). These can be associated with infections (hepatitis C, infectious mononucleosis, syphilis, Mycoplasma infection), autoimmune diseases, and lymphoreticular malignancy (Waldenström's macroglobulinemia, myeloma). Cold urticaria may precede these diseases by several years. Secondary cold urticaria can also be drug-related (penicillin, oral contraceptives, angiotensin-converting enzyme (ACE) inhibitors).

The diagnosis of cold urticaria is confirmed by an ice cube challenge, although some atypical cold-induced urticarias have a negative ice cube test.

The clinical workup in cold urticaria includes measurement of cryoproteins. Patients should be cautious about bathing or swimming in cold water, and consuming cold food or drinks. Antihistamine treatment is often helpful but does not prevent anaphylaxis caused by swimming in cold water. In severe cold urticaria tolerance induction may be attempted: this involves depletion of mast cell histamine by repeated cold exposure.

Heat urticaria

Heat-induced urticaria is very rare. It is induced by local heating of the skin at 38–50°C. A refractory period up to 24 hours is typical. Challenge test is done by application of hot water in a tube or beaker at up to 44°C for 4–5 minutes. Symptoms develop several minutes after exposure. Management of heat-induced urticaria presents some difficulties as the clinical efficacy of antihistamines is limited.

Other patterns of inducible urticaria
Cholinergic urticaria

Cholinergic urticaria is the second commonest physical urticaria and occurs mainly in adolescents, young adults, and atopic patients. Cholinergic urticaria usually follows a rise in core temperature due to physical exercise, fever, or external passive heat (hot bath, shower, sauna), but may also be provoked by emotional stress and spicy food. The characteristic lesions are highly pruritic pinpoint pale wheals of 1–3 mm surrounded by a red flare. They can occur anywhere except the soles and palms. Lesions usually begin on the trunk and neck, extending outwards to the face and limbs. As lesions progress, confluent areas of whealing and redness may develop. Severely affected patients can develop angioedema and even anaphylaxis. Most patients with mild disease do not seek medical help. The rash is triggered by activation of cholinergic sympathetic innervation of sweat glands but the mechanism of this remains unclear. Decreased blood protease inhibitor levels have been reported, and this is the rationale for using anabolic steroids to treat occasional severely affected individuals who are unresponsive to other measures. The prognosis is reasonably favorable, with spontaneous resolution within 8 years in most patients. However, 30% of patients are affected for >10 years.

Cholinergic urticaria can be confirmed by reproducing the rash with physical exercise or passive heating in a hot bath at up to 42°C. Treatment is primarily with antihistamines, but β-blockers, danazol, ketotifen, and montelukast have also been used. The condition is typically refractory for 24 hours and this may enable patients to prevent attacks by taking daily exercise.

Adrenergic urticaria

Adrenergic urticaria is very rare. The typical lesions are red papular wheals surrounded by a white areola, the opposite of cholinergic urticaria. It is thought that whealing is triggered by local release of norepinephrine. It is provoked by stress and may respond to β-blockers.

Solar urticaria

Solar urticaria affects >1% of all urticaria patients with slight female predominance. It can be associated with erythropoietic porphyria. Wheals are caused by electromagnetic wavelengths ranging from 290 and 760 nm (ultraviolet B, A, and visible spectrum). It develops within minutes or hours after sun exposure and fades within 24 hours. Lesions are usually confined to sun-exposed skin, although they can also develop under clothing. Severity of solar urticaria depends on the wavelength, intensity, and duration of irradiation. Short exposures induce flare and pruritus while longer exposures cause whealing. In patients sensitive to the visible spectrum, reactions can occur through window glass.

Solar urticaria is diagnosed by monochromator phototesting. Patients are advised to use creams with a high sun protection factor (SPF), protective clothing, and protective window shields and to limit time spent outdoors. Treatment of solar urticaria includes antihistamines, photochemotherapy and, occasionally, cyclosporine, or intravenous immunoglobulin.

Aquagenic urticaria and pruritus

Aquagenic urticaria is very rare. It occurs in women more often than men and is triggered by water contact but not after drinking water. Scattered small papular wheals, similar to cholinergic urticaria but with a larger flare, appear within 10–20 minutes of water contact and resolve in 30–60 minutes. Diagnosis is made by a challenge test with a wet compress at body temperature for up to 10 minutes on whichever part of the body is usually affected. Associations with HIV infection and hepatitis B have been described.

Aquagenic pruritus without skin lesions is associated with polycythemia, but most cases are idiopathic. Treatment is usually unsatisfactory; phototherapy and sodium bicarbonate in the bathwater have been used.

Contact urticaria

Contact urticaria occurs locally after skin or mucosal contact with the eliciting agent.[2,3] Reactions usually develop within a few minutes and resolve over 2 hours, although delayed-contact urticaria can occur with a latent period up to 48 hours. Contact urticaria can be caused by many organic and inorganic stimuli such as latex, animal danders and secretions, foods, plants, topical drugs, and cosmetics.

Allergic contact urticaria occurs mainly in atopic subjects. Sensitization can occur through skin, mucous membranes, respiratory, or gastrointestinal tracts. Foods are the most common cause. In ~15% of patients, contact with the allergen may induce anaphylaxis. The severity of contact reactions depends on many factors (area of exposure, duration of contact, amount and concentration of substance, patient reactivity, comorbidity, and concomitant treatment).

Nonallergic contact urticaria is commoner than allergic contact urticaria and is usually caused by low-molecular-weight chemicals. Contact urticaria to benzoic acid in food is thought to involve generation of eicosanoids because it can be blocked by NSAIDs, but for other substances (e.g., polyvinylchloride, polyethylene glycol) the mechanism remains unknown. Nonallergic contact urticaria may occur on first exposure and may depend on dose and concentration of the chemical.

Urticarial vasculitis

UV is characterized clinically by CU and histologically by leukocytoclastic vasculitis on lesional skin biopsy.[2,3,21] It is important to differentiate UV from chronic spontaneous urticaria in terms of prognosis, approach to diagnostic evaluation, and therapy.

UV affects ~5–10% patients with CU presenting to specialist clinics but is quite rare in the community. It often has a distinct clinical pattern with painful rather than itching wheals lasting over 24 hours leaving residual hyperpigmentation, but may be indistinguishable morphologically from spontaneous urticaria. In UV, skin lesions can be accompanied by systemic symptoms, including arthralgia or arthritis affecting mostly the small joints. Other systemic features include abdominal pain, diarrhea, nausea and vomiting, microscopic hematuria and proteinuria, and occasionally episcleritis, uveitis, or conjunctivitis.

The most common laboratory findings in UV are elevated ESR and hypocomplementemia. Circulating immune complexes, low-titer antinuclear antibodies, proteinuria, and hematuria may be present. Normocomplementemic UV is often idiopathic, limited to skin, and has a better prognosis than hypocomplementemic UV, in which systemic involvement is common. A combination of UV, hypocomplementemia, anti-C1q antibodies, and low serum C1q associated with SLE is termed the hypocomplementemic UV syndrome (HUVS).

Skin biopsy may reveal vascular injury with or without fibrinoid deposits in or around the vessel wall, endothelial swelling, perivascular neutrophilic infiltrate, leukocytoclasis (fragmentation of neutrophils with nuclear dust), and extravasation of red blood cells. Immunofluorescence reveals IgM, IgG immunoglobulins, C3, and fibrin deposition in and around the vessel wall.

Treatment of UV depends on severity of cutaneous involvement and the presence and pattern of systemic symptoms. Prednisolone is widely used but long-term therapy is not recommended because of side effects. Other therapeutic modalities include colchicine and dapsone. Hydroxychloroquine seems to be more efficient in HUVS. For severe UV, azathioprine, mycophenolate mofetil, and cyclosporine can be tried but evidence for these agents is mainly anecdotal.

Angioedema without wheals

Angioedema occurs in nearly half of CU patients, in whom the disease tends to be more severe and more difficult to treat. Angioedema without wheals occurs less frequently but needs specific investigation because it may be due to C1 inhibitor deficiency or drugs, although many cases remain unexplained (Fig. 40.7).

Angioedema due to C1 inhibitor deficiency

The diagnosis and clinical presentation of hereditary and acquired C1inh deficiency are covered in Chapter 20.

Fig. 40.7 Diagnostic pathway for the differential diagnosis of angioedema.

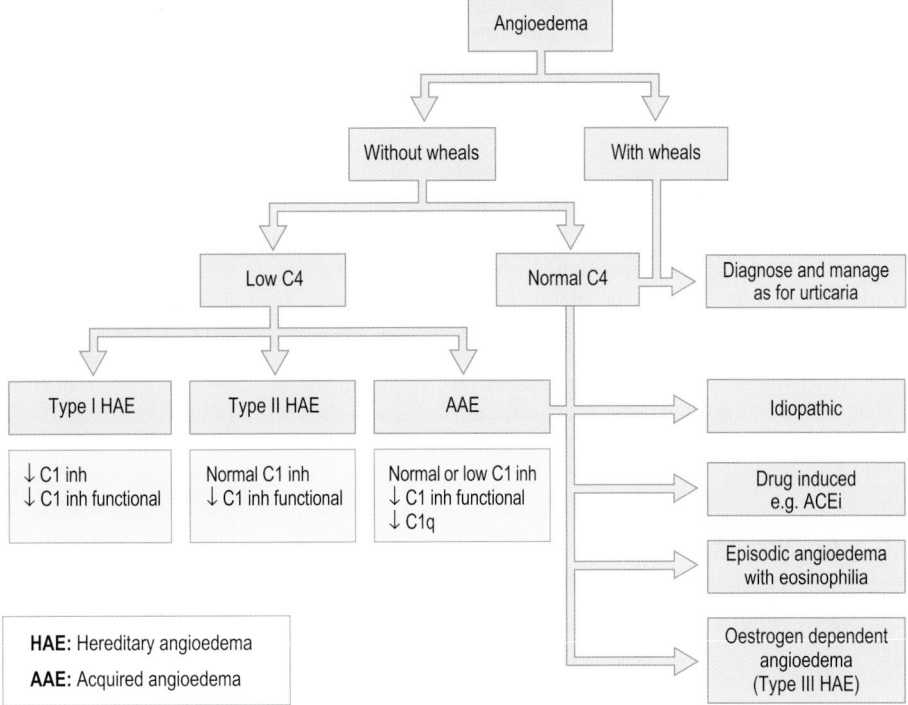

Angioedema with normal C1 inhibitor

Angioedema develops in 0.1–2% of patients on ACE inhibitors. It is thought to be due to inhibition of kininase II that breaks down bradykinin as well as converting angiotensin I to angiotensin II in the renin–aldosterone pathway. It usually presents with episodic and unpredictable swellings of the head and neck, especially of the tongue and oropharynx. Although in most cases angioedema develops within the first week of treatment with ACE inhibitors, the onset of symptoms may occur several years later. Treatment involves discontinuation of ACE inhibitor therapy. Angioedema often recurs on re-exposure to ACE inhibitors. ACE inhibitors can also precipitate angioedema in patients with angioedema due to other causes, including C1inh deficiency. Rare instances of angioedema have also been reported with angiotensin II receptor antagonists.

Angioedema without wheals occasionally occurs with NSAIDs, usually within several hours of intake.

Idiopathic angioedema is diagnosed when no cause can be established. It is generally self-limiting but can follow a prolonged course. Treatment of idiopathic angioedema is as for spontaneous urticaria. Antihistamines are the mainstay of therapy; corticosteroids (prednisolone 30–40 mg/day) are useful for up to 3 days to cover more severe episodes and epinephrine is life-saving in laryngeal angioedema. Tranexamic acid can help in idiopathic angioedema without wheals, but it is usually ineffective when angioedema occurs with urticarial wheals.

Autoinflammatory syndromes presenting with urticaria

Acquired Schnitzler's syndrome

Schnitzler's syndrome is a rare form of CU with intermittent fever, bone pain, high ESR, and monoclonal IgM or IgG gammopathy.[22] Clinically, patients present with nonpruritic or mildly pruritic CU, mainly affecting trunk and limbs. The wheals are resistant to antihistamines and angioedema is rare. Fever bouts may exceed 40°C, sometimes with chills and nocturnal sweating. Patients often suffer from bone pains, mainly in pelvis or tibias, arthralgia, and sometimes full-blown arthritis. Lymphadenopathy, hepato-, and splenomegaly may be present.

Kappa light-chain monoclonal IgM and, less commonly, IgG paraproteins are found on serum electrophoresis. The ESR is persistently elevated at 60–100 mm/h, with leukocytosis, elevated platelet count, and anemia. Skin histology shows neutrophilic urticaria in most cases; monoclonal IgM is deposited in the epidermis around the keratinocytes and along basement membranes on direct immunofluorescence. Bone examination may demonstrate hyperostosis on radiography and hyperfixation on bone technetium scanning. Bone marrow examination is normal in most patients, but shows nonspecific lymphocytic, plasmocytic, or polyclonal infiltration in about 20%.

The pathophysiology of Schnitzler's syndrome is still unclear and the severity of CU does not depend on the paraprotein level. Evidence of activation of IL-1, increased IL-6, and granulocyte–macrophage colony-stimulating factor and anecdotal reports of complete clinical responses to the IL-1 receptor antagonist anakinra suggest a leading role for cytokines in its pathogenesis.

The prognosis is generally benign. However, long-term follow-up is recommended because patients may develop B-cell lymphomas 10–20 years after its onset.

First-line treatment of Schnitzler's syndrome is with NSAIDs, and colchicine or dapsone. In severe cases with disabling fever or arthralgia, oral corticosteroids and immunosuppressive drugs (cyclosporine, cyclophosphamide, and interferon-α) have been used, but treatment of the paraprotein is not effective.

Hereditary (cryopyrin-associated) periodic syndromes

Several hereditary autoinflammatory urticarial syndromes show mutations of the NLRP-3 gene on chromosome 1q44. NLRP-3 encodes a protein called cryopyrin, which is involved in apoptosis and inflammation. These rare autosomal dominant disorders include familial cold autoinflammatory syndrome (FCAS), Muckle–Wells syndrome (MWS), and chronic infantile neurological cutaneous and articular syndrome (CINCA).[23]

Familial cold autoinflammatory syndrome

Periodic fever and urticaria are induced by generalized cold exposure.[20] Disease onset is usually at birth or within the first 6 months of life. Papular or plaque-like wheals develop in response to chilling but not local contact with cold water or an ice cube. Skin lesions occur after a few hours, subside in 24 hours, and are usually accompanied by fever, chills, conjunctival injection, sweating, headache, and arthralgia. During attacks there is marked leukocytosis, elevated ESR, and raised C-reactive protein.

Muckle–Wells syndrome

MWS develops in children or adolescents. It is characterized by CU, fever, aching, and malaise. Sensorineural deafness may develop in adulthood. Some MWS patients develop systemic amyloidosis (AA-type) with amyloid nephropathy. Laboratory findings in MWS include elevated ESR, C-reactive protein, IL-6, IL-1, and serum amyloid-associated protein.

Chronic infantile neurological cutaneous and articular syndrome

CINCA syndrome is more severe than FCAS or MWS, with neurological features and arthritis. Urticaria is rarely observed in infancy; other clinical features are lymphadenopathy, hepatosplenomegaly, dysmorphic features, developmental retardation, seizures, papilledema, neurological manifestations, and overgrowth of the distal femur and patella. Affected individuals are at risk of leukemia and other malignancies, infections, and systemic amyloidosis.

Recently, it has been shown that treatment with the IL-1 receptor antagonist anakinra leads to complete resolution of symptoms in FCAS and MWS with normalization of inflammatory indices. Canakinumab and rilonacept are now licensed for patients with CAPS.

Differential diagnosis

Several dermatoses may present with urticarial lesions, including erythema multiforme minor, bullous pemphigoid, and dermatitis herpetiformis.[2,3] These dermatoses can nearly always be distinguished clinically from urticaria on the basis of their polymorphic pattern, prolonged duration of individual lesions, lack of daily fluctuation, development of vesicles or blisters, and resistance to conventional therapy for urticaria. Very occasionally, skin biopsy, with or without indirect immunofluorescence, may be required to make the distinction.

Papular urticaria is an urticarial reaction to insect bites in sensitized individuals. The lesions are fixed rather than fluctuating, may take days or weeks to resolve fully, and may leave pigmentation or scars. Bites often occur asymmetrically in groups or lines. Although histamine is involved with the initial pruritic lesions, oral antihistamines are usually unhelpful and potent topical steroids may be required.

Workup in urticaria patients

Evaluation of patients with urticaria requires a detailed history and physical examination.[1–4,24] The history is particularly important in urticaria patients and should include a thorough search for all potential causes of the disorders, possible precipitating and aggravating factors, the timing of onset and duration of individual wheals, associated symptoms as well as travel history, recent infection, occupational exposure, food and drug intake, and co-morbidity. Patients can be asked to keep a diary of attacks, which may provide additional information about possible causes. The duration of individual lesions can be very helpful in distinguishing the different clinical patterns of urticaria.

> ### ● CLINICAL PEARLS
>
> **Diagnosis of clinical patterns of urticaria**
>
> - The duration of individual wheals can help to define the pattern of urticaria.
> - Wheals lasting an hour or less are usually triggered by a physical stimulus.
> - Localized wheals lasting up to 2 hours may be due to skin or mucosal contact with an allergen or a nonimmunological exposure.
> - Wheals that take 1–24 hours to fade are usually a presentation of the ordinary pattern of chronic spontaneous urticaria.
> - Wheals lasting more than 24 hours may be due to delayed-pressure urticaria or urticarial vasculitis.

Physical examination should focus on skin lesion morphology and careful systemic evaluation. If the patient is symptom-free at the time of evaluation, photographs may be helpful. The approximate duration of individual lesions can be assessed by outlining a particular lesion with a pen and observing it for a day. The appearance and distribution of skin lesions may suggest a diagnosis, e.g., the pinpoint lesions with a large flare in cholinergic urticaria or lesions on sun-exposed areas in solar urticaria. A thorough physical examination can also offer diagnostic clues for associated comorbidities, including thyroid dysfunction.

Further evaluation of patients with urticaria is guided by the patient's history and clinical pattern of disease. However, it must be remembered that there can be more than one cause for urticaria and that different clinical subtypes of urticaria can coexist in one patient.

Workup in acute urticaria

It is well established that allergies are common causes of acute urticaria. The culprit allergens can be suspected from the clinical history, including a close temporal relationship to the time of exposure to the allergen and a history of previous exposure and prompt resolution on allergy withdrawal. Therefore, patients with acute or episodic urticaria should undergo allergy evaluation by skin testing or fluoroenzymatic immunoassay (FEIA) – also known as CAP Phadiatop. In the case of food allergy, positive test results must also be verified by a trial of elimination diet followed by double-blind food challenge in supervised clinical settings.

Workup in physical urticarias

When physical urticaria is suspected, appropriate challenge testing should be performed to confirm the diagnosis. Generally, there is no need for further investigation, except for cold urticaria where plasma cryoproteins (cryoglobulin, cold agglutinin, or cryofibrinogen) should be assayed.

Workup in chronic ordinary urticaria

No laboratory workup is recommended for patients with mild ordinary CU that is easily controlled by antihistamines, unless the history points to an underlying disease. Studies have shown that random laboratory testing very rarely yields evidence of unsuspected internal diseases as a cause of CU and this should therefore be discouraged.[25]

Screening laboratory evaluation can be considered in patients with poor response to first-line treatment. A complete blood count with differential, ESR, thyroid-stimulating hormone, liver function tests, and urinalysis will exclude most diseases associated with urticaria.

Other evaluations should be guided by abnormal findings in the history and physical examination in patients with CU. Additional tests may include stool examination for ova and parasites, antinuclear antibody titer, thyroid function and antithyroid antibodies, hepatitis viral screen, skinprick tests, or CAP for IgE-mediated reactions in episodic urticaria. Tests for immediate hypersensitivities should not be undertaken in chronic continuous urticaria unless there are compelling reasons for doing so. Rarely, CU can be caused by a specific food additive, which should be confirmed by dietary exclusion and double-blind, placebo-controlled oral challenge.

The diagnosis of autoimmune CU

The diagnosis of autoimmune CU is not straightforward and involves *in vivo* and *in vitro* approaches. Autologous serum skin testing (ASST) is a simple and useful screening method for autoreactivity in CU patients. For skin testing, 0.05 mL of the patient's own serum should be injected intradermally into clinically uninvolved forearm skin together with an equal volume of saline and histamine (10 mg/mL) as controls at adjacent sites. The reaction is considered positive if the serum skin test forms a pink wheal at least 1.5 mm greater than the negative control at 30 minutes. The test is 80% specific and 70% sensitive for autoimmune CU as defined by a positive basophil histamine release assay.[13] A strongly positive ASST response (over 15 mm) was reported to be very specific for autoimmune CU (>96%) when a panel of basophil and mast cell donors was used for testing.[26]

The current diagnostic gold standard in autoimmune CU is functional release assays using basophils or mast cells, but these only give indirect evidence of functional autoantibodies. Being technically difficult and time-consuming, these assays remain confined to research centers. Moreover, immunoassays (Western blotting, ELISA) based on binding of autoantibodies to relevant antigens (FcεRIα or IgE) do not correlate well with the results of functional assays.[14]

Management of urticaria

Finding effective treatment for urticaria can be challenging for both clinician and patients. Treatment should be tailored to the clinical pattern, duration, and severity of the urticaria. Management should include nonpharmacological measures and drug therapy with a stepwise approach.[9,26,27]

THERAPEUTIC PRINCIPLES

Management of urticaria

- Eliminate infectious, drug, or food causes.
- Minimize nonspecific aggravators, including heat, stress, alcohol, nonsteroidal anti-inflammatory drugs, and pressure.
- Regular oral antihistamines are the first line of therapy for all spontaneous and inducible urticarias.
- Second-line treatments, including short courses of oral corticosteroids, may be necessary for specific clinical situations.
- Immunosuppressive therapies should be reserved for patients with severe autoimmune urticaria or steroid-dependent urticaria that has not responded to other first- and second-line measures.

General measures

Identification and avoidance of allergens, infections, and physical triggers are of primary importance. Patients with the ordinary pattern of CU should minimize exposure to nonspecific aggravating factors, identified by a thorough history that may include overheating, stress, alcohol, dietary pseudoallergens, and some drugs. NSAIDs aggravate CU in up to 30% of patients with the ordinary presentation and should generally be avoided. This probably does not apply to the physical urticarias, in particular DPU, where NSAIDs may be used as treatment. ACE inhibitors are contraindicated in angioedema without wheals and should be prescribed with caution in other patterns of urticaria. Although it is often recommended that CU patients should avoid codeine and penicillin, clinical experience suggests that this is not necessary. Cooling lotions and creams such as 1% menthol in aqueous cream may help to relieve pruritus. Some patients with ordinary but not physical CU appeared to respond to a low-pseudoallergen diet.[16] However, controlled clinical trials are lacking.

First-line therapy

Antihistamines are the cornerstone of treatment in urticaria. Second-generation antihistamines offer several advantages over classical H1 antihistamines, such as lack of sedation and impairment of performance, longer duration of action, and absence of anti-cholinergic side effects. Meta-analysis indicates that antihistamines are clinically effective in 40–90% of patients with CU. Second-generation antihistamines are inverse agonists of H1 receptors, which stabilize H1 receptors in the inactive conformation, and, therefore, are most effective in CU when taken regularly for prophylaxis. The timing of antihistamine intake should be adjusted to suit the diurnal pattern of urticaria. It has become common practice to increase second-generation antihistamines above their licensed doses when CU does not respond, because clinical experience shows that this achieves better control in some patients, although hard scientific evidence is still accruing. Although the evidence base for combining H1 and H2 antihistamines is poor, this may be helpful in some patients. Cimetidine (but not ranitidine) appears to increase the plasma concentration of H1 antihistamines by inhibiting hepatic cytochrome P450. H2 antihistamines also suppress the dyspepsia that often accompanies severe urticaria.

Second-line therapy

When urticaria does not respond to first-line measures, systemic corticosteroids are commonly used as short-term therapy for acute urticaria or severe exacerbations of CU. Long-term treatment with corticosteroids is not recommended because of safety concerns. In corticosteroid-dependent patients, an alternate-day dosing may be used and steroid-sparing drugs should also be considered. A wide variety of medications have been reported to be of benefit for antihistamine-unresponsive urticaria when oral corticosteroids might otherwise have to be considered but they are invariably used off-license and controlled trials are usually lacking. Where possible, these should be targeted at specific subgroups of urticaria patients; e.g., the leukotriene receptor antagonist montelukast has been shown to be effective in aspirin-sensitive CU patients, and there is limited evidence for a trial of thyroxine in biochemically euthyroid CU patients with thyroid autoimmunity.[28]

Third-line therapy

Immunosuppressive therapy is mainly considered for autoimmune CU.[3,13] However, clinical experience suggests it may also benefit therapy-resistant CU without evidence of circulating antibodies.

The best-studied immunosuppressive therapy is cyclosporine, shown to be effective at 4 mg/kg daily in CU patients. Patients must be monitored carefully for renal function and hypertension; treatment should normally be limited to 3 months. Cyclosporine is contraindicated for patients with previous malignant disease except non-melanoma skin cancer. Tacrolimus also appears to be effective in corticosteroid-dependent autoimmune CU.[18] There is some evidence for efficacy of plasmapheresis and immunoglobulins in chronic autoimmune urticaria, although these are expensive options and controlled clinical trials are needed. Methotrexate, mycophenolate mofetil and azathioprine have also been used alone or with corticosteroids.

Management of hereditary angioedema

The swellings of HAE are mediated by kinins rather than histamine so the management of HAE is completely different from mast cell dependent urticaria. The primary aim of therapy is to replace the missing functional C1 esterase inhibitor or stabilize the coagulation, fibrinolysis, complement and kallikrein-kinin pathways. Risk factors for attacks should be recognized and avoided were possible. ACE inhibitors should be avoided because ACE is a key enzyme involved in the breakdown of bradykinin. Angiotensin II receptor blocking drugs (ARA2) are probably safe alternatives. Exogenous estrogen (oral contraceptives and hormone replacement therapies) should be avoided in women since it appears to activate kallikrein through activated Factor XII. Lifestyle events that exacerbate HAE vary between

individuals in their importance, but may include local trauma (such as dental extraction), stress, tiredness and intercurrent infections, possibly including *Helicobacter pylori*. Attacks involving the extremities or abdomen are the most common. It is estimated that up to 50% of patients will develop an attack of oropharyngeal swelling over their lives so treatment must be rapidly available for emergencies in all patients as well as aiming to be preventative. The intention of treatment is to reduce or curtail the severity of a swelling and to reduce "downtime" if one occurs. Some patients with frequent peripheral swellings prefer to treat themselves symptomatically with analgesics and wait for spontaneous resolution over 3–4 days than have specific treatment since none are completely without risk of adverse effects, and potential problems with cost, availability or both. The management of types I and II HAE is better defined than the recently recognized type III but follows similar principles.[29]

Treatment of the acute attack

The "gold standard" treatment of oropharyngeal or gastrointestinal attacks in most countries (except the USA until recently) has been plasma-derived C1 esterase inhibitor (pd-C1inh) concentrate given by intravenous infusion.[30] It has proved to be effective and safe. The recommended dose is 20U/kg body weight in adults and children although smaller doses have been used in the past and may be effective. Up to 3 units of fresh frozen plasma (containing C1 inhibitor and its substrate, complement) may be given as an alternative in an emergency when pd-C1inh is not available, but will not have had the same stringent screening and production measures to eliminate the possibility of transmissible infection. Initial improvement in the swelling may be seen within 30–60 min and time to clearance is usually in the order of 24 hours after pd-C1inh. Self-administration can reduce the severity of attacks by allowing earliest treatment and should be encouraged. A recombinant C1inh is now licensed in Europe. Novel treatments currently marketed include icatibant (a bradykinin 2 receptor antagonist), that is licensed in Europe but not currently in the USA, and ecallantide (a kallikrein antagonist), which is currently licensed in the USA but not Europe. Both are given by subcutaneous injection, which provides an easier route for administration than intravenous infusion. Ecallantide should be given under medical supervision since there is a small risk of allergic reactions to it afterwards. Icatibant is now licensed for self-administration, which provides a potential advantage over the other treatments currently available. There have been no head-to-head studies of pdC1inh, ecallantide or icatibant, but in use experience suggests that the effectiveness of these products is comparable. It should be noted that antihistamines and steroids have no place in the management of HAE. Any improvement after epinephrine due to its effects on vasopermeability will be transient and there is no evidence that it changes the overall course of an attack.

Short-term prophylaxis

It has become common practice to give prophylactic treatment with pd-C1inh before procedures involving local trauma to the oropharynx, including dental extraction and intubation for general anaesthesia. The dose for prophylaxis may be less than that necessary for treatment of an acute attack. Common practice would be to give at least 500 units pd-C1inh within 1 hour before the procedure with an option of having a further dose available to give afterwards if a swelling develops. Other strategies include increasing the dose of prophylactic treatment with anabolic steroids (danazol or stanozolol) or plasmin inhibitors (tranexamic acid or epsilon aminocaproic acid) for at least 48 hours before and after the procedure. Specific guidance on dosing for adults and children can be found elsewhere.

Long-term prophylaxis

Anabolic steroids are the mainstay of long-term prophylaxis in countries where they are licensed for HAE. They increase the production of C1inh by the liver in heterozygotes with the remaining functioning allele. The dose should be titrated against the clinical response rather than blood levels of C1inh to the lowest that prevents or ameliorates the condition. Virilizing side effects can be problematic for women nevertheless and anabolic steroids are usually avoided in children because of concerns about growth retardation. Monitoring of liver function and lipid profiles should be undertaken periodically. Performing a liver ultrasound examination every 3 years to screen for development of hepatoma is usually recommended in patients on long-term prophylaxis. Plasmin inhibitors are generally less effective for prophylaxis than anabolic steroids but are preferred in children. Pd-C1inh infusions twice a week may be given as prophylaxis during pregnancy and in rare situations when alternative therapies are not appropriate.

Anaphylaxis

Anaphylaxis is a severe, life-threatening, systemic reaction of sudden onset involving respiratory compromise, cardiovascular collapse or both. Its clinical features and management have been well summarized in a recent World Allergy Organization guideline.[48]

Epidemiology of anaphylaxis

Estimates of the incidence of anaphylaxis in the general population vary from 3.2 cases per 100 000 inhabitants per annum in Denmark to 21 cases per 100 000 inhabitants per annum in the USA.[31] Lifetime personal risk estimate for anaphylaxis is believed to be 1–3%.[32] The mortality rate is estimated to be in the range of 1–2%.[33] In the UK anaphylaxis accounts for 20 deaths per year, which represents 1 death in 3 million people.[34] Anaphylaxis occurs more often in females than males[35] and in children more than adults.[36]

Hospital admissions for anaphylaxis nearly doubled in the UK in the 1990s.[37] Severe anaphylaxis was diagnosed in 1–9 per 10 000 people attending emergency departments in the UK, Australia, and the USA.[33] It is estimated that, in a 12-month period, 1 in 12 patients with previous anaphylaxis will have a recurrence, and 1 in 50 will require hospitalization or treatment with epinephrine.[36]

The pathophysiology of anaphylaxis

Although anaphylaxis is often subdivided into allergic or immunologic and non-immunologic groups, the clinical presentation is similar and most authorities no longer make a distinction. Immunologic anaphylaxis is further classified as IgE-mediated and non-IgE-mediated. In IgE-mediated anaphylaxis, allergen cross-links allergen-specific IgE antibodies on the surface of mast cells and basophils, leading to their degranulation. Release of mediators causes bronchoconstriction, mucus secretion, diminished cardiac contractility, increased vascular permeability, vasoconstriction of coronary and peripheral arteries, and vasodilation of venules, thereby producing clinical symptoms

of anaphylaxis. IgE-mediated reactions occur in presensitized patients (e.g., penicillin-, insulin-, latex- or peanut-induced anaphylaxis). In contrast, some substances such as opioids, radiocontrast media, vancomycin, and some muscle relaxants are capable of direct release of mediator (histamine) from basophils and mast cells without involvement of IgE. IgG- or IgM-related transfusion reactions should be classified as immunologic, non-IgE-mediated anaphylaxis. Although reactions to NSAIDs are considered to be pharmacological rather than immunological (due to the downstream effects of COX inhibition), an IgE-mediated mechanism has been suspected in a few patients but is difficult to prove. Apart from IgE, other antibodies may be involved: in murine models IgG-mediated FcγRIII-dependent anaphylaxis elicited by a high dose of allergen has been described. The key participating cells in this type of anaphylaxis are macrophages, with platelet-activating factor as the main mediator.[38]

The etiology of anaphylaxis

A cause of anaphylaxis can only be identified in about 60% of patients. Anaphylaxis is most commonly caused by foods, drugs, general anesthetic agents, insect stings, and latex. Rare causes include vaccines, semen, and aeroallergen inhalation. Exercise can occasionally cause anaphylaxis either on its own (exercise-induced anaphylaxis), or after prior ingestion of a food to which the individual is sensitized (food and exercise-induced anaphylaxis). Idiopathic anaphylaxis accounts for up to 40% of all cases.[38,39] Patients with idiopathic anaphylaxis should be investigated to exclude systemic mastocytosis.

The most common routes of allergen exposure are oral and parenteral, although inhalation of allergens (e.g., fish or legume allergens after cooking, latex particles in health care settings) or percutaneous penetration after skin contact can induce anaphylaxis in highly sensitized patients. The link with atopy is not clear, but anaphylaxis with predominant respiratory involvement elicited by skin and mucosal allergen contact is thought to be more often related to atopy than parenterally-induced anaphylaxis (e.g., insect stings or drug-induced anaphylaxis).[38]

Food-induced anaphylaxis

Food allergy is a common cause of anaphylaxis, with an annual incidence of 7.6 cases per 100 000 person-years.[38] Anaphylactic reactions to foods have been increasing over the last two decades: a fivefold increase in food allergy was reported in France from 1980 to 1995.[33] Food-induced anaphylaxis is the most common single cause of anaphylaxis treated in emergency departments in the USA, especially in the younger population, and accounts for 29 000 estimated emergency room visits and 150–200 deaths per year.[38] Over 60% of cases of food-induced anaphylaxis occur in patients younger than 30 years.[40] Peanuts and other nuts, fish, and shellfish are the most frequent culprits in food-induced anaphylaxis but almost any food can be implicated.[40] Many cases of severe anaphylaxis are caused by unintended exposure to hidden food allergens. In addition, alcohol, NSAIDs, exercise, or concurrent infection can increase the severity of a food-induced allergic reaction.

Drug-induced anaphylaxis

Drug-induced anaphylaxis is more common in hospitalized patients than in the community. Any drug can cause anaphylaxis, but the prevalence varies: one study found 5–15 cases per 100 000 patients for most NSAIDs and antibiotics, while for penicillin and contrast agents the figure was over 30 cases per 100 000.[41] Drugs are the leading cause of fatal anaphylaxis, comprising

43.5% of such deaths.[34] The mortality rate in drug-induced anaphylaxis is about one death per 50 000–100 000 treatment courses.[41] All routes of administration can be potentially fatal, including oral, intravenous, subcutaneous, intra-articular, intra-uterine, inhalational, rectal, or topical, but the risk is greatest after parenteral administration.

Anaphylaxis during anesthesia

The incidence of anaphylaxis in general anesthesia varies between 1:3500 and 1:20 000, significantly exceeding the overall prevalence of drug-induced anaphylaxis.[39] The French registry of anaphylaxis during general anesthesia reports a prevalence of one case in 13000 episodes of general anesthesia.[42] The incidence of anaphylaxis to local anesthetics is, by contrast, extremely rare. Most cases of suspected anaphylaxis to local anesthetics are probably due to vasovagal or panic attacks; a few adverse events may follow inadvertent intravascular injection.

A network of 38 French allergo-anesthesia outpatient clinics reported that around 60% of all cases were induced by muscle relaxants (rocuronium, suxemethonium, etc.), followed by latex and antibiotics.[42] Reactions to neuromuscular blocking agents mostly occur on first exposure and were associated with a 70% rate of cross-reactivity in this group. Latex, the next most important cause of anaphylaxis, accounted for 16% of intraoperative anaphylactic reactions.[42]

Insect sting-induced anaphylaxis

Severe anaphylaxis from insect stings causes approximately 40 deaths annually in the USA and nearly 100 in Europe.[27] The intensity of reaction depends on the type of insect, amount of venom, location of sting, and the patient's sensitivity. Allergen-specific immunotherapy with venom extracts has been shown to be safe and effective in patients with hymenoptera venom allergy, providing some clinical protection within the first 8 weeks of treatment and a long-lasting effect after 3–5 years of maintenance treatment (Chapter 41). It is noteworthy that patients with systemic mastocytosis are at risk of potentially fatal anaphylaxis to insect stings even if they are not presensitized to venom: this may be due to venom components, such as phospholipase A2, acting as mast cell liberators. Venom immunotherapy may be given to mastocytosis patients but there is quite a high risk of anaphylaxis during treatment.

Latex-induced anaphylaxis

The prevalence of latex allergy has been estimated to be as high as 1–6% in the general population, 8–17% in health care workers, and 67% in spina bifida patients.[31] Latex-induced anaphylaxis has been reported in surgery and dentistry and can be fatal. More than half of latex-allergic patients report allergic reactions to fruits such as banana, avocado, kiwi fruit, chestnut, pear, pineapple, grape, and papaya.

Other rare causes of anaphylaxis

Anaphylaxis occurs during 1 in 20 000–47 000 transfusions of blood or blood products, especially in patients with IgA deficiency.[43] IgA deficiency affects 1 in 500–700 Caucasians. One-third of these patients have circulating anti-IgA antibodies, which are associated with serious life-threatening anaphylactic reactions to blood products containing IgA.

Seminal fluid allergy is extremely rare, mostly affecting atopic young women, with 20% of cases developing life-threatening anaphylaxis. These reactions can be prevented with condom usage or intravaginal desensitization with seminal fluid.

Idiopathic anaphylaxis

Idiopathic anaphylaxis is a diagnosis of exclusion. Patients may have recurrent episodes of idiopathic anaphylaxis. Some patients with idiopathic anaphylaxis were shown to have evidence of an aberrant mast cell population carrying the activating point mutation (D816V) in *KIT*.[44]

The clinical diversity of anaphylaxis

In anaphylaxis, there is a remarkable range of clinical symptoms. Anaphylaxis can be preceded by prodromal symptoms such as tingling and redness of the palms and soles, anxiety, sense of impending doom, and disorientation. Anaphylaxis most commonly begins in the skin and mucous membranes, followed by involvement of the respiratory and gastrointestinal tracts, cardiovascular system and, finally, proceeding to cardiac and/or respiratory arrest. Generalized urticaria and angioedema are the most common manifestations of anaphylaxis observed in over 90% of cases, but may be absent. Respiratory symptoms may vary from rhinitis to laryngeal edema and airway obstruction, which are potentially life-threatening. Cardiovascular manifestations in anaphylaxis include hypotension and/or cardiac arrhythmias. In adults, reduced BP is regarded as systolic BP of <90 mmHg or >30% decrease from that person's baseline. Some patients present with only cardiovascular collapse in the absence of other signs of anaphylaxis, especially during general anesthesia.[45] Anaphylaxis is usually associated with tachycardia due to increased cardiac sympathetic drive in response to a decreased effective vascular volume, but bradycardia can also occur. Anaphylaxis can result in up to 35% of intravascular fluid leaking into extracellular space.[46] A two-phase reaction to the hypovolemia may present with tachycardia as a first phase followed by bradycardia when effective blood volume falls by 20–30%.[32] The differential diagnosis of anaphylaxis includes panic attacks and vasovagal episodes.

● CLINICAL PEARLS

Diagnosis of anaphylaxis

- Anaphylaxis is characterized by extreme difficulty with breathing due to airway obstruction from angioedema or bronchoconstriction, circulatory collapse, or both.
- It is nearly always accompanied by tachycardia, usually by flushing, urticaria, and panic, and sometimes by vomiting and diarrhea.
- Panic attacks do not involve airways obstruction, hypotension, or urticaria but may be accompanied by faintness or tetany of the hands due to rapid overbreathing.
- Vasovagal attacks present with fainting, nausea, slow pulse, and pallor without respiratory difficulty, diarrhea, or urticaria.

Four clinical patterns of anaphylaxis have been described: immediate, biphasic, protracted, and delayed.[38] Anaphylaxis can occur within seconds after allergen exposure: the more rapid the onset of anaphylaxis after allergen exposure, the more severe and life-threatening the reaction. Food-induced anaphylaxis takes slightly longer to develop than drug- or insect-induced anaphylaxis. Up to 20% of patients may have biphasic anaphylaxis, with recurrence 2–12 hours after the initial attack. Recurrent episodes do not differ clinically but may require more epinephrine. The occurrence of biphasic anaphylaxis cannot be predicted from the severity of the initial attack. Some patients may develop protracted anaphylaxis, which sometimes lasts longer than 24 hours, may be extremely severe, and is often resistant to treatment. Delayed onset of anaphylaxis has been reported anecdotally, but is very unusual in clinical practice.

The diversity and severity of symptoms in anaphylaxis depend on the dose of allergen, the route of allergen exposure, the extent of allergen absorption, the degree of sensitization, individual allergen threshold for a reaction, target tissue sensitivity, cofactor involvement, co-existing atopic diseases and their severity, and concomitant treatment. Recently, "summation anaphylaxis" has been recognized as occurring after simultaneous exposure to various stimuli (physical exercise, infection, stress or concomitant exposure to other allergens or treatment with NSAIDs, ACE inhibitors, or β-blockers).[38] Fatal reactions to foods are usually characterized by respiratory symptoms (bronchospasm and hypoxia). In contrast, anaphylaxis induced by insect stings is more likely to lead to cardiovascular collapse. Asthma sufferers are at higher risk of fatal anaphylaxis. The risk of relapse in anaphylaxis depends on the type of allergen, individual allergen threshold, success of allergen avoidance, and the availability of immunotherapy.

The most dangerous symptoms are laryngeal edema, respiratory failure, and circulatory collapse, which may lead to death. Deaths from acute asthma in anaphylaxis occur predominantly in patients with pre-existing unstable asthma. Rapidly fatal shock often occurs without other symptoms, while death from laryngeal angioedema is the least common cause of fatality. According to the UK fatal anaphylaxis registry, the earliest arrest in fatal food anaphylaxis develops within 25–35 minutes of exposure, slightly slower than for insect stings (10–15 minutes) or drugs (5 minutes or less in hospital and 10–20 minutes outside hospital).[34,38]

The diagnosis of anaphylaxis

The measurement of blood tryptase level is now widely used as a marker of mast cell degranulation for *in vitro* confirmation of anaphylaxis. Beta-tryptase is released from mast cells but not from basophils and diffuses more slowly than histamine. The concentration of tryptase peaks 1–2 hours after the onset of reaction and remains elevated with a half-life of 1.5–2.5 hours. The samples for tryptase testing should be collected within 6 hours of anaphylaxis onset and again after 24 hours to check that the value has returned to normal. Tryptase can also be detected in postmortem specimens after death from suspected anaphylaxis.[34]

Normally, mature tryptase is below detection limits in the serum of healthy subjects, while it is elevated in most cases of anaphylaxis with vascular compromise, especially if it is parenterally induced. A tryptase concentration $> 25 \, \mu g/L$ is highly suggestive of anaphylaxis.[42] However, a normal level of tryptase is often observed in food-induced anaphylaxis so a normal tryptase result does not exclude anaphylaxis.[38–40] The diagnostic value of other mast cell proteases in anaphylaxis is under investigation.

The management of anaphylaxis

Early recognition of anaphylaxis facilitates removal of the cause and prompt institution of treatment. The patient with anaphylaxis should lie down with the legs elevated in order to increase venous blood return and maintain cardiac output and intravenous fluids should be given. In drug-induced or insect-induced anaphylaxis a tourniquet may be placed proximal to the site of the injection or insect sting to slow absorption of injected antigens. The tourniquet should be released for 3 minutes at 5-minute intervals, with the total duration of application not exceeding 30 minutes. Epinephrine should be administered at the first sign of respiratory failure or cardiovascular collapse. Milder attacks of allergy are often treated with antihistamines as a first-line measure. Epinephrine auto-injectors for self-administration are available but a single pen may be insufficient to reverse severe reactions. Their use in anaphylaxis outside hospital can be life-saving. The earlier epinephrine is administered in anaphylaxis, the better the outcome and survival rate.[47] Overall, prompt diagnosis of anaphylaxis, early administration of epinephrine, and fast transport to emergency rooms are crucial factors for successful management of anaphylaxis.

Epinephrine is both an α- and β-adrenergic agonist with cyclic adenosine monophosphate (cAMP)-mediated pharmacological effects on target organs. In patients with anaphylaxis, stimulation of α_1-adrenergic receptors increases peripheral vascular resistance, thereby improving blood pressure and coronary perfusion, reversing peripheral vasodilation, and decreasing angioedema. Activation of β_1-adrenergic receptors increases myocardial contractility (inotropy, chronotropy) while stimulation of β_2-adrenoreceptors causes bronchodilation as well as decreasing the release of inflammatory mediators from mast cells and basophils.[38,47]

According to current recommendations, the intramuscular route for epinephrine administration is preferable to the subcutaneous route due to faster absorption and higher plasma level of epinephrine after intramuscular injection.[40] The appropriate dosage of epinephrine is 0.2–0.5 mL of a 1:1000 dilution for adults. Epinephrine has a rapid but short action, therefore the dose can be repeated every 5–15 minutes until symptoms improve. More than one dose is required in one in three patients. The intravenous administration of epinephrine (1:100 000 dilution, i.e., 1 mg in 100 mL saline; infusion at 30–100 mL/h) should be reserved for severe anaphylaxis with profound life-threatening hypotension that is refractory to other treatment because of a risk of potentially fatal cardiac arrhythmias and myocardial infarction.[46]

Common pharmacological adverse effects of epinephrine include anxiety, fear, headache, pallor, tremor, dizziness and palpitation. In the event of overdose, unwanted effects may include increased QTc interval on electrocardiography, ventricular arrhythmias, angina, myocardial infarction, increased blood pressure, pulmonary edema, and intracranial hemorrhage. Patients with cardiovascular diseases and thyrotoxicosis and cocaine users are particularly prone to adverse effects of epinephrine.

The efficacy of epinephrine can be decreased by concomitant therapy with β-blockers, which is associated with unopposed stimulation of α-adrenoreceptors and reflex vagotonic effects, leading to bradycardia, hypertension, coronary artery constriction, bronchoconstriction, and augmented mediator release. Anaphylaxis in patients on β-blockers can be severe, protracted, and unresponsive to treatment. Patients treated with β-blockers may require fluid replacement and treatment with glucagon, which increases intracellular cAMP independently of β-adrenergic receptors. Glucagon can be administered in an intravenous bolus of 1 mg, followed by infusion of 1–5 mg/hour. Glucagon may improve hypotension in 1–5 minutes with maximal effect at 5–15 minutes. Side effects of glucagon include nausea and vomiting.

Corticosteroids are often administered in anaphylaxis to minimize the risk of recurrent or protracted anaphylaxis. The beneficial effects of corticosteroids develop 6–12 hours after administration. Therefore, their main role in anaphylaxis is likely to be the prevention of relapse, but it is still unclear how they work.

If there is no response to epinephrine, life support measures should be instituted. The treatment choice depends on the clinical presentation. In resistant hypotension, large volumes of fluids (crystalloids) should be given rapidly to compensate for peripheral vasodilatation and for fluid loss into the extravascular space. Other vasopressors (dopamine, glucagon) may be needed to reverse severe hypotension. Oxygen should also be administered in circulatory or respiratory failure. Bronchospasm should be treated with nebulized or inhaled β_2-agonists. If there is severe laryngeal edema, endotracheal intubation and even emergency tracheostomy may be needed to maintain the airway. All patients should be observed in a hospital setting for at least 4 hours because of the risk of biphasic anaphylaxis. In severe cases, an observation period of 24 hours is advisable.

The prevention of anaphylaxis

The first step in prevention is to identify those at risk of anaphylaxis. Therefore, all patients with a history of anaphylaxis should be referred for assessment and undergo allergy evaluation. Patients should be instructed how to avoid culprit allergens and cross-reactive agents and should be advised on safe alternatives. The education of patients, their families and, in the case of children, caregivers and school staff about anaphylaxis and first-aid measures is of primary importance. Written treatment plans should be provided to patients at special risk. Emergency medications such as epinephrine auto-injectors should be dispensed and patients should receive training on their correct usage. Patients should be advised to carry an epinephrine auto-injector with them at all times. Immunotherapy is very effective for prophylaxis of bee and wasp venom-induced anaphylaxis in sensitized patients and can be life-saving. Drug-induced anaphylaxis can be prevented by avoidance of culprit drugs and cross-reacting agents, by premedication (for radio-contrast media) and in some cases by drug desensitization for antibiotics, chemotherapeutic agents, insulin, vaccines, etc. For food-induced anaphylaxis, oral immunotherapy may be available in some allergy centers. In idiopathic anaphylaxis, patients with frequent episodes (more than 6 episodes per year or two or more episodes within 2 months) can be treated with steroids to prevent further episodes. Prevention strategies for anaphylaxis should also involve public awareness and public health measures, such as appropriate food labeling, disclosure of food ingredients in restaurants, the withdrawal of peanuts from in-flight refreshments, first-aid training in anaphylaxis for school staff, and establishing national anaphylaxis registries.

Translational research opportunities

●ON THE HORIZON

- Defining the role of functional autoantibodies and understanding the mast cell activation signals in chronic "idiopathic" urticaria should improve clinical assessment and management of patient subgroups.
- Development of new bradykinin and kallikrein inhibitors for patients with hereditary angioedema should further improve the acute management of this rare but very important condition.
- Understanding the full clinical spectrum of patients with cryopyrin-associated periodic syndrome with *NLRP-3* mutations should allow earlier identification and treatment of these individuals with interleukin-1 blockers to improve quality of life and prevent later complications.

Ongoing research into the importance of functional autoantibodies in chronic urticaria and the cause or causes of mast cell activation in patients with "idiopathic" disease should help to refine clinical assessment and management pathways.

The recent commercialization of a bradykinin receptor antagonist and a kallikrein inhibitor for patients with acute hereditary angioedema has illuminated the key role of the kallikrein-kinnogen-kinin pathway in disease pathogenesis. Development of new inhibitors of this pathway may offer additional benefits to patients in the future.

Clarification of the phenotypic spectrum of patients with cryopyrin associated periodic syndrome with *NLRP-3* mutations will facilitate early detection of affected individuals presenting in childhood with persistent urticaria who would benefit from treatment with interleukin-1 blockers. Early treatment should improve quality of life and may prevent the development of systemic amyloidosis, nephropathy and deafness in adulthood.

References

1. Zuberbier T, Binslev-Jensen C, Canonica W, et al. EAACI/GA2LEN/EDF guideline: definition, classification and diagnosis of urticaria. Allergy 2006;61:316–20.
2. Henz BM, Zuberbier T, Grabbe J, et al., editors. Urticaria. Berlin: Springer-Verlag; 1998.
3. Greaves MW, Kaplan A, editors. Urticaria and angioedema. New York: Marcel Dekker; 2004.
4. Beltrani VS. An overview of chronic urticaria. Clin Rev Allergy Immunol 2002;23:147–69.
5. Aydogan K, Karadogan SK, Akdag I, et al. HLA class I and class II antigens in Turkish patients with chronic ordinary urticaria. Clin Exp Dermatol 2006;31:424–9.
6. O'Donnell BF, O'Neill CM, Francis DM, et al. Human leucocyte antigen class II associations in chronic idiopathic urticaria. Br J Dermatol 1999;140:853–8.
7. Oztas P, Onder M, Gonen S, et al. Is there any relationship between human leucocyte antigen class II and chronic urticaria (chronic urticaria and HLA class II)? Yonsei Med J 2004;45:392–5.
8. Kim SH, Choi JH, Lee KW, et al. The human leucocyte antigen-DRB1*1302-DQB1*0609-DPB1*0201 haplotype may be a strong genetic marker for aspirin-induced urticaria. Clin Exp Allergy 2005;35:339–44.
9. Grattan CEH. The urticaria spectrum: recognition of clinical patterns can help management. Clin Exp Dermatol 2004;29:217–21.
10. Maurer M, Metz M. The status quo and quo vadis of mast cells. Exp Dermatol 2005;14:923–9.
11. Hennino A, Berard F, Guillot I, et al. Pathophysiology of urticaria. Clin Rev Allergy Immunol 2006;30:3–11.
12. Church MK, el-Lati S, Caulfield JP. Neuropeptide-induced secretion from human skin mast cells. Int Arch Allergy Appl Immunol 1991;94:310–8.
13. Sabroe RA, Greaves MW. Chronic idiopathic urticaria with functional autoantibodies: 12 years on. Br J Dermatol 2006;154:813–9.
14. Kaplan AP. Chronic urticaria: pathogenesis and treatment. J Allergy Clin Immunol 2004;114:465–74.
15. Puccetti A, Bason C, Simeoni S, et al. In chronic idiopathic urticaria autoantibodies against Fc epsilonRII/CD23 induce histamine release via eosinophil activation. Clin Exp Allergy 2005;35:1599–607.
16. Zuberbier T. The role of allergens and pseudoallergens in urticaria. J Investig Dermatol Symp Proc 2001;6:132–4.
17. Grattan CE. Aspirin sensitivity and urticaria. Clin Exp Dermatol 2003;28:123–7.
18. Kozel MM, Sabroe RA. Chronic urticaria: aetiology, management and current and future treatment options. Drugs 2004;64:2515–36.
19. Buhner S, Reese I, Kuehl F, et al. Pseudoallergic reactions in chronic urticaria are associated with altered gastroduodenal permeability. Allergy 2004;59:1118–23.
20. Wanderer AA, Hoffman HM. The spectrum of acquired and familial cold-induced urticaria/urticaria-like syndromes. Immunol Allergy Clin North Am 2004;24:259–86.
21. Davis MD, Brewer JD. Urticarial vasculitis and hypocomplementemic urticarial vasculitis syndrome. Immunol Allergy Clin North Am 2004;24:183–213.
22. Frigas E, Nzeako UC. Angioedema. Pathogenesis, differential diagnosis, and treatment. Clin Rev Allergy Immunol 2002;23:217–31.
23. Almerigogna F, Giudizi MG, Capella F, et al. Schnitzler's syndrome: what's new? J Eur Acad Dermatol Venereol 2002;16:214–9.
24. Kozel MM, Bossuyt PM, Mekkes JR, et al. Laboratory tests and identified diagnoses in patients with physical and chronic urticaria and angioedema: a systematic review. J Am Acad Dermatol 2003;48:409–16.
25. Asero R, Lorini M, Chong SU, et al. Assessment of histamine-releasing activity of sera from patients with chronic urticaria showing positive autologous skin test on human basophils and mast cells. Clin Exp Allergy 2004;34:1111–4.
26. Grattan CE, Powell S, Humphreys F. British Association of Dermatologists. Management and diagnostic guidelines for urticaria and angioedema. Br J Dermatol 2001;144:708–14.
27. Zuberbier T, Binslev-Jensen C, Canonica W, et al. EAACI/GA2LEN/EDF guideline: management of urticaria. Allergy 2006;61:321–31.
28. Borzova E, Grattan C. Urticaria: current and future treatments. Expert Rev Dermatol 2007;2:317–34.

29. Zuraw BL. Hereditary angioedema. N Engl J Med 2008;359:1027–36.
30. Gompels MM, Lock RJ, Abinun M, et al. C1 inhibitor deficiency: consensus document. Clin Exp Immunol 2005;139:379–94.
31. Matasar MJ, Neugut AI. Epidemiology of anaphylaxis in the United States. Curr Allergy Asthma Rep 2003;3:30–5.
32. Kemp SF, Lockey RF. Pathophysiology and organ damage in anaphylaxis. In: Castells MC, editor. Anaphylaxis and hypersensitivity reactions. 1st ed. Humana Press; 2011. p. 33–46.
33. Moneret-Vautrin DA, Morisset M, Flabbee J, et al. Epidemiology of life-threatening and lethal anaphylaxis: a review. Allergy 2005;60:443–51.
34. Pumphrey R. Anaphylaxis: can we tell who is at risk of a fatal reaction? Curr Opin Allergy Clin Immunol 2004;4:285–90.
35. Sheikh A, Alves B. Age, sex, geographical and socio-economic variations in admissions for anaphylaxis: analysis of four years of English hospital data. Clin Exp Allergy 2001;31:1571–6.
36. Mullins RJ. Anaphylaxis: risk factors for recurrence. Clin Exp Allergy 2003;33:1033–40.
37. Sheikh A, Alves B. Hospital admissions for acute anaphylaxis: time trend study. Br Med J 2000;320:1441.
38. Novartis Foundation. Anaphylaxis 257. Chichester: Wiley; 2004.
39. Sampson HA, Munoz-Furlong A, Campbell RL, et al. Second symposium on the definition and management of anaphylaxis: summary report—Second National Institute of Allergy and Infectious Disease/Food Allergy and Anaphylaxis Network symposium. J Allergy Clin Immunol 2006;117:391–7.
40. Sampson HA. Anaphylaxis and emergency treatment. Pediatrics 2003;111:1601–8.
41. Leone R, Conforti A, Venegoni M, et al. Drug-induced anaphylaxis: case/non-case study based on an Italian pharmacovigilance database. Drug Safe 2005;28:547–56.
42. Mertes PM, Laxenaire MC, Lienhart A, et al. Reducing the risk of anaphylaxis during anaesthesia: guidelines for clinical practice. J Investig Allergol Clin Immunol 2005;15:91–101.
43. Salama A, Temmesfeld B, Hippenstiel S, et al. A new strategy for the prevention of IgA anaphylactic transfusion reactions. Transfusion 2004;44:509–11.
44. Akin C, Scott LM, Kocabas CN, et al. Demonstration of an aberrant mast-cell population with clonal markers in a subset of patients with "idiopathic" anaphylaxis. Blood 2007;110(7):2331–3.
45. Brown SG. Anaphylaxis: clinical concepts and research priorities. Emerg Med Australas 2006;18:155–69.
46. Bernstein DI. Pharmacological management of acute anaphylaxis. In: Castells MC, editor. Anaphylaxis and hypersensitivity reactions. 1st ed. Humana Press; 2011. p. 285–95.
47. Lieberman P. Use of epinephrine in the treatment of anaphylaxis. Curr Opin Allergy Clin Immunol 2003;3:313–8.
48. Simons FER, Ardusso LRF, Bilo MB, et al. World Allergy Organization anaphylaxis guidelines: summary. J Allergy Clin Immunol 2011;127:587–593.e22.

Ulrich R. Müller,
Gabrielle
Haeberli, Arthur
Helbling

Allergic reactions to stinging and biting insects

Insects can induce allergic reactions by stinging and biting. They sting humans to defend themselves; they bite to nourish. With regard to allergies, stings by insects of the order Hymenoptera (bees, wasps, or ants) are much more important than bites, which can be inflicted by various insects such as mosquitoes, horseflies, midges, fleas, and bed bugs. Stings by Hymenoptera can induce acute systemic allergic reactions that kill several hundred patients in Europe and America every year, whereas systemic allergic reactions to bites are very rare. Both stings and bites can induce local allergic or toxic reactions. Infections are only transmitted by bites.

Entomological aspects[1–4]

Stinging Hymenoptera all belong to the suborder Aculeatae (Fig. 41.1) with the families Apideae, Vespidae, Formicidae, and Myrmicidae. Latin and popular names in English, which partly differ in Europe and USA are given in Table 41.1.

Apidae

In this family the honeybee (*Apis mellifera*) (Fig. 41.2A) is clinically the most important cause of allergies. Stings occur either in the vicinity of beehives or when the insect feels threatened during human activities, such as cutting flowers or walking barefoot in the grass. Because the whole beehive survives over the winter, stings can occur not only in spring and summer, but occasionally also on warm winter days. Honeybees are brown and moderately hairy. In contrast to other Hymenoptera, when stinging they usually lose their barbed sting.

Bumblebees (e.g., *Bombus terrestris*) are increasingly used as pollinators in greenhouses and occasionally cause allergic sting reactions in greenhouse workers.[2] Bumblebees are distinctly larger and more hairy than honeybees, and most species have distinct yellow or white bands on their abdomen (Fig. 41.2B).

Vespidae

The vespids are divided into the subfamilies Vespinae and Polistinae, which differ morphologically in the junction between thorax and abdomen (Figs. 41.2C, D). Vespids are almost hairless, and in most species the abdomen is striped black and yellow. Vespids do not usually lose their sting when stinging and may therefore sting several times, even the same victim. Because only the queen survives over winter, larger populations develop only in summer and most stings occur in summer and fall. The subfamily Vespinae contains the three genera *Vespula*, *Dolichovespula*, and *Vespa*.

Vespula (*V. germanica* and *V. vulgaris* in Europe, *V. maculifrons* and *V. germanica* in USA) are called wasps in Europe and yellow jackets in the USA. They breed in the ground, in attics, or in shelters. The genus *Vespula* is by far the most aggressive. Stings occur not only near the nests, but more often while victims are eating outdoors.

Most species of *Dolichovespula* (*D. media*, *D. sylvestris*, *D. saxonica* in Europe, *D. maculata*, *D. arenaria* in USA) look very similar to *Vespula*, with black and yellow stripes on the abdomen and only a slightly larger size. They can be distinguished from *Vespula* by the larger distance between the eyes and the mandibles. Only *D. maculata*, the bald-faced hornet in the USA, is easy to distinguish from other vespids by its mostly black abdomen. *Dolichovespula* build their nests in tree branches or under the roofs of houses. They sting almost exclusively in the vicinity of their nests.

The genus *Vespa* (*V. crabro*, the European hornet, Fig. 41.2E, *V. orientalis*) is easy to distinguish from other vespids by its much larger size. The European hornet has been introduced to America. The oriental hornet is present in southeastern Europe, Asia, and Africa. Hornet stings are rare and occur almost exclusively in the vicinity of nests, which are usually in hollow tree trunks or bird nesting-boxes.

Polistinae (*P. annularis*, *P. exclamans*, *P. fuscatus*, paper wasp in USA; *P. dominulus*, *P. gallicus*, *P. nympha*, field wasp in Europe) live mostly in southern USA and in the Mediterranean area of Europe, but small colonies have been observed all over Europe except for the British Isles. Their small nests consist only of one womb and are built in trees or under roofs.

Ants (Myrmicinae, Formicinae)

In South and Central America, and in the southern states of the USA, fire ants (*Solenopsis invicta*, Fig. 41.2 F, *S. richteri*) are responsible for many systemic allergic sting reactions.[3] Fire ants build their mounds in yards, playgrounds, and fields. Occasional allergic sting reactions have been described to *Pogonomyrmex*, the North American harvester ant, and extremely rarely to the European red ant, *Formica rufa*. In contrast, species of Myrmecinae, especially *Myrmecia pilosula*, the jack-jumper ant, are an important cause of allergic sting reactions in southern Australia.[4] Another group of aggressive ants are the ponerinae of the genus *Pachycondyla*, including *P. chinesis* in the Far East and *P. senna arensis* in the Middle East, which may also cause systemic allergic reactions.[3]

Allergens in Hymenoptera venoms

All Hymenoptera venoms contain low-molecular-weight substances such as biogenic amines, phospholipids, amino acids and carbohydrates, and peptides such as melittin, apamin, or

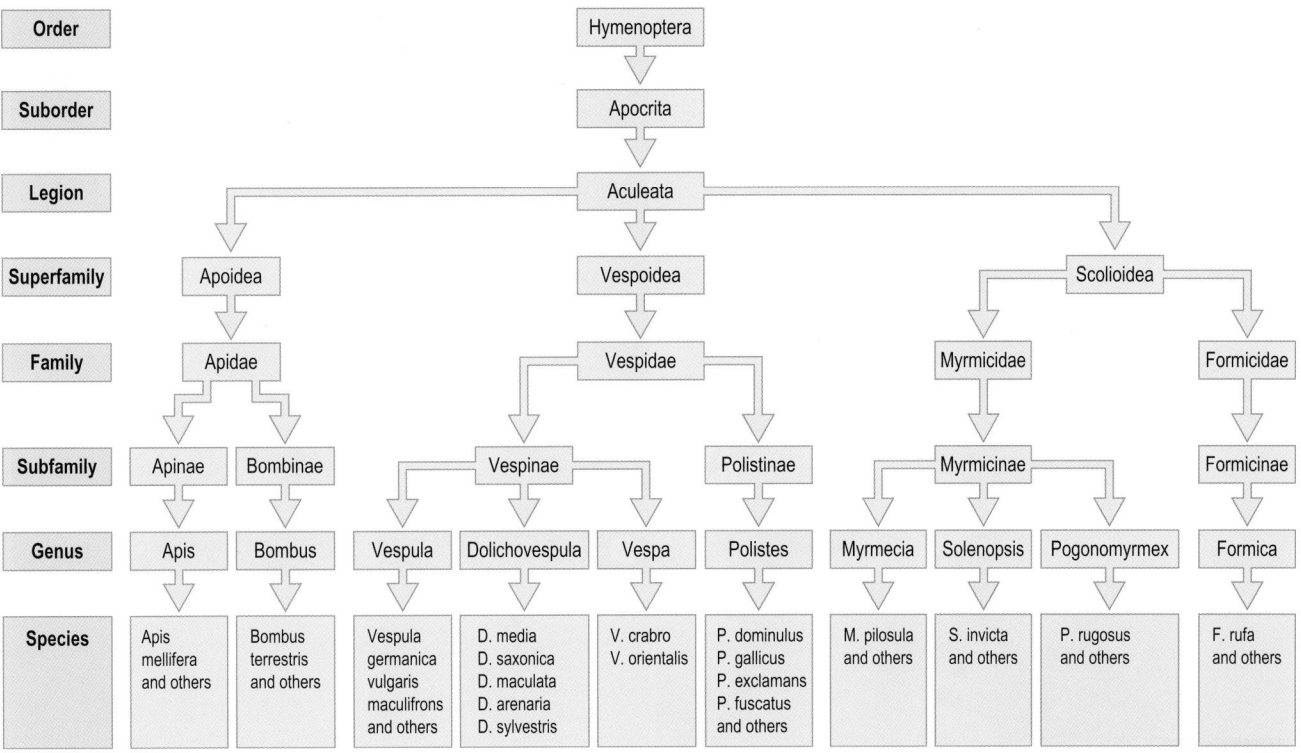

Fig. 41.1 **Taxonomy of Hymenoptera.**

Table 41.1 Popular names of the most frequent Hymenoptera in Europe and in USA

Latin name	Popular name Europe	Popular name USA
Apis mellifera	Honeybee	Honey bee
Bombus	Bumblebee	Bumble bee
Vespula ssp	Wasp	Yellow jacket
Dolichovespula maculata arenaria media	— — Median wasp	Bald faced hornet Yellow hornet —
Vespa crabro	Hornet	European hornet
Polistes spp	Field wasp	Paper wasp
Solenopsis invicta	—	Fire ant

Clinical picture

CLINICAL RELEVANCE

- Not every swelling after an insect sting relates to an allergy.
- Hymenoptera venom allergy generally reflects a systemic form of IgE-mediated allergy.
- While Hymenoptera venom allergy is not as prevalent as respiratory allergies, severe systemic reactions—even fatal—occur regularly all over the world.

Symptoms of venom hypersensitivity are most often due to IgE-mediated, but occasionally to non-IgE-mediated immunologic mechanisms. Rarely nonimmunologic mechanisms of mediator release play a role. The clinical presentation is classified into normal, large local, systemic allergic, systemic toxic, and unusual reactions.[1,2]

Normal local reactions

The normal local reaction of a nonallergic subject to a Hymenoptera sting consists of a painful, sometimes itchy, local wheal and flare reaction, followed by a swelling of up to 5–10 cm in diameter. Usually, local symptoms resolve within a few hours, by definition within 24 hours. The fire ant (*S. invicta*) attaches to the skin by means of its powerful mandibles and then stings, releasing venom that produces a characteristic fire like pain. If not removed, it will continue to rotate in a pivotal fashion, repeatedly injecting further small amounts of venom.[9] After it stings, a vesicle remains, which later develops into a pustule that only heals after 1–2 weeks.[3]

kinins, which contribute to the toxic effect but which—except for melittin—are probably irrelevant with regard to allergies. The allergens of the important stinging Hymenoptera are shown in Table 41.2. Most of them are glycoproteins of 10–50 kDa, some, e.g., dipeptidylpeptidases, up to 102 kDa. The major allergens in bee venom are phospholipase A2, hyaluronidase, and acid phosphatase; in vespid venoms antigen 5 and phospholipase A1. Ant venom from *S. invicta* contains a 37- and a 24-kDa allergen with some sequence homology to phospholipase A1 and to antigen 5 from vespid venom.[3] In ant venom from *M. pilosula* only pilosulin 1 has been identified as a major allergen so far. The genes of many major venom allergens have been cloned, and many of them have also been expressed as recombinant proteins comparable in allergenic activity and enzymatic function to their natural counterparts (Table 41.2)[5–8] The amount of venom injected during a sting varies between and within species, especially in vespids. Bees release 50–140 µg venom per sting; vespids much less: between 2 and 17 µg.[2]

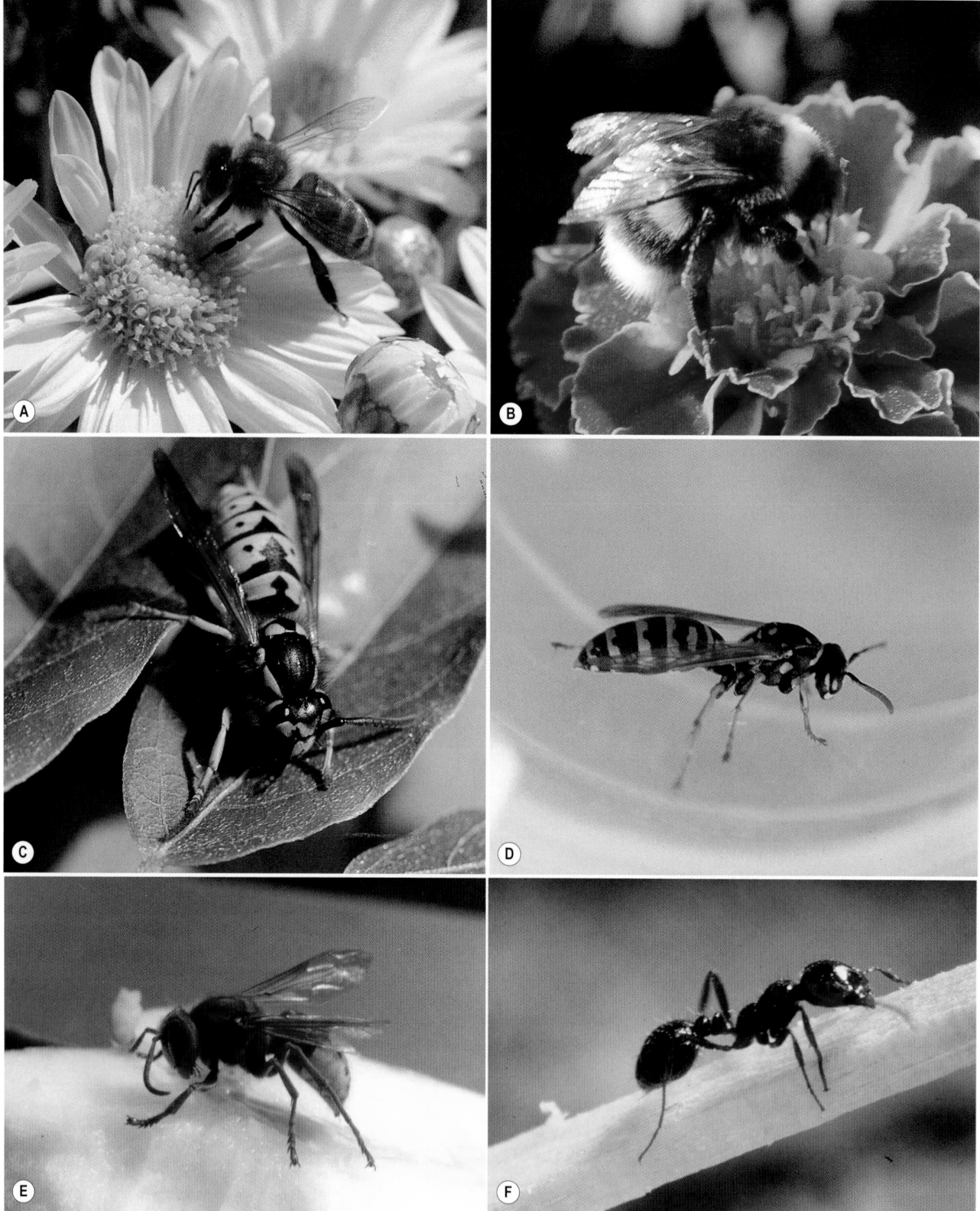

Fig. 41.2 Common Hymenoptera. (A) Honeybee (*Apis mellifera*), (B) bumblebee (*Bombus terrestris*), (C) wasp/yellow jacket (*Vespula* spp), (D) field wasp (*Polistes gallicus*), (E) European hornet (*Vespa crabro*), (F) fire ant (*Solenopsis invicta*).
Courtesy of the USA Department of Agriculture.

Table 41.2 Allergens of Hymenoptera venoms

Allergen	Molecular weight (kDa)	Glycosylation	Major/minor allergen[a]	Expressed as recombinant
Allergens in bee venom (*Apis mellifera*)				
Phospholipase A2 Api m1	16	Yes	Major	Yes
Hyaluronidase Api m2	45	Yes	Major	Yes
Acid phosphatase Api m3	49	Yes	Major?	Yes
Melittin Api m4	2.8	No	Minor	Yes
Dipeptidylpeptidase Api m5	102	Yes	Minor	Yes
Trypsin inhibitor Api m6	8	No	Minor	Yes
CUB serine protease Api m7	39	Yes	Major?	Yes
Carboxylesterase Api m8	70		Minor	
Carboxypeptidase Api m9	54		Minor	
Icarapin Api m10	29		Major?	Yes
Allergens of wasp/yellow jacket (*Vespula* spp, Ves v) and ant (*Solenosis invicta*, Sol i), *Myrmecia pilosula*, Myr p) venoms				
Vespula vulgaris Phospholipase A1 Ves v1	34	No	Major	Yes
Hyaluronidase Ves v2	38	Yes	Minor	Yes
Dipeptidylpeptidase Ves v3	100	Yes	?	Yes
Antigen 5 Ves v5	23	No	Major	Yes
Solenopsis Invicta Phospholipase A1 Sol i1	37	Yes	Major	Yes
Sol i2	14		Minor	Yes
Antigen 5 Sol i3	26		Major	Yes
Sol i4	20		Minor	
Myrmecia pilosula Myr p1	6.1		Minor	
Myr p2	5.6		Major	
Myr p3	8.2		Minor	

[a]Major allergen: ≥ 50% of allergic patients have specific IgE against. Minor allergen: < 50% of allergic patients have specific IgE against.

Large local reactions (LLR)

We define LLR as swellings around the sting site exceeding 10 cm in diameter, developing minutes to hours after the sting and lasting more than 24 hours.[1] LLR may be very disturbing, especially when they last for days or even weeks and involve a whole limb, eyelids, or lips. Sometimes they are accompanied by lymphadenopathy or lymphangitis. They may also be associated with nonspecific systemic inflammatory symptoms, such as malaise, fever, shivering, or headache. However, the development of a local infection, an abscess, or phlegmon at the sting site is inhibited

by the bacteriostatic effect of Hymenoptera venoms. In contrast, scratching after stings by the American fire ant or bites from blood-sucking insects, such as midges, can lead to skin infection.

The pathogenesis of LLR is thought to be based on IgE- and/or cell-mediated immune mechanisms, most likely a combination of both.[1,2]

Systemic allergic reactions (SR)

Systemic anaphylactic reactions are usually mediated by IgE. Affected organs can include the skin (pruritus, urticaria, flush, angioedema), the gastrointestinal tract (cramps, vomiting or diarrhea, dysphagia), the respiratory tract (laryngeal edema, bronchial obstruction, pulmonary edema), and the cardiovascular system (arterial hypotension, shock, arrhythmias, loss of consciousness with incontinence).

The most commonly used classification of SR was developed by Mueller.[10] Symptoms appear most often within a few minutes to 1 hour after the sting. The patient recovers usually within a few hours. A protracted course over more than a day or a biphasic course has been described as a rare event.

Lasting morbidity—e.g., myocardial or cerebrovascular infarction—as a consequence of SR, or even fatal reactions, can occur, but these are rare (see Epidemiological aspects).

Systemic toxic reactions

Toxic reactions are dose-dependent and a clinically significant toxic effect need only be considered after multiple stings—usually 50 to several hundred.[1,2] The main toxic effects develop within hours to days and comprise rhabdomyolysis and intravascular hemolysis leading to acute renal failure with tubular necrosis. Myocardial damage, hepatic dysfunction, coagulation disorders, and brain edema and/or necrosis may occur. The number of stings needed to cause a fatal reaction varies between 200 and 1000 in adults. In small children, however, fewer than 50 stings may be lethal. In most cases death occurs only after several days.

Unusual reactions

Unusual sting reactions are rare and appear after hours to days. More than half of them follow immediate local or systemic reactions.[1,11] Non-IgE-mediated immunologic mechanisms can play a role. The causal relation to the sting event often remains uncertain. Serum sickness-like syndromes with fever, arthralgias, exanthema, and lymphadenopathy are well documented. Less frequently reported complications following Hymenoptera stings include diseases of the nervous system (peripheral neuropathy, polyradiculomyelitis, extrapyramidal syndromes, acute disseminated encephalomyelitis), of the kidneys (glomerulonephritis, interstitial nephritis), of blood and blood vessels (hemolytic anemia, thrombocytopenia, Henoch–Schönlein syndrome and other forms of vasculitis). In these situations a causal relation to the sting is less well documented.

Epidemiological aspects

Prevalence of allergy to stings by flying Hymenoptera

KEY CONCEPTS

- Awareness of the most relevant insects, specifically Hymenoptera and their entomological subdivisions, causing IgE-mediated allergies.
- Assessment of clinical symptoms and classification of Hymenoptera venom allergy.
- Evaluation of persons and circumstances at risk for Hymenoptera venom allergy.
- Knowledge of appropriate diagnosis of Hymenoptera venom allergy, potential diagnostic and therapeutic control test tools.

Cumulative lifetime sting rates of 61–95% have been reported in people aged 16–65 years. Of course this can vary considerably in different regions of the world. Hymenoptera sting allergy can occur at any age. In general, due to their outdoor activities, men are more frequently stung than women, children more often than adults.[12]

The reported cumulative lifetime prevalence of LLR ranges from 2 to 26%, that of SR from 0.3 to 5%.[2] In beekeepers it varies between 14 and 43%.[13] In Europe and the USA SR are more frequently caused by vespids than by honeybees. In the southern states of the USA and in Australia ants are important causes of SR.

Risk factors for Hymenoptera allergy

The risk of developing a sting allergy increases with the number of stings. It is especially high if two stings occur within a short period (a few weeks to 2 months).[14] However, beekeepers stung less than 10 times a year have a much higher risk for SR than those stung more than 200 times a year.[13]

Cardiovascular diseases and their treatment with β-blocking drugs and ACE inhibitors are associated with more severe sting reactions, sometimes also with lasting morbidity due to cardiac or cerebrovascular infarction as a result of anaphylaxis.[1,15,16] However, β-blockers do not increase the overall risk of systemic sting reactions.[15] The presence of systemic mastocytosis, indicated by an elevated baseline serum tryptase, is a risk factor for severe or even fatal systemic sting reactions.[16] Atopy is no more frequent in Hymenoptera sting-allergic patients than in the general population. In an atopic patient with Hymenoptera venom allergy, however, systemic reactions may be more severe and more often affect the respiratory tract. About 50% of venom-allergic beekeepers are atopic. In atopic beekeepers sensitization may also occur by inhalation of dust containing venom during work on the beehives.[13]

Mortality due to Hymenoptera stings

Mortality from Hymenoptera stings varies from 0.09 to 0.48 deaths per million inhabitants per year.[17] The mean annual incidence of fatal Hymenoptera sting reactions over the past 40 years in Switzerland is 3.1, extrapolated to the whole of Europe about 200. The vast majority of fatal sting reactions occur in adults over 45 years of age.[2,17] Additional risk factors include a positive history of sting allergy, male gender, and stings on the head or neck. Autopsies have documented pre-existing cardiovascular disease in most cases.[17] Approximately half of the deaths occur in subjects with no known prior history of allergic sting reactions.

Natural history of Hymenoptera sting allergy

(Table 41.3)

In prospective clinical studies, the risk of developing a systemic reaction after a LLR is between 5 and 10%; after a mild SR between 15 and 30%; and after a severe SR between 50 and 75%.[18] The severity of an index sting reaction is an important factor determining the risk at re-exposure. Children are at a lower risk of re-sting SR than adults.[1] The re-sting SR risk is definitely lower in *Vespula*-allergic than in bee-venom-allergic patients, probably because of the smaller and more variable amount of venom injected.

Table 41.3 Natural history of Hymenoptera venom allergy based on prospective studies with sting re-exposure in patients without venom immunotherapy (summarized in reference[18])

Previous reaction	Author, year	Re-exposure by [a]	% with systemic reaction to re-exposure by			
			Bee or vespid	Bee	Vespid	Ant
Large local reactions	Müller, 1990	FS	6			
Systemic reactions (SR)	van der Linden, 1994	CH		51	25	
Mild SR children	Schuberth, 1983	FS	16			
Mild SR adults	Blaauw, 1985	CH		31	10	
Severe SR adults	Blaauw, 1985	CH	44	60	33	
SR in controls of controlled studies	Hunt, 1978 Müller, 1979 Brown, 2003	CH FS CH	61	75		72

[a]FS = field sting; CH = sting challenge.

Epidemiologic aspects of allergic reactions to ant stings

Nearly 50% of inhabitants of fire ant-endemic areas of the USA are stung each year.[3,9] Many report LLR, but up to 1% of patients who are stung by imported fire ants develop anaphylaxis, and some deaths have been reported. In Australia more than 90% of ant venom anaphylaxis is caused by *M. pilosula*. Age over 35 years, annual sting rate, and allergy to bee venom were predictors for more severe reactions.[20]

Diagnosis

History

The clinical history is the basis of the diagnosis of Hymenoptera sting allergy. This includes the date, number and circumstances of stings (e.g., environment, activities); kind and severity of symptom; sting site; retained or removed stinger; interval to onset of symptoms; emergency treatment; risk factors for a particularly severe reaction (e.g., comorbidity, drugs, elevated baseline serum tryptase); tolerated stings after the first systemic reaction; reduction of the quality of life;[21] and other allergies.[1,2] In individuals with only an LLR no further diagnostic tests are recommended. Basic diagnostic tests are skin tests, estimation of venom-specific serum IgE antibodies and, in case of severe SR, baseline serum tryptase.

Skin tests

Skin tests should be performed at least 3 weeks after a SR in order to avoid false-negative results during the refractory period. They are performed by intradermal or skin-prick endpoint titration;[2] 0.02 mL of venom solution are injected intradermally in increasing concentrations — from 0.00001 to 1 μg/mL — into the volar surface of the forearm. For skin-prick tests, concentrations of 0.01–300 μg/mL are used. However, even at 300 μg the sensitivity of skin prick is clearly lower than that of the intradermal test. We therefore prefer the intradermal test.

Venom-specific serum IgE antibodies (sIgE)

Several different *in vitro* immunoassays for the detection of sIgE have been derived from the original RAST (radio allergosorbent test) and are commercially available (Chapter 90). Immediately after a sting sIgE may be low or even undetectable, but usually increases within days or weeks after an SR. If no sIgE is detectable, the test should be repeated after 2–4 weeks.[2]

Sensitivity and specificity of skin tests and sIgE

The sensitivity of these tests is over 90% in patients with a history of SR within the past year, but decreases thereafter continuously, in patients both with and without venom immunotherapy, but may stay positive for many years. The specificity of both tests is, however, limited, since up to 20% of an unselected population have positive results while only 0.3–5% have a history of allergic sting reactions.[1,2] As a rule the intradermal test remains positive longer than sIgE. However, so far no reliable test exists to predict the risk of future SRs in untreated or treated patients. Despite a history of typical SRs to stings, a few patients have no detectable IgE and negative skin tests.[22] This may be due to insufficient sensitivity of the available tests, a long interval between SR and testing, with spontaneous decrease of sensitization, or non-IgE-mediated pathogenesis.

Specificity may cause problems: about 10–20% of people without a history of SR have a positive diagnostic test. Although sensitization following a previous sting is difficult to exclude, this positivity may reflect cross-reactivity (see below).

For the fire ant (*S. invicta*) only whole-body extracts are so far available for skin testing and venom immunotherapy. They have a good sensitivity but a low specificity. They should therefore only be done in patients with a history of systemic sting reactions and at least 30 days after the systemic reaction.[9] In contrast, venoms of *M. pilosula* have been shown to have an excellent sensitivity and specificity and also to be highly effective for venom immunotherapy.[4]

Cross-reactivity

Cross-reactivity between venom allergens is strong within a species, e.g., between *Vespula*, *Dolichovespula*, and *Vespa*, but only limited between *Vespinae* and *Polistinae* and honeybees and bumblebees. Between bee and vespid venom there is little cross-reactivity on protein basis, mainly due to an about 50% sequence identity between hyaluronidases and probably dipeptidyl-peptidases of the two families, but double-positivity with diagnostic tests to both venoms is frequently observed. This may reflect true double sensitization or cross-reactivity. Besides partial sequence homology of hyaluronidase, carbohydrate-containing epitopes are important. Cross-reacting carbohydrate determinants (CCDs) are present in many major Hymenoptera venom allergens, such as hyaluronidase, acid phosphatase, and phospholipase A2, but also in many plant proteins, e.g., in rapeseed pollen or bromelain. CCDs are certainly responsible for part of the double-positivity of diagnostic tests to bee and vespid venoms. They may also explain some of the positive tests in individuals with no history of SR. The CCDs are probably of no clinical relevance.[23] The RAST-inhibition test with venoms and CCDs is helpful in distinguishing between true double sensitization and cross-reactivity, and assisting in the choice of venoms for immunotherapy, but it is not always conclusive. Estimation of IgE antibodies to species-specific nonglycosylated, recombinant major allergens of both venoms, Api m1 (phospholipase A2) of bee venom and Ves v5 (antigen 5) of *Vespula* venom, reduce double-positivity to both venoms very significantly and is thus helpful for the choice of venoms for immunotherapy.[24]

Some crossreactivity between allergens Ves v1 and Ves v5 of vespid venoms and allergens of *S. invicta* have also been documented.[3]

Cellular tests

If routine tests in patients with a history of SR are negative, cellular tests may be helpful to demonstrate sensitization.[2]

In the *basophil histamine release test* peripheral blood leukocytes are incubated with venom allergens. The reaction with cell-bound IgE antibodies leads to histamine release from basophils. In the *cellular antigen stimulation test* (CAST) leukocytes of patients are pre-stimulated with IL-3 and exposed to venom allergens. The released sulfidoleukotrienes are determined by ELISA.

The *basophil activation test* (BAT) is based on flow-cytometric demonstration of an altered membrane phenotype of basophils stimulated by IL-3 and allergen exposure. At present the most commonly used expression marker is CD63. The sensitivity and specificity of the BAT seems to be superior to skin tests and venom-specifc serum IgE antibodies. It may also have a better predictive value. The test must, however, be performed in fresh blood; it is expensive and not yet well standardized: data on specificity and predictive value in relation to a sting re-exposure during or after venom immunotherapy are still scarce.

Allergen-specific IgG (sIgG)

The presence of specific IgG and IgG$_4$ primarily reflects exposure to the respective venom. sIgG titers increase after a sting, irrespective of the presence or absence of an allergic sting reaction. Venom immunotherapy induces a rise in sIgG. However, there is no close correlation between the concentration of sIgG or the sIgE/sIgG ratio and the clinical response to a re-sting during or after venom immunotherapy.[1] Routine assessment of sIgG is therefore not recommended, but may be helpful if the causing insect is unclear.

Baseline serum tryptase

Because of the association of an elevated baseline serum tryptase level (>11.4 µg/L) with especially severe, sometimes IgE-negative, systemic sting reactions and cutaneous or systemic mastocytosis, this enzyme should be determined in all patients with a history of SR.[16] The commercially available fluorescence immunoassay measures total tryptase. α-Tryptase is secreted continuously and reflects whole-body mast cell load. Elevated values are seen in cutaneous and systemic mastocytosis. β-Tryptase is released during mast cell activation, and is a marker of anaphylaxis.

Sting challenge tests

Sting challenge with a live insect is not recommended as a diagnostic tool in untreated patients, but a sting challenge under well-supervised clinical conditions may be helpful in evaluating the efficacy of venom immunotherapy.[18] A tolerated sting challenge does not, however, definitely exclude a reaction to future stings after immunotherapy, especially if these are repeated.

Prevention and treatment

Prevention

All patients with a history of SR should receive detailed instruction on the avoidance of future stings and measures to take if re-stung. Bee stings occur most often when walking barefoot on grass; wasp stings when eating outdoors, in orchards with fallen fruits, and near open waste-bins. The risk of a sting is especially high near beehives or vespid nests. While gardening, long trousers, shirts with long sleeves, and gloves are recommended. Strongly scented perfumes, suncreams, or shampoos, as well as brightly colored garments, should be avoided.

Treatment of large local reactions

Oral antihistamines and cooling of the sting site (e.g., with ice cubes) reduces local swelling, pain, and itching. Anti-inflammatory ointments or topical corticosteroids may diminish the local inflammatory process. In cases of severe swellings oral corticosteroids together with antihistamines over several days are recommended.[9]

Systemic allergic reactions

Sympathomimetics, antihistamines, and corticosteroids are the most effective drugs for symptomatic treatment of SR. All patients with SR should seek medical advice and should be medically observed until the symptoms resolve and the blood pressure is stable.

Mild reactions confined to the skin may be treated with rapidly acting oral antihistamines alone. If respiratory or cardiovascular symptoms occur, intramuscular epinephrine must be given immediately, intravenous access should be established, and antihistamines and corticosteroids given IV (Chapter 40). All patients with severe SR should be hospitalized and supervised until completely recovered. Patients with cardiovascular symptoms must be treated and transported in the supine position, and IV volume replacement is indicated.

Every patient with a systemic allergic sting reaction should be investigated with a view to prevention measures and immunotherapy.[9]

Emergency medication kit

All patients with a history of SR should carry an emergency kit for self-administration. After a sting patients should immediately take both antihistamines and corticosteroids, whether there are symptoms or not. If systemic symptoms such as urticaria, dyspnea, generalized weakness, or dizziness occur, epinephrine should be administered IM in the lateral thigh via an auto-injector Epipen (0.3 mg of epinephrine). In children below 30 kg bodyweight the Epipen junior (0.15 mg epinephrine) and half the dose of antihistamines and corticosteroids should be used. If any SR occurs, medical care must be sought.

Venom immunotherapy (VIT)[9]

Indications

VIT is indicated in children and adults with a history of severe systemic reactions (grade III/IV), provided sensitization to the relevant venom is demonstrated by skin and/or blood test. LLR or unusual reactions do not qualify for VIT. VIT is also recommended for patients with repeated mild, non-life-threatening reactions who are at high risk for re-exposure, such as beekeepers or their family members. Concomitant cardiovascular disease, mastocytosis, or strongly impaired quality of life due to the venom allergy are also indications for VIT in patients with non-life-threatening sting reactions.[16,21]

Contraindications for VIT are the same as for immunotherapy with other allergens (Chapter 91).

Dosage and treatment regimens

The recommended maintenance dose is 100 μg of the venom, for both children and adults. This maintenance dose is equivalent to approximately two bee stings or several vespid stings. A higher dose (e.g., 200 μg) is recommended when systemic reactions occur after re-exposure to a field sting or a sting challenge. In highly exposed subjects such as beekeepers or professional gardeners a maintenance dose of 200 μg is advised.

VIT may be initiated by a conventional or an ultra-rush protocol. The injection interval for maintenance VIT is 4 weeks for the first year. Afterwards intervals may be extended to 6 weeks if VIT is well tolerated.

Adverse reactions to VIT

The overall incidence of systemic adverse reactions to VIT varies between 5 and 40%. VIT with bee venom causes more side effects than with Vespula venom. Ultra-rush protocols are associated with a somewhat higher rate of side effects than conventional protocols. Most systemic side effects are mild; approximately one-third will require medical treatment.

Premedication with antihistamines reduces large local and other cutaneous reactions such as urticaria, but severe systemic reactions may not be suppressed. Many authors recommend giving antihistamines 2 hours before injections in the up-dosing phase of VIT until the maintenance dose has been repeatedly well tolerated.

Efficacy of VIT

In addition to three prospective controlled trials, the efficacy of VIT has been confirmed by well-tolerated sting challenges during VIT in a number of uncontrolled prospective studies. Treatment with bee venom results in full protection in 80–85% of patients; with Vespula venoms in 95–100%. The efficacy of immunotherapy with commercially available Solenopsis whole-body extract has not been documented in controlled studies. However, excellent results, comparable to those of VIT with Vespula venom, were obtained in a double-blind placebo-controlled study using *M. pilosula* venom.[4]

Duration of VIT

Lifelong treatment may be the safest recommendation, but in most allergy centers VIT is given for 5 years since after discontinuation of VIT of at least 3 years' duration protection persists in over 80% of both adults and children, when reassessed 1–7 years after discontinuation. Longer courses of treatment should be considered in high-risk patients such as those with very severe systemic sting reactions, coexisting cardiovascular or pulmonary disease, systemic allergic reactions to VIT or stings during VIT, and for subjects with elevated basal serum tryptase levels. Lifelong VIT is advised for patients with cutaneous or systemic mastocytosis.[9]

Risk factors for recurrence of systemic reactions after stopping VIT

A number of risk factors have been identified for relapse of Hymenoptera venom allergy after discontinuation of VIT: generally adults have a less favorable prognosis than children. Bee-venom-allergic patients have a higher relapse risk than those allergic to Vespula venom. The more severe the pre-treatment reactions were, the higher the risk for recurrence of systemic reactions following Hymenoptera stings. After VIT for 5 years, compared to only 3 years, the risk of relapse is reduced.

Allergic reactions to biting insects

Biting insects may cause local allergic reactions as a result of sensitization to their salivary proteins introduced during the process of blood sucking. Systemic reactions are very rare. The responsible insects belong to the orders Diptera, Hemiptera, and Siphonaptera (Fig. 41.3).[25]

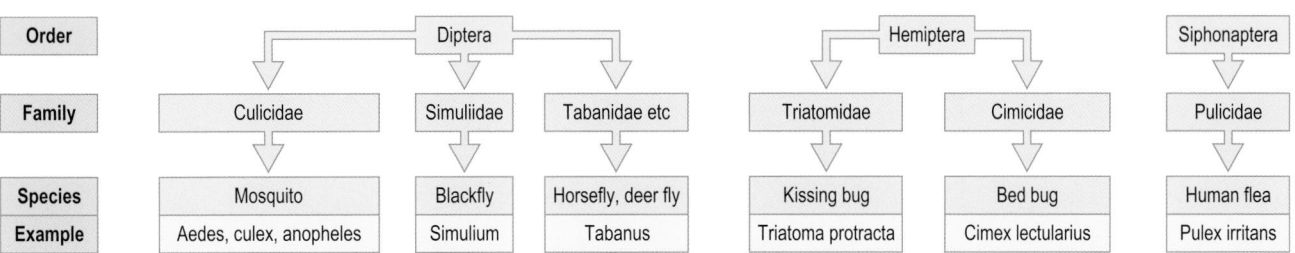

Order		Diptera			Hemiptera		Siphonaptera
Family	Culicidae	Simuliidae	Tabanidae etc	Triatomidae	Cimicidae		Pulicidae
Species	Mosquito	Blackfly	Horsefly, deer fly	Kissing bug	Bed bug		Human flea
Example	Aedes, culex, anopheles	Simulium	Tabanus	Triatoma protracta	Cimex lectularius		Pulex irritans

Fig. 41.3 Biting insects that may cause allergic reactions.

Clinical symptoms

Local reactions to insect bites may be characterized by immediate wheal and flare, or may be delayed, with pruritic erythema and papules developing after 12–24 hours and lasting for days to weeks; combined reactions can also occur. In delayed and combined reactions, vesicular, bullous, or even necrotic lesions may develop. Systemic reactions are much rarer than to Hymenoptera stings. They have, however, occasionally been described, especially following bites by horseflies (*Tabanus* spp.) and the kissing bug (*Triatoma protracta*).

Allergens

The salivary proteins involved have either digestive (amylases, esterases) or hemostatic function (e.g., factor Xa inhibition). Numerous IgE-binding proteins with a molecular weight of 15–81 kDa have been described, especially in the saliva of mosquitoes, but also in horseflies and kissing bugs; some of these have been cloned.[26]

Prevention and treatment

The application of insect repellents and prophylactic intake of antihistamines can prevent or mitigate outdoor exposure. Screens on windows and doors and mosquito nets over the beds are effective in homes. Bedbug infestation should be eliminated by appropriate pesticides; flea infestation of pet animals should be managed by a veterinarian. Local reactions may be treated with topical steroids or oral antihistamines.

Future perspectives

The availability of recombinant venom allergens offers several promising perspectives for both diagnosis and immunotherapy.[5–8] The specificity of these tests could be considerably improved by using recombinant cocktails with species-specific major allergens without CCDs for diagnosis instead of the whole venom. In patients with double-positive diagnostic tests using honeybee and *Vespula* venom, recombinant species-specific non-glycosylated major allergens from honeybee and *Vespula* venom make it possible to distinguish reliably between true double sensitization and cross-reactivity, an important issue for the choice of venoms for immunotherapy.

References

1. Müller U. Insect sting allergy. Stuttgart: Gustav Fischer Verlag; 1990.
2. Bilò MB, Ruëff F, Mosbech H, et al. Diagnosis of Hymenoptera venom allergy. Allergy 2005;60:1339–49.
3. Hoffmann DR. Ant venoms. Curr Opin Allergy Clin Immunol 2010;10:342–6.
4. Brown SGA, Franks RW, Baldo BA, Heddle RJ. Prevalence, severity, and natural history of jack jumper ant venom allergy in Tasmania. J Allergy Clin Immunol 2003;111:187–92.
5. Müller U. Insect venoms. In: Ring J, editor. Anaphylaxis, chemical immunol allergy. Basel: Karger; 2010. p. 141–56.
6. King TP, Guralnick M. Hymenoptera Allergens. In: Lockey R, Ledford D, editors. Allergens and allergen immunotherapy. 4th ed. Clin Allergy Immunol, vol. 21; 2008. p. 237–49.
7. Grunwald T, Bockisch B, Spillner E, et al. Molecular cloning and expression in insect cells of honeybee venom allergen acid phosphatase (Api m 3). J Allergy Clin Immunol 2006;117:848–54.
8. Seismann H, Blank S, Braren I, et al. Dissecting cross-reactivity in Hymenoptera venom allergy by circumvention of α-1,3-core fucosylation. Mol Immunol 2010;47:799–808.
9. Müller U, Golden DBK, Lockey RF, Byol S. Immunotherapy for *Hymenoptera* venom hypersensitivity. In: Lockey R, Ledford D, editors. Allergens and allergen immunotherapy. 4th ed. Clin Allergy Immunol, vol. 21. 2008. p. 377–92.
10. Mueller HL. Diagnosis and treatment of insect sensitivity. J Asthma Res 1966;3:331–3.
11. Reisman RE. Unusual reactions to insect stings. Curr Opin Allergy Clin Immunol 2005;5:355–8.
12. Graif Y, Confino-Cohen R, Goldberg A. Allergic reactions to insect stings: Results from a national survey of 10 000 junior high school children in Israel. J Allergy Clin Immunol 2006;117:1435–9.
13. Müller U. Bee venom allergy in beekeepers and their family members. Curr Opin Allergy Clin Immunol 2005;5:343–7.
14. Antonicelli A, Bilò MB, Bonifazi F. Epidemiology of Hymenoptera allergy. Curr Opin Allergy Clin Immunol 2002;2:341–6.
15. Müller U, Haeberli G. Use of beta-blockers during immunotherapy for *Hymenoptera* venom allergy. J Allergy Clin Immunol 2005;115:606–10.
16. Ruëff F, Przybilla B, Bilò M, et al. Predictors of severe anaphylactic reactions in patients with hymenoptera venom allergy: Importance of baseline serum tryptase. J Allergy Clin Immunol 2009;124:1047–55.
17. Sasvary T, Müller U. Fatalities from insect stings in Switzerland 1978 to 1987. Schweiz Med Wschr 1994;124:1887–94.
18. Ruëff F, Przybilla B, Müller U, et al. The sting challenge test in Hymenoptera venom allergy. Allergy 1996;51:216–25.
19. Golden DBK, Kagey-Sobotka A, Norman PS, et al. Outcomes of allergy to insect stings in children, with and without venom immunotherapy. N Engl J Med 2004;351:668–74.
20. Brown SG. Cardiovascular aspects of anaphylaxis: implications for treatment and diagnosis. Curr Opin Allergy Clin Immunol 2005;5:359–64.
21. Oude Elberink JN, Dubois AE. Quality of life in insect venom allergic patients. Curr Opin Allergy Clin Immunol 2003;3:287–93.
22. Golden DBK, Kagey-Sobotka A, Norman PS, et al. Insect sting allergy with negative venom skin test responses. J Allergy Clin Immunol 2001;107:897–901.
23. Hemmer W, Focke M, Kolarich D, et al. Antibody binding to venom carbohydrates is a frequent cause for double positivity to honey bee and yellow jacket venom in patients with stinging insect allergy. J Allergy Clin Immunol 2001;108:1045–52.
24. Müller U, Johansen N, Petersen A, et al. Hymenoptera venom allergy: Analysis of double positivity to honey bee and *Vespula* venom by estimation of species-specific major allergens Api m1 and Ves v5. Allergy 2009;64:543–8.
25. Hoffman DR. Allergic reactions to biting insects. In: Levine MI, Lockey RF, editors. Monograph on insect allergy. Pittsburgh: Dave Lambert Associates; 2003. p. 161–74.
26. Simons FER, Peng Z. Mosquito allergy. In: Levine MI, Lockey RF, editors. Monograph on insect allergy. Pittsburgh: Dave Lambert Associates; 2003. p. 175–203.

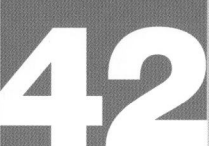

Atopic and contact dermatitis

Thomas Bieber,
Caroline Jagobi

Atopic dermatitis (AD) is a chronic and relapsing inflammatory skin disease affecting an increasing number of patients.[1,2] Characteristic features of AD include pruritus and chronic or chronically relapsing dermatitis, usually beginning during infancy. AD is a genetically complex disease and is often, but not always, accompanied by other atopic disorders such as allergic rhinoconjunctivitis or allergic bronchial asthma. These diseases may appear simultaneously or develop in succession during the course of AD. It characteristically starts during early childhood, whereas allergic rhinitis and asthma predominate in adolescence. This characteristic, age-dependent sequence has been termed the atopic march.[3] The cutaneous manifestation of atopy often represents the beginning of this atopic career while asthma is its full expression. Therapeutic strategies should be directed towards the delay or avoidance of this development, by early intervention against skin inflammation which may prevent subsequent sensitization and progression towards rhinitis and asthma.

AD is a genetically complex disease involving gene–gene and gene–environment interactions, but much progress in understanding its pathogenesis has been achieved in recent years. Genetic linkage studies have identified several chromosomal regions linked to epidermal barrier function, and genetic variants which favour the development of AD, but several candidate genes linked to the immune system have also been detected. A breakthrough has been the identification of loss of function mutations in the *filaggrin gene (FLG)* in patients with AD, which codes for an important epidermal structure protein.[4] The findings have been consistently replicated, and FLG mutations have been identified as the strongest risk factor for AD which is known so far.[5]

Stress, bacterial or viral infections, exposure to aero- or food allergens and hygienic factors have been implicated in aggravating the symptoms of AD. Although the so-called "hygiene hypothesis" is controversial, the importance of lifestyle and environment in the mechanisms of atopic disease is well accepted. Additionally, a generalized Th2-deviated immune response is closely linked to AD, but the skin disease itself is a biphasic inflammation with an initial Th2 phase, while chronic lesions harbour Th0/Th1 cells. Both regulatory T cells (Tregs) and the innate immune system have been shown to be altered in AD. The main treatment goals for AD include the elimination of inflammation and infection, preservation and restitution of barrier function, anti-pruritic management, and control of exacerbating factors. The long-term-strategy in AD aims to control skin inflammation and to improve the epidermal barrier function in order to prevent the emergence of sensitization.

KEY CONCEPTS

Pathophysiology of atopic dermatitis

- Atopic dermatitis is a genetic complex disease (gene–gene and gene–environment interactions).
- Defective epidermal barrier function and decreased epidermal innate immunity.
- Deviated immune response toward increased sensitization supported by skin inflammation.
- High microbial colonization that amplifies skin inflammation.
- Role of FcεRI/IgE-bearing dendritic cells.
- Role of IgE-mediated immune response to autoallergens.
- Decreased activity of regulatory T cells.

Definition

Over the last 120 years, AD has been given a multitude of different names, e.g., Besnier's prurigo, disseminated neurodermitis, or neurodermitis constitutionalis sive atopica, but atopic dermatitis and nonatopic dermatitis are currently the most widely used names. According to a recent consensus nomenclature by the World Allergy Organization (WAO), the term AD should be reserved for the eczematous condition with the typical clinical signs and associated with immunoglobulin E (IgE)-mediated sensitization to aeroallergens. Indeed, in 2004 a WAO consensus group proposed a revised terminology for atopy, restricting its use to conditions associated with IgE sensitization.[6] According to this classification, the term atopy should only be applied in combination with documented allergen-specific IgE antibodies in serum or with a positive skin prick test. This current terminology substitutes the former term of extrinsic AD and includes only patients who show IgE sensitization against inhalant and/or food allergens in skin tests or serum. A small group of approximately 20–30% of affected patients shows clinical signs of AD, without any IgE-sensitization. This group may be classified as having "nonatopic dermatitis," replacing the previous term intrinsic AD. Patients with nonatopic dermatitis show negative skin tests and have no other signs of IgE-mediated sensitization. Both atopic and nonatopic dermatitis are most probably highly related, in terms of natural history of the disease, as will be discussed below.

From an etymological perspective, dermatitis means any dermal inflammation, while eczema (from Greek Εκζειν = boiling) is more an epidermal acute inflammation with vesicles. Nevertheless, in order to be consistent and not to complicate the issue in this chapter, the term "dermatitis" will be used, although both "eczema" and "dermatitis" are used interchangeably by physicians worldwide.

Epidemiology

With an incidence of 15–30% in children and 2–10% in adults, AD has clearly increased by two- to threefold during the past three decades in industrialized countries.[7] AD usually presents during early infancy and childhood but may also persist into adulthood or start in adulthood. In 45% of affected children the onset of AD occurs during the first 6 months of life; during the first year 60% of the children are affected, and 85% of those who will be affected will show symptoms before the age of 5. The severity of AD seems to be linked to sensitization to foods, in particular hen's egg and cow's milk. Interestingly, however, more than 50% of children in the first 2 years of life do not display any sign of allergic sensitization even though they suffer from classical skin lesions.[6]

Clinical manifestations

It should be emphasized that nonatopic dermatitis and AD are not clinically different; both develop on dry skin that may in some instances resemble a mild form of ichthyosis. Intense pruritus is also a common feature of both forms of dermatitis. The clinical spectrum is wide, ranging from mild forms such as pityriasis alba, to major forms with erythrodermic variants. The dermatitis is polymorphic, with acute (oozing, crusted, vesicles, or papules on erythematous plaques), subacute (mainly excoriated plaques), and chronic (lichenified and excoriated plaques) forms. Although pruritus can occur throughout the day, it generally worsens at night and can profoundly affect the quality of life.

Clinical patterns usually vary with age. The first signs of inflammation typically occur during the third month of life and infants present with facial and patchy or generalized dermatitis (Fig. 42.1). Lesions generally first appear on the cheeks and are characterized by dry and erythematous skin with papulovesicular lesions. The term "milk crust" or "milk scurf" refers to the occurrence of yellowish crusts on the scalp that are similar to scalded milk. At a later age, the inner and outer parts of the arms

and legs may also be affected. The diaper area is usually spared. Itching and scratching are intense and promote the tendency to bacterial superinfection, mainly by *Staphylococcus aureus*. In childhood, sites of predilection of dermatitis are flexural areas and the dorsum of the feet and hands. They can either develop from the preceding neonatal phase or arise de novo. Rashes usually begin with papules that go on to become lichenified. The skin around the lips may be inflamed and constant licking of the area may lead to small, painful cracks in the perioral skin. For unknown reasons, in more than 60% of cases AD may enter into complete remission during puberty.

As in childhood, localized inflammation with lichenification of the flexural areas is the most common pattern of adult AD. Sites of predilection are the neck, upper chest, large joint flexures, and backs of the hands. If the face is affected, this is usually on the forehead, eyelids, and perioral region. Scalp involvement can occur and may even lead to diffuse hair loss. During adulthood, even if the inflammation has resolved, dry skin continues to be a persistent problem, especially in winter months. In adults some minimal variants of AD may occur such as hand dermatitis, nummular dermatitis, periocular inflammation, lichenification of the anogenital area, cheilitis sicca, nipple dermatitis, and pityriasis alba.

Complications

The most important complications of AD are due to secondary infections. It has been shown that deficiency in anti-microbial peptides (AMP: see below) for host defense and possibly a reduced cell-mediated immunity over years contribute to the occurrence of bacterial and viral complications. Nearly all AD patients have their skin heavily colonized by *S. aureus*, although clinical signs of infection are mostly lacking. In children with strong pruritus and excoriations, impetigo-like crusting can develop.

Patients with AD are at increased risk for fulminant herpes simplex virus infections (eczema herpeticum). The course of this complication can be severe, with high fever and widespread eruptions. Clinically, numerous vesicles in the same stage of development are characteristic. Patients feel systemically unwell and the diagnosis should be confirmed rapidly by polymerase chain reaction. It remains unclear whether the prevalence of viral warts or molluscum contagiosum is increased in AD.

Histology and immunohistology

The histology of both forms of dermatitis is similar to that of allergic contact dermatitis (ACD) and has no fundamental impact on the diagnosis of AD. Clinically normal appearing skin of AD patients contains a sparse perivascular T-cell infiltrate suggesting minimal inflammation.[8] Acute papular skin lesions are characterized by marked intercellular edema (spongiosis) of the epidermis (Fig. 42.2). Langerhans cells (LC), in lesional and, to a lesser extent, in nonlesional skin of AD frequently exhibit surface-bound IgE molecules. In acute lesions there is a marked perivascular T-cell infiltrate in the dermis with monocytes–macrophages. The lymphocytic infiltrate consists predominantly of activated memory T cells bearing CD3, CD4, human leukocyte antigen (HLA)-DR, CD25, and CD45RO. Eosinophils, basophils, and neutrophils are rarely present in acute AD. Mast cells are present in various stages of degranulation.

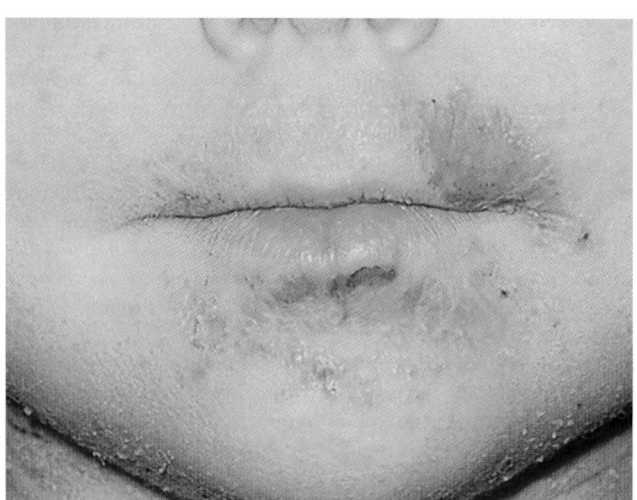

Fig. 42.1 Facial lesions in atopic dermatitis.

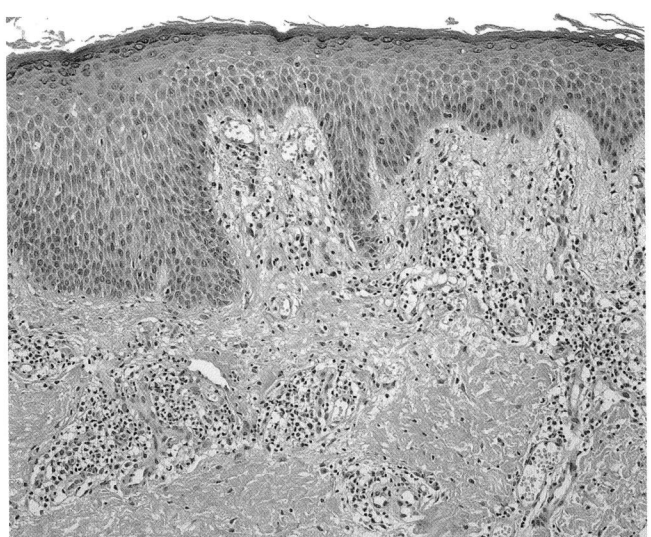

Fig. 42.2 Thickening of the epidermal compartment (acanthosis) with mild spongiosis. Lymphocytic and histiocytic inflammatory dermal infiltrate, mainly around the vessels.

Chronic lichenified lesions are characterized by a hyperplastic epidermis with elongation of the rete ridges, prominent hyperkeratosis, and minimal spongiosis. There is an increased number of IgE-bearing dendritic cells (DC) in the epidermis, and macrophages dominate the dermal mononuclear cell infiltrate. The number of mast cells is increased but the cells do not generally show evidence of degranulation. Although intact eosinophils are hardly visible histologically, they are implicated in the dermis of chronic AD skin lesions since their products, such as eosinophil major basic protein, eosinophil cationic protein, and eosinophil-derived neurotoxin can be detected by immunostaining. Thus eosinophils likely contribute to allergic skin inflammation by the secretion of cytokines and mediators that augment allergic inflammation and may induce tissue injury in AD through the production of reactive oxygen intermediates and release of toxic granule proteins.

Pathogenesis

Much insight has been achieved into the pathogenesis of AD in recent years. We have learned that development of the chronic skin inflammation underlying both forms of dermatitis requires a combination of a genetically determined intrinsic defect of the epidermal barrier, immunological abnormalities, and environmental factors.

Genetics

Parental atopy, in particular dermatitis, is significantly associated with the manifestation and severity of early AD in children.[11] Unexpectedly, other parental atopic diseases such as allergic asthma or allergic rhinitis seem to be a minor factor in the development of AD, suggesting the existence of genes specific to AD. Genome–wide linkage studies have identified candidate gene regions on chromosomes 3q14, 13q14, 15q14-15, 17q21,[9] 4q22, 3p24, 3q21,[10] 1q21, 17q25, 20p, 5q13, 11p, 3p, 4p, 18q, 15q21, and 1q24, but the results diverge strongly and only few of the loci could be replicated reliably. The regions of strongest linkage were found on chromosomes 1q21 and 17q25, although contradictory results have been found for the latter one.[11]

The other genetic approach is to screen variants, i.e., single nucleotide polymorphisms (SNPs), of candidate genes for possible association with the AD clinical phenotype (reviewed by Morar et al).[12] Several candidate genes have been identified in recent years, notably on chromosome 5q31-33, which contains genes for the Th2 cytokines interleukin (IL)-3, -4, -5, IL-13, and granulocyte–macrophage colony-stimulating factor (GM-CSF). Further studies have identified variants of the IL-13 coding region, functional mutations of the promoter region of the chemokine RANTES (17q11) and gain-of-function polymorphisms in the alpha subunit of the IL-4 receptor (16q12). Polymorphisms of the IL-4 subunit may have an influence on the IL-4-receptor-related synthesis of IgE. This could be linked to the incidence of nonatopic dermatitis, which occurs without any IgE sensitization. Similarly, a dysbalance between Th1 and Th2-immune responses in AD may be explained by polymorphisms of the IL-18-gene, resulting in a Th2 predominance. At a functional level, upon stimulation with superantigens, peripheral blood mononuclear cells (PBMC) from individuals with these polymorphisms respond with upregulation of IL-18 and downregulation of IL-12 and consequently show a Th2 predominance. A particularly severe course of AD with colonization of *S. aureus* may be associated with a SNP of the Toll-like receptor (TLR)-2 gene.

A hallmark in the genetic research in AD has been the identification of an association of "loss of function mutations" in the *filaggrin gen* (FLG) with AD. The gene is located in the epidermal differentiation complex (EDC) on chromosome 1q21.[4] It encodes for the epidermal structure protein FLG, which is a key protein in the terminal differentiation of the epidermis. A deficiency in FLG that affects about 10% of the European population causes a very dry skin. Carriers of two FLG-mutations suffer from ichthyosis, a hereditary skin disease characterized by extremely dry and scaly skin. In AD several loss of function mutations have been identified in various studies (e.g. R501X, 2282del4, R2447X, S3247X, 3702delG). These mutations highly vary depending on the populations considered. Studies on European cohorts have shown about 17 to 50% of AD patients to be carrier of at least one mutation. FLG-mutations have been shown to be related to an early onset of the disease, high IgE levels, increased food allergy and ultimately the development of allergic asthma. These findings strongly suggest that FLG mutations are determinant for the development of the so-called atopic march. However, it is expected that a number of yet-to-be-defined other genetic alterations may account for the remaining 30 to 70% of AD patients.

Disturbed epidermal barrier function

AD is characterized by dry skin affecting lesional and nonlesional skin areas. Altered skin barrier function, resulting in increased transepidermal water loss, is typical for this condition and may be, among others, an explanation for the facilitated penetration of allergens, bacteria, and viruses. The mechanisms behind this dryness are complex and closely related to the disturbed epidermal barrier function.[13] The loss of skin ceramides, which serve as the major water-retaining molecules in the extracellular space of the cornified envelope, has been proposed to cause this modification of the skin barrier. Furthermore, variations of the stratum corneum pH may impair lipid metabolism in the skin. Overexpression of enzymes such as chymotrypsin is also likely to contribute to the breakdown of the AD epidermal barrier. Further considerations include a D-6-desaturase deficiency and a decreased conversion of ω6-linoleic acids to prostaglandin in affected patients.

As mentioned above, recent studies underline the importance of a primary epithelial barrier defect in the pathogenesis of AD. Mutations of filaggrin (R510X and 2282del4), a key protein in terminal differentiation of the epidermis, have been shown to be important risk factors for AD and for AD in combination with asthma.[5] The skin barrier may be impaired due to an alteration of keratin aggregation and hence permit the penetration of allergens, including high-molecular-weight aeroallergens.

Immunological mechanisms

As mentioned above, both a disturbed epidermal barrier and defects in the immune system are mandatory for the development of AD (Fig. 42.3). Having focused over the last three decades on the mechanisms directing adaptive immunity, mainly orchestrated by T and B cells for cellular and humoral immunity respectively, scientists have tended to overlook the significance of the so-called innate immunity (Chapter 3).[14]

Innate immunity

In recent years there has been a radical transformation of our understanding of how mammalian organisms respond to microbial exposure. The innate immune system is able to react promptly to almost all kinds of microbial colonization and onslaught, while it is also involved in the initiation of the more specific but slower mechanisms of the adaptive immune response. Epithelial cells of the skin and cells residing at the interface between our environment and our organism are the first line of defense in the innate immune system.[14] They are equipped with highly conserved recognition structures, the so-called pattern recognition receptors (PRRs) such as the TLRs, which were initially described in the fruit fly. These TLRs can bind a variety of microbial structures due to highly conserved microbial surface molecules, the pathogen-associated molecular patterns (PAMP). At least 10 different TLRs have been described so far in humans and are more or less specialized in binding bacterial or fungal cell walls or viral nucleic acids (DNA or RNA with so-called CpG motifs). Hence, TLRs represent putative therapeutic targets to alter or modulate the adhesion of microbes to epithelial cells.

The binding of microbial products to the cell surface of epithelial cells leads to cellular activation, ultimately resulting in the production of molecules with anti-microbial activity: the so-called AMPs.[15] These belong to the family of defensins and cathelicidins. In human skin at least one cathelicidin (LL37) and three defensins, the human β-defensins 1, 2, and 3 (HBD1, HBD2, and HDB3) have been described.

In AD, skin is highly colonized by bacteria such as *S. aureus*. Much attention has been focused on the putative role of the innate immune system and particularly of AMPs in the control of these bacteria as well as of viruses. Recently it has been shown that AMPs are downregulated in the skin of human atopic individuals, probably due to the particular inflammatory micromilieu created by infiltrating cells and their cytokines. These mechanisms predispose AD patients to develop extensive herpes infections such as eczema herpeticum.[16]

Acquired immunity

T cells and the Th1/Th2 concept

A predominant systemic Th2 dysbalance with increased IgE levels and eosinophilia is widely accepted in the pathogenesis of atopic diseases.[17] The production of Th2 cytokines, notably IL-4, -5, and -13, can be detected in lesional and nonlesional skin during the acute phase of disease. IL-4 and -13 are implicated in the initial phase of tissue inflammation and in upregulating the expression of adhesion molecules on endothelial cells. IL-5 seems to increase the survival of eosinophils. A systemic eosinophilia and an increase of the eosinophilic cationic protein (ECP) are characteristic during high disease activity of AD.

However, although Th2 cytokines seem to be predominant in the acute phase of AD, they are less important during its chronic course. In chronic AD skin lesions an increase of interferon-γ (IFN-γ) and IL-12, as well as IL-5 and GM-CSF, could be detected, being characteristic for a Th1/Th0 dominance.

The maintenance of chronic AD involves the production of the Th1-like cytokines IL-12 and -18, as well as several remodeling-associated cytokines such as IL-11 and transforming growth factor (TGF)-β₁, expressed preferentially in chronic forms of the

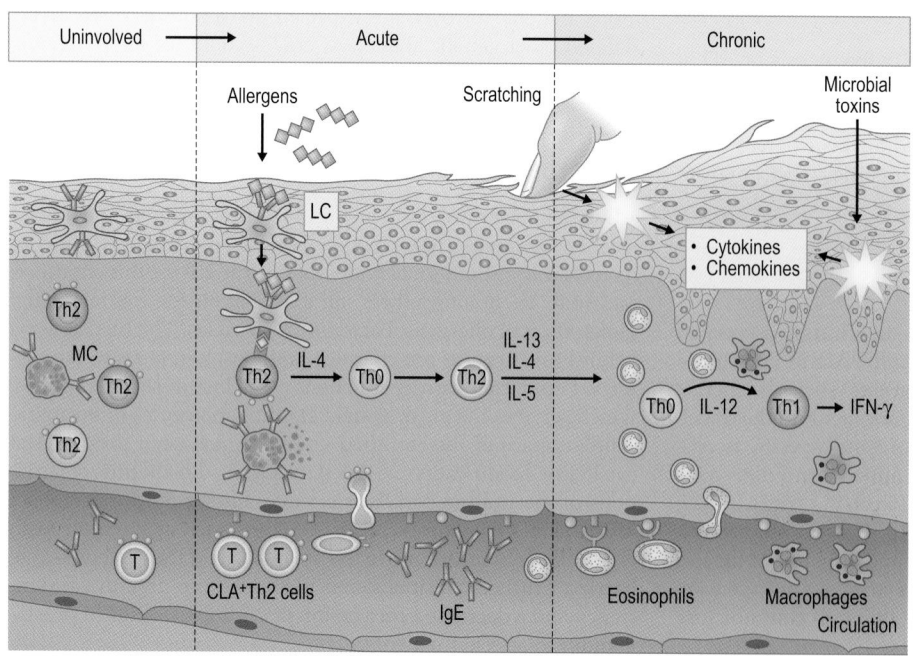

Fig. 42.3 Immunologic progression of atopic dermatitis.
Modified from Leung DYM. Atopic dermatitis: new insights and opportunities for therapeutic intervention. J Allergy Clin Immunol 2000; 105: 860.

disease. Th-1-mediated cells seem to be responsible for apoptosis of cells, although their pathomechanisms are yet not fully understood. Clearly, a generalized Th2-deviated immune response is closely linked to the condition of AD but the skin disease itself is a biphasic inflammation with an initial Th2 phase, while the chronic phase involves Th0/Th1 cells. This biphasic pattern of T-cell activation has also been demonstrated in studies of allergen patch test skin reaction sites.[18] Twenty-four hours after allergen application to the skin, increased expression of IL-4 mRNA and protein is observed, after which IL-4 expression returns to baseline levels. In contrast, IFN-γ mRNA expression is not detected in 24-hour patch test lesions, but is strongly expressed at the 48- to 72-hour time points. Interestingly, the increased expression of IFN-γ mRNA in atopic patch test lesions is preceded by a peak of IL-12 expression coinciding with the infiltration of macrophages and eosinophils.

Tregs are a diverse and complex family of cells with regulatory activities that became the focus of interest in the field of transplantation or tumor immunology as well as in allergy, since they have the ability to suppress T-cells (TH1 and TH2) (Chapter 16).[19] Special combinations of surface markers (CD25+/CD4+) as well as mutations of the nuclear factor Foxp3 are characteristic for these cells. It has been shown that mutations of Foxp3 result in hyper-IgE, food allergy, and dermatitis. In addition, staphylococcal superantigens can subvert the function of Tregs and may thereby augment skin inflammation (Fig. 42.4).[23]

Recently two new subclasses of T-cells has been identified, the so called TH17 and TH22 cells. They are generated under the influence of IL-23 and express the cytokines IL-17 and -22, respectively. TH17-cells have shown to play a key role in the pathogenesis of psoriasis, but in AD their importance is not clarified yet. In general IL-17 seems to play a role in the recruitment of neutrophils in acute AD, whereas IL-22 is thought to contribute to the induction of acanthosis and a defective terminal differentiation of keratinocytes in chronic AD.[20]

In skin biopsies from atopy-patch test lesions a subgroup of T-cells which expressed IL-4 and IL-17 on their surface, the so called Th2/Th17 cells could be identified.[21] They might be have an effect on the epidermal barrier, as it could be shown, that in FLG-deficient mice a percutaneous allergen challenge lead to a Th-17 dominated epidermal inflammation.[22]

Cytokines and chemokines

The defining characteristic of the atopic immune system is the expression of proinflammatory cytokines and chemokines.[23] Cytokines from resident cells (such as keratinocytes, mast cells, or DCs) bind to receptors on the vascular endothelium and activate cellular signaling. This results in an initiation of processes leading to the characteristic extravasation of inflammatory cells.

Several different chemokines have been implicated in the pathology of AD. Large amounts of chemokines such as MIP-4/CCL18, TARC/CCL17, PARC/CCL18, MDC/CCL22, and CCL1 seem to be involved in the development of acute and chronic skin manifestations. These chemokines play an important role in the amplification of allergic reactions to bacteria or allergens. C-C chemokines (MCP-4, RANTES, and eotaxin) contribute to the infiltration of macrophages, eosinophils, and T-cells into acute and chronic AD skin lesions. An increasing number of chemokines have been shown to be up- or downregulated in patients with AD but their exact role in the pathogenesis of AD is still not resolved.

IL-31 seems to play an important role in the development of pruritus in AD. I could be shown that T cells of patients which had been stimulated with *S. aureus* enterotoxin express IL-31, which induces pruritus after binding to the sensory nerve fibres.[24] There might be a connection between IL-31 and the H4 receptor. It has been demonstrated, that IDECs express the H-4 receptor on their surface[25] and the stimulation of the H4-receptor in AD has been shown to release the increase of IL-31.[26]

Dendritic cells

DCs are highly specialized professional antigen-presenting cells (APCs) and are essential for allergen uptake and its presentation to T cells in the context of primary and secondary immune responses (Chapter 7). The role of DC in AD has been extensively discussed elsewhere.[27] Two types of DC have been found in lesional skin of AD: myeloid (mDC) and, to a much lesser extent, plasmacytoid DCs (pDC). LC and inflammatory dendritic epidermal cells (IDEC) both belong to the group of mDC and express the high-affinity receptor for IgE (FcεRI) in lesional skin, suggesting a complex regulatory mechanism related to atopic status.

Fig. 42.4 Mechanisms of staphylococcal superantigen action in atopic dermatitis.
Modified from Leung DYM. Atopic dermatitis: new insights and opportunities for therapeutic intervention. J Allergy Clin Immunol 2000; 105: 860, with permission from Elsevier.

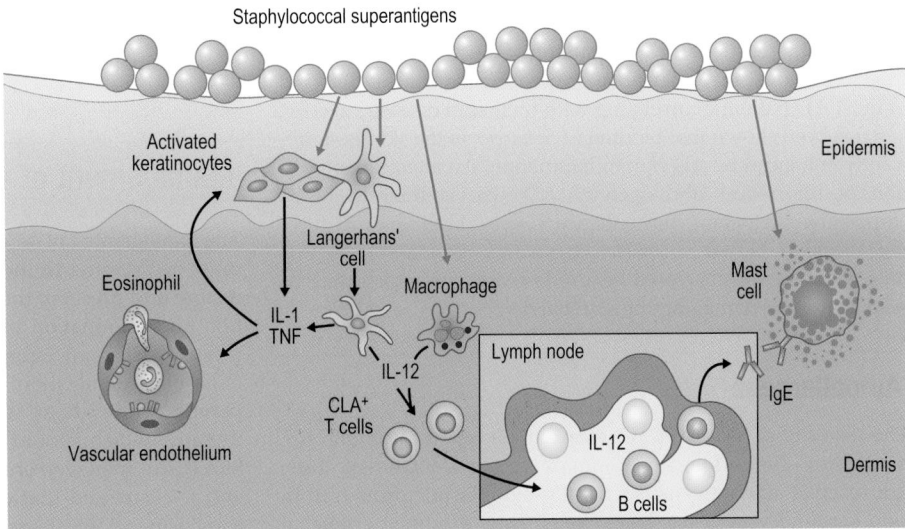

While LC are present in normal skin, IDEC are mainly detected in inflamed skin.

LC and IDEC play a central role in the uptake and presentation of antigens or allergens to Th1/Th2 cells and most probably also to Tregs. Interestingly, FcεRI-expression is detected on LC from normal skin during active flare-ups of other atopic diseases such as allergic asthma or rhinitis, while FcεRI$^+$ IDEC are confined to lesional skin. Although it remains to be definitely proven, there is some *in vitro* evidence that LC play a less dominant role than expected initially in the initiation of the allergic immune response. Nevertheless, they are active in priming naïve T cells to become T cells of Th2 type and produce distinct chemokines such MCP-1 upon receptor ligation. In contrast, the stimulation of FcεRI on IDEC leads to a switch to Th1 response and to the release of high amounts of proinflammatory signals that amplify the allergic immune response. The atopy patch test can be used as an experimental model for AD—skin biopsies of such patch tests show that, 72 hours after allergen challenge, high numbers of IDEC invade the epidermis while alterations of the phenotype of LC and IDEC occur, including the upregulation of FcεRI.

Compared to ACD, the number of pDC is dramatically decreased in the skin of AD patients. pDC have been shown to play a major role in the defense against viral infections by producing type 1 interferons. A lower density of pDC might contribute to the susceptibility towards viral skin infections such as eczema herpeticum in these patients. In contrast to LC and IDEC, pDC seem to express FcεRI constitutively and this is upregulated in AD patients. Activation of this receptor leads to altered surface expression of major histocompatibility complex (MHC) molecules, enhanced apoptosis of pDC, and a decrease in the secretion of type I interferons.

Microbial agents

Staphylococcus aureus is the predominant skin microorganism in AD lesions and is found in over 90% of AD patients.[28] This high colonization rate is probably due to a defect in the production of AMP by atopic keratinocytes. Infections often provoke exacerbation or aggravation of lesional skin. *S. aureus*-derived enterotoxins have been shown to play an important role in the pathogenesis of AD. Enterotoxins such as staphylococcal enterotoxin A (SEA), B (SEB), C (SEC), and D (SED) are frequently detected in patients and might provoke sensitization. Moreover, since *S. aureus* enterotoxins act as superantigens, they interact directly with the MHC–T-cell complex on APC and provoke antigen-independent proliferation of T cells. This results in an amplification of the inflammation and may lead to typical eczematoid skin reactions of AD patients. Specific IgE antibodies directed against staphylococcal superantigens can be detected in most AD patients, correlating with their skin disease severity.

It has been shown that binding of *S. aureus* to the skin is significantly enhanced by AD skin inflammation. An altered composition of fibrin and fibrinogen of AD skin is thought to be responsible. Scratching may enhance *S. aureus* binding by disturbing the skin barrier. *Staphylococcus aureus* isolated from AD patients possesses increased ceramidase activity, which may be responsible for damaging the skin barrier.

Autoallergens

The majority of sera from patients with severe AD contain IgE antibodies directed against human proteins.[29] One of these IgE-reactive autoantigens is a 55-kDa cytoplasmic protein from skin keratinocytes; it has been cloned from a human epithelial cDNA expression library and designated Hom s 1.[30] Although the autoallergens characterized to date have mainly been intracellular proteins, some have been detected in IgE immune complexes in sera of sensitized patients, suggesting that release of these autoallergens from damaged keratinocytes due to scratching could trigger IgE- or T-cell-mediated responses. A more recent study has shown that the emergence of IgE against self-proteins can be detected as early as 1 year of age.[31] These data suggest that, while IgE immune responses are initiated by environmental allergens in combination with skin inflammation, allergic inflammation can be maintained by human endogenous antigens in patients with severe AD. Thus, if the assumed pathophysiological role of these antibodies holds true, AD should be considered as a disease at the boundary between allergy and autoimmunity.

Nonatopic and atopic dermatitis in the context of the natural history of atopic dermatitis

As mentioned above, the new definition of AD requires the presence of IgE-mediated sensitization. However, this would imply that nonatopic dermatitis and AD represent two different diseases. Since dry skin is an important clinical sign of both conditions and is considered as a cardinal sign in atopic individuals as well, there is a great need for new concepts that reconcile these diverging ideas. Based on most recent genetic and immunological findings, a new picture emerges in which the natural history of AD seems to be divided into three phases: (1) an initial phase representing nonatopic dermatitis occurring in early infancy before any sensitization has taken place. This is then followed in 60–80% of cases by (2) sensitization to food and/or environmental allergens with the development of true AD (according to the new definition). In this phase, it is speculated that FcεRI$^+$ DC play a major role in controlling the inflammation. Consequently, these AD patients will benefit from allergen avoidance measures. Finally, (3) probably due to scratching, tissue damage, and molecular mimicry, an IgE sensitization to self-proteins is observed in about 25% of AD patients. Whether these specific IgE have a pathophysiological role or are just an epiphenomenon remains to be clarified. According to this concept, sensitization could be influenced by the intensity of skin inflammation, which would be in accord with the concept of the atopic march. Furthermore, attempts to control skin inflammation effectively as early as possible would putatively help to hamper the degree of subsequent sensitization.

Management of atopic dermatitis

The management of AD can be established on five main axes and must be adapted to the severity of the lesions: (1) skin care to restore and preserve the epidermal barrier function; (2) recognition and elimination of the provocation factors; (3) control of (even subclinical) inflammation and pruritus; (4) reduction of microbial colonization; and (5) education of patients and their parents. Throughout, topical treatment is preferred to systemic therapy, which should be reserved for the most severe forms. Successful management thus requires a multifaceted approach, and it is stressed that education of the patient is as important as pharmacological strategies.

Basis therapy

The regular use of emollients and skin hydration is essential to improve dryness, to prevent intense pruritus, and to control sub-clinical inflammation during periods of remission. The choice of emollients depends on the individual skin status. Water-in-oil or oil-in-water emulsions may be substituted to support the skin barrier function. Moisturizing factors, such as urea and glycerol allow an intensive hydration of the skin. In adult patients rather high concentrations (5–10%) of urea in emollients are tolerated, in children and on excoriated skin, urea should not be used at concentrations above 4% because it may burn on the skin. Recently novel emollients containing lipids, cholesterol fatty acids and ceramides have been developed which aim to substitute the missing components of the epidermis.[32]

Treatment with emollients is important both during the course of steroid treatment and as part of long-term management.

Patients should use mild soap-free detergents or oil-bath for washing and apply an emollient on the humid skin afterwards.

Elimination of provocation factors

The patient should be educated adequately to avoid provoking factors. Specific provocation factors, such as airborne and food allergens, have to be considered and identified by serum tests for allergen-specific IgE or skin prick tests. Because of the putative role of food allergens in children, diets directed by allergological tests can be of interest but blind extensive diets, which can be nutritionally deficient, are useless. Sensitized patients should avoid house dust mites; this may include use of house dust mite-proof encasings on pillows, mattresses, and box springs. Whether patients sensitized to animal dander should be discouraged from keeping household pets is still a matter of debate.

Food hypersensitivity affects 10–40% of children with AD. In children 90% of reactions are caused by only five allergens: eggs, milk, peanuts, soy, and wheat. Dietary restriction is only of value in patients whose allergies have been properly diagnosed, though any exclusion diets should be properly supervised by a pediatric dietician to ensure adequate nutrition.

Control of inflammation

Topical glucocorticosteroids

Topical steroids are safe and effective when used properly. Anxiety among both the general public and family physicians is often well out of proportion to the true risk. Aside from their anti-inflammatory effect, topical steroids contribute to a reduction of skin colonization with *S. aureus*. The strength and mode of application depend on disease activity and severity, the locations to be treated, and the age of the patient. In the treatment of AD topical steroids from the di-ester class which are characterized by a favourable therapeutical index such as prednicarbate, hydrocortisone butyrate, methylprenisolonaceponate, fluticasone, or mometasonfuroate should be favoured.

Only mild to moderately potent preparations should be used on facial, genital, or intertriginous skin areas. In children less than 1 year steroids with a low potency should be used and their application should be limited to short courses of about 2 weeks, no more than once a day. A number of different therapeutic schemes have been proposed: the initial treatment of acute phase can be with moderate- to high-potency steroids followed by a dose reduction or an exchange to a lower potency preparation.

However, our own experience has shown better compliance by tapering off the use of the same mid-potent topical steroid over several weeks.

Topical calcineurin inhibitors

Pimecrolimus and tacrolimus are immunosuppressive compounds that inhibit a calcium-activated phosphatase called calcineurin. They suppress the early phase of T-cell activation, degranulation of mast cells, and the expression of various cytokines required to activate cellular immunity. In contrast to topical steroids, which induce apoptosis of T cells and DC in the treated epidermis of patients with AD, calcineurin inhibitors do not affect LC numbers or function but effectively repress IDEC.[33]

Pimecrolimus cream (1%) and tacrolimus ointment (0.03%) are available for treatment of children 2 years of age and older. Tacrolimus ointment (0.1%) is only approved for use in adults. Side effects such as dermal atrophy or teleangiectasia are not seen, which therefore makes treatment of the face possible. Post-marketing surveillance of several million treated patients has not identified any particular problems as long as the drugs are used under medical supervision. Side effects include a transient burning sensation of the skin. While using calcineurin inhibitors, patients should avoid excessive exposure to natural or artificial sunlight (tanning beds or ultraviolet (UV) A/B treatment). Long-term safety studies analyzing a possible causal link between the topical use of calcineurin inhibitors and cancer as well as an increased incidence of viral infections are ongoing.

There has been concern because of reported cases of lymphoma and viral super-infections under the therapy with topical calcineurin inhibitors, which could not be confirmed by further investigation.

Proactive management

Proactive management of AD means to treat the acute flare with a topical steroid or a topical calcineurin inhibitor until the visible eczema has resolved. Afterwards the therapy is not tapered down completely, but continued once or twice weekly on prone areas, in order to reduce the pro-inflammatory infiltrate in the epidermis and therefore prevent new flare-ups.

This kind of management has been proven to reduce flares for up to 12 months with increased compliance and better overall disease control.[34] Studies comparing the proactive application of tacrolimus to a reactive therapy in adults as well as in children over a period of one year showed that the proactive therapy is effective to prevent new flares without a higher consumption of medication.[35,36]

Control of pruritus

Itch is often the most troublesome symptom for patients and is difficult to treat. Currently there is no specific anti-pruritic treatment except local applications of anti-inflammatory preparations and emollients. H1-receptor antagonists (alimemazine and promethazine) are predominantly used for their sedative effect and are given 1 hour before bedtime. Most studies conclude that non-sedating antihistamines have little or no value in AD. In fact, the most effective control of pruritus is still provided by an effective anti-inflammatory regimen.

Reduction of microbial colonization

As mentioned above, both the affected and nonaffected skin of AD patients is heavily colonized with *S. aureus*. Even in the absence of exudation and pustule formation, which imply a superinfection, topical antiseptics with a low sensitizing potential such as octenidin can be used since they show low resistance rates. If an antibiotic is needed to treat infection, fusidic acid is the agent of choice, due to high resistance rates of *S. aureus* to erythromycin. Intranasal eradication of methicillin-resistant *S. aureus*, frequently found in AD patients, can be achieved by the topical use of mupirocin.

When widespread bacterial secondary superinfection (primarily *S. aureus*) occurs, systemic antibiotic treatment is indicated. A short-course treatment (3–7 days) with cephalosporins (cephalexin) or semisynthetic penicillins (floxacillin or amoxicillin-clavulanate) has been shown to be effective. Due to the high frequency of resistance, erythromycin is less useful.

Managing severe forms of AD

It is well accepted that, in severe cases of AD, topical treatment alone will not allow sufficient control of the condition. In these cases, systemic therapy is indicated, at least for a limited period of time until topical regiment can be resumed.

Oral corticosteroids

Oral corticosteroids have a limited but definite role in the treatment of severe exacerbations of AD. A brief course may be used to control severe disease, but ongoing use of systemic corticosteroids carries significant adverse effects.

Despite its side effects, especially renal toxicity with hypertension and renal impairment, multiple studies have shown a beneficial effect of *Cyclosporine A (CyA)* in children and adults. Close monitoring of creatinine and CyA serum levels is essential. Exacerbation can occur after discontinuation, but posttreatment disease severity often does not return to baseline levels.[37] Treatment regimes are adjusted to body weight, with 3–5 mg/kg per day for a high-dose regime or 2.5 mg/kg per day as low-dose treatment. In order to minimize side effects, the lowest effective dose should be used.

Mycophenolate mofetil

Mycophenolate mofetil is an immunosuppressive purine biosynthesis inhibitor used for the treatment of moderate to severe AD.[38] The drug is generally well tolerated when given as short-term oral treatment with 2 g/day. After 5 weeks the dosage can be reduced to 1 g/day and continued for another 3 weeks. Occasional herpes retinitis has been recorded and should be watched for and treated appropriately.

Azathioprine

Azathioprine affects purine nucleotide synthesis and metabolism and has both anti-inflammatory and anti-proliferative effects. Controlled trials have not been reported; side effects are common, including myelosuppression, hepatotoxicity, gastrointestinal disturbances, increased susceptibility for infections, and possible development of skin cancer. As azathioprine is metabolized by thiopurine methyltransferase, a deficiency of this enzyme should be excluded before starting oral immunosuppression with azathioprine.[39]

Phototherapy

UVB (280–320 nm), narrow-band UVB (311–313 nm), UVA (320–400 nm), medium- and high-dose UVA1 (340–400 nm), and psoralen UVA (PUVA) have all undergone trials for the treatment of AD UVA1 irradiation seems to be superior to conventional UVA–UVB phototherapy in patients with severe AD, and has become established as a standard second-line treatment for adults with or without additional topical or systemic treatment. The use of UV therapy in children should be restricted since data about long-term side effects of UV therapy (e.g., skin cancer) are still not available. Bearing in mind a possible link between UV irradiation and photo-aging, skin carcinogenesis, or melanoma induction, the duration of therapy should be limited to about 4–6 weeks.

Immunotherapy

In older studies, no benefit could be shown from allergen-specific desensitization in AD. These findings have also suggested over years that AD is if anything a contraindication for immunotherapy. More recent studies using specific immunotherapy in AD patients sensitized to house dust mite (*Dermatophagoides pteronyssinus*) have led us to revise this opinion.[40] Further studies are now ongoing in order to validate this concept. Another promising area of study is the use of sublingual immunotherapy (SLIT), which has been established as efficient in rhinitis and asthma.[39]

Education of patients with atopic dermatitis

Patient education has proven to be of great benefit in the management of AD, especially for young patients and their parents. Knowledge about the disease and its therapeutic strategies lead to a higher level of compliance as well as psychological stability. The acceptance of the disease and its chronic course by the patient and those around the patient significantly improves their quality of life. Adequate educational programs are additionally effective when offered in a multidisciplinary context, with dermatologists, pediatricians, dieticians, psychologists, and nursing staff working with patients and their families.

● THERAPEUTIC PRINCIPLES

Management of atopic dermatitis

Principles and tools

1. Skin care to restore and preserve the epidermal barrier function
   - Individually adapted emollients and/or ointments with or without urea
2. Recognize and eliminate the provocation factors
   - Allergological diagnostic, food allergens and aeroallergens, encasing
3. Control of skin inflammation and pruritus
   - Topical steroids (first-line), topical calcineurin inhibitors
   - Phototherapy
   - Antihistamines
   - Systemic steroids, immunosuppressive agents (cyclosporine A, azathioprine, mycophenolate mofetil)
   - Specific immunotherapy
   - Biologicals
4. Reduce microbial colonization
   - Topical antiseptics
   - Systemic antibiotics only in severely infected cases
5. Education
   - Need for early intervention
   - Atopic dermatitis educational programs, atopic dermatitis schools

Translational research

We are currently experiencing a new and fascinating phase in AD research. Combining data from epidemiology, genetics, skin physiology, immunology, and allergy provides new areas of research that will certainly offer new perspectives and new concepts in the pathophysiology and management of this disease. The identification of FLG mutations as a strong risk factor for AD has emphasized the role of the epidermal barrier defect in AD. But as only a subgroup of AD patients carries FLG mutations, it may be suggested that among AD patients various subgroups with different genetic patterns exist. The idea of individualized medicine is to treat those subgroups individually, according to their special needs. Progress in genetics will provide the requested scientific background for this new and tailored approach in the management of AD.

Hopefully the pharmacological research will lead to the development of new biologics but also new antagonist molecules based on small-molecular-weight compounds, steroid analogues, and other treatments that are or will be in the pipeline over the next few years. Finally, beside these new pharmacological approaches, one of the most important aspects remains the strategy of very early treatment of young children by controlling skin inflammation at the earliest practical time point. This strategy may help us to control the emergence of sensitization and provide a rapid and hopefully definitive cure of the disease.

● ON THE HORIZON

- Early treatment of AD in children is essential to prevent sensitizations and further allergic diseases, i.e., the atopic march.
- Proactive therapy is effective for controlling flare-ups.
- Steroid analogs may enrich the range of topical therapies.
- New strategies aimed to overdrive a deficiency in filaggrin production will specifically improve the disturbed epidermal barrier function.
- Biologicals or small molecules targeting, e.g., IL-31 and IL-4 are warranted for the treatment of severe recalcitrant AD.

Allergic contact dermatitis

Definition

Contact dermatitis is an eczematous skin eruption caused by local exposure to allergic sensitizer or irritant/toxic substances. These include immunologic, chemical, protein, or physical agents but infectious agents are excluded. Contact dermatitis is a common cause of morbidity with a life prevalence of 15% and incidence of more than 7.9 per 1000. However, the sensitization rate is higher than this—studies in Scandinavia have shown that 15–20% of the population displays at least one positive patch test reaction to contact sensitizers. In the USA, occupationally related contact dermatitis is estimated to cost $250 million per year in lost productivity, medical care, and disability payments.

Pathophysiology
Genetics

ACD is a multifactorial condition in which genetic background plays an important part, as shown by twin and family studies. In case-control studies, SNPs in certain enzymes such as NAT2 (N-acetyltransferase) or the promoter region of IL-16 have been associated with multiple sensitization status.[41,42]

Interestingly an association between the loss of function mutations R501x and 2282del4 in the FLG gene with a clinical manifest sensitization against nickel II-sulfate combined with an intolerance to fashion jewellery could be shown , but it was not associated with a type IV-sensitization to other contact allergens.[43] The FLG mutations have further been shown to lower the age of onset of nickel dermatitis.[44]

The allergens

Most contact allergens are haptens, i.e., simple chemicals that bind to proteins (carrier) present in skin to form a complete antigen. The key to understanding the pathogenesis of contact allergy is an appreciation of the discriminate nature by which chemicals can serve as antigens (Chapter 6). Clearly, not all chemicals act as allergens. To be allergenic, the chemical must be able to penetrate the principal barrier in skin (the stratum corneum) and reach the living cells of the epidermis. Only molecules with molecular mass less than 500 Da are capable of penetrating the stratum corneum, and so most contact allergens are low-molecular-weight compounds. Lipid solubility promotes transit through the stratum corneum. Thus, most contact allergens are small, lipophilic molecules. The most common of these chemicals are listed in Table 42.1. Once in the epidermis, the nature of the protein carrier for the hapten is very important because if the contact sensitizer is complexed to nonimmunogenic carriers, this may induce tolerance rather than sensitization.[43]

The sensitization phase

The pathophysiology of ACD has been extensively reviewed elsewhere.[45] The principal event during sensitization is presentation of antigen to responder T cells by APC, culminating in activation and differentiation of T cells that proliferate in an antigen-specific clonal manner. LC are the principal APCs within the epidermis and are generally thought to be responsible for presentation of contact allergens in the primary (sensitization) phase as well as in the secondary (elicitation) phase of the immune response. However, recent studies in LC knockout animal models have seriously challenged this view.[46] Other DCs in skin, especially in the dermis, may also serve as APCs for contact allergens, including LC precursors, and dermal DCs, while macrophages may be important in the elicitation phase.

The clinical outcome of each exposure to antigen depends upon several factors. First and foremost is the integrity of the stratum corneum. An injured or diseased stratum corneum that allows greater penetration of exogenous substances will increase the chances of activating APCs in the skin. A second factor is the viability of APCs in skin, since these cells need to seek and bind appropriate responder T cells. Third is the presence or absence of extracellular factors, including cytokines produced by keratinocytes that can promote or hinder APC–T-cell engagement. The final factor is the pre-existing mix of T-cell subtypes specific for the antigen. The higher the frequency of cells of an effector subtype, the higher the likelihood that dermatitis will result,

Table 42.1 Most common contact allergens (listed in approximate order of decreasing frequency)

1. Nickel sulphate	Nickel-plated objects are omnipresent. Jewelry that looks like gold or silver has nickel in it. Gold greater than 18 carats is safe; so is aluminum; stainless steel contains nickel but it is not releasable.
2. Fragrance mix	Anything that smells good has fragrance chemicals in it (e.g., cinnamates, vanillin, oak moss, eugenol, geraniol). Also used as flavorings.
3. *P*-phenyldiamine	Preservative used in vaccines, antitoxins, eye and nasal medications.
4. Chromate	Sensitizer in wet cement. Used as an oxidizing agent and for its anticorrosion properties. Found in glues and adhesives, leather, paints, matches, detergents, and bleaches.
5. Methyldibromoglutaronitril/ phenoxyethanol (MDBGN/PE)	Preservatives, antimicrobial, and industrial biocides.
6. Thiuram mix	Rubber accelerator and vulcanizer. Fungicide and animal repellant. Also found in lubricating oils. Cross-reacts with disulfiram.
7. Methylchloroisothiazolinon/ methylisothiazolinon (Kathon CG)	Preservative in paints, glues, and cosmetics.
8. Formaldehyde	Preservative found in cosmetic products and topical medications; sterilizer in cleaning agents; fixative for tissues; tanning agent for leather; hardener for fabrics; fumigant, fungicide, and insecticide
9. Parabens	Used as sunscreen agent and preservative in cosmetic products

whereas a higher frequency of cells of a regulatory subtype may limit or prevent the development of dermatitis. Recently, in a mouse model of contact sensitization to Nickel, the role of the innate receptor TLR4 has been demonstrated.[47] Whether this is also relevant for humans remains to be determined.

The elicitation phase

The elicitation or efferent phase is characterized by invasion of the skin by antigen-specific memory T cells as well as other inflammatory cells, producing what is clinically recognized as ACD. Memory T cells and other inflammatory cells leave vessels and enter the skin through sequential activation of a number of adhesion molecules by cytokines. Memory T cells constitutively express cutaneous lymphocyte antigen (CLA). E-selectin, the ligand for CLA, is induced on vascular endothelium by inflammatory mediators such as IL-1 and tumor necrosis factor-α (TNF-α). This interaction causes memory T cells to slow down and roll along the endothelial surface as a prelude to migration to sites of inflammation. Firm adhesion and migration of leukocytes to the endothelium are mediated by T-cell VLA-4/LFA-1 and endothelial cell VCAM-1/ICAM-1, respectively. Subsequently, LFA-1[+] T cells migrate toward ICAM-1[+] epidermal cells.

Mast cells may also participate in the elicitation phase. In mice, mast cells can be activated by a T-cell-derived antigen-binding factor that induces release of serotonin, producing swelling 2 hours after challenge. In addition, mast cells contain preformed TNF-α, which may regulate the adhesion molecules involved in the early recruitment of helper T cells.[48]

The net result is an influx of T cells secreting IL-2 and IFN-γ into the area of allergen exposure. These cytokines enhance the immune response through activation and recruitment of more inflammatory cells, producing spongiosis and the inflammatory dermal infiltrate characteristic of ACD.

Clinical manifestations (Fig. 42.5)

As a rule, ACD takes several hours, days, or even weeks to develop, while irritant contact dermatitis may manifest within minutes to hours of contact, especially when due to strong agents. If left alone, most cases of contact dermatitis resolve completely. Unfortunately, this ideal situation is almost never realized because the accompanying itch results in scratching and attempts at topical treatment, which in turn lead to spread of the dermatitis, often with superimposed bacterial or dermatophytic infection. These and the effects of partial but incomplete treatment can produce diagnostic confusion.

The intensity of the dermatitis depends on the concentration of the inciting chemical and, in the case of ACD, on the sensitivity of the individual to the allergen. Acute inflammation is expressed as erythema, blistering, oozing, and crusting; rarely frank necrosis may ensue. Subacute inflammation manifests as erythema, scaling, fissuring, or a parched, scalded appearance. Chronic inflammation may have less erythema, but the skin becomes thickened with lichenification and excoriation. Itching is a cardinal feature of contact dermatitis, regardless of severity.

The location of the dermatitis also serves as an important clue to the source of the offending chemical (Table 42.2). Although ACD usually affects the site of principal exposure, it can spread to other more distant sites, either by inadvertent contact or by autosensitization. Furthermore, the scalp, palms, and soles are relatively resistant to ACD and may not exhibit pathology, while

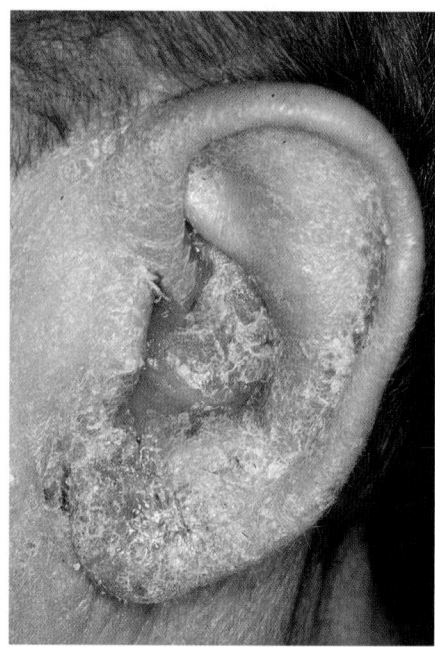

Fig. 42.5 Allergic contact dermatitis.

Table 42.2 Common causes of contact dermatitis by location

Scalp	Shampoos, hair dyes
Ears	Metal earrings, eyeglasses, hair care products
Eyelids	Nail polish, cosmetics, contact lens solution, airborne allergens
Face	Cosmetics, other topical preparations, including sunscreens, air-borne allergens
Neck	Necklaces, perfumes, air-borne allergens
Trunk	Topical preparations, clothing, including metal components and elastic in undergarments
Axillae	Deodorants, clothing
Hands	Soaps and detergents, occupational chemicals, metals, including jewelry, topical preparations, rubber gloves
Genitals	Topical preparations, condoms
Anal region	Fecal spillage, topical preparations
Legs	Topical preparations, elastic in socks
Feet	Rubber, leather, or synthetic materials in shoes

surrounding areas are severely affected. A geographic approach can be very helpful in identifying the causal allergen. Although the typical presentation is eczematous, contact dermatitis may occasionally present as urticaria (contact urticaria), altered pigmentation (either hyperpigmentation or hypopigmentation), erythema multiforme, or even purpura (usually on the legs). Widespread involvement, particularly of the face and of body areas unprotected by clothing, should raise suspicions of contact dermatitis produced by airborne allergens such as plant pollen, sprays, or fumes. Photocontact dermatitis can also have a similar diffuse presentation. Rarely, contact dermatitis may become generalized, presenting as exfoliative erythroderma. In some cases ACD can be induced by body contact (e.g., to perfumes or cosmetics).

ACD can occur at any age, but it is less frequently seen in the very old or very young. Older individuals have been shown to have various defects in the induction and/or elicitation of ACD. When ACD occurs in children, it is typically in older pediatric patients. The most common causes include poison ivy, nickel (jewelry), rubber (shoes), fragrance, formaldehyde (cosmetics and shampoo) and neomycin (topical antibiotics). In adults the most likely sources of ACD are allergens peculiar to the individual's occupation or hobbies. Piercings have been shown to be a strong risk factor for nickel allergy.[49]

Management of ACD

Diagnosis

The clinical and histological findings of ACD are characteristic, but not diagnostic. The most widely available method for confirming the diagnosis of ACD is patch testing. Patch tests are especially indicated in cases characterized by recurrent episodes of ACD, in cases in which there is a need to identify the offending allergen, and in cases recalcitrant to conventional therapy. Patch tests document the presence of delayed-type hypersensitivity; results are usually read at 48 and 96 hours after placement of the allergens. Systemic immunosuppressive agents or sunbathing can suppress T-cell-driven responses, and a 2- to 3-week washout period is advisable prior to performing patch tests in patients treated with these drugs.

The results of patch tests must be interpreted in the context of the patient's experience and exposure. A positive result does not definitively identify the cause of the ACD. False positives may be due to an irritant (rather than an allergic) effect. In these cases, patch testing in control individuals can be of great value. False negatives can occur because patch testing does not reproduce the actual environment in which the allergen is encountered. Failure to perform a second reading (between 4 and 7 days after allergen placement) may mean that late positive results are missed. Finally, only a limited number of chemicals may be tested, and although most series of allergens include the most common causes of ACD, they will not include all possible allergens. Thus a negative patch test may simply mean that the relevant allergen was not tested. Equally, some cases of contact dermatitis are due to irritants rather than to allergic sensitizers. Usually it will be clear from the history if irritant materials are being used, but if the patch tests are negative it is worth going back over the history with the patient to see whether any irritant exposures have been overlooked.

Allergen avoidance

The most important aspect of managing patients with ACD is to identify correctly the cause and provide instructions about avoiding further contact with the allergen(s). Many allergens cross-react with other compounds and thus patients should be informed of this possibility.

Symptomatic therapy

Acute forms of contact dermatitis, particularly those involving greater than 10% of the total body surface, respond well to systemic corticosteroid treatment. Topical therapy may suffice for less acute or less widespread forms of contact dermatitis.

Short courses of corticosteroids over 2–3 weeks are the definitive treatment. As mentioned previously, acute dermatitis and widespread involvement require systemic administration (e.g., oral prednisone, initially at a maximum dose of 1 mg/kg, tapered over at least 2 weeks). Less acute or less widespread dermatitis responds well to topical corticosteroids, the strength of which should be tailored to the age of the patient and the body part involved. As a rule, lotions and creams work best in the acute and subacute phases while ointments should be reserved for chronic and lichenified lesions.

Conclusion

ACD is a delayed-type, T-cell-mediated response following exposure to chemical sensitizers. The role of epidermal LC in the induction of ACD has recently been questioned and they may be more involved in inducing tolerance, while dermal DCs and other APC seem to play a more important role than previously believed. The association between loss-of-function mutations in the FLG gene with contact sensitization to nickel stresses the role of an impaired skin barrier for the development of a contact sensitization. Irritant contact dermatitis has a similar histology, but does not involve specific sensitization.

Patch testing is the procedure of choice to confirm the diagnosis of ACD and to identify the offending contact allergens. Despite international standardization, there are still concerns about the reproducibility of patch tests and their interpretation requires both experience and judgment. The keys to management are prevention by avoiding substances containing the allergens that have been identified, and the administration of topical and/or systemic corticosteroids to get rid of any ongoing dermatitis.

References

1. Akdis CA, Akdis M, Bieber T, et al. Diagnosis and treatment of atopic dermatitis in children and adults: European Academy of Allergology and Clinical Immunology/American Academy of Allergy, Asthma and Immunology/PRACTALL Consensus Report. Allergy 2006;61:969–87.
2. Bieber T, Novak N. Pathogenesis of atopic dermatitis: new developments. Curr Allergy Asthma Rep 2009;9:291–4.
3. Spergel JM, Paller AS. Atopic dermatitis and the atopic march. J Allergy Clin Immunol 2003;112:S118–27.
4. Palmer CN, Irvine AD, Terron-Kwiatkowski A, et al. Common loss-of-function variants of the epidermal barrier protein filaggrin are a major predisposing factor for atopic dermatitis. Nat Genet 2006;38:441–6.
5. Rodriguez E, Baurecht H, Herberich E, et al. Meta-analysis of filaggrin polymorphisms in eczema and asthma: robust risk factors in atopic disease. J Allergy Clin Immunol 2009;123:1361–70.
6. Johansson SG, Bieber T, Dahl R, et al. Revised nomenclature for allergy for global use: Report of the Nomenclature Review Committee of the World Allergy Organization, October 2003. J Allergy Clin Immunol 2004;113:832–6.
7. Bieber T. Atopic dermatitis. N Engl J Med 2008;358:1483–94.
8. Mihm Jr MC, Soter NA, Dvorak HF, et al. The structure of normal skin and the morphology of atopic eczema. J Invest Dermatol 1976;67:305–12.
9. Bradley M, Soderhall C, Wahlgren CF, et al. The Wiskott-Aldrich syndrome gene as a candidate gene for atopic dermatitis. Acta Derm Venereol 2001;81:340–2.
10. Christensen U, Moller-Larsen S, Nyegaard M, et al. Linkage of atopic dermatitis to chromosomes 4q22, 3p24 and 3q21. Hum Genet 2009;126:549–57.
11. Cookson WO. The genetics of atopic dermatitis: strategies, candidate genes, and genome screens. J Am Acad Dermatol 2001;45:S7–9.
12. Morar N, Willis-Owen SA, Moffatt MF, et al. The genetics of atopic dermatitis. J Allergy Clin Immunol 2006;118:24–34.
13. Proksch E, Folster-Holst R, Jensen JM. Skin barrier function, epidermal proliferation and differentiation in eczema. J Dermatol Sci 2006;43:159–69.
14. Maintz L, Novak N. Modifications of the innate immune system in atopic dermatitis. J Innate Immun 2011;3:131–41.
15. Schittek B. The antimicrobial skin barrier in patients with atopic dermatitis. Curr Probl Dermatol 2011;41:54–67.
16. Howell MD, Gallo RL, Boguniewicz M, et al. Cytokine milieu of atopic dermatitis skin subverts the innate immune response to vaccinia virus. Immunity 2006;24:341–8.
17. Ong PY, Leung DY. Immune dysregulation in atopic dermatitis. Curr Allergy Asthma Rep 2006;6:384–9.
18. Grewe M, Walther S, Gyufko K, et al. Analysis of the cytokine pattern expressed in situ in inhalant allergen patch test reactions of atopic dermatitis patients. J Invest Dermatol 1995;105:407–10.
19. Beissert S, Schwarz A, Schwarz T. Regulatory T cells. J Invest Dermatol 2006;126:15–24.
20. Souwer Y, Szegedi K, Kapsenberg ML, et al. IL-17 and IL-22 in atopic allergic disease. Curr Opin Immunol 2010;22:821–6.
21. Eyerich K, Pennino D, Scarponi C, et al. IL-17 in atopic eczema: linking allergen-specific adaptive and microbial-triggered innate immune response. J Allergy Clin Immunol 2009;123:59–66.
22. Oyoshi MK, Murphy GF, Geha RS. Filaggrin-deficient mice exhibit TH17-dominated skin inflammation and permissiveness to epicutaneous sensitization with protein antigen. J Allergy Clin Immunol 2009;124:485–93.
23. Homey B, Steinhoff M, Ruzicka T, et al. Cytokines and chemokines orchestrate atopic skin inflammation. J Allergy Clin Immunol 2006;118:178–89.
24. Sonkoly E, Muller A, Lauerma AI, et al. IL-31: a new link between T cells and pruritus in atopic skin inflammation. J Allergy Clin Immunol 2006;117:411–7.
25. Dijkstra D, Stark H, Chazot PL, et al. Human inflammatory dendritic epidermal cells express a functional histamine H4 receptor. J Invest Dermatol 2008;128:1696–703.
26. Gutzmer R, Mommert S, Gschwandtner M, et al. The histamine H4 receptor is functionally expressed on T(H)2 cells. J Allergy Clin Immunol 2009;123:619–25.
27. Bieber T, Novak N, Herrman N, Koch S. Role of dendritic cells in atopic dermatitis: an update. Clin Rev Allergy Immunol 2011;41(3):254–8.
28. Boguniewicz M, Leung DY. Atopic dermatitis: a disease of altered skin barrier and immune dysregulation. Immunol Rev 2011;242:233–46.
29. Zeller S, Glaser AG, Vilhelmsson M, et al. Immunoglobulin-E-mediated reactivity to self antigens: a controversial issue. Int Arch Allergy Immunol 2008;145:87–93.
30. Aichberger KJ, Mittermann I, Reininger R, et al. Hom s 4, an IgE-reactive autoantigen belonging to a new subfamily of calcium-binding proteins, can induce Th cell type 1-mediated autoreactivity. J Immunol 2005;175:1286–94.
31. Mothes N, Niggemann B, Jenneck C, et al. The cradle of IgE autoreactivity in atopic eczema lies in early infancy. J Allergy Clin Immunol 2005;116:706–9.
32. Katoh N. Future perspectives in the treatment of atopic dermatitis. J Dermatol 2009;36:367–76.
33. Wollenberg A, Sharma S, von BD, et al. Topical tacrolimus (FK506) leads to profound phenotypic and functional alterations of epidermal antigen-presenting dendritic cells in atopic dermatitis. J Allergy Clin Immunol 2001;107:519–25.
34. Berth-Jones J, Damstra RJ, et al. Twice weekly fluticasone propionate added to emollient maintenance treatment to reduce risk of relapse in atopic dermatitis: randomised, double blind, parallel group study. BMJ 2003;326:1367.
35. Thaci D, Reitamo S, Gonzalez Ensenat MA, et al. Proactive disease management with 0.03% tacrolimus ointment for children with atopic dermatitis: results of a randomized, multicentre, comparative study. Br J Dermatol 2008;159:1348–56.
36. Wollenberg A, Reitamo S, Girolomoni G, et al. Proactive treatment of atopic dermatitis in adults with 0.1% tacrolimus ointment. Allergy 2008;63:742–50.
37. Harper JI, Ahmed I, Barclay G, et al. Cyclosporin for severe childhood atopic dermatitis: short course versus continuous therapy. Br J Dermatol 2000;142:52–8.
38. Neuber K, Schwartz I, Itschert G, et al. Treatment of atopic eczema with oral mycophenolate mofetil. Br J Dermatol 2000;143:385–91.
39. Lear JT, English JS, Jones P, et al. Retrospective review of the use of azathioprine in severe atopic dermatitis. J Am Acad Dermatol 1996;35:642–3.
40. Werfel T, Breuer K, Rueff F, et al. Usefulness of specific immunotherapy in patients with atopic dermatitis and allergic sensitization to house dust mites: a multi-centre, randomized, dose-response study. Allergy 2006;61:202–5.
41. Schnuch A, Westphal GA, Muller MM, et al. Genotype and phenotype of N-acetyltransferase 2 (NAT2) polymorphism in patients with contact allergy. Contact Dermatitis 1998;38:209–11.
42. Westphal GA, Reich K, Schulz TG, et al. N-acetyltransferase 1 and 2 polymorphisms in para-substituted arylamine-induced contact allergy. Br J Dermatol 2000;142:1121–7.
43. Novak N, Baurecht H, Schafer T, et al. Loss-of-function mutations in the filaggrin gene and allergic contact sensitization to nickel. J Invest Dermatol 2008;128:1430–5.
44. Ross-Hansen K, Menne T, Johansen JD, et al. Nickel reactivity and filaggrin null mutations–evaluation of the filaggrin bypass theory in a general population. Contact Dermatitis 2011;64:24–31.
45. Krasteva M, Kehren J, Ducluzeau MT, et al. Contact dermatitis I. Pathophysiology of contact sensitivity. Eur J Dermatol 1999;9:65–77.
46. Kissenpfennig A, Malissen B. Langerhans cells–revisiting the paradigm using genetically engineered mice. Trends Immunol 2006;27:132–9.
47. Schmidt M, Raghavan B, Muller V, et al. Crucial role for human Toll-like receptor 4 in the development of contact allergy to nickel. Nat Immunol 2010;11:814–9.
48. Groves RW, Allen MH, Ross EL, et al. Tumour necrosis factor alpha is pro-inflammatory in normal human skin and modulates cutaneous adhesion molecule expression. Br J Dermatol 1995;132:345–52.
49. Thyssen JP. Nickel and cobalt allergy before and after nickel regulation—evaluation of a public health intervention. Contact Dermatitis 2011;65(Suppl. 1):1–68.

Food allergy | Barbara Bohle

In technical usage, the term "food allergy" means immune-mediated non-toxic adverse reactions to foods (Fig. 43.1).[1] The most common form of food allergy is mediated by immunoglobulin E (IgE) antibodies and reflects an immediate-type ("type 1 hypersensitivity") reaction, with acute onset of symptoms after ingestion or inhalation of foods. IgE-mediated food allergy can be further classified into primary (class 1) and secondary (class 2) food allergy on the basis of the affected group of patients (children or adults), clinical appearance, the disease-eliciting food allergens, and the underlying immune mechanisms. Primary (class 1) or "true" food allergy starts in early life and often represents the first manifestation of the atopic syndrome. The most common foods involved are cow´s milk, hen´s egg, legumes (peanuts and soybean), fish, shellfish, and wheat. Of note, allergens contained in these foods not only elicit allergic reactions in the gastrointestinal (GI) tract but often cause or influence urticaria and atopic dermatitis as well as bronchial obstruction. With a few exceptions (peanut and fish) most children outgrow class 1 food allergy within the first 3 to 6 years of life.

Secondary (class 2) food allergy mainly affects adolescent and adult individuals with established respiratory allergy, for example to the pollen of birch, mugwort, or ragweed, or to rubber latex, and results from cross-reactivity between respiratory and food allergens. In principle, IgE antibodies specific for inhaled allergens recognize structurally related proteins in foods and may induce clinical symptoms. Most secondary food allergens are rapidly degraded by gastric and intestinal enzymes. Therefore, clinical symptoms are mainly confined to the site of contact with fresh foods and severe systemic reactions are rare. However, some foods, particularly celery, nuts, and soy, can cause more severe, systemic reactions. At present, there is no curative treatment for class 1 and class 2 food allergies.

The pathophysiology of IgE-mediated food allergy

In IgE-mediated allergic disorders CD4 T helper (Th) lymphocytes play a major role. They provide help for antibody production by B lymphocytes and recruit neutrophils, eosinophils, and basophils to sites of inflammation through their production of cytokines and chemokines. Naïve CD4 Th lymphocytes are activated by professional antigen-presenting cells (APC), such as dendritic cells, recognizing small peptide fragments resulting from allergen processing bound to major histocompatibility complex (MHC) class II molecules (Chapter 6). Depending on key cytokines present during T-cell priming, i.e., the initial interaction with APC, naïve CD4 T cells differentiate into four different (and possibly even more) "classical" effector cell subsets. At present, the classical subsets comprise Th2, Th1, Th17 cells, and induced regulatory T (Treg) cells. The presence of interleukin (IL)-4 promotes T-cell differentiation into allergen-specific Th2 cells that produce high amounts of the signature cytokines IL-4, -5, -9, and -13 but little or no interferon (IFN)-γ (Chapter 16). IL-4 is the major switch factor for IgE synthesis in B cells. The presence of IL-12 and -27 during T-cell priming fosters the differentiation of Th1 cells that produce high amounts of the signature cytokine IFN-γ, which is a potent antagonist of IL-4 and inhibits the differentiation of Th2 cells. Human Th17 cells differentiate in the presence of IL-1β and -23. This subset synthesizes the signature cytokines IL-17a, -17f, -22, and -21. Th17 cells are important for the defense against extracellular bacteria and fungi and play a role in inflamed skin in atopic dermatitis. Moreover, Th17 cells have been shown to be involved in initiation and augmentation of inflammation in the airways and in the gut mucosa. Induced Treg cells suppress the differentiation and effector phases of other T-cell subsets either by cell–cell contact and/or by IL-10 and/or transforming growth factor (TGF)-β. Different subsets of Treg cells have been described. So-called Th3 cells producing high amounts of TGF-β have been implicated as mediators of oral tolerance. The term "Tr1 cells" was proposed for all IL-10-producing regulatory T-cell populations induced by IL-10. Additional subsets of Treg cells may exist as well as additional subsets of effector cells, e.g., the more recently described Th9 and Th22 cells.[2]

IgE-mediated disorders are believed to result from an imbalance between the different subsets of allergen-specific CD4 T cells. In contrast to non-allergic individuals, allergic subjects show an aberrant Th2-dominated response to allergens due to ineffective counter-regulation by allergen-specific Th1 and Treg cells. The overshooting allergen-specific Th2 response induces the production of allergen-specific IgE antibodies that subsequently are bound to the high affinity receptor (FcεRI) on the surface of effector cells such as mast cells and basophils. Cross-linking of IgE by allergen induces activation of these effector cells and the release of preformed mediators, most importantly, histamine, which cause immediate allergic symptoms. After 6–8 hours late phase reactions occur, which are mediated by eosinophils and allergen-specific T cells that have migrated to the site of inflammation. Allergen–IgE complexes bind to low affinity IgE receptors (FcεRII, CD23) expressed on lymphocytes, monocytes, macrophages, and platelets. Receptor-mediated endocytosis of allergens via FcεRII is an important way of allergen uptake by B lymphocytes, which is thought to increase allergic responses by promoting Th2 responses.

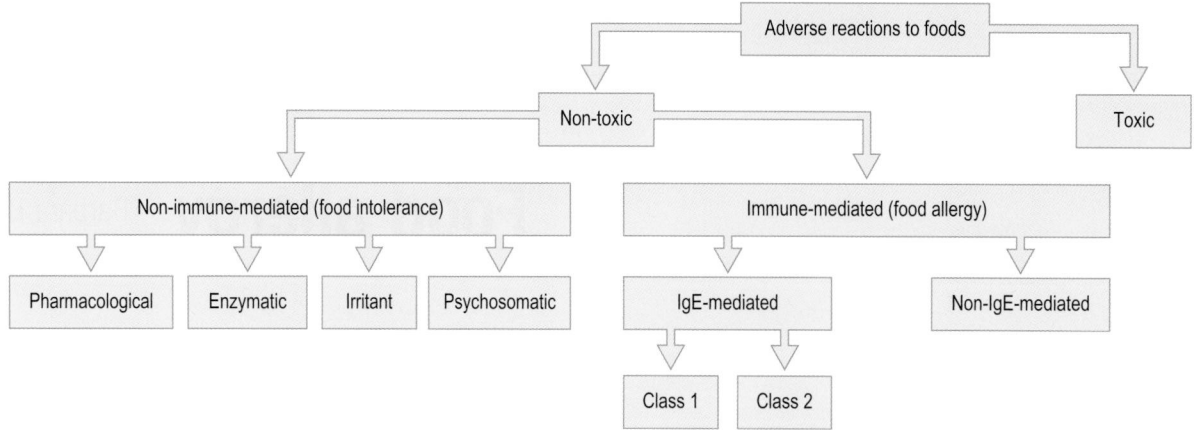

Fig. 43.1 Classification of adverse reactions to foods according to the pathophysiology.[1] Adverse reactions to foods comprise toxic and non-toxic reactions. The latter reactions are either non-immune-mediated or immune-mediated. IgE-mediated reactions constitute type I (immediate) hypersensitivity while non-IgE-mediated reactions are tentatively deemed to be mediated by IgG or IgM immune complex reactions or T-cell-mediated delayed-type reactions.

Sensitization to class 1 food allergens

Class 1 food allergy is characterized by the presence of IgE antibodies specific for "true" food allergens, which are resistant to degradation by gastric and intestinal enzymes, e.g., pepsin or trypsin. Thus, these allergens reach the intestine and are absorbed as intact proteins and consequently are capable of sensitizing atopy-prone individuals. The GI tract is constantly exposed to ingested proteins, commensal bacteria, and pathogens. A single layer of tightly connected intestinal epithelial cells separates the antigenic plethora of foreign antigens from lymphocytes, APC, stromal cells, and other immune cells located in the organized gut-associated lymphoid tissue (GALT) and in the lamina propria (Chapter 19). Complex interactions between these compartments are necessary to guarantee that the GALT can discriminate between pathogens, the GI flora, and harmless antigens, such as food protein. There is an extensive crosstalk between the gut lumen and the GALT. So-called M cells, which are specialized enterocytes located in the follicle-associated epithelium, constantly transport intact antigens to the lymphoid tissue underneath for antigen processing and presentation. Alternatively, luminal antigens can be sampled directly by dendritic cells across the mucosal epithelia. They either extend dendrites through the paracellular space between or interact directly with the epithelial cells. Antigen-loaded dendritic cells then migrate to the draining mesenteric lymph nodes where they prime naïve T lymphocytes. Moreover, increasing evidence suggests that the mucosal epithelium itself is not only an inert physical barrier but is involved in antigen recognition, processing, and presentation.[3] Epithelial cells express MHC class II molecules on their basolateral membranes and can act as nonprofessional APC that lack conventional co-stimulatory molecules, thereby favoring the induction of T-cell anergy or tolerance. Finally, in addition to active uptake, dietary protein antigens may also simply cross the epithelial layer and reach the GALT located beyond.

After intracellular processing by APC residing within the lamina propria luminal antigens are presented to diverse and highly specialized intestinal T-cell populations important for the decision between tolerance induction and activation.[4] For example, $CD8\alpha\alpha^+$ intraepithelial cells are crucial in maintaining and restoring barrier homeostasis by stimulating intestinal epithelial cell turnover. $CD8\alpha\beta^+$ intraepithelial cells contribute to the prevention of pathogen spreading by immediate and high cytolytic activity upon activation. Intraepithelial $CD4^+$ T cells produce cytokines that stimulate dendritic cells to synthesize different factors that influence priming of naïve $CD4^+$ T cells in mesenteric lymph nodes. Furthermore, dendritic cells seem to receive site-specific signals from the intestinal epithelium through interactions with E-cadherin, a ligand of CD103. For example, $CD103^-$ lamina propria dendritic cells are strongly pro-inflammatory, whereas $CD103^+$ dendritic cells are pro-tolerogenic and promote the differentiation of Treg cells in the presence of retinoic acid, a vitamin A analog, and TGF-β. On the other hand, the presence of IL-6 and TGF-β-activated dendritic cells supports the differentiation of Th17 cells. Thus, retinoic acid and IL-6 reciprocally regulate the pro- and anti-inflammatory immune deviation of Treg and Th17 cells. Finally, the lamina propria is also home to agonist-selected Foxp3-expressing naturally occurring Treg cells.

In addition to T lymphocytes, the intestinal mucosa contains a high number of plasma cells, most of which produce dimers or polymers of IgA antibodies.[5] The terminal differentiation of B cells to IgA-producing plasma cells occurs in the lamina propria where T cells produce TGF-β in response to antigen stimulation. TGF-β is an important switch factor for IgA. The locally produced antibodies are actively exported through secretory epithelia via the polymeric immunoglobulin receptor (pIgR). Secretory IgA performs so-called "immune exclusion." This term has been coined for antibody functions at the mucosal surface aiming to control both microbial colonization and penetration of noxious antigens through the epithelial barrier. IgA contributes with different anti-inflammatory mechanisms to the homeostasis within the mucosa. IgA does not activate complement and may prevent the attraction and activation of neutrophils and monocytes as well as the production of inflammatory cytokines, such as TNF-α. Moreover, IgA can trap luminal antigens in immune complexes that are subsequently cleared through the secretory epithelium via pIgR-mediated translocation to the lumen.

Usually, an initial antigen exposure through the GI tract induces a robust T-cell-mediated suppression termed oral tolerance (Fig. 43.2).[6] The induction and regulation of tolerance primarily takes place in the GALT and draining mesenteric lymph nodes, whereas the lamina propria and epithelial compartments principally constitute effector sites for intestinal immune responses.

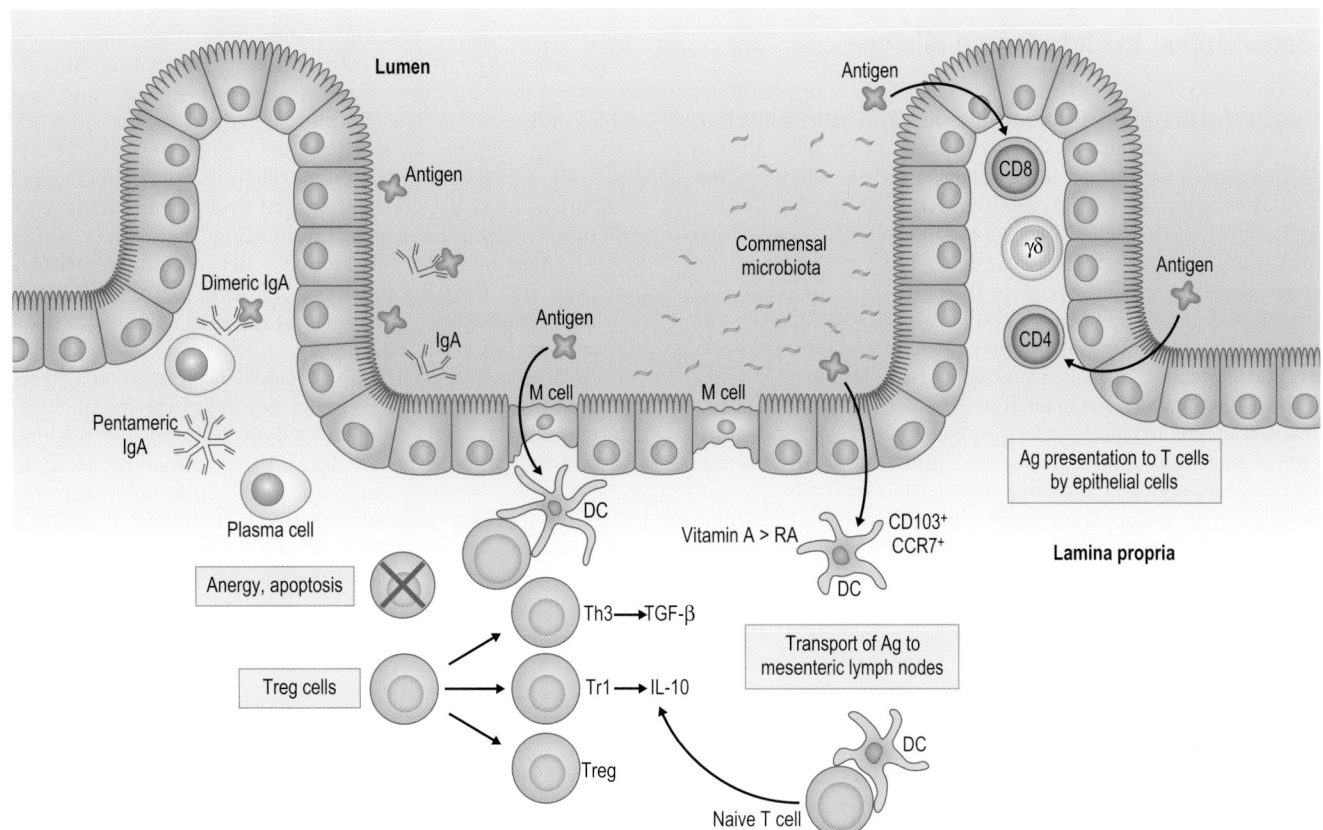

Fig. 43.2 Putative mechanisms of oral tolerance induction. Luminal antigen (Ag) is absorbed by membrane cells (M), dendritic cells (DC), or active transport through epithelial cells. Thereafter, Ag is presented to T cells located in the lamina propria or in mesenteric lymph nodes. Mucosal and peripheral activation of effector T cells is avoided by Treg cells, either via cell–cell contact by naturally occurring Treg cells or via suppressive cytokines (TGF-β, IL-10) produced by Th3 and Tr1 cells, respectively. In addition, immune suppression results from Ag presentation by epithelial cells (non-professional APC lacking co-stimulatory molecules) to CD4$^+$, CD8$^+$, and $\gamma\delta^+$ T cells. CD103$^+$CCR7$^+$ DC promote the differentiation of Treg cells in the presence of retinoic acid (RA) and TGF-β. Plasma cells produce dimers or polymers of IgA that can be actively exported into the gut lumen.
Adapted from Brandtzaeg P. Food allergy: separating the science from the mythology. Nat Rev Gastroenterol Hepatol 2010;7:380–400.

The immune suppressive T-cell events comprise anergy, clonal deletion, and the induction of Treg cells. Still, the development of oral tolerance is not fully understood but explained by the complex interplay of several variables including genetics, age, dose and timing of postnatal oral antigen administration, antigenic structures and composition, gut epithelial barrier integrity, and the degree of concurrent local immune activation. The leakiness of the intestinal epithelium seems particularly important for induction and maintenance of oral tolerance. Structural integrity is conferred by contact between intestinal epithelial cells through desmosomes, adherens junctions, and tight junctions.[7] The intestinal permeability is established and regulated by multiple factors, including epithelial apoptosis, cytokines, immune cells, commensal gut bacteria, and exogenous factors. In healthy children it may take years until this functional barrier is fully developed. For example, the cytokines IFN-γ and TNF-α can disrupt tight junctions and thereby increase intestinal permeability. On the other hand, Th2-cytokines and IL-10 are associated with a protective role in intestinal barrier function. A dysbalance of commensal microbiota caused by environmental influences, e.g., pathogens or antibiotics, can also impair the gut barrier. Other environmental factors that have been considered to influence tolerance induction are food ingredients, e.g., omega-3 polyunsaturated fatty acids or vitamin A and D.[8] In addition, an infectious inflammation can enhance the epithelial permeability, either persistently or temporarily, and results in increased absorption.

Inflammatory responses also abrogate the tolerogenic properties of intestinal CD103$^+$ DC that in normal circumstances promote the differentiation of Treg cells.

Primary food allergy can be considered as a failure to establish or maintain immunological tolerance against innocuous antigens in the gut. The fact that the immunosuppressive intestinal environment is controlled by a complex network of immunological interactions between epithelial cells, APC, and lymphocytes makes it difficult to unravel the precise mechanisms that underlie the development of food allergy. A dysfunction of any of the different steps of the complex interplay can cause disease in susceptible individuals. Moreover, the establishment of immune homeostasis depends on windows of opportunity during which innate and adaptive immunity are coordinated by APC orchestrated by microbial products and dietary constituents. In particular, the neonatal period is critical for the induction of the necessary homeostatic mechanisms because the mucosal epithelial barrier and the immunoregulatory network are poorly developed in newborns. Finally, intrinsic features of food allergens can be important for the development of food allergy. In the recent past extensive research has been performed to determine common features of relevant food and respiratory allergens. However, although molecular resemblance to Toll-like receptor ligands, intrinsic protease activity, and carbohydrate residues of allergens have been discussed, no generally applicable characteristics of allergenicity were found so far.

Sensitization to class 2 food allergens

In contrast to class 1 food allergens, class 2 food allergens do not pass the harsh conditions of the digestive system in intact form and thus, are incapable of sensitizing an individual via the gut. In most cases secondary food allergens induce allergic symptoms due to immunological cross-reactivity with respiratory allergens, which have originally sensitized the patient. A well-known and prevalent class 2 food allergy is birch pollen-associated food allergy, which affects more than 70% of individuals with established birch pollinosis.[9] The most common triggers are stone-fruits (apple, peach) and hazelnuts. In addition, particular vegetables (celery, carrot), peanuts, and soy products can also induce allergic reactions in birch pollen-allergic patients. Because many relevant birch pollen allergens have been characterized with regard to amino acid sequence and protein fold, the immune mechanisms underlying birch pollen-related food allergy could be studied in detail. Thus, birch pollen-related food allergy is an excellent disease-model to illustrate the pathophysiology of class 2 food allergy (Fig. 43.3).

Birch pollen contains one major allergen, Bet v 1, which is recognized by IgE antibodies from more than 95% of birch pollen-allergic patients. Bet v 1 was cloned and sequenced in 1989.[10] It belongs to the pathogenesis-related (PR) 10 protein family. Other members of this protein family are present in different foods, such as fruits of *Rosaceae* (e.g., Mal d 1 in apple, Pru p 1 in peach, Pru a 1 in cherry, Pyr c 1 in pear), vegetables of *Apiaceae* (e.g., Api g 1 in celery, Dau c 1 in carrot), hazelnut (Cor a 1), soybean (Gly m 4), mungbean (Vig r 1), and peanut (Ara h 8). Due to their high amino acid sequence similarity with Bet v 1 these proteins display the typical Bet v 1-fold.[11] As a consequence, IgE-antibodies specific for Bet v 1 can bind to these structurally related food homologs and cause IgE-mediated reactions. The most common manifestation of birch pollen-related food allergy is the oral allergy syndrome (OAS), consisting of itching, tickling, blistering, and/or angioedema confined to the oropharynx immediately after contact with fresh fruits or vegetables. However, systemic and more severe symptoms occur occasionally, in particular upon consumption of soy-containing food products. Typically, only fresh fruits and vegetables induce immediate symptoms. In contrast, cooked foods are usually tolerated by birch pollen-allergic patients. This is due to the fact that heat treatment destroys the 3-dimensional structure of most Bet v 1-related food proteins and the loss of structure results in the loss of IgE-binding.[12]

In addition to IgE cross-reactivity, Bet v 1 and its dietary homologs also cross-react at the T-cell level. Bet v 1-specific T cells may proliferate and produce cytokines in response to stimulation with Bet v 1-related dietary allergens. Bet v 1 contains various distinct T-cell-activating regions and the amino acid sequences of its food homologs match several of these sequences. Consequently, a T cell specific for a Bet v 1-epitope can respond to a similar peptide sequence derived from a food homolog. In particular, the immunodominant T-cell epitope of Bet v 1 located within amino acid 142-156 is involved in cellular cross-reactivity because this C-terminal region is highly conserved among various Bet v 1-isoforms and Bet v 1-related proteins. Clinically, T-cell cross-reactivity can cause late phase responses, e.g., a worsening of atopic eczema 12–48 hours after consumption of birch pollen-related foods. In such skin lesions Bet v 1-specific T cells were detected.[13] Thus, after consumption of birch pollen-related food and their passage through the GI tract, fragments of Bet v 1-homologous food allergens containing T-cell epitopes are absorbed and may activate Bet v 1-specific T cells to migrate into the skin and exert effector functions. Of note, this T-cell cross-reactivity still occurs after cooking of birch pollen-related foods because heat treatment destroys the 3-dimensional structure but not the amino acid sequence of Bet v 1-related food allergens. Heat-denatured food allergens are internalized and processed by APC and presented to T cells. Consequently, patients can develop a worsening of atopic eczema after consuming cooked birch pollen-related food without experiencing an IgE-mediated immediate reaction, e.g., an OAS.[12]

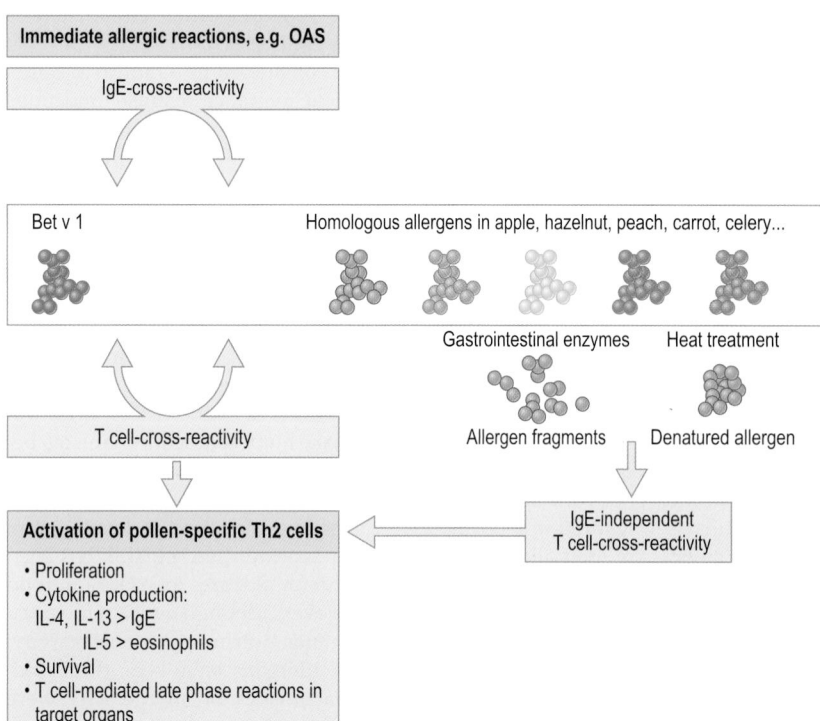

Fig. 43.3 Pathophysiology of birch pollen-related food allergy. Patients are sensitized to Bet v 1, the major birch pollen allergen. Due to sequence and structural similarity Bet v 1-specific IgE antibodies and T cells cross-react with homologous allergens in various foods. IgE-cross-reactivity induces immediate symptoms often confined to the site of allergen contact, i.e., an oral allergy syndrome (OAS). T-cell-cross-reactivity with food allergens activates Bet v 1-specific T cells to proliferate and produce cytokines. Clinically, T-cell-mediated late-phase reactions may occur in target organs, e.g., the skin. Cooking of birch pollen-related food allergens and gastrointestinal conditions destroy their IgE-binding capacity. However, Bet v 1-specific T cells can be activated in an IgE-independent manner.

Clinical and immunological data support the view that in secondary food allergy respiratory allergens are the primary sensitizing agents. Clinically, most patients develop food-induced allergic symptoms after the onset of respiratory allergy. Only a very limited number of individuals show IgE reactivity to Bet v 1-related food allergens in the absence of Bet v 1-specific IgE antibodies, in most cases children sensitized to the Bet v 1-homolog in hazelnut, Cor a 1. Immunologically, Bet v 1 dominates the IgE and T-cell response to its food homologs. For example, pre-incubation of patients´ sera with Bet v 1 totally abolishes their IgE-binding to Bet v 1-related food allergens. In contrast, pre-incubation with Bet v 1-related food allergens reduces IgE-binding to the major birch pollen allergen by only about 50%. These experimental findings indicate that Bet v 1 contains most IgE epitopes of its food homologs and binds IgE antibodies with a higher affinity. These humoral observations are also reflected by the T-cell response to Bet v 1-homologous food allergens. When these T cells were isolated from the peripheral blood of allergic patients and re-stimulated with the food allergen and Bet v 1, most cultures responded more strongly to the major birch pollen allergen. Together, these immunological findings underline that Bet v 1 is the primary cause for allergic sensitization in the patient.

KEY CONCEPTS

- The most common allergies to food are IgE-mediated reactions.
- Class 1 food allergy is considered as a failure to establish or maintain oral tolerance.
- Any event causing epithelial barrier defects may cause allergic sensitization to food allergens, not only in the gut, but also in the skin and airways.
- Successful tolerance induction depends on the dose and timing of enteric exposure to potential allergens, commensal microbiota, and dietary factors, such as vitamin A and D, or lipids.
- Class 2 food allergy is due to immunological cross-reactivity between food and respiratory allergens.
- At present no effective specific immunotherapy for IgE-mediated food allergy exists.

Allergen-specific immunotherapy of food allergy

Allergen-specific immunotherapy (SIT) is currently the only causative treatment for IgE-mediated allergy.[14] SIT consists in repeated administration of allergens to allergic patients with the aim to induce clinical tolerance to natural allergen exposure. Successful SIT is characterized by an improved quality of life, reduced allergic symptoms and reduced medication use. Moreover, SIT prevents the development of new allergic sensitizations and reduces progression of allergic rhinitis to asthma. SIT has an acceptable efficacy for the treatment of allergic rhinoconjunctivitis; however, SIT is not effective in a substantial fraction of patients. Successful SIT alters the allergic immune response and, therefore, shows long-term benefit that exceeds the treatment period.[15] Successful SIT has been associated with the shift from the disease-eliciting Th2 toward a more Th1-like response to allergens. The reduced allergen-specific Th2 cell response that has been shown in *in vitro* experiments is reflected by reduced T-cell-mediated late-phase responses *in vivo*. Another important factor that contributes to the downregulation of the allergen-specific Th2 response is the induction of allergen-

specific Treg cells that produce IL-10 and/or TGF-β. Both cytokines are important switch factors for B cells and promote the production of IgA, IgG1, and IgG4 antibodies. Among different IgG subclasses allergen-specific IgG4 antibodies rise most dramatically during SIT. Therefore, they are considered as "blocking" antibodies that compete with IgE for allergen binding. Indeed, in different *in vitro* experiments, sera of individuals who had received SIT were capable of inhibiting IgE-binding to allergens.[16] The removal of IgG4 antibodies from such sera resulted in an almost complete loss of the inhibition of binding of allergen–IgE complexes. This indicated that IgG4 antibodies bear highest blocking capacity among the different subclasses of IgG antibodies. Apart from the modulation of the adaptive immune response to allergens, SIT also modulates the function of APC and effector cells, e.g., reduction of the number of mast cells and their ability to release mediators. The recruitment of eosinophils and neutrophils to sites of allergen exposure is also reduced during SIT.

SIT and class 1 food allergy

At present, there is no approved SIT for IgE-mediated class 1 food allergy. First attempts to cure class 1 food allergy by conventional subcutaneous SIT had to be abandoned due to an unacceptable risk of severe anaphylactic reactions. Patients are instructed to strictly avoid the respective foods. However, a constant state of vigilance erodes the quality of life and accidental reactions are common even among the most cautious patients. Therefore, attempts aiming at safely bringing allergic patients to a maintenance dose equivalent to the amount of protein contained in a "bite" of the allergenic food are being pursued. In the recent past, evidence accumulated that oral (OIT) and sublingual immunotherapy (SLIT) may achieve this more safely than subcutaneous SIT.[17] OIT requires the individual to mix a powdered allergen dose in a vehicle food and ingest it each day at home for several months. Different OIT trials in egg and peanut allergy have been performed and demonstrated desensitization, i.e., the ability to raise the amount of food protein required for induction of a clinical reaction while still on daily immunotherapy. One study of six egg-allergic patients showed that the patients remained desensitized in a tolerance challenge after 4 weeks of abstinence from egg.[18] Immunological changes induced by OIT resembled those described for SIT for pollen allergies and comprised increased allergen-specific IgG and IgG4, decreased allergen-specific IgE and mast cell responses, and a shift away from the Th2 profile with increases of TGF-β and IL-10.

The second promising approach actively studied for the treatment of food allergy is SLIT. Drops of allergen extract are placed under the tongue and subsequently, are swallowed. Up to now, SLIT has been successful inducing clinical tolerance to Pru p 3 and Cor a 8, the non-specific lipid transfer proteins inducing severe systemic reactions to peach and hazelnut, respectively, as well as to peanut allergens.[19,20] The immune mechanisms induced by SLIT are similar to conventional, subcutaneous administration of allergen extracts. Oral Langerhans cells are thought to be involved in the tolerance induction during SLIT that induce Treg cells and the shift from Th2 towards Th1-like responses. As a consequence of the modulated T-cell response, allergen-specific blocking antibodies occur.[21]

It must be noted that the OIT and SLIT studies performed so far were all conducted in relatively small groups of patients at medical centers with appropriate support staff and are not yet ready to be implemented into normal clinical practice. Nevertheless, OIT and SLIT are viable approaches for the treatment of class 1 food allergy and future studies are required to make them safe and efficient for a broader application.

SIT and class 2 food allergy

Class 2 food allergy is the consequence of immunological cross-reactivity between structurally related respiratory and food allergens. Thus, one would assume that successful SIT of the respiratory allergy would concomitantly cure the associated food allergy. Unfortunately, this is not the case for the majority of patients. Although some studies have described a curative effect of birch pollen-SIT on birch pollen-associated food allergy, others have reported the opposite, namely the development of food allergy during the course of therapy. The limited benefit of birch pollen-SIT on birch pollen-associated food allergy is puzzling because it is not easily comprehensible why cross-reactivity can cause, but not cure, allergic disorders. Interestingly, patients who had received birch pollen extract either subcutaneously or sublingually did neither develop remarkable levels of food-specific IgG4 antibodies nor show a long-term shift of the food-specific Th2 response.[22,23] Thus, it seems that the administration of pollen extract does not alter the food-reactive immune response in a sufficient manner to develop tolerance. This makes birch pollen-related food allergy an interesting model to investigate the precise mechanisms that fail in patients who are successfully desensitized to birch pollen but not to the respective foods. Hopefully, future studies will bring insights into the complicated mechanisms underlying tolerance to food allergens. In view of the reports on successful desensitization of class 1 food allergy by SLIT with food extracts and the limited efficacy of SLIT with birch pollen extract, one may conclude that specific treatment of class 2 food allergy should be performed employing the involved food allergens. Indeed, a first trial in a limited number of patients showed an improvement of pollen-associated hazelnut-induced OAS in response to sublingual administration of hazelnut extract.[19] However, an effective treatment of secondary food allergy may require the administration of both, respiratory and food allergens. This issue still needs to be addressed in clinical trials. To obtain reliable results complex studies involving a large number of patients need to be performed. Furthermore, objective clinical measurements for food-induced allergic reactions are needed in order to assess the improvement or failure of the investigated allergy vaccines.

Concluding remarks

● ON THE HORIZON

- The development of safe and efficient vaccines for specific immunotherapy of food allergy needs to be promoted.
- The identification and characterization of relevant food allergens is one important basis for the development of vaccines with a reduced risk for side effects.
- Reliable and simple diagnostic procedures for food allergy are essential for early therapeutic intervention.
- The elucidation of immune mechanisms underlying food allergy contribute to the development of therapeutic strategies.

Class 1 and 2 food allergies are relevant forms of IgE-mediated allergic disorders. Class 1 food allergy primarily affects children, whereas class 2 food allergy is very abundant among adolescent/adult individuals with established respiratory allergy. It is, however, remarkable that only a limited number of different foods induce these diseases considering the plethora of non-self antigens to which the GI tract is persistently exposed. The top causes for class 1 food allergy are milk, egg, peanut, tree nuts, soybeans, wheat, fish, and shellfish. In secondary food allergy various foods may be involved that often are not biologically related to the allergen source originally causing the disease. Compared to respiratory IgE-mediated allergy, in many ways food allergy is special. It often manifests at different sites of the body apart from the GI tract, e.g., in the skin and lung. It is difficult to diagnose and also more difficult to cure than respiratory allergy. There is currently no effective treatment for food allergy.

Thus, at present the major challenge in the field of food allergy is the development of safe and efficient therapeutic approaches for primary and secondary food allergy. Indeed, various new strategies for treating food allergy are under investigation and increase the likelihood of success.[24] This development goes hand in hand with the development of a reliable and easy diagnosis. Currently, the golden standard for the diagnosis of food allergy is a double-blind placebo-controlled food challenge. However, this form of diagnosis is complicated and very time-consuming. Test substances need to be blinded by a dietician and the challenge must be performed in clinical settings. Thus, one requirement in the field of food allergy is the development of less complicated tests for proper diagnosis of food allergy. A more simplified diagnostic procedure will also cover larger numbers of patients. In parallel, the development of safe and effective allergen-specific vaccines needs to be promoted. Currently, no therapeutic options for patients suffering from food allergy can be offered. The investigation of basic immune mechanisms relevant for disease development and its cure are pivotal for the development of safe and efficient vaccines for specific immunotherapy for food allergy. In summary, basic research in the field of food allergy and its translation from "bench to bedside" should be promoted.

References

1. Bruijnzeel-Koomen C, Ortolani C, Aas K, et al. Adverse reactions to food. European Academy of Allergology and Clinical Immunology Subcommittee. Allergy 1995;50:623–35.
2. Eyerich S, Eyerich K, Pennino D, et al. Th22 cells represent a distinct human T cell subset involved in epidermal immunity and remodeling. J Clin Invest 2009;119:3573–85.
3. Henderson P, van Limbergen JE, Schwarze J, et al. Function of the intestinal epithelium and its dysregulation in inflammatory bowel disease. Inflamm Bowel Dis 2010;17:382–95.
4. van Wijk F, Cheroutre H. Intestinal T cells: facing the mucosal immune dilemma with synergy and diversity. Semin Immunol 2009;21:130–8.
5. Brandtzaeg P. Update on mucosal immunoglobulin A in gastrointestinal disease. Curr Opin Gastroenterol 2010;26:554–63.
6. du Pre MF, Samsom JN. Adaptive T-cell responses regulating oral tolerance to protein antigen. Allergy 2011;66:478–90.
7. Groschwitz KR, Hogan SP. Intestinal barrier function: molecular regulation and disease pathogenesis. J Allergy Clin Immunol 2009;124:3–20; quiz 21–22.
8. Lack G. Epidemiologic risks for food allergy. J Allergy Clin Immunol 2008;121:1331–6.
9. Geroldinger-Simic M, Zelniker T, Aberer W, et al. Birch pollen-related food allergy: Clinical aspects and the role of allergen-specific IgE and IgG(4) antibodies. J Allergy Clin Immunol 2011;127:616–22, e611.
10. Breiteneder H, Pettenburger K, Bito A, et al. The gene coding for the major birch pollen allergen Betv1, is highly homologous to a pea disease resistance response gene. EMBO J 1989;8:1935–8.
11. Radauer C, Lackner P, Breiteneder H. The Bet v 1 fold: an ancient, versatile scaffold for binding of large, hydrophobic ligands. BMC Evol Biol 2008;8:286.
12. Bohle B, Zwolfer B, Heratizadeh A, et al. Cooking birch pollen-related food: divergent consequences for IgE- and T cell-mediated reactivity in vitro and in vivo. J Allergy Clin Immunol 2006;118:242–9.

13. Reekers R, Busche M, Wittmann M, et al. Birch pollen-related foods trigger atopic dermatitis in patients with specific cutaneous T-cell responses to birch pollen antigens. J Allergy Clin Immunol 1999;104:466–72.

14. Bousquet J, Lockey R, Malling HJ. Allergen immunotherapy: therapeutic vaccines for allergic diseases. A WHO position paper. J Allergy Clin Immunol 1998;102:558–62.

15. Larche M, Akdis CA, Valenta R. Immunological mechanisms of allergen-specific immunotherapy. Nat Rev Immunol 2006;6:761–71.

16. James LK, Shamji MH, Walker SM, et al. Long-term tolerance after allergen immunotherapy is accompanied by selective persistence of blocking antibodies. J Allergy Clin Immunol 2011;127:509–16, e501–5.

17. Kulis M, Vickery BP, Burks AW. Pioneering immunotherapy for food allergy: clinical outcomes and modulation of the immune response. Immunol Res 2011;49:216–26.

18. Vickery BP, Pons L, Kulis M, et al. Individualized IgE-based dosing of egg oral immunotherapy and the development of tolerance. Ann Allergy Asthma Immunol 2010;105:444–50.

19. Enrique E, Pineda F, Malek T, et al. Sublingual immunotherapy for hazelnut food allergy: a randomized, double-blind, placebo-controlled study with a standardized hazelnut extract. J Allergy Clin Immunol 2005;116:1073–9.

20. Kim EH, Bird JA, Kulis M, et al. Sublingual immunotherapy for peanut allergy: Clinical and immunologic evidence of desensitization. J Allergy Clin Immunol 2011;127:640–6, e641.

21. Scadding GW, Shamji MH, Jacobson MR, et al. Sublingual grass pollen immunotherapy is associated with increases in sublingual Foxp3-expressing cells and elevated allergen-specific immunoglobulin G4, immunoglobulin A and serum inhibitory activity for immunoglobulin E-facilitated allergen binding to B cells. Clin Exp Allergy 2010;40:598–606.

22. Bohle B, Kinaciyan T, Gerstmayr M, et al. Sublingual immunotherapy induces IL-10-producing T regulatory cells, allergen-specific T-cell tolerance, and immune deviation. J Allergy Clin Immunol 2007;120:707–13.

23. van Hoffen E, Peeters KA, van Neerven RJ, et al. Effect of birch pollen-specific immunotherapy on birch pollen-related hazelnut allergy. J Allergy Clin Immunol 2011;127:100–1, 101, e101–3.

24. Nowak-Wegrzyn A, Sampson HA. Future therapies for food allergies. J Allergy Clin Immunol 2011;127:558–73.

25. Brandtzaeg P. Food allergy: separating the science from the mythology. Nat Rev Gastroenterol Hepatol 2010;7:380–400.

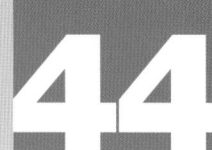

Petr L. Hruz,
Alex Straumann

Eosinophil-associated gastrointestinal disorders

The human gastrointestinal tract represents the largest host–environment interface of the body where the epithelial surface is exposed to an overwhelming load of diverse micro-organisms as well as dietary products, including potentially allergenic macromolecules. Several mechanisms are involved to maintain a physical and functional barrier to protect the interior of the body. Beside the physical barriers, the mucosal immune system with the "evolutionarily ancient" innate and the more specific and more diverse adaptive immunity is of particular importance. It needs to mount an inflammatory response against invading micro-organisms while persisting in a state of non-responsiveness or tolerance to innocuous substances such as commensal bacteria or food antigens. Each system of immunity relies on different cell types, gene products with characteristic modes of action.

Eosinophils—a cell type of the innate immune system—are present in the peripheral blood of healthy individuals and account for approximately 1–3% of the peripheral leucocytes with an upper limit of the normal range of 350 cells/μL of blood.[1] Tissue-dwelling eosinophils reside in the hematopoietic and lymphatic organs, such as the bone marrow, spleen, lymph nodes and thymus. However, based on a comprehensive analysis of normal human tissues from almost all body organs, we know that the only non-hematopoietic organ showing tissue-dwelling eosinophils under *resting conditions* is the gastrointestinal tract.[2] The distribution of the eosinophils is not homogeneous throughout the digestive tract with the highest density of cells in the cecal and appendiceal region.[3] Under physiological conditions the esophagus is the only segment of the digestive tract without tissue-dwelling eosinophils.[3,4] In addition to the resident eosinophils, a marked accumulation of eosinophils in the digestive tract can be seen under *inflammatory conditions*. Because eosinophils are non-specific late phase inflammatory cells an infiltration can occur in the context of any inflammation—e.g., bacterial and parasitic infections, celiac disease, Crohn's disease, ulcerative colitis—independently of its cause.[1]

Here, we focus exclusively on three *idiopathic* eosinophil-associated gastrointestinal disorders (EGID): idiopathic eosinophilic esophagitis (EoE), idiopathic eosinophilic gastroenteritis (EGE) and idiopathic hypereosinophilic syndromes (HES) with gastrointestinal manifestation (Table 44.1). The adjective "eosinophil-associated" denominates that the histological inflammatory response is characterized by an eosinophil-predominant tissue infiltration. Moreover, it is likely that eosinophils play a crucial role in the pathogenesis of these disorders. Because each of these conditions has different properties and likely its own pathogenesis, to subsume them into one single category is quite arbitrary and based exclusively on descriptive features. EoE is definitely an esophageal-restricted disease with a benign long-term prognosis.[4] In patients with EGE, the inflammatory process can involve several segments of the gastrointestinal tract but,

nevertheless, this chronic inflammation can also be considered clinically a benign disorder. In contrast, HES is primarily a multi-system disorder that may involve several organs, including the digestive tract, and often has a fatal outcome.[5,6] Despite these fundamental differences, all three conditions share the same features of being idiopathic and eosinophilic, and, as long as our understanding of the underlying mechanisms remains so fragmentary, we may take the liberty of classifying them into one single category.

EoE is by far the most common EGID. Because of its clinical relevance, EoE is discussed in this review in greater depth than the other two EGIDs.

Eosinophilic esophagitis

Definition

A recently updated consensus report proposed that: EoE represents a chronic, immune mediated esophageal disease, characterized clinically by symptoms related to esophageal dysfunction and histologically by an eosinophil-predominant inflammation.[7]

> ## CLINICAL PEARLS
>
> **Eosinophilic esophagitis**
>
> - Predominantly males present with persistent dysphagia and/or food impaction.
> - Often with coexisting allergic airway disease and less frequently with food allergies.
> - Structural changes may be observed at endoscopy.
> - Diagnosis based on the histological finding of >15 eosinophils/HPF (magnification ×400) on biopsy specimens.
> - Treatment includes topical and systemic steroids as well as individualized and allergen-specific diets.
> - Dilation treatment is reserved for disease involving structural changes.

Epidemiology

Epidemiological data are essential to determine the clinical and socioeconomic relevance of any disease; and thus, the knowledge of the epidemiologic parameters of a disease is crucial for identifying risk factors as well as pathogenetic mechanisms, for planning preventive measures and for determining optimal treatment approaches.

Table 44.1 Eosinophil-associated gastrointestinal disorders

Eosinophilic esophagitis (EoE)
Eosinophilic gastroenteritis (EGE)
Hypereosinophilic syndrome (HES)

Demographic cornerstones

Cases of EoE patients have been reported worldwide and identified in a variety of ethnic backgrounds, including Caucasian, African, Hispanic, and Asian. However, as there are no controlled data about geographic variations of prevalence, it remains unclear whether EoE is more common in any particular ethnic or racial group, especially as most of the reported data come from studies of Caucasian patients. EoE can be found in all age groups but most studies report an average age between 34 and 42 years with a male-to-female risk ratio of 3:1.[8-13] This suggests that EoE is predominantly a disease of middle-aged male adults.

Interestingly, age at diagnosis does not correlate with onset of EoE-attributed symptoms, which can be considered as onset of disease. Several studies report a substantial time lag between onset of symptoms and diagnosis (diagnostic delay), which in some cases can be attributed to unawareness of sentinel features at endoscopy (doctor's delay). Often patients develop specific eating strategies with careful chewing and avoidance of dry and rough food and bypass medical care, despite a substantial impairment of quality of life (patient delay). A diagnostic delay of several years for EoE diagnosis is not uncommon.[8,12,14]

Incidence and prevalence of eosinophilic esophagitis

Although it is considered a rare disease several epidemiological studies from geographically-confined regions implicate an increasing incidence and prevalence of EoE in the adult population during the last years.[8,11,12]

Probably the most conclusive epidemiological data originate from the geographically confined region of Olten County (Switzerland) where a prospective population-based assessment strategy with unchanged diagnostic and enrolment procedures for evaluation of EoE has been used systematically. Between 1989 and 2009, EoE was diagnosed in 46 patients (76% males; mean age 41 ± 16 years). An average annual incidence rate of 2.45/100 000 was calculated. In the face of a constant diagnostic delay and the lack of EoE awareness programs significantly more EoE cases were diagnosed between 2000 and 2009 compared to those between 1989 and 1999. In the same time period, the number of upper endoscopies increased markedly less (63%) than the incidence rate of EoE (153%). The cumulative EoE prevalence rose to 42.8/100 000 in 2009 (personal communication).

Prevalence of esophageal eosinophilia

In an analysis based mainly on histology, the prevalence of any eosinophils in the most distal parts of the esophagus was found to be 4.8% in the general population, predominantly among men (63%), with 54% of these subjects reporting reflux symptoms.[15] This finding suggests that the presence of esophageal eosinophils may be more common in the general population than expected, but may also be of ambiguous clinical significance, especially as there are no data about the prevalence of eosinophils in the mid- and proximal portions of the esophagus. The presence of eosinophils in the distal part of the esophagus was associated with erosive esophagitis, hiatus hernia, narrowing of the esophageal lumen, and esophageal ulcer, thereby suggesting that the presence of esophageal eosinophils, especially in the distal esophageal portions, may be predominantly a manifestation of reflux disease. EoE was suspected only in 4 cases (0.4% of the general population) with only one subject presenting with bronchial asthma and dysphagia, which would suggest that this patient was suffering from clinico-pathologically defined EoE.

Thus, the presence of eosinophils in the esophagus should be considered abnormal. Esophageal eosinophilia is unspecific and can be observed in a wide range of diseases, such as gastroesophageal reflux disease (GERD), Crohn's disease, vascular diseases, infectious esophagitis, drug-induced esophagitis, EGE, and hypereosinophilic syndrome. In particular, eosinophilic infiltration of the distal part of the esophagus has been reported in patients having GERD and therefore esophageal eosinophilia requires a process of differential diagnosis and cannot, *a priori*, be equated with EoE.[16]

● KEY CONCEPTS

Differential diagnosis of EoE

- Gastroesophageal reflux disease (GERD)
- Infectious esophagitis (Herpes, Candida)
- Parasitic disease
- Drug-induced esophagitis
- Autoimmune disease (vascular diseases)
- Eosinophilic gastroenteritis affecting the esophagus
- Hypereosinophilic syndrome affecting the esophagus
- Crohn's disease affecting the esophagus

Pathophysiology

Eosinophils' natural life cycle

Eosinophils reside predominantly in three anatomical compartments, the bone marrow, blood vessels, and organs with mucosal surfaces. Eosinophils originate in the bone marrow from pluripotent stem cells. Their differentiation process is mainly orchestrated under the influence of three cytokines, interleukin (IL)-3, IL-5, and granulocyte-macrophage colony stimulating factor (GM-CSF) to a fully granulated state before migration to the vascular space occurs. Especially, IL-5 is very specific for the eosinophil lineage and stimulates the release of eosinophils from the bone marrow and extends their survival once in target tissue. Mice lacking IL-5 develop a significant reduction in tissue eosinophilia, whereas mice overexpressing IL-5 show markedly increased peripheral eosinophilia.[17] A multistep process mediated by adhesion molecules on endothelial cells and corresponding ligands on eosinophils (P-selectin and β_1 and β_2 integrins) enables the migration from the vascular space into tissues. It is orchestrated by Th2 cytokines (IL-4 and IL-13) that induce expression of cell surface ligands of the β-integrin family, such as very late antigen (VLA)-4 (β_1 integrin) on the surface of eosinophils and their counter ligands on endothelia that include vascular cell adhesion molecule (VCAM)-1.[18] Various chemoattractants—released within local mucosal environments—including leukotriene B$_4$, platelet activating factor, chemokines (eotaxins), and bacterial products, provoke eosinophil migration.[19] Eotaxin is particularly important as it binds the chemokine receptor CCR-3 on eosinophils. Eosinophils are absent from the gastrointestinal tract in mice lacking eotaxin-1.

IgE-mediated activation of mast cells

The accumulation of eosinophils in the esophageal wall of EoE patients with specific patterns of cytokine expression resembles the findings of other allergic diseases. Indeed, in up to 70% of adult EoE patients a medical history of concomitant atopic diseases such as allergic rhinitis, bronchial asthma, atopic dermatitis and including immunglobulin E (IgE)-mediated food allergies is reported.[8,10–13] Elevated total serum IgE levels occur in up to 80% of pediatric and in up to 60% of adult EoE patients and total IgE levels were significantly higher in patients sensitized to food and/or aeroallergens. Therefore, food allergens as well as aeroallergens have been implicated as contributing factors in inducing and maintaining the eosinophilic inflammation.[20,21] In the pediatric population EoE patients show IgE sensitization to a wide variety of food including cow's milk, soy, peanuts, chocolate, wheat, and egg. In the skin prick test (SPT) and atopy patch test (APT) pediatric EoE patients revealed sensitization to food in 73 and 80%, respectively.[22] The most common food allergens detected by SPT were milk, eggs, soy, and peanuts, whereas positive APT reactions were frequently observed to corn, soy, wheat, and milk. After a successful diet (six-food elimination diet and elemental formula) with disease improvement in up to 80%, all patients redeveloped EoE symptoms following an open food challenge, suggesting that food allergens might be potent triggers of EoE.[23–25] In contrast, adults with EoE are more sensitized to aeroallergens as food elimination diet is not effective.[26] These observations indirectly suggest that IgE-mediated activation and degranulation of mast cells is involved in EoE pathogenesis (Fig. 44.1). Mast cells can promote inflammation through production of general inflammatory mediators such as tumor necrosis factor (TNF)-α or IL-1 and more eosinophil-specific cytokines such as IL-4 and IL-5. But non-IgE-mediated mechanisms are also involved in the pathogenesis of EoE as treatment with omalizumab (anti-IgE) leads only to symptomatic improvement of patients with EGID, with only a partial decrease in the absolute eosinophil count and tissue eosinophilia.[27]

Th2-mediated immune response

Besides the IgE-mediated activation of mast cells, EoE shows an infiltration with cells having a characteristic Th2-type inflammatory pattern (Fig. 44.1).[28] In esophageal biopsy specimens of EoE patients increased numbers of lymphocytes (T and B cells) and mast cells as well as increased expression of the important cytokines IL-5 and IL-13 were found.[28] The crucial role of IL-5 and -13 in the pathogenesis of EoE has been demonstrated in various experimental models.[29–31] As a proof of concept study of aeroallergen-induced esophageal eosinophilia, intranasal allergen challenge with *Aspergillus fumigatus* resulted in an infiltration of eosinophils in both the esophagus and the bronchi, whereas tissue eosinophilia did not develop in IL-5-deficient mice.[30] Direct delivery of IL-13—the other important cytokine of the Th2 immune response—into the pulmonary tree induced esophageal eosinophilia, which can be blocked by anti-human IL-13 antibody.[31] Interestingly, esophageal epithelial cells produce eotaxin-3—an important chemoattractant for eosinophils—after IL-13 stimulation through a transcriptional mechanism dependent on signal transducer and activator of transcription (STAT)-6.[32] Esophageal eotaxin-3 strongly correlates with tissue eosinophilia and *eotaxin-3* is one of the most induced genes in patients with EoE.[33] Moreover a single-nucleotide polymorphism (SNP 2496 T->G) in the *eotaxin-3* gene is linked to increased disease susceptibility for EoE.[34]

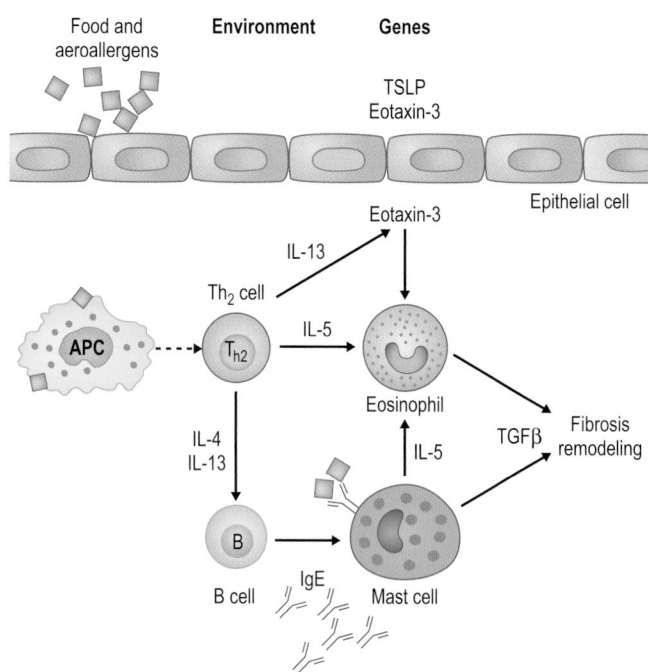

Fig. 44.1 The current understanding of cellular and molecular mechanisms in the pathogenesis of eosinophilic esophagitis (EoE) involves a complex interaction of genetic and environmental factors. EoE disease susceptibility is linked to single nucleotide polymorphisms (SNPs) in the eotaxin-3 and thymic stromal lymphopoietin (TSLP) gene. A sensitization to food and aeroallergens has been noted. Two possible pathways can lead to accumulation of eosinophils in the esophageal wall. First, allergens can be recognized by antigen presenting cells (APC), such as dendritic cells, and activate a type 2 helper T-lymphocyte (Th2) immune response to induce the release of eosinophil-specific cytokines such as IL-5 and IL-13 and subsequently the production of eotaxin-3, which is a very potent chemoattractant for eosinophils. Second, allergen exposure can result in the cross-linking of IgE on mast cells leading to release of specific inflammatory mediators, which boost directly or through stimulation of epithelial cells' accumulation of eosinophils in the esophageal layers. Both eosinophils and mast cells produce TGF-β – a potent cytokine involved in fibrosis and smooth muscle contraction which promotes tissue remodeling leading to loss of elasticity of the esophageal wall and luminal narrowing.

Accumulation and activation of eosinophils in the esophagus is followed by release of various granule proteins and cytokines. These mediators can exert cytotoxic effects (e.g., major basic protein (MBP), eosinophil-derived neurotoxin (EDN), eosinophil peroxidase (EPO)) or contribute to perpetuation of the inflammatory response through activation of a wide range of other inflammatory cytokines such as IL-1, IL-3, IL-4, IL-5, IL-13, IL-15, GM-CSF, TNF-α, RANTES, MIP1-α, transforming growth factor beta (TGF-β) pointing out complex pathophysiological mechanisms.

Esophageal remodeling

Unbridled eosinophilic inflammation leads to fibrosis and angiogenesis with an ensuing loss of elasticity of the esophageal wall and luminal narrowing. This phenomenon is called tissue remodeling and has been described in clinical studies as well as in animal models.[4,35,36] Although the exact mechanism is not known, eosinophils and subepithelial mast cells expressing tryptase are critically involved in this process via secretion of the cytokine TGF-β1. Recent data suggest that this cytokine is involved in numerous processes relevant to allergic inflammation, including regulation of profibrotic processes and modulation of smooth muscle contraction with increased contractility, thereby potentially contributing to clinical symptoms such as dysphagia and bolus obstruction in patients with EoE.[37] Furthermore, in murine models there is growing evidence that the two crucial cytokines involved in tissue eosinophilia IL-5 and IL-13 also induce esophageal remodeling.[36]

Under the influence of the topical corticosteroid budesonide, the expression of the fibrosis related markers such as TGF-β_1 and tenascin C markedly decreased in the esophageal tissue, suggesting that anti-inflammatory treatment can interrupt or even reverse the remodeling of the esophagus.[38]

Symptoms

The predominant symptom of adult EoE is dysphagia for solids, often leading to long-lasting food impaction with the necessity of endoscopic bolus removal. Because EoE patients rapidly develop specific eating strategies a careful evaluation of changes in eating habits is required. EoE patients tend to chew carefully, and avoid dry and rough food. Dysphagia and food impaction are reported increasingly with age. A minority of patients reports GERD-like symptoms, non-swallowing-related chest pain, and upper abdominal pain. In contrast, in neonates and infants, food refusal and failure to thrive may be observed as dysphagia cannot be easily expressed in this age group. Children often complain of GERD-like symptoms, such as heartburn and reflux, vomiting and abdominal pain, and less frequently, diarrhea (Table 44.2).

Endoscopy and histology

Endoscopy shows a heterogeneous mix of abnormalities: subtle reddish, longitudinal furrows and white exudates may occur and reflect local edema and acute inflammation, respectively. Signs of transient or fixed corrugated rings as well as crêpe paper mucosa may be observed due to a loss of mucosal elasticity and are likely a sequela of the chronic eosinophilic inflammation (Fig. 44.2A–D). However, as endoscopic features can be absent in EoE, histological evaluation is recommended. The diagnosis of EoE is based on typical esophageal symptoms and characteristic histological findings ($\geq$ 15 eosinophils/high power field ($\times$400)) after exclusion of other esophageal diseases associated with an eosinophilic infiltrate of the mucosa (e.g., GERD). Several biopsies in EoE are recommended as a patchy distribution of tissue eosinophils in EoE can be observed and the eosinophils appear superficially along the luminal surface. Because white exudates correspond to eosinophil aggregations and microabscesses (Fig. 44.3) biopsies should preferably be taken from these areas.

Treatment

As a result of recent advances in the understanding of the natural course of the disease there are several reasons to treat EoE: (1) Improvement of the quality of life after resolution of the swallowing disturbances; (2) reduction of the risk for severe esophageal injury by preventing long-lasting food impactions; and (3) prevention of esophageal remodeling. The current treatment options can be summarized with three D's for drugs, diet and dilation.

⬤ THERAPEUTIC PRINCIPLES

Current treatment options for eosinophilic esophagitis

Drugs
- Topical steroids (budesonide, fluticasone)
- Systemic steroids (prednisone)
- Biologics (monoclonal antibodies against IL-5 , IL-13, and IgE)
- Immunosuppressants (azathioprine, 6-mercaptopurine)
- Anti-allergic agents (leukotriene antagonists and CRTH2-blockers)

Diets
- Elimination diets (individualized, allergen-specific)
- "6-food" elimination diet (milk, soy, wheat, nuts, eggs, seafood)
- Elemental diet

Dilation
Dilation of strictures or stenosis

Drugs

Acid suppression with proton pump inhibitors (PPIs) is not usually effective in relieving symptoms and resolving eosinophilic inflammation in patients with EoE. However, patients with concomitant GERD, and a subgroup of EoE patients with PPI-responsive EoE may respond to treatment with PPIs. PPI therapy should therefore not be considered as a first-line treatment but used as co-therapy in patients who have secondary or coexisting GERD.

Systemic and topical corticosteroids show comparable effectiveness in resolving symptoms and signs of active EoE in children and in adults.[38,39] As topical steroids have fewer side effects they are recommended as first-line therapy. Short-term use of systemic corticosteroids may be limited to emergent cases, such as dysphagia requiring hospitalization, patients with dehydration due to swallowing difficulties, or patients with symptoms refractory to topical steroids. Discontinuation of topical and systemic corticosteroids is usually followed by recurrence of the disease within a few weeks.

So far, anti-allergic drugs have proven less effective in EoE treatment. Cromolyn sodium has no apparent therapeutic effect while leukotriene receptor antagonists have been shown to induce symptomatic relief, but without affecting esophageal eosinophilia.[40]

Only limited data are available for targeted therapy with novel biologic agents or immunosuppressants. Mepolizumab (anti-IL-5 antibody) led to a significant reduction of esophageal eosinophils in adult EoE patients, but with only minimal clinical improvement.[41] Treatment of EoE patients with the anti-TNF-α antibody infliximab was not effective either in reducing eosinophilic tissue infiltration or in improving symptoms, although in active EoE a massive expression of TNF-α in the squamous epithelium of the esophagus was shown. The immunosuppressants azathioprine and 6-mercaptopurine were effective in inducing and maintaining a remission in three corticosteroid-refractory EoE patients.[42] However, further evaluation of these alternatives for corticosteroid-refractory EoE is needed before they can be implemented into routine clinical practice.

Table 44.2 Symptoms of EoE

Adults	Children
Dysphagia	Food aversion / food refusal
Bolus obstruction	Vomiting / regurgitation
Non-swallowing related chest pain	Abdominal pain
	Failure to thrive
	Dysphagia
	Heartburn / reflux
	Bolus obstruction
	Diarrhea

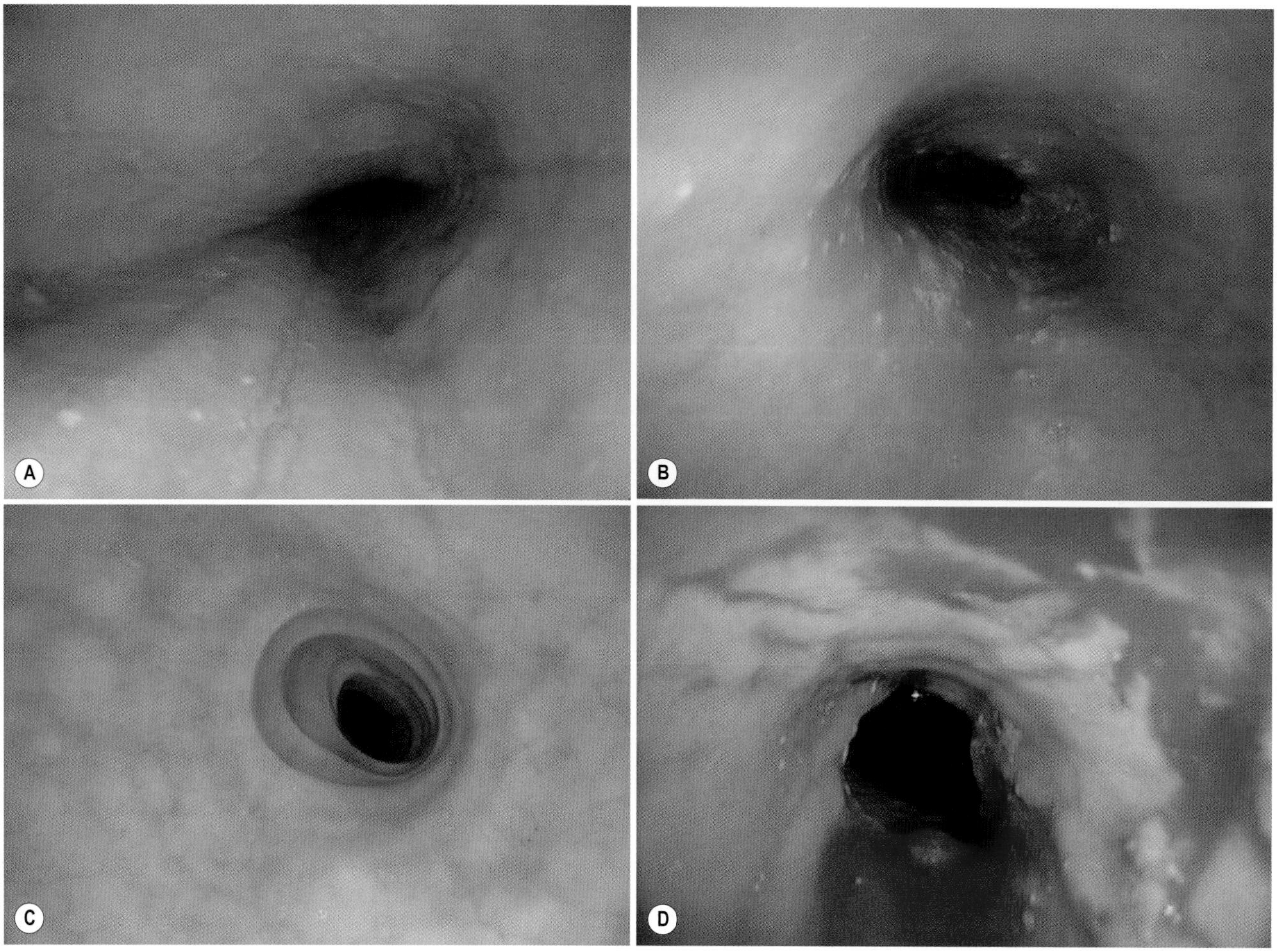

Fig. 44.2 Endoscopic findings in eosinophilic esophagitis: (A) red furrows, (B) whitish exudates, (C) corrugated rings, (D) crêpe paper mucosa.

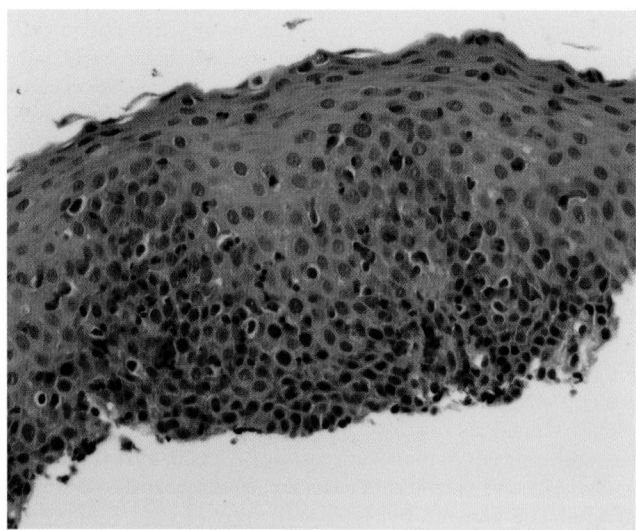

Fig. 44.3 On histological evaluation eosinophilic microabscesses can be found (representative picture ×40 magnification).

Diet

Mainly in pediatric patients, several trials have been conducted to assess the potential of different diets in treating EoE. Individually adjusted elimination diets, rigid 6-food elimination diet (removal of the 6 most common allergenic foods such as milk, eggs, wheat, soy, peanuts, fish/shellfish) and protein-free elemental diet have shown efficacy in the treatment of children with EoE.[22,23,43] When deciding on the use of a specific dietary therapy, the patient's lifestyle and family resources also need to be considered. So far, dietary treatment has been more effective in children than in adults. Overall, the value of dietary therapy in adults requires further evaluation.

Dilation

Esophageal dilation leads to long-lasting symptom relief but does not influence the underlying inflammation. It should therefore be reserved for patients who present with a functional narrowing (strictures, stenosis) of the esophagus refractory to adequate drug therapy. Endoscopic dilation should be performed with caution as it is associated with a certain risk of esophageal injury although recently published large series have demonstrated that this risk is not as great as originally thought.[44]

Idiopathic eosinophilic gastroenteritis

Definition and classification

EGE is a rare, heterogeneous, and poorly defined condition. It is characterized by a chronic-recurrent tissue infiltration of the gastrointestinal tract with eosinophils.[45] The diagnosis is based on the following three criteria:

(1) Non-specific gastrointestinal symptoms;
(2) Eosinophilic infiltration of one or more areas of the gastrointestinal tract;
(3) Exclusion of other causes for the intestinal eosinophilia.[46]

No consensus has yet been reached regarding the histological criteria for diagnosing EGE. This may be related to the fact that the healthy gastric and intestinal mucosa harbors eosinophils under physiological conditions and "normal" cell numbers are difficult to establish.

● CLINICAL PEARLS

Eosinophilic gastroenteritis (EGE)

- Rare, poorly defined clinical condition affecting males more than females.
- Patients present with non-specific gastrointestinal symptoms.
- Eosinophilic infiltration of one or more segments of the gastrointestinal tract can occur and can affect all layers of the intestinal wall.
- Diagnosis is based on exclusion of other causes for intestinal eosinophilia and histological evaluation of biopsy specimens.
- Treatment of the serosal type of EGE consists typically of systemic steroids while optimal treatment for the other forms is not yet defined.

EGE can be subclassified either according to the segments of the gastrointestinal tract affected by the process or according to the depth of the eosinophilic infiltration.[47] The latter, Klein's classification system, distinguishes among mucosal, muscular, and serosal forms of EGE.[48] Parasitic infections, inflammatory bowel disease, connective tissue diseases, side effects of drugs, and lymphoproliferative malignancies must be ruled out before a diagnosis of EGE can be established.[45]

Epidemiology and natural history

EGE is predominantly a male disorder that affects children as well as adults.[45] In contrast to EoE, EGE is a very rare disease. During the 70 years since it was first described by Kaijser in 1937, the literature has reported approximately 200 cases. Despite the fact that EGE is likely a chronic disorder, its natural course is still not defined.

Clinical presentation

The clinical manifestation of EGE depends on its location within the gastrointestinal tract and on its depth of infiltration of the intestinal wall. Mucosal involvement is typically associated with vomiting, diarrhea, abdominal pain, weight loss, failure to thrive, and occult or frank bleeding.[47] Affliction of the muscular layers can lead to signs and symptoms of intestinal obstruction, whereas patients with serosal involvement typically complain of bloating and can present with ascites.[49] Peripheral blood eosinophilia is observed in approximately two-thirds of EGE patients.[47]

Diagnostic measures

The mucosal form of the disease is easier to diagnose as alterations can be visualized by endoscopy. Typical findings include thickening of the intestinal folds with deformation of the luminal configuration, diminished peristalsis, and an erythematous and friable mucosa with lesions.[50] Additionally, conventional endoscopy enables representative biopsy samples to be taken for histologic confirmation of the diagnosis.[51] Patients with suspected serosal disease should be evaluated by laparoscopy, where the findings for this form of EGE include ascites, whitish nodules, and thickening of both the parietal and visceral peritoneum.[49]

The muscular form of EGE can be detected by CT scan or conventional radiological examinations. These methods are hampered by the difficulty encountered in taking histologic samples for diagnosis confirmation. Most reported cases of muscular disease were diagnosed after surgical resection of an intestinal obstruction or suspected malignancy.

Treatment

EGE is an uncommon disease and therefore no therapeutic studies are available. In the literature, case reports and small case series have reported treatment response to a variety of agents, including corticosteroids, proton pump inhibitors, mast cell stabilizers, antihistamines, leukotriene antagonists, and surgical resection of strictured segments.[51–55]

While patients with the serosal type typically respond to steroid therapy, optimal treatment is not yet defined for other EGE forms. Based on these limited data, first a treatment trial with proton pump inhibitors should be considered with a switch to systemic corticosteroids if there is no response. Unfortunately, the relapsing nature of the disease means there is a risk of corticosteroid side effects. Leukotriene inhibitors should be evaluated in patients with frequent flare-ups.

Hypereosinophilic syndrome with gastrointestinal involvement

Definition and classification

The hypereosinophilic syndrome (HES) represents a heterogeneous group of rare disorders, characterized in the past by:

(1) Persistent peripheral blood eosinophilia with more than 1500 cells/μL blood for a period of > 6 months;
(2) No known cause of eosinophilia; and
(3) Signs and symptoms of organ involvement.[6,56,57]

Recent efforts led to reclassification of this heterogeneous group of disorders according to the recognition of several clinical subtypes and new biomarkers. Currently recognized subtypes include fip1-like1/platelet-derived growth factor receptor α (FIP1L1-PDGFRA)-associated HES, lymphocytic variant HES, chronic eosinophilic leukemia, and familial eosinophilia.[5] Independent of this subclassification, the eosinophilic infiltration can affect the cardiovascular system (90%), the peripheral and central nervous systems (90%), including the retina, the coagulation system (80%), the skin (55%), the respiratory system (50%), the liver and spleen (35%), and the gastrointestinal tract (25%).

Hypereosinophilic syndrome (HES)

- A heterogeneous group of disorders characterized by persistent peripheral blood eosinophilia > 6 months of unknown etiology.
- Affects predominantly middle-aged males.
- Eosinophilic infiltration usually involves several organ systems.
- Symptoms are dependent on the organs involved.
- Intestinal and cardiac involvement is associated with a poor prognosis.
- Treatment strategies include regimens that potentially lower the eosinophil tissue infiltration including corticosteroids, cytotoxic agents, and interferon-α, and for the PDGFRA-associated HES sub-form imatinib mesylate.

Epidemiology and natural history

HES—similar to the other idiopathic eosinophilic disorders—affects predominantly middle-aged males with a male-to-female ratio of 3:1. The onset of the disease commonly occurs between the ages of 20 to 50 years. Data about its prevalence or incidence are not available.

Clinical presentation

HES has a gradual onset with initially general symptoms, such as anorexia, fatigue, weight loss, fever, abdominal pain, and night sweats. Throughout the course of the disease, the clinical manifestations depend on the organs involved. With gastrointestinal involvement abdominal pain and diarrhea with malabsorption have been reported, but the leading sign is hepatosplenomegaly, typically evoked by eosinophilic infiltration or secondary through congestive heart failure. During its long-term course, extraintestinal manifestations or lymphoproliferative conditions may appear and facilitate the definite diagnosis. The ultimate prognosis depends on the extent of end-organ damage. Intestinal manifestations and cardiac involvement is associated with poor prognosis and risk of fatal outcome, whereas patients with skin disease generally have a milder course.[56]

Immunopathogenesis

HES encompasses several disease processes with different pathogenic mechanisms. One form is characterized by a significant elevation of the eosinophilopoetic cytokine IL-5 in the serum.[58,59] Recently, an IL-5-independent form of HES has been described in which a tyrosine kinase is overexpressed as a consequence of gene fusion.[60] Heterogeneity of underlying mechanisms leads to the common clinical manifestation of HES and despite their apparent diverse etiologies, they share the common feature of eosinophil-mediated end-organ tissue damage.

Treatment

Comparable to EGE, HES is a rare disorder and no prospective treatment studies have been carried out to date. Treatment strategies for patients with HES include regimens that potentially lower the eosinophil tissue infiltration. Corticosteroids have been used for decades in the treatment of HES and, with the exception of PDGFRA-associated HES, remains first-line therapy.[61] Cytotoxic agents, such as hydroxyurea, vincristine, and chlorambucil, have been successfully used in corticosteroid-refractory patients.[6] Interferon-α is reported to be a useful agent in patients with mucosal ulcerations.[62] Recently, imatinib mesylate, a tyrosine kinase inhibitor, has shown to be an effective drug in inducing prolonged remissions in patients with PDGFRA-associated HES.[60] Future studies will show whether monoclonal antibodies against IL-5 could prove to be a valuable approach as patients with HES often present with high levels of IL-5.[63]

Summary

- Clinical research is needed:
  - to improve diagnostic criteria
  - to implement new diagnostic tools to achieve early diagnosis
  - to improve quality of life and avoid tissue remodeling in patients with EoE
- Multicenter clinical studies are needed: to evaluate alternative treatment strategies (biologics, immunosuppressants) for steroid-refractory EoE
- Translational research will help:
  - To identify cellular and molecular factors involved in fibrosis of the esophageal wall
  - To understand molecular mechanisms of tissue remodeling

It is clear that much remains to be learned about diagnosing and treating patients suffering from one of the three EGIDs.

EoE is a common disease but difficult to diagnose due to its confusing endoscopic features. Patients, usually males, present with recurrent dysphagia and food impaction as well as coexisting allergic airway diseases. Untreated EoE can induce relevant structural changes of the esophagus, finally leading to an extremely fragile and rigid esophageal wall structure with increased risk for complications, including perforation. Effective treatments for adult patients with EoE include systemic or topical corticosteroids, hypoallergenic diets, and esophageal dilation. Although the quality of life is substantially diminished in this chronic disorder, life expectancy is not affected.

EGE, a rare disorder that predominantly affects males, can involve the entire gastrointestinal tract or be restricted to isolated segments and affect the mucosal, muscular, and serosal layers of the intestinal wall. Clinical manifestation depends on location and depth of the infiltration. Mucosal involvement, the most frequent subtype, is typically associated with vomiting, diarrhea, abdominal pain, and weight loss. The muscular form can mimic intestinal obstruction or acute abdomen. Patients with the serosal form complain mainly of bloating and ascites, and usually respond dramatically to corticosteroids.

The HES is a heterogeneous group of rare disorders, characterized by persistent peripheral blood eosinophilia with more than 1500 cells/μL for longer than 6 months, no known cause of eosinophilia, and signs and symptoms of organ involvement. Prognosis depends on the degree and location of the eosinophil-mediated end-organ tissue damage.

References

1. Rothenberg ME. Eosinophilia. N Engl J Med 1998;338:1592–600.
2. Kato M, Kephart GM, Talley NJ, et al. Eosinophil infiltration and degranulation in normal human tissue. Anat Rec 1998;252:418–25.
3. Lowichik A, Weinberg AG. A quantitative evaluation of mucosal eosinophils in the pediatric gastrointestinal tract. Mod Pathol 1996;9:110–4.
4. Straumann A, Spichtin HP, Grize L, et al. Natural history of primary eosinophilic esophagitis: a follow-up of 30 adult patients for up to 11.5 years. Gastroenterology 2003;125:1660–9.
5. Klion AD, Bochner BS, Gleich GJ, et al. Approaches to the treatment of hypereosinophilic syndromes: a workshop summary report. J Allergy Clin Immunol 2006;117:1292–302.
6. Weller PF, Bubley GJ. The idiopathic hypereosinophilic syndrome. Blood 1994;83:2759–79.
7. Liacouras CA, Furuta GT, Hirano I, et al. Eosinophilic esophagitis: Updated consensus recommendations for children and adults. J Allergy Clin Immunol 2011;128:3–20.
8. Croese J, Fairley SK, Masson JW, et al. Clinical and endoscopic features of eosinophilic esophagitis in adults. Gastrointest Endosc 2003;58:516–22.
9. Kapel RC, Miller JK, Torres C, et al. Eosinophilic esophagitis: a prevalent disease in the United States that affects all age groups. Gastroenterology 2008;134:1316–21.
10. Mackenzie SH, Go M, Chadwick B, et al. Eosinophilic oesophagitis in patients presenting with dysphagia—a prospective analysis. Aliment Pharmacol Ther 2008;28:1140–6.
11. Prasad GA, Alexander JA, Schleck CD, et al. Epidemiology of eosinophilic esophagitis over three decades in Olmsted County, Minnesota. Clin Gastroenterol Hepatol 2009;7:1055–61.
12. Straumann A, Simon HU. Eosinophilic esophagitis: escalating epidemiology? J Allergy Clin Immunol 2005;115:418–9.
13. Veerappan GR, Perry JL, Duncan TJ, et al. Prevalence of eosinophilic esophagitis in an adult population undergoing upper endoscopy: a prospective study. Clin Gastroenterol Hepatol 2009;7:420–6, 426 e421–422.
14. Muller S, Puhl S, Vieth M, et al. Analysis of symptoms and endoscopic findings in 117 patients with histological diagnoses of eosinophilic esophagitis. Endoscopy 2007;39:339–44.
15. Ronkainen J, Talley NJ, Aro P, et al. Prevalence of oesophageal eosinophils and eosinophilic oesophagitis in adults: the population-based Kalixanda study. Gut 2007;56:615–20.
16. Ahmad M, Soetikno RM, Ahmed A. The differential diagnosis of eosinophilic esophagitis. J Clin Gastroenterol 2000;30:242–4.
17. Foster PS, Hogan SP, Ramsay AJ, et al. Interleukin 5 deficiency abolishes eosinophilia, airways hyperreactivity, and lung damage in a mouse asthma model. J Exp Med 1996;183:195–201.
18. Schnyder B, Lugli S, Feng N, et al. Interleukin-4 (IL-4) and IL-13 bind to a shared heterodimeric complex on endothelial cells mediating vascular cell adhesion molecule-1 induction in the absence of the common gamma chain. Blood 1996;87:4286–95.
19. Elsner J, Kapp A. Activation of human eosinophils by chemokines. Chem Immunol 2000;76:177–207.
20. Arora AS, Yamazaki K. Eosinophilic esophagitis: asthma of the esophagus? Clin Gastroenterol Hepatol 2004;2:523–30.
21. Rothenberg ME, Mishra A, Collins MH, et al. Pathogenesis and clinical features of eosinophilic esophagitis. J Allergy Clin Immunol 2001;108:891–4.
22. Spergel JM, Beausoleil JL, Mascarenhas M, et al. The use of skin prick tests and patch tests to identify causative foods in eosinophilic esophagitis. J Allergy Clin Immunol 2002;109:363–8.
23. Kagalwalla AF, Sentongo TA, Ritz S, et al. Effect of six-food elimination diet on clinical and histologic outcomes in eosinophilic esophagitis. Clin Gastroenterol Hepatol 2006;4:1097–102.
24. Kelly KJ, Lazenby AJ, Rowe PC, et al. Eosinophilic esophagitis attributed to gastroesophageal reflux: improvement with an amino acid-based formula. Gastroenterology 1995;109:1503–12.
25. Orenstein SR, Shalaby TM, Di Lorenzo C, et al. The spectrum of pediatric eosinophilic esophagitis beyond infancy: a clinical series of 30 children. Am J Gastroenterol 2000;95:1422–30.
26. Simon D, Straumann A, Wenk A, et al. Eosinophilic esophagitis in adults—no clinical relevance of wheat and rye sensitizations. Allergy 2006;61:1480–3.
27. Foroughi S, Foster B, Kim N, et al. Anti-IgE treatment of eosinophil-associated gastrointestinal disorders. J Allergy Clin Immunol 2007;120:594–601.
28. Straumann A, Bauer M, Fischer B, et al. Idiopathic eosinophilic esophagitis is associated with a T(H)2-type allergic inflammatory response. J Allergy Clin Immunol 2001;108:954–61.
29. Blanchard C, Mishra A, Saito-Akei H, et al. Inhibition of human interleukin-13-induced respiratory and oesophageal inflammation by anti-human-interleukin-13 antibody (CAT-354). Clin Exp Allergy 2005;35:1096–103.
30. Mishra A, Hogan SP, Brandt EB, et al. IL-5 promotes eosinophil trafficking to the esophagus. J Immunol 2002;168:2464–9.
31. Mishra A, Rothenberg ME. Intratracheal IL-13 induces eosinophilic esophagitis by an IL-5, eotaxin-1, and STAT6-dependent mechanism. Gastroenterology 2003;125:1419–27.
32. Blanchard C, Mingler MK, Vicario M, et al. IL-13 involvement in eosinophilic esophagitis: transcriptome analysis and reversibility with glucocorticoids. J Allergy Clin Immunol 2007;120:1292–300.
33. Blanchard C, Stucke EM, Rodriguez-Jimenez B, et al. A striking local esophageal cytokine expression profile in eosinophilic esophagitis. J Allergy Clin Immunol 2011;127:208–17, 217 e201–207.
34. Blanchard C, Wang N, Stringer KF, et al. Eotaxin-3 and a uniquely conserved gene-expression profile in eosinophilic esophagitis. J Clin Invest 2006;116:536–47.
35. Aceves SS, Newbury RO, Dohil R, et al. Esophageal remodeling in pediatric eosinophilic esophagitis. J Allergy Clin Immunol 2007;119:206–12.
36. Mishra A, Wang M, Pemmaraju VR, et al. Esophageal remodeling develops as a consequence of tissue specific IL-5-induced eosinophilia. Gastroenterology 2008;134:204–14.
37. Aceves SS, Chen D, Newbury RO, et al. Mast cells infiltrate the esophageal smooth muscle in patients with eosinophilic esophagitis, express TGF-beta1, and increase esophageal smooth muscle contraction. J Allergy Clin Immunol 2010;126:1198–204, e1194.
38. Straumann A, Conus S, Degen L, et al. Budesonide is effective in adolescent and adult patients with active eosinophilic esophagitis. Gastroenterology 2010;139:1526–37, 1537 e1521.
39. Schaefer ET, Fitzgerald JF, Molleston JP, et al. Comparison of oral prednisone and topical fluticasone in the treatment of eosinophilic esophagitis: a randomized trial in children. Clin Gastroenterol Hepatol 2008;6:165–73.
40. Attwood SE, Lewis CJ, Bronder CS, et al. Eosinophilic oesophagitis: a novel treatment using Montelukast. Gut 2003;52:181–5.
41. Straumann A, Conus S, Grzonka P, et al. Anti-interleukin-5 antibody treatment (mepolizumab) in active eosinophilic oesophagitis: a randomised, placebo-controlled, double-blind trial. Gut 2010;59:21–30.
42. Netzer P, Gschossmann JM, Straumann A, et al. Corticosteroid-dependent eosinophilic oesophagitis: azathioprine and 6-mercaptopurine can induce and maintain long-term remission. Eur J Gastroenterol Hepatol 2007;19:865–9.
43. Markowitz JE, Spergel JM, Ruchelli E, et al. Elemental diet is an effective treatment for eosinophilic esophagitis in children and adolescents. Am J Gastroenterol 2003;98:777–82.
44. Schoepfer AM, Gonsalves N, Bussmann C, et al. Esophageal dilation in eosinophilic esophagitis: effectiveness, safety, and impact on the underlying inflammation. Am J Gastroenterol 2010;105:1062–70.
45. Khan S, Orenstein SR. Eosinophilic gastroenteritis: epidemiology, diagnosis and management. Paediatr Drugs 2002;4:563–70.
46. Cello JP. Eosinophilic gastroenteritis—a complex disease entity. Am J Med 1979;67:1097–104.
47. Talley NJ, Shorter RG, Phillips SF, et al. Eosinophilic gastroenteritis: a clinicopathological study of patients with disease of the mucosa, muscle layer, and subserosal tissues. Gut 1990;31:54–8.
48. Klein NC, Hargrove RL, Sleisenger MH, et al. Eosinophilic gastroenteritis. Medicine (Baltimore) 1970;49:299–319.
49. Solis-Herruzo JA, de Cuenca B, Munoz-Yague MT. Laparoscopic findings in serosal eosinophilic gastroenteritis. Report of two cases. Endoscopy 1988;20:152–3.
50. Navab F, Kleinman MS, Algazy K, et al. Endoscopic diagnosis of eosinophilic gastritis. Gastrointest Endosc 1972;19:67–9.
51. Colon AR, Sorkin LF, Stern WR, et al. Eosinophilic gastroenteritis. J Pediatr Gastroenterol Nutr 1983;2:187–9.
52. Di Gioacchino M, Pizzicannella G, Fini N, et al. Sodium cromoglycate in the treatment of eosinophilic gastroenteritis. Allergy 1990;45:161–6.
53. Katz AJ, Goldman H, Grand RJ. Gastric mucosal biopsy in eosinophilic (allergic) gastroenteritis. Gastroenterology 1977;73:705–9.
54. Melamed I, Feanny SJ, Sherman PM, et al. Benefit of ketotifen in patients with eosinophilic gastroenteritis. Am J Med 1991;90:310–4.
55. Neustrom MR, Friesen C. Treatment of eosinophilic gastroenteritis with montelukast. J Allergy Clin Immunol 1999;104:506.
56. Chusid MJ, Dale DC, West BC, et al. The hypereosinophilic syndrome: analysis of fourteen cases with review of the literature. Medicine (Baltimore) 1975;54:1–27.
57. Hardy WR, Anderson RE. The hypereosinophilic syndromes. Ann Intern Med 1968;68:1220–9.
58. Owen WF, Rothenberg ME, Petersen J, et al. Interleukin 5 and phenotypically altered eosinophils in the blood of patients with the idiopathic hypereosinophilic syndrome. J Exp Med 1989;170:343–8.
59. Simon HU, Rothenberg ME, Bochner BS, et al. Refining the definition of hypereosinophilic syndrome. J Allergy Clin Immunol 2010;126:45–9.
60. Cools J, DeAngelo DJ, Gotlib J, et al. A tyrosine kinase created by fusion of the PDGFRA and FIP1L1 genes as a therapeutic target of imatinib in idiopathic hypereosinophilic syndrome. N Engl J Med 2003;348:1201–14.
61. Fauci AS, Harley JB, Roberts WC, et al. NIH conference. The idiopathic hypereosinophilic syndrome. Clinical, pathophysiologic, and therapeutic considerations. Ann Intern Med 1982;97:78–92.
62. Butterfield JH, Gleich GJ. Response of six patients with idiopathic hypereosinophilic syndrome to interferon alfa. J Allergy Clin Immunol 1994;94:1318–26.
63. Plotz SG, Simon HU, Darsow U, et al. Use of an anti-interleukin-5 antibody in the hypereosinophilic syndrome with eosinophilic dermatitis. N Engl J Med 2003;349:2334–9.

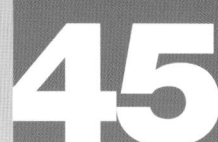

Virginia L. Calder,
Melanie
Hingorani, Sue L.
Lightman

Allergic disorders of the eye

Allergic disorders of the eye range from the common, milder conditions of seasonal allergic conjunctivitis (SAC) and perennial allergic conjunctivitis (PAC), to the less common but clinically more severe diseases, vernal keratoconjunctivitis (VKC) and atopic keratoconjunctivitis (AKC). The ocular allergic responses in SAC and PAC are confined to the conjunctival tissues, while the cornea can also be affected in VKC and AKC, leading to impaired vision. Much research has been conducted over the past few years to identify the inflammatory cells and molecules involved in allergic responses at the ocular surface, and their role in the pathogenesis of allergic eye diseases. Differential expression profiles of key cell adhesion molecules, cytokines, and cell types have been identified in each form of conjunctivitis, and various experimental models are being used to investigate the different immunopathogenic mechanisms.

KEY CONCEPTS

Predominating cell types in the conjunctival tissues

- In SAC, PAC mast cells predominate.
- In VKC, eosinophils, T cells, neutrophils, mast cells predominate.
- In AKC, T cells, eosinophils, neutrophils predominate.

Seasonal allergic conjunctivitis

Ocular allergy is the commonest ocular disorder seen in primary care, most with seasonal allergic conjunctivitis. SAC is a recurrent conjunctivitis manifesting only during the relevant pollen season with the timing of symptoms (spring, summer, or autumn) dependent on which particular pollen or pollens (e.g., tree, grass) are allergenic for that individual. SAC can occur at any age but is more frequently seen in children and young adults and tends to lessen in severity with increasing age.

Patients present with seasonally recurring itching, watering, redness, and swelling of the eyes and lids and there may be increased discharge. Rhinitis is commonly present and there is often a personal or family history of atopy. During the allergen season, the ocular signs range from mild to dramatic and are usually bilateral and symmetrical. Edema of the lids and conjunctiva may be mild and often outweighs the degree of hyperemia, giving a milky or pink appearance to the eye, but the swelling may be gross, with inability to open the lids and a ballooning out of the conjunctiva (chemosis), particularly after exposure to high allergen concentrations or after rubbing of the eye. Eversion of the lids to reveal the tarsal conjunctiva demonstrates some hyperemia and mild infiltration (loss of transparency and thickening) of the conjunctiva with diffuse small inflammatory excrescences known as papillae. Since there is no serious limbal disease or conjunctival scarring, and the cornea is not involved, visual acuity remains normal. Outside the pollen season there is nothing to find on eye examination.

Conjunctival immunostaining in SAC

SAC involves an immediate hypersensitivity response and mast cells are the main infiltrating cells in the conjunctiva (Fig. 45.1), with some neutrophils and eosinophils in less than half of symptomatic SAC patients but minimal T-cell influx.[1] Mast cells and their products (histamine, proteases, leukotrienes, chemokines, cytokines) primarily orchestrate the inflammatory response in SAC, although neutrophils and eosinophils are also able to secrete a wide range of pro-inflammatory mediators that could augment the inflammation. Immunohistochemical studies of tarsal and bulbar conjunctival biopsy specimens demonstrated increased expression of intercellular adhesion molecule-1 (ICAM-1) and E-selectin adhesion molecules in SAC in comparison with controls, but only in-season,[2] and levels returned to baseline outside the pollen season. This pattern of expression correlated with the degree of neutrophil or eosinophil infiltration in the bulbar tissue, suggesting a mast cell-mediated cell recruitment process.

Therapy

General measures can provide effective relief, particularly where the disease is not severe. Minimizing pollen exposure by avoiding grassy fields or rural areas, keeping windows shut, and remaining indoors, especially on high-pollen count days, is common sense. Cold compresses and ocular lubricants (artificial tears) relieve symptoms, particularly itching.

CLINICAL PEARLS

SAC

- Seasonal response to allergen (e.g., pollen)
- Mast cell-mediated.
- Antihistamines, mast cell inhibitors.

H1 antihistamine drugs, both oral and topical, provide rapid symptom reduction but are not preventative and have limited potency as they only address one part of the inflammatory mediator response. Oral antihistamines also treat any rhinitis, but the onset of ocular action is slower and the local effective concentration is less than for topical therapy, and they expose the

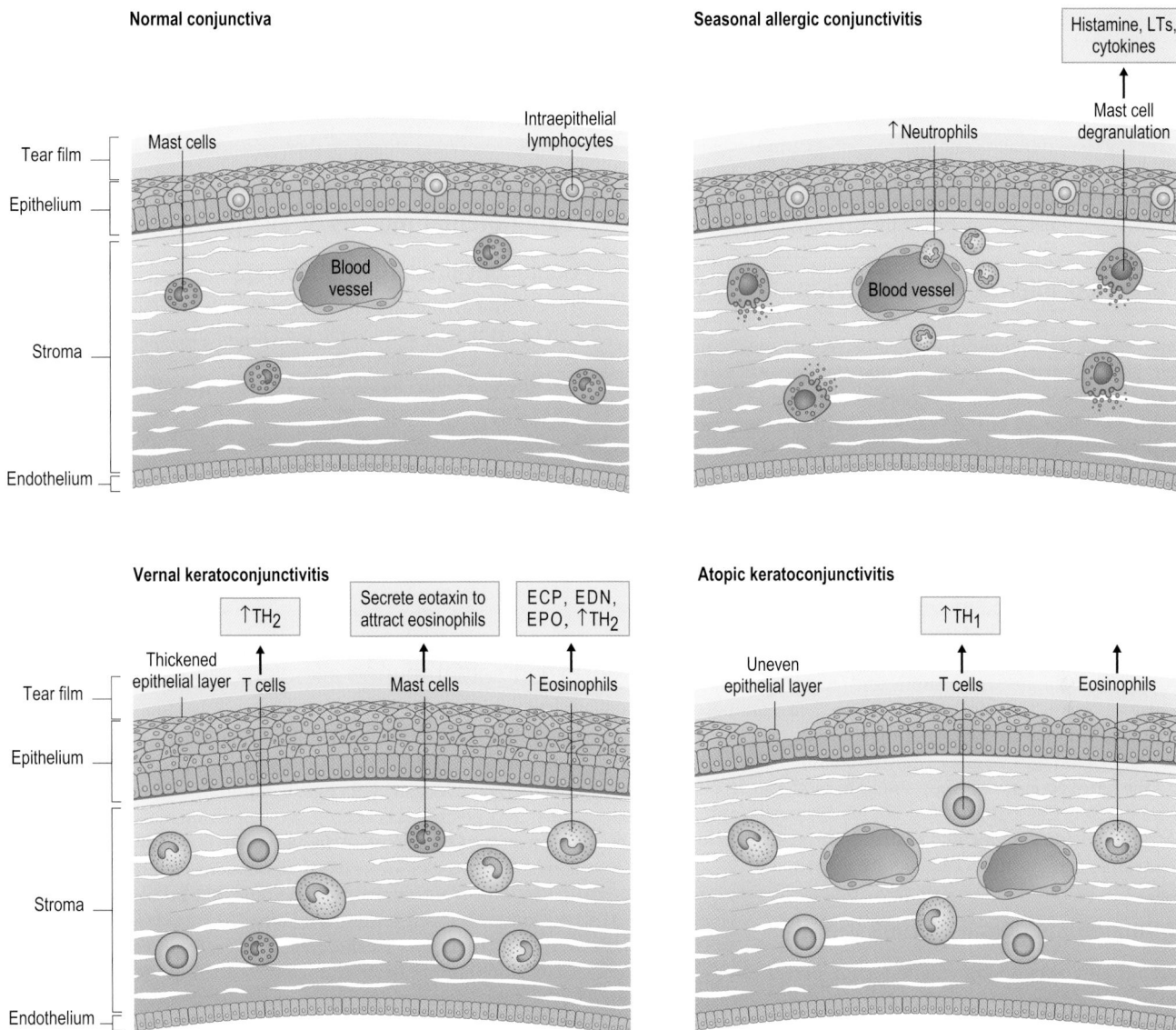

Fig. 45.1 A cross-section of conjunctival tissue biopsy, showing the cell processes involved in normal vs SAC vs VKC vs AKC affected tissues. ECP, eosinophil cationic protein; EPO, eosinophil peroxidase; EDN, eosinophil-derived neurotoxin.

patient to the risk of systemic unwanted effects. They are often used for children where drop use can be difficult and at night when any sedative effect can be advantageous. Topical antihistamines are available as lower potency in combination with a vasoconstrictor (where there is a synergistic action between the two components, e.g., antazoline-naphazoline) or as higher potency antihistamine-only preparations (e.g., levocabastine, emedastine, azelastine). The higher potency preparations provide a more rapid onset of symptom relief, have a more prolonged action after drop instillation, and avoid the problems of rebound vasodilatation and potential permanent dilatation of the conjunctival vessels that can occur with long-term vasoconstrictor use. Topical antihistamine drops, particularly in combination with vasoconstrictors, are a recognized cause of contact allergic conjunctivitis, which may limit their use in a number of patients.

Of the several topical non-steroidal anti-inflammatory drugs (NSAIDs) assessed in ocular allergy, ketorolac is the only one approved for ocular allergy. NSAIDs offer the advantage of safety, but there have been concerns that the efficacy is not well proven against other established remedies, and cost concerns. The use of NSAIDs is more common outside the UK, but has not gained widespread acceptance among UK ophthalmologists.

Topical mast cell inhibitors, the prototype being sodium cromoglycate, are the most useful drugs for non-sight-threatening ocular allergy. They have a number of actions (inhibition of other leukocytes, direct mediator antagonism) in addition to inhibiting one of the earliest mechanisms of the acute ocular allergic response (mast cell degranulation), which accounts for their potency and their ability to offer a preventative action if used early, and continued throughout, the allergen season. One limitation is the slower onset of symptom relief compared with antihistamines, although this is less of an issue with the newer, high potency preparations (lodoxamide, nedocromil), and some tendency to stinging after instillation (possibly less with lodoxamide). They are almost completely safe, though very occasionally can cause a local contact allergy.

Several of the newer topical antihistamines claim adjunctive mast cell inhibition and other mediator antagonism, in particular olopatadine, epinastine, and ketotifen. They offer the potential advantage of a rapid onset of action with the preventive and long-term effect of inhibiting mast cell mediator release.[3] Olopatadine and epinastine, in particular, seem to offer some clinical advantage over other antihistamines and compare well with mast cell inhibitors in allergen challenge models and, in some studies, in SAC.[4]

Topical steroids have a minimal role in SAC, due to their potential for ocular adverse effects (see below). They are occasionally used in short courses for severe disease to gain control of inflammation but their use must be supervised by an ophthalmologist.

Perennial allergic conjunctivitis

Perennial allergic conjunctivitis is the second most common ocular allergy.[5] It bears many similarities to SAC but the time course is different as the allergens responsible for PAC are present for most or all of the year and therefore the disease is not seasonal. Like SAC, PAC is most frequent and severe in children and young adults. House dust mite (*Dermatophagoides pteronyssinus*) is the most common sensitizing allergen but animal hair and dander, molds and other antigens may be responsible.

The symptoms are perennial ocular itch, discomfort, watering, redness, and some discharge. Patients may be able to correlate symptomatology with exposure to, for example, pets or a particular location. House dust mite allergy sufferers give a history of symptoms worse in the morning. Approximately one-third have an associated rhinitis, and a family and/or personal atopic history is very common. The clinical appearance is of a mild conjunctival inflammation and clinical signs may be very slight. The bulbar conjunctiva (on the eye globe) may be slightly red and edematous and the tarsal conjunctiva shows mild to moderate hyperemia, infiltration, and fine papillae. Lid edema is usually mild. As with SAC, there is no conjunctival scarring, corneal, or serious limbal involvement, so normal visual acuity is maintained.

Immunohistological studies in PAC

PAC also involves an immediate-type hypersensitivity response but, since the allergens are present continuously, the resultant inflammation is more chronic. Therefore the immunopathology may differ somewhat from that of SAC. Increased numbers of mast cells are detected in both tarsal conjunctival epithelium and in the substantia propria, with both mucosal and connective tissue type mast cell phenotypes.[2] Apart from mast cells, eosinophils, neutrophils, and some T cells are present, suggesting other cell-mediated processes are likely to be involved although it is not yet known whether these cells contribute to the chronic inflammation in PAC. In general, little is known about the basic immunological processes occurring within the conjunctival tissues in PAC and further research is needed.

Therapy

In house dust mite sensitivity, advice should be provided on mite reduction and allergy support groups can be helpful for this and in accessing equipment. Potential mite reduction maneuvers include removal of soft furnishings (e.g., carpet, curtains) in the bedroom, use of special vacuum cleaners, intensive and regular vacuuming including the curtains and mattress, mite-impermeable mattress and pillow covers, washing bedlinen and curtains at mitocidal temperatures (>55°C), and mitocidal chemicals. For mold sensitivity, the use of dehumidifying devices and mold-killing chemicals may help.

The drug treatment of PAC is essentially the same as for SAC (see above), but since the disease is usually prolonged, the continuing use of mast cell inhibitors assumes more importance and antihistamines tend to be used episodically for flare-ups of inflammation. Another consideration when using topical medication is the potential development of an ocular response to the preservatives, either an allergic response or damage to the ocular surface, so preservative-free therapy should be used if possible.

Experimental models of allergic conjunctivitis

Conjunctival allergen challenge

This model involves challenging the ocular surface with an allergen to artificially induce the ocular allergic response in sensitized individuals.[6] Symptoms are similar to those seen in SAC and therefore the model is useful for investigating the early and late phase allergic responses at the ocular surface. During the early phase (20 minutes) increased levels of histamine and tryptase can be detected in tears, suggesting the infiltrating cell population is predominantly mast cells. At 6 hours histamine and eosinophil cationic protein levels are increased, but not tryptase, suggesting that basophils and eosinophils infiltrate during the late phase.[7] T cells are also increased but only in bulbar biopsy specimens. The allergen challenge model is often used for testing the efficacy of eye drops.

Experimental murine allergic conjunctivitis

A mouse model of allergic conjunctivitis has been established,[8] in genetically susceptible hosts, by an initial footpad sensitization with short ragweed pollen followed, 7–10 days later, by conjunctival allergen challenge. Infiltration of mast cells, neutrophils, and eosinophils occurs, as well as increased conjunctival chemosis and lid edema. Although there is no significant infiltration of T cells, the model is IFN-γ-dependent since it could be inhibited by anti-IFN-γ antibody and could not be induced in IFN-γ knockout mice,[9] supporting a role for Th1 cytokines in this model. Furthermore, in γ/δ T-cell-deficient mice, there was significantly less eosinophilic infiltration and reduced Th2 cytokine production, suggesting a role for γ/δ T cells in allergic conjunctivitis.[10] A role for thymic stromal lymphopoietin (TSLP) has also been demonstrated in this model, with TSLP expression upregulated in allergen-challenged corneal and conjunctival epithelium and TSLP-containing conditioned medium from stimulated corneal epithelial cultures induced maturation of dendritic cells *in vitro*.[11]

Vernal keratoconjunctivitis

Vernal keratoconjunctivitis is a serious ocular allergy of childhood. It makes up 0.1 to 0.5% of ocular disease in the developed world but is more common and much more severe in hot dry countries, especially the Middle East, West Africa, and the Mediterranean. In the United Kingdom, VKC is an unusual, self-limiting, often seasonal ocular allergy that affects children and young adults, males (85%) in particular, many of whom have a personal or family history of atopy. The link with atopy and seasonality is less clearly defined in less temperate climates.

The symptoms are worse in the spring and summer but last all year in severe cases. Patients complain of marked itching, discomfort or pain, photophobia, stringy discharge, blurred vision, and difficulty opening their eyes in the morning. The ocular signs may be very asymmetrical. Conjunctival signs are maximal in the superior tarsal conjunctiva and limbus and the heavily inflamed lid may droop (ptosis). The conjunctival surfaces are hyperemic, edematous, and infiltrated, and a stringy mucoid discharge is present. The tarsal conjunctiva is densely infiltrated, with papillae that are often large (>1 mm in diameter, also known as cobblestone papillae). The limbus may show discrete swellings or, less often, diffuse hyperemia and infiltration; the presence of small white chalky deposits (Trantas' dots) is typical of vernal limbitis. In the later stages, fine reticular white scarring may be seen, but this does not lead to significant shrinkage and distortion of the ocular surface such as occurs in some cicatrizing conjunctival diseases (e.g., AKC, see below).

Visual acuity can be affected by involvement of the cornea (keratopathy), which is most marked in the upper third of the cornea: this is due to greater exposure to toxic inflammatory mediators, rather than mechanical rubbing by the papillae. At its mildest, there is a punctate disturbance of the epithelium that may coalesce to form a discrete epithelial defect (macroerosion). Deposition of mucus, fibrin, and inflammatory debris can then result in the formation of a shallow oval plaque (or shield) ulcer, which repels the hydrophilic tears and the epithelial healing response (Fig. 45.2A). Herpetic and bacterial corneal infection may occur. In the later stages, corneal scarring can lead to permanent visual reduction. Steroid treatment-related complications and sensory-deprivation amblyopia (because of the young age group) also contribute to the potential for long-term visual loss.

Immunological studies in VKC

Several studies have found that cells of both the innate and adaptive immune responses are activated during VKC. T lymphocytes and eosinophils predominate, with mast cells, neutrophils, and other activated cell types infiltrating the conjunctival epithelium and stroma (see Fig. 45.1). Increased numbers of activated CD4 T cells are found in tarsal conjunctival tissue, mainly in the subepithelial layer, and there is increased HLA-DR expression compared to normal subjects.[12] Increased numbers of Langerhans' cells and activated macrophages (CD68[+]) were also found. Cloned T cells,[13] derived from VKC conjunctival tissues, have been functionally characterized as Th2-type, while *in situ* hybridization staining demonstrated upregulation of interleukin-3 (IL-3), -4, and −5 mRNAs in areas of maximum T-cell infiltration in VKC, further supporting Th2 cell involvement (Chapter 16).[14] VKC tear samples have increased levels of IL-4, IL-10, IFN-γ, eotaxin, and tumor necrosis factor-α (TNF-α) compared to controls.[15] Increased expression of RANTES, eotaxin, monocyte chemotactic protein (MCP)-1 and MCP-3 has been detected in conjunctival biopsy specimens from VKC patients,[16] reflecting the range of inflammatory cells present. Conjunctival expression of the chemokine receptor CXCR3 was found to be specifically localized to T cells.[17]

Management of VKC

The treatment goals of VKC are to achieve adequate symptom control and to prevent both disease and iatrogenic complications that might permanently reduce visual acuity, bearing in mind that the disease is likely to remit spontaneously before adulthood. In cases where there appears to be pollen sensitivity, advice on pollen avoidance should be given similar to that for SAC (see above). Simple measures including cold compresses, ocular lubricants, and mucolytic drops may help. Antihistamines have a very limited role in the disease. Immunotherapy is not helpful.

Mast cell inhibitors are effective in VKC and should be maintained throughout the period of active inflammation, two to four times daily, depending on the severity of disease and which preparation is used. Lodoxamide and nedocromil can offer slight extra potency in clinical control. Patients with mild disease may be able to discontinue therapy during the winter months. It is important to emphasize to patients and parents that mast cell inhibitors are safe and must be continued when using steroids to minimize the dose of steroids required, and therefore the risk of steroid complications. Whether agents such as olopatadine are useful in VKC is not yet established.

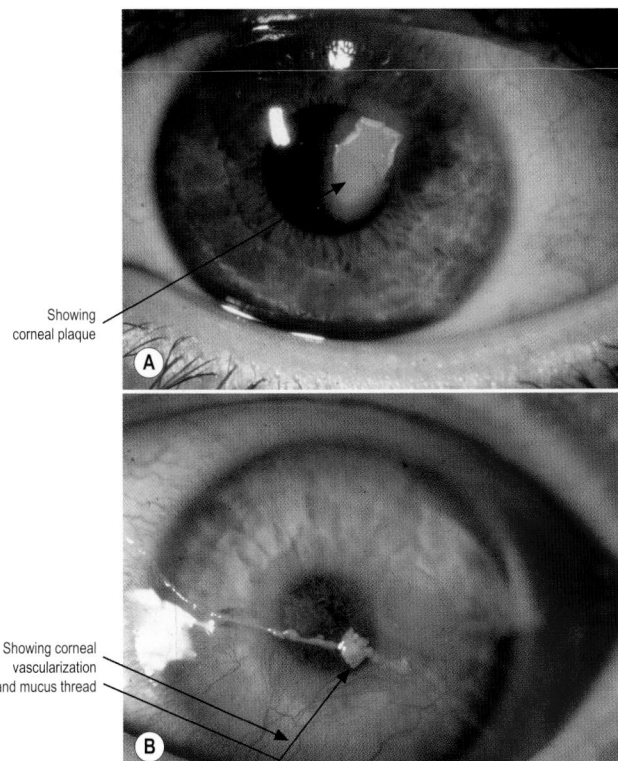

Showing corneal plaque

(A)

Showing corneal vascularization and mucus thread

(B)

Fig. 45.2 Two clinical pictures showing features of (A) VKC, corneal plaque formation, formation of giant papillae and (B) AKC, mucus thread, corneal vascularization.

> ### ● CLINICAL PEARLS
>
> **VKC**
>
> - A chronic conjunctival inflammation with seasonal exacerbations
> - Eosinophils and Th2 T cells infiltrate the conjunctival tissues
> - Usually affects young males
> - Cornea can be affected
> - Increased expression of Th2 cytokines, adhesion molecules, eotaxin
> - Often requires steroids and topical cyclosporine

Steroids are highly potent controllers of multiple features of allergic inflammation and are frequently required in VKC. Unfortunately they carry a significant risk of ocular adverse effects, including ocular hypertension, glaucoma, and cataract, and they worsen infective keratitis. This is a particular concern in children, where examination to detect these complications can be difficult (e.g., tonometry for intraocular pressure) and where iatrogenic adverse effects can have long-term visual consequences beyond the time when the disease has spontaneously regressed. To minimize the risk of adverse effects, other therapies should be used (especially mast cell inhibitors, but also cyclosporine) and steroids can be prescribed in short, sharp, rapidly tapering doses during episodes of high disease activity or significant keratopathy. In addition, the use of surface-acting preparations with a reduced intraocular action is advisable (e.g., fluoromethalone, rimexolone), although these are not available in the preservative-free formulations that may be required for high-frequency use. Systemic steroids are also sometimes utilized but expose the patient to numerous potential adverse effects. Supratarsal injections of steroids, either long-acting (triamcinolone) or short-acting (e.g., dexamethasone), can also be used to great effect but these are not surface-acting agents and therefore carry significant risks of local side effects; unlike drops, neither the treatment effect nor any adverse effects can be suddenly stopped if problems arise.

Cyclosporine is a specific T-cell inhibitor that has a number of other inhibitory effects (e.g., on eosinophils, mast cells) that are likely to contribute to its effectiveness in ocular allergic disease. Topical cyclosporine 2% dissolved in oil (usually maize) has been used to great effect in VKC.[18] and is particularly effective in treating corneal complications and as a steroid sparing agent. It has no systemic adverse effects and none of the serious ocular complications of steroids, so it can generally be used safely long term. It may cause temporary lid-skin and corneal-surface irritation that resolve on drug cessation. However, there are some difficulties with its use. It can produce intense post-instillation stinging, which can prevent ocular opening for some time, and the oil base can cause symptomatic visual smearing that may persist for some hours and be sufficiently severe to limit driving. Moreover, the eyedrop preparation is not available commercially at this concentration and needs to be obtained from one of the very few individual hospital pharmacies that make it on-site, in a labor- and time-intensive process. The commercially available and well-tolerated 0.05% cyclosporine emulsion, marketed for dry eye, has unfortunately not proven effective in VKC, although it can be useful in AKC (see below).[19] Some units have obtained the unlicensed 0.2% veterinary ointment on a named-patient basis and claim benefit.

Surgical interventions are sometimes required in VKC for the corneal manifestations: surgical or excimer laser superficial keratectomy can be used in conjunction with drug treatments for plaque ulcer; rarely corneal grafting may be required for scarring. Surgical removal of giant papillae or conjunctival reconstruction is not generally recommended.

Experimental model of VKC

In genetically susceptible rats and mice, an immune-mediated blepharo-conjunctivitis is inducible by subcutaneous immunization with short ragweed pollen followed by conjunctival allergen challenge at day 10. In this model a significant eosinophilia is found 24 hours after challenge and this model has therefore been used to study eosinophil infiltration in VKC. It can also be induced by adoptively transferring Th2, but not Th1, T cells, demonstrating that eosinophil infiltration is Th2-mediated.[20] Similarly, transfer of antigen-specific IgE is less potent at inducing conjunctival eosinophil infiltration than transfer of antigen-primed splenocytes.[21] Modulation of co-stimulatory molecules (4-1BB) significantly affected conjunctival eosinophil infiltration, suggesting a possible mode of therapy for VKC.[22]

Atopic keratoconjunctivitis

Atopic keratoconjunctivitis is the least common but most serious of the ocular allergies. AKC is a life-long condition that affects adults who have systemic atopic disease, particularly atopic dermatitis. The usual onset is in the late teens, but unlike VKC the disease is persistent and can be relentlessly progressive; occasionally the disease begins in childhood. AKC is a highly symptomatic disorder with severe itching, pain, watering, stickiness, and redness of the eyelids and eye.[23]

CLINICAL PEARLS

AKC

- The most severe form of allergic eye disease
- Affecting adults with atopic dermatitis or asthma
- Predominant infiltration of T cells expressing IFN-γ in severe cases
- Cornea can be affected, often due to secondary infections
- Requires steroids and cyclosporine

There is usually facial atopic dermatitis involving the eyelids. The lid margins show severe blepharitis (chronic inflammation of the lash follicles and meibomian glands) and are thickened and hyperemic, posteriorly rounded, sometimes keratinized, and the lid anatomy may be distorted with ectropion (outwardly turning eyelid), entropion (inwardly turning eyelid), trichiasis (inturning lashes), loss of lashes, and notching. The whole conjunctiva is affected and shows intense infiltration, papillae (that may be giant), and sometimes scarring with linear and reticular white scar tissue, lid to conjunctiva adhesions (symblepharon) and shrinkage or loss of the conjunctival sac and secondary lid distortions. Marked limbal inflammation may develop and Trantas' dots can occur. The disease may never affect the cornea, in which case it is sometimes referred to as atopic blepharoconjunctivitis (ABC); in this situation, the overall inflammation is generally less severe.

The cornea may be affected directly during inflammation or may be damaged secondarily following extensive changes to the protective ocular surface by continual mechanical trauma, reduced lid protection, or severe loss of conjunctival tear production. Significant visual acuity reduction occurs due to corneal involvement in 40 to 70% of cases. Keratopathy may consist of punctate and macroscopic epithelial defects, filamentary keratitis, plaque ulcer, progressive scarring, neovascularization (with or without lipid deposition), thinning, and secondary corneal infections (herpetic, bacterial, and fungal) (Fig. 45.2B). Associations between AKC and eye rubbing, keratoconus, atopic cataract, and retinal detachment are recognized.

Immunological studies in AKC

In AKC the predominant cell types that infiltrate the conjunctival tissues are T cells, eosinophils, and neutrophils (Fig. 45.1). As in VKC, increased numbers of activated CD4+ T cells, HLA-DR expression, and cells of the monocyte/macrophage lineage are found in conjunctival biopsy specimens in AKC.[12] as well as mRNA expression of IL-3, -4, and -5 in the stroma. However, in AKC, there is a significant increase in the expression of IL-2 mRNA, and in numbers of IFN-γ expressing T cells, suggesting a Th1-mediated inflammation in this severest ocular allergic disease.[14]

The production of pro-inflammatory cytokines by infiltrating cells could provide a mechanism whereby local tissue resident cells such as conjunctival fibroblasts become involved, since collagen deposition and conjunctival tissue remodeling are considerable in VKC and AKC. Tear levels of eosinophil cationic protein correlated well with the clinical severity of AKC when used as a biomarker for responsiveness to tacrolimus.[24]

Therapy

The therapy of AKC is not just symptomatic, but also attempts to modify and reduce serious sight-threatening sequelae and should therefore be aggressive. Topical treatment of the ocular surface is similar to VKC, in that some general therapy may help, antihistamines are not useful, mast cell inhibitors are continued long term, and steroid and cyclosporine drops are often required. However, AKC is generally less episodic than VKC and so long-term steroid use is more common and steroid-related complications are more problematic. In particular, herpetic keratitis, which is more common and severe in AKC, can be potentiated by topical steroids. Facial and lid dermatitis should be actively managed, if necessary in conjunction with a dermatologist, and lid margin inflammation (blepharitis) treated with hot compresses followed by lid hygiene, topical antibiotic and/or steroid preparations, and systemic low-dose antibiotics (especially tetracyclines), all of which will lessen the need for anti-inflammatory and immunosuppressive therapy.

Systemic therapy can be necessary in severe cases, and particularly when surgical therapy is undertaken, and includes steroids, cyclosporine, and sometimes other immunosuppressive agents such as mycophenolate mofetil, but all carry a risk of serious side effects and also affect the general atopic disease, so that consultation with the patient's physician is advisable.

A significant proportion of patients require ocular surgery, either as a consequence of the disease or because of the associated keratoconus. Surgery for AKC includes both elective procedures and emergency interventions and may consist of corneal gluing, patch grafts, corneal transplants (partial or full thickness), conjunctival reconstruction, amniotic membrane grafts, and limbal transplantation. These are generally high-risk procedures and often require support with systemic immunosuppression.

In summary, allergic disorders of the eye range in severity and duration, and recent studies have increased our understanding of the molecular mechanisms involved. VKC and AKC require immunosuppressive therapy, which can have serious side effects. Whilst the therapeutic options for treating mast cell-mediated forms of allergic conjunctivitis have improved, there is still a need to find alternative, safer therapies for the more severe and chronic forms.

Translational research

● ON THE HORIZON

- Improved clinical classification to ensure the relevant treatment strategy is applied.
- Development of biomarkers for use in clinical classification and in predicting response to treatment.
- Development of steroid-sparing therapies for clinically severe cases.

The challenge in the next 5–10 years is to take laboratory discoveries into the clinical arena of ocular allergy. The earlier the diagnosis, the sooner the correct course of action can be taken to avoid the long-term effects of the inflammation, in particular the corneal damage. Given the differing clinical features in different parts of the world, it is vital that an agreed classification be used to optimize therapy. Biomarkers should be identified that could be used for early diagnosis and in treatment choice. Steroids and cyclosporine can have very serious side effects for the eye, and future therapy should be aimed at reducing the need for these conventional immunosuppressives. Our understanding of the cells and cytokines driving the inflammation in the different subtypes of disease should allow for more specific therapeutic interventions in the near future. Tools for the early diagnosis of ocular allergy are sorely needed to improve the clinical outcome for the patients.

References

1. Anderson DF, MacLeod JD, Baddeley SM, et al. Seasonal allergic conjunctivitis is accompanied by increased mast cell numbers in the absence of leucocyte infiltration. Clin Exp Allergy 1997;27:1060.
2. Bacon AS, McGill JI, Anderson DF, et al. Adhesion molecules and relationship to leukocyte levels in allergic eye disease. Invest Ophthalmol Vis Sci 1998;39:322.
3. del Culvillo A, Sastre J, Montoro J, et al. The role of H1 antihistamines both topical and oral in non-sight threatening allergic rhinoconjunctivitis. J Invest Allergol Clin Immunol 2009;19(Suppl. 1):11–18.
4. Whitcup SM, Bradford R, Lue J, et al. Efficacy and tolerability of ophthalmic epinastine: a randomised, double-masked, parallel-group, active- and vehicle-controlled environmental trial in patients with seasonal allergic conjunctivitis. Clin Ther 2004;26:29.
5. Dart JK, Buckley RJ, Monnickendan M, Prasad J. Perennial allergic conjunctivitis: definition, clinical characteristics and prevalence. A comparison with seasonal allergic conjunctivitis. Trans Ophthalmol Soc U K 1986;105:513.
6. Friedlaender MH. Objective measurement of allergic reactions in the eye. Curr Opin Allergy Clin Immunol 2004;4:447.
7. Bacon AS, Ahluwalia P, Irani AM, et al. Tear and conjunctival changes during the allergen-induced early- and late-phase responses. J Allergy Clin Immunol 2000;106:948.
8. Magone MT, Whitcup SM, Fukushima A, et al. The role of IL-12 in the induction of late-phase cellular infiltration in a murine model of allergic conjunctivitis. J Allergy Clin Immunol 2000;105:299.
9. Stern ME, Siemasko K, Gao J, et al. Role of interferon-γ in a mouse model of allergic conjunctivitis. Invest Ophthalmol Vis Sci 2005;46:3239.
10. Reyes NJ, Mayhew E, Chen PW, Niederkorn JY. γ/δ T cells are required for maximal expression of allergic conjunctivitis. Invest Ophthalmol Vis Sci 2011;52:2211.
11. Zheng X, Ma P, de Paiva CS, et al. TSLP and downstream molecules in experimental mouse allergic conjunctivitis. Invest Ophthalmol Vis Sci 2010;51:3076.
12. Metz DP, Bacons AS, Holgate S, Lightman SL. Phenotypic characterization of T cells infiltrating the conjunctiva in chronic allergic eye disease. J Allergy Clin Immunol 1996;98:686.
13. Maggi E, Biswas P, Del Prete G, et al. Accumulation of Th2-like helper T cells in the conjunctiva of patients with vernal conjunctivitis. J Immunol 1991;146:1169.
14. Metz DP, Hingorani M, Calder VL, et al. T-cell cytokines in chronic allergic eye disease. J Allergy Clin Immunol 1997;100:817.
15. Leonardi A, Curnow SJ, Zhan H, Calder VL. Multiple cytokines in human tear specimens in seasonal and chronic allergic eye disease and in conjunctival fibroblast cultures. Clin Exp Allergy 2006;36:777.
16. Abu El-Asrar AM, Struyf S, Al-Kharashi SA, Missotten L, et al. Chemokines in the limbal form of vernal keratoconjunctivitis. Br J Ophthalmol 2000;84:1360.
17. Abu El-Asrar AM, Struyf S, Al-Mosallam AA, et al. Expression of chemokine receptors in vernal keratoconjunctivitis. Br J Ophthalmol 2001;85:1357.
18. Secchi AG, Tognon MS, Leonardi A. Topical use of cyclosporine in the treatment of vernal keratoconjunctivitis. Am J Ophthalmol 1990;110:641.
19. Donnenfeld E, Pflugfelder S. Topical ophthalmic cyclosporine: pharmacology and clinical uses. Surv Ophthalmol 2009;54:321.
20. Ozaki A, Seki Y, Fukushima A, Kubo M. The control of allergic conjunctivitis by suppressor of cytokine (SOCS)3 and SCOS5 in a murine model. J Immunol 2005;175:5489.
21. Fukushima A, Ozaki A, Jian Z, et al. Dissection of antigen-specific humoral and cellular immune responses for the development of experimental immune-mediated blepharoconjunctivitis in C57BL/6 mice. Curr Eye Res 2005;30:241.
22. Fukushima A, Yamaguchi T, Ishida W, et al. Engagement of 4-1BB inhibits the development of experimental allergic conjunctivitis in mice. J Immunol 2005;175:4897.
23. Foster CS, Calonge MD. Atopic kerato-conjunctivitis. Ophthalmol 1990;97:992.
24. Wakmatsu TH, Tanaka M, Satake Y, et al. Eosinophil cationic protein as a marker for assessing the efficacy of tacrolimus ophthalmic solution in the treatment of atopic keratoconjunctivitis. Mol Vis 2011;17:932.

Werner J. Pichler

Drug hypersensitivity

Drug-induced adverse reactions are common and can be classified into those that represent predictable side effects due to pharmacological actions of the drug and those that are not predictable, comprising idiosyncratic reactions due to some individual predisposition (e.g., an enzyme defect), and hypersensitivity reactions.[1] Drug hypersensitivity reactions account for about one-sixth of all adverse drug reactions. They comprise allergic and so-called pseudoallergic reactions, the latter involving direct stimulation of immune effector cells, and thus imitating an allergic reaction, but without detectable reactions of the adaptive immune system.

Drug hypersensitivity can present in many different ways, some of which are quite severe and even fatal.[2,3] The most common allergic reactions occur in the skin and are observed in about 2–3% of hospitalized patients.[4,5] Any drug can elicit hypersensitivity reactions, but antibiotics and antiepileptics are the drugs most frequently responsible. The risk of sensitization and the severity of clinical symptoms depend on the state of immune activation of the individual, the dose and duration of treatment, female sex, and immunogenetic predisposition (in particular human leukocyte antigen (HLA)-B-alleles), while a pharmacogenetic predisposition has seldom been detected.

Epicutaneous application of a drug clearly increases the risk of sensitization compared to oral or parenteral treatment. Atopy—defined as the genetic predisposition to mount an immunoglobulin E (IgE) response to inhaled or ingested innocuous proteins—is not normally associated with a higher risk of drug hypersensitivity, but an atopic predisposition can prolong the detectability of drug-specific IgE in the serum.[6]

Immune recognition of drugs

The hapten and prohapten concept

The recognition of small molecules, such as drugs, by B and T cells is usually explained by the hapten concept.[1,7] Haptens are chemically reactive small molecules (mostly < 1 kDa) that are able to undergo a stable, covalent binding to a larger protein or peptide (Chapter 6). Only by this modification of a protein or peptide does a small molecule become antigenic (Fig. 46.1). Modification can affect soluble autologous proteins (e.g., albumin), cell-bound proteins (e.g., integrins) or the peptide embedded in the antigen-binding groove of a major histocompatibility complex (MHC) molecule. Consequently, a wide array of immune responses can develop to a hapten, as many different antigens are formed, which induce different types of immune responses (Fig. 46.1A) This can lead to a great heterogeneity of clinical

pictures. Indeed, drug hypersensitivity is today the great imitator of diseases, having taken over this role from syphilis, which was the great imitator a century ago.

An immune response can only arise if the hapten is also able to stimulate innate immunity. This could occur by covalent binding to cell structures, which might induce expression of CD40 or CD80 on dendritic cells.

A typical hapten is penicillin G, which binds covalently to ε-amino groups on lysine residues within soluble or cell-bound proteins, thereby modifying them and eliciting B- and T-cell reactions. The hapten may also bind directly to the immunogenic peptide presented by the MHC-molecule. In this case no processing is required (Fig. 46.1A). Direct alteration of the MHC molecule is also possible, but evidence from mouse models suggests that this is less frequent.[8]

Many drugs are not chemically reactive but are still able to elicit immune-mediated side effects. The prohapten hypothesis tries to reconcile this phenomenon with the hapten hypothesis by stating that a chemically inert drug may become reactive upon metabolism (Fig. 46.1B).[1,7,9] Sulfamethoxazole is a prototype prohapten. It is not chemically reactive itself but intracellular metabolism by cytochrome p450 2 C9 leads to sulfamethoxazole-hydroxylamine. This can be found in the blood and urine and is easily transformed to the highly reactive sulfamethoxazole-nitroso by oxidation. The latter is chemically highly reactive and binds covalently to proteins/peptides (Fig. 46.1B), forming neoantigens. The resulting clinical picture can be as variable as with haptens: sulfamethoxazole is known to cause many different diseases, affecting many organs. These side effects are mediated by antibodies and/or T cells. On the other hand, transformation of a prohapten to the reactive hapten may occur exclusively in the liver or kidney and may thus cause an isolated hepatitis or interstitial nephritis.

The p-i concept

Recently, another possibility, namely a pharmacological interaction of drugs with immune receptors (p-i concept; Fig. 46.1C) has been elaborated.[10,11] According to this concept, chemically inert drugs, incapable of covalently binding to peptides or proteins, can nevertheless activate T cells: two possibilities exist: the drug might fit into any of the innumerable different T-cell receptors (TCRs) available and stimulate T cells, if an additional interaction with HLA occurs (p-i (TCR)). Or the drug loosely associates with a certain HLA-peptide complex, which is then recognized by T-cell receptors and stimulates T cells (p-i (HLA)). Both of these "pharmacological" interactions can result in selective T-cell stimulation, similar to the activation of T cells by peptide MHC. This drug binding to proteins does not require

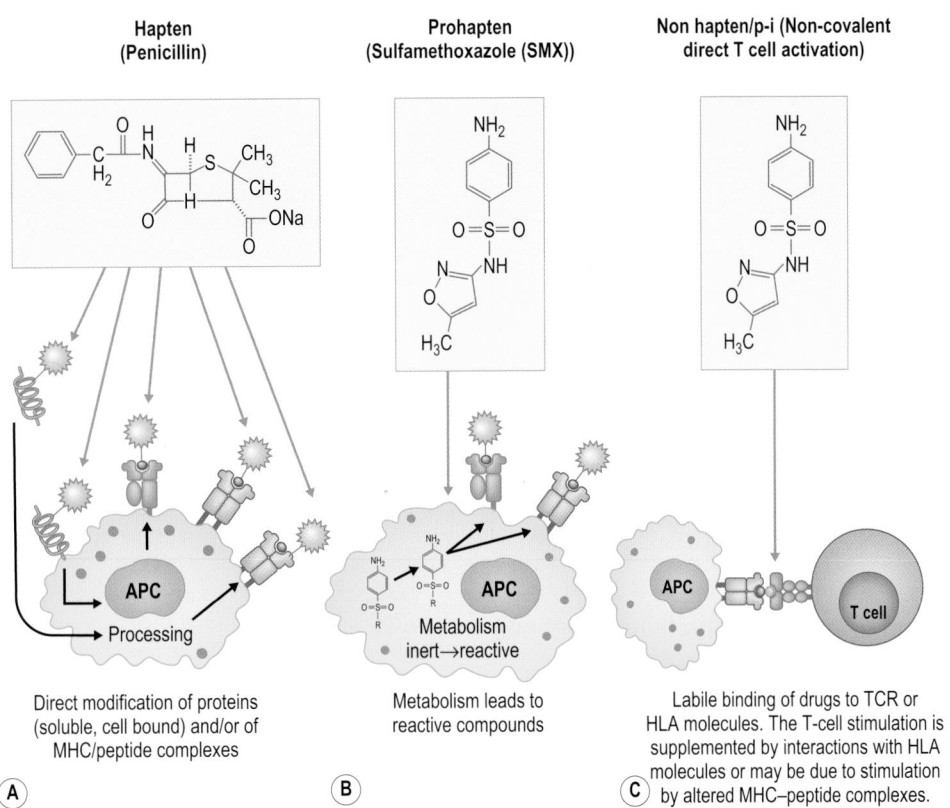

Fig. 46.1 Hapten and prohapten-concept and the noncovalent drug presentation to T cells. (A) Haptens: drugs are haptens if they can bind covalently to molecules, either soluble or cell-bound (e.g., penicillin G). They can even bind directly to the immunogenic major histocompatibility complex (MHC)–peptide complex on antigen-presenting cells (APC), either to the embedded peptide or to the MHC molecule itself. Thus, the chemical reactivity of haptens leads to the formation of many distinct antigenic epitopes, which can elicit both humoral and cellular immune responses. (B) Prohaptens: other drugs are prohaptens, requiring metabolic activation to become haptens (chemically reactive). The metabolism leads to the formation of a chemically reactive compound (e.g., from sulfamethoxazole (SMX) to the chemically reactive form SMX-NO). The resulting intake may lead to modification of cell-bound or soluble proteins by the chemically reactive metabolite, similar to a real hapten. (C) The p-i-concept (pharmacological interaction with immune receptors): drugs are often designed to fit into certain proteins/enzymes to block their function. Some drugs may happen also to bind into some of the available T-cell receptors. Under certain conditions (see text) this drug–T-cell receptor interaction can lead to an immune response of the T cell with a "fitting" T-cell receptor. For a full T-cell stimulation by such an inert drug, an interaction of the T-cell receptor with the MHC molecule is required. This type of drug stimulation results in an exclusive T-cell stimulation. Modified from Pichler WJ. Delayed drug hypersensitivity reactions. Ann Intern Med 2003; 139: 683–693, with permission from the American College of Physicians.

biotransformation (to a chemically reactive compound), it is solely based on *van der Waals* interactions between drugs and certain regions of a protein acting as an "immune-receptor." It is assumed that the drug activates previously primed memory T cells with a certain peptide specificity and a lower threshold of reactivity than naïve T cells. This threshold might be further lowered by a massive immune stimulation of T cells such as occurs during generalized herpes or human immunodeficiency virus (HIV) infection, but also during exacerbations of autoimmune diseases. This would explain the high occurrence of drug hypersensitivity in these diseases. The p-i (HLA) has recently been extended: in the abacavir model it was shown that abacavir binding to HLA-B*5701 results in exchange of peptides, allowing the presentation of novel peptides. The relevance of this finding needs more data, as it was observed with very high abacavir concentrations.[52-54]

The p-i concept radically changes our understanding of drug-induced hypersensitivity reactions, but may in fact explain some unusual features of drug hypersensitivity that are not explained by the hapten concept. According to the p-i concept, the symptoms are the consequence of a pharmacological reaction of immunologically competent cells, and not the result of a specific immune response. This can explain the symptoms at the first encounter with the drug without a sensitization phase, the lack of a memory response in weak drug stimulations, the higher risk of

drug hypersensitivity in generalized viral infections, and some peculiar *in vitro* and *in vivo* features of drug-elicited immune responses, which are reminiscent of superantigenic stimulation (Chapter 6) rather than a coordinated immune response leading to a massive overstimulation.[11] Detailed analysis of T-cell stimulation by sulfamethoxazole, phenytoin, and carbamazepine suggests that the hapten and p-i concepts can often occur together.

Classification of drug hypersensitivity reactions

Drug hypersensitivity reactions can cause many different diseases. To account for this heterogeneity and to explain the various clinical pictures, in 1976 Gell and Coombs[12] classified drug hypersensitivity as well as other immune reactions in four categories, termed type I–IV reactions.

This classification has been revised to take into account the heterogeneity of T-cell functions and the interdependence of these reactions since, for example, the maturation of B cells to IgE- or IgG-producing plasma cells depends on T-cell help. Thus, type I and type IVb reactions often occur together, as do type II or III with type IVa reactions, and the clinical picture is probably dominated by the prevalent immune reaction.

Table 46.1 Common causes of allergic and "pseudoallergic" drug reactions

Drugs involved in IgE-mediated allergies[a]	Drugs causing "pseudoallergic" reactions[a]
Foreign proteins (chimeric antibodies)	(Radio)contrast media[b]
Immunoglobulin preparations (IgE anti-IgA)	Plasma expanders
β-Lactam antibiotics Penicillin Cephalosporin	NSAID: acetylsalicylic acid, diclofenac, mefenamic acid, ibuprofen
Pyrazolones	Pyrazolones
Quinolones	Quinolones
Muscle relaxants	Muscle relaxants

[a]Not complete; only main groups mentioned.
[b]Some reactiions appear to be IgE mediated.
NSAID, nonsteroidal anti-inflammatory drug.

Antibody-mediated drug hypersensitivity reactions

As outlined above (Fig. 46.1), hapten-like features of a drug allow the modification of soluble and cell-bound proteins. The natural reaction of the immune system to such antigens is the development of a humoral immune response. Consequently, if a humoral immune response develops, the eliciting drug should have hapten-like features forming hapten–carrier complexes, or itself be protein-bearing "foreign" determinants (e.g., chimeric antibodies). Indeed, the majority of drugs able to elicit IgE-mediated allergies are known haptens, or contain foreign antigenic structures (Table 46.1).

Type I (IgE-mediated) allergies

The IgE system is geared to react to small amounts of antigens. It achieves this extraordinary sensitivity by the ubiquitous presence of mast cells armed with high-affinity Fcε receptors (FcεRI), to which allergen/drug-specific IgE is bound. Very small amounts of a drug are apparently sufficient to interact and stimulate these receptor-bound IgE molecules, as occasionally even skin tests with drugs can elicit systemic reactions. Upon cross-linking the FcεRI, various mediators (histamine, tryptase, leukotrienes, prostaglandins, tumor necrosis factor-α (TNF-α)) are released, which cause the symptoms (Chapters 22 and 42).

IgE-mediated reactions to drugs are usually thought to depend on the prior development of an immune response to a hapten-carrier complex: B cells need to mature into IgE-secreting plasma cells, and T cells help in this process by interacting with B cells (i.e., CD40–CD40L interaction) and by releasing interleukin-4 (IL-4)/IL-13, which are switch factors for IgE synthesis. This sensitization phase is asymptomatic and may have occurred during a previous course of treatment. Upon renewed contact with the drug, a hapten–carrier complex is formed again, which then cross-links preformed drug-specific IgE on mast cells. The drug itself is normally too small to cross-link two adjacent IgE molecules (Fig. 46.2A).

These reactions were at one time erroneously considered to be dose-independent, as sometimes very small amounts can already cause severe reactions. But further diminishing the dose—as done in desensitization procedures—demonstrates that these reactions are clearly dose-dependent.

In sensitized individuals the reaction can start within seconds after parenteral administration, and minutes after oral intake (Fig. 46.2A). Anaphylactic shock can occur within 15 minutes, and asphyxia due to laryngeal edema between 15 and 60 minutes. The initial symptoms can be palmar, plantar, genital, or axillary itch, which should be seen as an alarm sign, as it often heralds a possibly severe, anaphylactic reaction, following rapidly within minutes: The skin becomes red (diffuse erythema), often first affecting the trunk, and later the whole body. In the next ~30–60 minutes an urticaria may appear, together with swelling of the periorbital, perioral, and sometimes genital areas (Fig. 46.3). Asphyxia may account for 60% of anaphylaxis-related deaths: laryngeal swelling should be suspected if the voice

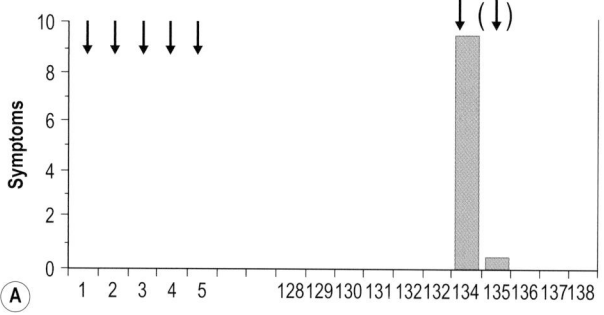

Possible scheme for IgE-mediated, immediate reactions after a previous, silent sensitization phase

X-axis: days;
Y-axis: relative frequency of appearance

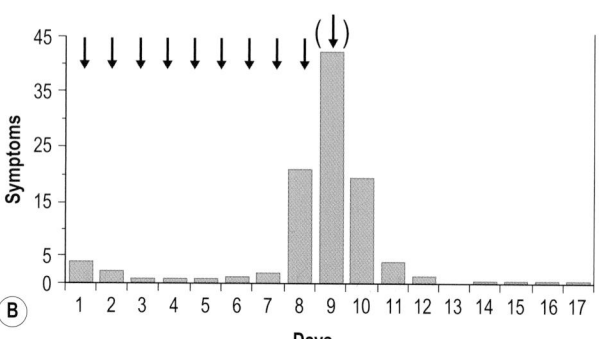

Appearance of maculopapular exanthem in gemifloxacin-treated 20–40-year-old females

X-axis: days;
Y-axis: number of affected patients (n=270)

Fig. 46.2 Kinetics of IgE and T-cell-mediated reactions. (A) Schematic representation of a sensitization phase, which was asymptomatic. At re-exposure at a later time point symptoms appeared rapidly, mostly within 1 hour. (B) Appearance of exanthem in gemifloxacin-treated healthy volunteers. The largest study undertaken to investigate drug-induced side effects was performed with gemifloxacin, a quinolone. Initial data revealed that rashes appeared more commonly in women under 40 years of age and in those patients submitted to longer treatment (> 7 days). A prospective study was performed in 987 healthy women aged 18–40; 790 (80%) were treated with gemifloxacin for 10 days while the remaining 197 (20%) received ciprofloxacin for 10 days. A mostly very mild exanthem appeared in 260/790 (31.7%) gemifloxacin-treated women but only in 7/197 (4.3%) ciprofloxacin-treated women, with a clear peak on days 8–10 after treatment onset. Aminopenicillin-induced exanthems have a similar time kinetic.
Data from Food and Drug Administration website: http://www.fda.gov/ohrms/dockets/ac/03/slides/3931S1_04_LFLife%20Sciences-Factive.pdf.

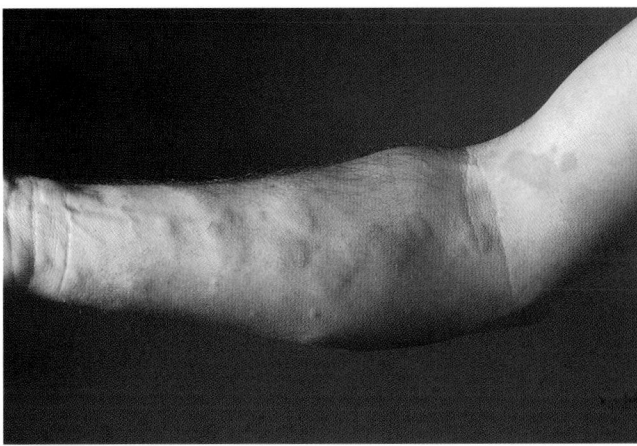

Fig. 46.3 Urticaria with itching wheals (nonsteroidal anti-inflammatory drug intolerance reaction).

becomes hoarse, and the patient has difficulty speaking and swallowing due to tongue swelling. Patients can also complain of chest tightness and dyspnea—signs of acute bronchospasm. Some patients develop gastrointestinal symptoms (nausea, cramps, vomiting, and fecal incontinence). The blood pressure may collapse, either just due to a shift of volume into the extravascular space or due to cardiac arrhythmia. The full syndrome is anaphylactic shock, which is lethal in ~1% of cases. Risk factors for a severe episode are fulminant appearance, pre-existing (undertreated) asthma, and older age, as myocardial infarction or cerebral hypoxia/damage can lead to death days after the acute event. Anaphylaxis is a severe event, and survivors not infrequently have some cognitive or intellectual impairment. Table 46.1 summarizes the main drugs causing anaphylaxis.

Most IgE-mediated reactions to drugs are less severe, and often only urticaria, angioedema, or a local wheal may develop. However, any IgE-mediated drug allergy can be potentially life threatening, as the mild symptoms might be due to a relatively low dose, and each treatment may boost the IgE response.

Many anaphylactic reactions to intravenously administered muscle relaxants, radio-contrast media, some β-lactam antibiotics, etc. clearly occur at the first encounter with the drug: the well documented formation of drug-reactive IgE must have been triggered by a cross-reactive compound, be it another chemical, drug, or even a protein. Thus, occurrence of IgE-mediated anaphylaxis on first exposure is clearly possible!

Pseudoallergy (nonimmune-mediated hypersensitivity)

An unsolved problem are so-called "pseudoallergic" reactions (nonimmune-mediated hypersensitivities), which in fact are as frequent as IgE-mediated reactions. The majority of these reactions imitate the most frequent clinical features of immediate reactions (erythema, urticaria) and are not dangerous, but some of these reactions cause anaphylaxis and can be lethal. They can appear at the first encounter with the drug and tend to arise less rapidly (often > 15 minutes) than true IgE-mediated allergies; they require higher doses, and the typical initial symptoms for anaphylaxis, namely palmar and/or plantar itch, are less common. High serum tryptase levels after some reactions underline the role of mast cell degranulation at least in some of these reactions.

"Pseudoallergic" reactions can be elicited by many drugs, but some drugs seem to elicit them more often (Table 46.1). *In vitro*, these drugs do not release mediators from basophils or mast

cells. Some people seem to be more prone to react in this way, and they develop similar, mostly mild symptoms to a quite heterogeneous range of drugs, with clearly distinct chemical and pharmacological features. Neither IgE nor T-cell reactions have been demonstrated, and only very few patients have constantly elevated tryptase levels as a sign of a mastocytosis. Some reactions can be suppressed by pretreatment with antihistamines.

● KEY CONCEPTS

The pharmacological interaction of drugs with immune receptors (p-i) concept postulates direct interaction of drugs with T-cell receptors [p-i (TCR)] or HLA molecules [p-i (HLA)][7,11]

Non-covalent binding of the drug with immune receptors can occur (1) to HLA-proteins (this is the case for strongly HLA-associated reactions as, e.g., abacavir and HLA-B*5701; or (2) to the T-cell receptor for antigen itself (no HLA-restriction detectable).

- Fixed antigen-presenting cells, unable to process antigens, can still present the drug and stimulate specific T cells.
- Stimulation of drug-specific T cells occurs also if drug metabolism or antigen processing in the antigen (drug) presenting cell is not possible or blocked.
- Drug-reactive T-cell clones react to the drug within seconds or minutes, long before metabolism and processing can take place.
- Some, limited T-cell reactivity to drugs can already be observed in the absence of antigen-presenting cells – drug binding to HLA can eventually lead to exchange of HLA-bound peptides: an otherwise not presented peptide might be presented, giving rise to an altered immune response (shown for abacavir).
- The p-i concept has been found to be relevant for such different drugs as sulfamethoxazole, lidocaine, mepivacaine, celecoxib, lamotrigine, carbamazepine and p-phenylendiamine, causing MPE, DiHS/DRESS, AGEP, TEN, and contact dermatitis.
- AGEP, acute generalized exanthematous pustulosis; DiHS, drug-induced hypersensitivity syndrome; DRESS, drug rash with eosinophilia and systemic symptoms; MPE, maculopapular exanthem; TEN, toxic epidermal necrolysis.

IgG-mediated reactions (cytotoxic mechanism, type II)

Type II and type III reactions rely on the formation of complement-fixing IgG antibodies (IgG$_1$, IgG$_3$). Occasionally, IgM is involved. They are similar, as both depend on the formation of immune complexes and interaction with complement and Fcγ receptor (FcγRI, IIa and IIIa) bearing cells (on macrophages, natural killer cells, granulocytes, platelets), but the target structures and physiological consequences are different.

In type II reactions, either the antibody is directed to cell structures on the membrane (rarely) or immune complex activation occurs on the cell surface. Both events can lead to cell destruction or sequestration. Affected target cells include erythrocytes, leukocytes, platelets, and probably hematopoietic precursor cells in the bone marrow. The mechanism of type II reaction is not as clear as originally thought, since a clear hapten-specific immune reaction can often not be documented.[13,14] One can distinguish two patterns:

1. Development of an IgG immune reaction to the hapten–carrier complex, mostly after longer duration of high-dose treatment. This is rather rare and best documented for high-dose penicillin and cephalosporin treatments. The immune reaction is due to complement-fixing antibodies (IgG$_1$, IgG$_3$,

rarely IgM). Some antibody reactivity may be directed to the carrier molecule itself (i.e., autoantibodies). Onset of this autoimmune form is less abrupt, but it lasts longer (weeks instead of days) after cessation of the drug.

2. Nonspecific adherence with autoantibody induction can occur when a drug or metabolite becomes adsorbed to the erythrocyte or thrombocyte membrane, creating a new antigenic complex in combination with the cell membrane. For example, quinine-induced immune thrombocytopenia is caused by IgG and/or IgM immunoglobulins that react with selected epitopes on platelet membrane glycoproteins, usually GPIIb/IIIa (fibrinogen receptor) or GPIb/IX (von Willebrand factor receptor) only when the drug is present in its soluble form.[13] Well-documented cases are due to quinine, quinidine, or sulfonamides. The antibodies are clearly not hapten-specific, and it remains enigmatic how a soluble drug can promote binding of an otherwise innocuous antibody to a membrane glycoprotein and cause platelet destruction.

The antibody-coated cells will be sequestered within the reticuloendothelial system in liver and spleen by Fc- or complement receptor binding. More rarely, intravascular destruction can occur by complement-mediated lysis.

Hemolytic anemia has been attributed to penicillin and its derivatives, cephalosporins, levodopa, methyldopa, quinidine, and some anti-inflammatory drugs. Today cephalosporins are the main cause. The clinical symptoms of hemolytic anemia are insidious and may be restricted to symptoms of anemia (fatigue, pallor, shortness of breath, tachycardia) and jaundice with dark urine. Laboratory investigation can reveal reduced erythrocyte and hemoglobin levels, increased reticulocytes, and positive direct and (if the drug is present during the test) indirect Coombs tests. Unconjugated bilirubin levels are elevated and haptoglobulin is decreased. Urinary hemoglobin and hemosiderin are increased.

Thrombocytopenia is a relatively common side effect of drug treatment. Acute, sometimes severe and life-threatening thrombocytopenia is a recognized complication of treatment with quinine, quinidine, sulfonamide antibiotics, and many other medications. It can also complicate treatment with biologicals, which often contain human Fc elements themselves. Drug-induced immune thrombocytopenia usually develops after 5–8 days of exposure to the sensitizing medication or after a single exposure in a patient exposed previously to the same drug. Patients often present with widespread petechial hemorrhages in the skin and buccal mucosa, sometimes accompanied by urinary tract or gastrointestinal bleeding. Intracranial hemorrhage is rare, but has been reported. After discontinuing the culprit medication, platelet counts usually return to normal within 3–5 days.

A special, intermediate form between type II and III reactions is heparin-induced thrombocytopenia: Platelets have low-affinity Fc-receptors (FcγRIIa) that can bind immune complexes, and activate platelets.[15] Heparin is a high-molecular-weight, sulfated, linear polysaccharide that inhibits blood coagulation by activating regulatory proteins such as anti-thrombin III. About 50% of patients anti-coagulated with heparin for >7 days produce antibodies that recognize complexes consisting of heparin and platelet factor 4, a CXC chemokine normally stored in platelet alpha granules. When a patient with such an antibody is given heparin, heparin–PF4 complexes are formed. These complexes react with antibodies to form immune complexes, which bind to the platelet FcγRIIa receptors, leading to platelet activation, additional PF4 release and eventually, platelet destruction. Thrombocytopenia occurs in about 5% of patients given heparin and is rarely severe enough to cause bleeding. However, about 10% of affected patients experience paradoxical thrombosis that can be life-threatening.

IgG-mediated reactions (immune complex deposition, type III)

Immune complex formation is a common event during a normal immune response and does not normally cause symptoms. Immune complexes can also be formed during drug treatment, either if the drug forms a hapten–carrier complex and thus gives rise to an immune reaction or if the drug is a (partly) foreign protein that elicits an immune reaction itself (e.g., chimeric antibodies). Such immune complexes will normally be rapidly cleared, by binding to FcγRI or complement receptor 1 (CR1) on reticuloendothelial cells. No symptoms arise, but the efficiency of treatment decreases.

Why immune complex disease develops under certain circumstances is not clear. Very high immune complex levels, a relative deficiency of some complement components, and thus lower capacity to eliminate immune complexes or an aberrant FcγR function might be responsible. Recently, a low copy number of FcγRIII were found to be associated with another immune complex disease, glomerulonephritis.[16]

Type III reactions can present as small-vessel vasculitis and/or serum sickness: Serum sickness was first described with heterogous or foreign serum used for passive immunization. Antibodies are generated within 4–10 days, which react with the antigen, forming soluble circulating immune complexes. Complement (C1q)-containing immune complexes are deposited in the postcapillary venules and attract leukocytes by interacting with their FcγRIII,[17] which then release proteolytic enzymes that mediate tissue damage.

Currently, nonprotein drugs are the most common cause of serum sickness, although the broader use of protein drugs (e.g. recombinant antibodies) may alter this picture in future. Hypersensitivity vasculitis reportedly has an incidence of 10–30 cases per million people per year. Most reports concern cefaclor, followed by trimethoprim-sulfamethoxazole, cephalexin, amoxicillin, nonsteroidal anti-inflammatory drugs (NSAIDs), and diuretics.

The main symptoms of immune complex diseases are arthralgia, myalgia, fever, and vasculitis. This may be localized mainly to the skin as "palpable purpura" — purplish, red spots, usually on the legs. In children, it is often diagnosed as Henoch-Schönlein purpura, often with arthritis. Lesions may coalesce to form plaques that occasionally ulcerate. The internal organs most commonly affected are the gastrointestinal tract, the kidneys, and joints. The prognosis is good when there is no internal involvement. Histology can reveal IgA-containing immune complexes, and the histology of kidney lesions is in fact identical to IgA nephropathy.

T-cell-mediated, delayed drug hypersensitivity reactions

The original Gell and Coombs classification was established before a detailed understanding of T-cell subsets and functions was available. Since then it has become clear that the three antibody-dependent types of reactions also require the involvement of helper T cells (Chapter 16). Moreover, T cells can orchestrate different forms of inflammation. Therefore T-cell-mediated type IV reactions have been further subclassified into IVa–IVd reactions, as shown in Fig. 46.4.[7] This subclassification considers the distinct cytokine production by T cells and thus incorporates the well-accepted Th1/Th2 distinction of T cells; it includes the cytotoxic activity of both CD4 and CD8 T cells (IVc); and it emphasizes the participation of different effector cells such as monocytes (IVa), eosinophils (IVb), or neutrophils (IVd), which cause the inflammation and tissue damage.

Type IVa

Type IVa reactions correspond to Th1-type immune reactions: Th1-type T cells activate macrophages by secreting large amounts of interferon-γ (IFN-γ), drive the production of complement-fixing antibody isotypes involved in type II and III reactions (IgG$_1$, IgG$_3$), and are co-stimulatory for pro-inflammatory responses (TNF, IL-12) and CD8 T-cell responses. The T cells promote these reactions by secretion of IFN-γ and possibly other cytokines (TNF-α, IL-18). An *in vivo* correlate would be monocyte activation, e.g., in skin tests to tuberculin or even granuloma formation, as seen in sarcoidosis. On the other hand, these

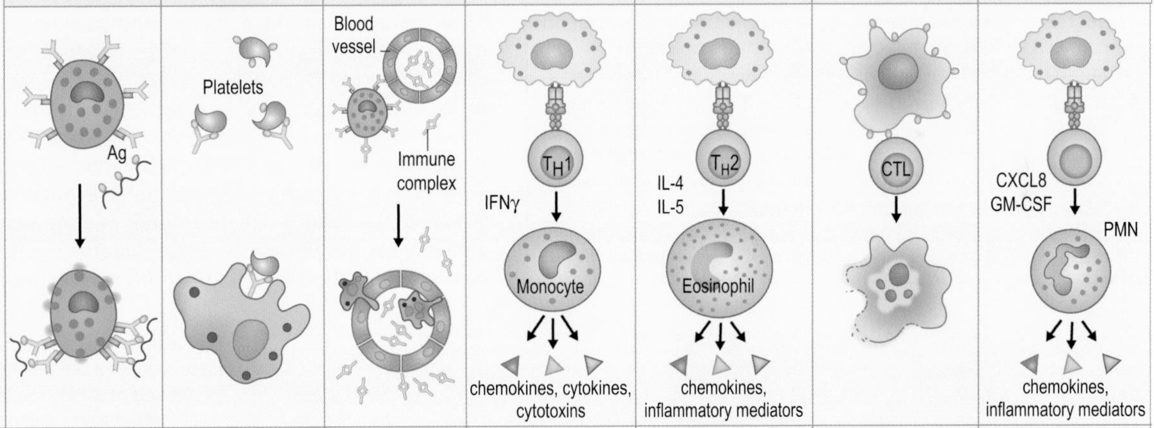

	Type I	Type II	Type III	Type IVa	Type IVb	Type IVc	Type IVd
Immune reactant	IgE	IgG	IgG	IFNγ, TNFα (T$_H$1 cells)	IL-5, IL-4/IL-13 (T$_H$2 cells)	Perforin/ GranzymeB (CTL)	CXCL-8. GM-CSF (IL-17) (T cells)
Antigen	Soluble antigen	Cell or matrix-associated antigen	Soluble antigen	Antigen presented by cells or direct T-cell stimulation	Antigen presented by cells or direct T-cell stimulation	Cell-associated antigen or direct T-cell stimulation	Soluble antigen presented by cells or direct T-cell stimulation
Effector	Mast-cell activation	FcR$^+$ cells (phagocytes, NK cells)	FcR$^+$ cells Complement	Macrophage activation	Eosinophils	T cells	Neutrophils
Example of hypersensitivity reaction	Anaphylaxis, allergic rhinitis, asthma (with IVb)	Hemolytic anaemia, thrombocytopenia	Serum sickness, Arthus reaction	Tuberculin reaction contact dermatitis (with IVc)	Maculopapular exanthema with eosinophilia, chronic asthma, allergic rhinitis	Contact dermatitis, maculopapular and bullous exanthem, hepatitis	AGEP Behçet disease, psoriasis

Fig. 46.4 Revised Gell and Coombs classification of drug reactions. Drugs can elicit all types of immune reactions. Although all reactions are T-cell-regulated, the effector functions are either predominantly antibody-mediated (type I–III) or rely more on T-cell/cytokine-dependent functions (type IVa–IVd). Type I reactions are IgE-mediated. Cross-linking IgE molecules on high-affinity IgE receptors (FcϵRI) on mast cells and basophilic granulocytes leads to degranulation and release of mediators, which cause a variety of symptoms (vasodilatation, increased permeability, bronchoconstriction, itch). Type II reactions are IgG-mediated, and cause cell destruction due to complement activation or interaction with Fcγ receptor-bearing killer cells. Type III reactions are also IgG-mediated. Complement deposition and activation in small vessels and recruitment of neutrophilic granulocytes via Fcγ receptor interaction lead to a local vascular inflammation. Type IVa corresponds to Th1 reactions with high IFN-γ/TNF-α secretion and involves monocyte/macrophage activation. Often, one can see also a CD8 cell recruitment (type IVc reaction). Type IVb reactions correspond to eosinophilic inflammation and to a Th2 response with high IL-4/IL-5/IL-13 secretion; they are often associated with an IgE-mediated type I reaction. Type IVc: the cytotoxic reactions rely on cytotoxic T cells (both CD4 and CD8 cells) themselves as effector cells. They seem to occur in all drug-related delayed hypersensitivity reactions. Type IVd reactions correspond to a T-cell-dependent, sterile neutrophilic inflammatory process. They are clearly distinct from the rapid influx of polymorphonuclear leukocytes in bacterial infections and seem to be related to high CXCL-8/granulocyte–macrophage colony-stimulating factor (GM-CSF) production by T cells (and tissue cells). The role of IL-17 in IVd reactions is not yet defined.

Modified from Pichler WJ. Immune mechanism of drug hypersensitivity. Immunol Allergy Clin North Am 2004; 24: 373–397, with permission from Elsevier.

Th1 cells are known to activate CD8 cells, which might explain the common combination of IVa and IVc reactions (e.g., in contact dermatitis).

Type IVb

Type IVb corresponds to the Th2-type immune response. Th2 T cells secrete the cytokines IL-4, -13, and -5, which promote B-cell production of IgE and IgG$_4$, macrophage deactivation and mast cell and eosinophil responses. The high production of the Th2 cytokine IL-5 leads to eosinophilic inflammation, which is the characteristic inflammatory cell type in many drug hypersensitivity reactions.[7] In addition, there is a link to type I reactions, as Th2 cells support IgE production by IL-4/IL-13 secretion. *In vivo* correlates include eosinophil-rich maculopapular exanthem (MPE), infestations with nematodes, or allergic inflammation of the bronchi or nasal mucosa (asthma and rhinitis).

⬤ KEY CONCEPTS

Immunological findings in drug-induced exanthema

- Drug-specific T cells are found in the blood, in affected skin, and in positive patch tests.
- Drug-specific T cells show a high frequency for many years after the reaction (1:250–1:3000 of CD4 T cells react with the drug).
- Both drug-specific CD4 and CD8 cells can kill in a drug-dependent manner. CD4-mediated killing is perforin/granzyme B-dependent and responsible for focal, hydropic degeneration of keratinocytes in maculopapular exanthema.
- The clinical picture of the exanthem is determined by the cytokine released by the T cells infiltrating the skin. Secretion of interferon-γ → macrophage activation; secretion of interleukin-5 → eosinophil activation; secretion of CXCL-8 and granulocyte–macrophage colony-stimulating factor → neutrophil activation and recruitment.
- A high number of drug-specific CD8 T cells causes more severe, bullous skin diseases, probably because all cells are targets for CD8-mediated cytotoxicity and because these cells can release the highly cytotoxic molecule granulysin.
- CD8-mediated severe reactions to carbamazepine, allopurinol, and abacavir show striking human leukocyte antigen (HLA)-B associations, which differ with different drugs.

Type IVc

T cells can also act as effector cells: they emigrate to the tissue and can kill tissue cells like hepatocytes or keratinocytes in a perforin/granzymeB and FasL-dependent manner (Fig. 46.5).[18,19] Recently a role for granulysin in severe drug allergies has been described.[20] Such reactions occur in most drug-induced delayed hypersensitivity reactions, mostly together with other type IV reactions (monocyte, eosinophil, or polymorphonuclear leukocyte recruitment and activation). Cytotoxic T cells thus play a role in maculopapular or bullous skin diseases as well as neutrophilic inflammation, such as acute generalized exanthematous pustulosis (AGEP), and in contact dermatitis. Type IVc reactions appear to be dominant in bullous skin reactions like Stevens–Johnson syndrome (SJS) and toxic epidermal necrolysis (TEN), where activated CD8 T cells kill keratinocytes,[7,18,19] but may also be dominant in drug-induced hepatitis or nephritis.

Type IVd

Another rather neglected possibility is that T cells can coordinate sterile neutrophilic inflammation. A typical example would be AGEP. In this disease CXCL8 and granulocyte–macrophage colony-stimulating factor (GM-CSF)-producing T cells recruit neutrophilic leukocytes via CXCL8 release, and prevent their apoptosis via GM-CSF release.[21] Besides AGEP, such T-cell reactions are also found in Behçet's disease and pustular psoriasis.[22] It is likely that Th17 cells and IL-17/-22 cytokines are also involved in these drug-driven, neutrophilic inflammations, but this has not yet been proven.

Tolerance mechanism

Most patients can take drugs without developing immune-mediated side effects. This could be because they lack precursor cells able to interact with the drug. But the great heterogeneity of the immune response to drugs,[7] a high precursor frequency in sensitized patients[23] and the finding that 2–4% of the normal population, but 30% to > 50% of HIV-infected patients, may react with sulfamethoxazole suggests that it is not a lack of precursor cells but other factors like the underlying immune status (preactivation of memory T cells) and "regulatory" mechanisms that may be important. The role of regulatory T cells in drug allergy has not

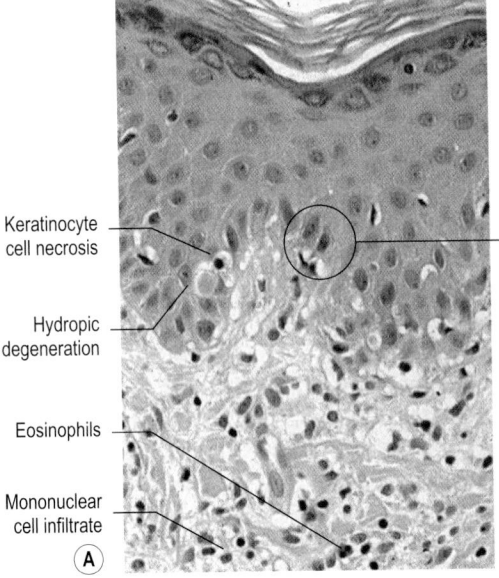

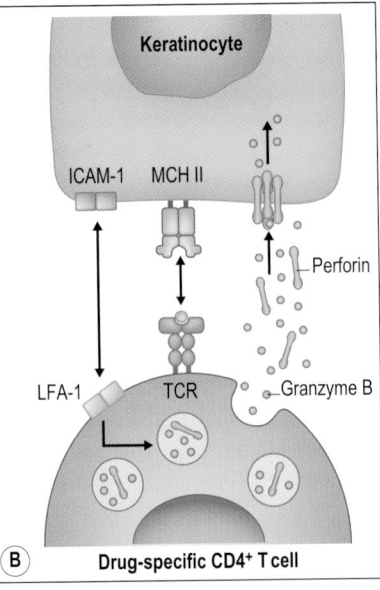

Fig. 46.5 (A) Typical histology of a maculopapular exanthem. Note the focal keratinocyte necrosis, often in close apposition of T cells (which have cytotoxic potential and are perforin-positive). (B) Schematic representation of CD4-mediated killing of activated keratinocytes, which express major histocompatibility complex (MHC) class II and ICAM1 molecules.

Modified from Pichler WJ. Delayed drug hypersensitivity reactions. Ann Intern Med 2003; 139: 683–693, with permission from the American College of Physicians.

Keratinocyte cell necrosis

Hydropic degeneration

Eosinophils

Mononuclear cell infiltrate

Keratinocyte

ICAM-1   MCH II

Perforin

LFA-1   TCR   Granzyme B

Drug-specific CD4+ T cell

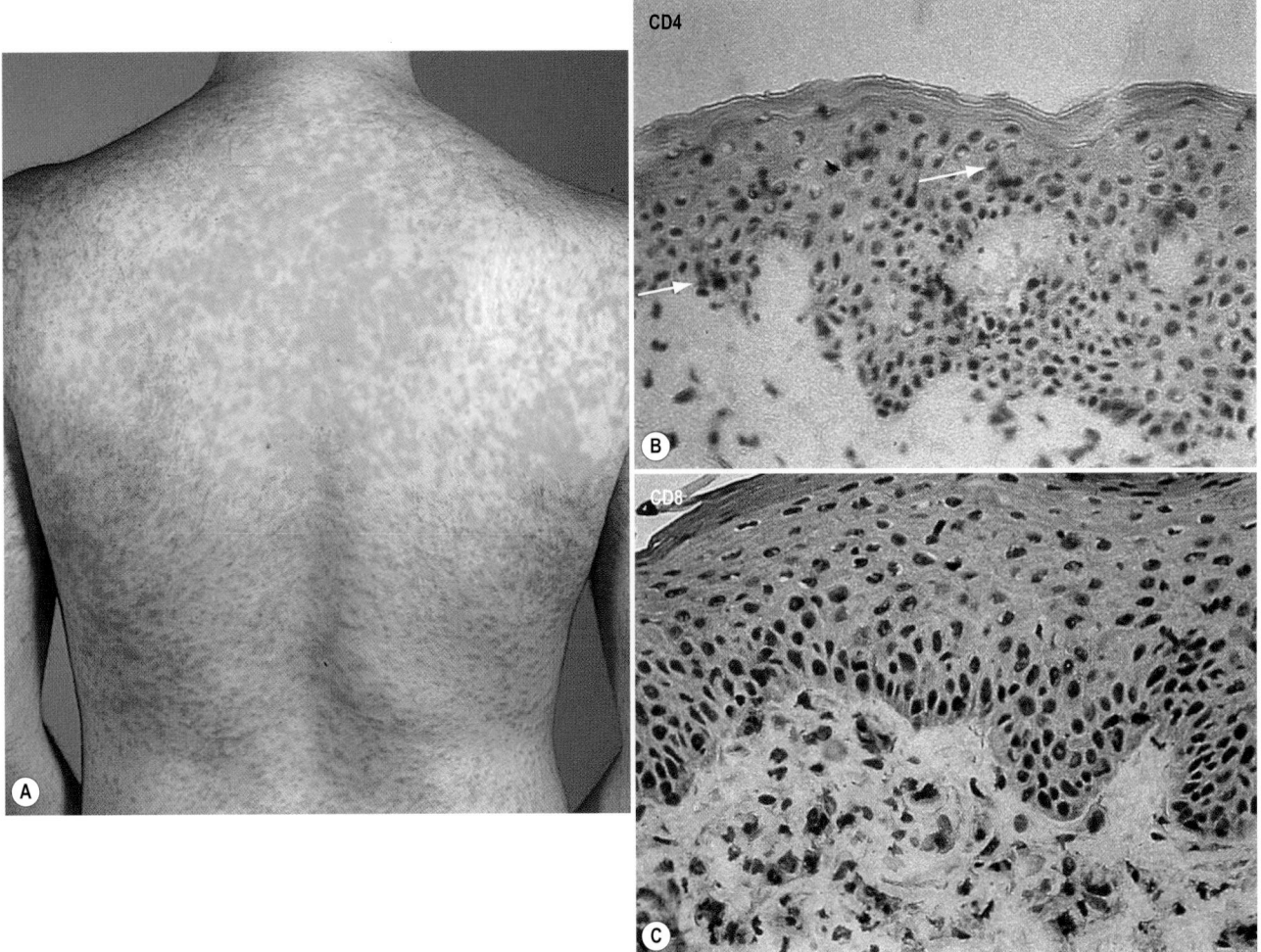

Fig. 46.6 Clinical pictures and immunohistologies of drug-induced exanthems. Maculopapular drug eruption (A): the immunohistology reveals infiltration of CD4 (B) and only a few CD8 T cells (C) in the dermis and epidermis. These cells express perforin and granzyme B, granulysin and, to a variable degree, FasL.
From Hari Y, Frutig-Schnyder K, Hunni M, et al. T cell involvement in cutaneous drug eruptions. Clin Exp Allergy 2001; 31: 1398–1408, with permission from Blackwell Publishing.

yet been investigated in detail—but preliminary data suggest that the distribution and function of regulatory T cells is normal.

Maculopapular exanthem (MPE)

The most frequent manifestations of drug allergies are delayed-appearing cutaneous reactions—so-called "rashes." They comprise a broad spectrum of clinical and distinct histopathological features that appear >6 hours to 10 days after drug intake (Fig. 46.2).

In all forms of delayed drug-induced reactions like exanthems, nephritis, and probably hepatitis, cytotoxic mechanisms seem to play an important role. The clinical picture is determined by the strength of cytotoxicity (amount of drug-specific cytotoxic T cells and tissue destruction), the generation of cytotoxic CD8 versus CD4 cells, and the type of associated effector mechanism (monocyte or activation of eosinophils and neutrophilic granulocytes).

MPE is the most frequent drug hypersensitivity reaction, affecting 2–8% of hospitalized patients, especially after treatment with β-lactams, sulfamethoxazole, quinolones, diuretics, and many more.[4,5] In most cases it appears 8–11 days after start of treatment (Fig. 46.2), but sometimes even 1–2 days after stopping treatment (Fig. 46.6). In previously sensitized individuals it can appear on the first day of treatment. It is clearly dose-dependent. A study investigating exanthemata after treatment with the quinolone gemifloxacin showed that females of childbearing age had a higher

risk of exanthema, suggesting an influence of estrogens on the clinical manifestation (Fig. 46.2B) (http://www.fda.gov/ohrms/dockets/ac/03/slides/3931S1_04_LFLife%20Sciences-Factive.pdf). Most MPE, particularly if caused by β-lactams or gemifloxacin, are rather mild, and treatment with an emollient cream, and possibly topical corticosteroids, or systemic antihistamines to treat pruritus is sufficient. Some patients can continue treatment without aggravation. The exanthema often heals with desquamation within 2–10 days after stopping the incriminated drug. It is unlikely that SJS/TEN will develop from MPE, as the cells involved are different. On the other hand, some drugs may induce a mixed CD4 and CD8 cell activation (Table 46.2). In such cases prolonged treatment may lead to confluence of the papules, the patient may complain of malaise and fever, and liver function tests indicate hepatitis (more than threefold increased transaminase levels). Eosinophilia (> 0.5 g/L) and activated CD8 cells are found in the blood.[24] This illustrates that even "mild" drug hypersensitivity reactions are systemic diseases, and that cutaneous manifestations may only be the tip of the iceberg.

Immunohistology reveals drug-specific CD4 cell infiltration (CLA[+], CCR6[+]) in perivascular areas of the dermis.[7,24] Some T cells progress into the dermoepidermal junction zone and epidermis, where they are reactivated (MHC class II[+] and CD25[+]) and kill keratinocytes in a contact-dependent way by releasing perforin/granzyme B. Some keratinocytes undergo hydropic degeneration, but this apoptosis is not as extensive as with CD8

Table 46.2 Drugs eliciting severe cutaneous or systemic reactions[a]

Acute generalized exanthematous pustulosis (AGEP)	Stevens–Johnson syndrome (SJS) and toxic epidermal necrolysis (TEN)	Drug-induced hypersensitivity syndrome/drug rash with eosinophilia and systemic symptoms (DiHS/DRESS)
Aminopenicillins[a]	**Allopurinol**[b]	**Carbamazepine**[b]
Cephalosporins	**Phenytoin**[b]	Phenytoin
Pristinamycin	**Carbamazepine**[b]	Lamotrigine
Celecoxib	**Nevirapine**	Minocycline
Quinolone	Lamotrigine	Allopurinol[b]
Diltiazem	Cotrimoxazole	Dapsone
Terbinafine	Barbiturate	Sulfasalazine
Macrolides	Nonsteroidal anti-inflammatory drug (oxicams)	Cotrimoxazole
		Abacavir[c]

[a]List incomplete: the most frequent elicitors are given in bold.
[b]The type of reaction might be determined by the presence of a certain human leukocyte antigen (HLA)-B phenotype.
[c]Abacavir-induced systemic reactions often lack eosinophilia and preferentially affect the respiratory and gastrointestinal tract.

T-cell-mediated killing (Fig. 46.5). In addition, the immigrating CD4 T cells exhibit a heterogeneous cytokine profile, including type 1 (IFN-γ) and type 2 (IL-4, IL-5) cytokines, suggesting that both Th1 and Th2 cells infiltrate the skin. The cytokine IL-5 is also detectable in the serum. Tissue and blood eosinophilia can be found.[24–26] The recruitment of eosinophils is also enhanced by expression of the chemokines eotaxin and RANTES in MPE lesions.

Acute generalized exanthematous pustulosis

Acute generalized exanthematous pustulosis (AGEP) is a rare disease (∼ 1:100 000 treatments) with an estimated incidence equal to severe bullous skin diseases (SJS and TEN combined).[21,27] It is caused by drugs in >90% of cases (Table 46.2). Its clinical hallmark is the rapid appearance of myriads of disseminated, sterile pustules in the skin (Fig. 46.7), often 3–5 days after starting treatment. Patients have fever and massive leukocytosis in the blood, sometimes with eosinophilia, but no involvement of mucous membranes. Epicutaneous patch test reactions can cause a similar pustular reaction locally.

Immunohistology of the acute lesion reveals subcorneal or intraepidermal pustules, which are filled with neutrophilic granulocytes and surrounded by activated, HLA-DR-expressing CD4

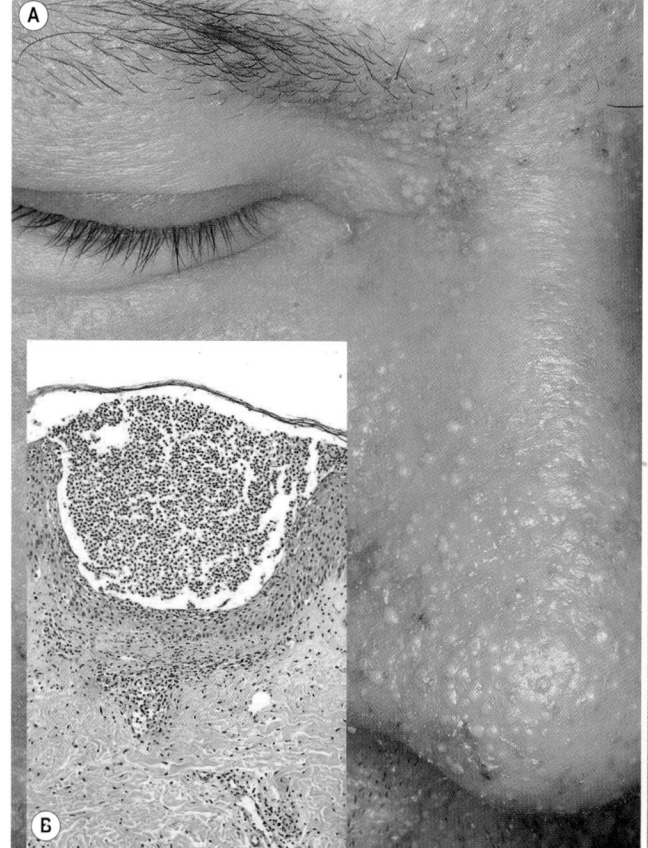

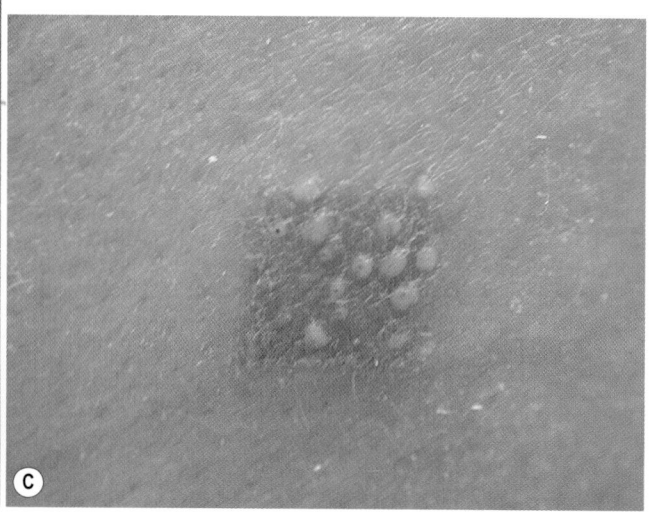

Fig. 46.7 Clinical pictures and immunohistologies of drug-induced exanthem. (A) Pustular drug eruption (acute generalized exanthematous pustulosis: AGEP). (B) Note the intraepidermal, nonfollicular pustules. (C) A patch test reaction leading to a pustular reaction is shown as well.
From Schaerli P, Britschgi M, Keller M, et al. Characterization of human T cells that regulate neutrophilic skin inflammation. J Immunol 2004; 173: 2151–2158. Copyright 2004, with permission from The American Association of Immunologists, Inc.

and CD8 T cells. Keratinocytes show elevated expression of the neutrophil-attracting chemokine IL-8 (CXCL-8), and even the T cells migrating into the epidermis express CXCL-8 and GM-CSF. Analysis of sequential patch test reactions at 48–96 hours suggests that drug-specific cytotoxic T cells emigrate first, causing formation of vesicles by killing keratinocytes. Subsequently T cells and keratinocytes release CXCL8, which recruits granulocytes into the vesicles that then transform into pustules.[19] Some pustules coalesce together and can form bullae. The condition is fatal in 2–4% of cases, mainly in older people. Healing occurs within 5 days after stopping the drug. This disease and the underlying T-cell reaction seem to be a model for sterile neutrophilic inflammations (type IVd) like pustular psoriasis and Behçet's disease.[22]

Bullous exanthemata, Stevens–Johnson syndrome, and toxic epidermal necrolysis

The most severe forms of drug-induced skin reactions involve formation of bullae (Fig. 46.8). The most severe bullous skin reactions are Stevens–Johnson syndrome (SJS) and toxic epidermal necrolysis (TEN). TEN and SJS are rare (~1:1 000 000 for TEN, ~1:100 000 for SJS). They are today considered to be the milder and more severe form of the same disease (SJS < 10% skin detachment, TEN > 30% detachment). They are graded according to SCORTEN, whereby age, underlying disease, and the amount of maximal skin detachment are the most important prognostic factors. According to the European study group of severe cutaneous drug reactions, SJS has a mortality of ~13%, and TEN of ~39%. The intermediate

form with 10–30% skin detachment is called SJS/TEN overlap syndrome and has a lethality of ~21%.

SJS/TEN are clearly different from erythema exudativum multiforme, which is mainly caused by viral infections,[3] is often recurrent, and affects younger persons (mean age 24 years). In ~6% no drug treatment was given in the week before SJS/TEN started and an infectious origin (*Mycoplasma pneumoniae, Klebsiella pneumoniae*) was suspected. SJS/TEN can also be due to graft-versus-host disease. Most reactions start within the first 8 weeks of treatment (mean onset of symptoms at about 17 days), with some differences according to the causing drug (e.g., it may appear later with sulfonamide antibiotics).

SJS/TEN can develop quite rapidly. Initially a macular, purple-red exanthem is often be observed, which can become painful—an ominous sign. Within 12–24 hours bullae may be seen, and the Nikolsky sign is positive (Table 46.3). Stopping drug treatment at this stage may not prevent SJS developing, but might prevent progression to an even more severe reaction (TEN). Mucous membranes (mouth, genitalia) are involved with blister formation, as well as a purulent keratoconjunctivitis with formation of synechiae, which may result in permanent eye damage.

The main causes for SJS/TEN are drugs (Table 46.2), which appear to differ in frequency in various regions due to genetic and ethnic background. Important risk factors are HIV infection (low CD4, high CD8 counts), renal disease, and active systemic autoimmune diseases such as systemic lupus erythematosus, Still's syndrome, Sjögren's disease, and rheumatoid arthritis. In biopsies of

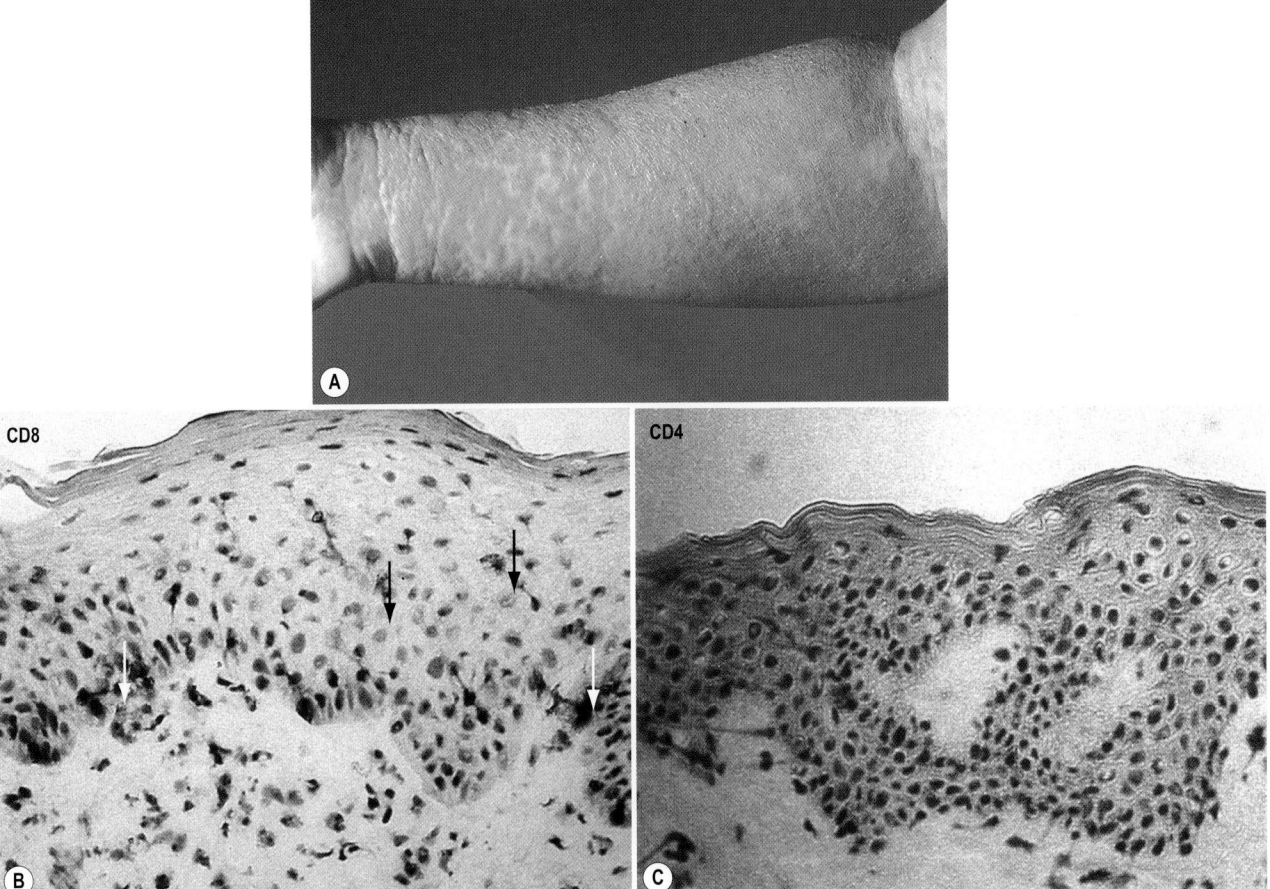

Fig. 46.8 Clinical pictures and immunohistologies of drug-induced exanthem. Bullous drug eruption (A) with some blisters exhibiting more intraepidermal CD8 cell infiltration (B) than CD4 T cells (C) by immunohistology.

From Hari Y, Frutig-Schnyder K, Hunmi M, et al. T cell involvement in cutaneous drug eruptions. Clin Exp Allergy 2001; 31: 1398–1408, with permission from Blackwell Publishing.

Table 46.3 Clinical and laboratory investigations and *danger signs*[a] in drug-induced exanthems

Clinic	Laboratory
Extent and type of exanthem (infiltration, *bullae, pustules*) *Pain of skin, Nikolsky sign*	Eosinophilia (> 1000–1200/μL[b]); *atypical (activated) lymphocytes in the circulation* (> 2%[b])
Involvement of mucous membranes	C-reactive protein elevation
Systemic symptoms (malaise, fever) *Lymphadenopathy, hepatosplenomegaly*	Liver enzymes (ALAT, ASAT, γGT, AP) (increase > 2–3 ×[b]) additional investigations depend on clinical signs, liver, kidney, lung, pancreas involvement (urine analysis, creatinine)

[a] *Danger signs in italics.*
[b] The cut-off values of the laboratory parameters are estimates, and are not based on prospective studies; severe reactions can also develop in the absence of these signs!

TEN lesions, many dead keratinocytes are found, but there is little cellular infiltration. However, the bullae may be filled by cytotoxic CD8 T cells, expressing CD56 and $\alpha\beta$-TCRs, which kill via granulysin and perforin/granzyme B but not via the Fas-mediated pathway at this stage of the disease.[18] On the other hand, the massive cell death of keratinocytes is hard to reconcile with a cell contact-dependent killing process. It has been proposed that the apoptosis of keratinocytes is due to FasL, a soluble molecule of the TNF family, which binds to keratinocytes via Fas and functions as a so-called death receptor.[28] Since blocking anti-Fas antibodies are found in immunoglobulin preparations, it has been proposed to treat patients with TEN with intravenous immunoglobulin, but the efficacy of this therapy is still unproven.[29]

Recent data have revealed striking HLA associations of severe, CD8-mediated drug hypersensitivity reactions.[30–32] These associations were found only with certain drugs: The HLA-allele B*1502 is common in Chinese/east Asian populations and strikingly associated with carbamazepine-induced SJS/TEN; in European and Japanese HLA-B*1502 is almost absent, and carbamazepine-allergic patients often carry HLA-A*3101.[33,34] Patients with severe allopurinol hypersensitivity reactions and/or SJS/TEN often (~70%) carry HLA-B*5801. It has been well documented that in these strongly HLA-related reactions the drug itself, and not a metabolite, binds to the HLA molecule (carbamazepine, but also abacavir). Recent data have suggested that a disease only develops if the patients expresses TCR with a certain CDR3 region.[35]

The extremely frequent association of certain HLA-alleles with hypersensitivity reactions to particular drugs is already being used to prevent such side effects in the case of reactions to carbamazepine and abacavir, since HLA-typing can be used to identify patients at risk.[36]

Systemic drug reactions – severe drug hypersensitivity syndromes

Some drugs are known to cause severe systemic disease, with fever, lymph node swelling, massive hepatitis, and various forms of exanthemata (Table 46.2). A few patients develop colitis, pancreatitis, or interstitial lung disease.[37] Over 70% have a marked eosinophilia (often > 10^{12}/L), and activated lymphocytes are often found in the circulation, similar to acute HIV or generalized herpes virus infections. This syndrome has many names. The most frequently used are drug (induced) hypersensitivity syndrome (DHS or DiHS) or drug rash with eosinophilia and systemic symptoms (DRESS). Importantly, the symptoms can begin up to

12 weeks after starting treatment, often after a dose increase, and may then persist and recur for many weeks, even after cessation of the culprit drug. The clinical picture resembles a generalized viral infection (e.g. acute Epstein–Barr virus infection), but it is distinguished by the prominent eosinophilia. Many patients have facial swelling, and some have signs of a capillary leak syndrome, similar to patients experiencing a cytokine release syndrome. Indeed, various cytokines are massively increased in the serum of these patients. As the clinical picture is quite dramatic and as the disease tends to persist in spite of stopping drug treatment, many patients *are not diagnosed correctly or in a timely manner.* However, physicians using anticonvulsants should be familiar with this syndrome, as it occurs in about 1:3000 treated patients. The mortality is ~10%, and some patients require emergency liver transplantation.

Patients with DHS/DRESS have many activated T cells in their circulation. These drug-specific T cells are stimulated by the parent compound (p-i concept) and they secrete large amounts of IL-5 and IFN-γ.[38] A peculiar feature of this syndrome is its long-lasting clinical course despite withdrawal of the causative drug. There can also be persistent intolerance to other, chemically distinct drugs, leading to flare-up reactions to what are normally innocuous drugs (e.g., acetaminophen) months after stopping the initial drug therapy, further adding to the confusion. Treatment often requires high doses of corticosteroids, particularly if the hepatitis is severe.

Recently it has been shown that in many patients with this syndrome, human herpes virus 6 DNA can be found during the third or fourth week of the disease (but not before), followed by a rising antibody titer to human herpes virus 6.[39] Other reports document reactivation of cytomegalovirus infection. Thus, similar to HIV, where T-cell activation can also enhance virus production, the drug-induced massive immune stimulation may somehow reactivate these latent lymphotropic herpes viruses, which subsequently replicate and possibly contribute to the chronic course and persistent drug intolerance in affected patients.

Many drugs can induce isolated hepatitis and some (penicillins, proton pump inhibitors, quinolones, disulfiram) can cause an isolated (interstitial) nephritis. Rarely interstitial lung diseases (furadantin), pancreatitis, isolated fever, or eosinophilia can present as the only symptom of a drug allergy. In drug-induced interstitial nephritis eosinophils can sometimes be detected in the urine (even in the absence of blood eosinophilia).

Multiple drug hypersensitivity syndrome

The term "multiple drug hypersensitivity" is used to describe different forms of side effects to multiple drugs. Some physicians use the term to characterize patients with multiple drug intolerance ("pseudoallergy" to NSAID), others reserve this term for well-documented repeated immune-mediated reactions to structurally unrelated drugs.[40] Cross-reactivity due to structural similarity is excluded from the definition.

In our experience, about 10% of patients with well-documented drug hypersensitivity (skin and/or lymphocyte transformation test positive) have multiple drug allergies.[41] For example, they may have reacted to injected lidocaine with angioedema and years later they develop contact allergy to corticosteroids. Alternatively, a patient reacts to amoxicillin, phenytoin, and sulfamethoxazole within a few months, but with different symptoms (MPE, DiHS/DRESS, erythroderma). Most of these patients have had rather severe reactions to at least one drug. An IgE-mediated reaction might be followed by a T-cell-mediated reaction. In a recent publication it was shown that patients with this syndrome have more circulating activated T cells, which contain the drug-reactive T cells. The cause for this *in vivo* activation is unknown.[55]

Multiple drug hypersensitivity should be differentiated from flare-up reactions.[42] In patients with systemic drug allergies, the T-cell immune system is massively activated, similar to acute viral infections. As in the latter, these patients seem to have a higher tendency to react to a new drug and might show a flare-up of their rash to a new antibiotic, but the second drug remains negative in skin tests and is later well tolerated, if the co-stimulatory conditions are no longer present.

Diagnosis of drug hypersensitivity

The diagnosis of drug hypersensitivity addresses three questions: (1) Is it a drug hypersensitivity? (2) Which mechanism might be involved? and (3) Which drug has caused it? The symptoms can be extremely heterogeneous, and in a patient with "bizarre" symptoms a drug hypersensitivity reaction should always be included in the differential diagnosis! On the other hand, some of the above-described skin exanthems are rather typical for drug hypersensitivity and easy to recognize.

Clinical diagnosis

Drug hypersensitivity is often suspected if a "rash" appears. Differential diagnosis of this rash includes viral exanthems, occasionally other infections, food allergy, and a graft-versus-host reaction. Pruritus, blood eosinophilia, and recent administration of a new drug argue for an allergic reaction.

It is important to document the severity of the presumed drug hypersensitivity, as this may determine whether the drug can be given again. Special attention should be paid to the type and extent of skin symptoms, the involvement of mucosal areas, lymph node enlargement, fever, and subjective symptoms like malaise, as this could indicate involvement of internal organs. A painful

---

⬤ THERAPEUTIC PRINCIPLES

Cross-reactivity

- The risk of cross-reactivity depends on the type of reaction.
- In nonsteroidal anti-inflammatory drug-induced "pseudoallergy," cross-reactivity seems to be due to the pharmacological action and not the structure.
- IgE-mediated reactions have a higher degree of cross-reactivity than T-cell reactions, probably because antibodies can recognize small molecular components, whereas T cells tend to recognize the complete structure.
- Cross-reactivity of T cell and antibodies is common within the same class of drugs (e.g., penicillins, quinolones, pyrazolones, cephalosporins).

Penicillin–cephalosporin cross-reactivity

- Not seen in T-cell-mediated reactions (maculopapular exanthem); in IgE-mediated reactions cross-reactivity might occur in ~4% of penicillin skin test-positive patients with first- and second-generation cephalosporins. The chance of cross-reactivity is very low if the second drug is negative in skin tests.

Sulfonamide cross-reactivity

- There is an extensive cross-reactivity between sulfonamide-containing antibacterials (sulfanilamides), which mainly induce sensitization, but not with other drugs containing a sulfonamide (e.g., furosemide, celecoxib, glibencamide).

---

skin and a positive Nikolsky sign might herald a severe bullous skin reaction, which can develop within hours. One should be aware of danger signs (Table 46.3) and the most important elicitors of SJS/TEN and DRESS (Table 46.2). Some patients have no skin involvement, but develop an isolated drug-allergic hepatitis or interstitial nephritis.

Different mechanisms can lead to drug hypersensitivity symptoms. They should be differentiated, as they need distinct diagnostic steps and can have a different prognosis; the combination of symptoms and time course usually helps to discriminate them. Immediate reactions start < 1 hour after drug intake and are usually IgE-mediated (or due to drug-induced mast-cell release). Occasionally, IgE-mediated reactions occur later than 1 hour. Typical symptoms are urticaria and anaphylaxis. Delayed reactions start >12 hours after drug intake and are mostly non-IgE-mediated, but involve T-cell orchestrated inflammation or IgG-mediated reactions. In highly sensitized individuals symptoms can arise as early as 2–4 hours after drug intake—the more drug-specific precursor T cells are present, the more rapidly symptoms may appear.

Laboratory investigations can also help to determine the severity of the reaction. In more severe acute reactions tryptase levels should be determined, optimally between 2 and 4 hours after the peak of the reaction to confirm mast cell involvement. The analysis should be repeated later (>2 days) to rule out a constitutively elevated tryptase level (mastocytosis). Such measurements are particularly important if anaphylaxis is suspected during anesthesia, where the sole sign of anaphylaxis might be cardiac arrest, without skin symptoms.

In delayed reactions a differential blood count may reveal activated lymphocytes and eosinophilia, which is common in drug hypersensitivity (observed in up to ~40% of patients with MPE, in 30% with AGEP (together with leukocytosis, and in > 70% in DiHS/DRESS). Measurements of liver enzymes (ALAT, ASAT, ALP, and γGT) should be done in patients with malaise, in those with extensive skin involvement, or if drugs known to cause DiHS/DRESS or hepatitis/cholestasis are involved. A transient mild hepatitis is not rare and seems to occur in ~25% of patients with more severe MPE.[24] Dependent on the symptoms other tests may also be indicated (creatinine, urinary analysis). C-reactive protein (CRP) may be elevated (e.g., in drug-induced interstitial lung or kidney diseases), but can be normal even in severe hypersensitivity reactions like DiHS/DRESS.

Identifying the culprit drug

The important questions are: Which drugs were taken, and since when? Was the dose increased? Are there co-medications? And could they possibly interfere with drug metabolism? How were the drugs tolerated previously? Were other drugs tolerated that are known to cause similar effects? What was the underlying disease? Have similar reactions already occurred previously without or with drugs? Books listing side effects, websites (e.g., http://www.pneumotox.com) and pharmaceutical companies can provide information about the known side effects of a drug. In many instances, the history and these sources may allow a rather conclusive allocation of symptoms and drug intake. However, many patients have taken several drugs and the history alone may be insufficient. In these cases further tests can be justified, although these are often not well validated.

The *in vivo* (skin test) and *in vitro* tests for drug allergy diagnosis are difficult to standardize. Although drug allergy is common it only occurs rarely for each individual drug; a single drug might elicit different symptoms, requiring different tests;

provocation tests—which would prove the allergy and the sensitivity of the test—are often not performed for ethical reasons, and for some tests living cells are needed rather than serum, which requires a greater logistic effort. Despite these obstacles, many groups perform tests, but two rules are important: (1) the test can only supplement the history; and (2) the sensitivity of the tests is generally low, while the specificity is high, so a positive test may be more meaningful than a negative test, which cannot rule out a drug allergy.

For investigating immediate reactions, both prick and intradermal tests are available. Penicillin tests are widely used. To form repetitive determinants able to cross-link two FcεRI-bound IgE molecules, the drug is coupled to poly-lysine, either by opening the penicillin-ring and forming penicilloyl-carriers, or by binding via the thiol structure (minor components). The pure substance (e.g., amoxicillin) can also be evaluated, since it frequently gives positive skin tests as well. The sensitivity of these tests is controversial: older studies from the USA suggested a sensitivity of > 95%; but more recent studies from Spain found only 70%.[43] Other drugs can be tested as well by prick or intradermal tests, but false-positive reactions (e.g., to quinolones) can occur and it is essential to test control individuals as well. Further information on test procedures and concentrations is available elsewhere.[44]

In vitro tests for immediate reactions include the determination of specific IgE. However, availability of such tests is very limited and the sensitivity of commercial assays for drug-specific IgE appears to be rather low. Various read-out systems for basophil degranulation/activation tests have been proposed to be usable for drug hypersensitivity diagnosis (e.g., Flow-Cast). Sensitivity in IgE-mediated reactions is reported to be ~40%.[45]

In Europe it is common to perform patch tests for delayed reactions (e.g., for contact dermatitis).[46] The overall sensitivity is considered to be < 50%[46] and depends on the disease (often negative in macular reactions, and delayed urticarial exanthems, but more useful in severe MPE, DiHS/DRESS, AGEP: Fig. 46.7). This is a reliable test for abacavir hypersensitivity, even if only hepatitis occurs.

⬤THERAPEUTIC PRINCIPLES

Treatment

- Stop drug(s).
- Avoid drugs, until culprit drug is identified.
- Avoid re-exposure to the drug class (cross-reactivity) in acute immunoglobulin E-mediated reactions, in acute "pseudoallergic" reactions, and in severe delayed reactions.
- Symptomatic treatment according to symptoms.
- Avoid treating through with drugs known to cause toxic epidermal necrolysis, drug-induced hypersensitivity syndrome or drug rash with eosinophilia and systemic symptoms, or if danger signs are present.

The lymphocyte transformation (proliferation/activation) test (LTT) relies on the activation and proliferation of T cells cultured in the presence of the drug.[47] Reactivity can be measured by ^{3}H-thymidine incorporation after 5- to 6-day culture, or by ELISPOT, CSFE staining, CD69 upregulation. LTT is cumbersome, but a clearly positive value is useful. The sensitivity of LTT depends on the pathophysiologic mechanism of the drug hypersensitivity and is > 90% for DiHS/DRESS, but lower in more cytotoxic reactions like SJS/TEN (<25%). LTT is positive in drugs sensitizing via the hapten mechanism or stimulated via the p-i concept.

Provocation tests are considered to be the gold standard for the diagnosis. They are useful for immediate reactions, but less so for

delayed reactions, since 7–10 days of treatment may be required to provoke the same allergy symptoms.[48,49] Co-factors are often important in the initial event, and these are absent during provocation, while the dose needed to elicit symptoms will often not be reached. Thus one might be able to exclude immediate reactions to the dose used in the provocation test, but treatment with higher doses can still cause symptoms.

Therapeutic aspects

The therapy of drug hypersensitivity diseases is dependent on the symptoms and ranges from the usual treatment of anaphylaxis to acute liver transplantation. Stopping the possible culprit drugs and avoiding them until clarity is achieved should be possible in most circumstances and might reduce the development of more severe symptoms. In some milder skin reactions (e.g., non-bullous exanthem due to sulfamethoxazole in HIV-positive patients), experience has shown that continuation of treatment may be possible, whereas reintroducing the drug after stopping it may actually precipitate more severe symptoms.

Desensitization

In certain circumstances a drug that causes allergic or "pseudoallergic" side effects is essential for treatment, for example, penicillin to treat syphilis during pregnancy or certain cytostatic drugs in cancer treatments (e.g., cisplatin). Most desensitization protocols refer to hypersensitivity reactions involving mast cell degranulation, and the procedure is best established for penicillin and NSAIDs.[50,51]

The starting dose for desensitization is determined by the dose the patient tolerated in skin testing. This dose generally translates to 1:10 000 of the therapeutic dose. Doubling doses are administered every 15 minutes (usually via I.V. administration) until the full dose is reached. Once desensitization is completed, the patient can receive the full therapeutic course via the desired route. If treatment is discontinued for more than 48 hours, the patient will once more be at risk of developing anaphylaxis and the full desensitization protocol must be repeated (e.g., before each chemotherapy course).

In dubious, skin test-negative cases, where one actually expects *no* allergy, *graded drug challenges* under careful supervision can be used, starting with ~1/100 or 1/20 of the standard dose, and increasing the dose stepwise (double or triple) every 30–60 minutes. The full dose may be achieved in 1 day and can be continued during the next days.

References

1. Naisbitt DJ, Gordon SF, Pirmohamed M, et al. Immunological principles of adverse drug reactions: the initiation and propagation of immune responses elicited by drug treatment. Drug Saf 2000;23:483–507.
2. Lazarou J, Pomeranz BH, Corey PN. Incidence of adverse drug reactions in hospitalized patients: a meta-analysis of prospective studies. JAMA 1998;279:1200–5.
3. Roujeau JC, Stern RS. Severe adverse cutaneous reactions to drugs. N Engl J Med 1994;331:1272–85.
4. Bigby M, Jick S, Jick H, et al. Drug-induced cutaneous reactions. A report from the Boston Collaborative Drug Surveillance Program on 15 438 consecutive inpatients, 1975 to 1982. JAMA 1986;256:3358–63.
5. Hunziker T, Kunzi UP, Braunschweig S, et al. Comprehensive hospital drug monitoring (CHDM): adverse skin reactions, a 20-year survey. Allergy 1997;52:388–93.
6. Manfredi M, Severino M, Testi S, et al. Detection of specific IgE to quinolones. J Allergy Clin Immunol 2004;113:155–60.
7. Pichler WJ. Delayed drug hypersensitivity reactions. Ann Intern Med 2003;139:683–93.
8. Martin S, Weltzien HU. T cell recognition of haptens, a molecular view. Int Arch Allergy Immunol 1994;104:10–6.

9. Griem P, Wulferink M, Sachs B, et al. Allergic and autoimmune reactions to xenobiotics: how do they arise? Immunol Today 1998;19:133–41.

10. Zanni MP, von Greyerz S, Schnyder B, et al. HLA-restricted, processing- and metabolism-independent pathway of drug recognition by human alpha beta T lymphocytes. J Clin Invest 1998;102:1591–8.

11. Pichler WJ. Pharmacological interaction of drugs with antigen-specific immune receptors: the p-i concept. Curr Opin Allergy Clin Immunol 2002;2:301–5.

12. Coombs RR, Gell PG. Classification of allergic reactions responsible for clinical hypersensitivity and disease. In: Gell PG, editor. Clinical aspects of immunology. Oxford: Oxford University Press; 1976 p. 575–96.

13. Aster RH. Drug-induced immune thrombocytopenia: an overview of pathogenesis. Semin Hematol 1999;36:2–6.

14. Arndt PA, Garratty G. The changing spectrum of drug-induced immune hemolytic anemia. Semin Hematol 2005;42:137–44.

15. Greinacher A, Warkentin TE. Recognition, treatment, and prevention of heparin-induced thrombocytopenia: review and update. Thromb Res 2006;118:165–76.

16. Aitman TJ, Dong R, Vyse TJ, et al. Copy number polymorphism in Fcgr3 predisposes to glomerulonephritis in rats and humans. Nature 2006;439:851–5.

17. Stokol T, O'Donnell P, Xiao L, et al. C1q governs deposition of circulating immune complexes and leukocyte Fcgamma receptors mediate subsequent neutrophil recruitment. J Exp Med 2004;200:835–46.

18. Nassif A, Bensussan A, Dorothee G, et al. Drug specific cytotoxic T-cells in the skin lesions of a patient with toxic epidermal necrolysis. J Invest Dermatol 2002;118:728–33.

19. Schnyder B, Frutig K, Mauri-Hellweg D, et al. T-cell-mediated cytotoxicity against keratinocytes in sulfamethoxazol-induced skin reaction. Clin Exp Allergy 1998;28:1412–7.

20. Chung WH, Hung SI, Yang JY, et al. Granulysin is a key mediator for disseminated keratinocyte death in Stevens-Johnson syndrome and toxic epidermal necrolysis. Nat Med 2008;14(12):1343–50.

21. Britschgi M, Steiner UC, Schmid S, et al. T-cell involvement in drug-induced acute generalized exanthemtous pustulosis. J Clin Invest 2001;107:1433–41.

22. Keller M, Spanou Z, Schaerli P, et al. T cell-regulated neutrophilic inflammation in autoinflammatory diseases. J Immunol 2005;175:7678–86.

23. Beeler A, Engler O, Gerber BO, et al. Long-lasting reactivity and high frequency of drug-specific T cells after severe systemic drug hypersensitivity reactions. J Allergy Clin Immunol 2006;117:455–62.

24. Hari Y, Frutig-Schnyder K, Hurni M, et al. T cell involvement in cutaneous drug eruptions. Clin Exp Allergy 2001;31:1398–408.

25. Pichler WJ, Zanni M, von Greyerz S, et al. High IL-5 production by human drug-specific T cell clones. Int Arch Allergy Immunol 1997;113:177–80.

26. Hari Y, Urwyler A, Hurni M, et al. Distinct serum cytokine levels in drug- and measles-induced exanthem. Int Arch Allergy Immunol 1999;120:225–9.

27. Roujeau J, Bioulac-Sage P, Bourseau C. Acute generalized exanthematous pustulosis: analysis of 63 cases. Arch Dermatol 1991;127:1333–8.

28. Viard I, Wehrli P, Bullani R, et al. Inhibition of toxic epidermal necrolysis by blockade of CD95 with human intravenous immunoglobulin. Science 1998;282:490–493.

29. Bachot N, Roujeau JC. Intravenous immunoglobulins in the treatment of severe drug eruptions. Curr Opin Allergy Clin Immunol 2003;3:269–74.

30. Mallal S, Nolan D, Witt C, et al. Association between presence of HLA-B*5701, HLA-DR7, and HLA-DQ3 and hypersensitivity to HIV-1 reverse-transcriptase inhibitor abacavir. Lancet 2002;359:727–32.

31. Chung WH, Hung SI, Hong HS, et al. Medical genetics: a marker for Stevens–Johnson syndrome. Nature 2004;428:486.

32. Hung SI, Chung WH, Liou LB, et al. HLA-B*5801 allele as a genetic marker for severe cutaneous adverse reactions caused by allopurinol. Proc Natl Acad Sci U S A 2005;102:4134–9.

33. McCormack M, Alfirevic A, Bourgeois S, et al. HLA-A*3101 and carbamazepine-induced hypersensitivity reactions in Europeans. N Engl J Med 2011;364(12):1134–1143.

34. Ozeki T, Mushiroda T, Yowang A, et al. Genome-wide association study identifies HLA-A*3101 allele as a genetic risk factor for carbamazepine-induced cutaneous adverse drug reactions in Japanese population. Hum Mol Genet 2011;20(5):1034–41.

35. Yang CW, Hung SI, Juo CG, et al. HLA-B*1502-bound peptides: implications for the pathogenesis of carbamazepine-induced Stevens-Johnson syndrome. J Allergy Clin Immunol 2007;120(4):870–7.

36. Mallal S, Phillips E, Carosi G, et al, PREDICT-1 Study Team. HLA-B*5701 screening for hypersensitivity to abacavir. N Engl J Med 2008;358(6):568–79.

37. Knowles SR, Shapiro LE, Shear NH. Anticonvulsant hypersensitivity syndrome: incidence, prevention and management. Drug Saf 1999;21:489–501.

38. Naisbitt DJ, Farrell J, Wong G, et al. Characterization of drug-specific T cells in lamotrigine hypersensitivity. J Allergy Clin Immunol 2003;111:1393–403.

39. Hashimoto K, Yasukawa M, Tohyama M. Human herpesvirus 6 and drug allergy. Curr Opin Allergy Clin Immunol 2003;3:255–60.

40. Sullivan T. Studies of the multiple drug allergy syndrome. J Allergy Clin Immunol 1989;83:270.

41. Gex-Collet C, Helbling A, Pichler WJ. Multiple drug hypersensitivity—proof of multiple drug hypersensitivity by patch and lymphocyte transformation tests. J Investig Allergol Clin Immunol 2005;15:293–6.

42. Pichler WJ, Daubner B, Kawabata T. Drug hypersensitivity: flare-up reactions, cross-reactivity and multiple drug hypersensitivity. J Dermatol 2011;38(3):216–21.

43. Torres MJ, Blanca M, Fernandez J, et al. Diagnosis of immediate allergic reactions to beta-lactam antibiotics. Allergy 2003;58:961–72.

44. Brockow K, Romano A, Blanca M, et al. General considerations for skin test procedures in the diagnosis of drug hypersensitivity. Allergy 2002;57:45–51.

45. Sanz ML, Gamboa P, de Weck AL. A new combined test with flowcytometric basophil activation and determination of sulfidoleukotrienes is useful for in vitro diagnosis of hypersensitivity to aspirin and other nonsteroidal anti-inflammatory drugs. Int Arch Allergy Immunol 2005;136:58–72.

46. Barbaud A, Goncalo M, Bruynzeel D, et al. Guidelines for performing skin tests with drugs in the investigation of cutaneous adverse drug reactions. Contact Dermatitis 2001;45:321–8.

47. Pichler WJ, Tilch J. The lymphocyte transformation test in the diagnosis of drug hypersensitivity. Allergy 2004;59:809–20.

48. Aberer W, Bircher A, Romano A, et al. Drug provocation testing in the diagnosis of drug hypersensitivity reactions: general considerations. Allergy 2003;58:854–63.

49. Borch JE, Bindslev-Jensen C. Full-course drug challenge test in the diagnosis of delayed allergic reactions to penicillin. Int Arch Allergy Immunol 2011;155(3):271–4.

50. Solensky R. Drug allergy: desensitization and treatment of reactions to antibiotics and aspirin. Clin Immunol 2004;18:585–606.

51. Cernadas JR, Brockow K, Romano A, et al. European Network of Drug Allergy and the EAACI interest group on drug hypersensitivity. General considerations on rapid desensitization for drug hypersensitivity—a consensus statement. Allergy 2010;65(11):1357–66.

52. Illing PT, Vivian JP, Dudek NL, et al. Immune self-reactivity triggered by drug-modified HLA-peptide repertoire. Nature 2012;486(7404):554–8.

53. Norcross MA, Luo S, Lu L, Boyne MT, et al. Abacavir induces loading of novel self-peptides into HLA-B*57: 01: an autoimmune model for HLA-associated drug hypersensitivity. AIDS 2012;26(11):F21–F29.

54. Ostrov DA, Grant BJ, Pompeu YA, et al. Drug hypersensitivity caused by alteration of the MHC-presented self-peptide repertoire. Proc Natl Acad Sci U S A 2012;109(25):9959–66.

55. Daubner B, Groux-Keller M, Hausmann OV, et al. Multiple drug hypersensitivity: normal Treg cell function but enhanced in vivo activation of drug-specific T cells. Allergy 2012;67(1):58–66.

Jean-Luc Malo | # Occupational asthma

While environmental allergens are ubiquitous and most often present from the very first breath that a human being takes at birth, occupational allergens are specific to a particular working environment and exposure to occupational allergens starts in adult life. Environmental allergens are generally proteins or protein derivatives, whereas occupational allergens can be proteins, protein derivatives (high-molecular-weight agents), or chemicals (low-molecular-weight allergens). Although the allergic mechanism has been elucidated in the case of proteinaceous materials, this generally remains uncertain for most occupational chemicals.

Rhinitis and asthma induced by occupational agents represent an interesting conceptual model of the development and natural history of asthma in humans: subjects can be assessed prospectively with the assessment of risk markers and factors before exposure starts, at the time of sensitization and onset of symptoms, and serially after ending exposure.[1,2] Such a model cannot be considered for environmental allergens because exposure begins at birth and cannot be interrupted nor controlled.

Historical aspects and definitions

● KEY CONCEPTS

Definitions and diagnosis

- Work-related asthma includes:
  - Asthma caused by occupational sensitization.
  - Asthma aggravated by workplace conditions.
- For some agents direct sensitization can be shown on skin tests.
- For others, there is no satisfactory allergen extract.
- Some causes do not involve IgE so no skin test is likely to become available.

The influence of the working environment on the onset of asthma was recognized long ago, especially by Ramazzini in the early eighteenth century who described the occurrence of respiratory symptoms in cereal handlers.[3] Several proteinaceous substances (flours, beans, gums, insects) and metallic agents (chromium, platinum) present in the workplace and causing asthma were described in the beginning of the twentieth century and it was recognized from the 1940s onwards that chemicals such as phthalic anhydride and diisocyanates can cause sensitization.[3] Reproduction of asthmatic reactions by exposing workers in the laboratory to agents present in their workplace was pioneered by Pepys and led to the identification of many causal agents as well as creating great interest in the occurrence of late asthmatic reactions, an important

cornerstone in the physiopathology of asthma.[4] Finally, it was in the twentieth century that the deleterious respiratory consequences of inhalational accidents in the workplace were recognized and their acute and long-term asthmogenic effects described.[5]

It has been estimated that nearly 10% of asthmatic workers report that their asthma gets worse in the workplace, loosely termed as "asthma in the workplace."[6] This label encompasses two distinct conditions, one in which pre-existing asthma is exacerbated in the workplace, and the other condition being true occupational asthma (OA), that is asthma caused by the workplace. A modern definition of occupational asthma is "a disease characterized by variable airflow limitation and/or airway hyper-responsiveness and/or airway inflammation due to causes and conditions attributable to a particular occupational environment and not to stimuli encountered outside the workplace."[7] Two types of OA are distinguished by whether they appear after a latency period. In the case of the immunologic type, there is a latency period between exposure and the development of symptoms; the immunologic mechanism has been identified for most high- and for some low-molecular weight agents (Table 47.1). The non-immunologic type encompasses irritant-induced asthma (IrIA) or reactive airways dysfunction syndrome (RADS), which may occur after single or multiple exposures, generally accidental, to nonspecific irritants at high concentrations.[8]

Physiopathology

OA can be differentiated into immunologically or non-immunologically mediated forms. Immunologically mediated OA is characterized by a latency period that is necessary for acquiring sensitization, whereas non-immunologically mediated OA has no latency period and follows inhalational accidents.

● KEY CONCEPTS

Pathogenesis of occupational asthma

- OA is caused by two main mechanisms: immunologic sensitization and irritant-induced inflammation.
- Most patients with allergic OA will have associated nasal and ocular symptoms.
- Allergic forms of OA involve the same cellular mechanisms as "ordinary" atopic asthma, with activation of mast cells, eosinophil, and T cells, together with mucous hypersecretion and epithelial damage.
- More than one mechanism may be triggered by a single inciting agent.
- Pathological changes associated with OA may improve or resolve fully after cessation of exposure.

Table 47.1 Major causes of immunologic and non-immunologic occupational asthma

Immunologic
High-molecular-weight agents
Plant-derived products: cereals, flour
Animal-derived allergens: laboratory animals, enzymes
Enzymes
Seafood
Low-molecular-weight agents
IgE-dependent causes
Acid anhydrides
Metals
Other potential immunologic mechanisms
Diisocyanates
Wood dusts
Amines and epoxy resins
Colophony
Acrylates
Pharmaceutical products
Formaldehyde, glutaradehyde, biocides
Persulfate salts
Acid anhydrides
Reactive dyes
Non-immunogic
Ammonia, chlorine

Immunologic, IgE-mediated OA

High-molecular-weight occupational agents act as complete antigens and induce specific IgE antibody production that can be documented by immediate skin reactivity and increased specific IgE levels. Some low-molecular-weight occupational agents, including platinum and other metal salts, various acid anhydrides, can also induce specific IgE and IgG antibodies. They probably act as haptens and bind with autologous proteins to form complete antigens. The modified proteins are processed and displayed on the surface of antigen-presenting cells as hapten-conjugated peptides bound to major histocompatibility molecules (Chapter 6), whereupon they induce a T-cell response that leads to production of several interleukins and consequent specific IgE antibody responses by B cells.[9]

Immunologic, non-IgE-mediated OA

Many low molecular weight agents, including diisocyanates and plicatic acid (the agent causing asthma due to Western red cedar), cause OA but these do not consistently induce specific IgE antibodies.[9] Diisocyanate-induced OA is associated with the presence of specific IgG and antigen-stimulated monocyte chemoattractant protein-1 synthesis.[10]

Bronchial biopsy specimens from subjects with OA obtained at the time of diagnosis have shown activation of T lymphocytes. Although asthma and OA have both been identified as diseases in which eosinophilic inflammation plays a key role, neutrophils are also present in the airways.[11]

Non-immunologic OA

OA resulting from non-immunologic mechanisms occurs without a latent period. The underlying mechanism of IrIA is not known. It has been postulated that the extensive denudation of the epithelium in these conditions leads to airway inflammation and airway hyper-responsiveness.[8] Sequential changes have been described in the airways of a subject with IrIA.[12] In the acute phase of IrIA, there is rapid denudation of the mucosa with fibrinohemorrhagic exudate in the submucosa, regeneration of the epithelium with proliferation of basal and parabasal cells, and subepithelial edema.[9] Similar events have been documented in animal models of IrIA.

The pathology in the airways of subjects with immunologic OA is the same as for non-occupational asthma either in the short term or in the long term after cessation of exposure. In the case of non-immunologic OA, there is more subepithelial fibrosis in either the short[8] or the long term,[13] which is probably responsible for the reduced reversibility of airflow obstruction observed in IrIA.[8]

Epidemiology of OA

Frequency

A meta-analysis of several large population-based studies of asthma, including information on the occupation, estimated that the median population attributable risk of asthma related to the workplace was 17.6%.[6] In the European Community Respiratory Health Survey,[14] the population-attributable risk for adult asthma due to occupational exposures ranges from 10 to 25%.[15] A study carried out in six communities in Canada showed that the frequency of possible and probable OA was as high as 36.1% (95%CI = 31.3–41.0%).[16] The major limitation of all population studies is the lack of objective confirmation of OA;[17] in other words the studies rarely ascertain the proportion of asthma in the workplace that really represents OA. At least two studies have also delineated the frequency of the immunologic and non-immunologic types of asthma in the workplace from population-based information.[15,18]

National registers are useful for assessing the frequency of OA as shown in studies carried out in Scandinavian countries.[19] Such studies have documented increased risks in occupations such as cleaners and construction workers. Data based on medicolegal agencies or compensation boards usually underestimate the true incidence of OA since some workers may not wish to apply to such agencies and the criteria used for accepting claims differ from one country to the next. In Quebec, where the diagnosis of OA is generally confirmed by specific inhalation challenges, the incidence of OA is 10–15 new cases/year per million workers.[20] Sentinel projects of self-reported cases by specialized physicians have been proposed. With the exceptions of the SWORD project in the UK and the SENSOR project in six of the United States, most have been in existence for a short time. The SWORD project has shown a stable incidence of OA in UK with some changes in the responsible agents.[21] IrIA represented 13.8% of all OA cases reported in four states included in the SENSOR project.[22] Another source of useful information on the frequency of OA is from medical practice. In a tertiary care clinic, approximately 15% of asthmatic subjects were probable cases of OA.[23]

Cross-sectional workforce-based surveys are the most common source of frequency estimates in at-risk workplaces. The prevalence of OA caused by high-molecular-weight agents is generally <5% and 5–10% by low-molecular-weight agents. Prospective studies offer a more satisfactory way for estimating frequency although they are more expensive and demanding.

Gautrin and co-workers have carried out several longitudinal studies of apprentices entering programs in which they were exposed to various high-[24,25] and low-molecular-weight occupational agents.[26,27] These investigators more recently described the long-term outcome of the apprentices 10 years after entering the workforce,[28] some of them losing sensitization acquired during their training and some being newly sensitized. Incident sensitization was less frequent than during the apprenticeship period, which suggests that surveillance programs should be advocated in the first years after starting exposure.

Exposure and host factors

There is a dose–response relationship between the degree of exposure and the development of OA. In recent years, assessment of the working environment has improved due to improvement in methodology (immunologic techniques) and the use of personal sampling.[29] The likelihood for a given low-molecular-weight agent to cause sensitization can be predicted by referring to a structure-activity index,[30] which is useful for new chemical agents that are steadily introduced in the working environment. Although the level of exposure is an essential factor for development of OA, given the same level of exposure only a small proportion of workers developed sensitization or OA. Several host susceptibility factors have been implicated. For high-molecular-weight agents, atopy has been found consistently to be associated with the development of OA although the level of association is generally low. Smoking has been associated with the development of OA in workers exposed to some occupational agents.

Genetic predisposition

Studies of OA due to high-molecular-weight allergens have not found any strong associations with HLA allelic inheritance. An excess of HLA-DR3 and a deficit of HLA-DR6 have been reported in skin test-positive platinum refinery workers compared with controls matched for intensity and duration of exposure and ethnic background.[31] Studies of laboratory animal workers have found twice the prevalence of HLA-DR4 and HLA-B15 in cases with laboratory animal allergy compared to healthy controls.[32] Studies in diisocyanate-induced asthma have shown that alleles within the HLA class II region appear to be associated with increased or decreased risk of disease although this finding has not been consistently reproduced.[33,34] Polymorphism of glutathione S-transferase P1 (GSTP1) has also been associated with diisocyanate-induced asthma.[35]

The natural history of OA is illustrated in Fig. 47.1. Sensitization to work-related allergens occurs mainly during the first 2 years after starting exposure in apprentices exposed to laboratory animals. The incidence–density of rhinoconjunctivitis symptoms is greater in years 1 and 2 after starting exposure, whereas onset of respiratory symptoms is greater in years 2 and 3.[1]

Clinical aspects

It is important to confirm OA by objective testing. An open questionnaire administered during a medical consultation has a reasonable sensitivity but lacks specificity. Diagnosing OA on the basis of a compatible history alone is unacceptable because the diagnosis of OA carries significant social and financial consequences. Unlike pneumoconiosis, subjects with OA tend to be young. Keeping at work a worker whose asthma is caused by the workplace leads to worsening of asthma, and deaths from asthma have been reported in subjects who continue to be exposed with symptoms. The longer a worker with OA remains exposed to the causal agent, the more likely he/she will be left with permanent asthma after removal from exposure.[20]

OA should be suspected in every adult with new-onset asthma. A good occupational history should cover not only the current job and exposure but also past jobs and exposures. In many cases the patient may not be aware of the exact chemical exposures at work. Material safety data sheets can be requested from the workplace and may be of help in clarifying the presence of a workplace sensitizer, although not all information is necessarily declared in this documentation. Rhinoconjunctivitis symptoms can precede the onset of asthma symptoms in workers who develop asthma due to high-molecular-weight agents, but this does not occur with the low-molecular-weight agents.[36] A typical history of OA includes the appearance or worsening of asthma symptoms at work and their disappearance or improvement away from work. However, this pattern is frequently obscured, especially when affected workers continue to be exposed to the sensitizing agent. Under such conditions, remission of symptoms in the evenings or during weekends tends to disappear, and much longer periods off work are necessary for improvement to take place. Thus, OA often remains unrecognized by the affected workers and their physicians, the diagnosis being usually made 2 to 4 years after the onset of symptoms.

There has been considerable literature on the diagnosis of OA and consensus guidelines have been proposed, although they are not necessarily followed.[37] Figure 47.2 shows an algorithm that

Stages:

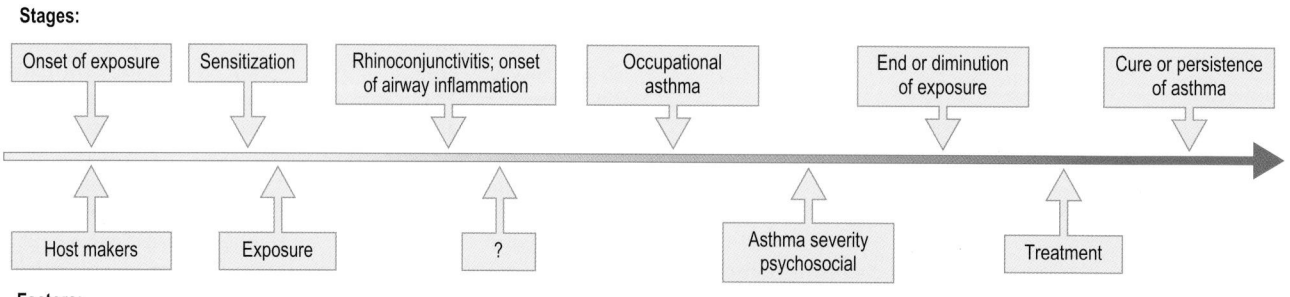

Factors:

Fig. 47.1 Stages in the development of occupational allergic sensitization and asthma, with factors shown that may influence the evolution or persistence of disease.

Fig. 47.2 Stepwise scheme of investigation of work-related asthma.

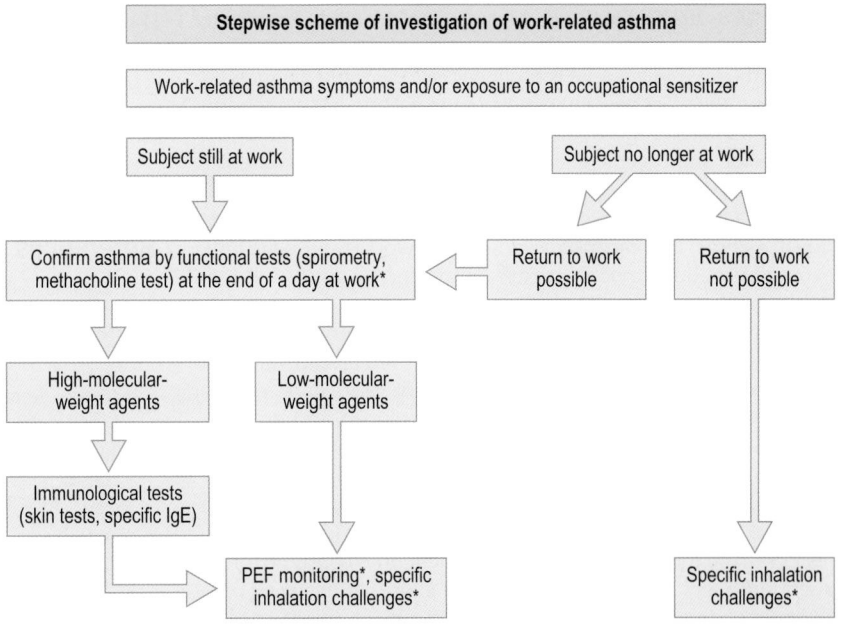

Stepwise scheme of investigation of work-related asthma

Work-related asthma symptoms and/or exposure to an occupational sensitizer

Subject still at work | Subject no longer at work

Confirm asthma by functional tests (spirometry, methacholine test) at the end of a day at work* ← Return to work possible | Return to work not possible

High-molecular-weight agents | Low-molecular-weight agents

Immunological tests (skin tests, specific IgE)

PEF monitoring*, specific inhalation challenges* | Specific inhalation challenges*

* Assessment of airway inflammation (sputum, exhaled NO) and nasal tests (lavage, rhinometry) can be added in the investigation process.

is proposed in approaching a patient with work-related asthmatic symptoms. A negative methacholine challenge test does not exclude OA if performed when the patient is off work and free of symptoms. However, if the challenge test is performed when the patient is working and symptomatic, the diagnosis of OA can be excluded, except in patients with eosinophilic bronchitis.[38]

Serial measurement of peak expiratory flows (PEF) with the subject at work and away from work with online interpretation of graphs has been found useful in obtaining objective information on OA,[39] although compliance can be poor and there is imperfect correspondence with results of specific inhalation challenges.[40]

Occupational-specific laboratory challenge tests are performed in relatively few centers. Although still considered a gold standard for diagnosis of OA, there is potential for false-positive and false-negative responses. A false-negative response can occur if the wrong agent is used, if the exposure conditions are not comparable to those in the workplace, or if the subject has been away from work for a long time (though complete desensitization is uncommon). Methods for specific challenge tests have been described in detail elsewhere[41] and improved equipment to make tests safer is available.[42]

Immunologic tests in the diagnosis of OA are limited by the lack of commercially available or standardized reagents for skin testing and assessment of specific IgE antibodies. Measurement of exhaled nitric oxide and induced sputum analysis have been tested in the investigation of OA. Evaluation of sputum eosinophil levels is a satisfactory adjunct to peak expiratory flow rate interpretation[40] and levels of nonspecific airway responsiveness.[43]

The diagnosis of IrI OA/RADS is entirely based on the clinical history and the demonstration of airway obstruction and/or hyper-responsiveness. There should be a history of a single (in some instances, multiple) high exposure to an irritant product with respiratory symptoms (mainly coughing) appearing shortly after the event.[44]

●KEY CONCEPTS

Implications of occupational asthma

Where possible, sensitization thresholds for major occupational agents that will reduce or abolish the likelihood of sensitization are needed.

Once established, occupational asthma has serious economic and psychological impacts on the patient. Accurate diagnosis is essential to make sure workers are removed when appropriate but not removed from the workplace incorrectly.

A diagnosis of occupational allergy is likely to be subjected to medicolegal scrutiny

Criteria for the diagnosis of irritant-induced asthma (reactive airways dysfunction syndrome)[44]

- Symptoms simulating asthma with wheeze, cough, and dyspnea
- Absence of preceding respiratory complaints
- Exposure to high concentrations of a gas, smoke, fume, or vapor with irritant properties
- Onset of symptoms, after single-exposure incident or accident
- Onset within 24 hours of exposure
- Persistence of symptoms for at least 3 months
- Airflow obstruction on pulmonary function tests and/or non-specific bronchial hyper-responsiveness
- Exclusion of all other pulmonary disease

Medicolegal aspects and surveillance

Medicolegal agencies should require objective testing before accepting a claim for OA. Once this essential step has been taken, proper rehabilitation programs should be offered with possible retraining in the first 2 years in the case of workers who cannot work in the same environment. The median cost of the program had been estimated to be CAN\$60 000 for each case of OA for the period 1988–2002.[45] Quality of life is only moderately inferior to asthma patients with the same severity of asthma although there are significant psychosocial consequences.[46] Once the diagnosis is made and the worker is removed from exposure, the early addition of inhaled steroids to the asthma treatment program may accelerate the improvement in bronchial hyper-responsiveness.[47] Keeping the worker at work with protective devices or inhaled steroid treatment can help, but commonly still leads to deterioration of asthma. In some instances, for those workers who are only exposed part-time to occupational sensitizers the use of full-face masks can be considered.

Approximately 75% of workers with OA are left with permanent bronchial hyper-responsiveness even after removal from exposure to the causal agent.[20] Scales for assessing impairment/disability for asthma have been developed and are now widely employed.[48] Three factors are considered in the assessment: airway caliber, airway responsiveness, and the need for medication to adequately control asthma. Workers should be assessed 2 years after cessation of exposure as improvement is faster during the first 2 years; improvement does continue thereafter, although at a slower pace.[49] The factor that has been consistently shown to be the most important in the persistence of asthma is the duration of exposure with symptoms.

Unlike subjects with immunologic OA, workers with acute IrIA may be able to continue in their usual jobs if the risk of accidental high-level exposures is prevented through engineering controls.

Primary prevention programs should be implemented for OA in high-risk workplaces just as they have been in the case of inorganic dusts (silica and asbestos fibers). The most important measure is to reduce the level of exposure. Permissible exposure limits should be established for all high-risk agents for OA,[50] as in bakeries,[51] for which a permissible exposure limit of 0.5 mg/m³ has been proposed. However, once a subject develops OA, he or she may react symptomatically to much lower levels of exposure than the level that led to sensitization.

Because of the low predictive value of atopy for the development of rhinoconjunctivitis and asthma and because nearly 50% of young adults are atopic, atopic subjects should not be excluded from high-risk workplaces. Smoking should be discouraged in all workplaces. Nasal symptoms should be considered as a concomitant or predisposing marker of the development of lower respiratory tract symptoms.[52]

Expected advances and research opportunities

● ON THE HORIZON

- Identification of genetic determinants that predispose to OA.
- Improved understanding of the irritant and potential long-term asthmagenic properties of pollutants and chemicals present in the workplace.
- Better ways of assessing airways inflammation and linking this to outcome.
- Online recording of lung function.
- Objective tests of nasal sensitization.
- Large-scale primary and secondary prevention programs for high-risk workplaces.
- Tools for assessing the psychosocial and economic consequences of occupational asthma in order to improve how we identify long-term sequelae and socioeconomic impact.

The efficacy of medical prevention programs in high-risk industries have been explored and found worthwhile.[53]

Major advances are anticipated in the next several years in the mechanistic, clinical, epidemiological, and prevention aspects of asthma in the workplace.[54]

References

1. Gautrin D, Ghezzo H, Infante-Rivard C, Malo JL. Natural history of sensitization, symptoms and diseases in apprentices exposed to laboratory animals. Eur Respir J 2001;17:904–8.
2. Walusiak J, Hanke W, Gorski P, Palczynski C. Respiratory allergy in apprentice bakers: do occupational allergies follow the allergic march? Allergy 2004;59:442–50.
3. Pepys J, Bernstein IL. Historical aspects of occupational asthma. In: Bernstein IL, Chan-Yeung M, Malo JL, Bernstein DI, editors. Asthma in the workplace. 3rd ed. New York: Taylor & Francis; 2006. p. 9–35.
4. Pepys J, Hutchcroft BJ. Bronchial provocation tests in etiologic diagnosis and analysis of asthma. Am Rev Respir Dis 1975;112:829–59.
5. Das R, Blanc PD. Chlorine gas exposure and the lung: a review. Toxicol Ind Health 1993;9:439–55.
6. Toren K, Blanc P. Asthma caused by occupational exposures is common - a systematic analysis of estimates of the population-attributable fraction. BMC Pulm Med 2009;9:7.
7. Bernstein IL, Bernstein DI, Chan-Yeung M, Malo JL. Definition and classification of asthma in the workplace. In: Bernstein IL, Chan-Yeung M, Malo JL, Bernstein DI, editors. Asthma in the workplace. 3rd ed. New York: Taylor & Francis; 2006. p. 1–8.
8. Gautrin D, Bernstein IL, Brooks SM, Henneberger PK. Reactive airways dysfunction syndrome and irritant-induced asthma. In: Bernstein IL, Chan-Yeung M, Malo JL, Bernstein DI, editors. Asthma in the workplace. 3rd ed. New York: Taylor & Francis; 2006. p. 579–627.
9. Frew A, Chan H, Dryden P, et al. Immunologic studies of the mechanisms of occupational asthma caused by Western red cedar. J Allergy Clin Immunol 1993;92:466–78.
10. Bernstein DI, Cartier A, Cote J, et al. Diisocyanate antigen-stimulated monocyte chemoattractant protein-1 synthesis has greater test efficiency than specific antibodies for identification of diisocyanate asthma. Am J Respir Crit Care Med 2002;166:445–50.
11. Lemière C, Romeo P, Chaboillez S, et al. Airway inflammation and functional changes after exposure to different concentrations of isocyanates. J Allergy Clin Immunol 2002;110:641–6.
12. Lemiere C, Malo JL, Boutet M. Reactive airways dysfunction syndrome due to chlorine: sequential bronchial biopsies and functional assessment. Eur Respir J 1997;10:241–4.
13. Takeda N, Maghni K, Daigle S, et al. Long-term pathologic consequences of acute irritant-induced asthma. J Allergy Clin Immunol 2009;124:975–81.
14. Burney PG, Luczynska C, Chinn S, Jarvis D. The European Community Respiratory Health Survey. Eur Respir J 1994;7:954–60.
15. Kogevinas M, Zock JP, Jarvis D, et al. Exposure to substances in the workplace and new-onset asthma: an international prospective population-based study (ECRHS-II). Lancet 2007;370:336–41.
16. Johnson AR, Dimich-Ward HD, Manfreda J, et al. Occupational asthma in adults in six Canadian communities. Am J Respir Crit Care Med 2000;162:2058–62.
17. Malo JL, Gautrin D. From asthma in the workplace to occupational asthma. Lancet 2007;370:295–7.
18. Demir A, Joseph L, Becklake MR. Work-related asthma in Montreal, Quebec: Population attributable risk in a communirty-based study. Can Respir J 2008;15:406–12.
19. Karjalainen A, Kurppa K, Martikainen R, et al. Work is related to a substantial portion of adult-onset asthma incidence in the Finnish population. Am J Resp Crit Care Med 2001;164:565–8.
20. Bersntein II, Keskinen H, Blanc PD, et al. Medicolegal aspects, compensation aspects, and evaluation of impairment/disability. In: Bernstein IL, Chan-Yeung M, Malo JL, Bernstein DI, editors. Asthma in the workplace. 3rd ed. New York: Taylor & Francis; 2006. p. 319–51.
21. McDonald JC, Keynes HL, Meredith SK. Reported incidence of occupational asthma in the United Kingdom, 1989–97. Occup Environ Med 2000;57:823–9.
22. Jajosky RA, Harrison R, Reinisch F, et al. Surveillance of work-related asthma in selected U.S. states using surveillance guidelines for state health departments-California, Massachusetts, Michigan and New Jersey. MMWR 1999;48(3):1–20.
23. Tarlo SM, Leung K, Broder I, et al. Asthmatic subjects symptomatically worse at work: Prevalence and characterization among a general asthma clinic population. Chest 2000;118:1309–14.
24. Gautrin D, Infante-Rivard C, Ghezzo H, Malo JL. Incidence and host determinants of probable occupational asthma in apprentices exposed to laboratory animals. Am J Respir Crit Care Med 2001;163:899–904.
25. Gautrin D, Ghezzo H, Infante-Rivard C, Malo JL. Incidence and host determinants of work-related rhinoconjunctivitis in apprentice pastry-makers. Allergy 2002;57:913–8.
26. El-Zein M, Malo JL, Infante-Rivard C, Gautrin D. Incidence of probable occupational asthma and of changes in airway calibre and responsiveness in apprentice welders. Eur Respir J 2003;22:513–8.
27. Dragos M, Jones M, Malo JL, et al. Specific antibodies to diisocyanate and work-related respiratory symptoms in apprentice car-painters. Occup Environ Med 2009;66:227–34.
28. Gautrin D, Ghezzo H, Infante-Rivard C, et al. Long-term outcomes in a prospective cohort of apprentices exposed to high-molecular-weight agents. Am J Respir Crit Care Med 2008;177:871–9.

29. Nieuwenhuijsen M, Baur X, Heederik D. Environmental monitoring: general considerations, exposure-response relationships, and risk assessment. In: Bernstein IL, Chan-Yeung M, Malo JL, Bernstein DI, editors. Asthma in the workplace. 3rd ed. New York: Taylor & Francis; 2006. p. 253–74.

30. Seed M, Agius R. Further validation of computer-based prediction of chemical asthma hazard. Occup Med 2010;60:115–20.

31. Newman Taylor AJ, Cullinan P, Lympany PA, et al. Interaction of HLA phenotype and exposure intensity in sensitization to complex platinum salts. Am J Respir Crit Care Med 1999;160:435–8.

32. Low B, Sjostdt L, Willirs S. Laboratory animal allergy-possible association with HLA B15 and DR4. Tissue Antigens 1988;32:224–6.

33. Balboni A, Baricordi OR, Fabbri LM, et al. Association between toluene diisocyanate-induced asthma and DQB1 markers: a possible role for aspartic acid at position 57. Eur Respir J 1996;9:207–10.

34. Rihs HP, Barbalho-Krolls T, Huber H, Baur X. No evidence for the influence of HLA Class II in alleles in isocyanate-induced asthma. Am J Ind Med 1997;32:522–7.

35. Mapp CE, Beghè B, Balboni A, et al. Association between HLA genes and susceptibility to toluene diisocyanate-induced asthma. Clin Exp Allergy 2000;30:651–6.

36. Malo JL, Lemière C, Desjardins A, Cartier A. Prevalence and intensity of rhinoconjunctivitis in subjects with occupational asthma. Eur Respir J 1997;10:1513–5.

37. Barber CM, Frank T, Walsh K, et al. Knowledge and utilisation of occupational asthma guidelines in primary care. Prim Care Respir J 2010;19(3):274–80.

38. Quirce S. Eosinophilic bronchitis in the workplace. Curr Opin Allergy Clin Immunol 2004;4:87–91.

39. Gannon PFG, Newton DT, Belcher J, et al. Development of OASYS-2: a system for the analysis of serial measurement of peak expiratory flow in workers with suspected occupational asthma. Thorax 1996;51:484–9.

40. Girard F, Chaboillez S, Cartier A, et al. An effective strategy for diagnosing occupational asthma. Induced sputum. Am J Respir Crit Care Med 2004;170:845–50.

41. Vandenplas O, Malo JL. Inhalation challenges with agents causing occupational asthma. Eur Respir J 1997;10:2612–29.

42. Caron S, Boileau JC, Malo JL, Leblond S. New methodology for specific inhalation challenges with occupational agents. Respir Res 2010;11:72.

43. Malo JL, Cardinal S, Ghezzo H, et al. Association of bronchial reactivity to occupational agents with methacholine reactivity, sputum cells and immunoglobulin E-mediated reactivity. Clin Exp Allergy 2011;41:497–504.

44. Bardana EJ. Reactive airways dysfunction syndrome (RADS): guidelines for diagnosis and treatment and insight into likely prognosis. Ann Allergy Asthma Immunol 1999;83:5836.

45. Malo JL, L'Archevêque J, Ghezzo H. Direct costs of occupational asthma in Quebec between 1988 and 2002. Can Respir J 2008;15:413–6.

46. Miedinger D, Lavoie KL, Larchevêque J, et al. Quality-of-life, psychological, and cost outcomes 2 years after diagnosis of occupational asthma. J Occup Environ Med 2011;53:231–8.

47. Malo JL, Cartier A, Côté J, et al. Influence of inhaled steroids on the recovery of occupational asthma after cessation of exposure: an 18-month double-blind cross-over study. Am J Crit Care Respir Med 1996;153:953–60.

48. Cocchiarella L, Andersson GBJ, editors. Guides to the evaluation of permanent impairment. 5th ed. Chicago: American Medical Association; 2001. p. 102–104.

49. Malo JL, Ghezzo H. Recovery of methacholine responsiveness after end of exposure in occupational asthma. Am J Respir Crit Care Med 2004; 169:1304–7.

50. Baur X, Chen Z, Liebers V. Exposure-response relationships of occupational inhalative allergens. Clin Exp Allergy 1998;28:537–44.

51. Houba R, Doekes G, Heederik D. Occupational respiratory allergy in bakery workers: A review of the literature. Am J Ind Med 1998;34:529–46.

52. Castano R, Gautrin D, Thériault C, et al. Occupational rhinitis in workers investigated for occupational asthma. Thorax 2009;64:50–4.

53. Tarlo SM, Liss GM. Can medical surveillance measures improve the outcome of occupational asthma? J Allergy Clin Immunol 2001;107:583–5.

54. Malo JL. Future advances in work-related asthma and the impact on occupational health. Occup Med 2005;55:606–11.

PART SIX
Systemic immune diseases

CHAPTERS

48.

Mechanisms of autoimmunity

Tricia Cottrell,
Antony Rosen

Human autoimmune diseases occur frequently (affecting in aggregate more than 5% of the population worldwide), and impose a significant burden of morbidity and mortality on the human population.[1] Autoimmune diseases are defined as diseases in which immune responses to specific self-antigens contribute to the ongoing tissue damage occurring in the disease. Both the specificity of the immune response and its role in tissue damage are central components of the definition. Autoimmune diseases can be either tissue-specific (e.g., thyroid, β-cells of the pancreas), where unique tissue- specific antigens are targeted, or can be more systemic, in which multiple tissues are affected, and a variety of apparently ubiquitously expressed autoantigens are targeted.[2] Although the definition appears relatively simple in concept, the complexity of this spectrum of disorders is enormous, and has greatly challenged elucidation of simple shared mechanisms. This complexity affects almost every domain, including genetics, phenotypic expression, and kinetics. In the latter case, there is frequently a prolonged period (weeks to months) between initial onset of symptoms and development of the diagnostic phenotype, and disease may vary in expression in the same individual over time. However, despite this enormous complexity, there is a striking association of the clinical phenotype with the targets of the autoimmune response. This association is, in fact, so strong that autoantibodies have been used for diagnosis and prognosis in the human autoimmune diseases.[2] For example, autoantibodies recognizing thyroid peroxidase are found in patients with autoimmune thyroiditis, autoantibodies to the Sm splicing ribonucleoprotein complex are diagnostic of systemic lupus erythematosus (SLE), and autoantibodies recognizing topoisomerase-1 are found in patients with the diffuse form of scleroderma. The immune response in autoimmune diseases has features of an adaptive immune response (usually directed against exogenous antigens), but its targets are autoantigens. Since the adaptive immune response is initiated when suprathreshold concentrations of molecules with structure not previously tolerized by the host are encountered in a pro-immune context, the association of specific autoantibodies with distinct clinical phenotypes provides critical clues to understanding the initiation and propagation of autoimmune diseases.

KEY CONCEPTS

Autoantibodies in autoimmune diseases

- Some autoantibodies precede the development of any symptoms by years (e.g., anti-nuclear antibodies and anti-phospholipid antibodies in SLE, anti-CCP in RA).
- Some autoantibodies only occur at around the time of onset of disease manifestations (e.g., anti-Sm and anti-RNP in SLE).
- There is a striking association of specific autoantibodies with distinct clinical phenotypes (e.g., anti-topoisomerase-1 with diffuse scleroderma and interstitial lung disease).

This chapter highlights some of the mechanistic principles that underlie autoimmune diseases. The extraordinary breadth and complexity of this disease spectrum means that the areas included cannot nearly encompass everything relevant.

The distinct phases in the development of autoimmunity

A major barrier to understanding mechanisms of autoimmunity comes from difficulty in defining early events in these diseases. Since diseases are only recognizable after development of the diagnostic phenotype, there has been the tendency to interpret findings at the time of disease diagnosis with events present at disease initiation. By studying the development of autoantibodies over time in patients who subsequently manifest an autoimmune disease, significant recent data have demonstrated that the onset of an autoimmune response and the development of clinical symptoms are generally separated in time. In the case of type I diabetes, development of islet cell autoantibodies frequently precedes diabetes, and additional islet cell autoantibodies accrue over time.[3] Similarly, autoantibodies recognizing citrullinated proteins (rheumatoid arthritis (RA)-specific autoantibodies; see below) frequently precede the development of RA.[4] These findings indicate that either a threshold needs to be exceeded in terms of tissue damage before symptoms manifest, or that there are two distinct phases in disease development, one marked by production of a group of autoantibodies, the second by auto-amplifying tissue damage. In a landmark study in SLE, Harley and colleagues have provided important insights into this issue.[5] They analyzed sera collected from patients in the US military who subsequently developed SLE. Strikingly, autoantibodies in SLE could be divided into two groups: (i) those that precede the diagnosis of SLE by several years—these included antinuclear and antiphospholipid antibodies; and (ii) those that occurred around the time of onset of symptoms—these included anti-Sm, anti-RNP, and to a lesser extent anti-DNA. The observation that one group of autoantibodies precedes symptoms in SLE, and that another group appears coincident with the phenotype strongly suggests that the groups mark distinct events in the development of autoimmune disease. Members of the first group are likely markers of disease initiation; members of the second group are likely markers of disease propagation. The antigens targeted by the immune system in this latter phase (i.e., associated with clinical disease) are more likely to have some function in disease propagation, possibly through their possession of pro-inflammatory or adjuvant functions (see below).[6]

Barriers to defining mechanisms of human autoimmune disease

- Genetic and phenotypic complexity
- Interval between initiating events and development of diagnostic phenotype
- Challenges in quantifying human immune responses

It is therefore useful to examine the development of autoimmune diseases in four phases (Fig. 48.1):

1. Susceptibility phase — before disease, but where one or several preconditions for later initiation are satisfied. This would include impaired tolerance induction, or altered immune signaling thresholds. The susceptibility phase could either be inherited or acquired, permanent or transient.

2. Initiation phase — before onset of clinical disease, but marked by the presence of an autoimmune response (e.g., in the case of SLE — antiphospholipid antibodies).

3. Propagation phase — this corresponds with the onset of clinical disease, marked by propagation-specific immune responses (e.g., in the case of SLE — anti-Sm antibodies).

4. Regulation/resolution phase — It should also be noted that in many cases during disease propagation, immunoregulatory pathways are also activated, which may result in natural inhibition of clinical disease over time. In rare cases, these inhibitory pathways can lead to permanent resolution. This resolution phase will not be discussed further here, but its existence provides important evidence that homeostasis can be re-established even after the amplified phenotype develops.

Phase I: Susceptibility

Although autoimmune diseases in humans are genetically complex, significant advances in understanding have occurred over the past several years. In some cases, advances have come from the study of autoimmunity with Mendelian patterns of inheritance (e.g., APECED, IPEX, C1q deficiency). Advances have also come from genetic association studies of various autoimmune phenotypes (e.g., SLE, type I DM). There have also been important advances in the genetics of autoimmunity in several mouse models. These studies highlight a critical role for pathways of tolerance induction, immunoregulation, and setpoints/thresholds for immune signaling in avoiding emergence of autoimmunity.

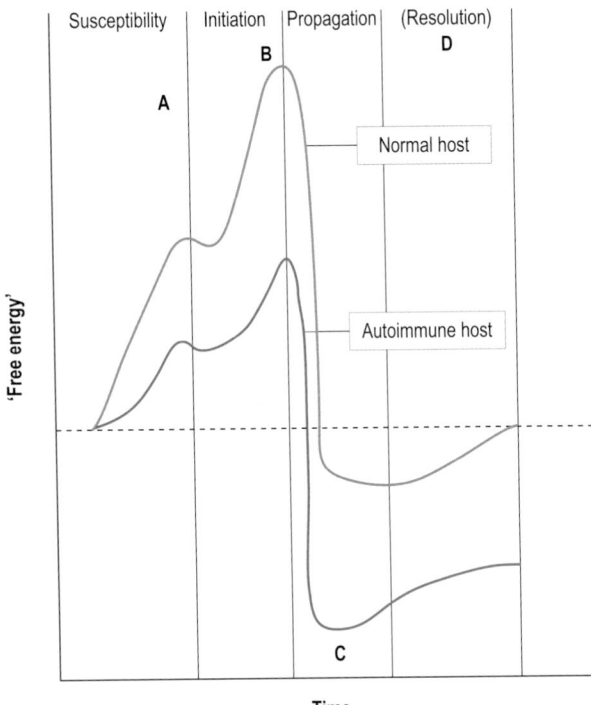

A	Susceptibility
• Impaired tolerance induction • Impaired production of regulatory T cells • Altered immune signaling thresholds	

B	Initiation
• Suprathreshold concentration of autoantigens • Non-tolerized structure • Pro-immune context – infection, malignancy, exposure to adjuvants	

C	Propagation
• Acquisition of adjuvant properties by disease specific autoantigens • Increased autoantigen expression in the target tissue • Immune effector pathways generate/expose autoantigen, which further drives the immune response	

Fig. 48.1 Mechanisms of autoimmunity. Autoimmune diseases result from a complex interplay of pathways and events that allow autoreactivity to manifest, and cause self-sustaining tissue damage. Mechanistically, it is useful to divide the process into 3 phases. (1) Susceptibility phase – this is present before disease, and is the phase in which one or several preconditions for later initiation are satisfied; (2) Initiation phase – this is marked by the presence of autoimmunity, but precedes the diagnostic clinical phenotype; (3) Propagation phase – this is marked by autoimmunity and tissue damage, in which immune effector pathways cause damage and provide antigen to drive the ongoing immune response.

Mechanisms underlying susceptibility to autoimmunity

- Incomplete induction of tolerance in the thymus to peripherally expressed autoantigens (AIRE deficiency causing APECED syndrome)
- Impaired clearance and tolerance induction by apoptotic cells (e.g., deficiency of C1q, C4, MFG-E8, Mer)
- Defective production of regulatory T cells (FOXP3 deficiency causing IPEX syndrome)
- Altered immune signaling thresholds (e.g., CTLA-4 polymorphisms, PTPN22 polymorphisms)

Incomplete thymic tolerance induction predisposes to autoimmunity

Significant insights into basic mechanisms can derive from the study of rare human phenotypes. This has been true for autoimmunity, where several monogenic disorders have defined important pathogenic principles. Autoimmune polyendocrine syndrome type I (APS1), also called autoimmune polyendocrinopathy candidiasis ectodermal dystrophy (APECED), is a rare disease in which patients develop multiple autoimmune diseases, often beginning in childhood.[7] While candidiasis and ectodermal dystrophy (including involvement of enamel and nails, as well as keratopathy) are features of the disease, the syndrome is characterized by striking autoimmunity directed against multiple different target tissues. Autoimmune processes include autoimmune hypoparathyroidism, Addison disease, autoimmune gastritis with pernicious anemia, type I diabetes, thyroid disease, autoimmune hepatitis, celiac disease, and gonadal failure. Numerous autoantigens have been defined as targets of autoimmunity in APS1, and include enzymes specifically expressed in various endocrine tissues (e.g., steroid 21-hydroxylase, specific for adrenal cortex; steroid 17α-hydroxylase, found in adrenal cortex and gonads; GAD65, found in pancreatic islets; and thyroid peroxidase). Moreover, antibodies to tissue-specific antigens have been associated with symptomatic tissue damage, such as anti-NALP5 antibodies found only in APS1 patients with hypoparathyroidism.[8] The genetic basis of APS1 was mapped to a gene on chromosome 21q22.3, subsequently termed *AIRE* (for autoimmune regulator). *AIRE* expression is highest in the thymus, where it is expressed in medullary thymic epithelial cells. Several predicted structural features of the AIRE protein, and its localization in nuclear dots, suggested that the protein might be a transcriptional regulator, and significant evidence for this proposal was obtained *in vitro*. Several *AIRE*-deficient mouse models were subsequently generated, which allowed the definition of important pathogenic pathways in APS1 that are likely broadly relevant to the mechanisms of autoimmunity in general. Thus, mice deficient for *AIRE* developed various autoimmune phenotypes, resembling those found in human APS1. These included multiorgan lymphocytic infiltration and autoantibodies, as well as autoimmune eye disease. In an elegant series of experiments, Mathis and colleagues demonstrated that AIRE regulates expression in thymic epithelial cells of various peripheral autoantigens normally expressed exclusively in endocrine target tissues.[9] Similarly, thymic expression of the mouse lung protein vomeromodulin is also AIRE-dependent, and loss of tolerance to this antigen is sufficient to cause interstitial lung disease in wild type mice.[10] Thus, AIRE appears to regulate the ectopic expression in the thymus of tissue-restricted autoantigens, and provide an antigen source against which to establish central tolerance.[9]

These data demonstrate that expression of peripheral autoantigens in the thymus constitutes a major barrier to the subsequent development of autoimmunity against these peripheral sites. Although it is likely that similar principles apply to ubiquitously expressed autoantigens targeted in systemic autoimmune diseases, there are currently few data directly addressing this issue.

Impaired clearance and tolerance induction by apoptotic cells: susceptibility defect in systemic autoimmunity

Although little is known in humans about the thymic pathways of tolerance induction to ubiquitously expressed autoantigens, there is accumulating evidence to suggest that in the periphery, apoptotic cells play an important role in providing a source of autoantigens against which the organism becomes tolerant.[11] Apoptotic cells are generally very efficiently cleared by phagocytic cells; these events are normally associated with the production of anti-inflammatory cytokines and result in tolerance induction.[12] Interestingly, early components of the classical complement pathway (e.g., C1q and C4) and C-reactive protein are required for efficient apoptotic cell clearance, with production of IL-10 and TGF-β. It is of particular note therefore that homozygous C1q deficiency is associated with a striking susceptibility to SLE in humans, suggesting that rapid, efficient, tolerance-inducing clearance of apoptotic cells may play a role similar to AIRE expression in the thymus in preventing subsequent emergence of autoimmunity to ubiquitously expressed

autoantigens.[13] Additional support for this model comes from recent studies of milk fat globule-EGF factor 8 (MFG-E8), a glycoprotein secreted from macrophages that is required for the efficient attachment and clearance of apoptotic cells by macrophages and immature dendritic cells. MFG-E8 is also expressed in tingible-body macrophages in the germinal centers of secondary lymphoid tissues. Interestingly, many unengulfed apoptotic cells are present in the germinal centers of the spleen in *MFG-E8*-deficient mice, which develop a striking lupus-like phenotype (reviewed in Rai and Wakeland).[12] Together, the data strongly suggest that efficient, anti-inflammatory clearance of apoptotic cells plays a central role in tolerance induction and prevention of autoimmunity.

Defective production of Treg cells

Although pathways exist that (i) regulate autoantigen expression at sites of tolerance induction, and (ii) guide autoantigens towards tolerance-inducing outcomes, these pathways alone are clearly insufficient to prevent the emergence of autoimmune disease. This fact is highlighted by the emergence of autoimmunity when regulatory T-cell (Treg) differentiation is abnormal in humans with immune dysregulation, polyendocrinopathy, enteropathy, X-linked (IPEX) syndrome, the human equivalent of the *scurfy* mouse. IPEX is a rare, X-linked recessive disorder characterized by type I diabetes, thyroiditis, atopic dermatitis, and inflammatory bowel disease (IBD), and is caused by mutations in the *FOXP3* gene.[14] FOXP3 is a member of the forkhead family of transcription factors, and is essential for the development of CD4+ Tregs, which have been shown to regulate the activation and differentiation of effector T cells at many different levels.

Preliminary investigations into the role of Tregs in human autoimmune diseases have produced mixed results, but these cells likely play important roles in regulating disease onset and amplitude. As additional cell subsets and details about function emerge, this area will clarify significantly.

Signaling thresholds and susceptibility to autoimmunity

Several modulators of T-cell signaling have been defined as important susceptibility determinants in autoimmunity.[15] For example, CTLA4 polymorphisms are associated with increased risk of a variety of autoimmune diseases, including type I diabetes, Graves disease, and RA. Similarly, a functional polymorphism in PTPN22 has been identified as a major risk factor for several human autoimmune diseases, including SLE, RA, and type I diabetes. Although the exact mechanisms underlying susceptibility to autoimmunity remain unclear, in both cases the polymorphisms appear to regulate the balance of stimulatory and inhibitory signaling in effector and regulatory T cells, favoring effector T-cell activation.

Recent genetic studies have also suggested a potential role for innate immune sensors in autoimmunity, focusing attention on the critical balance between activation of the immune response to mitigate infectious damage, and limiting the magnitude of the response to avoid immunopathology. Loss of function variants of both *DDX58* (encoding RIG-I) and *IFIH1* (encoding MDA5) are associated with protection from type I diabetes.[16] These RNA helicases are essential for the detection of cytoplasmic viral RNA and activation of type I IFN secretion by infected cells. The reduction of type I diabetes risk with reduced function of these anti-viral pathways suggests that excessive interferon signaling may facilitate the development of autoimmunity. Key immune signaling pathways that protect the host from deleterious infectious and malignant challenges, but potentially also enhance damage of self-tissues in the process may therefore be important susceptibility factors in autoimmune diseases.

There are thus many barriers to the development of autoimmunity, including effective tolerance induction in the thymus and periphery, tightly regulated immune signaling, and homeostatic pathways of immunoregulation to limit anti-self responses should these occur. It is likely that the genetic susceptibility to autoimmunity in outbred humans represents an integrated threshold involving genes that regulate these various pathways—upon which environmental and stochastic events act to accomplish disease initiation and propagation.

Phase 2: Initiation

Initiation of an adaptive immune response requires presentation to T cells of suprathreshold concentrations of molecules with structure not previously tolerized by the host. One of the more persuasive models proposed to explain the persistence of potentially autoreactive T cells within the repertoire of the host is that of immunodominance of T-cell epitopes. This model provides major insights into the pathogenesis of autoimmunity.[15,17]

● KEY CONCEPTS

Potential mechanisms that can alter antigen processing to reveal potentially cryptic epitopes

- Modification of autoantigen processing through high affinity binding to ligands or antibodies.
- Distinct proteolytic machinery in the thymus and periphery—or differential modification of proteolytic activity.
- Modification of autoantigen structure that modifies its processing by endogenous antigen presenting cell machinery, generally through post-translational modifications.
- Novel proteolytic events not present in the normal APC pathways—e.g., novel cleavage during cell death or damage or inflammation.
- Novel forms of autoantigens generated by mutation, truncation, or splicing.

Dominance and crypticity

Studies by Sercarz and colleagues[17] have stressed that while antigens contain numerous potential determinants that could be presented on major histocompatibility complex (MHC) class II molecules during antigen processing, not all determinants in a particular molecule are equally likely to be efficiently presented. Those determinants that are most efficiently presented are termed 'dominant'; those that are not loaded onto MHC class II to a significant degree are termed 'cryptic'. For self-antigens, it is likely that a constant set of dominant determinants are generated during antigen processing under most circumstances, with similar outcomes in the thymus and periphery. Antigens processed by the 'standard' pathway are therefore fully tolerized, with the T-cell repertoire purged of reactivity to the dominant self. However, the balance of dominant and cryptic epitopes presented during antigen processing is influenced significantly by changes of protein structure, that occur during various relevant physiological states.[18] Several potential mechanisms that may alter antigen processing to reveal potentially cryptic epitopes are summarized below.

High affinity binding of antigen to ligands or antibodies

Several studies have demonstrated that antigen processing can be dramatically altered when the antigen binds with high affinity to a ligand or antibody. Simitsek and colleagues (reviewed in Lanzavecchia)[18] demonstrated that presentation of T-cell determinants in tetanus toxin can be either enhanced or suppressed as a direct consequence of antibody modulation of antigen processing in human B lymphoblastoid cells. Remarkably, a single bound antibody can simultaneously enhance the presentation of one T-cell determinant by more than 10-fold while strongly suppressing the presentation of a different T-cell determinant. Biochemical analysis showed that both the suppressed and boosted determinants fall within an extended domain of antigen stabilized by this antibody during proteolysis. Thus, ligand-induced changes in processing can destroy dominant determinants or reveal cryptic self determinants. Similar observations have also been made with numerous other antigen-antibody partners.[18]

Tissue-specific protease expression

Watts and colleagues (reviewed in Darrah and Rosen)[19] showed that a principal HLA-DR2-restricted epitope in myelin basic protein (MBP amino acids 85–99) contains a processing site for asparagine endopeptidase (AEP), with cleavage by AEP abolishing the epitope. AEP activity is therefore a critical factor in presentation of this epitope.[19] In human antigen-presenting cells, presentation of MBP85-99 is inversely proportional to the amount of cellular AEP activity, and inhibition of AEP greatly enhances presentation of the MBP85-99 epitope. Interestingly, both MBP and AEP are expressed in the thymus, AEP at abundant levels. These data suggest that this major epitope in neurological autoimmunity may not be presented under normal circumstances in the thymus due to destruction by AEP, therefore raising the potential for later presentation in the periphery in the setting of decreased AEP activity.

Post-translational modification of autoantigen structure

Autoantigens undergo a variety of post-translational modifications, including phosphorylation, proteolytic cleavage, ubiquitination, transglutamination, citrullination, and isoaspartyl modification.[20] In several cases, autoantibodies recognize exclusively the modified form of the antigen (e.g., RNA polymerase-II large subunit, serine/arginine-rich [SR] proteins, citrullinated vimentin and other RA autoantigens), indicating that the modified forms of the molecules are important in driving the immune response. In addition, Doyle and Mamula[20] have demonstrated that post-translational modification of autoantigen structure may be more broadly relevant than can be appreciated by studying autoantibody specificity alone. They showed that while mouse immunization with a murine cytochrome c peptide (amino acids 90–104) resulted in no T- or B-cell response, immunization with the isoaspartyl form of this peptide resulted in strong T- and B-cell responses. Although the autoantibodies elicited recognized both the modified and the native form of the antigen, the T cells only recognized the isoaspartyl form. Similar observations have also been made for several SLE autoantigens. The difficulty detecting and quantifying antigen-specific T cells in various autoimmune diseases may reflect their preferential recognition of subtly modified forms of autoantigen. This is an important area for future study — currently there is no systematic way to generate the relevant autoantigen forms.

Novel antigen cleavage during cell damage, cell death, or inflammation

Recent studies have provided evidence that single proteolytic events early in antigen processing can play critical roles in defining the epitopes generated. For example, Watts and colleagues (reviewed in Darrah and Rosen)[19] have conclusively demonstrated that early cleavage by asparagine endopeptidase (AEP) determines subsequent proteolytic events. Modifications of the antigen that affect this early cleavage dramatically change the epitopes loaded onto MHC class II molecules.[19]

Inflammatory microenvironments can create significant potential to load distinct epitopes because unique proteolytic activities are present. Activated inflammatory cells constitute a major source of proteases, including various cytotoxic lymphocyte granule proteases (granzymes), as well as numerous neutrophil and monocyte granule proteases. It is of interest that numerous autoantigens targeted in systemic autoimmune diseases are substrates for these inflammatory proteases, and that unique autoantigen fragments are generated through the activity of granzyme B and potentially other similar proteases.[19] Such autoantigen forms are not generated during other forms of cell damage or death, and similar activity is not observed against non-autoantigens. Thus, novel proteolytic cleavage of intracellular autoantigens during activity of cytotoxic immune effector pathways may provide a source of cryptic epitopes not generated during homeostatic 'tolerance-inducing' tissue turnover. Direct evidence that inflammatory protease-mediated revelation of cryptic epitopes is relevant to initiation of autoimmunity *in vivo* is still needed.

Autoantigen alteration due to mutation, truncation or splicing

Since the final epitopes generated and loaded onto MHC class II can be profoundly influenced by single, early cleavage events during antigen processing, relatively minor but critically placed changes in the primary structure of autoantigens can have the capacity to influence peptide selection. A study of the melanoma and vitiligo-associated autoantigens, tyrosinase-related proteins (TRP) 1 and 2, has strikingly demonstrated that this mechanism may play an important role in generating immune responses to self and tumor antigens.[21] In this study, Houghton and colleagues examined whether mutated-self gene products are more likely to initiate immunity, and used a systematic approach to define some of the principles that determine this. They generated cDNA libraries encoding large numbers of random mutations in syngeneic TRP proteins. They then used a DNA immunization approach into black mice to test the immunogenicity of the altered proteins encoded by the pools of mutated cDNAs. Immunization with non-mutated proteins induced no detectable immune responses, consistent with establishment of tolerance to the full-length molecules. In contrast, the mutated cDNA pools elicited both autoimmune depigmentation and the ability to reject melanoma tumors. Additional analysis showed that autoimmunity resulted from mutations that altered autoantigen cell biology, particularly degradation rates and pathways. Mutations also created new helper T-cell epitopes, and induced recognition of non-mutated but previously cryptic epitopes. Interestingly, mutations themselves did not form part of CD8 epitopes that

drive the anti-self and anti-tumor immune responses. Mutated molecules that were immunogenic were frequently truncated, leading the authors to propose that inappropriately truncated self-proteins can provoke autoimmunity when present in a pro-inflammatory environment. Although there are not yet good examples where natural autoimmunity arises due to the progressive accumulation of somatic mutations over time, with the expression of mutant, truncated forms of autoantigens, this study does provide an important mechanistic underpinning for the proposal that accumulated mutations have a role in the initiation of autoimmunity.

Indeed, there are significant data that link autoimmunity and cancer. For example, cancer is present in ~20% of individuals with dermatomyositis, with a striking temporal clustering of cancer diagnosis around the time of diagnosis of the myositis.[22] A recent study of patients with scleroderma and cancer found an association between anti-RNA polymerase I/III antibodies and a cancer diagnosis within two years of scleroderma onset.[23] Moreover, the cancers of these patients expressed high levels of RNA polymerase I/III protein relative to the cancers of anti-RNA Pol I/III negative patients and normal tissues. Similarly, there is evidence for an association of SLE with cancer, particularly lymphoma, again clustered within the first 2 years of SLE diagnosis.[24] These associations, both with timing of diagnosis, as well as preferentially with specific tumor types, are strongly indicative of a non-random clustering of autoimmune processes and cancer, which is likely of mechanistic significance. There is also growing evidence that, when associated with 'paraneoplastic' autoimmune syndromes, cancers are frequently smaller at diagnosis and may have a better prognosis. Perhaps the most striking evidence for a potential mechanistic association between autoimmunity and effective anti-cancer immunity comes from studies showing that development of autoimmunity during immunotherapy for a variety of different cancers is a predictor of a better cancer outcome. This may target both (i) tissue-specific antigens (e.g., in metastatic melanoma, where development of vitiligo is a predictor of an effective anti-tumor response)[25] or (ii) non-tissue-specific autoantigens (e.g., systemic high dose adjuvant interferon α-2b therapy for metastatic melanoma inducing new autoantibodies).[26]

It is likely that somatic mutations acquired with age, and their association with malignancy, are important in the genesis of some forms of human autoimmunity. Additional studies to confirm this and elucidate the underlying mechanisms remain a high priority. However, the barriers to such studies in humans are very significant, as effective anti-cancer immunity may be phenotypically silent and convenient technologies to quantify somatic mutation and specific immune responses in normal individuals will be needed to draw conclusions of causality.

Antigen mimicry

The process of antigen mimicry (see below) has frequently been proposed as a potential initiator of autoimmune diseases.[27,28] This mechanism, particularly when isolated, is only likely relevant to those autoimmune processes clearly associated with antecedent infections, and particularly those that resolve spontaneously, and subsequently recur upon re-exposure to the offending agent. The mechanism may, however, also play a role in initiation of the autoimmune response in self-sustaining autoimmune processes, but in this case, requires that T-cell responses to the cross-reacting self-antigen are initiated.

Foreign antigens, which often differ from their homologous self-antigens in some areas, may nevertheless bear significant structural similarity to self-antigens in other regions. Initiation of an immune response to the foreign antigen may generate a cross-reactive antibody response that also recognizes the self-protein (antigen mimicry). When the antigen is a cell surface molecule, antibody-mediated effector pathways can lead to host tissue damage. Although the antibody response is cross-reactive with self-molecules, the T cells that drive this response are generally directed at the foreign antigen, at least initially (see below). Diseases involving this sort of "antigen mimicry" therefore tend to be self-limited, although they can recur upon re-exposure to the offending antigen. It is important to realize that antigen mimicry alone cannot explain self-sustaining autoimmune diseases, which are driven by self-antigens and autoreactive T cells. In these cases, there is a requirement for overcoming T-cell tolerance to the self protein. The central issues in this regard are (i) how T-cell tolerance to self antigens might initially be broken, and (ii) once this has occurred, why these antigens continue to drive the immune response to self. The simultaneous liberation of self-antigen in the presence of the cross-reactive antibody response has been proposed to play critical roles in this regard. For example, several studies suggest that when a humoral response to a foreign protein is induced that cross-reacts with the self-antigen, a strong helper T-cell response specific for the self-antigen can occur. The simultaneous liberation of significant amounts of self-antigen in the setting of a cross-reactive antibody response may allow effective presentation of cryptic epitopes in the self-antigen to autoreactive T cells by activated cross-reactive B cells. If continued release of self-antigen occurs, a specific, adaptive immune response to self will be sustained. Antigen release from tissues likely plays a critical role in driving this autoimmune process. Understanding the mechanisms of ongoing antigen release at sites of tissue damage in autoimmune disease (e.g., unique pathways of cell injury and death) is a high priority for future work, as it provides a novel target for therapy (see below).

It is clear from the above discussion that extraordinary complexity is operative in initiation of the human autoimmune diseases. The patient population is genetically heterogeneous, the human immune system is complex and extremely plastic, and it interacts with a plethora of environmental stimuli and stochastic events. The simultaneous confluence of susceptibility factors and initiation forces to set off the self-sustained and auto-amplifying process is therefore a rare occurrence. In contrast, once activation of autoreactive T cells has occurred, the ability of the immune system to vigorously respond to low concentrations of antigen, to amplify the specific effector response to those antigens, and to spread the response to additional antigens in that tissue, greatly reduces the stringency that must be met to keep the process going.

Phase III: Propagation

Principles of amplification

One of the central features of human autoimmunity is the tendency of the process to amplify progressively with the accumulation of significant immune-mediated tissue damage. Furthermore, in the vast majority of cases, once such amplification begins, the process is very unlikely to resolve spontaneously. Autoantigens themselves can be very important in this phase, both in terms of acquisition of adjuvant properties, as well as regulation of levels of expression. The essential features of amplification are a substrate cycle, in which antigen expression and

adjuvant properties induce an immune response, which induces increased antigen expression and tissue damage—and further drive the immune response. The importance of tissue-specific autoantigen expression in focusing such immune responses is only beginning to be recognized.

Acquisition of adjuvant properties by disease-specific autoantigens

In spite of the fact that tens of thousands of molecules could be targeted by the immune system in autoimmunity, the number of molecules that are frequently targeted in the different phenotypes are markedly restricted—limited perhaps to 100 or so. This has led to the proposal that frequently targeted autoantigens may themselves have properties that make them pro-immune. Work by Howard et al. provided important initial support for this proposal (reviewed in Plotz).[29] They observed that the autoantigenic histidyl aminoacyl tRNA synthetase (HRS), which is targeted in autoimmune myositis (but not non-autoantigenic lysyl- and aspartyl-aminoacyl tRNA synthetases), is a chemoattractant to immature dendritic cells and other leukocytes. The authors suggested that the selection of a self-molecule as a target for an autoantibody response may be a consequence of pro-inflammatory properties of the molecule itself. They further suggested that modification of autoantigen structure during processes of cell damage or death may be critical in recruiting these additional functions of autoantigens.

Role of innate immune receptors in amplification

Several innate immune receptor systems that sense and transduce the signals from pathogen-associated molecular patterns (PAMPs) (e.g., receptors of the Toll-like receptor [TLR] and RIG-I like receptor [RLR] families) may also play roles in transducing the pro-inflammatory properties of autoantigens.[6,30,31] Ligands for TLRs include both microbial and endogenous molecules, the latter group being particularly relevant to autoimmunity (see below). Microbial ligands include components of Gram-positive bacteria, Gram-negative bacteria, yeast, and protozoans. For example, lipoteichoic acid and fungal products (e.g., zymosan) signal through TLR-2, lipopolysaccharide activates TLR-4 signaling, dsRNA signals through TLR-3, flagellin through TLR-5, ssRNA through TLR-7 and TLR-8, bacterial or viral DNA through TLR-9, and *Toxoplasma* profilin through TLR-11.[32] Although viral and bacterial nucleic acids are the most likely ligands for TLRs, accumulating data demonstrate that complexes containing endogenous nucleic acids are able to signal through TLRs. Although the exact nature and source of endogenous ligands for TLRs *in vivo* remains unclear, recent studies have demonstrated that components from stressed, injured and dying cells may play critical roles in this regard.[6]

Working in several models, numerous investigators have now provided evidence that the frequent targeting of nucleoprotein autoantigens (which contain DNA or RNA) results from the ability of these nucleic acid components to ligate Toll-like receptors (TLRs) (reviewed in Kawasaki et al).[6] For example, anti-chromatin immune complexes can activate DCs and B cells through ligation of both FcγR and TLR-9. B-cell activation via TLR-7 ligation by RNA-containing immune complexes has also been demonstrated. *In vivo* studies have linked these *in vitro* findings to the development of autoimmunity. For example, when *TLR-9* deficiency is bred onto MRL-lpr mice—which are an excellent model of SLE—animals no longer get autoantibody responses to chromatin. Interestingly, these animals nevertheless manifest the SLE phenotype—in some cases, more severely than the *TLR-9*-sufficient animals. In another model, Ehlers et al. showed that *TLR-9* deficiency inhibits both anti-DNA responses and also abrogates the development of renal disease.[31] Similarly, when mice are rendered *TLR-7*-deficient, the autoantibody response to Sm is markedly inhibited, and severity of the SLE phenotype is improved. Reciprocally, over-expression of TLR-7 is sufficient to induce an SLE-like disease (reviewed in Kawasaki et al.).[6] These data confirm that autoantigens frequently selected in different autoimmune phenotypes likely have the dual property of being able to simultaneously activate the innate and adaptive immune systems. The source, form, and uptake of nucleic acids clearly influence adjuvant activity. For example, while bacterial and viral DNA, and oligonucleotides with CpG motifs have significant adjuvant activity,[33] mammalian genomic DNA, in which CpG is usually methylated, has very poor adjuvant activity. In contrast, human DNA present within immune complexes in SLE serum activates plasmacytoid DCs effectively, in a DNA-dependent way. Several potential explanations have been advanced to explain these observations.[6] First, that FcγR-mediated uptake effectively captures self-DNA bound by anti-DNA-antibodies and directs it to the correct endosomal compartment for TLR signaling. Second, that co-ligation of TLR-9 and either B-cell receptor or FcγR alters the signaling threshold of immune complexes. Last, that the difference lies in the nucleic acid itself, with additional modifications of DNA and RNA structure occurring in cells under different physiologic circumstances (e.g., cell death) and regulating nucleic acid binding to TLRs.[34] Recent studies suggest that other sensors of PAMPs (e.g., NOD-like receptors, RIG-like receptors) may play similar roles to TLRs in amplifying adaptive responses to specific intracellular autoantigens (e.g. MDA5, IFI-16), but definitive evidence is not yet available.

The TLR-interferon interface has been recognized as critical in the propagation phase of systemic autoimmune diseases (reviewed in Hall and Rosen,[35] and Swiecki and Colonna).[36] Much attention has been focused on plasmacytoid dendritic cells (pDCs), a relatively rare class of immature DC that can secrete large amounts of type I interferons upon TLR ligation, and that express TLR-7 and TLR-9 at high levels.[36] Recent studies in mouse models have demonstrated the ability of pDCs to alternately promote wound healing or chronic inflammation, depending on the predisposing genetic background. For example, non-specific skin injury in wild type mice (by tape stripping) leads to pDC recruitment, TLR-7 and TLR-9 recognition of nucleic acids, and transient expression of type I interferons with subsequent wound healing.[37] In contrast, the same skin damage in a lupus prone mouse strain results in chronic inflammation mediated by sustained type I interferon expression, which can be ameliorated with pDC depletion or TLR7/9 inhibition.[38] Extending these observations to human autoimmunity, IFN-α-inducing activity is abrogated by chloroquine or bafilomycin, agents that interfere with endosome acidification and TLR-7 and −9 signaling. In addition, Rönnblom and colleagues demonstrated that when added to material from apoptotic or necrotic cells, autoantibodies from SLE and Sjögren syndrome patients with specificity for DNA or RNA autoantigens induce striking interferon secretion (reviewed in Hall and Rosen).[35] Type I interferons have a broad set of functions that likely contribute to the feed forward, propagation phase of systemic autoimmune diseases.[6] For example, they (i) promote the differentiation of monocytes into mature DCs, which drive autoreactive T- and B-cell responses; (ii) increase target cell sensitivity to killing pathways; (iii) upregulate cytotoxic effector pathways; and (iv) upregulate expression of autoantigens like Ro52.

This general ability of autoantigens, particularly in the context of immune complexes, to stimulate interferon and other cytokine secretion, is likely an important principle in the initiation and propagation of autoimmunity.

Enhanced autoantigen expression in the target tissue

The striking association of specific autoantibody responses with distinct phenotypes suggests that autoantigen expression or form in specific target tissues may play an important role in both focusing the immune response and generating tissue damage. Unfortunately, very little is currently known about such parameters *in vivo* in relevant target tissues, both in normal and pathologic circumstances.

Recent studies on human autoimmune myopathies have begun to provide important insights into this problem. Myositis-specific autoantigens are expressed at very low levels in control muscle, but at high levels in myositis tissue, where antigen expression is at highest levels in regenerating muscle cells.[39] Interestingly, histidyl tRNA synthetase (HRS) expression is also found at high levels in lung and anti-HRS antibodies are associated with autoimmune myopathies with interstitial lung disease. Recently, 3-hydroxy-3-methylglutaryl-coenzyme A reductase (HMGCR) was identified as an autoantigen in patients with statin-associated autoimmune myopathy.[40] In addition to the induction of HMGCR protein expression by statin treatment of cultured cells, this group also demonstrated increased expression of this protein in regenerating muscle fibers of anti-HMGCR positive patients. These data suggest that enhanced autoantigen expression in the target tissue may be a feature of disease propagation, and that antigen expression during tissue repair may provide an ongoing antigen source to sustain and amplify tissue damage.

Defining whether similar principles are operating in other autoimmune diseases, and elucidating the pathways of antigen expression and modification in relevant target tissues is an important focus of future studies and may have important therapeutic potential.

●ON THE HORIZON

- Precise clinical and molecular phenotyping of patients at various disease stages is critical for improving diagnosis, monitoring, and treatment of autoimmune diseases.
- Understanding mechanisms of disease amplification, propagation, and regulation will enable the development of effective targeted therapies.
- Understanding the mechanisms of human autoimmunity will likely provide important insights into the normal functioning of the immune system, particularly with regard to natural cancer immunity.

Translational research

The challenge in the next decade is to continue elucidating the underlying mechanisms of autoimmunity in order to improve diagnosis, treatment, and enable more precise monitoring of these diseases. The existence of distinct phases in the development of autoimmune disease provides an opportunity to identify patients at risk of developing tissue damage before this occurs, and potentially to interdict the process before the amplification cycle is established. Understanding natural mechanisms of regulation of disease amplitude, or even in some circumstances of disease resolution, will provide important opportunities for disease therapy. The role of the target tissue as an active participant rather than a passive bystander in the ongoing destruction will likely be understood in molecular detail, and provide novel approaches to decreasing the amplitude of amplifying cycles. The identification of precise biomarkers of all these events requires exceptional clinical phenotyping of patients with early disease, longitudinal analysis by centers of excellence that follow large numbers of patients with similar phenotypes over time, with effective coupling to basic laboratory enterprise. Critical areas of future investigation relevant to diagnosis and therapy include clarifying the roles of genetic and epigenetic factors, interactions between the innate and adaptive immune responses, regulatory T cells, and focus on the target tissue and antigen contributions to ongoing amplification.

References

1. Davidson A, Diamond B. General features of autoimmune disease. In: Rose NR, Mackay IR, editors. The autoimmune diseases. St Louis: Elsevier Academic Press; 2006.
2. von Muhlen CA, Tan EM. Autoantibodies in the diagnosis of systemic rheumatic diseases. Semin Arthritis Rheum 1995;24(5):323–58.
3. Winter WE, Schatz DA. Autoimmune markers in diabetes. Clin Chem 2011;57(2):168–75.
4. Nielen MM, van Schaardenburg D, Reesink HW, et al. Specific autoantibodies precede the symptoms of rheumatoid arthritis: A study of serial measurements in blood donors. Arthritis Rheum 2004;50(2):380–6.
5. Arbuckle MR, McClain MT, Rubertone MV, et al. Development of autoantibodies before the clinical onset of systemic lupus erythematosus. N Engl J Med 2003;349(16):1526–33.
6. Kawasaki T, Kawai T, Akira S. Recognition of nucleic acids by pattern-recognition receptors and its relevance in autoimmunity. Immunol Rev 2011;243(1):61–73.
7. Peterson P, Nagamine K, Scott H, et al. APECED: A monogenic autoimmune disease providing new clues to self-tolerance. Immunol Today 1998;19(9):384–6.
8. Alimohammadi M, Bjorklund P, Hallgren A, et al. Autoimmune polyendocrine syndrome type 1 and NALP5, a parathyroid autoantigen. N Engl J Med 2008;358(10):1018–28.
9. Anderson MS, Venanzi ES, Klein L, et al. Projection of an immunological self shadow within the thymus by the aire protein. Science 2002;298(5597):1395–401.
10. Shum AK, DeVoss J, Tan CL, et al. Identification of an autoantigen demonstrates a link between interstitial lung disease and a defect in central tolerance. Sci Transl Med 2009;1(9) 9ra20.
11. Steinman RM, Turley S, Mellman I, Inaba K. The induction of tolerance by dendritic cells that have captured apoptotic cells. J Exp Med 2000;191(3):411–6.
12. Elliott MR, Ravichandran KS. Clearance of apoptotic cells: Implications in health and disease. J Cell Biol 2010;189(7):1059–70.
13. Manderson AP, Botto M, Walport MJ. The role of complement in the development of systemic lupus erythematosus. Annu Rev Immunol 2004;22:431–56.
14. Bennett CL, Christie J, Ramsdell F, et al. The immune dysregulation, polyendocrinopathy, enteropathy, X-linked syndrome (IPEX) is caused by mutations of FOXP3. Nat Genet 2001;27(1):20–1.
15. Rai E, Wakeland EK. Genetic predisposition to autoimmunity–what have we learned? Semin Immunol 2011;23(2):67–83.
16. Shigemoto T, Kageyama M, Hirai R, et al. Identification of loss of function mutations in human genes encoding RIG-I and MDA5: Implications for resistance to type I diabetes. J Biol Chem 2009;284(20):13348–54.
17. Sercarz EE, Lehmann PV, Ametani A, et al. Dominance and crypticity of T cell antigenic determinants. Annu Rev Immunol 1993;11:729–66.
18. Lanzavecchia A. How can cryptic epitopes trigger autoimmunity? J Exp Med 1995;181(6):1945–8.
19. Darrah E, Rosen A. Granzyme B cleavage of autoantigens in autoimmunity. Cell Death Differ 2010;17(4):624–32.
20. Doyle HA, Mamula MJ. Posttranslational modifications of self-antigens. Ann N Y Acad Sci 2005;1050:1–9.
21. Engelhorn ME, Guevara-Patino JA, Noffz G, et al. Autoimmunity and tumor immunity induced by immune responses to mutations in self. Nat Med 2006;12(2):198–206.
22. Hill CL, Zhang Y, Sigurgeirsson B, et al. Frequency of specific cancer types in dermatomyositis and polymyositis: A population-based study. Lancet 2001;357(9250):96–100.
23. Shah AA, Rosen A, Hummers L, et al. Close temporal relationship between onset of cancer and scleroderma in patients with RNA polymerase I/III antibodies. Arthritis Rheum 2010;62(9):2787–95.
24. Bernatsky S, Boivin JF, Joseph L, et al. An international cohort study of cancer in systemic lupus erythematosus. Arthritis Rheum 2005;52(5):1481–90.
25. Phan GQ, Yang JC, Sherry RM, et al. Cancer regression and autoimmunity induced by cytotoxic T lymphocyte-associated antigen 4 blockade in patients with metastatic melanoma. Proc Natl Acad Sci U S A 2003;100(14):8372–7.
26. Gogas H, Ioannovich J, Dafni U, et al. Prognostic significance of autoimmunity during treatment of melanoma with interferon. N Engl J Med 2006;354(7):709–18.
27. James JA, Harley JB, Scofield RH. Epstein-barr virus and systemic lupus erythematosus. Curr Opin Rheumatol 2006;18(5):462–7.
28. Fourneau JM, Bach JM, van Endert PM, Bach JF. The elusive case for a role of mimicry in autoimmune diseases. Mol Immunol 2004;40(14–15):1095–102.
29. Plotz PH. The autoantibody repertoire: Searching for order. Nat Rev Immunol 2003;3(1):73–8.
30. Christensen SR, Shupe J, Nickerson K, et al. Toll-like receptor 7 and TLR9 dictate autoantibody specificity and have opposing inflammatory and regulatory roles in a murine model of lupus. Immunity 2006;25(3):417–28.
31. Ehlers M, Fukuyama H, McGaha TL, et al. TLR9/MyD88 signaling is required for class switching to pathogenic IgG2a and 2b autoantibodies in SLE. J Exp Med 2006;203(3):553–61.
32. Kawai T, Akira S. Toll-like receptors and their crosstalk with other innate receptors in infection and immunity. Immunity 2011;34(5):637–50.
33. Krieg AM. CpG motifs in bacterial DNA and their immune effects. Annu Rev Immunol 2002;20:709–60.
34. Green NM, Marshak-Rothstein A. Toll-like receptor driven B cell activation in the induction of systemic autoimmunity. Semin Immunol 2011;23(2):106–12.
35. Hall JC, Rosen A. Type I interferons: Crucial participants in disease amplification in autoimmunity. Nat Rev Rheumatol 2010;6(1):40–9.
36. Swiecki M, Colonna M. Unraveling the functions of plasmacytoid dendritic cells during viral infections, autoimmunity, and tolerance. Immunol Rev 2010;234(1):142–62.
37. Gregorio J, Meller S, Conrad C, et al. Plasmacytoid dendritic cells sense skin injury and promote wound healing through type I interferons. J Exp Med 2010;207(13):2921–30.
38. Guiducci C, Tripodo C, Gong M, et al. Autoimmune skin inflammation is dependent on plasmacytoid dendritic cell activation by nucleic acids via TLR7 and TLR9. J Exp Med 2010;207(13):2931–42.
39. Casciola-Rosen L, Nagaraju K, Plotz P, et al. Enhanced autoantigen expression in regenerating muscle cells in idiopathic inflammatory myopathy. J Exp Med 2005;201(4):591–601.
40. Mammen AL, Chung T, Christopher-Stine L, et al. Autoantibodies against 3-hydroxy-3-methylglutaryl-coenzyme A reductase in patients with statin-associated autoimmune myopathy. Arthritis Rheum 2011;63(3):713–21.

49.

Interface of autoimmunity and immunodeficiency

Magda Carneiro-Sampaio, Antonio Coutinho

Next to the increased susceptibility to infections, autoimmune disease (AID) manifestations represent the most common group of clinical features in patients with primary immunodeficiency diseases (PIDs). While PID/AID associations were only sporadically noted in the past, they have recently received much attention.[1-3] Interestingly, clinical observations that brought forth this association were in apparent opposition to a prevalent view in the basic immunology community, i.e., that AID represent an exacerbation, rather than a failure, of immune mechanisms and pathways. This notion has now been significantly revised, in part because of this clinical evidence.

Several reasons justify the interest in PID/AID associations. Given our current limitations in the full understanding of autoimmune pathogenesis, the experiments of nature represented by PIDs may offer novel insights into molecular and cellular mechanisms of disease, particularly as we now have at hand the genetic basis for an increasing number of PIDs. Importantly in clinical practice, AID symptoms and signs may often represent the first clinical manifestations of PIDs, and clinicians would benefit from this understanding in their diagnostic considerations.

If PIDs and AIDs are considered together, there is an apparent asymmetry in conventional views. Thus, while PIDs have long been recognized as representing defects of either adaptive or innate immunity, AIDs have classically been considered as diseases of the adaptive immune system, a consequence of pathogenic autoantibodies, of autoreactive T cells, or of both. Yet, a large group of PIDs[5] that include auto-inflammatory disorders have revealed that deficits in components of innate immunity can also be at the origin of aggressive pathology. We suggest that these disorders are also appropriately classified as AIDs. Just as we group adaptive (aPID) and innate (iPID) immunodeficiencies, we shall then speak of adaptive (aAID) and innate (iAID) autoimmune diseases. Innate and adaptive mechanisms of immunity interact extensively and may well amplify or modulate each other's manifestations; in addition, genes related to innate immunity are often also expressed in lymphocytes (e.g., TLRs, cytokines, etc.). In many conditions, "adaptive" auto-reactivity seems to be necessary to amplify or maintain the disease process, even if the initial trigger is related to "non-immune" inflammation, or other forms of tissue damage. Yet, rather than defining AIDs by their targets or end results, it would appear that primary mechanisms provide a more consistent classification. Were this proposal to become generally accepted, PID/AID associations would have again contributed novel insights.

Beyond innate and adaptive immunity, a third and more primitive layer of defense mechanisms is represented by cellular stress responses and tissue-protective genes/pathways.[6] While the participation of this set of responses in modulating autoimmune manifestations is now clear,[7,8] no corresponding PIDs have been described, perhaps because of critical roles of these pathways in embryonic and fetal development.

Heterogeneity of PID/AID associations

The frequency at which PIDs appear in association with AIDs varies widely, both in cases of adaptive and of innate immunity. Certain PIDs are systematically associated with autoimmunity, to the extent that, whenever the genetic basis of PID has been identified, we may speak of "monogenic AIDs":[1,3] a unique gene/mechanism is sufficient to establish disease, even if pathogenesis clearly involves many other pathways of both innate and adaptive immunity. This is the case with the autoimmune endocrinopathies in autoimmune polyendocrinopathy, candidiasis, ectodermal dystrophy (APECED); with the neonatal enteropathy and type I diabetes in the immune dysregulation, polyendocrinopathy, enteropathy, X-linked (IPEX) syndrome; or with the lupus disease in C1q deficiency. In contrast, autoimmune manifestations have rarely or never been described in other PIDs, even in patients presenting recurrent and/or chronic infections.[1-3] Variability is likely to result either from "modifier genes," which modulate susceptibility to AID, from the nature of putative triggering or aggravating events (e.g., infections, stresses), or else, simply represent current limitations in a complete description of pathology. Heterogeneity of association extends to the "target" tissues, organs, or functions for the autoimmune aggression: certain PIDs associate with specific phenotypes, such as organ-specific endocrine diseases in patients with AIRE (autoimmune regulator) mutations, autoimmune cytopenias in patients with autoimmune lymphoproliferative syndrome (ALPS), or systemic lupus erythematosus as the only autoimmune manifestation of complement deficiencies. The reasons for such selective manifestations of autoimmunity are generally not clear.

A classification of PID/AID associations according to their frequency is shown in Tables 49.1–49.4. Naturally, analyses of AID association could only be performed for those PIDs with a significant number of patients already reported. More than 80% of patients in the first group of PIDs present clinical autoimmune manifestations, and we speak of innate or adaptive PIDs that are "systematically associated" with autoimmunity (Table 49.1). AID is systematically associated with aPIDs in:

(a) IPEX;

(b) APECED, also called autoimmune polyglandular syndrome type I (APS-I);

(c) Omenn syndrome; and

(d) ALPS.

Several of these were classified as "syndromes with autoimmunity" within the group "diseases of immune dysregulation" by the International Union of Immunological Societies (IUIS) committee of PID experts.[5] From the genetic point of view, all entities in this group could be seen as monogenic forms of autoimmunity, representing, respectively:

Table 49.1 PIDs *systematically* associated with adaptive AID and/or Innate AID manifestations*

PID	Defective gene or protein	Main AID features	Frequency (%)	References
Adaptive immunity				
IPEX[1]	FOXP3	Enteropathy (92**), diabetes mellitus (66), skin lesions (42-60), cytopenias (28), hypothyroidism (20)	100	32, 35
Omenn syndrome	RAG1, RAG2, Artemis, IL-7RA, 22q11.2 deletion, others	Extensive skin lesions (erythrodermia, exfoliative lesions), enteropathy, alopecia	100	10
APECED[2]	AIRE	Hypoparathyroidism (79-93), hypoadrenalism (73), ovarian (43-50) or testicular failure, hypothyroidism (10), type 1 diabetes mellitus (12), hepatitis (20), alopecia (29-37), vitiligo (15)	Almost 100	44, 47
ALPS[3]	TNFRSF6 (Fas), TNFSF6 (FasL), CASP10, NRAS, KRAS	Hemolytic anemia (29), thrombocytopenia (23), neutropenia (19), Evans'syndrome	More than 80	31, 33
Innate immunity				
Familial HLH[4]	PFR1, STX11, UNC13D	Systemic inflammation, hepatosplenomegaly, pancytopenia, neuropathy	100	11
Chediak–Higashi syndrome	LYST	Hemophagocytic syndrome in the accelerated phase	Almost all cases	11
Griscelli syndrome	RAB27A	Hemophagocytic syndrome	Almost all cases	11
XL-lymphoproliferative syndrome	SH2D1A	Hemophagocytic syndrome	Almost all cases	11
Autoinflammatory disorders	MEFV, TNFRSF1A, CIAS1, MVK, NOD2, PSTP1P1, LPIN2, IL1RA, others	Arthritis, urticarial rashes, serositis, sterile pyogenic abscesses, uveitis, granuloma formation, systemic inflammation	100	12, 45
C1q deficiency	C1Q	Systemic lupus erythematosus	93	14

*>80% of PID cases present AID manifestations.
**% of PID patients with the autoimmune disorder.
[1]Immunedysregulation polyendocrinopathy enteropathy X-linked.
[2]Autoimmune polyendocrinopathy candidiasis ectodermal dystrophy.
[3]Autoimmune lymphoproliferative syndrome.
[4]Familial hemophagocytic lymphohistiocytosis.

(a) Defects of Foxp3, essential for the development and functions of regulatory T cells (Treg);

(b) Defective lymphocyte selection in the thymus due to loss-of-function *AIRE* mutations;

(c) Severely restricted repertoires of T-cell receptors (TCR) and B-cell receptors (BCR), involving pauciclonality and compensatory clonal expansions, due to either hypomorphic mutations in genes involved in somatic rearrangements (RAG-1 or 2, Artemis), or to profound limitations in lymphocyte production (as in defects of cytokine pathways involved in lymphocyte production and/or development, or in those associated with atypical DiGeorge syndrome); and

(d) Defects of Fas-mediated and intrinsic pathway-related apoptosis.[1,4,9,10]

Innate immunity defects that are systematically associated with AID include:

(a) Familial hemophagocytic lymphohistiocytosis (HLH) forms (due to perforin, syntaxin 11 and UNC13D deficiencies) and other conditions associated with macrophage activation and hemophagocytic syndrome (Chediak–Higashi syndrome, Griscelli syndrome, X-linked lymphoproliferative syndrome);[5,11]

(b) Autoinflammatory disorders resulting from several defects in inflammatory pathways such as IL-1R antagonist;[12] and

(c) complete C1q deficiency, showing a unique association with SLE, the pathogenesis of which is yet to be fully understood, but may involve impaired clearance of apoptotic debris and immune complexes.[13,14]

It was recently demonstrated that C1q deficiency is associated with higher immune complex-induced interferon-α production.[15]

We designate as "strongly associated with autoimmunity" another group of PIDs including the most prevalent entities, in which 20 to 80% of all patients show autoimmune manifestations, a frequency that is 3-10 times higher than in the general population (Table 49.2). As in other groups, both aPIDs and iPIDs show AID associations, including IgA deficiency (IgAD), common variable immune deficiency (CVID), partial T-cell immunodeficiencies resulting from hypomorphic mutations of the same genes that cause severe T-cell defects,[16] deficiencies of early complement components in the classical pathway other than C1q (C1r, C1s, C4, and C2), NFκB essential modulator (NEMO) defects, and the Wiskott–Aldrich syndrome. Some reports suggest inclusion of the "syndrome of 22q11.2 deletion" (mainly the so called "incomplete" DiGeorge syndrome) as well.[1,10,14,17–20] We also include chronic granulomatous disease (CGD) in this group, because one-third of CGD patients present dysregulated inflammatory responses, with frequent granulomatous manifestations in hollow viscera of the gastrointestinal and urinary tracts, as well as clinical and endoscopic features of inflammatory bowel disease.[21] Again, there is

Table 49.2 PIDs *strongly* associated with AID manifestations*

PID	Defective gene or protein	Main AID features	Frequency (%)	References
Adaptive Immunity				
Wiskott–Aldrich syndrome	WASP	Cytopenias (14-36), arthritis (11-29), skin and cerebral vasculitis (13-22), renal disease (12), IBD[2] (9)	40–72	18
CVID[1]	Unknown in most cases, ICOS, TNFRSF13B (TACI), TNFRS13C (BAFF-R), CD19	Cytopenias (most frequent), rheumatoid-like arthritis, IBD, pernicious anemia, primary biliary cirrhosis, SLE-like syndrome, thyroiditis, myesthenia gravis, others	21–25	22, 43
XL-Hyper IgM syndrome	CD40L	Neutropenia (45-60), hemolytic anemia, thrombocytopenia, IBD, arthritis, sclerosing cholangitis, hepatitis	60	19
AID deficiency	AICDA	Cytopenias (most frequent), hepatitis, enteropathy	25	19
IgA deficiency	Unknown	Hypothyroidism, rheumatoid-like arthritis, cytopenias, SLE (5% of juvenile cases), pernicious anemia, celiac disease, Sjögren syndrome, type 1 diabetes mellitus, hepatitis, vitiligo, others	7–38	23
22q11.2 deletion (DiGeorge syndrome)	Polygenic disorder	Hemolytic anemia and/or thrombocytopenia (most frequent), arthritis, Graves disease	10–33	17, 20
Innate immunity				
C4, C1r/s, C2 deficiencies	C1R, C1S, C4A, and C4B, C2	Systemic lupus erythematosus	75, 57, and 20, respectively	13, 14
Chronic granulomatous disease (CGD)	CYBB, CYBA, NCF1, NCF2	IBD, inflammatory and granulomatous lesions in hollow viscera, mainly GI and urinary tracts, chorioretinitis, lupus-like features in patients and X-linked CGD female carriers, Behçet disease	33	21, 38
NEMO deficiency (XL-EDA with ID)[3]	IKBKG	IBD (most frequent), arthritis, hemolytic anemia	25	19

*Less than 80% and more than 20% of the PID patients with autoimmune manifestations.
[1]Common variable immunodeficiency.
[2]Inflammatory bowel disease.
[3]X-linked ectodermal dysplasia with immunodeficiency.

Table 49.3 Examples of PIDs that are *slightly* associated with AID manifestations*

PID	Defective gene or protein	Main AID features	Frequency (%)	References
Adaptive Immunity				
XL-agammaglobulinemia	BTK	Arthritis (most cases), dermatomyositis, scleroderma, alopecia, type 1 diabetes mellitus	11–15	26
AR-hyper-IgE syndrome	TYK2	Cytopenias**, systemic lupus erythematosus, cerebral vasculitis, anti-phospholipide syndrome, renal disease	Few cases	25
MHC class II deficiency	C2TA, RFX5, RFXAP, RFXANK	Hemolytic anemia	2/30 pts	48
Ataxia telangiectasia syndrome	ATM	Cytopenias	Few cases	24, 28
Innate immunity				
C3 and C5-C9 deficiency	C3, C5-C9	Systemic lupus erythematosus	~10	14
FcγRIIIb deficiency	FCGR3B	Thyroiditis	2/21 pts	49

*<20% of the PID patients with autoimmune manifestations.
**Clinical descriptions are suggestive of autosomal recessive-hyper-IgE syndrome, but genetic studies were not available in most cases.

Table 49.4 Examples of PIDs with no described association with autoimmune manifestations

PID	Defective gene	Reference
Adaptive immunity		
Autosomal dominant-hyper-IgE syndrome	STAT-3	27
IL-12/IL-23–IFN-γ axis deficiencies	IL12RB1, IL12B, IFNGR1, IFNGR2, STAT-1	30
Asplenia	Unknown	1
Innate immunity		
IRAK-4 deficiency	IRAK 4	29

some selectivity in "target" manifestations: CVID patients tend to develop immune thrombocytopenia or hemolytic anemia,[22] while those with IgAD are prone to both systemic (chronic arthritis, SLE) and organ-specific (hypothyroidism) disorders,[23] and CGD patients can also manifest inflammatory bowel disease and discoid lupus.

In the group of PIDs classified as "mildly associated with autoimmunity," less than 20% of the patients already described presented AID manifestations. This group includes agammaglobulinemia, deficiencies of C3 and MAC (membrane attack complex in the complement system) proteins, as well as autosomal recessive hyper-IgE syndrome, and ataxia-telangiectasia in which cytopenias were recently reported (Table 49.3).[14,24–28] A fourth group consists of PIDs in which AID manifestations have never been described, such as IL-12/IL-23-IFN-γ axis defects, and IRAK-4 deficiency, as well as rare conditions such as asplenia, factor D-deficiency, and WHIM (warts, hypogammaglobulinemia, infections, myelokatexis) syndrome (Table 49.4).[1, 29,30] Such "negative associations" could also be informative in guiding hypotheses on pathogenic mechanisms of AID.

● KEY CONCEPTS

Association between PIDs and autoimmune disorders

- Autoimmune phenomena are the second most common clinical features of PIDs, only after high susceptibility to infections.
- Autoimmune disease may be the initial manifestation of a PID, both in infants with severe conditions and in adults with milder ones.
- Diagnosis of an underlying PID should be considered in all early-onset autoimmune disorders, particularly in boys, and in the autoimmune patient whenever he/she presents:
  - Recurrent infections or a given infection;
  - Other signs of immune dysregulation, such as exaggerated inflammation, atopic-like features, high IgE levels, or enlarged lymphoid organs;
  - Multiple targets of autoimmunity.
- Treatment should aim at ultimately correcting the underlying immunodeficiency.

PID/AID associations contribute to understanding AID pathogenesis

The study of PIDs represents a most successful branch of "translational immunology"; thus, we now have satisfactory clinical descriptions of a few hundred such diseases, having identified the responsible genes and mutations in a large number of these, and derived rational and curative therapies through stem cell replacement and gene therapy. This represents an exceptional achievement in modern medicine. In sharp contrast, we continue to be severely limited in respect to AIDs: we have at hand few, if any, rational, curative therapies, such that the clinical management of patients continues to rely on symptomatic, nonspecific treatments, and we have made little progress in diagnosing AID before there is compromise of target organs or functions, let alone in advancing solid predictions of disease risks from genetic information. It is fair to say that our difficulties relate to the complexity of autoimmune pathogenesis and to current limitations in understanding all mechanisms involved in the natural acquisition of tolerance to body tissues. In this context, detailed consideration of PID/AID associations and respective clinical manifestations may contribute some insight.

Role of recurrent/chronic infections

It has been suggested that AID in PID patients may simply be the consequence of repeated infections, either by "overstimulation" of immune responses or by "antigenic cross-reactivity" (mimicry) between microbial antigens and those of "self." This is neither a satisfactory explanation for many such conditions, nor is it a valid general hypothesis. Thus, as seen above (Table 49.4), several PIDs that evolve with repeated and/or chronic infections do not lead to autoimmunity, possibly because the regulatory mechanisms that ensure self-tolerance are not compromised. Furthermore, some of the most serious autoimmune conditions (e.g., IPEX and ALPS) appear in PIDs where the frequency of infections is not particularly increased.[31–33] Finally, as pointed out previously,[34] AID cases that are thought to result from antigenic mimicry following infection, such as in the classical example of carditis after *Streptococcus* A infection, are rare: only a few percent of all infected patients develop AID, suggesting that infections merely operate to trigger the pathogenic process in patients that are already "autoimmune-prone."

Relative importance of recessive (deletional) versus dominant (regulatory) mechanisms in the establishment of natural tolerance

A major conceptual shift in putative mechanisms of natural tolerance has taken place in recent years. While, over the past few decades, tolerance was thought to be "recessive" and result from elimination of auto-reactive T and B lymphocytes, the role of "dominant" regulatory mechanisms, particularly Treg-dependent suppression, is currently given much importance. PID/AID associations are very informative in suggesting the relative importance of recessive (deletional) versus dominant (regulatory) mechanisms in natural tolerance. Thus, "pure" deficits in Tregs with conserved deletion of autoreactive lymphocytes, as in IPEX patients, result in very severe auto-aggressive disease.[32,35] In contrast, conditions where regulation is conserved but deletional mechanisms are impaired, as in IRAK-4 deficiency, do not result in AID, despite a very abundant autoreactive repertoire.[29] It would seem, therefore, that "dominant" tolerance represents the most critical of possibly many mechanisms involved in establishing self-tolerance.

Critical role of lymphocyte homeostatic peripheral expansion

T lymphocytopenia is often accompanied by autoimmunity, Omenn syndrome providing for the first and best characterized example.[10] A number of other genetic conditions, however, result in similar, if less severe phenotypes.[16] Deficits in T-cell production may result from limitations in:

(a) the gene recombination process (*RAG1*, *RAG2*, Artemis are already known, but others are likely to be discovered, for more genes and their protein products are required for V(D)J recombination); and

(b) the process of cellular production from precursors, which involves extensive, cytokine-dependent proliferation and differentiation, in a particular organ environment (thymus) that requires a multiplicity of cell types and respective interactions (stroma, epithelium, bone marrow-derived antigen-presenting cells of various types, lymphoid precursors themselves).

Not surprisingly, therefore, a variety of conditions can lead to deficits in T-cell production, "incomplete" DiGeorge syndrome being the most common, to which many hypomorphic mutations of genes involved in SCID have now been added.[16,20] Whatever the origin and precise mechanisms, these patients produce a limited number of TCRs and a restricted repertoire of specificities; that is, they suffer the consequences of "oligoclonality". Given the unpredictable nature of V(D)J gene recombination that produces TCR variable regions, restricted repertoires are unpredictable, and will harbor variable frequencies of both autoreactive effector T cells, and of autoreactive regulatory T cells. The relative balance between these two subsets, and the frequencies of any given specificity in either, will determine the severity and "targets" of the autoimmune syndrome. Yet one more factor may influence the outcome of such conditions, namely the fact that under conditions of lymphopenia, available T cells will expand in the periphery, often to numbers that do not differ much from the normal levels: peripheral repertoires, therefore, remain oligoclonal, but now contain very large clones of T cells. This process is known as "homeostatic expansion" and may be driven by productive autoreactivity of the expanding clones. Again, depending on the precise specificities that expand and on the relative levels of expansion in effector or regulatory cells, a clinical condition may ensue.

Given all this variability, a few "invariables" are remarkable. First, that thymic T-cell production assumes such a critical role in the prevention of autoimmunity; hence, it is advisable to investigate this parameter (by determining in peripheral T cells, the time-dependent dynamics of "TREC" levels, or the representation of recent thymic emigrants) in clinical cases compatible with this possibility. It is conceivable that deficient thymic production may originate or aggravate other forms of AID, and it would be useful for investigating interventions aimed at (re)establishing this process. Second, it is striking that in such PID/AID associations, the predominant target tissues are blood cells, skin, and intestine, i.e., tissues in constant renewal. Finally, the predominance of IgE production in these and other cases (e.g., IPEX, Omenn syndrome, Wiskott–Aldrich syndrome) where Tregs are limiting suggests that this may be a useful general indicator for immune dysregulation. When evaluating an AID patient suspected of having a PID, some laboratory parameters can provide critical information:

(a) TREC levels, or the representation of recent thymic emigrants, may reveal lower lymphocyte thymic production;

(b) Immunoscopy or spectratyping (or V-region sequencing) suggests or ascertains TCR oligoclonality; and

(c) Increased serum IgE levels may be a good marker of immune dysregulation.

Autoimmune "targets" in different PIDs

As shown in Tables 49.5–49.8, each autoimmune condition associated to PIDs is characterized by a limited set of "target" organs, tissues, and functions. This is not restricted to PID-dependent AID (e.g., the predominance of auto-antibodies to structural nucleolar components in SLE, or of anti-mitochondrial antibodies in autoimmune biliary cirrhosis), but remains a poorly understood phenomenon. We have no satisfactory explanation why, for instance, APECED patients develop endocrinopathies almost exclusively, or why IPEX patients—expected to develop generalized autoimmunity—present with enteropathy and type I diabetes preferentially, while ALPS patients exclusively develop autoimmune cytopenias, just as we do not understand why antibodies to acetylcholine receptors appear in association with thymoma. Elegant studies in mice have demonstrated that many genes are at play in determining "targeting" of autoimmunity, but most of these have not been characterized.

Cytopenias, particularly hemolytic anemia and thrombocytopenia, represent the most common autoimmune complication associated with several PIDs, mostly in the adaptive group (Table 49.5). In ALPS and CVID, cytopenia is often the first PID manifestation.[22,31] In contrast, autoimmune endocrinopathies (Table 49.6) have been associated with few aPIDs: multiple endocrinopathies are characteristic of APECED, persistent neonatal diabetes mellitus and hypothyroidism are observed in most IPEX babies, whereas thyroiditis is described as a very frequent autoimmune complication in IgAD patients. Table 49.7 describes the associations of PIDs with other "epithelial" AID. Enteropathy is the most frequent IPEX manifestation, including colitis features in some babies, and inflammatory bowel disease has been described as the most common autoimmune consequence of NEMO deficiency, but also in other iPIDs and aPIDs. Arthritis is another manifestation seen in both aPIDs

Table 49.5 PIDs that manifest as autoimmune cytopenias

	Frequency (%)*	References
Hemophagocytic lymphohistiocytosis (HLH)**	100	11
ALPS	>80	31, 33
X-linked IgM syndrome	44-60	19
Wiskott–Aldrich syndrome	36	18
IPEX	28	32, 35
CVID	20-25	22
Hyper-IgM syndrome due to AID*** deficiency	25	19
DiGeorge syndrome	10-33	17, 20
Selective IgA deficiency SCID due to PNP+ deficiency	3 Few cases	23, 50

*% of PID patients with any autoimmune cytopenia
**Cytopenias in HLH are not considered as classically antibody-mediated phenomena
***Activation-induced cytidine deaminase+ purine nucleoside phosphorylase

Table 49.6 PIDs associated with autoimmune endocrinopathies

	APECED	IPEX	IgA deficiency	Other
Thyroiditis	10%*	20	8	TACl** deficiency FcγRIIIb deficiency (10)
Hypoparathyroidism	79-93			DiGeorge syndrome*** (26)
Hypoadrenalism	73		rare	
Type 1 diabetes mellitus	12	66	rare	CVID (some cases)
Ovarian failure	43-50			
Testicular failure	14			
Hypophysitis	7			
References	44, 47	32, 35	23	17, 43, 49

*% of PID patients with the autoimmune disorder.
**Transmembrane activator and CAML interactor.
***Hypoparathyroidism results from a developmental defect and is not an autoimmune phenomenon

Table 49.7 PIDs associated with intestinal, cutaneous and other autoimmune epithelial disorders

	APECED	IPEX	CVID	IgA deficiency	Others
Enteropathy	15-18%*	92-97			AID** deficiency
Inflammatory bowel disease		Some cases	6-10	Some cases	CGD (33) NEMO deficiency (25) Wiskott–Aldrich syndrome (9) X-linked hyper-IgM syndrome IL-10R deficiency
Coeliac disease			1	4%	X-linked agammaglobulinemia (one case)
Alopecia	29-37		2-4		
Vitiligo	12-15		Some cases	<1%	
Other autoimmune skin disease		42-60			Omenn syndrome (100) Autoinflammatory disorders (almost all patients with the different entities)
Pernicious anemia	13-15		1-9	<1%	
Hepatitis	12-20	Some cases	Some cases	Some cases	X-linked hyper-IgM syndrome AID deficiency
Sclerosing cholangitis				<1%	X-linked hyper-IgM syndrome
References	44, 47	31, 35	22, 43	23	1,10,12,18,19,21,26,45,51

*(%) frequency of the PID patients with the autoimmune disorder.
**Activation-induced cytidine deaminase.

Table 49.8 PIDs associated with chronic or recurrent arthritis

	Frequency (%)*	References
Autoinflammatory disorders (particularly familial Mediterranean fever, TRAPS**, cryopyrinopathies, mevalonate kinase deficiency, others)	60-80	12, 45
Wiskott–Aldrich syndrome	10-29	18
X-linked agammaglobulinemia	11-15	26
CVID	1-10	43
Selective IgA deficiency	4	23
X-linked IgM syndrome	Few cases	19
DiGeorge syndrome	Few cases	20

*% of PID patients with different forms of chronic arthritis.
**TNF receptor associated periodic syndrome.

(agammaglobulinemia, CVID, IgA deficiency, Wiskott–Aldrich syndrome) and iPIDs, being an important feature of various autoinflammatory disorders (Table 49.8).

PID-AID associations also contribute to assessment of the notion that "pathogenic" or "disease-associated" autoantibodies differ from "natural autoantibodies" that can be systematically scored in healthy conditions, by their increased affinity, which is brought about by (auto)antigen-dependent selection following extensive somatic mutation.[36] This notion is related to the idea that, contrary to IgG autoantibodies, those of the IgM class are harmless and represent physiological autoreactivity.[36] Hyper-IgM syndromes, where somatic hypermutation does not occur at all (AID deficiencies) or to a limited extent only (CD40L mutations), nevertheless show autoimmune manifestations that seem to be mediated, at least in part, by "pathogenic" auto-antibodies. Interestingly, a recent report in the mouse model demonstrates that somatic hypermutation, rather than class switch, is critical for physiological neutralization of gut flora.[37]

PIDs may provide useful insights into SLE pathophysiology

Few PIDs have been described as consistently associated with SLE or lupus-like manifestations (Table 49.9):

(a) Homozygous deficiencies of early components of the classical complement pathway;

(b) Selective or partial immunoglobulin deficiencies, particularly isolated IgA and IgM deficiencies; and

(c) CGD, in both patients and female carriers of the X-linked CGD allele (Table 49.2).[13,14,21,38–41]

Complete deficiency of any of the early components of the classical complement pathway represents the strongest single genetic risk factor for the development of SLE identified to date. SLE or lupus-like manifestations have been detected in 93% of homozygous C1q-deficient, 75% of C4-deficient, 57% of C1r/C1s deficient, and 20-32% of C2-deficient individuals.[13,14,16] Yet, although complement deficiencies have contributed to new concepts on the mechanisms of SLE pathogenesis, the prevalence of homozygous deficiencies is currently estimated at less than 1% of SLE patients. The prevalence of IgAD among SLE patients is higher: 5.2% in 77 patients with juvenile SLE, and 2.6% in 152 adult onset SLE patients].[40] Isolated IgM deficiency (<30 mg %) in 3/72 patients, and low IgG2 (<15 mg%) levels in 4/72 patients all older than 10 years of age, were recently reported in juvenile forms of SLE,[42] but other antibody deficiencies have not been associated with this disease. Rather, severe antibody deficiencies (e.g., agammaglobulinemia and CVID) are thought to be incompatible with the development of SLE lesions, since pathogenic autoantibodies seem necessary for tissue damage.[26,43]

In a large CGD series (368 patients), Winkelstein et al.[38] found that 3.2% presented with discoid lupus erythematosus or SLE, and others reported this association not only in patients but also in female carriers of the X-linked CGD allele.[21,39]

In contrast, a number of PIDs that are systematically or strongly associated with autoimmune manifestations are selectively "deprived" of SLE or lupus-like clinical or laboratory manifestations. These include APECED, IPEX, ALPS, autoinflammatory disorders, Wiskott–Aldrich syndrome, X-linked-hyper-IgM syndrome (due to CD40L mutations), and DiGeorge syndrome.[12,17,18,31,33,35,41,44,45] "Monogenic PIDs" may contribute,

therefore, to unraveling some of the pieces of the "puzzle" represented by the pathophysiology of SLE, a prototypic polygenic autoimmune disease.

Translational research

The study of patients with monogenic PIDs and autoimmune manifestations represents a unique opportunity to unravel the pathophysiology of autoimmunity as well as the genetics of autoimmune diseases. Different PIDs or groups of PIDs prototypically are associated with distinct autoimmune disorders, e.g., AIRE mutations with organ-specific endocrinopathies, Foxp3 deficiency with enteropathy, complement deficiencies with SLE, autoinflammatory diseases with chronic arthritis, thus providing critical insights into pathogenesis of autoimmune disorders, notably on the "targeting" of the autoimmune process. In addition, the study of PID patients may open new therapeutic perspectives aimed at improving thymic function,[46] and development of new immunobiologicals.

● ON THE HORIZON

- The analyses of typical PID genes (sequencing and expression) in pediatric and adult patients with complex autoimmune diseases may lead to a better understanding of the pathogenesis of autoimmune disorders.

References

1. Carneiro-Sampaio M, Coutinho A. Tolerance and autoimmunity: lessons at the bedside of primary immunodeficiencies. Adv Immunol 2007;95:51–82.
2. Westerberg LS, Klein C, Snapper SB. Breakdown of T cell tolerance and autoimmunity in primary immunodeficiency—lessons learned from monogenic disorders in mice and men. Curr Opin Immunol 2008;20:646–54.
3. Arason GJ, Jorgensen GH, Ludviksson BR. Primary immunodeficiency and autoimmunity: lessons from human diseases. Scand J Immunol 2010;71:317–28.
4. Coutinho A, Carneiro-Sampaio M. Primary immunodeficiencies unravel critical aspects of the pathophysiology of autoimmunity and of the genetics of autoimmune disease. J Clin Immunol 2008;28(Suppl. 1):S4–10.
5. Notarangelo LD, Fischer A, Geha RS, et al. Primary immunodeficiencies: 2009 update. International Union of Immunological Societies Expert Committee on Primary Immunodeficiencies. J Allergy Clin Immunol 2009;124:1161–78.
6. Gozzelino R, Jeney V, Soares MP. Mechanisms of cell protection by heme oxygenase-1. Annu Rev Pharmacol Toxicol 2010;50:323–54.
7. Yoh K, Itoh K, Enomoto A, et al. Nrf2-deficient female mice develop lupus-like autoimmune nephritis. Kidney Int 2001;60:1343–53.
8. Chora AA, Fontoura P, Cunha A, et al. Sobel RAHeme oxygenase-1 and carbon monoxide suppress autoimmune neuroinflammation. J Clin Invest 2007;117:438–47.
9. Notarangelo LD, Gambineri E, Badolato R. Immunodeficiencies with autoimmune consequences. Adv Immunol 2006;89:321–70.
10. Milner JD, Fasth A, Etzioni A. Autoimmunity in severe combined immunodeficiencies (SCID): Lessons from patients and experimental models. J Clin Immunol 2008;28(Suppl. 1):S29–33.
11. Janka GE. Hemophagocytic syndromes. Blood Rev 2007;21:245–53.
12. Masters SL, Simon A, Aksentijevich I, et al. Horror autoinflammaticus: the molecular pathophysiology of autoinflammatory disease. Annu Rev Immunol 2009;27:621–68.
13. Pickering MC, Botto M, Taylor PR, et al. Systemic Lupus Erythematosus, complement deficiency, and apoptosis. Adv Immunol 2000;76:227–34.
14. Manderson AP, Botto M, Walport MJ. The role of complement in the development of systemic lupus erythematosus. Annu Rev Immunol 2004;22:431–56.
15. Santer DM, Hall BE, George TC, et al. C1q deficiency leads to the defective suppression of IFN-alpha in response to nucleoprotein containing immune complexes. J Immunol 2010;185:4738–49.
16. Liston A, Enders A, Siggs OM. Unravelling the association of partial T-cell immunodeficiency and immune dysregulation. Nat Rev Immunol 2008;8:545–58.
17. Gennery AR, Barge D, O'Sullivan JJ, et al. Antibody deficiency and autoimmunity in 22q11.2 deletion syndrome. Arch Dis Child 2002;86:422–5.
18. Schurman SH, Candotti F. Autoimmunity in Wiskott-Aldrich syndrome. Curr Opin Rheumatol 2003;15:446–53.
19. Jesus AA, Duarte AJ, Oliveira JB. Autoimmunity in hyper-IgM syndrome. J Clin Immunol 2008;28(Suppl. 1):S62–S66.
20. McLean-Tooke A, Barge D, Spickett GP, et al. Immunologic defects in 22q11.2 deletion syndrome. J Allergy Clin Immunol 2008;122:362–7.

Table 49.9 Association between PIDs and systemic lupus erythematosus (SLE) or lupus-like manifestations

Consistently associated	Not associated
*C1q deficiency (93%**)	APECED
*C4 deficiency (75%)	IPEX and female carriers of X-linked IPEX allele
*C1s/r deficiency (57%)	
*C2 deficiency (20-32%)	ALPS
IgA deficiency (5%)***	Wiskott–Aldrich syndrome
IgM deficiency (3/72)+	X-linked agammaglobulinemia
CGD++ and female carriers of X-linked CGD allele	X-linked hyper-IgM syndrome (CD40L deficiency)
	DiGeorge syndrome
	Autoinflammatory disorders
	FcγRIIIb deficiency

*Homozygous deficiency.
**% of the PID patients that developed SLE.
***Juvenile SLE patients with the PID.
+Serum IgM levels <30 mg in a juvenile SLE series.
++Chronic granulomatous disease.
References: 12–14,18,19,21,26,31–33,35,38–40,44,45,47,49.

21. Rosenzweig SD. Inflammatory manifestations in chronic granulomatous disease. J Clin Immunol 2008;28(Suppl. 1):S67–72.

22. Wang J, Cunningham-Rundles C. Treatment and outcome of autoimmune hematologic disease in common variable immunodeficiency (CVID). J Autoimmun 2005;25:57–62.

23. Jacob CM, Pastorino AC, Fahl K, et al. Autoimmunity in IgA deficiency: revisiting the role of IgA as a silent housekeeper. J Clin Immunol 2008;28(Suppl. 1):S56–61.

24. Meyts I, Weemaes C, De Wolf-Peeters C, et al. Unusual and severe disease course in a child with ataxia-telangiectasia. Pediatr Allergy Immunol 2003;14:330–3.

25. Renner ED, Puck JM, Holland SM, et al. Autosomal recessive hyperimmunoglobulin E syndrome: a distinct disease entity. J Pediatr 2004;144:93–9.

26. Howard V, Greene JM, Pahwa S, et al. The health status and quality of life of adults with X-linked agammaglobulinemia. Clin Immunol 2006;118:201–18.

27. Freeman AF, Holland SM. Clinical manifestations, etiology, and pathogenesis of the hyper-IgE syndromes. Pediatr Res 2009;65(5 Pt 2):32R–37R.

28. Heath J, Goldman FD. Idiopathic thrombocytopenic purpura in a boy with ataxia telangiectasia on immunoglobulin replacement therapy. J Pediatr Hematol Oncol 2010;32:e25–e27.

29. Isnardi I, Ng YS, Srdanovic I, et al. IRAK-4- and MyD88-dependent pathways are essential for the removal of developing autoreactive B cells in humans. Immunity 2008;29:746–57.

30. Beaucoudrey L, Samarina A, Bustamante J, et al. Revisiting human IL-12Rβ1 deficiency: a survey of 141 patients from 30 countries. Medicine (Baltimore) 2010;89:381–402.

31. Oliveira JB, Fleisher TA. Autoimmune lymphoproliferative syndrome. Curr Opin Allergy Clin Immunol 2004;4:497–503.

32. Torgerson T, Ochs HD. Immune dysregulation, polyendocrinopathy, enteropathy, X-linked: forkhead box protein 3 mutations and lack of regulatory T cells. J Allergy Clin Immunol 2007;120:744–50.

33. Oliveira JB, Bleesing JJ, Dianzani U, et al. Revised diagnostic criteria and classification for the autoimmune lymphoproliferative syndrome (ALPS): report from the 2009 NIH International Workshop. Blood 2010;116:e35–40.

34. Demengeot J, Zelenay S, Moraes-Fontes MF, et al. Regulatory T cells in microbial infection. Springer Semin Immun 2006;28:41–50.

35. Wildin RS, Smyk-Pearson S, Filipovich AH. Clinical and molecular features of Immune dysregulation, polyendocrinopathy, and X-linked inheritance (IPEX), a syndrome. J Med Genet 2002;39:537–45.

36. Coutinho A, Kazatchkine MD, Avrameas S. Natural autoantibodies. Curr Opin Immunol 1995;7:812–8.

37. Wei M, Shinkura R, Doi Y, et al. Mice carrying a knock-in mutation of Aicda resulting in a defect in somatic hypermutation have impaired gut homeostasis and compromised mucosal defense. Nat Immunol 2011;12:264–70.

38. Winkelstein JA, Marino MC, Johnston Jr RB, et al. Chronic granulomatous disease. Report on a national registry of 368 patients. Medicine (Baltimore) 2000;79:155–69.

39. Cale CM, Morton L, Goldblatt D. Cutaneous and other lupus-like symptoms in carriers of X-linked chronic granulomatous disease: incidence and autoimmune serology. Clin Exp Immunol 2007;148:79–84.

40. Cassidy JT, Kitson RK, Selby CL. Selective IgA deficiency in children and adults with systemic lupus erythematosus. Lupus 2007;16:647–50.

41. Carneiro-Sampaio M, Liphaus BL, Jesus AA, et al. Understanding SLE pathophysiology in the light of Primary Immunodeficiencies. J Clin Immunol 2008;28(Suppl. 1):S34–41.

42. Jesus AA, Liphaus BL, Silva CAA, et al. Complement and antibody primary immunodeficiency in juvenile systemic erythematosus lupus patients. Lupus 2011;20:1275–84.

43. Agarwal S, Cunningham-Rundles C. Autoimmunity in common variable immunodeficiency. Curr Allergy Asthma Rep 2009;9:347–52.

44. Husebye ES, Perheentupa J, Rautemaa R, et al. Clinical manifestations and management of patients with autoimmune polyendocrine syndrome type I. J Intern Med 2009;265:514–29.

45. Jesus AA, Oliveira JB, Hilário MO, et al. Pediatric hereditary autoinflammatory syndromes. J Pediatr (Rio J) 2010;86:353–66.

46. Holländer GA, Krenger W, Blazar BR. Emerging strategies to boost thymic function. Curr Opin Pharmacol 2010;10:443–53.

47. Betterle C, Greggio NA, Volpato M. Autoimmune polyglandular syndrome type 1. J Clin Endocrinol Metab 1998;83:1049–55.

48. Klein C, Lisowska-Grospierre B, LeDeist F, et al. Major histocompatibility complex class II deficiency: clinical manifestations, immunologic features, and outcome. J Pediatr 1993;123:921–8.

49. de Haas M, Kleijer M, van Zwieten R, et al. Neutrophil Fc gamma RIIIb deficiency, nature, and clinical consequences: a study of 21 individuals from 14 families. Blood 1995;86:2403–13.

50. Notarangelo LD. Primary immunodeficiencies (PIDs) presenting with cytopenias. Hematology Am Soc Hematol Educ Program 2009;139–43.

51. Glocker EO, Kotlarz D, Boztug K, et al. Inflammatory bowel disease and mutations affecting the interleukin-10 receptor. N Engl J Med 2009;361:2033–45.

50.

Systemic lupus erythematosus

Cynthia Aranow,
Betty Diamond,
Meggan Mackay

Systemic lupus erythematosus (SLE) is a systemic autoimmune disease characterized by the production of autoantibodies and a diversity of clinical manifestations. It most commonly presents in women during their child-bearing years. Although the etiology of SLE is unknown, both genetic and environmental factors contribute to loss of self-tolerance. Current therapeutic modalities are anti-inflammatory and immunosuppressive.

Epidemiology

The American College of Rheumatology (ACR) classification (Table 50.1),[1] created to identify SLE patients for clinical studies, is the most widely accepted instrument for "diagnosing" lupus; however, these criteria do not represent the full spectrum of disease. Patients fulfilling four out of the 11 criteria are classified with SLE with approximately 95% certainty, although many individuals who meet only two or three criteria are "diagnosed" with SLE. During the child-bearing years, the ratio of women to men with lupus is approximately 9:1. This ratio is less in younger and older populations, supporting a role for hormonal factors in disease induction. The majority of lupus presents during adulthood; approximately 20% are diagnosed in the pediatric population. Recent studies suggest that age at diagnosis may be increasing in some populations; mean ages at diagnosis reported since 2002 range from 31 in Martinique and Brazil to 51.7 in Wisconsin and 47 in Sweden.

Lupus occurs throughout the world; susceptibility is linked to race and ethnicity. Worldwide incidence rates vary from 1.9 to 8.7/100 000 and prevalence rates vary from 19.3 to 207/100 000;[2] however, incidence rates in African Americans, African Caribbeans, Hispanics, and Asians are approximately three times greater than in Caucasians. Clinical manifestations of disease are also modulated by ethnicity (Table 50.2).

Immunopathogenesis

The immune system is designed to protect the host against foreign pathogens and to remove cellular debris without damaging self. Clearly, with the universal production of autoantibodies and characteristic pathological findings of inflammation, vasculitis, vasculopathy, and immune complex deposition, SLE patients display a failure to downregulate autoreactivity. The heterogeneity of disease manifestations reflects the multiplicity of genetic, hormonal, and immune abnormalities contributing to clinical disease (Table 50.3). Progression from initial autoreactivity to clinical disease occurs over time (Fig. 50.1).

Autoantibodies

Antinuclear antibodies (ANA) are present in over 98% of patients diagnosed with SLE. Their presence is not specific to SLE as they are present in patients with other autoimmune diseases, malignancies, and viral (hepatitis) and parasitic (malaria) infections, as well as in response to environmental triggers such as therapeutic agents (see section on drug-induced lupus, below). Furthermore, ANA are found in low titer in 5% of the general population with prevalence increasing with age. Common ANA specificities found in lupus patients include dsDNA, ssDNA, extractable nuclear antigens (Sm, RNP, Ro and La), histones, and chromatin. Specific ANA are associated with disease subsets such as anti-Ro antibodies with subacute cutaneous and neonatal SLE, and anti-dsDNA antibodies with renal disease. Most autoantibody titers do not correlate with disease activity; anti-dsDNA antibodies are a notable exception. Their fluctuation with disease activity suggests a pathogenic role for this autoantibody and helps to predict impending disease flare in some patients.

The predisposed host: genetic contributions

SLE is a multigenic disease. Most disease-associated alleles are present in healthy individuals. Only when multiple alleles are present, as well as an appropriate environmental trigger, will a lupus-like phenotype arise. The degree of familial disease clustering and a higher disease concordance in monozygotic than dizygotic twins suggest both an underlying genetic susceptibility and the importance of environmental or epigenetic factors. Presumed susceptibility genes identified in humans include those affecting differentiation and survival of cells, lymphocyte activation, proliferation and apoptosis, cytokine production, antigen presentation, and clearance of apoptotic debris. Many of these genes are also implicated in susceptibility to other autoimmune diseases (e.g., *CTLA4* in Graves disease and type 1 diabetes, *PTPN22* polymorphisms in rheumatoid arthritis and type 1 diabetes).[3,4] More recently, genome-wide association studies (GWAS) and genome-wide linkage analyses have utilized high-throughput techniques to study hundreds of thousands of single nucleotide polymorphisms (SNPs) in individual patients with SLE. Six published studies in Caucasian and Asian lupus populations have yielded 31 SLE-associated susceptibility

Table 50.1 American College of Rheumatology criteria for systemic lupus erythematosus

Criteria	Description
Malar rash	Fixed malar erythema, flat or raised
Discoid rash	Erythematous raised patches with adherent keratotic scaling and follicular plugging; atrophic scarring may occur in older lesions
Photosensitivity	Skin rash as an unusual reaction to sunlight, by patient history or physician observation
Oral ulcers	Oral and nasopharyngeal ulcers, usually painless, observed by physician
Arthritis	Nonerosive arthritis involving two or more peripheral joints, characterized by tenderness, swelling, or effusion
Serositis	Pleuritis (convincing history of pleuritic pain or rub heard by physician or evidence of pleural effusion) *or* Pericarditis (documented by electrocardiogram or rub or evidence of pericardial effusion)
Renal disorder	Persistent proteinuria > 0.5 protein:creatinine ratio or > 3+ if quantification not performed *or* Cellular casts may be red cell, hemoglobin, granular, tubular, or mixed
Neurologic disorder	Seizures—in the absence of offending drugs or known metabolic derangements, e.g., uremia, ketoacidosis, or electrolyte imbalance *or* Psychosis—in the absence of offending drugs or known metabolic derangements, e.g., uremia, ketoacidosis, or electrolyte imbalance
Hematologic disorder	Hemolytic anemia – with reticulocytosis *or* Leukopenia (<4000/mm^3 total on two or more occasions) *or* Lymphopenia (<1500/mm^3 on two or more occasions) *or* Thrombocytopenia (<100 000/mm^3 in the absence of offending drugs)
Immunologic disorder	Anti-ds DNA: antibody to native DNA in abnormal titer *or* Anti-Sm: presence of antibody to Sm nuclear antigen *or* Positive finding of antiphospholipid antibodies based on: (1) an abnormal serum level of IgG or IgM anticardiolipin antibodies; (2) a positive test for lupus coagulant using a standard method; or (3) a false-positive serologic test for syphilis known to be positive for at least 6 months and confirmed by *Treponema pallidum* immobilization or fluorescent treponemal antibody absorption test
Antinuclear antibodies	An abnormal titer of antinuclear antibody by immunofluorescence or an equivalent assay at any point in time and in the absence of drugs known to be associated with "drug-induced lupus" syndrome

loci (reviewed in Deng and Tsao)[5] with associated ethnic and racial variation.

Genes associated with antigen presentation

Polymorphisms of major histocompatibility complex (MHC) genes determine the peptides of self and foreign antigens presented within the MHC that select the naïve T-cell repertoire. Human leukocyte antigen (HLA)-DR2 haplotypes in African American, African, Taiwanese, and Korean populations and HLA-DR3 haplotypes in Caucasian populations have been associated with a two- to three-fold increased risk for developing SLE.[6] Associations between anti-Ro antibodies with HLA-DR3 and anti-La antibodies with HLA-DR25 are consistent with the concept of an antigen-driven process involving T-cell recognition.

Genes associated with impaired clearance of apoptotic debris

Patients with severe deficiencies of C2, C4, and C1q display disease risks of 10, 75, and 90%, respectively, for SLE.[7] Reduced uptake of apoptotic cells has been implicated in disease initiation in murine models of SLE and is seen histopathologically in lymph nodes of lupus patients.[8] Though rare, individuals homozygous for null alleles of C2, C4, and C1q are at significantly increased risk. Polymorphisms of mannose-binding lectin (MBL) and C-reactive protein (CRP), acute-phase reactants that facilitate opsonization and phagocytosis of immune complexes, apoptotic debris and microbes, associate with SLE susceptibility; MBL haplotypes appear to be more important in Chinese and Spanish populations than in Caucasians. *TREX1* encodes a 3' repair exonuclease that monitors DNA synthesis and TREX1 deficiency leads to accumulation of endogenous DNA that is associated with increased expression of interferon (IFN) and autoimmunity. *ITGAM* encodes the alpha portion of an integrin adhesion molecule that binds C3b fragments and other pro-inflammatory molecules. GWAS have identified associations between *TREX1*, *ITGAM* and SLE susceptibility in European populations. *ITGAM* has also been reported as a susceptibility gene in African American and Hispanic populations but not in Asians (reviewed in Deng and Tsao).[5]

Genes associated with lymphocyte activation, proliferation, and function

The Fcγ receptors, FcγR1 (CD 64), FcγRII (CD32), and FcγRIII (CD16), have different binding affinities for immunoglobulin G (IgG) and immune complexes, as well as different cell-specific expression and function. FcγRI, FcγRIIa, and FcγRIIIa and IIIb are all activating receptors. Cross-linking results in degranulation, phagocytosis, antibody-dependent cellular cytotoxicity, cytokine gene transcription, and release of inflammatory mediators. In contrast, FcγRIIb is an inhibitory receptor. Cross-linking of FcγRIIb and the B-cell receptor (BCR) results in decreased intracellular calcium flux with decreased B-cell activation and proliferation. Engagement of FcγRIIb on dendritic cells also delivers an inhibitory signal. Deficiency in FcγRIIb results in a lower threshold for B-cell activation and unopposed activating FcR signaling in dendritic cells and macrophages. Substitutions of one or more amino acids in the activating FcγR genes—arginine (R) for histidine (H) at position 131 in FcγRIIA and phenylalanine (F) for valine (V) at position 158 in FcγRIIIA—results in decreased affinity for IgG immune complexes. Associations between the FcγRIIA R131H allele and disease susceptibility or nephritis occur in Brazilian, Thai, Korean, German, and

Table 50.2 Prevalence (%) of American College of Rheumatology criteria in different ethnic cohorts

	[†]Hispanic PROFILE cohort[a] (n = 78)	[†]Hispanic Puerto Rican[b] (n = 134)	[‡]Caucasian Spain[c] (n = 239)	[‡]Caucasian USA[d] (n = 46)	[†]Caucasian PROFILE cohort[a] (n = 260)	[‡]Caucasian Norwegian[e] (n = 346)	[‡]Caucasian Danish[f] (n = 513)	[†]African American PROFILE cohort[a] (n = 216)	[‡]Chinese[d] (n = 175)
Malar rash	64	72	NA	24	67	40	48	45	58
Discoid rash	6.	10.	27	24	12	13	14	33	6
Photosensitivity	59	77	29	46	72	41	43	46	31
Oral/nasal ulcers	58	30	18	7	57	1	11	46	15
Arthritis	91	67	71	54	87	83	67	89	54
Seizure/psychosis	12	9	6	4	9	8	13	16	9
Renal	59	30	23	54	23	17	45	54	29
Serositis	64	28	33	26	42	34	39	60	11
Cytopenias	85	77	55	83	62	36	67	82	58
Antinuclear antibody	97	93	100	83	97	99	98	97	95
Immunologic	83	NA	NA	57	65	57	98	79	81

[†]Cumulative data.
[‡]Inception data.
[a]Alarcon GS, et al. Baseline characteristics of a multiethnic lupus cohort: PROFILE. Lupus 2002; 11: 95–101.
[b]Vila LM, et al. Clinical and immunological manifestations in 134 Puerto Rican patients with systemic lupus erythematosus. Lupus 1999; 8: 279–286.
[c]Bujan S, et al. Contribution of the initial features of systemic lupus erythematosus to the clinical evolution and survival of a cohort of Mediterranean patients. Ann Rheum Dis 2003; 62: 859–865.
[d]Thumboo J, et al. A comparative study of the clinical manifestations of systemic lupus erythematosus in Caucasians in Rochester, Minnesota, and Chinese in Singapore, from 1980 to 1992. Arthritis Rheum 2001; 45: 494–500.
[e]Gilboe IM, Husby G. Application of the 1982 revised criteria for the classification of systemic lupus erythematosus on a cohort of 346 Norwegian patients with connective tissue disease. Scand J Rheumatol 1999; 28: 81–87.
[f]Jacobsen S, et al. A multicentre study of 513 Danish patients with systemic lupus erythematosus. I. Disease manifestations and analyses of clinical subsets. Clin Rheumatol 1998; 17: 468–477.

Table 50.3 Factors contributing to autoimmunity

Genetic factors
Loss of peripheral tolerance
• B-cell abnormalities
• T-cell abnormalities
• Dendritic cell abnormalities
Cytokine milieu
Hormonal influences
Environmental triggers

African-American populations and FcR polymorphisms may also predict a therapeutic response to immunobiologic agents such as rituximab.[9] FcγRIIIA F158V and FcγRIIIB NA2/NA2 polymorphisms are reported to associate with disease susceptibility in Dutch, Korean, Thai, and Caucasian populations. The FcγRIIb I232T allele leads to the inability of the receptor to enter lipid rafts and is associated with SLE in Asian populations.[10]

There are several genes associated with regulation or activation of lymphocytes. *BLK*, *LYN* and *BANK1* encode the tyrosine-kinase proteins BLK and LYN and B-cell scaffold protein with ankarin repeats; all are associated with intracellular signaling pathways. *ETS1* and *IKZF1* encode ftranscription factors, are involved with regulation of B-cell differentiation and self-tolerance, and differentiation of type 17 T-helper cells. CTLA-4 is upregulated on T cells after activation and dampens the inflammatory response. It has a higher affinity than CD28 for binding to B7.1 (CD80) and B7.2 (CD86), thereby competitively inhibiting engagement of CD28, and blocking the co-stimulatory signal required for activation. CTLA-4 ligation of B7 also activates indoleamine 2,3-dioxygenase (IDO) expression, an enzyme involved in tryptophan metabolism, and diminishes T-cell proliferation. Finally, CTLA-4 is critical for activation of regulatory T cells. In its absence, an uncontrolled, lethal inflammatory response occurs in mice. CTLA-4 alleles with decreased production of soluble CTLA-4 are implicated in the pathogenesis of several autoimmune diseases, including Sjögren's disease, ulcerative colitis, psoriasis, type 1 diabetes, and multiple sclerosis, as well as SLE.[11]

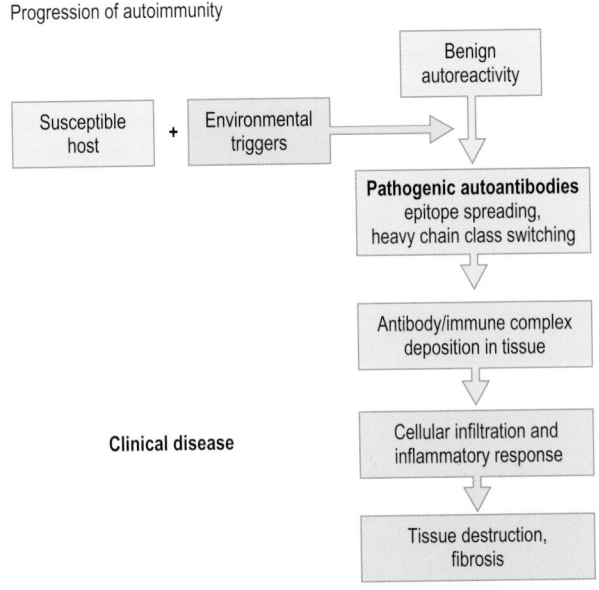

Progression of autoimmunity

Clinical disease

Fig. 50.1 Spectrum of autoimmunity.

The *PTPN22* gene encodes a tyrosine phosphatase responsible for downregulating T-cell receptor activation. A *PTPN22* polymorphism resulting in diminished ability to control T-cell receptor activation has been reported in SLE and other autoimmune diseases, suggesting a common mechanism of immune dysregulation.

Genes encoding cytokines and chemokines

Interferon regulatory factor 5 gene (*IRF5*) encodes a critical transcription factor in the type I IFN pathway; the IRF5 locus has the strongest association with SLE outside of the MHC region. Four allelic variants have been identified in multiple ethnically diverse populations. Variants of the signal transducer and activator of transcription factor 4 protein (*STAT4*) gene have also been associated with SLE susceptibility in GWAS studies of Caucasian and Asian populations. There are data suggesting interaction between IRF5 and STAT4 and the combinations of one or more risk alleles of the two genes confers increased susceptibility. IL-1 receptor-associated kinase 1 (*IRAK1*) and methyl-CPG-binding protein 2 (*MECP2*) genes are both found on the X chromosome and have been associated with SLE risk in GWAS studies. IRAK1 regulates multiple pathways in innate and adaptive immune responses including the link between immune complexes, Toll-like receptor (TLR) signaling, TCR signaling, and IFN production. Monocyte chemoattractant protein (MCP-1) is a potent chemoattractant for monocytes, memory T cells, and natural killer T cells. MCP-1 expression is upregulated in renal tubular cells and glomeruli in lupus nephritis and urine levels of MCP-1 are increased in patients with active lupus nephritis. A functional MCP-1 polymorphism resulting in increased production of MCP-1 has been associated with SLE nephritis.[12] Polymorphisms in the tyrosine kinase-2 (*TYK2*) gene are associated with increased expression of type I interferons (IFN-α, IFN-β) in SLE. IFN-α-regulated genes are highly expressed in peripheral blood cells from SLE patients compared to healthy controls (the interferon signature).[13] IFN-α mediates maturation of dendritic cells and monocytes, increasing the capacity for T-cell activation, and promotes B-cell differentiation and Ig class switching. However, in two murine models of lupus, decreases in type 1 interferons unexpectedly led to worsening disease, suggesting that the effect of IFN-α on autoimmunity is more complex than currently appreciated.

Multiple polymorphisms in the *IL10* gene have been reported, with conflicting results with respect to SLE susceptibility. A meta-analysis of 15 studies concluded that some *IL10* polymorphisms do associate with SLE but their importance is modulated by ethnic background.[14]

In the NZB/W murine model, a tumor necrosis factor (TNF) allele associated with low production is linked with disease, and treatment with TNF decreases autoantibody production. Consistent with this observation, TNF blockade for rheumatoid arthritis or inflammatory bowel disease leads to autoantibody production and infrequently to frank lupus. Several polymorphisms for genes encoding TNF-α and -β (lymphotoxin-α) have been associated with SLE; these associations are also influenced by ethnicity.[15]

Genes associated with cell survival

Fas ligand (expressed on activated T cells) binding to Fas (CD95) stimulates a signaling pathway resulting in apoptotic death of the Fas-expressing cell. Fas-induced apoptosis of activated cells contributes to the elimination of autoreactive B and T lymphocytes. Lymphopenia in SLE has been associated with increased Fas expression on lymphocytes and Fas and Fas ligand alleles have been linked to disease susceptibility.[16]

Bcl-2 family genes encode intracellular proteins that are either pro- or anti-apoptotic. Increased expression of Bcl-2, an anti-apoptotic molecule, leads to a lupus-like serology and nephritis in mice with certain genetic backgrounds. Increased intracellular levels of BCL-2 are reported in SLE; particularly in Chinese and Mexican populations. The combination of a BCL-2 susceptibility allele and interleukin-10 (IL-10) susceptibility allele confers a 40-fold increased risk of SLE, demonstrating that *infelicitous* combinations potentiate risk.[17]

Epigenetic contributions

Epigenetic regulation plays a determining role in gene activation. The major epigenetic influences in SLE involve DNA methylation at cytosine-guanine nucleotides (CpG methylation) and histone post-translational modifications (lysine acetylation or methylation, phosphorylation of serine or threonine, arginine methylation) (reviewed in Ballestar).[18] SLE is associated with DNA hypomethylation. Several drugs known to induce a lupus-like disease (procainamide, hydralazine) also cause decreased DNA methylation. A landmark study of high throughput analysis of DNA methylation in discordant twins demonstrated DNA hypomethylation in the affected siblings.[19] It is not surprising that genes encoding integrins, NGAL, CD40 ligand, IFN-γ receptor, and IL-6 are among the hypomethylated genes in SLE. Mechanisms for hypomethylation remain unclear; decreased efficacy of DNA methyltransferases (DNMTs) and over-expression of microRNAs (miRNAs) that interfere with DNMT activity have been proposed.

B cells

B-cell selection

The process of immunoglobulin variable region gene rearrangement produces large numbers of self-reactive B cells. Most B cells displaying self-reactive immunoglobulin are deleted centrally in the bone marrow and at subsequent checkpoints in the periphery (Fig. 50.2), so the frequency of autoreactive cells decreases from 75% in immature B cells in the bone marrow to 20% in the mature naïve B-cell population in healthy individuals. Several of these checkpoints appear deficient in SLE. The IgM cross-reactive autoantibodies made by these remaining autoreactive mature naïve B cells are thought to facilitate clearance of apoptotic cells, decreasing the development of potentially pathogenic T- and B-cell responses to self-antigens.

Another important peripheral checkpoint is entry into the T-cell-dependent, long-lived memory compartment. 9 G4 B cells express antibodies, encoded by the *VH4-34* gene, reactive with *N*-acetyllactosamine (NAL) determinants of glycoproteins on blood group antigens targeted by cold agglutinins, gangliosides, gastrointestinal mucins, glycolipids, and CD45 on B lymphocytes.[20] 9 G4 B cells are present in 5–10% of the naïve B-cell population in healthy donors as well as in the IgM memory compartment. However, 9 G4 B cells are excluded from the T-cell-dependent IgG memory and plasma cell populations, suggesting that these autoreactive cells fail to cross a developmental checkpoint following activation in normal individuals. Evaluation of tonsillar biopsies and spleens from healthy donors shows that the frequency of germinal centers with 9 G4⁺ cells is less than 1%, implying that negative selection of autoreactive cells occurs at the transition of naïve to germinal center cells. In contrast, tonsillar biopsies from SLE patients demonstrate that 15–20% of germinal centers are positive for autoreactive 9 G4 B cells. Autoreactive B cells surviving negative selection in the germinal center join the pool of long-lived antibody-producing plasma cells that home to the marrow.

Pathogenic B-cell autoimmunity

While studies demonstrate a failure to tolerize naïve autoreactive B cells, it is clear that some pathogenic autoantibodies are not derived from natural autoantibodies. Back mutation of a few anti-DNA antibodies to their germline-encoded precursors has identified non-autoreactive precursors. The failure of censoring mechanisms in germinal centers may reflect intrinsic B-cell abnormalities or abnormalities in co-stimulatory molecules, cytokines (such as BAFF, see below), dendritic cell, and T-cell interactions.

B-cell signaling

Hyperactive B-cell responses to immunologic stimulation are implicated in the production of pathogenic antibodies. SLE B cells have increased intracellular Ca^{2+} flux in response to BCR signaling.[21] This is attributable, in part, to FcγRIIb dysfunction, including defective upregulation of FcγRIIb on memory B cells, decreased availability of the FcRIIb-associated intracellular SHIP protein, and an FcγRIIb polymorphism (Ile 232 Thr) that prevents partitioning of the receptor into lipid rafts where it usually associates with the BCR.[10]

The intracellular protein tyrosine kinase Lyn has both positive and negative effects on BCR signaling. Decreased expression of Lyn results in increased intracellular Ca^{2+} flux and B-cell hyperactivity is present in Lyn-deficient mice. Correspondingly, LYN expression is decreased in resting and activated B cells in one-half to two-thirds of SLE patients, suggesting that LYN may modulate negative regulation of BCR signaling in human disease. In contrast, a mutation in mice leading to increased expression of Lyn also results in an autoimmune phenotype with autoantibody production and severe glomerulonephritis suggesting that Lyn expression is critical to tolerance pathways.

Fig. 50.2 Autoreactive B-cell checkpoints. There are tolerance checkpoints at every stage of B-cell activation and maturation. How many checkpoints need to be breached to achieve a pathogenic state and clinical disease is not known.

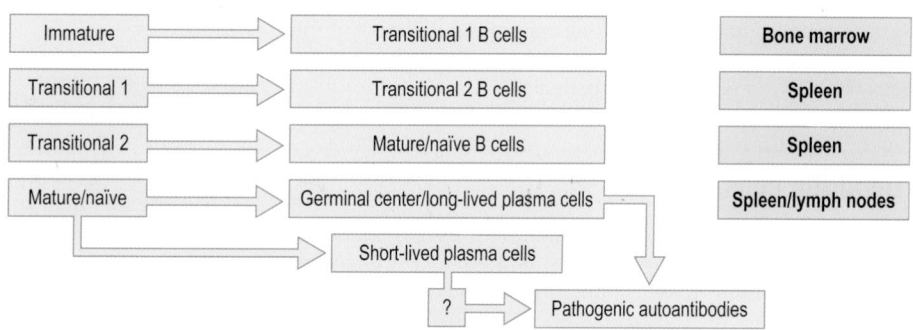

B-cell rescue

B lymphocyte stimulator (BAFF; also known as BLyS) is a member of the TNF family and participates in B-cell maturation and survival. BAFF enhances survival of B cells through ligation of several receptors—BCMA, BAFF-R, and TACI. High levels of this cytokine allow survival of autoreactive B cells in mice resulting in a lupus-like disease.[22] Evidence supporting a role for BAFF in autoreactive B-cell rescue and human SLE includes the elevated levels seen in lupus patients, associations of BAFF with autoantibody titers and, in some reports, correlations with disease activity.

Interactions between CD40 (B cell) and CD40 ligand (CD40L, T cell) are essential for B-cell proliferation, differentiation of memory cells into plasma cells and germinal center formation. Immature autoreactive B cells can be rescued from antigen-induced apoptosis by engagement of CD40 or by IL-4.[23] SLE T and B cells have upregulated CD40L, providing a critical molecule to mediate B-cell rescue. The combination of IL-17 and BAFF facilitates B lymphocyte proliferation and maturation. This combination can serve as an alternative stimulatory signal for B-cell activation and can replace CD40/CD40L interactions. Therefore, in a permissible and pro-inflammatory cytokine milieu, B-cell activation and autoantibody production may occur in the absence of cognate T-cell help.[24]

B-cell pathogenicity unrelated to antibody production

An essential role for B cells in SLE that is independent of antibody production is demonstrated by the T-cell activation, kidney inflammation, and increased mortality in MRL/lpr lupus-prone mice that lack the ability to secrete antibody and their absence in mice that lack B cells. B cells are efficient antigen-presenting cells; B cells with self-reactive specificity that have escaped tolerance are likely to present self-peptides to autoreactive T cells.

Neutrophils

An important link between neutrophils and autoimmunity has recently been established. Neutrophil extracellular traps (NETS) are chromatin filaments released from neutrophils to trap microbes. In addition to microbial peptides, NETS also contain neutrophil peptides including neutrophil-encoded antimicrobial peptide LL37 (cathelicidin). Circulating DNA-containing immune complexes from lupus patients have been shown to contain peptide LL37. These combined DNA/LL37 immune complexes are potent TLR-9 stimulants, resulting in production of IFN-α by plasmacytoid DCs (pDC).[25] Moreover, anti-RNP antibodies also induce "NETosis" in a process that is dependent on TLR7 and FcγRIIa signaling.[26] Thus, it is possible that autoantibodies accelerate NET formation, and increase formation of DNA/LL37 immune complexes and pDC production of IFN-α. These studies confirm earlier work that described a "granulocyte signature" with significant upregulation of granulocyte specific transcripts within peripheral blood mononuclear cells (PBMCs) in pediatric SLE patients.[27]

Dendritic cells

Dendritic cells (DCs) recognize pathogens through membrane pattern recognition receptors (PRRs) and are a critical component of the immune system connecting the innate and adaptive immune responses (reviewed in Kis-Toth and Tsokos).[28] They can be tolerogenic or highly inflammatory due to their high expression of costimulatory molecules. DCs function normally as surveillance cells, phagocytizing cellular debris and determining if there is cause for alarm. PRRs on DCs bind pathogen associated molecular patterns (PAMPs) and damage associated molecular patterns (DAMPs). Following internalization of the PAMPs and DAMPs, endosomal Toll-like receptors (TLRs) are activated by nucleic acids. The role of IFN-α in SLE pathogenesis is now well established and the primary cells responsible for IFN-α production are plasmacytoid DCs (pDCs). TLR7 or 9 activation with RNA and DNA respectively, induces immature DCs to differentiate to immunocompetent, IFN-α-producing DCs that have wide-reaching effects on T cells, B cells, neutrophils and monocytes. pDCs have been demonstrated in skin and renal lesions and upregulation of genes triggered by the presence of IFN-α (the "IFN signature") is observed in many SLE patients and has been associated with disease activity. A number of susceptibility genes identified through GWAS are associated with IFN pathways in SLE including *IRF5*, *IRF7* and *STAT4*.

T cells

T cells in lupus contribute to the abrogation of self-tolerance by providing help to autoreactive B cells and facilitating the production of somatically mutated, high-affinity, pathogenic autoantibodies. Lupus patients can exhibit T-cell phenotypes consisting of increased numbers of CD3+CD4-CD8- T cells, increased TH17 cells and T follicular helper (T$_{FH}$) cells and decreased numbers of regulatory T cells (Tregs) (reviewed in Crispin et al.).[29] Additionally, lupus T cells display increased expression of activation markers and abnormal T-cell receptor (TCR) signaling responses A substitution of TCR ζ-chain by the γ-chain of the Fc receptor results in increased intracellular influx of Ca^{2+} following TCR stimulation and a concomitant decrease in IL-2 production. Lupus T cells are additionally less susceptible to activation-induced cell death.

Self-tolerance is maintained in part by the suppressive actions of Tregs. "Natural" Tregs arise *de novo* in the thymus whereas "induced" Tregs evolve from naïve T cells exposed to IL-2 and TGF-β. These cells are characterized by high surface expression of the IL-2 receptor α chain, CD25 and high levels of FoxP3 intracellularly. Tregs act together with tolerogenic DCs to maintain a steady state of immature DCs. In contrast, effector T cells can secrete IFN-γ and IL-17 that promote immature DC differentiation to immunogenic DC capable of secreting IL-1, -6, -12, and TNF-α and can activate autoreactive T cells thereby establishing a feedback loop with impaired Tregs and activation of autoreactive T cells (reviewed in Scheinecker et al.).[30] Studies of Tregs in patients with SLE have demonstrated reduced numbers and altered function of peripheral CD4+CD25+ FoxP3+ cells in patients with active disease.[31]

Hormonal influences

The most compelling evidence for the role of sex hormones in SLE is the fact that lupus affects women of child-bearing age. The female-to-male ratio is 2:1 prior to menarche, 8–9:1 in the fourth decade, and 2:1 after menopause. Numerous case reports and studies of disease flares correlating with pregnancy, menstruation, and use of oral contraceptives containing high doses of estrogen suggest a role for estrogen in disease activity. A significant correlation between plasma levels of estradiol and clinical disease activity and increased α hydroxylation of estrogen in SLE yielding the more active metabolite 16α-hydroxyestrone are also reported.[32] No significant differences in levels of sex hormones (including estrogen, testosterone, prolactin) are noted in male SLE patients, suggesting that the development of SLE in females may be more closely related to sex hormones than in men. Randomized, controlled studies of estrogen in SLE suggest that the use of exogenous estrogen in patients with stable disease may be safe; however, a subset of patients appears to have an estrogen-sensitive disease. Mild to moderate flare rates were significantly increased in postmenopausal women treated with hormone replacement therapy.

Most of what we understand about hormonal modulation of B-cell development comes from mouse studies.[23] Estrogen treatment of NZB/W and MRL/lpr mice or castration of male lupus-prone mice exacerbates disease whereas oophorectomy of females ameliorates disease. Treatment of lupus-prone mice with the selective estrogen receptor modulator tamoxifen also ameliorates disease.

Estrogen and prolactin promote the loss of B-cell tolerance in non-autoimmune mice. Estrogen results in diminished B-cell responsiveness to BCR cross-linking and less stringent negative selection. Additionally, estrogen has also been reported to inhibit activation-induced T-cell death by downregulation of Fas ligand expression, thereby permitting increased numbers of autoreactive T cells.[33] There is also emerging data to suggest that estrogen receptor signaling promotes differentiation of DCs into immune competent DCs through increased expression of the transcription factor IRF4 (reviewed in Cunningham and Gilkeson).[34]

Elevated prolactin levels are reported in 20% of patients with SLE, and increased prolactin exposure in lupus-prone mice exacerbates disease activity. While treatment of patients with bromocriptine yielded equivocal results, treatment of NZB/W lupus mice with bromocriptine results in improved survival. Transmembrane prolactin receptors are present on a variety of cells, including T and B cells. Upregulation of both Bcl-2 and CD40 on B cells and CD40L on T cells occurs in response to prolactin, identifying pathways that may be involved in the prolactin-mediated rescue of autoreactive B cells.

Clinical manifestations

> ### ● CLINICAL PEARLS
>
> - SLE is a systemic disease with the potential to affect any organ system.
> - The differential diagnosis of a lupus flare mandates consideration of infection, drug toxicities, or other etiologies.
> - Corticosteroid exposure should be minimized.
> - In the absence of data from randomized trials, use of aggressive treatment must be balanced against associated toxicity.
> - SLE patients are at increased risk of developing atherosclerotic disease, osteoporosis, malignancy, DM, and HTN; screening for and reduction of modifiable risk factors is essential.
> - Appropriate vaccinations are advisable.

The prevalence of the diverse clinical and laboratory features of lupus varies in published reports (Table 50.2). Both genetic and environmental factors are likely to account for much of the variability between cohorts. Characteristics of published cohorts including inception vs long-standing lupus cohorts, community versus academic settings, socio-economic factors and ascertainment differences are also likely to contribute to observed differences in the prevalence of clinical manifestations. Over time, the course of lupus is characterized by flares and remissions of disease activity.

> ### ● KEY CONCEPTS
>
> - Continued heightened awareness of SLE to shorten the time between onset of symptoms and diagnosis will improve outcomes.
> - Lupus is a disease characterized by recurrent flares.
> - Attentive monitoring even during periods of disease remission leads to early recognition of impending flare, better control, and better prognosis.
> - Lupus is a chronic disease; the importance of a therapeutic partnership between physicians and patients, emotional/social support, and patient education cannot be overemphasized.

The most common features of lupus are constitutional and include fatigue, malaise, low-grade fever, anorexia, and lymphadenopathy. These symptoms may accompany other organ system manifestations of active disease or can occur alone. Although frequent, these symptoms are nonspecific and do not aid in making the diagnosis of SLE. Symptoms of fatigue and malaise may also represent fibromyalgia, which can co-occur with SLE or confound the diagnosis.[35]

Musculoskeletal involvement

The musculoskeletal system is the most common organ system affected in SLE; joint pain is the presenting symptom in approximately 50% of patients.

Arthritis and arthralgia

The pattern of joint involvement is usually symmetric, affecting the small joints of the hands, wrists, and knees. Pain in the ankles, elbows, shoulders, or hips or monoarticular involvement is less typical. In contrast to rheumatoid arthritis, morning stiffness is typically limited to several minutes. Frequently, the subjective complaints of pain are greater than the objective findings of warmth, swelling and erythema. Lupus arthritis is characteristically non-erosive on X-ray and non-deforming. Some lupus patients do develop a hand deformity with hypermobile joints secondary to tendon and ligamentous laxity (Jacoud's arthritis) (Fig. 50.3). Proliferative tenosynovitis, synovitis, small erosions not detectable on plain radiographs and capsular swelling are features of joint and soft-tissue involvement that may be seen on MRI.

Joint effusions, when they occur, are usually small. The fluid is clear, yellow with normal viscosity, and forms a mucin clot. It is typically non-inflammatory with a normal glucose level and a white blood cell (WBC) count of less than 2000 cells/mL that is predominantly lymphocytic. ANA performed on the synovial fluid may be positive and LE cells may be present. Synovial fluid complement levels may be normal or depressed. Synovial histology in lupus is not specific and shows synovial hyperplasia with

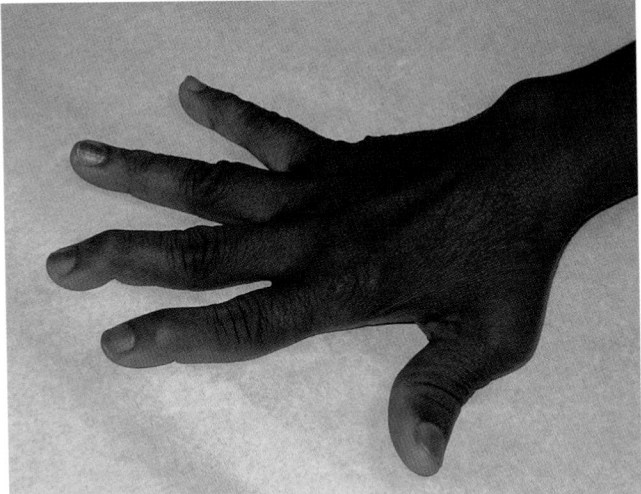

Fig. 50.3 **Jacoud's arthritis in systemic lupus erythematosus.**

fibrin deposition and microvascular changes that include a perivascular infiltrate in the majority of cases.

Tendinitis

Tendinitis is not usually attributed to SLE unless associated with tendon rupture. When present, it is usually located in the Achilles tendon or the tendons around the knee. Tendon ruptures are more common in males and have been associated with trauma, steroid use, and long disease duration.[35] Biopsy shows a mononuclear infiltrate with tendon degeneration and neovascularization. The diagnosis can be easily demonstrated on MRI.

Myositis/myalgia

Generalized myalgia is extremely common in lupus. It frequently affects the deltoids and quadriceps and occurs during flares of active disease. Muscle disease secondary to treatment with corticosteroids, statins, and anti-malarials or in association with hypothyroidism is also frequent and must be considered in the evaluation of a lupus patient with myalgia. Inflammatory muscle disease with weakness and an elevated creatine phosphokinase is less common and occurs in approximately 10% of lupus patients.[35] Electromyography may be normal or may be characteristic of the myositis observed in polymyositis or dermatomyositis. Muscle biopsy may also be normal or may show changes associated with dermatomyositis such as a perivascular or perifascicular infiltrate and immunoglobulin and complement deposition. Muscle atrophy, fiber necrosis, microtubular inclusions, and/or a mononuclear infiltrate have been documented. MRI findings are nonspecific.

Avascular necrosis

Avascular necrosis (AVN) has been reported in up to 30% of lupus patients, and is frequently asymptomatic.[36] The most commonly affected site is the femoral head. Groin pain exacerbated with weight-bearing is a common complaint. In addition to the hip, AVN can involve the knees, shoulders, and wrists. The majority of AVN is associated with administration of high doses of corticosteroids (> 30 mg/day). Bone biopsy in lupus patients affected by AVN does not reveal unique findings.

Mucocutaneous manifestations

Skin

The skin is commonly affected in SLE with numerous types of lesions; three of which are part of the diagnostic criteria. Though rarely life-threatening, cutaneous lesions can be quite disfiguring.

Acute cutaneous SLE

The malar rash typically occurs across the cheeks and nose but can include the forehead and chin, sparing the nasolabial folds (unlike seborrheic dermatitis) (Fig. 50.4). It usually begins as small discrete erythematous macules or papules that coalesce, is frequently associated with sun exposure and heals without scarring. Some patients additionally have facial swelling. The differential diagnosis includes acne rosacea, seborrheic dermatitis, erysipelas, dermatomyositis, and contact dermatitis. Microscopic analysis reveals a sparse inflammatory lymphocytic dermatitis with occasional histiocytes engulfing nuclear debris resembling LE cells found close to the dermoepidermal junction. Immunofluorescent staining for complement components and immunoglobulin at the dermoepidermal junction is positive in 70–80% of patients.

Many lupus rashes arise in sun-exposed areas and sun exposure can precipitate flares of systemic disease. Typically, a photosensitive rash erupts within hours of sun exposure and consists of tiny pruritic plaques and vesicles lasting several days. Ultraviolet (UV) light induces DNA damage and triggers apoptosis of keratinocytes, providing a rich source of antigen. SLE patients have increased numbers of apoptotic keratinocytes after exposure to UV light,[37] with increased chemotaxis of plasmacytoid dendritic cells and T cells to skin lesions and ensuing production of pro-inflammatory cytokines (IL-1, TNF-α, IL-10, IFN-γ).

Subacute cutaneous lupus (SCLE) is characterized by recurrent, non-scarring, non-indurated skin lesions. This distinctive rash consists of erythematous papules and plaques, with or without adherent pityriasiform scale, that erupt on the extremities and trunk, usually sparing the head and neck. These lesions may assume an annular polycyclic form with central pallor and tiny vesicles at the active margins and can be mistaken for erythema multiforme. The differential diagnosis also includes psoriasis, polymorphic light eruption, and tinea corporis. SCLE is exacerbated by UV light and a growing list of medications; including thiazides and calcium channel blockers. Biopsy reveals a lymphocytic dermatitis confined to the superficial and mid dermis, frequently with associated dermal edema, mucinosis, and degenerating keratinocytes. Both TNF-α and IL-6 have been demonstrated in active SCLE lesions. SCLE is most commonly seen in Caucasian populations. Genetic analyses have revealed

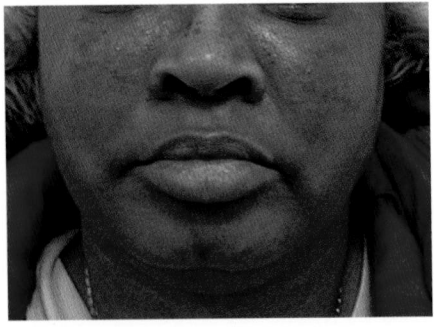

Fig. 50.4 **Malar rash in a systemic lupus erythematosus patient.**

associations with HLA-A1, -B8, and -DR3 haplotypes, as well as with deficiencies of C2, C4, and C1q. Sixty to 90% of SCLE patients have anti-Ro antibodies.

Chronic cutaneous SLE

Discoid lesions (DLE) are usually localized to the head and neck in photoexposed areas with a predilection for the ears and peri-orbital areas (Fig. 50.5). The lesions vary in size and result in scar tissue with significant disfigurement. Early lesions appear as erythematous plaques with or without follicular hyperkeratosis, plugging, and scale and progress to scarring annular lesions with an erythematous, indurated border, adherent scale, and a central area with atrophy and telangectasias. There are no autoantibody associations with DLE and only 5% of patients with DLE develop systemic lupus. High-titer ANA, Raynaud's phenomenon, and the presence of arthralgias may identify patients at risk for systemic evolution. Histopathology characteristically reveals a lymphocytic interface dermatitis with CD4 lymphocytes and plasmacytoid dendritic cells involving follicles and epidermis. There is vacuolar degeneration of the basal layer of epidermal keratinocytes and prominent keratotic follicular plugging. Dermal mucin deposition is also present and there is usually dense granular deposition of immunoglobulin (predominantly IgG) and C3 at the dermal–epidermal junction. Patients with C2, C4, and C1q deficiencies may be predisposed to DLE and promoter region polymorphisms leading to high IL-10 and low TNF-α are risk factors for DLE.

Lupus profundus typically presents as firm, tender, deep subcutaneous nodules that may atrophy over time. Overlaying epidermal changes include DLE, ulcerations, and dystrophic calcification. Biopsy reveals a lobular panniculitis with patchy lymphoplasmacytic infiltrate in subcutaneous fat lobules. Panniculitis occurs in 10–20% of patients and must be differentiated from a subcutaneous T-cell lymphoma, erythema nodosum, pancreatic panniculitis, and morphea.

Nonspecific skin lesions reported in SLE are typically seen during disease flares and are associated with greater disease severity. Theses lesions include, but are not limited to, entities such as cutaneous vasculitis (Fig. 50.6), urticaria, Raynaud's phenomenon, livedo reticularis, alopecia, sclerodactyly, calcinosis cutis, atrophie blanche, bullous lesions, erythema multiforme, lupus tumidus and leg ulcers.

The lupus band test (LBT) refers to the deposition of immunoglobulin (IgG, IgM, and/or IgA) and/or C3 along the dermoepidermal junction. Approximately 25% of normal individuals display weak IgM staining at the dermoepidermal junction; 70–80% of SLE patients have a positive LBT in sun-exposed, non-lesional skin. Half of SLE patients have a positive LBT in

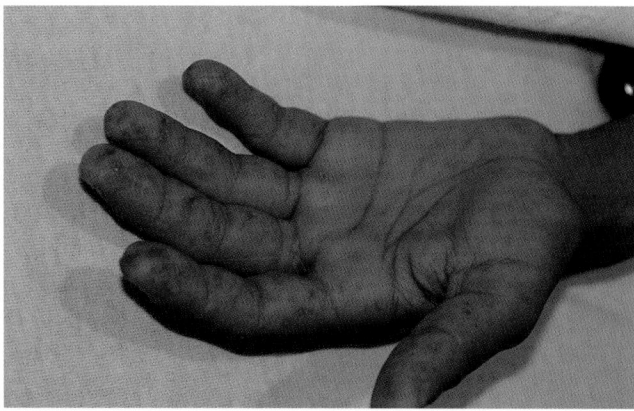

Fig. 50.6 Cutaneous vasculitis affecting the hands in a patient with active systemic lupus erythematosus.

non-sun-exposed, non-lesional skin. It is unclear if the LBT is a consequence of circulating ANA targeting denatured DNA from UV light-damaged keratinocytes, or immune complex deposition or anti-basement membrane antibodies. The test may be useful diagnostically and prognostically as it correlates with increased systemic disease severity.

Nonspecific cutaneous lesions such as cutaneous vasculitis or ulcers are associated with a more aggressive disease course than most of the SLE-specific lesions.

Hair and nail

Hair involvement in SLE includes scarring alopecia resulting in permanent hair loss, induced by DLE. This can be differentiated from other common forms of scarring alopecia by immunofluorescent studies. Patchy or diffuse nonscarring alopecia is frequently associated with disease activity. Histologically, there is a peribulbar lymphocytic infiltrate surrounding shrunken anagen hair bulbs similar to findings in alopecia areata. Non-scarring alopecia resolves with complete hair regrowth with control of disease activity.

A wide spectrum of nail abnormalities, including pitting, ridging, onycholysis, and dyschromia with blue or black hyperpigmentation, are reported in up to 30% of SLE patients but none are lupus-specific. Nailfold erythema with ragged cuticles and splinter hemorrhages resembling the changes of dermatomyositis are common.

Oral lesions

The spectrum of oral lesions reported in SLE includes cheilitis, ulcerations, erythematous patches, lichen planus-type plaques on the buccal mucosa and palate, and DLE.[38] Most oral lesions are asymptomatic and must be looked for on exam. Positive immunofluorescent staining on biopsy may be useful to differentiate DLE from lichen planus-like lesions and leukoplakia. Lupus mucosal ulcerations demonstrate an interface mucositis and not leukocytoclastic vasculitis.

Gastrointestinal manifestations

Gastrointestinal manifestations of SLE[39] are common; attribution is critical as it is often difficult to differentiate between disease activity, side effects of medications, and infectious complications.

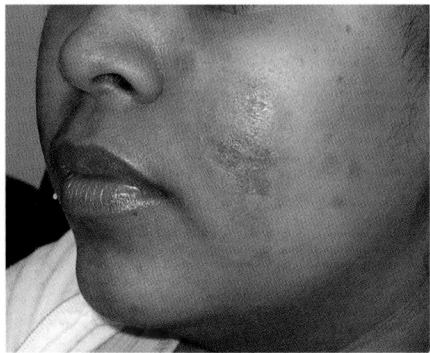

Fig. 50.5 Discoid lesion in systemic lupus erythematosus.

Esophagus

The prevalence of esophageal involvement varies. Many of the reviews citing a high incidence of dysphagia and odynophagia predate the advent of proton pump inhibitors and H_2 blockers and the relationship of medication use to symptoms is not clear. Dysphagia and heartburn are reported in 1–50% of patients, although dysmotility is observed in up to 72%. An inflammatory process involving esophageal muscle or vasculitic damage to the Auerbach plexus is thought to contribute to the esophageal dysmotility. Ulceration is rarely seen outside the context of infections such as invasive candidiasis, herpes simplex, or cytomegalovirus. SLE patients with a secondary Sjögren's syndrome may have salivary gland dysfunction resulting in decreased saliva contributing to dysphagia.

Abdominal pain/vasculitis

Abdominal pain is commonly seen in SLE with an incidence reported as high as 40%. The most catastrophic gastrointestinal disturbances are related to ischemia of the small and large intestines resulting from medium- and small-vessel vasculitis or thrombotic complications of anti-phospholipid antibodies. The mortality associated with intestinal ischemia is high and early consideration and intervention is critical. Increased SLEDAI scores reflecting increased disease activity have been correlated with intestinal ischemia in patients presenting with acute abdominal pain. Computed tomography (CT) and/or MR with or without angiography are the preferred imaging tests for evaluation of abdominal pathology and the radiographic signs of intestinal ischemia do not differ based on pathogenesis.

Intestinal vasculitis has a prevalence that varies from 0.2 to 53%. Its presentation may be acute, severe abdominal pain or an insidious, stuttering course, with nausea, vomiting, bloating, diarrhea, post-prandial fullness, anorexia, and weight loss. Mesenteric vasculitis preferentially affects the superior mesenteric artery, involving the small intestine more commonly than the large bowel. Vasculitis can occur in the esophagus, stomach, peritoneum, rectum, gallbladder, pancreas, and liver. In cases with an insidious clinical course, endoscopy and colonoscopy may provide evidence of ischemia demonstrating ulcerating or heaped-up lesions and overt vasculitis on biopsy. The lesions are segmental and focal. Histologically, there is a small-vessel arteritis and venulitis with neutrophilic, lymphocytic, and macrophage infiltrates and fibrinoid necrosis of the vessel walls, associated thrombosis, and mononuclear infiltrate in the lamina propria. There may be immunoglobulin, C3, and fibrin deposition in the adventitia and media.

Treatment of acute abdominal pain in SLE is tailored to the underlying cause. Most patients are treated with high-dose intravenous corticosteroids (1–2 mg/kg per day) with good response. There are no randomized trials of immunosuppressive agents to date for the treatment of intestinal vasculitis.

Peritonitis

Inflammation of serosal membranes is well described in SLE; despite evidence of peritoneal inflammation in 63% of autopsy studies, clinical pericarditis and pleuritis occur far more commonly than peritonitis. Acute peritonitis is attributed to peritoneal vasculitis or ischemia and presents with abdominal pain (see above). The finding of ascitic fluid by CT scan or ultrasound mandates an evaluation of the fluid to exclude infection and malignancy. Rarely, ascites may be attributable to hepatic or portal vein thrombosis. Chronic peritonitis characterized by large amounts of painless ascites attributable to SLE and not to heart failure, constrictive pericarditis or severe hypoalbuminemia due to nephrotic syndrome, liver disease, or a protein-losing enteropathy is rare. In lupus peritonitis, the ascitic fluid is generally exudative with a predominance of lymphocytes; LE cells, autoantibodies and low complement levels are frequent. On biopsy, the peritoneum is usually edematous, and sometimes hemorrhagic with lymphocytic perivascular infiltrates.

Pancreatitis

Pancreatitis attributable to SLE is rare, with an annual reported incidence $\leq 1/1\ 000$. Although corticosteroids and azathioprine are medications known to trigger pancreatitis, 34% of reported cases are not on these medications at the onset of pancreatitis and most patients respond to steroid therapy. The clinical presentation of pancreatitis and diagnosis is similar in patients with and without SLE. Specific to SLE, leukopenia, thrombocytopenia, and anemia are commonly observed. Histologic findings show inflammation and necrosis; there is a single report of pancreatic vasculitis. Mortality rates are reported from 18 to 27%; poor outcome is associated with increased systemic SLE activity (particularly low complement and thrombocytopenia).

Liver

Controversy continues over the existence of "lupoid hepatitis."[40] Analysis of SLE liver pathology from 52 autopsies in Japan revealed a variety of findings, including congestion (40/52), fatty liver (38/52), arteritis (11/52), cholestasis (9/52), and a few cases each of chronic persistent hepatitis, nodular regenerative hyperplasia, hemangioma, and cholangiolitis. Cirrhosis is an extremely rare complication of liver involvement in SLE. The distinction between subclinical liver inflammation related to SLE (lupus hepatitis/LH) and autoimmune hepatitis (AIH) is important since therapy and prognosis are different. In contrast to the mild enzyme abnormalities associated with lupus hepatitis, AIH is a progressive disease frequently leading to hepatic failure. Both conditions share a predilection for young women and both demonstrate features of autoimmunity, including hypergammaglobulinemia, arthralgias, and serum autoantibodies. Histologically, biopsies of LH reveal lobular and periportal lymphocytic infiltrates, in contrast to the periportal and piecemeal necrosis with dense lymphocytic infiltrates seen in AIH with progression to panlobular or multilobular necrosis and cirrhosis. Serologically, anti-ribosomal P antibodies are associated with liver disease in LH but not AIH; AIH is associated with antibodies to liver and kidney microsomes. Anti-smooth-muscle antibodies are observed in 60–80% of patients with AIH compared to 30% of patients with LH. Although both have a favorable response to steroids, AIH usually requires additional immunosuppressive agents.

Distinguishing LH from hepatitis C (HCV) can be difficult. Up to 30% of patients chronically infected with HCV have low titers of ANA and other autoantibodies (anti-DNA, anti-cardiolipin antibodies, and rheumatoid factor). They can also have cryoglobulins and associated cryoglobulinemic vasculitis. It is necessary to confirm a positive enzyme-linked immunosorbent assay (ELISA) for HCV with polymerase chain reaction (PCR) in patients presenting with arthritis, cutaneous vasculitis, and a positive ANA as SLE patients may have false-positive serological tests for HCV.

Protein-losing enteropathy

Profound hypoalbuminemia in the absence of severe nephrotic syndrome, liver disease, or constrictive pericarditis should trigger a consideration of protein-losing enteropathy (PLE). The diagnosis is confirmed with an increased α_1-antitrypsin level in a 24-hour stool collection. A review of the 31 cases reported prior to 2002 found that only half the patients experienced diarrhea; endoscopy was either normal or revealed edematous bowel.[41] In biopsies from 22 patients, normal or edematous villi were seen in 12 patients, lymphangiectasia in 2, dilated lymphatic vessels in 2, inflammation in 2, and venulitis in 1. Biopsy results suggest a role of TNF-α and IFN-γ in the increased vascular and enterocyte permeability in PLE.

Pulmonary involvement

Lupus affects the lungs in diverse ways involving the pleura, lung parenchyma, and blood vessels. The most frequent and important complicating feature is infection.

Pleuritis

Pleuritis is the most common pulmonary manifestation of SLE, reported in 40–56% of patients.[42] Pleural involvement in up to 93% of lupus patients at autopsy suggests that much pleuritis may be asymptomatic. Clinically, patients note typical pleuritic pain. On physical exam, the most frequent abnormality is tachypnea; a pleural friction rub is present in some cases and pleural effusions occur in more severe cases. Pleural fluid is usually exudative with normal glucose and pH and elevated protein levels. The leukocyte count can range from several hundred to 20 000 cells/μL; both a lymphocytic and neutrophilic predominance are reported. Immunologic testing on pleural fluid may show reduced complement levels and the presence of ANA, anti-DNA antibodies, and LE cells. Although these tests are commonly obtained, these results are neither sensitive nor specific to diagnose lupus pleuritis.

Lupus pneumonitis

Lupus pneumonitis is uncommon, occurring in up to 10% of patients. Patients present with dyspnea, cough, mild pleuritic chest pain, and fever. Pulmonary infiltrates are present on plain radiograph or CT. This presentation must be distinguished from an infectious etiology. Histologic examination of affected lung tissue shows alveolar edema and hemorrhage with hyaline membrane formation; immunofluorescent staining reveals immune complex deposition.

Pulmonary hemorrhage

Pulmonary hemorrhage is a rare but potentially fatal complication of SLE. Symptoms include shortness of breath and hemoptysis accompanied by a fall in hemoglobin, usually occurring in the context of multiorgan involvement from SLE. Imaging may show patchy infiltrates. Pulmonary function testing is marked by an increased diffusion capacity (DLCO) secondary to the presence of alveolar blood while arterial O_2 saturation is decreased. Histopathology shows bland intra-alveolar hemorrhage and hemosiderin-laden macrophages, although microangiitis with an inflammatory infiltrate and necrosis of the alveolar septa can occur. As hemorrhage into the lung may be secondary to thrombotic thrombocytopenia, demonstration of an inflammatory process in the pulmonary vessels or tissue is helpful to establish a diagnosis of primary pulmonary hemorrhage.

Chronic diffuse interstitial lung disease

Chronic diffuse interstitial lung disease is a relatively uncommon manifestation of SLE occasionally associated with anti-Ro antibodies. It usually has a progressive course with a chronic nonproductive cough, dyspnea and pleuritic chest pains. Physical exam is frequently remarkable for basilar rales with diminished diaphragmatic movement. Pulmonary function tests demonstrate a restrictive pattern with decreased diffusion capacity; oxygen saturation is decreased. Imaging often shows interstitial fibrosis that is more prominent at the lung bases. High-resolution CT (HRCT) is a sensitive technique used for detection of parenchymal abnormalities that may also help determine the extent of treatable disease, i.e., fibrosis (honeycombing) versus inflammation (ground glass). However, the most reliable method to assess the extent of pulmonary inflammation in comparison to fibrotic damage is histologic examination. Evaluation of bronchial alveolar lavage fluid helps to exclude infection.

Pulmonary hypertension

Pulmonary hypertension unrelated to chronic pulmonary emboli or interstitial lung disease occurs in SLE. Severe cases are rare; the recent recognition of milder cases may be partially attributed to the availability of newer effective therapies. Patients note progressive dyspnea commonly occurring in the absence of infiltrates on chest radiographs or significant hypoxemia. Chest pain and a chronic nonproductive cough are also frequently present. Pulmonary function testing reveals a reduced DLCO. Elevated pulmonary artery pressure is documented with cardiac angiogram or echocardiogram. Biopsy or autopsy specimens of the lung reveal "plexiform" lesions that resemble those seen in primary pulmonary hypertension.

Shrinking-lung syndrome

The shrinking-lung syndrome refers to the rare findings of shortness of breath occurring in the absence of pleuritis or interstitial lung disease plus a chest X-ray showing elevated hemidiaphragms. Pulmonary function testing shows a restrictive pattern with loss of lung volume. It is generally accepted that this syndrome results from diaphragmatic weakness (from a myopathic process) or chest wall restriction. There is no definitive therapy, although immunosuppressive therapy with cytotoxic agents usually results in an improvement of lung function and respiratory symptoms.

Cardiac involvement

There are a number of ways in which lupus affects the cardiovascular system; targets include the myocardium, valves, pericardium, and vessels.

Myocardium

Myocardial dysfunction in SLE is likely to be secondary to factors other than lupus, including hypertension, medications, or coronary artery disease (CAD). However, a cardiomyopathy resulting from immune-mediated myocardial inflammation does occur, either in isolation or concomitant with systemic disease, including myositis. Inflammatory myocarditis is often associated with anti-RNP antibodies. Histopathology typically shows a mononuclear, inflammatory cell infiltrate. Perivascular or myocardial wall deposits of immune complexes and complement also occur. Myocardial biopsy is useful for diagnosis as well as for determination of the extent of active inflammatory disease and fibrosis. Symptoms and signs of myocarditis include unexplained tachycardia, an abnormal electrocardiogram (with ST and T-wave abnormalities), cardiomegaly; and heart failure. Echocardiography may show systolic and diastolic ventricular dysfunction. Myocardial involvement without overt clinical signs occurs commonly and may be documented using Doppler echocardiography. A non-inflammatory cardiomyopathy may be seen in association with high-dose cyclophosphamide.

Valvular heart disease

Valvular abnormalities, with thickening, regurgitation, or verrucous vegetations, occur commonly in SLE and are documented by transesophageal echocardiograpy in 50–60% of patients.[43] The characteristic Libman–Sacks lesion, nonbacterial verrucous vegetations, is observed at autopsy in 15–60% of patients. Mitral, aortic, and tricuspid valves are most frequently involved. Clinically these lesions are usually asymptomatic, and hemodynamic compromise, rupture of the chordae tendinae, or infection are rare events. On histologic examination, mononuclear cells, hematoxylin bodies, fibrin and platelet thrombi, and immune complexes are present. Anti-phospholipid antibodies can be associated with the development of valvular heart disease, although their pathogenic role remains unproven.

Pericarditis

Pericardial inflammation is a frequent manifestation of SLE. While asymptomatic pericarditis occurs in more than 50% of patients, clinically apparent pericarditis occurs in only 25% and cardiac tamponade and constrictive pericarditis are infrequent. Pericardial fluid and thickening are easily detected by echocardiography; cardiac silhouette enlargement on plain films is seen in the presence of large effusions. There are no unique signs and symptoms of pericarditis in lupus patients. The histologic findings of acute pericarditis in lupus are inflammation with a monuclear cell infiltrate accompanied by immunoglobulin and complement deposition. Results of pericardial fluid analysis are neither sensitive nor specific; the fluid is usually an exudate with elevated protein concentrations, normal or low glucose levels, and an elevated WBC count that is primarily neutrophilic. Complement levels in the fluid are low and autoantibodies (ANA, dsDNA) and LE cells have been reported.

Coronary artery disease

Myocardial infarction, angina, and sudden death resulting from CAD are well described in SLE. Estimates of the prevalence of CAD vary widely; however, the risk of myocardial infarction is 50-fold greater in young women with lupus than in normal age-matched controls.[44] Coronary artery vasculitis is a potential cause of CAD but is exceedingly rare and surgical and postmortem specimens commonly show atherosclerotic plaque. The prevalence of traditional risk factors for CAD, such as hypertension, diabetes, and hyperlipidemia, is increased in lupus patients. An increased prevalence of the metabolic syndrome in SLE likely contributes additional risk. Lupus-related risk factors include duration of SLE, duration of corticosteroid use, renal disease and absence of use of hydroxychloroquine. The potential

contributing influence of antibodies to phospholipids or disease activity continues to be explored. There is a growing body of evidence supporting a risk conferred by inflammation per se. The atherosclerotic plaque is infiltrated by activated monocytes, macrophages, and T cells that produce proinflammatory cytokines. Inflammation drives both the formation and the rupture of atherosclerotic plaque. In SLE, the pathology of acute events seems to focus on unstable plaque. If endothelial dysfunction and vascular injury are the events triggering atherosclerosis, there are multiple potentially responsible processes in lupus, including autoantibodies directed to endothelial cells, immune complexes, and enhanced cleavage of membrane endothelial protein C receptor.[45]

Renal involvement

Lupus nephritis is a common manifestation of disease with significant impact on morbidity and mortality. The prevalence of nephritis ranges from 50 to 75% overall, with increased prevalence of proliferative nephritis and more aggressive disease in African Americans and Hispanics compared to Caucasians. Low socioeconomic status, independent of ethnicity, is predictive of poor prognosis. Additionally pediatric lupus and male lupus are both associated with a greater incidence of, and more aggressive, nephritis. Onset of nephritis occurs at any time and monitoring for potential renal activity is an ongoing obligation. Clinically, patients are asymptomatic unless they are nephrotic or have developed end-stage renal disease. Detection typically relies on examination of the urine, although a rising creatinine or hypertension may herald renal involvement. The development of proteinuria on urinalysis or the presence of hematuria (>5 red blood cells (RBCs)/high-power field) or pyuria (>5 WBCs/high-power field) in the absence of other etiologies should prompt an evaluation for nephritis. A 24-hour urine collection remains the most accurate measurement of urinary protein loss; however, the protein/creatinine ratio in a spot urine is useful for following a patient with existing proteinuria. Monitoring serum creatinine as a surrogate for the glomerular filtration rate is standard; however, creatinine is an insensitive marker of lupus renal disease and should be used in conjunction with other assays. Renal activity is usually preceded or accompanied by serologic activity. Antibodies to dsDNA are almost always elevated or rising whereas measurements of serum complement ($C3$, $C4$, or CH_{50}) are usually low or dropping.

The traditional World Health Organization (WHO) classification of lupus nephritis has been modified by the International Society of Nephrology/Renal Pathology Society (ISN/RPS).[46] In general, membranous nephritis (class V) presents with a bland urinary sediment (i.e., no RBCs, WBCs, or casts), nephritic-range proteinuria, a normal to mildly elevated creatinine, a normal blood pressure and normal serologies. Patients with mesangial disease (class II) present with a bland or minimally active sediment, low-grade proteinuria (less than 500 mg/24 hours) and a normal serologic profile. Class III (focal) and class IV (diffuse) proliferative nephritis are characterized by active urinary sediment, proteinuria (>500 mg/24 hours), active serologies, and frequently hypertension and elevated serum creatinine. Class III is defined as ≤50% glomerular involvement and class IV is defined as >50%. The extent of proteinuria, urinary sediment activity, serologic abnormalities, and creatinine elevation is often less in class III than in class IV renal disease. Most cases of class II nephritis do not require initiation of cytotoxic therapy and progression to end-stage kidney disease is rare. The prognosis of class III disease is dependent upon the degree of activity; patients with 40–50% of glomerular involvement have a prognosis similar to that of patients with class IV disease. In addition to the number of involved glomeruli, renal biopsy assessment includes measures of activity (proliferative response) and chronicity (sclerotic response). Therapeutic intervention in class III or IV disease usually requires cytotoxic therapy in addition to high-dose corticosteroids provided the chronicity index is not too high, indicating irreversible damage. Even with potent immunosuppressant therapy such as cyclophosphamide or mycophenolate mofetil, a complete response is induced in only approximately 20% and a partial response in about 80% of patients. Relapses and flares of renal disease are not infrequent, particularly when tapering corticosteroids or discontinuing immunosuppressive treatment. Potential therapies that maintain podocyte integrity or prevent activation of renal endothelial cells as well as agents directed against inflammatory cytokines, B cells or T cells may offer therapeutic advantage and improved renal outcome (see Chapter 67).[47]

Hematologic

Hemocytopenias occur frequently in SLE and prevalence varies among lupus cohorts (Table 50.4). Evaluation for medication effects is essential before attributing a cytopenia to an immune-mediated mechanism.

Anemia

Antibody-mediated peripheral destruction of red blood cells, autoimmune hemolytic anemia (AHA), occurs in 5–14% of SLE patients (Table 50.4). The anti-erythrocyte antibody is usually an opsonizing IgG. The specificities of the anti-erythrocyte antibodies in SLE have not been clearly defined; the only non-rhesus-specific antigen reported in SLE is the membrane band 3 anion transporter protein. The presence of AHA is associated with increased disease severity and decreased survival and is readily diagnosed by a positive Coombs test, elevated lactate dehydrogenase and total bilirubin, and the presence of spherocytes on the peripheral smear. There are also reports of an association between AHA and anti-phospholipid antibodies, which may reflect cross-reactivity with erythrocyte membrane antigens.[48]

Anemia of chronic disease is the most common cause of anemia in SLE; however, if the hemoglobin is less than 10 g/dL, another cause of anemia should be considered. The inhibitory effects of pro-inflammatory cytokines on erythrocyte production can be compounded by increased hepcidin levels and an inadequate erythropoietin response. Low erythropoietin levels in SLE may be attributable to renal disease as well as anti-erythropoietin antibodies. Although hemophagocytosis of hematopoietic cells is frequently noted on bone marrow biopsies, the hemophagocytic syndrome characterized by spiking fevers, tender hepatosplenomegaly, anemia, leukopenia, and markedly elevated serum ferritin is rare.

Lupus is also associated with a thrombotic microangiopathic hemolytic anemia with schistocytes, helmet cells, and triangular fragments of red blood cells. The clinical constellation of high fever, renal insufficiency, neurologic symptoms, and thrombocytopenia is characteristic of thrombotic thrombocytopenic purpura (TTP). Coexistent TTP and SLE is a rare and frequently fatal phenomenon that has been associated with antibodies to ADAMTS 13 (von Willebrand factor cleaving protease) and anti-phospholipid antibodies.

Leukopenia

Leukopenia, either neutropenia or lymphopenia, occurs in 15–50% of patients (Table 50.4). Both neutropenia and lymphopenia can reflect disease activity and predispose to infection. Anti-neutrophil antibodies directed against membrane components of mature and progenitor cells resulting in decreased phagocytosis and accelerated apoptosis are implicated as are antibodies against granulocyte colony-stimulating factor (G-CSF) and hyposensitivity of myeloid cells to G-CSF. Binding of TNF-related apoptosis-inducing ligand (TRAIL) to TRAIL receptors on neutrophils accelerates neutrophil apoptosis.[49] One of four known TRAIL receptors is unable to transduce the death signal and functions as a decoy receptor; this receptor is reduced in SLE patients with neutropenia and is upregulated by steroid therapy.

Lymphopenia with reduced numbers of circulating CD4 T cells and a decreased CD4-to-CD8 ratio occurs with a reported incidence of 19–62% (see Table 50.4). Lymphocytotoxic antibodies, increased apoptosis related to Fas and Fas ligand upregulation, and increased serum IL-10 levels have all been implicated

Table 50.4 Prevalence (%) of cytopenias in different ethnic cohorts

	Caucasian/ British[a]	Hispanic/ Texas[b]	Hispanic/ Puerto Rican[b]	Latin American GLADEL[c]	Caucasian/ Danish[d]	African American[e]	Caucasian/ USA[e]
Leukopenia		27	33	42	25	20	15
Lymphopenia		62	54	59	42	23	19
Thrombocytopenia	17	21	3.7	19	24	10	12
Hemolytic anemia	5	9	3.7	12	11	14	7

[a]Sultan SM, Begum S, Isenberg DA. Prevalence, patterns of disease and outcome in patients with systemic lupus erythematosus who develop severe haematological problems. Rheumatol (Oxf) 2003; 42: 230–234.
[b]Vila LM, Alarcon GS, McGwin G Jr, et al. Early clinical manifestations, disease activity and damage of systemic lupus erythematosus among two distinct US Hispanic subpopulations. Rheumatol (Oxf) 2004; 43: 358–363.
[c]Pons-Estel BA, Catoggio LJ, Cardiel MH, et al. The GLADEL multinational Latin American prospective inception cohort of 1,214 patients with systemic lupus erythematosus: ethnic and disease heterogeneity among "Hispanics". Medicine (Baltimore) 2004; 83: 1-17.
[d]Jacobsen S, Petersen J, Ullman S, et al. A multicentre study of 513 Danish patients with systemic lupus erythematosus. I. Disease manifestations and analyses of clinical subsets. Clin Rheumatol 1998; 17: 468–477.
[e]Cooper GS, Parks CG, Treadwell EL, et al. Differences by race, sex and age in the clinical and immunologic features of recently diagnosed systemic lupus erythematosus patients in the southeastern United States. Lupus 2002; 11: 161–167.

in pathogenesis. B cells expressing the 9 G4 idiotype found on V_H 4.34 heavy chains may be responsible for production of anti-lymphocyte antibodies. In the absence of recurrent infection, leukopenia in SLE rarely warrants treatment. Increased steroids can increase the leukocyte count but also contribute to the risk of infection.

Thrombocytopenia

Low platelet counts are seen in approximately 25% of patients, although severe thrombocytopenia is reported in fewer than 10% (see Table 50.4). Immune-mediated consumption is the most frequent cause, but rarely thrombocytopenia occurs with micro-angiopathic hemolytic anemia, TTP, disseminated intravascular coagulation (DIC) or as part of the hemophagocytic syndrome; all of which are associated with high mortality and morbidity. A pathogenic role for antibodies against platelet membrane gly-coproteins (IIb/IIIa antigen) is well established.[50] Other possible mechanisms include antibodies to thrombopoeitin, and anti-phospholipid and anti-CD40-ligand antibodies that bind to platelets, resulting in platelet sequestration.

Central and peripheral nervous system

Neurologic and psychiatric manifestations of SLE are diverse and frequently occur irrespective of systemic disease activity. Neuropsychiatric symptoms can be focal or diffuse, peripheral or central, isolated or complex.

In 1999 a consensus committee established by the ACR developed reporting standards, case definitions, and recommendations for laboratory and imaging studies for 19 neurologic, psychiatric, and cognitive syndromes (Table 50.5). Diagnosis of a neuropsychiatric syndrome attributable to SLE (NPSLE) requires the exclusion of infections, metabolic disturbances, bleeding disorders, malignancy, and medication toxicities.

Table 50.5 Neuropsychiatric syndromes in systemic lupus erythematosus

Headache
Cerebrovascular disease
Seizures
Acute confusional state
Anxiety disorder
Cognitive dysfunction
Mood disorder
Psychosis
Aseptic meningitis
Autonomic disorder
Demyelinating syndrome
Mononeuropathy
Movement disorder
Myasthenia gravis
Myelopathy
Cranial neuropathy
Plexopathy
Polyneuropathy
Polyradiculopathy

Using this new nomenclature, NPSLE is common, with a prevalence of 57–95%. Headache, mood disorders, cerebrovascular events, cognitive dysfunction and seizures are frequent; polyneuropathy, demyelinating disease, mononeuritis, myasthenia gravis, chorea, cranial neuropathy, myelopathy, and Guillain–Barré syndrome are uncommon.

Focal presentations attributable to specific central nervous system (CNS) lesions occur frequently in association with anti-phospholipid (APL) antibodies. These presentations include strokes, transient ischemic attacks, seizures, movement disorders, and cranial neuropathies. In contrast, global dysfunction presents as intractable headaches, coma, delirium, cognitive dysfunction, and psychiatric syndromes, e.g., psychosis, mania, anxiety and depression. Ischemic strokes associated with APL antibodies are treated with anticoagulation whereas immuno-suppression in combination with neuroleptic and anti-seizure medications are generally required for treatment of the diffuse CNS events.

The diagnosis of CNS NPSLE is frequently difficult and the clinical evaluation of a patient with presumed CNS NPSLE mandates an exhaustive search for other potential causes. Cerebrospinal fluid (CSF) examination is useful for excluding infection or malignant cells. While CSF in NPSLE can be characterized by a lymphocytosis and increased immunoglobulin with elevated total protein, IgG index, and oligoclonal bands, these abnormalities are not consistently present. Numerous autoantibodies (ANA, anti-dsDNA, anticardiolipin, anti-ribosomal P, anti-N-methyl D-aspartate receptor (NMDAR), anti-neuronal) and various cytokines have been identified in the CSF of patients with SLE; however, none is specific for active NPSLE and routine testing is not recommended. MRI is extremely sensitive for detection of structural lesions and new ischemic lesions, but is frequently not helpful in diagnosing active NPSLE with diffuse manifestations; MRI studies may be normal in patients with psychiatric syndromes and global dysfunction.[51] Imaging studies of neuronal function, positron emission tomography (PET) and single-photon emission computed tomography (SPECT) scans measuring cerebral glucose uptake and blood flow, respectively, magnetic resonance spectroscopy and functional MRI (fMRI) correlate to a limited extent with diffuse NPSLE. These scans must be interpreted carefully since atrophy with neuronal cell loss leads to changes in metabolism and blood flow. Cerebral angiograms can be helpful if a diagnosis of cerebral vasculitis is considered; however, central nervous system vasculitis is rare with true vasculitis in only 5–8% of autopsies. More commonly, a bland vasculopathy with degenerative and proliferative changes in small vessels, perivascular infiltrates, microinfarcts, and microhemorrhages is present.

There are no serologic tests specific for CNS NPSLE. Serologic evidence of disease activity (elevated anti-DNA antibodies and low complement) may help to diagnose CNS NPSLE, particularly if combined with other clinical signs of active disease. However, CNS NPSLE may also flare in the absence of serologic and clinical disease activity. Cognitive impairment in particular, tends to develop insidiously irrespective of peripheral disease activity. Recent data from murine models and *in vitro* studies strongly support the role of specific autoantibodies directed against NMDAR, phospholipid, α tubulin and ribosomal P in NPSLE.[52] Anti-NMDAR and anti-P antibodies have been identified in the sera, CSF, and brain of SLE patients and are associated with cognitive and depressive syndromes in some SLE patients. The current challenge is to identify easily accessible, sensitive and specific serologic or imaging biomarkers for the diagnosis of CNS NPSLE syndromes that can also be used to monitor therapy.

Peripheral nervous system events attributable to NPSLE are recognized on the basis of clinical presentation with diagnostic studies such as EMG and peripheral nerve biopsy. Because there is no blood brain barrier intervening, peripheral nerves are more accessible to circulating complement, autoantibodies and inflammatory molecules and vasculitis of epineural arteries is a common finding.

Antiphospholipid antibody syndrome is described in detail in Chapter 60.

Drug-induced lupus

Until recently, drug-induced lupus referred to a clinical syndrome characterized by constitutional, musculoskeletal symptoms and serositis that resembles mild lupus and occurs following exposure to a number of drugs (most notably procainamide, hydralazine, chlorpromazine, and methyldopa). Drug-induced lupus has been associated with ANA and anti-histone antibodies whereas generation of more specific autoantibodies has been rare. Symptoms generally begin weeks to months following initiation of the inciting therapeutic agent and resolve within weeks after the drug is discontinued; autoantibodies can persist for up to 12 months. Host factors affecting drug metabolization (e.g., slow acetylation of procainamide and hydralazine) contribute to the risk of developing drug-induced lupus. Multiple potential mechanisms resulting in the loss of self-tolerance have been suggested for this classic model. One of the most extensively explored is inhibition of DNA methylation with TLR activation, resulting in overexpression of co-stimulatory molecules such as LFA-1 on T cells and enhanced T-cell help.[53]

Since the introduction of anti-TNF agents, a different type of drug-induced lupus has been recognized. Up to 30% of patients receiving TNF blockade develop autoantibodies, including a positive ANA and antibodies to dsDNA. A minority develops anti-DNA antibodies, nephritis, and vasculitis. The pathogenesis of the immunologic deregulation is not known, although low TNF is present in the NZB/W mouse model of lupus.[54]

Treatment

> ●THERAPEUTIC PRINCIPLES
>
> I. Suppression of inflammation
> ■ Induction of remission
> ■ Maintenance of remission
> ■ Preservation of organ function
> II. Suppression of immune activation
> ■ Modulation of the immune response
> III. Treatment/prevention of drug-related toxicities

The goals of lupus treatment are to stop and reverse ongoing organ inflammation, prevent or limit irreversible organ damage, and to suppress the immune response driving the inflammation, and prevent flares. Therapeutic agents, and combinations thereof, can be used for induction of remission, maintenance of remission or prevention of flare. The efficacy of therapeutic agents must be balanced against their potential toxicity. Thus, treatment must be tailored to the individual patient based on disease manifestations. In general, milder disease requires treatment with less potent or lower doses of anti-inflammatory and immunosuppressive medications than more active, severe disease affecting major organs such as the kidney or brain (Table 50.6). Individual patient responses to a given medication will vary and patients must be monitored closely for response as well as toxicity.

Some genetic factors predicting risk of toxicity or therapeutic benefit for individual agents have been identified. Polymorphisms of a key enzyme in the metabolism of azathioprine, thiopurine methyltransferase (TPMT), are common; 0.3 and 11% of Caucasians are homozygous and heterozygous (respectively) for mutations associated with altered expression of TPMT.[55] TPMT-deficient patients are especially susceptible to leukopenia and pancytopenia associated with azathioprine. Cyclophosphamide is metabolized to its active form by cytochrome P450. Individuals heterozygous or homozygous for a specific cytochrome P450 polymorphism (*CYP2C19*2*) have a lower probability of developing premature ovarian failure, but also show a poorer response to therapy.[56]

Table 50.6 Treatments for systemic lupus erythematosus disease manifestations

	NSAIDs	Antimalarials[†]	Low-dose corticosteroids (<0.5 mg/kg per day)	High-dose corticosteroids (>0.5 mg/kg per day)[‡]	Azathioprine	MMF	CTX
Constitutional	+	+	+		+		
Musculoskeletal	+	+	+		+	+	
Mucocutaneous		+	+				
Serositis	+	+	+		+		
Hematologic			+	+	+		
Renal			+	+	+	+	+
Central nervous system				+			+
Vasculitis			+	+		+	+

[†]Antimalarials should be given to all patients to sustain remission and reduce damage.
[‡]High-dose corticosteroids are required for remission induction or an inadequate response to low dose therapy.
CTX, cyclophosphamide; MMF, mycophenolate mofetil; NSAIDs, nonsteroidal anti-inflammatory drugs.

Although corticosteroids are the foundation of treatment, exposure must be minimized to the greatest extent given their multiple and frequent side effects, including hypertension, diabetes mellitus, increased susceptibility to infection, bone loss, and weight gain. Additional disease modifying agents that are also steroid-sparing include antimalarials (hydroxychloroquine), anti-metabolites such as azathioprine (1–2.5 mg/kg per day), methotrexate (7.5–25 mg/week), leflunomide (10–20 mg/day), and mycophenolate mofetil (MMF; 2–3 g/day) and alkylating agents such as cyclophosphamide (monthly pulse 0.5–1.0 g/m²). When more conventional therapies have failed, anecdotal reports, case series, and open-label studies suggest the use of intravenous immunoglobulin (2 g/kg over 2–5 days), thalidomide (50–100 mg/day) or cyclosporine (3–5 mg/kg/day). Medications such as dapsone, danazol, and chlorambucil may be efficacious in cutaneous disease, hematologic disease, and in severe refractory disease respectively, but in general these medications are not commonly used due to their toxicity, and the introduction and availability of better-tolerated, efficacious agents. Belimumab, a monoclonal antibody directed against BAFF, was approved by the FDA for treatment of SLE in 2011 and represents a therapeutic option for patients with non-renal, non-CNS active disease. How and when this agent will be used remains to be determined.

There are a number of newer agents on the horizon for treatment of SLE. Some are currently available but approved for other indications, whereas others are still in developmental stages. These therapies, in general, have more specific immunologic targets than standard treatments. Although there are multiple agents that have been tested in animal models of disease, we will only focus on therapies that have been given to humans. Several of these agents have been recently evaluated in phase III clinical trials and have been unable to demonstrate superiority over treatment with placebo or standard of care. Although imperfect trial design may account for some of these failures, the possibility remains that these agents are not effective treatments for SLE. Rituximab (anti-CD20 antibody) a B-cell directed therapy approved for use in rheumatoid arthritis, targeting all B cells except plasma cells, failed to demonstrate improved performance over standard of care in trials of patients with active SLE or in patients with active lupus nephritis added to a background therapy of MMF and corticosteroids. Abatacept (CTLA4-Ig) which is also approved for use in rheumatoid arthritis and blocks T-cell activation, was no better than placebo in trials of active lupus and of lupus nephritis, again added to background therapy of corticosteroids and MMF. Although treatment with abetimus sodium (LJP 394), a B-cell toleragen, resulted in decreased titers of anti dsDNA antibodies, associated clinical efficacy was not demonstrated.

Despite the failure of rituximab in two clinical trials, B-cell-directed therapies remain an attractive approach. Several uncontrolled studies using B-cell depletion with rituximab in combination with cyclophosphamide for patients with active disease resistant to standard of care have demonstrated significant efficacy suggesting the importance of drug combinations and timing. Epratuzumab (anti-CD22 antibody) targeting all B cells and other agents targeting BAFF are under development. TACI-Ig, which blocks both BAFF and April is undergoing clinical study although two previous clinical trials were terminated prematurely because of infectious complications. Tociluzumab, an antibody to the IL-6 receptor, a cytokine involved in B-cell survival and activation as well as differentiation of TH17 and T_{FH} cells, which is approved for RA, are under study in SLE. Other agents in earlier clinical development are inhibitors of intracellular B-cell signaling molecules designed to block B-cell activation; R406, a SYK inhibitor and Janus tyrosine kinase (JAK) inhibitors

are being studied using topical administration for discoid lupus and have recently shown efficacy when given orally in RA.

Potential therapies aimed at the dendritic cells include vitamin D, which blocks dendritic cell maturation and T-cell activation, and inhibitory oligodeoxynucleotides, which block TLR9 signaling and dendritic cell maturation. Hydroxychloroquine, a standard agent for lupus, interferes with TLR7 and TLR9 signaling by preventing acidification of the endosomal compartment.

Other potential therapies are directed against IFN-α, IFN-γ, IL-1, or IL-12. Multiple studies of monoclonal antibodies against IFN-α are underway in lupus. The monoclonal antibody against IL-12 has demonstrated efficacy in Crohn's disease.

Novel interventions directed at T cells include anti-CD40 antibodies, abtacept (CTLA4-Ig) in combination with cyclophosphamide for proliferative nephritis and studies targeting ICOS, an inducible T-cell co-stimulator.

Therapies in development for other autoimmune diseases may also prove useful in SLE. Eclizumab, currently approved for paroxysmal nocturnal hemoglobinuria, is an antibody directed against C5 that blocks cleavage of C5 and the subsequent triggering of the complement cascade. Alicaforsen, an antisense oligodeoxynucleotide that inhibits ICAM-1 expression, decreases inflammation in both rheumatoid arthritis and Crohn's disease. Efalizumab, a monoclonal antibody against CD11a (an LFA-1 subunit that interacts with ICAM-1), benefits patients with psoriasis. Although there are no chemokine targeted therapies in clinical trial in lupus, a CCR1 antagonist slowed disease progression in a mouse model of lupus and has been tested in patients with rheumatoid arthritis. FTY720, an agonist for the sphingosine-1 phosphate receptor that prevents egress of lymphocytes from secondary lymphoid organs and inflamed tissues, has beneficial effects in the MRL/lpr mouse model of lupus; it has been given to transplant recipients and to patients with multiple sclerosis. The use of anti-TNF-α agents for SLE is inhibited by its lupus-like effects in some patients. Paradoxically, TNF-α is involved in renal inflammation in SLE and short-term treatment with monoclonal antibody to TNF-α appears to improve lupus nephritis, showing that agents can abort inflammation and yet exacerbate autoimmunity

Translational research

● ON THE HORIZON

- Increased understanding of the functional consequences of single nucleotide polymorphisms identified as susceptibility loci in SLE may provide insight into:
  - Dysregulation of tolerance mechanisms and pathogenesis of disease in different ethnic populations
  - Predictors of response to therapy
  - New therapeutic targets
- Development of organ-specific biomarkers, perhaps through use of microarray techniques and imaging, will allow for improved use of immunomodulating and immunosuppressive therapies and possibly for use of preventive therapies

Laboratory research continues to inform us about dysregulated immunologic pathways in SLE. The current challenge of translational medicine is to shed light on the clinical relevance of these altered pathways. Increased understanding of the qualitative and quantitative differences of these molecular perturbations should not only result in improved diagnostic capabilities and biomarkers for disease, but will lead to the ability to subset patients for prognosis and response to therapy. Improved organ-specific biomarkers and methods for subsetting patients on a molecular level are likely to result in improved use of immunobiologic therapies. In particular, the brain which has been relatively inaccessible to mechanistic and diagnostic probing is likely to be an organ to be more fully explored. Ultimately, advances in translational studies should result in more effective and less toxic therapeutic interventions.

Conclusions

In the past several years much has been learned about genetic susceptibility to SLE and it is encouraging that many of the genes identified are associated with pathways that also have been implicated in disease pathogenesis. The role of B cells in disease pathogenesis has been confirmed but recent studies have also highlighted the role of T cells, dendritic cells and neutrophils. Enhanced understanding of each of these contributing factors and the cross-talk between them has allowed identification of numerous potential therapeutic targets. The disappointing results from clinical trials of immunobiologic agents for lupus have highlighted the critical importance of study design. The overall goal in therapy must be to eliminate autoreactivity while maintaining immunocompetence. Among the challenges we now face are the careful phenotyping of patients to identify etiopathologically distinct subpopulations and new clinical trial designs to allow the use of combinations of agents, each of which alone may have a negligible effect on disease course.

References

1. Tan EM, Cohen AS, Fries JF, et al. The 1982 revised criteria for the classification of systemic lupus erythematosus. Arthritis Rheum 1982;25:1271–7.
2. Borchers AT, Naguwa SM, Shoenfeld Y, Gershwin ME. The geoepidemiology of systemic lupus erythematosus. Autoimmun Rev 2010;9:A277–87.
3. Gregersen PK, Olsson LM. Recent advances in the genetics of autoimmune disease. Annu Rev Immunol 2009;27:363–91.
4. Ueda H, Howson JM, Esposito L, et al. Association of the T-cell regulatory gene CTLA4 with susceptibility to autoimmune disease. Nature 2003;423:506–11.
5. Deng Y, Tsao BP. Genetic susceptibility to systemic lupus erythematosus in the genomic era. Nat Rev Rheumatol 2010;6:683–92.
6. Orozco G, Sanchez E, Gonzalez-Gay MA, et al. Association of a functional single-nucleotide polymorphism of PTPN22, encoding lymphoid protein phosphatase, with rheumatoid arthritis and systemic lupus erythematosus. Arthritis Rheum 2005;52:219–24.
7. Manderson AP, Botto M, Walport MJ. The role of complement in the development of systemic lupus erythematosus. Annu Rev Immunol 2004;22:431–56.
8. Baumann I, Kolowos W, Voll RE, et al. Impaired uptake of apoptotic cells into tingible body macrophages in germinal centers of patients with systemic lupus erythematosus. Arthritis Rheum 2002;46:191–201.
9. Anolik JH, Barnard J, Cappione A, et al. Rituximab improves peripheral B cell abnormalities in human systemic lupus erythematosus. Arthritis Rheum 2004;50:3580–90.
10. Floto RA, Clatworthy MR, Heilbronn KR, et al. Loss of function of a lupus-associated FcgammaRIIb polymorphism through exclusion from lipid rafts. Nat Med 2005;11:1056–8.
11. Wong M, Tsao BP. Current topics in human SLE genetics. Springer Semin Immunopathol 2006;28:97–107.
12. Tucci M, Barnes EV, Sobel ES, et al. Strong association of a functional polymorphism in the monocyte chemoattractant protein 1 promoter gene with lupus nephritis. Arthritis Rheum 2004;50:1842–9.
13. Crow MK. Interferon pathway activation in systemic lupus erythematosus. Curr Rheumatol Rep 2005;7:463–8.
14. Nath SK, Harley JB, Lee YH. Polymorphisms of complement receptor 1 and interleukin-10 genes and systemic lupus erythematosus: a meta-analysis. Hum Genet 2005;118:225–34.
15. Schotte H, Willeke P, Tidow N, et al. Extended haplotype analysis reveals an association of TNF polymorphisms with susceptibility to systemic lupus erythematosus beyond HLA-DR3. Scand J Rheumatol 2005;34:114–21.
16. Wu J, Metz C, Xu X, et al. A novel polymorphic CAAT/enhancer-binding protein beta element in the FasL gene promoter alters Fas ligand expression: a candidate background gene in African American systemic lupus erythematosus patients. J Immunol 2003;170:132–8.
17. Mehrian R, Quismorio Jr. FP, Strassmann G, et al. Synergistic effect between IL-10 and bcl-2 genotypes in determining susceptibility to systemic lupus erythematosus. Arthritis Rheum 1998;41:596–602.
18. Ballestar E. Epigenetic alterations in autoimmune rheumatic diseases. Nat Rev Rheumatol 2010;7:263–71.
19. Javierre BM, Fernandez AF, Richter J, et al. Changes in the pattern of DNA methylation associate with twin discordance in systemic lupus erythematosus. Genome Res 2010;20:170–9.
20. Milner EC, Anolik J, Cappione A, Sanz I. Human innate B cells: a link between host defense and autoimmunity? Springer Semin Immunopathol 2005;26:433–52.
21. Pugh-Bernard AE, Cambier JC. B cell receptor signaling in human systemic lupus erythematosus. Curr Opin Rheumatol 2006;18:451–5.
22. Mackay IR. The hepatitis-lupus connection. Semin Liver Dis 1991;11:234–40.
23. Grimaldi CM, Hill L, Xu X, et al. Hormonal modulation of B cell development and repertoire selection. Mol Immunol 2005;42:811–20.
24. Doreau A, Belot A, Bastid J, et al. Interleukin 17 acts in synergy with B cell-activating factor to influence B cell biology and the pathophysiology of systemic lupus erythematosus. Nat Immunol 2009;10:778–85.
25. Lande R, Ganguly D, Facchinetti V, et al. Neutrophils activate plasmacytoid dendritic cells by releasing self-DNA-peptide complexes in systemic lupus erythematosus. Sci Transl Med 2011;3: 73ra19.
26. Garcia-Romo GS, Caielli S, Vega B, et al. Netting neutrophils are major inducers of type I IFN production in pediatric systemic lupus erythematosus. Sci Transl Med 2011;3: 73ra20.
27. Bennett L, Palucka AK, Arce E, et al. Interferon and granulopoiesis signatures in systemic lupus erythematosus blood. J Exp Med 2003;197:711–23.
28. Kis-Toth K, Tsokos GC. Dendritic cell function in lupus: Independent contributors or victims of aberrant immune regulation. Autoimmun 2010;43:121–30.
29. Crispin JC, Kyttaris VC, Terhorst C, Tsokos GC. T cells as therapeutic targets in SLE. Nat Rev Rheumatol 2010;6:317–25.
30. Scheinecker C, Bonelli M, Smolen JS. Pathogenetic aspects of systemic lupus erythematosus with an emphasis on regulatory T cells. J Autoimmun 2010;35:269–75.
31. Miyara M, Amoura Z, Parizot C, et al. Global natural regulatory T cell depletion in active systemic lupus erythematosus. J Immunol 2005;175:8392–400.
32. McMurray RW. Bromocriptine in rheumatic and autoimmune diseases. Semin Arthritis Rheum 2001;31:21–32.
33. Zhang W, Wu K, He W, et al. Transforming growth factor beta 1 plays an important role in inducing CD4(+)CD25(+)forhead box P3(+) regulatory T cells by mast cells. Clin Exp Immunol 2010;161:490–6.
34. Cunningham M, Gilkeson G. Estrogen receptors in immunity and autoimmunity. Clin Rev Allergy Immunol 2011;40:66–73.
35. Zoma A. Musculoskeletal involvement in systemic lupus erythematosus. Lupus 2004;13:851–3.
36. Aranow C, Zelicof S, Leslie D, et al. Clinically occult avascular necrosis of the hip in systemic lupus erythematosus. J Rheumatol 1997;24:2318–22.
37. Tebbe B. Clinical course and prognosis of cutaneous lupus erythematosus. Clin Dermatol 2004;22:121–4.
38. Orteu CH, Buchanan JA, Hutchison I, et al. Systemic lupus erythematosus presenting with oral mucosal lesions: easily missed? Br J Dermatol 2001;144:1219–23.
39. Hallegua DS, Wallace DJ. Gastrointestinal manifestations of systemic lupus erythematosus. Curr Opin Rheumatol 2000;12:379–85.
40. Kaw R, Gota C, Bennett A, et al. Lupus-related hepatitis: complication of lupus or autoimmune association? Case report and review of the literature. Dig Dis Sci 2006;51:813–8.
41. Yazici Y, Erkan D, Levine DM, et al. Protein-losing enteropathy in systemic lupus erythematosus: report of a severe, persistent case and review of pathophysiology. Lupus 2002;11:119–23.
42. Lawrence E. Systemic lupus erythematosus and the lung. New York: Wiley; 1987.
43. Moder KG, Miller TD, Tazelaar HD. Cardiac involvement in systemic lupus erythematosus. Mayo Clin Proc 1999;74:275–84.
44. Manzi S, Meilahn EN, Rairie JE, et al. Age-specific incidence rates of myocardial infarction and angina in women with systemic lupus erythematosus: comparison with the Framingham Study. Am J Epidemiol 1997;145:408–15.
45. Sesin CA, Yin X, Esmon CT, et al. Shedding of endothelial protein C receptor contributes to vasculopathy and renal injury in lupus: in vivo and in vitro evidence. Kidney Int 2005;68:110–20.
46. Weening JJ, D'Agati VD, Schwartz MM, et al. The classification of glomerulonephritis in systemic lupus erythematosus revisited. J Am Soc Nephrol 2004;15:241–50.
47. Davidson A, Aranow C. Lupus nephritis: lessons from murine models. Nat Rev Rheumatol 2010;6:13–20.
48. Sultan SM, Begum S, Isenberg DA. Prevalence, patterns of disease and outcome in patients with systemic lupus erythematosus who develop severe haematological problems. Rheumatology (Oxford) 2003;42:230–4.
49. Matsuyama W, Yamamoto M, Higashimoto I, et al. TNF-related apoptosis-inducing ligand is involved in neutropenia of systemic lupus erythematosus. Blood 2004;104:184–91.
50. Michel M, Lee K, Piette JC, et al. Platelet autoantibodies and lupus-associated thrombocytopenia. Br J Haematol 2002;119:354–8.
51. Govoni M, Castellino G, Padovan M, et al. Recent advances and future perspective in neuroimaging in neuropsychiatric systemic lupus erythematosus. Lupus 2004;13:149–58.

52. Karassa FB, Afeltra A, Ambrozic A, et al. Accuracy of anti-ribosomal P protein antibody testing for the diagnosis of neuropsychiatric systemic lupus erythematosus: an international meta-analysis. Arthritis Rheum 2006;54:312–24.

53. Kaplan MJ, Deng C, Yang J, Richardson BC. DNA methylation in the regulation of T cell LFA-1 expression. Immunol Invest 2000;29:411–25.

54. Jacob CO, McDevitt HO. Tumour necrosis factor-alpha in murine autoimmune 'lupus' nephritis. Nature 1988;331:356–8.

55. Yates CR, Krynetski EY, Loennechen T, et al. Molecular diagnosis of thiopurine S-methyltransferase deficiency: genetic basis for azathioprine and mercaptopurine intolerance. Ann Intern Med 1997;126: 608–614.

56. Takada K, Arefayene M, Desta Z, et al. Cytochrome P450 pharmacogenetics as a predictor of toxicity and clinical response to pulse cyclophosphamide in lupus nephritis. Arthritis Rheum 2004;50:2202–10.

51

Rheumatoid arthritis | Andrew P. Cope

Rheumatoid arthritis (RA) is one of the most common chronic inflammatory diseases, and in modern times has become a prototype disease entity for defining the molecular and pathological basis of chronic inflammatory syndromes. The term "rheumatoid arthritis" was coined by Garrod in 1859. However, this was probably an inappropriate use of the term because it encompassed polyarticular osteoarthritis, as well as inflammatory polyarthritis. For many years, there has been considerable debate as to whether RA is in fact a new disease, an hypothesis based largely on negative data and inconclusive deductions from archive material, including the visual arts and archaeological artifacts. In spite of references to inflammatory afflictions of joints by the likes of Galen, Sydenham and Heberden, the first convincing case reports of the disease, described in terms that would be recognizable today, were published in 1800 by Landré-Beauvais, who labelled the disease *"la goutte asthénique primitive."*[1] This description was distinct since all patients were female, an observation that was significant when the most important differential diagnosis at that time was polyarticular gout, a disease predominantly of males.

Today we recognize RA as a chronic inflammatory disorder of joints of unknown etiology in which the major target tissue is the synovial lining of joints, bursae and tendon sheaths.[2] While traditionally considered an autoimmune disease, RA differs from organ specific autoimmune disease entities in several respects. From the outset of clinically apparent disease, the systemic immuno-inflammatory process, driven by cytokines and other inflammatory mediators, promotes the activation and proliferation of stromal joint tissues, in particular the fibroblastic synovial lining layer. This appears to contrast with organ specific autoimmune diseases such as type I diabetes or autoimmune thyroiditis that are characterized by an antigen driven inflammatory process *in situ* leading to targeted cellular destruction of pancreatic β-islet or thyroid tissue cells. In RA, once the inflammatory process is established, the inflammatory synovium, or pannus, can invade and erode underlying cartilage and bone, at least in a subset of patients. Unlike some autoimmune diseases that target single organs or tissues, RA is a systemic inflammatory disease that likely encompasses a heterogeneous syndrome with marked variations in clinical expression that most clinicians today would acknowledge is more than one disease entity. Indeed, over a period of several decades it has become increasingly apparent that the disease is heterogeneous not only clinically, but also pathologically, serologically and genetically, presenting a major challenge to the immunologist and physician alike.

Epidemiology

The incidence of RA (the rate of new cases arising in a given period) is 0.1–0.2 per 1000 of the population for males, and 0.2–0.4 per 1000 for females.[3] These rates plateau between the ages of 45 and 75 years in some series but can increase steadily with age until the seventh decade, declining thereafter. The largest difference in incidence between the sexes occurs in those under 50 years of age. Past evidence indicates that the incidence may be in decline, at least for seropositive disease. Public health measures and their impact on the environment, might account for this, at least in part. The disease prevalence should ideally include all past and inactive cases. For RA, large cross-sectional population samples indicate that the figure ranges from 0.5 to 2% for Caucasian European and North American populations over the age of 15, with a female to male excess of 2–4.[3] Despite similar prevalence estimates for these geographically diverse populations, greater diversity has been documented for rural African populations, where the prevalence has been reported to be as low as 0.1%, and Native Americans (including the Pima, Yakima and Chippewa tribes) where the prevalence may be as high as 5%. Such variance across geographical borders likely reflects distinct environmental factors and socio-demographic determinants, as well as a spectrum of genetic admixture.

Complex polygenic autoimmune syndromes like RA are diseases of low penetrance, where thresholds of disease expression may be higher in males. This is based in part on the observation that the increased risk of disease in siblings of probands (denoted λs) is rather small; the λs for RA (risk to sibling divided by population risk) is estimated to be 3, while the λs for SLE may be as high as 30, and for celiac disease the λs is closer to 50. Twin studies provide perhaps the most compelling evidence for genetic effects given the excess concordance rates for monozygotic (12–15%) as compared to dizygotic twins (< 5%, and probably nearer to 3.5%).[4] When compared to a background prevalence of 1% in outbred populations, these figures translate to a significant contribution of genetic factors, calculated to be of the order of 60%; more recent estimates return values of 68% for those patients carrying antibodies to citrullinated protein antigens (ACPA⁺) and 66% for those who do not (ACPA⁻).[5] HLA is thought to contribute approximately 40% of this value. This leaves a substantial contribution for disease susceptibility from environmental factors, influenced by occupation, socioecomonic status, exposure to infectious pathogens and lifestyle factors, a conglomeration of factors termed the "exposome."

● KEY CONCEPTS

Important risk factors for developing RA

- Female gender; impact of X chromosome, microchimerism, lifestyle
- Age; associated with immune senescence
- Inheritance of genetic variants; *HLADRB1* and *PTPN22*
- Autoantibodies; to citrullinated protein antigens (ACPA), rheumatoid factor
- Family history; first degree relatives have higher prevalence of genetic and serological risk factors
- Hormonal factors; nulliparity, the first 3 months postpartum, low androgen or high estrogen status (in males); longer duration breastfeeding
- Smoking status; > 25 cigarettes/day for > 20 years confers a 15-fold risk in subjects who carry disease associated HLA-DRB1 alleles
- Alcohol intake
- Environmental antigens (the "exposome"); dietary factors, exposure to infectious (and non-infectious/microbiota) pathogens at mucosal surfaces such as the lung, periodontium, and gut, non-inherited maternal antigens (NIMA)
- Urban dwelling

Two of the more intriguing factors contributing to disease occurrence are age and gender. Age-associated changes in susceptibility to infection, neoplastic disease and autoimmunity suggest that a common mechanism could be responsible. Immune senescence is one possibility, where age-related decline in host immunity is characterized at the cellular and molecular level by massive expansions of lymphocyte clones, corresponding contractions of the naïve T- and B-cell repertoires and telomere erosion of leukocytes, indicative of an extensive proliferative history.[6] When combined with oxidative stress and a range of biochemical derangements of pathways integral to antigen responsiveness and immune regulation, these factors may combine to (1) increase susceptibility to foreign pathogens, (2) augment reactivity to self tissue antigens (modified post-translationally as a consequence of the ageing process), and to (3) generate a repertoire of lymphocytes defective in terms of tumor surveillance. Thus, immune senescence should be considered a risk factor for RA.

The female sex preponderance implies that hormonal and reproductive factors strongly influence risk. On the one hand, nulliparity is a risk factor for RA. Women entering the first 3 months of the postpartum period are also at increased risk. By contrast, oral contraceptive use, pregnancy and hormonal replacement therapy have all been associated with reduced risk or less severe disease.[7] Extended periods of breastfeeding appears to increase risk. Several possible immune mechanisms have been proposed. For example, materno-fetal mismatch at the MHC locus has been associated with higher disease remission rates during pregnancy. In contrast, non-inherited HLA-DRB1 DERAA-positive (occupying the same amino acid positions as the QQRAA/QKRAA/KKRAA shared epitope motif) antigens (NIMA) expressed on maternal cells constitute a novel environmental factor that is protective to a DERAA-negative child, perhaps through mechanisms relating to microchimerism. In mouse models pregnancy has been associated with quantitative changes in the numbers of regulatory T cells. An influence of hormonal factors is further suggested in studies of men where disease is associated with lower androgenic testosterone and dehydroepiandrosterone (DHEA) levels and increased estradiol, when compared to a cohort of healthy control male subjects.

Etiology and pathogenesis

Environmental and non-genetic factors

Most, but not all, studies have reported an association between RA and smoking. One of the largest studies comprising over 370 000 women from Women's Health Cohort Study reported a relative risk of 1.4 for women who smoked more than 25 cigarettes per day for more than 20 years, when compared to non-smokers.[8] The association appears to be more closely related to duration rather than the amount of tobacco exposure, and may influence severity since smokers are more likely to have seropositive, erosive disease with extra-articular manifestations. The effect may be fully reversible in those individuals who stop smoking for ten years or more. Further evidence of gene-environment interactions with respect to smoking have been documented more recently in a population based case–control study of Swedish RA patients.[9] In this study the relative risk of developing rheumatoid factor positive (RF$^+$) RA was calculated according to smoking status and HLA-DRB1 genotype. The relative risk of developing RA increased from 2.5 in non-smokers with disease associated HLA-DRB1 genes to 7.5 and 15.7 in smokers who carried one or two copies of the susceptibility alleles, respectively. The association between smoking and seropositive disease was explored further in a follow up study that demonstrated more robust associations with smoking, HLA-DRB1 status and the presence of autoantibodies to citrullinated protein antigens (ACPA).

Being female, a smoker and carrying specific disease associated genes may be necessary but not sufficient to initiate chronic inflammatory arthritis. Other environmental triggers may be involved. Not least among these are exposure to foreign pathogens. This association has gained much credibility because of the presumed link between not only infection and autoimmunity but also immunodeficiency and autoimmune disease. Nonetheless, no single pathogen or group of pathogens has been defined. This could imply that aberrant host responses (either exaggerated innate inflammatory responses, or failure to terminate such responses) can occur following a wide range of infectious insults. Indeed bacterial products including superantigens, mycoplasma species, viruses (including herpes family, parvovirus and retroviruses) and fungi have all been implicated but data have been insufficient to prove causation. Epstein–Barr virus (EBV) infection has been a particularly attractive candidate as infection is common; antibodies to EBV nuclear antigens have been reported in patients with RA, EBV is a polyclonal activator of B lymphocytes, EBV-specific T cells reactive to EBV gp110 have been identified in RA synovial joints, and EBV RNA has been isolated from the synovium. More recently, evidence has been provided for an intriguing link between infection with *Porphyromonas gingivalis*, which expresses its own enzymatic machinery capable of generating bacterial or host derived citrullinated proteins, severe periodontitis (which shares risk factors for RA) and RA.[10] According to this model, molecular mimicry may arise through the development of autoimmune responses to bacterial derived proteins such as enolase and cross-reactivity to the human orthologue α-enolase, expressed in abundance by myeloid cells in inflamed periodontium and synovium. Finally, recent data from mouse models of autoimmune arthritis, comparing the microbial genomes from the colon of animals housed in conventional versus germ free facilities, suggest that a single gut residing species, in this case filamentous bacteria, can profoundly influence the clinical expression of inflammatory arthritis. Mechanisms include the generation of IL-17 expressing T cells in lamina propria.[11]

Immunogenetics

RA is a clinically heterogeneous disease and so comprehensive identification of disease susceptibility genes has been challenging, in spite of heritability estimates of up to 60%. With the exception of the MHC, where extensive gene polymorphism contributes about one-third of genetic susceptibility, and *PTPN22* (odds ratio 1.8), these genes confer low to moderate risk and have low penetrance (odds ratios in the range of 1.1–1.5). Nevertheless, five genome-wide linkage scans of multiplex families with RA have established an important contribution of the MHC.[12] This lends support to a wealth of epidemiological and genetic data describing associations between RA and specific HLA-DRB1 alleles, in particular HLA-DR4 subtypes. While this association was first described by Stastny in the 1970s, it was shown more than a decade later that susceptibility to RA across different ethnic populations correlated closely with the expression of a specific consensus amino acid sequence (referred to as the "shared epitope," hereafter SE) within the HLA-DR β chain α helix (Fig. 51.1).[13] This sequence was subsequently shown by several groups of investigators to be encoded by HLA-DRB1 alleles, including HLA-DR4 (*0401, *0404, *0405, and *0408), but also HLA-DR1 (*0101), DR6 (*1402), and DR10 (*1001) alleles, among others. HLA-DR9 (*09) is associated but not in Caucasians. According to this model, RA is associated with the RA shared epitope sequence (72–74 positions) and the association is modulated by the amino acids at positions 70 and 71, resulting in six genotypes with RA risks varying from 4.4 to 22.2. On the other hand, the finding of DERAA encoding HLA-DRB1 alleles (DRB1*0103, *0402, *1102, *1103, *1301, *1302, and *1304) conferring lower disease risk, and more importantly reduced radiographic progression in RA even in the presence of one copy of the SE, raises the possibility that specific subsets of MHC class II genes may confer an independent protective role.[14] The studies of non-inherited maternal antigens are consistent with this notion.

Specific genotypes co-segregate with distinct clinical features.[15] For example, in population based studies, different HLA-DRB1 alleles influence the severity of disease, with DRB1*0401

being found in patients with severe, seropositive, erosive RA (often with extra-articular features such as vasculitis and Felty's syndrome in *0401 homozygous or *0401/*0404 compound homozygote individuals), while DRB1*0101 and *1001 are observed at a higher frequency in patients with less severe, seronegative, non-erosive disease. Inheriting two copies of alleles expressing the consensus sequence increases disease penetrance, time of onset and severity. Thus, rather than a hierarchy of phenotypes of a single disease, these genetic associations, which are by no means uniform, are reflected clinically as distinct disease entities.

On the basis of early observations, two principal models were proposed to account for the association between RA and the consensus DR β-chain sequence.[16] Both were based on the assumption that the shared epitope is the critical genetic element linked directly to disease. The first model proposed that the shared epitope determines specific peptide binding, and that "pathogenic" peptides bind only to disease-associated HLA class II molecules (Fig. 51.1). This model predicted that a gradient of affinities of disease inducing peptide for MHC class II molecules might account for the differences in susceptibility and/or severity conferred by different HLA-DR molecules. Along the same lines, disease associated alleles may preclude the binding of peptides required for the generation of naturally occurring regulatory T cells specific for self-peptide antigens. The second model proposed that the shared epitope influences T-cell receptor (TCR) recognition by binding and selecting autoreactive T cells during thymic maturation, and expanding these populations in the peripheral compartment; again perturbations of a repertoire of regulatory T cells could arise through opposing influences of the shared epitope sequence.

Two recent lines of experimental evidence provide further insights into HLA-disease associations. The first is the association between HLA-DR4 subtypes and telomere erosion in RA patients and healthy donors, detectable before the age of 20.[6] Telomere loss has been associated with ageing and immune senescence. Whether this implies a direct contribution of HLA-DR4 expression to accelerated differentiation of hematopoietic cells in the context of a chronic inflammatory process is intriguing, but certainly warrants further investigation. The second line of evidence pointing to specific functions of SE⁺ alleles has arisen through analysis of autoantibodies in RA patients typed at the HLA-DRB1 locus.[17] These studies, replicated in European and

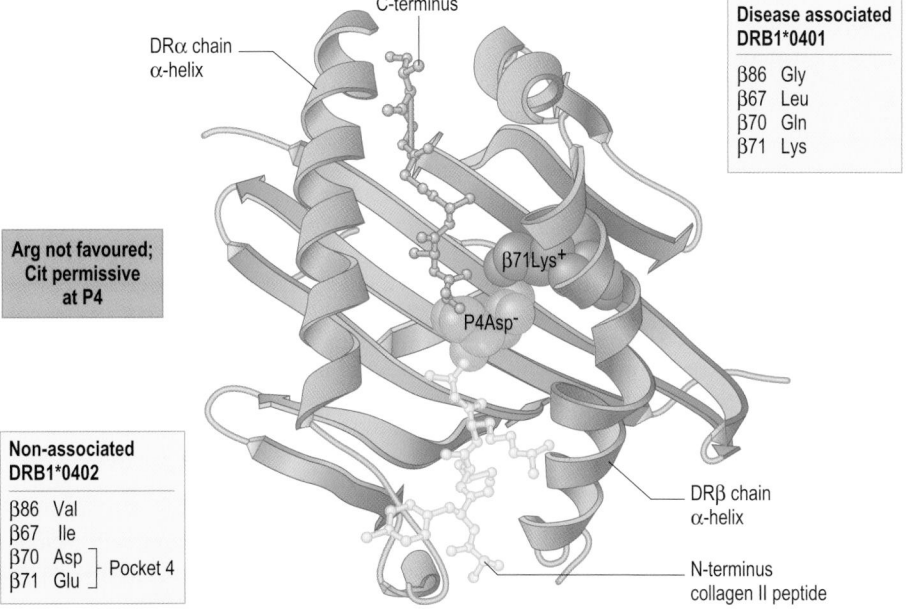

Fig. 51.1 Crystal structure of a collagen II peptide/HLA-DR4 complex. Ribbon model of an immunodominant collagen II peptide (1168–1180) complexed to HLA-DR4 (DRA*0101/DRB1*0401); a view of the MHC/peptide complex as seen from the T-cell surface. DRα and DRβ chain helices are shown in red, while the β-pleated sheet comprising the floor of the peptide binding grove is shown in blue. Residues 67 to 74 of the DRβ chain, components of the third hypervariable region, derive the "shared epitope." The ball and stick model of the CII peptide is shown. Interacting residues of the peptide position 4 (Asp, orange) and DRβ chain residue (β71Lys, green), which make up part of pocket 4, are depicted as van der Waal's spheres. Differences in amino acid sequence between the closely related disease associated DRB1*0401 and non-associated DRB1*0402 gene products are illustrated. Note that while Arg would not be favored at position 4 in the peptide, modification of Arg → Cit by deimination would be permissive. Figure generated by R. Visse and A. Cope, based on crystal data derived by Wiley and colleagues (Dessen et al, Immunity 1997; 7: 473).

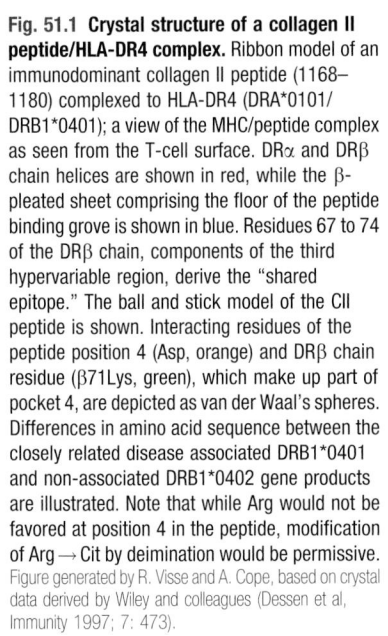

Disease associated DRB1*0401	
β86	Gly
β67	Leu
β70	Gln
β71	Lys

Arg not favoured; Cit permissive at P4

Non-associated DRB1*0402		
β86	Val	
β67	Ile	
β70	Asp	Pocket 4
β71	Glu	

US RA cohorts, demonstrated associations between SE frequencies and antibodies to cyclic citrullinated peptides (anti-CCP), as opposed to rheumatoid factor (RF). Specifically, when compared to healthy controls, the odds ratio for the association between one or two copies of the SE and anti-CCP positivity was 4.4 and 11.8, respectively. These findings point to SE associating not with RA per se, but with a clinical phenotype, in this case autoantibodies to modified proteins.[17] An additional pathogenetic link between HLA and citrullination is supported by the observation that peptides carrying citrulline (neutral), as opposed to arginine (positive charge), in the pocket four binding motif of the HLA-DRαβ binding grove (see Fig 52.1) convert a poorly binding peptide to a high affinity epitope that induces robust T- and B-cell responses *in vivo*. Indeed, citrullinated human fibrinogen, but not the non-derivatized protein, induces chronic inflammatory arthritis in HLA-DR4 transgenic mice but not their non-transgenic C57BL/6 littermates. The importance of citrulline as a molecular feature of human T-cell-specific autoantigenic determinants has yet to be established.

Genome wide association studies (GWAS) of large patient cohorts, stratified by autoantibody serology, have contributed significantly to our understanding of RA genetics.[12] Recent meta-analyses have identified more than 30 susceptibility loci that have been subsequently validated. Among the strongest associations outside HLA is *PTPN22*, initially identified in candidate gene association studies. *PTPN22* encodes the hematopoietic protein tyrosine phosphatase LYP. Combining all studies, the odds ratio is now higher than 1.8. Some, but not all, studies have revealed an association between the RA-associated variant *PTPN22* (R620W) with RF and anti-CCP positivity, which is also independent of SE. The data suggest that *PTPN22* may influence autoantibody production and be involved in the initiation of disease, as distinct from regulating severity. *PTPN22* mutations have also been described in type I diabetes, a subset of systemic lupus erythematosus patients, oligoarticular juvenile idiopathic arthritis, vitiligo, Addison's disease and autoimmune thyroid disease, but not multiple sclerosis or psoriasis, pointing to a more generic link with pathogenic autoantibodies in a range of syndromes.[12] Recently, the disease associated LYP 620W variant was shown to be a gain-of-function mutant, leading to hyporesponsiveness to TCR engagement through attenuated receptor proximal signaling, reduced IL-2 production and proliferative responses. Although the genetic data suggest that the impact of this mutation may be weak relative to MHC genes, this hyporesponsive phenotype could alter thymic selection, or mechanisms of peripheral tolerance that are critically dependent on TCR signaling.[18]

Scrutiny of other, non-MHC susceptibility loci, point to genes whose products are involved in proximal signaling pathways that regulate T-cell activation, differentiation, and persistence. Besides *HLA* and *PADI4*, which influence the molecular determinants of T-cell "input signals," these include *CD28*, *CTLA4*, and *CD2-CD58* (regulation of T-cell co-stimulation), *CD3Z*, *PTPN22*, *PRKCQ*, and *REL* (transducer modules of TCR signaling), *STAT4* and *TNFRSF14* (inducers of lineage specific cytokine gene expression and persistence of memory T cells), *REL*, *IL2-IL-21*, *IL2RA* and *IL2RB* (regulators of IL-2 gene expression and IL-2R signaling). Notable overlap with these and other allelic variants have been reported in other autoimmune diseases, indicating that susceptibility to RA is linked to fundamental perturbations of immune tolerance.

Synovial pathology

RA targets diarthrodial joints, structures characterized by hyaline cartilage lining opposing articulating surfaces and a cavity of viscous synovial fluid lined by synovial membrane lacking a basement membrane, but encased by a fibrous joint capsule. Normal synovial tissue comprises a lining layer, no more than a few cells in depth, of stromal fibroblast-like synoviocytes (FLS—also known as type B synoviocytes) and sublining macrophages (type A synoviocytes). The synovium serves to line non-cartilaginous surfaces, and although blood vessels are sparse, it functions to provide essential nutrients to avascular structures including cartilage, tendons and bursae.

Increased vascularity and cell migration

The range of pathology observed in patients with RA perhaps most convincingly underscores the heterogeneity of the disease (reviewed in Manzo et al.[19]). The earliest changes observed relate to increases in vascularity characterized by vascular congestion and thrombosis with obliteration of small vessels in association with perivascular inflammatory infiltrates. Hyperplasia of the synovial lining layer is a typical early finding. These changes are rather non-specific and certainly not diagnostic.

A key checkpoint defining the switch from acute to chronic persistent inflammation is the sustained activation of microvascular endothelium, phenotypic changes in the high endothelial venules (reminiscent of tissue injury) and the concomitant upregulation of adhesion molecules such as intercellular adhesion molecule (ICAM)-1 and vascular cell adhesion molecule (VCAM)-1. According to current thinking the expression of chemoattractants derived from synovial stromal cells heralds the rolling, adhesion and transmigration of mononuclear cells through endothelial barriers into the synovial membrane, and contributes to the progressive synovial hypertrophy and hyperplasia, sometimes with villous-like projections more typical of chronic, established inflammation. Intravital imaging of synovial joints of mice injected with arthritogenic antibodies derived from the serum of $K/B \times N$ mice indicates that enhanced vasopermeability at sites destined to become arthritic is a crucial early event, at least in antibody-induced disease. This process is dependent on mast cells and neutrophils, and the release of the vasoactive amines histamine and serotonin.[20]

Neovascularization further promotes influx of inflammatory cells. To what extent this is driven by the hypoxic environment is not entirely clear, but angiogenic growth factors such as vascular endothelial growth factor (VEGF) and hypoxia inducible factor (HIF) make important contributions. It has been proposed that influx of inflammatory lymphocytes and cells of monocytic lineage far outweighs the egress of cells from synovial tissue, possibly due to chemokine gradients. Once in the synovium egress may be promoted by specific mediators such as sphingosine-1-phosphate, which actively promotes cellular egress, or blocked through integrin/adhesion molecule interactions, e.g., between antigen-specific T cells and dendritic cells/APC, through TCR-dependent signals that abrogate chemokine responsiveness, or perhaps through highly selective and specific inactivation of chemokines by proteolysis, e.g., stromal derived factor (SDF)-1 cleavage by cell surface dipeptidyl peptidase CD26. The abundance of lymphatic vessels in inflamed synovium, as determined by expression of podoplanin and CD31, suggests that there exists active lymphangiogenesis that may promote efflux of cells and fluid from the synovium.[19] Interestingly, enhanced proliferation of lymphatic vessels and lymphatic drainage has been documented following TNF blockade. Lymphatic growth factors such as VEGF-C (which signal through VEGFR-3/Flt-4) have been implicated in promoting this joint protective effect.

Organization of lymphoid tertiary microstructures

Tissue microstructure dictates and facilitates immune responses in secondary lymphoid organs and mucosa-associated lymphoid tissues (MALT). These structures have evolved to coordinate responses to pathogens, and direct lymphocyte recirculation, and while their role in immune homeostasis is established, quite how they contribute to pathological states is less well understood. Thus, in established disease in mouse and, in which lymphadenopathy may be a characteristic feature, the inflamed synovium appears to be uniquely suited to supporting distinct patterns of cellular infiltrates—non-capsulated, as opposed to capsulated—inducible lymphoid structures, that could play a role in pathways of cell activation, differentiation and survival.[19,21] These include diffuse, rather disorganized, lymphocytic infiltrates, and comprise the most common form of synovitis, occurring in ~30% in prospective cohort studies; up to 70% has been described in late stage disease (at arthroscopy, joint replacement surgery). In 40–50% of patients there may exist more organized follicular structures (Fig. 51.2). Based on immunohistochemical analysis, approximately 25% of these follicular structures include organized germinal centers in which there are zones of proliferating B cells with affinity maturation, in addition to a distinct T-cell zone. In aggregates lacking germinal centers, follicular dendritic cells are also absent.

A fourth histological pattern has been described in a much smaller subset of patients characterized by granulomatous reactions. The cellular and molecular determinants of these structures include the homeostatic lymphoid chemokines CXCL13 and the CCR7 ligands CCL21 and CCL19, VCAM-1$^+$ICAM-1$^+$LTβR$^+$ mesenchymal organizer cells, and hematopoeitic derived CD3$^-$CD4$^+$IL-7R$^+$RANK$^+$ lymphoid inducer cells. Lymphoid tissue inducer cells produce LTβ, which is required for high endothelial venule differentiation, lymphoid chemokine expression amplification, and stromal architecture development. The mechanisms that sustain these lymphoid structures over time are not fully characterized but could involve persistence of antigen and augmented antigen presenting function through the differentiation of follicular dendritic cells, localized and autonomous expression of cytokines and growth factors,

chemokine gradients favoring cellular interactions, and dysregulation of leukocyte homing and/or egress. Documentation of class switch recombination and somatic mutation of immunoglobulin genes *in situ* is further evidence of active adaptive immunity within synovial lymphoid follicles, and suggests that supporting *in situ* production of pathogenic antibodies is of considerable pathobiological importance.

From a clinical standpoint, it has been suggested from cross-sectional studies that these distinct patterns not only reflect the heterogeneity of the disease, but also a spectrum of disease severity. More recent prospective studies, however, seem to indicate that the presence of lymphoid aggregates is a rather dynamic process and while associated with the degree of synovial tissue cellularity and vascularity, it is not diagnostic for RA, nor does it predict radiographic outcome such as joint erosions. This observation is not inconsistent with the idea that organized immuno-inflammatory responses can play a role in the tissue response – and in particular the process of repair. The dynamic nature of these lymphoid structures is further supported by their dissolution following therapy with rituximab (anti-CD20) and TNF inhibitors, in the latter case enhancing lymphatic flow.

Gene expression signatures

Gene array technology has now permitted analysis of synovial tissue at the whole genome level, and, like genetic, serological and histological analysis, provides further evidence of disease heterogeneity. This strategy makes the assumption that each disease phenotype should be represented in gene expression signatures of multiple genes. Remarkable variation in gene expression signatures has been observed, although initial analyses seem to suggest that these signatures can be divided broadly into two groups.[22] The first is characterized by upregulation of immune response and inflammatory genes; these tissues are enriched for MHC and immunoglobulin gene products. In some tissues this signature may resemble an anti-viral response consistent with prior infectious insult, and, more specifically, a STAT-1 dependent gene signature (promoting protective or pro-inflammatory effects).[22] This has also been observed in peripheral blood lymphocytes (PBL) from patients. The second group is more indicative of tissue remodelling, more reminiscent of that seen in osteoarthritis. Most interestingly, distinct fibroblast-like synoviocytes (FLS) genotypes and phenotypes match the type of RA tissue from which they derived. For example, FLS signatures from high intensity inflammatory tissue resemble that of TGFβ/Activin A induced expression profiles in myofibroblasts, while growth factors such as insulin-like growth factor 2 and insulin-like growth factor binding protein 5 characterize FLS from tissues with low intensity inflammation. These data support the notion of RA heterogeneity being reflected in FLS as a stable, if not transformed, trait. They would also be consistent with a model of T-cell-dependent RA that progresses with time to a relatively T-cell-independent process, characterized by autonomous, invasive and aggressive FLS.[23]

Gene expression signatures may have clinical utility. For example, a type I IFN signature in peripheral blood cells negatively predicts the response to B-cell-depleting therapy rituximab. TNF blockade induces changes in the expression of multiple genes involved in inflammation, angiogenesis, B- and T-cell activation, regardless of clinical response indicating that there are TNF-dependent and -independent pathways that contribute to disease expression in different patient subgroups. By analyzing 459 446 single nucleotide polymorphisms (SNPs) in 566 patients with RA, a recent GWAS identified class as opposed to drug-specific genetic predictors of anti-TNF response (based on

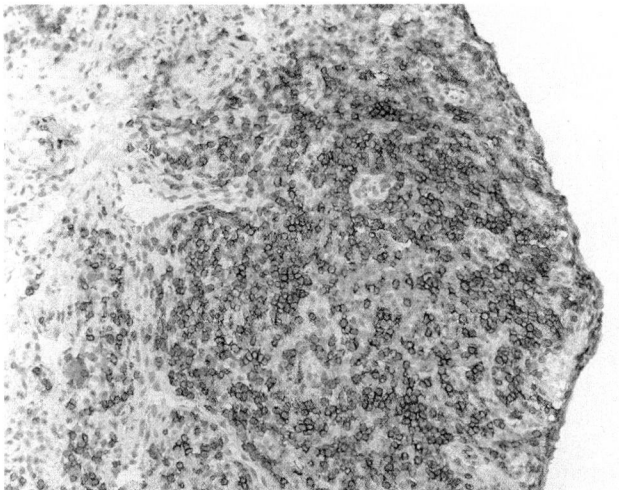

Fig. 51.2 Lymphoid follicular structures in inflamed RA synovial tissue.
A characteristic, hematoxylin and eosin stained tissue section from a patient with active RA showing a large follicular-like structure (original magnification × 100). This section is also stained with monoclonal antibodies to CD3e, followed by a 3-step immunoperoxidase staining protocol (CD3$^+$ T cells stained dark red).

disease activity score of 28 joints). Among seven variants, minor alleles of *PDZD2* and *EYA4* had the strongest associations with reduced and improved response, respectively. *EYA4* is of interest because it encodes a nuclear factor that regulates the expression of type I IFN (IFN-β) and the chemokine CXCL10.[24]

Immunobiology of RA

Initiation of the immune response

Synovial fibroblasts are exquisitely sensitive to inflammatory cytokines such as IL-1, TNF-α and IL-6.[23] Accumulating evidence indicates that FLS also express a range of Toll-like receptors (TLRs) that can respond to exogenous, pathogen-associated molecular patterns (PAMPs) or indeed a growing range of self-tissue proteins, some of which could be considered damage associated molecular patterns (DAMPS).[25] Endogenous ligands especially relevant to inflammatory arthritis include heat shock proteins, fibrinogen fragments, antibody-DNA complexes, high mobility group box (HMGB)-1 and hyaluronan oligosaccharides. Recent data suggest that synovial FLS, as well as synovial macrophages, express TLR2 *in situ*. Expression is upregulated following stimulation with IL-1 and the TLR2 ligand peptidoglycan. TLR2 engagement induces cytokines such as IL-6, matrix metalloproteinases, adhesion molecules and an array of chemokines including granulocyte chemotactic protein (GCP)-2, RANTES, monocyte chemoattractant protein (MCP)-2, IL-8, growth-related oncogene-2, and to a lesser extent, macrophage-inflammatory protein 1α, MCP-1, EXODUS, and CXCL-16. Data suggest that TLR3, TLR4, TLR7, and TLR9 are also expressed at mRNA and possibly protein level,[25] and may augment inflammatory cytokine expression by dendritic cells from patients with RA.

Dendritic cells are likely to be important antigen presenting cells in RA. Indeed, the proinflammatory environment would certainly favor DC maturation in regional lymph nodes as well as inflamed tissue.[26] Thus, in peripheral blood, dendritic cell precursors express either an immature CD33^{dim}CD14-^{dim}CD16$^-$ phenotype or a more mature HLA-DR/DQ^{bright} CD11c$^+$CD33^{bright}CD14^{dim} surface phenotype typical of myeloid DC (mDC); neither population expresses co-stimulatory molecules. In contrast, synovial fluid and tissue mDC subsets resemble mature peripheral blood cells but in addition a subset expresses high levels of CD86 and can support allogeneic mixed leukocyte reactions. More recent data indicate that they may differentiate further *in situ* as suggested by nuclear translocation of RelB in DC localized within perivascular infiltrates, consistent with prior cytokine receptor or TLR engagement *in vivo*. Perivascular RA synovium also contains populations of HLA-DR$^+$CD11c$^-$CD123$^+$ plasmacytoid DC (pDC); in contrast to the myeloid DC subset, these are RelB$^-$ and comprise ~30% of all synovial DC. A subset of pDC express BDCA2, capable of producing IFNα *in situ*. Unlike their PB counterparts, synovial pDC efficiently activate allogeneic T cells to proliferate as well as to produce IFN-γ, TNF-α, and IL-10.

While the common myeloid precursor cell is the precursor for all myeloid cells, including DC and tissue macrophages, the precise role of monocytes, namely CD14$^+$CD16$^-$, CD14$^+$CD16$^+$, and the more recently described CD14^{dim}CD16$^+$ subset, in synovial inflammation is uncertain. They are good candidates as persistence factors through their capacity to activate and polarize T-cell subsets, to respond to the environment through TLR expression and their production of a wide range of inflammatory mediators including IL-1, TNF, IL-6, IL-8, CCL2, NO, and type I IFN. In contrast a more recently described CD14^{dim}CD16$^+$ subset may

function to sense damage, scavenge cell debris and higher order molecular complexes and to promote angiogenesis and tissue repair. More work is needed to establish the contribution of these distinct functional subsets to the chronic inflammatory process. Nonetheless, multiple cellular and molecular determinants exist in RA synovium that could serve to both initiate and to perpetuate the immune inflammatory response.

This initial wave of inflammation has two major consequences. First, inflammatory cytokines will promote the activation of vascular endothelium, changes that occur very early in disease (see above and Fig. 51.3). Under the influence of locally generated cytokines and chemokines synovial post-capillary venules undergo morphological changes to an extent that they resemble high endothelial venules (HEV) similar to those observed in secondary lymphoid organs. The second major consequence is the migration of inflammatory leukocytes including polymorphonuclear leukocytes and immature or undifferentiated monocytes, orchestrated by chemokines produced by resident stromal as well as infiltrating cells (Fig. 51.3). CXC, CC, C, and CX$_3$C chemokines all play a role, exerting chemotactic activity towards neutrophils, lymphocytes, and monocytes, but also influencing the topology of inflammatory infiltrates, as discussed above. They are invariably early activation genes (e.g., type I IFN response genes), in response to inflammatory stimuli. Besides homeostatic chemokines described above, the key players include IL-8/CXCL8, RANTES/CCL5, MIP-1α/CCL3, SDF-1/CXCL12, IP-10/CXCL10, and MCP-1/CCL2.[27] Upregulation on endothelium of cell surface adhesion molecules, including ICAM-1, VCAM-1, and E-selectin permits the rolling and adhesion of leukocytes, as they migrate. In synovial joints, resident stromal cells and infiltrating macrophages are a dominant source of such factors. Crucially, the expression of cognate chemokine receptors such as CCR4, CCR5, CCR6, CXCR3, and CX3CR1 on inflammatory cell subsets will provide selectivity of cellular recruitment.[27] Within the T-cell compartment, there exist distinct profiles of chemokine receptor expression, patterns evolved perhaps to facilitate eradication of pathogens. For example, Th1 cells preferentially express CCR5, Th2 express CCR3, Th17 cells express CCR6 and CCR4, and TFH express CXCR5. These events characterize the acute phase of an innate immune response, a key checkpoint that precedes the progression to subsequent events that herald the onset of the chronic inflammatory phase.

Autoantigens in RA

Although current models of adaptive immune responses would suggest that DC carry antigens derived from damaged or dying synovial tissue, the molecular nature of disease-associated antigens has, until recently, remained an enigma. Many RA-associated autoantigens have been described (Table 51.1 for examples), and for some there exist *in vivo* arthritis model correlates.[28] The best described are collagen II, proetoglycans, HCgp-39, glucose-6-phosphate isomerase, and, more recently, citrullinated fibrinogen. However, when used as recombinant native antigen, few have been found to elicit reproducible and/or robust PB or SF T- or B-cell responses in a significant proportion of patients, as opposed to healthy donors. There are several plausible explanations for this. The most obvious are that antigens that drive autoimmune arthritis are not the same in mouse and man, or that effector T-cell responses are more important very early and are blunted in established disease, or are just present at very low frequency. Another possibility is that the autoantigens used to test lymphocyte reactivity *in vitro* do not carry the post-translational modifications (i.e., the neo-epitopes) recognized by autoantibody or antigen receptor. Good examples

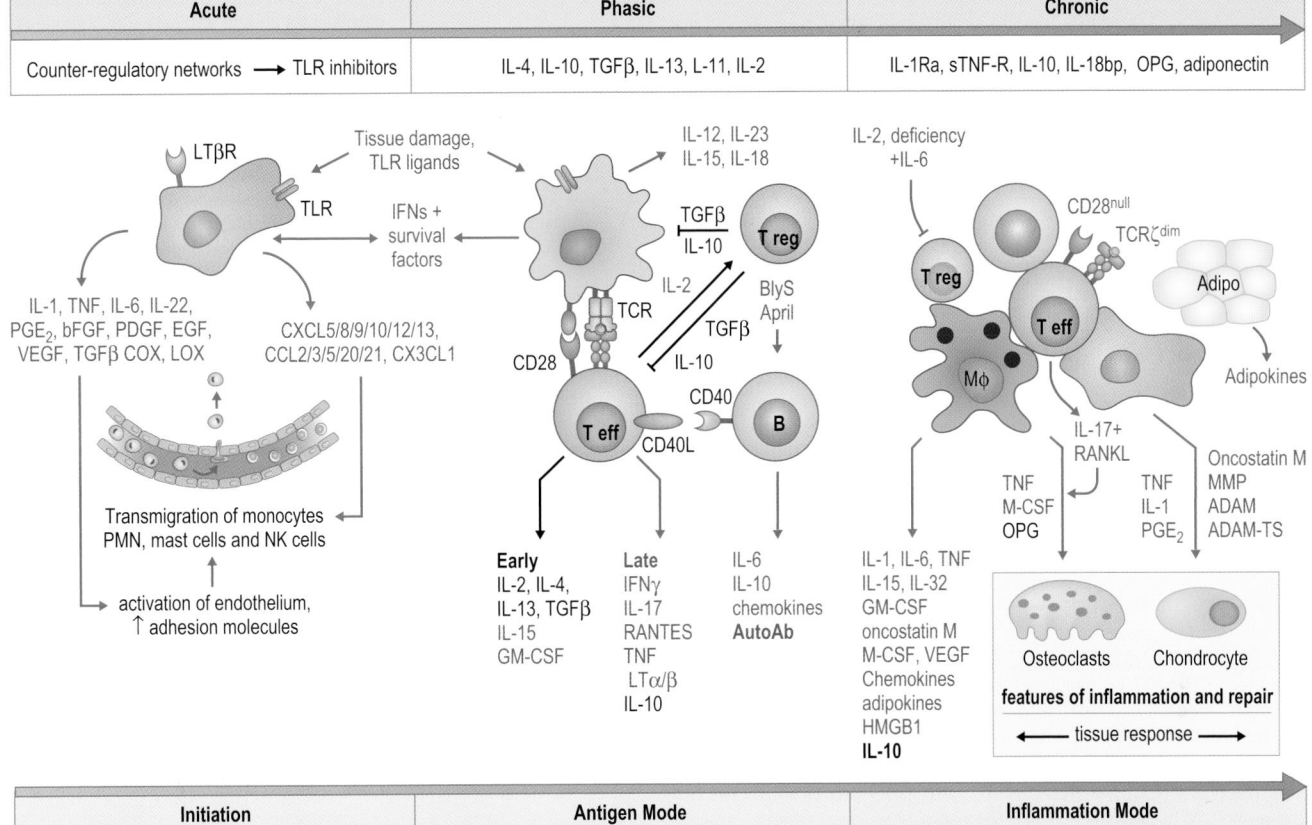

Acute	Phasic	Chronic
Counter-regulatory networks ⟶ TLR inhibitors	IL-4, IL-10, TGFβ, IL-13, L-11, IL-2	IL-1Ra, sTNF-R, IL-10, IL-18bp, OPG, adiponectin

| Initiation | Antigen Mode | Inflammation Mode |

Fig. 51.3 Cytokine networks in RA. The pathogenesis of RA can be thought of as a series of complex and closely related pathways temporally and spatially regulated. These include (1) an acute insult that may trigger the disease, characterized by stimulation of fibroblast-like synoviocytes (FLS) by inflammatory stimuli and the generation of cytokines and chemokines that promotes the migration and infiltration by cells of the innate immune system; (2) repeated episodes of antigen-specific adaptive immune responses (in lymph node, bone marrow, and *in situ*). Failure to resolve adaptive immunity is a key checkpoint that may lead to (3) a cytokine-driven chronic inflammatory phase where multiple cellular and molecular components sustain the response. Through multiple pathways acting on many cell types, this process leads to tissue injury. Pro-inflammatory pathways are shown in blue (text) and red (arrows), while anti-inflammatory, counter-regulatory pathways are shown in black (text and arrows). FLS, fibroblast-like synoviocytes; DC, dendritic cell; T_eff, effector T helper cell; TCR, T-cell antigen receptor; Treg, regulatory T cell; B, B cell; AutoAb, autoantibodies; MΦ, macrophage; Adipo, adipocyte.

Table 51.1 Autoantigens in RA

Established	T or B cell[a]	Molecular specificity	Assay
Immunoglobulin G	B	Human Fc IgG	Rheumatoid factor
Cyclic peptides	B	Citrullinated peptides	Anti-CCP
Fibrin	B	α and β chain epitopes	Research[b]
Fibrinogen	Both	Multiple epitopes	Research
Enolase	B	CEP-1 dominates	Research
Vimentin	B	Citrullinated vimentin	MCV assay
Collagen II	Both	Multiple epitopes	Research
HnRNPA2	Both	Multiple epitopes	Research
Aggrecan	Both	Multiple epitopes	Research
HCgp-39	Both	Multiple epitopes	Research
Glucose-6-phosphate isomerase	Both	Multiple epitopes	Research

[a]Denotes autoantigens defined experimentally to be recognized by T or B cells, or both.

[b]Assay is either not commercially available, or not in routine clinical use. Details of assays may be found in primary research communications.

are the carbohydrate moieties of collagen II epitopes that serve as key TCR contacts in collagen II immunity, or the citrullination of key arginine residues in triple helical CII or fibrinogen peptides that appear to be the immunodominant autoantibody epitopes. The lack of good reagents to detect antigen reactive T cells, such as class II MHC tetramers or pentamers, has also hindered progress.

Generation of neoepitopes by deimination

In 1998, van Venrooij and colleagues first reported that patients with RA carried antibodies that recognized deiminated peptides of fillagrin, the substrate that was found to be the antigen recognized in rat keratinized epithelium.[29] This substrate formed the basis of the anti-perinuclear factor (APF) assay. Using new generation anti-cyclic citrullinated peptide based assays, the presence of these antibodies, now collectively termed antibodies to citrullinated protein antigens (ACPA), have now been shown by many groups to be both sensitive (up to 80%) and highly specific (> 95%) for the diagnosis of RA.[29] Indeed, serum anti-CCP levels are stable with disease, they have been detected as early as 14 years prior to disease onset and have been shown to be predictors of radiographic progression. Citrullination is not specific for RA. Indeed, citrullination may be inflammation specific, since it has been documented in inflamed synovium derived from patients with reactive arthritis and psoriatic arthritis, as well as RA, but not OA. What appears specific for RA is the

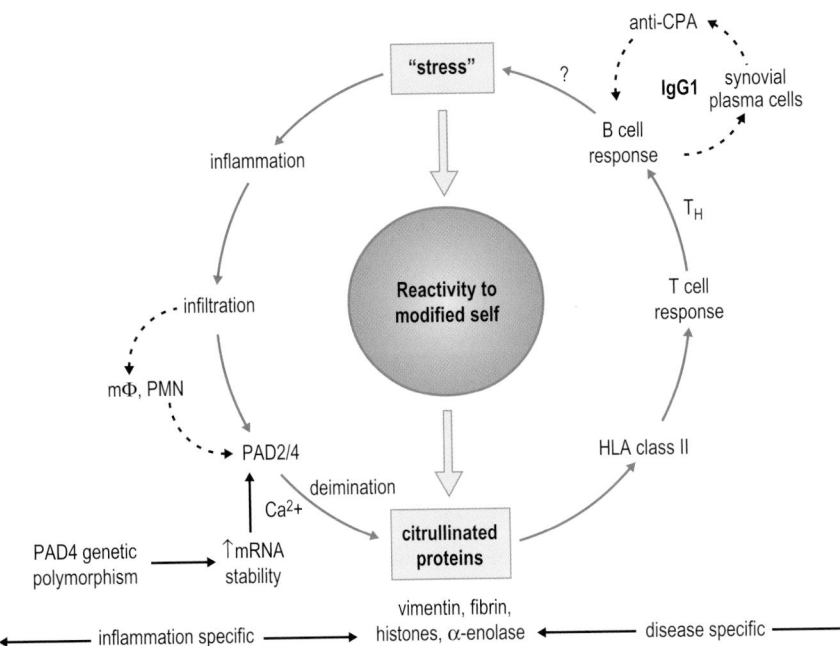

Fig. 51.4 The generation of autoantibodies to citrullinated protein antigens. The stressed and inflamed synovium is characterized by an influx of inflammatory cells including macrophages and neutrophils that express peptidyl-arginine deiminases (PAD). In the presence of sufficient $[Ca^{2+}]$, PAD deiminate target proteins including, among others, vimentin, fibrin, histones, and α-enolase. This is inflammation but not disease specific. The combination of environmental stimuli (including inflammation and tobacco smoke) and the inheritance of specific HLA-DRB1 alleles favor T- and B-cell immune responses to the host's derivatized neo-epitope peptide antigens. T_H, T helper effector cell; anti-CPA, autoantibodies to citrullinated protein antigens.

immune response to citrulline (Fig. 51.4). As outlined above, a link between ACPA and HLA-DRB1 alleles, specifically SE$^+$ alleles, has now been established.[17] Linkage analysis across chromosome 6 has documented a peak with LOD scores in excess of 10 for ACPA$^+$ patients but not for those that do not carry these antibodies. This relationship is independent of RF status since the SE allele frequencies in ACPA$^+$ patients are twice those of ACPA$^-$ patients, even those patients who are RF$^+$. Indeed, the risk of carrying SE in RF$^+$ACPA$^-$ patients is no different from the healthy control population. These data would be consistent with a model where T cells from patients with RA can recognize peptide autoantigens modified by citrullination if they carry SE$^+$ DRB1 alleles. Studies in HLA-DR4 transgenic mice suggest that the conversion of positively charged arginine at key residues in antigenic peptides from candidate autoantigens such as fibrinogen to neutral citrulline is permissive for peptide binding and the induction of antigen specific, arthritogenic immune responses *in vivo*.

Finally, citrullination is widespread in multiple tissues in response to appropriate provocations. Although the molecular basis for these triggers is poorly understood, recent data point to a link between smoking, an environmental exposure known to be linked with RA, citrullination and individuals carrying SE.[30] Thus, cells derived from bronchoalveolar lavage from smokers, but not from non-smokers, express citrulline. The association between the development of RA and smoking has now been linked to ACPA$^+$ patients whose relative risk increases to 20 if they smoke and carry two copies of the SE$^+$ DRB1 alleles, as compared to ACPA$^-$ patients where there appears to be a much weaker or no such relationship. A second example relates to the fact that *P. gingivalis*, a pathogen associated with severe periodontitis, expresses its own deiminating enzyme, and has the capacity to modify host proteins such as fibrinogen and α-enolase in inflamed gingival tissue. Molecular mimicry is suggested by the finding that anti-α-enolase autoantibodies from patients with RA cross react with *P. gingivalis* derived α-enolase. The link between autoantibodies to the immunodominant α-enolase epitope CEP1, smoking, SE$^+$DRB1 and disease associated *PTPN22* alleles remains the strongest defined to date. These data are the first to show a direct link between environmental exposure and disease specific immune responses governed by immune response genes.

ACPA are clinically significant because at the outset of disease they provide useful predictors of patients who are more likely to progress to develop severe erosive joint disease.

Lymphocyte biology

Flow cytometric analysis of dissociated synovial mononuclear cell cultures indicates that infiltrating T lymphocytes make up approximately 10–35% of cells in inflamed tissue. The ratio of CD4 to CD8 T cells seen in peripheral blood is skewed in favor of the CD4 subset. Much of the information of phenotype and function is derived from detailed analyses of synovial fluid, and, to a lesser extent, synovial tissue subsets. Similar enrichment of these subsets is commonly detected in PBL. The majority of synovial T cells express phenotypic markers of antigen experienced, terminally differentiated T cells with enhanced migratory capacity. Thus synovial T cells would typically carry cell surface markers such as HLA-DR$^+$, LFA-1$^+$, VLA-1$^+$, CD69$^+$, CD45RO$^+$, CD45RA$^-$, CD45RB^{dim}, CD29^{bright}, CD27^{neg}, and CD25^{neg}. Synovial B cells also express a typical memory/differentiated phenotype. Indeed, the analysis of the variable (V) regions of the Ig heavy and light chains confirm that an antigen specific activation and differentiation of B cells into plasma cells takes place in the chronically inflamed synovial tissue of patients with RA.

Analysis of synovial T cells reveals that expression of the TCR invariant chain subunits CD3ε and TCRζ is found at lower density than that found in corresponding peripheral blood T cells, evidence of prior antigen engagement. While synovial fluid T cells are also FasL$^+$, Bcl2$^-$, Bax^{bright}, favoring a pro-apoptotic state, it is thought that environmental cues transduced through common γ chain receptor signaling cytokines such as IL-2, IL-7, and IL-15, as well as type I interferons prevent apoptois of T cells *in situ*.[31] Synovial tissue derived lymphocytes may be different. Consistent with their state of terminal differentiation, synovial T cells comprise populations with a contracted oligoclonal repertoire, based on assessment of TCR gene rearrangements.[6] A subset of these cells are CD28^{null}, while at the same time expressing a range of NK cell surface receptors that are thought to contribute to effector function independently of cognate antigen. Nevertheless, to date there exists no common TCRVβ family that might suggest expansion of such clones by a common RA specific antigen. A subset of IFN-γ producing CD56^{bright}TCRζ^{neg} NK cells also appears to accumulate in RA synovial joints.

For over a decade it has been known that one of the dominant cytokines expressed in synovial T cells from patients with established disease is IFN-γ. Somewhat surprisingly, a significant proportion of IFN-γ^+ cells also express IL-10. Recent data support a model in which there exists, during differentiation, a transition from IFNγ^+ Th1 T cells through an IFN-γ^+IL-10$^+$ double-positive stage to a single-positive IL-10$^+$ stage. This last phase could represent part of the normal lifecycle of an effector T cell, where IL-10 expression promotes the resolution of the adaptive immune response, attenuating the function of dendritic cells. Interestingly data indicate that this Th1 lifecycle involving a switch from IFN-γ to IL-10 production may be defective in patients with active RA, providing an important mechanism for persistence of effector responses *in vivo*.[32]

Emerging evidence, supported by pre-clinical models, points to a role for IL-17 in the pathogenesis of inflammatory arthritis.[33] Immuno-histochemistry of RA synovium indicate that the dominant source are CD4 T cells, although $\gamma\delta$ T cells, NK cells, and mast cells also contribute. Flow cytometric analysis reveals that the frequency of IL-17$^+$ T cells is less than IFN-γ^+ T cells, and that a subset expresses both IL-17 and IFN-γ. The TNF$^+$IL-6$^+$IL-1$^+$-rich synovial environment is capable of supporting the differentiation of Th17 cells, while sustained IL-17 expression and stimulation of IL-17R expressing stromal cells, macrophages, chondrocytes, and osteoclast precursors is implicated in promoting local tissue responses, including induction of chemokines, matrix metalloproteinases, nitric oxide, cyclo-oxygenase, and promotion of osteoclastogenesis, key pathways that underpin pathways of cartilage destruction and bone erosion.

Molecular basis of persistence

Understanding the molecular basis of persistence is of major importance in diseases such as RA. It is now well established that enhanced expression of inflammatory cytokines is one of the hallmarks of chronic inflammatory diseases such as RA.[34] With few exceptions most cytokines are expressed in inflamed synovium at mRNA or protein levels. For example, unlike PBL from healthy donors, explants of synovial mononuclear cells constitutively express IL-1, IL-6, IL-8, GM-CSF, a vast array of chemokines as well as growth factors including FGF, VEGF and PDGF (Fig. 51.3). While anti-inflammatory or immunoregulatory cytokines, including IL-4, IL-10, IL-11, TGFβ as well as specific naturally occurring inhibitors of IL-1α/β (IL-1Ra) and TNFα (soluble TNF-R) may also be detected, functional bioassays suggest that the over-riding response is an inflammatory one. Indeed, levels of IL-1Ra and solubleTNF-R are significantly upregulated in synovial fluid compared to serum from patients with RA, and yet IL-1 and TNF bioactivity persists in spite of this, suggesting that attempts to suppress cytokine bioactivity are insufficient. The specific activity of subsets of cytokines, their networks and how they can contribute to RA is illustrated in see Fig. 51.3. In many cases, the pathogenic roles of cytokines have been established in rodent models, either by selectively blocking their function (e.g., with specific monoclonal antibodies or soluble receptor fusion proteins) or by gene-targeting approaches. Perhaps the best documented include the inflammatory arthritides documented in transgenic mice over-expressing human TNF-α in IL-6 signaling gp130 mutant mice and ZAP-70 mutant SKG mice.[35] Disruption of immunoregulatory or inhibitory cytokines, including IL-1Ra, IL-10, and TGF-β, each leads to severe auto-inflammatory syndromes targeting different organs depending on genotype.

A major challenge has been to identify the pathways that promote persistence of cytokine and chemokine expression *in vivo*. One possible mechanism is that of cell contact dependent stimulation of macrophages and fibroblasts by activated T cells (see Fig. 51.3).[36] Physical contact of activated but not resting T cells induces abundant TNF-α, IL-1β, IL-8, MCP-1, and MMP production by monocytes. This can be reproduced using T-cell plasma membrane preparations and prevented by interrupting cell contact. Interestingly, the effector response depends on the nature of the T-cell stimulus. Thus, Th2 T cells produce relatively more monocyte dependent IL-1Ra than IL-1β and higher ratios of TIMP compared to MMP. Contact between T cells and synovial fibroblasts has also been shown to induce IL-6, MMPs and PGE$_2$, each of which can contribute to distinct aspects of downstream effector pathways.

Immune regulation

Investigation of regulatory cell subsets and their anti-inflammatory properties has perhaps more firmly established the concept that failure of the host's intrinsic mechanisms of immune regulation can underpin autoimmune diseases. Experiments in gene deficient mice (e.g., Foxp3, IL-2, IL-2R, IL-2R signaling, STAT5, IL-10, TGF-β) lend support to this concept. In RA the data remain less clear.[37] For example, there is *in vitro* evidence for a relative deficiency of constitutive IL-10 expression in synovial cell cultures, and yet clinical trials of IL-10 were rather disappointing; TGF-β is yet to be tested. These results may reflect the complex role of these cytokines in disease pathogenesis. The identification of defective numbers and/or function of CD4$^+$CD25^{bright} regulatory T cells (Tregs) has been suggested by several investigators, but reports are conflicting.[37] Some studies have shown clear reduction in the numbers of peripheral blood Tregs in patients with RA, while others have shown no difference; interestingly Tregs appear deficient in cell number in subsets of children with JIA whose disease tends to progress. In synovial joints, the data are more consistent, with many reports showing substantial increases in Treg numbers in synovial tissue and fluid compared to paired PB. However, some studies have reported normal function at a cellular level, while others have shown depressed regulatory function. An alternative explanation, yet to be proven, is that synovial effector T cells are refractory to regulatory pathways.

Reports of Treg phenotype and function in patients receiving anti-TNF therapy have provided some insight into the relationship between inflammation and defective regulatory function. Ehrenstein and colleagues demonstrated that while PB Tregs from patients with active RA could suppress the proliferation of CD4$^+$CD25$^-$ effector T cells, they failed to suppress IFNγ and TNFα production.[37] Treatment with infliximab reversed this defect, but also conferred the capacity of CD4$^+$CD25$^-$ precursors to become regulatory cell subsets. A second study demonstrated that TNF at high doses suppresses the expression of Foxp3, a helix-loop-helix transcription factor family member whose deficiency causes Scurfy disease and IPEX in mice and man, respectively, and is expressed relatively selectively in Tregs (more specific for mouse than human Tregs). In this study, infliximab treatment restored FOXP3 expression in PB T cells. The data provide a crucial link between inflammation and failure of immune regulation, and may go some way to explain the immunomodulatory properties and sustained clinical benefit of anti-TNF not only in RA but in a wide range of other chronic inflammatory diseases.

Impact of the immune response on cartilage and bone

For many years it was considered that the terminal effector phase of chronic inflammation that led to cartilage destruction and bone resorption was driven almost exclusively by inflammatory cytokines and proteinases. IL-1, MMPs (MMP1, 3, 8, 13) and aggrecanases (ADAMTS 4 and 5) were, and remain, major culprits. Attempts to establish more directly a link between adaptive immunity and destruction of target tissue failed, not least because of the lack of a direct physical link between lymphocytes, chondrocytes and bone. A breakthrough came in the late 1990s with the identification of the TNF/TNFR family member receptor for activation of NF-κB ligand (RANKL)/TRANCE/ODF and its counter receptor RANK, and the dissection of the molecular and cellular components required for osteoclast differentiation from monocyte precursors.[38] According to contemporary paradigms, RANKL is necessary and sufficient for osteoclast differentiation. TNF, M-CSF, IL-1, and IL-17 contribute, while RANKL independent pathways may also play a role. RANKL is expressed on synovial fibroblasts and osteoblasts but also on activated T cells, its counter receptor being expressed on myeloid lineage cells including monocytes, osteoclast precursors and dendritic cells. Its expression is regulated by inflammatory mediators including TNF and PGE$_2$. RANKL is shed, probably through the action of several membrane associated proteases including MT1-MMP (MMP14). Gene targeting of RANKL or RANK in mice leads to inhibition of osteoclastogenesis and a profound osteoporotic bone phenotype. Deletion of OPG, the naturally occurring decoy soluble receptor for RANK, leads to unbridled osteoclast differentiation and bone resorption, and substantially reduced bone mass. A good example of the link between adaptive immunity and bone resorption comes from CTLA4$^{-/-}$ mice, characterized by sustained chronic T-cell activation.[39] T cells from these mice over express RANKL. Importantly, the bone but not the inflammatory phenotype is rescued by inhibition of RANK/RANKL signaling. In RA several studies have demonstrated perturbations of serum RANKL/OPG ratios, a parameter currently under investigation as a biomarker for bone homeostasis. Recent clinical experience with denosumab, a fully humanized monoclonal antibody that binds to RANKL, demonstrates increased bone mineral density and reduced bone turnover in patients with RA.

Distinct from enhanced bone resorption, bone formation is impaired in RA, although until recently the pathways involved were rather obscure. The inflammatory process itself and its effects on osteoblast maturation and function has been directly implicated, since bone formation at surfaces adjacent to bone marrow, as opposed to inflamed synovium, are relatively well preserved.[40] Evidence now points to the canonical Wingless (*Wnt*) signaling pathway as being an essential control point in osteoblast function, based on the observation that in animal models of RA antibodies to dickkopf homologue 1 (DKK1), a secreted antagonist of *Wnt* blocking signals at the level of its cognate receptor *Frizzled*, promote bone formation and inhibit bone resorption indirectly by increasing production of OPG (reviewed in Walsh and Gravallese).[40] This indicates that *Wnt* signals negatively regulate osteoclastogenesis. Oxidative stress and hypoxia within the synovial compartment may contribute to attenuation of osteoblast promoting *Wnt* signals. Together these data support the view that bone and joint integrity are regulated by a delicate balance of catabolic and anabolic immune and inflammatory mediators influencing the maturation and function of osteoblasts (Wnt:DKK1) and osteoclasts (RANKL:OPG). How these pathways function to promote bone integrity in health remains a topic of great interest.

Disease onset

RA is a heterogeneous disease that does not conform to a single clinical entity.[2] While 10% of patients may have an acute severe onset and 20% a more subacute onset, the onset of signs and symptoms may be insidious in up to 70% of patients. A more episodic or palindromic onset has also been described. A common presentation, more likely during the winter months, will be that of a female in her fifth to sixth decade of life who complains of diffuse symmetrical joint pain, swelling and stiffness of peripheral joints. Patients may complain that they can no longer make a fist, especially in the early morning. The targeting of afflicted synovial joints may be symmetrical in most but not all cases, typically affecting small joints of the hands and feet, as well as wrists. Less frequent are those presenting with slow onset monoarticular disease. Patients not fulfilling the diagnostic classification criteria for RA (see below) may, at this point, be ascribed the more appropriate diagnostic label of undifferentiated arthritis, since in a proportion of cases signs and symptoms may resolve spontaneously. At one year approximately 30% will progress to develop the syndrome we call RA. Systemic disease is much less common in current clinical practice, in part through application of earlier, more intensive treatment regimens (see below). Nonetheless, the systemic nature of the disease may be manifest through a wide array of systemic, extra-articular clinical features that may occur in patients with disease at the more severe end of the spectrum (Table 51.2).

Table 51.2 Systemic and extra-articular features of RA

General	Neurological
Fever, sweats	Myelopathy
Lymphadenopathy	Entrapment neuropathy
Weight loss	Peripheral neuropathy
Fatigue, weakness	Mononeuritis multiplex

Dermatological	Haematological
Palmar erythema	Anemia
Subcutaneous nodules	Thrombocytosis
Vasculitis	Lymphocytosis or lymphopenia
Ulceration, neutrophilic dermatoses	FELTY'S syndrome
	Large granular lymphocytes
	Lymphoproliferative disease

Ophthalmic	Renal
Episcleritis	Interstitial nephritis
Scleritis	Renal tubular acidosis
Choroid and retinal nodules	Amyloidosis
Keratoconjunctivitis sicca	

Pulmonary	Gastrointestinal
Pleuritis	Xerostomia
Nodules	Transaminitis
Interstitial pneumonitis	NSAID enteropathy
Bronchiolitis obliterans	
Arteritis	
Pulmonary hypertension	

Cardiac	Musculoskeletal
Pericarditis	Myositis, muscle weakness
Myocarditis	Steroid myopathy
Coronary vasculitis	Osteoporosis
Atheromatous disease	
Valvular nodulosis	

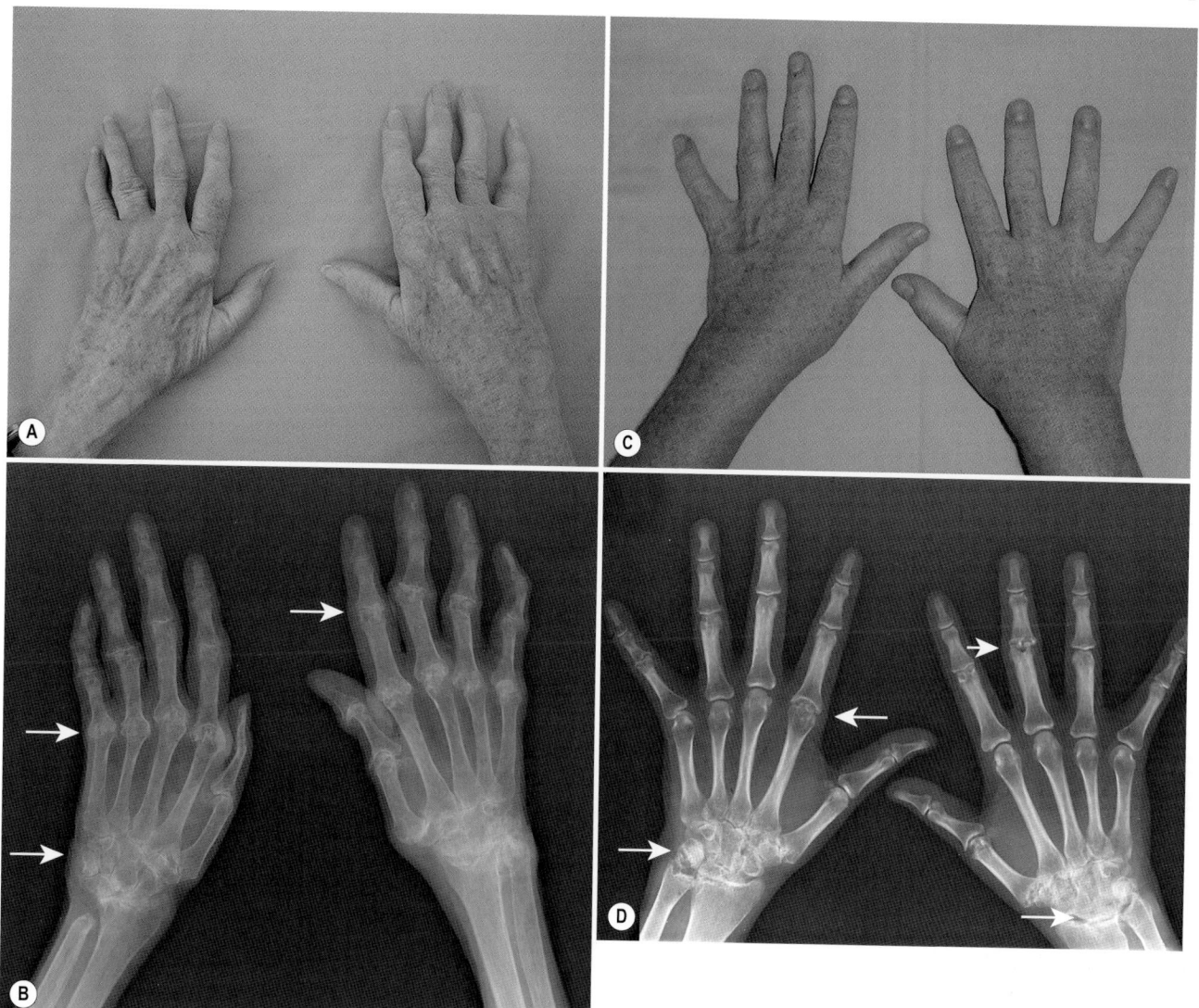

Fig. 51.5 Photomicrographs and radiographs of the rheumatoid hand. A comparison of chronic, severe, and erosive RA, refractory to treatment, showing joint swelling and classical deformities (A and B) with that of erosive disease whose progression has been attenuated by combination and biological therapy (C and D). White arrows indicate major areas of bone and cartilage destruction.
Reproduced with kind permission from the patients.

A spectrum of disease severity may also be evident from hand radiographs; examples are shown in Fig. 51.5.

Diagnosis

Classification criteria

The American College of Rheumatology criteria for the classification of RA are a set of clinical and laboratory parameters, serving as a guide for the diagnosis of RA, which were established largely for epidemiological purposes. They are relatively straightforward and easy to apply, especially to patients with established disease. However, failure of a patient with early signs and symptoms of an inflammatory arthropathy to fulfil them does not mean that she or he does not have RA. The 1987 criteria were simplified further by removing the "probable," "definite," and "classic" subclassifications.[41] These criteria returned a sensitivity for RA of 91–94% and a specificity of 89% in the clinical setting. New criteria, established by a steering group comprising members of the American College of Rheumatology (ACR) and the

European League Against Rheumatism (EULAR), and published in 2010,[42] are based on a weighted score around four domains, including extent of joint involvement (scoring 0–5 points), serology (0–3) that includes RF or ACPA and is weighted according to antibody levels, duration of synovitis (0–1), and acute phase reactants (0–1), where a score of 6 or above is indicative of an early disease state requiring initiation of disease-modifying antirheumatic drugs, such as methotrexate (Table 51.3).[42]

Laboratory findings

Until the late 1990s, IgM rheumatoid factors, autoantibodies that recognize the Fc subunit of IgG, remained one of the few parameters of value in the clinical setting, forming the basis of the seropositive versus seronegative RA stratification, and identifying those patients more likely to progress to erosive disease with or without extra-articular features. Nevertheless, RF can be detected in up to 5% of the healthy population and between 10–20% of the elderly population (> 65 years of age), and is found in a range of rheumatic conditions including Sjögren's syndrome, SLE, cryoglobulinemia, as well as in acute infectious

Table 51.3 2010 ACR/EULAR classification criteria for RA

Domain	Score
Joint involvement (0–5)	
1 medium to large joint	0
2–10 medium to large joints	1
1–3 small joints	2
4–10 small joints	3
> 10 joints (with at least one small joint)	5
Serology (0–3)	
Neither RF or ACPA positive ($\leq$ ULN)	0
At least one test, low positive titer ($> 1 \leq 3 \times$ ULN)	2
At least one test, high positive titer ($> 3 \times$ ULN)	3
Duration of synovitis (0–1)	
< 6 weeks	0
$\geq$ 6 weeks	1
Acute phase reactants (0–1)	
Neither ESR or CRP abnormal	0
Abnormal ESR or CRP	1
TOTAL ($\geq$ 6 indicates *definite* RA):	_____

RF, rheumatoid factor; ACPA, antibodies to citrullinated protein antigens; ULN, upper limit of normal; ESR, erythrocyte sedimentation rate; CRP, C-reactive protein.

Table 51.4 Biomarkers in RA and clinical association

Biomarker	Clinical association
Autoantibodies	
IgM RF	May antedate disease; associated with more severe +/− extra-articular disease; predictor of radiographic progression
IgA RF	Extra-articular disease; risk factor for disease in pre-clinical phase
ACPA*	May antedate disease onset for 10+ years;
(Anti-cit vimentin,	HLA-DRB1 (SE$^+$) status; smoking
Anti-cit αenolase,	Predictor of radiographic progression
Anti-cit fibrin)	Felty's syndrome, vasculitis
Acute phase response	
ESR and CRP	Active disease; time integrated levels associated with radiographic progression
IL-6, SAA	Active disease
Synovial vascularity	
VEGF	Radiographic progression
Cartilage metabolism	
MMP1 and 3	Radiographic damage
COMP	High levels in early RA associated with more severe disease in large and small joints
Aggrecan cleavage fragments	Slow onset destructive disease in small and large joints
C-terminal/helical	Urinary levels associated with radiographic progression
Cross-linked	
CII peptides	
Bone metabolism	
Pyridinoline cross-links	Disease activity
Carboxy-terminal	Predictor of joint damage in early RA
CI telopeptides	

RF, rheumatoid factor; ACPA, antibodies to citrullinated protein antigens; *previously known as APF, anti-perinuclear factor, and AKA, anti-keratin antibodies; VEGF, vascular endothelial growth factor; MMP, matrix metalloproteinase; COMP, cartilage oligomeric protein; CI/II, collagen type I/II.

and neoplastic disease entities, influencing its diagnostic utility. In general RF is not of value for monitoring responses to therapy.

The discovery of ACPA has had a major impact on diagnostic practice as the assays have become more widely available, not least because they are found very early in disease (Table 51.4).[30] They also have prognostic value in terms of radiographic progression, and titers may alter with therapy. The new generation anti-CCP kits have demonstrated diagnostic sensitivity of 80% and specificity of 98%. It is likely that as the range of RA-associated autoantigens expands, and as the repertoire of deiminated target autoantigens is defined, multiplex assay of serum autoantibodies will play an increasingly important role in the diagnosis and prognosis of subsets of inflammatory arthritides.

Insights into the pre-clinical phase of disease

The identification of a pre-clinical phase of RA, through the detection in serum of autoantibodies up to 14 years prior to disease onset, has sparked considerable interest in characterizing the RA prodrome in more detail. Work has focused around evaluation of acute phase proteins, which appear to rise 1–2 years before onset of clinical disease, whole blood gene expression analysis, which shows similarities to patients with established disease (including type I interferon-inducible gene signatures in a subset) and imaging by MRI and ultrasonographic modalities with variable results. To date, the strongest predictors of progression from this early pre-clinical phase are best characterized in those at risk subjects by the presence of high titer ACPA and RF autoantibodies, joint pains (arthralgia) without clinically detectable

● CLINICAL PEARLS

Predictors of poor outcome in RA

- Chronic, unremitting disease onset, especially at advanced age
- High disease activity scores at baseline
- Female gender
- Poor functional status determined by validated functional disability indices such as the Stanford Health Assessment Questionnaire (HAQ) and the Arthritis Impact Measurement Scale (AIMS)
- Low socioeconomic status
- Systemic and extra-articular features
- Co-morbidity, e.g., infection, cardiovascular disease, renal impairment
- Early erosive disease (in first 6–12 months; may be associated with ACPA autoantibodies)
- Persistent acute phase response (e.g., time integrated CRP levels)
- Autoantibodies (RF and ACPA) and HLA-DRB1 status (SE$^+$)
- Significant delay in early use of DMARD and corticosteroids

ACPA, antibodies to citrullinated protein antigens; CRP, C-reactive protein; RF, rheumatoid factor; SE, shared epitope; DMARD, disease modifying anti-rheumatic drugs.

Pre-RA

- Targeting those individuals at risk of developing RA with preventative strategies provides the best chance of achieving cure.
- In-depth molecular and cellular studies for characterizing the pre-clinical phase of disease will be critical to the success of this endeavor.
- Models for progression to RA have identified the following phases:
    - (I) Genetic risk
    - (II) Genetic risk with autommunity (e.g., ACPA, RF)
    - (III) Genetic risk with autoimmunity and arthralgia (but absence of clinically apparent synovitis)
    - (IV) Undifferentiated arthritis (clinically apparent synovitis, not fulfilling RA classification criteria)
    - (V) Early RA (fulfilling disease criteria; need for DMARDs)
- Stratification of risk, including genetic, serological, and demographic factors, will permit the identification of subjects most suitable for intervention studies.
- Studying the impact of lifestyle modifications, e.g., diet, stopping smoking, would be of great interest.
- Success with pharmacological intervention will depend on identification of those at highest risk and the acceptability to patients of therapy during the pre-clinical phase of disease.
- Re-establishing immune homeostasis and/or induction of immune tolerance may provide the best chance of achieving cure in subjects during the pre-clinical phase of disease.
- Regardless of the approach, success will depend on establishing robust assays for immune signatures (e.g., immune phenotyping by flow cytometry, extended autoantibody serotyping, multiplex assays for detection of inflammatory mediators in serum, whole blood transcriptomic profiles) that reflect a healthy immune system

Treatment paradigms in RA

- Education and counseling through early involvement of multidisciplinary team, including specialist nurse; appropriate balance of rest and exercise during disease flares
- Adequate nutrition (especially important with severe, active disease)
- Comprehensive assessment of disease activity especially during early phase of disease to achieve disease control
- Complete suppression of inflammation early in disease, with tight control through regular and frequent re-assessments focused around disease activity scores
- Yearly imaging assessments, e.g., X-rays or ultrasound examination of hands and feet to monitor disease progression
- Early use of DMARD/SAARDs
- Early use of corticosteroids (e.g., low doses ∼7.5 mg/day), including use of intra-articular joint injections to suppress inflammation, and use of step-up combination therapy in severe disease
- Appropriate use of biologics, e.g., early use of anti-TNF in severe disease
- Early relief of pain with judicious use of NSAID or COX2 inhibitors according to safety/risk profile
- Monitoring for drug toxicity
- Effective contraception, where appropriate
- Bone protection
- Monitoring for risk factors of cardiovascular disease
- Prevention of infection through vaccination (preferably before instituting immunosuppressive agents)

NSAID, non-steroidal anti-inflammatory drugs; COX, cyclo-oxygenase; DMARD, disease modifying anti-rheumatic drugs; SAARD, slow acting anti- rheumatic drugs.

synovitis. Genetic markers, such as HLA-DRB1 shared epitope, have not contributed further to risk estimates, although this may be due to the small size of the cohorts under observation, and the enrichment of ACPA$^+$ subjects in these studies. Progression rates for ACPA$^+$ arthralgia patients with subclinical synovitis detected by ultrasound examination are of the order of 20% over a median of 28 months.[43] This rate of progression is considered to be sufficient to justify secondary prevention intervention studies.[44]

Treatment

Disease modifying anti-rheumatic drugs

Over the last two decades there has been a dramatic paradigm shift in the therapy of RA from control of symptoms to the control of the disease process. This shift has come about through a growing appreciation of the relationship between joint inflammation and joint destruction, and the development of imaging technology that has documented evidence of erosive changes within the first 6–12 months of disease. The impact of this paradigm shift in therapeutic terms is striking. Traditional "go-low, go-slow" regimens of the 1970s and 1980s included the initiation of non-steroidal anti-inflammatory drugs (NSAIDs), followed by implementation of disease modifying anti-rheumatic drugs only after destructive disease became evident. Depending on the clinical response, sequential monotherapy was the norm. While this strategy may still be appropriate for patients with mild disease, current practice now dictates aggressive combination therapy (two or more conventional DMARDs) from the outset for patients with poor prognostic factors, with preference for the faster acting DMARDs such as methotrexate, leflunomide and sulfasalazine (onset 3–6 weeks) over slower acting agents, hydroxychloroquine, gold and D-penicillamine (onset 3–6 months), but with the addition of low dose prednisolone (< 10 mg/day).

The rationale for combination therapy is far from clear, and is currently the objective of a large number of clinical trials, but could relate to the targeting of distinct pathogenic pathways by different agents, a strategy favored by oncologists for decades. Corticosteroids have a major place in clinical practice when administered as a single intramuscular injection either as therapy for disease flares, as bridging therapy until DMARDs take effect, or when administered as an intra-articular injection for treating isolated joint synovitis. Some regimens favor high initial dose step-down corticosteroid protocols. Regardless of the route of administration, evidence points to the value of corticosteroid usage early in the disease process. Alternative DMARDs such as cyclosporine, azathioprine and leflunomide are valuable adjuncts, but used less often as first line therapy in some countries. Regardless of the specific agent, meta-analyses have demonstrated better response and retention rates when multiple DMARDs are used early. Adverse events appear to be more frequent with combination therapy. More recent data suggest that the specific choice of therapy may be less important than the strategy. For example, the TICORA and BeST studies both indicate that intensive treatment when combined with intensive control most convincingly influences outcome measures including clinical response, retention, functional status and radiographic progression.[45,46]

The immunobiology of DMARD therapy

The traditional paradigm of antigen driven lymphocyte effector responses in RA promoted the application of a range of immunosuppressive drugs for treating RA. These contrast with more anti-inflammatory DMARDs such as sulfasalazine (a scavenger of reactive oxygen intermediates with effects on prostanoid synthesis), gold (an inhibitor of AP-1 and NF-κB transcription factor DNA binding and/or transcriptional activity), D-penicillamine (a modulator of sulfhydryl groups with impacts on surface receptor function, intracellular signaling and transcription factor binding), anti-malarials (which perturb lysosome acidification and intracellular trafficking) and low dose corticosteroids (with anti-inflammatory actions related to transactivation and transrepression of inflammatory gene expression as well as effects on inflammatory gene mRNA stability). The best characterized immunosuppressive agents include methotrexate (a dihydrofolate reductase inhibitor that targets T cells and the production of inflammatory cytokines as well as IL-2), azathioprine (the active metabolite of which, 6-mercaptopurine, suppresses lymphocyte proliferative and cytokine responses as well as immunoglobulin synthesis), cyclosporine (an inhibitor of the phosphatase calcineurin and NFAT transcriptional activity), and leflunomide (an inhibitor of dihydro-orotate dehydrogenase a rate limiting step in *de novo* pyrimidine synthesis that inhibits lymphocyte proliferative responses, which may favor Th2 differentiation). Somewhat paradoxically, most though not all of these DMARDs can restore cell mediated immune responses under circumstances where there is robust suppression of inflammation. On the other hand, significant changes in autoantibody titers, especially rheumatoid factor, are less frequently observed.

The immunobiology of biological therapy

Anti-cytokine therapy

The introduction of targeted therapy to the clinic using biological agents (e.g., chimeric or fully humanized antibodies to ligands or receptors, soluble receptor fusion proteins, or recombinant receptor antagonists) has transformed the treatment of RA. The prototype is TNF-α blockade.[47] The rationale for inhibiting TNF-α bioactivity is based upon its pleiotropic effects on cell activation, cellular adhesion and migration, induction of cytokine and inflammatory gene mRNA and protein, and the regulation of cartilage catabolic factors such as IL-1 and matrix metalloproteinases (Fig. 51.3). TNFα and other inflammatory cytokines such as IL-1, IL-6, IL-15, and IL-17 are expressed constitutively in inflamed synovial tissue at mRNA and protein level. In many cases the expression of their high affinity cognate receptors is upregulated and the functional activity of the corresponding naturally occurring inhibitors (e.g., soluble TNF-R or IL-1Ra) is reduced (although levels of protein may be increased, reflecting an attempt at restoring homeostasis). As proof of principle, inhibition of cytokine activity, including TNF-α, IL-1, IL-6, IL-15, and IL-17

have all been shown to have benefit in animal models of arthritis. Further, mice overexpressing human TNF-α as a transgene develop a spontaneous inflammatory destructive arthritis with 100% penetrance.[28]

Chimeric anti-TNF monoclonal antibodies (infliximab) were first used to treat RA in open label clinical trials in 1992.[47] Humanized antibodies (adalimumab) and the soluble p75 TNF-R IgG fusion protein (etanercept) were tested subsequently with comparable therapeutic effects; golimumab and a construct comprising a PEGylated anti-TNF antibody Fab fragment (certolizumab) are also licensed for use in patients with RA. TNFα blockade leads to dramatic and rapid reductions in symptoms (pain, stiffness and fatigue) and signs (joint pain and swelling) of arthritis in a dose dependent fashion, and in a significant proportion of patients (∼60–70%) who have failed conventional DMARDs.[47] These biological agents can be used repeatedly and when used in combination with methotrexate, are superior to either drug alone. The mechanism is not clear but may be related to reductions in immunogenicity of the therapeutic antibody (i.e., the anti-chimeric antibody response), or perhaps the effects of combining anti-cytokine and anti-T-cell agents. Radiographic progression may be attenuated for more than 3 years, even in subsets of patients with poor clinical responses, and in some patients radiographic scores improve suggesting that healing of joint tissues may take place. TNF-α blockers when used early demonstrate superior remission rates. Some studies have shown that a significant proportion of patients remain in remission even after withdrawal of anti-TNF. Possible evidence of immune modulation.[37,46] The contribution of TNF to host defense is further suggested by an approximately two-fold increased risk especially during the first 6 months, of serious infections of the upper respiratory tract, skin, and joint, as well as a significantly increased risk of reactivation of latent tuberculosis, regardless of the TNF inhibitor used. The global risk of malignancy, particularly lymphoma, which is already increased in the RA population as a whole, does not appear to be increased with anti-TNF therapy, although much of the data are derived from meta-analysis of relatively short-term controlled clinical trials; an increased risk of melanoma has been reported by some registries. While these data are encouraging, large, longer term observational studies are required to address this key issue. The development of anti-nuclear antibodies in 8–15% patients, as well as rare cases of demyelination, point to effects that may be related to restoration of autoimmune responses in predisposed subjects, following TNF-α inhibition.

The clinical benefit of TNF-α blockade has prompted extensive mechanism of action studies.[47] Anti-TNF reduces the acute phase response, including IL-6 serum levels. Leukocyte trafficking is inhibited, as demonstrated through an early (within hours) and dramatic rise in lymphocyte counts through demargination, a more prolonged and sustained exclusion of leukocytes based on reductions in cellularity of synovial tissue biopsies after treatment and suppression of markers of angiogenesis, including VEGF. The effects of anti-TNF on cell viability and apoptosis remain controversial, however. TNF-α blockade has also been shown to downregulate markers of cartilage and bone destruction, including the collagenases MMP1 and 3, and to reduce the ratio of RANKL and OPG in serum, effects that might explain in part the joint preserving effects of anti-TNF *in vivo*. Finally, there is additional evidence of anti-TNF-induced immune homeostasis, based on restoration of cell mediated immune responses to recall antigens, as well as mitogens, but also an increase in both the numbers and function of CD4+CD25high regulatory T cells, at least in some studies.[37] This effect could be explained in part by the effect of TNF blockade on restoring the expression of the Treg associated transcription factor FOXP3. Given that, at least in mice, IL-2 is a critical factor for maintaining Treg metabolic fitness, enhanced IL-2 production by effector T cells may contribute to immune homeostasis.

The IL-1 receptor antagonist (IL-1Ra) is the only IL-1 inhibitor currently licensed for use in RA.[48] It has good effects in animal models of arthritis, with potent joint protection, but has proven less effective in patients with RA compared to anti-TNF. Nevertheless, it has been used effectively to treat patients who have failed TNF-α blockade, and has been shown to slow radiographic progression. Anti-IL-6R blockade (tocilizumab) is now licensed for use in patients with established RA. Evidence suggests that in early disease it is as effective as monotherapy, as it is when combined with methotrexate, suppressing signs and symptoms of RA, mediated through effects of blocking IL-6 on the immune response, the acute phase response, osteoclastogenesis, B-cell activation and immunoglobulin production, angiogenesis and cell adhesion (reviewed in Kishimoto).[49] Clinical responses are comparable to those observed with TNF blockade. Inhibition of IL-17 in RA seems a biologically plausible approach;[33] the outcomes of phase III studies are eagerly awaited.

Finally, the impact of using small molecule inhibitors of cytokine signals, transduced through receptors that utilize members of the Janus kinase (JAK) family of tyrosine kinases,[50] has been recently evaluated.[51] Tofacitinib has high affinity for JAK3, but is also able to partially inhibit JAK1 and, to a lesser extent, JAK2. In a phase II study of RA patients who had failed previous therapy, including synthetic and biological DMARDs, this orally active inhibitor (also known as CP-690,550) demonstrated up to 81% ACR20 improvement when compared to 29% in the placebo group; ACR70 responses were achieved by 28% compared to 3% of patients receiving placebo. Tofacitinib also appears to be well tolerated when used in combination with methotrexate. Inhibition of another kinase, spleen tyrosine kinase (Syk) with R788 (fostamatinib) has also shown clinical efficacy in RA.

Anti-T-cell therapy

Although methotrexate, cyclosporine and other immunosuppressive agents have claimed a place in the armamentarium for treating established RA, T-cell-targeted therapeutic agents have been relatively disappointing as a group. Depleting anti-CD4 monoclonal antibodies were among the first specific agents to target this cell subset. Clinical efficacy was observed with responder rates consistently less than 30%, perhaps because of ineffective depletion of CD4 T cells in synovial joints, or because the antibody would not distinguish between T-cell effector and regulatory subsets. Theoretically, non-depleting anti-CD4 should be more effective, but this has yet to be confirmed in large phase III studies.

In contrast, the contribution of costimulatory signals ("signal 2") transduced through CD28 to priming and activation of naïve cells and amplification of cytokine gene expression and proliferative responses has provided a rationale for testing costimulatory blockade in patients. This has been achieved using a non-depleting humanized IgG1-CTLA4 fusion protein that prevents CD80 and CD86 (B7 family members) from engaging CD28 (but also CTLA4) expressed on T cells. Initial studies confirmed that the agent was safe and well tolerated.[52] When administered as an intravenous infusion on days 1, 14, and 28, and then monthly thereafter at a 10 mg/kg dose in combination with methotrexate, 60% of patients achieved ACR20 compared to 35.3% controls; ACR50 responses were 36.5 versus 11.8%, respectively. CTLA4-Ig (licensed as abatacept) has since been shown

to inhibit radiographic progression and structural damage by ~50%, and is also effective in treating those patients who have had inadequate responses to TNF blockade as well as to methotrexate. From an immunological standpoint the data are interesting in several respects. First, the time to peak effect, which may take up to one year for some patients, is longer than for anti-TNF or anti-IL-6R therapy. This could reflect the presence of a significant number of costimulation independent T cells (e.g., CD4$^+$CD28^{null}) involved in disease progression, or perhaps the cumulative impact of blocking the activation and differentiation of naïve T-cell precursors over time. Second, inhibition of CD28 signals does not block development of regulatory T cells, as might have been predicted from mouse studies.

Anti-B-cell therapy

Rituximab is a humanized monoclonal antibody that recognizes human CD20, a 33- to 37-kDa membrane-associated phosphoprotein expressed on pre-B, immature and mature B cells but not plasma cells. While CD20 ligation promotes B-cell activation, differentiation and cell cycle progression, the function of CD20 is still poorly understood. The therapeutic effects of anti-CD20 are related to B-cell depletion, which can vary between patients, due to antibody dependent cell cytotoxicity, complement mediated cell lysis and/or triggering of intracellular pathways for apoptotic cell death.[53]

The initial open label studies in RA patients combined rituximab with cyclophosphamide and steroids, and so the precise contribution of rituximab to the clinical response was unclear. A pivotal placebo-controlled trial of rituximab therapy randomized 161 patients with rheumatoid factor positive RA compared the efficacy and safety of methotrexate alone (standard therapy) versus methotrexate plus rituximab (1000 mg on days 1 and 15), rituximab alone or rituximab plus cyclophosphamide.[54] All groups received a 17-day course of steroids, which may facilitate B-cell depletion. Up to 43% of patients receiving combination of rituximab with methotrexate achieved 50% improvement in clinical and laboratory parameters after 24 weeks (based on American College of Rheumatology response criteria—the ACR50), and this was at least as good as the rituximab/cyclophosphamide combination (41% achieving ACR50) and superior to methotrexate (13%) or rituximab alone (33%). The overall incidence of infection was similar across treatment groups, but seven serious infections were reported in rituximab treated patients. Post marketing surveillance has documented progressive multifocal leukoencephalopathy in a small number of patients.

Detailed analysis of this and subsequent studies in RA patients indicate that the B-cell depletion, which may depend on *FCGR3* allelic variants, is profound (< 2%), with no major differences in infection rates between groups with the possible exception of lower respiratory tract infections. Repopulation occurs at a mean of 8 months after treatment, comprises immature IgD$^+$CD38$^+$CD27$^-$CD5$^+$ B cells, and is associated with increased serum BLyS levels. Early relapse is associated with reconstitution of CD27$^+$ memory B cells. The effects on serum immunoglobulin levels are modest with levels remaining in the normal range, unless patients undergo repeated cycles of B-cell depletion. Selective and rapid decreases in pathogenic IgM, IgG, and IgA rheumatoid factor (~60%) and IgG anti-CCP autoantibodies have been documented; these changes are more striking in rituximab responders. Antibody titers to tetanus toxoid or to pneumococcal capsular polysaccharides were only modestly affected (~25%). These changes are intriguing given that terminally differentiated plasma cells do not express CD20. One possibility is that germinal center and marginal zone B cells may be resistant to anti-CD20. These encouraging results have prompted alternative B-cell-targeted therapies,[55] of which anti-IL-6R should be included, as well as, TACI-Ig, and monoclonal antibodies to BLyS/BAFF.

Future prospects for therapy

There remain unmet needs in the treatment of RA. Principal among these are the fact that treatment is invariably lifelong for the majority of patients imposing greater risk of toxicity and, as the immune system senesces, increased risk of infection or lymphoproliferative disease. There is little doubt that early treatment with tight control offers the best outcome. From an immunological perspective, there remains a pressing need to develop immunological tools or immune biomarkers that can redefine disease subsets, and measure effector and regulatory cell subsets using technology readily accessible to routine clinical laboratories in ways that will inform disease activity states at a biological level. While such tools may provide better insights into disease pathogenesis, they can also be adapted to monitor the impact of therapeutic intervention, whether this turns out to be cell based therapy or the application of novel immune modulators. It is possible that similar approaches to developing immune signatures could be used in the future to identify those ACPA+ arthralgia patients, who have a genetic predisposition to RA and are at highest risk of developing disease.

References

1. Snorrason E. Landre-Beauvais and his goutte asthénique primitive. Acta Med Scand 1952;142:115.
2. Harris ED. Rheumatoid arthritis; pathophysiology and implications for therapy. N Engl J Med 1990;322:1277.
3. Silman AJ, Hochberg MC. Epidemiology of rheumatic diseases. Oxford: Oxford University Press; 1993.
4. Silman AJ, MacGregor AJ, Thomson W, et al. Twin concordance rates for rheumatoid arthritis: results from a nationwide study. Br J Rheumatol 1993;32:903.
5. van der Woude D, Houwing-Duistermaat JJ, Toes RE, et al. Quantitative heritability of anti-citrullinated protein antibody-positive and anti-citrullinated protein antibody-negative rheumatoid arthritis. Arthritis Rheum 2009;60:916.
6. Weyand CM, Goronzy JJ. Stem cell aging and autoimmunity in rheumatoid arthritis. Trends Mol Med 2004;9:426.
7. Spector TD, Roman E, Silman AJ. The pill, parity, and rheumatoid arthritis. Arthritis Rheum 1990;33:782.
8. Karlson EW, Lee IM, Cook NR, et al. A retrospective cohort study of cigarette smoking and risk of rheumatoid arthritis in female health professionals. Arthritis Rheum 1999;42:910.
9. Padyukov L, Silva C, Stolt P, et al. A gene-environment interaction between smoking and shared epitope genes in HLA-DR provides a high risk of seropositive rheumatoid arthritis. Arthritis Rheum 2004;50:3085.
10. Lundberg K, Wegner N, Yucel-Lindberg T, Venables PJ. Periodontitis in RA—the citrullinated enolase connection. Nat Rev Rheumatol 2010;6:727.
11. Wu HJ, Ivanov II, Darce J, et al. Gut-residing segmented filamentous bacteria drive autoimmune arthritis via T helper 17 cells. Immunity 2010;32:815.
12. Gregersen PK. Recent advances in the genetics of autoimmune disease. Annu Rev Immunol 2005;27:363.
13. Gregersen PK, Silver J, Winchester RJ. The shared epitope hypothesis. An approach to understanding the molecular genetics of susceptibility to rheumatoid arthritis. Arthritis Rheum 1987;30:1205.
14. Van der Helm-van Mil AH, Huizinga TW, Schreuder GM, et al. An independent role of protective HLA class II alleles in rheumatoid arthritis severity and susceptibility. Arthritis Rheum 2005;52:2637.
15. Weyand CM, McCarthy TG, Goronzy JJ. Correlation between disease phenotype and genetic heterogeneity in rheumatoid arthritis. J Clin Invest 1995;95:2120.
16. Nepom GT. Major histocompatibility complex-directed susceptibility to rheumatoid arthritis. Adv Immunol 1998;68:315.
17. Huizinga TW, Amos CI, van der Helm-van Mil AH, et al. Refining the complex rheumatoid arthritis phenotype based on specificity of the HLA-DRB1 shared epitope for antibodies to citrullinated proteins. Arthritis Rheum 2005;52:3433.
18. Burn GL, Svensson L, Sanchez-Blanco C, et al. Why is PTPN22 a good candidate susceptibility gene for autoimmune disease? FEBS Lett 2011;585(23):3689–98.
19. Manzo A, Bombardieri M, Humby F, Pitzalis C. Secondary and ectopic lymphoid tissue responses in rheumatoid arthritis: from inflammation to autoimmunity and tissue damage/remodeling. Immunol Rev 2010;233:267.
20. Binstadt BA, Patel PR, Alencar H, et al. Particularities of the vasculature can promote the organ specificity of autoimmune attack. Nat Immunol 2006;7:284.
21. Goronzy JJ, Weyand CM. Rheumatoid arthritis. Immunol Rev 2005;204:55.
22. van der Pouw Kraan TC, van Gaalen FA, Kasperkovitz PV, et al. Rheumatoid arthritis is a heterogeneous disease: evidence for differences in the activation of the STAT-1 pathway between rheumatoid tissues. Arthritis Rheum 2003;48:2132.
23. Firestein GS. Evolving concepts of rheumatoid arthritis. Nature 2003;423:356.
24. Plant D, Bowes J, Potter C, et al., Wellcome Trust Case Control Consortium, British Society for Rheumatology Biologics Register. Barton A. Genome-wide association study of genetic predictors of anti-tumor necrosis factor treatment efficacy in rheumatoid arthritis identifies associations with polymorphisms at seven loci. Arthritis Rheum 2011;63:645.
25. Sacre SM, Drexler SK, Andreakos E, et al. Could toll-like receptors provide a missing link in chronic inflammation in rheumatoid arthritis? Lessons from a study on human rheumatoid tissue. Ann Rheum Dis 2007;66(Suppl. 3):81.
26. Pettit AR, Thomas R. Dendritic cells: the driving force behind autoimmunity in rheumatoid arthritis? Immunol Cell Biol 1999;77:420.
27. Szekanecz Z, Kim J, Koch AE. Chemokines and chemokine receptors in rheumatoid arthritis. Semin Immunol 2003;15:15.
28. Kollias G, Papadaki P, Apparailly F, et al. Animal models for arthritis: innovative tools for prevention and treatment. Ann Rheum Dis 2011;70:1357.
29. van Venrooij WJ, Vossenaar ER, Zendman AJ. Anti-CCP antibodies: the new rheumatoid factor in the serology of rheumatoid arthritis. Autoimmun Rev 2004;3(Suppl. 1):S17.
30. Klareskog L, Rönnelid J, Lundberg K, et al. Immunity to citrullinated proteins in rheumatoid arthritis. Annu Rev Immunol 2008;26:651.
31. Salmon M, Scheel-Toellner D, Huissoon AP, et al. Inhibition of T cell apoptosis in the rheumatoid synovium. J Clin Invest 1997;99:439.
32. Cope A, Le Friec G, Cardone J, Kemper C. The Th1 life cycle: molecular control of IFN-γ to IL-10 switching. Trends Immunol 2011;32:278.
33. Miossec P, Korn T, Kuchroo VK. Interleukin-17 and type 17 helper T cells. N Engl J Med 2009;361:888.
34. McInnes IB, Schett G. Cytokines in the pathogenesis of rheumatoid arthritis. Nat Rev Immunol 2007;7:429.
35. Sakaguchi S, Sakaguchi N. Animal models of arthritis caused by systemic alteration of the immune system. Curr Opin Immunol 2005;17:589.
36. Dayer JM, Burger D. Cell-cell interactions and tissue damage in rheumatoid arthritis. Autoimmun Rev 2004;3(Suppl. 1):S14.
37. Miyara M, Gorochov G, Ehrenstein M, et al. Human FoxP3(+) regulatory T cells in systemic autoimmune diseases. Autoimmun Rev 2011;10(12):744–55.
38. Schett G, Hayer S, Zwerina J, et al. Mechanisms of disease: the link between RANKL and arthritic bone disease. Nat Clin Pract Rheumatol 2005;1:47.
39. Theill LE, Boyle WJ, Penninger JM. RANK-L and RANK: T cells, bone loss, and mammalian evolution. Annu Rev Immunol 2002;20:795.
40. Walsh NC, Gravallese EM. Bone remodeling in rheumatic disease: a question of balance. Immunol Rev 2010;233:301.
41. Arnett FC, Edworthy SM, Bloch DA, et al. The American Rheumatism Association 1987 revised criteria for the classification of rheumatoid arthritis. Arthritis Rheum 1988;31:315.
42. Aletaha D, Neogi T, Silman AJ, et al. 2010 Rheumatoid arthritis classification criteria: an American College of Rheumatology/European League Against Rheumatism collaborative initiative. Arthritis Rheum 2010;62:2569.
43. Bos WH, Wolbink GJ, Boers M, et al. Arthritis development in patients with arthralgia is strongly associated with anti-citrullinated protein antibody status: a prospective cohort study. Ann Rheum Dis 2010;69:490.
44. Bykerk VP. Strategies to prevent rheumatoid arthritis in high-risk patients. Curr Opin Rheumatol 2011;23:179.
45. Grigor C, Capell H, Stirling A, et al. Effect of a treatment strategy of tight control for rheumatoid arthritis (the TICORA study): a single-blind randomised controlled trial. Lancet 2004;364:263.
46. Goekoop-Ruiterman YP, de Vries-Bouwstra JK, Allaart CF, et al. Clinical and radiographic outcomes of four different treatment strategies in patients with early rheumatoid arthritis (the BeSt study): a randomized, controlled trial. Arthritis Rheum 2005;52:3381.
47. Feldmann M, Maini RN. Anti-TNF alpha therapy of rheumatoid arthritis: what have we learned? Annu Rev Immunol 2001;19:163.
48. Jiang Y, Genant HK, Watt I, et al. A multicenter, double-blind, dose-ranging, randomized, placebo-controlled study of recombinant human interleukin-1 receptor antagonist in patients with rheumatoid arthritis: radiologic progression and correlation of Genant and Larsen scores. Arthritis Rheum 2000;43:1001.
49. Kishimoto T. Interleukin-6: from basic science to medicine—40 years in immunology. Annu Rev Immunol 2005;23:1.
50. Ghoreschi K, Laurence A, O'Shea JJ. Janus kinases in immune cell signaling. Immunol Rev 2009;228:273.
51. Cohen S, Fleischmann R. Kinase inhibitors: a new approach to rheumatoid arthritis treatment. Curr Opin Rheumatol 2010;22:330.
52. Kremer JM, Westhovens R, Leon M, et al. Treatment of rheumatoid arthritis by selective inhibition of T-cell activation with fusion protein CTLA4Ig. N Engl J Med 2003;349:1907.
53. Edwards JC, Cambridge G. B-cell targeting in rheumatoid arthritis and other autoimmune diseases. Nat Rev Immunol 2006;6:394.
54. Edwards JC, Szczepanski L, Szechinski J, et al. Efficacy of B-cell-targeted therapy with rituximab in patients with rheumatoid arthritis. N Engl J Med 2004;350:2572.
55. Dörner T, Kinnman N, Tak PP. Targeting B cells in immune-mediated inflammatory disease: a comprehensive review of mechanisms of action and identification of biomarkers. Pharmacol Ther 2010;125:46.

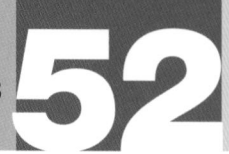

Juvenile idiopathic arthritis

Randy Q. Cron,
Peter Weiser,
Timothy
Beukelman

Epidemiology

Juvenile idiopathic arthritis (JIA) is a collection of conditions that manifest with chronic arthritis in childhood. By definition, JIA occurs prior to the 16th birthday (juvenile), has no known causes (idiopathic), and has evident chronic (>6 weeks duration) swelling/inflammation of a joint or joints (arthritis).[1] The nomenclature and subcategorization of JIA was published, with a second revision in 2004, in part, to unify the American (juvenile rheumatoid arthritis, JRA) and European (juvenile chronic arthritis, JCA) classification schemes.[2] Removal of the word "rheumatoid" was also important to distinguish these unique disorders from adult rheumatoid arthritis (RA) (Chapter 51). The new classification of JIA also includes the HLA-B27-associated spondyloarthropathies (Chapter 56), which occur frequently during childhood (Table 52.1).

Because JIA is a diagnosis of exclusion, other causes of childhood chronic arthritis need to be excluded. For example, sarcoidosis (Chapter 72), Sjögren disease (Chapter 53), systemic lupus erythematosus (Chapter 50), Lyme disease (Chapter 26), dermatomyositis (Chapter 55), and a variety of vasculitides (Chapters 57 and 58) can all present as chronic arthritis in childhood.[1] JIA by definition is idiopathic; however, chronic arthritis as part of inflammatory bowel disease (IBD) (Chapter 74), or associated with psoriasis (Chapter 63), are categorized under the JIA umbrella. When considering the seven categories of JIA together, the estimated prevalence of JIA is roughly 1 in 1,000 children with rates varying throughout different regions of the world, likely due to genetic risk factors and/or environmental triggers.[3] Moreover, the relative rates of JIA categories vary in different regions of the world (e.g., oligoarticular JIA is very common in Scandinavia, and enthesitis related JIA is more typical in Latin America).

Etiology and pathogenesis

Genetic contribution

Because JIA is an eclectic group of disorders with joint inflammation, is far less common than RA, and is classified into unique categories based largely on subjective clinical phenotypes, the ability to understand its genetic causes is extremely difficult. Indeed, the relatively arbitrary distinction of having four clinically arthritic joints or less to be considered as oligoarticular JIA is influenced by whether temporomandibular joint (TMJ)

arthritis (or in essence any other suspected joint involvement) is screened for by MRI.[4] Distinctions based on the types and location of joints manifesting arthritis may prove useful in developing more homogeneous subtypes. Thus, the criteria will likely continue to evolve and benefit from more precise clinical, laboratory, and genetic distinctions. One such suggested re-classification of JIA categories is based on shared similarities among children with JIA who are anti-nuclear antibody (ANA) positive[5] regardless of total joint count. Nevertheless, there have been several attempts to characterize the genetics of the JIA categories using a variety of approaches.[6]

Polygenic disorder

Like most autoimmune conditions, JIA is a polygenic disorder with 20 or more potential genes contributing to the phenotypes of chronic arthritis presenting during childhood. An exception is the systemic JIA (sJIA) category, which resembles an autoinflammatory disorder.[7] Unlike autoimmunity, which is believed to be the result of an imperfect adaptive immune system, autoinflammatory conditions are thought to result from genetic perturbations in the innate immune response. Many autoinflammatory recurrent fever syndromes have been identified as resulting from single gene defects, such as pyrin in familial Mediterranean fever (FMF), and tumor necrosis factor (TNF) receptor in TRAPS (Chapter 59).[8] Whether sJIA is the result of a single gene defect, or one of many potential single gene defects in the same immune pathway, is currently unknown. However, a common complication of sJIA is the life-threatening condition of macrophage activation syndrome (MAS), which resembles familial hemophagocytic lymphohistiocytosis (fHLH) (Fig. 52.1). MAS may be present in ~50% of children with sJIA in either an overt or occult/subclinical fashion.[9] Recently, genetic polymorphisms and heterozygous (single copy) mutations in genes associated with fHLH when present as homozygous defects, have been identified in children with sJIA and overt MAS.[9] Protein products of these genes, including perforin 1 and MUNC 13-4, are critical in the pathway leading to cytolysis by CD8 T cells and natural killer (NK) cells (Chapter 17). This cytolysis is crucial to the ability to shut down an immune response following control of infection. Defects in this pathway can result in a hyper-inflammatory state (cytokine storm) leading to pancytopenia, coagulopathy, and multi-system organ failure.[10] The most common condition resulting in MAS during childhood is sJIA. Therefore, sJIA may be genetically related to fHLH, but associated with heterozygous, rather than homozygous, mutations in genes critical for cytolysis.[7,9]

Table 52.1 Clinical and laboratory features of the JIA categories

| Classifications | JIA (juvenile idiopathic arthritis) | | | | | |
| | Former JRA (juvenile rheumatoid arthritis) | | | | Spondyloarthropathy | |
JIA categories/ features	Systemic	RF (-) poly	RF (+) poly	Oligo (persistent & extended)	Psoriatic (early & late onset)	ERA (including AS & IBD)
HLA	DRB1*11	DRB1*08	DRB1*04	A2	DRB1*01	B27
Sex	Equal	F>>M	F>>M	F>>M	F>M	M>>F
Onset age	Peak 2 yrs	Dual peaks	Teenage	1–3 yrs	Dual peaks	Teenage
ANA	Rare	Yes	Yes	Yes	Yes	Rare
Uveitis	Rare	Yes	Yes	Yes	Yes	Non-silent
TMJ	Yes	Yes	Yes	Yes	Yes	Yes
Enthesitis	No	No	No	No	Older age	Yes
Arthritis	Erosive	Symmetric	Erosive	Mixed	Dactylitis	Axial

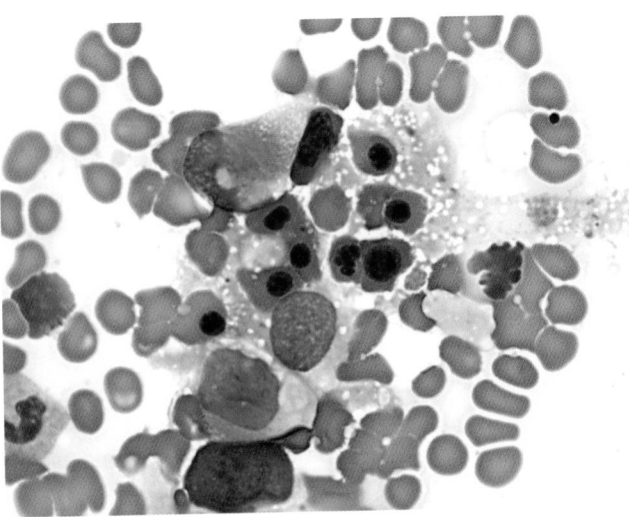

Fig. 52.1 Hemophagocytosis as part of MAS. A centrally located, vacuolated histiocyte is pictured engulfing numerous nucleated immune cells and non-nucleated mature red blood cells. Wright stain at 198 × magnification.
Courtesy of Dr. David Kelly.

HLA associations

For all other JIA categories, polygenic influences, including the major histocompatibility complex (MHC), contribute to disease pathology. The MHC is complex and densely packed (>200 genes) with immune-associated genes (Chapter 5). The MHC is also the most polymorphic region of the human genome and gives rise to MHC class I and class II genes, complement proteins, TNF, and others. The critical role of MHC proteins in preventing autoimmunity by shaping the T-cell repertoire (Chapter 8) likely explains why the MHC is the most consistently and strongly associated genetic locus for most JIA categories. However, weak MHC associations, together with the lack of a sex predilection for children developing sJIA, are additional arguments to consider sJIA as autoinflammatory rather than autoimmune.

By contrast, the enthesitis related arthritis (ERA) JIA category, along with a subset of children with psoriatic JIA, share one of the strongest known MHC associations, HLA-B27, for any described autoimmune disorder. HLA-B27 is present in 70–90% of Caucasian children with the ERA JIA category. Inheritance of ERA follows an autosomal dominant pattern and is the only JIA category likely to have similarly afflicted first degree relatives. The pathophysiologic explanation for the association of HLA-B27 remains unknown but hypotheses vary from molecular mimicry of pathogens presented by HLA-B27 (Chapter 48) to the unfolded protein response.[11] The remaining JIA categories have all been linked to various other MHC proteins to lesser degrees (Table 52.1).

Non-HLA associations

Genes outside of the MHC have also been linked to developing JIA. Genetic approaches have highlighted the importance of genetic differences in the development of JIA, but at most 11% of the contribution can be linked to the MHC.[6] Recent developments in high throughput genetic sequencing combined with the identification of densely present restriction fragment length polymorphisms (RFLPs) throughout the human genome have allowed for powerful new genetic approaches. These include genome-wide association studies (GWAS) designed to identify genes associated with a variety of disorders, including autoimmune diseases like RA.[12] The greater numbers of RA patients available to study along with a more homogeneous disorder than JIA have allowed for identification of genes linked to RA development. Nevertheless, several genes have been reported to be associated with JIA.[6]

Strong evidence that genetic factors contribute to JIA susceptibility include twin and family studies. Data from a JIA national registry reported monozygotic twin pairs have a higher than expected proportion of twins with JIA. Moreover, siblings of children with JIA have as high as a 30-fold increased risk of developing JIA compared to the general population. Interestingly, siblings with JIA typically share the same JIA category, age of onset, and disease course.[6] Polymorphisms in MHC class II genes have been estimated to account for less than 20% of the recurrence risk of JIA in siblings and thus support the concept that JIA is a complex genetic trait. JIA likely shares general or common autoimmunity gene risk factors with many autoimmune disorders, but likely is also influenced by specific JIA risk associated genes.[13]

Using linkage and association studies, researchers have identified a variety of potentially JIA-associated genes. However, outside of the HLA genes, only a small percentage of these genes have been independently confirmed by other investigators.

A few of the independently confirmed JIA associated genes/gene products include *PTPN22* (a phosphatase involved in inhibition of T-cell activation), *WISP3* (a signaling protein), interleukin-1α (a pro-inflammatory cytokine), TNF-α (another pro-inflammatory cytokine), MIF (macrophage migratory inhibitory factor), and *SLC11A1* (a resistance factor to intracellular pathogens in macrophages).[6] Thus, gene products linked to both the innate and adaptive immune response likely contribute to JIA disease susceptibility. Ongoing GWAS studies will likely help validate the importance of these genes, and should help identify other candidate gene risk factors for JIA in the near future. Eventually, epigenetic (covalent modifications to DNA nucleotides rather than changes in the DNA sequence) risk factors that confer susceptibility to JIA will be explored.[14]

Environmental factors

In addition to genetic factors, there are likely a variety of environmental triggers for developing JIA in genetically susceptible hosts. A number of infectious agents have been explored as risk factors for development of JIA. Perhaps two of the best studied have been parvovirus and rubella virus infections.[1] However, replication of these associations has been difficult. In addition, some scientists have suggested that heat shock proteins, resulting from cells undergoing environmental stress, may contribute to the development of JIA.[15] There is also a clear link of gut pathogens, and potentially commensal organisms (gut microbiome), and the development of the HLA-B27 associated spondyloarthropathies.[16] Lastly, prior to the identification of *Borrelia* as a cause of childhood arthritis, Lyme disease associated arthritis was difficult to distinguish from oligoarticular JIA.[17] Perhaps, because there a variety of potential environmental triggers for JIA, combined with the number of different JIA categories, no single environmental trigger has been conclusively identified as contributing to the development of JIA.

Immune abnormalities

Autoantibodies

As JIA is considered an autoimmune disease, except for sJIA as discussed earlier, there have been a variety of explorations into the role of various components of the immune system involved in JIA pathogenesis. The importance of the immune system in JIA pathology is highlighted by the increased incidence of childhood chronic arthritis among children with various immunodeficiencies. For example, children with IgA deficiency are at increased risk of developing chronic arthritis.[18] By contrast, the presence of specific autoantibodies is associated with various forms of JIA. ANAs are present in up to 40% of JIA patients, particularly those with the oligoarticular category, and are associated with silent uveitis (Chapter 73).[19] Similarly, antibodies to the nuclear oncoprotein, DEK, have been associated with uveitis as well as joint inflammation in children with JIA.[20] By comparison, IgM rheumatoid factor (RF) is present in a small subset of children with polyarticular JIA and is associated with a more aggressive/erosive form of arthritis as in adults with rheumatoid factor positive (RF[+]) RA (Chapter 51).[21] More recently,

identification of anti-cyclic citrullinated peptide (CCP) antibodies have been found in a partially overlapping subset of children with RF[+] poly JIA.[21] Thus, a variety of B-cell-derived autoantibodies are associated with JIA.

T helper cells

T lymphocytes are also thought to play a major role in the development of JIA as evidenced by their relative predominance among mononuclear cells in synovial fluid of chronically inflamed joints in children with JIA. CD4 T helper (Th) cells have been categorized into a variety of cytokine producing subsets (Chapter 16). CD4 Th1 cells characterized by the production of interferon-γ (IFN-γ) have been identified in chronically inflamed joints in children with JIA, whereas IL-4-producing Th2 CD4 T cells are associated more commonly in oligoarticular (generally less aggressive arthritis) than polyarticular JIA joints. More recently, two relatively newly described CD4 Th subsets, regulatory T cells (Tregs) and Th17 cells, have taken center stage in the hypothesized pathogenesis of JIA disease pathology.

CD4[+], CD25[high] Tregs are characterized by the transcription factor, FoxP3, and by the ability to suppress immune activation (Chapter 15).[22] The ability of Tregs to suppress other T cells likely occurs by both cell contact dependent (through the surface protein, CTLA-4) and independent (via suppressive cytokines) mechanisms.[23] Tregs secrete the anti-inflammatory cytokines, IL-10 and tumor growth factor-β (TGF-β), whereas Th17 cells, characterized by the transcription factor, RORγT, produce the pro-inflammatory cytokine, IL-17.[24] IL-17 is thought to contribute to a variety of autoimmune disorders, including JIA. The balance between these two juxtaposed Th subsets may determine whether autoimmunity develops (Th17-dominant) or a state of immune tolerance to self (Chapter 12) persists (Treg dominant). Indeed, recent studies have identified a predominance of Th17 cells and associated pro-inflammatory cytokines in the inflamed joints of children with JIA.[25] Thus, a balance of pro-inflammatory cytokines and suppressive cytokines may dictate the expression of autoimmunity in the form of JIA.

Cytokines

Cytokines (Chapter 9), and particularly their inhibition, have taken a prominent status in the pathology and treatment of chronic arthritis, including JIA. The bench to bedside translation of anti-TNF-α therapy to the treatment of chronic arthritis has revolutionized the care of adults with chronic arthritis, as well as children with JIA.[26] Inhibition of this pro-inflammatory cytokine in the circulation (via specific monoclonal antibodies (mAb) or receptor fusion proteins) rapidly and effectively treats most forms of JIA. The one exception is sJIA, which may or may not respond to anti-TNF-α treatment. However, other pro-inflammatory cytokines, including IL-1, -6, and -18, are thought to be central to sJIA pathogenesis.[7] Indeed, serum from sJIA patients was shown to induce transcription of a variety of innate immunity genes, including IL-1, in normal peripheral blood mononuclear cells.[27] Fortunately, novel therapies that target either IL-1 or -6 have proven highly successful in treating even the severest forms of sJIA, including associated MAS.[28]

Macrophage activation syndrome (MAS)

● KEY CONCEPTS

Macrophage activation syndrome (MAS)

- MAS is present in up to 50% of children with sJIA in a subclinical or overt (10%) form.
- MAS manifests as fever, liver dysfunction, pancytopenia, central nervous system disturbance, hyperferritinemia, hemophagocytosis, and coagulopathy.
- MAS resembles hemophagocytic lymphohistiocytosis (HLH) and is thought to result from defects in cytolysis by CD8 T cells and NK cells.
- Patients with sJIA and MAS have been noted to have NK cell defects and mutations in perforin-1 and polymorphisms in MUNC 13-4 cytolytic pathway genes.
- MAS can be fatal if not recognized and treated early. Mainstays of therapy include high dose corticosteroids and cyclosporine.
- Recently, interleukin-1 (IL-1) blockade with biologic therapies has been found to be quickly and dramatically beneficial in treating MAS associated with sJIA.

The sometimes fatal complication, MAS, is most commonly seen in sJIA among rheumatic diseases. Clinically, MAS resembles many features of a sJIA disease flare, and it has been suggested that MAS may be inherent to sJIA disease pathology in up to half of all patients with sJIA.[9] MAS is likely part of the spectrum of HLH disorders. Primary or fHLH typically presents in infancy following infection and results from homozygous mutations in genes involved in the cytolytic pathway employed by NK cells and CD8 T cells. Recent evidence suggests that sJIA patients with MAS have heterozygous defects in these same cytolytic pathway genes.[9] MAS can be triggered by a variety of infectious organisms, particularly members of the herpes virus family, but the precise role of infectious triggers of MAS in children with sJIA remains unknown. Nevertheless, the inability to effectively shut down an immune response via cytolytic mechanisms results in a "storm" of pro-inflammatory cytokines, such as IL-1, -6, -18, TNF-α, and IFN-γ.[10] Mouse models of MAS/HLH have suggested that IFN-γ is the pivotal cytokine in MAS. Practically speaking, inhibition of IL-1, and potentially IL-6, as well, has proven rather effective at treating MAS in children with sJIA.[28] It is quite remarkable how dampening of one critical cytokine can help restore the immune imbalance of multiple pro-inflammatory cytokines and rapidly reverse the life-threatening clinical scenario of MAS.

Juvenile idiopathic arthritis clinical subtypes

As already mentioned, JIA is a group of chronic inflammatory joint diseases lasting at least six weeks and commencing prior to the age of 16 with no identifiable cause. There is heterogeneity of clinical presentation and progression of the various subtypes which is largely addressed by the ILAR classification schema (Table 52.1). Nevertheless, as more information becomes available from multi-center studies about genetic factors, response to medication and subsequent outcomes, revisiting the classification in the near future seems inevitable. Along these lines, some have recently suggested that children with JIA and a positive ANA should be categorized separately.[5]

The current classification of JIA relies heavily on the number of the joints involved (four and fewer in oligoarticular; five and more in polyarticular, with or without the presence of RF).[2] Other categories of JIA are also classified based on associated symptoms and signs like fever, rash, and laboratory indicators of inflammation in sJIA, or associated diseases like psoriasis. There is a separate JIA category affecting more boys than girls, ERA, with inflammation of the entheses, attachments of the tendons and ligaments to bone (see Table 52.1). An important finding of recent years is that imaging (MRI or ultrasound) can identify ongoing inflammation in clinically quiet joints. This has led to screening for TMJ inflammation primarily by MRI. TMJ arthritis in JIA is frequently clinically silent but capable of resulting in facial dysmorphism from micrognathia in all JIA categories, including oligoarticular JIA.[4]

Oligoarticular JIA

Oligoarticular JIA is likely the most common category of JIA, affecting children who have 1–4 joints inflamed, most commonly the knee, the ankle, and the fingers.[1] The archetype of this group is a preschool-aged, blonde-haired, blue-eyed girl who limps with a swollen knee. The diagnosis of arthritis may be delayed as it is often painless.[1] Due to this fact, by the time she is seen in the medical office, she may already have developed bony hypertrophy and limb length discrepancy,[29] as chronic articular inflammation stimulates the osteoblasts of the nearby growth plates. In addition, there is often notable muscle wasting around the arthritic joint which can last into adulthood. The oligoarticular JIA category has highest percentage of positive ANA blood tests and associated potentially damaging silent uveitis.[19] Monoarticular involvement calls for a careful differential diagnosis. JIA rarely presents with isolated hip involvement; toxic synovitis, septic hip, and malignancy need to be ruled out.[30] Oligoarticular JIA is also quite uncommon in middle and high school aged children, where the diagnosis of reactive arthritis, IBD-related arthritis, and Lyme disease should be entertained. The ILAR classification has a separate sub-category for children who develop additional joint involvement after the first 6 months based on clinical presentation, extended oligoarticular JIA,[2] which might be a variant of the RF-negative polyarticular category. Wrist involvement is considered to be a bad prognostic factor, as is the extended oligoarticular phenotype.

Polyarticular JIA

Arthritis of five or more joints includes two main JIA categories (see Table 52.1) based on the presence of serum RF, an IgM antibody against the IgG Fc receptor.

RF-positive serum on two occasions at least 3 months apart is required for a child to be diagnosed with RF⁺ polyarticular JIA. Joint involvement is typically bilateral and symmetric, involving the small joints of the hands and feet.[1] However, large joints and cervical involvement are often present. RF⁺ polyarticular JIA usually presents in adolescent girls and is considered to be a form of early onset adult RA.[1] It is a relatively infrequent category of JIA with <5 % of all JIA patients classified in this category. Antibodies to CCP are much less common in children with polyarticular JIA than in adults,[29] but these children usually have active arthritis for many years. The presence of RF predicts more destructive/erosive disease calling for early aggressive therapy.[31] As in adult RA, arthritis of the wrists and fingers can lead to ulnar deviation and boutonniere and swan neck deformities. Destructive TMJ involvement is also common.[1]

Similar to adult RA, children with RF$^+$ polyarticular JIA commonly have extraarticular manifestations such as low grade fever and occasionally rheumatoid nodules over bony surfaces.

The *RF-negative* polyarticular JIA category usually presents with asymmetrical involvement of the large joints, mostly the knees, wrists, and ankles. Like in psoriatic JIA, small joint involvement tends to occur later in life. In another similarity to psoriatic JIA, RF$^-$ polyarticular JIA has a bimodal distribution with preschool children and early adolescent patients.[1] There is more silent uveitis in the former group, and it is often difficult to distinguish from ERA in the latter. TMJ inflammation leading to condylar damage and facial dysmorphism is frequent.[4]

Psoriatic arthritis

Arthritis with concurrent psoriasis, or arthritis with two of either: dactylitis, psoriatic nail changes, or family history of a first degree relative with psoriasis, comprises a separate category of JIA. There seems to be a bimodal distribution of age of onset for psoriatic JIA.[32] Preschool aged children have mostly large joint involvement like the oligoarticular category, but also may have dactylitis, whereas middle school-aged patients resemble ERA with enthesitis, sacroiliac joint involvement (albeit milder), and even spondylitis.[32] In general, there is asymmetric involvement of the joints, and, if untreated, it will progress to polyarticular joint disease. Since up to 50% of the patients develop psoriatic skin findings several years after arthritis presentation, it is often difficult to diagnose this condition at onset. It is important to carefully examine children with JIA for dactylitis (tenosynovitis causing swelling of the digit beyond the joint capsule) and nail pits and onycholysis. Psoriatic JIA seems to be more resistant to therapy and approximately 40% of children have active disease into adulthood while on medications. Insidious onset of anterior uveitis is more typical for the younger age group while those with enthesitis resemble the adult type of psoriatic arthritis with an associated HLA-B27 genotype and chronic symptomatic eye disease (see Table 52.1).

Enthesitis-related arthritis

ERA affects more boys than girls[1] and may sometimes be a manifestation of IBD. Entheses are the attachments of the tendons, ligaments or joint capsules to the bone. These can be tender even in healthy children, but usually three or more tender entheses are associated with disease (Table 52.1). ERA often occurs in boys 8 years of age and older.[1] They typically complain of joint pain with sports, but there is also morning stiffness and pain that gets better during the day and worsens after a lot of activities. Many consider ERA a potential prelude to ankylosing spondylitis, a HLA-B27 associated inflammatory condition resulting in currently irreversible fusion of the vertebrae.[33] Recent therapeutic efforts are focusing on preventing the calcifying hypercorrection of inflamed vertebral edges using TNF-α blockade. Outcomes are still under investigation.

Systemic JIA

Approximately 10% of children with chronic arthritis belong to the sJIA category, also known as Still disease. The peak incidence of sJIA is between ages 1 and 5, but it can present in adulthood. The ILAR criteria to classify sJIA require fever for 2 weeks, with at least 3 episodes of daily spiking (quotidian) fever, with at least one of the following: fleeting pink macular rash, arthritis, lymphadenopathy, and hepatosplenomegaly.[2] During the fever children act rather ill, and the rash is more prominent and can be evoked by contact (Koebner phenomenon).[1] Typically, fever subsides and children feel visibly better in the morning hours. High levels of systemic inflammation are typical at onset and may subside later in the disease. Arthritis is often very aggressive and frequently involves wrists, ankles, and knees, but also causes ankylosis of the hip and neck leading to long-term damage and gait abnormalities. Occasionally, joint involvement begins months after fever onset making sJIA diagnosis more difficult. Initial presentation mimics that of infections and malignancies, which need to be considered, as sJIA is a diagnosis of exclusion. Fifty percent of children can develop (only 10% clinically overt) MAS, a serious and grave complication resembling consumptive coagulopathy.[9]

Laboratory evaluation

There is no one laboratory indicator that will establish or rule out chronic arthritis itself.

The complete blood count (CBC) is largely normal in oligoarticular involvement, as is the erythrocyte sedimentation rate (ESR). White blood cells (WBCs) are highly elevated in sJIA, but mostly within normal limits in other groups. Anemia of chronic disease presents as normocytic and normochromic and is often found in polyarticular involvement. In those cases, the ESR can also be elevated. Intermittent joint effusion of a single large joint with an elevated ESR asks for further evaluation, and IBD should be considered, especially if there is a low serum albumin level and/or growth delay. Of note, elevated ESR on presentation predicts a worse outcome.

The platelet count, as a marker of inflammation, can be elevated in polyarticular disease and substantially so in sJIA.

Liver function tests are used for monitoring certain disease modifying anti-rheumatic drugs (DMARDs), such as methotrexate and leflunomide. They can be elevated due to prolonged, and frequently concomitant, use of non-steroidal anti-inflammatory drugs (NSAIDs).

As mentioned above, 10% of sJIA patients can progress to overt MAS. Ferritin, an acute phase reactant, is a very sensitive indicator of this condition. A sudden drop of at least two cell lines in the CBC, a rising C-reactive protein with decreasing ESR, elevated liver transaminases, prolonged prothrombin or partial thromboplastin times, high D-dimer levels, elevated triglycerides, and low fibrinogen should all alert the caretakers about the likelihood of MAS in a child with sJIA.[9]

While 75–85% of adult RA patients have either a RF or CCP antibody, less than 5% of JIA patients have RF, and those are mostly the early onset RA patients, often teenage girls with symmetric small joint involvement. Another rather frequently ordered test is the serum ANA titer. Similar to the RF, the ANA is not suited for screening, as it is of no diagnostic utility in either making or excluding the diagnosis of JIA.[34] The ANA is useful for identifying already diagnosed JIA patients at highest risk for developing uveitis.[19] In addition, the ANA may alert the clinician to the possibility of juvenile Sjögren disease or lupus as the etiology of the chronic arthritis.

The prevalence of the HLA-B27 antigen is 8% in the general Caucasian population but nearly 90% in the ankylosing spondylitis group. HLA-B27 is useful to predict axial involvement in ERA, psoriatic and IBD-related arthritis patients, but should be evaluated in patients with clinically established arthritis and/or enthesitis rather than as a routine screening test during a work-up for back pain.

Additional laboratory indicators can be helpful. Elevated serum lactate dehydrogenase and uric acid levels can point toward malignancy. Elevated angiotensin converting enzyme (ACE) and lysozyme levels can both be useful when considering sarcoidosis as the etiology of childhood arthritis and uveitis, but non-caseating granulomas seen on biopsy are much more revealing.[1] In addition, a wide variety of imaging techniques are available for diagnosing arthritis and evaluating treatment.[35]

Differential diagnosis

A wide variety of conditions can mimic symptoms and signs of JIA.[29] While both acute and chronic arthritis can present with joint pain, tenderness, swelling, and warmth, a single acutely involved joint at onset should be considered septic until proven otherwise.[1] Septic arthritis frequently has an erythematous discoloration of the skin while JIA does not. Prompt evaluation with arthrocentesis is necessary, especially in indeterminate cases. Infection of the joint may lead not only to rapid destruction but also to dissemination of infection systemically.

Parainfectious arthritis, often due to viral disease, is usually short-lived and typically requires only NSAID treatment. In contrast, Lyme disease is characterized by a chronic extensively swollen joint(s), commonly the knee.[1] It appears several weeks to months after the usually unnoticed tick bite and should be considered in areas of high incidence (e.g., northeastern United States). There are a few diseases associated with migratory arthritis, including malignancy, gonococcal arthritis, and rheumatic fever arthritis, the latter having a typically very tender, red, hot joint persisting in each location for a couple of hours before moving to another.

As sJIA is a diagnosis by exclusion, multiple other etiologies of systemic inflammation should be considered. Fever and elevated WBCs, platelets, and ESR can also accompany polyarteritis nodosa, Kawasaki disease, Henoch-Schönlein purpura, and other vasculitides.[1] Ehrlichiosis and recurrent fever syndromes (e.g., familial Mediterranean fever, TNF receptor-associated periodic fever syndrome) can also manifest as systemic inflammation, arthralgias, and rashes. A typically non-erosive symmetric arthritis can occur in systemic lupus erythematosus (SLE),[1] often with cytopenias. Arthritis is also seen in related diseases (e.g., mixed connective tissue disease (MCTD)), and evidence of antibodies to extractable nuclear antigens are common in SLE (anti-Smith, anti-double-stranded DNA) and MCTD (anti-ribonuclear protein).

Patients presenting with joint pain only, without associated swelling or morning stiffness, most commonly have overuse syndromes or benign hypermobility syndrome.[1] Little league shoulder and elbow are rather common in middle school aged baseball players; wrist pain occurs in gymnasts frequently. Pain in the hip without morning stiffness can indicate Legg-Calve-Perthes disease or slipped capital femoral epiphysis. Relentless knee pain in teenagers without improvement can be due to osteochondritis dissecans. Other common causes of teenage knee pain include Osgood-Schlatter disease and patello-femoral syndrome.[1]

Clinically silent complications

There are two common findings that present insidiously during the course of JIA yet can cause major damage/morbidity, namely, uveitis and TMJ arthritis.

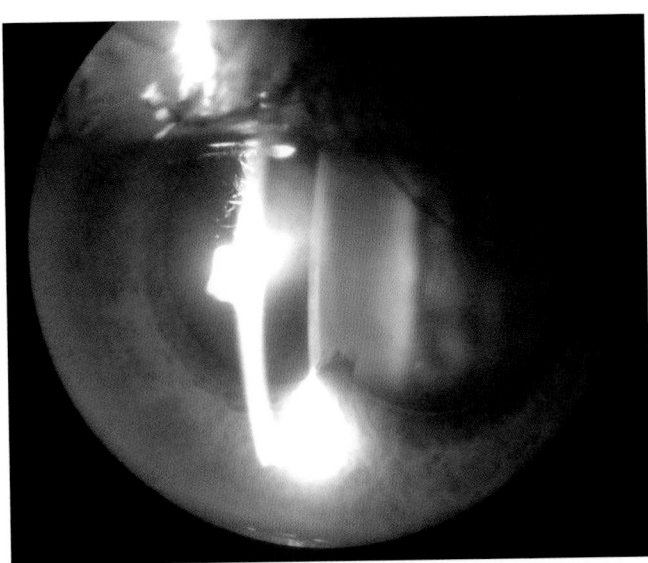

Fig. 52.2 Posterior synechia, a complication of chronic anterior uveitis, is associated with several categories of JIA. The irregularities of the inner margins of the iris reflect fibrous adhesions between the iris and lens capsule.
Courtesy of Dr. Scott Olitsky.

Uveitis is a relatively common complication of JIA with potentially long-term morbidity. It usually presents as iridocyclitis but the choroid can also be affected. While extremely rare in sJIA, approximately 20% of oligoarticular and 5% of polyarticular JIA patients develop eye inflammation.[19] Some children with psoriatic JIA are also at risk of developing silent uveitis. Uveitis can lead to a great deal of morbidity including cataracts, increased intraocular pressure, band keratopathy, and posterior synechiae (Fig. 52.2), with up to 40% developing decreased vision.[36] The danger of most JIA-associated uveitis is the asymptomatic presentation, with the exception of symptomatic uveitis in children with ERA. Considering that the highest prevalence is in oligoarticular JIA, which is most common in preschool and younger children, it is not surprising that many of them go unnoticed. A routine ophthalmologic exam may fail to detect uveitis, and children need to have a formal slit lamp exam to look for inflammatory cells.[19] The most common presenting signs are synechiae (an irregular iris border due to adhesions to the lens), hypopyon, and band keratopathy (Fig. 52.2). Uveitis may develop many months or years after joint presentation which warrants close follow-up. ANA positivity and young age are associated with increased incidence; thus ANA+ oligoarticular children need to be screened the most often, but other categories are suggested to follow a set schedule as well.[37] Failure to do so and missed eye involvement can lead to cataracts, glaucoma, impaired vision, and even blindness.

KEY CONCEPTS

Temporomandibular joint (TMJ) arthritis

- TMJ arthritis is extremely common, present in up to 80% of children with JIA. It is typically asymptomatic and thus requires early screening by MRI with contrast.
- TMJ arthritis is often active despite therapy with DMARDs and biologics (e.g., methotrexate plus TNF inhibitors) and thus requires treatment with intra-articular long-acting corticosteroids to help prevent mandibular growth damage and associated micrognathia and facial dysmorphology.

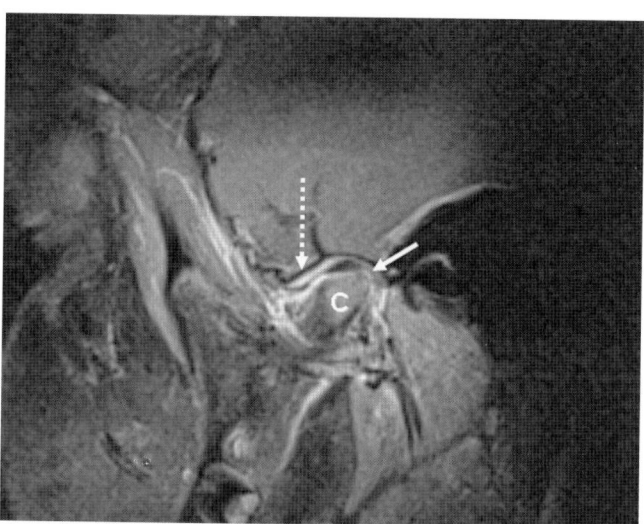

Fig. 52.3 Acute and chronic TMJ arthritis in a child with JIA. Synovial thickening and enhancement (long dashed arrow) and mandibular condyle ("C") flattening with contour irregularity/erosion (short arrow) are noted in this parasagittal post-contrast T1-weighted MRI image.
Courtesy of Dr. Dan Young.

Another frequently asymptomatic complication of JIA is TMJ arthritis. TMJ arthritis in children with JIA has been recognized increasingly in recent years as a joint inflammation leading to silent destruction and facial deformity despite systemic therapy.[38] TMJ arthritis is quite common with 40–80% of all JIA patients affected.[4] The overall true prevalence is likely closer to the higher range since not all children with JIA receive TMJ MRI screening (Fig. 52.3) at disease onset, and pre-micrognathic arthritis may be missed.[4] The highest rates of TMJ arthritis have been found in the extended oligoarticular and RF-negative polyarticular groups, as well as those children with upper extremity and neck involvement, and with an elevated ESR.[39] Currently, intra-articular corticosteroid injection seems to be the most effective therapy, whereas TMJ arthritis often develops despite systemic use of methotrexate and TNF inhibitors.[4,38] TMJ arthritis needs to be recognized early in children with JIA so it can be treated prior to growth disturbance.

Treatment

Overview

Despite significant advances in the understanding of the pathogenesis of JIA, there are currently no curative treatments. JIA frequently persists into adulthood and may result in significant morbidity including physical disability. The objective of treatment is to prevent disability and preserve normal growth and development while providing relief of symptoms and improved quality of life by controlling the inflammatory process.[40]

Over the past 15 years, remarkable advances in the treatment of JIA have been made. Chief among these advances was the advent of targeted biologic therapeutic agents (Table 52.2). These agents have been shown to be quite beneficial against active disease and generally well tolerated.[41] The early initiation of biologic therapeutic agents may in fact alter and improve the subsequent disease course.[42] These new breakthroughs have prompted pediatric rheumatologists to "invert the treatment pyramid," that is to rapidly incorporate more effective therapeutic agents instead of slowly progressing to them in a stepwise fashion.[43]

● THERAPEUTIC PRINCIPLES

Early aggressive therapy

■ Accumulating evidence suggests that early aggressive therapy that includes targeted biologic agents near the time of clinical diagnosis (during the "window of opportunity") may possibly permanently improve the future disease course.

In response to the growing number of treatment options for JIA and the advent of the biologic therapeutics, the American College of Rheumatology (ACR) issued Recommendations for the Treatment of JIA in 2011.[44] These recommendations were developed using a rigorous methodology to produce evidence- and consensus-based guidance that reflected the current state of the field.

Table 52.2 Biologic therapeutic agents used in the treatment of JIA

Biologic target	Name	Structure	Frequency of administration	Route of administration
Tumor necrosis factor	Etanercept	Receptor-IgG fusion protein	Twice weekly to weekly	SQ injection
	Infliximab	Monoclonal antibody (chimeric)	Every 4 to 8 weeks	IV infusion
	Adalimumab	Monoclonal antibody (humanized)	Every 1 to 2 weeks	SQ injection
	Golimumab	Monoclonal antibody (humanized)	Every 4 weeks	SQ injection
	Certolizumab pegol	Monoclonal antibody (humanized and PEGylated)	Every 2 weeks	SQ injection
CD80/86	Abatacept	CTLA-4-IgG fusion protein	Every 4 weeks	IV infusion
IL-1	Anakinra	Receptor antagonist	Daily	SQ injection
	Canakinumab	Monoclonal antibody (humanized)	Every 8 weeks	SQ injection
	Rilonacept	Receptor-fusion protein	Weekly	SQ injection
IL-6 receptor	Tocilizumab	Monoclonal antibody (humanized)	Every 2 weeks	IV infusion
CD20+ B-cells	Rituximab	Monoclonal antibody	2 infusions 2 weeks apart, repeat every 6 months	IV infusion

With new and effective therapies continuing to be introduced to the therapeutic armamentarium, treatment goals have become elevated and more stringent. The current goal is to attain clinically inactive disease,[45] that is, the absence of any significant signs or symptoms of active arthritis. Though this is not always currently possible for all children, until there is curative therapy for JIA attainment of inactive disease status for as many children as possible remains the goal.

Despite recent advances, the treatment of JIA is not currently influenced by some of the distinct categories of JIA. For example, there are no specific therapies directed at psoriatic arthritis as opposed to oligoarthritis or RF-negative polyarthritis. Accordingly, the discussion of treatment in this chapter will not detail all categories of JIA, but will focus rather on the "treatment groups" as defined by the 2011 ACR JIA Recommendations.[44]

Non-steroidal anti-inflammatory drugs

NSAIDs formed the foundation of the treatment of JIA for decades, and numerous NSAIDs have been shown to have beneficial effects. In the absence of significant numbers of head-to-head trials, it is believed that in general all NSAIDs are similarly effective,[31] although indomethacin is considered by some to be the most effective NSAID (especially in sJIA). One NSAID may be found to be more effective for a particular individual child than a different NSAID.

In general, NSAIDs are not considered to be disease modifying agents, that is, they are not felt to slow the progression of disease or prevent the appearance of radiographic damage. For this reason, monotherapy with NSAIDs initially began to decline in favor with the advent of agents, such as methotrexate, that have been shown to modify the disease process. NSAIDs are frequently used for symptomatic relief, but most children who require daily chronic use of NSAIDs would likely benefit from the addition of systemic immunosuppression, such as from DMARDs.

Gastrointestinal discomfort is a frequent adverse effect of NSAID therapy,[1] though frank gastrointestinal bleeding appears to occur at a lower incidence than in adults. Scarring pseudoporphyria of sun exposed skin is another risk of NSAIDs.[1] The long-term cardiovascular effects of NSAIDs in children have not been studied.

Glucocorticoids

As for many rheumatologic diseases, JIA has been shown to respond to treatment with glucocorticoids (Chapter 87). Intra-articular glucocorticoid injections typically result in a near immediate decrease in inflammation that is maintained for many months.[46] Accordingly, intra-articular injections may form the foundation of therapy for children with mild or limited oligoarthritis. In addition, intra-articular injections can be effective in children with more extensive arthritis and in those who are receiving concurrent systemic therapy. Randomized trials have shown unequivocally that triamcinolone hexacetonide has the longest duration of effect following injection.[46]

JIA also may be effectively treated with systemic glucocorticoids. They are frequently used in the treatment of systemic features of JIA and may form the foundation of the treatment for the sJIA category. The use of systemic glucocorticoids for the treatment of synovitis in children with JIA is not an uncommon practice. However, the risks, benefits, and appropriate use of this approach are less clear. The recent 2011 ACR JIA Recommendations remain silent on this use of systemic glucocorticoids due to the near complete absence of any published evidence.[44] In general, most pediatric rheumatologists would agree that the use of DMARD agents is preferable to the use of moderate- or high-dose systemic glucocorticoids for the treatment of synovitis in JIA. The anticipated adverse effects of long-term use of moderate doses of glucocorticoids can include growth failure, osteoporosis, cataract formation, glaucoma, hyperglycemia, hypertension, avascular necrosis of bone, striae, and others.[1]

Non-biologic disease modifying anti-rheumatic drugs

The use of DMARDs was introduced in the 1980s (Chapter 88). The most widely used and studied is methotrexate, which has been shown to be efficacious for treatment of JIA in randomized clinical trials.[31] Following these studies, methotrexate became the cornerstone of therapy for many children with JIA. Methotrexate is typically administered weekly through either the oral or subcutaneous route, though studies have shown subcutaneous methotrexate to be better absorbed and more effective.[31]

Methotrexate can be associated with several typically minor adverse effects, such as nausea and fatigue. Occasionally, methotrexate can cause liver toxicity, necessitating periodic measurement of serum aminotransferase levels for routine monitoring.[1]

Leflunomide has been shown to be similarly to slightly less efficacious than methotrexate in the treatment of JIA.[31] It may serve as an alternative therapy for children who are intolerant of methotrexate. Sulfasalazine is used to a varying degree among pediatric rheumatologists and may be of particular benefit to children with the ERA JIA category.[31] Hydroxychloroquine monotherapy has been demonstrated inefficacious in treating JIA.[31]

Biologic disease modifying anti-rheumatic drugs

The use of biologic DMARDs for the treatment of JIA began in the late 1990s (Chapter 92). Etanercept, a TNF-α inhibitor, was the first studied and was shown to be efficacious in a randomized clinical trial.[41] Additional TNF-α inhibitors have been introduced and used in the treatment of JIA; adalimumab was also shown to be efficacious in a randomized clinical trial.[41] Notable differences have been discovered regarding the effectiveness of the TNF receptor fusion protein (etanercept) and the monoclonal antibodies (adalimumab, infliximab, others). MAb TNF-α inhibitors have been shown to be effective against two important JIA-associated conditions: anterior uveitis and IBD. Receptor fusion proteins have been shown to be far less effective for these conditions. The precise mechanism for these differences in treatment effectiveness is not clear, but may be related to the ability of etanercept to bind TNF-β (lymphotoxin) or the ability of the mAb to bind surface membrane-bound TNF-α.[47]

Because the TNF-α inhibitors are large proteins, they must be administered parenterally, either by subcutaneous injection or intravenous infusion (Table 52.2). TNF-α inhibitors are not generally associated with common medication adverse effects, such as headache or nausea, though they may result in injection site or infusion reactions. There appears to be a modest increase in the incidence of bacterial infections associated with TNF-α inhibitor use, but a significant risk of re-activation of latent tuberculosis.[41] Therefore, individuals should be screened for tuberculosis infection prior to initiating treatment with TNF-α inhibitors.[44]

The possible association between TNF-α inhibitors and an increased rate of malignancy in JIA remains an open question;[48] however, currently there is no convincing evidence of a strong increased risk of overall malignancy.

In addition to TNF-α inhibitors, the T-cell co-stimulation modulator, abatacept, has been shown to be efficacious for the treatment of JIA in a randomized clinical trial.[23,41] At present, it remains to be seen how this agent will be best used to treat JIA.

The B-cell depleting agent, rituximab, has been minimally studied in the treatment of JIA.[41] However, it appears effective in some instances, particularly for those children who appear to have early onset RA (teenagers with RF[+] and CCP[+] polyarthritis).

The IL-1 inhibitor, anakinra, has been shown to be particularly effective in the treatment of sJIA in uncontrolled studies.[49] Similar to the experience in adults with RA, anakinra appears less effective in treating synovitis among children with the other categories of JIA.[41] Additional IL-1 inhibitors (rilonacept, canakinumab) are now commercially available. It remains to be seen how these agents will be best used in treating JIA.

The IL-6 inhibitor tocilizumab has been shown in randomized clinical trials to be efficacious in the treatment of sJIA,[50] but only recently became commercially available in the United States and Europe. It may prove to be a valuable therapeutic agent in the treatment of synovitis in children with other categories of JIA as well.

There are numerous other investigational agents currently being evaluated for the treatment of RA. It is likely that many of these newer agents will prove effective in the treatment of JIA as well.

Treatment of oligoarthritis (arthritis of 4 or fewer joints)

Due to fewer involved joints, oligoarthritis may generally be viewed as a milder form of JIA. However, significant disability can still occur and children with this condition should not be assumed to experience good clinical outcomes without proper evaluation and therapy. The foundation of treatment for this JIA phenotype is intra-articular glucocorticoid injections. These injections may be performed in multiple joints concurrently and may be repeated as needed.[46] A good response typically results in resolution of clinical signs and symptoms of arthritis for 4 to 12 months. Children who do not respond as desired to injections or who have more significant arthritis should initiate DMARD therapy.[44] Methotrexate is typically the first choice. Significant arthritis that does not respond adequately to methotrexate can be treated with TNF-α inhibitors.[44]

Treatment of polyarthritis (arthritis of 5 or more joints)

Methotrexate is currently recommended for nearly all children with polyarthritis.[44] If a brief trial of methotrexate proves inadequate to control the arthritis, then TNF-α inhibitors are frequently recommended.[44] If there is not an adequate response to the initial TNF-α inhibitor, then switching to another of the TNF-α inhibitors or switching to abatacept is currently recommended.[44] The precise role of other biologic DMARDs, such as rituximab and tocilizumab (Table 52.2), in the treatment of JIA is yet to be defined.

Treatment of arthritis involving specific joints

Arthritis involving the TMJ, hip, and sacroiliac joints may deserve special therapy. Destructive arthritis of the TMJ among children with JIA has been noted for decades. Clinical evaluation of this joint is particularly challenging, as symptoms are often absent initially and physical examination findings may be normal.[4] Accordingly, the optimal treatment of TMJ arthritis is unclear. Most authors recommend targeted therapy with intra-articular glucocorticoid injections, similar to the treatment of arthritis in other joints.[4] Increased systemic therapy is likely also appropriate, though TMJ arthritis has been known to demonstrate radiographic progression despite treatment with systemic TNF-α inhibitors and in the absence of signs of active synovitis of other joints.[38]

The presence of hip arthritis in JIA has been shown in several studies to portend a poor prognosis.[44] Accordingly, many authors advocate early intra-articular glucocorticoid injections and increased systemic therapy when active hip arthritis is identified.

Sacroiliac arthritis is strongly associated with the development of ankylosing spondylitis. Because axial arthritis has been shown to be less responsive to methotrexate therapy, current recommendations suggest a lower threshold for the initiation of TNF-α inhibitors when sacroiliac arthritis is present.[44] However, some recent evidence suggests that TNF-α inhibitors may not be the optimal choice for the treatment of ankylosing spondylitis due to the apparent inability to prevent progression of ankylosis in all affected individuals.[51]

Treatment of erosive arthritis

It appears that not all children with JIA have the propensity to develop an erosive arthritis that is similar to that frequently seen in adults with RA. Children who develop erosions visualized on plain radiographs are considered to have a worse prognosis, and the current recommendation is to increase the intensity of their treatment accordingly.[44]

Treatment of systemic features of systemic arthritis

For decades, the mainstay of therapy for sJIA has been systemic glucocorticoids and NSAIDs. Nearly all children with sJIA will respond favorably to systemic glucocorticoids, if given in sufficient doses. However, often children become "steroid-dependent" and efforts to decrease the glucocorticoid burden to minimize adverse effects are unsuccessful.

Presumably due to its different pathogenesis, sJIA has not been shown to respond to TNF-α inhibitors as favorably as the other categories of JIA. Instead, IL-1 and -6 appear to be key cytokines in the disease process. Treatment with the IL-1 inhibitor, anakinra, is currently recommended for children who require a second-line therapy in addition to systemic glucocorticoids.[44] IL-6 inhibition is likely to play a key future role in the treatment of many children with sJIA (Table 52.2).

The appearance of clinically significant MAS generally requires directed therapy. The typical treatment approach involves increased systemic glucocorticoids. The calcineurin inhibitor, cyclosporine, is frequently added,[52] and some authors advocate IL-1 and -6 inhibitors for treatment of MAS.[28] In severe refractory cases, cytotoxic chemotherapeutic agents, such as cyclophosphamide or etoposide, may be warranted.[9]

Treatment of arthritis of systemic arthritis

Some children with sJIA will develop a chronic course of polyarthritis with a relative absence of concurrent systemic features. In general, it is recommended these children be treated similarly to children with polyarthritis who did not have systemic features at onset.[44] Indeed, these children have been included in clinical trials of biologic agents for the treatment of polyarthritis.

Treatment of uveitis

JIA-associated anterior uveitis frequently requires directed therapy. Topical glucocorticoid eye drops, such as prednisolone acetate 1%, are frequently initiated at the time of diagnosis by the treating ophthalmologist.[53] Though effective in decreasing the inflammation of uveitis, glucocorticoid eye drops cannot be tolerated in high doses for extended periods of time due to the development of cataracts and glaucoma.[53] For this reason, systemic medications are frequently employed in the treatment of JIA-associated uveitis. Methotrexate has been shown to be effective for uveitis and is the most commonly used systemic medication.[53] The mAb TNF-α inhibitors (infliximab, adalimumab, and others) have been shown highly effective in the treatment of anterior uveitis in uncontrolled studies, and they are a frequent choice for children in whom methotrexate proves inadequate to control the disease.[53] Other biologic agents (rituximab and abatacept) appear to be effective in some children with refractory uveitis but their overall role remains unclear.

Duration of therapy

As stated, the current goal of therapy is the attainment of clinically inactive disease. However, once this goal is attained, the appropriate next steps in management are less clear. Though none of the currently available therapies are believed to be curative, many children are able to successfully decrease or discontinue therapies after attaining inactive disease status without immediate recurrence of active disease. Many pediatric rheumatologists will consider decreasing the level of therapy if inactive disease status is maintained for a prolonged period, such as 12 months, though this is arbitrary. A recent randomized study showed no difference in the rate of disease flare following discontinuation of methotrexate after approximately 9 versus 15 months of inactive disease prior to discontinuation.[54] The further study of the appropriate management of children who attain prolonged inactive disease status will be an important future focus.

Translational research

The explosion in advances in immunology and genetics are leading to major breakthroughs in therapy for rheumatic diseases, including JIA. Challenges remain, however, in diagnosing and treating MAS complicating sJIA. To distinguish sJIA disease flare from MAS, expert opinion and Delphi techniques are currently exploring novel criteria for diagnosing MAS among children with sJIA. Data collection regarding clinical, laboratory, and pathologic features of children with sJIA, with and without

---

ON THE HORIZON

- Novel criteria for identifying MAS among children with sJIA will rely on clinical features and timely and available laboratory findings for early diagnosis.
- Genetic screening for mutations in cytolytic pathway genes will help identify those individuals at risk for developing MAS.
- Murine models are paving the way for better understanding of MAS immunopathology and potential pathways for clinical intervention.
- Clinical trials involving treatment of MAS with inhibitors of pro-inflammatory cytokines are just around the corner.

MAS, are being used to further refine the preliminary diagnostic criteria. Furthermore, genetic mutations and polymorphisms in genes linked to the defective cytolytic pathway in lymphocytes from MAS patients are being explored to identify sJIA patients with propensity to develop MAS. Mouse models of MAS are helping to better understand MAS immunopathology and the role of pro-inflammatory cytokines in the process. Early recognition of MAS and a better understanding of the role of various cytokines in the pathogenesis of MAS will allow for improved targeted therapy for this often fatal condition.

References

1. Weiss JE, Ilowite NT. Juvenile idiopathic arthritis. Rheum Dis Clin North Am 2007;33(3):441–70 vi.
2. Petty RE, Southwood TR, Manners P, et al. International League of Associations for Rheumatology classification of juvenile idiopathic arthritis: second revision, Edmonton, 2001. J Rheumatol 2004;31(2):390–2.
3. Berkun Y, Padeh S. Environmental factors and the geoepidemiology of juvenile idiopathic arthritis. Autoimmun Rev 2010;9(5):A319–24.
4. Ringold S, Cron RQ. The temporomandibular joint in juvenile idiopathic arthritis: frequently used and frequently arthritic. Pediatr Rheumatol Online J 2009;7:11.
5. Ravelli A, Varnier GC, Oliveira S, et al. Antinuclear antibody-positive patients should be grouped as a separate category in the classification of juvenile idiopathic arthritis. Arthritis Rheum 2011;63(1):267–75.
6. Prahalad S, Glass DN. A comprehensive review of the genetics of juvenile idiopathic arthritis. Pediatr Rheumatol Online J 2008;6:11.
7. Vastert SJ, Kuis W, Grom AA. Systemic JIA: new developments in the understanding of the pathophysiology and treatment. Best Pract Res Clin Rheumatol 2009;23(5):655–64.
8. Goldbach-Mansky R, Kastner DL. Autoinflammation: the prominent role of IL-1 in monogenic autoinflammatory diseases and implications for common illnesses. J Allergy Clin Immunol 2009;124(6):1141–9; quiz 50–1.
9. Grom AA, Mellins ED. Macrophage activation syndrome: advances towards understanding pathogenesis. Curr Opin Rheumatol 2010;22(5):561–6.
10. Behrens EM. Macrophage activation syndrome in rheumatic disease: what is the role of the antigen presenting cell? Autoimmun Rev 2008;7(4):305–308.
11. Colbert RA, DeLay ML, Klenk EI, Layh-Schmitt G. From HLA-B27 to spondyloarthritis: a journey through the ER. Immunol Rev 2010;233(1):181–202.
12. de Vries R. Genetics of rheumatoid arthritis: time for a change!. Curr Opin Rheumatol 2011;23(3):227–32.
13. Angeles-Han S, Prahalad S. The genetics of juvenile idiopathic arthritis: what is new in 2010? Curr Rheumatol Rep 2010;12(2):87–93.
14. Hewagama A, Richardson B. The genetics and epigenetics of autoimmune diseases. J Autoimmun 2009;33(1):3–11.
15. Prakken BJ, Albani S. Using biology of disease to understand and guide therapy of JIA. Best Pract Res Clin Rheumatol 2009;23(5):599–608.
16. Stoll ML. Interactions of the innate and adaptive arms of the immune system in the pathogenesis of spondyloarthritis. Clin Exp Rheumatol 2011;29(2):322–30.
17. Steere AC, Drouin EE, Glickstein LJ. Relationship between immunity to Borrelia burgdorferi outer-surface protein A (OspA) and Lyme arthritis. Clin Infect Dis 2011;52(Suppl. 3):s259–65.
18. Davies K, Stiehm ER, Woo P, Murray KJ. Juvenile idiopathic polyarticular arthritis and IgA deficiency in the 22q11 deletion syndrome. J Rheumatol 2001;28(10):2326–34.
19. Wright T, Cron RQ. Pediatric rheumatology for the adult rheumatologist II: uveitis in juvenile idiopathic arthritis. J Clin Rheumatol 2007;13(4):205–10.
20. Mor-Vaknin N, Kappes F, Dick AE, et al. DEK in the synovium of patients with juvenile idiopathic arthritis: characterization of DEK antibodies and posttranslational modification of the DEK autoantigen. Arthritis Rheum 2011;63(2):556–67.

21. Syed RH, Gilliam BE, Moore TL. Rheumatoid factors and anticyclic citrullinated peptide antibodies in pediatric rheumatology. Curr Rheumatol Rep 2008;10(2):156–63.
22. Ochs HD, Gambineri E, Torgerson TR. IPEX, FOXP3 and regulatory T-cells: a model for autoimmunity. Immunol Res 2007;38(1–3):112–21.
23. Cron RQ. A signal achievement in the treatment of arthritis. Arthritis Rheum 2005;52(8):2229–32.
24. Weaver CT, Hatton RD. Interplay between the TH17 and TReg cell lineages: a (co-) evolutionary perspective. Nat Rev Immunol 2009;9(12):883–9.
25. Nistala K, Wedderburn LR. Th17 and regulatory T cells: rebalancing pro- and anti-inflammatory forces in autoimmune arthritis. Rheumatology (Oxford) 2009;48(6):602–606.
26. Shenoi S, Wallace CA. Tumor necrosis factor inhibitors in the management of juvenile idiopathic arthritis: an evidence-based review. Paediatr Drugs 2010; 12(6):367–77.
27. Pascual V, Allantaz F, Patel P, et al. How the study of children with rheumatic diseases identified interferon-alpha and interleukin-1 as novel therapeutic targets. Immunol Rev 2008;223:39–59.
28. Miettunen PM, Narendran A, Jayanthan A, et al. Successful treatment of severe paediatric rheumatic disease-associated macrophage activation syndrome with interleukin-1 inhibition following conventional immunosuppressive therapy: case series with 12 patients. Rheumatology (Oxford) 2011;50(2):417–9.
29. Boros C, Whitehead B. Juvenile idiopathic arthritis. Aust Fam Physician 2010;39(9):630–6.
30. Houghton KM. Review for the generalist: evaluation of pediatric hip pain. Pediatr Rheumatol Online J 2009;7:10.
31. Hashkes PJ, Laxer RM. Medical treatment of juvenile idiopathic arthritis. JAMA 2005;294(13):1671–84.
32. Stoll ML, Nigrovic PA. Subpopulations within juvenile psoriatic arthritis: a review of the literature. Clin Dev Immunol 2006;13(2–4):377–80.
33. Colbert RA. Classification of juvenile spondyloarthritis: Enthesitis-related arthritis and beyond. Nat Rev Rheumatol 2010;6(8):477–85.
34. McGhee JL, Kickingbird LM, Jarvis JN. Clinical utility of antinuclear antibody tests in children. BMC Pediatr 2004;4:13.
35. McKay GM, Cox LA, Long BW. Imaging juvenile idiopathic arthritis: assessing the modalities. Radiol Technol 2010;81(4):318–27.
36. Kump LI, Castaneda RA, Androudi SN, et al. Visual outcomes in children with juvenile idiopathic arthritis-associated uveitis. Ophthalmology 2006;113(10):1874–7.
37. Cassidy J, Kivlin J, Lindsley C, Nocton J. Ophthalmologic examinations in children with juvenile rheumatoid arthritis. Pediatrics 2006;117(5):1843–5.
38. Arabshahi B, Cron RQ. Temporomandibular joint arthritis in juvenile idiopathic arthritis: the forgotten joint. Curr Opin Rheumatol 2006;18(5):490–5.
39. Cannizzaro E, Schroeder S, Muller LM, et al. Temporomandibular joint involvement in children with juvenile idiopathic arthritis. J Rheumatol 2011;38(3):510–5.
40. Beresford MW. Juvenile idiopathic arthritis: new insights into classification, measures of outcome, and pharmacotherapy. Paediatr Drugs 2011;13(3):161–73.
41. Hayward K, Wallace CA. Recent developments in anti-rheumatic drugs in pediatrics: treatment of juvenile idiopathic arthritis. Arthritis Res Ther 2009;11(1):216.
42. Cush JJ. Early rheumatoid arthritis—is there a window of opportunity? J Rheumatol Suppl 2007;80:1–7.
43. Prince FH, Otten MH, van Suijlekom-Smit LW. Diagnosis and management of juvenile idiopathic arthritis. BMJ 2010;341:c6434.
44. Beukelman T, Patkar NM, Saag KG, et al. 2011 American College of Rheumatology recommendations for the treatment of juvenile idiopathic arthritis: Initiation and safety monitoring of therapeutic agents for the treatment of arthritis and systemic features. Arthritis Care Res (Hoboken) 2011;63(4):465–82.
45. Wallace CA, Ruperto N, Giannini E. Preliminary criteria for clinical remission for select categories of juvenile idiopathic arthritis. J Rheumatol 2004;31(11):2290–4.
46. Scott C, Meiorin S, Filocamo G, et al. A reappraisal of intra-articular corticosteroid therapy in juvenile idiopathic arthritis. Clin Exp Rheumatol 2010;28(5):774–81.
47. Rigby WF. Drug insight: different mechanisms of action of tumor necrosis factor antagonists-passive-aggressive behavior? Nat Clin Pract Rheumatol 2007;3(4):227–33.
48. Cron RQ, Beukelman T. Guilt by association—what is the true risk of malignancy in children treated with etanercept for JIA? Pediatr Rheumatol Online J 2010;8:23.
49. Nigrovic PA, Mannion M, Prince FH, et al. Anakinra as first-line disease-modifying therapy in systemic juvenile idiopathic arthritis: report of forty-six patients from an international multicenter series. Arthritis Rheum 2011;63(2):545–55.
50. Yokota S, Imagawa T, Mori M, et al. Efficacy and safety of tocilizumab in patients with systemic-onset juvenile idiopathic arthritis: a randomised, double-blind, placebo-controlled, withdrawal phase III trial. Lancet 2008;371(9617):998–1006.
51. Haibel H, Sieper J. Editorial review: how early should ankylosing spondylitis be treated with a tumor necrosis factor-blocker? Curr Opin Rheumatol 2010;22(4):388–92.
52. Deane S, Selmi C, Teuber SS, Gershwin ME. Macrophage activation syndrome in autoimmune disease. Int Arch Allergy Immunol 2010;153(2):109–20.
53. Simonini G, Cantarini L, Bresci C, et al. Current therapeutic approaches to autoimmune chronic uveitis in children. Autoimmun Rev 2010;9(10):674–83.
54. Foell D, Wulffraat N, Wedderburn LR, et al. Methotrexate withdrawal at 6 vs 12 months in juvenile idiopathic arthritis in remission: a randomized clinical trial. JAMA 2010;303(13):1266–73.

Gabor Illei,
Sarfaraz A. Hasni,
Ilias Alevizos

Sjögren's syndrome

Sjögren's syndrome (SS) is a chronic systemic autoimmune disease characterized by lachrymal and salivary gland dysfunction. It was named after the Swedish ophthalmologist Henrik Sjögren after he reported 19 cases of keratoconjunctivitis in 1933.[1] The hallmark feature of SS is deficient tear and saliva production due to lymphocytic infiltration of the salivary and lachrymal glands leading to *xerostomia* (dry mouth) and *xerophthalmia* (dry eyes). In addition, SS can involve any organ system and present with a wide spectrum of clinical features. The autoimmune process seems to primarily affect the lining epithelium of various organs; in fact some experts propose the term "autoimmune epithelitis" to be used instead of SS.[2]

Epidemiology

Sjögren's syndrome predominantly effects females (female:male ratio 9:1) in their fourth and fifth decades of life. However, symptoms can be present for much longer time and there is usually a 5- to 10-year delay in the diagnosis of SS. The reported prevalence of SS varies widely from 0.1 to 4.8%.[3] This variation may be due to the use of different classification criteria, geographical and environmental influences, and study size and target population. When a more strict definition is applied to the available data the true prevalence of SS is estimated to be around 1%,[4] making it the second most common systemic rheumatic disease after rheumatoid arthritis.

Immunopathogenesis

The pathogenesis of SS is still largely unknown. In a genetically predisposed individual, various environmental factors, such as viral infections, may lead to epithelial cell activation and a protracted inflammatory response with features of autoimmunity. Autoreactive lymphocytes and autoantibodies are considered important in this process, although the pathogenic role of any particular autoantibody is still undefined.[5]

Immunogenetic factors

There is a well-established association between SS with HLA class II genes. The first HLA class II associations described with primary SS were with DR3 and DR2 in European populations. This genetic association predominantly involves antibody-positive but not antibody-negative Sjögren patients. Several small studies suggested an association between anti-Ro/SSA and anti-La/SSB antibodies and molecularly defined HLA-DR and HLA-DQ alleles, especially *DRB1*0301*, *DRB1*15*, and *DQB1*0201*. Several genetic polymorphisms previously linked to other autoimmune diseases are also associated with SS. From these, two transcription factors, STAT4 (signal transducer and activator of transcription 4) and IRF5 (interferon regulatory factor 5), which were both independently associated with SS showed an additive effect increasing the risk of SS from around 1.6–1.9 for one risk allele to 6.7 when both risk alleles were present.[6] Ongoing large genome-wide association studies will soon provide better insight in the genetic basis of SS.

Environmental factors

The inciting event in the pathogenesis of SS is not known, and it may not be a single event. The strong predominance of females suggests gender-specific predisposing factors. Although sex hormones are obvious targets, there is no conclusive proof yet that the difference in the pathogenesis between males and females is due to sex hormones alone. Estrogens are considered contributors to autoimmunity, whereas androgens are thought to be protective. But since the peak age of onset in SS occurs around menopause, characterized by a decrease in estrogens, the increased risk may be due to a change in the androgen–estrogen ratio rather than absolute levels of estrogens. Ovaries produce low levels of testosterone, which decrease at the time of menopause. The other significant source of androgens is the adrenal cortex, which produces dehydroepiandrosterone (DHEA), a weak androgen prohormone that can be converted to either androgens or estrogen locally in target organs. This intracrine conversion of DHEA to active sex steroids accounts for a significant proportion of all sex steroids produced in humans. Patients with SS have low systemic DHEA levels as well as a defective intacrine processing of DHEA in salivary glands, suggesting both a systemic and local androgen deficient state. Women may be particularly vulnerable to local androgen deficiency in the salivary gland in SS since their local dihydrotestosterone production is completely dependent on local conversion of DHEA, whereas in men systemic androgens may satisfy the local requirement.[7]

Viral infections have also been proposed as inciting events. This theory is strongly supported by the fact that chronic inflammation of the salivary glands has been observed with chronic hepatitis C, HTLV-1, and human immunodeficiency virus infections, and such infections cause a disease with a clinical spectrum very similar to that of SS. The fact that some viruses, such as Epstein–Barr virus (EBV), are known to replicate in oropharyngeal and lachrymal glands led to the hypothesis that these viruses may be involved in the pathogenesis of SS. In fact, genetic material from EBV was detected by DNA hybridization in SS salivary tissue, but it was also found in normal individuals. Other viruses, such as coxsackievirus or endogenous retroviruses, have also been proposed as causative agents. However, there is no proof, to date, that any of these viruses play a pathogenic role in SS.

Epithelial cell activation and chronic inflammation

The histologic hallmark of SS is a periductal mononuclear infiltrate in salivary and lachrymal glands (Fig. 53.1). The majority of the infiltrating cells are CD4 T lymphocytes, whereas CD8 cytotoxic T cells are found in smaller numbers. Activated B lymphocytes are also present, including autoantibody-secreting plasma cells.

Epithelial cell activation, such as the expression of HLA class II molecules and various activation markers on the surface of acinar and ductal salivary epithelial cells, is key in initiating the recruitment of the inflammatory infiltrate. The expression of these molecules along with upregulation of adhesion molecules and chemokines contributes to the recruitment of inflammatory cells, such as T and B lymphocytes, macrophages, and dendritic cells and suggests that epithelial cells act as antigen-presenting cells and actively participate in lymphocyte activation.[8] The ensuing chronic inflammatory process is characterized by a complex interaction between activated epithelial cells, the innate and acquired immune system. In the most severe forms of inflammation the characteristic periductal infiltrates can progress to the formation of germinal centers, which is associated with a higher risk of lymphoma development. Extraglandular manifestations occur as a result of similar lymphocytic infiltrations at other organs. This is described by some as *autoimmune epithelitis* to better reflect the systemic nature of the disease.[8] In most patients, only partial destruction of the glands is noted. Local production of cytokines, autoantibodies, metalloproteinases, and other inflammatory mediators may contribute to the dysfunction of the remaining epithelial cells. It is increasingly recognized that the innate immune system plays a crucial rule in the immunopathogenesis of SS.[9] Increased expression of interferon-regulated genes was described in the salivary glands and peripheral blood of SS patients. One of the cytokines upregulated by IFN-α is BAFF (B-cell-activating factor), which promotes B-cell survival and thus contributes to B-cell hyperactivity seen in SS.

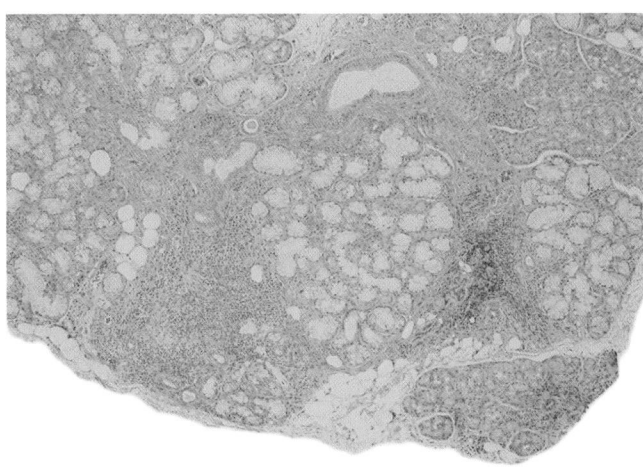

Fig. 53.1 Minor salivary gland biopsy with characteristic periductal inflammation.

Autoantibodies

Autoantibodies are the hallmarks of systemic autoimmune diseases, including SS. The best defined autoantibodies in SS are the anti-Ro/SSA and anti-La/SSB antibodies.[10] Both are targeted against ribonucleoprotein antigens. Anti-Ro/SSA recognizes two RNA binding proteins (the 52- or the 60-kDa protein), whereas anti-La/SSB antibodies recognize RNA polymerase III. Anti-Ro/SSA antibodies are found in over 70% of patients with SS, but are also frequently found in SLE and other autoimmune diseases even in the absence of oral or ocular dryness. Anti-La/SSB is more specific; it is present in 50% of patients with primary SS or SS/SLE but is rarely seen in other diseases. The pathogenic role of these antibodies is not yet defined except in newborns born to women with anti-Ro/SSA and/or anti-La/SSB antibodies. These antibodies can cross the placenta and bind to Ro and La antigens located on the cell surface of fetal myocardial tissue, leading to fetal heart block. Other autoantibodies, such as anti-nuclear antibodies and rheumatoid factor, are frequently present in patients with both primary and secondary SS. Although they lack specificity, they are markers of a systemic autoimmune response and thus can help distinguish SS from other causes of salivary or lachrymal gland dysfunction.

In recent years, research has focused on identifying antibodies more specific for SS, such as anti-α-fodrin and anti-muscarinic acetylcholine receptor antibodies, but the results have been controversial. The major stimulus for saliva production is the binding of acetylcholine to muscarinic acetylcholine receptors. The hypothesis that oral and ocular dryness could result from antibodies antagonizing the muscarinic acetylcholine receptor-3 is intriguing. These antibodies have been demonstrated to play an essential role in eliciting glandular dysfunction in the NOD mouse model of SS, possibly through an inhibitory effect on the receptor. In humans, however, results are still contradictory as multiple attempts to detect these antibodies with conventional immunologic methods have been fruitless. The best evidence for their existence comes from functional studies, where IgG from SS patients inhibited acetylcholine-induced bowel or bladder contraction or acetylcholine-induced Ca^{2+} influx in human salivary gland cells.[11]

Autonomic nervous system

Autonomic nervous system (ANS) abnormalities are common in SS and may play an etiologic role in its pathogenesis. Xerostomia and xerophthalmia, the cardinal SS manifestations, are features of cholinergic parasympathetic ANS dysfunction, whereas sympathetic cholinergic failure results in xerosis and decreased sweating, which are frequently reported by SS patients.

The complexity of the ANS along with differences in methodology and studied populations has resulted in variable results but abnormalities in SS have been reported in both sympathetic and parasympathetic ANS domains. Delayed gastric emptying is common in SS and is consistent with involvement of the enteric ANS. The underlying cause of these ANS abnormalities has not yet been defined but they may potentially be mediated through interference with muscarinic receptor signaling. Recently, it was shown that IgG from SS patients blocks acetylcholine-mediated contraction of smooth muscle preparations from various parts of the gastrointestinal tract and that this effect was specific to interference with the muscarinic acetylcholine receptor-3.[12] Although other mechanisms cannot be excluded, anti-muscarinic acetylcholine receptor autoantibodies would provide a link between autoimmunity and ANS dysfunction in SS.

Clinical manifestations

Clinical manifestations due to salivary and lachrymal glands dysfunction are the dominant features of Sjögren syndrome. Symptoms secondary to other exocrine gland dysfunction such as skin and vaginal dryness and chronic cough from tracheal dryness are frequently present. Multiple extraglandular manifestations can also be present, reflecting the systemic nature of the autoimmune process.[5]

Constitutional symptoms

One of the most common extraglandular manifestations of Sjögren syndrome is excessive fatigue. Approximately 70% of patients with Sjögren syndrome report disabling fatigue leading to reduced quality of life.[13] Attempts to identify a biological basis for fatigue failed to reveal any correlations with levels of inflammatory markers, cytokines, or autoantibodies. This fatigue is commonly associated with arthralgia, malaise, and mental cloudiness (brain fog), resulting in diagnosis of these patients as having fibromyalgia or chronic fatigue syndrome. Less commonly patients also experience low grade fever and weight loss.

Ocular involvement

Lachrymal gland dysfunction leads to constellation of symptoms such as dry, sandy eyes with foreign body sensation. Frequently there is a history of intolerance to contact lenses. Patients often complain of sticky eyes and accumulation of thickened mucus as a result of loss of aqueous component of tears.

Enlarged lachrymal glands can be noted at the onset of disease. In the initial stages injected conjunctivae with strands of thickened mucus at the inner canthus can be found. In more advanced stages conjunctivae lose their normal luster and become edematous. Corneal involvement results in punctuate keratitis due to

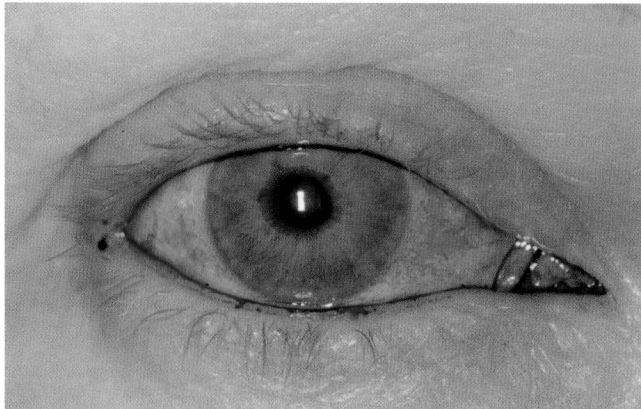

Fig. 53.2 Punctate keratititis due to dry eye. Lissamine green stains dead or degenerated corneal epithelial cells green.
(Courtesy of Manuel Datiles, MD.)

epithelial cell death (Fig. 53.2). Initially it may be limited to the lower quadrants of cornea and later on involves the entire cornea. If left untreated, corneal ulcers can develop with rapid thinning of cornea. In addition to reduced tear production there is also evidence of inflammation of the ocular surface epithelium as shown by the presence of inflammatory cell infiltrate and elevated levels of inflammatory cytokines.

Oral involvement

Saliva plays a critical role in maintaining oral health and comfort. Saliva has antibacterial, lubricating, remineralizing, digestive, buffering, and cleansing properties. Therefore decreased salivary production or altered salivary composition can result in numerous conditions affecting oral health, comfort, and quality of life. Symptoms and signs of salivary gland dysfunction include oral dryness (xerostomia); oral pain and sensitivity; difficulty chewing, swallowing, and speaking; diminished taste; inflamed, morphologically altered, or infected mucosal tissues; and increased tooth decay.

The oral symptoms associated with SS mainly result from salivary gland hypofunction leading to dryness of the oral cavity, which necessitates the use of fluids throughout the day and night. It is not uncommon for SS patients to wake up at night to drink fluids to relieve dryness and also to use fluids to be able to speak, chew, and swallow. A burning sensation along with taste alterations and decreased tolerance to spicy foods is described by a significant percentage of patients.

Head and neck examination often reveals dry and chapped lips, angular cheilitis, and swollen major salivary glands (Fig. 53.3), which may be recurrent or chronic. Acute swelling might occur due to blockage of the salivary ducts by thick mucus that forms plugs, and can also lead to infections. Intraoral findings include decreased salivary pooling under the tongue, and depapillated tongue often associated with erythematous candidiasis (Fig. 53.4). Vasculitis can also manifest in the oral cavity. The teeth often exhibit an increased rate of caries with characteristic decay affecting the roots and cusp tips (Fig. 53.5).

Musculoskeletal involvement

Musculoskeletal complaints are present in the majority of patients with SS. The incidence of arthralgia is between 50 and 75% in various studies and precedes sicca symptoms in up to

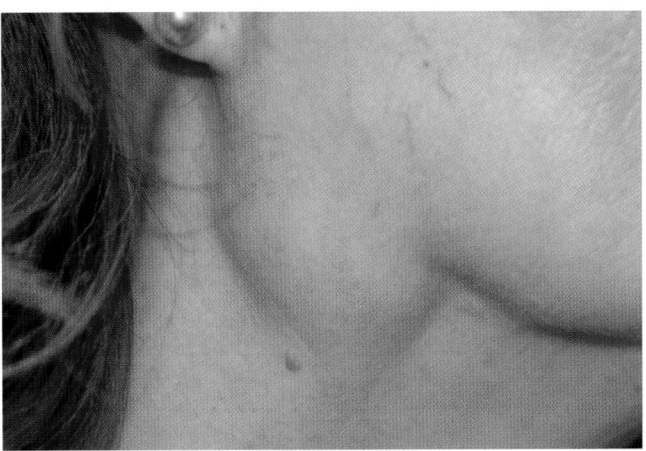

Fig. 53.3 Parotid enlargement.

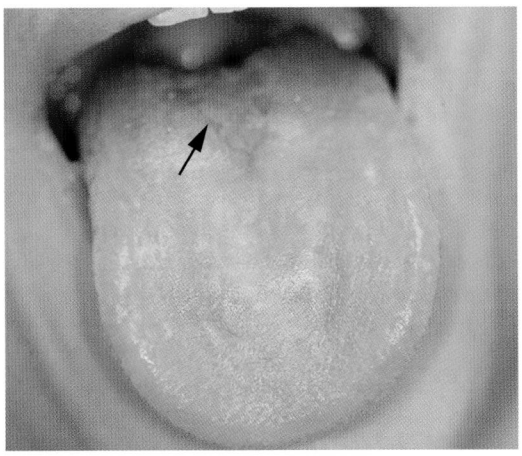

Fig. 53.4 Papillary atrophy and candidiasis of the tongue. The loss of filiform papillae results in a smooth surface of the tongue. Oral candidiasis is common in SS and can present as erythema only with minimal or no exudate (arrow).

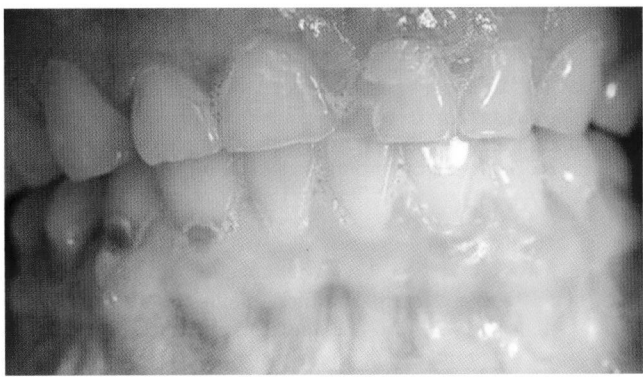

Fig. 53.5 Root caries on the anterior teeth is a common finding due to the loss of the protective functions of saliva. The cusp tips of the posterior teeth are also commonly affected.

30% of patients. Arthralgia is symmetrical usually without evidence of synovitis or erosions. Large and small joint involvement is equally reported and 10–20 % of patients have recurrent monoarthritis or oligoarthritis.

From a clinical perspective it is often difficult to differentiate between primary SS patients with symmetrical joint involvement and those with rheumatoid arthritis presenting with sicca symptoms. Anti-cyclic citrullinated peptide (anti-CCP) antibodies can be found in up to 10% of primary SS patients, mainly in those with articular manifestations. Patients with positive anti-CCP antibodies did not develop joint erosions and no progression to RA was found in a large cohort.[14]

Neuropsychiatric manifestations

Primary SS is associated with multiple neurological manifestations involving both central and peripheral nervous systems. Peripheral nervous system (PNS) manifestations are more common and are present between 5 and 20% of SS patients.[15] PNS involvement in SS can present as sensory neuropathy, small fiber neuropathy, cranial neuropathy, inflammatory myopathies, and autonomic neuropathy. Small fiber neuropathy is increasingly being recognized as the most common PNS manifestation of SS. It presents as a subacute to chronic development of excruciating burning pain. There is selective impairment of pinprick and temperature sensation with preserved vibratory sense and proprioception. Diagnosis is made by skin biopsy.[15]

Symptoms suggestive of autonomic dysfunction such as orthostatic hypotension, temperature intolerance, constipation, urinary frequency or hesitancy, or delayed gastric emptying are present in up to half of the SS patients.[16] Central nervous system involvement is rare and can present as white matter lesions suggestive of multiple sclerosis, myelopathy, optic neuritis as well as cognitive dysfunction, seizures, and encephalopathy.[16] Anxiety and depression is commonly seen in SS patients perhaps due to severe impact of the symptoms on their quality of life.

Dermatological involvement

Skin is involved in about 50% of SS patients.[17] Lesions can either be vasculitic or non-vasculitic. Most common non-vasculitic involvement is dry, itchy skin (xerosis) and angular cheilitis. Other less common non-vasculitis lesions include alopecia, vitiligo, eyelid dermatitis, and erythema nodosum-like lesions. Annular erythema, a rash similar to subacute cutaneous lupus, has been reported in SS. However, the rash is less photosensitive and histologically has deeper perivascular and periappendageal lymphocytic infiltration.

Vasculitic lesions include non-palpable purpura due to hypergammaglobinemia, palpable purpura, and uritcarial vasculitis.[17] Patients with vasculitis have higher prevalence of positive ANA, anti-Ro/SSA antibodies, and rheumatoid factors as compared to non-vasculitic skin involvement. Palpable purpura is histologically characterized by leukocytoclastic vasculitis and may indicate presence of underlying cryoglobulinemia. The presence of palpable purpura may be associated with central nervous system and pulmonary involvement requiring more aggressive treatment. Such patients should be tested for hepatitis C infection.

Raynaud phenomenon is also seen in 30–50% of SS patients and frequently precedes the development of sicca symptoms.

Gastrointestinal involvement

Dysphagia is common due to dryness of pharynx and esophageal dysmotility. Nausea, epigastric pain, and constipation are also common. GI tract dysmotility can be seen as a result of autonomic nervous system involvement by SS. Pancreatic dysfunction is present in 25% of SS patients. Commonly exocrine function is affected with reduced production of amylase and lipase.

Pulmonary involvement

Cough is a common complaint in SS patients resulting from tracheobronchitis sicca (tracheal and bronchial dryness). Clinically significant pulmonary involvement is reported in 9–12% of SS patients.[18] Pulmonary manifestations include large and small airway disease, bronchial hyper-responsiveness, and recurrent respiratory infections. Interstitial lung disease, pulmonary hypertension, pleuritis, and pulmonary amyloidosis are less commonly seen.

Cardiac involvement

Clinically significant cardiac involvement is uncommon in primary SS. Patients may develop pericarditis, thickened pericardium, or left ventricle diastolic dysfunction. Rhythm abnormalities due to autonomic dysfunction may be encountered. Placental transfer of anti-SSA/Ro and anti-SSB/La antibodies from pregnant SS patients can cause lesions in the cardiac conducting system of the fetus. Pregnant women with positive anti-SSA/Ro and anti-SSB/La antibodies have a 2.5% risk of delivering a baby with congenital heart block.

Genitourinary and renal involvement

Renal involvement is frequently due to tubulointerstitial nephritis often presenting as distal (type1) renal tubular acidosis, renal calculi, and hypokalemia. Glomerular disease is rare. Urinary bladder epithelium can be involved in SS. Its inflammation leads to interstitial cystitis in SS patients. Vaginal dryness leading to dyspareunia is observed in 40% of women.

Clinical manifestations in children

Primary SS is rarely diagnosed in children, but many adult SS patients recall presence of symptoms since childhood. Clinical presentation in children is more insidious with predominant recurrent parotitis and less common, sicca symptoms.[19]

Associated autoimmune conditions

Autoimmune thyroiditis is seen in more than one-third of patients with SS. Celiac disease is also increasingly being recognized in SS patients, with a prevalence 10 times higher than general population.

Lymphoma associated with SS

Sjögren's syndrome is associated with increased risk of lymphoma, with about 5% of SS patients developing lymphoma. In a meta-analysis of 20 studies the standardized incidence rate of lymphoma was 18.9% (confidence interval, 9.4–37.9).[20] Most of these are low grade marginal zone lymphomas of MALT (mucosa-associated lymphoid tissue) type. Only 10% of lymphomas in SS patients evolve into a less differentiated cell (more aggressive) variety. Risk factors for development of lymphoma include persistent enlargement of parotid glands, palpable purpura, and leg ulcers secondary to vasculitis, mixed cryoglobunemia, and low C4 level.

Diagnosis and classification criteria

MANAGEMENT OF SJÖGREN'S SYNDROME

Ocular manifestations
- Symptomatic relief with artificial tear drops and lubricating ointments.
- Topical cyclosporine eyedrops
- Blockage of nasolacrimal duct by punctual plug placement or surgical cautery.

Oral manifestations
- Symptomatic relief with water and artificial saliva preparations.
- Physical measures to increase saliva production: sugar-free candies and gum.
- Maintain meticulous oral hygiene, use fluoride toothpaste.
- Sialogogues: pilocarpine, or cevimeline.

Systemic manifestations
- Hydroxychloroquine most commonly used to alleviate fatigue and arthralgia.
- Other immunosuppressive medications may be considered in more severe internal organ involvement.
- Anti-TNF blocking agents not recommended.
- Rituximab showed limited efficacy.

Patient education
- Avoid extreme dry environments such as proximity to open fire places.
- Wear protective eye glasses or goggles.
- Use of sugar-free sour candies or gum.
- Maintain good ocular and oral hygiene.
- Avoid use of medications and substances causing sicca symptoms.
- Women of child-bearing age with positive anti-SSA or anti-SSB antibodies should be counseled about the risk of congenital heart block.
- Educate patient about increased risk of lymphoma associated with Sjögren's syndrome.
- Safety precautions due to smoke and gas leakage in patients with loss of smell.
- Information regarding focus groups such as Sjögren's Syndrome Foundation (http://www.sjogrens.com/) and the British Sjögren's Syndrome Association.

Patients with SS can present with heterogeneous combinations of sicca symptoms and extraglandular manifestations. Moreover, various clinical syndromes and medications can lead to similar symptoms and mimic SS. The diagnosis of SS is based on the combination of subjective symptoms of dryness (sicca symptoms), objective evidence of lachrymal, or salivary gland hypofunction and evidence of autoimmunity or salivary gland inflammation. The most recent classification criteria were proposed by an American-European consensus group in 2002,[21] primarily for classification of patients for clinical studies. These criteria are widely accepted and are frequently used as a guide for clinical diagnosis. Application of these criteria to classify primary SS patients has a sensitivity of 89.5% and specificity of 95.2%, whereas for secondary SS its sensitivity is 97.2% and specificity is 90.2%.[21] The American–European consensus classification scheme is based on a set of two subjective and four objective criteria as listed in Fig. 53.6.

Patients are classified as having primary SS in the absence of any other systemic autoimmune disease, whereas in secondary SS sicca manifestations are present in conjunction with other underlying autoimmune diseases, such as systemic lupus erythematosus, rheumatoid arthritis, polymyositis/dermatomyositis or systemic sclerosis. SS is excluded if patients use anticholinergic medications or have other conditions that can mimic SS, such as chronic viral infections, graft versus host disease or irradiation of the head and neck region.

Patients presenting with sicca symptoms suggestive of SS should undergo specialized testing to confirm the diagnosis. Lachrymal function can be assessed by the Schirmer's test to quantify the amount of tear production, whereas corneal and conjunctival damage due to dryness can be measured by fluorescein and lissamine green staining. Salivary gland evaluation is done by collection of unstimulated saliva or salivary scintigraphy. Laboratory workup should include testing for auto-antibodies to SSA/Ro and SSB/La antigens, which are detected in sera of 45–70 and 20–50%, respectively, of SS patients. Rheumatoid factor is also commonly positive in Sjögren patients.

Treatment

Symptomatic treatment of sicca symptoms

The mainstay of treatment in SS is providing symptomatic relief. Use of artificial tears is often helpful. In patients with sticky mucus or strands over the eyes use of mucolytic agents is indicated. Blockage of lachrymal ducts with punctual plugs or surgically can be beneficial.

Artificial saliva available as spray or lozenges provides only limited relief. Local activation of salivary glands (in patients with preserved function) with sugar-free sour candies or gums provides relief of symptoms.

Cholinergic agonists such as pilocarpine and cevimeline provide good symptomatic relief in selected patients. Cevimeline is a more selective muscarinic agonist predominantly affecting M1 and M3 receptors; hence it is associated with fewer side effects than pilocarpine.[4]

I. Ocular symptoms: Positive response to at least one question:

1. Have you had daily, persistant, troublesome dry eyes for more than 3 months?
2. Do you have a recurrent sensation of sand or gravel in the eyes?
3. Do you use tear subsitutes more than three times a day?

III. Ocular signs: Positive results for at least one of the following two tests:

1. Schirmer's I test, performed without anesthetsia (≤5 mm in 5 minutes)
2. Rose bengal score or other ocular dye score (≥4 according to van Bijsterveld's scoring system).

V. Salivary gland involvement:

Objective evidence of salivary gland involvement defined by a positive result for at least one of the following diagnostic tests:

1. Unstimulated whole salivary flow (≤1,5 ml in 15 minutes)
2. Parotid sialography revealing diffuse sialectasias (punctate, cavitary or destructive pattern) without evidence of obstruction in the major ducts
3. Salivary scintigraphy showing delayed uptake, reduced concentration and/or delayed excretion of tracer.

Primary Sjögren syndrome:

Patients fulfilling 4 out of 6 items are classified as having primary Sjögren syndrome with compulsory presence of a positive biopsy (item IV) or anti-SSA or anti-SSB autoantibodies (item VI). Alternatively patients with three of the four objective items (III, IV, V or VI) may also be classified with Sjögren's syndrome.

Exclusion criteria:

To avoid incorrectly diagnosing such patients with Sjögren syndrome, the presence of the following are considered as exclusion criteria: past head and neck radiation treatment, hepatitis C infection, acquired immunodeficiency disease (AIDS), pre-existing lymphoma, sarcoidosis, graft versus host disease and the use of anticholinergic drugs (within 4 half-lives of the drug).

II. Oral symptoms: Positive response to at least one question:

1. Have you had a daily feeling of dry mouth for more than 3 months?
2. Have you had recurrently or persistant swollen salivary glands as an adult?
3. Do you frequently drink liquids to aid in swallowing dry food?

IV. Histopathology:

In minor salivary glands (obtained through normal-appearing mucosa) focal lymphocytic sialadentis, evaluated by an expert histopathologist with focus score of ≥1 defined as a number of lymphocytic foci (which are adjacent to normal-appearing mucous acini and contain more than 50 lymphocytes) per 4mm 2 of glandular tissue.

VI. Autoantibodies:

Presence in the serum of the following autoantibodies:
1. Antibodies to Ro(SSA) or La(SSB) antigens or both.

Secondary Sjögren syndrome:

Patients diagnosed with another systemic autoimmune disease are classified as having secondary Sjögren syndrome if they have either subjective dry eye (item I) or dry mouth (item II) and any two from items III, IV and VI.

Fig. 53.6 American–European Consensus Group classification criteria for Sjögren's syndrome.
(Modified from Vitali C, Bombardieri S, Jonsson R, et al. Classification criteria for Sjogren's syndrome: a revised version of the European criteria proposed by the American-European Consensus Group. Ann Rheum Dis 2002; 61(6): 554-558.)

Immune modulating medications

Cyclosporine eye drops are frequently prescribed to reduce a local immune response involving conjunctiva and cornea. Use of topical non-steroidal anti-inflammatory and steroid-based eyedrops provide short-term benefits and should be used cautiously.

Hydroxychloroquine is commonly prescribed for patients with SS even though trials showed significant laboratory improvement with no beneficial effects on symptoms.

Other immune modulating agents such as azathioprine, cyclosporine, methotrexate, and mycophenolate mofetil showed only limited benefits in treating sicca symptoms and are used primarily for extraglandular manifestations.[22]

Trials using biologic agents such as infliximab and etanercept failed to show any significant improvement in the primary outcomes of oral and ocular dryness.[22]

The data on rituximab are controversial with some studies showing some benefit.[22]

Treatment for lymphoma associated with SS

 LYMPHOMA IN SJÖGREN SYNDROME

Risk factors

- Risk increases with time. Cumulative risk 3.4% at 5 years and 9.8% at 15 years after diagnosis of Sjögren's syndrome.
- Persistent enlargement of parotid glands.
- Splenomegaly and lymhpadenopathy.
- Palpable purpura.
- Leg ulcers secondary to vasculitis.
- Mixed cryoglobunemia.
- Low complement levels.
- CD4 lymphocytopenia.

Staging and management (in collaboration with an oncologist)

- CT scan of neck, thorax, and abdomen.
- Laboratory tests: LDH, serum and urine electrophoresis and immunofixation, HIV, and hepatitis C serology.
- Bone marrow biopsy.
- Localized low grade MALT lymphoma (most common): careful monitoring.
- Multiple extra-nodal site involvement: single agent chemotherapy.
- High grade transformation or aggressive lymphoma at presentation: rituximab and CHOP.

As discussed above lymphoma associated with SS is usually low grade with 5-year survival rates of 86–100%. In a study of SS patients overall survival rates of patients with MALT lymphoma was similar in both treated and untreated groups.[23] However, patients with disseminated and more aggressive lymphoma showed reduced overall survival.

Future direction

As no effective treatment is currently available to treat SS patients, several medications and other non-drug-based modalities are being studied. B-cell-depleting agents (rituximab, epratuzumab) and anti-B cell-activating factor (belimumab) therapy are currently in clinical trials. Use of steroids locally in the salivary glands showed some promising initial results, which should be confirmed in independent studies.

Patient education

Due to its significant impact on quality of life, educating patients and their families is of utmost importance. Excellent resources for patient education are available through focus groups such as the Sjögren's Syndrome Foundation (http://www.sjogrens.com/) and the British Sjögren's Syndrome Association.

In general patients are advised to avoid dry environments, protect eyes from bright sunlight, maintain good dental hygiene, and be aware of symptoms suggestive of lymphoma. They should avoid medications and substances that may worsen sicca symptoms. Women of child-bearing age with positive anti-SSA/Ro and anti-SSB/La antibodies should be counseled regarding the risk of congenital heart block in fetuses. Patients with loss of smell associated with SS are at an increased risk of injury in the event of gas leakage. Alternate methods to detect gas leakage in the patient's environment should be employed.

Translational research

● ON THE HORIZON

- Genome-wide association studies will lead to better understanding of genetic risk factors.
- Further studies are needed to better understand the interaction between immune and non-immune abnormalities leading to Sjögren's syndrome.
- Pilot clinical studies are needed to identify candidates for larger efficacy trials.
- There is a pressing need to identify and to validate clinically relevant biomarkers.

Sjögren's syndrome is the clinical manifestation of a complex interplay between genetic factors, environmental and stochastic events that involve innate and adaptive immunity, hormonal mechanisms, and the autonomic nervous system. A better understanding of these elements is necessary to develop more effective treatments. Two large genome-wide association studies are currently underway to better delineate the genetic risk factors of SS. Pilot treatment trials targeting key cells (B and T lymphocytes) and mediators (Blyss, lymphotoxin, interferon) of autoimmune/inflammatory pathways are expected to identify the most promising molecule(s) that can be tested in larger efficacy studies. There is a clear and present need to identify and validate biomarkers that can be used in clinical trials as well as everyday clinical practice to improve the management of Sjögren patients.

References

1. Venables PJ. Sjogren's syndrome. Best Pract Res Clin Rheumatol 2004;18:313–29.
2. Skopouli FN, Moutsopoulos HM. Autoimmune epitheliitis: Sjogren's syndrome. Clin Exp Rheumatol 1994;12(Suppl. 11):S9–11.
3. Mavragani CP, Moutsopoulos HM. The geoepidemiology of Sjogren's syndrome. Autoimmun Rev 2010;9(5):A305–10.
4. Venables PJ. Sjogren's syndrome. Best Pract Res Clin Rheumatol 2004;18(3):313–29.
5. Fox RI. Sjogren's syndrome. Lancet 2005;366(9482):321–31.
6. Scofield RH. Genetics of systemic lupus erythematosus and Sjogren's syndrome. Curr Opin Rheumatol 2009;21(5):448–53.
7. Porola P, Laine M, Virtanen I, et al. Androgens and integrins in salivary glands in Sjogren's syndrome. J Rheumatol 2010;37(6):1181–7.
8. Voulgarelis M, Tzioufas AG. Pathogenetic mechanisms in the initiation and perpetuation of Sjogren's syndrome. Nat Rev Rheumatol 2010;6(9):529–37.
9. Nikolov NP, Illei GG. Pathogenesis of Sjogren's syndrome. Curr Opin Rheumatol 2009;21(5):465–70.
10. Hernandez-Molina G, Leal-Alegre G, Michel-Peregrina M. The meaning of anti-Ro and anti-La antibodies in primary Sjogren's syndrome. Autoimmun Rev 2011;10(3):123–5.
11. Dawson LJ, Allison HE, Stanbury J, et al. Putative anti-muscarinic antibodies cannot be detected in patients with primary Sjogren's syndrome using conventional immunological approaches. Rheumatology (Oxford) 2004;43(12):1488–95.
12. Park K, Haberberger RV, Gordon TP, Jackson MW. Antibodies interfering with the type 3 muscarinic receptor pathway inhibit gastrointestinal motility and cholinergic neurotransmission in Sjogren's syndrome. Arthritis Rheum 2011;63(5):1426–34.
13. Bowman SJ. Patient-reported outcomes including fatigue in primary Sjogren's syndrome. Rheum Dis Clin North Am 2008;34(4):949–62 ix.
14. Fauchais AL, Ouattara B, Gondran G, et al. Articular manifestations in primary Sjogren's syndrome: clinical significance and prognosis of 188 patients. Rheumatology (Oxford) 2010;49(6):1164–72.
15. Birnbaum J. Peripheral nervous system manifestations of Sjogren syndrome: clinical patterns, diagnostic paradigms, etiopathogenesis, and therapeutic strategies. Neurologist 2010;16(5):287–97.
16. Chai J, Logigian EL. Neurological manifestations of primary Sjogren's syndrome. Curr Opin Neurol 2010;23(5):509–13.
17. Fox RI, Liu AY. Sjogren's syndrome in dermatology. Clin Dermatol 2006;24(5):393–413.
18. Hatron PY, Tillie-Leblond I, Launay D, et al. Pulmonary manifestations of Sjogren's syndrome. Presse Med 2011;40(1 Pt 2):e49–64.
19. Houghton K, Malleson P, Cabral D, et al. Primary Sjogren's syndrome in children and adolescents: are proposed diagnostic criteria applicable? J Rheumatol 2005;32(11):2225–32.
20. Voulgarelis M, Moutsopoulos HM. Mucosa-associated lymphoid tissue lymphoma in Sjogren's syndrome: risks, management, and prognosis. Rheum Dis Clin North Am 2008;34(4):921–33 viii.
21. Vitali C, Bombardieri S, Jonsson R, et al. Classification criteria for Sjogren's syndrome: a revised version of the European criteria proposed by the American-European Consensus Group. Ann Rheum Dis 2002;61(6):554–8.
22. Ramos-Casals M, Tzioufas AG, Stone JH, et al. Treatment of primary Sjogren syndrome: a systematic review. JAMA 2010;304(4):452–60.
23. Tzioufas AG, Voulgarelis M. Update on Sjogren's syndrome autoimmune epithelitis: from classification to increased neoplasias. Best Pract Res Clin Rheumatol 2007;21(6):989–1010.

John Varga,
Fredrick M.
Wigley

Scleroderma-systemic sclerosis

Systemic sclerosis (SSc) is a chronic multisystem connective tissue disease characterized by autoimmunity and inflammation, widespread functional and structural abnormalities in small blood vessels, and progressive fibrosis of the skin and visceral organs. Multiple cell types and their products interact to mediate the pathogenetic processes that underlie the diverse clinical manifestations of SSc.

Prevalence and epidemiology

Systemic sclerosis is a sporadic disease with worldwide distribution. Incidence estimates in the United States range from 9 to 19 cases per million per year, and prevalence rates range from 28 to 253 cases per million. However, a community-based survey of SSc yielded a prevalence estimate of 286 cases per million population.[1] Age, gender and ethnicity are important factors determining disease susceptibility.[2] Like other connective tissue diseases, SSc is more prevalent in women, with the most common age of onset in the range 30–50 years. Disease onset occurs at an earlier age among patients of African descent than among whites. Furthermore, black patients are more likely to have diffuse skin involvement, digital ulcers, pulmonary hypertension, and pulmonary fibrosis, and have a worse prognosis.

Etiology and pathogenesis

Genetic factors

Systemic sclerosis is not inherited in a Mendelian fashion, and disease concordance rates among both monozygotic and dizygotic twin pairs are relatively low (<5%). Nonetheless, 1.6% of SSc patients have a first-degree relative with the disease, representing a relative risk of 13, indicating an important role for genetic background in disease susceptibility. In contrast to other rheumatic tissue diseases, HLA linkages with SSc are weak, although specific HLA haplotypes do associate with distinct autoantibody responses. Genetic investigations in SSc have focused on candidate genes and genome-wide association studies (GWAS). Candidate genes shown to be associated with SSc (generally weak associations) include *STAT4, IRF4, PTPN22, BANK1*, HLA Class II, angiotensin-converting enzyme (ACE) and endothelin-1. A recent GWAS of European ancestry cases identified multiple susceptibility loci outside the MHC region, including *CD247, IRF5*, and *STAT4*. It is remarkable that several of these genes are involved in immune regulation and innate immune responses, highlighting the potential importance of immune dysregulation in the pathogenesis of SSc.[3]

Environmental factors

While the etiology if SSc is unknown, Viruses and exposure to environmental and occupational agents and drugs have been implicated as potential triggering factors. Patients with SSc have increased serum levels of antibodies directed against the human cytomegalovirus (hCMV). Furthermore, autoantibodies to topo-isomerase-I in a subset of SSc patients cross-react with antigenic epitopes on hCMV-derived proteins, suggesting that molecular mimicry may mechanistically link hCMV infection and SSc. Evidence of human parvovirus B19 infection has also been presented. These studies need confirmation and the etiologic role of virus in SSc remains conjectural. Although reports of apparent geographic clustering of SSc cases suggest shared environmental exposures, careful investigations have failed to substantiate these clusters. Epidemic outbreaks of apparently novel multi-systemic illnesses with SSc-like features have been linked to environmental exposures such as contaminated rapeseed cooking oils in Spain (the toxic oil syndrome), and L-tryptophan dietary supplements in the United States (eosinophilia-myalgia syndrome). While both of these apparently novel syndromes were characterized by chronic scleroderma-like skin induration, they showed clinical and pathological features clearly distinguishing them from SSc.[4] The incidence of SSc is increased among miners, and others with occupational exposure to silica. Additional occupational exposures linked with increased risk of SSc include polyvinyl chloride, trichloroethylene and organic solvents. Drugs potentially implicated in SSc-like illnesses include bleomycin, pentazocine and cocaine, and appetite suppressants associated with pulmonary hypertension. The apparent association of SSc with silicone breast implants originally raised concern, but epidemiologic investigations failed to substantiate an increased risk.[5]

Pathology

The hallmark pathological features of SSc are a non-inflammatory microangiopathy in multiple vascular beds and fibrosis of the skin and internal organs. In relatively early-stage disease, cellular infiltrates may be found in many organs. In the skin, the infiltrates are located predominantly around blood vessels. With disease progression, inflammatory infiltrates become sparse.

Vascular injury is likely to be the earliest and possibly primary event in the pathogenesis of SSc. Patients with established SSc show widespread vascular lesions characterized by bland in-

© 2013 Elsevier Ltd.

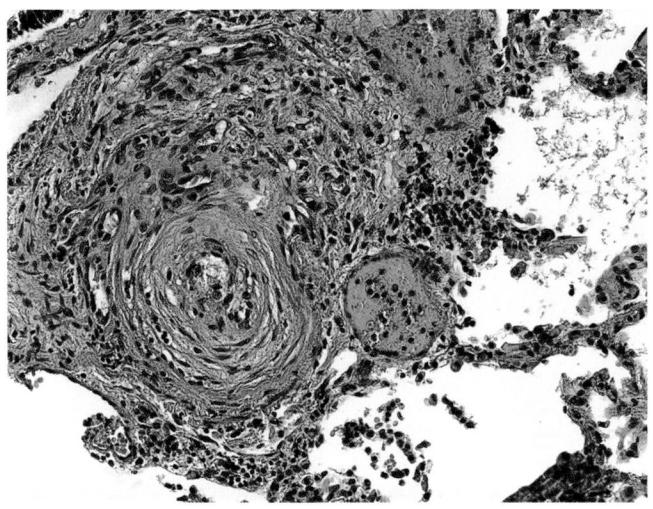

Fig. 54.1 Pulmonary arterial involvement. Significant intimal layer hyperplasia is seen, leading to narrowing of the vascular lumen.
Courtesy of Dr Anjana Yeldandi.

timal proliferation in the small and medium-sized arteries (Fig. 54.1). The heart, lungs, kidneys and intestinal tract are most prominently affected. Vasculitic lesions are virtually never found. In late stages, perivascular adventitial fibrosis is prominent.

Fibrosis affects multiple organs. Prominent fibrotic changes are seen in the skin, lungs, gastrointestinal tract, heart, tendon sheath, and perifascicular tissue surrounding skeletal muscle. Accumulation of collagen-rich connective tissue composed of fibronectin, elastin, proteoglycans and other structural macromolecules in these organs leads to disruption of tissue architecture, resulting in progressive functional impairment. In the skin, fibrosis causes massive dermal expansion with obliteration of the hair follicles, sweat and sebaceous glands. Collagen deposition invades the subjacent adipose layer with entrapment of fat cells. The lungs show patchy infiltration of the alveolar walls with lymphocytes, plasma cells, macrophages and eosinophils in early disease, whereas in later stages fibrosis and vascular damage predominate, often coexisting in the same lesions. However, in patients with limited cutaneous SSc, the vascular lesions may predominate. Intimal thickening of the pulmonary arteries, best seen with elastin stain, is associated with pulmonary hypertension, and at autopsy is often associated with multiple pulmonary emboli.

In the lungs, progressive fibrous thickening of the alveolar septae results in obliteration of the air spaces with a characteristic nonspecific interstitial pneumonia (NSIP) pattern, and less commonly honeycombing, and loss of pulmonary blood vessels. This process impairs gas exchange, and contributes to worsening of pulmonary hypertension. In the gastrointestinal tract, prominent pathological changes can occur at any level from the mouth to the rectum. The esophagus shows atrophy of the lamina propria, submucosa and muscular layers with modest fibrosis, and characteristic vascular lesions. Replacement of the normal intestinal architecture results in disordered peristaltic activity, with gastroesophageal reflux, small bowel dysmotility, and bacterial overgrowth. Chronic gastroesophageal reflux leads to esophageal inflammation, ulcerations and stricture formation, and in some cases premalignant Barrett's metaplasia.

The heart is frequently affected, with prominent myocardial contraction band necrosis reflecting ischemia-reperfusion injury, and patchy areas of myocardial fibrosis. In the kidneys vascular lesions predominate, and glomerulonephritis is rare. Chronic renal ischemia is associated with shrunken glomeruli. Scleroderma renal crisis is associated with dramatic changes in small renal arteries. Prominent findings include reduplication of elastic lamina, marked intimal proliferation and narrowing of the lumen (onion skinning), often with microangiopathic hemolysis.

Pathogenesis

A comprehensive picture of the pathogenesis of SSc must integrate the vasculopathy, immune dysregulation, and fibrosis of multiple organs. As illustrated in Fig. 54.2, complex and dynamic interplay among these distinct processes initiates, amplifies and sustains tissue damage in SSc.[6]

Microangiopathy

Evidence of vascular involvement is an early and widespread feature of SSc, and vascular damage has major impact on the course of the disease. Vascular endothelial cell injury is initially associated with purely functional and reversible alterations. There is abnormal blood flow response to vasomotor or cold challenge, and altered production of and responsiveness to factors mediating vasodilatation (nitric oxide and prostacyclins) and vasoconstriction (endothelins). Microvessels show increased permeability, enhanced trans-endothelial leukocyte migration, activation of fibrinolytic cascades and platelet aggregation culminating in thrombosis. Activated endothelial cells express surface adhesion molecules, and release endothelin-1, which further promotes leukocyte adhesion, smooth muscle cell proliferation, and endothelial-mesenchymal transition. Ensuing intimal and medial hypertrophy and fibrosis of the adventitial layers leads to vessel stiffening and luminal narrowing. Combined with endothelial cell apoptosis, the process culminates in the characteristic striking absence of blood vessels seen on angiograms of the hands and kidneys in late-stage disease. Paradoxically, the process of re-vascularization appears to be defective in SSc, possibly due to a defect in bone marrow-derived CD34[+] circulating endothelial progenitor cells.[7]

Cellular and humoral immune responses

In the early stages of SSc, activated T cells and macrophages accumulate in lesional skin and lung, where they secrete proinflammatory and profibrotic mediators including transforming growth factor-β (TGF-β), cytokines and chemokines. These molecules can activate fibroblasts as well as endothelial cells, and initiate the fibrotic response. Because TGF-β in particular can induce its own production as well as that of other growth factors such as connective tissue growth factor (CTGF), an initial cytokine burst could result in amplified cytokine production and sustained autocrine and paracrine signaling. Additionally, as the matrix undergoes remodeling, it increases its stiffness, which itself triggers biomechanical activation of resident fibroblasts, further amplifying the fibrotic response.

Virtually all patients with SSc have serum antinuclear and other autoantibodies. These autoantibodies are highly specific for SSc and are mutually exclusive (see below). Moreover, the SSc-specific autoantibodies show strong association with individual disease phenotypes, and their titers can fluctuate with disease activity. Multiple mechanism(s) have been proposed to account for autoantibody generation in SSc. B cells from SSc patients overexpress the surface receptor CD19, resulting in

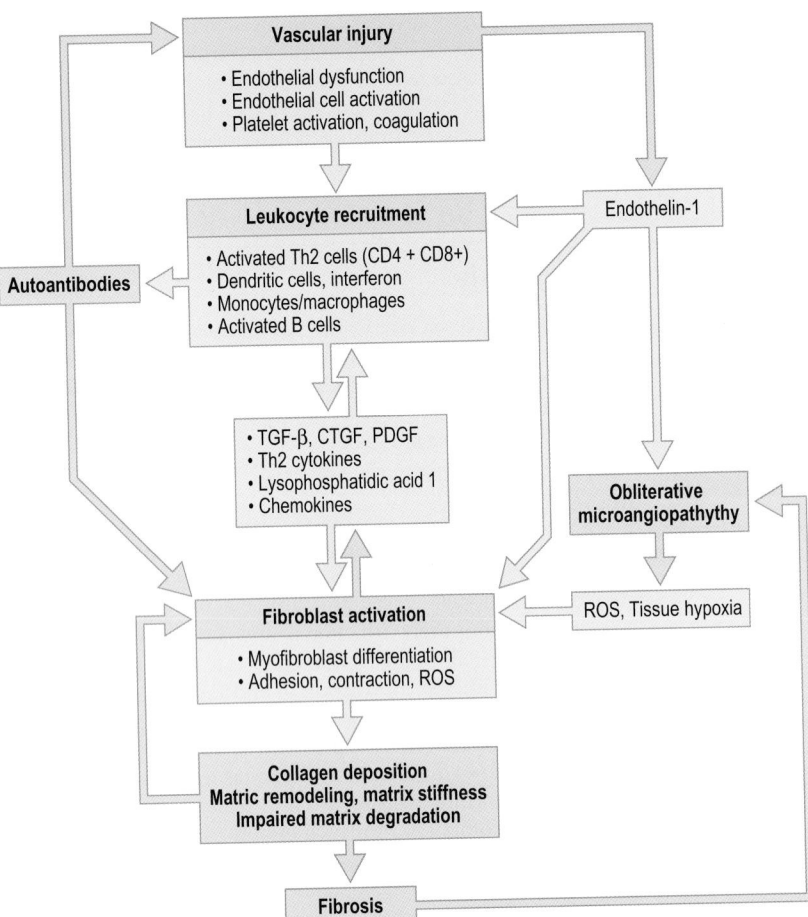

Fig. 54.2 Pathogenesis of SSc. Interactions of cellular and molecular events triggered by injury that underlie the pathogenesis of vascular and immune dysfunction, culminating in fibrosis.

their hyperresponsivess.[8] Additionally, it has been proposed that in SSc, specific self antigens undergo post-translational modifications such as proteolytic cleavage, increased expression or misdirected subcellular localization that create neoepitopes recognized as non-self by the immune system. While SSc-associated autoantibodies have well-established clinical utility as diagnostic markers, their direct role in disease manifestations remains uncertain.[9] Some SSc patients also have antibodies directed against fibroblasts and endothelial cells, the PDGF receptor, and matrix metalloproteinases.

Fibrosis: cellular and molecular components

Interstitial and vascular fibrosis, the hallmark of SSc, is characterized by replacement of normal tissue architecture with dense connective tissue. Fibrosis in multiple tissues accounts for much of the late morbidity and mortality of SSc. Fibroblasts and related mesenchymal cells are key effector cells responsible for the development of fibrosis. In response to extracellular signals such as TGF-β, CTGF, chemokines, endothelin-1, lysophosphatidic acid (LPA1), reactive oxygen species (ROS), and hypoxia, as well as integrin-mediated biomechanical signals from a stiff extracellular matrix, these cells proliferate, migrate, produce a broad array of matrix macromolecules, adhere to and remodel connective tissue, secrete growth factors and cytokines and express surface receptors for them, and undergo transdifferentiation into contractile myofibroblasts. Together, these biosynthetic, contractile, and adhesive functions enable fibroblasts to execute effective

wound healing. Whereas under physiologic conditions the fibroblast repair program is tightly regulated and self-limited, under pathological conditions fibroblast activation is sustained and amplified, resulting in exaggerated matrix deposition and remodelling. Uncontrolled activation of fibroblasts, combined with their relative resistance to apoptosis, is a fundamental pathogenetic alteration underlying fibrosis in SSc. In addition to fibroblasts normally residing in tissues, bone marrow-derived mesenchymal progenitor cells called fibrocytes also participate in the fibrotic response. Moreover, peripheral blood mononuclear cells can also differentiate into fibroblasts *in vitro*. The factors that govern the mobilization of mesenchymal progenitor cells from the bone marrow, and their trafficking to lesional tissue, and *in situ* differentiation into matrix-producing adhesive and contractile fibroblasts, remain unknown.

Fibroblasts explanted from lesional SSc tissues display an abnormal phenotype when cultured *ex vivo*. These cells display enhanced synthesis of collagen and other extracellular matrix molecules, express alpha smooth muscle actin and cell surface adhesion molecules, spontaneously generate ROS and resist induction of apoptosis. The activated scleroderma phenotype persists during the serial passage of lesional fibroblasts *in vitro*. Cell-autonomous persistence of the abnormal fibroblast phenotype could reflect epigenetic modifications of these cells due to chromatin remodeling, DNA methylation, or altered expression of microRNA such as miR21 or miR29; or may be due to autocrine TGF-β signaling. Multiple abnormalities in TGF-β pathways have been identified in SSc. Lesional fibroblasts secrete TGF-β, and exhibit TGF-β hyper-responsiveness due to elevated TGF-β surface receptors and integrin-mediated activation of latent TGF-β. Furthermore, SSc fibroblasts show evidence of activated intracellular signaling, with constitutive phosphorylation of Smads and other key kinase pathways that might contribute to the persistence and progression of fibrosis.[10] Targeted therapies that block TGF-β signaling and abrogate other fibrogenic pathways mediated by chemokines, endothelins, and CTGF are under development.

Clinical features

Overview

Systemic sclerosis is highly variable in its clinical expression and thus represents a broad spectrum of disease. Whereas the disease process targets the skin, blood vessels, lungs, heart, gastrointestinal tract, kidneys, and musculoskeletal system, subsets of patients exist with unique clinical features and distinct clinical outcomes. Raynaud phenomenon is virtually universal in SSc, suggesting that perturbation of the terminal arteries of the circulation is a fundamental process that links the different subsets of the disease. Thickening of the skin distinguishes SSc from other rheumatic diseases (Table 54.1): scleroderma (hard skin) is the most specific and prominent physical finding. Patients vary in the expression of the skin changes, and are classified into two major subsets defined by the degree of clinically involved skin. In the diffuse skin variant called diffuse cutaneous SSc (dcSSc), fibrosis of the skin is widespread, and the illness is more violent in expression, with rapid onset and increased risk of serious and internal organ disease. In contrast, the limited skin variant called limited cutaneous SSc (lcSSc) presents with long-standing Raynaud phenomenon, skin fibrosis limited to the fingers or distal limbs, and a generally indolent disease course. Limited SSc is less likely to be associated with organ failure or shortened life expectancy. Predictors of elevated mortality rates among SSc patients include diffuse skin disease and internal organ involvement, female gender, black race, and later age of disease onset.[11,12]

Although classification of SSc as diffuse and limited cutaneous has utility, disease expression is far more complex and several distinct phenotypes are recognized within each of the two subsets. For example, 10–15% of patients with lcSSc develop severe pulmonary arterial hypertension without significant lung fibrosis. Other patients develop systemic features of SSc without appreciable skin involvement, a phenotype that is termed systemic sclerosis sine scleroderma. Unique clinical phenotypes of SSc associate with specific autoantibodies (Table 54.2). For example, anti-centromere antibodies associate with lcSSc, while anti-topoisomerase-I antibodies associate with the presence of interstitial lung disease. The presence of anti-RNA polymerase antibodies associate with rapid and widespread skin disease and an increased risk of a scleroderma renal crisis. Some patients with SSc have "overlap" features, where SSc coexists with clinical and laboratory evidence of another autoimmune disease such as polymyositis, autoimmune thyroid disease, Sjögren's syndrome, polyarthritis, autoimmune liver disease or systemic lupus erythematosus (Table 54.2).

> ● KEY CONCEPTS
>
> **Clinical patterns of systemic sclerosis**
>
> **Limited cutaneous scleroderma**
> - Distal skin sclerosis (sclerodactyly)
> - Severe Raynaud phenomenon with digital ischemia
> - Numerous telangiectasia
> - Isolated pulmonary arterial hypertension
>
> **Diffuse cutaneous scleroderma**
> - Rapidly progressing widespread skin involvement
> - Scleroderma renal crisis
> - Interstitial lung disease
> - Severe gastrointestinal dysmotility
> - Cardiomyopathy

Table 54.1 Classification of systemic sclerosis

Diffuse cutaneous scleroderma—skin thickening on the trunk in addition to the face, proximal and distal extremities

Limited cutaneous scleroderma—skin thickening limited distal to the elbow and knee; may also involve the face and neck

CREST syndrome (subcutaneous calcinosis; Raynaud phenomenon; esophageal dysmotility; sclerodactyly; telangiectasis)

Sine scleroderma—no apparent skin thickening but characteristic visceral organ involvement, vascular and serologic features

Overlap syndrome—criteria for SSc, coexisting with features of systemic lupus erythematosus, rheumatoid arthritis or inflammatory muscle disease

Mixed connective tissue disease—overlap syndrome with anti-U1RNP antibodies

Early disease—Raynaud phenomenon with clinical and/or laboratory features of SSc; specific autoantibodies, abnormal nailfold capillaroscopy, finger edema, and ischemic injury

Table 54.2 Autoantibody/phenotype association in SSc

Antigen	Subtype	Clinical phenotype
Topoisomerase I (Scl-70)	Diffuse	Pulmonary fibrosis, cardiac involvement and cancer
RNA polymerase III	Diffuse	Severe skin involvement, renal crisis
Centromere proteins B, C	Limited (CREST)	Ischemic digital loss, sicca
U3-RNP (fibrillarin, Mpp 10, hU3-55 K)	Diffuse or limited	Pulmonary arterial hypertension, cardiac and skeletal muscle involvement
B23	Diffuse or limited	Pulmonary arterial hypertension, lung disease
Th/To-RNP	Limited	Lung disease, small bowel involvement, renal crisis
PM/Scl	Overlap	Myositis
U1-RNP	Overlap	SLE, myositis, polyarthritis

CREST, calcinosis, Raynaud phenomenon, esophageal dysfunction, sclerodactyly, telangiectasia syndrome; RNP, ribonucleoprotein particle; SLE, systemic lupus erythematosus.
From Harris ML, Rosen A. Autoimmunity in scleroderma: the origin, pathogenetic role, and clinical significance of autoantibodies. Curr Opin Rheumatol 2003; 15(6): 778-784.

Table 54.3 Classification of localized scleroderma

Plaque types of morphea
• Circumscribed plaques
• Guttate
• Keloid/nodular
• Bullous
Generalized morphea
• Three or more locations
• Pansclerotic morphea
Linear scleroderma
• Frontoparietal linear morphea (en coup de sabre)
• Parry–Romberg syndrome (progressive hemifacial atrophy)
• Linear streaks on limbs or trunk
Deep morphea

In contrast to SSc, the term "scleroderma" is now properly used to describe patients with localized disease, a group of related fibrosing skin disorders that occurs with similar frequency in both children and adults (Table 54.3). Localized scleroderma is infrequently associated with significant systemic involvement. Morphea, a form of localized scleroderma, can occur as solitary or multiple lesions (generalized morphea) of expanding circular patches of thickened skin. The most common form of localized scleroderma in children is linear scleroderma. It presents as a streak of thickened skin, generally in one or both lower extremities. Linear scleroderma often involves the subcutaneous tissues with fibrosis and atrophy of supporting structures, muscle and bone, and radiographs may show melorheostosis of the long bones. In children with linear scleroderma, the growth of affected tissues, muscles and long bones can be retarded. When the lesions cross joints, significant contractures of the affected joint can develop. Linear scleroderma can occur on the head leaving severe facial deformity. When this occurs it is called "*en coup de sabre.*" This should be distinguished from Perry-Rhomberg syndrome or facial hemiatrophy that also affects the face, usually unilaterally, with atrophy of skin rather than fibrosis. Both *en coup de sabre* and Perry-Rhomberg syndrome can be associated with central nervous system involvement presenting as headaches, visual disturbance or a seizure disorder. Uncommon forms of localized scleroderma include pansclerotic morphea, keloid morphea, deep morphea presenting as a fasciitis and bullous morphea with blistering. Morphea lesions can be seen in patients with SSc and often lichen sclerosus is seen in association with morphea.

Symptoms

Characteristically, the earliest symptoms of SSc are non-specific, and include fatigue, musculoskeletal distress (stiffness or pain), and feeling ill. Cold sensitivity and Raynaud phenomenon occur early in the disease and may be the only clinical clue. Symptoms of esophageal dysfunction with heartburn are common, and along with Raynaud phenomenon, can precede other manifestations of SSc by years. Visible capillary abnormalities at the nailfold (dilatation and loss or dropout of capillaries) are almost a universal finding in SSc, and precede other manifestations of the disease. An individual presenting with Raynaud phenomenon, abnormal nailfold capillaries, and the presence

of an SSc-specific autoantibody can be suspected of having SSc even before other more obvious manifestations are noted.[13]

● CLINICAL PEARLS

Clinical features of early systemic sclerosis

- Definite Raynaud phenomenon
- Gastroesophageal reflux with heartburn
- Swelling of the fingers and hands
- Musculoskeletal pain and stiffness
- Dilated nailfold capillaries
- Hyper- or hypopigmentary changes of the skin

Diffuse SSc

In general, patients with dcSSc have a short interval between the onset of Raynaud phenomenon and other signs and symptoms. Soft tissue swelling, intense pruritus and burning, and non-pitting edema are signs of the early inflammatory or "edematous" phase of the diffuse cutaneous form of the disease. The skin of the fingers, hands, distal limbs and face are usually affected first and more severely than other body areas (Fig. 54.3). Carpal tunnel syndrome can be present as a consequence of soft tissue inflammation around the hands and wrists. Patients may note skin hyperpigmentation (patches or generalized tanning). Other early skin changes include vitiligo-like hypo-pigmentation ("salt and pepper" appearance), often on the chest or the back (Fig. 54.4). Escalating musculoskeletal symptoms are common, and are associated with muscle weakness and decreased joint mobility. Significant finger and hand/wrist disease limits the patient from doing simple chores or providing self-care.

The early edematous phase of dcSSc has prominent inflammatory features, with significant skin edema and erythema, and is associated with inflammatory cell infiltration in the dermis. After a period of weeks to months, the inflammatory phase evolves into the "fibrotic" phase as increased collagen and extracellular material is deposited in the skin causing the skin to feel thickened and lose flexibility. The fibrotic process starts in the dermis, and is associated with loss of body hair, reduced production of skin oils and a decline in sweating capacity as these cutaneous structures atrophy. Gradually, the

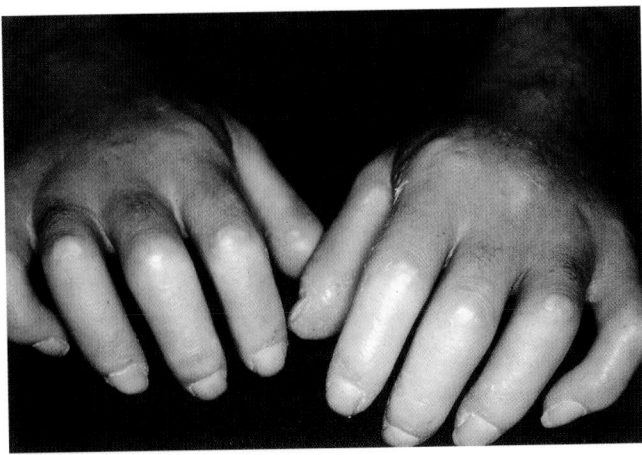

Fig. 54.3 Skin fibrosis in systemic sclerosis. Severe fibrosis of the skin of the hands and forearms causing joint contractures and skin ulcerations in a woman with diffuse cutaneous systemic sclerosis.

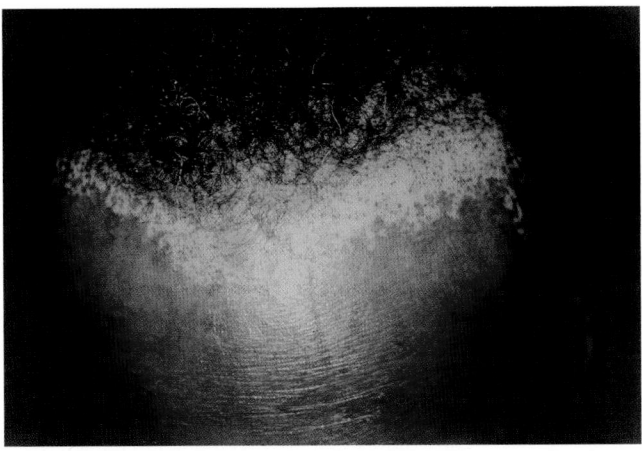

Fig. 54.4 Pigmentation changes in the skin. Vitiligo (salt-and-pepper) appearance of the involved skin in a patient of African descent with diffuse cutaneous systemic sclerosis.

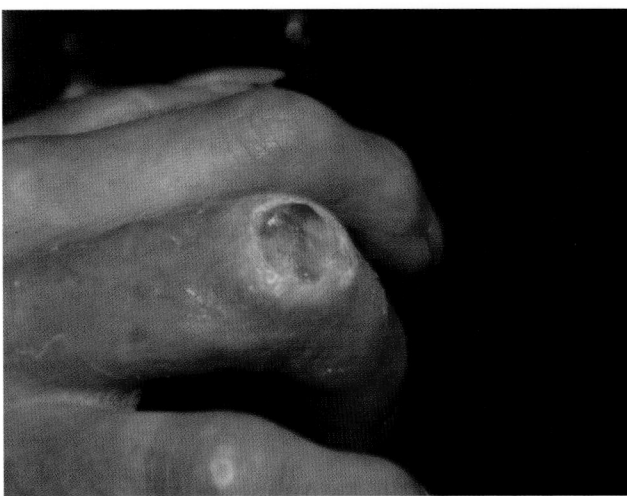

Fig. 54.5 Traumatic digital ulcer. Ulceration of atrophic skin over the metacarpal joint of patient with diffuse scleroderma.

subcutaneous tissue becomes affected, with atrophy of subcutaneous fat and fibrosis extends to the underlying fascia, muscle and other soft tissue structures. During the fibrotic phase patients note pain, progressive loss of flexibility, distressing disfigurement and profound weight loss. Progressive flexion contractures of the finger joints ensue. Other joints, including wrist, elbow, shoulder, hip girdle, knees, and ankle can also also be affected due to fibrosis of the supporting joint structures (Fig. 54.3). Thick ridges at the neck due to firm adherence of the skin to the underlying platysma muscle interfere with neck extension. Tendon friction rub is a prominent crepitance that can be felt or even heard over tendons of the lower and upper extremity. Tendon friction rubs are due to fibrosis in the tissues surrounding the affected joints; they are associated with rapidly progressive skin disease and are linked to an overall poor prognosis. Fibrosis of the skin of the face yields a characteristic facial appearance with diminished oral aperture, loss of facial expression, vertical lines around the lips, loss of lip thickness and protrusion of the teeth.

The natural history of skin disease in SSc tends to be monophasic, and relapse after the edematous and active fibrotic phase is uncommon. The duration of active skin disease from the first signs of skin involvement to its maximal extent is characteristically less than three years; cutaneous inflammation and progressive fibrosis gradually subsides and regression of skin involvement begins. However, this time frame is highly variable from one patient to another, with many patients demonstrating rapid skin regression while other showing chronically active disease over years. In the late stages of dcSSc, skin remodeling can be dramatic with return to normal-appearing skin in those areas spared from severe end-stage fibrosis. In more severely affected areas the skin becomes thin or atrophic and can be bound down to underlying structures. Skin ulcerations or dystrophic calcification often complicate the fibrotic, atrophic, and avascular skin (Fig. 54.5).

While the skin involvement is generally the most dramatic and visible manifestation of dcSSc, internal organ involvement occurs during the early active stage of advancing skin disease. Patients with dcSSc have a significant risk for interstitial lung disease, severe gastrointestinal dysfunction, SSc renal crisis, progressive heart disease and recurrent digital ulcers during the initial active inflammatory and fibrotic phases of the skin disease. In practical terms, this means that in dcSSc, the initial 3–4 years is the period that the systemic process is most active;

if organ failure does not occur during this period, the systemic process then may stabilize without further progression.

Limited cutaneous SSc

The disease course in the limited cutaneous variant of SSc is more indolent and often relatively benign. After the onset of Raynaud phenomenon, several years may pass before additional symptoms or signs are recognized. The most common non-Raynaud symptoms in patients with lcSSc are those of upper gastrointestinal disease with dysphagia and gastroesophageal reflux. Dilated capillaries form visible erythematous vascular lesions (telangiectasia), seen most commonly on the fingertips, nailfold areas of the digit, palms, face, lips, and inside the oral cavity (Fig. 54.6). The CREST (subcutaneous *c*alcinosis, *r*aynaud phenomenon, *e*sophageal dysfunction, *s*clerodactyly, and *t*elangiectsia) syndrome is a subtype of lcSSc with distinctive features, an overall good prognosis and an association with the presence of anti-centromere antibodies. Subcutaneous calcinosis, due to deposition of calcium hydroxyapatite crystals, occurs commonly at sites of tissue ischemia and recurrent trauma such as the fingertips, forearm, or elbow.

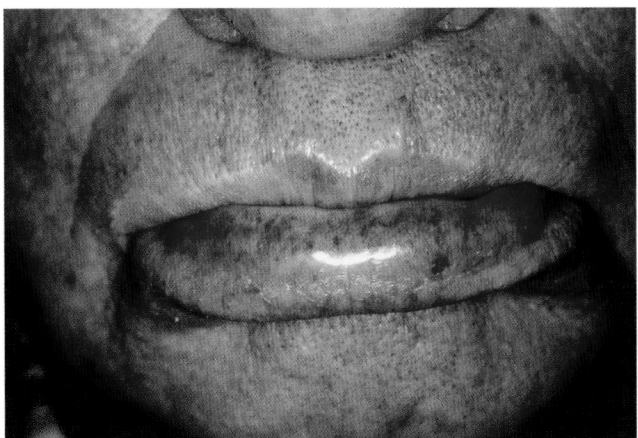

Fig. 54.6 Telangiectasia. Characteristic telangiectasia on the lip in a woman with limited cutaneous systemic sclerosis.

Although significant internal organ disease occurs with lower frequency in patients with lcSSc, isolated pulmonary arterial hypertension (PAH) develops in 10–15% of patients and may be life-threatening.[14] Significant interstitial lung disease can occur in a subset. Severe Raynaud phenomenon with macrovascular occlusive involvement occurs more frequently in lcSSc than in dcSSc, and can be associated with critical digital ischemia, ischemic ulcerations, gangrene, and amputation. Overlap with other autoimmune syndromes including the sicca complex, polyarthritis, cutaneous vasculitis, and autoimmune liver disease such as biliary cirrhosis, is seen primarily in the lcSSc subset of SSc.

Raynaud phenomenon

The skin has a unique vascular architecture designed to help maintain a stable central body temperature. This system has superficial and deep vascular plexuses connected by arteriovenous shunts that allow shunting of blood away from the skin surface during cold exposure and increases surface blood flow during hot ambient temperatures. Temperature-activated receptor ion channels on the ends of unmyelinated nerve fibers located in the skin sense the ambient temperature and then send impulses to the dorsal root ganglion and the central nervous system. Following this input, efferent signals via the sympathetic nervous system directly determine vascular reactivity in the skin. Raynaud phenomenon-associated increase in vascular tone is due in part to a defect in the vascular response to normal sympathetic signals. Recent studies find that α-2c adrenergic receptors on smooth muscle cells of cutaneous vessels are responsive to cold temperature and can be over-expressed in patients with Raynaud phenomenon.[15]

Raynaud phenomenon is clinically defined as cold- or emotional stress-induced vascular constriction of arteriovenous shunts, arterioles, and small arteries in the skin and tissues of the digits. Raynaud phenomenon is manifested as pallor of the digits (the phase of complete loss of blood flow) followed by cyanosis of the skin (low flow with deoxygenated blood) and hyperemia as blood flow rebounds after re-warming the skin. Raynaud phenomenon affects as much as 3–5% of the general population. Raynaud phenomenon is considered to be primary when there is no other associated disease state. In these cases, it is thought to represent a genetic trait with cold sensitivity due to abnormal cutaneous vessel reactivity to environmental temperatures. In SSc, the disease process targets thermoregulatory blood vessels, and alters the normal vascular responses to ambient temperature, thus presenting clinically with Raynaud phenomenon. Patients with SSc often have severe Raynaud phenomenon with multiple and often prolonged daily episodes associated with critical ischemia, leading to digital infarction or tissue gangrene. There is evidence that abnormal vascular reactivity in SSc is systemic, with recurrent bouts of vasospasm in the pulmonary, renal, gastrointestinal and coronary circulations.

Treatment of Raynaud phenomenon must be individualized and adjusted according to its severity. Initial therapy should include avoidance of cold exposure and methods of stress reduction. The best studied medications to treat Raynaud phenomenon are the calcium channel blockers (e.g., nifedipine) and they remain the recommended first choice of therapy. Other vasoactive drugs reported to be helpful include the α-1 adrenergic receptor blocker prazosin, phosphodiesterase inhibitors including sildenafil, serotonin re-uptake inhibitors such as fluoxetine, nitrates including topical nitroglycerine, and intravenous prostaglandins.[16] Bosentan, an endothelin-1 receptor inhibitor was recently shown to reduce the occurrence of new digital ulcers in patients with SSc, but not to alter the frequency of Raynaud's events.[17] Statins may also protect peripheral blood vessels and prevent ischemic digital ulcers and anti-oxidants have the potential of reducing oxidative stress to tissues.

Gastrointestinal involvement

Gastrointestinal disease is the most frequent initial symptom after Raynaud phenomenon. Patients with lcSSc and dcSSc are equally at risk. Gastrointestinal involvement is characterized by abnormal motility of the esophagus, stomach, small and large bowel, and rectum. Pathological studies show that the smooth muscle (circular greater that longitudinal) of the bowel atrophies without significant fibrosis, vascular injury or inflammation.[18] Functional and pharmacological studies have shown that a neurogenic process precedes smooth muscle dysfunction. Virtually every patient with SSc demonstrates evidence of distal esophageal dysfunction. Clinically, this may present with dysphagia and dyspepsia typical of gastroesophageal reflux disease. Esophageal manometric evaluation reveals the characteristic triad of low or absent primary and secondary peristalsis activity in the distal esophagus, normal proximal esophageal (striated muscle) motility, and the loss of the lower esophageal sphincter tone. Complications include reflux esophagitis, esophageal strictures, mucosal erosions and bleeding; Barrett's metaplasia or very rarely, adenocarcinoma may also develop.

Early satiety, bloating, nausea, periodic vomiting and decreased appetite with weight loss are common, and may be secondary to poor gastric emptying and retention of food and liquids in the stomach. Gastroparesis commonly associates with esophageal dysfunction and aggravates reflux disease. Dilatation of mucosal capillaries is common in the gastrointestinal tract, particularly in the gastric antrum. Gastric antral vascular ectasia (GAVE), also known as watermelon stomach, is the major gastric manifestation, which may lead to occult bleeding and significant anemia. Intestinal dysmotility can involve the small and large bowel. Patients may note a change in bowel habits or present with episodes of pseudo-obstruction with severe abdominal pain, bloating, abdominal distension, and vomiting. Persistent diarrhea may be a manifestation of malabsorption of fats due to bacterial overgrowth in atonic small bowel, and can be associated with dramatic weight loss and malnutrition. In the late stages the bowel wall thins out and traps air (pneumatosis cystoides intestinalis). Wide mouth diverticuli develop in the colon or the bowel, and may rupture. Incontinence of stool can occur due to dysfunction of anal sphincters.

Pulmonary involvement

Lung disease is now the leading cause of death in patients with SSc, and accounts for significant lifetime morbidity. Even in patients without respiratory symptoms, sensitive methods of pulmonary function testing reveal pulmonary abnormalities, and 40% of SSc patients have clinically significant lung involvement. The most common and serious forms of lung involvement are interstitial lung disease (ILD) and pulmonary vascular disease. Risk factors for severe ILD include black race, diffuse skin involvement, and presence of topoisomerase-I autoantibodies. Additional pulmonary manifestations of SSc include aspiration pneumonitis, pulmonary hemorrhage due to endobronchial telangiectasia, bronchiolitis obliterans with organizing pneumonia, pleural reactions and pneumothorax. The risk of lung cancer is increased in patients with SSc.

Interstitial lung disease

In patients with SSc, intersitital lung disease is most commonly characterized by the nonspecific interstitial pneumonia (NSIP) histologic pattern.[19] Inflammatory alveolitis and subsequent tissue fibrosis causes restrictive ventilatory defect and abnormal gas exchange. Patients with ILD may experience rapid initial decline in lung function during the early period of active skin disease. About 20% of patients with ILD continue to progress to severe end-stage disease. If there is only minor impairment in forced vital capacity (FVC) on lung function after more than five years of disease duration then is it much less likely to develop severe lung fibrosis later in the disease course. In early disease, most patients have no respiratory symptoms. The most sensitive method to detect early lung disease is pulmonary function testing. Imaging by high resolution computed tomography (HRCT) can be used to demonstrate fibrosis and ground glass opacities, and may provide an indication of the activity of the process; the degree of fibrosis correlates with decline in forced vital capacity. When the extent of disease defined by HRCT is <20%, the 10 year survival is reported to be 67%, whereas the group with HRCT-defined disease extent of >20%, 10 year survival was considerably poorer at 43%.[20] Likewise, a FVC of less than 70% associates with a poor lung prognosis. Until recently, bronchoalveolar lavage (BAL) was often performed to determine level of activity, to predict outcome, and to rule out occult pulmonary infection. The presence of a BAL neutrophilia was originally thought to predict risk of disease progression,[21] but likely increased neutrophils in the BAL fluid is a reflection of more extensive fibrotic disease and does not clearly define prognosis or response to therapy. Multicenter clinical trials comparing cyclophosphamide versus placebo demonstrated statistically significant stabilization of lung function (forced vital capacity), along with improvement in skin score and a variety of clinical measures, in the active treatment group.[22,23] Case series suggest that mycophenolate can also stabilize lung function in scleroderma patients with active ILD and a variety of anti-fibrotic agents are being tested.[24]

Pulmonary arterial hypertension

Pulmonary arterial hypertension is increasingly recognized as a frequent and severe complication of SSc. Pulmonary arterial hypertension is detected in 8–15% of SSc patients, and may occur as sole pulmonary manifestation of the disease, or in association with ILD.[25] The natural history of PAH is highly variable. In many patients with SSc, it follows a relentless downhill course with right heart failure and significant mortality. The estimated 3-year survival among patients with untreated PAH associated with SSc is approximately 50%. It is thought to be a late (9–12 years after onset of RP) complication in patients with limited scleroderma; but now it is recognized that many patients have PAH from disease onset, particularly in scleroderma with onset in older patients. Risk factors for PAH in SSc include late age at disease onset, history of severe Raynaud phenomenon, numerous skin telangiectasias, reduced nailfold capillaries, the presence

of anti-centromere, U1 RNP, anti-fibrillarin or anti-B23 antibodies. A worse prognosis with increased mortality is associated with increased blood brain naturetic protein (BNP), echocardiographic signs of right heart disease and decreased diffusion capacity (DLCO) on lung testing, Current therapy for SSc-associated PAH is focused on supportive care, reduction of cardiac work load and vasoactive drugs.[26] Short-acting prostacyclin analogues, including intravenous (epoprostenol or treprostinil) or inhaled (iloprost) prostaglandins, are in use for severe disease. Selective and non-selective endothelin-1 receptor inhibitors (bosentan, ambrisentan), and phosphodiesterase type 5 inhibitors (sildenafil, tadalafil) alone or in combination are helpful for milder disease. In relatively short-term clinical trials, each of these treatments improve exercise tolerance and hemodynamics, with variable benefit on disease progression. Lung transplantation remains an option for some SSc patients with severe lung disease.

Cardiac involvement

Cardiac involvement is common but often there are no signs or symptoms until late in the disease course. When heart disease is symptomatic or evident by objective testing, the prognosis is poor. SSc can affect virtually any cardiac structure including myocardial fibrosis with associated left ventricular (LV) systolic dysfunction and/or LV diastolic dysfunction, conduction abnormalities with arrhythmias, myocardial microvascular disease, and pericardial disease with large or small effusions. Valvular heart disease is usually not directly related. Cardiac disease can be secondary to other organ disease including PAH, ILD, or scleroderma renal crisis. Risk factors for scleroderma heart disease include dcSSc, longstanding disease and the presence of myositis.[27] While generally asymptomatic, pericardial disease can cause typical pericarditis, and rarely significant hemodynamic compromise and tamponade. Myocarditis is less common but can respond to anti-inflammatory drugs. Modern techniques for detecting occult heart disease are providing opportunities for early intervention such as the use of vasodilator therapy. These methods include tissue Doppler imaging, speckle-tracking echocardiography, cardiac magnetic resonance imaging (MRI), and blood biomarkers such as BNP.

Renal involvement

The most dreaded complication of SSc is acute renal involvement called scleroderma renal crisis (SRC). It develops in 10–15% of patients, most commonly those with dcSSc, and is generally a relatively early (<3 years) complication of the disease.[28] The presence of tendon friction rubs, pericardial effusion, new unexplained anemia, and presence of RNA polymerase III autoantibodies also increase the risk of renal crisis. The use of corticosteroids is thought to increase the risk of a SRC. Scleroderma renal crisis characteristically presents as malignant hypertension and rapidly progressive oliguric renal failure. Proteinuria, microhematuria, and evidence of a microangiopathic hemolytic process with thrombocytopenia are present. Patients with SRC who present with a creatinine > 3 mg/dL have a poor outcome, with permanent hemodialysis and high mortality. Prompt and aggressive intervention with angiotensin converting enzyme (ACE) inhibitors to achieve good blood pressure control before evidence of renal dysfunction significantly improves prognosis. Introduction of ACE inhibitors dramatically improved survival from a 10% 1-year survival to 60% 5-year survival. All patients with a SRC should be treated with an ACE inhibitor, but other vasodilators can be helpful including calcium channel blockers, endothelin receptor inhibitors and prostaglandins. Recovery can occur months after renal failure caused by a SRC. Renal transplantation is an option with outcome similar to other causes of renal failure. While SRC is the most important renal complication, other processes that need to be considered in scleroderma include interstitial nephritis, glomerulonephritis and renal vasculitis.

● CLINICAL PEARLS

Recommend approach to systemic sclerosis

- Determine scleroderma skin score to define clinical subtype
- Frequent clinical reassessment to define disease activity
- Careful clinical history to evaluate for gastrointestinal dysmotility
- Monitor for new onset hypertension: prevent renal crisis
- Pulmonary function test: early detection of interstitial lung disease
- Doppler echocardiography: screen for pulmonary arterial hypertension
- Obtain serology profile to help predict clinical outcome

Musculoskeletal complications

While musculoskeletal complaints are among the earliest symptoms of SSc, inflammatory erosive polyarthritis is uncommon. Joint involvement is usually due to fibrosis of the overlying skin, the supporting joint structures and the joint capsule itself. Flexion contractures associated with "friction rubs" over tendons are typical of advanced dcSSc, most prominent over the ankles, knees, shoulders and wrist. Muscle weakness is common, and may reflect deconditioning or disuse, malnutrition and weight loss, as well as inflammatory myositis and muscle fibrosis and atrophy.

Other disease manifestations

Many patients develop dry eyes and dry mouth (sicca complex). Unlike Sjögren's syndrome, in SSc these manifestations are due to fibrosis rather than lymphocytic infiltration of the minor salivary and tear glands. Furthermore, in SSc the sicca complex is associated with anticentromere antibodies. Primary biliary cirrhosis is a rare complication of lcSSc, and is associated with antimitochondrial antibodies. Autoimmune hepatitis can also occur. Up to 20% of SSc patients are hypothyroid, due to direct thyroid fibrosis or a consequence of autoimmune thyroiditis. The central nervous system is generally spared in SSc, but cases of trigeminal neuralgia have been reported. Erectile dysfunction frequently develops, and is due to a combination of microvascular disease and corporeal fibrosis. In some patients with SSc, erectile failure is the initial manifestation of the disease. Because SSc impacts on every aspect of a patient's life and is disfiguring, it is not surprising that significant depression is common.[29] Chronic pain and the lack of social support are major causes of depression and, therefore, vigorous pain control and anti-depressive medication are important considerations in the management of SSc.

Treatment

● THERAPEUTIC PRINCIPLES

Treatment of systemic sclerosis

Organ-specific therapy

- Vasodilator therapy for Raynaud phenomenon
- Proton pump inhibitor for gastroesophageal reflux
- ACE inhibitor for scleroderma renal crisis
- Vasodilator therapy for pulmonary arterial hypertension
- Anti-inflammatory therapy for arthritis
- Immunosuppressive therapy for interstitial lung disease

Disease-modifying agents

- No ideal treatment available; immunomodulatory, anti-inflammatory, vasoactive and anti-fibrotic agents are used and/or under study.

To date, no drug or intervention has been shown to be effective and safe for modifying disease course. Most successful SSc treatments are directed to the specific organ(s) involved. Therapy is focused on an organ-specific disease process (e.g., ACE inhibitor in SRC), or to aid a failing organ (e.g., proton pump inhibitors or metoclopramide for gastroesophageal reflux disease). Therefore, it is important to carefully characterize the patient's clinical phenotype and define the level of disease activity before deciding on therapy. For example, a patient with lcSSc who has no evidence of visceral organ involvement is likely to have a benign course requiring only symptomatic therapy (e.g., treatment of GERD and RP); disease modifying drugs would not be indicated. It is also important to distinguish disease activity from severity or advanced cumulative organ damage. For example, a patient with late-stage dcSSc is unlikely to benefit from aggressive immunosuppressive or anti-inflammatory therapy. Intervention with currently available drugs should be initiated early, ideally during the edematous active inflammatory phase of the disease. It is during the early disease that immunosuppression, anti-inflammatory and anti-fibrotic agents have the greatest potential to control disease progression. Clinical experience teaches that once the edematous phase of the disease shifts to the more indolent fibrotic phase, current treatments are ineffective to control the progression and tissue damage. Few well-designed controlled studies have been carried out for the treatment of early active disease; most reports are anecdotal uncontrolled experiences complicated by investigator bias and the highly variable natural course of SSc.

Evidence-based management of SSc is helpful,[30] while innovative therapies are being studied in clinical trials.[31] Medications that have been used in SSc but appear to have little or no benefit include colchicine, DMSO, para-aminobenzoic acid, interferon gamma, photopheresis, minocycline, and anti-tumor necrosis factor alpha agents. Controlled clinical trials have failed to provide evidence for the efficacy of D-penicillamine, a drug long in widespread use for SSc, or for relaxin. Immunosuppressive drugs are used to control *early active* dcSSc because of the evidence that the SSc is an autoimmune disease initiated and/or propagated by an immune process. However, no rigorous trials have evaluated the efficacy of popular approaches to dcSSc. Drugs reported to have benefit include methotrexate, cyclophosphamide and mycophenolate mofetil. Additional reports suggest benefit with cyclosporine, intravenous immunoglobulin, anti-thymocyte globulin, rapamycin, and anti-IL-6. The use of cyclophosphamide is limited by bone marrow suppression and bladder toxicity; mycophenolate mofetil by the issue of long-term immunosuppression; intravenous immunoglobulin by its expense; cyclosporine by frequent renal toxicity; and methotrexate by its potential to induce or exacerbate liver or lung fibrosis. Treatments targeting B cells with rituximab and inhibitors of interferon are under way. Multicenter clinical trials of immunoablative therapy with high-dose cyclophosphamide alone or with radiation, followed by stem cell rescue, are in progress. High-dose cyclophosphamide without stem rescue is also used in a variety of autoimmune diseases including scleroderma.[32] The use of novel biologic agents such as anti-cytokines (TGF-β), anti-chemokines (CCR2) or inhibitors of growth factors (CTGF) is being explored. Physicians are encouraged to refer patients with early dcSSc to specialty centers focusing on clinical trials.

● ON THE HORIZON

Novel therapeutic approaches to SSc management in clinical trials

- Targeted therapies to block TGF-β
- Development of anti-fibrotic agents, including new approaches to blocking of fibrogenic pathways
- Use of biologic agents, including anti-cytokines, anti-chemokines, and growth factor inhibitors

---

Other fibrosing diseases

Several disorders can cause skin fibrosis and mimic SSc or scleroderma.[33] These include localized forms of scleroderma (Table 54.3), eosinophilic fasciitis, the eosinophilia-myalgia syndrome, scleromyxedema (papular mucinosis) and scleredema (Table 54.4). Nephrogenic systemic fibrosis is described in patients with end-stage renal disease who were exposed to gadolinium-based contrast agents.[34] Eosinophilia-myalgia syndrome (EMS) is an apparently new disease first described occurring as an epidemic outbreak in 1989. The syndrome is characterized by acute onset of myalgia and eosinophilia, followed by more gradual evolution of diffuse scleroderma-like skin fibrosis, often accompanied by peripheral neuropathy and myopathy. Fibrosis in the skin spares the fingers, distinguishing it from the skin changes of SSc. The EMS outbreak was associated with consumption of L-tryptophan as dietary supplement, and largely subsided following the ban of L-tryptophan. However, sporadic cases of EMS continue to occur.[35] SSc can be distinguished from these scleroderma-like fibrosing conditions by its characteristic clinical, pathological and laboratory features. These include evidence of widespread vasculopathy with abnormal skin capillaries and Raynaud phenomenon, the characteristic distribution pattern of skin changes and typical dermatopathological features, the unique pattern of visceral organ involvement, and presence of SSc-specific serum autoantibodies.

Table 54.4 Differential diagnosis of SSc and scleroderma

Disorders characterized by similar presentations
Systemic lupus erythematosus
Sjögren's syndrome
Rheumatoid arthritis
Polymyositis/dermatomyositis
Primary Raynaud phenomenon

Disorders characterized by similar visceral features
Primary pulmonary hypertension
Primary biliary cirrhosis
Idiopathic intestinal hypomotility
Idiopathic pulmonary fibrosis
Malignant hypertension

Disorders characterized by skin thickening
Scleromyxedema
Scleredema (of Buschke), diabetic scleredema
Nephrogenic fibrosing dermatopathy
Eosinophilic fasciitis/diffuse fasciitis with eosinophilia
Eosinophilia-myalgia syndrome
Generalized morphea
Chronic graft versus host disease
POEMS syndrome
Amyloidosis
Carcinoid syndrome
Pentazocine-induced scleroderma
Diabetic digital sclerosis
Vinyl chloride disease
Toxic oil syndrome
Bleomycin exposure
Werner's syndrome
Phenylketonuria
Porphyria cutanea tarda
Vibration white finger syndrome
Chronic reflex sympathetic dystrophy

References

1. Maricq HR, Weinrich MC, Keil JE, et al. Prevalence of scleroderma spectrum disorders in the general population of South Carolina. Arthritis Rheum 1989;32(8):998–1006.
2. Mayes MD, Lacey Jr JV, Beebe-Dimmer J, et al. Prevalence, incidence, survival, and disease characteristics of systemic sclerosis in a large US population. Arthritis Rheum 2003;48(8):2246–55.
3. Radstake TR, Gorlova O, Rueda B, et al. Genome-wide association study of systemic sclerosis identifies CD247 as a new susceptibility locus. Nat Genet 2010;42(5):426–9.
4. Hummers LK. The importance of recognizing scleroderma-type disorders in clinical practice. Nat Clin Pract Rheumatol 2008;4(12):638–40.
5. Janowsky EC, Kupper LL, Hulka BS. Meta-analyses of the relation between silicone breast implants and the risk of connective-tissue diseases. N Engl J Med 2000;342(11):781–90.
6. Abraham DJ, Varga J. Scleroderma: from cell and molecular mechanisms to disease models. Trends Immunol 2005;26(11):587–95.
7. Kuwana M, Okazaki Y, Yasuoka H, et al. Defective vasculogenesis in systemic sclerosis. Lancet 2004;364(9434):603–10.
8. Sato S, Fujimoto M, Hasegawa M, Takehara K. Altered blood B lymphocyte homeostasis in systemic sclerosis: expanded naive B cells and diminished but activated memory B cells. Arthritis Rheum 2004;50(6):1918–27.
9. Harris ML, Rosen A. Autoimmunity in scleroderma: the origin, pathogenetic role, and clinical significance of autoantibodies. Curr Opin Rheumatol 2003;15(6):778–784.
10. Mori Y, Chen SJ, Varga J. Expression and regulation of intracellular SMAD signaling in scleroderma skin fibroblasts. Arthritis Rheum 2003;48(7):1964–78.
11. Krishnan E, Furst DE. Systemic sclerosis mortality in the United States: 1979–1998. Eur J Epidemiol 2005;20(10):855–61.

12. Ioannidis JP, Vlachoyiannopoulos PG, Haidich AB, et al. Mortality in systemic sclerosis: an international meta-analysis of individual patient data. Am J Med 2005;118(1):2–10.

13. LeRoy EC, Medsger Jr. TA. Criteria for the classification of early systemic sclerosis. J Rheumatol 2001;28(7):1573–6.

14. Tyndall AJ, Bannert B, Vonk M, et al. Causes and risk factors for death in systemic sclerosis: a study from the EULAR Scleroderma Trials and Research (EUSTAR) database. Ann Rheum Dis 2010;69(10):1809–15.

15. Flavahan NA. Regulation of vascular reactivity in scleroderma: New insights into Raynaud's phenomenon. Rheum Dis Clin North Am 2008;34(1):81–7, vii.

16. Boin F, Wigley FM. Understanding, assessing and treating Raynaud's phenomenon. Curr Opin Rheumatol 2005;17(6):752–60.

17. Korn JH, Mayes M, Matucci Cerinic M, et al. Digital ulcers in systemic sclerosis: prevention by treatment with bosentan, an oral endothelin receptor antagonist. Arthritis Rheum 2004;50(12):3985–93.

18. Roberts CG, Hummers LK, Ravich WJ, et al. A case-controlled study of the pathology of oesophageal disease in systemic sclerosis (scleroderma). Gut 2006;55(12):1697–703.

19. Veeraraghavan S, Nicholson AG, Wells AU. Lung fibrosis: new classifications and therapy. Curr Opin Rheumatol 2001;13(6):500–4.

20. Goh NS, Desai SR, Veeraraghavan S, et al. Interstitial lung disease in systemic sclerosis: a simple staging system. Am J Respir Crit Care Med 2008;177(11):1248–54.

21. White B, Moore WC, Wigley FM, et al. Cyclophosphamide is associated with pulmonary function and survival benefit in patients with scleroderma and alveolitis. Ann Intern Med 2000;132(12):947–54.

22. Tashkin DP, Elashoff R, Clements PJ, et al, Scleroderma Lung Study Research Group. Cyclophosphamide versus placebo in scleroderma lung disease. N Engl J Med 2006;354(25):2655–66.

23. Hoyles RK, Ellis RW, Wellsbury J, et al. A multicenter, prospective, randomized, double-blind, placebo-controlled trial of corticosteroids and intravenous cyclophosphamide followed by oral azathioprine for the treatment of pulmonary fibrosis in Scleroderma. Arthritis Rheum 2006;54(12):3962–70.

24. Koutroumpas A, Ziogas A. Mycophenolate mofetil in systemic sclerosis-associated interstitial lung disease. Clin Rheumatol 2010;29:1167–8.

25. Le Pavec JL, Humbert M, Mouthon L, Hassoun PM. Systemic sclerosis-associated pulmonary arterial hypertension. Am J Respir Crit Care Med 2010;181:1285–93.

26. Mathai SC, Hassoun PM. Therapy for pulmonary arterial hypertension associated with systemic sclerosis. Curr Opin Rheumatol 2009;21(6):642–8.

27. Follansbee WP, Zerbe TR, Medsger Jr. TA. Cardiac and skeletal muscle disease in systemic sclerosis (scleroderma): a high risk association. Am Heart J 1993;125(1):194–203.

28. Denton CP, Lapadula G, Mouthon L, Muller-Ladner U. Renal complications and scleroderma renal crisis. Rheumatology 2009;48:iii32–5.

29. Haythornthwaite JA, Heinberg LJ, McGuire L. Psychologic factors in scleroderma. Rheum Dis Clin North Am 2003;29(2):427–39.

30. Khanna D, Denton CP. Evidence-based management of rapidly progressing systemic sclerosis. Best Pract Res Clin Rheum 2010;24:387–400.

31. Ong VH, Denton CP. Innovative therapies for systemic sclerosis. Curr Opin Rheumatol 2010;22:264–72.

32. DeZern AE, Petri M, Drachman DB, et al. High-dose cyclophosphamide without stem cell rescue in 207 patients with aplastic anemia and other autoimmune diseases. Medicine 2011;90(2):89–98.

33. Boin F, Hummers LK. Scleroderma-like fibrosing disorders. Rheum Dis Clin North Am 2008;34(1):199–220.

34. Jalandhara N, Arora R, Batuman V. Nephrogenic systemic fibrosis and gadolinium-containing radiological contrast agents: an update. Clin Pharmacol Ther 2011;89(6):920–3.

35. Allen J, Peterson A, Sufit R, et al. Post-epidemic eosinophilia myalgia syndrome associated with L-tryptophan. Arthritis Rheum 2011;63(11):3633–9.

55

Inflammatory muscle diseases

Lisa Christopher-Stine, Sabiha Khan

The idiopathic inflammatory myopathies (IIM)—dermatomyositis (DM), polymyositis (PM), and inclusion body myositis (IBM)—constitute the largest subgroup of the acquired myopathies. They are a heterogeneous group and are rare among immunologic illnesses. However, the IIM share many clinical features and laboratory abnormalities, including related autoantibodies, and are closely related to major autoimmune diseases. Because their presentation and major clinical manifestations are weakness and/or rash, the differential diagnosis includes many more common diseases familiar to neurologists and dermatologists.

Clinical features

The clinical hallmark of polymyositis and dermatomyositis is the gradual onset of symmetrical proximal muscle weakness over weeks to months. In some cases, myalgia may be the presenting or most bothersome symptom, but more often the patient is evaluated for the physical limitations imposed by weakness: difficulty arising from a low chair or bed, or combing and brushing hair. Rash is the first feature in a considerable proportion of patients who have dermatomyositis, but muscle weakness usually follows within a few months. A subset of patients with dermatomyositis, clinically amyopathic dermatomyositis (C-ADM), may present only with rash in the absence of muscle weakness throughout the course of their illness. These patients are also at risk for pulmonary involvement, as are those with classic DM. The prevalence of interstitial pneumonitis in C-ADM can approach 5–10%—as compared to 40% of patients with classic DM.[1] Arthritis, Raynaud's phenomenon, fever, or lung disease presenting as cough or dyspnea may dominate the clinical picture. Cardiac and gastrointestinal symptoms other than dysphagia in severe cases are rarely early manifestations. Renal and central nervous system (CNS) involvement are almost never a part of the IIM.

Some of the rashes of dermatomyositis are virtually pathognomonic; others are not disease specific (Fig. 55.1). The heliotrope rash, a violaceous discoloration of the eyelids, is sometimes no more than a line along the margin of the upper lid, but may also affect both upper and lower lids completely, and can be associated with edema mimicking thyroid disease. A reddish, sometimes raised and/or scaly eruption over the metacarpophalangeal joints is known as Gottron's papules. In some cases, the metatarsophalangeal joints, elbows, knees, and malleoli show a similar rash. Both heliotrope and Gottron's rashes can occur rarely in cases of frank systemic lupus erythematosus (SLE) without muscle involvement. Other common rashes include a flat red blanching eruption of the upper chest (often in a V distribution), the upper back (where a shawl would touch), and sometimes the extensor surfaces of the upper arms and thighs. Another rash that mimics the malar rash of lupus on the face may be present, but, in contrast to lupus, does not spare the nasolabial folds. Although found on sun-exposed parts of the body, these rashes are often not photosensitive in nature. As in other connective tissue diseases, nailfold capillary dilatation, infarcts, and cuticular overgrowth occur. A roughening and cracking of the radial sides of the fingers and the palm, resembling a condition found in people who labor with their hands (mechanic's hands), is characteristic of a subset of myositis patients with the "antisynthetase syndrome" and can also be seen in patients with PM-Scl and U1-RNP autoantibodies.

Classification

In the past 40 years, several investigators have proposed diagnostic classification criteria for IIM. The criteria proposed by Bohan and Peter three decades ago remain the most familiar and accepted definitions of PM and DM.[2,3] They combine clinical, laboratory, electrodiagnostic, and pathological features. These criteria currently serve as the gold standard for clinical diagnosis and for inclusion in clinical trials. However, they are limited by their poor specificity in distinguishing PM from other entities, including late-onset muscular dystrophies. The resultant misclassification limits the homogeneity of the patients included in previous observational and interventional studies. Additionally, the Bohan and Peter criteria completely omit the diagnosis of IBM, the most frequent type of IIM in patients over 50 years of age.[4]

Additional classification criteria have been proposed by Tanimoto et al.[5] and by Targoff et al.[6] (Table 55.1), but neither classification has been widely used. The Targoff classification scheme suggests the incorporation of MRI and myositis-specific antibodies (MSAs), but the sensitivity and specificity of this

KEY CONCEPTS

Definition and incidence of idiopathic inflammatory myopathies (IIM)

- Polymyositis, dermatomyositis, and related inflammatory muscle diseases are called IIM.
- Indistinguishable muscle inflammation may accompany other autoimmune connective tissue diseases or limb-girdle muscular dystrophies.
- The annual incidence in the USA is 5–10 cases per million. DM and PM are more common in women than men in all age groups; IBM is more common in men.

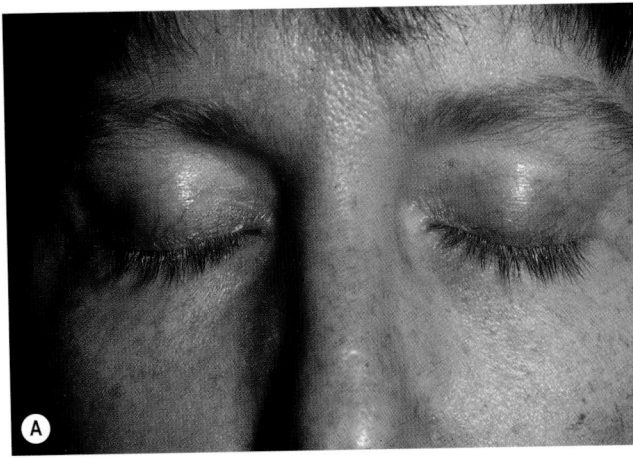 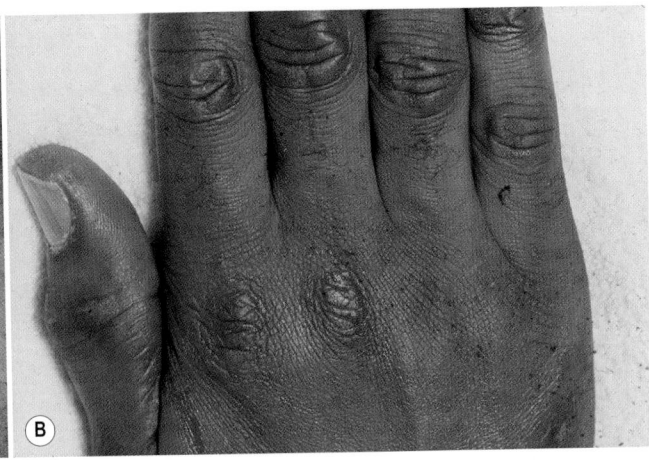

Fig. 55.1 Dermatomyositis rash. (A) In addition to the heliotrope rash on the eyelids of this patient with dermatomyositis, there is a flat red rash on the nose and cheeks. (B) A raised shiny red rash—Gottron's papules—is apparent on the interphalangeal and the second and third metacarpophalangeal joints of this man with dermatomyositis.

Table 55.1 Current idiopathic inflammatory myopathy: diagnostic criteria

Bohan and Peter criteria	Targoff proposed criteria	Tanimoto proposed criteria
1. Symmetrical proximal muscle weakness	1. Symmetrical proximal muscle weakness	1. Symmetrical proximal muscle weakness
2. Skeletal muscle enzyme elevation	2. Skeletal muscle enzyme elevation	2. Skeletal muscle enzyme elevation
3. Abnormal EMG[a]	3. Abnormal EMG[a]	3. Abnormal EMG[a]
4. Muscle biopsy abnormalities	4. Muscle biopsy abnormalities[b]	4. Muscle biopsy abnormalities[b]
5. Typical skin rash of DM[c]	5. Typical skin rash of dermatomyositis[c]	5. Typical skin rash of dermatomyositis[c]
	6. One of the myositis specific antibodies (MSAs)	6. Muscle pain
	7. MRI may substitute for criterion 1 or 2	7. Positive Anti-Jo-1 antibody
		8. Nondestructive arthritis/arthralgia
		9. Systemic inflammatory signs[d]

[a]Polyphasic, short, small motor-unit potentials; fibrillation, positive sharp waves, increased insertional irritability; bizarre, high-frequency, repetitive discharges.
[b]Degeneration/regeneration, perifascicular atrophy, necrosis, phagocytosis, fiber size variation, and mononuclear inflammatory infiltrate.
[c]Gottron's sign, heliotrope rash.
[d]Fever > 37 °C, elevated CRP, elevated ESR > 20 mm by Westergren method.

For the Bohan and Peter criteria
Possible PM = any two of the first four criteria; possible DM = criterion 5 (rash) + any two criteria.
Probable PM = any three of the first four criteria: probable DM = criterion 5 (rash) + any three criteria.
Definite PM = all four of the first four criteria; definite DM = criterion 5 (rash) + all four other criteria.

For the Targoff criteria
Possible IIM = any two criteria.
Probable IIM = any three criteria.
Definite IIM = any four criteria.
MRI results consistent with inflammation may be substituted for criterion 1 or 2.

For the Tanimoto criteria
Rash + at least four of the other eight items = DM.
Four of the items excluding rash = PM.
(There are no definite/probable/possible categories.)

Table 55.2 Proposed diagnostic criteria for inclusion body myositis

Pathologically defined IBM:
None of the other clinical or laboratory features are mandatory if muscle biopsy features are diagnostic. Muscle biopsy must show invasion of non-necrotic fibers by mononuclear cells and rimmed vacuoles, and either intracellular amyloid deposits or 15- to 18-nm filaments.

Clinically defined IBM
Clinical features
Duration of weakness > 12 **months**
Age > 35 **years**
Weakness of distal muscles greater than proximal muscles:
Finger flexion **weakness** > shoulder abduction **weakness**
AND
Knee extension **weakness** > hip f006Cexion weakness
Pathologic features
Invasion of non-necrotic fibers by mononuclear cells or rimmed vacuoles or increased MHC-1, but no intracellular amyloid deposits or 15- to 18-nm filaments

Possible IBM
Clinical criteria
Duration of weakness > 12 months
Age > 35 years
Weakness of distal muscles greater than proximal muscles:
Finger flexion weakness > shoulder abduction weakness
OR
Knee extension weakness > hip flexion weakness
Pathologic criteria
Invasion of non-necrotic **fibers by mononuclear cells** or rimmed vacuoles or increased MHC-1, but no **intracellular amyloid deposits** or 15- to 18-nm filaments

scheme have not been validated.[5] The Tanimoto criteria lack quantification or specific requirements for satisfying some criteria, and do not include MRI.[6] Separate classification criteria systems for IBM have been devised (Table 55.2), but characteristic muscle biopsy changes remain the defining feature in IBM.

It has been useful for some purposes to divide cases into groups: polymyositis, dermatomyositis, juvenile myositis, myositis associated with another connective tissue disease (usually systemic sclerosis, SLE, or Sjögren syndrome), cancer-associated myositis (usually cases in which the diagnoses are made within 6–12 months of one another), inclusion body myositis, and a miscellaneous group that includes such rare entities as eosinophilic myositis (Table 55.3). This classification has allowed recognition

Table 55.3 Traditional classification of idiopathic inflammatory myopathies

Type I	Primary idiopathic polymyositis
Type II	Primary idiopathic dermatomyositis
Type III	Dermatomyositis or polymyositis associated with malignancy
Type IV	Childhood dermatomyositis or polymyositis
Type V	Myositis associated with another connective tissue disease
Type VI	Inclusion body myositis
Type VII	Miscellaneous: eosinophilic myositis, localized nodular myositis, etc.

Table 55.4 Clinical features associated with myositis-specific autoantibodies

Autoantibodies	Characteristic clinical features
Anti-Jo-I and other antisynthetases	Relatively acute onset of myositis, frequent interstitial lung disease, fever, Raynaud's phenomenon, arthritis, mechanic's hands, moderate response to therapy, persistent disease. Patients sometimes meet criteria for SLE or RA, but muscle disease or lung disease dominate the clinical picture and prognosis
Anti-SRP	Very acute onset of myositis, often in autumn, severe weakness, no rash, palpitations, females predominate, poor response to therapy
Anti-Mi-2	Relatively acute onset of myositis, classic dermatomyositis rashes with V sign and shawl sign, cuticular overgrowth, good response to therapy
Anti-200/100	Necrotizing myopathy, preceded by statin therapy, very high CK levels, minimal muscle wasting
Anti-CADM-140	Clinically amyopathic dermatomyositis with interstitial lung disease
Anti-155/140	Juvenile dermatomyositis and cancer-associated dermatomyositis

SRP, signal recognition particle.

of unique clinical and pathogenetic features and response to therapy. In the case of cancer-associated myositis, a more rational approach to workup based on recognition of groups at risk is now possible.

More recently, it has been proposed that immune-mediated necrotizing myopathy is a separate category of myositis. Though it may have primary inflammation, the predominant features on histology are degeneration, regeneration, and necrosis. A specific antibody, anti-200/100-kDa, has been associated with a large subset of patients with necrotizing myopathy. Clinically, these patients present with subacute onset of proximal muscle weakness, irritable myopathic changes on EMG, elevated muscle enzymes, and edema on MRI. However, they differ from other autoimmune myopathies by evidence of very high creatine kinase (CK) levels, and only minimal muscle wasting. They are also frequently associated with preceding statin therapy.[7]

KEY CONCEPTS

Characteristic hallmarks of inflammatory myositis

- The clinical hallmark is proximal limb and neck weakness, rarely associated with muscle pain.
- The laboratory hallmarks are elevated serum levels of creatine kinase (CK), aldolase, lactic dehydrogenase, and the transaminases, and a characteristic pattern ("irritable myopathy") on electromyography (EMG). Elevated serum levels of autoantibodies are common.
- The pathologic hallmarks are focal muscle necrosis, degeneration, regeneration, and inflammation.

There are several other autoantibodies unique to myositis—called "myositis-specific autoantibodies." These have allowed a useful alternative classification (Table 55.4).[8] For example, patients with antibodies to the aminoacyl-tRNA (transfer RNA) synthetases, of which Jo-1 is the best known, have a characteristic syndrome called anti-synthetase syndrome, which usually includes interstitial lung disease, nondeforming inflammatory arthritis, fevers, mechanic's hands, and Raynaud's phenomenon, in addition to myositis. Those with antibodies to the signal recognition particle (anti-SRP) have severe disease of abrupt onset, often in the autumn, unaccompanied by rash. Recent work has shown that cardiac involvement is less common and survival is better in patients with anti-SRP than has previously been reported.[9] Those with antibodies to the nuclear antigen Mi-2 almost always have the V and shawl rashes and cuticular overgrowth in addition to myositis. As mentioned, anti-200/100 is a unique subset of necrotizing myositis in which

patients frequently have had previous statin exposure, and respond to immunosuppressive therapy. Each of the different autoantibody-associated groups also has a predominant histocompatibility type and clinical course (Table 55.4).[2,8]

Inclusion body myositis is different from other inflammatory myopathies. It is not associated with MSAs. Patients with IBM rarely improve in strength with immunosuppressive therapy. They tend to be older than others with myositis, and in contrast to patients with PM and DM, who are predominantly women, IBM patients are commonly men. They have gradual, painless, progressive weakness and focal atrophy that develop over years, and may complain of frequent falls. The forearms of these patients exhibit a scalloped appearance, attributed to muscle atrophy. Difficulty with swallowing can occur with any inflammatory myopathy, and is frequently a major problem in patients with IBM. The CK and other skeletal muscle-associated serum enzymes are normal in about one-quarter of patients with IBM, and only moderately elevated in the remainder. The electromyogram in IBM frequently demonstrates both myogenic and neurogenic features secondary to the effective denervation of some muscle cells by inflammation and necrosis.

Proposed criteria for the diagnosis of IBM rely on both pathologic and clinical features. In the clinical setting of an inflammatory myopathy, the presence of the characteristic inclusions or rimmed vacuoles is diagnostic. Among the inflammatory myopathies, IBM is distinguished by substantial numbers of rimmed cytoplasmic vacuoles with tubulofilamentous material within myofibers. A variety of proteins have been found by immunohistochemistry in the muscle cells in IBM, including ubiquitin, β-amyloid precursor protein, and the transcription factor NF-kB, but it is not yet possible to tie them to the pathogenesis of the illness.[10] The infiltrates in the muscle of patients with IBM are composed predominantly of CD8 lymphocytes, closely resembling those found in the inflammatory infiltrate in the muscles of patients with polymyositis.[10] MHC-1 expression is also seen in the muscles of patients with IBM.[11] Most recently, criteria have been proposed by Hilton-Jones et al. to better classify IBM.[12]

IBM must be distinguished from other chronic myopathies. These include acquired myopathies, such as those caused by toxins, and genetically determined myopathies, such as some muscular dystrophies and the metabolic myopathies. There are several important differences between IBM and these other myopathies. The distinction, however, is not as well defined as might be expected. Although some of the familial forms of IBM have a distinctive clinical presentation, often early in life, there have been several families with the typical late onset and inflammatory picture of the presumed sporadic cases. Several genetic loci have been identified in familial IBM, so it will be important to assess any identified mutations in familial IBM-associated genes in sporadic cases.[14] A further complexity is that IBM has been described occurring decades after typical dermatomyositis.

Etiology

Immunologic clues to origin

The implications of myositis-specific autoantibodies that bind to and inhibit the function of native human enzymes involved in the formation of new proteins are tantalizing and probably significant. These autoantibodies appear to develop before symptomatic weakness or serum CK elevation, suggesting a close link to an initiating factor. Some of the clinical features, such as fever, arthritis, and lung disease, and the apparent seasonality in onset of disease in patients with anti-SRP, are reminiscent of some viral infections. In patients with autoantibodies against one of the aminoacyl-tRNA synthetases, such as Jo-1 (histidyl-tRNA synthetase), the possible connection to a viral inciting agent appeared compelling, as certain picornaviruses, which are closely related to viruses long suspected of causing myositis, such as coxsackie viruses, can mimic tRNA in acting as a substrate for an aminoacyl-tRNA synthetase.[15] Direct proof connecting picornaviruses to human myositis, however, has not been obtained.[16] A rare example of a viral myopathy seen in conjunction with the West Nile Virus (WNV) has been observed.[16,17] Symptoms in addition to the neurological manifestations included a myositis characterized by a T-lymphocyte infiltration of nerve fibers, leading the authors to conclude that the virus may reach the central nervous system via peripheral nerves. Evidence for a viral trigger has also been observed with HIV or HTLV-1. In infected individuals, the development of IBM has been noted. However, it is not always the first manifestation in these cases. There is no evidence of viral replication within the muscles, but instead the chronic infection triggers an inflammatory response.[18]

Drugs and toxins

A large number of environmental agents have been associated with myopathies. Drug-induced myopathy should be considered particularly in cases where no other cause has been identified. Sometimes the illness strikingly resembles the spontaneous disease. d-Penicillamine, for example, can induce a variety of autoimmune phenomena, including an inflammatory myopathy that closely resembles polymyositis. A number of drugs can also produce myopathies that can be clinically confused with IIM but are histologically distinct. This large group includes 3-hydroxy-3-methylglutaryl-coenzyme A (HMG-CoA) reductase inhibitors, corticosteroids, colchicine, and zidovudine (AZT).

The HMG-CoA reductase inhibitors can produce elevated CK and myalgias in some patients. Rhabdomyolysis is rare. Muscle biopsy may be normal, or can show ragged red fibers and deficiency of cytochrome C oxidase.[19] In corticosteroid-induced myopathy, type II muscle fiber atrophy is prominent on muscle biopsy and weakness improves when the dose is lowered. Colchicine can cause myopathy and painful neuromyopathy. The CYP3A4 system metabolizes colchicine, and taking another drug metabolized by the same pathway can result in myopathy.[19] Muscle biopsy shows autophagic vacuoles that stain for acid phosphatase. Discontinuation of colchicine usually results in improvement. AZT produces a characteristic mitochondrial myopathy. The myopathy associated with HIV infection can be distinguished from that caused by AZT by muscle biopsy, as characteristic mitochondrial abnormalities are found in the latter. Amiodarone rarely causes proximal and distal muscle weakness, along with tremor and distal sensory loss. Muscle biopsy reveals autophagic vacuoles with myeloid inclusions and debris. This is seen more commonly in patients with chronic kidney disease.[19] The antimalarial drugs chloroquine and hydroxychloroquine produce a vacuolar myopathy, possibly by raising the intralysosomal pH so that the acid cathepsins that digest waste products in the lysosome are inoperable, and waste products accumulate in vacuoles.

For most other drugs, the mechanism of toxicity is unknown. The claims that injections of type I collagen or silicone breast implants can cause inflammatory myositis were initially unsupported by epidemiological data, but more recent work by NIH investigators concluded from a case series study that women who develop IIM after receiving silicone breast implants constituted an immunologically distinct group of patients. Those with silicone implants and myositis were reported to have an increased frequency of HLA-DQA1*0102 and a decreased frequency of DRB1*0301 compared to patients with IIM in the absence of implants.[20]

Bacterial and parasitic diseases

Certain parasitic diseases can produce an illness by direct invasion of muscle. Weakness, fever, and eosinophilia are usually present. Bacterial pyomyositis is uncommon in North America, but occurs more commonly in other parts of the world. It is attended by the signs of local infection and is often asymmetrical. A recent report, however, details two cases of pyomyositis initially diagnosed as polymyositis. Patients presenting with disseminated pyomyositis may be difficult to distinguish clinically from those with IIM, especially in immunosuppressed individuals who may not mount a systemic response.[21]

Pathogenesis

The precise mechanisms of cell damage and death in the IIM are unknown. Apoptosis is absent in IIM biopsies, but infiltrating CD8 T cells in polymyositis do appear to release perforin and granzyme into targeted muscle cells. After damage, a muscle fiber, which is a syncytium, can regenerate. Initially, on light microscopy one can appreciate loss of striations leading to a homogeneous appearance, fiber size variation, atrophy, and centralization of the nuclei. In the inflammatory myopathies, mononuclear cell invasion is a primary method of destruction.

Macrophages and cytotoxic T cells invade the myofibers. The myocyte cytoplasm in the region of the invaginated cells appears vacuolated and swollen. Other regions of the same cell may show intense regeneration, as seen histologically by aggregates of nuclei with prominent nucleoli and fiber splitting. Thus, degeneration and regeneration can coexist in the same fiber.

The inflammatory milieu in inflamed muscle has been studied. Proinflammatory cytokines were not always detectable, although the chemokines MIP-1a and RANTES were present in most biopsies,[22,23] and IL-1b was also usually present.[24] TGF-β is constitutively present in muscle. The muscle cells and inflammatory cells present in IIM often have co-stimulatory molecules on their surfaces, reinforcing the picture of a direct interaction between them.[25] Tissue culture observations of muscle cells have demonstrated that they can both produce and respond to a considerable range of cytokines.

Engel and colleagues[13] have demonstrated several important pathologic distinctions between dermatomyositis and polymyositis, and have suggested that, in dermatomyositis, the initial point of injury may be the capillaries. A model of disease has been proposed in which capillaries are primarily damaged and myocytes are secondarily involved. Complement and immunoglobulins may be found in the walls of the capillaries even where the remainder of the muscle is normal. The membrane attack complex of complement deposits there, and endothelial cells are swollen and pale. Even in unaffected regions of muscle, special staining reveals a marked decrease in capillary numbers.[26] More advanced changes include microtubular endothelial inclusions and microvacuoles. Evaluation of lymphocyte populations in dermatomyositis shows a high percentage of B cells in the perivascular regions and an increasing frequency of T cells towards the perimysium and endomysium. T cells found within the muscle are mostly CD4+. In dermatomyositis, especially the juvenile-onset form, inflammation and necrosis followed by atrophy appear in a perifascicular pattern. Perivascular lymphocytic infiltrates, typical of later disease, have not been described as an early change. As in SLE, interferon-α/β-inducible gene and protein expression may contribute to the pathogenesis of DM. This innate immune response is characterized by plasmacytoid dendritic cell invasion.[27] Consistent with the importance of immune complexes, histological abnormalities in the skin in dermatomyositis are indistinguishable from the changes in lupus.

In contrast to dermatomyositis, polymyositis and IBM do not demonstrate marked capillary changes, perivascular infiltrates are less pronounced, and T-cell infiltrates in the perimysial and endomysial regions are more pronounced. Nonnecrotic fibers may be surrounded by T lymphocytes and macrophages. The T cells are enriched for the CD8 subset. Attempts to culture these cells and look for lysis of autologous myocytes have met with limited success. There is negligible evidence of NK cell-like activity. Should cytotoxic T cells prove to be the major effector cells, it will be necessary to clone T cells to identify the antigenic targets. Most cytotoxic T cells are of the CD8 phenotype and therefore recognize their antigenic peptide in association with MHC class I molecules. Although resting normal muscle has very low class I expression, it is upregulated in regenerating and degenerating fibers found in both inflammatory and noninflammatory myopathies. Interestingly, in dermatomyositis, class I expression is upregulated predominantly in the perifascicular regions, around sites of atrophy, and near sites of cellular invasion. In contrast, in polymyositis, class I expression may be diffusely upregulated even where there is no cellular infiltrate. IBM shows a more focal class I distribution in regions of T-cell invasion. The presence of focal regions of MHC class I expression in nonnecrotic fibers at the site of activated CD8 T cells is compatible with cytotoxicity as a prime mechanism of myocyte necrosis in IBM and polymyositis. A pivotal study using transgenic mice demonstrated that abnormal accumulation of MHC class I molecules in the endoplasmic reticulum (ER) of muscle may initiate the ER stress response.[28]

> **KEY CONCEPTS**
>
> **Differential features of myositis**
>
> - In dermatomyositis the earliest changes involve vessel walls, and B cells and CD4 T cells predominate in the muscle biopsy.
> - In polymyositis and inclusion-body myositis the dominant pathologic feature is targeting and invasion of muscle cells by CD8 cytotoxic cells.

Proposed pathogenic mechanisms for the development of both the familial and the sporadic forms of IBM include the concept of increased transcription and accumulation of the β-amyloid precursor protein and its proteolytic fragments; abnormal accumulations of the components of lipid metabolism, including cholesterol; and oxidative stress.[29] These characteristics, in concert with the theory of misfolded or unfolded proteins in the context of a cellular aging milieu, appear to contribute to the pathogenesis of IBM. One of the most intriguing steps forward in the study of IBM in recent years has been the identification of mutations in the UDP-N-acetylglucosamine 2-epimerase/N-acetylmannosamine kinase gene in the recessive familial quadriceps-sparing IBM first described in Iranian Jews, but now more extensively recognized.

The role of MHC class II molecules remains to be clarified. Cultured myoblasts constitutively express high levels of class I and are negative for class II. Class II has been found to be upregulated in the endothelial cells of patients with dermatomyositis, but its expression on T cells, a marker of activation, is more prominent in polymyositis.

Finally, γδ T lymphocytes have been cloned from the muscle biopsy of one patient with polymyositis. Subsequent evaluation of his biopsy demonstrated γδ T cells and a 65-kDa heat shock protein in the endomysial region. The relative importance of γδ T cells in the spectrum of IIM is unknown.

The role of B cells within affected muscles is not understood. It is not yet known whether they produce any autoantibodies, particularly the myositis-specific antibodies, or whether they play a role in antigen presentation for the T cells.

In necrotizing autoimmune myositis, there is necrosis of muscle fibers, which is mediated by macrophages. There is no expression of MHC-1 or T-cell infiltration. There has also been evidence of complement deposition on blood vessels. Antibodies against 200/100-kDa and SRP have been found.[18]

The pathogenic role of the autoantibodies found in patients with IIM remains uncertain. MSAs are found in 30–40% of patients, appear to delineate specific clinical entities, and each group has a strong but not absolute HLA association. In a patient with myositis and antihistidyl-tRNA synthetase (Jo-1) autoantibodies, sera available from long before the onset of symptoms or biochemical damage to muscle tissue contained the autoantibodies, suggesting that the autoantibodies were not merely a response to release of tissue antigens. The extraordinary specificity of myositis-specific antibodies for IIM and the lack of evidence for strong polyclonal stimulation in these diseases suggest that MSA are related to the fundamental causative process in IIM. Although 80–90% of patients with IIM are found to have antibodies to myosin or myoglobin, these antibodies are also found in patients with noninflammatory myopathies.

The structures bound by MSA are mostly intracellular ribonucleoproteins involved in protein synthesis, such as the aminoacyl-tRNA synthetases and the signal recognition particle (SRP). These autoantigens are found in every nucleated cell. The antibodies in general bind to conformational epitopes and, at least in the case of the antisynthetases, block enzymatic activity. It is possible that a structural property of muscle allows these particular proteins to be presented to the immune system when the cells are damaged, or, alternatively, the capacity of muscle fibers to degenerate alongside intense regeneration within the same fiber may allow these proteins to be efficiently displayed.[30] Recent experiments have suggested that some aminoacyl-tRNA synthetases have a direct proinflammatory role through a subsidiary chemokine-like action.[31]

A landmark study recently determined that cultured myoblasts express high levels of autoantigens, which are strikingly downregulated as cells differentiate into myotubes *in vitro*. These data strongly associate regenerating rather than mature muscle cells as the source of continuous autoantigen supply in autoimmune myositis.[30]

Genetics

The IIM do not exhibit a simple mode of inheritance, and the rare familial cases mostly reflect IBM of early onset. As noted above, there are HLA associations for particular MSAs. Specifically, HLA-DR52 has a strong association (90%) with antisynthetase-positive myositis in people of both European and African descent.[32]

Natural history

The prognosis for patients with IIM varies greatly with clinical type, autoantibodies, extraskeletal muscle involvement, and the interval between diagnosis and the start of treatment.

Patients with dermatomyositis or myositis accompanying another connective tissue disease are likely to recover most of their strength with prompt and adequate therapy. Although recurrences are common, persistent profound weakness does not usually occur. Most patients with anti-Mi-2 autoantibodies also usually respond well to therapy. Strength usually recovers well in patients whose myositis is cancer related, but overall mortality due to the tumor is high. Indeed, an accompanying tumor remains one of the most frequent causes of death in patients with an IIM. The diagnostic value of serum tumor markers (CEA, CA125, CA19-9 and CA15-3) was investigated in a study that demonstrated that serial CA125 and CA19-9 assessment could be useful markers in predicting which patients will develop cancer, especially in the subset of patients without interstitial lung disease.[33]

Patients with polymyositis fare less well, even when those with IBM are rigorously excluded. A return to normal strength is very unusual, and each recurrence is likely to be followed by greater residual weakness, even if inflammation is fully controlled. IBM has a poorer prognosis, but it is possible that the gradual decline in strength can be halted for long periods by corticosteroid and/or cytotoxic therapy if continuing inflammation is present. Severe muscle weakness and atrophy are prominent features in patients with anti-SRP autoantibodies. They have traditionally had the worst prognosis because there is rampant muscle destruction at the very outset. Those with anti-Jo-1 autoantibodies or antibodies to another synthetase are likely to respond to therapy initially, but to require continuing immunosuppression to treat frequent recurrences. In this group

morbidity and mortality are heavily influenced by the progression of lung involvement. Longitudinal studies of outcomes in DM and PM patients are few. Cardiac involvement, respiratory involvement, and cancer were the main causes of death in several cohort analyses.[33–35] Disease course is monocyclic in approximately 20% of patients, polycyclic in 20%, and chronic in the remainder.[35] Relapses have been noted in the initial years of therapy and after prolonged disease-free intervals; therefore, periodic surveillance is warranted for at least 2 years following remission.[36,37]

Patient management

The treatment of myositis is based on controlling skeletal muscle inflammation and damage. Immunosuppressive therapy is used in the initial stages of the disease to reduce inflammation and muscle damage. There are very few randomized controlled trials of any of the immunosuppressive agents used; thus, therapeutic regimens and responses have remained largely anecdotal. Clinical trials to assess the efficacy of TNF-α inhibitors, tacrolimus, and rituximab are currently under way. After the initial inflammation is controlled, strengthening exercises are useful in improving functional capabilities.

Corticosteroids

Corticosteroids are the main immunosuppressive agents used in the treatment of myositis. An initial course of pulses of methylprednisolone may be helpful, particularly in disease of acute onset, and may also be helpful in managing disease flares. If active muscle inflammation persists or the side-effects of corticosteroids are severe, other immunosuppressive treatments are employed.

Second-line immunosuppressive therapies

The most frequently used second-line agents in the treatment of myositis are azathioprine and methotrexate. Azathioprine has been shown to reduce long-term disability.[38] Methotrexate is useful in patients with little or no response to corticosteroid therapy.[39,40] Combination therapies, such as methotrexate with azathioprine, are useful even if patients have failed to respond to one of the agents alone.[41] High-dose intravenous immunoglobulin is of proven benefit in dermatomyositis.[42] Its usefulness in polymyositis is less predictable. Apheresis proved ineffective in a controlled blinded study.[43] Both cyclosporine and tacrolimus have been effective in some cases, as have cyclophosphamide and chlorambucil. The most recent therapeutic options include mycophenolate and rituximab. Rituximab has been reported to be effective in some cases of polymyositis, dermatomyositis, and necrotizing autoimmune myositis.[44] A controlled study looking at the effects of rituximab is nearing completion. Thus far, there has been no effective therapeutic regimen for IBM. However, IVIg has been reported to provide a transient response.[18]

Monitoring disease activity

Improvement in strength and normalization of serum CK activity are the best indirect measures of disease activity. A decrease in serum CK activity may herald clinical improvement, but corticosteroid treatment alone can reduce CK activity without associated clinical improvement. A lack of improvement in strength in a corticosteroid-treated patient may be due to the resistance of the inflammatory process, the presence of a corticosteroid-induced myopathy, and/or misdiagnosis. A diagnostic and therapeutic taper of the corticosteroids may then be warranted. If inflammation is present concurrently, other immunosuppressive agents are useful as the dosage of corticosteroids is lowered. If the CK value begins to rise, even if it is still within the normal range, and the symptoms of myositis are worsening in a patient whose disease has previously been controlled with corticosteroids, an increase in the dose may be warranted.

Treatment-resistant myositis

Some treatment-resistant polymyositis patients have another disease. In such cases IBM or a limb girdle muscular dystrophy should be suspected. Unlike other myositis patients, those with IBM rarely, if ever, improve in strength with immunosuppressive therapy, but stabilization of strength can be achieved in some IBM patients with immunosuppressive agents.[45,46] Patients with limb-girdle muscular dystrophies may mimic polymyositis clinically. They may have inflammation on muscle biopsy, and occasionally have associated autoantibodies. Thus, patients with a suspected IIM who do not respond to immunosuppressive therapy should undergo further evaluation, including genetic testing, to search for a limb-girdle muscular dystrophy.

Nonskeletal muscle involvement

Other organs frequently involved in myositis include the skin, lungs, and joints. Such organ involvement and the systemic features of myositis (fever and weight loss) usually improve with immunosuppressive therapy that controls inflammation in the skeletal muscle. Hydroxychloroquine and other antimalarials are useful in controlling the rashes associated with myositis.

Diagnostic tools, evaluation, and differential diagnosis

CLINICAL PEARLS

Clinical features that suggest a non-IIM diagnosis

- Family history of a similar illness
- Weakness related to exercise, eating, or fasting
- Sensory, reflex, or other neurologic signs
- Cranial nerve involvement
- Fasciculations
- Muscle cramping (severe)
- Myasthenia (increasing weakness with repeated contractions)
- Myotonia (difficulty relaxing a contracted muscle)
- Significant atrophy or hypertrophy early in the illness
- Marked asymmetry
- Dyspnea due to diaphragmatic weakness with normal chest X-ray

Clinical, laboratory, pathologic, and electrodiagnostic findings contribute to the proper diagnosis of IIM. Even in individuals with typical clinical features of IIM, it is essential to exclude other diseases that may have similar symptoms and signs (Table 55.5). Certain clinical features should suggest a different diagnosis.

Table 55.5 Differential diagnosis of IIM

Neuromuscular disorders
Genetic muscular dystrophies
Metabolic myopathies
Disorders of carbohydrate metabolism: McArdle disease, phosphofructokinase deficiency, adult acid maltase deficiency, and others
Disorders of lipid metabolism: carnitine deficiency, carnitine palmitoyl transferase deficiency
Disorders of purine metabolism: myoadenylate deaminase deficiency
Mitochondrial myopathies
Spinal muscular atrophies
Neuropathies: Guillain–Barré and other autoimmune polyneuropathies, diabetes mellitus, porphyria
Myasthenia gravis and Eaton–Lambert syndrome
Amyotrophic lateral sclerosis
Myotonic dystrophy and other myotonias
Familial periodic paralysis

Endocrine and electrolyte disorders
Hypokalemia, hypercalcemia, hypocalcemia, hypomagnesemia
Hypothyroidism, hyperthyroidism
Cushing syndrome, Addison's disease

Toxic myopathies (partial list)
Alcohol
Amiodarone
Chloroquine and hydroxychloroquine
Cocaine
Colchicine
Corticosteroids
D-Penicillamine
Ipecac
Statins and other lipid-lowering agents
Zidovudine (AZT)

Infections
Viral: HIV, HTLV-1, influenza
Bacterial: staphylococcus, streptococcus, clostridia
Parasitic: toxoplasmosis, trichinosis, schistosomiasis, cysticercosis

Miscellaneous
Polymyalgia rheumatica
Vasculitis
Eosinophilia myalgia syndrome
Paraneoplastic syndromes

These include a family history of a similar illness; sensory, reflex, or other neurologic changes; fasciculations; a relationship of the weakness to exercise, food intake, or fasting; major muscle cramping, myotonia (difficulty relaxing a contracted muscle), or myasthenia (increasing weakness with repeated contractions); significant early muscle atrophy or hypertrophy; marked asymmetry; weakness in the distribution of the cranial nerves; and dyspnea due to diaphragmatic weakness rather than lung fibrosis.

The single most useful laboratory feature of muscle destruction is elevation of the serum CK, although this is nonspecific, and a small proportion of patients—probably < 5%—have a bona fide inflammatory muscle disease without ever having an elevated CK. Elevations of the serum levels of aldolase, serum glutamic-oxaloacetic transaminase (SGOT), serum glutamate pyruvate transaminase (SGPT), and lactate dehydrogenase (LDH) are as frequent but less specific for muscle disease. Unlike other autoimmune inflammatory diseases, inflammatory markers such as the erythrocyte sedimentation rate and C-reactive protein are often not elevated. Although some studies have shown ESR to be elevated in 50% of patients, most experts find a substantially lower proportion of IIM patients to have an elevated ESR, even with active disease.[47] Likewise, hematologic abnormalities, including anemia, are uncommon and rarely related to the underlying myopathy. If a significant abnormality is found, the physician should be alert to another cause for it.

Electromyographic (EMG) abnormalities are frequently present. Although the test is useful for excluding some neurologic diseases that resemble IIM, it is painful for many patients and not useful for following the course of the illness.

Magnetic resonance imaging (MRI), especially a combination of the T1 and the fat-suppressed T2 (STIR) sequences, is remarkably useful in defining the extent of involvement and planning a biopsy (Fig. 55.2). Whole-body MRI has been shown to facilitate the characterization of inflammatory myopathy, as certain patterns of muscle and subcutaneous tissue inflammation were predictive of the IIM subset (DM, PM, or IBM).[48] MRI can also help differentiate active disease from chronic disease, with active myositis being notable for changes consistent with muscle edema on T2-weighted images, and chronic myositis revealing decrease in muscle bulk and replacement by adipose on T1-weighted images.[49] Although not specific, the changes of inflammatory myopathy on imaging can provide considerable assistance in confusing cases, as well as help in choosing a site to biopsy.

A muscle biopsy should be performed in every suspected case of myositis (Fig. 55.3). Although the patchy involvement means that the biopsy can occasionally miss inflammation, confounding diagnoses, for example amyloidosis, eosinophilic myositis, dystrophy, or some metabolic myopathies as well as the important variant IBM, can only be diagnosed definitively by biopsy. The identification of autoantibodies, particularly the myositis-specific autoantibodies, has distinct clinical and prognostic use. MSAs are highly specific for myositis compared to other neuromuscular diseases, and are not simply associated with muscle inflammation.[50]

At present, of these autoantibodies only anti-Jo-1 is commercially available, but tests for the others are carried out in research centers, and some will eventually become more widely available.

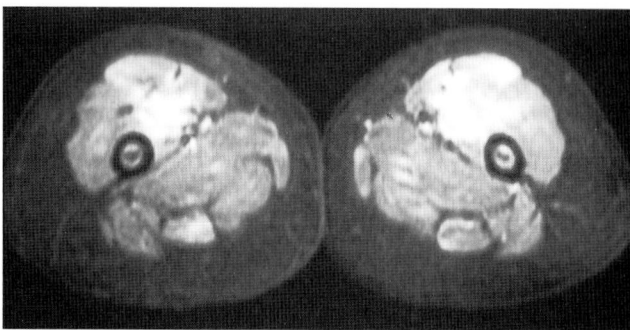
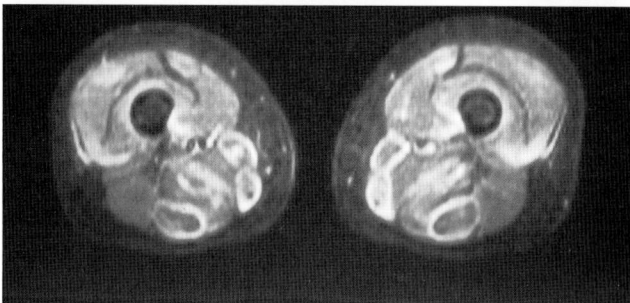

Fig. 55.2 Magnetic resonance images of the upper and lower thighs of a patient with dermatomyositis using the fat-suppressed T2 (STIR) technique. With this technique inflammation appears as a bright signal; normal muscle is gray; and bone, fat, fascia, and normal skin are dark. Blood vessels may appear as bright spots. Note the remarkable symmetry of the inflammation. In this patient most of the involvement is in the quadriceps in the upper thighs and around the periphery of the hamstring muscle group.

ON THE HORIZON

- Development of revised and updated classification criteria for inflammatory myopathies is needed.
- Improved diagnostic classification of cases through novel autoantibodies as well as immunohistochemistry.
- Recognition of immune-mediated necrotizing myopathy (IMNM) as a new phenotype among the inflammatory myopathies.
- This proposed entity is characterized by a lack of primary inflammation, but rather necrosis and regeneration with myophagocytosis.
- Patients may develop autoantibodies directed against signal recognition particle (SRP) and HMGCoA reductase.

Pitfalls

It is increasingly apparent that the boundary between IIM and some genetically determined myopathies cannot be cleanly drawn. In the last several years, dystrophies with an extraordinary variety of

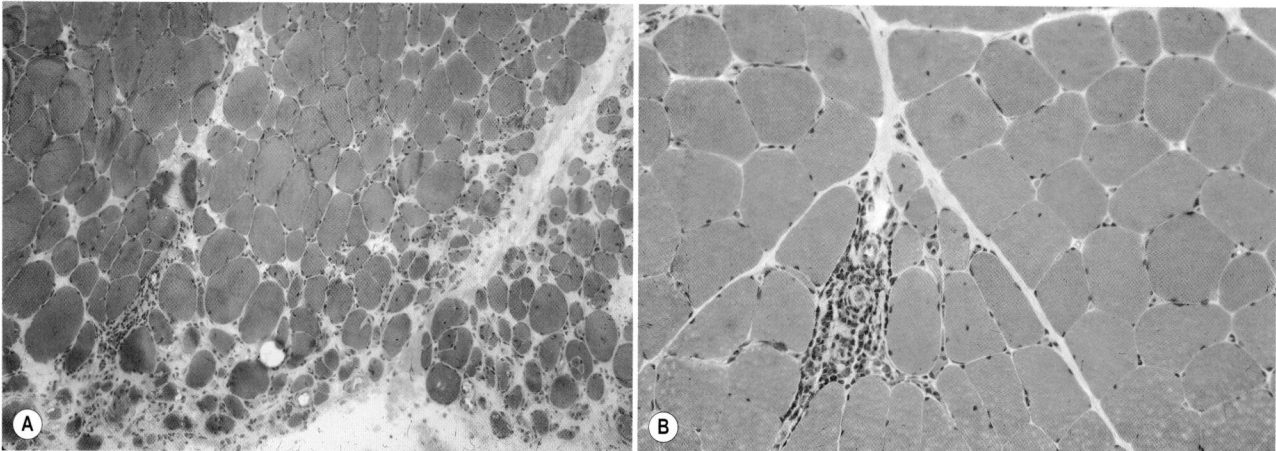

Fig. 55.3 Biopsy in dermatomyositis. (A) Low-power (original magnification × 100) view of a muscle biopsy from a patient with dermatomyositis. Note the marked variation in fiber size and the large number of atrophic myocytes, particularly at the periphery of the fascicles. (B) High-power (original magnification × 200) view of inflammation around the vessels in the muscle biopsy of a patient with dermatomyositis. There are nearby atrophic cells and cells whose nuclei have moved away from the periphery of the cell (centralized nuclei).

clinical manifestations (with regard to age and distribution of weakness) have also been described.[51] Not only can inflammation be seen on biopsy in some patients, but a partial clinical response to corticosteroids can occur. Furthermore, it is increasingly recognized that mitochondrial abnormalities can be limited to groups of skeletal muscles, leading to confusion with IIM. Toxic myopathies, of course, will continue to occur with the release of new drugs, and will continue to be a possible source of diagnostic confusion.

Thus, not only must the history, physical examination, and biopsy be performed and interpreted with compulsiveness and care, but molecular diagnostic techniques must be employed by clinicians in pursuit of an accurate diagnosis and appropriate therapy. The correct response to disease that persists in the face of powerful immunosuppressive therapy is a careful re-thinking of the diagnosis, including, on occasion, re-biopsy and molecular consultation.

References

1. Sontheimer RD. Dermatomyositis: an overview of recent progress with emphasis on dermatologic aspects. Dermatol Clin 2002;20:387–408.
2. Bohan A, Peter JB. Polymyositis and dermatomyositis (second of two parts). N Engl J Med 1975;292:403–7.
3. Bohan A, Peter JB. Polymyositis and dermatomyositis (first of two parts). N Engl J Med 1975;292:344–7.
4. Badrising UA, Maat-Schieman M, van Duinen SG, et al. Epidemiology of inclusion body myositis in the Netherlands: a nationwide study. Neurology 2000;55:1385–7.
5. Tanimoto K, Nakano K, Kano S, et al. Classification criteria for polymyositis and dermatomyositis. J Rheumatol 1995;22:668–74.
6. Targoff IN, Miller FW, Medsger Jr TA, Oddis CV. Classification criteria for the idiopathic inflammatory myopathies. Curr Opin Rheumatol 1997;9:527–35.
7. Christopher-Stine L, Casciola-Rosen LA, Hong G, et al. A novel autoantibody recognizing 200-kd and 100-kd proteins is associated with an immune-mediated necrotizing myopathy. Arthritis Rheum 2010;62(9):2757–66.
8. Zong M, Lundberg IE. Pathogenesis, classification and treatment of inflammatory myopathies. Nat Rev Rheumatol 2011;5:1–10.
9. Kao AH, Lacomis D, Lucas M, et al. Anti-signal recognition particle autoantibody in patients with and patients without idiopathic inflammatory myopathy. Arthritis Rheum 2004;50:209–15.
10. Yang CC, Askanas V, Engel WK, Alvarez RB. Immunolocalization of transcription factor NF-kappa B in inclusion-body myositis muscle and at normal human neuromuscular junctions. Neurosci Lett 1998;254:77.
11. Needham M, Mastaglia FL. Inclusion body myositis: current pathogenetic concepts and diagnostic and therapeutic approaches. Lancet Neurol 2007;6(7):620–31.
12. Hilton-Jones D, Miller A, Parton M, et al. Inclusion body myositis. MRC Centre for Neuromuscular Diseases. IBM workshop, London, 13 June 2008. Neuromuscul Disord 20:143.
13. Engel AG, Arahata K, Emslie-Smith A. Immune effector mechanisms in inflammatory myopathies. Res Publ Assoc Res Nerv Ment Dis 1990;68:141.
14. Argov Z, Eisenberg I, Mitrani-Rosenbaum S. Genetics of inclusion body myopathies. Curr Opin Rheumatol 1998;10:543.
15. Mathews MB, Bernstein RM. Myositis autoantibody inhibits histidyl-tRNA synthetase: a model for autoimmunity. Nature 1983;304:177.
16. Leff RL, Love LA, Miller FW, et al. Viruses in idiopathic inflammatory myopathies: absence of candidate viral genomes in muscle. Lancet 1992;339:1192.
17. Smith RD, Konoplev S, DeCourten-Myers G, Brown T. West Nile virus encephalitis with myositis and orchitis. Hum Pathol 2004;35:254–8.
18. Dalakas M. Pathophysiology of inflammatory and autoimmune myopathies. Presse Med 2011;e237–247.
19. Mor A, Wortmann RL, Mitnick HJ, Pillinger MH. Drugs causing muscle disease. Rheumatic Dis Clin N Am 2011;37(2):219–31.
20. OHanlon T, Koneru B, Bayat E, et al. Environmental Myositis Study Group. Immunogenetic differences between Caucasian women with and those without silicone implants in whom myositis develops. Arthritis Rheum 2004;50:3646–50.
21. Walji S, Rubenstein J, Shannon P, Carette S. Disseminated pyomyositis mimicking idiopathic inflammatory myopathy. J Rheumatol 2005;32:184–7.
22. Adams EM, Kirkley J, Eidelman G, et al. The predominance of beta (CC) chemokine transcripts in idiopathic inflammatory muscle diseases. Proc Assoc Am Phys 1997;109:275.
23. Lundberg I, Brengman JM, Engel AG. Analysis of cytokine expression in muscle in inflammatory myopathies, Duchenne dystrophy, and non-weak controls. J Neuroimmunol 1995;63:9.
24. Lundberg I, Ulfgren AK, Nyberg P, et al. Cytokine production in muscle tissue of patients with idiopathic inflammatory myopathies. Arthritis Rheum 1997;40:865.
25. Nagaraju K, Raben N, Villalba ML, et al. Costimulatory markers in muscle of patients with idiopathic inflammatory myopathies and in cultured muscle cells. Clin Immunol 1999;92:161.
26. Estruch R, Grau JM, Fernandez-Sola J, et al. Microvascular changes in skeletal muscle in idiopathic inflammatory myopathy. Hum Pathol 1992;23:888.
27. Greenberg SA, Pinkus JL, Pinkus GS, et al. Interferon a/b mediated innate immune mechanisms in dermatomyositis. Ann Neurol 2005;57:664–78.
28. Nagaraju K, Casciola-Rosen L, Lundberg I. Activation of the endoplasmic reticulum stress response in autoimmune myositis: potential role in muscle fiber damage and dysfunction. Arthritis Rheum 2005;52:1824–35.
29. van der Pas J, Hengstman GJ, ter Laak HJ, et al. Diagnostic value of MHC class I staining in idiopathic inflammatory myopathies. J Neurol Neurosurg Psychiatry 2004;75:136–9.
30. Casciola-Rosen L, Nagaraju K, Plotz P, et al. Enhanced autoantigen expression in regenerating muscle cells in idiopathic inflammatory myopathy. J Exp Med 2005;201:591–601.
31. Wakasugi K, Schimmel P. Two distinct cytokines released from a human aminoacyl-tRNA synthetase. Science 1999;284:147.
32. Goldstein R, Duvic M, Targoff IN, et al. HLA-D region genes associated with autoantibody responses to histidyl-transfer RNA synthetase (Jo-1) and other translation-related factors in myositis. Arthritis Rheum 1990;33:1240.
33. Amoura Z, Duhaut P, Huong DTL, et al. Tumor antigen markers for the detection of solid cancers in inflammatory myopathies. Cancer Epidemiol Biomarkers Prev 2005;14:1279–82.
34. Danko K, Ponyi A, Constantin T, et al. Long-term survival of patients with idiopathic inflammatory myopathies according to clinical features. Medicine 2004;83:35–42.
35. Bronner IM, van der Muelen MFG, de Visser M, et al. Long-term outcome in polymyositis and dermatomyositis. Ann Rheum Dis 2006;65:1456–61 Epub 2006; Apr 10.
36. Ponyi A, Constantin T, Balogh Z. Disease course, frequency of relapses and survival of 73 patients with juvenile or adult dermatomyositis. Clin Exp Rheumatol 2005;23:50–6.
37. Agarwal SK, Monach PA, Docken WP. Characterization of relapses in adult idiopathic inflammatory myopathies. Clin Rheumatol 2005;25:1–6.
38. Bunch TW. Prednisone and azathioprine for polymyositis: long-term followup. Arthritis Rheum 1981;24:45.
39. Metzger AL, Bohan A, Goldberg LS, et al. Polymyositis and dermatomyositis: combined methotrexate and corticosteroid therapy. Ann Intern Med 1974;81:182.
40. Joffe MM, Love LA, Leff RL, et al. Drug therapy of the idiopathic inflammatory myopathies: predictors of response to prednisone, azathioprine, and methotrexate and a comparison of their efficacy. Am J Med 1993;94:379.
41. Villalba L, Hicks JE, Adams EM, et al. Treatment of refractory myositis: a randomized crossover study of two new cytotoxic regimens. Arthritis Rheum 1998;41:392.
42. Dalakas MC, Illa I, Dambrosia JM, et al. A controlled trial of high-dose intravenous immune globulin infusions as treatment for dermatomyositis. N Engl J Med 1993;329:1392–3.
43. Miller FW, Leitman SF, Cronin ME, et al. Controlled trial of plasma exchange and leukapheresis in polymyositis and dermatomyositis. N Engl J Med 1992;326:1380.
44. Valiyil R, Casciola-Rosen L, Hong G, et al. Rituximab therapy for myopathy associated with anti-signal recognition particle antibodies: a case series. Arthritis Care Res 2010;62:1328–34.
45. Leff R, Miller F, Hicks J, et al. The treatment of inclusion body myositis (IBM): A retrospective review and a randomized, prospective trial of immunosuppressive therapy. Medicine (Baltimore) 1993;72:225.
46. Sayers ME, Chou SM, Calabrese LH. Inclusion body myositis: analysis of 32 cases. J Rheumatol 1992;19:1385.
47. Rider LG, Miller FW. Laboratory evaluation of the inflammatory myopathies. Clin Diagn Lab Immunol 1995;2:1–9.
48. Goodwin DW. Imaging of skeletal muscle. Rheum Dis Clin N Am 2011;37:245–51.
49. Cantwell C, Ryan M, O'Connell M, et al. A comparison of inflammatory myopathies at whole-body turbo STIR MRI. Clin Radiol 2005;60:261–7.
50. Hengstman GJ, van Brenk L, Vree Egberts WT, et al. High specificity of myositis specific autoantibodies for myositis compared with other neuromuscular disorders. Neurology 2005;252:534–7.
51. Emery AE. The muscular dystrophies. Br Med J 1998;317(7164):991–5.

John D. Reveille

Spondyloarthritis

The term spondyloarthritis (SpA) (otherwise known as spondyloarthropathy) encompasses a heterogeneous group of inflammatory diseases characterized by spinal and peripheral joint oligoarthritis, inflammation of the attachments of ligaments and tendons to bones (enthesitis) and, at times, mucocutaneous, ocular, and/or cardiac manifestations. These disorders show familial aggregation and are typically associated with genes of the major histocompatibility complex (MHC), particularly human leukocyte antigen (HLA)-B271 (Chapter 5). The SpA include: (1) ankylosing spondylitis (AS); (2) reactive arthritis (ReA) — known previously as Reiter's syndrome; (3) psoriatic arthritis (PsA) and/or spondylitis; (4) enteropathic arthritis and/or spondylitis associated with the inflammatory bowel diseases (IBD), ulcerative colitis (UC), or Crohn's disease; and (5) undifferentiated SpA, which encompasses patients expressing elements of, but failing to fulfill, accepted criteria for one of the above diseases. In addition, isolated acute anterior uveitis (AAU)[1] and spondylitic heart disease (complete heart block and/or lone aortic regurgitation)[2] associated with HLA-B27 may also be classified within the spectrum of SpA.

Classification of spondyloarthritis

There are no diagnostic criteria for any of the SpA. Classification criteria have been developed in order to provide greater specificity in clinical studies. The European Spondyloarthropathy Study Group (ESSG) criteria for SpA were developed in 1991, have been validated in numerous population groups, and remain the basis of many clinical and epidemiologic studies (Table 56.1).[3] The modified New York criteria, developed in 1966 and modified in 1984, remain the "gold standard" for AS.[4] However, this depends on the presence of radiographic sacroiliitis, which takes up to 10 years to develop after the onset of inflammatory back pain. New criteria have been developed for axial SpA based on the presence of inflammatory back pain that take advantage of diagnostic innovations such as magnetic resonance imaging (MRI) and HLA-B27 typing.[5] More recently, criteria have also been developed for peripheral spondyloarthritis based on the presence of peripheral arthritis, enthesitis, or dactylitis, which utilize these innovations.[6]

For PsA, the classification criteria for psoriatic arthritis (CASPAR) criteria have been developed (see Table 56.1),[7] stemming from the perception that the ESSG criteria were not "sensitive" enough.

The International League Against Rheumatism (ILAR) juvenile idiopathic arthritis classification criteria for enthesitis-related arthritis (ERA) have been proposed for juvenile SpA (JSpA: Table 56.1). No criteria have been validated for enteropathic arthritis.

Epidemiology

The frequency of SpA in general and AS in particular varies in different populations and parallels the frequency of HLA-B27. The prevalence of AS varies between 0.2 and 0.7% among people of European ancestry,[8–11] and has been reported in similar frequencies in eastern Asia (Table 56.2). Higher prevalences have been reported in Eskimo groups from Siberia and Alaska as well as in groups from Scandinavia, and as high as 4.3% in male Haida Indians of Canada, where the frequency of HLA-B27 is 50%.[9–11] AS is much less frequent in Africans and Japanese, where HLA-B27 is rare.

The prevalence of ReA is unknown and probably varies over time depending on endemic rates of the sexually acquired (*Chlamydia*) and enteric (*Shigella*, *Salmonella*, *Campylobacter*) infections that trigger it. It appears that the frequency of ReA has dramatically declined in the wake of the human immunodeficiency virus (HIV) epidemic, at least in Western countries, and with the adoption of safer sexual practices and better sanitation.

Psoriasis affects 1–3% of the general population. The frequency of PsA is less clear, and is higher in those with more severe disease; population studies among Caucasians estimate a frequency of approximately 0.1%.[11]

The prevalence of IBD is 100–200 per 100 000 in Caucasians, with equal male-to-female ratio.[8,12] It is rare in people of African and Asian descent. The risk of spondylitis and peripheral arthritis varies in different reports, perhaps reflecting the subspecialty of the observer. Spondylitis occurs in as many as 15–20% of those with IBD. In general, peripheral arthritis occurs less frequently in those with UC (up to 10%) than in those with Crohn's disease (up to 20%), although its frequency tends to be higher in series where the assessor was a rheumatologist.[9,11,12]

Pathogenesis

Genetics of spondyloarthritis
Familial aggregation

Susceptibility to AS is clearly attributable to genetic factors, with a sibling recurrence risk ratio as high as 82 and twin-based studies estimating disease heritability to exceed 90%.[12,13] The concordance rate for AS in identical twins has been reported to be as high as 63%, compared to 23% in non-identical twins.[12] The concurrence rate for psoriasis in monozygotic twins is 70 versus

15–30% in dizygotic twins. Recurrence risk for parents and sibs of patients with Crohn's disease is 4.8 and 7%, respectively, and for UC 0.9 and 1.2%, respectively.[13]

KEY CONCEPTS

The genetic basis of spondyloarthritis

- Human leukocyte antigen (HLA)-B27 comprises nearly half of the overall susceptibility to ankylosing spondylitis (AS), and contributes heavily to susceptibility to reactive arthritis, psoriatic, and enteropathic spondylitis.
- Additional influences seem to come from other major histocompatibility complex (MHC) genes, including C*0602 for psoriasis, whose identification has been confounded by linkage to HLA-B27.
- Genetic modeling has suggested up to six additional non-MHC influences.
- Genome-wide association studies utilizing dense SNP mapping have located at least 14 genes or genetic regions in AS susceptibility.
- Over 26 genes have been identified thus far in psoriasis pathogenesis.
- Genome-wide association studies utilizing dense SNP mapping will likely locate many of the remaining genes in AS susceptibility.

HLA-B27 and spondyloarthritis

HLA-B27, which is encoded in the MHC class I region, confers the greatest known risk for AS, and is found in up to 90% of AS patients of European ancestry[12,13] (Table 56.3), as opposed to 6–8% of white normal.[14] The prevalence of HLA-B27 in the USA is 6.1% overall, highest in younger individuals (7.5% before age 50), falling rapidly over age 50 (3.3%).[14]

Approximately 70% of patients with ReA have HLA-B27, except in Africa, where no association of HLA-B27 is seen in those with HIV-associated SpA.[12,13]

HLA-B27 is found in 60–70% of patients with psoriatic spondylitis and in 25% of those with peripheral PsA.[12,13] Up to 70% of those with IBD-associated spondylitis have HLA-B27, although no HLA-B27 association is seen with asymptomatic sacroiliitis. Approximately 50% of patients with AAU alone are HLA-B27-positive.[13]

Table 56.1 Current classification criteria for spondyloarthritis

A. European Spondyloarthropathy Study Group (ESSG) criteria for spondyloarthritis
1. Inflammatory back pain or synovitis (asymmetric, lower extremity) *plus* one of the following:
   (a) Alternating buttock pain
   (b) Sacroiliitis
   (c) Heel pain (enthesitis)
   (d) Positive family history
   (e) Psoriasis
   (f) Crohn's, disease, ulcerative colitis
   (g) Urethritis or cervicitis or acute diarrhea in the preceding 4 weeks

B. The modified New York criteria for ankylosing spondylitis[4]
1. Clinical criteria:
   (a) Low-back pain and stiffness for more than 3 months which improves with exercise, but is not relieved by rest
   (b) Limitation of motion of the lumbar spine in both the sagittal and frontal planes
   (c) Limitation of chest expansion relative to normal values correlated for age and sex
2. Radiological criterion:
   (a) Sacroiliitis grade 2 bilaterally or grade 3–4 unilaterally
   (b) *Definite ankylosing sponylitis* if the radiological criterion is associated with at least one clinical criterion

C. The classification criteria for psoriatic arthritis (CASPAR) criteria for psoriatic arthritis
1. Inflammatory joint disease plus at least three points from the following features:
   (a) Current psoriasis (assigned a score of 2; all others assigned a score of 1)
   (b) History of psoriasis
   (c) Family history of psoriasis
   (d) Dactylitis
   (e) Juxta-articular new bone formation
   (f) Rheumatoid factor seronegativity
   (g) Nail dystrophy

D. ASAS Criteria for axial spondyloarthritis in patients with chronic low back pain for at least three months
1. Sacroiliitis on imaging (either MRI findings of inflammatory disease in the sacroiliac joints or sacroiliitis on standard pelvic X-rays by New York criteria) plus ONE of the following OR HLA-B27 positivity plus TWO of the following:
   (a) Inflammatory low back pain
   (b) Arthritis
   (c) Enthesitis
   (d) Dactylitis
   (e) Psoriasis
   (f) Crohn's disease or ulcerative colitis
   (g) Good response to nonsteroidal anti-inflammatory agents
   (h) Positive family history of SpA
   (i) Presence of human leukocyte antigen (HLA)-B27
   (j) Elevated C-reactive protein

E. ASAS Criteria for Peripheral Spondyloarthritis—Arthritis or enthesitis or dactylitis with at least one of:
a. Uveitis
b. Psoriasis
c. Crohn's disease or ulcerative colitis
d. Previous infection
e. Presence of HLA-B27
f. Sacroiliitis on imaging
OR
with at least two of:
a. Inflammatory low back pain
b. Arthritis
c. Enthesitis
d. Dactylitis
e. Positive family history of SpA

F. The International League Against Rheumatism (ILAR) Juvenile Idiopathic Arthritis Classification Criteria for Enthesitis-Related Arthritis (ERA)
Arthritis and enthesitis
OR
Arthritis or enthesitis with at least two of:
1. Sacroiliac joint tenderness and/or inflammatory spinal pain
2. Presence of HLA-B27
3. Family history in at least one first- or second-degree relative of medically confirmed HLA-B27-associated disease
4. Anterior uveitis that is usually associated with pain, redness, or photophobia
5. 5. Onset of arthritis in a boy after 8 years of age

Exclusions
Psoriasis confirmed by a dermatologist in at least one first- or second-degree relative
Presence of systemic arthritis

Table 56.2 The epidemiology of spondyloarthritis

Ethnic group	HLA-B27 frequency (%)	Prevalence of AS	Prevalence of PsA	Prevalence of SpA
Circumpolar groups				
Eskimos (Alaska)	40	0.4	1.5	1.5
Sami (North Norway)	24	1.8	0.23	n.a.
Asia				
China	2-9	0.11–0.26	n.a.	0.5-1.0
Taiwan	5.7	0.19–0.54	n.a.	n.a.
Vietnam	n.a.	0.05	n.a.	0.28
Thailand	4.0	n.a.	n.a.	0.12
Japan	< 1	0.007	n.a.	0.01
Europe and North America				
Norway	16	1.1–1.4	0.195	n.a.
Moravia	16	0.5	n.a.	n.a.
Greece	5.4	0.24	0.17	0.49
France	8	0.2	0.19	0.3
Italy	n.a.	0.37	0.42	n.a.
Germany	9	0.7	1.9	1.9
USA	6.1%	0.5	0.1	1.4

AS, ankylosing spondylitis; HLA, human leukocyte antigen; n.a., not available; PsA, psoriatic arthritis; SpA, spondyloarthritis

Table 56.3 Genetic factors implicated in spondyloarthritis

Factor	Ankylosing spondylitis (%)	Reactive arthritis (%)	Psoriasis/psoriatic arthritis/spondylitis (%)	IBD/enteropathic arthritis/spondylitis (%)
HLA-B27 frequency	90%	70%	24/60/70	7/7/70
Other MHC genes	B*60 (B*4001	DRB1*04	C*0602, B*38, B*39, DRB1*04, DRB1*07	None/DRB1*0103/none
Shared Non-MHC genes	ERAP1, IL23R, KIF21B, IL1R2, IL1A, IL12B, CDKAL1, PTGER4, CARD9, STAT3		ERAP1, IL23R, IL1A, IL12B, REL, CDKAL1,TYK2, PTPN22, DEFB4	IL23R, KIF21B, IL1R2, REL, IL12B, CDKAL1, PTGER4, CARD9, TYK2, STAT3, PTPN22, DEFB4
Unique Non-MHC genes	RUNX3, ANTXR2, TFRS1/LTBR, TRADD		IL28RA, LCE, IF1H, IL2/IL21, IL4/IL13, TNIP1, LIRF, MICA, TRAF3IP2, TNFAIP3, IL23A, NFBKIA, NOS2, ADAM33, RNF114	FCGR2A, DENND1B, IL10, PUS10, IL18RAP, ATG16L1, IL8RA, IL7R, ERAP2, IRGM, PRDM1, CCR6, TAGAP, IRF5, JAK2, TNSF15, IL2RA, NKX2-3, LSP1, NOD2, ORMDL3, PTPN2, TFRSF15, ICOSLG, NCF4

HLA, human leukocyte antigen; MHC, major histocompatibility complex; TNF, tumor necrosis factor.

Over 80 molecular subtypes of HLA-B27 have been described this far. The most common subtypes (HLA-B*2705, B*2702, B*2704, B*2707, B*2714) are clearly associated with SpA. Two subtypes of HLA-B27, HLA-B*2706 and B*2709, found in Southeast Asia and Sardinia, respectively, appear not to be associated with AS,[13] possibly due to amino acid differences in the "B" pocket of the HLA antigen-binding cleft at positions 114 and 116 that could alter the composition and anchoring of peptides presented by these HLA-B27 subtypes. The other subtypes of HLA-B27 are too rare to have had disease associations established. These subtypes evolved from the parent allele HLA-B*2705 along three lines (Fig. 56.1) in three distinct geographic regions.

The exact mechanism underlying the effect of HLA-B27 on disease susceptibility has still not been determined. One theory suggests that SpA results from a unique set of antigenic peptides, either bacterial or self, that are bound and presented by all disease-associated HLA-B27 subtypes (but not by other HLA class I molecules) to CD8 T cells, resulting in an HLA-B27-restricted cytotoxic T-cell response found only in joints and other affected tissues (the so-called arthritogenic peptide hypothesis). In fact, recent gene association data showing interaction between HLA-B27 and a loss-of-function variant of endoplasmic reticulum-associated aminopeptidase I (ERAP1) suggest that aberrant antigen processing may play a central role in AS susceptibility.[15] However, a specific "arthritogenic peptide" has yet to be demonstrated.

An alternative concept focuses on self-association as a unique property of the HLA-B27 molecule. HLA-B27 heavy chains can form homodimers in vitro that are dependent on disulfide binding through their cysteine-67 residues in the extracellular α1 domain (as well as other cysteine residues in other domains) (Fig. 56.2).[13,16] This occurs as a result of B27 misfolding within the endoplasmic reticulum. The accumulation of misfolded protein results in a pro-inflammatory intracellular stress response through the stimulation of interferon-β secretion. Also,

Fig. 56.1 The three major families of human leukocyte antigen (HLA)-B27 subtypes (HLA-B*2713 and B*2718 are assumed to have evolved separately) are denoted in relationship to the "parent" subtype HLA-B*2705. Most B27 subtypes have evolved through three patterns of evolution along geographic lines. The first group, including HLA-B*2703-B*2723 (and B*2730), appears to have evolved in Africa and Europe, and entails anywhere from one to seven amino acid substitutions in the first (α_1) domain, and has the second (α_2) domain identical to B*2705. The second group, including HLA-B*2704-B*2744, evolved in Asia and includes a uniform amino acid substitution in the α_1 domain and anywhere from one to seven substitutions in the α_2 domain. The third group, including HLA-B*2709-B*2707, evolved in southern Asia, the Middle East, and Sardinia and has an α_1 domain identical to B*2705 and an α_2 domain with one to seven amino acid substitutions. Notable exceptions include HLA-B*2713, which has an amino acid substitution outside α_1 and α_2, B*2718, B*2740 and B*2744, which appear to have evolved separately in Asia, and B*2730, which shares features of the first and third groups. Not shown are B27 subtypes whose ethnic origin is not designated in http://www.ebi.ac.uk/cgi-bin/imgt/hla/allele.cgi

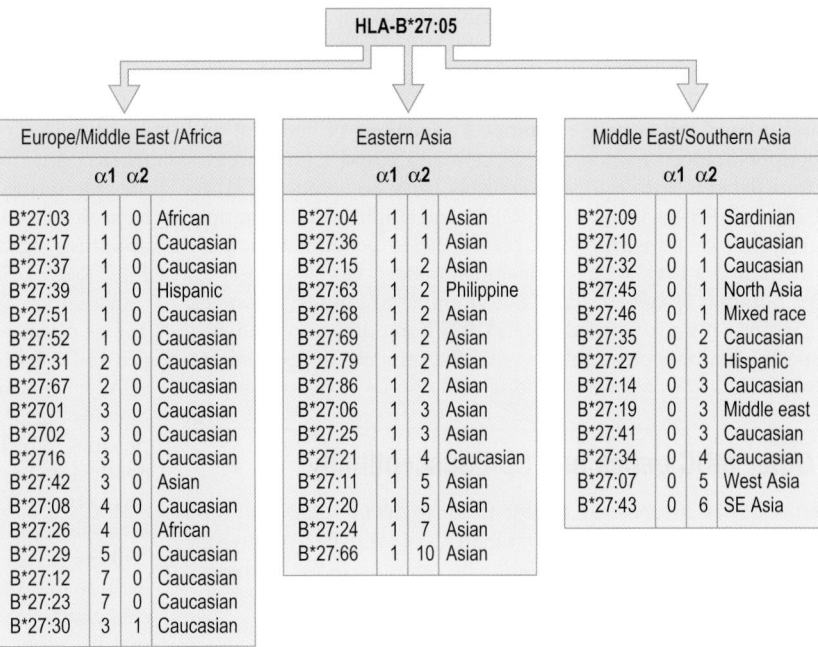

HLA-B*27:05

Europe/Middle East /Africa	α1	α2	
B*27:03	1	0	African
B*27:17	1	0	Caucasian
B*27:37	1	0	Caucasian
B*27:39	1	0	Hispanic
B*27:51	1	0	Caucasian
B*27:52	1	0	Caucasian
B*27:31	2	0	Caucasian
B*27:67	2	0	Caucasian
B*2701	3	0	Caucasian
B*2702	3	0	Caucasian
B*2716	3	0	Caucasian
B*27:42	3	0	Asian
B*27:08	4	0	Caucasian
B*27:26	4	0	African
B*27:29	5	0	Caucasian
B*27:12	7	0	Caucasian
B*27:23	7	0	Caucasian
B*27:30	3	1	Caucasian

Eastern Asia	α1	α2	
B*27:04	1	1	Asian
B*27:36	1	1	Asian
B*27:15	1	2	Asian
B*27:63	1	2	Philippine
B*27:68	1	2	Asian
B*27:69	1	2	Asian
B*27:79	1	2	Asian
B*27:86	1	2	Asian
B*27:06	1	3	Asian
B*27:25	1	3	Asian
B*27:21	1	4	Caucasian
B*27:11	1	5	Asian
B*27:20	1	5	Asian
B*27:24	1	7	Asian
B*27:66	1	10	Asian

Middle East/Southern Asia	α1	α2	
B*27:09	0	1	Sardinian
B*27:10	0	1	Caucasian
B*27:32	0	1	Caucasian
B*27:45	0	1	North Asia
B*27:46	0	1	Mixed race
B*27:35	0	2	Caucasian
B*27:27	0	3	Hispanic
B*27:14	0	3	Caucasian
B*27:19	0	3	Middle east
B*27:41	0	3	Caucasian
B*27:34	0	4	Caucasian
B*27:07	0	5	West Asia
B*27:43	0	6	SE Asia

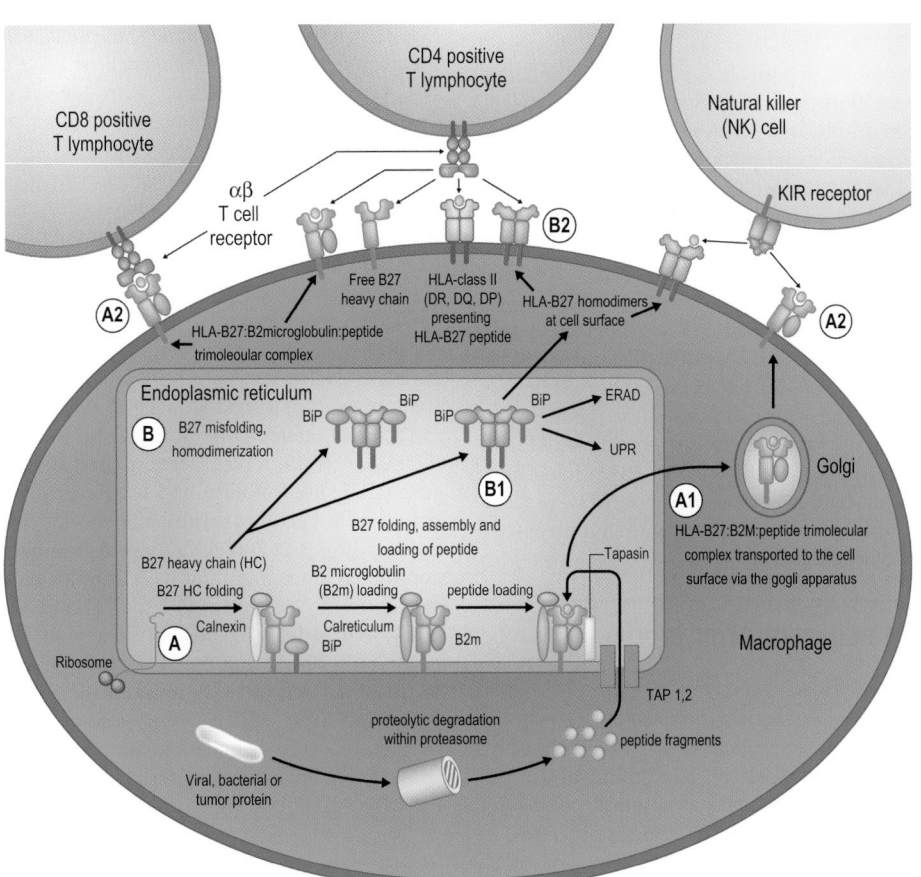

Fig. 56.2 After transcription of the human leukocyte antigen (HLA)-B27 heavy chain on ribosomes in macrophages, it is inserted into the endoplasmic reticulum (ER), glycosylated, and two pathways ensue. (A) The B27 heavy chain is retained through binding with calnexin and ERp57, folded into its tertiary structure and bound to β_2-microglobulin. After that calnexin releases the complex and it is associated with calreticulum, which in turn chaperones the formation of the peptide loading on to the complex of heavy chain, β_2-microglobulin and antigenic peptide, via the TAP proteins and tapasin. The antigenic peptide is derived from intracellular proteins from viruses, bacteria, tumors, etc., that have been degraded in proteasomes, and then the peptides are trimmed for optimal length for peptide loading by endoplasmic reticulum-associated aminopeptidase (ERAP1). Then the trimolecular peptide complex (HLA-B27 heavy chain, β_2-microglobulin and peptide) travels through the Golgi apparatus (A1) to the cell surface, where the antigenic peptide is presented either to the $\alpha:\beta$ T-cell receptor on CD8$^+$ T lymphocytes or to the killer immunoglobulin (KIR) receptor on natural killer (NK) cells (A2); or (B) the HLA-B27 heavy chain misfolds in the ER, forming B27 homodimers and other misfoldings which are bound to the ER chaperone BiP. Then, they either (B1) accumulate there, causing either ER-associated degradation (ERAD) or a proinflammatory ER unfolded protein response (UPR); or (B2) the B27 homodimers migrate to the cell surface where they either become antigenic themselves or present peptide to receptors on T cells and natural killer (NK) cells.

HLA-B27 homodimers are detectable at the cell surface in patients with SpA, are capable of peptide binding, and are more abundantly expressed when the cell's antigen-presenting function is impaired. They are ligands for a number of natural killer (NK) and related cell surface receptors. Populations of synovial and peripheral blood monocytes, NK cells and B and T lymphocytes from patients with SpA and controls carry receptors for HLA-B27 homodimers, including KIR3DL1 and KIR3DL2 and immunoglobulin-like transcript 4 (ILT4).[13–15] It is possible that these homodimers may act as a pro-inflammatory target or receptor for humoral or cell-mediated autoimmune responses. However, it is not yet known whether HLA-B27 homodimer formation is specific for, or even correlates with, the presence of SpA; in fact, most HLA-B27-positive individuals do not develop disease.

Other MHC genes and SpA susceptibility

HLA-B27 is not the only genetic factor involved in AS and SpA susceptibility (Table 56.3). Fewer than 5% of HLA-B27-positive individuals in the general population become affected,[12,13] whereas up to 20% of HLA-B27-positive relatives of AS patients will develop SpA. Family studies have suggested that HLA-B27 contributes less than 40% of the overall genetic risk for SpA12 while the entire effect of the MHC, on the other hand, is about 50%.[12,13]

HLA-B60, a serologically defined HLA specificity that correlates with HLA-B*4001 on DNA analysis, has been described as augmenting the risk for AS in both HLA-B27-positive and negative individuals from Europe and Taiwan.[12,13] Other MHC genes have also been implicated in AS in addition to B27, although their identification is complicated by the tight linkage disequilibrium found within the MHC, and many of the associations described thus far might be better explained by linkage to B27. These include MICA, located adjacent to HLA-B27, which encodes a marker of "stress" in epithelial cells, and acts as a ligand for cells expressing a common activator NK receptor (NKG2D), as well as tumor necrosis factor (TNF), heat shock protein (HSP)-70, LMP-2 and LMP-7, HLA-DRB1*01, and DRB1*04 alleles.[13] In addition, HLA-DRB1*08 has been implicated both in susceptibility to uveitis in the setting of AS and to juvenile-onset AS.[1,13,14] In psoriasis, the primary MHC association is with HLA-Cw6 (HLA-C*0602). Both HLA-DRB1*04 and *07 alleles have been implicated in PsA. There is not a significant MHC association with IBD per se, although HLA-DRB1*0103 has been associated with enteropathic peripheral arthritis.[13]

Non-MHC genes in susceptibility to spondyloarthritis

Recent genomewide association studies (GWAS) in AS from the UK and North America[15,17] have implicated up to 14 genes in AS susceptibility (Table 56.3). The most consistent (and best replicated) association is with ERAP1, which acts as a molecular ruler in the endoplasmic reticulum in trimming peptides processed in proteasomes to optimal length on nine amino acids for MHC class I binding and presentation. Recently it has been observed that HLA-B27 negative AS patients lack an association with ERAP115. A number of genes whose products are operative in the Th17 pathway have also been implicated, including the *interleukin 23 receptor (IL23R)*, which pairs with IL12RB1 gene product to confer IL23 (but not IL12) responsiveness on cells expressing both subunits.; *prostaglandin E Receptor 4 (PTGER4)*, which stimulates dendritic cell production of IL-23, and, in turn, Th17 expansion, and is overexpressed in SpA synovium; *Signal Transducer and Activator of Transcription 3 (STAT3)*, a key regulatory factor in Th17 responses and *interleukin 12 beta (IL12B)*, which encodes the IL12p40 protein, a component of both IL-12 and IL-23, is also associated with AS susceptibility.

Other immunologically relevant genes that have been implicated in AS susceptibility include the *Interleukin 1 Receptor 2 (IL1R2)* gene, which encodes a protein that acts as a decoy receptor, interfering with the binding of IL-1 to IL-1R1; *Caspase recruitment domain-containing Protein 9 (CARD9)*, which participates in apoptosis signaling and induces nuclear factor kappa-B (NFκB); *Runt-Related Transcription Factor 3 (RUNX3)*, which encodes a transcription factor involved in CD8 lymphocyte differentiation; *Tumor Necrosis Factor Receptor Type 1-Associated Death Domain (TRADD)*, which is a negative regulator of interferon-γ-induced STAT1 DNA binding, activation, and function; and the *Tumor Necrosis Factor Receptor Superfamily, Member 1A (TNFRS1)* gene product, which associates with the MADD protein through a death domain-death domain interaction, providing a physical link between TNFR1 and induction of mitogen-activated protein kinase activation and arachidonic acid release (Table 56.3).

Other genes associated with AS of less clear disease relevance include the *Anthraxin receptor 2 (ANTXR2* gene), which binds to collagen IV and laminin and may be involved in extracellular matrix adhesion. *CDK5 Regulatory Subunit-Associated Protein 1-Like 1 (CDKAL1)* gene, associated with type I diabetes, of unknown immunologic function, and *Kinesin Family Member 21B (KIF21B)*, a member of a family of plus end directed kinesin motor proteins of unclear relevance to AS. Of particular note are well replicated associations with gene deserts at chromosome 2p15 and 21q22, which may contain other as yet uncharacterized regulatory factors.[17]

Genome-wide association studies in psoriasis and PsA have identified over 26 genes implicated in disease susceptibility outside the MHC.[18] These include those in common with AS (IL23R, IL12B, CDKAL1, and ERAP1, the latter showing interaction with HLA-Cw6 similar to that seen with HLA-B27). Detailing all the non-MHC genes associated with psoriasis is outside the scope of this chapter. Non-MHC genes implicated in PsA susceptibility include IL-1A, as well as the IL-2/IL-21 and the IL-4/IL-13 gene complexes (both important in Th2-associated autoimmunity) (Fig. 56.3).

The first gene to be implicated in IBD susceptibility was *NOD2/CARD15*, which accounts for about 20% of Crohn's disease (CD) susceptibility and whose protein product serves as a receptor for bacterial products in monocytes that transduces signals leading to NFκB activation. A number of GWAS have been conducted since then that have implicated over 99 genes in IBD susceptiblity,[19] including 71 for CD and 47 for ulcerative colitis (UC), and at least 28 shared genes between CD and UC. The autophagy 16-like 1 gene (ATG16L1), which is highly expressed in intestinal cell likes, is linked to CD susceptibility. Dendritic cells from those with CD with susceptibility variants in NOD2 or ATG16L1 are deficient in autophagy induction, suggesting these genes influence bacterial degradation and interact with the MHC class II antigen presentation machinery.

Genes and severity of SPA

Disease severity in AS also has a hereditary component.[12,13] Defining severity by disease activity and loss of function, the Oxford group demonstrated that these traits are highly heritable.[13,14] A region on chromosome 18 was linked to disease activity, age at symptom onset with a region of chromosome 11p, and functional impairment with a region on chromosome 2q (outside the IL-1 region). No evidence was found for an MHC contribution to severity.

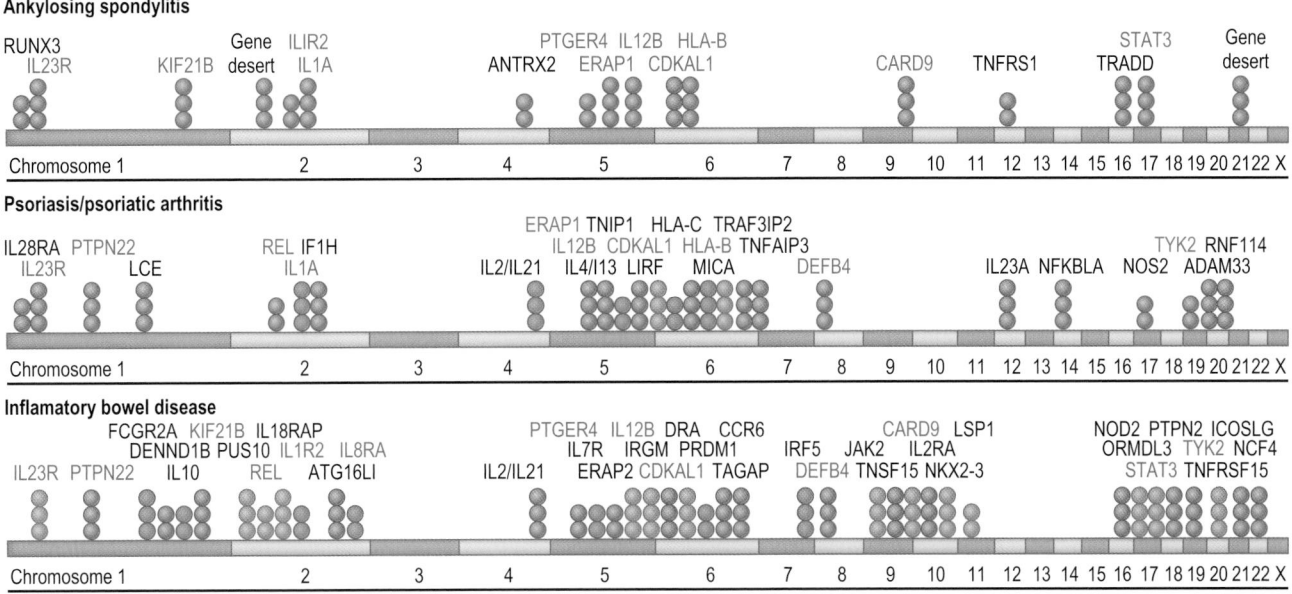

Fig. 56.3 The innate immunity, antigen presentation and the TH17 pathway all implicated in AS, psoriasis/PsA and IBD susceptibility. Three red balls over the chromosome indicate a gene identified in a GWAS and/or multiple case:control studies and extensively replicated. Two red balls indicate relatively novel GWAS findings not yet replicated elsewhere or genes well replicated in case:control studies not seen in GWAS. For other abbreviations, see Tables 56.1–56.4. For the psoriasis/PsA chromosomal depiction, the red balls indicate genes associated with psoriasis alone, the blue balls genes associated with psoriatic arthritis alone, and the purple balls genes associated with both. For the IBD chromosomal depiction, the red balls indicate genes associated with Crohn's disease alone, the blue balls genes associated with ulcerative colitis alone, and the purple balls genes associated with both diseases. Other genes of less clear functional relevance to psoriasis not shown in Fig. 56.2 include such as *Pituitary Tumor-Transforming Gene 1* (*PTTG1*-5q35.1), *Cub And Sushi Multiple Domains 1* (*CSMD1*-8p23.2), *Gap Junction Protein, Beta-2* (*GJB2*-13q11), *Serpin Peptidase Inhibitor, Clade B, Member 8* (*SERPINB8*) at 18q21.3, and *Zinc Finger Protein 816 A* (*ZNF816A*). Similarly, genes whose functional relevance to Crohn's disease or UC has not been established, such as, for Crohn's and UC, *MST1- Macrophage Stimulating 1* at chr. 3p21 and *Proteasome Assembly Chaperone 1* (*PSMG1*) at chr21q22.3; for Crohn's disease, *DNA Methyltransferase 3A* (*DNMT3A*) at chr. 2p23, *Paired-Like Homeobox 2b* (*PHOX2B*) at chr. 4p12, *BTB and CNC homology 2* (*BACH2*) at chr. 6q15, and *Chromosome 11 Open Reading Frame 30*-c11orf30-at chr.11q13.5; and for UC, *OTU Domain-Containing Protein 3* (*OTUD3*) at chr.1p36.13, *Death-Associated Protein* (*DAP*) at chr.5p15, *LYR Motif-Containing Protein 4* (*LYRM4*) at chr. 6q25, *Guanine Nucleotide Binding Protein* (*GNA12*) at 7p22.2, *Laminin, Beta 1* (*LAMB1*) at chr. 7q22, *Cyclin Fold Protein-1* (*CCNY*) at chr. 10p11, *Cullin 2* (*CUL2*) at chr. 10p11.21, and *HECT Domain and RCC1-like Domain 2* (*HERC2*) at chr. 15q13.1 are not shown.

Infection

A role for triggering infections has been better documented in SpA than in most other rheumatic diseases. The most frequent type of ReA in developed countries follows urogenital infections with *Chlamydia trachomatis* (endemic ReA). Postdysenteric ReA, more commonly encountered in "less technologically advanced countries," follows various *Shigella* and *Salmonella* (especially *S. typhimurium* and *S. enteriditis*), *Campylobacter jejuni* and *C. fetus* and, in Europe, *Yersinia enterocolitica* species. Micro-organisms implicated in ReA share common biologic features: (1) they can invade mucosal surfaces and replicate intracellularly; and (2) they contain lipopolysaccharide in their outer membrane. Of particular note, antigens from *Salmonella*, *Yersinia*, and *Chlamydia* have been found in synovial tissues and fluids of patients with ReA, often many years after the initial infection. While only bacterial fragments of the enteric pathogens have been found, evidence for viable *C. trachomatis* and perhaps *C. pneumoniae* have been demonstrated in several studies. *Chlamydia* and other organisms have also been reported in the joints of healthy individuals, thus questioning the pathogenic significance of these findings.[13] Other data, however, support the likelihood that bacterial persistence plays an important role in ReA, including the finding of specific IgA antibodies and synovial T-cell proliferation to the initiating infectious agent.

The contribution of infection to other types of SpA is less clear. In older studies *Klebsiella pneumoniae* was implicated in the pathogenesis of AS, although recent data have not borne this out.[13] It may also be significant that there are high serum IgA levels in AS, although studies seeking significant IgA antibodies to a variety of organisms have been unrewarding. In fact, it has been proposed that there might be no specific infectious trigger in AS; that this may result from gut flora and may thus be "ubiquitous."

The gut and spondyloarthritis

In studies from Belgium and from Scandinavia, up to 50% of patients with AS have microscopic ileal inflammation seen on ileocolonoscopy. Moreover, two-thirds of patients with undifferentiated SpA have histologic gut inflammation. Gut inflammation in AS appears to be immunologically related to that seen in Crohn's disease. These observations have raised speculation that the inciting event in the SpA may be a breakdown of the gut–blood barrier to intestinal bacteria, although such has yet to be proven. It has been established that patients with AS and their relatives have increased intestinal permeability compared to healthy controls.

Pathology of SPA

One of the biggest problems with studies of the synovium in SpA and PsA is that most lesions are examined late in the course of disease, i.e., in the hips, and this only at joint replacement. Few data exist from early disease, and the difficulty with tissue access further complicates this.[20,21] Nonetheless, striking advances have occurred. For the most part the synovium in SpA resembles that of rheumatoid arthritis, with some notable differences. The synovium in SpA displays a tortuous vascular morphology compared to rheumatoid synovium, which is linear, and has diminished lymphoid aggregates. This may be due to vascular endothelial growth factor (VEGF) and the angiogenic growth factor Ang2, the mRNA of which have been observed at higher levels in the synovium in PsA compared to rheumatoid arthritis. VEGF is particularly interesting because it can synergize with RANK ligand (RANKL) to induce bone resorption and also synergize with bone morphogenetic proteins to trigger bone formation, both processes typical of the altered bone remodeling seen in PsA and SpA.[20,21]

Increased production of the scavenger receptor CD163 by macrophages in both the lining and sublining layers is seen in SpA compared to rheumatoid arthritis.[20] Local production of soluble CD163 inhibits synovial T-cell activation, and levels of synovial CD163 fall with effective treatment. Increased expression of Toll-like receptors 2 and 4 (TLR2, 4) has been shown in SpA on CD163+ peripheral blood mononuclear cells in patients with synovitis, which decreases with TNF-α blockade. This leads to the speculation that SpA represents an exaggerated inflammatory response of the innate immune system in genetically susceptible patients.[21]

Osteoclasts also appear to have a role, and have also been observed at the bone–pannus junction in PsA. In addition, CD14+ monocytes that are committed to becoming osteoclasts or osteoclast precursors are increased in the circulation of PsA patients compared to healthy controls, and decline rapidly following treatment with TNF antagonists. The clinical improvement is accompanied by a MRI-defined reduction of bone marrow edema.

Even fewer data exist on enthesitis (the enthesium being the insertion of tendons, ligaments, joint capsules, or fascia into bone). Pathological examination of enthesitis in AS demonstrates local inflammation, fibrosis, erosion, and ossification. Immunohistochemical staining for phosphorylated smad1/5 in entheseal biopsies of patients with SpA reveals active bone morphogenetic protein signaling.[20]

The pathology of psoriasis consists of an inflammatory cell infiltration in the dermis, with localized increased cytokine production and hyperproliferation of keratinocytes (Chapter 63). CD4 cells are prominent in the dermis, CD8 in the epidermis; Langerhans cells function as antigen-presenting cells. The synovium is infiltrated with CD8 T cells, but demonstrates less pronounced intimal lining layer hyperplasia and fewer synovial T cells and is more vascular than rheumatoid arthritis, contains numerous B cells and macrophages, and has upregulation of adhesion molecules such as ICAM-1 and E-selectin and overexpression of proinflammatory cytokines such as TNF-α, IL-1β, -6, and -18.[21]

Clinical features

Ankylosing spondylitis
Musculoskeletal symptoms

> ● **KEY CONCEPTS**
>
> **Clinical features of inflammatory back pain**
>
> - Low-back pain that is present every day for at least 3 months
> - Age of onset at less than 45 years
> - Morning stiffness in the back lasting at least 30 minutes
> - Pain that is relieved by exercise and worsened by rest
> - Alternating-buttock pain
> - Relief with nonsteroidal anti-inflammatory agents

The first symptoms of AS usually appear in adolescence or early adulthood and usually start before the age of 45. The hallmark of AS is the presence of inflammatory back pain.[5] This is a dull, persistent ache, usually described by the patient in the buttocks or hips, that is worst in the early-morning hours (between 2 and 5 a.m.), and is associated with morning stiffness lasting more than 30 minutes (and sometimes several hours to all day). The pain is classically worsened by rest or recumbency, and improves with activity. One important component of inflammatory back pain is the striking improvement that results from the use of nonsteroidal anti-inflammatory drugs (NSAIDs: usually in high doses). Although the pain may be unilateral or intermittent at first (in fact, alternating buttock pain is a cardinal feature of the disease),[5] within a few months it usually becomes persistent and bilateral, and the lower lumbar area becomes stiff and painful.[4,5] Occasionally the first symptom of AS comes from extraspinal sources, such as AAU, peripheral arthritis, or enthesitis, especially in patients with disease onset in childhood.

The most commonly affected joints in AS patients outside the spine are in the hips and shoulders (in up to 50% of patients),[23] with rapidly progressive destructive arthritis that necessitates joint arthroplasty at an early age. A characteristic radiographic finding is a fairly characteristic osteophytic collar that forms at the junction of the femoral head and the neck.[22] Peripheral arthritis other than in the hips and shoulders is uncommonly seen in AS patients, but when present is typical of that seen in other types of SpA, with an asymmetric oligoarthritis presenting predominantly in the lower extremities.

Chest pain, often pleuritic, can be seen in patients with AS due to involvement of the costovertebral and manubriosternal joints. This and progressive thoracic spinal involvement can result in fusion of the costovertebral joints, with loss of chest expansion and a mechanical restrictive ventilatory defect.

Enthesitis (inflammation of the origin and insertion of ligaments, tendons, aponeuroses, annulus fibrosis, and joint capsules) is a classic feature of AS and other SpA (Fig. 56.4). The most common (and most disabling) sites for enthesitis are in the foot, at the insertion of the Achilles tendon, and of the plantar fascia on to the calcaneus.[23]

Three physical measurements have been validated and recommended by the Assessment in Ankylosing Spondylitis (ASAS) working group as useful for evaluating patients with AS specifically and with inflammatory back pain in general. The Schober test is measured as the increase with maximal forward spinal flexion with locked knees of a 10-cm segment marked on the patient's back with the inferior mark at the level of the posterior superior iliac spines. The measured distance should increase from 10 cm to at least 13.5 cm in an adult. Chest wall expansion with inspiration is measured with a tape measure placed circumferentially around the chest wall at the fourth intercostal space. Normal chest expansion in an adult is greater than 5 cm, although this may vary with age and gender. An occiput-to-wall distance of more than 2.5 cm is definitely abnormal. To measure the occiput-to-wall distance, the patient stands with heels and buttocks touching the wall behind and with the knees straight. The patient is asked how far back he/she can get the head, still keeping the chin in the normal position. In the straight position, the distance between the posterior convexity of the occiput and the wall is measured to the nearest 0.1 cm. The better of two attempts is recorded. Anything greater than zero is regarded as abnormal.

Another measure that is increasingly commonly employed is the measurement of lateral bending. Here the patient stands with the heels and back against the wall. There is no flexion of the knees, nor bending forward. The distance between the patient's middle fingertip and the floor is measured. The patient then

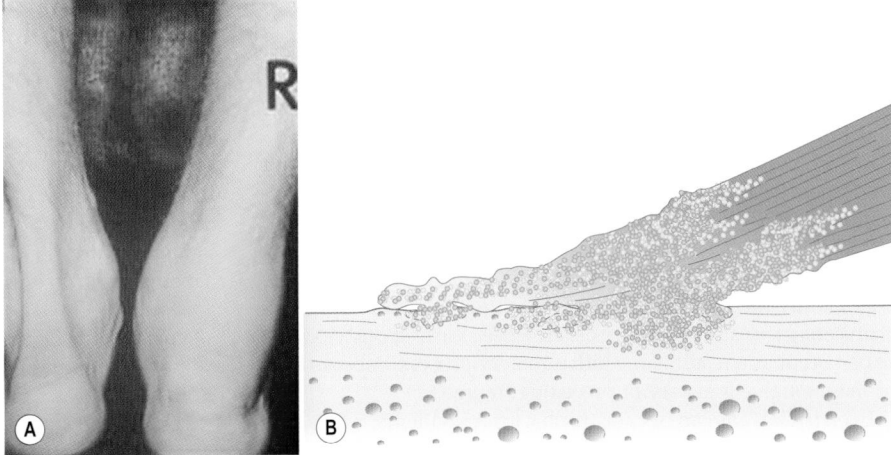

Fig. 56.4 (A) Achilles tendinitis/enthesitis in a patients with reactive arthritis. (B) Schematic drawing of enthesitis, showing periosteal new bone formation, and subchondral bone inflammation and resorption.

bends sideways without bending the knees or lifting the heels. A second reading is taken and the difference between the two is recorded. The best of two tries is recorded for left and right. The mean of left and right gives the final result (in centimeters to the nearest 0.1 cm). Normal is greater than 10 cm.

Extra-articular manifestations

Uveitis

The anterior portion of the uvea consists of the iris and ciliary body while the posterior portion is known as the choroid. Inflammation of the anterior uveal tract is known as anterior uveitis or iritis. When the adjacent ciliary body is also inflamed, the process is known as iridocyclitis. AAU represents the typical uveitis found in SpA, occurring in about 40% of patients with AS,[1] of whom approximately 90% are HLA-B27-positive (Table 56.2).[1] Typically, AAU presents unilaterally with sudden onset, is self-limiting, and tends to be recurrent. Symptoms may include redness, pain, blurred vision, increased lacrimation, photophobia, and miosis. The diagnosis is characteristically confirmed by slit-lamp examination, which is also useful in monitoring response to treatment.

Prognosis is favorable in AAU, with resolution of symptoms within a few weeks. However, if treatment is delayed or inadequate, complications can occur; these include anterior synechiae (adherence of the iris to the cornea), posterior synechiae (adherence of the iris to the lens), which can lead to cataracts, and cystoid macular edema.[1] Rarely, increased ocular pressure is seen.[1] Macular edema has been shown to be the main factor that determines visual outcome in cases of uveitis.[1] Although AAU is the most common uveitis associated with AS, posterior uveitis has been reported and tends to be more severe, especially in those with coexistent IBD.[1]

Cardiac manifestations

The characteristic cardiac abnormalities in AS are aortitis, aortic regurgitation and conduction abnormalities that are seen in up to 9% of patients with AS followed over many years. Less commonly associated cardiac conditions include pericarditis, cardiomyopathy, and mitral valve disease. HLA-B27 is an important genetic risk factor for these cardiac conditions. Aortic regurgitation is well characterized and distinguished from aortic valvular dysfunction in other disorders. Three factors contribute to the development of incompetent aortic valves: dilatation of the aortic root, fibrotic thickening and downward retraction of the bases of the cusps, and inward rolling of the edges or margins of the cusps. Aortic regurgitation is present in 2–10% of patients with AS and increases in likelihood with greater disease duration.

Cardiac conduction abnormalities, including atrioventricular and intraventricular blocks, have been regarded as the most common cardiac complication in patients with AS. Complete heart block has been found in 1–9% of patients with AS. Electrophysiologic studies show that the preferential level of block is in the atrioventricular node itself, which is in contrast with most cases of acquired complete heart block, where 80% are within or below the bundle of His. Rare complications include myocardial involvement, mitral regurgitation, and pericarditis.

Pulmonary manifestations

The incidence of pleuropulmonary involvement in AS is estimated to be 1%. The most frequently recognized manifestations are upper-lobe fibrosis, mycetoma formation, and pleural thickening. Fusion of the costovertebral joints caused by inflammation and ankylosis of the thoracic spine can lead to restrictive ventilatory impairment on pulmonary function testing. The upper-lobe fibrosis tends to be progressive. Another common finding is the presence of bilateral symmetric apical pleural thickening. Several recent studies have demonstrated that high-resolution computed tomography is more sensitive than chest radiography in detecting the presence of pulmonary abnormalities in AS, suggesting that pulmonary involvement in AS is more common than once thought. The clinical implications of these observations remain unclear as lung involvement in AS is usually asymptomatic.

Renal manifestations

Renal involvement in AS, although uncommon, may include secondary renal amyloidosis (AA type), NSAID nephropathy, and glomerulonephritis.

Osteoporosis

Measuring bone mineral density in patients with spondylitis is complicated by false increases in spinal density from dense syndesmophyte formation, leading some to recommend quantitative computer tomography over standard dual-energy X-ray absorptiometry (DEXA) for bone mineral density measurements. Nevertheless, up to half of patients with long-standing AS have been reported as having osteopenia or osteoporosis.[24] This has been attributed to the impact of inflammation on bone remodeling, due to aberrant activation of bone morphogenic protein and Wnt signaling. This can be further worsened by treatment factors and decreased mobility or physical activity, in addition to osteoclast/osteoblast imbalance.[24]

Spondylodiscitis and spinal fractures

An uncommon but well-recognized complication of AS is spondylodiscitis, a destructive discovertebral lesion also called Andersson lesion.[25] Typically, these lesions are confined to the thoracic and lumbar spine, sometimes with multiple-level involvement; however, cervical spondylodiscitis has been reported. Pain and tenderness localized to the affected disk are the most common presenting features of spondylodiscitis, although it can be asymptomatic and only detected on routine radiographic examination many years later. Spondylodiscitis usually occurs at an advanced stage of AS under the form of an erosive condition related to both mechanical factors and osteoporosis. However, early spondylodiscitis can occur as a result of the inflammatory process. Patients may or may not give a history of preceding trauma.

Even trivial falls can be catastrophic for AS patients, who are at risk for spinal fractures due to their spinal rigidity and osteoporosis. The estimated prevalence of vertebral fractures in AS varies from 4 to 18%. Fractures through the disk space, the weakest point in the ankylosed spine, are most common, with the cervical spine being the most frequently affected region, followed by the thoracolumbar junction, and may, or may not, be complicated by injury to the spinal cord ranging from mild sensory loss to quadriplegia. Spontaneous atlantoaxial subluxation is also rarely seen.

Neurological manifestations

Neurological involvement in AS is most often related to spinal fracture, atlantoaxial subluxation, or cauda equina syndrome. The cauda equina syndrome in AS is characterized by a slow insidious progression and a high incidence of dural ectasia, although a rapid onset secondary to a traumatic event has been reported. It tends to be a late manifestation of AS, often when the disease is no longer active. The prevalence of neurologic findings in cauda equina syndrome in AS is very high, presenting with a prodrome of sensory, motor, or reflex loss before the progression to sphincter disturbance. About half of patients have pain in the rectum or lower limbs that is presumably neurogenic in origin. Case reports have also been published about the occurrence of AS with a multiple sclerosis-like syndrome and transverse myelitis, although the association is not conclusive.

Fatigue and psychosocial manifestations

Fatigue is a common problem in patients with AS and seems to be associated with more severe disease. Sleep disturbance has also recently been reported to be as high as nearly 81% of female AS patients and 50% of male AS patients. The disturbance is closely related to pain during the night characteristic of active disease. A high level of depressive symptoms has been reported in approximately one-third of patients with AS, with women reporting more depression than men. Pain was found to be a major determinant of depression for women, but was of lesser importance for men.

AS in women

AS in women may not be as severe as it is in men, and may present with isolated neck pain in the absence of typical back pain.[26] There tends to be a greater delay in the diagnosis of AS in women compared to men. Women tend to have less severe involvement of the spine, with peripheral joint involvement. A large review of the impact of AS on reproductive events on women concluded that AS did not adversely affect the ability to conceive, pregnancy outcome, or neonatal health.[26]

Reactive arthritis

The classic triad of arthritis, urethritis, and conjunctivitis, representing what was formerly known as Reiter's syndrome, is a presenting feature of only a minority of patients with ReA (comprising only a third of the cases in some series). In ReA, the clinical features are today viewed more as a spectrum ranging from the classic triad to undifferentiated SpA. In fact, the manifestations vary among patients, depending on the genetic makeup, the triggering event, and the sequential immunologic reaction.

Typically, the features start 1–4 weeks after a triggering event, frequently identified as an enteric or urogenital infection, but often the event passes unnoticed without any specific symptoms. The syndrome starts with constitutional symptoms such as fatigue, malaise, and fever, and then is typically manifested by asymmetric, additive lower-extremity oligoarticular inflammatory arthritis along with an array of different extra-articular features, including a sterile oligoarticular or monoarticular and asymmetric arthritis of the lower extremities, especially the knees, ankles, and, occasionally, hips. Upper-extremity involvement is encountered less commonly. Dactylitis occurs in the toes or fingers, resulting in the "sausage digits," which represent inflammation not only of the interphalangeal joints of the hands and feet, but also of the surrounding soft-tissue structures including the tendons and subcutaneous tissue.

Sacroiliitis and spondylitis are less common than peripheral arthritis, although inflammatory back pain does occur. Unilateral and bilateral sacroiliac involvement and even spondylitis occur, especially in those with chronic or long-standing disease. The most common sites for enthesitis are the Achilles tendon and plantar fascia insertions, although tenderness over the symphysis pubis, iliac crest, ischial tuberosity, greater trochanters, and thoracic cage ribs can also occur.

Mucocutaneous lesions also occur that can be difficult to distinguish from PsA, especially *circinate balanitis* and *keratoderma blenorrhagica*. Circinate balanitis is an ulcerative mucosal lesion over the glans or shaft of the penis that is demarcated by a serpiginous erythematous border. The lesion is usually painless and sterile unless a superimposed infection occurs. Keratoderma blenorrhagica is a painless desquamative psoriatic-like papulosquamous eruption and is sometimes referred to as pustulosis palmoplantaris and occurs on the palms and soles of the feet. Oral lesions have been described as shallow, painless ulcers or patches on the palate and tongue, or mucositis of the soft palate and uvula. Conjunctivitis and AAU also occur, as described in AS. Conjunctivitis may be unilateral or bilateral and is usually an early feature manifesting with irritation, erythema, and lacrimation. It is usually associated with a sterile discharge unless a superimposed infection occurs due to eye rubbing. It can be severe and occasionally progresses to episcleritis, scleritis, or keratitis. Other findings seen in AS, such as cardiac involvement, rarely occur. Although renal involvement is mainly described in the context of the urogenital triggering infectious process, sterile pyuria in conjunction with proteinuria and microscopic hematuria are sometimes encountered. Documented glomerulonephritis is rarely described.

Juvenile spondyloarthritis

Basically there are two clinical subsets of JSpA. Undifferentiated JSpA, which includes peripheral arthritis and enthesitis, primarily affects the lower limbs, may also present with sacroiliac tenderness and/or inflammatory spinal pain, and also includes isolated episodes of arthritis, enthesitis, tendinitis, dactylitis, and seronegative enthesopathy and arthropathy (SEA) syndrome.[27] Differentiated JSpA (juvenile AS, PsA, IBD-related arthropathy) includes peripheral arthritis and enthesitis plus evidence of structural changes in JAS (radiographic sacroiliitis, spinal disease, or tarsal ankylosis) and/or specific extra-articular symptoms (e.g., psoriasis or IBD). The SEA syndrome was originally referred to the combination of enthesitis and arthritis or arthralgia as an idiopathic disease or as part of a well-defined SpA.[27]

Psoriatic arthritis

Skin involvement exhibits four clinical patterns.[28] The most common type is psoriasis vulgaris. Nearly as common is guttate psoriasis. The most severe type is the erythrodermic variety. Finally, pustular psoriasis is the type most closely associated with HLA-B27. Usually the disease appears coincident with or after the onset of skin manifestations, although approximately 15–20% of patients will have pre-existent arthritis. The joint disease likewise occurs in different subtypes, as defined by the Moll and Wright classification (Fig. 56.5), including oligoarticular, asymmetric, polyarticular, symmetric, distal interphalangeal (DIP)-predominant, spondylitis (sacroiliitis), arthritis mutilans, inflammation of DIP joints (often with nail involvement (~80%)), dactylitis: "sausage digits," and enthesitis.[26] Extra-articular features include nail pitting (which correlates best with DIP involvement) and uveitis (which occurs in some series as high as 33% but in most far less). Radiographically, large eccentric erosions are encountered.

Enteropathic arthritis

The arthritis associated with IBD (enteropathic arthritis) is most commonly nondestructive and reversible. Two patterns have been recognized (Table 56.4): type 1 is oligoarticular, involving the knees and ankles more than the upper extremities. It tends to resolve in < 6 weeks. The second type has a polyarticular presentation, is more likely to involve the metacarpophalangeal

Table 56.4 Extraintestinal manifestations of inflammatory bowel disease

Feature	Crohn's disease (%)	Ulcerative colitis (%)
Peripheral arthritis	15	10
Axial arthritis	15–20	10–15
Septic arthritis	Rare	No association
Skin	< 9	< 1
Aphthous ulcers	Rare	8
Nephrolithiasis	< 15	No association
Liver disease	3–5	7
Uveitis	13	4
Vasculitis	Takayasu's arteritis	< 5
Clubbing of fingers	4–13	1–5

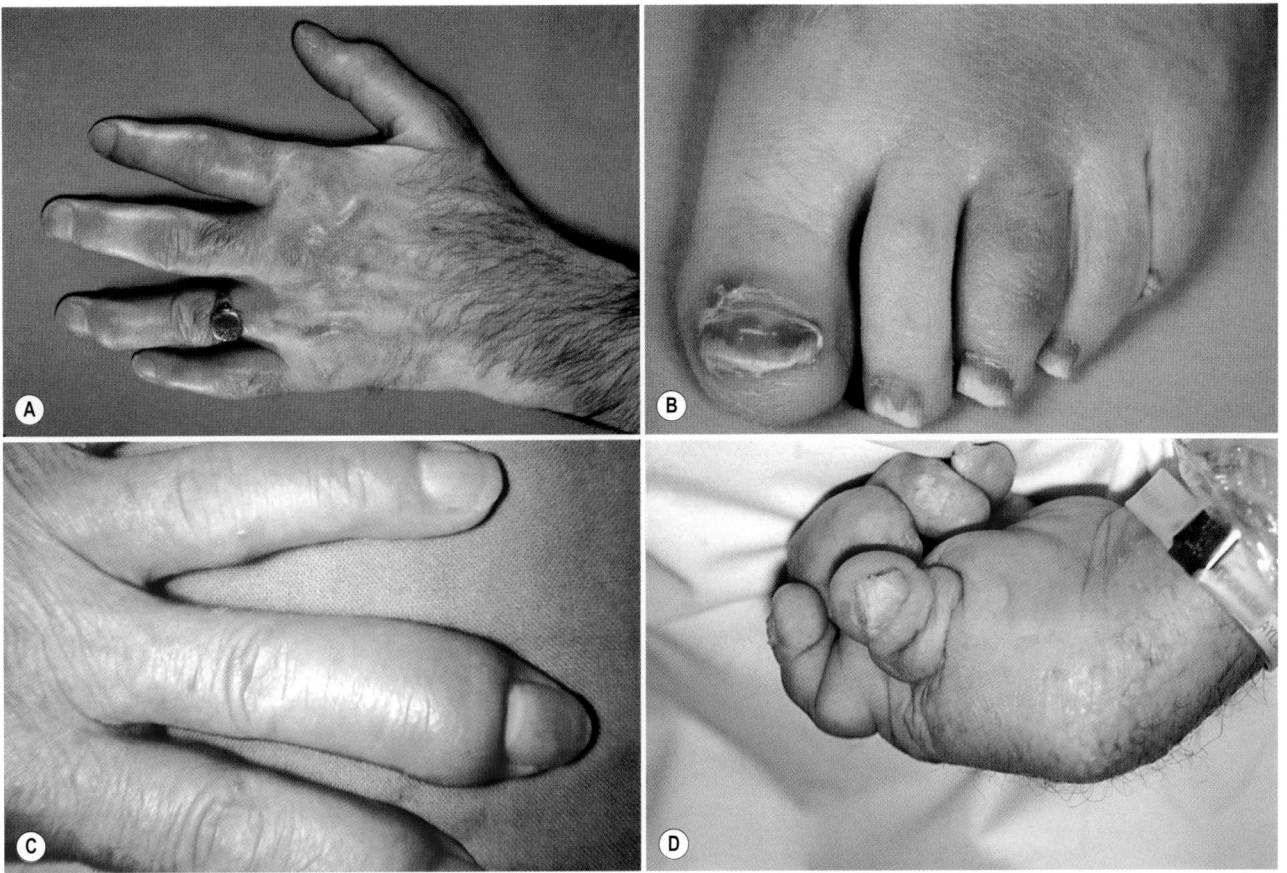

Fig. 56.5 Patterns of psoriatic arthritis, showing (A) rheumatoid-like distribution; (B) sausage digits; (C) distal interphalangeal involvement; and (D) psoriatic arthritis mutilans.

(MCP) and proximal interphalangeal (PIP) joints than the lower extremities, and is more likely to have a chronic course. The symptoms of peripheral arthritis tend to coincide with activity of the bowel disease in UC but not in Crohn's disease. Total colectomy is associated with remission of arthritis in half of patients. In contrast, axial involvement may precede the development of IBD, has no gender predilection, and resembles the development of AS. The axial symptoms do not parallel activity of bowel disease. In addition to spondylitis, an isolated sacroiliitis occurs that is often asymmetric and not associated with HLA-B27.

Mucocutaneous complications of IBD include erythema nodosum, which occurs in fewer than 10% of those with Crohn's disease and is rare in UC; pyoderma gangrenosum, seen in slightly over 1% of those with Crohn's disease and rarely occurring in those with UC; and, rarely, erythema multiforme. Painful aphthous ulcers occur in about 8% of those with UC and are rare in Crohn's disease.

The uveitis with IBD that is bilateral, posterior, insidious in onset, and/or chronic in duration contrasts with the uveitis associated with other types of SpA, which is predominantly anterior, unilateral, sudden in onset, and limited in duration. Only 46% of patients with uveitis associated with IBD are HLA-B27-positive, as opposed to 89% of the patients with SpA. Episcleritis, scleritis, and glaucoma are more common among patients with IBD than in those with SpA.

Undifferentiated spondyloarthritis

Patients are regarded as having undifferentiated SpA who do not meet criteria or clinical features of the "classic" spondyloarthritides. Generally, at presentation, about 40% of patients will be classified as having undifferentiated SpA,[29] and the frequency of HLA-B27 reaches around 80% in Caucasians (Table 56.5). Follow-up studies suggest that over time about one-third will go into remission and more than half will develop a "classical" SpA, usually AS.[29]

Laboratory Investigations

The most useful investigations in SpA come from musculoskeletal imaging, but some laboratory tests can be informative.

Data on the correlation of erythrocyte sedimentation rate (ESR) and C-reactive protein (CRP) in the assessment of disease activity in SpA show ambiguous results, although most studies suggest that CRP performs better. A recent literature review on the validity of ESR and CRP in AS concluded that ESR and CRP do not comprehensively represent the disease process and thus do not have the same validity as in rheumatoid arthritis.[13,29] Generally, it is felt that patients with peripheral joint involvement or with IBD more often have elevated ESR and CRP than those patients with axial disease.[13] However, a normal ESR and/or CRP does not exclude the presence of clinically active AS. Synovial fluid does not differ in appearance or cytology from that of any inflammatory joint disease.

Diagnosis

In most cases, SpA is largely diagnosed, or at least initially suspected, on clinical grounds. Current criteria for AS demand that the patient have radiographic sacroiliitis (at least

Table 56.5 Frequencies of different symptoms and signs in patients with undifferentiated spondyloarthritis

Feature	Percent (%)
Demographic	
Males	62–88
Mean age at onset (years)	16–23
Clinical	
Low-back pain	52–80
Peripheral arthritis	60–100
Polyarthritis	40
Enthesopathy	56
Heel pain	20–28
Mucocutaneous involvement	16
Conjunctivitis	33
Genitourinary disease	28
Inflammatory bowel disease	4
Cardiac abnormalities	8
Laboratory	
Elevated erythrocyte sedimentation rate	19–30
Human leukocyte antigen (HLA)-B27 positive	80–84
Radiographic	
Sacroiliitis	16–30
Spinal radiographic changes	20

Adapted from Chen CH, Lin KC, Yu DT, et al. Serum matrix metalloproteinases and tissue inhibitors of metalloproteinases in ankylosing spondylitis: MMP-3 is a reproducibly sensitive and specific biomarker of disease activity. Rheumatol (Oxf) 2006; 45: 414–420.

grade II bilaterally or grade III unilaterally) in conjunction with clinical signs of inflammatory back pain and limitation of spinal mobility. However, given that up to 10 years can pass from the onset of inflammatory back pain and the development of radiographic sacroiliitis, many of those with inflammatory back pain might not have radiographic evidence of sacroiliitis. With the development of effective treatments (i.e., anti-TNF blockers), criteria have been developed for earlier diagnosis of axial SpA that take into account recent advances in MRI scanning as well as the added benefit provided in HLA-B27 testing.[5,6]

CLINICAL RELEVANCE

Utility of human leukocyte antigen (HLA)-B27 testing in the evaluation of inflammatory back pain and spondyloarthritis

- Not indicated where the diagnosis is unquestionable, as it has little value in prognosis.

- Although patients with spondyloarthritis of African and Middle Eastern ancestry are more likely to be HLA-B27-negative, the finding of HLA-B27 in these patients has higher predictive value.

- Most useful in patients with either inflammatory back pain without radiographic changes or with other features of spondyloarthritis (unexplained lower extremity arthritis in a young adult, uveitis, etc.).

- If serologic testing is used to ascertain HLA-B27, ensure the blood sample arrives in the laboratory within 24 hours of being drawn (false negatives due to cell death).

Measures of SpA activity and severity

In the past few years, outcome measures have been developed and validated to quantitate disease activity and severity; these are summarized in Table 56.6. These instruments are extensively validated and easy to administer in clinical practice, and have been shown to perform well in clinical trials. The Ankylosing Spondylitis Disease Activity Scale (ASDAS) has recently been developed to gauge disease activity.

Radiographic imaging of spondyloarthritis
Axial spondyloarthritis

The bottom line in the diagnosis of AS is the demonstration of radiographic sacroiliitis (Fig. 56.6).[4] Two outcome instruments

---

Table 56.6 Measurements of disease outcome in spondyloarthritis

Ankylosing spondylitis
1) **Disease activity**
  (a) Bath Ankylosing Spondylitis Disease Activity Index (BASDAI)
  (b) Ankylosing Spondylitis Disease Activity Score (ASDAS)
  (c) Patient and Physician Global Assessments
2) **Function**
  (a) Bath Ankylosing Spondylitis Functional Index (BASFI)
  (b) Dougados Functional Index
3) **Quality of Life**
  (a) SF-36
  (b) Ankylosing Spondylitis Quality of Life Index (ASQOL)
4) **Metrometry**
  (a) Schober's test (lumbar flexion)
  (b) Chest expansion\
  (c) Occiput-to-wall distance
  (d) Lateral bending
  (e) Bath Ankylosing Spondylitis Metrology Index (BASMI) lateral ending
5) **Imaging**
  (a) Standard radiographs
  (b) Computed tomography scanning
  (c) Magnetic resonance imaging
6) **Assessment in Ankylosing Spondylitis (ASAS) 20**
  (a) An improvement of > 20% and absolute improvement of 10 units on a 0–100 scale in three of the following four domains:
    i. Patient global assessment (by visual analog scale (VAS) global assessment)
    ii. Pain assessment (the average of VAS total and nocturnal pain scores)
    iii. Function (represented by BASFI)
    iv. Inflammation (the average of the BASDAI's last two VAS concerning morning stiffness, intensity, and duration)
    v. Absence of deterioration in the potential remaining domain (deterioration is defined as 20% worsening)

Psoriatic arthritis
1) *Arthritis*
  (a) ACR response criteria
  (b) Psoriatic Arthritis Response Criteria (PsARC)
  (c) Ritchie Articular Index
2) *Skin response*
  (a) Psoriasis Area and Severity Index (PASI)
  (b) Target lesion score
  (c) Static global assessment
3) **Quality of life (HAQ, SF-36, DLQI)**
4) **Radiographic**

---

have been introduced in the assessment of disease damage and progression in AS: the Bath Ankylosing Spondylitis Radiographic Index (BASRI) and the modified Stokes Ankylosing Spondylitis Scoring System (mSASSS).[30] As a rule, they have a low sensitivity to change (7.5% over 2 years), have been validated in long-duration disease only, and their predictive effect for disease activity is not yet ascertained.

One problem with radiographic imaging is the average decade-long interval from the onset of inflammatory back pain to the appearance of radiographic sacroiliitis.[5] The introduction of MRI imaging of the spine and entheses has allowed not only correct anatomic description of spinal structures, but also differentiation of AS-related and unrelated inflammatory spinal lesions earlier than is possible by standard radiographs.[31] MRI of the sacroiliac joints and spine is currently the only imaging tool to localize and quantify spinal inflammation accurately (Fig. 56.7), and is being developed as a measure of disease activity and treatment response.

Psoriatic arthritis

PsA has some rather characteristic radiographic manifestations, including asymmetric involvement, involvement of the DIP joints, and the classical "pencil-in-cup" deformities. Also seen are periostitis, bony ankylosis, and bony erosions with new bone formation. Radiographic severity is quantitated by the modified Sharp scoring method used in rheumatoid arthritis.

The measures used in PsA to assess disease severity include the ACR response criteria, the Psoriatic Arthritis Response Criteria (PsARC), which entail improvement in at least two of the following four criteria: (1) physician; and (2) patient global assessments (on 0–5 visual analog scales); (3) tender and swollen joint scores (> 30% improvement), with improvement in at least one of these two joint scales; and (4) no worsening in any criteria. The Ritchie Articular Index is also used. The Psoriasis Area and Severity Index (PASI) is used to assess the extent of skin involvement, as well as general measures such as the target lesion score, and the static global assessment. The PASI is a composite index of skin disease severity, including an overall evaluation and quantitation of the extent of scaling, erythema, and induration weighted: (1) by severity; and (2) by body surface area. A target lesion is a single lesion > 2 cm in diameter evaluated over time by a dermatologist and that is graded for size, elevation, erythema, and scaling.

Disease course and prognosis

Ankylosing spondylitis

AS impacts significantly on the lives of those affected. Recent data suggest that patients with AS are more likely to be work disabled or even not participate in the labor force compared with population controls, especially in older patients and in those with longer disease duration. Moreover, in the same study, AS patients were more likely to have never married or to be divorced. Women with AS were less likely than expected to have had children.[32]

Although AS is a chronic condition that can frequently have an unpredictable course, some studies suggest that those with higher levels of disease activity early in the course of the disease are more likely to have active disease in the future (Fig. 56.8).[32] Hip involvement has been shown to be a predictive factor for severe disease.[32] Other factors that may be suggestive of severe

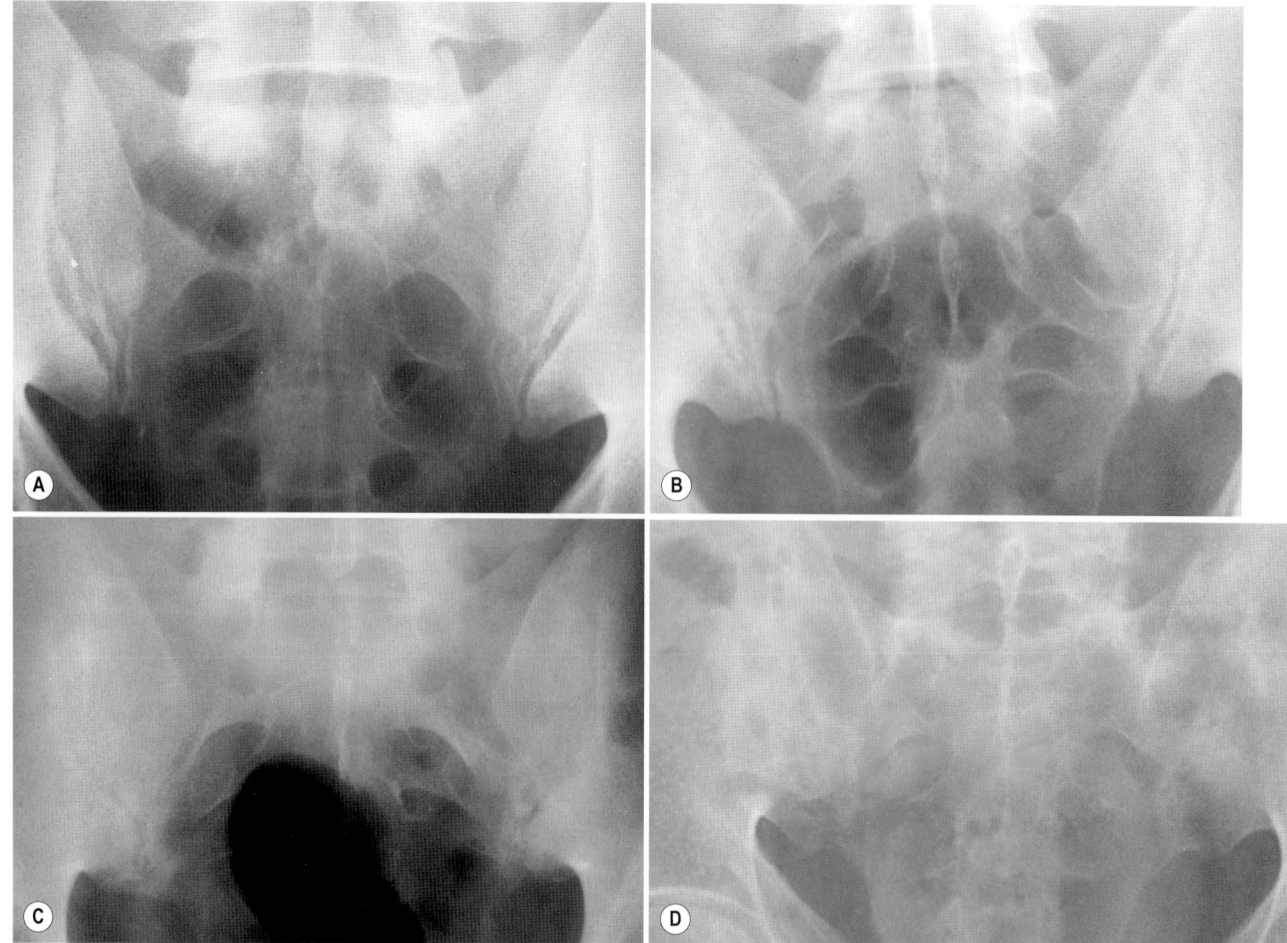

Fig. 56.6 Grading of radiographic sacroiliitis, including: (A) grade 0–1 (normal); (B) grade 2–3, with sclerosis and small erosions; (C) advanced grade 3, with joint space narrowing and large erosions; and (D) grade 4 (total sacroiliac fusion).

disease and severe outcome include: ESR > 30 mm/hr, unresponsiveness to NSAIDs; limitation of lumbar spine; "sausage" digits; oligoarthritis; or onset at < 16 years.[32] Longitudinal studies in patients with AS revealed that deformities and disability occur within the first 10 years of disease.[30] Most of the loss of function occurred during the first 10 years, and correlated significantly with the occurrence of peripheral arthritis, radiographic changes of AS in the spine, and the development of "bamboo" spine.[32]

Significant risk factors for work disability from several studies include older age, longer disease duration, lower level of education, reduced physical functioning, pain, and more physically demanding jobs. Patients with AS have an overall frequency of disability and economic costs similar to that of rheumatoid arthritis, with a threefold greater rate of disability than the general population, a higher rate of sick leave episodes (up to 50% more), and an overall 8% loss of productivity.[33] Moreover, a growing body of data has shown that AS patients are at risk for early cardiovascular mortality.[34] However, the impact of newer agents, such as anti-TNF drugs, on the natural history of this disease remains to be seen.

Reactive arthritis

Early studies of outcome in ReA suggested a relatively poor prognosis. More recent studies, however, have found that, in general, the prognosis of ReA is fairly good.[35] Most cases appear to remit within 6 months of onset. Given the introduction of highly effective biologic agents such as anti-TNF blockers, it is likely that the long-term prognosis in ReA will improve even further.

Psoriatic arthritis

Recent studies—although before the introduction of biologic treatments—have shown that the prognosis of PsA is worse than previously suggested.[1,22,36] In one large cohort, 40–57% of patients had deforming arthritis, 17% had[3] five deformed joints, and up to 19% of patients had disability. Overall, more rapidly progressive disease was associated with a greater number of actively inflamed joints, the early use of disease-modifying agents, and the presence of HLA-B27 and B39. Patients with PsA have also been shown to have increased mortality, which is associated with a high ESR, high "advanced" medication usage, and early radiographic damage.

Juvenile spondyloarthritis

Although not extensively studied, the prognosis in JSpA is guarded.[28] Available data suggest that children with disease activity for more than 5 years are more likely to be disabled. In fact, the probability of remission was only 17% after 5 years of disease. Nearly 60% of children with JSpA have moderate to severe limitation after 10 years of disease. What is not clear is the extent to which the outcome in juvenile-onset AS is different from that in adult-onset disease.

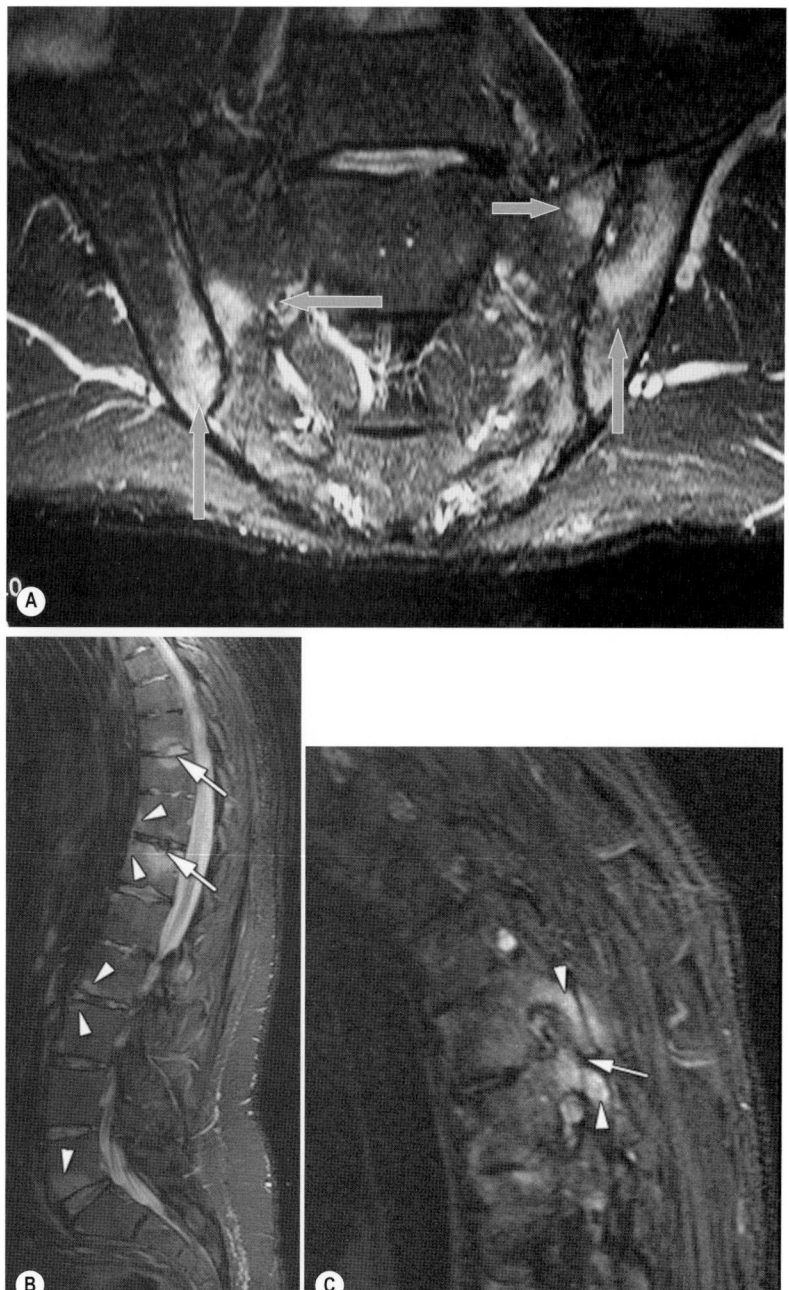

Fig. 56.7 (A) Magnetic resonance imaging of the sacroiliac joints, showing areas of marrow edema (indicated by arrows) on STIR sequences. (B) Lateral spine, showing enhancement of the insertion of the annulus fibrosis on the disk (arrowheads) and subchondral bone (arrows). (C) Involvement of the subchondral bone of the apophyseal joints.

Fig. 56.8 The "classical" course of ankylosing spondylitis, showing disease progression from shortly after disease onset in 1947 until just before the patient's death in 1973. The slight improvement between 1972 and 1973 was due to his having gotten total hip arthroplasties.

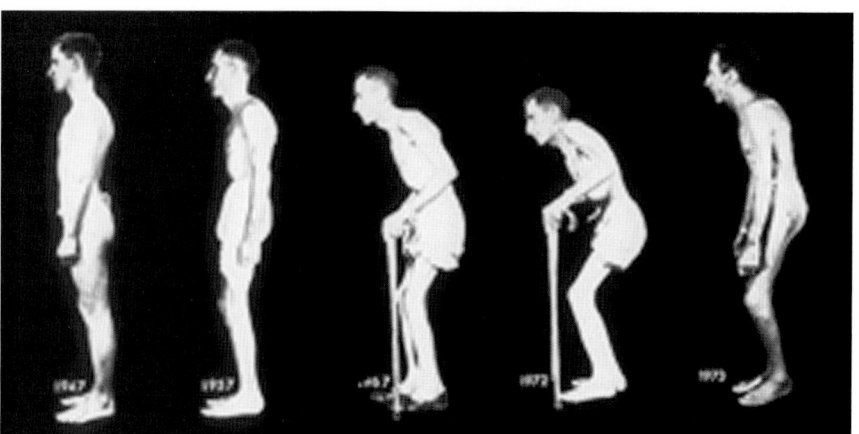

Table 56.7 Treatment of spondyloarthritis

Patient education
Physiotherapy
Medications
Nonsteroidal anti-inflammatory drugs
Disease-modifying antirheumatic drugs
  • Sulfasalazine (especially for peripheral arthritis)
  • Methotrexate (especially for psoriatic arthritis, psoriasis)
  • Leflunomide
Corticosteroids
  • Systemic
  • Intra-articular, intralesional
Biologic agents
  • Tumor necrosis factor blockers
  • Alefacept (psoriasis)
  • Ustekinumab (psoriasis)
Treatment of osteoporosis
Surgery
Hip replacement
Corrective spinal surgery

Treatment (Table 56.7)

Patient education and physiotherapy

A great deal of educational information is available for patients (http://www.spondylitis.org and http://www.arthritis.org). Unsupervised recreational exercise improves pain and stiffness, and back exercise improves pain and function in patients with AS and other types of SpA, but these effects differ with disease duration. Health status is improved when patients perform recreational exercise at least 30 minutes per day and back exercises at least 5 days per week.

Medical treatment

◖THERAPEUTIC PRINCIPLES

Treatment principles for medical management of spondyloarthritis

- Patient education and physiotherapy should be initiated early in the disease course.
- Nonsteroidal anti-inflammatory drugs (NSAIDs) remain 'first-line' treatment.
- Disease-modifying anti-inflammatory drugs (DMARDs: sulfasalazine, methotrexate) for peripheral arthritis.
- Intra-articular/intralesional corticosteroidal injections.
- Anti-tumor necrosis factor agents for axial disease refractory to NSAIDs, peripheral arthritis refractory to DMARDs, and entheseal lesions refractory to NSAIDs.
- Don't forget to treat coexistent/complicating conditions (inflammatory bowel disease, psoriasis, osteoporosis).

Nonsteroidal anti-inflammatory drugs

NSAIDs remain the starting point of treatment, and many patients will attain satisfactory symptom control with these agents alone. There are no strong data to suggest the superiority of any specific NSAID in patients with SpA. NSAIDs when taken regularly (not on an as-needed basis) and at full anti-inflammatory doses retard the radiographic progression of AS,[37] an observation that has recently been replicated. Cyclooxygenase-2 antagonists are recommended mainly for patients with proven peptic ulcer disease. Of concern is the association of the use of NSAIDs with flares of colitis, suggesting they should be used with care in this setting.

Disease-modifying anti-inflammatory drugs (DMARDs)

Sulfasalazine

The efficacy of sulfasalazine in the treatment of peripheral joint involvement in AS and other SpA has been shown in several controlled trials, including two large multicenter studies in the USA and France.[38] It is not efficacious in axial disease. Coincident with improvement in peripheral arthritis is a fall in acute-phase reactants such as the ESR and CRP.

Other DMARDs

Although less well studied than sulfasalazine, methotrexate has been shown to be effective in the treatment of peripheral arthritis and psoriasis in patients with AS and other SpA. Its efficacy in treating axial arthritis has not been established.

The use of leflunomide in patients with SpA has not been well examined. Limited data suggest it is useful in the treatment of peripheral joint involvement in SpA as well as PsA, although not for axial involvement.

Corticosteroids

Although not well studied in patients with AS, many clinicians add low-dose glucocorticoids to the management of active SpA where NSAIDs or DMARDs fail to achieve a satisfactory response. On occasion pulse steroids have also been utilized. Given the lack of controlled data as to their effectiveness, the side effects of long-term glucocorticoid therapy (including osteoporosis, a major cause of morbidity in AS patients, and possible worsening of psoriasis) and the emergence of more effective treatments, their use is not recommended unless more effective treatments are not available.

Intra-articular/intralesional corticosteroids

Intra-articular and peritendinous injections of depot steroid preparations are frequently employed by clinicians for symptomatic relief of local flares, although they have not been extensively studied in controlled trials. Injecting around the Achilles tendon is generally not recommended because of the risk of tendon rupture.

Antibiotics

Early data suggested that a 3-month course of antibiotics in the acute phase after disease onset may have a beneficial effect on the course of ReA, specifically in those with *Chlamydia trachomatis*-triggered ReA, but not in other patients. Recent long-term follow-up data, however, suggest that tetracycline treatment did not change the natural history of the disease. In another recent study, however, a six-month course of azithromycin and rifampin in the acute phase was found to have a beneficial effect on the long-term prognosis.[39] It is clear that early antibiotic therapy for chlamydial genital infections can prevent ReA, although the same is not true for enteric pathogens. For patients at risk for enteric infections and ReA, prophylactic antibiotics should be considered. There is no evidence that antibiotics have any place in the management of other SpA.

TNF-α blockers

With the initial clinical trials dating back as far as 2000, this category of medications has been shown to be highly effective in controlling inflammation and improving function in patients with AS. There are currently five agents that are in clinical use for the treatment of AS, four of which having been approved for use by the Food and Drug Administration. What these agents do not retard is the progression of spinal fusion.

The use of TNF blockers in the treatment of AAU is less clear, however. Recent data suggest they are useful, at least those comprised of monoclonal antibodies.[1]

Infliximab

An infusion of a chimeric monoclonal antibody to TNF-α (infliximab) at 5 mg/kg of infliximab every 6 weeks has been shown to be beneficial in both the axial and peripheral manifestations of AS in both open-label and in placebo-controlled clinical trials.[40] The onset of action is quite rapid, usually following the first infusion, with over 80% of patients achieving > 20% improvement in measures of disease activity. Improvement was seen not only clinically but also radiographically, with clearing of lesions suggestive of disease activity on MRI.

Etanercept

The soluble TNF-α receptor, etanercept, given 25 mg subcutaneously twice weekly, has been shown to be effective in the treatment of AS in patients in a 4-month randomized double-blind placebo-controlled study of 40 AS patients.[40] Improvement was sustained in an open-label extension of this study for over 10 months. Similar positive results were seen in another longitudinal study of 10 SpA patients studied in the UK, with statistically significant improvement seen not only in all clinical and functional parameters, but also in MRI-detectable entheseal lesions, of which 86% either regressed completely or improved.[41] Similar positive results have been reported in PsA,[42] where substantial improvement was seen in both the joint and entheseal involvement as well as in the extent and severity of the psoriatic skin lesions. The Food and Drug Administration has approved the use of etanercept in the treatment of both AS and PsA.

Adalimumab and golimumab

Adalimumab and golimumab are fully human monoclonal antibodies against TNF α that have been approved by the Food and Drug Administration for the treatment of AS and psoriatic arthritis. Adalimumab is used at a dose of 40 mg every other week.[43] In patients in whom biweekly dosing does not suffice, weekly administration may be necessary. Recent data have also shown adalimumab to be effective in pre-radiographic axial SpA.[44] Golimumab is used at a dose of 50 mg administered subcutaneously monthly.[45]

ASAS guidelines for the use of TNF blockers

Because of the high cost and potential side-effect profiles of TNF blockers, as well as the finding that many patients with AS are well controlled with NSAIDs or sulfasalazine alone, the ASAS working group formulated and subsequently revised guidelines for the use of TNF blockers. These take into account both the patient's and physician's assessments of disease activity (Table 56.8).[46]

Table 56.8 International Assessment in Ankylosing Spondylitis (ASAS) consensus statement for the use of anti-tumor necrosis factor (TNF) agents in patients with ankylosing spondylitis (AS) and axial spondyloarthritis (ASpA)

1. For the initiation of anti-TNF-α therapy:
(a) A diagnosis of definitive AS or axial SpA
(b) Presence of active disease for at least 4 weeks as defined by both a sustained Bath AS Disease Activity Index (BASDAI) of at least 4 *and* an expert opinion based on clinical features, acute-phase reactants, and imaging modalities
(c) Presence of refractory disease defined by failure of at least two nonsteroidal anti-inflammatory drugs during a single 4-week period, failure of intra-articular steroids if indicated, and failure of a disease-modifying anti-rheumatic drug, preferably sulfasalazine, in patients with peripheral arthritis
(d) Application and implementation of the usual precautions and contraindications for biological therapy
2. For the monitoring of anti-TNF-α therapy: both the BASDAI and the ASAS core set for clinical practice should be followed regularly
3. For the discontinuation of anti-TNF-α therapy: in nonresponders, consideration should be made after 12 weeks' treatment. Response is defined as improvement of:
(a) At least 50% or 2 units (on a 0–10 scale) of the BASDAI
(b) Expert opinion that treatment should be continued

Surgical treatment of AS complications

Because the hip is the joint most commonly involved in patients with AS, total hip arthroplasty is the most common surgical procedure.[24] Heterotopic new bone formation can be a potential problem.

Limited prevalence data suggest that patients with AS, even those with mild disease, are at increased risk for vertebral fracture, often resulting in neurologic compromise.[25] In general, halo vest immobilization is recommended. Surgical intervention may be necessary when neurological impairment is seen. The fixed kyphotic deformities seen in patients with advanced AS are of considerable distress to patients and can result in substantial functional impairment. A small minority of AS patients will seek surgical correction of their spinal deformities. In general, open, polysegmental, and closing wedge osteotomies are employed. Loss of correction is seen least commonly in closing wedge osteotomy. In a meta-analysis of the literature between 1945 and 1998, an average correction of 37°–40° was seen, with perioperative mortality of 4% due to pulmonary, cardiac, and intestinal problems.[47]

Conclusions and research opportunities

● ON THE HORIZON

Research opportunities in spondyloarthritis

- Improved understanding of pathogenetic mechanisms of SpA
- Elucidation of the roles of non-MHC genes in SpA
- Definition of the link between gut inflammation and AS triggering
- Improved measures of treatment outcomes
- Advances in biologic therapies of SpA

Great progress has been made in the classification and epidemiology of SpA, particularly in the elucidation of the factors involved in the SpA pathogenesis in recent years. It has become clear that HLA-B27, the primary genetic factor identified in the pathogenesis of SpA, functions in a variety of roles, including "classical" antigen presentation. How these lead to disease remains to be seen. Genome-wide scans have identified a number of regions that may contain other susceptibility genes for SpA, and these are being examined. Non-MHC genes that contribute to SpA susceptibility are currently being elucidated and a number of promising candidates have been identified.

On the other hand, less recent progress has been made in nongenetic factors. Despite what has been learned in ReA, no infectious trigger has been identified in AS (and in fact there might be no specific trigger). The link of gut inflammation to the triggering of AS is strongly suggested by data thus far, but has still not been defined. This is clearly an area of promise for further investigation.

Novel outcome measures have been developed that will help us to care better for our patients, especially in the area of imaging. Most exciting has been the advances in treatment, particularly in the development of biologic treatments, which hold promise for a better future for patients with these diseases.

References

1. Monnet D, Breban M, Hudry C, et al. Ophthalmic findings and frequency of extraocular manifestations in patients with HLA-B27 uveitis: a study of 175 cases. Ophthalmology 2004;111:802–9.
2. Bergtfeldt L. HLA-B27 associated cardiac disease. Ann Intern Med 1997;127:621–9.
3. Dougados M, van der Linden S, Juhlin R, et al. The European Spondylarthropathy Study Group preliminary criteria for the classification of spondylarthropathy. Arthritis Rheum 1991;34:1218–27.
4. van der Linden S, Valkenburg HA, Cats A. Evaluation of diagnostic criteria for ankylosing spondylitis. A proposal for modification of the New York criteria. Arthritis Rheum 1984;27:361–8.
5. Rudwaleit M, van der Heijde D, Landewe R, et al. The development of Assessment of SpondyloArthritis International Society classification criteria for axial spondyloarthritis (part II): validation and final selection. Ann Rheum Dis 2009;68:777–83.
6. Rudwaleit M, van der Heijde D, Landewe R, et al. The Assessment of SpondyloArthritis International Society classification criteria for peripheral spondyloarthritis and for spondyloarthritis in general. Ann Rheum Dis 2011;70:25–31.
7. Taylor W, Gladman D, Helliwell P, et al. Classification criteria for psoriatic arthritis: development of new criteria from a large international study. Arthritis Rheum 2006;54:2665–73.
8. Helmick CG, Felson DT, Lawrence RC, et al. Estimates of the prevalence of arthritis and other rheumatic conditions in the United States. Arthritis Rheum 2008;58:15–25.
9. Maurer K. Basic data on arthritis: knee, hip and sacroiliac joints in adults ages 25–74 years, United States, 1971–1975. Vital Health Stat 1979;11:213.
10. Reveille JD. Epidemiology of spondyloarthritis in North America. Am J Med Sci 2011;341:284–6.
11. Loftus EV. Clinical epidemiology of inflammatory bowel disease: incidence, prevalence, and environmental influences. Gastroenterology 2004;126:1504–17.
12. Brown MA, Kennedy LG, MacGregor AJ, et al. Susceptibility to ankylosing spondylitis in twins: the role of genes, HLA, and the environment. Arthritis Rheum 1997;40:1823–8.
13. Reveille JD. The genetic basis of spondyloarthritis. Ann Rheum Dis 2011;70(Suppl. 1): i44–50.
14. Reveille JD, Hirsch R, Dillon CF, et al. The Prevalence of HLA-B27 in the United States: Data from the U.S. National Health and Nutrition Examination Survey, 2009. Arthritis Rheum; 2011, Dec 2. doi:10.1022/art.33503.
15. Australo-Anglo-American Spondyloarthritis Consortium (TASC) and the Wellcome Trust Case Control Consortium 2 (WTCCC2) Genome-wide association study in ankylosing spondylitis identifies further non-MHC associations, and demonstrates that the *ERAP1* association is restricted to HLA-B27 positive cases implicating peptide presentation as the likely mechanism underlying the association of HLA-B27 with the disease. Nat Genet 2011;43:761–7.
16. Delay ML, Turner MJ, Klenk EI, et al. HLA-B27 misfolding and the unfolded protein response augment interleukin-23 production and are associated with Th17 activation in transgenic rats. Arthritis Rheum 2009;60:2633–43.
17. Reveille JD, Sims AM, Danoy P, et al. Genomewide association study of ankylosing spondylitis identifies multiple non-MHC susceptibility loci. Nat Genet 2010;42:123–7.
18. Genetic Analysis of Psoriasis Consortium and The Wellcome Trust Case Control Consortium 2. A genomewide association study identifies new psoriasis susceptibility loci and an interaction between HLA-C and ERAP1. Nat Genet 2010;42:985–90.
19. Laukens D, Georges M, Libioulle C, et al. Evidence for significant overlap between common risk variants for Crohn's disease and ankylosing Spondylitis. PLoS One 2010;5:e13795.
20. Melis L, Elewaut D. Progress in spondylarthritis. Immunopathogenesis of spondyloarthritis: which cells drive disease? Arthritis Res Ther 2009;11(3):233.
21. van Kuijk AWR, Tak PP. Synovitis in psoriatic arthritis: immunohistochemistry, comparisons with rheumatoid arthritis, and effects of therapy. Curr Rheumatol Rep 2011;13:353–9.
22. Sweeney S, Gupta R, Taylor G, et al. Total hip arthroplasty in ankylosing spondylitis: outcome in 340 patients. J Rheumatol 2001;28:1862–6.
23. McGonagle D, Gibbon W, Emery P. Classification of inflammatory arthritis by enthesitis. Lancet 1998;352:1137–40.
24. Carter S, Lories RJ. Osteoporosis: a paradox in ankylosing spondylitis. Curr Osteoporos Rep 2011;9:112–5.
25. Mitra D, Elvins DM, Speden DJ, et al. The prevalence of vertebral fractures in mild ankylosing spondylitis and their relationship to bone mineral density. Rheumatol (Oxf) 2000;39:85–9.
26. Lee W, Reveille JD, Davis JC, et al. Are there gender differences in the severity of ankylosing spondylitis: results from the PSOAS cohort. Ann Rheum Dis 2007;66:633–8.
27. Colbert R. Classification of juvenile spondyloarthritis: Enthesitis-related arthritis and beyond. Nat Rev Rheumatol 2010;6:477–85.
28. Ritchlin C. Psoriatic disease—from skin to bone. Nat Clin Pract Rheumatol 2007;3:698–706.
29. Zeidler H, Brandt J, Schnarr S. Undifferentiated spondyloarthritis. In: Weisman MH, Reveille JD, van der Heijde D, editors. Ankylosing spondylitis and the spondyloarthropathies. Philadelphia: Elsevier; 2006. p. 75–93.
30. van der Heijde D, Landewe S, van der Linden S. How should treatment effect on spinal radiographic progression be measured? Arthriits Rheum 2005;52:1979–85.
31. Maksymowych WP, Inman RD, Salonen D, et al. Spondyloarthritis Research Consortium of Canada magnetic resonance imaging index for assessment of sacroiliac joint inflammation in ankylosing spondylitis. Arthritis Rheum 2005;53:703–9.
32. Ward MM, Reveille JD, Learch TJ, et al. Impact of ankylosing spondylitis on work and family life: comparisons with the US population. Arthritis Rheum 2008;59:497–503.
33. Boonen A, Brinkhuizen T, Landewe R, et al. Impact of ankylosing spondylitis on sick leave, presenteeism and unpaid productivity, and estimation of the societal cost. Ann Rheum Dis 2010;69:1123–8.
34. Szabo SM, Levy AR, Rao SR, et al. Increased risk of cardiovascular and cerebrovascular diseases in individuals wih ankylosing spondylitis: a population-based study. Arthritis Rheum 2011;63:3294–304.
35. Sairanen E, Paronen I, Mahonen H. Reiter's syndrome: a follow-up study. Acta Med Scand 1969;185:57–63.
36. Gladman DD, Chandran V. Review of clinical registries of psoriatic arthritis: lessons learned?: value for the future? Curr Rheumatol Rep 2011;13:346–52.
37. Wanders A, van der Heijde D, Landewe R, et al. Nonsteroidal anti-inflammatory drugs reduce radiographic progression in patients with ankylosing spondylitis: a randomized clinical trial. Arthritis Rheum 2005;52:1756–61.
38. Clegg DO, Reda DJ, Abdellatif M. Comparison of sulfasalazine and placebo for the treatment of axial and peripheral articular manifestations of the seronegative spondylarthropathies: a Department of Veterans Affairs cooperative study. Arthritis Rheum 1999;42:2325–9.
39. Carter JD, Espinoza LR, Inman RD, et al. Combination antibiotics as a treatment and for chronic Chlamydia-induced reactive arthritis: a double blind, placebo-controlled, prospective trial. Arthritis Rheum 2010;62:1298–307.
40. Braun J, Brandt J, Listing J, et al. Treatment of active ankylosing spondylitis with infliximab: a randomised controlled multicentre trial. Lancet 2002;359:1187–93.
41. Gorman J, Sack KE, Davis Jr. JC. Treatment of ankylosing spondylitis by inhibition of tumor necrosis factor α. N Engl J Med 2002;346:1349–56.
42. Mease PJ, Goffe BS, Metz J, et al. Etanercept in the treatment of psoriatic arthritis and psoriasis: a randomised trial. Lancet 2000;356:385–90.
43. Van der Heijde D, Kivitz A, Schiff MH, et al. Efficacy and safety of adalimumab in patients with ankylosing spondylitis: results of a multicenter, randomized, placebo-controlled trial. Arthritis Rheum 2006;54:2136–46.
44. Haibel H, Rudwaleit M, Listing J, et al. Efficacy of adalimumab in the treatment of axial spondylarthritis without radiographically defined sacroiliitis:results of a twelve-week randomized, double-blind, placebo-controlled trial followed by an open-label extension up to week fifty two. Arthritis Rheum 2008;58:1981–91.
45. Inman RD, Davis JC, van der Heijde D, et al. Efficacy and safety of golimumab in patients with Ankylosing Spondylitis: results of a randomized double-blind, placebo-controlled, phase III trial. Arthritis Rheum 2008;58:3402–12.
46. Van der Heijde D, Sieper J, Maksymowych WP, et al. 2010 Update of the international ASAS recommendations for the use of anti-TNF agents in patients with axial spondyloarthritis. Ann Rheum Dis 2011;70:905–8.
47. Van Royen BJ, De Gast A. Lumbar osteotomy for correction of thoracolumbar kyphotic deformity in ankylosing spondylitis. A structured review of three methods of treatment. Ann Rheum Dis 1999;58:399–406.

Small and medium vessel primary vasculitis

John H. Stone

Vasculitis is defined as inflammation within blood vessel walls. Inflamed blood vessels are prone to stenosis, thrombosis, or rupture, with the result that tissues served by those vessels undergo ischemic damage. Vasculitides often begin with nonspecific symptoms and signs, unfolding in an enigmatic fashion. Thus, vasculitis is one of the great diagnostic challenges in medicine. Treatment of these diseases can be daunting because of the need to apply potentially toxic immunosuppressive therapies for prolonged periods. However, most patients improve with therapy, some enter disease remissions, and a substantial portion—variable according to disease type—are cured. Rapidly expanding knowledge of the pathophysiology of vasculitides has recently led to improved mechanism-based therapies in some conditions and promises further developments in the future.

Classification of vasculitis

More than 20 different forms of vasculitis are recognized and distinguished by their clinicopathologic differences.[1] The causes of most types of vasculitis remain unknown. Classification schemes have traditionally categorized the different forms of vasculitis according to the size of blood vessels affected (Table **57.1**). Beyond vessel size, the vasculitides can also be distinguished by such considerations as the typical host (e.g., the elderly as opposed to the very young, or individuals infected by known disease-casuing viruses), the organs most commonly affected, and the presence of certain pathologic features. For example, within the small-vessel vasculitides, Henoch–Schönlein purpura (HSP/IgA vasculitis) most commonly occurs in children, typically affects the gut, skin, joints, and kidneys, and produces vasculitis characterized by deposition of IgA. In contrast, granulomatosis with polyangiitis (formerly Wegener's granulomatosis, herein abbreviated GPA) usually strikes adults, has a predilection for the upper airways, lungs, and kidneys, and causes granulomatous inflammation. Finally, disorders in which vasculitis is the central cause of the symptoms and signs are designated "primary." "Secondary" forms of vasculitides are those in which vasculitis complicates another type of disease, such as systemic lupus erythematosus (SLE) (Chapter 50) or rheumatoid arthritis (RA) (Chapter 51). This chapter focuses on primary vasculitides.

Pathogenesis

The precise knowledge of how the various effector cells of the immune system, the endothelial cells, cytokines, and other mediators interact to cause vascular inflammation is incomplete. Nevertheless, discussion of what is known about a few forms of vasculitis provides a framework for considering how perturbations of the immune system might play a role. The mechanisms described below are models of disease pathophysiology that have been proposed to explain ANCA-associated and immune complex-mediated vasculitis, respectively.

ANCA model

Anti-neutrophil cytoplasmic antibodies (ANCA) are directed against different enzymes contained within primary granules of neutrophils and macrophages. In vasculitis, two main patterns of immunofluorescence (IF) are seen: a cytoplasmic pattern (C-ANCA) (Fig. 57.1) or a perinuclear pattern (P-ANCA). The C-ANCA pattern, usually caused by antibodies to serine proteinase 3 (PR-3), has a specificity for GPA.[2] The P-ANCA pattern, typically caused by antibodies to myeloperoxidase (MPO), is much less specific, being found in some patients with GPA, microscopic polyangiitis, the eosinophilic granulomatosis with polyangiitis (EGPA; the Churg–Strauss syndrome), and other diagnoses.

Two murine models of ANCA-associated vasculitis (AAV) reveal that adoptive transfer of autoantibody alone is sufficient to induce a necrotizing vasculitis that resembles human disease. These models involved two types of genetically altered mice: the MPO knockout mouse, and the recombinase-activating gene 2 (RAG-2)-deficient mouse. The latter species lacks both T- and B-cells (Chapter 4). These models provide *in vivo* evidence for the pathogenic potential of ANCA. In the MPO-knockout model,[3] mice were initially immunized with mouse MPO, resulting in the formation of anti-MPO T cells and B cells and anti-MPO antibodies. RAG-2 deficient mice were subsequently injected with either anti-MPO splenocytes or control splenocytes, which did not produce anti-MPO antibodies. RAG-2-deficient mice that received anti-MPO splenocytes developed clinical features of AAV, including crescentic glomerulonephritis and systemic necrotizing vasculitis. By comparison, RAG-2-deficient mice that received non-MPO antibody producing splenocytes displayed only a relatively mild immune complex glomerulonephritis. In the RAG-2 model, RAG-2 deficient and wild-type mice were injected with anti-MPO or control immunoglobulins. Only mice receiving anti-MPO antibodies developed a pauci-immune glomerulonephritis.

Potential disease triggers in humans

For AAV in humans, a variety of infectious, genetic, and environmental risk factors (and combinations of all three) have been considered as triggers. Because the symptoms of GPA at disease onset overlap substantially with those due to infectious processes, research efforts have focused upon the identification of

Table 57.1 Major categories of primary vasculitis

Large-vessel vasculitis
Giant-cell arteritis
Takayasu's arteritis
Medium-vessel vasculitis
Polyarteritis nodosa
Kawasaki's disease
Primary central nervous system vasculitis
Buerger's disease
Small-vessel vasculitis
Anti-neutrophil cytoplasmic antibody (ANCA)-associated small-vessel vasculitis: • Microscopic polyangiitis • Wegener's granulomatosis • Churg–Strauss syndrome • Drug-induced ANCA-associated vasculitis Immune-complex small-vessel vasculitis: • Hypersensitivity vasculitis • Cryoglobulinemic vasculitis • Connective tissue disorders • Urticarial vasculitis • Behçet's disease • Goodpasture's syndrome • Serum sickness • Infection-induced vasculitis Paraneoplastic small-vessel vasculitis Inflammatory bowel disease vasculitis

Adapted from Jennette J, Falk R. Small vessel vasculitis. N Engl J Med 1997; 337: 1512.

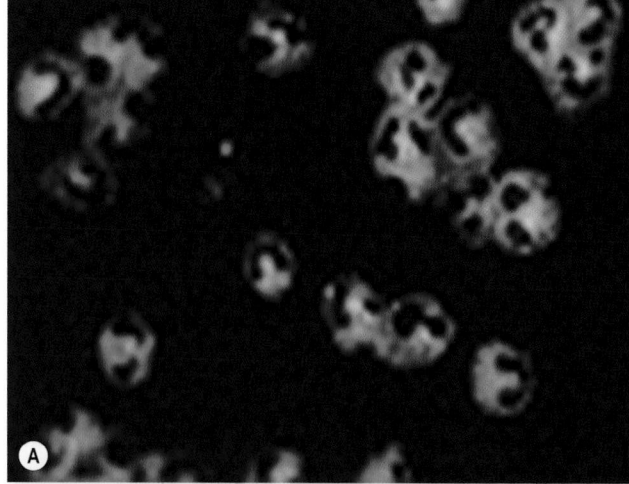
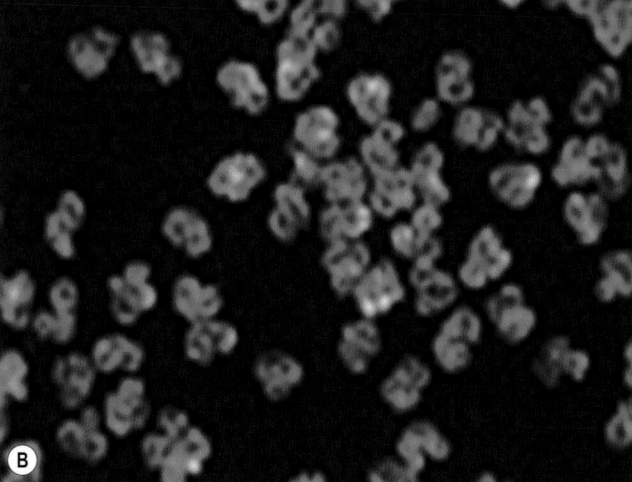

Fig. 57.1 ANCA patterns. (A) Immunofluorescence study of serum on the substrate of human neutrophils, demonstrating cytoplasmic immunofluorescence (a positive ANCA assay, C-ANCA pattern). (B) Perinuclear immunofluorescence (P-ANCA pattern).

pathogens that may precipitate GPA in individuals of the proper genetic background. However, attempts to identify an infectious cause(s) for GPA have not been fruitful. Efforts to define genetic risk factors have also met with limited success.[4–6]

Given the frequency with which the first symptoms of GPA occur in the respiratory tract, exposure to noninfectious agents or toxins via the inhalational route is another possible inciting event. One such candidate is silica dust. The odds ratio of exposure to silica dust has been reported to be 4.4 times higher for patients with AAV than in a comparison group of patients with renal disease caused by lupus or other conditions.[7] However, exact relationships between environmental exposures and vasculitis are complicated by difficulties in obtaining reliable measurements of exposures, the likelihood of recall bias among patients who are diagnosed with AAV, and the choice of appropriate control groups.

Because alpha-1 antitrypsin (AAT) is the primary *in vivo* inhibitor of PR3, the observation that patients with AAT deficiency are at increased risk for GPA suggests a potential pathogenic role in this disease for deficient PR3 clearance from sites of inflammation.[8,9] Decreased local concentrations of AAT caused by genetic polymorphisms or alterations in the enzyme's functionality induced by inflammation may therefore lead to protease/antiprotease imbalance in the disease microenvironment. Although unproven, these events may be responsible for generating immunogenic forms of PR3 in these patients.

Mechanisms of ANCA production

Autoantibodies reactive to ANCA are probably generated against newly exposed epitopes (i.e., cryptic sites) of the target autoantigen. Following the production of ANCA, the antibody response may generalize to the rest of the molecule or to other components of a macromolecular protein complex via the process of epitope

spreading. With GPA, these neoepitopes may arise at the sites of initial tissue injury. Since it is an antigen-driven process, the disease may heavily depend upon help from T cells.

This hypothesis is supported by the finding that T lymphocytes have a significant role in AAV:

- Patients with active GPA have much higher levels of activated CD4 T cells and monocytes than do patients in remission or healthy controls.[10]
- High levels of the Th1 cytokines TNF-α and interferon (IFN)-γ are observed in patients with active GPA. Monocytes from these patients release large quantities of interleukin-12 (IL-12), a major inducer of Th1 cytokines.
- Population-based studies of GPA patients reveal a diminished frequency of a major inhibitory CTLA-4 allele.[11] This may contribute to increased T-cell activation in these patients.

These findings suggest that IL-10, a known antagonist of monocyte activation, may inhibit the Th1 pathway in this disease by impairing the production of IL-12. In one study, for example, IL-10 treatment of peripheral blood mononuclear cells from active GPA patients impaired the production of IFN-γ *in vitro*.[10]

The role of B cells

B cells can also play an important role in AAV. The number of activated B cells in the circulation correlates with disease activity scores in AAV.[12] Furthermore, B-cell depletion is an effective therapy in AAV.[13,14] The rationale for why B-cell depletion may be effective in AAV is not clear, but possibilities include the complete removal or substantial reduction of ANCA production; diminution of the contribution of B cells to antigen presentation and cytokine production; and the inhibition of B-cell/T-cell cross-talk. The notion that ANCA have a direct role in inducing disease, however, is questioned by the poor relationship between ANCA titers and clinical disease flares (see below).

The roles of ANCA isotypes and Fc receptors

In theory, the isotype of ANCA in a given individual may have pathophysiological importance. Most patients with AAV, for example, produce isotype-switched IgG ANCA, implying a T-cell dependent immune response. However, studies regarding the relative importance of IgG subtypes and other types of ANCA (e.g., IgM, IgA) have been inconclusive and contradictory. Presently, there is no clear evidence that particular ANCA isotypes influence the susceptibility to or clinical expression of AAV. The magnitude of enhanced neutrophil activation by ANCA may also be influenced by antibody specificity for different PR3 epitopes, IgG subclass, and the type of Fcγ-R engaged. The Fcγ-RIIIB allele polymorphism NA1, which allows more efficient neutrophil activation by ANCA, is overrepresented in patients with severe forms of GPA.[15]

ANCA and neutrophil activation

The significant role described above for lymphocytes in AAV does not exclude an important role for ANCA themselves. Because Th1 cytokines are effective stimuli of both neutrophils and monocytes, the production of ANCA may further enhance tissue injury by augmenting the damage caused by mononuclear cells. The effects of ANCA are determined by the state of neutrophil activation. PR3 and MPO, located in the cytosol, can be relatively inaccessible to antibody binding. However, neutrophils primed with tumor necrosis factor (TNF) as well as those undergoing apoptosis express increased quantities of membrane-associated PR3,[16] a process known as neutrophil "priming."

Once neutrophils have been activated by priming, ANCA are able to bind relevant membrane-bound antigens, causing abnormal constitutive activation via either the crosslinking of MPO or PR3 or the binding of Fc receptors.[17] Persistent ANCA binding to neutrophils on the endothelial surface can enhance the degree of vascular injury. The rate at which primed neutrophils degranulate and release chemoattractants and cytotoxic oxygen free-radical species into the local tissue environment is also increased by ANCA. In addition, primed neutrophils can adhere to and damage vascular endothelial cells and attract additional neutrophils to the site of damage, thereby creating an auto-amplifying loop.

Patients with AAV have increased numbers of primed neutrophils in renal biopsy specimens, paralleling the activity of the disease. In addition, persistent membrane expression of PR3 during periods of disease remission is associated with an increased risk of relapse in GPA patients. Enhanced generation of reactive oxygen species by circulating neutrophils in these patients compared to controls may occur.

ANCA-associated activation can induce neutrophil actin polymerization, resulting in increased neutrophil rigidity.[18] Such activated neutrophils can become sequestered in small sized vessels since they are unable to adapt morphologically to arterioles; this may help explain the predilection for small blood vessels in ANCA-associated disease.

Role of the endothelial cell

Whether endothelial cells produce PR3 and display this molecule upon activation is controversial. In the early stages of AAV, however, endothelial cells are known to recruit inflammatory cells and enhance their adhesion to sites of vascular injury. The subsequent release of PR3 (from infiltrating leukocytes, at a minimum) and other neutrophil proteases may induce endothelial synthesis and secretion of IL-8, a potent neutrophil chemoattractant, thereby attracting additional neutrophils. PR3 released by neutrophils can also enhance the adhesion of accumulating neutrophils and mononuclear cells to the endothelial surface via the induction of adhesion molecules, such as vascular cell adhesion molecule-1 (VCAM-1). VCAM-1 is known to be expressed *in situ* within the renal lesions of patients with AAV. The soluble endothelial protein C receptor binds activated neutrophils via interactions with PR3, providing a link between neutrophil priming, vascular inflammation, and the coagulation cascade. This may explain, in part, the increased risk of venous thrombotic events in observed in GPA.[19] Organ-specific antiendothelial antibodies have also been reported, albeit the precise antigens and role in disease development are unclear.

Immune complex model

Another established mechanism for causing vasculitis is the deposition of circulating immune complexes (ICs). ICs are known to contribute substantially to a number of types of vasculitis in humans. IC deposition is thought to be the prevailing disease mechanism, for example, in Henoch-Schönlein purpura (IgA vasculitis), hypersensitivity vasculitis, mixed cryoglobulinemia, and hepatitis B-associated polyarteritis nodosa. After the formation of soluble ICs, the complexes are deposited in the subendothelium, an event facilitated by the release of vasoactive amines (e.g., histamine) from platelets and basophils. Once trapped in the subendothelial space, ICs fix complement and generate chemotactic factors for the recruitment and activation of neutrophils. Degranulation of these neutrophils leads to the release of oxygen radicals and lysosomal enzymes, which in turn damage the blood vessel walls.

The IC model is compatible with the transient vasculitis known as serum sickness that develops following exposure to some foreign antigens. Antigens as varied as the horse serum formerly used in immunizations, antibiotics (e.g., penicillin), virus-associated antigens (e.g., hepatitis B or C) or self-antigens (e.g., double-stranded DNA) are capable of causing immune complex-mediated vasculitis in humans. In cases involving a "one-shot" antigen exposure, the vasculitis resolves as the antigen is cleared. However, when the antigen persists—e.g., in chronic viral hepatitis, SLE, or RA—the vasculitis can be chronic (albeit the precise antigen is not always known).

Formation of ICs is common, even in healthy individuals, but the occurrence of vasculitis is relatively rare. Several factors determine the pathogenicity of ICs. Antigen load is one determinant, as only amounts of antigen large enough to overwhelm the reticuloendothelial system (RES) provoke a pathologic IC response. Another important factor is solubility of the immune complex, which changes with the ratio of antigen to antibody. When the antigen:antibody ratio is very high, for example, complexes of antibody and antigen do not form. Conversely, when antibody is present in large excess compared to the antigen, the RES clears the antigen rapidly. ICs formed in slight antigen excess are most likely to be pathogenic, because they are both soluble and of sufficient size to deposit in blood vessel walls. Finally, physical forces such as pressure within the blood vessel (which can damage vessels), temperature (certain ICs such as cryoglobulin form at colder temperatures), or locations of vascular branch points (where turbulence favors immune complex deposition) are believed to influence the development of vasculitis.

General clues to detecting vasculitis

Inflamed vessels produce clinical symptoms and signs either by being associated with the release of inflammatory cytokines that cause malaise, fever, and weight loss, or by causing direct ischemic damage to specific tissues, such as the induction of digital gangrene. Because the vasculitides demonstrate predilections for certain tissues and organs, their presenting manifestations vary greatly. However, most of the vasculitides share four general features: first, they unfold in a subacute fashion, over weeks or months; second, pain is often a prominent feature of a vasculitis, be it from mononeuritis multiplex, scleritis, migratory oligoarthritis/arthralgias, myalgias, mesenteric ischemia, or another consequence of vascular inflammation; third, signs of inflammation, such as fever, rashes, and weight loss are prominent; fourth, evidence of multiorgan system dysfunction is common.

> ● **KEY CONCEPTS**
>
> ### ANCA patterns and associations with antigens and diseases
>
> | Pattern | Antigen | Disease association |
> |---------|---------|---------------------|
> | C-ANCA | Proteinase-3 | Granulomatosis with polyangiitis (Wegener's) |
> | P-ANCA | Myeloperoxidase | Granulomatosis with polyangiitis (Wegener's) Microscopic polyarteritis Eosinophilic granulomatosis with polyangiitis/ Churg-Strauss syndrome |

The "ANCA-associated" vasculitides

In a landmark 1954 paper, Godman and Churg[20] noted similar pathological features among three clinically distinct disease entities: GPA, microscopic polyangiitis (MPA), and eosinophilic

granulomatosis with polyangiitis (EGPA; Churg–Strauss). These diseases, Godman and Churg noted, "group themselves into a compass, ranging from necrotizing and granulomatous processes with angiitis, through mixed forms, to vasculitis without granulomata." Over the past 15 years GPA, MPA, and EGPA (Churg–Strauss) have become recognized as the cardinal forms of vasculitis associated with ANCA. They are commonly termed ANCA-associated vasculitides (AAV), although not all patients who meet the clinical definitions of these diseases have ANCA. The hallmarks of GPA, MPA, and EGPA (Churg–Strauss) are displayed in Table 57.2.

> ● **CLINICAL PEARLS**
>
> ### General clues to detecting vasculitis
>
> - Clinical symptoms and signs in vasculitis relate to:
>   - The release of inflammatory cytokines that cause malaise, fever, and weight loss.
>   - Direct ischemic damage to specific tissues.
> - Most of the vasculitides share four general features:
>   - Disease manifestations usually unfold in a subacute fashion, over weeks or months.
>   - Pain is often a prominent feature.
>   - Signs of inflammation, such as fever, rashes, and arthritis, are prominent
>   - Evidence of multi-organ system dysfunction is common.

Serologic testing for ANCA

Two types of ANCA tests, immunofluorescence (IF) and enzyme immunoassay (EIA), are now in common use. IF tests are highly operator-dependent, require a high degree of experience for proper interpretation, and are not antigen-specific. They are, however, generally superior to EIA in terms of sensitivity. In contrast to IF assays, EIAs are antigen-specific and demonstrate substantially higher positive predictive values for AAV. A widely-adopted strategy for optimizing the utility of ANCA tests, therefore, is to screen patients with potential AAV by IF testing, and then to perform EIAs on patients who test

Table 57.2 Hallmarks of granulomatosis with polyangiitis (GPA), Wegener's granulomatosis (WG), microscopic polyangiitis (MPA), and eosinophilic granulomatosis with polyangiitis (EGPA)

	GPA	MPA	EGPA
ANCA positive	80–90%	75%	50%
Typical immunofluorescence/Enzyme immunoassay results	C-ANCA/PR-3	P-ANCA/MPO	P-ANCA/MPO
Upper respiratory tract	Nasal septal perforation Saddle-nose deformity Subglottic stenosis	Mild	Nasal polyps Allergic rhinitis
Lung	Nodules Cavitary lesions	Alveolar haemorrhage	Asthma Fleeting infiltrates
Kidney	NCGN, occasional granulomatous features	NCGN	NCGN (severe renal disease unusual)
Distinguishing feature	Destructive upper airway disease	No granulomatous inflammation	Allergy Eosinophilia

ANCA, anti-neutrophil cytoplasmic antibody; C-ANCA, cytoplasmic ANCA; MPO, myeloperoxidase; NCGN, necrotizing crescentic glomerulonephritis; P-ANCA, perinuclear ANCA; PR-3, proteinase 3.
Adapted from Rao JY, Weinberger M, Oddone EZ, et al. The role of antineutrophil cytoplasmic antibody (C-ANCA) testing in the diagnosis of Wegener's granulomatosis. Ann Intern Med 1995; 123: 425.

positively.[21] Capture EIAs, available at some centers, do not have clear advantages over these other assays.

GPA, MPA, and EGPA (Churg–Strauss) have variable strengths of association with ANCA (Table 57.2). The strength of association for each disease is affected by several factors, including disease activity, disease extent, and intensity of therapy. Even in GPA, the disease for which the association with ANCA is the strongest, most series indicate that 10–20% of patients with active, "disseminated," and untreated disease are ANCA negative. One study of ANCA in patients with severe GPA in which all of the ANCA assays were performed in an excellent central laboratory indicated that 96% of patients were ANCA-positive.[22] However, for GPA patients with "limited" GPA, defined as the absence of an immediate threat to either the function of a vital organ or the patient's life, 30% or more of patients lack ANCA. Comparatively fewer studies have examined the presence of ANCA in MPA and EGPA (Churg–Strauss), but existing data suggest that the prevalences of ANCA-positivity in MPA and EGPA (Churg–Strauss) are approximately 70 and 50%, respectively.

●CLINICAL PEARLS

Vasculitides associated with antineutrophil cytoplasmic antibodies (ANCA)

- Granulomatosis with polyangiitis (formerly Wegener's), microscopic polyangiitis (MPA), and eosinophilic granulomatosis with polyangiitis/Churg–Strauss syndrome (EGPA (Churg–Strauss)) have become recognized as the types of vasculitis associated with ANCA.

- Shortcomings of reliance upon ANCA to define this group of complex diseases:
  - The role (if any) of ANCA in the pathogenesis of these conditions is unclear.
  - Not all patients with these diseases have a positive test for ANCA.
  - A variety of systemic illnesses, including infections, malignancies, and other conditions may be associated with a positive ANCA test, particularly when positive immunoflourescence tests are not confirmed by enzyme immunoassay.
  - Even when ANCA are present, they are unreliable indicators of disease activity. They are poor predictors of disease flares.

When carefully employed and properly interpreted, ANCA assays constitute an important, albeit imperfect, adjunct to diagnosis. In rare instances, in the setting of classic clinical presentations and highly consistent ANCA test results (e.g., C-ANCA immunofluorescence and PR3-ANCA), the combination of clinical findings and ANCA assays may preclude the need for tissue biopsies to confirm the diagnosis. Despite advances in ANCA testing techniques, however, histopathology remains the cornerstone of diagnosis in AAV. When the diagnosis is unconfirmed, all reasonable attempts to obtain a "tissue diagnosis" should be pursued.

With regard to predicting disease flares, several studies indicate that elevations in ANCA titers do not predict disease flares; i.e., the temporal relationship between an increase in ANCA and the development of a clinical disease flare is poor.[23] Moreover, disease flares can also occur in the absence of an ANCA titer elevation. In summary, ANCA assays are helpful for diagnosis, but highly unreliable in gauging disease activity and predicting disease flares.

Granulomatosis with polyangiitis (formerly Wegener's granulomatosis)

In 1936 a German pathologist, Friedrich Wegener, reported three patients in their mid-30s, whose innocuous presentations were those of a "common cold."[24] Within 7 months, all had succumbed to systemic inflammatory illnesses that culminated in uremia. Three years later, Wegener provided a more detailed description of this disease, which he referred to as "a peculiar rhinogenic granuloma with particular involvement of the arterial system and the kidney."[25]

Godman and Churg recognized the three pathologic hallmarks of GPA[20]: (1) necrotizing granulomas in the upper and/or lower respiratory tract; (2) necrotizing vasculitis affecting arteries or veins; and (3) segmental glomerulonephritis, associated with necrosis and thrombosis of capillary loops, with or without granulomatous lesions. GPA is one of the most common forms of systemic necrotizing vasculitis, with an annual incidence of 8.5 cases/million.[26] Although the disease occurs among individuals of all races, there is a strong predilection for individuals of northern European heritage. "Classic" GPA involves the upper respiratory tract, the lungs, and the kidneys, but distinctive features of this disease can also occur in the eye, ear, and other organs. Involvement of tissues as diverse as the prostate gland and meninges has been reported.

The numerous disease manifestations of GPA throughout the respiratory tract have long engendered suspicion that the disease results from interactions between an inhaled microbial pathoallergen(s) and a susceptible host. Approximately 90% of patients with GPA have nasal involvement.[27] The nasal manifestations of GPA include crusting, bleeding, and obstruction. Cartilaginous inflammation can lead to nasal septal perforation and even to collapse of the nasal bridge, a condition known as a "saddlenose" deformity (Fig. 57.2). Most patients with nasal (or sinus) disease eventually develop secondary infections of these tissues.

Erosive sinus disease is highly characteristic of GPA. Among the AAV, only GPA is likely to cause destructive lesions of the bony sinuses. Subglottic stenosis, resulting from a peculiar predilection of GPA to cause scarring inflammation in the region of the trachea inferior to the vocal cords, is a potentially disabling disease feature. Subglottic involvement is often asymptomatic

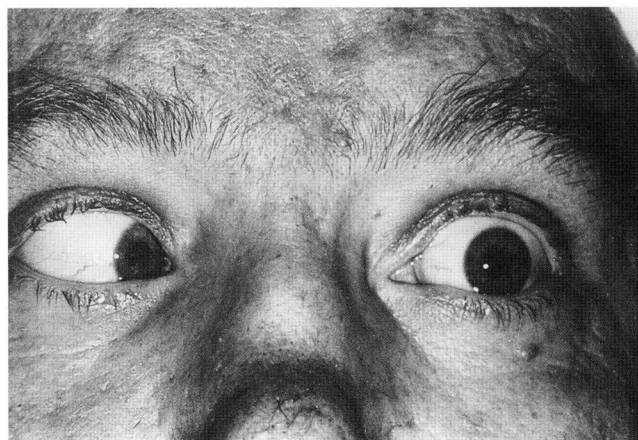

Fig. 57.2 Saddle-nose deformity in granulomatosis with polyangiitis (formerly Wegener's granulomatosis). Saddle-nose deformity and a left sixth cranial nerve lesion (the latter caused by meningeal inflammation) in a patient with granulomatosis with polyangiitis (formerly Wegener's).

(Reproduced with permission from Jinnah H, Dixon A, Brat D, Hellmann D. Chronic meningitis with cranial neuropathies in Wegener's granulomatosis: Case report and review of the literature. Arthritis Rheum 1997; 40: 573.)

and may manifest itself only as a subtle hoarseness. However, some patients present with the subacute onset of respiratory stridor. With time, airway scarring occurs, sometimes accompanied by profound tracheal narrowing. Severe cases require tracheostomy. Subglottic stenosis, particularly when associated with scarring and fibrosis, often responds poorly to immunosuppressive therapy. The most effective therapeutic approach to subglottic stenosis in these cases is usually mechanical, i.e., surgical dilatations to enlarge the airway narrowing, combined with local glucocorticoid injections.

Two principal forms of ear disease, conductive and sensorineural hearing loss, are typical of GPA. "Mixed" hearing loss, the conjoint occurrence of both auditory lesions, is also common. Conductive hearing loss results from granulomatous involvement of the middle ear cavity, most often leading to serous otitis media. In contrast, the mechanism of inner ear disease in GPA is poorly understood. Granulomatous inflammation in the middle ear may compress the seventh cranial nerve (which courses through the middle ear cavity), leading to a peripheral facial nerve palsy. Less commonly, vasculitic neuropathy infarcts the nerve at some point during its path through the temporal bone.

GPA can be associated with several clinically important ocular lesions (Fig. 57.3). Retro-bulbar masses, among the most treatment-refractory GPA lesions, may lead to proptosis and

visual loss through ischemia of the optic nerve. Scleritis, which causes eye pain and an angry, purplish scleral hue, may lead to scleromalacia perforans and visual loss (Chapter 73). Other ocular manifestations of GPA include episcleritis, peripheral ulcerative keratitis, uveitis, conjunctivitis, nasolacrimal duct obstruction (characteristically leading to wet rather than dry eyes), and, occasionally, occlusion of the retinal arteries or veins.

Although the histological features of pulmonary GPA are similar to those found in specimens from other tissues, lung biopsy specimens are more likely to reveal the full pathologic spectrum than are biopsies from other organs (Fig. 57.4). Both vasculitic and necrotizing granulomatous features, which do

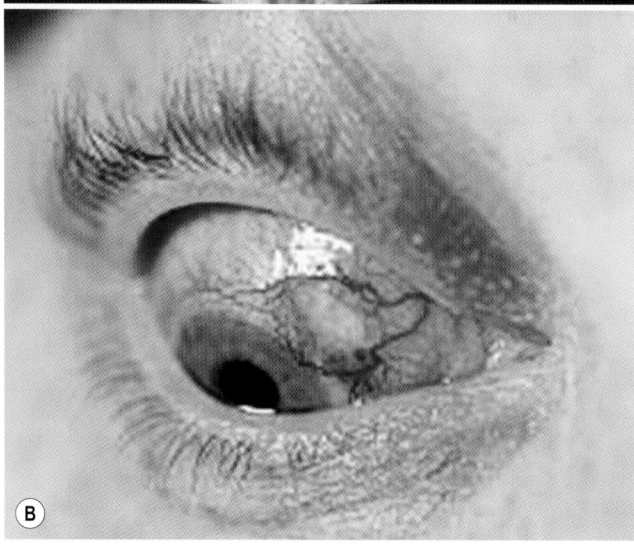

Fig. 57.3 The cardinal ocular manifestations of granulomatosis with polyangiitis (formerly Wegener's granulomatosis). (A) bilateral retro-orbital masses, causing proptosis of the left eye; (B) necrotizing scleritis.

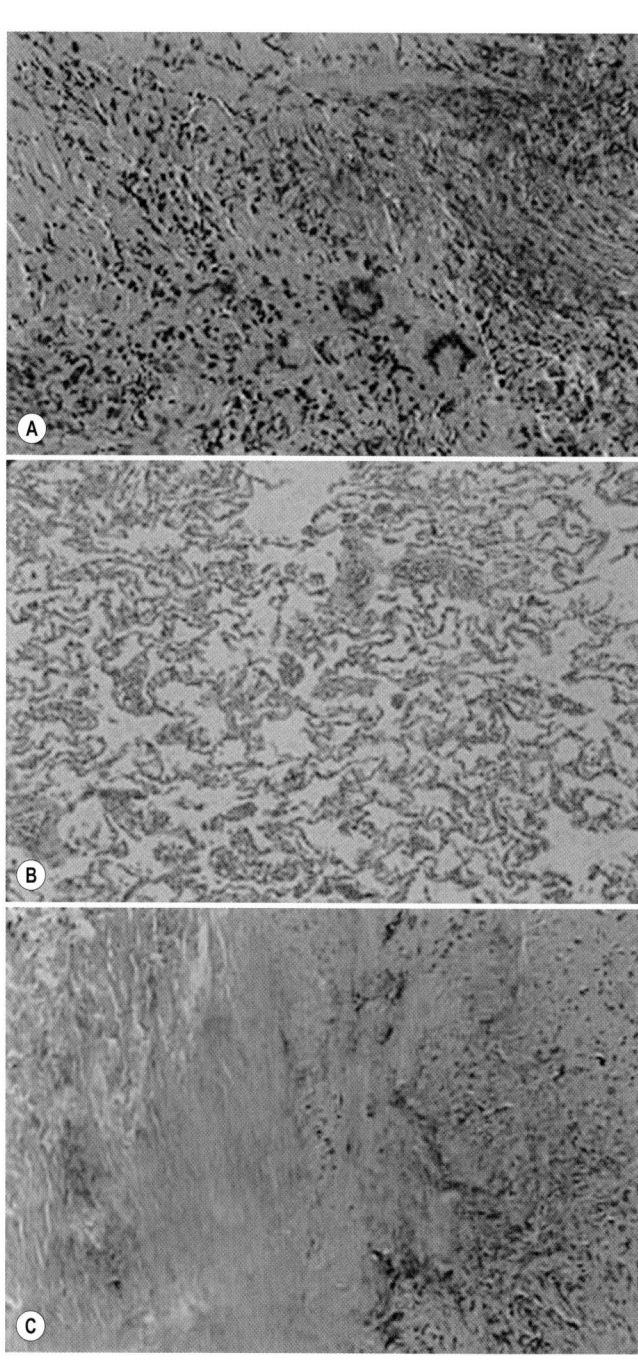

Fig. 57.4 Histopathology of granulomatosis with polyangiitis (formerly Wegener's granulomatosis). The pathologic features of granulomatosis with polyangiitis (formerly Wegener's): (A) Langerhans giant cells and palisading granulomatous inflammation; (B) small-vessel vasculitis and fibrinoid necrosis of the lung; (C) "geographic" necrosis.

not invariably coexist, may be confirmed in lung biopsy specimens. In addition to these two processes, pulmonary GPA frequently demonstrates an extensive, nonspecific inflammatory background. The leukocytoclastic vasculitis in the lung can involve arteries, veins, and capillaries, with or without granulomatous features. Vascular necrosis begins as clusters of neutrophils within the blood vessel wall (microabscesses) that degenerate and become surrounded by palisading histiocytes. Coalescence of such neutrophilic microabscesses leads to extensive regions of "geographic" necrosis. The range of granulomatous inflammation found in GPA can include palisading granulomas, scattered giant cells, and poorly formed granulomas.

The clinical manifestations of pulmonary GPA are equally diverse, ranging from asymptomatic lung nodules to fulminant alveolar hemorrhage. The most common radiographic findings are pulmonary infiltrates and nodules. The infiltrates, which may wax and wane, are often misdiagnosed initially as pneumonia. Nodules are usually multiple and bilateral, and often result in cavitation (Fig. 57.5). Hilar and/or mediastinal adenopathy is not a classic feature of GPA but can often be appreciated on computed tomography scans of the chest more readily than on chest radiographs.

Renal involvement is the most ominous clinical manifestation of GPA. The typical lesion of GPA (indeed, of all forms of AAV) is segmental necrotizing glomerulonephritis, usually associated with the formation of glomerular crescents (Chapter 67). The histopathology of renal disease in AAV—in contrast to mixed cryoglobulinemia, Henoch-Schönlein purpura (IgA vasculitis), and systemic lupus erythematosus, for example—is pauci-immune in nature (i.e., scant immunoglobulin or complement deposition). Thrombotic changes in the glomerular capillary loops are among the earliest histologic changes evident in AAV. Granulomatous changes, although frequently present in other organs, are identified only rarely in renal biopsies. The clinical presentation of renal disease in GPA is that of rapidly progressive glomerulonephritis: hematuria, red blood cell casts, proteinuria (usually non-nephrotic), and progressive renal insufficiency. Without appropriate therapy, end-stage renal disease ensues within days to weeks. A commonly observed clinical occurrence is acceleration of the overall disease process once renal involvement is evident.

Less classic but nevertheless common features in GPA are involvement of the musculoskeletal system, skin, and nervous system. Approximately half of all patients with GPA are rheumatoid factor positive, and RA is a common misdiagnosis early in the disease course when nonspecific arthralgias and arthritis may occur. The risk of an RA misdiagnosis is compounded by the frequent occurrence of cutaneous extravascular necrotizing granulomata (Churg–Strauss granulomas)—nodules that occur typically over the extensor surfaces of the elbows. Migratory oligoarthralgias and arthritis are a common presentation of disease flares. Unlike RA, the arthritis of GPA tends to involve large joints and to spare the small joints of the hands,. Splinter hemorrhages, digital ischemia, and digital gangrene resulting from inflammation in large digital arteries are under-appreciated as manifestations of GPA. Skin lesions in GPA include the full panoply of lesions associated with cutaneous vasculitis (see Hypersensitivity vasculitis). Although involvement of the brain parenchyma with GPA has been reported, meningeal inflammation presenting as excruciating headaches and cranial neuropathies are more common central nervous system manifestations of this disease. Finally, devastating mononeuritis multiplex can accompany GPA, but this feature is less characteristic of GPA than of the other major forms of AAV—MPA and EGPA (Churg–Strauss).

The clinical course of GPA is marked by a tendency to recur following tapering or cessation of treatment. In one clinical trial, somewhat less than half of patients achieved disease remissions and maintained them throughout the trial, which had a mean follow-up of approximately two years.[28] Even with therapy strategies such as B-cell depletion with rituximab, remission induction followed by eventual disease flare is the rule much more often than the exception. The requirement for repeated administration of the potentially toxic treatments in GPA can lead to substantial long-term morbidity. It is not clear yet whether newer therapeutic approaches, such as rituximab plus a 5- to 6-month glucocorticoid taper are less toxic over the long term as long-term follow-up studies are still awaited.

Microscopic polyangiitis

In 1948, Davson et al.[29] suggested the division of polyarteritis nodosa (PAN) patients into two groups based on the presence or absence of glomerulonephritis. One group of patients, Davson noted, demonstrated renal vasculitis only in medium-sized vessels of the kidneys (sparing the glomerulus). In contrast, patients in the other group had glomerular inflammation (i.e., small-vessel vasculitis, with or without medium-sized vessel involvement). This subset of patients with small-vessel vasculitis of the kidney was designated as having "microscopic polyarteritis nodosa." More recently, microscopic PAN has been renamed "microscopic polyangiitis" (MPA), in recognition of the tendency of MPA to involve not only arteries but also capillaries and veins as well.

The distinction of MPA from PAN was emphasized by the 1994 Chapel Hill Consensus Conference on the nomenclature of vasculitides,[1] which defined MPA as a process: (1) involving necrotizing vasculitis with few or no immune deposits; (2) affecting small blood vessels (capillaries, venules, or arterioles) as well as (perhaps) medium-sized arteries; and (3) demonstrating a tropism for the kidneys (glomerulonephritis) and lungs (pulmonary capillaritis). Table 57.3 compares the principal features of MPA to those of classic PAN.

As with GPA, a dominant feature of MPA is necrotizing glomerulonephritis with crescent formation (Fig. 57.6). In one study of 34 MPA patients with glomerulonephritis, the percentage of patients with functioning kidneys was only 55% and the actuarial survival only 65% at 5 years of follow-up,

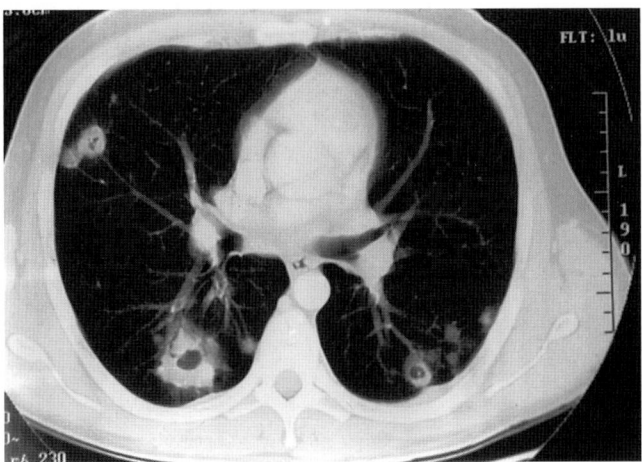

Fig. 57.5 Chest CT abnormalities in granulomatosis with polyangiitis (formerly Wegener's granulomatosis). Multiple, bilateral pulmonary nodules, several of which have cavitated.

Table 57.3 Features of microscopic polyangiitis versus classic polyarteritis nodosa

Feature	Microscopic polyangiitis	Classic polyarteritis nodosa
Granulomas	No	No
Vessel size	Small (and medium)	Medium
Renovascular hypertension	No	Yes
Rapidly progressive glomerulonephritis	Yes	No
Lung involvement	Alveolar haemorrhage	No
Mononeuritis multiplex	Yes	Yes
Anti-neutrophil cytoplasmic antibody (ANCA)-positive	P-ANCA (anti-myeloperoxidase)	Rare
Hepatitis B association	No	Sometimes (10%)
Vascular aneurysms	Occasionally	Commonly

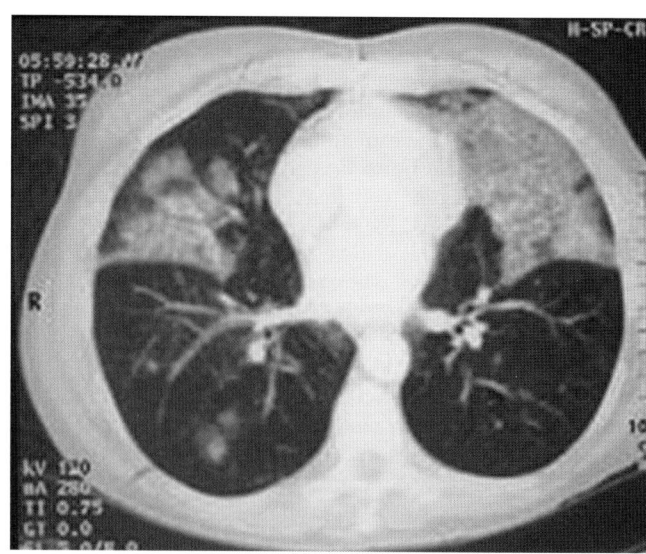

Fig. 57.7 Alveolar hemorrhage in microscopic polyangiitis.

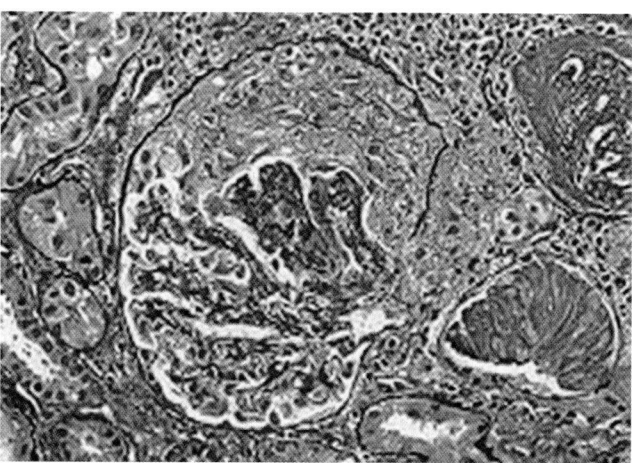

Fig. 57.6 Crescentic glomerulonephritis in microscopic polyangiitis. Glomerular crescent in a patient with rapidly progressive glomerulonephritis secondary to microscopic polyangiitis.

despite aggressive immunosuppressive therapies.[30] Pulmonary capillaritis, most typical of MPA, may lead rapidly to life-threatening hemorrhage from the lungs, requiring prompt, aggressive treatment (Fig. 57.7). In aggregate, the AAV constitute a far more common cause of these pulmonary-renal syndromes than does anti-glomerular basement membrane (GBM) disease. In some cases, both ANCA and anti-GBM antibodies occur in the same patient, with disease outcomes generally worse than with either antibody alone.

In one series of MPA patients,[31] renal manifestations (79%), weight loss (73%), mononeuritis multiplex (58%), and fever (55%) were the most common disease manifestations. Alveolar hemorrhage occurred in 12%. Upper respiratory tract symptoms in MPA are much milder than those associated with GPA. MPA is not associated with erosion of the bony sinuses, scarring of the subglottic region, or saddle-nose deformities. The essential difference between MPA and GPA, however, is the absence of granulomatous inflammation in MPA.

Eosinophilic granulomatosis with polyangiitis (Churg-Strauss syndrome)

In 1951, Churg and Strauss reported a series of 13 patients with "periarteritis nodosa" who demonstrated severe asthma and an unusual constellation of symptoms: "fever ... hypereosinophilia, symptoms of cardiac failure, renal damage, and peripheral neuropathy, resulting from vascular embarrassment in various systems of organs."[32] The investigators believed the syndrome to represent a new disease entity, which they termed "allergic angiitis and allergic granulomatosis." Three histologic criteria for this disorder, now known as eosinophilic granulomatosis with polyangiitis (EGPA; the Churg–Strauss syndrome), were specified: (1) presence of necrotizing vasculitis; (2) tissue infiltration by eosinophils (Fig. 57.8); and (3) extravascular granulomas. Today the diagnosis is often made on the basis of more loose clinical criteria, because finding all three criteria in a single patient is challenging in the absence of a post-mortem examination.

The 1990 American College of Rheumatology criteria for the classification of EGPA (Churg–Strauss)[33] are intended to distinguish patients with EGPA (Churg–Strauss) from those with

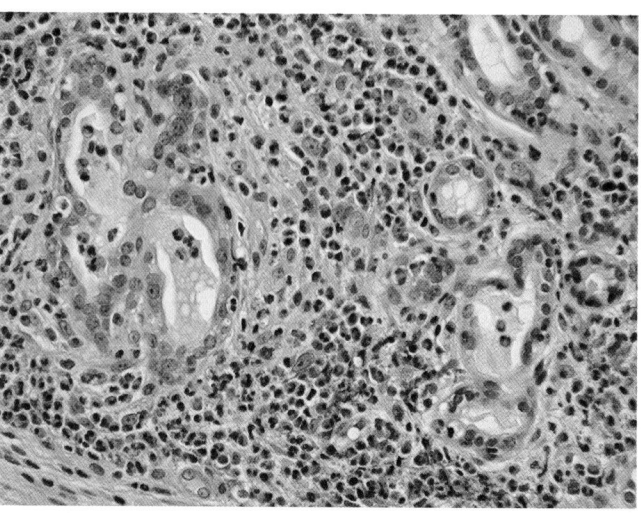

Fig. 57.8 Eosinophilic infiltration of a salivary gland.

Table 57.4 American College of Rheumatology classification criteria for Churg–Strauss syndrome

Criterion	Definition
Asthma	History of wheezing or diffuse high-pitched rales on expiration
Eosinophilia	Eosinophilia >10% on white blood cell differential count
Mononeuropathy or polyneuropathy	Development of mononeuropathy, multiple mononeuropathies, or polyneuropathy (i.e., stocking/glove distribution)
Pulmonary infiltrates, nonfixed	Migratory or transitory pulmonary infiltrates on radiographs
Paranasal sinus abnormality	History of acute or chronic paranasal sinus pain or tenderness, or radiographic opacification of the paranasal sinuses
Extravascular eosinophils	Biopsy including artery, arteriole, or venule, showing accumulations of eosinophils in extravascular areas

From Masi A, Hunder G, Lie J, et al. The American College of Rheumatology 1990 criteria for the classification of Churg–Strauss syndrome (allergic granulomatosis and angiitis). Arthritis Rheum 1990; 33: 1094.

other vasculitic disorders (Table 57.4). The presence of four or more of the six disease criteria yielded a sensitivity and specificity of 85 and 99.7% for EGPA (Churg–Strauss), respectively. The Chapel Hill Consensus Conference defined EGPA (Churg–Strauss) as the presence of eosinophil-rich, granulomatous inflammation involving the respiratory tract, with necrotizing vasculitis of small to medium-sized vessels, associated with asthma and eosinophilia.[1] In addition to the other vasculitides, EGPA (Churg–Strauss) must be distinguished from a group of hypereosinophilic disorders: Löffler syndrome, eosinophilic gastroenteritis, chronic eosinophilic pneumonia, the hypereosinophilic syndrome, eosinophilic fasciitis, and eosinophilic leukemia (Chapter 23).

More than 90% of EGPA (Churg–Strauss) patients have histories of asthma. Their asthma is typically either of new onset or constitutes a significant exacerbation of long-standing disease. Upon encroachment of the vasculitic phase of EGPA (Churg–Strauss), patients' asthma may improve substantially, even before therapy for vasculitis is begun. Following successful treatment of the vasculitic phase, however, glucocorticoid-dependent asthma persists in many patients.

● CLINICAL PEARLS

Three phases of eosinophilic granulomatosis with polyangiitis/Churg–Strauss syndrome

- Prodromal phase, characterized by the presence of allergic disease (typically asthma or allergic rhinitis), which may last from months to many years.
- Eosinophilia/tissue infiltration phase, in which remarkably high peripheral eosinophilia may occur and tissue infiltration by eosinophils is observed in the lung, gastrointestinal tract, and other tissues.
- Vasculitic phase, in which systemic necrotizing vasculitis afflicts a wide range of organs, ranging from the heart and lungs to peripheral nerves and skin.

Chest radiographs are normal in the majority of EGPA (Churg–Strauss) patients. Radiographic abnormalities are usually limited to fleeting pulmonary infiltrates, detected in one third of

patients. Pulmonary hemorrhage is unusual, and cavitary lesions should suggest the alternative diagnosis of GPA. The pathological features of lung disease in EGPA (Churg–Strauss) vary according to the disease phase: in the prodromal phase, there is extensive eosinophilic infiltration of the alveoli and interstitium; during the vasculitic phase, necrotizing vasculitis and granulomas are evident. Upper airway disease in EGPA (Churg–Strauss) usually takes the form of nasal polyps or allergic rhinitis. A high percentage of patients have histories of nasal polypectomies, often long before the diagnosis is considered. Although pansinusitis occurs frequently, destructive upper airway disease is not characteristic of EGPA (Churg–Strauss).

In contrast to GPA, mononeuritis multiplex occurs with a remarkable frequency in EGPA (Churg–Strauss). This potentially disabling complication was evident in 74 of the 96 patients (77%) in one series.[34] Cardiac involvement (usually congestive heart failure) also occurs with a disproportionate frequency in EGPA (Churg–Strauss); cardiac complications are a common mode of death in this condition. Renal disease in EGPA (Churg–Strauss) has been described as less common and less malignant compared to that associated with other AAV. When it occurs, histopathological findings are often indistinguishable from those of GPA, MPA, and other forms of pauci-immune glomerulonephritis, with the possible exception of increased eosinophils in biopsies from EGPA (Churg–Strauss) patients.

Peripheral blood eosinophilia is a hallmark of this disorder, with eosinophils accounting for up to 60% of the white blood cell count (before treatment). Approximately 50% of EGPA (Churg–Strauss) patients test positive for ANCA, which is usually directed to myeloperoxidase.

Although clinical remissions are obtained in more than 90% of patients with EGPA (Churg–Strauss), disease recurrences are common upon cessation of therapy (as with other AAVs). In the largest series reported to date, flares were detected in more than 25% of the patients.[34] In most cases, relapses were heralded by the return of eosinophilia. Many patients develop glucocorticoid-dependent asthma after the vasculitic phase of their disease appears to have subsided. Distinguishing simple asthma flares from EGPA (Churg–Strauss) recurrences is often challenging in such cases.

Treatment of the ANCA-associated vasculitides

Patients with GPA, MPA, or EGPA (Churg–Strauss) whose symptoms constitute immediate threats to either the function of vital organs or to the patient's life urgently require treatment with intensive immunosuppression. The treatment of GPA and MPA will be considered separately from that of EGPA (Churg–Strauss).

Until 2010, cyclophosphamide (an alkylating agent) combined with high-dose glucocorticoids was the cornerstone of therapy for severe GPA or MPA but two recent randomized controlled trials have compared cyclophosphamide plus glucocorticoids to B-cell depletion with rituximab plus glucocorticoids.[35,36]

The investigators of the European trial (ref Jones et al) concluded that the rituximab-based regimen was not superior to standard intravenous cyclophosphamide for severe ANCA-associated vasculitis and was not associated with reductions in early severe adverse events. The RAVE Trial[35] indicated that the rituximab-based regimen is not inferior to the cyclophosphamide-based regimen for remission induction.[37] Moreover, rituximab was superior for patients who presented with relapsing disease. The rituximab regimen employed in this trial was that used traditionally in the treatment of lymphoma (375 mg/m² weekly times four doses). However, it is usually more convenient to administer two 1000 mg rituximab infusions approximately 15 days apart. Follow-up of the RAVE cohort out to 18 months indicated that one course of rituximab was as effective as continuous conventional immunosuppression with 3–6 months of cyclophosphamide followed by azathioprine.[38] Many patients will require periodic re-treatment with rituximab in order to maintain disease remission. Baseline risk factors for disease flare include a history of relapsing disease at baseline, a diagnosis of GPA as opposed to MPA, and positivity for PR3-ANCA. Disease flares are uncommon and always mild if they occur in patients whose B cells are absent and ANCA assays remain negative.[38] Rituximab-based induction strategies are an attractive alternative in patients at high risk for infertility.

While the risk and benefits of cyclophosphamide as an immunosuppressive have been recognized for decades, much less is known about the long-term efficacy and safety of rituximab-mediated B-cell depletion. Obviously, killing of CD20$^+$ B cells is a strongly immunosuppressive intervention and serious, sometimes fatal, side effects (e.g., progressive multifocal leukoencephalopathy) have been described in patients with other autoimmune diseases treated with rituximab.[39] Additional studies exploring the recovery capacity of the immune system after B-cell depletion are necessary, particularly so in elderly patients.

The cyclophosphamide regimen is still used in many parts of the world where rituximab is not approved for the treatment of GPA and MPA and where costs of therapy are major considerations. The typical regimen is cyclophosphamide for 3–6 months, followed by azathioprine for an additional 18 months.[40,41] Cyclophosphamide can be administered on either an intermittent basis intravenously or a daily basis by mouth. The latter route is more likely to induce sustained remissions but may be associated with a higher risk of adverse effects.[42]

Practice regarding the use of either daily or intermittent cyclophosphamide varies from center to center. Remission is induced with either daily or intermittent regimens of cyclophosphamide (combined with glucocorticoids) in high percentages of patients. Regardless of the route by which cyclophosphamide is administered, however, the medication is associated with potential hazards. Careful monitoring, particularly of the white cell count, is essential. Complete blood counts every 2 weeks are advised for patients on cyclophosphamide. The induction of neutropenia is not required to achieve a therapeutic effect in AAV, and avoidance of this side-effect is highly desirable as a strategy to prevent opportunistic infections. Cyclophosphamide should be withheld temporarily if the WBC count falls below $4.0 \times 10^6/\mu L$.

"Limited" forms of GPA may respond to the combination of glucocorticoids and methotrexate, thus sparing patients the potential side-effects of cyclophosphamide or B-cell depletion. Increasing experience with methotrexate and prednisone has demonstrated, however, that durable remissions of GPA with this regimen are rare, and smoldering or recurrent disease that reactivates upon taper of the medications is the rule as in many patients with AAV.

A substantial number of patients with EGPA (Churg–Strauss) achieve satisfactory responses with glucocorticoids alone, and monotherapy is a reasonable first approach for many of these patients. However, patients with evidence of rapidly progressive glomerulonephritis or symptoms of mononeuritis multiplex should be treated promptly with both cyclophosphamide and glucocorticoids to halt these devastating disease manifestations. The efficacy of rituximab in the setting of EGPA (Churg–Strauss) is not clear. Despite the numerous overlaps between EGPA (Churg–Strauss) and the other AAV, EGPA (Churg–Strauss)

has the distinctive feature of a tissue and peripheral eosinophilia, and the impact of B-cell depletion in that setting remains relatively unexplored. Alpha-interferon therapy for EGPA (Churg–Strauss) has appeared promising in small studies,[43] but studies of sufficient size to evaluate this treatment fully are lacking. Inhibitors of IL-5 appear to be relatively well tolerated and may play an important role in the treatment of EGPA (Churg–Strauss) in the future, but there remains a dearth of data from clinical trials.

◉ THERAPEUTIC PRINCIPLES

Treatment of ANCA-associated vasculitides

- The presence of symptoms that constitute immediate threats to either function of vital organs or to survival requires urgent treatment with high doses of glucocorticoids and a second immunosuppressant. Alternatives for the second immunosuppressant include rituximab and cyclophosphamide. Data on long-term efficacy, safety, and cost-effectiveness are awaited to further refine the optimal immunusuppressive regimen for each patient.

- Limited forms of granulomatosis with polyangiitis (Wegener's) may respond to a combination of glucocorticoids and methotrexate, but durable remissions with this regimen are rare and rituximab may be a better choice for remission induction in these patients.

- In eosinophilic granulomatosis with polyangiitis/Churg–Strauss syndrome patients without serious organ involvement, treatment with glucocorticoids is a reasonable first approach. However, the presence of glomerulonephritis or mononeuritis multiplex requires immediate treatment with cyclophosphamide and glucocorticoids.

Polyarteritis nodosa

Polyarteritis nodosa (PAN), the grandfather of all the vasculitides, was described in 1866 by Kussmaul and Maier.[44] The patient was a 27-year-old journeyman tailor who died from a multisystem illness characterized by fever, weight loss, polyneuropathy, and abdominal pain. The nodular swellings found along the course of muscular arteries at autopsy prompted Kussmaul and Maier to term the disease "periarteritis nodosa." The term was unfortunate because in fact the inflammatory process consists of a panarteritis that involves the entire thickness of the vessel wall. Subsequent authors have adopted the more accurate name "polyarteritis nodosa."

PAN can begin in childhood or in the eighth decade of life, but the average age of onset is about 40–45 years. Series vary in the proportion of men and women afflicted. Ten to 30% of patients develop the disease related to infection with hepatitis B, due to the deposition of ICs containing viral antigens.[45] In the remainder of the cases, the etiology remains unknown. No genetic susceptibility to PAN has been identified, and familial PAN is exceedingly rare.

Clinical features

The initial symptoms of PAN are usually nonspecific, such as malaise, fatigue, fever, and extremity pain from myalgia or arthralgia (Table 57.5). Typically it is not until weeks or months

Table 57.5 Clinical features in patients with polyarteritis nodosa

Clinical feature	Percentage with finding
General	
Fever	71
Weight loss	54
Organ system involvement	
Kidney	70
Musculoskeletal system:	64
• Arthritis/arthralgia	53
• Myalgias	31
Hypertension	54
Peripheral neuropathy	51
Gastrointestinal tract	44
• Abdominal pain	43
• Nausea/vomiting	40
• Cholecystitis	17
• Bleeding	6
• Bowel perforation	5
• Bowel infarction	1
Skin	43
• Rash/purpura	30
• Nodules	15
• Livedo reticularis	4
Cardiac	36
• Congestive heart failure	12
• Myocardial infarction	6
• Pericarditis	4
Central nervous system	23
• Cerebral vascular accident	11
• Altered mental status	10
• Seizure	4

From Cupps T, Fauci A. Systemic necrotizing vasculitis of the polyarteritis nodosa group. In: Smith LH (ed) The vasculitides major problems in internal medicine, vol. 21. Philadelphia: WB Saunders; 1981: 26.

later that patients develop signs of vasculitis. The most helpful clinical clues often come from the skin and peripheral nerves because these areas are affected relatively early, and their manifestations of vasculitis are distinctive. Skin lesions of PAN include livedo reticularis, subcutaneous nodules, leg ulcers, palpable purpura, and digital gangrene.[46]

Mononeuritis multiplex, a peripheral neuropathy characterized by the segmental infarction of named nerves, is both one of the most specific clues to vasculitis and a hallmark of PAN. Mononeuritis multiplex affects the peroneal, tibial, ulnar, median, and radial nerves most often, leading to foot or hand symptoms (e.g., foot or wrist drop). Mononeuritis multiplex almost always causes sensory abnormalities, particularly painful dysesthesias. Motor involvement occurs in one-third of patients. Sometimes patients with PAN appear to have a (nonspecific) symmetrical polyneuropathy. In such cases, electrodiagnostic testing may unmask greater asymmetry to the process than is evident clinically, and also confirm that the pattern of nerve injury is one of axonal degeneration.

The gastrointestinal tract is also frequently involved in PAN.[47] The classic manifestation is "intestinal angina"—periumbilical pain starting 30–60 minutes after eating. The pain results from intestinal ischemia occurring because the increased metabolic demands of the bowel after eating cannot be met by the limited blood flow in inflamed mesenteric vessels. Ischemic bowel can be difficult to recognize, especially in patients receiving

glucocorticoids, which blunt the signs of an acute abdomen. Vasculitis of individual organs can mimic cholecystitis and appendicitis.

Renal involvement is nearly universal at autopsy in PAN, but tends to produce few clinical symptoms. The new onset of hypertension, hematuria, and rising serum creatinine are the most common signs. Renin-mediated hypertension, a hallmark of PAN, is rare in AAV, which tends to involve smaller vessels and glomeruli rather than medium-sized interlobar renal arteries.

Cardiac involvement, often striking at autopsy, is usually inconspicuous during life. Pericardial effusions, cardiomyopathy, and myocardial infarctions are the most common manifestations. Central nervous system disease usually results from hypertension rather than intracranial vasculitis, but involvement of cerebral blood vessels sometimes occurs. Scleritis is the most common ocular manifestation. Testicular infarction can occur early in the course, causing acute pain and swelling that mimics torsion of the testicle. Remarkably—as noted by Kussmaul and Maier—PAN spares the lung parenchyma.

Although PAN typically involves multiple organs, "limited" forms have been described. "Cutaneous PAN" is a medium-vessel vasculitis limited to the skin, causing nodules or ulcers. Over time, some of these patients develop systemic disease. Some cases of cutaneous PAN are induced by drugs (especially minocycline) and are associated with ANCA that do not have specificities for either proteinase-3 or myeloperoxidase.

The laboratory features of PAN, although frequently strikingly abnormal, are nonspecific. Anemia, mild thrombocytosis, elevation of the erythrocyte sedimentation rate (ESR), and microscopic hematuria are common.

The pathologic changes in PAN involve small and medium-sized arteries and may be macroscopic and microscopic. Involved arteries may show readily visible aneurysmal bulges of the vessel wall. Infarctions, ruptured aneurysms, and gangrenous tissue may be easily visible. Histological sections show inflammatory cells infiltrating the vessel wall (Fig. 57.9), leading to fibrinoid necrosis. Varying degrees of intimal proliferation and thrombosis occur. Lesions tend to be segmental and to favor branch points. In the acute phase of the illness, the inflammatory infiltrate consists chiefly of neutrophils, whereas mononuclear cells predominate in the chronic phase. Granulomas are absent in PAN, and eosinophils rarely present.

Diagnosis

Criteria for the classification of PAN have been developed by the American College of Rheumatology (ACR) (Table 57.6).[48] Diagnostic certainty requires a positive biopsy or an angiogram demonstrating characteristic microaneurysms (Fig. 57.10). Biopsies of symptomatic sites such as nerve, muscle, or testicle are often useful (sensitivity, 60–70%; specificity, ~97%). In the absence of a symptomatic site to biopsy, mesenteric angiography may demonstrate telltale microaneurysms (sensitivity ~60%; specificity, 99%).

Treatment and prognosis

For patients with idiopathic PAN, treatment usually consists of prednisone and cyclophosphamide. In the precorticosteroid era, only 13% of patients survived 5 years. With high doses of glucocorticoids, it is estimated that approximately half of all patients can achieve remission with prednisone alone. Although there have been few controlled trials (and even case series of PAN are contaminated by patients with other diagnoses, such as

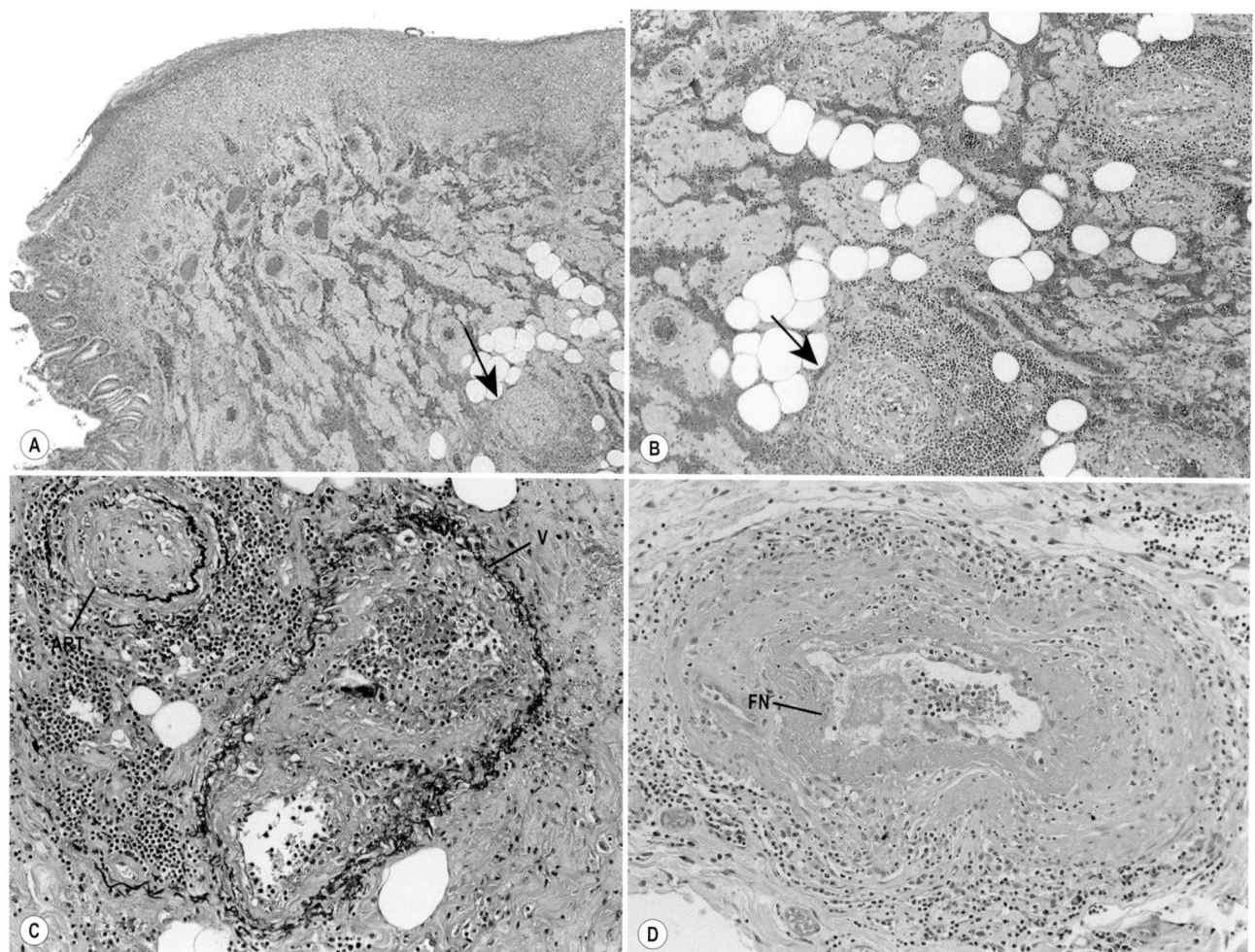

Fig. 57.9 Polyarteritis nodosa histopathology. Photomicrographs of a jejunal specimen obtained at laparotomy from a 74-year-old man who died of complications of mesenteric ischemia related to polyarteritis nodosa. (A) Viable appearing jejunal mucosa with the loss of villi is seen in the lower left corner of the photomicrograph. In the remainder of the visible lumen, the mucosa is replaced by a highly inflamed, ischemia-induced ulcer. In the lower right corner, there is a narrowed, chronically inflamed, medium-sized artery (arrow) surrounded by a lymphocytic infiltrate. (B) Higher powered view of the artery shown in (A) (arrow), along with several other inflamed arteries. The extensive lymphocytic infiltrate indicates the chronic nature of the inflammatory process. (C) Elastin stain of an artery (ART) and a vein (V) within the wall of the jejunum. The internal elastic lamina of the artery has been disrupted focally by the inflammatory process, and fibrinoid necrosis is present. (D) Medium-sized muscular artery from the jejunum, characterized by chronic lymphocytic inflammation, abundant fibrinoid necrosis (FN), and luminal narrowing.

Reproduced with permission from Levine SM, Hellmann DB, and Stone JH. Gastrointestinal involvement in polyarteritis nodosa [1986–2000]: Presentation and outcomes in 24 patients. Am J Med 2002; 112 386.

Table 57.6 Criteria for classification of polyarteritis nodosa

1. Weight loss ≥ 4 kg
2. Livedo reticularis
3. Testicular pain or tenderness
4. Myalgias, weakness, or leg tenderness
5. Mononeuropathy or polyneuropathy
6. Diastolic blood pressure > 90 mmHg
7. Elevated blood urea nitrogen or creatinine
8. Hepatitis B virus
9. Arteriographic abnormalities
10. Biopsy of small or medium-sized artery containing polymorphonuclear cells in the vessel wall

For classification purposes, a patient shall be said to have polyarteritis nodosa if at least 3 of these 10 criteria are present.
From Lightfoot R, Michel B, Bloch D, et al. The American College of Rheumatology 1990 criteria for the classification of polyarteritis nodosa. Arthritis Rheum 1990; 33: 1088.

microscopic polyangiitis or the Churg–Strauss syndrome), the only randomized controlled trial comparing prednisone alone with prednisone and cyclophosphamide showed no difference in 10-year survival: approximately 70% in both treatment groups.[49] Patients treated with cyclophosphamide, however, experienced fewer relapses than those treated with prednisone alone (9 vs. 38% of patients). Thus, for severe PAN or for cases that are refractory to initial therapy with prednisone, the combination of glucocorticoids and cyclophosphamide is the standard of care. When using cyclophosphamide to treat PAN, achieving leukopenia is neither required nor desirable. Indeed, frequent monitoring of the white blood cell count (e.g., every 2 weeks) is advisable so that leukopenia can be detected early and cyclophosphamide reduced or stopped as needed. The relative efficacy of daily versus intermittent (e.g., monthly) cyclophosphamide is not clear.

Most patients begin to improve within 2–4 weeks of starting treatment. Tapering of prednisone may begin after the first month and is continued slowly until the drug is stopped after

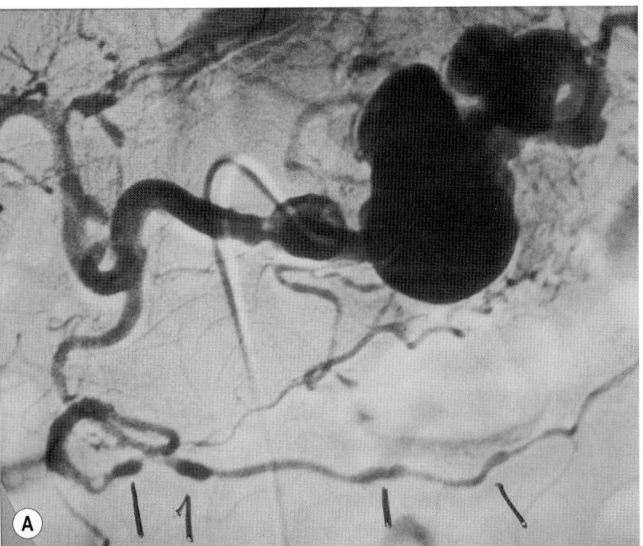

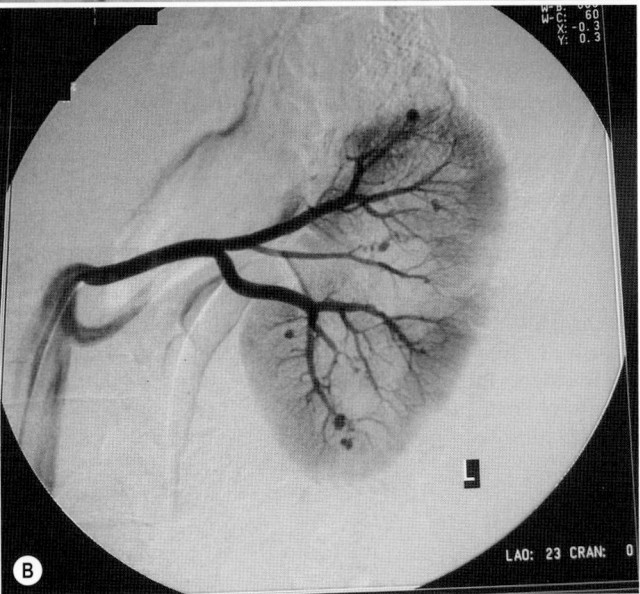

Fig. 57.10 Angiograms in polyarteritis nodosa. (A) Large aneurysms in the distribution of the splenic artery in a 60-year-old woman with polyarteritis nodosa. The largest of these aneurysms ruptured, requiring an emergent laparotomy. (B) Microaneurysms within the kidney of a 20-year-old man with PAN.
Reproduced with permission from Levine SM, Hellmann DB, Stone JH. Gastrointestinal involvement in polyarteritis nodosa [1986–2000]: Presentation and outcomes in 24 patients. Am J Med 2002; 112 386.

6–12 months. Whenever possible, cyclophosphamide should be discontinued after 6 months and replaced by a less toxic medication (e.g., azathioprine) for the completion of one full year of therapy.

Antiviral agents have revolutionized the treatment of PAN associated with hepatitis B. Before the availability of antiviral agents, all survivors of PAN treated with immunosuppression alone became chronic carriers of hepatitis B and assumed the risks of cirrhosis and hepatoma. The availability of antiviral agents permitted a treatment strategy based on an understanding of disease pathogenesis.[45] Initially patients are treated with prednisone (1 mg/kg/day) to suppress the inflammation. After the first week, prednisone is rapidly tapered and then discontinued over 3–7 days, and antiviral therapy (e.g., entecavir 0.5 mg/day) is started. For several weeks throughout this period, plasma exchange is carried out 2–3 times a week for an average of about 20 exchanges per patient, depending on clinical response. With this regimen, 80% of patients survive the vasculitis and 56% no longer demonstrate serologic evidence of hepatitis B replication.

Mixed cryoglobulinemia

Wintrobe discovered cryoglobulins in 1931 when, in the course of evaluating a 56-year-old woman with anemia, Raynaud's phenomenon, and symptoms of hyperviscosity who ultimately turned out to have myeloma—he refrigerated a tube of the patient's blood and noted the formation of a precipitate in her plasma.[50] To share his discovery with colleagues, he placed the tube in his coat pocket and walked to the wards. Pulling the tube from his warm pocket he was startled to see that his discovery had vanished. This experience helped to define the hallmark of cryoglobulins—antibodies that precipitate under conditions of cold and solubilize on re-warming (see below).[51]

Cryoglobulins are classified into three types (I, II, or III) (Table 57.7) based on whether they (a) are monoclonal, and (b) demonstrate rheumatoid factor activity.[51] Type I cryoglobulins, characteristically found in hematopoietic malignancies, are monoclonal but do not have rheumatoid factor activity. Cryoglobulin types II and III, which occur typically in autoimmune disorders and infections, are designated "mixed" cryoglobulins (MC), because they consist of both IgG and IgM. The IgM component in type II and type III cryoglobulinemia has rheumatoid factor activity. In type II cryoglobulinemia, the IgM is monoclonal, whereas in type III it is polyclonal. Not all patients with cryoglobulins have symptoms. Indeed, half of all patients with

Table 57.7 Classification of cryoglobulins and their immunochemical features and clinical associations

Type	Rheumatoid factor activity	Monoclonality	Clinical syndrome	Disease present
I	Yes (usually IgG)	No	Hyperviscosity	Malignancy
II	Yes (IgM)	Yes	Vasculitis	Hepatitis C Rheumatic diseases Malignancy Idiopathic
III	No	Yes	Vasculitis	Hepatitis C Rheumatic diseases Idiopathic

Ig, immunoglobulin.

hepatitis C have demonstrable cryoglobulins, yet vasculitis occurs in <1%. Vasculitis results when ICs containing cryoglobulins and antigenic components deposit in blood vessel walls and activate complement.

The clinical syndrome and underlying disease can be predicted from the type of cryoglobulin present. For example, monoclonal cryoglobulins without rheumatoid factor activity (type I) do not activate complement effectively and are more likely—as in Wintrobe's patient—to cause hyperviscosity than vasculitis. In contrast, the mixed cryoglobulins (types II and III) often activate complement efficiently, and are prone to cause vasculitis.

After the discovery of hepatitis C virus (HCV), it quickly became evident that this infection accounted for more than 80% of the cases of "essential" mixed cryoglobulinemia (EMC). The precise mechanism by which HCV and other infections induce cryoglobulins and the syndrome of EMC is not clear.

Among patients with HCV and mixed cryoglobulinemia, approximately one third have type II cryoglobulins and two thirds have type III. Type II MC developed a mean of 7.6 years after infection, and type III MC after a mean of 13.7 years following infection.[52] The genetic susceptibility of individual patients to EMC, the duration of HCV infection, and the genotype of particular HCV subspecies may explain why only some patients with HCV develop EMC.

MC causes small-vessel vasculitis with a predilection for the skin, peripheral nerves, and kidney. The most common manifestation is recurrent crops of palpable purpura on the legs (Fig. 57.11). Other common manifestations are dysesthesias and mononeuritis multiplex caused by vasculitic neuropathy, glomerulonephritis, arthralgias, malaise, and fatigue. Some patients develop mesenteric vasculitis, Raynaud's phenomenon, livedo reticularis, or secondary Sjögren's syndrome. Lung and heart disease are uncommon. Some patients with MC develop a severe medium-vessel vasculitis with large, painful ulcerations that are clinically indistinguishable from those of PAN.

Most patients with MC have anemia, an elevated ESR, and elevated liver transaminases. Those with type II MC usually show an IgM-κ monoclonal spike. Ninety percent of patients with MC vasculitis are hypocomplementemic, with C4 levels characteristically more depressed than C3. Biopsies of petechial lesions in the skin or gastrointestinal tract show leukocytoclastic vasculitis, with immunofluorescence studies revealing IgG and IgM deposition in both medium and small blood vessels. Renal

biopsies in patients with type II MC typically show membranoproliferative glomerulonephritis (Chapter 67). The diagnosis of cryoglobulinemic vasculitis is established by isolating type II or type III cryoglobulins following refrigeration at 4 °C for several days and by demonstrating vasculitis pathologically (usually by skin biopsy).

The treatment of MC is often challenging. For patients with mild symptoms such as infrequent crops of purpura, no therapy is required. For those with HCV-associated MC, frequent purpura, and a mild vasculitic neuropathy, pegylated interferon (1.5 mcg/kg/week) and ribavirin (1000–1200 mg/day) may be effective.[53] Fewer than half of patients with HCV-associated MC respond to antiviral therapy. Patients younger than 60 who do not have HCV genotype 1 (the most common in Americans) are more likely to respond. This regimen eliminates purpura, reduces the cryocrit, normalizes complement levels, and eliminates HCV-RNA in 30–60% of patients. Unfortunately, up to 90% of patients relapse (clinically or serologically) if the therapy is discontinued. For this reason, antiviral therapy is sometimes continued indefinitely (albeit at lower doses). Newer-generation HCV therapies are likely to be more effective in the setting of MC because of their more potent anti-viral effect. Moreover, an important recent advance in therapy has been the addition of B-cell depletion strategies to antiviral therapies.[54] These treatment approaches appear to be highly synergistic.

Hypersensitivity vasculitis

The proliferation of names for cutaneous vasculitis is principally due to the fact that, compared to the relatively limited number of disorders that cause large- or medium-vessel arteritis, a host of disorders can be associated with small-vessel vasculitis of the skin. These disorders include both primary vasculitides and secondary causes of vasculitic inflammation. Whereas some of these conditions cause only cutaneous vasculitis, others can also cause organ- or life-threatening involvement of vital organs, such as the lungs or kidney. This section focuses on types of small-vessel vasculitis confined to the skin. Other prominent causes of cutaneous vasculitis, e.g., cryoglobulinemia, Henoch–Schönlein purpura (IgA vasculitis), urticarial vasculitis, the ANCA-associated disorders, and cutaneous polyarteritis nodosa (PAN), are discussed in other sections of this chapter.

In 1952, in the first classification scheme ever devised for the vasculitides, Zeek[55] coined the term "hypersensitivity vasculitis." The purpose of this term was to distinguish a form of necrotizing arteritis that involved only small blood vessels from PAN, which has a predilection for larger vessels. The word "hypersensitivity" stemmed from animal models of vasculitis induced by the administration of horse serum, sulfonamides, and other drugs. These vasculitis models—attempts to develop an animal model of PAN—differed from PAN in their prominent cutaneous involvement, their involvement of the venous as well as the arterial circulation, and their involvement of "small" blood vessels, i.e., arterioles, venules, and capillaries. Moreover, in contrast to PAN, all of the lesions in hypersensitivity vasculitis tended to occur in "crops," and thus were approximately the same age. Finally, in contrast to the characteristically unrelenting nature of PAN, hypersensitivity vasculitis was self-limited.

Since Zeek's first description of hypersensitivity vasculitis, the term has been narrowed to denote small-vessel vasculitis confined principally to the skin and not associated with any other primary vasculitis (e.g., Henoch–Schönlein purpura (IgA vasculitis), GPA, or cryoglobulinemia). The identification of an inciting antigen for the vasculitis is not a prerequisite to the

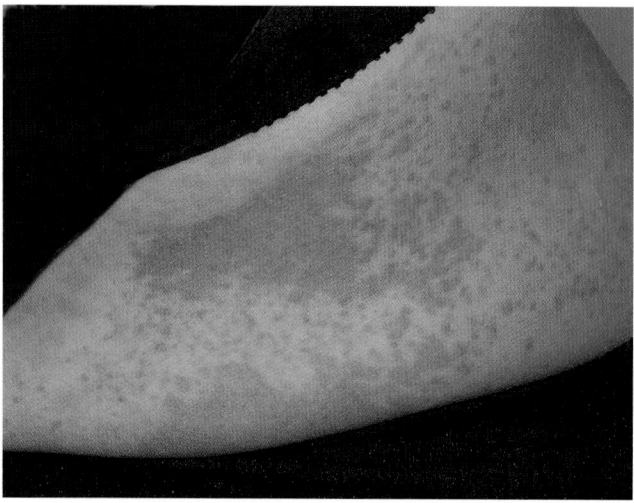

Fig. 57.11 Purpura in vasculitis. Palpable purpura in a patient with cryoglobulinemic vasculitis.

diagnosis, because no such provocation is found in many patients who fit the clinical and pathological picture of the disease.

The ACR formulated criteria for the classification of hypersensitivity vasculitis included: (1) age of onset greater than 16 years; (2) medication at disease onset; (3) palpable purpura; (4) maculopapular rash; and (5) biopsy of arteriole or venule showing granulocytes in a perivascular or extravascular location.[56] The presence of three of five criteria resulted in sensitivity of 71% and specificity of 84%.

The 1994 Chapel Hill Consensus Conference on nomenclature of the vasculitides proposed an alternative term for hypersensitivity vasculitis—"cutaneous leukocytoclastic angiitis"—because of the frequent failure to identify a precipitant (no manifest cause of "hypersensitivity"). This designation is also problematical, however, because although most lesional skin biopsies demonstrate a neutrophil predominance, others show a primarily lymphocytic infiltration. Moreover, these two histopathological patterns do not appear to represent different evolutionary stages of the same process, but rather (at a minimum) two distinct processes, underscoring the difficulty of using a single term to define all patients with this clinical phenotype.

Regardless of the name, certain similarities exist among patients who present with symptoms and signs of cutaneous vasculitis. First, the lesions typically occur first in dependent regions, i.e., the lower extremities or buttocks. Second, the lesions may be asymptomatic, but are usually accompanied by a burning or tingling sensation. A wide array of skin lesions can occur, including palpable purpura, papules, urticaria/angioedema, erythema multiforme, vesicles, pustules, ulcers, and necrosis. The simultaneous occurrence of livedo reticularis usually indicates the involvement of medium-sized arteries as well. Most cases with a clearly identified precipitant resolve over a period over 1–4 weeks, often with some residual hyperpigmentation or (in the case of ulcerated lesions) scars. A subset of patients, however, have recurrent disease that remains confined to the skin and requires prolonged therapy.

The pleiomorphic lesions of cutaneous vasculitis and the large number of mimics of vasculitis make confirmation of the diagnosis by skin biopsy essential. Biopsy of an active lesion (< 48 hours old, if possible) usually demonstrates leukocytoclastic vasculitis of the postcapillary venules (Fig. 57.12). Immunofluorescence shows variable quantities of immunoglobulin and complement deposition, confirming the importance of ICs to the underlying disease process but not demonstrating a diagnostic pattern. The performance of immunofluorescence studies, however, is

Table 57.8 Workup for patient with possible cutaneous vasculitis

Skin biopsy with immunofluorescence
Complete blood count
Serum creatinine
Liver transaminases
Serum and urine electrolytes
Urinalysis with microscopy
Chest radiograph
Antinuclear antibody assay
Serum complement levels
Anti-neutrophil cytoplasmic antibodies
Cryoglobulins
Hepatitis C antibody

Erythrocyte sedimentation rate.

an important (and often neglected) part of the workup, critical for the exclusion of Henoch–Schönlein purpura (IgA vasculitis), hypocomplementemic urticarial vasculitis, and cryoglobulinemia.[57] The workup for a patient with possible hypersensitivity vasculitis includes a number of other laboratory studies to exclude internal organ involvement and to differentiate from other diseases (Table 57.8).

Treatment strategies for hypersensitivity vasculitis are largely empiric. The type, intensity, and duration of therapy are based on the degree of disease severity in an individual patient. For cases in which a precipitant can be identified, removal of the offending agent usually leads to resolution of hypersensitivity vasculitis within days to weeks. Mild cases may be treated simply with leg elevation and the administration of nonsteroidal anti-inflammatory drugs (and/or H_1 antihistamines). Colchicine, hydroxychloroquine, or dapsone can be tried for persistent disease that does not lead to cutaneous gangrene. For refractory or more severe disease, immunosuppressive agents may be indicated, generally beginning with glucocorticoids. Failure of the patient to tolerate a steroid taper over some weeks or the requirement for excessive glucocorticoids dictates the use of an additional immunosuppressive agent. Azathioprine is commonly used for this purpose.

Henoch–Schönlein purpura (IgA vasculitis)

Henoch–Schönlein purpura (HSP/IgA vasculitis) is a distinct form of small-vessel vasculitis characterized by nonthrombocytopenic purpura, arthritis, abdominal pain, and renal disease.[58,59] The histopathologic findings are those of a leukocytoclastic vasculitis with IgA deposition. HSP/IgA vasculitis can develop at any age, but occurs most frequently in children. Indeed, HSP/IgA vasculitis is the most common form of vasculitis in children. The mean age of children with HSP/IgA vasculitis is 5.9 years, and 93% of affected children are less than 9 years old. The disease often remits spontaneously but sometimes causes life-threatening or chronic complications, most notably gastrointestinal hemorrhage (especially in children) and nephritis (especially in adults). Although the cause is unknown, an infectious trigger is suggested by the fact that two thirds of patients experience an acute, virus-like, upper respiratory illness an average of 10 days before the onset of HSP/IgA vasculitis.

The central role of IgA in the pathogenesis of this condition is emphasized by the demonstration that most patients have increased serum IgA levels, IgA-containing circulating immune complexes, and IgA deposition in inflamed blood vessels. Two

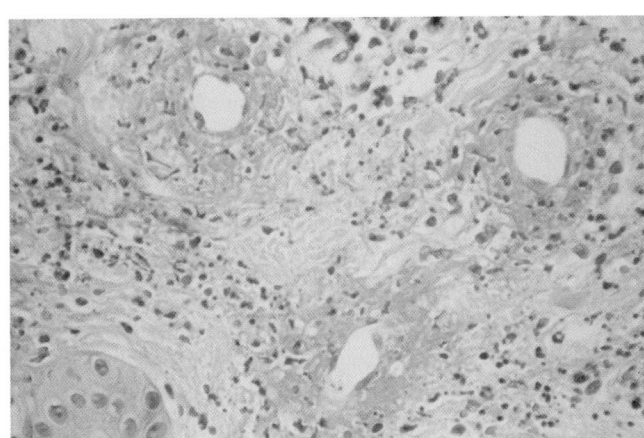

Fig. 57.12 Histopathology of hypersensitivity vasculitis. Necrotizing vasculitis of a small cutaneous vessel, with fibrinoid necrosis.

subclasses of IgA exist in humans, IgA1 and IgA2. The IgA subclass associated with both HSP/IgA vasculitis and IgA nephropathy (the most common form of immune-mediated glomerulonephritis in humans) is entirely IgA1.[60] This link to IgA1 stems from an aberrant glycosylation of IgA1 that is inherited as a genetic risk factor for both HSP/IgA vasculitis and IgA nephropathy.

HSP/IgA vasculitis patients have a heritable predisposition to aberrant glycosylation of O-linked glycans in the hinge region of a fraction of their IgA1 molecules. The aberrant galactose-deficient O-glycans end with N-acetylgalactosamine (GalNAc) rather than galactose. This terminal GalNAc moiety can be recognized by anti-glycan antibodies, leading to the formation of immune complexes. High serum galactose-deficient IgA1 levels are clearly a risk factor for HSP/IgA vasculitis but elevated concentrations of this immunoglobulin are not sufficient to cause the disease, as high concentrations can also be found in asymptomatic first-degree relatives of affected patients. Thus, a "second hit" appears to be required in the form of other heritable risk factors, an environmental exposure, or both in order to induce clinical disease.

Patients with HSP/IgA vasculitis present with the acute onset of fever, palpable purpura on the lower extremities and buttocks, abdominal pain, arthritis, and hematuria (Table 57.9). The purpura tends to be extensive, producing lesions too numerous to count. Although the purpura is most extensive on the legs and buttocks, it can involve the arms and, infrequently, the trunk. In some patients, the cutaneous involvement takes the form of maculopapular lesions, blisters, and ulcers. The abdominal pain is often colicky and may worsen after eating (i.e., intestinal angina). Some patients experience nausea, vomiting, and upper or lower gastrointestinal bleeding. Joint disease manifests as arthralgias or arthritis in large joints, especially the knees and ankles, and to a lesser degree, the wrists and elbows. Migratory patterns can be seen.

The clinical hallmark of nephritis in HSP/IgA vasculitis is hematuria, which is usually microscopic. Proteinuria almost never occurs in the absence of hematuria. Unlike gastrointestinal disease and arthritis, which occasionally precede the onset of purpura, nephritis almost always follows the appearance of skin disease. Other organs are rarely involved, but pulmonary involvement can be manifested by hemoptysis, and central nervous system involvement can result in subarachnoid or intracerebral bleeding. With the exception of renal disease, HSP/IgA vasculitis is self-limited, lasting an average of 4 weeks (range, 3 days–2 years).

The manifestations of HSP/IgA vasculitis vary with age. Among children with this condition, infants have milder disease. Children under the age of 2 are less likely than older children to develop nephritis or abdominal complications. As a group, children differ from adults with HSP/IgA vasculitis in having more frequent gastrointestinal symptoms and less frequent renal disease. Gastrointestinal involvement in children can cause intussusception, which rarely occurs in adults. Renal disease, which affects 50–85% of adult patients, is also more likely to lead to renal insufficiency compared to children.

Routine blood tests show few abnormalities other than a mild leukocytosis. The ESR is elevated only in about a third of patients. Urinalysis reveals hematuria, proteinuria, and red cell casts, but the serum creatinine is usually normal. Approximately 60% of patients have an elevated total serum IgA. Serum complement levels are usually normal.

Leukocytoclastic vasculitis is the dominant finding in most affected organs, including the skin and gut. Deposition of IgA can be demonstrated in most lesional skin biopsies. Renal lesions range from minimal change disease to focal or diffuse proliferative glomerulonephritis with crescents. Immunofluorescence studies characteristically demonstrate IgA deposition in the mesangium.

Classification criteria for HSP have been established by the ACR to help differentiate this disease from other vasculitides.[61] The differential diagnosis of HSP includes other disorders that cause leukocytoclastic vasculitis. Cryoglobulinemia shares the predilection of HSP for producing purpura, hematuria, and abdominal pain. Cryoglobulinemia is more likely than HSP to recur chronically. Tests for cryoglobulin and HCV help to distinguish the two conditions, and the finding of IgA deposition within lesional biopsies strongly favors HSP. Hypersensitivity vasculitis, unlike HSP, should not be associated with hematuria or gastrointestinal complaints. Unlike the ANCA-associated vasculitides, which can also produce purpura, hematuria, and arthritis, HSP seldom affects the lungs. Patients with AAV also differ from those with HSP/IgA vasculitis in that the glomerulonephritis is pauci-immune, not associated with substantial IgA deposition. Infrequently, bacterial endocarditis and other infections can produce purpura and hematuria that resemble HSP/IgA vasculitis. The purpuric lesions associated with thrombocytopenia are usually extremely fine, very small (albeit diffuse), and not palpable.

Treatment of HSP/IgA vasculitis has not been studied extensively. Most patients, especially children, have a self-limited disease course. Nonsteroidal anti-inflammatory drugs may alleviate arthralgias but can aggravate gastrointestinal symptoms and should be avoided in any patient with renal disease. Although glucocorticoids have not been evaluated rigorously in HSP, they appear to ameliorate joint and gastrointestinal symptoms. Glucocorticoids do not appear to improve the rash, however, and their effectiveness in renal disease is controversial.[59] Uncontrolled trials suggest that high-dose methylprednisolone followed by oral prednisone or high-dose prednisone combined with azathioprine or cyclophosphamide may help patients with severe nephritis (i.e., nephrotic syndrome and >50% crescents). Chronic renal failure is rare except in adults with more than 50% crescents on renal biopsy.

Table 57.9 Clinical features in 100 children with Henoch–Schönlein purpura

Feature	Percentage
Purpura	100
Arthritis	82
Abdominal pain	63
Gastrointestinal bleeding	33
• Occult bleeding	23
• Gross bleeding	10
Nephritis	
• Hematuria	40
• Gross hematuria	7
• Proteinuria	25
• Nephrotic syndrome	3
Miscellaneous	
• Orchitis	5 (9% of boys)
• Duodenal obstructions	1
Recurrence of symptoms	33

From Saulsbury F. Henoch–Schonlein purpura in children. Medicine 1999; 78: 395.

Behçet's disease

The triad of recurrent mouth ulcers, genital ulcers, and eye inflammation was first recognized as a distinct syndrome in 1937 by the Turkish dermatologist, Dr Hulusi Behçet.[62] In addition to these manifestations, Behçet's disease can affect non-mucosal surfaces of skin, the central nervous system, the gastrointestinal tract, and other organs. Most of the tissue damage in Behçet's disease results from vasculitis. Although Behçet's disease most commonly affects small and medium arteries, it can involve larger arteries and has a proclivity—in contrast to polyarteritis nodosa, for example—to involve veins as well as arteries. The cause is unknown. Most patients are in their 20s or 30s at disease onset. Behçet's disease is rare in North America, where it affects only 1 out of 500 000 people, but is 100 times more common along the ancient Silk Route, which includes Greece, Turkey, Saudi Arabia, Iran, Korea, China, and Japan. Genetic factors also affect susceptibility to the disease, especially in Asia where up to 80% of patients have the HLA-B51 allele.

The diagnosis of Behçet's disease rests upon a set of established criteria (Table 57.10). No single clinical or laboratory feature is pathognomonic, but the diagnosis is untenable in the absence of recurrent aphthous ulcers of the mouth (Fig. 57.13). The mouth ulcers usually number 2–10 and can affect the tongue, buccal mucosa, gums, and pharynx. The oral ulcers can cause such severe odynophagia that some patients lose weight and become dehydrated. Most patients also experience intermittent, painful genital ulcers. Ocular disease, which most commonly presents as anterior or posterior uveitis, can cause substantial disability in Behçet's disease. The anterior uveitis, typically associated with a red, photophobic eye, may be so intense that pus in the anterior chamber produces a white meniscus, called a hypopyon, evident on examination (Chapter 73). Scar tissue or synechiae formation between the iris and the lens can lead to distortion of the pupil.

With posterior uveitis, essentially a retinal vasculitis, lesions may be subclinical until significant portions of the retina have

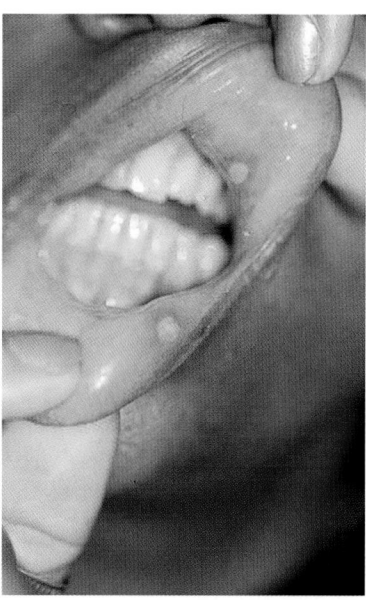

Fig. 57.13 Aphthous oral ulcers in a patient with Behçet's disease.

been damaged. Skin lesions (Table 57.10) may include folliculitis and erythema nodosum, which (in contrast to the erythema nodosum of sarcoidosis and inflammatory bowel disease) has a tendency to ulcerate. In most cases, the "erythema nodosum" of Behçet's disease is actually a medium-vessel vasculitis, rather than a septal panniculitis. The phenomenon of pathergy—the development of pustules at the sites of sterile needle pricks—can be an important clue to the diagnosis but is not specific and does not occur in every patient.[63]

Manifestations of Behçet's disease are not limited to those encompassed by the diagnostic criteria. For example, meningoencephalitis, which produces recurrent "sterile meningitis" with fever and encephalopathy, rivals uveitis as the most common cause of permanent disability. Strokes can also complicate Behçet's disease. Additional features seen in some patients include peripheral arthritis (usually nondeforming, oligoarticular, involving large joints in an asymmetrical pattern), sacroiliitis, thrombophlebitis (often migratory), gastrointestinal disease (mimicking Crohn's disease), epididymitis, coronary angiitis, and large vessel vasculitis.

Laboratory tests during active disease usually show mild leukocytosis, thrombocytosis, and an elevated erythrocyte sedimentation rate. The cerebrospinal fluid of patients with meningoencephalitis shows a lymphocytosis and elevated protein. Biopsies of the ulcers in the mouth, genital area, or colon show ulcerations and infiltration with mononuclear cells. Granulomas are not seen, a feature that helps to distinguish Behçet's disease of the bowel from Crohn's disease. Biopsies in other affected organs may reveal vasculitis.

Treatment depends on the type and severity of the disease. Severe disease in any organ system almost always requires high doses of prednisone (e.g., 1 mg/kg/day). Tumor necrosis factor inhibitors have also proven to be effective for patients with severe ocular manifestations or central nervous system disease,[64] but controlled trials of this approach are lacking. Because of the striking efficacy of TNF inhibitors, medications such as cyclophosphamide and chlorambucil are now employed sparingly. Azathioprine has also been proven to be effective in Behçet's disease.[65] Because disease activity in Behçet's disease tends to remit and relapse, drug therapy is slowly tapered once the patient improves.

Table 57.10 Criteria for the diagnosis of Behçet's disease

Finding	Definition
Recurrent oral ulceration	Minor aphthous, major aphthous, or herpetiform ulcers observed by the physician or patient, which have recurred at least three times over a 12-month period
Recurrent genital ulceration	Aphthous ulceration or scarring observed by the physician or patient
Eye lesions	Anterior uveitis, posterior uveitis, or cells in the vitreous on slit-lamp examination; or retinal vasculitis detected by an ophthalmologist
Skin lesions	Erythema nodosum observed by the physician or patient, pseudofolliculitis, or papulopustular lesions, or acneiform nodules observed by the physician in a postadolescent patient who is not receiving corticosteroids
Positive pathergy test	Test interpreted as positive by the physician at 24–48 hours

The criteria were drawn up by the International Study Group for Behçet's disease. Criteria for diagnosis of Behçet's disease. Lancet 1990; 335(8697): 1078–1080.
For the diagnosis to be made, a patient must have recurrent oral ulceration plus at least two of the other findings in the absence of other clinical explanations.

Buerger's disease

In 1908, Dr Leo Buerger reported pathological studies on the blood vessels obtained from 11 amputated lower extremities of patients with a disorder he termed "thrombo-angiitis obliterans."[66] Buerger wrote that the disorder usually occurred in young adults between the ages of 25 and 40, and was characterized by a thrombotic process in the arteries and veins, followed by organization and re-canalization. Portions above and below the diseased segment appear normal.

Buerger proceeded to describe the typical presentation and evolution of this disorder, from the onset of "indefinite pains in the foot, in the calf of the leg, or in the toes, and particularly of a sense of numbness or coldness whenever the weather is unfavorable." The initially nonspecific symptoms of Buerger's disease sometimes suggest a primary neuropathic process. Buerger observed that "Some of these cases give the typical symptoms of intermittent claudication." Upon the development of critical limb ischemia by the patient, Buerger described the development of a "blister, hemorrhagic bleb, or ulcer … near the tip of one of the toes …, and when this condition ensues the local pain becomes intense." Finally, Buerger reported, the condition resulted in dry gangrene and often in amputation because of unbearable pain.

Except for the remarkably strong association of Buerger's disease with the use of tobacco (see below), relatively little has been learned of this peculiar condition since the time of Buerger's original description. The classic patient with Buerger's disease is a young male who smokes cigarettes heavily. However, in populations where smoking is highly prevalent among females, Buerger's disease can afflict women as well. Although Buerger's disease has a predilection for the distal lower extremities, the distal upper extremities can also be involved severely.

Angiography of the extremities may suggest the diagnosis, but the findings are not pathognomonic (Fig. 57.14). The vessels most commonly involved are the digital arteries of the fingers and toes, as well as the palmar, plantar, tibial peroneal, radial, and ulnar arteries. Obliteration of these vessels leads to the development of collaterals that frequently have a "corkscrew" appearance. Examination of the proximal vasculature by aortography is essential to exclude embolic sources and to demonstrate normality of the proximal vessels, which is characteristic of Buerger's disease.

Buerger's disease is unusual among the vasculitides in several respects: (1) the disease involves veins as well as arteries (even though the most striking symptoms are secondary to arterial involvement); (2) despite the intense involvement of medium-sized arteries, there is virtually no involvement of internal organs or any tissues besides the extremities; (3) although associated with the formation of a highly inflammatory thrombus, compared to other vasculitides there are fewer inflammatory changes within blood vessel walls, and fibrinoid necrosis is absent; and finally (4) Buerger's disease is poorly responsive to immunosuppression.

Buerger's disease does not occur in the absence of exposure to tobacco, usually large accounts of cigarette smoking. Once established, the disease may be maintained by even small exposures to tobacco (even smokeless tobacco or second-hand smoke), so cessation of smoking is essential in the treatment of this disease. Failure to stop smoking is associated with a dramatic increase in the risk of limb loss by amputation.[67] Although smoking is necessary, it is clearly not sufficient on its own to cause Buerger's disease. Other factors, including genetic factors and

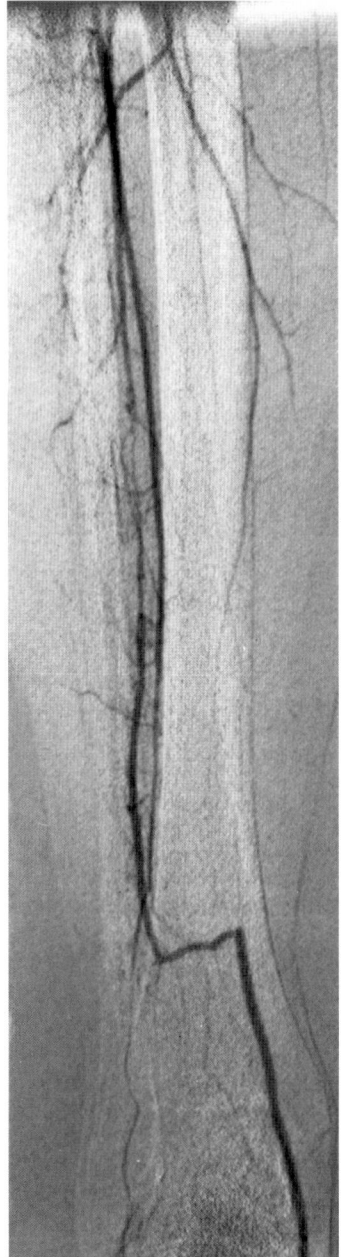

Fig. 57.14 Angiogram in Buerger's disease. Lower extremity arteriogram in a 20-year-old woman with Buerger's disease. The anterior tibial artery attenuates in the mid-calf. The posterior tibial artery is occluded proximally, but is reconstituted above the ankle by collateral circulation from the peroneal artery. Distal to its reconstitution, the posterior tibial artery appears normal, consistent with the segmental nature of Buerger's disease.

abnormalities of cellular and humoral immunity are currently under investigation.

In addition to encouraging cessation of smoking in the strongest possible terms, the therapy of Buerger's disease requires meticulous local wound care, avoidance of trauma to the involved areas, and ample use of narcotic analgesia. A variety of empiric therapies may be employed, including calcium channel blockers, pentoxifylline, iloprost, and sympathectomy, but there is currently little evidence to support their efficacy. The impact of anti-coagulation appears to be minimal. Thrombolytic therapies have not been studied in detail.

Cogan syndrome

In 1945, Cogan reported four young patients (aged 20–35) who presented with either nonsyphilitic interstitial keratitis (bilateral eye pain, erythema, and photophobia) or symptoms of severe inner ear dysfunction (disabling vertigo, tinnitus, and progressive bilateral deafness).[68] Regardless of which organ (eye or ear) became involved first, the onset of symptoms in one was followed within days to weeks by the development of symptoms in the other. Interstitial keratitis in the patients reported by Cogan waxed and waned, with only mild long-term ocular morbidity. In contrast, 3 of the 4 patients reported by Cogan suffered inexorable declines in auditory function, leading to deafness.

The combination of inflammatory eye disease and vestibulo/auditory dysfunction is the *sine qua non* of Cogan syndrome. The classic presentation is that of interstitial keratitis and sensorineural hearing loss. This disorder afflicts young adults, with no gender predominance. In approximately 10% of cases, eye and ear inflammation is associated with arthritis of medium- and large-sized vessels (including aortitis).[69] The ocular manifestations (and presumably the inner ear disease) of Cogan syndrome are also vasculitic in nature.

Interstitial keratitis leads to the sensation of ocular irritation, excessive lacrimation, and photophobia, and is accompanied by moderate reductions (generally reversible) in visual acuity. The eye findings may be evanescent, and often require repeated examination for detection. Examination of the cornea by slit lamp (Fig. 57.15) reveals stromal clouding in the anterior and middle cornea. Pathologically, the cornea shows lymphocyte and plasma cell infiltration into the deep layers of the cornea, with varying degrees of neovascularization. Although non-syphilitic interstitial keratitis is the ophthalmological hallmark of Cogan syndrome, virtually any type of inflammatory eye disease can occur in this disease, including conjunctivitis, uveitis, episcleritis, scleritis, exophthalmos, papilledema, retinal vasculitis, and inflammation of the optic papilla that suggests optic neuritis.

The greater cause of long-term morbidity in Cogan syndrome is the ear manifestations. Failure to recognize the nature of the problem promptly and institute appropriate therapy leads to more than half of the patients with Cogan syndrome suffering some degree of irreversible hearing loss. A substantial percentage become profoundly deaf in at least one if not both ears, and become candidates for cochlear implantation. Audiologic testing reveals sensorineural hearing loss. The vestibular manifestations may also be severe, and usually present with the abrupt onset of vertigo, ataxia, tinnitus, and nausea and vomiting. The severity of these symptoms is often sufficiently great to confine patients to bed. Vestibular dysfunction can lead to the disabling visual complaint of oscillopsia, in which patients perceive objects to jiggle back and forth.

Access to tissue at any stage of ear involvement in Cogan syndrome is rare. Consequently, knowledge of the pathology of this disorder stems mostly from temporal bone specimens from patients with long-standing, intensively treated disease. These findings include endolymphatic hydrops, acute labyrinthitis resulting in atrophy of the hair cells and their supporting structures, focal or diffuse proliferation of fibrous tissue and bone ("neo-osteogenesis"), and neuronal degeneration. Definitive evidence of vasculitis in these tissues is absent.

Medium- and large-vessel arteritis can lead to a host of complications in patients with Cogan syndrome, including aortitis, aortic regurgitation, coronary artery inflammation, mesenteric vasculitis, and limb claudication. The large vessel disease of Cogan's syndrome must be distinguished from that of Takayasu's arteritis (Chapter 58).

Interstitial keratitis generally responds well to topical steroid therapy, which often must be administered chronically. In contrast, sensorineural hearing loss must be treated early and aggressively, with high doses of systemic glucocorticoids. Failure to institute such therapy within the first 2 weeks of symptoms frequently results in irreversible hearing loss. Most patients who will respond generally do so within 2 weeks. Cytotoxic agents such as cyclophosphamide may also be considered for either the eye or ear manifestations if sufficiently severe. Because of the recurrent nature of Cogan syndrome in many cases, the cumulative morbidity from treatment may be substantial. Once the disease is controlled, a moderate remission maintenance regimen should be considered, particularly in patients who have experienced disease flares before.

Primary angiitis of the central nervous system

Primary angiitis of the central nervous system (PACNS), a rare disease of unknown etiology, is characterized by small- and medium-sized vessel vasculitis limited to the brain or spinal cord.[70,71] The once commonly used label—"granulomatous angiitis"—has dropped out of favor because not all patients with vasculitis limited to the central nervous system demonstrate granulomatous inflammation, and other forms of vasculitis, including systemic diseases such as sarcoidosis and GPA, can cause granulomatous vasculitis in the brain. Vasculitis limited to the central nervous system is the most difficult form of vasculitis to diagnose accurately. The protean manifestations of the disease, the unreliability of noninvasive diagnostic tests, and the difficulty of obtaining adequate brain biopsies all contribute to the diagnostic conundrum of PACNS.

Patients with PACNS classically manifest the triad of headache, encephalopathy, and multifocal strokes. However, only a minority of patients present with all three features, and many develop a wide range of other neurological manifestations. Most patients present in the fourth or fifth decade of life, but can range in age from 3 to 74. The disease affects women and men equally often. The disease can begin suddenly or develop slowly. The first symptom is usually headache, often severe and sometimes associated with nausea and vomiting. Almost all patients eventually develop encephalopathy with lethargy, confusion, and memory loss. Some develop multifocal strokes, seizures,

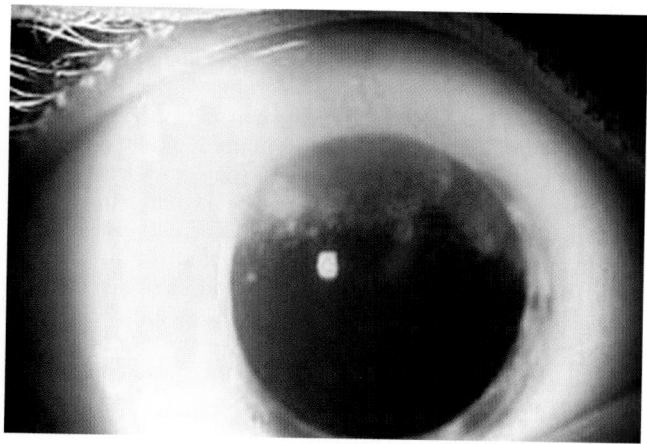

Fig. 57.15 Interstitial keratitis in Cogan syndrome. Nonsyphilitic interstitial keratitis, demonstrated by slit-lamp examination in a patient with Cogan syndrome.

evidence of increased intracranial pressure, or myelopathy. Constitutional symptoms, a hallmark of most forms of vasculitis, are notably absent in patients with PACNS.

In keeping with the isolated nature of the inflammation of PACNS, routine laboratory tests are usually normal. The majority of patients do not have anemia or an elevated erythrocyte sedimentation rate. The lumbar puncture yields abnormal cerebrospinal fluid in approximately 80% of cases; the most common abnormalities are a modest CSF monocytosis and an increased CSF protein. Oligoclonal bands and elevated IgG indices in the cerebrospinal fluid do not appear to be either sensitive or specific for PACNS.

The clinical and laboratory features described above apply to patients who are diagnosed by brain biopsy. Over the past 30 years, an increasing number of cases have been reported in which the diagnosis is based on CNS angiography alone, without the performance of a brain biopsy.[71,72] These patients differ from those with biopsy-confirmed cases in that the majority are women, the onset tends to be more abrupt, the neurological signs less severe, and the lumbar puncture normal.

Of the noninvasive imaging tests, magnetic resonance imaging (MRI) is more sensitive than computed tomography (CT).[73] The false negative rate of MRI appears to be less than 10% in most series. Most commonly the MRI shows multiple, bilateral, bland infarctions, distributed in the subcortical white matter, cortical gray matter, deep gray matter, deep white matter, or cerebellum. Hemorrhagic lesions and mass lesions also occur. No MRI pattern is specific for PACNS. The classic abnormality on angiography is the "string of beads" pattern produced by segmented arterial narrowing alternating with dilatations (Fig. 57.16). Vascular occlusions, collateral formation, and prolonged circulation time may also be seen. Microaneurysms, frequently seen on visceral angiograms in patients with PAN, rarely occur in PACNS. Unfortunately, no angiographic pattern is pathognomonic, and other disorders, including intravascular lymphoma, systemic infections, and vasospasm can produce similar angiographic abnormalities (see below).

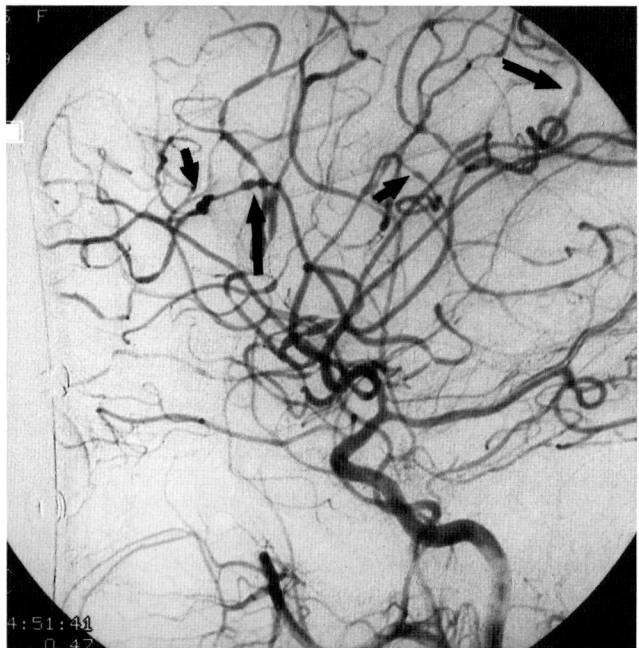

Fig. 57.16 Cerebral angiogram in primary angiitis of the central nervous system. The angiogram illustrates the dilatations and narrowing of arteries typical of PACNS.

The diagnosis of PACNS is definite if the patient: (1) presents with multifocal strokes or encephalopathy accompanied by headache; (2) has a cerebral angiogram showing changes consistent with vasculitis; (3) has no evidence of systemic infection, neoplasm, or toxic exposure; and (4) has a biopsy of the leptomeninges or brain cortex demonstrating vasculitis in the absence of other causes. The diagnosis of PACNS should be considered possible when the patient meets all criteria except that of a positive brain biopsy. In patients not having a positive biopsy, systemic vasculitides and other diseases that can mimic vasculitis must be excluded.

Histological specimens in PACNS show vasculitis of small and medium-sized leptomeningeal and cortical arteries. Veins and venules are involved less often. The inflammatory infiltrate varies, but consists predominantly of lymphocytes admixed with histiocytes. Langerhans and foreign body giant cells occur in about half of the cases. The inflammation usually targets the intima and media and produces variable degrees of necrosis.

The rarity of PACNS has prevented prospective treatment trials. Prednisone and cyclophosphamide are recommended for patients who have severe neurological deficits and a positive brain biopsy. Prednisone alone (beginning at 1 mg/kg/day) appears to be adequate therapy for some patients, especially those who experience a sudden onset of mild to moderate abnormalities that are not progressive, have a normal CSF, and whose diagnosis is supported by an angiogram in the absence of a brain biopsy. Mortality rates, once as high as 95% in untreated patients, have plummeted to less than 10% for treated patients. Most patients improve with treatment; the degree of recovery correlates inversely with the severity of deficits at diagnosis and the age of the patient.

An important (and much more common) mimic of PACNS is reversible cerebral vasoconstriction syndrome (RCVS).[74] RCVS, generally a self-limited condition, is frequently misdiagnosed as PACNS. In contrast to PACNS, RCVS has a sudden onset, typically with a thunderclap headache. Strokes are uncommon in RCVS and MRI studies are generally normal, but re-perfusion bleeds following intense vasoconstriction can sometimes occur. Watershed infarctions are also observed in some patients. The lumbar puncture is usually normal in RCVS, another characteristic that distinguishes it from PACNS. RCVS has multiple causes, particularly medications such as cold medications or other agents with the potential for inducing vasoconstriction.

Hypocomplementemic urticarial vasculitis

In 1973, Mayo Clinic investigators described 4 patients with recurrent attacks of urticarial lesions and combinations of synovitis, abdominal symptoms, and glomerulonephritis.[75] Although transient, urticaria in these patients generally persisted for at least 24 hours (longer than the 6–8 hours typically associated with chronic idiopathic urticaria) and sometimes left traces of hyperpigmentation, indicative of red blood cell extravasation through damaged capillaries. Low complement levels were present in all of the patients during periods of active disease, and skin biopsies demonstrated evidence of an immune complex-mediated disease process. Investigations excluded SLE and mixed cryoglobulinemia, leading to the report of a previously undescribed disorder now known as the hypocomplementemic urticarial vasculitis syndrome (HUVS).

HUVS is now recognized as one of a group of disorders known as urticarial vasculitis. At least three subtypes of urticarial vasculitis are known[76]: (1) a normocomplementemic form, which is generally idiopathic and benign; (2) a hypocomplementemic form, which is often associated with a systemic inflammatory disease; and (3) HUVS, a potentially severe condition usually associated with autoantibodies to the collagen-like region of C1q. Most patients with urticarial vasculitis have the hypocomplementemic subtype and demonstrate low C3, C4, and CH50. Patients with urticarial vasculitis who show evidence of complement activation are much more likely to manifest signs of a systemic disorder than those with normal complement levels. The majority of urticarial vasculitis patients (80–90%) have an underlying systemic disorder, usually SLE, Sjögren's syndrome, or cryoglobulinemia.

The lesions of urticarial vasculitis must be distinguished from chronic idiopathic urticaria, which is encountered far more commonly in clinical practice. Only about 10% of patients with chronic urticaria have urticarial vasculitis. In contrast to chronic idiopathic urticaria (the principal symptom of which is pruritus), urticarial lesions associated with vasculitis are often accompanied by stinging or burning. Urticarial vasculitis affects the capillaries and postcapillary venules, and the classic features of leukocytoclastic vasculitis may be evident on light microscopy. Immunofluorescence reveals both immunoglobulin and complement deposition in or around blood vessels of the upper dermis and/or the dermal—epidermal junction (Fig. 57.17).

HUVS frequently mimics SLE. As with SLE, HUVS has a striking female predominance, with a female:male ratio of 8:1. However, SLE-specific antibodies (e.g., those to dsDNA and the Sm antigen) do not occur in HUVS, and there are several distinguishing clinical features. For example, HUVS may be associated with angioedema, ocular inflammation, and chronic obstructive pulmonary disease (COPD), all of which are highly atypical of SLE. Although exacerbated by tobacco use, COPD may occur in the absence of any history of cigarette smoking, and may be severe. The few cases of lung biopsies in patients with this complication have not demonstrated vasculitis, but rather shown panacinar emphysema. As in SLE, kidney biopsies in HUVS patients may reveal mesangial inflammation or membranoproliferative glomerulonephritis, but progression to end-stage renal disease in HUVS is unusual. Severe cardiac valve disease and Jaccoud's arthropathy have also been reported in HUVS.

Most patients with HUVS make C1q "precipitins," i.e., IgG autoantibodies to the collagen-like region of C1q.[76] Whether or not anti-C1q antibodies contribute to the pathogenesis of HUVS remains unclear. Anti-C1q antibodies are also detected in up to one third of patients with SLE, and in more than 80% of SLE patients with glomerulonephritis. Despite the prevalence of these antibodies in SLE, few patients who are seropositive for anti-C1q antibodies develop urticarial lesions. Glomeruli from patients with lupus nephritis may contain large quantities of anti-C1q antibodies.

The natural history of urticarial vasculitis is difficult to predict. Some cases, particularly those with normal complement levels during attacks, are self-limited and require little therapy. Other cases, especially HUVS, may cause life-threatening involvement of the lungs or other organs, and require periods of intensive immunosuppression. The rarity of HUVS means that there exists little consensus regarding the optimal therapeutic strategy, and treatment decisions must be individualized according to each patient's clinical status. For hypocomplementemic urticarial vasculitis limited to the skin, antimalarial agents, dapsone, and low doses of glucocorticoids may be useful. Anecdotal experience suggests that tumor necrosis factor inhibition can be an effective strategy in patients with HUVS whose disease is refractory to conventional medications.[77]

Kawasaki's disease

The first case of the disease now known as Kawasaki's disease was described in 1939[78,79] and involved a 5-year-old girl who presented with high fever, sore throat, and rash and subsequently died from rupture of a coronary artery aneurysm. In 1961, Tomisaku Kawasaki evaluated a Japanese child with similar disease features, and also noted prominent cervical adenopathy. Over the next 6 years he performed a careful clinical and epidemiological study of the new disorder, and eventually reported the disease in the Japanese literature as "mucocutaneous lymph node syndrome" in 50 patients.[79,80] Formal diagnostic criteria for Kawasaki's disease have been developed.[81] The disease has a predilection for Asian children, but occurs in all races. Eighty percent of all cases occur in children younger than 5 years of age. The annual attack rate in Japan is approximately 80–90 cases per 100 000 children under the age of 5,[82] compared to roughly 10 per 100 000 among Caucasian children in the USA.[83]

In all of the patients described initially by Kawasaki, the symptoms resolved without sequelae within one month. In subsequent years, however, mortality from cardiac complications (usually coronary artery thrombosis) was reported. Cardiac complications of Kawasaki's disease result from a severe panvasculitis, leading to narrowing of the coronary lumina by the migration of myointimal cells from the media through the fragmented internal elastic lamina. Although catastrophic heart complications occur in only a small minority of patients, evidence suggests that the preponderance of patients with Kawasaki's disease have at least some cardiac involvement. Heart lesions can include myocarditis, pericarditis, aneurysmal dilatation and thrombosis of the coronary arteries, and myocardial infarction (Fig. 57.18). The tropism of the vascular inflammation for coronary arteries and its unusual propensity to cause aneurysm formation remain unexplained. The prompt institution of high-dose intravenous immunoglobulin (IVIg) may prevent this complication (see treatment, below).

Certain clinical features of Kawasaki's disease (fever, conjunctivitis, stomatitis, erythema multiforme-like rash, and the overwhelming predominance of the disease in young children) bear strong resemblance to a number of childhood exanthems. Moreover, the disease epidemiology of Japanese outbreaks is reminiscent of the classic spread of infectious agents. However,

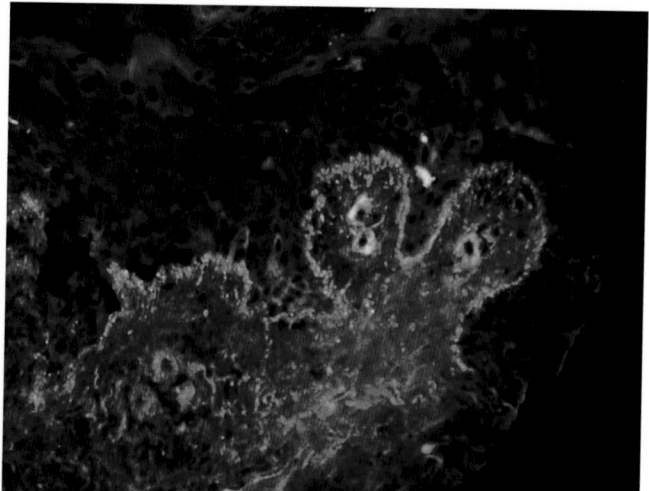

Fig. 57.17 Immunofluorescence study of a skin biopsy from a patient with hypocomplementemic urticarial vasculitis syndrome (HUVS). There is positive staining for IgG along the basement membrane and around small arteries in the dermal papillae.

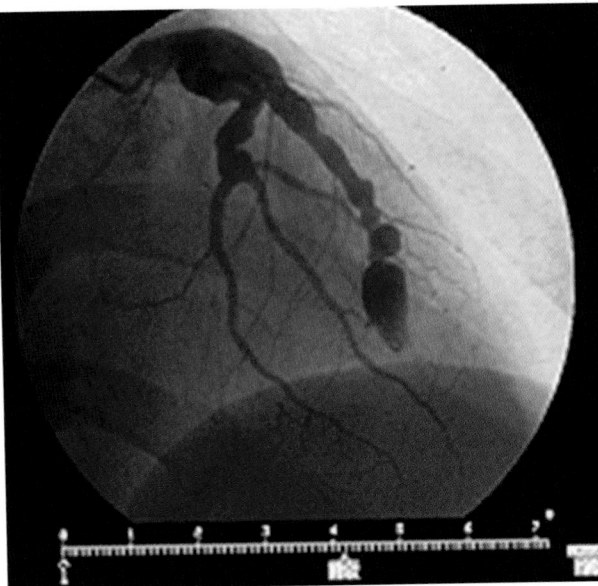

Fig. 57.18 Coronary angiogram in 38-year-old patient with history of Kawasaki's disease as a child. Febrile illness at the age of 4 led to coronary artery aneurysms, one of which thrombosed at the age of 38, leading to a myocardial infarction.

the profound disturbances of immunoregulation in Kawasaki's disease, e.g., the unusual degree of T-cell and monocyte activation, far exceed the abnormalities accompanying most other febrile childhood illnesses. Skewing of the T-cell receptor Vβ distribution has been reported by some investigators, but not confirmed by others. The degree of immune activation in Kawasaki's disease and the acute but generally self-limited nature of the illness have been discussed as supporting a role of superantigens in the disease pathogenesis (Chapter 6). Substantial attention has focused on toxic shock syndrome toxin-1 (TSST-1), an exotoxin produced by *S. aureus*, but the true relationship of this and other potential superantigens to the etiology of Kawasaki's disease remains unclear.

Before the availability of effective therapy, at least 20% of patients with Kawasaki's disease developed coronary aneurysms and 2% succumbed to the disease. To confirm earlier reports of efficacy of IVIg in Kawasaki's disease, seven pediatric centers in the USA enrolled 168 children with acute disease into a randomized trial. Half of the patients received IVIg 400 mg/kg/day on four consecutive days plus high-dose aspirin (100 mg/kg/day), and the other half received aspirin alone.[83] IVIg reduced the incidence of coronary aneurysms by 78% and relieved the symptoms of Kawasaki's disease with dramatic swiftness, establishing the combination of IVIg and aspirin as the standard for therapy of Kawasaki's disease. The mechanism of action of IVIg in this disorder remains unknown. The optimal dose of IVIg in Kawasaki's disease has not been defined: meta-analyzes suggest a lower rate of coronary aneurysms in patients who receive higher IVIg doses.

References

1. Jennette J, Falk R, Andrassy K, et al. Nomenclature of systemic vasculitides. Proposal of an international consensus conference. Arthritis Rheum 1994;37:187.
2. Hoffman G, Specks U. Antineutrophil cytoplasmic antibodies. Arthritis Rheum 1998;41:1521.
3. Xiao H, Heeringa P, Hu P, et al. Antineutrophil cytoplasmic autoantibodies specific for myeloperoxidase cause glomerulonephritis and vasculitis in mice. J Clin Invest 2002;110:955.
4. Huang D, Giscombe R, Zhou Y, Lefvert AK. Polymorphisms in CTLA-4 but not tumor necrosis factor-alpha or interleukin 1beta genes are associated with Wegener's granulomatosis. J Rheumatol 2000;27:397.
5. Stassen PM, Cohen-Tervaert JW, Lems SP, et al. HLA-DR4, DR13(6) and the ancestral haplotype A1B8DR3 are associated with ANCA-associated vasculitis and Wegener's granulomatosis. Rheumatology (Oxford) 2009;48(6):622–5.
6. von Vietinghoff S, Busjahn A, Schönemann C, et al. Major histocompatibility complex HLA region largely explains the genetic variance exercised on neutrophil membrane proteinase 3 expression. J Am Soc Nephrol 2006;17(11):3185–91.
7. Hogan SL, Satterly KK, Dooley MA, et al. Silica exposure in anti-neutrophil cytoplasmic autoantibody-associated glomerulonephritis and lupus nephritis. J Am Soc Nephrol 2001;12:134.
8. Mahr AD, Edberg JC, Stone JH, et al. for the WGGER Research Group. Alpha 1-antitrypsin deficiency-related alleles Z and S and the risk for Wegener's granulomatosis. Arthritis Rheum 2010;62:3760–7.
9. Mahr AD, Neogi T, Merkel PA. Epidemiology of Wegener's granulomatosis: Lessons from descriptive studies and analyses of genetic and environmental risk determinants. Clin Exp Rheumatol 2006;24(2 Suppl. 41):S82–S91.
10. Ludviksson BR, Sneller MC, Chua KS, et al. Active Wegener's granulomatosis is associated with HLA-DR+ CD4+ T cells exhibiting an unbalanced Th1-type T cell cytokine pattern: Reversal with IL-10. J Immunol 1998;160:3602.
11. Zhou Y, Huang D, Paris PL, et al. An analysis of CTLA-4 and proinflammatory cytokine genes in Wegener's granulomatosis. Arthritis Rheum 2004;50:2645.
12. Popa ER, Stegeman CA, Bos NA, et al. Differential B- and T-cell activation in Wegener's granulomatosis. J Allergy Clin Immunol 1999;103(5 Pt 1):885–94.
13. Stone JH, Merkel PA, Spiera R, et al. Rituximab compared with cyclophosphamide for remission induction in ANCA-associated vasculitis. N Engl J Med 2010;363:221–32.
14. Keogh KA, Ytterberg SR, Fervenza FC, et al. Rituximab for refractory Wegener's granulomatosis: report of a prospective, open-label trial. Am J Respir Crit Care Med 2006;173:180–7.
15. Tse WY, Abadeh S, Jefferis R, et al. Neutrophil FcgammaRIIIb allelic polymorphism in anti-neutrophil cytoplasmic antibody (ANCA)-positive systemic vasculitis. Clin Exp Immunol 2000;119:574.
16. Falk R, Terrell R, Charles L, et al. Anti-neutrophil cytoplasmic autoantibodies induce neutrophils to degranulate and produce oxygen radicals in vitro. Proc Natl Acad Sci U S A 1990;87:4115.
17. Lepse N, Abdulahad WH, Kallenberg CG. Heeringa P. Immune regulatory mechanisms in ANCA-associated vasculitides. Autoimmun Rev 2011;11(2):77.
18. Tse WY, Nash GB, Hewins P, et al. ANCA-induced neutrophil F-actin polymerization: implications for microvascular inflammation. Kidney Int 2005;67:130.
19. Merkel PA, Lo GH, Holbrook JT, et al. for the WGET Research Group. Incidence of venous thrombotic events among patients with Wegener's granulomatosis. Ann Intern Med 2005;142:620.
20. Godman G, Churg J. Wegener's granulomatosis: Pathology and review of the literature. Arch Pathol Lab Med 1954;58:533.
21. Hagen E, Daha M, Hermans J, et al. Diagnostic value of standardized assays for anti-neutrophil cytoplasmic antibodies in idiopathic systemic vasculitis. Kidney Int 1998;53:743.
22. Finkielman JD, Lee AS, Hummel AM, et al. WGET Research Group. ANCA are detectable in nearly all patients with active severe Wegener's granulomatosis. Am J Med 2007;120(7):643.e9–643.e14.
23. Finkielman JD, Merkel PA, Schroeder D, et al. WGET Research Group. Antiproteinase 3 antineutrophil cytoplasmic antibodies and disease activity in Wegener granulomatosis. Ann Intern Med 2007;147(9):611–9.
24. Wegener F. Ueber generalisierte, septische Gefässerkrankungen. Verh Dtsch Ges Pathol 1936;29:202.
25. Wegener F. Ueber eine eigenartige rhinogene Granulomatose mit besonderer Beteiligung des Arteriensystems und der Nieren. Beitr Pathol Anat Allg Pathol 1939;36:36.
26. Watts R, Carruthers D, Scott D. Epidemiology of systemic vasculitis: changing incidence or definition? Semin Arthritis Rheum 1995;25:28.
27. Hoffman G, Kerr G, Leavitt R, et al. Wegener's granulomatosis: An analysis of 158 patients. Ann Intern Med 1992;116:488.
28. The WGET Research Group . Etanercept in addition to standard therapy in patients with Wegener's granulomatosis. N Engl J Med 2005;352(4):351–61.
29. Davson J, Ball J, Platt R. The kidney in periarteritis nodosa. Q J Med 1948;17:175.
30. Savage C, Winearls C, Evans D, et al. Microscopic polyarteritis: presentation, pathology and prognosis. Q J Med 1985;56:467.
31. Guillevin L, Durand-Gasselin B, Cevallos R, et al. Microscopic polyangiitis. Arthritis Rheum 1999;42:421.
32. Churg J, Strauss L. Allergic granulomatosis, allergic angiitis, and periarteritis nodosa. Am J Pathol 1951;27:277.
33. Masi A, Hunder G, Lie J, et al. The American College of Rheumatology 1990 criteria for the classification of Churg–Strauss syndrome (allergic granulomatosis and angiitis). Arthritis Rheum 1990;33:1094.
34. Guillevin L, Cohen P, Gayraud M, et al. Churg–Strauss syndrome: Clinical study and long-term follow-up of 96 patients. Medicine 1999;78:26.
35. Specks U, Merkel PA, Hoffman GS, et al. for the RAVE-ITN Research Group. Design of the rituximab in ANCA-associated vasculitis (RAVE) trial. Open Arthritis J 2011;4:1–18.
36. Jones RB, Tervaert JW, Hauser T, et al. European Vasculitis Study Group. Rituximab versus cyclophosphamide in ANCA-associated renal vasculitis. N Engl J Med 2010;363(3):211–20.
37. Stone JH, Merkel PA, Spiera R, et al. and Specks U for the RAVE-ITN Research Group. Rituximab compared with cyclophosphamide for remission induction in ANCA-associated vasculitis. N Engl J Med 2010;363:221–32.

38. Stone JH, Merkel PA, Spiera R, et al. and Specks U for the RAVE-ITN Research Group. Long-term results of the RAVE Trial: Which disease subsets are at greatest risk for disease flare? Arthritis Rheum 2011;63(10):S946 [Abstract].

39. Tavazzi E, Ferrante P, Khalili K. Progressive multifocal leukoencephalopathy: an unexpected complication of modern therapeutic monoclonal antibody therapies. Clin Microbiol Infect 2011;17(12):1776–80.

40. Jayne D, Rasmussen N, Andrassy K, et al. A randomized trial of maintenance therapy for vasculitis associated with antineutrophil cytoplasmic autoantibodies. N Engl J Med 2003;349:36.

41. Wung PK, Stone JH. Therapeutics of Wegener's granulomatosis. Nature Clinical Rheum 2006;2:192.

42. de Groot K, Harper L, Jayne DR, et al. EUVAS (European Vasculitis Study Group). Pulse versus daily oral cyclophosphamide for induction of remission in antineutrophil cytoplasmic antibody-associated vasculitis: a randomized trial. Ann Intern Med 2009;150(10):670–80.

43. Tatsis E, Schnabel M, Gross W. Interferon-alpha treatment of four patients with the Churg–Strauss syndrome. Ann Intern Med 1998;129:370.

44. Kussmaul A, Maier R. Ueber eine bisher nicht beschriebene eigenthumliche arterienerkrankung (periarteritis nodosa), die mit morbus brightii und rapid fortschreitender allgemeiner muskellahmung einhergeht. Dtsch Arch Klin Med 1866;1:484.

45. Guillevin L, Mahr A, Callard P, et al. Hepatitis B virus-associated polyarteritis nodosa: clinical characteristics, outcome, and impact of treatment in 115 patients. Medicine 2005;84(5):313–22.

46. Stone JH. Polyarteritis nodosa. JAMA 2002;288(13):1632–9.

47. Levine SM, Hellmann DB, Stone JH. Gastrointestinal involvement in polyarteritis nodosa (1986–2000): presentation and outcomes in 24 patients. Am J Med 2002;112:386.

48. Lightfoot R, Michel B, Bloch D, et al. The American College of Rheumatology 1990 criteria for the classification of polyarteritis nodosa. Arthritis Rheum 1990;33:1088.

49. Guillevin L, Jarrousse B, Lok C. Longterm followup after treatment of polyarteritis nodosa and Churg–Strauss angiitis with comparison of steroids, plasma exchange and cyclophosphamide to steroids and plasma exchange. A prospective randomized trial of 71 patients. J Rheumatol 1991;18:567.

50. Wintrobe M, Buell M. Hyperproteinemia associated with multiple myeloma. Bull Johns Hopkins Hospital 1933;52:156.

51. Ramos-Casals M, Stone JH, Cid MC, Bosch X. The cryoglobulinaemias. Lancet 2012;379(9813):348–60.

52. Lunel F, Musset L, Cacoub P, et al. Cryoglobulinemia in chronic liver diseases: role of hepatitis C virus and liver damage. Gastroenterology 1994;106:1291.

53. Cacoub P, Saadoun D, Limal N, et al. PEGylated interferon alfa-2b and ribavirin treatment in patients with hepatitis C virus-related systemic vasculitis. Arthritis Rheum 2005;52:911.

54. Ferri C, Cacoub P, Mazzaro C, et al. Treatment with rituximab in patients with mixed cryoglobulinemia syndrome: Results of multicenter cohort study and review of the literature. Autoimmun Rev 2011;11(1):48–55.

55. Zeek P. Periarteritis nodosa: A critical review. Am J Clin Path 1952;221:777.

56. Calabrese L, Michel B, Bloch D, et al. The American College of Rheumatology 1990 criteria for the classification of hypersensitivity vasculitis. Arthritis Rheum 1990;33:1108.

57. Stone JH, Nousari HC. "Essential" cutaneous vasculitis: What every rheumatologist should know about vasculitis of the skin. Curr Opin Rheumatol 2001;13:23–34.

58. Gairdner D. The Schönlein–Henoch syndrome (anaphylactoid purpura). Q J Med 1948;17:95.

59. Saulsbury FT. Henoch-Schönlein purpura. Curr Opin Rheumatol 2010;22(5):598–602.

60. Kiryluk K, Moldoveanu Z, Sanders JT, et al. Aberrant glycosylation of IgA1 is inherited in both pediatric IgA nephropathy and Henoch-Schönlein purpura nephritis. Kidney Int 2011;80(1):79–87.

61. Mills J, Michel B, Bloch D, et al. The American College of Rheumatology 1990 criteria for classification of Henoch–Schonlein purpura. Arthritis Rheum 1990;33:1114.

62. Behçet H. Ueber rezidivierende Aphthose, durch ein Virus verursachte Gerschwure am Mund, am Auge und der Genitalie. Dermatol Wochenschr 1937;105:1552.

63. Yazici Y, Yurdakul S, Yazici H. Behçet's syndrome. Curr Rheumatol Rep 2010;12(6):429–35.

64. Arida A, Fragiadaki K, Giavri E, Sfikakis PP. Anti-TNF agents for Behçet's disease: analysis of published data on 369 patients. Semin Arthritis Rheum 2011;41(1):61–70.

65. Saadoun D, Wechsler B, Terrada C, et al. Azathioprine in severe uveitis of Behçet's disease. Arthritis Care Res (Hoboken) 2010;62(12):1733–8.

66. Buerger L. Thromboangiitis obliterans: a study of the vascular lesions leading to presenile spontaneous gangrene. Am J Med Sci 1908;136:567.

67. Piazza G, Creager MA. Thromboangiitis obliterans. Circulation 2010;121(16):1858–61.

68. Cogan DG. Corneoscleral lesions in periarteritis nodosa and Wegener's granulomatosis. Trans Am Ophthalmol Soc 1955;53:321–42.

69. Gluth MB, Baratz KH, Matteson EL, Driscoll CL. Cogan syndrome: a retrospective review of 60 patients throughout a half century. Mayo Clin Proc 2006;81(4):483–8.

70. Hajj-Ali RA, Singhal AB, Benseler S, et al. Primary angiitis of the CNS. Lancet Neurol 2011;10(6):561–72.

71. Salvarani C, Brown Jr RD, Calamia KT, et al. Primary central nervous system vasculitis: analysis of 101 patients. Ann Neurol 2007;62(5):442–51.

72. Calabrese L, Gragg L, Furlan A. Benign angiopathy: A distinct subset of angiographically define primary angiitis of the central nervous system. J Rheumatol 1993;20:2046.

73. Zuccoli G, Pipitone N, Haldipur A, et al. Imaging findings in primary central nervous system vasculitis. Clin Exp Rheumatol 2011;29(1 Suppl. 64):S104–9.

74. Calabrese LH, Dodick DW, Schwedt TJ, Singhal AB. Narrative review: reversible cerebral vasoconstriction syndromes. Ann Intern Med 2007;146(1):34–44.

75. McDuffie F, Sams Jr W, Maldonado J, et al. Hypocomplementemia with cutaneous vasculitis and arthritis. Mayo Clin Proc 1973;48:430.

76. Wisnieski J, Baer A, Christensen J, et al. Hypocomplementemic urticarial vasculitis syndrome: Clinical and serological findings in 18 patients. Medicine 1995;74:24.

77. Kroshinsky D, Stone JH, Nazarian RM. Case records of the Massachusetts General Hospital. Case 22-2011. A 79-year-old man with a rash, arthritis, and ocular erythema. N Engl J Med 2011;365(3):252–62.

78. Spector S. Scarlet fever, periarteritis nodosa, aneurysm of the coronary artery with spontaneous rupture, hemopericardium. Arch Pediat 1939;25:319.

79. Kawasaki T. Acute febrile mucocutaneous syndrome with lymphoid involvement with specific desquamation of the fingers and toes in children. Jpn J Allerg 1967;178. [in Japanese].

80. Kawasaki T, Kosaki F, Okawa S, et al. A new infantile acute febrile mucocutaneous lymph node syndrome (MLNS) prevailing in Japan. Pediatrics 1974;54:271.

81. Centers for Disease Control. Kawasaki disease. MMWR 1980;29:61.

82. Yanagawa H, Yashiro M, Nakamura Y, et al. Epidemiologic pictures of Kawasaki disease in Japan: from the nationwide incidence survey in 1991 and 1992. Pediatrics 1995;95:475.

83. Newburger J, Takahashi M, Burns J, et al. The treatment of Kawasaki syndrome with intravenous gamma globulin. N Engl J Med 1986;315:341.

Cornelia M.
Weyand, Jörg
J. Goronzy

Large-vessel vasculitides

Whereas most tissues have compensatory mechanisms that allow them to sustain the damaging effects of acute and chronic inflammation, medium and large arteries are organs without redundancy and limited regenerative capacity. Life is unsustainable unless the major arteries have uncompromised function. Accordingly, inflammatory damage to such arterial vessels leads to severe clinical consequences, immediately posing a threat for the loss of vital organ function. When affected by inflammation, the aorta and its branches have two possible response patterns: inflammatory destruction of the vessel wall leads to dilatation, aneurysm formation, and, infrequently, dissection and hemorrhage; or the inflammation initiates an injury response that results in luminal occlusion, disruption of blood supply, and ischemic damage of dependent organ structures.

In contrast to other vasculopathies, especially those related to atherosclerosis, vasculitides of the larger blood vessels are almost always associated with a syndrome of intense systemic inflammation.[1] Recent evidence has challenged the traditional view that systemic inflammation represents a spillover of inflammatory mediators from the vasculitic lesions. Instead, systemic activation of the innate immune system appears to be a pinnacle event that initiates the processes leading to vessel wall inflammation. The coincidence of malaise, fever, wasting, and myalgias with signs of ischemia due to vascular failure remains a critical clue for the physician when diagnosing and treating large-vessel vasculitis.

The two major forms of large-vessel vasculitis are giant-cell arteritis (GCA) and Takayasu arteritis (TA). In addition, aortitis can infrequently be seen in other diseases, such as infections, connective tissue diseases, sarcoidosis, and inflammatory bowel disease; and, occasionally, is diagnosed as an idiopathic syndrome. Polymyalgia rheumatica (PMR) is a condition closely related to GCA; it occurs in the same patient population and often precedes or follows the clinical diagnosis of GCA.[2] Patients with PMR do not have typical vascular lesions; consequently PMR is not classified as a vasculitis. However, PMR patients do have a systemic inflammatory syndrome indistinguishable from GCA and about 10% of PMR patients eventually progress to full-blown vasculitis. Similarities in the vascular lesions of GCA and TA have been interpreted as revealing parallels in the immunopathogenesis of these vasculitides. However, a comparative analysis of disease-relevant cells, molecular mediators and signalling abnormalities in GCA and TA is currently not available. Whether the systemic inflammatory reactions accompanying GCA, TA, and PMR have disease-specific elements remains unanswered, but opens the possibility of developing biomarkers that are urgently needed for the monitoring of affected patients. Excellent progress has been made in unraveling the pathogenesis of GCA, and this will inevitably lead to improvements in diagnosis, long-term management, and broadening of the therapeutic armamentarium.

Epidemiology

GCA may be a very old disease, as suggested by historic evidence that more than 1000 years ago removal of the temporal artery was recommended by a physician in Baghdad. In 1932, Horton and colleagues at the Mayo Clinic in Minnesota recognized that GCA was an inflammatory vasculopathy when they found dense inflammation in the temporal arteries of two systemically ill patients with severe headaches. The first reports of TA, or "pulseless disease," in young women surfaced in Japan in the nineteenth century. The syndrome was named after Dr. Takayasu, an ophthalmologist who in 1905 described peculiar optic fundus abnormalities caused by ischemia-driven collateral formation.

The strongest risk factor for GCA, TA, and PMR is age.[3,4] GCA and PMR are essentially absent in individuals younger than 50 years of age, and their incidence climbs continuously during the seventh and eighth decades of life. TA is almost exclusively diagnosed in individuals younger than 40 years of age, with peak incidence during the second and third decades of life. All three syndromes affect women much more often than men, with a 2:1 ratio in PMR and GCA and a 9:1 ratio in TA.[3,4]

Marked geographic variations in the incidence and prevalence of GCA, TA, and PMR have given rise to speculations about environmental exposures as key factors in disease pathogenesis. GCA is the most frequent vasculitis in the Western world, with yearly incidence rates reaching 10–20 cases per 100 000 persons over 50 years of age.[3] In general, PMR is diagnosed three- to fourfold more frequently, with a prevalence of up to 1 case per 133 individuals older than 50.[2] Iceland, Norway, Sweden, and Denmark are high-risk areas; also, higher incidence rates are maintained in Scandinavian immigrant populations in the USA. The risk is significantly lower in Hispanics and African-Americans. Although TA can afflict all races, a predilection exists for individuals of Asian, and Central and South American origins. Japan, Thailand, India, Turkey, and nations in Central and South America are considered high-incidence regions. TA is a rare disease with an annual incidence of 1–2 cases/million. The typical patient is a female in her 20s to 30s. In middle-aged men and women, it can be challenging to differentiate TA from rapidly progressing atherosclerotic disease, especially as both disease processes may coexist.[5]

Etiology and pathogenesis

Medium- and large-vessel vasculitides are caused by dysregulated immune responses.[1,6,7] Studies from the last decade have revealed that vasculitis involves a combination of multiple effector mechanisms mediated by both the innate and adaptive arms of the immune system. Inflammation is a critical host-defense response protecting against infection and tissue injury, but it invariably triggers collateral damage to the very tissue site in which it intends to destroy microbes and remove the injured cells. If initiated in the absence of an instigator or if the triggering stimulus persists, inflammation eventually becomes the cause of disease as tissue damage accumulates and, in the case of vasculitis, leaves the host with malfunctional arteries.

The similarities in tissue tropisms and histologic lesions of GCA and TA suggest overlapping disease pathways and many aspects of immune pathogenesis may be transferrable from one syndrome to the other. Marked progress has been made in understanding early and late events in GCA with studies in human artery-severe combined immunodeficiency (SCID) mice yielding valuable insights. The etiopathogenesis of PMR is less well understood, but experimental evidence suggests that it represents a forme fruste of GCA in which inflammatory attack to the vessel wall remains below a threshold, and standard histology describes noninflamed arteries.

The human artery-SCID model of vasculitis

The prototypic components of GCA/TA pathogenesis are chronically persistent inflammatory infiltrates settled within vascular walls that have three distinct layers and well-developed elastic membranes. To overcome limitations encountered in animal models of vasculitis, which cannot mimic the vessel size, vessel wall structure, or aging component of the host, a novel experimental model for GCA was established by implanting GCA-affected or normal human arteries into immunodeficient mice. Within 1 week, the human arteries are engrafted and supplied with blood through their vasa vasorum trees.[8] Chimeras can then be treated with cell-depleting antibodies, anti-cytokine reagents, or with adoptive transfer of immuno-inflammatory cells. This model has been extremely helpful in deciphering which cells and mediators sustain vasculitis. Equally importantly, the model has allowed for vasculitis induction in normal arteries, thereby illustrating the early pathogenic steps that precede establishment of granulomatous mural lesions.[9]

Early steps in vasculitis

KEY CONCEPTS

- Medium and large human arteries have multiple wall layers and a wall structure substantial enough to be the target of transmural inflammation.

- Vasculitis causes the rapid and concentric growth of hyperplastic intima, leading to luminal occlusion and ischemia of dependent tissues. Intramural inflammation of the aorta can result in wall damage followed by aneurysm formation and rupture.

- Due to the vital function and nonregenerative nature of large human arteries, the threshold for the induction and persistence of innate and adaptive immune responses in the wall structures of such arteries must be explicitly high.

- Inflammatory infiltrates typical for granulomatous vasculitis enter the vessel from the "back door," the adventitia, and not from the lumen.

- Besides their critical role in securing blood flow, medium and large blood vessels also possess immunoregulatory functions mediated by dendritic cells indigenous to the vascular wall. Dendritic cells in each vascular territory express a distinctive pattern of Toll-like receptors, giving each vessel its own immunological identity.

Recognition that normal human arteries of the medium and large categories harbor immunocompetent cells and participate in immunosurveillance has fundamentally changed the concepts of how arteries and the immune system interact. Three-layered human arteries possess a population of dendritic cells that have been named vascular dendritic cells (vasDC).[10] Such vasDC are strategically positioned at the media–adventitia border and have been implicated in initiating wall inflammation.[11] In contrast to other DC-containing tissues, normal human arteries do not stimulate T cells when implanted into SCID mice. This immunologic quiescence, despite being equipped with DC networks, has given rise to the hypothesis that the primary function of vascular DCs lies in maintaining a very high threshold for induction and persistence of adaptive immune responses. A principal role for vascular DCs in functioning as tolerance inducers fits well with the host's need to avoid inflammatory damage in critical and nonregenerative organs such as arteries.

The tolerant state of vascular DCs can, however, be broken if the artery is exposed to danger signals, such as microbial-derived products (Fig. 58.1). Pathogen-associated molecular patterns (PAMPs) and danger-associated molecular patterns (DAMPs) are rapidly detected by human arteries, in principle by activating Toll-like receptors (TLR) expressed on vascular DCs.[12] Injection of lipopolysaccharide, a moiety conserved across Gram-negative bacteria, into human artery-SCID chimeras, leads to robust activation of the vasDCs residing in the human arteries and is sufficient to initiate wall inflammation[13] Specifically, vasDC triggering causes CD4 T-cells recruitment to the vessel, orchestrates T-cell migration toward the adventitia–media junction, and instigates T-cell in situ activation and clonal expansion. Arteries harvested from patients with PMR, despite having no sign of inflammation, have pre-activated DCs and do not require exposure to lipopolysaccharide. Spontaneously, they recruit and activate T cells from co-implanted GCA arteries.[9] Thus, vasDC stimulation is a very early step in the initiation of vasculitis, occurring long before the chronic phase of wall inflammation.

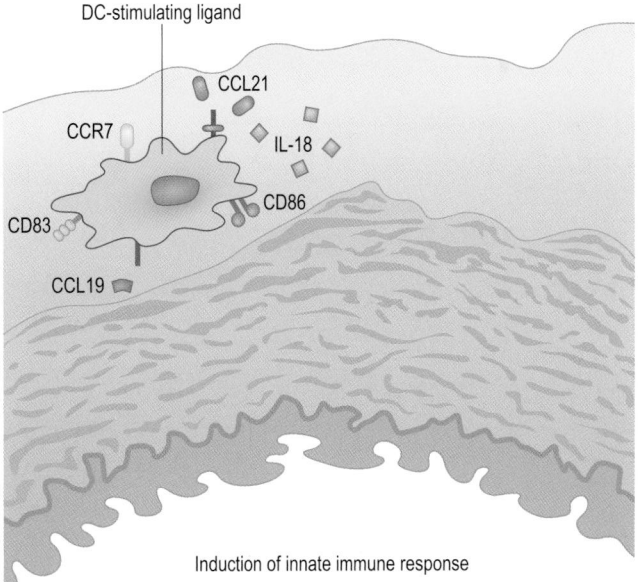

Fig. 58.1 Pathogenic pathways in giant-cell arteritis (GCA). Under physiologic conditions, dendritic cells (DCs) in the adventitia are immature and resting. In polymyalgia rheumatica and GCA, adventitial DCs sense danger signals and undergo activation with the induction of co-stimulatory ligands and chemokines. Under experimental conditions, adventitial DCs can be triggered with pathogen-associated molecular patterns that interact with Toll-like receptors.

Remarkably, the immune sensing function of human arteries is a vessel-specific feature.[13] In a study of six different human arteries (arteria temporalis, a. mesenterica, a. iliaca, a. carotis, a. subclavia and aorta) each vascular territory expressed a distinctive pattern of danger-recognizing Toll-like receptors; supporting the concept that each artery has an immunological identity. Given the checkpoint function of vasDC in vasculitis these findings provide a biologic basis for selective susceptibility of vascular regions to vasculitis.

The potential of pathogen-derived molecules to start inflammatory responses in arterial tissues has rekindled old discussions on whether vasculitis is elicited by infection. In this context it is important to mention that recurring reports of finding infectious organisms in inflamed temporal arteries from GCA patients have not been confirmed in more comprehensive studies. As stimulation of adventitial vasDCs by microbial products is sufficient to induce vascular inflammation, the presence of the organism in the affected artery is obviously not necessary, but infections located elsewhere in the patient may still have a facilitating role.

Adaptive immune responses in giant-cell arteritis

Chronic inflammatory infiltrates occupying all layers of the affected artery are comprised of CD4 T cells, a few CD8 T cells, and macrophages, all arranged in granulomas. Multinucleated giant cells are found in about 50% of patients and are often localized close to the intima–media border adjacent to the lamina elastica interna. Fragmentation of that elastic membrane is a hallmark of GCA. The CD4 T-cell composition depends on the disease stage. In a recent study of repeated temporal artery biopsies harvested before and after steroid treatment, early arteritis was characterized by the combination of IL-17-producing Th17 cells and IFN-γ-producing Th1 cells (Fig. 58.2).[14] Lesions in

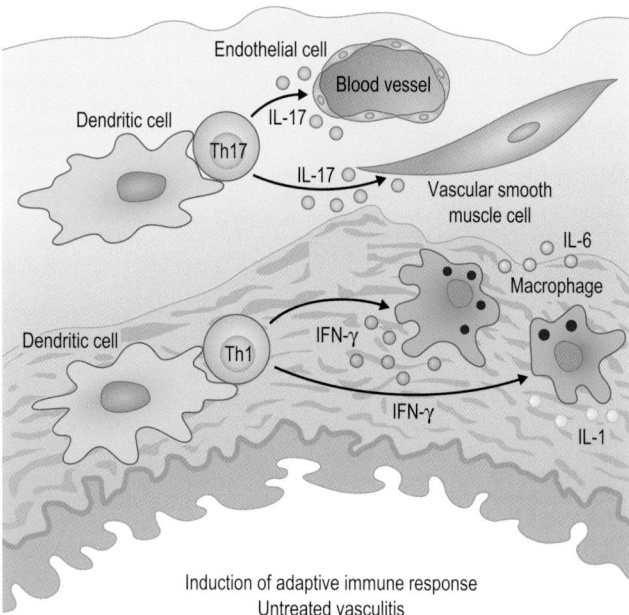

Fig. 58.2 Pathogenic pathways in giant-cell arteritis (GCA). In untreated arteritis, CD4 T cells are recruited to the adventitia by activated dendritic cells and undergo *in situ* activation. Release of IL-1β, -6, and -23 promotes the differentiation of IL-17-producing Th17 cells. IL-17 exerts its pro-inflammatory actions by regulating endothelial cells, vascular smooth muscle cells and fibroblasts. Other CD4 cells committed to the Th1 lineage differentiate when stimulated with IL-12 and secret IFN-γ. The main effect of IFN-γ lies in the stimulation of macrophages.

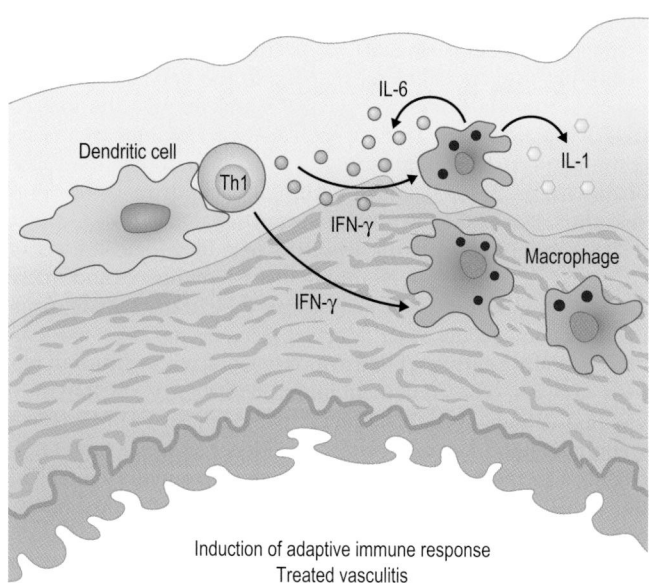

Fig. 58.3 Pathogenic pathways in giant-cell arteritis (GCA). In patients that have been treated with corticosteroids Th17 cells are rapidly suppressed whereas Th1 cells are resistant to this therapy. IFN-γ-releasing Th1 cells persist and maintain arteritis.

treated patients persisted and were maintained almost exclusively by IFN-γ-secreting T cells (Fig. 58.3). Tissue levels of IFN-γ correlate closely with patterns of clinical manifestations.[15] For example, tissue IFN-γ levels predict the density of neocapillaries that sustain the growth of the lumen occlusive neointima.[16] In TA, direct cytotoxic function of CD8 T cells, natural killer cells, and γδ T cells has been implicated in local tissue injury.[17]

CD4 T cells continue to receive instructive signals from DCs even in chronically established disease since DC depletion effectively disrupts granulomatous inflammation.[9] In mature vasculitic lesions, DCs are the sole producers of CCL19 and CCL21, chemokines implicated in T-cell recruitment. Also, they express CD86 and thus provide necessary co-stimulatory signals to maintain T-cell responses.[11] The nature of the initial DC activating signal has important consequences for the evolving inflammation. Triggering with Toll-like receptor 4 ligands leads to the formation of panarteritis, whereas stimulation with Toll-like receptor 5 ligands results in periarteritis.[18]

Naturally, the question of whether a unique antigen exists that drives adaptive immune responses in GCA has been raised. Studies with T-cell lines established from inflamed temporal arteries have suggested that the T-cell populations are nonrandom and clonally selected. Identical CD4 T cells dominating the inflammatory infiltrate in the right and left temporal arteries of patients with bilateral biopsies have added weight to these findings.[19] The spectrum of possible antigens includes microbes, products of injured or stressed cells, and altered self. An alternative hypothesis puts emphasis on the uniqueness of the tissue compartment and the dysfunction of T-cell homeostasis and T-cell regulation in the aged host, and considers ordinary self-antigens as sufficient to drive these misplaced immune responses.[1,12]

Gene expression profiling of temporal artery lesions has discovered a role for the NOTCH-NOTCH ligand pathway in initiating and sustaining vasculitis.[20] Arteritis-affected temporal arteries had abundant expression of the NOTCH receptor and its ligands, Jagged1 and Delta1. Disrupting the translocation of NOTCH into the nucleus through γ-secretase inhibitors had strong anti-vasculitic effects in human artery-SCID chimeras.

Immune-mediated tissue injury and the artery's contribution to vascular failure

Accumulated data support the premise that a major part of the tissue injury in the arterial wall is actually mediated by macrophages (Fig. 58.4).[1] Remarkably, wall-invading macrophages commit to selected pathways of maturation according to their placement in the wall structure.[21] Macrophages positioned in the adventitia mainly produce proinflammatory monokines, such as interleukin-6 (IL-6) and IL-1 (Fig. 58.2). Their major function may lie in supporting on-going T-cell responses. Intimal macrophages express nitric oxide synthase and peroxynitrite generation has been associated with endothelial dysfunction.[22] Macrophages captured in the medial smooth-muscle cell layer have a portfolio of tissue-damaging functions (Fig. 58.3).[23,24] They release metalloproteinases, likely contributing to digestion of the elastic structures. They are potent in secreting reactive oxygen species, facilitating oxidative damage to smooth-muscle cells and endothelial cells. Most importantly, they are the source for platelet-derived growth factor and vascular endothelial growth factor,[16,25] supporting wall-resident cells in their injury response pattern. Myofibroblasts migrate towards the intima, proliferate, and release matrix proteins. The unfortunate consequence is intimal hyperplasia, the essential mechanism underlying luminal stenosis and vascular failure. Notably, in both GCA and TA, destruction of the arterial wall with subsequent rupture and hemorrhage is the exception. Instead, a fast, concentric, and almost complete intimal hyperproliferation leads to obstruction of the lumen and ischemic damage of dependent organs. Not all GCA patients develop vascular stenosis. In some patients mural inflammation does not lead to intimal hyperplasia and the lumen is maintained. Patients with nonobstructive vasculitis have a distinct clinical presentation; vascular malfunction is not noticeable but they have intense systemic inflammation, coming to medical attention with fever-of-unknown-origin.

Failure of the inflamed arteries, presenting as lumen obstruction, would not be possible without the active contribution of the arterial wall residents. Proliferating myofibroblasts, rather than immune cells, build the scaffold of the lumen-obstructive neotissue.[25] Also, neoangiogenesis effectively supports the artery's response-to-injury reaction, supplying oxygen and nutrients to the thickening wall.[16] In essence, the immune system emerges as an instructor to a maladaptive response of the vessel itself. The critical participation of vascular components may provide an explanation for the stringent tissue tropism of large-vessel vasculitides, which selectively target certain vascular territories. Alternatively, the vessel-specific distribution of vasDC introduces a unappreciated level of vascular diversity.[13] As vasDc have checkpoint function in vasculitis, their specification in each vascular territory will determine whether an artery is susceptible to large-vessel arteritis.

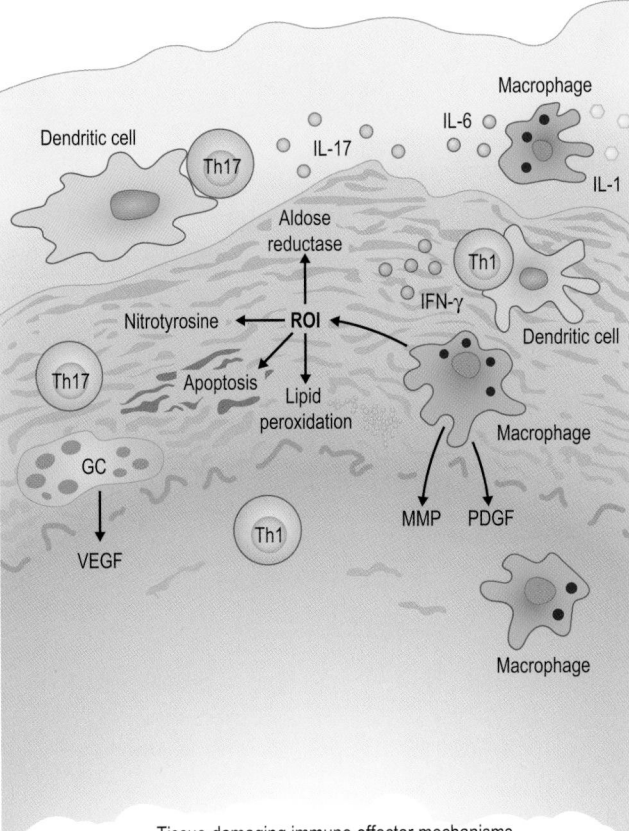

Fig. 58.4 Pathogenic pathways in giant-cell arteritis (GCA). Fully developed GCA is a panarteritis with transmural T-cell and macrophage infiltrates. Macrophages in different wall layers commit to distinct damage pathways involving production of proinflammatory cytokines, reactive oxygen intermediates (ROI), metalloproteinases, or growth factors. Multinucleated giant cells also provide growth and angiogenic factors that promote intimal hyperplasia and luminal occlusion.

Clinical features in Giant-Cell Arteritis

● CLINICAL PEARLS

Clinical and epidemiologic clues in giant-cell arteritis

- Patient older than 50 years of age
- Female
- Northern European heritage
- Laboratory findings of a highly activated acute-phase response
- Insidious onset of nonspecific symptoms (weight loss, night sweats, malaise, fever)
- Ischemia of ocular structures, cranial muscles, scalp, or upper extremities

Clinical manifestations of GCA reflect the combination of a systemic inflammatory syndrome with vascular insufficiency (Table 58.1).[2,26] Depending on the preferred target of vascular inflammation, patients fall into the category of either cranial GCA or large-vessel GCA. In addition, there exists another subpopulation of patients in whom the clinical consequences of arterial inflammation are minimal, and they come to clinical attention with a wasting syndrome.

In cranial GCA, symptoms result from vascular stenosis of the neck and head arteries, most prominently in the branches of the external carotid artery. Arteritis of the scalp arteries leads to the typical presentations of headaches and scalp tenderness. Patients report difficulties with wearing glasses or combing their hair. The headaches are often intense and unresponsive to standard analgesics. Headaches are a nonspecific clinical symptom, yet in an elderly individual with other findings of an inflammatory syndrome, physicians need to rule out GCA. Insufficient blood flow to the masseter muscles and the tongue causes jaw

Table 58.1 Clinical features of giant-cell arteritis (GCA), polymyalgia rheumatica (PMR), and Takayasu arteritis (TA)

Organ system	Clinical features	Frequencies		
		GCA	PMR	TA
Vascular	Headaches	***		*
	Limb claudication	*		***
	Scalp tenderness	**		
	Jaw claudication	**		
	Absent or asymmetric pulses	*		***
	Asymmetric blood pressure readings	*		***
	Bruit	*		***
	Tongue claudication	*		
	Tissue gangrene	*		
	Abdominal angina			*
	Cough (dry, nonproductive)	*		*
Constitutional	Malaise	**	**	***
	Failure-to-thrive	*	**	*
	Weight loss	**	**	**
	Fever	*	*	*
Central nervous system	Ocular symptoms	**		*
	Stroke/transient ischemic attack	*		*
	Ischemia of the central nervous system	*		*
Peripheral nervous system	Peripheral neuropathy	*		
Cardiac	Aortic dilatation and regurgitation	*		*
	Myocardial infarction	*		*
	Congestive heart failure			*
Musculoskeletal	Proximal stiffness/ muscle pain	**	***	
	Synovitis of peripheral joints		*	
Others	Intense acute-phase response	***	***	***
	Normochromic or hypochromic anemia	**	*	**

Key: *** = high frequency (>70%); ** = moderate frequency (20–70%); * = low frequency (<20%).

Chronic nonproductive cough can be related to arteritis in branches of the bronchial arteries. If the vertebral and basilar arteries develop vasculitic stenosis, ischemia of the central nervous system manifests with transient ischemic attacks or frank stroke.

In patients with large-vessel GCA, cranial symptoms may be minimal, and temporal artery biopsy can be negative.[27] Instead, vascular insufficiency is focused on the upper-extremity vessels and the aorta. In rare cases, lower extremities are affected. Typically, patients have asymmetric blood pressure readings or totally lose upper-extremity blood pressures and pulses. The underlying lesions are occlusions in the distal subclavian arteries, often extending into the axillary sections (Fig. 58.5). Patients with subclavian GCA are on average about 10 years

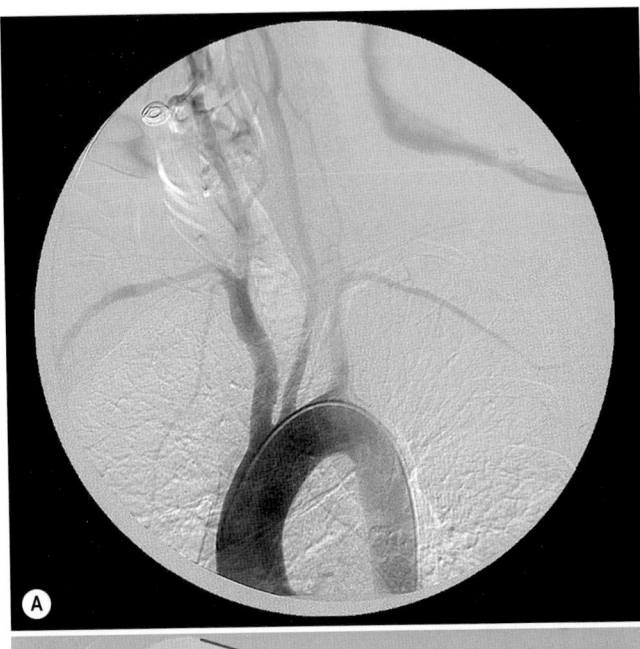

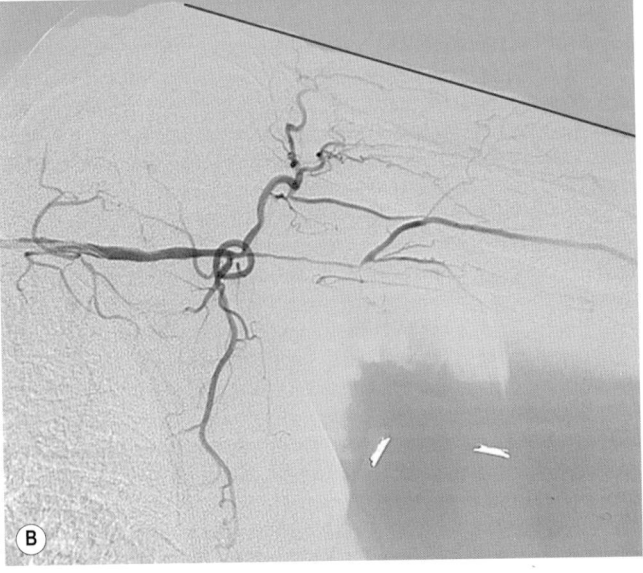

Fig. 58.5 Involvement of the subclavian axillary artery in giant-cell arteritis. Angiography of the aortic arch and its primary branches shows luminal irregularities in both distal subclavian arteries (A). The digital subtraction angiogram focuses on the left subclavian axillary junction and demonstrates a high-degree, long-segment stenosis that is smooth-walled and tapered (B). Newly formed collateral vessels branching off the distal subclavian artery supply blood to the arm.

or tongue claudication, elicited by prolonged chewing and talking. Although this type of claudication is present in less than 30% of patients, it is clinically helpful as it rarely occurs outside GCA. Similarly, painful dysphagia can be a useful clinical clue.

The orbita and the optic nerve are strictly dependent on blood supply from the external carotid system, particularly the ophthalmic artery. GCA in branches of the ophthalmic artery, specifically the posterior ciliary arteries, leads to anterior ischemic optic neuropathy, presenting as sudden and painless vision loss. Typically patients lose vision in the early-morning hours or wake up blind. Involvement of one eye may be followed by visual loss in the partner eye if the disease is not diagnosed and treated promptly. Besides anterior optic neuropathy, GCA can cause a number of ischemic complications in the orbits and along the visual axis, which may present as diplopia or partial vision loss. If recognized and treated immediately, vasculitis-associated sight loss is preventable, thus making GCA an ophthalmologic emergency.

younger at disease onset than are those with dominant cranial manifestations. Diagnosis of large-vessel GCA can be delayed as symptoms are nonspecific and the systemic inflammatory component is less pronounced. Ischemic pain in the hands when using the arms is often combined with coolness and bluish discoloration. Gangrene of the fingertips is rare. Disability can be significant, as patients have difficulties with activities of daily living. With stenotic lesions of the subclavian arteries, blood pressure readings can be unreliable or totally absent, requiring alternative strategies for blood pressure monitoring. Although carotid involvement is considered infrequent, it can be challenging to distinguish atherosclerotic and vasculitic disease. Patients with carotid GCA are at high risk for cerebral ischemic events. Aortic involvement preferentially targets the thoracic aorta and infrequently the abdominal aorta (Fig. 58.6). Dilation of the aortic root can lead to aortic insufficiency. Aortic aneurysms are often clinically silent. The diagnosis may first be made from tissue obtained surgically during aortic aneurysm repair. In extreme cases, the aortic wall ruptures.

The response pattern of arteries to inflammation may not include intimal hyperplasia, thus eluding luminal compromise and vascular failure. In such patients, the systemic inflammatory component dominates the clinical presentation. Fever, fatigue, malaise, weight loss, and depression are often intense enough to prompt a workup for a malignancy. GCA needs to be on the list of differential diagnosis in all cases of fever-of-unknown-origin, particularly in elderly individuals. Whereas patients with cranial GCA have abnormally thick and tender temporal arteries exhibiting nodularity and loss of pulses, clinical findings in nonstenosing GCA can be bland and unremarkable. Temporal artery biopsy should be pursued even if clinical examination does not suggest the diagnosis.

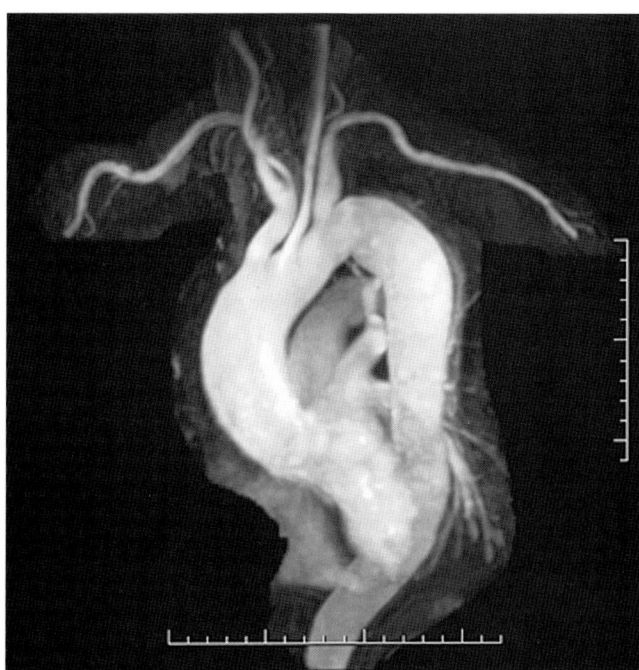

Fig. 58.6 Aortic aneurysm in giant-cell arteritis. A three-dimensional reconstruction of a magnetic resonance angiography demonstrating wall irregularities and ectasia throughout the thoracic aorta of a 63-year-old female with biopsy-proven giant-cell arteritis is shown. The ascending aorta appears most affected. The origins of the subclavian and innominate arteries are dilated, indicating inflammatory damage of the wall. Mild irregularities of the subclavian apex are seen, without evidence for stenosis.

Clinical features in Polymyalgia Rheumatica

PMR is diagnosed in patients presenting with pronounced stiffness and pain in the shoulder and pelvic girdle muscles (Table 58.1).[2] Laboratory testing shows a systemic inflammatory syndrome; arterial biopsy is negative for arteritis. It is estimated that about 10% of PMR patients who have no signs of vascular inflammation will eventually develop full-blown vasculitis. Notably, PMR often occurs in patients with GCA and is present in about 40% of GCA patients at disease onset. Tapering of immunosuppressive therapy in GCA is frequently associated with new or remittent PMR symptoms.[26] Complaints are focused on muscle pain and stiffness, classically affecting the neck, the shoulder girdle, and the pelvic girdle. Muscles of the torso may be involved. Peripheral arms and legs are spared. Muscle pain is most intense in the early morning and improves during the day. Inability to get out of bed, stand up from a chair, or get off the toilet seat should alert the physician to consider PMR. Some patients with PMR have synovitis or bursitis in their shoulder and hip joints,[2,28] making them difficult to distinguish from those with seronegative rheumatoid arthritis. No diagnostic procedure is available that allows for the diagnosis of PMR; the syndrome remains an exclusion diagnosis in cases of myalgia combined with laboratory signs of systemic inflammation. On clinical examination, passive motion of shoulder and hip joints is maintained, but active motion is restricted due to pain. Muscle strength is often normal. Careful evaluation of the temporal arteries is warranted to avoid missing fully developed GCA.

Clinical features in Takayasu Arteritis

The clinical manifestations of TA are diverse and depend on the affected vascular territory (Tables 58.1 and 58.2).[29,30] Initial symptoms are usually nonspecific, such as fever, cough, malaise, weight loss, night sweats, myalgias, and arthralgias. Signs of vascular deficiency

Table 58.2 Takayasu arteritis: relationship between clinical symptoms and affected vascular territories

Vascular bed involvement	Approximate frequency (%)	Predominant clinical symptoms
Subclavian	90	Arm claudication, pulselessness
Common carotid	60	Visual defects, stroke, transient ischemic attack, syncope
Abdominal aorta	45	Claudication, hypertension, abdominal angina
Renal	35	Hypertension
Aortic arch/root	35	Aortic insufficiency, congestive heart failure
Vertebral	35	Dizziness, visual impairment
Celiac axis	20	Abdominal angina
Superior mesenteric	20	Abdominal angina
Iliac	20	Claudication
Pulmonary	10	Dyspnea, chest pain
Coronary	10	Myocardial infarction, angina

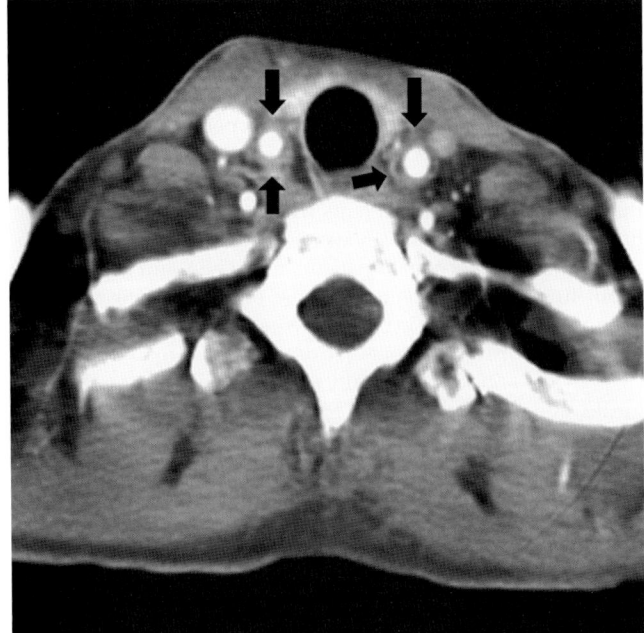

Fig. 58.7 Diagnosis of vascular involvement of Takayasu arteritis by computed tomography angiography. Axial images show marked thickening of the circumferential wall of both common carotid arteries (arrows). The vessel lumen is patent without evidence for hemodynamic stenosis. Lumen and wall of the vertebral arteries are normal.

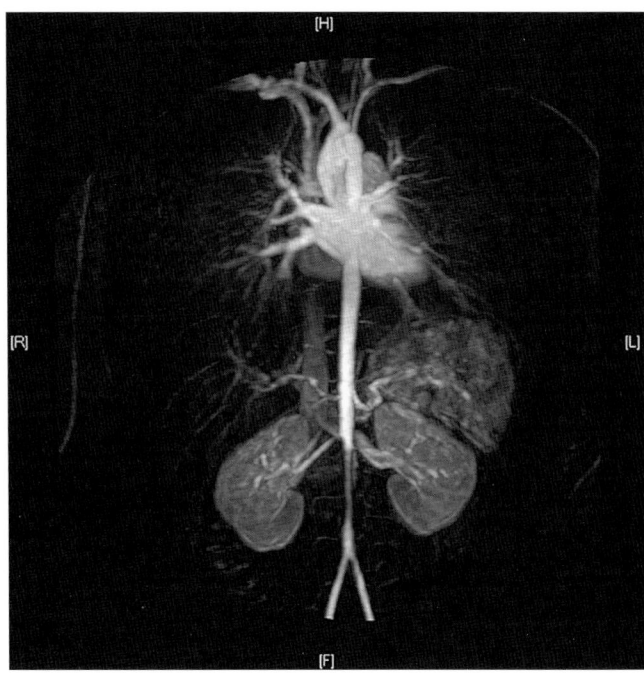

Fig. 58.8 Magnetic resonance angiography of Takayasu arteritis. The three-dimensional reconstruction shows normal caliber of the ascending and descending aorta in a 16-year-old female with Takayasu arteritis. The infrarenal abdominal aorta is narrowed diffusely over a 7-cm segment with the residual lumen measuring only 5 mm. There is mild narrowing of the common iliac arteries bilaterally, just distal to the aortic bifurcation.

develop later in the disease course and generally are ischemic in nature. Geographical variations in disease pattern have been reported, likely reflecting the interplay between host risk genes and dysfunctional immunity. In North American, Japanese, and Korean patients, the aortic arch and its primary cervical and upper extremity branches are preferentially targeted, giving rise to aortic insufficiency, cerebral ischemia, face and neck pain, ocular ischemia, and the typical presentation of "pulseless disease" (Fig. 58.7). In India, the abdominal aorta and renal arteries are more commonly affected, causing renovascular hypertension and the long-term risk of cardiac failure (Fig. 58.8).[31]

Nonspecific complaints of headaches, syncope, and face and neck pain are often misinterpreted as stress-related problems, particularly in young women. Consequently, the diagnosis can be missed for months. Only a few patients come to clinical attention with catastrophic neurological symptoms related to brain ischemia. Helpful clues are differences in blood pressure, loss of pulses, and vascular bruits heard on clinical examination. Retinal neoangiogenesis, induced by hypoperfusion of the eye, is now relatively rare, but fleeting visual abnormalities may indicate transient ischemic attacks. Signs of aortic insufficiency are unlikely to be encountered in early disease, but continuous monitoring for aortic dilation is an essential part of follow-up care. Coronary artery stenosis in a young patient must prompt the physician to rule out TA. In a subset of patients, the origins of mesenteric arteries are involved by stenosing vasculitis. Clinical consequences include weight loss, nausea, vomiting, diarrhea, and abdominal claudication, typically elicited by the increased intestinal blood demand following a meal.

Renal artery stenosis may be clinically silent and is often noticed in routine screening. Correct measurement of blood pressures can represent a pressing clinical problem if the upper-extremity arteries are affected. Involvement of the infrarenal aorta can lead to lower-extremity claudication. Musculoskeletal examinations are usually unrevealing, although joint and muscle pains are common complaints.

Diagnosis

Classification criteria have been developed for GCA and TA in order to differentiate patients with large-vessel vasculitis from those with other vasculitic entities (Tables 58.3–58.5).[32-34] Age at disease onset and the pattern of arteritis are clearly important for establishing the diagnosis and distinguishing between these two related vasculopathies. Diagnostic criteria for PMR remain a challenge (Table 58.3) as they rely on nonspecific symptoms, such as muscle pain and stiffness and elevated erythrocyte sedimentation rate (ESR), all of which can occur in many diseases.[2] No pathogenic test is currently available to diagnose PMR. Therapeutic responsiveness of PMR patients to low-dose corticosteroids is clinically helpful but stresses the need for objective diagnostic criteria.

Table 58.3 American College of Rheumatology 1990 classification criteria for giant-cell arteritis[a] and polymyalgia rheumatica

Age at disease onset ≥ 50 years
New onset or new type of headache
Temporal artery tenderness or decreased artery pulse
Elevated erythrocyte sedimentation rate (≥ 50 mm/hr)
Histologic incidence of arteritis (characterized by a predominance of mononuclear cell infiltrates or a granulomatous process with multinucleated giant cells)

[a]A patient is classified as having giant-cell arteritis if at least three of the five criteria are present.
Reprinted from Hunder GG, Bloch DA, Michel BA, et al. The American College of Rheumatology 1990 criteria for the classification of giant cell arteritis. Arthritis Rheum 1990; 33: 1122–1128, with permission of Wiley-Liss, Inc., a subsidiary of John Wiley & Sons, Inc. ©1990.

Table 58.4 Provisional classification criteria for polymyalgia rheumatica

Age ≥ 50 years	required
Bilateral shoulder aching	required
Abnormal CRP and/or ESR	required
Morning stiffness > 45 min	2
Hip pain or limited range of motion	1
Absence of RF or ACPA	2
Absence of other joint involvement	1
A score of 4 or more is categorized as polymyalgia rheumatica	

Reprinted from Dasgupta B, et al. Provisional classification criteria for polymyalgia rheumatica: a European League Against Rheumatism/American College of Rheumatology collaborative initiative. Arthritis Rheum 64:943–954, 2012 (doi: 10.1002/art.34356).

Table 58.5 American College of Rheumatology 1990 criteria[a] for the classification of Takayasu arteritis

Disease onset at ≤ 40 years
Claudication of an extremity
Decreased brachial artery pulse
> 10 mmHg difference in systolic blood pressure between arms
Bruit over the subclavian arteries or the aorta
Arteriographic evidence of narrowing or occlusion of the entire aorta, its primary branches, or large arteries in the proximal upper or lower extremities

[a]For purposes of classification, a patient is classified as having Takayasu arteritis if more than three of the six criteria are fulfilled.
Reprinted from Arend WP, Michel BA, Bloch DA, et al. The American College of Rheumatology 1990 criteria for the classification of Takayasu arteritis. Arthritis Rheum 1990; 33: 1129–1134, with permission of Wiley-Liss, Inc., a subsidiary of John Wiley & Sons, Inc. ©1990.

Laboratory tests

In all three conditions, GCA, PMR, and TA, the vast majority of patients have laboratory findings of an intense acute-phase response.[2,26,29] Generally, this is captured by measuring ESR or C-reactive protein (CRP). It is important to note, however, that a subset of GCA patients has normal ESR readings, even before initiation of immunosuppressive therapy. A normal ESR or CRP reading is not sufficient to exclude the diagnosis, and further diagnostic workup is required if clinical presentation is suspicious for vasculitis. Other acute-phase proteins, such as fibrinogen and serum amyloid A, have been reported to be elevated as well. IL-6 is a potent inducer of acute-phase proteins in the liver and has been found to be a sensitive marker of continuous systemic inflammation.[35,36] Other laboratory abnormalities, such as elevation of alkaline phosphatase, thrombocytosis, and anemia, are in line with a robust acute-phase response.

Autoantibody measurements are not helpful beyond excluding differential diagnoses, such as rheumatoid arthritis, systemic lupus erythematosus, or anti-neutrophil cytoplasmic antibody (ANCA)-related vasculitides. No disease-specific autoantibodies for GCA and TA have been discovered , emphasizing that B cells are not involved in the pathogenic events leading to granulomatous inflammation of large vessels.

Tissue biopsy

In patients with TA, tissue biopsies are rarely available unless the patient had to undergo vascular reconstructive surgery. In most patients, the diagnosis is made based on imaging procedures revealing luminal and wall abnormalities in affected blood vessels.

In contrast, arterial biopsy remains a critical diagnostic approach in patients with GCA. Temporal arteries are easily accessible, and a segment of these arteries can be removed in an outpatient setting. Recommendations include harvesting 2–3 cm of the temporal artery, starting at the most symptomatic side. Frozen tissue sections can lead to a quick diagnosis of granulomatous vasculitis. Whether the second side should be biopsied during the same surgical procedure remains a matter of debate. In cohorts including several hundred patients, vasculitis was detected in 2–3% of tissue samples from the second side if the first side was negative. If the clinical suspicion is strong, biopsy confirmation can be sought from a second-side biopsy immediately after the first biopsy or after careful monitoring of the patient several weeks later. Negative findings on temporal artery biopsy do not exclude the diagnosis of GCA. In a retrospective cohort study, about half of all patients with subclavian GCA had no evidence of vasculitis in the temporal arteries, emphasizing that the disease may display clear preference for certain vascular territories.[37]

Corticosteroid therapy does not eradicate pathologic findings of vascular wall infiltrates and biopsy can still be valuable in making the diagnosis in patients on steroids.[37] Nevertheless, it is possible that treatment with steroids leads to a false-negative biopsy result in some patients.

Histomorphologic reports describe mononuclear cell infiltrates penetrating through all layers of the vessel wall (Fig. 58.9).[1] Since the disease process enters the vessel wall through the adventitia, this may be the only site of inflammation. The finding of isolated inflammatory cell clusters in the adventitia, although not diagnostic, should at least be considered as highly suspicious. Multinucleated giant cells may or may not be found. They tend to lie along the internal elastic lamina, at the junction between the media and the intima. Media destruction is not unusual, but findings of fibrinoid necrosis should prompt a search for a different vasculitic entity. The vessel lumen is more or less compromised by hyperplastic intima formed from proliferating fibroblasts, smooth-muscle cells, and deposition of acid mucopolysaccharides.

Histology of TA is similar to that in GCA, making it difficult to dissect both syndromes in tissue samples derived from the aorta or its primary branches.[38] Lymphocytes and plasma cells accumulate around vasa vasorum. Marked wall thickening with inflammatory tissue extending into perivascular structures is typical for TA (Fig. 58.10). Destruction of elastic membranes is often extensive and combined with patchy areas of media necrosis. Weakening of the vessel wall can lead to aneurysm formation. Notably, inflammatory lesions can be arranged in a "skipped" pattern with normal vessel wall segments alternating with stretches of intense destructive inflammation.

Physicians can be confronted with morphologic findings of granulomatous aortitis in patients undergoing aortic aneurysm repair without any prior diagnosis of vasculitis. Detailed workup of these patients is necessary to identify those with undiagnosed PMR, GCA, or TA. Rare causes of aortitis, including inflammatory bowel disease, sarcoidosis, syphilis, relapsing polychondritis and connective tissue disease, should

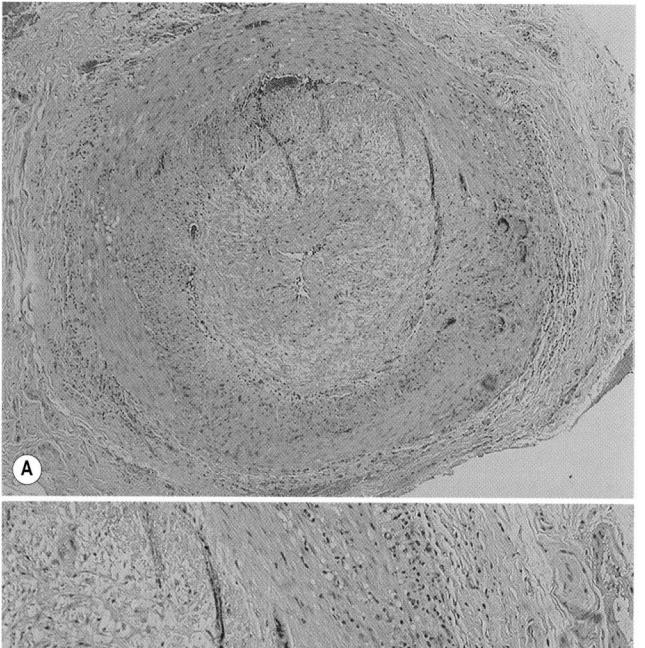

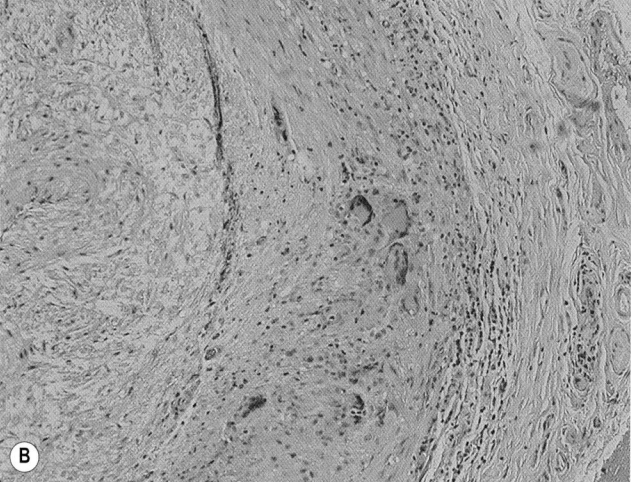

Fig. 58.9 Histomorphology of giant-cell arteritis. (A) Temporal artery cross-section with mononuclear infiltrates throughout all wall layers. The adventitia is infiltrated by round cells with cuffing of vasa vasorum by lymphocytes. The vessel lumen is occluded by intimal hyperplasia. (B) Higher magnification showing intense granulomatous inflammation with multinucleated giant cells in the proximal media and at the media–intima junction.

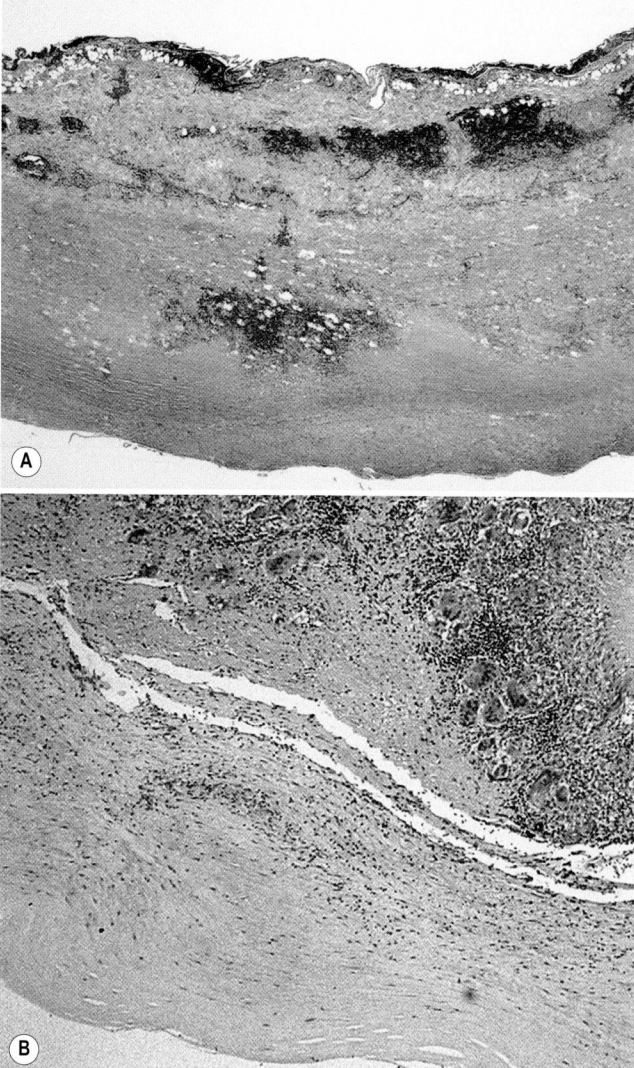

Fig. 58.10 Histopathology of Takayasu arteritis. (A) Full-thickness section of the aortic wall shows dense mononuclear infiltrates in the adventitia and media. The intima is thickened and wavy; hematoxylin and eosin (H&E). (B) Florid granulomatous inflammation along the media–intima junction with numerous giant cells; H&E.

be ruled out. Isolated granulomatous aortitis is diagnosed as idiopathic aortitis. The pathogenesis and prognosis of this condition are essentially unknown, but relatively good outcomes have been described in patients who did not receive immunosuppressive therapy.

Diagnostic imaging

Modern imaging modalities have fundamentally changed the diagnostic approach to large-vessel vasculitis.[26] Indeed, diagnosing TA mostly depends on identifying vascular lesions in typical distribution by imaging.[39]

Conventional angiography still has its place in presurgical planning and can be combined with intravascular interventions. It provides ideal visualization of the vascular lumen not only for large but also for medium-sized arteries such as the axillary and brachial arteries (Fig. 58.5). Ultrasound (US)-based methods are extremely useful for screening carotid arteries but also emerge as the method of choice for initial assessment of the distal

subclavian arteries, vertebral arteries, renal arteries, and femoral arteries. Also, US examination is the optimal method for long-term monitoring of vessel bypasses in patients who have undergone revascularization surgical procedures. Magnetic resonance (MR) imaging and MR angiography, as well as computed tomography (CT), are now widely used for evaluating the vascular tree. Both methods provide excellent information on abnormalities of the vascular lumen and wall, but are still limited to larger vessels and provide insufficient information about the distal subclavian arteries or the second to fifth branches of the aorta. CT imaging is fast, well tolerated by claustrophobic patients, and allows excellent assessment of the aorta and its wall (Fig. 58.7). However, it has the disadvantages of contrast loading and radiation exposure. With its inherent multiplanar imaging capabilities, MR is used to examine neck vessels, the aorta, and its primary branches (Figs. 58.6 and 58.8). Great hope was placed on its potential to measure wall edema and intramural vascularity, which would make MR a useful tool in estimating disease burden and responses to therapy. However, a carefully conducted study comparing imaging results with laboratory parameters of inflammation to results from surgically harvested vessel biopsies has been disappointing, cautioning that edema-weighted MR should not be used as a sole means of measuring disease activity and therapeutic responsiveness.[40]

Therapeutic management

THERAPEUTIC PRINCIPLES

- To prevent vision loss, patients with giant-cell arteritis (GCA) require immediate treatment. Similarly, with the threat of catastrophic cerebral ischemia in Takayasu arteritis (TA), prompt initiation of therapy is imperative.
- Corticosteroids are the immunosuppressive drug of choice for large-vessel vasculitis. Often, they must be given over a period of several years but may be clinically effective at very low doses.
- Clinical trials have failed to show convincing steroid-sparing effects for either methotrexate or tumor necrosis factor (TNF)-α blockade in GCA.
- Molecular studies of the inflammatory infiltrate in GCA have shown that early and untreated disease is characterized by two functional T-cell lineages; Th1 and Th17 cells. Th17 cells are rapidly responsive to corticosteroids, whereas Th1 cells persist and promote chronic, smoldering vasculitis.
- It is not known whether the smoldering activity persisting beyond the acute phase of disease requires immunosuppressive therapy or whether the benefits of chronic immunosuppressive therapy outweigh the potential risks.
- Clinical experience (not evidence-based therapeutic trials) suggests that a combination of methotrexate, mycophenolate mofetil, or TNF-α-blocking agents with corticosteroids may be beneficial in controlling disease in some patients with TA.
- Close monitoring for diabetes, hypertension, and hyperlipidemia combined with bone-saving therapy should be part of the treatment regime in patients with large-vessel vasculitis on long-term corticosteroids.

With increasing knowledge of the disease process and refinement of diagnosis and long-term treatment, the prognosis for large-vessel vasculitis patients has significantly improved. Life expectancy of patients with GCA is not shorter than of age-matched controls. Follow-up studies of Japanese patients with TA suggest good control of disease activity in about 75% of patients, with only 25% experiencing serious complications and cardiac manifestations that dominate long-term outcome. Recent discussions have focused on the question of whether vasculitis predisposes patients to accelerated atherosclerotic disease, given the combination of chronic inflammation and injury to vessel wall structures. It is not known whether progression of atherosclerosis and its complications require a different management approach or whether standard vaso-protective measures (such as treating hypertension and hyperlipidemia and advising patients to avoid smoking) are sufficient.[5]

ON THE HORIZON

- Human medium and large arteries sense danger signals through wall-embedded cells; changing the understanding of how the immune system interacts with the vascular system.
- The multi-lineage nature of vasculitic T cells, which display differential therapeutic responsiveness, almost certainly will require more complex therapies, adapted to disease stage and immune status of the host.
- The immune system changes profoundly with age. Seek age-appropriate management of each patient and avoid overtreatment of the elderly.
- Current therapies in large-vessel vasculitis induce partial remission. Appropriately designed studies are required to explore whether partial remission is sufficient and whether the risk–benefit ratio is maintained if complete remission is attempted.

Pathogenic studies have pointed out that the traditional view of GCA as a self-limiting disease is incorrect.[36] To the contrary, granulomatous vasculitis has shown surprising resistance to immunosuppression in models of the disease, such as the temporal artery-SCID chimeras.[41] The paradigm of GCA as a chronic smoldering condition is supported by studies showing that sensitive markers of systemic inflammation remain elevated even in patients who are clinically asymptomatic and are weaned off immunosuppression. Based on examination of subsequent temporal artery biopsies collected from untreated and treated patients it is now clear that arteritis persists, albeit sustained by a immune network distinct from that in untreated patients.[14] It is currently unknown whether this persistent smoldering process needs to be treated. Unchanged life expectancy in this population of elderly patients with an average age of 75 years at disease onset suggests that current management may be adequate. It could be argued that intensification of immunosuppressive therapy is necessary to prevent long-term complications, such as aortic aneurysm/dissection from GCA aortitis. However, the number of patients developing such complications is low, and there is no evidence to indicate that therapy can stop progression of aortic wall destruction. The ultimate decision depends on the cost–benefit analysis comparing the risk from smoldering disease with the risks imposed by long-standing immunosuppression. In that context it is important to remember the profound impact of the immune aging process, which leaves the patient with an impaired immune system and amplifies the risk of immunosuppression.[42]

The immunosuppressants of choice in GCA, TA, and PMR are corticosteroids. Modern anti-cytokine reagents have not shown therapeutic efficacy in GCA and PMR; however, they may be helpful for some TA patients.[43] Methotrexate appears to lack steroid-sparing action in GCA and PMR,[44] but may have a limited effect in TA.[43] Commensurate with low tumor necrosis factor (TNF)-α production in the vascular lesions of GCA, TNF-α blockade has been disappointing and lacks steroid-sparing efficacy.[45] The unparalleled response pattern of patients with large-vessel vasculitis to corticosteroids emphasizes disease-specific pathogenic pathways in these syndromes that are distinct from most other autoimmune entities. Equally remarkable is the fact that patients with GCA, PMR, and TA improve within hours after being started on steroid therapy. The response is usually dramatic, with improvements within 24–48 hours. The promptness of clinical improvement is so exceptional that it has been suggested as a diagnostic criterion for PMR. Data from a study in untreated and treated GCA patients suggest that the acute clinical benefit may be due to suppressing the effects of IL-17, whereas IFN-γ production continues unabated.[46] Signs and symptoms of vascular stenosis are much less responsive, compatible with the persistence of IFN-γ-induced vessel wall inflammation.[14] Reduction in wall edema may help to re-establish some blood flow. Over time, formation of collateral blood vessels is an important mechanism for dealing with tissue ischemia.

Patients with GCA are started on a daily prednisone dose of 40–60 mg (about 1 mg/kg body weight). Once stabilized, steroid tapering is guided by close monitoring of the clinical presentation as well as laboratory markers of inflammation. In general, steroids should be reduced 10–20% every 2 weeks. Monthly monitoring of ESR and CRP is mandatory to adjust therapy. Patients frequently return with signs or symptoms of recurrent disease as immunosuppression is lowered. Fortunately, disease exacerbations causing vision loss are infrequent. Disease flares typically present with PMR symptoms or nonspecific manifestations of malaise and failure to thrive. In most patients, disease control can be reinstated by a transient small increase in the steroid dose.

A recent study has suggested that initial treatment of vasculitis can alter the patients' long-term course. Guided by experiments in human artery-SCID chimeras, patients with biopsy-proven GCA were treated with pulse corticosteroids as induction therapy.[47] After receiving pulses of 1000 mg methylprednisolone for three consecutive days, therapy was continued on oral prednisone, and daily doses were swiftly tapered. Compared to patients in the control arm of the study, those who received the three initial steroid pulses had lower likelihoods of disease flares. Particularly, once they reached steroid doses close to 10 mg/day, these patients could tolerate steroid withdrawal significantly better, and the majority were taking 5 mg/day prednisone at 36 weeks.[47] The benefit from initial pulse therapy continued over subsequent months, suggesting potential benefit of intense immunosuppression during early disease.

When given to human artery-SCID chimeras, acetylsalicylic acid (aspirin) has marked anti-inflammatory activities, with suppression of IFN-γ in vascular lesions.[48] Clinical trials are needed to test whether this immunosuppressive action can translate into corticosteroid sparing. Because arteries are the primary target of large-vessel vasculitis, the use of aspirin as an anti-platelet agent should be routinely recommended.

There is no evidence that immunosuppressants such as azathioprine and cyclophosphamide reduce the need for prednisone, prevent vascular complications, or shorten the duration of corticosteroid use. An integral part of chronic immunosuppression with prednisone is regular monitoring for diabetes and hypertension. Patients should be encouraged to increase physical activity, as steroid-induced myopathy occurs frequently. A major issue of chronic steroid treatment, particularly in elderly individuals, is the potential of excessive bone loss, possibly as a result of both increased bone resorption and impaired bone formation. A number of effective and safe therapies for osteoporosis are available. Calcium and vitamin D supplementation should be part of the therapeutic regimen.

Many, but not all patients can be discontinued from immunosuppressive treatment 18–24 months after diagnosis. Markers of systemic inflammation may remain elevated, and continuous monitoring for aortic involvement and recurrence of cranial arteritis is recommended.

In patients with PMR who have no evidence for frank vasculitis, much lower doses of steroids are necessary to induce prompt relief of symptoms. Most patients are sufficiently treated with an initial dose of 20 mg of prednisone per day. In some patients, 10 mg of prednisone can induce and sustain a clinical response. Steroids should be titrated to minimally needed doses to avoid side effects; tapering usually needs to be slow, over many months.

In TA, initial therapy is similar to that in GCA, but long-term management should be tailored to individual patient conditions.[43] It has been discussed that patients should be maintained on a low dose of corticosteroids, such as 5–7 mg prednisone daily, even after successful control of active disease.

Given the age at disease onset in TA, preventive measures to counteract accelerated atherosclerosis and optimize blood pressure control are important aspects of management.

It has been suggested that up to 50% of TA patients may require a second immunosuppressive agent.[43] Steroid-sparing effects of methotrexate have been reported for some patients. Similarly, mycophenolate mofetil may have clinical efficiency, although published data are only available on a small patient cohort. Empirically, azathioprine may have a place in maintenance therapy of TA patients who may require anti-inflammatory management over many years. Finally, there may be a place for agents blocking TNF-α in patients with persistent disease activity. Results from well-designed placebo-controlled treatment trials testing the efficiency of such immunosuppressive drugs are awaited.

Detecting and treating hypertension is an essential component of caring for patients with TA. Untreated hypertension leads to acceleration of atherosclerosis and cardiac insufficiency. In patients with upper-extremity involvement, obtaining accurate blood pressure measurements is a challenge and requires education of the patient and caregivers.

Besides pharmacologic therapy, revascularization procedures—including both surgical and endovascular interventions—have vastly broadened therapeutic options in patients with TA and large-vessel GCA.[43] To minimize the risk of complications, such as rapid reocclusion, an effort should be made to suppress vascular wall inflammation optimally before subjecting the patients to revascularization treatment. Conventional bypass grafts are still considered the method of choice. Percutaneous transluminal angioplasty can be useful in managing renal artery stenosis or other short-segment lesions. Bypass surgery is needed in patients with cerebrovascular ischemia in whom catastrophic strokes may be prevented by bypassing critical stenosis of cervical vessels with grafts originating from the aortic arch. Re-establishing flow in upper- and lower-extremity arteries can be complicated by multiple and long-segment stenosis, and arterial reconstructions with prosthetic graft materials or veins may be the only alternative to obtain long-term patency. Placing of conventional stents can be complicated by eliciting rapid restenosis, and it is not known whether outcomes can be improved by drug-eluting stents. Occlusive disease of the coronary arteries usually represents a challenging clinical scenario, and most physicians opt for conventional bypass surgery. Depending on symptoms, patients with aortic regurgitation may require repair of the weakened aortic wall.

References

1. Weyand CM, Goronzy JJ. Medium- and large-vessel vasculitis. N Engl J Med 2003;349:160–9.
2. Salvarani C, Cantini F, Boiardi L, et al. Polymyalgia rheumatica and giant-cell arteritis. N Engl J Med 2002;347:261–71.
3. Nordborg E, Nordborg C. Giant cell arteritis: epidemiological clues to its pathogenesis and an update on its treatment. Rheumatology (Oxford) 2003;42:413–21.
4. Vanoli M, Bacchiani G, Origg L, et al. Takayasus arteritis: a changing disease. J Nephrol 2001;14:497–505.

5. Numano F, Kishi Y, Tanaka A, et al. Inflammation and atherosclerosis. Atherosclerotic lesions in Takayasu arteritis. Ann N Y Acad Sci 2000;902:65–76.
6. Seko Y. Takayasu arteritis: insights into immunopathology. Jpn Heart J 2000;41:15–26.
7. Weyand CM, Ma-Krupa W, Goronzy JJ. Immunopathways in giant cell arteritis and polymyalgia rheumatica. Autoimmun Rev 2004;3:46–53.
8. Weyand CM, Goronzy JJ. Arterial wall injury in giant cell arteritis. Arthritis Rheum 1999;42:844–53.
9. Ma-Krupa W, Jeon MS, Spoerl S, et al. Activation of arterial wall dendritic cells and breakdown of self-tolerance in giant cell arteritis. J Exp Med 2004;199:173–83.
10. Weyand CM, Ma-Krupa W, Pryshchep O, et al. Vascular dendritic cells in giant cell arteritis. Ann N Y Acad Sci 2005;1062:195–208.
11. Krupa WM, Dewan M, Jeon MS, et al. Trapping of misdirected dendritic cells in the granulomatous lesions of giant cell arteritis. Am J Pathol 2002;161:1815–23.
12. Ma-Krupa W, Kwan M, Goronzy JJ, et al. Toll-like receptors in giant cell arteritis. Clin Immunol 2005;115:38–46.
13. Pryshchep O, Ma-Krupa W, Younge BR, et al. Vessel-specific Toll-like receptor profiles in human medium and large arteries. Circulation 2009;118:1276–84.
14. Deng J, Younge BR, Olshen RA, et al. Th17 and Th1 T-cell responses in giant cell arteritis. Circulation 2010;121:906–15.
15. Weyand CM, Tetzlaff N, Bjornsson J, et al. Disease patterns and tissue cytokine profiles in giant cell arteritis. Arthritis Rheum 1997;40:19–26.
16. Kaiser M, Younge B, Bjornsson J, et al. Formation of new vasa vasorum in vasculitis. Production of angiogenic cytokines by multinucleated giant cells.. Am J Pathol 1999;155:765–74.
17. Seko Y, Minota S, Kawasaki A, et al. Perforin-secreting killer cell infiltration and expression of a 65-kD heat-shock protein in aortic tissue of patients with Takayasus arteritis. J Clin Invest 1994;93:750–8.
18. Deng J, Ma-Krupa W, Gewirtz AT, et al. Toll-like receptors 4 and 5 induce distinct types of vasculitis. Circ Res 2009;104(4):488–95.
19. Weyand CM, Schonberger J, Oppitz U, et al. Distinct vascular lesions in giant cell arteritis share identical T cell clonotypes. J Exp Med 1994;179:951–60.
20. Piggott K, Deng J, Warrington K, et al. Blocking the NOTCH pathway inhibits vascular inflammation in large vessel vasculitis. Circulation 2011;123:309–18.
21. Wagner AD, Goronzy JJ, Weyand CM. Functional profile of tissue-infiltrating and circulating CD68 + cells in giant cell arteritis. Evidence for two components of the disease. J Clin Invest 1994;94:1134–40.
22. Borkowski A, Younge BR, Szweda L, et al. Reactive nitrogen intermediates in giant cell arteritis: selective nitration of neocapillaries. Am J Pathol 2002;161:115–23.
23. Rittner HL, Hafner V, Klimiuk PA, et al. Aldose reductase functions as a detoxification system for lipid peroxidation products in vasculitis. J Clin Invest 1999;103:1007–13.
24. Rittner HL, Kaiser M, Brack A, et al. Tissue-destructive macrophages in giant cell arteritis. Circ Res 1999;84:1050–8.
25. Kaiser M, Weyand CM, Bjornsson J, et al. Platelet-derived growth factor, intimal hyperplasia, and ischemic complications in giant cell arteritis. Arthritis Rheum 1998;41:623–33.
26. Weyand CM, Goronzy JJ. Giant-cell arteritis and polymyalgia rheumatica. Ann Intern Med 2003;139:505–15.
27. Brack A, Martinez-Taboada V, Stanson A, et al. Disease pattern in cranial and large-vessel giant cell arteritis. Arthritis Rheum 1999;42:311–7.
28. Salvarani C, Cantini F, Olivieri I, et al. Proximal bursitis in active polymyalgia rheumatica. Ann Intern Med 1997;127:27–31.
29. Kerr GS, Hallahan CW, Giordano J, et al. Takayasu arteritis. Ann Intern Med 1994;120:919–29.
30. Numano F, Kobayashi Y. Takayasu arteritis—beyond pulselessness. Intern Med 1999;38:226–32.
31. Kobayashi Y, Numano F. 3. Takayasu arteritis. Intern Med 2002;41:44–6.
32. Hunder GG, Bloch DA, Michel BA, et al. The American College of Rheumatology 1990 criteria for the classification of giant cell arteritis. Arthritis Rheum 1990;33:1122–8.
33. Dasgupta B, et al. Provisional classification criteria for polymyalgia rheumatica: a European League Against Rheumatism/American College of Rheumatology collaborative initiative. Arthritis Rheum 2012;64:943–54 (doi: 10.1002/art.34356).
34. Arend WP, Michel BA, Bloch DA, et al. The American College of Rheumatology 1990 criteria for the classification of Takayasu arteritis. Arthritis Rheum 1990;33:1129–34.
35. Roche NE, Fulbright JW, Wagner AD, et al. Correlation of interleukin-6 production and disease activity in polymyalgia rheumatica and giant cell arteritis. Arthritis Rheum 1993;36:1286–94.
36. Weyand CM, Fulbright JW, Hunder GG, et al. Treatment of giant cell arteritis: interleukin-6 as a biologic marker of disease activity. Arthritis Rheum 2000;43:1041–8.
37. Achkar AA, Lie JT, Hunder GG, et al. How does previous corticosteroid treatment affect the biopsy findings in giant cell (temporal) arteritis? Ann Intern Med 1994;120:987–92.
38. Johnston SL, Lock RJ, Gompels MM. Takayasu arteritis: a review. J Clin Pathol 2002;55:481–6.
39. Steeds RP, Mohiaddin R. Takayasu arteritis: role of cardiovascular magnetic imaging. Int J Cardiol 2006;109:1–6.
40. Tso E, Flamm SD, White RD, et al. Takayasu arteritis: utility and limitations of magnetic resonance imaging in diagnosis and treatment. Arthritis Rheum 2002;46:1634–42.
41. Brack A, Rittner HL, Younge BR, et al. Glucocorticoid-mediated repression of cytokine gene transcription in human arteritis-SCID chimeras. J Clin Invest 1997;99:2842–50.
42. Mohan SV, Kao YJL, Kim JW, et al. Giant cell arteritis – Immune and vascular aging as disease risk factors. Arthritis Res Ther 2011;13:231.
43. Liang P, Hoffman GS. Advances in the medical and surgical treatment of Takayasu arteritis. Curr Opin Rheumatol 2005;17:16–24.
44. Hoffman GS, Cid MC, Hellmann DB, et al. A multicenter, randomized, double-blind, placebo-controlled trial of adjuvant methotrexate treatment for giant cell arteritis. Arthritis Rheum 2002;46:1309–18.
45. Hoffman GS, Cid MC, Rendt-Zagar KE, et al., for the Infliximab-GCA Study Group. Infliximab for maintenance of glucocorticosteroid-induced remission of giant cell arteritis. A randomized trial. Ann Intern Med 2007;146:621–30.
46. Weyand CM, Younge BR, Goronzy JJ. IFN-γ and IL-17: the two faces of T-cell pathology in giant cell arteritis. Curr Opin Rheumatol 2011;23:43–9.
47. Mazlumzadeh M, Hunder GG, Easley KA, et al. Treatment of giant cell arteritis using induction therapy with high-dose glucocorticoids: a double-blind, placebo-controlled, randomized prospective clinical trial. Arthritis Rheum 2006;54:3310–8.
48. Weyand CM, Kaiser M, Yang H, et al. Therapeutic effects of acetylsalicylic acid in giant cell arteritis. Arthritis Rheum 2002;46:457–66.

Jeroen C.H. van
der Hilst, Jos
W.M. van der
Meer, Anna Simon

Systemic autoinflammatory syndromes

"Autoinflammatory" is a term that was coined more than 10 years ago to indicate disorders characterized by too much inflammation, without obvious signs of dysregulation of the adaptive immune system, such as autoantibodies or antigen-specific T cells, thus making the term "autoimmune" less applicable.[1] It is clear that autoinflammation and autoimmunity have several common features, and they are seen as two ends of a spectrum of what could be called an "over-active immune system." At the extreme "autoinflammatory end" of the spectrum are the (Mendelian) inherited autoinflammatory syndromes that are the main subject of this chapter.

KEY CONCEPTS

Autoinflammatory versus autoimmune disorder

- Common features:
  - Too much inflammation through dysregulation of immune system
  - Phenotype characterized by exacerbations and remissions
- Distinctive features:
  - Autoinflammation: dysregulation of innate immunity, no high-titer autoantibodies or antigen-specific T cells
  - Autoimmunity: dysregulation of adaptive immunity, defect in lymphocytes and/or autoantibodies
- Many immunological disorders have features of both autoinflammation and autoimmunity, which has led to the concept of a continuous spectrum including the two entities.

Hereditary autoinflammatory syndromes, also known as hereditary periodic fever syndromes, encompass a group of genetic disorders characterized by lifelong recurrent inflammatory attacks of noninfectious origin. Each syndrome is characterized by a mix of symptoms that may include fever, abdominal symptoms, arthralgias, arthritis, lymphadenopathy, and skin manifestations. Inflammatory attacks are always accompanied by an intense acute phase response with elevated C-reactive protein (CRP), serum amyloid A (SAA), and leukocytosis.[2]

The mutated genes in these syndromes all code for proteins with a role in the regulation of innate immunity. Some of these were already known regulators (e.g., TNF-receptor type 1 or interleukin-1 receptor antagonist (IL-1ra)), but some were previously unknown proteins that have since been shown to be central in inflammation (e.g., NLRP3 or pyrin). In one case, the mutated protein was already very familiar, though the direct link with regulation of inflammation has only partly been unraveled so far (mevalonate kinase). This dysregulation of inflammation results in the inappropriate and increased secretion of inflammatory cytokines, particularly IL-1β.

Apart from these strict hereditary autoinflammatory syndromes, there is a growing number of disorders that are now recognized to have characteristics fitting in this category which are either acquired or probably have a complex genetic background.

In this chapter, the details of four of the hereditary autoinflammatory disorders (Table 59.1) and two systemic autoinflammatory disorders that have no monogenic inheritance pattern are described. Characteristics of a number of other autoinflammatory disorders are also highlighted in a separate paragraph.

The cornerstone of the diagnosis of the autoinflammatory diseases is clinical assessment. This includes a detailed medical and family history and preferably, observation of an inflammatory episode. The first step is to exclude other, more common, causes of inflammation, including infections, malignancies (paraneoplastic phenomena) and autoimmune diseases (see for extensive list of differential diagnoses, Bodar et al.[3])

Based on age of onset of symptoms, family history, ethnic background, accompanying symptoms, and duration of fever, a first differentiation can be made (Table 59.2), which will indicate the appropriate further diagnostic tests.

Epidemiology

It is important to realize that the hereditary autoinflammatory diseases are generally quite rare and that the incidence depends on the background population, since gene distribution is associated to some extent with ethnicity. Familial Mediterranean fever (FMF) is the most prevalent of these diseases, with more than 10 000 persons affected worldwide. It is found in persons originating from the Mediterranean basin, including Turks, Jews (primarily non-Ashkenazi), Armenians, and Arabs. However, sporadic cases in other ethnic groups have been described. With the discovery of the mutated gene, the *Me*diterranean *fe*ver gene (MEFV), it was appreciated that FMF is also relatively common in Italians and Ashkenazi Jews, although often with a less severe phenotype than in the high-prevalence populations. In selected populations, the carrier frequency can be as high as 1 in 3 to 1 in 6.[3] The high carrier rate suggests that carriers of the MEFV gene in the founder population may have had an evolutionary selection advantage, possibly due to protection against an infectious agent by an exaggerated inflammatory response.

The first patients with hyperimmunoglobulin D and periodic fever syndrome (HIDS) were described in 1984 in the Netherlands.[4] At present, over 200 patients have been reported. The majority of patients come from Western Europe, particularly the Netherlands and France. This observation is partly explained by the increased awareness among physicians in these countries, but a founder effect has been described for the most prevalent mutation as well.[4]

Table 59.1 The autoinflammatory syndromes: names, acronyms and alternative names

Name	Acronym	Alternatives
Familial Mediterranean fever	FMF	Hereditary periodic fever (old abandoned name)
Cryopyrin-associated periodic syndrome	CAPS	Clinical syndromes: Familial cold autoinflammatory syndrome (FCAS) Muckle–Wells syndrome (MWS) Neonatal-onset multisystemic inflammatory disease (NOMID); also known as chronic infantile neurologic cutaneous and articular syndrome (CINCA)
Tumor necrosis factor receptor-associated periodic syndrome	TRAPS	Familial Hibernian fever (FHF), Autosomal dominant periodic fever [both old abandoned names]
Hyperimmunoglobulin D and periodic fever syndrome	HIDS	Mevalonate kinase deficiency (MKD)
Periodic fever, aphthous stomatitis, pharyngitis and adenitis	PFAPA	

Two mutations in the mevalonate kinase gene (V377I and I268T) account for almost 90% of the patients described to date. Almost all patients are of Caucasian origin, though cases from India and Japan have been described. Men and women are equally affected.

Tumor necrosis factor (TNF) receptor-associated periodic syndrome (TRAPS) was originally named familial Hibernian fever after the first family described, a Scottish–Irish family with periodic fever. Though TRAPS has been reported in families from Central America, Australia, and Central Europe, most families originate from North-western Europe. So far, a few dozen families and over 200 sporadic cases have been reported.[3]

The prevalence of the cryopyrin-associated periodic syndrome (CAPS) is unknown, but availability of good treatment options has improved disease awareness and recognition.

Periodic fever, aphthous stomatitis, pharyngitis and adenitis (PFAPA) was first reported by Marshall et al. in 1987.[5] It is difficult to estimate the incidence of PFAPA. There seems to be a great variability between different countries; this may also depend greatly on patient and pediatrician awareness of the disorder. At one children's hospital in the USA, 122 patients fulfilled the diagnosis PFAPA in a period of 10 years;[6] it is more commonly diagnosed than the hereditary monogenic autoinflammatory syndromes (except for FMF in certain populations).[7]

Schnitzler syndrome—first described by dermatologist Schnitzler in 1972[8]—appears to be an acquired disorder, manifesting itself at a median age of 51 years. There have been less than 150 cases reported in the literature worldwide.

Pathogenesis

Familial Mediterranean fever

The MEFV gene responsible for FMF was discovered in 1997 by two international collaborative groups and is located on the short arm of chromosome 16.[2] So far, more than 70 mutations have been reported in a central registry (http://fmf.igh.cnrs.fr/ISSAID/infevers/), most of which are clustered in exon 10 of the gene. The six most prevalent mutations (M694V, V726A, M680I, M694I, V694I, E148Q) represent some 80% of all cases. The gene encodes a 781-amino-acid protein termed pyrin that is primarily expressed in peripheral blood leukocytes, especially

Table 59.2 Hereditary autoinflammatory syndromes

	FMF	CAPS	TRAPS	HIDS
Mode of inheritance	Autosomal recessive	Autosomal dominant	Autosomal dominant	Autosomal recessive
Age of onset (years)	<20	Generally <1, in MWS/FCAS <20 possible	Variable, most <10	<1
Main ethnic distribution	Turks, Arabs, Jews, Armenians	European	All	North-west European (Dutch, French)
Gene involved	*MEFV*	*CIAS1 (=NLRP3)*	*TNFRSF1A*	*MVK*
Protein involved	Pyrin	NLRP3 (traditional name: cryopyrin)	TNF-receptor type 1	Mevalonate kinase
Duration of typical attack	2–3 days	Variable; hours–days or continuous inflammation	Days–weeks	4–6 days
Distinguishing symptoms	Peritonitis, pleuritis, erysipelas-like skin lesions	Aseptic meningitis; sensorineural deafness; bone lesions, dysmorphic features; cold-induced	severe myalgia, periorbital edema	Lymphadenopathy, attacks induced by vaccination
Risk of amyloidosis[a]	Up to 75%	Up to 33%	25%	<5%
Treatment (see text)	Colchicine (if resistant: IL-1 inhibition, TNF-inhibition)	IL-1 inhibition	Mild disease: NSAIDs; Severe disease: IL-1 inhibition, TNF-inhibition	IL-1 inhibition

FMF, familial Mediterranean fever; HIDS, hyperimmunoglobulin D and periodic fever syndrome; CAPS, cryopyrin-associated periodic syndrome; TRAPS, tumor necrosis factor (TNF) receptor-associated periodic syndrome.
[a]In patients that do not receive appropriate treatment.

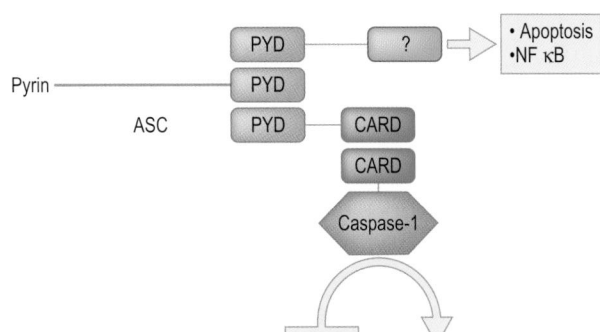

Fig. 59.1 Inflammatory mechanism of pyrin. Pyrin contains a PYD domain that can bind to apoptosis-associated speck-like protein (ASC). ASC in turn, can recruit caspase-1 via the CARD domain. Caspase-1 is capable of cleaving inactive proIL-1β into active IL-1β.

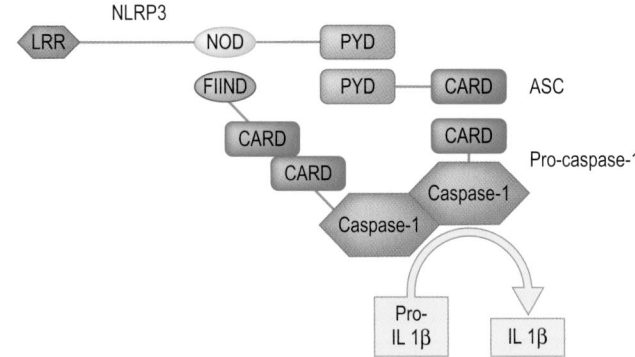

Fig. 59.2 The NLRP3 inflammasome. NLRP3 (or cryopyrin) is the central component of this inflammasome. NLRP3 contains three domains: a pyrin domain (PYD), a nucleoside oligomerization domain (NOD), and a domain of leucine-rich repeats (LRR). Cryopyrin binds ASC through its PYD domain and through the NOD domain. The association of these proteins ultimately leads to the release of active caspase-1, which in turn activates IL-1β through the cleavage of proIL-1β. Upon its secretion into the extracellular milieu, IL-1β sets off a series of events that result in inflammation.

neutrophils and monocytes. Pyrin is a cytosolic protein and its expression is upregulated during myeloid differentiation. Several proinflammatory cytokines upregulate transcription of the MEFV gene.[9]

Pyrin is the first of a new class of proteins discovered that play an important role in the regulation of inflammation and apoptosis. These *Pyrin domain* (PYD)-containing proteins can bind to the PYD domain of other proteins like the apoptosis-associated speck-like protein (ASC), forming complexes that activate caspase-1 to produce IL-1β. Possibly, pyrin can also bind to other PYD proteins that can initiate apoptosis or activate NF-κB (Fig. 59.1). Pyrin can also itself be cleaved by caspase-1 and the cleaved N-terminal fragment translocates to the nucleus and enhances ASC-independent nuclear factor (NF)-κB activation through interactions with p65 NF-κB and IκB-α.[10]

Cryopyrin-associated periodic syndrome (CAPS)

The mutated gene in cryopyrin-associated periodic syndrome (CAPS) encodes another member of the PYD protein family, which was unknown at the time of the discovery of the disease association.[2] In analogy with pyrin in FMF, and to indicate the influence of cold in this syndrome, the protein was named cryopyrin—however, the official name is now NLRP3 (other previous designations for the protein that can make the literature confusing: NALP3, PYPAF1). NLRP3 is predominantly expressed in monocytes and granulocytes. NLRP3 is able to associate with other proteins to form a complex termed the inflammasome. In the NLRP3 inflammasome, NLRP3 associates with the adaptor protein ASC, which in turn recruits the proinflammatory caspase precursor procaspase-1 (Fig. 59.2). The conversion of procaspase-1 into caspase-1 leads to the conversion of pro-IL-1β into IL-1β. IL-1β is a key mediator of inflammation, with a wide variety of effects ranging from induction of fever and extravasation of leukocytes to enhanced expression of adhesion molecules on endothelial cells and induction of bone resorption.[11]

Tumor necrosis factor receptor-associated periodic syndrome (TRAPS)

TRAPS is caused by mutations in TNFRSF1A, located on chromosome12p13. The gene encodes TNF receptor superfamily 1A (TNFRSF1A), the main surface receptor for TNF.[12] TNFRSF1A has three important domains: an extracellular ligand-binding

domain, a transmembrane portion, and an intracellular effector domain (DD) belonging to the DD superfamily. More than 50 different TNFRSF1A mutations have been described that cause TRAPS. The TRAPS-associated mutations are all located within the extracellular domain of the molecule. The TNF receptor forms trimers after binding to its ligand. This triggers the recruitment of adaptor proteins, which can initiate a downstream signaling cascade leading to NF-κB and MAPK activation, and caspase-induced apoptosis (Fig. 59.3). Furthermore, upon receptor activation through TNF, the extracellular domain of the TNF receptor is shed from the membrane. This shedding of receptors leads to a pool of soluble TNF receptors that is thought to mitigate the immune response.

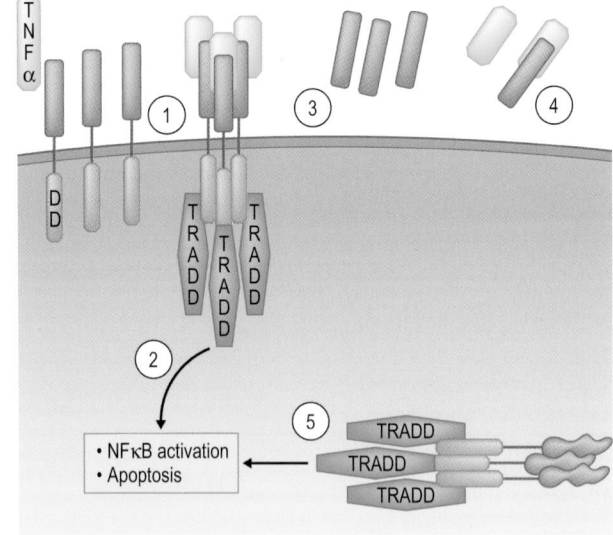

Fig. 59.3 Proposed pathophysiology of tumor necrosis factor receptor-associated periodic syndrome (TRAPS). (1) Tumor necrosis factor (TNF) binds to the TNF receptor on the surface of inflammatory cells (2). After receptor triggering, TRADD is recruited and a signal leads to apoptosis and cytokine production (3). In healthy individuals the receptors are shed from the surface, leading to a pool of receptors that dampen immune response (4). In patients with TRAPS there is diminished shedding, which may lead to a proinflammatory state by ongoing stimulation of retained cell surface receptors. Alternatively, the deficiency of soluble TNF receptors reduces scavenging of excess TNF. (5) Other research has shown that mutated TNF receptors form aggregates and are retained intracellularly. These aggregated receptors are capable of binding TRADD and stimulate ligand-independent cytokine production.

Two hypotheses are offered to explain the inflammatory phenotype of TRAPS. The shedding hypothesis was first coined after the initial observation that patients with TRAPS have reduced serum levels of soluble TNF receptors. Furthermore, in vitro experiments showed that some mutated cell lines exhibit impaired shedding of TNF receptors. The defective shedding would lead to a deficiency of soluble TNF receptors that can scavenge excess TNF and diminish the immune response. Furthermore, since receptors remain present on the membrane, there is ongoing stimulation of the cells. However, the shedding hypothesis fails to explain the complete phenotype, as not all TRAPS patients have defective shedding and TNF-inhibition does not block all TRAPS symptoms. Recently an alternative explanation, the so-called misfolding hypothesis, was proposed.[12] The mutations in the extracellular domain of TNFRSF1A lead to misfolding of the molecule. The misfolded receptors are not expressed at the surface, but are retained intracellularly. in vitro results show that the aggregated TNFRSF1A retain signal function and can induce ligand-independent reactive oxygen species (ROS) production and MAPK signaling, resulting in inflammation.

Two mutations in TNFRSF1A, R92Q and P46L, form an exception. These are present in low frequency in the general population, and do not result in misfolding of the receptor. These mutations do confer a phenotype with increased inflammation, though it differs from classical TRAPS.[12,13] They will not be discussed further here.

Hyperimmunoglobulin D and periodic fever syndrome (HIDS)

HIDS is caused by mutations in the mevalonate kinase gene (MVK), located on the long arm of chromosome 12 (12q24). Mevalonate kinase is a key enzyme in the isoprenoid pathway and follows 3-hydroxy-3methylglutaryl-coenzyme A reductase (HMG coA reductase). In patients with HIDS, the activity of mevalonate kinase is reduced to 5–15% of normal levels — thus, the disease is also known as "mevalonate kinase deficiency."

In the isoprenoid pathway cholesterol is produced in addition to a number of nonsterol isoprenoids. Isoprenoids are essential compounds in diverse cellular function and include ubiquinone, heme A, farnesyl, and geranyl. The direct link between reduced activity of mevalonate kinase and an autoinflammatory condition is not fully understood, but seems to be mediated through geranylgeranylation of small GTP-ases and caspase-1 activation.[2,14] Proinflammatory cytokine production by mononuclear cells of patients with HIDS is strongly enhanced. Furthermore, a defect in apoptosis of HIDS lymphocytes has been detected. It has been hypothesized that this leads to an inability to curtail an excessive cytokine response after a trivial stimulus.

Periodic fever, aphthous stomatitis, pharyngitis, adenitis (PFAPA)

PFAPA does not appear to have a Mendelian inherited genetic background but may be linked to a complex genetic trait. A positive family history has been described in PFAPA,[15,16] although in some of these cases, the hereditary autoinflammatory diseases were not excluded. As in the hereditary syndromes described above, fever episodes are thought to be triggered by external stimuli, possibly microbial in origin,[17,18] despite the fact that the disease flares can occur with great regularity. PFAPA is also distinguished from the other disorders in this chapter because in

the overwhelming majority, symptoms cease during or before adolescence.[6,15] The cause for this spontaneous resolution is unknown (the symptom complex is now also recognized in adults with episodic fever of unknown origin but it is debatable whether the term PFAPA should be used there; see below). Whole-blood RNA microarray studies in 6 PFAPA patients showed upregulation of complement genes during flares, as well as genes in the interferon pathway and in the IL-1 pathway,[17] which fits with the increase of serum concentration of the cytokine IP10.[7,17] During PFAPA flares, a relative neutrophilia and lymphopenia can be observed.[7,17]

Schnitzler syndrome

The etiology of Schnitzler syndrome remains unknown. Involvement of autoreactive antibodies has been suggested but could generally not be confirmed in other studies.[19] This makes the inclusion of Schnitzler syndrome as an autoinflammatory syndrome still a question of debate. A central role of IL-1β is evidenced by ex vivo observations,[20] but especially by the efficacy of anti-IL-1 therapy in clinical practice.[19,21] This disorder is seen as a paraneoplastic syndrome by some; in long-term follow-up, patients have a 15% risk of developing Waldenström's macroglobulinemia after 10 years.[19]

Laboratory investigations

During inflammatory attacks or exacerbations of the hereditary autoinflammatory syndromes, patients invariably show a strong acute-phase response with high CRP concentrations and (polymorphonuclear) leukocytosis. Indeed, if at time of disease exacerbation there is no raised CRP, a hereditary autoinflammatory syndrome can be excluded. During remission, laboratory analysis may show signs of persistent inflammation despite the fact that patients are clinically well, although results can also be normal. In periods of frequent inflammatory attacks, thrombocytosis and anemia of chronic disease may be seen. No cold agglutinins, ANA or any autoantibodies or cryoglobulins are present, or are found only at low titers. Proteinuria (more than 0.5 g of protein per 24 hours) is highly suggestive of amyloidosis. Hyper-IgD syndrome (or mevalonate kinase deficiency) has certain specific biochemical abnormalities, which are discussed in that section; similarly, the paraprotein characteristic of Schnitzler syndrome is discussed in that section.

Clinical features and diagnosis

Familial Mediterranean fever

Clinical features

FMF is an autosomal recessive disease. More than 90% of patients become symptomatic within the first two decades of life. Typically an attack has an abrupt onset with high fever, reaching a peak soon after onset, lasting from 12 hours to 3 days and then rapidly subsiding.[3] There are no consistent triggers, but in some patients vigorous exercise, emotional stress, or menstruation precedes an attack. The frequency of attacks varies greatly between patients, from 2 or 3 times a month to once a year. Even in a given patient the frequency can vary greatly over the years.

Signs of painful serositis accompanying the fever are the hallmark of the disease. Abdominal pain of two to three days'

(HPLC) are necessary for detection. Measurement of mevalonate kinase enzyme activity (e.g., in cultured fibroblasts) is mainly done in research settings.

It has previously been suggested to designate patients with inflammatory attack and raised IgD, without signs of mevalonate kinase deficiency (i.e., no mutation in the *MVK* gene and no increase in mevalonic acid during attacks) as "variant type HIDS." However, this is currently not recommended. A raised IgD can be found in almost any inflammatory condition, and the group of patients designated "variant type HIDS" is very diverse with few common characteristics. It seems preferable to give such patients in which other diagnoses have been excluded a tentative diagnosis of "systemic autoinflammatory syndrome of unknown origin," thus making clear that a further diagnosis might be possible in the future.

Periodic fever, aphthous stomatitis, pharyngitis, adenitis (PFAPA)

Clinical features

PFAPA is described as a childhood disease. Age of onset is before the age of 5 years. Patients present with recurring episodes of fever that generally last 3–6 days and recur every 3–6 weeks; in many children the episodes recur with great regularity.[6,25] Additional symptoms during a fever episode include aphthous stomatitis (38%), pharyngitis (85%), and cervical adenitis (62%), as included in the name of this syndrome.[6] Other symptoms can include headache (44%), vomiting (27%), and mild abdominal pain (41%). Arthralgia and myalgia can also occur. In between fever episodes, children are well, and have normal growth and development. In the majority of patients, symptoms resolve after a number of years without sequelae, generally before or during adolescence.[15]

Lately, it has been suggested that a diagnosis of PFAPA can also be made in adults[26–28] and that it should be considered in patients with recurrent fever of unknown origin. Since PFAPA is still mainly a descriptive diagnosis, this seems currently to be used primarily as a possibility of offering patient and physician a label (instead of the less satisfactory "autoinflammatory syndrome not otherwise specified"), and it should be used with discretion.

Diagnosis

The diagnosis of PFAPA is based on recognition of clinical characteristics; for these, a version of the modified criteria by Thomas et al. is frequently used (Table 59.5),[29] sometimes supplemented by numeric limits, such as minimum number of experienced episodes and number of days of fever.[6] Exclusion of other causes, including the monogenic hereditary autoinflammatory syndromes, is important. There is no diagnostic test.

Schnitzler syndrome

Clinical features

Patients typically present with a chronic, recurrent urticarial rash as the first symptom, commonly without pruritus (in 65% of cases). The full symptom complex (Table 59.6) includes fever, arthralgia or frank arthritis and bone pain. Symptoms progress over the years, and will eventually if left untreated lead to general malaise, fatigue, and weight loss. Mean age of onset is 51 years.[19]

Table 59.5 Diagnostic criteria used for PFAPA

- Regularly recurring fevers with an early age of onset (< 5 years of age)
- Constitutional symptoms in the absence of upper respiratory infection with at least 1 of the following clinical signs:
  - Aphthous stomatitis
  - Cervical lymphadenitis
  - Pharyngitis
- Exclusion of cyclic neutropenia
- Completely asymptomatic interval between episodes
- Normal growth and development

From Thomas et al., Diagnostic criteria used for PFAPA Periodic fever syndrome in children, J Pediatrics,1999;135(1):15–21.

Table 59.6 Diagnostic criteria for Schnitzler syndrome {de Koning Semin Arthritis Rheum 2011}

Major
(Chronic) urticarial rash
Monoclonal IgM (or IgG: variant type)

Minor
Intermittent fever
Arthralgia or arthritis
Bone pain
Lymphadenopathy
Hepato- and/or splenomegaly
Elevated ESR and/or leukocytosis
Bone abnormalities (on radiological or histological examination)
Diagnosis requires a combination of both major criteria and 2 or more minor criteria after exclusion of other causes.

From de Koning, Diagnostic Criteria for Schnitzler Syndrome, Semin Arthritis Rheum, 2007:37(3):137–148.

A retrospective study of 94 patients, in which 40 patients had a follow-up of at least 10 years, indicated a normal life expectancy compared with the general population (91% survival after 15 years). Eleven patients of this group had developed Waldenström's macroglobulinemia, or an incidence of 15% at 10 years follow-up.[19]

Diagnosis

Diagnosis is based on clinical criteria (Table 59.6). Exclusion of other causes, particularly other causes of the paraproteinemia, is of paramount importance. Onset of symptoms can precede the appearance of a detectable concentration of paraprotein by several years, and symptom severity is not dependent on the amount or type of paraprotein.[19] Characteristic for Schnitzler syndrome is an IgM type paraprotein; when an IgG paraprotein is found the term "variant type" Schnitzler syndrome is sometimes used.

Other hereditary autoinflammatory syndromes

A few other hereditary autoinflammatory syndromes with a clear Mendelian inheritance pattern are discussed briefly.

Pyogenic arthritis, pyoderma gangrenosum and acne (PAPA) syndrome

PAPA syndrome is characterized by the features that are in its name. Age of onset is in childhood, and it is inherited in an autosomal dominant pattern; (minor) trauma is often a triggering factor for the sterile erosive pyogenic arthritis and pyoderma gangrenosum. Fever is not a major symptom. It is caused by a mutation in the gene for the protein PSTPIP1 (also known as CD2BP1), which can interact with pyrin. This suggests that it would share a pathogenic pathway with FMF, although the phenotype is very different.[3,30]

Blau syndrome (BS)

Blau syndrome, which is also known as familial or pediatric granulomatous arthritis or early-onset sarcoidosis (EOS), is a granulomatous disease with an autosomal dominant inheritance pattern. The typical sites that are affected are skin, including a maculopapular skin rash, joints, with a polyarticular granulomatous arthritis, and eyes, with a granulomatous uveitis. In severe cases, the granulomatous inflammation can disseminate to liver, lung and kidney. Diagnosis is made by a combination of medical history, histologic evidence of (non-caseating) granulomas at the site of inflammation and genetic testing for mutations in the *NOD2/CARD15* gene.[3]

Deficiency of the interleukin-1–receptor antagonist (DIRA)

In 2009 a new autoinflammatory syndrome was described in nine patients from six families arising from Canada, the Netherlands, Puerto Rico, and Lebanon. The syndrome is characterized by neonatal onset of pustular skin rash and sterile multifocal osteomyelitis and periostitis. Empirical therapy with anakinra proved very successful, leading to a search for mutations in the IL-1 pathway. Indeed, homozygous mutations were identified in the IL-1 receptor antagonist gene (*IL1RN*). The *IL1RN* mutations result in a truncated protein of the natural occurring IL-1 receptor antagonist that is not secreted. Thus, cells are hyper-responsive to IL-1β stimulation.[31] The severe proinflammatory phenotype and the strong clinical response to substitution of IL-1RA (anakinra) stress the importance of a balance in the IL-1 response and the central role of this cytokine in the pathogenesis of the auto-inflammatory diseases.

NLRP12-associated periodic fever syndrome

NLRP12-associated periodic fever syndrome is, as its name suggests, caused by a mutation in NLRP12 protein (previously known as NALP12, MONARCH1 or PYPAF7). It has been described in two families, with a phenotype consisting of episodic fever, arthralgia and skin lesions, triggered by cold exposure. Therefore, the name "familial cold autoinflammatory syndrome type 2" is also used.[32]

Deficiency of IL-36 receptor antagonist (DITRA) in generalized pustular psoriasis

Deficiency of IL-36 receptor antagonist (DITRA) in generalized pustular psoriasis was most recently genetically identified by two groups, who published almost simultaneously in 2011.[33,34] This disorder is characterized by episodic generalized pustular skin inflammation that can be accompanied by fever, general malaise. It can be lethal. Through homozygosity mapping in nine Tunisian multiplex families[33] and through exome-sequencing in five unrelated individuals from European ancestry,[34] respectively, two research groups identified missense mutations in the gene for IL-36 receptor antagonist, resulting in deficiency of this protein. The IL-36 receptor antagonist inhibits IL-36α, -36β, and -36γ, three cytokines belonging to the IL-1 cytokine family—underlining similarities with DIRA (see above), although DITRA seems to have less extracutaneous organ involvement.

Autoinflammatory disease of unknown origin

Despite the fact that clinical assessment allows the identification of a number of syndromes, we fail to make a classifiable diagnosis in a large proportion of patients who consult us with periodic fever. It is therefore expected that study of the pathogenesis of the various autoinflammatory syndromes will identify new proteins and pathways implicated in hitherto unrecognized syndromes.

Amyloidosis

Reactive or type AA amyloidosis is a serious complication of all autoinflammatory syndromes.[35] It is caused by the deposition of insoluble fibrils in the extracellular matrix of organs and tissues, most notably the kidneys, spleen, and liver. The fibrils are composed of a degradation product of SAA. Since SAA is an acute-phase reactant there is a close relationship between the continuous elevation of SAA and the development of amyloidosis. Before the recognition of colchicine as an effective treatment for FMF, amyloidosis occurred in up to 75% of patients. Even before the advent of effective treatment, not all FMF patients developed amyloidosis, suggesting that other factors contribute to the risk of developing amyloidosis.

In FMF there is a strong correlation between ethnicity and risk of amyloidosis, with the highest risk for Sephardic Jews. Another identified risk factor for developing amyloidosis is single nucleotide polymorphisms (SNPs) in the *SAA* gene. Two SNPs define three different SAA proteins: SAA 1.1, 1.3, and 1.5. Patients with the *SAA 1.1/1.1* genotype have a three- to sevenfold increased risk of developing amyloidosis.

Up to a quarter of TRAPS patients develop amyloidosis, if the disease is left untreated. There seems to be a strong family predilection. In some families almost all adults are affected whereas in other families no cases of amyloidosis are found. In CAPS, an estimated one-third of patients develop amyloidosis if the disease is left untreated, although exact numbers are missing.

Patients with HIDS have a relatively small risk of developing amyloidosis: only 4–5 cases of HIDS patients with amyloidosis are known world-wide. This is a remarkably lower incidence of amyloidosis in HIDS compared to the other periodic fever syndromes, despite a similar acute-phase response.[36]

A diagnosis of amyloidosis is confirmed by Congo red staining of affected tissues, showing a typical apple-green birefringence under polarized light microscopy (Fig. 59.5). Biopsy of subcutaneous fat or rectal tissue can be used to detect amyloid fibrils. If these are negative and there is a high index of suspicion, a direct biopsy from an affected organ can be considered.

The natural history of amyloidosis is progression to renal failure. If inflammation cannot be controlled, amyloid deposits in a variety of organs (liver, spleen, gastrointestinal tract, heart) occur. As a consequence malabsorption with severe diarrhea may ensue. Cardiac failure and rhythm disturbances are typical manifestations of cardiac involvement. The prognosis of patients with established amyloidosis is grave, with a median survival of 24–53 months. However, the progression of amyloidosis is strongly dependent on the ability to control the underlying inflammatory process.

Antiplatelet agents other than aspirin, long-term LMWH treatment, or direct/indirect thrombin inhibitors, empirically used, have not been formally tested in clinical trials. Platelet glycoprotein IIb/IIIa specific antagonists, P38MAPK inhibitors, thromboxane A2 inhibitors, tissue factor expression inhibitors, complement inhibitors, and synthetic peptides, may be candidates for future clinical trials.

Conclusions and translational research

● ON THE HORIZON

Translational research in antiphospholipid syndrome

- A better understanding of the cellular mechanisms of antiphospholipid antibody (aPL)-mediated clinical events that will help us design more specifically targeted treatments.
- Identification of patients who are at risk for future aPL-related events.
- Controlled studies of theoretically useful medications such as hydroxychloroquine, statins, complement inhibitors, or anti-B-cell therapies.

APS is a systemic autoimmune systemic disease consisting of thromboses, pregnancy losses, and persistent high-titer aPL. Inflammation and complement activation are established mechanisms of aPL-related manifestations in murine models; however, definitive studies in humans do not exist. The disease is too variable clinically, and its mechanisms too diverse, to expect that a single mechanism defined in a single model will apply to all aspects of this disease. Given that the mechanisms of aPL-induced thrombosis are not well understood, thrombosis is multifactorial, and controversies exist about the strength of association between aPL and clinical events, the drug development specific for aPL-positive patients has been challenging. Anticoagulation is the primary treatment today, but a future therapeutic approach will likely include immunomodulatory agents.

References

1. Miyakis S, Lockshin MD, Atsumi T, et al. International consensus statement on an update of the classification criteria for definite antiphospholipid syndrome (APS). J Thromb Haemost 2006;4:295.
2. Wilson WA, Gharavi AE, Koike T, et al. International consensus statement on preliminary classification criteria for definite antiphospholipid syndrome: report of an international workshop. Arthritis Rheum 1999;42:1309.
3. Koike T, Ichikawa K, Kasahara K. Epitopes on beta2-GPI recognized by anticardiolipin antibodies. Lupus 1998;7(Suppl 2):S14.
4. Manfredi AA, Rovere P, Heltai S, et al. Apoptotic cell clearance in systemic lupus erythematosus. II. Role of b2-glycoprotein I. Arthritis Rheum 1998;41:215.
5. Petri M. Epidemiology of the antiphospholipid antibody syndrome. J Autoimmun 2000;15:145.
6. Olech E, Merrill JT. The prevalence and clinical significance of antiphospholipid antibodies in rheumatoid arthritis. Curr Rheumatol Rep 2006;8:100.
7. Ginsburg JS, Liang MH, Newcomer L, et al. Anticardiolipin antibodies and the risk for ischemic stroke and venous thrombosis. Ann Intern Med 1992;117:997.
8. The Antiphospholipid Antibody Stroke Study (APASS) Group. Anticardiolipin antibodies are an independent risk factor for first ischemic stroke. Neurology 1993;43:2069.
9. Levine SR, Brey RL, Sawaya KL, et al. Recurrent stroke and thrombo-occlusive events in the antiphospholipid syndrome. Ann Neurol 1995;38:119.
10. Stephenson MD. Frequency of factors associated with habitual abortion in 197 couples. Fertil Steril 1996;66:24.
11. Erkan D, Lockshin MD. What is antiphospholipid syndrome? Curr Rheumatol Rep 2004;6:451.
12. Gharavi AE, Pierangeli SS, Harris EN. Origin of antiphospholipid antibodies. Rheum Dis Clin North Am 2001;27:551.
13. Blank M, Krause I, Fridkin M, et al. Bacterial induction of autoantibodies to beta2-glycoprotein-I accounts for the infectious etiology of antiphospholipid syndrome. J Clin Invest 2002;109:797.
14. Gharavi AE, Sammaritano LR, Wen J, et al. Induction of antiphospholipid antibodies by immunization with beta 2 glycoprotein I (apolipoprotein H). J Clin Invest 1992;90:1105.
15. Kamboh MI, Manzi S, Mehdi H, et al. Genetic variation in apolipoprotein H (beta2-glycoprotein I) affects the occurrence of antiphospholipid antibodies and apolipoprotein H concentrations in systemic lupus erythematosus. Lupus 1999;8:742.
16. Bancsi LFJMM, Van der Linden IK, Bertina RM. b2-glycoprotein I deficiency and the risk of thrombosis. Thromb Haemost 1992;67:649.
17. Sheng Y, Reddel SW, Herzog H, et al. Impaired thrombin generation in beta 2-glycoprotein I null mice. J Biol Chem 2001;276:13817.
18. Nojima J, Suehisa E, Kuratsune H, et al. Platelet activation induced by combined effects of anticardiolipin and lupus anticoagulant IgG antibodies in patients with systemic lupus erythematosus-possible association with thrombotic and thrombocytopenic complications. Thromb Haemost 1999;81:436.
19. Smirnov MD, Triplett DT, Comp PC, et al. On the role of phosphatidylethanolamine in the inhibition of activated protein C activity by antiphospholipid antibodies. J Clin Invest 1995;95:309.
20. Rand JH, Wu XX, Guller S, et al. Antiphospholipid immunoglobulin G antibodies reduce annexin-V levels on syncytiotrophoblast apical membranes and in culture media of placental villi. Am J Obstet Gynecol 1997;177:918.
21. Roubey RA. New approaches to prevention of thrombosis in the antiphospholipid syndrome: hopes, trials, and tribulations. Arthritis Rheum 2003;48:3004.
22. Girardi G, Berman J, Redecha P, et al. Complement C5a receptors and neutrophils mediate fetal injury in the antiphospholipid syndrome. J Clin Invest 2003;112:1644.
23. Roman MJ, Shanker B-A, Davis A, et al. Prevalence and correlates of accelerated atherosclerosis in systemic lupus erythematosus: a case-control study. N Engl J Med 2003;349:2399.
24. Oshiro BT, Silver RM, Scott JR, et al. Antiphospholipid antibody and fetal death. Obstet Gynecol 1996;87:489.
25. Asherson RA, Cervera R, de Groot P, et al. Catastrophic antiphospholipid syndrome (CAPS): International Consensus Statement on Classification Criteria and Treatment Guidelines. Lupus 2003;12:530.
26. Erkan D, Espinosa G, Cervera R. Catastrophic Antiphospholipid Syndrome: Updated Diagnostic Algorithms. Autoimmun Rev 2010;10(2):74–9.
27. Horbach DA, Vanoort E, Derksen RHWM, et al. The contribution of anti-prothrombin-antibodies to lupus anticoagulant activity-Discrimination between functional and non-functional anti-prothrombin antibodies. Thromb Haemost 1998;79:790.
28. Erkan D, Bateman H, Lockshin MD. Lupus-anticoagulant - Hypoprothrombinemia syndrome associated with systemic lupus erythematosus: report of 2 cases and review of literature. Lupus 1999;8:560.
29. Ortel TL. The antiphospholipid syndrome: what are we really measuring? How do we measure it? And how do we treat it? J Thromb Thrombolysis 2006;21:79.
30. Pengo V, Tripodi A, Reber G, et al. Update of the guidelines for lupus anticoagulant detection. Subcommittee on Lupus Anticoagulant/Antiphospholipid Antibody of the Scientific and Standardisation Committee of the International Society on Thrombosis and Haemostasis. J Thromb Haemost 2009;7:1737.
31. Galli M, Luciani D, Bertolini G, Barbui T. Lupus anticoagulants are stronger risk factors for thrombosis than anticardiolipin antibodies in the antiphospholipid syndrome: a systematic review of the literature. Blood 2003;101:1827.
32. Erkan D, Derksen WJ, Kaplan V, et al. Real world experience with antiphospholipid antibody tests: how stable are results over time? Ann Rheum Dis 2005;64:1321.
33. Erkan D, Lockshin MD. New approaches to the management of Antiphospholipid Syndrome. Nat Clin Pract Rheumatol 2009;5(3):160.
34. Vero S, Asherson RA, Erkan D. Critical care review: catastrophic antiphospholipid syndrome. J Intensive Care Med, in press.
35. Crowther MA, Ginsberg JS, Julian J, et al. Comparison of two intensities of warfarin for the prevention of recurrent thrombosis in patients with the antiphospholipid antibody syndrome. N Engl J Med 2003;349:1133.
36. Finazzi G, Marchioli R, Brancaccio V, et al. A randomized clinical trial of high-intensity warfarin vs. conventional antithrombotic therapy for the prevention of recurrent thrombosis in patients with the antiphospholipid syndrome (WAPS). J Thromb Haemost 2005;3:848.
37. Levine SR, Brey RL, Tilley BC, et al. Antiphospholipid antibodies and subsequent thrombo-occlusive events in patients with ischemic stroke. JAMA 2004;291:576.
38. Barbhaiya M, Erkan D. Primary thrombosis prophylaxis in antiphospholipid antibody patients: where do we stand? Curr Rheumatol Rep 2011;13(1):59.
39. Erkan D, Harrison MJ, Levy R, et al. Aspirin for primary thrombosis prevention in the antiphospholipid syndrome: a randomized, double-blind, placebo-controlled trial in asymptomatic antiphospholipid antibody-positive individuals. Arthritis Rheum 2007;56:2382.
40. Derksen RH, Khamashta MA, Branch DW. Management of the obstetric antiphospholipid syndrome. Arthritis Rheum 2004;50:1028.
41. Erkan D, Leibowitz E, Berman J, Lockshin MD. Perioperative medical management of antiphospholipid syndrome: Hospital for Special Surgery experience, review of the literature and recommendations. J Rheumatol 2002;29:843.
42. Ridker PM, Danielson E, Fonseca FA, et al. JUPITER Trial Study Group. Reduction in C-reactive protein and LDL cholesterol and cardiovascular event rates after initiation of rosuvastatin: a prospective study of the JUPITER trial. Lancet 2009;373:1175.
43. Glynn RJ, Danielson E, Foseca FA, et al. A randomized trial of rosuvastatin in the prevention of venous thromboembolism. N Engl J Med 2009;360:1851.

PART SEVEN

Organ-specific inflammatory disease

Table 61.1 Classification of immune hemolytic disorders

Autoimmune
Warm antibody-mediated Idiopathic
Secondary
Drugs, lymphoid malignancies, infections
Other autoimmune diseases
Cold antibody-mediated Cold agglutinin disease
Idiopathic
Secondary
Infection, lymphoid malignancies
Paroxysmal cold hemoglobinuria Idiopathic
Secondary to infections
Alloimmune
Secondary to red cell transfusions (alloantibodies, isoantibodies)
Secondary to fetomaternal hemorrhage
Secondary to transplanted lymphocytes

Thermal amplitude describes the temperature dependence of its binding to red cells: for example, antibodies that exclusively bind at 4°C are only active *in vitro*, whereas those that bind at > 30°C can bind to red cells in the peripheral circulation and begin the process of complement fixation, which can be continued as the cells return to body core temperatures. The activity of the IgM is also determined by its relative affinity for the I- and i-antigens, which varies from one individual to the next.

Two general types of cold agglutinin disease are recognized: a chronic idiopathic disease presenting in patients over age 50 and caused by monoclonal IgM (monoclonal anti-I), and a transient disease secondary to certain infections (e.g., mycoplasma, Epstein–Barr virus, cytomegalovirus) and caused by polyclonal IgM (polyclonal anti-i and anti-I) (Table 61.1). Avoidance of cold environments is important in both categories of cold agglutinin disease. In addition, cold agglutinin disease can be associated with lymphoproliferative disorders and this typically is responsive to rituximab as well as the combination of rituximab with fludarabine.[6]

Paroxysmal cold hemoglobinuria

Paroxysmal cold hemoglobinuria (PCH) is caused by anti-P IgG that is very effective in fixing complement and producing intravascular hemolysis.[2] Although rare, it is most common in children following a viral illness and can be managed by avoidance of cold. In the past it was more commonly associated with syphilis (Table 61.1). There is also an autoimmune variety of PCH that may require immunosuppression with corticosteroids. As a consequence of the fact that the hemolysis is intravascular, splenectomy is not helpful.

Hemolytic transfusion reactions

Because individuals with group O red cells have preformed iso-anti-A and -B, they must only be transfused with group O cells. Similarly, individuals with group A red cells with preformed anti-B isoantibodies must only receive group A red cells, and individuals with group B red cells must only receive group B red cells. Because of the absence of either group A or B antigens on the surface of group O red cells, such cells can be used in transfusion of A, B, or AB individuals in emergency situations. Failure to abide by these rules results in acute intravascular hemolysis that can cause renal failure, disseminated intravascular coagulation and death.

Other hemolytic transfusion reactions are caused by alloantibodies, predominantly IgG. Therefore, a multiply transfused patient is at risk for hemolysis from alloantibodies if the patient receives incompatible blood. Multiparous women are at similar risk because of exposure to paternal fetal red cell antigens. Fortunately, for unclear reasons, most red cell antigens do not elicit an immune response although Rh, Kell, Kidd, and Duffy are clearly immunogenic. Exposure particularly to Kidd or Duffy antigens may stimulate alloantibody formation that can rise to sufficient titer to cause hemolysis with an onset typically delayed by approximately one week. Such delayed transfusion reactions may be subtle or cause an abrupt drop in hemoglobin with jaundice and hemoglobinuria.

Immune hemolysis associated with transplantation

Any transplanted tissue may contain "passenger" lymphocytes that will survive if the recipient is sufficiently immunosuppressed.[7] When the red cells of the recipient carry A- or B-antigen and the donor is ABO-incompatible, the transplanted lymphocytes will respond to the recipient red cells as foreign, and allogeneic anti-A or anti-B antibodies will be produced that can lead to significant hemolysis. If the transplant involves hematopoietic stem cells, this dilemma will resolve once the donor's erythropoiesis prevails and the donor lymphocytes are no longer exposed to recipient red cells.

Immunopathogenesis

The antigens for anti-erythrocyte IgG are usually proteins, including the clinically important antigens (D, C, c, E, e) on the Rh-associated glycoprotein (RhAG).[8] In contrast, anti-erythrocyte IgM is directed at polysaccharides, which include the ABO and I-antigens (I, i) found on the anion and glucose transporter proteins in the red cell membrane.[9,10]

IgG and IgM antibodies are distinguished by being "warm-" and "cold-" reactive respectively, meaning that they can bind to their antigens at core body temperature (warm) or they bind preferentially at lower temperatures (cold) in the peripheral circulation or *ex vivo*. This distinction results from the different thermodynamics of binding to protein (hydrophobic) and polysaccharide (electrostatic) antigens.[10]

IgG and IgM also differ in their ability to fix complement, and this affects the resulting mechanism of hemolysis. In order to attach the first component of the classical complement pathway, two IgG molecules must bind to the red cell in close proximity. However, because of its pentameric structure, a single IgM molecule can initiate complement activation.

Erythrocyte-bound IgG becomes attached to the Fc receptors of splenic macrophages, which may engulf all or part of the cell or release lysosomal enzymes that digest its membrane (antibody-dependent cell-mediated cytotoxicity or ADCC).[11] Red cell fragments escaping from this encounter lose more membrane than cytoplasm and become spherical (spherocytes) to compensate for this change in their surface-to-volume ratio. If IgG has initiated complement activation on the cell surface, binding of

C3b to splenic macrophages will augment erythrocyte phagocytosis in the spleen.[12]

When IgM fixes complement, the process begins in the cooler peripheral circulation, which facilitates IgM binding to red cells. If the amount of IgM bound is relatively high with at least some of it remaining on the cell at 37°C (e.g., anti-A or anti-B isoantibodies), the cascade of complement activation goes to completion. Doughnut-shaped holes are formed in the cell membrane that allow the influx of water and sodium, inducing intravascular osmotic rupture of the cell.[11] However, if the IgM elutes from the red cell as it returns to body core temperature, the complement reaction diminishes. In these circumstances the components remain on the cell but do not cause intravascular hemolysis. Instead, the cells are cleared by hepatic macrophages via complement-binding sites.[13]

Antibody-mediated hemolysis causes variable degrees of anemia and reticulocytosis. Intravascular hemolysis releases hemoglobin into the circulation. However, the amount of hemoglobin swept away as macrophages are engulfing red cells is generally too small to cause measurable hemoglobinemia, although it will result in consumption of haptoglobin, which quickly becomes depleted. In contrast, when hemolysis results from complement-mediated lysis, such as follows an ABO-incompatible blood transfusion, hemoglobinemia becomes massive, overcoming the scavenging capacity of plasma hemoglobin binders (haptoglobin, hemopexin, albumin) and resulting in hemoglobinuria. Because hemoglobin is toxic to the renal tubular epithelium, renal function may become impaired. Red cell membrane fragments released by massive intravascular hemolysis are procoagulant and can cause disseminated intravascular coagulation.

In contrast, the consequences of extravascular hemolysis (i.e., via phagocytosis) are much less severe. In macrophages iron is removed from the hemoglobin and recycled to the circulation to support a compensatory reticulocytosis while the heme porphyrin is metabolized to bilirubin.

Patients with immune-mediated anemia have an increased incidence of venous thromboembolism and detection of a lupus anticoagulant in these patients places them at a particularly high risk for this complication.[14]

Diagnosis

With few exceptions, if the mechanism is immune-mediated, an anti-red cell antibody can be demonstrated, either on the red cell surface, in the serum or in both samples.[1,2] With autoimmune hemolysis immunoglobulin (IgG or IgM) and/or complement components can be identified by a direct antibody test (DAT), originally known as a direct Coombs test (Fig. 61.1). For this assay a patient's red cells are washed and suspended in buffer. Surface-bound IgG is detected by adding anti-IgG antibody, which, being divalent, can bind to IgG on adjacent red cells and agglutinate them into visible aggregates. Because of its pentameric structure, IgM on the cells can cause agglutination without the addition of a second antibody. Even when IgM has previously eluted from the cell surface, its earlier presence *in vivo* can be detected by telltale remnants of complement that are fixed to the red cell. In this setting detection requires the addition of anti-complement (e.g., anti-C3dg) antibody.

Alloantibodies can also be detected by the DAT if allogeneic red cells are still circulating from a previous transfusion. If these have been cleared, however, red cell antibodies can be identified in the patient's serum by adding the serum to a panel of red cells carrying different antigens. Agglutination is detected as described above; this constitutes the indirect antibody test.

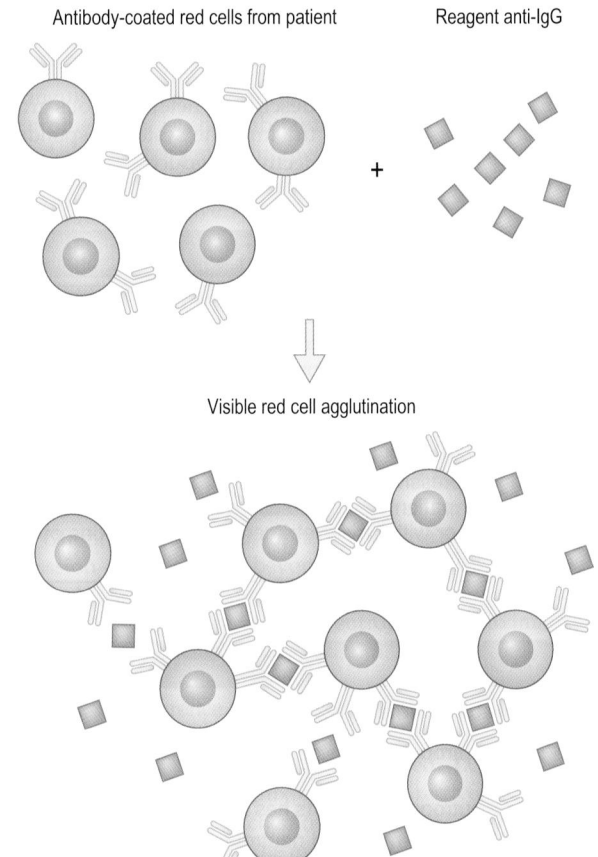

Fig. 61.1 The direct antibody test (DAT). The test is positive when immunoglobulin G (IgG: light blue triangles)-coated red cells are cross-linked by anti-IgG antibody (dark blue triangles) to form visible cell aggregates. Cell-bound complement and/or IgM can be detected by using anti-complement or anti-IgM reagent antibodies.

Therapy

The first line of therapy is corticosteroids and 80% of patients achieve a partial or complete response to 1 mg/kg/d of prednisone (orally). Once a response is achieved the prednisone dose is weaned slowly. Approximately 50% of patients require prednisone at a dose of 15 mg/d or less to maintain the hemoglobin level > 10 g/dL and it may take up to 3 weeks for patients to achieve a response. Patients who do not respond in 3 weeks should be started on second-line therapy. It is estimated that long-term complete responses not requiring prednisone can be achieved in 20% of patients.[15]

Splenectomy and anti-CD20 antibody (rituximab) are considered second-line therapy. Splenectomy is associated with short-term partial or complete responses in two-thirds of patients. The overall response rate to rituximab is approximately 80% but rituximab is contraindicated in patients with untreated hepatitis B. The rare, but most severe long-term complication of rituximab therapy is progressive multifocal leukoencephalopathy.[15]

Danazol, a synthetic anabolic steroid, has been used as a first-line agent in conjunction with prednisone; its effectiveness appears to be less in relapsed or refractory disease. The role of high-dose intravenous immunoglobulin remains controversial; its effectiveness remains to be determined in larger trials. Third-line therapy consists of immunosuppressive agents (e.g., azathioprine, cyclophosphamide, alemtuzumab, mycophenolate mofetil, cyclosporine).[1,15]

Khaled M. Hassan, Russell P. Hall III

Bullous diseases of the skin and mucous membranes

Pemphigus

Pemphigus is the term used to describe a group of diseases that have in common superficial blistering of the skin and mucous membranes. Pemphigus can be separated into four distinct groups: pemphigus vulgaris (PV), pemphigus foliaceus (PF), paraneoplastic pemphigus, and intraepidermal immunoglobulin A (IgA) neutrophilic dermatosis.

Pemphigus vulgaris

PV is the most severe form of pemphigus. PV presents most often in the fourth to sixth decades, but has been reported to occur at any age. Clinically, PV is characterized by the presence of flaccid blisters and erosions of the skin and mucous membranes. Virtually all patients with PV will develop oral erosions at some point during the course of their disease. Most present with oral erosions and many have oral erosions as their only disease manifestation for months to years (Fig. 62.1). These lesions are often persistent, shaggy erosions that can involve all areas of the oral mucosa, extending into the esophagus. In severe cases other mucous membranes, such as the conjunctiva, nasal, anal, cervical, or urethral mucosa, can also be affected.

The blisters seen in patients with PV are flaccid, easily ruptured, and can occur on either inflamed or noninflamed skin. The ease with which these blisters rupture is the origin of the Nikolsky sign, which is elicited when lateral traction on the skin results in desquamation of the superficial layer of the skin. This sign, although helpful, is not unique to PV. Once broken these blisters leave large, nonhealing erosions. Blisters can occur on any area of the skin, most often beginning on the head and neck or trunk. Generalized blistering is not uncommon, especially if diagnosis and/or treatment has been delayed (Fig. 62.2).

Pemphigus vegetans is an unusual variant of PV in which lesions develop primarily in the axilla, groin, and other flexural areas. The lesions are characteristically plaques of hypertrophic granulation tissue with occasional pustules. This presentation can occur *de novo* or after healing of PV lesions. The etiology of this unusual clinical presentation is not known.

Before the advent of systemic glucocorticoid therapy, PV was almost uniformly fatal, with patients developing large areas of denuded skin and dying from overwhelming sepsis. Since the introduction of systemic glucocorticoids the mortality rate has fallen to approximately 10%. The residual mortality is due largely to side effects of the high doses of systemic glucocorticoids required to treat the disease, particularly in debilitated or elderly patients.

Histologically, PV is characterized by the presence of an intraepithelial blister, with acantholysis or breaking apart of the suprabasilar portion of the epidermis. Biopsy of an early lesion of PV reveals that the basal cells of the epidermis remain attached to the dermis, forming a 'row of tombstones,' with loss of attachment of individual keratinocytes to each other, resulting in the formation of an intraepidermal blister.

A major advance in the understanding of PV occurred in the early 1960s, when investigators found IgG antibodies bound to the epithelial keratinocyte cell surface in the skin of patients with PV and showed that serum of patients with PV contained IgG antibodies that bound in an identical pattern to normal human skin.[1] These findings demonstrated that PV is an autoimmune disease directed against a normal component of stratified squamous epithelium.

Pemphigus foliaceus

PF is characterized by blisters within the epidermis, resulting in the development of superficial erosions with scaling and crusting

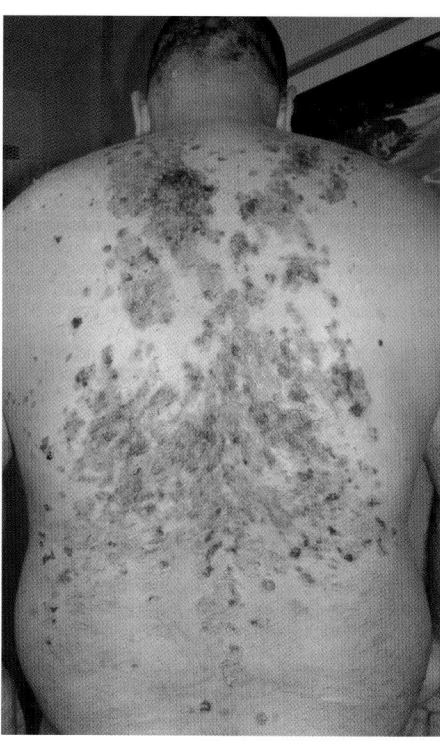

Fig. 62.1 Patient with pemphigus vulgaris showing ulcerative plaques and crust involving the back.

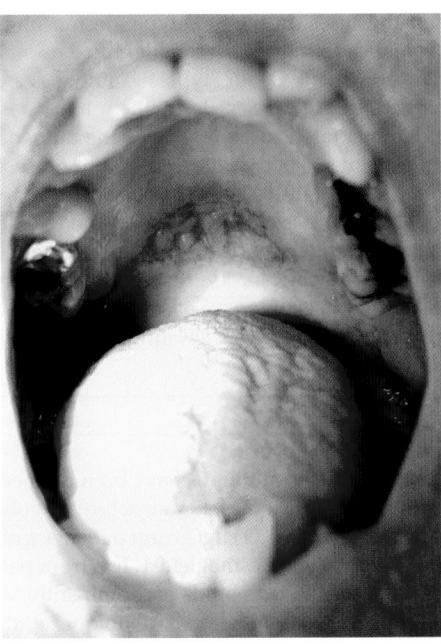

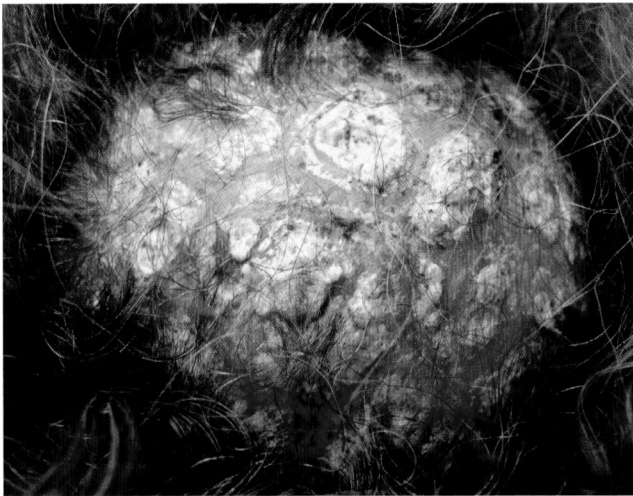

Fig. 62.4 Patient with pemphigus foliaceus showing involvement of the scalp with erosions and adherent crust with alopecia. The patient's hair fully regrew after initiation of treatment.

Fig. 62.2 Patient with pemphigus vulgaris showing ulceration of the soft palate.

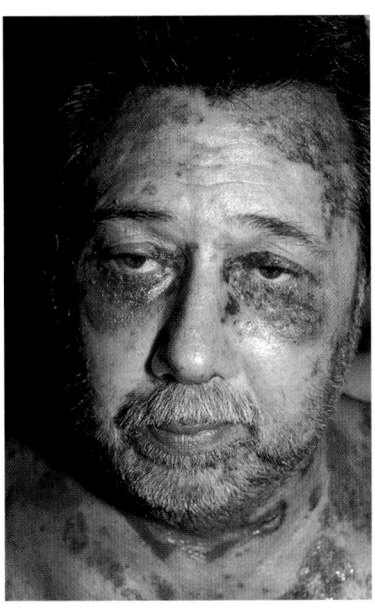

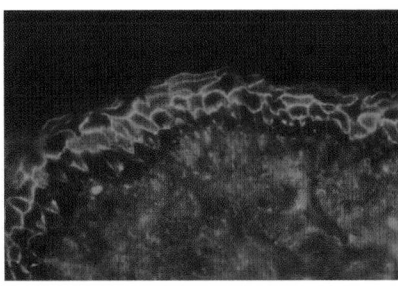

Fig. 62.5 Direct immunofluorescence of perilesional normal-appearing skin from a patient with pemphigus foliaceus using antibodies directed against human immunoglobulin G (IgG). Cell surface IgG deposits are seen on the epidermal keratinocytes. A similar pattern is seen in patients with pemphigus vulgaris.

Fig. 62.3 Patient with pemphigus foliaceus showing superficial erosions and crust formation on the head and neck.

(Fig. 62.3). Unlike patients with PV, those with PF rarely develop mucous membrane lesions. Because of the superficial nature of the blister many patients present with only erythematous, scaling, and crusted plaques on the head, neck, and trunk (Fig. 62.4). The prognosis for patients with PF is markedly better than for those with PV, although patients with severe disease do occasionally die as a result of infections and/or therapy. The better prognosis is likely secondary to the more superficial nature of the blistering process.

An unusual variant of PF is the endemic form of the disease, fogo selvagem (Portuguese for "wild fire").[2] Although clinically identical to the sporadic form of PF, fogo selvagem occurs only in certain rural areas of South America. The epidemiology suggests an infectious etiology, and preliminary data suggest that an arthropod vector may be involved in spreading the disease.

Pemphigus erythematosus, or Senear–Usher syndrome, is another variant of PF. These patients have typical features of PF with additional characteristics suggestive of systemic lupus erythematosus, such as malar involvement and antinuclear antibodies. The clinical course tends to parallel that of PF, and most patients do not develop systemic lupus erythematosus. The pathogenesis of this form of PF is poorly understood.

PF can also be associated with drugs. The most common agents that induce pemphigus are D-penicillamine and angiotensin-converting enzyme inhibitors.[3] Although these drugs can induce a PV-like picture, the clinical manifestations are most often similar to those of PF. Patients with drug-induced pemphigus have autoantibodies directed against the keratinocyte cell surface but the pathogenetic mechanisms that lead to formation of these antibodies are unknown. It has been postulated that reactive sulfhydryl or amide groups on the drugs associated with drug-induced pemphigus may be important elements in this reaction.[3]

The histology of a PF blister reveals a superficial, intraepidermal blister with acantholysis of only the most superficial portion of the skin. This blistering occurs in the region of the granular cell layer of the skin, with the result that blisters have a base of epithelium and not the single basal cell layer that is seen in patients with PV.

The immunohistologic features of PF are indistinguishable from those seen in PV (Fig. 62.5). Cell surface deposits of IgG are seen in the skin of patients with PF, and IgG antbodies which

Therapy

The mainstay of therapy for BP is systemic glucocorticoids, with the majority of patients responding rapidly to 0.5–2.0 mg/kg/day of oral prednisone. Mild or localized disease can sometimes be managed by the use of potent topical corticosteroids, but this form of BP may progress to more severe involvement, necessitating systemic therapy. When new blister formation has stopped and healing has begun, a slow taper of the systemic steroids can commence. The speed of the taper is dictated by the severity of the patient's initial disease and the minor flares that may occur during the taper. The majority of patients can be tapered off systemic steroids completely within 6–18 months but recurrence of disease activity is not uncommon. These episodes should be managed with the lowest dose of systemic steroids possible and can occasionally be treated just using topical corticosteroid therapy. In general, BP is a self-limiting process, which usually lasts between 1.5 and 5 years, and responds promptly to treatment with systemic glucocorticoids.[28]

A minority of patients requires prolonged high-dose systemic glucocorticoids. In these individuals, adjunctive use of immunosuppresive agents such as azathioprine, cyclophosphamide, or methotrexate will often allow tapering or discontinuation of systemic steroid therapy. Few prospective, controlled studies have been done to determine which of these drugs, if any, is superior as a steroid-sparing agent. One controlled study reported a benefit to using plasma exchange in addition to prednisone over one month of treatment. Other studies have failed to replicate this finding, or to demonstrate any substantial benefit from using prednisone plus mycophenolate mofetil, niacinamide with tetracycline, or azathioprine.[28] It is important to note, however, that these data do not address the utility of these agents in patients who were unable to discontinue therapy with systemic glucocorticoids. Other unproven adjunctive therapies that may help in some patients include dapsone, cyclosporine and rituximab. When additional therapy is needed, we favor the use of azathioprine at doses of 1–2 mg/kg/day. Analysis of controlled trials concluded that very potent topical steroids may be effective and safe and that starting doses of prednisolone above 0.75 mg/kg/day do not offer any greater benefit.[28]

IVIg has been used at varying dosages, with varying success rates, in the treatment of BP. A recent review of data using IVIg concluded that 70% of patients showed a positive clinical response; in the remaining patients no clinical benefit was observed. A minimum dose of 2 g/kg given over 5 days at monthly intervals for 3 months has been commonly used, and typically more than one cycle has been necessary to prevent recurrence. Occasional side-effects include headache, nausea, and vomiting. In some patients the use of IVIg appears to permit a reduction in systemic corticosteroiddose. Longer use of IVIg has led to sustained clinical remission in some patients. IVIG was ineffective in patients who received low-dose IVIg or who only received a single infusion.[29]

The anti-CD20 chimeric murine monoclonal antibody rituximab, a target-specific therapy used in treatment for BP, eliminates CD20[+] B cells through complement- and antibody-dependent cell-mediated cytotoxicity, as well as by inducing structural changes and apoptosis. The targeted B cells remain absent from the circulation for 6–12 months. Several groups have reported clinical success using rituximab for pemphigus, but it has only had limited success in the treatment of BP.[30]

Epidermolysis bullosa acquisita

EBA is a chronic subepidermal blistering disease that typically presents in the fourth to sixth decades. EBA usually presents in one of two forms—a classic, non-inflammatory type with blisters on distal extremities, and an inflammatory type that closely resembles bullous pemphigoid. Patients with the classic form of EBA present with peripherally-distributed blisters that heal with scarring and milia formation. The skin of these patients is extremely fragile, often resulting in numerous erosions in areas of mechanical trauma, such as the hands, feet, elbows, and knees. Oral mucous membrane lesions, including esophageal involvement, are often seen. Patients with classic EBA may also develop ocular, vaginal, urethral, and rectal mucosal lesions. Ocular changes are common, and these patients may clinically resemble those with MMP. Other cutaneous manifestations include scarring alopecia and variable degrees of nail dystrophy. Patients with the nonclassic inflammatory type of EBA often display a similar clinical presentation to that seen in BP, with widespread tense bullae on an erythematous base, which heal without scarring (Fig. 62.10).[31]

EBA has been associated with a variety of diseases, particularly inflammatory bowel disease and bullous systemic lupus erythematosus. These associations may partly result from the association of EBA with HLA-DR2.[32]

Skin biopsies of early lesions from patients with EBA reveal subepidermal blisters with variable degrees of inflammation. In patients with classic EBA, lesional skin biopsies often have a minimal inflammatory cell infiltrate. In contrast, patients with the inflammatory variant may have substantial collections of inflammatory cells in the superficial dermis, usually consisting of mononuclear cells, PMN, and eosinophils.

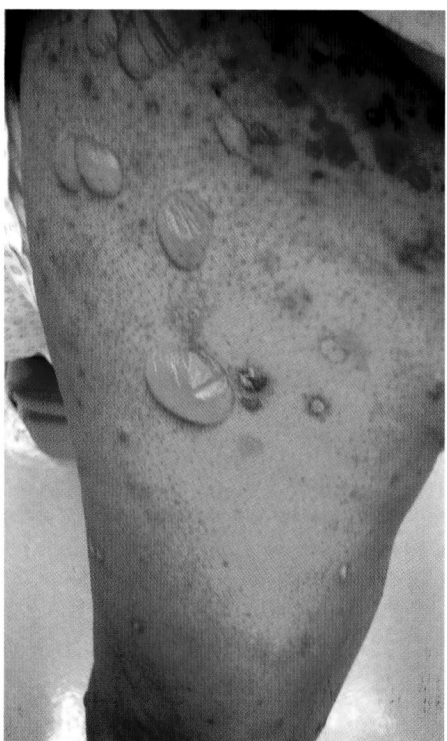

Fig. 62.10 Patient with epidermolysis bullosa acquisita showing extremity involvement with tense bullae. Note the similarity to lesions of bullous pemphigoid, with somewhat less inflammation surrounding the base of bullae.

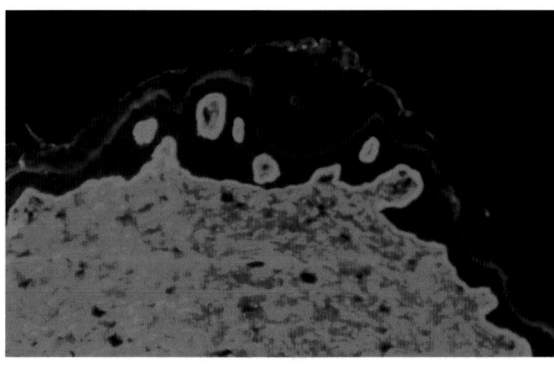

Fig. 62.11 Direct immunofluorescence sample of normal-appearing uninvolved skin from a patient with epidermolysis bullosa acquisita, showing linear deposition of IgG at the dermal-epidermal junction.

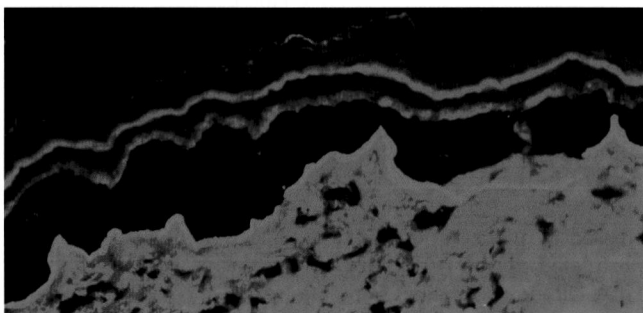

Fig. 62.12 Direct immunofluorescence sample from a patient with EBA after incubation with 1 mol/L NaCl, showing localization of IgG immunoreactants to the floor (dermal side) of the blister cavity.

Direct immunofluorescence of perilesional skin biopsies from patients with EBA displays a similar pattern to BP, with linear deposits of IgG at the DEJ. Linear deposits of C3, IgM, IgA, and fibrinogen have also been reported in patients with EBA (Fig. 62.11).[31] However, these deposits are localized differently from those found in the skin of patients with BP. In EBA, the deposits are localized exclusively below the lamina lucida. This distinctive pattern can be visualized by incubating the patient's skin biopsy with 1 mol/L NaCl, which splits the skin at the basement membrane zone. Direct immunofluoresence testing of this "split skin" from patients with EBA will show IgG in the floor of the blister, whereas in patients with BP, the IgG is in the blister roof (Fig. 62.12).

Indirect immunofluorescence using stratified squamous epithelia such as normal human skin shows circulating anti-basement membrane-zone antibodies in 30–50% of patients with EBA. However, when NaCl-treated split skin is used as a substrate, IgG antibody can be detected in up to 85% of patients, making this a more sensitive and specific substrate for clinical testing. As would be expected from the *in vivo* deposition pattern, IgG from patients with EBA localizes to the blister floor. Sera from patients with EBA recognize the 300-kDa protein, type VII collagen, primarily targeting its immunodominant NC1 domain, as shown by immunoblotting with normal human dermal extracts.

Pathogenesis

Immunoelectron microscopy has shown immunoglobulin deposits in patients with EBA localized to the lamina densa zone of the basement membrane, below the lamina lucida. Standard transmission electron microscopy of lesional skin of patients with EBA shows that the anchoring fibrils are decreased or absent. These findings may be relevant in the development of the clinically evident skin fragility, as anchoring fibrils are postulated to play a role in epidermal–dermal adherence via the linkage of the hemidesmosome through the basement membrane. The lack of an inflammatory infiltrate in many patients with EBA suggests that autoantibodies may disrupt the interaction between anchoring fibrils and dermal matrix proteins.

The target antigen for the IgG autoantibodies present in the sera of patients with EBA is type VII collagen, a 300-kDa glycoprotein composed of a 145-kDa noncollagenous domain (NC1) at the amino-terminal end, an 18-kDa noncollagenous domain (NC2) at the carboxy-terminus, and a central collagenous domain. IgG antibodies from patients with EBA appear to be specific for epitopes within the NC1 noncollagenous domain of the protein. Type VII collagen is the major structural component of anchoring fibrils and is produced by both epithelial keratinocytes and dermal fibroblasts. Passive transfer experiments in mice, as well as active immune models, have provided additional support for the critical role of antibodies directed against type VII collagen in the pathogenesis of EBA.[31] Recently, researchers have shown that induction of specific types of antibodies is linked to the MHC haplotype in experimental mouse-model EBA, setting the stage for future attempts at identifying non-MHC EBA susceptibility genes.[33]

Treatment

Spontaneous resolution is infrequent in EBA, and management is difficult. The main goals of therapy are to minimize blistering and scar formation, with particular concern for ocular and oral mucosal lesions. Systemic glucocorticoids are the mainstay of therapy, especially for patients with the inflammatory variant of EBA. Unfortunately, even high-dose systemic steroids do not usually affect fragility and trauma-induced blister formation of the skin. Mucosal lesions often respond to systemic steroids in doses of 0.5–1.5 mg/kg/day, but may recur with tapering and/or discontinuation of steroids. Several agents have been proposed as adjunctive agents, including azathioprine, cyclophosphamide, colchicine, dapsone, hydroxychloroquine, and plasmapheresis. However, none has been consistently demonstrated to be effective. Cyclosporine has been used to treat patients with EBA with some success, although toxicity can limit therapy. Photophoresis and IVIg have also been reported effective in some patients with refractory EBA. Rituximab has shown promise in otherwise recalcitrant cases of EBA.[31] Mucous membrane lesions can prove particularly difficult to manage and may necessitate systemic therapy. Patients with ocular lesions should be followed by an ophthalmologist and may require systemic glucocorticoids to prevent conjunctival scarring. Oral mucous membrane lesions can sometimes be managed with frequent application of potent topical steroid ointments or gels (0.05% clobetasol propionate, 0.05% fluocinonide). If this fails and the degree of oral erosions is inhibiting the maintenance of appropriate nutrition, systemic glucocorticoid therapy may be required. In addition, clinicians should be aware of possible involvement of the esophageal and/or tracheal mucosa and involve appropriate specialists to monitor and treat these potentially severe complications.

The management of chronic skin wounds is vitally important in EBA. Protection of the skin from trauma and the early use of topical and systemic antibiotics when infections develop are critical to improving the rate of healing. The development of new biological dressings for chronic ulcers has also proved helpful in the management of these wounds.

therapy alone. If this fails, management techniques such as those discussed for patients with BP are usually successful.[43]

Linear IgA bullous disease

Linear IgA bullous disease (LABD) is a clinically heterogeneous blistering disease in which direct immunofluorescence of perilesional skin biopsies reveals the presence of a linear band of IgA at the basement membrane zone. The majority of patients with LABD present with pruritic vesicles and papules, localized primarily to the extensor surfaces, similar to the clinical pattern seen in patients with dermatitis herpetiformis (DH). Patients with LABD do not, however, have an associated gluten-sensitive enteropathy, are not able to control their disease by a gluten-free diet, and do not have the characteristic HLA associations of patients with DH.

Other patients with linear IgA deposits present with a clinical picture more suggestive of BP, with pruritic tense blisters on an erythematous base. Other clinical presentations have been described with clinical as well as histologic and immunopathologic overlap between patients with LABD and MMP or EBA. Children can develop a subepidermal blistering disease with linear IgA basement membrane deposits, a process previously termed chronic bullous disease of childhood. In these juvenile cases, the blisters occur mainly in flexural surfaces, around the genitalia, and on the face, especially the perioral region.[45]

Histopathology of lesional skin of patients with LABD reflects the clinical heterogeneity seen in these patients. Biopsy usually reveals collections of neutrophils in the dermal papillary tips in a pattern virtually identical to that seen in biopsies from patients with DH. However, subepidermal blisters with eosinophils may also be seen, similar to those observed in patients with BP.

Direct immunofluorescence of perilesional skin in patients with LABD reveals a linear band of IgA, almost exclusively IgA1, at the basement membrane zone.[46] Further characterization of these IgA deposits in the skin has revealed that both κ and λ light chains are present, indicating that the antibodies are polyclonal. In addition, J chain has not been detected, suggesting that the IgA is monomeric and may not be of gut origin. Immunoelectron microscopic localization of the immunoreactants most often reveals IgA deposits in the lamina lucida; however, sublamina densa IgA deposits have also been noted. Circulating IgA antibodies against the basement membrane zone of stratified squamous epithelium are detected in only 10–30% of patients (children and adults) with linear IgA deposits. Other immunoreactants, especially IgG and C3, have been found in 30–40% of these patients.[46]

Pathogenesis

The paucity and heterogeneity of circulating antibody has made it difficult to determine the antigenic target in LABD. Zone et al. reported that sera from both adults and children with linear IgA deposits within the lamina lucida reacted with a 97-kDa protein that is identical to a portion of the 180-kDa BP antigen BPAG2.[47] In patients with LABD or linear IgA disease of childhood and who have sublaminar densa IgA deposits, investigators have identified reactivity to type VII collagen and to an unknown 285-kDa dermal protein.[47] These findings support the hypothesis that the target antigens in LABD, including linear IgA disease of childhood, are heterogeneous. Regardless of the location of the IgA deposits or the specific antigenic target, the mechanism of lesion formation in patients with LABD remains unknown.

Therapy

Dapsone is the mainstay of therapy of patients with all forms of LABD. The mechanism of its action is not known, but it seems most useful in cases with marked neutrophil infiltrates in lesional skin. The dosage needed to control the cutaneous eruption ranges from 25 to 200 mg/day. Most patients can be controlled with 100 mg/day, with minimal side effects. Although dapsone is well tolerated by most patients, it does have significant pharmacologic and idiosyncratic adverse effects and should only be used by physicians experienced in its use. Occasionally patients may not respond to dapsone alone. In these cases the addition of low doses of systemic glucocorticoids (prednisone 10–20 mg/day) may result in significant improvement. If patients cannot tolerate dapsone, systemic glucocorticoids in doses of 40–60 mg/day are usually effective. However, as most adult patients with LABD require long-term therapy, treatment with prednisone alone should be avoided when possible.

Dermatitis herpetiformis

Clinical features

DH is an intensely pruritic blistering disease that classically presents in the second or third decade with erythematous papules and/or vesicles localized over the extensor surfaces (Fig. 62.13). Patients often present with a broad spectrum of lesions. The severe pruritus leads to patients scratching the small papules and vesicles, resulting in erosions that may be the presenting feature.

Patients can also present with urticarial plaques or, less commonly, frank bullae. Lesions are usually symmetrically distributed over the extensor surfaces, especially the elbows, knees, buttocks, back, and posterior hairline. Symptomatic mucous membrane lesions are rarely present. A clinical hallmark of DH is the extreme pruritus that patients experience. They characteristically report feeling a severe burning or stinging 12–24 hours before the appearance of a lesion, which persists until the vesicle is broken and the crust forms. Although the clinical manifestations of DH can wax and wane, it is generally a life-long dermatosis. The wide variety of clinical presentations

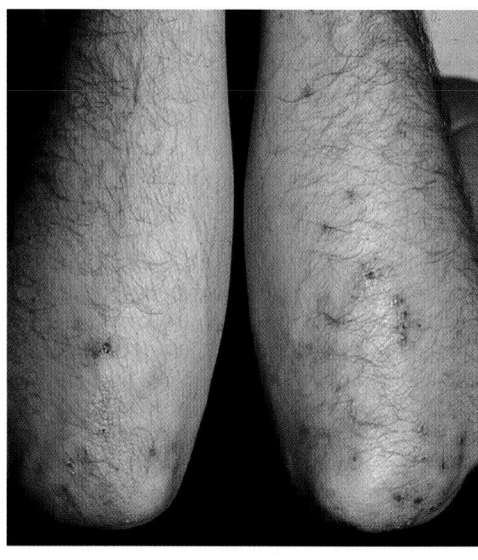

Fig. 62.13 Patient with dermatitis herpetiformis showing erythematous papules with crusts on the elbows. Rare intact vesicles are present.

of DH often suggests a long differential diagnosis, including erythema multiforme, HG, BP, transient acantholytic dermatitis, papular urticaria, scabies, bug bites, and neurotic excoriations.

The frequency of DH varies in different ethnic groups. In Anglo-Saxon and Scandinavian populations it has been estimated to be between 10 and 39 per 100 000 persons, whereas DH occurs much less frequently in other populations, such as African-Americans and Asians. This relates in part to differing frequencies of the DH-associated HLA antigens in different populations, as detailed below.

Biopsy of an early lesion of DH reveals a characteristic neutrophilic infiltrate in the dermal papillae with the presence of fibrin, neutrophilic fragments, edema, and variable numbers of eosinophils. This histologic pattern is not specific and has been reported in patients with BP, linear IgA disease, the bullous eruption of systemic lupus erythematosus, and leukocytoclastic vasculitis. When older bullous lesions are biopsied in patients with DH, the histologic features are often indistinguishable from those seen with other blistering disorders.

IgA is present at the DEJ of the skin of patients with DH when tested with direct immunofluorescence (Fig. 62.14). Two patterns of IgA deposition were initially described in patients with identical clinical findings: 85–90% of patients had granular deposits of IgA at the DEJ, and 10–15% had a linear band of IgA at the DEJ. These patterns, consistent within a given individual, have now been shown to distinguish between two different diseases. Patients with linear IgA deposits have LABD, whereas patients with granular deposits of IgA are considered to have true DH. The granular deposits of IgA at the DEJ are specific for patients with DH and have not been found in those with isolated gluten-sensitive enteropathy (GSE) or asymptomatic relatives of patients with DH.[48]

Granular deposits of IgA are found in both involved and uninvolved skin of patients with DH, including the oral mucosa. Consistent regional variations in the amount of IgA in the skin of patients with DH have not been reported. However, Zone and co-workers reported that IgA was either markedly decreased or absent in skin in which the patient reported never having had any lesions.[49] These observations suggest that biopsies taken for direct immunofluorescence studies should be obtained from normal-appearing perilesional skin in order to maximize the diagnostic yield.

IgG, IgM, and IgE are not usually found in the skin of patients with DH. C3, along with early components of the alternative complement pathway, may be present in skin biopsies of

patients with DH. The neoantigens of the C5–C9 membrane attack complex have also been reported in normal-appearing skin of patients with DH. However, the co-localization of vitronectin with the C9 neoantigen suggests that the C5–C9 neoantigen is deposited in DH skin as part of the nonlytic C5–C9 complex, and that the lytic membrane attack complex of complement may not play a primary role in the development of DH skin lesions.[50]

Characterization of IgA in DH skin has shown that it contains both κ and λ light chains, indicating that the IgA is polyclonal. Secretory component, a transport protein bound to secretory IgA, has not been found in these IgA deposits. IgA1 is the predominant subclass found in the skin of patients, with either minimal or no deposits of IgA2 detected.[51] Although this would seem to suggest that the IgA in DH skin may not be mucosal in origin, IgA1 is also the predominant subclass in the gastrointestinal secretions of patients with DH.[52]

In 1966 Marks and co-workers noted a gastrointestinal abnormality in 60–70% of patients with DH, which was histologically similar to that seen in isolated GSE.[53] This abnormality was reversible with the avoidance of dietary gluten, confirming that DH was a gluten-sensitive disease (Chapter 74). The histologic changes seen in the small bowel of patients with DH are characterized by flattening of the normal villous architecture of the jejunal epithelium, with elongation of the intestinal crypts and a mononuclear cell infiltrate both within the lamina propria and in an intraepithelial location. These findings are often patchy in character in both DH and isolated GSE, and in general the findings in patients with DH are less severe than those seen in isolated GSE. Essentially all patients with the clinical features of DH and granular IgA deposits have associated GSE.

Despite the morphological similarity of the intestinal abnormality seen in patients with DH and those with isolated GSE, most patients with DH have no gastrointestinal symptoms. Only 10% of patients with DH have the typical symptoms of isolated GSE, such as bloating, diarrhea, and malabsorption, whereas 20–30% may have mild steatorrhea. However, many patients with DH do have abnormal intestinal function, as documented by abnormal absorption of D-xylose, iron, folate, glucose, water, and bicarbonate.

Despite the asymptomatic nature of the GSE associated with DH, it is clear that it plays a critical role in the pathogenesis of DH. Patients with DH who adhere to gluten-free diets can control their skin disease, normalize the morphologic changes of the small intestine, and after years of gluten avoidance lose the cutaneous IgA deposits. However, the exact relationship between the skin disease, the cutaneous IgA deposits, and the associated GSE remains unknown.

Initial studies of HLA associations in patients with DH and granular deposits of IgA revealed that 70–90% of those with DH express the HLA class I antigen B8, compared to only 20–30% of control subjects. Subsequent studies showed that 90–95% of patients with DH express HLA-DR3, compared to about 23% of controls. In addition, 95–100% of DH patients express HLA-DQ2 (which is in linkage disequilibrium with HLA-B8 and -DR3), compared to 40% of controls. The HLA-DR and HLA-DQ alleles involved in the pathogenesis of DH are DQB1*0201, DQA1*0501, and DRB1*0301 and are essentially identical to those that have been described for patients with isolated GSE.

In addition to the striking association of DH with gluten-sensitive enteropathy, a number of other disease associations have been noted. For example, patients with DH have an increased frequency of gastric atrophy and gastric hypochlorhydria. Thyroid abnormalities, including hypothyroidism, hyperthyroidism, thyroid nodules, and thyroid cancer, also occur

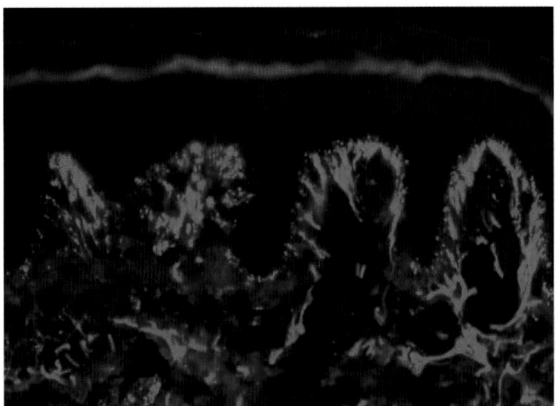

Fig. 62.14 Direct immunofluorescence of normal-appearing perilesional skin of a patient with dermatitis herpetiformis using antibodies against human immunoglobulin A (IgA). Granular deposits of IgA are present at the dermal-epidermal junction.

45. Patrício P, Ferreira C, Gomes M, et al. Autoimmune bullous dermatoses: a review. Ann N Y Acad Sci 2009;1173:203–10.

46. Wojnarowska F, Whitehead P, Leigh IM, et al. Identification of the target antigen in chronic bullous disease of childhood and linear IgA disease of adults. Br J Dermatol 1991;124(2):157–62.

47. Zone JJ, Taylor TB, Meyer LJ. The 97 kDa linear IgA bullous disease antigen is identical to a portion of the extracellular domain of the 180 kDa bullous pemphigoid antigen, BPAg2. J Invest Dermatol 1998;110:207–10.

48. Lawley TJ, Strober W, Yaoita H, et al. Small intestinal biopsies and HLA types in dermatitis herpetiformis patients with granular and linear IgA skin deposits. J Invest Dermatol 1980;74:9–12.

49. Zone JJ, Meyer LJ, Peterson MJ. Deposition of granular IgA relative to clinical lesions in dermatitis herpetiformis. Arch Dermatol 1996;132:912–8.

50. Dahlback K, Lofberg H, Dahlback B. Vitronectin colocalizes with Ig deposits and C9 neoantigen in discoid lupus erythematosus and dermatitis herpetiformis, but not in bullous pemphigoid. Br J Dermatol 1989;120:725–33.

51. Olbricht SM, Flotte TJ, Collins AB, et al. Dermatitis herpetiformis. Cutaneous deposition of polyclonal IgA1. Arch Dermatol 1986;(122):418–21.

52. Hall RP, McKenzie KD. Comparison of the intestinal and serum antibody response in patients with dermatitis herpetiformis. Clin Immunol Immunopathol 1992;62:33–41.

53. Marks J, Shuster S, Watson AJ. Small bowel changes in dermatitis herpetiformis. Lancet 1966;2:1280–2.

54. Viljamaa M, Kaukinen K, Pukkala E, et al. Malignancies and mortality in patients with coeliac disease and dermatitis herpetiformis: 30-year population-based study. Dig Liver Dis 2006;38(6):374–80.

55. Hall RP, Lawley TJ, Heck JA, et al. IgA-containing circulating immune complexes in dermatitis herpetiformis, Henoch–Schönlein purpura, systemic lupus erythematosus and other diseases. Clin Exp Immunol 1980;40:431–7.

56. Dieterich W, Laag E, Bruckner-Tuderman L, et al. Antibodies to tissue transglutaminase as serologic markers in patients with dermatitis herpetiformis. J Invest Dermatol 1999;113(1):133–6.

57. Zone JJ, Schmidt LA, Taylor TB, et al. Dermatitis herpetiformis sera or goat anti-transglutaminase-3 transferred to human skin-grafted mice mimics dermatitis herpetiformis immunopathology. J Immunol 2011;186(7):4474–80.

58. Molberg O, McAdam SN, Korner R, et al. Tissue transglutaminase selectively modifies gliadin peptides that are recognized by gut-derived T cells in celiac disease. Nat Med 1998;4:713–7.

59. Smith AD, Bagheri B, Streilein RD, et al. Expression of interleukin-4 and interferon-gamma in the small bowel of patients with dermatitis herpetiformis and isolated gluten-sensitive enteropathy. Dig Dis Sci 1999;44(10):2124–32.

60. Hall RP, Takeuchi F, Benbenisty K, et al. Cutaneous endothelial cell activation in normal skin of patients with dermatitis herpetiformis associated with increased serum levels of IL-8, sE-Selectin and TNF-g. J Invest Dermatol 2006;126:1331–7.

61. Leonard J, Haffenden G, Tucker W, et al. Gluten challenge in dermatitis herpetiformis. N Engl J Med 1983;308:816–9.

Immunology of psoriasis | Cristina Albanesi

Clinical and histologic features of psoriasis

Psoriasis is a common chronic, relapsing immune-mediated disease involving the skin and small joints of genetically predisposed individuals. It affects approximately 2% of the general population and in >50% of patients presents in the first three decades of life. There is a wide spectrum of cutaneous manifestations of psoriasis. Individual lesions vary from pinpoint to large plaques, or even generalized erythroderma. More specifically, the clinical spectrum of psoriasis includes the plaque, guttate, small plaque, inverse, erythrodermic, and pustular variants.[1,2] The most common and well-recognized morphologic presentation of psoriasis is that of the plaque type (Fig. 63.1). The disease is characterized by the formation of demarked erythematous plaques with large scaling. The scales are a result of a hyperproliferative epidermis with premature maturation of keratinocytes and incomplete cornification with retention of nuclei in the stratum corneum (parakeratosis). The mitotic rate of the basal keratinocytes is increased as compared with that of normal skin. As a result, the epidermis is thickened (acanthosis), with

elongated rete ridges that form finger-like protrusions into the dermis.[3] The granular layer of the epidermis, the starting site of terminal keratinocyte differentiation, is strongly reduced or missing. The epidermis is infiltrated by neutrophils and activated CD8 T lymphocytes and within the dermis, an inflammatory infiltrate composed mainly of CD3$^+$ T cells, dendritic cells (DC), macrophages, mast cells, and neutrophils is observed. Elongated and dilated blood vessels in the dermal papillae represent a further histological hallmark of psoriatic skin lesions (Fig. 63.2).

Immune-related genetic factors predisposing to psoriasis

The genetic basis of psoriasis has long been recognized, since family members of patients with psoriasis are at greater risk of developing the disease. The mode of inheritance is complex. It is thought that there is not a single disease gene, but rather a complex set of gene variants resulting in an aberrant response to environmental factors.[4] At least nine chromosomal loci with statistically significant linkage to psoriasis have been identified, termed psoriasis susceptibility 1 through 9 (PSORS1 through PSORS9). PSORS1 is the major genetic determinant of psoriasis and is located within the HLA complex on chromosome 6p (Chapter 5). An association with HLA-B13 was first identified and later with other class I antigens HLA-B17, -B37, -B57, -Cw6 and Cw7, and class II antigens HLA-DR4 and -DR7. Among these, the highest and most consistently reported relative risk is for HLA-Cw6 haplotype. A significantly higher frequency of HLA-Cw6 is associated with early-onset (type I) psoriasis as compared with late-onset psoriasis (type II). Current data suggest that HLA-Cw6 is the susceptibility allele within PSORS1; however, no disease-specific mutations have been identified, and variants in regulatory sequences potentially affecting several downstream genes cannot be ruled out. HLA-C might be involved in immune responses at the levels of both antigen presentation and natural killer (NK)-cell regulation. Recently, compelling evidence has emerged for an interaction between the HLA-C and ERAP1 (involved in major histocompatibility complex (MHC) class I peptide processing) loci in psoriasis.[5] ERAP1 variants only influenced psoriasis susceptibility in individuals carrying the HLA-C risk allele.

Other predisposing polygenes were found in the PSORS2 region, on chromosome 17q25. Two distinct regions harbouring susceptibility loci have been identified: the first contains the genes SLC9A3R1 and NAT9 and the second the gene RAPTOR.[6] The SLC9A3R1 gene encodes a PDZ domain-containing phosphoprotein, implicated in several biological processes occurring in T cells. NAT9 encodes an N-acetyltransferase involved in MHC class I antigen-presentation and in immunological

KEY CONCEPTS

- Psoriasis is a common chronic-relapsing immune-mediated skin disease affecting approximately 2% of the general population.

- There is strong evidence that psoriasis is determined by genetic predisposition. There is not a single disease gene, but rather a complex set of gene variants responsible for an aberrant response to environmental factors.

- Psoriasis is a disease caused by the infiltration of effector immune cells in both the epidermis and dermis, which determines hyperproliferation of the epidermis with premature maturation of keratinocytes and incomplete cornification. As a result, the epidermis is thickened, with elongated rete ridges forming protrusions into the dermis.

- Primary effector cells are dermal dendritic cells (DC), in particular plasmacytoid DC, whose activation can depend on DNA-LL-37 complexes released by injured keratinocytes and leads to a massive production of IFN-α.

- pDC-released IFN-α activates myeloid DC, which in turn induces type-1 and -17 T-cell responses. T helper 22 response is also pathogenetically induced.

- Pathologic cytokines include T-cell-derived lymphokines such as IFN-γ, TNF-α, IL-17, IL-22, IL-21, and antigen presenting cell-derived cytokines such as IL-12 and -23.

- Intrinsic alterations of keratinocytes in the activation of signal tranduction pathways (i.e., STAT3, IKK-2, AP1, etc.) are fundamental for the amplification of psoriatic processes.

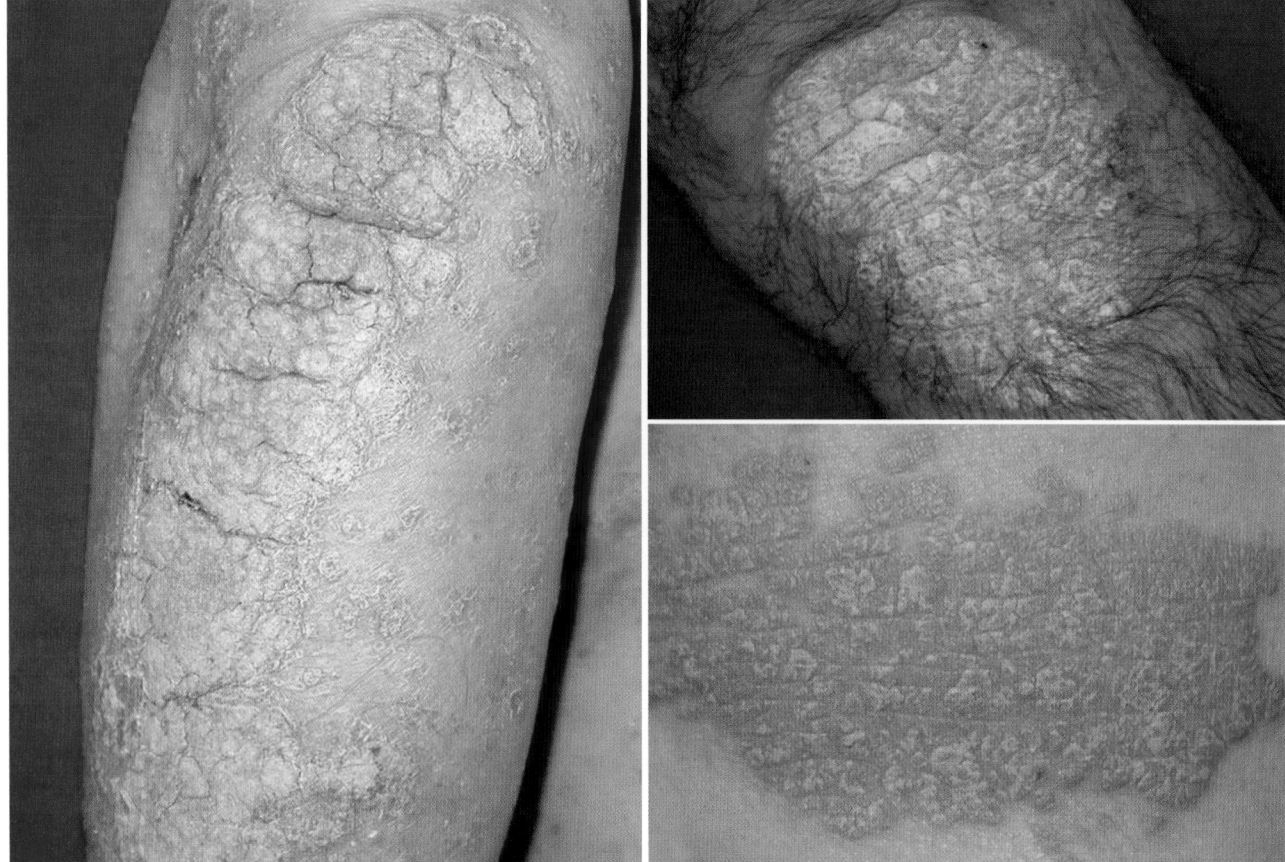

Fig. 63.1 Clinical aspect of plaque psoriasis. Scaly, erythematous, sharply demarcated plaques in different sizes and shapes are hallmarks of psoriasis.

processes related to autoimmune diseases. Additionally, between *SLC9A3R1* and *NAT9* is a polymorphism for the binding site of a transcription factor RUNX1 that may affect regulation of the immune synapse.[7] Associations with alleles of IL-12, IL-23 receptor (IL-23R), IL-19/20, and IRF2 have also been described. Interestingly, IL-12 and IL23R single nucleotide polymorphisms do not have interactions with HLA-Cw6.[8]

Effector cells and immune mechanisms operating in psoriasis

Even though successful treatment regimens for the therapy of psoriasis are long-established, the primary pathogenetic mechanism and the cell type(s) involved in the onset of the disease are still under debate. Psoriasis is classically responsive to trigger factors that can induce psoriasis *de novo* or exacerbate skin lesions.[9] Trigger factors range from nonspecific stimuli such as skin trauma to more specific triggers such as pathogens (i.e., streptococci) or drugs (i.e., lithium, interferon (IFN)-α). All of these factors generate a pathogenetic cascade culminating in the expansion of lesional and/or circulating T cells in the psoriatic skin (Fig. 63.3). Much effort has been devoted to understanding the link between the trigger stimuli and the pathogenic T-cell cascade that leads to psoriasis. Recent evidence suggests that type-1 IFN may represent the missing link. The prototypical type I IFN, IFN-α, is produced by plasmacytoid dendritic cells (pDC) during the early phase of psoriasis developmenty (Fig. 63.3A).[9,10] In turn, IFN-α indirectly stimulates the pathogenic T-cell cascade by promoting the activation and maturation of myeloid DC

(mDC) or by direct stimulation of IFN-α-sensitive pathogenic T cells (Fig. 63.3B). T-cell infiltrate present in active psoriatic skin establishes a cytokine milieu that dictates specific and pathogenetic gene signatures in resident skin cells. Thus, cytokine-activated keratinocytes overexpress a number of inflammatory mediators that aberrantly amplify and sustain the psoriasiform tissue reactions (Fig. 63.3C). Intrinsic defects and/or alterations of keratinocytes in their immune response to pro-inflammatory cytokines are fundamental to the induction of psoriatic processes, as demonstrated in genetically manipulated mouse systems.

Plasmacytoid dendritic cells as inducers of primary immune responses in psoriasis

pDC are characterized by a plasma cell morphology and a distinctive surface phenotype (CD4+, CD45RA+, CD123+, BDCA-2+, BDCA-4+, CD62L+, cutaneous lymphocyte-associate antigen (CLA)+ and CD11c-). They are considered as key effector cells in antiviral defense because of their ability to produce large amounts of type I IFN.[11] Upon viral stimulation, pDC differentiate into a unique type of mature DC and induce an IFN-α-dependent activation of bystander mDC with the ability to induce T helper (Th) 1 responses, thus providing a necessary link between innate and adaptive immunity.[11,12] Several studies have demonstrated that pDC infiltrate psoriatic skin, and that pDC-derived IFN-α initiate the expansion of autoimmune T cells, leading eventually to the skin lesions of psoriasis.[13–15] Blocking of type I IFN signaling with neutralizing antibodies to IFN-α/β receptors inhibited the development of psoriasis in symptomless pre-psoriatic skin engrafted onto immunodeficient AGR129

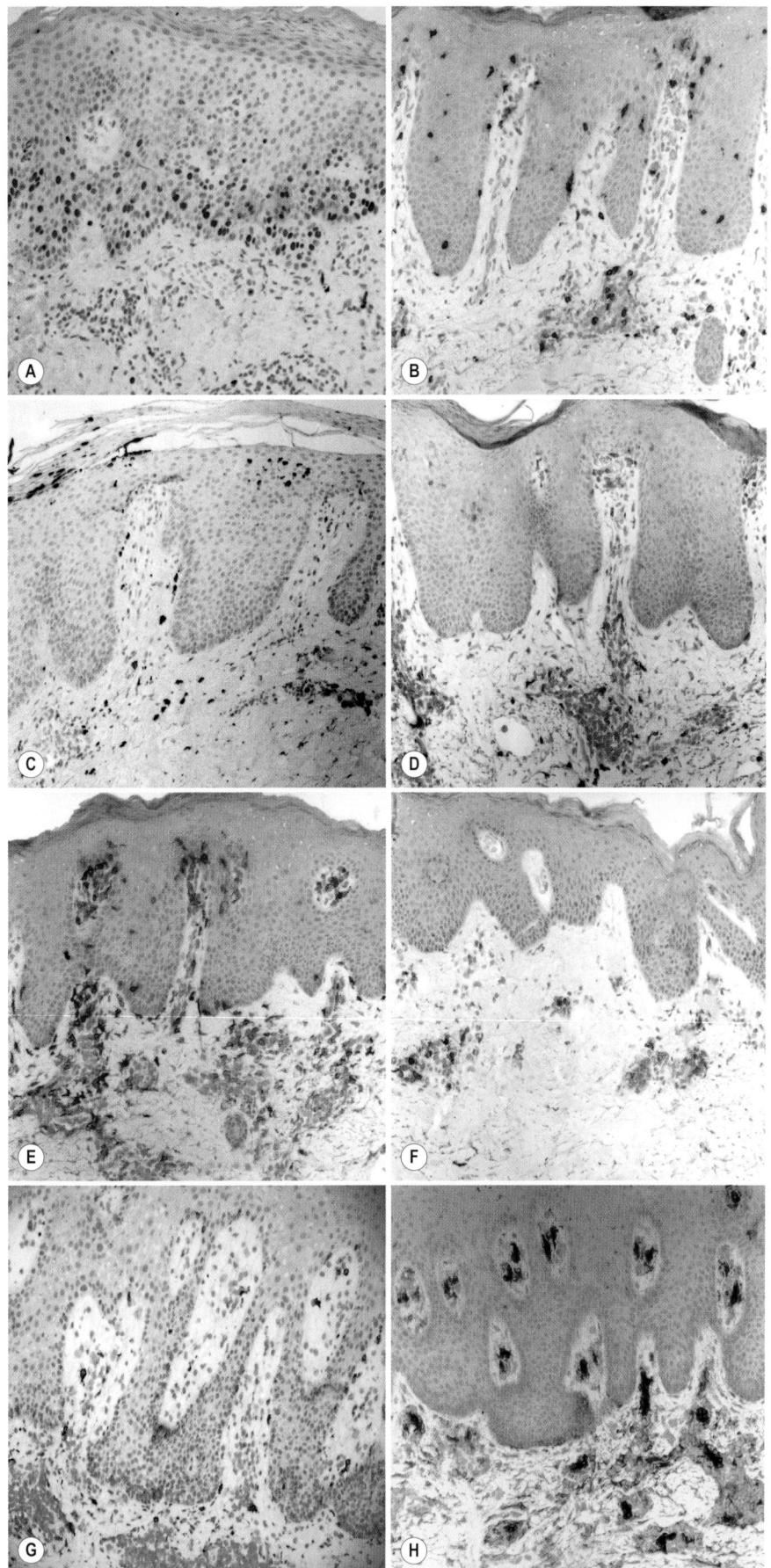

Fig. 63.2 Histological components of a mature psoriatic plaque. Psoriatic skin lesions are characterized by a hyperproliferative epidermis showing an increased mitotic rate of the basal keratinocytes (A, Ki67 immunostaining). As a consequence, the epidermis is thickened, with elongated rete ridges that form typical finger-like protrusions into the dermis. The epidermis becomes infiltrated by activated CD8 T lymphocytes and neutrophils (B and C, immunostaining for CD8 and CD15, respectively). Within the dermis, an inflammatory infiltrate mainly composed of CD3$^+$ T cells (D), CD11c$^+$ dendritic cells (E), BDCA-2$^+$ plasmacytoid dendritic cells (F), c-kit$^+$ mast cells (G), and neutrophils (C) is observed. Elongated and dilated ICAM-1$^+$ (H) blood vessels in the dermis represent another histological hallmark of psoriatic skin.

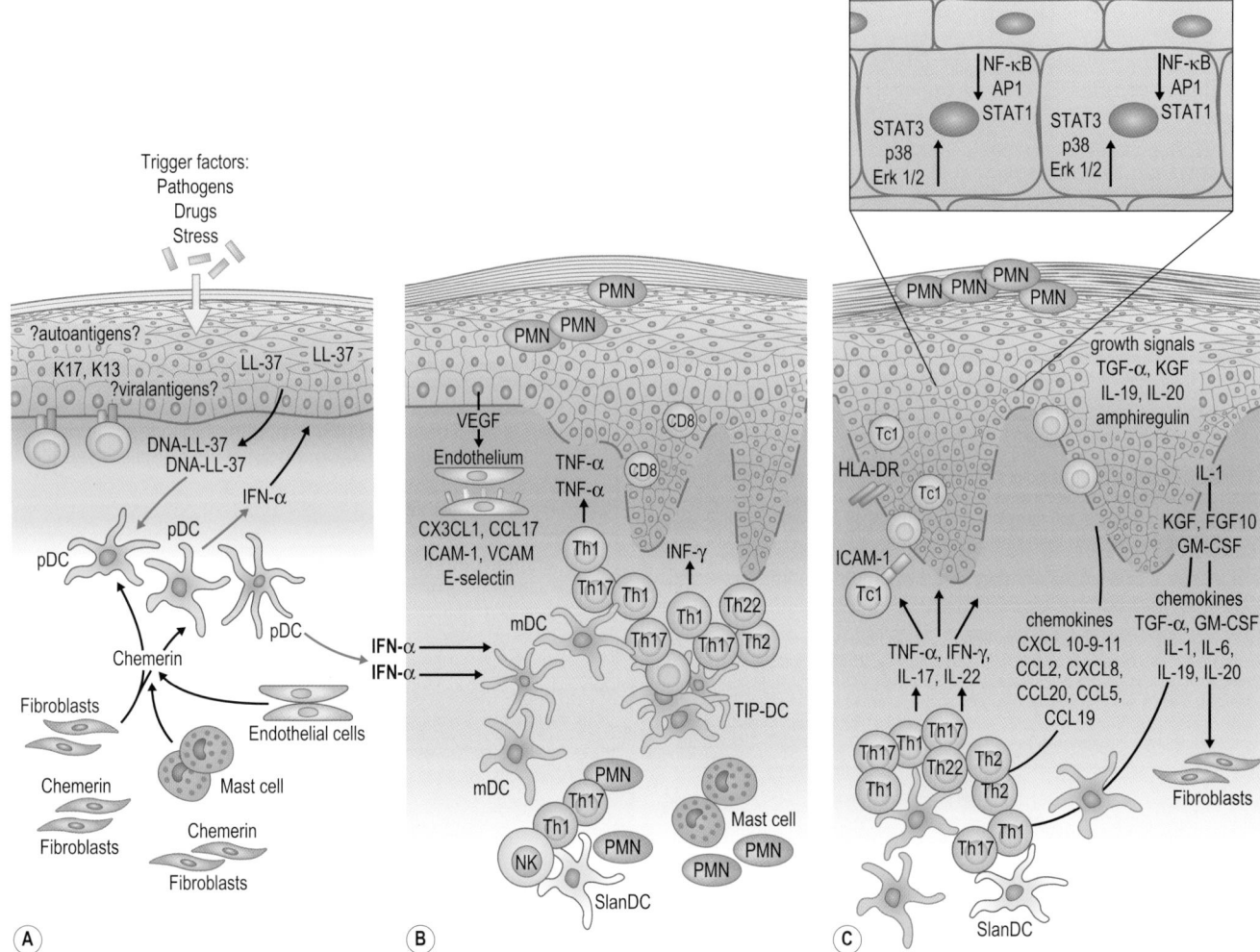

Fig. 63.3 Scheme of pathogenic mechanisms operating in psoriasis. The psoriatic lesion starts to evolve after keratinocytes are injured, for instance by physical trauma or bacterial products. Thereafter, a cascade of events including the formation of complexes formed by keratinocyte-derived DNA and the cathelicidin LL-37 leads to the activation of plasmacytoid dendritic cells (pDC), which routinely patrol psoriatic skin (A). Other pDC are recruited in the early phase psoriasis development by the chemokine chemerin, derived primarily from dermal fibroblasts, and to lesser extent from mast cells and endothelial cells, and induced to release high amounts of IFN-α. IFN-α locally activates keratinocytes and participates in the activation processes undergoing myeloid dendritic cells. In turn, DC migrate into draining lymph nodes and induce the differentiation of naïve T cells into effector cells, such as type 17 T helper (Th) 17 or type 17 T cytotoxic (Tc) cells and type 1 Th1 or Tc1 cells. Effector cells recirculate and proliferate into psoriatic skin, and produce massive amounts of pro-inflammatory cytokines, such as IFN-γ and TNF-α (B). The latter cytokine is also abundantly released by dermal DC, mainly represented by TNF-α and inducible nitric oxide synthase-producing-DC (TIP-DC). SlanDC also reinforce immunity in psoriasis by interacting with and potentiating the activity of both neutrophils and NK cells, as well as inducing Th1 and Th17 responses. IFN-γ and TNF-α are responsible for the activation of resident skin cells, in particular keratinocytes, which respond to cytokines with a stereotypical set of genomic responses leading to synthesis of inflammatory mediators (C). Keratinocytes are also targets of T-cell-derived IL-22, which induces proliferation and de-differentiation of psoriatic keratinocytes in a STAT3-dependent manner. Keratinocyte-derived chemokines, cytokines, and membrane molecules have a major role in maintaining the recruitment of leukocytes into inflammatory sites. Because of their intrinsic defects, psoriatic keratinocytes aberrantly respond to cytokines and show altered intracellular signaling pathways, including STAT3 cascade (C). The uncontrolled hyperproliferation and differentiation observed in psoriatic skin could also derive from a dysregulated production of tissue growth factors and regulators, such as TGF-α, KGF, amphiregulin, GM-CSF, FGF-10, IL-19, and IL-20 produced by keratinocytes and fibroblasts. It is unclear whether psoriatic keratinocytes produce autoantigens (i.e., keratin (K) 17 and K13) capable of inducing clonal T-cell responses. Finally, the inflammatory cytokine milieu also influences the immune functions of fibroblasts and endothelium, with the latter being critical for leukocyte trafficking and extravasation.

mice.[14] Moreover, inhibition of IFN-α release by pDC through anti-BDCA-2 antibody prevented the activation and expansion of pathogenetic T cells and the development of a psoriatic phenotype. The detailed mechanisms responsible for the IFN-α-induced expansion of T cells in psoriasis are currently unknown, but it appears that IFN-α favors cross-presentation of sequestered tissue-specific autoantigens by mDC.[16] pDC-derived IFN-α may also enhance the survival of autoreactive T cells through the induction of IL-15 or by promoting a Th1 cell bias through the induction of T-bet and IL-12Rβ2 expression.[17] The pathogenetic role of IFN-α is also suggested by the observations that its signaling signature is present in resident skin cells of psoriatic plaques,[18] and that the treatment of psoriatic patients

with recombinant IFN-α for unrelated conditions (i.e., viral infections or tumors), or with imiquimod, a Toll-like receptor (TLR) agonist that induces production of IFN-α by pDC, exacerbates psoriasis.[19] In addition, excessive activation of type I IFN signaling in mice deficient for IFN regulatory factor (IRF)-2, a transcriptional repressor of IFN signaling, causes an inflammatory skin disease resembling psoriasis.[17] Recently, a genome-wide analysis conducted on paired lesional and non-lesional psoriatic skin and on the skin of healthy donors revealed a significant overexpression of many components of the IFN-α pathway in psoriatic patients, including the receptor subunits for type I IFN, IFNAR1, and IFNAR2, the transcriptional activators of IFN-α-inducible genes, signal transducer and activator of transcription (STAT) 1, IRF1, and IRF7.[18] All of these molecules are master regulators of IFN-α-mediated immune responses.

The molecular mechanisms leading pDC to produce type I IFN involve the activation of TLR7 and TLR9, intracellular receptors that recognize viral/microbial nucleic acids within endosomal compartments. pDC do not normally respond to self-DNA, but this restriction is broken down in some human autoimmune diseases. In psoriatic skin, pDC can be activated to produce massive amounts of type I IFN in response to extracellular self-DNA fragments.[20] However, this process requires the coupling of self-DNA to the endogenous antimicrobial peptide LL-37, known to be overexpressed in psoriatic skin. LL-37 breaks innate tolerance to self-DNA by forming aggregated and condensed structures that can trigger a robust IFN-α induction via TLR9 activation.[20] This suggests a fundamental role for LL-37 in alerting resident skin pDC of tissue damage associated with cell death and the release of self-DNA. pDC are typically absent in unperturbed skin and peripheral tissues under homeostatic conditions, but can enter secondary lymphoid organs through the expression of CD62L and chemokine receptors (CXCR4, CXCR3, CCR5, and ChemR23).[21] pDC can also infiltrate inflamed tissue of immune-mediated skin diseases, and, in particular, accumulate in the skin of psoriatic patients early during disease development.[13,14] Many studies have shown an evident IFN-α signature (e.g., increased expression of IRF-7 and the presence of MxA, markers for IFN-α activity) in primary psoriatic plaques in the absence of detectable levels of the IFN-α cytokine. Indeed, IFN-α expression was detected early and transiently during the development of the psoriatic phenotype, whereas its effect persisted until lesions became chronic. Paralleling IFN-α expression, BDCA-2+ pDC were detected only during the early developmental stages of psoriasis.[14] In fact, pDC infiltration in psoriatic skin correlates with the expression of markers typical of early phases of psoriasis (CD15+ neutrophils and c-kit+ mast cells localized in the mid and papillary dermis, and few CD8+ T lymphocytes or ICAM-1+ keratinocytes), whereas they are almost absent in long-lasting lesions.[13] Importantly, pDC recruitment in psoriatic skin is strictly associated with the expression of the chemokine chemerin, which is temporally produced by dermal fibroblasts and active during psoriatic plaque development.[13] pDC migration towards fibroblast-derived chemerin is completely dependent on the expression of ChemR23 receptor on pDC. Compared to other chemokines potentially active on pDC (CXCL10 and CXCL12), chemerin is the main, if not the only, protein responsible for the pDC chemotactic activity released by fibroblasts in psoriatic skin.[13]

DC driving of T-cell responses in psoriatic skin

Although pDC are responsible for triggering psoriasis, mDC are the main amplifiers of local inflammation. Dermal mDC are dramatically increased in psoriasis, while targeted immunotherapy reduces their quantity in psoriatic patients, supporting the concept that mDC have a key pathogenetic role.[22–25] Dermal mDC are found at the dermal–epidermal junction as well as throughout the whole dermis. mDC are able to capture extracellular antigens for presentation to T cells and also intracellular antigens from adjacent cell types via cross-presentation. In addition, mDC within psoriatic lesions are intrinsically stronger stimulators of T-cell proliferation than DC derived from peripheral blood or from the skin of healthy patients. mDC uniformly express CD11c, and they can be further subdivided based on expression of CD1c (BDCA-1). Steady-state skin has a predominance of CD11c+ CD1c+ resident DC while CD11c+ CD1c− mDC predominate in psoriatic inflammation.[25] A small fraction of CD11c+ CD1c+ DC bear

"maturation" markers, such as DC-LAMP, CD83, and endocytic receptor DEC-205/CD205, suggesting that they could function as conventional DC and present antigens to T cells to trigger acquired immune responses.[25] These rare, phenotypically mature cells, often aggregating in dermal clusters, could be required for rapid antigen presentation to local T cells, or for ongoing "micro" immune responses. During psoriasis development, dermal CD11c+ DC mature and acquire a CD1c− HLA-DR+ CD45+ CD14− dendritic cell-specific ICAM-3-grabbing nonintegrin (DC-SIGN)+ phenotype.[25] These inflammatory mDC are CCR7+ and respond to the chemokine CCL19, suggesting that they may migrate to draining lymph nodes for antigen presentation. CD11c+ CD1c− inflammatory DC express very high levels of tumor necrosis factor (TNF)-α and the enzyme inducible nitric oxide synthase (iNOS) and can be considered as the human equivalent of TIP-DC (TNF-α and iNOS-producing DC), which have been shown in mice to have effector functions in clearing some bacterial infections.[26] The pro-inflammatory nature of TNF-α in psoriasis and other inflammatory diseases is well established, and the receptors TNFR1 and TNFRII are expressed on a wide range of cells in psoriatic skin, including keratinocytes and endothelial cells. TNF-α induces expression of ICAM-1 on keratinocytes, facilitating the adhesion of circulating leukocytes. Moreover, TNF-α can stimulate keratinocytes and dermal fibroblasts to produce the potent neutrophil chemoattractant CXCL8, as well as the pro-inflammatory cytokines IL-6 and -1, which help generate and maintain Th17 cells. The role of TNF-α in psoriasis is underlined by the therapeutic success of anti-TNF-α therapies in psoriasis.[26] In addition, polymorphisms of the TNF-α promoter region have been associated with psoriasis. On the other hand, iNOS production by inflammatory DC leads to nitric oxide (NO) release, inducing vasodilation, inflammation, and antimicrobial effects in psoriatic skin. Interestingly, NO inhibitors (e.g., statins) can have a beneficial effect on psoriasis, although this has not been studied in a randomized prospective manner. Inflammatory DC also produce other cytokines, e.g., IL-23 and -12, linked to psoriasis. IL-12 mainly induces IFN-γ production, whereas IL-23 also stimulates IL-17 and -22 release by T cells, as shown in mice.[27] Other evidence for a role of IL-23 in psoriasis includes the clinical efficacy of an anti-p40 monoclonal antibody against psoriasis and the association of a single nucleotide polymorphism in the IL-23R gene in psoriasis patients.[28] mDC of psoriatic lesions also release the pro-inflammatory cytokine IL-15 that induces T-cell proliferation and monocyte activation as well as skin hyperplasia by protecting keratinocytes from apoptosis.

Recently, a distinct population of inflammatory mDC, defined by the selective expression of the 6-sulfo LacNAc residue on the P-selectin glycoprotein ligand 1 membrane molecule, has been identified in psoriatic skin.[29,30] 6-Sulfo LacNAc+ DC (slanDC) have a well-defined phenotype (CD1c−, CD11c+, CD16+, CD14−) that clearly distinguishes them from classic CD1c+ blood DC (CD1c+, CD11c+) or pDC (BDCA-2, BDCA-4). SlanDC produce more TNF-α, IL-23, IL-12, IL-1β, and IL-6, and can thus induce Th1/Th17 cells. SlanDC also reinforce innate immunity in psoriasis by interacting with and potentiating the activity of neutrophils and NK cells.[29]

The function of another DC subset, the Langerhans cell, is still controversial. Langerhans cells are only found in the epidermal compartment where they are similar in number and phenotype in lesional and non-lesional skin, but they fail to migrate in response to pro-inflammatory stimuli.[31] These findings and data from Langerhans cell ablation models suggest that Langerhans cells may help sustain immune tolerance in psoriasis. In psoriatic skin, the epidermis contains an additional DC subset, known as inflammatory dendritic epidermal cells and distinguishable from Langerhans cells by the expression of the macrophage mannose receptor CD206.

Activation of T lymphocytes and establishment of the cytokine milieu influencing keratinocyte proliferation and immune functions

Psoriasis lesional skin shows many inflammatory T cells in both the papillary dermis and the epidermis.[32] Immunophenotyping of T cells shows that these are mainly activated memory T cells expressing HLA-DR, CD25, CD27, and cutaneous lymphocyte antigen (CLA). Although there is differential T-cell receptor usage in T cells from psoriatic skin, the causative antigens responsible for T-cell activation in psoriasis remain unknown. Exposure of altered autoantigens from keratinocytes could be responsible for the activation and expansion of distinct T-cell subpopulations in psoriatic skin.[32] These autoantigens might include keratin 17 (patients with active psoriasis have an increased frequency of circulating Th1 cells reacting to peptides from keratin 17),[33] and corneodesmosin, an attractive candidate for psoriasis susceptibility based on its putative biological function in keratinocyte adhesion.[34] Keratinocytes could also be responsible for the activation of pathogenetic T cells by viral or bacterial products. For example, a significant prevalence of human papillomavirus 5 (HPV-5) DNA and antibodies to HPV-5 virus-like particles have been found in psoriasis.[35] Streptococcal infections are also frequently associated with psoriasis, and streptococcal superantigens could be presented to T cells by binding MHC class II molecules expressed by lesional keratinocytes. Putative psoriatic antigens are assumed to be keratinocyte proteins that might share structural homology with streptococcal proteins and might thereby induce cross-reactive T-cell responses against skin components.[36]

T-cell migration from the dermis into the epidermis is a key event in psoriasis. It is controlled by the interaction of $\alpha_1\beta_1$ integrin (very late antigen 1) on T cells with collagen IV in the basement membrane of the epidermis. Blockade of this interaction inhibits the development of psoriasis in clinically relevant models.[37] Based on the analysis of infiltrating cell types, their secreted products, and genetic signatures present in lesional skin, psoriasis has been considered for many years as a type-1 (i.e., Th1)-mediated reaction with IFN-γ playing a prominent role.[38] Consistent with Th1 pattern of response, CCR10 is preferentially expressed by skin homing CLA$^+$ memory T cells, which secrete TNF-α and IFN-γ but minimal amounts of IL-10 and -4 upon activation. However, other cytokines and T-cell subsets have also been identified during inflammatory responses in psoriasis. These include Th17 cells and the recently identified Th22 cells.[39] Both IL-17 and -22 belong to a class of cytokines with predominant effects on epithelial cells. Keratinocytes are strongly influenced by IL-17, and upregulate chemokines and immunomodulatory molecules in response to this cytokine.[40,41] A functional role of Th17 cells in psoriasis is suggested by their reduction during successful anti-TNF-α treatment. IL-22 also acts pathogenetically in psoriatic skin by inducing proliferation and de-differentiation of keratinocytes, as well as promoting their production of antimicrobial peptides and chemokines including CXCL8 and CXCL1.[42,43] Binding of IL-22 to its receptor, the expression of which in the skin is confined to keratinocytes, mediates epidermal acanthosis through the activation of STAT3.[27] These observations may explain the increased STAT3 expression in the epidermal compartment and the pathogenicity of STAT3 overexpression in the epidermis of transgenic mice (see below).[44] The demonstration that T cells are the primary

regulators of keratinocyte proliferation and differentiation in psoriasis came from studies showing that supernatants from lesional skin-derived T cells transformed β-integrin$^+$ keratin 1/keratin 10$^-$ PCNA$^-$ stem cells of patients with psoriasis, but not stem cells of healthy subjects, into PCNA$^+$ active cycling cells. T-cell-derived supernatants contained high levels of granulocyte macrophage colony-stimulating factor (GM-CSF) and IFN-γ, and low levels of IL-3 and TNF-α.[45] However, among these cytokines, only IFN-γ affects the proliferation of psoriatic stem cells. *In vivo*, IFN-γ injection into pre-lesional psoriatic skin triggers keratinocyte proliferation and plaque development. Considering that IFN-γ is an anti-proliferative cytokine and an inducer of squamous differentiation, these latter findings are paradoxical. This discrepancy may reflect an intrinsic defect in the response of psoriatic keratinocytes to IFN-γ, and/or altered localization and expression of the IFN-γ receptor complex in the epidermis of psoriatic skin.[46]

Another T-cell-derived cytokine that has been shown to regulate keratinocyte proliferation in psoriatic skin is IL-21, which is mainly released by CD4 T cells and NKT cells. IL-21 contributes to epidermal hyperplasia, and neutralization of IL-21 reduces both skin thickening and expression of inflammatory molecules. Interestingly, IFN-γ is necessary for IL-21-induced epidermal hyperplasia, while abrogation of IL-21 signals reduces IFN-γ expression in psoriatic T cells.[47]

Finally, the importance of T regulatory (Treg) lymphocytes in psoriasis has been examined in the peripheral blood and the inflamed skin of patients. The number of Treg cells (defined by expression of the transcription factor FOXP3) in the peripheral blood of individuals with psoriasis is increased, and this increase is positively correlated with the disease activity index. CD4$^+$CD25$^+$FOXP3$^+$ Treg cells are also present in psoriatic lesions with more in lesional skin biopsies than in control or uninvolved skin biopsies. However, these Treg cells may be less functional in that Treg cells from both the peripheral blood and psoriatic skin lesions showed reduced ability to suppress effector T cells. This impairment may be dependent on IL-6 as blockade of IL-6 reversed the impairment in suppression observed in co-cultures of Treg cells and effector T cells from patients with psoriasis.[48]

Intrinsic defects of keratinocytes are fundamental for the amplification of psoriatic processes

Endogenous defects in keratinocytes may be pathogenically relevant for psoriasis, as shown in mice with engineered epidermal phenotypes. Transgenic animals that overexpress the transcription factor STAT3 or that lack the inhibitor of NF-κB kinase-2 (IKK-2) in their epidermis develop skin lesions that closely resemble human psoriasis.[44,49] Similarly, the abrogation of JunB in keratinocytes triggers a skin phenotype with the histological features of psoriasis, including marked hyperplasia of the epidermis and dense dermal inflammatory cell infiltrates.[50] The hyperplasia observed in these models may, in part, depend on overexpression of S100A8 and S100A9, two antimicrobial peptides with chemotactic activity and a recognized role in keratinocyte maturation and proliferation. The development of psoriatic lesions in mice with an epidermal deletion of STAT3 depends on the presence of activated T cells, whereas the inflammatory responses occurring in the skin of IKK2-transgenic mice are mediated by TNF-α. This implicates an intrinsically dysregulated interrelation between keratinocytes and cells of both the innate and acquired immune response in the pathogenesis of psoriasis. Within psoriatic lesions, alterations are observed in the levels of expression of several growth factors, such as insulin-like growth factor, keratinocyte growth factor, TGF-α, and amphiregulin, all of which stimulate basal cell proliferation in an autocrine fashion.[38] Other cytokines aberrantly elevated in psoriasis include members of the inhibitory TGF-β family, and cytokines such as IL-19 and -20 that stimulate keratinocyte proliferation and inflammation.[38,40,51] Finally, two anti-inflammatory molecules (suppressors of cytokine signaling (SOCS)1 and SOCS3) are dysregulated in psoriatic keratinocytes.[52,53] These efficiently suppress the IFN-γ- and TNF-α-dependent molecular cascades in keratinocytes, and it has been hypothesized that strengthening of the action of SOCS1 in keratinocytes could be a valid therapeutic approach for treatment of IFN-γ- and TNF-α-dependent skin diseases, including psoriasis.[38]

Conclusions

A complex interplay between environmental and genetic factors triggers a cascade of events that leads to psoriasis expression. Early upstream events occurring in the disease include activation of DC, and the generation of effector T cells that migrate and expand into the psoriatic skin lesions. Cross-talk between keratinocytes and immune cells amplifies inflammation and is responsible for chronicity. Recent research has implicated many immunological mechanisms in psoriasis progression, and this has led to the development of new, pathogenesis-based therapies. Although this progress is remarkable, much remains unknown, especially how to prevent the condition and how to develop drugs with appropriate risk-benefit and long-term profiles. Future work must take into account these aspects in order to establish therapeutic and preventive approaches that lead to improved patient outcomes.

References

1. Griffiths CE, Barker JN. Pathogenesis and clinical features of psoriasis. Lancet 2007;370:263–71.
2. Schon MP, Boehncke WH. Psoriasis. N Engl J Med 2005;352:1899–912.
3. Heidenreich R, Rocken M, Ghoreschi K. Angiogenesis drives psoriasis pathogenesis. Int J Exp Pathol 2009;90:232–48.
4. Bowcock AM, Krueger JG. Getting under the skin: the immunogenetics of psoriasis. Nat Rev Immunol 2005;5:699–711.
5. Strange A, Capon F, Spencer CC, et al. A genome-wide association study identifies new psoriasis susceptibility loci and an interaction between HLA-C and ERAP1. Nat Genet 2011;42:985–90.
6. Capon F, Helms C, Veal CD, et al. Genetic analysis of PSORS2 markers in a UK dataset supports the association between RAPTOR SNPs and familial psoriasis. J Med Genet 2004;41:459–60.
7. Helms C, Cao L, Krueger JG, et al. A putative RUNX1 binding site variant between SLC9A3R1 and NAT9 is associated with susceptibility to psoriasis. Nat Genet 2003;35:349–56.
8. Cargill M, Schrodi SJ, Chang M, et al. A large-scale genetic association study confirms IL12B and leads to the identification of IL23R as psoriasis-risk genes. Am J Hum Genet 2007;80:273–90.
9. Nestle FO, Kaplan DH, Barker J. Psoriasis. N Engl J Med 2009;361:496–509.
10. Albanesi C, Scarponi C, Bosisio D, et al. Immune functions and recruitment of plasmacytoid dendritic cells in psoriasis. Autoimmunity 2010;43:215–9.
11. Colonna M, Trinchieri G, Liu YJ. Plasmacytoid dendritic cells in immunity. Nat Immunol 2004;5:1219–26.
12. Sapoznikov A, Fischer JA, Zaft T, et al. Organ-dependent in vivo priming of naive CD4+, but not CD8+, T cells by plasmacytoid dendritic cells. J Exp Med 2007;204:1923–33.
13. Albanesi C, Scarponi C, Pallotta S, et al. Chemerin expression marks early psoriatic skin lesions and correlates with plasmacytoid dendritic cell recruitment. J Exp Med 2009;206:249–58.
14. Nestle FO, Gilliet M. Defining upstream elements of psoriasis pathogenesis: an emerging role for interferon alpha. J Invest Dermatol 2005;125:xiv–xv.
15. Wollenberg A, Wagner M, Gunther S, et al. Plasmacytoid dendritic cells: a new cutaneous dendritic cell subset with distinct role in inflammatory skin diseases. J Invest Dermatol 2002;119:1096–102.
16. Le Bon A, Etchart N, Rossmann C, et al. Cross-priming of CD8+ T cells stimulated by virus-induced type I interferon. Nat Immunol 2003;4:1009–15.
17. Hida S, Ogasawara K, Sato K, et al. CD8(+) T cell-mediated skin disease in mice lacking IRF-2, the transcriptional attenuator of interferon-alpha/beta signaling. Immunity 2000;13:643–55.
18. Yao Y, Richman L, Morehouse C, et al. Type I interferon: potential therapeutic target for psoriasis? PLoS One 2008;3:e2737.
19. Ketikoglou I, Karatapanis S, Elefsiniotis I, et al. Extensive psoriasis induced by pegylated interferon alpha-2b treatment for chronic hepatitis B. Eur J Dermatol 2005;15:107–9.
20. Lande R, Gregorio J, Facchinetti V, et al. Plasmacytoid dendritic cells sense self-DNA coupled with antimicrobial peptide. Nature 2007;449:564–9.
21. Diacovo TG, Blasius AL, Mak TW, et al. Adhesive mechanisms governing interferon-producing cell recruitment into lymph nodes. J Exp Med 2005;202:687–96.
22. Alshenawy HA, Hasby EA. Immunophenotyping of dendritic cells in lesional, perilesional and distant skin of chronic plaque psoriasis. Cell Immunol 2011;269:115–19.
23. Johnson-Huang LM, McNutt NS, Krueger JG, et al. Cytokine-producing dendritic cells in the pathogenesis of inflammatory skin diseases. J Clin Immunol 2009;29:247–56.
24. Nestle FO, Di Meglio P, Qin JZ, et al. Skin immune sentinels in health and disease. Nat Rev Immunol 2009;9:679–91.
25. Zaba LC, Krueger JG, Lowes MA. Resident and "inflammatory" dendritic cells in human skin. J Invest Dermatol 2009;129:302–8.
26. Lowes MA, Chamian F, Abello MV, et al. Increase in TNF-alpha and inducible nitric oxide synthase-expressing dendritic cells in psoriasis and reduction with efalizumab (anti-CD11a). Proc Natl Acad Sci U S A 2005;102:19057–62.
27. Zheng Y, Danilenko DM, Valdez P, et al. Interleukin-22, a T(H)17 cytokine, mediates IL-23-induced dermal inflammation and acanthosis. Nature 2007;445:648–51.
28. Nestle FO, Conrad C. The IL-12 family member p40 chain as a master switch and novel therapeutic target in psoriasis. J Invest Dermatol 2004;123:xiv–xv.
29. Costantini C, Calzetti F, Perbellini O, et al. Human neutrophils interact with both 6-sulfo LacNAc + DC and NK cells to amplify NK-derived IFN{gamma}: role of CD18, ICAM-1, and ICAM-3. Blood 2011;117:1677–86.
30. Hansel A, Gunther C, Ingwersen J, et al. Human slan (6-sulfo LacNAc) dendritic cells are inflammatory dermal dendritic cells in psoriasis and drive strong T(h)17/T(h)1 T-cell responses. J Allergy Clin Immunol 2011;787–94.
31. Cumberbatch M, Singh M, Dearman RJ, et al. Impaired Langerhans cell migration in psoriasis. J Exp Med 2006;203:953–60.
32. Bos JD, de Rie MA, Teunissen MB, et al. Psoriasis: dysregulation of innate immunity. Br J Dermatol 2005;152:1098–107.
33. Gudmundsdottir AS, Sigmundsdottir H, Sigurgeirsson B, et al. Is an epitope on keratin 17 a major target for autoreactive T lymphocytes in psoriasis? Clin Exp Immunol 1999;117:580–6.
34. Trembath RC, Clough RL, Rosbotham JL, et al. Identification of a major susceptibility locus on chromosome 6p and evidence for further disease loci revealed by a two stage genome-wide search in psoriasis. Hum Mol Genet 1997;6:813–20.
35. Majewski S, Jablonska S. Possible involvement of epidermodysplasia verruciformis human papillomaviruses in the immunopathogenesis of psoriasis: a proposed hypothesis. Exp Dermatol 2003;12:721–8.
36. Prinz JC. Psoriasis vulgaris—a sterile antibacterial skin reaction mediated by cross-reactive T cells? An immunological view of the pathophysiology of psoriasis. Clin Exp Dermatol 2001;26:326–32.
37. Conrad C, Boyman O, Tonel G, et al. Alpha1beta1 integrin is crucial for accumulation of epidermal T cells and the development of psoriasis. Nat Med 2007;13:836–42.
38. Albanesi C, Pastore S. Pathobiology of chronic inflammatory skin diseases: interplay between keratinocytes and immune cells as a target for anti-inflammatory drugs. Curr Drug Metab 2010;11:210–27.
39. Eyerich S, Eyerich K, Pennino D, et al. Th22 cells represent a distinct human T cell subset involved in epidermal immunity and remodeling. J Clin Invest 2009;119:3573–85.
40. Albanesi C, De Pita O, Girolomoni G. Resident skin cells in psoriasis: a special look at the pathogenetic functions of keratinocytes. Clin Dermatol 2007;25:581–8.
41. Albanesi C, Scarponi C, Cavani A, et al. Interleukin-17 is produced by both Th1 and Th2 lymphocytes, and modulates interferon-gamma- and interleukin-4-induced activation of human keratinocytes. J Invest Dermatol 2000;115:81–7.
42. Sestito R, Madonna S, Scarponi C, et al. STAT3-dependent effects of IL-22 in human keratinocytes are counterregulated by sirtuin 1 through a direct inhibition of STAT3 acetylation. FASEB J 2011;25:916–27.
43. Wolk K, Haugen HS, Xu W, et al. IL-22 and IL-20 are key mediators of the epidermal alterations in psoriasis while IL-17 and IFN-gamma are not. J Mol Med 2009;87:523–36.
44. Sano S, Chan KS, Carbajal S, et al. Stat3 links activated keratinocytes and immunocytes required for development of psoriasis in a novel transgenic mouse model. Nat Med 2005;11:43–9.
45. Bata-Csorgo Z, Hammerberg C, Voorhees JJ, et al. Kinetics and regulation of human keratinocyte stem cell growth in short-term primary ex vivo culture. Cooperative growth factors from psoriatic lesional T lymphocytes stimulate proliferation among psoriatic uninvolved, but not normal, stem keratinocytes. J Clin Invest 1995;95:317–27.
46. Jackson M, Howie SE, Weller R, et al. Psoriatic keratinocytes show reduced IRF-1 and STAT-1alpha activation in response to gamma-IFN. FASEB J 1999;13:495–502.
47. Caruso R, Botti E, Sarra M, et al. Involvement of interleukin-21 in the epidermal hyperplasia of psoriasis. Nat Med 2009;15:1013–15.
48. Goodman WA, Levine AD, Massari JV, et al. IL-6 signaling in psoriasis prevents immune suppression by regulatory T cells. J Immunol 2009;183:3170–6.
49. Pasparakis M, Courtois G, Hafner M, et al. TNF-mediated inflammatory skin disease in mice with epidermis-specific deletion of IKK2. Nature 2002;417:861–6.
50. Zenz R, Eferl R, Kenner L, et al. Psoriasis-like skin disease and arthritis caused by inducible epidermal deletion of Jun proteins. Nature 2005;437:369–75.
51. Albanesi C, Scarponi C, Giustizieri ML, et al. Keratinocytes in inflammatory skin diseases. Curr Drug Targets Inflamm Allergy 2005;4:329–34.
52. Madonna S, Scarponi C, De Pita O, et al. Suppressor of cytokine signaling 1 inhibits IFN-gamma inflammatory signaling in human keratinocytes by sustaining ERK1/2 activation. FASEB J 2008;22:3287–97.
53. Madonna S, Scarponi C, Sestito R, et al. The IFN-gamma-dependent suppressor of cytokine signaling 1 promoter activity is positively regulated by IFN regulatory factor-1 and Sp1 but repressed by growth factor independence-1b and Kruppel-like factor-4, and it is dysregulated in psoriatic keratinocytes. J Immunol 2010;185:2467–81.

Arnold I. Levinson

Myasthenia gravis

Myasthenia gravis (MG) is a disease characterized by weakness of striated muscles. The weakness is due to impaired neuromuscular transmission resulting from a reduction in the number of receptors for the neurotransmitter acetylcholine (ACh) at the postsynaptic myoneural junction. This reduction is caused by the action of anti-acetylcholine receptor (anti-AChR) antibodies. The disease occurs with a reported prevalence of 0.5–5/100 000 and an incidence of 0.4/100 000/year. Although MG can occur at any age, it typically presents in the second and third decades of life, with a later peak occurring after age 50 (late-onset disease). A female preponderance (3:1–4:1) has been reported in the first 40 years of life; thereafter the incidence is comparable between the sexes.

Classification

MG patients have traditionally been divided into two categories: those with generalized disease and those presenting with disease limited to the ocular muscles.[1] Within these two groups, patients can be further subdivided on the basis of age of onset. Neonatal MG affects 10–20% of offspring born to myasthenic mothers. Disease manifestations are those of generalized MG (see below) but are transient, dissipating with the metabolism of maternal anti-AChR antibodies that had been transmitted across the placenta during the third trimester of pregnancy. Several congenital myasthenic syndromes have been described. For the most part, these manifest during the neonatal period, persist into adulthood, and are not considered to have an autoimmune basis.[2] Juvenile MG describes patients who present with disease between 1 year of age and puberty. Apart from the age of onset, juvenile myasthenics behave like adult MG patients.

Adults can present with ocular involvement or signs of more generalized disease. The ocular involvement is characterized by impaired ocular muscle motility and lid weakness, manifesting as diplopia and ptosis, respectively. The vast majority of MG patients will experience ocular involvement, with roughly 50% of patients presenting with ocular signs at the time of diagnosis. Those generally at risk of disease progression are: (1) patients with evidence of subclinical disease affecting limb muscles on electrophysiological testing; and (2) patients who have markedly elevated titers of anti-AChR antibodies. Typically, patients with ocular symptoms for longer than 2 years will not progress to a more generalized form of disease.

In the generalized disease group patients can be classified into mild, moderate and severe on the basis of clinical activity. Any skeletal muscle group can be affected, but typically the palatal, pharyngeal and upper esophageal muscles are involved. This results in dysarthria, dysphagia and difficulty in handling secretions. Involvement of the diaphragm and intercostal muscles produces dyspnea and can lead to respiratory failure. Involvement of the muscles of the extremities and trunk occurs in 20–30% of patients at initial presentation and causes difficulties with activities of daily living. The hallmark of all muscle involvement in MG is its variability over time, with weakness usually exacerbated by repetitive use.

CLINICAL PEARLS

Telltale signs of myasthenia gravis

- Variable muscle weakness
- Weakness in cranial nerve distribution
- Normal reflexes and sensation

Diagnosis

The differential diagnosis is extremely broad, encompassing neuropathies, primary and secondary myopathies, muscular dystrophy, demyelinating disorders, degenerative diseases, cerebrovascular accidents, mass lesions and infectious diseases. The clinical features that point to a diagnosis of MG include the variable nature of the muscle weakness, normal sensation and normal deep tendon reflexes. The diagnosis can usually be confirmed by pharmacologic and electrophysiologic testing. A decremental pattern is characteristically seen following repetitive nerve stimulation (Fig. 64.1) and this pattern is normalized following treatment with the anticholinesterase agent tensilon. Further confirmation rests on detecting anti-AChR antibodies, which are found in 85–90% of patients with generalized disease. In the standard assay, sera are reacted with a nicotinic AChR preparation labeled with ^{125}I-α-bungarotoxin, a snake venom polypeptide that binds irreversibly to the receptor. Bound antibodies are immunoprecipitated by an anti-immunoglobulin reagent or staphylococcal protein A, and the quantity of antibodies detected is expressed in terms of the amount of α-bungarotoxin bound.

AChR structure

The nicotinic acetylcholine receptor (nAChR) is a member of a larger family of ligand-gated ion channels. The muscle-type receptor, which is involved in myasthenia, can be subclassified further into mature junctional receptors, and immature, extrajunctional or denervated receptors. The nAChR at a mature myoneural junction is composed of four subunits, labeled α, β, δ, and ε (Fig. 64.2). In fetal muscle and adult denervated muscle or nonjunctional membrane, a γ subunit replaces the ε subunit found in

Fig. 64.1 Neuromuscular transmission in normal and myasthenic subjects. With repetitive stimulation there is a reduction in the efficiency of ACh release, with a subsequent recovery in efficiency as the train of stimuli continues. Although the endplate potential (EPP) fluctuates at the normal junction, sufficient current is generated to stimulate an action potential of constant magnitude. At the myasthenic junction, however, the amplitude of the EPP in response to a given amount of ACh is reduced. Under conditions of inefficient ACh release, e.g., repetitive stimulation, the minimum current for conduction is not generated, resulting in a profile of action potentials that shows a progressive decline or "decrement" with subsequent recovery.

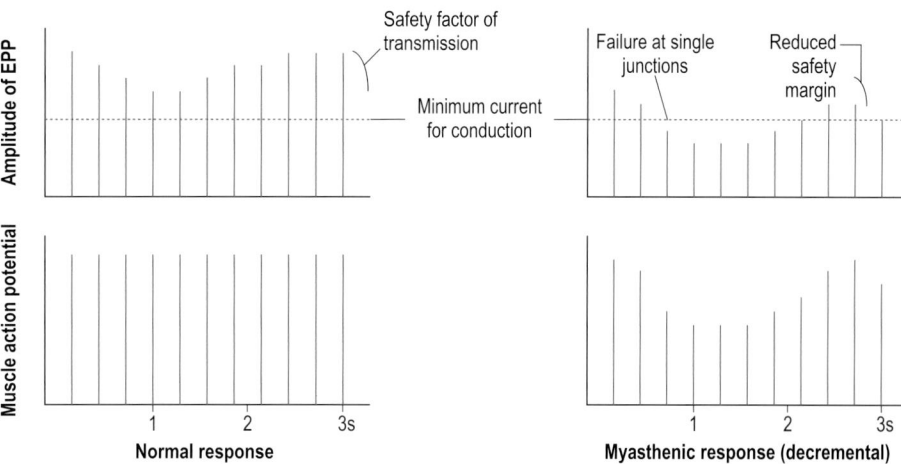

Fig. 64.2 The acetylcholine receptor. The subunits of the acetylcholine receptor – α, β, δ, and γ or ε – are arranged like barrel staves around the central ion pore. Each subunit winds through the junctional membrane four times (sites M1, M2, M3, and M4). In the unfolded view of the α subunit, the amino-terminal end of the α subunit is extracellular, where it is accessible to acetylcholine, which binds at the site shown (amino acids 192 and 193). In myasthenia gravis, autoantibodies may bind to various epitopes of all subunits, but a high proportion of antibodies bind to the main immunogenic region of the α subunit.

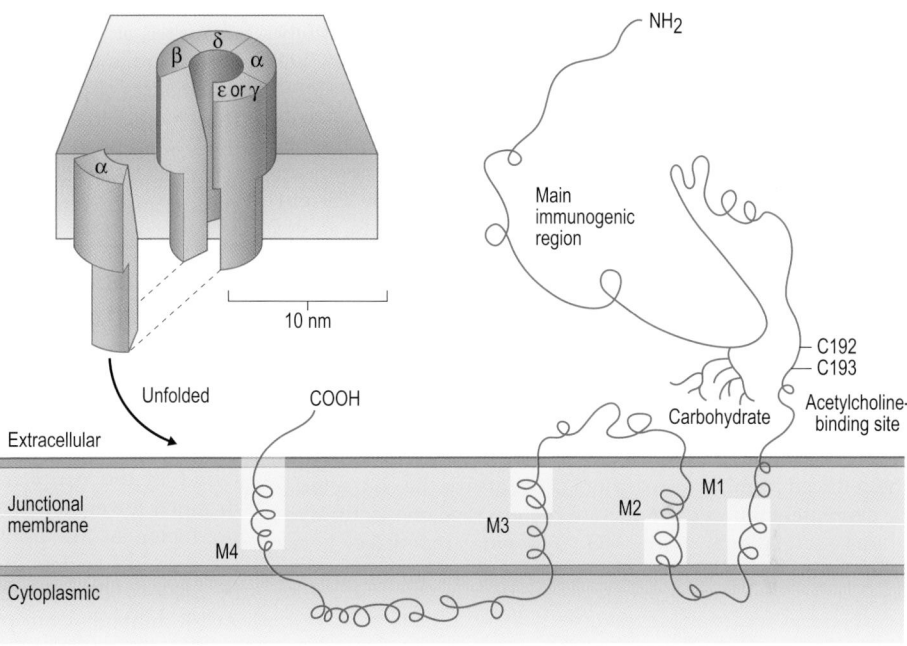

mature innervated muscle endplates. This form of the receptor differs from the mature junctional form by its lower density (500 receptors/mm²) and its distribution over most of the surface of the sarcolemma. The immature receptor also has a lower conductance, a longer open time, a more rapid turnover and a decreased half-life.

The genes for the α, δ, and γ subunits are located on chromosome 2 in humans, and subunits β and ε on chromosome 17. There are two isoforms of the α subunit, which are generated by alternative splicing.[3] The larger, which includes an additional sequence of 25 amino acids between exons 3 and 4, is found only in humans and other primates. The subunits of the AChR are homologous to each other and to their counterparts across species, with the greatest conservation of sequence being in the α subunit. Two α subunits and one of each of the other subunits are assembled to form an asymmetric hourglass channel spanning the membrane. Each subunit has a large amino terminus located extracellularly, four transmembrane regions and a short cytoplasmic tail formed by a loop between the third and fourth

transmembrane domains. The receptor appears as a dimer owing to disulfide bonding between the δ subunits of two receptors. The two α subunits are not contiguous in each receptor but are separated by another subunit. One ACh-binding site is found on each of the α subunits around the pair of cysteines at amino acids 192 and 193. The binding of ACh to the α subunits is believed to engender a conformational change, possibly resulting in rearrangement of charged groups. The binding of ACh to both α subunits increases the probability of transition of the channel to an open conformation. Binding of curare or α-bungarotoxin to the α subunits blocks this channel.

In normal innervated neuromuscular junctions there are two forms of the AChR, the predominant form having a long half-life, and a small subset that is rapidly turned over.[4] The rapidly turned-over receptors are precursors of the stable receptors. It is not clear how these two types differ, or how they are regulated. The receptors are concentrated at the top of the folds in the muscle endplate, adjacent to the nerve terminus, at a density of 10 000/mm². This localization reflects the action of agrin, a nerve-derived synaptic organizing molecule.[5] The AChRs are organized into clusters by rapsyn, a 43-kDa cytoplasmic protein.[5] The clustered AChRs are linked to the cytoskeleton by connections between rapsyn and a dystrophin–glycoprotein complex.

Neuromuscular transmission

When an impulse is transmitted along an axon terminal it results in the release of the neurotransmitter ACh across its pre-synaptic membrane (Fig. 64.3). ACh diffuses across a 50-nm synaptic cleft, where it interacts with AChRs that are displayed in greatest density at the tops of the junctional folds of the post-synaptic muscle membrane or endplate. This interaction leads to a local depolarization or endplate potential caused by increased membrane permeability to sodium and potassium. The endplate potential is terminated by acetylcholinesterases, which are present in highest concentrations in the synaptic cleft around the junctional folds. If the summation of endplate potentials attains a prescribed threshold it produces an action potential that depolarizes the surrounding sarcolemma and causes muscle contraction. In a healthy individual the arrival of an impulse at the presynaptic membrane of a motor nerve releases considerably more ACh than is required to generate an action potential. This reserve, roughly four times the current needed for propagation of the impulse, is referred to as the safety factor of neuromuscular transmission. Because of the severe reduction in receptor number in MG, the electrical threshold for propagation of an action potential cannot be attained and muscle contraction is prevented. With a less severe reduction in receptor numbers neuromuscular transmission may proceed normally unless the efficiency of presynaptic vesicle release is compromised, as occurs with repetitive use of muscles. The combination of decreasing availability of ACh and the reduced number of receptors accounts for the characteristic decremental nerve conduction pattern seen on electromyograms of patients with MG following repetitive nerve stimulation (Fig. 64.1).

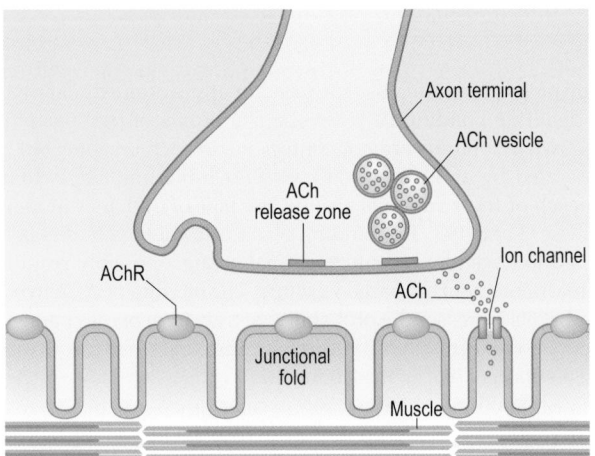

Fig. 64.3 Schematic representation of the myoneural junction. Vesicles of ACh release their contents at active zones across from AChRs in response to impulses conducted down nerve axons. ACh diffuses across synaptic cleft and binds to AChRs, with opening of the ion channel and the generation of endplate potential. Action potential is propagated to muscle when sufficient amplitude of summated endplate potentials is attained.

Immunopathogenesis of MG

● KEY CONCEPTS

Involvement of anti-acetylcholine receptor (AChR) antibodies in the pathogenesis of myasthenia gravis (MG)

- Anti-AChR antibodies found in the serum of 85–90% of MG patients
- Infants born to myasthenic mothers sometimes develop MG
- IgG and complement deposited at the postsynaptic junction
- Transfer of serum IgG from MG patients to mice induces neuromuscular blockade

Anti-AChR antibodies are detected in 85-90% of MG patients and are responsible for the impaired neuromuscular transmission.[6] IgG, along with C3 and the terminal attack complex (C5–C9) is deposited at AChR-containing areas of the postsynaptic membrane, and anti-AChR/AChR complexes can be extracted from the muscles of patients with MG. Transfer of myasthenic serum from mother to fetus, or from human to mouse, results in symptoms or signs of myasthenia in the recipient. Plasmapharesis, which decreases anti-AChR antibody levels, is associated with clinical improvement.

Properties of anti-AChR antibodies and characterization of B-cell epitopes

Anti-AChR antibodies are produced by a small subset of B cells in affected people. The frequency of IgG-producing AChR-specific peripheral blood mononuclear cells is estimated to be 1 in 15 000–70 000.[7] IgG anti-AChR-secreting cells are also found in the peripheral blood of healthy volunteers, albeit in much lower numbers. The proportion of immunoglobulin-producing AChR-specific B cells or plasma cells is greater in the germinal centers of hyperplastic thymuses, but still only 1 in 1000–10 000 antibodies produced is AChR specific. Anti-AChR antibodies are predominantly IgG1 and IgG3 but IgG2 and IgG4 isotypes have also been found. IgA and IgM anti-AChR antibodies are present in some patients, but never in the absence of IgG anti-AChR. IgA and IgM anti-AChR tend to appear in patients whose disease is of longer duration and greater severity, and in association with high IgG titers.

The pathogenic anti-AChR antibodies in MG are thought to be directed to conformationally-dependent structures. Immunization of animals with irreversibly denatured AChR leads to the formation of anti-AChR capable of binding to native AChR, but the antibodies are not capable of causing disease. This observation indicates that conformationally-dependent epitope(s) are important in the induction of disease. Many of the anti-AChR antibodies are directed against the α subunit, particularly to a small region on the extracellular portion referred to as the main immunogenic region (Fig. 64.2).[8] Approximately 60% of the anti-AChR antibodies are directed against this region, which encompasses a set of overlapping epitopes clustered around amino acids 67–76 of the α subunit.[9] The reason for the predominant role of the α chain in the antibody response in myasthenia is not known. Not all disease-producing antibodies in humans or rats are directed to this region. Many patients also have antibodies recognizing the γ-containing embryonic form of AChR. This observation has spawned speculation about a nonmuscle source of sensitization.

Anti-AChR antibody levels and relationship to disease activity

The relationship of anti-AChR antibody and disease activity in MG is complicated. In general, serum levels of anti-AChR or anti-AChR/AChR complexes correlate poorly with disease severity. Among patients within one clinical grade, anti-AChR levels can vary by several orders of magnitude. In addition, approximately 10–15% of patients with clinical MG have no anti-AChR antibody by standard assays. Anti-AChR antibodies are more likely to be present if the disease is generalized or severe, and there is a tendency for higher levels of anti-AChR to correlate with more severe disease. Also, in an individual patient an increase or decrease in anti-AChR levels often accompanies deterioration or improvement, respectively, in clinical activity.

As the quantity of anti-AChR produced does not fully explain disease severity, studies have also focused on qualitative differences in these antibodies among different patients. These studies, however, have not distinguished properties of anti-AChR antibodies that lead to greater pathogenicity. Differences in specificity and avidity of binding to AChR have not been associated with particular functional effects or disease severity. Anti-AChR antibodies that bind or compete for the same region of AChR can have different functional effects. Anti-AChR antibodies show extensive heterogeneity by isoelectric focusing, but this characteristic also does not correlate with pathogenic potential.

As noted above, 10–15% of MG patients are persistently antibody negative. A subset of these patients has serum IgG antibodies specific for muscle tyrosine kinase (MuSK).[10] This skeletal muscle receptor tyrosine kinase is activated by agrin and is critical for formation of the neuromuscular junction. Affected patients tend to be young adult females with bulbar, neck, or respiratory muscle weakness. They frequently have muscle atrophy (particularly tongue and bulbar muscles) and variable responses to cholinesterase inhibitors. They benefit from plasmapharesis and although they typically lack thymus pathology, thymectomy is often associated with clinical improvement. Although MuSK antibodies affect AChR clustering on cultured myotubes, their contribution to the pathogenesis of MG remains unclear.

More recently, patients previously classified as seronegative have been found to have low affinity AChR-specific IgG when their sera were tested with very sensitive assays that rely on tissue substrates on which the receptors are aggregated.[11] Antibody binding was facilitated by the high concentrations of AChRs, which compensate for the low affinity of the autoantibodies. Like the anti-AChR antibodies in classical anti-AChR antibody positive MG, these antibodies belong to the IgG1 subclass. Also similar to the conventional antibodies, the low affinity antibodies bind complement. These properties differ from the anti-MuSK antibodies, which are predominantly IgG4 and are not associated with complement deposition *in vivo*.

Patients with myasthenia gravis associated with thymoma show distinct patterns of antibody production. Almost all patients with thymoma are anti-AChR antibody positive and most produce anti-striational antibodies.[12] These antibodies react with titin, a giant filamentous protein of striated muscle. Titin filaments are involved in muscle assembly and contribute to the muscle's ability to recoil following stimulation. Such anti-striational antibodies are also found in approximately 50% of the sera of older, non-thymoma MG patients who have thymic

atrophy, but are not frequently detected in patients with early-onset disease and thymic hyperplasia. The finding of anti-striational antibodies in an MG patient less than 40 years old strongly suggests the presence of thymoma. There is no evidence that anti-striational antibodies are involved in muscle weakness.

MG sera also contain antibodies reacting with the ryanodine receptor.[12] These receptors, which are critically involved in muscle contraction, are Ca^{2+} release channels located in the sarcoplasmic reticulum of striated muscles. Antibodies to ryanodine receptors are found in 50% of MG patients with thymoma, and patients with high levels have a worse prognosis than do antibody-negative MG patients with thymoma. *In vitro* studies have suggested a pathogenic role for these autoantibodies in MG.

Anti-rapsyn antibodies have been detected in a small subset of MG patients.[13] Seropositive patients with MG are indistinguishable from seronegative patients with regard to clinical and laboratory features of disease. The presence of this autoantibody specificity is not specific for MG, having been detected in the sera of an occasional MS patient and a majority of the lupus patients tested.

Pathogenic effects of anti-AChR antibodies

> ● **KEY CONCEPTS**
>
> **Effects of anti-acetylcholine receptor (AChR) antibodies in myasthenia gravis pathology**
>
> - Reduced number of receptors
> - Widening of the synaptic cleft
> - Distorted geometry of the synaptic membrane
>
> **Mechanism of damage**
>
> - Complement-dependent damage to muscle endplate
> - Enhanced rate of AChR degradation
> - Block cholinergic binding sites

Complement-mediated damage

The critical problem in MG is the anti-AChR antibody-mediated reduction in the number of nAChRs at the myoneural junction. There are several possible mechanisms by which anti-AChR antibodies could lead to impaired neuromuscular transmission.[14] Ultramicroscopy shows marked destructive changes in some endplates, particularly at the peaks of the postsynaptic folds, where AChR is usually present in greatest concentration. The architecture of the muscle endplate is simplified, with loss of junctional folds and widening of the synaptic cleft that contains membrane debris. C3, C9 and the membrane attack complex are deposited at the muscle endplate, suggesting a role for complement in membrane destruction.[15] Indeed, the anti-AChR antibodies in many patients can fix complement *in vitro* when bound to skeletal muscle, and can damage cultured rat myotubes with a resultant decrease in AChR content.

Although antibody-directed complement-mediated destruction is important in the pathophysiology of MG, it is not the entire story. The rapid clinical improvement in MG following certain therapeutic interventions and the lack of destructive changes in many neuromuscular junctions of symptomatic areas despite prominent immunoglobulin deposition suggest that a more readily reversible process is also likely to be involved in the neuromuscular block.

Acceleration of AChR degradation

In vitro and *in vivo* studies have shown that anti-AChR antibodies can accelerate the rate of degradation of extrajunctional and junctional receptors, respectively.[16] This reaction is complement independent and is due to the endocytosis of AChRs via shallow depressions, presumably clathrin-coated pits. Other membrane receptors are not affected. Both stable and rapidly turned-over receptors appear to be affected, thereby explaining the greater than expected antibody-mediated loss of AChRs observed at neuromuscular junctions. The reaction requires cross-linking of adjacent AChRs, as it can be mediated by F(ab)₂ fragments, but not Fab fragments, of anti-AChR antibodies. The effect of antibody on the synthesis of new AChR is controversial.

Receptor blockade

The inhibition of ACh binding has been assessed by studying the effects of MG serum on the binding of the neurotoxin α-bungarotoxin to AChRs. Such blocking antibodies are found in a variable number of MG sera. Blockade has been generally attributed to steric hindrance of the ligand-binding site, rather than direct binding to the ACh-binding site.[17] The importance of these antibodies in the pathophysiology of MG remains unclear. However, in one study the functional ability of an individual serum to accelerate degradation and cause blockade of AChRs paralleled most closely the clinical status of the patient. The *in vivo* significance of such antibodies has also been demonstrated by passive transfer of certain rat monoclonal anti-AChR antibodies into chicks. Complete paralysis was observed within 1 hour of the transfer, presumably before there was time for complement-mediated damage. In MG patients it has been reasoned that such blocking antibodies could further diminish synaptic function already decreased owing to complement-mediated damage and/or accelerated receptor degradation. This could result in acute clinical deterioration or a rapid clinical improvement after plasmapharesis, before the repair of damaged membrane and regeneration of new AChRs.

Role of T cells

An overwhelming body of data indicates that anti-AChR antibody production in MG patients and rodents with experimental autoimmune myasthenia gravis is dependent on the activity of CD4 T cells. Researchers have used freshly isolated CD4 T cells, T-cell lines, and T-cell clones stimulated with AChR purified from the electric organs of the electric eel *Torpedo californica* (T-AChR), recombinant human AChR, human AChR concentrated on immunomagnetic beads, and synthetic AChR peptides. Most of the T cells derived from MG patients have responded to the complete AChR or the α subunit, but responses to the δ, ε, and γ subunits have also been demonstrated.[18] Unlike experimental autoimmune myasthenia gravis, a T-cell immunodominant epitope has not been found in humans. However, T cells from most patients recognize a limited number of AChR sequences. In an individual patient, T cells reactive with a particular AChR epitope can show limited TCR Vβ usage, but the same TCR Vβ usage has not been observed for different patients. A range of major histocompatibility complex (MHC) class II molecules can present AChR epitopes. This is not surprising, given the degenerate binding capabilities of MHC molecules needed to present an extremely large and diverse group of peptides to the immune system. T cells from normal controls respond to some of the same epitopes to which MG patient's T cells respond, albeit in smaller numbers and less vigorously.

Experimental autoimmune myasthenia gravis

The serendipitous discovery that rabbits injected with purified AChR developed not only anti-AChR antibodies but signs of myasthenia gravis provided the evidence for the pivotal role of antibodies in this disease, and paved the way for development of an experimental model of human MG.[19] Experimental autoimmune myasthenia gravis (EAMG) has been studied in a number of different animal species.[20] It is generally induced by immunizing animals with AChR purified from the electric organs of *Torpedo californica* that is emulsified in adjuvant. Disease may also be passively transferred by immunoglobulin from affected animals or from patients with myasthenia. Animals suffer from fatigue, hypoactivity, weight loss, paralysis, difficulty in breathing and dysphagia; these signs are reversible with anticholinesterases. There is a decremental response to repetitive nerve stimulation on electromyography in EAMG as in MG. Anti-AChR antibodies are present and most are directed against the main immunogenic region (Fig. 64.2). They are deposited along with complement at the muscle endplate. Similar to the pathology in humans, there is simplification of the muscle endplate and a loss of AChR content of muscles in the experimental disease. A major difference between the induced rodent models of EAMG and spontaneous human MG is the absence of thymic pathology in the former.

In murine models there are disease-resistant and disease-susceptible strains. The MHC determines this susceptibility in part, with specific H-2 alleles associated with susceptibility or resistance. However, even in the high-responder strains only 50–70% of immunized animals manifest disease. This lack of concordance remains to be fully explained. Differences in the level of complement activation and the physiologic safety factor of neuromuscular transmission may partly account for the variability in disease expression.

Most immunized animals demonstrate anti-AChR antibodies whether or not they develop EAMG. Induction of pathogenic antibody production requires the integrity of the three-dimensional structure of the receptor, as immunization with denatured AChR elicits antibody production but not disease, even in susceptible animals. Anti-AChR antibody levels correlate with anti-AChR/AChR complexes and with the AChR content of the muscle, but not with clinical disease severity. No characteristic feature distinguishing disease-producing and nonpathogenic autoantibodies has been defined. Antibodies in rats with and without disease are predominantly of the same immunoglobulin isotype and subclass, express similar clonotypic heterogeneity, and show similar avidities. The percentage of antibodies that recognize the native receptor (as opposed to the foreign eel receptor immunogen) is low (0.2–2%), but similar between the symptomatic and the asymptomatic mice. The percentage of antibody directed against the main immunogenic region of AChR is also similar. The antibodies that develop in asymptomatic animals can bind and cause a decrease in receptor half-life, as well as those that develop in paralyzed animals. In fact, EMG abnormalities can be demonstrated in mice that appear disease free.[21] An analogous situation in humans may be the high frequency of single-fiber EMG abnormalities in asymptomatic family members of patients with MG. Importantly, antibodies from affected animals will cause disease in resistant strains, indicating that disease differences between strains is not caused by differences in the AChR receptor itself.

Although EAMG is mediated by autoantibodies, it is a T-cell-dependent process. Examination of T-cell responses in rats and mice has shown that EAMG requires the action of CD4 T cells. These cells recognize immunodominant T-cell epitopes located on the α subunit.[20] The T-cell responses to the immunodominant epitope in rats involve a variety of TCRVβ and Jβ gene segments. However, in susceptible C57BL/6 mice there is a predominant use of the TCRVβ6 family in the CD4 T-cell response. CD4 T cells in susceptible and resistant strains recognize different immunodominant AChR α-chain epitopes.[22]

Early reports suggested that AChR-reactive T-cell clones did not fit neatly into T-helper 1 (Th1) and Th2 subsets. However, later studies suggested that interferon-γ production by Th1 cells is essential for the development of disease and that IL-4 may subserve a protective role.[20,23] In addition to IFN-γ, TNF-α, IL-6, -12, -18, -1, -5, and -10 have been reported to promote the development of EAMG. However, a more recent publication indicated that C57BL/6 mice genetically deficient in IL-12/-23 and IFN-γ are susceptible to experimental EAMG, suggesting a pathogenic role of non-Th1 cells. This result led the authors to suggest that AChR-specific Th17 cells may also contribute to the pathogenesis of this experimental autoimmune disease.[24]

The roles of several co-stimulatory factors have also been investigated in EAMG. CD28/B7 and CD40/CD40L appear to be required for development of the primary immune response to AChR. An interaction between ICOS and B7RP.1 may play an important role in the secondary response and/or in the maintenance of the immune response to this autoantigen.

The thymus in myasthenia gravis

Several lines of evidence have implicated the thymus in the pathogenesis of MG.

Pathology

● KEY CONCEPTS

Pathogenic roles of the thymus in myasthenia gravis

Pathological
- 65–75% of patients have follicular hyperplasia; 10% have thymoma

Clinical
- Improvement following thymectomy

Immunological
- nAChR subunits expressed on myoid cells and thymic epithelial cells
- nAChR-reactive T and B cells localized in the thymus
- Anti-AChR antibody secreted by thymic B-lineage cells
- IL1-β, IL-6, CXCL13, and CCL21 overexpressed in thymus

Early observations from autopsy material and later analyses of thymectomy specimens indicated that the thymus is pathologically abnormal in 80–90% of MG patients.[25] The majority of patients (65–75%) have thymic follicular hyperplasia. This histologic picture is seen most frequently in women with a relatively early disease onset and with HLA-B8 and DR3 haplotypes. The architecture of the hyperplastic thymi is generally preserved, with well demarcated cortical and medullary regions. However, the medulla is crowded by numerous germinal centers

that display the architectural features and cellular constituents of germinal centers in the secondary follicles of peripheral lymph nodes from normal individuals. Although these germinal centers in patients are generally thought to occupy an intraparenchymal position, some observers feel that they may actually lie extraparenchymally in the perivascular space. The appearance of thymic germinal centers is not unique to MG. They have been observed in the thymi of healthy subjects who have died suddenly from traumatic injury, and in autopsy specimens of patients with SLE, thyrotoxicosis and multiple sclerosis. Nevertheless, they are widely regarded to be larger and more numerous in patients with MG.

Patients with MG and associated thymomas tend to be older and show no gender predominance or HLA associations. Histologic sections show neoplastic epithelial cells admixed with thymocytes and a loss of the normal corticomedullary definition. The affected epithelial cells belong to the cortical epithelial compartment, and the thymocytes have the immunophenotypic properties of normal immature cortical thymocytes.

Clinical

The demonstration of thymic pathology prompted empiric trials of thymectomy in patients with MG. Although no controlled study has been performed, there is general agreement that removal of the thymus, particularly in young patients with follicular hyperplasia, leads to clinical improvement. This topic is considered in more detail in the discussion on therapy below.

Intrathymic AChR

For some time there has been evidence that nAChR is expressed in the thymus.[25,26] This finding, in conjunction with the thymic pathology, has raised the hypothesis that thymic expression of AChR may be involved in the initiation or perpetuation of the autoimmune response in MG. At the protein level, the AChR α chain is expressed on thymic myoid cells and epithelial cells. Most of the current evidence is consistent with the expression of a fetal receptor on myoid cells and an adult receptor on thymic epithelial cells. In addition, an epitope localized to residues 373–380 of the AChR α-chain cytoplasmic domain has been detected on neoplastic epithelial cells of thymomas and thymic carcinomas, and is most often seen in thymomas associated with MG. This epitope is also found in smaller amounts on normal thymic medullary cells. The source of the epitope is not AChR but a cross-reactive protein with a molecular weight of 153 kDa.[27] The overexpression of this protein in thymomas may trigger an anti-AChR antibody response, leading to the development of MG.

Studies relying on molecular probes of AChR expression indicate that both major isoforms of the α subunit are expressed in human thymus.[26,28] The smaller P3A⁻ isoform is present in approximately a fivefold excess in both MG and control thymic tissue,[28] which differs from the equivalent expression of these isoforms in control and MG muscle. These observations suggest that the expression of mRNAs encoding the P3A⁻ and P3A⁺ isoforms is regulated differently in human thymus compared to muscle. As the same disproportionate expression of P3A⁻ was observed in control and MG thymus, the differential pattern of expression observed in thymus relative to muscle is probably not a manifestation of thymic pathology in MG. Rather, this pattern may reflect control processes that are unique to these two distinct tissue compartments. It is currently not known whether the disproportionate expression of P3A⁻ and P3A⁺ isoforms has pathogenic significance. Notably, the expression of both P3A$^+$ and P3A$^-$ mRNAs is increased in MG thymus relative to control thymus. This finding parallels that reported for skeletal muscle, where AChR mRNA expression is greater in MG muscle than in control muscle. The finding of increased AChRα mRNA expression in MG thymus may represent an attempt to compensate for the destructive action of locally secreted anti-AChR antibodies. The increased AChR mRNA expression may also reflect the antecedent action of other local environmental factors, e.g., cytokines.

In this regard, we have found that IFN-γ enhances the expression of AChRα mRNA on human thymic epithelial cells *in vitro*.[28] It is known that IFN-γ upregulates the expression of MHC class II molecules on thymic epithelial cells.[29,30] This dual effect of IFN-γ on AChRα and MHC class II molecules raises the possibility that this cytokine, and perhaps others, can alter expression of thymic AChRα *in vivo* in a manner that leads to the development or perpetuation of MG. Additional evidence supporting the potential contribution of IFN-γ to intrathymic events in MG comes from recently reported microarray data derived from MG hyperplastic thymus.[31] Although genes encoding interferons and interferon receptors were not upregulated, evidence for increased expression of type-1 and -2 inducible interferon genes was obtained. These results suggest an antecedent action by type I and/or type II interferon. Interestingly, it has been reported that interferon regulatory factor-8, one of the genes induced by IFN-γ, upregulates the transcription of *CHRNA1*, the gene that encodes the alpha subunit of AChR.[32] This finding provides a molecular explanation for the IFN-γ upregulated thymic epithelial cell expression of AChRα. Taken together, these findings support a pivotal role for the local action of IFN in development of thymic pathology and possibly MG.

Sequencing of P3A$^+$ and P3A$^-$ cDNA clones recovered from control and MG thymi indicates that they share the same nucleotide sequence as their respective counterparts at the myoneural junction.[28,33] Therefore, unless there are post-translational changes, the structure of the AChRα proteins expressed in the thymus and the periphery are likely to be identical. These results provide a structural basis for proposing that an immune response directed at thymic nAChRα is indeed responsible for initiating or perpetuating disease.

Immunologic

From an immunologic standpoint the MG thymus has unique features that could reflect pathogenic involvement and help explain some of the histologic abnormalities.[25] Although B cells and Ig-secreting cells are rare intramedullary inhabitants of normal thymi, they are increased in cell suspensions of MG thymus, particularly hyperplastic thymus relative to control thymus (obtained from subjects undergoing elective cardiothoracic surgery). When stimulated *in vitro* with the polyclonal B-cell activator pokeweed mitogen, both MG and normal thymus cell suspensions produced surprisingly large amounts of immunoglobulin, with the IgG isotype greatly exceeding IgM.

There has been great interest in determining whether the heightened B-cell activity in MG thymus reflects local immune events. Single cell suspensions from thymi of MG patients with follicular hyperplasia secrete anti-AChR *in vitro* without addition of B-cell activators.[25] However, the thymic B-cell repertoire also includes anti-influenza and anti-tetanus toxoid specificities. The latter is only detected when patients are booster immunized to tetanus toxoid 3–4 weeks prior to thymectomy. Thus, the

B-cell repertoire in the MG thymus may reflect systemic as well as local immune events.

AChR-reactive CD4 T cells have been detected and propagated as long-term lines and clones from MG thymus (both thymoma and hyperplasia), but not from normal thymus. These antigen-specific T cells seem to be enriched in the thymus relative to the blood of the same MG patient. Migration of T cells reactive to foreign antigen into the thymus is known to occur.[34] Therefore, it is not clear whether AChR-reactive T cells in MG thymus are sensitized in the periphery with subsequent intrathymic localization, or are sensitized *in situ*. The state of intrathymic T regulatory cells is less clear with reports of both decreased and normal numbers of CD4$^+$CD25$^+$ Foxp3$^+$ cells associated with decreased *in vitro* activity.

Hyperplastic MG thymus shows increased numbers of IL-1- and -6-producing cells. These cells are found largely in the perifollicular areas and connective tissue adjacent to the septae of disrupted cortex. Cells producing IL-2 are less prominent and confined largely to perifollicular areas. This distribution of cytokine production is not seen in normal thymus or in hyperplastic lymph nodes.

Using DNA microarray, overexpression of CXCL13 and CCL21 in hyperplastic MG thymus was detected.[31] These chemokines are involved in germinal center formation in the peripheral lymphoid system. Expression of these genes as well as others encoding pro-inflammatory cytokines was less prominent in thymi from patients receiving corticosteroid treatment. It was suggested that the overexpression of CXCL13 and CCL21 served to attract B cells and activated T cells to the thymus. In addition, a proliferation-inducing ligand (APRIL) and B-cell activating factor of the tumor necrosis factor family (BAFF), two B-cell-survival factors secreted by macrophages and dendritic cells, were detected in hyperplastic MG thymi.[35]

Together, these studies indicate that MG thymus contains the components necessary for an antibody response directed against AChR. These include AChR-reactive B cells and helper T cells, cytokines that can facilitate B-cell activation and promote their survival, chemokines that attract immigrant lymphocytes, possibly decreased CD4$^+$CD25$^+$ T regulatory cell function and a local source of the autoantigen. Impaired thymic T-regulatory cell function could impede the development or maintenance of T-cell tolerance to locally expressed AChR. Nevertheless, it is not known whether autosensitization occurs in the thymus with spillover to the myoneural junction, or whether the thymic pathology is causally related to the pathogenesis of MG. Of note, thymic pathologic changes are not typically seen in the thymi of rodents with actively or passively induced MG. Thus, the pathologic changes seen in MG thymus are not secondary to the systemic autoimmune response and may be linked to the etiopathogenesis of this disease. The cause of the putative intrathymic sensitization is unknown, although the totality of findings are consistent with an antecedent pro-inflammatory event in the thymic medulla.[36]

Etiologic factors

Genetic factors

Similar to most autoimmune diseases, the MHC is an important genetic susceptibility locus for the development of MG. The MHC haplotype HLA-B8, DR3 DQ2 is associated with early-onset MG and hyperplastic thymus in Caucasians. An association with HLA-B7 and DR2, although weaker, has also been described for patients with MG onset after age 40 associated with atrophic thymic histology. In mice the MHC class II molecules I-A^b and I-E^k have been associated with susceptibility to EAMG.[20] In EAMG the permissive MHC class II molecules are capable of binding AChR peptides that are recognized by antigen-specific CD4 T cells.

The potential contributions of other immune system-related genes in the pathogenesis of MG include a reported association for a particular IL-1β allele and MG[37] with increased serum levels of this cytokine. This was most pronounced in patients lacking disease-predisposing HLA genes. An association between MG and the presence of particular TNF-α polymorphisms has been reported.[38–40] The expression of a high-transcription TNF-α allotype correlated with early-onset MG and the absence of anti-titin antibodies. In this regard, MG patients demonstrate increased serum levels of TNF-α and their peripheral blood mononuclear cells display increased expression of TNF-α mRNA.[40] Polymorphisms in the IL-10 promoter region are said to be associated with distinct patterns of thymic histology.[41] No correlations have been made between IL-4 alleles and MG. Allotypic markers on IgG and FcγRIIA receptors have been associated with the coexistence of MG and thymoma.[42] A single nucleotide polymorphism in the gene encoding the intracellular tyrosine phosphatase PTPN22, which has been associated with the risk of developing other autoimmune diseases, has been identified in both a subgroup of anti-titin antibody positive nonthymomatous MG patients and patients with thymomatous MG.[43,44] The risk of developing MG has also been linked to a polymorphism in the promoter region of *CHRNA1*, the gene that encodes the alpha subunit of AChR.[32] In this case, it was postulated that the variant genotype causes reduced expression of AChRα on thymic medullary epithelial cells, thereby impairing central deletion of AChRα-specific thymocytes.

Exogenous factors

Whether or not sensitization to AChR occurs in the thymus or the periphery, the stimulus for this autoimmune response remains a conundrum. Moreover, it remains to be determined whether the stimulus is self-antigen (AChR) or a foreign antigen that mimics the receptor's molecular structure. In this regard, several examples of molecular mimicry between AChRα chain and other molecules have been reported. Use of certain monoclonal anti-AChR antibodies demonstrated epitope sharing between the receptor and several bacteria, including *Klebsiella pneumoniae*, *Escherichia coli*, *Proteus vulgaris*, and *Yersinia enterocolitica*.[45] However, for the most part no difference was observed in the binding of polypeptides from these organisms by either MG patient or control sera. A computer search of protein banks revealed a sequence homology between AChRα chain and a short peptide in herpes simplex glycoprotein D,[46] although the significance of this finding is unknown. Finally, similarities were reported between idiotypic determinants on anti-AChR antibodies and antibodies reactive with α1,3 dextran. Interestingly, anti-dextran antibodies were detected in approximately 13% of MG patients but rarely in normal controls.[47] α1,3 dextran is found in the cell walls of several common enteric pathogens and thus represents a potential ubiquitous source of immunogen. This type of idiotypic network connectivity led to postulation that an unregulated anti-idiotypic response to anti-α1,3 dextran antibodies might lead, in certain individuals, to an anti-AChR antibody response. Unfortunately, there has been no follow-up to these observations.

A striking association has been reported between the development of MG and treatment with the drug penicillamine,[48,49] particularly in individuals with HLA-DR1. MG developed in patients with rheumatoid arthritis and patients with Wilson's disease treated with this agent. After discontinuation of penicillamine, resolution of MG symptoms was reported in some patients but not others. Penicillamine treatment was associated with the development of anti-AChR antibodies that appeared to have the same specificity profile as found in idopathic myasthenia. Additional evidence suggests that penicillamine may directly interfere with neuromuscular transmission. Although penicillamine has been shown to have diverse effects on the immune response in the normal host, and has reactive sulfhydryl groups capable of modifying self-antigens, its role in the development of MG is unknown.

Treatment of myasthenia gravis

THERAPEUTIC APPROACHES

- Anticholinesterase agents
- Thymectomy
- Plasmapheresis
- Corticosteroids
- Immunosuppressive agents
- Intravenous γ-globulin

Therapeutic intervention in MG usually proceeds in a stepwise manner, beginning with anticholinesterase agents.[50]

Anticholinesterases

Anticholinesterases are the mainstay of treatment. These agents protect acetylcholine from hydrolysis by cholinesterase, thereby increasing the amount of neutrotransmitter and the number of contacts with the reduced number of receptors in MG at the postsynaptic junction. This in turn raises the probability of attaining the necessary threshold for neuromuscular transmission. In addition, some of the anticholinesterases are direct agonists at the postsynaptic junction. The three most popular such agents are neostigmine bromide (Prostigmin), pyridostigmine bromide (Mestinon) and ambenonium chloride (Mytelase). Although there are only slight differences between these agents, pyridostigmine bromide is the most commonly used. It has an onset of action of 30–60 minutes, peak action at about 2 hours, and loss of activity after 4 hours. The drug is usually initiated at a dose of 60 mg every 3–4 hours and increased if necessary in 30–60 mg increments. Additional benefit is usually not seen at doses higher than 240 mg every 3–4 hours or 120 mg every 2 hours. It is important to individualize the dosing schedule for each patient. For example, a patient with bulbar symptoms should be instructed to take anticholinesterase 30 minutes to 1 hour before meals. Adverse effects of these agents reflect excessive stimulation of nicotinic and muscarinic receptors. The nicotinic side effects include fasciculations, muscle cramps, and increased weakness. Muscarinic side effects include diarrhea, abdominal cramps, palpitations, increased sweating, and nasal and bronchial secretions. Adding atropine or an atropine analog to the regimen can minimize the latter group of reactions. This provides a cushion for increasing the amount of drug, and hence, its effect at the postsynaptic junction. Ephedrine and xanthine derivatives (theophylline) are thought to increase the presynaptic release of ACh. However, their minimal added benefit has not warranted common usage.

Thymectomy

Another mainstay in the therapy of adults with generalized MG is thymectomy.[51,52] The benefit is greatest in younger patients and those with thymic hyperplasia, although many centers also include older patients. Although no controlled study has been published, the accumulated clinical experience indicates that thymectomy is associated with an excellent outcome, measured as either remission or an improvement in clinical symptoms. In one study 90% of patients were asymptomatic or in complete remission within a few years of thymectomy, and 46% were off all medications. Currently there is a randomized, single-blind-controlled trial underway that is evaluating the value of adding thymectomy to prednisone monotherapy. With improvements in preoperative care, anesthesia, surgical technique, and postoperative care, thymectomy has become a very safe procedure, but its value and safety in children and older patients is less well established. The mechanism responsible for the salutary effect of thymectomy is unknown. No obvious effects on immunoregulatory mechanisms have been demonstrated, although anti-AChR titers tend to fall months after the procedure. Thymectomy is also the recommended treatment for patients of all ages suspected of having thymoma.

Corticosteroids

Corticosteroids are used in patients with generalized MG who fail to respond to anticholinesterase agents or thymectomy, and in patients needing optimization of their clinical condition in preparation for thymectomy.[53] They are generally not used as a first-line agent to replace thymectomy. They are also used in patients with ocular myasthenia who fail to respond to anticholinesterases. Corticosteroids are initially given on a daily basis, with therapy begun in hospital. This cautious approach is followed because of the fear of clinical deterioration that occurs in some patients during the introduction of corticosteroids. Because of this concern, some groups advocate starting patients on alternate-day therapy, which is not typically associated with clinical deterioration and can be carried out on an outpatient basis. Daily corticosteroids are usually started in patients with generalized MG at a dose > 1 mg/kg prednisone. Patients should be continued on this dose until clinical improvement is maintained for several days, and then gradually converted to alternate-day therapy. With improvement sustained over several months, an effort should be made to reduce the dose (usually in 5-mg decrements) administered on the alternate day. Although a Cochrane review underscored the dearth of controlled trials, the improvement rate is generally estimated to be 60–90%.[54] Complete remission is rare and most patients will require some dose of steroids indefinitely. Anticholinesterase requirements may decrease as the patient responds to corticosteroids.

Plasmapheresis

Plasmapheresis has enjoyed popularity since its introduction as an auxiliary treatment modality in 1976, particularly as a temporizing measure.[55] It appears most beneficial in patients in myasthenic crisis and in those experiencing progressive deterioration despite treatment with anticholinesterases and corticosteroids. Plasmapheresis has also proved useful in preparing patients for thymectomy when the course is complicated by involvement of the bulbar and respiratory musculature. Such patients may also require short-term plasmapheresis during the postoperative period. There is no long-term benefit of plasmapharesis when added to prednisone. Although there are no clear rules, the average exchange is 1–2 L/day for 7–14 days. Improvement is usually observed within a few days of concluding the treatment course, although patients in crisis often benefit more quickly. The mechanism of action most likely involves removal of the pathogenic autoantibody, as a reduction in titer of anti-AChR correlates with clinical improvement. However, it is also possible that the removal of other phlogistic humoral factors contributes to clinical efficacy.

Intravenous immunoglobulins

The efficacy of intravenous immunoglobulin (IVIG) in MG was suggested by several uncontrolled clinical trials. Interest in the use of IVIG grew out of its demonstrated efficacy in other autoimmune diseases, particularly autoimmune thrombocytopenia. Subsequent randomized double-blind placebo-controlled trials provided proof of clinical efficacy. Conventional dosing is infusion of 2 g/kg divided over five days although some practitioners prefer to administer this dose over two days. In a randomized, controlled trial a total dose of 1 g/kg was as efficacious as a dose of 2 g/kg. IVIG therapy is generally associated with rapid clinical improvement in responsive patients, independent of whether they had undergone thymectomy or were being treated concurrently with corticosteroids or immunosuppressive agents. In some patients improvement was sustained over a period of several weeks. The mechanism(s) of this apparent salutary effect is unknown although a recent report highlighted the possible action of antibodies in IVIG directed against the idiotypes of anti-AChR antibodies. Improvement has not always been accompanied by a consistent reduction in anti-AChR titers. In general, IVIG and plasmapheresis appear equivalent in efficacy.[56] However, IVIG may be preferable because of better tolerance and lower cost.

Immunosuppressive agents

Immunosuppressive drugs have been tried primarily in patients who have failed treatment with anticholinesterases, thymectomy, plasmapheresis, and corticosteroids.[57] Most of the experience has been obtained with azathioprine, which has strong anti-inflammatory effects as well as immunosuppressive activity. The dose of azathioprine has varied between 1 and 3 mg/kg/day, with improvement seen between 5 and 20 weeks. The drug is usually started at a lower dose and escalated weekly to achieve the maintenance dose. Patients should be followed with complete blood counts, particularly during therapy initiation, as azathioprine has a suppressive effect on the bone marrow. A white blood cell count below 2500/μL or a neutrophil count below 1500/μL should prompt a reduction or termination of the dosage. The results of a randomized double-blind placebo-controlled trial indicated that the addition of azathioprine (2.5 mg/kg) to alternate-day prednisolone was associated with a reduction of the prednisolone dose, fewer treatment failures, longer remissions, and fewer side effects.[58] There is considerably less experience in treatment of steroid-unresponsive patients with cyclophosphamide. It is associated with more adverse effects and does not appear to offer significant advantage over azathioprine when used in standard dosing regimens. High-dose intravenous cyclophosphamide therapy of MG patients refractory to conventional immunosuppressive agents has been investigated as an approach to immunoablate the bone marrow and allow for subsequent repopulation by endogenous stem cells. Although durable responses were seen in some patients in an early trial, this regimen is not readily available and should only be utilized in refractory patients under treatment in specialized centers. Methotrexate has been used in some uncontrolled studies but there is no information to indicate that it is more efficacious or safer than azathioprine and its onset of action may take as long as several months. As is true for corticosteroid therapy, it is the rare patient who enjoys a permanent remission following institution of immunosuppressive therapy, and those who show some improvement often require treatment indefinitely.

Cyclosporine has been investigated because it interferes with IL-2-mediated T-cell proliferation and thus would be expected to interfere with the generation of T cells that would "help" the anti-AChR antibody response. A retrospective study suggested that cyclosporine provided benefit in patients whose disease was refractory to corticosteroids and azathioprine. Serious renal toxicity and treatment withdrawal, which plagued earlier studies, were reduced by careful selection of patients. In a 12-month European trial, cyclosporine appeared to be as efficacious as azathioprine in producing clinical improvement. Tacrolimus has a similar mechanism of action to cyclosporine. When used in low dosage, it has proved as effective as cyclosporine as a corticosteroid-sparing agent, and with fewer side effects. Nevertheless, most practitioners reserve these agents for use in patients refractory to the combination of azathioprine and prednisone.

Mycophenolate mofetil (MMF), another immunosuppressive agent that affects both T and B cells, was widely touted following the completion of early trials as a steroid-sparing agent in patients with MG. That experience suggested that it was effective 70–75% of the time although probably less so in refractory MG. It has an acceptable safety profile with adverse effects largely related to gastrointestinal intolerance. Benefit may require many weeks of administration. However, two recent randomized, placebo-controlled trials have challenged the early optimism. In one, the addition of MMF at the initiation of a 36-week schedule of prednisone tapering was not found superior to placebo in maintaining myasthenia control.[59] In the second, the co-administration of MMF and prednisone provided no better control of myasthenic weakness than prednisone alone in the initial management of generalized MG.[60] However, none of the patients included in these two studies were known to be steroid-resistant. Thus, whether MMF has long-term benefits with respect to myasthenic weakness or steroid-sparing effects in the population of steroid-resistant patients remains unanswered.

Possible future therapeutic options

There are a number of possible experimental avenues of approach that have been spawned by studies in EAMG. These are aimed at interrupting the sensitization process of helper CD4 T cells, interrupting their effector function, or interdicting the downstream action of pro-inflammatory molecules. Studies directed at CD4 T-cell-orchestrated responses include blocking the presentation of immunogenic AChR peptides by antigen presenting cells with nonimmunogenic forms of peptides, impeding activation by inhibitors of the co-stimulatory molecules CD28 and ICOS, the induction of anergy or apoptosis of AChR-reactive T cells, and suppression of AChR-specific Th1 responses by the induction of T regulatory cells. In addition, inhibition of the cytokines TNF or IL-1 by anti-TNF reagents and an IL-1 receptor

antagonist, respectively, have shown efficacy in EAMG. Additional studies directed at AChR-specific B cells or IgG anti-AChR antibodies include the use of (1) AChR-Fc fusion proteins that induce apoptosis of AChR-specific B cells in vitro and ex vivo by cross-linking their AChR receptors and inhibitory FcγRIIBs and (2) non-cross-linking IgG4 anti-AChR antibodies that inhibit pathogenic IgG autoantibody-induced antigenic modulation. Complement inhibition has shown efficacy in the treatment of EAMG and represents a target in MG patients now that complement inhibitors have demonstrated benefit in the treatment of a number of human disorders.

Three biologics that have begun to receive attention in clinical MG trials are rituximab, etanercept, and infliximab. The former is a monoclonal antibody specific for CD20, a protein expressed on B lymphocytes. Etanercept is a fusion protein consisting of the human p75 TNF receptor and Fc fragment of IgG while infliximab is an anti-TNF monoclonal antibody. Rituximab, developed as a therapeutic for B-cell malignancies, has shown efficacy in a number of autoimmune disorders including some in which T cells, rather than B cells, are regarded as the principal effector mechanism. Anecdotal reports and small uncontrolled case series have shown improvement of MG following administration of rituximab. Responsive patients in one study did not demonstrate a reduction in anti-AChR antibodies. Although most treated patients have been anti-AChR antibody positive, benefit has also been observed in anti-MuSK positive anti-AChR antibody negative patients. Etanercept also appears promising as a type of immunomodulatory agent in MG. However, rare patients treated with this agent for inflammatory arthritis have developed MG that improved following cessation of treatment. Clinical improvement has been reported in a few MG patients treated with infliximab.

Acknowledgment

This work was supported by National Institutes of Health (NIH) Grant NS19546.

References

1. Lisak RP, Barchi RL. Myasthenia gravis. In: Walton JN, editor. Major problems in neurology, vol. 11. Philadelphia: WB Saunders; 1982. p. 5.
2. Engel A. The investigation of congenital myasthenic syndromes. Ann N Y Acad Sci 1993;681:425.
3. Beeson D, Vincent A, Morris A, et al. cDNA and genomic clones encoding the muscle acetylcholine receptor. Ann N Y Acad Sci 1993;681:165.
4. Karlin A. Explorations of the nicotinic acetylcholine receptor. Harvey Lect 1991;85:71.
5. Sanes JR, Apel ED, Gautam M, et al. Agrin receptors at the skeletal neuromuscular junction. Ann N Y Acad Sci 1998;841:1.
6. Levinson AI, Zweiman B, Lisak RP. Immunopathogenesis and treatment of myasthenia gravis. J Clin Immunol 1987;7:187.
7. Yi Q, Pirskanen R, Lefvert AK. Human muscle acetylcholine receptor reactive T and B lymphocytes in the peripheral blood of patients with myasthenia gravis. J Neuroimmunol 1993;42:215.
8. Tindal RSA. Humoral immunity in myasthenia gravis: biochemical characterization of acquired anti-receptor antibodies and clinical correlations. Ann Neurol 1981;10:437.
9. Papadouli I, Sakarellos C, Tzartos SJ. High-resolution epitope mapping and fine antigenic characterization of the main immunogenic region of the acetylcholine receptor. Eur J Biochem 1993;211:227.
10. Sanders DB, Juel VC. MuSK-antibody positive myasthenia gravis: questions from the clinic. J Neuroimmunol 2008;201–202:85–9.
11. Leite MI, Jacob , Viegas S, Cossins J, et al. IgG1 antibodies to acetylcholine receptors in "seronegative" myasthenia gravis. Brain 2008;131:1940–52.
12. Aarli JA, Skeie GO, Mygland A, et al. Muscle striation antibodies in myasthenia gravis. Ann N Y Acad Sci 1998;841:505.
13. Agius MA, Zhu S, Kirvan CA, et al. Rapsyn antibodies in myasthenia gravis. Ann N Y Acad Sci 1998;841:516.
14. Drachman DB, Adams RN, Josifek LF, et al. Antibody-mediated mechanisms of ACh receptor loss in myasthenia gravis: clinical relevance. Ann N Y Acad Sci 1981;377:175.
15. Engel AG, Sahashi K, Fumagalli G. The immunopathology of acquired myasthenia gravis. Ann N Y Acad Sci 1981;377:158.

16. Drachman DB, Angus CW, Adams RN, et al. Myasthenic antibodies cross-link acetylcholine receptors to accelerate degradation. N Engl J Med 1978;298:1116.

17. Richman DP, Wollmann RL, Maselli RA, et al. Effector mechanisms of myasthenic antibodies. Ann N Y Acad Sci 1998;681:264.

18. Conti-Fine B, Navaneetham D, Karachunski PI, et al. T cell recognition of the acetylcholine receptor in myasthenia gravis. Ann N Y Acad Sci 1998;841:283.

19. Patrick J, Lindstrom J. Autoimmune response to acetylcholine receptor. Science 1973;180:871.

20. Christadoss P, Poussin M, Deng C. Animal models of myasthenia gravis. Clin Immunol 2000;94:75.

21. Pachner AR, Kantor FS. The relation of clinical disease to antibody titre, proliferative response and neurophysiology in murine experimental autoimmune myasthenia gravis. Clin Exp Immunol 1983;51:543.

22. Bellone M, Ostile N, Lei S, Conti-Tronconi BM. Experimental myasthenia gravis in congenic mice. Sequence mapping and H-2 restriction of T helper epitopes on the a subunits of Torpedo californica and murine acetylcholine receptors. Eur J Immunol 1991;21:2303.

23. Karachunski PI, Ostlie NS, Okita DK, Conti-Fine BM. Interleukin-4 deficiency facilitates development of experimental myasthenia gravis and precludes its prevention by nasal administration of CD4+ epitope sequences of the acetylcholine receptor. J Neuroimmunol 1999;95:73.

24. Wang W, Milani M, Ostlie N, et al. C57BL/6 mice genetically deficient in IL-12/IL-23 and IFN-{gamma} are susceptible to experimental autoimmune myasthenia gravis, suggesting a pathogenic role of non-Th1 cells. J Immunol 2007;178:7072.

25. Levinson AI, Wheatley LM. The thymus and the pathogenesis of myasthenia gravis. Clin Immunol Immunopathol 1995;78:1.

26. Wheatley LM, Urso D, Zheng Y, et al. Molecular analysis of intrathymic nicotinic acetylcholine receptor. Ann N Y Acad Sci 1993;681:74.

27. Schultz A, Hoffacker V, Wilisch A, et al. Neurofilament is an autoantigenic determinant in myasthenia gravis. Ann Neurol 1999;46:167.

28. Zheng Y, Wheatley LM, Liu T, Levinson AI. Acetylcholine receptor alpha subunit mRNA expression in human thymus: augmented expression in myasthenia gravis and upregulation by interferon-g. Clin Immunol 1999;91:170.

29. Galy AHM, Spits H. IL-1, IL-4 and IFN-g differentially regulates cytokine production and cell surface molecule expression in cultured human thymic epithelial cells. J Immunol 1991;147:3283.

30. Berrih-Aknin S, Arenzana-Seisdedos F, Cohen S, et al. Interferon-gamma modulates MHC class II expression on cultured human epithelial cells. J Immunol 1985;35:1165.

31. Cizeron-Clairac G, Le Panse R, Frenkian-Cuvelier M, et al. Thymus and Myasthenia Gravis: what can we learn from DNA microarrays? J Neuroimmunol 2008;57:201–2.

32. Giraud M, Taubert R, Giraud M, et al. An IRF8-binding promoter variant and AIRE control CHRNA1 promiscuous expression in thymus. Nature 2007;448:934.

33. Wheatley L, Urso D, Tumas K, et al. Molecular characterization of the nicotinic acetylcholine receptor alpha chain in mouse thymus. J Immunol 1992;148:3105.

34. Naparstek Y, Ben-Nun A, et al. T lymphocyte lines producing or vaccinating against autoimmune encephalomyelitis (EAE). Functional activation induces peanut agglutinin receptors and accumulation in the brain and thymus of line cells. Eur J Immunol 1983;13:418.

35. Thangarajh M, Masterman T, Helgeland L, et al. The thymus is a source of B-cell-survival factors–APRIL and BAFF–in myasthenia gravis. J Neuroimmunol 2006;178:161.

36. Levinson AI, Zheng Y, Gaulton G, et al. Intrathymic expression of neuromuscular acetylcholine receptors and the immunpathogenesis of myasthenia gravis. Immunol Res 2003;27:399.

37. Huang D, Pirskanen R, Hjelmstrom P, Lefvert AK. Polymorphisms in IL-1beta and IL-1 receptor antagonist genes are associated with myasthenia gravis. J Neuroimmunol 1998;81:76.

38. Skeie GO, Pandey JP, Aarli JA, Gilhus NE. TNFA and TNFB polymorphisms in myasthenia gravis. Arch Neurol 1999;56:457.

39. Hjelmstrom P, Peacock CS, Giscombe R, et al. Polymorphism in tumor necrosis factor genes associated with myasthenia gravis. J Neuroimmunol 1998;88:137.

40. Huang DR, Pirskanen R, Matell G, Lafvert AK. Tumour necrosis factor-alpha polymorphism and secretion in myasthenia gravis. J Neuroimmunol 1999;94:165.

41. Huang DR, Zhou YH, Xia SQ, et al. Markers in the promoter region of interleukin-10 (IL-10) gene in myasthenia gravis: implications of diverse effects of IL-10 in the pathogenesis of the disease. J Neuroimmunol 1999;94:82.

42. Raknes G, Skeie GO, Gilhus NE, et al. FcgammaRIIa and FcgammaRIIIB polymorphisms in myasthenia gravis. J Neuroimmunol 1998;81:173.

43. Chuang WY, Strobel P, Belharazem D, et al. The PTPN22gain-of-function+1858T(+) genotypes correlate with low IL-2 expression in thymomas and predispose to myasthenia gravis. Genes Immun 2009;10:667.

44. Greve B, Hoffmann P, Illes Z, et al. The autoimmunity-related polymorphism PTPN22 1858C/T is associated with anti-titin antibody-positive myasthenia gravis. Hum Immunol 2009;70:540.

45. Stefansson K, Dieperink ME, Richman DP, Marton LS. Sharing of epitopes by bacteria and the nicotinic acetylcholine receptor: a possible role in the pathogenesis of myasthenia gravis. Ann N Y Acad Sci 1987;505:451.

46. Schwimmbeck PL, Dyrberg T, Drachman DB, Oldstone MB. Molecular mimicry and myasthenia gravis: an autoantigenic site of the acetylcholine receptor a-subunit that has biologic activity and reacts immunochemically with herpes simplex virus. J Clin Invest 1989;84:1174.

47. Dwyer DS, Vakil M, Bradleg RT, et al. A possible cause of myasthenia gravis: Idiotypic networks involving bacterial antigens. Ann N Y Acad Sci 1987;505:461.

48. Bever Jr. CT, Chang HW, Penn AS, et al. Chemical alteration of acetylcholine receptor by penicillamine: a mechanism for induction of myasthenia gravis. Neurology 1982;32:1077.

49. Penn AS, Jacques JJ. Cells from mice exposed chronically to D-penicillamine show proliferative responses to D-penicillamine-treated self (macrophage/dendritic cells): a graft-versus-host response? Ann N Y Acad Sci 1993;681:319.

50. Kumar V, Kaminski HJ. Treatment of myasthenia gravis. Curr Neurol Neurosci Rep 2011;11:89.

51. Olanow CW, Wechsler AS, Sirotkin-Roses M, et al. Thymectomy as primary therapy in myasthenia gravis. Ann N Y Acad Sci 1987;505:595.

52. Sonnett JR, Jaretzki III A. Thymectomy for nonthymomatous myasthenia gravis a critical analysis. Ann N Y Acad Sci 2008;1132:315.

53. Johns TR. Long-term corticosteroid treatment of myasthenia gravis. Ann N Y Acad Sci 1987;505:568.

54. Schneider-Gold C, Gadjos P, Toyka K, et al. Corticosteroids for myasthenia gravis. Cochrane Database Syst Rev 2005;18: CD002828.

55. Seybold M. Plasmapheresis in myasthenia gravis. Ann N Y Acad Sci 1987;505:58.

56. Miller RG, Barohn RJ, Dubinsky R. Expanding the evidence base for therapeutics in myasthenia gravis. Ann Neurol 2010;68:776.

57. Sanders DB, Evoli A. Immunosuppressive therapies in myasthenia gravis. Autoimmunity 2010;43:428.

58. Palace J, Newsom-Davis J, Lecky B. A randomized double-blind trial of prednisolone alone or with azathioprine in myasthenia gravis. Myasthenia Gravis Study Group. Neurology 1998;50:1778.

59. Sanders DB, Hart IK, Mantegazza R, et al. An international, phase III, randomized trial of mycophenylate mofetil in myasthenia gravis. Neurology 2008;71:400.

60. The Muscle Study Group. A trial of mycophenylate mofetil with prednisone as initial immunotherapy in myasthenia gravis SYMBOL. Neurology 2008;71:394.

65

Multiple sclerosis

Tanuja Chitnis,
Samia J. Khoury

Multiple sclerosis (MS) is a disease of the central nervous system characterized by inflammatory cell infiltration, demyelination, and axonal damage. Clinically, it is characterized by neurological deficits disseminated in time and space. MS is generally considered to be an autoimmune disease, and many of the effective therapies for MS target the immune system.

MS is a major cause of disability in the adult population in North America. Women are predominantly affected at a ratio of 2:1. The disease is characterized by a varying array of neurological deficits. There are four main disease types, classified on the basis of the clinical disease course: relapsing-remitting (RR), secondary progressive (SP), primary progressive (PP), and progressive relapsing (PR). RR disease affects 80% of patients and is characterized by onset of neurological deficits that remit over a period of weeks to months. After 15 years, most RR patients go on to have an SP form of disease, in which neurological deficits become fixed and accumulate. A primary progressive form of MS affects approximately 15% of patients. PP patients accumulate permanent neurological deficits from the onset of disease. PR is rare and disease is characterized by a combination of progressive and stepwise deficits. Disease onset generally occurs in the early 20s for RR disease and in the mid-30s for PP disease, although childhood-onset MS is becoming increasingly recognized.[1]

Patients with MS can experience a variety of symptoms including relapses of optic neuritis affecting vision, transverse myelitis affecting spinal cord functions including gait, and brainstem attacks affecting eye movements, coordination, or speech or swallowing. Fatigue, depression, and bladder and bowel dysfunction are also common symptoms of MS. Magnetic resonance imaging (MRI) typically demonstrates hyperintense lesions on T2 imaging (Fig. 65.1A) and in more advanced disease brain atrophy and T1 black holes (Fig. 65.1B) may be present. A diagnosis of MS can be confirmed using the new revised McDonald criteria that require a combination of specific clinical and MRI features (Table 65.1). Cerebrospinal fluid testing for oligoclonal bands is no longer required for a diagnosis of MS; however, it is supportive particularly in cases of PPMS.

● CLINCAL PEARLS

- Relapsing remitting (RR) MS
  - Affects 80% patients with presentation in early 20s
  - Neurologic deficits remit over weeks to months
- Secondary progressive (SP) MS
  - Develops in most RRMS after 15 years
- Primary progressive (PP) MS
  - Affects 15% patients
  - Permanent neurologic deficit from onset
- Progressive relapsing (PR) MS
  - Rare form begins in mid-30s
  - Combination of progressive and stepwise deficits

Pathology

Pathologically, MS is characterized by inflammatory infiltrates in the central nervous system (CNS) white matter with resultant demyelination and axonal transections[2] producing sclerotic plaques. Inflammation is generally perivenular, and lesions typically occur in the periventricular subcortical white matter, corpus callosum, optic nerve, brainstem, cerebellum, and spinal cord. Cortical lesions have also been described.[3] Recently, the pathology of MS lesions has been classified into four distinct subtypes with the following predominant features: (1) cellular infiltration, (2) antibody deposition, (3) oligodendrocyte apoptosis, and (4) oligodendrocyte death without apoptosis.[4] The observations to date show a single subtype of lesion in each patient, raising the possibility of distinct MS disease pathogenetic types. Activated microglia have been demonstrated in normal-appearing white matter (NAWM), and appear to play an important role in axonal damage and disease progression.[5] B-cell follicles have been demonstrated at autopsy in patients with chronic MS,[6] and may play a role in facilitating an autonomous inflammatory response within the CNS. Cortical demyelination is also associated with progressive forms of MS.[5]

● KEY CONCEPTS

- There is significant heterogeneity in the pathology of MS.
- Inflammatory cell infiltration and demyelination are the hallmarks of disease.
- Both demyelination and axonal damage are present in the early phases of diseases.
- Diffuse axonal damage and cortical demyelination may play key roles in progressive MS.

Risk factors

The etiology of MS remains elusive; however, it is assumed that both a complex genetic background and environmental factors contribute to disease manifestations. Monozygotic twins carry a concordance rate of 27%, whereas dizygotic twins of the same gender display a 2.3% concordance rate. The incidence for first-degree relatives of MS patients is 2–5%, whereas the incidence for the general population is under 0.1%. Genetic linkage studies have been performed and several regions of interest have been found, with the most robust association in the HLA region. There is an increased incidence of MS in patients with the HLA-DR2 (DR1501) haplotype.[7-9] The HLA class II extended haplotype HLA-DRB5*0101-HLADRB11501-HLA-DQA1

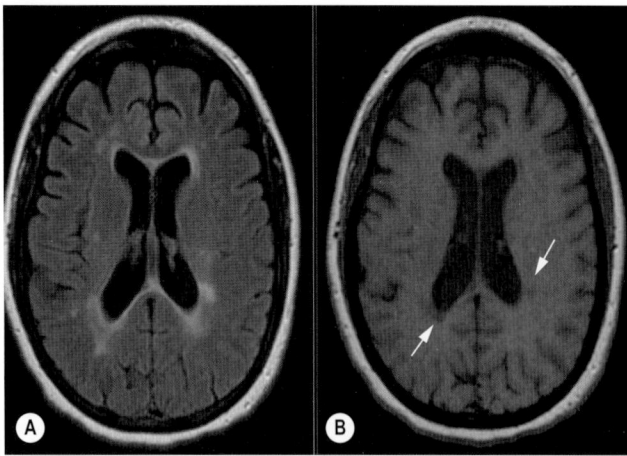

Fig. 65.1 (A) T2-weighted FLAIR MRI image of the brain of an MS patient showing hyperintense T2 lesions located in the periventricular and subcortical white matter. (B) T1-weighted MRI image showing T1-black holes (arrows) and generalized atrophy with enlarged ventricles.

Table 65.1 McDonald 2010 criteria for the diagnosis of multiple sclerosis

Clinical presentation	Additional data needed for an MS diagnosis
≥2 attacks; objective clinical evidence of ≥2 lesions or objective clinical evidence of 1 lesion with reasonable historical evidence of a prior attack	None
≥2 attacks; objective clinical evidence of 1 lesion	Dissemination in space demonstrated by ≥1 T2 lesion in at least 2 or 4 MS-typical regions (periventricular, juxtacortical, infratentorial, or spinal cord)
1 attack; objective clinical evidence of ≥2 lesions	Simultaneous presence of asymptomatic gadolinium-enhancing and nonenhancing lesions at any time; or a new T2 and/or gadolinium-enhancing lesion(s) on follow-up MRI, irrespective of its timing with reference to a baseline scan; or Await a second clinical attack
1 attack; objective clinical evidence of 1 lesion (clinically isolated syndrome)	Dissemination in space and time, demonstrated by: *For DIS:* ≥1 T2 lesion in at least 2 of 4 MS-typical regions of the CNS (periventricular, juxtacortical, infratentorial, or spinal cord); or Await a second clinical attack implicating a different CNS site; and *For DIT:* Simultaneous presence of asymptomatic gadolinium-enhancing and nonenhancing lesions at any time; or A new T2 and/or gadolinium-enhancing lesion(s) on follow-up MRI, irrespective of its timing with reference to a baseline scan; or Await a second clinical attack
Insidious neurological progression suggestive of MS (PPMS)	1 year of disease progression (retrospectively or prospectively determined) plus 2 of 3 of the following criteria: 1. Evidence for DIS in the brain based on ≥1 T2 lesions in the MS-characteristic (periventricular, juxtacortical, or infratentorial) regions 2. Evidence for DIS in the spinal cord based on ≥2 T2 lesions in the cord 3. Positive CSF (isoelectric focusing evidence of oligoclonal bands and/or elevated IgG index)

From Polman CH, Reingold SC, Banwell B, et al. Diagnostic criteria for multiple sclerosis: 2010 revisions to the McDonald criteria. Ann Neurol 2011; 69(2): 292–302.

*0102- HLA-DQB1*0602 accounts for approximately 50% of the genetic risk for MS. The whole genome scan effort has identified genes outside the HLA region as solid candidates for MS genetic risk although with weaker effects. More recently, a large genome-wide study identified single nucleotide polymorphism of IL-2R and IL-7R alleles as risk alleles for multiple sclerosis.[10] MS remains most prevalent among people of Northern European descent. There is a lower prevalence in other populations, such as Arabic and Mediterranean people, but among those with disease there is a higher incidence of other disease-associated haplotypes such as DR4 and DR6.

Gender is one of the most important genetic determinants associated with autoimmune disease. Many autoimmune diseases are more frequent in females; systemic lupus erythematosus (SLE) is 10 times more common in women, and MS twice as common in females. Evidence from animal models has shown that females are more resistant to infections and reject foreign skin grafts sooner than their male counterparts. This is especially true during periods of high estrogen availability. Estrogen levels decrease after ovulation or during pregnancy, and are associated with a progesterone surge. The lowering of estrogen ensures immunological tolerance toward sperm and subsequently toward the fetus. Therefore estrogen's effects on the immune system may predispose women toward autoimmune diseases. This is reflected in experimental disease models of autoimmunity. Only female (NZB X NZW)F₁ mice develop the SLE-like disease, and this is abrogated by androgen treatment. Similarly, in experimental autoimmune encephalomyelitis, an experimental model for MS, female SJL mice are more susceptible to disease induction and are protected with testosterone. Preliminary studies testing the effectiveness of a testosterone gel in males with multiple sclerosis have shown encouraging results, but require additional validation. Initial studies investigating estriol effects in women with multiple sclerosis have shown a potent effect on reduction of new MRI lesion formation.[11]

Viral and other microbial agents have been proposed as MS risk factors, although none of them is a necessary condition for the disease. This is true also for the Epstein–Barr virus (EBV), which appears to play a role in the majority of MS patients: (1) Seropositivity for EBV is almost universal in MS patients; (2) individuals with a history of infectious mononucleosis as teens have two- to threefold increased risk of developing MS compared with individuals who acquired EBV earlier in life; and

(3) years before MS onset, individuals at risk present increased titers of antibodies to the EBV nuclear antigen (EBNA) complex and EBNA-1, antigens that are mainly expressed during latent infection. Interestingly, epitopes of EBV resemble myelin basic protein, supporting a role for molecular mimicry in disease

pathogenesis. Despite these associations, however, it is clear that the majority of individuals infected with EBV do not have auto-immune sequelae. Recent studies have integrated risk factors in the pathogenesis of MS, and have found that the relative risk of MS among DR15-positive women who have elevated ($>$1:320) anti-EBNA-1 titers was nine-fold higher than that of DR15-negative women with low ($<$1:80) anti-EBNA-1 titers.[12]

Epidemiological studies have shown that residence in certain geographical areas and migration to these areas before the age of 15 increases the incidence of MS. In addition, there is a diminishing north-to-south gradient in MS prevalence in the Northern Hemisphere, with an opposite trend in the Southern Hemisphere. This led to the hypothesis and demonstration of an inverse association between sunlight exposure and MS.[13]

An extension of the "sunlight" hypothesis has led to the exploration of the role of vitamin D in MS since vitamin D is metabolized in the skin by UV irradiation. A prospective study in army recruits found that 25-hydroxyvitamin D levels in the highest quintile (above 99.1 nmol/L) were associated with a lower risk of MS (OR 0.38).[14] Treatment of animal models of MS with vitamin D ameliorates disease and several studies have shown that the active form of vitamin D, calcitriol, can downregulate pro-inflammatory dendritic cells (DC) and reduce Th1 lymphocyte responses, while promoting anti-inflammatory Th2 lymphocyte responses.[15]

Smoking is another important modifiable risk factor that contributes to the risk of developing MS[16] and cigarette smoke has been shown to enhance macrophage activation. In addition, there are emerging data suggesting that smoking can accelerate disease progression. A prospective study of 179 patients with relapsing-remitting MS (RRMS) demonstrated that even smokers with RRMS converted to secondary progressive MS (SPMS) at a faster rate than never smokers.[17] In contrast, a recent retrospective study including 364 patients (164 of whom had RRMS) found that cigarette smoking was not significantly associated with the development of SPMS or progression of clinical disability as measured by the expanded disability status scale (EDSS).[18] We have recently conducted a large prospective study of over 1400 MS patients from our Partners MS Center cohort showing that a history of smoking was associated with an accelerated rate of conversion to SPMS.[19]

● KEY CONCEPTS

Risk factors for MS include:

- Female gender
- Early exposure to Epstein–Barr virus
- Low vitamin D levels
- Smoking

Genetic risk alleles include:

- HLA DRB1*1501
- IL-2 receptor and IL-7 receptor

Peripheral immune changes

The hypothesis that MS is an autoimmune disease mainly stems from the similarities observed between MS and the animal model of the disease, experimental autoimmune encephalomyelitis (EAE). EAE is induced by immunizing animals with myelin-derived proteins (or peptides) such as proteolipid protein (PLP), myelin oligodendrocyte glycoprotein (MOG), and myelin basic protein (MBP), and the disease is largely driven by myelin-specific CD4 T cells. Similar to MS, animals can develop RR or chronic-progressive disease courses that pathologically are characterized by CNS inflammation and demyelination. Myelin-specific autoreactive T cells are found in the peripheral blood and cerebrospinal fluid (CSF) of MS patients, although they are also observed in healthy controls with similar frequencies. However, myelin-reactive T cells from MS patients are more activated and have a memory phenotype compared to the resting naïve phenotype found in controls.[20,21] This "activated state" of myelin-reactive T cells observed in MS patients is also associated with upregulation of adhesion molecules that make these cells more prone to interact with and cross the blood–brain barrier (BBB) and drive an inflammatory response directed against myelin antigens within the CNS.

How these autoreactive T cells from MS patients become activated in the periphery is still a matter of debate, and processes such as molecular mimicry, wherein T cells generated against non-self epitopes (viral or microbial antigens) cross-react with self-myelin epitopes of similar sequence,[22] or T-cell activation triggered by myelin antigens constitutively presented in cervical lymph nodes,[23,24] have been postulated as potential mechanisms. The fact that myelin-specific T cells from MS patients are more activated in the periphery has given rise to the hypothesis that deficient immunoregulatory control rather than increased generation of autoreactive T cells occurs in MS patients due to failure of central tolerance mechanisms.[25]

Migration to the CNS

Migration to the CNS of activated lymphocytes is the next step in the immunopathogenic cascade. Transmigration of lymphocytes across the BBB is a sequential process mainly mediated by adhesion molecules, chemokines, and matrix metalloproteinases (MMPs). Initial steps in the migration through the BBB involve interactions between adhesion molecules expressed on endothelial cells and immune cells (Chapter 11). A key adhesion molecule implicated in leukocyte extravasation is the $\alpha_4\beta_1$ integrin (VLA-4, very late activation antigen-4), which is expressed on the surface of activated lymphocytes and interacts with the vascular cell adhesion molecule 1 (VCAM-1) expressed on capillary endothelial cells. The importance of this interaction in MS pathogenesis is further underscored by the observation that the therapeutic blockade of the α_4-integrin subunit of VLA-4 by the humanized monoclonal antibody natalizumab inhibits migration of immune cells into the CNS, and is associated with significant reductions in both clinical and radiological MS disease activity.[26]

MMPs are proteolytic enzymes involved in BBB disruption by degrading the extracellular matrix and basement membranes but also have roles in demyelination, cytokine activation, and axonal damage. CSF and peripheral blood levels of MMP-9 have consistently been reported to be elevated in MS patients compared with healthy controls and found to correlate with clinical and radiological disease activities.[27]

Chemokines are low-molecular-weight cytokines that regulate recruitment and migration of immune cells from peripheral blood into the CNS (Chapter 10). Chemokines displayed at the endothelial lumen bind chemokine receptors expressed on circulating leukocytes and determine which leukocyte subsets will extravasate and enter the CNS. Several studies have reported altered levels of chemokines and their receptors in peripheral blood, CSF, and brain lesions from MS patients,[28] findings that emphasize the role of chemokines in the neuropathogenesis of the disease.

Perivascular dendritic-like cells have been shown to play a role in T-cell reactivation in animal models of MS;[29] however, their role in the human disease is unclear. The invasion of activated T cells into the brain and reactivation within the CNS initiates a cascade of cytokines. IL-2, IFN-γ, and TNF-α activate macrophages, which in turn produce nitric oxide and TNF-α. In experimental models, myelin damage is mediated by nitric oxide lipid peroxidation, direct TNF-α damage, and complement-induced pore formation. As mentioned previously, Th2 cytokines can induce B-cell activation and antibody production that further damage myelin. Each of these steps in the pathogenesis may be targeted for therapeutic intervention.

Cellular players of the immune response in MS

CD4 T cells

During the past years, MS research has mostly focused on the role of CD4 T cells in disease pathogenesis. The notion that MS is primarily a CD4 T-cell-mediated disease arises from EAE studies wherein the disease is driven by myelin-specific CD4 T cells and can be adoptively transferred to unaffected animals by injection of these myelin-reactive T cells.

Within the CNS, myelin-specific CD4 T cells are reactivated *in situ* by myelin antigens presented in the context of HLA class II molecules in conjunction with accessory molecules on the surface of antigen-presenting cells (APCs; macrophages, microglia). Reactivation triggers the release of pro-inflammatory cytokines and soluble mediators that will disrupt further the BBB and stimulate chemotaxis, resulting in a second larger wave of inflammatory cell recruitment into the CNS. The reactivation of T cells heralds an inflammatory response within the CNS, resulting in more tissue damage and release of secondary antigens. Subsequent T-cell reactivity to secondary antigens is termed "epitope spreading" (Fig. 65.2). Evidence of epitope spreading has been

demonstrated in animal models of MS,[30] and may play an important role in the pathogenesis of the human disease.

Upon exposure to an antigen, antigen-specific T cells proliferate and differentiate into effector T cells. The vast majority of effector T cells undergo apoptosis as the immune response progresses, and the few lymphocytes that survive become long-lived memory T cells. Memory T cells are specific to the antigen encountered during the primary immune response and react rapidly and vigorously on re-encounter with the same antigen. Functionally, in terms of activation requirements, memory T cells can be activated by lower concentrations of anti-CD3, require less costimulation by anti-CD28, and readily secrete more effector cytokines than their naïve T-cell counterparts, indicating a state of hyper-responsiveness. In MS patients, T cells that can be activated in the absence of CD28 have been detected.[31] This suggests that memory T cells play a role in MS pathogenesis, and are an important consideration when designing immunomodulatory therapies.

New research has focused on the different roles played by subsets of CD4 T cells in MS. Following activation, naïve T cells differentiate into various T-cell populations with different effector functions. Th1 cells produce pro-inflammatory cytokines such as IFN-γ that activate macrophages to kill intracellular pathogens. On the other hand, Th2 cells secrete anti-inflammatory cytokines such as IL-4 and are important in clearing extracellular pathogens. A dysregulation in the balance between Th1 and Th2 cytokines has long been implicated in MS immunopathogenesis.

Th17 cells represent a distinct lineage of effector T cells. IL-23 produced by macrophages and dendritic cells is critical for expansion of Th17 cells that synthesize the pro-inflammatory cytokines IL-17A and IL-17F. Studies in EAE have shown that suppression of Th17 cells is associated with a reduction of disease severity, although this is becoming an area of debate. Interestingly, the Th17-to-Th1 ratio appears to be a critical determinant of CNS inflammation, and high Th17-to-Th1 ratios are associated with T-cell infiltration and inflammation in the brain parenchyma.[32] Pathological studies in MS patients and in the EAE model demonstrated that cells expressing IL-17 or IFN-γ

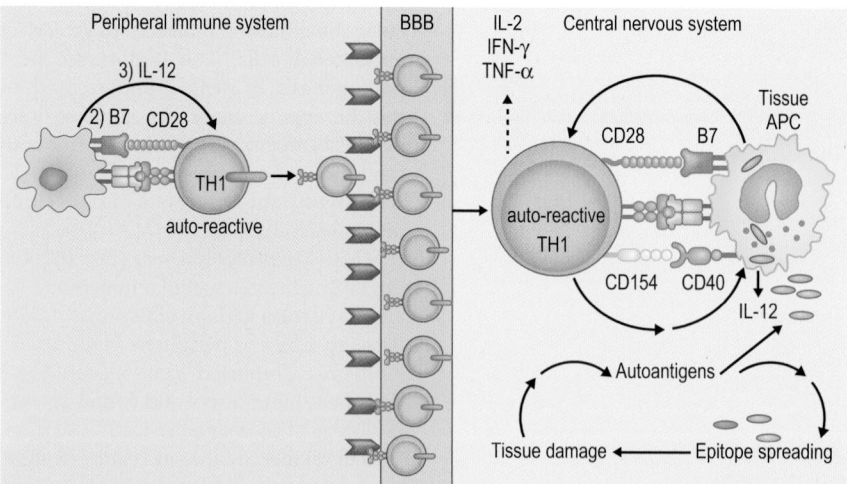

Fig. 65.2 T cell in the initiation and propagation of autoimmune disease in MS. In the peripheral immune system, a foreign antigen is presented to T cells via the TCR by the MHC molecule present on antigen-presenting cells (APCs). The presence of co-stimulatory signals facilitates T-cell activation, while IL-12 cytokine facilitates Th1 differentiation. These activated T cells traverse the blood–brain-barrier (BBB) and reach the CNS tissue. Within the CNS, T cells are re-activated by presentation of cross-reactive myelin antigens by local APCs. The inflammatory environment can induce upregulation of additional co-stimulatory molecules, and can facilitate presentation of antigens to T cells by CNS APCs. Re-activation of T cells induces production of cytokines, in particular TNF-α as well as recruitment of macrophages into the CNS, which facilitates tissue damage. This results in a release of additional tissue antigens, which can be taken up by potential APCs in the CNS, such as macrophages/microglia, and astrocytes and presented to T cells (epitope spreading), thus, inciting further T-cell activation and tissue damage.
Redrawn from Chitnis T, Khoury SJ. T-cell-based therapies for multiple sclerosis. In: Cohen JA, Rudick RA, eds, Multiple sclerosis therapeutics, 4th edition. Cambridge: Cambridge University Press, 2011; pp. 472–482.

efficiently cross the BBB and accumulate within the brain.[33] Increased expression of IL-17 was reported in blood, CSF, and brain tissue of MS patients.[34] The frequency of Th17 cells in CSF from MS patients has been reported to be higher at the time of clinical exacerbations than that of clinical remission phases of the disease.[35] Additionally, phenotypic characterization of Th17 T-cell clones revealed higher expression of activation markers and co-stimulatory and adhesion molecules in these cells than in Th1 T-cell clones,[35] pointing to a high pathogenic potential of Th17 cells. In addition to CD4$^+$IL-17$^+$ Th17 cells, a new putative subtype of IL-17-producing CD4 T cells with CD4$^+$IL-17$^+$IFNγ^+ (Th17-1 cells) double-positive phenotype has also been identified. In addition to Th17 cells, Th17-1 cells are also present in MS and EAE.[36,37] Th17-1 cells infiltrate the brain prior to the development of clinical symptoms of EAE and this coincides with activation of CD11b$^+$ microglia and local production of IL-1β, TNF-α, and IL-6 in the CNS. Based on these observations many investigators consider Th17 and Th17-1 cells central in MS pathogenesis.

Naturally occurring regulatory T cells (CD4$^+$CD25$^+$ Treg) comprise a small subset of CD4 T cells that have also been implicated in MS pathogenesis. Although the number of Treg cells in peripheral blood and CSF appears to be similar between MS patients and healthy controls, several studies point to defects in the capacity of Tregs from MS patients to suppress the activation of myelin-specific T cells in the periphery.[38,39] The *in vitro* suppressive capacity of Tregs was reported to be compromised in RRMS patients but not in those from SPMS patients.[40] It should be emphasized that the above-mentioned studies have focused on the suppressive properties of Tregs obtained from peripheral blood, but their actual role in preventing inflammation within the CNS is controversial. In fact, FOXP3$^+$ Treg cells were not detected in MS brain tissue,[34] an absence that may indicate either a lack of Treg-mediated suppression within the CNS or defects in the migration or survival of Tregs in the CNS. These findings contrast with studies in EAE, in which disease-relevant Tregs accumulate in the CNS, but, however, fail to suppress autoimmune inflammation.[41]

CD8 T cells

There are several lines of evidence suggesting an important role of CD8 T cells in MS immunopathogenesis: (1) CD8 T cells are prominent in the inflammatory infiltrate in CNS lesions, and in some studies CD8 T cells outnumber CD4 T cells;[42] (2) infiltrating CD8 T cells are clonally expanded and may persist in the CSF for many years;[43] (3) CD8 T cells may promote CNS vascular permeability;[44] (4) adoptive transfer of activated myelin-specific CD8 T-cell clones has been shown to induce EAE, suggesting a role for CD8 T cells as effector cells in MS pathogenesis;[45] (5) axonal damage was correlated with the number of CD8 T lymphocytes infiltrating the lesion;[46] and (6) *in vitro* studies have shown that CD8 T cells can transect neurites in an MHC class I/peptide-restricted fashion, indicating that CD8 T cells may participate in the axonal damage observed in MS lesions by directly attacking neurons.[47]

B cells

Humoral immunity is considered to play an important role in MS pathogenesis as indicated by: (1) B cells isolated from CSF and MS brain lesions are clonally expanded;[48] (2) there is a persistent intrathecal production of oligoclonal immunoglobulins in the CSF from MS patients, a finding that is part of the diagnostic criteria for the disease;[49] (3) B cells may directly participate in the demyelination process by secreting pathogenic antibodies that

target oligodendrocytes with or without the presence of complement;[50] (4) the presence of follicle-like aggregates with germinal centers in the meninges of some patients with a chronic progressive disease course, which suggests that B-cell responses such as proliferation, antigen-driven affinity maturation selection, and differentiation into antibody-producing plasma cells can be maintained locally within the CNS and may contribute to the pathogenic process;[51] and (5) B-cell ablative therapy with rituximab, an anti-CD20 monoclonal antibody that efficiently depletes naïve and memory B cells, was recently shown to reduce MS inflammatory brain lesions and clinical relapses,[52] presumably by decreasing antigen-presenting capacity and cytokine production by B cells.

Neuronal degeneration

Demyelination has long been considered a primary pathological feature of MS. However, axonal loss is an important pathological finding in MS that correlates with disease progression and permanent neurologic disability in patients.[2] It is important to highlight that axonal transection is an early and persistent finding in MS that is even present in CIS patients.[53] Mechanisms for axonal damage in MS are manifold and include a specific immunologic attack on axons; the presence of soluble mediators such as proteases, cytokines, and free radicals released as part of the inflammatory environment taking place in the CNS of MS patients; and a lack of neurotrophic factors provided to the axon by oligodendrocytes as result of chronic demyelination.[54] These observations underline the importance of therapeutic strategies in MS designed to protect axons and neurons and provide compelling evidence for their administration in early phases of the disease.

Progressive disease

There is mounting evidence indicating that T cells play a key role in the RR phase of MS. However, recent work has demonstrated that disease progression in MS may be due to distinct mechanisms.[55] Epitope spreading can occur within the CNS, and in animal models can be facilitated by microglia, macrophages, and DCs.[30] Activated microglia are found in progressive forms of the disease and have been associated with axonal damage and demyelination.[5] B-cell follicles have been demonstrated at autopsy in patients with chronic MS,[6] and may play a role in facilitating an autonomous inflammatory response within the CNS. Cortical demyelination is also associated with progressive forms of MS.[5] Targeting these mechanisms may ultimately delay or prevent irreversible disability in MS patients.

MS therapies

Immunological mechanisms of currently used medications, as well as experimental therapeutic strategies, are described.

Beta-interferon(IFN-β)

IFN-β therapy for MS is one of the most important advances in the treatment of this disease. It is available in three different forms—subcutaneous IFN-β-1b (Betaseron), subcutaneous IFN-β-1a (Rebif), and intramuscular IFN-β-1a (Avonex). Interferons have many properties including suppressing proliferation of viruses and T cells. The mechanisms of IFN-β action in MS include increased production of IL-10 by macrophages that downregulates the number of Th1 cells. IFN-β has also been shown to decrease production of IL-12 by DCs, potential CNS APCs, further inhibiting Th1 cell formation. In addition, IFN-β modulates adhesion molecule expression, primarily by facilitating the conversion of cell-associated VCAM-1 into soluble VCAM-1. These drugs also downregulate costimulatory molecule expression, thus decreasing T-cell activation and migration to the CNS.[56]

Glatiramer acetate (GA)

GA also known as copolymer-1 or Copaxone is another class of drug used in the treatment of MS. GA is a synthetic molecule originally designed to resemble MBP. It is composed of random repetitive sequences of the amino acids glutamic acid, lysine, alanine, and tyrosine (G-L-A-T). Its mechanism of action is unclear; however, it is thought to bind with high affinity to the MHC groove, leading to the generation of GA-specific T cells. Several studies have suggested that GA-specific T cells display a Th2 bias,[57] and animal models have demonstrated that these cells can migrate to the CNS and ameliorate EAE through a local downregulation of the immune responses.[58] It has also been demonstrated that GA-specific T cells protect from optic nerve crush injuries, possibly mediated by the production of brain-derived neurotrophic factor (BDNF).[59]

Natalizumab

Natalizumab is a monoclonal antibody that targets $\alpha_4\beta_1$-integrin. It is approved for the treatment of relapsing-forms of multiple sclerosis,[26] and effectively blocks T- and B-cell migration across the BBB. However, blockade of CNS immune surveillance has produced profound adverse effects, as evidenced by the development of progressive multifocal leukoencephalopathy (PML) with a frequency of approximately 1:1000. The experience with natalizumab (Tysabri) has highlighted the importance of balancing potential adverse effects such as infection and tumorigenicity with therapeutic efficacy.

Fingolimod

A novel strategy for suppressing immune responses in MS is by fingolimod, a small molecule that targets the sphingosine-1-phosphate receptor necessary for lymphocyte egress from lymph nodes.[60–62] This drug may specifically target Th17 central memory cells.[63]

Rituximab

Rituximab, an antibody that primarily targets activated B cells has recently been shown to reduce disease activity in relapsing-remitting[52] and in a subset of primary progressive MS patients.[64] Interestingly, open-label studies have suggested that rituximab treatment is effective in patients with neuromyelitis optica, which is increasingly thought of as an antibody-mediated disease.

Cell cycle inhibitors

Many therapeutic strategies that have been used in the past non-specifically target components of the immune response. Nonspecific strategies include cyclophosphamide, mitoxantrone, and cladribine, which depress bone marrow production of cells, including T cells. Cyclophosphamide can also function by inducing a cytokine switch with a decrease in IL-12 and an increase in IL-4, IL-5, and TGF-β.[65]

Experimental therapies
Altered peptide ligands (APL)

APL resembling MBP have been used in phase I trials for MS, with little success. Two concurrent trials were initiated using the same compound CGP77116. One showed an increased number of lesions on MRI in some patients after the initiation of treatment.[66] In the other trial, 9% of patients developed allergic-type reactions associated with a Th2 deviation.[67] Both trials were stopped because of safety concerns.

Alemtuzumab

Alemtuzumab is a monoclonal antibody targeting the CD52 receptor present on lymphocytes and monocytes. Phase II studies have shown potent effects in MS, with depletion of peripheral lymphocytes. However, a quarter of treated patients develop autoimmune thyroid disease, and rarely immune thrombocytopenic purpura during the immune reconstitution phase, suggesting immune dysregulation may occur due to slower recovery of regulatory cells.[68,69]

Daclizumab

Daclizumab is a monoclonal antibody that blocks the IL-2Rα chain (CD25) present in the high affinity IL-2 receptor on T cells, thus inhibiting T-cell replication and making more IL-2 available to the low affinity CD25 receptor present on NK cells, which induces a regulatory NK cell population.[70] Phase III studies examining a subcutaneous form of anti-IL-2 receptor are ongoing.

CTLA4Ig

CTLA4Ig is a fusion protein that blocks B7-CD28 co-stimulatory signals on T cells and may induce T-cell anergy *in vivo*. A phase I study was recently completed,[71] and it is currently being studied in a phase II clinical trial.

Other therapies including ocrelizumab, which targets B cells, and fumaric acid are in late stage clinical trials for MS.

Future directions

The understanding of MS immunopathogenesis has advanced significantly over the past 15 years, which has led to major therapeutic developments. MS patients with relapsing forms of disease now have several effective treatment options, and clinical trials for additional agents are ongoing. The next challenge for the MS field is the control of disease progression, which may have immunologic mechanisms distinct from the relapsing form of disease. Additional therapeutic challenges include induction of remyelination and repair within the CNS, perhaps through the mobilization of neural stem cells. Further progress on the identification of MS risk factors may ultimately lead to strategies to prevent the development of disease.

● ON THE HORIZON

- There have been significant advances in anti-inflammatory therapies for MS during the past 15 years that reduce relapse rates.
- Newer strategies will need to focus on prevention of disease progression.
- Regenerative therapies including remyelination and neural repair may help to restore function to patients.
- Further work to identify and clarify risk factors for MS may eventually lead to strategies for preventing disease.

References

1. Chitnis T, Krupp L, Yeh A, et al. Pediatric multiple sclerosis. Neurol Clin 2011;29:481–505.
2. Trapp BD, Peterson J, Ransohoff RM, et al. Axonal transection in the lesions of multiple sclerosis. N Engl J Med 1998;338:278–85.
3. Lucchinetti CF, Popescu BFG, Bunyan RF, et al. Inflammatory cortical demyelination in early multiple sclerosis. N Engl J Med 2011;365:2188–97.
4. Lucchinetti C, Bruck W, Parisi J, et al. Heterogeneity of multiple sclerosis lesions: implications for the pathogenesis of demyelination. Ann Neurol 2000;47:707–17.
5. Kutzelnigg A, Lucchinetti CF, Stadelmann C, et al. Cortical demyelination and diffuse white matter injury in multiple sclerosis. Brain 2005;128:2705–12.
6. Serafini B, Rosicarelli B, Magliozzi R, et al. Detection of ectopic B-cell follicles with germinal centers in the meninges of patients with secondary progressive multiple sclerosis. Brain Pathol 2004;14:164–74.
7. Stewart GJ, McLeod JG, Basten A, Bashir HV. HLA family studies and multiple sclerosis: A common gene, dominantly expressed. Hum Immunol 1981;3:13–29.
8. Haines JL, Terwedow HA, Burgess K, et al. Linkage of the MHC to familial multiple sclerosis suggests genetic heterogeneity. The Multiple Sclerosis Genetics Group. Hum Mol Genet 1998;7:1229–34.
9. Sawcer S, Goodfellow PN. Inheritance of susceptibility to multiple sclerosis. Curr Opin Immunol 1998;10:697–703.
10. Hafler DA, Compston A, Sawcer S, et al. Risk alleles for multiple sclerosis identified by a genomewide study. N Engl J Med 2007;357:851–62.
11. Sicotte NL, Liva SM, Klutch R, et al. Treatment of multiple sclerosis with the pregnancy hormone estriol. Ann Neurol 2002;52:421–8.
12. De Jager PL, Simon KC, Munger KL, et al. Integrating risk factors: HLA-DRB1*1501 and Epstein-Barr virus in multiple sclerosis. Neurology 2008;70:1113–8.
13. van der Mei IA, Ponsonby AL, Dwyer T, et al. Past exposure to sun, skin phenotype, and risk of multiple sclerosis: case-control study. BMJ 2003;327:316.
14. Munger KL, Levin LI, Hollis BW, et al. Serum 25-hydroxyvitamin D levels and risk of multiple sclerosis. JAMA 2006;296:2832–8.
15. Penna G, Amuchastegui S, Giarratana N, et al. 1,25-Dihydroxyvitamin D3 selectively modulates tolerogenic properties in myeloid but not plasmacytoid dendritic cells. J Immunol 2007;178:145–53.
16. Ascherio A, Munger KL. Environmental risk factors for multiple sclerosis. Part II: Noninfectious factors. Ann Neurol 2007;61:504–13.
17. Hernan MA, Jick SS, Logroscino G, et al. Cigarette smoking and the progression of multiple sclerosis. Brain 2005;128:1461–5.
18. Koch M, van Harten A, Uyttenboogaart M, De Keyser J. Cigarette smoking and progression in multiple sclerosis. Neurology 2007;69:1515–20.
19. Healy BC, Ali EN, Guttmann CR, et al. Smoking and disease progression in multiple sclerosis. Arch Neurol 2009;66:858–64.
20. Zhang J, Markovic-Plese S, Lacet B, et al. Increased frequency of interleukin 2-responsive T cells specific for myelin basic protein and proteolipid protein in peripheral blood and cerebrospinal fluid of patients with multiple sclerosis. J Exp Med 1994;179:973–84.
21. Lovett-Racke AE, Trotter JL, Lauber J, et al. Decreased dependence of myelin basic protein-reactive T cells on CD28-mediated costimulation in multiple sclerosis patients. A marker of activated/memory T cells. J Clin Invest 1998;101:725–30.
22. Wucherpfennig KW, Hafler DA, Strominger JL. Structure of human T-cell receptors specific for an immunodominant myelin basic protein peptide: positioning of T-cell receptors on HLA-DR2/peptide complexes. Proc Natl Acad Sci U S A 1995;92:8896–900.
23. Zhang H, Podojil JR, Luo X, Miller SD. Intrinsic and induced regulation of the age-associated onset of spontaneous experimental autoimmune encephalomyelitis. J Immunol 2008;181:4638–47.
24. Furtado GC, Marcondes MC, Latkowski JA, et al. Swift entry of myelin-specific T lymphocytes into the central nervous system in spontaneous autoimmune encephalomyelitis. J Immunol 2008;181:4648–55.
25. Lisak RP, Zweiman B. In vitro cell-mediated immunity of cerebrospinal-fluid lymphocytes to myelin basic protein in primary demyelinating diseases. N Engl J Med 1977;297:850–3.
26. Polman CH, O'Connor PW, Havrdova E, et al. A randomized, placebo-controlled trial of natalizumab for relapsing multiple sclerosis. N Engl J Med 2006;354:899–910.
27. Lee MA, Palace J, Stabler G, et al. Serum gelatinase B, TIMP-1 and TIMP-2 levels in multiple sclerosis. A longitudinal clinical and MRI study. Brain 1999;122(Pt 2):191–7.
28. Holman DW, Klein RS, Ransohoff RM. The blood-brain barrier, chemokines and multiple sclerosis. Biochim Biophys Acta 2011;1812:220–30.
29. Greter M, Heppner FL, Lemos MP, et al. Dendritic cells permit immune invasion of the CNS in an animal model of multiple sclerosis. Nat Med 2005;11:328–34.
30. McMahon EJ, Bailey SL, Castenada CV, et al. Epitope spreading initiates in the CNS in two mouse models of multiple sclerosis. Nat Med 2005;11:335–9.
31. Markovic-Plese S, Cortese I, Wandinger KP, et al. CD4+CD28- costimulation-independent T cells in multiple sclerosis. J Clin Invest 2001;108:1185–94.
32. Stromnes IM, Cerretti LM, Liggitt D, et al. Differential regulation of central nervous system autoimmunity by T(H)1 and T(H)17 cells. Nat Med 2008;14:337–42.
33. Kebir H, Ifergan I, Alvarez JI, et al. Preferential recruitment of interferon-gamma-expressing TH17 cells in multiple sclerosis. Ann Neurol 2009;66:390–402.
34. Tzartos JS, Friese MA, Craner MJ, et al. Interleukin-17 production in central nervous system-infiltrating T cells and glial cells is associated with active disease in multiple sclerosis. Am J Pathol 2008;172:146–55.
35. Brucklacher-Waldert V, Stuerner K, Kolster M, et al. Phenotypical and functional characterization of T helper 17 cells in multiple sclerosis. Brain 2009;132:3329–41.
36. Abromson-Leeman S, Bronson RT, Dorf ME. Encephalitogenic T cells that stably express both T-bet and ROR gamma t consistently produce IFNgamma but have a spectrum of IL-17 profiles. J Neuroimmunol 2009;215:10–24.
37. Suryani S, Sutton I. An interferon-gamma-producing Th1 subset is the major source of IL-17 in autoimmune encephalitis. J Neuroimmunol 2007;183:96–103.
38. Tsaknaridis L, Spencer L, Culbertson N, et al. Functional assay for human CD4+CD25+ Treg cells reveals an age-dependent loss of suppressive activity. J Neurosci Res 2003;74:296–308.
39. Viglietta V, Baecher-Allan C, Weiner HL, Hafler DA. Loss of functional suppression by CD4+CD25+ regulatory T cells in patients with multiple sclerosis. J Exp Med 2004;199:971–9.
40. Venken K, Hellings N, Hensen K, et al. Secondary progressive in contrast to relapsing-remitting multiple sclerosis patients show a normal CD4+CD25+ regulatory T-cell function and FOXP3 expression. J Neurosci Res 2006;83:1432–46.
41. Korn T, Reddy J, Gao W, et al. Myelin-specific regulatory T cells accumulate in the CNS but fail to control autoimmune inflammation. Nat Med 2007;13:423–31.
42. Babbe H, Roers A, Waisman A, et al. Clonal expansions of CD8(+) T cells dominate the T cell infiltrate in active multiple sclerosis lesions as shown by micromanipulation and single cell polymerase chain reaction. J Exp Med 2000;192:393–404.
43. Skulina C, Schmidt S, Dornmair K, et al. Multiple sclerosis: brain-infiltrating CD8+ T cells persist as clonal expansions in the cerebrospinal fluid and blood. Proc Natl Acad Sci U S A 2004;101:2428–33.
44. Johnson AJ, Suidan GL, McDole J, Pirko I. The CD8 T cell in multiple sclerosis: suppressor cell or mediator of neuropathology? Int Rev Neurobiol 2007;79:73–97.
45. Huseby ES, Liggitt D, Brabb T, et al. A pathogenic role for myelin-specific CD8(+) T cells in a model for multiple sclerosis. J Exp Med 2001;194:669–76.
46. Bitsch A, Schuchardt J, Bunkowski S, et al. Acute axonal injury in multiple sclerosis. Correlation with demyelination and inflammation. Brain 2000;123(Pt 6):1174–83.
47. Medana IM, Gallimore A, Oxenius A, et al. MHC class I-restricted killing of neurons by virus-specific CD8+ T lymphocytes is effected through the Fas/FasL, but not the perforin pathway. Eur J Immunol 2000;30:3623–33.
48. Obermeier B, Mentele R, Malotka J, et al. Matching of oligoclonal immunoglobulin transcriptomes and proteomes of cerebrospinal fluid in multiple sclerosis. Nat Med 2008;14:688–93.
49. Polman CH, Reingold SC, Edan G, et al. Diagnostic criteria for multiple sclerosis: 2005 revisions to the "McDonald Criteria" Ann Neurol 2005;58:840–6.
50. O'Connor KC, Appel H, Bregoli L, et al. Antibodies from inflamed central nervous system tissue recognize myelin oligodendrocyte glycoprotein. J Immunol 2005;175:1974–82.
51. Magliozzi R, Howell O, Vora A, et al. Meningeal B-cell follicles in secondary progressive multiple sclerosis associate with early onset of disease and severe cortical pathology. Brain 2007;130:1089–104.
52. Hauser SL, Waubant E, Arnold DL, et al. B-cell depletion with rituximab in relapsing-remitting multiple sclerosis. N Engl J Med 2008;358:676–88.
53. Rovaris M, Gallo A, Falini A, et al. Axonal injury and overall tissue loss are not related in primary progressive multiple sclerosis. Arch Neurol 2005;62:898–902.
54. Chitnis T, Imitola J, Khoury SJ. Therapeutic strategies to prevent neurodegeneration and promote regeneration in multiple sclerosis. Curr Drug Targets 2005;5:11–26.
55. Weiner HL. The challenge of multiple sclerosis: how do we cure a chronic heterogeneous disease? Ann Neurol 2009;65:239–48.
56. Yong VW. Differential mechanisms of action of interferon-beta and glatiramer aetate in MS. Neurology 2002;59:802–8.

57. Duda PW, Schmied MC, Cook SL, et al. Glatiramer acetate (Copaxone) induces degenerate, Th2-polarized immune responses in patients with multiple sclerosis. J Clin Invest 2000;105:967–76.

58. Aharoni R, Teitelbaum D, Sela M, Arnon R. Copolymer 1 induces T cells of the T helper type 2 that crossreact with myelin basic protein and suppress experimental autoimmune encephalomyelitis. Proc Natl Acad Sci U S A 1997;94:10821–6.

59. Kipnis J, Yoles E, Porat Z, et al. T cell immunity to copolymer 1 confers neuroprotection on the damaged optic nerve: possible therapy for optic neuropathies. Proc Natl Acad Sci U S A 2000;97:7446–51.

60. Comi G, O'Connor P, Montalban X, et al. Phase II study of oral fingolimod (FTY720) in multiple sclerosis: 3-year results. Mult Scler 2010;16:197–207.

61. Cohen JA, Barkhof F, Comi G, et al. Oral fingolimod or intramuscular interferon for relapsing multiple sclerosis. N Engl J Med 2010;362:402–15.

62. Kappos L, Radue EW, O'Connor P, et al. A placebo-controlled trial of oral fingolimod in relapsing multiple sclerosis. N Engl J Med 2010;362:387–401.

63. Mehling M, Lindberg R, Raulf F, et al. Th17 central memory T cells are reduced by FTY720 in patients with multiple sclerosis. Neurology 2010;75:403–10.

64. Hawker K, O'Connor P, Freedman MS, et al. Rituximab in patients with primary progressive multiple sclerosis: results of a randomized double-blind placebo-controlled multicenter trial. Ann Neurol 2009;66:460–71.

65. Comabella M, Balashov K, Issazadeh S, et al. Elevated interleukin-12 in progressive multiple sclerosis correlates with disease activity and is normalized by pulse cyclophosphamide therapy. J Clin Invest 1998;102:671–8.

66. Bielekova B, Goodwin B, Richert N, et al. Encephalitogenic potential of the myelin basic protein peptide (amino acids 83–99) in multiple sclerosis: results of a phase II clinical trial with an altered peptide ligand. Nat Med 2000;6:1167–75.

67. Kappos L, Comi G, Panitch H, et al. Induction of a non-encephalitogenic type 2 T helper-cell autoimmune response in multiple sclerosis after administration of an altered peptide ligand in a placebo-controlled, randomized phase II trial. The Altered Peptide Ligand in Relapsing MS Study Group. Nat Med 2000;6:1176–82.

68. Coles AJ, Compston DA, Selmaj KW, et al. Alemtuzumab vs. interferon beta-1a in early multiple sclerosis. N Engl J Med 2008;359:1786–801.

69. Jones JL, Phuah CL, Cox AL, et al. IL-21 drives secondary autoimmunity in patients with multiple sclerosis, following therapeutic lymphocyte depletion with alemtuzumab (Campath-1H). J Clin Invest 2009;119:2052–61.

70. Bielekova B, Catalfamo M, Reichert-Scrivner S, et al. Regulatory CD56(bright) natural killer cells mediate immunomodulatory effects of IL-2Ralpha-targeted therapy (daclizumab) in multiple sclerosis. Proc Natl Acad Sci U S A 2006;103:5941–6.

71. Khoury S, Viglietta V, Buckle G, et al. A Phase I Trial of CTLA4Ig Treatment in MS. In: American Academy of Neurology. 57th Annual Meeting; 2005. Miami, FL, USA; 2005.

66.

Autoimmune peripheral neuropathies

Marinos C.
Dalakas

Autoimmune peripheral neuropathies (APN) occur when immunologic tolerance to peripheral nerve components (myelin, Schwann cell, axon, and motor or ganglionic neurons) is lost. In some of these neuropathies there is direct evidence for autoimmune reactivity mediated by specific antibodies or autoreactive T lymphocytes against peripheral nerve. In others, the underlying immune-mediated mechanism is secondary or indirect, and an autoimmune cause is suspected when the neuropathy coexists with another systemic autoimmune disease or viral infection.

This chapter reviews the most common autoimmune neuropathies (Table 66.1), their clinical features and diagnostic criteria, the prevailing autoimmune phenomena that govern each neuropathy, and the most effective therapeutic approach.

Acute inflammatory polyneuropathy: the Guillain–Barré syndrome(s)

Guillain–Barré syndrome (GBS) is an acute demyelinating polyneuropathy characterized by acute (within 1 week) or subacute (within 4 weeks) ascending motor weakness, areflexia, and mild or moderate sensory abnormalities.[1,2] It is a disease of all ages and occurs sporadically, although occasional outbreaks have been noted. In typical cases the maximum deficit is reached by the fourth week, a sign conventionally used to separate GBS from chronic inflammatory demyelinating polyneuropathy (CIDP), in which the disease begins slowly and usually reaches a nadir after at least two months. There are, however, CIDP patients (perhaps up to 16%) with sub-acute onset and monophasic course who fall between the two time-frame periods and still others with an even more acute onset, reaching a nadir within 6-8 weeks and resembling GBS.[3] Distinguishing GBS from acute-onset CIDP is challenging as the distinction in most cases becomes evident in retrospect, although recent criteria may help separating the two early in the disease.[3]

GBS is not one, but several syndromes reflecting the varying degree of involvement of the motor or sensory nerve fibers and the myelin sheath or the axon. The GBS syndromes, or GBS[1,2] variants, include:

- *Acute inflammatory demyelinating polyneuropathy (AIDP)* accounts for the majority of patients. In classic cases, the weakness starts from the legs and spreads up to the arms, the intercostal and diaphragmatic muscles, and the facial or bulbar muscles, causing dysphagia and dysarthria. At times the weakness may be limited to one or two limbs or to cranial nerves.[1,2] Patients need to be monitored for impending respiratory failure, hence the need for early admission to intensive care units (ICUs). Varying degree of autonomic dysfunction occurs in up to 65% of patients; if severe, it can be life-threatening due to cardiac arrhythmias or hemodynamic changes such as hypertension, orthostatic hypotension, and reduced peripheral vascular tone.

- *Acute, motor axonal neuropathy (AMAN)* exhibits primary axonal damage due either to massive acute demyelination and inflammation, as occurs in experimental allergic neuritis when the animals are immunized with a high dose of myelin antigen,[4] or to a primary axonal event mediated by macrophages. These patients have a fulminant course with severe paralysis and complete electrical inexcitability of motor nerves as early as 3–5 days after onset. Recovery of motor function may be incomplete. Infection with *Campylobacter jejuni* appears to be responsible for the majority of these cases.[4–6] A number of patients also have high levels of anti-ganglioside GM1 antibodies.

- *Acute motor–sensory axonal neuropathy (AMSAN)* is like AMAN but with involvement of the sensory axons.

- *C. Miller-Fisher syndrome* is characterized by acute onset of ophthalmoplegia, gait ataxia, normal sensation, and areflexia.[1,2] In a third of patients there is muscle weakness with pharyngeal, facial, trunk, and respiratory muscle involvement.[1,5,6] The C. Miller-Fisher syndrome is a distinct variant due to the presence of a unique IgG antibody against GQ1b ganglioside.[5–7]

- *Sensory ataxic GBS* is due to involvement of roots and ganglionic neurons. Some of these patients have antibodies to GD1b ganglioside and they probably form a continuum with Miller-Fisher syndrome because they share autoantibodies with the same sialic groups.[6–9]

- *Acute pandysautonomic neuropathy*, where the target antigen is in the ganglionic neurons as discussed later.

Diagnosis

The classic laboratory abnormalities in GBS patients are elevated cerebrospinal fluid (CSF) protein and abnormal nerve conduction studies consistent with active demyelination.

The CSF protein may be normal in the early phase of the disease, but it can be as high as 1000 mg/dL by the sixth week. The elevation of CSF protein may be due to involvement of the roots related to inflammation, but, as the blood–nerve barrier becomes impaired, serum albumin and IgG may enter freely into the CSF, contributing further to protein elevation. The CSF cell count is normal unless GBS occurs in conjunction with viral infections, such as HIV, CMV, Epstein–Barr virus (EBV), or associated with Lyme disease. When the CSF protein is very high, papilledema can develop because of impaired reabsorption of CSF and raised intracranial pressure. Oligoclonal IgG bands can be also seen.

Table 66.1 Common autoimmune neuropathies

- Guillain–Barré syndrome(s)
- Chronic inflammatory demyelinating polyneuropathy (CIDP) and its variants
- Polyneuropathy associated with paraproteinemias
  - IgM monoclonal gammopathies
  - IgG and IgA monoclonal gammopathy
  - Polyneuropathy, organomegaly, endocrinopathy, myeloma, and skin changes (POEMS) syndrome
  - Cryoglobulinemic polyneuropathy
- Multifocal motor neuropathy with conduction block
- Paraneoplastic neuropathies associated with anti-Hu antibodies
- Autoimmune autonomic neuropathies
- Vasculitic neuropathies
- Infectious neuropathies (HIV, CMV, EBV, herpes, Lyme, leprosy, Chagas' disease, diphtheria, others)

The differential diagnosis of GBS should include other forms of acute flaccid paralysis, such as brainstem stroke; brainstem encephalitis; acute motor neuron involvement due to poliomyelitis or West Nile virus infection; acute myelopathy; disorders of neuromuscular transmissions such as myasthenia gravis or botulism; disorders of muscles such as hypokalemia, inflammatory myopathy, acute rhabdomyolysis, or periodic paralysis; and other causes of acute neuropathy such as due to porphyria, vasculitis, or critical illness neuropathy.

Antecedent illnesses or events

Two-thirds of patients with GBS give a history of a flu-like illness or acute dysenteric episodes that precede the development of GBS by 1–3 weeks.[1,2] Among the implicated viruses are cytomegalovirus, EBV, herpes, hepatitis A, and HIV. Among bacteria, infection with *Mycoplasma pneumoniae* and, most importantly, *Campylobacter jejuni* may be present in 15–20% of patients.[5–8] *Campylobacter* is of special interest because it contains glycoconjugates that share epitopes with the peripheral myelin, as discussed later. Two vaccines—one against rabies and the other against the swine flu A/New Jersey influenza strain that caused an outbreak of GBS in 1976[1]—have been convincingly connected with the development of GBS. Rabies vaccine that contains brain material is followed by GBS in about one in 1000 cases. Apart from these vaccines, however, there is no convincing evidence that the incidence of GBS is increased in connection with other vaccines, despite anecdotal reports.

Surgery can precede the development of GBS in some patients.[1] Surgical stress, the release of nerve autoantigens, and infections have been proposed as possible explanations for this association. There are three drugs causally associated with acute demyelinating neuropathy: gold, perhexiline, and suramin at high doses. GBS has occurred in patients who suffer from neoplasms, especially lymphoma, melanoma, and Hodgkin's disease.[1] Interestingly, GBS is rarely seen as part of another connective tissue disorder.

Immunopathology

GBS is an inflammatory demyelinating polyneuropathy in which the peripheral myelin, the axon, or the Schwann cells are the putative target antigens of an immune attack, possibly triggered by the various antecedent events. Both the cellular and the humoral components of the immune system have been implicated.[5]

Cellular factors

There are two prominent histologic features in GBS: (1) perivascular and endoneurial inflammatory infiltrates throughout the nerves, roots or plexuses;[1,5] and (2) segmental demyelination in areas associated with the lymphoid infiltrates and especially macrophages, which are the most dominant cells. The macrophages break through the basement membrane of healthy Schwann cells and make direct contact with the outermost myelin lamellae, leading finally to lysis of the superficial myelin sheath. Cytokines and chemokines released by the activated T cells or complement activation may increase capillary permeability and facilitate transmigration of additional macrophages. When the demyelination is extensive, it is followed by axonal degeneration.[1,5] The degree and effectiveness of remyelination and axonal regeneration dictate the degree of clinical recovery.

The role for a T-cell-mediated process in GBS is mostly derived by analogy to the animal model of experimental allergic neuritis (EAN), which resembles GBS in both its pathology and its clinical course.[1,5] Animals sensitized to whole human nerve or to various myelin proteins such as Po, P2, and the neutral glycolipid galactocerebroside develop segmental demyelination with mononuclear cell infiltrates consisting of macrophages and T cells. In EAN, the T cells are sensitized against myelin and can passively transfer the disease to healthy animals. Increased levels of IL-2 and soluble IL-2 receptors are noted in the serum during the acute phase of GBS suggesting ongoing T-cell activation. Further, lymphocytes from GBS patients exert myelinotoxic activity when applied to cultures of myelinated axons.

Humoral factors and anti-ganglioside antibodies

There is much stronger evidence that circulating serum factors are responsible for GBS. On clinical grounds, this is supported by the beneficial effect of plasmapheresis, presumably by removing putative antibodies. On laboratory grounds it is supported by the variety of autoantibodies detected in the patients' serum. Serum from the acute phase of GBS can demyelinate rodent dorsal root ganglionic extracts in a complement-dependent manner. Further, GBS serum injected into rat sciatic nerves causes demyelination and conduction block. Immunocytochemical studies on the peripheral nerves of GBS patients show deposits of IgG, IgM, and membranolytic attack complex, implying complement-fixing antibody activity of the serum immunoglobulin.[1,5] Further, complement-fixing IgM antibodies against a human peripheral nerve myelin glycolipid that contains carbohydrate epitopes as well as high-titer antibodies against various sulfated or acidic glycosphingolipids are present in several GBS patients.[6,7]

IgG antibodies that react with GM1, GD1a, GalNAc-GD1a, and GM1b are found in 80% of cases with the motor axonal form of GBS (AMAN and AMSAN). In the common AIDP subtype, however, these antibodies are not frequent. Among the gangliosides, the one that clearly correlates with a specific clinical syndrome is the GQ1b.[6–9] IgG anti-GQ1b antibodies appear to be specifically associated with the C. Miller-Fisher variant of GBS because they are present in more than 90% of these patients. In contrast, IgM anti-GQ1b antibodies can be found in patients with IgM paraproteinemic polyneuropathies.[9] Anti-GQ1b IgG antibodies are also found in post-infectious ophthalmoplegias as well as in GBS patients with ophthalmoplegia, but not in GBS patients without ophthalmoplegia or under other autoimmune conditions.[8] Of interest, anti-GQ1b antibody immunostains the paranodal regions of oculomotor nerves III, IV, and VI, suggesting that damage to

Fig. 66.1 Sequence of events in the mechanisms of immune-mediated demyelinating polyneuropathy. Cytokines lead to increased expression of major histocompatibility complex (MHC) class I and intercellular adhesion molecules, allowing the sensitized T cells and macrophages to exit the endothelial cell wall and traffic to the peripheral nerve. There, they recognize myelin antigen and induce a macrophage-mediated demyelination. The antigen-presenting cells (probably Schwann cells or macrophages), in concert with MHC class II expression, interact with CD4 T cells and lead to clonal expansion of B cells, producing antibodies against various peripheral nerve antigens.

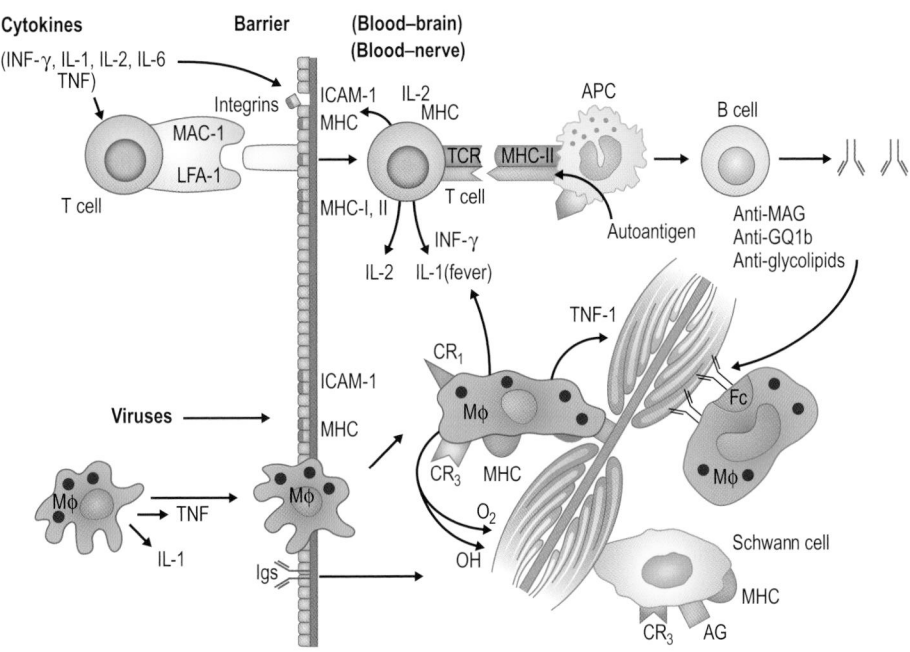

these regions blocks impulse generation at the nodes of Ranvier, resulting in a conduction block that is characteristic for GBS. Many patients with antibodies to GQ1b also have antibodies to GD1a.

Gangliosides are present in all tissues but are especially abundant in the nervous system. Their lipid portion lies in the cell membrane, and their signature sugar residues are exposed at the extracellular surface bearing one or more sialic acid molecules, such as one sialic acid ganglioside (GM1), two (GD1a), three (GT1a), or four (GQ1b).[6–9] Although they do not form a common "GBS antigen" different gangliosides are involved in different GBS subtypes. They are of pathogenic relevance because immunization of rabbits with GM1 and GDIb induces acute neuropathy with histological features of AMAN.[8] Their pathogenicity was also confirmed by an inadvertent experiment in humans who had received ganglioside injections for various maladies and developed AMAN with GM1 antibodies.[10] Additionally, antibodies to GQ1b or GD1a cause conduction block at the motor nerve terminals in a preparation of mouse phrenic nerve.[6–8] Similarly, antibodies to GalNAc-Gd1a from a patient with AMAN blocked neuromuscular transmission in a mouse spinal cord muscle co-culture system.

The reasons for different clinical syndromes in connection with specific gangliosides remains unclear, but distribution, accessibility and density or configuration of ganglioside at different sites may be critical factors. For example, there is more GM1 in ventral than in dorsal roots, hence the predominantly motor neuropathy seen with GM1 antibodies; there is also more GQ1b in the ocular motor nerves, which explains the eye involvement in Miller-Fisher syndrome. How these antibodies induce disease remains unclear. Current evidence suggests that antibodies against different acidic glycolipids or sulfatides may be related to the different viral or bacterial antecedent factors. Molecular mimicry between epitopes of viral proteins (which trigger the disease) and myelin components may result in sensitization of cross-reactive T cells that could mediate the demyelinating process as discussed below. The activated T cells may then stimulate B cells to produce specific antibodies directed against myelin components, or may recruit

macrophages as effector cells. A combination of cellular and humoral factors therefore seems to participate in the cause of the disease.[5] Circulating cytokines triggered by the initiating event (virus, bacteria) could also upregulate intercellular adhesion molecule (ICAM)-1 expression on the endothelial cells and facilitate the entrance of activated T cells or antibodies to the endoneurial parenchyma. It is relevant, therefore, that ICAM-1 has been found to be increased in GBS patients.[5] A scheme summarizing the immunopathogenic mechanism is shown in Fig. 66.1.

Molecular mimicry as a pathogenic factor: relationship between *C. jejuni* or other microbial agents with gangliosides

Antecedent infection with *Campylobacter jejuni* has been associated with certain GBS subtypes, more commonly AMAN. The strain of *C. jejuni* associated with AMAN (Penner D: 19 Serogroup) is different from those causing common enteritis and more likely to have the genes for enzymes that synthesize sialic acid in the bacterial wall mimicking ganglioside GM1, GD1a, or GQ1b.[6–8,11] These patients have a higher incidence of anti-GM1 antibodies suggesting a cross-reactivity between epitopes in the lipo-oligosaccharide in the bacterial wall and ganglioside.[11] Further, injection of lipo-oligosaccharides extracted from *C. jejuni* into rabbits induced an acute neuropathy with GM1 antibodies identical to those of AMAN,[6–8,11] while immunization of mice with these lipo-oligosaccharides generated a monoclonal antibody that reacted with GM1 and bound to human peripheral nerve. This GM1 monoclonal antibody as well as the anti-GM1 IgG extracted from GBS patients block muscle action potentials in muscle–spinal cord co-culture. Carbohydrate mimicry between the bacterial lipo-oliogosaccharide and human GM1 is therefore an important cause of AMAN. Because *C. jejuni* is a common cause of a diarrheal illness worldwide, and diarrhea has been an antecedent event in up to 50% of GBS patients, *Campylobacter* appears to trigger the disease in some patients. Isolation of *Campylobacter* from stools early in acute GBS varies from 44 to 88% of patients, and IgG or IgM *Campylobacter*-specific antibody titers are seen in a higher percentage (36%) of GBS patients than in controls (10%).

Molecular mimicry may not be limited to *C. jejuni* because GM1 and GQ1b epitopes are also found in the bacteria wall of *Hemophilus influenzae*, which is also a triggering factor in GBS. GBS triggered by CMV infection has been also associated with the presence of IgM anti-GM2 antibodies. Another potential factor for molecular mimicry is *Mycoplasma pneumoniae*, which precedes GBS in 5% of cases and is known to stimulate antibodies against human carbohydrate antigens, including galactocerebroside, the main glycolipid antigen in peripheral nerves.[1,5–8,11]

● KEY CONCEPTS

Autoimmunity in Guillain–Barré syndrome

Cellular factors

- The peripheral myelin or the Schwann cells are target antigens.
- Activated macrophages are the dominant endoneurial cells and lift the outermost myelin lamellae, lysing the superficial myelin sheaths.
- Peripheral blood lymphocytes exert myelinotoxic activity *in vitro*.
- Levels of IL-2 and soluble IL-2 receptors are increased during the acute phase of the disease and decline during recovery.

Humoral factors

- Serum exerts a complement-dependent demyelination *in vitro*.
- Intraneural injections of serum from acute GBS patients cause demyelination and conduction block.
- IgG, IgM, and membranolytic attack complex are detected immunocytochemically on the patients' nerves.
- High titers of IgG antibodies against peripheral nerve acidic glycolipids (GM1, GQ1b) are detected in the serum of AMAN and Miller-Fisher's syndrome. The GQ1b ganglioside is a specific antigen for Miller-Fisher's syndrome.
- High incidences of antibodies to *Campylobacter jejuni* and GM1, with molecular mimicry between *Campylobacter* and nerve gangliosides.
- Injection of lipooligosaccharides extracted from *Campylobacter jejuni* cause AMAN and elicit GM1 antibodies in rabbits.
- Anti-ganglioside antibodies extracted from GBS patients block muscle action potentials *in vitro*.

Chronic inflammatory demyelinating polyneuropathy

Chronic inflammatory demyelinating polyneuropathy (CIDP) is the most common form of chronic APN with prevalence as high as 9/100 000.[3] It is also the most important and gratifying chronic neuropathy because it is treatable in the majority of the cases. It can be considered as the chronic counterpart of GBS because of their various clinical, electrophysiologic, histologic, and laboratory similarities. CIDP differs from GBS predominantly by its tempo, mode of evolution, prognosis, and responsiveness to steroids. First described as steroid-responding relapsing polyneuropathy, CIDP shares with GBS a variety of common autoimmune features.

Clinical features and disease variants

The typical CIDP is characterized by a progressive, symmetrical, proximal and distal muscle weakness, paresthesias, sensory dysfunction and impaired balance that evolve slowly over at least 2 months.[3,12–14] The tendon reflexes are absent or reduced. Cranial nerves may be rarely affected. The course is often monophasic with stepwise progression; at times the disease is relapsing with spontaneous remissions necessitating the need to evaluate periodically the usefulness of continuing immunotherapeutic interventions. Because the demyelination is multifocal affecting spinal roots, plexuses, and proximal nerve trunks,[3,12] the clinico-pathological picture can vary according to the distribution of symptoms and signs.[3,12–15] The most notable CIDP variants include *the asymmetric, unifocal or multifocal motor-sensory form (Lewis-Sumner syndrome); the pure motor; the pure sensory; the sensory ataxic;* and *the pure distal*.

Diagnosis

In CIDP, the CSF protein is elevated, up to six-fold, without pleocytosis (except if an infection coexists). The nerve biopsy shows demyelination and remyelination, occasional epineurial or endoneurial T cells and macrophages either scattered or in small perivascular clusters in the endoneurium (Fig. 66.2).[3,12–15] Electrophysiologic testing is fundamental for the diagnosis of CIDP by demonstrating the following typical features of demyelination in motor and sensory fibers: (a) slow conduction velocity; (b) prolonged distal motor or sensory latencies; (c) prolonged F waves latencies; and (d) conduction block with dispersion of the compound muscle action potentials. An associated axonal loss is not unusual in the majority of CIDP cases. A variety of diagnostic criteria have been proposed to capture the most pertinent of the aforementioned features; the revised EFNS/PNS guidelines seem the most appropriate because they offer 81% sensitivity and 96% specificity to capture patients more likely to respond to therapies.[14,15] Routine CSF testing and nerve biopsy are not mandatory for the diagnosis,[3,14] but they can be helpful when the electrophysiology is not convincing, or there is a need to exclude hereditary and vasculitic neuropathies. Other diseases causing neuropathy that should be excluded include severe diabetes (although CIDP seems more frequent in diabetics), neoplasms, amyloidosis, IgM paraproteinemia (IgG or IgA MGUS can be seen in CIDP), myelomas, vasculitis, alcoholism, exposures to neurotoxic drugs, or family history of neuropathy.

● KEY CONCEPTS

Autoimmunity in CIDP

- Activated macrophages are the predominant endoneurial cell, displacing the Schwann cell cytoplasm, disrupting myelin, and lysing superficial myelin lamellae.
- Complement-fixing IgG and IgM antibodies are deposited on the myelin sheath.
- IgG antibodies to acidic glycolipids LM1, GM1, or GD1b and against the 28-kDa Po myelin proteins are detected in the serum of some patients.
- There is upregulation of DR and B-7 co-stimulatory molecules in the Schwann cells and macrophages.
- The serum IgG can induce conduction block when injected into rat nerves.

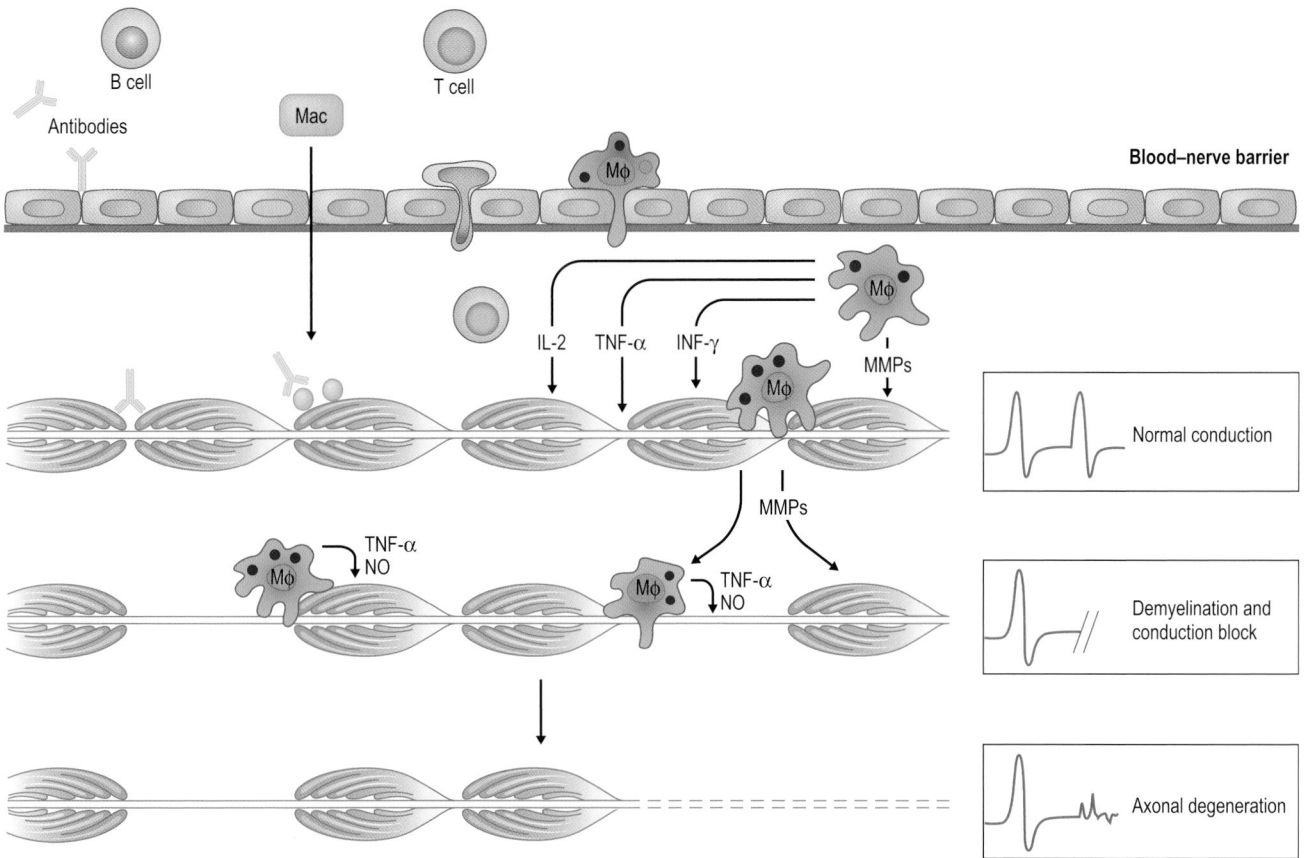

Fig. 66.2 Diagrammatic scheme of the main cellular elements that seem to play a major role in the demyelinating process of CIDP. Activated macrophages (Mϕ) and T cells cross the endothelial cell wall of the blood–nerve barrier and reach the myelinated fibers. Activated, TNF-α-positive Mϕ invade the myelin sheath, causing Mϕ-mediated segmental demyelination. Axonal loss secondary to demyelination, probably enhanced by TNF-α and metalloproteinases, may become prominent in the chronic phases of the disease. Other cytokines, T cells sensitized to unidentified antigens, and putative antibodies may participate. IL, interleukin; INF, interferon; MMP, metalloproteinase; Mϕ, activated macrophage; TNR, tumor necrosis factor.

Immunopathogenesis

Based on the immunopathologic similarities with GBS and the relapsing–remitting experimental allergic neuritis, in CIDP activated T cells, macrophages, complement and autoantibodies seem to work in concert with each other to induce an immune attack against peripheral nerve antigens[3,12,13] No pathogenic autoantibody or a single triggering antigen have been so far identified.

The predominant endoneurial mononuclear cell in CIDP is the macrophage; T cells are sparse.[3,12,13] The demyelinating process is always associated with the presence of macrophages, presumably activated by cytokines, which sequentially penetrate the basement membrane of the Schwann cell, displace the cytoplasm, and finally disrupt the myelin by focal lysis of the superficial myelin lamellae.[12] In CIDP, macrophages and Schwann cells may serve as antigen-presenting cells because they express HLA-DR and co-stimulatory molecules B7-1, B7-2, whereas their counter-receptors CTLA-4 and CD28 are expressed on rare endoneurial CD4 T cells.[16] B7-2-deficient mice also develop CIDP.[17] Elevated soluble adhesion molecules, chemokines, cytokines, and metalloproteinases are detected in the sera and CSF, probably facilitating lymphoid cell transmigration across the blood–nerve barrier.

Humoral factors may play a major role but the target antigens remain still elusive. The beneficial effect of plasmapheresis provides indirect evidence that some circulatory factors are pathogenetic. Complement-fixing IgG and IgM are deposited on the patient's myelin sheath, indicative of anti-myelin antibodies.[18]

Antibodies to glycolipids LM1, GM1, or GD1b are also seen in some patients, but less frequently than in GBS and more frequently than in controls.[3,12,13] Passive transfer experiments have demonstrated that serum IgG can induce conduction block in rat nerve. The 28-kDa myelin protein Po was identified as a putative antigen in up to 20% of the patients. Recent studies suggest that adhesion molecules within the non-compact myelin and the Schwann cell/axonal interactions, such as those against neurofascins, gliomedin, contactins [i.e., TAG-1 (Transient Axonal Glycoprotein-1 or Caspr), connexin, NCAM, cadherin, ankyrin, and others] rather than the compact myelin, may be targets of an immune attack.[3,19] The immunopathogenetic scheme proposed for GBS (Fig. 66.1) is also appropriately applied to CIDP, with some modification to denote the frequent axonal loss that accompanies demyelination (Fig. 66.2). Molecular mimicry can be implicated in rare CIDP patients associated with melanoma because the carbohydrate myelin epitopes GM3, GM2, and GD3 are also expressed on melanoma cells and antibodies against melanoma cells react with myelin glycoproteins.[20]

Multifocal motor neuropathy (MMN) with conduction block

MMN is a distinct disease that should be recognized early because it is treatable. It affects males more than females, and is more common in those under 50 years of age. MMN presents with progressive weakness, atrophy, and areflexia that often begins in the hands and is prominent in distal muscle groups supplied by many individual peripheral nerves (multifocal).[21] It differs from vasculitic neuropathy because it is slow and painless, and by affecting only motor nerve fibers. It also differs from the motor variant of CIDP because it is multifocal and asymmetric. Because patients with MMN can experience cramps and fasciculations, the disease is often erroneously diagnosed as lower motor neuron disease and treatment is delayed. In contrast to lower motor neuron disease however, MMN progresses very slowly, the weakness is within distributions of peripheral nerves and not multisegmental, and the cranial musculature is often spared. The CSF protein is normal, an important finding that distinguishes MMN from the motor variant of CIDP.

MMN has distinct electrophysiologic criteria, namely, multifocal conduction block in motor nerves. In contrast to CIDP, in which sensory conduction block is also present, in MMN the sensory conduction remains normal across the nerve segments that have motor block. The reason for a selective motor involvement is unclear. Differences in the antigenic specificities in the myelin components between the motor and the sensory fibers are suspected because the ceramide composition of gangliosides differs between sensory and motor fibers. Although the immunopathology of the disease is unclear, MMN patients respond remarkably well to immunotherapy, as discussed later. Up to 50% of patients have high GM1 antibody titers but their role is uncertain. IgM GM1 antibodies can be also seen in other dysimmune neuropathies and in up to 25% of ALS patients who do not have conduction block.

Polyneuropathies associated with monoclonal gammopathies of undetermined significance (MGUS)

A distinct subset of acquired polyneuropathies has been associated with a circulating monoclonal protein (Chapter 80). Although neuropathy occurs in a setting of myeloma, plasmacytoma, or Waldenström's macroglobulinemia, the majority of patients with paraproteinemic neuropathies do not have a lymphoproliferative disease and the monoclonal gammopathy is of undetermined significance (MGUS). A benign monoclonal gammopathy may occur in up to 1% of normal people over age 50.[22] The incidence increases to 1.7% above age 70 and reaches up to 6% above the age of 90. Monoclonal gammopathies, however, are 10 times more frequent in patients with polyneuropathy than in an age-matched control population, and almost 10% of patients with acquired polyneuropathy have MGUS.[23] If one categorizes these gammopathies into subclasses, the incidence of polyneuropathy among patients with IgM monoclonal proteins can be as high as 50%,[23,24] implying that almost 50% of patients with IgM MGUS may have or will develop polyneuropathy. The association of monoclonal gammopathy with peripheral neuropathy is not therefore fortuitous. Today, polyneuropathies with MGUS comprise 10% of patients with acquired neuropathy,[23,24] and paraproteinemic polyneuropathy is a potentially treatable APN.[25]

Patients with demyelinating polyneuropathy associated with IgG or IgA MGUS are indistinguishable from CIDP and respond to immunotherapy. In these patients the causal relationship between the IgG or IgA paraprotein and neuropathy has not been established. In contrast, the demyelinating polyneuropathy associated with IgM MGUS is a distinct clinicopathologic entity and

the IgM is considered pathogenic as it is often directed against myelin glycoproteins or glycolipids.[9,24]

Some patients with paraprotein may have an associated amyloidosis derived from the variable region of the immunoglobulin light chain. When amyloidosis is present, the neuropathy is painful and the sensorimotor deficits are accompanied by autonomic symptoms consisting of orthostatic hypotension, impotence, impaired gastric motility, or frequent diarrhea. Amyloid neuropathy is difficult to treat, and, apart from symptomatic therapy (mostly opiates), immunosuppressive therapies have been largely unsuccessful.

IgM MGUS polyneuropathies with myelin-associated ganglioside antibodies (anti-MAG)

Most patients present with a sensory, large-fiber, demyelinating polyneuropathy that manifests as sensory ataxia.[24–26] Other patients have a sensorimotor polyneuropathy with mixed features of demyelination and axonal loss. The CSF protein is elevated, up to 250 mg/dL (normal is ≤50 mg/dL). Nerve conduction studies demonstrate slow conduction velocity and a rather characteristic prolonged distal motor and sensory latency. Sural nerve biopsy demonstrates a diminished number of myelinated axons (Fig. 66.3). On electron microscopy there is splitting of the outer myelin lamellae, linked to the presence of IgM deposits in the same area of the split myelin sheath.

Sera from approximately 50% of these patients react with myelin-associated glycoprotein (MAG), a 100-kDa glycoprotein of the central and peripheral nerve myelin, as well as other glycoproteins or glycolipids that share antigenic determinants with MAG.[27] The antigenic determinant for the anti-MAG IgM resides in the carbohydrate component of the MAG molecule.[28] The anti-MAG IgM paraproteins co-react with an acidic glycolipid in the

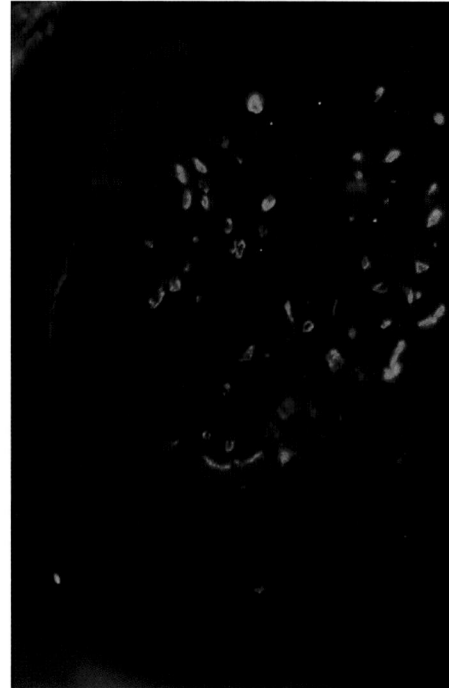

Fig. 66.3 Cross-section of a sural nerve from a patient with IgM paraproteinemia and demyelinating polyneuropathy. Fresh-frozen nerve specimen stained with FITC-conjugated antibodies to human IgM reveals IgM deposits in many myelinated fibers.

ganglioside fraction of human peripheral nerves, identified as a sulfoglucuronyl glycosphingolipid (SGPG).[29] In contrast to MAG, which is mostly present in the CNS, SGPG is found only in the peripheral nerves. The sera of some IgM-MGUS patients with sensory ataxia may not react with MAG, but with various gangliosides, most commonly those that contain either a disialosyl moiety, such as GD1b, GQ1b, GT1b, the GalNac-GM1b and GalNAc-GD1a, or two gangliosides that share epitopes with GM2, or a combination of GM2 and GM1, GM1 and GD1b.[9,29,30] More than half of the IgM paraproteins recognize MAG and SGPG, and 75% of the rest recognize ganglioside antigens, indicating that acidic glycolipids are the most common antigenic epitopes.[9,29,30]

Human anti-MAG antibodies can be detected readily in sera by ELISA, or preferably by standard western blot. Because anti-MAG-reacting sera always recognize the SGPG glycolipid, the assay has been often performed using SGPG as antigen instead of purified human MAG. It is preferable, however, to use MAG as the target antigen rather than SGPG, because the IgM binds to MAG 10–100 times more strongly than to SGPG and low-affinity anti-MAG antibodies can be missed if SGPG is used as the antigen. The glycolipids implicated as antigens in immune-mediated neuropathies are depicted in Fig. 66.4.[9]

The following factors suggest that these antibodies are related to the cause of the neuropathy:

a. IgM and complement are deposited on the myelinated fibers on the patient's sural nerve biopsy,[25,31] suggesting that activated complement may be needed in the induction of demyelination (Fig. 66.3).

b. The IgM recognizes neural cell adhesion molecules and co-localizes with MAG on the areas of the split myelin lamellae, suggesting involvement in myelin disadhesion. Skin biopsies from these patients have also confirmed the presence of IgM, complement C3d, and MAG deposition on the dermal myelinated fibers and the concurrent loss of nerve fibers.[32]

c. Injection of serum from patients with IgM anti-MAG/SGPG paraprotein supplemented with fresh complement into feline peripheral nerve causes complement-dependent demyelination and conduction block within 2–9 days of the injection.[33] The IgM injected intraneurally localizes to the outer layer of the myelin sheath, and

d. Systemic transfusion of anti-MAG IgM paraproteins produces segmental demyelination in chickens,[34] with

deposition of IgM on to the outer lamellae of the myelin along with splitting of the myelin lamellae, similar to that observed in the human neuropathy.

Polyneuropathy, organomegaly, endocrinopathy, myeloma, and skin changes (POEMS)

A subset of patients with malignant IgG or IgA MGUS have polyneuropathy with osteosclerotic myeloma. Most of them comprise the POEMS syndrome (*p*olyneuropathy, *o*rganomegaly, *e*ndocrinopathy, *M* protein, and *s*kin changes).[35] Not included in the acronym are several features such as sclerotic bone lesions, giant lymph node hyperplasia (Castleman's disease), papilledema, pleural effusion, edema, ascites, and thrombocytosis.[35] More than 50% of patients with osteosclerotic myeloma of IgA or IgG type have a sensorimotor, symmetric polyneuropathy with mixed demyelinating and axonal features and high (usually

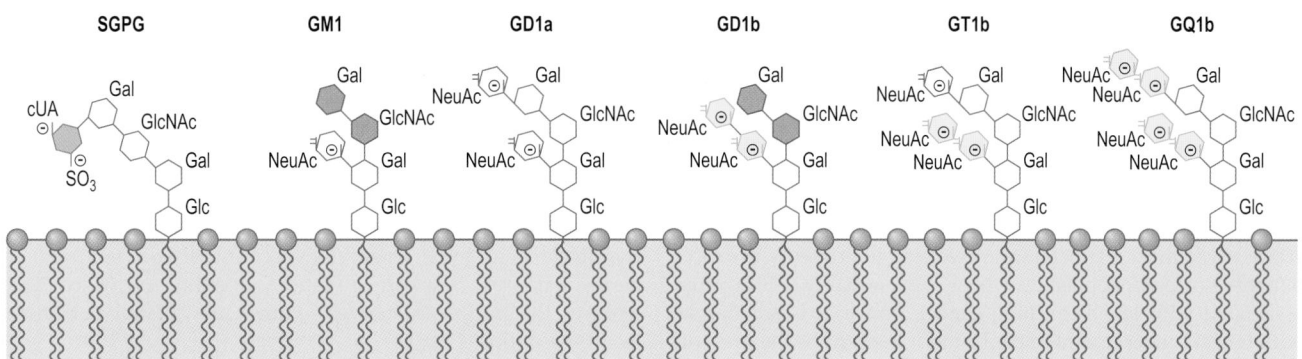

Fig. 66.4 Glycolipids implicated as antigens in immune-mediated neuropathies. Sulfate-3-glucuronyl paragloboside (SGPG) is the glycolipid sharing a carbohydrate epitope with myelin-associated glycoprotein (MAG), and the terminal sulfated glucuronic acid is a key part of the epitope. GM1 is the ganglioside implicated in motor nerve disorders, and in most cases the terminal Gal (β1-3) GalNAc epitope, which is shared with GD1b, is involved. The disialosyl moiety implicated in sensory neuropathies consists of NeuAca2-–8NeuAc– and is present in GD1b and GT1b gangliosides, as well as the simpler GD2 and GD3 gangliosides (not shown). GQ1b ganglioside, which is the target antigen in C. Miller-Fisher syndrome, has two disialosyl moieties. Although GD1a ganglioside has two sialic acid residues they are not linked to each other, so antibodies to GD1a do not cross-react with the anti-GD1b antibodies. The color-coded sugar moieties represent key aspects of the various epitopes, but carbohydrate sequences recognized by the antibodies may include additional sugar residues. GlcUA, glucuronic acid; Gal, galactose; G1cNAc, N-acetylglucosamine; Glc, glucose; GalNAc, N-acetylgalactosamine; NeuAc, N-acetylneuraminic acid (sialic acid).

200 mg/dL) CSF protein.[35] Pure axonal neuropathies can be also seen. In POEMS the neuropathy tends to be associated with edema in the legs, with hyperpigmentation, sclerodermatous thickening or papular angiomas of the skin, and hypertrichosis with dark hair. Endocrinopathy most often includes gonadal failure, amenorrhea, impotence, gynecomastia, hypothyroidism, diabetes, or elevated prolactin levels. The IgG class is slightly more common than the IgA class, but the λ light chain is present in the majority of the patients.[35] The bone lesions can be sclerotic, solitary, or multiple, sparing the skull and the extremities. When sclerotic lesions are absent, patients are said to have Crow–Fukase syndrome.[36] Pathologic changes in the lymph nodes resemble those of Castleman's disease, which can also be associated with polyneuropathy.[35] In POEMS there is an imbalance of proinflammatory cytokines with increased IL-1b, IL6, and TNF-α. Vascular endothelial growth factor (VEGF) may play a major role because it induces a rapid increase in vascular permeability and is a growth factor important in angiogenesis and endothelial cells.[35]

The neuropathy in some patients responds to steroids, tamoxifen, or alkylating agents. In others, it may respond to the removal or irradiation of the solitary sclerotic lesion, suggesting that the tumor may secrete neurotoxic factors. IVIG and plasmapheresis are ineffective. The median survival is 165 months.[35]

Cryoglobulinemic neuropathy

Cryoglobulins are proteins that precipitate in the cold and redissolve when heated (Chapter 57). There are three types of cryoglobulin: type I, which is monoclonal often of the IgM and IgG class; type II, which is mixed polyclonal with one monoclonal (often monoclonal IgM with polyclonal IgG); and type III, which is polyclonal (often IgM and IgG). Polyneuropathy occurs most often with mixed cryoglobulinemias and presents as distal, sensory, symmetric polyneuropathy or as mononeuropathy multiplex. These patients also have purpura, polyarthralgias, cutaneous vasculitis, Raynaud's phenomenon, renal involvement with proteinuria, and polyneuropathy. Type II cryoglobulinemia may be associated with an underlying lymphoproliferative process. There is an increased incidence (up to 90%) of hepatitis C virus infection in patients with mixed cryoglobulinemia. The nerve biopsy shows perivascular inflammatory cuffing with axonal degeneration.

Paraneoplastic peripheral neuropathies with anti-Hu antibodies

Peripheral neuropathy is not an uncommon complication of cancer, related either to the systemic effects of the tumor or, more often, to various neurotoxic chemotherapeutic agents. It usually affects the small nerve fibers causing numbness or painful dysethesias The most distinct immune-related neuropathy in cancer patients is a paraneoplastic sensory neuronopathy (PSN), often associated with small-cell lung cancer, and to a lesser degree with breast cancer or other neoplasms.[37] It might be the presenting symptom preceding the discovery of the tumor by months. PSN has a unique clinical picture, characterized by burning or aching paresthesias; sensory loss of the large fibers, causing sensory gait ataxia and chorioathetotic movements related to loss of proprioception in the feet and hands; normal strength; and areflexia. Some patients may have autonomic dysfunction, encephalopathic symptoms, or cerebellar disturbances. The CSF protein is increased, electrophysiologic testing shows an axonal sensory

neuropathy and nerve biopsy demonstrates axonal degeneration with rare mononuclear cell infiltrates. PSN is a ganglionopathy (sensory neuronopathy) due to a variable degree of inflammation in the dorsal root ganglionic neurons. The patients have specific IgG anti-Hu autoantibodies directed against a closely spaced group of proteins with a molecular weight of 35–40 kDa.[37] The antibodies are found in higher titers in the CSF, suggesting intrathecal synthesis. The Hu protein is also present in the tumors of patients with PSN. Further, low titers of anti-Hu antibodies can be seen in up to 20% of patients with small-cell lung cancer even without neurologic symptoms, suggesting that PSN may be the result of an autoimmune reaction against antigens shared by both the tumor cells and the dorsal root ganglionic neurons. Although the role of anti-Hu antibodies in the causation of PSN is unclear, these antibodies are specific markers to detect an occult small-cell lung cancer in patients who present with sensory ataxic neuropathy.

Autoimmune autonomic neuropathies

Autoimmune autonomic neuropathy (AAN) is highlighted by circulating antibodies against the ganglionic nicotinic acetylcholine receptors (AChR).[38] These patients present with a subacute (within 4 weeks) or chronic (within months) onset of neurogenic orthostatic hypotension, defined as a systolic blood pressure reduction of at least 30 mmHg or mean blood pressure reduction of at least 20 mmHg that occurs within 3 minutes of head tilting. The subacute onset is often preceded by a viral infection. In addition, patients demonstrate three or four parasympathetic/enteric symptoms: sicca (dry eyes and dry mouth); abnormal pupillary response to light; upper gastrointestinal symptoms (early satiety, postprandial nausea and vomiting that lead to severe weight loss); and neurogenic bladder. Patients with more severe cholinergic impairment have higher titer antibodies against ganglionic AChR. Some of these symptoms can be passively transferred to mice injected with the patient's IgG suggesting that these antibodies may be pathogenic. Further, rabbits immunized with a fragment of ganglionic AChR protein exhibit autonomic failure, similar to the human disease.[39] Because ganglionic AChR have also been found in small-cell lung carcinoma cell lines, cancer may be a potential initiator of ganglionic AChR autoimmunity.

Localized, isolated vasculitis of the peripheral nerves

Polyneuropathy is a common manifestation of systemic vasculitis.[40] It occurs in patients with polyarteritis nodosa; with connective tissue diseases, such as rheumatoid arthritis or Sjögren's syndrome; with hypersensitivity vasculitis; or with temporal arteritis. There is, however, a distinct vasculitic entity localized only to the peripheral nerve,[40] known as isolated peripheral nerve vasculitis (PNV).

PNV involves the small and medium-sized arteries of the epineurium and perineurium and causes ischemic changes within the peripheral nerve. The presentation is similar to the vasculitic neuropathy seen in systemic vasculitis—the only difference is the lack of systemic organ involvement. The diagnosis is confirmed with nerve biopsy either of the sural, the superficial peroneal, or the superficial radial nerve. When nerve biopsy is combined with a muscle biopsy, the diagnostic yield is higher.

PNV has a better prognosis than the systemic vasculitides and is a treatable form of neuropathy.

An evaluation for PNV should include all the tests needed to exclude systemic vasculitis and cryoglobulinemia, as well as hepatitis B and C infection, which is often associated with PNV.

Neuropathy with viruses and HIV

Neuropathy can be seen in a setting of infectious, viral, or bacterial processes. In patients with Lyme disease, various neuropathies, including Guillain–Barré syndrome and mononeuritis (Bell's palsy), have been noted. Other infections, such as CMV, hepatitis, herpes, leprosy, Chagas disease, and diphtheria, can affect peripheral nerves, triggering an autoimmune peripheral neuropathy.

The most common neuropathies seen today in a setting of a viral infection are those associated with HIV. The immune-mediated neuropathies, including GBS, CIDP, acute ganglioneuritis, or mononeuritis multiplex, occur early in the infection or they are the presenting manifestation of unsuspected HIV infection.[41] HIV has been cultured from peripheral nerves and HIV viral RNA has been amplified from sural nerve biopsies of some

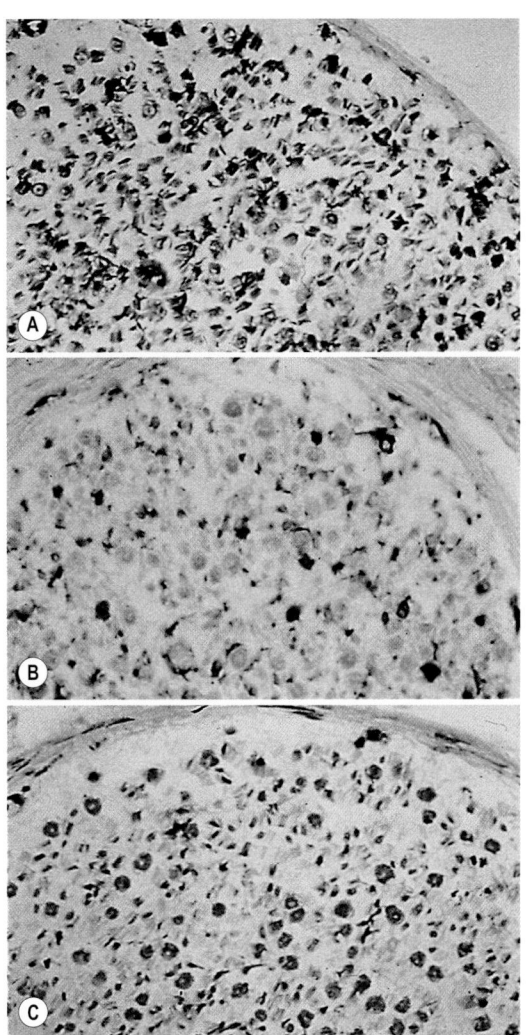

HLA-DR,
Macrophages,
CD8(+)T cells

Fig. 66.5 Serial sections of a nerve biopsy from a patient with HIV-chronic inflammatory demyelinating polyneuropathy stained for (A) HLA-DR, (B) macrophages, and (C) CD8 T shows that the majority of the endoneurial cells are macrophages. Only rare CD8 cells are noted.

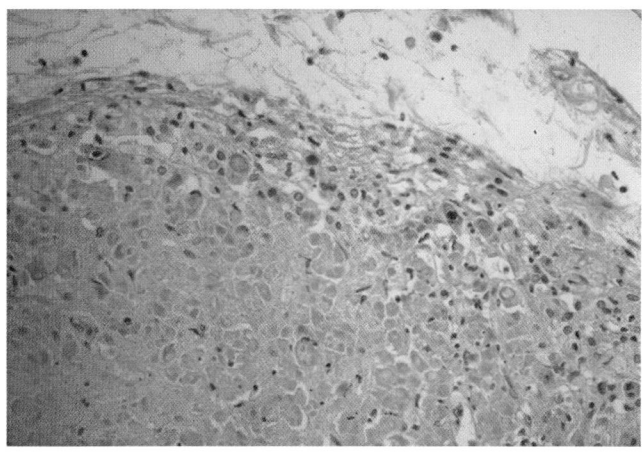

Fig. 66.6 Cross-section of a root from a patient with HIV-associated Guillain–Barré syndrome shows cytomegalovirus inclusions within the Schwann cell.

patients in the author's laboratory. However, there is no convincing evidence that the neuropathy results from direct infection of peripheral nerves with the virus. Immunocytochemical studies have shown that HIV is present only in rare endoneurial macrophages, but not within the Schwann cells or the axons. A strong expression of HLA class I and class II molecules on Schwann cells, endothelial cells, and/or macrophages, but sparse presence of CD8 and CD4 T cells, is also noted (Fig. 66.5). It is possible that systemic viral infection or rare HIV-infected endoneurial lymphoid cells may release lymphokines and cytokines that expose new nerve antigens against which there is no self-tolerance, generating a tissue-specific autoimmune attack.

A rare neuropathy seen in later-stage HIV infection is a lumbosacral polyradiculoneuropathy related to CMV infection that affects roots and sensory ganglia. It presents with lower-extremity muscle weakness, sacral and distal paresthesias, areflexia, and atrophy, mostly of the legs, associated with sphincteric dysfunction resembling a cauda equina syndrome. CMV inclusions can be found within Schwann cells or endothelial cells (Fig. 66.6). Early recognition is important because anti-CMV therapy with ganciclovir or foscarnet can be helpful.

Today the most common neuropathy in AIDS patients is a painful sensory axonal neuropathy that affects up to 70% of adults with AIDS and occurs later in the disease.[42] It is due to a cumulative effect on the peripheral nerves of various endogenous or exogenous neurotoxins related to a multisystem disease and dysfunction of many organs along with toxicity from various anti-retroviral drugs. Clinical findings include distal painful dysethesias, sensory loss or hypesthesia, areflexia, and, in advanced cases, distal weakness. Despite the relative lack of motor involvement, the severity of neuropathic pain can be disabling.

Treatment

APN are clinically important because they are potentially treatable with various immunosuppressive, immunomodulating, or chemotherapeutic agents. The selection of an effective protocol is based on the results of experimental therapeutic trials, clinical experience, and the risk–benefit ratio of available therapies. The author's approach to the treatment of these disorders is described below.

Guillain–Barré syndrome

Supportive care

The dramatic reduction in the mortality of GBS is mainly due to the availability of ICUs, improvement of respiratory support, antibiotic therapy, and control of autonomic cardiac dysregulation. A GBS patient is best monitored in an ICU, even if respiratory compromise is not evident at the time of admission. When forced vital capacity (FVC) drops or bulbar weakness is severe, intubation is in order. A team approach provides the best results.

Plasmapheresis

In several double-blind studies[43] plasmapheresis has been shown to be effective if performed within the first week from onset of the illness. A series of five or six exchanges, with one exchange every other day, is sufficient. Early relapses can occur in up to 20% of patients, who may require a second series of plasma exchanges. Plasmapheresis has been shown to be effective even in mild cases of GBS; two exchanges are sufficient for mild GBS and four are optimal for moderate cases, but there is no difference between those who receive four plasma exchanges and those who receive six.

High-dose intravenous immunoglobulin (IVIG)

Based on two controlled studies,[43] IVIG given at 2 g/kg over 2–5 days has been shown to be equally effective as plasmapheresis, with no added benefit when the two procedures were combined. The decision as to which treatment to choose is governed by circumstances, availability of the treatment modality, experience, age of the patient, and other associated conditions. Early relapses can also occur with IVIG, as often as with plasmapheresis. Because IVIG is easy to administer and more readily available, and because time to initiate treatment is of the essence, IVIG has become the therapeutic choice worldwide.

Steroids are ineffective in GBS and may even increase the incidence of future relapses. Combining IVIG with IV methylprednisolone shows no significant added benefit.

CIDP

Prednisone

CIDP is a classically steroid-responsive polyneuropathy. The efficacy of steroids was proven in a controlled study, albeit with inadequate blinding, and reconfirmed in another.[3] A high-dose regimen of 80–100 mg prednisone daily is preferred, followed by a taper to every other day dosing. Azathioprine, cyclosporine, or mycophenolate can be used as steroid-sparing agents, but their efficacy, although not tested in controlled studies, is overall disappointing.[3,14]

IVIG

In several controlled studies[3] IVIG has been effective in the majority of patients with CIDP. The more chronic the disease and the more severe the axonal degeneration that has taken place, the fewer the chances that the recovery will be complete or significant. IVIG has been shown an effective first-line therapy while mainatainance therapy can prevent relapses.[44]

Plasmapheresis

Plasmapheresis has been also effective in controlled studies.[3,14] After a series of six plasma exchanges, maintenance therapy, with one exchange at least every 8 weeks, may be required if this therapy is beneficial. IVIG has now replaced plasmapheresis, although in the author's experience some patients may benefit more from steroids, others more from IVIG, and still others more after plasmapheresis.

Polyneuropathy with paraproteinemias

Patients with benign IgG or IgA demyelinating polyneuropathies respond like CIDP patients. Patients with malignant paraproteinemias should be treated with chemotherapy as needed for the underlying disease. When the neuropathy is axonal, treatments are generally disappointing.

For the IgM anti-MAG demyelinating polyneuropathies, treatments with prednisone plus chlorambucil, plasmapheresis, and IVIG[45] has shown a variably marginal benefit. Rituximab, a monoclonal antibody against CD20, is the most promising therapy,[46] providing efficacy in almost 40% of the patients in a small double-blind study.

Multifocal motor neuropathy

This neuropathy responds very well only to IVIG, which is the treatment of choice based on controlled trials. In difficult cases, cyclophosphamide or rituximab may be promising but no controlled studies have been carried out.[21]

Paraneoplastic anti-Hu neuropathy

Anecdotally, some of these patients have responded to plasma exchange or IVIG, but overall this neuropathy has not been easily responsive to available therapies.

Vasculitic neuropathies

For isolated peripheral nerve vasculitis a combination of prednisone 1.5 mg/kg/day with cyclophosphamide 2 mg/kg/day orally, or 1 g/m^2 intravenously monthly for 6 months, are the treatments of choice; specific treatment protocol may vary between patients. The administration of cyclophosphamide may not be necessary for more than 6 months as in systemic vasculitis. Plasmapheresis has been tried in cryoglobulinemic neuropathies, with variable results.

HIV neuropathies

The demyelinating neuropathies GBS and CIDP are treated with the same immunomodulatory therapies as used in HIV-negative patients. Ganciclovir may be helpful in CMV-related polyradiculoneuropathy. Painful sensory neuropathy can be quite disabling because of intractable pain. Tricyclic antidepressants, nonsteroidal anti-inflammatory drugs, anticonvulsants (carbamazepine, gabapentin, topiramate), and topical capsaicin in various combinations provide some relief from neuropathic pain.

Acknowledgments

The author thanks the various Neurology Fellows who provided excellent care to his patients; and Drs Amjad Ilyas and Richard Quarles for help with immunochemistry.

References

1. Hughes RA, Cornblath DR. Guillain–Barré syndrome. Lancet 2005;366:1653–66.
2. Winer JB. Guillain-Barré syndrome: clinical variants and their pathogenesis. J Neuroimmunol 2011;231(1–2):70–2.
3. Dalakas MC. Advances in the diagnosis, pathogenesis and treatment of CIDP. Nat Rev Neurol 2011;7(9):507–17.
4. Feasby TE, Hahn AF, Brown WF, et al. Severe axonal degeneration in acute Guillain–Barré syndrome: evidence of two different mechanisms? J Neurol Sci 1993;116:185–92.
5. Hartung HP, Kieseier BC, Kiefer R. Progress in Guillain-Barré syndrome. Curr Opin Neurol 2001;14(5):597–604.
6. Yuki N, Susuki K, Koga M, et al. Carbohydrate mimicry between human ganglioside GM1 and *Campylobacter jejuni* lipooligosaccharide causes Guillain–Barré syndrome. Proc Natl Acad Sci U S A 2004;101:11404–11409.
7. Willison HJ, Yuki N. Peripheral neuropathies and anti-glycolipid antibodies. Brain 2002;125:2591–625.
8. Kusunoki S, Kaida K. Antibodies against ganglioside complexes in Guillain-Barré syndrome and related disorders. J Neurochem 2011;116(5):828–32.
9. Dalakas MC, Quarles RH. (Editorial) Autoimmune ataxic neuropathies (sensory ganglionopathies): Are glycolipids the responsible autoantigens? Ann Neurol 1996;39:419–22.
10. Illa I, Ortiz N, Gallard E, et al. Acute axonal Guillain–Barré syndrome with IgG antibodies against motor axons following parenteral gangliosides. Ann Neurol 1995;38:218–24.
11. Ang CW, Jacobs BC, Laman JD. The Guillain–Barré syndrome: a true case of molecular mimicry. Trends Immunol 2004;25:61–6.
12. Koller H, Kieseier BC, Jander S, Hartung HP. Chronic inflammatory demyelinating polyneuropathy. N Engl J Med 2005;352:1343–56.
13. Dalakas MC. Advances in chronic inflammatory demyelinating polyneuropathy: disease variants and inflammatory response mediators and modifiers. Curr Opin Neurol 1999;12:403–409.
14. Van den Bergh PYK, Hadden RD, Bouche P, et al. Joint Task Force of the EFNS and the PNS: European Federation of Neurological Societies/Peripheral Nerve Society Guideline on management of chronic inflammatory demyelinating polyradiculoneuropathy. First revision. Eur J Neurol 2010;17:356–63.
15. Rajabally YA, Nicolas G, Piéret F, et al. Validity of diagnostic criteria for chronic inflammatory demyelinating polyneuropathy: a multicentre European study. J Neurol Neurosurg Psychiatry 2009;80:1364–8.
16. Murata K, Dalakas MC. Expression of the co-stimulatory molecule BB-1, the ligands CTLA-4 and CD28 and their mRNAs in chronic inflammatory demyelinating polyneuropathy. Brain 2000;123:1660–6.
17. Salomon B, Rhee L, Bour-Jordan H, et al. Development of spontaneous autoimmune peripheral polyneuropathy in B7-2-deficient NOD mice. J Exp Med 2001;194:677–84.
18. Dalakas M, Engel WK. Immunoglobulin deposits in chronic relapsing polyneuropathies. Arch Neurol 1980;37:637–40.
19. Pollard JD, Armati PJ. CIDP—the relevance of recent advances in Schwanncell/axonal neurobiology. J Peripher Nerv Syst 2011;16:15–23.
20. Weiss MD, Luciano CA, Semino-Mora C, et al. Molecular mimicry in chronic inflammatory demyelinating polyneuropathy and melanoma. Neurology 1998;51:1738–41.
21. Van Asseldonk JT, Franssen H, Van den Berg-Vos RM, et al. Multifocal motor neuropathy. Lancet Neurol 2005;4:309–19.
22. Kyle RA, Therneau TM, Rajkumar SV, et al. Prevalence of monoclonal gammopathy of undetermined significance. N Engl J Med 2006;354:1362–9.
23. Kelly JJ, Kyle RA, O'Brien PC, Dyck PJ. The prevalence of monoclonal gammopathy in peripheral neuropathy. Neurology 1981;31:1480–3.
24. Latov N, Hays A, Sherman WH. Peripheral neuropathy and anti-MAG antibodies. Crit Rev Neurobiol 1988;3:301–32.
25. Dalakas MC, Engel WK. Polyneuropathy and monoclonal gammopathy: studies of 11 patients. Ann Neurol 1981;10:45–52.
26. Dalakas MC. Chronic idiopathic ataxic neuropathy. Ann Neurol 1986;19:545–54.
27. Latov N, Braun PE, Gross RB, et al. Plasma cell dyscrasia and peripheral neuropathy: identification of the myelin antigens that react with human paraproteins. Proc Natl Acad Sci U S A 1981;78:7139.
28. Ilyas AA, Quarles RH, McIntosh TD, et al. IgM in a human neuropathy related to paraproteinemia binds to a carbohydrate determinant in the myelin-associated glycoprotein and to a ganglioside. Proc Natl Acad Sci U S A 1984;81:1225–9.
29. Ilyas AA, Quarles RH, Dalakas MC, Brady RO. Polyneuropathy with monoclonal gammopathy: glycolipids are frequently antigens for IgM paraproteins. Proc Natl Acad Sci U S A 1985;82:6697–6700.
30. Duane GC, Farrer RG, Dalakas MC, Quarles RH. Sensory neuropathy associated with monoclonal IgM to GD1b ganglioside. Ann Neurol 1992;31:683–5.
31. Monaco S, Bonetti B, Ferrari S, et al. Complement dependent demyelination in patients with IgM monoclonal gammopathy and polyneuropathy. N Engl J Med 1990;322:844–52.
32. Lombardi R, Erne B, Lauria G, et al. IgM deposits on skin nerves in anti-myelin-associated glycoprotein neuropathy. Ann Neurol 2005;57:180–7.
33. Willison HJ, Trapp BD, Bacher JD, et al. Demyelination induced by intraneural injection of human antimyelin associated glycoprotein antibodies. Muscle Nerve 1988;11:1169–76.
34. Tatum AH. Experimental paraprotein neuropathy; demyelination by passive transfer of human IgM anti-MAG. Ann Neurol 1993;33:502–506.
35. Dispenzieri A, Kyle RA, Lacy MQ, et al. POEMS syndrome: definitions and long-term outcome. Blood 2003;101:2496–2506.
36. Nakanishi T, Sobue I, Toyokura Y, et al. The Crow–Fukase syndrome: a study of 102 cases in Japan. Neurology 1984;34:712–20.
37. Darnell RB, Posner JB. Paraneoplastic syndromes affecting the nervous system. Oncology 2006;33:270–98.
38. Vernino S, Low PA, Fealey RD, et al. Autoantibodies to ganglionic acetylcholine receptors in autoimmune autonomic neuropathies. N Engl J Med 2000;343:847–55.
39. Lennon VA, Ermilov LG, Szurszewski JH, Vernino S. Immunization with neuronal nicotinic acetylcholine receptor induces neurological autoimmune disease. J Clin Invest 2003;111:907–13.
40. Chalk CH, Dyck PJ, Conn DL. Vasculitic neuropathy. In: Dyck PJ, Thomas PK, Griffin JW, et al., editors Peripheral neuropathy. Philadelphia: WB Saunders; 1993. p. 1424–36.
41. Dalakas MC, Pezeshkpour GH. Neuromuscular diseases associated with human immunodeficiency virus infection. Ann Neurol 1988;23:38–48.
42. Dalakas MC. Peripheral neuropathy and antiretroviral drugs. J Peripher Nerv Syst 2001;6:14–20.
43. Hughes RA, Wijdicks EF, Barohn R, et al., Quality Standards Subcommittee of the American Academy of Neurology. Practice parameter: immunotherapy for Guillain-Barré syndrome: report of the Quality Standards Subcommittee of the American Academy of Neurology. Neurology 2003;61(6):736–40.
44. Hughes RA, Donofrio P, Bril V, et al. Intravenous immune globulin (10% caprylate-chromatography purified) for the treatment of chronic inflammatory demyelinating polyradiculoneuropathy (ICE study): a randomised placebo-controlled trial. Lancet Neurol 2008;7:136–44.
45. Dalakas MC, Quarles RH, Farrer RG, et al. A controlled study of intravenous immunoglobulin in demyelinating neuropathy with IgM gammopathy. Ann Neurol 1996;40:792–5.
46. Dalakas MC, Rakocevic G, Salajegheh M, et al. Placebo-controlled trial of rituximab in IgM anti-myelin associated glycoprotein antibody demyelinating neuropathy. Ann Neurol 2009;65:286–93.

67

James E. Balow,
Monique E. Cho,
Meryl Waldman,
Howard A.
Austin III

Immunologic renal diseases

There is compelling clinical, pathologic and experimental evidence that most forms of glomerulonephritis result from some form of immune mediated injury.[1,2] The primary events or inciting factors that instigate the host immune responses that are directly or indirectly pathogenic to the kidney are largely unknown. In some conditions, normal or allergic immune responses to exogenous infectious agents or drugs can lead to incidental nephropathic injury (e.g., post-infectious glomerulonephritis, serum sickness). In the case of autoimmune diseases, nephropathic responses range from loss or lack of self tolerance to specific constitutive renal (e.g., anti-GBM disease) or non-renal (e.g., antineutrophil cytoplasmic autoantibodies) to unregulated polyclonal immune responses and immune complex disease (e.g., lupus nephritis). The molecular targets of the abnormal immune response are unknown for the majority of human glomerular diseases, but recent advances have begun to uncover candidate antigens involved in the pathogenesis of immune mediated renal diseases (e.g., some subsets of membranous nephropathy). It has become increasingly apparent that the immune system does not operate in isolation and that there are complex interactions among vast networks involving components of native and adaptive humoral immunity, cell-mediated immune systems, small molecular weight mediators derived from lymphoid and other cell types, complement factors and their regulatory proteins, and other inflammatory amplification and coagulation system pathways that will be unravelled with the emerging tools of modern systems biology and bioinformatics.[3]

Appropriate evaluation of patients with immune-mediated kidney diseases requires particular attention to the findings of urinalysis, tests of renal functions, and renal biopsy.[4,5] Urine microscopy plays a pivotal role in the assessment of urinary disorders. The physician should be mindful of the many "false negative" urinalyses reported by practice-oriented clinical pathology laboratories pressured by high sample throughput. As a general rule, reports of positive findings are much more likely to be accurate than are negative reports. The thorough clinician should personally review microscopic urinalysis in any case in which there is a reasonable index of suspicion of immune-mediated renal disease.

Hematuria

Evaluation of hematuria should begin with determination of whether the bleeding is due to upper urinary tract (glomerular and/or tubulointerstitial) pathology or to lower urinary tract abnormalities. Urinary erythrocyte morphology helps to determine the cause of hematuria. Red blood cells that emanate from lesions of the calices, ureters, bladder or urethra tend to maintain their normal morphology; when non-dysmorphic red blood cells are present, it is usually appropriate to refer the patient to urology for further evaluation. Red blood cells that result from glomerular or tubulointerstitial pathology are more likely to appear dysmorphic (abnormal shapes and sizes, fragmented); when dysmorphic red blood cells are present, it is usually appropriate to refer the patient to nephrology for further evaluation. Erythrocyte and/or leukocyte casts are indicative of glomerulonephritis (or interstitial nephritis). Cellular casts can be formed from erythrocytes and/or leukocytes that enter the tubular lumen because of glomerular or tubular inflammation (Fig. 67.1).

Proteinuria

Proteinuria is a cardinal feature of renal parenchymal disease and may indicate glomerular or tubular pathology. Glomerular proteinuria results from a loss of the size-selective and/or charge-selective properties of the glomerular capillary wall and disruptions of the glomerular epithelial cells (podocytes), allowing plasma proteins (especially albumin) to leak into the filtrate. Tubulointerstitial nephropathy often leads to impaired tubular absorption of other normally filtered low molecular weight proteins; this so-called "tubular proteinuria" exhibits a characteristic pattern on urine protein electrophoresis (low fraction of albumin), rarely exceeds 2 g/day, and is often associated with other manifestations of tubular dysfunction.

The validity of 24-hour urine collections for determination of quantitative proteinuria is often an issue; under- and over-collections are common and must be countered with explicit instructions to patients regarding urine collection procedures. Owing to the high prevalence of collection errors, many clinicians have turned to estimates of proteinuria based on the protein-to-creatinine concentration ratio in random urine samples. Normally, the urine protein-to-creatinine ratio is less than 0.1. This random urine sample method has steadily gained favor as an efficient, cost-effective method to monitor proteinuria in both children and adults.

Filtration of abnormal plasma proteins can be responsible for proteinuria (e.g., multiple myeloma or immunoglobulin light-chain disease). This type of proteinuria (paraproteinuria) may be undetected by albumin-sensitive dipstick screening. Paraproteinemia may also be undetected or underestimated by standard plasma electrophoresis or even plasma immunofixation electrophoresis; however, a new highly sensitive assay for free light chains for detecting low levels of plasma light chain paraproteins

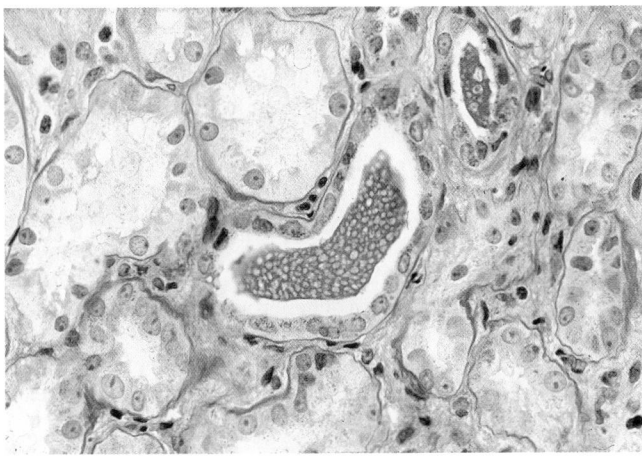

Fig. 67.1 Red blood cell cast. Cast present *in situ* within the lumen of a distal renal tubule. (PAS stain.)

has recently become available.[6] Confirmation of light chain paraproteinuria requires urine immunofixation electrophoresis.

Nephrotic syndrome

The nephrotic syndrome is characterized by substantial degrees of proteinuria (> 3.5 g/day) resulting in hypoalbuminemia, edema, hyperlipidemia and lipiduria. The degree of proteinuria can offer a helpful diagnostic clue because some immune-mediated conditions with typically diffuse glomerular disease (e.g., membranous nephropathy, systemic lupus, amyloidosis) are more likely than others with typically focal disease (e.g., IgA nephropathy, microscopic polyangiitis, granulomatosis with polyangiitis – Wegener's granulomatosis) to be associated with the nephrotic syndrome.

Acute nephritic syndrome

The acute nephritic syndrome is characterized by hematuria (dysmorphic cells), erythrocyte casts, abnormal proteinuria, fluid retention, azotemia and hypertension. Histologically, this constellation of clinical findings is due to proliferative glomerulonephritis. A variant of this syndrome, called rapidly progressive glomerulonephritis, is defined by 50% or greater loss of glomerular filtration rate over 3 months, along with cellular crescents on renal biopsy. It is important to recognize that rapidly progressive glomerulonephritis can present subtly as hematuria and/or proteinuria without oliguria, edema, hypertension or azotemia, yet become an explosive manifestation of several immunologic renal diseases, particularly granulomatosis with polyangiitis, microscopic polyangiitis, Henoch–Schönlein nephritis, and proliferative lupus nephritis.

Chronic glomerulonephritis

Chronic glomerulonephritis is not a diagnosis, but rather is a stage in the evolution of immune-mediated renal disease. The urinalysis often provides valuable clues regarding the duration of glomerular disease. Broad and waxy casts are features of chronic renal disease that are not likely to be seen in recent-onset acute glomerulonephritis.

Renal biopsy

After extensive clinical and laboratory evaluations, a renal biopsy may be indicated to establish or confirm a tissue diagnosis, to clarify the precise type of renal involvement, to formulate a prognosis, and to direct therapy. Some of the more important indications for renal biopsy are listed in Table 67.1. To assist the reader in recognizing patterns of glomerular diseases addressed in subsequent discussions, a normal glomerulus is illustrated in Fig. 67.2. Excellent color atlases of glomerular diseases are available.[7,8]

Table 67.1 Indications for renal biopsy

1. Active 'nephritic' urine sediment
    Dysmorphic erythrocytes: > 10 per high-power field
    Cellular casts: erythrocyte or leukocyte

2. Proteinuria > 2 g/day

3. Abnormal renal function
    Associated with the above features of active nephritis
    Particularly important if the duration of renal disease and/or rate
    of change are unknown

4. Document indications for use of high risk therapeutic interventions

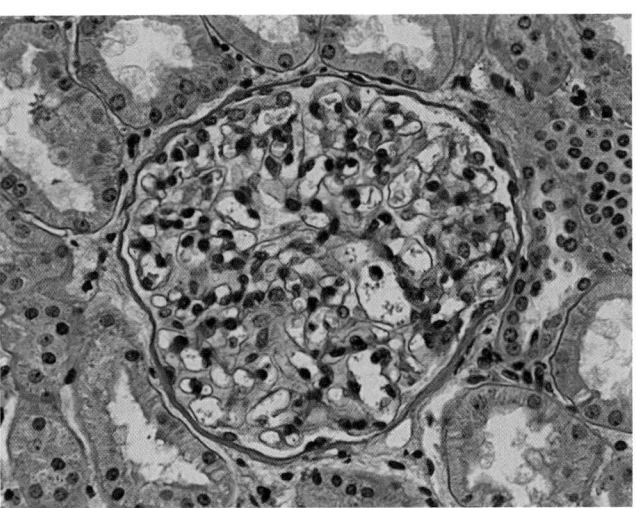

Fig. 67.2 Normal glomerular architecture. Note the thin, delicate capillary walls. Neither cells nor matrix encroach upon the patency of the capillary lumina. (PAS stain.)

Minimal change nephropathy (lipoid nephrosis)

● KEY CONCEPTS

Minimal change nephropathy

- Most common cause of nephrotic syndrome in children
- High rate of response to glucocorticoids
- Cyclophosphamide is useful for frequent relapsers
- Renal prognosis is characteristically excellent
- Subset may evolve to focal segmental glomerulosclerosis

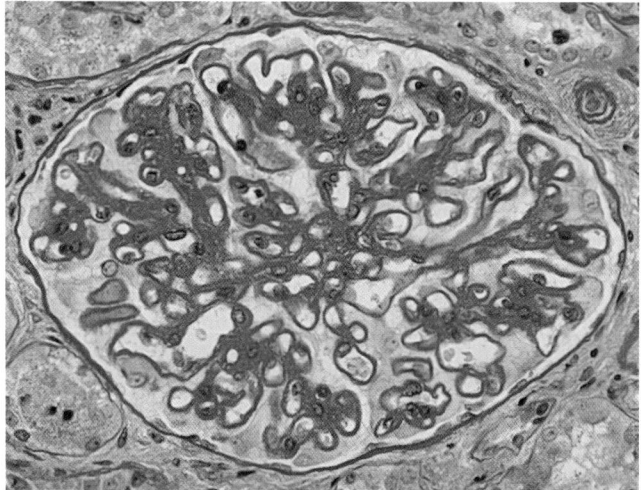

Fig. 67.4 Membranous nephropathy. Capillary walls are nearly uniformly thickened but remain widely patent. Cellularity of the glomerulus is normal. (PAS stain.)

Diagnosis of secondary membranous nephropathy depends on concurrent abnormalities in clinical and laboratory data.

Natural history

The clinical course of idiopathic membranous nephropathy is highly variable. On average, about one-quarter of adult patients progress to end-stage renal failure within 10 years. Another quarter experience a spontaneous remission of proteinuria. The majority are likely to have persistent proteinuria and moderately impaired renal function over an extended period of observation. Patients with sustained hyperlipidemia are at risk for premature cardiovascular disease. Reduction of cardiovascular risk may be as important an element in the rationale for treatment as is preserving kidney function.

It is difficult to predict the clinical course of individual patients with membranous nephropathy. Baseline characteristics such as severe nephrotic syndrome, hypertension and azotemia have been associated with poor outcomes. Protracted high-grade nephrotic-range proteinuria is a relatively strong predictor of an adverse renal outcome. On the other hand, complete or partial remission of proteinuria is associated with excellent long-term prognosis.

Treatment

Management of patients with membranous nephropathy usually includes diuretics to reduce edema, lipid-lowering drugs (for severe hyperlipidemia), anticoagulant therapy for thromboembolic complications, and antihypertensive agents. Angiotensin antagonists have been shown to have a substantial antiproteinuric effect. Whereas patients with severe nephrotic syndrome due to membranous nephropathy are often treated with high-dose alternate-day prednisone, it is generally considered that prednisone does not significantly reduce the risk of progression to renal failure. There is evidence that a combination of prednisone and cytotoxic drug therapy is more effective than prednisone alone. Azathioprine has not been widely used for the treatment of membranous nephropathy. Several small case series and randomized studies of the related drug, mycophenolate mofetil, have shown conflicting results. The most compelling

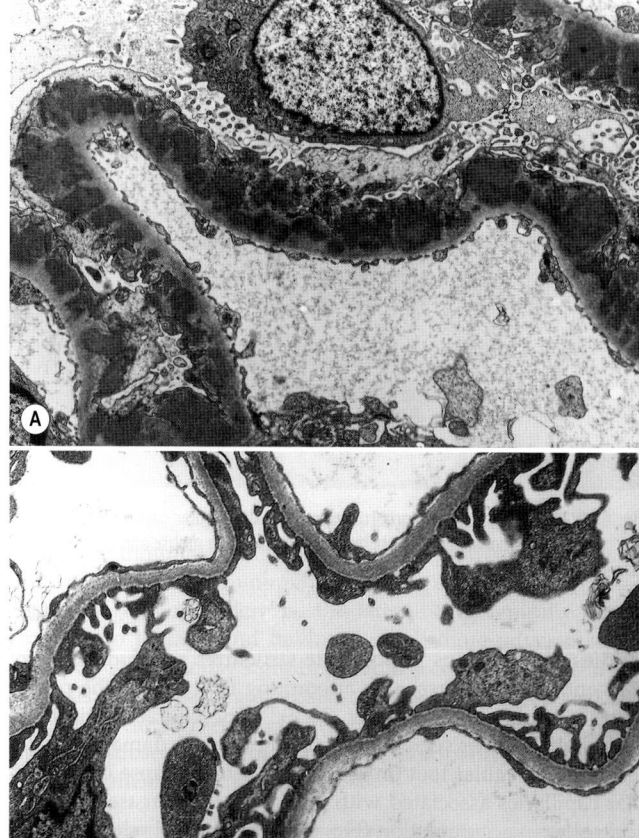

Fig. 67.5 Membranous nephropathy (ultrastructure). (A) Electron micrograph demonstrates heavy, dark-staining immune complex deposits along the outer surface of the glomerular basement membrane and beneath the epithelial foot processes (hence the terms subepithelial or epimembranous deposits). Note the thickening and projections of the gray-staining basement membrane between the electron-dense deposits. (B) Ultrastructure of a normal glomerular capillary wall for comparison.
Electron micrographs courtesy of Dr S. Sabnis, Armed Forces Institute of Pathology; Washington, DC.

results from controlled trials have shown that patients with membranous nephropathy treated with alternating monthly courses of pulse methylprednisolone and chlorambucil or cyclophosphamide were more likely than controls to experience a remission of the nephrotic syndrome and achieve stable renal function.

Several anecdotal series and controlled trials of cyclosporine in membranous nephropathy have suggested a moderate benefit on proteinuria and renal function. Relapses of proteinuria are common, particularly after a short course of cyclosporine therapy. Preliminary studies suggest that rituximab (which depletes CD20 B lymphocytes) may be a useful alternative for treatment of membranous nephropathy.[16]

Membranoproliferative glomerulonephritis

● KEY CONCEPTS

Membranoproliferative glomerulonephritis (MPGN)

- Rare form of chronic nephritis mostly discovered as asymptomatic hematuria, variable proteinuria, and/or insidious chronic renal insufficiency
- Type I MPGN: subendothelial immune complex deposits
- Type II MPGN: dense intramembranous deposits (containing C3 complement)
- Hypocomplementemia associated with C3 nephritic factor, an autoantibody to C3 convertase of the alternative complement pathway
- Response to immunosuppressive drug treatment generally poor
- Both types MPGN tend to recur in renal allografts

Membranoproliferative glomerulonephritis (MPGN) is a rare condition that is sometimes referred to as mesangiocapillary glomerulonephritis (Fig. 67.6). Besides the presence of pathologic immunoreactants in glomerular sites, the immune-mediated nature of this disease is suggested by the high frequency of persistent hypocomplementemia. It is of interest that both congenital complement deficiencies (e.g., C3 and factor H deficiencies) and sustained hypocomplementemia induced by nephritic factor autoantibodies or circulating immune complexes have all been associated with MPGN.[3,17,18]

Pathologic variants

The nomenclature of MPGN includes two main pathological subsets: type I, MPGN with subendothelial deposits (Fig. 67.7A), and type II, MPGN with dense intramembranous deposits (Fig. 67.7B).[19] Although most cases of MPGN are of unknown etiology, studies over the past decade have shown that chronic hepatitis C infection, particularly when accompanied

Fig. 67.6 Membranoproliferative glomerulonephritis (MPGN). Glomerulus exhibits the typical lobulated appearance of this disease. Markedly increased mesangial cells and matrix in all of the lobules. Mesangium extends outward into the capillary loops and forms double contours with the glomerular basement membrane. (PAS stain.)

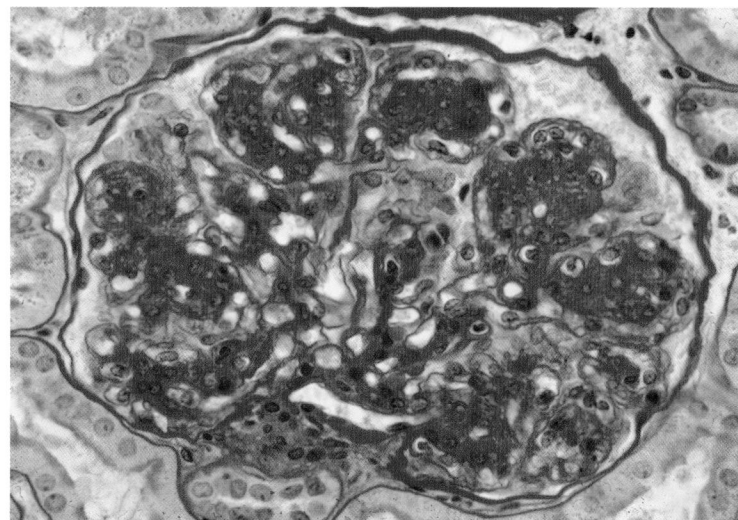

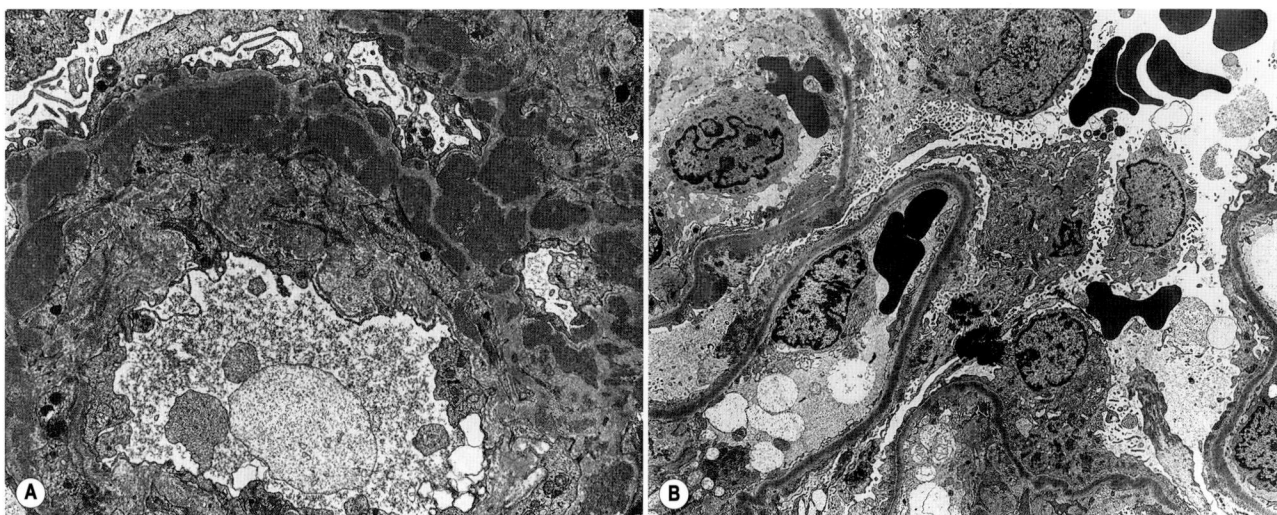

Fig. 67.7 Membranoproliferative glomerulonephritis (MPGN) ultrastructure. (A) Type I MPGN: capillary wall is markedly thickened and contains heavy, dark-staining electron dense immune complexes in the subendothelial space. Mesangium (lighter material) extends into the capillary loop, where it is interposed between the basement membrane and the endothelium; the process gives the appearance of a massively thickened capillary loop on hematoxylin and eosin staining, and the split appearance by PAS and silver stains. (B) Type II MPGN (dense intramembranous deposit disease): capillary loops contain smooth, continuous linear dense material within the basement membrane.

Electron micrographs courtesy of Dr S. Sabnis, Armed Forces Institute of Pathology; Washington, DC.

by cryoglobulinemia, is associated with massive subendothelial immune complex deposition and accounts for a substantial portion of cases of type I MPGN.

Types I and II idiopathic MPGN are clinically indistinguishable. Typically, asymptomatic hematuria and proteinuria are discovered incidentally. Judging from the chronicity found on initial renal biopsies, MPGN probably goes undetected for long periods in most patients. Although it is characteristically a chronic low-grade nephropathy, some patients experience complicated nephrotic syndrome and even rapidly progressive and crescentic disease phases.

Nephritic factors

Patients with type II MPGN, and to a lesser extent type I, exhibit a complement-activating antibody called nephritic factor. The typical nephritic factor is an IgG autoantibody that binds to the alternative pathway convertase called C3bBb. Nephritic factor stabilizes and prolongs the activity of the enzyme by interfering with normal factors controlling the convertase activity. This leads to sustained activation and severe depletion of serum C3 levels, which is a hallmark of MPGN. Whether or how C3 nephritic factor plays a role in the pathogenesis of either form of MPGN is unknown. Interestingly, in type II MPGN there are no immunoglobulin components in the dense intramembranous deposits, although there are heavy linear deposits of C3 complement, possibly indicating an effect of the prolonged C3 activation.

Treatment

There is no consensus about the treatment of MPGN. The overwhelming opinion is that no therapy is effective in inducing remission or in protecting against progressive renal failure. Overall, renal survival is approximately 50% at 10 years from diagnosis, although a subset of patients have a rapidly progressive course if they develop superimposed crescentic glomerulonephritis. Alternate-day prednisone is commonly tried in children with MPGN, but no controlled trials are available and the long-term prognosis remains unfavorable. The efficacy of cytotoxic drug therapy, anticoagulants, and anti-platelet drugs are similarly unproven. A more targeted approach using eculizumab, a monoclonal antibody that blocks activation of C5 complement, is being explored. Both forms of MPGN tend to recur in renal allografts; recurrences of both types of MPGN have a detrimental effect on graft survival.[20]

POSTINFECTIOUS NEPHROPATHIES

An ever-expanding list of infectious agents has been implicated in the pathogenesis of immune-mediated nephropathies. Some are acute and self-limited, but many of the nephritogenic infections are protracted and are associated with circulating immune complexes, cryoglobulins, high-titer rheumatoid factor, and hypocomplementemia.

Viral infections

Hepatitis B

Hepatitis B-associated nephropathy most frequently presents as nephrotic syndrome accompanied by microscopic hematuria; only rarely is there evidence of renal functional impairment or progressive liver disease on presentation. Renal biopsy most commonly shows membranous nephropathy. Immunofluorescence studies usually show immunoglobulin, C3 and viral antigens, particularly HBsAg and HBeAg. Electron microscopy shows subepithelial and intramembranous deposits, but unlike in idiopathic membranous nephropathy there may also be mesangial and even some subendothelial deposits.

Therapy for hepatitis B renal disease has focused on antiviral drugs, as glucocorticoids and cytotoxic agents may promote viral replication. Currently, the three drugs approved for hepatitis B infection in adults are recombinant human IFN-α, lamivudine and adefovir. IFN-α has been shown to produce remission of both liver and kidney disease. Lamivudine should be used for at least 1 year, and continued for at least 6 months after HBeAg seroconversion. Adefovir and other nucleoside analogues may have a role for those patients who are resistant to lamivudine.[21]

Hepatitis C

Hepatitis C virus (HCV) is a major cause of both transfusion-associated and sporadic chronic hepatitis. Persistent infection occurs in approximately 50% of patients and can result in chronic active hepatitis, cirrhosis, cryoglobulinemia, and MPGN. The pathogenesis of the renal disease is unknown, but may relate to deposition within glomeruli of immune complexes containing HCV, anti-HCV antibody and virus-related (or unrelated) cryoglobulins.

Treatment of hepatitis C includes combination therapy with IFN-α and ribavirin which can be effective in reducing viral replication and improving renal and liver disease.[22] Newer antiviral drugs, particularly combination therapies, hold considerable promise for improving response rates and averting the morbidity of current therapies for hepatitis C. Rituximab and plasma exchange are currently under investigation for the treatment of patients with severe refractory cryoglobulin-related renal disease or vasculitis.

Human immunodeficiency virus (HIV)

Patients with the acquired immunodeficiency syndrome (AIDS) develop a wide variety of renal abnormalities, including focal segmental glomerulosclerosis, immune complex glomerulonephritis with lupus-like features, and drug-induced interstitial nephritis.[23] Black patients and intravenous drug abusers are more likely to develop an aggressive form of glomerular disease, currently designated HIV-associated nephropathy (HIVAN). HIVAN is characterized by focal segmental glomerulosclerosis (collapsing type) with extensive tubular ectasia and interstitial fibrosis. Treatment with highly active antiretroviral therapies has somewhat ameliorated the otherwise poor renal prognosis of HIVAN, although complications of the drug therapy itself have been observed. The use of standard immunosuppressive drug therapies for HIVAN is controversial.

Bacterial infections

Post-streptococcal glomerulonephritis

Post-streptococcal glomerulonephritis is the result of skin or throat infection with nephritogenic strains of group A streptococci. Nephritic syndrome characteristically appears around 2 weeks after the infection. Whereas the role of streptococcal infection in causing the disease is widely accepted, the demonstration of streptococcal antigens and antibodies in glomeruli has been controversial.

Infection-related nephropathies

- *Viral:* Hepatitis B—membranous nephropathy; hepatitis C—cryoglobulinemic membranoproliferative glomerulonephritis; HIV—focal segmental glomerulosclerosis (HIV nephropathy)
- *Bacterial (mainly Gram-positive):* Nephritogenic streptococcal infections, prosthetic device (shunt) infections, subacute bacterial endocarditis, chronic deep tissue abscesses – mainly diffuse or focal proliferative glomerulonephritis; secondary syphilis – membranous nephropathy
- *Parasitic: Schistosomiasis mansoni* (chronic hepatosplenic form)—focal segmental glomerulosclerosis and membranoproliferative glomerulonephritis
- Effective control of renal disease under most conditions (except perhaps schistosomiasis) depends on eradication of the organism; immunosuppressive or anti-inflammatory drug therapies are rarely indicated

Post-streptococcal glomerulonephritis is characterized by a nephritic syndrome consisting of smoky or rust-colored urine, generalized edema, hypertension, and nephritic urine sediment. Proteinuria is typically mild. Patients have rising titers of anti-streptolysin and depressed C3 levels early in nephritis but normal or minimally depressed C4 levels, indicating activation of the alternative complement pathway.

Complete clinical resolution of nephritis is the rule, and therefore renal biopsy is not usually indicated in children. In adults, biopsy is often necessary for diagnosis. Proliferative glomerulonephritis with polymorphonuclear leukocyte and monocyte infiltration, granular immune deposits of IgG and C3, and dome-shaped electron-dense subepithelial deposits (humps) are characteristic. The prognosis is excellent: almost all children will recover with supportive care. Progressive renal failure accompanied by severe hypertension appears to be more common in adults.

Glomerulonephritis associated with focal infections

Renal disease has been associated with infective endocarditis, infection of artificial vascular devices, and localized chronic abscesses.[24] A variety of organisms have been implicated in the pathogenesis of renal disease, which seems to be immune-complex mediated. Overlap with renal vasculitic diseases is common. Renal biopsy findings in fulminant infections resemble those of acute post-streptococcal glomerulonephritis. In subacute forms (e.g., endocarditis), focal segmental proliferative glomerulonephritis is more common. The course and prognosis are variable. Antibiotic therapy in most cases is associated with improvement in the renal lesions.

Syphilis

Nephropathy can occur in both congenital and acquired syphilis. In acquired syphilis the nephropathy usually becomes apparent during the secondary phase of the infection. Most patients present with nephrotic syndrome and have membranous nephropathy on renal biopsy. Patients with concurrently positive syphilis serologies and antinuclear antibodies may have lupus-related rather than syphilis-associated membranous nephropathy. Following the institution of antimicrobial therapy most, but not all, patients with syphilis-associated nephropathy recover.

Parasitic diseases

Schistosomiasis

Schistosomal infections affect millions of patients in tropical countries. Nephropathy usually occurs after the development of the chronic hepatosplenic infection with *Schistosoma mansoni* and is characterized by proteinuria, hypertension and chronic renal failure. Renal biopsy usually demonstrates focal segmental glomerulosclerosis or membranoproliferative glomerulonephritis. Long-standing schistosomiasis rarely produces secondary renal amyloidosis. Treatment of the underlying schistosomiasis or the nephropathy with corticosteroids and immunosuppressive therapy do not seem to affect the progression of the schistosomiasis-associated nephropathy.

IGA nephropathy

IgA nephritis

- Common cause of asymptomatic microscopic hematuria, recurrent macroscopic hematuria, and/or low-grade proteinuria
- Spectrum of disease, including idiopathic IgA nephritis and Henoch–Schönlein purpura nephritis; IgA in skin and renal biopsies
- Mostly benign prognosis, especially in children
- Patients with progressive renal insufficiency and/or crescentic glomerulonephritis warrant trial of glucocorticoids and/or cytotoxic drug therapy

Idiopathic IgA nephropathy (also known as Berger's disease) is among the most common forms of glomerular disease in many parts of the world, especially southern Europe, Australia, and Asia. The high frequency of IgA nephropathy in these countries appears partly to reflect widespread routine screening of healthy schoolchildren and military recruits for urinary abnormalities, and frequent use of renal biopsy to evaluate asymptomatic, isolated hematuria. Renal histologic features and aspects of immunopathogenesis are comparable to those of Henoch–Schönlein nephritis.[25,26]

Clinical features

IgA nephropathy can affect patients of all ages, especially children and young adults, with a male preponderance. Unexplained is the fact that IgA nephropathy is rare in black patients. This observation and examples of familial clustering of IgA nephropathy favor an important element of genetic susceptibility. IgA nephropathy may be discovered as asymptomatic microscopic hematuria. Alternatively, patients (especially children) can present with recurrent episodes of macroscopic hematuria that occur within 24–48 hours after an intercurrent infection, usually an upper respiratory or gastrointestinal tract infection. A transient elevation in serum creatinine has been associated with macroscopic hematuria in about one-third of cases. This has been attributed to tubular injury and obstruction caused by intraluminal red blood cell casts. An episode of macroscopic hematuria is occasionally associated with extensive cellular crescent formation, rapidly deteriorating renal function, hypertension and nephrotic syndrome.

Natural history

IgA nephropathy typically has a benign renal prognosis. However, it is recognized that at least one-third of patients with IgA nephropathy eventually progress to end-stage kidney failure. Twenty years after apparent disease onset the probability of renal failure is 25%, and the probability of some renal dysfunction is 50%. Hypertension occurs frequently as the disease progresses and forebodes a poor prognosis.

Other clinical features that have been associated with a poor prognosis include older age at apparent disease onset, persistent proteinuria (>1 g/day), and persistent azotemia. On renal biopsy evaluation extensive cellular crescents, endocapillary proliferation, and extension of immune deposits to the peripheral glomerular capillary walls are indicative of severe immune-mediated glomerulonephritis and a poor prognosis. Evidence of irreversible renal parenchymal injury (glomerular sclerosis, interstitial fibrosis and tubular atrophy) also identifies high-risk patients.

Treatment

The treatment of progressive IgA nephropathy remains undefined and controversial.[27] Angiotensin antagonists are recommended to achieve blood pressure control, to reduce proteinuria, and to slow the rate of deterioration of renal function.[28] There are conflicting data about the value of fish oil dietary supplements (eicosanoids) in preventing renal progression in patients with IgA nephropathy. The risk–benefit of corticosteroids is unclear, but these agents are generally used in patients with persistent proteinuria >1 g/day despite maximally tolerated angiotensin antagonist therapies. Cytotoxic drugs are indicated in a small subset of patients with crescentic rapidly progressive IgA glomerulonephritis.

Henoch–Schönlein nephritis (Chapter 57)

Henoch–Schönlein purpura (HSP) is a generalized vasculitis that usually affects children and typically involves the skin, joints, kidneys and gastrointestinal tract. Classic Henoch–Schönlein disease, manifested as purpuric rash with features of joint, kidney, and/or gastrointestinal involvement, is readily recognized. Characteristic skin and renal biopsy findings can support the diagnosis. Skin biopsies reveal leukocytoclastic vasculitis with granular deposits of IgA along dermal vessels of purpuric and uninvolved skin.

Whereas in most patients the disease remits spontaneously, some patients develop serious renal and/or gastrointestinal complications. Evidence of immune complex causation has prompted recommendations for immunosuppressive treatment of severe Henoch–Schönlein nephritis, but the data are uncontrolled and controversial.

Clinical features

Urinary abnormalities were seen in about one-third of a largely unselected sample of children with Henoch–Schönlein purpura. Microscopic hematuria is detected in nearly all cases of Henoch–Schönlein nephritis, and is accompanied by variable proteinuria in more than 90% of cases. Approximately 40% of patients reported from referral centers had nephrotic-range proteinuria, and in two-thirds of those there were complicating features, including various

combinations of hypertension, azotemia, and hypoproteinemia. Renal biopsy findings range from mild mesangial proliferation to crescentic glomerulonephritis. Immune deposits are predominantly mesangial and characteristically contain IgA.

Natural history

Most patients with Henoch–Schönlein nephritis follow a relatively benign clinical course. The probability of maintaining life-supporting renal function is nearly 90% at 10 years. It is debated whether adults are at greater risk for renal failure than children. Patients who present with microscopic hematuria without proteinuria rarely progress to renal failure. Approximately 80% of patients who initially manifest hematuria and proteinuria have normal renal function with little or no urinary abnormality after extended observation; another 10% are likely to progress to renal failure. Patients who present with proteinuria >1 g/day, impaired renal function and hypertension are at considerable risk for end-stage kidney failure. The renal biopsy also provides useful prognostic information. Widespread cellular crescents, interstitial fibrosis and tubular atrophy portend an increased risk of renal failure.[29]

Therapy

Decisions regarding the treatment of Henoch–Schönlein nephritis are made difficult by a lack of compelling data from prospective randomized therapeutic trials and by the highly unpredictable nature of this disease. Corticosteroids and cytotoxic drugs should be reserved for the high-risk patients described above. Pulse intravenous methylprednisolone seems to offer additional benefit. Uncontrolled observations also suggest that azathioprine, cyclosporine, plasma exchange, anticoagulants, dipyridamole and urokinase may be useful, but additional studies are needed. Renal transplantation is a reasonable option for patients who progress to terminal renal failure, provided the disease has been in remission for several months preoperatively.

Nephropathies associated with anti-neutrophil cytoplasmic antibodies (classic polyarteritis, microscopic polyangiitis, granulomatosis with polyangiitis (Wegener's granulomatosis), and idiopathic necrotizing crescentic glomerulonephritis) (Chapters 57 and 58)

● KEY CONCEPTS

Renal vasculitis

- Renal vasculitis with glomerular involvement includes microscopic polyangiitis, granulomatosis with polyangiitis, and necrotizing crescentic glomerulonephritis (renal-limited vasculitis)
- Associated with anti-neutrophil cytoplasmic antibodies (ANCA)
- Rapidly progressive glomerulonephritis is common; early treatment includes pulse methylprednisolone, cyclophosphamide (possibly adjunctive plasma exchange)
- Maintenance therapy: azathioprine, mycophenolate, methotrexate

Clinical and pathologic features

Renal involvement is common in the systemic vasculitides but varies in type and severity.[30] In classic polyarteritis nodosa the vasculitis primarily affects arteries outside the glomerulus, producing ischemia, hypertension, segmental infarctions, and renal failure. In microscopic polyangiitis, granulomatosis with polyangiitis and renal-limited necrotizing and crescentic glomerulonephritis, the vasculitis occurs mainly within the glomerulus. The glomerular abnormalities are similar among these groups (Fig. 67.8). The lesions are characteristically focal and segmental in distribution, with fibrinoid necrosis and crescent formation but few, if any, immune deposits (some use the term pauci-immune glomerulonephritis). Clinically, rapidly progressive glomerulonephritis is a common manifestation of these renal vasculitides, making early detection of glomerulonephritis critically important in management.

Another common feature of the renal vasculitides is the presence of autoantibodies to neutrophil cytoplasmic antigens. As shown in Table 67.2, microscopic polyangiitis, granulomatosis with polyangiitis and idiopathic necrotizing crescentic glomerulonephritis all express anti-neutrophil cytoplasmic antibodies (ANCA), but in somewhat different patterns. There is a strong correlation between the presence of ANCA and glomerular involvement in systemic vasculitis. Recent murine models with anti-myeloperoxidase antibodies have demonstrated the role of ANCA in the pathogenesis of the vasculitic diseases.[31]

Treatment and prognosis

Renal vasculitis tends to be severe and fulminant. Even with early diagnosis, approximately one-third of patients will progress to renal failure within 5 years. Relapsing courses are common in patients with microscopic polyangiitis, and particularly granulomatosis with polyangiitis. Glucocorticoids are important in the early treatment of renal vasculitis, but their efficacy is limited and maintenance should include alternate-day therapy whenever possible.

In patients with severe pulmonary hemorrhage or rapidly progressive glomerulonephritis due to renal vasculitis, pulse methylprednisolone followed by prednisone and daily cyclophosphamide are clearly indicated. Adjunctive plasma exchange

Table 67.2 Prevalence of anti-neutrophil cytoplasmic antibodies (ANCA) in renal vasculitis

Type of renal vasculitis	ANCA test positivity (%)	
	P-ANCA or Anti-MPO	C-ANCA or Anti-PR3
Polyarteritis nodosa	10–20	10–20
Microscopic polyangiitis	50–80	10–20
Granulomatosis with polyangiitis (Wegener's granulomatosis)	10–20	80–90
Necrotizing and crescentic GN	50–80	10–20

MPO = myeloperoxidase; PR3 = proteinase 3.

is commonly used in cases of aggressive pulmonary–renal syndrome.

Although controversial, some recent experience indicates that intermittent pulse cyclophosphamide may be substituted for daily cyclophosphamide in order to reduce the toxicity of extended therapy in ANCA-associated glomerulonephritis. Granulomatosis with polyangiitis is generally considered an exception, in which case most investigators advocate daily cyclophosphamide for remission induction therapy with conversion to azathioprine, mycophenolate, methotrexate, or more recently, rituximab for maintenance.[32] Cyclosporine has not proved to be an effective alternative to conventional cytotoxic drug therapy, either as primary therapy or in preventing renal relapse following kidney transplantation.

Anti-GBM antibody-mediated nephritis: Goodpasture's disease

● KEY CONCEPTS

Goodpasture's disease

- Circulating anti-GBM antibody
- Pulmonary hemorrhage: treated mostly with pulse methylprednisolone
- Rapidly progressive glomerulonephritis with cellular crescents and linear deposits of IgG
- Treated with high-dose steroids, cyclophosphamide, plasma exchange

Goodpasture's disease is a rare but classic immune-mediated cause of severe pulmonary–renal syndrome.[33] Its essential components include pulmonary hemorrhage and rapidly progressive glomerulonephritis, both of which are characteristically (but not universally) fulminant. The cardinal pathogenic factor is autoantibody to a component of type IV collagen present in the capillary basement membranes of the lung and kidney.[34]

The genesis of anti-GBM antibodies in sporadic cases is unknown. Iatrogenic cases have occurred when normal kidneys have been transplanted into patients with hereditary Alport's nephropathy (who lack normal Goodpasture antigen and tolerance thereto); thus, recipients mount an anti-GBM antibody response to the new donor Goodpasture antigen. It appears that anti-GBM antibodies are expressed for a limited duration (weeks to months) in sporadic cases of Goodpasture's disease. This is of little consolation because of the devastating nature of the disease during the height of the pulmonary–renal syndrome. Hence,

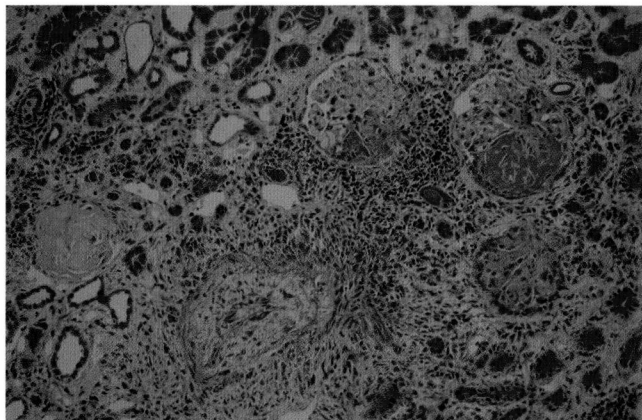

Fig. 67.8 Renal vasculitis showing both glomerular and arteriolar lesions. Small renal vessel shows healing arteritis with proliferation, edema, and fibrosis that severely compromise the lumen. Lesions in the four glomeruli include segmental fibrinoid necrosis (upper right), cellular crescent (lower right) and hyalinized glomerulus (middle left). Tubular atrophy and interstitial fibrosis are prominent. (Masson stain.)
Micrograph courtesy of Dr S. Sabnis, Armed Forces Institute of Pathology; Washington, DC.

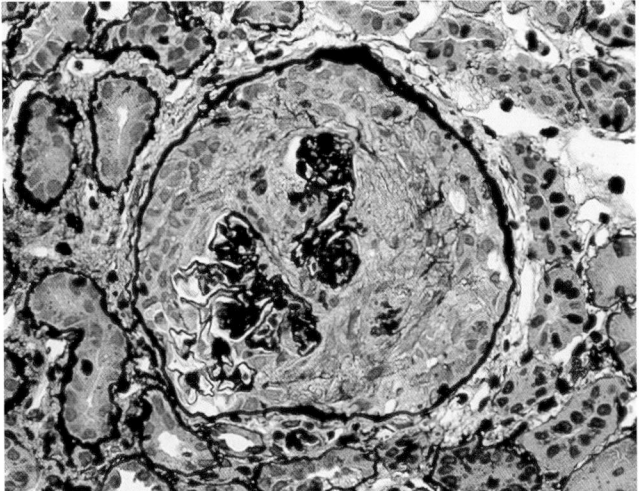

Fig. 67.9 Goodpasture's disease. Circumferential cellular crescent fills Bowman's capsule and compresses the glomerular tuft. (Silver stain.)

aggressive treatments with pulse methylprednisolone, cyclophosphamide and plasma exchange are indicated early in the course of Goodpasture's disease. Reversibility of renal disease is unlikely if renal function is substantially impaired or oliguria ensues before treatment is begun. Immunosuppressive treatment is normally continued until the patient has been in sustained clinical remission and anti-GBM titers are minimal or absent for at least 3 months.

Lupus nephritis (Chapter 50)

● KEY CONCEPTS

Lupus nephritis

- Class II, mesangial: no treatment indicated unless transforms to class III or IV disease
- Class III, focal nephritis and class IV, diffuse nephritis: high-dose prednisone for induction with alternate-day maintenance with adjunctive immunosuppressive therapy options of: (a) pulse cyclophosphamide or (b) mycophenolate mofetil; azathioprine may be used as more cost effective maintenance therapy
- Membranous nephropathy: alternate-day prednisone with bimonthly pulse cyclophosphamide or low-dose daily cyclosporine

Glomerular disease affects the majority of patients with SLE, but lupus nephritis has a wide spectrum of disease expression and outcomes among different patient populations; in particular, lupus nephritis generally exhibits a substantially more ominous prognosis and a poorer response to treatment in black patients than in white patients. Nephritis is a major cause of morbidity and mortality, and accounts for a large portion of all hospital admissions in lupus patients. The majority experience chronic renal disease with remissions and exacerbations. Patients rarely enter permanent remission or achieve complete cure of SLE.

Pathogenesis

Several different mechanisms appear to be involved in the pathogenesis of lupus nephritis, resulting in a wide spectrum of renal lesions. Deposition of immune complexes from the circulation

into the kidney appears to be the initiating event in proliferative lupus nephritis; however, only a subset of immune complexes appears to be nephritogenic. DNA and anti-DNA antibodies are known to be concentrated in glomerular deposits in the subendothelial location and are likely to play a central role in the pathogenesis of proliferative lupus nephritis. Unfortunately, there are fewer insights into the pathogenesis of lupus membranous nephropathy with its characteristic epimembranous immune deposits. Although T cells are almost certainly involved in autoantibody production, it is unknown whether they have a direct role in the pathogenesis of lupus nephritis.

Clinical features

Asymptomatic hematuria or proteinuria may be the presenting features, but they often progress to nephritic and/or nephrotic syndromes. Nephrotic syndrome is seen in both severe proliferative and membranous forms of lupus nephritis. Hypertension, azotemia, nephritic urine sediment (with hematuria and cellular casts), hypocomplementemia and high anti-dsDNA titers are more commonly found in patients with proliferative lupus nephritis. Rapidly progressive glomerulonephritis is usually associated with the appearance of cellular crescents and may be superimposed on severe proliferative or membranous forms of lupus nephritis.

Diagnosis

Proper evaluation of the urinary sediment is very helpful in assessing and monitoring renal disease activity. Active glomerulonephritis is indicated by hematuria (with dysmorphic erythrocytes) as well as cellular casts. Broad and/or waxy casts indicate long-standing or advanced glomerulonephritis. Serum complement levels (especially C3 and C4) have been found to correlate with activity of glomerular disease on renal biopsy. Falling levels of complement components may indicate a flare of lupus nephritis; other tests (including anti-dsDNA antibodies) are less reliable. Therapeutic decisions should not be based on serologic tests alone, because none of these tests have adequate sensitivity or specificity to justify treatment decisions. Renal biopsy is indicated only if the patient has laboratory evidence of urinary abnormalities.

The former World Health Organization (WHO) classification of renal biopsy in lupus nephritis has recently been revised by an international committee (Figs. 67.9–67.12).[35] A summary of the histologic features in each class of lupus nephritis can be found in Table 67.3.

Treatment

Treatment of mesangial lupus nephritis is usually not indicated unless protein excretion exceeds 2 g/day. However, the distinction between early mesangial lesions that are in transition to more ominous classes from those that reflect mild and stable nephropathy is difficult. Patients with focal or diffuse proliferative glomerulonephritis and a relative paucity of activity and/or chronicity features on renal biopsy may benefit from oral glucocorticoids or monthly pulses of intravenous methylprednisolone. A prolonged course of intravenous cyclophosphamide pulses is more efficacious than pulses of methylprednisolone in patients with severe focal or diffuse proliferative nephritis.[36] Plasmapheresis does not offer any significant advantage over

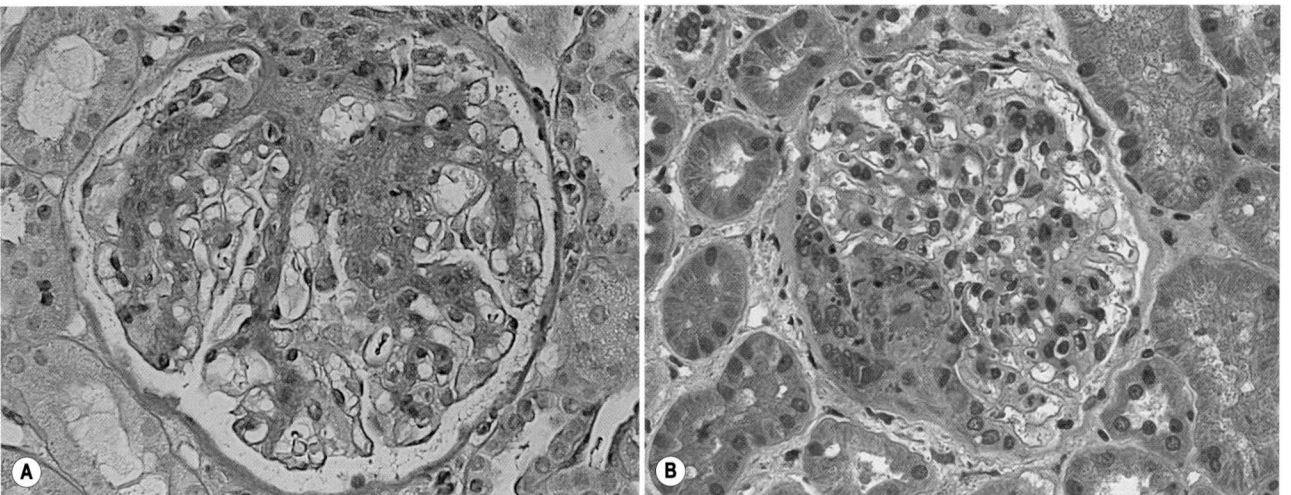

Fig. 67.10 Classes of the pathology of lupus nephritis (1). (A) Class II, mesangial proliferative lupus nephritis. Mesangial areas are expanded by cells and matrix but the peripheral capillary loops remain widely patent. PAS stain. (B) Class III, focal lupus nephritis. Solid lesion at the lower right portion of this glomerulus demonstrates segmental fibrinoid necrosis. Note the nuclear fragments (karyorrhexis) in the fibrinous exudate. (Hematoxylin and eosin stain.)

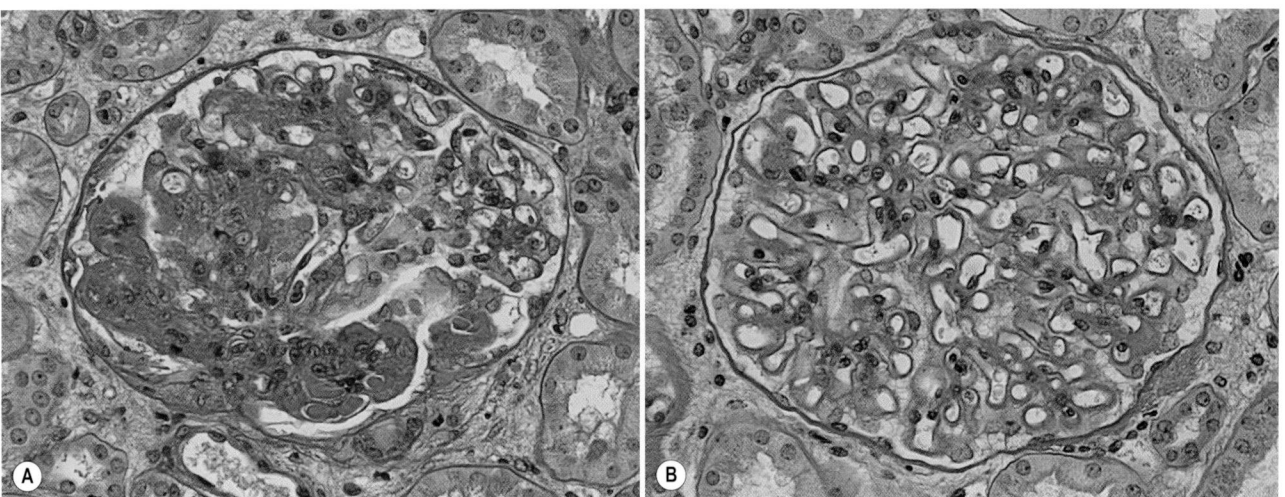

Fig. 67.11 Classes of the pathology of lupus nephritis (2). (A) Class IV, diffuse lupus nephritis. Glomerulus with irregular but nearly global changes including obliteration of many capillary loops due to endocapillary hypercellularity, "wire loop" thickening and hyaline thrombi. (PAS stain.) (B) Class V, membranous lupus nephritis. Glomerulus shows minimally increased mesangial cellularity with thickened but widely patent capillary loops. (PAS stain.)

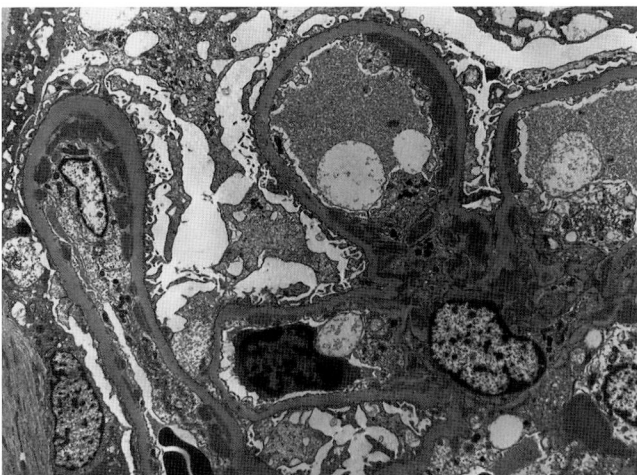

Fig. 67.12 Ultrastructure of proliferative lupus nephritis. Electron micrograph demonstrates the characteristic mesangial deposits (dark materials interspersed within the centrally located amorphous, gray mesangial matrix) and subendothelial deposits (dark materials extending along the peripheral capillary loops).

cytotoxic therapy. Controlled studies have shown that intermittent pulse cyclophosphamide is more efficacious than either high-dose conventional prednisone or extended courses of pulse methylprednisolone.[37,38] In general, treatment should continue for at least 1 year after remission of renal disease to prevent exacerbations. Recent short-term studies have shown that mycophenolate is equivalent to cyclophosphamide for both induction and maintenance therapy in lupus nephritis.[39–41]

Neither pulse cyclophosphamide nor mycophenolate is universally effective in the management of lupus nephritis, hence the search for more efficacious alternative treatment regimens, including rituximab, immunoablation without or with stem cell reconstitution, and immunological co-stimulation inhibitors (e.g., CTLA4-Ig), continues.[42]

No definitive therapeutic guidelines have been established for lupus membranous nephropathy. High-dose alternate-day glucocorticoids, cyclophosphamide, and cyclosporine have been used, with mixed results. Results of a prospective controlled trial indicate that both cyclophosphamide and cyclosporine are more effective than steroids alone in inducing complete remission of proteinuria in lupus membranous nephropathy.[43]

Table 67.3 International Society of Nephrology/Renal Pathology Society 2004 Classification of Lupus Nephritis

Class	Histologic features/comments
I. Minimal mesangial	Normal light microscopy (LM); mesangial deposits by immunofluorescence (IF) and electron microscopy (EM)
II. Mesangial proliferative	Pure mesangial hypercellularity and matrix expansion; *IF* and *EM*: mesangial immune deposits
III. Focal	Glomerular capillary obliteration in < 50% of nephrons owing to proliferation or sclerosis; *LM*: Increased numbers of mesangial, endothelial, and/or hematogenous cells. Active inflammatory lesions (karyorrhexis, fibrinoid necrosis, adhesion to Bowman's capsule, cellular crescents, interstitial inflammatory infiltrates). Wire loop lesions. Hyaline thrombi; *IF* and *EM*: Mesangial and peripheral capillary loop (subendothelial) immune complex deposits
IV. Diffuse	Qualitatively similar histologic lesions as in class III. Glomerular capillary obliteration involving > 50% of nephrons. Subsets defined as primarily global (class IV-G) or primarily segmental (class IV-S) involvement
V. Membranous	*LM*: Regular thickening of the peripheral capillary loops of the glomerulus. Mesangial expansion; *EM*: Subepithelial, intramembranous, mesangial (but no or very rare subendothelial) immune complex deposits
VI. Advanced sclerosis	More than 90% global sclerosis without residual active lesions

Scleroderma (systemic sclerosis) (Chapter 54)

● KEY CONCEPTS

Nephropathies of selected connective tissue diseases

- *Scleroderma renal crisis*: Predominantly renal vasculopathy; severe (high renin) hypertension with progressive renal failure—treated with angiotensin-converting enzyme inhibitors or receptor antagonists
- *Sjögren's syndrome*: Distal renal tubular acidosis with nephrocalcinosis, interstitial nephritis or pseudolymphoma; glomerulonephritis rare
- *Rheumatoid arthritis*: Mild mesangial proliferative glomerulonephritis, membranous nephropathy, or necrotizing renal vasculitis

Renal disease occurs in the diffuse form of systemic sclerosis and is a major cause of morbidity and mortality in these patients.[44] Patients with early (within the first year of disease onset) renal disease may experience rapidly progressive disease and early death. Acute scleroderma renal crisis is particularly ominous. Proteinuria, urine sediment abnormalities (hematuria or pyuria), hypertension and renal insufficiency are clinical markers of renal disease. Renal disease is more common in the first 5 years of the disease, especially if there is rapid progression of skin disease. A significant decrease in renal function, proteinuria in excess of 500 mg/day, or urinary sediment abnormalities should alert the physician. Plasma renin activity increases with the onset of renal injury, but there is no convincing evidence that the rise precedes the onset of scleroderma renal crisis.

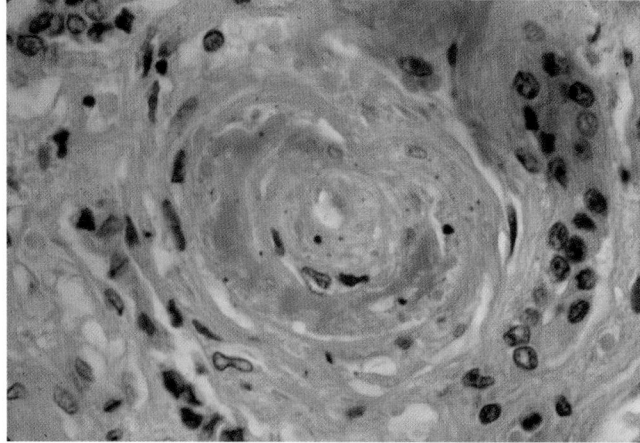

Fig. 67.13 Scleroderma renal crisis. Renal arteriole demonstrates extensive fibrin deposition (dark material) within multiple layers of its wall. The lumen is further compromised by severe swelling and intimal hyperplasia. (Masson trichrome stain.)

Scleroderma renal crisis is characterized by renin-mediated malignant hypertension, rapid deterioration of renal function, and proteinuria (usually nonnephrotic). The primary pathogenic process appears to be a renal vasculopathy involving predominantly the interlobular arteries and arterioles. Marked intimal thickening with an attendant "mucoid" appearance, and fibrinoid necrosis in the absence of vasculitis, are common and characteristic of the disease (Fig. 67.13). Immune deposits are rarely observed by fluorescence or electron microscopy studies.

Although a variety of treatments have been proposed for patients with scleroderma, none has been proved to be consistently efficacious. The most significant therapeutic advance in the treatment of renal involvement is the use of angiotensin antagonists, which have dramatically increased the 1-year survival of patients with scleroderma renal crisis. Despite this initial improvement, approximately half will subsequently progress to death or renal failure. Survival of patients requiring renal replacement therapy for end-stage renal disease due to scleroderma has been poor but generally survival is better with renal transplantation.

Sjögren's syndrome (Chapter 53)

A variety of renal manifestations occur in approximately one-third of patients with primary Sjögren's syndrome, including tubular dysfunction (distal or proximal tubular acidosis, nephrogenic diabetes insipidus), nephrocalcinosis, interstitial nephritis, pseudolymphoma, necrotizing vasculitis and glomerulopathy.[44] Mild, nonspecific glomerular changes are common in patients with Sjögren's syndrome. However, overt primary glomerular disease is rare. Membranous nephropathy and proliferative glomerulonephritis (focal or diffuse, and membranoproliferative) have been reported in primary Sjögren's syndrome. In such cases the possibility of overlap with systemic lupus should be considered.

Rheumatoid arthritis (Chapter 51)

Mild mesangial proliferative glomerulonephritis has been described in patients with rheumatoid arthritis who had renal biopsy because of hematuria and/or proteinuria; mesangial nephropathy is usually mild and follows a relatively benign course. Membranous nephropathy, formerly seen as a complication of gold or D-penicillamine therapies, is rarely seen in patients receiving contemporary therapies for rheumatoid arthritis. Segmental necrotizing glomerulonephritis, often associated with ANCA, can be a component of rheumatoid vasculitis. Secondary amyloidosis (AA amyloid), formerly common in advanced rheumatoid arthritis, has become a rare complication under the salutary effects of contemporary therapies.[44]

RENAL DISEASES IN DYSPROTEINEMIAS AND PARAPROTEINEMIAS (CHAPTER 80)

● KEY CONCEPTS

Renal diseases associated with dysproteinemias and paraproteinemias

- *Multiple myeloma:* Cast nephropathy; distal renal tubular acidosis; AL amyloidosis
- *Light-chain disease:* Light-chain crystalline deposits along basement membranes
- *Amyloidosis:* Glomerular and vascular deposition of characteristic amyloid fibrils
- *Cryoglobulinemia:* Occlusive microvascular and glomerular "thrombi" composed of cryoprecipitable protein

Multiple myeloma

Multiple myeloma results from a neoplastic proliferation of plasma cells that produce one or more abnormal monoclonal proteins (M-proteins). Abnormal bands of light or heavy chains of immunoglobulin are present in the urine of 50–70% of patients with myeloma. These paraproteins have a predilection to precipitate in the tubular lumina to produce the so-called cast nephropathy or myeloma kidney. Acute renal failure (precipitated by dehydration or contrast dyes) and chronic renal failure can result from the cast tubulopathy. Distal renal tubular acidosis is also a common manifestation of myeloma protein deposition in renal tubules. Myeloma paraproteins are not detected by urine protein dipstick methods because dipsticks only detect abnormal levels of urine albumin. Urinary protein electrophoresis and immunofixation electrophoresis are critically important for diagnosis.[45]

Light-chain deposition disease

In this systemic disease, monoclonal immunoglobulin light chains, usually κ type, are commonly deposited in the vessel walls of multiple organs, especially the renal glomeruli.[45] Proteinuria (accompanied by nephrotic syndrome in about 30% of cases), microscopic hematuria, hypertension and progressive renal failure are common. Renal biopsy shows nodular sclerosing glomerulonephritis (Fig. 67.14) similar in light-microscopic appearance to diabetic glomerulosclerosis and amyloidosis. Diagnosis depends on finding monoclonal light chains by immunofluorescence studies of renal biopsy tissue. Treatment with prednisone and alkylating agents may halt or reverse the progression of renal failure. Stem cell transplantation has been successful in advanced cases.

Amyloidosis

The glomerular and renal vasculature is a common locus for deposition of amyloid fibrils in patients with systemic amyloidosis. Both immunoglobulin-associated (primary, AL) and protein

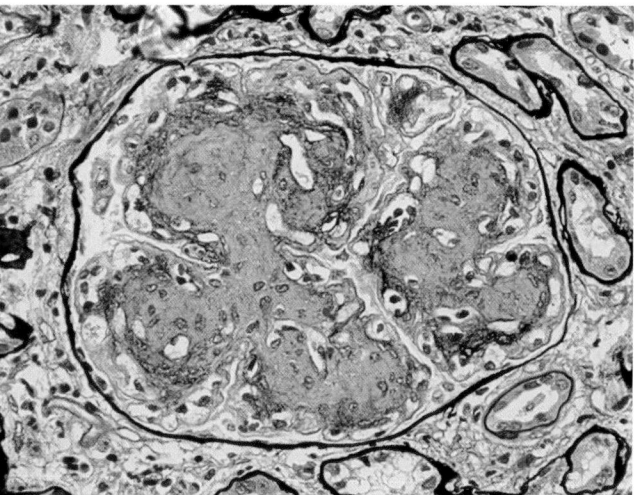

Fig. 67.14 Light-chain nephropathy. Glomerulus has the characteristic appearance of an extrinsic deposition disease. The mesangial areas are filled with pale-staining material that produces a lobular pattern and severely compromises the capillary loops. Immunofluorescence studies are needed to distinguish the light-chain deposits from amyloid infiltration. (Silver stain.)

A-associated (secondary, AA) amyloid have been associated with renal involvement.

Proteinuria (often within the nephrotic range) is the most frequent indicator of renal involvement. Hematuria and hypertension are uncommon. Long-standing amyloidosis is regularly accompanied by autonomic neuropathy and postural hypotension. Glomerular involvement is found in nearly all cases of AA amyloidosis, whereas in AL amyloidosis glomerular disease is present in only half of patients.

Deposition of amyloid protein is recognized by the characteristic staining with metachromatic dyes such as Congo red, which exhibits birefringence on polarized light microscopy. Involvement is typically generalized and diffuse in distribution, and not associated with any significant cellular proliferation or glomerular inflammation (Fig. 67.15A). Immunohistochemical staining can be used to define the type of amyloid deposit (Fig. 67.15B). Amyloid deposits initially involve the mesangium, but with disease progression they extend on to the glomerular capillary surfaces (which become markedly and irregularly thickened); this ultimately results in capillary luminal occlusion, glomerular obliteration, and end-stage renal disease. Amyloid deposits are also found in the intrarenal vasculature, resembling hyaline arteriosclerosis on hematoxylin and eosin-stained sections. Electron microscopic findings of fibrillar material of characteristic morphology confirm the diagnosis.

Treatment of primary AL amyloidosis with cytotoxic agents has generally not resulted in a favorable long-term outcome. However, there are some recent very encouraging reports of salutary effects of aggressive cytotoxic drug therapy followed by stem cell reconstitution.[46–49] For patients with secondary amyloidosis control of the underlying diseases may prevent, stabilize or even reverse this process.[41] Colchicine and anti-tumor necrosis factor therapies can prevent deposition of amyloid if started early in familial Mediterranean fever.

Cryoglobulinemia

Cryoglobulins (immunoglobulins which reversibly precipitate on cooling) are present in the serum of patients with a wide variety of autoimmune, lymphoproliferative and infectious

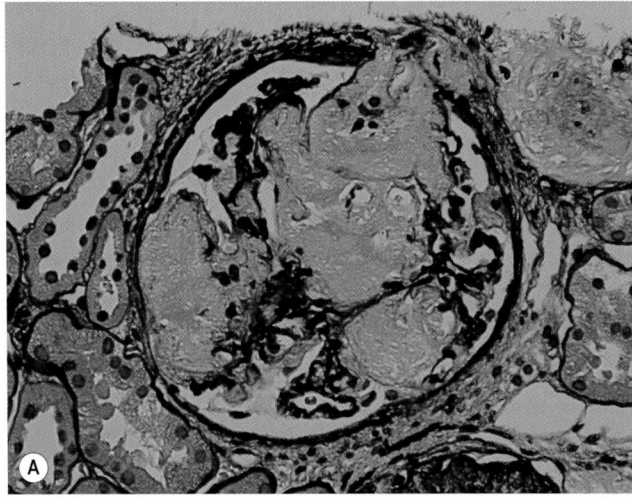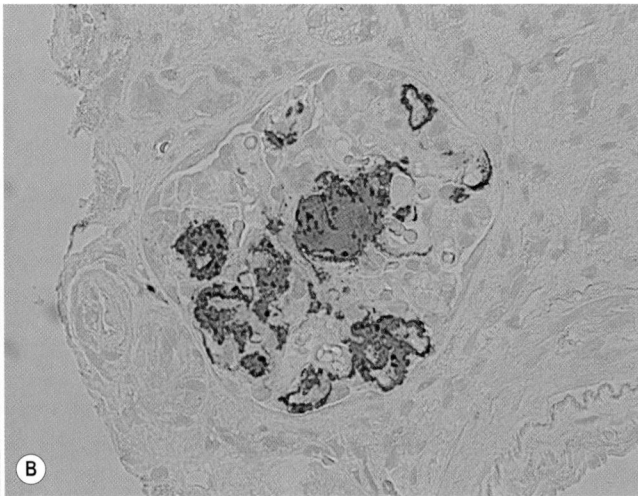

Fig. 67.15 Amyloidosis of the kidney. (A) Glomerulus contains nodules of pale-staining amorphous material distorting and compromising the capillary loops. (Silver stain.) (B) Immunohistochemistry of glomerular amyloid deposits demonstrated by peroxidase-labeled antibody specific for AA proteins. (Immunoperoxidase technique.)

diseases. Cryoglobulinemia with MPGN is commonly associated with chronic hepatitis C.[50] Essential mixed cryoglobulinemia (ECM) refers to an idiopathic clinical syndrome consisting of recurrent episodes of palpable purpura involving the lower extremities, constitutional symptoms, arthralgias, vasculitis, hepatosplenomegaly, lymphadenopathy, and neuropathy.

Renal complications are common with mixed cryoglobulinemia. A waxing and waning course is characteristic of this disease. Glomerular involvement may develop acutely, particularly after dehydration or exposure to cold, and may be associated with oliguric acute renal failure. Other clinical syndromes can also occur, including nephrotic syndrome, hematuria, renal insufficiency, and chronic or rapidly progressive glomerulonephritis. Deposition of cryoglobulins usually occurs in the glomerular subendothelial space, and these deposits exhibit a unique fibrillar appearance on electron microscopy (Fig. 67.16). The glomerulonephritis is typically membranoproliferative and/or crescentic

in nature. Large eosinophilic, PAS-positive intraluminal deposits ("thrombi") are found in more than one-third of patients.

Treatments with combinations of glucocorticoids, cytotoxic drugs, rituximab and plasma exchange have been successful in controlling cryoglobulinemic nephritis. IFN-α has been shown in small, nonrandomized studies to be efficacious even in patients refractory to conventional therapy.

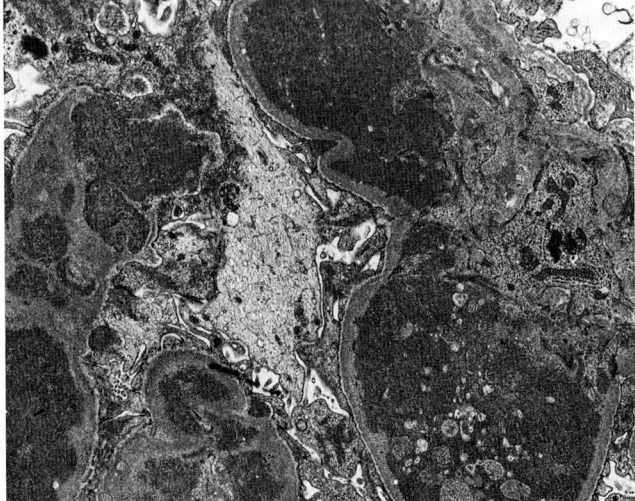

Fig. 67.16 Cryoglobulinemic nephropathy. Electron micrograph demonstrates dense material completely filling the glomerular capillary lumina. On light microscopy these capillary "plugs" have the appearance of microvascular thrombi, but ultrastructural studies show the crystalline structure of immune aggregates, not fibrin tactoids.
Electron micrographs courtesy of Dr S. Sabnis, Armed Forces Institute of Pathology; Washington, DC.

References

1. Segelmark M, Hellmark T. Autoimmune kidney diseases. Autoimmun Rev 2010;9:A366–71.
2. Nangaku M, Couser WG. Mechanisms of immune-deposit formation and the mediation of immune renal injury. Clin Exp Nephrol 2005;9:183–91.
3. Pickering M, Cook HT. Complement and glomerular disease: new insights. Curr Opin Nephrol Hypertens 2011;20:271–7.
4. Greenberg A, Chung AK, editors. Primer on kidney diseases. 5th ed. London: Elsevier-Saunders; 2009.
5. Rosner MH, Bolton WK. Renal function testing. Am J Kidney Dis 2006;47:174–83.
6. Davids MS, Murali MR, Kuter DJ. Serum free light chain analysis. Am J Hematol 2010;10:787–90.
7. Churg J, Bernstein J, Glassock RJ. Renal disease: classification and atlas of glomerular diseases. 2nd ed. New York: Igaku-Shoin; 1995.
8. Fogo AB, Kashgarian M. Diagnostic Atlas of Renal Pathology. 2nd ed. London: Elsevier; 2012.
9. Waldman M, Crew RJ, Valeri A, et al. Adult minimal change disease: clinical characteristics, treatment and outcomes. Clin J Am Soc Nephrol 2007;2:445–53.
10. Kistler AD, Peev V, Forst AL, et al. Enzymatic disease of the podocytes. Pediatr Nephrol 2010;25:1017–23.
11. Kopp JB, Nelson GW, Sampath K, et al. APOL1 genetic variants in focal segmental glomerulosclerosis and HIV-associated nephropathy. J Am Soc Nephrol 2011;22:2129–37.
12. Thomas DB, Franceschini N, Hogan SL, et al. Clinical and pathologic characteristics of focal segmental glomerulosclerosis pathologic variants. Kidney Int 2006;69:920–6.
13. McCarthy ET, Sharma M, Savin VJ. Circulating permeability factors in idiopathic nephrotic syndrome and focal segmental glomerulosclerosis. Clin J Am Soc Nephrol 2010;5:2115–21.
14. Beck LH, Salant D. Membranous nephropathy. Kidney Int 2010;77:765–70.
15. Ronco P, Debiec H. Membranous glomerulopathy: the evolving story. Curr Opin Nephrol Hypertens 2010;19:254–9.
16. Waldman M, Austin III HA. Controversies in the treatment of idiopathic membranous nephropathy. Nat Rev Nephrol 2009;5:469–79.
17. Walport MJ. Complement. N Engl J Med 2001;344:1058–66.
18. Fakhouri F, Fremeaux-Bacchi V, Noel LH, et al. C3 glomerulopathy: a new classification. Nat Rev Nephrol 2010;6:494–9.
19. Appel GB, Cook HT, Hageman G, et al. Membranoproliferative glomerulonephritis type II (dense deposit disease): an update. J Am Soc Nephrol 2005;16:1392–403.
20. Ponticelli C, Glassock RJ. Post-transplant recurrence of primary glomerulonephritis. Clin J Am Soc Nephrol 2010;5:2363–72.
21. Yi Z, Jie YW, Nan Z. The efficacy of anti-viral therapy on hepatitis B virus-associated glomerulonephritis: a systematic review and meta-analysis. Ann Hepatol 2011;10:165–73.
22. Rosen HR. Chronic hepatitis C. New Engl J Med 2011;364:2429–38.
23. Phair J, Palella F. Renal disease in HIV-infected individuals. Curr Opin HIV AIDS 2011;6:285–9.

24. Montseny JJ, Meyrier A, Kleinknecht D, et al. The current spectrum of infectious glomerulonephritis: experience with 76 patients and review of the literature. Medicine (Baltimore) 1995;74:63–73.
25. Glassock RJ. The pathogenesis of IgA nephropathy. Curr Opin Nephrol Hypertens 2011;20:153–60.
26. Davin JC, Ten Berge IJ, Weening JJ. What is the difference between IgA nephropathy and Henoch–Schönlein purpura nephritis? Kidney Int 2001;59:823–34.
27. Appel GB, Waldman M. The IgA nephropathy treatment dilemma. Kidney Int 2006;69: 1939–44.
28. Locatelli F, Del Vecchio L, Pozzi C. IgA glomerulonephritis: beyond angiotensin-converting enzyme inhibitors. Nat Clin Pract Nephrol 2005;2:24–31.
29. Coppo R, Andrulli S, Amore A, et al. Predictors of outcome in Henoch–Schönlein nephritis in children and adults. Am J Kidney Dis 2006;47:993–1003.
30. Jennette JC. Nomenclature and classification of vasculitis: lessons learned from granulomatosis with polyangiitis (Wegener's granulomatosis). Clin Exp Immunol 2011;164(Suppl. 1):7–10.
31. Wilde B, van Paassen P, Wiltzke O, Cohen-Tervaert JW. New pathophysiological insights and treatment of ANCA-associate vasculitis. Kidney Int 2011;79:599–612.
32. Rhee EP, Laliberte KA, Niles JL. Rituximab as maintenance therapy for antineutrophil cytoplasmic antibody-associated vasculitis. Clin J Am Soc Nephrol 2010;5:1394–400.
33. Bolton WK. Goodpasture's syndrome. Kidney Int 1996;50:1753–61.
34. Pedchenko V, Vanacore R, Hudson B. Goodpasture's disease: molecular architecture of the autoantigen provides clues to etiology and pathogenesis. Cur Opin Nephrol Hypertens 2011;20:290–5.
35. Weening JJ, D'Agati VD, Schwartz MM, et al. The classification of glomerulonephritis in systemic lupus erythematosus revisited. J Am Soc Nephrol 2004;15:241–50.
36. Austin HA, Klippel JH, Balow JE, et al. Therapy of lupus nephritis: controlled trial of prednisone and cytotoxic drugs. N Engl J Med 1986;314:614–19.
37. Boumpas DT, Austin HA, Vaughan EM, et al. Controlled trial of pulse methylprednisolone versus two regimens of pulse cyclophosphamide in severe lupus nephritis. Lancet 1992;340:741–55.
38. Illei GG, Austin HA, Crane M, et al. Combination therapy with pulse cyclophosphamide plus pulse methylprednisolone improves long-term renal outcome without adding toxicity in lupus nephritis. Ann Intern Med 2001;135:248–57.
39. Contreras G, Pardo V, Lecleercq B, et al. Sequential therapies for proliferative lupus nephritis. N Engl J Med 2004;350:971–80.
40. Ginzler EM, Dooley MA, Aranow C, et al. Mycophenolate mofetil or intravenous cyclophosphamide for lupus nephritis. N Engl J Med 2005;353:2219–28.
41. Chan TM, Tse KC, Tang CS, et al. Long-term study of mycophenolate mofetil as continuous induction and maintenance treatment for diffuse proliferative lupus nephritis. J Am Soc Nephrol 2005;16:1076–84.
42. Bomback AS, Appel GB. Updates on the treatment of lupus nephritis. J Am Soc Nephrol 2010;21:2028–35.
43. Austin 3rd HA, Illei GG, Braun MJ, Balow JE. Randomized, controlled trial of prednisone, cyclophosphamide, and cyclosporine in lupus membranous nephropathy. J Am Soc Nephrol 2009;20:901–11.
44. Waldman M, Balow JE, Austin 3rd HA. Systemic sclerosis, rheumatoid arthritis, Sjögren syndrome and polymyositis/dermatomyositis. In: Schrier RW, editor. Diseases of the kidney and urinary tract. 9th ed. Philadelphia: Lippincott Williams & Wilkins; in press.
45. Ronco P, Plaisier E, Aucouturier P. Ig-related renal disease in lymphoplasmacytic disorders: an update. Semin Nephrol 2010;30:557–69.
46. Dember LM. Modern treatment of amyloidosis: unresolved questions. J Am Soc Nephrol 2009;20:469–74.
47. Gertz A, Leung N, Lacy MQ, et al. Myeloablative chemotherapy and stem cell transplantation in myeloma or primary amyloidosis with renal involvement. Kidney Int 2005;68:1464–71.
48. Gillmore JD, Hawkins PN. Drug insight: emerging therapies for amyloidosis. Nature Clin Pract 2006;2:263–70.
49. Merlini G, Seldin DC, Gertz MA. Amyloidosis: pathogenesis and new therapeutic options. J Clin Oncol 2011;29:1921–33.
50. Alpers CE, Smith KD. Cryoglobulinemia and renal disease. Curr Opin Nephrol Hypertens 2008;17:243–9.

Prediman K. Shah

Inflammation and atherothrombosis

Arterial occlusive disorders include atherosclerosis of native arteries, accelerated atherosclerosis involving vein grafts and arteries of transplanted organs, and restenosis following angioplasty and stenting. Atherosclerotic vascular disease is a leading cause of death and disability throughout the United States and other industrialized nations and consumes enormous fiscal resources. An improved understanding of the pathophysiology of atherosclerosis and thrombosis is likely to lead to improved prevention, diagnosis, and treatment of this common disorder.

Atherosclerosis involves the development of a plaque composed of variable amounts of lipoproteins, extracellular matrix (collagen, proteoglycans, glycosaminoglycans), calcium, vascular smooth muscle cells, inflammatory cells (chiefly monocyte-derived macrophages, T lymphocytes, mast cells, dendritic cells), and new blood vessels (angiogenesis). A body of evidence now suggests that atherosclerosis represents a chronic inflammatory response to vascular injury caused by a variety of agents that activate or injure endothelium and promote lipoprotein infiltration, retention, and modification, combined with leukocyte entry, retention, proliferation, and activation.[1] One of the key early steps in atherogenesis appears to be the trapping of atherogenic lipoproteins within the subendothelial vascular matrix due to interaction with proteoglycans that is initially mediated through a charge-based interaction and later through enzymatic modification induced by macrophage-derived phospholipases.[2] Over-expression of human low-density lipoprotein (LDL) containing apo B100 protein variants with reduced proteoglycan binding significantly reduces murine atherosclerosis despite severe hyperlipidemia, suggesting the potential importance of LDL retention in atherogensis (the so-called response-to-retention hypothesis).[2] The interaction between apo B100 on atherogenic lipoproteins with proteoglycans in subendothelial matrix are charge-based in the beginning but further accentuated and sustained through secretion of lipoprotein lipase and sphingomyelinases produced locally by macrophages in the lesion.[3]

● KEY CONCEPTS

Pathophysiology

- Atherosclerosis is a chronic immuno-inflammatory disease.
- Immune activation and inflammation are involved in initiation, progression, and destabilization of atherosclerosis.
- Most lethal consequences of atherosclerosis result from thrombosis superimposed on a ruptured or eroded atherosclerotic plaque.
- Plaque composition rather than the luminal stenosis severity is the major determinant of vulnerability to plaque rupture.
- Plaques that rupture are generally large with a large acellular lipid-core, intimal and adventitial inflammation, enhanced plaque neovascularity, hemorrhage and outward adventitial remodeling.

Shear stress and endothelial inflammatory gene activation at sites of predilection

The sites of predilection for atherosclerosis are characterized by low and oscillatory shear stress, evidence of endothelial activation with expression of pro-inflammatory genes such as leukocyte adhesion molecules, and increased influx and/or prolonged retention of lipoproteins (Table 68.1; Fig. 68.1).[4] Specific arterial sites, such as branches, bifurcations, and curvatures, cause characteristic alterations in the flow of blood, including decreased shear stress and increased turbulence. Changes in flow alter the expression of genes that have elements in their promoter regions that respond to shear stress. For example, the genes for intracellular adhesion molecule 1, platelet-derived growth factor B chain, and tissue factor have these elements, and their expression is increased by reduced shear stress.[5-7] Recent studies have suggested that athero-promoting flow patterns activate inflammatory and prothrombotic endothelial phenotype by inhibiting a key flow-sensitive transcription factor KLF2 (Kruppel like factor 2),[8] perhaps accounting for the lipid-rich inflamed phenotype of such plaques in animal models.[9] In fact, there is evidence of pro-inflammatory priming of atherosclerosis-prone vascular sites in mice long before hyperlipidemia or atherosclerosis is induced.[10] Rolling and adherence of inflammatory cells (monocytes and T cells) occur at these sites as a result of the upregulation of adhesion molecules on both the endothelium and the leukocytes. At these sites, specific molecules form on the endothelium that are responsible for the adherence, migration, and accumulation of monocytes and T cells. Such adhesion molecules, which act as receptors for glycoconjugates and integrins present on monocytes and T cells, include several selectins, intercellular adhesion molecules, and vascular-cell adhesion molecules.[5-7] Molecules associated with the migration of leukocytes across the endothelium, such as platelet-endothelial-cell adhesion molecules, act in conjunction with chemoattractant molecules generated by the endothelium, smooth muscle, and monocytes—such as monocyte chemotactic protein-1 (MCP-1), osteopontin, and modified LDL—to attract monocytes and T cells into the artery.[4-7] Chemokines may be involved in the chemotaxis and accumulation of macrophages in fatty streaks.[11] Activation of monocytes and T cells leads to upregulation of receptors on their surfaces, such as the mucin-like molecules that bind selectins, integrins that bind adhesion molecules of the immunoglobulin superfamily, and receptors that bind chemoattractant molecules. These ligand–receptor interactions further activate mononuclear cells, induce cell proliferation, and help define and localize the inflammatory response at the site of lesions.

Table 68.1 Key steps in atherogenesis highlighting role of inflammation at various steps

1. Endothelial activation with increased infiltration of atherogenic lipoproteins at sites of low or oscillating shear stress (branch points and flow dividers).
2. Subendothelial retention and modification of atherogenic lipoproteins (low-density lipoprotein/very-low-density lipoprotein).
3. Endothelial activation with increased mononuclear leukocyte (inflammatory cell) adhesion, chemotaxis, and subendothelial recruitment.
4. Subendothelial inflammatory cell activation with lipid ingestion through monocyte scavenger receptor expression resulting in foam cell formation.
5. Intimal migration and proliferation of medial/adventitial smooth-muscle cells/myofibroblasts in response to growth factors released by activated monocytes with matrix production and formation of fibrous cap and fibrous plaque.
6. Abluminal plaque growth with positive (outward) arterial adventitial remodeling preserving lumen size in early stages; later, plaque growth or negative remodeling results in luminal narrowing.
7. Neoangiogenesis due to angiogenic stimuli produced by inflammatory cells (macrophages) and other arterial wall cells (vascular endothelial growth factor, interleukin-8).
8. Death of foam cells by necrosis/apoptosis leading to necrotic lipid core formation.
9. Plaque disruption (rupture of fibrous cap or endothelial erosion) due to inflammatory cell-mediated matrix degradation and death of matrix-synthesizing smooth-muscle cells.
10. Exposure of thrombogenic substrate (lipid core-containing tissue factor derived from inflammatory cells) following plaque disruption with arterial thrombosis.

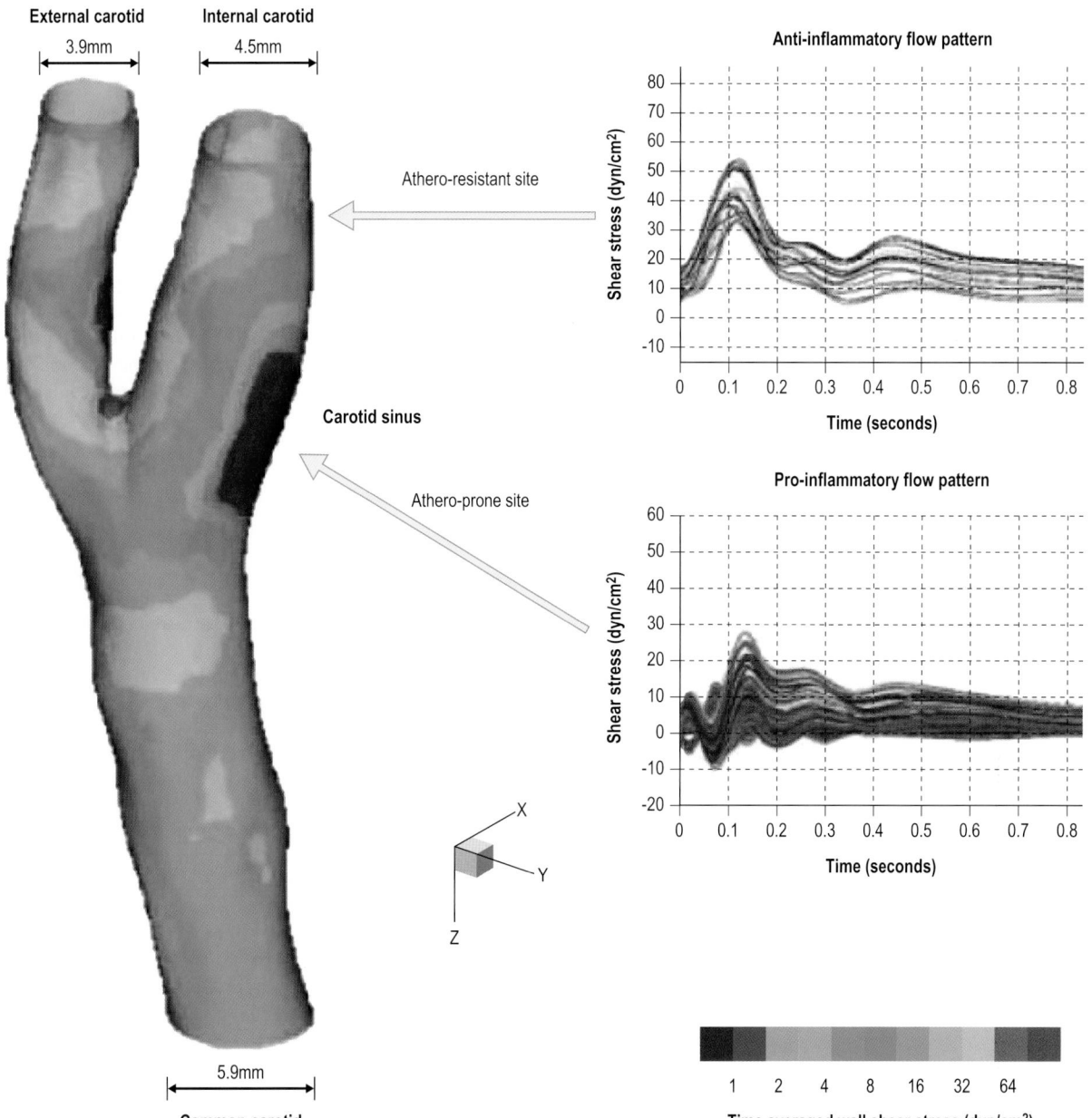

Fig. 68.1 Different shear stress patterns resulting from different flow patterns in the athero-prone segment versus athero-resistant segment of a human carotid artery, as measured by ultrasound technique. Note that the low shear stress flow pattern in athero-prone segments is able to induce inflammatory genes in endothelial cells in culture; this may contribute to propensity for lesion localization at athero-prone sites.

(Adapted from: Dai G, Kaazempur-Mofrad MR, Natarajan S, et al. Distinct endothelial phenotypes evoked by arterial waveforms derived from atherosclerosis-susceptible and -resistant regions of human vasculature. Proc Natl Acad Sci USA 2004; 101(41): 14871-14876.)

In genetically modified mice that are deficient in apolipoprotein E (and have hypercholesterolemia), intercellular adhesion molecule-1 (ICAM-1) is constitutively increased at lesion-prone sites long before the lesions develop.[6] In contrast, vascular cell adhesion molecule 1 (VCAM-1) is absent in normal mice but is present at the same sites as ICAM-1 in mice with apolipoprotein E deficiency.[6] Mice that are completely deficient in ICAM-1, P-selectin, CD18, or combinations of these molecules, have reduced atherosclerosis in response to lipid feeding. Proteolytic enzymes may cleave adhesion molecules such that in situations of chronic inflammation, it may be possible to measure the "shed" molecules in plasma as markers of a sustained inflammatory response to help identify patients at risk for atherosclerosis or other inflammatory diseases.[12]

Key role of endothelial activation/dysfunction and inflammation in atherogenesis

Several studies have suggested that one of the earliest steps in atherogenesis is endothelial activation or injury/dysfunction with infiltration and retention and modification of atherogenic lipoproteins (predominantly the apo B containing lipoproteins) in the subendothelial space of the vessel wall (Table 68.2).[13–15]

Various factors contribute to endothelial activation or the development of endothelial injury/dysfunction predisposing to atherosclerosis, including risk factors such as elevated and modified atherogenic lipoproteins (apo B100 containing lipoproteins) such as LDL/VLDL/IDL cholesterol; reduced HDL cholesterol; oxidant stress caused by cigarette smoking, hypertension, and diabetic mellitus; genetic alterations; elevated plasma homocysteine concentrations; infectious microorganisms such as herpes viruses or *Chlamydia pneumoniae*; estrogen deficiency; and

Table 68.2 Endothelial activation/dysfunction in atherosclerosis

Phenotypic features
Reduced vasodilator and increased vasoconstrictor capacity
Enhanced oxidant stress with increased inactivation of nitric oxide
Increased expression of endothelin
Enhanced leukocyte (inflammatory cell) adhesion and recruitment
Increased adhesion molecule expression (ICAM, VCAM)
Increased chemotactic molecule expression (MCP-1, IL-8)
Increased prothrombotic and reduced fibrinolytic phenotype
Increased growth-promoting phenotype

Factors contributing to endothelial activation/dysfunction
Dyslipidemia and atherogenic lipoprotein modification
Elevated LDL, VLDL, LP(a)
LDL modification (oxidation, glycation)
Reduced HDL
Increased angiotensin II and hypertension
Insulin resistance and diabetes
Estrogen deficiency
Smoking
Hyperhomocysteinemia
Advancing age
Infection?

HDL, high-density lipoprotein; ICAM, intercellular adhesion molecules; IL-8, interleukin-8; LDL, low-density lipoprotein; LP, lipoprotein; MCP-1, monocyte chemotactic protein-1; VCAM, vascular adhesion molecules; VLDL, very-low-density lipoprotein.

advancing age.[15] Endothelial activation and injury/dysfunction can manifest as:

(a) Increased adhesiveness of the endothelium to inflammatory cells (leukocytes) or platelets;
(b) Increased vascular permeability;
(c) Change from an anticoagulant to a procoagulant phenotype;
(d) Change from a vasodilator to a vasoconstrictor phenotype; or
(e) Change from a growth-inhibiting to a growth-promoting phenotype through elaboration of cytokines.

Abnormal vasomotor function has been one of the most well-studied manifestations of endothelial dysfunction in subjects either with established atherosclerosis or with risk factors for atherosclerosis. Normal healthy endothelium produces nitric oxide from arginine through the action of a family of enzymes known as nitric oxide synthases.[15] Nitric oxide acts as a local vasodilator by increasing smooth muscle cell cyclic guanosine monophosphate (GMP) levels while at the same time inhibiting platelet aggregation and smooth muscle cell proliferation.[15] In the presence of risk factors, a reduced vasodilator response to endothelium-dependent vasodilator stimuli or even paradoxical vasoconstrictor response to such stimuli has been observed in large vessels as well as in the microcirculation, even in the absence of structural abnormalities in the vessel wall.[15] These abnormal vasomotor responses have been attributed to reduced bioavailability of endothelium-derived relaxing factor(s), specifically nitric oxide, due to rapid inactivation of nitric oxide by oxidant stress or excess generation of asymmetric dimethylarginine and/or increased production of vasoconstrictors such as endothelin.[15]

One of the major contributors to endothelial injury is LDL cholesterol modified by processes such as oxidation, glycation (in diabetes), aggregation, association with proteoglycans, or incorporation into immune complexes.[15,16] Oxidized LDL has been shown to be present in the atherosclerotic lesions of both experimental animals and humans.[17] Subendothelial retention of LDL particles results in progressive oxidation and its subsequent internalization by macrophages through the scavenger receptors. The internalization leads to the formation of lipid peroxides and facilitates the accumulation of cholesterol esters, even finally resulting in the formation of foam cells. Once modified and taken up by macrophages, LDL activates the foam cells. In addition to its ability to injure these cells, modified LDL is chemotactic for other monocytes and can upregulate the expression of genes for macrophage colony-stimulating factor (M-CSF) and monocyte chemotactic protein derived from endothelial cells.[18] Thus, it may help expand the inflammatory response by stimulating the replication of monocyte-derived macrophages and the entry of new monocytes into lesions. Continued inflammatory response stimulates migration and proliferation of smooth muscle cells that accumulate within the areas of inflammation to form an intermediate fibroproliferative lesion resulting in thickening of the artery wall.

The inflammatory and immune response in atherosclerosis consists of accumulation of monocyte-derived macrophages and specific subtypes of T lymphocytes at every stage of the disease.[19,20] The fatty streak, the earliest type lesion, common in infants and young children, consists of monocyte-derived macrophages, macrophage-derived foam cells, and T lymphocytes. The critical role of the macrophage in atherogenesis is supported by the virtual absence (or drastic reduction) of atherosclerosis when M-CSF null genotype is introduced in murine models of severe dyslipidemia induced by diet or genetic manipulation.[21]

Continued inflammation results in increased numbers of macrophages and lymphocytes, which both emigrate from the blood and multiply within the lesion. Activation of these cells leads to the release of proteolytic enzymes, cytokines, chemokines, and growth factors that can induce further damage and eventually lead to focal necrosis. Necrosis and/or apoptosis of foam cells results in the formation of the necrotic lipid core in the plaque. Thus, cycles of accumulation of mononuclear cells, migration and proliferation of smooth muscle cells, and formation of fibrous tissue lead to further enlargement and restructuring of the lesion, so that it becomes covered by a fibrous cap that overlies a core of lipid and necrotic tissue, resulting in the formation of an advanced and complicated atherosclerotic plaque.

The inflammatory response itself can influence lipoprotein transfer within the vessel wall. Pro-inflammatory cytokines, such as tumor necrosis factor-α (TNF-α), interleukin-1 (IL-1), and M-CSF increase binding of LDL to endothelium and smooth muscle and increase the transcription of the LDL-receptor gene.[1] After binding to scavenger receptors *in vitro*, modified LDL initiates a series of intracellular events that include the induction of proteases and inflammatory cytokines.[1] Thus, a vicious circle of inflammation, modification of lipoproteins, and further inflammation can be maintained in the artery by the presence of these modified lipoproteins.

Monocyte-derived macrophages are present in various stages of atherosclerosis and act as scavenging and antigen-presenting cells. They produce cytokines, chemokines, growth-regulating molecules, tissue factor, metalloproteinases, and other hydrolytic enzymes. The continuing entry, survival, and replication of monocytes/macrophages in lesions depend in part on growth factors, such as M-CSF and granulocyte-macrophage colony-stimulating factor (GM-CSF), whereas IL-2 is involved in a similar manner for T lymphocytes. Recent experimental observations suggest that in and out trafficking of macrophages within the atherosclerotic vascular wall may be regulated by the microenvironment within the lesion with ingress and retention being promoted by a pro-inflammatory milieu related to oxidized lipids. Whereas egress via the lumen or via transformation into migratory dendritic cells and subsequent immigration to regional lymph nodes is associated with reduced pro-inflammatory lipids in the lesion, an environment promoted by high levels of high-density lipoprotein (HDL) favoring lesion regression.[22] Dendritic cells have been identified within the subendothelium and the adventitia of normal blood vessels. An increase in the number and activity of subendothelial dendritic cells has been observed in the atherosclerotic lesion, raising the possibility that dendritic cells may be involved in the pathophysiology of atherosclerosis.[23]

Activated macrophages as well as lesional smooth muscle cells express class II histocompatibility antigens such as HLA-DR that allow them to present antigens to T lymphocytes.[1,19,20] Atherosclerotic lesions contain both CD4 and CD8 T cells, implicating the immune system in atherogenesis.[19,20] T-cell activation, following antigen processing, results in production of various cytokines, such as interferon-γ (INF-γ) and TNF-α and -β, which can further enhance the inflammatory response.[1] Antigens presented include oxidized LDL and heat shock protein 60 that may participate in the immune response in atherosclerosis.[4,19,20]

Macrophages, T cells, endothelial and smooth muscle cells in the atherosclerotic lesions express CD40 ligand and its receptor, which may play a role in atherogenesis by regulating the function of inflammatory cells.[24] The anti-atherogenic effects of CD40 blocking antibodies in the murine model of atherosclerosis suggest that CD40-mediated signaling may play an important role in atherogenesis.[25]

Monocyte–macrophage heterogeneity

A number of recent studies have shown that there exists a considerable degree of monocyte–macrophage heterogeneity when various macrophage markers are used to identify macrophage subsets.[26] An over-simplified generalization of this concept recognizes M1 macrophages (classically activated) that have largely pro-inflammatory effects as compared to M2 macrophages (alternatively activated) that are more likely to be involved in healing and possibly inflammation resolution.[26] The mechanisms for macrophage polarization into various subsets and the pathophysiologic significance of the monocyte–macrophage heterogeneity remains to be determined, although recent experimental studies suggest that apolipoprotein A-1 therapy modulates the circulating or lesional monocyte macrophages into a dominantly M2 phenotype.[27,28]

Macrophage efferocytosis

Macrophages in atherosclerosis undergo apoptosis at various stages of evolution of the atherosclerotic lesion and the apoptotic macrophages are rapidly cleared by another subset of macrophages using various receptors such as MERTEK in a process called efferocytosis, thereby preventing post-apoptotic necrosis and consequent activation of inflammatory pathways.[29,30] Early in the course of lesion formation, efferocytosis is efficient preventing necrotic debris accumulation; however, in advanced lesions, there is evidence that efferocytosis is impaired, contributing to necrotic debris accumulation and further activation of the inflammatory cascade. In fact, deletion of the MERTEK receptor gene has been shown to expand the necrotic lipid-rich core in animal models of atherosclerosis.[29,30] Similarly partial deletion of the *Npc1* gene, which is involved in free cholesterol-induced macrophage apoptosis, is associated with more lesion cellularity and less necrotic core formation in animal models.[31] These data suggest that certain macrophage subsets may actually play a favorable role in atherosclerosis by participating in efferocytosis.[29]

Cholesterol crystals and NLRP Inflammasome mediated inflammation in atherosclerosis

It has recently been demonstrated that cholesterol crystals, commonly observed in experimental as well as human atherosclerotic lesions, may play an important role in plaque inflammation.[32,33] Following macrophage activation by a first signal, such as might be delivered by oxidized LDL and Toll-like receptor-mediated signaling, cholesterol crystal uptake induces a pro-inflammatory cytokine activation leading to secretion of active IL-1β, which plays a pro-atherogenic role.[32,33] The activation of inflammatory cytokine secretion by ingested cholesterol crystals has been shown to involve the NLRP3 inflammasome complex, analogous to urate crystal-induced inflammatory responses.[32,33]

Platelet adhesion and mural thrombosis are ubiquitous in the initiation and generation of the lesions of atherosclerosis in animals and humans.[1] Platelets can adhere to dysfunctional endothelium, exposed collagen, and macrophages. When activated, platelets release their granules, which contain cytokines and growth factors that, together with thrombin, can contribute to the migration and proliferation of smooth muscle cells and monocytes. Activation of platelets leads to the formation of free arachidonic acid, which can be transformed into prostaglandins such as thromboxane A2, one of the most potent vasoconstricting and platelet-aggregating substances known, or into leukotrienes, which can amplify the inflammatory response.

Angiotensin II, a potent vasoconstrictor, may also contribute to atherogenesis by stimulating the growth of smooth muscle, increasing oxidant stress, inducing LDL oxidation, and promoting an inflammatory response.[1,25,34]

Elevated plasma homocysteine concentrations, resulting from enzymatic defects or vitamin deficiency, can facilitate atherothrombosis by inducing endothelial dysfunction with reduction in vasodilator capacity and enhanced prothrombotic phenotype and smooth muscle replication.[35,36] Hyperhomocysteinemia is associated with an increased risk of atherosclerosis of the coronary, peripheral, and cerebral arteries.[35,36] However, it should be noted that clinical trials testing the effects of reduction of plasma homocysteine levels by vitamins such as folic acid, B6, and B12, have been negative and largely disappointing.[37]

Potential role of infection, oral and gut microflora, in atherosclerosis

It is likely that a number of stimuli are responsible for provoking and sustaining a chronic inflammatory response in the vessel wall in atherosclerosis. Among the key potential culprits are modified lipoproteins, cholesterol crystals, and infectious agents. Oxidatively modified lipoproteins can induce a variety of pro-inflammatory genes in the vessel wall that are responsible for recruiting and activating inflammatory cells such as ICAM- and VCAM-type adhesion molecules, chemotactic cytokines such as MCP-1, IL-8, and colony-stimulating factors such as M-CSF. In addition to modified lipoproteins, there is now a body of evidence suggesting that arterial wall infections with organisms such as *Chlamydia pneumoniae*, CMV/herpes virus, as well as remote infections such as chronic bronchitis, gingivitis, and *Helicobacter pylori* infection can affect inflammation, thereby contributing to atherogenesis and/or plaque disruption and thrombosis in the presence of pre-existing atherosclerosis (Table 68.3).[38–44] Increased titers of antibodies to these organisms

have been used as a predictor of further adverse events in patients who have had a myocardial infarction. Organisms, particularly *C. pneumoniae*, have been identified in atheromatous lesions in coronary arteries and in other organs obtained at autopsy. The case for *C. pneumoniae* is of particular interest since both in the hypercholesterolemic rabbit and in genetically hyperlipidemic mice, acceleration of atherosclerosis with *C. pneumoniae* infection has been demonstrated.[42] In addition, pilot clinical trials of anti-chlamydial macrolide antibiotics have raised the possibility that such therapy may reduce the risk of recurrent coronary events.[43,44] *In vitro* studies have suggested that *C. pneumoniae* can trigger proatherogenic events, such as foam cell formation, procoagulant activity, and metalloproteinase activity in monocytes, probably mediated by its heat shock protein 60 (HSP60). Molecular antigenic mimicry between certain chlamydia antigens and myosin has also raised the additional possibility that such antigenic mimicry could be involved in an immune-mediated vascular and myocardial injury. However, recent large-scale clinical trials have failed to demonstrate any clinical benefit of using antibiotics targeting *C. pneumonia*, raising serious doubts about a causal link between infection and atherothrombosis.[45–48]

Recent studies have implicated oral and gut microflora in the pathogenesis of human and experimental atherosclerosis.[49,50] The investigators employed 454 pyrosequencing of 16 S rRNA genes to determine the microbial composition of atherosclerotic plaques and test the hypothesis that the oral or gut microbiota can contribute to atherosclerosis in humans; they identified *Chryseomonas* genes in all atherosclerotic plaque samples, and *Veillonella* and *Streptococcus* genes in the majority.[49] Interestingly, the combined abundances of *Veillonella* and *Streptococcus* genes in atherosclerotic plaques correlated with their abundance in the oral cavity.[49] Moreover several bacterial taxa in the oral cavity and the gut correlated with plasma cholesterol levels, and the overall results of the study suggest that bacteria from the oral cavity, and perhaps even the gut, may correlate with disease markers of atherosclerosis.[49] The precise mechanisms by which specific patterns of gut microflora contribute to pathogenesis of atherosclerosis remains unresolved, but it has been suggested that by-products of phosphatidylcholne metabolism generated by gut microflora (such as choline) and subsequent hepatic metabolism of absorbed products (such as trimethylamine N-oxide) may lead to enhanced foam cell formation by increasing scavenger receptors on monocytes.[50]

Table 68.3 Potential role of infection in atherosclerosis and thrombosis

Infectious organisms implicated
Viruses Herpes virus Cytomegalovirus
Bacteria *Chlamydia pneumoniae* *Helicobacter pylori* *Porphyromonas gingivalis?*
Mechanism(s) by which infections may contribute to atherothrombosis
Direct infection of the vascular wall with endothelial injury, inflammatory cell recruitment, and activation (*Chlamydia pneumoniae*, herpes virus, cytomegalovirus) Immune-mediated vascular injury through molecular mimicry (*Chlamydia pneumoniae*) Remote infections with systemic activation of the inflammatory response (*Helicobacter pylori*, *Porphyromonas gingivalis*)

Toll-like receptors, innate Immunity, and Atherosclerosis

Toll-like receptors (TLR) are a family of transmembrane receptors that serve as signaling receptors in the innate immune system; their ligation by exogenous and possibly endogenous ligands triggers a pro-inflammatory signaling cascade in various cells linking innate immunity to inflammation (Chapter 3). Recent studies have shown that TLRs are expressed in murine and human atherosclerotic lesions, that hyperlipidemia induces pro-inflammatory signaling, in part through these receptors, and that in murine models their downstream adaptor molecules such as MyD88 (myeloid differentiation factor) contribute to vascular inflammation, neointimal hyperplasia, and atherosclerosis.[51–53]

Angiogenesis in atherosclerosis

Angiogenesis or neovascularization is an essential process that supports chronic inflammation and fibroproliferation, processes that are involved in atherogenesis. Several studies have demonstrated increased neoangiogenesis in atherosclerotic lesions and hypercholesterolemia has been shown to increase adventitial neovascularity in porcine arteries before the development of an atherosclerotic lesion.[54,55] Pro-inflammatory chemokines such as IL-8 and other angiogenic growth factors such as vascular endothelial growth factor (VEGF) have been demonstrated in atherosclerotic lesions, where they could contribute to angiogenesis. Angiogenesis may contribute to plaque progression by providing a source of intraplaque hemorrhage, which in turn may provide red cell membrane-derived cholesterol contributing to the expansion of the necrotic lipid core. In addition, neovascular channels may also provide access for inflammatory cells into the vessel wall; thus, angiogenesis and inflammation appear to be linked pathophysiologic processes. Perivascular accumulation of mast cells has been identified as a potential contributor to adventitial neovascularity, capillary leaks, and intraplaque hemorrhage; furthermore, substance P derived from local nerve endings in the perivascular space has been suggested as a potential trigger for mast cell activation and degranulation.[56]

Recently, the ability of macrophages to undergo transdifferentiation into functional endothelial cells has been demonstrated, suggesting a more direct link between inflammation and angiogenesis.[57] Data demonstrating an inhibitory effect of angiostatin in murine models of atherosclerosis suggest a potential proatherogenic role for angiogenesis.[58]

Role of inflammation in plaque rupture, plaque erosion, and thrombosis

●THERAPEUTIC PRINCIPLES

Management of atherothrombosis

- Atherothrombotic clinical events can be reduced or prevented by:
  - Prevention of progression of atherosclerosis
  - Stabilization of lesions by changing plaque composition
  - Facilitating regression of pre-existing lesions.
- Traditional risk factor modification, including LDL lowering, reduces atherothrombotic events largely by slowing or preventing lesion progression or by lesion stabilization through change in lesion composition (reduced plaque lipid and plaque inflammation).
- Increasing quantity or functional quality of HDL can regress atherosclerotic lesions and reduce plaque inflammation by promoting egress of plaque lipid and inflammatory cells.
- Direct immune modulation to suppress pro-inflammatory aspects or stimulate anti-inflammatory aspects of the immune system can also inhibit atherothrombosis.

Thrombosis-complicating atherosclerosis is the mechanism by which atherosclerosis leads to acute ischemic syndromes of unstable angina, non-Q- and Q-wave myocardial infarction, and many cases of sudden cardiac death.[59–62] In most cases, coronary thrombosis occurs as a result of uneven thinning and

rupture of the fibrous cap, often at the shoulders of a lipid-rich lesion where macrophages and T cells accumulate, and are activated, and where apoptosis may occur (Figs. 68.2, 68.3, 68.4).[59–62] Thinning of the fibrous cap may result from elaboration by inflammatory cells (chiefly macrophages) of matrix-degrading

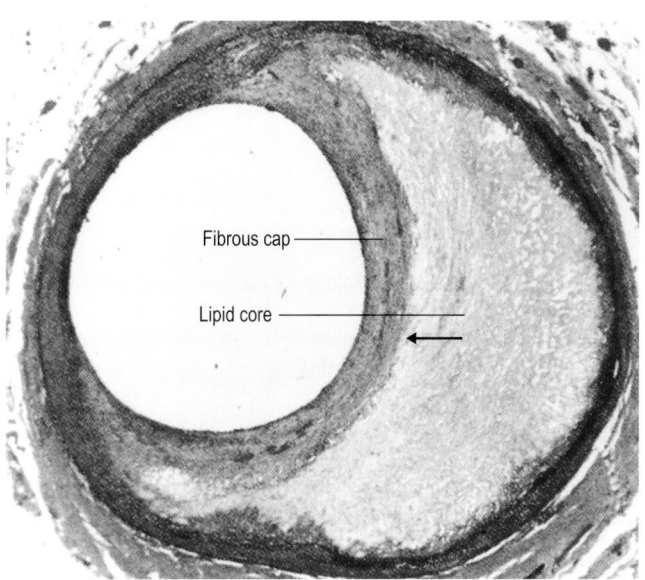

Fibrous cap

Lipid core

Composition of Fibrous
1, Extracellular matrix Collagen Elastin Proteoglycans Glycoseaminoglycans
2, Smooth muscle cells
3, Inflammatory cells

Fig. 68.2 An atherosclerotic plaque in a human coronary artery depicting various components of the lesion.

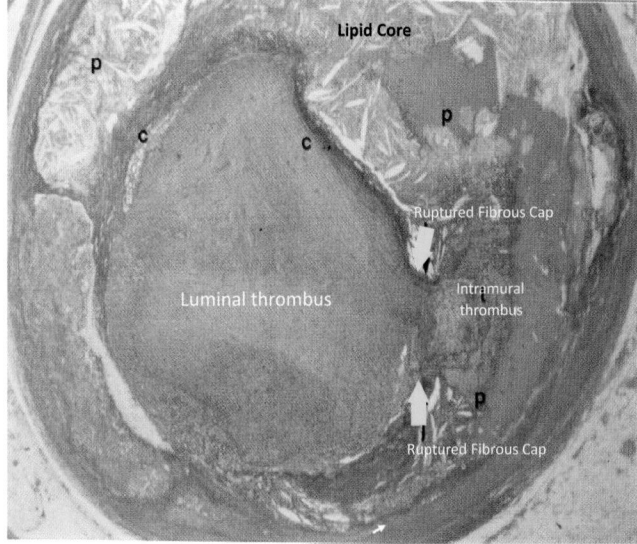

Lipid Core

p

c

c

p

Ruptured Fibrous Cap

Intramural thrombus

Luminal thrombus

p

Ruptured Fibrous Cap

Fig. 68.3 Coronary thrombosis resulting from rupture of the fibrous cap of a lipid-rich coronary artery plaque (Plaque rupture) (p = plaque, c = cap).

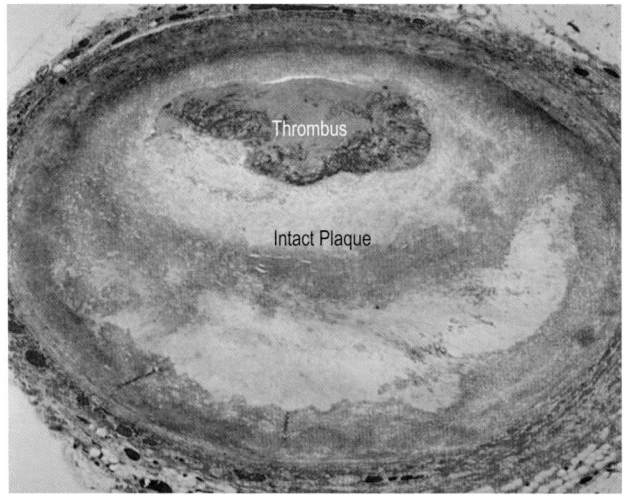

Fig. 68.4 Coronary thrombosis resulting from superficial endothelial erosion without rupture of the plaque (Plaque erosion).

metalloproteinases (MMPs) such as collagenases (MMP-1, MMP-13), gelatinases (MMP-2, MMP-9), elastases (MMP-12), and stromelysins (MMP-3), and/or other proteases such as cathepsins.[59–62] These proteases may be induced or activated by oxidized LDL, cell-to-cell interaction between macrophages and activated T cells, CD40 ligation, mast cell-derived proteases, oxidant radicals, matrix proteins such as tenascin-C, and infectious agents.[59–62] Thinning may also result from increased smooth muscle cell death by apoptosis/necrosis and consequent reduced matrix production; increased smooth muscle cell death may result from oxidized LDL, cleavage products of tenascin-C, or direct contact with plaque infiltrating CD 4 T cells expressing TNF-related apoptosis inducing ligand (TRAIL).[63–65]

Inflammatory cells, specifically macrophages, are also the main source of tissue factor in the atherosclerotic plaque.[66] Tissue factor, when exposed to circulating blood, interacts with activated factor VII to generate activated factor X; activated factor X in turn cleaves thrombin from prothrombin. Thrombin is involved in recruiting and activating platelets as well as the clotting cascade, thereby initiating thrombus formation. Tissue factor expression is increased in atherosclerotic plaques, particularly in unstable coronary syndromes.[66] The lipid core of the atheromatous lesion is heavily impregnated with tissue factor derived from dead (possibly apoptotic) macrophages and foam cells, accounting for its high thrombogenicity. Macrophage tissue factor expression can be induced by a variety of signals in the atherosclerotic plaque, including various cytokines, infectious agents, and oxidized lipoproteins. Thrombosis can also occur on a proteoglycan-rich matrix without a large lipid core, and in such cases, evidence of superficial endothelial erosion is found.[67] This plaque erosion may account for thrombosis in a relatively higher proportion of young victims of sudden death, particularly in women and smokers.[68] The molecular basis for these plaque erosions is not clear although endothelial desquamation through activation of basement membrane-degrading MMP may be involved.[62]

Plaques with a large core, activated inflammatory infiltration, and a thinned fibrous cap are therefore considered vulnerable or unstable plaques. Their identification can be particularly difficult because they may not produce symptoms because of lack of flow-limiting stenoses, and may thus escape detection by stress testing and even angiography. Inflammation in atherosclerosis can be accompanied by elevation of circulating pro-inflammatory markers such as C-reactive protein (CRP), IL-6, serum amyloid A, and a variety of soluble leukocyte adhesion molecules.[68,69] Elevated CRP levels have been shown to predict an increased risk of adverse cardiac events in patients with symptomatic vascular disease, as well as in asymptomatic subjects at risk for vascular disease.[68]

Conclusions and translational research

● ON THE HORIZON

Ongoing clinical trials of the agents described below should clarify their role for the prevention of atherothrombotic cardiovascular events.

- Novel HDLA-based therapies that exploit the known beneficial effects of HDL on the vasculature (potential agents include novel cholesteryl ester transfer protein (CETP) inhibitors, apo A-I or apo A-I Milano infusion, HDL delpidation and reinfusion, apo A-I mimetic peptides, apo A-I or apo A-I Milano gene-therapy, endothelial lipase antagonists, nuclear hormone receptor agonists)
- Anti-inflammatory agents that target inflammatory mediators relevant to the progression and destabilization of atherosclerosis (such as darapladib that inhibits LpPLA2 (lipoprotein-associated phospholipase A2), anti-IL1B antibody)
- Immunomodulating therapies such as apo B100-related peptide vaccines and anti-oxidized LDL antibodies.
- Non-statin LDL lowering agents for patients that either do not respond or do not tolerate statin therapy (such as microsomal transfer protein (MTP) inhibitors, Apo B 100 antisense oligonucleotides, anti- PCSK9 antibodies)

Atherosclerosis is a complex disease process that involves lipoprotein influx, lipoprotein modification, increased pro-oxidant stress, and inflammatory, angiogenic, and fibroproliferative responses intermingled with extracellular matrix and lipid accumulation, resulting in the formation of an atherosclerotic plaque. Endothelial activation/dysfunction is common in atherosclerosis and often manifests as a reduced vasodilator or enhanced vasoconstrictor phenotype that contributes to luminal compromise. Thrombosis resulting from plaque rupture or superficial erosion complicates atherosclerosis, often resulting in abrupt luminal occlusion with resultant acute ischemic syndromes (Fig. 68.5). Infectious agents may contribute to the inflammatory response and thus to destabilization of lesions.

Although risk factor modification with adoption of a heart-healthy lifestyle and statins have significantly contributed to the reduction in atherothrombotic cardiovascular events, a substantial residual risk remains. In fact, despite aggressive preventive therapies, nearly 50% of adverse atherothrombotic cardiovascular events continue to occur. An improved understanding of the pathophysiology of atherosclerosis is providing novel directions for its prevention and treatment. In particular, the recognition of the important role of inflammation could lead to novel therapeutic interventions directed at selective inhibition of the inflammatory cascade in the vessel wall. Targeting inflammatory triggers such as lipoproteins, angiotensin II, possible infectious agents, and others is likely to lead to improved outcomes in patients with atherosclerosis.

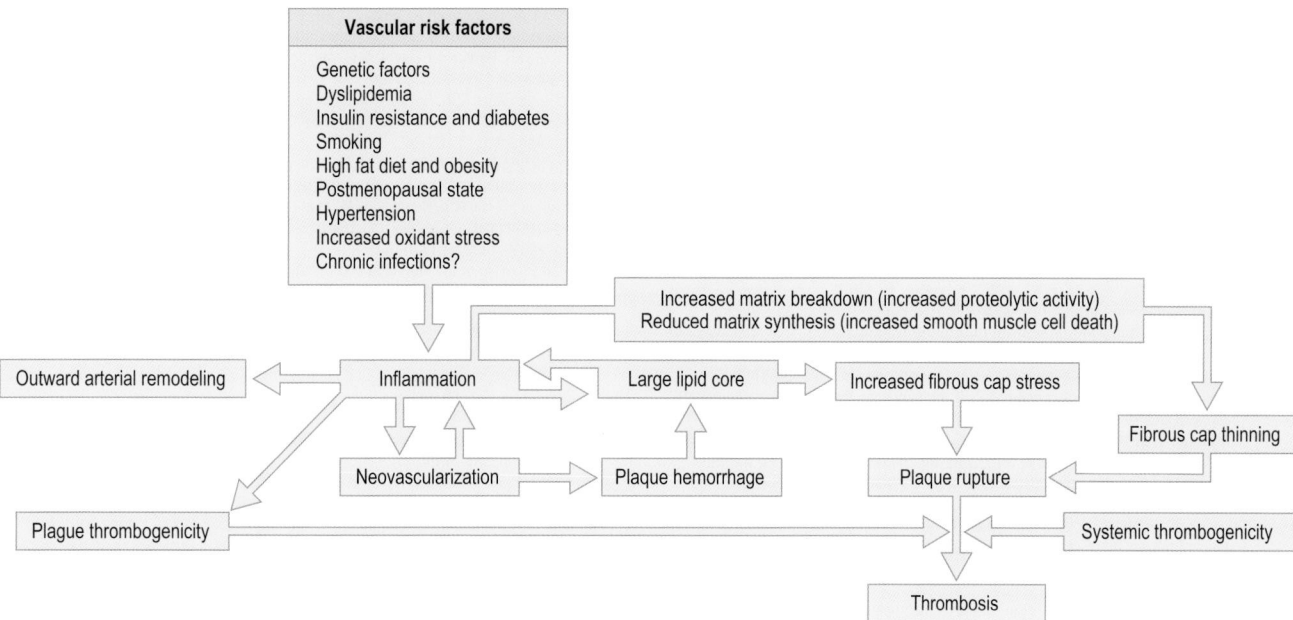

Fig. 68.5 Schematic showing the pathophysiology of plaque rupture and thrombosis.

References

1. Ross R. Atherosclerosis: An inflammatory disease. N Engl J Med 1999;340:115–26.
2. Skålén K, Gustafsson M, Rydberg EK, et al. Subendothelial retention of atherogenic lipoproteins in early atherosclerosis. Nature 2002;417(6890):750–4.
3. Gustafsson M, Levin M, Skålén K, et al. Retention of low-density lipoprotein in atherosclerotic lesions of the mouse: evidence for a role of lipoprotein lipase. Circ Res 2007;101(8):777–83.
4. McMillian DE. Blood flow and the localization of atherosclerotic plaques. Stroke 1985;16:582–7.
5. Resnick N, Collins T, Atkinson W, et al. Platelet-derived growth factor B chain promoter contains a cis-acting fluid shear-stress-responsive element. Proc Natl Acad Sci U S A 1993;90:4591–5.
6. Nakashima Y, Raines EW, Plump AS, et al. Upregulation of VCAM-1 and ICAM-1 at atherosclerosis-prone sites on the endothelium in the ApoE-deficient mouse. Arterioscler Thromb Vasc Biol 1998;18:842–51.
7. Giachelli CM, Lombardi D, Johnson RJ, et al. Evidence for a role of osteopontin in macrophage infiltration in response to pathological stimuli in vivo. Am J Pathol 1998;152:353–8.
8. Parmar KM, Larman HB, Dai G, et al. Integration of flow-dependent endothelial phenotypes by Kruppel-like factor 2. J Clin Invest 2006;116(1):49–58.
9. Cheng C, Tempel D, van Haperen R, et al. Atherosclerotic lesion size and vulnerability are determined by patterns of fluid shear stress. Circulation 2006;113(23):2744–53.
10. Jongstra-Bilen J, Haidari M, Zhu SN, et al. Low-grade chronic inflammation in regions of the normal mouse arterial intima predisposed to atherosclerosis. J Exp Med 2006;203(9):2073–83.
11. Boisvert WA, Santiago R, Curtiss LK, Tekeltaub RA. A leukocyte homologue of the IL-8 receptor CXCR-2 mediates the accumulation of macrophages in atherosclerotic lesions of LDL receptor-deficient mice. J Clin Invest 1998;101:353–63.
12. Hwang S-J, Ballantyne CM, Sharrett AR, et al. Circulating adhesion molecules VCAM-1, ICAM-1, and E-selectin in carotid atherosclerosis and incident coronary heart disease cases: the Atherosclerosis Risk in Communities (ARIC) study. Circulation 1997;96:4219–25.
13. Napoli C, D'Armiento FP, Mancini FP, et al. Fatty streak formation occurs in human fetal aortas and is greatly enhanced by maternal hypercholesterolemia: intimal accumulation of low density lipoprotein and its oxidation precede monocyte recruitment into early atherosclerotic lesions. J Clin Invest 1997;100:2680–90.
14. Stary HC, Chandler AB, Glagov S, et al. A definition of initial, fatty streak, and intermediate lesions of atherosclerosis: A report from the Committee on Vascular Lesions of the Council on Atherosclerosis, American Heart Association. Circulation 1994;89:2462–78.
15. Kinlay S, Ganz P. Role of endothelial dysfunction in coronary artery disease and implications for therapy. Am J Cardiol 1997;80:111–61.
16. Griendling KK, Alexander RW. Oxidative stress and cardiovascular disease. Circulation 1997;96:3264–5.
17. Yla-Herttuala S, Palinski W, Rosenfeld ME, et al. Evidence for the presence of oxidatively modified low density lipoprotein in atherosclerotic lesions of rabbit and man. J Clin Invest 1989;84:1086–95.
18. Quinn MT, Parthasarathy S, Fong LG, Steinberg D. Oxidatively modified low density lipoproteins: A potential role in recruitment and retention of monocyte/macrophages during atherogenesis. Proc Natl Acad Sci U S A 1987;84:2995–8.
19. Hansson GK, Jonasson L, Siefert PS, Stemme S. Immune mechanisms in atherosclerosis. Arteriosclerosis 1989;9:567–78.
20. Stemme S, Faber B, Holm J, et al. T lymphocytes from human atherosclerotic plaques recognize oxidized low density lipoprotein. Proc Natl Acad Sci U S A 1995;92:3893–7.
21. Qiao J-H, Tripathi J, Mishra NK, et al. Role of macrophage colony-stimulating factor in atherosclerosis: studies of osteopetrotic mice. Am J Pathol 1997;150:1687–99.
22. Llodra J, Angeli V, Liu J, et al. Emigration of monocyte-derived cells from atherosclerotic lesions characterizes regressive, but not progressive, plaques. Proc Natl Acad Sci U S A 2004;101(32):11779–1184.
23. Lord RS, Bobryshev YV. Clustering of dendritic cells in athero-prone areas of the aorta. Atherosclerosis 1999;146:197–8.
24. Schonbeck U, Mach F, Sukhova GK, et al. Regulation of matrix metalloproteinase expression in human vascular smooth muscle cells by T lymphocytes: A role for CD40 signaling in plaque rupture? Circ Res 1997;81:448–54.
25. Mach F, Schonbeck U, Sukhova GK, et al. Reduction of atherosclerosis in mice by inhibition of CD40 signaling. Nature 1998;394:200–3.
26. Hristov M, Weber C. Differential role of monocyte subsets in atherosclerosis. Thromb Haemost 2011;106(5):757–62.
27. Tian F, Wang L, Yang M, et al. Favorable modulation of atherosclerosis and monocyte phenotype by intravenous AAV 8 mediated Apo A-I Milano gene transfer in mice. Circulation 2010;122:A17407 (abst).
28. Feig JE, Rong JX, Shamir R, et al. HDL promotes rapid atherosclerosis regression in mice and alters inflammatory properties of plaque monocyte-derived cells. Proc Natl Acad Sci U S A 2011;108(17):7166–71.
29. Tabas I. Consequences and therapeutic implications of macrophage apoptosis in atherosclerosis: the importance of lesion stage and phagocytic efficiency. Arterioscler Thromb Vasc Biol 2005;25:2255–64.
30. Ait-Oufella H, Pouresmail V, Simon T, et al. Defective mer receptor tyrosine kinase signaling in bone marrow cells promotes apoptotic cell accumulation and accelerates atherosclerosis. Arterioscler Thromb Vasc Biol 2008;28:1429–31.
31. Feng B, Zhang D, Kuriakose G, et al. Niemann-Pick C heterozygosity confers resistance to lesional necrosis and macrophage apoptosis in murine atherosclerosis. Proc Natl Acad Sci U S A 2003;100(18):10423–8.
32. Duewell P, Kono H, Rayner KJ, et al. NLRP3 inflamasomes are required for atherogenesis and activated by cholesterol crystals that form early in disease. Nature 2010;464(7293):1357–61.
33. Rajamaki1 K, Lappalainen J, Oorni1 K, et al. Cholesterol crystals activate the NLRP3 inflammasome in human macrophages: a novel link between cholesterol metabolism and inflammation. PLoS ONE 2010;5(7):e11765.
34. Lacy F, O'Connor DT, Schmid-Schonbein GW. Plasma hydrogen peroxide production in hypertensive and normotensive subjects as genetic risk of hypertension. J Hypertens 1998;16:291–303.
35. Nygard O, Nordrehaug JE, Refsum H, et al. Plasma homocysteine levels and mortality in patients with coronary artery disease. N Engl J Med 1997;337:230–6.
36. Omenn GS, Beresford SSA, Motulsky AG. Preventing coronary heart disease: B vitamins and homocysteine. Circulation 1998;97:421–4.
37. Debreceni B, Debreceni L. Why do homocysteine-lowering B vitamin and antioxidant E vitamin supplementations appear to be ineffective in the prevention of cardiovascular diseases? Cardiovasc Ther 2011 Apr 1;doi:10.1111/j.1755-5922.2011.00266.x Epub ahead of print].
38. Hendrix MG, Salimans MM, van Boven CP, Bruggeman CA. High prevalence of latently present cytomegalovirus in arterial walls of patients suffering from grade III atherosclerosis. Am J Pathol 1990;136:23–8.
39. Jackson LA, Campbell LA, Schmidt RA, et al. Specificity of detection of *Chlamydia pneumoniae* in cardiovascular atheroma: Evaluation of the innocent bystander hypothesis. Am J Pathol 1997;150:1785–90.

40. Nicholson AC, Hajjar DP. Herpesviruses in atherosclerosis and thrombosis: etiologic agents or ubiquitous bystanders? Arteriocler Thromb Vasc Biol 1998;18:339–48.

41. Shah PK. Plaque disruption and coronary thrombosis: new insight into pathogenesis and prevention. Clin Cardiol 1997;20(II):38–44.

42. Muhlestein JB, Anderson JL, Hammond EH, et al. Infection with *Chlamydia pneumoniae* accelerates the development of atherosclerosis and treatment with azithromycin prevents it in a rabbit model. Circulation 1998;97:633–6.

43. Gurfinkel E, Bozovich G, Daroca A, et al. Randomized trial of Roxithromycin in non-Q-wave coronary syndromes: ROXIS Pilot Study. ROXIS Study Group [see comments]. Lancet 1997;350:404–7.

44. Gupta S, Leatham EW, Carrington D, et al. Elevated *Chlamydia pneumoniae* antibodies, cardiovascular events, and azithromycin in male survivors of myocardial infarction. Circulation 1997;96:404–7.

45. Cercek B, Shah PK, Noc M, et al., AZACS Investigators. Effect of short-term treatment with azithromycin on recurrent ischemic events in patients with acute coronary syndrome in the Azithromycin in Acute Coronary Syndrome (AZACS) trial: a randomised controlled trial. Lancet 2003;361(9360):809–13.

46. O'Connor CM, Dunne MW, Pfeffer MA, et al., Investigators in the WIZARD Study. Azithromycin for the secondary prevention of coronary heart disease events: the WIZARD study: a randomized controlled trial. JAMA 2003;290(11):1459–66.

47. Cannon CP, Braunwald E, McCabe CH, et al., Pravastatin or Atorvastatin Evaluation and Infection Therapy-Thrombolysis in Myocardial Infarction 22 Investigators. Antibiotic treatment of *Chlamydia pneumoniae* after acute coronary syndrome. N Engl J Med 2005;352(16):1646–54.

48. Grayston JT, Kronmal RA, Jackson LA, et al., ACES Investigators. Azithromycin for the secondary prevention of coronary events. N Engl J Med 2005;352(16):1637–45.

49. Koren O, Spor A, Felin J, et al. Human oral, gut, and plaque microbiota in patients with atherosclerosis. PNAS 2011;108(Suppl. 1):4592–8.

50. Wang Z, Klipfell E, Bennett BJ, et al. Gut flora metabolism of phosphatidylcholine promotes cardio-vascular disease. Nature 2011;472:57–63.

51. Michelsen KS, Doherty TM, Shah PK, Arditi M. TLR signaling: an emerging bridge from innate immunity to atherogenesis. J Immunol 2004;173:5901–7.

52. Michelsen KS, Wong MH, Shah PK, et al. Lack of Toll-like receptor 4 or myeloid differentiation factor 88 reduces atherosclerosis and alters plaque phenotype in mice deficient in apolipoprotein E. Proc Natl Acad Sci U S A 2004;101:10679–84.

53. Bjorkbacka H, Kunjathoor VV, Moore KJ, et al. Reduced atherosclerosis in MyD88-null mice links elevated serum cholesterol levels to activation of innate immunity signaling pathways. Nat Med 2004;10:416–21.

54. Barger AC, Beeuwkes R, Iainey LL, Silverman KJ. Hypothesis: Vasa vasorum and neovascularization of human coronary arteries. N Engl J Med 1984;310:175–7.

55. O'Brien ER, Garvin MR, Dev R, et al. Angiogenesis in human atherosclerotic plaques. Am J Pathology 1994;145:883–94.

56. Bot I, de Jager SCA, Bot M, et al. The neuropeptide substance P mediates adventitial mast cell activation and induces intraplaque hemorrhage in advanced atherosclerosis. Circ Res 2010;106:89–92.

57. Sharifi BG, Zeng Z, Wang L, et al. Pleiotrophin induces transdifferentiation of monocytes into functional endothelial cells. Arterioscler Thromb Vasc Biol 2006;26(6):1273–80.

58. Moulton KS, Heller E, Konerding MA, et al. Angiogenesis inhibitor endostatin or TNP-470 reduces intimal neovascularization and plaque growth in apolipoprotein E deficient mice. Circulation 1999;99:1726–32.

59. Shah PK. Role of inflammation and metalloproteinases in plaque disruption and thrombosis. Vasc Med 1998;3:199–206.

60. Shah PK. Plaque disruption and thrombosis. Potential role of inflammation and infection. Cardiol Clin 1999;17:271–81.

61. Xu XP, Meisel SR, Ong JM, et al. Oxidized low-density lipoprotein regulates matrix metalloproteinase-9 and its tissue inhibitor in human monocyte-derived macrophages. Circulation 1999;99:993–8.

62. Rajavashisth TB, Xu XP, Jovinge S, et al. Membrane type 1 matrix metalloproteinase expression in human atherosclerosis plaques: Evidence for activation by proinflammatory mediators. Circulation 1999;99:3103–9.

63. Wallner K, Chen Li, Shah PK, et al. The EGF-L domain of tenascin-C is pro-apoptotic for cultured smooth muscle cells. Arterioscler Thromb Vasc Biol 2004;24:1416–21.

64. Sato K, Niessner A, Kopecky SL, et al. Trail expressing T cells induce apoptosis of vascular smooth muscle cells in atherosclerotic plaque. J Exp Med 2006;203(1):239–50.

65. Pryschep S, Sato K, Goronzy JJ, Weyand CM. T cell recognition and killing of vascular smooth muscle cells in acute coronary syndromes. Circ Res 2006;98(9):1168–76.

66. Moreno PR, Bernardi VH, López-Cuéllar J, et al. Macrophages, smooth muscle cells, and tissue factor in unstable angina. Implications for cell-mediated thrombogenicity in acute coronary syndromes. Circulation 1996;94:3090–7.

67. Burke AP, Farb A, Malcom GT, et al. Effect of risk factors on the mechanism of acute thrombosis and sudden coronary death in women. Circulation 1998;97(21):2110–6.

68. Ridker PM, Cushman M, Stampfer MJ, et al. Inflammation, aspirin, and the risk of cardiovascular disease in apparently healthy men. N Engl J Med 1997;336:973–9.

69. Haverkate F, Thompson SG, Pyke SD, et al. Production of C-reactive protein and risk of coronary events in stable and unstable angina: European Concerted Action on Thrombosis and Disabilities Angina Pectoris Study Group. Lancet 1997;349:462–6.

Autoimmune thyroid diseases

Anna L. Mitchell,
Simon H.S.
Pearce

The autoimmune thyroid diseases are common in all societies, forming, as a group, the most prevalent autoimmune disorders in man. Despite many common underlying features, such as a marked female preponderance, shared susceptibility alleles and common autoantigens, Graves' disease and autoimmune hypothyroidism have contrasting clinical characteristics. Over recent years, our knowledge about the underlying pathogenesis has increased owing to advances in human genomics, molecular immunology and in the availability of tractable murine models of disease. Novel therapies are now emerging, based on this increased understanding.

KEY CONCEPTS

Classification of autoimmune thyroid disease

Autoimmune hyperthyroidism	Graves' disease
Autoimmune thyroiditis	Hashimoto's thyroiditis
	Atrophic thyroiditis
	Post-partum thyroiditis

Graves' hyperthyroidism

Introduction

Graves' disease (GD) is a common autoimmune condition that accounts for the majority of cases of hyperthyroidism in the developed world. Its pathogenesis is unique among the autoimmune endocrinopathies, as a key feature is the presence of stimulating autoantibodies directed against the thyrotropin (TSH) receptor, which mimic the action of TSH to drive thyroid overactivity. Interestingly, thyroid dysfunction is commonly associated with other extrathyroidal manifestations of GD, the most common being ophthalmopathy.

Epidemiology

GD is one of the most common autoimmune diseases, with a prevalence of approximately 1% in women in the developed world.[1] It is more common in iodine sufficient countries, where it accounts for between 60 and 90% of cases of hyperthyroidism.[2] GD is seven times more common in women than in men and may affect individuals at any age; however, the peak incidence occurs between the ages of 35 and 40 years.

Etiology

GD is a complex genetic condition, implying that environmental stimuli precipitate disease in individuals with one or more susceptibility alleles. A large twin study estimated that about 80% of the propensity to develop GD is attributable to genetic factors.[3] Further evidence for the heritability of GD comes from the observation that it clusters within families. Up to one quarter of individuals with GD have a first degree relative with the condition or with another autoimmune thyroid disease such as autoimmune hypothyroidism.[4] Should an individual have a sibling with GD, it is estimated that the relative risk (λ_s) of that individual developing GD is around 10, which is comparable to that of other heritable autoimmune conditions, such as type 1 diabetes which has a λ_s of 15.

A number of genetic loci have been shown to contribute to the susceptibility to GD (Fig. 69.1). These genes encode proteins in biological pathways that regulate immune system activity or thyroid biology.[4,5] The major histocompatibility (MHC) region on chromosome 6p21 has long been associated with multiple autoimmune conditions. HLA genes found within the MHC region play a vital role in pathogen and self-peptide recognition, and therefore have a clear role in immunity and in establishing and maintaining immune tolerance. In European populations the primary association between MHC and GD is with alleles of the class II MHC genes. The *HLA-DR3* allele is detected twice as frequently in GD subjects as in healthy controls (i.e., 50% of GD subjects vs 25% of controls). At the protein level, neutral amino acids alanine or glutamine are substituted for positively charged arginine at position 74 in the HLA-DR peptide-binding pocket, which alters the binding-pocket configuration, more readily allowing self-peptides to enter the antigen binding site.[5] Importantly, 50% of individuals with GD do not have the *HLA-DR3* allele, implying that there is unlikely to be a single antigenic epitope responsible for GD.

The cytotoxic T lymphocyte-antigen 4 (*CTLA-4*) gene (chromosome 2q33) encodes a co-stimulatory molecule expressed on the surface of activated T cells, which plays a role in downregulating T-cell responses and checking T-cell activation. The *CT60* single nucleotide polymorphism (SNP) downstream from the 3'UTR was found to influence GD susceptibility (odds ratio 1.5) and has been suggested as a possible etiological variant;[6] however, the functional effects of this variant remain poorly defined and contributions from other variants such as at codon 17 in the CTLA-4 signal peptide remain likely. About 50% of individuals from healthy European populations carry the autoimmune "susceptible" *CTLA-4* haplotype; therefore, other important factors are clearly also at play. CTLA-4 polymorphisms also contribute to susceptibility to type 1 diabetes, celiac disease, and several other autoimmune conditions.

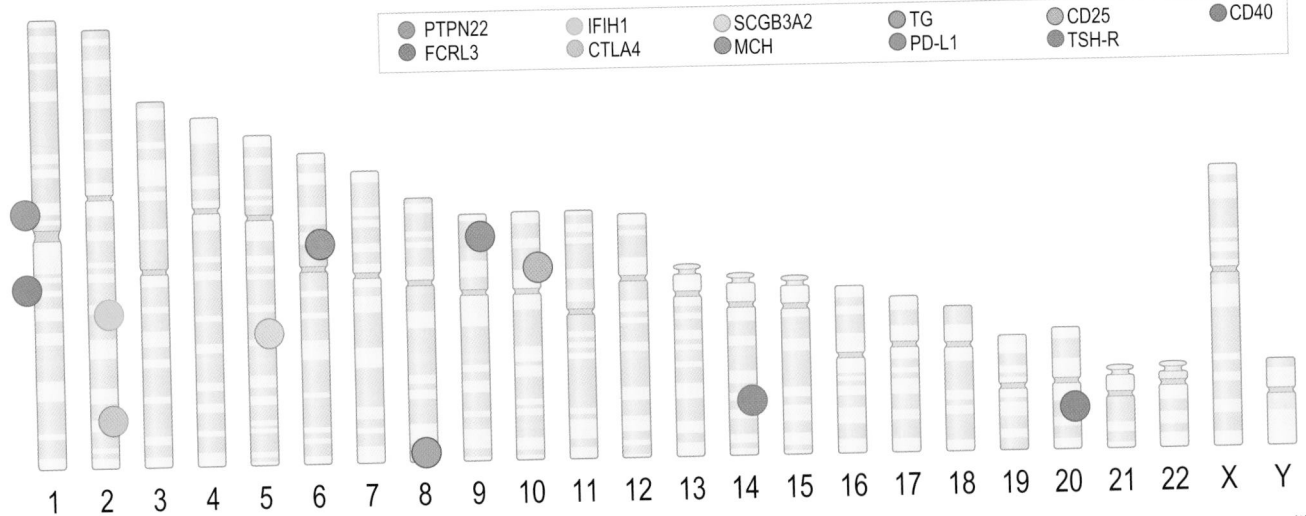

Fig. 69.1 Schematic diagram to illustrate the loci that have been associated with Graves' disease to date. Each locus is shown on its respective chromosome, with chromosome 1 depicted on the left and chromosome Y on the right. Loci discovered using a genome-wide approach are depicted with yellow text while loci discovered using the candidate gene approach are depicted with white text.

The protein tyrosine phosphatase-22 (*PTPN22*) gene on chromosome 1p13 encodes the lymphoid tyrosine phosphatase (LYP) molecule, which, like CTLA-4, is involved in the regulation of T-cell activation. In GD, a coding variant (R620W) was found more frequently in Caucasians with GD than in controls (13 vs 7% respectively, odds ratio 1.8).[7] However, this variant has recently been shown to be hypomorphic, resulting in a short-lived enzyme, producing inhibition of T-cell receptor signaling compared to the wild-type protein. The PTPN22*620 W variant is very rare in non-Caucasian populations, but different *PTPN22* alleles have been associated with autoimmunity in Asian populations.

Genes for several other molecules involved in immunoregulation have also been demonstrated to have allelic variants associated with GD including CD25, CD40, PD-L1, IFIH1, and FCRL3. The replication of these associations has been patchy, suggesting that they may have relatively weak effects or contribute to susceptibility in some but not all populations.

In addition to the above variants in immune regulatory pathways, loci specific to GD have been identified based on known thyroid pathophysiology. The gene encoding the TSH receptor (TSH-R) on chromosome 14q31 is an obvious candidate for GD, as the TSH-R is directly stimulated by autoantibodies in affected individuals. While initial studies reported conflicting results, a definite association between a number of SNPs in intron 1 of the *TSH-R* gene and GD has now been confirmed in Caucasians.[5] The mechanism by which these intronic SNPs confer disease susceptibility is unknown. Another GD candidate is the *thyroglobulin* (*Tg*) gene (8q24). This encodes the Tg protein, the precursor for the thyroid hormones triiodothyronine (T3) and thyroxine (T4). SNPs in the *Tg* gene have been associated with GD in some Caucasian cohorts and an epistatic interaction between a SNP in *Tg* exon 33 and *HLA-DR* has been suggested. This interesting interaction has raised the possibility that Tg polymorphisms predispose to GD by alternating Tg peptide presentation by antigen presenting cells on HLA class II molecules to T cells.

Despite years of research into the genetic etiology of GD, 30 to 40% of the inherited susceptibility has yet to be accounted for. This "hidden" heredity is a common theme in genetically complex traits, but it is likely to be owing to rare genomic variants, polymorphisms in regulatory DNA sequences, and/or epigenetic factors.

GD is one of the few autoimmune conditions where links to environmental factors have been definitively established.[8]

● KEY CONCEPTS

Environmental factors known to influence Graves' disease susceptibility

- Smoking
- Iodine
- Stress
- Immune system reconstitution states
  - Pregnancy
  - Successful treatment of HIV with HAART
  - T-cell depletion therapy, e.g., alemtuzumab
- Infections e.g., hepatitis C

Iodine is one of the most common precipitants of thyroid dysfunction. With regard to GD, more cases are observed in iodine sufficient areas. This was observed in a study where the incidence of GD was noted to be more than twice as common among younger individuals in Iceland, where iodine intake is high, compared to age-matched individuals in East Jutland, Denmark, where iodine intake is low.[2]

Cigarette smoking influences GD susceptibility and severity, in particular of Graves' ophthalmopathy (GO). Meta-analysis of eight studies showed an odds ratio for developing GD was 3.3 for current smokers compared to lifelong non-smokers.[9] The same study also revealed that current smokers are more likely to develop GO when compared to non-smokers (odds ratio 4.4). The mechanism for this interaction remains to be fully elucidated; however, cigarette smoke extract has been shown, *in vitro*, to stimulate adipogenesis and glycosaminoglycans production by orbital fibroblasts, which accumulate in the orbital tissues in GO.[10]

Stress also appears to influence both GD disease onset and clinical course. In one study, individuals with Graves' disease retrospectively reported more negative life events in the preceding year compared to matched controls.[11] This finding is replicated even when a group of "non-autoimmune" hyperthyroid individuals are used as controls, suggesting that stress is truly a precipitant for autoimmune GD.[12]

Changes in immune system function appear to influence the onset of GD. During pregnancy, hyperthyroid GD is often mild and manageable with smaller antithyroid drug doses. However, in the postpartum period, when the immune system normalizes, there is typically worsening or relapse of GD. A similar phenomenon is seen in individuals who have been significantly immunosuppressed and then recover. For example, new-onset GD has been reported in people who have been successfully treated with highly active antiretroviral therapy (HAART) for HIV infection. During treatment, naïve T cells are produced as the immune system recovers, and these are re-exposed to thyroid antigens resulting in an autoimmune response at the time of immune reconstitution.[13] A similar phenomenon has been seen in individuals with multiple sclerosis treated experimentally with the lymphocyte-depleting anti-CD52 antibody, alemtuzumab (Campath-1 H).

Immunopathogenesis

Histologically, the thyroid in GD is characterized by a diffuse lymphocytic infiltrate, consisting of both T and B cells, associated with thyrocyte hyperplasia (Fig. 69.2). While the T cells play a major role in inflammatory cell recruitment, cytokine secretion, antigen recognition, and thyrocyte damage, infiltrating B cells also produce antibodies including those that drive the hyperthyroidism. The major autoantigens in GD are the TSH-R, the thyroid peroxidase (TPO) enzyme, and Tg. More than 95% of GD patients have detectable circulating TSH-R autoantibodies,[14] and these are likely to be necessary for hyperthyroidism, while approximately 90% have detectable TPO autoantibodies.[15] Antibodies directed against the sodium iodide symporter and the apical iodide transporter, pendrin, have been reported in smaller numbers of patients.[15]

GD is unique among autoimmune conditions in that the TSH-R autoantibodies directly stimulate thyroid gland activity. This is exemplified by neonatal GD, where maternal TSH-R autoantibodies cross the placenta resulting in transient hyperthyroidism in the newborn. However, while TSH-R autoantibodies are sufficient to result in transient hyperthyroidism in these infants, they are not sufficient, per se, to result in the persistent thyroid autoreactivity of true GD. TSH-R antibodies are classically IgG1 subclass and target an epitope in the amino-terminal region of the leucine-rich repeat motif in the extracellular domain of the TSH-R16 (Fig. 69.3).[16] When the autoantibody binds to the TSH-R, this activates intracellular

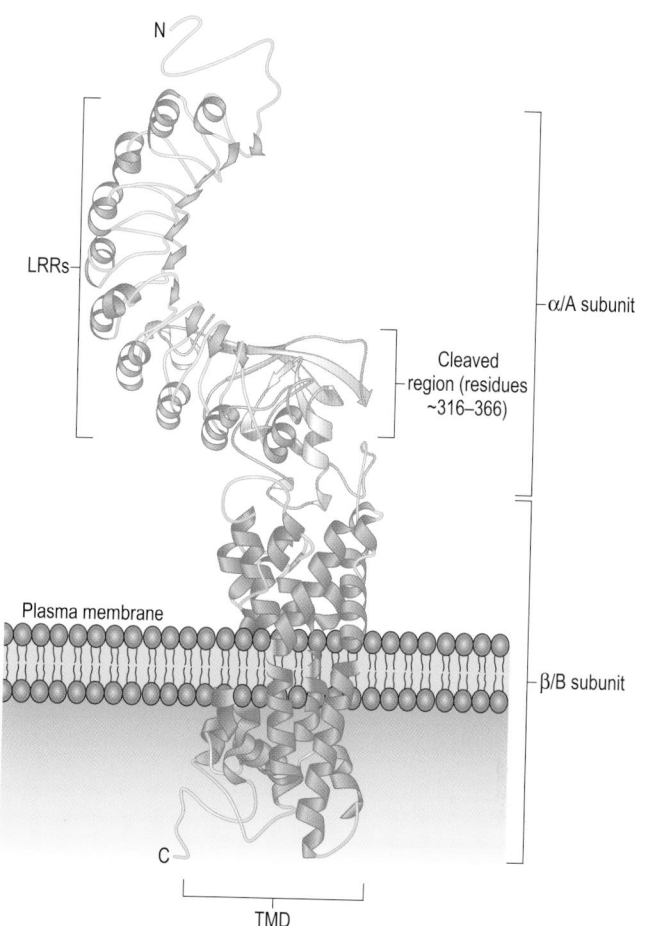

N

LRRs

Cleaved region (residues ~316–366)

α/A subunit

Plasma membrane

β/B subunit

C

TMD

Fig. 69.3 Structure of the TSH receptor.
Courtesy of R Latif; adapted from Davies et al[30]

G proteins, which in turn induce transcription of genes such as TPO and Tg, via the cyclic-AMP and phospholipase-C pathways. This results in thyrocyte hyperplasia and increased thyroid hormone synthesis. The TSHR-Ab-induced expression of TPO and Tg, which are also thyroid antigens, may be a mechanism for disease perpetuation. TSH-R autoantibodies can also be "blocking" in nature and prevent receptor activation. This may result in hypothyroidism. These two types of autoantibodies can also coexist, resulting in fluctuating thyroid function. Thus while it is common to equate GD with hyperthyroidism, individuals with GD may occasionally be hypothyroid or euthyroid (presenting with GO).

TPO antibodies can be of IgG subclass 1, 2, or 4 and typically circulate in concentrations 1000-fold higher than that of TSHR Abs. They are directed against two structurally complex regions of the TPO molecule, the epitopes involving residues from both the myeloperoxidase-like and the complement control protein-like domains. TPO antibodies may have pathogenic significance in that they can fix complement and target the thyrocyte for cell-mediated cytotoxicity.[17] In contrast to TSH-R antibodies, they do not appear to either stimulate or block the enzymatic activity of TPO.

Clinical presentation

Hyperthyroid GD can present with manifestations affecting almost any organ system in the body, and as with many endocrine conditions, affected individuals may report a gradual onset of non-specific symptoms, typically over a period of months. This

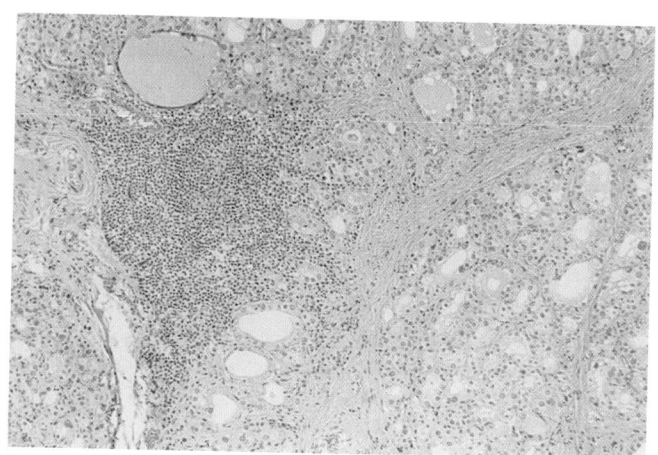

Fig. 69.2 Diffuse lymphocyte infiltrate and thyrocyte hyperplasia in a patient with Graves' disease.

often leads to a delay in seeking medical attention and in making the initial diagnosis. The signs and symptoms of GD can be divided into those associated with hyperthyroidism in general and those specific to GD. These are summarized in Table 69.1.

Investigation and diagnosis of GD

The diagnosis of GD is a clinical one, supported by laboratory investigations. Imaging is occasionally required if the diagnosis is in doubt.

Table 69.1 Common and rarer clinical manifestations of hyperthyroidism

Common	Rare
Neuropsychiatric	
Anxiety	Chorea
Fatigue and exhaustion	Collapse (periodic paralysis)
Fine tremor	Pseudobulbar palsy
Restlessness and fidgeting	Spasticity
Gastrointestinal	
Increased appetite	Hepatosplenomegaly
Loose stools	
Increased frequency of defecation	
Nausea	
Weight loss	
Cardiorespiratory	
Palpitations	Congestive cardiac failure
Shortness of breath on exertion	
Tachycardia (sinus, atrial fibrillation)	
Peripheral vasodilation, flushing	
Systolic hypertension	
Genitourinary	
Menstrual irregularities	
Cutaneous	
Itch	Thyroid acropachy*
Heat intolerance	Pretibial myxedema*
Hair loss	Onycholysis
Musculoskeletal	
Hyperreflexia	
Proximal muscle weakness	
Ophthalmic	
Lid lag	Optic neuropathy*
Lid retraction	
Exophthalmos and proptosis*	
Eye dryness	
Chemosis*	
Ophthalmoplegia*	
Miscellaneous	
Thirst	
Thyroid bruit*	
Manifestations marked with an * are specific to Graves' disease.	

Thyrotoxicosis is diagnosed biochemically on the basis of an elevated serum free T3 (fT3) or free T4 (fT4) in the presence of a completely suppressed TSH. If thyrotoxicosis is found in a patient with extrathyroidal signs, such as GO or pretibial myxedema, the diagnosis of hyperthyroid GD is clear and further investigations are not required. If no extrathyroidal signs are present, the presence of serum autoantibodies should be sought. TSH-R antibodies are highly sensitive for GD; however, the TSH-binding inhibitory immunoglobulin (TBII), an indirect assay of TSH-stimulating antibodies, is commonly assayed. TPO antibodies are often measured as a surrogate for thyroid autoimmunity, as the presence of either TBII or TPO antibodies has more than 90% sensitivity for GD.

Imaging is reserved for individuals in whom the diagnosis is not clear. A radionuclide scan, for example ^{99}Tc or ^{123}I, is favored over an ultrasound scan, as this gives functional information on the activity of the thyroid gland (Fig. 69.4). In GD, there is diffuse uptake in the thyroid gland.

Management of GD

The management of hyperthyroid GD can be divided into three broad categories: medical management, radioiodine treatment, and surgery.[18]

Medical management – antithyroid drugs

The thionamide drugs (carbimazole, its metabolite methimazole, and propylthiouracil) compete with Tg to act as substrates for iodination by TPO. Once iodinated, they are metabolized peripherally, depleting thyroid iodine stores. When the thyroid iodine stores are depleted and the intra-thyroidal thionamide concentration is high enough, thyroid hormone synthesis is abrogated. Most individuals become euthyroid following 4 to 8 weeks of treatment; however, euthyroidism may take longer to achieve in those with poor medication compliance or with a history of recent iodide exposure. Following initial treatment, thionamides may either be administered as a fixed high dose,

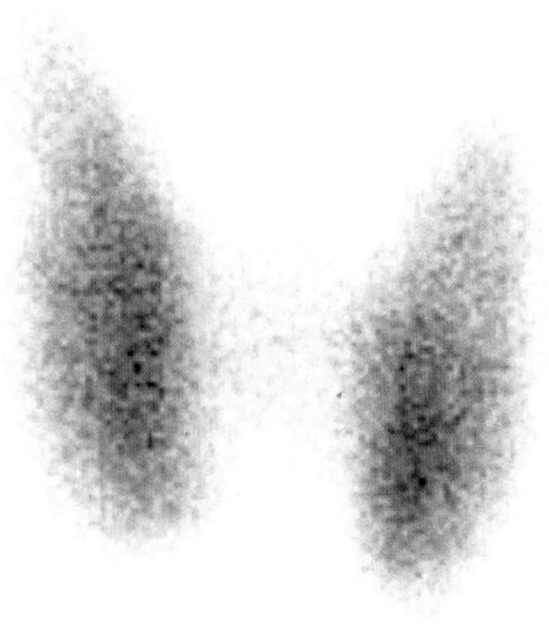

Fig. 69.4 ^{99}Tc pertechnetate radionuclide scan image from an individual with Graves' disease showing diffuse uptake throughout the thyroid gland.

with levothyroxine supplementation to prevent hypothyroidism (known as block-replace regimen) or at progressively lower doses, titrated to allow adequate thyroid hormone generation. Following 6 to 18 months of thionamide treatment about 50% of patients will remain in remission following cessation of therapy. There is no improvement in remission rate in individuals with GD who are treated for longer than 18 months. The mechanism of the thionamide-induced remission in GD remains obscure; however, the lymphocytic infiltrate in the GD thyroid is rapidly abolished by thionamide treatment. Serum TSH-R and TPO autoantibodies also decrease during treatment. It is telling that several induced murine models of thyroiditis can be ameliorated by thionamide treatment, suggesting an immunomodulatory role that is distinct from the anti-thyroid hormone synthesis action. If the patient relapses following medical treatment, definitive treatment should be considered, as a second course of thionamide treatment rarely induces prolonged remission.

Definitive treatment

Radioiodine therapy and surgical thyroidectomy are both efficacious treatments for GD, effectively removing functional thyroid tissue and leaving the patient hypothyroid. Radioiodine (^{131}I, RAI) therapy takes advantage of the thyroid's ability to concentrate iodine. RAI is administered orally and concentrates in the thyroid, primarily emitting beta radiation to produce local thyrocyte DNA damage. These cells then undergo necrotic change and the thyroid atrophies over the subsequent year. RAI renders more than 80% of those with GD hypothyroid and needing long-term thyroid hormone replacement. RAI is generally well-tolerated and long-term follow-up studies in adults are reassuring with regards to carcinogenicity. RAI is absolutely contraindicated in pregnancy and is best avoided in those with active, inflammatory GO.

Total or near-total thyroidectomy is also an effective treatment for GD and is particularly suitable for individuals with a large goiter, those with severe hyperthyroidism who cannot tolerate thionamides or with active GO in whom RAI is relatively contraindicated. The complications of thyroidectomy include change in voice due to intraoperative damage to the recurrent laryngeal nerve and hypocalcemia (often transient) due to parathyroid gland damage.

Graves' ophthalmopathy

Epidemiology

Graves' ophthalmopathy (GO) is the most common extrathyroidal manifestation of GD. It is clinically apparent in 25–50% of people presenting with GD, although almost all patients have radiological changes consistent with GO. The peak age of incidence is in the fifth and seventh decades of life. GO precedes thyroid gland dysfunction in about 20% of people, arises at the same time in 40%, and occurs after diagnosis of thyroid dysfunction in the other 40% of people. Males, the elderly, and smokers are more likely to have severe disease. Ninety-three percent of cases of GO occur in people with hyperthyroid GD. However, 3% of GO occurs in hypothyroid and 4% in euthyroid patients. A proportion of these "euthyroid Graves'" patients will eventually become hyperthyroid; however, some will remain hypothyroid or euthyroid despite the presence of TSH-R antibodies.

Etiology

GO shares many etiological factors with GD. Smoking is the major environmental risk factor for GO, with smokers or ex-smokers 4 times more likely to develop GO than lifelong non-smokers. In addition, the number of cigarettes smoked per day correlates with the risk of developing eye disease. RAI therapy is also known to occasionally cause flare-ups of GO, particularly if uncontrolled post-RAI hypothyroidism occurs. Smokers, and those with active GO, seem particularly susceptible to this complication.[19]

Immunopathogenesis

The molecular mechanism that links thyroid dysfunction with GO remains incompletely understood. The TSH-R is widely believed to be the primary autoantigen linking the thyroid and the orbit. Orbital fibroblasts (OFs) have been shown to express cell-surface TSH-R, and these are thought to be functional (TSH stimulation *in vitro* results in an increase in intracellular cAMP). Mechanistically, the orbital changes that occur in GO are better understood. TSH-R autoantibodies that bind to the TSH-R on OFs (or possibly other OF receptors such as the insulin-like growth factor receptor; IGF-1R) are believed to activate OFs to secrete cytokines and chemokines, which attract lymphocytes and other inflammatory cells. These infiltrate the orbital tissues, augmenting further the proinflammatory cytokine environment, causing OFs to proliferate and to secrete excessive glycosaminoglycans (GAGs).[20] GAGs accumulate in the extraocular muscles, increasing their size. These matrix molecules are also osmotically active, resulting in edema and swelling of surrounding tissues. In addition, the adaptive arm of the immune system is thought to interact via HLA and CD40 molecules expressed by the OFs to increase the presentation of autoantigens, perpetuating the cycle. The OFs are also thought to differentiate into adipocytes, resulting in increased retro-orbital fat deposition. The resulting inflammation gives rise to redness and edema of the orbital tissues, with the cellular proliferation and GAG accumulation producing proptosis, increased intraorbital pressure, and restriction of extraocular eye movements.[20]

Diagnosis and clinical presentation

When the clinical signs of GO are associated with thyroid dysfunction and/ or circulating thyroid autoantibodies the diagnosis is generally straightforward. If proptosis is completely unilateral, or GO features occur without upper lid retraction then the diagnosis needs to be confirmed by imaging. The patient may complain of gritty, watery or uncomfortable eyes, with or without a change in appearance (upper eyelid retraction, soft tissue swelling, redness of the eyes and proptosis) (Fig. 69.5). Diplopia occurs if eye movements are restricted by stiffness of the extraocular muscles or high intraorbital pressure. Deteriorating visual acuity and color desaturation are sinister symptoms in GO, indicating incipient optic neuropathy.

GO has a predictable and generally monophasic natural history (Fig. 69.6). There is an early phase of increasing disease activity at which medical therapy can be targeted, followed by a plateau phase. Then follows a gradual improvement until a stable, inactive phase is reached. GO manifestations can be classified in two ways: severity, which indicates the extent of functional, anatomical and cosmetic features; and activity, which

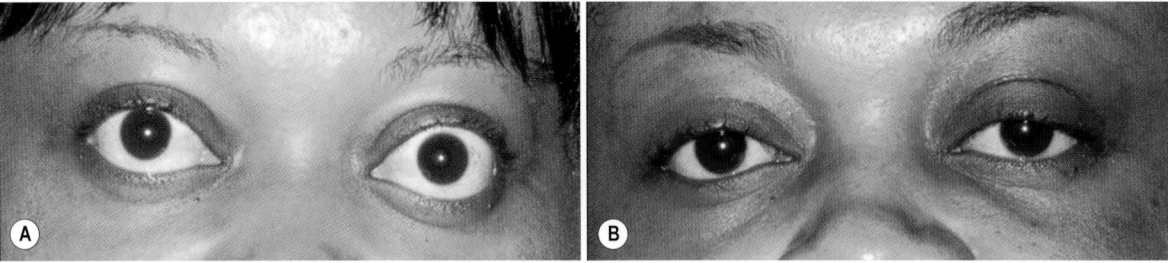

Fig. 69.5 (A) Clinical photograph of the eyes of an individual with Graves' ophthalmopathy prior to treatment. (B) Clinical photograph of the same patient's eyes following surgical orbital decompression and rehabilitative surgery.

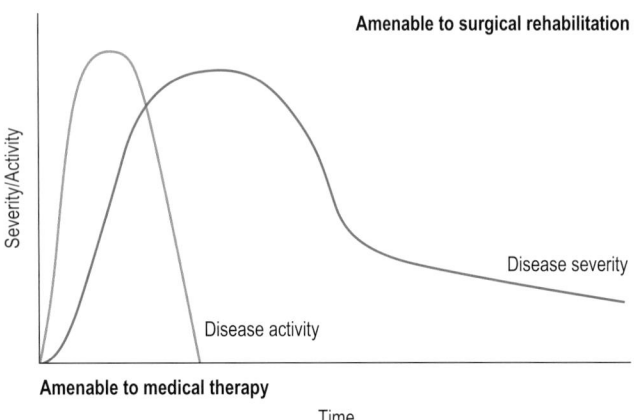

Fig. 69.6 Rundle's curve illustrating the natural history of GO.

denotes the intensity of any acute inflammatory reaction. Severity of GO is assessed using the "NO SPECS" classification system (Table 69.2, panel A). Activity is assessed using the clinical activity score (CAS) (Table 69.2, panel B). A score of 3 or more indicates active GO.[19] These classifications allow determination of which patients require treatment and which therapy is most appropriate.

Treatment

Patients with GD (with and without GO) should be strongly encouraged to stop smoking and offered smoking cessation support. The general health benefits are numerous and, in addition, smokers are more likely to relapse after a course of medical therapy compared to non-smokers. In parallel to restoring and maintaining euthyroidism, the successful treatment of GO depends on staging the activity and severity of the disease.

In patients with mild, active GO, an observational policy can be employed with symptomatic measures, such as artificial tears and dark glasses. In those with moderate, active and progressive GO, a course of oral or intravenous (IV) glucocorticoids is indicated. Orbital radiotherapy is also efficacious in people with active inflammation and diplopia. In people with optic neuropathy high dose IV steroids are used, and orbital pressure is relieved by urgent orbital decompression surgery. Eye ointments and protective eye pads are essential for patients whose eyelids do not close completely to protect against corneal damage and ulceration. Once disease activity has burned out, rehabilitative surgery can greatly improve the function and cosmetic appearance of the eyes. Orbital decompression, strabismus correction and eyelid surgery are commonly used procedures.[21]

Table 69.2 (A) The "NO SPECS" classification system to assess the severity of Graves' ophthalmopathy. (B) The Clinical Activity Score (CAS) to assess activity of Graves' ophthalmopathy

A: NO SPECS classification
Class 0—No signs or symptoms
Class 1—Only signs (limited to upper lid retraction and stare, with or without lid lag)
Class 2—Soft tissue involvement (edema of conjunctivae and lids, conjunctival injection, etc.)
Class 3—Proptosis
Class 4—Extraocular muscle involvement (usually with diplopia)
Class 5—Corneal involvement (primarily due to lagophthalmos, the inability to completely close the eyelids)
Class 6—Sight loss (due to optic nerve involvement)

B: CAS scoring system
A single point is scored for each of the features present. Each feature has equal weighting. A higher score indicates more active disease. 1. Spontaneous orbital pain 2. Gaze evoked orbital pain 3. Eyelid swelling that is considered to be due to active GO 4. Eyelid erythema 5. Conjunctival redness that is considered to be due to active GO 6. Chemosis 7. Inflammation of caruncle or plica 8. Increase of > 2 mm in proptosis 9. Decrease in uniocular ocular excursion in any one direction of > 8° 10. Decrease of acuity equivalent to 1 Snellen line

Future developments for Graves' hyperthyroidism and orbitopathy

Novel approaches to modulating the immune response in GD are starting to be considered. One trial has employed B-cell depletion therapy in individuals with relapse of hyperthyroid GD following conventional thionamide therapy. Other studies have employed either anti-TNF agents, such as etanercept,[22] or B-cell depletion therapy in patients with active GO, and from the limited available data these approaches seem potentially efficacious. Two randomized trials of B-cell depletion in GO are currently recruiting. A longer-term goal is the development of an anti-TSHR antibody or small molecule antagonist that could block binding of stimulatory TSHR Abs, or inhibit TSHR signaling, thus ameliorating the cause of hyperthyroidism.

Autoimmune hypothyroidism

The most common cause of autoimmune hypothyroidism (AH) is chronic (or lymphocytic) autoimmune thyroiditis. There are two variants, atrophic and goitrous (Hashimoto's thyroiditis).

Epidemiology

In populations living in iodine sufficient areas, AH is common, affecting between 1 and 10% of the population. The prevalence increases with age, with 3–20% of individuals over 75 years old being hypothyroid. AH is more common in women than in men. In a UK community survey, the incidence of hypothyroidism in women was 3.5/1000/year which increased to 13.7/1000/year in women aged between 75 and 80 years. In men, the incidence was just 0.6/1000/year.[23]

Etiology

AH, like GD, is a complex genetic condition. Familial clustering provides evidence for a genetic etiology, which in several studies appears stronger than that for GD. The λs for AH is estimated to be between 10 and 45. Families frequently have different individuals affected by AH and GD, suggesting some shared genetic factors. The differing prevalences of AH in different ethnic groups, with AH being more common in Caucasian than in black populations also supports a genetic background. Knowledge about the genetics of AH is limited, with the majority of studies carried out being small and under-powered, and putative associations at several loci have not been replicated in follow-up studies. The loci that have been associated with AH to date are summarized below.

The MHC class II *DR3*, *DR4*, and *DR5* alleles have been associated with AH in Caucasians only. Conflicting results have been reported for *HLA-DQ* alleles. One study reported that the *HLA-DQ* alleles *DQA1*0301* and *DQB1*0201* confer susceptibility to AH in Caucasians, with certain *HLA-DQ* alleles (*DQA1*0102* and *DQB1*0602*) reported to confer a protective effect. These data highlight the need to further investigate the MHC region to clarify its role in AH susceptibility.

In common with GD, the *CTLA-4* gene also appears to influence AH susceptibility. Three *CTLA-4* polymorphisms have been associated with AH in a number of populations. An A/G SNP located downstream of the 3'UTR (designated CT60), an A/G polymorphism at codon 17, and a 106-bp microsatellite repeat in the 3'UTR of exon 3. A locus on Chr. 8q24 containing the thyroglobulin gene was linked to AH and number of SNPs were subsequently studied in AH individuals with modest reported odds ratios for association of between 1.32 and 1.56. Other loci implicated in AH susceptibility include the tumour necrosis factor (TNFα) gene, *PTPN22*, *CYP27B1*, T-cell receptor (TCR) genes, and several immunoglobulin genes and cytokine regulatory genes.

In contrast to GD, environmental factors in AH susceptibility have been challenging to identify. However, the role of iodine is widely accepted, since population studies have reported an increase in the prevalence of thyroid lymphocytic infiltration and autoantibodies following public health salt iodization programs. Infectious agents have also been implicated in susceptibility to AH. Several studies have identified an increased prevalence of IgG and/or IgA antibodies to virulence-associated outer membrane proteins of *Yersinia enterocolitica* in AH patients and in relatives of people with AH, suggesting that susceptibility genes for *Yersinia* infection may also confer risk for AH.

The effect of radiation, either "internal" (nuclear "fallout" or from RAI treatment) or "external" (radiotherapy or direct exposure during a nuclear accident), on AH susceptibility has been extensively studied. Following the Chernobyl accident, a rise in thyroid autoantibodies was noted 15 years following exposure; however, this was not accompanied by thyroid dysfunction.[24] Long-term follow-up studies of thyroid function in Japanese survivors of Nagasaki and Hiroshima have demonstrated a clear link between radiation exposure and thyroid cancer; however, the association with AH remains disputed. One study, at 40 years follow-up, demonstrated a significant relationship between dose of radiation exposure at Nagasaki and AH. However, a further study, at more than 50 years of follow-up, showed that radiation exposure did not correlate with either the occurrence of thyroid autoantibodies or AH.[25]

Immunopathogenesis

The mechanisms by which tolerance to thyroid antigens is lost in the first instance remain obscure. It appears that both a susceptible genetic background and a permissive environment are required before AH develops. Notably, AH is much more frequent in the autoimmune polyendocrinopathy type 1 (APECED) syndrome than GD, suggesting that central thymic T-cell selection, and therefore central tolerance, may be more important in AH than in GD. Histologically, lymphocytic infiltrates can be seen in the thyroid, consisting of both T and B cells (Fig. 69.7). These infiltrates can be diffuse or focal. Scarring and fibrosis may also be seen, with destruction of the normal thyroid architecture and an absence of colloid in thyroid follicles.

Both cell-mediated and humoral immune mechanisms are important in the continuing thyroid damage seen in AH. T cells are known to play a pivotal role in both the initiation and perpetuation of AH. Studies in which researchers induced hypothyroidism in *Rag1*-deficient transgenic mice that were unable to produce autoantibodies confirm this.[26] T cells respond to antigen presenting cells (APCs) and release cytotoxic and lytic factors, which result in thyrocyte death. Thyroid follicular cells have themselves been demonstrated to express HLA class II molecules, suggesting that they may also have a direct role in antigen presentation.

The humoral immune response is also important in AH. More than 90% of individuals with AH have detectable TPO antibodies. Autoantibodies directed against Tg, and to a lesser degree the TSH-R, are also commonly detected. *In vitro*, TPO

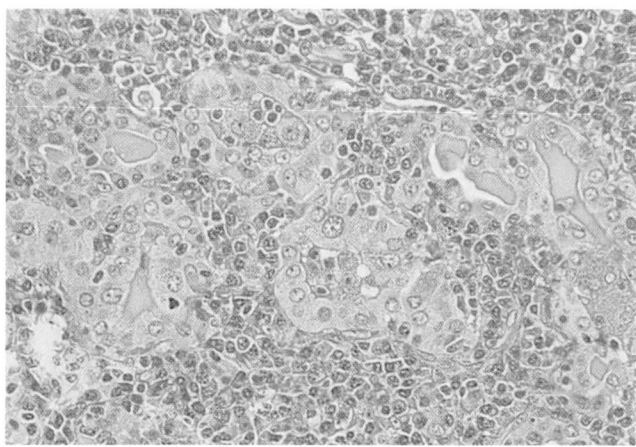

Fig. 69.7 Lymphocytic infiltration of the thyroid in a patient with autoimmune hypothyroidism.

antibodies can fix complement and directly induce cell damage.[17] Their presence within thyroid follicles in AH patients suggests they may have the same effect *in vivo*, although the thyrocyte destruction found in the *Rag1*-deficient mouse suggests TPO antibodies are not necessary for AH. Interestingly, the epitopes toward which TPO antibodies are directed in both GD and AH are overlapping and there is no disease specificity for the targeted TPO domain.[17] The TSH-R autoantibodies found in some patients with AH are likely to exert a blocking or antagonist effect, thus inducing hypothyroidism. As thyroid hormone secretion falls, increasing thyrocyte stimulation by elevation of serum TSH may induce or augment thyroid auto-antigen expression (e.g., TPO, Tg), thereby perpetuating the autoimmune response.

Clinical presentation

Hypothyroidism can result in changes in almost every organ system in the body (Table 69.3). Initially, the signs and symptoms may be subtle and non-specific and hypothyroidism is frequently diagnosed incidentally following blood tests for another problem.

The typical goiter palpable in Hashimoto's thyroiditis is moderate in size and firm with a finely granular surface. Individuals often report a gradual increase in size over a number of years. However, rapid growth is unusual. In atrophic AH, the size of the thyroid gland is reduced.

Investigation and diagnosis

Hypothyroidism is detected biochemically by a raised serum TSH with reduced fT4. AH is differentiated from other forms of hypothyroidism by the presence of circulating autoantibodies, including TPO and Tg. On ultrasound scanning, the thyroid gland appears homogeneous and hypoechoic; a change that predates serum autoantibody positivity in some. A fine needle aspirate demonstrates lymphocytes and Hürthle cells, but this investigation is generally only indicated if a discrete nodule is present.

Reflecting the effects of hypothyroidism on multiple organ systems, many biochemical and hematological abnormalities are also commonly detected in patients with AH, such as mild anemia, hyponatremia or elevated serum creatine kinase, transaminases, lactate dehydrogenase, and low-density lipoprotein (LDL) cholesterol.

Management

AH requires lifelong treatment with thyroid hormone replacement therapy. The most commonly prescribed is synthetic thyroxine, levothyroxine (L-T4), which is widely available and inexpensive. Except for individuals with known heart disease or the very elderly, a full, weight-related replacement dose (~1.6 µg/kg/d) should be started. Once the patient is on a stable dose, thyroid function should be assessed annually to ensure that the patient continues to receive the appropriate dose. Some commonly prescribed medications such as calcium and iron supplements, and proton pump inhibitors interfere with the absorption of L-T4, and patients should be advised to take these at least 4 hours before or after their L-T4 to ensure maximum absorption.

Table 69.3 Common and rare clinical manifestations of hypothyroidism

Common	Rare
Neuropsychiatric	
Lethargy	Cerebellar ataxia
Impaired cognitive function	Deafness
Slow speech	Psychosis
Depression	
Gastrointestinal	
Anorexia	Ascites
Weight gain	
Constipation and bloating	
Abnormal liver function tests	
Cardiorespiratory	
Shortness of breath on exertion	Pericardial effusion
Reduced exercise tolerance	
Bradycardia	
Diastolic hypertension	
Cardiomegaly	
Low voltage ECG	
Peripheral edema (non-pitting)	
Genitourinary	
Oligomenorrhea, amennorhea, menorrhagia	
Reduced libido	
Early fetal loss	
Impotence	
Cutaneous	
Cold intolerance	
Skin dryness and thickening	
Malar flush	
Edema of the face, hands and feet	
Change in face shape	
Pallor	
Nail abnormalities	
Alopecia	
Musculoskeletal	
Bradykinesia	
Joint and muscular pains	
Delayed relaxation of tendon reflexes	
Miscellaneous	
Goiter (in Hashimoto's thyroiditis)	
Reduced basal metabolic rate	
Increased sensitivity to exogenous insulin	
Abnormal lipid metabolism	

Subclinical hypothyroidism

While the need to treat individuals with overt AH is universally accepted, it is unclear whether thyroid hormone replacement is beneficial in individuals with persistent subclinical hypothyroidism (serum TSH raised, but fT4 and fT3 within the normal reference range on at least two separate occasions). Progression to overt hypothyroidism from this state occurs in about 2% of individuals per year who are TPO antibody negative, rising to 5% per year if antibodies are present. Observational data confirm an increase in vascular disease mortality in population cohorts with subclinical hypothyroidism. However, no large randomized trials of thyroxine treatment have been carried out, and smaller studies have generally failed to show a convincing benefit of treating those with subclinical disease. Due to the lack of evidence for treating those with subclinical disease, a pragmatic approach is often applied by clinicians. For example, many endocrinologists offer a trial of L-T4 to those who appear to be symptomatic to determine if their symptoms improve. In addition, all patients with an elevated TSH should be treated during pregnancy and many physicians elect to treat patients with goiter, severe dyslipidemia or other significant cardiovascular risk factors.[27]

Future developments

The genetics of AH remain understudied considering its frequency as the commonest autoimmune disease in man. Considerable work remains to be done on whether treatment of subclinical hypothyroidism is beneficial. Given the insidious nature of the development of AH, it remains a good target for a preventative immunotherapeutic intervention, if a safe and economic treatment can be found.

Other forms of thyroiditis

The term thyroiditis relates to conditions resulting in inflammation of the thyroid gland. A number of etiologies have been described, including infection, radiation exposure, drug-induced, and autoimmune. A common pattern to the natural history of several thyroiditides is frequently seen, involving an initial thyrotoxic phase of 1 to 3 months, followed by a rapid drop in serum thyroid hormones and a transient hypothyroid phase, often lasting another 1 to 4 months. During the thyrotoxic phase, pre-formed thyroid hormone stores are released from the thyroid follicles, leading to thyrotoxicosis, which may be severe. The hypothyroid phase follows when these pre-formed stores are exhausted and the thyroid has become depleted of hormones. In about 90% of cases this hypothyroidism is transient, but in some cases it never resolves.

Post-partum thyroiditis

Post-partum thyroiditis (PPT) is a common endocrine condition, which manifests within 1 year following pregnancy. It affects between 5 and 10% of women in the general population.[28] PPT is classically a biphasic disorder, consisting of a period of transient thyrotoxicosis (median onset 12–14 weeks post-partum) followed by a period of transient hypothyroidism (median onset 18–20 weeks post-partum); however, a monophasic (thyrotoxicosis or hypothyroidism alone) or reversed biphasic (hypothyroidism then thyrotoxicosis) pattern can also occur. During pregnancy, there is a state of relative immune tolerance, followed by a rebound in immune function following delivery, coinciding with the occurrence of PPT. The presence of thyroid autoantibodies and a lymphocytic infiltrate on thyroid biopsy supports an autoimmune basis for this condition.[28]

Clinically, the thyrotoxic phase of PPT is often mild, resulting in symptoms of fatigue and irritability, which can be misdiagnosed as postnatal depression. If the thyrotoxic episode is short, it may even go unnoticed. Neck pain is not a feature. Women with PPT who are thyrotoxic may benefit from a beta-blocker such as propranolol for symptom relief. Anti-thyroid drugs are not effective as the thyrotoxicosis is due to release of preformed thyroid hormones. Following the episode of thyroid dysfunction, 10 to 20% of women remain permanently hypothyroid.[28] In women who have had PPT and then recovered, an annual assessment of thyroid function is recommended, as their risk of long-term hypothyroidism is considerable.[29] In those women who return to being euthyroid, there is a 75% risk of PPT in subsequent pregnancies and a 50% risk of permanent hypothyroidism at 7 years.[29]

Translational research

ON THE HORIZON

New approaches to therapy of Graves' disease

- Novel immunotherapeutic agents for Graves' orbitopathy.
- Anti-TSH receptor blocking antibodies for control of hyperthyroid Graves' disease.
- Small molecule TSH receptor antagonists for management of hyperthyroidism in Graves' disease.

The major challenge of the next 5–10 years is to take novel immunotherapeutic agents, including "biologicals" that have been developed for rheumatic disorders into the clinical arena for autoimmune thyroid diseases. The primary target of these efforts should be Graves' orbitopathy, which remains a disfiguring condition, often with substantial functional impairment of vision and associated low quality of life. While there are currently trials of B lymphocyte-depleting agents underway, other powerful agents need to be investigated as this remains a disorder with no wholly satisfactory treatment. Early diagnosis of Graves' orbitopathy and development of markers that predict progressive or severe disease will also be helpful in identifying people for early intervention.

The development of anti-TSH receptor blocking antibodies as a therapeutic agent for hyperthyroid Graves' disease seems likely. These agents might have a role in people unlikely to gain medical remission from thionamide antithyroid drugs, or in those for whom rapid control of hyperthyroidism is desirable. Small molecule TSH receptor antagonists may also come to the clinic, with a similar role.

References

1. Tunbridge WM, Evered DC, Hall R, et al. The spectrum of thyroid disease in a community: the Whickham survey. Clin Endocrinol (Oxf) 1977;7(6):481–93.
2. Laurberg P, Pedersen KM, Vestergaard H, Sigurdsson G. High incidence of multinodular toxic goitre in the elderly population in a low iodine intake area vs. high incidence of Graves' disease in the young in a high iodine intake area: comparative surveys of thyrotoxicosis epidemiology in East-Jutland Denmark and Iceland. J Intern Med 1991;229(5):415–20.
3. Brix TH, Kyvik KO, Christensen K, Hegedüs L. Evidence for a major role of heredity in Graves' disease: a population-based study of two Danish twin cohorts. J Clin Endocrinol Metab 2001;86(2):930–4.
4. Vaidya B, Kendall-Taylor P, Pearce SH. The genetics of autoimmune thyroid disease. J Clin Endocrinol Metab 2002;87(12):5385–97.
5. Eschler DC, Hasham A, Tomer Y. Cutting edge: the etiology of autoimmune thyroid diseases. Clin Rev Allergy Immunol 2011;41(2):190–7.

6. Ueda H, Howson JM, Esposito L, et al. Association of the T-cell regulatory gene CTLA4 with susceptibility to autoimmune disease. Nature 2003;423(6939):506–11.

7. Velaga MR, Wilson V, Jennings CE, et al. The codon 620 tryptophan allele of the lymphoid tyrosine phosphatase (LYP) gene is a major determinant of Graves' disease. J Clin Endocrinol Metab 2004;89(11):5862–5.

8. Brent GA. Environmental exposures and autoimmune thyroid disease. Thyroid 2010;20(7):755–61.

9. Vestergaard P. Smoking and thyroid disorders—a meta-analysis. Eur J Endocrinol 2002;146(2):153–61.

10. Cawood TJ, Moriarty P, O'Farrelly C, O'Shea D. Smoking and thyroid-associated ophthalmopathy: A novel explanation of the biological link. J Clin Endocrinol Metab 2007;92(1):59–64.

11. Winsa B, Adami HO, Bergström R, et al. Stressful life events and Graves' disease. Lancet 1991;338(8781):1475–9.

12. Matos-Santos A, Nobre EL, Costa JG, et al. Relationship between the number and impact of stressful life events and the onset of Graves' disease and toxic nodular goitre. Clin Endocrinol (Oxf) 2001;55(1):15–9.

13. Chen F, Day SL, Metcalfe RA, et al. Characteristics of autoimmune thyroid disease occurring as a late complication of immune reconstitution in patients with advanced human immunodeficiency virus (HIV) disease. Medicine (Baltimore) 2005;84(2):98–106.

14. Smith BR, Bolton J, Young S, et al. A new assay for thyrotropin receptor autoantibodies. Thyroid 2004;14(10):830–5.

15. Czarnocka B. Thyroperoxidase, thyroglobulin, Na(+)/I(-) symporter, pendrin in thyroid autoimmunity. Front Biosci 2011;16:783–802.

16. Costagliola S, Bonomi M, Morgenthaler NG, et al. Delineation of the discontinuous-conformational epitope of a monoclonal antibody displaying full in vitro and in vivo thyrotropin activity. Mol Endocrinol 2004;18(12):3020–34.

17. McLachlan SM, Rapoport B. Thyroid peroxidase as an autoantigen. Thyroid 2007;17(10):939–48.

18. Hegedus L. Treatment of Graves' hyperthyroidism: evidence-based and emerging modalities. Endocrinol Metab Clin North Am 2009;38(2):355–71 ix.

19. Cawood T, Moriarty P, O'Shea D. Recent developments in thyroid eye disease. BMJ 2004;329(7462):385–90.

20. Bahn RS. Graves' ophthalmopathy. N Engl J Med 2010;362(8):726–38.

21. Bartalena L, Baldeschi L, Dickinson A, et al. Consensus statement of the European Group on Graves' orbitopathy (EUGOGO) on management of GO. Eur J Endocrinol 2008;158(3):273–85.

22. Paridaens D, van den Bosch WA, van der Loos TL, et al. The effect of etanercept on Graves' ophthalmopathy: a pilot study. Eye 2005;19(12):1286–9.

23. Vanderpump MP, Tunbridge WM, French JM, et al. The incidence of thyroid disorders in the community: a twenty-year follow-up of the Whickham Survey. Clin Endocrinol (Oxf) 1995;43(1):55–68.

24. Agate L, Mariotti S, Elisei R, et al. Thyroid autoantibodies and thyroid function in subjects exposed to Chernobyl fallout during childhood: evidence for a transient radiation-induced elevation of serum thyroid antibodies without an increase in thyroid autoimmune disease. J Clin Endocrinol Metab 2008;93(7):2729–36.

25. Imaizumi M, Usa T, Tominaga T, et al. Radiation dose-response relationships for thyroid nodules and autoimmune thyroid diseases in Hiroshima and Nagasaki atomic bomb survivors 55-58 years after radiation exposure. JAMA 2006;295(9):1011–22.

26. Quaratino S, Badami E, Pang YY, et al. Degenerate self-reactive human T-cell receptor causes spontaneous autoimmune disease in mice. Nat Med 2004;10(9):920–6.

27. Vaidya B, Pearce SH. Management of hypothyroidism in adults. BMJ 2008;337:a801.

28. Landek-Salgado MA, Gutenberg A, Lupi I, et al. Pregnancy, postpartum autoimmune thyroiditis, and autoimmune hypophysitis: intimate relationships. Autoimmun Rev 2010;9(3):153–7.

29. Stagnaro-Green A. Clinical review 152: Postpartum thyroiditis. J Clin Endocrinol Metab 2002;87(9):4042–7.

30. Davies TF, Ando T, Lin RY, et al. Thyrotropin receptor-associated diseases: from adenomata to Graves' disease. J Clin Invest 2005;115:1972–83.

70

Diabetes and related autoimmune diseases

George
S. Eisenbarth

Diabetes mellitus is a heterogeneous group of disorders characterized by glucose intolerance and hyperglycemia. The clinical manifestations of this disease are the result of either an absolute or a relative deficiency of insulin secretion. An expert committee of the American Diabetes Association proposed four categories of diabetes, based on etiology rather than the age of disease onset (e.g., juvenile-onset versus adult-onset) or the requirement for insulin therapy (insulin-dependent versus noninsulin-dependent) (Table 70.1).[1] Type 1 diabetes is divided into types 1A (immune mediated) and 1B (idiopathic loss of insulin secretion), depending primarily on the presence or absence respectively of anti-islet autoantibodies.

The subject of this chapter is type 1A or immune-mediated diabetes, and there is now convincing evidence that this form results from immune-mediated destruction of the cells that produce insulin. Despite older designations for this category, approximately the same number of adults develop type 1A diabetes as do children, and many individuals early in the course of type 1A diabetes are not "insulin dependent" but can transiently be treated with oral hypoglycemic agents. The incidence of type 2 diabetes increases dramatically with age, whereas that of type 1A changes relatively little with age (less than three-fold).[2] Thus, when a child develops diabetes they usually (>90% for non-Hispanic white children) have type 1A diabetes mellitus. The information indicating that type 1A diabetes is an immune-mediated autoimmune illness has greatly increased. The recognition that there might be a form of "juvenile" or insulin-dependent diabetes of autoimmune origin came from the observation that diabetes was often associated with disorders thought to be of autoimmune origin, such as Addison's disease, Graves' disease and thyroiditis.

KEY CONCEPTS

Type 1A diabetes is an autoimmune disease

- Genetic and familial clustering of diabetes and additional autoimmune disorders.
- Presence of high-affinity autoantibodies and T cells reactive to islet cell autoantigens.
- Strong HLA association (DR3/DR4)
- Ability to transfer the disease in animal models through adoptive transfer of islet cell-reactive T-cell clones.
- Recurrence of disease in pancreas transplanted between identical twins.
- Regulatory T cells important; their loss in IPEX syndrome leads to neonatal diabetes.

Studies of monozygotic twins with diabetes revealed very different patterns of inheritance for insulin-dependent and noninsulin-dependent diabetes mellitus, and two major forms of the disease were proposed. Specific HLA alleles were found to be associated with the insulin-dependent form,[3] and in 1974 cytoplasmic islet cell autoantibodies were found for diabetic patients with polyendocrine autoimmunity (e.g., Addison's disease).[4] Islet cell autoantibodies were then found to be present prior to the development of diabetes, and studies of monozygotic twins of patients with type 1 diabetes led to the observation that this was a chronically progressive autoimmune disorder. In identical twins developing diabetes, islet cell autoantibodies and loss of insulin secretion preceded the development of diabetes by years. As discussed below, the measurement of anti-islet autoantibodies has improved dramatically during the past two decades, and for many individuals the development of type 1A diabetes can now be predicted.

Despite the emphasis on anti-islet autoantibodies, most investigators believe that T cells, and not autoantibodies, mediate the immune destruction of insulin-producing cells.[5] Studies of T cells have benefited from the discovery of two animal models of type 1A diabetes, the NOD mouse and the BB rat.[5] In animal models diabetes can be transferred to nondiabetic animals by T-cell clones. In addition, a clinical observation by Sutherland and co-workers was particularly informative in terms of demonstrating the importance of T cells in this disease.[6] They transplanted the tail of the pancreas from monozygotic twins who had not developed diabetes into their respective twin mates with more than a decade of diabetes. The transplanted islets were invaded by lymphocytes, and islet β cells (the cells that produce insulin) were specifically and rapidly destroyed.

Despite considerable progress in studies of type 1A diabetes, a series of basic and clinical questions remain unanswered or have only partial answers (Table 70.2). This chapter reviews current knowledge concerning many of these questions.

Diagnosis

The demonstration of elevated plasma glucose and/or HbA1c is the *sine qua non* for diagnosis of diabetes mellitus. Recent recommendations by the American Diabetes Association have lowered the diagnostic level of fasting glucose from 140 mg/dL (7.8 mmol/L) to 126 mg/dL (7.0 mmol/L). Other diagnostic criteria include a random plasma glucose level >200 mg/dL (11.1 mmol/dL) or a plasma glucose level >200 mg/dL (11.1 mmol/dL) 2 hours after ingestion of 75 g oral glucose (the oral glucose tolerance test—OGTT). In addition, HbA1c ≥7.5 (glycosylated hemoglobin reflecting 3 month average glucose level) is diagnostic of diabetes.

Table 70.1 Classification of diabetes mellitus (DM)

Diabetes mellitus	Previous designations	Etiologic distinctions	Clinical distinctions
Type 1 A. Immune-mediated B. Idiopathic	Fulminant Juvenile onset/IDDM Type 1.5/Flatbush DM	β-cell destruction Immune Unknown	Both result in insulin deficiency, with loss of β-cells
Type 2	NIDDM	Insulin resistance and relative insulin deficiency	Oral hypoglycemic agents are effective early in the disease
Other specific types	MODY/Monogenic secondary diabetes	Specific genetic defects Pancreatic disease Endocrinopathies Chemical induced Infection related Immune-mediated forms Genetic syndromes	Specific mutations identified and defined clinical syndromes
Gestational	Unchanged		Onset during pregnancy

IDDM, insulin-dependent diabetes; MODY, maturity-onset diabetes of youth; NIDDM, non-insulin dependent diabetes.

Table 70.2 Key questions in type 1A diabetes

Basic science questions

What genes determine type 1A diabetes susceptibility?
What triggers or suppresses the activation of autoimmunity?
What are the major target molecules and is there a primary autoantigen?
What are the effector mechanisms for islet destruction?

Clinical questions

Is type 1A diabetes predictable?
Is the rate of progression to overt diabetes predictable?
Is type 1A diabetes preventable?

The clinical signs and symptoms associated with hyperglycemia and osmotic diuresis (e.g., polyuria and polydipsia) are recognized by clinicians and lay people alike, making the diagnosis relatively straightforward. Insulin deficiency, if untreated, leads to the utilization of fats for fuel, with subsequent metabolism of fatty acids and the production of ketoacids. Thus, the presentation of ketonuria, ketonemia, and ketoacidosis, often associated with nausea or hyperventilation, is an important clinical feature. Unexplained weight loss, along with the classic signs and symptoms mentioned above, is highly suggestive of the diagnosis of diabetes. Despite the classic signs and symptoms, approximately 1 in 200 children die at the onset of type 1 diabetes. If the first healthcare provider to see the child fails to make a diagnosis of diabetes, the child may subsequently present with severe ketoacidosis and may develop cerebral edema, which is often fatal.

CLINICAL PEARLS

- Type 1A diabetes can occur at any age. Testing of islet cell autoantibodies identifies 10% of adults (thought to have type 2 diabetes) as having type 1A diabetes.
- Half of African American and Hispanic American children are negative for anti-islet autoantibodies and have type 2 or type 1B diabetes.
- Organ-specific autoimmunity (in particular celiac disease, thyroid disease, Addison's disease and pernicious anemia) is greatly increased in patients with type 1A diabetes.
- The more common the organ-specific autoimmune disease in the general population, the more common the disease in patients with type 1A diabetes. For example, thyroid autoimmunity is common and routine TSH testing is advised.
- In diabetic patients with decreasing insulin need or severe hypoglycemia, rule out Addison's disease.

The diagnosis of specific diabetic syndromes, including type 1A diabetes, requires further information. Several clinical criteria increase or reduce the probability that an individual has type 1A diabetes (e.g., increase: onset at age <35, nonobese, presence of ketoacidosis, immediate therapy with insulin required, family or personal history of organ-specific autoimmunity; decrease: age of onset >35, effective therapy with oral hypoglycemic agents, African American or Hispanic American child, obesity). These clinical criteria are, however, imprecise guidelines at best. For example, as many as 10% of obese white adults presenting with diabetes have type 1A. The hallmark of type 1 versus type 2 diabetes is the early (several years after diagnosis) development of severe insulin deficiency. The connecting peptide (C-peptide) of the proinsulin molecule is secreted in equimolar quantity to insulin by pancreatic β cells. Within 3 years of the onset of type 1A diabetes, most children have a severe impairment of insulin secretion with low C-peptide. The range of C-peptide secretion, however, is large at the onset in both types 1 and 2 diabetes. Secretion is influenced by metabolic control, such that determination of C-peptide at onset has limited diagnostic utility in distinguishing type 1 from type 2 diabetes. The maintenance of C-peptide secretion can also be used as a measure of effective immunotherapy in clinical trials.

It should be recognized that both type 1A and type 2 diabetes are relatively common disorders, and thus individuals might have both diseases. Type 2 diabetes would be manifested by resistance to insulin, such that overt hyperglycemia will present earlier in the course of the islet β-cell destruction associated with type 1A diabetes. It has been proposed ("accelerator hypothesis") that type 1A and type 2 diabetes both result from metabolic changes associated with insulin resistance, and that type 1A represents a more severe form of diabetes with anti-islet autoimmunity. Data leading to this hypothesis are slightly faster growth and higher body mass index (BMI) in children who develop type 1A diabetes. Given the improved knowledge of the genetics of type 1A diabetes with multiple immune genetic polymorphisms influencing risk, it is unlikely that insulin resistance is a major factor in the initiation of islet autoimmunity,[7] although insulin resistance is likely to reveal overt hyperglycemia earlier in the course of immune-mediated β-cell destruction

The best immunologic marker for distinguishing type 1A from other forms of diabetes is the presence of islet cell autoantibodies. Diagnostic accuracy depends on the sensitivity and specificity of the autoantibody assays employed. Assays for autoantibodies reacting with insulin, glutamic acid decarboxylase (GAD65), ICA512 (IA-2), and ZnT8, when performed with fluid-phase assays (not ELISA), can be set such that fewer than 1 in 100 non-diabetic individuals are positive. One or another of these three autoantibodies is present in approximately 95% of children with recent-onset type 1A diabetes. However, approximately half of Hispanic American children presenting with diabetes do not express any of the four anti-islet antibodies (compared to approximately 10% of non-Hispanic white children). We believe that the majority of the antibody-negative population represent a type 2 diabetes variant, although there are important genetic variants, including half of neonatal diabetes determined by mutations of the sulfonylurea receptor Kir6.2 gene and multiple MODY (maturity onset diabetes of the young) genes.[8] Approximately 10% of children lacking all islet autoantibodies at diagnosis have non-autoimmune monogenic forms of diabetes.

Epidemiology/incidence

KEY CONCEPTS

Epidemiology and incidence of type 1A diabetes

- One of the most common chronic diseases of childhood and the most common type of diabetes in persons under 40 years of age.
- A leading cause of blindness, amputations, and end-stage renal disease, and contributes to premature death.
- Peak age of onset is 12–13 years, but may occur at any age, in all racial groups, with equal prevalence between males and females.
- More children are diagnosed in the fall and winter months, but it is likely that this reflects factors that bring children to medical attention.
- The incidence of type 1A diabetes has been increasing in many countries.
- No conclusive evidence exists for an association between vaccination and incidence of type 1A diabetes.

Type 1A diabetes is one of the most common chronic diseases of childhood and is the most common type of diabetes in persons under 40. Diabetes is the leading cause of blindness, amputations and end-stage renal disease, and is a major factor contributing to cardiovascular disease and premature death. It typically presents in children (with a peak onset at 12–13 years of age), but it may occur at any age and in all racial groups, with approximately similar prevalence in both females and males.

The annual incidence of type 1A diabetes varies dramatically. In children the incidence is approximately 15/100 000 in the United States, 35/100 000 in Finland, and fewer than 1/100 000 in Japan. The prevalence in the USA is approximately 1/300, and 90% of children developing diabetes do not have a first-degree relative with the disorder. Approximately 1/20 first-degree relatives of patients develop the disease. The risk to offspring of a father with type 1A diabetes is approximately twice that of offspring of an affected mother. In the US, non-Hispanic white Americans are approximately 1.5 times more likely to develop type 1A diabetes than are other groups.

The prevalence of type 1A diabetes is greatest in countries where the predominant population is Caucasian. For example, it is most prevalent in Finland and Sardinia and rare in Japan, Korea, and China. A child in Finland has a 35 times greater risk of developing diabetes than a child in Japan. In Japan, for example, monozygotic twins of patients with type 1A diabetes and their first-degree

relatives have a risk of diabetes similar to that of twins and relatives in the USA. This suggests that the bulk of differences between countries relates to genetic differences and not environmental factors. Studies of migrant populations from developed countries have failed to reveal major differences in the incidence of diabetes based on migration from a high-incidence to a lower-incidence country. Nevertheless, there are less well characterized populations where the incidence may have changed dramatically with migration, e.g., Yemenite Jews migrating to Israel.

Seasonal variations in the incidence of type 1A diabetes have been well documented, with more children presenting with the disease in the fall and winter months. This seasonal variation has been ascribed to potential viral infections that destroy β cells; however, with increased knowledge of the natural history of type 1A diabetes it is more likely that such seasonal variation may simply reflect factors (such as viral infections) that either bring children to medical attention or produce insulin resistance when limited islet β-cell mass remains.

Natural history

Studies over the past decade in humans are defining details of the chronology of development of type 1A diabetes. In addition, studies in animal models have contributed to a greater understanding of the pathogenesis of the disease. At present, there are three major hypotheses (described below) concerning the natural history of type 1A diabetes, with a fourth having almost no supporters. The fourth hypothesis, which was prominent two decades ago, was that type 1A diabetes was an acute disorder induced by viral infection. If the development of diabetes is acute it is likely to be extremely rare, given studies of both relatives and the general population. Anti-islet autoantibodies almost always precede diabetes by years, as does the loss of first-phase insulin secretion.[9] In Asian countries, approximately 10% of type 1 patients have fulminant diabetes with near normal HbA1c at diagnosis and severe hyperglycemia likely resulting from viral infection and immune-mediated β-cell destruction despite usual lack of islet autoantibodies.[10]

- Hypothesis 1: Type 1A diabetes is a chronic and progressive disorder resulting from immune-mediated destruction of islet β cells.[11] A corollary of this hypothesis is that as immunologic and immunogenetic assays are refined, one should be able to predict both the risk of diabetes and the approximate time of progression to diabetes, with different individuals progressing at different rates. This hypothesis is encapsulated in the division of type 1A diabetes into a series of stages (I, genetic susceptibility; II, triggering of autoimmunity; III, active immunity; IV, loss of insulin secretion; and V, overt diabetes) (Fig. 70.1).[11]
- Hypothesis 2: Type 1A diabetes is preceded by a long prodromal phase of autoimmunity, but actual islet β-cell destruction is acute and occurs at the end of the process.
- Hypothesis 3: Type 1A diabetes results from "multiple" hits, perhaps viral, and thus develops slowly, but would be difficult to predict as the "hits" are not predictable.[12]

It is possible that a combination of all three hypotheses will eventually be found to apply to different individuals developing diabetes. For example, an identical twin with diabetes who receives half of the pancreas from their non-diabetic twin rapidly develops recurrent diabetes within several weeks.[6] Thus, the immune system has the potential to rapidly destroy human β cells. Nevertheless, there is considerable evidence that the first hypothesis is generally applicable. It reflects the progressive loss

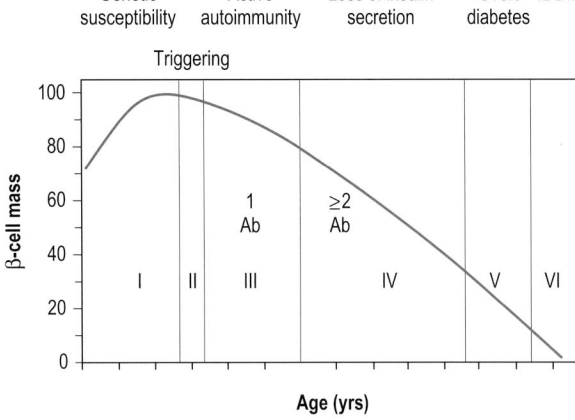

Fig. 70.1 Stages in the development of type 1A diabetes.
From Eisenbarth GS. Type I diabetes mellitus. A chronic autoimmune disease. N Engl J Med 1986; 314: 1360.

Table 70.3 High-risk and protective HLA haplotypes

High risk			
DR3	DRB1*0301	DQA1*0501	DQB1*0201
DR4	DRB1*0401	DQA1*0301	DQB1*0302
	DRB1*0402	DQA1*0301	DQB1*0302
	DRB1*0405	DQA1*0301	DQB1*0302
Moderate risk			
DR1	DRB1*01	DQA1*0101	DQB1*0501
DR8	DRB1*0801	DQA1*0401	DQB1*0402
DR9	DRB1*0901	DQA1*0301	DQB1*0303
Protective			
Strong protection			
DR2	DRB1*1501	DQA1*0102	DQB1*0602
DR6	DRB1*1401	DQA1*0101	DQB1*0503
DR7	DRB1*0701	DQA1*0201	DQB1*0303
Moderate protection			
DR5	DRB1*1101	DQA1*0501	DQB1*0301
Weak protection			
DR4	DRB1*0401	DQA1*0301	DQB1*0301
	DRB1*0403	DQA1*0301	DQB1*0302
DR7	DRB1*0701	DQA1*0201	DQB1*0201

of first-phase insulin secretion that precedes diabetes, and the chronic loss of C-peptide secretion (over years) after the diagnosis of diabetes. This hypothesis is also consistent with recent analysis of β-cell loss and regeneration in NOD mice prior to diabetes.[13]

Despite evidence for progressive loss of β cells in the NOD mouse,[13] there is evidence for important changes in the immune system at the onset of diabetes. In the NOD mouse, splenocytes from recently diabetic—but not non-diabetic—mice transfer diabetes. Close to the time of diabetes, but not at early ages, NOD mice destroy islet transplants. Finally, anti-CD3 therapy produces long-term improvement in blood sugar levels if given at the onset of disease, but not with early treatment.[14]

Stage I: genetic susceptibility

Twin studies

Monozygotic twins of patients with type 1A diabetes have approximately a 50% concordance rate for type 1A diabetes. This concordance is markedly different from that of dizygotic twins (5–10%). This difference reflects a significant role for genetic factors, but suggests that environmental and possibly somatic mutations or other stochastic events may also play a significant role in the pathogenesis. Although the risk of a discordant twin progressing to type 1A diabetes decreases proportionately with the duration of discordance, twins can become concordant after many years. In a prospective study involving 187 monozygotic twins from the UK and the USA who were discordant at the time of enrolment, 47 became concordant, with a range of time of onset of 0.4–39 years. The median discordance time of the twin pairs was 4.2 years, and 25% became concordant after 14 years of discordance.[15]

HLA genes

A major determinant of genetic susceptibility resides in the MHC class II region (IDDM1). HLA class II molecules, particularly DR and DQ, account for approximately 50% of the genetic risk for type 1A diabetes. As the MHC region displays a significant degree of linkage disequilibrium (e.g., specific DQ and DR alleles are non-randomly associated with each other; Chapter 5) associations of HLA with disease must be thought of as haplotype specific and not allele specific. Class I HLA alleles can also influence disease, and it is possible that unknown genes linked to the HLA region are important. Nevertheless, the identification of HLA class II alleles associated with high, moderate, low risk and even "protection" is useful in disease prediction (Table 70.3).

Individuals with the highest risk for type 1A diabetes in the USA express both DQA1*0501-DQB1*0201 (DQ2), which is almost always inherited with DRB1*0301, and DQA1*0301-DQB1*0302 (DQ8), inherited with DRB1*0401 or *0404. These individuals have been referred to as DR3/DR4 or DQ2/DQ8 heterozygotes. The genotype, DQ2/DQ8 (DR3/DR4), is commonly observed in type 1A diabetics. Although only 2% of children in the USA have this genotype, they constitute approximately 30% of those developing diabetes. Observations of transmission frequencies of particular haplotypes have helped illustrate the importance of certain haplotypes in contributing to diabetes susceptibility. For example, analysis of the Human Biological Data Interchange (HBDI) family collection has revealed that DQA1*0501-DQB*0201 and DQA1*0301-DQB1*0302 are transmitted to more than 80% of diabetic children. DQB1 alleles without an aspartic acid at position 57 of the β chain have been proposed to determine diabetes risk. However, no simple amino acid rule adequately describes the risk associated with DQ alleles.

HLA DQ alleles have also been associated with dominant protection from type 1A diabetes. Approximately 20% of the general population have DQA1*0102-DQB1*0602, the HLA haplotype that provides dominant protection from type 1A diabetes. Interestingly, autoantibody-positive relatives of affected individuals who express the HLA haplotype DQA1 0102, DQB1*0602 are protected from progression to diabetes, albeit not completely.

HLA class I and DP alleles are also associated with diabetes risk. For example, the A24 allele is associated with early age of onset of type 1A diabetes,[16] and HLA-B39 confers increased risk.

Non-HLA genes

Genome-wide screens for loci linked with diabetes (using microsatellite markers from all of the chromosomes) have led to the identification of more than 40 genetic loci contributing to

Table 70.4 Two genetic forms of type 1A diabetes inheritance

Monogenic model
Susceptibility to type 1A diabetes and other endocrine and nonendocrine autoimmune diseases can be determined by a mutation in a single gene. Two examples are the autoimmune polyendocrine syndrome type I (APS-I) with a mutation in the autoimmune regulator (AIRE) gene, and mutation of FOXP3 gene (IPEX syndrome: immune dysregulation, polyendocrinopathy, enteritis, X-linked), both of which are rare.[48]
Polygenic model
A major role for class II molecules (DQ, DR) in determining susceptibility for type 1A diabetes is well recognized. In the NOD mouse model more than 15 non-MHC loci have been found to contribute to diabetes risk. The idea that multiple genetic polymorphisms, each contributing a small component to disease susceptibility, is a popular model.

Table 70.5 Spontaneous animal models of type 1A diabetes

BB rat (oligogenic inheritance)
Homozygosity lymphopenia gene (Ian gene)
RT1-U MHC class II alleles
Additional loci
BB-DR No lymphophenia & DM induction with kilhem rat virus infection or poly IC
NOD mouse (polygenic inheritance of diabetes)
I-A^{97}; I-Eα deletion; class I allele
IL-2 polymorphism
More than 15 additional IDDM loci
Tokushima rat (oligogenic inheritance)
RT1-U MHC alleles
Homozygosity chromosome 11 (Cblb gene)

diabetes in humans, with variable statistical significance. However, for the great majority of these putative loci no actual genes have been identified.

Because the autoimmune response against the β cell-specific molecule insulin is a major component of type 1A diabetes, the insulin gene would be an ideal candidate locus. In fact, polymorphisms in the 5′ flanking sequence (promoter region) of the insulin gene have been associated with diabetes risk, and account for about 10% of the familial aggregation of type 1A diabetes.[17] The insulin gene is located on the short arm of chromosome 11 and has been termed IDDM2. Polymorphisms in the 5′ sequence leading to alterations in insulin gene expression could be envisaged as potentially modulating the development of tolerance in the thymus or yolk sac. A low level of insulin gene expression in the thymus may allow insulin-reactive T cells to escape negative selection. The insulin gene polymorphism (larger repeat region), which results in greater thymic expression of proinsulin, is associated with protection.[18] The mutated gene underlying the autoimmune polyendocrine syndrome type I (APS-I), namely AIRE (autoimmune regulator gene) appears also to control insulin expression in the thymus and hence diabetes risk.[19]

The third most important gene is PTPN22 where an arginine replacing a tryptophan enhances the phosphatase activity of the molecule and decreases T cell receptor signaling. Two potential patterns of inheritance for diabetes will be addressed: monogenic and polygenic (Table 70.4).

Rodent models

Studies in animal models have contributed greatly to our understanding of the pathogenesis of type 1A diabetes. Numerous models exist, both induced (e.g., with alloxan, streptozotocin treatment) and spontaneous (e.g., NOD mouse, BB rat) (Table 70.5). Some important advantages of an autoimmune model include access to the pancreas at various stages in the immunopathology; ability to breed and genetically manipulate the animals; and intervention strategies that can be employed at various disease stages (e.g., preinsulitis, insulitis/presymptomatic stage etc.).

NOD mouse

The best-studied animal model for type 1A diabetes is the non-obese diabetic (NOD) mouse, which develops diabetes spontaneously. In the NOD mouse, cellular and humoral immune responses specific for β cells are present, anti-insulin autoantibodies precede overt diabetes, and disease is associated with specific MHC alleles. Pancreatic insulitis in the NOD mouse can be detected as early as 2 weeks with electron microscopy, and becomes detectable by light microscopy at 4–5 weeks of age. Approximately 80% of female mice and 20% of male mice progress to diabetes by 30 weeks of age. The reason for the excess of female cases is unknown, but may be related to the effects of sex hormones.

Multiple genetic loci in this mouse determine disease susceptibility, with the MHC (termed Idd1) being necessary but not sufficient for disease. The class II region in NOD mice encodes the I-Ag7 molecule, the ortholog of the human class II DQ8 and DQ2. I-Ag7 is unique among the known I-A molecules in that it has a serine instead of an aspartic acid at position 57 of the β chain. Like a number of normal strains, NOD mice do not express I-E (the murine ortholog of HLA-DR) because of a mutation in the Eα promoter. The introduction of a normal I-Eα gene inhibits the development of diabetes in the NOD mouse, implying that its absence is important. Transgenic NOD mice expressing a "normal" I-A, or with amino acid substitutions at positions 56 and 57 of the NOD I-Ag7, are protected from disease. Recent studies suggest that insulin may be a primary autoantigen for the disorder, and mutation of a single amino acid of insulin prevents the development of diabetes (Table 70.6).[20]

BB rat

The BB rat also develops diabetes spontaneously, with equal frequency among males and females.5 Ninety percent of both sexes developing insulitis progress to overt diabetes between 50 and 90 days of age. Selective breeding of BB rats resulted in the production of a diabetes-prone (DP) and a diabetes-resistant (DR) strain.

Genetic susceptibility for type 1A diabetes in the BB rat is also determined in part by the MHC genes. In the BB rat, diabetes is independent of class I alleles but requires the MHC class II haplotype RT-1U (Iddm2), in which at least one allele must be present for diabetes to develop. A second locus (Iddm1) is inherited in an autosomal recessive manner and is responsible for T-cell lymphopenia in these animals, determined by a frameshift mutation of an Ian (immune associated nucleotide) gene.[21]

The DR-BB rats are non-lymphopenic and diabetes can be induced either by the administration of RT6 monoclonal antibodies or by infection with the Kilham rat virus. The Kilham

Table 70.6 Summary of transgenic and knockout studies on the NOD background

Transgene/Retrogene	Observation	Conclusion
I-Eα	Diabetes prevented	Class II alleles dominant
I-Aβ proline 56, Asp57	Diabetes prevented	I-A sequence around B57 is important
Proinsulin with class II promoter	Diabetes prevented	Insulin "key" autoantigen
GAD65 with class II promoter	No decrease in diabetes	GAD65 not essential
IL-2 B6 variant	Diabetes decreased	IL-2 polymorphisms contribute to diabetes
TCR TRAV 5D-4 alpha chain	Insulin autoimmunity	V alpha chain anti B:9-23
Multiple TCR retrogene	Insulitis if target islet	Only specific TCR invade islet
Expression in β cells		
TNF-α	Accelerated diabetes	Neutrophil infiltration induced
IL-10	Accelerated diabetes	
FasL	Accelerated diabetes	
B7.1	Accelerated diabetes	B7.1 co-stimulation CD8 T cell
TGF-β	Decreased diabetes	TGF-β may suppress islet-reactive T cells
IL-4	Diabetes prevention	IL-4 may induce a 'protective' Th2 response
Expression in T cells		
IL-10	Protection with limited diabetes	"Tr1" regulatory
Expression in α cells (paracrine effect)		
TGF-β	Protected against diabetes	Paracrine TGF-β is important for suppressing autoimmunity, perhaps through induction of regulatory T cells
In vitro		
Bcl-2 transgenic islet cells	Protected from IL-1β, TNF-α, IFN-γ-induced destruction	Bcl-2 antiapoptotic factor blocks Cytokine-induced apoptosis
Knockout/inactivating mutation		
Rag, SCID, TCR Cd	Diabetes prevented	T-cell receptors are essential
Mu chain of immunoglobulin	Diabetes prevented	B cells important
Class II deficient B lymphocytes	Diabetes prevented	B-cell expression of class II important
β2-microglobulin ('class I knockout')	Diabetes prevented	Class I and CD8 T cells are important
CIITA 'Class II transactivator'	Pancreatic infiltration/seldom	CD4 T cells essential
Perforin	Decreased diabetes	Perforin-dependent cytotoxicity important
Fas	Fas$^{-/-}$ prevents diabetes	Fas is important
Knockout insulin 1 and 2 gene	Diabetes prevented	Insulin B:9-23 essential
IA-2, IA-2β, GAD65, IAPP	Diabetes unchanged	Multiple antigens not essential
IFN-γ	Diabetes unchanged	IFN-γ not essential
TNF Receptor 1	Diabetes prevented	TNFR1 signal important
IL-12	Diabetes unchanged	Other cytokines may substitute
IL-4	Diabetes unchanged	Other cytokines may substitute

rat virus does not infect β cells but is believed to alter immune regulation.[22] Table 70.5 lists several animal models of type 1A diabetes.

Stage II: triggering of autoimmunity (potential environmental factors)

Environmental factors suggested to influence the development of type 1A diabetes include viral infections, bacterial and/or viral superantigens, dietary components and environmental toxins. Many investigators support a viral etiology for type 1A diabetes. However, so far there has been no formal demonstration that viral infections directly cause type 1A diabetes in humans.

The mechanism by which microbial infections might influence the autoimmune process of type 1A diabetes is poorly defined. Hypotheses include: (1) microbial-specific T and B cells may cross-react with self-antigens (molecular mimicry); (2) virally infected β cells may be directly destroyed by cytotoxic T lymphocytes reacting to viral epitopes displayed on MHC class I; (3) indirect or "bystander" activation of autoreactive lymphocytes

may occur owing to a local increase in inflammatory cytokines associated with viral infection; (4) the effects of congenital infection (e.g., rubella) on the developing immune system may contribute to disease susceptibility; and (5) changes in the GI tract microbiome may alter risk. Without convincing epidemiological evidence for relevant environmental factors, it is difficult to test these hypotheses.

Rubella virus

Congenital rubella infection is a well-defined environmental factor contributing to the development of type 1A diabetes in humans. Approximately 12–20% of individuals infected with rubella in utero develop diabetes in 5–20 years, in what appears to be an autoimmune process. One hypothesis to explain this association involves molecular mimicry, suggested by a shared epitope between a rubella viral noncapsid protein and a 52-kDa islet autoantigen. Alternatively, the rubella virus may alter β-cell antigens as it buds from the membrane, resulting in the formation of a novel antigenic determinant. A separate hypothesis is that rubella infection might modulate T-cell development and result in abnormal immunologic tolerance to islet and thyroid tissues.

Coxsackie B viruses

Coxsackie viruses are RNA-containing picornaviruses that have been implicated in the etiology of type 1A diabetes. Sequence similarity exists between the coxsackie viral protein 2 C (P2-C) and the glutamic acid decarboxylase (GAD65) autoantigen expressed in the pancreas. This homology is highly conserved in coxsackie B4 isolates, and the relevant peptide binds to HLA-DR3 but not DR4, giving rise to speculation that the molecular mimicry may be limited to the HLA-DR3 subpopulation of type 1A diabetics. In another study, a GAD-peptide AA 247-279 similar to the coxsackie B virus was shown to stimulate Th1 lymphocytes derived from children with recent-onset type 1A diabetes. Lymphocytes from these patients had increased IFN-γ mRNA expression, which was not seen in lymphocytes derived from HLA-matched controls.

Attempts to relate antibodies to coxsackie viruses to the development of type 1A diabetes revealed both positive and negative results. Because these viruses are ubiquitous in the environment, it has been difficult to definitively associate viral infection with the disease. One alternative hypothesis is that a coxsackie B viral infection might act as a final insult and induce hyperglycemia in individuals who have already lost a substantial amount of β-cell mass.

In addition to the coxsackie and rubella viruses, numerous other viruses have been implicated in the etiology of type 1A diabetes, including cytomegalovirus, herpes viruses, mumps, retroviruses, rotaviruses, Epstein–Barr viruses and echoviruses.[2]

Milk proteins

Milk proteins, namely bovine serum albumin (BSA), cereals and omega-3 fatty acids, have received the most attention as possible dietary components important for the development of type 1A diabetes, and a pilot trial of bovine milk elimination was associated with a decrease in cytoplasmic islet cell antibodies.[23] Studies from Scandinavia found a correlation between reduction in breastfeeding and an increase in the incidence of type 1A diabetes while studies from the US found no association.[24] Antibodies against BSA have been found in humans, NOD mice and BB rats. One hypothesis is that a peptide of BSA, homologous to the islet antigen ICA-69, results in the activation of autoimmunity through molecular mimicry. Most of the studies associating the ingestion of milk with the development of diabetes are retrospective and with relatively small effects (odds ratio of 1.6). Importantly, several prospective studies examining the possible association between the expression of anti-islet autoimmunity and early infant exposure to cow's milk in high-risk first-degree relatives failed to find an association.[24] A recent pilot trial of a casein hydrolysate formula in infants was associated with a decrease in a subset of islet autoantibodies.[25]

Stage III: active immunity

Islet-cell autoantibodies can be detected in sera prior to the development of type 1A diabetes and in new-onset patients prior to insulin therapy.[26] For four of the autoantigens (glutamic acid decarboxylase (GAD65), insulin, ICA512/IA2, and ZnT8) the frequency of positive autoantibody tests is high, and the assays are in a form that allow the testing of thousands of samples (Table 70.7). However, there is no evidence that autoantibodies

Table 70.7 Assays for anti-islet autoantibodies using recombinant antigens

Antigen	Sensitivity (%)	(Specificity) (%)	Comment
Insulin	40–95	(99)	Prevalence inversely correlated with the age of onset
GAD	70	(99)	Prevalence increases with age
ICA512 (IA-2)	60	(99)	Islet tyrosine phosphatase homolog
IA2β (Phogrin)	55	(99)	These autoantibodies are predominantly a subset of ICA512/ IA2/autoantibodies
ZnT8	70	(99)	One of the last antibodies to develop

play a pathogenic role in the immunopathogenesis of type 1A diabetes, and one study found less development of islet autoimmunity for infants with transplacental GAD65 autoantibodies.[27,28] Evidence against autoantibodies contributing directly to β-cell damage comes from studies of infants born to mothers with type 1A diabetes. Anti-islet autoantibodies of mothers are transferred to the infant transplacentally, yet these infants do not develop disease. As discussed above, the lack of an influence exerted by autoantibodies does not rule out an important role for B lymphocytes in the pathogenesis of diabetes. Studies from B-cell-deficient NOD mice indicate that the development of diabetes is markedly suppressed in such animals, and other studies indicate that transplacental autoantibodies are important in the NOD mouse model. Administration of anti-CD20 antibodies prevent diabetes in NOD mice and delayed loss of C-peptide in a Trial-Net study.[29]

Autoantigens/autoantibodies

Insulin

The insulin molecule is the only β-cell-specific autoantigen so far associated with type 1A diabetes, and antibodies against insulin are one of the earliest clinical markers of pre-diabetes. Insulin autoantibodies (IAA) can be detected in the sera of approximately 60% of newly diagnosed type 1A patients prior to insulin therapy. The presence of IAA is inversely correlated with age of diabetes onset, with almost 100% of newly diagnosed children less than 5 years of age expressing IAA, compared to less than 20% of those diagnosed after 15 years of age. Moreover, the levels of IAA are associated with the rate of the autoimmune destruction of the β cells, making their detection an important aspect of diagnosis and prevention. Recent studies indicate that insulin autoantibodies are of high affinity when first detected in young infants, and high-affinity insulin autoantibodies are indicators of high risk. Insulin antibodies develop after about 2 weeks of insulin injections.

GAD65

Glutamic acid decarboxylase (GAD) is an enzyme that converts glutamate to γ-amino butyric acid (GABA). Two isoforms, GAD65 and GAD67, named for their molecular weights in kilodaltons, have been identified. GAD65 is expressed in human β cells (but is also expressed by α and δ cells of islets) and is a major target autoantigen in type 1A diabetes. Although antibodies to GAD65 can be detected in the sera of 70% of new-onset type 1A patients, only 10% of GAD antibody-positive relatives progress to type 1A diabetes (with long-term follow-up) if no other islet antibodies are expressed.

ICA512 (IA-2)

ICA512 was identified by screening an islet cDNA library with sera from new-onset type 1A diabetics. The gene encodes a putative tyrosine phosphatase-related molecule expressed in the pancreas (associated with the β-cell secretory granules) and the brain. The antigen appears to be produced in two alternative splice variants, with the variant lacking the transmembrane exon 13 domain termed ICA512 bdc. Autoantibodies usually react with both variants, although approximately 10% of sera from new-onset patients react with one or the other.

The above-mentioned autoantibodies appear in a sequential manner rather than simultaneously, with insulin and GAD65 usually appearing first.

ZnT8

Autoantibodes to the zinc transporter ZnT8 is an important autoantigen with up to 70% of patients with new onset diabetes having anti-ZnT8 autoantibodies.[30] The transporter brings zinc into insulin secretory granules to form zinc-insulin "storage" crystals.

Stage IV: loss of insulin secretion

Given the presence of anti-islet autoantibodies, the loss of first-phase insulin secretion following the administration of intravenous glucose and abnormalities on oral glucose tolerance testing are parameters that aid in defining the time to development of overt diabetes. Prospective studies indicate that identification of risk greatly decreases hospitalization and ketoacidosis. In children closely followed to development of diabetes, a rise in HbA1c of 0.4% (e.g., 6.1 to 6.5%) indicates increased near-term risk.[31]

Stage V: overt diabetes

By the time overt diabetes develops in humans, most (80–90%) of the β cells are apparently destroyed. In patients who die shortly after the onset of type 1A diabetes, insulitis can be found within the islets that still contain β cells. After β-cell destruction has occurred in humans and in the various animal models, islets with no β cells remain and the insulitis resolves. The decrease in β-cell mass accompanying the onset of overt diabetes is associated with a lack of first-phase insulin secretion, which is not restored even if patients are treated with cyclosporine. At the time of diagnosis anti-islet autoantibodies can still be detected in the sera of these patients, and probably reflects the insulitis and β-cell destruction that is still ongoing. Newly diagnosed type 1A diabetes is often associated with a brief metabolic remission, termed the "honeymoon phase," in which low doses of insulin are required or, in some cases, patients may be transiently insulin independent. This brief metabolic remission usually lasts for less than 1 year. It is likely that this period reflects decreased insulin resistance after treatment of severe hyperglycemia. The ability to induce this temporary remission makes the search for an agent that can maintain long-term remission an important goal.

Effector mechanisms of β-cell destruction

An important feature supporting the conclusion that type 1A diabetes is an autoimmune disorder is the finding of a lymphocytic infiltrate in the islets. The mechanism by which these cells gain access to the islets and mediate the selective destruction of the insulin-secreting β cells, while leaving other islet cells intact, is still unclear. It is believed by many investigators that the destruction of β cells occurs through apoptosis in a process that requires B lymphocytes and CD4 and CD8 T lymphocytes. Studies in which B cells or macrophages are depleted in the NOD model show that these antigen-presenting cells are important in the disease process.

Although some studies have shown that either CD4 or CD8 T cells may, under certain experimental conditions, be sufficient to cause β-cell destruction, it would be difficult to imagine that these cells are acting in isolation. It is more likely that there is a complex interaction between antigen-presenting cells (dendritic cells, macrophages and B cells), T lymphocytes and numerous cytokines that brings about the destruction of the β cells. Studies have supported the role of proinflammatory cytokines, including TNF-α, IL-1, IL-6, and IFN-γ, as well as Fas–FasL interactions, perforin and granzymes and reactive oxygen intermediates (e.g., nitric oxide). Despite numerous reports describing the involvement of many of these molecules, the extent to which each of them participates in β-cell destruction is controversial.

CD4 T cells

CD4 T cells appear to be critical in the pathogenesis of type 1A diabetes. In NOD mice depletion of CD4 T cells using anti-CD4 antibodies, or NOD mice engineered to be genetically deficient in CD4, diabetes does not develop. Islet-specific T-cell clones have been isolated from the spleen, lymph nodes and islets of Langerhans of NOD mice, and such islet-specific T cells can induce diabetes after adoptive transfer. Nearly all of these T-cell clones are CD4[+] and require peptide presentation in the context of the NOD class II I-A^{g7} molecule. Of the CD4[+] T-cell clones isolated from NOD islets, 55% have been found to be insulin reactive and the remainder reactive to molecules such as chromogranin and islet-associated polypeptide (IAPP). More than 95% of the insulin-reactive clones recognize a single peptide of insulin that spans the amino acid residues 9–23 of the insulin B chain. This epitope is termed B9-23, or the B2 peptide. Molecular characterization of the known B9-23 reactive CD4[+] T-cell clones derived from the NOD islet reveals that the TCR α chain is highly restricted to Vα13 and Jα45 or Jα34.[32] This TCR motif is expressed in up to 60% of insulin-reactive T-cell clones.

CD8 T cells

Studies of knockout mice have confirmed the importance of CD8 T cells in islet cell pathology. In β2-microglobulin-null NOD mice, which are deficient in CD8 T cells, neither diabetes nor insulitis occurs. A similar finding is observed when NOD mice are treated with a monoclonal antibody against CD8. Wong and colleagues identified insulin as the autoantigen recognized by a NOD-derived pathogenic CD8 T cell. Interestingly, the region recognized by the CD8 T cells overlapped with the portion of the insulin B chain recognized by the majority of the insulin-reactive CD4 T cells.

Despite the importance of T lymphocytes for the development of type 1A diabetes, both in humans and in animal models, T-cell assays useful for the prediction or follow-up of the diabetes process are not yet specific or sensitive enough for diabetes prediction. There is evidence that ELISPOT or tetramer assays can detect autoreactive T lymphocytes,[33] but a major limitation is likely to be the frequency of autoreactive T cells outside the islets that are available for study.

Histopathology

Studies in the NOD model have provided the opportunity to examine the islets at various stages of the natural history of the disease. Through these studies it has become clear that intra-islet infiltration evolves from a stage of peri-insulitis and MHC class I hyperexpression in the NOD islet β cells. The perivascular and periductal T-cell infiltration, termed peri-insulitis, is usually observed at 4–6 weeks of age. Animals at this stage have been described as being in a state of "benign autoimmunity," in which case the peri-insulitis is thought to be nondestructive. The conversion to invasive insulitis and β-cell destruction ("malignant autoimmunity") in these mice was reported to occur abruptly and unpredictably as the mice aged. However, O'Brien and colleagues reported that apoptosis in the NOD islets was detectable throughout the period of peri-insulitis.[34] Apoptotic death of the islets preceded lymphocytic infiltration and then declined when progression to overt diabetes occurred. In another study, NOD mice were observed to have an early increased "compensatory" β-cell proliferation. This was unable to keep pace with the progressive β-cell destruction and resulted in a reduction in β-cell mass that became worse with time and correlated with a decrease in the insulin secretory response.[13]

Histological analyses of the islets in humans have been limited for several reasons, which include the relative inaccessibility of the pancreas for biopsy; the fact that the islets make up only 2–3% of the pancreatic tissue; and the fact that histologic examination of the islets at the time of disease onset (which precedes clinical presentation) has not been possible. Histological evaluation of pancreases from children who have died at disease onset also suggests a slowly evolving autoimmune process. Foulis and colleagues[35] described three histologically distinguishable types of islet in patients with new-onset diabetes: insulin-deficient islets (pseudoatrophic), which make up the largest fraction (approximately 70%); insulin-containing islets with a chronic inflammatory cell infiltrate; and insulin-containing islets that appear normal. T cells make up most of the infiltrate, with CD8 T cells comprising a larger fraction than CD4 in some studies. Bingley and colleagues described greatly decreased numbers of β cells in pancreases from long-term patients, but nevertheless evidence of β-cell apoptosis.[36] The destruction of β cells occurs in a lobular fashion with large areas of "normal" islets and large areas of only pseudoatrophic islets.[29]

In contrast to the characteristic peri-insulitis associated with the early stages of immunopathology in the NOD mouse, peri-insulitis does not appear to be a common feature in humans. Another distinction is that insulitis in the NOD mouse is associated with massive mononuclear cell infiltrates not typically seen in humans. The mechanisms that underlie these differences remain unclear. It is, however, a good reminder that the NOD mouse, albeit an excellent model, is clearly not identical to humans.

Type 1A diabetes prediction

By the time a diagnosis of type 1A diabetes is made, approximately 80–90% of the β cells may have been destroyed. Therefore, the ability to predict who will develop type 1A diabetes among high-risk individuals (siblings of type 1A diabetics) has become an important goal. Using HLA haplotype analysis and "combinatorial" autoantibody analyses, clinicians should be able to identify high-risk individuals. Because the autoimmune process in type 1A diabetes begins years before the progression to overt symptoms, the chance of early intervention is feasible. Furthermore, if a definable environmental trigger exists for type 1A diabetes, as it does for celiac disease (wheat gliadin), preventing exposure may be important.

The most important risk factor for disease development is the expression of multiple anti-islet autoantibodies,[36] particularly two or more of GAD65, ICA512 (IA-2), ZnT8 or insulin autoantibodies (Fig. 70.2). However, there is a subset of relatives who express a single autoantibody, and an even smaller subset expressing multiple autoantibodies, who have the "protective" HLA alleles DQA1*0102, DQB1*0602. In individuals with DQB1*0602 the risk of progressing to diabetes is low, but still present. Approximately 1% (versus 20% of the general population) of patients with type 1A diabetes have this allele.

⬤THERAPEUTIC PRINCIPLES

- Autoantibody testing in combination with HLA testing can be used to predict type 1A diabetes.
- Insulin therapy is mandatory in type 1A patients who are ketosis prone. Testing of islet cell autoantibodies identifies 10% of adults (thought to have type 2 diabetes) as having type 1A diabetes.
- Prevention of microvascular diabetic complications is feasible; it requires routine screening for retinal lesions and microalbuminuria.

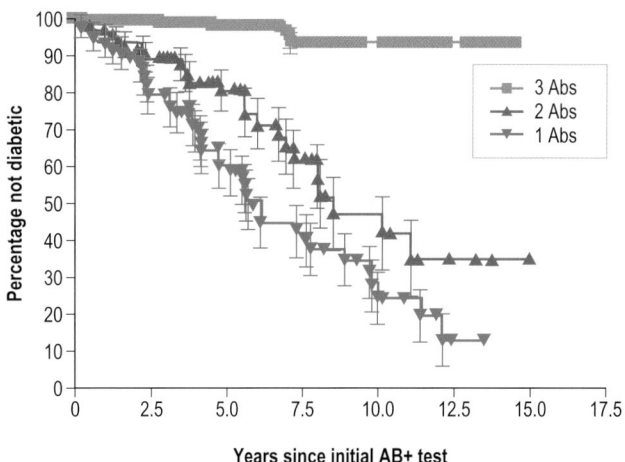

Fig. 70.2 Life table analysis of progression to type 1A diabetes in relatives of affected patients subdivided by the number of autoantibodies (GAD65, insulin, ICA512) expressed.

Prevention

Immunosuppression

The first major trial of general immunosuppressive therapy for newly diagnosed subjects involved the administration of cyclosporin A (CyA).[37] CyA was effective in prolonging insulin secretion when treatment lasted 1 year and was initiated during the first 6 weeks of insulin therapy. Long-term benefit was limited, however, with relapse of hyperglycemia occurring within 3 years despite continued CyA therapy, and despite continued maintenance of improved insulin secretion as measured with C-peptide. When CyA was discontinued, insulin secretion was rapidly lost. Because of the potential for nephrotoxicity and the risk of malignancy associated with long-term treatment, CyA therapy has not been adopted. Other immunosuppressive agents have been studied, including prednisone, anti-CD5, anti-CD25, anti-thymocyte globulin and anti-T12, but so far they have had little success in providing long-term protection. Recent studies of anti-T cell antibodies (in particular modified anti-CD3 antibodies) have shown promise but again only transient efficacy.[38,39]

Autoantigen administration

The administration of certain islet cell autoantigens, such as insulin and GAD, and derivatives of these autoantigens can prevent diabetes in animal models. For example, in the NOD mouse long-term (up to 1 year) oral ingestion of these autoantigens has been reported to delay the onset and/or reduce the incidence of disease. Subcutaneous and intranasal administration of the insulin B chain B9-23 can prevent diabetes in the NOD mouse. Although the precise mechanism by which subcutaneous administration of the insulin peptide mediates immunoprotection is unknown, the isolation of B9-23-reactive CD4 T-cell clones expressing TGF-β suggests that protection may be mediated by regulatory T cells. Much evidence exists that in type 1A diabetes a Th1-dominant response enhances β-cell destruction, whereas a Th2 response is protective (Chapter 16). Autoantigen administration appears to dampen the autoimmune response via bystander suppression through the generation of regulatory T cells secreting a Th2 cytokine profile. In the USA individuals at moderate risk for type 1A diabetes were randomized to receive oral insulin in the NIH TrialNet Study. Insulin therapy did not overall decrease progression to diabetes, but there was evidence in a subgroup (those with high levels of insulin autoantibodies) of a significant delay in progression.[40]

Adjuvants

In the NOD mouse a single injection of complete Freund's adjuvant prevents the development of diabetes[41] but not insulitis. A single injection of incomplete Freund's adjuvant (IFA) is unable to induce this effect. However, when combined with an injection of B chain of insulin or the B9-23 peptide, IFA is able to prevent diabetes in the NOD mouse. Vaccination with the bacillus Calmette–Guérin (BCG) strain of *Mycobacterium bovis* has also been found to prevent diabetes in the NOD mouse. In several randomized double-blinded placebo-controlled trials intradermal BCG vaccination did not alter remission rate or protect β cells.

Nicotinamide

In the NOD mouse large doses of the vitamin nicotinamide delayed the development of diabetes, and preliminary uncontrolled trials suggested that such therapy might also be successful in humans. In light of this, two randomized controlled trials of nicotinamide, the small German DENIS (Deutsche Nicotinamide Trial) trial and the larger ENDIT (European Nicotinamide Trial) trial in Europe, were initiated and no protection was found.[42]

Treatment with insulin

Insulin is administered subcutaneously to millions of individuals with diabetes. Over the past three decades, not only has the purity of the insulin preparations improved, but in developed countries human insulin has replaced the use of porcine or bovine insulin. Porcine insulin differs from human insulin by only one amino acid, whereas bovine insulin differs by three amino acids. Multiple recombinant forms of human insulin have been introduced into clinical practice. For fast-acting insulins the change in the insulin molecule disrupts the natural ability of insulin to form hexamers and speeds subcutaneous absorption. Although the insulin is modified, modifications have not been associated with an increase in insulin antibodies or greater immunologic reactions to insulin.

Essentially, all patients treated with insulin, even human insulin, develop a low level of antibodies that cross-react with native insulin. These antibodies are of relatively low affinity compared to the insulin autoantibodies of pre-diabetic patients, and do not usually interfere with insulin action. Insulin resistance due to induced insulin antibodies (defined as patients requiring more than 200 U of insulin per day, and insulin antibodies with a capacity that usually exceeds 50 U of insulin per liter of serum) was always rare and appears to be nearly disappearing as human insulin replaces animal insulins. Allergic or hypersensitivity reactions to insulin and (in the past) lipoatrophy or lipohypertrophy at the site of insulin injection, are also very rare at present. Such allergic reactions can be treated by changing the formulation of insulin used (e.g., NPH insulin to Lente insulin) or, for delayed hypersensitivity, adding small amounts of glucocorticoids to the insulin preparation.

Associated autoimmune disorders

Type 1A diabetes is associated with several autoimmune diseases, including Addison's disease, thyroiditis, Graves' disease, pernicious anemia, celiac disease, myasthenia gravis and vitiligo.[43] The association with other organ-specific autoimmune diseases points to the importance of screening for these diseases in type 1A patients. Several commonly associated diseases or unique syndromes are discussed in this section.

Autoimmune polyendocrine syndromes

Polyendocrine syndromes are characterized by multiple autoimmune disorders. Two distinct forms have been described: autoimmune polyendocrine syndrome I (APS-I) and II (APS-II).

Autoimmune polyendocrine syndrome type I (APS-I)

APS-I consists of a triad of chronic mucocutaneous candidiasis, hypoparathyroidism and Addison's disease, which often present in that order. Other endocrine and nonendocrine disorders can

Table 70.8 Autoimmune polyendocrine syndrome types I and II

	APS-I[a]	APS-II[b]
Inheritance	Autosomal recessive AIRE gene 21q22.3	Autosomal dominant polygenic/ oligogenic
HLA association	None but DR2 decreases DM	HLA DR3 and DR4
Immunodeficiency	Mucocutaneous candidiasis (anti-IL-17 and -22) asplenism	
Age of onset	Infancy or early childhood	Adulthood (peak 20–60)
Sexual prevalence	Equal among males and females	Greater in females (by two- to threefold)
Mucocutaneous candidiasis[a]	73–100%	Not associated
Hypoparathyroidism[a]	80–89% (Nalp5 auto Ab)	Not associated
Addison's disease[a,b]	60–72% (21 hydroxylase auto Ab)	70%
Type 1 diabetes[b]	4–15%	52%
Autoimmune thyroid disease[b]	10–40%	70%
Gonadal failure	38–60% of females	3.5–10% of females
	7–14% of males	5–50% of males
Vitiligo	4–9%	4.5%
Hepatitis	10–15%	Rare
Pernicious anemia	12–15%	<1%
Malabsorption	18%	With celiac disease

[a]Classic triad for APS-I.
[b]Classic triad for APS-II.
Ab = autoantibody

also be present or develop later in patients with this syndrome (Table 70.8). Eighteen percent of patients develop type 1A diabetes. APS-I is also known as autoimmune polyendocrinopathy candidiasis ectodermal dystrophy (APECED), and is an autosomal recessive disorder in which males and females are equally affected. In contrast to APS-II, in which the manifestations of disease usually occur in middle age, APS-I usually manifests in infancy or early childhood. In both syndromes the detection of autoantibodies against endocrine and nonendocrine tissues precedes overt disease.

APS-I is of considerable importance in that it has a defined monogenic etiology. The gene underlying the pathogenesis of APS-I is localized to the long arm of chromosome 21 (21q22.3) and is termed autoimmune regulator (*AIRE*). AIRE has two zinc-finger motifs and a DNA-binding domain, and is localized to the nucleus, suggestive of a role in modulating transcription. Studies by Anderson and colleagues have led to the hypothesis that AIRE is important for induction of tolerance to "peripheral" antigens such as insulin, expressed at low levels in the thymus.[44] Autoantibodies to Type 1 interferons are diagnostic and autoantibodies to Th17 cytokines (IL17 and IL22) are associated with mucocutaneous candidiasis (Chapter 18).[45]

Autoimmune polyendocrine syndrome type 2 (APS-II)

APS-II, or Schmidt's syndrome, is the most common of the polyendocrine syndromes and, in contrast to APS-I, the incidence is two to three times higher in females than in males, with onset typically in adulthood. The classic triad of APS-II involves Addison's disease, autoimmune thyroid disease and type 1A diabetes, but other endocrine and nonendocrine disorders can be seen in affected patients. Unlike APS-I, APS-II is strongly associated with HLA alleles and susceptibility is probably determined by an interaction between multiple genetic loci and environmental factors. The class II HLA alleles associated with most of the component disorders of APS-II are DR3 (DQB*0201) with HLA-B8 and DR4 (DRBI*0404) with (DQB1*0302).

Addison's disease

Addison's disease, or primary adrenocortical insufficiency, is an autoimmune disease characterized by the presence (in 70% of patients) of autoantibodies directed predominantly against 21-hydroxylase, a key regulator of mineralocorticoid and glucocorticoid synthesis. The myriad clinical manifestations of Addison's disease, including muscle weakness and fatigue, hypotension and hyponatremia, and loss of axillary and pubic hair in women, are the result of cortisol, aldosterone and sex hormone deficiencies, respectively. Addison's disease is the principal component disorder of APS-II.

In "DR4" patients with Addison's disease DRB1*0404 is the DR4 allele most often carried. Individuals with type 1A diabetes have a 100 times greater risk of developing Addison's disease. This significant increase justifies anti-21-hydroxylase autoantibody screening in type 1A diabetics. HLA-B8 and the MICA-5.1 allele are additionally associated with Addison's disease.

Celiac disease

Celiac disease is a common autoimmune disease (incidence >1% with screening in the USA) characterized by immune-cell-induced intestinal lesions which may lead to malabsorption and growth failure (Chapter 74). The highest incidence occurs in type 1A diabetics and their relatives, with most of these patients expressing DQA1*0501; DQB1*0201 (DR3, DR3/3, or DR5/7). Of the autoimmune diseases, celiac disease is unique in that intestinal pathology is entirely dependent on the ingestion of cereal proteins, namely wheat, rye and barley. Remarkably, the removal of gliadin from the diet resolves the intestinal lesions and also leads to the disappearance of autoantibodies associated with the disease.

Tissue transglutaminase (tTG), an enzyme that catalyzes the cross-linking of proteins via glutamyl–lysine bonds, has been shown to be the primary autoantigen of the autoantibodies directed to the intestinal tissues (anti-endomysial antibodies).[46] Glutamine residues make up over 40% of the amino acid residues of the gliadin protein, making it a good substrate for transglutaminase. It is postulated that gliadin may become cross-linked to transglutaminase, creating a novel antigenic determinant that is then recognized by T cells.

Tissue transglutaminase IgA antibodies have been assessed using both an enzyme-linked immunoabsorbent assay (ELISA) and a radioisotope-binding assay.[47] Ten percent of all type 1A diabetics are positive for tTG autoantibodies. Using the radioisotope-binding assay, 22 of 68 (32%) of type 1A diabetics homozygous for HLA-DQ2 express tTG autoantibodies, as opposed to <2% of those lacking DQ2 or DQ8.[47] Approximately

70% of anti-glutaminase-positive individuals have celiac disease on biopsy if high levels of the antibody are present (e.g., 10 times 99th percentile normals).

Pitfalls/controversies

General population screening

Current trials that target individuals at increased risk for the development of type 1A diabetes, such as the large multicenter randomized trial headed by the National Institutes of Health (TrialNet), are aimed at intervening in the pre-diabetic stage with the hope of either delaying or preventing disease onset. The success of such trials relies partly on our ability to reliably detect at-risk individuals (e.g., siblings of affected patients). However, 90% of patients with type 1A diabetes do not have an affected first-degree relative, making prediction in the general population an important goal.

General population screening depends on the development of effective interventions that can be instituted prior to the development of diabetes, and potentially prior to autoimmunity. Given the natural history of type 1A diabetes (for many individuals), this will mean that treatment would need to be initiated in infancy. Further complicating this strategy is that only a subset of genetically susceptible individuals progress to diabetes. This subset is highest (40–50%) for DQ8/DQ2 heterozygous first-degree relatives of patients with type 1A diabetes. Trials can be designed that will determine whether autoantibodies, and subsequently disease, are preventable. Because only 10% of first-degree relatives of patients with type 1A diabetes are DQ8/DQ2 heterozygous, such trials will require the screening of more than 1000 neonates. This is obviously a logistical hindrance to such trials, but the major impediment is likely to be the consideration that antigen-based trials have some possibility of activating disease. Thus, it is likely that therapies will initially be evaluated in patients with recent-onset type 1A diabetes, and in individuals expressing autoantibodies and progressing to diabetes, before instituting trials involving individuals with genetic susceptibility alone.

Distinguishing various forms of diabetes

Not all children presenting with diabetes mellitus have type 1A diabetes. Whereas only 10% of non-Hispanic white children do not express GAD65, ICA512, ZnT8 or insulin autoantibodies, as many as 50% of Hispanic and African-American children do not express these antibodies. For patients with type 2 diabetes oral hypoglycemic agents may be the more appropriate therapy. In such cases, clinicians need to carefully monitor these patients for possible decompensation requiring insulin treatment.

In a fraction of adults presenting with what appears to be type 2 diabetes, anti-islet autoantibodies can be detected.[48] When these patients are followed, most eventually require exogenous insulin for control of glycemia. It is likely that such patients, who represent approximately 5–10% of adults presenting with diabetes mellitus, actually have type 1A diabetes. One goal for clinicians is to identify both of the groups described above to ensure that they receive the appropriate therapy in a timely fashion.

Large quantities of antibodies to insulin can occur separately from treatment with insulin as part of the insulin autoimmune syndrome (also termed Hirata syndrome). The two forms of this syndrome, both very rare, are characterized by high-titer anti-insulin antibodies. In the rarest form, monoclonal insulin autoantibodies are produced. The form of the syndrome with polyclonal anti-insulin autoantibodies is frequently associated with ingestion of sulfhydryl-containing drugs such as methimizole (treatment for Graves' disease) in East Asian patients. In both syndromes hypoglycemia and not insulin resistance is the usual presenting abnormality. The polyclonal syndrome is strongly associated with a specific DRB1 allele (DRB1*0406) and usually resolves with discontinuation of the inciting drug. Ninety-six percent of Japanese patients (48/50) were found to have DR4, and 42 of these had DRB1*0406.[49]

Autoantibodies to the insulin receptor are present in a rare syndrome characterized by both hypoglycemia and hyperglycemia in the same patient at different times. It is thought that the anti-insulin receptor antibodies can act as agonists or antagonists. Patients with this syndrome frequently have systemic autoimmune disorders such as lupus erythematosus, rheumatoid arthritis and Sjögren's syndrome. There are reports of a favorable response to immunosuppression (e.g., with anti-CD20).[50]

On the horizon

● ON THE HORIZON

- Panels of islet autoantibodies (GAD65, IA-2, ZnT8, insulin) for diagnosing type 1A (autoimmune diabetes) applied at onset in all diabetic patients.
- Pilot programs of population-based HLA typing to define high risk for a series of autoimmune disorders (e.g., type 1A diabetes, celiac disease, Addison's disease) followed by periodic antibody determination and early diagnosis.
- Development of autoimmune T-cell assays to facilitate diabetes prediction and, more importantly, serve as potential biomarkers for therapeutic trials.
- Islet transplantation as alternative to pancreatic transplantation for diabetic patients receiving a kidney transplant.
- Continuous glucose monitors controlling insulin pumps to improve the lives of patients living with type 1A diabetes.

There are both immunologic advances and metabolic therapies that will potentially impact type 1 diabetes and associated autoimmune disorders in the next five years. In particular the bar will be raised for consideration of immunotherapies or islet transplantation as continuous glucose monitoring systems are introduced, providing feedback control of insulin pumps. The first iteration will be systems that discontinue insulin administration when hypoglycemia is detected.

Research assays are now available for a series of islet autoantibodies as well as assays for celiac disease (transglutaminase) and Addison's disease (21-hydroxylase). Commercial non-radioactive versions of these assays will likely be widely available. Since the autoantibodies characteristically decline (except for insulin, where insulin injections induce antibodies) after onset, measurement at onset will facilitate proper diagnosis. A longer term development will likely be defining genetic risk of multiple autoimmune disorders followed by periodic testing for relevant autoantibodies to allow early diagnosis or entry into preventive trials. It is estimated that approximately fifty children per year die at the onset of type 1A diabetes associated with delayed diagnosis, while many more have life-threatening ketoacidosis. Both are prevented by knowledge of islet autoimmunity.

It is known that a large percentage of children have undiagnosed celiac disease (approximately 1% of Colorado children). Knowledge of the genetics and natural history of multiple autoimmune disorders provides opportunity to develop translational medical programs dealing with multiple diseases.

References

1. Gavin JR, Alberti G, Davidson MB, et al. Report of the Expert Committee on the Diagnosis and Classification of Diabetes Mellitus. Diabetes Care 1997;20:1183.
2. Rewers M, Norris JM, Kretowksi A. Epidemiology of type I diabetes, In: Eisenbarth GS, editor. Type I diabetes: molecular, cellular, and clinical immunology. Denver, CO: publisher Barbara Davis Center; July 14, 2006, Web book at, http://www.barbaradaviscenter.org.
3. Johnston C, Pyke DA, Cudworth AG, Wolf E. HLA-DR typing in identical twins with insulin-dependent diabetes: difference between concordant and discordant pairs. BMJ 1983;286:253–5.
4. Bottazzo GF, Florin-Christensen A, Doniach D. Islet-cell antibodies in diabetes mellitus with autoimmune polyendocrine deficiencies. Lancet 1974;2:1279.
5. Mordes JP, Bortell R, Doukas J, et al. The BB/Wor rat and the balance hypothesis of autoimmunity. Diabetes Metab Rev 1996;12:103.
6. Sutherland DE, Sibley R, Xu XA, et al. Twin-to-twin pancreas transplantation: reversal and reenactment of the pathogenesis of type I diabetes. Trans Assoc Am Physicians 1984;97:80.
7. Ladner MB, Bottini N, Valdes AM, Noble JA. Association of the single nucleotide polymorphism C1858T of the PTPN22 gene with type 1 diabetes. Hum Immunol 2005;66:60–4.
8. Porter JR, Barrett TG. Monogenic syndromes of abnormal glucose homeostasis: clinical review and relevance to the understanding of the pathology of insulin resistance and beta cell failure. J Med Genet 2005;42:893–902.
9. Bingley PJ, Bonifacio E, Williams AJK, et al. Prediction of IDDM in the general population: strategies based on combinations of autoantibody markers. Diabetes 1997;46:1701.
10. Hanafusa T, Imagawa A. Fulminant type 1 diabetes: a novel clinical entity requiring special attention by all medical practitioners. Nat Clin Pract Endocrinol Metab 2007;3(1):36–45.
11. Eisenbarth GS. Prediction of type I diabetes: the natural history of the pre-diabetic period. In: Eisenbarth GS, editor. Type I diabetes: molecular, cellular, and clinical immunology. Denver: publisher Barbara Davis Center. Web book at http://www.barbaradaviscenter.org 11/1/10.
12. Greenbaum CJ, Sears KL, Kahn SE, Palmer JP. Relationship of B-cell function and autoantibodies to progression and nonprogression of subclinical type 1 diabetes. Diabetes 1999;48:170.
13. Sreenan S, Pick AJ, Levisetti M, et al. Increased β-cell proliferation and reduced mass before diabetes onset in the nonobese diabetic mouse. Diabetes 1999;48:989.
14. Chatenoud L, Thervet E, Primo J, Bach JF. Anti-CD3 antibody induces long-term remission of overt autoimmunity in nonobese diabetic mice. Proc Natl Acad Sci U S A 1994;91:123.
15. Redondo MJ, Yu L, Hawa M, et al. Heterogeneity of type 1 diabetes: analysis of monozygotic twins in Great Britain and the United States. Diabetologia 2001;44:354–62.
16. Nakanishi K, Kobayashi T, Murase T, et al. Human leukocyte antigen-A24 and -DQA1*0301 in Japanese insulin-dependent diabetes mellitus: independent contributions to susceptibility to the disease and additive contributions to acceleration of beta-cell destruction. J Clin Endocrinol Metab 1999;84:3721.
17. Bennett ST, Lucassen AM, Gough SCL, et al. Susceptibility to human type I diabetes at IDDM2 is determined by tandem repeat variation at the insulin gene minisatellite locus. Nat Genet 1995;9:284.
18. Pugliese A, Zeller M, Fernandez A, et al. The insulin gene is transcribed in the human thymus and transcription levels correlate with allelic variation at the INS VNTR-IDDM2 susceptibility locus for type I diabetes. Nat Genet 1997;15:293.
19. Su MA, Anderson MS. Aire: an update. Curr Opin Immunol 2004;16:746–52.
20. Nakayama M, Abiru N, Moriyama H, et al. Prime role for an insulin epitope in the development of type 1 diabetes in NOD mice. Nature 2005;435:220–3.
21. Moralejo DH, Park HA, Speros SJ, et al. Genetic dissection of lymphopenia from autoimmunity by introgression of mutated Ian5 gene onto the F344 rat. J Autoimmun 2003;21:315–24.
22. Zipris D, Lien E, Xie JX, et al. TLR activation synergizes with Kilham rat virus infection to induce diabetes in BBDR rats. J Immunol 2005;174:131–42.
23. Akerblom HK, Virtanen SM, Ilonen J, et al. Dietary manipulation of beta cell autoimmunity in infants at increased risk of type 1 diabetes: a pilot study. Diabetology 2005;48:829–37.
24. Couper JJ, Steele C, Beresford S, et al. Lack of association between duration of breast-feeding or introduction of cow's milk and development of islet autoimmunity. Diabetes 1999;48:2145.
25. Knip M, Virtanen SM, Seppa K, et al. Dietary intervention in infancy and later signs of beta-cell autoimmunity. N Engl J Med 2010;363(20):1900–8.
26. Palmer JP, Asplin CM, Clemons P, et al. Insulin antibodies in insulin-dependent diabetics before insulin treatment. Science 1983;222:1337.
27. Achenbach P, Bonifacio E, Koczwara K, Ziegler AG. Natural history of type 1 diabetes. Diabetes 2005;54:S25–31.
28. Koczwara K, Bonifacio E, Ziegler AG. Transmission of maternal islet antibodies and risk of autoimmune diabetes in offspring of mothers with type 1 diabetes. Diabetes 2004;53:1–4.
29. Gianani R, Campbell-Thompson M, Sarkar SA, et al. Dimorphic histopathology of long-standing childhood-onset diabetes. Diabetologia 2010;53:690–8.
30. Wenzlau JM, Moua O, Sarkar SA, et al. SIC30A8 is a major target of humoral autoimmunity in type 1 diabetes and a predictive marker in prediabetes. Ann N Y Acad Sci 2008;1150:256–9.
31. Stene LC, Barriga K, Hoffman M, et al. Normal but increasing hemoglobin A1c levels predict progression from islet autoimmunity to overt type 1 diabetes: Diabetes Autoimmunity Study in the Young (DAISY). Pediatr Diabetes 2006;7(5):247–53.
32. Simone E, Daniel D, Schloot N, et al. T cell receptor restriction of diabetogenic autoimmune NOD T cells. Proc Natl Acad Sci U S A 1997;94:2518.
33. Mallone R, Nepom GT. Targeting T lymphocytes for immune monitoring and intervention in autoimmune diabetes. Am J Ther 2005;12:534–50.
34. O'Brien BA, Harmon BV, Cameron DP, Allan DJ. Apoptosis is the mode of β-cell death responsible for the development of IDDM in the nonobese diabetic (NOD) mouse. Diabetes 1997;46:750–7.
35. Itoh N, Hanafusa T, Miyazaki A, et al. Mononuclear cell infiltration and its relation to the expression of major histocompatibility complex antigens and adhesion molecules in pancreas biopsy specimens from newly diagnosed insulin-dependent diabetes mellitus patients. J Clin Invest 1993;92:2313.
36. Bingley PJ, Christie MR, Bonifacio E, et al. Combined analysis of autoantibodies improves prediction of IDDM in islet cell antibody-positive relatives. Diabetes 1994;43:1304.
37. Stiller CR, Dupre J, Gent M, et al. Effects of cyclosporine immunosuppression in insulin-dependent diabetes mellitus of recent onset. Science 1984;223:1362.
38. Herold KC, Hagopian W, Auger JA, et al. Anti-CD3 monoclonal antibody in new-onset type 1 diabetes mellitus. N Engl J Med 2002;346:1692–8.
39. Keymeulen B, Vandemeulebroucke E, Ziegler AG, et al. Insulin needs after CD3-antibody therapy in new-onset type 1 diabetes. N Engl J Med 2005;352:2598–608.
40. DPT Study Group . Effects of Oral Insulin in Relatives of Patients With Type 1 Diabetes: The Diabetes Prevention Trial-Type 1. Diabetes Care 2005;28:1068–76.
41. Sadelain MW, Qin H-Y, Lauzon J, Singh B. Prevention of type I diabetes in NOD mice by adjuvant immunotherapy. Diabetes 1990;39:583.
42. Bingley PJ, Gale EA. Progression to type 1 diabetes in islet cell antibody-positive relatives in the European Nicotinamide Diabetes Intervention Trial: the role of additional immune, genetic and metabolic markers of risk. Diabetology 2006;49:881–90.
43. Eisenbarth GS, Gottlieb PA. Autoimmune polyendocrine syndromes. N Engl J Med 2004;350:36–47.
44. Anderson MS, Venanzi ES, Klein L, et al. Projection of an immunological self shadow within the thymus by the aire protein. Science 2002;298:1395–401.
45. Kisand K, Boe Wolff AS, Podkrajsek KT, et al. Chronic mucocutaneous candidiasis in APECED or thymoma patients correlates with autoimmunity to Th17-associated cytokines. J Exp Med 2010;207(2):299–308.
46. Dietrich W, Ehnis T, Bauer M, et al. Identification of tissue transglutaminase as the autoantigen of celiac disease. Nat Med 1997;3:797.
47. Bao F, Yu L, Babu S, et al. One third of HLA DQ2 homozygous patients with type 1 diabetes express celiac disease associated transglutaminase autoantibodies. J Autoimmun 1999;13:143.
48. Turner R, Stratton I, Horton V, et al. UKPDS 25: autoantibodies to islet-cell cytoplasm and glutamic acid decarboxylase for prediction of insulin requirement in type 2 diabetes. UK Prospective Diabetes Study Group. Lancet 1997;350:1288.
49. Uchigata Y, Hirata Y. Insulin autoimmune syndrome (IAS, Hirata disease). In: Eisenbarth G, editor. Molecular mechanisms of endocrine and organ specific autoimmunity. Austin, TX: RG Landes; 1999. p. 133.
50. Malek R, Chong AY, Lupsa BC, et al. Treatment of type B insulin resistance: a novel approach to reduce insulin receptor autoantibodies. J Clin Endocrinol Metab 2010;95(8):3641–7.

71

Andrew P.
Fontenot, Philip
L. Simonian

Immunologic lung diseases

The lung serves as an interface between the environment and the sanctuary of the body. The defense systems of the upper airways clear the majority of inhaled particulates. Those that evade the upper-airway defenses are combated by the innate and acquired immune responses. Essentially all autoimmune diseases are dependent on the inappropriate activation of autoreactive CD4 T cells as well as autoreactive B cells responsible for pathogenic autoantibodies. Immunologic lung diseases develop when the normal mechanisms of immune self-tolerance fail. This chapter deals with the pulmonary manifestations of these disorders.

Inflammation in the pathogenesis of interstitial lung disease

In the normal host, the macrophage is the predominant cell type in fluid from bronchoalveolar lavage (BAL). Macrophages serve as scavenger cells, ingesting and degrading the inhaled antigenic load. In addition, these cells serve as antigen-presenting cells for T lymphocytes. Relatively few lymphocytes are present in the normal lung parenchyma. However, after stimulation by the relevant antigen in the surrounding lymphoid tissues, antigen-specific lymphocytes migrate to the lung and participate in the inflammatory response.

In addition to lymphocytes, other inflammatory and immune cells accumulate in the lung of patients with immunologic lung disease including neutrophils, eosinophils and other mononuclear cells, depending on the underlying disease. Within the normal alveolus, the major cellular constituents are alveolar macrophages and epithelial cells. An initial insult typically involves the alveolar epithelial cell. Damage to type I alveolar epithelial cells results in release of chemokines that recruit and activate inflammatory cells, allowing for resolution of inflammation and repair of injured tissue (Fig. 71.1). With either prolonged exposure or failure to adequately clear an inhaled antigen, persistent inflammation results in extracellular matrix deposition with subsequent tissue remodelling and permanent lung dysfunction. With ongoing inflammation, progressive collagen deposition results in scarring of the lungs (pulmonary fibrosis), resulting in impaired ventilation and gas exchange with consequent patient morbidity and mortality. With destruction of type I alveolar epithelial cells, exposure of the underlying basement membrane can cause further inflammation. Proper restoration of the epithelial barrier is critical for resolution of lung inflammation. Type II alveolar epithelial cells can serve as progenitor cells that migrate and differentiate into type I alveolar epithelial cells to re-establish an intact lung epithelium.

Macrophages and lymphocytes have also been localized to areas of pulmonary fibrosis in patients with immunologic lung diseases including idiopathic pulmonary fibrosis (IPF), systemic sclerosis, and rheumatoid arthritis.[1] In the lung, macrophages have been divided by their location into alveolar or interstitial macrophages. Alveolar macrophages are phagocytic cells in epithelial surfaces and lining fluid of the alveoli and airways. With relatively poor antigen-presenting ability, they function to remove inhaled particles and bacteria. Interstitial macrophages are located in the tissue spaces between the alveoli. In the context of lung injury, interstitial macrophages increase greatly in number. Although interstitial macrophages have less phagocytic activity than alveolar macrophages, they have increased capability to present antigens to T cells.[2] Upon activation, these macrophages express a variety of cytokines including tumor necrosis factor-α (TNF-α) and monocyte chemotactic protein-1 (MCP-1). In addition to antigen presentation to T cells, macrophages are important for lung fibrosis and tissue remodelling in immunologic lung diseases through secretion of specific growth factors such as transforming growth factor-β (TGF-β), insulin-like growth factor-1 (IGF-I), platelet-derived growth factor (PDGF), and fibroblast growth factor (FGF).

T cells are also associated with lung fibrosis. For example, T cells have been located in areas of interstitial fibrosis and honeycombing with relative sparing in areas of normal lung in patients with IPF.[3] In connective tissue disease-associated interstitial lung disease (ILD), T cells are diffusely distributed throughout the lung and within focal lymphoid aggregates.[4] In animal models, depending on their phenotype, T cells can be either pro-fibrotic or anti-fibrotic. γδ T cells decrease lung inflammation and fibrosis in multiple mouse models.[5] CD8 T cells have been found in high proportion in BAL and surgical lung biopsy samples from patients with IPF, as well as patients with systemic sclerosis but their role in these immunologic lung diseases is not well understood.

Different subsets of CD4 T cells (Chapter 16) have been implicated in the pathogenesis of immunologic lung diseases. T helper type 1 (Th1) cells express IFN-γ. Although IFN-γ is a potent pro-inflammatory cytokine, it has anti-fibrotic effects through inhibiting fibroblast proliferation and collagen expression.[6] Th2 cells are defined by expression of interleukin-4 (IL-4), -5, and -13. In contrast to IFN-γ, Th2 cytokines have been shown to promote lung fibrosis. Therefore, the balance between Th1/Th2 T cells through expression of different cytokines affects the development of pulmonary fibrosis. Th17 cells express IL-17A and -17F, which are potent inflammatory cytokines important for the recruitment of neutrophils to areas of inflammation.[7] Th17 cells have been implicated in the development of lung fibrosis in murine models.[8,9] Conversely, regulatory T cells (Tregs) suppress pathogenic T cell responses that promote inflammation (Chapter 15). In patients with IPF, Tregs may be less able to

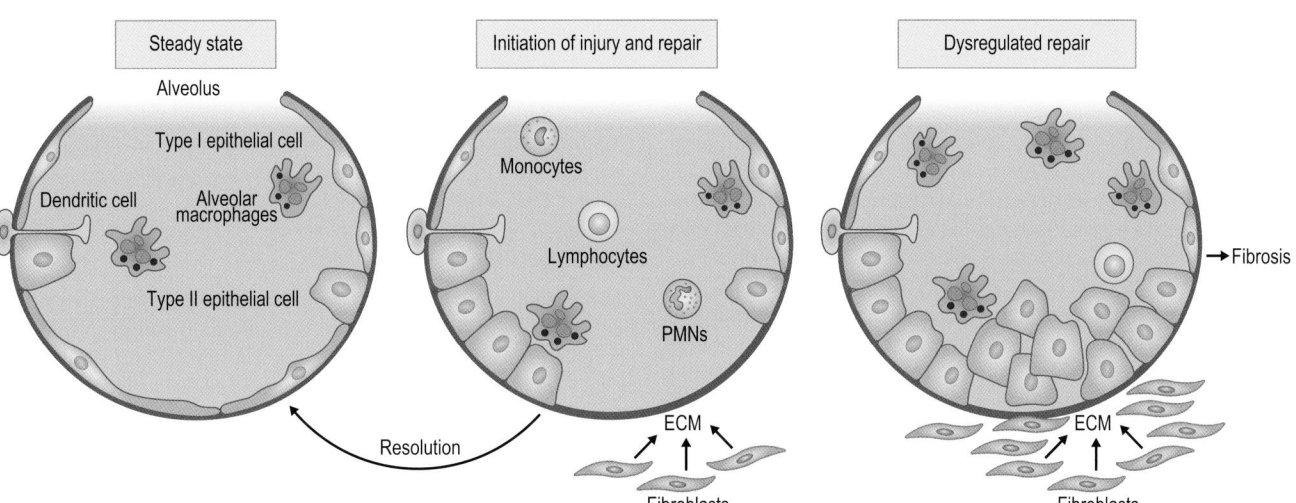

| Steady state | Initiation of injury and repair | Dysregulated repair |

1. Denudation of barrier
2. Cytokine/chemokine expression
3. Recruitment of inflammatory cells
4. Proliferation of type II epithelial cells
5. DC maturation
6. Fibroblasts express ECM

Fig. 71.1 Pathogenesis of interstitial lung disease. In the healthy lung, the alveoli maintain an anti-inflammatory state to prevent unwanted inflammation. The predominant cells in the healthy alveolus are macrophages and types I and II epithelial cells. Upon injury, there is denudation of the epithelial barrier, resulting in the expression of cytokines/chemokines, recruitment of inflammatory cells, proliferation of type II epithelial cells, dendritic cell (DC) maturation, and expression of extracellular matrix (ECM) by fibroblasts. This inflammatory milieu leads to the resolution of inflammation and repair of lung injury. Conversely, in the presence of either prolonged antigen exposure or an inability to clear antigen, persistent inflammation ensues, resulting in extracellular matrix deposition with subsequent tissue remodelling, fibrosis, and permanent lung dysfunction.

suppress expression of cytokines by Th1 and Th2 cells suggesting that Tregs may be important in regulating inflammatory lung disease and pulmonary fibrosis.[10]

Idiopathic interstitial pneumonias

● KEY CONCEPTS

Classification of the idiopathic interstitial pneumonias

- The idiopathic interstitial pneumonias comprise a group of seven histologically distinct disorders.
- The distinction is important since response to treatment and prognosis differs:
  - Idiopathic pulmonary fibrosis (IPF) with histopathology labeled as usual interstitial pneumonitis (UIP): the pathology of UIP can occur in other diseases such as collagen vascular diseases
  - Acute interstitial pneumonitis (AIP)
  - Desquamative interstitial pneumonitis (DIP)
  - Respiratory bronchiolitis-associated interstitial lung disease (RB-ILD)
  - Nonspecific interstitial pneumonitis (NSIP)
  - Lymphocytic interstitial pneumonitis (LIP)
  - Cryptogenic organizing pneumonia (COP)
- In order to differentiate between these diseases, a thorascopic lung biopsy is often required.

The clinical syndromes known collectively as IPF or idiopathic interstitial pneumonias comprise a group of histologically distinct disorders. The classical form of IPF has a histological appearance termed usual interstitial pneumonitis (UIP). Other histological and clinical forms include acute interstitial pneumonitis (AIP), desquamative interstitial pneumonitis (DIP), respiratory bronchiolitis-associated interstitial lung disease (RB-ILD), nonspecific interstitial pneumonitis (NSIP), and cryptogenic organizing pneumonia (COP). In order to differentiate between these diseases, a thoracoscopic lung biopsy is often required. The distinction between these disorders is important since response to treatment and outcome differs.

Idiopathic pulmonary fibrosis

The usual form of IPF, also known as cryptogenic fibrosing alveolitis, is the commonest diffuse parenchymal lung disease of unknown etiology.[11] It is characterized by progressive clinical deterioration despite available therapy. Although IPF has characteristic clinical, radiographic, and histologic appearances, other interstitial lung diseases, including the collagen vascular diseases (CVD), drug reactions, and environmental exposures, can mimic these findings.

Clinical manifestations

● CLINICAL PEARLS

Idiopathic pulmonary fibrosis (IPF)

- IPF is one of the most common causes of diffuse parenchymal lung disease of unknown etiology and is characterized by insidious onset of cough and dyspnea.
- The histopathologic pattern of IPF is usual interstitial pneumonitis.
- A confident diagnosis of IPF based on high-resolution computed tomography can only be made in two-thirds of cases.
- IPF is generally a fatal disorder, characterized by relentless progression and a 5-year survival of 30–50%.

The incidence and prevalence of IPF are uncertain, although prevalence rates for men and women of 20.2 per 100 000 and 13.2 per 100 000, respectively, have been reported.[12] Both the incidence and prevalence of IPF increase with age, with most patients presenting between 40 and 70 years of age. Although the clinical features of IPF are variable, most patients present with the insidious onset of exertional dyspnea and a dry, nonproductive cough. Physical examination typically reveals dry, end-inspiratory crackles; clubbing is present in 25–50% of patients.

The chest radiograph typically shows diffuse reticular opacities, predominantly in the peripheral lower lung zones. Ground-glass opacities, small cysts (honeycombing), and reduced lung volumes may also be seen (Fig. 71.2A). These radiographic changes often precede the onset of symptoms, and serial chest radiographs usually reveal progressive loss of lung volume. High-resolution computed tomography (HRCT) findings include bibasal peripheral reticular opacities (Fig. 71.2B).[13] Honeycombing, traction bronchiectasis, and subpleural fibrosis can also be present. The finding of ground-glass opacities on the initial HRCT suggests alveolar inflammation and may identify patients with IPF who are more likely to respond to glucocorticoid therapy.

The typical physiologic abnormalities in IPF are those of a restrictive lung disease with a low diffusing capacity for carbon monoxide and severe gas exchange abnormalities exacerbated by exercise.

Histopathology

The gross appearance of the lungs in IPF shows a nodular pleural surface while histopathologic examination reveals UIP. UIP is characterized by nonuniform and variable distribution of the interstitial changes. At low magnification, alternating zones of interstitial fibrosis, inflammation, honeycombing, and normal lung can be seen (Fig. 71.3A). At higher magnification, findings include derangement of alveolar walls with edema, fibrinous exudate, fibroblast proliferation, and fibrosis. Honeycomb change refers to enlarged airspaces lined by metaplastic bronchial epithelium and surrounded by walls thickened with

collagen (Fig. 71.3B). The earliest finding in UIP is thought to be the fibroblast focus, a lesion consisting of distinct clusters of fibroblasts and myofibroblasts in a loose connective tissue matrix within the alveolar wall, with minimal interstitial inflammation or intra-alveolar macrophage accumulation (Fig. 71.3C).[14] Tables 71.1 and 71.2 compare the clinical and pathologic features of UIP, DIP, RB-ILD, and NSIP.

Pathogenesis

The pathogenesis of IPF is poorly understood, but current evidence suggests that the disease is mediated through an interplay between immunologic, genetic, environmental and viral factors (Fig. 71.4).[11] Some cases of IPF are familial, inherited as an autosomal dominant trait with variable penetrance.[15] A recent study suggested that dysregulated expression of a mucin gene, *MUC5B*, may be involved in the pathogenesis of familial IPF.[16] Mutations in the telomerase ribonucleoprotein complex associated with telomere shortening have also been linked with familial interstitial pneumonitis.[17,18] In addition, surfactant protein C mutations have been rarely associated with IPF.[19]

In the normal lung, the interstitium is thin and delicate with few lymphoid cells and fibroblasts. Following the initiation of the inflammatory process, damage to the alveolar epithelium occurs, followed by infiltration of the interstitium with activated immune cells. In addition, immune complexes have been identified in the serum and lungs of IPF patients.[20] Activated alveolar macrophages secrete IL-1, IL-8, TNF-α, PDGF, and IGF-1. This cytokine milieu promotes the activation and recruitment of neutrophils and lymphocytes to the area of alveolitis.

T lymphocytes, which accumulate in the alveolar space and interstitium, express an activated phenotype, including the expression of HLA-DR and IL-2 receptor. Following activation, CD4 T cells evolve into three major subsets distinguished by the cytokines produced (Chapters 10 and 17).[21] In IPF, T cells expressing a Th2-type phenotype predominate, producing IL-4, -5, and -13. It appears that a switch to Th2-type cells may be important in the development of fibrosis through the deposition of matrix components and by attracting the influx of fibroblasts.

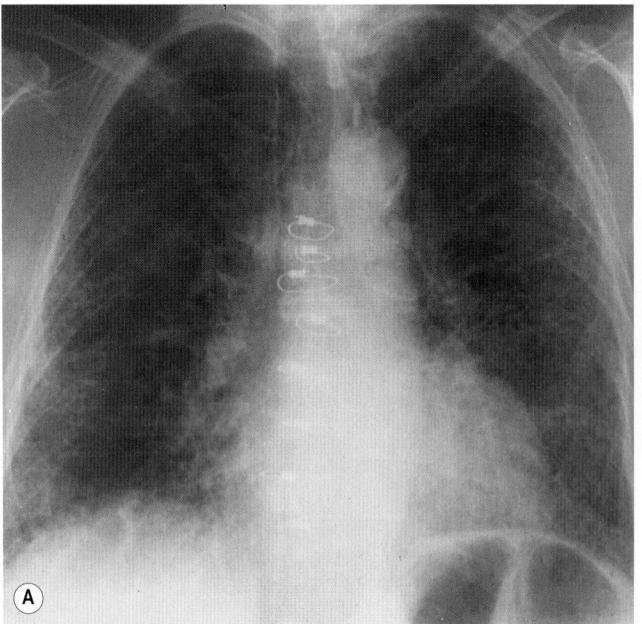

(A)

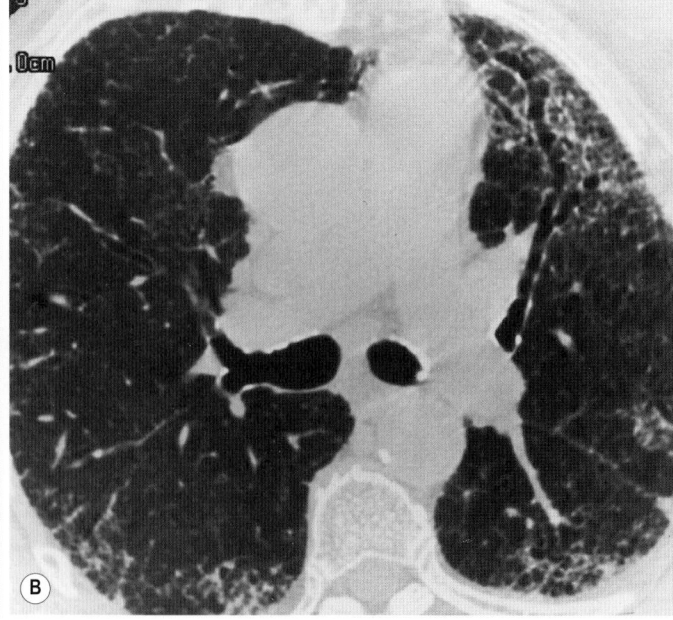

(B)

Fig. 71.2 Radiographic manifestations of idiopathic pulmonary fibrosis. (A) Chest radiograph in a patient with idiopathic pulmonary fibrosis showing diffuse, coarse reticular opacities with a lower lung zone predominance. Cystic radiolucencies, consistent with honeycombing, are evident. (B) High-resolution computed tomography shows peripheral reticular opacities, honeycombing, and traction bronchiectasis.

Table 71.1 Clinical features of the idiopathic interstitial pneumonias

	UIP	DIP	RB-ILD	AIP	NSIP
Mean age (years)	57	42	36	49	49
Childhood	No	Rare	No	Rare	Occasionally
Onset	Insidious	Insidious	Insidious	Acute	Subacute, insidious
Mortality (mean survival)	68% (5–6 years)	27% (12 years)	0%	62% (1–2 months)	11% (17 months)
Response to steroids	Poor	Good	Good	Poor	Good
Recovery possible	No	Yes	Yes	Yes	Yes

AID, acute interstitial pneumonitis; DIP, desquamative interstitial pneumonitis; NSIP, nonspecific interstitial pneumonitis; RB-ILD, respiratory bronchiolitis-associated interstitial lung disease; UIP, usual interstitial pneumonitis.
Adapted from Katzenstein AL, Myers JL. Idiopathic pulmonary fibrosis: clinical relevance of pathologic classification. Am J Respir Crit Care Med 1998; 157: 1301.

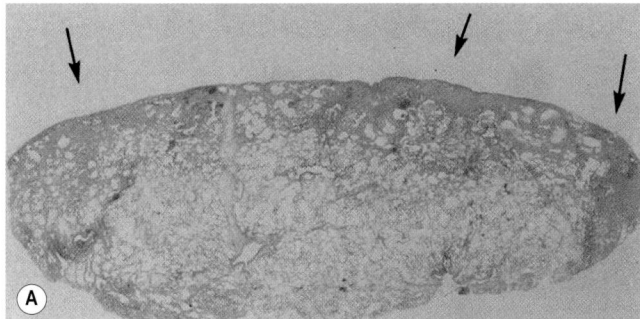
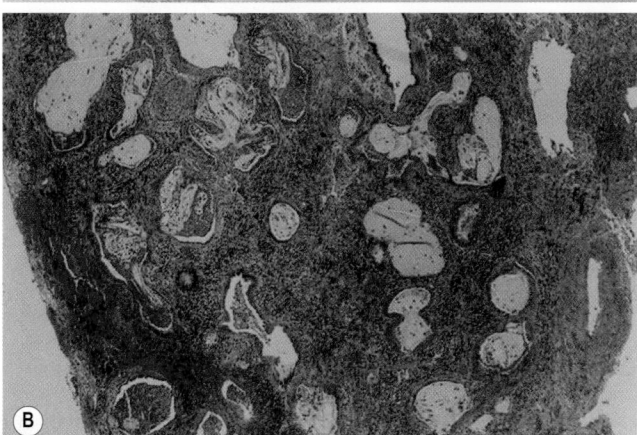
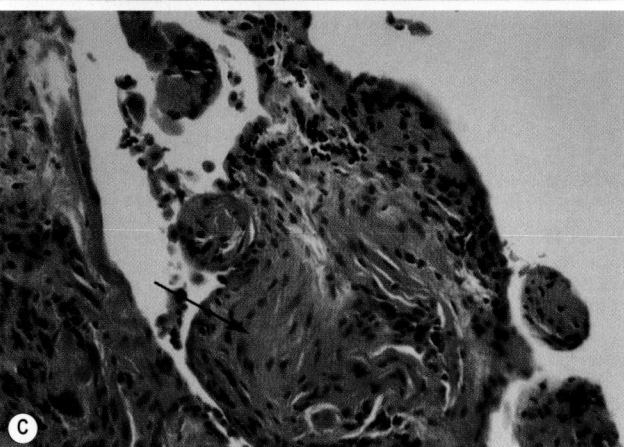

Fig. 71.3 Histopathology of usual interstitial pneumonitis (UIP). (A) Low-magnification photomicrograph of UIP showing the variegated appearance from one field of view to the next with areas of dense subpleural fibrosis (arrows) separated from other areas of normal lung. (B) High-magnification photomicrograph of UIP showing honeycomb change characterized by enlarged airspaces filled with mucin and separated by fibrosis. (C) Fibroblast focus in UIP is characterized by clusters of spindle-shaped fibroblasts (arrow) in a loose connective tissue matrix within the alveolar wall.

In addition, the Th17 cytokine, IL-17A, has been linked to the development of bleomycin-induced lung injury and collagen deposition.[8,9] Evidence also suggests that IPF patients have oligoclonal CD4 T cell expansions that proliferate in response to antigens present in diseased tissue.[22] Finally, regulatory T-cell function may be impaired in patients with IPF.[10] Taken together, these findings implicate T-cell-mediated immune function in IPF pathogenesis.

In addition to their role as scavengers, alveolar macrophages are vital in the repair phase of inflammation. However, the distinguishing feature between a self-resolving inflammatory process and a fibrotic response, as seen in IPF, is the accumulation of collagen. Current evidence suggests that the fibrotic process in IPF is a consequence of dysregulation of both collagen synthesis and degradation. Macrophage-derived growth factors, including TGF-β, PDGF, and IGF-1, stimulate fibroblast proliferation and collagen deposition.[23] Adequate resolution of an inflammatory process requires matrix degradation. Matrix metalloproteases produced by macrophages and fibroblasts are involved in matrix

Table 71.2 Histopathologic features of the idiopathic interstitial pneumonias

	UIP	DIP/RB-ILD	AIP	NSIP
Temporal appearance	Variegated	Uniform	Uniform	Uniform
Interstitial inflammation	Scant	Scant	No	Prominent
Collagen/fibrosis	Patchy	Diffuse (DIP) Focal (RB-ILD)	No	Diffuse
Fibroblast proliferation	Fibroblast foci prominent	No	Diffuse	Rare
BOOP	No	No	No	Focal
Honeycomb change	Yes	No	No	Rare
Intra-alveolar macrophages	Focal	Diffuse (DIP) Focal (RB-ILD)	No	Patchy
Hyaline membranes	No	No	Focal	No

AIP, acute interstitial pneumonitis; BOOP, bronchiolitis obliterans organizing pneumonia; DIP, desquamative interstitial pneumonitis; NSIP, nonspecific interstitial pneumonitis; RB-ILD, respiratory bronchiolitis-associated interstitial lung disease; UIP, usual interstitial pneumonitis.
Adapted from Katzenstein AL, Myers JL. Idiopathic pulmonary fibrosis: clinical relevance of pathologic classification. Am J Respir Crit Care Med 1998; 157: 1301.

degradation, and control of metalloprotease production involves substances known as tissue inhibitors of metalloproteases (TIMPs). TIMPs are elevated in the lungs of patients with IPF. In addition, TGF-β can markedly augment TIMP production. Thus, there appears to be a loss of balance between the events mediating resolution and those mediating perpetuation of the inflammatory response, setting the stage for lung injury, tissue remodeling, and the development of irreversible pulmonary fibrosis.

● KEY CONCEPTS

Pathogenesis of the idiopathic interstitial pneumonias

- Although the inciting event(s) is unknown in the different diseases, a common result is a dysregulated fibroproliferative response (similar to wound healing), which leads to excessive extracellular matrix production and lung remodeling.

- A genetically determined inability to repair and re-epithelialize the denuded basement membranes adequately may be a contributing factor and may relate to the familial occurrence of some cases of idiopathic pulmonary fibrosis.

- The presence of a chronic stimulus (autoantigen), as is seen in the pneumoconioses, may result in a persistent inflammatory and immune response and lead to a failure in the normal healing process.

- The release of transforming growth factor-β following epithelial injury stimulates collagen synthesis and the prevention of apoptosis of proliferating fibroblasts in the lung and may impair collagen degradation by inhibiting the production of metalloproteases.

- A predominant Th2 response in the lung and the absence of interferon-γ favor the development of a fibrotic response.

Diagnosis

The diagnostic evaluation of a patient with diffuse parenchymal lung disease includes a thorough history and physical examination with particular attention to symptoms and signs that could indicate collagen vascular disease, occupational and environmental exposures, or medication and drug usage. A careful family history is also important.

The history and physical findings in IPF are nonspecific. However, extrapulmonary involvement does not occur: the presence of fever, arthralgias, myalgias, or pleuritis should suggest a collagen vascular disorder. Antinuclear antibodies and rheumatoid factor are present in 10–20% of IPF patients, but titers greater than 1:160 should suggest an alternative diagnosis.

The majority of patients with IPF have an abnormal chest radiograph at the time of presentation. Basal peripheral reticular opacities are the characteristic radiographic findings. A confident diagnosis of IPF from HRCT of the lung requires the presence of patchy, peripheral bibasal reticular abnormalities.[12] The presence of extensive ground-glass opacities on HRCT should suggest an alternative diagnosis, such as DIP, hypersensitivity pneumonitis, bronchiolitis obliterans organizing pneumonia (BOOP), or NSIP.

A surgical lung biopsy is recommended in suspected IPF patients without a definitive HRCT appearance and who do not have contraindications to the procedure. This is especially important in patients with atypical clinical or radiographic findings, which could suggest the possibility of one of the other histologic patterns of the idiopathic interstitial pneumonias and an improved prognosis. Biopsy may be omitted in elderly patients with cardiovascular disease, or those with evidence of extensive honeycomb change. Video-assisted thoracoscopic (VATS) biopsy is the preferred surgical technique and has been associated with less morbidity and a decreased hospital stay compared with open lung biopsy.

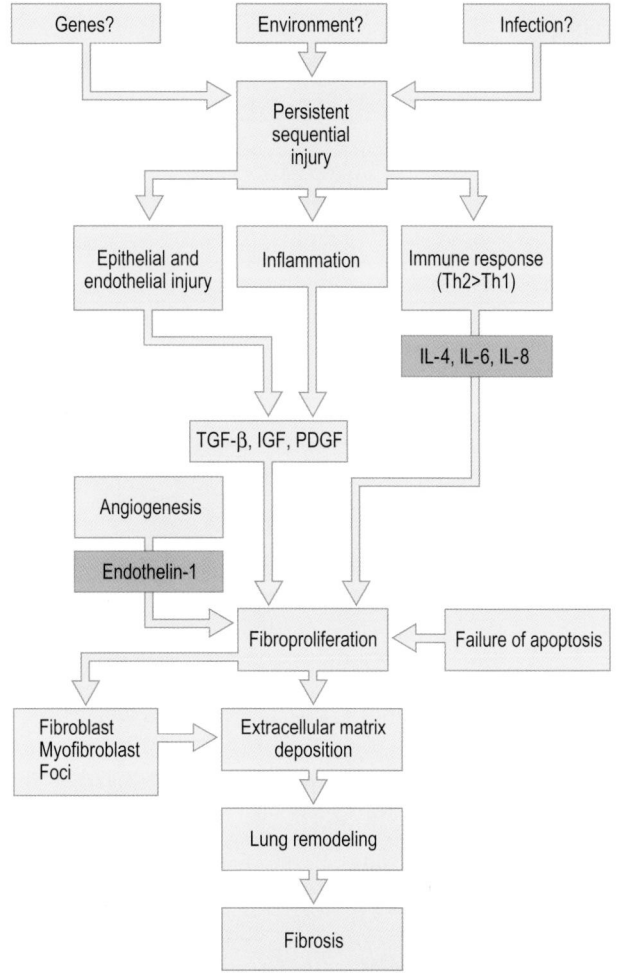

Fig. 71.4 Events hypothesized to be involved in the pathogenesis of idiopathic pulmonary fibrosis. The initiating event(s) leading to persistent lung injury remains poorly understood. The interaction between genetic factors, environmental exposures, and infectious agents leads to epithelial and endothelial injury, resulting in the secretion of macrophage-derived growth factors, including transforming growth factor-β (TGF-β), insulin-like growth factor-1 (IGF-1), and platelet-derived growth factor (PDGF). This cytokine milieu stimulates fibroblast proliferation and collagen deposition. In addition, the resulting Th2 immune response stimulates extracellular matrix production and fibroblast proliferation, resulting in lung remodeling and, eventually, lung fibrosis.

Treatment and outcome

The usual course of IPF is relentless progression without spontaneous remission, commonly with a fatal outcome. The most common cause of death in patients with IPF is progression of the underlying disease[24] with two-thirds of deaths due to respiratory failure, or cardiovascular complications. Other causes of death in IPF include bronchogenic carcinoma (10%), infection (7%), and pulmonary embolism (3%). Recent studies in patients with biopsy-proven IPF indicate a shorter survival than previously thought (30–50% 5-year survival).[25] This change in survival rate could be real or result from changes in clinical practice (i.e., which patients go for biopsy). Currently available treatment options include glucocorticoids or immunosuppressant drugs, either alone or in combination. However, numerous clinical trials using different therapies have failed to show a significant survival benefit.[26] Thus, there is no good evidence to support the use of any specific therapy in the management of IPF. Lung transplantation should be considered in patients with progressive clinical and physiologic deterioration who meet established criteria. Early listing is crucial since the waiting time may exceed 2 years.

Acute interstitial pneumonia

Acute interstitial pneumonia (AIP) is a fulminant form of idiopathic interstitial pneumonia. Although it was previously thought to represent an acute phase of UIP, recent studies suggest it is a distinct entity.[27] However, patients with documented UIP/IPF experiencing acute exacerbations can have the pathology of AIP superimposed on the features of UIP.[28,29]

Clinical manifestations

AIP usually presents with acute onset of dyspnea followed by rapid progression to respiratory failure. The clinical, radiographic, physiologic, and histologic features are identical to those of the acute respiratory distress syndrome (ARDS) but without any identifiable cause. Most patients are previously healthy individuals over 40 years of age. Men and women are equally affected. A viral prodrome is common, with symptoms including fever, nonproductive cough, and dyspnea. Laboratory studies are nonspecific. Chest radiographs show diffuse, bilateral airspace opacities, and on HRCT there is ground-glass attenuation. A similar presentation may complicate or represent the initial manifestation of a CVD.

Histopathology

AIP is characterized by diffuse interstitial fibrosis that is temporally uniform (Fig. 71.5).[30] The changes are identical to the organizing phases of diffuse alveolar damage, as seen in ARDS. Within the thickened interstitial space, there is active, diffuse fibroblast proliferation similar to the focal fibroblast foci seen in UIP. If this is progressive, honeycomb change occurs. However, these airspaces are lined with alveolar epithelium as opposed to the bronchiolar epithelium lining honeycomb spaces. Other features of acute lung injury, which are frequently seen in AIP, are intra-alveolar hyaline membranes.

Diagnosis

The diagnosis of AIP is based on a clinical syndrome of idiopathic ARDS and the presence of organizing diffuse alveolar damage on lung biopsy.[31] Lung biopsy is recommended to secure the diagnosis and exclude other causes of acute interstitial lung disease.

Treatment and outcome

No effective therapy exists for patients with AIP. Glucocorticoids are utilized in most cases, but no survival benefit has been shown. One study found that the additional use of anticoagulation improves survival. Overall, the prognosis of patients with AIP is poor, with mortality rates ranging from 50 to 88%. Half of patients die within 6 months of disease onset. However, those who survive may have complete recovery of lung function. Once recovered, AIP rarely recurs.

Desquamative interstitial pneumonitis

DIP represents fewer than 3% of all cases of interstitial lung disease.[32] However, it is a distinct clinicopathological entity that differs substantially from UIP.

Clinical manifestations

DIP affects individuals in their fourth to fifth decades of life with a male predominance in most studies. It occurs predominantly in cigarette smokers. Clinically, most individuals present with subacute onset of a dry, nonproductive cough and dyspnea. Clubbing is present in approximately 50% of DIP patients. Laboratory evaluation is usually nonspecific.

The chest radiograph shows non-specific bibasal ground-glass opacities. Reticulonodular interstitial infiltrates have also been reported. The chest radiograph can be normal in up to 20% of symptomatic individuals. HRCT confirms the presence of ground-glass attenuation in the periphery of the lower lung zones (Fig. 71.6). Pulmonary function testing shows a restrictive defect with hypoxemia and an associated decrease in diffusion capacity.

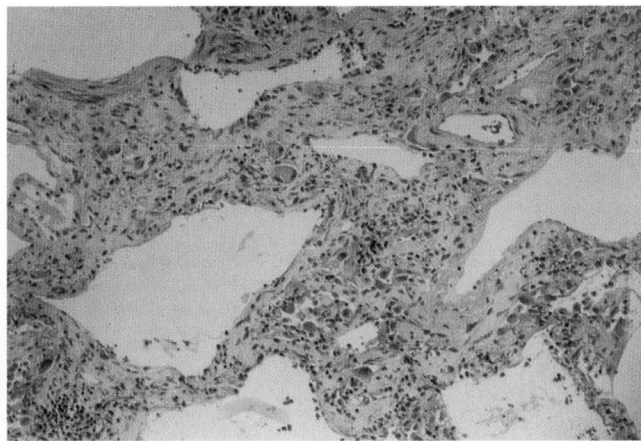

Fig. 71.5 Histopathology of acute interstitial pneumonitis. Diffuse thickening of the alveolar septum with an infiltration of mononuclear cells is the characteristic abnormality. The temporal uniformity of this process is also apparent.

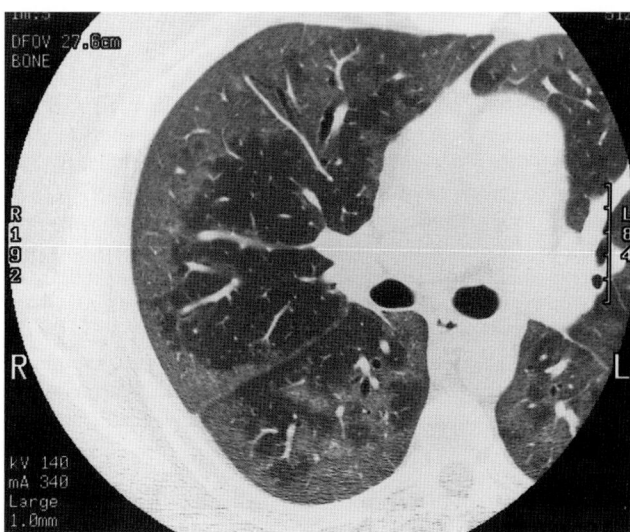

Fig. 71.6 Radiographic manifestations in desquamative interstitial pneumonitis. High-resolution computed tomography in a patient with desquamative interstitial pneumonitis shows ground-glass attenuation in the periphery of the upper and lower lung fields.

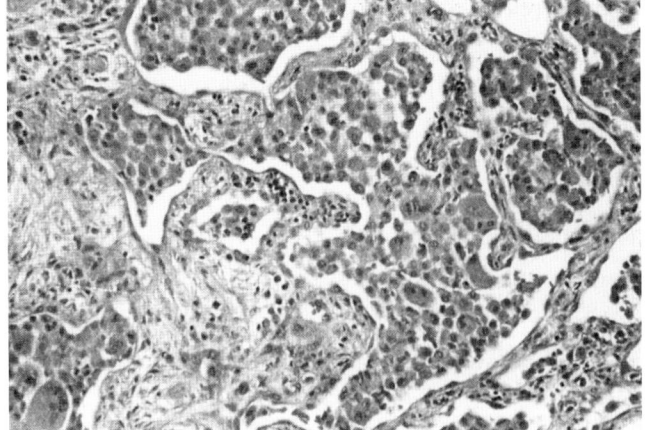

Fig. 71.7 Histopathology of desquamative interstitial pneumonitis. A high-magnification photomicrograph of desquamative interstitial pneumonitis shows the uniform, diffuse accumulation of macrophages within the alveolar space with associated thickening of the alveolar septum. These aggregates of macrophages almost completely fill the alveolar spaces.

Histopathology

DIP is a misnomer. It was initially thought that the intra-alveolar cells represented sloughed or desquamated alveolar epithelial cells. However, DIP is pathologically characterized by uniform, diffuse accumulation of macrophages in the alveolar space (Fig. 71.7).[16] At low magnification, the overall appearance is one of uniformity from one field of view to the next as opposed to the variegated appearance of UIP. In addition, there is scant interstitial inflammation with varying degrees of fibrosis of the alveolar septum.

Diagnosis

The diagnosis of DIP requires tissue confirmation of the pathologic lesion. This is important since DIP has a better prognosis and response to therapeutic intervention compared to IPF. A DIP-like pattern is frequently seen in the other idiopathic interstitial pneumonias as well as in eosinophilic granuloma, collagen vascular diseases, drug reactions, and other unrelated conditions. Thus, the diagnosis of DIP requires careful correlation of pathologic findings with clinical and radiologic findings.

Treatment and outcome

The primary intervention in DIP is smoking cessation. Since this is a rare condition with relatively few published cases, it is unclear whether glucocorticoids alter the natural history of this disease. A mortality rate of 28% with a mean survival of 12 years has been reported, compared to a 66% mortality and a mean survival of 5.6 years in UIP. Of note, 22% patients improved spontaneously and 60% responded to glucocorticoid therapy. This picture is dramatically different from IPF, in which spontaneous improvement rarely, if ever, occurs and a response to glucocorticoids is seen in only 10–15% of patients. There are, however, a significant minority of DIP patients who fail to respond to treatment and progress to respiratory failure, secondary to advanced fibrosis.

Respiratory bronchiolitis-associated interstitial lung disease

RB-ILD is a distinct clinical entity that occurs in current or former cigarette smokers. It is unclear whether RB-ILD and DIP represent different diseases or different ends of the spectrum of the same disease process.[32] DIP occurs predominantly and RB-ILD occurs exclusively in cigarette smokers, suggesting a common pathogenesis related to cigarette smoke.

Clinical manifestations

The mean age at presentation with RB-ILD is 36 years. Males are more often affected, and all individuals with RB-ILD were cigarette smokers. The most common symptoms are a dry, non-productive cough and dyspnea. Clubbing is absent in RB-ILD, whereas it is frequently present in DIP. Laboratory evaluation is nonspecific.

The chest radiograph typically shows diffuse, fine reticular or nodular interstitial opacities with normal lung volumes. Additional findings include bronchial wall thickening and a prominent peribronchovascular interstitium. HRCT may reveal ground-glass opacification as well as emphysema.

Pulmonary function tests most commonly reveal a mixed restrictive–obstructive pattern with a reduced diffusing capacity and mild hypoxemia. The residual volume may be increased with no change in other spirometric parameters.

Histopathology

The pathology of RB-ILD is similar to DIP. However, in RB-ILD, the intra-alveolar macrophages accumulate primarily within the peribronchiolar airspaces and are associated with thickening of the alveolar septum in these areas (Fig. 71.8). The differentiation of this lesion from DIP requires sparing of distal airspaces with the lesion confined to the peribronchiolar airspaces in RB-ILD.

Diagnosis

RB-ILD should be suspected in young individuals with a history of cigarette use who complain of cough and dyspnea with a chest radiograph or HRCT showing nodular and/or reticular interstitial opacities. The diagnosis requires tissue confirmation of the pathologic findings noted above.

Treatment and outcome

The key therapeutic intervention in RB-ILD is cessation of smoking. The use of glucocorticoids has been associated with favorable results. At present, the clinical course and prognosis of patients with RB-ILD are unknown. In most clinical series, patients either improved or stabilized, and mortality is uncommon.[32,33]

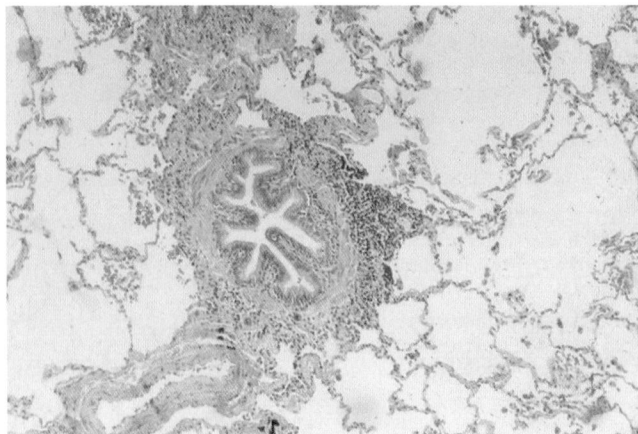

Fig. 71.8 Histopathology of respiratory bronchiolitis—interstitial lung disease. An ectatic bronchiole with a thickened wall is shown, with a mononuclear infiltrate extending into the immediately surrounding alveoli.

Nonspecific interstitial pneumonitis

The term NSIP was first used to describe cases of interstitial pneumonia that did not demonstrate a pattern of UIP, AIP, or DIP.[34] Currently, the term NSIP is applied to an idiopathic interstitial pneumonia or to a similar histologic pattern that occurs in collagen vascular disease, hypersensitivity pneumonitis, infection or drug-induced lung disease. Thus, the diagnosis of NSIP should prompt investigation for a causative agent.[27] In fact, 16% of patients in the original description of NSIP had one of the collagen vascular diseases.[34]

Clinical manifestations

Idiopathic NSIP is most often seen in middle-aged individuals, with a slight female predominance. A dry, nonproductive cough and exertional dyspnea are the most common symptoms, although fever is present in 25% of patients. Symptoms are usually present for 6–10 months prior to diagnosis. As in other interstitial pneumonias, the laboratory evaluation is nonspecific.

The chest radiograph usually shows bilateral interstitial infiltrates and sometimes can be normal in a symptomatic patient. HRCT characteristically shows bilateral, patchy ground-glass attenuation indistinguishable from DIP or RB-ILD.[13]

Histopathology

NSIP is characterized by varying but temporally uniform degrees of fibrosis and inflammation of the alveolar septum, without histopathologic features indicative of UIP, AIP, or DIP (Fig. 71.9). NSIP has been divided into three groups depending on the presence or absence of interstitial fibrosis: interstitial lymphoplasmacytic inflammation (48% of cases); inflammation and fibrosis (38%); and fibrosis (14%).[19] Although the changes are temporally uniform, they may be patchy with intervening areas of normal lung.

This temporal uniformity is in contrast to the variegated pattern seen in UIP. Fibroblast foci, the earliest lesion seen in UIP, are found in 20% of patients with NSIP, making the differentiation of fibrotic NSIP from UIP difficult. The key feature in this circumstance is the temporal uniformity of the lesion in NSIP.

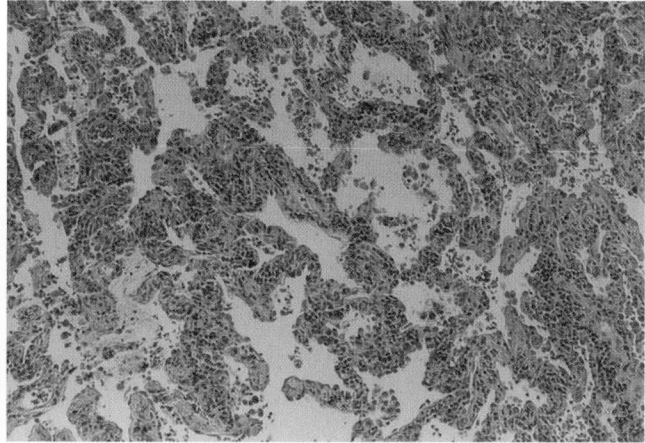

Fig. 71.9 Histopathology of nonspecific interstitial pneumonitis. Low-magnification photomicrograph of cellular nonspecific interstitial pneumonitis shows diffuse uniform thickening of the alveolar septum due to the presence of a lymphoplasmacytic infiltrate.

Treatment and outcome

Unlike patients with UIP, individuals with NSIP have a favorable prognosis. In the original description of the disease, 45% of subjects completely recovered while another 42% remained stable or improved.[34] Only 11% of patients died, with a mean survival of 16 months. All of the individuals with an aggressive course were in the fibrotic group. Ten-year survival in the cellular group was 90%, compared to 35% in patients with the fibrotic pattern. Despite the worse prognosis of NSIP with a fibrosing pattern, this is still significantly better than the 10-year survival rate of UIP patients (15%).[35]

Cryptogenic organizing pneumonia

Cryptogenic organizing pneumonis (COP) or idiopathic bronchiolitis obliterans organizing pneumonia (BOOP) is a specific clinicopathologic disorder of unknown etiology characterized by excessive proliferation of granulation tissue within the lumen of the distal airspaces.[36] The term COP is reserved for cases demonstrating BOOP without an obvious cause, since this histologic appearance of BOOP occurs in a variety of inflammatory lung disorders, including collagen vascular diseases, malignancy, infections, and those caused by medications.

Clinical manifestations

The onset of disease is usually in the fifth to sixth decades of life; men and women are affected equally. Most individuals have symptoms for less than 2 months prior to diagnosis. The initial presentation is usually with a dry, nonproductive cough and flu-like symptoms, including fever, sore throat, and malaise. This is followed by progressive dyspnea and cough. Routine laboratory evaluation is nonspecific.

The chest radiograph shows diffuse, often patchy alveolar opacities in the setting of normal lung volumes (Fig. 71.10A). These opacities can be migratory and usually have a peripheral distribution similar to those seen in chronic eosinophilic pneumonia. Rarer radiographic manifestations include linear or nodular interstitial opacities and honeycombing. The presence of a pleural effusion or pleural thickening should suggest an associated collagen vascular disease.

HRCT shows patchy airspace consolidation especially in the lung periphery with a lower-lung zone predominance (Fig. 71.10B). Other findings include ground-glass attenuation, small nodular opacities, and bronchial wall thickening.

As in other interstitial lung diseases, a restrictive ventilatory defect is the most common pulmonary function abnormality. Gas exchange abnormalities are common and are accompanied by decreased diffusing capacity, widening of the alveolar-arterial gradient, and exercise-induced hypoxemia.

Histopathology

The histopathology of COP is characterized by excessive proliferation of granulation tissue in the small airways and alveolar ducts with associated chronic inflammation in the alveolar walls (Fig. 71.11).[36] The intraluminal fibrotic buds (Masson bodies) consist of loose collagen-embedding fibroblasts and myofibroblasts and have a tendency to extend from one alveolus to the next, giving a characteristic "butterfly" pattern. The lesions are patchy in nature and have a uniform temporal appearance at low magnification with preservation of the underlying lung parenchyma. COP has been described as the prototypical healing response of the lung to a variety of insults.

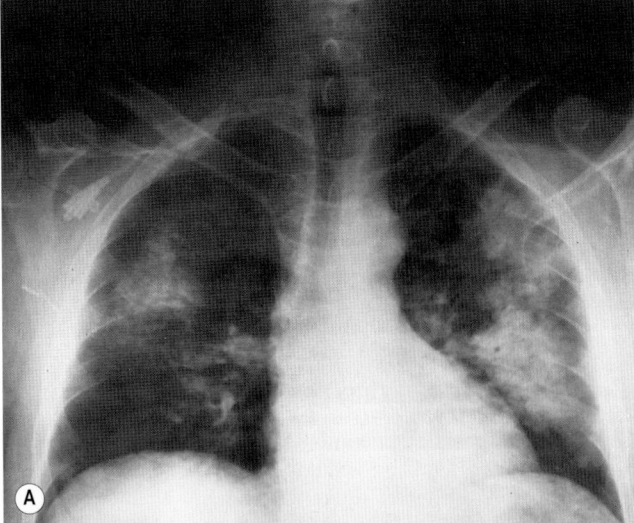

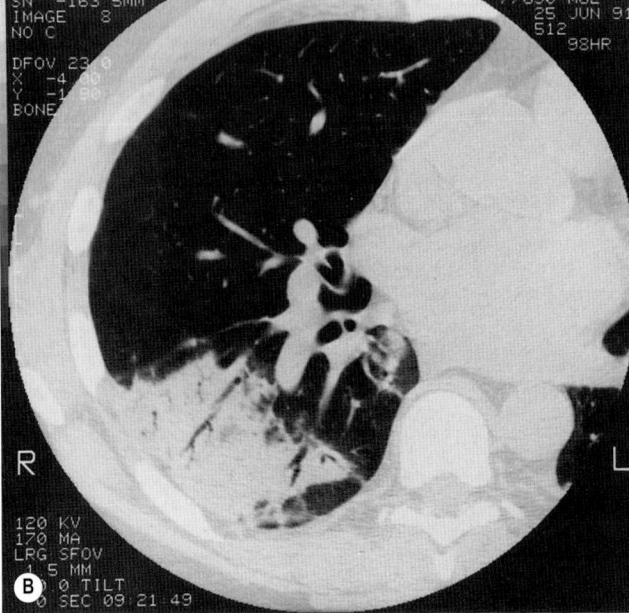

Fig. 71.10 Radiographic findings in cryptogenic organizing pneumonia.
(A) Chest radiograph in a patient with cryptogenic organizing pneumonia shows bilateral patchy alveolar opacities with a peripheral distribution in the setting of normal lung volumes. (B) Chest computed tomography shows a dense right lower lung consolidation with the presence of air bronchograms.

Diagnosis

The presence of BOOP in a lung biopsy does not necessarily represent COP since this is a diagnosis of exclusion. Organizing pneumonia is a nonspecific response to many lung injuries and may occur in conjunction with another pathologic process or as a component of other primary pulmonary disorders such as infections, irradiation, collagen vascular disease, hypersensitivity pneumonitis, Wegener's granulomatosis (WG), or chronic eosinophilic pneumonia (Table 71.3).

Treatment and outcome

Treatment with glucocorticoids usually offers dramatic clinical and radiographic improvement within days to weeks.[36] Complete clinical, physiologic, and radiographic recovery occurs in two-thirds of cases. However, in the remainder, persistent disease with progression to fibrosis occurs. It is common for relapses to occur with glucocorticoid tapering, followed by

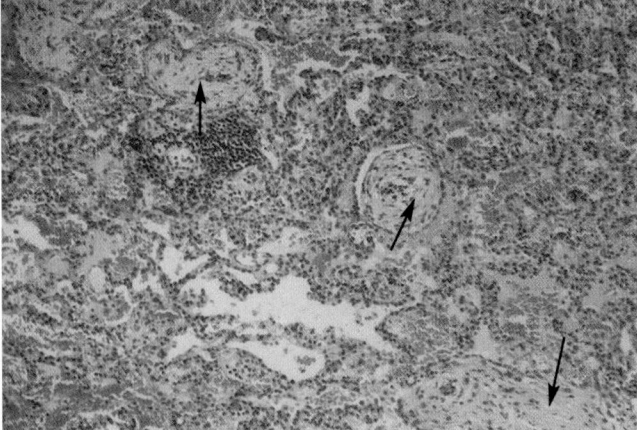

Fig. 71.11 Histopathology of cryptogenic organizing pneumonia.
A photomicrograph of cryptogenic organizing pneumonia shows intra-alveolar fibroblast proliferation (arrows) and early collagen production. In addition, thickening of the alveolar septa with a lymphoplasmacytic infiltrate consistent with cellular nonspecific interstitial pneumonitis is present.

Table 71.3 Disorders associated with a bronchiolitis obliterans organizing pneumonia (BOOP) pattern

Idiopathic BOOP (cryptogenic organizing pneumonia)
Collagen vascular diseases
•Systemic lupus erythematosus
•Rheumatoid arthritis
•Polymyositis/dermatomyositis
•Sjögren syndrome
Hypersensitivity pneumonitis
Chronic eosinophilic pneumonia
Drug-induced
•Gold
•Penicillamine
•Amiodarone
•Bleomycin
•Sulfa drugs
Wegener's granulomatosis
Bone marrow transplantation
Lung transplantation/rejection
Inhalational injury
Neoplasms
Lung irradiation
Virus-associated
•Human immunodeficiency virus (HIV)
•Influenza
•Adenovirus

improvement with reintroduction of treatment; consequently at least 6 months of therapy is recommended. The 5-year survival in COP is 73%, compared to 5-year survival rates of 44% in patients with BOOP due to other causes (e.g., collagen vascular disease) or 30% for IPF.

Lung involvement in collagen vascular diseases

CVD are a heterogeneous group of systemic autoimmune diseases that frequently involve the lungs. The pleuropulmonary manifestations of these diseases are diverse, affecting all parts

Table 71.4 Pleuropulmonary manifestations of collagen vascular diseases

	SLE	RA	SSc
Pulmonary hypertension	+	+	+++
Vasculitis	+	±	±
Pleural disease	+++	+++	+
Bronchiolitis obliterans	±	++	+
Aspiration pneumonia	−	−	++
Diaphragmatic dysfunction	++	−	−
Lung nodules	−	++	−
Diffuse alveolar damage	+	±	±
BOOP	±	+	±
UIP	+	++	+++
Capillaritis	++	+	±
LIP	+	+	+
NSIP	+	++	+

BOOP, bronchiolitis obliterans organizing pneumonia; LIP, lymphocytic interstitial pneumonitis; NSIP, nonspecific interstitial pneumonitis; RA, rheumatoid arthritis; SLE, systemic lupus erythematosus; SSc, systemic sclerosis; UIP, usual interstitial pneumonitis.

of the respiratory tract (i.e., airways, alveoli, blood vessels, and pleura) (Table 71.4). Although pulmonary complications generally occur in patients with well-established disease, occasionally the lung involvement is the first manifestation of the autoimmune disorder. This section discusses the pleuropulmonary manifestations of systemic lupus erythematosus (SLE), rheumatoid arthritis (RA), and systemic sclerosis (SSc) (for a discussion of other manifestations in these diseases, see Chapters 50–54).

Systemic lupus erythematosus

SLE is a disease of unknown etiology characterized by the presence of autoantibodies directed against various nuclear antigens. These autoantibodies and the resultant immune complexes mediate many of the manifestations of SLE (Chapter 50). This disease primarily affects young women (female-to-male ratio > 8:1) and may involve virtually every organ system. Pleuropulmonary involvement occurs at some point in the disease course in 38–89% of cases.[37] Thus, the respiratory system is affected more commonly in SLE than in any other CVD. However, infectious pneumonia remains the commonest cause of pulmonary disease and death in these patients. Thus, in SLE patients presenting with a febrile illness and pulmonary infiltrates, a community-acquired or opportunistic infection must be promptly excluded.

Acute lupus pneumonitis

Acute lupus pneumonitis is an uncommon pulmonary manifestation of SLE, occurring in fewer than 5% of cases.[37] The clinical presentation mimics that of an infectious pneumonia with the abrupt onset of fever, cough, and dyspnea. Serum complement levels are often low and the chest radiograph typically shows diffuse alveolar opacities. It can be accompanied by pericarditis and often pleuritis and pleural effusion.

It can be difficult to distinguish acute lupus pneumonitis from an infectious pneumonia. BAL followed by thoracoscopic lung biopsy is often recommended prior to instituting corticosteroid therapy. The histopathology varies and includes diffuse alveolar damage, BOOP, NSIP, or a combination of these.

There are no controlled trials of therapy for acute lupus pneumonitis. Treatment includes high-dose glucocorticoids (1–2 mg/kg/day) with or without accompanying cytotoxic drugs, such as cyclophosphamide. Mortality rates as high as 50% have been reported. In those patients who fail to respond to treatment, respiratory failure is the usual cause of death.

Diffuse alveolar hemorrhage

DAH occurs in fewer than 5% of patients with SLE, and it represents the initial manifestation of disease in 11–20% of those cases.[38] However, most cases develop in individuals with well-established diagnoses of SLE, usually with pre-existing lupus nephritis.

The symptoms of DAH mimic those of infectious pneumonia and acute lupus pneumonitis.[39] Hemoptysis is present in 42–66% of patients at presentation. Therefore, the absence of hemoptysis does not exclude the diagnosis, particularly in the setting of a falling hematocrit, diffuse pulmonary infiltrates, and blood-stained BAL fluid. DAH in SLE is most often due to pulmonary capillaritis, but it can also be caused by diffuse alveolar damage. Immunofluorescence studies show granular deposits of IgG and C3 along alveolar walls, interstitium, and capillary endothelial cells.

There are no controlled trials for the treatment of alveolar hemorrhage in SLE. Glucocorticoids, cytotoxic drugs, and plasmapheresis have been used in various combinations. The mortality rate associated with DAH is approximately 50%. Poor prognostic factors include the need for mechanical ventilation, presence of infection, and prior treatment with cyclophosphamide.

Lupus pleuritis

The pleura are the most common site of respiratory involvement in SLE, with pleurisy and pleural effusions occurring in 50–80% of patients. Lupus pleuritis can be the presenting manifestation of disease, but, more commonly develops in patients with established SLE. It is often recurrent. The clinical manifestations include chest pain, fever, and dyspnea, and the chest radiograph typically shows bilateral pleural effusions. The pleural fluid is serous or serosanguineous and exudative in nature. Compared to effusions in RA, the glucose is higher and the lactate dehydrogenase level is lower. The most helpful measurement is a pleural fluid antinuclear antibody titer greater than 1:160. Examination of the pleura reveals infiltration with plasma cells and lymphocytes accompanied by pleural thickening and fibrosis. Treatment with nonsteroidal anti-inflammatory drugs and/or glucocorticoids is usually effective for relief of pleural discomfort.

Interstitial lung disease

The presence of ILD in SLE was once thought to be uncommon, especially when compared to SS or RA.[40] However, minor interstitial abnormalities can be found on HRCT in approximately one-third of SLE patients who have a normal chest radiograph and physiological testing. The significance and natural history of these subclinical findings are uncertain. The presence of anti-SSA (Ro) has been noted in approximately 80% of lupus patients with interstitial changes. In addition, the prevalence of ILD is increased in a subset of SLE patients with sclerodermatous skin changes.

The diagnosis of SLE is usually well established in the subgroup of patients who develop the insidious form of ILD. The disease course is characterized by progressive dyspnea and cough; the chest radiograph shows reduced lung volumes and reticular interstitial infiltrates. A restrictive lung function pattern with reduced diffusing capacity and exercise-induced hypoxemia are typical. The histopathology of chronic interstitial disease in SLE resembles UIP, although cases of BOOP, lymphocytic interstitial pneumonitis (LIP), and NSIP have been described. Response to therapy depends on the underlying histopathology, with the UIP-like form being least responsive.

Pulmonary vascular disease

In acutely ill SLE patients, a syndrome of acute reversible hypoxemia has been described. These patients have hypoxemia and a widened alveolar–arterial oxygen gradient with a normal chest radiograph and ventilation–perfusion scan. The etiology of this syndrome is unknown, but complement-mediated intravascular neutrophil aggregation has been suggested. The hypoxemia usually resolves with glucocorticoid treatment.

Although previously thought to be unusual, the development of pulmonary hypertension has been increasingly noted in SLE, with an incidence ranging from 0.5 to 14%. Pulmonary hypertension in SLE has been associated with the presence of Raynaud syndrome, serositis, digital vasculitis, and antiphospholipid antibodies.[41] Dyspnea and fatigue, despite a normal chest radiograph, is the most common presentation. The majority of SLE patients with pulmonary hypertension are female, with 3- and 5-year survival rates of 45 and 17%, respectively, which represent a much worse prognosis than patients with idiopathic pulmonary hypertension. The vascular changes of SLE-associated pulmonary hypertension are similar to those seen in idiopathic pulmonary hypertension with intimal hyperplasia, smooth muscle hypertrophy and medial thickening. Several pathologic mechanisms have been proposed for the development of pulmonary hypertension including vasoconstriction in addition to vasculitis and thrombosis with an association with antiphospholipid and anticardiolipin antibodies. Serum endothelin levels are elevated in patients with SLE-associated pulmonary hypertension and correlate with pulmonary arterial pressures.

As the pulmonary hypertension advances, the central pulmonary arteries enlarge. Pulmonary function testing shows an isolated decrease in the diffusing capacity for carbon monoxide. Patients with SLE-associated pulmonary hypertension may respond to immunosuppressive therapy. In a small study, 5 of 12 patients with SLE responded to monthly intravenous bolus doses of cyclophosphamide in addition to systemic glucocorticoids. A positive response was indicated by sustained hemodynamic improvement after at least 1 year of treatment without the need for additional pulmonary hypertension-specific therapies. Patients that responded to immunosuppression could be maintained on azathioprine or mycophenolate mofetil to avoid potential adverse effects of cyclophosphamide. SLE patients treated with bosentan did not have clinical worsening and showed an improvement in 6-minute walk distance.[42] However, the optimal treatment regimen for SLE-associated pulmonary hypertension is still unknown.

Respiratory muscle dysfunction

The shrinking or vanishing-lung syndrome is due to diaphragmatic weakness as well as weakness of other respiratory muscles.[43] This entity accounts for the findings of dyspnea without evidence of interstitial infiltrates or pulmonary vascular disease. It is estimated to occur in 25% of patients with SLE. The chest radiograph typically shows elevated diaphragms and basilar atelectasis. The pathogenesis of respiratory muscle weakness is unknown, but it is not associated with generalized muscle weakness. Glucocorticoids are frequently ineffective in the treatment of this syndrome. Improvement has been noted with inhaled β-agonist and

theophylline therapy. Despite a variable response to therapy, it is unusual for this manifestation of SLE to be progressive.

Rheumatoid arthritis

RA is an autoimmune disease associated with autoantibodies directed against citrullinated antigens[44] and characterized by the presence of a symmetric, inflammatory polyarthritis (Chapter 51). It occurs more frequently in women, with a 2:1 female-to-male ratio. Disease onset is most commonly in the fourth to fifth decades of life. The pleuropulmonary complications of RA occur more commonly in individuals with subcutaneous nodules, high titers of rheumatoid factor, and more severe chronic articular involvement. Although RA itself is more common in women, the pleuropulmonary manifestations have a higher incidence in men. The pleuropulmonary complications of RA are numerous, but the treatment-related lung toxicity and pulmonary infections are difficult to differentiate from the primary pleuropulmonary manifestations of the disease.

Pleuritis and pleural effusions

As in SLE, pleural abnormalities are one of the most common pulmonary complications of RA. Pleural effusion is clinically evident in approximately 5% of patients, and this can occur prior to the development of arthritis. Pleural disease is often discovered as an incidental finding on routine chest radiographs, but nonspecific chest pain, dyspnea, and fever are not unusual. The effusion can be unilateral or bilateral and can coexist with interstitial lung disease.

Typically, the effusion is an exudate, with a glucose level less than 30 mg/mL in 70–80% of cases. The mechanism underlying the low pleural fluid glucose is impaired membrane transport of glucose. A low pleural fluid pH is thought to occur secondary to impaired carbon dioxide exit from the pleural space. If the effusion is chronic, the cholesterol concentration can be increased, and the pleural fluid can have a milky appearance (pseudochylothorax). Cytologic examination typically reveals multinucleated giant cells, spindle-shaped macrophages, and necrotic debris.

Most rheumatoid effusions are small and asymptomatic and require no treatment. They resolve over several months without complications. The use of glucocorticoids for active articular disease hastens the resolution of the pleural process.

● CLINICAL PEARLS

Lung involvement in rheumatoid arthritis (RA)

- RA is more common in women, but pleuropulmonary complications occur more frequently in men.
- Factors associated with pleuropulmonary complications of RA include more severe articular involvement, subcutaneous nodules, and high levels of rheumatoid factor.
- Pleural effusions are the most common complication, characterized by an exudate and a low glucose and low pH.
- The differentiation of rheumatoid nodules from malignant lesions can be difficult.
- The rapid growth of a nodule should prompt aggressive investigation for a malignant cause.

Rheumatoid nodules

Rheumatoid or necrobiotic nodules are the only pleuropulmonary manifestation specific for RA. These nodules are most commonly seen in men with active articular disease, high rheumatoid factor titers, and subcutaneous nodules. Most individuals are asymptomatic and are diagnosed on routine chest radiograph. Radiographically, these nodules can be singular or multiple with an upper to mid-lung zone predominance. Cavitation occurs in approximately 50% of cases. High-resolution chest CT indicates a higher frequency of nodules than previously thought. Rarely, subpleural necrobiotic nodules can erode into the pleural space, resulting in a pneumothorax with a complicating bronchopleural fistula. It can be difficult to differentiate these nodules from malignant lesions, and frequently open-lung biopsy is necessary. Evidence on chest radiograph of rapid growth should prompt an aggressive diagnostic evaluation.

Caplan syndrome refers to the rapid development of pulmonary nodules with an upper-lung-zone predominance, originally described in Welsh coalminers with RA. Histologically, these nodules are identical to necrobiotic nodules. Other occupational dust exposures have also been associated with this syndrome.

Airway disease

Airflow limitation is a common finding in patients with RA, being present in approximately one-third of patients. The mechanism(s) responsible for airway disease is poorly understood. The interplay of cigarette smoking and RA may play a role.

A life-threatening complication of RA is upper-airway obstruction, resulting from synovitis of the cricoarytenoid joint. Common presenting complaints include a sore throat, hoarseness, and fullness in the throat. It can progress to inspiratory stridor and upper-airway obstruction. This complication occurs more commonly in women, particularly in those with advanced RA. Seventy-five percent of patients were found to have cricoarytenoid abnormalities when screening with direct or indirect laryngoscopy and computed tomography was utilized. The treatment of cricoarytenoid arthritis includes anti-inflammatory medications.

Bronchiolitis obliterans is a progressive form of obstructive lung disease that is being increasingly recognized as a complication of RA.[45] This entity was thought to develop secondary to the use of penicillamine for the treatment of RA, but most cases occur in the absence of this therapy. The histopathologic lesion of bronchiolitis obliterans is constrictive bronchiolitis, which is characterized by concentric submucosal and peribronchiolar fibrosis resulting in extrinsic compression and obliteration of the bronchiolar lumen. The typical clinical presentation is with insidious onset of cough and dyspnea, with a normal or hyperinflated chest radiograph. This complication occurs more commonly in women than in men. Pulmonary function studies show airflow limitation with hyperinflation and a reduced diffusing capacity. Expiratory high-resolution CT shows multiple areas of air trapping (mosaic pattern). Some individuals respond to high-dose glucocorticoids and cytotoxic drugs, but most patients with bronchiolitis obliterans progress to respiratory failure.

Bronchiectasis occurs at an increased frequency in RA, usually in individuals with long-standing articular disease. Productive cough and dyspnea are the most common respiratory symptoms. In most patients, bronchiectasis is not clinically significant. Recurrent pneumonia and respiratory failure are potentially fatal complications of this problem.

Interstitial lung disease

Although ILD is a common complication of RA, the incidence is difficult to determine, since different methods of detection have been employed and dissimilar populations of patients have been studied. However, clinically significant ILD occurs in approximately 14% of patients.[46] The development of ILD in relation to the onset of arthritis is variable. Most often, the ILD develops subsequent to arthritis, but, in approximately 20% of patients, the lung disease precedes the onset of arthritis and is associated with cigarette smoking, presence of the shared HLA-DR4 epitope, and RA-specific anti-citrullinated protein antibodies.

The most common histopathologies identified in this patient population are UIP, LIP, NSIP, and BOOP. The clinical manifestations of ILD in RA resemble those seen in idiopathic disease and include a dry, nonproductive cough and dyspnea on exertion. The chest radiograph and high-resolution CT show increased reticular markings with a predilection for the peripheral lower-lung zones. Often, pleural abnormalities accompany the interstitial changes. With advanced disease, progression to honeycomb lung occurs. LIP usually occurs in cases of RA complicated by Sjögren syndrome: the presence of keratoconjunctivitis sicca and xerostomia in a patient with RA and ILD should suggest this histologic type.

In general, ILD in RA appears more indolent than in idiopathic interstitial pneumonitis. Thus, due to uncertain treatment benefits and possible adverse effects, the decision to institute therapy should be based on clinical, radiographic, and physiologic deterioration.

Drug-induced lung disease

Methotrexate and gold are the two main anti-RA drugs capable of causing lung injury. Methotrexate administered weekly (10–20 mg/week) is associated with the development of interstitial changes in 1–5% of patients with RA.[47] No correlation with age, sex, disease duration, or cumulative dose has been identified. The clinical presentation is subacute, with fever, cough, and dyspnea occurring 1–5 months after initiation of the drug. The chest radiograph shows mixed interstitial–alveolar infiltrates. Nonspecific laboratory abnormalities include leukocytosis, sometimes with mild eosinophilia, and an elevated erythrocyte sedimentation rate. In most cases, BAL reveals a lymphocytosis. Histologically, cellular NSIP is seen with areas of organizing pneumonia. Noncaseating, granulomatous inflammation similar to that seen in hypersensitivity pneumonitis may also be present. The primary treatment of methotrexate-induced pneumonitis is withdrawal of methotrexate, plus appropriate supportive care.

Gold-induced pneumonitis occurs in fewer than 1% of RA patients treated with gold. Dyspnea and cough usually begin after 4–6 weeks of therapy; eosinophilia occurs in a minority of patients. The chest radiograph typically reveals mixed alveolar–interstitial opacities with an upper-lung zone predilection. The histology is similar to that seen in RA patients with ILD. Thus, the differentiation of gold-induced pneumonitis from RA-associated interstitial lung disease can only be established when discontinuation of the medication results in remission.

Systemic sclerosis (scleroderma)

SSc is characterized by excessive deposition of extracellular matrix in the skin and internal organs, and vascular involvement (Chapter 54). The degree of visceral organ involvement determines morbidity and mortality. Pulmonary involvement occurs in 70–100% of patients with SSc. There is no correlation with the degree of extrapulmonary disease. Interstitial lung disease is the most common pulmonary manifestation of SSc. Of note, with the improved mortality associated with renal involvement in SSc, lung disease has become the most important cause of morbidity and mortality.

Interstitial lung disease

The incidence of ILD in SSc depends on the method of detection. Autopsy studies have reported an ILD incidence of 60–100% of cases, whereas studies based on chest radiographs have noted interstitial changes in 14–66% of cases.

Cough and dyspnea on exertion are the most common symptoms. Physical examination reveals bibasalar rales. Radiographic findings include basal reticulonodular infiltrates, enlargement of pulmonary arteries, and progressive volume loss with associated honeycomb change. Pulmonary function testing reveals restrictive lung disease, preservation of flow rates, and decreased diffusing capacity. A disproportionate decrease in diffusing capacity compared to lung volume changes should suggest pulmonary hypertension, especially in individuals with limited scleroderma (calcinosis, Raynaud's phenomenon, esophageal dysmotility, sclerodactyly, telangectasia (CREST) syndrome). The predominant histopathologic abnormality is UIP with honeycomb changes and is identical to that seen in IPF. Rarely, LIP may complicate cases of SSc associated with Sjögren syndrome. Although the 5-year survival for SSc patients with ILD is 38–45%, it is better than that of patients with IPF.[48]

Pulmonary vascular disease

Pulmonary hypertension is a frequent complication of SSc, occurring in approximately 30% of patients with diffuse scleroderma and in 10–50% of those with limited scleroderma (Chapter 54). Pulmonary hypertension can either be associated with interstitial fibrosis or result from involvement of small and medium-sized arteries and arterioles with smooth-muscle hyperplasia, medial hypertrophy, and intimal proliferation (plexogenic). Direct involvement of the pulmonary circulation is more common with limited scleroderma while pulmonary hypertension in patients with diffuse scleroderma is more likely associated with ILD.

The clinical presentation is characterized by the insidious onset of fatigue and dyspnea on exertion. Physical examination and chest radiographs show signs typical of pulmonary hypertension, while decreased diffusing capacity is seen on pulmonary function testing. Risk factors for developing SSc-associated pulmonary hypertension include limited skin involvement, duration of disease greater than 10 years, onset of SSc at older age and severity and duration of Raynaud phenomenon.

The pathogenesis of SSC-associated pulmonary hypertension is poorly understood. Vascular changes occur at an early stage in SSc, which include apoptosis, endothelial cell activation with increased expression of cell adhesion molecules, inflammatory cell recruitment, intimal proliferation and adventitial fibrosis leading to vessel obliteration.[49] Endothelial injury is reflected by increased levels of soluble cell adhesion molecules, disturbances of angiogenesis with increased levels of circulating vascular endothelial growth factor and presence of angiostatic factors. It remains unclear to what extent dysregulated angiogenesis in SSc-associated pulmonary hypertension is driven by an inflammatory process or other as yet unidentified mechanisms.[50]

Treatment of SSc-associated pulmonary hypertension has been largely disappointing. Calcium channel blockers are not usually indicated for patients with SSc-associated pulmonary hypertension, although often used at lower doses for Raynaud phenomenon. Continuous intravenous epoprostenol improves exercise capacity and hemodynamics but does not have a significant effect on survival. Randomized clinical trials with phosphodiesterase inhibitors including sildenafil showed a modest effect on exercise capacity, hemodynamic parameters and

functional class after 12 weeks of treatment.[51] Carefully selected patients may be considered for heart–lung transplantation but are often excluded due to postoperative complications arising for SSc-related gastrointestinal reflux disease and renal dysfunction.

References

1. Luzina IG, Todd NW, Iacono AT, Atamas SP. Roles of T lymphocytes in pulmonary fibrosis. J Leukoc Biol 2008;83:237–44.
2. Gharaee-Kermani M, Phan SH. Molecular mechanisms of and possible treatment strategies for idiopathic pulmonary fibrosis. Curr Pharm Des 2005;11:3943–71.
3. Parra ER, Kairalla RA, Ribeiro de Carvalho CR, et al. Inflammatory cell phenotyping of the pulmonary interstitium in idiopathic interstitial pneumonia. Respiration 2007;74:159–69.
4. Wells AU, Lorimer S, Majumdar S, et al. Fibrosing alveolitis in systemic sclerosis: increase in memory T-cells in lung interstitium. Eur Respir J 1995;8:266–71.
5. Simonian PL, Wehrmann F, Roark CL, et al. γδ T cells protect against lung fibrosis via IL-22. J Exp Med 2010;207:2239–53.
6. Atamas SP, White B. Cytokine regulation of pulmonary fibrosis in scleroderma. Cytokine Growth Factor Rev 2003;14:537–50.
7. Park H, Li Z, Yang XO, et al. A distinct lineage of CD4 T cells regulates tissue inflammation by producing interleukin 17. Nat Immunol 2005;6:1133–41.
8. Sonnenberg GF, Nair MG, Kirn TJ, et al. Pathological versus protective functions of IL-22 in airway inflammation are regulated by IL-17A. J Exp Med 2010;207:1293–305.
9. Wilson MS, Madala SK, Ramalingam TR, et al. Bleomycin and IL-1beta-mediated pulmonary fibrosis is IL-17A dependent. J Exp Med 2010;207:535–52.
10. Kotsianidis I, Nakou E, Bouchliou I, et al. Global impairment of CD4+CD25+FOXP3+ regulatory T cells in idiopathic pulmonary fibrosis. Am J Respir Crit Care Med 2009;179:1121–30.
11. Meltzer EB, Noble PW. Idiopathic pulmonary fibrosis. Orphanet J Rare Dis 2008;3:8.
12. Coultas DB, Zumwalt RE, Black WC, Sobonya RE. The epidemiology of interstitial lung diseases. Am J Respir Crit Care Med 1994;150:967–72.
13. Lynch DA, David Godwin J, Safrin S, et al. High-resolution computed tomography in idiopathic pulmonary fibrosis: diagnosis and prognosis. Am J Respir Crit Care Med 2005;172:488–93.
14. Cool CD, Groshong SD, Rai PR, et al. Fibroblast Foci are Not Discrete Sites of Lung Injury/Repair: the Fibroblast Reticulum. Am J Respir Crit Care Med 2006;174:654–8.
15. Lee HL, Ryu JH, Wittmer MH, et al. Familial idiopathic pulmonary fibrosis: clinical features and outcome. Chest 2005;127:2034–41.
16. Seibold MA, Wise AL, Speer MC, et al. A common MUC5B promoter polymorphism and pulmonary fibrosis. N Engl J Med 2011;364:1503–12.
17. Alder JK, Chen JJ, Lancaster L, et al. Short telomeres are a risk factor for idiopathic pulmonary fibrosis. Proc Natl Acad Sci U S A 2008;105:13051–6.
18. Armanios MY, Chen JJ, Cogan JD, et al. Telomerase mutations in families with idiopathic pulmonary fibrosis. N Engl J Med 2007;356:1317–26.
19. Lawson WE, Grant SW, Ambrosini V, et al. Genetic mutations in surfactant protein C are a rare cause of sporadic cases of IPF. Thorax 2004;59:977–80.
20. Dreisin RB, Schwarz MI, Theofilopoulos AN, Stanford RE. Circulating immune complexes in the idiopathic interstitial pneumonias. N Engl J Med 1978;298:353–7.
21. Weaver CT, Hatton RD, Mangan PR, Harrington LE. IL-17 family cytokines and the expanding diversity of effector T cell lineages. Annu Rev Immunol 2007;25:821–52.
22. Feghali-Bostwick CA, Tsai CG, Valentine VG, et al. Cellular and humoral autoreactivity in idiopathic pulmonary fibrosis. J Immunol 2007;179:2592–9.
23. Lee CG, Homer RJ, Zhu Z, et al. Interleukin-13 induces tissue fibrosis by selectively stimulating and activating transforming growth factor beta₁. J Exp Med 2001;194:809–21.
24. Martinez FJ, Safrin S, Weycker D, et al. The clinical course of patients with idiopathic pulmonary fibrosis. Ann Intern Med 2005;142:963–7.
25. Ley B, Collard HR, King Jr. TE. Clinical course and prediction of survival in idiopathic pulmonary fibrosis. Am J Respir Crit Care Med 2011;183:431–40.
26. Raghu G, Collard HR, Egan JJ, et al. An official ATS/ERS/JRS/ALAT statement: idiopathic pulmonary fibrosis: evidence-based guidelines for diagnosis and management. Am J Respir Crit Care Med 2011;183:788–824.
27. American Thoracic Society/European Respiratory Society International Multidisciplinary Consensus Classification of the Idiopathic Interstitial Pneumonias . This joint statement of the American Thoracic Society (ATS), and the European Respiratory Society (ERS) was adopted by the ATS board of directors, June 2001 and by the ERS Executive Committee, June 2001. Am J Respir Crit Care Med 2002;165:277–304.
28. Olson AL, Huie TJ, Groshong SD, et al. Acute exacerbations of fibrotic hypersensitivity pneumonitis: a case series. Chest 2008;134:844–50.
29. Hyzy R, Huang S, Myers J, Flaherty K, Martinez F. Acute exacerbation of idiopathic pulmonary fibrosis. Chest 2007;132:1652–8.
30. Katzenstein AL, Myers JL, Mazur MT. Acute interstitial pneumonia. A clinicopathologic, ultrastructural, and cell kinetic study. Am J Surg Pathol 1986;10:256–67.
31. Vourlekis JS, Brown KK, Schwarz MI. Acute interstitial pneumonitis: current understanding regarding diagnosis, pathogenesis, and natural history. Semin Respir Crit Care Med 2001;22:399–408.
32. Ryu JH, Myers JL, Capizzi SA, et al. Desquamative interstitial pneumonia and respiratory bronchiolitis-associated interstitial lung disease. Chest 2005;127:178–84.
33. Portnoy J, Veraldi KL, Schwarz MI, et al. Respiratory bronchiolitis-interstitial lung disease: long-term outcome. Chest 2007;131:664–71.
34. Katzenstein AL, Fiorelli RF. Nonspecific interstitial pneumonia/fibrosis. Histologic features and clinical significance. Am J Surg Pathol 1994;18:136–47.

35. Travis WD, Matsui K, Moss J, Ferrans VJ. Idiopathic nonspecific interstitial pneumonia: prognostic significance of cellular and fibrosing patterns: survival comparison with usual interstitial pneumonia and desquamative interstitial pneumonia. Am J Surg Pathol 2000;24:19–33.

36. Cordier JF. Cryptogenic organising pneumonia. Eur Respir J 2006;28:422–46.

37. Kamen DL, Strange C. Pulmonary manifestations of systemic lupus erythematosus. Clin Chest Med 2010;31:479–88.

38. Santos-Ocampo AS, Mandell BF, Fessler BJ. Alveolar hemorrhage in systemic lupus erythematosus: presentation and management. Chest 2000;118:1083–90.

39. Badsha H, Teh CL, Kong KO, et al. Pulmonary hemorrhage in systemic lupus erythematosus. Semin Arthritis Rheum 2004;33:414–21.

40. Cheema GS, Quismorio Jr. FP. Interstitial lung disease in systemic lupus erythematosus. Curr Opin Pulm Med 2000;6:424–9.

41. Hassoun PM. Pulmonary arterial hypertension complicating connective tissue diseases. Semin Respir Crit Care Med 2009;30:429–39.

42. Mok MY, Tsang PL, Lam YM, et al. Bosentan use in systemic lupus erythematosus patients with pulmonary arterial hypertension. Lupus 2007;16:279–85.

43. Oud KT, Bresser P, ten Berge RJ, Jonkers RE. The shrinking lung syndrome in systemic lupus erythematosus: improvement with corticosteroid therapy. Lupus 2005;14:959–63.

44. van Venrooij WJ, van Beers JJ, Pruijn GJ. Anti-CCP antibodies: the past, the present and the future. Nat Rev Rheumatol 2011;7:391–8.

45. Schwarz MI, Lynch DA, Tuder R. Bronchiolitis obliterans: the lone manifestation of rheumatoid arthritis? Eur Respir J 1994;7:817–20.

46. Gabbay E, Tarala R, Will R, et al. Interstitial lung disease in recent onset rheumatoid arthritis. Am J Respir Crit Care Med 1997;156:528–35.

47. Barrera P, Laan RF, van Riel PL, et al. Methotrexate-related pulmonary complications in rheumatoid arthritis. Ann Rheum Dis 1994;53:434–9.

48. Kocheril SV, Appleton BE, Somers EC, et al. Comparison of disease progression and mortality of connective tissue disease-related interstitial lung disease and idiopathic interstitial pneumonia. Arthritis Rheum 2005;53:549–57.

49. Cerinic MM, Valentini G, Sorano GG, et al. Blood coagulation, fibrinolysis, and markers of endothelial dysfunction in systemic sclerosis. Semin Arthritis Rheum 2003;32:285–95.

50. Choi JJ, Min DJ, Cho ML, et al. Elevated vascular endothelial growth factor in systemic sclerosis. J Rheumatol 2003;30:1529–33.

51. Badesch DB, Hill NS, Burgess G, et al. Sildenafil for pulmonary arterial hypertension associated with connective tissue disease. J Rheumatol 2007;34:2417–22.

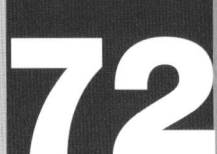

David R. Moller

Sarcoidosis

Sarcoidosis is a multisystem disorder of unknown etiology characterized by noncaseating epithelioid granulomas in affected organs.[1,2] The disease most commonly affects the lungs and intrathoracic lymph nodes, although granulomatous inflammation may involve any organ system. The clinical manifestations and course of sarcoidosis varies greatly. An estimated 30–60% of patients with sarcoidosis are asymptomatic, usually with isolated bilateral hilar adenopathy. Symptomatic manifestations most frequently involve the respiratory system, with symptoms of cough, dyspnea and chest discomfort.[3] Löfgren syndrome is a form of acute sarcoidosis characterized by erythema nodosum, bilateral hilar adenopathy, polyarthritis and often uveitis. Other clinical manifestations depend on the range and extent of extrapulmonary involvement (Table 72.1).

Epidemiology

Sarcoidosis is found worldwide, though there are striking differences in the prevalence of the disease in different geographic areas and racial groups.[4] In Europe and North America the prevalence is estimated to range from 10–64 cases per 100 000 with higher rates in African-American populations. Worldwide there is a slight female preponderance. Although all ages can be affected, more than 80% of cases are diagnosed between the ages of 20 and 50 years, with a later incidence peak after age 55.

The frequency of different clinical manifestations and disease severity varies among different groups. Löfgren syndrome has a particularly high frequency in Scandinavian countries and Ireland, but occurs in less than 5% of African American patients with sarcoidosis. Lupus pernio, a disfiguring nodular facial condition associated with chronic sarcoidosis, is more frequent in patients of African descent. Cardiac sarcoidosis may affect over 50% of Japanese patients with sarcoidosis, but 10–25% of European and North American patients. Retrospective studies suggest that sarcoidosis is the direct cause of death in <1–6% of cases, usually from pulmonary, cardiac or neurologic involvement.

Genetics

There is substantial evidence for a genetic predisposition to sarcoidosis. Small cases series suggest higher concordance among monozygotic than dizygotic twins. Familial clustering is noted in 5–16% of patients. A recent US-based multicenter study of sarcoidosis called ACCESS (A Case Control Etiologic Study of Sarcoidosis) compared 706 newly diagnosed, biopsy-proven sarcoidosis cases to age-, sex-, and race-matched relatives and found an approximate fivefold increased relative risk in siblings of sarcoidosis cases and in parents.[5]

Genetic association studies support the view that MHC class II alleles are the major contributor to disease susceptibility across different ethnic populations in sarcoidosis.[6] HLA- DR3 is associated with increased sarcoidosis risk in Scandinavian and European populations while HLA-DR1 and -DR4 alleles are associated with disease protection. The ACCESS study found a significant association between HLA-DRB1*1101 in both African-Americans and Caucasians, while HLA-DRB1*1501 was associated with sarcoidosis risk only in Caucasians.[7] One study found that residues forming pocket 4 of HLA-DR and pocket 9 of HLA-DQ influence sarcoidosis risk suggesting specific antigenic peptides are involved in sarcoidosis etiology.[8] MHC class I alleles have also been associated with sarcoidosis risk in different populations.

HLA class I and II alleles are associated with clinical course. HLA DRB1*0301 or the closely linked DQB1*0201 alleles are associated with favorable outcomes (Löfgren syndrome, acute arthritis, stage I chest radiograph, or remission within 2 years) whereas DR14 and DR15 are associated with severe, chronic disease in European and Japanese populations. DRB1*150101 or the closely linked DQB1*0602 alleles were associated with more severe or chronic disease sarcoidosis in another study.[9]

Studies of non-HLA polymorphisms have yielded few clues to the genetic basis of sarcoidosis. A meta-analysis found tumor necrosis factor-α (TNF-α) was associated with a 1.5-fold increased risk of developing sarcoidosis.[10] Isolated studies report associations with sarcoidosis and the CC chemokine receptors CCR2 and CCR5 and the Receptor for Advanced Glycation Endproducts (RAGE), though wider confirmation is lacking. Other studies find no association of sarcoidosis with serum angiotensin converting enzyme, vitamin D converting enzyme, the *CARD15/NOD2* gene involved in Blau syndrome or *NRAMP1* gene linked to tuberculosis.

Genome-wide association scans in both familial and sporadic sarcoidosis incident cases have identified chromosomal regions both inside and outside the MHC that contribute to sarcoidosis susceptibility. German and US investigators report that the butyrophilin-like 2 (*BTNL2*) gene within the MHC locus is associated with sarcoidosis risk in Caucasians and to a lesser extent, African-American populations.[11,12] BTLN2 is a member of the B7 receptor family that functions in T-cell costimulation, leading to the hypothesis that this gene plays a role in the polarized Th1 granulomatous response in sarcoidosis. The gene-encoding annexin A11, a molecule involved in apoptosis and cellular proliferation, has also been identified potentially increasing susceptibility by this approach.

Table 72.1 Major clinical features of systemic sarcoidosis

Organ system (approx. % involvement)	Major clinical features
Pulmonary (90)	Bilateral hilar adenopathy, restrictive and obstructive disease, fibrocystic disease, bronchiectasis, mycetomas
Upper airway (5–10)	Hoarseness, laryngeal or tracheal obstruction, nasal congestion, sinusitis, saddle nose deformity
Ocular (25)	Anterior and posterior uveitis, chorioretinitis, conjunctivitis, optic neuritis, glaucoma, lacrimal gland enlargement
Skin (20)	Erythema nodosum, chronic nodules and plaques, lupus pernio, alopecia
Hepatic (10)	Hepatomegaly, pruritus, jaundice, cirrhosis
Cardiac (5–10)	Arrhythmias, heart block, cardiomyopathy, sudden death
Central nervous system (5–10)	Cranial neuropathy, e.g., Bell's palsy, aseptic meningitis, brain mass, seizures, obstructing hydrocephalus, myelopathy, polyneuropathy, mononeuritis multiplex
Salivary and parotid gland (10)	Salivary and parotid gland enlargement, sicca syndrome
Hematologic (30–50)	Lymphadenopathy, splenomegaly, hypersplenism, anemia, lymphopenia, thrombocytopenia
Joints/ musculoskeletal (10–20)	Polyarthritis, bone cysts, Achilles' tendonitis, heel pain, myopathy
Endocrine (< 10)	Hypercalciuria (more common), hypercalcemia, hypopituitarism, diabetes insipidus
Renal (< 5)	Renal calculi, nephrocalcinosis, renal failure, epididymitis, testicular mass

Environmental factors

Environmental factors have been implicated in the etiology of sarcoidosis with reports of time–space clustering and a higher incidence of disease in the springtime months. Occupations such as healthcare workers, military personel and firefighters have also been suggested to have a higher incidence of sarcoidosis.

The largest study of sarcoidosis etiology (ACCESS) found weak positive associations (O.R. ~ 1.5) with insecticide use at work, mold/mildew exposures at work, and musty odors suggesting possible links to microbial-rich environments.[13] Sarcoidosis was not found to be associated with exposure to heavy metals including beryllium, wood dusts, or rural residence. The ACCESS study found a robust negative association of smoking and sarcoidosis risk. Studies of rescue workers and others exposed to the heavy dust burden from the World Trade Center disaster found an increased incidence of a sarcoidosis-like granulomatous pulmonary disease (SLGPD) in these groups, suggesting certain dust or smoke exposures can trigger sarcoidosis.[14]

Role of infectious agents

Since the initial descriptions of sarcoidosis, investigators have postulated an infectious cause of the disease based on its clinical similarities to other infectious diseases, most notably tuberculosis. There is evidence for prior mycobacterial infection in sarcoidosis from studies using polymerase chain reaction to detect mycobacterial DNA in sarcoidosis tissues. A meta-analysis concludes there is a 10- to 20-fold greater likelihood of detecting mycobacterial DNA in sarcoidosis tissues than control tissues.[15] A study by the author and his colleagues used a limited proteomic approach to identify potential pathogenic antigens in sarcoidosis tissues based on the biochemical properties of the Kveim reaction and not on *a priori* hypotheses regarding specific infectious or autoimmune causes.[16] The Kveim reaction, first studied in the 1940s, involves the intradermal inoculation of a suspension of sarcoidosis tissue which results in the development 2–4 weeks later of a nodular skin reaction with sarcoid-like granulomas in patients with suspected sarcoidosis.[17] Using mass spectrometry methods and protein immunoblotting, we detected the mycobacterial catalase-peroxidase protein (mKatG) in over 50% of sarcoidosis tissues. IgG responses to mKatG were detected in ~50% of sarcoidosis patients, supporting the premise that mKatG is a pathogenic antigen. Several groups have now demonstrated lung and blood CD4 and CD8 T-cell responses to multiple mycobacterial antigens in sarcoidosis including KatG, *M. tuberculosis* ESAT-6, Ag85, superoxide dismutase, and heat shock proteins.[18,19] These studies provide evidence that mycobacterial organisms trigger sarcoidosis in a subgroup of patients.

Studies from Japanese investigators report the presence of *Proprionibacterium acnes* or *P. granulosum* genomes in 80–98% of sarcoidosis tissues from Japan and Europe but also in 0–60% of control tissues tissues.[20] In animal models *P. acnes* proteins have been shown to induce Th1-driven granulomatous inflammation in part, via TLR9 stimulation.[21] Given that these organisms are part of the normal skin and upper airway flora, a pathogenic role for these organisms remains uncertain.

Many other microbial organisms, including cell wall-deficient organisms, have been proposed to cause sarcoidosis but none have been confirmed by other centers. Although direct demonstration of an infectious etiology remains unproven, most investigators favor the hypothesis that certain classes of microbial organisms trigger sarcoidosis in those with genetic susceptibility.

Autoimmunity

Sarcoidosis patients often express low titer autoantibodies that may be part of the generalized hypergammaglobulinemia observed in many patients resulting from the effects of T-cell activation. Whether autoimmunity plays a role in sarcoidosis is unknown given the absence of disease-specific autoantibodies. Recent studies from Sweden identified several potential autoantigens such as ATP synthase that bound to HLA-DRB1*0301 molecules derived from alveolar macrophages of Swedish sarcoidosis patients, but whether these autoantigens play a pathogenic role remains uncertain.[22]

Immunology/pathogenesis

● KEY CONCEPTS

Immunopathogenesis of sarcoidosis

- Pathology of non-caseating epithelioid granulomas
- Genetic susceptibility determined primarily by HLA genes of MHC
- Oligoclonal expansion of T-cell receptor specific T cells consistent with antigen driven inflammation
- Th1 polarization at sites of disease
- Decrease in regulatory T-cell function contributes to Th1-mediated inflammation
- Etiology involves microbial triggers with mycobacterial or propionibacterial organisms most commonly implicated
- Misfolded serum amyloid A within granulomas leading to self-aggregation of SAA provides a mechanism for chronic disease
  - Nidus for granuloma formation
  - Feed-forward amplification of local Th1 responses in part through TLR2

The histologic hallmark of sarcoidosis is the presence of discrete, compact noncaseating granulomas (Fig. 72.1). The dominant cell in the central core is the epithelioid cell, thought to be a differentiated form of a mononuclear phagocyte. CD4 T cells and mature macrophages are interspersed throughout the epithelioid core, whereas both CD4 and CD8 T cells are seen around the periphery of the granuloma. Multinucleated giant cells are scattered throughout the inflammatory locus. In the lung, granulomas tend to form along areas that are rich in lymphatic vessels, such as bronchovascular, bronchial submucosal, and interlobular septal regions.

The concept of sarcoidosis as a disorder of enhanced cell-mediated immune processes at sites of granulomatous inflammation was based on landmark studies in the 1980s using bronchoalveolar lavage (BAL). These studies demonstrated increased proportions and numbers of activated CD4 BAL lymphocytes in pulmonary sarcoidosis. Prior to these findings, sarcoidosis was thought to be a disease of immune depression

exemplified by circulating lymphopenia and cutaneous anergy. Researchers reported BAL T cells are CD4$^+$ with a CD45RO$^+$ "memory" phenotype expressing high levels of activation molecules DR and VLA-1 (very late activation antigen-1, CD49a).

Direct evidence that sarcoidosis is an antigen driven disorder is provided by studies analyzing T-cell receptor (TCR) gene expression. These studies document the expansion of oligoclonal populations of lung (BAL), blood or skin (Kveim biopsy) T cells expressing specific α/β or γ/δ TCR. The most compelling data derive from HLA-DRB1*0301-positive Swedish patients who have greatly expanded numbers of AV2S3 Th1 cells in the lung. Sequence analyses demonstrate that expanded oligoclonal αβ$^+$ T-cell subsets in sarcoidosis often contain shared amino acid motifs in the CDR3 region of their Vβ or Vα/Jα genes, consistent with a conventional antigen-driven T-cell response. Despite intense efforts, the specificities of these expanded T-cell clones have yet to be identified.

Th1 polarization in sarcoidosis

An immunologic hallmark of sarcoidosis at time of diagnosis is a highly polarized Th1 cytokine profile (Chapter 16) at sites of disease (Fig. 72.2).[23] BAL studies demonstrate expression of IFN-γ and TNF in pulmonary sarcoidosis. Consistent with a polarized type 1 process, Th1-promoting cytokines IL-12, -18, -2, -15, and -27, are upregulated in sarcoidosis-affected tissues. Chemokines and chemokine receptors such as CXCR3, CCR5, monocyte chemotactic protein (MCP)-1, RANTES, macrophage inflammatory protein (MIP)-1, MIG (monokine-induced by IFN-γ) and osteopontin (early T-lymphocyte activation protein) that are typically associated with Th1 responses are also upregulated in sarcoidosis. The Th1-differentiation transcription factor STAT-1 and its phosphorylated form are upregulated in sarcoidosis. In contrast, low or undetectable levels of Th2 effector cytokines IL-4 and -5 and Th2-associated chemokines and chemokine receptors are found in the sarcoidosis lung.

Clinical evidence supports the importance of polarized Th1 immunity in sarcoidosis. Biologic therapies with Th1-promoting effects such as IFN-α, IFN-γ, and IL-2 have been associated with new onset or recrudescent sarcoidosis. Sarcoidosis has also been

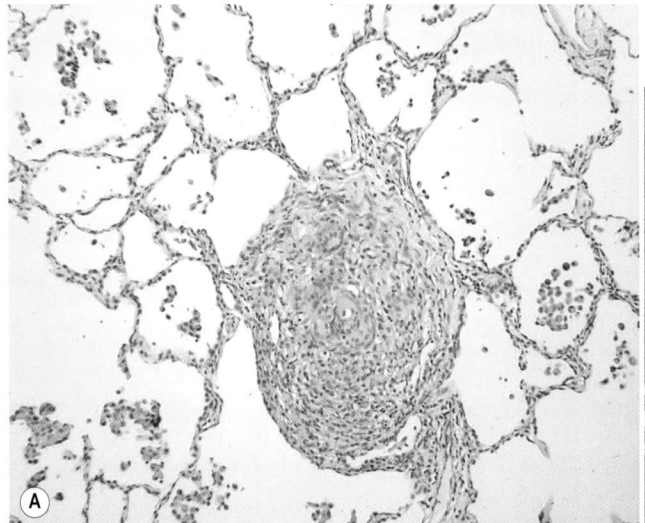

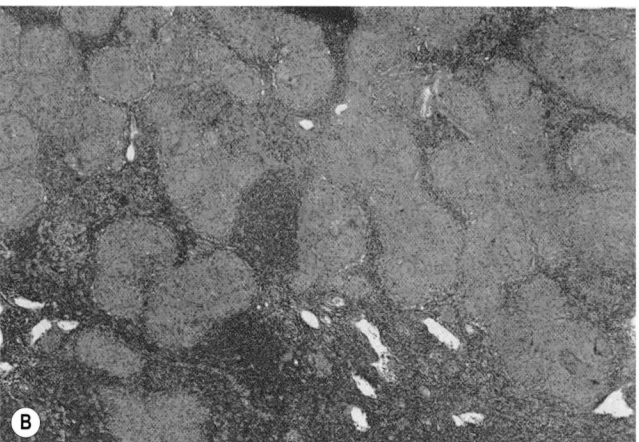

Fig. 72.1 (A) Open lung biopsy showing typical noncaseating epithelioid granuloma, giant cells, and lymphocytic infiltrates in lung parenchyma in sarcoidosis. (B) Lymph node biopsy showing extensive replacement with well-defined epithelioid granulomas in a patient with sarcoidosis.

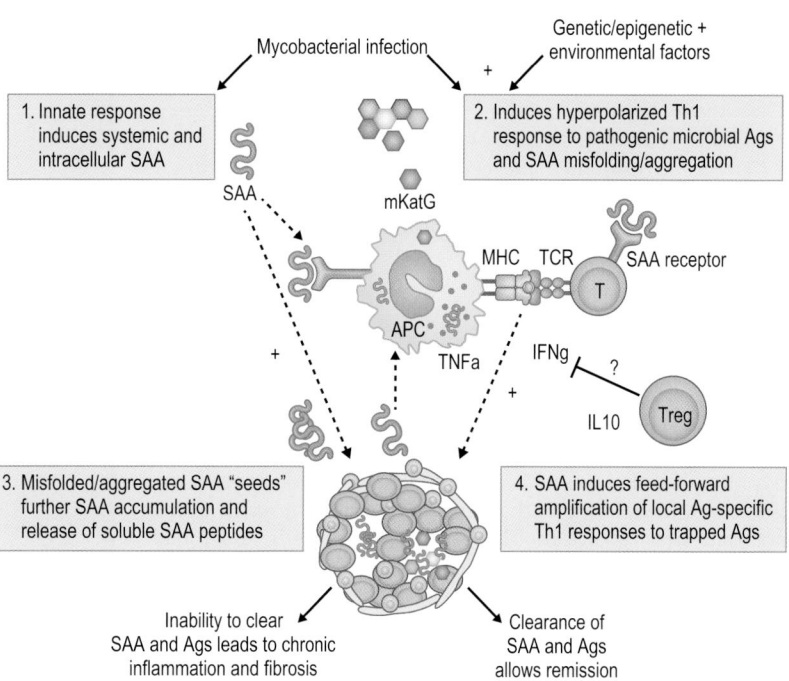

Fig. 72.2 Conceptual model of the immunopathogenesis of sarcoidosis. Granuloma formation in sarcoidosis results from stimulation by poorly soluble antigens that evoke a hyperimmune Th1 response with stimulation of INF-γ, along with TNF, IL-12, IL-10, and other cytokines from mononuclear phagocytes and dendritic cells. As a consequence of this response, misfolded SAA aggregates in an amyloid-like process to provide a persistent poorly soluble nidus and a template for further SAA aggregation within sarcoidosis granulomas. SAA and SAA peptides released from the granulomas stoke a feed-forward stimulation of macrophages and T cells that amplifies polarized Th1 responses to local tissue antigens. This course continues to progress unless there is removal of stimulating antigen(s) and clearance of SAA, allowing remission of Th1-driven granuloma formation. The model depicts mycobacterial organisms as the etiologic trigger, though other microbes or environmenal agents might trigger a similar pathogenic pathway.

described in patients with 5q-myelodysplasia with deletion of Th2 genes (IL-4, IL-13, CSF2).

A potential role for Th17 effector responses in driving the granulomatous response in sarcoidosis remains unclear. One study found that expression of IL-17a mRNA was reduced in BAL T cells from patients with Löfgren syndrome compared to healthy controls, but there was no difference between controls and non-Löfgren patients. Another study reported that a subset of CD4 T cells in sarcoidosis lung tissue and bronchoalveolar lavage expressed Th17 polarization. The overall contribution of these T17 cells in driving granulomatous inflammation in sarcoidosis remains uncertain.

The role of immunoregulatory cells and cytokines in sarcoidosis is poorly understood. One study found that patients with active sarcoidosis who underwent spontaneous remission within 6 months had significantly greater production of transforming growth factor-β (TGF-β) from their cultured BAL cells at the time of initial evaluation than did patients who later required therapy or who demonstrated progressive disease. Because TGF-β is a potent endogenous inhibitor of IL-12 and CD4 Th1 development, these observations suggest that TGF-β may downregulate Th-1 driven granulomatous responses in sarcoidosis. Other studies find a reduced number of immunoregulatory CD1d-restricted Vα24 natural-killer T (NKT) cells in the blood of patients with non-remitting sarcoidosis suggesting a deficiency of these cells may play a role in chronic sarcoidosis.

Different subsets of regulatory T cells (Tregs) maintain immune homeostasis by inhibiting antigen presenting cells and effector T-cell function (Chapter 15). One group reports that FOXP3+ natural Tregs (nTreg) expressing CD4+CD25^bright FOXP3+ T cells accumulate at the periphery of sarcoidosis granulomas, in bronchoalveolar lavage fluid, and in peripheral blood of patients with active disease but were functionally deficient with a reduced ability to inhibit *in vitro* granuloma formation.[24] Other studies report FOXP3 expression in T cells is reduced in sarcoidosis, consistent with reduced regulatory function. Whether alterations inTreg function are critical to the imbalanced Th1 effector

responses in sarcoidosis remains under active investigation. A report that nebulized Vasoactive Intestinal Peptide significantly reduced TNF production by lung cells in sarcoidosis and increased the frequency of lung CD4+CD127-CD25+ Tregs, possibly by converting naïve CD4+CD25- T cells to Tregs, suggests inhaled VIP as a possible treatment for sarcoidosis.[25]

Alveolar macrophages are thought to play a central role in the development of granulomatous inflammation in sarcoidosis by presenting disease-specific antigens and producing cytokines that regulate granuloma formation. Alveolar macrophages from patients with sarcoidosis express higher levels of surface class II MHC molecules, leukocyte function associated-antigen-1 (LFA-1), intracellular adhesion molecule-1 (ICAM-1) and the accessory molecules CD86 (B7.2), CD80 (B7.1) and CD40 than do alveolar macrophages from healthy controls. These characteristics are consistent with an M1-phenotype (induced by type 1 cytokines) and likely contribute to the enhanced ability of sarcoidosis alveolar macrophages as antigen presenting cells compared to normal alveolar macrophages. Sarcoidosis alveolar macrophages produce proinflammatory cytokines TNF-α, IL-6, -1a, and -15 and increased amounts of lysozyme, angiotensin-converting enzyme, reactive oxygen species, fibronectin and insulin-like growth factor-1 (IGF-1).

Sarcoidosis patients with pulmonary fibrosis may have alveolar macrophages that express an alternative (non-M1) phenotype expressing chemokines such as CCL18, perhaps from local exposure to IL-10 and/or -13.[26] These macrophages may promote pulmonary fibrosis along with locally expressed TGF-β, IGF-1, fibronectin and matrix metalloproteinases that are present in the sarcoidosis lung.

Serum amyloid A misfolding hypothesis

Despite evidence that sarcoidosis is triggered by infectious agents such as mycobacterial organisms, there is no clinical or pathologic evidence of an active infection or reactivation of a latent mycobacterial or other microbial infection in sarcoidosis. This clinical observation holds for patients undergoing years of corticosteroid, immunosuppressive, or anti-TNF therapy. Thus, the mechanisms causing chronic, progressive granulomatous inflammation in sarcoidosis are uncertain.

Our group examined the expression of amyloid precursor proteins in sarcoidosis tissues because of our recognition that the granuloma-inducing component in the clinically validated Kveim reaction had biophysical properties that closely resemble amyloid or prion proteins.[27] Within sarcoidosis granulomas we found the expression of serum amyloid A (SAA), the amyloid precursor of AA amyloid and an acute phase reactant, was typically several orders of magnitude greater than in other granulomatous disorders. SAA-stimulated expression of TNF, Th1-related cytokines and immunoregulatory IL-10 by lung cells from sarcoidosis patients through TLR2. With these findings, we hypothesized that the pathobiology of sarcoidosis involves the induction, misfolding, and aggregation of SAA, a result of the aberrant hyperpolarized Th1 response to specific microbial antigens (Fig. 72.2). Misfolded SAA promotes progressive self-aggregation in an amyloid-like process, with SAA and its peptides stimulating a feed-forward amplification of Th1 responses to antigens present within sarcoidosis granulomas. This mechanism offers an explanation for the cardinal clinical feature of progressive inflammation in the absence of any tissue infection.

Patient evaluation and differential diagnosis

Pulmonary sarcoidosis

The most common symptoms of pulmonary sarcoidosis are progressive shortness of breath, cough and ill-defined, variably severe chest discomfort (Table 72.1). Chronic sputum production and hemoptysis are more frequent in advanced fibrocystic disease. Typically, there are few physical findings in pulmonary sarcoidosis. Lung crackles are heard in less than 20% of patients and clubbing is rare. Findings of pulmonary hypertension or cor pulmonale are seen in 1–4% of patients, usually from severe fibrocystic sarcoidosis or, rarely, a granulomatous vasculitis of the pulmonary vessels.

Chest radiographs are abnormal in more than 90% of patients with sarcoidosis. By international convention, the chest radiograph is divided into the following stages:

Stage 0:
Normal chest radiograph
I: Bilateral hilar adenopathy
II: Bilateral hilar adenopathy + interstitial infiltrates
III: Interstitial infiltrates only (non-fibrotic)
IV: Fibrocystic interstitial lung disease.

Stage I is initially seen in 40–50% of cases. Typically, the hilar adenopathy is discrete, symmetric, and often accompanied by right paratracheal adenopathy. A stage II chest radiograph, often with mid- or upper-zone infiltrates, is initially seen in 20–30% of cases (Fig. 72.3). A stage III radiograph is initially seen in 10–20% of cases. Chest radiographs with fibrotic changes are frequently placed in a separate subgroup, stage IV, in recognition of the poor outcome of this group of patients (Fig. 72.4). Mycetomas are mobile fungus balls that colonize pre-existing cystic spaces in fibrocystic sarcoidosis. More unusual patterns of pulmonary sarcoidosis include large, well defined nodular infiltrates, miliary disease, or a pattern of patchy air-space consolidation

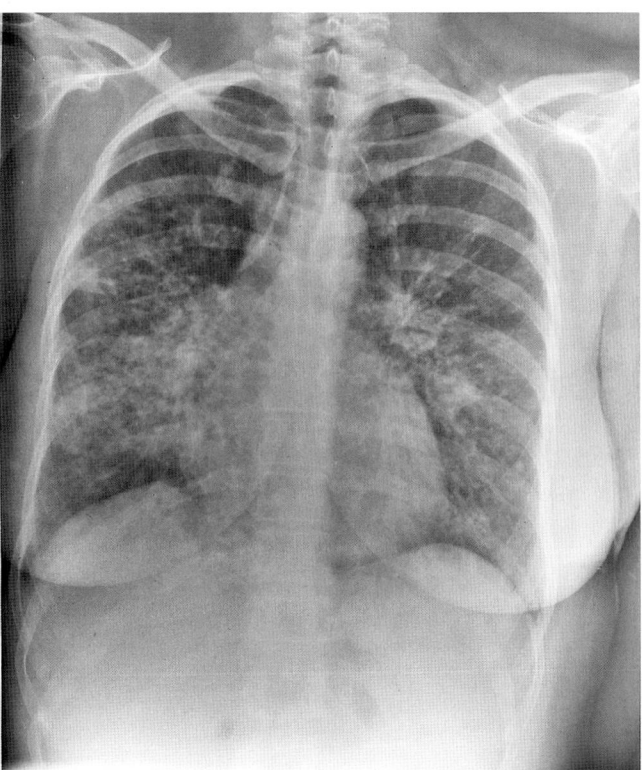

Fig. 72.3 Chest radiograph demonstrating a stage II pattern with bilateral hilar adenopathy and reticulonodular infiltrates.

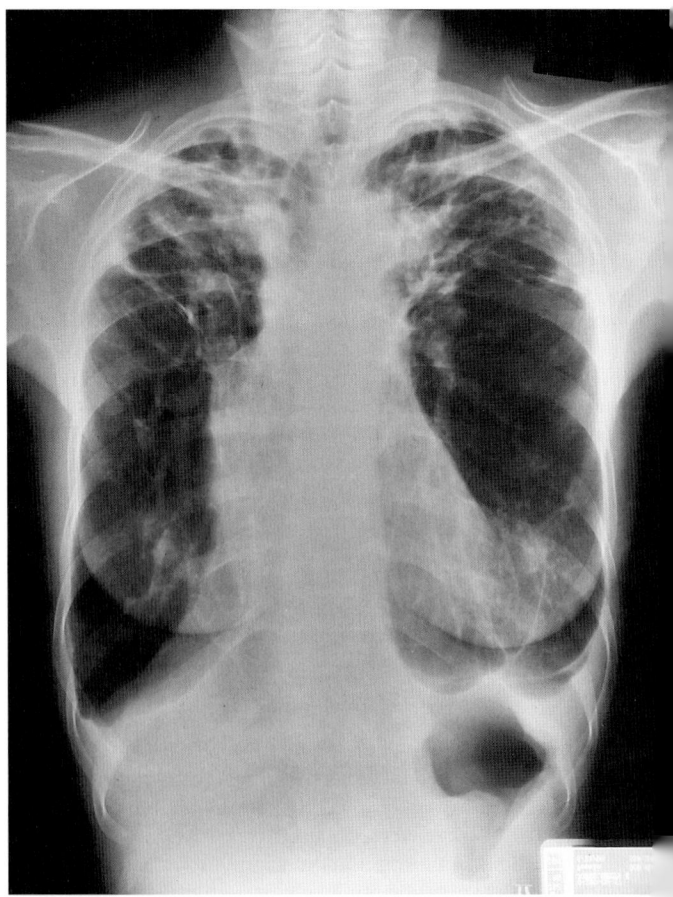

Fig. 72.4 Fibrocystic (stage IV) pulmonary sarcoidosis with typical upward hilar retraction and multiple cystic and bullous changes.

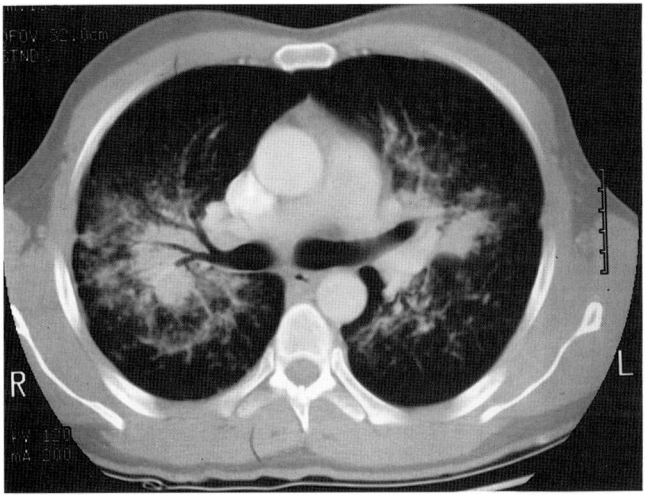

Fig. 72.5 CT scan of the chest in a patient with biopsy-proven pulmonary sarcoidosis, demonstrating bilateral hilar, paratracheal and paraaortic lymphadenopathy with interstitial infiltrates in a dominantly central bronchovascular distribution.

with air bronchograms, termed "alveolar sarcoidosis." Pleural effusions and pneumothorax are rare.

Computed tomography (CT) of the chest is more sensitive than plain radiography in demonstrating enlarged lymph nodes and pulmonary infiltrates. Chest CT typically demonstrates nodular infiltrates that follow central bronchovascular structures (Fig. 72.5).

Pulmonary function tests do not correlate well with chest radiographs. In patients with stage I chest radiographs pulmonary function tests are normal in about 80% of cases, or have only an isolated reduction in diffusing capacity for carbon monoxide (DL_{CO}). When pulmonary infiltrates are present on chest radiography, restrictive impairment with reduction in lung volumes, FVC and FEV_1, or a reduction in DL_{CO} is found in 40–70% of cases. Obstructive impairment is found in <30–50% of patients, most often in advanced fibrocystic sarcoidosis. Bronchial hyperreactivity is present in 10–30% of patients. Gas exchange is usually preserved until extensive fibrotic changes are evident.

Pulmonary hypertension is seen in approximately 5% of patients, although this proportion increases to 50% in those patients with dyspnea that is not explained by the level of pulmonary function impairment. Screening for pulmonary hypertension is indicated in patients with advanced lung disease due to the increased mortality associated with this manifestation.

Extrapulmonary sarcoidosis

Most patients have clinically important involvement of more than one organ, either with or without pulmonary sarcoidosis (Table 72.1).

Sarcoidosis of the upper respiratory tract

Sarcoidosis of the upper respiratory tract can cause nasal congestion, crusting, epistaxis, anosmia, rhinorrhea, sinusitis, nasal septal perforation, a "saddle nose" deformity or palatal perforation or bone erosion may occur. Laryngeal sarcoidosis with hoarseness, dysphonia, dysphagia, dyspnea or, rarely, stridor and acute respiratory failure occurs in <1–5% of patients.

Ocular sarcoidosis

Unilateral or bilateral anterior uveitis is the most common manifestation of ocular sarcoidosis and is often associated with bilateral hilar adenopathy. Chronic uveitis occurs in as many as 20% of patients with chronic sarcoidosis, more frequently in Black populations. Other manifestations include posterior uveitis, granulomatous conjunctivitis, severe chorioretinitis, or optic neuritis that can cause blindness.

Cutaneous sarcoidosis

Erythema nodosum is a component of Löfgren syndrome, and may recur. Chronic skin sarcoidosis usually manifests as nontender and nonpruritic plaques and subcutaneous nodules around the hairline, eyelids, ears, nose, mouth, and the extensor surfaces of the arms and legs. Lupus pernio is a disfiguring form of cutaneous sarcoidosis of the face, with violaceous plaques and nodules covering the nose, nasal alae, malar areas, and around the eyes.

Cardiac sarcoidosis

Cardiac involvement is clinically apparent in <5–10% of patients with sarcoidosis in North America and Europe, although autopsy studies suggest the prevalence may be higher than 25%. In Japan, cardiac involvement may be present in >50% of patients. Complete heart block, ventricular arrhythmias, bundle branch blocks, sudden death, cardiomyopathy, supraventricular arrhythmias and valvular dysfunction can occur. One study has suggested "palpitations" is a predictor of cardiac sarcoidosis that warrants further assessment to test for its presence.[28]

Hepatic sarcoidosis

Symptomatic hepatic sarcoidosis manifests with fever, tender hepatomegaly or pruritis. Characteristically, the serum alkaline phosphatase and γ-glutamyl transferase are elevated proportionately higher than the aspartate aminotransferase (AST) and alanine aminotransferase (ALT) and bilirubin, although all patterns can be seen. The term "abdominal sarcoidosis" is often used for patients manifesting with liver, spleen and abdominal lymph node involvement, often with hypercalcemia; pulmonary involvement may not be evident.

Joints and bones

Arthralgias are common in multisystem sarcoidosis, although joint radiographs are usually negative. Acute, often incapacitating, polyarthritis involving the ankles, feet, knees and wrists can be seen in Löfgren syndrome. Persistent joint disease with pain, swelling and tenderness of the phalanges of the hands and feet is found in less than 5% of patients with chronic sarcoidosis. Joint radiographs may demonstrate "punched-out" lesions with cystic changes without erosive chrondritis. Cystic lesions of the long bones, pelvis, sternum, skull, and vertebrae rarely occur.

Neurosarcoidosis

Neurosarcoidosis occurs in 5–15% of patients with sarcoidosis. The most common manifestation is cranial neuropathy, most frequently bilateral or unilateral seventh-nerve (Bell) palsy. The palsy may resolve spontaneously or with corticosteroids, but sometimes recurs years later. Optic neuritis can result in blindness. Manifestations of central nervous system (CNS) involvement include mass lesions, aseptic meningitis, obstructive hydrocephalus and hypothalamic/pituitary dysfunction. Seizures, headache, change in mental status, confusion and diabetes insipidus can be presenting symptoms. Myelopathy with paraparesis, hemiparesis and back and leg pain have been described. Peripheral neuropathies account for about 15% of cases of neurosarcoidosis, often presenting as mononeuritis multiplex or a primary sensory neuropathy. Small fiber neuropathy with or without autonomic neuropathy are increasingly recognized in sarcoidosis patients, particularly in patients with pain and chronic disease.

Salivary, parotid, and lacrimal gland sarcoidosis

Parotid or lacrimal gland enlargement or sicca syndrome may be the dominant clinical manifestations of sarcoidosis. Herefordt syndrome, also known as uveoparotid fever, manifests as fever, parotid and lacrimal gland enlargement, uveitis, bilateral hilar adenopathy and sometimes cranial neuropathies, usually facial palsy.

Hematologic sarcoidosis

Peripheral lymph node enlargement occurs in 20–30% of patients as an early manifestation of sarcoidosis, but then typically undergoes spontaneous remission. Persistent, bulky lymphadenopathy occurs in less than 10% of patients. Splenomegaly, occasionally massive, occurs in less than 5% of cases and is often associated with hepatomegaly or hypercalcemia. Polyclonal hypergammaglobulinemia is present in 25% or more of patients.

Sarcoidosis myopathy

Although random muscle biopsies in autopsy series demonstrate muscle granulomas in a majority of patients with sarcoidosis, symptomatic myopathy with weakness and tenderness is uncommon. Rarely, sarcoidosis can present as a polymyositis with profound weakness and elevated serum creatine kinase and aldolase.

Hypercalcemia, hypercalciuria, and renal disease

Hypercalcemia is present in 2–5% of patients; hypercalciuria is more common. Chronic hypercalcemia or hypercalciuria most commonly manifest as kidney stones or nephrocalcinosis. Abnormal calcium regulation is thought to be due to an increased conversion of 25-OH vitamin D_3 to the active 1,25-(OH)2 vitamin D_3 by macrophages and epithelioid cells in granulomas with increased expression of 1α-hydroxylase-25-hydoxyvitamin-D. Thus, in sarcoidosis patients, a low 25-OH vitamin D_3 level obtained to screen for vitamin D deficiency can be associated with elevated active vitamin D_3 levels, placing a patient at risk for nephrocalcinosis with renal failure if provided vitamin D replacement therapy.

Psychosocial manifestations

Depression and/or fatigue have been found in 30–60% of symptomatic patients with sarcoidosis. In the ACCESS study, depression was associated with female sex, lower socioeconomic status, poor access to care and increased disease severity, but not race.

Associated conditions

Sarcoidosis and pregnancy

There is usually little effect on the course of sarcoidosis from pregnancy, although some patients experience spontaneous improvement. In these patients, exacerbations frequently follow several months after delivery. The temporary clinical improvement may relate to suppressed Th1 immunity during pregnancy.

Th1-promoting therapeutics

The administration of Th1-promoting therapeutics such as IFN-α, IFN-γ, IL-2, and IFN-β have been linked to initiation or recrudescence of sarcoidosis.

Common variable immunodeficiency

Sarcoidosis is associated with common variable immunodeficiency (CVID) in both adult and pediatric sarcoidosis. A high index of suspicion must be maintained for this condition in sarcoidosis patients who have recurrent infections.

Human immunodeficiency virus (HIV)

Sarcoidosis may develop in HIV-infected patients with immune reconstitution following initiation of highly active antiretroviral therapy, perhaps from reconstituted Th1 immunity. Granulomatous inflammation of the lungs or skin is most often reported.

Autoimmune disorders

Sarcoidosis has been described in association with autoimmune diseases such as Crohn disease, ulcerative colitis, primary biliary cirrhosis, scleroderma, Sjögren syndrome, autoimmune hemolytic anemia, and autoimmune endocrinopathies. These associations could be the result of a common, predisposing altered Th1 immunity.

Cancer

Multisystem sarcoidosis may develop in patients with a recent history of cancer or following chemotherapy treatment, perhaps related to a rebound in immunologic responsiveness following successful treatment.

Diagnosis

A diagnosis of sarcoidosis is based on a compatible clinical picture, histologic evidence of noncaseating granulomas and the absence of other known causes of this pathologic response.[1] Chronic beryllium disease and hypersensitivity pneumonitis must be excluded when there is a compatible history and clinical findings are confined to the lung. In the absence of defined multisystem disease a diagnosis of sarcoidosis should be presumed, as local "sarcoid" reactions can occur in response to infection, tumor or foreign material. Biopsy confirmation of sarcoidosis is usually not necessary in Löfgren syndrome, except in regions where histoplasmosis is endemic.

In general, biopsy of the easiest, most accessible abnormal tissue site is used to confirm the diagnosis. Biopsy of a skin nodule, superficial lymph node, lacrimal gland, nasal mucosae, conjunctivae or salivary gland (lip biopsy) can establish a diagnosis.

Biopsy by fiberoptic bronchoscopy is frequently used to diagnose pulmonary sarcoidosis because of its relative safety and high yield. The yield of transbronchial biopsy is operator dependent, but approaches 50–85% of patients when pulmonary infiltrates are present. Endoscopic bronchial ultrasound has improved the diagnostic yield of sampling intrathoracic lymph nodes over standard bronchoscopy in sarcoidosis. Mediastinoscopy or surgical lung biopsy is considered when lymphoma or other intrathoracic malignancy cannot be reasonably excluded. Imaging techniques such as gadolinium-enhanced MRI, ^{18}F-fluorodeoxyglucose (FDG)-PET scanning or gallium 67 scanning are non-specific, but can assist in assessing the presence of inflammation in the heart, brain, and bone, or to direct a biopsy approach.

● CLINICAL PEARLS

Tests recommended for an initial evaluation of a patient with sarcoidosis

- Chest radiograph
- Pulmonary function tests
  - Spirometry
  - Diffusing capacity
  - Lung volumes
  - Flow–volume loop (if suspected upper airway obstruction)
- Slit-lamp examination (to exclude subclinical uveitis)
- Liver and renal function tests
- Calcium level
- Complete blood count
- Electrocardiogram
- Purified protein derivative skin test

An initial diagnostic evaluation of a patient with possible sarcoidosis should consist of tests to evaluate the presence and extent of pulmonary involvement and screen for extrathoracic disease. In the presence of cardiac symptoms such as palpitations, a 2D echocardiogram and Holter monitor are usually indicated as screening tests. Cardiac MR or cardiac PET have greater sensitivity in demonstrating patchy inflammation or scar than gated technetium-99 m sestamibi or echocardiogram.[28] Endomyocardial biopsy is positive in <10–25% of cases of cardiac sarcoidosis, owing to the patchiness of the granulomatous inflammation; thus, a negative biopsy never excludes the diagnosis. A diagnosis of cardiac sarcoidosis is usually made by biopsy confirmation of a site other than the heart in association with compatible cardiac imaging or conduction abnormalities or arrhythmias.

When CNS or spinal cord sarcoidosis is considered, MRI with gadolinium enhancement is the optimal test to detect the characteristic inflammatory lesions, particularly in the periventricular and leptomeningeal areas. A normal scan does not exclude neurosarcoidosis, particularly for cranial neuropathies or during corticosteroid therapy. Cerebral spinal fluid characteristically demonstrates lymphocytic pleocytosis and/or elevated protein levels. A diagnosis of neurosarcoidosis is usually confirmed by biopsy of a non-CNS site, generally by bronchoscopic or lymph node biopsy. Rarely, brain biopsy is needed to exclude infectious or malignant disease. In suspected cases of peripheral neuropathy or myopathy, EMG or nerve conduction studies should be considered.

Other diagnostic studies

There are no noninvasive tests that have been shown to be useful in assisting the clinician in making a diagnosis of sarcoidosis. Serum angiotensin-converting enzyme (SACE) levels are elevated in 40–90% of patients with clinically active disease, but are non-specific and can be found in other inflammatory and granulomatous diseases.

Clinical course and patient management

The clinical course of sarcoidosis is highly variable. Overall, 50–65% of patients undergo spontaneous remission, usually within the first 2–3 years. Löfgren syndrome is associated with spontaneous remission in >70–80% of patients. Peripheral adenopathy, salivary and parotid gland enlargement and Bell palsy generally subside spontaneously or with treatment, and do not recur. Elevated serum liver function tests also can revert to normal without treatment. Approximately 50–80% of patients with a stage I chest radiograph, 30–60% with a stage II radiograph and 20–30% with a stage III radiograph undergo remission. Patients with a stage IV chest radiograph with fibrocystic changes rarely (<5%) experience remission. Extrapulmonary disease that is severe on presentation tends to persist and require treatment. The major causes of mortality in sarcoidosis are from advanced pulmonary, cardiac and neurologic involvement with overall mortality ranging from 1–6%.[1]

The intensity of surveillance of sarcoidosis depends on the severity of clinical presentation, but should include serial tests of organ-specific function. When sarcoidosis undergoes remission, the disease rarely recurs; exceptions often involve neurologic or ocular manifestations. There are no biomarkers that have been shown to be useful in management decisions.

Treatment

Current treatment approach

> ⬤ THERAPEUTIC PRINCIPLES
>
> **Indications for corticosteroid therapy in patients with sarcoidosis**
>
> - Pulmonary involvement
>   - Moderate or severe, symptomatic pulmonary disease
>   - Progressive, symptomatic pulmonary disease
>   - Persistent pulmonary infiltrates or abnormal lung function for 1–2 years with mild symptoms to assess reversibility
>   - Advanced fibrocystic disease
> - Extrapulmonary involvement
>   - Threatened organ failure: severe ocular, cardiac, or CNS disease
>   - Posterior uveitis or anterior uveitis not responding to local steroids
>   - Persistent hypercalcemia
>   - Persistent renal or hepatic dysfunction
>   - Pituitary disease
>   - Myopathy
>   - Palpable splenomegaly or evidence of hypersplenism such as thrombocytopenia
>   - Severe fatigue and weight loss
>   - Painful lymphadenopathy
>   - Disfiguring skin disease

Consensus statements on the treatment of sarcoidosis have been published.[29] Current therapies are non-specific and largely unproven. When there is not serious or organ-threatening involvement, a period of observation is often indicated to evaluate whether the patient will undergo spontaneous remission.

Corticosteroids remain the mainstay of therapy for the intial treatment of progressive organ-threatening or life-threatening manifestations of sarcoidosis.[1,29] The optimal doses and duration of corticosteroid treatment have not been established by rigorous clinical studies. Initial treatment with corticosteroids usually employs no more than 20–40 mg/day of prednisone for 2–4 weeks, followed by a slow tapering regimen over several months to a maintenance dose of 5–15 mg/day. Alternate-day therapy is suggested by some investigators, although such a regimen may not be effective in a subgroup of patients who then respond to daily dosing. Treatment is ordinarily continued for a minimum of 6–12 months, as premature tapering is likely to result in relapse. Recurrent, progressive pulmonary disease occurs in 16–74% of patients as corticosteroid therapy is tapered; those patients with repetitive relapses usually benefit from chronic suppressive therapy to minimize loss of lung function. Inhaled corticosteroids may be helpful in reducing symptoms of cough or airway irritability, but have not been proven useful as sole agents in pulmonary sarcoidosis. Weight gain, hypertension, hyperglycemia, glaucoma, and osteoporosis are serious potential complications. Bisphosphonate therapy is recommended for patients on chronic corticosteroid therapy.

Pentoxifylline, a phosphodiesterase inhibitor, was found to be beneficial in one study of mild pulmonary sarcoidosis, though wider experience suggests only a small minority of patients respond to the drug. Gastrointestinal side effects often limit the dose that is tolerated.

Alternative cytotoxic therapies

Corticosteroid-sparing therapies are frequently employed for chronic, progressive sarcoidosis when corticosteroid adverse effects significantly degrade quality of life.[3,30] Methotrexate in low weekly doses (10–20 mg/week) is recommended as an alternative therapy in corticosteroid-recalcitrant pulmonary, cardiac, ocular (panuveitis), cutaneous and neurologic sarcoidosis. Success rates range from 50–70%, but may take 6 months or longer to show effectiveness. Potential serious complications include hepatotoxicity, opportunistic infections, bone marrow suppression and pulmonary toxicity. Azathioprine can also be useful in corticosteroid-recalcitrant sarcoidosis with 50–70% response rates, often with low doses of corticosteroids. Mycophenylate mofetil has been used with anecdotal benefit, particularly in neurologic and ocular sarcoidosis. Potential drug toxicities in these latter two drugs include bone marrow suppression, gastrointestinal symptoms, skin rashes, and an increased risk of malignancy. Small case series suggest leflunomide may be effective in sarcoidosis. Cyclophosphamide has been used in steroid-recalcitrant sarcoidosis, particularly refractory neurosarcoidosis, though its use is severly limited because of its oncogenic potential. Cyclosporine inhibits T-cell activation, but appears to be ineffective and cannot be recommended.

Clinical trials support the effectiveness of anti-TNF therapy in sarcoidosis. One multicenter study found infliximab to improve pulmonary function or extrapulmonary manifestations after 24 weeks of therapy. Case series suggest adalimumab may also be effective in some patients with sarcoidosis. Etanercept was reported to be ineffective in a small clinical trial of pulmonary sarcoidosis and cannot be recommended at this time. Further studies are needed to define their role in sarcoidosis since these therapies carry an increased risk of serious, life-threatening infections and malignancy.

Specific situations

Löfgren syndrome

Nonsteroidal anti-inflammatory drugs are recommended for the relief of constitutional symptoms and joint pains. For disabling arthritis or severe constitutional symptoms, corticosteroids are almost immediately effective and can be tapered over a few weeks to months.

Mucocutaneous and joint sarcoidosis and hypercalcemia

Hydroxychloroquine is often tried as a first-line treatment for cutaneous, joint, nasal or sinus manifestations when corticosteroids are not immediately needed. Hypercalcemia may also respond to hydroxychloroquine as maintenance therapy. Chloroquine can be effective in some patients unresponsive to hydroxychloroquine, but has a greater potential for ocular toxicity and is rarely used. Minocycline and doxycycline have been reported to be effective in a small number of patients with cutaneous sarcoidosis.

Ocular sarcoidosis

Anterior uveitis is usually treated with topical corticosteroids. Oral or IV corticosteroids are used initially for posterior uveitis, chorioretinitis or optic neuritis.

Pulmonary hypertension

Small retrospective case series suggest that pulmonary vasodilator treatment is associated with reductions in pulmonary artery pressure and improvements in exercise dyspnea and 6-minute walk distance in sarcoidosis patients with pulmonary hypertension.[31] The benefit of vasodilator therapy on survival rates remains uncertain.

Cardiac sarcoidosis

Initial treatment consists of cardiac medications (antiarrhythmic therapy, diuretics, afterload-reducing agents) along with corticosteroid therapy that may reverse heart block, reduce arrhythmias and improve cardiac function. Corticosteroids are recommended in moderate doses based on studies that suggest no difference in 5-year survival rates for patients treated with prednisone >30 versus <30 mg/day. Initial therapy for intractable arrhythmias or heart block often begin with higher doses. Patients with significant cardiomyopathy may require long-term treatment and often cytotoxic drugs are used as steroid-sparing drugs. Small case series suggest TNF inhibitors may also be useful, but caution is advised since these therapies have been shown to worsen congestive heart failure (CHF) in non-sarcoidosis cardiomyopathy. Automatic implantable defibrillators (ICDs) or pacemakers are indicated in patients at risk for sudden death from serious arrhythmias or heart block, though indications for their prophylactic placement are controversial. The effectiveness of radiofrequency ablation for prevention of arrhythmias in cardiac sarcoidosis remains uncertain.

Neurosarcoidosis

High doses of oral corticosteroids (60–80 mg/day) or high-dose pulse intravenous therapy are often employed for serious CNS involvement. Tapering should be performed over several months after evidence of suppression of inflammation by objective criteria (e.g., serial MRI scans). With the exception of cranial neuropathies, neurosarcoidosis tends to be chronic and requires long-term therapy.

Depression/fatigue/pain

Small case series highlight the existence of small fiber neuropathy and autonomic neuropathy in sarcoidosis, particularly in those patients with pain. A few case reports suggest anti-TNF therapies may be beneficial in small fiber neuropathy, but their role in sarcoidosis remains undefined. One study suggested the stimulant dexmethylphenidate hydrochloride may be helpful in treating chronic fatigue in sarcoidosis. Therapies directed at treating depression may improve quality of life in these patients, though clinical trials are lacking.

Role of transplantation in sarcoidosis

Lung, heart, kidney and liver transplantations have been performed successfully in patients with sarcoidosis. Recurrent granulomas are found in the transplanted organs of some patients but are generally responsive to an increase in immunosuppression. Overall, the survival rate for lung and cardiac transplantation in sarcoidosis appears to be similar to that of other organ-specific diseases.

Opportunities for progress in sarcoidosis

● ON THE HORIZON

- Diagnostic tools based on immunologic reactivity to specific microbial proteins.
- Prognostic tools based on genotyping and genomic/microbiomic/proteomic signatures at time of diagnosis.
- Improvements in imaging tools to assist in assessment of organ involvement.
- Multicenter clinical trials of newer immune-based therapies for treatment of sarcoidosis.

The foundations for making rapid progress in understanding sarcoidosis appear to be in place. Although there is tremendous clinical heterogeneity, clinical phenotypes are well established, from acute sarcoidosis (Löfgren syndrome) to chronic progressive organ disease. It is known that the genetic basis of sarcoidosis predominantly resides within the MHC. Immunologic hallmarks of the disease include non-caseating granulomas, highly polarized Th1 immunity and proinflammatory cytokines such as TNF at sites of disease, and possibly, reduced regulatory T-cell immunity. Evidence from multiple centers suggest microbial organisms such as mycobacterial and possibly propionibacterial organisms, may trigger sarcoidosis. Recent identification of innate immune pathways, one of which involves serum amyloid A, suggest mechanisms that may explain the pathogenesis of chronic sarcoidosis in the absence of evidence for any active chronic infection. The challenge in the next 5–10 years is to translate these laboratory discoveries into clinical tools to assist the clinician in the diagnosis and prognosis of individual patients. Newer therapies are sorely needed for the treatment of sarcoidosis patients, particularly those with chronic disease who require long-term maintenance therapy. The potential for curing this disease is suggested by a remission rate of over 50%, although progress towards this goal awaits a better understanding of the relevant mechanisms that allow remission to occur. Research that integrates assessment of clinical phenotype, genetic background, individual immunophenotypic and environmental triggers in different subgroups of patients may offer the best chance for rapid progress.

References

1. Statement on sarcoidosis. Joint Statement of the American Thoracic Society (ATS), the European Respiratory Society (ERS) and the World Association of Sarcoidosis and Other Granulomatous Disorders (WASOG) adopted by the ATS Board of Directors and by the ERS Executive Committee, February 1999. Am J Respir Crit Care Med 1999;160:736–55.
2. Chen ES, Moller DR. Sarcoidosis—scientific progress and clinical challenges. Nat Rev Rheumatol 2011;7:457–67.
3. Baughman RP, Culver DA, Judson MA. A concise review of pulmonary sarcoidosis. Am J Respir Crit Care Med 2011;183:573–81.
4. Rybicki BA, Iannuzzi MC. Epidemiology of sarcoidosis: recent advances and future prospects. Semin Respir Crit Care Med 2007;28:22–35.
5. Rybicki BA, Iannuzzi MC, Frederick MM, et al. Familial aggregation of sarcoidosis. A case-control etiologic study of sarcoidosis (ACCESS). Am J Respir Crit Care Med 2001;164:2085–91.
6. Muller-Quernheim J, Schurmann M, Hofmann S, et al. Genetics of sarcoidosis. Clin Chest Med 2008;29:391–414 viii.
7. Rossman MD, Thompson B, Frederick M, et al. HLA-DRB1*1101: a significant risk factor for sarcoidosis in blacks and whites. Am J Hum Genet 2003;73:720–35.
8. Voorter CE, Amicosante M, Berretta F, et al. HLA class II amino acid epitopes as susceptibility markers of sarcoidosis. Tissue Antigens 2007;70:18–27.
9. Voorter CE, Drent M, Hoitsma E, et al. Association of HLA DQB1 0602 in sarcoidosis patients with small fiber neuropathy. Sarcoidosis Vasc Diffuse Lung Dis 2005;22:129–32.

10. Medica I, Kastrin A, Maver A, Peterlin B. Role of genetic polymorphisms in ACE and TNF-alpha gene in sarcoidosis: a meta-analysis. J Hum Genet 2007;52:836–47.

11. Valentonyte R, Hampe J, Huse K, et al. Sarcoidosis is associated with a truncating splice site mutation in BTNL2. Nat Genet 2005;37:357–64.

12. Rybicki BA, Walewski JL, Maliarik MJ, et al. The BTNL2 gene and sarcoidosis susceptibility in African Americans and Whites. Am J Hum Genet 2005;77:491–9.

13. Newman LS, Rose CS, Bresnitz EA, et al. A case control etiologic study of sarcoidosis: environmental and occupational risk factors. Am J Respir Crit Care Med 2004;170:1324–30.

14. Izbicki G, Chavko R, Banauch GI, et al. World Trade Center "sarcoid-like" granulomatous pulmonary disease in New York City Fire Department rescue workers. Chest 2007;131:1414–23.

15. Gupta D, Agarwal R, Aggarwal AN, Jindal SK. Molecular evidence for the role of mycobacteria in sarcoidosis: a meta-analysis. Eur Respir J 2007;30:508–16.

16. Song Z, Marzilli L, Greenlee BM, et al. Mycobacterial catalase-peroxidase is a tissue antigen and target of the adaptive immune response in systemic sarcoidosis. J Exp Med 2005;201:755–67.

17. Teirstein AS. Kveim antigen: what does it tell us about causation of sarcoidosis? Semin Respir Infect 1998;13:206–11.

18. Chen ES, Wahlstrom J, Song Z, et al. T cell responses to mycobacterial catalase-peroxidase profile a pathogenic antigen in systemic sarcoidosis. J Immunol 2008;181:8784–96.

19. Drake WP, Dhason MS, Nadaf M, et al. Cellular recognition of *Mycobacterium tuberculosis* ESAT-6 and KatG peptides in systemic sarcoidosis. Infect Immun 2007;75:527–30.

20. Eishi Y, Suga M, Ishige I, et al. Quantitative analysis of mycobacterial and propionibacterial DNA in lymph nodes of Japanese and European patients with sarcoidosis. J Clin Microbiol 2002;40:198–204.

21. Tchaptchet S, Kirberg J, Freudenberg N, et al. Innate, antigen-independent role for T cells in the activation of the immune system by *Propionibacterium acnes*. Eur J Immunol 2010;40:2506–16.

22. Wahlstrom J, Dengjel J, Winqvist O, et al. Autoimmune T cell responses to antigenic peptides presented by bronchoalveolar lavage cell HLA-DR molecules in sarcoidosis. Clin Immunol 2009;133:353–63.

23. Zissel G, Prasse A, Muller-Quernheim J. Sarcoidosis—immunopathogenetic concepts. Semin Respir Crit Care Med 2007;28:3–14.

24. Taflin C, Miyara M, Nochy D, et al. FoxP3+ regulatory T cells suppress early stages of granuloma formation but have little impact on sarcoidosis lesions. Am J Pathol 2009;174:497–508.

25. Prasse A, Zissel G, Lutzen N, et al. Inhaled vasoactive intestinal peptide exerts immunoregulatory effects in sarcoidosis. Am J Respir Crit Care Med 2010;182:540–8.

26. Prasse A, Pechkovsky DV, Toews GB, et al. A vicious circle of alveolar macrophages and fibroblasts perpetuates pulmonary fibrosis via CCL18. Am J Respir Crit Care Med 2006;173:781–92.

27. Chen ES, Song Z, Willett MH, et al. Serum amyloid A regulates granulomatous inflammation in sarcoidosis through Toll-like receptor-2. Am J Respir Crit Care Med 2010;181:360–73.

28. Mehta D, Lubitz SA, Frankel Z, et al. Cardiac involvement in patients with sarcoidosis: diagnostic and prognostic value of outpatient testing. Chest 2008;133:1426–35.

29. Bradley B, Branley HM, Egan JJ, et al. Interstitial lung disease guideline: the British Thoracic Society in collaboration with the Thoracic Society of Australia and New Zealand and the Irish Thoracic Society. Thorax 2008;63(Suppl. 5):v1–v58.

30. Baughman RP, Costabel U, du Bois RM. Treatment of sarcoidosis. Clin Chest Med 2008;29:533–48 ix–x.

31. Barnett CF, Bonura EJ, Nathan SD, et al. Treatment of sarcoidosis-associated pulmonary hypertension. A two-center experience. Chest 2009;135:1455–61.

73

Immunologic ocular disease

James T.
Rosenbaum,
Justine R. Smith

The immune system can induce disease in virtually any portion of the eye. Examples include conjunctivitis, keratitis, keratoconjunctivitis, uveitis, scleritis, optic neuritis, and orbital inflammation. The anatomy of the eye is depicted schematically in Fig. 73.1. Two relatively common immunologically mediated ocular diseases discussed elsewhere in this volume are sicca syndrome secondary to Sjögren's syndrome (Chapter 54) and anterior ischemic optic neuropathy secondary to giant cell arteritis (Chapter 59). Before considering those additional ocular disorders that are the most common and visually significant, it is critical to review some unique considerations related to ocular immunology.

Ocular immune privilege

Many of the mechanisms that drive inflammation in the eye are identical to those operating at other tissue sites. The major difference between the immunopathology of intraocular inflammation and that of systemic inflammatory disease relates to the fact that the eye, like the brain and the testis, is an immunologically privileged site. During uveitis, keratitis, and scleritis, as well as following corneal transplantation, a variety of local immunosuppressive mechanisms act to limit the damage caused by infiltrating leukocytes, and, consequently, to influence the patient's clinical course. One of the most important factors is the constitutive expression of Fas ligand (FasL) within the eye. In addition, normal ocular tissues produce relatively high levels of immunomodulatory cytokines and immunosuppressive neuropeptides, as well as complement regulatory proteins. Other factors include the blood–aqueous and blood–retinal anatomical barriers, limited MHC expression, a paucity of lymphatic drainage channels within the eye, and, in the case of the cornea, the complete absence of blood vessels. Anterior chamber-associated immune deviation (ACAID) describes the suppression of a cell-mediated immune response when soluble antigen is directly injected into the aqueous humor. ACAID presumably results from some or all of the above factors.

Fas ligand

Many immune cells, including neutrophils, monocytes, macrophages, and lymphocytes, express Fas (CD95) on their surface. The interaction between Fas and its receptor FasL (CD95L) triggers apoptosis of the Fas-bearing cell. FasL is constitutively expressed within the eye, being detected in normal cornea, anterior uvea and retina. The importance of FasL to ocular immune privilege has been demonstrated primarily in experimental models of ocular inflammation. Corneal allografts from FasL-negative mice into recipients of normal phenotype are rejected in all cases, whereas approximately half of FasL-positive grafts survive.[1] When injected into the eyes of FasL-deficient mice, herpes simplex virus causes a severe invasive infection. A similar procedure in normal phenotype control animals results in relatively minor inflammation. Levels of FasL in aqueous humor during human acute anterior uveitis are capable of inducing apoptosis in Fas-positive lymphoid cells. In this self-limiting condition, as well as in relevant rodent models, apoptosis of infiltrating T cells is observed early in the course of the inflammation. In addition to FasL, the local expression of tumor necrosis factor (TNF)-related apoptosis-inducing ligand (TRAIL) by corneal endothelium also contributes to enhanced apoptosis and immune privilege within the eye.[2]

Cytokine network, neuropeptides, and complement

Tissues in both the anterior and the posterior segments of the human eye constitutively express the immunomodulatory cytokine transforming growth factor-β (TGF-β).[3] The concentration of TGF-β in the aqueous humor is sufficient to inhibit T-cell activation and proliferation in a variety of assays.[4] As might be anticipated, significantly lower levels of this activated cytokine are measured in the aqueous humor of patients with a variety of uveitis syndromes compared to levels present in normal eyes. The inflammatory cytokine interleukin (IL)-1 has been implicated in

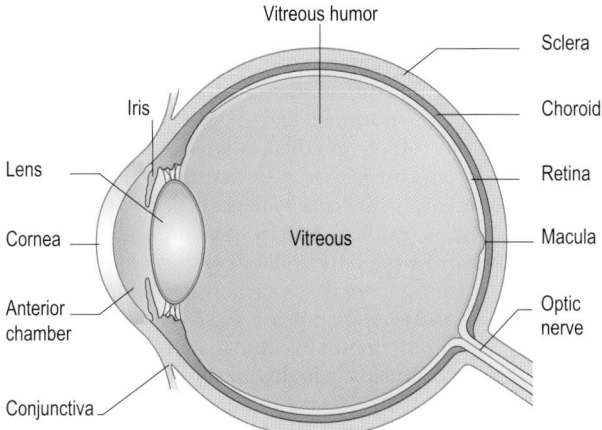

Vitreous humor
Sclera
Choroid
Iris
Retina
Lens
Macula
Cornea
Vitreous
Anterior chamber
Optic nerve
Conjunctiva

Fig. 73.1 Schematic representation of the eye.

the pathogenesis of various ocular inflammatory diseases. There is expression of IL-1 receptor antagonist (IL-1Ra) in normal cornea[5] and retinal pigment epithelium, implying that this tissue contains a control mechanism for responses mediated by IL-1. Interestingly, topical application of IL-1Ra has a significantly positive effect in promoting experimental corneal allograft survival. The aqueous humor contains neuropeptides, including α-melanocyte stimulating hormone, vasoactive intestinal peptide, and calcitonin gene-related peptide, that inhibit the activities of T cells and macrophages. Complement is active at low levels in the healthy eye, regulated by complement regulatory proteins that are expressed both on intraocular cell membranes and within the intraocular fluid; this system may participate in the destruction of pathogens invading the eye.[6] However, interestingly, iC3b, generated because of this activation, appears to inhibit antigen-specific delayed-type hypersensitivity.

Anterior chamber-associated immune deviation

Anterior chamber-associated immune deviation is "a stereotypic, systemic immune response to antigens placed in the anterior chamber (of the eye) in which delayed hypersensitivity is avoided and suppressed." The molecular events that are responsible for this phenomenon include the following:[7] Entry of an antigen into the eye stimulates production of TNF-α, and hence the upregulation of cell adhesion molecules; secretion of IL-10 by the infiltrating T cells; and sensitization of these cells for FasL-mediated killing. TGF-β also induces ocular antigen-presenting cells to secrete IL-10 during antigen processing.[8] Apoptotic T cells pass in the bloodstream to the spleen, where they are phagocytosed and induce activation of Th2-type CD4 T cells. The Th2-type cells control Th1 function by secreting various immunomodulatory cytokines. T-cell receptor α-chain fragments from apoptotic cells are presented in the class I pathway. This event generates CD8 killer cells, which are capable of deleting the CD4 T cells that would otherwise mediate a delayed-type hypersensitivity response. CD8 T cells that secrete immunomodulatory cytokines, including IL-10 and TGF-β, are also generated. ACAID is also dependent on the presence of invariant natural killer T cells.

Immobility of dendritic cells within the anterior chamber

The vast majority of cells that phagocytose foreign antigen within the iris fail to migrate after antigen uptake. This is clearly demonstrable by intravital microscopy and correlates with the failure of these antigen-bearing cells to migrate to the local lymph nodes.[9] The inability to migrate is consistent with the known lack of lymphatics within the eye, and must mean that soluble antigen injected into the anterior chamber is not presented in the regional lymph node in a manner that is comparable to what follows antigen exposure in an organ such as the skin.

Interleukin-17

Lymphocytes that synthesize IL-17 have been strongly implicated in some animal models of uveitis.[10] However, uveitis in laboratory rodents can also be induced by either a Th1 or Th2

response. The heterogeneity of uveitis means that different clinical entities should vary with regard to pathogenesis. Monoclonal antibodies to IL-17 have been tested in several clinical trials to treat uveitis. Evidence strongly implicates IL-17 in Behçet's disease, but a clinical trial using anti-IL-17 for this indication was withdrawn.

Uveitis

Uveitis as a diagnostic entity

The uveal tract is the middle layer of the eye, divided into the anterior uvea (iris, ciliary body) and posterior uvea (choroid). The uvea is sandwiched between an outer layer (sclera) and an inner layer (retina). The anterior segment is separated from the posterior segment by the lens. Uveitis is an extremely variable spectrum of different diseases that includes a variety of infections and immune-mediated diseases (Table 73.1). It is the third leading cause of preventable blindness worldwide. Inflammatory disorders of the retina (retinitis) and sclera (scleritis) frequently involve the adjacent uveal tract. Many different immune mechanisms could result in uveitis, as evidenced in animal models. These mechanisms include an immune response to a sequestered self-antigen, molecular mimicry, immune complex deposition, and the response to a toxin.

The differential diagnosis of uveitis is facilitated by identifying characteristic clinical features. Uveitis can be classified by location: anterior (iritis, iridocyclitis), intermediate (pars planitis, vitritis), or posterior (retinitis, choroiditis, retinochoroiditis, chorioretinitis, retinal vasculitis). Some forms of uveitis involve all portions of the uveal tract (panuveitis). Uveitis can be classified by course (self-limited, chronic, or recurrent); by onset (sudden, insidious); by symmetry (unilateral, bilateral); by associated complications such as glaucoma, cystoid macular edema (Figs 73.2–73.4), synechiae (for example, adhesion of the iris to the lens) (Fig. 73.5), retinal detachment, or band keratopathy (the deposition of calcium in the epithelium of the cornea) (Fig. 73.6); and by the appearance of inflammatory keratic precipitates on the endothelium of the cornea within the eye (granulomatous, nongranulomatous) (Fig. 73.7). Granulomatous diseases with large cellular concretions on the cornea or nodules within the iris include tuberculosis, syphilis, sarcoidosis, Vogt–Koyanagi–Harada disease, and sympathetic ophthalmia. The group of nongranulomatous diseases includes ankylosing spondylitis, reactive arthritis, and juvenile idiopathic arthritis. Table 73.2 shows how these parameters contribute to the differential diagnosis. Additionally, ethnic and geographic considerations factor into the differential diagnosis. For example, sarcoidosis, Behçet's syndrome, and Vogt–Koyanagi–Harada disease have strong ethnic predispositions, whereas certain infections such as cytomegalovirus in association with AIDS, leprosy, or onchocerciasis vary in prevalence based on geographic area. Together with a medical history, gender, and age, these findings help to narrow the differential diagnosis of uveitis.

The following case vignettes illustrate how important a precise and critical history and examination are. A 22-year-old man with low back pain and a red painful eye due to episodic, unilateral, sudden onset anterior uveitis is highly likely to have a spondyloarthropathy (Chapter 57). A 6-year-old girl with no ocular complaints but biomicroscopic findings of bilateral band keratopathy and leukocytes in the anterior chamber is likely to suffer from the pauciarticular subset of juvenile idiopathic arthritis (Chapter 53).

Table 73.1 Diagnostic categories of uveitis

Diagnostic group		Diagnosis
Infectious causes	Viral	Herpes simplex
		Herpes zoster
		Cytomegalovirus
		Chikungunya
		HTLV-1
		Mumps
		West Nile
	Bacterial or spirochetal	Atypical *Mycobacterium*
		Bacterial endocarditis
		Bartonella
		Brucellosis
		Leprosy
		Leptospirosis
		Lyme disease
		Propionibacterium
		Tuberculosis
		Leprosy
		Syphilis
		Whipple's disease
	Parasitic (protozoan or helminthic)	*Acanthamoeba*
		Cysticercosis
		Onchocerciasis
		Pneumocystis jiroveci
		Toxoplasmosis
		Toxocariasis
	Fungal	Histoplasmosis
		Coccidioidomycosis
		Candidiasis
		Aspergillosis
		Sporotrichosis
		Blastomycosis
		Cryptococcosis
Immune mediated		Ankylosing spondylitis
		Behçet's disease
		Crohn's disease
		Drug or hypersensitivity reaction (such as rifabutin or cidofovir)
		Familial granulomatous synovitis with uveitis
		Interstitial nephritis
		Juvenile idiopathic arthritis
		Kawasaki disease
		Multiple sclerosis
		Psoriatic arthritis
		Reactive arthritis
		Relapsing polychondritis
		Rheumatic fever
		Sarcoidosis
		Scleritis
		Sjögren's syndrome
		Sweet's syndrome
		Systemic lupus erythematosus
		Ulcerative colitis
		Vasculitis
		Vogt–Koyanagi–Harada syndrome

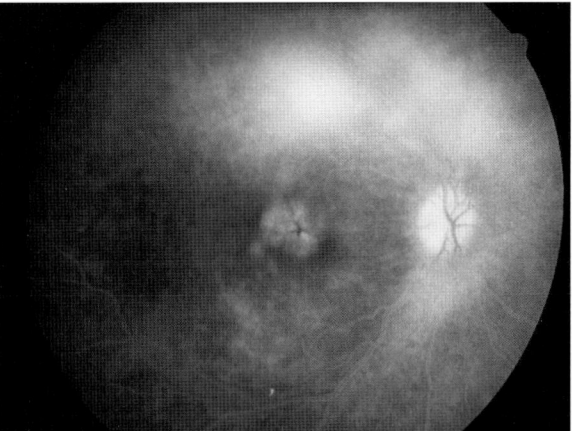

Fig. 73.2 Fundus fluorescein angiogram showing cystoid macular edema. Fluorescein, which appears as a white stain, should be absent from the center of this photograph because the macular area is avascular.

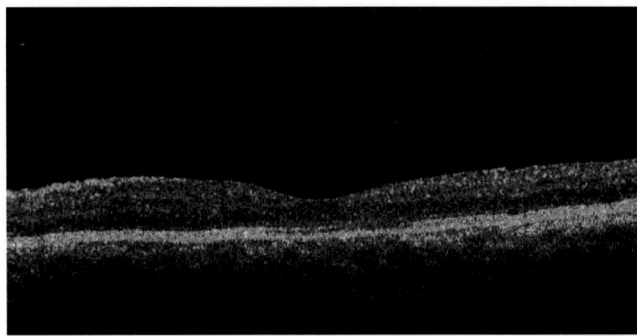

Fig. 73.3 Optical coherence tomogram (OCT). This is an image of a normal eye. An OCT allows precise quantification of macular thickening. In this image, the macula shows a normal dimple or indentation.

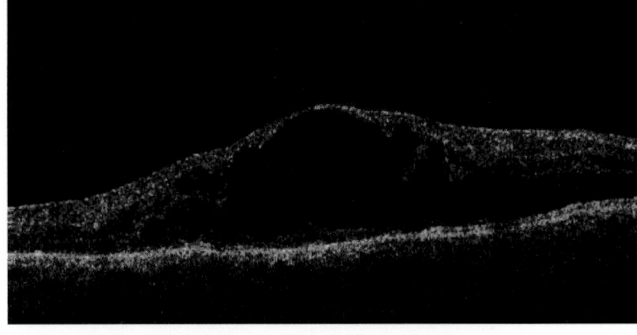

Fig. 73.4 OCT image showing marked macular edema. The macula is markedly elevated.

The most obvious sign of uveal inflammation is the presence of biomicroscopically visible leukocytes in the anterior chamber or the vitreous humor of the eye. Most patients with anterior uveitis will experience pain, redness, photophobia, miosis, and a variable degree of visual loss. In contrast, many forms of uveitis that affect the posterior segment will cause no redness, no pain, no change in pupil size (no macroscopically apparent signs of an inflamed eye). Instead, disturbances in visual acuity may vary from normal vision to seeing floaters, to blurred vision to blindness.

Epidemiology

The incidence and prevalence of the different types of uveitis varies among regions of the world, depending on numerous factors: level of development, HLA distribution, prevalence of different infectious diseases in each region, and also the methodology employed by each physician to evaluate and classify uveitis (Table 73.3).[11] Using a northern California database for enrolees in a health maintenance study, Gritz and Wong[12]

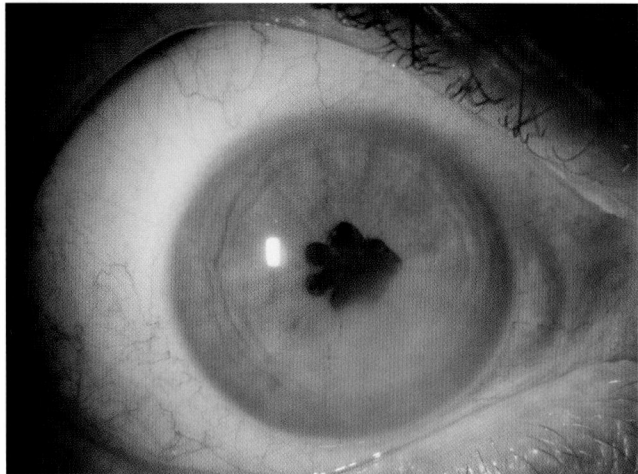

Fig. 73.5 Posterior synechiae. The cloverleaf appearance of the pupil is due to the iris adhering to the lens.

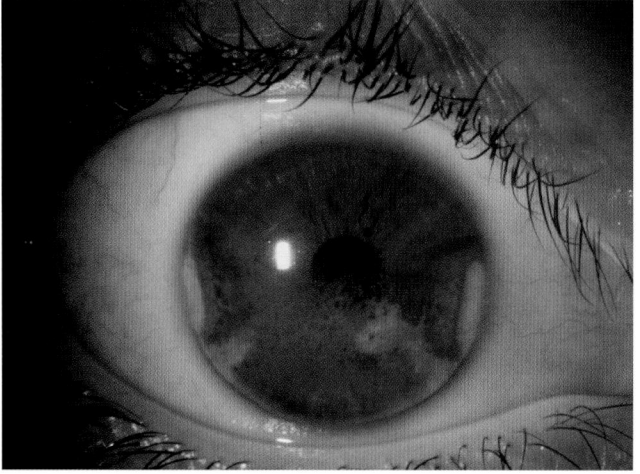

Fig. 73.6 Band keratopathy. Calcium deposition in the corneal endothelium complicates the iridocyclitis in a patient with juvenile idiopathic arthritis.

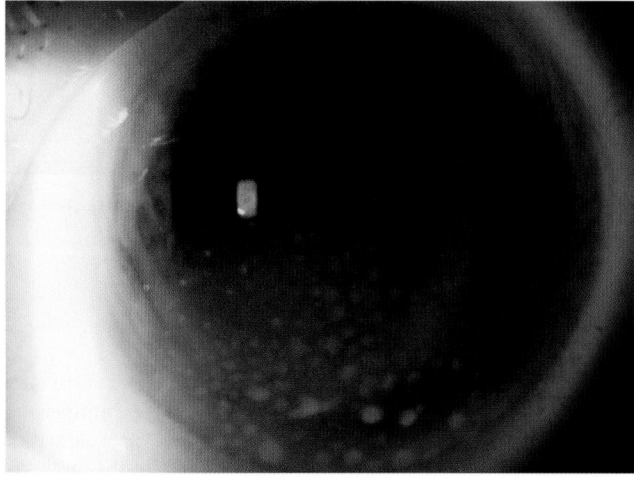

Fig. 73.7 Granulomatous keratic precipitates. Round white dots are scattered in a triangular shape. The dots represent concretions of leukocytes adherent to the corneal endothelium.

Table 73.2 Characteristic features of common forms of uveitis

Parameter	
Location	**Anterior:** Ankylosing spondylitis, reactive arthritis, juvenile idiopathic arthritis **Intermediate:** Pars planitis **Posterior:** Vogt–Koyanagi–Harada syndrome
Onset	**Sudden:** Ankylosing spondylitis, reactive arthritis **Insidious:** Pars planitis, juvenile idiopathic arthritis
Symmetry	**Unilateral:** Ankylosing spondylitis, toxoplasmosis **Bilateral:** Pars planitis, lymphoma, juvenile idiopathic arthritis
Course	**Self-limited:** Toxoplasmosis **Recurrent:** Behçet's disease, ankylosing spondylitis **Chronic:** Pars planitis

Table 73.3 Likelihood of developing uveitis in association with a specific disease

Diagnosis	Likelihood (%)
Ankylosing spondylitis	30
Sarcoidosis	25–50
Behçet's disease	80
Inflammatory bowel disease	1–9
Psoriatic arthritis	7
Juvenile idiopathic arthritis	<2–53
Multiple sclerosis	<1–2

recently reported an incidence of 52.4 per 100 000 per year and a prevalence of 115.3/100 000. Anterior uveitis is much more common than intermediate or posterior uveitis.

Prevention and patient management

Uveitis can be the first sign of occult, potentially severe, systemic disease (for example, sarcoidosis, syphilis, or central nervous system lymphoma). Despite the difficulty of successful systemic anti-inflammatory/immunosuppressive treatment, there are some diagnoses that can be treated to complete recovery, such as syphilis. Therefore it is essential to identify as accurately as possible the cause of uveitis. A targeted approach is preferable, with a limited work-up guided by the type and severity of uveitis and the presence of systemic findings. The history assumes greater importance than in any other ophthalmic entity. The minimal work-up for uveitis of unknown etiology requires an extensive and careful review of systems, a syphilis serology, and a chest X-ray.[13]

Most practitioners use a stepladder approach to the treatment of uveitis. The first step is treatment with corticosteroids for all patients with noninfectious uveitis (topical, especially for anterior uveitis, local peribulbar injection, intravitreal injection, or systemic administration). A surgically implantable intravitreal device to release fluocinolone continuously for approximately 2.5 years is an additional option that is limited by cost and complications, which can include cataract, glaucoma, and scleral thinning.[14] New delivery approaches include injectable corticosteroids complexed with slowly dissolving polymers to prolong the beneficial effects; iontophoresis to deliver medication across the sclera and into the vitreous humor; and topical light chain antibodies or small molecules which seem to have a much broader biodistribution within the eye compared to topical prednisolone. Systemic immunosuppressive therapy should be used in cases of inadequate benefit from corticosteroids or unacceptable steroid side effects. Immunosuppression is usually reserved for bilateral forms of uveitis with a severity sufficient to alter activities of daily living, and is frequently chosen for eye involvement with Behçet's disease. Immunosuppression may be contraindicated by active infection in the eye or elsewhere.

The role for biologic therapy to treat uveitis is being actively assessed by randomized controlled trials. In an open label trial, infliximab has proven effective but had frequent severe toxicities for this indication. The authors frequently prescribe infliximab to treat the uveitis associated with Behçet's disease (see below). Biologic therapy for uveitis might also have a strong rationale if the underlying disease such as Crohn's disease or psoriatic arthritis is responsive to the biologic.

Overview of the most common uveitis diagnoses

Ankylosing spondylitis (AS) is the most common systemic diagnosis associated with uveitis in Western nations. A genetic predisposition with the HLA-B27 marker is found in 88–96% of patients with AS. About 30% of AS patients develop anterior uveitis transiently during their lifetime; conversely 30% of anterior uveitis patients have AS. Approximately 50% of patients with a sudden onset anterior uveitis are HLA-B27 positive. In some studies, 80–90% of individuals with HLA B27-associated iritis have a systemic disease, either ankylosing spondylitis or reactive arthritis. Ankylosing spondylitis should be considered in any patient with sudden onset, primarily anterior, unilateral uveitis associated with redness and pain. Recurrent disease, fibrin in the anterior chamber, posterior synechiae, relatively brief inflammation that resolves in less than 2 months, and lowered intraocular pressure are additional hallmarks that sometimes help to distinguish HLA-B27-associated iritis from other categories of intraocular inflammation.[15] Cells can be seen in the anterior chamber by slit lamp examination. Inflammation is sometimes so severe that a hypopyon (Fig. 73.8) develops. The posterior segment of the eye is not commonly involved in this disease except for the development of a vision-reducing cystoid macular edema (see Figs 73.2, 73.4), which is a more frequent complication than with other forms of anterior uveitis. The

disease usually shows a good response to topical corticosteroids. In frequently recurrent cases, therapy with sulfasalazine or TNF inhibitors has been shown to be effective in reducing the frequency and severity of the attacks.

Ocular manifestations of inflammatory bowel disease (IBD) (Crohn's disease and ulcerative colitis; Chapter 74) include iritis, episcleritis, and scleritis (1–9% of all cases). Twenty percent of patients with IBD may have sacroiliitis; 60% of these are HLA-B27 positive. The anterior uveitis in patients with IBD is often similar to that seen with the HLA-B27 spectrum of joint diseases (ankylosing spondylitis): sudden in onset, unilateral, and self-limited. But Crohn's disease is a granulomatous process: like sarcoidosis, it may result in intraocular inflammation that is insidious in onset, bilateral, posterior to the lens, chronic, or associated with a retinal vasculitis.[16]

Crohn's disease is a complex genetic disease, meaning that multiple genes undoubtedly contribute to susceptibility to this inflammation. One of the best characterized of these genes is NOD-2, which is also known as CARD-15. This gene functions as an intracellular Toll-like receptor that recognizes muramyl dipeptide from both Gram-negative and -positive bacteria. The NOD-2 gene has homology to genes implicated in autoinflammatory diseases such as familial cold urticaria. A mutation in the portion of the NOD-2 gene known as the nucleotide-binding domain results in a rare autosomal dominant form of uveitis known as Blau syndrome.

One to 2% of the population has psoriasis; roughly 10% of psoriasis patients have arthritis;[17] and 7% of patients with psoriasis and arthritis have uveitis. The diagnosis is made clinically with the typical findings of cutaneous changes (erythematous, hyperkeratotic rash) and joint disease. Patients with sacroiliac disease and psoriatic arthritis are especially likely to develop uveitis.

Ocular disease is the initial manifestation of sarcoidosis (Chapter 72) in 20% of patients. The systemic illness begins as ocular inflammation almost as often as it initially presents as pulmonary disease. Between 25 and 50% of patients with systemic sarcoidosis exhibit ocular inflammatory disease during the course of the illness. In most case series sarcoidosis accounts for 3–10% of all patients with uveitis, and it therefore follows spondyloarthropathy as the second most common systemic illness associated with uveitis in North America and Europe. The diagnosis of sarcoidosis should always be considered in any patient presenting with a uveitis of unknown etiology. Sarcoidosis has a strong ethnic association: it occurs in the USA 10 times more frequently among African Americans than among whites. Because it can affect almost every part of the eye, symptoms of ocular sarcoidosis vary widely depending on the distribution of pathology. Most commonly, patients will have a bilateral chronic granulomatous iridocyclitis.[18] The disease often regresses clinically, with two-thirds of patients symptom-free after 10 years. Typical findings include "mutton-fat" keratic precipitates of the cornea (Fig. 73.7), Koeppe and Busacca iris nodules, posterior synechiae (Fig. 73.5), and white clumps of cells ("snowballs") in the inferior anterior vitreous. A chest X-ray (or CT scan of the chest [19]) should be included in every basic workup of patients with uveitis of unknown cause. The diagnosis is most reliably established by a biopsy that demonstrates the noncaseating granuloma in the absence of an infection or beryllium exposure. Possible biopsy sites include lymph nodes, lung, skin, oral mucosa, and conjunctiva. Serological abnormalities are not sufficiently unique to establish a diagnosis. They include elevated serum angiotensin-converting enzyme and lysozyme levels. In general, the combination of uveitis and symmetrical hilar adenopathy is specific for sarcoidosis. It is therefore not necessary to obtain tissue confirmation when this presentation

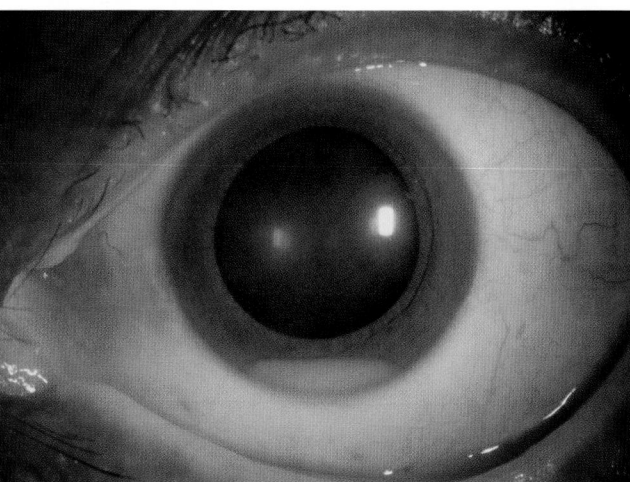

Fig. 73.8 Hypopyon. Intense inflammation has resulted in a creamy exudate (pus), seen as whitening over the inferior portion of the anterior chamber. In this example, hypopyon was secondary to rifabutin, not ankylosing spondylitis.

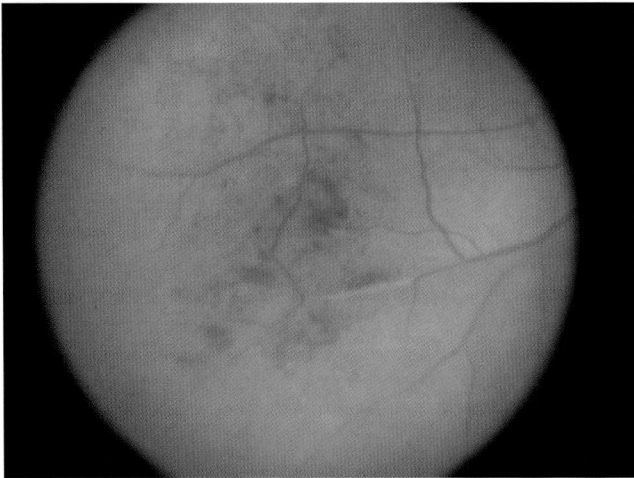

Fig. 73.9 Fundus photograph showing retinal vasculitis. The scattered hemorrhages are secondary to the vasculitis. The patient has Behçet's syndrome.

occurs. Topical, periocular, and systemic corticosteroids are the mainstay of therapy.

Behçet's syndrome is a generalized occlusive vasculitis of unknown cause (Chapter 58). It accounts for about 2.5% of patients at a North American referral uveitis clinic, and has a strong ethnic relationship. It is most common in Japan (20% of uveitis patients) and prevalent in Middle Eastern countries along the Silk Road.

The classic complex includes aphthous stomatitis, genital ulceration and iritis, sometimes with hypopyon (30% of patients), and skin lesions. The posterior segment is more commonly involved than the anterior and includes an occlusive retinal vasculitis (Fig. 73.9).[20] Extraocular manifestations most commonly include arthritis, erythema nodosum, diarrhea (mimicking inflammatory bowel disease), and sterile meningitis. There is a strong tendency for the symptoms to remit and exacerbate spontaneously. HLA-B5 or its subset, B51, is more commonly found among Behçet patients. Behçet's syndrome may lead to blindness if ischemic optic neuropathy and retinopathy are not adequately treated. Patients are often inadequately managed by corticosteroids alone: a regimen with immunosuppressive drugs (cyclosporine A or azathioprine) has been proved useful. Some investigators advocate the use of α-interferon.[21] Infliximab has demonstrated dramatic benefit in studies reported from Europe and Japan.[22] It is now approved for this indication in Japan.

Although retrobulbar optic neuritis is the ocular inflammation most clearly associated with multiple sclerosis, both intermediate uveitis (pars planitis) and a bilateral granulomatous anterior uveitis are well described in association with this demyelinating central nervous system disease (Chapter 65).[23] The granulomatous inflammation is typically bilateral and may indicate a worse prognosis for the neurologic disease. The HLA-DR2 antigen, strongly associated with MS, is also associated with uveitis.

Patients with juvenile idiopathic arthritis (JIA; Chapter 53) need special consideration as the disease often does not present with a "red eye": The uveitis is often a smoldering, silent inflammation with a quiet, white eye. These young patients need to be screened on a routine basis to avoid structural damage to the eye from even low-grade inflammation with resulting blindness. In 20% of all JIA cases the joint involvement is pauciarticular (five or fewer joints affected). Uveitis occurs far more commonly in this pauciarticular subset, and these patients require ophthalmic screening every 3–4 months. Girls are affected four times more

often than boys, although boys may be more likely to develop complications.[24] Eighty percent of uveitis cases are positive for anti-nuclear antibodies (ANA) and negative for rheumatoid factor. The onset of ocular disease is usually within 5 years of arthritis. Biomicroscopically, bilateral fine keratic precipitates, band keratopathy (Fig. 73.6), flare and cells in the anterior chamber, posterior synechiae, glaucoma, and cataract formation can be found. Topical and periocular corticosteroid treatment with a slow taper is the mainstay of therapy. Systemic therapy with methotrexate can be used as a substitute for corticosteroids and may be indicated to reduce the morbidity of chronic corticosteroid use. The TNF inhibitor such as adalimumab is useful in selected patients.[25] Cataract surgery is a special challenge and may require intense perioperative immunosuppression.

> ● **KEY CONCEPT**
>
> Immune-mediated diseases can affect virtually any portion of the eye. Uveitis, scleritis, keratoconjunctivitis sicca, conjunctivitis, optic neuritis, keratitis, and orbital inflammation are examples of eye diseases that are frequently immune mediated.

> ● **CLINICAL PEARL**
>
> The immune privilege of the eye does not prevent immune-mediated eye disease.

Scleritis

Description/natural history

Scleritis is a relatively uncommon inflammation that affects the sclera, the white tunic that encases the posterior eye. Scleritis is usually presumed to represent a vasculitis of scleral vessels. At least one-third of patients with scleritis will have clinical evidence for a systemic vasculitis elsewhere in the body.[26] The most common systemic diseases are Wegener's granulomatois (often in a limited form) or rheumatoid arthritis (RA; Chapter 52). The subset of patients with RA who develop scleritis are especially likely to develop rheumatoid nodules, high-titer rheumatoid factor, and pleuropericarditis as well as small vessel vasculitis of the lower extremities. Other systemic diseases commonly associated with scleritis are listed in Table 73.4. The epidemiology of scleritis has not been adequately reported. However, rheumatoid arthritis accounts for about one-third of all cases of scleritis. Because only 1% of patients with rheumatoid arthritis develop scleritis and about 1% of the population has

Table 73.4 Systemic immune-mediated diseases associated with scleritis

Rheumatoid arthritis
Wegener's granulomatosis
Inflammatory bowel disease
Polyarteritis nodosa
Temporal arteritis/giant cell arteritis
Systemic lupus erythematosus
Ankylosing spondylitis
Relapsing polychondritis

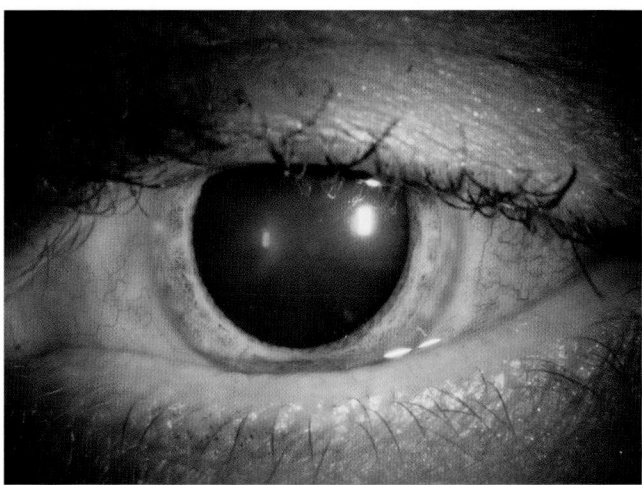

Fig. 73.10 Diffuse anterior scleritis. The red patch of vessels temporally is secondary to scleritis.

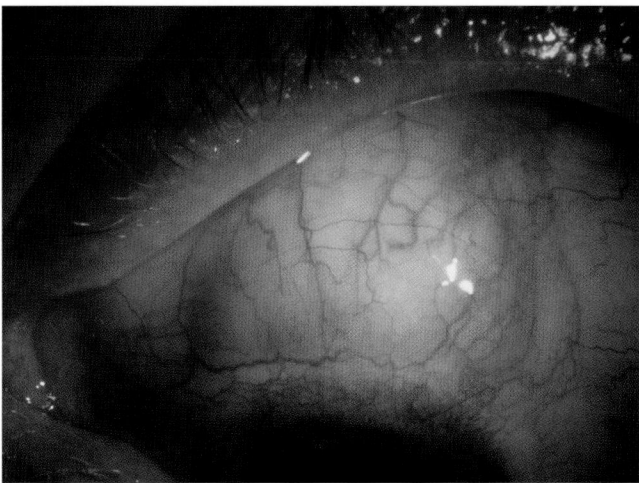

Fig. 73.11 Scleromalacia perforans. Blue sclera is visible secondary to inflammation, resembling a rheumatoid nodule in the eye.

RA, one can estimate that the prevalence of scleritis is $0.01 \times 0.01 \times 3$, or 3/10 000.

Scleritis is frequently divided into five subsets based on the clinical presentation: diffuse anterior (Fig. 73.10); nodular anterior; necrotizing; scleromalacia perforans (Fig. 73.11); and posterior.[27] Scleromalacia perforans is also known as necrotizing without inflammation. The clinical presentation will vary according to the type, but scleritis is usually a very painful and persistent condition. Even with treatment, median duration reaches 5 years.

Genetic/environmental factors

Genetic factors affecting scleritis have not been adequately studied. Genes that affect the associated systemic diseases, such as RA, Wegener's granulomatosis, and polyarteritis, presumably also influence susceptibility to scleritis. Environmental triggers for scleritis have not been defined, except that some cases of scleritis can be a manifestation of infection, such as herpes zoster ophthalmicus, syphilis, or Lyme disease, as well as other bacterial and fungal infections.

Immunology/pathology

Biopsy of the sclera entails some risk. Accordingly, many of the published histological observations are based on end-stage or extremely severe disease. In one pathology study of 55 examples of necrotizing scleritis the histology was divided into four types: zonal necrotizing granulomatous; nonzonal diffuse; necrotizing with microabscess; and sarcoidal granulomatous.[28] Eighty-five percent of patients with zonal necrotizing granulomatous pathology had a systemic disease, usually rheumatoid arthritis. The pathology associated with RA was not distinct from other systemic diseases such as Wegener's granulomatosis. None of 19 patients with nonzonal diffuse scleral inflammation had a systemic disease. Just over half of the patients with microabscesses had an identifiable infection as the cause of scleritis. Only one patient had "sarcoidal granulomatous inflammation," and that patient had sarcoidosis.

Prevention/management

Topical medications are only slightly beneficial for most patients with scleritis. Topical nonsteroidal anti-inflammatory drugs (NSAIDs), such as ketorolac, have not been proved efficacious. A topical corticosteroid can sometimes help in symptomatic control but also has risk, especially the promotion of cataract formation and elevation of intraocular pressure. The role for topical cyclosporine has not been adequately evaluated, but the authors' clinical experience has not been favorable.

Although most forms of scleritis represent a vasculitis, oral NSAIDs can be immensely beneficial. Although not all patients derive adequate control from NSAIDs, a subset will benefit sufficiently such that no other medication is required. We speculate that the subset responsive to an NSAID might have a pathogenesis other than vasculitis, but this hypothesis is unproven. Indomethacin has most frequently been reported to be effective, but other NSAIDs have simply not been tested in a sufficiently large sample population. Selective cyclooxygenase-2 inhibitors may control scleritis, but use must be weighed against relatively higher cost and risk of cardiovascular toxicity.

Many patients with scleritis will not benefit adequately from a nonsteroidal agent and will require immunosuppression. In general, for those with an associated systemic disease the control of that disease will lead to control of the scleritis. For those without a systemic illness, oral corticosteroids are an accepted initial approach to treatment. For example, therapy might begin with a dose of prednisone of 1 mg/kg bodyweight per day. The use of calcium and vitamin D, and other measures to preserve bone mineral density, should be considered for any patient who will be receiving corticosteroid on a chronic basis. If prednisone is not adequate for disease control, or if the medication is toxic, poorly tolerated, and cannot be safely tapered to a modest dosage, it is reasonable to add a steroid-sparing medication such as methotrexate, azathioprine, cyclosporine, mycophenolate, or even an alkylating agent such as cyclophosphamide. There is considerable interest in the use of biologic agents as corticosteroid-sparing agents in patients with scleritis. Multiple recently published case reports and small case series describe the successful use of drugs, including TNF blockers and rituximab, in some patients with resistant disease.[29]

Locally injected, subconjunctival or periocular, corticosteroids may be very effective for uveitis, but they are contraindicated for patients with necrotizing scleritis. The corticosteroid probably promotes reduced wound healing and thus enhances the likelihood that the necrotic sclera might perforate as a result of the inflammation. On the other hand, for non-necrotizing anterior scleral inflammation, there is accumulating evidence that subconjunctivally injected corticosteroid is safe and may be highly effective.[30] Scleral inflammation limited to the posterior sclera can probably be safely treated with a periocular corticosteroid injection.

In choosing to treat with oral corticosteroid or an immunosuppressive, the clinician will, of course, weigh the risk/benefit ratio. The rationale for aggressive therapy is much stronger if the disease is bilateral and is affecting activities of daily living, because of either pain or a reduction in visual acuity.

> ## CLINICAL PEARL
>
> Uveitis and scleritis are frequently associated with a systemic illness. These illnesses can usually be diagnosed by history without resorting to extensive laboratory testing.

Evaluation/differential diagnosis

Patients with scleritis generally have characteristic findings that allow an accurate diagnosis; scleritis can usually be readily distinguished from other causes of a red, painful eye. The most difficult distinction is between scleritis and episcleritis. The episclera overlies the sclera. In general patients with episcleritis do not experience pain, do not have an associated systemic disease, do not have complications such as iritis or glaucoma, and have an excellent prognosis, with complete resolution usually within weeks. The differences between scleritis and episcleritis are highlighted in Table 73.5.

The scleritis associated with a systemic vasculitis is often more severe than scleritis not associated with a systemic illness.[31] The scleritis associated with Wegener's granulomatosis may be particularly destructive and refractory to therapy. Scleritis in association with rheumatoid arthritis is often a poor prognostic sign for the joint disease. For example, prior to the routine use of disease-modifying anti-rheumatic drugs, the small subset of patients with scleritis in association with rheumatoid arthritis had a shortened life expectancy compared to other patients with RA and no evidence for scleritis.

Posterior scleritis can be an extremely difficult disease to diagnose. If the anterior sclera is uninvolved, no redness is present. Pain with posterior scleritis is much more variable. The examination may show elevation of the adjacent retina and choroid. The diagnosis can be confirmed with an ultrasound examination or, less commonly, with a CT scan of the orbit demonstrating thickening of the sclera. Posterior scleritis is treated similarly to anterior scleritis.

Pitfalls/controversy

Some experts believe that scleritis is often a *forme fruste* of Wegener's granulomatosis. It clearly occurs in association with Wegener's granulomatosis, and patients with scleritis, a positive ANCA test, and no other evidence for Wegener's granulomatosis have been well described.[32]

With the exception of the ANCA, laboratory studies are generally selected according to the history and general physical examination. For example, although rheumatoid arthritis is associated with scleritis, the patients almost always have long-standing severe RA. A rheumatoid factor and/or anti-cyclic citrullinated peptide antibody titer would not be appropriate tests if no joint disease were present clinically. The findings from one recent study, however, do support screening patients with scleritis with serologic tests to detect RA.[33] Similarly, systemic lupus can be associated with scleritis, but one would not diagnose lupus on the basis of a positive ANA, scleritis, and the absence of other findings to suggest lupus. An erythrocyte sedimentation rate can sometimes be helpful in reassuring that a systemic process is not present. Other laboratory tests are largely dictated by the medication that is chosen to treat the scleritis, and how that medication is monitored.

Keratitis

The cornea is the anteriorly situated window to the eye. Normally it should be clear. It can become opacified due to trauma, exposure to toxins, infection, dryness, calcium deposition, or genetic diseases such as corneal dystrophies. The three main immune-mediated diseases that affect the cornea are corneal melt, Mooren's ulcer, and Cogan's syndrome.

Corneal melt is also known as marginal keratolysis (Fig. 73.12). The majority of patients have an associated systemic form of vasculitis and usually scleritis. The medical therapy is basically the same as that described for scleritis, with emphasis on controlling the underlying systemic illness and the use of immunosuppression. Corneal melt often leads to perforation of the eye. This is usually treated surgically with tissue adhesives, conjunctival flaps, or corneal transplantation, in addition to aggressive systemic immunosuppression. Corneal melt is fortunately a very rare disease. A melt must also be distinguished from some other causes of corneal thinning, such as Terrien's marginal

Table 73.5 Contrasting features of scleritis and episcleritis

	Scleritis	**Episcleritis**
Pain	Prominent	Minimal
Duration	Years	Days to months
Association with systemic disease	Frequent	Uncommon
Vessels blanch with topical vasoconstrictor	No	Yes
Associated ocular complications including visual loss	Sometimes present	Rarely present
Vessel color	Violaceous	Light pink

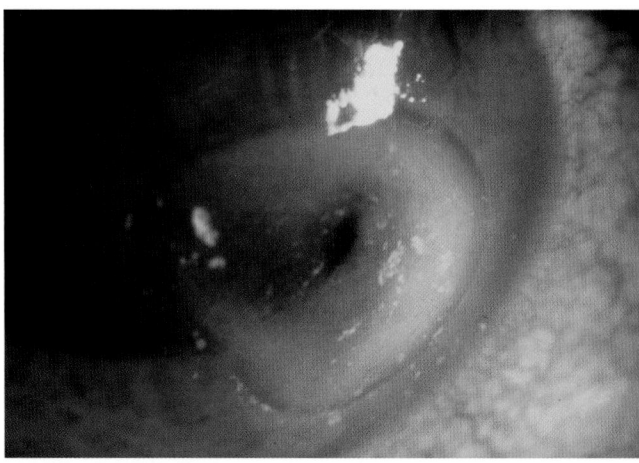

Fig. 73.12 Corneal melt. A pie-shaped wedge of the cornea is thinned. The eye is red secondary to an associated scleritis.

degeneration or a senile marginal furrow, both of which are generally more benign and rarely lead to perforation.

Mooren's ulcer is clinically very similar to a melt, except that there is no accompanying scleritis and no evidence for a systemic illness. The superior cornea is especially likely to be involved. Mooren's ulcer is too rare for therapeutic options to be studied with randomized clinical trials. It may respond to oral immunosuppression, which is warranted if the severity threatens visual acuity because of impending perforation of the eye. One small study, not confirmed by subsequent investigations, suggested that Mooren's ulcer is frequently associated with evidence of previous infection with hepatitis C. Some patients with Mooren's ulcer have an autoantibody to calgranulin C. This antigen is expressed in cornea, in neutrophils, and by filarial nematodes.

The cornea is divided into five layers: the epithelium facing the atmosphere, Bowman's membrane, the stroma, Descemet's membrane, and the endothelium abutting the aqueous humor. Opacification of the stroma is known as interstitial keratitis. Congenital syphilis and other infections such as herpes simplex are important causes of this. Cogan's syndrome is defined as an autoimmune disease of the eighth nerve combined with interstitial keratitis, presumably also on an autoimmune basis.[34] Some ophthalmologists also recognize autoimmune eighth-nerve disease associated with other forms of ocular inflammation, such as uveitis, as examples of Cogan's disease. The pathogenesis of Cogan's syndrome is presumed to be a vasculitis, and many patients will have evidence for vasculitis elsewhere in the body. The treatment usually requires aggressive use of systemic immunosuppressive medications.

Corneal transplantation and transplant rejection

Corneal transplantation involves the repair of a diseased cornea with healthy cadaver tissue. Since the 1970s, advances in microsurgical techniques and eye banking procedures have led to widespread acceptance of this procedure. Currently corneal transplantation is performed more than 40 000 times annually in the USA alone. The usual indication for a corneal graft is poor vision, although the operation may also be undertaken to relieve ocular pain. Keratoconus, a condition in which myopic astigmatism develops as the cornea becomes progressively more conical in shape, corneal edema following intraocular surgery, and a failed previous corneal graft are the commonest medical conditions leading to corneal transplantation.[35]

Although the eye is an immune privileged site, and corneal transplants enjoy a 91% 1-year survival as shown by Kaplan–Meier survival analyses, only 62% of grafts are functional at 10 years.[30] The commonest cause of transplant failure is immunologic rejection.[35] Corneal allograft rejection rarely occurs within 2 weeks, and may occur as late as 20 years following surgery. Animal studies using monoclonal antibodies directed against different T-cell subsets indicate that CD4 T cells play a critical role in the rejection response. However, the exact mechanisms responsible for this process continue to be studied.

Early recognition of a rejection episode is the most important factor in achieving survival of the corneal transplant. In its most florid form, the anterior eye is obviously inflamed, with intense conjunctival injection, a cellular anterior chamber reaction and a Khodadoust line. This line, which is visible with the slit-lamp biomicroscope, is a classic sign of corneal graft rejection. It appears as a linear formation of inflammatory precipitates stretching across the corneal endothelium and represents a wave of lymphocytes marching across the cornea and destroying the endothelium in their path.[36] As endothelial pump function is lost, the cornea becomes waterlogged and opaque. At an early stage of rejection the patient may be asymptomatic, but later, ocular redness, photophobia, halos and blurred vision are frequent complaints.

An intensive and extended course of topical corticosteroids is the mainstay of treatment for a rejecting corneal graft, and in severe cases intravenous and/or oral corticosteroids may also be administered. Patients considered to be at high risk of transplant rejection, such as those with corneal neovascularization or a history of other anterior segment inflammation, are often given perioperative systemic immunosuppression. The ideal prophylactic regimen has not been defined, although various combinations of prednisone, cyclosporine and azathioprine may be used. Despite the critical influence of donor–recipient histocompatibility matching for solid organ transplant survival, the chance of corneal graft survival is not significantly improved by HLA matching.

Cancer-associated retinopathy

Cancer-associated retinopathy (CAR) is a rare paraneoplastic syndrome that is most commonly induced by small cell carcinoma of the lung.[37] In addition, the disease has been documented in association with various tumors of the female reproductive tract, carcinoma of the breast and neuroendocrine bronchial carcinoma. For 50% of patients, CAR is the presenting feature of their malignancy. Interestingly, there are now reports of retinopathy mimicking CAR, but occurring in an apparently healthy individual. Melanoma-associated retinopathy is a related syndrome, occurring in patients with metastatic cutaneous melanoma.

Histopathological examinations of postmortem specimens taken from patients with CAR consistently demonstrate loss of inner and outer segments of the retinal photoreceptors. This destruction was initially attributed to the release of a hormone-like substance by the malignant cells, but evidence has now accumulated in support of an autoimmune etiology. Affected individuals produce antibodies against one or more retinal photoreceptor antigens.[38] These antibodies induce experimental CAR when injected into laboratory animals. Although over 15 antigens have been described in relation to CAR, the commonest is the so-called CAR antigen.[38] This 23-kDa protein has been identified as recoverin, a photoreceptor protein that participates in visual adaptation. Experimental work supports the hypothesis that a single mutational event simultaneously activates the recoverin gene and eliminates functional p53, a tumor suppressor protein.[39] Consequently, there is development of a tumor that encodes for CAR antigen and stimulates formation of anti-recoverin antibody. Anti-recoverin antibodies are capable of inducing photoreceptor apoptosis, leading to the characteristic loss of both rods and cones.

Cancer-associated retinopathy generally occurs after the age of 60. Patients usually complain of decreased vision, although other symptoms may include transient visual obscurations, various positive visual phenomena, night blindness, scotomata, glare and photosensitivity. Although visual acuity may be dramatically reduced, other clinical signs are often subtle. Color vision can be impaired. An afferent pupillary defect can be present if the retinopathy is asymmetric. There may be mild iridocyclitis and/or vitritis, narrowing of retinal arterioles, mottling of retinal pigment epithelium and optic disc pallor. Visual field abnormalities occur, the most common being several midperipheral scotomata that later join up as a ring scotoma or central defect. Electroretinography shows either reduced or completely flattened amplitudes. The disease must be differentiated from optic neuritis which, unlike CAR, typically occurs in younger persons, some of whom suffer from multiple sclerosis, and is painful. In contrast to CAR, optic neuritis typically has an abrupt onset. In patients with malignancy, direct tumor spread and the effects of drugs, including chemotherapy agents, must be excluded before CAR is diagnosed.

The natural history of CAR is one of progressive visual loss, although this occurs over a variable period. Treatment directed towards curing or palliating the malignancy does not appear to prevent this loss. Corticosteroid and other immunosuppressive drugs have been successfully used to treat the ocular disease, however.[40] It is suggested that monitoring serum antibody levels can be used to guide therapy, although, in some cases, advanced photoreceptor damage may be irreversible despite therapy.

Immunologic etiological factors in "nonimmunologic" ocular disease

The eye contains many unique proteins that are sequestered from the immune system in early development, and which, if released systemically during adulthood, could act as autoantigens. Autoantibodies directed against certain ocular proteins have been detected in the serum of patients with a variety of ocular diseases traditionally regarded as nonimmunologic. Examples of such conditions include cataract, glaucoma, age-related macular degeneration (AMD), and retinal degenerative diseases such as retinitis pigmentosa (RP). The unanswered question is whether these antibodies contribute to the pathogenesis of the disease or merely coexist as an epiphenomenon.

Cataract is an opacification of the crystalline lens of the eye. It is the most frequent cause of blindness worldwide, most commonly occurring as an age-related phenomenon. The prevalence of cataract is approximately 70% in those over 75 years of age. The pathogenesis is poorly understood, and many varied mechanisms, including autoimmunity, have been hypothesized. Autoantibodies to sequestered lens proteins termed crystallins are present in some normal individuals, but occur significantly more frequently in patients with cataract. Immune complexes have been demonstrated in human cataractous lenses. Immunization of rabbits with human lens protein can induce cataract formation, which is suppressed by systemic corticosteroid therapy. Human sera containing autoantibodies against lens proteins are cytotoxic for lens epithelial cells in culture.[41] On the other hand, it has not been possible to demonstrate T-cell-mediated immune responses to lens proteins experimentally, suggesting that a process of active tolerance might prevent these autoantigens from inducing significant inflammation.

In glaucoma, a relative elevation of intraocular pressure is associated with optic nerve damage and visual field loss. More than 3 million people in the world are irreversibly blind owing to this disease, the basic mechanisms of which continue to puzzle clinicians and scientists despite very extensive research. There is recent evidence that autoimmunity may play a role in glaucoma. Increased titers of antibodies directed against retinal, optic nerve and optic nerve head antigens, have been measured in patients with primary angle-closure glaucoma, as well as normal-tension glaucoma, in which there is not apparent elevation of intraocular pressure above population normal levels.[42] It is postulated that these antibodies may contribute to the neurodegeneration that

is characteristic of glaucoma, or might represent a stress response of retinal neurons.

Age-related macular degeneration is the leading cause of irreversible visual loss for elderly persons in Western nations. A spectrum of pathologies may occur at the macula, ranging from relatively benign focal hypo- and hyperpigmentation of the retinal pigment epithelium to sinister subretinal neovascularizations, which may leak serous fluid and blood. The pathogenic stimulus for these aging changes is unknown. Genetic polymorphism of the complement regulatory protein, complement factor H, influences the susceptibility to AMD, suggesting that this disease is related to chronic inflammation.[43] Subretinal scar tissue removed from patients with advanced, neovascular disease may contain immunoglobulins and complement components. The histopathology of AMD includes inflammatory cells, including lymphocyte subsets, and local cell populations may express class II MHC antigens. Mouse models of retinal changes that resemble macular degeneration can be induced by the deletion of chemokines or chemokine receptors. Macular drusen, seen early in the course of AMD, may also contain immunoglobulin.

Retinitis pigmentosa is a hereditary pigmentary degeneration of the retina. Just under half of patients have no family history. Various anti-retinal antibodies have been detected in approximately half of patients with this disease, including antibodies directed against the enzymes carbonic anhydrase II and enolase. Interestingly, there is a significant association between the occurrence of cystoid edema at the macula, a dreaded vision-threatening complication of RP, and the presence of the circulating anti-retinal antibodies. The complication has been reported in 90% of affected individuals with antibodies, compared to only 13% of patients who are antibody negative.[44]

● ON THE HORIZON

Innovative delivery techniques using polymers and local injection may ultimately markedly reduce the need for systemic immunosuppression to treat uveitis.

References

1. Stuart PM, Griffith TS, Usui N, et al. CD95 ligand (FasL)-induced apoptosis is necessary for corneal allograft survival. J Clin Invest 1997;99:396–402.
2. Wang S, Boonman ZF, Li HC, et al. Role of TRAIL and IFN-gamma in CD4+ cell-dependent tumor rejection in the anterior chamber of the eye. J Immunol 2003;171:2789–96.
3. Pasquale LR, Dorman-Pease ME, Lutty GA, et al. Immunolocalization of TGF-beta1, TGF-beta2, and TGF-beta3 in the anterior segment of the human eye. Invest Ophthalmol Vis Sci 1993;34:23–30.
4. Cousins SW, McCabe MM, Danielpour D, Streilein JW. Identification of transforming growth factor-beta as an immunosuppressive factor in aqueous humor. Invest Ophthalmol Vis Sci 1991;32:2201–11.
5. Kennedy MC, Rosenbaum JT, Brown J, et al. Novel production of interleukin-1 receptor antagonist peptides in normal human cornea. J Clin Invest 1995;95:82–8.
6. Poli V, Balena R, Fattori E, et al. Interleukin-6 deficient mice are protected from bone loss caused by estrogen depletion. EMBO J 1994;13:1189–96.
7. Ferguson TA. The molecular basis of anterior associated immune deviation (ACAID). Ocul Immunol Inflamm 1997;5:213–5.
8. D'Orazio TJ, Niederkorn JY. A novel role for TGF-beta and IL-10 in the induction of immune privilege. J Immunol 1998;160:2089–98.
9. Dullforce PA, Garman KL, Seitz GW, et al. APCs in the anterior uveal tract do not migrate to draining lymph nodes. J Immunol 2004;172:6701–8.
10. Luger D, Silver PB, Tang J, et al. Either a Th17 or a Th1 effector response can drive autoimmunity: conditions of disease induction affect dominant effector category. J Exp Med 2008;205:799–810.
11. Vadot E, Barth E, Billet P. Epidemiology of uveitis-preliminary results of a prospective study in Savoy. In: Saari KM, editor. Uveitis Update. Amsterdam: Excerpta Medica; 1984. p. 13–6.
12. Gritz DC, Wong IG. Incidence and prevalence of uveitis in Northern California; the Northern California Epidemiology of Uveitis Study. Ophthalmology 2004;111:491–500.
13. Rosenbaum JT. An algorithm for the systemic evaluation of patients with uveitis: guidelines for the consultant. Semin Arthritis Rheum 1990;19:248–57.
14. Lim LL, Smith JR, Rosenbaum JT. Retisert (Bausch & Lomb/Control Delivery Systems). Curr Opin Investig Drugs 2005;6:1159–67.

15. Rosenbaum JT. Acute anterior uveitis and spondyloarthropathies. Rheum Dis Clin North Am 1992;18:143–51.
16. Lyons JL, Rosenbaum JT. Uveitis associated with inflammatory bowel disease compared with uveitis associated with spondyloarthropathy. Arch Ophthalmol 1997;115:61–4.
17. Ibrahim G, Waxman R, Helliwell PS. The prevalence of psoriatic arthritis in people with psoriasis. Arthritis Rheum 2009;61:1373–8.
18. James DG. Ocular sarcoidosis. Ann N Y Acad Sci 1986;465:551–63.
19. Kosmorsky GS, Meisler DM, Rice TW, et al. Chest computed tomography and mediastinoscopy in the diagnosis of sarcoidosis-associated uveitis. Am J Ophthalmol 1998;126:132–4.
20. Michelson JB, Chisari FV. Behcet's disease. Surv Ophthalmol 1982;26:190–203.
21. Kotter I, Zierhut M, Eckstein AK, et al. Human recombinant interferon alfa-2a for the treatment of Behcet's disease with sight threatening posterior or panuveitis. Br J Ophthalmol 2003;87:423–31.
22. Van Staa TP, Leufkens HGM, Abenhaim L, et al. Use of oral corticosteroids and risk of fractures. J Bone Miner Res 2000;15:993–1000.
23. Lim JI, Tessler HH, Goodwin JA. Anterior granulomatous uveitis in patients with multiple sclerosis. Ophthalmology 1991;98:142–5.
24. Edelsten C, Lee V, Bentley CR, et al. An evaluation of baseline risk factors predicting severity in juvenile idiopathic arthritis associated uveitis and other chronic anterior uveitis in early childnood. Br J Ophthalmol 2002;86:51–6.
25. Simonini G, Taddio A, Cattalini M, et al. Prevention of flare recurrences in childhood-refractory chronic uveitis: an open-label comparative study of adalimumab versus infliximab. Arthritis Care Res (Hoboken) 2011;63:612–8.
26. Raiji VR, Palestine AG, Parver DL. Scleritis and systemic disease association in a community-based referral practice. Am J Ophthalmol 2009;148:946–50.
27. Watson PG, Hayreh SS. Scleritis and episcleritis. Br J Ophthalmol 1976;60:163–91.
28. Riono WP, Hidayat AA, Rao NA. Scleritis: a clinicopathologic study of 55 cases. Ophthalmology 1999;106:1328–33.
29. Butler NJ, Lim LL, Giles TR, et al. Rituximab in the treatment of refactory scleritis and non-infectious orbital inflammation: 24 week outcomes from a phaseI/II prospective, randomized study. Invest Ophthalmol Vis Sci 2011. (electronic abstract).
30. Albini TA, Zamir E, Read RW, et al. Evaluation of subconjunctival triamcinolone for nonnecrotizing anterior scleritis. Ophthalmol 2005;112:1814–20.
31. Sainz de la Maza M, Foster CS, Jabbur NS. Scleritis associated with rheumatoid arthritis and with other systemic immune mediated diseases. Ophthalmology 1994;101:1281–6.
32. Soukiasian SH, Foster CS, Niles JL, Raizman MB. Diagnostic value of anti-neutrophil cytoplasmic antibodies in scleritis associated with Wegener's granulomatosis. Ophthalmology 1992;99:125–32.
33. Lin P, Bhullar SS, Tessler HH, Goldstein DA. Immunologic markers as potential predictors of systemic autoimmune disease in patients with idiopathic scleritis. Am J Ophthalmol 2008;145:463–71.
34. Cogan DG. Syndrome of nonsyphilitic interstitial keratitis and vestibuloauditory symptoms. Arch Ophthalmol 1945;33:144–9.
35. Williams KA, Muehlberg SM, Lewis RF, Coster DJ. Long-term outcome in corneal allotransplantation. Australian Corneal Graft Registry 1997;29:983.
36. Khodadoust AA, Silverstein AM. Transplantation and rejection of individual cell layers of the cornea. Invest Ophthalmol 1969;8:180–95.
37. Weleber RG, Watzke RC, Shults WT, et al. Clinical and electrophysiologic characterization of paraneoplastic and autoimmune retinopathies associates with antienolase antibodies. Am J Ophthalmol 2005;139:780–94.
38. Thirkill CE, Keltner JL, Tyler NK, Roth AM. Antibody reactions with retina and cancer-associated antigens in 10 patients with cancer-associated retinopathy. Arch Ophthalmol 1993;111:931–7.
39. McGinnis JF, Austin B, Klisak I, et al. Chromosomal assignment of the human gene for the cancer-associated retinopathy protein (recoverin) to chromosome 17p13.1. J Neurosci Res 1995;40:165–8.
40. Ferreyra HA, Jayasundera T, Khan NW, et al. Management of autoimmune retinopathies with immunosuppression. Arch Ophthalmol 2009;127:390–7.
41. Ibaraki N, Lin LR, Dang L, et al. Anti-beta-crystallin antibodies (mouse) or sera from humans with age-related cataract are cytotoxic for lens epithelial cells in culture. Exp Eye Res 1997;64:229–38.
42. Joachim SC, Pfeiffer N, Grus FH. Autoantibodies in patients with glaucoma: a comparison of IgG serum antibodies against retinal, optic nerve, and optic nerve head antigens. Graefes Arch Clin Exp Ophthalmol 2005;243:817–23.
43. Edwards AO, Ritter RI, Abel KJ, et al. Complement factor H polymorphism and age-related macular degeneration. Science 2005;308:421–4.
44. Heckenlively JR, Jordan BL, Aptsiauri N. Association of antiretinal antibodies and cystoid macular edema to patients with retinitis pigmentosa. Am J Ophthalmol 1999;127:565–73.

Peter J. Mannon

Immunologic diseases of the gastrointestinal tract

The gastrointestinal tract accommodates the largest mass of immune cells of any organ in the body. Moreover the gut is continuously exposed to dietary and microbial antigens and employs a number of strategies that contribute to the immune tolerance that characterizes the healthy state. These strategies include secreted IgA antibodies, epithelial-produced antimicrobial peptides, a physical barrier (the tight junction) between the lumen and the lamina propria, a specialized epithelial cell (the M cell) that directs particulate antigen processing, and a dendritic cell network that provides for induction of inflammatory and regulatory (suppressive) immune responses (Chapter 19). Despite these immune adaptations, the gastrointestinal tract is uniquely susceptible to chronic immune-mediated inflammation. These conditions arise from genetically determined antigen responsiveness and defects in the adaptive and innate immune systems that confer loss of regulation of the immune response and susceptibility to chronic infection. This chapter discusses some of the most frequent immunologic diseases of the gastrointestinal tract likely to be encountered in the clinic (Fig. 74.1).

Gastritis

Gastritis is a histologic description of stomach inflammation that can result from toxic exposures, infection, idiopathic inflammation, and autoimmunity. While symptoms tend to be very non-specific, the etiology and pathogenesis of gastritis can be extremely specific, especially for *Helicobacter pylori* infection, with important implications for treatment and natural history.

Atrophic gastritis/pernicious anemia

Among the most classic autoimmune diseases of the GI tract is atrophic gastritis resulting in loss of the oxyntic (acid-producing) mucosa of the gastric body and leading to pernicious anemia (PA). The autoimmune basis of this disease is linked to the detection of anti-intrinsic factor and anti-parietal cell antibodies and an association with other autoimmune diseases such as autoimmune thyroiditis, vitiligo and type I diabetes.[1] While the typical presentation is in elderly females (there is a 2:1 female preponderance of PA) of European ethnicity, 25% of cases occur in persons below age 50 and atrophic gastritis is also noted in African and Asian ethnicity.[2] The detection of both anti-intrinsic factor and anti-parietal cell serum antibodies has 73% sensitivity and 100% specificity for PA.[3]

The etiology of the atrophic gastritis lesion in PA, however, has been challenged as to its strict primary autoimmune origins. While it is clear that classical oxyntic mucosa-restricted inflammation and atrophy associated with anti-parietal cell antibodies, an intact antral mucosa, and no evidence of *H. pylori* infection does exist, other observations raise questions about a role for *H. pylori* infection. Among these observations are the frequency of antral inflammation (up to 92%) and mucosal atrophy (up to 30%) and histologic evidence of *H. pylori* infection (up to 30%) in case series of PA.[2] In addition, not only are autoantibodies to H^+-K^+-ATPase (the parietal cell membrane protein that secretes H ions into the gastric lumen) more frequent in *H. pylori*-associated chronic gastritis, but there are gastric mucosa CD4 T cells with cross-reactivity to H^+-K^+-ATPase and *H. pylori* antigens.[4,5] In this scenario, *H. pylori* infection could begin in the antrum and could advance to involve the gastric body with eventual atrophy and loss of oxyntic mucosa. The actual linkage of *H. pylori* infection to pernicious anemia has not been settled, but it is known that *H. pylori* chronic gastritis can involve the oxyntic mucosa. If there is a role for antigenic mimicry between *H. pylori* infection and PA pathophysiology, it is likely related to patients with susceptible HLA backgrounds.

The gastric oxyntic mucosa contains the acid-producing parietal cells that additionally make intrinsic factor, a vitamin B_{12}-binding protein critical for vitamin B_{12} absorption by the distal ileum. Therefore the loss of the oxyntic mucosa results in the two major pathophysiologic features of atrophic gastritis/PA, namely gastric achlorhydria and eventual vitamin B_{12} deficiency. The achlorhydric state has consequences for digestion (impaired non-heme iron absorption, protein degradation) as well as for innate immunity (loss of gastric barrier against ingested microbes). Lastly, because of the lack of acid production, patients with atrophic gastritis often have increased serum gastrin levels mimicking those seen in gastrinoma patients (the major difference being that atrophic gastritis patients have no acid production and gastrinoma patients have excessive acid production, a finding easily determined by measurement of gastric pH or basal acid output). The hypergastrinemia stimulates proliferation of enterochromaffin cells resulting in hyperplasia detected by biopsy. This ECL cell hyperplasia is considered a risk factor for gastric carcinoid development, but there are no firm guidelines for carcinoid screening in atrophic gastritis/PA at this time. Treatment approaches for atrophic gastritis/PA focus on B_{12} and iron replacement.

Helicobacter pylori gastritis

Helicobacter pylori infection of the gastric mucosa has been established as the leading cause of peptic ulcer disease as well as being a WHO-designated class I carcinogen for gastric carcinoma.[6] While the epidemiology is not precisely known, current data consistently shows that primary infection is largely acquired in childhood, that poor sanitation is associated with lower age and higher frequency

Fig. 74.1 Endoscopic biopsy specimen histology in health and disease. (A) Normal duodenal histology. (B) Celiac disease with blunted villus, increased plasma cell infiltrate, increased intraepithelial lymphocytes. (C) CD3 staining in celiac disease showing increased intraepithelial lymphocytes. (D) Crohn's colitis showing mucosa expanded with lymphoplasmacytic infiltrate and two granulomata. (E) Ulcerative colitis showing crypt dropout, cryptitis, crypt abscess, and lymphoplasmacytic infiltrate. (F) CVID enteropathy showing villous blunting, increased intraepithelial lymphocytes, and epithelial apoptosis. Photomicrographs courtesy of Dr. Leona Council, UAB Dept. of Pathology.

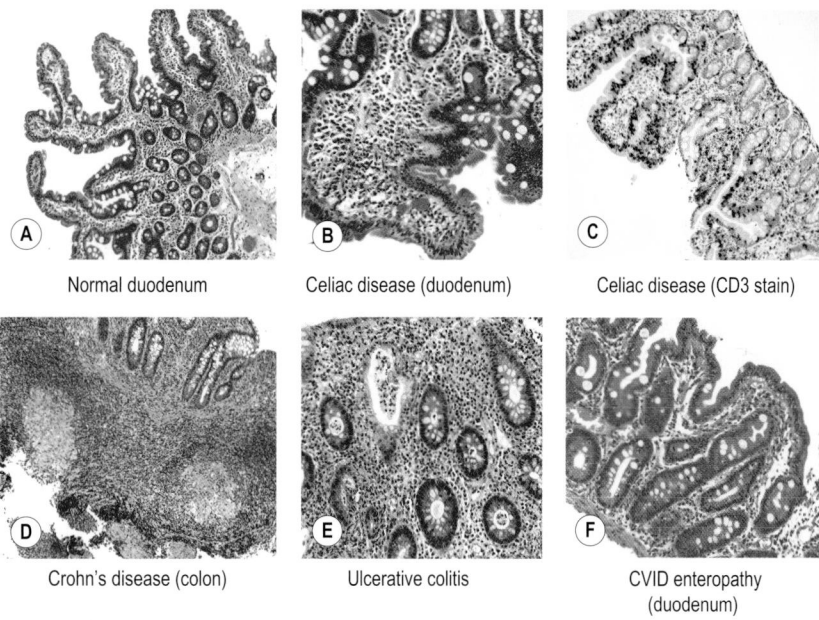

Normal duodenum   Celiac disease (duodenum)   Celiac disease (CD3 stain)

Crohn's disease (colon)   Ulcerative colitis   CVID enteropathy (duodenum)

of acquisition and that infection is likely via fecal/gastro-oral pathways instead of person-to-person.[7] There is an acute phase of infection characterized by abdominal pain and dyspepsia observed during deliberate infection in the research setting, but there is little actual clinical recognition of acute infection itself. The significance of *H. pylori* is its ability to establish chronic infection of the stomach that is thought to persist in most persons unless they are exposed to antibiotics. *H. pylori* is uniquely adapted to the acidic environment of the stomach by its ability to produce ammonia from urea, which can provide a buffered environment (ammonium ions using up the hydrogen protons). This mechanism allows prolonged asymptomatic colonization, and 15% of chronically infected persons can develop chronic gastric and duodenal ulcers and up to 1% can develop gastric adenocarcinoma. Several injurious mechanisms of ulcer development have been proposed including *H. pylori* infection lowering of the mucus pH adjacent to the gastric epithelium, increased permeability of the mucus to hydrogen ions, inhibition of bicarbonate secretion by the epithelium, expression of cytotoxins (vaculolating cytotoxin, VacA) and up-modulation of the mucosal inflammatory response by virulence factors such as CagA.[8,9] The recognition of *H. pylori* as a causative agent in the vast majority of recurrent peptic ulcers, and that its elimination could cure this disease, led to the awarding of the Nobel Prize in Medicine or Physiology to Marshall and Warren in 2005.

The development of peptic ulcer disease and adenocarcinoma as a result chronic *H. pylori* infection seems to segregate according to different anatomic distributions of inflammation. *H. pylori* chronic gastritis can occur either as predominantly affecting the antrum, in which case there is an association with duodenal ulcers, increased serum gastrin levels and excess acid production, and no gastric mucosal atrophy.[10] Alternatively, the chronic gastritis can also present as a pangastritis affecting the body and the antrum in a confluent or patchy manner, with the development of intestinal metaplasia, oxyntic mucosa atrophy, and decreased acid production; this type of *H. pylori* chronic gastritis is associated with gastric ulcerations and increased risk for adenocarcinoma and mucosa-associated lymphoid tissue (MALT) B-cell lymphoma. In this setting while eradication of *H. pylori* can reverse the mucosal atrophy and restore acid production, this occurs in a minority of patients and does not seem to reverse the intestinal metaplasia. Histologically, this form of atrophic gastritis is differentiated from

autoimmune atrophic gastritis by the presence of *H. pylori* organisms in the specimen (and concurrent involvement of the antrum, see above). Specific immunohistochemical methods for detecting *H. pylori* may be required when organisms are not seen on hematoxylin and eosin staining, when intestinal metaplasia is seen widely (*H. pylori* does not colonize intestinal metaplasia heavily), or when confirming eradication after treatment.[11] While there are many pieces of evidence to support immune mechanisms for persistence of *H. pylori* infection in the stomach (reviewed in Ernst et al.[7]), it is not clear how the inhibition of T-cell proliferation, promotion of T-cell apoptosis and interference with antigen presentation contribute to evasion from immune eradication. Nonetheless, preclinical and clinical trials are being pursued aiming to develop a vaccine to prevent chronic infection from occurring.

The indications for diagnosis and treatment of active *H. pylori* infection include patients with active gastroduodenal ulcer disease, gastric MALT lymphoma, and, in highly endemic areas, dyspepsia symptoms (upper abdominal pain, bloating, early satiety, and nausea).[12] Active disease can be diagnosed by endoscopic biopsy (angularis plus greater curve of body and antrum) that, though invasive, has high sensitivity and specificity (using immunohistochemical staining or rapid urease testing of biopsies) while allowing for additional diagnostic confirmation of extent and activity of inflammation as well as detection of peptic or malignant complications.[12] Non-invasive testing includes serum antibody detection (best used in highly endemic areas to predict active infection), urea breath testing (limited by expense), and fecal antigen testing (which has potential advantages in the setting of intestinal metaplasia and after antibiotic treatment). There are many effective eradication therapies for *H. pylori* infection that need to be tailored to patient tolerance and allergy as well as local antibiotic resistance patterns, but in general a 14-day course of a proton pump inhibitor (H2 blockers may be substituted) and two antibiotics (clarithromycin with amoxicillin or metronidazole) is recommended as first-line treatment.[12,13] Alternative regimens including bismuth or sequential therapy may be needed in cases of antibiotic resistance. Eradication of infection can be confirmed by either invasive or non-invasive (not serum antibody) methods. In addition to the cure of recurrent gastroduodenal ulcer disease, eradication of *H. pylori* can cause regression of gastric MALT lymphoma in a majority of co-infected patients.

Celiac disease

Celiac disease (also known as gluten enteropathy) is the most prevalent immune-mediated disease of the human GI tract. It is a chronic inflammation due to activation of gluten-specific T cells resulting in specific autoantibody formation, small intestinal villous atrophy, and malabsorption. Celiac pathophysiology and genetics are understood in some detail due to the identification of the antigen-presenting HLA molecules and the gluten peptide cognate ligands that drive the immune activation of T cells. In this respect therapeutic approaches beyond the avoidance of gluten are being pursued along the lines of modulating the processing of the gluten antigen and enhancing gut epithelial barrier function.

Presentation

The classic clinical presentation of celiac disease reflects the sequelae of damage to the absorptive surface of the small intestine: chronic diarrhea, weight loss, and abdominal bloating. However, this symptomatic presentation is in fact encountered in only a minority of affected patients. Celiac disease patients are more likely to present with complications of malabsorption (anemia, osteoporosis, failure to thrive in children) without overt GI complaints. Celiac disease can also present largely with a gluten-responsive skin disease (dermatitis herpetiformis), cerebellar ataxia, infertility and miscarriage, chronic fatigue, and associated autoimmune disorders such as diabetes and thyroiditis, Addison's disease, Sjögren syndrome, autoimmune hepatitis and primary biliary cirrhosis.[14,15] Celiac disease is also reported to occur at higher incidence in selective IgA deficiency and Down and Turner syndromes. To make matters more difficult in terms of choosing whom to screen for celiac disease, non-specific gastrointestinal symptoms such as abdominal pain and constipation are reported in over one-fifth of newly diagnosed subjects.[16] In any case, the gradation of presenting symptoms reflects several features of celiac disease: (1) celiac disease severity follows a dose effect of risk alleles; (2) celiac disease expression requires additional genetic and environmental factors beyond the well-characterized HLA molecules; (3) celiac disease expression can depend on the quantity and quality of gluten exposure; and (4) celiac disease manifestations reflect the severity of the inflammation and the length of involved bowel.[17,18] The concept of a vast subclinical celiac disease prevalence has lead to an "iceberg model" where the visible tip is the group with symptomatic gastrointestinal disease and the characteristic gut mucosal lesion, and below the surface are those with silent disease (no overt symptoms but gut mucosal lesions) and latent disease (no symptoms or mucosal lesions but genetic susceptibility possibly with positive serology).

The key to diagnosing celiac disease is simply to consider it in the differential of not only classical malabsorption but also with subtle manifestations of malabsorption; conversely, the differential diagnosis of villous blunting or intraepithelial lymphocytosis includes small intestinal bacterial overgrowth, tropical sprue, autoimmune enteropathy, common variable immune deficiency enteropathy, and *H. pylori* gastritis, remembering that celiac disease is not solely a histologic diagnosis.

Immune pathophysiology

Celiac disease is caused by the immune activation of T cells by gluten peptides offered by antigen-presenting cells expressing specific HLA molecules in the lamina propria of the gut (primarily the small intestine). In the absence of dietary gluten or the specific HLA molecules HLA-DQ2 or DQ8, celiac disease can theoretically not occur. Dietary gluten, largely from wheat, barley, and rye, exists in polymeric (glutenin) and monomeric (gliadin) form and is incompletely digested to small peptides by gut luminal enzymes due to a high glutamine and proline content.[17] These large gluten peptides cross the epithelial barrier and can bind to the pocket of the specific HLA-DQ2 or DQ8 molecules. It has been demonstrated that the enzyme tissue transglutamidase can deamidate the gluten peptide, and the resulting negative charge actually increases the affinity of the gluten peptide for the HLA binding site. When the gluten peptide is presented to cognate T-cell receptors, the activated T cells produce pro-inflammatory cytokines IFNγ, IL-18, tumor necrosis factor-alpha (TNF-α), and IL-21. These activated T cells can induce B-cell maturation to plasma cells producing antibodies to gluten peptides as well as tissue transglutaminase; how the production of anti-gliadin as well as anti-tissue transglutaminase (anti-TTG) autoantibodies occurs is unknown. However, it is also unknown whether the autoantibodies contribute to gut disease pathology, but anti-tTG6 autoantibodies have been suggested as a cause of ataxia and anti-tTG3 autoantibodies are believed to cause dermatitis herpetiformis and infertility (inducing trophoblast apoptosis).

According to animal models, the activated T cells are not sufficient to induce the epithelial damage and villous blunting. The characteristic villous atrophy is induced by gut antigen-presenting cell- and epithelial cell-produced IL-15 that enhances infiltration of CD8 T cells into the epithelium and upregulates NKG2D receptors on intraepithelial lymphocytes (to confer cytotoxicity against the epithelium). IL-17 also may be an important component to the inflammatory response. These inflammatory activities contribute to degradation of the epithelial barrier, further exposing the lamina propria to gluten peptides and other luminal contents.

Diagnosis

The ultimate diagnosis of celiac disease is based on a constellation of findings. The diagnostic work-up of celiac disease is initiated by both suggestive symptoms and signs (weight loss, chronic diarrhea) as well as by atypical presentations, such as isolated complications of chronic malabsorption or unexplained hyperamylasemia or hypertransaminasemia. Initial tests include measuring serum IgA antibodies against tissue transglutamidase and endomysial proteins; these have estimated specificity/sensitivity of 98/98% and 95/99%, respectively.[19] It is advisable to measure a total serum IgA level as well in order to be certain that these IgA-based screening tests are not falsely negative. However, in the setting of IgA deficiency, elevated anti-TTG IgG levels and identification of celiac disease susceptibility HLA genes can help determine the risk and presence of disease. The introduction of deamidated gluten peptide IgG antibody testing can also support the diagnosis of celiac disease in the presence of IgA deficiency.

In any case, an important part of celiac diagnosis is biopsy of the upper small intestine mucosa, typically 3–4 endoscopic biopsies both from the duodenal bulb and the distal duodenum. While the absolute requirement for histologic diagnosis of celiac disease may be debated (and cannot be used alone due to a lack of specificity), it remains important for several reasons. One, currently the serologic markers should only be used as a screening test, indicating which patients are at highest risk for the disease and appropriate for biopsy. Two, even in possession of celiac-susceptibility HLA genes, only a minority of persons will develop celiac disease (latent disease), so that evaluating non-specific symptoms will require histologic examination. Three, because the treatment can be life-altering, the most comprehensive information is needed to make a definitive diagnosis.

Beyond celiac disease, a true gluten-induced enteropathy, other entities have been identified, namely gluten sensitivity and gluten allergy. Gluten sensitivity includes a set of poorly characterized gut and extra-intestinal disorders that lack the defining features of celiac disease yet respond to a gluten-free diet.[20] Gluten allergy is the presence of an IgE response to wheat peptides that also can be associated with non-specific gastrointestinal complaints but is not at all related to celiac disease.

Treatment

The treatment of celiac disease is avoidance of gluten, specifically foods containing wheat, barley and rye. While easier said than done, a gluten-free diet can be accomplished, and with the increased awareness of food sensitivities, gluten free processed foods and meals are increasingly available. The expected response to gluten restriction is the resolution of symptoms including malabsorption that typically precedes the restoration of the mucosal histology. In fact, follow-up endoscopy for repeat biopsy to assess response to therapy should be done only after 6–12 months of a strict gluten-free diet (GFD). There are no accurate biomarkers to monitor adherence to a gluten free diet although one indication may be a fall in the pre-treatment level IgA anti-TTG serum antibodies; it is useful therefore to do a follow-up endoscopy with biopsy to document improvement in the inflammation and restoration of the villous architecture. Symptom improvement, correction of malabsorption, and regrowth of villi (seen by endoscopy or video capsule) may not reflect complete histologic healing, but the long-term risk of this is unknown.

As reported, about 5% of celiac patients do not respond to a GFD, but that number is probably higher. Ensuring a strict adherence to a GFD is important to discern the reasons for non-response, whether through inadvertent gluten exposure or whether the inflammation is refractory to even a strict GFD. One group of so-called refractory celiac disease patients with polyclonal intra-epithelial lymphocyte (IELs) populations may respond to corticosteroids and immunosuppressant treatment; another group with monoclonal IELs do not, and are at increased risk of lymphoma.

The majority of celiac patients can respond positively to a GFD with return of normal gut absorption. However, ongoing inflammation is associated with risk of small bowel lymphoma so that ensuring adherence to a GFD and documenting mucosal healing can affect the natural history of this disease. Finally, since first-degree relatives are at increased risk of celiac disease, patients should be advised about serum antibody screening of these family members.

KEY CONCEPTS

Celiac disease

- Celiac patients present more often with complications of malabsorption than chronic diarrhea and weight loss.
- HLA DQ2 or DQ8 alleles are necessary but not sufficient for celiac disease to develop.
- IgA antibodies to tissue transglutamidase and endomysial proteins should be used for screening only (not diagnosis) and should be measured along with total IgA for validity.
- The goals of gluten-free diet treatment are relief of symptoms, reversal of malabsorption, and restoration of villi.

ON THE HORIZON

- Development of new diagnostic criteria and validated non-invasive blood-based testing (genetics, serology, immune response parameters) that will avoid need for endoscopic biopsy.
- Discovery of additional genetic and environmental factors that unequivocally determine whether persons with the HLA DQ2 and DQ8 risk alleles will actually develop celiac disease leading to strategies to modify or eliminate that risk.
- Novel therapies that modify gluten to non-immunogenic forms or that induce tolerance to gluten in persons at risk for or suffering from celiac disease.

Crohn's disease

Crohn's disease is a chronic idiopathic inflammation of the gut characterized by transmural involvement of the bowel wall (mucosa, muscle layer and serosa). While earlier referred to as "terminal ileitis," the majority of Crohn's patients actually have colitis coexisting or by itself. Crohn's disease runs a predominantly chronic, relapsing course often complicated by bowel obstruction from fibrous strictures as well as bowel wall perforation leading to abscesses and fistulae. Crohn's disease is treated with corticosteroids and immunosupressants and more recently with antibodies targeting TNF-α and the integrin molecule $\alpha4$.

The cause of Crohn's disease is unknown, but it is thought to result from a dysregulated immune response to gut microbes. There is clear evidence for heritable disease susceptibility in twin and multiplex family studies, and several genes involved in innate immune function, notably mutations in *NOD2*, have been linked to Crohn's disease risk.

Presentation

While the presentation of Crohn's disease can be protean, most often patients come to medical attention because of abdominal pain, altered bowel habits, and rectal bleeding.[21] Abdominal pain can be an indication of bowel obstruction (especially if it is post-prandial), an inflamed viscus, or a penetrating complication such as an abscess or fistula. Diarrhea is related to inflammatory (cytokine effects on absorption and secretion) and non-inflammatory mechanisms (e.g., bile salt wasting, small intestinal bacterial overgrowth), and bleeding is from mucosal friability and ulceration. Constipation in Crohn's disease is often a sign of stricturing of the bowel, particularly the small intestine. In addition, signs and symptoms such as fever, unexplained weight loss, fatigue, anemia, and growth retardation (in children) can accompany the gastrointestinal complaints or be the primary presentation. Extra-intestinal manifestations of Crohn's disease include arthritis, uveitis, inflammatory skin lesions, and stomatitis. The arthritis can affect the axial (spine and pelvis) and articular skeleton, with the latter more often mirroring the activity of the gut disease. The joint complaints range from arthralgias to frank synovitis with swelling and tenderness (typically characterized by non-specific findings on arthrocentesis and without erosive joint destruction). The uveitis most commonly occurs as episcleritis and iritis and the skin lesions include erythema nodosum and pyoderma gangrenosum. Many of these lesions will subside with effective therapy aimed at the gut but they can also have independent courses that require site-targeted treatment.

The incidence of Crohn's disease has been estimated in North American populations to be around 3.1–14.6 cases/100 000 person-years.[22] Ashkenazi Jewish heritage confers increased risk in Caucasians, while African-Americans seem to have similar rates to non-Jewish Caucasians, and Hispanic and Asians have much lower rates.[23,24] There is a genetic risk with up to tenfold increased rates of inflammatory bowel disease in relatives of Crohn's patients and a 30% concordance rate in monozygotic twin pairs.[25] The typical patient will be diagnosed in their second or third decade and there is no significant gender preference. The only environmental exposure to be reproducibly linked to risk of Crohn's disease has been tobacco use.

Most Crohn's patients (up to 70%) experience a remitting and relapsing course, but some have chronically active symptoms refractory to medical remission. There are recognized phenotypes of disease including inflammatory disease (manifested primarily by intestinal edema and ulceration), fibro-stenotic disease (luminal narrowing by fibrous strictures dominate with symptoms of painful obstruction), and fistulizing disease (inflammatory tracts between the bowel and other intestines, the bladder, vagina, skin, and other structures). While the majority of patients have predominantly inflammatory disease at the time of diagnosis, over time this evolves so that after 20 years of disease duration 70 and 18% of Crohn's patients report penetrating or fibrostenotic complications, respectively.[26] Accompanying this change in phenotype is the need for surgical treatment. Most Crohn's patients will at some point require surgical treatment for their disease with estimates of 80% by 20 years of disease duration.

Immune pathophysiology

The current paradigm of Crohn's disease inflammatory origins is a dysregulated immune response to microbial components (antigens and pathogen-associated molecular patterns), likely from gut commensal organisms themselves. Much of what we infer about Crohn's disease comes from animal models of induced and spontaneous colitis.[27–29] In the TNBS model of colitis, results showed a predominant Th1 inflammation with antigen presenting cells secreting IL-12 and effector T cells producing interferon-γ; the colitis could be blocked or reversed by treating animals with anti-IL-12 antibodies. This model was further refined with the discovery of IL-23 and its control of IL-17 production. While IL-12 induces Th1 T cells, IL-23 is more important for the maintenance and function of IL-17-secreting cells (Th17 cells);[30] Th17 T cells are induced by IL-6 and TGF-β, whereupon Th17 cells begin to express cell surface IL-23 receptor making them responsive to IL-23 stimulation (Chapter 16). In fact, roles for IL-23 and IL-17 in Crohn's disease have also been suggested by certain animal models. In the IL-10 deficient mouse model of spontaneous colitis and the cell transfer model of induced colitis, where colitogenic naïve CD4$^+$CD45RB^{high} T cells from wild type mice are infused into T-cell-deficient mice, the inflammation was more dependent on the IL-23/IL-17 pathway.[31,32] However, despite the important role of the IL-23/IL-17 axis in the transfer model of colitis, blockade of IFNγ activity also prevented development of gut inflammation.[33] In the transfer model of colitis there is evidence that a functioning IL-23/IL-17 cytokine axis can limit inflammation since transferring IL-17-deficient T cells caused earlier onset weight loss and higher expression of inflammatory cytokines in the gut, while IL-23-deficient mice had more severe induced colitis.[34,35] Studies of Crohn's disease confirm that production of IL-12, IL-23, IFN-γ, and IL-17 are significantly elevated.[36,37] In light of this, the hierarchy of cytokine control of Crohn's inflammation is currently being examined by a number of ongoing clinical trials that are testing the clinical effectiveness of targeting both IL-12 and IL-23, IL-23 alone, and IL-17 in Crohn's disease.

While the mechanisms of the susceptibility to gut inflammation in Crohn's disease are not entirely clear, work on the genetic risk factors and the gut microbiome are providing data to generate hypotheses. For example, a polymorphism in the coding region of the IL-23 receptor gene found in 14% of healthy controls is associated with protection from Crohn's disease (and ulcerative colitis).[25] Two other Crohn's disease-associated susceptibility polymorphisms affect the *NOD2* and *ATG16L1* genes, both involved with innate immune responses to microbes. The *NOD2* gene product is an intracellular protein that binds muramyl dipeptide (MDP), a component of the TLR2 ligand peptidoglycan derived from bacterial cell walls. Intact NOD2 responds to microbial products and regulates the inflammatory reactivity. Disease-associated mutations not only disrupt this pathway, but because NOD2 is also expressed by small intestinal epithelial Paneth cells, mucosal production of anti-microbial defensins is decreased potentially compromising barrier function. The *ATG16L1* autophagy gene product is important for the metabolism of autologous cell proteins as well as intracellular microbes. Expression of the Crohn's-associated polymorphic ATG16L1 by a colon cancer cell line *in vitro* showed inhibition of packaging of intracellular *Salmonella* into autophagosomes, supporting the hypothesis that this mutation could lead to impaired clearance of microbes and chronic inflammation.[38] Finally, Crohn's disease has been associated with an intestinal dysbiosis, particularly with a reduction in the butyrate-producing *Faecalibacterium prausnitzii* compared to healthy controls, but it is not known whether this is a cause or effect of the gut inflammation.[39,40]

Diagnosis

The diagnosis of Crohn's disease depends on a number of findings from radiographic, endoscopic, and histologic examinations. In general, a combination of colonoscopy (with ileal intubation if possible) and small bowel exam (barium small bowel follow through, CT or MR enterography, and video endoscopy) is usually sufficient to demonstrate active inflammatory disease of the colon and small bowel. Endoscopically, mucosal ulceration and friability in a patchy distribution separated by unaffected mucosa ("skip areas") are hallmarks of the disease. Radiographically, evidence of patchy bowel wall thickening, mucosal hyperemia, stricturing, and penetrating complications such as fistulae, abscesses, and extraintestinal inflammatory masses involving the bowel all suggest Crohn's disease. Histologically, while the appearance of non-caseating granulomata is highly supportive of a Crohn's diagnosis, in practice they are not often detected by endoscopic biopsy, particularly in adults. More often evidence of chronic inflammation such as architectural crypt distortion and basal lymphoplasmacytosis are sought to differentiate the inflammation from an acute, self-limited colitis or enteritis. Other findings such as fecal leukocytes or elevated fecal calprotectin can indicate an inflammatory colitis, but is not specific for diagnosis of a chronic idiopathic inflammatory bowel disease (IBD) such as Crohn's or ulcerative colitis. In the setting of supportive imaging or endoscopic findings, the measurement of certain serum antibodies can further strengthen the diagnosis of Crohn's disease and even help differentiate it from ulcerative colitis, but they should not be used by themselves as a diagnostic test.[41] It has been shown that up to 68% of Crohn's patients are seropositive for antibodies targeting microbial antigens such as anti-*Saccharomyces cerevesiae* antibody (up to 16% of UC patients are seropositive). Additional anti-microbial antibodies such as anti-OmpC, anti-I2, and anti-CBir can also be seen in Crohn's disease.

Finally, Crohn's disease may need to be differentiated from other conditions including ulcerative colitis, chronic ischemic colitis, infectious enteritis/colitis (amebiasis, *Yersinia enterocolitica, Mycobacterium tuberculosis*), intestinal lymphoma, celiac disease, diverticula-associated colitis, and radiation- and NSAID-induced enteropathy.

Treatment

The treatment of Crohn's disease includes medical and surgical approaches. Since there is no cure for Crohn's disease, the principles of therapy are to first make sure that any symptoms are due to the underlying idiopathic inflammation, and not infectious or non-inflammatory causes such as coexisting irritable bowel syndrome, and then to attempt quick induction of remission from symptoms and establish therapy to maintain the remission. A traditional approach to therapy has been to use corticosteroids and mesalamine preparations to start, then to add immunosuppressants (azathioprine, 6-mercaptopurine, and methotrexate) if symptoms persist, and finally to start anti-TNF-α agents for recalcitrant disease.[42] Only corticosteroids and the anti-TNF agents are reliable for inducing clinical responses in short periods of time, within days to weeks. Therefore corticosteroid use may need to be prolonged while immunosuppressants are begun concomitantly, since the latter's clinical effects may not be maximized until months later. For maintenance of remission, only immunosuppressants and anti-TNF agents reliably exert long-term control of symptoms. In this way they may be used for years as long as the Crohn's disease is responding. Currently, medically refractory inflammatory disease can be treated with natalizumab, an anti-α4 integrin antibody. An emerging approach to immunosuppressant- and biologic-naïve patients is to begin with a combination of azathioprine and infliximab, as this has been shown to be superior to either single agent alone for inducing remission, especially at one year later.[43] This "top-down" approach continues to be studied for long-term efficacy.

Surgery is required in cases of bleeding, pain/obstruction, and fistula complications that are refractory to medical therapy. Surgery typically involves resection limited to inflamed segments of small intestine and colon; small strictures can be treated *in situ* by stricturoplasty. In addition surgery is required for treatment of intestinal adenocarcinoma that also complicates the chronic inflammation of the bowel.[44] There is a high incidence of endoscopic and symptomatic recurrence of inflammation by two years after surgery, but no consensus about prevention is currently available.

● KEY CONCEPTS

Crohn's disease

- Crohn's disease affects the full thickness of the bowel wall resulting in fistulae and abscesses in 70% of patients by 20 years' disease duration.
- Th1 and Th17 cytokine pathways mediate disease in animal models, but the hierarchy of these effects in human disease is being tested by targeted monoclonal antibodies in clinical trials.
- Several gene mutations and many genetic loci are associated with disease risk, including *NOD2* and *ATG16L1*, which are important in innate immune function.
- Crohn's disease is a chronic, relapsing inflammation of the bowel and up to 80% of patients will require surgical treatment at some point.

● ON THE HORIZON

- Defining the actual mechanisms of inflammation for disease susceptibility genes such as *NOD2* and *ATG16L1*, and designing gene therapy approaches for selected subgroups of Crohn's disease patients.
- Describing the immune and pharmacologic mechanisms of primary non-response to conventional and novel biologic therapy in order to stratify patients for additional GWAS analysis and design prospective studies for optimizing therapeutic outcomes for specific agents.

Ulcerative colitis

Ulcerative colitis (UC) also is a chronic idiopathic inflammation of the gut limited to the mucosal layer of the colon. It can affect the rectum alone (ulcerative proctitis), the distal transverse colon to rectum (left-sided colitis) or the entire colon (pancolitis). Because it lacks transmural inflammation of Crohn's disease, penetrating complications like fistulae and abscesses are generally not features of UC. Oral and topical (per rectum) mesalamine preparations are most often used to treat UC, although patients also can require corticosteroids, immunosuppressants, and anti-TNF antibody agents to induce and maintain remission. Unlike Crohn's disease, total colectomy eliminates the disease; however, there can be ongoing complications of the surgery such as pouchitis when an ileal-pouch anal anastomosis is performed. Over 40% of UC patients require surgery to treat medically refractory symptoms or development of dysplasia over their lifetime.[45]

The cause of ulcerative colitis is not known. It has inherited risk but not as strongly as in Crohn's disease. While it shares some polymorphic risk alleles with Crohn's, there also are disease susceptibility loci unique to UC. Probably the most distinguishing biologic factor observed in this inflammation is the Th2-like inflammatory cytokines that are produced, in comparison to the dominant Th1 and Th17 profile of Crohn's disease.

Presentation

The presentation of ulcerative colitis reflects the primary involvement of the rectum and varying amounts of colitis extending proximally.[21] While rectal bleeding and diarrhea (including nocturnal) are common symptoms, proctitis-specific complaints of rectal urgency and incomplete evacuation are also prominent. Crampy abdominal pain can accompany the diarrhea but obstructive-type pain is not common. As in Crohn's disease, fever, unexplained weight loss, fatigue, and anemia can accompany the gastrointestinal complaints or be the primary presentation. Extra-intestinal manifestations also can include arthritis, uveitis, inflammatory skin lesions, and stomatitis.[46] An interesting genetic connection exists between UC and HLA B27-positive spondyloarthropathy with 60% of ankylosing spondylitis patients showing inflammation on colonoscopy.[47] UC is also closely associated with primary sclerosing cholangitis (PSC); while up to 3% of UC patients develop PSC, up to 75% of all patients with PSC have ulcerative colitis.[48]

With an incidence up to 20.3 cases per 100 000 person-years, the typical UC patient will be diagnosed in their second or third decade and there is no significant gender preference.[22]

Approximately 6–15% of first-degree relatives of UC patients have a history of UC, but in general the genetic contribution to risk is thought to be lower than in Crohn's disease. There appears to be a higher incidence of UC in European and North American populations compared to Asian and Latin American countries. The only environmental exposures linked to risk of ulcerative colitis are a protective effect of tobacco use and of appendectomy in the first decade of life.

The natural history of ulcerative colitis shows that most patients experience a remitting and relapsing course (60%), but some can have prolonged remission after their first episode of disease (20%) and others have chronically active symptoms refractory to medical remission (20%). Total colectomy is done for refractory symptoms or development of epithelial dysplasia. Chronic inflammatory ulcerative colitis (and Crohn's colitis) is accompanied by an increased incidence of colorectal cancer (18% after 30 years disease duration), so much so that recurring colonoscopic surveillance for dysplasia with biopsy is recommended starting 8–10 years after diagnosis.[49]

Immune pathophysiology

Ulcerative colitis has been characterized as a Th2-like disease (Chapter 16) because of the increased IL-5 and IL-13 production in inflamed gut tissue seen in an animal model of UC, oxazolone-induced colitis, as well as from patient specimens.[50] Oxazolone applied to the colon produces a gut injury similar to human disease where inflammation is limited to the mucosal layer. In the animal model, not only were mucosal natural killer T (NKT) cells the source of excess IL-13, but the colitis was reversed by immunoneutralizing IL-13.[51,52] When translated to humans, UC patients also were found to have high capacity for IL-13 production also by type II NKT cells. It turns out that IL-13 is a biologically plausible effector cytokine in UC injury because it disrupts the epithelial tight junction by upregulating claudin-2 and has a direct toxic effect on human gut epithelial cells *in vitro*.[53]

Data from genetic susceptibility studies in UC have provided less compelling examples of disease-specific mechanisms compared to Crohn's disease, but there are clear associations with HLA class II genes distinct from Crohn's.[54] Furthermore, other associated gene loci contain genes involved in epithelial barrier function such as *GNA12* for tight junction formation, *CDH* for epithelial cadherin-1, and *LAMB1* for the laminin constituent of basement membranes.[25] So there may be defects overrepresented in barrier function versus innate immune response that favor the development of UC, but this remains to be rigorously tested.

Diagnosis

The diagnosis of ulcerative colitis is based on establishing the presence of colitis that typically involves the rectum and adjacent proximal colonic segments in a confluent inflammatory injury. This is primarily and best accomplished by colonoscopy (ileal intubation can confirm that the inflammation is limited to the colon). Biopsies should contain histologic features of chronic inflammation including crypt distortion, crypt dropout, and lymphoplasmacytosis. The presence of acute inflammatory features alone (polymorphonuclear cells, crypt abscess and cryptitis) may also be seen, but when in isolation indicates other etiologies such as infectious, drug-induced, ischemic and toxic exposures. While no blood test can be used to diagnose UC, the presence of high titer perinuclear anti-neutrophil cytoplasmic antibodies (pANCA) can be seen in up to 70% of UC patients; this information can help support an established diagnostic impression or help differentiate a chronic indeterminate colitis from Crohn's colitis when coupled with anti-*Saccharomyces cerevisiae* antibody (ASCA) serologies (see above).[41] At all times, acute infections from enteric pathogens including *Clostridium difficile* should also be excluded as these can also occur in IBD and mimic an exacerbation of disease. Evaluation for cytomegalovirus infection should also be done especially in the setting of UC seemingly refractory to immunosuppressants. Once a diagnosis is established, elevations in transaminases or alkaline phosphatase should prompt an examination of the biliary tree for PSC starting with a magnetic resonance cholangiopancreatogram.

Treatment

Treatment can be tailored to the extent and activity of disease.[55] For instance, mild to moderate proctitis can often be treated with topical corticosteroids or mesalamine alone (enemas and/or suppositories). Most often with more extensive colonic involvement, oral mesalamine is required, which can be useful for induction and maintenance of remission. In severe disease, corticosteroids may be required to induce rapid responses while immunosuppressants such as azathioprine or 6-mercaptopurine are used for remission. Maximal therapeutic effect may take months such that steroids serve as a bridge to this late effect, and the immunosuppressant is used for eventual "steroid-sparing" maintenance of response. Anti-TNF-α agents also are used to induce fairly rapid clinical responses and remission as single agents, as well as for maintenance therapy.

Mesalamine-based drugs are a cornerstone of therapy in UC and are generally included in most ongoing UC medical regimens. There is controversy about whether use of mesalamine even in quiescent disease confers chemoprotection from developing dysplasia, but due to their low adverse event rate and high tolerance long-term use is a reasonable choice.

As discussed, surgery has a definite role in treating medically refractory disease or addressing dysplasia discovered by surveillance colonoscopy (dysplasia surveillance is done every 1–2 years after 8–10 years of disease by taking 4-quadrant biopsies every 10 cm). When total colectomy is performed the options include an ileal pouch anal anastomosis or a permanent end ileostomy.

● KEY CONCEPTS

Ulcerative colitis

- Ulcerative colitis is a chronic, relapsing inflammation of the colon that is limited to the mucosa and is not transmural.
- Animal models and human disease show the dominant cytokines to be IL-5 and IL-13, suggesting a Th2-like (no IL-4) inflammatory response.
- Though less strongly associated with genetic inheritance compared to Crohn's disease, several disease susceptibility loci are associated with epithelial barrier function.
- Over the course of the disease up to 40% of patients will undergo total colectomy for refractory symptoms or detection of epithelial dysplasia.

Other idiopathic inflammatory bowel diseases

Microscopic colitis

Microscopic colitis is an increasingly recognized condition that links chronic watery diarrhea with intraepithelial lymphocytosis alone (lymphocytic colitis) or accompanied by increased subepithelial collagen deposition (collagenous colitis). It differs from Crohn's disease and ulcerative colitis because it does not display endoscopic mucosal damage or show evidence of histologic chronicity (no architectural crypt distortion, lymphoplasmacytosis, or loss of Goblet cells). However, it causes significant morbidity and can require chronic immunosuppression for treatment. While its etiology remains elusive, there are associations with autoimmune conditions as well as with certain drug exposures.

The hallmark symptom of microscopic colitis is chronic, watery, non-bloody diarrhea. This frequently is accompanied by marked complaints of poor quality of life. Fatigue, arthralgias, and weight loss may also be reported. Microscopic colitis has its typical onset in the sixth to seventh decade, has a female gender predominance, and is associated with a history of autoimmunity especially thyroid diseases, rheumatoid arthritis and the limited cutaneous form of scleroderma (CREST syndrome; Chapter 54).[56] A connection between microscopic colitis and celiac disease has also be observed, where lymphocytosis of the colonic epithelium was observed in 31% of patients with typical malabsorption symptoms and small bowel lesions of celiac disease.[57] This may be a sequela of gluten antigen reactivity and epithelial response but it becomes important to address as an independent process of microscopic colitis if diarrhea and colonic lymphocytosis persist despite a gluten-free diet. Conversely, while celiac-like villous blunting may be seen in <10% of microscopic colitis patients, celiac serologies are not positive, indicating that in this setting gluten enteropathy is not playing a role.

There is no current information on the immune mechanism of microscopic colitis. In particular there are no data on the factors driving or sustaining the inflammation nor have the key effector cells and inflammatory mediators been identified. Activated NFκB is seen in the mucosa of microscopic colitis, consistent with the general inflammatory picture. Excess nitric oxide and prostaglandin production have also been measured, possibly contributing more to the diarrhea rather than the inflammation. Excess TGF-β has also been measured in collagenous colitis, consistent with its role in collagen production and fibrosis. Interestingly, medications have been associated with microscopic colitis, including H2 blockers, proton pump inhibitors, selective serotonin reuptake inhibitors, and ticlopidine, among others.[58] Reports also suggest that long-term use of NSAIDs can induce or sustain microscopic colitis, although whether concomitant NSAID use is a confounder in the association with microscopic colitis or induces a similar mucosal injury remains to be proven.[59]

The diagnosis of microscopic colitis is a histologic one, that is, when coupled with appropriate symptoms. The *sine qua non* of microscopic colitis is increased numbers of intraepithelial lymphocytes on colonic mucosal biopsy, usually > 20 lymphocytes/100 epithelial cells. This can be accompanied by a chronic inflammatory infiltrate in the lamina propria and less often a limited appearance of neutrophils (especially cryptitis), the latter finding suggesting that the etiology of the microscopic colitis may actually be related to an injurious drug effect such as NSAID exposure. In collagenous colitis, a prominent subepithelial collagen band ≥ 10 µm is seen in addition to the intraepithelial lymphocytosis. Biopsies should be obtained proximal to the rectosigmoid junction (preferentially throughout colon) to avoid false-negative results due to reports of milder changes in the rectum.

As a general treatment approach to the patient with microscopic colitis, the clinician should review and eliminate suspect concomitant medications such as NSAIDs. As discussed, co-existing celiac disease should be considered where appropriate and addressed with gluten withdrawal. Overall the choice of treatment begins with low risk medications in mild or moderate disease in an attempt to settle on a regimen that delivers the most relief of symptoms with the lowest side effects.[59] Therefore treatment can begin with anti-diarrheals (loperamide, diphenoxylate/atropine), adding a trial of cholestyramine as bile salt malabsorption has been hypothesized to play a role in microscopic colitis. Despite inconsistent findings relative to bile salt malabsorption, use of cholestyramine has been reported to be successful in some patients. Bismuth sulfate has been reported to benefit a minority of patients with microscopic colitis. In patients with refractory or initially severe symptoms, corticosteroids have been very effective. In particular oral budesonide, 9 mg taken once per day, has reliably improved diarrhea and induced remission, a result supported by several small placebo-controlled studies. The challenge is managing the relief of symptoms with the long-term side effects of corticosteroid use, to which budesonide is also subject. Emerging strategies include use of lower doses of budesonide (3–6 mg/day) while monitoring for side effects or using immunosupressive medications such as azathioprine and methotrexate for long-term maintenance. Occasionally, patients may need colectomy and ileostomy to manage refractory symptoms or drug intolerance.

Eosinophilic esophagitis

Eosinophilic esophagitis is a recently characterized disease of the esophagus defined by symptomatic idiopathic eosinophilic inflammation in the absence of other known causes, especially chronic gastroesophageal reflux disease (GERD).[60] While its patho-etiology is unclear, there are specific genetic associations and data from animal models and human observations that implicate central roles for loss of tolerance to food antigens and the Th2 cytokines IL-5 and IL-13 in the inflammation. What is clear is that eosinophilic esophagitis is being recognized with increasing frequency most likely due to enhanced awareness against a background of an increased frequency of allergic diseases.

Eosinophilic esophagitis (EE) is estimated to occur at 4–5 cases/10 000 children and has a male predominance (up to 70%) and peak incidence in 0- to 3-year-old children. Symptoms include failure to thrive and feeding difficulty (e.g., food refusal, limited variety diet, prolonged feeding times) and abdominal pain and vomiting in older children and adolescents. In adults, the primary symptom is typically intermittent dysphagia and the first presentation may even be a food impaction in the esophagus. In addition, adult patients may report gastroesophageal reflux symptoms that do not respond to adequate acid-suppression therapy. Patients can report a high rate (>50%) of atopy (rhinoconjunctivitis, wheezing, or family history of atopy) as well as food allergies (including positive skin-prick or RAST test or anaphylactic response to a dietary allergen).[61] There is also an association of esophageal disease (strictures or EE) in 8–10% of parents of patients.[62]

The diagnosis of EE requires endoscopic biopsy of the esophagus since the presence of increased eosinophils in the esophageal epithelium is required to make the diagnosis. The endoscopic appearance of the esophagus can show multiple thin rings ("feline esophagus") with linear longitudinal furrows and whitish papules that represent eosinophilic microabscesses at the surface of the squamous epithelium. The biopsy should show an infiltrate of eosinophils in the epithelium of at least 15–20 eosinophils/hpf. These often concentrate just under the epithelial surface and also form microabscesses of groups of 4 or more eosinophils. It is important to take at least 3 biopsies since involvement can be variable and patchy; in addition it is advisable to take biopsies from the distal and mid to upper esophagus (to help differentiate changes seen in GERD that can be limited to the distal esophagus). In addition, biopsies from the gastric and duodenal mucosae are useful to show that the eosinophilic infiltration is limited to the esophagus and doesn't represent a diffuse process such as found in eosinophilic gastroenteritis or hypereosinophilic syndrome. In terms of GERD, it is important to make sure that any excess acid reflux is treated and controlled; persistent symptoms (and persistent biopsy abnormalities) may prompt a 24-hour ambulatory pH study of the distal esophagus to ensure that the acid-suppression treatment results in a normal acid-contact time. In terms of the dysphagia, a fixed stricture or narrowing is usually not seen by endoscopy, suggesting that a motility disturbance contributes to the dysphagia; in fact multiple types of esophageal dysmotility, often reversible with treatment, have been described in EE.[63] Systemic eosinophilia can be seen in over 70% of EE patients.

As noted, the pathogenesis of EE seems to be linked to allergen hypersensitivity. Clearly given the familial association of EE, atopy, and food allergy, a genetic component seems to be contributing to disease susceptibility. Several gene/gene loci have been identified as risk variants in EE by a candidate gene approach, including the 3' untranslated region of eotaxin (*CCL26*), the TGF-β_1 promoter, a Filaggrin (*FLG*) exon, and a thymic stromal lymphopoietin (*TSLP*) intron and TSLP receptor (*CRLF2*) exon.[64] These associations are biologically plausible since eotaxin is excessively expressed in EE mucosa, filaggrin is a structural skin protein that helps to maintain barrier function (and is downregulated by IL-13), and TSLP has been shown to stimulate IL-13 production by innate helper cells in the lamina propria. Moreover, the inflammation in EE is characterized by increased IL-13 and IL-5 production; in animal models of aeroallergen induction of an EE-like lesion, both IL-13-deficient and STAT6-deficient (an intracellular molecule important for IL-13 receptor α_1 signaling) animals are protected from developing the inflammation. These data support the model that IL-13 secretion induces production of eotaxin from epithelial cells that together with IL-5 drives the local eosinophilic infiltration. Finally, the association with food allergy has led to successful therapy of EE by using strict elimination diets (sometimes informed by skin testing) or even the use of elemental diet tube feedings.

Given the strong association with food allergies, strict elimination of suspect foods or those identified by RAST or skin prick testing may be done first, though it can be difficult to precisely identify offending antigens or they may be widely distributed among a number of foods. Lack of improvement in symptoms would lead to a trial of an amino acid-based elemental liquid diet, necessitating nasogastric (or later percutaneous gastrostomy) placement. But this can be uncomfortable, impractical, and expensive. If this dietary approach is successful, then after several weeks, individual foods can be added back every 5 to 7 days.[65] For patients not responding to dietary therapy or with no identifiable dietary allergens, corticosteroid treatment has been used successfully. Both systemic oral and swallowed topical (e.g., fluticasone propionate metered dose inhalers,) corticosteroids for 4–6 weeks have been shown to relieve symptoms and resolve histologic inflammation. However, relapse rates are high over the year following a course of steroids. Lastly, endoscopic therapy to treat strictures using dilation incurs higher risk of mucosal tears so that conservative treatment (smaller dilators, assessment for tears during the procedure before proceeding further) is encouraged.

Gastrointestinal complications of primary immunodeficiencies

Certain primary immunodeficiency diseases can result in gastrointestinal complications. These complications fall into three main categories of etiology, infectious, idiopathic inflammatory/autoimmune, and neoplastic. Common variable immunodeficiency and chronic granulomatous disease have some of the most frequent and significant gut manifestations, and these are discussed in detail. However, a variety of inherited conditions of broad lymphocyte or innate immune cell dysfunction can affect the gut.

Common variable immunodeficiency

Common variable immunodeficiency (CVID) is a syndrome of hypogammaglobulinemia (levels of IgG and IgA or IgM that are more than two standard deviations below the age-adjusted mean) and recurrent suppurative sino-pulmonary infections (Chapter 34). Patients cannot mount an adequate antibody response to immunizing antigens. In general, replacement of immunoglobulin treats the sinopulmonary infections, but other complications such as autoimmune disease and gastrointestinal symptoms, including intestinal infections, do not respond well or at all to this treatment. Many genetic defects resulting in deficient activities have been described with the CVID phenotype including inducible costimulator (ICOS), transmembrane activator and calcium-modulator and cyclophilin ligand interactor (TACI), B-cell activating factor of the tumor necrosis factor family receptor (BAFF-R) and even CD19 genes.[66] Case series of CVID patients show that up to 60% of patients experience gastrointestinal symptoms.[67] When considering the differential diagnostic possibilities for the etiology of the gastrointestinal complications of CVID, it is helpful to separate them into infectious, immune-mediated, and neoplastic processes. Among the infectious agents, *Giardia lamblia*, non-typhoidal *Salmonella*, and *Campylobacter jejuni* are frequently seen, but *Cryptosporidium* and *Clostridium difficile* as well as viral agents (cytomegalovirus) can be encountered. In addition, there is a high rate of gastric *H. pylori* infection, and small intestinal bacterial overgrowth (SIBO) has been seen in up to 30% of CVID patients, and should be kept in mind. The immune-mediated GI complications of CVID include inflammatory lesions such as idiopathic enteropathy (villous atrophy, increased intraepithial lympho-cytes/microscopic colitis, nodular lymphoid hyperplasia) man-ifesting as severe malabsorption (see below) and less-frequently ulcerating disease resembling UC and Crohn's disease.[67] CVID-associated autoimmune disease involving the GI tract also includes type II gastritis that can lead to achlorhydria and vitamin B_{12} defi-ciency ("pernicious anemia") and even autoimmune hepatitis and primary biliary cirrhosis. Lastly, neoplastic complications of intestinal lymphoma and gastric adenocarcinoma (related to achlorhydric autoimmune gastritis) have been reported.

Presentation

The most common symptom of GI complications of CVID is epi-sodic or chronic diarrhea, regardless of the etiology. This can be ac-companied by weight loss if the mechanism of the diarrhea involves significant maldigestion or malabsorption (along with bloating and crampy abdominal discomfort). In the setting of pro-longed malabsorption with subclinical symptoms, suspicion of a GI complication may be raised by lab abnormalities such as iron deficiency, macrocytic anemia, osteoporosis, or other vitamin de-ficiencies. In addition, patients can present with abdominal pain related to splenomegaly (with or without portal hypertension) or ascites (portal hypertension secondary to hepatic nodular regen-erative hyperplasia is a known complication of CVID). Lastly, symptoms of weight loss, fever, intestinal obstruction, and GI bleeding may indicate the development of small bowel lymphoma.

Immune pathophysiology

It is not clear that the lack of immunoglobulins alone causes sus-ceptibility to gut infections and inflammation because X-linked agammaglobulinemia patients rarely report gastrointestinal dis-ease. Even persons lacking IgA alone, the predominant secreted mucosal surface antibody, have little in the way of a stereotypic GI disease, including infections (although the possibility of in-creased production and secretion of IgM is cited as a possible compensatory mechanism). In fact the T-cell dysfunction that of-ten accompanies CVID may contribute substantially to suscepti-bility to gastrointestinal disease.

In terms of an increased gastrointestinal infection risk, autoim-mune gastritis-induced achlorhydria could increase small bowel exposure to swallowed commensals and pathogens escaping this innate barrier to infection. In addition, while the loss of secreted IgA alone is not enough to meaningfully increase susceptibility to intestinal infections, perhaps the additional of loss of IgG and IgM and presence of T-cell dysfunction is more permissive, al-though no mechanism for this has been established. Mucosal nodular lymphoid hyperplasia, characterized by disorganized secondary lymphoid nodules with poorly formed germinal cen-ters, is likely related to the inability of B cells to undergo class switching when presented with antigen *in situ*. Lastly the enter-opathy characterized clinically by severe malabsorption and histologically by blunted villi, increased intraepithelial lympho-cytes, and epithelial apoptosis is associated with excess Th1 cy-tokine secretion (IL-12 and IFN-γ).[68] These cytokines themselves can cause acute damage to the small intestinal mucosa when ad-ministered directly to mice, and their overproduction can induce the histologic changes seen in CVID enteropathy. It remains un-known why this inflammatory lesion occurs in the first place.

Diagnosis

The work-up of GI complications of CVID often takes place on multiple occasions over time as symptoms are usually first epi-sodic but can eventually turn into chronic, progressive complaints. The cornerstone of diagnosis is the reliable evaluation of treatable infectious causes. This requires stool collection for as-say and culture techniques to detect bacterial (especially *Campylo-bacter*) and protozoal agents. In addition hydrogen breath testing can detect small intestinal bacterial overgrowth (SIBO) and so un-cover another antibiotic-responsive etiology of the symptoms.

Negative results for infectious causes require endoscopy for biopsy of the proximal small intestine and colon. Routine histol-ogy will detect the features of enteropathy including blunted villi and increased IELs that are often interpreted as celiac disease. However, unlike celiac disease, there usually is a lack of plasma cell infiltrate and crypt hyperplasia, as well as a preserved brush border and Goblet cells, and there is often an increase in epithe-lial cell apoptosis particularly in the colon.[69] In fact some of the villous changes in CVID enteropathy can be mimicked by SIBO, which should be investigated as above. If the diagnosis of celiac disease must be ruled out, then genetic testing for celiac suscep-tibility HLA alleles should be done; the absence of combinations of A and B alleles for DQ2 or DQ8 that confer risk will rule this out. However, even if celiac disease gene alleles are detected, it still does not indicate that this is a celiac or gluten-driven lesion, but will require a trial of gluten-free diet nonetheless. The functional significance of any histologic lesion in the small intestine can be evaluated by a measure of steatorrhea (fecal fat excretion) and small bowel absorption (d-xylose absorption test), values that can be used to track improvement following treatments (NB: not all appearances of villous blunting confers actual malabsorption).

Treatment

None of the GI complications of CVID are treated by administra-tion of intravenous immunoglobulin (IVIg), and in fact many oc-cur in patients who would be considered replete with IgG. Any detected bacterial or protozoal pathogens should be treated with a recommended course of conventional antibiotics. This includes *C. difficile* toxin-positive patients. SIBO should also be treated with any number of evidence-based courses of antibiotics, and recurrent SIBO may need to be treated with cycling antibiotic regimens.[70]

The treatment of the enteropathy is very challenging. While this seems to be a late complication in a subset of patients, it can be devastating and fatal. In the early stages it may be respon-sive to a short course of oral corticosteroids, either prednisone or even budesonide. Case reports attest to the efficacy of in-fliximab, but this cannot be routinely advised. It is possible that immunosuppressants can be used to control the inflamma-tory response underlying the small bowel mucosal damage, but this should only be done in a closely observed clinical setting, monitoring for infections. At all times the patient's nutritional status should be maintained, balanced calories as well as vita-mins and micronutrients, initially using the oral route but administering parenteral nutrition to complement oral nutri-tion and when oral feedings are not adequately absorbed and exacerbating the diarrhea.

The portal hypertension that can complicate CVID can come from the nodular regenerative hyperplasia; there is little fibrosis that occurs. In addition it needs to be established that the portal hypertension is not exacerbated by excessive splenic vein flow due to splenomegaly (induced by antibody-mediated autoim-mune cytopenias) that might be ameliorated by splenectomy if in fact the splenomegaly is not actually secondary to the portal hypertension. In any scenario, the management of such late complications requires an especially skilled team of internists, surgeons, and nutritionists.

CVID

- The majority of GI complications of CVID are infectious and generally do not respond to IVIg therapy (compared to sinopulmonary suppurative infections).
- CVID enteropathy is a rare immune-mediated complication of CVID that also does not respond to IVIg.
- CVID enteropathy is often confused with celiac disease due to similar villous damage on biopsy but additional features (lack of plasma cells, increased epithelial apoptosis, absence of celiac gene risk alleles) can help differentiate them.
- CVID enteropathy has no established therapy though judicious use of short courses of oral steroids or conventional immunosuppression may relieve the malabsorption and diarrhea temporarily.

Chronic granulomatous disease

Chronic granulomatous disease (CGD) results from defects in members of the NADPH oxidase complex, thereby diminishing the ability of phagocytic cells to produce the reactive oxygen species required to kill bacteria and fungi in phagosomes (Chapter 21). Multiple gene mutations have been found to contribute to the clinical phenotype including the most common, the X-linked recessive defect in *CYBB* encoding the gp91^{phox} unit of NADPH oxidase (affecting about 65% of CGD patients), and four autosomal recessive mutations in other NADPH oxidase subunits (*CYBA* gene encoding p22phox (<5%), *NCF1* encoding p47phox (about 30%), *NCF2* encoding p67phox (<5%), and *NCF4* encoding p40phox.[71] Commonly, CGD patients have recurrent infections of the skin and lungs, but nearly half develop gut inflammatory complications affecting the mouth to the anus. Interestingly, the frequency of GI disease in CGD is higher in the X-linked gp91^{phox} defect but the most recently described p40phox defect occurred in a young male patient who presented with granulomatous colitis alone.[72,73]

Presentation

The most common gastrointestinal complaints are abdominal pain and diarrhea (with or without rectal bleeding). Most frequently, GI symptoms begin in the first decade of life and can even precede the severe infections and diagnosis of CGD. While infectious diarrhea (especially *Salmonella* spp.) and antibiotic-associated colitis occur, an idiopathic granulomatous inflammatory disease causes site-specific symptoms: in the mouth, granulomatous stomatitis (coupled with conjunctivitis), ulcers and dental abscesses cause pain and difficulty feeding;[72,74] in the esophagus, dysphagia, chest pain, and vomiting can result from narrowing by strictures or stenosis (sometimes with proximal dilatation) and loss of motility related to granulomatous inflammation and fibrosis; in the stomach, loss of motility and capacity due to thickened walls and narrowed lumen, especially in the antrum, leads to vomiting (as in gastric outlet obstruction), epigastric pain, and weight loss due to feeding difficulty; in the small and large intestine, diarrhea (including protein losing enteropathy), bowel obstruction (pain and vomiting), rectal bleeding and tenesmus can reflect the presence of active colitis/enteritis with mucosal ulceration, large granulomata compromising the size of the lumen, and the presence of anal fissures and perianal abscesses. In addition, due to the transmural nature of the granulomatous inflammation, penetrating complications such as fistulae and abscesses can occur. Feeding difficulties

and the chronic inflammatory state itself predispose to growth delay that often afflicts the pediatric CGD patient.

Hepatic abscesses represent another frequent complication in CGD[72,75] occurring in up to 45% of patients. These patients most often present with fever, as well as abdominal pain, fatigue, and, less often, abdominal tenderness and hepatomegaly on exam. The sedimentation rate and alkaline phosphatase level are elevated in half of affected patients. However, a high level of suspicion, especially in the setting of fever with or without abdominal pain, should instigate a search for hepatic abscess.

Immune pathophysiology

Given the difficulty of phagocytic cells in killing ingested bacterial and fungal organisms, pathogens and possibly commensals, it is thought that the exuberant granulomatous response is due to delayed antigenic clearance or persistent infection. In this way granulomata continue to multiply and grow as other mechanisms that normally deal with the microbes or induced by cytokines are stimulated. This process of granulomatous inflammation is most evident in tissues rich in macrophages and reticulo-endothelial cells such as the lamina propria, liver, lymph nodes and spleen.

Diagnosis

The symptoms and signs will dictate the initial diagnostic exams. For diarrheal complaints, stool culture and examination for *C. difficile* toxin are required; in the setting of hypoalbuminemia, fractional fecal excretion of α_1-antitrypsin (> 50 mg/24 hour) can detect protein-losing enteropathy due either to diffuse mucosal inflammation or lymphangiectasia. For complaints of dysphagia, vomiting, or epigastric pain, upper endoscopy is required to document macroscopic and microscopic involvement with granulomatous inflammation by imaging and histology. Radiological studies using oral contrast can be helpful in showing narrowing, strictures, and motility and mucosal abnormalities of the esophagus and stomach but cannot provide for histologic confirmation. However, radiologic imaging studies may be the primary diagnostic tools to evaluate obstructive symptoms coming from the small intestine, including barium small bowel studies and CT enterography. Images may show lumen narrowing, bowel wall thickening, mucosal abnormalities including ulceration, and penetrating complications such as fistulization. Finally, for lower abdominal and perianal pain and rectal bleeding, anoscopy, colonoscopy and pelvic CT or MR will help diagnose granulomatous inflammation of the colon and its complications including perirectal and perianal abscesses. In the case of hepatic abscess detection (generally 1–6 cm), CT, MR, and ultrasound have been reported to have similar sensitivity, around 60%.[75] Active abscesses appear to be solid, hypoechoic lesions on ultrasound and post-contrast ring-enhancing lesions on CT and MR images.

The gastrointestinal histologic diagnosis hinges on the presence of non-caseating granulomata, both gross and microscopic. These granulomata are often seen against a background of acute inflammation (acute focal colitis, crypt abscesses, cryptitis) and chronic inflammation (lymphocytic infiltrate, Paneth cell metaplasia in the colon) that can be mild to severe. The histologic picture may resemble Crohn's disease except that the granulomata of CGD are well-defined, often large collections of epithelioid histiocytes that can expand the mucosa and even deform the overlying epithelium to make it look flattened in the case of the villous mucosa of the small intestine. Like Crohn's disease, the inflammation can affect the three layers of the gut wall, but unlike Crohn's disease CGD biopsies also show prominent lipid-laden macrophages that have PAS-positive cytoplasmic granules.

Treatment

Current clinical practice for CGD includes using prophylactic antimicrobials to prevent infections, typically trimethoprim-sulfamethoxazole for bacterial and itraconazole for fungal infections. Some clinicians also use IFN-γ to prevent infections, although this is not a universal practice.[76] Obviously, discovery of potential infectious etiologies of diarrhea should be treated appropriately.

Once infections are ruled out and granulomatous inflammation of the GI tract is established, with or without complications such as stricturing of the bowel, treatment with corticosteroids is indicated; beginning doses up to 1 mg/kg/day tapering over 12 to 20 weeks to maintenance doses of 2.5–5 mg on alternate days has been reported to induce rapid improvement in symptoms. Use of sulfasalazine for colitis may have limited benefit for some patients. Isolated reports of successful use of cyclosporine and infliximab are best reserved for refractory cases due to the potential for infectious side effects. Similarly both G-CSF and GM-CSF have been used with therapeutic benefit for CGD GI complications, because of their success in the granulomatous colitis of glycogen-1-β storage disease.[77,78] Though there are no data to suggest that IFN-γ worsens established disease, it also may not prevent it as over 40% of one cohort developed GI manifestations of granulomatous inflammation after starting it; on the other hand, isolated reports attribute improvement of GI inflammation to IFNγ.[79,80] Finally, it cannot be overstated that surgical drainage of complicating abscesses and resection of fibrotic or refractory strictures needs to be pursued when indicated. While there can be considerable postoperative complications due to ongoing fistula formation and wound breakdown, this may be managed by administration of corticosteroids. In addition judicious use of endoscopic therapy to dilate narrowed esophageal or pyloric regions is an option for symptomatic strictures.

Treatment of hepatic abscesses typically requires diligent, often repeated surgical debridement and long-term parenteral antibiotics, usually beyond 8 weeks. Few patients can be managed with antibiotics alone, although antibiotics alone likely treat small abscesses below the limit of radiographic detection (possibly discovered by intraoperative ultrasonography). Percutaneous aspiration of hepatic abscesses may be attempted pre-operatively to identify an organism, but empiric antibiotics can be started until a surgical specimen can be sent for culture (up to 60% yield on isolates). The surgical management is quite different from suppurative hepatic abscesses in immunocompetent patients and the operating surgeon needs to be aware of the specialized approach.[75]

● KEY CONCEPTS

CGD

- Half of CGD patients develop GI involvement with granulomatous inflammation
- Symptoms are due to both obstructive complications of stricture formation and mucosal inflammation.
- A resemblance to Crohn's disease is suggested by the granulomatous inflammation, the transmural bowel involvement, and underlying innate immune defect, but unlike Crohn's there are also prominent skin and lung infections and PAS-positive lipid-laden macrophages in the lamina propria.
- Complicated hepatic abscesses require specialized medical and surgical intervention.

● ON THE HORIZON

- Post-hematopoietic stem cell transplantation with immune reconstitution follow-up regarding resolution of bowel disease.
- Gene therapy to correct defect on CGD and follow-on improvement in GI complications.

GI complications occurring in other primary immunodeficiency states

Severe combined immunodeficiency covers a wide phenotype of low to absent T cells, NK cells, and dysfunctional B cells reflecting the mechanisms of the genetic defect: IL2RG in X-linked SCID, adenosine deaminase deficiency, RAG-1 and RAG-2 mutations preventing V(D)J recombination in Omenn syndrome, JAK3 kinase, Artemis/DCLRE1C also preventing V(D)J recombination and global DNA repair, as well as defects involving CD45, ZAP70, and IL-7Rα among others (Chapter 35). Recurrent infectious diarrhea and thrush are common before a diagnosis of SCID in newborns and neonates.[81] After a diagnosis and treatment with bone marrow transplantation, gastrointestinal graft-versus-host disease is not uncommon.

The rare X-linked recessive Wiskott–Aldrich syndrome results from WASP protein gene mutations, a signaling protein largely restricted to hematopoietic cells, and leads to a syndrome of eczema, thrombocytopenia, and infections related to combined immunodeficiency (impaired antibody responses and T-cell function). An interesting aspect of the gut complication in this immunodeficiency is that patients can develop a noninfectious colitis resembling ulcerative colitis with confluent mucosal inflammation with ulceration, crypt abscesses and no granulomata plus bleeding exacerbated by the thrombocytopenia.[82] Patients can respond to mesalamine drugs but use of steroids and immunosuppressive must be done cautiously due to exacerbating infection risk. Successful bone marrow transplantation can treat the colitis as well.

The hyper-IgM syndrome (type 1) is an X-linked condition resulting from mutations in CD40 ligand leading to defective antibody class switching (Chapter 34). Cryptosporidial infectious diarrhea is seen, and sclerosing cholangitis, cirrhosis and neoplasms of the hepatobiliary system complicate the course in teenagers and young adults.[83] Rarely non-infectious colitis has been reported. Bone marrow transplant, preferably performed before chronic complications occur, is the only potential for cure.

Lastly the immune dysregulation, polyendocrinopathy, enteropathy, X-linked (IPEX) syndrome is interesting in that it results from a defect in FOXP3 expression and function thereby inhibiting the suppressive effect of regulatory T cells (Chapter 35). In this case, rather than an immunodeficiency there is a lack of regulation and enhanced immune responses occur. The gut mucosa is a major site affected by inflammation, and this complication presents with a watery, sometimes bloody diarrhea and malabsorption. Biopsies show villous blunting and atrophy, increased intraepithelial lymphocytes, lamina propria infiltration with T cells, eosinophils, and neutrophils.[84] Treatment requires bone marrow transplantation, but the gut disease may be managed temporarily with corticosteroids and immunosuppressants.

References

1. Toh BH, van Driel IR, Gleeson PA. Pernicious anemia. N Engl J Med 1997; 337:1441–8.
2. Lahner E, Annibale B. Pernicious anemia: new insights from a gastroenterological point of view. World J Gastroenterol 2009;15:5121–8.

3. Lahner E, Norman GL, Severi C, et al. Reassessment of intrinsic factor and parietal cell autoantibodies in atrophic gastritis with respect to cobalamin deficiency. Am J Gastroenterol 2009;104:2071–9.

4. Amedei A, Bergman MP, Appelmelk BJ, et al. Molecular mimicry between *Helicobacter pylori* antigens and H+, K+-adenosine triphosphatase in human gastric autoimmunity. J Exp Med 2003;198:1147–56.

5. Claeys D, Faller G, Appelmelk BJ, et al. The gastric H+, K+-ATPase is a major autoantigen in chronic *Helicobacter pylori* gastritis with body mucosa atrophy. Gastroenterology 1998;115:340–7.

6. Schistosomes, liver flukes and *Helicobacter pylori*. IARC Working Group on the Evaluation of Carcinogenic Risks to Humans. Lyon, 7–14 June 1994. IARC Monogr Eval Carcinog Risks Hum 1994;61:1–241.

7. Ernst PB, Peura DA, Crowe SE. The translation of Helicobacter pylori basic research to patient care. Gastroenterology 2006;130:188–206; quiz 212–213.

8. Fukuda Y, Bamba H, Okui M, et al. *Helicobacter pylori* infection increases mucosal permeability of the stomach and intestine. Digestion 2001;63(Suppl. 1):93–6.

9. Atherton JC. *H. pylori* virulence factors. Br Med Bull 1998;54:105–20.

10. Egan BJ, Holmes K, O'Connor HJ, et al. *Helicobacter pylori* gastritis, the unifying concept for gastric diseases. Helicobacter 2007;12(Suppl. 2):39–44.

11. Sepulveda AR, Patil M. Practical approach to the pathologic diagnosis of gastritis. Arch Pathol Lab Med 2008;132:1586–93.

12. Chey WD, Wong BC. American College of Gastroenterology guideline on the management of *Helicobacter pylori* infection. Am J Gastroenterol 2007;102:1808–25.

13. Fock KM, Katelaris P, Sugano K, et al. Second Asia-Pacific Consensus Guidelines for *Helicobacter pylori* infection. J Gastroenterol Hepatol 2009;24:1587–600.

14. Chand N, Mihas AA. Celiac disease: current concepts in diagnosis and treatment. J Clin Gastroenterol 2006;40:3–14.

15. Fasano A. Systemic autoimmune disorders in celiac disease. Curr Opin Gastroenterol 2006;22:674–9.

16. Fasano A, Berti I, Gerarduzzi T, et al. Prevalence of celiac disease in at-risk and not-at-risk groups in the United States: a large multicenter study. Arch Intern Med 2003;163:286–92.

17. Abadie V, Sollid LM, Barreiro LB, Jabri B. Integration of genetic and immunological insights into a model of celiac disease pathogenesis. Annu Rev Immunol 2011;29:493–525.

18. Ensari A. Gluten-sensitive enteropathy (celiac disease): controversies in diagnosis and classification. Arch Pathol Lab Med 2010;134:826–36.

19. Leffler DA, Schuppan D. Update on serologic testing in celiac disease. Am J Gastroenterol 2010;105:2520–4.

20. Troncone R, Jabri B. Coeliac disease and gluten sensitivity. J Intern Med 2011;269:582–90.

21. Sands BE. From symptom to diagnosis: clinical distinctions among various forms of intestinal inflammation. Gastroenterology 2004;126:1518–32.

22. Loftus Jr EV. Clinical epidemiology of inflammatory bowel disease: Incidence, prevalence, and environmental influences. Gastroenterology 2004;126:1504–17.

23. Hou JK, El-Serag H, Thirumurthi S. Distribution and manifestations of inflammatory bowel disease in Asians, Hispanics, and African Americans: a systematic review. Am J Gastroenterol 2009;104:2100–9.

24. Mahid SS, Mulhall AM, Gholson RD, et al. Inflammatory bowel disease and African Americans: a systematic review. Inflamm Bowel Dis 2008;14:960–7.

25. Cho JH, Brant SR. Recent insights into the genetics of inflammatory bowel disease. Gastroenterology 2011;140:1704–12.

26. Cosnes J, Cattan S, Blain A, et al. Long-term evolution of disease behavior of Crohn's disease. Inflamm Bowel Dis 2002;8:244–50.

27. Liu Z, Geboes K, Heremans H, et al. Role of interleukin-12 in the induction of mucosal inflammation and abrogation of regulatory T cell function in chronic experimental colitis. Eur J Immunol 2001;31:1550–60.

28. Simpson SJ, Shah S, Comiskey M, et al. T cell-mediated pathology in two models of experimental colitis depends predominantly on the interleukin 12/Signal transducer and activator of transcription (Stat)-4 pathway, but is not conditional on interferon gamma expression by T cells. J Exp Med 1998;187:1225–34.

29. Neurath MF, Fuss I, Kelsall BL, et al. Antibodies to interleukin 12 abrogate established experimental colitis in mice. J Exp Med 1995;182:1281–90.

30. McGeachy MJ, Chen Y, Tato CM, et al. The interleukin 23 receptor is essential for the terminal differentiation of interleukin 17-producing effector T helper cells in vivo. Nat Immunol 2009;10:314–24.

31. Uhlig HH, McKenzie BS, Hue S, et al. Differential activity of IL-12 and IL-23 in mucosal and systemic innate immune pathology. Immunity 2006;25:309–18.

32. Yen D, Cheung J, Scheerens H, et al. IL-23 is essential for T cell-mediated colitis and promotes inflammation via IL-17 and IL-6. J Clin Invest 2006;116:1310–6.

33. Powrie F, Leach MW, Mauze S, et al. Inhibition of Th1 responses prevents inflammatory bowel disease in scid mice reconstituted with CD45RBhi CD4+ T cells. Immunity 1994;1:553–62.

34. Becker C, Dornhoff H, Neufert C, et al. Cutting edge: IL-23 cross-regulates IL-12 production in T cell-dependent experimental colitis. J Immunol 2006;177:2760–4.

35. O'Connor Jr W, Kamanaka M, Booth CJ, et al. A protective function for interleukin 17A in T cell-mediated intestinal inflammation. Nat Immunol 2009;10:603–9.

36. Fujino S, Andoh A, Bamba S, et al. Increased expression of interleukin 17 in inflammatory bowel disease. Gut 2003;52:65–70.

37. Fuss IJ, Becker C, Yang Z, et al. Both IL-12p70 and IL-23 are synthesized during active Crohn's disease and are down-regulated by treatment with anti-IL-12 p40 monoclonal antibody. Inflamm Bowel Dis 2006;12:9–15.

38. Kuballa P, Huett A, Rioux JD, et al. Impaired autophagy of an intracellular pathogen induced by a Crohn's disease associated ATG16L1 variant. PLoS One 2008;3:e3391.

39. Joossens M, Huys G, Cnockaert M, et al. Dysbiosis of the faecal microbiota in patients with Crohn's disease and their unaffected relatives. Gut 2011;60(5):631–7.

40. Sokol H, Pigneur B, Watterlot L, et al. Faecalibacterium prausnitzii is an anti-inflammatory commensal bacterium identified by gut microbiota analysis of Crohn disease patients. Proc Natl Acad Sci U S A 2008;105:16731–6.

41. Reese GE, Constantinides VA, Simillis C, et al. Diagnostic precision of anti-Saccharomyces cerevisiae antibodies and perinuclear antineutrophil cytoplasmic antibodies in inflammatory bowel disease. Am J Gastroenterol 2006;101:2410–22.

42. Baumgart DC, Sandborn WJ. Inflammatory bowel disease: clinical aspects and established and evolving therapies. Lancet 2007;369:1641–57.

43. Colombel JF, Sandborn WJ, Reinisch W, et al. Infliximab, azathioprine, or combination therapy for Crohn's disease. N Engl J Med 2010;362:1383–95.

44. Triantafillidis JK, Nasioulas G, Kosmidis PA. Colorectal cancer and inflammatory bowel disease: epidemiology, risk factors, mechanisms of carcinogenesis and prevention strategies. Anticancer Res 2009;29:2727–37.

45. Farmer RG, Easley KA, Rankin GB. Clinical patterns, natural history, and progression of ulcerative colitis. A long-term follow-up of 1116 patients. Dig Dis Sci 1993;38:1137–46.

46. Kethu SR. Extraintestinal manifestations of inflammatory bowel diseases. J Clin Gastroenterol 2006;40:467–75.

47. Mielants H, Veys EM, Cuvelier C, De Vos M. Course of gut inflammation in spondylarthropathies and therapeutic consequences. Baillieres Clin Rheumatol 1996;10:147–64.

48. Loftus Jr EV, Harewood GC, Loftus CG, et al. PSC-IBD: a unique form of inflammatory bowel disease associated with primary sclerosing cholangitis. Gut 2005;54:91–6.

49. Eaden JA, Abrams KR, Mayberry JF. The risk of colorectal cancer in ulcerative colitis: a meta-analysis. Gut 2001;48:526–35.

50. Fuss IJ, Strober W. The role of IL-13 and NK T cells in experimental and human ulcerative colitis. Mucosal Immunol 2008;1(Suppl. 1):S31–3.

51. Heller F, Fuss IJ, Nieuwenhuis EE, et al. Oxazolone colitis, a Th2 colitis model resembling ulcerative colitis, is mediated by IL-13-producing NK-T cells. Immunity 2002;17:629–38.

52. Fuss IJ, Heller F, Boirivant M, et al. Nonclassical CD1d-restricted NK T cells that produce IL-13 characterize an atypical Th2 response in ulcerative colitis. J Clin Invest 2004;113:1490–7.

53. Heller F, Florian P, Bojarski C, et al. Interleukin-13 is the key effector Th2 cytokine in ulcerative colitis that affects epithelial tight junctions, apoptosis, and cell restitution. Gastroenterology 2005;129:550–64.

54. Stokkers PC, Reitsma PH, Tytgat GN, van Deventer SJ. HLA-DR and -DQ phenotypes in inflammatory bowel disease: a meta-analysis. Gut 1999;45:395–401.

55. Kornbluth A, Sachar DB. Ulcerative colitis practice guidelines in adults: American College Of Gastroenterology, Practice Parameters Committee. Am J Gastroenterol 2010;105:501–23; quiz 524.

56. Kao KT, Pedraza BA, McClune AC, et al. Microscopic colitis: a large retrospective analysis from a health maintenance organization experience. World J Gastroenterol 2009;15:3122–7.

57. Wolber R, Owen D, Freeman H. Colonic lymphocytosis in patients with celiac sprue. Hum Pathol 1990;21:1092–6.

58. Beaugerie L, Pardi DS. Review article: drug-induced microscopic colitis - proposal for a scoring system and review of the literature. Aliment Pharmacol Ther 2005;22:277–84.

59. Pardi DS, Kelly CP. Microscopic colitis. Gastroenterology 2011;140:1155–65.

60. Furuta GT, Liacouras CA, Collins MH, et al. Eosinophilic esophagitis in children and adults: a systematic review and consensus recommendations for diagnosis and treatment. Gastroenterology 2007;133:1342–63.

61. Noel RJ, Putnam PE, Rothenberg ME. Eosinophilic esophagitis. N Engl J Med 2004;351:940–1.

62. Rothenberg ME. Biology and treatment of eosinophilic esophagitis. Gastroenterology 2009;137:1238–49.

63. Nurko S, Rosen R. Esophageal dysmotility in patients who have eosinophilic esophagitis. Gastrointest Endosc Clin N Am 2008;18:73–89; ix.

64. Sherrill JD, Rothenberg ME. Genetic dissection of eosinophilic esophagitis provides insight into disease pathogenesis and treatment strategies. J Allergy Clin Immunol 2011;128:23–32; quiz 33–34.

65. Spergel JM, Brown-Whitehorn T, Beausoleil JL, et al. Predictive values for skin prick test and atopy patch test for eosinophilic esophagitis. J Allergy Clin Immunol 2007;119:509–11.

66. Park MA, Li JT, Hagan JB, et al. Common variable immunodeficiency: a new look at an old disease. Lancet 2008;372:489–502.

67. Malamut G, Verkarre V, Suarez F, et al. The enteropathy associated with common variable immunodeficiency: the delineated frontiers with celiac disease. Am J Gastroenterol 2010;105:2262–75.

68. Mannon PJ, Fuss IJ, Dill S, et al. Excess IL-12 but not IL-23 accompanies the inflammatory bowel disease associated with common variable immunodeficiency. Gastroenterology 2006;131:748–56.

69. Washington K, Stenzel TT, Buckley RH, Gottfried MR. Gastrointestinal pathology in patients with common variable immunodeficiency and X-linked agammaglobulinemia. Am J Surg Pathol 1996;20:1240–52.

70. Cunningham-Rundles C, How I. treat common variable immune deficiency. Blood 2010;116:7–15.

71. Matute JD, Arias AA, Wright NA, et al. A new genetic subgroup of chronic granulomatous disease with autosomal recessive mutations in p40 phox and selective defects in neutrophil NADPH oxidase activity. Blood 2009;114:3309–15.

72. Barton LL, Moussa SL, Villar RG, Hulett RL. Gastrointestinal complications of chronic granulomatous disease: case report and literature review. Clin Pediatr (Phila) 1998;37:231–6.

73. Marciano BE, Rosenzweig SD, Kleiner DE, et al. Gastrointestinal involvement in chronic granulomatous disease. Pediatrics 2004;114:462–8.

74. Wysocki GP, Brooke RI. Oral manifestations of chronic granulomatous disease. Oral Surg Oral Med Oral Pathol 1978;46:815–9.

75. Lublin M, Bartlett DL, Danforth DN, et al. Hepatic abscess in patients with chronic granulomatous disease. Ann Surg 2002;235:383–91.

76. Marciano BE, Wesley R, De Carlo ES, et al. Long-term interferon-gamma therapy for patients with chronic granulomatous disease. Clin Infect Dis 2004;39:692–9.

77. Huang A, Abbasakoor F, Vaizey CJ. Gastrointestinal manifestations of chronic granulomatous disease. Colorectal Dis 2006;8:637–44.

78. Wang J, Mayer L, Cunningham-Rundles C. Use of GM-CSF in the treatment of colitis associated with chronic granulomatous disease. J Allergy Clin Immunol 2005;115:1092–4.

79. Born M, Willinek WA, Hassan C. Gastric outlet obstruction in chronic granulomatous disease. Z Gastroenterol 2002;40:511–6 [in German].

80. Hague RA, Eastham EJ, Lee RE, Cant AJ. Resolution of hepatic abscess after interferon gamma in chronic granulomatous disease. Arch Dis Child 1993;69:443–5.

81. Buckley RH. Primary cellular immunodeficiencies. J Allergy Clin Immunol 2002;109:747–57.

82. Hsieh KH, Chang MH, Lee CY, Wang CY. Wiskott-Aldrich syndrome and inflammatory bowel disease. Ann Allergy 1988;60:429–31.

83. Winkelstein JA, Marino MC, Ochs H, et al. The X-linked hyper-IgM syndrome: clinical and immunologic features of 79 patients. Medicine (Baltimore) 2003;82: 373–384.

84. Patey-Mariaud de Serre N, Canioni D, Ganousse S, et al. Digestive histopathological presentation of IPEX syndrome. Mod Pathol 2009;22:95–102.

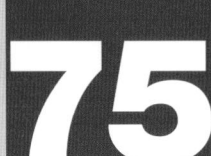
Carlo Selmi,
Michael P.
Manns, M. Eric
Gershwin

Inflammatory hepatobiliary diseases

Inflammatory hepatobiliary disease is a generic term that comprises conditions presenting a complex noninfectious etiopathogenesis characterized by chronic inflammatory infiltrate and autoimmune features. Among these, the main distinction is based on the target tissue, whether this is the hepatocyte (as in the case of autoimmune hepatitis (AIH)) or the bile duct cell (intrahepatic small and medium sized in the case of primary biliary cirrhosis (PBC) or any level in the case of primary sclerosing cholangitis (PSC)). In between, there is a series of conditions sharing characteristics of both groups coined overlap syndromes with unique features as to clinical management. Regardless of the subgroup, all conditions eventually lead to liver cirrhosis and ultimately liver failure; however, progression rates vary widely and are likely determined by unknown genetic factors while intermediate complications and putative pathogenetic mechanisms are quite common to these conditions.[1,2]

KEY CONCEPTS

Inflammatory hepatobiliary diseases

- An autoimmune pathogenesis is recognized for autoimmune hepatitis, reasonably implied for primary biliary cirrhosis, and suggested for primary sclerosing cholangitis.

- In all cases, the etiology remains enigmatic, although the roles of genetic susceptibility and environmental factors are well established and genome-wide association studies have recently been completed for PBC and PSC.

- The diagnosis of autoimmune hepatitis, primary sclerosing cholangitis, and primary biliary cirrhosis is based on criteria comprising clinical, imaging, and histological factors.

- Overlap syndromes can ensue between the diseases and with autoimmune pancreatitis, possibly modifying the natural history and the therapy approach.

Autoimmune hepatitis

Clinical features and diagnostic challenge

AIH is a chronic disease of unknown etiology resulting from the immune-mediated destruction of hepatocytes secondary to a loss of immune tolerance against liver tissues.[3] AIH's major features[4] include striking female predominance, presence of hypergammaglobulinemia, significant association with the HLA alleles DR3 and DR4, good clinical response to steroids and other immunosuppressive treatments, and detection of serum autoantibodies. In some cases, the diagnosis can be challenging due to the presence of confounding factors or features mimicking other conditions. For these reasons, a scoring system has been developed to account for all criteria that influence the likelihood of AIH diagnosis. The system, first introduced in 1992 and then modified in 1999, is a practical tool for clinical management and allows a high sensitivity and specificity in the diagnosis (Table 75.1). Factors taken into account in this system include sex, plasma biochemical variables, serum autoantibodies, liver histology, possible co-factors (drugs, alcohol, viruses), and response to medical treatment. The sum of all factors produces a score to be used for determining the likelihood of the AIH diagnosis either prior to or after medical treatment; in particular, a score >15 prior to therapy or >17 after treatment is associated with a definite diagnosis of AIH while scores in the 10–15 (pre-treatment) or 12–17 (post-treatment) ranges characterize a probable case. The 1992 version of the scoring system allowed high sensitivity (89%) with a relatively low specificity, particularly in cases of chronic hepatitis C with autoimmune features (80%) or chronic cholestatic liver diseases (61%). The revised 1999 criteria appear to give a better distinction between PSC and AIH; however, conflicting data support the need for prospective validation studies.

AIH is a rare disease estimated to have a prevalence of 170/million persons in Europe. It affects women of any age more commonly than men, but the female-to-male ratio in AIH is lower compared to PBC. The onset is typically indolent and asymptomatic. Individuals diagnosed with AIH following a screening examination currently represent the majority of cases. On the other hand, if symptoms are present at diagnosis, these are nonspecific or secondary to end-stage liver disease (jaundice, pruritus, ascites, upper digestive bleeding).

CLINICAL PEARLS

Autoimmune hepatitis

- Autoimmune hepatitis is most commonly diagnosed in symptomless patients during routine blood work.
- A scoring system is available to make the diagnosis of autoimmune hepatitis likely or definitive.
- Several types of serum autoantibodies can be detected, in some cases with high specificity.
- Three types are recognized based on clinical, epidemiological, and serological characteristics.

Blood tests

Plasma biochemical evaluation commonly reveals a frank elevation of aminotransferases often accompanied by a cholestatic pattern

Table 75.1 Revised 1999 diagnostic scoring system for autoimmune hepatitis (AIH)

Parameters/features	Score
Female sex	+2
Alkaline phosphatase (ALP)/aspartate aminotransferase (or alanine aminotransferase) ratio	
< 1.5	+2
1.5–3.0	0
> 3.0	−2
Serum globulins or immunoglobulin G above normal	
> 2.0	+3
1.5–2.0	+2
1.0–1.5	+1
< 1.0	0
Antinuclear antibody, SMA, or LKM1	
> 1:80	+3
1:80	+2
1:40	+1
< 1:40	0
AMA-positive	−4
Hepatitis virus markers	
Positive	−3
Negative	+3
Drug history	
Positive	−4
Negative	+1
Average alcohol intake	
< 25 g/day	+2
> 60 g/day	−2
Liver histology	
Interface hepatitis	+3
Predominantly lymphoplasmacytoid infiltrate	+1
Rosetting of liver cells	+1
None of the above	−5
Biliary changes	−3
Other changes	−3
Other autoimmune diseases	+2
Optional additional parameters	
Other defined autoantibodies	+2
Human leukocyte antigen (HLA) DR3 or DR4	+1
Response to therapy	
Complete	+2
Relapse	+3

A score > 15 or > 17 indicates a definite diagnosis of AIH pre- or post-treatment, respectively. On the other hand, scores between 10 and 15, and 12 and 17 indicate a probable diagnosis, pre- or post-therapy, respectively. AMA, anti-mitochondrial autoantibodies; LKM-1, anti-liver–kidney microsomal antibodies; SMA, anti-smooth-muscle antibodies.

Table 75.2 Synopsis comparing clinical, serological, epidemiological, and genetic characteristics of autoimmune hepatitis (AIH) subtypes

Clinical features	Type 1	Type 2	Type 3
Diagnostic antibodies	SMA, ANA Anti-actin	Anti-LKM P450 IID6	Anti-soluble liver–kidney Ag, AK 8, CK18
Age (years)	Bimodal (10–20, 45–70)	Pediatric (2–14)	Adults (30–50)
Women (%)	78	89	90
Autoimmune comorbidity (%)	41	34	58
Gamma-globulin ↑	+++	+	++
Immunoglobulin A ↓	No	Occasional	No
Human leukocyte antigen (HLA) association	B8, DR3, DR4	B14, DR3, C4AQ0	Uncertain
Steroid response	+++	++	+++
Progression to cirrhosis (%)	45	82	75

Ag, antigens; ANA, antinuclear antibodies; Ig, immunoglobulin; LKM, anti-liver–kidney microsomal antibodies; SMA, anti-smooth-muscle antibodies.

scoring system. Furthermore, serum globulins, particularly of the γ type, are commonly increased in AIH cases regardless of the histological stage. Lastly and most importantly, serum autoantibodies are invariably positive (defined as titer ≥1:80) in patients with AIH and allow a finer distinction of the three disease subtypes. In fact, type I is characterized by the presence of antinuclear (ANA) and/or anti-smooth-muscle (SMA, directed against actin) autoantibodies, type II by anti-liver–kidney microsomal antibodies (LKM-1, directed at cytochrome P450 2D6 or UDP-glucuronosyltransferases), and type III by autoantibodies against soluble liver antigens (SLA/LP). Apart from antibody patterns, these three subtypes are associated with other important clinical, epidemiological, and biochemical differences, as presented in Table 75.2.

Liver histology

The role of liver histology in the management of AIH remains critical and all suspect cases should undergo a liver biopsy. In fact, although no typical feature can be sufficient to prove the diagnosis, histology remains the gold standard for grading and staging, particularly to determine the response to therapy. Common findings include periportal hepatitis with lymphocyte and plasma cell infiltrate and piecemeal necrosis. Fibrosis is usually observed and bridging necrosis ultimately indicates advanced disease evolving into frank cirrhosis. Importantly, the presence of granulomas, bile duct damage, or iron or copper accumulation should not be overlooked since these signs point towards other diagnoses. On the other hand, steatosis is a nonspecific finding that does not rule out AIH.

Serum autoantibodies

In 2004, the International Autoimmune Hepatitis Group established procedures and reference guidelines for more reliable serum autoantibody testing to overcome the lack of

(increased alkaline phosphatase, bilirubin). It is of note, however, that a ratio between the elevations of alkaline phosphatase and either transaminases > 3 is considered indicative of chronic cholestatic disease and not of AIH, as also represented in the proposed standardization.[5] In fact, routine tests for serum ANA, SMA, and LKM are critical in the diagnosis of AIH, as indicated by the diagnostic scoring system (Table 75.1). Other sets of autoantibodies should also be tested in suspected cases and include those against liver-cytosol type 1 (LC1), perinuclear anti-neutrophil cytoplasmic antibodies (pANCA), SLA/LP, and the asialoglycoprotein receptor. Finally, other less specific autoantibodies are also detected in a subgroup of patients, i.e., antibodies against cardiolipin, chromatin, and Saccharomyces cerevisiae, but are of limited clinical impact.

Antibodies to nuclear antigens

ANA were the first autoantibodies observed in AIH sera over 50 years ago and remain the most sensitive marker of AIH, most frequently producing a homogeneous or speckled pattern. The test is not specific for AIH, since ANA positivity is not uncommon in sera from patients with viral or other autoimmune liver diseases, as well as in as many as 15% of healthy subjects. This latter percentage has recently been reduced by abandoning Hep2 cells as a substrate for indirect immunofluorescence, which remains the most widely used ANA screening method. The nature of AIH-associated ANA autoantigens is incompletely understood; these include centromers, ribonucleoproteins, cyclin A, histones, and other antigens. Similar to most autoantibodies, ANA positivity, pattern, or titer does not reflect different AIH phenotypes nor can they predict the disease's course.

Antibodies to smooth-muscle antigen

Serum SMA react with different proteins (actin, tubulin, vimentin, desmin, cytokeratins) of the cytoskeletal components (microfilaments, microtubuli, intermediate filaments). Their presence characterizes both autoimmune (type 1 AIH, celiac disease) and viral diseases (chronic hepatitis C, infectious mononucleosis). When detected at titers >1:80, they are considered a sensitive marker for type 1 AIH, being found in up to 80% of cases. Within the spectrum of SMA, anti-actin antibodies are the most specific for the diagnosis of type 1 AIH. At present, immunomorphological techniques are still the gold standard for SMA testing; recently, however, new immunochemical tests with purified antigens have been demonstrated to be reliable. A pathogenic role for SMA in AIH has not been demonstrated and, to date, this is still controversial. Finally, SMA-positive type 1 AIH sera also frequently react by counterimmunoelectrophoresis with an unknown antigen, provisionally called XR1, which is present in the heterogeneous antigenic "cocktail" derived from the aqueous extract of rabbit thymus that is currently used to detect antibodies to extractable nuclear antigens.

Autoantibodies to liver–kidney microsomal antigens

Autoantibodies against microsomal proteins form a heterogeneous group and are associated with several immune-mediated diseases, including AIH and drug-induced hepatitis. Serum autoantibodies against LKM-1 are the main serological markers of type 2 AIH and recognize the proximal renal tubule and hepatocellular cytoplasm. The 50-kDa autoantigen was identified as the cytochrome P450 2D6 (CYP2D6). Interestingly, the sequence between amino acids 316 and 327, which is most likely exposed on the surface of the molecule, appears to be a region capable of differentiating LKM-1 activity in AIH and hepatitis C virus and may represent a key target for autoimmunity. The mechanisms of onset remain enigmatic and solid evidence of a causative role of hepatitis C virus cross-reactivity is still awaited. Similarly, the

pathogenic role of anti-LKM-1 and their prognostic significance are debated, despite the development of type 2 AIH animal models following immunization with human CYP2D6 or with adenoviruses in mice transgenic for human CYP2D6. Finally, two other types of serum anti-LKM have been described in patients with ticrynafen-associated hepatitis (anti-LKM-2, directed against CYP2C9) and in 10% of patients with type 2 AIH (anti-LKM-3, directed against UGT1A), either alone or in combination with LKM-1 antibodies.

Autoantibodies to soluble liver antigen/liver pancreas antigen

Anti-SLA/LP antibodies are detectable by radioimmunoassay and enzyme-linked immunosorbent assay but not by immunofluorescence and are directed against different epitopes of a UGA tRNA suppressor. Serum anti-SLA/LP antibodies are occasionally found in patients with AIH who are negative for ANA, SMA, or anti-LKM and are cumulatively detected in 10–30% of cases of type 1 and type 2 AIH. Recent data indicate that anti-SLA/LP antibodies are also detectable in subgroups of pediatric patients with autoimmune cholangitis or adult patients with hepatitis C virus infection when tested with sensitive methods.

Antibodies to liver-cytosol type 1

Anti-LC1 antibodies are detected by indirect immunofluorescence in sera from up to 50% of patients with type 2 AIH and less frequently in type 1 AIH or chronic hepatitis C. Importantly, however, anti-LC1 are the only detectable markers in 10% of AIH cases.

The LC1 autoantigen is the liver formiminotransferase cyclodeaminase, an enzyme involved in folate metabolism. Interestingly, serum anti-LC1 antibodies correlate with AIH severity and progression.

Other autoantibodies

Antibodies to the asialoglycoprotein receptor are observed in up to 90% of all patients with AIH and often coexist with other autoantibodies while lacking specificity for the disease. Similar to anti-LC1, however, anti-asialoglycoprotein titers are associated with a more florid inflammatory disease activity and may change with treatment response.

Antibodies to neutrophil cytoplasmic antigens (pANCA) can be detected by indirect immunofluorescence in sera from patients with type 1 AIH but also in a subgroup of patients with PSC or chronic viral hepatitis.

Pathogenesis

Similar to most autoimmune diseases, the current hypothesis states that environmental factors trigger autoimmunity onset in genetically susceptible individuals. Several microorganisms, particularly viruses, have been suggested as triggers but sound evidence is lacking. The proposed mechanism is based on molecular mimicry between infectious agent epitopes and human liver antigens.[3] Most recently, experimental data suggested that $CD25^+$ T cells are quantitatively impaired in AIH thus suggesting that the expansion of this crucial regulatory pool may hold promise for the treatment of patients.[6]

From a genetic standpoint, AIH is considered a complex disease not following a strictly hereditary pattern.[4] In fact, conclusive data of a single genetic locus causing AIH onset have not been obtained and multiple genes are likely to contribute to disease susceptibility.

The best evidence for genetic risk in AIH comes from the study of major histocompatibility complex (MHC) alleles, critical molecules in the T-cell recognition process (Chapters 5, 6) while we wait for genome-wide association studies in this rare condition. Data from Caucasian patients in northern Europe and the USA reported an association with HLA DRB1*0301 and DRB*0401 although most reported associations appear to be limited to specific geographical areas or ethnicities. Nevertheless, the association of AIH with DR3 and DR4 alleles is solid to the point of being included in the diagnostic scoring system currently in use. The scenario is further complicated by the possibility that different environmental factors trigger AIH in different areas. HLA alleles associated with AIH not only confer susceptibility towards AIH but also appear to influence the course of the disease. Most strikingly, patients with DRB1*0301 are younger at disease onset and have a lower frequency of response to treatment. HLA DR3 is further associated with a lower probability of remission, more frequent relapses and need for liver transplantation. Furthermore, associations have also been reported between AIH and tumor necrosis factor-α and carbonic anhydrase gene polymorphisms, although these genes might not represent primary susceptibility genes but rather markers of MHC associations. Outside the MHC cluster, polymorphisms of genes involved in the regulation of immune responses have been investigated, leading to inconclusive data. These include the genes for cytotoxic T-lymphocyte antigen 4 (CTLA-4), cytokines, vitamin D receptor, CD45, and Fas receptor.

Natural history

Data on the natural course of AIH are limited, particularly due to the paucity of clinical trials during the past decades when hepatitis C became manifest as a common confounding factor significantly influencing the disease progression. Accordingly, older studies reported that AIH had a very poor prognosis and 5- and 10-year survival rates of 50 and 10% without treatment while immunosuppressants could significantly improve survival to 10-year rates as high as 90%. At the time of diagnosis, approximately 30% of adult patients have histological evidence of cirrhosis; when appropriately treated, however, only a small number of patients develop cirrhosis during follow-up if an anti-inflammatory response is achieved. Nevertheless, having cirrhosis at presentation significantly increases the risk of liver-related death or the need for liver transplantation.[4]

The scenarios are different when pediatric or elderly cases are studied. In fact, almost 50% of children with AIH manifest cirrhosis at diagnosis and the majority of patients require long-term immunosuppressive treatment until adulthood. In elderly patients a more severe initial histology grade should be expected, alongside a similar response rate to immunosuppression. It is still debated if these patients should be treated with higher or lower doses of steroids. Beside age at presentation, race also affects disease progression. In fact, cirrhosis is more frequent at younger age in African American patients with AIH compared to Caucasian subjects from the same areas.

The occurrence of hepatocellular carcinoma in patients with AIH is a rare event and only develops in long-standing cirrhosis. In the absence of solid data on large numbers of cases, primary liver neoplasia incidence should be regarded as similar to other nonviral cases of cirrhosis.

Therapy

Different from the other autoimmune liver diseases described herein, immunosuppressants are the treatment of choice for AIH, based on the good response in terms of biochemistry, histology, and survival.[7] Corticosteroids (prednisone), as monotherapy or in combination with azathioprine, are the first line of treatment and should be started in patients with aminotransferase levels >5 times the upper normal limit or histological evidence of bridging or multilobular necrosis. Prednisone and azathioprine appear equally effective. Treatment follows guidelines (Table 75.3) but tailored schedules are encouraged in selected cases. In asymptomatic patients with milder presentation, the need for treatment is still a matter of debate since the survival of these patients without treatment is similar to the overall AIH population. Nevertheless, a close follow-up is required in these patients since symptoms develop in 25% of cases. The goal of a biochemical and histological resolution of inflammation as well as the clinical remission of symptoms is observed in up to 80% of patients treated with steroids within the first 3 years, most commonly during the first few months. It should be noted, however, that subgroups of patients manifest disease progression (approximately 10%) or are intolerant to standard therapy (13%). Relapses following therapy discontinuation are common since only 20% of patients remain in sustained remission. Second-choice therapies include cyclosporine, tacrolimus, cyclophosphamide, mercaptopurine, mycophenolate mofetil, or deflazacort, thus far tested in small populations of patients. Ursodeoxycholic acid (UDCA) is a well-tolerated drug; its efficacy in AIH therapy or in combination with immunosuppressive therapy remains debated, particularly in terms of survival or histological improvement. Finally, patients with end-stage liver disease or fulminant presentation who do not respond to immunosuppressive therapy should be promptly considered for liver transplantation. Patients with AIH undergoing liver transplant have overall

Table 75.3 Treatment guidelines for autoimmune hepatitis

Therapeutic stages	Single-drug regimen	Combination regimen
Induction therapy		
Week 1	40–60 mg prednisone/day[a]	40–60 mg prednisone/day + 1–2 mg azathioprine/kg body weight
Week 2	40 mg prednisone/day	15 mg prednisone/day + 1–2 mg azathioprine/kg body weight
Week 3	30 mg prednisone/day	15 mg prednisone/day + 1–2 mg azathioprine/kg body weight
Week 4	Taper down 5 mg every week, until maintenance therapy	
Maintenance therapy	5–15 mg prednisone/day are common	10 mg prednisone/day + 1–2 mg azathioprine/kg body weight dosages. *Alternative option*: 2 mg/kg azathioprine as monotherapy
Upon relapse	Like induction therapy	Like induction therapy

[a]Prednisolone may be taken instead of prednisone.

5- and 10-year survival rates of 90 and 75%, respectively, although infectious complications and disease recurrence are common.[8]

Primary biliary cirrhosis

CLINICAL PEARLS

Primary biliary cirrhosis

- Primary biliary cirrhosis is an autoimmune disease, affecting middle-aged women more commonly than men.
- Genetic factors are considered critical in the pathogenesis of the disease but proposed genetic associations are found only in a minority of patients; environmental factors are important, possibly infectious or chemical.
- The serum hallmark is serum anti-mitochondrial antibodies (AMA), found in >90% of cases.
- At presentation, patients most commonly manifest early stages and have limited or nonspecific symptoms.

PBC is a chronic cholestatic liver disease of unknown etiology characterized by high-titer serum anti-mitochondrial autoantibodies (AMA) and an autoimmune-mediated destruction of the small and medium-sized intrahepatic bile ducts.[9] It affects women more frequently than men, with a female-to-male ratio of 9:1, the average age at diagnosis is within the fifth and sixth decades of life, and it presents a geographical pattern of prevalence with widely variable prevalence and the highest rate in the USA described in Minnesota with a point prevalence of 402 per million in the general population. Sporadic cases of PBC onset in pediatric ages have recently been reported. The diagnosis of PBC is based on the presence of two out of three internationally accepted criteria, i.e., detectable serum AMA (titer >1:40), increased enzymes indicating cholestasis (i.e., alkaline phosphatase) for longer than 6 months, and a compatible or diagnostic liver histology.[10] The classification proposed to indicate a definite diagnosis only when all criteria are met may be too narrow as, for example, patients lacking serum AMA appear to follow a similar natural history when compared to their AMA-positive counterparts. Although it remains critical for the assessment of the histological stage, the issue of whether a liver biopsy is needed for the diagnosis of PBC is still highly debated. Currently, performing a liver biopsy seems not to be indicated when the other two diagnostic criteria are met. In a large number of cases (20–60%) the diagnosis of PBC is established in the absence of symptoms indicating a liver condition or cholestasis, and the proportion of asymptomatic cases at diagnosis has been increasing since the first series were reported.

Clinical features

Symptoms most commonly accompanying PBC at presentation are classically defined as fatigue and pruritus while physical findings may include skin hyperpigmentation, hepatosplenomegaly, and (rarely) xanthelasmas. End-stage symptoms are those of all types of liver cirrhosis, including ascites, jaundice, hepatic encephalopathy, and upper digestive bleeding. Fatigue is an incompletely defined, nonspecific symptom that affects up to 70% of patients with PBC and that is often overlooked, particularly in middle-aged women. Importantly, the severity of fatigue is independent of the stage of PBC or its other features (pruritus or severe cholestasis), nor does it depend on psychiatric factors. No medical treatment has been shown to be effective in alleviating this symptom, although fatigue has never been included as an endpoint in any of the large controlled clinical trials.

As many as 70% of patients with PBC and jaundice suffer from pruritus. Longitudinal data show that the vast majority of patients experience this symptom during their lifetime; pruritus might long precede jaundice onset. Typically, pruritus worsens at night, following contact with wool, or in warm climates. The bases of PBC-associated pruritus are not clear and two hypotheses have been proposed: serum bile acid retention secondary to chronic cholestasis or amplified release of endogenous opioids. Treatment of pruritus can be challenging. The use of cholestyramine (4 g two or three times a day) ameliorates pruritus. In cases poorly responsive to resins, rifampicin has been used to achieve rapid symptom relief; its prolonged use, however, should be avoided. Based on the opioid theory of pruritus, treatment with opiate antagonists such as naltrexone (50 mg/day) is currently being used, with limited adverse effects. The recently proposed use of sertraline is encouraged by promising preliminary data but warrants further evaluation.

Portal hypertension is frequently found in patients with PBC and, importantly, does not imply the presence of liver cirrhosis. Over half of untreated patients eventually develop portal hypertension over a 4-year period. The prevention and treatment of PBC-associated portal hypertension are not different from other chronic liver diseases.

Although there are conflicting data, it appears that accelerated bone loss accompanies long-standing cholestasis in PBC compared to sex- and age-matched healthy individuals. It has been coined metabolic bone disease secondary to reduced bone deposition. Current treatment of bone loss includes oral calcium supplementation, weight-bearing activity, and oral vitamin D replacement, if deficiency is found. Postmenopausal hormone replacement therapy should be considered but jaundice and other signs of liver failure should be evaluated during the first months of treatment. Efficacy and safety of other treatments are being evaluated.

Hyperlipidemia is common in up to 85% of patients with PBC and high levels of both serum cholesterol and triglyceride can be observed. Interestingly, however, such alterations are not accompanied by a proportionally increased incidence of cardiovascular events or atherosclerosis and do not correlate with disease stage. Treatment with bile acid helps reduce blood lipids levels via unknown mechanisms.

Comorbidity is an important feature of PBC. Various disorders, particularly other autoimmune syndromes, are associated with PBC at various degrees. Our epidemiological study of 1032 patients with PBC has demonstrated that one-third of cases are affected by another autoimmune disease, most commonly Sjögren's syndrome, Raynaud's phenomenon, autoimmune thyroid disease, scleroderma, and systemic lupus erythematosus, while the prevalence of rheumatoid arthritis did not differ from controls. Interestingly, recent data demonstrated that patients affected by both PBC and scleroderma manifest a less aggressive liver disease, thus suggesting an active interaction between the two conditions. Similarly to other types of cirrhosis, end-stage PBC can be complicated by the occurrence of hepatocellular carcinoma and patients with intense nodular liver structure at ultrasound should be monitored by computed tomography. Importantly, PBC appears not to be associated with cholangiocarcinoma (CCA) or breast cancer.

Blood tests

At presentation, PBC is suspected if a biochemical cholestatic pattern represented by increased plasma alkaline phosphatase or γ-glutamyltransferase is present. Such increase is typically not accompanied by an increase of similar magnitude in plasma aminotransferase levels. Serum IgM levels are typically elevated in PBC cases without being correlated with AMA titers or levels of other Ig subtypes. Data suggest that this phenomenon might be secondary to an aberrant response of the patients' memory B cells to bacterial stimuli, but its clinical significance remains enigmatic. Once cirrhosis has developed, biochemical alterations are similar to other types of cirrhosis.

Liver histology

According to the classification of Ludwig et al.,[11] histology identifies four PBC stages. Stage I manifests with portal tract inflammation with predominantly lymphoplasmacytic infiltrates, resulting in vanishing septal and interlobular bile ducts (diameter <100 μm). At this stage, bile duct obliteration and granulomas (possibly found at all stages) are strongly suggestive of PBC. In stage II a periportal inflammatory infiltrate is observed and signs of cholangitis, granulomas, and florid proliferation of ductules are typical. Stage III demonstrates septal or bridging fibrosis, with ductopenia (over half of the visible interlobular bile ducts having vanished), and copper deposition in periportal and paraseptal hepatocytes can be seen. Stage IV corresponds to frank cirrhosis. The observation of eosinophils in the portal tract is a specific finding in PBC histology. Finally, the possibility of a sampling error should be considered when evaluating histology in PBC and, in case of variable staging within one biopsy, the highest stage should be accepted. Figure 75.1 illustrates the histological findings in representative cases of early PBC.

Serum autoantibodies

Anti-mitochondrial antibodies

AMA are highly specific for PBC and can be detected in nearly 100% of patients when sensitive diagnostic methodologies based on recombinant antigens are used.[11] In most clinical settings, however, indirect immunofluorescence techniques are used for initial screening of cases and might provide false-positive or -negative results. AMA are directed against components of the 2-oxoacid dehydrogenase (2-OADC) family of enzymes within the mitochondrial respiratory chain, most frequently the E2 and E3-binding protein (E3BP) components of the pyruvate dehydrogenase complex and the E2 components of the 2-oxo glutarate dehydrogenase and branched-chain 2-oxo acid dehydrogenase complexes. In all three antigens epitopes contain the motif DKA, with lipoic acid covalently bound to the lysine (K) residue. The role of lipoic acid in epitope recognition by AMA is unclear. The pathogenic role of AMA is debatable, since no clinical correlation can be found and animal models developing serum AMA do not develop PBC-like liver lesions.

Antinuclear antibodies

As many as 50% of patients with PBC have detectable serum ANA, most commonly producing "nuclear rim" or "multiple nuclear dots" patterns. The pattern is based on the recognition by the autoantibodies of gp210 and nucleoporin 62 (within the nuclear pore complex) and Sp100 and promyelocytic leukemia protein (PML) (possibly also cross-reacting with small ubiquitin-like modifiers, SUMO), respectively.[11] ANA-positive patients are more frequently AMA-negative, possibly because of the lack of a masking effect of these latter antibodies in such sera. The pathogenic role of ANA in PBC remains enigmatic, although

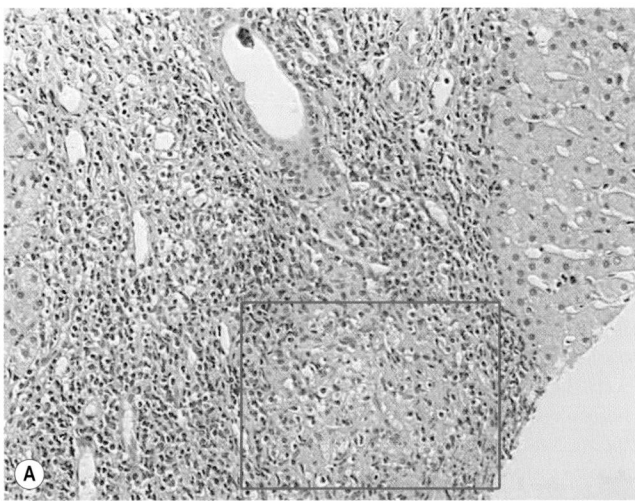
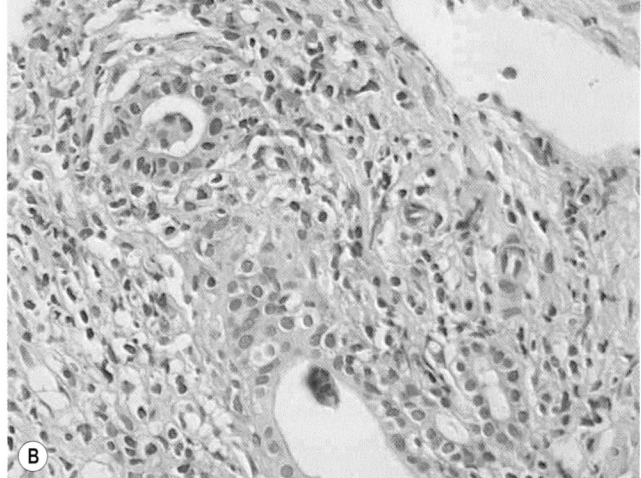

Fig. 75.1 Histological findings in early stages of primary biliary cirrhosis, i.e., nonsuppurative destructive cholangitis, following hematoxylin and eosin staining. (A) Mixed lymphocytic and plasma cell periductular inflammation with bile duct infiltration and granulomatous reaction (square). Magnification × 200. (B) Detail of bile duct disruption with lymphocytic and plasmacellular periductular and intraepithelial infiltration. Magnification × 400.
Courtesy of Dr. Marco Maggioni, Human Pathology Service, San Paolo Hospital, Milan, Italy.

cross-sectional and longitudinal data demonstrate an association between ANA positivity and a worse prognosis. Finally, patients with PBC and limited systemic sclerosis have detectable serum anti-centromere antibodies in 10–15% of cases.

Pathogenesis

Several clinical and experimental findings strongly imply an autoimmune pathogenesis for PBC while two components are necessary for disease onset: a permissive genetic background and an environmental trigger and these are discussed below. Nevertheless, recent years have witnessed a growing amount of evidence to support the role of peculiar apoptotic features of the biliary epithelial cells that may constitute the mechanism for the tissue-specific autoimmune injury in PBC.[12]

Genetics

PBC is more frequent in relatives of affected individuals and the term "familial PBC" has been coined to indicate families that have more than one case. Our data indicate 6% of cases have a first-degree relative that is also affected.[13] More importantly, the concordance rate observed among monozygotic twins for PBC is 63%, among the highest reported in autoimmunity, reinforcing the idea of an important role of genetics in disease susceptibility.[14] Several association studies have attempted to identify genes associated with PBC although no family study of genetic linkage has been performed. Associations are often not applicable to all populations but suggest that a multi-hit genetic model seems to apply to PBC, with different genetic variants conferring susceptibility (first hit) and others influencing disease progression (second hit). The study of the variants of MHC (including type I, II, and III loci) have produced associations that are often weak or limited to specific geographical areas. Similar findings were also reported from the study of the genetic variants of immunomodulatory molecules (such as chemokines and their receptors), enzymes producing vasoactive compounds, and bile acid transporters that have recently been reviewed elsewhere. Following the numerous association studies reported over the past decades for candidate genes in PBC, the first genome-wide case-control association studies were reported in 2009 and 2010 in patients and controls from Canada, the US, and Italy and demonstrated significant associations of PBC with IL-12A, IL-12RB2, and STAT4 polymorphisms.[15,16] The importance of IL-12 was recently supported by data in a PBC animal model. IL-12p40 seems to be crucial to autoimmunity development thus providing a link between genomic studies and disease pathogenesis with potential therapeutic implications. Furthermore, the growing field of microRNA effects on immune modulation has been investigated also in PBC where a specific signature was described for the first time.[17]

Of note, an age-dependent enhanced monosomy X was reported in peripheral white blood cells of women with PBC,[18] suggesting that PBC might ensue from a polygenic model with an X-linked major locus of susceptibility in which genes escaping inactivation are the major candidates. On the other hand, it can also be hypothesized that susceptibility to PBC is the result of a multigenic complex inheritance model where Y-linked genes might exert a protective role.

Environmental factors

Although genetics should be regarded as a major determinant in susceptibility to PBC, several other factors have been proposed. Our epidemiological study has demonstrated that a high risk of developing PBC is associated with a positive family history for PBC, a history of urinary or vaginal infections, comorbidity with other autoimmune diseases, lifestyle factors, such as smoking, and previous pregnancies (Table 75.4). Furthermore, we observed that the frequent use of nail polish also slightly increased the risk of having PBC. Experimental studies have focused on two main classes of agents possibly triggering PBC: infectious (bacteria and viruses) and chemical (xenobiotics). Most evidence has been reported for *Escherichia coli*, while contrasting data have been obtained on the role of *Chlamydia pneumoniae*. Finally, we have provided experimental evidence suggesting that *Novosphingobium aromaticivorans*, a ubiquitous xenobiotic-metabolizing Gram-negative bacterium, is the best candidate yet for the induction of PBC.[19] Figure 75.2 illustrates our bacterial theory.

Xenobiotics are foreign compounds that may either alter or complex to defined self or non-self proteins, inducing a change in the molecular structure of the native protein sufficient to induce an immune response. Such immune responses may then result in the cross-recognition of the self form, which could in turn perpetuate the immune response, thus leading to chronic autoimmunity. Interestingly, most xenobiotics are metabolized in the liver, thereby increasing the potential for liver-specific

Table 75.4 Risk/protective factors (expressed as odd ratios, OR) for primary biliary cirrhosis

	OR	95% CI
Medical/family history		
Family history of PBC	10.736	4.227–27.268
Family history of SLE	2.234	1.261–3.957
Family history of Sjögren's	5.814	1.279–26.435
History of urinary tract infections	1.511	1.192–1.915
Lifestyle factors		
Ever smoked > 100 cigarettes/day	1.569	1.292–1.905
No passive smoke at work	0.820	0.582–1.155
Don't have a job	1.369	1.095–1.712
Uses of nail polish/year	1.002[a]	1.000–1.003
Number of cigarettes smoked	0.999	0.998–1.000
Each additional smoker in household	0.5078	0.3167–0.8143
Reproductive history[b]		
Ever used hormonal replacement	1.548	1.273–1.882
Never pregnant	0.6118	0.4489–0.8338
Age of first pregnancy	0.9541	0.9331–0.9755

Results of multiple logistic regression models obtained from 1032 patients and 1041 controls are presented.[13]
CI, confidence interval; PBC, primary biliary cirrhosis; SLE, systemic lupus erythematosus
[a]Calculated for each additional use of nail polish/year.
[b]For female cases and controls only.

alteration of proteins. Data from our laboratory at University of California—Davis demonstrate that certain chemical compounds can induce AMA or are in fact recognized by patients' sera with higher affinity compared to self proteins and that specific ones are found in common-use products.[20]

Natural history

The progression of PBC varies widely, as represented by patients who remain asymptomatic and others who progress to liver failure at young ages. The factors influencing the severity and progression of the disease are largely unknown, although data seem to indicate that genetic factors other than those inducing the disease ("second hit") might play a role. In general terms, the natural history of the disease is divided into three time periods preceding liver failure, i.e., asymptomatic, symptomatic, and pre liver failure. The duration of these periods can vary significantly but the first step might last for decades, while the third is usually very rapid. The diagnosis of PBC is most commonly made within the first stage; patients presenting with symptoms or advanced disease are now less frequent compared to older reports.

Having symptoms at presentation is considered the major factor determining survival rates of patients with PBC. In fact, symptomless PBC is accompanied by 10-year survival rates similar to the general population. On the other hand, 67% of precirrhotic patients will develop liver cirrhosis over a 7-year observation period while 70% of asymptomatic patients will develop symptoms. Accordingly, more recent regression models indicate that asymptomatic patients with PBC have significantly lower survival than the general population. Based on conflicting data, it has been hypothesized that survival rates of asymptomatic patients with PBC are shorter than the general population if symptoms develop during follow-up. An additional

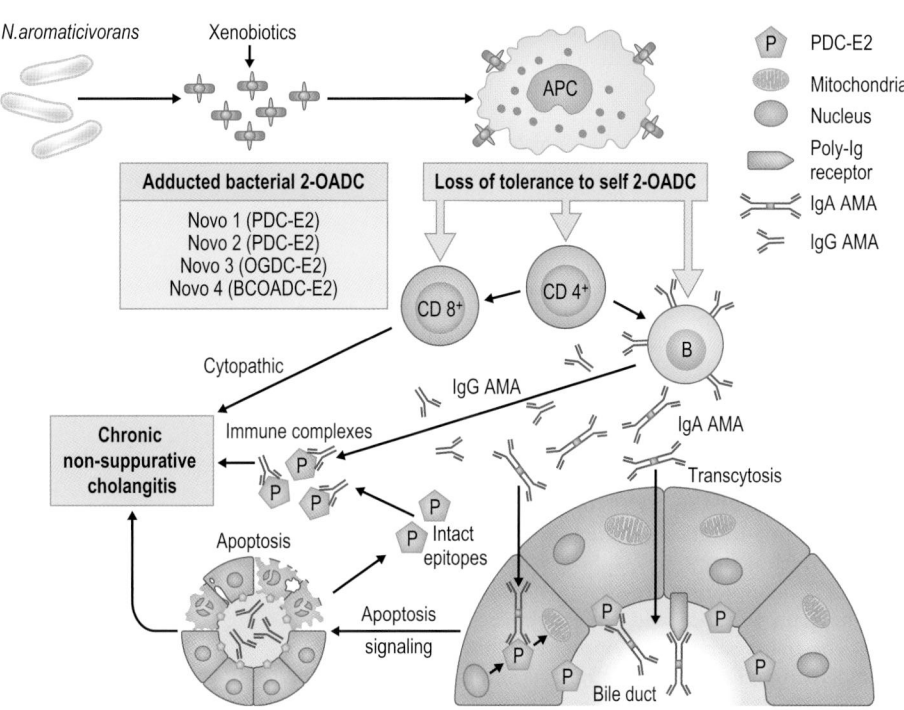

Fig. 75.2 Representation of the proposed theory on the etiopathogenesis of primary biliary cirrhosis based on the suggested role of *Novosphingobium aromaticivorans* in combination with individual susceptibility and environmental factors. The bacterium enters the mucosal system and its lipoylated proteins (Novo) are modified by xenobiotics, thus creating immunoreactive molecules. Modified proteins are then processed by antigen-presenting cells (APC) in the mucosa, thus activating autoreactive T and B cells. While T cells exert a cytopathic effect directly and/or recruit additional lymphocytes, B cells secrete anti-mitochondrial autoantibodies (AMA) of the IgG and IgA isotypes. IgA enters the lumen of biliary epithelial cells (BECs) by transcytosis and then reacts with molecules mimicking pyruvate dehydrogenase ED (PDC-E2), thus initiating apoptosis. The intact PDC-E2 liberated from apoptotic cells forms immune complexes with circulating AMA IgG. Such immune complexes, the enhanced apoptosis, the direct cytopathic effect of T cells, and possibly AMA eventually lead to the appearance of the histological signs of primary biliary cirrhosis, i.e., chronic nonsuppurative cholangitis.

confounding factor is provided by the rate of non-liver-related deaths that appears to cause the reduced survival of asymptomatic patients. Further studies on large populations and longer follow-up periods are clearly warranted.

Patients with symptomatic PBC show a more rapid progression to late-stage disease and a worse prognosis than their asymptomatic counterparts with survival times of 6–10 years.[21] Older age at diagnosis and signs of advanced disease (clinical, histological, or biochemical) are associated with a worse prognosis. The establishment of accurate prognostic models to predict survival in patients with PBC is of obvious importance in clinical practice. The model based on the Mayo score is the only one validated and is the most widely utilized;[22] it is calculated based on clinical (age, presence of ascites) and biochemical variables as represented by cholestasis (bilirubin levels) and liver function (prothrombin time, albumin). This model is a static representation of a dynamic entity and has a lower accuracy for patients with early disease. Most recently, Invernizzi and colleagues reported that PBC-specific serum ANA, albeit found in a minority of patients, can predict more aggressive disease, as suggested by longitudinal data collected during long follow-up periods.[23]

Therapy

The only approved treatment for PBC is the hydrophilic bile acid UDCA. The mechanism of action of UDCA in PBC is incompletely understood. It has been hypothesized that it is based on a number of factors, including modification of the bile acid pool, reduction in proinflammatory cytokines, effects on apoptosis and on vasoactive mediators.[24] Doses ranging from 13 to 15 mg/kg of UDCA are currently used and lead to optimum bile enrichment. A meta-analysis demonstrated that an increased survival is only obtained when a dose >13 mg/kg is prescribed,[25,26] despite the fact that a complete biochemical response to UDCA (i.e. normalization of alkaline phosphatase) is achieved in approximately 50% of treated patients. Immunosuppressive drugs have also been used in PBC with poor efficacy,

including corticosteroids, azathioprine, cyclosporine, methotrexate, penicillamine, and colchicine. Their use is currently encouraged only in combination with UDCA in selected cases (i.e., when features of AIH are found). Definitive data are still awaited on the efficacy of UDCA plus bezafibrate, mycophenolate mofetil, budesonide, and tamoxifen while new biologics are currently undergoing evaluations in phase II clinical trials. Liver transplantation is the ultimate treatment for end-stage PBC, with survival rates of 92 and 85% at 1 and 5 years after transplant, respectively. Recurrence is common and its rates seem to be influenced by certain immunosuppressive regimens, while the use of UDCA for recurrence is safe and recommended.

Primary sclerosing cholangitis

● KEY CONCEPTS

Primary sclerosing cholangitis

- Primary sclerosing cholangitis is a cholestatic liver disease of unknown etiology that is more common in men.
- It might affect any section of the biliary tree, usually producing strictures and dilations.
- Primary sclerosing cholangitis is significantly associated with inflammatory bowel diseases, particularly ulcerative colitis in an often indolent form.
- An increased risk of extrahepatic cholangiocarcinoma is observed and the diagnosis is often challenging.
- Autoimmune pancreatitis with increased IgG4 levels may coexist with sclerosing cholangitis.

PSC is a progressive cholestatic liver disease of unknown etiology presenting with autoimmune features and associated with significant morbidity and mortality. Different from PBC, PSC can affect all tracts of the biliary tree, including the extra-hepatic bile ducts. Epidemiological data indicate that annual incidence rates are not increasing over time despite earlier ages at diagnosis and, possibly, longer survival, similar to what was observed in PBC. Recent data from the northern USA (Olmstead County, MN) reported a disease prevalence of 20.9 per 100 000 men and 6.3 per 100 000 women.[27] In fact, different from the vast majority of autoimmune diseases, PSC is more commonly diagnosed in men, with a female-to-male ratio estimated as 1:2.

Clinical features

PSC is diagnosed most commonly in the absence of symptoms and during routine blood tests in healthy individuals or patients with inflammatory bowel disease (IBD). In fact, PSC is strongly associated with IBD, particularly ulcerative colitis (UC) with prevalence rates as high as 4%. Conversely, patients with PSC are affected by IBD in >75% of cases (more commonly UC). The other important association is with cholangiocarcinoma (CCA), which is found in 7–13% of patients with PSC. At early stages, PSC symptoms are generally nonspecific and include abdominal pain, jaundice, and fever in the case of bacterial cholangitis. The management of symptoms, which include pruritus, bone density reduction, and fatigue, is similar to that described for PBC. At more advanced stages, symptoms include those of all types of decompensated cirrhosis or neoplasia. Commonly, PSC is further complicated by episodic bacterial cholangitis favored by biliary strictures. Subgroups of patients manifest the "small-duct" variant or overlap syndrome.

Diagnosis

PSC is characteristically accompanied by a biochemical cholestatic pattern, as represented by elevated serum alkaline phosphatase and γ-glutamyltransferase, while tests of liver function are normal until late stages. Autoantibodies are of limited use in the diagnosis of PSC due to low sensitivity and specificity. A variable percentage of patients (as low as 33%) have detectable serum atypical p-ANCA, which can also be found in patients with AIH or IBD without PSC. More useful in the diagnosis of PSC are the imaging techniques that demonstrate strictured and dilated tracts within the intrahepatic or extrahepatic bile ducts. Among the imaging approaches in use, endoscopic retrograde cholangiopancreatography (ERCP) and magnetic resonance cholangiopancreatography (MRCP) are currently considered equal for sensitivity but their results are influenced by the operator's skills and experience. Liver histology is crucial in establishing the diagnosis in the case of small-duct PSC (typically characterized by the absence of ERCP or MRCP alterations) or PSC-AIH overlap syndrome.

Liver histology

Although not necessary for establishing the diagnosis, liver histology is essential for the staging of PSC or when the small-duct variant, an overlap syndrome, or CCA is suspected. The histological picture varies widely, from minimal alterations to cirrhosis with portal inflammation, concentric "onion-skin" periductal fibrosis, and periportal fibrosis developing into septal and bridging necrosis. Similar to PBC, sampling errors should be considered in the liver sample collection. Histological findings are only diagnostic in one-third of patients. Figure 75.3 illustrates the histological findings in two representative cases of early and advanced PSC.

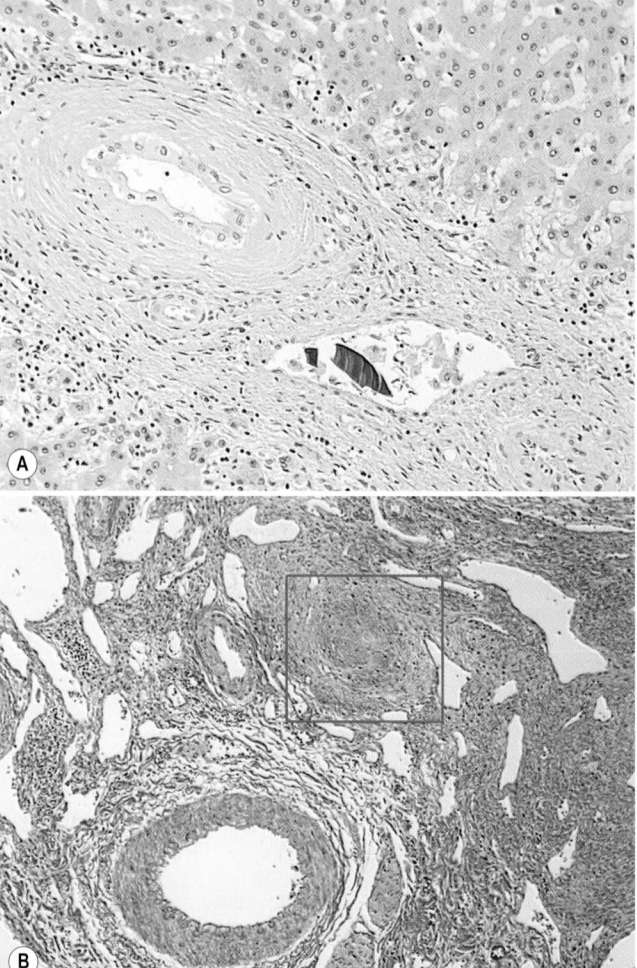

Fig. 75.3 Histological findings in primary sclerosing cholangitis. (A) Early disease and periductular fibrosis. Magnification × 200, hematoxylin and eosin staining. **(B)** Advanced disease with cirrhosis and bile duct substitution by fibrous scar (square). Magnification × 200, Masson staining.
Courtesy of Dr. Marco Maggioni, Human Pathology Service, San Paolo Hospital, Milan, Italy.

Inflammatory bowel disease

As mentioned above, the majority of patients with PSC are also affected by IBD, often at asymptomatic stages.[29] Alongside the varying genetic background for IBD in different areas, the prevalence of IBD in patients with PSC changes in various parts of the world. Accordingly, asymptomatic patients with PSC should undergo endoscopic evaluation with appropriate histological sampling. When IBD is found in this setting, IBD symptoms can ensue several years after diagnosis. Importantly, UC in patients with PSC is clinically different from UC without PSC in that it is often quiescent and rectum-sparing. PSC in UC increases the risk of colon dysplasia or carcinoma compared to UC alone.

Pathogenesis

The etiopathogenesis of PSC is unknown, despite growing evidence that (auto)immune-mediated mechanisms play a role.[30] This is indicated by the association with IBD in the majority of patients, the presence of serum autoantibodies, and the reported HLA susceptibility associations. It has been hypothesized that PSC is either an atypical autoimmune disease or an immune-mediated inflammatory disease. From a genetic standpoint, PSC occurs in susceptible individuals, as indicated by several association studies, particularly with HLA haplotypes. Family and twin studies are not available for PSC but a recent genome-wide association study has reported HLA as the only major association, albeit in a minority of patients and in some cases overlapping with IBD-associated genes.[28,29] Experimental insights into the disease pathogenesis have demonstrated a multistep pathway where innate immunity and microorganisms (possibly derived from an IBD-affected gut) play a role. Specifically, cholangiocytes are first activated by bacterial stimuli in the presence of gut-specific chemokines and endothelial cell adhesion molecules. Further, gut-primed T cells migrate into the portal tracts and peribiliary spaces where focal lesions subsequently appear. Finally, chronic inflammation and progressive fibrosis of the biliary epithelium lead to chronic cholestasis secondary to vanishing bile ducts and ultimately to biliary cirrhosis.

Natural history

Cumulatively, data on the natural history of PSC indicate that the median timespan from diagnosis to liver-related death or liver transplantation can be estimated at 18 years.[30] It is still debated whether medical treatment with UDCA in fact produces a longer survival. The prognosis is clearly influenced by the possible onset of CCA. In most cases, an early diagnosis of CCA is problematic since its clinical presentation is not distinguishable from benign dominant biliary strictures and cytology is not 100% sensitive in the diagnosis of the neoplasia.[31] Similar to forms not associated with PSC, the prognosis of PSC-related CCA at 1 year is extremely poor, with the exception of selected patients undergoing liver transplantation.

Another important distinction in predicting the natural history is small-duct PSC. In fact, the clinical course of this subgroup of patients is relatively benign and only a minority (12%) of patients progresses to develop classical PSC.[32] Importantly, no CCA occurrence was reported in these cases, although IBD comorbidity was equally common (with possibly a higher representation of Crohn's disease), compared to classical PSC.

Therapy

● THERAPEUTIC PRINCIPLES

Inflammatory hepatobiliary diseases

- Despite common putative pathological mechanisms (i.e., autoimmunity), the treatment of early stages of autoimmune hepatitis (AIH), primary biliary cirrhosis (PBC), and primary sclerosing cholangitis (PSC) differs significantly.
- Immunosuppressants (steroids, azathioprine) are the only effective treatments for AIH.
- Ursodeoxycholic acid (13–15 mg/kg per day) is the only effective treatment for PBC.
- Ursodeoxycholic acid at high doses (15-20 mg/kg per day) for PSC might influence disease progression while endoscopic treatments may ameliorate cholestasis.
- Expanding T regulatory cells and cytokine targeting may hold potential as new therapeutic strategies.
- Once liver cirrhosis ensues, treatment of complications (ascites, digestive bleeding) does not differ from other types of cirrhosis.
- Liver transplantation is the only effective treatment for all three conditions, with good survival rates; relapses are common.

The treatment of PSC includes medical and endoscopic measures, as well as liver transplantation.[33] Most clinical trials in PSC have investigated the effects of UDCA, with conflicting results (Table 75.5). Taken together, the available evidence suggests that UDCA is not proven to produce a substantial change in the course of PSC, despite remaining the most prescribed drug. However, it appears that high-dose UDCA might reduce the rate of progression and might prevent the development of colon cancer in patients with PSC and UC, while longer-term observations advise against UDCA doses exceeding 20 mg/kg/day in PSC.[34] Endoscopic measures are indicated to treat complicated PSC through the opening of short- and long-segment stenoses of the common bile duct and short-segment stenoses of the hepatic ducts near the bifurcation.[35] The

Table 75.5 Available data on ursodeoxycholic acid (UDCA) efficacy for primary sclerosing cholangitis (PSC)[33]

Author	Year	No. of patients	Daily UDCA dose	Duration (months)	Biochemical improvement	Symptom improvement	Histology improvement
O'Brien et al.	1991	12	10 mg/kg	30	Y	Y	–
Beuers et al.	1992	6	13–15 mg/kg	12	Y	N	Y
Lo et al.	1992	23	10 mg/kg	24	Y	N	N
Stiehl et al.	1994	20	750 mg	12–48	Y	N	Y
De Maria et al.	1996	59	600 mg	24	N	–	–
Lindor et al.	1997	105	13–15 mg/kg	34	Y	N	N
Van Hoogastraten et al.	1998	48	10 mg/kg	24	Y	N	–
Mitchell et al.	2001	26	20–25 mg/kg	24	Y	N	Y
Harnois et al.	2001	30	25–30 mg/kg	12	Y	–	–
Okolicsanyi et al.	2003	86	8–13 mg/kg	–	Y	Y	N
Olsson et al.	2004	110	17–23 mg/kg	60	Y	N	–

treatment can be repeated over time once restenoses ensue and resulting survival rates are higher compared to patients not treated endoscopically. Finally, PSC represents an important indication for liver transplantation since patients are commonly younger compared to other autoimmune liver diseases.[36,37] Indication is made in the absence of biliary neoplasias (ruled out by bile duct brushing) and timing is challenging due to the variable disease course. Survival rates at 1 year are approximately 90% and are only slightly lower in patients in whom CCA is diagnosed on the explanted liver. Recurrence of disease is common and affects 20–40% of transplanted patients during prolonged follow-up.

Autoimmune cholangitis

The term "autoimmune cholangitis" was first introduced to indicate AMA-negative PBC, possibly with serum ANA.[38] However, more recently a broader significance has been suggested to include: (1) serum ANA and/or SMA positivity and/or hypergammaglobulinemia; (2) serum AMA negativity by immunofluorescence; (3) biochemical and/or histological features of cholestatic and hepatocellular injury; and (4) exclusion of chronic viral, metabolic, or toxic liver disease. This definition possibly includes PBC with atypical presentation, small-duct PSC, idiopathic adulthood ductopenia, and transitional stages of the classic diseases. Consensus is still awaited on this issue.

Overlap syndromes

It is currently estimated that as many as 18% of patients with autoimmune liver disease also manifest features of a second autoimmune liver disease. These patients are considered to have overlap syndromes.[39] Patients with overlap syndromes usually present with both hepatocellular and cholangiocellular injury with biochemical and histological features of AIH and PBC or PSC. When not treated, these patients show a progressive course toward liver cirrhosis and failure. More specifically, AIH–PBC overlap syndrome is found in 10% of adults with AIH or PBC and AIH–PSC overlap syndromes in 6–8% of children, adolescents, and young adults with AIH or PSC. Besides overlaps, transitions are also possible in rare cases from PBC to AIH, AIH to PBC, or AIH to PSC. The pathogenesis of overlap syndromes is poorly understood, and few data are available regarding the clinical characteristics and outcome of these syndromes. Thus, the clinical management of overlap syndromes is based on that of single diseases and medical treatment is empiric. Therefore, UDCA is used for chronic cholestasis and immunosuppressants (steroids and azathioprine) for AIH, while liver transplantation is indicated for end-stage disease.

IgG4-related pancreatitis/cholangitis

There have been numerous reports of a new clinical entity coined autoimmune pancreatitis/IgG4-associated sclerosing cholangitis with peculiar clinical and therapeutic characteristics.[40] Autoimmune pancreatitis features raised serum levels of IgG4 (in >70% of cases), and an IgG4-positive lymphoplasmacytic tissue infiltrate along with a rapid response to steroids. The biliary phenotype is defined as IgG4-associated cholangitis mimicking PSC at imaging techniques. Elevated serum IgG4 is not uncommon in PSC being found in almost 10% of patients and may represent the sign of rapidly evolving disease.

Translational research

● ON THE HORIZON

- New modified antigens may increase the sensitivity and specificity of serum autoantibody tests.
- Discovering pathogenetic mechanisms could provide new targets for novel treatments, as in the case of cholangiocyte apoptosis in primary biliary cirrhosis.
- Biologics being used in other autoimmune or chronic inflammatory conditions are expected to prove helpful in inflammatory and autoimmune liver disease.
- Studies of cytokine/chemokines, microRNA, epigenetic changes, and nuclear receptors may provide new therapeutic targets.

A challenge for the the next 5-10 years is to determine the ideal diagnostic tools to identify earlier stages of autoimmune liver diseases in which medical treatments are most effective. In particular, we can expect that monoclonal antibodies being utilized in other immunological conditions may apply also to autoimmune hepatitis, primary biliary cirrhosis, and primary sclerosing cholangitis, although we are skeptical that one approach will fit all three conditions. First, we can hypothesize that targeting specific cytokines or chemokines may prove beneficial in primary biliary cirrhosis along with proposed treatments with farnesoid X receptor agonists such as obeticholic acid. Second, translational research is expected to determine whether unique apoptotic features of bile duct cells may provide a culprit to tackle autoimmune injury in primary biliary cirrhosis. Third, we should also expect that newest developments in epigenetics and microRNA will identify novel target pathways for future treatments. Nevertheless, the rarity of these conditions constitutes a major challenge for investigation of new treatments and we are convinced that only a rigorous clinical classification and a multicenter effort will allow the design of persuasive clinical studies.

Concluding remarks

As indicated, several aspects of inflammatory hepatobiliary diseases remain enigmatic. Moreover, it appears that PBC, PSC, and AIH share limited features and should be considered as separate diseases in clinical practice as well as in bench research. Specifically, medical treatment of those diseases has substantial differences in response and outcomes. Finally, while it appears straight-forward in many cases, the diagnosis of these conditions is often challenging. Overlap syndromes and antibody-negative forms are commonly difficult to define and can only be resolved through a collaborative effort by radiologists, pathologists, and hepatologists. We foresee that data produced by genome-wide association studies will eventually translate into new molecular mechanisms and new therapeutic targets.

References

1. Selmi C. The worldwide gradient of autoimmune conditions. Autoimmun Rev 2010;9: A247–A250.
2. Meda F, Folci M, Baccarelli A, Selmi C. The epigenetics of autoimmunity. Cell Mol Immunol 2011;8:226–36.
3. Vergani D, Mieli-Vergani G. Cutting edge issues in autoimmune hepatitis. Clin Rev Allergy Immunol 2011 Jan 6. [Epub ahead of print].

4. Czaja AJ, Manns MP. Advances in the diagnosis, pathogenesis, and management of autoimmune hepatitis. Gastroenterology 2010;139:58–72 e54.
5. Vergani D, Alvarez F, Bianchi FB, et al. Liver autoimmune serology: a consensus statement from the committee for autoimmune serology of the International Autoimmune Hepatitis Group. J Hepatol 2004;41:677–83.
6. Longhi MS, Hussain MJ, Kwok WW, et al. Autoantigen-specific regulatory T cells, a potential tool for immune-tolerance reconstitution in type-2 autoimmune hepatitis. Hepatology 2011;53:536–47.
7. Montano Loza AJ, Czaja AJ. Current therapy for autoimmune hepatitis. Nat Clin Pract Gastroenterol Hepatol 2007;4:202–14.
8. Schramm C, Bubenheim M, Adam R, et al. Primary liver transplantation for autoimmune hepatitis: a comparative analysis of the European Liver Transplant Registry. Liver Transpl 2010;16:461–9.
9. Selmi C, Bowlus CL, Gershwin ME, Coppel RL. Primary biliary cirrhosis. Lancet 2011;377:1600–9.
10. Lindor KD, Gershwin ME, Poupon R, et al. Primary biliary cirrhosis. Hepatology 2009;50:291–308.
11. Selmi C, Zuin M, Bowlus CL, Gershwin ME. Anti-mitochondrial antibody-negative primary biliary cirrhosis. Clin Liver Dis 2008;12:173–85 ix.
12. Lleo A, Shimoda S, Ishibashi H, Gershwin ME. Primary biliary cirrhosis and autoimmune hepatitis: apoptes and epitopes. J Gastroenterol 2011;46(Suppl. 1):29–38.
13. Gershwin ME, Selmi C, Worman HJ, et al. Risk factors and comorbidities in primary biliary cirrhosis: a controlled interview-based study of 1032 patients. Hepatology 2005;42:1194–202.
14. Selmi C, Mayo MJ, Bach N, et al. Primary biliary cirrhosis in monozygotic and dizygotic twins: genetics, epigenetics, and environment. Gastroenterology 2004;127:485–92.
15. Hirschfield GM, Liu X, Xu C, et al. Primary biliary cirrhosis associated with HLA, IL12A, and IL12RB2 variants. N Engl J Med 2009;360:2544–55.
16. Liu X, Invernizzi P, Lu Y, et al. Genome-wide meta-analyses identify three loci associated with primary biliary cirrhosis. Nat Genet 2010;42:658–60.
17. Padgett KA, Lan RY, Leung PC, et al. Primary biliary cirrhosis is associated with altered hepatic microRNA expression. J Autoimmun 2009;32:246–53.
18. Selmi C. The X in sex: how autoimmune diseases revolve around sex chromosomes. Best Pract Res Clin Rheumatol 2008;22:913–22.
19. Selmi C, Balkwill DL, Invernizzi P, et al. Patients with primary biliary cirrhosis react against a ubiquitous xenobiotic-metabolizing bacterium. Hepatology 2003;38:1250–7.
20. Rieger R, Gershwin ME. The X and why of xenobiotics in primary biliary cirrhosis. J Autoimmun 2007;28:76–84.
21. Pares A, Rodes J. Natural history of primary biliary cirrhosis. Clin Liver Dis 2003;7:779–94.
22. Grambsch PM, Dickson ER, Kaplan M, et al. Extramural cross-validation of the Mayo primary biliary cirrhosis survival model establishes its generalizability. Hepatology 1989;10:846–50.
23. Invernizzi P, Selmi C, Ranftler C, et al. Antinuclear antibodies in primary biliary cirrhosis. Semin Liver Dis 2005;25:298–310.
24. Lazaridis KN, Gores GJ, Lindor KD. Ursodeoxycholic acid 'mechanisms of action and clinical use in hepatobiliary disorders'. J Hepatol 2001;35:134–46.
25. Gluud C, Christensen E. Ursodeoxycholic acid for primary biliary cirrhosis. Cochrane Database Syst Rev 2002; CD000551.
26. Gong Y, Huang ZB, Christensen E, Gluud C. Ursodeoxycholic acid for primary biliary cirrhosis. Cochrane Database Syst Rev 2008; CD000551.
27. Bowlus CL. Cutting edge issues in primary sclerosing cholangitis. Clin Rev Allergy Immunol 2011;41:139–50.
28. Melum E, Franke A, Schramm C, et al. Genome-wide association analysis in primary sclerosing cholangitis identifies two non-HLA susceptibility loci. Nat Genet 2011;43:17–9.
29. Janse M, Lamberts LE, Franke L, et al. Three ulcerative colitis susceptibility loci are associated with primary sclerosing cholangitis and indicate a role for IL2, REL, and CARD9. Hepatology 2011;53:1977–85.
30. Levy C, Lindor KD. Primary sclerosing cholangitis: epidemiology, natural history, and prognosis. Semin Liver Dis 2006;26:22–30.
31. Charbel H, Al-Kawas FH. Cholangiocarcinoma: epidemiology, risk factors, pathogenesis, and diagnosis. Curr Gastroenterol Rep 2011;13:182–7.
32. Bjornsson E, Boberg KM, Cullen S, et al. Patients with small duct primary sclerosing cholangitis have a favourable long term prognosis. Gut 2002;51:731–5.
33. Cullen SN, Chapman RW. Review article: current management of primary sclerosing cholangitis. Aliment Pharmacol Ther 2005;21:933–48.
34. Lindor KD, Kowdley KV, Luketic VA, et al. High-dose ursodeoxycholic acid for the treatment of primary sclerosing cholangitis. Hepatology 2009;50:808–814.
35. Stiehl A. Primary sclerosing cholangitis: the role of endoscopic therapy. Semin Liver Dis 2006;26:62–8.
36. Goldberg DS, French B, Thomasson A, et al. Current trends in living donor liver transplantation for primary sclerosing cholangitis. Transplantation 2011;91:1148–52.
37. Bowlus CL, Li CS, Karlsen TH, et al. Primary sclerosing cholangitis in genetically diverse populations listed for liver transplantation: unique clinical and human leukocyte antigen associations. Liver Transpl 2010;16:1324–30.
38. Czaja AJ, Carpenter HA, Santrach PJ, Moore SB. Autoimmune cholangitis within the spectrum of autoimmune liver disease. Hepatology 2000;31:1231–8.
39. Boberg KM, Chapman RW, Hirschfield GM, et al. Overlap syndromes: the International Autoimmune Hepatitis Group (IAIHG) position statement on a controversial issue. J Hepatol 2011;54:374–85.
40. Webster GJ, Pereira SP, Chapman RW. Autoimmune pancreatitis/IgG4-associated cholangitis and primary sclerosing cholangitis—overlapping or separate diseases? J Hepatol 2009;51:398–402.

PART EIGHT
Immunology of neoplasia

76.

Principles of tumor immunology

Theresa L. Whiteside, Bruce W.S. Robinson, Carl H. June, Michael T. Lotze

Tumor immunology has emerged as a distinct scientific discipline relatively recently, and only upon the realization that most adult tumors arise in the setting of chronic inflammation, tumor-associated antigens (TA) are immunogenic, and immune responses to TA are detectable in most tumor-bearing hosts.[1-3] Although rare, spontaneous cancer regression occurs in humans, e.g., in patients with melanoma and renal cancer,[2] and adaptive and innate immune responses can eliminate abnormal cells.[1] Immune cells accumulating at the tumor site can also contribute to its growth.[3] Thus, the immune system can either mediate tumor rejection or promote tumor progression.

Interactions between developing tumors and the immune system

Tumor development from a single transformed cell to the mass of malignant cells is a multi-step process involving genetic changes that culminate in the appearance of an established tumor.[4] In humans, this occurs over a period of many years and includes several distinct genetic modifications that are now well known. Solid tumors are characterized by genomic instability and generate multiple mutational neo-epitopes that can be recognized by the host immune system, leading to tumor elimination. The ability of the host to survey for abnormal cells was recognized many years ago by F. M. Burnet[5] and is referred to as "tumor immunosurveillance." An expanded, modern version of this concept is known as the "cancer immunoediting" hypothesis.[6] The hypothesis postulates that a developing tumor engages the immune system from its very beginning (Fig. 76.1). As tumor cells are recognized by immune effectors and eliminated, they are replaced by immunoresistant genetic variants. The result of "editing" or "immunoselection" is emergence of the tumor consisting of a heterogeneous population of rapidly proliferating, immunoresistant, and genetically unstable cells that continue to undergo further genetic modifications. These selected tumor cells cannot be destroyed by the host immune system and represent the "immune evasion" phase of tumor progression.[6] However, to be fully successful, the tumor now develops mechanisms designed to promote "epithelial reconstitution" and protect it from immune elimination. In effect, the tumor subverts anti-tumor responses by silencing immune cells, entering the phase known as "immune deviation," or "immune subversion." This, as all immune editing phenomena, actually represents a mechanism by which damaged epithelia limit further damage, allowing development of the barrier function central to their role, and should be considered a normal response to stress, perpetuated within the tumor microenvironment.

KEY CONCEPTS

"Immune editing" of tumors

- *Immune selection*: tumor cells sensitive to immune intervention are eliminated and are replaced by immunoresistant tumor cells.
- *Immune evasion*: mechanisms to enable tumor escape from the immune system are established.
- *Immune subversion or deviation*: the tumor actively eliminates/suppresses the host anti-tumor immune responses.

The tumor induces immune suppression, which is mediated by tumor-derived soluble factors, microvesicles (TMV/exosomes), or suppressor cells, such as regulatory T cells (Treg), plasmacytoid dendritic cells, or myeloid-derived suppressor cells (MDSC), and is a characteristic feature of most human tumors. Because it is difficult to counter various escape mechanisms adopted by human tumors, immune subversion, also known as "tumor counterattack," has been a major proposed problem limiting effective cancer therapy.

KEY CONCEPTS

The host immune system and cancer

- The host immune system has the potential to either attenuate tumor growth or to promote tumor progression.

Interactions between the tumor and immune cells are complex, bidirectional, and influenced by the local microenvironment. Depending on the tumor's capability to shape its milieu and disarm the immune system, these interactions might result in the tumor demise or the demise of tumor-reactive immune cells. Recognizing the dual capability of the immune system to both promote and attenuate tumor growth, current therapeutic strategies are designed to promote or restore anti-tumor activity of immune cells in cancer while simultaneously inducing death of tumor cells.

Recognition of tumor targets by immune cells or antibodies

The presence of TA, which induce tumor-specific immune responses, has been well documented in mouse and human tumors.[7] Cloning of the first gene encoding a human melanoma

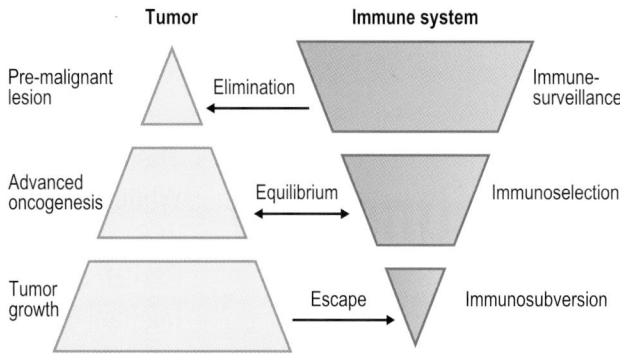

Tumor   Immune system

Pre-malignant lesion — Elimination — Immune-surveillance

Advanced oncogenesis — Equilibrium — Immunoselection

Tumor growth — Escape — Immunosubversion

Fig. 76.1 The concept of cancer immunosurveillance predicts that the immune system can recognize cancer precursor cells and, in most cases, destroy these cells before they become clinically apparent. Although tumors induce at least transient immune responses, cancer can still develop. This is due to cellular immune responses being unable to prevent the development of cancer either because tumor cells that successfully evade the immune system are selected (immunoselection) or because tumor-antigen specific immune tolerance is induced. Immunosubversion is a manifestation of tumor-induced tolerance. The goal of cancer immunotherapy is to shift the balance back in favor of the immune system, so that it can recognize the tumor, eliminate it, and prevent its recurrence. Reproduced with permission from Zitvogel L et al., Cancer despite immunosurveillance: immunoselection and immunosubversion, Nat Rev Immunol 2006; 6(10): 721-727.

antigen recognized by T cells, MAGE-1, in 1991 provided the molecular proof for the existence of TA.[8] and a subsequent search for additional TA has yielded a long list of well-defined common antigens, many of which have been tested in clinical trials as targets for immunotherapy (Table 76.1).[9] The development of therapeutic cancer vaccines has been facilitated by the availability of

Table 76.1 Human tumor-associated antigens (TA) commonly used in translational research[a]

Tumor antigen category	Examples
Oncofetal antigens	Glypican 3 (heparan sulfate proteoglycan) Alpha-fetoprotein (AFP) Carcinoembryonic antigen (CEA)
Oncogenes	Ras-mutant (e.g., RasG12D) p53-mutant ; p53 non-mutant Her2/neu WT-1
Cancer-testis antigens	MAGE-1, BAGE, GAGE, SAGE, NY-ESO-1
Human melanoma antigens	MelanA/MART-1, gp-100, Tyrosinase Tyrosinase related proteins (TRP) 1 and 2 Chondroitin sulfate proteoglycan 4 (CSGP4)
Human glioblastoma antigens	Ephrin (Eph) A2 IL-13Ralpha 2 Survivin Epidermal growth factor receptor (EGFRv III)
Head and neck cancer antigens	EGFR Human papilloma virus (HPV E6,E7) Aldehyde dehydrogenase A1 (ALDH A1) CSGP4
Overexpressed or modified antigens	MUC-1 Cyclin-B1 Prostate-specific antigen (PSA) Prostate membrane-specific antigen (PSMA) Disialoganglioside (GD2) Epithelial cell adhesion molecule (EpCAM)

[a]A more complete list of human TA prioritized by the NCI Pilot Project for the Acceleration of Translational Research can be found in Cheever et al.[9]

these TA, which are delivered to patients as proteins or peptides with or without adjuvants, viruses containing TA-coding sequences, or antigen-presenting cells (APC) loaded with TA. There are two main types of tumor antigens, self-antigens (e.g., cancer-testis, differentiation) and neoantigens (e.g., mutations and viruses). Most TA are derived from self-proteins that are either mutated or differentially expressed in tumor and normal cells, as exemplified by oncogenes, oncofetal antigens, or cancer-testis antigens (Table 76.1), though it is predicted that many neoantigens are present in established tumors.[10]

Most tumor antigens appear to be unique to the tumor (argued to be at least 75% of the T cells and antibodies recognizing tumor antigens as distinct from the common antigens). The immune system mediates adaptive immunity via anti-TA antibodies (Abs) or anti-TA-specific $CD3^+$ T cells. The initial innate signal, the so-called "Signal 0" by the late Charles Janeway, recruits inflammatory cells based on the response to pathogen-associated or damage-associated molecular pattern molecules (PAMPs and DAMPs). A fundamental difference exists between the subsequent adaptive immune response with the TA recognition process mediated by Abs and that mediated by T cells. The former respond to TA expressed on the surface of tumor cells. T cells recognize epitopes derived from intracellular proteins that are processed by antigen processing machinery (APM) components and presented by major histocompatibility complex (MHC) class I molecules on tumor cells or cross-presented by MHC class II molecules expressed on antigen-presenting cells (APC) such as dendritic cells (DC) or B cells (Chapter 6). For an adaptive immune response to occur, T cells expressing cognate T-cell receptors (TCR) must be present. Tri-molecular complexes (a nanopeptide-β_2-microglobulin (β_2m)-MHC class I heavy chain) presented on the surface of APC are recognized by memory T cells. Binding of the peptide presented by APC to the variable domains of the TCR initiates signaling (*Signal 1*) and induces clonal expansion of the peptide-specific cytolytic effector T cells. Because this series of events involves expansion of pre-existing memory T cells, it is called a recall or anamnestic response. Alternatively, precursor T cells expressing the correct TCR can be primed by the tri-molecular complexes presented by DC, and the subsequent development of TA-specific T effector cells (Teff) represents a primary immune response. DC are the only APC able to prime naïve T cells. In either case, *Signal 2* provided by co-stimulatory molecules and *Signal 3*, promoting polarization of the immune response and mediated by cytokines, are necessary for an immune response to proceed.[11] *Signal 4* represents the largely integrin-mediated signal defining to which tissues the T cells should emigrate (skin, lung, gut, etc.). *Signal 5* represents the fine integration of signals within the tumor microenvironment that allows an integrated immune response. In cancer, cross-presentation of tumor antigens is quite efficient, but the signals necessary for APC functions can also be either missing or incomplete, and the process of TA presentation is altered by tumor-derived factors.[12]

In addition, exogenous proteins taken up by APC can be processed and presented by MHC class II molecules, leading to induction of CD4 Treg.[11] The molecular signals directing APC to execute tolerogenic versus immunogenic programs in response to TA are not yet fully understood. TA-specific responses, like all immune responses, do not continue indefinitely, but peak and then contract, restoring the pre-activation homeostatic balance. The mechanisms responsible for immune contraction have not been defined, but Treg and other suppressive mechanisms probably regulate ongoing immune reactivity. It also appears that events in the tumor and tissue microenvironment such as the continued presence of DAMPs, e.g., the high

KEY CONCEPTS

Antigen presentation and antigen-presenting cells (APC) in cancer

- Dendritic cells (DC) infiltrate tumors and tumor-draining lymph nodes; high DC density in the tumor is associated with prolonged OS.
- Fewer DC are found in metastatic than primary lesions and in lethal cancers such as pancreatic cancer, found at very few numbers.
- TA can be processed and cross-presented by DC to T cells.
- DC exposed to tumor cells and DC found in tumors experience signaling defects:
  - (a) Downregulate expression of MHC class I molecules and β_2-microglobulin, i.e., lack signal 1 (TA presentation)
  - (b) Downregulate expression of co-stimulatory molecules, i.e., lack signal 2 (display of co-stimulatory molecules)
  - (c) Lack sufficient IL-2 and IFN-γ and instead are exposed to IL-10 and TGF-β, i.e., experience altered signal 3 (a need for stimulatory cytokines)
- DC found in the tumor have defects if expression of antigen processing machinery (APM) components.
- DC in the peripheral circulation of cancer patients are less mature and are functionally deficient relative to DC in the blood of healthy donors.
- Tumor-derived VEGF and IL-10 have been identified as "anti-dendropoietic factors."
- Most of the phenotypic and functional defects in DC are reversible.

mobility group box 1 protein (HMGB1), as well as the cytokine milieu, play a key role in the control of immune expansion or contraction.

In addition to Abs and T cells responsible for acquired or adaptive immunity, anti-tumor immune responses involving innate or natural immunity are mediated by cells or soluble factors that naturally exist and can be recruited into tissues. Among hematopoietic cells, monocytes/macrophages, granulocytes, CD3[-]CD56[+] natural killer (NK) cells, CD3[+]CD56[-] non-MHC-restricted T cells, and γ/δ T cells have the natural capacity to eliminate stress-receptor-expressing (e.g., MICA/MICB, etc.) tumor cell targets. Natural Abs with specificities directed at surface components of tumor cells are present in sera of patients with cancer.[13] Other factors commonly present in sera such as the complement components, C-reactive protein, mannose-binding protein, or serum amyloid protein can also interfere with tumor cell growth or survival.

Damage-associated molecular pattern molecules and anti-tumor immunity

Many human tumors arise and develop in the setting of chronic microbial or viral infections. Examples include human papilloma virus (HPV) and cervical or head and neck cancers, hepatitis B or C and hepatocellular carcinoma, *Helicobacter pylori* infections and gastric cancer or Epstein–Barr virus and Burkett lymphoma. It has been suggested that intracellular pathogens induce inflammatory responses in the host that then become chronic. These chronic tissue inflammatory infiltrates are thought to contribute to tumor development by creating a microenvironment permissive or supportive of tumor growth.[3]

Immune cells detect pathogens due to expression of pattern-recognition receptors (PRRs), which enable them to detect PAMPs. The best studied of these receptors, Toll-like receptors (TLRs), are widely distributed on immune and non-immune cells.[14] Recognition by immune cells of PAMPs promotes generation of vigorous cellular and antibody responses to pathogens.[15] At the same time, signaling via TLRs expressed on human tumor cells has been shown to promote tumor growth.[14] Immune cells are also able to recognize endogenous danger signals, which are typically released from cells undergoing necrosis or late apoptotic death.[15] These cells recognize DAMP molecules such as heat shock proteins (HSP), the S100 family of molecules, purine metabolites including uric acid and ATP, hyaluronan, and heparan sulfate.[16] The prototype of DAMPs is a HMGB1, which is present within the nuclei (and cytoplasm at about 10% of the levels in the nucleus) of nearly all cell types.[16] It is the second most abundant protein in the nucleus and is released from cells following autophagy or necrotic, but not apoptotic, cell death. Cytolytic effector T cells or effectors of innate immunity promote its release from tumor cells. Thus, immune recognition and tumor elimination by immune cells unleashes DAMPs and PAMPs (in the setting of pathogen-associated carcinogenesis), which play an important role in tumor progression.

KEY CONCEPTS

DAMPs and PAMPs in tumor progression

- Immune cells are found in the tumor stroma and parenchyma and their density and location correlate with clinical outcome.
- Linkage between pro-inflammatory cytokine production, infiltrating immune cells, micro-organisms, and tumor progression (e.g., colon carcinoma).
- Human tumors express TLRs, and TLR signaling promotes tumor progression.
- Increased expression of HMGB1, a prototype DAMP, and its receptor, RAGE, are associated with cancer progression.
- Release of DAMPs occurs in cancer and is associated with disease progression.
- Hepatitis B vaccinations decrease incidence of hepatoma.

TA-specific immune responses and tumor cell elimination

The presence of TA-specific T cells in the peripheral circulation of cancer patients and/or TA-specific Abs in their sera begs a question of why tumors progress when they are recognized by the host immune system. However, the frequency of such T cells and Ab titers are generally low (i.e., significantly lower than antiviral responses in the same hosts) and do not seem to influence clinical outcome or responses to therapy. Difficulties in detecting robust anti-tumor immunity in cancer patients are not due to methodological problems. They instead reflect suppression of host-cell anti-tumor immunity that has been promoted by tumor cells. Cancer patients who have not been treated with chemotherapy or radiotherapy generally have intact immune responses to bacterial and viral antigens, although they are often unable to respond robustly to their own TA.

In contrast to human studies, evidence derived from pre-clinical studies in murine models of cancer suggests that the immune system can prevent tumor growth or lead to its rejection.[17] In both the prevention and therapeutic settings, most immune anti-tumor therapies used in mice result in tumor rejection and the establishment of long-lasting TA-specific immunological memory.[17] This has been a consistent pattern observed with carcinogen-induced, virally-induced or spontaneously-arising tumors in mice, suggesting a fundamental difference in immune responses to TA between mice and humans. This difference might reflect:

(a) greater immunogenicity of murine TA, which largely consist of virus- or carcinogen-related epitopes and thus are foreign rather than "self";

(b) a short period of tumor development in mice relative to extended periods of silent tumor growth in humans, which leaves little opportunity for immune selection and the development by a tumor of escape mechanisms; and

(c) the tolerogenic nature of human TA, which are "self" or "altered self."

To minimize this difference, transgenic murine cancer models have been developed, allowing for genetically driven "spontaneous" tumor development. Transgenic mice have been especially useful in the design of prophylactic cancer vaccines,[18] providing encouraging results, potentially translatable to the future development of tumor immunoprophylaxis in humans. To date, however, it has not been possible to translate positive therapeutic anti-tumor effects observed in transgenic mice to immunotherapy of established solid tumors in humans. Murine tumors grow rapidly and are eliminated by therapy in a very short time, leaving little room for the development of escape routes, while human tumors are diagnosed and treated after many years of silent coexistence with the host, which creates an ample opportunity for nominal immune editing and perfecting escape pathways. Most of these concepts are proven in mice rather than in humans. Immune anti-tumor responses in humans are influenced by the gradual deterioration of the immune system with age.[19] The increased incidence of cancer in the elderly might be due to immunosenescence, which could interfere with the patients' ability to mount and sustain anti-tumor immune responses or with the effectiveness of cancer immunotherapies. Weak and ineffective immune responses to TA, which are "self" or "altered-self," might be exacerbated by the lack of DAMPs similar to those induced by PAMPs within the tumor milieu.[14] However, DAMPs are likely continuously released into the tumor microenvironment through a process that we have termed a chronic tumor lysis syndrome. A rational explanation may be that in cancer, as opposed to autoimmune diseases, tolerance to self prevents the development of effective immune responses to TA, and breaking tolerance is necessary for generating strong anti-tumor immunity. Mutated epitopes are the only "unique" TA known to elicit robust immune responses. However, only a handful of such epitopes are known, while the vast majority of TA are poorly immunogenic or tolerogenic.

Another explanation for the lack of robust anti-tumor immunity in cancer patients is the immunosuppressive nature of the tumor microenvironment.[20] Immune subversion is a well-recognized attribute of human tumors, which attract immune suppressor cells and produce a broad array of inhibitory factors responsible for the downregulation of TA-specific responses. As these suppressive effects are not only local but also systemic, it is not surprising that anti-tumor immunity is weak, inefficient, or perhaps even absent in patients with aggressively growing tumors.

● KEY CONCEPTS

Tumor microenvironment

- Immunoedited tumors successfully create a unique microenvironment dominated by immunosuppressive tumor-derived cytokines and other soluble factors that exert local as well as systemic inhibitory effects on the host immune system.

Immune cells infiltrating human tumors

Immune cells are frequently found in the tumor stroma and infiltrating among tumor cells. T lymphocytes, referred to as tumor-infiltrating lymphocytes (TIL), are the most prominent cell type found in tumors along with tumor-associated macrophages (TAM), DC, granulocytes, and occasionally B cells. These infiltrating immune cells are in an intimate contact with tumor cells, stromal fibroblasts, extracellular matrix (ECM) components, and blood vessels. They can mediate pro-tumor or anti-tumor functions, depending on signals received in the tumor microenvironment (Table 76.2). Among them, $CD3^+TCR^+$ TIL thought to be enriched in TA-specific T cells and responsible for tumor cell elimination have received the most attention (Table 76.3). TIL have variable but reversible functional impairments. Clearly, the tumor microenvironment exerts negative effects on anti-tumor activities of TIL, especially those present within advanced or metastatic lesions.[20] CD4 helper T cells present in tumors also mediate anti-tumor activities, and their frequency may be associated with an improved prognosis. Immune responses to TA are controlled by the balance of cytokines produced by distinct helper T-cell subsets, Th1, Th2,[21] Tregs, Th17, and Th22 cells. Generally only the Th1-type signature (Tbet[+], IL-2, and IFN-γ producing Th cells) is associated with a favorable clinical outcome, while the Th2-type profile (GATA3[+], IL-4, IL-5, IL-13 producing Th cells) predicts a poor prognosis. Thus, Th1-type helper cells play a critical role in anti-tumor immunity, and a higher ratio of Th2GATA3[+] to Th1Tbet[+] TIL is a negative predictive marker of patients' survival in cancer.

Table 76.2 Immune cells infiltrating humor tumors mediate pro-tumor and anti-tumor functions, depending on locally generated signals

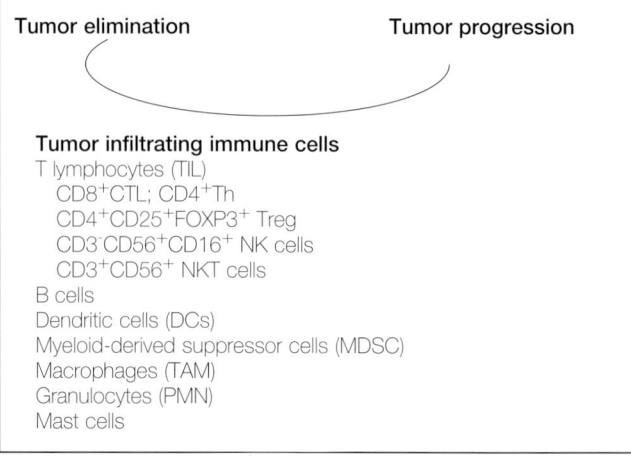

Tumor elimination   Tumor progression

Tumor infiltrating immune cells

T lymphocytes (TIL)
  $CD8^+$CTL; $CD4^+$Th
  $CD4^+CD25^+$FOXP3$^+$ Treg
  $CD3^-CD56^+CD16^+$ NK cells
  $CD3^+CD56^+$ NKT cells
B cells
Dendritic cells (DCs)
Myeloid-derived suppressor cells (MDSC)
Macrophages (TAM)
Granulocytes (PMN)
Mast cells

Table 76.3 Characteristics of TIL found within human solid tumors[a]

Morphology	Small to large lymphocytes
Phenotype	CD3$^+$TCRαβ$^+$; few CD3$^-$CD56$^+$ NK cells CD3$^+$CD8$^+$ and CD3$^+$CD4$^+$; variable CD4/CD8 ratio CD45RO$^+$CCR7$^-$ memory T cells CD25$^+$, CD69$^+$ >95% CD95$^+$ (Fas$^+$) Most are PD-1$^+$ Increased % of CD4$^+$CD39$^+$FOXP3$^+$ Treg Increased % of CD4$^+$IL-17$^+$ (Th17) cells
Clonality	Oligoclonal; restricted TCR Vβ gene expression
Specificity	TA-specific T cells detectable at a variable frequency
Functions	Decreased locomotion, proliferation, cytotoxicity
Signaling via TCR	Reversibly altered Low CD3ζ expression Decreased Ca mobilization Low pAkt expression Low pErk expression Suppressed NFκB activation
Cytokine profile	Largely GATA3$^+$ Th2-type (IL-4, IL-5, IL-13) Low or no IL-2 or IFN-γ production Expression of TGF-β and/or IL-10
In vitro response to IL-2	Variable but lower than that of PBL TIL from metastatic lesions respond poorly
AICD	High % of TUNEL$^+$ANX$^+$CD8$^+$TIL

AICD, activation-induced cell death; TUNEL, terminal deoxynucleotidyl transferase-mediated dUTP nick end labeling; ANX, Annexin.
[a]A list of human TIL properties based on the data available in the literature (reviewed in Nagaraj and Gabrilovich).[23]

Tumor-associated macrophages (TAM) are CD14$^+$ and differ from normal tissue macrophages. They are programmed or selected by the tumor to release inhibitory cytokines, such as IL-10, reactive oxygen species (ROS), or prostaglandin E$_2$ (PGE$_2$).[22] A related subset of myeloid-derived cells, myeloid-derived suppressor cells (MDSC), are less well differentiated than TAM, recognized by expression of the IL4Rα chain as well as CD14, also accumulate within tumors and mediate immune suppression.[23]

Dendritic cells largely found in tumor-draining lymph nodes (LN) are also present among immune cells infiltrating tumors, often with limited expression of co-stimulatory molecules.[24] DC exposed to tumor cells or tumor-derived factors *in vitro* and DC isolated directly from tumors have impaired maturation and antigen-presenting functions.[24] Tumor-associated gangliosides inhibit DC generation and their functions. Furthermore, these DC are programmed to support the expansion of Treg in addition to limiting numbers of T effector cells. Similar to T cells and TAM, DC present within the tumor microenvironment are co-opted to mediate tolerogenic rather than immunogenic signals.

NK cells (CD3$^-$CD56$^+$CD16$^+$) are rarely found among TILs[24] except in the setting of renal cancer, despite the fact that tumor cells frequently downregulate MHC antigen expression and are enriched in MICA and MICB, the two activating ligands for the NKG2D receptor on NK cells. The *in vivo* role of NK cells in anti-tumor immunity is not entirely clear, although their absence in

mice is associated with a more rapid and higher rate of tumor formation and with an improved prognosis in patients with colorectal cancer.

Granulocytes (PMN), which are a major cellular component of most murine tumors, are also infrequently seen in infiltrates of human solid tumors. They are largely replaced by MDSC or TAM, possibly because these inflammatory infiltrates are chronic rather than acute. Mast cells are numerous in tumor tissues, and might substantially contribute to re-structuring of the extracellular matrix by secretion of cytokines (e.g., IL-9) and metaloproteinases.

B cells (CD19$^+$, CD20$^+$) are rare in human tumors, with the exception of medullary breast carcinomas and melanomas, where distinct, follicle-like accumulations of B cells may be found.[24] The presence in most patients with cancer of TA-specific Abs suggests that B cells and plasma cells play an important role in host defense against cancer.

The composition, intensity, and activation state of cells in inflammatory infiltrates change as tumors progress. Initially, the recruitment and influx into tumors of phagocytic macrophages, which depend on the glycolytic pathway for survival, is favored by tumor hypoxia. They process dying tumor cells, producing ROS. The subsequent vessel growth and oxygenation of the tumor milieu is accompanied by lymphocyte infiltration and secretion of pro-inflammatory cytokines.[24] Responding to cytokine cascades, the tumor and stromal cells release soluble factors with a wide range of biologic effects that benefit the tumor and mediate tumor cell migration, matrix remodeling, and angiogenesis.[24] In some circumstances carcinogens can directly inhibit NK cell function,[25] possibly leading to emergence of the tumor without an effective immune response. The tumor's ability to drive remodeling of its environment, including functions of inflammatory cells, determines the success of tumor progression. Cancer development and progression are associated with chronic inflammation.[3] Inflammatory cells in solid tumors are strongly, but not irreversibly, conditioned to support tumor growth and to suppress the tumor immunity.

● KEY CONCEPTS

Inflammation and cancer development

- Cancer is characterized by genomic instability.
- Genomic instability results from genetic (e.g., mutations) and/or epigenetic (i.e., non-genetically driven) events.
- Pre-malignant lesions are associated with immune infiltrates consisting of activated immune cells producing cytokines, chemokines, and enzymes able to modify the local microenvironment.
- Human tumors often contain inflammatory infiltrates enriched in T lymphocytes and DC that are capable of mediating anti-tumor functions.
- Elimination of abnormal cells by anti-tumor CTL leads to immune selection of tumor cells resistant to immune intervention.
- Tissue changes occurring in growing tumors ("host reaction") resemble the process of chronic inflammation.
- Immune deviation (re-programming of immune cells) with accumulations of Th2 and suppressor cells (Treg and/or MDSC) promotes tumor escape ("ineffective inflammation").
- Immune activity is sustained by accumulating Th1 cells and tumor-reactive CD8 T cells ("effective inflammation").

The prognostic impact of tumor-infiltrating immune cells

Despite the immunosuppressive milieu of most human tumors, it appears that not all immune cells present *in situ* are devoid of the ability to mediate anti-tumor functions. In fact, the presence of CD3⁺CD8⁺ T cells within human solid tumors is associated with improved patient survival, recently re-examined using modern immunopathologic methods.[26] When TIL are removed from the suppressive tumor milieu and placed in the presence of IL-2, they tend to recover their function.

The density and cellular composition of tumor infiltrates are potentially significant in predicting tumor prognosis.[26] Although the TNM classification (*t*umor size, lymph *n*ode involvement, distant *m*etastasis) has been traditionally used to predict cancer patients' prognosis, recent use of systems biology methods for the analysis of interactions between tumor and infiltrating immune cells has led to the development of immunologically based classification.[26] This new immunologic classification of cancer patients, which considers variables such as the cell type, density, localization, activation, and the functional status of immune cells within the tumor, seems to be as effective as the TNM system in predicting patients' disease-free survival (DFS) and overall survival (OS). The multiparameter techniques of systems biology confirm the prognostic significance of immune infiltrates into human tumors and indicate that immune biomarkers and immune reactivity at the tumor site influence clinical outcome (Table 76.4).

Immune effector cells in the peripheral circulation of patients with cancer

In humans, peripheral blood is a convenient source of immune cells for phenotypic and functional studies. All immune cell subsets have been extensively examined and compared with their equivalents in the blood of normal age- and sex-matched human

Table 76.4 Prognostic impact of immune infiltrates in human solid tumors

Tumor type	Infiltrate profile	Prognostic value
Primary colorectal Ca	High density of CD8⁺ and CD45RO⁺ memory T cells	Low relapse risk Prolonged DFS
	High density of Th1 cells	High relapse risk
	High density of Th17⁺ cells	Better OS
	High density of Treg	None
	Th1 cell clusters	Short OS
	Expression of p-STAT3	
Breast Ca	High CD8 T-cell count in tumor stroma	Longer OS
	High TAM counts	Shorter DFS; reduced OS
Oral Ca	Low density of DC	Low OS
	High density of T cells expressing TcR ζ chain and high DC counts	Longer OS
Ovarian Ca	High levels of IL-17 in tumor ascites	Longer OS
	High CD8/ Treg ratio	Longer OS
Primary melanoma	"Brisk" TIL infiltrations	Longer OS

Table 76.5 T cells in the peripheral circulation of patients with cancer versus T cells of healthy donors[a]

Phenotype	CD3⁺TCR⁺ T lymphocytes CD8⁺/CD4⁺ ratio: variable Increased % of CD3⁺CD25⁺, CD3⁺CD95⁺, CD3⁺PD-1⁺ Increased % of CD8⁺ANX⁺
Differentiation	CD8⁺ and CD4⁺ Decreased naïve (CD45RO⁻CCR7⁺), central memory (CDRO⁺CCR7⁺), and peripheral memory (CD45RO⁺CCR7⁻) Increased effector/terminally differentiated (CD45RO⁻CCR7⁻)
Regulatory T cells (Treg)	Increased % of CD4⁺CD25^high FOXP3⁺
Clonality	Polyclonal with various restricted TCR Vβ specificities
Specificity	TA-specific/tetramer⁺CD8⁺ cells detectable at a various frequency
Functions	Variably suppressed; impairments are similar to those in autologous TIL but less evident Rapid lymphocyte turnover

[a]Characteristics of peripheral blood T cells in cancer patients were compared with those obtained from the blood of age- and sex-matched healthy subjects. The data are obtained from the literature reports.[23]

subjects. Interestingly, functional and phenotypic abnormalities observed in tumor-infiltrating cells are also present within the peripheral blood cells of cancer patients (Table 76.5). The proportions of CD8⁺CD95⁺ T cells that bind Annexin V (Anx⁺) but are 7-amino-actinomycin D (7-AAD)- or propidium iodide (PI)-negative are significantly greater in the peripheral circulation of cancer patients than in controls.[24] CD8 T cells, nearly all of which are CD95⁺ and PD-1⁺ in cancer patients, are particularly sensitive to activation-induced cell death (AICD). The Fas/FasL and/or PD-1/PD-L1 pathways also likely contribute to the demise of CD8 T cells. Some human tumors express FasL and PD-L1 and can export these death ligands to the periphery via TMV (exosomes); this mechanism of targeting activated CD8 T cells might be one of the major mechanisms responsible for tumor escape from the host immune system.[24]

A loss of activated CD8 T cells responsible for anti-tumor activity can have serious consequences for lymphocyte homeostasis. Circulating Vβ-restricted and tumor-peptide-specific, tetramer-positive CD8 T cells are especially sensitive to spontaneous apoptosis and may be at risk for elimination.[24] Rapid lymphocyte turnover is another consequence of enhanced T-cell apoptosis in tumor-bearing individuals.[27] Using the T-cell receptor excision circle (TREC) analysis, a PCR-based technology allowing for quantification of recent thymic emigrants in the peripheral circulation, it was observed that cancer patients have significantly fewer recent thymic-derived naïve T cells than age-matched healthy individuals.[27] This suggests a lower thymic output or faster peripheral differentiation of naïve T cells. A loss of activated effector T cells combined with a decreased thymic output could severely compromise anti-tumor functions and contribute to tumor progression. While the clinical significance of rapid CD8 T-cell turnover in cancer is not broadly appreciated, data suggest that it may be prognostically important as it discriminates healthy subjects from cancer patients and also patients with active disease from disease-free patients following oncological therapies. Expression on T cells of CCR7, a chemokine receptor and a lymphocyte differentiation marker, emerges as a significant correlate of T-cell resistance to apoptosis. CCR7 signaling upregulates type I PI3 kinase activity, enhances Bcl-2 expression, and lowers Bax and Fas expression in T cells.[24] The frequency of CCR7+ T cells in the peripheral blood may be a readily measurable biomarker predictive of longer survival in patients with cancer.

NK cells are also dysfunctional in the circulation of cancer patients. NK cells have the capability to eliminate circulating tumor cells and thus prevent distant metastasis formation. In addition to mediating perforin- or granzyme-mediated lysis of susceptible targets, NK cells produce a variety of cytokines, notably IFN-γ. They constitutively express the TNF family ligands and can induce death of TNF receptor-positive tumor targets. In the presence of IL-2, NK cells readily differentiate into cells with lymphokine-activated killer cell (LAK) activity, enriched in cytotoxic granules with the ability to kill NK cell-resistant targets.[28] Killer-inhibitory (KIRs) or killer-activating receptors (KARs) expressed on NK cells endow them with the ability to survey tumor targets and discriminate between normal and abnormal cells. Tumor cells that downregulate expression of HLA class I molecules and upregulate that of MICA/MICB, ligands for NKG2D receptor, on their surface are excellent NK-cell targets. However, endogenous NK cells in patients with cancer are partly inhibited from killing tumor targets. The inhibition of cytotoxicity is attributable to tumor-derived factors, such as TGF-β, and is especially evident in patients with a large tumor burden or those with metastatic disease.[24]

Other immune cells present in the peripheral circulation of cancer patients, monocytes, DC, NKT cells, and granulocytes, are also variously influenced by the tumor and show phenotypic and/or functional alterations. Cytolytic CD3+CD56+ invariant (i)NKT cells with the potential to eliminate tumor cells are a minor but potentially important subset of circulating lymphocytes that expands in patients with cancer.[29] They recognize glycolipid antigens in the context of CD1d, which is expressed by many cells including APC. Because iNKT cells are also armed with a lethal arsenal of molecules such as perforin, granzymes, TNF-α, FasL, and TRAIL, they are likely to be involved in destroying malignant cells. When activated, they are avid secretors of several cytokines, especially IFN-γ, and transactivate downstream effector cells, including DC, monocytes, NK, T, and B cells. Their expansion and activation in cancer has been linked to improved patient survival.[29] In contrast to NKT cells, the frequency of circulating DC is decreased in cancer patients, and their phenotype and functions are altered.[30] The molecular mechanisms involved in DC dysfunction are under intense scrutiny, and remain unclear, but a lack of adequate maturation and IL-12 secretion mediated by tumor-derived factors clearly are the main reasons for DC malfunction in cancer.[30] PMN in cancer patients' circulation are often increased, and an increased neutrophil-to-lymphocyte ratio (NRL) is an independent prognostic factor for short survival in patients with ovarian carcinoma. It has also been observed that tumor-derived macrophage migration inhibitory factor (MIF) leads to accumulation of PMN in the tumor and promotes tumor-growth. Tumors not only modulate numbers and functions of immune cells *in situ,* but exert significant effects on immune cells in the peripheral circulation.

Mechanisms responsible for tumor escape from the immune system

Although the abundant presence of immune cells at tumor sites has been associated with improved prognosis in many studies, most tumors progress, metastasize, and recur after therapy

Table 76.6 Mechanisms of tumor escape from the host immune system

Mechanism	Result
A loss or downregulation of TA in tumors	Change in a tumor antigenic profile
Selection of epitope-loss tumor variants	Tumor not recognized by immune cells
Downregulation of APM components	Antigen processing is impaired
HLA class I antigen loss/low expression in tumor cells and APC	Failure in epitope presentation to T cells (low Signal 1)
Tolerance to TA that are "self"	No or low-avidity T cell generated
Low expression of co-stimulatory molecules in tumor cells and APC	Signal 2 is missing or low
Production of inhibitory cytokines in the tumor milieu	Signal 3 is missing or low
Defects in expression of vascular adhesion receptors or integrins on tumor vessels	Inhibition of lymphocyte trafficking to the tumor with lack of Signal 4 allowing targeting of cells
Release by the tumor of microvesicles (TMV/exosomes)	Induce apoptosis of activated T cells/DC; promote Treg and MDSC generation
Accumulations of regulatory cells	Increased % of Treg, MDSC, and others
Activation-induced cell death of CD8 T cells	Depletion of tumor-reactive CD8 T cells
Mobilization of dormant stem cells in the tumor	Initiation of new tumors; resistance to therapy

despite the existence of anti-tumor immunity. It has been suggested that "immune editing" by TA-specific effector cells enables tumors to escape by the selection of immunoresistant tumor cells.[6] The net effect of attempts by the immune system to control malignancy is tumor escape resulting from tumor-driven "counterattack" aimed at immune effector cells. Tumors use many different mechanisms to engineer their escape from the host immune system (Table 76.6).[20] Numerous tumor-derived factors responsible for altering functions of immune cells have been identified to date (Table 76.7). The targets of these factors can interfere with generation, proliferation, differentiation, or function of TA-specific immune cells. The factors mediating various escape mechanisms appear to be unique for individual tumors rather than "global." They are responsible in part for the limited success of current cancer immunotherapies, and it now appears that it might be necessary to *a priori* identify the "immunologic profile" of each tumor in order to select therapies likely to block the relevant inhibitors and restore vigorous anti-tumor immunity. Among these inhibitors, two are of special current interest: PD-L1 (B7-H1) and IL-17. The first is broadly expressed on tumor cells and signals to its receptor, PD-1, present on T cells and other immune cells and inhibiting their functions. Blockade of PD-1/PD-Ll signaling promotes TA-specific T-cell generation and protects Teff from Treg-mediated suppression.[31] The second, IL-17, is produced by CD4 T cells (Th17+ TIL), which accumulate in many human tumors. When IL-17 binds to IL-17 receptors expressed on tumor cells, it initiates IL-6 production, oncogenic STAT3 activation, and activation of pro-angiogenic genes.[32] Thus, Th17+ cells promote tumor growth in part through activation of the IL-6/STAT3 pathway in tumor

Table 76.7 Tumor-derived factors responsible for immune suppression in cancer[a]

Factors	Immunoinhibitory activity
Small molecules	
Adenosine	Signals via A1, A2a, A2b, or A3R, upregulates 3'5'-cAMP levels in leukocytes and inhibits functions
Prostaglandin E$_2$ (PGE$_2$)	Signals via Ep1-Ep4R, upregulates 3'5'-cAMP levels in leukocytes and inhibits functions
Reactive oxygen species (ROS)	Superoxide generation and inhibition of TA-specific T- and NK-cell-mediated cytotoxicity
Cytokines	
TGF-β (membrane-bound in TMV)	Inhibits T-/NK-cell functions, promotes Treg expansion
IL-10	Has multiple pro- and anti-tumor effects; promotes Treg expansion
GM-CSF	Promotes expansion of TAM, recruits MDSC to the tumor
IL-6 and other pro-inflammatory cytokines (IL-8, TNF-α, IL-1β)	Promote chronic inflammation, create pro-inflammatory cytokine/chemokine cascades
IL-17	Produced by Th17 in the tumor; binds to its receptors on tumor cells initiating oncogenic IL-6/STAT3 cascade
Enzymes	
Arginase I	Metabolizes L-arginine, an essential amino acid for T-cell proliferation
Indoleamine-2, 3 dioxygenase (IDO)	Depletes tryptophan, an essential amino acid for T-cell growth
iNOS	Produces immunosuppressive nitric oxide
COX-2	Produces immunosuppressive PGE2
Ectonucleotidases (CD39, CD73)	Hydrolyze ATP to immunosuppressive adenosine
Death receptor ligands	
FasL, TRAIL, TNF-α	Induce apoptosis of immune cells expressing the relevant receptor
Immunoregulatory ligands	
PD-L1 (B7-H1)	Binds to PD-1 on T cells and DC, inhibits functions
MICA/MICB	Bind to NKG2D on NK cells, inhibit cytotoxicity
Tumor-associated gangliosides	Inhibit IL-2-induced proliferation, interfere with DC maturation, induce T-cell apoptosis, suppress NFκB activation
Tumor-associated galectins-1, -3, -9	Inhibit T-cell proliferation, induce T-cell apoptosis
Tumor-derived MV (exosomes)	Carry membrane-bound death ligands, TGF-β, and other suppressive factors, induce T-cell apoptosis, promote Treg and MDSC generation/functions
Virus-related factors	
P15E (CKS-17, synthetic peptide)	Inhibits Th1-type cytokines, upregulates IL-10 production
BBI-3 (homologue of IL-12p40)	Inhibits lymphocyte proliferation and DC differentiation

[a]A partial list of tumor-derived immunoinhibitory factors. It illustrates the diversity of molecular strategies evolved by the tumor to inhibit anti-tumor immunity. The above listed factors may be produced and released individually by different tumors or several different factors might be simultaneously released in the tumor microenvironment. Most are found in the body fluids of patients with cancer.

cells. On the other hand, Th17$^+$ cells can be converted to IFN-γ-producing Th1 cells that mediate tumor rejection, and numbers of Th17$^+$ cells infiltrating ovarian cancers positively predict survival.[32] Thus, the role Th17$^+$ cells in tumor promotion versus tumor rejection remains open, but it illustrates the capabilities of tumors to regulate functions of immune cells found within the microenvironment.

Regulatory immune cells in patients with cancer

Suppressor cells can be broadly defined as regulatory elements necessary for maintaining homeostasis within host tissues and the immune system. More than 35 years ago, Gershon coined the term to describe CD8 T lymphocytes capable of blocking functions of other T cells.[33] Today, it is clear that various immune cells can acquire and exercise regulatory function. While Treg and MDSC are the two regulatory cell types most commonly associated with immune suppression in cancer, other immune cells, including plasmacytoid DC (pDC), PMN, and NK and B cells, are also capable of suppression in the tumor microenvironment. Accumulations of activated suppressor cells in tumors and the peripheral blood of cancer patients have been associated with tumor progression and poor prognosis.[34] Also, these regulatory cells are considered to be responsible in part for a limited clinical efficacy of immune therapies, because they downregulate therapy-induced anti-tumor responses.

Treg are a small subset of CD4 T cells (~5%) that suppress functions of Teff cells by various mechanisms.[35] They comprise several subsets of phenotypically similar cells that mediate suppression via distinct and often unexpected mechanisms.[35] At least two Treg subsets have been recognized in humans:

(a) natural Treg (nTreg), which originate in the thymus, mediate suppression by cell contact-dependent mechanisms involving the granzyme B/perforin or Fas/FasL pathways, and constitute the major regulatory T-cell subset responsible for maintaining peripheral tolerance to self; and

(b) inducible Treg (iTreg) also referred to as type 1 regulatory T cells (Tr1), which are induced in the periphery following chronic antigenic stimulation in the presence of IL-10 derived from tolerogenic antigen-presenting cells (Chapter 15).

They differentiate into active suppressor cells that mediate suppression via contact-independent mechanisms largely involving TGF-β1, IL-10, or other soluble immunoinhibitory factors such as adenosine or PGE$_2$. The phenotype of human Treg is not firmly defined. Most nTreg are CD3$^+$CD4$^+$CD25^{high}FOXP3$^+$, while Tr1 cells have a somewhat different phenotype characterized by high expression levels of inhibitory cytokines, TGF-β1 and IL-10, and the absence of IL-4. Treg recruited to the tumor site appear to be resistant to death and mediate higher levels of suppression than Treg in the peripheral circulation. Considerable controversy exists as to the phenotype and the role of Treg in tumor progression. It is important to remember that Treg-mediated regulation of activated immune cells represents a physiologically normal response designed to maintain a homeostatic balance and prevent undesirable immune activation. Treg found in pathologic conditions, such as cancer or chronic infections, may be recruited to affected tissues and conditioned to suppress excessive activation of immune cells, including anti-tumor Teff, thus favoring tumor growth. If Treg play a role in tumor progression, then their silencing could eliminate tumor escape. For example, by directly inhibiting adenosine and PGE$_2$ production by the tumor and/or Treg or by protecting Teff from inhibitory effects of these factors, it might be possible to restore effective anti-tumor immunity in patients with malignancies.

The second major subset of regulatory cells in tumor-bearing hosts MDSC are potent suppressors of T-cell- and NK-cell-mediated immunity through a broad variety of mechanisms.[23] They are a heterogeneous population of immature myeloid cells defined by expression of common myeloid markers, CD33 and/or CD11b, IL4Rα, and the absence of lymphoid lineage markers (LIN-), such as CD3, CD19, or CD56. In cancer patients, several subsets of phenotypically distinct MDSC exist in the peripheral circulation, which may functionally differ from one another. The frequency of LIN-DR-CD33$^+$, LIN-DR-CD11b$^+$, LIN-DR-CD14$^+$, and LIN-DR-CD15$^+$ cell subsets may be variously increased in the peripheral blood of patients with cancer, depending on the cytokine milieu established by the tumor. A large number of potential MDSC-inducing or-activating factors are known, including vascular endothelial growth factor (VEGF), IL-6, PGE$_2$, stem cell factor (SCF), macrophage- or granulocyte-colony stimulating factors (M-CSF and GM-CSF), TGF-β, and others.[23] MDSC are also heterogenous in respect to mechanisms they employ for suppression. In the peripheral blood, only MDSC in the LIN-DR-CD15$^+$ subset released arginase I, while all other subsets, except the granulocytic LIN-DR-CD15$^+$ cells, could inhibit proliferation of autologous CSFE (5,6-carboxyfluorescein diacetate succinimidyl ester)-labeled CD4 T cells stimulated via the TCR. MDSC produce cytokines and chemokines that can interfere with T-cell homing, promote generation of Treg, suppress NK-cell functions, and promote angiogenesis. In addition, they are a rich source of nitrogen and ROS, which inhibit TA-specific T-cell- and NK-cell-mediated cytotoxicity.[33] MDSC also produce indoleamine-2,3-dioxygenase, an enzyme involved in catabolism of tryptophan, an amino acid essential for T-cell proliferation and

differentiation. Tumors recruit MDSC from the bone marrow through tumor-derived soluble factors such as TGF-β, VEGF, GM-CSF, or IL-10. Accumulating in LN, they interfere with DC cross-priming of T cells, while at the tumor site they inhibit TA-specific cytotoxicity.

PMNs also contribute to tumor progression by secretion of enzymes, chemokines, and cytokines that can alter the tumor microenvironment, including migration and anti-tumor functions of immune cells. PMNs found within the tumor or in the peripheral circulation have been linked to poor prognosis in patients with cancer.[36] PMNs recruited to the tumor by chemokines such as IL-8 demonstrate enhanced production of ROS, NADPH oxidase, and myeloperoxidase (MPO) as well as lactoferrin and metalloproteinases. The production of these factors by infiltrating PMNs converts the tumor microenvironment into an intensely inflammatory site, potentially promoting cancer growth.[37]

● KEY CONCEPTS

Regulatory immune cells in cancer

- Recruited from the precursors in the bone marrow or induced in the periphery by cytokine-driven conversion.
- Accumulate in the tumor and the peripheral circulation.
- Exert their effects in the draining lymph node and/or within the tumor itself.
- Different immune cell types can become regulatory cells (immune cell plasticity).
- Suppress functions (proliferation, differentiation, cytokine production, cytotoxicity) of anti-tumor effector cells.
- Utilize different contact-dependent or -independent mechanisms of suppression.
- The tumor microenvironment drives regulatory cell generation, accumulation, and suppressor activity.
- May be induced by certain immunotherapies and may be responsible for limited success of cancer therapies.
- Treg and MDSC are best characterized regulatory cells, but molecular events controlling their suppressor activities remain unknown.

In the tumor, accumulating immune regulatory cells, whether they are lymphocytes, monocytes, or PMNs, acquire capabilities for downregulating functions of other immune cells. While this process is orchestrated by the tumor and mediated by factors produced by the tumor (Table 76.7), it illustrates a tremendous plasticity of immune cells, which allows them to respond to changes occurring in the environment. In cancer, these changes almost always benefit the tumor.

Chemotherapy and anti-tumor immunity—cancer treatment can enhance anti-tumor immunity

Although it was initially assumed that chemotherapy drugs would block anti-cancer immunity, this has recently been shown to be erroneous. In some circumstances, individual chemotherapy drugs can boost anti-tumor immune responses

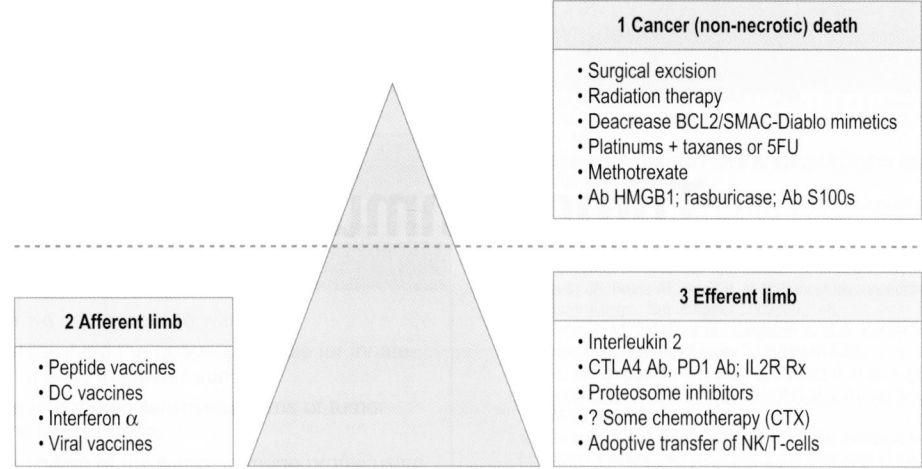

Fig. 77.1 Immunotherapeutic triangle. Traditional therapies for cancer (shown above the dotted line) have involved those designed to primarily (1) kill the tumor cell, largely by mediating necrotic cell death, taking the tumor out or treating with chemotherapy. More recently, it has become apparent that how the tumor cell dies, normally with apoptosis or autophagic death versus necrotic death, is of likely importance. More modern strategies have included use of platinums, which sequester HMGB1 in the cytosol, typically in conjunction with taxanes or fluoropyrimidines such as 5FU; radiation therapy, which induces oxidative strand breaks in DNA, limiting necrosis; use of agents such as methotrexate that promote metabolic/autophagic death; or use of means to block anti-apoptotic factors such as BCL2. Antibodies to HMGB1 or S100 proteins or blockade of purine metabolites such as uric acid with enzyme therapies such as rasburicase recognize the critical role of cell death. Below the dotted line are the postulated role of emergent immunotherapies for cancer, which typically focus on enhancing (2) the afferent limb of the immune response through vaccination strategies or application of immune stimulants such as IFN-α, or (3) the efferent limb of the immune response with IL-2 promoting delivery of immune effectors into the tumor microenvironment, potentiating their cytolytic activity, or use of agents that directly (CTLA4 antibody or antibodies to other inhibitory pathways) or indirectly (some chemotherapy) limit means of escape from immune detection.

heating the skin of the tumor. This was the first clinical experiment in which a purposeful bacterial infection was intended to cure cancer. Subsequently, a New York surgeon, William B. Coley, used a bacterial vaccine to treat inoperable sarcoma, with a reported cure rate of better than 10%.[27]

- **Passive immunotherapy (PI).** PI is defined as the direct delivery to the host of immunologically effective agents including antibodies and antibody conjugates as well as cells including T and NK cells. Köhler and Milstein described a method for developing antibodies with defined specificity, winning the Nobel prize for their efforts.[28] Croce and Koprowski demonstrated that such antibodies could be used therapeutically, ushering in the application for infectious diseases and cancer.[29-31] Anti-CD20 monoclonal antibodies (Rituximab) were approved by the FDA for the treatment of B-cell non-Hodgkin's lymphoma.[32-36] Addition of rituximab to standard CHOP chemotherapy provided improvement in survival.[37-41] Application of antibodies to the CTLA-4 inhibitory molecule (Ipilimumab) expressed on T cells has now been associated with remarkable durable responses in patients with melanoma and this approach has recently been approved.[19,43] Problematic immune-mediated toxicities including panhypophysitis, hepatitis, and colitis are now well recognized and controlled with medical therapy including steroids. Early exciting studies targeting PD1 with antibodies,[15] promoting anti-tumor responses in patients with melanoma, kidney cancer, and lung cancer, have been recently reported.
- Transfer of IL-2-activated NK cells to patients with melanoma and other tumors were initially promising,[44] but were found to be no more effective in randomized trials than IL-2 alone; however, they have had a renaissance in treatment of leukemias.[45] More recently, pioneering studies with the adoptive transfer of genetically modified T cells has had demonstrable success with elimination of large, progressively growing tumors when coupled with lymphodepletion.[46,47] Dendritic cell therapies have been associated with anecdotal

responses in patients with lymphoma and melanoma[48,49] and are approved for the treatment of patients with prostate cancer (Sipuleucel-T).[20,21] This is the first cellular immunotherapy to prolong the life of patients with hormone-refractory prostate cancer (HRPC).

- **Limiting inhibitory factors.** The notion that immunosuppression and regulatory cells (Table 77.1) play a critical role in cancer has been recognized for many years.[50-52] The suppressive role of tumor-derived factors (now molecularly defined as TGF-β and DAMPs) was presaged by Revesz (Fig. 77.2), in pioneering studies performed over half a century ago at the Karolinska Institute.[53-56] He demonstrated that tumors failed to grow in murine recipients unless irradiated tumors were added to limiting numbers of tumor cells. He suggested that the growth promoting effect was due to: (1) specific stimulation by homologous cell products; (2) provision of a "feeder effect" in which the dead cells released essential nutrients; or (3) stimulation that provoked an inflammatory response and/or vascularization from the host. More recent promising strategies include the use of antibodies to CTLA-4 and PD1, thus enabling clonal expansion of T-cell effectors and overcoming limitation of host effector mechanisms, respectively.[42,43] Ipilimumab (anti-CTLA4) was approved by the FDA for patients with melanoma.

Transferable tumor immunity is dependent on T cells, and less dependent on humoral factors. Thus a generation of immunotherapies predicated on active immunization with antigens and various adjuvants ensued with some recent successes. Passive immunotherapies with the application of monoclonal antibodies targeting cell surface molecules and the role of innate immune cells, although thought to be of less importance in previous studies, is now re-emerging with Toll-like receptors (TLRs), NOD-like receptors (NLRs), RIG-like receptors (RLRs), and AIM-like receptors (ALRs) signaling cell death pathways.[57] Recently the application in clinical trials of histone deacetylase (HDAC) inhibitors to alter gene expression, heat shock protein (HSP) 90 inhibitors, and small molecules to inhibit the mammalian target of rapamycin suggests that modern small

Table 77.1 Darwinian selection and coevolution of cancer in its host: means of escape from immune control

Host	Tumor	Stroma
Immunosuppressive cytokines/factors (TGF-β, IL-10, PGE2), VEGF	Immunosuppressive cytokines/factors (TGF-β, IL-10, PGE2), VEGF	Vascular endothelium in tumor-limiting recruitment of host effectors; lack of responsiveness to TNF
Suppressor macrophages	Downregulation of receptors (e.g., TGFβR)	Non-senescent fibroblasts
Plasmacytoid dendritic cells producing indoleamine 2,3-dioxygenase	Specific downregulation of antigens	Reducing tumor microenvironment
Granulocytes promoting acute inflammatory response	Individual allelic class I MHC molecule expression	Wound repair response to DAMPs
Basophils promoting immunosuppression and angiogenesis	B$_2$ microglobulin loss	Release of IL-9 to promote mast cell recruitment
Regulatory T cells limiting immune effectors	Shedding stress receptors such as MICA/MICB	Production of and response to TGF-β
Blocking antibodies	Tumor antigen loss variants	Matrix proteins regulating cytokine and antibody capture, modification
Th2–Th4 biased response	Reduced tumor microenvironment	IL-23, IL-27, IL-35 production

molecule therapies with defined targets could join biologic agents driving important immune-mediated antitumor effects. Caveats involve the possible development of regulatory T (Treg) cells (Chapter 15) in this setting.[58]

Pathogen-associated molecular pattern molecules (PAMPs) and tumor immunotherapy

Perhaps the most effective strategies for preventing cancer are those designed to limit infections and resultant chronic inflammation. Indeed immunization to hepatitis B has been shown to limit hepatoma[59] with a risk ratio of 0.36 for incidence of hepatocellular carcinoma (HCC) in Taiwanese children born after initiation of the vaccine program. Moreover, in hepatitis B carrier children born after the immunization program was initiated, HCC development was primarily linked either to a poor vaccine response or to a failure to use hepatitis B immunoglobulin at birth. Vaccination to human papilloma virus has also led to substantial decreases in cervical carcinoma precursor lesions[60] and in vulvar intraepithelial neoplasia.[61]

Damage-associated molecular pattern molecules (DAMPs) and tumor immunotherapy

DAMPs are typically released following necrotic and late apoptotic tumor death (Fig. 77.3). DAMPS include the small calcium-binding S100 family of molecules, purine metabolites including uric acid and ATP, hyaluronan, HSPs, heparin sulfate, and syndecan.[24] An interesting member of the DAMP family that has cytokine-like properties is the evolutionarily conserved nuclear protein high mobility group box 1 (HMGB1). HMGB1 is

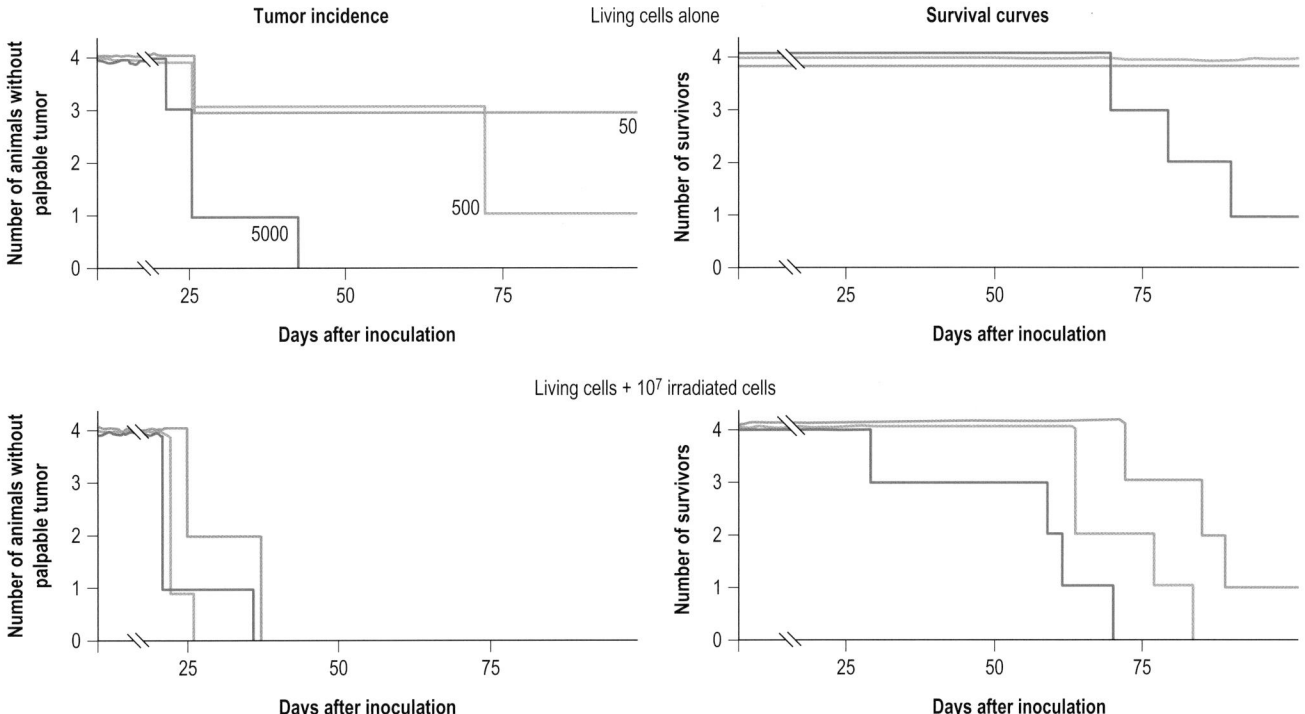

Fig. 77.2 Tumor cell death promotes tumor cell growth. Over 50 years ago, it was recognized that limiting numbers of tumor cells failed to grow in murine hosts unless additional irradiated cells were added. The role of these added cells was considered at the time to mediate its effects by: (1) specific stimulation by homologous cell products; (2) a "feeder effect" in which the dead cells release essential nutrients; or (3) stimulation through provoking an inflammatory response and/or vascularization from the side of the host. Thus the role of inflammation and immune mechanisms was suggested early as an important part of tumor biology, promoting resultant growth of both primary and metastatic tumors. The factors mediating these effects are recognized today as damage-associated molecular pattern molecules (DAMPs). Data from Revesz L. Effect of tumour cells killed by x-rays upon the growth of admixed viable cells. Nature 1956; 178: 1391-1392.

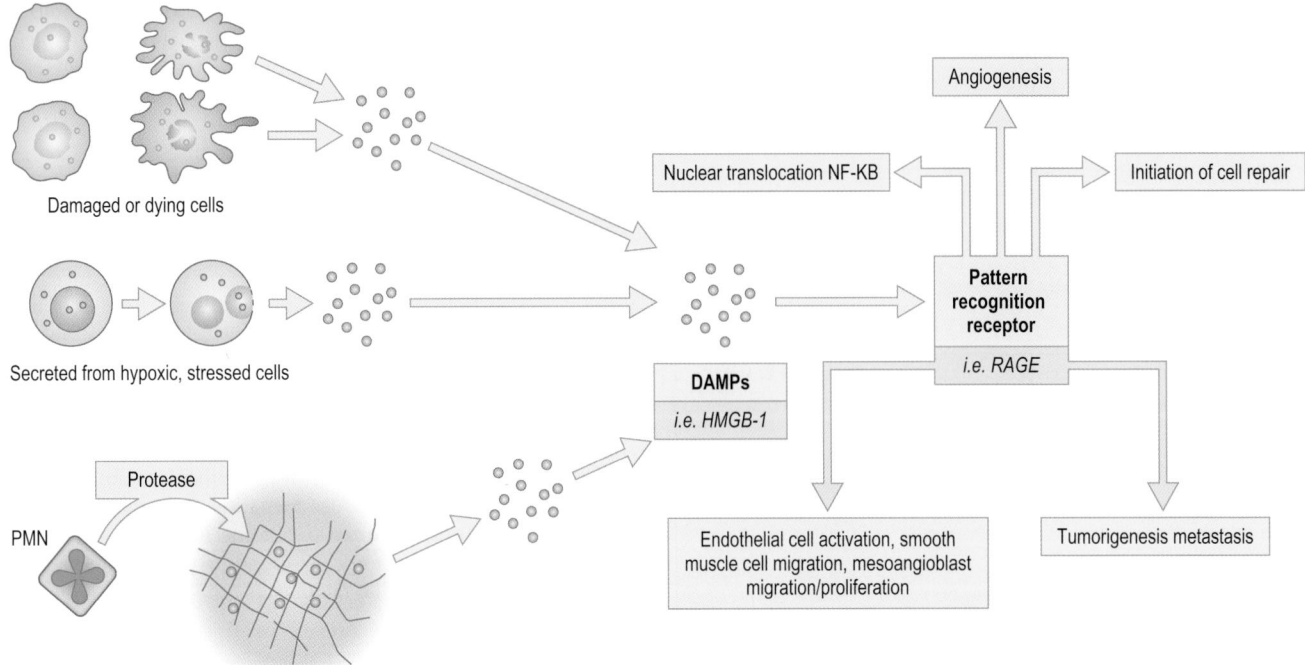

Fig. 77.3 Tumor sources of endogenous damage-associated molecular pattern molecules (DAMPs). In the setting of tumor growth and death, release of DAMPs by damaged or dying cells leads to recruitment and recognition by innate immune effectors of these products. Together, these changes lead to enhanced survival in viable epithelial cells through upregulation of NF-κB, angiogenesis and stromagenesis, and intiation of a wound repair pheontoype, and are associated with enhanced tumorigenesis, migration, and metastasis.

present in the nuclei and cytoplasm of nearly all cell types.[23] It is released upon necrotic but not apoptotic death (Fig. 77.4), and cytolytic effectors promote release from tumor cells.[22] Successful therapeutic strategies for established tumors may involve induction of release of these molecules via selected chemotherapies to boost the host response to tumor antigens.[15]

⬤ THERAPEUTIC PRINCIPLES

Immunotherapy of cancer

- Assess immune reactivity, presence of infiltrating immune cells in the peripheral blood and tumor when available; assess presence of necrosis in the tumor.
- General immune status, DTH reactivity to recall antigens.
- Baseline serum and peripheral blood to assess pretreatment immunity to nominal target antigens in the tumor (e.g., MART1/Melan A, NY-ESO1).
- Determine evidence of DAMPs in the peripheral blood (HMGB1, uric acid, LDH) and DAMP-Rs/induced (sRAGE, IL1RA, neopterin)

Immunotherapy of cancer

Active immunotherapy with vaccination strategies

Long-term survival in patients with cancer has changed little in the past 30 years and introducing effective vaccination to cancer patients remains a major therapeutic challenge. Although cancer vaccines have been practiced in animal models for over 50 years, such immunotherapy in patients remains a novel and experimental approach in most instances (other than the approved use of a dendritic cell (DC)-based vaccine in prostate cancer). Active specific immunotherapy in patients with various solid tumors has been carried out for 10 years with emergent evidence of response to nominal common tumor antigens (Table 77.2), such as the melanoma gp100 and the antigen prostatic acid phosphatase (PAP), which is present in 95% of prostate cancer cells. The use of long synthetic peptides from the human papilloma virus (HPV)-16 oncoproteins E6 and E7 has been unusually effective in women with preneoplastic vulvar intraepithelial neoplasia;[61] complete responses correlated with induction of HPV-16-specific immunity.

Each tumor also has its own immunodominant antigens, distinct from histologically similar tumors arising in other individuals, best demonstrated with the recent successes in use of idiotype vaccines in the setting of lymphoma.[62] Similarly, overall survival obtained by systemic chemotherapy in patients with advanced cancer has been poor, comparable to the low improvement observed with cancer vaccines.[63] In such trials involving 440 patients conducted at the NIH Surgery Branch, the objective response rate was low (2.6%), comparable to the poor results obtained by others. Perhaps the greatest experience has been in patients with melanoma as a consequence of the identification of many melanoma antigens recognized by T cells. Clinical trials performed with various vaccination strategies, including whole tumor cells, antigen peptides, antigen-pulsed DCs, recombinant viruses, plasmids or naked DNA, and HSPs, failed to demonstrate efficacy in the few large Phase III randomized clinical trials performed to date, although the results of the pivotal Phase III clinical trials of MAGE 3 vaccination in patients with melanoma and lung cancer are awaited. Recently two vaccines, one in melanoma and another in childhood neuroblastoma, have been reported to be effective.[63,64] Interestingly, chemotherapy is itself also a "vaccine" in that its use results in the delivery of tumor antigens, including unknown neo-antigens, into the antigen-presentation pathway.[17]

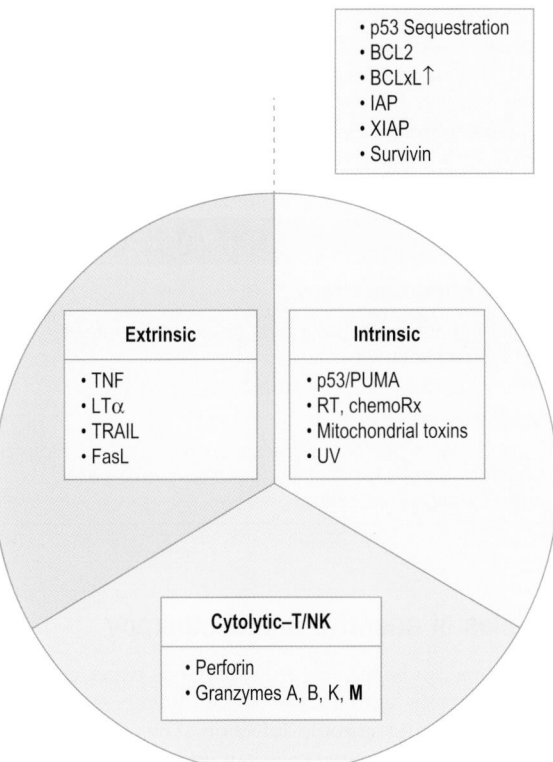

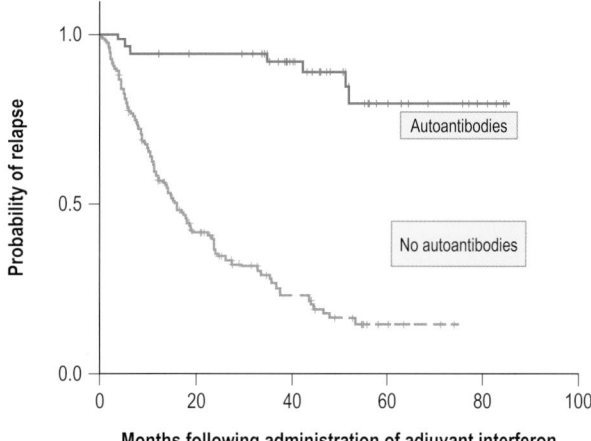

Fig. 77.4 Apoptosis and necrosis in tumor immunobiology. The chevron diagram of apoptotic death involves: (1) intrinsic pathways induced by p53-sensitive induction of cell cycle arrest, and in the absence of genomic repair, upregulation of the BH3 domain containing proteins, PUMA and NOXA, which promote mitochondrial-mediated cell death and release of SMAC/Diablo and cytochrome C. These are typically induced by radiation therapy, some chemotherapeutic agents, toxins, and ultraviolet (UV) irradiation; (2) extrinsic pathways mediated by members of the tumor necrosis factor (TNF) family including lymphotoxin α (LTα), TNF-related apoptosis-inducing ligand (TRAIL), or Fas ligand (FAS L); or by (3) cytolytic effectors, specifically NK and T cells. Paradoxically, in the setting of p53 sequestration, often mediated by mutation, in the cytosol, upregulation of the antiapoptotic proteins, BCL2, BCLxL, IAP, XIAP, and surviving, tumor cells fail to undergo apoptosis or autophagy but rather under conditions of genomic, nutrient, or endoplasmic reticulum stress, undergo necrotic cell death. The consequences are release of DAMPs (Fig. 77.3) and resultant recruitment of inflammatory cells.
Zeh HJ, 3rd, Lotze MT. Addicted to death: invasive cancer and the immune response to unscheduled cell death. J Immunother 2005; 28: 1-9.

Fig. 77.5 Time to progression by auto-antibody status in melanoma patients receiving adjuvant interferon-alpha. Immunotherapy for patients with advanced melanoma induces both serologic and clinical manifestations of autoimmunity. Serum was obtained from 200 patients before the initiation of adjuvant intravenous IFN-α therapy, after 1 month of therapy, and at 3, 6, 9, and 12 months following therapy. It was tested for antithyroid, antinuclear, anti-DNA, and anticardiolipin auto-antibodies, and patients were examined for vitiligo. After a median duration of follow-up of 45.6 months, relapse was observed in 115 patients, and 82 patients died. Auto-antibodies and vitiligo were detected in 52 patients (26%). The median relapse-free survival was 16.0 months among patients without autoimmunity (108/148 relapsed) and was not reached among patients with autoimmunity (7/52 relapsed). In multivariate regression analyses, autoimmunity independently predicted relapse-free and overall survival ($p < 0.001$). The appearance of auto-antibodies/autoimmunity during treatment with IFN-α2b was associated with statistically significant improvements in relapse-free and overall survival in patients with melanoma.
Gogas H, Ioannovich J, Dafni U, et al. Prognostic significance of autoimmunity during treatment of melanoma with interferon. N Engl J Med 2006; 354(7): 709-718.

Active immunotherapy with cytokine treatment

Cytokine therapies are designed to alter immune homeostasis with the tumor and provoke or disinhibit immune effectors. Although both IFN-α (Fig. 77.5) and IL-2 (Fig. 77.6) have been approved for the treatment of patients with metastatic renal cell carcinoma and melanoma, no randomized studies have demonstrated substantial (>10%) efficacy and the high doses necessary to mediate anti-tumor effects have considerable toxicities that have precluded widespread acceptance. Other systemic therapies, including administration of IFN-γ, IL-1, IL-3, GM-CSF/IL-3 fusion protein, IL-4, -7, -10, -12, -18, and TNF-α, have not been demonstrably effective as systemic therapies or as gene therapies when tested. Marked expansion of T cells was recently noted with infusion of IL-7 into patients with refractory malignancies.[65] Further studies of both IL-7 and -15 to support lymphocyte expansion and activation are planned by the National Cancer Institute (NCI) and the Cancer Immunotherapy Trials Network. IL-21 is currently in clinical testing and given the increasing numbers of IL-1 family members, IL-17 family members, and other cytokines, there are numerous additional factors suitable

Table 77.2 Examples of tumor antigens applied in cancer immunotherapy

Altered self	Viral antigens	Oncofetal antigens	Autoantigens
K-ras, p53 mutants Products of normally unexpressed genes (MAGE, BAGE, GAGE) Proteins of alternative reading frame, - of post-translational modification Melanosomal antigens (MART1/Melan A, gp100, tyrosinase) hTERT Proteins with altered glycosylation, (mucin-CA125, MUC1)	EBV- EBNA HPV E-6,-7 SV40 T Ag	Carcinoembryonic antige (CEA α-fetoprotein (AFP) Prostate-specific membrane antigen (PSMA) and PSA Pancreatic oncofetal antigen	Overexpression c-myc in lymphomas, leukemias HER-2/neu epidermal growth factor receptor—breast cancer (Herceptin) CD19 in CLL Prostate acid phosphatase Idiotype on malignant B cells

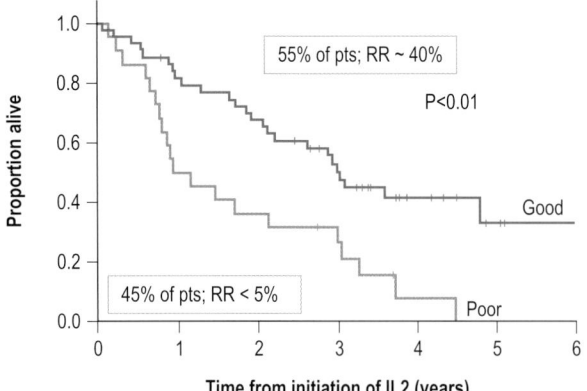

Fig. 77.6 IL-2 treatment-related survival in patients with renal cell carcinoma (RCC) defined by pathologic appearance and carbonic anhydrase IX (CAIX) expression. In patients with RCC, a refined pathology definition of poor risk along with low CAIX expression was associated with nonresponse to therapy (21/39) in 54% of patients and only 4% of responses. Renal cancer response to IL-2 therapy and patient survival correlates with tumor histology and CAIX expression. Tissue specimens were obtained from 66 patients, 27 of whom (41%) had responded to IL-2-based therapy. Fifty-eight specimens were assessed as clear cell, with 56, 33, and 4 having alveolar, granular, and papillary features, respectively. Twenty-four (36%), 31 (47%), and 11 (17%) were classified into good, intermediate, and poor prognosis groups according to the Upton pathology model. Median survival was prolonged ($p = 0.04$) and survival >5 years was only seen in high CAIX expressers. CAIX expression is a predictor of outcome in renal cell carcinoma patients receiving IL-2 therapy and enhances information obtained from pathology. Atkins M, Regan M, McDermott D, et al. Carbonic anhydrase IX expression predicts outcome of interleukin 2 therapy for renal cancer. Clin Cancer Res 2005; 11(10): 3714-3721.

for testing. Still, it seems unlikely that advanced neoplasms will bow to individual or combination cytokine therapies based on the broad experience acquired to date. Prophylactic or adjuvant therapies have not been conducted in sufficient numbers to know whether they might be more effective in this setting.

Passive immunotherapy with adoptive transfer of T cells, NK cells, or DCs

Based on an assumption that the endogenous lymphocyte or DC repertoire is insufficient, inappropriate, or blocked, a number of strategies involving *ex vivo* growth and transfer of these cells into patients have been used. We initially applied IL-2 expanded T and NK cells for therapy over 25 years ago.[44] Transfer of IL-2-activated NK cells was initially promising,[44] but was ineffective in randomized trials. They have received renewed interest based on *in vivo* expansion of human haploidentical NK cells to treat patients with cancer.[45] Isolation of antigen-specific cells, *ex vivo* expansion, and subsequent autologous administration continues to be practiced at a few centers; molecular monitoring of the persistence and transport of transferred cells has afforded highly selected patients with metastatic cancer some benefit. More recently, pioneering studies with the adoptive transfer of genetically altered T cells demonstrates rather conclusively that most patients are not benefited, but in rare patients elimination of large, progressively growing tumors was possible when coupled with aggressive lymphodepletion.[46,47] DC therapies, which we have championed, have led to responses in patients with lymphoma and melanoma.[48,49] DCs can be derived from progenitors in the blood or from bone

marrow using combinations of cytokines, particularly granulocyte macrophage-colony-stimulating factor (GM-CSF) (e.g., sargramostim) and IL-4. *In vivo* expansion or mobilization with GM-CSF promotes antigen presentation of DCs in the setting of therapeutic cancer vaccine. Once stimulated, DCs can present tumor antigen to naïve T cells to initiate an immune response.

THERAPEUTIC PRINCIPLES

Adoptive immunotherapy

- Avoid induction of immune response to adoptively transferred cells
- Prevent or delay cellular immunosenescence
- Maximize helper effects
- Lymphopenia promotes therapeutic effects of adoptively transferred cells by facilitating niche creation and homeostatic proliferation

Principles of adoptive immunotherapy

Many lessons can be learned from previous experiments in rodents and humans with adoptive T-cell therapies for the treatment of cancer and chronic infection. The idea that passive transfer of primed immune cells can generate immunity in the recipient is a relatively old idea. First proposed by Billingham, Brent, and Medewar in 1954, who coined the term "adoptive immunity," numerous animal studies have demonstrated its effectiveness in the treatment of cancer and infectious disease. Moreover, adoptive immune cell transfer has the potential to induce long-standing effects via the establishment of immunologic memory.

Two basic approaches have been tested for adoptive immunotherapy (Fig. 77.7). The first approach has been to isolate and activate antigen-specific T cells from peripheral blood or tumor specimens and then clonally expand the antigen-specific cells *in vitro*. In the second approach, polyclonal *ex vivo* activation of the input T cells is done, based on the assumptions that antigen-specific T cells are present in the patient and have been primed *in vivo*. The first approach will guarantee antigen specificity but is costly and labor intensive while the second approach is technically more facile. Both approaches have been strengthened by the realization that homeostatic expansion of transferred lymphocytes can improve engraftment and effector functions *in vivo*. Studies conducted during the past several decades have uncovered a number of principles of adoptive immunotherapy: (1) avoid the induction of immunogenicity of the infused cells; (2) prevent or delay cellular immunosenescence; (3) maximize help; and (4) choose lymphopenic rather than lymphoreplete hosts. Given that the immune system is such an efficient biosensor system, it is not surprising that seemingly trivial modifications to cell culture technologies can have large differences in their immunogenicity and subsequent engraftment of the adoptively transferred cells. Lymphodepletion eliminates regulatory T cells and other competing elements of the immune system that act as "cytokine sinks," enhancing the availability of cytokines such as IL-7 and -15.[66] This hypothesis has been tested clinically in patients with metastatic melanoma and myeloma, and initial results suggest that the efficacy of adoptive transfer is improved in patients rendered immunodeficient by cytotoxic chemotherapy and radiation therapy.

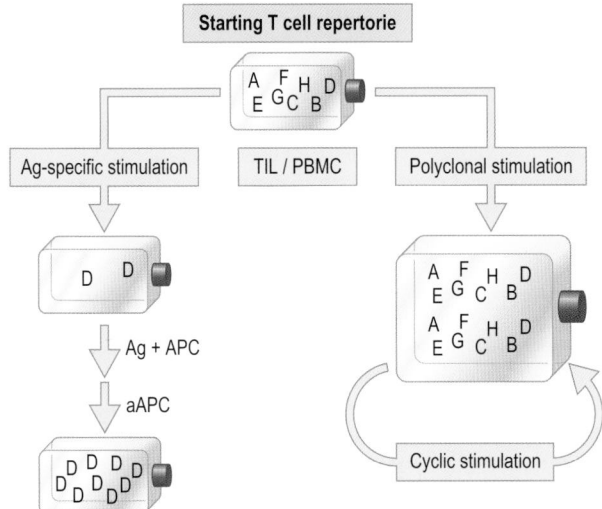

Fig. 77.7 General approaches for *ex vivo* T-cell expansion. Antigen-specific T cells can be generated from the input repertoire by selection of cells with desired specificity with tetramers or antigen-pulsed antigen-presenting cells (APC) and repeated stimulation with APC. This process usually requires several rounds of stimulation (left). Alternatively, the starting T-cell repertoire can be expanded and by polyclonal stimulation to generate polyclonal effector T cells. During the culture process, the cells can be manipulated to increase or decrease effector T cells or Tregs. In addition, cells can be genetically modified during culture. At least 27 cell divisions are required from a single precursor T cell in order to generate 1 billion clonal T cells. TIL: tumor infiltrating lymphocytes; PBMC: peripheral blood mononuclear cells.

Adoptive transfer of effector T cells

Virally induced lymphomas

Virally induced lymphomas that retain some expression of the inciting viral genome are likely to present a good target for adoptive cellular therapy. Unlike most spontaneous tumors, the repertoire of T-cell receptors contains T cells with high-affinity receptors for the viral protein, reflecting a lack of deletion of these T cells in the thymus. In patients recovering from allogeneic bone marrow transplantation, a severe defect in the cellular immune system exists, and this often results in the death of the patients from reactivation of systemic cytomegalovirus (CMV) or Epstein–Barr virus (EBV) infection. Donor-derived, CMV antigen-specific CD8[+] cytotoxic T lymphocytes (CTL) have been administered to the patients with a promising restoration of immune function noted.[67] Recent studies indicate that even relatively modest doses of T cells (1×10^6 cells/kg) were effective in treatment or prophylaxis of EBV-associated lymphoma, with complete remissions recorded in most patients.[68] Pneumonitis and tumor swelling with respiratory obstruction have been reported as adverse events following CTL infusion for lymphoma. EBV-specific CTLs are safe and have significant anti-tumor activity in patients with Hodgkin's disease and nasopharyngeal carcinoma associated with EBV infection.[68]

T cells directed to self antigens

Recent technical advances permit the generation of tumor-specific CTLs, but their clinical utility has not yet been extensively evaluated. Unlike viral-specific T cells, a high degree of tolerance is present for T cells that target self antigens; most CTLs therefore have

low avidity for non-viral-associated tumors. Tumor-specific CTLs generated *ex vivo* with the rapid expansion method appear to have substantial activity in melanoma.[69] However, recent studies at the NCI suggest that host conditioning with chemotherapy and radiation therapy can increase the response to adoptive immunotherapy with tumor-infiltrating lymphocytes (TILs).[66] Adverse effects included opportunistic infections, and the frequent induction of vitiligo and uveitis, presumably due to autoimmunity mediated by the transferred cells. If confirmed, these results indicate that prior host immunosuppression is useful for improving anti-tumor efficacy of adoptive immunotherapy for solid tumors.

Turning off the immune response with suppressor T cells

Suppressor or Tregs can prevent a number of autoimmune disorders in mice. A congenital deficiency of the transcription factor FOXP3 in humans leads to a deficiency of Tregs and is associated with a variety of autoimmune immunopathologies.[70] Tregs were initially thought to be hypoproliferative; however, recent studies show that they can be expanded *in vitro* sufficiently for potential adoptive therapy approaches.[71] In adults with hematologic malignancies, the adoptive administration of cord-blood-derived Tregs demonstrated safety and potential efficacy.[72]

> ### ● KEY CONCEPTS
>
> **Adoptive immunotherapy with genetically modified lymphocytes**
>
> - Antigen specificity can be assured by transduction of chimeric artificial receptors or natural antigen receptors.
> - T-cell lifespan can be regulated by incorporation of conditional suicide genes or genes to delay senescence.
> - T cells are efficiently transduced with retroviruses, lentiviruses, and transposon/transposase systems.
> - Genetically modified T cells can be used to study engraftment and trafficking of adoptively transferred T cells.
> - Genetically modified T cells have been shown to persist for years in patients after adoptive transfer.
> - T cells expressing chimeric antigen receptors targeting CD19 can expand significantly in patients in response to patient tumor cells and normal B cells.

Genetically modified lymphocytes

Genetic modification of T cells *ex vivo* to engineer an improved anti-tumor effect is an attractive strategy for many settings including lymphoma[73] and synovial sarcoma.[74] Advances in basic science have presented numerous approaches for engineering lymphocytes at the genomic, RNA, and protein levels.[75]

A number of issues can be addressed with genetically modified T cells to overcome limitations of natural lymphocytes. The first use of genetically modified T cells was to demonstrate that adoptively transferred cells could persist in the host and traffic to tumor. The next step has been to address a principal limitation of cancer immunotherapy: tumor-induced tolerance that results in few natural T cells having high avidity for tumor-specific antigens (Fig. 77.8). To deal with this problem, some clinical trials in progress attempt to endow T cells with novel receptor constructs by introducing high-affinity TCRs or "T bodies"—chimeric antigen receptors (CAR) that have antibody-based external receptor structures and cytosolic domains that encode signal transduction modules of the T-cell receptor.[76,77] This approach has proved remarkably effective in patients with chronic lymphoid leukemia. These constructs can function to retarget T cells *in vitro* in an MHC-unrestricted manner.

Adoptive transfer with T-cell receptor-modified T cells

Bispecific T cells with specificity conferred by the endogenous TCR and by a transgenic TCR can be created (Fig. 77.8). Important factors for consideration during the selection of TCRs for potential use in TCR gene therapy include the degree to which the cognate antigen is expressed among cells within a particular cancer; the affinity of the TCR for cognate peptide–MHC complex; the ability of the TCR to bind independently of CD8 or CD4 co-receptors; and its ability to properly assemble and pair on the T-cell surface. Transfer of both the α and β chains of the TCR directs expression of the transgenic TCR; however,

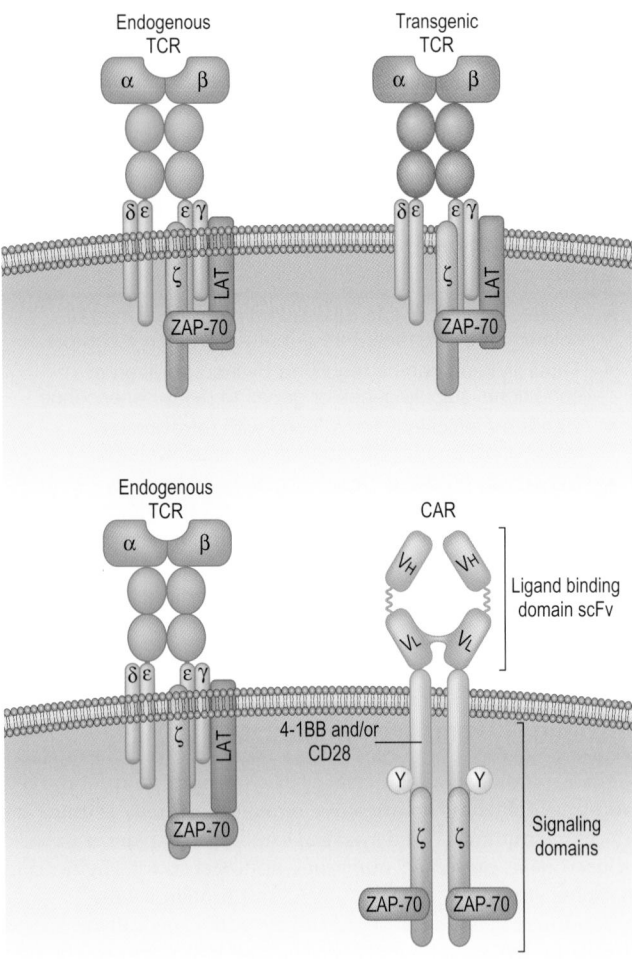

Fig. 77.8 Approaches to engineer lymphocytes. Endogenous T cells express a single heterodimeric T-cell receptor (TCR). Bispecific retargeted T cells are created by the introduction of genes that encode proteins that recognize target antigens. These genes can encode natural TCRs or TCRs with enhanced affinity that function in the same MHC-restricted manner as endogenous TCRs (top). Alternatively, these genes can encode chimeric antigen receptors (CAR) that target surface antigens in an MHC-independent fashion. CARs express an extracellular ligand generally derived from an antibody and intracellular signaling modules derived from T-cell-signaling proteins (bottom).

Modified from June CH. Adoptive T cell therapy for cancer in the clinic. J Clin Invest 2007; 117: 1466–1476.

mispairing with endogenous TCR α and β chains can occur, thereby reducing the surface density of antigen-specific TCRs and increasing the potential for inducing novel autoreactive heterodimeric TCRs.[75] A phase I trial testing engineered MART-1 and HLA0A*0201-specific T cells in patients with melanoma showed that higher affinity TCRs are preferable and generated promising cancer regression in patients. A number of early stage trials testing TCR engineered T cells are currently underway.

Engineered T cells with conditional survival

Graft-versus-host disease (GvHD) is associated with a potent anti-tumor effect. The ability to terminate GvHD at will without use of pharmacologic immunosuppressants following allogeneic T-cell infusions would be useful. Furthermore, genetic strategies that enhance the life span of T cells, interfering with their homeostasis, or modify their antigen specificity to recognize "self" antigens carry an inherent safety risk due to excessive lymphoproliferation or toxicity to normal organs. Integrating viral vectors used for gene modification carries the risk of insertional mutagenesis. These risks could be obviated by the elimination of infused cells. Genetically modified T cells that have an inducible "suicide switch" have been tested in patients after allogeneic hematopoietic stem cell transplantation. Another problem is ascertaining that a rapid means for eradicating cells can be developed in the event of toxicity. Straathof and colleagues modified a late-stage apoptosis pathway molecule, caspase 9, and showed that this suicide gene could be stably expressed in human T cells without compromising their functional and phenotypic characteristics. The T cells demonstrated acute sensitivity to a chemical inducer of dimerization, which caused apoptosis in 99% of transduced cells, and in principle, should be non-immunogenic.[78]

Natural killer (NK) cells

Unlike T cells, natural killer (NK) cells are cytolytic for targets even in the absence of MHC class I expression. Another hallmark of NK cells is their use of a variety of non-rearranging receptors to initiate cytolytic activity and cytokine production. The ability of NK cells to kill tumors that have diminished MHC class I expression predicts that immunotherapies based on adoptive NK-cell transfer should be synergistic with T-cell-based therapies, in that MHC loss variants that emerge as a result of tumor immunoediting by T cells could theoretically be "cleaned up" by NK-cell-based approaches.

The availability of recombinant IL-2 enabled the first clinical trials of adoptively transferred autologous NK cells. Due to poor efficacy, adoptive therapy with NK cells was largely abandoned until recently. However, given the recent appreciation that NK cells express both activating and inhibitory (KIR) receptors, a resurgence of interest has occurred. Infusions of "alloreactive" NK cells have been shown to mediate antileukemic effects against acute myelogenous leukemia in the setting of mismatched transplantation when KIR ligand incompatibility existed in the direction of GvHD, i.e., MHC class I KIR ligand that is absent in the recipient but present in the donor.[79] Recent studies indicate that alloreactive NK cells are cytotoxic for melanoma and renal cell cancer cells *in vitro*, suggesting that HLA-mismatched hematopoietic stem cell transplantation may be an attractive setting for exploiting NK-cell adoptive therapies for patients with solid tumors. Myeloablative therapy and NK-cell infusions with recombinant IL-2 were ineffective although testing in T-cell-replete patients may still be in order.[80]

Passive immunotherapy with bone marrow transplantation

The power of cellular immunotherapy for the treatment of malignancies has been demonstrated clinically by the success of allogeneic hematopoietic stem cell transplantation and its associated graft-versus-leukemia effects (GvL).[81] In particular this has been shown by the success of administration of donor lymphocyte infusions (DLI) for the treatment of relapsed chronic myelogenous leukemia following allogeneic hematopoietic stem cell transplantation. However, this GvL effect is frequently coupled to the development of GvHD, indicating the relevance of alloantigen versus tumor-associated or tumor-specific antigen recognition by donor T cells as the driving force of GvL reactivity. HLA-identical siblings invariably differ at multiple minor histocompatibility antigen loci, resulting in an immune response of greater magnitude than that directed against a single or small number of tumor antigens. Since many of these minor histocompatibility antigens are shared by leukemia cells, it is not surprising that these GvH alloresponses against minor histocompatibility antigens are associated with GvL. T cells recognizing allogeneic MHC molecules, as in the setting of non-HLA-identical bone marrow transplantation, are present at an even higher frequency (approximately 7%) in the unprimed T-cell repertoire of a normal individual.[82]

MHC-mismatched transplantation

Clinical data support the conclusion that T-cell-mediated alloresponses directed against MHC alloantigens lead to even stronger GvL effects than those detected in the setting of MHC identity and minor histocompatibility differences only. Unfortunately, the powerful alloresponse against extensive HLA disparities is associated with an unacceptably high incidence of severe GvHD,[83] thus far greatly limiting the ability to exploit this alloresponse for the achievement of maximal graft-versus-tumor (GvT) effects. However, it has been recently proposed that transplantation across HLA barriers is clinically feasible and can result in potent GvL effects in the absence of GvHD. The strategy ("megadose therapy") that was developed to overcome these barriers and led to the successful transplantation of multiple HLA-mismatched grafts in the absence of GvHD was based on the administration of very large doses of rigorously T-cell-depleted $CD34^+$ hematopoietic progenitor cells following a highly intensive conditioning regimen. Thus, the GvL effects observed in haploidentical transplantations were achieved in the absence of donor T cells and were thought to be mediated by alloreactive donor NK cells.

Passive immunotherapy with bone marrow transplantation

The successful introduction of monoclonal antibody therapy for the treatment of lymphomas as demonstrated by anti-CD20 therapy has proven that immunotherapy of tumors has become a reality. However, in contrast to monoclonal antibody-mediated immunotherapy, induction of autochthonous T-cell-mediated tumor immunity has been less successful and remains a formidable challenge. The major reasons for this failure to induce or maintain T-cell-dependent anti-tumor responses involves different mechanisms of immune escape including (but not limited to)

downregulation of MHC molecules, direct tolerization of effector cells, and induction of Treg cells.

Allogeneic hematopoietic stem cell transplantation is currently the most successful form of cellular immunotherapy for the treatment of malignant hematopoietic diseases despite the clinical problems associated with GvHD or the sequelae of immunosuppression needed to control GvHD. However, allogeneic hematopoietic stem cell transplantation continues to serve as a model for manipulation of the immune response in the clinical situation and has paved the way for various novel treatment approaches currently being explored in non-transplant immunotherapeutical settings for the treatment of malignancies (e.g., induction of host lymphopenia using non-myeloablative conditioning for Treg depletion and allowing homeostatic expansion of adoptively transferred tumor reactive T cells).

Improving the success of cancer immunotherapy by "removing the brakes"

There are a variety of factors and cells that limit the natural anti-tumor response and hence the effectiveness of immunotherapies. Reversing these brakes is a logical and effective strategy. Blocking CTLA4 using a monoclonal antibody (ipilimumab) improved the median overall survival of melanoma patients by 3.6 months.[19] A variety of strategies for blocking the PD1 system are being tested with early promising results.[84] Tregs, particularly the most suppressive ones, can be blocked in animals and patients using low-dose cyclophosphamide as an "immunotherapy."[85]

Conclusions and desirable advances in tumor immunotherapy

● ON THE HORIZON

- PD1/PDL1 antagonists—enhance T-cell effector mechanisms
- HMGB1 antagonism (sRAGE, Ab, ethyl pyruvate)— decrease Tregs, myeloid-derived suppressor cells (MDSCs)
- Chimeric T-cell receptors for T-cell transfection and administration (leukemia, Ewing's sarcoma, possibly breast and prostate cancer)
- Targeting the epithelial–mesenchymal transition with immunotherapies to transcriptional repressors
- Autophagy inhibitors (hydroxychloroquine and others) to promote effectiveness of immune T and NK cells
- CD40 agonists to decrease myeloid-derived suppressor cells
- Applying chemo- and radiotherapy to enhance calreticulin exposure; HMGB1 and ATP release to promote immunogenicity
- Targeting therapies based on pathologic assessment of immune infiltrate
- Targeting antigen to host DCs *in vivo* (e.g., $DEC205^+$ TLR ligand)

Cancer in adults represents the end-stage of mutation accumulation following chronic inflammation, often subclinical and thus without symptoms. As such, three strategies focusing on mediating and enhancing apoptotic or autophagic death of tumors, inducing an afferent immune response, and enhancing and promoting an effective or disinhibited efferent response represent the three mainstays of cancer immune-based therapy. Combinations of selected cytolytic agents, cytokines, adoptive transfer of T cells/dendritic cells or bone marrow, informed by understanding of the mechanism of cell death with afferent and efferent immunotherapy strategies will promote tumor elimination and drive resultant homeostasis in the host.

Within the next 3–5 years, laboratory discoveries in cancer biology and tumor immunology need to be integrated. This will require extraordinary advances in cancer biology associated with deep understanding of cell cycle regulation, the role of the epithelial barrier, apoptosis and necroptosis, coupled with emergent understanding of autophagy in tumor cells as a means of resistance to chemo-, radiation, and immunotherapies. The critical roles of both innate and adaptive immunity must be appreciated by the cancer biology community in order to integrate effectively with more established therapies and to this end there are several promising agents and strategies on the horizon.

References

1. Tang D, Lotze MT, Kang R, Zeh HJ. Apoptosis promotes early tumorigenesis. Oncogene 2011;30(16):1851–4.
2. Vakkila J, Lotze MT. Inflammation and necrosis promote tumour growth. Nat Rev Immunol 2004;4(8):641–8.
3. Galon J, Costes A, Sanchez-Cabo F, et al. Type, density, and location of immune cells within human colorectal tumors predict clinical outcome. Science 2006;313(5795):1960–4.
4. Pages F, Berger A, Camus M, et al. Effector memory T cells, early metastasis, and survival in colorectal cancer. N Engl J Med 2005;353(25):2654–66.
5. Maeurer MJ, Martin D, Walter W, et al. Human intestinal Vdelta1+ lymphocytes recognize tumor cells of epithelial origin. J Exp Med 1996;183(4):1681–96.
6. Woo EY, Chu CS, Goletz TJ, et al. Regulatory CD4(+)CD25(+) T cells in tumors from patients with early-stage non-small cell lung cancer and late-stage ovarian cancer. Cancer Res 2001;61(12):4766–72.
7. Zhang L, Conejo-Garcia JR, Katsaros D, et al. Intratumoral T cells, recurrence, and survival in epithelial ovarian cancer. N Engl J Med 2003;348(3):203–13.
8. Trautmann K, Terdiman JP, French AJ, et al. Chromosomal instability in microsatellite-unstable and stable colon cancer. Clin Cancer Res 2006;12(21):6379–85.
9. Kim GJ, Fiskum GM, Morgan WF. A role for mitochondrial dysfunction in perpetuating radiation-induced genomic instability. Cancer Res 2006;66(21):10377–83.
10. Grady WM, Markowitz S. Genomic instability and colorectal cancer. Curr Opin Gastroenterol 2000;16(1):62–7.
11. Segal NH, Parsons DW, Peggs KS, et al. Epitope landscape in breast and colorectal cancer. Cancer Res 2008;68(3):889–92.
12. Kurts C, Robinson BWS, Knolle PA. Cross-priming in health and disease. Nat Rev Immunol 2010;10(6):403–14.
13. Stumbles PA, Himbeck R, Frelinger JJ, et al. Tumour-specific CTL are constitutively cross-armed in draining lymph nodes and transiently disseminate tumor regression following systemic cd40 activation. J Immunol 2004;173:5923–8.
14. Yuan J, Adamow M, Ginsberg BA, et al. Integrated NY-ESO-1 antibody and CD8+ T-cell responses correlate with clinical benefit in advanced melanoma patients treated with ipilimumab. Proc Natl Acad Sci U S A 2011;108(40):16723–8.
15. Brahmer JR, Drake CG, Wollner I, et al. Phase I study of single-agent anti-programmed death-1 (MDX-1106) in refractory solid tumors: safety, clinical activity, pharmacodynamics, and immunologic correlates. J Clin Oncol 2010;28(19):3167–75.
16. Green DR, Ferguson T, Zitvogel L, Kroemer G. Immunogenic and tolerogenic cell death. Nat Rev Immunol 2009;9(5):353.
17. Lake RA, Robinson BWS. Immunotherapy and chemotherapy- a practical partnership. Nat Rev Cancer 2005;5:397–405.
18. Broomfield S, Currie A, van der Most RG, et al. Partial, but not complete, tumor-debulking surgery promotes protective antitumor memory when combined with chemotherapy and adjuvant immunotherapy. Cancer Res 2005;65:7580–4.
19. Hodi FS, O'Day SJ, McDermott DF, et al. Improved survival with ipilimumab in patients with metastatic melanoma. N Engl J Med 2010;363:711–23.
20. Cha E, Fong L. Immunotherapy for prostate cancer: biology and therapeutic approaches. J Clin Oncol 2011;29(27):3677–85.
21. Kantoff PW, Higano CS, Shore ND, et al. IMPACT Study Investigators, Sipuleucel-T immunotherapy for castration-resistant prostate cancer. N Engl J Med 2010;363(5):411–22.
22. Ito N, DeMarco RA, Mailliard RB, et al. Cytolytic cells induce HMGB1 release from melanoma cell lines. J Leukoc Biol 2007;81(1):75–83.
23. Lotze MT, Tracey KJ. High-mobility group box 1 protein (HMGB1): nuclear weapon in the immune arsenal. Nat Rev Immunol 2005;5(4):331–42.
24. Zeh 3rd HJ, Lotze MT. Addicted to death: invasive cancer and the immune response to unscheduled cell death. J Immunother 2005;28(1):1–9.
25. Mishra B. Intelligently deciphering unintelligible designs: algorithmic algebraic model checking in systems biology. J R Soc Interface 2009;6(36):575–97.
26. Busch W. VII. Verhandlungen Arztlicher Gesellschaften. Berliner Klinische Wochenschrift 1868;5:137–8.
27. Wiemann B, Starnes CO. Coley's toxins, tumor necrosis factor and cancer research: a historical perspective. Pharmacol Ther 1994;64(3):529–64.
28. Köhler G, Milstein C. Continuous cultures of fused cells secreting antibody of predefined specificity. Nature 1975;256(5517):495–7.
29. Gilliland DG, Steplewski Z, Collier RJ, et al. Antibody-directed cytotoxic agents: use of monoclonal antibody to direct the action of toxin A chains to colorectal carcinoma cells. Proc Natl Acad Sci U S A 1980;77:4539–43.
30. Koprowski H, Steplewski Z, Herlyn D, Herlyn M. Study of antibodies against human melanoma produced by somatic cell hybrids. Proc Natl Acad Sci U S A 1978;75(7):3405–9.
31. Croce CM, Linnenbach A, Hall W, et al. Production of human hybridomas secreting antibodies to measles virus. Nature 1980;288(5790):488–9.
32. Press OW, Appelbaum F, Ledbetter JA, et al. Monoclonal antibody 1F5 (anti-CD20) serotherapy of human B cell lymphomas. Blood 1987;69(2):584–91.
33. Maloney DG, Liles TM, Czerwinski DK, et al. Phase I clinical trial using escalating single-dose infusion of chimeric anti-CD20 monoclonal antibody (IDEC-C2B8) in patients with recurrent B-cell lymphoma. Blood 1994;84(8):2457–66.
34. Reff ME, Carner K, Chambers KS, et al. Depletion of B cells in vivo by a chimeric mouse human monoclonal antibody to CD20. Blood 1994;83(2):435–45.
35. Press OW, Eary JF, Appelbaum FR, et al. Radiolabeled-antibody therapy of B-cell lymphoma with autologous bone marrow support. N Engl J Med 1993;329:1219–24.
36. Kaminski MS, Zasadny KR, Francis IR, et al. Radioimmunotherapy of B-cell lymphoma with anti-B1 (anti-CD20) antibody. N Engl J Med 1993;329(7):459–65.
37. Coiffier B. Standard treatment of advanced-stage diffuse large B-cell lymphoma. Semin Hematol 2006;43(4):213–20.
38. Sehn LH, Donaldson J, Chhanabhai M, et al. Introduction of combined CHOP plus rituximab therapy dramatically improved outcome of diffuse large B-cell lymphoma in British Columbia. J Clin Oncol 2005;23(22):5027–33.
39. Feugier P, Van Hoof A, Sebban C, et al. Long-term results of the R-CHOP study in the treatment of elderly patients with diffuse large B-cell lymphoma: a study by the Groupe d'Etude des Lymphomes de l'Adulte. J Clin Oncol 2005;23(18):4117–26.
40. Czuczman MS, Weaver R, Alkuzweny B, et al. Prolonged clinical and molecular remission in patients with low-grade or follicular non-Hodgkin's lymphoma treated with rituximab plus CHOP chemotherapy: 9-year follow-up. J Clin Oncol 2004;22(23):4711–6.
41. Coiffier B, Lepage E, Briere J, et al. CHOP chemotherapy plus rituximab compared with CHOP alone in elderly patients with large-B-cell lymphoma. N Engl J Med 2002;346(4):235–42.
42. Robert C, Thomas L, Bondarenko I, et al. Ipilimumab plus dacarbazine for previously untreated metastatic melanoma. N Engl J Med 2011;364(26):2517–26.
43. Curran MA, Kim M, Montalvo W, et al. Combination CTLA-4 blockade and 4-1BB activation enhances tumor rejection by increasing T-cell infiltration, proliferation, and cytokine production. PLoS One 2011;6(4):e19499.
44. Lotze MT, Line BR, Mathisen DJ, Rosenberg SA. The in vivo distribution of autologous human and murine lymphoid cells grown in T cell growth factor (TCGF): implications for the adoptive immunotherapy of tumors. J Immunol 1980;125:1487–93.
45. Miller JS, Soignier Y, Panoskaltsis-Mortari A, et al. Successful adoptive transfer and in vivo expansion of human haploidentical NK cells in patients with cancer. Blood 2005;105(8):3051–7.
46. Morgan RA, Dudley ME, Wunderlich JR, et al. Cancer regression in patients after transfer of genetically engineered lymphocytes. Science 2006;314(5796):126–9.
47. Muranski P, Boni A, Wrzesinski C, et al. Increased intensity lymphodepletion and adoptive immunotherapy - how far can we go? Nat Clin Pract Oncol 2006;3(12):668–81.
48. Grover A, Kim GJ, Lizee G, et al. Intralymphatic dendritic cell vaccination induces tumor antigen-specific, skin-homing T lymphocytes. Clin Cancer Res 2006;12(19):5801–8.
49. Palucka AK, Ueno H, Connolly J, et al. Dendritic cells loaded with killed allogeneic melanoma cells can induce objective clinical responses and MART-1 specific CD8+ T-cell immunity. J Immunother 2006;29(5):545–57.
50. Hattler Jr B, Amos B. The immunobiology of cancer: tumor antigens and the responsiveness of the host. Monogr Surg Sci 1966;3(1):1–34.
51. Morton DL. Acquired immunologic tolerance and carcinogenesis by the mammary tumor virus. Surg Forum 1966;17:107–8.
52. Schwartz RS, Beldotti L. Malignant lymphomas following allogenic disease: transition from an immunological to a neoplastic disorder. Science 1965;149:1511–4.
53. Revesz L, Klein G. Quantitative studies on the multiplication of neoplastic cells in vivo. II. Growth curves of three ascites lymphomas. J Natl Cancer Inst 1954;15:253–73.
54. Klein G, Revesz L. Quantitative studies on the multiplication of neoplastic cells in vivo. I. Growth curves of the Ehrlich and MC1M ascites tumors. J Natl Cancer Inst 1953;14:229–77.
55. Revesz L. Effect of lethally damaged tumor cells upon the development of admixed viable cells. J Natl Cancer Inst 1958;20(6):1157–86.
56. Revesz L. Effect of tumour cells killed by x-rays upon the growth of admixed viable cells. Nature 1956;178(4547):1391–2.
57. Horvath GL, Schrum JE, De Nardo CM, Latz E. Intracellular sensing of microbes and danger signals by the inflammasomes. Immunol Rev 2011;243(1):119–35.
58. Rosborough BR, Castellaneta A, Natarajan S, et al. Histone deacetylase inhibition facilitates GM-CSF-mediated expansion of myeloid-derived suppressor cells in vitro and in vivo. J Leukoc Biol 2011. [Epub ahead of print].
59. Chang MH, Chen TH, Hsu HM, et al. Taiwan Childhood HCC Study Group. Prevention of hepatocellular carcinoma by universal vaccination against hepatitis B virus: the effect and problems. Clin Cancer Res 2005;11(21):7953–7.
60. Harper DM, Franco EL, Wheeler CM, et al. HPV Vaccine Study Group. Sustained efficacy up to 4.5 years of a bivalent L1 virus-like particle vaccine against human papillomavirus types 16 and 18: follow-up from a randomized control trial. Lancet 2006;367(9518):1247–55.
61. Kenter GG, Welters MJ, Valentijn AR, et al. Vaccination against HPV-16 oncoproteins for vulvar intraepithelial neoplasia. N Engl J Med 2009;361(19):1838–47.

62. Schuster SJ, Neelapu SS, Gause BL, et al. Vaccination with patient-specific tumor-derived antigen in first remission improves disease-free survival in follicular lymphoma. J Clin Oncol 2011;29(20):2787–94.

63. Schwartzentruber DJ, Lawson DH, Richards JM, et al. gp100 peptide vaccine and interleukin-2 in patients with advanced melanoma. N Engl J Med 2011;364(22):2119–27.

64. Yu AL, Gilman AL, Ozkaynak MF, et al. Children's Oncology Group. Anti-GD2 antibody with GM-CSF, interleukin-2, and isotretinoin for neuroblastoma. N Engl J Med 2010;363(14):1324–34.

65. Sportès C, Babb RR, Krumlauf MC, et al. Phase I study of recombinant human interleukin-7 administration in subjects with refractory malignancy. Clin Cancer Res 2010;16(2):727–35.

66. Rosenberg SA, Yang JC, Sherry RM, et al. Durable complete responses in heavily pretreated patients with metastatic melanoma using T-cell transfer immunotherapy. Clin Cancer Res 2011;17(13):4550–7.

67. Riddell SR, Watanabe KS, Goodrich JM, et al. Restoration of viral immunity in immunodeficient humans by the adoptive transfer of T cell clones. Science 1992;257:238–41.

68. Cohen JI, Jaffe ES, Dale JK, et al. Characterization and treatment of chronic active Epstein-Barr virus disease: a 28-year experience in the United States. Blood 2011;117(22):5835–49.

69. Yee C, Thompson JA, Byrd D, et al. Adoptive T cell therapy using antigen-specific CD8+ T cell clones for the treatment of patients with metastatic melanoma: in vivo persistence, migration, and antitumor effect of transferred T cells. Proc Natl Acad Sci U S A 2002;99:16168–73.

70. Gambineri E, Torgerson TR, Ochs HD. Immune dysregulation, polyendocrinopathy, enteropathy, and X-linked inheritance (IPEX), a syndrome of systemic autoimmunity caused by mutations of FOXP3, a critical regulator of T-cell homeostasis. Curr Opin Rheumatol 2003;15:430–5.

71. Brunstein CG, Miller JS, Cao Q, et al. Infusion of ex vivo expanded T regulatory cells in adults transplanted with umbilical cord blood: safety profile and detection kinetics. Blood 2011;117:1061–70.

72. Hippen KL, Merkel SC, Schirm DK, et al. Massive ex vivo expansion of human natural regulatory T cells (Tregs) with minimal loss of in vivo functional activity. Sci Transl Med 2011;3:83ra41.

73. Kochenderfer JN, Wilson WH, Janik JE, et al. Eradication of B-lineage cells and regression of lymphoma in a patient treated with autologous T cells genetically engineered to recognize CD19. Blood 2010;116(20):4099–102.

74. Robbins PF, Morgan RA, Feldman SA, et al. Tumor regression in patients with metastatic synovial cell sarcoma and melanoma using genetically engineered lymphocytes reactive with NY-ESO-1. J Clin Oncol 2011;29(7):917–24.

75. Johnson LA, Morgan RA, Dudley ME, et al. Gene therapy with human and mouse T cell receptors mediates cancer regression and targets normal tissues expressing cognate antigen. Blood 2009;114:535–46.

76. Kalos M, Levine BL, Porter DL, et al. T cells with chimeric antigen receptors have potent antitumor effects and can establish memory in patients with advanced lleukemia. Sci Transl Med 2011;3(95):95ra73.

77. Porter DL, Levine BL, Kalos M, et al. Chimeric antigen receptor-modified T cells in chronic lymphoid leukemia. N Engl J Med 2011;365(8):725–33.

78. Di Stasi A, Tey SK, Dotti G, et al. Inducible apoptosis as a safety switch for adoptive cell therapy. N Engl J Med 2011;365(18):1673–83.

79. Ruggeri L, Capanni M, Urbani E, et al. Effectiveness of donor natural killer cell alloreactivity in mismatched hematopoietic transplants. Science 2002;295(5562):2097–100.

80. Parkhurst MR, Riley JP, Dudley ME, Rosenberg SA. Adoptive transfer of autologous natural killer cells leads to high levels of circulating natural killer cells but does not mediate tumor regression. Clin Cancer Res 2011;17(19):6287–6297.

81. Wingard JR, Majhail NS, Brazauskas R, et al. Long-term survival and late deaths after allogeneic hematopoietic cell transplantation. J Clin Oncol 2011;29(16):2230–9.

82. Jagasia M, Arora M, Flowers ME, et al. Risk factors for acute GVHD and survival after hematopoietic cell transplantation. Blood 2012;119(1):296–307.

83. Lucas CL, Workman CJ, Beyaz S, et al. LAG-3, TGF-β, and cell-intrinsic PD-1 inhibitory pathways contribute to CD8 but not CD4 T-cell tolerance induced by allogeneic BMT with anti-CD40L. Blood 2011;117(20):5532–40.

84. Brahmer JR, Drake CG, Wollner I, et al. Phase I study of single-agent anti-programmed death-1 (MDX-1106) in refractory solid tumors: safety, clinical activity, pharmacodynamics, and immunologic correlates. J Clin Oncol 2010;28(19):3167–75.

85. van der Most RG, Currie AJ, Mahendran S, et al. Tumor eradication after cyclophosphamide depends on concurrent depletion of regulatory T cells: a role for cycling TNFR2-expressing effector-suppressor T cells in limiting effective chemotherapy. Cancer Immunol Immunother 2009;58(8):1219–1228.

Moshe E. Gatt,
Dina Ben-Yehuda,
Shai Izraeli

Lymphoid leukemias

The leukemias are a group of hematologic malignant clonal diseases arising in the bone marrow that present with differing clinical and laboratory features. The focus of this chapter is on acute lymphoblastic leukemia, which is the most common leukemia of lymphoid precursors; and on chronic lymphocytic leukemia, which is the most common type of leukemia of mature lymphoid cells in adults. A special emphasis is given to immunological aspects of both diseases.

Acute lymphoblastic leukemia

Acute lymphoblastic leukemia (ALL) manifests with the clonal proliferation and accumulation of malignant lymphoid progenitors. ALL can be viewed as a developmental disease of the lymphoid system as it often arises as a "developmental accident" during normal fetal lymphopoiesis. Studies of chromosomal translocations in ALL cells have identified key genes involved in normal lympho- and hematopoiesis. Conversely, basic studies of the development of the immune system and the immune receptors have provided important tools for diagnosis and management of ALL. These achievements in basic and clinical research have led to the remarkable transformation of ALL from a uniformly fatal disease several decades ago to a disease which is currently curable in more than 80% of children. Adults, however, remain a challenge.[1]

Epidemiology and etiology

ALL is the most common malignancy of childhood. One of every 2 000 children will develop leukemia by 15 years of age. In contrast ALL accounts for less than 20% of leukemias in adults. In developed countries, the incidence of ALL peaks at 2–5 years of age and then rises again in individuals older than 65 years. Males are generally affected more often than females. The low age peak is characteristic of affluent societies and explains the higher rate of childhood ALL in whites when compared to blacks, and in Northern America and Europe when compared with Asia and Africa.[2]

Most ALLs are sporadic, with less than 5% associated with hereditary or constitutional syndromes. For example, children with Down syndrome have about 20-fold increased risk of ALL. This higher risk may reflect the leukemogenic role of chromosome 21, as extra copies of chromosome 21 are frequently observed in leukemic blasts of sporadic ALL. Other diseases associated with increased risk are inherited genomic instability syndromes such as ataxia–telangiectasia, Bloom and Li-Fraumeni syndromes. Similarly ALL is more common in patients with other congenital immunodeficiencies, such as X-linked agammaglobulinemia, IgA deficiency, and common variable immunodeficiency.

Studies of leukemia in identical twins have shed light on the etiology of childhood ALL. Although ALL is not hereditary, there is markedly increased risk of leukemias in identical twins. If leukemia occurs in one identical twin, the other twin generally has a 10–20% chance of developing the disease by the age of 10 years. This phenomenon has promoted the hypothesis that at least two genetic hits are required for the development of ALL (Fig. 78.1).[2] The first occurs during fetal lymphopoiesis and results in clonal proliferation of a pre-leukemic clone. Intrauterine metastasis of such a pre-leukemic clone from one twin to the other via their shared placental circulation is responsible for the concordant leukemia. Additional genetic hits in the pre-leukemic cells occur after birth and are required for the development of full-blown leukemia. The initial findings in identical twins with leukemia have been extended to sporadic ALL; in at least 70% of patients the preleukemic clone can be detected molecularly in the neonatal blood samples collected after birth (known as Guthrie cards). More recently, careful molecular analysis of the cord blood of normal infants has demonstrated that the occurrence of a preleukemic clone carrying a leukemia-defining chromosomal translocation is relatively common. However, only 1% of children born with such a preleukemic clone will develop leukemia, implying the impracticality of a molecular screen for the early diagnosis of childhood ALL.

● CLINICAL PEARLS

Environmental factors in the epidemiology of childhood ALL. Roles for infection and immunity?

"Common" B cell precursor ALL at the preschool age is the most common type of ALL in the suburban regions of affluent countries. The causes for this phenomenon are unknown. A popular hypothesis suggests a modified immune response to delayed infections during infancy.

The causes of the relatively rare postnatal leukemogenic genetic hits are unknown. Although environmental agents such as ionizing radiation and chemical mutagens have been implicated in the induction of ALL, almost all cases lack discernible etiologic factors. As the risk of B-cell precursor ALL during early childhood is markedly increased by higher socioeconomic status and suburban style of living in which the exposure of children to infectious pathogens is typically delayed beyond the neonatal period, Greaves hypothesized that many childhood cases are the consequence of an abnormally late immunologic response to common infections. One proposed mechanism is that growth inhibitory factors, such as interferon or TGF-β, secreted during

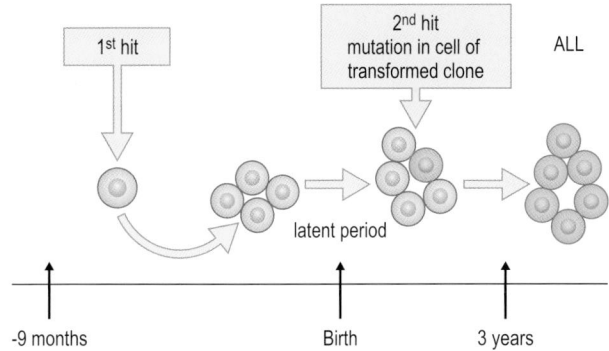

Fig. 78.1 A model for the development of childhood acute lymphoblastic leukemia (ALL). The first acquired genomic hit (e.g., chromosomal translocation or change in chromosomal copy number) occurs during fetal hematopoiesis and results in clonal proliferation of a preleukemic clone. This event is common, occurring in up to 1 in every 20 children. Additional genetic aberrations occurring after birth are required for the development of ALL. These events are rare and are estimated to occur in about 1% of children born with a preleukemic clone.[5]

this immune response provide a survival advantage to a preleukemic clone, setting the stage for additional leukemogenic mutations.[2,3]

Immunologic and molecular classification of ALL

Immunologic classification

The subtypes of ALL are usually identified by their immunophenotype, which tends to resemble the lymphoid developmental stage in which the leukemic cell was arrested (Table 78.1).[4]

B-cell precursor leukemias

These are the most common childhood leukemias. Pro-B ALL is characterized by expression of CD19 and CD34 without CD10. This is the most common leukemia of infants that usually contains rearrangements of the histone methyltransferase *MLL* gene on chromosome 11q23 and is associated with a poor outcome. Leukemic blast cells of early pre-B ALL resemble normal B-lymphoid cell precursors. They express CD19, CD22, and CD79a. CD10 and terminal deoxynucleotidyl transferase (TdT) are detectable in 90% of cases, and CD34 in more than 75% of cases. This is the most common type of ALL, and thus often called "common ALL" (cALL). In pre-B ALL cases lymphoblasts accumulate cytoplasmic immunoglobulin heavy chains, but have no detectable surface immunoglobulins. This subtype also expresses CD19, CD22 and CD79a. pre-B ALL often contains a translocation that fuses the *E2A* gene on chromosome 19 with the *PBX1* gene on chromosome 1.[5] Leukemic cells that express both cytoplasmic and surface immunoglobulin heavy chains have been designated transitional pre-B ALL. The surface μ chains on these leukemic cells associate with surrogate-light chain (VpreB λ5[λ14.1]) as well with CD79a and CD79b.

Mature B-cell ALL is the leukemic form of Burkitt's lymphoma (Chapter 79). As the treatment of mature B-cell ALL is dramatically different from that of B-cell precursor ALL, this condition must be specifically ruled out as part of the immunophenotypic evaluation of the leukemia. These mature cells express surface immunoglobulin μ heavy chains in association with conventional κ or λ light chains. In most cases these cells have L3 morphology and express CD19, CD22, and CD20. CD10 is also frequently expressed, but CD23 and CD34 are absent.

T-cell ALL

In affluent countries, T-ALL occurs in 10–15% of children with ALL. It is more prevalent in non-affluent countries; probably as a reflection of a lower incidence of the common B-lineage early childhood peak. T-ALL is also more common in adults.

T-cell ALL cells express CD7 and cytoplasmic CD3 (cCD3) antigens on their surface; and more than 90% of T lymphoblasts express CD2, CD5, and TdT. Three stages of immunophenotypic differentiation can be determined: early (CD7+, cCD3+, surface CD3−, CD4−, and CD8−), intermediate (cCD3+, surface CD3−, CD4+, CD8+, and CD1+) and late (surface CD3+, CD1−, and either CD4+ or CD8+). However, in as many as 25% of T-lineage ALL cases, the immunophenotype does not conform to any of these maturation stages. T-cell receptor (TCR) proteins are heterogeneously expressed in T-lineage ALL. In approximately two-thirds of cases membrane CD3 and TCR proteins are absent.

Table 78.1 Immunophenotypic classification of ALL

| Subtype | Leukocyte antigen expression (% of cases positive) | | | | | | | | | | Frequency (%) | |
	CD19	cCD22	CD79a	CD10	CD7	CD2	cCD3	clg μ	slg μ	slg κ or γ	Children	Adults
Pre-pre-B	100	>95[a]	>95	0	0	0	0	0	0	0	5	10
Early pre-B	100	>95[a]	>95	95	5	<5	0	0	0	0	60–65	50–55
Pre-B	100	100[a]	100	>95	0	0	0	100	0	0	20–25	10
Transitional pre-B	100	100[a]	100	50	0	0	0	100	100	0	1–3	?
B	100	100[a]	100	50	0	0	0	>95	>95	>95	2–3	4
Pre-T	<5	0	0–20	45	100	0	100	0	0	0	1	5
T	<5	0	0–20	45	100	95	100[a]	0	0	0	10–15	15–20

c, cytoplasmic; clg μ, cytoplasmic immunoglobulin μ chain; slg μ, surface immunoglobulin μ chain; slg κ or λ, surface immunoglobulin κ or λ chains.
[a]Detectable on the cell surface membrane in some cases.

In half of these cases, however, TCR proteins (TCRβ, TCRα, or both) are present in the cytoplasm. When membrane CD3 and TCR chains are expressed, the αβ form of the TCR predominates. Only a minority of cases express TCR γδ proteins.

The expression of myeloid-associated antigens, such as CD13, CD15, CD33, or CD65, in leukemic lymphoblasts confounded leukemia classification in early studies. However, the diagnosis of B-lineage ALL should be made when leukemic cells express cytoplasmic immunoglobulin, CD79a, or CD19 plus CD22, regardless of myeloid-associated antigen expression. Likewise, the diagnosis of T-lineage ALL should be made when leukemic cells express CD7 plus either surface or cytoplasmic CD3.

Recently a genetically and immunophenotypic distinct form of T-ALL originating from early T-cell precursors (ETPs) has been recognized. It is characterized by low or absent CD1a and CD5 coupled with the expression of at least one myeloid marker.[6]

Genetic and molecular classification

Virtually every leukemic cell contains acquired alterations in multiple genes. These alterations are often manifested by gross numerical or structural aberrations that frequently define a specific clinical subtype of ALL. The common and/or clinically significant genetic aberrations that are typically found in ALL are reviewed in[7] and summarized in Table 78.2.

Numerical chromosomal aberrations

Deviation from the normal chromosomal modal number is called aneuploidy and is the most common chromosomal aberration in cancer. High hyperdiploid ALL (Fig. 78.2A), containing between 50 and 60 chromosomes, is the most common type of B-lineage ALL in children and is associated with about a 90% cure rate. Typically there is an excess of specific chromosomes, most commonly chromosomes 6, 10, 14, 17, 18, 21, and X.

Hypodiploid ALL (Fig. 78.2B), which contains less than 45 chromosomes, is much rarer and is associated with a very bad prognosis.

Table 78.2 Frequencies of major, clinically important genetic aberrations in childhood and adult ALL

Genetic aberration	Children	Adults
B-cell lineage		
Hyperdiploidy (>50 chromosomes)	30%	9%
Hypodiploid (<45 chromosomes)	1%	2%
Amplified 21q	2%	?
TEL-AML1 (t12;21)	25%	3%
MLL rearrangements	9%	13%
BCR-ABL	4%	33%
E2A-PBX1	5%	4%
MYC rearrangements	2%	5%
CRLF2 rearrangements	8%	10%
T-cell lineage		
Notch1 mutations	60%	70%
IL-7R mutations	10%	?
PTEN mutations	10%	?
TAL1 (SCL) cluster	58%	33%
HOX11 (TLX1) cluster	3%	33%
HOX11L2 (TLX3) cluster	20%	5%
LYL1 cluster	12%	37%
MLL-ENL	2%	2%
NUP214-ABL	6% (?)	6% (?)
MYB rearrangements	5%	

Modified from Armstrong SA, Look AT. Molecular genetics of acute lymphoblastic leukemia. J Clin Oncol. 2005; 23: 6306-6315.

Structural genetic aberrations

Chromosomal translocations can be divided into two general subtypes.[8] The first results from a translocation of an oncogene into the proximity of a strong regulatory region, resulting in its marked overexpression. Often these translocations are mediated by the V(D)J recombination machinery (Chapter 4) and can be therefore viewed as an unfortunate developmental "accident" caused by the physiologic lymphocyte specific genomic instability that is necessary for the creation of the astronomic diversity required to recognize novel antigens. Examples of these translocations include the activation of the MYC oncogene by the t(8;14) translocation in Burkitt's lymphoma and of the gene by a t(1;14) translocation or a SIL gene translocation on chromosome 1p32 in T-ALL. Most of the chromosomal translocations observed in T-ALL are of this type. The second type of translocation creates a novel fusion protein consisting of parts of the genes that participate in the chromosomal translocation. The mechanisms that underlie these translocations remain unclear. Most of the translocations characteristic of B precursor ALL are of this type, for example the t(12;21) fusing of the TEL (ETV6) gene on chromosome 12 with the AML1 (RUNX1) gene on chromosome 21.

Amplification and deletion of a small chromosomal region is another type of structural aberration that is often detected in leukemias. For example deletions of the INK4A locus or PAX5 are commonly detected in T- and B-cell precursor ALLs, respectively.

Oncogenic activating mutations in ALL are reported with an increasing frequency. For example the Notch pathway, which plays a role in T-cell development, has been recently reported to be activated by acquired mutations in more than 60% of T-ALL.[9] This finding is of potential therapeutic significance since novel γ-secretase inhibitors, originally developed for treatment of Alzheimer's disease, block the Notch pathway.

Many of the genes modified by chromosomal translocations, amplification, deletions or point mutations function in normal lymphoid or hematopoietic development (Table 78.3). The acquired aberrations promote malignant transformation by either over- or mis-expression (in the wrong cell or in the wrong developmental stage) of the developmental gene. A recent discovery involving IL-7Rα is a good example. Loss of function mutations in this receptor cause $T^-B^+NK^+$ severe combined immunodeficiency (Chapter 35) and activating mutations are found in 10% of T-ALL.[10] One common mutation introduces cysteine into the IL-7Rα juxtamembranous domain, inducing homodimerization with ligand independent activation of the receptor.

An example involving both mis-expression and activation of an immune receptor is the aberrant activation of the receptor to Thymic Stromal Lymphopoietin (TSLP). This receptor, which is created by heterodimerization of IL-7Rα and CRLF2, is normally expressed in dendritic and some CD4 T cells. It is involved in allergy and inflammation. Activation of this receptor in B lineage ALL is multi-staged: first, chromosomal translocations likely mediated by aberrant V(D)J cause the mis-expression of CRLF2 in a B-cell precursor. This is followed by activating mutations in the TSLP receptor components—either CRLF2, IL-7Rα, or the downstream signaling enzymes JAK2 or JAK1.[11,12] Aberrant expression and activation of the TSLP receptor is found in 10% of sporadic B-ALLs (in 60% of DS-ALLs) and is associated with a bad prognosis. It may also be a amenable to targeted therapy. Conversely, the acquired genetic aberration may block the normal developmental function of the involved gene(s). Good examples are genomic deletions or inactivating mutations in B-cell differentiation genes such as PAX5, EBF, or IKZF1, which are detected in about 50% of B lineage ALLs.[13]

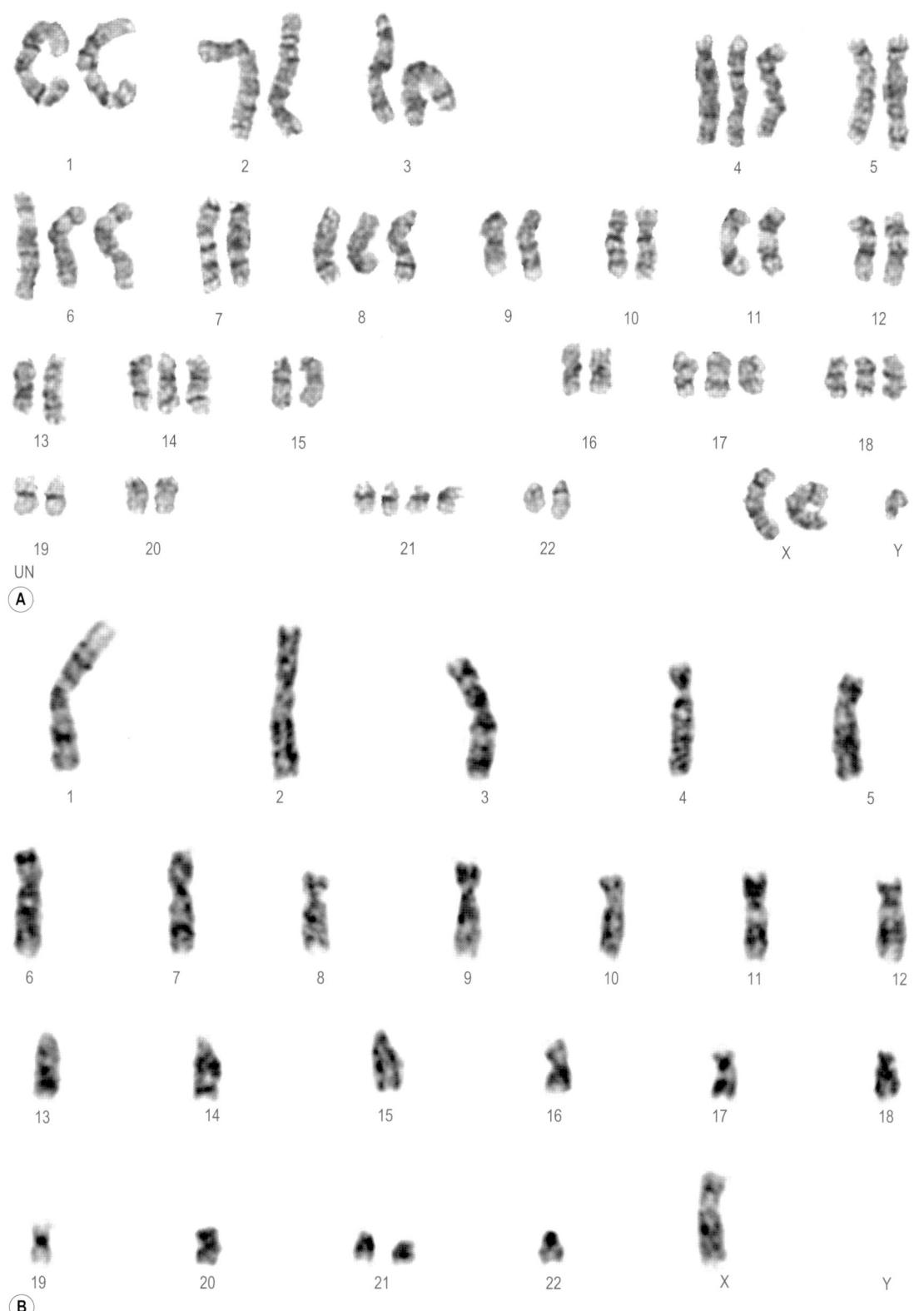

Fig. 78.2 Chromosomal aneupoloidy in acute lymphoblastic leukemia (ALL). A typical karyotype of (A) hyperdiploid and (B) hypodiploid ALL.
(Courtesy of B. Stark and D. Betts.)

Table 78.3 Example of hematopoietic genes involved in the pathogenesis of leukemia

Gene(s) names	Normal hematopoietic development	Leukemic involvement
SCL (TAL1)	Hemangioangioblast specification. Erythro- and megakaryopoiesis	T-ALL
LMO1/2	Similar to SCL	T-ALL
NOTCH1	T lymphocytes	T-ALL
HOX11	Spleen	T-ALL
E2A	T and B lymphocytes	BCP-ALL
PAX5	B lymphocytes	BCP-ALL, B-NHL
SLP-65	B lymphocytes	BCP-ALL
TEL	Bone-marrow hematopoietic stem cells	BCP-ALL, T-ALL rarely myeloid malignancies
RUNX1 (AML1, CBFA2)	Definite hematopoiesis. Megakaryopoiesis and T lymphocytes	BCP ALL, AML (M0-M1) Hereditary FPD/AML
CBFB	Same as RUNX1	AML (M4e)
C/EBP 1-3	Myeloid cells	AML (M1, M2)
PU.1	Myeloid and lymphoid stem cells	AML
GATA1	Erythropoiesis, megakaryopoiesis and mast cells	AML (M7) associated with trisomy 21
FLT3	Hematopoiesis and lymphopoiesis	AML and ALL
MLL	Hematopoiesis stem cells	AML and ALL
IL7R	T lymphocytes	ALL

Major, clinically relevant, molecular subtypes of ALL (Table 78.2)

B-lineage ALL

Hyperdiploid and TEL-AML1 ALL comprise the majority of "common ALL" leukemias typical of young children, and are rare in adults with ALL. Both are associated with an extremely good prognosis. In contrast the much less common hypodiploidy (less than 45 chromosomes) and the internal amplification of chromosome 21q (iAMP 21q) are associated with bad prognosis.[14] Another bad prognosis aberration is the BCR-ABL fusion created by the t(9;22) "Philadelphia chromosome." Its frequency is low in children (3–5%) and much higher in adults (at least 30%). These differences may explain the poorer outcome of ALL in adults compared with children. The MLL gene located on chromosome 11q23 is involved in fusion translocations with more than 80 different partner genes. The most common translocation in ALL fuses the MLL with the AF4 gene on chromosome 4. This t(4;11) translocation is characteristic of infant leukemia and is associated with poor prognosis. The clinical significance of the E2A-PBX1 fusion caused by the t(1;19) translocation, occurring in less than 5% of childhood ALL, is uncertain. It was associated with a worse prognosis on treatment protocols which were mainly based on anti-metabolite chemotherapy. With newer protocols that incorporate anthracyclines, this prognostic significance has been lost. Indeed, this type of ALL may be associated with a better outcome. The change in the prognostic

significance of this particular translocation as a result of improved therapy exemplifies the general principle that the prognostic impact of a clinical or biological parameter is highly dependent on the specific treatment protocol.[1] The E2A gene is rarely fused with the HLF gene in the t(17;19) translocation. This is an extremely rare translocation that is associated with a clinical presentation of diffuse intravascular coagulation (DIC) and hypercalcemia and an extremely poor prognosis.

Several secondary genetic lesions (lesions that may be associated with some of the abnormalities described above) have prognostic significance and maybe included in risk stratification in future treatment protocol. Examples are deletions of Ikaros (IKZF1)[15] and CRLF2 aberrations.[16]

T-lineage ALL

Although multiple genetic and molecular subtypes of T-ALL have been described recently, at present their clinical significance is unclear[7,17] except for the bad prognosis of ETP ALL.[6] Most of the genetic aberrations in T-ALL result in the abnormal expression of transcription factors. Examples include SCL (TAL1) that forms a complex with LMO1 or LMO2, HOX11L2 (TLX3) or HOX11 (TLX1), and LYL1 and MYB. Other abnormalities include MLL-ENL fusions and amplification of the ABL oncogene. Cooperating mutations are activating mutations in NOTCH1 or IL-7R and inactivating mutations in the E3 ligase FBW7 or the PTEN phosphatase.

Clinical features

The clinical signs and symptoms relate to the replacement of bone marrow cells by leukemic blasts and to the infiltration of extramedullary sites. Anemia, thrombocytopenia and neutropenia caused by bone marrow involvement may manifest with pallor, fatigue, petechiae or bleeding and fever. Bone pain and arthralgias, the onset of limp and refusal to walk, and even frank arthritis are not uncommon. The musculoskeletal symptoms may be confused with osteomyelitis or juvenile rheumatoid arthritis and this may delay the diagnosis. Uncommonly, central nervous system (CNS) involvement may present with the signs and symptoms of increased intracranial pressure, such as headaches and papilledema; by cranial nerve palsies or nuchal rigidity; and rarely with hyperphagia and obesity caused by infiltration of the hypothalamus. Overt testicular leukemia at diagnosis is rare and manifests with painless testicular enlargement. Mediastinal involvement, common in T-ALL, can cause dyspnea and superior vena cava syndrome, or frank respiratory failure.

Clinical laboratory findings often reveal anemia and thrombocytopenia. Approximately 20% of children present with leukocyte counts greater than 50 000/μL. Importantly, approximately 40% of children have leukocyte counts of less than 10 000/μL and leukemic blasts may or may not be seen on peripheral smears. Therefore the diagnosis of leukemia may occasionally be missed in a routine automated blood count. Elevated serum lactate dehydrogenase activity, and uric acid and phosphorus concentrations are common in patients with a large leukemic cell burden.

The diagnosis of ALL is established by examination of the bone marrow. The normal bone marrow contains less than 5% blasts. A minimum of 25% lymphoblasts on differential examination of the bone marrow aspirate is necessary for the diagnosis of ALL. Most children with ALL have a hypercellular marrow with blasts constituting 60 to 100% of the nucleated cells.

Traditionally, CNS leukemia is defined by the presence of at least 5 leukocytes per microliter of CSF and the detection of leukemic blast cells, or by the presence of cranial nerve palsy or by retinal involvement as detected by ophthalmoscopy. While overt CNS leukemia is relatively rare, submicroscopic CNS involvement in the absence of any neurological symptoms is present at diagnosis in at least half of the patients. Therefore CNS directed therapy is routinely included in ALL therapy (see below).

The differential diagnosis of ALL includes both neoplastic and non-neoplastic diseases. Because children with ALL present with a variety of nonspecific symptoms, several pediatric non-malignant conditions can be confused with leukemia. Since treatment with steroids can mask the presence of ALL, serious consideration of the diagnosis of ALL must be given before starting treatment with steroids to any pediatric non-malignant disorder. Bone marrow examination is recommended in uncertain cases. Idiopathic thrombocytopenic purpura (ITP) is a common cause of bruising and petechiae in children. ITP is characterized by the absence of other hematological abnormalities. The bone marrow should be examined if anemia or hepatosplenomegaly are present. Infectious mononucleosis may present with fever, malaise, adenopathy, splenomegaly, rash, and lymphocytosis. Lymphocytosis accompanied by thrombocytopenia and immunohemolytic anemia can further confuse the diagnosis. The atypical lymphocytes may morphologically resemble the leukemic lymphoblasts, although an experienced hematologist can usually easily distinguish between the two conditions. Rarely, flow cytometry may be necessary to distinguish between the activated atypical lymphocytes and the immature leukemic lymphoblasts. Occasionally bone marrow examination is needed. A leukemoid reaction, observed in sepsis, acute hemolysis and other disorders, is usually easy to distinguish from ALL by morphological examination of the peripheral blood smear. Since occasionally ALL presents with pancytopenia, aplastic anemia is also on the differential diagnosis list.

CLINICAL PEARLS

ALL and rheumatoid disorders

ALL can mimic juvenile idiopathic arthritis (JIA) and other musculoskeletal disorders. Because leukemic blasts be absent from the peripheral blood, bone marrow examination should be considered in any child with JIA, especially prior to commencement of steroid therapy.

Between 5–10% of children with ALL are first evaluated at pediatric rheumatology clinics. Fever, arthralgias, arthritis, or a limp accompanied by anemia, mild splenomegaly and lymphadenopath can frequently be confused with juvenile idiopathic arthritis (JIA) or osteomyelitis. Some of these patients receive antibiotics and anti-inflammatory agents for several weeks to months before the diagnosis of ALL is made. An examination of the bone marrow should be seriously considered in such patients.

As leukemic lymphoblasts are small round blue cells when stained with hematoxylin and eosin, they can rarely be confused with metastatic small round cell pediatric tumors, including neuroblastoma, rhabdomyosarcoma and retinoblastoma.

Special diagnostic tests

The classification and the risk stratification for treatment protocols of ALL is based on detailed immunophenotyping and genotyping analysis.[18] Immunophenotyping by flow cytometry is required for confirmation of the diagnosis of ALL and for determination of the specific immunophenotype (Chapter 94). Flow cytometry of propidium iodide stained lymphoblasts can be used to determine the DNA index for the diagnosis of numerical chromosomal aberrations. A high DNA index (>1.16) is typical for the good prognosis high hyperdiploid ALL, while a low DNA index reflects hypodiploidy associated with poor outcome. Cytogenetic analysis is required for determination of the major genetic subtypes. In most centers classical cytogenetics techniques are used to establish the karyotype (Fig. 78.2). However, due to a paucity of metaphases, the karyotypic yield in ALL is often less than 70%. Because leukemic blasts coexist with normally dividing bone marrow cells, karyotype analysis may yield normal results despite the presence of ALL. These technical difficulties can be avoided through use of interphase fluorescent in-situ hybridization (FISH; Chapter 98), a method that does not require metaphases, because all clinically relevant structural and numerical chromosomal aberrations can be detected by the use of commercially available FISH probes (Fig. 78.3). In addition, fusion translocations, such as *BCR-ABL*, *TEL-AML1* and *MLL-AF4* can be detected by RT-PCR (Chapter 98).

The continuing decline in the cost of genome sequencing and the clinical implementation of developing genomic technologies are likely to revolutionize the diagnostics of leukemias in the near future. While the diagnostic power of microarray-based gene expression analysis of ALL has been demonstrated,[19] these newer methodologies of whole genome analysis are likely to transform both the understanding of leukemia biology and the diagnostic approach to these diseases.

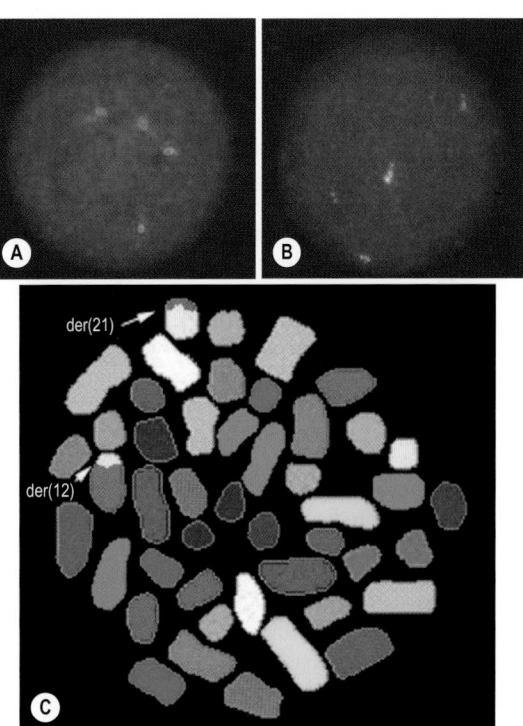

Fig. 78.3 Molecular cytogenetic techniques for the diagnosis of chromosomal translocations in acute lymphoblastic leukemia (ALL). (A) and (B) display interphase fluorescent in-situ hybridization (FISH) with probes to the AML1 (RUNX1) gene on chromosome 21 (red) and to the TEL (ETV6) gene on chromosome 12 (green). (A) displays a normal cell, and (B) displays a leukemic cell that has undergone a fusion TEL-AML1 translocation (arrow). (C) displays the same translocation as depicted in B, but on metaphase chromosomes. It uses a molecular cytogenetic technique called spectral karyotyping (arrows). Classical cytogenetic analysis often misses this translocation.
(Courtesy of Dr. L. Trakhtenbrot.)

Principles of therapy[1]

Supportive therapy is given before the initiation of leukemia-specific therapy. This includes hydration, treatment and preventive therapy of hyperuricemia, blood and platelet transfusion, and treatment of emergencies such as respiratory insufficiency associated with mediastinal leukemia.

It is highly recommended that children and adults with ALL be treated in specialized centers as a part of clinical prospective studies. Over the past several decades, such clinical trials have led to dramatic improvements in the treatment and outcome of ALL.

Treatment of ALL is initiated with an intensive remission induction regimen. This is usually followed by risk stratification into several treatment arms based on molecular studies and the response to initial therapy. An intensification course may be followed by a reinduction phase. All protocols include a prolonged maintenance phase, which consists of low-dose oral chemotherapy continued for a total 2 or 3 years. Continuous chemotherapy for at least 2 years is a unique feature of treatment for ALL because treatments for mature B-cell or acute myeloid leukemias are characterized by several very intensive courses for a relatively short time. This empiric evolution of vastly different treatment protocols to B-cell precursor ALL and mature B-cell leukemias probably reflects the different biologic properties of the progenitors of these leukemic cells.

Typical remission induction regimens include a glucocorticoid (prednisone, prednisolone or dexamethasone), vincristine, and L-asparaginase, with or without anthracycline. The rate of complete remission now ranges from 97 to 99% in children and from 75 to 90% in adults. Intensification therapy uses either high doses of multiple agents not used during the induction phase or repeats the induction regimen. Regimens used for children include high-dose methotrexate with or without 6-mercaptopurine; high-dose L-asparaginase given for an extended period; an epipodophyllotoxin plus cytarabine; or a combination of dexamethasone, vincristine, L-asparaginase, doxorubicin and thioguanine, with or without cyclophosphamide. Another integral component of many protocols is reinduction therapy. This treatment employs drugs similar to those used during the initial phase of induction therapy and has improved the outcomes of both children and adults with ALL. Maintenance therapy consists of a combination of methotrexate administered weekly and mercaptopurine administered daily. Some protocols add intermittent pulses of vincristine and dexamethasone.

CNS prophylactic therapy consisting of cranial irradiation plus intrathecal chemotherapy, introduced after the induction of complete remission, became one of the cornerstones of ALL therapy in the 1970s. More recently, because of concerns about neurotoxicity and the occurrence of brain tumors, intensive intrathecal and systemic chemotherapy are used instead for most patients.

Allogeneic stem cell transplantation (SCT) is reserved for patients with relapsed or refractory leukemia and for those with a very high-risk leukemia that manifests a slow response to therapy. With modern therapy, including targeted therapy with imatinib for BCR-ABL, there is almost no indication for SCT in first remission. With improvements in the prevention of transplant-related toxicities, suitable marrow donors can include matched unrelated donors and, in some situations, two- and three-antigen mismatched family members in addition to HLA-identical siblings or single-antigen mismatched family members. Umbilical cord blood and peripheral blood stem cells have also been used successfully.

Prognostic factors (Table 78.4)

Modern therapy for ALL is based on adjustment of the intensity of therapy to the risk assessment of the relapse hazard.[1]

The two major clinical parameters of prognostic significance are age at diagnosis and leukocyte count. Favorable prognostic factors include an age of presentation of one to nine years and a leukocyte count of less than $50 \times 10^9/L$. In adults, the outcome of therapy worsens with increasing age and leukocyte count. Patients older than 60 years of age and/or with a leukocyte count $>100 \times 10^9/L$ have a particularly poor treatment response. Girls fare somewhat better than boys and in some protocols boys are treated for three years instead of two. Hyperdiploidy (> 50 chromosomes), in particular trisomies of chromosomes 4 and 10, and a TEL–AML1 fusion translocation are favorable prognostic factors that strongly correlate with age and white cell count.

Poor biologic prognostic factors are MLL gene rearrangements, especially the MLL–AF4 fusion. This fusion translocation is detected mostly in infant leukemia. The presence of the Philadelphia chromosome encoding the BCR-ABL fusion also confers a poor prognosis. Patients with either of these abnormalities are stratified into a high-risk treatment arm in all current protocols. Recently the outcome of BCR-ABL ALL has been dramatically improved with the combination of chemotherapy and specific inhibitors of the BCR-ABL tyrosine kinase.[20] Hypodiploidy and amplification of the AML1 region on chromosome 21 are also associated with a bad prognosis. T-ALL has traditionally done worse than B lineage ALL; however, in many modern protocols these differences have been eliminated.

The most significant prognostic factor is the initial response to therapy. A rapid clearance of leukemic cells from the blood or bone marrow confers a favorable prognosis. The prognosis of a child with BCR-ABL positive ALL who presented with a low leukocyte count and in whom all blasts disappeared from peripheral blood after one week of steroids tends to be better than a similar child with hyperdiploid leukemia who has not reduced significantly the blast count after two weeks of therapy. More recently, the level of minimal residual disease after the induction of clinical remission has emerged as a powerful tool for gauging treatment response and predicting outcome.

Table 78.4 Major prognostic factors in ALL[a]

Prognostic factor	Good prognosis	Worse prognosis
Age at diagnosis	1<age<10 (children) years	<1 yr; >10 yr (children) >60 yrs (adult)
Peripheral blood WBC[b]	<50 000 cells per µL	> 100 000 cells per µL
Response to therapy	Early response to therapy; Negative MRD at the end of induction	Slow response to therapy. High MRD
Genetic abnormalities	Hyperdiploidy (>50 chr.); TEL/AML1 (ETV6/RUNX1)	BCR/ABL MLL/AF4 Hypodiploidy <45 chr.

[a]The most important prognostic factor is the *treatment protocol*. Thus the prognostic significance of various clinical and laboratory variables may differ between protocols. Here, the significant parameters common to most studies are listed.
[b]Abbreviations: WBC, white blood cells; MRD, minimal residual disease; chr., chromosomes.

Where immunology meets oncology—minimal residual disease

Modern treatment protocols lead to morphological complete remission, defined as less than 5% blasts in the bone marrow examination, in the majority of patients. If treatment is discontinued at that stage, most patients will eventually relapse. Indeed all prospective clinical studies have shown that ALL should be treated for at least 2 years. These facts indicate that at the completion of remission induction, not all clonigenic malignant lymphoblasts are destroyed even though most of the patients are in clinical and morphological remission. Indeed, patients may have as many as 10^{10} undetectable neoplastic cells when in remission by this criterion. Since leukemic cells have to constitute at least 1–5% of the nucleated cells in the bone marrow in order to be detected by microscopic examination, morphological examination is clearly inadequate for evaluation of the quality of remission in patients with ALL. The need for more sensitive techniques for detection of rare leukemic cells has led to the incorporation of modern techniques of detection of minimal residual disease (MRD) into treatment protocols of childhood ALL.

Real time PCR is an extremely sensitive technique for the detection of residual leukemic cells that carry fusion translocations (such as *BCR-ABL* and *TEL-AML*). However, the majority of the leukemias lack these translocations. During the last decade, two general methodologies for sensitive detection of submicroscopic residual leukemic cells have been developed. These methodologies are the fruit of years of basic research studies that have led to definition of the developmental phenotype of immune cells (Chapters 7 and 8) and of the elaborate process of immunoglobulin gene rearrangements (Chapter 4).

The most widely studied DNA-based MRD methodology is based on the identification of clonospecific rearrangements of immunoglobulin genes or T-cell receptors (IgTCR-PCR).[21] This approach exploits the physiologic process of somatic rearrangement of Ig and TCR gene loci that occur during early differentiation of any lymphocyte. Basic research studies have shown that any single lymphocyte carries a unique rearrangement that is shared only by other daughters of the same original cell that arose in the primary lymphoid organs. This process ensures the level of diversity of the immune response against an unlimited number of antigens. Since leukemia is clonal, that is, each leukemic cell descends from only one original leukemic precursor cell, all the leukemic cells of a particular person carry the same Ig and/or TCR rearrangements. Because leukemic cells are genetically unstable, they often (>90% of the cases) carry multiple rearrangements, a fact that facilitates the usefulness of using these rearrangements as a clonal marker for MRD detection. The major advantages of this technique are the exquisite sensitivity (at least 10^{-5}), reliability, reproducibility, and its applicability to more than 90% of children with ALL. Its biggest disadvantages are the costs and complexity.

Current strategies for flow cytometric detection of MRD rely on combinations of leukocyte markers that do not normally occur in cells of the peripheral blood and bone marrow. Such leukemia-associated phenotypes can be identified by two-, three- or four-color staining techniques (Fig. 78.4). Flow cytometric analysis of these immunophenotypes allows the detection of one leukemic cell among 10^4 or more normal cells. The advantages of flow cytometry for MRD detection are adequate sensitivity and the presence of immunophenotyping facilities in most major centers, which facilitate timely performance the analysis on fresh cells at a reasonable cost. There are a few disadvantages, however. First, immunophenotyping requires a flow cytometry operator with a high level of expertise and it is more difficult to standardize compared to PCR. And second, it can be difficult to distinguish between regenerating B-cell progenitors and leukemic blasts. Thus Flow MRD is most reliable and sensitive at very early stages (up to four weeks) of therapy.[22]

Many clinical studies on relatively small numbers of patients (which include a total of several hundred patients) enrolled on ALL treatment protocols revealed strikingly similar results. Fast clearance of leukemic blasts to below 10^{-4} cells within the first 2–4 weeks of therapy is detected in about 40% of children with ALL and is associated with an extremely good prognosis.

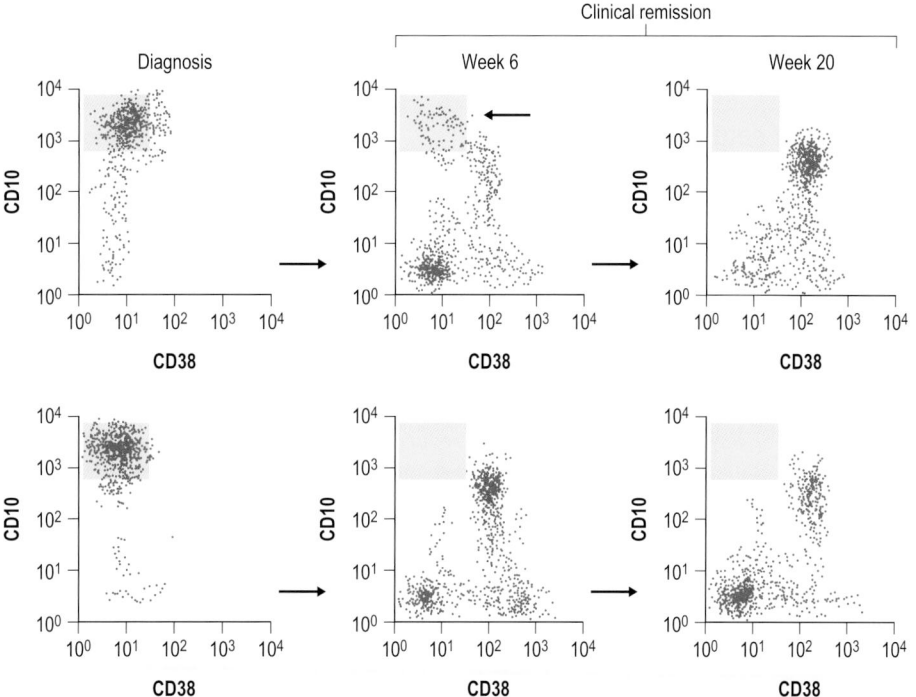

Fig. 78.4 Different kinetics of leukemia cytoreduction revealed by minimal residual disease (MRD) studies with flow cytometry.[51] The left panels illustrate the leukemia-specific immunophenotype (CD10+, CD38−) determined at diagnosis in two children with ALL. This phenotype is not found in normal bone marrow. Bone marrow samples were collected during clinical remission from both patients. In one patient (top panels), 0.04% of mononuclear cells expressed the leukemia-specific phenotype at week 6. MRD was undectable by week 20. In the other patient (bottom panels), a profound remission (MRD < 0.01%) was achieved by week 6 and maintained at week 20.

Conversely, the presence of more than 0.1% blasts after two or three months of therapy defines a very high-risk group.[23,24] These initial findings led the BFM-AEIOP study group to initiate a prospective study on children with ALL that utilize the MRD level determined by IgTCR-PCR for risk classification. This study, which involved 3,184 patients, confirmed the strength of PCR MRD over genetic classification as a prognostic marker.[25]

MRD studies are incorporated into most current treatment protocols. Patients with high MRD are stratified into a high-risk arm and receive more intensive chemotherapy. A few protocols are also testing whether therapy can be reduced for patients with no detectable MRD after 2–4 weeks of therapy, irrespective of their clinical presentation. While the robustness of MRD as the most sensitive and reliable prognostic indicator in ALL has been confirmed, at present it is unclear if adjustments to therapy based on the MRD level will improve survival for higher risk patients.

Course and prognosis

Under current protocols, the cure rate of children with ALL is about 80%. This reflects a greater than 90% cure rate for children with low risk leukemia coupled with an approximate cure rate of 70% for high-risk leukemia. The cure rates for adults is significantly lower (around 35–40%).[26] This likely reflects increased prevalence of poor prognosis genetic subtypes.

Most relapses occur during treatment or within the first two years after completion of therapy, although late relapses (even 10 years after diagnosis) are increasingly seen, especially in patients with the *TEL-AML1* genotype. The clinical relapse can occur in an extramedullary site, most often the CNS and the testes. Leukemic relapse occasionally occurs at other sites, including the eye, ear, ovary, uterus, bone, muscle, tonsil, kidney, mediastinum, pleura and paranasal sinuses. The prognosis of relapse depends on the time from diagnosis (earlier is worse), leukocyte count, immunophenotype and genotype (similar to the prognostic factors at diagnosis). Isolated extramedullary relapse carries a better prognosis. Although some relapses can be treated by chemotherapy only, most are being treated by stem cell transplantation. The most important prognostic factor which has emerged is the MRD level before transplant. More than half of the late relapses in patients with "good prognosis" ALL are curable. The prognosis of early relapses and relapsed T-ALL is grim.

Treatment sequelae

In the 1990s, improvements in supportive care reduced the rate of early death to less than 2%. However, the death rate among elderly patients during remission induction therapy remains as high as 30% due to hematological, hepatic and cardiac toxicity.

Long term toxicity is of major concern for children cured from ALL. Aseptic necrosis of various bones is a common late toxicity of glucocorticoids, especially in adolescent girls treated with dexamethasone.[27] The dose of anthracyclines used in most ALL protocols is unlikely to produce severe cardiomyopathy. The rate of long term neurotoxicity has been reduced due to replacement of cranial irradiation with high dose and intrathecal methotrexate. However at present it is unclear whether intensive methotrexate therapy will lead to very late neurodegeneration effects. Secondary cancers are a major concern. The development of therapy-related acute myeloid leukemia has been linked to the use of topoisomerase II inhibitors (teniposide and etoposide), and the risk is apparently dependent on the treatment schedule and the concomitant use of other agents (e.g., L-asparaginase, alkylating agents, and perhaps antimetabolites). Children who received cranial irradiation at 6 years of age or younger are most susceptible to the development of brain tumors. This risk is increased by the intensive use of antimetabolite drugs before and during cranial irradiation.[28]

Recent long-term follow-up studies of Scandinavian children cured of ALL confirm excellent long term outcome, as judged by their socio-educational achievements and by reproductive success resulting in healthy children.[29]

Current controversies and future perspectives

High cure rates in patients with ALL (nearly 80% of children and 40% of adults) attest to the steady progress that has been made in treating this disease. A further increase in cure rates will require efforts to maximize the efficacy and minimize the toxicity of current therapy. Currently MRD measurement can reliably distinguish between low and high-risk patients. However, about half of the patients belong to an "intermediate risk" group in which most relapses occur. Optimization of diagnosis and treatment of this group of patients is one of the current major challenges in the field. Improvement in risk classification among this group would help optimize therapy for individual patients.

Advanced genomic technologies carry the promise of discovering the full spectrum of leukemogenic pathways and the identification of targets for new therapies. Genomic analysis has also discovered marked subclonal heterogeneity.[30] Most of the relapses apparently arise from a minor subclone present at diagnosis. The identification and specific targeting of these resistant cells is a major focus of current clinical research.

The development of new targeted treatments for ALL is another major challenge, especially for high-risk patients.[31] Specific inhibitors of the BCR-ABL tyrosine kinase have already proven effective in combination with chemotherapy. The recent discovery of CRLF2-IL7R-JAK-STAT pathway activation has led to phase I/II studies with JAK and mTOR inhibitors and may also indicate a potential future role of antibodies against TSLPR and IL-7R. New immunological approaches to therapy are emerging. For example exciting preliminary results have been obtained with a novel bispecific antibody engaging autologous T-cells against CD19 positive leukemic cells.[32]

● ON THE HORIZON

Translational research of ALL

- Whole genomic analyses will discover all leukemia genetic abnormalities, enabling further personalization of treatment.
- Novel therapies targeting specific leukemia-associated abnormalities will be implemented.
- Immunotherapy utilizing antibodies directed against lymphoid antigens and conjugated either to toxins or to T-cell engaging molecules will be implemented in treatment of high-risk ALL.

Chronic lymphocytic leukemia

Chronic lymphocytic leukemia (CLL) is an indolent lymphoproliferative neoplasm of mature peripheral circulating B cells. It is the most common leukemia in adults of the western hemisphere. According to the WHO classification, CLL and small lymphocytic lymphoma (SLL), are considered to be one disease at different stages.[33] CLL originates from a clonal lymphoid evolved mature stem cell that can be identified by its distinct B-cell immunoglobulin gene rearrangement. Both clinically and at the molecular level it is a heterogeneous disease. Some patients have an indolent course with distinct genetic markers, whereas others have a more rapid and aggressive disorder with its own molecular signature. During its progression, CLL may be associated with significant immune deficiencies and autoimmune phenomena, which complicate its course and treatment. These abnormalities may be of sufficient severity to alter the nature of the disease, and they are attributed to the clonal nature of its B-cell origin. Less than 5% of patients have T CLL. All other patients have a B-cell phenotype.

Epidemiology

The clinical diagnosis of CLL requires absolute lymphocytosis of more than 5,000/μL mature lymphocytes in the peripheral blood. The extensive use of automated peripheral blood lymphocyte counts has increased the rate of diagnosis of asymptomatic patients with CLL. The incidence rate of CLL increases logarithmically from age 35, with a median age at the time of diagnosis of 65 years. There is a male predominance, and the disease appears to have a geographic and ethnic variation in incidence. In the USA, CLL is reported to occur with equal incidence among those of African and European descent, but it is uncommon in those of Asian descent. The incidence reported is 4.3 per 100 000 per year. Because many of these patients may never require tissue diagnosis or inpatient treatment, they are not likely to be recorded by a tumor registry thus making the true annual incidence of the disease higher than previously thought (6.8 per 100 000 population).[34] With sensitive techniques, a monoclonal population of B lymphocytes that is indistinguishable from CLL cells may be found in the blood of 3.5% of persons older than 40 years of age.[35] The presence of fewer than 5 000 B-lymphocytes/μL showing clonality is defined as monoclonal B-lymphocytosis (MBL). MBL is an indolent disorder that may progress to frank CLL at a rate of 1 to 2% per year.[36,37] Prospective studies of patients with CLL show that almost all previously demonstrated MBL with

evidence of clonal B-cell amplification as defined by IgH rearrangement studies.[38]

The etiology of CLL is largely unknown; however, as with other forms of malignancy, there is increasing evidence for the role of inherited factors in its development. Family surveys show a genetic predisposition in first degree relatives. Anticipation, i.e., the phenomenon of earlier onset and more severe phenotype in successive generations, has been reported in CLL families.[39]

Pathogenesis and the biology of leukemic lymphocytes

CLL has been considered a single homogeneous disease of accumulating immature, immune-competent, minimally self-renewing B cells. It is now viewed as two related entities, originating from B lymphocytes according to differences in activation, and the maturation state of the cellular subgroup.[35]

Normal B lymphocytes mature in the bone marrow, and in the process undergo rearrangement of the immunoglobulin variable (V) gene segments to create the code for an immunoglobulin molecule that serves as the B-cell receptor for antigen. When an antigen of adequate affinity engages the receptor, the cell enters a germinal center located in a lymphoid follicle, where, as a centroblast, it rapidly divides and its V genes undergo somatic hypermutation. This process introduces mutations in the rearranged gene segments that code for the binding site of the receptor. Through these mutations, the receptors of the descendant B cells, called centrocytes, acquire new properties. Cells with receptors that have enhanced antigen-binding affinity proliferate in the presence of the antigen, whereas centrocytes with receptors that no longer bind the antigen (or bind autoantigens) are normally eliminated. Once the centrocytes are selected, they become plasma or memory B cells (Fig. 78.5). The CLL cell population may originate from a clone of few or no V-gene mutations or from a more mature clone where these genes are hypermutated, thus creating two related entities, both originating from

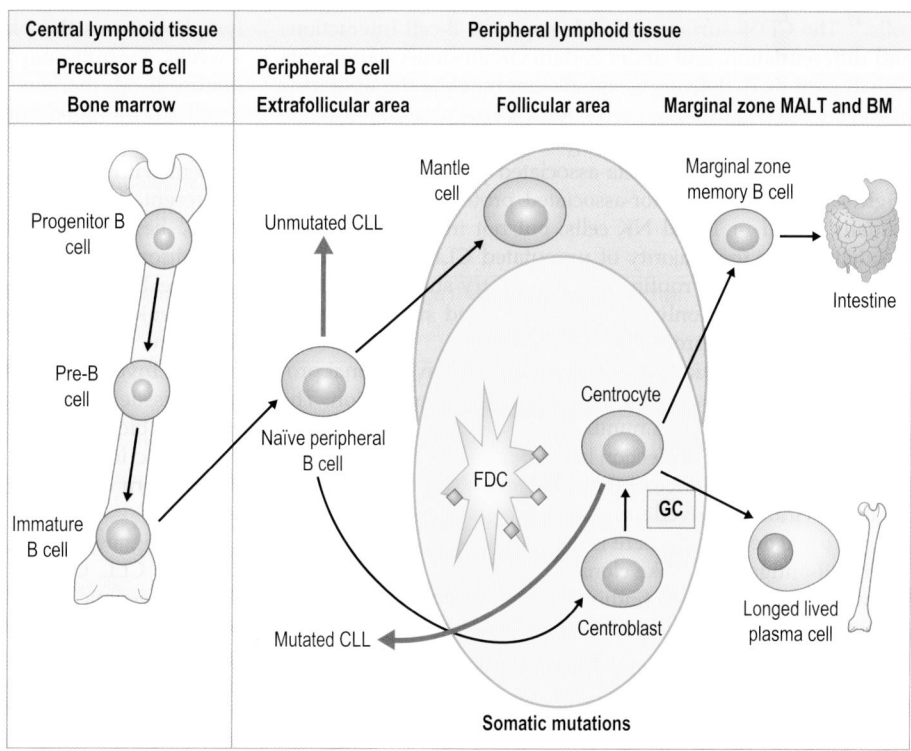

Fig. 78.5 Chronic lymphocytic leukemia (CLL) and B-cell development. The phenotype displayed by a B-cell lymphoproliferative disorder reflects the stage of normal B-cell development it achieved prior to its final transformation. Development begins in the fetal liver and in fetal and adult bone marrow. Maturing B cells exit to the peripheral blood, but typically require entry into the germinal center (GC) in order to undergo somatic hypermutation. The CLL cells that express unmutated immunoglobulin variable domains thus likely underwent final transformation prior to entry into the GC, whereas those that express mutated variable domains likely transited the GC and then underwent final transformation. Transformation in pro- and pre-B cells typically gives rise to acute lymphoblastic leukemia. Transformation of intermediate stages can give rise to mantle-zone lymphomas. Transformation at later stages can give rise to marginal-zone lymphomas and plasma cell-derived multiple myeloma.

Central lymphoid tissue	Peripheral lymphoid tissue		
Precursor B cell	Peripheral B cell		
Bone marrow	Extrafollicular area	Follicular area	Marginal zone MALT and BM

Progenitor B cell

Pre-B cell

Immature B cell

Unmutated CLL

Mantle cell

Naïve peripheral B cell

FDC

Marginal zone memory B cell

Intestine

Centrocyte

GC

Mutated CLL

Centroblast

Longed lived plasma cell

Somatic mutations

are relatively uncommon (2–14%) and are characterized by progressive lymphadenopathy and constitutional symptoms. The prognosis is generally ominous.

Treatment

As CLL remains an incurable tumor, treatment may be delayed and the patient monitored until becoming symptomatic.[35,50,51] Guidelines for treatment include the development of symptoms, worsening anemia and/or thrombocytopenia, autoimmune cytopenias, progressive splenomegaly, progressive lymphadenopathy, or a lymphocyte doubling time of 6 months or less. No prospective data exist yet to support the early treatment of the patients with asymptomatic adverse prognostic features, although clinical trials are being performed. On the other hand, many patients will be treated with supportive care only due to advanced age and co-morbidities.

Chlorambucil, alone or combined with corticosteroids, has been the most commonly used drug. It is advantageous in relieving symptoms, even in advanced disease. However, several randomized trials have failed to demonstrate improved survival, and hardly any patient achieves complete remission (CR). Purine analogues (most commonly fludarabine) with or without cyclophosphamide have been shown to induce higher response rates when compared to chlorambucil, with some patients achieving CR.

The CD52 antigen is present on lymphocytes (B,T, and NK cells), monocytes, and some granulocytes. The humanized monoclonal anti-CD52 antibody (alemtuzumab) has been shown to have an effect against B-CLL cells. Studies have demonstrated high activity of this drug in previously treated and even refractory CLL patients, as well as in eliminating minimal residual disease especially in the bone marrow.[53] Nevertheless, patients are exposed to severe infectious complications due to significant B- and T-cell depletion, particularly in the case of CMV reactivation.[54] Anti-CD20 (rituximab) as single agent shows limited efficacy in CLL, possibly because of the weak receptor expression on CLL cells. However, in combination with chemotherapy, particularly fludarabine and cyclophosphamide, it appears to act synergistically and to achieve high rates of response including molecular CR and prolongation of both disease-free and overall survival.[51,55-57] The combination of alemtuzumab with rituximab had a good but limited overall response.[53,58] A newer fully

human monoclonal antibody targeting CD20 (ofatumumab) has been shown to have a very potent effect as a single agent in both naïve and rituximab-treated patients.[58] It targets a different epitope on the CD20 antigen. Other immune-based therapies include lumiliximab (anti CD23), apolizumab (anti HLA-DR) and anti CD40 which are all B-cell molecules, which are being tested with or without the addition of chemotherapy. Other investigational agents include lenalidomide (an immune modulator related to thalidomide), which has shown efficacy albeit in association with an interestingly initial flare-up phenomenon of disease enlarged lymph nodes. Clinical trials with specific inhibitors of oncogenic pathways such as PI3kinase delta, flavopiridol and small molecules targeting BCL2 also have shown promising results.[58]

Some immunologic novel futuristic approaches include expanded auto-reactive activated T cells, which have shown a safe profile and modest clinical improvements in phase I trials, as well as vaccination strategies utilizing autologous leukemic cells transduced with different pro-apoptotic receptors (i.e., CD40 and CD95).[53]

Allogeneic hematopoietic stem cell transplantation (HSCT) is the only curative CLL treatment. Allogeneic HSCT relies on myeloablative doses of chemoradiotherapy, which makes this treatment unacceptably risky for the majority of CLL patients. In non-myeloablative, or reduced intensity approaches, rates of engraftment are similar to fully ablative conditioning regimens, with lower rates of early toxicity. Early evidence suggests that the graft-versus-leukemia (GVL) effect is present against the disease. Patients with deletion 17p (p53 involvement), who show extremely bad prognosis, and are physically fit are candidates for allo-HSCT.[59,60] Studies involving autologous transplantation and high-dose chemotherapy for CLL have a limited survival advantage. Relapses are frequent and there is a high incidence of secondary myelodysplastic syndrome and acute myeloid leukemia.

The present treatment criteria do not identify patients in early stages with adverse prognostic high-risk features. Nevertheless, the overall survival of CLL patients has globally improved from 5 to 8 years for Binet stage B patients and from 2 to 5 years for stage C patients. This consistent improvement could be due to subsequent treatment advances provided to patients failing to respond to initial treatment.[60] Thus, pending ongoing clinical trials, it may become feasible to treat patients with good performance and early stage status according to unfavorable prognostic features.[61]

Immunologic aspects of CLL

CLL is characterized by multiple immune deficiencies and auto-immune phenomena. It is reasonable to hypothesize that immune incompetence and autoimmunity are two sides of the same coin.[62]

The pathophysiologic rationale

CLL cells secrete TGF-β, which is a potent inhibitor of B-cell proliferation, and release high levels of circulating IL-2 receptor, which downregulates T helper function. Furthermore, B-CLL cells (as do anergic normal B cells) fail to present soluble antigen and alloantigens, whereas normal, activated B cells are very effective antigen-presenting cells.[62] There is increasing evidence of T-cell dysfunction in CLL, which may contribute to the etiology and progress of the disease. An absolute CD8 lymphocytosis correlates with disease progression. Also, as found in autoimmune diseases, low expression of CD4 and CD8 is seen with abnormal expression of other surface molecules. In addition, the T cells in CLL patients were found to have profound abnormalities of their antigen receptor (TCR) repertoire, and appear dysfunctional in terms of cytokine secretion. Aberrant levels of IFNγ, IL-2, 4, and 6 production have been described,[63] and are dependent on the number of leukemic B cells and disease stage. This suggests that as the disease progresses T-cell function declines, B cells exert greater negative feedback on T cells, B cells use the cytokine production to an increasing extent, or a combination of these factors occurs. This cytokine imbalance may be the cause of upregulation of BCL-2 anti-apoptotic activity. T-cell dysfunction could also explain the higher incidence of autoimmune complications, such as autoimmune hemolytic anemia, among patients receiving purine analogs therapy, which induces T-cell depletion. Assuming that certain T-cell subsets prevent the development of autoreactive B cells, loss of these cells after treatment with purine analogs may permit autoreactive B-cell clones to emerge and expand. However, this last complication is mainly observed among heavily pretreated patients who are receiving purine analogs as salvage therapy.[61]

Immunologic deficiencies

Patients with CLL are extremely sensitive to various infectious agents. A monoclonal immunoglobulin peak, usually of the IgM type, is found in 5% of CLL, and a small amount of a monoclonal component can be identified in the serum or urine of 60% of patients. Hypogammaglobulinemia occurs in at least 60% of B-CLL cases and may include all three classes (IgG, IgA, IgM). The pathogenesis of hypogammaglobulinemia in B-CLL is poorly understood as this phenomenon is rare in other B-cell malignancies except for multiple myeloma. Regulatory abnormalities in T cells may play a role in the induction of hypogammaglobulinemia, but may also result as a consequence of dysfunction of nonclonal normal B cells.[61] Low Ig levels correlate with recurrent infections with encapsulated organisms. Patients who receive intravenous immune globulin (IVIG) have a decrease in the incidence of major bacterial infections.[64] Although costly, patients who have demonstrated a pattern of repeated serious infections should be treated with prophylactic IVIG.

Infections are a major cause of morbidity and mortality in CLL patients. Impaired humoral and cellular immunity, defects in the complement systems and variable neutropenia, depending on marrow infiltrates, all contribute to the high rate of infections.[54] It is estimated that up to 50% of patients have recurrent infections, some severe. Bacterial infections are the principal risk in patients treated with conventional therapies. Opportunistic infections are initially uncommon as the result of the relative preservation of cellular immunity early in the disease. *Pneumocystis jirovecii* pneumonia and other fungal infections, listeriosis, mycobacterial infections, respiratory syncytial and herpes virus infections occur in heavily pretreated patients receiving combination chemotherapy. This presumably reflects the cumulative effects of numerous immune suppressive therapies. The risk of infection is increased following purine analog therapy because of the side effects of myelosuppression and marked lymphopenia with T-cell depletion. The combination of purine analogs with steroids substantially increases this infection risk. Patients with fludarabine-resistant or partially responsive disease are at highest risk of infection. The addition of rituximab, the anti-B-cell marker CD20 antibody, to nucleoside analog-based therapy does not appear to increase the risk of early or late infections, but may increase the rate of neutropenia. The addition of the anti-B- and T-cell marker CD52 antibody alemtuzumab in pretreated patients and as first line therapy is also associated with high levels of infections, particularly in non-responders. Active immunization with vaccines is hampered by the patient's inability to generate or retain a long and significant immune response.

Autoimmune phenomenon

Autoimmune-associated features are frequently observed in CLL. These manifestations are mainly directed against hematopoietic cells. The most common known cause of autoimmune hemolytic anemia (AIHA) is CLL.[65] A positive direct antiglobulin test (direct Coomb's test) has been reported to be as high as 7–35% of CLL patients, and AIHA itself occurs in 10–25% of patients during the course of their disease. AIHA occurs twice as often in patients with unmutated genes as in those with mutated ones. Tumor cells secrete small amounts of idiotypic IgM that may react with autoantigens as the Fc region of IgG, single- and double-stranded DNA, histones, cardiolipin, and other proteins. In most cases, however, autoantibodies against red blood cells are warm-reactive polyclonal IgG and are not secreted by the malignant clone, but rather from normal B cells.[61,65] Cold agglutinins are rare. AIHA is thought to arise from an imbalance among lymphocyte subsets, contributed in part by therapy, resulting in the emergence of the autoimmune clone. Men, aged patients, and patients with a higher lymphocyte count have shown a significantly higher rate of AIHA. It is usually observed in advanced stages of the disease, correlating with a poor prognosis, and has a close relationship with the activity of CLL. After therapy, autoimmune antibodies may disappear in up to 70% of patients.[66]

Immune thrombocytopenic purpura (ITP) is observed in about 2–3% of cases, with increased megakaryocytes in the bone marrow. It should be distinguished from thrombocytopenia induced by marrow infiltration, which is very common in up to 50% of patients at presentation.[65] Two thirds of CLL-associated ITP also have AIHA. This combination is termed Evan's syndrome. Pure red cell aplasia and autoantibodies against neutrophils are only rarely observed, but are part of the CLL related autoimmunity repertoire. The appearance of autoantibodies may be due to a defect of T-cell subsets controlling the autoantibody producing B cells. This approach is supported by the observation that autoimmunity is much more common in patients treated with fludarabine, a drug known to induce profound suppression of circulating CD4 T cells. Autoimmune phenomena in patients treated with purine analogs (mostly fludarabine-related) are of a more severe nature, and generally trigger AIHA, although ITP and possibly pure red cell aplasia (PRCA) and neutropenia are also seen.

Other rare entities are reported as paraneoplastic autoimmune disorders with connective tissue disease manifestations, including polymyositis, dermatopolymyositis, focal myositis,[67,68] pemphigus vulgaris,[69] and acquired angioedema. These autoimmune disorders are once again related to T-cell dysfunction and may be associated with purine analog treatment. Paraneoplastic pemphigus is reported to occur in up to 30% of CLL patients and may be triggered by chemo- and radiotherapy.[63] Glomerulonephritis and the nephrotic syndrome are seldom reported, although when present are related to different mechanisms including cryoglobulins and anti-neutrophil cytoplasmic antibodies (ANCA).

Therapy of autoimmune phenomena includes high-dose steroids and disease control.[65,66] For patients refractory to or relapsing after steroid therapy, further treatment is warranted. High-dose immunoglobulins offer amelioration in some patients, but only with a transient response. Splenectomy may induce some remission, especially in patients with AIHA due to IgG alone and no complement component. Splenic irradiation can substitute for splenectomy in older and sicker patients. Cytotoxic agents or cyclosporine may represent valid rescue approaches. In patients where the AIHA has been triggered by fludarabine, further exposure is hazardous, although courses combining cyclophosphamide with fludarabine are much less prone to develop AIHA. Withholding treatment to patients with a positive direct antiglobulin (Coomb's) test is controversial. Rituximab may be an alternative agent for the treatment of CLL-associated autoimmune diseases,[70] and in rare autoimmune phenomena as pemphigus and PRCA.

Conclusion

CLL is a common indolent lymphoid neoplasm with a wide clinical heterogeneity. It is currently suspected and diagnosed more commonly because of routine blood tests. Diagnosis is made with simple immunophenotyping, but it is common to perform other advanced laboratory evaluations including cytogenetics and molecular diagnostic techniques in order to determine prognosis. The origin of CLL is yet to be elucidated, but as data accumulate two related entities emerge, both originating from antigen-stimulated mature B lymphocytes but with different clinical behaviors. The complications of CLL appear to be unique to this neoplasm and are part of a failing immune system with T- and B-cell dysregulation. This predisposes patients to recurrent infections and autoimmune diseases. New molecular and protein markers that identify patients at a high risk for progressive disease may provide clues for effective targeted therapies.

References

1. Pui CH, Evans WE. Treatment of acute lymphoblastic leukemia. N Engl J Med 2006;354:166–78.
2. Greaves M. Infection, immune responses and the aetiology of childhood leukaemia. Nat Rev Cancer 2006;6:193–203.
3. Einav U, Tabach Y, Getz G, et al. Gene expression analysis reveals a strong signature of an interferon-induced pathway in childhood lymphoblastic leukemia as well as in breast and ovarian cancer. Oncogene 2005;24:6367–75.
4. Campana D, Coustan-Smith E. Advances in the immunological monitoring of childhood acute lymphoblastic leukaemia. Best Pract Res Clin Haematol 2002;15:1–19.
5. Izraeli S, Henn T, Strobl H, et al. Expression of identical E2A/PBX1 fusion transcripts occurs in both pre-B and early pre-B immunological subtypes of childhood acute lymphoblastic leukaemia. Leukemia 1993;7:2054–6.
6. Coustan-Smith E, Mullighan CG, Onciu M, et al. Early T-cell precursor leukaemia: a subtype of very high-risk acute lymphoblastic leukaemia. Lancet Oncol 2009;10:147–56.
7. Armstrong SA, Look AT. Molecular genetics of acute lymphoblastic leukemia. J Clin Oncol 2005;23:6306–15.
8. Look AT. Oncogenic transcription factors in the human acute leukemias. Science 1997;278:1059–64.
9. Weng AP, Ferrando AA, Lee W, et al. Activating mutations of NOTCH1 in human T cell acute lymphoblastic leukemia. Science 2004;306:269–71.
10. Shochat C, Tal N, Bandapalli OR, et al. Gain-of-function mutations in interleukin-7 receptor-{alpha} (IL7R) in childhood acute lymphoblastic leukemias. J Exp Med 2011;208:901–8.
11. Hertzberg L, Vendramini E, Ganmore I, et al. Down syndrome acute lymphoblastic leukemia, a highly heterogeneous disease in which aberrant expression of CRLF2 is associated with mutated JAK2: a report from the International BFM Study Group. Blood 2010;115:1006–17.
12. Russell LJ, Capasso M, Vater I, et al. Deregulated expression of cytokine receptor gene, CRLF2, is involved in lymphoid transformation in B-cell precursor acute lymphoblastic leukemia. Blood 2009;114:2688–98.
13. Mullighan CG, Goorha S, Radtke I, et al. Genome-wide analysis of genetic alterations in acute lymphoblastic leukaemia. Nature 2007;446:758–64.
14. Strefford JC, van Delft FW, Robinson HM, et al. Complex genomic alterations and gene expression in acute lymphoblastic leukemia with intrachromosomal amplification of chromosome 21. Proc Natl Acad Sci U S A 2006;103:8167–72.
15. Mullighan CG, Su X, Zhang J, et al. Deletion of IKZF1 and prognosis in acute lymphoblastic leukemia. N Engl J Med 2009;360:470–80.
16. Cario G, Zimmermann M, Romey R, et al. Presence of the P2RY8-CRLF2 rearrangement is associated with a poor prognosis in non-high-risk precursor B-cell acute lymphoblastic leukemia in children treated according to the ALL-BFM 2000 protocol. Blood 2010;115:5393–7.
17. Ferrando AA, Neuberg DS, Staunton J, et al. Gene expression signatures define novel oncogenic pathways in T cell acute lymphoblastic leukemia. Cancer Cell 2002;1:75–87.
18. Harrison CJ, Haas O, Harbott J, et al. Detection of prognostically relevant genetic abnormalities in childhood B-cell precursor acute lymphoblastic leukaemia: recommendations from the Biology and Diagnosis Committee of the International Berlin-Frankfurt-Munster study group. Br J Haematol 2010;151:132–42.
19. Haferlach T, Kohlmann A, Wieczorek L, et al. Clinical utility of microarray-based gene expression profiling in the diagnosis and subclassification of leukemia: report from the International Microarray Innovations in Leukemia Study Group. J Clin Oncol 2010;28:2529–37.
20. Schultz KR, Bowman WP, Aledo A, et al. Improved early event-free survival with imatinib in Philadelphia chromosome-positive acute lymphoblastic leukemia: a children's oncology group study. J Clin Oncol 2009;27:5175–81.
21. Szczepanski T, Orfao A, van der Velden VH, et al. Minimal residual disease in leukaemia patients. Lancet Oncol 2001;2:409–17.
22. Basso G, Veltroni M, Valsecchi MG, et al. Risk of relapse of childhood acute lymphoblastic leukemia is predicted by flow cytometric measurement of residual disease on day 15 bone marrow. J Clin Oncol 2009;27:5168–74.
23. Borowitz MJ, Pullen DJ, Shuster JJ, et al. Minimal residual disease detection in childhood precursor-B-cell acute lymphoblastic leukemia: relation to other risk factors. A Children's Oncology Group study. Leukemia 2003;17:1566–72.
24. van Dongen JJ, Seriu T, Panzer-Grumayer ER, et al. Prognostic value of minimal residual disease in acute lymphoblastic leukaemia in childhood. Lancet 1998;352:1731–8.
25. Conter V, Bartram CR, Valsecchi MG, et al. Molecular response to treatment redefines all prognostic factors in children and adolescents with B-cell precursor acute lymphoblastic leukemia: results in 3184 patients of the AIEOP-BFM ALL 2000 study. Blood 2010;115:3206–14.
26. Wrzesien-Kus A, Robak T, Pluta A, et al. Outcome of treatment in adults with Philadelphia chromosome-positive and/or BCR-ABL-positive acute lymphoblastic leukemia-retrospective analysis of Polish Adult Leukemia Group (PALG). Ann Hematol 2006;85:366–73.
27. Nachman JB. Adolescents with acute lymphoblastic leukemia: a new "age" Rev Clin Exp Hematol 2003;7:261–9.
28. Relling MV, Rubnitz JE, Rivera GK, et al. High incidence of secondary brain tumours after radiotherapy and antimetabolites. Lancet 1999;354:34–9.
29. Koch SV, Kejs AM, Engholm G, et al. Leaving home after cancer in childhood: a measure of social independence and early adulthood. Pediatr Blood Cancer 2006;47:61–70.
30. Anderson K, Lutz C, van Delft FW, et al. Genetic variegation of clonal architecture and propagating cells in leukaemia. Nature 2011;469:356–61.
31. Bourquin JP, Izraeli S. Where can biology of childhood ALL be attacked by new compounds? Cancer Treat Rev 2010;36:298–306.
32. Topp MS, Kufer P, Gokbuget N, et al. Targeted therapy with the T-cell-engaging antibody blinatumomab of chemotherapy-refractory minimal residual disease in B-lineage acute lymphoblastic leukemia patients results in high response rate and prolonged leukemia-free survival. J Clin Oncol 2011;29:2493–8.
33. Harris NL, Jaffe ES, Diebold J, et al. World Health Organization classification of neoplastic diseases of the hematopoietic and lymphoid tissues: report of the Clinical Advisory Committee meeting—Airlie House, Virginia, November 1997. J Clin Oncol 1999;17:3835–49.
34. Zent CS, Kyasa MJ, Evans R, Schichman SA. Chronic lymphocytic leukemia incidence is substantially higher than estimated from tumor registry data. Cancer 2001;92:1325–30.
35. Chiorazzi N, Rai KR, Ferrarini M. Chronic lymphocytic leukemia. N Engl J Med 2005;352:804–15.
36. Mulligan CS, Thomas ME, Mulligan SP. Monoclonal B-cell lymphocytosis and chronic lymphocytic leukemia. N Engl J Med 2008;359:2065–6 author reply 2066.
37. Rawstron AC, Bennett FL, O'Connor SJ, et al. Monoclonal B-cell lymphocytosis and chronic lymphocytic leukemia. N Engl J Med 2008;359:575–83.
38. Landgren O, Albitar M, Ma W, et al. B-cell clones as early markers for chronic lymphocytic leukemia. N Engl J Med 2009;360:659–67.
39. Yuille MR, Matutes E, Marossy A, et al. Familial chronic lymphocytic leukaemia: a survey and review of published studies. Br J Haematol 2000;109:794–9.
40. Damle RN, Wasil T, Fais F, et al. Ig V gene mutation status and CD38 expression as novel prognostic indicators in chronic lymphocytic leukemia. Blood 1999;94:1840–7.
41. Oscier DG, Gardiner AC, Mould SJ, et al. Multivariate analysis of prognostic factors in CLL: clinical stage, IGVH gene mutational status, and loss or mutation of the p53 gene are independent prognostic factors. Blood 2002;100:1177–84.

42. Dohner H, Stilgenbauer S, Benner A, et al. Genomic aberrations and survival in chronic lymphocytic leukemia. N Engl J Med 2000;343:1910–16.

43. Orchard JA, Ibbotson RE, Davis Z, et al. ZAP-70 expression and prognosis in chronic lymphocytic leukaemia. Lancet 2004;363:105–11.

44. Herishanu Y, Perez-Galan P, Liu D, et al. The lymph node microenvironment promotes B-cell receptor signaling, NF-kappaB activation, and tumor proliferation in chronic lymphocytic leukemia. Blood 2011;117:563–74.

45. Caligaris-Cappio F. Role of the microenvironment in chronic lymphocytic leukaemia. Br J Haematol 2003;123:380–8.

46. Messmer BT, Messmer D, Allen SL, et al. In vivo measurements document the dynamic cellular kinetics of chronic lymphocytic leukemia B cells. J Clin Invest 2005;115:755–64.

47. Cukierman T, Gatt ME, Libster D, et al. Chronic lymphocytic leukemia presenting with extreme hyperleukocytosis and thrombosis of the common femoral vein. Leuk Lymphoma 2002;43:1865–8.

48. Rai KR, Sawitsky A, Cronkite EP, et al. Clinical staging of chronic lymphocytic leukemia. Blood 1975;46:219–34.

49. Binet JL, Lepoprier M, Dighiero G, et al. A clinical staging system for chronic lymphocytic leukemia: prognostic significance. Cancer 1977;40:855–64.

50. Shanafelt TD, Geyer SM, Kay NE. Prognosis at diagnosis: integrating molecular biologic insights into clinical practice for patients with CLL. Blood 2004;103:1202–10.

51. Abbott BL. Advances in the diagnosis and treatment of chronic lymphocytic leukemia. Hematol Oncol 2005;23:34–40.

52. Tsimberidou AM, Keating MJ. Richter syndrome: biology, incidence, and therapeutic strategies. Cancer 2005;103:216–28.

53. Wierda WG, Kipps TJ, Keating MJ. Novel immune-based treatment strategies for chronic lymphocytic leukemia. J Clin Oncol 2005;23:6325–32.

54. Thursky KA, Worth LJ, Seymour JF, et al. Spectrum of infection, risk and recommendations for prophylaxis and screening among patients with lymphoproliferative disorders treated with alemtuzumab*. Br J Haematol 2006;132:3–12.

55. Badoux XC, Keating MJ, Wang X, et al. Fludarabine, cyclophosphamide, and rituximab chemoimmunotherapy is highly effective treatment for relapsed patients with CLL. Blood 2011;117:3016–24.

56. Bryan J, Borthakur G. Role of rituximab in first-line treatment of chronic lymphocytic leukemia. Ther Clin Risk Manag 2011;7:1–11.

57. Robak T, Dmoszynska A, Solal-Celigny P, et al. Rituximab plus fludarabine and cyclophosphamide prolongs progression-free survival compared with fludarabine and cyclophosphamide alone in previously treated chronic lymphocytic leukemia. J Clin Oncol 2010;28:1756–65.

58. Abou-Nassar K, Brown JR. Novel agents for the treatment of chronic lymphocytic leukemia. Clin Adv Hematol Oncol 2010;8:886–95.

59. Stilgenbauer S, Zenz T. Understanding and managing ultra high-risk chronic lymphocytic leukemia. Hematology Am Soc Hematol Educ Program 2010;2010:481–8.

60. Gribben JG. How I treat CLL up front. Blood 2010;115:187–97.

61. Dighiero G. Unsolved issues in CLL biology and management. Leukemia 2003;17:2385–91.

62. Caligaris-Cappio F, Hamblin TJ. B-cell chronic lymphocytic leukemia: a bird of a different feather. J Clin Oncol 1999;17:399–408.

63. Scrivener S, Goddard RV, Kaminski ER, Prentice AG. Abnormal T-cell function in B-cell chronic lymphocytic leukaemia. Leuk Lymphoma 2003;44:383–9.

64. Molica S, Musto P, Chiurazzi F, et al. Prophylaxis against infections with low-dose intravenous immunoglobulins (IVIG) in chronic lymphocytic leukemia. Results of a crossover study. Haematologica 1996;81:121–6.

65. Hamblin TJ. Autoimmune complications of chronic lymphocytic leukemia. Semin Oncol 2006;33:230–9.

66. Mauro FR, Foa R, Cerretti R, et al. Autoimmune hemolytic anemia in chronic lymphocytic leukemia: clinical, therapeutic, and prognostic features. Blood 2000;95:2786–92.

67. Terrier B, Lavie F, Miceli-Richard C, et al. Focal myositis with fasciitis and vasculitis revealing chronic lymphocytic leukaemia. Rheumatology (Oxford) 2005;44:1324–6.

68. Cabuk M, Inanir I, Turkdogan P, et al. Cyclic lymphocytic vasculitis associated with chronic lymphocytic leukemia. Leuk Lymphoma 2004;45:811–13.

69. Hohwy T, Bang K, Steiniche T, et al. Alemtuzumab-induced remission of both severe paraneoplastic pemphigus and leukaemic bone marrow infiltration in a case of treatment-resistant B-cell chronic lymphocytic leukaemia. Eur J Haematol 2004;73:206–9.

70. Zaja F, Vianelli N, Sperotto A, et al. Anti-CD20 therapy for chronic lymphocytic leukemia-associated autoimmune diseases. Leuk Lymphoma 2003;44:1951–5.

Stefania Pittaluga,
Elaine S. Jaffe

Lymphomas

The classification of the malignant lymphomas has undergone significant reappraisal over the past 50 years. These changes have resulted from insights gained through the application of immunological and molecular techniques, as well as a better understanding of the clinical aspects of lymphoma through advances in diagnosis, staging, and treatment. Early classifications were based on morphological characteristics of the neoplastic elements; however, with increasing knowledge of the complexity of the immune system a more functional approach was sought. Differentiation schemes provided a useful starting point for understanding lymphomas (Fig. 79.1). Recently, genomic-scale gene expression profiling (GEP) has been applied to lymphomas to define their molecular signatures with the aim of improved understanding of oncogenic pathways and their clinical implications.[1] These studies have led to new prognostic and diagnostic tools and as a result we are beginning to see the implementation of more targeted therapies.[2]

● KEY CONCEPTS

Lymphoma

- Classification consists of a list of individual disease entities defined by morphologic, immunophenotypic, genetic, and clinical features.
- Neoplastic cells are related to the postulated normal counterpart, when possible.
- Histologic grade should be applied within individual diseases.
- Clinical factors for individual patients, as measured by the International Prognostic Index (IPI) and gene expression profiling, are useful in predicting clinical outcome.

The guiding principles of the World Health Organization (WHO) classification of neoplasms of the hematopoietic and lymphoid tissues, published in 2001 and updated in 2008[3] (Table 79.1) were based on the Revised European-American Classification of lymphoid neoplasms (REAL) published by the International Lymphoma Study group in 1994. The focus was on the identification of individual disease entities based on an integration of morphologic, immunophenotypic, genetic, and clinical features. The recent application of GEP in lymphomas has generated distinct molecular "signatures" for a variety of disease entities, in some cases corresponding more closely to different stages of lymphoid differentiation, and in other instances offering insights into mechanisms of neoplastic transformation with delineation of alterations in specific pathways.

The advent of whole genome sequencing will likely contribute additional new insights into pathogenetic mechanisms.[4]

● KEY CONCEPTS

Somatic mutation in relation to normal B-cell development

- Premutational stage: circulating naïve B cells (immunoglobulin (Ig)M⁺/D⁺) prior to antigen exposure.
- Stage of somatic mutation, clonal expansion, and isotype switch: at the germinal center.
- Postmutational stage: selected B cells move to the periphery (postgerminal center) or to the recirculating pool (memory B cells), or undergo terminal differentiation (plasma cells).

This chapter focuses on the classification of neoplasms derived from mature B cells, T cells, and natural killer (NK) cells, with emphasis on malignant lymphomas. Other chapters in this volume cover the lymphoid leukemias (Chapter 78) and the immunosecretory disorders, including plasma cell neoplasms (Chapter 80). Special attention is devoted to newly emerging areas of interest, such as the impact of clinical features (e.g., age and anatomic site) on disease definition and a greater appreciation of early events in neoplastic transformation. These early lesions can sometimes be detected in otherwise healthy individuals, and may or may not progress to overt lymphoma or leukemia. They appear to carry fewer genetic aberrations than the conventional forms of the disease, perhaps explaining their indolent clinical behavior.[5]

● CLINICAL RELEVANCE

Indolent lymphomas

- Natural history: survival measured in years
- Least sensitive to therapy
- Good response to low-dose oral alkylating agents, radiotherapy, and steroids, but no curability
- Higher response rate and complete remission with combination of standard chemotherapy and anti-CD20 monoclonal antibody
- Gene expression profiling can help to identify patients who might benefit from high-dose chemotherapy and autologous stem-cell transplantation, which is a potentially curative modality.

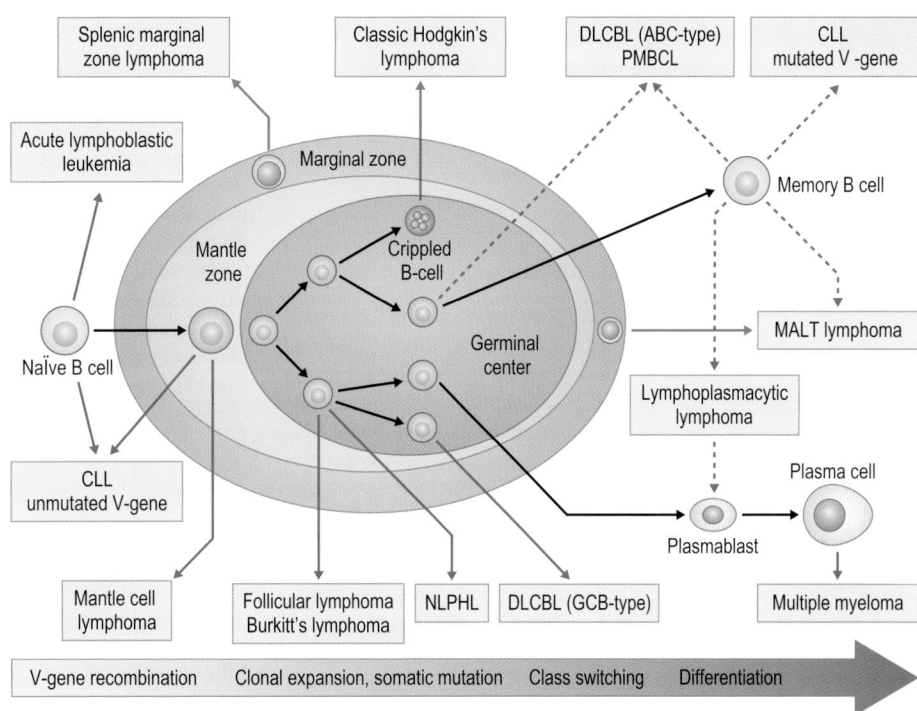

Fig. 79.1 Normal B-cell differentiation in relation to a secondary B follicle, mutational stages of the immunoglobulin genes, and cellular counterparts for B-cell lymphomas. Simplified version of B-cell development indicates points at which V-gene recombination, clonal expansion, and somatic mutations occur in relation to a secondary B follicle. B-cell lymphomas are related to different stages of B-cell differentiation and function. ABC-type, activated B-cell-like type; CLL, chronic lymphocytic leukemia/lymphoma; DLCBL, diffuse large B-cell lymphoma; GCB-type, germinal center B-cell-like type; MALT lymphoma, marginal-zone B-cell lymphoma of mucosa-associated lymphoid tissue (MALT) type; NLPHL, nodular lymphocyte-predominant Hodgkin lymphoma; PMBCL, primary mediastinal B-cell lymphoma.

Table 79.1 WHO classification of tumors of hematopoietic and lymphoid tissues (2008)

B-cell neoplasm

Precursor B-cell lymphoblastic leukemia/lymphoma
  B lymphoblastic leukemia/lymphoma, not otherwise specified
  B lymphoblastic leukemia/lymphoma with recurrent genetic abnormalities

Mature B-cell neoplasm

Chronic lymphocytic leukemia/small lymphocytic lymphoma
B-cell prolymphocytic leukemia
Splenic B-cell marginal zone lymphoma
Hairy cell leukemia
Splenic B-cell lymphoma/leukemia, unclassifiable
  Splenic diffuse red pulp small B-cell lymphoma
  Hairy cell leukemia-variant
Lymphoplasmacytic lymphoma
Heavy chain diseases
Plasma cell myeloma
Solitary plasmacytoma of bone
Extraosseous plasmacytoma
Extranodal marginal zone lymphoma of mucosa-associated lymphoid tissue (MALT lymphoma)
Nodal marginal zone lymphoma
  Pediatric nodal marginal zone lymphoma
Follicular lymphoma
  Pediatric follicular lymphoma
  Primary intestinal follicular lymphoma
  Other extranodal follicular lymphoma
  Intrafollicular neoplasia/"in situ" follicular lymphoma
Primary cutaneous follicle centre lymphoma
Mantle cell lymphoma
Diffuse large B-cell lymphoma (DLBCL), NOS
T-cell/histiocyte rich large B-cell lymphoma
Primary DLBCL of the CNS
Primary cutaneous DLBCL, leg type
EBV positive DLBCL of the elderly
DLBCL associated with chronic inflammation
Lymphomatoid granulomatosis
Primary mediastinal (thymic) large B-cell lymphoma
Intravascular large B-cell lymphoma
ALK positive large B-cell lymphoma
Plasmablastic lymphoma
Large B-cell lymphoma arising in HHV8-associated multicentric Castleman disease
Primary effusion lymphoma
Burkitt lymphoma

B-cell lymphoma unclassifiable, with features intermediate between diffuse large B-cell lymphoma and Burkitt lymphoma
B-cell lymphoma unclassifiable, with features intermediate between diffuse large B-cell lymphoma and classical Hodgkin lymphoma

T-cell neoplasm

Precursor T-cell lymphoblastic leukemia/lymphoma

Mature T- and NK-cell neoplasms

T-cell prolymphocytic leukemia
T-cell large granular lymphocytic leukemia
Chronic lymphoproliferative disorder of NK cells
Aggressive NK leukemia
EBV positive T-cell lymphoproliferative disorders of childhood
  Systemic EBV positive T-cell lymphoproliferative disease of childhood
  Hydroa vacciniforme-like lymphoma
Adult T-cell leukemia/lymphoma
Extranodal NK/T-cell lymphoma, nasal type
Enteropathy-associated T-cell lymphoma
Hepatosplenic T-cell lymphoma
Subcutaneous panniculitis-like T-cell lymphoma
Mycosis fungoides
Sézary syndrome
Primary cutaneous CD30 positive T-cell lymphoproliferative disorders
  Primary cutaneous anaplastic large cell lymphoma
  Lymphomatoid papulosis
Primary cutaneous peripheral T-cell lymphomas, rare subtypes
  Primary cutaneous gamma-delta T-cell lymphoma
  Primary cutaneous CD8 positive aggressive epidermotropic cytotoxic T-cell lymphoma
  Primary cutaneous CD4 positive small/medium T-cell lymphoma
Peripheral T-cell lymphoma, NOS
Angioimmunoblastic T-cell lymphoma
Anaplastic large cell lymphoma, ALK positive
Anaplastic large cell lymphoma, ALK negative

Hodgkin lymphoma

Nodular lymphocyte-predominant Hodgkin lymphoma
Classical Hodgkin lymphoma
Nodular sclerosis Hodgkin lymphoma
Lymphocyte-rich classical Hodgkin lymphoma
Mixed cellularity classical Hodgkin lymphoma
Lymphocyte-depleted classical Hodgkin lymphoma

Provisional entities in italics
Data from Swerdlow SH, Campo E, Harris, et al. WHO classification of tumours of haematopoietic and lymphoid tissue, 4th edn. WHO 2008.

Mature B-cell neoplasms

Lymphoplasmacytic lymphoma

The definition of lymphoplasmacytic lymphoma (LPL) is still controversial as specific genetic and immunophenotypic markers have not yet been identified. Moreover, many B-cell neoplasms occasionally show maturation to plasmacytoid or plasma cells containing cytoplasmic immunoglobulin (cIg). The term LPL should be restricted to tumors lacking features of other well-defined disease entities (e.g., chronic lymphocytic leukemia (CLL) or mantle cell lymphoma), which may on occasion manifest plasmacytoid differentiation. Many but not all patients with LPL may have clinical evidence of Waldenström's macroglobulinemia (WM), which, as defined by the second international workshop on WM, is based on the detection of an IgM monoclonal gammopathy of any concentration associated with bone marrow involvement by LPL (Chapter 80).

LPL is a disease of adult life (median age in the 60s) that usually presents with generalized lymphadenopathy, vague constitutional symptoms, anemia, and splenomegaly. The tumor consists of a diffuse proliferation of small lymphocytes, plasmacytoid lymphocytes, and plasma cells, with or without Dutcher bodies. The growth pattern is often interfollicular, with sparing of the sinuses. The cells have surface and cytoplasmic Ig, usually IgM and usually lacking IgD, and express B-cell-associated antigens (CD19, 20, 22, 79a). They are generally negative for CD5 and CD10. CD25 or CD11c may be weakly expressed in some cases. The lack of CD5 and the presence of strong cytoplasmic Ig are useful in distinguishing LPL from CLL. The postulated normal counterpart is thought to be a post-follicular medullary cord B-cell-based in part on the presence of somatic mutations in the Ig heavy- and light-chain variable region genes.

Mantle-cell lymphoma

Mantle-cell lymphoma (MCL) cytologically is composed of small lymphoid cells with finely clumped chromatin, scant cytoplasm, inconspicuous nucleoli, and irregular nuclear contours. Blastoid and pleomorphic variants are associated with a more aggressive clinical course. The molecular hallmark of MCL is the t(11;14)(q13;q32) involving cyclin D1 (*CCND1*) and the *IGH*μ gene. Cyclin D1 overexpression is believed to be essential in the pathogenesis of MCL. However, rare variants negative for Cyclin D1 with similar immunomorphology and gene expression signature have been identified.[6] Cyclin D1 negative forms usually express either Cyclin D2 or Cyclin D3, which may functionally substitute for Cyclin D1. SOX11 is overexpressed in most cyclin D1 positive and negative cases.[7,8]

The postulated normal counterpart is the CD5+ "naïve" B cell, sIgM+, and sIgD+, that can be found in the peripheral blood and in the mantle of reactive germinal centers. These cells usually do not carry somatic mutations in their rearranged immunoglobulin genes; however, similarly to CLL a subset of MCL have mutated *IG* genes challenging the view that the cell of origin is indeed a pregerminal center cell.

MCL occurs in adults (median age 62), with a high male-to-female ratio. Most patients present with advanced-stage disease. Common sites of involvement include the lymph nodes, spleen, bone marrow, peripheral blood, and lymphoid tissue of Waldeyer's ring. Gastrointestinal tract involvement is common and is associated with the picture of lymphomatous polyposis. In data collated from several retrospective studies the prognosis is poor, with a median survival ranging from 3-5 years and a high relapse rate following initial remission.[9]

The proliferation rate was previously identified as prognostically important based on scoring of Ki67+ cells. More recently GEP, using genes involved in cell cycle progression and DNA synthesis, has identified a proliferation signature that defines different prognostic groups, which correlate to some extent with cytological subtype.[10] For example, the blastoid variant has a high proliferation rate.

In situ MCL is the term used to describe a clonal proliferation of cyclin D1 positive cells restricted to the follicular mantle zone in an otherwise reactive lymph node or lymphoid tissue. Most often these represent an incidental finding, but some cases will eventually progress to overt MCL.[3] In some cases *in situ* MCL is detected in a lymph node involved by another lymphoma type, such as follicular lymphoma. The risk of progression of *in situ* MCL is difficult to ascertain, as the number of reported cases is few.

● CLINICAL RELEVANCE

Aggressive lymphomas

- Natural history: survival measured in months
- Successful therapy can be achieved with combination chemotherapy.
- Relapses from chemotherapy-induced remission may be cured with high-dose chemotherapy with hematopoietic support.
- In addition to the International Prognostic Index (IPI), gene expression profiling can be useful in predicting prognosis and survival of individual patients.

Another newly identified variant is an indolent form characterized by a leukemic phase without nodal disease but often long-standing splenomegaly. These patients have an indolent clinical course and do not appear to require aggressive chemotherapy.[11] These cases carry t(11;14) with few additional chromosomal abnormalities, and lack expression of SOX11 in contrast to conventional MCL.[11]

The treatment approach to newly diagnosed patients with MCL depends on the patient's eligibility for stem-cell transplantation (SCT). However, because of the frequent bone marrow involvement, purging of the neoplastic cells is difficult to achieve and SCT has proven not be curative. The addition of rituximab to standard chemotherapy regimens has provided a good initial response, but inability to sustain it; therefore, new drug regimens are needed.[12] Novel therapies such as proteosome inhibitors, immunomodulatory agents and mTOR inhibitors, are being tested based on the better understanding of the signaling pathways involved in MCL.[9]

Besides the *CCND1/IGH*μ translocation, additional alterations involving other cell cycle regulatory molecules (RB, p53, CDK inhibitors) have been described in the more aggressive forms of MCL. *INK4a/ARF* deletions occur in approximately 20% of cases. In recent years the research focus has shifted towards the understanding of the signaling pathways in MCL downstream from the B-cell receptor (BCR), such as PI3K/AKT/mTOR, NF-κB, WNT and Hedgehog pathways, which offer new potential therapeutic targets.[9]

Follicular lymphoma

Follicular lymphoma (FL) is the most common subtype of non-Hodgkin lymphoma in the USA and accounts for approximately 45% of all newly diagnosed cases. It has a peak incidence in the fifth and sixth decades, and is rare under the age of 20. Men and women are equally affected. FL is found less commonly in African American and Asian populations. Most patients have stage 3 or 4 disease at diagnosis, with generalized lymphadenopathy and staging evaluation that usually reveals bone marrow involvement. Approximately 10% of patients have circulating malignant cells. However, careful immunophenotypic or molecular analyses may disclose peripheral blood involvement in a higher proportion of patients.

FL is indolent, but still incurable with available therapeutic modalities. Clinical parameters have been used to develop prognostic indexes (e.g., the FLIPI, adjusted from the IPI for aggressive B-cell lymphoma). Other prognostic models have examined biological features using GEP or immunohistochemistry to evaluate the tissue microenvironment and nature of the infiltrating inflammatory cells.[13,14]

The natural history of the disease is associated with histologic progression in both pattern and cell type (Fig. 79.2). FL is composed of varying proportions of follicle center type cells, centrocytes and centroblasts, with centroblasts representing the proliferative component. According to the WHO classification, all low grade FL are combined into a single category, Grade 1-2, all containing overall a predominance of centrocytes with fewer than 15 centroblasts/high power field. FL grade 3 (with > 15 centroblasts/hpf) is further subdivided in 3A and 3B based on the presence or absence of centrocytes in the background. Biologically many Grade 3B FL appear more closely related to diffuse large B-cell lymphoma (DLBCL) than FL; however, more data are needed to confirm this hypothesis.[5]

The vast majority of FL (approximately 90%) are associated with a t(14; 18) involving rearrangement of the *BCL2* gene. This translocation appears to result in constitutive expression of BCL-2 protein, which is capable of inhibiting apoptosis in lymphoid cells. The cells of FL accumulate and are at risk for secondary mutations, which may be associated with histologic progression. It is thought that the *BCL2* translocation occurs at a very early stage of B-cell development, during immunoglobulin gene rearrangement. This fact may contribute to the difficulty of eradicating the neoplastic clone with chemotherapy. The small subset of grade 3B FL is less commonly associated with the *BCL2* translocation, but carries genetic aberrations more commonly seen in DLBCL.

The 2008 WHO classification recognizes several variants of FL, namely p*ediatric FL, primary intestinal FL* and other *extranodal FL*. Pediatric FL is also often extranodal at presentation and usually of large-cell type (grade 3), suggesting an alternate molecular pathogenesis.[15] When these tumors are localized (without lymph node involvement) they usually have a good prognosis. Complete remissions may be obtained with either surgical excision or local radiation therapy. Pediatric FL is more common in males than females.

The WHO classification recognizes "*In situ FL*" (also termed *intrafollicular neoplasia*) as a distinctive lesion. It should be distinguished from partial involvement of FL. "*In situ*" FL shows involvement of germinal centers by CD10 and BCL2 positive cells carrying t(14;18) in an otherwise reactive lymph node and often represents an incidental finding.[16] Patients lacking evidence of FL at staging have a low risk of developing the disease, and this phenomenon appears to represent the tissue counterpart of circulating clonal B cells carrying t(14;18) as detected in healthy individuals.[17] The term "FL-like B-cell of unknown significance" was recently proposed for this lesion.[5]

Primary cutaneous follicle center lymphoma, which frequently lacks the *BCL2* translocation and BCL2 expression, is now considered by the WHO classification as a separate entity. However, when BCL2 expression is detected, the possibility that this may represent a secondary site of involvement should be considered.

The neoplastic cells in FL have a mature B-cell phenotype with expression of the B-cell antigens CD19, CD20, and CD22. Surface Ig is positive, most commonly with IgM expression, but IgG or IgA can be seen in many cases. CD10, BCL-6 stains are positive, but CD5 is negative.

FL represents the neoplastic counterpart of the reactive germinal center cells. Consistent with their normal counterparts, intraclonal heterogeneity with high numbers of somatic mutations and ongoing mutations of the Ig genes was detected in the neoplastic cells.

Mucosa-associated lymphoid tissue (MALT) lymphomas

Most lymphomas of marginal-zone derivation present in extranodal sites and have histopathologic and clinical features that are part of the spectrum of MALT lymphomas. MALT lymphomas are characterized by a heterogeneous cellular composition including centrocyte-like cells, monocytoid B cells, small lymphocytes, and plasma cells. In most cases large transformed cells are uncommon, but reactive germinal centers are nearly always present. The distinction from reactive lesions has historically been problematic. Clonality can be established based on light chain restriction or molecular studies. When follicular colonization by the neoplastic cells occurs the process can simulate FL.

MALT lymphomas have been described in nearly every anatomic site, but are most frequent in the stomach, lung, thyroid, salivary gland, and lacrimal gland. Other less common sites of involvement include the orbit, breast, conjunctiva, bladder, kidney, and thymus. The clinical course is usually quite indolent. MALT lymphomas tend to relapse in other MALT-associated sites. MALT lymphomas of the salivary gland and thyroid are usually associated with a history of autoimmune diseases. There is a strong association between chronic infection with *Helicobacter*

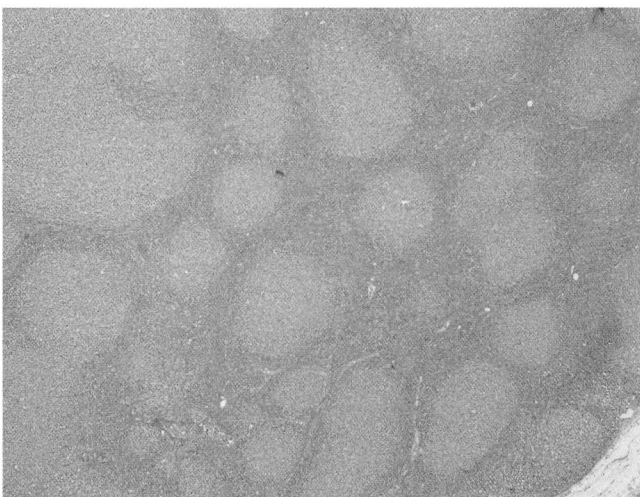

Fig. 79.2 Follicular lymphoma. The neoplastic follicles are similar in size and are partially surrounded by lymphoid cuffs. In contrast to reactive germinal centers, they lack polarization and tingible body macrophages ("starry-sky pattern").

pylori and gastric MALT lymphoma. Other infectious agents have been described in MALT lymphomas involving skin (*Borrelia burgdorferi*), ocular adnexae (*Chlamydia psittaci*), and small intestine (*Campylobacter jejuni*); however, a causal relationship has not yet been demonstrated. Chronic antigen stimulation is critical to both the development of a MALT lymphoma and the maintenance of the neoplastic state. Indeed, in some cases antibiotic therapy and the eradication of *H. pylori* has led to the spontaneous remission of gastric MALT lymphoma in cases lacking genetic aberrations.

MALT lymphomas are positive for B-cell-associated antigens CD19, CD20, and CD22, but are negative for CD5 and CD10. BCL-6 and CD10 are helpful markers to identify residual reactive germinal center cells. MALT lymphomas also have several recurring cytogenetic abnormalities, including t(11;18)(q21;q21), t(1;14)(p22;q32), t(14;18)(q32;q21), t(3;14)(q27;q32), and t(3;14)(p14.1;q32), which are observed with variable frequency, often depending upon the anatomical site.[18] Although several genes are involved in these translocations, at least three of them— t(11;18), t(1;14), and t(14;18)—share a common pathway, which leads to the activation of NFκB and its downstream targets.[18]

By genome-wide DNA profiling integrated with GEP, differences were detected among the three different main types of marginal zone lymphomas, lending support to the current WHO classification, which separates these three entities.[19]

The translocation t(11;18)(q21;q21) is associated exclusively with low-grade extranodal MALT and is not detected in cases with simultaneous low- and high-grade tumors, or in primary extranodal large-cell lymphomas, raising the question of whether these primary extranodal lymphomas are in fact related to low-grade MALT. In the WHO Clinical Advisory Committee, the term extranodal marginal-zone lymphoma (MZL) of MALT type applies only to low-grade MALT, and it was recommended that the term high-grade MALT not be used for extranodal large-cell lymphomas in a MALT site. The putative cell of origin of MZL is a memory B cell (postgerminal center).

Nodal marginal zone lymphoma

Nodal marginal zone lymphoma (NMZL) is a primary nodal disease, which resembles other marginal zone lymphomas, extranodal or splenic types. Adult patients often present with bone marrow involvement and tend to have a more aggressive clinical course than those with extranodal MALT. In contrast, when NMZL occurs in children, it shows a striking male predominance, presents with localized disease and can be managed with local therapies.[20]

The neoplastic proliferation is mostly composed of small- to medium-sized B cells, often with pale cytoplasm. The immunophenotype is similar to that of other marginal-zone B-cell lymphomas, CD20$^+$, CD5$^-$, CD10$^-$, with variable IgD expression (weak to negative). Some NMZL have a morphology and immunophenotype similar to those of splenic marginal zone (see below) and in these cases the tumor cells are IgD$^+$.

● **CLINICAL RELEVANCE**

Highly aggressive lymphomas

- More common in children
- Natural history similar to acute leukemia
- Successful treatment includes high-dose chemotherapy (induction, consolidation, and maintenance phases) with central nervous system prophylaxis.

Splenic marginal-zone lymphomas

Splenic marginal-zone lymphomas (SMZL) present in adults and are slightly more common in women than in men. The clinical presentation is splenomegaly, usually without peripheral lymphadenopathy. The majority of patients have bone marrow involvement, but there is usually only a modest lymphocytosis, with elevations in the lymphocyte count usually less than in CLL. Some evidence of plasmacytoid differentiation may be seen and patients may have a small M protein. The abundant pale cytoplasm evident in tissue sections may also be seen in peripheral blood smears. The cytologic features may be mistaken for those of hairy-cell leukemia. The course is reported to be indolent, and splenectomy may be followed by a prolonged remission.[21]

Histologically, the spleen shows expansion of the white pulp, but usually some infiltration of the red pulp is present as well. A characteristic biphasic pattern in the neoplastic white pulp has been described in which a central zone of small lymphocytes is surrounded by a peripheral zone of larger cells that resemble marginal-zone cells. In this instance the residual polytypic mantle is no longer present. The phenotype of these cells resembles that of the other marginal-zone B-cell lymphomas; however, sIgD expression is more frequently positive.

Deletion of 7q31 has been described in SMZL and although it can be seen in isolated cases of splenic B-cell lymphoma/leukemia unclassifiable, it has not been detected in other splenic lymphomas.[22] Studies of the Ig variable genes have also revealed the presence of somatic mutations, suggesting a postfollicular origin; however, similar to CLL cases, a more complex picture with cases of SMZL lacking somatic mutations has been reported.

Splenic lymphoma with villous lymphocytes

Splenic lymphoma with villous lymphocytes (SLVL) shares many features with SMZL, and is one of a group of variants of splenic lymphoma, grouped under the heading splenic B-cell lymphoma/leukemia unclassifiable.

Diffuse large B-cell lymphoma, not otherwise specified

Diffuse large B-cell lymphoma, not otherwise specified (DLBCL, NOS) is one of the more common subtypes of non-Hodgkin lymphoma, representing up to 40% of cases. It has an aggressive natural history but responds well to chemotherapy. The complete remission rate with modern regimens is 75–80%, with long-term disease-free survival approaching 50% or more in most series. This diagnosis is used both for primary DLBCL as well transformed cases from a low grade lymphoma. DLBCL may be nodal or involve extranodal sites, including bone, skin, thyroid, gastrointestinal tract, and lung.

DLBCL is one of the most heterogeneous categories in the WHO classification, in terms of morphology and phenotype and currently several morphologic variants are recognized as well as specific subtypes.[3] Because of the variation in the response to chemotherapy and the frequency of DLBCL, there has been great interest in identifying morphologic or immunophenotypic features that might be prognostically important. To address these issues, which were traditionally not resolved by morphology and phenotype, DLBCL was among the first lymphomas to be analyzed by cDNA microarray. Three groups were identified based on the differential expression of a large set of genes, namely germinal center-like group (GCB), *activated B-cell-like* group (ABC), and *primary mediastinal (thymic) large B-cell lymphoma* (PMBCL).[23] GCB DLBCLs express a set of genes that are associated with normal germinal center B cells, whereas ABC DLBCLs show downregulation of these genes and share similarities with postgerminal center B cells. A unique signature was identified by GEP in PMBCL and shared similarities with Hodgkin lymphoma (HL) cell lines, including constitutive activation of the NF-κB and recurrent gains and amplification of c-Rel.[24,25]

The t(14;18) translocation involving *BCL-2* and immunoglobulin heavy-chain gene has been detected in the GCB, but not in the other subtypes. By contrast, ABC cases express high levels of BCL-2 protein due to gene amplification and not to the *BCL-2* translocation. Indeed, previous studies have also shown reduced disease-free survival in cases of DLBCL with overexpression of BCL-2 (irrespective of the presence of the translocation). GEP identified differences in outcome in patients treated with anthracycline-based chemotherapy regimens, particularly between GCB and ABC subtypes (with a 5-year survival rate of 59 and 31%, respectively),[23] while PMBCL behaved similarly to the GCB group, with a 5-year survival rate of 64%.[25] This stratification is statistically independent of the IPI in predicting survival, and therefore probably reflects true biological differences. However, not all heterogeneity can be explained based on expression profiling;[26] clinical factors also have an impact on survival, as shown by the IPI stratification of patients with aggressive lymphomas.

DLBCL, NOS is composed of large transformed lymphoid cells with nuclei at least twice the size of a small lymphocyte (Fig. 79.3). The nuclei generally have vesicular chromatin, prominent nucleoli, and basophilic cytoplasm, and resemble either centroblasts or immunoblasts, but with greater overall cellular pleomorphism. Although there is no absolute correlation between morphology and GEP, the majority of centroblastic DLBCL falls into the GCB group, and the majority of immunoblastic DLBCL into the ABC group.

Algorithms based on immunophenotype have been proposed as surrogates for cDNA microarray using CD10/BCL-6 positivity for GCB and Mum-1/IRF-4 for ABC with the addition of BCL-2 in combination with IPI. This approach could improve the stratification of DLBCL. However, there is as yet no consensus for the best model to address the heterogeneity of DLBCL and immunohistochemistry based algorithms should be used with caution.[27]

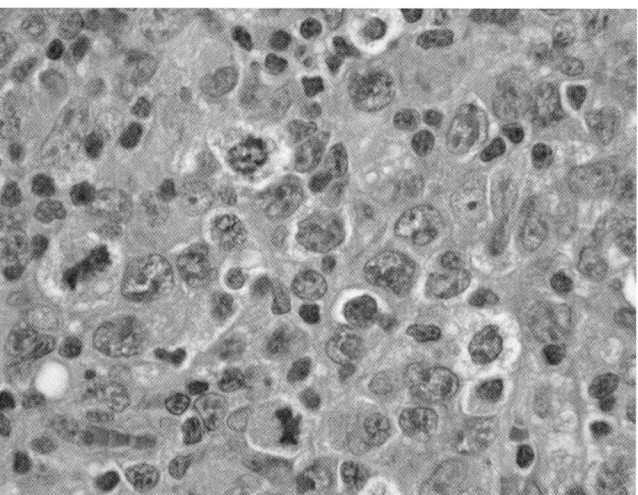

Fig. 79.3 Diffuse large-cell lymphoma. The neoplastic cells have large round to oval nuclei with vesicular chromatin and multiple eosinophilic nucleoli. Numerous mitoses are also present.

T cell/histiocyte rich large B-cell lymphoma (THRLBCL), as currently defined, is now considered a distinct clinical pathologic entity rather than a morphologic variant. THRLBCL has an aggressive clinical behavior, it tends to occur in younger patients compared to other DLBCL, NOS, and often presents with advanced stage and bone marrow involvement. The relevance of the microenvironment and recruitment mechanism of the inflammatory cells, which are the main histological component, have been the focus of recent studies.[28]

The WHO classification recognizes that some lymphomas arising in certain anatomic sites may have distinctive features both clinically and biologically. Among these are *primary DLBCL of the central nervous system* (CNS) and *primary cutaneous DLBCL, leg type*. Primary DLBCL of the CNS has some distinctive features based on GEP, and shares some similarities with DLBCL arising in other immune privileged sites such as the testis.[29] Primary cutaneous DLBCL, leg type, has a GEP resembling the ABC type of DLBCL, presents most often in elderly females, and generally has an aggressive clinical course.[30]

There are several EBV-positive B-cell lymphoproliferations that are often grouped with DLBCL. *EBV-positive DLBCL of the elderly* is a provisional entity in the 2008 WHO classification. It appears to develop as a consequence of decreased immune surveillance.[31,32] The morphological spectrum is broad and includes polymorphous and more monomorphic tumors. Most cases have an aggressive clinical course, and should be distinguished from atypical hyperplasia associated with EBV, and lesions with a self-limited course, such as EBV-positive mucocutaneous ulcer.[33] *Lymphomatoid granulomatosis* is an EBV-positive B-cell lymphoproliferative disorder (LPD) associated with an inflammatory background rich in T cells. The lung is nearly always involved, with skin, kidney, liver and brain being frequently affected as well. *DLBCL associated with chronic inflammation* was first described in association with chronic pyothorax, but now has been associated with EBV-driven large B-cell proliferations in diverse clinical settings, usually associated with a confined anatomic space and a background of chronic inflammation. These cases appear to have a good prognosis if successfully resected.

There are several LPDs associated with HHV-8/KSHV. These include *primary effusion lymphoma (PEL)* and *multicentric Castleman disease (MCD)*, as well as lymphomas arising in the context of (MCD). The cells of PEL are usually coinfected with EBV, and the disease is most often diagnosed in the setting of HIV infection and immunosuppression. While pleural or peritoneal effusions are most common, extracavitary PEL can present as a tumor mass, usually in extranodal sites. PEL has a phenotype resembling that of terminally differentiated B cells, i.e., plasmablastic.

Two other lymphomas with a plasmablastic phenotype include *plasmablastic lymphoma (PBL)*, and *ALK-positive large B-cell lymphoma*. PBL is usually positive for EBV, most often extranodal, and associated with immunosuppression from either HIV infection or advanced age. Recent studies have identified a high incidence of *MYC* translocation in PBL. ALK-positive large B-cell lymphomas show overexpression of ALK, usually as a consequence of translocation. They mainly affect older individuals, but can occur at any age. Interestingly, IgA is most often expressed.[34]

Primary mediastinal large B-cell lymphoma

Primary mediastinal large B-cell lymphoma (PMBCL) is considered a distinct clinicopathologic entity. The diagnosis is usually made by a constellation of clinical and morphological features.

A common feature is relatively abundant pale cytoplasm with distinct cytoplasmic membranes, and fine compartmentalizing sclerosis. The tumor appears to be derived from medullary B cells within the thymus gland. These cells express CD20 and CD79a, but not surface Ig. Recently, the expression of the *MAL* gene has been detected in PMBCL and not in other DLBCL.[35]

Clinically, PMBCL shows marked female predominance. It is common in adolescents and young adults, with a median age at presentation in the fourth decade. The clinical presentation is that of a rapidly growing anterior mediastinal mass with frequent superior vena cava syndrome and/or airway obstruction. Nodal involvement is uncommon at presentation and also at relapse. Frequent extranodal sites of involvement, particularly at relapse, include the liver, kidneys, adrenal glands, ovaries, gastrointestinal tract, and central nervous system. The treatment approach includes aggressive systemic chemotherapy, plus rituximab, with radiation therapy used in some centers.[36]

A new aspect of the 2008 WHO classification is the inclusion of borderline categories, one of which manifests features intermediate between DLBCL, especially PMBCL, and classic HL (CHL). These tumors are sometimes referred to as *gray-zone lymphomas*.[37] A close relationship between PMBCL and CHL was supported by gene expression profiling.[24,25] TRAF1 expression and c-REL amplification also were seen in both types of neoplasms and could be detected with suitable immunohistochemical studies.[38]

Gray-zone lymphomas are more common in males than females, present with bulky mediastinal masses, and appear to have a more aggressive clinical course than PMBCL or CHL. A recent study using methylation profiling identified gray-zone lymphomas as having a signature distinct from both CHL and PMBCL.[39] However, by fluorescence *in situ* hybridization, gray-zone lymphomas, PBMCL and cHL share a number of common cytogenetic aberrations including gains at 2p16.1 (*REL/BCL11A* locus), 9p24.1 (*JAK2/PDL2*) and rearrangements of 16p13.13 (*CIITA*).[40] It is not clear how these patients should be managed clinically, but they appear to benefit from combined modality therapy.

Burkitt lymphoma

Burkitt lymphoma (BL) is most common in children and accounts for up to one-third of all pediatric lymphomas in the USA. It is the most rapidly growing of all lymphomas, with 100% of the cells in cell cycle at any time. It usually presents in extranodal sites. In nonendemic regions, such as the USA, common sites of presentation are the ileocecal region, ovaries, kidneys, or breasts. Jaw presentations, as well as the involvement of other facial bones, are common in African or endemic cases and are occasionally seen in nonendemic regions. Bone marrow involvement is a poor prognostic sign.

BL is one of the more common tumors associated with the human immunodeficiency virus (HIV). It can present at any time during the clinical course. In some patients with HIV infection BL is the initial AIDS-defining illness.

The pathogenesis of BL is undoubtedly related to the translocations involving the *c-MYC* oncogene, which are seen in virtually 100% of cases. Most of the translocations involve the Ig heavy-chain gene on chromosome 14. Less commonly the light-chain genes on chromosomes 2 and 22 are involved. The *MYC* translocation is considered a primary event and often is the sole karyotypic abnormality detected. This is in contrast with other aggressive lymphomas in which the *MYC* translocation occurs as a secondary event in a more complex karyotype.[41,42]

African BL occurs in regions endemic for malaria, and it has been postulated that immunosuppression associated with malarial infection puts patients at increased risk. In this regard, the pathogenesis appears similar to that seen with HIV infection; recent GEP data also support a common pathogenetic mechanism.[43]

Epstein–Barr virus (EBV) is closely linked to BL in endemic regions but is less frequently seen (15–20%) in Europe and North America. In other regions, characterized by low socioeconomic status and EBV infection at an early age, BL is often EBV-positive, in the range of 50–70%. These data support the concept the EBV is a cofactor for the development of BL. Differences in the proportion of cases associated with the two EBV strains (types 1 and 2) have also been shown in sporadic and endemic EBV-positive BL.

Cytologically, BL is monomorphic with cells of medium size, round nuclei, and multiple (2–5) basophilic nucleoli. The cytoplasm is deeply basophilic and moderately abundant. These cells contain cytoplasmic lipid vacuoles, which are probably a manifestation of the high rates of proliferation and spontaneous cell death. The starry-sky pattern characteristic of BL is a manifestation of the numerous benign macrophages that have ingested karyorrhectic or apoptotic tumor cells. BL has a mature B-cell phenotype. The cells express CD19, CD20, CD22, CD79a, and monoclonal surface Ig, nearly always IgM. CD10 is positive in nearly all cases, and CD5, CD23, and BCL-2 are consistently negative.

Historically it has been difficult for pathologists to distinguish some DLBCL with a very high growth fraction from BL with atypical cytology. In addition, there are cases that have a molecular GEP of BL, but carry additional cytogenetic abnormalities, most often involving *BCL2* or *BCL6*.[44] These double hit and triple hit lymphomas have a very aggressive clinical course. In order to recognize and delineate these cases this borderline category was created in the 2008 WHO classification.[3] However, it should not be utilized for otherwise typical DLBCL with a *MYC* translocation. The clinical impact of *MYC* overexpression in DLBCL has not been fully resolved, but in some series has been associated with a more aggressive clinical course.[45]

T-cell and putative NK-cell neoplasms

Overview of the classification of T-cell neoplasms

Whereas the definition of T-lymphoblastic neoplasms is straightforward, the classification of *peripheral T-cell lymphoma* (PTCL) has been controversial. These are uncommon, representing fewer than 15% of all non-Hodgkin lymphomas. Most previously published classification schemes for the malignant lymphomas in the USA or Europe have been based on the far more common B-cell malignancies. In addition, the molecular pathogenesis of most peripheral T-cell neoplasms has not been defined, and immunophenotypic markers are less specific for apparently distinct disease entities. For these reasons, the WHO classification relies to a considerable extent on clinical presentation to subdivide these tumors.[3]

Extranodal NK/T-cell lymphoma, nasal type

Extranodal NK/T-cell lymphoma, nasal type, is a distinct clinicopathologic entity highly associated with EBV. It is much more common in Asians than in those of European background. Clusters of the disease have also been reported in Central and

South America in individuals of Native American heritage, suggesting that ethnic background may play a role in the pathogenesis of these lymphomas. It affects adults (median age 50) and the most common clinical presentation is a destructive nasal or midline facial lesion. Palatal destruction, orbital swelling, and edema can be prominent. NK/T-cell lymphomas have been reported in other extranodal sites, including the skin, soft tissue, testis, upper respiratory tract, and gastrointestinal tract. The clinical course is usually aggressive, with a slightly improved median survival in patients with localized disease, in which local radiation therapy may be useful.[46] A hemophagocytic syndrome is a common clinical complication, and adversely affects survival.

Extranodal NK/T-cell lymphoma, nasal type, is characterized by a broad cytologic spectrum. Although the cells express some T-cell-associated antigens, most commonly CD2, other T-cell markers, such as surface CD3, are usually absent. Cytoplasmic CD3 is positive but most cases lack clonal T-cell gene rearrangement. In favor of an NK-cell origin, the cells are nearly always CD56$^+$, although CD16 and CD57 are usually negative. EBV is invariably positive by *in situ* hybridization. Emerging oncogenic pathways have been identified by GEP.[47]

Aggressive NK-cell leukemia is a closely related entity. It presents at a younger age than extranodal NK/T-cell lymphoma, is associated with systemic disease, and a fulminant clinical course. It has a similar phenotype, EBV association, and epidemiology.[46]

There are other EBV$^+$ T-cell and NK-cell proliferations that are seen mainly in children. These include *systemic EBV$^+$ T-cell lymphoproliferative disease*, *hydroa vacciniforme-like lymphoma*, and *mosquito bite allergy*, the latter usually being derived from NK-cells. All are seen most often in Asian children. The latter two conditions affect mainly the skin and have a more indolent clinical course, whereas the systemic disease has a very aggressive clinical course with survival measured in weeks. Systemic EBV$^+$ T-cell LPD may arise in a background of chronic active EBV-infection.[48,49]

Angioimmunoblastic T-cell lymphoma

Angioimmunoblastic T-cell lymphoma (AILT) was initially proposed as an abnormal immune reaction, but later considered a variant of T-cell lymphoma. The majority of cases show clonal rearrangements of T-cell receptor genes, but proliferation of B cells also contributes to the histologic and clinical picture The median survival is usually less than 5 years.

The nodal architecture is generally effaced, but peripheral sinuses are often open and even dilated. Follicles are typically regressed, but there is a proliferation of dendritic cells often surrounding the high endothelial venules (HEV). Proliferation of HEV is often prominent.

The atypical lymphoid cells have clear cytoplasm and are admixed with small lymphocytes, immunoblasts, plasma cells, and histiocytes, with or without eosinophils. The abnormal cells are T cells usually positive for CD4, CD10, and PD-1, a phenotype characteristic of follicular T-helper cells (T$_{FH}$). CXCL-13, a chemokine involved in B-cell trafficking into the germinal centers, is also expressed. A relationship to T$_{FH}$ has been confirmed by GEP.[50,51] In keeping with a proposed derivation from T$_{FH}$, B-cell proliferation including marked polyclonal plasmacytosis is often present. In some cases the plasma cells may be monoclonal. EBV-positive B cells are nearly a constant factor in the background, and progression to an EBV-positive B-cell lymphoma may occur. The exact role of EBV in AILT is uncertain; theories include expansion due to decreased immune surveillance or a more direct but uncertain role in pathogenesis.

AILT presents in adults; most patients have generalized lymphadenopathy with prominent systemic symptoms, including fever, weight loss, and skin rash. There is usually a polyclonal hypergammaglobulinemia. Patients may initially respond to steroids or mild cytotoxic chemotherapy, but progression usually occurs. More aggressive combination chemotherapeutic regimens have led to a higher remission rate but patients are prone to secondary infectious complications.[52]

Peripheral T-cell lymphomas, not otherwise specified

Peripheral T-cell lymphomas, not otherwise specified (PTCL, NOS) is a diagnosis of exclusion and is admittedly a heterogeneous category with most cases being nodal in origin. PTCL are characterized by a heterogeneous cellular composition, and may or may not include an inflammatory background. Cases with abundant epithelioid histiocytes are categorized as the lymphoepithelioid cell variant. Cases composed mostly of smaller lymphoid cells restricted to the paracortex are recognized under the T-zone variant. There is also a rare follicular variant composed of T$_{FH}$ cells that are restricted to the lymphoid follicles.[53]

Clinically, PTCL most often presents in adults. Most patients exhibit generalized lymphadenopathy, hepatosplenomegaly, and frequent bone marrow involvement. The clinical course is generally aggressive, with a lower response rate than that seen for aggressive B-cell lymphomas.

PTCL, as defined in the WHO classification, remains heterogeneous. It is likely that individual clinicopathologic entities will be delineated in the future from this broad group of malignancies. Thus far, immunophenotypic criteria have not been helpful in delineating subtypes. Most cases have a mature T-cell phenotype and express one of the major subset antigens, with CD4 expression seen more frequently than CD8. These are not clonal markers, and antigen expression can change over time. Loss of one of the pan-T-cell antigens (CD3, CD5, CD2, or CD7) is seen in 75% of cases, with CD7 most frequently being absent. GEP studies have shown some cases with a profile resembling AILT.[53] Cases with a high proliferation signature appear to have a more aggressive clinical course, but GEP has not led to the delineation of distinctive subtypes as independent entities.[54]

Anaplastic large-cell lymphoma

Anaplastic large-cell lymphoma (ALCL) is characterized by pleomorphic or monomorphic cells that have a propensity to invade lymphoid sinuses. Because of the sinusoidal location of the tumor cells and their lobulated nuclear appearance, this disease was previously interpreted as a variant of malignant histiocytosis. A consistent feature is the expression of the CD30 antigen, which is a hallmark of this disease. However, CD30 expression is not specific for ALCL and may also be seen in other forms of malignant lymphoma, including CHL. ALCL-ALK$^+$ is associated with a characteristic chromosomal translocation, t(2;5)(p23;q35), involving *ALK/NPM* genes, respectively. A variety of other partners of ALK has been identified and monoclonal antibodies to the ALK protein have been made, and are able to identify tumor cells regardless of the underlying translocation. In the majority of cases the neoplastic cells show both nuclear and cytoplasmic staining. The presence of cytoplasmic staining for ALK suggests a variant translocation.[55,56]

The cells of classic ALCL have large, often lobulated nuclei with small basophilic nucleoli. In some cases the nuclei may be round. The cytoplasm is usually abundant and amphophilic, with distinct cytoplasmic borders. A prominent Golgi region is generally visible.

Immunohistochemistry is very valuable in the correct diagnosis of ALCL. The prominent Golgi region usually shows intense staining for CD30 and epithelial membrane antigen (EMA).

The cells exhibit an aberrant phenotype with loss of many of the T-cell-associated antigens. Both CD3 and CD45RO, the most widely used pan-T-cell markers, are negative in more than 50% of cases. CD2 and CD4 are positive in the majority of cases, whereas CD8 is usually negative. ALCL cells, despite the CD4$^+$/CD8$^-$ phenotype, often express the cytotoxic-associated antigens TIA-1, granzyme B, and perforin. In addition clusterin is generally present in ALCL and represents another useful diagnostic marker. Molecular studies in most cases demonstrate T-cell receptor rearrangement, confirming a T-cell origin.

ALCL is most common in children and young adults, and more common in males than females. While nodal presentations are most common, a variety of extranodal sites can be involved including skin, soft tissue, bone, and more rarely the central nervous system. Overall survival and disease-free survival are significantly better in ALK$^+$ than in ALK$^-$ cases. Both ALK$^+$ and ALK$^-$ ALCL have a better prognosis than other PTCLs, with a plateau in the survival curve seen in both groups.[57]

It has been controversial whether ALCL, ALK negative (ALCL-ALK$^-$) is a separate entity or part of the spectrum of PTCL, NOS. Part of the controversy relates to the lack of absolute criteria to recognize these cases. They should be morphologically and phenotypically similar to ALK$^+$ ALCL, with strong CD30 expression and a cytotoxic phenotype. They occur in an older age group than the ALK$^+$, and as noted above, appear to have a better prognosis than other PTCL,NOS.[57]

Primary cutaneous ALCL

Primary cutaneous ALCL is closely related to lymphomatoid papulosis and differs clinically, immunophenotypically, and at the molecular level from the systemic form. Indeed, lymphomatoid papulosis and cutaneous ALCL appear to represent a histologic and clinical continuum of CD30$^+$ cutaneous lymphoproliferative diseases. Small lesions are likely to regress, whereas patients with large tumor masses may develop disseminated disease with lymph node involvement. However, primary cutaneous ALCL is a more indolent disease than other T-cell lymphomas of the skin. Most patients with primary cutaneous ALCL have multiple skin lesions. Because the skin nodules may show spontaneous regression, a period of observation is usually warranted before the institution of any chemotherapy. Cutaneous ALCL is CD30$^+$, but usually ALK-1- and EMA-negative, and also lacks the t(2;5) translocation.

Subcutaneous panniculitis-like T-cell lymphoma

Subcutaneous panniculitis-like T-cell lymphoma (SPTCL) usually presents with subcutaneous nodules, primarily affecting the extremities and ranging in size from 0.5 cm to several centimeters in diameter. In its early stages the infiltrate may appear deceptively benign, and lesions are often misdiagnosed as panniculitis. However, histologic progression usually occurs and subsequent biopsies show more pronounced cytologic atypia. The neoplastic cells are CD8$^+$ cytotoxic α/β T cells that are also positive for the cytotoxic proteins perforin, granzyme B, and TIA-1. These proteins may be responsible for the cellular destruction seen in these tumors. EBV is negative in SPTCL. Some PTCL

of γ/δ T-cell derivation may show similar features, but differ from SPTCL in clinical behavior (more aggressive) and histological pattern, as they are often not confined to the subcutis.[58]

Some patients with SPTCL have a history of autoimmune disease, and in particular, the differential diagnosis of SPTCL with lupus profundus panniculitis can be challenging. Lupus panniculitis usually contains abundant plasma cells, which are generally rare in SPTCL.

A hemophagocytic syndrome can be a complication of SPTCL, but is more often associated with γ/δ T-cell lymphomas involving the subcutaneous tissue. Patients present with fever, pancytopenia, and hepatosplenomegaly. It is most readily diagnosed in bone marrow aspirate smears, where histiocytes containing erythrocytes, platelets, and other blood elements may be observed. The hemophagocytic syndrome usually heralds a fulminant downhill clinical course.[59]

Primary cutaneous γ/δ T-cell lymphomas

Primary cutaneous γ/δ T-cell lymphomas can present with disease involving the subcutis, the dermis, or with epidermal infiltration. These are clinically aggressive tumors. The cells have a cytotoxic phenotype, and like normal γ/δ T cells, lack CD5, and express cytotoxic molecules. They may be CD8$^+$, or more often, double-negative for CD4 and CD8. While skin is the most common presenting site, similar lymphomas of γ/δ T-cell origin can present in other extranodal sites, including gastrointestinal tract and lung.[60]

Mycosis fungoides (MF) and Sézary syndrome (SS)

Mycosis fungoides (MF) and Sézary syndrome (SS) are now regarded as separate diseases, but are closely related and often considered together from a clinical and biological standpoint. Both are primary cutaneous T-cell malignancies derived from mature skin homing CD4$^+$ T cells. Epidermotropism is the hallmark of MF; the cells have a tendency to infiltrate the epidermis, producing Pautrier microabscesses. However, early in the course Pautrier microabscesses may be absent and patients may have clinical manifestations for some years prior to a definitive diagnosis. The cutaneous lesions are categorized as patches, plaques, and tumors, based on the extent of the infiltrate.

SS presents with exfoliative erythroderma and circulating cerebriform lymphocytes known as Sézary cells. Clinically SS is more aggressive than MF.[61]

Enteropathy-associated T-cell lymphoma

Enteropathy-associated T-cell lymphoma (EATL) is highly associated with celiac diseaes, and shows a similar epidemiology on a world-wide basis. The small bowel usually shows ulceration, frequently with perforation, and a mass may or may not be present. The infiltrate shows a varying cytologic composition with an admixture of small, medium, and larger atypical lymphoid cells. Anaplastic cells strongly positive for CD30 can be present. The adjacent small bowel usually shows villous atrophy associated with celiac disease. The neoplastic cells are CD3$^+$, CD7$^+$ T cells that also express the homing receptor CD103 (HML-1). The cells express cytotoxic molecules, a feature shared by nearly all extranodal T-cell lymphomas.[62]

This disease occurs in adults, the majority of whom have either overt or clinically silent gluten-sensitive enteropathy. Ulcerative jejunitis may precede the development of overt EATL, and may share a common T-cell gene rearrangement pattern with the subsequent lymphoma. Patients usually present with abdominal symptoms such as pain, small-bowel perforation, and associated peritonitis. The clinical course is aggressive. Other PTCL can present with intestinal disease, and should be distinguished from EATL. These include the EBV-positive extranodal T/NK-cell lymphomas, and γ/δ T-cell lymphomas.

The majority of peripheral T lymphocytes belong to the αβ T-cell receptor subset, whereas only a minority express the γδ T-cell receptor. Similarly, most PTCLs are of αβ T-cell derivation. However, there is a unique subtype of PTCL that in most cases is derived from γδ T cells.

Hepatosplenic T-cell lymphoma

Hepatosplenic T-cell lymphoma (HSTCL) presents with marked hepatosplenomegaly. The homing pattern manifested by the malignant cells is similar to that of normal γδ T cells, which also populate the sinusoidal areas of the spleen.[60]

HSTCL shows a marked male predominance and most patients are young adults. The clinical presentation is that of marked hepatosplenomegaly in the absence of lymphadenopathy. Abnormal cells are usually present in the bone marrow but may be difficult to identify. They selectively infiltrate the bone marrow sinusoids and can be most easily recognized with immunohistochemical stains.

The cells of HSTCL are usually moderate in size, with a rim of pale cytoplasm. The nuclear chromatin is loosely condensed, with small inconspicuous nucleoli, and usually some irregularity of the nuclear contour can be seen. The liver and spleen show marked sinusoidal infiltration, with sparing of both portal triads and white pulp, respectively. The neoplastic cells have a phenotype that resembles that of normal γδ T cells, usually expressing neither CD4 nor CD8. CD56 is often positive. *In situ* hybridization for EBV is negative. The cells are positive for the cytotoxic protein TIA-1, but are not activated and generally lack granzyme B and perforin. Isochromosome 7 is a consistent cytogenetic abnormality, usually seen in conjunction with trisomy 8. Rare cases with similar morphological and biological features are derived from αβ T cells.[63]

Clinically, HSTCL is aggressive. Although patients may respond initially to chemotherapy, relapse occurs in the vast majority of cases and the median survival is less than 3 years. Allogeneic bone marrow transplantation is required for sustained remission.

Adult T-cell leukemia/lymphoma

Adult T-cell leukemia/lymphoma (ATLL) is a distinct form of T-cell lymphoma associated with the retrovirus HTLV-1, and the worldwide distribution of the virus mimics the incidence of ATLL. The highest areas of incidence include Southwestern Japan and the Caribbean basin. The disease has a long latency, and affected individuals usually are exposed to the virus very early in life. The virus may be transmitted in breast milk, and through exposure to blood and blood products. The cumulative incidence of ATLL is estimated to be 2.5% among HTLV-1 carriers. The virus is monoclonally integrated into tumor DNA.

The cells are often markedly polylobated, and have been referred to as flower cells. Peripheral blood involvement is very common, but often in the absence of bone marrow disease. Cutaneous involvement is seen in the majority of patients. The cells have a characteristic phenotype that resembles T regulatory (Treg) cells: CD3+, CD4+, CD25+. Some cases express FoxP3, but

usually in a minority of tumor cells. The function of the tumor cells as Treg cells may correlate with the associated immunodeficiency.[64]

Hodgkin lymphomas

● CLINICAL RELEVANCE

Hodgkin lymphoma

- B-cell lineage established in nearly all cases.
- Reed–Sternberg cell, the hallmark of the disease, represents a "crippled" germinal-center B cell.
- Nodular lymphocyte-predominant Hodgkin lymphoma considered a related but distinct entity.
- Eighty percent of patients are curable with current therapy.
- Stage of disease guides the choice of therapy; even patients with advanced-stage disease may be cured.
- Late complications from treatment include acute leukemia (alkylating agents with extended-field radiation therapy), second solid tumors (radiation therapy), and premature atherosclerotic coronary artery disease (radiation therapy).
- Cause of death in the first 5–10 years is mainly Hodgkin lymphoma; after 10 years, mainly secondary malignant tumors.

Hodgkin lymphoma (HL) and non-Hodgkin lymphoma have long been regarded as distinct disease entities based on their differences in pathology, phenotype, clinical features, and response to therapy. It is now accepted the malignant cell of HL is an altered B cell.[65] Therefore, it is not surprising that both biological and clinical overlaps should occur between these two lymphoma groups, as also shown by GEP in PMBCL and classic Hodgkin cell lines.[24,25] Although we have become aware of this closer relationship from the histogenetic point of view (hence the name Hodgkin lymphoma), these disorders are still treated with different modalities.

The diagnosis of classic HL (CHL) depends on the identification of Hodgkin/Reed–Sternberg (HRS) cells in an appropriate inflammatory background composed of small T lymphocytes, plasma cells, histiocytes, and granulocytes (often eosinophils). All cases of CHL share certain immunophenotypic and genotypic features. The phenotype is CD30+, CD15+/−, CD45−, and EMA−. Expression of B-cell-associated antigens is seen in up to 75% of cases. However, when present, CD20 staining is weaker than that seen in normal B cells with variable in intensity among individual tumor cells. CD79a is usually negative. Ig and T-cell receptor genes are usually germline, due to the paucity of tumor cells in the inflammatory background, but using microdissection and polymerase chain reaction (PCR) amplification for clonal rerrangement of the *IG* genes can generally be shown. In addition, the presence of somatic mutations indicates transit through the germinal center.[65]

Sufficient evidence has emerged in recent years to warrant the recognition of nodular lymphocyte-predominant HL as a distinct entity. Although it resembles other types of HL in having a minority of putative neoplastic cells on a background of benign inflammatory cells, it differs morphologically, immunophenotypically, and clinically from classic HL. The preferred term of Hodgkin lymphoma over Hodgkin disease reflects current knowledge concerning the nature of the neoplastic cell as a lymphocyte.

Nodular lymphocyte-predominant Hodgkin lymphoma

Nodular lymphocyte-predominant Hodgkin lymphoma (NLPHL) usually has a nodular growth pattern, with or without diffuse areas; it is rarely purely diffuse. Nodularity may be more easily recognized using immunohistologic stains with anti-B-cell or anti-follicular dendritic cell (FDC) antibodies. Progressively transformed germinal centers are often seen in partially involved lymph nodes or other lymph node sites. The atypical cells have vesicular, polylobated nuclei and small nucleoli. These had been called lymphocytic and/or histiocytic (L&H) cells, or "popcorn" cells, but the term LP cell is now preferred. Although these cells may be very numerous, usually no diagnostic HRS cells are found. The background is predominantly lymphocytes with or without epithelioid histiocyte clusters. Plasma cells are infrequent, and eosinophils and neutrophils are rarely seen. Occasionally sclerosis may cause lesions to resemble nodular sclerosis.

The atypical cells are CD45$^+$-expressing B-cell-associated antigens (CD19, 20, 22, 79a), CDw75$^+$, EMA$^{+/-}$ CD15$^-$, CD30$^{-/+}$ and usually sIg$^-$ by routine techniques, although one study reported light-chain restriction. J chain has been demonstrated in many cases. Small lymphocytes in the nodules are predominantly B cells with a mantle-zone phenotype. However, numerous T cells are present, with CD57$^+$ T cells surrounding the LP cells. The proportion of T cells tends to increase over time in sequential biopsies. A prominent meshwork of FDC is present within the nodules. LP cells, when isolated by microdissection, have clonally rearranged IG genes with evidence of somatic hypermutation.[66]

NLPHL occurs at all ages, in adults more commonly than in children, and in males more than in females. It usually involves peripheral lymph nodes, with sparing of the mediastinum. It is usually localized at diagnosis, but rarely may be disseminated. Survival is long, with or without treatment, for localized cases. However, when disseminated the prognosis is often poor. Patients with advanced stage disease may benefit from treatment regimens used for aggressive B-cell lymphomas. Late relapses have been reported to be more common than in other types of HL; it may be associated with, or progress to, large B-cell lymphoma. Progression to a process resembling T-cell/histiocyte-rich large B-cell lymphoma may also be seen.

Classic Hodgkin lymphoma, nodular sclerosis

The variant of HL termed classic Hodgkin lymphoma, nodular sclerosis (NSCHL) is most common in adolescents and young adults, but can occur at any age; female cases equal or exceed those in males. The mediastinum is commonly involved; stage and bulk of disease have prognostic importance. NSCHL is often curable; however, in long-term survivors the risk of secondary malignancies is increased, especially in those receiving both radiation and chemotherapy. NSCHL of the mediastinum is thought to be closely related to PMBCL, and both types of tumors can be seen in the same patient, either as composite malignancy, or sequentially.[37]

The tumor has at least a partially nodular pattern, with fibrous bands separating the nodules in most cases. Diffuse areas may be present, as is necrosis. The characteristic cell is the lacunar-type RS cell, which may be very numerous. Diagnostic RS cells are usually also present. The background contains lymphocytes, histiocytes, plasma cells, eosinophils, and neutrophils. It can be graded according to the proportion of the tumor cells and the presence of necrosis: Grades I and II. However, grading is considered optional. The immunophenotype and genotype are characteristic of CHL. However, EBV is infrequently positive, less than 15% of cases.

Classic Hodgkin lymphoma, mixed cellularity

Patients with classic Hodgkin lymphoma, mixed cellularity (CHLMC) are usually adults; males outnumber females and the stage is often advanced. The course is moderately aggressive but is often curable. CHLMC has a bimodal age distribution, with a peak in young children, and again in older adults. It is often EBV-positive, seen in up to 75% of cases. Both CHLMC and the lymphocyte depleted form can be associated with underlying HIV-infection. The infiltrate is diffuse, without band-forming sclerosis, although fine interstitial fibrosis may be present (Fig. 79.4). HRS cells are of the classic type.

Classic Hodgkin lymphoma, lymphocyte depletion

Classic Hodgkin lymphoma, lymphocyte depletion (HLLD) is the least common variant of CHL and is most common in older people, in HIV-positive individuals, and in nonindustrialized countries. It frequently presents with abdominal lymphadenopathy, spleen, liver, and bone marrow involvement, without peripheral adenopathy. The stage is usually advanced at diagnosis.

The infiltrate is diffuse and often appears hypocellular, owing to the presence of diffuse fibrosis and necrosis. Relative to the number of normal lymphocytes there are large numbers of HRS cells and occasional bizarre "sarcomatous" variants, with a paucity of other inflammatory cells. The immunophenotype is characteristic of CHL. Since the histologic differential diagnosis often includes B- or T-large-cell lymphoma or ALCL, immunohistochemistry should be performed in most cases. EBV is positive in the majority of cases.

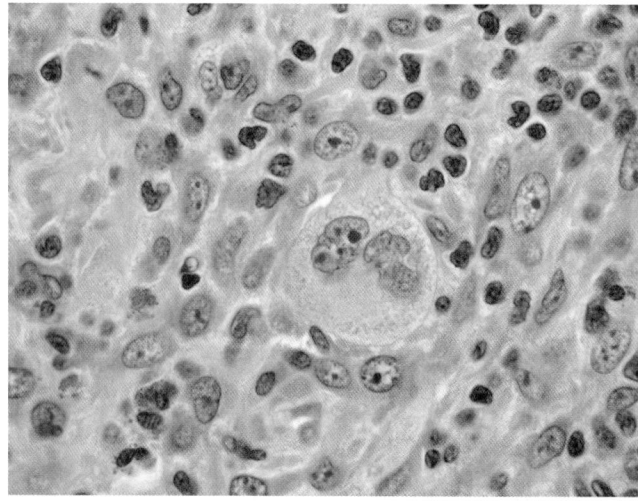

Fig. 79.4 Classic Hodgkin lymphoma, mixed cellularity subtype. A classic Reed–Sternberg cell is shown in a mixed inflammatory background with eosinophils, plasma cells, histiocytes, and small lymphocytes.

Classic Hodgkin lymphoma, lymphocyte-rich

Classic Hodgkin lymphoma, lymphocyte-rich (CHLLR) may be nodular or diffuse and contains relatively infrequent HRS cells, which are of the classic type, rather than the LP variants seen in NLPHL. There are infrequent eosinophils or plasma cells. In the nodular form the HRS cells are seen at the periphery of B-cell-rich nodules, mainly in the marginal zone. The neoplastic cells have the immunophenotype of classic HRS cells, but morphologically may be difficult to distinguish from LP cells in some cases. Thus, in the past many cases were misdiagnosed as NLPHL. The genetic features are similar to those of the other variants of CHL. Patients usually present with localized disease, and tend to be older than patients with NLPHL.

● ON THE HORIZON

- In recent years there has been a greater appreciation of early events in lymphoid neoplasia.

- These early lesions can in some ways be considered equivalent to benign neoplasms in the epithelial system.

- These are clonal proliferations of B or T cells that carry genetic aberrations associated with specific forms of lymphoid neoplasia: CLL, multiple myeloma, follicular lymphoma, mantle cell lymphoma.

- Examples include MGUS, MBL, follicular lymphoma *in situ*, and mantle cell lymphoma, lymphomatoid papulosis, patch stage of mycosis fungoides.

- Early lesions appear to lack the secondary and tertiary "hits" seen in lymphoid neoplasms that are clinically significant, and most patients have a very low risk of clinical progression.

- Challenges for the future are:
  - To define the precise genetic features that distinguish early lesions from lymphoma
  - To assess the risk of clinical progression, and
  - To determine how these patients should be managed clinically.

References

1. Staudt LM, Dave S. The biology of human lymphoid malignancies revealed by gene expression profiling. Adv Immunol 2005;87:163–208.
2. Nogai H, Dorken B, Lenz G. Pathogenesis of non-Hodgkin's lymphoma. J Clin Oncol 2011;29(14):1803–11.
3. Swerdlow SH, Campo E, Harris NL, et al. WHO classification of tumours of haematopoietic and lymphoid tissues. 4th ed. Lyon: International Agency for Research on Cancer; 2008.
4. Puente XS, Pinyol M, Quesada V, et al. Whole-genome sequencing identifies recurrent mutations in chronic lymphocytic leukaemia. Nature 2011;475:101–5.
5. Campo E, Swerdlow SH, Harris NL, et al. The 2008 WHO classification of lymphoid neoplasms and beyond: evolving concepts and practical applications. Blood 2011;117(19):5019–32.
6. Fu K, Weisenburger DD, Greiner TC, et al. Cyclin D1-negative mantle cell lymphoma: a clinicopathologic study based on gene expression profiling. Blood 2005;106(13):4315–21.
7. Ek S, Dictor M, Jerkeman M, et al. Nuclear expression of the non B-cell lineage Sox11 transcription factor identifies mantle cell lymphoma. Blood 2008;111(2):800–5.
8. Mozos A, Royo C, Hartmann E, et al. SOX11 expression is highly specific for mantle cell lymphoma and identifies the cyclin D1-negative subtype. Haematologica 2009;94(11):1555–62.
9. Perez-Galan P, Dreyling M, Wiestner A. Mantle cell lymphoma: biology, pathogenesis, and the molecular basis of treatment in the genomic era. Blood 2011;117(1):26–38.
10. Rosenwald A, Wright G, Wiestner A, et al. The proliferation gene expression signature is a quantitative integrator of oncogenic events that predicts survival in mantle cell lymphoma. Cancer Cell 2003;3(2):185–97.
11. Fernandez V, Salamero O, Espinet B, et al. Genomic and gene expression profiling defines indolent forms of mantle cell lymphoma. Cancer Res 2010;70(4):1408–18.
12. Williams ME, Connors JM, Dreyling MH, et al. Mantle cell lymphoma: report of the 2010 Mantle Cell Lymphoma Consortium Workshop. Leuk Lymphoma 2011;52(1):24–33.
13. Dave SS, Wright G, Tan B, et al. Prediction of survival in follicular lymphoma based on molecular features of tumor-infiltrating immune cells. N Engl J Med 2004;351(21):2159–69.
14. Gribben JG. Implications of the tumor microenvironment on survival and disease response in follicular lymphoma. Curr Opin Oncol 2010;22(5):424–30.
15. Oschlies I, Salaverria I, Mahn F, et al. Pediatric follicular lymphoma–a clinico-pathological study of a population-based series of patients treated within the Non-Hodgkin's Lymphoma–Berlin-Frankfurt-Munster (NHL-BFM) multicenter trials. Haematologica 2010;95(2):253–9.
16. Cong P, Raffeld M, Teruya-Feldstein J, et al. In situ localization of follicular lymphoma: description and analysis by laser capture microdissection. Blood 2002;99(9):3376–82.
17. Roulland S, Navarro JM, Grenot P, et al. Follicular lymphoma-like B cells in healthy individuals: a novel intermediate step in early lymphomagenesis. J Exp Med 2006;203(11):2425–31.
18. Farinha P, Gascoyne RD. Molecular pathogenesis of mucosa-associated lymphoid tissue lymphoma. J Clin Oncol 2005;23(26):6370–8.
19. Rinaldi A, Mian M, Chigrinova E, et al. Genome-wide DNA profiling of marginal zone lymphomas identifies subtype-specific lesions with an impact on the clinical outcome. Blood 2011;117(5):1595–604.
20. Swerdlow SH. Pediatric follicular lymphomas, marginal zone lymphomas, and marginal zone hyperplasia. Am J Clin Pathol 2004;122(Suppl.):S98–109.
21. Thieblemont C, Davi F, Noguera ME, Briere J. Non-MALT marginal zone lymphoma. Curr Opin Hematol 2011;18(4):273–9.
22. Watkins AJ, Huang Y, Ye H, et al. Splenic marginal zone lymphoma: characterization of 7q deletion and its value in diagnosis. J Pathol 2010;220(4):461–74.
23. Rosenwald A, Wright G, Chan WC, et al. The use of molecular profiling to predict survival after chemotherapy for diffuse large-B-cell lymphoma. N Engl J Med 2002;346(25):1937–47.
24. Savage KJ, Monti S, Kutok JL, et al. The molecular signature of mediastinal large B-cell lymphoma differs from that of other diffuse large B-cell lymphomas and shares features with classical Hodgkin lymphoma. Blood 2003;102(12):3871–9.
25. Rosenwald A, Wright G, Leroy K, et al. Molecular diagnosis of primary mediastinal B cell lymphoma identifies a clinically favorable subgroup of diffuse large B cell lymphoma related to Hodgkin lymphoma. J Exp Med 2003;198(6):851–62.
26. Scholtysik R, Kreuz M, Klapper W, et al. Detection of genomic aberrations in molecularly defined Burkitt's lymphoma by array-based, high resolution, single nucleotide polymorphism analysis. Haematologica 2009;95(12):2047–55.
27. Gutierrez-Garcia G, Cardesa-Salzmann T, Climent F, et al. Gene-expression profiling and not immunophenotypic algorithms predicts prognosis in patients with diffuse large-B-cell lymphoma treated with immunochemotherapy. Blood 2011;117(18):4836–43.
28. Van Loo P, Tousseyn T, Vanhentenrijk V, et al. T-cell/histiocyte-rich large B-cell lymphoma shows transcriptional features suggestive of a tolerogenic host immune response. Haematologica 2010;95(3):440–8.
29. Rubenstein JL, Shen A, Batchelor TT, et al. Differential gene expression in central nervous system lymphoma. Blood 2009;113(1):266–7 author reply 7–8.
30. Hoefnagel JJ, Dijkman R, Basso K, et al. Distinct types of primary cutaneous large B-cell lymphoma identified by gene expression profiling. Blood 2005;105(9):3671–8.
31. Asano N, Yamamoto K, Tamaru J, et al. Age-related Epstein-Barr virus (EBV)-associated B-cell lymphoproliferative disorders: comparison with EBV-positive classic Hodgkin lymphoma in elderly patients. Blood 2009;113(12):2629–36.
32. Dojcinov SD, Venkataraman G, Pittaluga S, et al. Age-related EBV-associated lymphoproliferative disorders in the Western population: a spectrum of reactive lymphoid hyperplasia and lymphoma. Blood 2011;117(18):4726–35.
33. Dojcinov SD, Venkataraman G, Raffeld M, et al. EBV positive mucocutaneous ulcer—a study of 26 cases associated with various sources of immunosuppression. Am J Surg Pathol 2010;34(3):405–17.
34. Laurent C, Do C, Gascoyne RD, et al. Anaplastic lymphoma kinase-positive diffuse large B-cell lymphoma: a rare clinicopathologic entity with poor prognosis. J Clin Oncol 2009;27(25):4211–6.
35. Copie-Bergman C, Plonquet A, Alonso MA, et al. MAL expression in lymphoid cells: further evidence for MAL as a distinct molecular marker of primary mediastinal large B-cell lymphomas. Mod Pathol 2002;15(11):1172–80.
36. Savage KJ, Al-Rajhi N, Voss N, et al. Favorable outcome of primary mediastinal large B-cell lymphoma in a single institution: the British Columbia experience. Ann Oncol 2006;17(1):123–30.
37. Traverse-Glehen A, Pittaluga S, Gaulard P, et al. Mediastinal gray zone lymphoma: the missing link between classic Hodgkin's lymphoma and mediastinal large B-cell lymphoma. Am J Surg Pathol 2005;29(11):1411–21.
38. Rodig SJ, Savage KJ, LaCasce AS, et al. Expression of TRAF1 and nuclear c-Rel distinguishes primary mediastinal large B-cell lymphoma from other types of diffuse large B-cell lymphoma. Am J Surg Pathol 2007;31(1):106–12.
39. Eberle FC, Rodriguez-Canales J, Wei L, et al. Methylation profiling of mediastinal gray zone lymphoma reveals a distinctive signature with elements shared by classical Hodgkin's lymphoma and primary mediastinal large B-cell lymphoma. Haematologica 2011;96(4):558–66.
40. Green MR, Monti S, Rodig SJ, et al. Integrative analysis reveals selective 9p24.1 amplification, increased PD-1 ligand expression, and further induction via JAK2 in nodular sclerosing Hodgkin lymphoma and primary mediastinal large B-cell lymphoma. Blood 2010;116(17):3268–77.
41. Dave SS, Fu K, Wright GW, et al. Molecular diagnosis of Burkitt's lymphoma. N Engl J Med 2006;354(23):2431–42.
42. Hummel M, Bentink S, Berger H, et al. A biologic definition of Burkitt's lymphoma from transcriptional and genomic profiling. N Engl J Med 2006;354(23):2419–30.
43. Piccaluga PP, De Falco G, Kustagi M, et al. Gene expression analysis uncovers similarity and differences among Burkitt lymphoma subtypes. Blood 2011;117(13):3596–608.
44. Salaverria I, Siebert R. The gray zone between Burkitt's lymphoma and diffuse large B-cell lymphoma from a genetics perspective. J Clin Oncol 2011;29(14):1835–43.

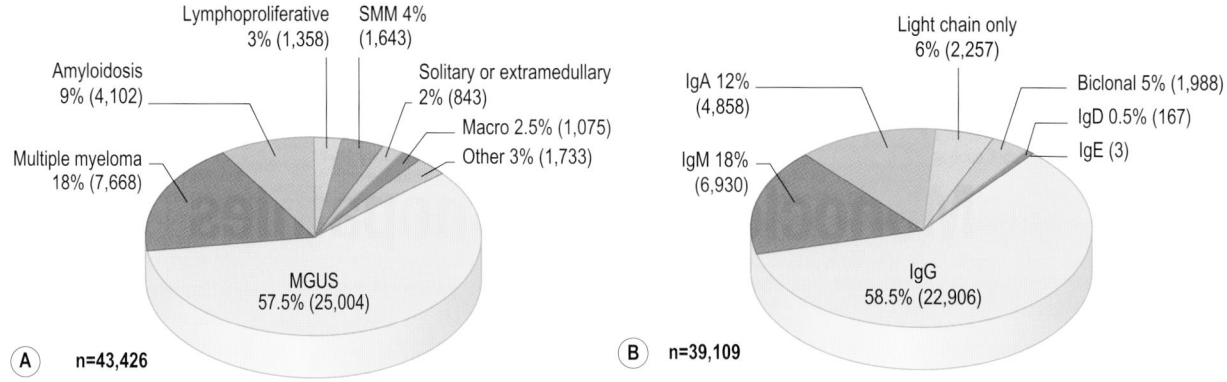

Fig. 80.1 (A) Monoclonal gammopathies Mayo Clinic 1960–2010. (B) Monoclonal serum proteins Mayo Clinic 1960–2010.

Monoclonal gammopathy of undetermined significance

MGUS is characterized by an M-protein concentration < 3 g/dL; fewer than 10% plasma cells in the bone marrow; no or only small amounts of M protein in the urine; and absence of lytic bone lesions, anemia, hypercalcemia, and renal insufficiency related to the plasma cell proliferative process. Although this disorder has been considered benign, it is known that symptomatic MM or related disorders can develop in many patients and for this reason the term MGUS is more appropriate.

MGUS has been reported in 3% of patients over 70 years and 1% of persons older than 50. In order to determine the prevalence, serum samples were obtained from 21 463 (77%) of the 28 038 enumerated residents of Olmsted County, Minnesota, who were 50 years of age or older.[4] MGUS was identified in 694 (3.2%) of these persons. Age-adjusted rates were higher in men than in women (4 vs 2.7%; p = 0.001). The prevalence of MGUS was 5.3% among persons 70 years of age or older and 7.5% among those 85 years of age or older. In both genders the prevalence increased with advancing age and was almost four times as high among persons 80 years of age or older than among those 50–59 years of age (Table 80.1). The isotype of the

monoclonal protein was IgG in 69% of the 694 with MGUS, IgM in 17%, IgA in 11%, and biclonal in 3%. The concentration of immunoglobulins was less than 1.0 g/dL in 63.5% and at least 2.0 g/dL in only 4.5% of the 694 persons; the median value was 0.5 g/dL. The level of uninvolved (normal, polyclonal) immunoglobulins was reduced in 28% of the 447 patients in whom quantitative immunoglobulins were measured. Urine from 70 persons with MGUS showed a monoclonal κ protein in 16.5% or λ in 5%.[4] The incidence of MGUS was higher in African Americans, as well as West Africans, when compared to Caucasians.[5]

Because of its frequency, it is of great importance to know whether the M protein will remain stable or will progress to MM, WM, AL, or other related disorders. At Mayo Clinic, 241 patients with an apparently benign monoclonal gammopathy have been followed for 3579 person-years (median, 13.7 years; range 0–39 years).[6] The bone marrow contained 1–10% plasma cells (median, 3%).

The actuarial risk of malignant transformation was 17% at 10 years, 34% at 20 years, and 39% at 25 years. The interval from recognition of M protein to the diagnosis of serious disease ranged from 1 to 32 years (median, 10.4 years). In 10 patients, MM was diagnosed more than 20 years after detection of the M protein. The mode of development of MM was variable, in that some patients remained stable for many years and MM developed gradually or suddenly, whereas in others there was a steady increase in the M-protein level until they became symptomatic. The median duration of survival after the diagnosis of MM was 33 months, which is not different from those who develop myeloma de novo.

In order to confirm the findings of the 241 Mayo Clinic patients from the USA and other countries, which may be subject to referral bias, a population-based study was conducted of a group of 1384 patients with MGUS from the 11 counties of southeastern Minnesota evaluated at the Mayo Clinic from 1960 to 1994.[7] The median age at diagnosis of MGUS was 72 years compared to 64 years in the 241-patient cohort. Fifty-four percent of patients were men and only 2% were < 40 years of age at diagnosis.[7] The size of the M protein at diagnosis ranged from unmeasurable to 3.0 g/dL (median 1.3 g/dL). The M protein was IgG in 70%, IgM in 15%, IgA in 12%, and biclonal in 3%. The uninvolved (normal or background) immunoglobulins were reduced in 38% of 840 patients who were evaluated. Of the 418 patients who had immunofixation of urine, 31% had a monoclonal light chain. In each case anemia or renal insufficiency, when present, was not attributable to the monoclonal plasma cell process.

The 1384 patients were followed for a total of 11 009 person-years (median, 15.4 years; range, 0–35 years), during which time 963 (70%) died. During follow-up, MM, AL, WM, chronic

Table 80.1 Prevalence of monoclonal gammopathy of undetermined significance (MGUS) according to age group and sex among residents of Olmsted County, Minnesota

| Age (years) | Number/total number (percent)[a] | | |
	Women	Men	Total
50–59	59/4335 (1.4)	82/4038 (2.0)	141/8373 (1.7)
60–69	73/3155 (2.3)	105/2864 (3.7)	178/6019 (3.0)
70–79	101/2650 (3.8)	104/1858 (5.6)	205/4508 (4.6)
≥ 80	111/1854 (6.0)	59/709 (8.3)	170/2563 (6.6)
Total	344/11994 (2.9)[b]	350/9469 (3.7)[b]	694/21463 (3.2)[b,c]

[a]The percentage was calculated as the number of patients with MGUS divided by the number who were tested.
[b]Prevalence was age-adjusted to the 2000 US population as follows: men, 4.0% (95% CI, 3.5–4.4); women, 2.7% (95% CI, 2.4–3.0), and total, 3.2% (95% CI, 3.0–3.5).
[c]Prevalence was age- and sex-adjusted to the 2000 US total population.
From Kyle RA, Therneau TM, Rajkumar SV, et al. Prevalence of monoclonal gammopathy of undetermined significance. N Engl J Med 2006; 354: 1362–1369, with permission from the Massachusetts Medical Society.

Table 80.2 Risk of progression among 1384 residents of southeastern Minnesota in whom monoclonal gammopathy of undetermined significance was diagnosed in 1960 through 2010[a]

Type of progression	No. of patients		Relative risk (95% CI)
	Observed	Expected	
Multiple myeloma	75	3.0	25.0 (20–32)
Lymphoma	19[b]	7.8	2.4 (2–4)
Primary amyloidosis	10	1.2	8.4 (4–16)
Macroglobulinemia	7	0.2	46.0 (19–95)
Chronic lymphocytic leukemia	3[c]	3.5	0.9 (0.2–3)
Plasmacytoma	1	0.1	8.5 (0.2–47)
Total	115	15.8	7.3 (6–9)

CI, confidence interval.
[a]Expected numbers of cases were derived from the age- and sex-matched white population of the Surveillance, Epidemiology, and End Results program in Iowa,[7] except for primary amyloidosis, for which data are from Kyle et al.[8]
[b]All 19 patients had serum immunoglobulin M (IgM) monoclonal protein. If the 30 patients with IgM, IgA, or IgG monoclonal protein and lymphoma were included, the relative risk would be 3–9 (95% confidence interval, 2.6–5.5).
[c]All 3 patients had serum IgM monoclonal protein. If all 6 patients with IgM, IgA, or IgG monoclonal protein and chronic lymphocytic leukemia were included, the relative risk would be 1.7 (95% confidence interval, 0.6–3.7).
From Kyle RA, Therneau TM, Rajkumar SV, et al. A long-term study of prognosis in monoclonal gammopathy of undetermined significance [see comment]. N Engl J Med 2002; 346: 564–569, with permission from the Massachusetts Medical Society.

lymphocytic leukemia, or plasmacytoma developed in 115 patients (8%) (Table 80.2). The cumulative probability of progression to one of these disorders was 10% at 10 years, 21% at 20 years, and 26% at 25 years (Fig. 80.2). The overall risk of progression was about 1% per year, but it must be emphasized that patients were at risk for progression even after 25 years or more of stable MGUS. In addition, there were 32 patients in whom the monoclonal protein value increased to more than 3 g/dL or the percentage of plasma cells increased to more than 10% but in whom symptomatic MM did not develop. At 20 years, the risk of death for patients with MGUS was 10% from plasma cell disorders and 72% from non-plasma cell disorders.

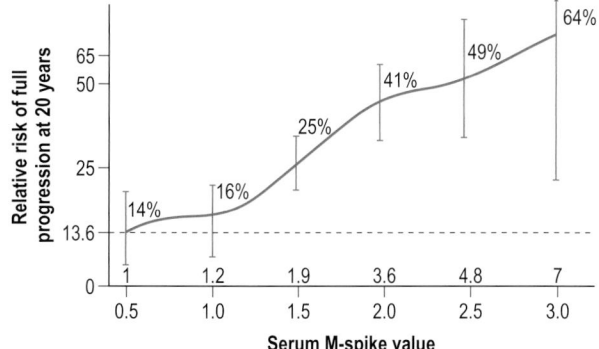

Fig. 80.2 Actuarial risk of full progression by serum monoclonal protein (M protein) value at diagnosis of monoclonal gammopathy of undetermined significance (MGUS) in persons from southeastern Minnesota.
From Kyle et al. Immunological Reviews, 2003; 194: 112–139, with permission of Blackwell Publishing.

The number of patients with progression to a plasma cell neoplasm or a related disorder (115 patients) was more than seven times expected on the basis of incidence rates for those conditions in the general population (Table 80.2). The risk of developing MM, WM, or AL was increased 25-, 46-, and 8.4-fold respectively.

MM was diagnosed more than 10 years after the detection of the monoclonal protein in 24 (32%) of the 75 patients, and after 20 years of follow-up in 5 (7%) patients. Characteristics of these 75 patients were comparable with those of the 1027 patients with newly diagnosed MM who were referred to the Mayo Clinic from 1985 to 1998, except that the southeastern Minnesota MGUS population was older (median 72 vs 66 years) and had a smaller percentage of men (46 vs 60%).[8]

Similar findings have been reported in other series: the actuarial risk was 8.5 and 19.2% at 5 and 10 years, respectively, in one series of 128 patients with MGUS. In a report of 335 patients with MGUS, the frequency of progression after a median follow-up of 70 months was 6.8%.

● CLINICAL PEARLS

Monoclonal gammopathies

- Monoclonal gammopathy of undetermined significance (MGUS) (benign monoclonal gammopathy) accounts for nearly 60% of all patients with a monoclonal gammopathy.
- MGUS occurred in 3.2% of persons older than 50 years and in 5.3% of those older than 70 years in a population-based study of 21 463 residents of Olmsted County, Minnesota.
- The risk of MGUS developing multiple myeloma, primary systemic amyloidosis, macroglobulinemia, or related disorders is 1% per year during long-term follow-up.

Progression of MGUS

The sequence of events responsible for progression of MGUS to myeloma or a related disorder is poorly understood.[9] Almost one-half of patients with MGUS have immunoglobulin heavy-chain translocations consisting of t(11;14), t(4;14), or t(14;16). These translocations lead to dysregulation of putative oncogenes. Deletions of chromosome 13 have also been found in MGUS.

Risk factors for progression consist of the level of the M protein at diagnosis, type of M protein, presence of abnormal serum FLC ratio, and bone marrow plasma cell involvement. In a series of 1384 patients with MGUS from southeastern Minnesota, the level of the M protein at diagnosis was the most important predictor of progression. The risk of progression to MM or a related disorder 20 years after the diagnosis of MGUS was 14% for patients with an initial M protein value of 0.5 g/dL and 49% for those presenting with an M spike of 2.5 g/dL. The risk of progression of a serum M protein of 1.5 g/dL was almost twice the risk of progression with a value of 0.5 g/dL and the risk of progression with 2.5 g/dL was 4.6 times that of a value of 0.5 g/dL. Patients with IgM or IgA protein had an increased risk of progression compared with those with IgG monoclonal protein ($p = 0.001$).

An abnormal FLC ratio was detected in 379 (33%) of 1148 patients from the 1384 patients with MGUS in this study and the risk of progression with an abnormal FLC ratio was significantly higher than that in patients with a normal ratio (hazard ratio 3.5; $p < 0.001$) and was independent of the level and type of serum M protein. From this a new stratification model for determining the risk of progression of MGUS was developed.[10] The number of plasma cells in the bone marrow may also help predict progression.[11]

In our experience, age; gender; levels of hemoglobin, serum creatinine, and serum albumin; presence, type, and amount of monoclonal urinary light chain; and reduction of uninvolved immunoglobulins have not helped to determine the risk of progression.

Management of MGUS

Despite the results of sophisticated laboratory tests, MM is differentiated from MGUS on the basis of clinical factors such as symptoms, anemia, hypercalcemia, renal insufficiency, and lytic bone lesions. The serum and urine M proteins must be measured periodically and a clinical evaluation conducted to determine whether MM, AL, WM, or a lymphoproliferative disorder has developed.

If a patient has no features of MM or AL, the serum protein value (IgG type) is less than 1.5 g/dL and FLC ratio is normal, the serum protein electrophoresis should be repeated in 6–12 months and, if the results are stable, every 2 years.

If the patient has an M-protein value of >1.5 g/dL, a 24-hour urine specimen should be collected for electrophoresis and immunofixation. A metastatic bone survey and bone marrow aspiration and biopsy should also be done. Determination of the plasma cell labeling index (PCLI), search for circulating plasma cells in the blood, and cytogenetic studies should be performed if possible. Levels of β₂-microglobulin and C-reactive protein should also be determined. Serum protein electrophoresis should be performed in 3–6 months and if stable it should be repeated in 6 months and then annually or sooner if symptoms develop. Patients should be instructed to contact their physician if there is any change in clinical condition.

Association of monoclonal gammopathies with other diseases

Although MGUS frequently exists without any other abnormalities, certain diseases are associated with it, as would be expected in an older population. There may be an apparent association because of differences in the referral practices or in other selected patient groups. Appropriate control populations are essential for determining whether the association is merely a coincidence. We studied the association of MGUS in a population-based cohort from Olmsted County, Minnesota.[12]

M proteins have been noted in lymphoproliferative disorders, leukemia, other hematologic diseases, connective tissue disorders, and neurologic conditions such as peripheral neuropathy. Dermatologic diseases, including lichen myxedematosus, pyoderma gangrenosum, necrobiotic xanthogranuloma, and plane xanthomatosis, have been associated with an M protein. M proteins have also been found after renal, bone marrow, or liver transplantation as a result of immunosuppressive therapy. More detailed reviews of the association of monoclonal gammopathy with nonplasma cell disorders have been published.[9]

Variants of MGUS

IgM MGUS

IgM MGUS comprises 15–20% of all patients with MGUS. IgM MGUS was diagnosed in 213 Mayo Clinic patients in the southeastern Minnesota study.[13] Non-Hodgkin's lymphoma (*n*=17), WM (*n*=6), chronic lymphocytic leukemia (*n*=3), or AL (*n*=3) developed in 29 (14%) for relative risks of 15, 262, 6, and 16, respectively. The risk of progression was 14%, 26%, 34%, and 41% for MGUS concentrations of 0.5, 1.5, 2.0, and 2.5 g/dL, respectively. Progression occurred at a rate of approximately 1.5%/year.

Light-chain MGUS

Light-chain MGUS is defined as an abnormal FLC ratio with no heavy-chain expression plus increased concentration of the involved light chain. The prevalence is 0.8% and is the precursor of light-chain MM. Risk of progression is 0.3% per 100-person years.[14]

Biclonal gammopathies

Biclonal gammopathies occur in approximately 4–6% of patients with monoclonal gammopathies and have similar clinical features. Two-thirds of cases of biclonal gammopathy are of undetermined significance.[15] The remainder have MM, AL, WM, or other lymphoproliferative disorders. More than 25 cases of triclonal gammopathy have been reported.

Idiopathic Bence Jones proteinuria

In most patients, the presence of Bence Jones proteinuria indicates MM, AL, WM, or other lymphoproliferative disorders. However, it may follow a benign course for many years. Patients with "idiopathic" Bence Jones proteinuria must be observed indefinitely, because MM or AL will eventually develop in most of those with >1 g of Bence Jones proteinuria/24 hours.[15]

Multiple myeloma

MM (myelomatosis, Kahler's disease) is characterized by the neoplastic proliferation of a single clone of plasma cells producing an M protein. This proliferation often results in skeletal destruction, with osteolytic lesions or pathologic fractures producing pain, hypercalcemia, and anemia. An excess of M protein can contribute to renal failure, the hyperviscosity syndrome, or recurrent bacterial infections.

Epidemiology

The annual incidence of MM is 4.3 per 100 000.[16] The apparent increased incidence during the past few decades is probably related more to the increased availability and use of medical facilities in the elderly and to improved diagnostic techniques rather than an actual increased incidence. MM represents 1% of all malignant disease and slightly more than 10% of hematologic malignancies. Its incidence in African Americans is twice that in Caucasians, and it is slightly more frequent in men than in women. MM occurs in all races and all geographic regions, but rates are lower in Asian populations. Only 10% of patients are younger than 50 years and 2% are younger than 40 years; the median age is 66 years.[8]

Biologic aspects

Plasma cells are cytoplasm Ig⁺ (cIg⁺) and express surface CD38. A small subset of myeloma cells express CD10 and 15–20% express CD20. CD56 (N-CAM) is expressed on the majority of malignant plasma cells, but CD34 is not. The clonogenic cell in MM has not been demonstrated with certainty. There is evidence that plasma cell precursors of myeloma circulate in the peripheral blood. The current hypothesis is that, by means of adhesion molecules, circulating clonogenic myeloma cells home to the bone marrow, where they find an appropriate microenvironment to differentiate and expand further.

Approximately 50% of patients have translocations that involve the immunoglobulin heavy-chain locus on chromosome 14q32 and one of five partner chromosomes.

Conventional cytogenetic studies show abnormal karyotypes in 30–40% of patients. Deletion of chromosome 13 or hypodiploidy are the most important abnormalities. Patients with 17p deletion, $t(4;14)$, $t(14;16)$, and $t(14;20)$ are considered to have high-risk disease.

Clinical manifestations

Bone pain, usually in the back or chest, is present at the time of diagnosis in about 60% of patients and is usually aggravated by movement.[8] Weakness and fatigue are common and usually associated with anemia. The major symptoms may result from an acute infection, renal failure, hypercalcemia, or amyloidosis. Pallor is the most frequent physical finding.

Renal involvement

The serum creatinine level is 2 mg/dL or more in one-fifth of MM patients at diagnosis. Two major causes of renal failure are "myeloma kidney" and hypercalcemia. Myeloma kidney is characterized by the presence of large, dense, waxy, laminated casts in the distal and collecting tubules. Hypercalcemia, which is present in 15% of patients initially, is a major and treatable cause of renal insufficiency. Dehydration, infections, or nonsteroidal antiinflammatory agents may all contribute to renal failure.

Skeletal involvement

Almost 80% of MM patients have lytic lesions, osteoporosis, or fractures with conventional radiographs at diagnosis. Magnetic resonance imaging (MRI) or computed tomography (CT) is most helpful in the detection of extramedullary plasmacytomas compressing the spinal cord in patients with severe back pain but no abnormalities on routine radiographs.

Neurologic involvement

Radiculopathy from nerve compression by an extradural plasmacytoma or by the collapsed bone itself is the most frequent neurologic complication of MM. Compression of the spinal cord occurs in about 5% of patients and must be recognized and treated without delay. Peripheral neuropathy is rare, and when present is usually due to amyloidosis. Leptomeningeal myelomatosis is uncommon but is being recognized more frequently while intracranial plasmacytomas are rare.

Other systemic involvement

The incidence of infections is increased in MM with impairment of antibody responses, reduction of normal immunoglobulin levels, neutropenia, and treatment with glucocorticoids all contributing to increased susceptibility to infection. Hepatomegaly from plasma cell infiltration is rare. Plasmacytomas of the ribs are often present. Diffuse pulmonary involvement and pleural effusion from plasma cell infiltration are rare and usually occur late in the course of the disease.

Laboratory findings

In a series of 1027 myeloma patients, approximately three-fourths had a normocytic, normochromic anemia at diagnosis (Table 80.3).[8] Hypercalcemia (> 11 mg/dL) occurred in 13% and 19% had an increase in the serum creatinine to ≥ 2.0 mg/dL. The serum protein electrophoretic pattern showed a spike

Table 80.3 Laboratory tests in 1027 patients with multiple myeloma

	n	Median	Range	Distribution of results	% of patients
Hemoglobin (g/dL)	1025	10.9	2.7–17.2	≤ 8 8.1–10.0 10.1–12 > 12	7 28 37 28
Creatinine (mg/dL)	1020	1.2	0.5–18.2	< 1.3 1.3–1.9 ≥ 2	52 29 19
Calcium (mg/dL)	1018	9.6	7.0–17.2	≤ 10.1 10.2–10.9 ≥ 11	72 15 13
Cholesterol (mg/dL)	364	173	52–433	≤ 100 > 250	10 9
Triglyceride (mg/dL)	332	124	25–640	≤ 100 > 250	33 12
β_2-microglobulin	735	3.9	0.8–82	≤ 2.7 2.8–4.0 4.1–6.0 > 6	25 28 21 26
C-reactive protein	285	0.4	0.01–49	< 0.8 > 5.0	66 10

From Kyle RA, Gertz MA, Witzig TE, et al. Review of 1027 patients with newly diagnosed multiple myeloma [see comment]. Mayo Clin Proc 2003; 78: 21–33, with permission from the Mayo Clinic.

or localized band in over 80% of patients at diagnosis. An M protein is found in the serum in 93% of patients, of which about half had an IgG monoclonal protein and approximately a fifth had IgA, and more than 15% had a free monoclonal light chain (Bence Jones proteinemia). Immunofixation of the urine revealed an M protein in 78% of patients. An M protein is found in the serum or urine in 97% of patients with MM at the time of diagnosis and the relative frequency of $\kappa{:}\lambda$ is 2:1. Plasma cells usually constitute more than 10% of all nucleated cells in the MM bone marrow, but the number may range from less than 5 to almost 100%.

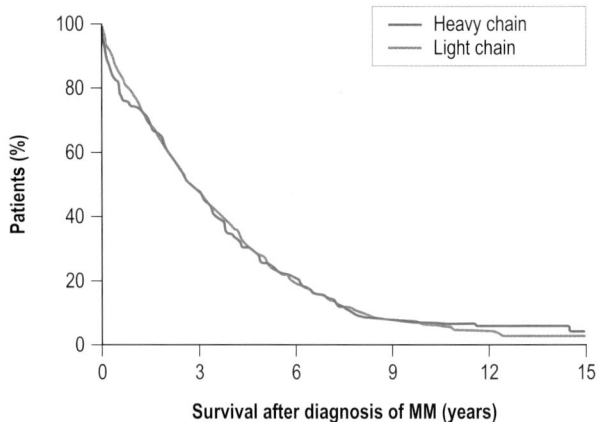

Fig. 80.3 Duration of survival in patients with light-chain myeloma and those with heavy-chain myeloma after diagnosis of multiple myeloma (MM). From Kyle et al. Review of 1027 patients with newly diagnosed multiple myeloma. Mayo Clinic Proceedings, 2003; 78: 21–33, with permission from the Mayo Clinic.

> ### CLINICAL PEARLS
>
> **Multiple myeloma**
>
> - At the time of diagnosis 97% of patients have a monoclonal protein in the serum or urine.
> - The most important prognostic factors are cytogenetic changes, plasma cell labeling index, and β_2-microglobulin level.

Differential diagnosis

The diagnosis of MM depends on the presence of an increased number of plasma cells in the bone marrow (usually > 10%), and an M protein in the serum (often > 3 g/dL), or a monoclonal light chain in the urine and end-organ damage (CRAB – hypercalcemia, renal insufficiency, anemia or bone lesions).[17] Clinical features of MM must also be present. Metastatic carcinoma, connective tissue disorders, and lymphoma must be considered in the differential diagnosis.

The concentration of the serum M protein, the amount of urine M protein, the number of bone marrow plasma cells, the hemoglobin, calcium, and creatinine levels and presence of lytic lesions are all helpful in differentiating MGUS and SMM from MM. The level of uninvolved serum immunoglobulins is not helpful because in one-third of the patients with MGUS they are reduced. The PCLI, which measures the synthesis of DNA, is helpful in differentiating MGUS or SMM from MM. Monoclonal plasma cells can be detected in the peripheral blood of 80% of patients with active MM. In contrast, patients with MGUS or SMM have few or no circulating plasma cells.

Differentiation of AL and MM is arbitrary because both diseases are plasma cell-proliferative disorders with different manifestations. In AL, the proportion of bone marrow plasma cells is usually less than 20%, there are no osteolytic lesions, and the amount of Bence Jones proteinuria is modest.

No single test reliably differentiates a patient with MGUS from one in whom MM or other malignant disease will subsequently develop. The most reliable means of differentiation is serial measurement of the M-protein value in the serum and urine and periodic evaluation of the pertinent clinical and laboratory features.

Prognostic factors

The median duration of survival in MM is approximately 5 years, but there is a great deal of variability between patients. There is no difference in survival of light- or heavy-chain (IgG or IgA) myeloma (Fig. 80.3).

The Durie–Salmon clinical staging system is based on a combination of factors that correlate with the myeloma cell mass. However, the unreliability of this system and its many shortcomings led to the search for other prognostic factors. The International Staging System, a collaborative effort by investigators from 17 institutions worldwide and data on 11 171 patients divides patients into three stages on the basis of β_2-microglobulin and albumin levels at diagnosis.[18]

Treatment

Most patients with MM have symptomatic disease at diagnosis and require chemotherapy. However, not all patients who fulfill the minimal criteria for the diagnosis of MM should be treated, and patients with SMM or MGUS should be observed until progression occurs. An increasing level of the M protein in the serum or urine, development of anemia, hypercalcemia, renal insufficiency, or the occurrence of lytic bone lesions or extramedullary plasmacytomas are all indications for therapy. If there is doubt about whether to begin the therapy, the most reasonable approach is to re-evaluate the patient in 2-3 months and delay treatment until progressive disease is evident. There is no evidence that early treatment of MM is advantageous.

Patients with symptomatic MM may be classified into high-risk or standard-risk disease.[19] We utilize a risk stratification system termed mSMART (Mayo Stratification of Myeloma and Risk Adapted Therapy), which is based upon fluorescence *in situ* hybridation (FISH), metaphase cytogenetics and the plasma cell labeling index (PCLI). High-risk disease accounts for 15–20% of MM patients and is characterized by deletion 17p, t(4;14) or t(14;16) by FISH, deletion of chromosome 13 or hypodiploidy by metaphase cytogenetics or a PCLI ≥ 3%. Patients who have none of the high-risk features are classified as standard-risk MM. Most standard-risk MM patients have hyperdiploidy (which is found in 50 to 60% of all myeloma patients), t(11;14) or t(6;14) by FISH studies. In addition to the risk factors listed above, lactate dehydrogenase and β_2-microglobulin levels are additional risk factors.

Clinical trials are strongly recommended, but if the patient is not eligible or if clinical trials are not available, one may separate the patients into those who are autologous stem-cell transplantation (ASCT) eligible or ineligible. Criteria for diagnosis, staging, risk stratification, response assessment and therapy of MM have been described in detail.[20,21]

Treatment of multiple myeloma

- Consider an autologous peripheral blood stem-cell transplant in newly diagnosed patients.
- Autologous peripheral blood stem-cell transplantation is not curative.
- Combinations of alkylating agents produce a higher response rate without improved survival compared to melphalan and prednisone.
- Allogeneic bone marrow transplant has a significant early mortality and is not recommended.
- Novel agents for multiple myeloma include thalidomide, bortezomib, and lenalidomide.

Initial therapy for transplant eligible patients

Eligibility for ASCT varies from country to country. In general, ASCT is offered to patients < 65 years of age, while in the United States decisions are made depending upon "physiologic age." Patients older than 70 years, serum creatinine > 2.5 mg/dL, ECOG performance status grade 3 or 4 or New York Heart Association functional status Class III or IV are generally ineligible for ASCT. Patients with renal failure may undergo ASCT but the morbidity and mortality is higher.

Those considered eligible for ASCT receive four cycles of induction therapy consisting of lenalidomide and weekly dexamethasone or bortezomib and dexamethasone.[22] Alkylating agents must be avoided prior to stem cell collection because they may damage stem cells. Melphalan (Alkeran) 200 mg/m[2] is the most widely used preparative regimen for ASCT. In two studies from France and the UK, ASCT was superior to combination conventional chemotherapy. Progression-free survival was longer, and the median overall survival was increased by approximately 1 year in the transplant group. Tandem (double) ASCT patients receive a second planned ASCT after recovery from the first transplant. The benefit of a second ASCT is limited to patients in whom complete response or very good partial response (> 90% reduction in M-protein level) was not achieved with the first procedure.[23]

Maintenance therapy

Maintenance therapy with interferon-α_2 is of limited value and is seldom used. Although progression-free survival (PFS) is prolonged with lenalidomide maintenance there is no evidence that overall survival (OS) is prolonged in a meaningful fashion. Adverse side effects, quality of life and cost must also be considered.[24]

Allogeneic bone marrow transplantation

Bone marrow transplantation from an identical-twin donor (syngeneic) is the treatment of choice if a donor is available.

Allogeneic bone marrow transplantation is advantageous because the graft contains no tumor cells and there may be a significant graft-versus-tumor effect. However, there is a mortality rate of at least 25%. Thus, conventional allogeneic transplantation cannot be recommended. Nonmyeloablative allogeneic transplantation (reduced intensity or mini-allogeneic) stem cell transplantation regimens have been used. In a recent study of 710 patients with MM randomized to a tandem autologous stem cell transplant or to an ASCT followed by an HLA matched sibling non-myeloablative allogeneic transplant revealed a 3-year PFS of 46% for the auto-auto regimen and 43% for the auto-allo groups.[25]

Patients not eligible for ASCT

There are many options for MM patients ineligible for ASCT. These include melphalan, prednisone, and thalidomide (MPT)[26,27] bortezomib, melphalan, and prednisone (VMP);[28] and lenalidomide[22] plus low-dose dexamethasone as the most commonly used regimens.

Is progress being made?

The median survival of MM was < 1 year prior to the introduction of melphalan more than a half century ago. Autologous stem cell transplantation was introduced in the 1980s and the novel agents, thalidomide, bortezomib, and lenalidomide have become available in the last decade.

In a series of 2981 MM patients from the Mayo Clinic the median survival was 29.9 months for those seen between 1971 and 1996, but increased to 44.8 months in those diagnosed after 1996. Median survival following relapse after an ASCT was 14.8 months in 226 patients who did not receive thalidomide, bortezomib, or lenalidomide, compared to a median survival of 30.9 months for those who did receive one of the novel agents.[29]

Treatment of complications of multiple myeloma

Local therapy

Radiation is reserved for spinal cord compression or solitary plasmacytoma. Rarely, palliative radiation in a dosage of 20–30 Gy may be given to patients with disabling pain who have a well-defined focal process that has not responded to chemotherapy.

Hypercalcemia

Hypercalcemia (> 11 mg/dL) is present in about 15% of patients at diagnosis. It should be suspected in the presence of anorexia, nausea, vomiting, polyuria, polydipsia, constipation, confusion, or stupor. Hypercalcemia also contributes to the development of renal insufficiency. Hydration and prednisone, 25 mg q.i.d., are effective in many cases. If not, a bisphosphonate such as zoledronic acid should be given. Patients with MM should be encouraged to be as active as possible because prolonged bedrest contributes to osteopenia and hypercalcemia.

Skeletal lesions

Complications related to lytic skeletal lesions are common in MM. Patients should be encouraged to be as active as possible but to avoid trauma. Fixation of fractures or impending fractures of long bones with an intramedullary rod and methyl methacrylate has produced good results.

In a prospective placebo-controlled study, pamidronate showed a significant reduction in skeletal events (pathologic fractures, need for radiation or surgery to treat or prevent pathologic fractures, or spinal cord compression associated with compression fractures).[30]

Intravenous bisphosphonates should be given to all patients who have lytic lesions, including pathologic fractures, or severe osteopenia. A recent randomized trial demonstrated that treatment with zoledronic acid in patients with newly diagnosed multiple myeloma was useful for prevention of skeletal-related events and also for potential antimyeloma benefits.[31] Zoledronic acid (Zometa) 4 mg intravenously over 15–30 minutes every 4 weeks and pamidronate (Aredia)

90 mg intravenously over 2–3 hours every 4 weeks are equally efficacious. Pamidronate should be reduced in patients with renal insufficiency while zoledronic acid is best avoided in those with severe renal insufficiency. Because renal insufficiency or nephrotic-range proteinuria can occur, serum creatinine and 24-hour urine protein monitoring are necessary. One may consider stopping bisphosphonates after 1 to 2 years if the patient has responded to therapy. They must be reinstituted in the event of relapsed MM with progressive skeletal involvement. It is advisable to have a comprehensive dental examination and appropriate preventive dentistry before bisphosphonate therapy is started because osteonecrosis of the jaw is a potential complication. Patients should practice oral hygiene and avoid invasive dental procedures while on bisphosphonate therapy.

Both vertebroplasty (injection of methyl methacrylate into a collapsed vertebral body) and kyphoplasty (introduction of an inflatable balloon tamp into the vertebral body and, after inflation, the injection of methyl methacrylate into the cavity) have been used successfully to decrease pain and help restore height.

Renal insufficiency

Cast nephropathy from excessive production of monoclonal light chains and hypercalcemia are the two major causes of renal failure. Dehydration may also precipitate acute renal failure. Bortezomib and dexamethasone is the favored therapeutic regimen. Plasmapheresis is a consideration for patients with acute renal failure. Renal transplantation for myeloma kidney may also be useful. Maintenance of a high (3 L/day) urine output is important for preventing renal failure in patients with Bence Jones proteinuria.

Anemia

Anemia occurs in almost all patients during the course of MM. Iron, folate or vitamin B_{12} deficiencies must be treated if present. Erythropoietin often increases the haemoglobin level. It should not be given unless the haemoglobin is <10 g/dL and should be discontinued when the haemoglobin reaches 11 g/dL. Guidelines for the use of erythropoietin have been published.[32] Blood transfusions are indicated for severe anemia.

Infections

Prompt and appropriate therapy for bacterial infection is essential. Pneumococcal and influenza vaccines should be given to all patients despite their suboptimal antibody response. Intravenous immunoglobulin may be helpful for patients with recurrent infections but is very expensive. Herpes zoster is common and requires antiviral therapy to prevent dissemination. Guidelines for the management of infections have been published.[33]

Spinal cord compression

Spinal cord compression should be suspected in patients with back pain, weakness, or paresthesias of the lower extremities, or bowel dysfunction. MRI or CT must be done immediately. Radiation therapy and dexamethasone are usually helpful and surgical compression is rarely necessary.

Thromboembolic risks

Patients receiving single-agent thalidomide or lenalidomide do not require anticoagulation unless they are at increased risk because of a prior thromboembolic event, obesity or bedrest.

If low-dose dexamethasone or prednisone is given with thalidomide or lenalidomide, aspirin in a dose of 325 mg daily is advised. If thalidomide or lenalidomide is given with high-dose dexamethasone, doxorubicin, liposomal doxorubicin or erythropoietin, full-dose warfarin or low-molecular-weight heparin should be given. Bortezomib does not produce greater risk of thromboembolic events.

Variants of multiple myeloma

Smoldering multiple myeloma

SMM is characterized by the presence of an M protein >3 g/dL and/or more than 10% plasma cells in the bone marrow but no evidence of anemia, hypercalcemia, skeletal lesions, or renal insufficiency. SMM accounts for 10–15% of all cases with newly diagnosed MM. The risk of progression to MM is approximately 10% per year for the first 5 years, 3% per year for the next 5 years and then 1 to 2% annually for the next 10 years[34] compared to 1% per year for MGUS. Treatment should not be given unless symptomatic MM develops.

Plasma cell leukemia

Plasma cell leukemia is defined as the presence of more than 20% plasma cells in the peripheral blood or an absolute plasma cell count $> 2 \times 10^9$/L. When it presents de novo (60% of cases) it is classified as primary, and when it presents as a leukemic transformation of a previously recognized MM it is secondary (40%). Patients with primary plasma cell leukemia are younger and have a greater incidence of hepatosplenomegaly and lymphadenopathy, fewer bone lesions, a lower serum M component and a longer survival than patients with secondary plasma cell leukemia.[35] Cytogenetic abnormalities are more common than in patients with MM. Poor survival was predicted by *MYC* translocation.[36] ASCT after response to high-dose chemotherapy has been beneficial for some patients. Those with secondary plasma cell leukemia rarely respond to chemotherapy because they have already received treatment for MM and are refractory.

Nonsecretory myeloma

Patients with nonsecretory myeloma have no M component in either the serum or the urine and account for only 3% of patients with MM. The FLC assay is abnormal in more than 60% of patients and is useful for monitoring response to therapy. The diagnosis is established by identification of an M protein in the plasma cells by immunofluorescence or immunoperoxidase. The behavior of nonsecretory myeloma is similar to MM, except there is less renal insufficiency.

Solitary plasmacytoma of bone

The diagnosis of solitary plasmacytoma of bone is based on the presence of a skeletal plasma cell tumor without evidence of MM. The incidence of solitary plasmacytoma of bone is 0.15/100 000 compared to 5.35/100 000 for MM in the SEER Program from 1992 to 2004.[37] The hemoglobin, calcium, and creatinine values are normal, there are no other bone lesions, and the bone marrow contains no increase in monoclonal plasma cells. Small amounts of M protein can be present in the serum or urine, but they usually disappear after tumoricidal radiation (40–50 Gy). MRI is useful because of the high incidence of MM if additional lesions are seen, in contrast to patients with no additional lesions on MRI.[38] Overt MM develops in approximately 55% of patients during long-term follow-up. New bone lesions or local recurrences develop in about 10%. There is no convincing evidence that chemotherapy affects the incidence of conversion to MM. Progression, when it occurs, is usually evident within 3–4 years.

Extramedullary plasmacytoma

The diagnosis is based on the finding of a plasma cell tumor in an extramedullary location and the absence of MM on bone marrow examination, radiography, and appropriate studies of serum and urine. The incidence of extramedullary plasmacytoma is 0.10/100 000 person years.[37] Approximately 80% of cases involve the upper respiratory tract, producing epistaxis, nasal discharge, or nasal obstruction.[39]

Treatment consists of tumoricidal radiation.[40] Adjuvant chemotherapy does not appear to lower the relapse rate or increase disease-free survival. Local recurrence is approximately 5% or less if tumoricidal radiation is given. A review of 400 publications between 1905 and 1997 found 800 cases. Patients who had combined surgery and radiation had better results than those who had only surgery or only radiation. There was local recurrence in 22% of patients whereas MM developed in 15%.[39] In a recent series of 68 patients, local recurrence was noted in 19% and MM developed in 23%.[41]

POEMS syndrome (osteosclerotic myeloma)

The major clinical findings in POEMS syndrome are characterized by polyneuropathy, organomegaly, endocrinopathy, M protein, and skin changes (POEMS).[42] Castleman's disease can also be present. The major clinical findings are chronic inflammatory demyelinating polyneuropathy with predominantly motor disability and sclerotic skeletal lesions. Papilledema, hepatosplenomegaly, and lymphadenopathy may be present. Skin hyperpigmentation and hypertrichosis can be prominent. Gynecomastia, testicular atrophy, and clubbing of the fingers and toes can occur. Pulmonary hypertension has been recognized in several instances. Ascites, pleural effusion, and peripheral edema are uncommon. The hemoglobin level is usually normal or elevated and thrombocytosis is common. Hypercalcemia and renal insufficiency rarely occur, and the bone marrow usually contains less than 5% plasma cells. Most patients have a λ protein, and IgA is common. The diagnosis is confirmed by the presence of monoclonal plasma cells in an osteosclerotic lesion. Radiation to the localized osteosclerotic lesion usually produces improvement of the neuropathy, but if the lesions are widespread, ASCT should be seriously considered.[43] About one-half of patients develop the engraftment syndrome following ASCT.[44]

Waldenström's macroglobulinemia

WM is a consequence of a malignant proliferation of plasma cells and B cells producing a monoclonal IgM protein. In a study from the USA, the incidence of WM was 0.3/100 000 in white men and 0.17/100 000 in white women, with approximately 1400 new cases occurring each year. The median age at diagnosis is 63 years; fewer than 1% of our patients are younger than 40 years and approximately 60% are males.

Clinical manifestations

The onset of WM is usually insidious and characterized by weakness and fatigue. There can be oozing from the oronasal area or blurring of vision. Weight loss, fever, and night sweats resembling lymphoma can occur. Peripheral neuropathy, pulmonary infiltration with cough, and dyspnea or skin lesions are uncommon. Dyspnea and congestive heart failure can be an initial finding. In contrast to MM, renal failure, osteolytic lesions, and AL are rare.

Pallor is a frequent finding on physical examination. Hepatomegaly, splenomegaly, or lymphadenopathy occurs in about a third of patients. Hyperviscosity is often present in WM and can produce oronasal bleeding, blurred vision, headache, vertigo, dizziness, sudden deafness, diplopia, or ataxia. Confusion, dementia, and disturbances of consciousness can occur. Clinical manifestations are rarely due to hyperviscosity if the serum viscosity is less than 4 centipoises (normal ≤1.8). The correlation between the serum viscosity and clinical manifestations is not precise. Clinical symptoms and retinal lesions, including hemorrhages, exudates, and venous congestion, are more important in making a therapeutic decision.

Laboratory findings

A normocytic, normochromic anemia occurs in almost all cases during the course of the disease. The hemoglobin and hematocrit values are often spuriously reduced because of the increased plasma volume. The serum cholesterol value is often low. Serum protein electrophoresis reveals a sharp narrow spike or dense localized band consisting of monoclonal IgM. A bone marrow aspirate is often hypocellular, but the biopsy specimen is hypercellular and extensively infiltrated by lymphocytes, plasma cells, lymphoplasmacytoid cells and mast cells. In contrast to MM, lytic lesions and fractures are rarely found.

Differential diagnosis

Diagnosis depends on the presence of typical symptoms, physical findings, IgM protein in the serum, and a lymphoplasma cell proliferation of more than 10% in the bone marrow. It must be differentiated from MGUS of the IgM type, smoldering WM, lymphoma, other lymphoproliferative diseases, MM, and chronic lymphocytic leukemia.

Prognosis

The median survival is approximately 5 years. Morel and colleagues developed an international prognostic scoring system in 587 patients with WM. They identified age > 65 years, hemoglobin ≤ 11.5 g/dL, platelets ≤ 100 × 10⁹/L, β₂-microglobulin > 3 mg/L and serum monoclonal protein > 7.0 g/dL as adverse features. Low-risk patients had zero or one adverse characteristic, intermediate-risk had two adverse characteristics, and high-risk patients had more than two adverse characteristics with 5-year survivals of 87, 68, and 36%, respectively.[45] Ghobrial et al[46] developed a prognostic model based on age more than 65 years and the presence of organomegaly as well as β_2-microglobulin.

Treatment

Therapy should be withheld until the patient has constitutional symptoms such as weakness, fatigue, night sweats, weight loss, features of hyperviscosity, anemia, significant hepatosplenomegaly, or lymphadenopathy. Plasmapheresis should be performed based on the patient's symptoms and physical findings, rather than on the magnitude of the viscosity measurement. Therapy includes rituximab, the nucleoside analogues, fludarabine, and cladribine (2-chlorodeoxyadenosine), akylating agents such has chlorambucil or cyclophosphamide, corticosteroids, and ASCT. Thalidomide has been disappointing but bortezomib and bendamustine are undergoing evaluation. A detailed approach to the management of WM has recently been published.[47]

Heavy-chain diseases

The heavy-chain diseases (HCD) are lymphoplasma cell-proliferative disorders characterized by the production of an M protein consisting of an incomplete heavy chain devoid of light chains. There are three major types: α, γ, and μ.[48]

α-Heavy-chain disease

α-HCD is the most common type and is characterized by the presence of a monoclonal α-chain with extensive internal deletions encompassing the VH region and the entire first constant domain.[49] It usually occurs in the second or third decade of life, and about 60% of patients are male. Most have been from the Mediterranean region and Middle East. Gastrointestinal tract involvement is most common and is manifested by malabsorption, with weight loss, diarrhea, and steatorrhea. It is similar to immunoproliferative small intestinal disease (IPSID), but patients with IPSID do not synthesize α-heavy chains. Poor hygiene and low socioeconomic status are important risk factors. Rarely, the respiratory tract is involved.

The serum protein electrophoretic pattern shows a broad band in the α_2 or β regions in half of patients and is normal in the remainder with no visible spike. The diagnosis depends on the recognition of a monoclonal α-heavy chain in the serum, jejunal fluid, or the lymphocytes and plasma cells. The amount of α-chain in the urine is small and Bence Jones proteinuria is absent. The bone marrow is normal. The course of α-HCD is variable but generally progressive. Surprisingly, antibiotics may produce remission. In patients who do not respond to antibiotics and in those with extensive intestinal or mesenteric involvement, chemotherapy with cyclophosphamide, doxorubicin (Adriamycin), vincristine, and prednisone should be given.

γ-Heavy-chain disease

In γ-HCD, the γ-chain is incomplete, with large deletions of amino acids, including the CH1 domain and a portion of the VH1 of the constant region. The median age at diagnosis is over 60 years but several patients younger than 20 years have been recognized. Its clinical picture has been described as a lymphoma-like illness, but its features are variable, ranging from an aggressive lymphoproliferative process to an asymptomatic state.[50] The most frequent presenting symptoms are weakness, fatigue, and fever. Autoimmune disorders such as rheumatoid arthritis, Sjögren's syndrome, systemic lupus erythematosus, Hashimoto's thyroiditis and myasthenia gravis have been noted.

Normocytic, normochromic anemia is found in 80% of cases. The amount of γ-heavy-chain protein in the urine ranges from nondetectable to 20 g/24 hours; more than half of patients excrete less than 1 g/24 hours of protein. Bence Jones proteinuria is not found. The bone marrow and lymph nodes contain an increased number of plasma cells, lymphocytes, and lymphoplasmacytoid cells. The diagnosis depends on demonstration of a monoclonal γ-heavy chain in the serum or urine.

The median duration of survival in a series of 23 patients from a single institution was 7.4 years (range 1 month to more than 21 years).[50] Therapy with cyclophosphamide, vincristine, and prednisone is a reasonable choice, but if there is no response, doxorubicin should be added.

μ-Heavy-chain disease

μ-HCD is characterized by a monoclonal μ-heavy chain in which the VH domain is absent. Other deletions can also occur. Most patients have a chronic lymphoproliferative process resembling chronic lymphocytic leukemia or lymphoma. A monoclonal peak is found in the serum of 40% of patients. Two-thirds have Bence Jones proteinuria. Increases in lymphocytes, plasma cells, and lymphoplasmacytoid cells in the bone marrow are common. Vacuolization of the plasma cells is an important clue for the diagnosis of μ-HCD, which depends on the demonstration of a μ-heavy chain in the serum. The course of the disease is variable; the duration of survival ranges from less than 1 month to 11 years (median, 24 months). Treatment with corticosteroids and alkylating agents has shown benefit.

Primary systemic amyloidosis

Amyloid consists of rigid, linear, nonbranching fibrils segregated in a β-pleated sheet conformation that stains with Congo red and shows apple-green birefringence under polarized light. It is composed of the variable portion of a monoclonal light chain, or rarely, an intact monoclonal light chain, and is the result of a clonal plasma cell proliferative disorder.[51]

Diagnosis

The diagnosis requires the demonstration of amyloid deposits that are composed of monoclonal light chains. Laser microdissection of clinical biopsy specimens followed by mass spectrometry is a highly specific and sensitive test for determining the type of amyloidosis.[52] It should be suspected in patients with nephrotic syndrome, cardiomyopathy with congestive heart failure, axonal peripheral neuropathy, or orthostatic hypotension, and the presence of a monoclonal light chain in the serum or urine. The source of tissue for diagnosis includes subcutaneous fat aspirate (75% positive), bone marrow biopsy (55% positive), or rectum (75% positive). Biopsy of the liver, kidney, heart, or sural nerve is almost 100% positive. The median age is 65 years. Macroglossia, carpal tunnel syndrome, and purpura involving the periorbital area, face, and neck can occur. Immunofixation of the serum and urine reveals a positive result in almost 90% of patients at diagnosis. The FLC ratio is abnormal in almost all patients with a negative immunofixation.

Prognosis

The median survival was 13 months in 474 patients seen at the Mayo Clinic within 1 month of diagnosis. On the other hand, the estimated median survival was 40 months for amyloid patients eligible for peripheral stem-cell transplantation.[53] Median survival of patients with detectable cardiac troponin T ($\geq$ 1 µg/L) was significantly shorter than those with undetectable levels (6 vs 22 months, respectively) (Table 80.4).

Treatment

Melphalan and prednisone have been the mainstays of treatment, but the results are not satisfactory. Patients who are not eligible for a stem-cell transplant (three or more organs involved, advanced cardiac amyloidosis, major comorbidities, or poor performance) are offered therapy with melphalan plus high-dose dexamethasone. Bortezomib as a once-weekly regimen appears to be as efficacious as the conventional schedule and is associated with sensorimotor peripheral neuropathy.[54] The conditioning regimen for transplantation consists of intravenous melphalan ($100–200$ mg/m^2).

Organ improvement can be achieved in 50% of patients treated with an ASCT. The mortality is approximately 5% compared to 1% for patients with MM. Patients with end-stage cardiomyopathy may be treated with a heart transplant followed by a stem-cell transplant. Treatment options have recently been summarized.[55]

Table 80.4 Risk stratification model to predict progression of primary amyloidosis

	Median survival	
Risk group	Patients undergoing stem-cell transplantation (months)	Patients not undergoing stem-cell transplantation (months)
Low risk (cardiac troponin level < 0.035 µg/L and NT-proBNP level < 332 ng/L)	Not reached at 40 months	26.4
Intermediate risk (any one factor abnormal)	Not reached at 40 months	10.5
High risk (cardiac troponin level ≥ 0.035 µg/L and NT-proBNP level ≥ 332 ng/L)	8.4	3.5

NT-proBNP, N-terminal pro-brain natriuretic peptide.
From Rajkumar SV, Dispenzieri A, Kyle RA. Monoclonal gammopathy of undetermined significance, Waldenström macroglobulinemia, AL amyloidosis, and related plasma cell disorders: diagnosis and treatment. Mayo Clin Proc 2006; 81:653–703, with permission.

ON THE HORIZON

- Approval of new agents such as carfilzomib and pomalidomide.
- Use of gene expression profiling to improve prognostic factors.
- Selection of better therapy for the individual patient.

References

1. Katzmann JA, Kyle RA. Immunochemical characterization of immunoglobulins in serum, urine, and cerebrospinal fluid. In: Detrick B, Hamilton R, Folds J, editors. Manual of molecular and clinical laboratory immunology. 7th ed. ASM Press; 2006. p. 88–100.
2. Katzmann JA, Kyle RA, Benson J, et al. Screening panels for detection of monoclonal gammopathies. Clin Chem 2009;55:1517.
3. Katzmann JA, Abraham RS, Dispenzieri A, et al. Diagnostic performance of quantitative κ and λ free light chain assays in clinical practice. Clin Chem 2005;51(5):878–81.
4. Kyle RA, Therneau TM, Rajkumar SV, et al. Prevalence of monoclonal gammopathy of undetermined significance. N Engl J Med 2006;354(13):1362–9.
5. Landgren O, Katzmann JA, Hsing AW, et al. Prevalence of monoclonal gammopathy of undetermined significance among men in Ghana. Mayo Clin Proc 2007;82(12):1468–73.
6. Kyle RA, Therneau TM, Rajkumar SV, et al. Long-term follow-up of 241 patients with monoclonal gammopathy of undetermined significance: the original Mayo Clinic series 25 years later. [see comment]. Mayo Clin Proc 2004;79(7):859–66.
7. Kyle RA, Therneau TM, Rajkumar SV, et al. A long-term study of prognosis in monoclonal gammopathy of undetermined significance. N Engl J Med 2002;346(8):564–9.
8. Kyle RA, Gertz MA, Witzig TE, et al. Review of 1027 patients with newly diagnosed multiple myeloma. [see comment]. Mayo Clin Proc 2003;78(1):21–33.
9. Kyle RA, Rajkumar SV. Monoclonal gammopathy of undetermined significance. Clin Lymphoma Myeloma 2005;6(2):102–14.
10. Rajkumar SV, Kyle RA, Therneau TM, et al. Serum free light chain ratio is an independent risk factor for progression in monoclonal gammopathy of undetermined significance. Blood 2005;106(3):812–7.
11. Cesana C, Klersy C, Barbarano L, et al. Prognostic factors for malignant transformation in monoclonal gammopathy of undetermined significance and smoldering multiple myeloma. J Clin Oncol 2002;20(6):1625–34.
12. Bida JP, Kyle RA, Therneau TM, et al. Disease associations with monoclonal gammopathy of undetermined significance: a population-based study of 17,398 patients. Mayo Clin Proc 2009;84(8):685–93.
13. Kyle RA, Therneau TM, Rajkumar SV, et al. Long-term follow-up of IgM monoclonal gammopathy of undetermined significance. Blood 2003;102(10):3759–64.
14. Dispenzieri A, Katzmann JA, Kyle R, et al. Prevalence and risk of progression of light-chain monoclonal gammopathy of undetermined significance: a retrospective population-based cohort study. Lancet 2010;375(9727):1721–8.
15. Kyle RA, Robinson RA, Katzmann JA. The clinical aspects of biclonal gammopathies. Review of 57 cases. Am J Med 1981;71(6):999–1008.
16. Kyle RA, Therneau TM, Rajkumar SV, et al. Incidence of multiple myeloma in Olmsted County, Minnesota—trend over 6 decades. Cancer 2004;101(11):2667–74.
17. Criteria for the classification of monoclonal gammopathies, multiple myeloma and related disorders: a report of the International Myeloma Working Group. Br J Haematol 2003;121(5):749–57.
18. Greipp PR, San Miguel J, Durie BG, et al. International staging system for multiple myeloma. J Clin Oncol 2005;23(15):3412–20.
19. Kumar SK, Mikhael JR, Buadi FK, et al. Management of newly diagnosed symptomatic multiple myeloma: updated Mayo Stratification of Myeloma and Risk-Adapted Therapy (mSMART) consensus guidelines. Mayo Clin Proc 2009;84(12):1095–110.
20. Kyle RA, Rajkumar SV. Criteria for diagnosis, staging, risk stratification and response assessment of multiple myeloma. Leukemia 2009;23(1):3–9.
21. Kyle RA, Rajkumar SV. Multiple myeloma. N Engl J Med 2004;351(18):1860–73.
22. Rajkumar SV, Jacobus S, Callander NS, et al. Lenalidomide plus high-dose dexamethasone versus lenalidomide plus low-dose dexamethasone as initial therapy for newly diagnosed multiple myeloma: an open-label randomised controlled trial. Lancet Oncol 2010;11(1):29–37.
23. Attal M, Harousseau JL, Facon T, et al. Single versus double autologous stem-cell transplantation for multiple myeloma.[see comment]. N Engl J Med 2003;349(26):2495–502 (Erratum appears in N Engl J Med. 2004;350(25):2628).
24. Kyle RA. Role of maintenance therapy after autologous stem cell transplant for multiple myeloma: lessons for cancer therapy. Mayo Clin Proc 2011;86(5):419–20.
25. Krishnan A, Pasquini M, Ewell M, et al. Tandem autologous hematopoietic stem cell transplants (AuHCT) with or without maintenance therapy (auto-auto) versus single AuHCT folllowed by HLA matched sibling non-myeloablative allogeneic HCT (auto-allo) for patients with standard risk (SR) multiple myeloma (MM): results from the blood and marrow transplant clinical trials network (BMT CTN) 0102 trial. Blood (Abstract #41) 2010;116(21):24–5.
26. Palumbo A, Bringhen S, Caravita T, et al. Oral melphalan and prednisone chemotherapy plus thalidomide compared with melphalan and prednisone alone in elderly patients with multiple myeloma: randomised controlled trial. Lancet 2006;367(9513):825–31.
27. Facon T, Mary JY, Hulin C, et al. Melphalan and prednisone plus thalidomide versus melphalan and prednisone alone or reduced-intensity autologous stem cell

transplantation in elderly patients with multiple myeloma (IFM 99-06): a randomised trial. Lancet 2007;370(9594):1209–18.

28. San Miguel JF, Schlag R, Khuageva NK, et al. Bortezomib plus melphalan and prednisone for initial treatment of multiple myeloma. N Engl J Med 2008;359(9):906–17.

29. Kumar SK, Rajkumar SV, Dispenzieri A, et al. Improved survival in multiple myeloma and the impact of novel therapies. Blood 2008;111(5):2516–20.

30. Berenson JR, Lichtenstein A, Porter L, et al. Long-term pamidronate treatment of advanced multiple myeloma patients reduces skeletal events. Myeloma Aredia Study Group. J Clin Oncol 1998;16(2):593–602.

31. Morgan GJ, Davies FE, Gregory WM, et al. First-line treatment with zoledronic acid as compared with clodronic acid in multiple myeloma (MRC Myeloma IX): a randomised controlled trial. Lancet 2010;376(9757):1989–99.

32. Rizzo JD, Somerfield MR, Hagerty KL, et al. Use of epoetin and darbepoetin in patients with cancer: 2007 American Society of Clinical Oncology/American Society of Hematology clinical practice guideline update. J Clin Oncol 2008;26(1):132–49.

33. Smith A, Wisloff F, Samson D. Guidelines on the diagnosis and management of multiple myeloma 2005. Br J Haematol 2006;132(4):410–51.

34. Kyle RA, Remstein ED, Therneau TM, et al. Clinical course and prognosis of smoldering (asymptomatic) multiple myeloma. N Engl J Med 2007;356(25):2582–90.

35. Garcia-Sanz R, Orfao A, Gonzalez M, et al. Primary plasma cell leukemia: clinical, immunophenotypic, DNA ploidy, and cytogenetic characteristics. Blood 1999;93(3):1032–7.

36. Tiedemann RE, Gonzalez-Paz N, Kyle RA, et al. Genetic aberrations and survival in plasma cell leukemia. Leukemia 2008;22(5):1044–52.

37. Dores GM, Landgren O, McGlynn KA, et al. Plasmacytoma of bone, extramedullary plasmacytoma, and multiple myeloma: incidence and survival in the United States, 1992–2004. Br J Haematol 2009;144(1):86–94.

38. Liebross RH, Ha CS, Cox JD, et al. Solitary bone plasmacytoma: outcome and prognostic factors following radiotherapy. Int J Radiat Oncol Biol Phys 1998;41(5):1063–7.

39. Alexiou C, Kau RJ, Dietzfelbinger H, et al. Extramedullary plasmacytoma: tumor occurrence and therapeutic concepts. Cancer 1999;85(11):2305–14.

40. Creach KM, Foote RL, Neben-Wittich MA, Kyle RA. Radiotherapy for extramedullary plasmacytoma of the head and neck. Int J Radiat Oncol Biol Phys 2009;73(3):789–94.

41. Bachar G, Goldstein D, Brown D, et al. Solitary extramedullary plasmacytoma of the head and neck—long-term outcome analysis of 68 cases. Head Neck 2008;30(8):1012–9.

42. Dispenzieri A, Kyle RA, Lacy MQ, et al. POEMS syndrome: definitions and long-term outcome. Blood 2003;101(7):2496–506.

43. Dispenzieri A, Moreno-Aspitia A, Suarez GA, et al. Peripheral blood stem cell transplantation in 16 patients with POEMS syndrome, and a review of the literature. Blood 2004;104(10):3400–7.

44. Dispenzieri A, Lacy MQ, Hayman SR, et al. Peripheral blood stem cell transplant for POEMS syndrome is associated with high rates of engraftment syndrome. Eur J Haematol 2008;80(5):397–406.

45. Morel P, Duhamel A, Gobbi P, et al. International prognostic scoring system for Waldenström macroglobulinemia. Blood 2009;113(18):4163–70.

46. Ghobrial IM, Fonseca R, Gertz MA, et al. Prognostic model for disease-specific and overall mortality in newly diagnosed symptomatic patients with Waldenström macroglobulinaemia. Br J Haematol 2006;133(2):158–64.

47. Ansell SM, Kyle RA, Reeder CB, et al. Diagnosis and management of Waldenström macroglobulinemia: Mayo stratification of macroglobulinemia and risk-adapted therapy (mSMART) guidelines. Mayo Clin Proc 2010;85(9):824–33.

48. Wahner-Roedler DL, Kyle RA. Heavy chain diseases. Best Pract Res Clin Haematol 2005;18(4):729–46.

49. Rambaud JC, Halphen M, Galian A, Tsapis A. Immunoproliferative small intestinal disease (IPSID): relationships with alpha-chain disease and "Mediterranean" lymphomas. Springer Semin Immunopathol 1990;12(2–3):239–50.

50. Wahner-Roedler DL, Witzig TE, Loehrer LL, Kyle RA. Gamma-heavy chain disease: review of 23 cases. Medicine 2003;82(4):236–50.

51. Gertz MA, Lacy MQ, Dispenzieri A, Hayman SR. Amyloidosis. Best Pract Res Clin Haematol 2005;18(4):709–27.

52. Vrana JA, Gamez JD, Madden BJ, et al. Classification of amyloidosis by laser microdissection and mass spectrometry-based proteomic analysis in clinical biopsy specimens. Blood 2009;114(24):4957–9.

53. Dispenzieri A, Lacy MQ, Kyle RA, et al. Eligibility for hematopoietic stem-cell transplantation for primary systemic amyloidosis is a favorable prognostic factor for survival. J Clin Oncol 2001;19(14):3350–6.

54. Bringhen S, Larocca A, Rossi D, et al. Efficacy and safety of once-weekly bortezomib in multiple myeloma patients. Blood 2010;116(23):4745–53.

55. Merlini G, Seldin DC, Gertz MA. Amyloidosis: pathogenesis and new therapeutic options. J Clin Oncol 2011;29(14):1924–33.

PART NINE
Transplantation

81

Concepts and challenges in organ transplantation: rejection, immunosuppression, and tolerance

Kathryn Wood,
Sushma Shankar,
Shruti Mittal

The clinical era of transplantation began on December 23, 1954, when Dr. Joseph Murray and colleagues performed the first successful renal transplant on the genetically identical Herrick twins.[1] Solid organ transplantation has since transformed the landscape of modern medicine, offering dramatic improvements in patient survival and quality of life in many end-stage diseases. The development of powerful immunosuppressive regimens and cutting edge biological agents represents an elegant proof of concept, translating seminal work from the laboratory bench to the patient's bedside. However, this ground-breaking field within clinical immunology is not without setbacks. Rejection of transplanted organs and tissues can result in devastating problems for the patient and potent immunosuppression is associated with substantial comorbidity, including exposure to infection, malignancy and cardiovascular risks that may be fatal. Theoretically, immunosuppression withdrawal and allograft-specific protection against host responses is the ultimate treatment to offer a transplant recipient. Undoubtedly this is challenging, but may be realized in defined subgroups o recipients within the next decade. This chapter examines the rejection response, outlines the mainstay of current immunosuppressive therapy and discusses the latest advances in the search for transplantation tolerance.

Rejection

The immune system is complex and has evolved in order to protect the individual from harm. This harm may be either in the form of foreign pathogenic microorganisms or premalignant mutations in the individual's own cells. Clearly to achieve this safely, the immune system must have the ability to distinguish "self" from "non-self" or "altered-self" to avoid damaging the host itself. If a specific adaptive immune response is mounted against self-antigens, autoimmune disease results. To prevent this from happening T cells specific to self-antigen are deleted in the thymus or controlled in the periphery. Any immune response that is generated must also be proportional to the threat and thus antigens encountered in the context of inflammation will prime T cells and evoke a more aggressive immune response. While an effective immune response is essential to survival in the context of infection or malignancy it can represent significant management challenges in the transplantation setting.

Some elements of the immune system respond to the general trauma associated with organ retrieval, perfusion and surgery, while others respond following specific recognition of antigenic differences between the donor and the recipient. If this destructive process continues uncontrolled, this inevitably leads to loss of the graft. Thus autografts (grafting of tissue from one site on an individual to another site) and isografts or syngeneic grafts (grafting of tissue between two genetically identical individuals such that there are no antigenic differences) provide fewer complications, whereas an allograft (transplantation of tissues from genetically different individuals) usually evokes an aggressive immune response as a result of the antigenic differences between donor and recipient. Tissue transplanted between individuals of different species, a xenograft, is also possible but is not yet in clinical use as xenografts usually trigger a more rapid and aggressive immune response compared to an allograft. This section considers the processes involved in allorecognition and graft destruction.

Innate immunity and ischemia-reperfusion injury

Trauma to the graft is initiated during, or even before, retrieval since donor brainstem death induces hemodynamic and neuroendocrine responses; in addition, organs from donors after cardiac death suffer a period of warm ischemia. During cold storage, loss of intracellular potassium and cell injury continues. This leads to graft damage through cell swelling and a build up of toxic metabolites, leaving the graft susceptible to further ischemia-reperfusion injury on rapid warming following revascularization. Efforts are made during storage and the organ implantation surgery to reduce the metabolic rate through storage on ice and perfusion with specialized cold perfusion fluids. This approach aims to minimize the accumulation of toxic metabolites and resultant pH changes in order to reduce the effect of cold ischemic time on post-transplant outcomes such as delayed graft function.[2]

Tissue injury leads to the expression of damage-associated molecular patterns (DAMPS), such as heparin sulphate, heat shock proteins, nucleic acids and high mobility group box protein 1 (HMGB1). These are identified by invariant pattern-recognition receptors of the innate immune system, e.g., Toll-like receptors (TLRs) (Chapter 3). This process results in the local production of inflammatory mediators, such as interleukin-1 (IL-1) and -6, chemokines, and expression of adhesion molecules within the graft. These early innate responses are seen in autografts as well isografts and are not alloantigen specific. In turn, this triggers activation of macrophages and dendritic cells (DCs) via cell surface and internal pattern recognition receptors,[3] causing macrophages and DCs to show greater antigen-presenting capacity and to enter a cytocidal state. Endogenous signals such as stress can also activate the complement cascade to generate several products including complement component C3 in the graft, which promotes DC maturation and subsequently their ability

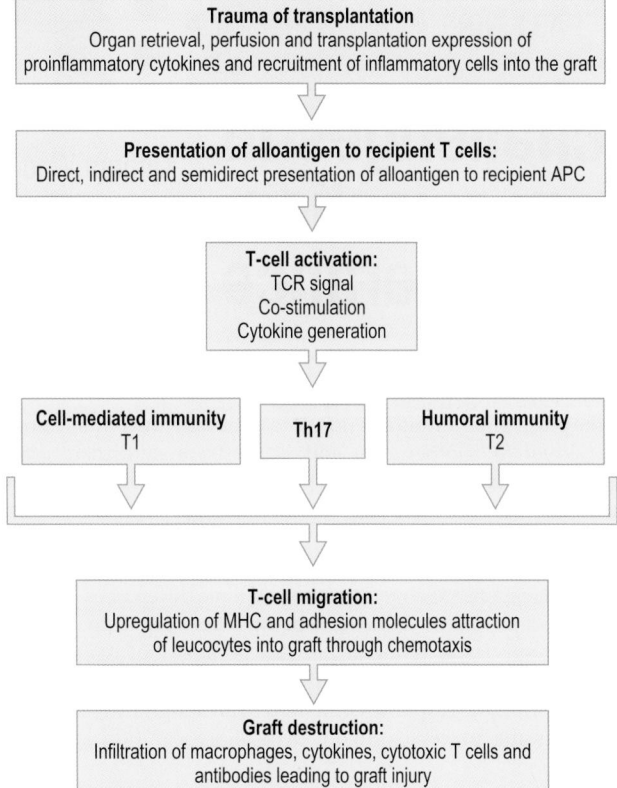

Fig. 81.1 Mechanisms leading to graft injury. Interplay of innate and adaptive immune responses results in eventual graft destruction.

to activate T cells. DCs are also activated by interferon-gamma (IFN-γ) produced by natural killer (NK) cells. In one or more of these ways the innate immune system, initiated by local tissue injury, promotes the initiation of adaptive immune responses when antigenic differences exist between the donor and the recipient. Activation of the adaptive immune system results in a series of mechanisms, both cell and antibody mediated, leading to further graft injury (Fig. 81.1).

A severely damaged graft will initiate a more aggressive immune response and this may explain the superior outcomes in living donor grafts compared to deceased donor grafts, even in the presence of significant major histocompatibility complex (MHC) mismatches.[4] The immune response evoked by the damaged tissue also helps to account for the higher rates of rejection observed in individuals with delayed graft function.[5]

Initiation of the adaptive immune system

Rejection is a complex process initiated due to recognition of differences between donor and recipient major and/or minor histocompatiblity (miH) molecules or antigens by T cells. The extensive polymorphism of MHC genes (Chapter 5) makes complete matching of unrelated individuals rare and therefore, almost inevitably, transplantation of cells or organs between genetically unrelated individuals occurs across an MHC mismatch. Knowledge of the MHC and the structure of MHC molecules have contributed significantly to our understanding of how rejection is triggered and has facilitated the development of novel immunosuppressive drugs. Additionally, transplantation between MHC-identical siblings has shown that differences in miH antigens can also be significant, particularly for example in bone marrow transplantation, leading to activation of the

adaptive immune system and subsequently to graft-versus-host disease (GVHD). These miH antigens may be derived from a wide variety of polymorphic proteins and are encoded for a vast array of genes distributed throughout the genome.

Signal 1: Recognition of alloantigen

Class I MHC molecules are cell surface glycoproteins expressed on most nucleated cells that are recognized by T-cell receptors (TCR) expressed by CD8 T cells; so-called class I restricted CD8 T cells. Class II MHC molecules are not expressed by every cell in the body, rather they are found on B lymphocytes, macrophages, DCs and, in humans, endothelial cells. MHC class II molecules are recognized by T cells bearing the CD4 surface glycoprotein, so-called MHC class II restricted T cells. Expression of both class I and II MHC molecules can be increased, or in the latter case induced, during inflammation such as can occur as a result of ischemia and reperfusion injury in the setting of transplantation (see above).

The structure of both class I and II MHC proteins is such that a highly polymorphic groove or cleft, that can bind peptides, is formed on a platform of beta strands, flanked by two alpha helices. Antigen processing within antigen presenting cells (APC) results in the production of peptides that can bind in these grooves producing a MHC–peptide complex that can be recognized by T cells (Chapter 6). These peptides may be of self origin or derived from foreign molecules, e.g., from an allograft following a transplant or a virus following an infection. In general, peptides derived from molecules present inside the cell are processed and loaded into MHC class I molecules, whereas molecules present outside the cell in the extracellular environment are processed into peptides that load into class II molecules. However, cross-presentation can also occur whereby some APCs, notably DCs, can process extracellular proteins such that they can be loaded onto MHC class I molecules and presented to CD8 T cells.[6]

The TCR is composed of two chains that confer MHC–peptide specificity and is associated with a complex of polypeptides referred to collectively as CD3 (Chapter 4). On antigen recognition by TCR, CD3 delivers signals to the T cell (Chapter 12). Recognition of antigen by the TCR/CD3 complex is the first step in T-cell activation and commonly referred to as "signal 1." This initial meeting between host naive and memory T cells and alloantigen from the foreign transplant is believed to take place in secondary lymphoid organs rather than in the transplanted graft itself, as rejection does not occur in naïve mice that lack secondary lymphoid tissues.[7] The inflammatory response triggered in the allograft by retrieval and implantation of the organ or tissue, as outlined above, not only initiates the migration of donor-derived passenger leukocytes but also their maturation into functional APCs expressing high levels of donor MHC molecules.

The presentation of intact allogeneic MHC molecules by donor-derived passenger leukocytes to T cells is known as the direct pathway of allorecognition. This is the dominant pathway through which the immune reaction to the graft is initiated, and T cells responding to direct antigen presentation constitute a vast majority of the alloreactive immune repertoire.[8] After a time, the donor lymphocytes transplanted with the graft are depleted; however, this does not abrogate rejection. The immune response against an allograft is maintained by recipient APCs, largely consisting of DCs and B cells, which process and present peptides derived from allogeneic MHC molecules shed from the graft (soluble MHC molecules or apoptotic cells) as well as miH antigens. This second route of allorecognition is known as the

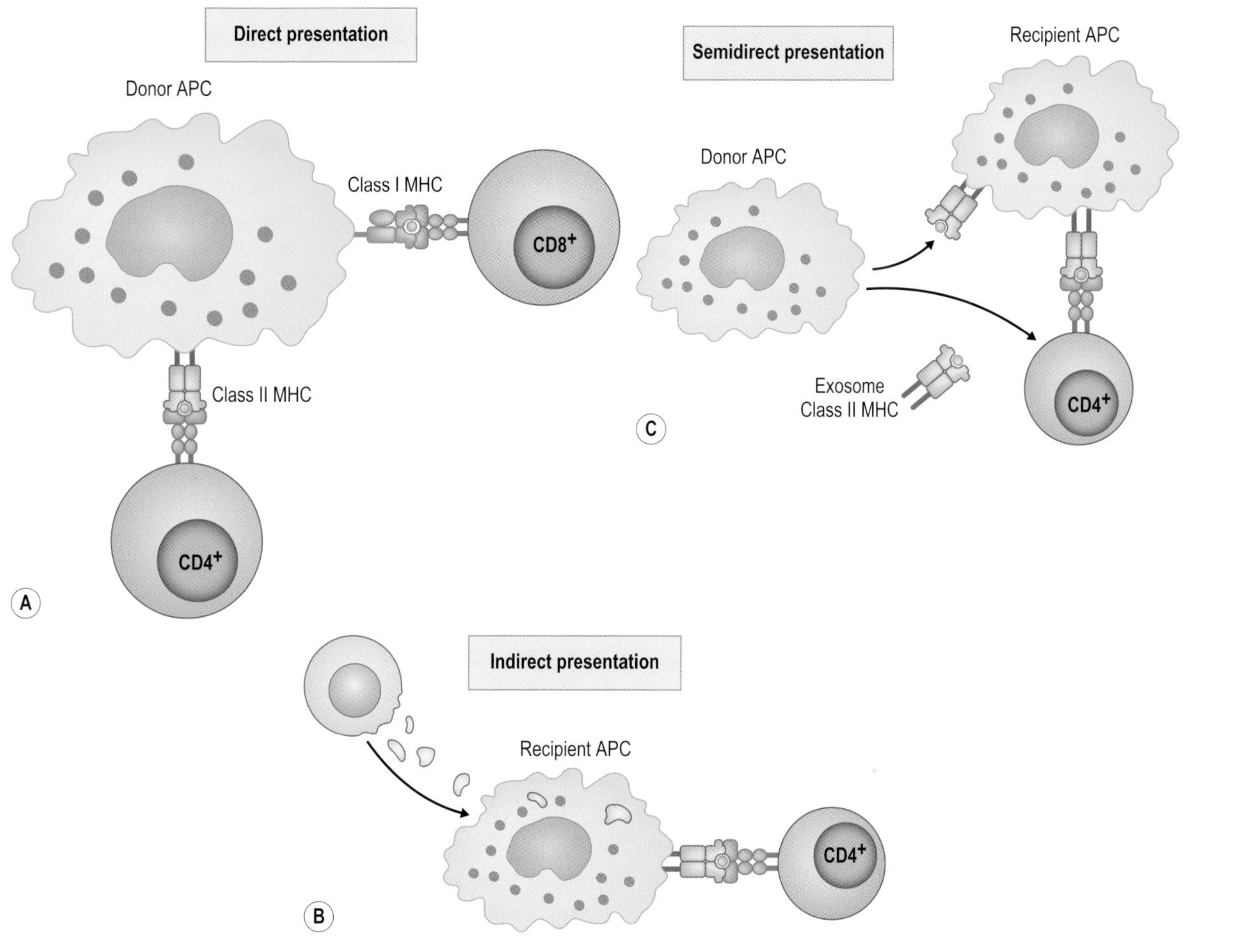

Direct presentation

Donor APC

Class I MHC

CD8⁺

Class II MHC

CD4⁺

(A)

Semidirect presentation

Recipient APC

Donor APC

Exosome
Class II MHC

CD4⁺

(C)

Indirect presentation

Recipient APC

CD4⁺

(B)

Fig. 81.2 Antigen presentation. (A) Direct presentation: passenger donor APCs present alloantigen to recipient T cells in lymphoid tissue; (B) indirect presentation: alloantigen from donor cells is processed and presented by recipient APCs via MHC class II to recipient CD4⁺ cells; (C) semi-direct presentation: donor MHC class I and class II may be transferred to the surface of recipient APCs enabling presentation of alloantigen to recipient T cells.

indirect pathway. Experimental models have shown that indirect presentation of donor antigens plays a greater role in rejection than direct presentation overall, as it continues for as long as the graft remains *in situ*.[9] It is also now known that the direct and indirect pathways of allorecognition interact as a third pathway referred to as the semi-direct pathway of antigen presentation. In the semi-direct pathway of allorecognition, donor MHC proteins are transferred intact to recipient APCs enabling them to present allogeneic MHC–peptide complexes intact to recipient T cells. This MHC transfer is temperature and energy dependent and requires close cell-to-cell contact. Both MHC class I and class II may be transferred, although class II MHC appears to be transferred more efficiently.[10] These three modes of antigen presentation are illustrated in Fig. 81.2.

Signal 2: Co-stimulation

T lymphocyte activation relies not only on contact of the TCR/ CD3 complex with its specific MHC–peptide complex (signal 1) but also on signals delivered by the interaction of several co-stimulatory receptors and their ligands, known collectively as signal 2 (Fig. 81.3). During T-cell activation, the membrane of the T cell reorganizes such that the TCR/CD3 complex and co-stimulatory molecules are brought together in the cell membrane to form the immunological synapse. While signal 1 is specific for the antigen involved, co-stimulation is not.

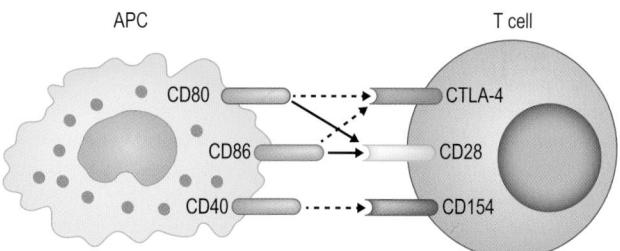

Fig. 81.3 Co-stimulation. Co-stimulation follows binding to MHC class I and class II on APCs and involves signal transduction via intracellular proteins and increased interaction affinity via the binding of several cell surface proteins. Several co-stimulatory molecule pairs have been identified.

Co-stimulatory receptors fall into two major families, the B7 family (e.g., CD28 and CD152) and the tumour necrosis factor (TNF) family (e.g., CD40) (Chapter 12). Although several co-stimulatory molecule pairs have been identified, the CD28 and CD40 pathways have been the most clearly defined to date. CD80 and CD86 are receptor ligands on the surface of DCs and other cells that can bind to CD28 on T cells, resulting in the activation of additional signal transduction pathways within the T cell. This has a number of effects: lowering the threshold for T-cell activation; increasing glucose metabolism, as well as cytokine and chemokine expression including IL-2 production; reducing T-cell death through apoptosis; and expanding the number of T cells that respond through proliferation.

CD80 and CD86 are also linked to an inhibitory receptor, CD152 or cytotoxic T lymphocyte-associated antigen-4 (CTLA-4), which inhibits T-cell activation possibly by competing with CD28 to bind with CD80 or CD86. CTLA-4 has a tenfold higher receptor affinity compared to CD28 and is rapidly upregulated following T-cell activation. Additionally, CD152 activates tryptophan catabolism in DCs, which results in the inhibition of proliferation and promotes apoptosis of the responding T cells. Related to this pathway are other pathways involving members of the B7–CD28 family of molecules, including ICOS/B7h, PD1/PD-L1/PD-L2, and B7-H3. Each of these can play a role in T-cell co-stimulation, but for the early phase of the response the CD28 pathway dominates. CD40 belongs to the TNF receptor family, expressed on all APCs, and binds to CD154 or CD40L, which is present on activated CD4 cells, a subset of CD8 cells and NK cells. CD40 stimulation causes triggering signals for antibody production and induces CD28 and MHC expression on APCs, so amplifying antigen presentation.[11]

In clinical transplantation, treatment with calcineurin inhibitors to block signal 1 and/or T-cell depleting agents has been highly successful in the prevention and reversal of rejection episodes. More recently blockade of costimulatory pathways has also been shown to be effective. These approaches are discussed in the section on Immunosuppression.

Signal 3: Proliferation and differentiation of effector T cells

Following alloantigen recognition by the TCR/CD3 complex and co-stimulation, a process begins resulting in "signal 3." This is the complex process involving the recruitment and phosphorylation of a series of signalling molecules, which in turn result in intracellular biochemical processes leading to the activation of three signal-transduction pathways: the calcium-calcineurin pathway, the Ras- and Rac-mitogen-activated protein kinase pathways and the protein kinase C nuclear factor kappa B (NF-κB) pathway. These pathways interact with inositol triphosphate (IP3) and diacylglycerol (DAG), formed from the hydrolysis of phosphatidylinositol 4,5-bisphosphonate, to activate transcription factors: nuclear factor of activated T cells (NFAT), activating protein 1 (AP-1), and NF-κB, respectively. These transcription factors cause the expression of many genes leading to upregulation of growth factors and cytokines, in particular, IL-2 and CD25 (IL2Rα). Growth signals are then delivered through the phosphoinositide-3-kinase (PI-3 K) and molecular-target-of-rapamycin (mTOR) pathways to promote cell cycle progression and initiate clonal expansion and differentiation of activated T cells to express effector functions. These mechanisms are targeted by various immunosuppressive agents discussed in the section on Immunosuppression and illustrated in Fig. 81.5.

The pattern of cytokine production through the interaction of the combination of signalling processes determines the nature of the response, in which either cell-mediated or antibody-mediated immunity is seen to dominate (Chapter 16). The T cells known to promote a cell-mediated response, and the cytokines they produce, are termed Th1 cells. These cells are associated with the production of IFN-γ. T cells promoting a humoral response are referred to as Th2 and are associated with the generation of IL-4, -5, and -6. Additionally, a Th17 population has been identified, characterized by the production of IL-17 and promoting the infiltration of neutrophils.[12] A subset of CD4 cells called T regulatory cells (Treg) can also be induced following antigen exposure in the periphery (Chapter 15).[13] These cells secrete IL-10 or TGF and have suppressive or regulatory functions

against effector cells and APC. The balance of these responses results in either graft injury or the induction of tolerance (discussed below).

Memory T cells

Following exposure to an antigen, antigen-specific memory T and B cells are generated. These memory cells are then able to produce a more rapid and intense immune reaction if the antigen is encountered on a second occasion, as they have a lower activation threshold and are less dependent on co-stimulation. Transplant recipients, particularly older patients or who have had previous antigen exposure through previous transplantation, blood transfusion, or pregnancy, may therefore have specific anti-donor memory cells. Memory-type responses may also occur as a result of antigen receptor cross-reactivity known as heterologous immunity.

Cell migration

Following activation, chemotactic cytokines, or chemokines, generated at the site of inflammation attract leukocytes that have been primed in secondary lymphoid tissue to the graft (Chapter 10). Once activated, leukocytes upregulate chemokine receptors enabling their migration along a chemokine gradient. Vessels in proximity to the graft become dilated, allowing increased blood flow, and the endothelium becomes activated. Activated endothelial cells externalize Weibel-Palade bodies containing P-selectin, and chemokines generated in the graft, such as IL-8, RANTES, and MCP-1, stick to the vascular endothelium (Chapter 11). This signals to passing leukocytes that an inflammatory process is occurring within the tissue, attracting activated leukocytes in post-capillary venules to leave laminar flow of blood and move closer to the vessel edge so that they can interact with the activated endothelial cells. Extravasation then occurs in a multistep process, involving molecules on the surface of activated leukocytes called Sialyl-Lewis moieties that interact with endothelial P-selectin and form temporary bonds that form and break causing the leukocytes to "roll." Chemokines on the endothelial surface then induce a conformational change in leukocyte integrin molecules allowing high-affinity binding to endothelial adhesion molecules such as ICAM-1. When this occurs, the leukocytes stop rolling, allowing them to extravasate and follow the chemokine gradient further into the graft, where damage then occurs

The effector response and graft destruction

The immune system generates many different effector mechanisms depending both on the challenge it meets and the microenvironments that are present. In transplantation, this response may be modified by the type of transplanted tissue, graft site and immune status of the recipient at time of transplantation. Although initiation of rejection in a non-sensitized recipient is principally T-cell-dependent, many components of the immune system contribute to the subsequent destruction of the transplanted tissue. Graft destruction may be alloantigen-specific, or there may be bystander tissue destruction. The nature of the immune cells involved in the effector response is reflected in the characteristics of the resulting damage and in the speed of onset of tissue destruction.

Acute antibody-mediated rejection

Alloantigen-specific antibodies or alloantibodies are secreted by plasma cells. Alloantibodies can be produced specifically following alloantigen-driven B-cell activation in the presence of T-cell help, such as can occur during rejection or following a blood transfusion. Antibodies that cross-react with alloantigens can also be generated as a result of infections that result in heterologous immunity. In the former case, in addition to DCs, the B cells themselves can act as APC. MHC class II molecules are presented to and bind to immunoglobulins on the surface of B cells enabling the B cell to internalize the alloantigen and process it into peptides that can be presented at the cell surface with MHC class II molecules to T cells (Chapter 6). The activated T cells produce cytokines that can activate the B cells enabling them to differentiate into alloantibody-producing plasma cells. When allospecific antibodies encounter their specific antigen, antibody-mediated rejection occurs. Antibody binding activates endothelial cells within the graft resulting in the expression of adhesion molecules, cytokines and chemokines and synthesis of tissue factor. Antibody binding can trigger complement activation that may result in cell lysis and graft damage directly or indirectly by the binding of complement components to the graft and the recruitment of macrophages and neutrophils to the graft. Additionally damage is caused by a second mechanism whereby effector cells such as NK cells and macrophages bind to the Fc non-antigen-specific portion of the antibody. This encourages NK cells and macrophages to kill any target cells with antibody bound to their surface. This is a non-specific process termed antibody-dependent cell-mediated cytotoxicity and can contribute to graft rejection.[14]

When donor-specific alloantibodies exist in a recipient prior to transplantation, e.g., due to previous transplant, blood transfusion or pregnancy, a dramatic response is seen on perfusion of the transplanted graft. Coagulation and complement cascades are activated resulting in extensive thrombosis and graft infarction within minutes. This so-called hyperacute rejection is now very rarely seen in clinical practice due to advances in screening and cross-matching techniques.

Acute cellular rejection

As described above, following the non-antigen specific, innate response to organ retrieval and implantation, an inflammatory environment is created within the graft thus promoting an adaptive cellular response over the ensuing days. Naïve cytotoxic T cells, activated by CD4 cells clustering with APCs, migrate to the graft where they recognize allogeneic class I MHC molecules. This causes them to release cytotoxic molecules such as perforin and granzyme B, upregulate surface Fas ligand and secrete soluble mediators such as TNF-α. Perforins insert into the target cell membrane to form pores allowing granzyme to enter the cell causing proteolysis and activating the caspase cascade. Fas ligand binds to Fas on the target cell and also initiates the caspase cascade. These processes induce target cell apoptosis and acute cellular rejection, and typically occur 1 week to 3 months after transplantation.

Additionally, a non-specific delayed-type hypersensitivity response occurs, usually mediated by CD4 cells that are attracted to the graft and involving the release of multiple proinflammatory cytokines, including Il-1, IFN-γ, and TNF-α. This leads to the recruitment and activation of further leukocytes, affects graft cell permeability and vascular smooth muscle tone so affecting graft physiology and contributing to acute and chronic rejection. CD4 alloreactive T cells responding to donor-derived peptides bound to recipient MHC class II have also been correlated with chronic allograft dysfunction.[15]

As acute allograft rejection is initiated by the recognition of polymorphic donor MHC molecules by recipient T cells, it follows that transplantation of MHC incompatible tissues will elicit a strong, T-cell-dependent immune response to donor tissues. In general, mismatches for only class I MHC result in slower rates of rejection than grafts with differences in class II MHC or both class I and II.[16] Rejection can still occur when transplantation has occurred between MHC-matched siblings due to T-cell recognition of minor histocompatibility antigens.

Chronic rejection and chronic allograft dysfunction

Chronic rejection has been mentioned previously and comprises a number of mechanisms, It is characterized by a cellular infiltrate comprised of macrophages, eosinophils, NK cells, and T cells where the primary target is the vascular endothelium.[17] Damaged endothelium allows platelet deposition on the arterial wall and growth factor production. This in turn leads to smooth muscle proliferation in the arterial wall media. Proliferating muscle cells invade the intima and contribute to intimal fibrosis. These changes are concentric, affecting all graft arteries.

Clinical implications

Clinically, acute graft rejection is suspected with a sudden deterioration in allograft function. Biopsy of the transplanted tissue is undertaken and histological evaluation performed, resulting in diagnosis of rejection and numerical grading of severity. Specific severity grading schemes, such as the Banff criteria shown in Fig. 81.4 have been developed dependent on the transplanted organ and, on the basis of this, further clinical management is guided and decisions to treat with high dose steroids or other immunosuppressive medications are made.

To prevent hyperacute rejection, patients on the transplant waiting list are monitored routinely for the development of anti-human leukocyte antigen (HLA) antibodies as a marker of sensitization. Immediately before transplantation a further check is performed by mixing recipient serum and donor splenocytes and observing for cell lysis.[18] The extent of the risk of hyperacute rejection is determined by the antibody target and quantitative titer of the anti-donor antibodies.[19] Highly sensitized recipients can remain on the waiting list for extended periods, but may be successfully transplanted following "desensitization" by removal of existing antibodies using plasma exchange or adsorption, or depletion of B cells with immunosuppressive agents such as rituximab. Despite the extensive screening performed to detect donor HLA antibodies before transplantation, preformed antibodies against donor non-MHC antigens may exist and have the ability to induce vascular rejection. There is increasing interest in determining the impact of such antibodies on graft outcome.

Acute graft rejection is suspected when there is a sudden deterioration in allograft function. Biopsy of the transplanted tissue is undertaken and histological evaluation performed, resulting in diagnosis of rejection and numerical grading of severity. Grading schemes, such as the Banff criteria, which provide semi-quantitative measures for histopathological assessment of the inflammatory response, have been developed for specific organs and form the basis on which further clinical management is guided; decisions to treat with high-dose steroids or other

1. Normal

2. Antibody-mediated rejection

Acute antibody-mediated rejection

I. ATN-like – C4d+, minimal inflammation
II. Capillary - margination and/or thromboses, C4d+
III. Arterial – v3, C4d+

Chronic active antibody-mediated rejection
Glomerular double contours and/or peritubular capillary basement membrane multilayering and/or interstitial fibrosis/tubular atrophy and/or fibrous intimal thickening in arteries, C4d

3. Borderline changes: 'suspicious' for acute T-cell-mediated rejection This category is used when no intimal arteritis is present, but there are foci of tubulitis

4. T-cell-mediated rejection

Acute T-cell-mediated rejection

IA. Cases with significant interstitial infiltration (>25% of parenchyma affected, i2 or i3) and foci of moderate tubulitis (t2)
IB. Cases with significant interstitial infiltration (>25% of parenchyma affected, i2 or i3) and foci of severe tubulitis (t3)
IIA. Cases with mild to moderate intimal arteritis (v1)
IIB. Cases with severe intimal arteritis comprising >25% of the luminal area (v2)
III. Cases with 'transmural' arteritis and/or arterial fibrinoid change and necrosis of medial smooth muscle cells with accompanying lymphocytic inflammation (v3)

Chronic active T-cell-mediated rejection
'Chronic allograft arteriopathy' (arterial intimal fibrosis with mononuclear cell infiltration in fibrosis, formation of neo-intima)

5. Interstitial fibrosis and tubular atrophy, no evidence of any specific etiology

I. Mild interstitial fibrosis and tubular atrophy (<25% of cortical area)
II. Moderate interstitial fibrosis and tubular atrophy (26–50% of cortical area)
III. Severe interstitial fibrosis and tubular atrophy/loss (>50% of cortical area) (may include non-specific vascular and glomerular sclerosis, but severity graded by tubulointerstitial features)

6. Other: Changes not considered to be due to rejection-acute and/or chronic

Fig. 81.4 Banff diagnostic criteria for renal allografts. Histological criteria have been developed and are regularly reviewed to aid diagnosis of the cause of chronic allograft dysfunction. Determining the cause of dysfunction aids decision-making regarding pathology and management.

immunosuppressive medications can thus be made following structured analysis of a transplant biopsy.

In addition to the diagnosis of cell-mediated rejection, modern staining techniques have enabled the identification of complement component 4d (C4d) in biopsy specimens from rejecting tissues, thus providing indirect evidence of antibody deposition and complement fixation in not only late but also early rejection. Antibody-mediated rejection is frequently seen following heart, lung, and kidney transplantation; however, greater resilience appears to be observed in liver allografts.[20] This is explored further in the discussion below on tolerance in the liver (see Fig. 81.7).

Although improved immunosuppression regimens have led to a reduction in the occurrence of acute rejection, chronic rejection has become more evident and remains a significant contributor to late graft loss. Non-immunological factors, including calcineurin inhibitor- induced toxicity, advanced donor age, ischemic injury during implantation, hypertension and infection, also contribute to chronic allograft dysfunction, and modifying these factors can improve graft outcome.[21] However, immunological processes play a significant role with increased levels of pre-transplant anti-HLA antibodies, de novo post-transplant donor-specific antibodies and antibodies against non-HLA antigen

MHC class I polypeptide-related sequence A (MICA) being seen to affect allograft survival.

The correlation between late acute rejection, chronic allograft dysfunction and graft loss has been consistently reported and there is increasing evidence that subclinical rejection may represent an important factor in predicting graft loss.[22] Establishing a clear link between subclinical rejection and development of chronic allograft dysfunction may be difficult, however, due to the interplay of other factors, including calcineurin toxicity.[21]

Immunosuppression

In recent years, substantial advances in immunosuppressive strategies and their translation to routine clinical practice have revolutionized management and outcomes in solid organ transplantation (SOT); an option that has become the therapy of choice for many end-stage organ diseases. Short-term outcomes such as patient and allograft survival at 1 year, acute rejection rates as well as time-course of disease progression and symptom-control have steadily improved since the first successful transplants performed over 50 years ago.

Fig. 81.5 Current immunosuppressive drugs and their targets. Signal 1 results from MHC:antigen recognition through the TCR:CD3 complex, a process blocked by anti-CD3 mAbs & indirectly by Rituximab. **Signal 2** results in co-stimulation, a process which can be blocked by Belatacept. Co-stimulation results in full activation of the TCR:CD3 complex, initiating signal transduction, **Signal 3:** Downstream signalling pathways result in calcineurin activation, a stage which can be inhibited by Tacrolimus & Cyclosporine. Activated calcineurin dephosphorylates NF-AT, allowing IL-2 transcription, a process which can be inhibited by steroids. IL-2 receptor stimulation, a step which can be blocked by Basiliximab, activates the mTOR signalling cascade, which can be inhibited by Sirolimus. This pathway induces the T cell to enter cell cycle & proliferate, which in turn can be blocked by Mycophenolate & Azathioprine. rATG exerts polyclonal affects while Alemtuzumab binds to CD52, both resulting in immunodepletion

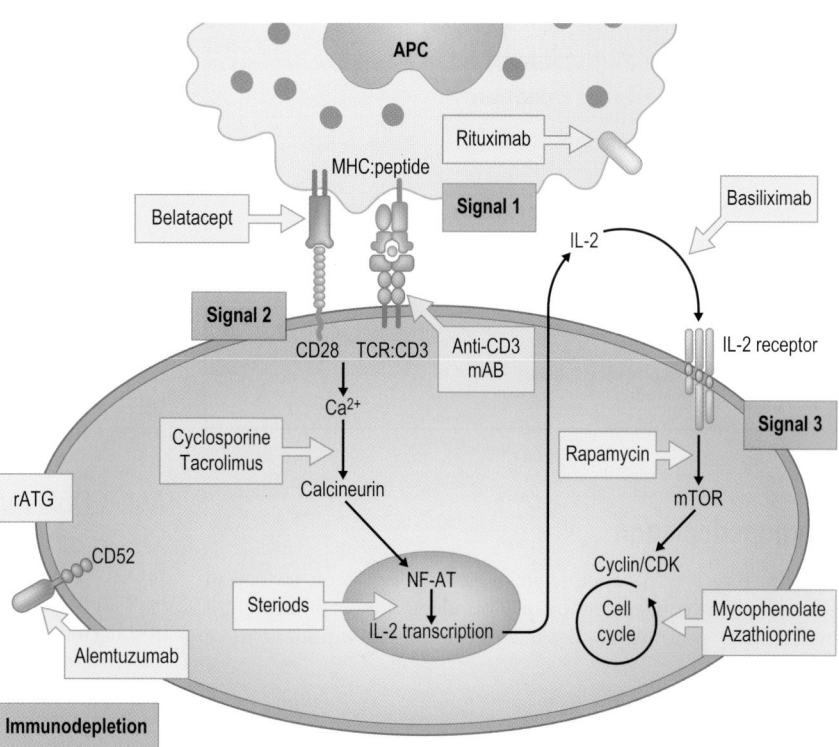

Therapeutic regimens implemented in clinic today are focused on targeting the various steps involved in the T-cell-mediated immune response to alloantigen. As outlined earlier, there are three main stages in this pathway, namely recognition of allo- or self-antigen, co-stimulation, and proliferation/differentiation of effector T cells. The current clinical paradigm is based on blockade of at least one of these stages and/or by total immuno-depletion therapy as well as by alterations in lymphocyte trafficking (Fig. 81.5).

The risk of acute graft rejection is greatest during the initial three months following transplantation; therefore current immunosuppression strategies are primarily based on a potent induction regimen using a monoclonal or polyclonal antibody, followed by "maintenance immunosuppression" often consisting of calcineurin inhibitors (CNIs—cyclosporine or tacrolimus), an antiproliferative agent (mycophenolate mofetil, MMF), and low-dose corticosteroids (prednisolone). Provided there are no episodes of acute rejection, the doses of these agents are gradually reduced and then maintenance immunosuppression is continued indefinitely (Fig. 81.6). This dose reduction is based on the concept that as graft inflammation subsides and donor-derived APCs are cleared, the immunogenicity and risk of rejection decreases.

Chronic immunosuppression is associated with several undesirable sequelae (Table 82.1), in particular an increased relative risk of infections and malignancy, cardiovascular morbidity (the leading cause of death with a functioning graft in transplant recipients), and target organ damage.

Many different immunosuppressive regimens for SOT are in clinical use, and a detailed discussion of these is beyond the scope of this chapter. What follows is an introduction to the immunosuppressive agents in widespread use currently.

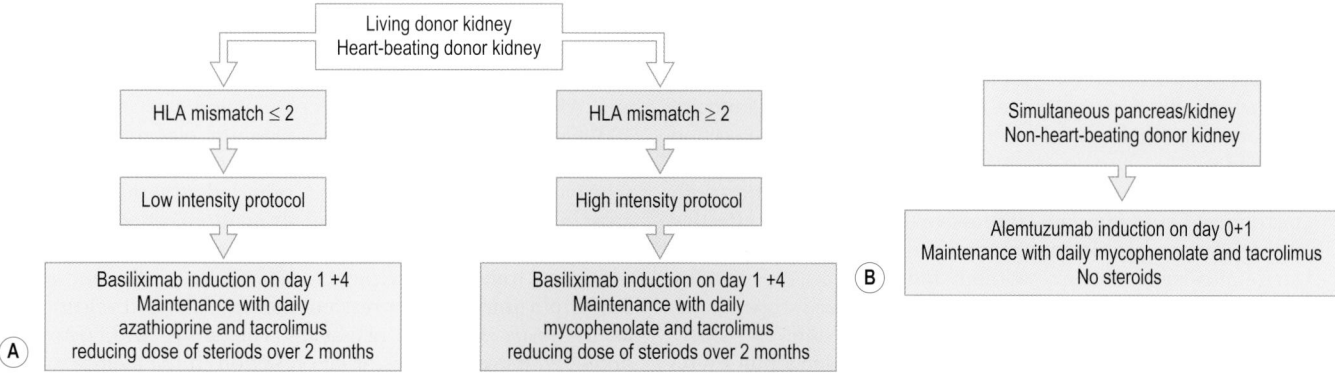

Fig. 81.6 Examples of immunosuppressive protocols in clinical use* (A) Patients receiving a renal transplant from a living donor or heart-beating donor are stratified according to HLA Mismatch. When HLA mismatch $\leq$ 2, the patient is treated with a low intensity protocol; When HLA mismatch $\geq$ 2, the patient is treated with a high intensity protocol. (B) Pancreas and non-heart-beating donor kidneys have higher immunogenicity and so induction is with a potent monoclonal antibody, Alemtuzumab; therefore steroids are not required. *Simplefied oxford transplant centre protocol.*

Treatment options for rejection

Acute cellular rejection
• High dose steroids

Rejection refractory to steroid treatment
• Anti-thymocyte globulin
• Alemtuzumab

Acute humoral rejection
• Plasmapharesis
• Intravenous immunoglobulin
• Rituximab

Immunodepletion

The more recent therapeutic strategies are based on induction therapies that concentrate on profound immune cell depletion at the time of transplant, when immune activation is most intense.

Anti-thymocyte globulin (ATG)

rATG (rabbit-derived) is a lymphocyte-depleting polyclonal IgG preparation with specificity towards human thymocytes. It binds primarily to peripheral blood lymphocytes, as well as to those from lymph nodes, spleen and thymus as demonstrated by *in vivo* studies in monkeys. The agent's polyclonal nature enables it to display specificity towards a wide variety of antigens expressed on the surface of T cells, B cells, DCs, NK cells, and endothelial cells, including those antigens involved in T-cell activation, proliferation, apoptosis, signal transduction, cell adhesion and trafficking.

The precise mechanism of action underlying the immunosuppressive efficacy of rATG in SOT recipients is unknown at present, although has been primarily attributed to T-cell depletion. Data from *in vitro* studies suggest that rATG modulates the expression of various lymphocyte surface antigens resulting in apoptosis, antibody-dependent cytolysis or complement-dependent lysis. Lymphocyte depletion with rATG has been further demonstrated in adult renal transplant patients in several randomized, comparative clinical studies, with repopulation reported to take at least 3 months.[23] More recently, data from preclinical and clinical studies suggest that rATG therapy may induce the expansion and enrichment of certain Treg subsets, such as CD4+CD25+ Forkhead box P3+ (FOXP3+), CTLA-4+, and glucocorticoid-induced TNF receptor+ Treg cells from human peripheral blood lymphocytes or peripheral blood mononuclear cells *in vitro*;[24] these Treg subsets are key to immune response modulation and are further discussed in the section Tolerance.

In terms of clinical use, rATG induction in combination with tacrolimus-based immunosuppressive therapy is more effective in preventing episodes of acute renal graft rejection than with tacrolimus-based therapy without induction, as reported by primary endpoint data from two, randomized, open-label, multicenter trials.[25,26] Moreover, the median time to biopsy-proven acute rejection (BPAR) was >1 week longer in rATG induction than in non-induction recipients; however, it should be noted that there was no significant difference between induction and non-induction regimens in terms of patient or graft survival.

Several randomized, multicenter studies report that the efficacy of rATG induction therapy is generally no different from that of basiliximab or low-dose daclizumab (IL-2R monoclonal antibodies, which are an alternative induction agent discussed later in this section) with regard to the incidence of BPAR, graft loss or death at 6 and 12 months post-transplantation, in the context of renal transplant recipients receiving triple immunosuppressive maintenance therapy. These trials, however, were not powered to show overall superiority of one agent over the other, were powered to address safety rather than efficacy parameters or used a limited daclizumab dosage regimen.[24] More robust studies are needed that are designed to evaluate the efficacy of rATG relative to IL-2R monoclonal antibodies (mAbs) specifically, in order to definitively establish the use of rATG with respect to these monoclonal agents.

Anti-CD52 mAb (alemtuzumab)

Anti-CD52 monoclonal antibody (alemtuzumab) is a humanized rat IgG2b directed against the CD52 antigen, which is expressed on 95% of peripheral blood lymphocytes, NK cells, macrophages and thymocytes;[27] thus almost all mononuclear cells are affected. The profound and long-lasting lymphopenia produced after the administration of one or two doses of alemtuzumab is probably partly explained by such abundance on monocyte cell surfaces. It should be noted that examination of peripheral blood lymphocytes from human recipients post-alemtuzumab induction has identified a subset of T cells, predominantly CD4 central memory cells that survive despite alemtuzumab induction and appear largely resistant to depletion; these memory T cells were found to express lower CD52 levels than naïve T cells.[28,29] CD52 is not present on granulocytes, platelets, erythrocytes, or hematopoietic stem cells.

After binding to CD52, alemtuzumab causes cell death through several mechanisms: complement-mediated cytolysis, antibody-mediated cytotoxicity and apoptosis. While the plasma elimination half-life is approximately 12 days, its clinical effects are far more persistent. Lymphocyte depletion of >99% can be seen after a single dose, with lymph node depletion taking up to 3–5 days compared with <1 hour seen in peripheral lymphocytes. Different subpopulations display varying rates of recovery depending on the subpopulation of interest: NK cells are almost unaffected and decrease only transiently (a population of CD52⁻ NK cells has also been identified); monocytes and B-cell recovery can be seen at 3 and 12 months, respectively; T cells levels recover to only 50% of baseline at 36 months.[30]

Alemtuzumab is being used with increasing frequency for induction in SOT, with the aim of minimizing maintenance immunosuppression. It was first used in transplantation as an induction agent in 1998,[31] in 13 renal transplant recipients who received low-dose cyclosporine alone as maintenance therapy. At 6–12 months follow-up, patient and graft survival were 100% and there were 2 episodes of acute rejection. The 5-year results of the initial series,[32] together with another 20 patients who were subsequently enrolled, reported no significant difference in graft or patient survival, or acute rejection rates when compared to a retrospective, contemporaneous control group of 66 renal transplant recipients who had received no induction, but triple immunosuppression therapy alone (cyclosporine, azathioprine and prednisolone). The study did also find, however, more episodes of late rejection in the alemtuzumab-treated group. Indeed, severe lymphopenia and homeostatic cytokines are known to drive the rapid homeostatic proliferation of naïve and memory T cells, and lymphocytes generated under such conditions have been previously found to be potent alloreactive cells, inevitably triggering rejection in animal models.[33] Investigation of this phenomenon in human recipients[28] illustrated that the recovery of the immune system post-alemtuzumab induction differed with respect to CD4 and CD8 T cells. While CD8 T cells recovered to pre-transplant levels by 6 months after alemtuzumab induction, the number of CD4 T cells remained low, even at 1-year post-transplant. Re-populating CD8 T cells were mainly of the immunosenescent CD28- CD8+ phenotype, and the percentage of this population was lower in those recipients who underwent rejection compared to those who did not mount an immune response to allograft. A series of *in vitro* experiments demonstrated that the expanded CD28- CD8+ T cells compete for immune space with CD4 T cells, suppressing their proliferation and therefore delaying CD4 T-cell recovery. This delay might be associated with the clinical outcome as CD4 T cells, notably CD4 T effector memory cells, have been shown to be associated with rejection.[34]

Despite considerable experience with this agent, largely in renal transplantation, there are few, relatively small randomized controlled trials available and thus interpretation of evidence is limited. In two such widely cited studies,[35,36] acute rejection rates, renal function, and patient and graft survival in alemtuzumab-treated recipients were comparable to other induction or no-induction regimens at up to 15 months follow-up. In addition, up to 80% of alemtuzumab-treated recipients remained steroid free. Subsequent randomized trials and larger retrospective studies corroborate these earlier findings, supporting the use of alemtuzumab as an induction agent with corticosteroid-free/withdrawal regimens.[37] However, similar to ATG, alemtuzumab cannot be used as a solitary immunosuppressive therapy, and requires chronic maintenance immunosuppression to prevent allograft rejection. Furthermore, recent work has demonstrated that patients with preformed donor-specific antibody (DSAb) despite a negative crossmatch, are at high risk of adverse outcomes when receiving a minimal immunosuppressive regime incorporating alemtuzumab induction; these patients may thus benefit from augmented immunosuppression.[38]

Review of rejection episodes which have occurred with alemtuzumab induction, particularly in the absence of CNIs, has highlighted some interesting findings. Several authors have reported that a number of these rejections demonstrate positive staining for C4d, indicative of acute antibody-mediated rejection. Furthermore, examination of acute rejection biopsies taken from patients who have received both alemtuzumab induction and tacrolimus, revealed none that were humoral in origin.[27] Immune profiles of renal transplant recipients receiving alemtuzumab induction, 60 days of a CNI and subsequent sirolimus monotherapy displayed a general increase in the naïve B-cell population.[39] Bloom et al. subsequently showed that B-cell activating factor (BAFF), a B-cell survival cytokine influencing the threshold of B-cell activation, substantially increased in renal transplantation following treatment with alemtuzumab.[40] This observation may, in fact, explain the prevalent development of alloantibody in patients treated with depleting antibody therapy at the time of SOT.

Signal 1: Blockade of antigen recognition

Activation of the rejection response to an allograft hinges on the recognition of antigen by the host immune system. Targeting signal 1 through the use of monoclonal antibodies has been used in both transplantation and autoimmunity.

Anti-CD3 mAb

Muromonab-CD3 (OKT3), a mouse mAb binding to the CD3 component of the TCR signal-transduction complex, has been successfully used as an induction agent for high-risk patients or for the treatment of corticosteroid-resistant acute rejection episodes. However, severe adverse effects of muromonab-CD3 such as cytokine-release syndrome (owing to the propensity of muromonab-CD3 to initially activate T cells, releasing TNF-α and IL-2) have now resulted in preference for rATG and anti-CD52 agents. Furthermore, OKT3 treatment may be limited by host production of human anti-mouse antibodies (HAMA) that bind to circulating reagent molecules, neutralizing their activity. Non-activating, therefore less toxic, humanized Fc-receptor-non-binding anti-CD3 mAbs, such as teplizumab and visilizumab, are currently being tested in phase I and II clinical trials in autoimmune disease settings (type 1 diabetes, Crohn's disease) as well as in renal and pancreatic islet transplantation.[41] Indeed, recent studies have suggested a further mechanism of action regarding anti-CD3 antibodies: circulating CD8 T cells isolated from type I diabetic patients, after treatment with anti-CD3 mAb, may have regulatory function *ex vivo*; recent data have demonstrated functional human CD8 Treg *in vivo* after administration of anti-CD3 mAb.[42] Further work is needed to elucidate the action of such agents on the immune response, in order to realize their full potential.

Anti-CD20 mAb (rituximab)

Rituximab is an anti-CD20, chimeric mAb that eliminates most B cells from the circulation. Originally approved to treat B-cell lymphoproliferative diseases in non-transplant patients as well as post-transplant lymphoproliferative disease (PTLD), it is also now used in SOT as a treatment of antibody-mediated rejection and to desensitize patients who are receiving ABO-incompatible transplants or re-transplants. Depletion of antibody-producing cells may be incomplete, however, as rituximab cannot target CD20+ plasmacytes. It has been hypothesized that the action of rituximab in allograft rejection is not only due to depletion of plasma cells, but to the effective depletion of APCs, which thus limits indirect pathway T-cell activation and a sustained immune response. Clinical administration is in conjunction with maintenance immunosuppressive agents, plasmapheresis, intravenous immunoglobulin and even splenectomy in some protocols.[43]

Recent work with non-human primate (NHP) models has shown that pre-emptive B-cell depletion with rituximab prevents both acute cellular rejection and antibody-mediated rejection of cardiac allograft: alloantibody was prevented from developing in the blood, and complement-mediated graft injury was avoided. Not only was the B-cell response inhibited, but acute cellular rejection was also reduced by the combination of cyclosporine and rituximab, suggesting that B cells may play a role in acute cellular rejection as well. There may be a role for targeting B cells pre-emptively in SOT, and additional strategies to downregulate the B-cell response are under evaluation. Promising targets include BAFF and its receptor, as well as co-stimulatory molecules such as CD28, CD154, and CD40.[44]

Signal 2: Blockade of co-stimulation

In the absence of appropriate co-stimulation, partially activated T cells either become hyporesponsive to subsequent antigen-specific TCR signals (donor-specific anergy) or die by apoptosis. The inhibition of full T-cell activation by co-stimulatory blockade rather than total T-cell depletion might more selectively target effector T cells and spare beneficial Treg cells, while avoiding the many adverse effects of non-specific immunodepletion.

CD28:B7 (CD80/CD86) blockade

CTLA-4 is an inducible, T-cell surface antigen that when bound to CD80/86 receptor:ligand (B7 molecules) on APCs, delivers inhibitory signals to the activated T cell. Belatacept (LEA29Y) is a fusion protein combining the extracellular binding domain of CTLA-4 with the Fc portion of IgG1, with specificity for CD80/86 expressed on APCs. Ligation of CD80/86 by CD28 (a surface antigen constitutively expressed on T cells) usually lowers the activation threshold of T cells. Belatacept has a higher affinity and slower dissociation rate from human B7 molecules (i.e., CD80/86) than CD28, resulting in inhibition of the co-stimulation required for effective T-cell activation.[43]

The complexities of the human immune system present significant difficulties to the translation of such agents into clinical practice: *in vivo* work indicates memory and cytotoxic CD8 T cells have different co-stimulation requirements for complete activation when compared with CD4 naïve T cells and may therefore be more resistant to some tolerance induction strategies. Such blockade may also affect the function of Treg as the CD28:B7 pathway has been shown to be important for the expansion and survival of Tregs. However, reassuringly, data from a phase II belatacept renal transplant study, albeit with small patient numbers, indicates that co-stimulation blockade does not interfere with Treg homeostasis.[45,46]

In NHP models, CTLA-4 immunoglobulin prolonged pancreatic islet survival, and in combination with CD154:CD40 pathway blockade, induced indefinite acceptance of renal and heart allograft. Phase II clinical trials with belatacept report promising short-term results, in terms of efficacy and safety within the first year in SOT, but longer follow-up data are needed to establish this agent's ability to prevent chronic allograft dysfunction or to induce tolerance. BENEFIT (belatacept evaluation of nephroprotection and efficacy as first line immunosuppression trial) is a 3-year, Phase III clinical trial that randomized patients to three groups: cyclosporine, less-intensive belatacept, and more-intensive belatacept. Patients received induction with basiliximab and were maintained on MMF and corticosteroids. Patient and graft survival were similar across the three groups at both one and two years post-transplant. At the end of one year, although the incidence of acute rejection was greater for more-intensive and less-intensive belatacept compared with cyclosporine, no apparent impact on graft survival was demonstrated. At the end of two years, however, glomerular filtration rate continued to be significantly higher (15–17 mL/min) in the belatacept-treated patients. Encouragingly, belatacept-treated patients also had sustained benefits in their cardiovascular and metabolic risk profile in comparison to cyclosporine, supporting the potential role of belatacept as a non-nephrotoxic alternative to CNIs.[47,48] Longer term data are needed to evaluate further chronic renal function and the incidence of chronic allograft dysfunction, as well as studies comparing belatacept to tacrolimus, an agent that has largely become the CNI of choice in recent years.

Owing to concerns about an increased PTLD risk in Epstein–Barr virus (EBV)-seronegative patients, current belatacept trial protocols have now been modified to enrol EBV-seropositive patients only. Unfortunately, this exclusion will complicate the introduction of this drug for young patients, who might derive the maximum long-term benefit from non-nephrotoxic regimens. A significant limitation to note is that administration of belatacept requires an intravenous infusion; this is not an ideal characteristic for a maintenance immunosuppressant and raises issues of patient compliance. Indeed, patient non-compliance has become the third leading cause of graft loss in renal transplantation in some series, after chronic allograft nephropathy and death with a functioning graft.[49] Furthermore, the agent has a long half-life of 8–10 days and so may be difficult to appropriately titrate in transplant recipients suffering with life-threatening infections.

Signal 3: Blockade of proliferation/differentiation

Activated T cells produce IL-2 which in turn binds to IL-2 receptors (IL-2Rs) that are expressed only on the surface of activated cells and are not present on resting T cells. IL-2R is composed of three high-affinity transmembrane protein subunits: α- (CD25), β- (CD122), and γ- (CD132) subunits, which are covalently linked. The α-subunit is specific to IL-2R only, and it is the binding of α- and β-subunits that is crucial to the IL-2 signal transduction and T-cell activation that subsequently leads to proliferation and clonal expansion of T and B cells specific to allo- or self-antigen. These cells are also stimulated to release more IL-2, further magnifying the immune response.

Anti-IL-2R mAb (basiliximab and daclizumab)

Basiliximab (chimeric form) and daclizumab (humanized form) are now commonly used in renal transplantation in low-risk recipients (as defined as first allograft, living-related donor, no delayed graft function).[50,51] As these drugs specifically target activated T cells, they do not cause significant lymphocyte depletion and are not associated with major adverse effects when compared to lymphocyte-depleting agents. However, it is important to remember that other types of T cells, including Treg cells, also express CD25 and therefore the use of these agents may also impact some of the natural mechanisms of immunoregulation.

Basiliximab binds to IL-2R with similar affinity as IL-2, thereby effectively competing with IL-2 and subsequently inhibiting IL-2 driven T-cell proliferation. Basiliximab has a high volume of distribution, almost completely saturating IL-2R on peripheral lymphocytes within 24 hours of a single dose of 2.5–25 mg in renal transplant recipients. The half-life in adults is approximately 13.4 days, and IL-2R saturation and suppression can last for 4–6 weeks.

Two meta-analyses evaluating the efficacy and safety of basiliximab in renal transplant recipients have been published.[51,52] Both studies showed that basiliximab was more effective than placebo in reducing acute cellular rejection 6 months after transplantation. However, both meta-analyses illustrated no significant differences in patient or graft survival rates between basiliximab and placebo groups at 1 year after transplantation. These findings are echoed in other randomized, double-blind placebo-controlled trials.

Several randomized trials have examined the safety profile of basiliximab, and have all reported no significant difference in type, incidence and severity of adverse events in patients who received basiliximab compared with placebo. The mAb is minimally immunogenic and rates of adverse events, malignancy and infection are all comparable to placebo, and even reduced when compared to other induction agents. However, studies involving high-risk transplant recipients comparing basiliximab to other induction agents such as rATG, indicate that while incidence of acute rejection is comparable with IL-2R mAb and rATG in kidney transplant recipients at low-immunological risk, the risk of rejection may be higher with IL-2R mAb in patients at high risk (i.e., high HLA-mismatch).[53]

Table 81.1 Immunosuppressive therapies in transplantation: maintenance and induction agents

Drugs	Mechanisms	Adverse effects
Maintenance agents		
Azathioprine	Inhibits purine & DNA synthesis, inhibits cell proliferation	Bone marrow depression, opportunistic infection, macrocytosis, liver toxicity
Cyclosporine	Binds to cyclophilin, inhibits calcineurin-phosphatase, blocks NF-AT dephosphorylation, blocks IL-2 transcription & T-cell activation	Hypertension, hyperlipidemia, nephrotoxicity, hepatotoxicity, pancreatitis, peptic ulcers, thrombotic microangiopathy, opportunistic infection, neurotoxicity, tremor, gingival hyperplasia, hirsutism
Mycophenolate mofetil	Inhibits inosine-monophosphate-dehydrogenase, inhibits purine synthesis & blocks cell proliferation	Gastrointestinal symptoms, bone marrow depression, opportunistic infection in particular CMV & BK nephropathy
Rapamycin	Binds to FKBP12, inhibits mTOR & blocks IL-2-driven cell proliferation	Delayed graft function, delayed wound healing, mouth ulcers, pneumonitis, increased proteinuria, peripheral edema, hyperlipidemia
Steroids	Induces phospholipase A_2 inhibitory proteins, inhibits arachidonic acid synthesis, inhibits prostaglandins & leukotrienes	Diabetes, delayed wound healing, peptic ulcers, psychosis, osteoporosis, infection, blurred vision, fluid retention, weight gain, acne, constipation
Tacrolimus	Binds to FKBP12, inhibits calcineurin-phosphatase and blocks T-cell activation	Post-transplantation diabetes mellitus, nephrotoxicity, thrombotic microangiopathy, neurotoxicity
Induction agents		
Anti-thymocyte globulin	Polyclonal effects not well characterized; immunosuppressive efficacy attributed to T cell depletion through apoptosis, antibody-dependent cytolysis and complement-dependent lysis	Polyclonal effects: Cytokine release syndrome, serum sickness, leukopenia, thrombocytopenia. De novo tumors & opportunistic infection: CMV & HSV.
Alemtuzumab	Binds to CD52 Ag, (expressed on 95% of peripheral blood lymphocytes, NK cells, macrophages & thymocytes). Results in profound lymphopenia.	Opportunistic infection: disseminated candidal & CMV infection
Basiliximab	Binds to IL-2R with similar affinity as IL-2, thereby inhibiting IL-2-driven T cell proliferation	Occasional hypersensitivity reactions, inadequate immunosuppression in immunologically high-risk recipients

IL-2, interleukin-2; NF-AT, nuclear factor of activated T cells; DHFR, dihydrofolate reductase; mTOR, mammalian target of rapamycin; CMV, cytomegalovirus; HSV, herpes simplex virus.

The highly selective and short-term immunosuppressive effects of basiliximab, which are confined to the highly immunogenic period immediately post-transplantation, makes this class of drug a useful substitute to steroids in early steroid-withdrawal/steroid-free regimens, as illustrated in studies with liver transplantation. Several prospective clinical trials using basiliximab induction to facilitate early steroid withdrawal or complete steroid avoidance after kidney transplantation were tried and proven safe. However, similar to alemtuzumab, the use of complete CNI avoidance protocols should be practiced with extreme caution; in several studies that withheld CNIs for any more than a very short period, despite adequate immunosuppression with IL-2R mAbs, MMF, and steroids, the acute cellular rejection rates after renal transplantation were much higher than with CNI use.[54] Thus, in kind with ATG and alemtuzumab, patients receiving basiliximab are still exposed to chronic administration of maintenance immunosuppression and its associated comorbidities.

Glucocorticoids

Corticosteroids were developed in the 1950s and have complex immunosuppressive as well as anti-inflammatory effects (Chapter 87). They act principally by binding to cytoplasmic glucocorticoid receptors, although at higher doses they can exhibit receptor-independent effects as well. The steroid–receptor complex translocates to the nucleus where it is able to alter the expression of multiple cytokines through DNA-binding and by targeting transcription factors such as AP-1 and NF-κB. Corticosteroids reduce the expression of many molecules important in the immune response including IL-1, -2, -3, and -6, TNF-α, IFN-γ, and chemokines. By inhibiting cyclooxygenase, corticosteroids are also able to reduce the production of inflammatory mediators such as leukotrienes and prostaglandins.

Corticosteroids have been the mainstay of maintenance immunosuppression regimens for several decades. However, due to the agents' wide-ranging effects, not only involving the immune response but also a multitude of organ systems (including nephrotoxic and diabetes-inducing properties, which can adversely affect a target allograft), modern immunosuppressive regimens look to avoid or withdraw corticosteroids at the earliest possible moment post-transplantation (Table 81.1).

Antiproliferative agents

Azathioprine and MMF interfere with DNA synthesis and prevent cell cycle progression. In the context of allograft rejection this impairs the clonal expansion of alloreactive T cells.

The introduction of azathioprine into clinical practice in the 1960s and its use in conjunction with corticosteroids allowed transplantation to progress from an experimental procedure into a practical therapy for patients with organ failure. It is metabolized in the liver to the purine analogue 6-mercaptopurine and incorporated into DNA. By inhibiting purine nucleotide synthesis (and therefore DNA and RNA synthesis), azathioprine reduces gene transcription and prevents cell cycle progression. The effects of azathioprine are not lymphocyte-specific and patients must be monitored closely for bone marrow suppression.

MMF is metabolized in the liver to mycophenolic acid, which is a non-competitive, reversible inhibitor of inosine monophosphate dehydrogenase (IMPDH). Cells are able to generate purines either *de novo* by converting inosine monophosphate to guanosine monophosphate (catalysed by IMPDH) or from guanine via the salvage pathway. The salvage pathway is less active in lymphocytes and therefore they are relatively dependent on the *de novo* pathway of purine synthesis compared to other cell types. As a result the effects of MMF are more lymphocyte-specific than azathioprine and it is less myelosuppressive. Both agents are commonly used in modern maintenance immunosuppression regimens.

Calcineurin inhibitors (CNIs)

The introduction of cyclosporine in the early 1980s presented a great step forward in transplant immunosuppression as this was the first drug able to selectively block T-cell activation. Subsequently a second CNI, the macrolide antibiotic tacrolimus, has also been developed. Similar to corticosteroids, CNIs have become a principle agent in maintenance immunosuppressive regimens: by the end of 2007, almost 99% of renal transplant recipients were discharged on CNIs.[55] Both cyclosporine and tacrolimus bind cytoplasmic immunophilins (cyclophilin in the case of cyclosporine and FK506-binding protein 12 (FKBP12) in the case of tacrolimus) to form complexes that can inhibit the calcium-dependent phosphatase calcineurin, a rate limiting enzyme in the T-cell receptor signal transduction pathway. By preventing translocation of the transcription factor NFAT to the nucleus, calcineurin inhibition impairs upregulation of many molecules important for T-cell proliferation and the generation of an effective immune response including the cytokines IL-2, IL-4, TNF-α, and IFN-γ and co-stimulatory molecules such as CD154 (CD40L). However, CNIs are well known for their nephrotoxic properties, and are thought to be major contributors to chronic allograft dysfunction (a leading cause of graft failure) in renal transplantation. Thus modern immunosuppressive regimens are looking to minimize or even replace this drug class with less harmful yet equally effective agents.

mTOR inhibitors

Sirolimus (rapamycin) and everolimus bind to the same immunophilin as tacrolimus (FKBP12) although the complexes they form are unable to interact with calcineurin. Instead they bind to the regulatory kinase mammalian target of rapamycin (mTOR), which has a critical role in cytokine receptor signal transduction. The usual actions of mTOR are to activate the ribosomal enzyme p70 S6 kinase and block an inhibitory protein 4E-BP1, both of which are required for translation of proteins necessary for progression from the G_1 (growth) phase to the S (DNA synthesis) phase of the cell cycle. Therefore inhibition of this pathway in T cells blocks the action of cytokines such as IL-2, -4, and -15, preventing cell cycle progression and clonal expansion.

In addition to inhibiting clonal expansion of effector T cells, there is growing evidence supporting the role of rapamycin in promoting the generation of Treg, which have been shown in several animal models to be capable of preventing allograft rejection.[56] For instance, rapamycin promotes the *de novo* conversion of alloantigen-specific Treg.[44] This is contrast to CNIs, which inhibit such conversion. This property makes rapamycin an attractive agent to potentially promote tolerance as discussed further in the following section.

Tolerance

Billingham, Brent and Medawar first introduced the term transplantation tolerance in 1953, with the report that inoculation of fetal mice with lymphoid cells from an allogeneic adult donor mouse of a different strain led to later acceptance of skin grafts from the original donors of skin graft:[57] seminal work for which Medawar received the Nobel Prize for Medicine in 1960. Murray and colleagues went on to perform the first successful renal transplant on the Herrick twins in 1954.[1] As a result of the genetic identity between the brothers, the recipient receives no immunosuppression after the operation, thus representing the very first case of clinical tolerance in humans, in the field of solid organ transplantation.

● THERAPEUTIC PRINCIPLES

Mechanisms of tolerance

Deletion

Deletion of allo- or auto-reactive T cells can be achieved centrally in the thymus or in the periphery. Infusion of donor bone marrow into a recipient who has been conditioned by non-myeloablative irradiation or immunotherapy enables APCs to access the thymus and trigger the deletion of maturing thymocytes. In the periphery, deletion can be triggered by alloantigen recognition under suboptimal conditions, including co-stimulation blockade, as well as immunodepletion by activation of apoptotic cell death and cytolysis.

Anergy

This is the functional inactivation of the T-cell response to restimulation by allo- or self-antigen, and has been described both *in vivo* and *in vitro*. Some forms of T cell anergy are also reported to result in the development of regulatory activity. Co-stimulation blockade, as well as inhibition of downstream proliferative pathways can trigger anergic states in T cells.

Immunoregulation

This active process results in the regulation of one cell population by the activity of another cell population. Various populations of leukocytes have been described as having the ability to control immune responsiveness to alloantigen stimulation in both the innate and adaptive immune responses. This mechanism, although well described in experimental models, is yet to be introduced therapeutically in a sustained, clinical setting.

Clonal exhaustion

This can occur as a result of chronic antigen stimulation or antigen recognition under suboptimal conditions. The consequence is either deletion or functional inactivation of the cells responding to the recognized antigen. An example of such exhaustion can be seen in liver transplantation, where the large number of donor-derived APCs migrating from the liver to draining lymphoid tissues after transplantation can trigger this type of response.

Ignorance

This is an uncommon mechanism in the induction phase of unresponsiveness to alloantigen as it is difficult to introduce donor cells or tissue without alerting the immune system to their presence, in transplantation. This mechanism, however, does describe the natural state of some self-reactive CD4 T-cell populations found in healthy individuals with no autoimmune pathology.

Technically, the condition in which an SOT recipient exhibits a well-functioning graft and lacks histological signs of rejection after receiving no immunosuppression for at least 1 year is referred to as *clinical operational tolerance* (COT).[58] Importantly, the patient in question is an immune-competent host capable of responding to other immune challenges, including infections. Over recent years, experimental models have shown that it is possible to exploit the processes by which immune homeostasis and tolerance to self-antigens are maintained in order to induce tolerance to alloantigen (Chapter 12). The optimal outcome for patients after transplantation would be to harness these mechanisms to induce specific immunological unresponsiveness or tolerance to the graft, thus avoiding the adverse side effects associated with current immunosuppressive regimens (Table 81.1).

Unfortunately, more than 5 decades of clinical experience in SOT have demonstrated that COT in humans is extremely difficult to achieve. Many successful experimental techniques can produce durable hyporesponsiveness to mismatched allografts in rodent models, but so far few of these have been successfully translated into large animal models or clinical trials. Progress in the field of transplantation tolerance is also hampered by the lack of definitive laboratory parameters able to give a clear indication of whether a particular recipient is tolerant of his or her graft. Furthermore, COT appears to be somewhat organ dependent. Recipients of a liver graft are more capable of developing COT because of the immune-privileged status of the liver (Fig. 81.7). Clinical experience in liver transplantation now demonstrates clear evidence that a permanent and stable immunosuppressive-free state can be safely attempted and sometimes achieved in patients who have received a liver transplant for non-immunological liver diseases.[59] However, COT has never been reported after intestinal, islet or whole organ pancreas transplantation, whereas two exceptional cases of COT have been described after lung and heart transplantation.[60,61] Since the first renal transplant over 55 years ago, only sporadic cases of COT have been documented after renal transplantation in the absence of genetic identity between donor and recipient.[59]

● CLINICAL PEARLS

Liver transplantation

- Positive cross-match or blood type incompatibility has little effect on graft survival.
- HLA-matching is not a prerequisite to liver transplantation.
- Reduced incidence of hyperacute rejection compared to other organs in solid organ transplantation.
- Frequent spontaneous recovery after severe rejection.
- Acute rejection does not impact severely on long-term graft and patient survival.
- Liver allograft protects other extra-hepatic allograft from rejection if derived from the same donor.
- Lower overall incidence of chronic rejection that is reversible in up to 30% cases.
- Clinical operational tolerance has been achieved most reliably and frequently in liver transplantation than with any other solid organ.

Tolerogenesis in the Liver	Clinical Observations
The liver is an important site for primary T cell activation, but this takes place in an environment biased toward tolerance: • Liver endothelium expresses adhesion molecules that facilitate the sequestration of circulating activated T cells, particularly CD8 T cells. This gives the liver a role in systemic immunoregulation. • These activated T cells may undergo apoptosis owing to FasL and TRAIL expressed on Kupffer cells (KC) and may also be phagocytosed. • Constitutive exposure of liver cells to traces of endotoxin and other microbial products via blood from the systemic circulation and intestine results in down-modulation of costimulatory molecules and the synthesis of IL-10 by Kupffer cells (KC) and liver sinusoidal endothelial cells (LSECS). • Non haematopoietic liver cells, including LSECs and hepatic stellate cells (HSC) act as APCs, presenting antigen to T cells in the presence of immunosuppressive cytokines (IL-10 and TGF-β1) and inhibitory cell surface ligands (PD-L1). Anergy, rather than activation is promoted. Thus immune responses to liver antigens can often result in tolerance.	• Positive cross-match or blood type incompatibility has little affect on graft survival • HLA matching is not a prerequisite to liver transplantation • Reduced incidence of hyperacute rejection ompared to other organs in SOT • Frequent spontaneous recovery after severe rejection • Acute rejection does not impact severely on long-term graft and patient survival • Liver allograft protects other extra-hepatic allograft from rejection if derived from the same donor • Lower overall incidence of chronic rejection that is reversible in up to 30% cases • COT has been achieved most reliably and frequently in liver transplantation than with any other solid organ

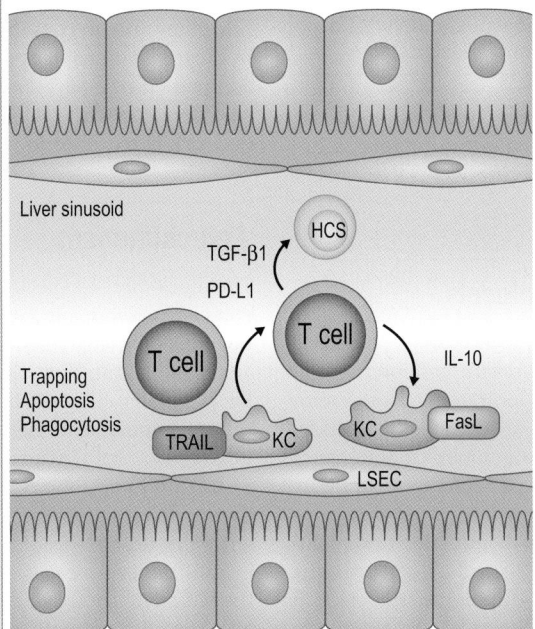

Fig. 81.7 Tolerogenesis in the liver The liver is an important site for primary T-cell activation, but this takes place in an environment biased toward tolerance. Liver endothelium expresses adhesion molecules that facilitate the sequestration of circulating activated T cells, particularly CD8 T cells. This gives the liver a role in systemic immunoregulation. These activated T cells may undergo apoptosis owing to FasL and TRAIL expressed on Kupffer cells (KCs) and may also be phagocytosed. Constitutive exposure of liver cells to traces of endotoxin and other microbial products via blood from the systemic circulation and intestine results in down-modulation of co-stimulatory molecules and the synthesis of IL-10 by KCs and liver sinusoidal endothelial cells (LSECS). Non-hematopoietic liver cells, including LSECs and hepatic stellate cells (HSC), act as APCs, presenting antigen to T cells in the presence of immunosuppressive cytokines (IL-10 and TGF-β₁) and inhibitory cell surface ligands (PD-L1). Anergy, rather than activation, is promoted. Thus immune responses to liver antigens can often result in tolerance.

Barriers to transplantation tolerance

T-cell memory

- Pre-sensitization—direct exposure to alloantigen, i.e., pregnancy or blood transfusion
- Heterologous immunity—cross-reactivity in the T-cell repertoire between antiviral, antibacterial, environmental, and transplantation antigen
- Homeostatic proliferation—induced by immunodepletory antibodies, i.e., alemtuzumab

Memory T cells generated by the above mechanisms can result in rapidly formed effector immune responses upon re-challenge. These T cells are less sensitive to T-cell depleting antibodies and co-stimulatory blockade, thus may be more resistant to some tolerance induction strategies.

B-cell response

- Recipients treated with immunodepletory antibodies display a general increase in the naïve B-cell population.
- There is a prevalent development of alloantibody in recipients treated with depleting antibody therapy.

Much focus of tolerogenic strategies is on the T-cell response. However, recent data suggest the humoral immune system may play a more significant role than previously thought, possibly contributing to more long-term outcomes. Further work in this area continues.

Lack of tolerance signature

- An episode of acute rejection can severely affect graft survival in most transplanted organs.
- Absence of validated biomarkers of tolerance or predictors of rejection.

Thus it is clinically difficult to justify often high-risk tolerogenizing strategies in patients who would otherwise do moderately well with standard immunosuppression.

In the next section, we discuss the current clinical strategies for tolerance induction as well as much-needed future approaches to produce more short acting, antigen-specific agents that can optimize outcomes in the clinic.

Molecule-based tolerogenic protocols

The induction of COT through the administration of presumed tolerogenic drugs and subsequent immunosuppression minimization is one such strategy currently under investigation. Promising results of the first use of alemtuzumab in human subjects by Calne et al.[31,62] with low-dose cyclosporine alone as maintenance therapy introduced the concept of "prope" tolerance: graft acceptance with reduced immunosuppression. Several groups have subsequently looked at alemtuzumab induction and maintenance therapy without nephrotoxic CNI agents. Unfortunately, results of pilot studies have been poor, with high acute rejection rates, (as much as 36% of recipients in one study). An attempt to induce donor allograft tolerance using alemtuzumab alone as an induction therapy with no maintenance immunosuppression at all resulted in 100% of patients developing acute rejection within the first month post-transplantation.[31] Encouragingly, physicians from the University of Wisconsin have demonstrated excellent long-term graft survival in 90% of patients maintained with only low-dose rapamycin monotherapy; these recipients had undergone alemtuzumab induction and an initial 60-day-only treatment with a CNI post-transplantation to prevent acute

rejection. It should be noted, however, that 50% of the patients developed alloantibody to either HLA class I or II and 40% demonstrated C4d$^+$ graft biopsies indicative of subacute humoral responses to allograft.[39]

In 2003, investigators at the University of Pittsburgh published the results of a seminal trial in which they administered an immunosuppressive regimen deemed to be tolerogenic to 82 adult kidney, liver, pancreas, and intestinal transplant recipients.[63] Their working hypothesis was that the need for continuous high-dose immunosuppression could be avoided in most cases with the use of a strong lymphocyte-depleting regimen before engraftment, followed by the administration of low-dose tacrolimus monotherapy. The goal of the induction treatment was the nonspecific removal of clones of immune cells responsible for rejection before contact with foreign donor antigens occurred, while minimizing exposure to maintenance immunosuppression.

After a mean follow-up of 18 months, overall 1-year patient and graft survival rates were 95 and 82%, respectively, immunosuppression-related morbidity was virtually eliminated, and 48 of 72 surviving patients were receiving spaced doses of tacrolimus monotherapy. These results were described as ground-breaking, as 64% renal, 70% liver, 42% pancreas, and 54% intestinal transplant recipients were on spaced doses at the time of publication. Despite the finding that no patient could be weaned completely off immunosuppression, the striking reduction in daily dosing should be regarded in itself as an outstanding achievement for two reasons; first, it was obtained after transplantation of organs considered highly immunogenic, and second, it led to a significant reduction in overall immunosuppression-related morbidity.

It is important to note that other protocols based on a similar strategy have since been attempted, including post-liver transplantation (an organ more capable than any other of developing COT). However, none of these protocols have achieved COT, nor have they shown convincingly any impact on overall outcomes. In most situations, it appears that leukocyte depletion is not accompanied by a permanent and complete deletion of alloaggressive donor-reactive cells, and the establishment of a regulatory network is required to maintain tolerance.

Full chimerism

The more robust experimental strategies for the induction of tolerance to foreign antigen utilize the mechanisms of central deletion to eliminate T-cell clones with specificity for the foreign antigens in question, thereby preventing them from entering the periphery. This can be reliably achieved by the establishment of hematopoietic chimerism through bone marrow transplantation (BMT). Stable engraftment of donor hemopoietic stem cells results in repopulation of the recipient thymus with donor-type thymic dendritic cells, with the result that developing T cells with anti-donor specificity are deleted by negative selection.

Full chimerism can be obtained rapidly through the ablation of the recipient's marrow and immune system with high dose radiation and/or chemotherapy; in addition it can be induced more slowly by non-ablative conditioning regimens, followed by the infusion of donor's marrow to colonize the recipient completely. This phenomenon paves the way for the onset of tolerance in the case of a subsequent SOT from the same donor.[64]

As proof of concept, there are a number of patients who have undergone successful BMT for hematological indications and have subsequently been successfully transplanted with a kidney from the same donor, without the requirement for increased immunosuppression.

It is important to highlight that in all these cases, the use of BMT was justified on the basis of the need for treatment of hematological malignancies. The establishment of full donor chimerism is not acceptable for the majority of recipients on the transplant waiting list as the risk profile, i.e., the toxicity and mortality associated with myeloablative conditioning regimens and the high incidence of GVHD with its potentially fatal complications, are not acceptable when compared to the alternative, i.e., life-long immunosuppression with the agents described above.

Mixed chimerism

A more promising approach is the induction of mixed hemopoietic chimerism, which can be achieved in experimental models with far less toxic induction therapy. Non-myeloablative conditioning regimens have been applied in the clinical setting for patients who have developed renal failure as a consequence of multiple myeloma. Further refinements of such protocols are being explored in experimental models. Examples of these include either a combination of depleting anti-CD4 and anti-CD8 antibodies together with mild, non-myeloablative total body irradiation or co-stimulatory blockade with anti-CD154 and/or CTLA-4-Ig. When these induction protocols are followed by BMT, the result is mixed chimerism (the continued survival of both donor and recipient hematopoietic progenitor cells). Animals that have undergone these therapies demonstrate durable tolerance to donor-type allografts, and have a much lower incidence of GVHD compared to full chimeras.

In particular, the Massachusetts General Hospital (MGH) transplantation group showed in mice and NHP that nonmyeloablative regimens could result in transient mixed chimerism with accompanying long-term transplantation tolerance.[65] Indeed, the same group has very recently reported the long-term follow-up of human recipients, with combined HLA-matched bone marrow and kidney transplantation for multiple myeloma with end-stage renal disease.[66] To achieve potent anti-myeloma responses and induce tolerance for the renal allograft, patients underwent a combined HLA-matched kidney and BMT with lead follow-up time of more than 12 years. Preparative therapy for the transplant consisted of high-dose cyclophosphamide, equine-derived antithymocyte globulin (eATG), and pretransplant thymic irradiation. Cyclosporine, as the sole post-transplant immunosuppressive therapy, was tapered and discontinued as early as day 73 post-transplant. All patients achieved mixed chimerism, over 70% had normal or near-normal renal function without needing systemic immunosuppression, and up to 50% of patients had no evidence of myeloma recurrence. These long-term follow-up data are encouraging, as they show that sustained renal allograft tolerance and prolonged anti-myeloma responses are achievable after combined HLA-matched kidney and BMT, and the induction of mixed lymphohematopoietic chimerism.

A very recent phase 2 clinical study reports for the first time,[77] the realisation of durable macrochimerism and tolerance, whilst avoiding GVHD or engraftment syndrome, in HLA-*mis*matched unrelated stem cell/renal transplant human recipients. Results were achieved with the introduction of a bioengineered, mobilised cellular product enriched for tolerogenic graft facilitating cells (FCs) as well as haematopoietic stem cells (HSCs – together with FCs, the treatment is termed FCRx), rather than just bone marrow graft alone. These bone marrow-derived FCs, which are CD8[+] but do not express TCR, potently enhance engraftment of allogeneic HSCs in conditioned recipients. FCs are composed predominantly of a plasmocytoid precursor dendritic cell subpopulation, induce the generation of antigen-specific Treg *in vitro* and *in vivo*, and have been found to effectively prevent GVHD in the mouse. In this clinical study, 8 HLA-mismatched kidney transplant recipients were treated with FCRx and nonmyeloablative conditioning during the peri-transplant period. One year later, 5 recipients exhibited durable macrochimerism with no incidence of GVHD or engraftment syndrome, and were immunosuppression-free i.e. these patients were clinically operationally tolerant. *In vitro* studies indicated that chimeric donor lymphocytes were tolerised to the recipient, and a significant increase in the CD4[+] Treg/T effector cell population ratio was observed in these patients when compared to those who had lost chimerism. The ability to establish high levels of donor multi-lineage chimerism in haploidentical and highly mismatched unrelated donor/recipient pairs without the development of GVHD or engraftment syndrome through the use of novel cellular therapies could have exciting therapeutic implications for disorders for which HSC transplantation can provide a 'functional cure,' including inherited metabolic disorders, haemoglobinopathies and autoimmune disease, as well as in solid organ transplantation.

Several other immunomodulatory cell groups are currently under investigation as potential tolerogenic therapies, such as mesenchymal stromal cells (MSCs) and transplant-acceptance inducing cells (TAICs). MSCs were originally isolated from the bone marrow but can now be isolated from almost any human tissue, and possess fascinating tissue repair and immunoregulatory properties. Preclinical models indicate that MSCs can promote engraftment of allogeneic cells/tissues/organs as well as prevent and/or treat rejection. Although there are no published reports to date on their potential in the setting of clinical SOT, it is expected that in the near future we will see numerous reports using MSCs as immune modulators after SOT.[64] TAICs were originally identified as the principal derivative of a rat embryonic stem cell line that is able to induce tolerance to allogeneic heart grafts.[67] As TAICs are able to influence recipient anti-donor activity through unknown mechanisms, they have been used in two safety trials (labelled as TAIC I and TAIC II studies). Overall, although these trials demonstrated that infusion of TAIC is feasible, major concerns remain regarding the efficacy and safety of such an approach. Further work is needed to establish whether this form of cell-based therapy can be used in the clinic to establish minimization of immunosuppression and COT.

Regulatory T cells (Treg)

There is now abundant evidence for the existence of populations of regulatory lymphocytes with the ability to suppress immune responses by other leukocytes (Chapter 15). Treg can be divided into two populations: thymic-derived naturally occurring CD25[+]CD4[+] cells (nTreg) and induced or adaptive Treg (iTreg) that are either differentiated from CD25[-]CD4[+] non-regulatory cells or expanded from CD25[+]CD4[+] cells in response to antigen. Expression of the transcription factor FOXP3 is essential for the development and function of Treg; however, nTreg and iTreg differ in origin, antigen experience, methylation patterns of FoxP3 and suppressive mechanisms. Both nTreg and iTreg have been demonstrated to play important roles in transplant tolerance.

nTreg develop within the thymus under the direction of FoxP3 and have a critical role in limiting immune responses to self-antigens, as demonstrated by experimental models where mice depleted of CD25[+]CD4[+] cells subsequently develop inflammatory bowel disease and widespread autoimmune phenomena. Mutation of FOXP3 in humans is responsible for the immune dysregulation, polyendocrinopathy, enteropathy, X-linked (IPEX) syndrome. There is evidence for the involvement of Treg in the downregulation of immune responses to tumors and chronic infections, as well as allogeneic transplants.[68]

Many strategies exist for the *in vivo* or *ex vivo* generation and/or expansion of Treg. The most common *in vivo* approaches are based on the fact that exposure to antigen increases Treg frequency and/or potency by either expanding naturally occurring Treg or inducing the generation of adaptive Treg from cells that do not originally possess regulatory activity. A well characterized strategy in mouse pre-clinical models, involves either co-receptor (CD4 or CD8) blockade or co-stimulation blockade using monoclonal antibodies, administered either at the time of transplantation or prior to transplantation in conjunction with donor antigen (such as a donor specific blood transfusion). $CD25^+CD4^+$ Treg play a critical role in both the induction and maintenance of transplantation tolerance in these models.[68]

Another approach to enrich mouse Treg *in vivo* is to create Treg-favoring conditions. In the transplantation setting, patients are treated with diverse immunosuppressive drug combinations, which may have a different impact on Treg. As mentioned in the previous section it has been demonstrated that CNIs, in particular cyclosporine, are detrimental to Treg, whereas the mTOR inhibitor rapamycin was shown to be beneficial for Treg both in terms of *in vivo* generation and function in mouse models and *in vitro* cultures of human Treg. It was recently demonstrated that adoptive transfer of a low number of alloantigen-specific Treg under a cover of low-dose rapamycin induced long-term survival of heart transplants in an un-manipulated host, an outcome otherwise difficult to obtain.[69]

Human Treg are currently less well characterized and understood than mouse Treg, and thus a thorough understanding of their biology is essential before clinical applications can be implemented. It is also important to appreciate the substantial differences between human and mouse Treg, in particular the differences in FOXP3 expression: in human, FOXP3 is also expressed by activated non-regulatory T cells as well as by Treg, and activated non-regulatory cells also upregulate CD25 expression. Thus not all $CD25^+FOXP3^+CD4^+$ cells will be genuine Treg and therefore isolation strategies based on $CD25^{hi}CD4^+$ are likely to be imperfect. Other markers are therefore needed to enrich Treg from human peripheral blood mononuclear cells (PBMC). Recently it has been demonstrated that $CD127^{lo}CD25^+CD4^+$ T cells are characterized by a higher percentage of $FOXP3^+$ cells with a more pronounced suppressive capacity,[70] and when expanded, this subset resulted in high yields of Treg that maintained high FOXP3 expression.[71] Importantly, as was recently demonstrated in a clinically relevant humanized model of transplant arteriosclerosis, *ex vivo* expanded $CD25^{hi}CD4^+$ and $CD127^{lo}CD25^+CD4^+$ Treg cells have been very effective in inhibiting vasculopathy, with $CD127^{lo}CD25^+CD4^+$ T cells being five-times more efficient than conventional Treg.[56]

A number of different strategies for the isolation/enrichment of human Treg have been described in the literature, but to date there is no consensus as to which strategy produces the optimal population for use in cell therapy applications. The most commonly used expansion protocol at present is based on stimulation by anti-CD3/anti-CD28 beads in the presence of high doses of recombinant Il-2, supplemented in some protocols with rapamycin. Despite the generation of sufficient numbers of Treg for cellular therapy, however, this mode of expansion is antigen non-specific without any enrichment step for the cells of interest. The concept of expanding or generating donor alloantigen-reactive Treg is much more appealing for clinical application in the setting of transplantation. Further work also needs to be

done to ascertain the long-term stability and plasticity of Treg *in vivo*, as well as the potential effects of Treg in anti-tumor and anti-viral immunity—theoretically, infusion of large numbers of potent suppressor cells may compromise the immune response towards infectious pathogens and tumor cells. There are several ongoing clinical trials examining the application of Treg cellular therapy, largely in the prevention and treatment of GVHD, and further clinical studies are being planned to apply Treg therapy in SOT.

Biomarkers of rejection or tolerance

Strategies that have shown tolerogenic effects in animal models and are currently in the process of clinical translation include the introduction of chimerism, Treg cell therapy as well as the combination of co-stimulatory blockade reagents, T-cell depletion and withdrawal of maintenance immunosuppression. Concerns have been raised about testing these approaches in recipients of organs such as kidney, heart or pancreas; an episode of acute rejection could severely affect graft survival. In these settings, most physicians are reluctant to withdraw immunosuppressive drugs in the absence of validated biomarkers of transplantation tolerance and rejection prediction. Biomarkers are thus needed to better evaluate the immune status of transplant recipients, determine the "tolerance signature" of recipients, predict and diagnose graft rejection non-invasively and individualize immunosuppressive therapy.

Technical advances in multi-parameter flow cytometry, antigen-specific lymphocyte assays and genome-wide analyses have led to the development of powerful and more standardized immunomonitoring techniques to characterize alloimmune responses. Histological analysis remains the gold standard method by which to detect graft rejection, but graft biopsy is an invasive procedure with inherent risks and so cannot be routinely performed for surveillance purposes; it is also associated with sampling error and interpretation biases.

Molecular or cell-based biomarkers are thus being developed as alternative surveillance methods. Following the original report by Vasconcellos et al.,[72] showing increased levels of messenger RNA (mRNA) transcripts derived from cytotoxic T cells in PBMCs collected from kidney recipients undergoing graft rejection, many laboratories have investigated the use of blood and urine cell transcriptional biomarkers to non-invasively detect acute rejection of kidney.[20] mRNA biomarkers of acute rejection have also been investigated in PBMCs from recipients of heart and pancreas allografts. In heart transplantation, the Cardiac Allograft Rejection Gene Expression Observation Studies[73] led to the development of a non-invasive commercially available diagnostic test for acute rejection.[74] Cell-based functional assays are more cumbersome and difficult to standardize than molecular tests, although they have been used to assess the risk of rejection, before or after transplantation through quantification of allospecific T cells.[20]

At present, it is striking that for the many biomarkers identified, discrepancies exist between data from different laboratories investigating the same parameter. This is likely due to differences in recipient and donor populations, clinical management and the actual laboratory techniques used to perform the assays. Therefore, it is of great importance that the assays used to detect biomarkers are optimized, validated and standardized and subsequently candidate biomarkers are investigated in large patient cohorts from different transplant centers using the same, validated, assays.[75] International research networks such as the RISET, ITN, and Genome Canada networks have already begun this process and are invaluable for discovering and validating biomarkers to enable them to be introduced into clinical practice.[76]

● ON THE HORIZON

Initiatives in clinical utilization of tolerance

- Clinical introduction of antigen-specific Treg therapy
- Identification of tolerance signatures and predictors of rejection
- Use of immunomodulatory stem cell populations, i.e., Mesenchymal stromal cells

---

References

1. Merrill JP, Murray JE, Harrison JH, Guild WR. Successful homotransplantation of the human kidney between identical twins. J Am Med Assoc 1956;160(4):277–82.
2. Salahudeen AK, Haider N, May W. Cold ischemia and the reduced long-term survival of cadaveric renal allografts. Kidney Int 2004;65(2):713–8.
3. Andrade CF, Waddell TK, Keshavjee S, Liu M. Innate immunity and organ transplantation: the potential role of toll-like receptors. Am J Transplant 2005;5(5):969–75.
4. Hart DN, Fabre JW. Kidney-specific alloantigen system in the rat. Characterization and role in transplantation. J Exp Med 1980;151(3):651–66.
5. Qureshi F, Rabb H, Kasiske BL. Silent acute rejection during prolonged delayed graft function reduces kidney allograft survival. Transplantation 2002;74(10):1400–4.
6. Whitelegg A, Barber LD. The structural basis of T-cell allorecognition. Tissue Antigens 2004;63(2):101–8.
7. Lakkis FG, Arakelov A, Konieczny BT, Inoue Y. Immunologic "ignorance" of vascularized organ transplants in the absence of secondary lymphoid tissue. Nat Med 2000;6(6):686–8.
8. Afzali B, Lombardi G, Lechler RI. Pathways of major histocompatibility complex allorecognition. Curr Opin Organ Transplant 2008;13(4):438–44.
9. Auchincloss Jr H, Sultan H. Antigen processing and presentation in transplantation. Curr Opin Immunol 1996;8(5):681–7.
10. Smyth LA, Herrera OB, Golshayan D, et al. A novel pathway of antigen presentation by dendritic and endothelial cells: Implications for allorecognition and infectious diseases. Transplantation 2006;82(1 Suppl.):S15–18.
11. Clarkson MR, Sayegh MH. T-cell costimulatory pathways in allograft rejection and tolerance. Transplantation 2005;80(5):555–63.
12. Heidt S, Segundo DS, Chadha R, Wood KJ. The impact of Th17 cells on transplant rejection and the induction of tolerance. Curr Opin Organ Transplant 2010;15(4):456–61.
13. Feng G, Chan T, Wood KJ, Bushell A. Donor reactive regulatory T cells. Curr Opin Organ Transplant 2009;14(4):432–8.
14. Gill RG. NK cells: elusive participants in transplantation immunity and tolerance. Curr Opin Immunol 2010;22(5):649–54.
15. Nath DS, Basha HI, Mohanakumar T. Antihuman leukocyte antigen antibody-induced autoimmunity: role in chronic rejection. Curr Opin Organ Transplant 2010;15(1):16–20.
16. Rosenberg AS. The T cell populations mediating rejection of MHC class I disparate skin grafts in mice. Transpl Immunol 1993;1(2):93–9.
17. Cramer DV, Wu GD, Chapman FA, et al. Lymphocytic subsets and histopathologic changes associated with the development of heart transplant arteriosclerosis. J Heart Lung Transplant 1992;11(3 Pt 1):458–66.
18. Gebel HM, Bray RA. The evolution and clinical impact of human leukocyte antigen technology. Curr Opin Nephrol Hypertens 2010;19(6):598–602.
19. Leffell MS, Zachary AA. Antiallograft antibodies: relevance, detection, and monitoring. Curr Opin Organ Transplant 2010;15(1):2–7.
20. Sanchez-Fueyo A, Strom TB. Immunologic basis of graft rejection and tolerance following transplantation of liver or other solid organs. Gastroenterology 2011;140(1):51–64.
21. de Fijter JW. Rejection and function and chronic allograft dysfunction. Kidney Int Suppl 2010;(119):S38–41.
22. Veronese FV, Noronha IL, Manfro RC, et al. Prevalence and immunohistochemical findings of subclinical kidney allograft rejection and its association with graft outcome. Clin Transplant 2004;18(4):357–64.
23. Shapiro R, Basu A, Tan H, et al. Kidney transplantation under minimal immunosuppression after pretransplant lymphoid depletion with Thymoglobulin or Campath. J Am Coll Surg 2005;200(4):505–15; quiz A59–61.
24. Deeks ED, Keating GM. Rabbit antithymocyte globulin (thymoglobulin): a review of its use in the prevention and treatment of acute renal allograft rejection. Drugs 2009;69(11):1483–512.
25. Charpentier B, Rostaing L, Berthoux F, et al. A three-arm study comparing immediate tacrolimus therapy with antithymocyte globulin induction therapy followed by tacrolimus or cyclosporine A in adult renal transplant recipients. Transplantation 2003;75(6):844–51.
26. Mourad G, Garrigue V, Squifflet JP, et al. Induction versus noninduction in renal transplant recipients with tacrolimus-based immunosuppression. Transplantation 2001;72(6):1050–5.
27. Morris PJ, Russell NK. Alemtuzumab (Campath-1H): a systematic review in organ transplantation. Transplantation 2006;81(10):1361–7.
28. Trzonkowski P, Zilvetti M, Chapman S, et al. Homeostatic repopulation by CD28-CD8 + T cells in alemtuzumab-depleted kidney transplant recipients treated with reduced immunosuppression. Am J Transplant 2008;8(2):338–47.
29. Pearl JP, Parris J, Hale DA, et al. Immunocompetent T-cells with a memory-like phenotype are the dominant cell type following antibody-mediated T-cell depletion. Am J Transplant 2005;5(3):465–74.
30. Lopez M, Clarkson MR, Albin M, et al. A novel mechanism of action for anti-thymocyte globulin: induction of CD4+CD25+Foxp3+ regulatory T cells. J Am Soc Nephrol 2006;17(10):2844–53.
31. Calne R, Friend P, Moffatt S, et al. Prope tolerance, perioperative campath 1H, and low-dose cyclosporin monotherapy in renal allograft recipients. Lancet 1998;351(9117):1701–1702.
32. Watson CJ, Bradley JA, Friend PJ, et al. Alemtuzumab (CAMPATH 1H) induction therapy in cadaveric kidney transplantation—efficacy and safety at five years. Am J Transplant 2005;5(6):1347–53.
33. Wu Z, Bensinger SJ, Zhang J, et al. Homeostatic proliferation is a barrier to transplantation tolerance. Nat Med 2004;10(1):87–92.
34. Trzonkowski P, Zilvetti M, Friend P, Wood KJ. Recipient memory-like lymphocytes remain unresponsive to graft antigens after CAMPATH-1H induction with reduced maintenance immunosuppression. Transplantation 2006;82(10):1342–51.
35. Vathsala A, Ona ET, Tan SY, et al. Randomized trial of Alemtuzumab for prevention of graft rejection and preservation of renal function after kidney transplantation. Transplantation 2005;80(6):765–74.
36. Ciancio G, Burke GW, Gaynor JJ, et al. A randomized trial of three renal transplant induction antibodies: early comparison of tacrolimus, mycophenolate mofetil, and steroid dosing, and newer immune-monitoring. Transplantation 2005;80(4):457–65.
37. Shyu S, Dew MA, Pilewski JM, et al. Five-year outcomes with alemtuzumab induction after lung transplantation. J Heart Lung Transplant 2011;30(7):743–54.
38. Willicombe M, Brookes P, Santos-Nunez E, et al. Outcome of patients with preformed donor-specific antibodies following alemtuzumab induction and tacrolimus monotherapy. Am J Transplant 2011;11(3):470–7.
39. Knechtle SJ, Pascual J, Bloom DD, et al. Early and limited use of tacrolimus to avoid rejection in an alemtuzumab and sirolimus regimen for kidney transplantation: clinical results and immune monitoring. Am J Transplant 2009;9(5):1087–98.
40. Bloom D, Chang Z, Pauly K, et al. BAFF is increased in renal transplant patients following treatment with alemtuzumab. Am J Transplant 2009;9(8):1835–45.
41. Chatenoud L, Bluestone JA. CD3-specific antibodies: a portal to the treatment of autoimmunity. Nat Rev Immunol 2007;7(8):622–32.
42. Ablamunits V, Bisikirska B, Herold KC. Acquisition of regulatory function by human CD8(+) T cells treated with anti-CD3 antibody requires TNF. Eur J Immunol 2010;40(10):2891–901.
43. Golshayan D, Pascual M. Tolerance-inducing immunosuppressive strategies in clinical transplantation: an overview. Drugs 2008;68(15):2113–30.
44. Knechtle SJ. Immunoregulation and tolerance. Transplant Proc 2010;42(9 Suppl.):S13–15.
45. Tang Q, Henriksen KJ, Boden EK, et al. Cutting edge: CD28 controls peripheral homeostasis of CD4+CD25+ regulatory T cells. J Immunol 2003;171(7):3348–52.
46. Bluestone JA, Liu W, Yabu JM, et al. The effect of costimulatory and interleukin 2 receptor blockade on regulatory T cells in renal transplantation. Am J Transplant 2008;8(10):2086–96.
47. Vincenti F, Charpentier B, Vanrenterghem Y, et al. A phase III study of belatacept-based immunosuppression regimens versus cyclosporine in renal transplant recipients (BENEFIT study). Am J Transplant 2010;10(3):535–46.
48. Larsen CP, Grinyó J, Medina-Pestana J, et al. Belatacept-based regimens versus a cyclosporine A-based regimen in kidney transplant recipients: 2-year results from the BENEFIT and BENEFIT-EXT studies. Transplantation 2010;90(12):1528–35.
49. Karam VH, Gasquet I, Delvart V, et al. Quality of life in adult survivors beyond 10 years after liver, kidney, and heart transplantation. Transplantation 2003;76(12):1699–704.
50. Vincenti F, de Andrés A, Becker T, et al. Interleukin-2 receptor antagonist induction in modern immunosuppression regimens for renal transplant recipients. Transpl Int 2006;19(6):446–57.
51. Webster AC, Playford EG, Higgins G, et al. Interleukin 2 receptor antagonists for renal transplant recipients: a meta-analysis of randomized trials. Transplantation 2004;77(2):166–76.
52. Keown P, Balshaw R, Khorasheh S, et al. Meta-analysis of basiliximab for immunoprophylaxis in renal transplantation. BioDrugs 2003;17(4):271–9.
53. Brennan DC, Schnitzler MA. Long-term results of rabbit antithymocyte globulin and basiliximab induction. N Engl J Med 2008;359(16):1736–8.
54. McKeage K, McCormack PL. Basiliximab: a review of its use as induction therapy in renal transplantation. BioDrugs 2010;24(1):55–76.
55. Carvalho-Gaspar M, Jones ND, Luo S, et al. Location and time-dependent control of rejection by regulatory T cells culminates in a failure to generate memory T cells. J Immunol 2008;180(10):6640–8.
56. Nadig SN, Wieckiewicz J, Wu DC, et al. In vivo prevention of transplant arteriosclerosis by ex vivo-expanded human regulatory T cells. Nat Med 2010;16(7):809–13.
57. Billingham RE, Brent L, Medawar PB. Actively acquired tolerance of foreign cells. Nature 1953;172(4379):603–6.
58. Ashton-Chess J, Giral M, Brouard S, Soulillou JP. Spontaneous operational tolerance after immunosuppressive drug withdrawal in clinical renal allotransplantation. Transplantation 2007;84(10):1215–9.
59. Orlando G, Soker S, Wood K. Operational tolerance after liver transplantation. J Hepatol 2009;50(6):1247–57.
60. Tzakis AG, Reyes J, Zeevi A, et al. Early tolerance in pediatric liver allograft recipients. J Pediatr Surg 1994;29(6):754–6.
61. Mazariegos GV, Sindhi R, Thomson AW, Marcos A. Clinical tolerance following liver transplantation: long term results and future prospects. Transpl Immunol 2007;17(2):114–9.

62. Calne R, Moffatt SD, Friend PJ, et al. Campath IH allows low-dose cyclosporine monotherapy in 31 cadaveric renal allograft recipients. Transplantation 1999;68(10):1613–6.

63. Starzl TE, Murase N, Abu-Elmagd K, et al. Tolerogenic immunosuppression for organ transplantation. Lancet 2003;361(9368):1502–10.

64. Orlando G, Hematti P, Stratta RJ, et al. Clinical operational tolerance after renal transplantation: current status and future challenges. Ann Surg 2010;252(6):915–28.

65. Turka LA, Wood K, Bluestone JA. Bringing transplantation tolerance into the clinic: lessons from the ITN and RISET for the Establishment of Tolerance consortia. Curr Opin Organ Transplant 2010;15(4):441–8.

66. Spitzer TR, Sykes M, Tolkoff-Rubin N, et al. Long-term follow-up of recipients of combined human leukocyte antigen-matched bone marrow and kidney transplantation for multiple myeloma with end-stage renal disease. Transplantation 2011;91(6):672–6.

67. Hutchinson JA, Riquelme P, Brem-Exner BG, et al. Transplant acceptance-inducing cells as an immune-conditioning therapy in renal transplantation. Transpl Int 2008;21(8):728–41.

68. Wieckiewicz J, Goto R, Wood KJ. T regulatory cells and the control of alloimmunity: from characterisation to clinical application. Curr Opin Immunol 2010;22(5):662–8.

69. Raimondi G, Sumpter TL, Matta BM, et al. Mammalian target of rapamycin inhibition and alloantigen-specific regulatory T cells synergize to promote long-term graft survival in immunocompetent recipients. J Immunol 2010;184(2):624–36.

70. Liu W, Putnam AL, Xu-Yu Z, et al. CD127 expression inversely correlates with FoxP3 and suppressive function of human CD4+ T reg cells. J Exp Med 2006;203(7):1701–11.

71. Putnam AL, Brusko TM, Lee MR, et al. Expansion of human regulatory T-cells from patients with type 1 diabetes. Diabetes 2009;58(3):652–62.

72. Vasconcellos LM, Schachter AD, Zheng XX, et al. Cytotoxic lymphocyte gene expression in peripheral blood leukocytes correlates with rejecting renal allografts. Transplantation 1998;66(5):562–6.

73. Deng MC, Eisen HJ, Mehra MR, et al. Noninvasive discrimination of rejection in cardiac allograft recipients using gene expression profiling. Am J Transplant 2006;6(1):150–60.

74. Lopez AS, Alegre E, LeMaoult J, et al. Regulatory role of tryptophan degradation pathway in HLA-G expression by human monocyte-derived dendritic cells. Mol Immunol 2006;43(14):2151–60.

75. Poste G. Bring on the biomarkers. Nature 2011;469(7329):156–7.

76. Sarwal MM, Benjamin J, Butte AJ, et al. Transplantomics and Biomarkers in Organ Transplantation—A report from the 1st International Conference. Transplantation 2011;91(4):379–82.

77. Leventhal J, et al. Chimerism and tolerance without GVHD or engraftment syndrome in HLA-mismatched combined kidney and hematopoietic stem cell transplantation. Sci Transl Med 2012;4(124):124ra28.

82.

Stem cell transplantation and immune reconstitution in immunodeficiency

Luigi D. Notarangelo, Sung-Yun Pai

Following the discovery of the major human leukocyte antigens (HLA) in 1958, hematopoietic stem cell transplantation (HSCT) came into practice to provide treatment for a variety of congenital and acquired disorders. Cure of an infant with severe combined immunodeficiency (SCID) in 1968 was the first successful experience in HSCT, marking the beginning of a new era in medicine.[1]

For many years, the successful use of HSCT in severe primary immune deficiencies was largely restricted to HLA-identical transplants, as HSCT from mismatched related family donors (usually represented by haploidentical parents) was followed by severe complications, graft-versus-host disease (GvHD) in particular. In the late 1970s it was demonstrated in animal models that removal of mature T lymphocytes from the graft obtained from mismatched related marrow allowed successful reconstitution upon injection into lethally irradiated recipient animals. This important achievement opened the way to a broader use of HSCT in severe forms of primary immune deficiency (PID). More recently, the availability of stem cells from volunteer matched unrelated donors (MUD) and from cord blood has further increased the successful application on HSCT in individuals with PID (Table 82.1).

Hematopoietic Stem Cell Transplantation: General Considerations

Sources of hematopoietic stem cells for transplantation

Several sources of hematopoietic stem cells are available for transplantation (Table 82.2). Hematopoietic stem cells can be retrieved from bone marrow, peripheral blood or from cord blood (Chapters 2, 32, 33). Bone marrow stem cells are most commonly obtained by multiple aspirations along the iliac crests, usually while the donor is under general anesthesia. The volume of bone marrow that is obtained may vary between 500 ml and 1 liter or even more, depending on the type of transplant (HLA-identical or T-cell depleted) and the weight of the recipient. Blood group matching for ABO antigens is not required for HSCT as mature red cells or anti-ABO antibodies can be removed by red blood cell depletion or plasma depletion respectively. In the case of HLA-identical transplantation, the marrow stem cells are then injected intravenously without further manipulation into a central line in the recipient. In the case of mismatched transplantation, bone marrow cells are T-cell depleted *in vitro* (see below); stem cells are then enumerated and injected intravenously.

Hematopoietic stem cells can also be retrieved from peripheral blood, following *in vivo* administration of granulocyte-colony stimulating factor (G-CSF) to the donor, usually at the dosage of 10 µg/kg/day for 5 days, which allows mobilization of stem cells. In this case, stem cells can also be purified by positive selection (see below), enumerated and injected.

Finally, cord blood is another rich source of hematopoietic stem cells. At birth, cord blood is collected in heparinized medium and stored in liquid nitrogen, with small aliquots preserved for HLA-typing. Whenever sufficient compatibility is identified between a patient and a stored cord blood, the latter

● KEY CONCEPTS

Sources of stem cells and selection of donors for hematopoietic stem cell transplantation in primary immunodeficiencies

- Sources of hematopoietic stem cells for transplantation include bone marrow, peripheral blood, and cord blood.

- If the donor is a genotypically HLA-identical sibling, unmanipulated bone marrow is used as source of stem cells.

- Whenever the donor is HLA-mismatched to the recipient, T-cell depletion must be performed to eliminate mature T lymphocytes from the graft. Methods for T-cell depletion of the bone marrow include use of soybean lectin agglutination (± E-rosetting), depletion with monoclonal antibodies plus complement, and positive selection of stem cells.

- Cord blood is a rich source of stem cells. However, the volume of cord blood is limited, so that its use is mainly restricted to young patients.

- The number of volunteers included in Bone Marrow Donor Registries is expanding. Consequently, there is a continuous increase in the number of Matched Unrelated Donor (MUD) transplantations performed for patients with primary immunodeficiencies.

- Whenever cord blood or MUD stem cells are used, conditioning regimen must be given to the recipient prior to transplantation, in order to facilitate engraftment of donor stem cells.

- Therapeutic options for patients with SCID include transplantation from HLA-genotypically identical donor, or from mismatched related donors. Recently, transplant from matched unrelated donor (MUD) has also been successfully used in SCID infants under stable conditions.

- For other forms of primary immunodeficiencies, whenever no related HLA-identical donor is available, search for a MUD or an unrelated cord blood should be started, since the results of such transplants are better than from related mismatched donors.

Table 82.1 Hematopoietic stem cell transplantation for Primary Immune Deficiencies in Europe. 1968–2004

Type of Immunodeficiency	Patients with genotypically-identical related donor	Patients with phenotypically-identical related donor	Patients with mismatched related donor	Patients with matched unrelated donor	Total number of patients
SCID	126	61	367	58	612
Omenn syndrome	14	9	29	10	62
MHC class II deficiency	20	10	26	5	61
PNP deficiency	2	1	1	1	5
CD40L deficiency	9	0	1	21	31
Other forms of CID	35	7	44	29	115
Di George syndrome	1	0	0	1	2
Other T cell deficiencies	5	1	5	4	15
WAS	45	8	47	50	150
FHL	26	6	37	19	88
XLP	3	0	1	7	11
Chediak-Higashi syndrome	10	5	3	4	22
Griscelli syndrome	6	2	1	1	10
Agranulocytosis	3	0	2	3	3
CGD	25	0	0	5	30
LAD	13	2	16	1	32
IFN-γ receptor deficiency	2	1	1	0	4
Other phagocytic disorders	2	0	0	1	3
All defects	347	113	581	220	1261

SCID: Severe Combined Immune Deficiency; MHC: Major Histocompatibility Complex; PNP: purine nucleoside phosphorylase; CID: Combined Immune Deficiency; WAS: Wiskott-Aldrich Syndrome; FHL: Familial Hemophagocytic Lymphohistiocytosis; XLP: X-linked lymphoproliferative disease; CGD: chronic granulomatous disease; LAD: Leukocyte adhesion deficiency.
(Data from the European SCETIDE Registry, courtesy of Paul Landais and Alain Fischer)

Table 82.2 Sources of hematopoietic stem cells for transplantation

HSCT from a related donor
•Bone marrow from an HLA-genotypically-identical sibling
•Bone marrow from an HLA-phenotypically-identical family member
•Bone marrow from a haploidentical parent
•T cell-depleted by negative selection with soybean lectin agglutination/SRBC
•T cell-depleted by negative selection with monoclonal antibodies
•Positive selection of CD34 + cells (± CD133 + cells)
HSCT from a Matched Unrelated Donor
•Unmanipulated bone marrow
•T cell-depleted bone marrow by means of positive selection of CD34+/CD133+ cells
•Positively selected peripheral blood CD34 + cells
HSCT from an unmanipulated related or unrelated cord blood

is thawed and injected into the recipient without further manipulation. With this procedure, the number of stem cells that can be transplanted is dictated by their concentration in the cord blood sample, and by the volume of the sample itself. More recently, *in vitro* expansion of cord blood stem cells and transplants with multiple cord blood units have been attempted in order to overcome this limitation.

Donor selection and manipulation of the graft

HSCT from a related HLA-identical donor

The use of unfractionated stem cells from an HLA-identical sibling offers the best chance of rapid engraftment and immune reconstitution. In such cases, the HLA-identity between recipient and donor minimizes the risk of GvHD. Furthermore, the mature T cells contained in the graft, especially in the case of HSCT for SCID, provide a first line of immune reconstitution after transplant, as they may expand and lead to a rapid increase in the number of circulating T lymphocytes as early as 2 weeks after HSCT. Finally, a relatively low number of stem cells is required to achieve engraftment and immune reconstitution following related HLA-identical HSCT, although even in this setting a larger cell dose may facilitate immune reconstitution.

HSCT from a haploidentical donor

Unfortunately, the option of related HLA-identical HSCT is limited only to a minority of patients. When no such donor is available, stem cell transplantation from a haploidentical parent should be considered, particularly in infants with SCID.

The rationale for haploidentical HSCT is based on the ability of donor-derived stem cells to repopulate the recipient's vestigial thymus, and give rise to fully mature T lymphocytes. Indeed, this is a life-saving procedure that has been successfully applied to several hundreds of infants with SCID.[2,3]

However, this procedure requires careful removal of T lymphocytes from the graft, as these would otherwise cause severe GvHD. Several methods are now available to attain T cell-depletion.[3]

Soybean lectin allows agglutination of the majority of mature marrow cells, which can be removed by sedimentation. This step is followed by further depletion of T lymphocytes by rosetting with sheep erythrocytes (E-rosetting technique) and density gradient centrifugation. Importantly, T-cell depletion by soybean lectin agglutination and E-rosetting maintains all immature marrow cells in the final preparation. In general, the procedure requires a relatively large collection (approximately 1 liter) of bone marrow from the donor.

T-cell depletion can also be achieved by incubation of the marrow with monoclonal antibodies to T lymphocytes plus complement. Campath-1 G, Leu 1 and other monoclonal antibodies have been used for this purpose, but the degree of T-cell depletion that is achieved is often less effective than with the soybean lectin and E-rosetting, possibly because of modulation of antigen expression on the surface of T lymphocytes. Consequently, there is a higher probability that GvHD may develop.

Positive selection of CD34[+] cells using monoclonal antibody affinity columns or immunomagnetic beads has been widely used in recent years. However, this approach removes immature CD34- cells and other cells (especially stromal marrow cells) that can facilitate stem cell engraftment. Following the recognition that CD133 is expressed on primitive hematopoietic progenitors, positive selection of CD133[+] cells with immunomagnetic beads has been also proposed.

Selection of the best donor is another important aspect of T cell-depleted haploidentical HSCT for SCID. In general, the donor is represented by one of the parents, since the volume of bone marrow that can be collected is much higher than it would be in case a haploidentical sibling were to serve as donor. It is also important to recognize that maternal T cell engraftment is a common finding in infants with SCID. In a survey of 121 SCID patients, Müller et al. identified 48 cases (or 39.7%) with maternally-derived T lymphocytes.[4] In such cases, T cell-depleted HSCT should be performed using the mother as donor if possible, since transplantation from the father might cause a graft-versus-graft reaction.

In utero haploidentical HSCT

The identification of a growing number of immunodeficiency-causing genes has resulted in continuous improvement in prenatal diagnosis, which in most cases of severe immunodeficiency can now be accomplished on chorionic villi DNA at 10-11 weeks of gestation. This has prompted prenatal transplantation of parental positively-selected CD34[+] stem cells in fetuses affected with SCID. This novel strategy has improved upon the previous largely unsatisfactory experience with fetal liver and other stem cells.

The technique used for in utero HSCT includes injection of purified CD34[+] cells into the fetal peritoneum under ultrasound guidance.

The rationale underlying in utero HSCT is based on a lower risk of graft rejection due to decreased fetal immunocompetence (although this consideration is not relevant in the case of fetuses with SCID), a presumed induction of tolerance to paternal antigens (which might favor successful engraftment after post-natal transplantation from the same donor), the predicted competition between donor and autologous stem cells at a time when several empty niches should be available for stem cell engraftment, the potential ability to provide pre-emptive treatment (thus reducing the risk of post-natal infection), and the lower cost of the procedure that does not require prolonged hospitalization. On the other hand, in utero HSCT is associated with the potential risks of fetal loss and of GvHD. Finally, if maternal T cells had engrafted into the fetus with SCID, transplantation of paternal CD34[+] cells might cause graft-versus-graft reaction.

In utero HSCT has been attempted in several infants with severe immunodeficiencies, most notably SCID.[5] Five of these transplants have been performed at the University of Brescia, Italy. All three cases with B[+] SCID (two of which due to γc deficiency, and one to IL-7Rα-deficient SCID; Chapter 35) have survived with evidence of T cell reconstitution; of the 2 cases with B- SCID, one has failed to achieve immune reconstitution, in spite of two additional boosting transplants from the same donor (the father) after birth. This patient eventually died of Bcell lymphoproliferative disease (BLPD) after a MUD HSCT. In the fifth patient (with B- SCID due to RAG2 mutation), thymopoiesis rapidly declined, and the patient remains profoundly lymphopenic. While the overall results of the procedure appear to be influenced by the nature of the underlying disease, the use of in utero HSCT for SCID is now largely unjustified, in consideration of the fact that early post-natal HSCT for SCID leads to long-term survival in 97% of the cases.[3,6] Furthermore, the observation that engraftment is restricted only to cell lineages that were missing in the affected fetus is a strong argument against the use of in utero HSCT for treatment of PID other than SCID.

HSCT from matched unrelated donors

Since the first successful experience, performed in 1977 in an infant with SCID,[7] HSCT from MUD has been increasingly used to treat severe primary immunodeficiencies. MUD HSCT has been shown to be more effective than T cell-depleted HSCT in patients with immunodeficiencies other than SCID,[2] and more recently, it has also been successfully used in infants with SCID.[8,9]

Transplantation from MUD has been facilitated by the increasing number of volunteer donors included in registries worldwide. In addition, advances in the quality of the techniques used for HLA typing permits t identification of an optimal MUD, and reduction in the risk of GvHD. As of July 2011, more than 18 million donors were included in the Bone Marrow Donors Worldwide (BMDW) registry. At present, it takes 3-4 months on average to identify a MUD. However, the probability of finding a suitable donor is lower for selected ethnic or racial groups that are poorly represented among volunteer donors.

Importantly, MUD HSCT requires use of a preparative chemotherapy regimen in the recipient (even in the case of SCID) and graft-versus-host prophylaxis (because of likely disparity between donor and recipient at minor histocompatibility loci), whereas neither one is necessary for related HLA-identical HSCT in SCID infants.

HSCT using unmanipulated cord blood

As opposed to MUD HSCT, which requires identification, willingness and medical clearance of an adult volunteer, stored cord blood is readily available as a source of stem cells for transplantation. In addition, the risk of GvHD at any given degree of HLA matching is lower when using cord blood than MUD HSCT, so that greater HLA disparity with the recipient can be tolerated. On the other hand, a major limitation of cord blood remains the number of cells contained in any defined unit. Low cell dose is not usually a problem for transplants performed in infants with SCID or other severe forms of immune deficiency, due to the low weight of the recipient. Indeed, unrelated umbilical cord stem cell transplantation has been successfully used in dozens of patients with severe primary immune deficiencies.[2,3,9,10] In practice, an unrelated hematopoietic stem cell donor should be simultaneously searched for in cord blood banks and in bone marrow donor registries for patients lacking an HLA-identical sibling hematopoietic stem cell donor. The option of performing cord blood transplants should be based on urgency of the transplant, the cell dose required, and the number of HLA disparities.

As for HSCT from MUD, transplantation using cord blood usually requires pretransplant conditioning and GvHD prophylaxis, irrespective of the underlying disease.

Complications of hematopoietic stem cell transplantation

A variety of complications can compromise the success of HSCT. Among these, incompatibility between donor and recipient can lead to graft rejection by the host immune system or, alternatively, to GvHD, caused by alloreactivity of donor-derived lymphocytes to the recipient's cells. Furthermore, conditioning regimens can cause toxicity of several organs. Myeloablative regimens cause anemia, thrombocytopenia, and leukopenia. Consequently, supportive treatment with red blood cell and platelet transfusions is necessary during the aplastic phase. Finally, the leukopenia predisposes the patient to an increased risk of life-threatening bacterial or fungal infections.

The frequency and severity of these complications depend on the type of transplant, the possible use of a conditioning regimen, and specific considerations related to the underlying disorder and to the clinical status of the recipient prior to transplantation.

● KEY CONCEPTS

Rejection of donor stem cells by the host immune system and reaction of donor's T lymphocytes to the host

- The host T cells are responsible for the elimination of donor stem cells, regardless of the degree of HLA compatibility. Under these circumstances, other than in patients with SCID, a chemotherapy-based conditioning regimen must be used prior to transplantation in order to allow for donor stem cell engraftment.

- If T cells are present in the graft, and especially is there is HLA-incompatibility between the donor and the recipient, the donor's T lymphocytes may react to host alloantigens, and cause graft-versus-host disease (GvHD).

- Risk factors for GvHD include HLA-mismatch between donor and recipient, older age at transplantation, gender mismatch, and previous viral infections.

- GvHD may develop early after transplantation (acute GvHD), or at 100 days or more after transplant (chronic GvHD). GvHD is one of the major causes of death and long-term disability after stem cell transplantation.

- Prevention is the best approach to the management of GvHD. Prevention of GvHD is based on selection of optimal donor and vigorous T-cell depletion in the case of HLA-mismatch between the donor and the recipient. Immunosuppressive drugs, such as cyclosporine, are another potent form of GvHD prevention.

Graft rejection

Graft rejection reflects the presence of immunocompetent cells in the host that specifically recognize and react to donor-derived stem cells. Several factors influence the likelihood of graft rejection, in particular: a) the degree of immunocompetence of the host; b) the degree of HLA disparity between donor and recipient; c) the number and source of stem cells infused; d) the type of conditioning regimen used; e) the possible pre-sensitization of the host to donor histocompatibility antigens; and f) the presence and source of donor T cells in the graft.

In the case of infants with SCID, graft rejection is an unlikely event, because of the profound immune deficiency that characterizes these conditions. Conversely, in other forms of primary immunodeficiency there is sufficient immune function in the host to allow for rejection of donor-derived stem cells, unless an appropriate conditioning regimen is used prior to HSCT

In children with nonmalignant disease, the most commonly used preparative regimen consists of busulfan and cyclophosphamide, with or without the addition of anti-thymocyte globulin (ATG). In some forms of congenital immunodeficiencies, such as phagocytic or hemophagocytic cell disorders, a more aggressive conditioning regimen, including additional drugs, may be used.

On the other hand, infants and children with pre-existing organ damage are highly sensitive to the toxic effects of drugs conventionally used in the conditioning regimen. In these cases, nonmyeloablative or reduced intensity regimens (e.g., fludarabine, melphalan and alemtuzumab) have been preferred.[11] A more vigorous GvHD prophylaxis is often necessary if nonmyeloablative conditioning is used, because of a higher risk of GvHD.

Acute graft-versus-host disease

Acute GvHD (aGvHD) is the result of alloreactivity of donor-derived T lymphocytes versus the recipient's antigens, and is one of the most severe complications of HSCT. It may occur as early as one week after HSCT, and is potentially fatal. Clinical manifestations of aGvHD include maculopapular skin rash (that tends to be confluent), diarrhea, and liver abnormalities (hepatomegaly, elevated liver enzymes, increased levels of conjugated bilirubin).[12] The disease may progress to severe skin manifestations, with exfoliative dermatitis, and significant liver and gut damage (with intractable watery or bloody diarrhea, protein-losing enteropathy, and abdominal pain). In the most severe cases, leakage of intravascular fluids into the interstitium (so-called "third space filling"), leads to generalized edema. Bone marrow aplasia, and a high susceptibility to infections (including reactivation of herpesvirus infections) are also often observed in severe aGvHD.

The severity of aGvHD is evaluated according to grading (Table 82.3). Major risk factors for aGvHD include: HLA-mismatch between donor and recipient, older age of the recipient or donor, gender mismatch, stem cell source.[12] However, aGvHD may also be observed following related HLA-identical HSCT, particularly when a conditioning regimen is used.

Finally, transfusion-associated aGvHD is a very severe complication after HSCT, that can be effectively prevented by using irradiated (1500-3000 rads) and filtered blood derivatives.

Chronic graft-versus-host disease

Chronic GvHD (cGvHD) has traditionally been defined as symptoms that persist or appear after 100 days since the time of transplantation. As the types of donor, stem cell sources

Table 82.3 Staging and grading of acute graft-versus-host disease (aGvHD)

Stage	Skin	Liver (Bilirubin)	GI (Stool output)
0	None	<2 mg/dL	Adult: <500 ml/day Child: < 10 ml/kg/day
1	Rash <25% BSA	2-3 mg/dL	Adult: 500-999 ml/day Child: 10-19.9 ml/kg/day or persistent nausea, vomiting, or anorexia, with a positive upper GI biopsy
2	Rash 25-50% BSA	3-6 mg/dL	Adult: 1000-1500 ml/day Child: 20-30 ml/kg/day
3	Rash >50% BSA	6.1-15 mg/dL	Adult: >1500 ml/day Child: >30 ml/kg/day
4	Generalized erythroderma with bullous formation	>15 mg/dL	Severe abdominal pain with or without ileus

Overall clinical grade of aGvHD is determined by combination of skin, liver and GI stage.
Grade 0: No stage 1-4 of any organ
Grade 1: Stage 1-2 skin rash only
Grade 2: Stage 3 skin rash, or stage 1 liver or stage 1 GI
Grade 3: Stage 2-3 liver or stage 2-3 GI with any skin stage except stage 4
Grade 4: Stage 4 skin or stage 4 liver or stage 4 GI

and conditioning regimens have changed, it is now recognized that symptoms of aGvHD can present later than 100 days and that cGvHD is better defined by its distinct clinical manifestations rather than the time of onset alone. These clinical manifestations include skin changes (scleroderma-like lesions, hyperpigmentation, hyperkeratosis, skin atrophy, ulcerations), tissue fibrosis and limitation of joint motility, fibrosis of exocrine glands ("sicca syndrome"), fibrosis of lungs and liver, increased susceptibility to infections, immune dysregulation and autoimmunity.[12] Consequently, cGvHD poses a major burden on the patients' quality of life, and can be fatal.

Although the incidence of cGvHD is lower in children than in adults treated by allogeneic HSCT, the risk factors and the spectrum of clinical manifestations are similar.

Acute GvHD represents a major risk factor for cGvHD, yet cGvHD can be observed even without preceding aGvHD, and when present, it does not represent merely the continuation of aGvHD. Older age of the recipient at HSCT, transplantation from a multiparous female donor into a male recipient (with reactivity to Y chromosome-associated antigens), and incompatibility at minor histocompatibility loci represent additional risk factors for cGvHD.[12] Furthermore, use of peripheral blood stem cells carries an increased risk of cGvHD as compared with use of bone marrow stem cells.

Prevention of GvHD

Prevention is the most effective approach to GvHD, and use of a fully matched donor remains the best method of prevention. Alternatively, if a related HLA-mismatched donor is used for transplantation, it is essential that the graft is vigorously T cell-depleted.

Whenever a conditioning regimen is used in the transplantation protocol, pharmacological prophylaxis of GvHD must

also be included, even in the case of HSCT from a related HLA-identical donor.

Long standing approaches to prevention of GvHD include cyclosporine daily for 6 months or methotrexate (15 mg/m² on the first day after HSCT, and then 10 mg/m² at days +3, +6, and +11 after transplant), or a combination of the two. Newer regimens substitute another calcineurin inhibitor, tacrolimus, for cyclosporine. ATG and alemtuzumab are also commonly used to prevent GvHD.

Attempts to prevent cGvHD have been less satisfactory. In particular, use of a prolonged immune suppression after transplant does not decrease the incidence of cGvHD.

Treatment of GvHD

Once GvHD has developed, treatment is mainly based upon the use of immunosuppressive drugs. Corticosteroids remain the first line therapy. Second line therapy includes ATG, mycophenolate mofetil, cyclosporine or tacrolimus, and a variety of monoclonal antibodies directed to human T lymphocyte antigens (such as anti-CD3) or to Th1-type cytokines (anti-TNF-α) and cytokine receptors (anti-CD25, daclizumab). Corticosteroids are usually effective for mild and moderate forms of aGvHD, but the efficacy of second line agents in severe or steroid unresponsive aGvHD is limited.

Treatment of cGvHD is also based on immunosuppression, but with limited efficacy.[13,14] Topical steroids and calcineurin inhibitors may alleviate mucosal and skin symptoms. Systemic steroids have been shown to improve survival, but at the risk of significant adverse effects. Ursodeoxycholic acid may be useful in cGvHD with significant liver involvement. Extracorporeal photopheresis can be used with the goal to induce tolerance; typically, its benefits, if present, are delayed until 2-3 months after initiation of treatment. Use of hydroxychloroquine, mycophenolate mofetil, anti-TNF-α monoclonal antibody, and etanercept (a recombinant form of soluble TNF-receptor) and anti-CD20 antibody (rituximab) remains at present investigational.

Infections

Infections represent one of the major complications following HSCT. Patients with severe primary immune deficiency are intrinsically highly susceptible to infections. For infants with SCID and with other forms of combined immune deficiency, viral and opportunistic infections can develop prior to transplantation and are one of the factors that adversely affect the outcome of HSCT itself.[2] Similarly, treatment-refractory bacterial and especially fungal infections can compromise survival after HSCT in children with phagocytic disorders.[15] Regardless of the type of underlying primary immunodeficiency, T-cell depleted HSCT carries a high risk of infections because of the longer time required to achieve immune reconstitution. Furthermore, use of a pretransplant conditioning regimen resulting in myeloablation and immune suppression, and GvHD prophylaxis contribute to the increased susceptibility to infections after HSCT.

Strict isolation of the patients during and after HSCT, and prophylactic administration of antibiotics have been associated with a better survival rate, particularly after related HLA-mismatched transplantation for SCID.[2] In spite of this, infections remain the major cause of death. Challenging viruses in infants with SCID include adenovirus, cytomegalovirus (CMV), parainfluenza type III virus, and Epstein-Barr virus (EBV), although several antiviral drugs (acyclovir, ganciclovir, foscarnet, cidofovir) are now available, with good results, especially against CMV.[16] Filtering of blood derivatives removes leukocytes, and thus reduces the risk of transfusion-associated infections, such as CMV. Viral infection after HSCT can cause interstitial pneumonia, enteritis, hepatitis and encephalitis. EBV can also cause BLPD, especially after T cell-depleted HLA-mismatched transplantation, in particular in patients with Wiscott-Aldrich syndrome (WAS) (Table 82.1). This complication is now often treated successfully with *in vivo* administration of anti-CD20 monoclonal antibody (rituximab).

Pneumocystis jiroveci is a common cause of pneumonia in severely immunocompromised patients. Treatment is based on intravenous co-trimoxazole (20 mg/kg/day).

Aspergillus infection is a severe complication in patients with chronic granulomatous disease (CGD) and in profoundly neutropenic patients.[15] Voriconazole offers some advantage as compared to liposomal amphotericin B for treatment of invasive aspergillosis, whereas prophylactic itraconazole reduces the incidence of fungal infections in patients with CGD prior to transplantation.

Bacterial infections are usually amenable to successful treatment, if the pathogen is identified, and appropriate and aggressive use of antibiotics is initiated. Prophylactic administration of immunoglobulins following HSCT also reduces the frequency and severity of infections.

Finally, the clinical manifestations of an infection tend to be more severe when initial signs of immune reconstitution appear, as the latter facilitates development of inflammatory reactions both at the site of infection and systemically.

Toxicity related to conditioning regimen

Chemotherapeutic agents that are used in the conditioning regimen of HSCT often cause significant short-term and long-term toxicity. Chemotherapeutic drugs that damage the liver vascular endothelium, particularly busulfan but also cyclophosphamide, can cause veno-occlusive disease (VOD) that is clinically marked by painful hepatomegaly, jaundice, ascites, fluid retention, and weight gain, and that can ultimately result in fatal multi-organ failure (MOF). Defibrotide is the most effective agent studied to date in the treatment of VOD.[17] Busulfan can also cause lung damage that is difficult to distinguish from pulmonary infection, and can induce seizures. Cyclophosphamide can cause hemorrhagic cystitis, a syndrome of inappropriate anti-diuretic hormone secretion, or rarely cardiac disturbances.

Long-term hormonal complications are more common when total body irradiation (TBI) is used. However, the busulfan and cyclophosphamide regimen can cause delayed puberty or sterility, and thyroid dysfunction is frequently observed, even in patients who have not received TBI. Effects on final height and growth, as well as long-term neurocognitive effects, are emerging as more children are treated and followed.

HSCT for the treatment of primary immunodeficiency disorders

In 1968, the first successful experience with HLA-identical HSCT in SCID was reported.[1] Shortly thereafter, partial success was achieved also with HSCT in a child with WAS.[18] Since then, over 1800 transplants have been performed in patients with primary immunodeficiencies, most of them in children with SCID.[2,3] The increasing number of transplants over the years reflects improved outcome as a result of advances in supportive and critical care before and after HSCT, increasingly improved strategies for T-cell depletion applied for related HLA-mismatched HSCT, and greater availability of MUD and cord blood for transplantation.

● CLINICAL PEARLS

Considerations of stem cell transplantation unique to SCID

- Patients with SCID are strongly impaired in their ability to reject allogeneic cells, including stem cells. Therefore, no chemotherapy is required in these patients in order to achieve T-cell reconstitution following stem cell transplantation.
- The quality and the kinetics of T-cell reconstitution following stem cell transplantation depend on the type of transplant.
- If unmanipulated bone marrow from genotypically HLA-identical related donor is used, mature T cells contained in the graft expand as early as 2 weeks after transplantation and provide a rapid source of immune competence.
- A similar phenomenon is also observed following unmanipulated MUD transplantation. In this case, however, drugs used in conditioning regimen decrease the degree of early expansion of donor-derived T cells.
- In contrast, appearance of naïve T cells occurs only at 3 months or more after transplantation, regardless of degree of HLA-matching between donor and recipient. Consequently, following haploidentical transplantation, there is a prolonged period during which the recipient remains lymphopenic and at high risk of infections.
- In the absence of pre-transplant conditioning, following haploidentical transplantation for SCID, engraftment is usually restricted to T lymphocytes. This may cause persistent B cell dysfunction. Furthermore, patients with NK$^+$ SCID may show some ability to reject stem cells from HLA-mismatched donors.

For these reasons, several centers (particularly in Europe) include pre-transplant conditioning for haploidentical transplantation for SCID. Conditioning regimen is typically used for MUD- or unrelated cord blood-HSCT.

HSCT for SCID

General considerations

SCID is a medical emergency, and is uniformly fatal, unless promptly diagnosed and successfully treated. With few exceptions in which alternative strategies (gene therapy, enzyme replacement therapy) can be used, allogeneic HSCT represents the most effective form of treatment (i.e., cure) for these disorders.

SCID is also a unique situation in which the virtual lack of T lymphocytes strongly impairs the ability of the recipient to reject the graft. Furthermore, donor-derived lymphoid progenitor cells have a striking advantage for *in vivo* T cell differentiation. Consequently, use of pre-transplant chemotherapy and immune suppression is not required in SCID infants who have a related HLA-identical donor. A similar strategy can also be used for T cell-depleted mismatched HSCT. However, this remains controversial and several centers prefer to use a conditioning regimen whenever an HLA-identical related donor is not available. Avoiding the use of a conditioning regimen eliminates the risk of drug-related toxicity, and reduces the chance of developing GvHD. On the other hand, use of a conditioning regimen favors the engraftment of donor-derived stem cells, and may lead to a better recovery of humoral immunity. Chemotherapy is typically used for "leaky" forms of SCID with a significant number of autologous, partially functioning T lymphocytes.

Survival following HSCT for SCID

The two largest series of SCID patients treated by HSCT in Europe and at a single center in the United States include 699 and 166 cases, respectively.[2,3]

In the European study, which includes transplants performed between 1968 and 2005, 203 patients had received HSCT from a genotypically (n=135) or phenotypically (N=68) identical related donor, with 10-year overall survival rates of 84% and 64%, respectively. This figure is clearly superior to the 54% survival rate observed among 415 patients who had received related HLA-mismatched HSCT. Finally, in this report 81 patients had received HSCT from a MUD, and 66% were alive.[2] At the University of Brescia, Italy (former institution of one of us, LDN), among 69 infants with SCID treated by HSCT, overall survival rates following related HLA-identical, MUD, and T cell-depleted haploidentical HSCT were 100%, 94%, and 52%, respectively (Fig. 82.1a). In the most recent report from Dr. Rebecca Buckley of Duke University, USA, the overall survival rate after HSCT for SCID was 76%.[3] In particular, all 17 recipients of related HLA-identical HSCT were reported to be alive, as were 109 of 149 (i.e., 73%) recipients of T cell-depleted related HLA-mismatched HSCT.

Survival after HSCT for SCID has improved over the years,[2] reflecting more effective treatment and prevention of disease-related and transplantation-associated complications, such as infections and GvHD. In particular, the current survival rate after HSCT from HLA-identical related donors is 90%, whereas 3-year survival after HSCT from related HLA-mismatched donors has improved from 49% in transplants performed up to 1994 to 69% in those performed between 1995 and 1999.[2] However, no further improvement in survival has been observed since that time.

Several factors influence survival after HSCT for SCID. In particular, younger age at transplantation leads to superior survival. Among 48 infants who were treated by Buckley and collaborators before 3.5 months of life, 45 (94%) survive[3] Importantly, the vast majority of these infants received T cell-depleted HLA-mismatched HSCT from a parent, without any conditioning or GvHD prophylaxis. In Europe, among SCID infants who received HLA-identical transplantation, 10-year survival was better when HSCT was performed at less than 6 months of age (68% survival rate) than at 12 months or more (survival rate: 51%).[2]

Other factors that affect outcome include: prophylaxis with trimethoprim-sulfamethoxazole, isolation in a protected environment and lack of pre-existing respiratory infection.[2]

Infants with B[+] SCID have a better 10-year survival after HSCT than infants with B[−] SCID (70 vs. 51%, respectively).[2] The poorer outcome observed in infants with B[−] SCID may reflect the presence of autologous NK cells detectable in most of these infants, which may increase the risk of rejection. Alternatively, many forms of B[−] SCID are due to genetic defects that cause a later block in T cell development than in the majority of patients with B[+] SCID. This may lead to a stronger competition between donor-derived vs. autologous T cell progenitors in patients with B[−] SCID who receive unconditioned HSCT. Finally, some forms of B[−] SCID are caused by genetic defects that affect ubiquitous pathways of DNA repair; such patients are more prone to complications, especially if chemotherapy is used. Consistent with these data, among 41 infants with SCID treated by haploidentical HSCT at the University of Brescia, Italy,, survival was better for infants with B[+] SCID than in those with B[−] SCID (59. 3% vs. 40%) (Fig. 82.2).

Recently, HSCT from MUD has been shown to be an effective treatment also for SCID. In a series of 41 patients treated with MUD HSCT at two centers (the Hospital for Sick Children in Toronto, and the University of Brescia Hospital in Italy), 33 (or 80%) have survived, as compared to 52% survival among 40 patients treated by related T cell-depleted HLA-mismatched transplantation.[8] In this study, use of MUD HSCT was reported to lead to sustained engraftment and better immune reconstitution as compared to T cell-depleted haploidentical HSCT. Similar favorable data have been reported in a smaller series of transplants performed at a single center in Japan, with all seven recipients of MUD HSCT reported to be alive, as compared to only one of eight patients treated by T cell-depleted haploidentical HSCT.[9] However, data from the largest cumulative European series do not support improved survival after MUD- vs. mismatched-related HSCT for SCID.[2]

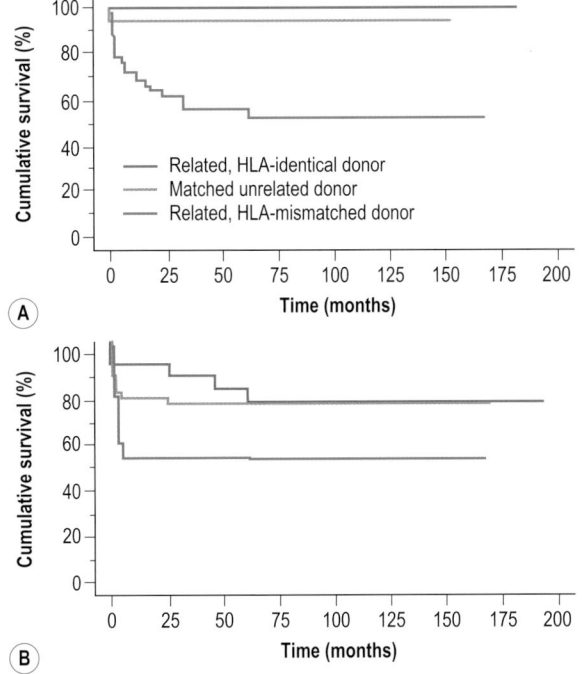

Fig. 82.1 Kaplan-Meyer survival curve for 148 consecutive children with primary immunodeficiency who have received hematopoietic stem cell transplantation (HSCT) at the University of Brescia, Italy. **(A)** Survival after HSCT in 69 infants with SCID, 12 of which have received related HLA.identical HSCT, 41 a mismatched related transplant, and 16 a MUD HSCT. **(B)** Survival after HSCT in 79 children with immunodeficiency other than SCID. Of these patients, 23 have received related HLA-identical HSCT, 13 a mismatched related HSCT, and 43 a MUD HSCT.

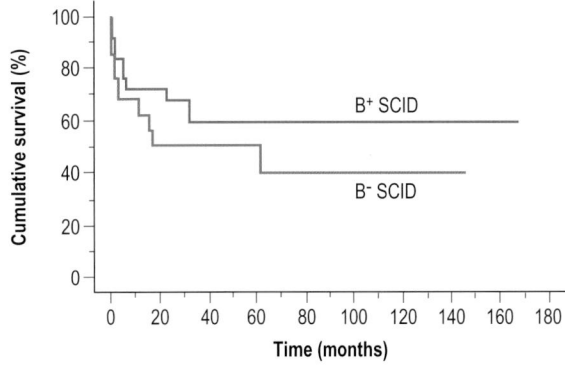

Fig. 82.2 Kaplan-Meyer survival curve in 25 infants with B[+] SCID and 16 infants with B[−] SCID, treated by mismatched related HSCT at the University of Brescia, Italy.

Outcome of stem cell transplantation for primary immunodeficiencies

- For SCID, the overall survival rate of patients transplanted since1968 is over 70%, and is higher for patients treated by HLA-identical transplantation. Moreover, there has been a continuous improvement in the outcome of the procedure. Currently, survival rates are over 90% for HLA-identical transplantation, and 75% for haploidentical transplantation.

- Improvements in clinical care (both in critical care and in prevention/treatment of infections) have recently led to increased use of MUD transplantation for SCID, also with excellent results. The decision to attempt a MUD transplantation for SCID must be weighed against the risks associated with the time interval required to identify such a donor.

- Factors influencing survival after transplantation for SCID include younger age at transplant, prevention of GvHD, and control of infections. For the latter, isolation in a protected environment, and prophylactic use of antibiotics are effective measures.

- The decline of T-cell function that is observed at 10 years or more after transplantation remains a concern, and may cause clinical problems. Therefore, there is a need for improvements in the procedures used to facilitate and sustain stem cell engraftment, and/or to boost donor-derived immunity.

- For primary immunodeficiencies other than SCID, there has been a progressive improvement in the outcome following stem cell transplantation. In particular, results are good both for HLA-identical transplants (with a survival rate of 70% or more, depending on the disease), and for MUD or cord blood transplantations. Reduced-intensity conditioning regimens have been often used in these patients, in the attempt to reduce the risks of drug-related toxicity.

Complications following HSCT for SCID

Despite advances in prophylaxis and treatment, infections (especially those caused by viruses) remain a significant cause of death after HSCT for SCID. In a report of 166 transplants performed at their center, Buckley and collaborators indicate that viral infections accounted for 30 of the 40 deaths observed. CMV and adenovirus were responsible for nine deaths each, and 18 additional deaths were due to infections caused by EBV, enteroviruses, parainfluenza virus type 3, varicella, herpes simplex and respiratory syncytial virus.[3]

Viral and opportunistic infections are more common early after HSCT, especially in recipients of T-cell depleted haploidentical HSCT, because of the delay in achieving immune reconstitution. Incomplete recovery of immune function at one year after HSCT is associated with a higher risk of late infections. In a single center study of 90 patients with SCID treated by HSCT, 11 (12%) developed significant infectious complications 2 to 17 years after transplantation.[19] Among late infections, chronic skin warts, due to papilloma virus, have been observed in a significant fraction of infants with γc or JAK3 deficiency after HSCT.[19,20] This complication may occur also in patients who attain robust immune function, and probably results from signaling defects that involve extra-hematopoietic cells such as keratinocytes.

GvHD is another major complication of HSCT for SCID. Buckley reported that GvHD occurred in 45/149 (30.2%) patients given T cell-depleted mismatched parental bone marrow, 8/17 (47%) given unfractionated HLA-identical marrow, and 4/5 given placental blood.[3] In most cases, GvHD occurred when there was presence of transplacentally acquired T lymphocytes. Most of the GvHD observed was mild (grade I or II) and required no treatment, however eleven patients developed GvHD grade III or IV, and required treatment with steroids, cyclosporine,

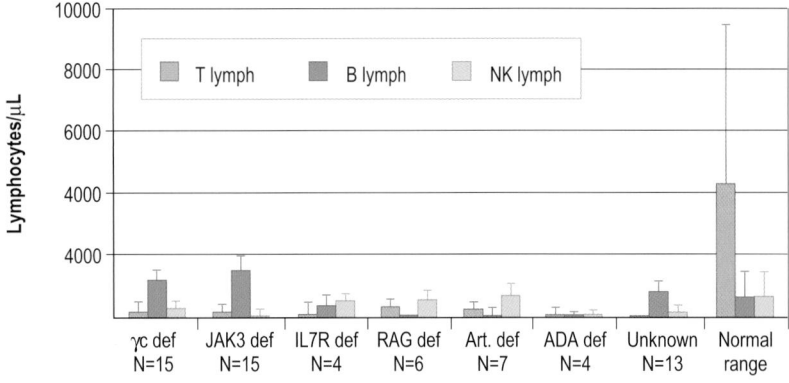

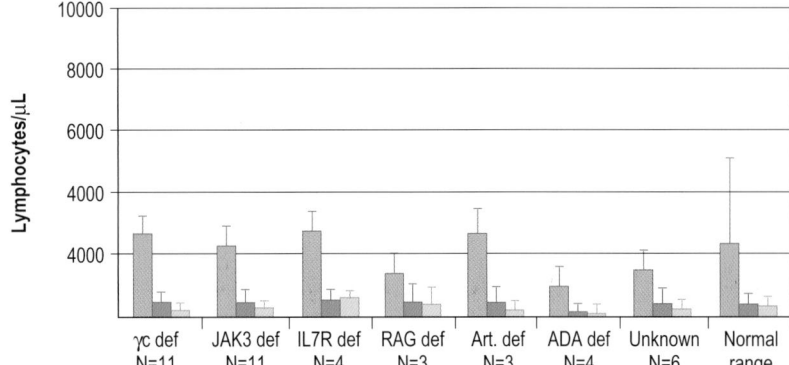

Fig. 82.3 Mean ($\pm$SE) numbers of CD3$^+$ T cells, CD19$^+$ B cells, and CD16$^+$ natural killer cells before transplantation (**A**) and at the most recent evaluation after transplantation (**B**) performed at the University of Brescia, Italy, according to the type of SCID.

and/or tacrolimus. None of these patients have died, but one has developed cGvHD.

In their article describing experience of HSCT for SCID at two centers (Brescia, Italy; and Toronto, Canada), Grunebaum et al., have reported that aGvHD developed in 4/13 patients (31%) who received related HLA-identical HSCT, 18/40 (45%) patients treated by T cell-depleted haploidentical transplantation, and 30/41 (73%) of patients receiving MUD HSCT.[8] Thus, unfractionated HSCT from MUD appears to increase the risk of aGvHD, possibly reflecting mismatch at minor histocompatibility loci. In spite of this difference, the incidence of aGvHD grade III or IV was similar (15-22%) among recipients of T-cell depleted mismatched HSCT or of MUD HSCT. While continuous improvement in HLA typing has already resulted in a progressively lower incidence of GvHD, these data illustrate the need for careful monitoring of infants treated with other than related HLA-identical HSCT, and call for adhering to guidelines on the use of immune suppression for GvHD prophylaxis after MUD HSCT or after conditioned T-cell depleted haploidentical transplantation.

Chronic GvHD disease has been reported in 10 of 90 patients (11%) who have survived for at least 2 years after receiving HSCT for SCID in Paris. Six of them developed disseminated cGvHD, and 3 died of cGvHD and related infectious complications.[19]

Immune dysregulation and autoimmunity represent additional complications of HSCT for SCID. In a joint series of 94 SCID infants transplanted in Brescia and Toronto, we have reported that 6/41 patients who received MUD HSCT, and 5/40 children treated by T cell-depleted haploidentical transplantation developed autoimmune cytopenias. These complications

may develop at few months after HSCT (when skewing of the T cell repertoire may be observed), or may persist, particularly in infants with delayed and incomplete immune reconstitution. In particular, Neven et al. have reported that among 90 long-term survivors after HSCT for SCID, 12 patients suffered from autoimmune and inflammatory complications at more than 2 years after HSCT for SCID, and in 6 of them the onset of such complications was within the first 2 years after transplantation. These late manifestations of immune dysregulation are often associated with incomplete immune reconstitution and may lead to poor outcome.[19]

Finally, prolonged nutritional support has been reported after HSCT for SCID. This complication was more frequent among patients treated by mismatched related or unrelated donor HSCT, especially if cGvHD, immune dysregulation or poor immune reconstitution are also present. Infants with Artemis deficiency (leading to impaired DNA repair) were at particularly high risk for this complication.[19]

Quality and kinetics of T-cell immune reconstitution

The effectiveness of HSCT in SCID is well illustrated by the normalization of the number and function of T lymphocytes that is achieved after transplantation (Fig. 82.3 and 82.4). The efficacy of the procedure has been demonstrated in all forms of SCID, although T lymphocyte count after HSCT tends to be lower in patients with adenosine deaminase (ADA) deficiency, possibly reflecting irreversible thymic damage. Moreover, normalization of T lymphocyte count after HSCT demonstrates the ability of the stem cells to seed and differentiate in a vestigial thymus.

Fig. 82.4 Number of TRECs (A) and *in vitro* proliferative response to phytohemagglutinin (PHA) (**B**) before transplantation and at the last follow-up after transplantation in a series of 42 SCID infants treated at the University of Brescia, Italy, according to the type of SCID.

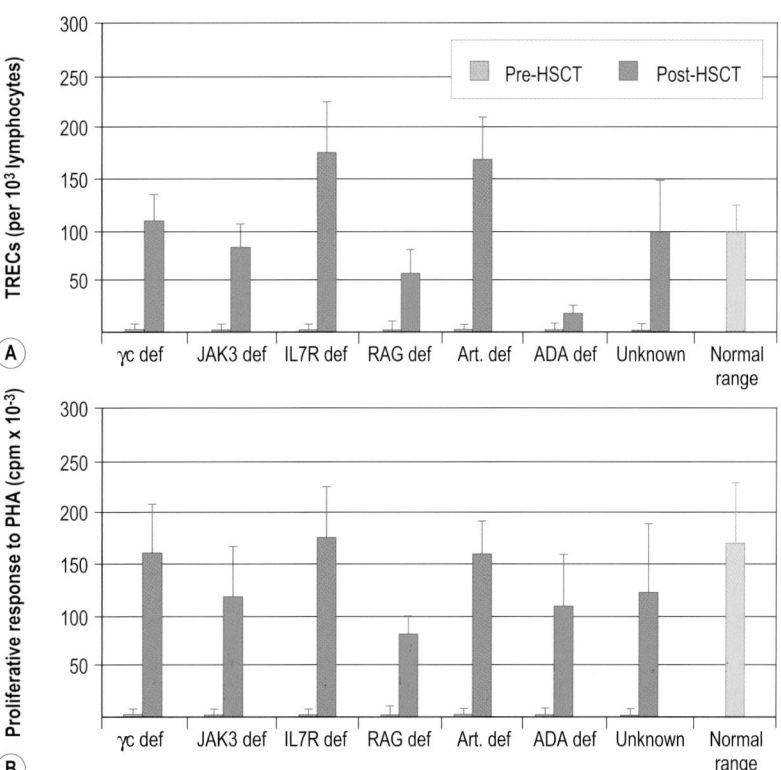

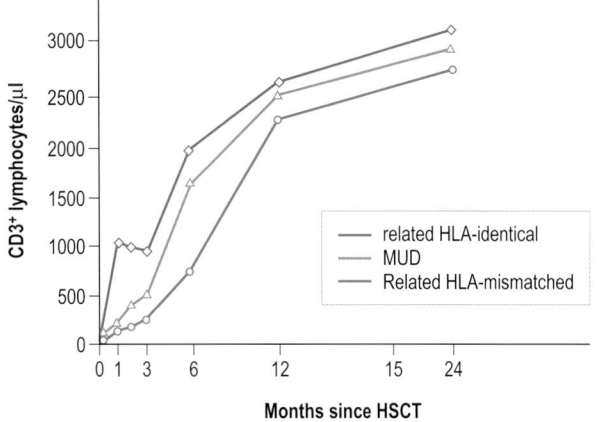

Fig. 82.5 Kinetics of CD3$^+$ T lymphocytes reconstitution in 48 SCID infants following HLA-identical (n = 12), MUD (n = 15) or haploidentical (n = 21) HSCT, performed at the University of Brescia, Italy. Geometric mean CD3$^+$ T cell counts are shown.

The kinetics of T lymphocyte reconstitution differs substantially depending on the type of transplantation. The unmanipulated graft from a related HLA-identical donor contains mature T lymphocytes. Homeostatic as well as antigen-driven expansion of these mature T cells occurs as early as 2 weeks after transplantation (Fig. 82.5).[20] These T cells have a memory (CD45RO) phenotype, are fully competent, and in fact provide the recipient with functional immunity.[21]

Mature T cells are present also in the bone marrow graft collected from MUDs. However, the use of conditioning in MUD HSCT impairs, at least in part, immune development in such transplants, as compared to unconditioned HSCT from related HLA-identical donors (Fig. 82.5).

In contrast, newly generated, naïve (CD45RA$^+$ CD31$^+$) T lymphocytes do not appear in circulation until 3-6 months after HSCT, irrespective of the type of transplant (HLA-identical or mismatched), and their number tends to peak at approximately one year after HSCT, when a fully polyclonal T cell repertoire is usually observed.[21] These naïve T lymphocytes are the product of ongoing active thymopoiesis, as shown by the fact that they contain T cell receptor excision circles (TRECs). TRECs are extrachromosomal DNA episomes, that are generated during V(D)J recombination (Chapter 4), and are not duplicated during mitosis. Therefore, TRECs identify newly generated naïve T lymphocytes.

The kinetics of T cell reconstitution is influenced by the recipient's age. Transplants performed early in life (at less than 3.5 months of age) lead to superior thymic output.[6] This may reflect lack of thymic damage (which is often observed in older infants after infections); alternatively, it is possible that a younger thymus has intrinsic superior ability to support active thymopoiesis.

Quantitation of TRECs sequentially after HSCT is an accepted approach to assess engraftment of *bona fide* stem cells and to monitor persistence of immunity. Although an earlier study had shown that levels of TRECs tended to decline at 10 years after HSCT in recipients of unconditioned mismatched-related transplantation,[22] more recent observations from the same group indicate that robust thymopoiesis and generation of a diversified repertoire of T lymphocytes were maintained long-term after HSCT.[23]

Reconstitution of B and NK cell immunity

In contrast to what is observed for T lymphocytes, the engraftment of B cells after HSCT for SCID is often problematic and delayed.

In their series, Buckley and collaborators reported that only 5/17 survivors of HLA-identical and 33/109 survivors of unconditioned haploidentical HSCT had evidence of donor derived B lymphocytes; overall, 63/126 survivors were requiring intravenous immunoglobulins.[3] Booster transplants have been used to overcome these problems; 33 of 49 patients who received such booster transplants at Dr. Buckley's institution were reported to be alive with improved immune function.[3]

In Europe, use of pre-transplant conditioning has been advocated in haploidentical HSCT with the goal of facilitating engraftment of stem cells and thus also of B lymphocytes. Mazzolari et al. have reported that donor B cell engraftment was achieved in only 1 of 11 survivors after unconditioned HSCT, vs. 26 of 29 patients who received myeloablative conditioning regimen.[24]

In patients with B$^+$ SCID, the difficulty to achieve B-cell engraftment after unconditioned HLA-identical HSCT may reflect competition between host and donor early B-cell precursors.[25] Finally, attainment of normal B-cell function may also depend on the nature of the genetic defect, as shown by the fact that among infants with B$^+$ SCID, those who have an *IL-7RA* gene defect usually develop normal Bcell immunity after HSCT even if no donor-derived B cells are present, whereas patients with γc or JAK3 deficiency (both of which compromise Bcell function) often remain dependent on immunoglobulin substitution therapy if engraftment of donor-derived B cells is not achieved.[3]

More limited data are available about reconstitution of NK cell function. In patients with NK$^-$ SCID, NK cells are often the first cells to appear after haploidentical HSCT.[3] Lower NK cell counts have been reported at long-term follow-up after HSCT in patients with γc orJAK3 defects.[3]

HSCT for immunodeficiencies other than SCID

Immunodeficiencies other than SCID are characterized by residual T cell-mediated immunity that may impede engraftment of donor-derived stem cells. Although these disorders are often severe, they rarely represent a medical emergency. For this reason, and because results of T cell-depleted haploidentical transplant are less satisfactory than in typical SCID, use of alternative donors (MUD and cord blood) has been explored, whenever an HLA-identical related donor is not available. In any case, the residual number and function of autologous T lymphocytes represents a common indication to use of a pre-transplant conditioning regimen in order to facilitate donor engraftment and immune reconstitution.

In a series of 79 patients with immunodeficiency other than SCID who received HSCT at the University of Brescia, Italy, overall survival rate after HLA-identical, T cell-depleted haploidentical, and MUD HSCT was 78.5%, 53.8%, and 78.1%, respectively (Fig. 82.1b).

Combined immunodeficiencies other than SCID

Omenn syndrome is a fatal disorder, unless treated with HSCT. Satisfactory results have been obtained with transplantation from related HLA-identical donors, but less so from haploidentical donors. However, improved outcome has been observed in the last decade. Mazzolari et al. have reported that 9 of 11 patients with Omenn syndrome were alive after HSCT; importantly, of these only one had a matched sibling, whereas two infants had a phenotypically-identical related donor, three were treated by MUD HSCT, and five received a haploidentical HSCT.[26]

HSCT has been attempted also in other predominant T cell immunodeficiencies, such as purine nucleoside phosphorylase deficiency, cartilage hair hypoplasia, and other forms of T cell activation deficiency, with an overall survival rate of approximately 50%.[2,3]

Major histocompatibility complex (MHC) class II deficiency remains a very difficult disease to transplant. In the European series, cumulative survival after HSCT performed in the period 1995-2005 remains around 40%.[2] Many patients fail to reconstitute the number of circulating CD4$^+$ T lymphocytes, probably because the lack of expression of HLA class II molecules on thymic epithelial cells prevents positive selection of CD4$^+$ lymphocytes.

The mainstay of treatment for patients with complete DiGeorge syndrome is represented by thymic transplantation. However, HSCT or even transplantation of unmobilized peripheral blood mononuclear cells may be attempted if an HLA-identical donor is available; in such cases, immune reconstitution is provided by T lymphocytes contained in the graft.[27]

Patients with CD40 ligand (CD40L) deficiency suffer from recurrent bacterial and opportunistic (*Pneumocystis jiroveci, Cryptosporidium parvum*) infections, resulting in only 46% survival rate at 25 years of age according to the European Registry (Notarangelo, unpublished). This has prompted use of HSCT in the treatment of this disease. In a series of 38 patients transplanted in Europe, 26 (68.4%) survived.[28] Early age at transplantation and lack of pre-existing pulmonary disease were associated with a more favorable outcome. Successful outcome has been also reported after HSCT for CD40 deficiency.[29]

Wiskott–Aldrich syndrome

Bone marrow transplantation for correction of WAS was attempted as early as 1968, with partial success.[18] Full correction following HSCT was first reported in 1978, when a more robust conditioning regimen was used.[30] Since then, results of related HLA-identical HSCT in WAS have been consistently good, with continuous improvement in recent years, and excellent results have been also achieved with MUD HSCT. A multi-institutional study of 194 WAS patients treated by HSCT has shown an overall survival of 84%, and a 5-year survival as high as 89.1% for transplants performed since year 2000. For patients treated with MUD-HSCT, younger age (<5 years) at transplantation was associated with improved outcome. Patients with pre-existing autoimmunity or recurrent/severe infections had a higher rate of complications post-transplant. Mixed chimerism was associated with the presence of immunological abnormalities and increased risk of autoimmunity, and myeloid chimerism <50% was associated with persistent thrombocytopenia.[31]

Cytotoxicity defects

Familial hemophagocytic lymphohistiocytosis (FHL) comprises a genetically heterogeneous group of disorders of T- and NK-cell-mediated cytotoxicity. While chemotherapy may induce remission, patients with FHL tend to relapse and ultimately die, mostly due to multi organ failure observed in the accelerated phase of the disease. At present, HSCT is the only curative approach to FHL. Unfortunately, allogeneic HSCT for patients with FHL is often complicated by critical illness, extensive organ involvement, active infections, or refractory disease. For these reasons, patients are unusually prone to developing transplant-related toxicities and complications. In the European series, 10-year survival after HSCT was only 58%.[2] Recently, significantly improved outcome has been reported after HSCT using a reduced-intensity conditioning regimen.[32] In a series of 40 patients treated at Cincinnati Children's Hospital between 2003 and 2009, 3-year survival was only 43% for 14 patients receiving myeloablative conditioning, but was as high as 92% for patients treated with a reduced-intensity regimen.[32]

Selection of optimal family donors is an important issue for HSCT in FHL. Functional and genetic studies should be used to screen potential family donors in order to avoid transplant from a genetically-affected, but as yet asymptomatic subject.

Excellent results have been reported also after HSCT for X-linked lymphoproliferative disease (XLP). In an international series of 91 patients with XLP due to *SH2D1A* gene defect, survival was 81.4% in 43 patients treated by HSCT vs. 62.5% in 48 untransplanted patients.[33] Furthermore, the majority of untransplanted survivors required immunoglobulin replacement therapy, whereas good immune reconstitution was achieved in most transplanted patients.[33] Ideally, the transplant should be performed before EBV infection.

Chediak-Higashi syndrome (CHS) can be cured by bone marrow transplantation.[34] In a series of 35 patients, 5-year survival after HSCT was 62%.[34] Mortality was higher in patients who were in life-threatening accelerated phase of the disease at the time of transplantation and in those who received HSCT from alternative related donor.[34] Use of MUD represents a valid option for HSCT in patients with CHS. On the other hand, the long-term outcome of CHS patients treated by HSCT remains unclear, especially since neurological deterioration has been consistently observed several years after transplant.[35]

Griscelli syndrome type 2 (GS2) is a genetic disease characterized by hemophagocytic lymphohistiocytosis and a high risk of neurological complications. Correction of the cytotoxicity defect after HSCT has been reported in a small series of GS2 patients, but neurologic sequelae remain a challenge, and may develop even in patients without pre-existing neurological problems.[36]

Phagocytic cell disorders

Although regular administration of prophylactic antibiotics and anti-fungal agents (± interferon-γ) has clearly improved the outcome in patients with chronic granulomatous disease (CGD), this remains a severe disorder, with a rather high risk of complications and death. Therefore, there has been a renewed interest for HSCT in CGD. In a survey of the European experience from 1985 to 2000, 27 patients with CGD were treated by HSCT; most of them received unmodified bone marrow from an HLA-identical sibling after myeloablative conditioning. Overall, 23/27 patients were reported to be alive, and the disease had been cured in 22 of them.[15] In this study, all 18 patients who were infection-free at the time of transplantation survived. Another single-center study from Newcastle, UK, reported that 18 of 20 CGD patients treated with matched related (n=10) or MUD (n=10) HSCT survived with normal neutrophil function and marked clinical improvement, in spite of the fact that many of them had significant pre-transplant complications (*Aspergillus* infection, inflammatory colitis).[37]

HSCT is a successful and life-saving procedure also in patients with the complete from of leukocyte adhesion deficiency type 1 (LAD1). A multicenter study of 36 such patients who underwent HSCT between 1993 and 2007 showed an overall survival of 75%, with similar results when matched related or unrelated donors were used. Mortality was higher (4 out 8 cases) after haploidentical HSCT. Stable mixed multilineage chimerism is sufficient to cure the disease.[38]

Administration of recombinant G-CSF is the treatment of choice for patients with severe congenital neutropenia (SCN). However, a subgroup of these patients fail to respond to G-CSF, and some of them are at high risk for development of myelogenous leukemia. Data from the SCN International

Registry reported that from 1976 to 1998 11 SCN patients were treated with HSCT for reasons other than malignant transformation[39] Of these, 7/8 who had a matched sibling survived with engraftment, and one rejected and had autologous reconstitution. Of the three patients treated by mismatched transplantation, two died, and one developed very severe GvHD. Data from the French SCN Registry indicate that nine patients were transplanted (seven from a MUD and two from a matched sibling). Engraftment occurred in all but one of the patients. Three patients died and six are alive in complete remission.[40]

Other primary immune deficiencies

Interferon-γ receptor 1 (IFN-γR1) deficiency leads to severe mycobacterial infections, with a high mortality rate early in life. Although HSCT should theoretically correct the disease, results of HSCT have been disappointing, with few exceptions. An international survey of eight patients transplanted, showed that only two were in full remission five years after transplant.[41] The high level of IFN-γ in these patients inhibits development of IFN-γR1-expressing donor-derived hematopoietic cells, accounting for the high rejection rate.[42]

Immunodysregulation, polyendocrinopathy, enteropathy, X-linked (IPEX) syndrome often leads to early death in. Successful outcome has been reported after HSCT using reduced-intensity conditioning.[43]

DOCK8 deficiency is a recently described form of combined immunodeficiency with elevated serum IgE, cutaneous viral infections and a high risk of malignancy. HSCT represents an effective form of treatment for this disease.[44]

Future translational research for HCST in the treatment of primary immunodeficiencies

While HSCT has clearly shown its efficacy in patients with severe forms of primary immunodeficiencies, several goals remain to be met. In particular, the main areas of interest for future development include: a) methods to improve and sustain engraftment of stem cells; b) strategies to facilitate engraftment and to reduce the incidence of GvHD in recipients of mismatched or matched unrelated transplants; c) attempts to improve thymopoiesis, with the goal to accelerate immune reconstitution and to avoid or postpone long-term decline of immunity; and, d) design strategies to reduce the burden of infections after HSCT.

Generation of a diversified pool of naïve T lymphocytes after HSCT depends on thymic function. Use of cytotoxic drugs and GvHD are significant risk factors for post-transplant T cell deficiency as they interfere with normal thymic function.[45] Strategies aimed at improving thymic function after HSCT (reviewed.[46]) may include: a) protection of thymic stroma that supports thymopoiesis; b) direct stimulation of early T-cell progenitors. Keratinocyte growth factor (KGF) is potentially attractive because it protects the thymic stroma. Administration of KGF before HSCT has been shown to enhance thymopoiesis and peripheral T cell numbers, and to reduce the incidence and severity of GvHD in murine models of HSCT.[46] However, more has to be learned about the long-term outcome of this treatment before clinical trials can be started.

Attempts to accelerate immune reconstitution might be based on the use of cytokines that promote T cell development and maturation in the thymus, such as IL-7. However, experience in severely immunodeficient mice has shown that infusion of IL-7 provides limited benefit in the MHC-compatible or partially compatible setting, whereas it has facilitated T cell development in a fully mismatched setting.[47]

Infusion of donor T cells that have anti-infective activity but no GvHD activity might help reduce infection-related mortality after HSCT. Such strategy could be based on removal of alloreactive cells by negative selection using anti-CD25 or anti-CD69 antibodies.

Recognition that B cell engraftment after HSCT is hampered by competition between host and donor early B cell precursors[25] may prompt novel forms of conditioning regimen targeted to host pro-B lymphocytes, with the attempt to facilitate development of donor-derived B cells, even in the unconditioned HLA-identical setting.

Furthermore, it has been demonstrated in a murine model that endogenous stem cells impair the engraftment of donor-derived stem cells, and that recipient's CD4 T lymphocytes inhibit productive engraftment, possibly by recognizing subtle histocompatibility differences.[48] Novel strategies aimed at interfering more specifically with the mechanisms involved in graft rejection, without requiring full myeloablation, could therefore be envisaged, at least for some severe T cell immunodeficiency disorders.

● ON THE HORIZON

- Methods to improve and sustain engraftment of stem cells
- Strategies to facilitate engraftment and reduce the occurrence of GvHD in patients with mismatched or MUD transplant
- Approaches to increase thymopoiesis and accelerate immune reconstitution
- Design of therapeutic strategies to reduce the infectious complications of HSCT

References

1. Gatti RA, Meuwissen HJ, Allen HD, et al. Immunological reconstitution of sex-linked lymphopenic immunological deficiency. Lancet 1968;2:1366–9.
2. Gennery AR, Slatter MA, Grandin L, et al. Transplantation of hematopoietic stem cells and long-term survival for primary immunodeficiencies in Europe: entering a new century, do we do better? J Allergy Clin Immunol 2010;126:602-10.e1–11.
3. Buckley RH. Transplantation of hematopoietic stem cells in human severe combined immunodeficiency: longterm outcomes. Immunol Res 2011;49:25–43.
4. Müller SM, Ege M, Pottharst A, et al. Transplacentally acquired maternal T lymphocytes in severe combined immunodeficiency: a study of 121 patients. Blood 2001;98:1847–51.
5. Muench MO. In utero transplantation: baby steps towards an effective therapy. Bone Marrow Transplant 2005;35:537–47.
6. Myers LA, Patel DD, Puck JM, Buckley RH. Hematopoietic stem cell transplantation for severe combined immunodeficiency in the neonatal period leads to superior thymic output and improved survival. Blood 2002;99:872–8.
7. O'Reilly RJ, Dupont B, Pahwa S, et al. Reconstitution in severe combined immunodeficiency by transplantation of marrow from an unrelated donor. N Engl J Med 1977;297:1311.
8. Grunebaum E, Mazzolari E, Porta F, et al. Bone marrow transplantation for severe combined immunodeficiency. JAMA 2006;295:508–18.
9. Tsuji Y, Imai K, Kajiwara M, et al. Hematopoietic stem cell transplantation for 30 patients with primary immunodeficiency diseases: 20 years experience of a single team. Bone Marrow Transplant 2006;37:469–77.
10. Gennery AR, Cant AJ. Cord blood stem cell transplantation in primary immune deficiencies. Curr Opin Allergy Clin Immunol 2007;7:528–34.
11. Veys P. Reduced intensity transplantation for primary immunodeficiency disorders. Immunol Allergy Clin North Am 2010;30:103–24.
12. Ferrara JL, Levine JE, Reddy P, Holler E. Graft-versus-host disease. Lancet 2009;373:1550–61.
13. Wolff D, Gerbitz A, Ayuk F, et al. Consensus conference on clinical practice in chronic graft-versus-host disease (GVHD): first-line and topical treatment of chronic GVHD. Biol Blood Marrow Transplant 2010;16:1611–28.
14. Wolff D, Schleuning M, von Harsdorf S, et al. Consensus Conference on Clinical Practice in Chronic GVHD: Second-Line Treatment of Chronic Graft-versus-Host Disease. Biol Blood Marrow Transplant 2011;17:1–17.

15. Seger RA, Gungor T, Belohradsky BH, et al. Treatment of chronic granulomatous disease with myeloablative conditioning and an unmodified allograft: a survey of the European experience, 1985–2000. Blood 2002;100:4344–50.
16. Tomblyn M, Chiller T, Einsele H, et al. Guidelines for preventing infectious complications among hematopoietic cell transplantation recipients: a global perspective. Biol Blood Marrow Transplant 2009;15:1143–238. Erratum in: Biol Blood Marrow Transplant 2010;16:294.
17. Richardson PG, Murakami C, Jin Z, et al. Multi-institutional use of defibrotide in 88 patients after stem cell transplantation with severe veno-occlusive disease and multisystem organ failure: response without significant toxicity in a high-risk population and factors predictive of outcome. Blood 2002;100:4337–43.
18. Bach FH, Albertini RJ, Joo P, et al. Bone marrow transplantation in a patient with the Wiskott-Aldrich syndrome. Lancet 1968;2:1364–6.
19. Neven B, Leroy S, Decaluwe H, et al. Long-term outcome after hematopoietic stem cell transplantation of a single-center cohort of 90 patients with severe combined immunodeficiency. Blood 2009;113:4114–24.
20. Fischer A, Le Deist F, Hacein-Bey S, et al. Severe combined immunodeficiency. A model disease for molecular immunology and therapy. Immunol Rev 2005;203:98–109.
21. Sarzotti M, Patel DD, Li X, et al. T cell repertoire development in humans with SCID after nonablative allogeneic marrow transplantation. J Immunol 2003;170:2711–8.
22. Patel DD, Gooding ME, Parrott RE, et al. Thymic function after hematopoietic stem-cell transplantation for the treatment of severe combined immunodeficiency. N Engl J Med 2000;342:1325–32.
23. Sarzotti-Kelsoe M, Win CM, Parrott RE, et al. Thymic output, T-cell diversity, and T-cell function in long-term human SCID chimeras. Blood 2009;114:1445–53.
24. Mazzolari E, Forino C, Guerci S, et al. Long-term immune reconstitution and clinical outcome after stem cell transplantation for severe T-cell immunodeficiency. J Allergy Clin Immunol 2007;120:892–9.
25. Liu A, Vosshenrich CA, Lagresle-Peyrou C, et al. Competition within the early B cell compartment conditions B cell reconstitution after hematopoietic stem cell transplantation in non-irradiatedrecipients. Blood 2006;108:1123–8.
26. Mazzolari E, Moshous D, Forino C, et al. Hematopoietic stem cell transplantation in Omenn syndrome: a single-center experience. Bone Marrow Transplant 2005;36:107–14.
27. Janda A, Sedlacek P, Hönig M, et al. Multicenter survey on the outcome of transplantation of hematopoietic cells in patients with the complete form of DiGeorge anomaly. Blood 2010;116:2229–36.
28. Gennery AR, Khawaja K, Veys P, et al. Treatment of CD40 ligand deficiency by hematopoietic stem cell transplantation: a survey of the European experience, 1993–2002. Blood 2004;103:1152–7.
29. Mazzolari E, Lanzi G, Forino C, et al. First report of successful stem cell transplantation in a child with CD40 deficiency. Bone Marrow Transplant 2007;40:279–81.
30. Parkman R, Rappeport J, Geha R, et al. Complete correction of the Wiskott-Aldrich syndrome by allogenic bone marrow transplantation. N Engl J Med 1978;342:1325–32.
31. Moratto D, Giliani S, Bonfim C, et al. Long-term outcome and lineage-specific chimerism in 194 Wiskott–Aldrich Syndrome patients treated by hematopoietic cell transplantation between 1980–2009: an international collaborative study. Blood 2011;118:1675–84.
32. Marsh RA, Vaughn G, Kim MO, et al. Reduced-intensity conditioning significantly improves survival of patients with hemophagocytic lymphohistiocytosis undergoing allogeneic hematopoietic cell transplantation. Blood 2010;116:5824–31.
33. Booth C, Gilmour KC, Veys P, et al. X-linked lymphoproliferative disease due to SAP/SH2D1A deficiency: a multicenter study on the manifestations, management and outcome of the disease. Blood 2011;117:53–62.
34. Eapen M, DeLaat CA, Baker KS, et al. Hematopoietic cell transplantation for Chediak-Higashi syndrome. Bone Marrow Transplant 2007;39:411–5.
35. Tardieu M, Lacroix C, Neven B, et al. Progressive neurologic dysfunctions 20 years after allogeneic bone marrow transplantation for Chediak-Higashi syndrome. Blood 2005;106:40–2.
36. Pachlopnik Schmid J, Moshous D, Boddaert N, et al. Hematopoietic stem cell transplantation in Griscelli syndrome type 2: a single-center report on 10 patients. Blood 2009;114:211–8.
37. Soncini E, Slatter MA, Jones LB, et al. Unrelated donor and HLA-identical sibling haematopoietic stem cell transplantation cure chronic granulomatous disease with good long-term outcome and growth. Br J Haematol 2009; 145:73–83.
38. Qasim W, Cavazzana-Calvo M, Davies EG, et al. Allogeneic hematopoietic stem-cell transplantation for leukocyte adhesion deficiency. Pediatrics 2009;123:836–40. Erratum in: Pediatrics 2009;123(5):1436.
39. Zeidler C, Welte K, Barak Y, et al. Stem cell transplantation in patients with severe congenital neutropenia without evidence of leukemic transformation. Blood 2000;95:1195–8.
40. Ferry C, Ouachéè M, Leblanc T, et al. Hematopoietic stem cell transplantation in severe congenital neutropenia: experience of the French SCN Registry. Bone Marrow Transplant 2005;35:45–50.
41. Roesler J, Horwitz ME, Picard C, et al. Hematopoietic stem cell transplantation for complete IFN-gamma receptor 1 deficiency: a multi-institutional survey. J Pediatr 2005;145:806–12.
42. Rottman M, Soudais C, Vogt G, et al. IFN-gamma mediates the rejection of haematopoietic stem cells in IFN-gammaR1-deficient hosts. PLoS Med 2008;5:e26.
43. Rao A, Kamani N, Filipovich A, et al. Successful bone marrow transplantation for IPEX syndrome after reduced-intensity conditioning. Blood 2007;109:383–5.
44. Bittner TC, Pannicke U, Renner ED, et al. Successful long-term correction of autosomal recessive hyper-IgE syndrome due to DOCK8 deficiency by hematopoietic stem cell transplantation. Klin Padiatr 2010;222:351–5.
45. Krenger W, Blazar BR, Holländer GA. Thymic T-cell development in allogeneic stem cell transplantation. Blood 2011;117:6768–76.
46. Wils E-J, Cornelissen JJ. Thymopoiesis following allogenic stem cell transplantation : new possibilities for improvement. Blood Rev 2005;19:89–98.
47. Andre-Schmutz I, Bonhomme D, Yates F, et al. IL-7 effect on immunological reconstitution after HSCT depends on MHC incompatibility. Br J Haematol 2004;126:844–51.
48. Bhattacharya D, Rossi DJ, Bryder D, Weissman IL. Purified hematopoietic stem cell engraftment of rare niches corrects severe lymphoid deficiencies without host conditioning. J Exp Med 2006;203:73–85.

Scott D. Rowley,
Thea Friedman,
Robert Korngold

Hematopoietic stem cell transplantation for malignant diseases

Hematopoietic stem cell transplantation (HSCT) is effective treatment for most hematological malignancies, including leukemia, lymphoma, and multiple myeloma, and the clonal but non-malignant myelodysplastic and myeloproliferative disorders. Autologous HSCT (Auto-HSCT) is commonly used as salvage therapy for patients with malignancies sensitive to chemo/radiotherapy in a dose-responsive manner. These patients receive intensive cytoreductive regimens designed to eliminate all tumor cells, but, which in so doing, also destroy the patient's hematopoietic function needed for blood formation. Infusion of previously collected HSC will rescue the patient from the marrow-ablative effects of this treatment. Allogeneic HSCT (Allo-HSCT), in addition to reconstitution of bone marrow function, achieves an immunotherapeutic benefit from donor T cells infused with the graft attacking residual tumor cells persisting after the conditioning regimen, greatly reducing the risk of later relapse of the disease. Thus, Allo-HSCT, in contrast to Auto-HSCT, does not require administration of dose-intensive regimens to achieve complete tumor cell kill, and non-myeloablative regimens may be used to "condition" the host for transplantation.

Auto-HSCT (including syngeneic twins) is justified by the dose-sensitivity of most hematological malignancies. Although there is some evidence that a more robust immunological recovery after Auto-HSCT predicts for a lower risk of relapse,[1] possibly opening an area of research in graft modification to enhance such recovery, treatment of the disease is primarily a result of the dose-intense, myeloablative chemo/radiotherapy administered. Infusion of cells is only required to recover hematopoiesis, and the stem cell infusion is, therefore, intended to treat the deleterious effect of chemotherapy on bone marrow function and not the disease itself. The primary complications of Auto-HSCT result from the administration of a dose-intense regimen and include a period of marrow hypoplasia, possibly requiring blood transfusions and antibiotics. Non-hematological toxicities, including mucositis resulting in inanition and diarrhea, and damage to other organs such as lung, liver, and kidney, limit the amount of chemotherapy that can be administered. Relapse of disease, particularly for patients who come to transplantation with chemotherapy-refractory disease, is the primary cause of failure of Auto-HSCT. Improvements in the outcome of Auto-HSCT will require new conditioning regimens with greater tumor cell kill or strategies (e.g., tumor vaccines) to induce an effective immune responsiveness to the residual disease after transplantation.

Allo-HSCT has a much lower relapse risk compared to Auto-HSCT as a result of a beneficial immunological graft-versus-tumor (GvT) effect achieved by engraftment of the donor immune system. Allograft recipients face a much higher risk of treatment-related mortality (TRM) from the identical but detrimental immunological graft-versus-host response against healthy tissues of the patient. The principal complication of

THERAPEUTIC PRINCIPLES

Autologous versus allogeneic HSCT

Autologous transplantation

- Based on chemo/radiotherapy dose-sensitivity of disease being treated
- Requires collection and storage of adequate HSC, preferably before extensive alkylating agent or purine analog therapy
- Lower risk of graft failure (no immunologic rejection)
- No routine post-transplant immunosuppression
- Minimal risk of GvHD
- No GvT effect
- Quicker post-transplant immune reconstitution
- Risk of tumor cell contamination in HSC product
- Not useful for diseases in which normal HSC cannot be collected (e.g., chronic myelogenous leukemia, myelodysplasia)

Allogeneic transplantation

- Rescues bone marrow function after dose-intense therapy
- Effective with reduced-intensity conditioning regimens
- Achieves a GvT effect in many malignancies
- Risk of GvHD but also accompanying GvT effect
- Higher risk of transplant-related complications that may offset the benefit of the GvT effect
- Risk of immunological graft rejection
- Slow post-transplant immune reconstitution
- No risk of tumor cell contamination

allogeneic HSCT is graft-versus-host disease (GvHD), which can occur early (within days; acute GvHD) or late (months to several years; chronic GvHD) after transplantation. The overall incidence of moderate to severe acute GvHD (aGVHD) is between 35-80% for all patients receiving an HLA-matched related or unrelated donor stem cell transplant, and aGvHD is a primary cause of death in 10-20% of these patients. Chronic GvHD (cGVHD), a clinicopathologically distinctive form of this alloreaction, is another form of this immunological complication and occurs in up to 80% of recipients, may involve aspects of regulatory T-cell (Treg) dysfunction and autoimmune-like responses, and may require years of therapy before tolerance is achieved allowing withdrawal of immunosuppressants.[2] Other significant complications of Allo-HSCT relate to problems of inadequate reconstitution of the immune system of the patient and the concomitant risk of opportunistic infections. Despite the apparent risks associated with Allo-HSCT, this treatment holds great promise as a curative therapy for several tumor types, particularly with strategies to either enhance the efficacy of the GvT effect or decrease the toxicity of the GvH response. Efforts have been made in recent years to make HSCT less toxic by development of low-dose, non-myeloablative conditioning regimens that allow the treatment of older patients or patients with co-morbid health issues otherwise precluding treatment with high doses of chemotherapy.

Immune mechanisms related to Allo-HSCT

Histocompatibility

The HLA major histocompatibility complex (MHC) (Chapter 5) is the primary consideration in selection of a donor for Allo-HSCT, since its loci contribute significantly to a host-versus-graft response (HvG), leading to immunological rejection of donor HSC, and to a graft-versus-host response (GvH), leading to GvHD and GvT reactions. HLA antigens are classified as class I (HLA-A, B, C) and class II (HLA-DR, DQ, DP) molecules and typing of donors and patients can be performed using low- or high-resolution techniques. The low-resolution serological techniques can determine a phenotypic mismatch (e.g., A02 vs A03), whereas high-resolution molecular techniques can identify allelic genotypic differences (e.g., A0201 vs A0202). The risks of aGVHD, cGvHD, and transplant-related mortality increase with the number of HLA mismatches, and ideally, genotypically-matched unrelated donors are sought for patients lacking an HLA-identical sibling. Disparity at HLA-A, -B, -C, and DRB1 alleles are definite risk factors for survival after unrelated donor transplantation, whereas single HLA-DQ or -DP mismatches appear to be better tolerated.[3] Complicating the analysis of HLA mismatching on transplant outcomes, however, are the differing frequencies of common alleles in various ethnic populations. Consequently, analysis of transplant outcomes based on broad classifications (e.g., HLA-A match vs mismatch) instead of analysis of specific allelic mismatching may obscure or enhance the ability to detect an effect on survival after transplantation. Not all mismatches result in a deleterious clinical outcome. Algorithms accounting for possible permissive mismatching in the selection of unrelated donors are currently being developed and tested.[3]

GvHD occurring after HLA-compatible transplantation, and the increased risk observed with matched unrelated donors, demonstrate the importance of minor histocompatibility antigens (miHA) on the outcome of Allo-HSCT.[4] MiHA are derived from polymorphic sites in normal proteins between individuals that are constantly processed by proteosome activity and presented on the cell surface by MHC molecules, and can thus be recognized by T cells from a HLA-matched donor. As a result, there may be hundreds of miHA variably expressed on host tissues that can trigger an alloresponse from donor T cells, and thereby causing GvHD. Unfortunately, only a few miHA have been identified, and miHA matching other than choosing a male donor for a male recipient is not a component of current algorithms for donor selection.

Mismatching for the killer-cell immunoglobulin-like receptor ligand (KIR-ligand) in the GvH direction appears to result in lower risk of relapse after Allo-HSCT.[5] This effect appears to be more evident in haploidentical transplantation using HSC grafts depleted of T-cells and in umbilical cord blood transplantation. The benefit of KIR-ligand mismatching is less obvious (and more controversial) after transplantation with T-cell replete grafts in which the anti-tumor effects of NK cells may be obscured by GvH reactions mediated by T cells.

GvHD

GvHD is caused by mature donor T cells contaminating the HSC inoculum, which can recognize HLA or miHA differences expressed by host antigen presenting cells and tissues (Fig. 83.1).[6] Cytokines released from host cells after a patient has received dose-intense tumor cytoreductive chemo/radiotherapy conditioning create an inflammatory environment that enables the generation of a response of infused donor T cells against host antigens. This initiates a cascade of T-cell activation events that results in proliferation, release of additional inflammatory cytokines, and the generation of effector T cells that can infiltrate target tissue, particularly the lymphoid system, intestinal tract, skin, and liver, and mediate destruction of host cells in those organs. Both CD4 and CD8 T cells can be involved in GvHD, depending upon the specific class I or class II HLA or miHA disparities involved.

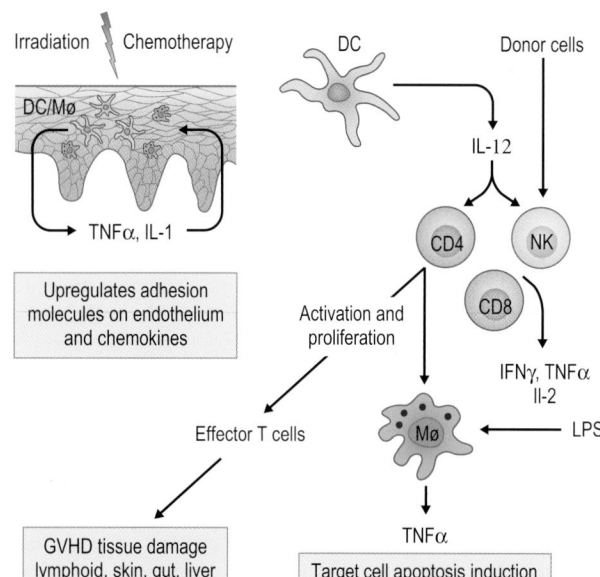

Fig. 83.1 Development of GvHD. Cytoreductive preconditioning treatment of patients with hematological malignancies with whole body irradiation or chemotherapeutic drugs causes damage to epithelium in the skin and gastrointestinal tract and activates the release of inflammatory cytokines by dendritic cells (DC) and macrophages (Mφ) in those tissues. These cytokines include tumor necrosis factor-alpha (TNFα) and interleukin (IL)-1, which upregulate adhesion molecules and chemokine release in the vascular endothelium of the tissues. Activated DC also migrate to the lymphoid system where they can present recipient histocompatibility antigens to infused donor T cells that are in the hematopoietic stem cell graft. The DC release IL-12 which helps to activate CD4 and CD8 T cells, as well as natural killer (NK) cells. These responding cells proliferate and produce additional inflammatory cytokines, including interferon-gamma (IFNγ), TNFα, and IL-2. Mφ are activated by both IFNγ and lipopolysaccharide (LPS) produced by bacteria found in the intestinal tract, and these cells then produce high levels of more TNFα. TNFα has many properties, including direct induction of apoptosis on cells in the tissues of target organs of GvHD, but it also helps effector T cells to home to and enter tissue sites through the vascular endothelium. Effector T cells specific for host histocompatibility antigens then get re-activated and perform their effector functions, including release of inflammatory and cytolytic cytokines and direct killing of recipient-type cells in the lymphoid compartment and in the skin, gut, and liver.

Graft-versus-host disease (GvHD)

- Caused by donor/recipient differences in:
  - Major histocompatibility complex (MHC) molecules
  - Minor histocompatibility antigens (miHA)
- Mediated by mature donor CD4 and/or CD8 T cells
- Requires inflammatory cytokines
- Primary target organs include lymphoid system, skin, gastrointestinal tract, and liver
- Acute and chronic forms

Table 83.1b Clinical Grading of Acute GvHD

Overall grade	Skin	Liver	Gut	Functional impairment
0 (none)	0	0	0	0
1 (mild)	1-2	0	0	0
2 (moderate)	1-3	1	1	1
3 (severe)	2-3	2-3	2-3	2
4 (life-threatening)	1-4	1-4	1-4	3

Adapted from Glucksberg H, Storb R, Fefer A, et al. Clinical manifestations of graft-versus-host disease in human recipients of marrow from HLA-matched sibling donors. Transplantation 1974;18:295-304.

The simplest way to avoid the development of GvHD is to deplete the donor HSC graft of T cells before infusion to a dose below 10^5 cells/kg.[7] This approach has succeeded in significantly diminishing the incidence of GvHD, but other complications related to the ensuing delay in immune reconstitution of recipients, an increased risk of relapse from loss of the GvT effect, and a higher rate of engraftment failure (also from loss of the GvH effect) have resulted in little improvement in long-term survival, compared to T-replete products. The conundrum is that the same alloreactive donor T cells that mediate GvHD may also provide a GvT response, although there may also be additional tumor-specific T cells. Thus, the overriding goal is to be able to manipulate the donor HSC inoculum in such a way as to avoid GvHD, but to still be able to mediate a GvT effect.[8,9]

Clinical aspects of aGvHD

Usually developing within the first three months after transplantation, aGVHD is a clinical diagnosis with characteristic but non-diagnostic pathological findings. The most common presenting manifestations include skin rash; nausea, anorexia, and diarrhea; and jaundice, depending upon the target organ(s) most affected.[10–14] The severity of aGVHD is graded and staged according to the extent of involvement of these organ systems (Tables 83.1a and 83.1b). In addition to the increased risks of developing aGVHD related to the extent of HLA and miHA disparity, additional factors include the increasing age of either the donor or recipient, gender disparity (female donor/male recipient), donor parity (female donors), and infusion of T-cell-replete HSC products. Conditioning with reduced-intensity regimens, with lower regimen-related toxicities to non-hematological tissues, also results in a lower risk of

aGvHD, and may delay the onset of its initial manifestation. Interactions between microbial-associated molecules and innate immune receptors (e.g., Toll-like receptors) appear to be involved in GvHD pathogenesis, as demonstrated in both murine models and human transplantation.[15] Protective isolation with gut decontamination may decrease the risk of developing aGvHD, but is no longer widely practiced because of poor patient acceptance, cost, and increased risk of colonization with antibiotic-resistant pathogenic bacteria.

Pharmacological agents are the mainstay of aGvHD prophylaxis. Most patients receive a combination of a calcineurin inhibitor (tacrolimus or cyclosporine) along with an anti-metabolite, such as methotrexate or mycophenylate mofetil (MMF).[7,16] Methotrexate is associated with delayed engraftment, mucositis, idiopathic pneumonia syndrome, and other transplant-related complications, prompting the development of other combination regimens, such as a calcineurin inhibitor in combination with sirolimus or MMF, or reduced doses of methotrexate. The addition of anti-thymocyte globulin (ATG) to the conditioning regimen lowers the incidence of both GvH and HvG reactions because of the persistence of this agent for several days after HSC infusion.[16] However, patients treated with ATG may face higher risks of infectious complications, including EBV-associated post-transplant lymphoproliferative disorder, as a result of the greater immunosuppression achieved. Novel combinations of agents continue to be explored to reduce the cost and morbidity of aGvHD and its treatments.

Glucocorticoids with a calcineurin inhibitor remain the standard approach to initial systemic management of clinically significant aGvHD.[13,17] About 30-50% of patients will respond to initial therapy,[14] and patients who fail to respond have a poor prognosis, as additional agents added for control increase the risk of opportunistic infections and other complications. The use of higher doses of corticosteroids, or the addition of ATG, for example, in the initial treatment of aGvHD have not improved the outcomes of patients and should be reserved for patients who are refractory to initial therapy. The infusion of regulatory cells such as mesenchymal stem cells is an interesting approach to the treatment of aGvHD.[18] A variety of clinical studies have shown differing outcomes in the management of aGvHD using this biological agent, which could be a consequence of the use of different cell sources, cell-dose infused, and treatment schedule. A number of drugs, including ATG, pentastatin, switching to tacrolimus from cyclosporine, and newer monoclonal antibodies have shown limited activity in the salvage treatment of patients with steroid-refractory aGvHD.[19] Extracorporeal exposure of peripheral blood mononuclear cells (PBMC) to the photosensitizing agent 8-methoxypsoralen and UV-A radiation (photopheresis) has been shown to be effective in the treatment of selected diseases mediated by T cells, including both aGvHD and cGvHD, and is a novel approach to the

Table 83.1a Clinical Staging of Acute GvHD

Stage	Skin	Liver	Gut
1	Maculopapular rash < 25% BSA	Bilirubin 2-3 mg/dL	Diarrhea 500-1000 ml/day, or Persistent nausea
2	Maculopapular rash 25-50% BSA	Bilirubin 3-6 mg/dL	Diarrhea 1000-1500 ml/day
3	Generalized erythroderma	Bilirubin 6-15 mg/dL	Diarrhea > 1500 ml/day
4	Desquamation and bullae formation	Bilirubin > 15 mg/dL	Pain ± ileus

Adapted from Glucksberg H, Storb R, Fefer A, et al. Clinical manifestations of graft-versus-host disease in human recipients of marrow from HLA-matched sibling donors. Transplantation 1974;18:295-304.

treatment of patients with steroid-refractory GvHD, although the mechanism of this effect remains to be elucidated.[20]

Autologous GvHD

A form of aGvHD may also occur after Auto-HSCT, probably as a manifestation of immune system dysregulation during reconstitution of the immune system after dose-intense therapy.[21] Initially studied in murine models of Auto-HSCT, it was demonstrated that the abrupt withdrawal of cyclosporine could induce clinical features non-distinguishable from that observed after Allo-HSCT transplantation. A mechanism has been proposed that involves the depletion of central memory cells, although depletion of Treg with inhibition of peripheral tolerance may also be involved. Autologous GvHD is also reported in patients not receiving post-transplant immunomanipulations (spontaneous GvHD). Based on the clinical benefits of GvT observed in Allo-HSCT, several clinical trials with administration of cyclosporine with or without interferon were performed in patients undergoing Auto-HSCT without obvious GvT effect. Both induced and spontaneous autologous aGvHD are, usually, self-limited complications, and easily managed with a course of corticosteroids for patients with more extensive involvement, in contrast to the more extensive and difficult-to-manage aGvHD that occurs after Allo-HSCT. Furthermore, cGvHD does not occur after Auto-HSCT.

Spontaneously occurring severe and sometimes fatal autologous GvHD involving the GI system with severe diarrhea has been reported for multiple myeloma patients treated with Auto-HSCT.[22] The presentation is clearly distinct from the spontaneous or induced GvHD previously observed in patients undergoing Auto-HSCT, and may be a consequence of prior treatments with immunomodulatory drugs such as lenalidomide or thalidomide, the proteosome inhibitor bortezomib, or high doses of potent glucocorticoids before collection and storage of autologous HSC. Patients with this complication may require intensive treatment with corticosteroids and a calcineurin

inhibitor, with courses more similar to those experienced by patients undergoing Allo-HSCT.

Clinical aspects of cGvHD

cGvHD is the leading cause of late TRM among Allo-HSCT recipients, and resembles autoimmune disorders such as scleroderma, Sjögren syndrome, and primary biliary cirrhosis. Diagnosis is, as with aGvHD, based on clinical observations with secondary laboratory or pathological confirmation (Table 83.2).[2] A falling performance status, progressive weight loss, or recurrent infections are usually signs of severe cGvHD. About 50% of long-term survivors will develop cGVHD at a median of 9 months post-transplantation, and patients must be monitored closely for this complication for at least three years so that appropriate treatment can be initiated before extensive target end-organ damage ensues. Permanent ocular or oral sicca syndrome and pulmonary dysfunction can result if cGvHD is not appropriately treated, with a marked deterioration in quality of life.

Factors predicting for the development of cGvHD again include degree of HLA and miHA disparity, but also include prior aGvHD, older patient age, the source of HSC (greater risk after peripheral blood stem cells than bone marrow transplantation), gender (female donor/ male recipient), and donor lymphocyte infusion (DLI) post-transplantation. Inflammatory events such as sunburn or surgical procedures can precipitate cGvHD. Patients who develop cGvHD have a higher risk of TRM, but lower risk of relapse as a result of the immunological GvT effect.[23] T-cell depletion of the graft or treatment with ATG may decrease the risk of cGvHD, although this has not been demonstrated in all studies. Most patients require at least two drugs for treatment of cGvHD, with the standard initial treatment again being glucocorticoids and a calcineurin inhibitor. About half of the patients do not achieve a complete remission with first-line therapy, although the manifold signs and symptoms of cGvHD complicate the definition of response to treatment.[24] There are no clear

Table 83.2 Staging of chronic GvHD

Target organ	Score 0	Score 1	Score 2	Score 3
Performance score	KPS 100%	KPS 80-90%	KPS 60-70%	KPS <60%
Skin	No Symptoms	<18% BSA	19-50% or sclerotic, still able to pinch	>50% or "Hidebound"
Mouth	No Symptoms	Mild symptoms, no limitations	Moderate symptoms, decreased oral intake	Severe symptoms with major decrease in intake
Eyes	No Symptoms	Mild dry eyes	Moderate dry eyes, drops >3x/day	Severe dry eyes affecting daily activities
GI Tract	No Symptoms	Symptoms without weight loss	Symptoms with moderate weight loss (5-15%)	Symptoms with weight loss >15%
Liver	Normal LFTs	LFTs elevated <2x upper limits of normal	LFTs elevated 2-5x upper limits of normal	LFTs elevated >5x upper limits of normal
Lungs	No Symptoms	Mild symptoms FEV 60-79%	Moderate symptoms FEV 40-59%	Severe symptoms FEV <40%
Joints and Fascia	No Symptoms	Mild tightness not affecting daily activities	Tightness affecting daily activities	Contractures with significant loss of range of motion
Female Genital Tract	No Symptoms	Symptomatic with middle signs on exam	Symptomatic with dispareunia	Symptomatic with strictures

At least one diagnostic and one distinctive sign is necessary to make a diagnosis of cGvHD. KPS, Karnofsky performance score; LFT, liver function tests. Adapted from Filipovich AH, Weisdorf D, Pavletic S, et al. National Institutes of Health consensus development project on criteria for clinical trials in chronic graft-versus-host disease: I. Diagnosis and staging working group report. Biol Blood Marrow Transplant 2005; 11: 945-955.

recommendations regarding second-line treatments and a variety of pharmacologic and immunologic techniques have been used.[25] Re-transplantation is ineffective but a single-center report of low-dose thoracoabdominal irradiation described an 82% response rate with the best responses observed for patients with fasciitis or oral involvement.[25] Photopheresis has an overall response rate of 50-60% with many patients achieving complete remission.[20] At least transient responses can be achieved with rituximab treatment, an anti-CD20 chimeric antibody, which illustrates the humoral immunity contribution to cGvHD.[25]

GvT responses

Although recognized in mouse models of transplantation in the 1950's, the first clinical report of a relationship between GvHD and GvT was published in 1979.[26] This relationship has been observed in Allo-HSCT patients between the incidence (but not the severity) of aGVHD or cGvHD and the relapse rate of chronic myeloid leukemia (CML), and to a lesser extent acute myeloid leukemia (AML), acute lymphocytic leukemia (ALL) and multiple myeloma.[23,26] Relapses after HSCT are thought to occur because of survival of malignant cells harboring in the bone marrow after administration of the pre-transplant conditioning regimen, and their outgrowth several months later. Relapse remains a major cause of failure after Allo-HSCT, and the survival rate after is relapse poor, despite the intended GvT effect of this treatment modality. The ability to mediate an effective GvT response likely depends on several factors, including: the presentation of appropriate antigens by MHC class I and/or class II molecules on the tumor cells that can be recognized by effector CD4 or CD8 T cells; the lack of strong Treg activity that may be induced by cytokines from the tumor cells; tumor cell susceptibility to lysis by effector T cells (e.g., the level of Bcl-2 expression and the ability to resist apoptosis induction); ability of T cells to home to sites of tumor growth; and the direct effect of immunosuppressive cytokines, such as TGF-β, produced by the tumor cells.[27] Many types of tumor cells downregulate expression of MHC on their surface, and perhaps CML and AML are most susceptible to GvT responses because the myeloid lineage is adapted for antigen presentation and high MHC expression. A number of novel immunotherapeutic approaches are being developed to overcome these obstacles and enhance GvT responses, keeping in mind that GvHD has to also be avoided or minimized to improve outcomes (Fig. 83.2). One example for the prevention of relapse is the use of delayed DLI, administered weeks or months post-HSCT, at a time when the recipient cytokine environment is less conducive to GvHD induction.[8]

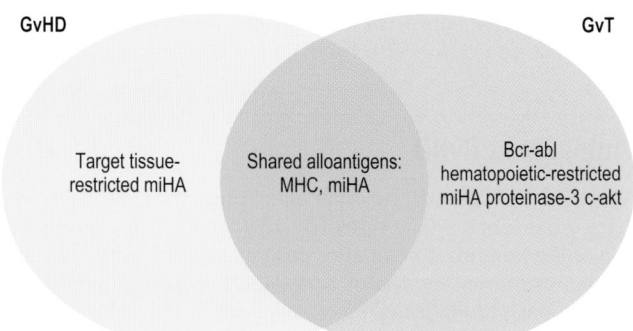

Fig. 83.2 GvHD and GvT responses. Donor T-cell responses to recipient antigens can cause GvHD, but can also target residual leukemia cells. T cells causing GvHD can recognize ubiquitous or tissue-restricted antigens (either MHC or miHA). Many of these recipient antigens can also be expressed by the leukemia cells, allowing for a GvT response. Additional leukemia-specific (e.g., bcr-abl, proteinase 3, or c-akt) or tissue-restricted antigens (some miHA, as those expressed only by certain lineages of hematological cells) may be dominantly expressed by the tumor cells and can be targeted by donor T cells without causing GvHD.

Immunomodulation is frequently the first treatment option for patients in relapse after Allo-HSCT, with rapid withdrawal of immunosuppressive medications and infusion of donor T-cells.[8,9] This treatment approach requires that donor T-cell chimerism be sustained to avoid rejection of effector cells through a HvG mechanism. Patients with low-grade lymphoid malignancies, such as CLL, indolent non-Hodgkin lymphoma (NHL), mantle cell NHL, and CML have the highest likelihood of response. A survey of 25 transplant programs identified 140 patients who had received DLI and reported a complete response rate of 60% in patients with CML. Response rates were higher in patients with cytogenetic and chronic-phase relapse (75.7%) than in patients with accelerated-phase (33.3%) or blastic-phase (16.7%) relapse, and almost 90% of these patients remained in remission at two years after treatment.[28] Complete remission rates in AML and ALL patients, who had not received pre-DLI chemotherapy, were 15.4% and 18.2%, respectively. Complications of DLI included aGvHD (60%), cGvHD (60.7%), and pancytopenia (18.6%). The development of GvHD after DLI was highly correlated with disease response (P <.00001). Patients with rapidly proliferative diseases such as acute leukemia will require systemic chemotherapy for disease management during the development of the GvT effect.

The number of lymphocytes infused is important in achieving the DLI effect, although it may be possible to induce GvT using doses of lymphocytes that are less likely to result in GvHD. However, a clear distinction between the cells responsible for inducing GvT and those causing GvHD has not been found, although several novel approaches, including the use of T-cell repertoire analysis, are in the developmental stage.[29] The delay in response between DLI and the development of a GvT effect suggests that only a minority of the cells infused recognize the tumor cell antigens and must undergo *in vivo* expansion before therapeutic effect is achieved. It may be possible to develop leukemia-specific cytotoxic T cells in the laboratory, decreasing the delay in effect, and possibly increasing the GvT potential in the more rapidly proliferative acute leukemias.[30] Donor immunity can be transferred, at least transiently, to the host, as demonstrated by delayed-type transfusion reactions to host red blood cells, mediated by donor lymphocytes transfused along with the HSC product.[31] Adoptive transfer of donor immunity against specific targets can be achieved, but its persistence requires immunization of both the donor and the recipient. A clinical utility for such manipulation of the immune system has not yet been demonstrated, but is clearly of interest as a technique to prevent post-transplant infections and/or disease relapse.

Adjuvant therapy with auto-HSCT

The relatively higher incidence of relapse after high-dose therapy leads to the hypothesis that chemo-ablation therapy with Auto-HSCT, although well-tolerated and able to prolong life, could be viewed as a platform for other approaches that may be effective in eliminating the minimal residual disease (MRD) of patients destined to relapse. Additional or yet higher-dose chemo/radiotherapy, unless directly targeted to the tumor target, increases the risk of non-hematopoietic toxicity and TRM from causes other than relapse. The correlation of more rapid lymphocyte recovery with a decreased risk of relapse, while likely a reflection of host factors and not direct evidence of a GvT effect after Auto-HSCT,[1] supports attempts to use HSCT as a tumor-debulking platform for post-transplant immunotherapies. Immunotherapies are of interest in this regard, and include administration of post-transplant cytokines; the addition of tumor-specific antibodies, used before and/or after HSCT as an "*in vivo* purge" and the development of tumor-specific vaccines, such as with tumor-antigen-pulsed dendritic cells (DC).[32] The immunoglobulin idiotype found in most patients with multiple myeloma and indolent NHL, which is unique to the malignant clone, can serve as a unique tumor-associated antigen for DC pulsing. The treatment appeared to be well tolerated,[33] and after vaccination, idiotype-specific responses were observed, characterized by T-cell-proliferative responses with cytokine release and the production of anti-idiotype antibodies, although again, a clinical benefit remains elusive.

Clinical HSCT

Sources of HSC

Bone marrow, peripheral blood stem cells (PBSC), or umbilical cord blood (UCB) are each appropriate sources of HSC for transplantation, with the primary differences being the quantities of HSC in each product and the quantities and functions of other blood cells that may influence the immunological outcomes of transplantation. PBSC have virtually replaced bone marrow as the HSC source for Auto-HSCT and are widely used for Allo-HSCT. Transplantation of PBSC (compared to bone marrow) achieves more rapid hematological recovery in both the Auto- and Allo-HSCT settings, resulting in lower complication rates and lower costs of treatment. PBSC appear to improve overall and disease-free survivals for allogeneic recipients with advanced hematological malignancies, although at the cost of a significant risk of extensive cGvHD.[34] In regard to immunological reconstitution, allogeneic PBSC transplantation results in a decreased CD4 Th1/Th2 ratio, which can adversely affect the ability to counteract infections and can favor cGvHD development.[35] It is also interesting to note that PBSC tend to contain about ten times more T cells than bone marrow product, yet those T cells are less functional, possibly because of inhibition by granulocytes activated by the G-CSF used for HSC mobilization.[36]

UCB is a rich source of HSC, with the major limitation for clinical use being the small quantity of cells collected, resulting in slower recovery of hematological function and increased risk of failure of sustained engraftment. A very significant advantage is the lower risk of GvHD because of the relative immaturity

of the donor immune system, allowing for the use of HLA-mismatched units without a prohibitory increase in transplant complications.[37] In general, as with other sources of HSC, outcomes of UCB transplantation reflect patient characteristics with lower survival probabilities for patients with advanced diseases or poorer performance status at time of transplantation. A number of investigators have proposed combining units of UCB in order to increase the cell dose infused into the patient, possibly increasing the speed of hematological recovery, but, more importantly, potentiating the GvT effect and reducing the risk of relapse.[38] *Ex vivo* expansion of one or more UCB units is also being studied as a mechanism to achieve more rapid hematological recovery.[39]

● THERAPEUTIC PRINCIPLES

Selection of HSC products for transplantation

Bone marrow
- Adequate quantities of cells can be obtained from most patients and donors
- Cytokine administration before harvesting may increase the quantities of HSC collected and the number and function of accessory cells affecting transplant outcomes
- Lower risk of chronic GvHD than PBSC

PBSC
- Faster hematological recovery than bone marrow or cord blood
- Better survival after related-donor HSCT for patients with advanced malignancy
- Lower tumor cell contamination than bone marrow collected from autologous patients
- Cytokine administration before harvesting may increase the quantities of HSC collected and the number and function of accessory cells affecting transplant outcomes

Umbilical cord blood (UCB)
- Relative immaturity of donor immune system permits multiple-antigen mismatched transplantation
- Transplant outcomes similar to mismatched unrelated bone marrow transplantation
- Slower hematological recovery than either PBSC or bone marrow
- Availability of stored units facilitates transplantation for patients with immediate need

---

Cell dose is an important predictor of outcome for both Auto- and Allo-HSCT and HSC comprise a very small portion (generally <1%) of the marrow, PBSC, or UCB product. It is now recognized that successful establishment of donor cell chimerism after Allo-HSCT is a complex interplay of pre- and post-transplant suppression of the host immune system, dose of HSC and accessory cells (including donor lymphocytes) contained in the graft, and donor HLA compatibility (Fig. 83.3). HLA-mismatching, T-cell depletion, and less intensive pre-transplant conditioning regimens all raise the risk of graft failure. Auto-HSCT does not present a likely risk of engraftment failure if the viability of the HSC is maintained during processing and storage, and adequate quantities of cells are infused. Instead, the speed of hematological recovery is related to the quantity of HSC re-infused in an exponential relationship.[40] For marrow-ablative regimens, increasingly higher CD34[+] cell (a surrogate marker of immature HSC) doses results in greater likelihood of rapid recovery of peripheral blood counts.[41] Autologous

Influence of graft, donor, and host factors on allogeneic HSC engraftment

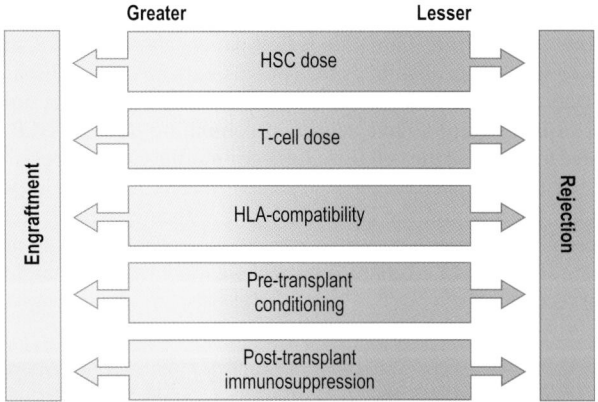

Fig. 83.3 Effect of donor and graft characteristics on Allo-HSCT. Hematological engraftment requires that the HvG reaction be overwhelmed, either by administration of a more intensive conditioning regimen before transplantation, use of more immunosuppressive medications after transplantation, closer matching of donor with host, or infusion of donor lymphocytes that can affect development of GVHD.

recipients who receive a dose of CD34$^+$ cells above an undefined threshold will engraft. At lower doses, there is considerable heterogeneity in engraftment speed, especially for platelet recovery, with some patients experiencing quick engraftment despite low doses of PBSC.[41] Products containing $\geq 2 - 3 \times 10^6$ CD34$^+$ cells/kg recipient weight have more consistent rapid granulocyte and platelet engraftment. Importantly, the duration of aplasia predicts the incidence of TRM after Auto-or Allo-HSCT.[42]

Similarly, cell dose is a predictor of outcome for patients undergoing Allo-HSCT.[43] The actuarial 5-year TRM, overall survival, and disease-free survival significantly favored patients receiving grafts with $>5 \times 10^8$ nucleated cells/kg. The cell-dose effect was more pronounced in patients >30 years of age, with advanced disease, a diagnosis of CML, and with alternative donors (other than HLA-compatible siblings). A similar study reported an association between CD34$^+$ cell dose and outcome of Allo-HSCT with either marrow or PBSC.[44]

HSC products are not uniform in characteristics and the relative contributions of CD34 + cell dose and the doses of accessory cells, including CD4, CD8, and NK cell populations, on the outcome of transplantation remain unsettled. Whether or not this is clinically significant, the ratio and quantity of cell populations collected will be affected by changes in the cytokines and chemokines, used singly or in combination, to mobilize HSC into the peripheral blood for collection or to alter bone marrow products collected from patients and donors.[45]

Purging of cell populations

For Auto-HSCT, attempts to purge tumor cells from the graft after collection have yet to demonstrate a survival advantage for the transplant recipient. On the other hand, T-cell depletion of donor HSC by various methods has proven an effective means of reducing aGvHD or cGvHD incidence, but increases the risk of graft failure, opportunistic infections, and relapse, effectively nullifying any advantage. Higher doses of HSC, which can be achieved by the use of large quantities of PBSC or combining marrow and PBSC components, reduce the risk of graft failure. Fixed doses of lymphocytes, as opposed to maximal T-cell depletion can also reduce the risk of graft failure. Some centers are

exploring partial T-cell depletion or post-transplant T-cell add-back in an effort to maintain the GvT effect while still reducing GVHD morbidity and mortality.

Expansion of HSC products

Ex vivo expansion of UCB HSC is one potential mechanism to offset the low cell dose and delayed hematological recovery post-transplantation. However, no expansion technique has yet achieved this goal, and such endeavors are complicated by the difficulty in identifying the pluripotent HSC in comparison to lineage-committed progenitor cells. Furthermore, it is likely that expansion techniques effective for HSC expansion will result in T-cell depletion, resulting in other complications described above.

Hematological recovery

HSC engraftment encompasses two concepts: recovery of hematopoietic and immunological function, and the rate at which this recovery occurs. Delay in or failure of sustained engraftment after myeloablative-conditioning regimen administration greatly increases treatment morbidity and cost.[42] Engraftment failure can occur as a result of inadequate HSC quantity from poor collection or loss in post-collection processing, inadequate host support of the infused cells, post-transplant events or medications, or by HvG rejection (Fig. 83.3). Engraftment failure is a very rare complication of Auto-HSCT, and is likely only with poor preservation of HSC after collection. For Allo-HSCT, the risk of engraftment failure is proportional to the donor HLA/miHA disparity, occurring more commonly in unrelated than in sibling donor transplantation, and with HLA-mismatched transplants. Engraftment failure is also increased by T-cell depletion of the marrow inoculum because of the loss of the GvH effect against residual host immune cells.

Chimerism assessment is important in evaluating poor marrow function after Allo-HSCT. A fall in peripheral blood counts could indicate HvG rejection of the graft or early relapse post-transplantation, or could result from GvHD or viral infection. Documentation of stable persistence of donor cells helps to discriminate between these possibilities. It is also important that sustained lymphoid chimerism be demonstrated if DLI is to be used in the treatment of disease relapse post-transplantation. The level of donor-host chimerism after Allo-HSCT is best demonstrated through evaluation of single nucleotide tandem repeats (STR) using molecular analysis. Obviously, such studies are of no value in assessing engraftment after Auto- (syngeneic) HSC.

Much of the emphasis in transplantation has been on myeloid engraftment, because initial patient survival depends on recovery of phagocytes and, to a lesser extent, platelets. Immune reconstitution, and in particular donor T-cell reconstitution, in HSCT patients is often hampered by recipient age, functional status of the thymus, cytokine milieu at the time of transplant, and post-transplant immunosuppressive treatments. The thymus involutes rapidly during childhood and, in a normal adult, is only able to contribute a very small portion to the mature T-cell compartment. The thymic tissue may be damaged as a result of a myeloablative conditioning regimen, or it can also be a target of alloreactive donor T cells mediating GvHD. As a result, restoration of the T-cell compartment in patients is often slow, particularly for CD4$^+$ T cells, and may be at suboptimal levels for many months to over a year. This situation, of course, endangers the ability of the patient to stave off opportunistic infections, and common complications arise from the herpes family of viruses, and fungal pathogens. If donor T cells are provided in the HSC inoculum, some reconstitution of the T-cell repertoire, mostly consisting of CD8 T cells, is provided by the mechanism of non-thymic homeostatic expansion, although the level of diversity may be limited. Experimentally, administration of cytokines, such as IL-7, post-HSCT, can enhance thymic function and help donor T-cell reconstitution. B cell reconstitution, on the other hand, is not that problematic in terms of the regeneration of the immune repertoire, although the ability to actually respond effectively to an infection with antibody production may still depend on the availability of antigen-specific CD4 T cells. Administration of immunoglobulin to patients with low IgG levels can prevent some of the infectious complications. HSCT patients who are conditioned with myeloablative regimens usually attain high levels of donor chimerism in their lymphoid compartment within a few months of transplant. This often correlates with the ability of alloreactive donor T cells, capable of mediating GvHD, to target residual recipient HSC elements so that the primary source of *de novo* lymphoid reconstitution will be from donor origin. By the same token, high donor chimerism is also associated with a lower incidence of malignant relapse.

Conditioning regimens

Dose-intensive and reduced intensity chemotherapy

The pre-transplant regimen is intended to accomplish two goals: ablate the tumor and achieve adequate immunosuppression to allow donor engraftment. Cancers treatable by HSCT are usually those that exhibit a strong dose-sensitivity, justifying the treatment of patients with dose-intense regimens. Bone marrow is also exquisitely sensitive to many of the agents used in the pre-transplant conditioning regimens, which is the basis for infusion of HSCT. For Auto-HSCT, only the dose-sensitivity of the tumor being treated need be considered. Lower-dose, non-myeloablative regimens, are not used in Auto-HSCT because with such regimens, infusion of HSC to reconstitute marrow function would not be needed. Total body irradiation (TBI) was initially used for conditioning of transplant recipients. This modality achieves tumor cytotoxicity, treatment of sanctuary sites of disease such as the central nervous system, and profound immunosuppression. TBI is usually combined in sequence with chemotherapy agents such as cyclophosphamide or etoposide. The non-hematopoietic toxicities of TBI are reduced by fractioning the dose over several days, allowing higher total doses, which decreases the risk of relapse.[46] Busulfan-based regimens were developed as alternatives to TBI for patients who had received prior dose-limiting radiotherapy, to avoid the effects of TBI on growth and development in children, and to eliminate the difficulty in scheduling patients to limited radiation resources. A review of several studies that compared the use of busulfan and TBI found no statistically significant difference in survival or disease-free survival for patients with CML or AML.[47] Other regimens are used in the treatment of certain malignancies such as dose-intense melphalan in the treatment of multiple myeloma and BCNU-containing regimens used in the treatment of lymphoma.

● KEY CONCEPTS

Conditioning regimens for HSCT transplantation

Autologous HSCT
- Allows dose-intensive therapy
- Allows use of marrow-toxic agents
- Regimens designed for optimal tumor cytotoxicity

Allogeneic HSCT
- Must achieve adequate patient immunosuppression (reduce HvG reaction) to achieve engraftment
- Allows, but does not require, dose-intensive therapy
- Allows, but does not require, marrow-toxic agents
- Need not be tumor specific

The myeloablative conditioning regimens currently used have been tested in dose-escalation studies to achieve the maximally-tolerated doses in otherwise healthy patients. Non-marrow toxicities such as pneumonitis, mucositis, and hepatic venocclusive disease limit further dose escalation of standard TBI- or chemotherapy-based regimens. New approaches include the addition of targeted therapies to the conditioning regimen, such as tumor-directed monoclonal antibodies or radioimmunoconjugates, that will not increase the toxicity to other organs. Tandem transplantation with the combination of a dose-intense regimen with Auto-HSCT followed, after recovery from the immediate regimen-related toxicities, by Allo-HSCT using a reduced-intensity regimen is a novel approach to combine the benefits of each transplant modality.

The hematological malignancies are predominantly diseases of the elderly. The potent GvT effect that is observed after Allo-HSCT allows allograft recipients to be treated with lower-dose non-myeloablative regimens with the immunosuppressive properties of the regimen to reduce HvG reactions and facilitate engraftment becoming more important than direct cancer cytotoxicity. Use of a reduced intensity regimen decreases the risks of regimen-related toxicities, allowing the treatment of a greater number of patients. The primary requirement in developing a reduced-intensity regimen is the need to achieve adequate immunosuppression to permit the development of hematopoietic chimerism, which became feasible with the development of the purine analog family of drugs. A variety of regimens are available, including combinations of fludarabine with melphalan, and fludarabine with busulfan. Among the least toxic are regimens that involve a single fraction of TBI. Storb et al., proposed that the HvG reaction leading to HSC rejection and the GvH reaction could both be modified by an appropriate immunosuppressive regimen administered after transplantation, allowing a reduction in the intensity of the pre-transplant conditioning regimen.[48] This group demonstrated in both canine models and human trials the ability to achieve durable donor cell engraftment with low levels of TBI (2 Gy), if high-concentrations of cyclosporine and mycophenolate mofetil were maintained after transplantation.[49]

HSCT for individual diseases

The treatment of diseases by Auto- or Allo-HSCT continues to evolve as the understanding of the biology of these diseases becomes more clearly understood (Chapter 78). Improvements in non-transplant treatments available to patients, such as the development of targeted tyrosine kinase inhibitors, which are very effective in the initial treatment of chronic myelogenous leukemia (CML), will reduce the numbers of patients requiring HSCT in the management of their disease. Patients are more likely, as a result of improving non-transplant treatments, to come to HSCT with refractory disease. Improvements in transplant medicine make this treatment modality available to greater patient populations including patients of older age or other health issues that previously were viewed as exclusion to HSCT. Organizations such as the American Society of Blood and Marrow Transplantation have published guidelines for treatment and reviews of the efficacy of treatment, identifying areas requiring additional research.[50-55]

Acute myelogenous leukemia (AML)

The primary clinical questions regarding use of HSCT in the treatment of AML are of patient selection and timing of treatment. Most patients with AML will achieve a remission with initial chemotherapy, but even with appropriate post-remission consolidation therapy, the majority of patients (~65%) will relapse within one to two years. Older age, the presence of defined cytogenetic abnormalities, inability to achieve a complete remission (CR) with the initial course of therapy, and a history of a preceding marrow disorder or receipt of prior chemotherapy (secondary AML) are predictors for failure of non-transplant therapy. Patients with these adverse-risk factors may be offered HSCT in first remission in place of non-transplant consolidation chemotherapy. Numerous studies of patients entering first remission compared standard consolidation therapy to dose intensification with Auto- or Allo-HSCT.[54] In general, Auto-HSCT was not shown to be more effective than non-transplant consolidation chemotherapy. Allo-HSCT had the lowest risk of relapse. Despite the higher transplant-related complications, in at least two major studies, patients assigned to Allo-HSCT achieved a significantly better disease-free survival (DFS) compared to patients assigned to either chemotherapy or Auto-HSCT. Allo-HSCT in first remission is particularly beneficial for patients with adverse-risk features, achieving about a 50-70% DFS regardless of cytogenetic changes, and is the treatment of choice for patients with adverse risk cytogenetics or leukemia that arises from prior chemotherapy or other marrow diseases.[54] Transplantation of patients with refractory disease or in a later remission has a lower probability of DFS. A number of phase II studies of Auto-HSCT for patients in second or later remission reported survival probabilities of 25-35%, which is higher than what would be expected with standard chemotherapy regimens, but still lower than is likely to be achieved with Allo-HSCT.[54]

Myelodysplastic syndromes (MDS)

MDS comprise a heterogeneous group of clonal hematological disorders characterized by expansion of abnormal HSC engendering variable degrees of cytopenia and frequent evolution to AML. Currently, Allo-HSCT is the only modality of treatment that can achieve long-term control of disease; Auto-HSCT is usually not feasible because of the inability to collect normal HSC from these patients.[55] The best results are seen in patients with earlier stage disease, although for patients with earlier stage MDS, a careful "watchful waiting" approach with transplantation performed at the time of disease progression may be appropriate.

Chronic myelogenous leukemia (CML)

Allo-HSCT is an appropriate treatment for CML with long-term survival rates >80% for younger patients undergoing related-donor transplantation within the first year after diagnosis. However, newly developed inhibitors of the tyrosine kinase (TK) encoded by the Philadelphia chromosome have relegated transplantation to the treatment of patients with advanced disease or the rare patient with CML not responsive to that targeted therapy. The probability of long-term survival falls for patients who undergo Allo-HSCT more than one year after diagnosis and for patients with more advanced diseases. The effect of prior therapy with a TK inhibitor on the outcome of transplantation is not known. CML is highly responsive to the immunologic GvT effect and many patients in relapse after transplantation can be salvaged by the administration of donor lymphocyte infusion. CML is a stem cell disease and the collection of normal HSC is unlikely for most patients, precluding Auto-HSCT. Of speculative interest is the collection of autologous cells after cytogenetic remission is achieved using a TK inhibitor, for subsequent use at the time of disease relapse.

Myeloproliferative diseases (MPD)

MPD are clonal stem cell diseases and include CML (discussed above), polycythemia vera, primary myelofibrosis, essential thrombocytosis, chronic myelomonocytic leukemia, and MPD not otherwise characterized. These disorders display overlapping clinical features, and may also show features more characteristic of MDS, but exhibit different natural histories and different therapeutic requirements. Allo-HSCT is effective in ablating the abnormal clone in these disorders. The timing of treatment is important because of the frequently long natural history of these diseases. Anemia, older age, and cytogenetic abnormalities all predict for poor survival in primary myelofibrosis, for example, suggesting that patients with anemia and an abnormal karyotype should proceed to Allo-HSCT. The extent of fibrosis of the marrow cavity appears irrelevant in the long-term success of treatment, and the fibrosis is frequently reversed within a few months of transplantation. Myeloablative Allo-HSCT results in a high rate of durable engraftment and cure in approximately 50% of patients. Transplant-related complications associated with more advanced disease and older age rather than disease recurrence accounts for the majority of treatment failures.

Acute lymphoblastic leukemia (ALL)

In contrast to treatment of the pediatric patient with ALL, only a small minority of adults with ALL are currently cured with non-transplant induction and consolidation regimens. As with AML, adverse risk features include certain cytogenetic changes and the inability to achieve remission with initial remission-induction chemotherapy. Allo-HSCT in first remission is clearly effective in the management of patients with defined adverse-risk cytogenetics such as translocation involving chromosome 4 and 11, or 9 and 22 (Philadelphia chromosome).[53] Recent randomized studies also demonstrate a survival advantage for patients with intermediate risk disease undergoing Allo-HSCT, especially since current salvage regimens for patients in relapse have a very low likelihood of achieving a second remission. There is little evidence to support the effectiveness of Auto-HSCT, despite its theoretical potential. The lack of a prominent GvT effect in the treatment of ALL suggests that reduced-intensity regimens will be much less effective than fully-ablative TBI-based regimens.

Chronic lymphocytic leukemia (CLL)

Many patients and physicians are reluctant to support aggressive treatment of CLL with Allo-HSCT because of the frequently indolent nature, long natural history, and the advanced age of most patients. Yet, disease progression is inevitable, and the aggressiveness of this disease can be predicted by various features including chromosome 17p and 11q deletions and detection of ZAP-70 mutation and CD38 expression. Therefore, HSCT should be considered as a treatment choice, especially for younger patients, or those with adverse features.

Allo-HSCT is very effective in the control of CLL.[56] The exquisite sensitivity of CLL cells to the GvT effect allows the use of reduced-intensity regimens with lower risks of regimen-related mortality in these, generally, older patients. Durable control of disease can be achieved for about 50% of patients. The extensive infiltration of bone marrow by malignant lymphocytes and the lack of the GvT effect preclude effective Auto-HSCT. In the few clinical studies that have been reported, high CR responses have been obtained with Auto-HSCT but relapses were the frequent cause of treatment failure.

Multiple myeloma (MM)

MM is a malignancy of plasma cells (Chapter 80) with a median age at time of diagnosis of 65 years, and in which dose-intense melphalan with Auto-HSCT can achieve about a 40% complete response rate.[52] Tandem Auto-HSCT with two cycles of dose-intense therapy at 2-6 month intervals doubles the overall survival of patients. Ultimately, most patients relapse and succumb to the disease. Although Auto-HSCT is not considered curative for this disease, the median duration of time without treatment is 2-3 years, and ~15% of patients may not need treatment for progressive disease for 5 years or longer, greatly improving their quality of life. Allo-HSCT after dose-intense therapy in the treatment of myeloma is characterized by unacceptable TRM, approaching 40% by day 100. Use of a reduced-intensity conditioning regimen decreases the risk of TRM to less than 10%, but patients with advanced disease are unlikely to respond to this treatment. The lower risk of complications with non-myeloablative conditioning regimens has led to studies of tandem Auto-HSCT, using an intensive chemotherapy regimen to achieve tumor debulking, followed 2-6 months later by Allo-HSCT using a reduced-intensity regimen to achieve the GvT effect.[57] This approach to the treatment of MM is being studied in large multi-center trials, and a clearly defined recommendation regarding Allo-HSCT in the management of patients with this disease is still elusive.

Non-Hodgkin lymphoma (NHL)

The lymphomas (Chapter 79) represent a diverse group of malignant diseases of B and T lymphocytes, comprising some of the slowest to fastest growing human malignancies, with a range of curability achieved by non-transplant therapies. As a group, the lymphomas exhibit a strong dose-response relationship to chemo/radiotherapy, and the benefit of dose-intense treatment with Auto-HSCT is well established.[50,51] Auto-HSCT avoids the morbidity of Allo-HSCT and is the preferred approach for the majority of patients, with some prominent exceptions discussed below. Popular chemotherapy regimens include cyclophosphamide, BCNU, and etoposide (CBV) and BCNU, etoposide, cytarabine, and melphalan (BEAM). However, no single chemotherapeutic or radiation-based regimen has emerged as a superior treatment.

Low-grade NHL

Low-grade NHL, in general, exhibits a variable and prolonged natural course, with many patients not requiring treatment until symptoms or organ toxicity appear. Therefore, most of the experience with HSCT has been in patients after initial relapse rather than at the time of initial diagnosis.[50] Few randomized studies comparing Auto-HSCT to other non-transplant therapies for patients have been reported. A number of phase II and registry data have been published for Auto-HSCT, and although response rates are high, a continuing pattern of relapse has been observed. In contrast, patients who undergo Allo-HSCT experience a higher probability of TRM, but a lower risk of relapse after transplantation. Indolent B-cell NHL, similar to other low-grade diseases such as CLL, appears to be very sensitive to the GvT effect of Allo-HSCT, and using reduced-intensity regimens will result in lower transplant-related complications. The difference in relapse rates between Auto-and Allo-HSCT could result from the possible reintroduction of lymphoma cells in the HSC product, but is more likely from the lack of a GvT effect of Auto-HSCT.

Aggressive NHL

Auto-HSCT is the standard of care for patients with B-cell NHL in first "chemotherapy-sensitive" relapse.[51] The success of this therapy reflects the extent and the responsiveness of the disease to chemotherapy at the time of transplantation, with relapse the major cause of treatment failure. The Parma randomized trial for high-dose therapy followed by Auto-HSCT reported a significantly higher event-free survival for patients treated with Auto-HSCT than for the group receiving standard-dose treatment (46% versus 12%). Furthermore, it is notable that no patients assigned to the conventional-dose salvage therapy could be rescued at the time of second relapse with a delayed transplant. The efficacy of Auto-HSCT is diminished for patients previously treated with rituximab, an anti-B-cell chimeric antibody, and who relapse within 12 months of initial therapy.[58] Other circumstances in which HSCT may be indicated, include treating patients who either respond slowly to initial therapy, have high-risk disease, are resistant to initial therapy, or are in relapse with chemotherapy-insensitive disease.[52] Results for patients with truly chemotherapy-refractory disease are poor, however, and such patients should be considered for Allo-HSCT.

Mantle cell lymphoma is known for its unremitting clinical course when treated conventionally and has proven relatively resistant to dose-intense treatment, especially when used for management of relapsed disease. Mantle cell NHL appears to be very sensitive to the GvT effect of Allo-HSCT allowing treatment with reduced-intensity regimens.

Burkitt lymphoma, Burkitt-like lymphomas, and lymphoblastic lymphomas are high-grade NHL associated with relatively poor long-term survival rates. The role of both Auto-and Allo-HSCT in these disorders remains unclear. There are no convincing risk models that identify clear indications for transplantation as part of the initial therapy. The lack of a clear contributory benefit of GvT in these disorders suggests that for patients without bone marrow involvement, Auto-HSCT may provide a reasonable treatment. Transplant registry data suggest that disease status at the time of transplant is the most important predictor of outcome in patients with high-grade disease.[59] For Burkitt and Burkitt-like lymphoma, the three year actuarial overall survival rate was 72% for patients transplanted during first remission, compared with 37% in those with chemotherapy-sensitive relapse, and 7% in patients with disease that was unresponsive to chemotherapy. For patients with lymphoblastic lymphoma, the six-year actuarial survival rate ranged from 63% in patients who were in first remission to 15% in those who had resistant disease. Patients in second remission had an intermediate survival rate of 31% at six years. These results with transplantation appear to be superior to conventional-dose salvage therapy.

T-cell lymphomas are less common than B-cell lymphomas. There is no well-defined management strategy for these disorders and treatment is based on the disease stage and immunopathologic grade. The relative results of treatment compared to the more common B cell type treatment regimens is lower, although the comparison may not be appropriate, as T-cell diseases present at more advanced stages than B cell diseases. The GvT effect may be more evident in T-cell NHL, and particularly for virus-associated NHL, Allo-HSCT is the preferred treatment approach.

Hodgkin lymphoma

Many patients with Hodgkin lymphoma will achieve durable remissions with non-transplant chemotherapy and/or radiation therapy, and algorithms for staging and treatment of this disease are well-defined. Dose-intense therapy with Auto-HSCT is available to those patients who do not achieve a remission or who relapse after initial therapy. The outcome for patients whose remission lasted less than one year is dismal with standard-dose second-line treatments, and these patients are best treated with dose-intense chemotherapy with stem cell rescue. Approximately 40-50% of patients with Hodgkin lymphoma who suffer a relapse within one year will achieve durable remissions after Auto-HSCT. Several studies have demonstrated that this approach can overcome drug resistance and lead to an overall survival rate of 34-50% for patients with chemotherapy-refractory disease.

Allo-HSCT is not a first choice for the treatment of relapsed Hodgkin lymphoma because of the higher transplant-related complications, despite the evidence of an effective GvT effect. With the regimen-related mortality of conventional myeloablative Allo-HSCT approaching 60% in some reports of dose-intense regimens used to salvage patients after a failed prior Auto-HSCT, nonmyeloablative approaches are being actively studied as an alternative.[60]

Solid tumors

Skin and colonic mucosa are primary targets of both acute and cGvHD, and this would suggest that Allo-HSCT would be effective therapy in the treatment of cancers of these organs. Yet, Allo-HSCT has not been shown to be effective in the control of these cancers, illustrating the discrimination between target antigens of normal tissues in GvH, such as the colonic crypt cells, compared to antigens expressed by tumors derived from these tissues targeted by GvT. With the exception of Allo-HSCT in the treatment of renal cell cancer, in which a graft-versus-tumor effect is clinically evident in some but not all studies,[61,62] transplantation in the treatment of solid tumors such as neuroblastoma, Wilm's tumor, and germ cell tumors is limited to Auto-HSCT with one or more cycles of dose-intense chemotherapy.

Future directions

Advances in HLA typing, chemotherapy-conditioning regimens, supportive care, and our understanding of the biology of the HvG and GvH reactions have greatly reduced the toxicity of both Auto- and Allo-HSCT. Although the diseases treatable by HSCT are those characterized by dose-sensitivity, currently available dose-intense conditioning regimens have been pushed to maximal tolerable doses. Newer approaches to the treatment of these malignancies will likely include the addition of therapies that are targeted to the malignancy, such as radioimmunoconjugates that will add minimal toxicity to other organs. The availability of reduced-intensity regimens permits tandem transplantation, using dose-intense therapy with Auto-HSCT to achieve maximal tumor-cell debulking, followed after recovery from transplant-related toxicities by Allo-HSCT, using a reduced-intensity regimen to achieve an immunological GvT effect. Finally, the ability to use HSCT as a platform for protein or cellular-based vaccination strategies is the subject of considerable interest.

ON THE HORIZON

Allogeneic HSCT
- Donor selection algorithms
  - Maximize GvT
  - Minimize GvH
- Combination conditioning regimens
  - Regimens with lower toxicities
  - Post-transplant maintenance
- Cellular therapies
  - Platform for other treatments
  - Enhance GvT

Autologous HSCT
- Tumor-specific conditioning regimens
  - Improve ratio of toxicity to tumor cell cytotoxicity
- Post-transplant vaccination strategies

References

1. Porrata LF, Inwards DJ, Ansell SM, et al. Early lymphocyte recovery predicts superior survival after autologous stem cell transplantation in non-Hodgkin lymphoma: a prospective study. Biol Blood Marrow Transpl 2008;14:807–16.
2. Filipovich AH, Weisdorf D, Pavletic S, et al. National Institutes of Health consensus development project on criteria for clinical trials in chronic graft-versus-host disease: I. Diagnosis and staging working group report. Biol Blood Marrow Transplant 2005;11:945–55.
3. Shaw BE, Arguello R, Garcia-Sepulveda CA, et al. The impact of HLA genotyping on survival following unrelated donor haematopoietic stem cell transplantation. Br J Haematol 2010;150:251–8.
4. Brickner AG. Mechanisms of minor histocompatibility antigen immunogenicity: the role of infinitesimal versus structurally profound polymorphisms. Immunol Res 2006;36:33–41.
5. Moretta L, Locatelli F, Pende D, et al. Killer Ig-like receptor-mediated control of natural killer cell alloreactivity in haploidentical hematopoietic stem cell transplantation. Blood 2011;117:764–71.
6. Socie G, Blazar BR. Acute graft-versus-host disease: from the bench to the bedside. Blood 2009;114:4327–36.
7. Messina C, Faraci M, de Fazio V, et al. Prevention and treatment of acute GvHD. Bone Marrow Transplant 2008;41(Suppl. 2):S65–S70.
8. Kolb H-J. Graft-versus-leukemia effects of transplantation and donor lymphocytes. Blood 2008;112:4371–83.
9. Porter DL, Alyea EP, Antin JH, et al. NCI First International Workshop on the biology, prevention, and treatment of relapse after allogeneic hematopoietic stem cell transplantation: report from the committee on treatment of relapse after allogeneic hematopoietic stem cell transplantation. Biol Blood Marrow Transplant 2010;16:1467–503.
10. Glucksberg H, Storb R, Fefer A, et al. Clinical manifestations of graft-versus-host disease in human recipients of marrow from HLA-matched siblings. Transplantation 1974;18:295–304.

11. Prezpiorka D, Weisdorf D, Martin P, et al. 1994 consensus conference on acute GvHD grading. Bone Marrow Transpl 1995;15:825–8.

12. Leisenring WM, Martin PJ, Petersdorf EW, et al. An acute graft-versus-host disease activity index to predict survival after hematopoietic cell transplantation with myeloablative conditioning regimens. Blood 2006;108:749–55.

13. Deeg HJ, Antin JH. The clinical spectrum of acute graft-versus-host disease. Semin Hematol 2006;43:24–31.

14. Weisdorf D. GVHD—the nuts and bolts. Hematology Am Soc Hematol Educ Program 2007;62–7.

15. Penack O, Holler E, van den Brink MRM. Graft-versus-host disease: regulation by microbe-associated molecules and innate immune receptors. Blood 2010;115:1865–72.

16. Storb R, Antin JH, Cutler C. Should methotrexate plus calcineurin inhibitors be considered standard of care for prophylaxis of acute graft-versus-host disease? Biol Blood Marrow Transpl 2010;16(Suppl 1):S18–27.

17. Paczesny S, Choi SW, Ferrara JL. Acute graft-versus-host disease: new treatment strategies. Curr Opin Hematol 2009;16:427–36.

18. Nauta AJ, Fibbe WE. Immunomodulatory properties of mesenchymal stromal cells. Blood 2007;110:3499–506.

19. Chao NJ, Chen BJ. Prophylaxis and treatment of acute graft-versus-host disease. Semin Hematol 2006;43:32–41.

20. Couriel D, Hosing C, Saliba R, et al. Extracorporeal photopheresis for acute and chronic graft-versus-host disease: does it work? Biol Blood Marrow Transplant 2006;12(Suppl. 2):37–40.

21. Kline J, Subbiah S, Lazarus HM, et al. Autologous graft-versus-host disease: harnessing anti-tumor immunity through impaired self-tolerance. Bone Marrow Transplant 2008;41:505–13.

22. Cogbill CH, Drobyski WR, Komorowski RA. Gastrointestinal pathology of autologous graft-versus-host disease following hematopoietic stem cell transplantation: a clinicopathological study of 17 cases. Mod Pathol 2011;24:117–25.

23. Lee SJ, Klein JP, Barrett AJ, et al. Severity of chronic graft-versus-host disease: association with treatment-related mortality and relapse. Blood 2002;100:406–14.

24. Pavletic SZ, Martin P, Lee SJ, et al. Measuring therapeutic response in chronic graft-versus-host disease: National Institutes of Health Consensus Development Project on Criteria for Clinical Trials in Chronic Graft-versus-Host Disease: IV. Response Criteria Working Group Report. Biol Blood Marrow Transplant 2006;12:252–66.

25. Wolff D, Schleuning M, von Harsdorf S, et al. Consensus conference on clinical practice in chronic GvHD: second-line treatment of chronic graft-versus-host disease. Biol Blood Marrow Transplant 2011;17:1–17.

26. Weiden PL, Flournoy N, Thomas ED, et al. Antileukemia effect of graft-versus-host disease in human recipients of allogeneic-marrow grafts. N Engl J Med 1979;300:1068–73.

27. van den Brink MRM, Porter DL, Giralt S, et al. Relapse after allogeneic hematopoietic cell therapy. Biol Blood Marrow Transplant 2010;16:S138–S145.

28. Collins Jr RH, Shpilberg O, Drobyski WR, et al. Donor leukocyte infusions in 140 patients with relapsed malignancy after allogeneic bone marrow transplantation. J Clin Oncol 1997;15:433–44.

29. Patterson AE, Korngold R. Infusion of select leukemia-reactive TCR Vβ+ T cells provides graft-versus-leukemia responses with minimization of graft-versus-host disease following murine hematopoietic stem cell transplantation. Biol Blood Marrow Transplant 2001;7:187–96.

30. Choudhury A, Gajewski JL, Liang JC, et al. Use of leukemic dendritic cells for the generation of antileukemic cellular cytotoxicity against Philadelphia chromosome-positive chronic myelogenous leukemia. Blood 1997;89:1133–42.

31. Rowley SD, Donato ML, Bhattacharyya P. Red blood cell incompatible allogeneic hematopoietic progenitor cell transplantation. Bone Marrow Transplant 2011;46(9):1167–85.

32. Palucka K, Ueno J, Banchereau J. Recent developments in cancer vaccines. J Immunol 2011;186:1325–31.

33. Leitch HA, Connors JM. Vaccine therapy for non-Hodgkin's lymphoma and other B-cell malignancies. Curr Opin Investig Drugs 2005;6:597–604.

34. Stem Cell Trialists Collaborative Group . Allogeneic peripheral blood stem-cell compared with bone marrow transplantation in the management of hematologic malignancies: an individual patient data meta-analysis of nine randomized trials. J Clin Oncol 2005;23:5074–87.

35. Endo T, Sato N, Koizumi K, et al. A preliminary analysis of the balance between Th1 and Th2 cells after CD34+ cell-selected autologous PBSC transplantation. Cytotherapy 2005;6:337–43.

36. Vasconcelos ZF, Santos BM, Costa ES, et al. T-lymphocyte function from peripheral blood stem-cell donors is inhibited by activated granulocytes. Cytotherapy 2003;5:336–45.

37. Rocha V, Gluckman E, Eurocord and European Blood and Marrow Transplant Group . Clinical use of umbilical cord blood hematopoietic stem cells. Biol Blood Marrow Transplant 2006;12(1 Suppl. 1):34–41.

38. Verneris MR, Brunstein CG, Barker J, et al. Relapse risk after umbilical cord blood transplantation: enhanced graft-versus-leukemia effect in recipients of 2 units. Blood 2009;114:4293–9.

39. Shpall EJ, Quinones R, Giller R, et al. Transplantation of ex vivo expanded cord blood. Biol Blood Marrow Transplant 2002;8:368–76.

40. Rowley SD, Zuehlsdorf M, Braine HG, et al. CFU-GM content of bone marrow graft correlates with time to hematologic reconstitution following autologous bone marrow transplantation with 4-hydroperoxycyclophosphamide purged bone marrow. Blood 1987;70:271–5.

41. Weaver CH, Hazelton B, Birch R, et al. An analysis of engraftment kinetics as a function of the CD34 content of peripheral blood progenitor cell collections in 692 patients after the administration of myeloablative chemotherapy. Blood 1995;86:3961–9.

42. Offner F, Schoch G, Fisher LD, et al. Mortality hazard functions as related to neutropenia at different times after marrow transplantation. Blood 1998;88:4058–62.

43. Dominietto A, Lamparelli T, Raiola AM, et al. Transplant-related mortality and long-term graft function are significantly influenced by cell dose in patients undergoing allogeneic marrow transplantation. Blood 2002;100:3930–4.

44. Ringden O, Barrett AJ, Zhang MJ, et al. Decreased treatment failure in recipients of HLA-identical bone marrow or peripheral blood stem cell transplants with high CD34 cell doses. Br J Haematol 2003;121:874–85.

45. Lonial S, Hicks M, Rosenthal H, et al. A randomized trial comparing the combination of granulocyte-macrophage colony-stimulating factor plus granulocyte colony-stimulating factor versus granulocyte colony-stimulating factor for mobilization of dendritic cell subsets in hematopoietic progenitor cell products. Biol Blood Marrow Transplant 2004;10:848–57.

46. Demirer T, Petersen FB, Appelbaum FR, et al. Allogeneic marrow transplantation following cyclophosphamide and escalating doses of hyperfractionated total body irradiation in patients with advanced lymphoid malignancies: a Phase I/II trial. Int J Radiat Oncol Biol Phys 1995;32:1103–9.

47. Socie G, Clift RA, Blaise D, et al. Busulfan plus cyclophosphamide compared with total-body irradiation plus cyclophosphamide before marrow transplantation for myeloid leukemia: long-term follow-up of 4 randomized studies. Blood 2001;98:3569–74.

48. Storb R, Yu C, Wagner JL, et al. Stable mixed hematopoietic chimerism in DLA-identical littermate dogs given sublethal total body irradiation before and pharmacological immunosuppression after marrow transplantation. Blood 1997;89:3048–54.

49. McSweeney PA, Niederwieser D, Shizuru JA, et al. Hematopoietic cell transplantation in older patients with hematologic malignancies: replacing high-dose cytotoxic therapy with graft-versus-tumor effects. Blood 2001;97:3390–400.

50. Oliansky DM, Gordon LI, King J, et al. The role of cytotoxic therapy with hematopoietic stem cell transplantation in the treatment of follicular lymphoma: an evidence-based review. Biol Blood and Marrow Transplant 2010;16:443–68.

51. Oliansky DM, Czuczman M, Fisher RI, et al. The role of cytotoxic therapy with hematopoietic stem cell transplantation in the treatment of diffuse large B cell lymphoma: update of the 2001 evidence-based review. Biol Blood and Marrow Transplant 2011;17:20–47.

52. Hahn T, Wingard JR, Anderson KC, et al. The role of cytotoxic therapy with hematopoietic stem cell transplantation in the therapy of multiple myeloma: an evidence-based review. Biol Blood Marrow Transplant 2003;9:4–37.

53. Hahn T, Wall D, Camitta B, et al. The role of cytotoxic therapy with hematopoietic stem cell transplantation in the therapy of acute lymphoblastic leukemia in adults: an evidence-based review. Biol Blood Marrow Transplant 2006;12:1–30.

54. Oliansky DM, Appelbaum F, Cassileth PA, et al. The role of cytotoxic therapy with hematopoietic stem cell transplantation in the therapy of acute myelogenous leukemia in adults: an evidence-based review. Biol Blood Marrow Transplant 2008;14:137–80.

55. Oliansky DM, Antin JH, Bennett JM, et al. The role of cytotoxic therapy with hematopoietic stem cell transplantation in the therapy of myelodysplastic syndromes: an evidence-based review. Biol Blood Marrow Transplant 2009;15:137–72.

56. Pavletic SZ, Khouri IF, Haagenson M, et al. Unrelated donor marrow transplantation for B-cell chronic lymphocytic leukemia after using myeloablative conditioning: results from the Center for International Blood and Marrow Transplant research. J Clin Oncol 2005;23:5788–94.

57. Lokhorst H, Einsele H, Vesole D, et al. International Myeloma Working Group consensus statement regarding the current status of allogeneic stem-cell transplantation for multiple myeloma. J Clin Oncol 2010;28:4521–30.

58. Gisselbrecht C, Glass B, Mounier N, et al. Salvage regimens with autologous transplantation for relapsed large B-cell lymphoma in the rituximab era. J Clin Oncol 2010;28:4184–90.

59. Sweetenham JW, Pearce R, Taghipour G, et al. Adult Burkitt's and Burkitt-like non-Hodgkin's lymphoma – outcome for patients treated with high-dose therapy and autologous stem-cell transplantation in first remission or at relapse: results from the European Group for Blood and Marrow Transplantation. J Clin Oncol 1996;14:2465–72.

60. Peggs KS, Hunter A, Chopra R, et al. Clinical evidence of a graft-versus-Hodgkin's-lymphoma effect after reduced-intensity allogeneic transplantation. Lancet 2005;365:1934–41.

61. Childs R, Chernoff A, Contentin N, et al. Regression of metastatic renal-cell carcinoma after nonmyeloablative allogeneic peripheral-blood-stem-cell transplantation. N Engl J Med 2000;343:750–8.

62. Rini BI, Halabi S, Barrier R, et al. Adoptive immunotherapy by allogeneic stem cell transplantation for metastatic renal cell carcinoma: a CALGB intergroup phase II study. Biol Blood Marrow Transplant 2006;12:778–85.

Mary Louise
Markert, Blythe
H. Devlin,
Elizabeth A.
McCarthy

Thymic reconstitution

Thymus transplantation is a promising investigational procedure for reconstitution of thymic function in infants with congenital athymia. Thymus transplantation was initiated in the 1960s and 1970s as a means of reconstituting the T-cell population and function in infants who presented with infections and low T-cell numbers. Although there were some reports of success, most of the infants died.[1] The poor results at that time may have been secondary to the difficulty in distinguishing athymic infants from those with a genetic defect in bone marrow stem cells. In addition, at the time, reagents such as monoclonal antibodies reactive with thymic epithelium were not available to evaluate the quality of thymus tissue. In the 1990s, with the ability to identify appropriate infants for treatment and with better reagents for assessing graft quality, the feasibility of using thymus transplantation was readdressed.

A summary of results of thymus transplantation by the authors is presented. The clinical trials involve infants with complete DiGeorge anomaly (DGA). The transplants are performed under an Investigational New Drug (IND) application with the Food and Drug Administration. With follow-up times of up to 17 years, the safety profile and resulting T-cell function are excellent.[2,3] The transplant recipients continue to be followed to assess the persistence of T-cell numbers and function and to monitor for potential autoimmune disorders.

Patient populations

Patients who may benefit from thymus transplantation include infants with congenital athymia as a consequence of complete DGA. This is a heterogeneous congenital anomaly in which infants present with variable defects in the heart, parathyroid gland and thymus.[4–7] Of these, approximately 1 in 100 have severe immunodeficiency and thus are categorized as having "complete" DGA.[8] Based on 74 infants with complete DGA enrolled in transplantation protocols, 61 of whom received thymic transplants, the main genetic and syndromic risk factors for complete DGA include 22q11 hemizygosity, CHARGE (coloboma, heart anomaly, choanal atresia, retardation, and genital and ear anomalies) association and diabetic embryopathy (Table 84.1).[9,10] It is notable that less than half of infants with complete DiGeorge anomaly are hemizygous at chromosome 22q11. All athymic infants present at birth with very low T-cell counts ($<50/mm^3$). They are consequently profoundly immunodeficient and susceptible to infections.

Athymic infants with complete DGA can develop oligoclonal T-cell populations at varying times after birth, usually within the first 12 months of life. The oligoclonal T cells can infiltrate the skin and other organs. Figure 84.1A shows a typical rash associated with circulating oligoclonal T cells. The rash is similar to severe atopic dermatitis, graft-versus-host disease, or Omenn's syndrome. On biopsy, the rash appears to be spongiotic dermatitis with T-cell infiltration.[11] Lymphadenopathy develops subsequent to the rash. Upon biopsy, the lymph nodes are typically given the diagnosis of dermatopathic lymphadenopathy. The term atypical DGA is used to characterize these infants. Athymic infants who develop circulating oligoclonal T cells remain susceptible to infections.

Recently two athymic infants with Foxn1 deficiency have undergone thymus transplantation.[12] These infants had no hair and have defects in the gene that leads to the nude phenotype in mice. One of these infants had no circulating T cells; the other infant had circulating oligoclonal T cells as in atypical complete DiGeorge anomaly, but did not have a rash.[12]

Diagnosis of athymia

Infants that may benefit from thymic transplantation require prompt diagnosis of athymia for effective treatment. The absence of a typical thymic shadow on chest X-ray, CT scan, or magnetic resonance imaging (MRI) cannot be used to diagnose athymia. The thymus may be embedded in the thyroid, for instance (unpublished findings). A small mass in the location where one anticipates finding the thymus may be a lymph node instead. Therefore, one must rely on blood tests to assess thymic function.

In normal infants, thymic function is revealed by the presence in blood of recent thymic emigrants, also called "naïve T cells." All T cells express the CD3 proteins, but naïve T cells also express the cell surface proteins CD45RA and CD62L. The co-expression of these molecules can be assessed by flow cytometry. Over 50% of a normal infant's T cells are naïve, reflecting active thymic function. Another characteristic of good thymic function is the presence of a broad T-cell receptor repertoire in the blood. The assays to assess these characteristics and the interpretation of the data in the differential diagnosis of athymia in infants with DiGeorge anomaly are described below.

> ● **CLINICAL PEARLS**
>
> Perform a T-cell count to diagnose complete DiGeorge anomaly in all infants with the following:
> - 22q11 hemizygosity
> - Coloboma, heart anomaly, choanal atresia, retardation, and genital and ear anomalies (CHARGE)
> - Primary hypoparathyroidism
> - Truncus arteriosus
> - Interrupted aortic arch type B

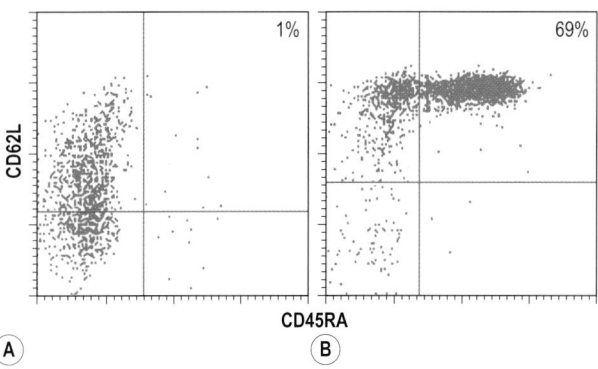

Fig. 84.2 **Naïve CD45RA⁺CD62L⁺ T cells pre and post thymus transplantation.** (A) Naïve CD3 T cells (1%) on day 8 pre thymus transplantation and (B) naïve CD4 T cells (69%) on day 550 (year 1.5) post transplantation in a patient with atypical complete DiGeorge anomaly. This is the same patient whose data are illustrated in Figs. 84.6D–F. On day 8 pre transplantation, the patient had 7684/mm³ total T cells with 585/mm³ CD4 T cells, 4594/mm³ CD8 T cells, and 2506/mm³ double-negative T cells. On day 550 post transplantation the patient had 1013/mm³ T cells with 674/mm³ CD4 T cells, 251/mm³ CD8 T cells, and 82/mm³ double-negative T cells.

Table 84.1 Syndromic associations in complete DiGeorge anomaly

Genetic or syndromic associations	Percentage*
22q11 hemizygosity	46
CHARGE	27
Infant of diabetic mother	15
Ectodermal dysplasia	1
None	11

*Data based on 74 patients with complete DiGeorge anomaly enrolled in protocols.

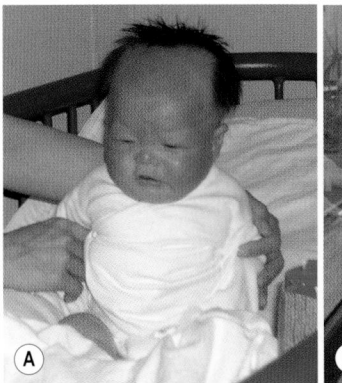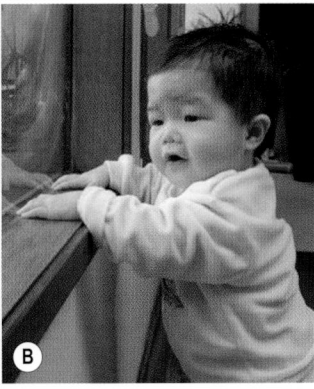

Fig. 84.1 **Dermatologic findings in patient with atypical complete DiGeorge anomaly.** (A) Rash before and (B) skin after thymus transplantation. Note hair loss with rash and regrowth after thymus transplantation.

In typical complete DGA, the total number of T cells (and hence the number of naïve T cells) is usually <50/mm³ and thus thymic function is considered to be absent. These T-cell numbers are profoundly depressed compared to a normal infant's T-cell count of >2000/mm³, with over 50% being naïve. The evaluation of thymic function is more difficult in infants with atypical complete DiGeorge anomaly because clonal expansion of T cells may lead to significantly elevated T-cell numbers.[2,3,11] The lack of thymic function in these infants is demonstrated when less than 5% of total T cells are found to be naïve by flow cytometry. Figure 84.2 presents an example of an infant with fewer than 5% naïve T cells prior to transplantation when the T-cell count was 2113/mm³. The very low percentage (<5%) of T cells co-expressing the markers CD45RA and CD62L confirms the diagnosis of athymia. It should be noted that clonally expanded T cells present in athymic infants may proliferate in response to the mitogen phytohemagglutinin (PHA). Thus, a T-cell proliferative response to mitogens such as PHA cannot be used to confirm the presence of a thymus.[2,3,11] The T cells that respond to PHA in infants with atypical complete DGA do not protect against pathogens, and the infant remains susceptible to infections.

Although the chest X-ray, CT scan, or MRI scan can be used to detect the lack of a thymus gland in an infant suspected of the DiGeorge anomaly, immune tests of the blood cells are necessary to confirm the diagnosis. These tests include measurements of total (CD3) T cells and naïve (CD45RA⁺CD62⁺) T cells by flow cytometry and assessment of the T-cell receptor β chain variable segment (TCRBV) repertoire by spectratyping or flow cytometry.

A broad polyclonal T-cell receptor (TCR) repertoire is found in infants with normal thymic function. Circulating T cells in athymic infants are usually oligoclonal. To support the diagnosis of athymia in infants who have circulating T cells, diversity of the TCR repertoire is evaluated by spectratyping or flow cytometry. Spectratyping assesses the repertoire of the TCR β chain variable segment (TCRBV) usage.[2] Most T cells express the TCRαβ receptor. Spectratyping uses PCR to amplify the TCRBV-containing mRNAs for different TCRBV families. In a normal individual with a diverse TCRBV repertoire, a quasi-Gaussian distribution of lengths of the mRNAs utilizing each TCRBV segment is present because of the variability of recombination joints between the variable (V), diversity (D), and joining (J) gene segments in the chromosome. Figure 84.3A presents a spectratype from a 4.5-month-old infant with atypical complete DGA who has an oligoclonal repertoire. Figure 84.3B illustrates a normal quasi-Gaussian spectratype from a patient with typical complete DGA 4.5 years after thymus transplantation. When an infant with DGA has normal numbers of T cells and very few naïve T cells, as in Figure 84.2, the TCRBV repertoire will be oligoclonal as in Figure 84.3A. Flow cytometry evaluation performed on the same infant on the same day as in Figure 84.3A is shown in Figure 84.3C. Expansions of TCRBV 3, 14, and 17 are detected. The advantage of flow cytometry over spectratyping is that the relative numbers of cells in each TCRBV family can be assessed. All infants with atypical complete DGA have had oligoclonal TCRBV repertoires.

Characteristics of naïve T cells

- Co-expression of CD45RA and CD62L
- Broad T-cell receptor repertoire

Thymus transplantation

Preparation of thymus tissue for transplantation

Thymus tissue is often removed by pediatric cardiac surgeons in order to access the surgical field necessary to repair the heart. For thymus transplantation, informed consent is obtained from the

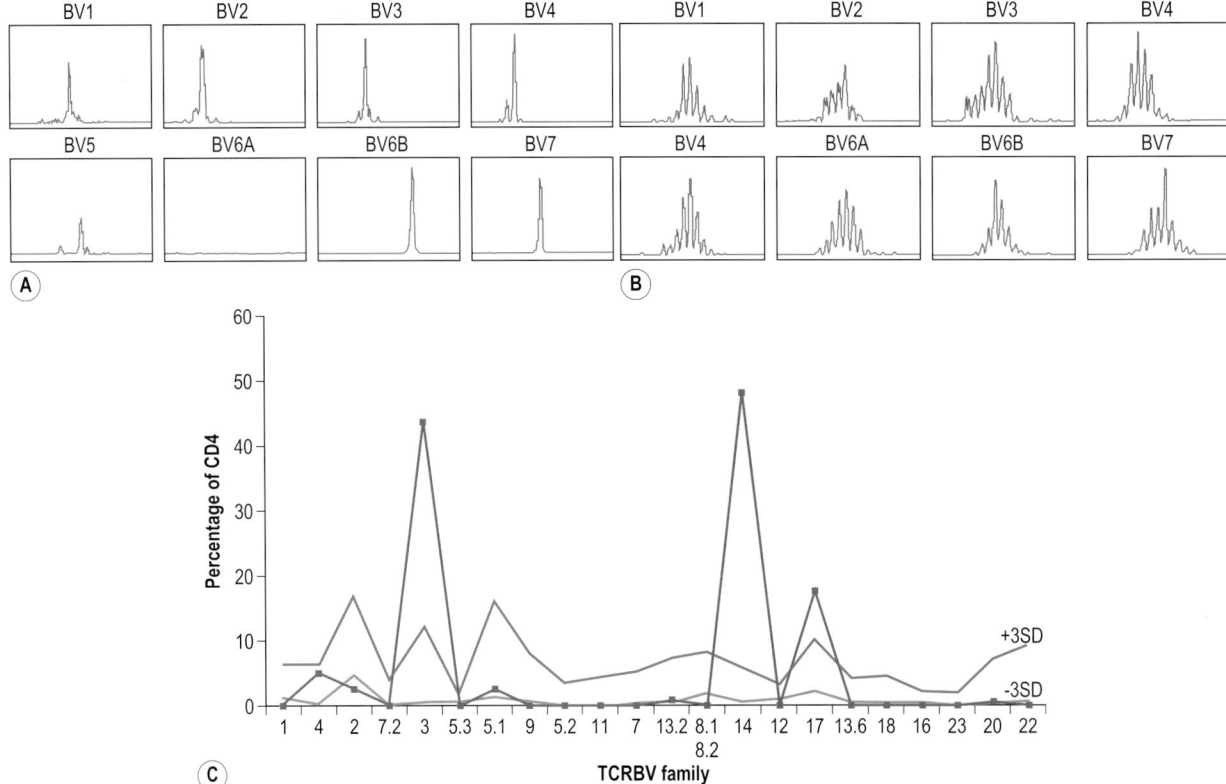

Fig. 84.3 Evaluation of TCRBV repertoire. (A) Eight panels from an oligoclonal CD4 spectratype from an infant with atypical complete DiGeorge anomaly who had 5897/mm³ circulating T cells with 2726/mm³ CD4 T cells. (B) Post transplantation CD4 T-cell spectratype in a patient with typical complete DiGeorge anomaly 4.5 years after transplantation, when the T-cell count was 998/mm³ with 729/mm³ CD4 T cells. The TCRBV family designation is above each panel. The Y axis indicates frequency and the X-axis the length of the CDR3 region. (C) CD4 TCRBV clonality assessed by flow cytometry using the same blood sample as that for the patient in (A).

parent(s) of the infant undergoing heart surgery in order to collect discarded tissue. The thymus is collected aseptically and processed in the laboratory. Based on the procedures initially described by Hong and Moore,[13] the thymus is sectioned and the slices are maintained in tissue culture for 2–3 weeks. Donor screening includes testing and screening for risk factors as recommended for all cell and tissue products (Code of Federal Regulations Title 21; Part 1270). HLA matching has not been shown to improve outcomes;[14] HLA matching is therefore not required.

Use of immunosuppression

Table 84.2 shows the number of infants who were transplanted without immunosuppression and the number given immunosuppression. No immunosuppression was used in 27 infants with typical complete DGA and 1 with Foxn1 deficiency who had very low T-cell numbers and very depressed T-cell proliferative responses to the mitogen PHA; these infants do not reject transplants.[2,3] Another 8 typical DGA infants, one with Foxn1 deficiency and all 26 atypical DGA were immunosuppressed. For most infants, the suppression included calcineurin inhibitors and pre-transplantation rabbit anti-thymocyte globulin.[2,3] Steroids were given with rabbit anti-thymocyte globulin and for longer courses in some patients.[2,3] Infections and deaths did not increase in the infants who received immunosuppression compared to those who did not.

Immunosuppression is given if an infant has atypical complete DGA, or if there is an elevation in the T-cell responses to mitogens in infants with typical complete DGA. The T cells of these infants can reject allografts, even though they do not protect against infection. Cyclosporine is often started when the

Table 84.2 Use of immunosuppression for thymus transplantation

Diagnosis	Treatment*	
	No suppression # surviving/ total	**Suppression # surviving/ total**
Typical complete DiGeorge anomaly	19/27 (70%)	6/8 (75%)
Atypical complete DiGeorge anomaly	0/0	18/26 (69%)
Foxn1 deficiency	1/1 (100%)	1/1 (100%)
Total	20/28 (71%)	25/35 (71%)

*Data based on 63 transplanted patients.

diagnosis of atypical complete DGA is made because the oligoclonal T cells can be very aggressive. The rash associated with these cells can be debilitating. The T cells can infiltrate other organs such as the liver and the gut. Cyclosporine is started at least 1 week prior to the rabbit anti-thymocyte globulin therapy. Rabbit anti-thymocyte globulin is currently used in all infants who receive immunosuppression. Seven infants with typical complete DGA and all those with atypical complete DGA were treated prior to thymus transplantation using three doses of the anti-thymocyte globulin at 2 mg/kg over 3 days. The cyclosporine is usually continued in infants with atypical complete DGA after transplantation until naïve T cells emerge in the blood. The Foxn1-deficient patient who had oligoclonal T cells was also treated with immunosuppression.[12]

Operative procedure

Thymus transplantation is an open procedure under general anesthesia. The surgeon creates furrows in the quadriceps muscle and places the slices of cultured thymus tissue individually into pockets in the muscle.[15] To allow the thymus to become vascularized in the first weeks after transplantation, steroids are limited to doses of methylprednisolone $\leq 2\ mg/kg/day$.

Results of thymus transplantation

Survival

Survival rate after thymus transplantation is 70% (43 of 61) in patients with complete DGA (Fig. 84.4). Thirty-six of the 43 surviving transplanted complete DGA patients are 3 or more years from transplantation. Of these 43 patients, the mean survival is 6.3 years and the median survival is 5.5 years (range 11 days to 17 years). Early deaths were not related to the transplantation but were predominantly secondary to infection. Deaths after one year were related to pre-existing medical issues such as cardiac defects, complications from tracheostomies and coagulation abnormalities. Both infants with Foxn1 deficiency survive.[12]

Immune outcomes

Thymus graft biopsy

Biopsies of the thymus graft 2–3 months post transplantation confirm thymopoiesis (Fig. 84.5). The biopsy illustrated was taken from an infant diagnosed with atypical complete DGA who was treated with immunosuppression. Analysis of the biopsy shows that immunosuppression does not prevent thymopoiesis. This infant had $5151/mm^3$ T cells 8 days prior to transplantation associated with rash and lymphadenopathy. The infant received pre-transplantation cyclosporine, rabbit

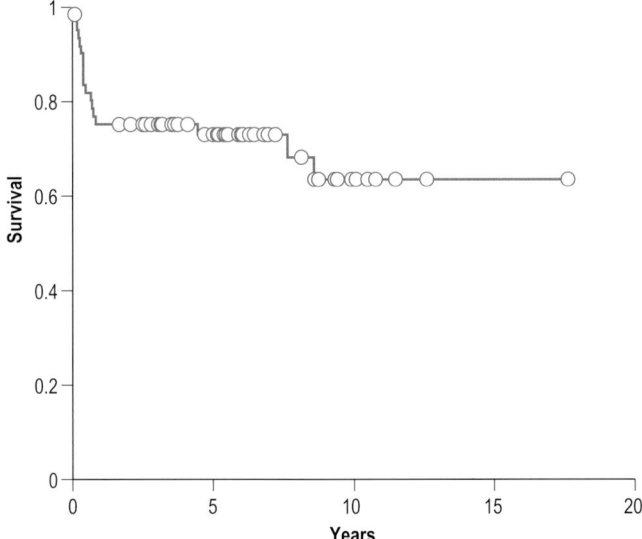

Fig. 84.4 Survival after thymus transplantation in complete DiGeorge anomaly. Forty three of 61 (71%) patients treated with thymus transplantation survive.

anti-thymocyte globulin, and steroids and post-transplantation cyclosporine and steroids. The biopsy, done 66 days after transplantation while the infant was still on cyclosporine, shows tissue that appears to be normal thymus with cortex and medulla (Fig. 84.5). Thus, pre-transplantation anti-thymocyte globulin and peri-transplantation cyclosporine does not prevent the development of T cells in transplanted thymus tissue.

T-cell numbers

Typical complete DiGeorge anomaly

Immune findings in the first year after transplantation vary depending on whether the infant has typical or atypical complete DiGeorge anomaly. In infants with typical complete DGA, T cells are first observed in the peripheral blood about 3–4 months post transplantation. Naïve T cells appear by 5–6 months. CD4 T cells predominate initially; CD8 T cells develop more slowly. By 2 years post transplantation, a stable total T-cell count reaches the 10th percentile in some patients, but is usually lower. CD8 numbers remain below the 10th percentile in all patients. The CD4:CD8 ratio remains >1 in all patients; only occasional evaluations in some patients have shown an inverted ratio. A typical pattern of T-cell development is shown in Figures 84.6A–C. By 9 months after thymus transplantation, T-cell proliferative responses to mitogens are normal. At that time patients are immunized with tetanus toxoid. Antigen-specific proliferative responses have developed by 2 years in all except two patients. The repertoire of TCRBV chain usage becomes polyclonal by 6–9 months. Composite data from these patients have been published elsewhere.[2,3]

Atypical complete DiGeorge anomaly

The time course of T-cell development in infants with atypical complete DGA is similar to that in typical infants, except that such infants may have predominantly CD4 single-positive, CD8 single-positive or double-negative ($CD3^+CD4^-CD8^-$) cells prior to transplantation. An example of an infant with a prominent CD8 single-positive population (greater than the CD4 single-positive or double-negative population) in the peri-transplant period is shown in Fig. 84.6D. As observed in other infants, by 4 months post-transplantation the number of CD4 T cells equalled the numbers of CD8 and double-negative cells, and by 5 months CD4 T cells outnumbered the sum of CD8 single-positive and double-negative T cells. As in other atypical and typical infants 6 months post transplantation, the presence of naïve CD4 T cells indicated thymic function (Fig. 84.6). For the infants who achieved immune reconstitution, the infants treated with immunosuppression developed normal proliferative responses and normal TCRBV repertoires over a time course similar to that of typical infants who did not receive immunosuppression. Composite data have been published on these patients elsewhere.[2,3]

TCRBV repertoire

Spectratyping and flow cytometric evaluation of the TCRBV repertoire provides supportive evidence for thymic function, as polyclonal repertoires are seen in the presence of thymic function. As a polyclonal repertoire develops, naïve T cells are detected in the peripheral blood by flow cytometry. Almost all infants develop a polyclonal TCRBV repertoire within 9 months of transplantation.[2] The TCRBV repertoire remains polyclonal in patients for many years, as illustrated in Fig. 84.3B.

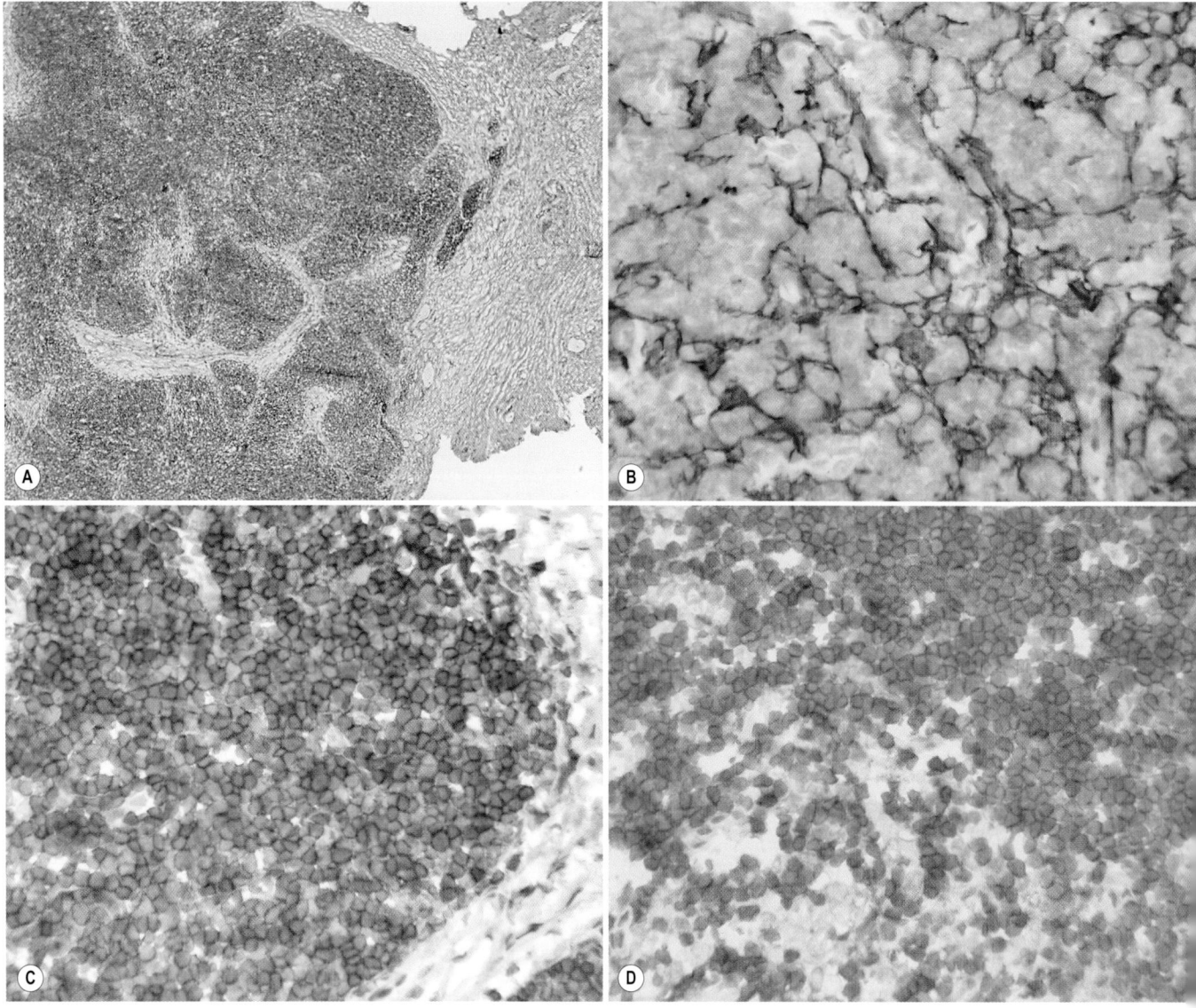

Fig. 84.5 Biopsy of thymus graft. (A) Hematoxylin and eosin staining showing cortex and medulla. Fibrous tissue and striated muscle can be seen on the right. (B) Cytokeratin staining reveals lacy patterns of cytokeratin. Hassall bodies were identified on other sections. (C) CD1 staining shows expression of this marker of normal cortical thymocytes. (D) CD3 staining shows many T cells. This biopsy was obtained 66 days after thymus transplantation. As expected, there were no circulating naïve T cells at this early time point. Cyclosporine had been started 14 days prior to thymus transplantation and was still being used at the time of this biopsy.

B-cell function

Immunoglobulin replacement is stopped after 9 months post transplantation when the infant is off immunosuppression, the proliferative response to PHA is normal, and the IgG trough level remains in the normal range. Patients are then given the normal childhood vaccines, but no live vaccines are used. Future research studies include plans to evaluate memory B-cell function by measuring antibody titers to secondary immunizations and the persistence of titers after immunization.

Safety

No serious adverse events have been associated with the transplantation or biopsy procedures. Most infants on cyclosporine developed hypertension that required therapy until the cyclosporine was discontinued. No thymus recipient developed graft-versus-host disease although thymus donor T cells were

detected in 3 infants, 2 of whom died in the first 3 months after transplantation, both from infection. The third infant, after thymus donor T cells developed, was diagnosed with Artemis deficient severe combined immunodeficiency (SCID) in addition to the infant's 22q11.2 deletion. The diagnosis of SCID likely explains the inability of this infant to develop genetically host T cells.

Clinical issues after transplantation

Rashes

Rashes can develop after transplantation prior to the development of naïve T cells in the blood. Skin biopsies of these post transplantation rashes have been diagnosed as spongiotic dermatitis with T cells identified infiltrating the skin, similar to the rashes seen with the development of oligoclonal T cells prior

Fig. 84.6 T-cell phenotype and function after thymus transplantation. A patient with typical complete DiGeorge anomaly who was not given immunosuppression is shown in (A–C). A patient with atypical complete DiGeorge anomaly who was given immunosuppression is shown in (D–F). (A, D) Absolute numbers of T-cell subsets in cells per cubic millimeter (mm³), (■) CD3, (o) CD4, (▲) CD8, (x) double negative, CD4⁻CD8⁻, T cells. (B, E) Naïve CD4 (■) and naive CD8 (o) T-cell development. (C, F) Proliferative responses in counts per minute (cpm) to the mitogen phytohemagglutinin (■) and the background of cells without mitogen (o). In (D), the number of pre-transplantation oligoclonal T cells was 7684/mm³ prior to administration of rabbit anti-thymocyte globulin. Composite graphs for patients receiving transplants with and without immunosuppression have been published.[2,3]

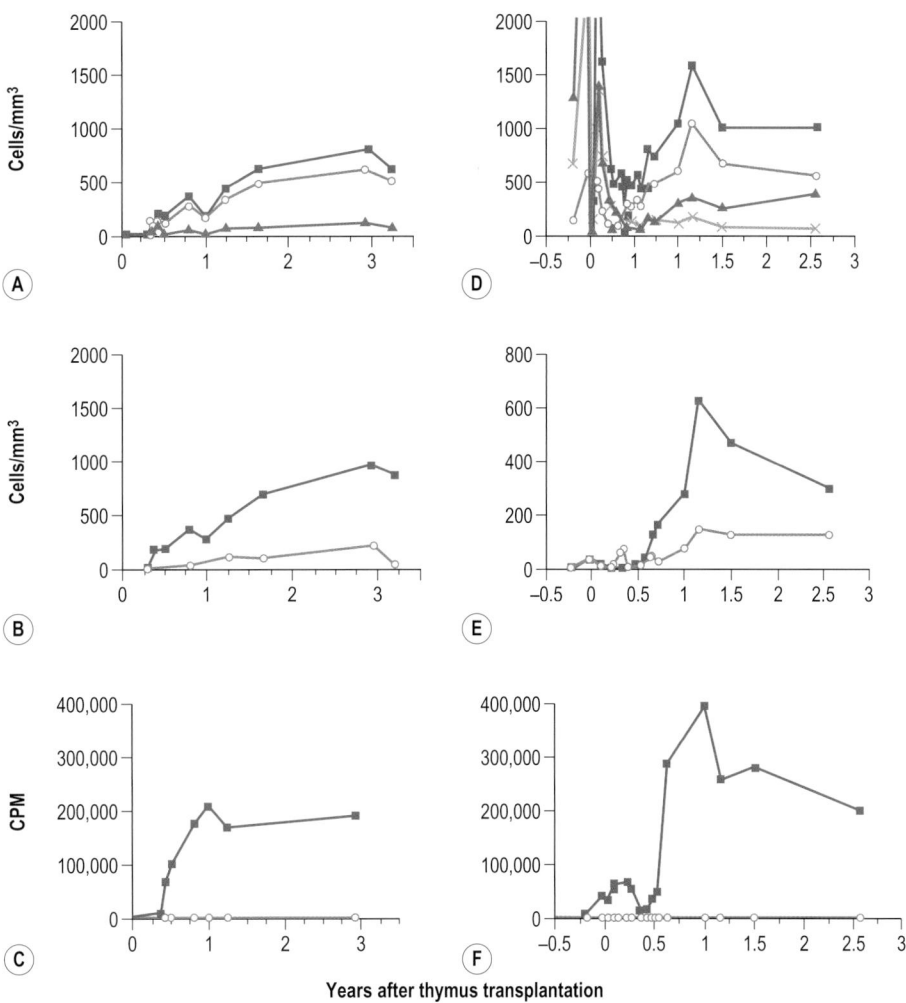

Years after thymus transplantation

to transplantation. The rashes are usually managed with cyclosporine. The rashes resolve in 3–4 months when naïve T cells emerge from the thymus. In one infant, maternal T cells were associated with a post-transplantation rash.

Infections

To prevent infections, the infants are maintained in reverse isolation and kept on prophylaxis for *Pneumocystis jiroveci* pneumonia. The prophylaxis for pneumocystis is continued for at least 9 months after transplantation and is then stopped when the patient is off immunosuppression, has over 200/mm³ CD4 T cells, and has a normal proliferative response to PHA. Prophylaxis for fungal or other viral infections is not used; however, specific infections are treated if they develop.

After T cells develop, infants clear infections that were present in the post-transplantation period, including infections with parainfluenza virus, respiratory syncytial virus, adenovirus, and rotavirus. Patients who contract viral infections after T cells develop are able to rapidly clear these viruses, including respiratory syncytial virus, parainfluenza virus, and adenovirus. One patient with ectodermal dysplasia was unable to mount an antigen-specific T-cell response and required hospitalization for several infections.

Autoimmune disease

Fourteen surviving complete DGA patients and one of the two Foxn1 deficient patients developed autoimmune-mediated thyroid disease that required hormone replacement.[2,3,12] Several patients developed autoimmune cytopenias within the first 2 years after transplantation.[2,3] Individual patients developed nephrotic syndrome (which resolved after a brief course of steroids), alopecia totalis, autoimmune hepatitis, and severe enteritis/colitis (that resulted in death).[2,3]

Oligoclonal T cells may develop in the first 3 months post transplantation prior to the development of naïve T cells. These oligoclonal T cells can cause autoimmune-like conditions. Three patients had mild wheezing or hypoxemia associated with the development of these cells.[2] These respiratory problems were controlled with steroids.

Long-term outcome

The long-term function of the grafted thymus tissue is unknown and is the focus of ongoing studies. To date, all patients have more CD4 than CD8 T cells, as expected. The T-cell receptor repertoire remains polyclonal (Fig. 84.3).

The patients have remained relatively healthy after transplantation. Most are growing along the growth curves at approximately the third percentile. Children who aspirate have ongoing aspiration-related respiratory infections. It is encouraging that some patients who had significant aspiration or general swallowing problems in the first few years of life have learned how to swallow, and now are taking all food by mouth. Quality of life and developmental outcomes are a current focus of research. Some children are fully functional and test at grade level, whereas others have severe developmental delays. The infants of diabetic mothers tend to perform the best functionally; those with CHARGE have more severe delays.

Other therapies

Other therapies that have been used for T cell reconstitution of complete DGA include bone marrow transplantation, infusion of peripheral blood mononuclear cells, and cord blood transplantation. None of these hematopoietic cells are T cell depleted. The mechanism for reconstitution is transfer of mature T cells into the athymic recipient. The hematopoietic cell donors have been siblings, parents, and unrelated individuals. In each case the matching of HLA to the recipient has been as close as possible. One survey[16] published in 2010 included 17 patients who had not been previously reported. A supplemental table accompanying the article included an additional 9 patients who had been reported previously. Taking the 26 patients together, the survival after use of hematopoietic cells from HLA matched siblings was 9/13 (69%). The survival using other donors was 4/13 (31%). The survey data must be interpreted carefully as it is not known how many other patients with complete DGA have undergone these procedures but have not been reported in the literature. To address this lack of data on hematopoietic transplantation for complete DGA, the Center for International Blood and Marrow Transplant Research (CIBMTR) has initiated new data collection methods with respect to complete DGA patient treatment outcomes. As all hematopoietic transplants must be reported to CIBMTR, the collection of data relevant to complete DGA outcomes will allow meaningful assessments of the efficacy of these treatments.

Future research directions

One potential future application of thymus transplantation is tolerance induction for solid organ transplantation. Initial research toward this goal has been performed by Chinn et al.[17] Four infants with complete DGA and profound hypoparathyroidism were transplanted with parental parathyroid and unrelated thymus.[17] One of the recipients developed long-term tolerance to the parental parathyroid despite maturation of host T cells in an unrelated thymus.[17] HLA typing of the subject, parent and thymus donor revealed that the thymus donor expressed all the HLA class II alleles in the parent that were not inherited by the subject.[17] Presumably the expression of the noninherited parental HLA antigens in the donor thymus led to deletion of T cells that could have rejected the parathyroid. Applying this approach to immunocompetent subjects will be a challenge and is being investigated in animal models.

Conclusion

Combining the data from the complete DGA and the Foxn1 deficient patients, thymus transplantation has resulted in survival in 45 of 63 infant patients (71%). Survival is directly attributable to the immune reconstitution of T-cell numbers and function. Research studies are being conducted to learn how long the transplanted thymus will function. It is hoped that further research will permit the application of this procedure to other clinical situations in which improved T-cell function is desirable.

References

1. Hong R. Reconstitution of T-cell deficiency by thymic hormone or thymus transplantation therapy. Clin Immunol Immunopathol 1986;40:136–41.
2. Markert ML, Devlin BH, Alexieff MJ, et al. Review of 54 patients with complete DiGeorge anomaly enrolled in protocols for thymus transplantation: Outcome of 44 consecutive transplants. Blood 2007;109:4539–47.
3. Markert ML, Devlin BH, McCarthy EA, et al. Thymus transplantation. Clin Immunol 2010;135:236–46.
4. Conley ME, Beckwith JB, Mancer JF, et al. The spectrum of the DiGeorge syndrome. J Pediatr 1979;94:883–90.
5. Thomas RA, Landing BH, Wells TR. Embryologic and other developmental considerations of thirty-eight possible variants of the DiGeorge anomaly. Am J Med Genet 1987;(Suppl. 3):43–66.
6. Muller W, Peter HH, Wilken M, et al. The DiGeorge syndrome. I. Clinical evaluation and course of partial and complete forms of the syndrome. Eur J Pediatr 1988;147:496–502.
7. Hong R. The DiGeorge anomaly. Immunodefic Rev 1991;3:1–14.
8. Ryan AK, Goodship JA, Wilson DI, et al. Spectrum of clinical features associated with interstitial chromosome 22q11 deletions: a European collaborative study. J Med Genet 1997;34:798–804.
9. Driscoll DA, Budarf ML, Emanuel BS. A genetic etiology for DiGeorge syndrome: consistent deletions and microdeletions of 22q11. Am J Hum Genet 1992;50:924–33.
10. Pagon RA, Graham Jr. JM, Zonana J, et al. Coloboma, congenital heart disease, and choanal atresia with multiple anomalies: CHARGE association. J Pediatr 1981;99:223–7.
11. Markert ML, Alexieff MJ, Li J, et al. Complete DiGeorge syndrome: development of rash, lymphadenopathy and oligoclonal T cells in five cases. J Allergy Clin Immunol 2004;113:733–40.
12. Markert ML, Marques JG, Neven B, et al. First use of thymus transplantation therapy for Foxn1 deficiency (nude/SCID): a report of two cases. Blood 2011;117:688–96.
13. Hong R, Moore AL. Organ culture for thymus transplantation. Transplantation 1996;61:444–8.
14. Markert ML, Devlin BH, Chinn IK, et al. Factors affecting success of thymus transplantation for complete DiGeorge anomaly. Am J Transplant 2008;8:1729–36.
15. Rice HE, Skinner MA, Mahaffey SM, et al. Thymic transplantation for complete DiGeorge syndrome: medical and surgical considerations. J Pediatr Surg 2004;39:1607–15.
16. Janda A, Sedlacek P, Honig M, et al. Multicenter survey on the outcome of transplantation of hematopoietic cells in patients with the complete form of DiGeorge anomaly. Blood 2010;116:2229–36.
17. Chinn IK, Olson JA, Skinner MA, et al. Mechanisms of tolerance to parental parathyroid tissue when combined with human allogeneic thymus transplantation. J Allergy Clin Immunol 2010;126:814–8205.

PART TEN
Prevention and therapy of immunologic diseases

CHAPTERS

Immunoglobulin therapy: replacement and immunomodulation

Mark C. Ballow

A cold ethanol fraction of plasma that contained an enriched fraction of gamma globulin was used intramuscularly (IM) over 70 years ago as passive immunotherapy for the treatment and protection of infectious pathogens, and subsequently as antibody replacement therapy for patients with primary immune deficiency (PID). This Cohn ethanol plasma fraction of IgG remained the principal form of therapy until 1981 when an intravenous preparation, i.e., immune globulin, intravenous or IVIG, became available. Subsequently, Imbach observed that thrombocytopenia resolved when immune deficiency patients were treated with IVIG. This observation led to the use of IVIG in patients with autoimmune idiopathic thrombocytopenia purpura, and an expansion on the use of IVIG as immunomodulatory therapy in a number of autoimmune disorders (Table 85.1).

KEY CONCEPTS

Properties of IVIG

- Plasma fractionation (1st step) by cold ethanol/Cohn–Oncley modification (fraction II)
- >98% IgG; >90% monomeric IgG
- Traces of other immunoglobulins, i.e., IgA and IgM, and serum proteins
- Addition of sugar, amino acids or albumin stabilizes IgG from aggregation
- Intact Fc receptor important for biological function
  - Opsonization and phagocytosis
  - Complement activation
  - Antibody dependent cytotoxicity
- Half-life comparable to serum IgG
- Normal proportion of IgG subclasses
- Broad spectrum of antibodies to bacterial and viral agents

Most IVIG preparations are derived from plasma by Cohn's ethanol fractionation method or the Cohn–Oncley modification. IVIG products are modified to prevent the formation of IgG aggregates to make IVIG suitable for the intravenous route. Excipients such as sugars, amino acids, or albumin stabilize the IgG molecules from reaggregation. Treatment with solvent and detergent, pasteurization or nanofiltration alone or in combination is used as a final step for viral inactivation and removal. Commercial IVIG preparations are derived from ~10 000 (range 10 000 to 60 000) donors. Each lot must contain adequate levels of antibody to measles. These products may vary slightly from each manufacturer and from lot to lot but they are generally comparable for clinical efficacy, but perhaps not tolerability. The characteristics of IVIG preparations available in the United States are reviewed in Table 85.2.

This chapter reviews the application of IVIG as replacement therapy in patients with primary immune deficiency and in the treatment of autoimmune and inflammatory diseases. The mechanism(s) by which IVIG modulates the immune or inflammatory process in certain disease is discussed. For more information the reader is referred to an evidence-based medicine review of the topic elsewhere.[1]

Replacement therapy with immune globulin, intravenous (IVIG)

Several early trials in the 1980s have been conducted to examine the efficacy of IVIG with IM gamma globulin, and a comparison of low dose with high dose IVIG therapy. Quartier and associates[2] performed a retrospective study of the clinical features and outcomes of 31 patients with X-linked agammaglobulinemia receiving replacement IVIG therapy between 1982 and 1997. Although early treatment with IVIG and achieving a trough serum IgG level of >500 mg/dL was effective in preventing severe acute bacterial infections, these levels did not prevent pulmonary disease, sinusitis or meningoencephalitis. The authors suggested that more intensive therapy to maintain a higher serum IgG trough level (e.g., >800 mg/dL) may improve pulmonary outcome.

Several studies have shown that pulmonary abnormalities are the most important factors associated with morbidity and mortality in patients with primary immunodeficiencies.[3] The number of infections, days on antibiotic therapy, days missed from school or at work and hospitalized days may not be sufficient indicators of adequate treatment. Therefore, the improvement or maintenance of pulmonary function is an important measure of the success of therapy. Orange and co-workers[4] examined the impact of serum IgG trough levels on pneumonia incidence in patients with PID receiving replacement IVIG therapy in a meta-analysis of published clinical studies. The results of their analysis showed that trough IgG levels increased 121 mg/dL for every 100 mg/kg increase in dose, which resulted in a decrease in pneumonia incidence by 27%. There was a strong correlation between increasing trough IgG levels and a decrease in pneumonia. Bonagura et al.[5] discussed the value of "biological" trough levels for the serum IgG related to the patient's clinical course, i.e., frequency of infections instead of arbitrarily choosing a trough value of 500 mg/dL. A study of 90 patients with CVID with follow-up of 22 years showed that the dose of IVIG needed to keep a patient free of infection varied between patients emphasizing that the goal of replacement therapy should be to improve clinical outcome and not a specific IgG trough level.[6]

Table 85.1 FDA-approved indications for IVIG

- Patients with primary immunodeficiency disease: replacement therapy
- Idiopathic thrombocytopenia: prevent severe bleeding
- Children with HIV/AIDS and recurrent infections: prevent serious bacterial infections
- B-cell chronic lymphocytic leukemia with recurrent infections and humoral immune deficiency: prevent bacterial infection
- Kawasaki disease: prevent coronary artery aneurysms
- Bone marrow transplantation: decreased risk of infection, interstitial pneumonia, and graft vs host disease in the first 100 days after transplantation
- Chronic inflammatory demyelinating polyneuropathy: arrest and reverse disease progression

The consensus among clinical immunologists is that an IVIG dose of 400–600 mg/kg/month is a good *starting point*. But immunologists may need to re-think these dosages in light of the studies cited above.[2-6] Individuals vary in their catabolism of infused immunoglobulin. The rate of elimination of IgG may be higher during a period of active infection. For persons with a higher catabolism of infused IgG or more frequent infections, infusions every 2–3 weeks with smaller doses may be more efficacious. In the final analysis trough levels are only a general guide and the clinical well being of the patient is a more important parameter. Clearly, with higher trough levels the incidence of pneumonia and comorbid conditions, e.g., bronchiectasis, and meningoencephalitis are reduced.[3-6]

For replacement therapy in patients with primary immune deficiency all brands of IVIG are probably equivalent, although there are differences in viral inactivation processes (Table 85.1). The choice of brands may be dependent on the hospital, payer, or home care formulary, and the distributor availability and cost. The dose, manufacturer, and lot number should be recorded for each infusion in order to perform look-back procedures for adverse events or other consequences. It is crucial to record all side effects that occur during the infusion Monitoring liver and renal function tests periodically, approximately once or twice yearly, is also recommended.

Table 85.2 Characteristics of IVIG preparations commercially available in the USA

Brand (Manufacturer)	Manufacturing process	pH	Stabilizer/ sodium	Parenteral form and final concentrations	IgA content	Anti-viral steps
Intravenous IgG						
Gammagard S/D (Baxter Healthcare Corp)	Cohn–Oncley cold ethanol fractionation, followed by ultracentrafiltration and ion exchange chromatography	6.4–7.2	Albumin, glycine, glucose; 0.85–1.7% sodium	Lyophilized powder 5%, 10%	<2.2 µg/mL (5% solution)	PEG precipitation, solvent detergent treated
Gammagard (Baxter Healthcare Corp)	Cohn–Oncley cold ethanol fractionation, followed by ultracentrafiltration and ion exchange chromatography	4.6–5.1	Glycine; trace sodium	10% solution	37 µg/mL	Solvent detergent treated, 35 nm nanofiltration, low pH incubation
Gamunex-C (Grifols)	Cold ethanol fractionation, diafiltration and depth filtration; caprylate/anion-exchange chromatography	4.0–4.5	Glycine; trace sodium	10% solution	46 µg/mL	Caprylate precipitation, depth filtration, low pH incubation
Privigen (CSL Behring)	Cold alcohol fractionation, filtration, fractionation and depth filtration	4.6–5.0	L-Proline; trace sodium	10% solution	≤25 µg/mL	Depth filtration, pH 4 incubation, nanofiltration
Flebogamma DF (Grifols)	Cold alcohol fractionation, ion exchange chromatography, PEG precipitation,	5.0–6.0	5% D-Sorbitol	5 and 10% solution	<50 µg/mL	PEG precipitation, pasteurization, S/D treatment, nanofiltration, pH 4 treatment
Octagam (Octapharma)	Cohn-Oncley cold ethanol fractionation, chromatography	5.1–6.0	Maltose	5% solution	<200 µg/mL	Solvent/detergent, pH 4 incubation
Gammaplex (Bio Products Laboratory)	Cold ethanol fractionation, chromatography	4.8–5.1	5% D-Sorbitol	5% solution	<10 µg/mL	Solvent detergent treated, nanofiltration, low pH incubation
Subcutaenous IgG						
Hizentra (CSL Behring)	Cold alcohol fractionation, octanoic acid fractionation, anion exchange chromatography	4.6–5.2	L-Proline; trace sodium	20%	≤50 µg/mL	Depth filtration, pH 4 incubation, nanofiltration
Gamunex-C (Talecris Biotherapeutics)	Cold ethanol fractionation, diafiltration and depth filtration; caprylate/anion exchange chromatography	4.0–4.5	Glycine; trace sodium	10%	46 µg/mL	Caprylate precipitation, depth filtration, low pH incubation

Contents of table summarized from: manufacturers' literature.

In patients with active infection, especially patients with common variable immunodeficiency (CVID) the initial (first) dose can be halved, i.e., 200-300 mg/kg, with the dose repeated two weeks later to achieve a full dose. To minimize cost and inconvenience, self-administration and home treatment have been studied and used successfully. For home therapy, patients need to be selected carefully. Infusions should be done only in the presence of a responsible adult who is ready to provide assistance. Home treatment has been reported to be as effective as hospital treatment in terms of the frequency of infections, days missed from school or work, antibiotics used, and immunoglobulin level achieved. Patients receiving home treatment should be seen as regularly as patients on hospital-based treatment to monitor clinical status, liver function, and serum IgG level.

Berger and colleagues were the first to describe the use of the subcutaneous (SC) route for immunoglobulin replacement therapy in 1980. It was reported to be safe, well tolerated, and effective in achieving adequate serum IgG levels. In a multicenter study of 165 patients with hypogammaglobulinemia receiving subcutaneous infusions (27 030 infusions at home) a significant reduction in adverse systemic reactions compared with intramuscular or intravenous administration was observed. Anaphylactoid reactions did not occur. Several studies have shown enhancements in quality of life measurements.[7-9] Local tissue reactions occur with subcutaneous immunoglobulin (SCIG) including swelling, soreness, redness, induration, local heat, itching, and bruising. A comparison of the advantages and disadvantages of subcutaneous and intravenous routes of replacement IgG therapy is shown in Table 85.3. Thus, SCIG is a suitable alternative to IVIG and may present certain opportunities for optimizing care for patients with PID.

The calculated dose for SC administration is generally 100 to 150 mg/kg weekly. Depending on the weight of the patient and the concentration of the SCIG, i.e. 10-20%, infusions may need to be given more frequently than every 7 days.

Pharmacokinetic studies in clinical trials suggest that upward adjustments in the dose ranging from 37 to 50% of the IVIG dose may be needed to achieve a comparable bioavailability. Each subcutaneous infusion requires a small portable syringe-driver type pump together with a 10- to 20-mL syringe and an infusion set with a specialized SC 25- to 27-gauge needle. The length of the needle may need to be adjusted for the thickness of the subcutaneous tissue of each patient. Before infusion, the line needs to be checked to ensure that there is no blood return. Infusions need to be given weekly at multiple sites or more often if needed to maintain adequate serum IgG levels. Infusion sites are usually on the abdominal wall and lateral thigh. Twenty to 35 mL can be infused into a single site in adults depending on the amounts of subcutaneous tissue. A general guideline for infusion rate is 15 to 25 mL/hour per site. The SCIG schedule should be started 1 week after the last dose of IVIG, or as a new patient loaded with 4 or 6 doses of SCIG. Before home treatment, patients need to be instructed on the correct technique under close supervision, and the recognition of possible side effects. The US Food and Drug Administration has approved several new IgG preparations ranging in concentration from 10 to 20% for SC administration. Currently, standard SC delivery of Ig is limited to frequent low volume (15-35 ml) infusions using multiple sites. A new innovative approach to SC infusion uses the addition of human recombinant hyaluronidase to facilitate a full monthly dose of Ig at a single site.[92] SCIG infusion is safer, better tolerated, and preferred by some patients. Several studies in Europe and Canada have shown that overall costs of SCIG therapy are lower than IVIG; similar pharmacoeconomic studies need to be done in the United States.[7,10] It should be considered as an alternative, especially in those patients with systemic adverse reactions from the intravenous route. More details about subcutaneous infusions can be found in several reviews.[9,11,12]

Adverse events associated with IVIG therapy

Table 85.3 Comparison of routes of immunoglobulin administration

Intravenous route
Advantages
• Achieve rapid plasma levels
• Can use this route in patients with bleeding disorders
• 3-4 week intervals
Disadvantages
• Need intravenous access
• Interrupt patient's schedule for 3- to 5-hr period
• Often needs to come to a hospital or infusion center
• Systemic side effects may be more frequent in some patients
Subcutaneous route
Advantages
• Intravenous access not needed for those patients with poor venous access
• Eliminate trough levels
• Achieve a stable serum level of IgG
• May eliminate 3rd–4th week fatigue prior to next infusion
• Fewer systemic adverse effects than IV route
• More flexibility for patient's (parent's) schedule
• Distance from infusion center or hospital
• Young adults going to college
Disadvantages
• Minor local reactions at the site of infusion
• Patient reliability
• Need for a pump

● KEY CONCEPTS

IVIG treatment of patients with primary immune deficiency

- Starting dose – 400–600 mg/kg every 4 weeks
- Maintain trough level of >500 mg/dL or a serum IgG level 300 mg/dL over baseline
- Higher trough levels (>800 mg/dL) may be necessary to prevent chronic pulmonary changes and enteroviral meningoencephalitis
- Depending on the rate of IgG catabolism and/or control over infections may need to decrease infusion interval to every 2-3 weeks
- It may take 3 or more months to achieve a steady state after a change in dose
- Monitor serum BUN, creatinine, and liver function tests every 6-12 months
- Keep a log of dose, manufacturer, lot number, and reactions for each infusion
- For patients with rate-related adverse side effects consider pre-treatment with:
  - Acetaminophen
  - Diphenhydramine
  - Non-steroidal anti-inflammatory medications
  - Corticosteroids
- Consider alternate route of subcutaneous IVIG in patients with frequent adverse reactions

Rate-related

Typical rate-related adverse reactions with IVIG include tachycardia, dyspnea, chest tightness, back pain, arthralgia, myalgia, hypertension or hypotension, headache, pruritus, rash and low-grade fever (Table 85.4). Mild to moderate reactions occur in 5-15% of infusions; severe reactions occur in less than 1% of patients. Of course, with higher doses used in patients with autoimmune disorders adverse reaction rates are higher. Patients with more profound immunodeficiency or patients with active infections tend to have more severe reactions. Other factors that contribute to adverse reactions include a change in IVIG product, concomitant infections, higher concentrations or lyophilized products, and rapid infusion rates. The cause of the reactions is thought to be related to the anti-complementary activity of IgG aggregates in the IVIG in which immune complexes form between infused antibodies and antigens of infectious agents in the patient. The other possible mechanism is that the formation of oligomeric or polymeric IgG complexes interacts with Fc receptors and triggers the release of inflammatory mediators. These rate-related reactions occur less frequently with the newer IVIG products that are liquid and iso-osmolar. Headaches are the most frequent symptom associated with IVIG infusions, occurring in 5-20% of infusions and

one-third of patients. Slowing the infusion rate or discontinuing therapy until symptoms subside may diminish the reaction. Pretreatment with nonsteroidal anti-inflammatory medications (NSAIDs), acetaminophen (15 mg/kg/dose), diphenhydramine (1 mg/kg/dose), and/or hydrocortisone (6 mg/kg/dose, maximum 100 mg) 1 hour before the infusion may prevent the adverse reactions. Oral hydration prior to the infusion is often helpful.

CNS-related adverse events

Aseptic meningitis has been reported as one of the complications of IVIG, especially with large doses and rapid infusions, and in the treatment of patients with autoimmune disease.[13] Interestingly, this rarely occurs in immunodeficient subjects. Symptoms, including headache, stiff neck, and photophobia, usually develop within 24 hours after completion of the infusion and may last 3-5 days. Spinal fluid pleocytosis occurs in most patients.[13] Long-term complications are minimal. The etiology of aseptic meningitis is unclear but migraine has been reported as a risk factor and may be associated with recurrence despite the use of different IVIG preparations and slower rates of infusion.

Renal adverse events

Acute renal failure is a rare but significant complication of IVIG treatment. Histopathologic findings of acute tubular necrosis, vacuolar degeneration, and osmotic nephrosis were suggestive of osmotic injury to the proximal renal tubules. Most patients (95%) had received large doses for the treatment of autoimmune disease. The majority of the cases were treated successfully with conservative therapy, but deaths were reported in 17 patients who had serious underlying conditions. Most cases of this adverse event were associated with IVIG products containing sucrose as a stabilizer. Risk factors include preexisting renal insufficiency, diabetes mellitus, dehydration, age greater than 65, sepsis, paraproteinemia and concomitant use of nephrotoxic agents. Newer IVIG products are using alternative stabilizers, e.g. amino acids instead of sucrose.

Thromboembolic events

This adverse effect is likely due to increased plasma viscosity or vasoactive contaminants in the IVIG in patients receiving large doses of IVIG for autoimmune diseases.[14,15] Patients with elevated serum viscosity, e.g. cryoglobulinemia, hypergammaglobulinemia, and hypercholesterolemia, are at risk for developing a critical increase in serum viscosity with IVIG; high doses especially predispose them to thromboembolic events. These changes can result in myocardial infarction, stroke, deep vein thrombosis, or pulmonary embolism. Recently, it has been postulated that small amounts of contaminating procoagulant factors, especially Factor XIa, may play a role in these thromboembolic events. Besides cerebral infarction, reversible posterior leukoencephalopathy syndrome has also been seen in several patients receiving high-dose IVIG. Patients at risk are older, on multiple drugs and have comorbidities. Patients at risk should be hydrated well, and the administration of the IVIG should be at lower rates, with products selected with low sodium and an osmolality in the physiological range.

Table 85.4 Adverse events associated with IgIV therapy

Rate-related
Chills
Headache
Back pain
Myalgia
Malaise, fatigue
Fever
Pruritus
Rash – urticaria
Nausea, vomiting
Tachycardia
Chest pain or tightness
Dyspnea
Hypotension/hypertension
Central nervous system
Severe headaches
Aseptic meningitis*
Renal
Azotemia
Renal failure
Thromboembolic events*
Thrombosis/Cerebral infarction
Myocardial infarction
Pulmonary embolism
Posterior leukoencephalopathy syndrome
Anaphylaxis from anti-IgE antibodies to IgA
Rare (isolated reports)
Cardiac rhythm abnormalities
Coagulopathy
Hemolysis – alloantibodies to blood type A/B
Cryoglobulinemia
Neutropenia
Alopecia
Uveitis
Noninfectious hepatitis

*See text for predisposing risk factors.

Transfusion reaction due to antibodies against IgA

There are a few reports of true anaphylaxis in patients with selective IgA deficiency and common variable immunodeficiency who developed IgE antibodies to IgA after treatment with immunoglobulin.[16] However, this adverse event appears to be much less frequent than originally thought. Patients with common variable immunodeficiency have IgG antibodies (10-22% in various studies) to IgA but there is no correlation between the presence of these antibodies and adverse reactions. Patients with anti-IgA antibodies who have had reactions with IVIG have tolerated SCIG.

Other adverse reactions

Other less common adverse reactions have been reported in association with IVIG infusions. These side effects are discussed in more detail elsewhere.[17]

Summary on use of IVIG in treatment of PID

● KEY CONCEPTS

Proposed mechanisms of action of IVIG in autoimmune idiopathic thrombocytopenic purpura

- Fc receptor blockade of reticuloendothelial system
- Fcγ receptor downregulation
- Idiotype–anti-idiotype interaction between anti-platelet GPIIb/IIa autoantibodies and the anti-idiotypic antibodies in IVIG
- Activation of inhibitory receptor FcγRIIB
- Saturation of FcRn receptor to accelerate the catabolism of anti-platelet autoantibodies

Immunoglobulin replacement is the mainstay of treatment for primary humoral immune deficiency. The goal of treatment is to provide a broad spectrum of antibodies to prevent infections and chronic long-term complications. The usual dose is 400–600 mg/kg/month but this may vary individually, and some patients may require higher doses. A serum trough level above 500 mg/dL has been shown to be effective in the prevention of serious bacterial infections. However, recent studies have suggested that even higher doses, e.g., a "biological" trough level and achieving trough levels of IgG in the range of 750–900 mg/dL, may be desirable.[6] Immunoglobulin can be given intramuscularly, intravenously, or subcutaneously. SC administration has proved to be safe, and is a good alternative in some patients, especially those experiencing side effects by the IV route. Generally, IVIG replacement therapy is considered safe in the majority of patients. Side effects are usually mild and treatable by premedication. Good manufacturing practices, improved screening of plasma donors, testing of the source plasma, and additional viral inactivation and removal steps has made IVIG a better and safer plasma-derived product.

The use of IVIG in autoimmune and inflammatory diseases and mechanisms of action

Although we still don't understand all the mechanisms by which IVIG has immunomodulatory effects, knowledge of how IVIG exerts its actions in these diseases will allow us to define appropriate indications and schedules of administration of IVIG, and to design a new generation of IVIG products that are better able to target the immune perturbations in these autoimmune and inflammatory processes. Furthermore, additional multicenter placebo-controlled clinical trials are needed to confirm clinical efficacy. This chapter does not review all the possible indications for IVIG therapy; the reader will be directed to more comprehensive reviews and practice-based guidelines for more details about the various indications for IVIG therapy in autoimmune and inflammatory disorders.

Autoimmune cytopenias

Idiopathic thrombocytopenic purpura

Idiopathic thrombocytopenic purpura (ITP) results from accelerated platelet destruction attributable to an immunologic process that could result in bleeding sometimes life threatening. A number of studies in childhood ITP have shown that IVIG leads to the reversal of the thrombocytopenia. IVIG as a single dose at 0.8 g/kg was similar to 1 g/kg on 2 consecutive days, but was more rapid than intravenous anti-D or oral corticosteroids. A meta-analysis of 13 controlled trials of acute ITP comparing high dose (2 g/kg) with low dose (< 2 g/kg) IVIG, found no difference in treatment efficacy but less side effects in the low dose IVIG treatment groups.[18] Studies have shown that intravenous anti-D immunoglobulin is as effective as IVIG in acute childhood ITP.[19] Anti-D IVIG therapy is FDA approved for the treatment of ITP in Rho(D) positive, nonsplenectomized children, children and adults with chronic ITP, and ITP secondary to HIV infection. The main side effect from anti-D IVIG therapy is anemia due to immune hemolysis. Rarely, patients may experience acute hemoglobinemia, hemoglobinuria, acute renal failure, or disseminated intravascular coagulation.[20] Anti-D IVIG therapy has the advantage of ease of administration and lower costs, and most hematologists prefer this form of therapy over IVIG.

Mechanisms of action of IVIG in ITP

● KEY CONCEPTS

Proposed mechanisms of action of IVIG in Kawasaki syndrome

- Neutralization or elimination of staphylococcal and streptococcal superantigens
- Inhibition of leukocyte adhesion to vascular endothelium
- Inhibition of cytokine production or blocking of cytokine action
- Enhancing the function of FoxP3+ regulatory T cells
- Inhibition of the differentiation of Th17 cells and their effector cytokines

IVIG treatment responses in ITP are due to a blockade of the reticuloendothelial system (RES). In a study of children with acute

ITP, treatment with intravenous Fcγ fragments resulted in a rapid increase in platelet counts. The efficacy of Fcγ fragment therapy strengthens the hypothesis that Fcγ receptor blockade is the main mechanism of action of IVIG in ITP. Other studies have suggested that Fcγ receptor downregulation or change in receptor affinity may also be involved. In addition, idiotype–anti-idiotype interactions between anti-platelet GPIIb/IIIa autoantibodies and IVIG could affect autoantibody production in ITP. However, in a murine model of ITP anti-idiotypic antibodies in the IVIG were not required for the increase in platelet counts. Most experimental systems have shown that the Fc portion of IgG is more important in the immune modulating effects of IVIG in ITP.

The FcRn receptor (neonatal Fc receptor) has been identified as the receptor responsible for protecting IgG from catabolism in the endocytotic vesicles of the endosome, and explains the relatively long half-life of this plasma protein. IVIG may accelerate the catabolism of IgG autoantibodies by saturating these protective receptors in direct proportion to the relative concentration of exogenous plasma levels of IgG from the IVIG.[21] Hansen and Balthasar showed in a rat model of immune thrombocytopenia that IVIG enhanced the clearance of anti-platelet antibodies in a dose dependent manner by saturation of the FcRn receptor.[22] They estimate that approximately 50% of the overall effect of IVIG in ITP may be due to IVIG-mediated acceleration of the elimination of anti-platelet antibodies by the FcRn saturation mechanism.[23]

Samuelsson et al., using a murine model of ITP, showed that the administration of IVIG prevented platelet destruction by a pathogenic monoclonal autoantibody.[24] Protection was associated with the induction of FcγRIIB receptors on splenic macrophages. This inhibitory FcγRIIB receptor was required for the protection of the animals against the monoclonal autoantibody since disruption of the receptor by either genetic deletion or a blocking monoclonal antibody reversed the therapeutic effects of IVIG. Kaneko et al. showed that that the inhibitory properties of IVIG was linked to the sialylation of the glycan component of the Fc fragment.[25] The important glycan moiety in the IgG molecule is located at the asparagine site (Asn^{297}) in the second domain of the constant region. Using a K/BxN serum-induced arthritis model in mice, Kaneko et al. showed that IVIG at 1 g/kg inhibited the inflammatory arthritic process.[25] Deglycosylated or neuraminidase-treated IVIGs were unable to inhibit this inflammation. IVIG enriched for the sialylated glycan moiety had comparable inhibitory effects on the inflammatory process at only 1/10th of the dosage used with intact IVIG. This inhibitory activity was dependent on FcγRIIB expression on effector macrophages. Recently, Anthony et al. engineered a recombinant/sialylated human IgG1 Fc protein that had a 35-fold enhanced immune modulating activity compared to native IVIG.[26] Anthony et al. performed studies to examine the mechanism by which the sialylated Fc fragment could mediate its anti-inflammatory activity, and to identify the target cell that initiates this anti-inflammatory pathway.[27] A splenic marginal zone macrophage expressing a C-type lectin receptor, e.g., SIGN-R1, was required for the anti-inflammatory activity of IVIG in concert with its ability to bind to sialylated Fc domains. The authors proposed that the interaction between sialylated IgG Fc and SIGN-R1 leads to the upregulation of the inhibitory FcγRIIB receptor on effector cells. They suggest that DC-SIGN, the human orthologue of SIGN-R1, has a comparable role for the anti-inflammatory effects of IgG Fc fragment on human macrophages and dendritic cells. The production of IL-33 by DC-SIGN+ macrophages or dendritic cells induces the expansion of IL-4 producing basophils that increases the expression of the FcγRIIB receptor on effector macrophages.[93]

The long-term effects of IVIG in patients with ITP could be due to other effects on antibody production. Using purified mouse B cells Proulx et al. reported that IVIG inhibited both B-cell receptor-dependent and -independent antigen presentation.[28] This inhibitory effect was not mediated through the FcγRIIB receptor, but was mediated by intracellular events. Further studies are needed to clarify these other mechanisms.

Kawasaki syndrome

Kawasaki syndrome (KS) is an acute multisystem disease of unknown etiology that primarily affects infants and young children (Table 85.5; Chapter 57). Although KS occurs worldwide in children of all racial groups, it is most prevalent in Japan and in children of Japanese ancestry. Although the acute illness is generally self-limited, coronary artery abnormalities related to a generalized inflammation and immune activation of small and medium sized blood vessels develop in up to 25% of untreated patients. Although the etiology remains unknown the clinical features and laboratory findings suggest an infectious or post-infectious process.

The administration of high dose IVIG together with aspirin is the standard of care in the treatment of KS.[29] A meta-analysis of published studies on the treatment of KS showed a dose response for IVIG with a threshold for decreased incidence of coronary artery aneurysm with IVIG dosages of >1 g/kg, and that low-dose aspirin (≤80 mg/kg) was comparable to high-dose aspirin (>80 mg/kg) when combined with high-dose IVIG.[30] However, 10-20% of patients have recrudescent or persistent fever 36 hours after their first dose of IVIG. These patients are at higher risk for development of coronary artery abnormalities. A retrospective analysis of re-treatment of patients who remained febrile after IVIG suggested improved outcome with 2 g/kg compared with 1 g/kg of IVIG. Other treatment modalities include intravenous methylprednisolone, oral corticosteroids, immunosuppressive drugs, and more recently infliximab.[31] Tsai et al. compared the

Table 85.5 Clinical features of Kawasaki syndrome*

Diagnostic criteria for complete Kawasaki syndrome
1. Fever of at least 5 days duration
2. Presence of at least 4 of the 5 following conditions: • Bilateral non-exudative conjunctival injection   • One of the following changes in the oropharynx: injected or fissured lips, injected pharynx, or "strawberry tongue"   • One of the following extremity changes: erythema of the palms or soles, edema of the hands or feet, or periungual desquamation   • Polymorphous rash   • Acute nonsuppurative cervical lymphadenopathy
3. Cardiovascular abnormalities: • Myocarditis, arterial aneurysms, pericarditis, aortic or mitral regurgitation, ventricular arrhythmias
4. Other: • Arthralgia and arthritis, urethritis with sterile pyuria, hydrops of the gallbladder, diarrhea, vomiting, or abdominal pain, sensorineural hearing loss

Diagnostic criteria for incomplete (atypical) Kawasaki syndrome
1. Fever of at least 5 days duration
2. At least two of the clinical criteria
3. Absence of any other reasonable explanation for the illness
4. Laboratory findings consistent with severe systemic inflammation

*Points 1 and 2 constitute the primary diagnostic criteria for KS.

clinical responses of patients with KS to four different brands of IVIG.[32] Two of the brands of IVIG were associated with significantly more non-responsiveness and more coronary artery abnormalities; these brands are no longer commercially available.

> ## ● KEY CONCEPTS
>
> ### Proposed mechanisms of action of IVIG in neuromuscular diseases
>
> - Modulation of pro-inflammatory cytokines, e.g., TNF-α, IL-1β in GBS
> - Reduction in muscle levels of ICAM-1, TGF-β, and TGF-β mRNA in dermatomyositis
> - Neutralization by anti-idiotypic antibodies in IVIG of potentially pathogenic autoantibodies, e.g., anti-Gm1 antibodies in GBS and CIDP, and anti-AchR in MG
> - IVIG saturation of FcRn receptors to accelerate degradation of IgG autoantibodies
> - Inhibition of complement deposition and formation of MAC on endomysial capillaries in dermatomyositis
>
> GBS—Guillain-Barré syndrome
> CIDP—chronic inflammatory demyelinating polyneuropathy
> MG—myasthenia gravis
> AchR—acetylcholine nicotinic receptor
> FcRn—neonatal Fc receptor
> MAC—membranolytic attack complex

KS is associated with marked activation of T-cells and monocytes-macrophages.[33] Based on the immunologic and clinical features overlapping with a bacterial toxic shock-like syndrome, studies were carried out to determine if KS is associated with exposure to a superantigen such as a bacterial toxin.[34] The mechanism by which a superantigen can lead to the clinical manifestations of KS remains to be elucidated. However, acute KS is associated with marked immune activation and increased circulating cytokine levels including IL-1, -6, -8, -4, -10, and TNF-α.[34] Some of these cytokines elicit proinflammatory and prothrombotic responses by inducing the expression of leukocyte adhesion molecules, which localize inflammatory cells to vascular endothelial cells. The expression of endothelial-leukocyte adhesion molecules has been demonstrated in acute KS and its downregulation correlates with favorable response to IVIG treatment.[33] The magnitude and persistence of proinflammatory cytokine synthesis have been reported to constitute a risk for the development of coronary artery abnormalities.

IVIG contains high titers of specific antibodies inhibitory to the activation of T cells by staphylococcal and streptococcal superantigens. These findings may account for the observation that treatment of acute KS with IVIG results in a marked reduction of macrophage and T-cell activation.[34] In this regard, the efficacy of IVIG in suppressing the immune activation associated with KS, and more importantly, its ability to prevent the development of coronary artery abnormalities in this illness may relate to the neutralizing antibody activity of IVIG against these bacterial toxins.[33] Toxin neutralization is not likely the only beneficial effect of IVIG in KS. Leung postulated that cytokines in KS stimulate local inflammatory responses of the blood vessels by modifying leukocyte adhesion after increasing the expression of cell surface determinants on vascular endothelial cells.[34]

Vassilev et al. showed that IVIG contains specific antibodies to a 10-peptide sequence including the RGD (Arg-Gly-ASP) motif that is expressed in adhesion molecules on a variety of cell surfaces.[35] Most integrins bind to this RGD sequence. Gill and co-workers reported that IVIG inhibits leukocyte recruitment into inflammatory tissues by inhibiting selectin and integrin binding.[36] In a mouse model of sickle cell vaso-occlusive crisis IVIG inhibited neutrophil adhesion to the vascular endothelium resulting in an increase in capillary blood flow and reversal of the vessel occlusion.[37] IVIG could modulate this cytokine-mediated endothelial cell activation by neutralizing the effects of the cytokines, by inhibiting endothelial cell responses to the cytokines, or alternatively, inhibiting the production of cytokines and growth factors. These mechanisms of IVIG may be playing an important role in preventing coronary artery abnormalities.

Another mechanism by which IVIG could modulate the immune system is by expanding and enhancing the function of FoxP3+ regulatory T cells (Tregs). Furuno et al. reported that clinical improvement in patients with KS was correlated with an increase in the number and function of Tregs.[38] In a mouse model of multiple sclerosis, experimental autoimmune encephalomyelitis, animals treated with IVIG had less severe disease and expanded their population of CD4+CD25+ FoxP3+ Treg cells.[39] This protective effect was lost in mice depleted of Tregs. Kessel et al. reported that IVIG added *in vitro* to human CD4+CD25hi Treg cells increased the intracellular expression of TGF-β, IL-10, and FoxP3, and enhanced the suppressive function of these Tregs.[40] Maddur et al. showed that IVIG enhanced FoxP3+ Tregs while inhibiting the differentiation of Th17 cells and their effector cytokines.[41] Thus, modulation of T-cell function, perhaps through enhancement of Treg cells, could be an important function of IVIG.

Autoimmune neuromuscular diseases

The autoimmune neuropathies (Chapters 55, 64–66) represent the largest group of autoimmune diseases that are treated with IVIG. In fact, autoimmune neurological diseases account for ~30–40% of all IVIG use for "recommended off-label" indications. The autoimmune neuropathies fall into 4 categories: the *inflammatory demyelinating polyneuropathies* which include the Guillain-Barré syndrome (GBS), chronic progressive or relapsing-remitting inflammatory demyelinating polyneuropathy (CIDP), and multifocal motor neuropathy; the *autoimmune neuromuscular junction defects* such as myasthenia gravis and Lambert-Eaton syndrome; the *inflammatory myopathies* which include dermatomyositis, polymyositis and inclusion body myositis; and the *central nervous system diseases* such as multiple sclerosis, stiff person syndrome, and Alzheimer's disease. More information about the use of IVIG in the autoimmune neuromuscular diseases can be found in reviews on this topic elsewhere.[1,42–44]

The inflammatory demyelinating polyneuropathies

Although the etiology of GBS is not known, the pathogenesis of GBS is thought to be an autoimmune process with destruction of peripheral nerve myelin. Patients present with a rapid ascending paralysis often with autonomic and sensory involvement. Most cases are preceded by an upper respiratory or diarrheal illness. About 80% of GBS patients recover satisfactorily from their disease process. The principal approach to the treatment of these patients has been supportive therapy. In 1992 a Dutch group showed in a randomized trial comparing plasma exchange (PE) and IVIG (0.4 g/kg/day for 5 days) that muscle strength improved and the median time to improvement was 41 and 27 days, respectively. Early recognition and treatment are important for the long term prognosis of patients who have severe disease and rapid progression.[45] Because IVIG treatment is more readily available, easier, and has less side effects than PE, this modality of treatment is more useful in GBS patients at the early stage of disease, especially in patients who have evidence of rapid progression, older age, or a history of diarrhea.[45] Several studies looking at optimal dosing showed that IVIG was most beneficial when given in a full dose of 2 g/kg (in 2–5 days), especially in patients who needed ventilatory assistance. Patients with antibodies to ganglioside GM1 or GM1b recovered faster when treated with IVIG than those treated with plasma exchange.[46]

CIDP is an inflammatory neurologic disease resembling GBS that may cause prolonged disability. As for GBS, an immune mediated mechanism for myelin destruction has been postulated in CIDP. A number of randomized controlled trials have been performed with IVIG and have been summarized in a Cochrane analysis.[47] A more recent clinical trial has led to FDA approval for this indication.[48] However, not all patients respond to IVIG and certainly not all patients respond to the same extent. Improvement is usually noticed within the first week of treatment and may last for 6–8 weeks. Many patients can be maintained on IVIG pulse therapy of 1 g/kg body weight prior to the expected relapse. A beneficial response to IVIG was found to be more likely in patients with acute relapse or with disease duration of 1 year or less. In stable patients on intermittent IVIG, the dose should be reduced before the frequency of administration is changed. Patients with an IgM monoclonal paraprotein associated with a demyelinating peripheral neuropathy may also have a modest response to IVIG treatment. In contrast, patients with a paraneoplastic neurological syndrome and antineuronal autoantibodies (anti-Hu and anti-Yo) did not respond to IVIG therapy.

These autoimmune demyelinating polyneuropathies are considered to be immunologically mediated disorders of the peripheral nervous system.[49] An initial lymphocytic infiltration, and later an influx of macrophages, lead to demyelination. A variety of cellular and humoral immune perturbations have been described in patients with GBS. Elevated serum levels of several proinflammatory cytokines including TNF and IFN-γ have been reported. Other cytokines have been reported elevated in the spinal fluids of GBS patients, including IL-1β and -6. Antibodies reactive against myelin components, e.g., ganglioside-specific antibodies such as GM1, GD1b, and GQ1b, are found in the sera of many patients with GBS. Anti-GM1 antibodies are more prominent in GBS patients lacking sensory symptoms and in those patients who have a prodromal diarrheal disease.

The autoimmune neuromuscular junction defects

Myasthenia gravis (MG) is an antibody-mediated autoimmune disease directed against the acetylcholine nicotinic receptor (AChR) of the post-synaptic neuromuscular membrane that results in abnormalities of neuromuscular transmission leading to fluctuating weakness and fatigability (Chapter 64). Improvement in muscle weakness following IVIG treatment has been shown in several controlled studies.[50,51] A controlled trial comparing the efficacy and side effects of IVIG (using two dosages) to PE in MG patients during disease exacerbation showed similar efficacy, but fewer side effects in the IVIG group.[52] Dosing of the IVIG is similar to other autoimmune neurologic diseases. The overall response rate is about 74% with improvement occurring within 3 weeks from the start of therapy. The duration of the response is variable and seems to be longer if patients are also receiving steroids. AChR antibody titers generally do not change; the clinical response does not appear to correlate with AChR antibody levels. Repeated courses of IVIG may be needed to maintain improvement but controlled studies have not been done.

The inflammatory myopathies

Polymyositis, dermatomyositis, and inclusion-body myositis are inflammatory muscle disorders characterized by muscle weakness and cellular infiltrates within the skeletal muscles (Chapter 55). Although the pathogenetic mechanisms in these diseases are thought to be similar, each inflammatory myopathy group has characteristic clinical and immunopathologic features that sets each apart. Dermatomyositis (DM) affects the proximal muscles and is associated with a violaceous rash on the face and extremities.

Dalakas and co-workers conducted a double blind, placebo-controlled study of 15 patients (age 18–55 years) with treatment resistant DM.[53] Patients were randomly assigned to receive IVIG therapy (2 g/kg) or placebo every month for 3 months. The patients receiving IVIG had significant improvements in muscle strength, neuromuscular symptoms related to daily living, and skin rash. Serum creatine kinase fell by 50% after the first infusion with further decreases toward normalization in subsequent infusions. Unfortunately, continued improvement of these patients was variable. Some patients continued to get IVIG less frequently along with low-dose steroids and were able to maintain improvement. Some patients who were unresponsive to steroids during their initial treatment regimen became steroid-responsive following IVIG infusion.

Muscle biopsies showed marked improvement in muscle histology after IVIG treatment.[54] The mean muscle fiber diameter and the mean number of capillaries increased. Immunological activation markers such as MHC class I and ICAM-1 expression diminished after IVIG therapy. TGF-β, which is upregulated in the muscle tissues of patients with DM, was markedly downregulated. Finally, in muscle biopsies after IVIG therapy, the complement-mediated damage was diminished.[54]

The central nervous system diseases

Multiple sclerosis (MS) is the most common demyelinating disorder of the central nervous system, and studies have suggested that the pathogenesis of multiple sclerosis is related to an autoimmune process (Chapter 65). Four randomized studies with IVIG (0.15–0.2 g/kg) administered every 4 weeks showed a pronounced reduction in relapse rate. Other studies using larger doses of IVIG showed beneficial effects on development of new gadolinium-enhancing lesions on MRI. A meta-analysis of four controlled trials in patients with relapsing-remitting MS showed that IVIG significantly reduced the annual relapse rate, increased the proportion of relapse free patients, and reduced disease progression as measured by the change in Kurtzke expanded disability status scale.[55] However, the prevention of relapses with IVIG trial (PRIVIG) of patients given 0.2 and 0.4 g/kg monthly did not show efficacy in relapse rate or MRI activity compared to placebo treated patients.[56]

10 to 20% of childhood epilepsies are intractable, and do not respond adequately with first line conventional anti-epileptic drug therapy. Children with drug-resistant epilepsy, who were treated with IVIG for recurrent respiratory tract infections, had a decrease in the frequency and severity of their seizures. A number of investigators have suggested that immune mechanisms are important in the pathogenesis of epilepsy, particularly those that are associated with infections or vaccination. A number of reports have appeared on the responsiveness of certain patients with childhood epilepsy to IVIG therapy. The favorable effects of IVIG treatment were especially seen in children with West

syndrome, Landau–Kleffner syndrome, Lennox–Gastaut syndrome, and Rasmussen encephalitis. Placebo-controlled studies showed significant reductions in seizure episodes with IVIG treatment. Additional multicenter placebo-controlled trials are needed to further define the subpopulation of children with intractable seizures who would benefit from IVIG treatment, although the best candidates appear to be those patients with West syndrome and Lennox–Gastaut syndrome, and those patients who have post-infectious epileptic encephalopathies.

Mechanisms of action of IVIG in neuromuscular diseases

> ● KEY CONCEPTS
>
> **Proposed mechanisms of action of IVIG in inflammatory and autoimmune skin diseases**
>
> - Fas antibodies in IVIG inhibit Fas-mediated keratinocyte apoptosis in toxic epidermal necrolysis
> - Anti-idiotypic neutralization of autoimmune antibodies in autoimmune mucocutaneous blistering diseases
> - Enhanced degradation of autoantibodies through the FcRn receptor pathway
> - Inhibition of cytokine production
> - Inhibition of B-cell function and decreased autoantibody production through activation of the FcγRIIB receptor (signaling through ITIM)
>
> ITIM—Immunoreceptor tyrosine inhibitory motif

The autoimmune neurologic diseases and inflammatory myopathies provide a broad group of immunologically mediated diseases in which many inflammatory and immune-mediated effector pathways lead to tissue destruction. These neurological and myopathic diseases provide models for the study of the mechanisms of action by which IVIG modulates these autoimmune and inflammatory processes. Several mechanisms have been proposed for the immune-modulating effects of IVIG. IVIG may modulate the inflammatory response by the suppression of cytokine production. Pro-inflammatory cytokines, e.g., TNF-α and IL-1β, in GBS patients decrease with IVIG therapy. Dalakas documented reduction in muscle levels of ICAM-1, TGF-β, and TGF-β mRNA in patients with inflammatory myopathies after IVIG treatment.[54] Although IVIG may contain antibodies to certain cytokines, other studies suggested that IVIG downregulates cytokine production by inhibiting gene expression. Of interest, PE was not associated with a decrease in these proinflammatory cytokines, suggesting that the mechanisms of action of PE and IVIG in GBS may be different.

A number of studies have shown that IVIG contains antibodies with idiotypic specificities that can bind and neutralize potentially pathogeneic autoantibodies such as anti-GM1 antibodies in GBS and CIDP and anti-AchR in MG.[54] Malik and co-workers showed that anti-idiotypic antibodies in the IVIG directed against idiotopes located on the anti-GM1 immunoglobulin molecule blocked the binding of the anti-GM1 antibodies to its target antigen.[57] Support for a similar mechanism in MG comes from the fact that IgG or F(ab')₂ fragments in the IVIG preparations are capable of binding to AChR antibodies *in vitro*.[58] Using *in vitro* nerve-muscle preparations Buchwald et al. showed that the F(ab')₂ portion of IVIG neutralized the "blocking" effect of serum from patients with acute GBS.[59]

As discussed above for ITP, the administration of large amounts of IgG could saturate the FcRn receptor and accelerate the degradation of the IgG autoantibodies found in many of the autoimmune neuropathies. This mechanism may be applicable to antibody-mediated neuromuscular diseases such as MG, Lambert–Eaton myasthenia syndrome, GBS, stiff-person syndrome, CIDP and multi-focal motor neuropathy.

The principal inflammatory mechanism in DM is complement (C)-dependent microangiopathy with activation of C3 and deposition of the complement C5b-9 membranolytic attack complex (MAC) on the endomysial capillaries.[54] Basta and colleagues have shown that IVIG can inhibit the uptake of C components on target tissues.[60] In DM patients treated with IVIG, C3 deposition was reduced with corresponding decreases in MAC expression on endomysial capillaries in the muscle tissues.[54,60] Consequently, IVIG allowed neovascularization to occur and reversal of the ischemic process, resulting in muscle tissue healing. This effect of IVIG on complement deposition may be relevant to other autoimmune neurological diseases such as in patients with MG, GBS and CIDP in which complement may be playing a role in the tissue damage.[54,60,61] Arumugam et al. showed that IVIG protects the brain against ischemic injury mediated by complement in a mouse model of experimental stroke.[62]

Rheumatologic diseases

Systemic vasculitis

IVIG has been shown to be useful as adjunct therapy in patients with anti-neutrophil cytoplasmic antibody (ANCA)-positive systemic vasculitis (Chapter 58). High-dose IVIG, e.g., 400 mg/kg/dose over 5 consecutive days, may benefit the disease activity and may be associated with reduced circulating ANCA levels. Response rates vary between 60% and 100%, and may be related in some patients to a chronic parvovirus B19 infection. Further placebo-controlled studies are needed.

Rheumatoid arthritis

There have been mixed results on the use of high-dose IVIG in adult patients with rheumatoid arthritis. In children not responding to conventional therapy, randomized controlled studies of high dose IVIG has been reported to be of benefit for severe juvenile idiopathic arthritis.[63]

Systemic lupus erythematosus

The clinical studies, mostly case reports and open labeled studies, of IVIG therapy in patients with systemic lupus erythematosus (SLE) have suggested some benefit especially for cutaneous lesions, arthritis and fever.[1] A controlled study of 20 patients showed a beneficial response in 17. SLE patients at increased risk of thromboembolic events or with renal compromise should not be treated with IVIG.

Further review of the literature for the treatment of autoimmune disorders can be found in the review by Kivity et al.[64]

Mechanisms of action of IVIG in rheumatic diseases and vasculitides

A number of mechanisms of action have been proposed to explain the immunoregulatory effects of IVIG in patients with vasculitis. Immune complexes are felt to be a major component in the pathophysiology of these inflammatory diseases. Several studies have suggested that IVIG can solubilize immune complexes making them less nephritogenic. This suggestion is supported by observation of decreases in circulating immune complexes in SLE patients treated with IVIG.

IVIG contains anti-idiotypic antibodies to anti-DNA, anti-factor VIII, ANCA autoantibodies, anti-thyroid autoantibodies and others.[65] The proposed mechanism of action of IVIG in ANCA positive vasculitis is binding or neutralization of the ANCA autoantibodies by anti-idiotypic antibodies in the IVIG. These anti-idiotypic antibodies may also act in concert with their effects on the FcγRIIB receptor on B-cells to produce a negative "off signal" to the B cells synthesizing these autoimmune antibodies.[66] Thus, it is postulated that the anti-idiotypic antibodies in IVIG may be beneficial by restoring the idiotypic control network in these autoimmune diseases.

IVIG contains a number of natural autoantibodies that may have immune modulating activities, e.g., antibodies to CD4, MHC class I, cytokines, and more recently, antibodies to Siglec-8 and -9 that can induce the death of eosinophils and neutrophils, respectively. Siglecs are a lectin family of inhibitory receptors that mediate cytokine-dependent cell death and anti-proliferative activities, and inhibit cellular activities. The presence of anti-Siglec antibodies in IVIG may have important immune modulating activities in cytokine-rich inflammatory and autoimmune disorders.[67] The "natural" antibodies in IVIG have also been shown to bind to a number of plasma and tissue proteins including BAFF, GM-CSF, liver antigens, and β-amyloid peptide. The binding of native IgG can be significantly increased by mild denaturing conditions, e.g., mild pH treatment and cold ethanol precipitation used during the manufacturing process of IVIG. St-Amour et al. suggest that these industrial fractionation processes for IVIG could contribute to the therapeutic anti-inflammatory effects.[68]

Antibody-mediated graft rejection

Antibody-mediated organ rejection (AMR) is a significant and unique form of graft rejection that does not respond well to standard immunosuppressive therapy directed at T-cell responses. AMR is particularly a problem in those patients who are highly HLA-sensitized or have ABO-incompatible transplants. Anti-HLA (donor-specific) antibodies and anti-endothelial cell antibodies are often associated with AMR. Rapid onset of allograft dysfunction in a high risk patient may indicate AMR, and is characterized by C4d deposition in the peritubular capillaries. IgG complement-fixing antibody to donor HLA antigens or an IgG-positive T-cell cross match indicate a high risk for AMR. Jordan and colleagues have shown that pretreatment with high dose IVIG decreases anti-HLA donor-specific antibodies, and is an effective treatment for AMR episodes.[69] Others have used IVIG in combination with rituximab.[70] Complement activation is an important factor in AMR, and as discussed above, IVIG can inhibit complement activation and neutralize or "scavenge" anaphylatoxins (C3a/C5a).[71,72] The use of IVIG therapy in patients undergoing solid organ transplantation is reviewed elsewhere.[73]

Toxic shock syndrome

IVIG may have therapeutic value in the treatment of patients with toxic shock syndrome secondary to *Staphylococcus aureus* or *Streptococcus pyogenes* exotoxins. In an open study by the Canadian Streptococcal Study Group IVIG appeared to be beneficial in patients with streptococcal toxic shock syndrome.[74] In a meta-analysis of IVIG treatment of neonatal sepsis there was a six-fold decrease in mortality. IVIG inhibits *Staphylococcus* exotoxin induced T-cell activation, and contains antibodies against exotoxins responsible for toxic shock syndromes. Great variations in neutralizing activity against streptococcal pyrogenic exotoxins of different brands and even among different lots of IVIG can be found. However, these findings suggest that it is possible to select one IVIG preparation that contains high levels of neutralizing activity against a wide variety of Group A streptococcal superantigens, which could be used in the treatment of streptococcal toxic shock syndrome. The neutralizing capacity of IVIG for these bacterial superantigens is important because of their potential to stimulate the production of proinflammatory cytokines that lead to clinical disease. A number of *in vitro* studies have shown that IVIG can inhibit the production of, or bind to and neutralize, a number of cytokines and growth factors from various cell types.[75-79] Thus, IVIG may exert its anti-inflammatory effects in many of these diseases by interrupting or modifying a number of different steps in the inflammatory cascade, from the inhibition of effector cell function to reduction in cytokine-induced endothelial cell activation, or the "neutralization" of cytokines.

Inflammatory and autoimmune skin diseases

Toxic epidermal necrolysis (TEN) and Stevens–Johnson syndrome (SJS)

Toxic epidermal necrolysis (TEN) and Stevens–Johnson syndrome (SJS) are severe drug induced skin diseases (reviewed in Letko et al).[80] TEN results in apoptotic epidermal cell death in which there is separation of large areas of the skin at the epidermal junction, producing the appearance of scalded skin. Keratinocyte apoptosis that precedes epidermal detachment is an early event in TEN. A number of drugs can cause TEN and SJS, including sulfonamides, anticonvulsants, and non-steroidal anti-inflammatory medications. The mortality rate can be as high as 30%. Viard et al. studied serum samples from patients who had TEN and found that the serum of these patients had very high levels of soluble Fas ligand (sFasL).[81] Keratinocytes normally express the death receptor Fas. The keratinocytes of patients with TEN also express very high levels of active Fas ligand. In a small pilot study, Viard and co-workers administered IVIG (0.2–0.75 g/kg for 4 consecutive days) to 10 patients with TEN.[81] In all 10 patients, the progression of skin disease was rapidly interrupted within 24–48 hours with rapid skin healing and no adverse effects. In *in vitro* studies, IVIG completely inhibited Fas-mediated keratinocyte apoptosis. This effect was related to the presence of naturally occurring Fas blocking antibodies in the IVIG that inhibited Fas-mediated keratinocyte cell death. Faye and Roujeau examined nine studies (156 patients) in which high-dose IVIG was used in the treatment of TEN and SJS.[82] Variations in dosages, time to initiation of therapy and duration of therapy precluded a meta-analysis. These authors concluded that although IVIG may be beneficial in TEN and SJS, the effects might be small. Any firm conclusions will have to await randomized placebo-controlled trials.

Risk factors for adverse events associated with IVIG therapy

- Pre-existing renal insufficiency
- Diabetes mellitus
- Age—elderly
- Dehydration with volume depletion
- Paraproteinemia or other causes of hyperviscosity
- Cardiac or peripheral vascular disorders

Autoimmune mucocutaneous blistering diseases

Autoimmune mucocutaneous blistering diseases are a group of diseases, e.g., pemphigus foliaceus, pemphigus vulgaris, bullous pemphigoid,, mucous membrane pemphigoid, epidermolysis bullosa acquisita, that involve the skin and mucous membranes that are immunologically mediated most often by tissue-specific antibodies (Chapter 62). These diseases are treated with high-dose systemic steroids and immunosuppressive agents. There is now a growing literature on the use of high-dose IVIG therapy in patients with autoimmune blistering disease.[83–85] In a randomized controlled trial of pemphigus Amagai et al. reported that higher doses of IVIG gave longer clinical responses, and decreased anti-desmoglein antibodies compared to the other treatment groups.[86] Often concomitant therapy with steroids or other immunosuppressive drugs could be reduced or even discontinued. However, like other autoimmune disorders the response to IVIG can be variable. In two other studies of pemphigus vulgaris and pemphigus foliaceus patients were disease free by approximately five months of monthly infusions of IVIG.[87] Immunosuppressive therapy was reduced or discontinued on average after 18–19 cycles of IVIG over 27–30 months.

The rapid decrease in autoantibodies is consistent with a mechanism related to the FcRn pathway of antibody catabolism. FcRn-deficient mice are resistant to developing experimental pemphigus in a passive transfer blister formation assay, and IVIG was not protective.[88] In contrast, the administration of high dose IVIG to normal mice prevented blister formation in this model. Mimouni et al. showed that the anti-idiotypic antibodies in IVIG to the anti-desmoglein antibodies ameliorate this experimental pemphigus disease model in mice.[89]

IVIG in atopic diseases

Asthma

A number of advances and new drugs have been introduced over the past 15 years for the treatment of asthma. IVIG has been used in some asthma patients as a steroid-sparing treatment modality. In an open label study of IVIG (2 g/kg at monthly intervals) in 8 children (ages 6–17) who had severe steroid dependent asthma, the average alternate day steroid dose decreased, with improvements in peak-flow rates and symptom scores. The serum IgE levels decreased from 324 IU prior to therapy to 133 IU after 6 months on IVIG. Immediate hypersensitivity skin testing to inhalant allergens decreased by 100-fold. However, other studies including a multicenter placebo-controlled study

did not show any differences between the IVIG treatment groups and the placebo groups. Perhaps IVIG can be useful in a subgroup of severe asthmatic patients who require high doses of oral steroids. A larger placebo-controlled trial of carefully selected patients who are oral steroid dependent or may have steroid resistance is needed to determine the efficacy of IVIG therapy in steroid-dependent asthmatics.

Several studies have shown that IVIG can modulate the synthesis of cytokines. Spahn et al. showed that the addition of IVIG to PHA-stimulated lymphocytes shifted the dexamethasone dose–response curve, rendering the cells more sensitive to the suppressive effects of steroids in patients with glucocorticoid-insensitive asthma.[90] In addition, IVIG significantly improved glucocorticoid receptor binding affinity that may be responsible for the steroid-sparing effects of IVIG.

The mechanism(s) by which IVIG suppresses immunoglobulin synthesis of B cells has been postulated to occur by inhibiting cytokine production and by directly suppressing B-cell function through the Fcγ RIIB receptor. Zhuang and Mazer reported that both intact IVIG and fractionated IVIG inhibited anti-CD40- and IL-4-stimulated IgE production of purified B-cells.[91] F(ab')₂ fragments were more potent than Fc fragments in inhibiting IgE production. Thus, through pathways that modulate cytokine production and decrease B-cell Ig synthesis, i.e., diminished serum levels of IgE antibodies, IVIG may have both anti-inflammatory and immunmodulating effects in allergic diseases.

Translational research

● ON THE HORIZON

Translational research opportunities related to IVIG therapy

- Elucidation of multiple mechanisms of action likely working together in mediating beneficial effects of IVIG in multiple clinical disorders.
- Development of "designer" IVIG products through the use of molecular biology based on improved understanding of IVIG ligands with their receptors that may provide an alternative to the use of human plasma.
- Enhanced understanding of pathogenetic mechanisms involved in IVIG-responsive autoimmune and inflammatory diseases that should lead to more effective therapy with IVIG or to more specific, modified forms of this product for treatment of these complex disorders.

IVIG has been found to be an effective treatment as replacement therapy for patients with primary immune deficiency and for a wide spectrum of autoimmune and inflammatory diseases. The "reintroduction" of the subcutaneous route of Ig replacement therapy has been a major advance in patients with PID. Changes in the formulation of the Ig product, e.g., 20% IgG concentration for SC administration, and future advances will make it easier for immunologists to treat their patients with PID.

At present, IVIG is FDA approved for only a few autoimmune and inflammatory diseases, e.g., ITP, CIDP and KS. However, even in ITP, CIDP and KS, the exact mechanism of action of IVIG remains to be fully elucidated. While no single mechanism can explain the beneficial effects of IVIG, it is likely that several mechanisms of action working together are responsible for the effects of IVIG in the many clinical disorders. The studies of Ravetch and colleagues have opened a new "chapter" in understanding the mechanisms of action of IVIG in patients with autoimmune disease. These exciting studies define an important mechanism by which IVIG may modulate immune processes mediated through sialylated Fc on the IgG molecule and the receptors, e.g., FcγRIIB and SIGN-R1, involved in this anti-inflammatory process. Activation of the inhibitory FcγRIIB receptor on effector macrophages and the saturation of the FcRn receptor may act together to reduce the levels of autoantibodies. These types of studies may lead to "designer" IVIG products through the use of molecular biology as published by Anthony et al.[26] A molecular-engineered product will save on a precious human commodity of plasma that is often in short supply, and provide a more specific product to modulate the immune system and control the autoimmune and inflammatory disease. Translational research focused on better understanding of the pathogenic mechanisms involved in these diseases will undoubtedly lead to more effective therapy with IVIG or more specific, modified forms of this product.

References

1. Orange JS, Hossny EM, Weiler CR, et al. Use of intravenous immunoglobulin in human disease: a review of evidence by members of the Primary Immunodeficiency Committee of the American Academy of Allergy, Asthma and Immunology. J Allergy Clin Immunol 2006;117:S525–S553.
2. Quartier P, Debre M, DeBlie J, et al. Early and prolonged intravenous immunoglobulin replacement therapy in childhood agammaglobulinemia: A retrospective survey of 31 patients. J Pediatrics 1999;134:589–96.
3. Busse PJ, Razvi S, Cunningham-Rundles C. Efficacy of intravenous immunoglobulin in the prevention of pneumonia in patients with common variable immunodeficiency. J Allergy Clin Immunol 2002;109:1001–4.
4. Stiehm ER, Orange JS, Ballow M, Lehman H. Therapeutic use of immunoglobulins. Adv Pediatr 2010;57:185–218.
5. Bonagura VR, Marchlewski R, Cox A, Rosenthal DW. Biologic IgG level in primary immunodeficiency disease: the IgG level that protects against recurrent infection. J Allergy Clin Immunol 2008;122:210–2.
6. Lucas M, Lee M, Lortan J, et al. Infection outcomes in patients with common variable immunodeficiency disorders: relationship to immunoglobuin therapy over 22 years. J Allergy Clin Immunol 2010;125:1354–60.
7. Fasth A, Nystrom J. Quality of life and health-care resource utilization among children with primary immunodeficiency receiving home treatment with subcutaneous human immunoglobulin. J Clin Immunol 2008;28:370–8.
8. Gardulf A, Nicolay U, Math D, et al. Children and adults with primary antibody deficiencies gain quality of life by subcutaneous IgG self-infusions at home. J Allergy Clin Immunol 2004;114:936–42.
9. Nicolay U, Kiessling P, Berger M, et al. Health-related quality of life and treatment satisfaction in North American patients with primary immune deficiency diseases receiving subcutaneous IgG self-infusions at home. J Clin Immunol 2006;26:65–72.
10. Misbah S, Sturzenegger MH, Borte MN, et al. Subcutaneous immunoglobulin: opportunities and outlook. Clin Exp Immunol 2009;158(Suppl. 1):51–9.
11. Berger M. Subcutaneous immunoglobulin replacement in primary immunodeficiencies. Clin Immunology 2004;112:1–7.
12. Bonilla FA. Pharmacokinetics of immunoglobulin administered via intravenous or subcutaneous routes. Immunol Allergy Clin North Am 2008;28(4):803–19.
13. Brannagan TH, Nagle KJ, Lange DJ, Rowland LP. Complications of intravenous immune globulin treatment in neurologic disease. Neurology 1996;47:674–7.
14. Dalakas MC. High-dose intravenous immunoglobulin and serum viscosity: risk of precipitating thromboembolic events. Neurology 1994;44(2):223–6.
15. Reinhart WH, Berchtold PE. Effect of high-dose intravenous immunoglobulin therapy on blood rheology. Lancet 1992;339:662–4.
16. Burks A, Sampson H, Buckley R. Anaphylactic reactions after gammaglobulin administration in patients with hypogammaglobulinemia. Detection of IgE antibodies to IgA. N Engl J Med 1986;314:560.
17. Thampakkul S, Ballow M. Replacement intravenous immune serum globulin therapy in patients with antibody immune deficiency. Allergy Immunol Clin North Am 2001;21:165–84.
18. Qin YH, Zhou TB, Su LN, et al. The efficacy of different dose intravenous immunoglobulin in treating acute idiopathic thrombocytopenic purpura: a meta-analysis of 13 randomized controlled trials. Blood Coagul Fibrinolysis 2010;21:713–21.
19. Tarantino MD, Madden RM, Fennewald DL, et al. Treatment of childhood acute immune thrombocytopenic purpura with anti-D immune globulin or pooled immune globulin. J Pediatr 1999;134(1):21–6.
20. Gaines AR. Disseminated intravascular coagulation associated with acute hemoglobinemia or hemoglobinuria following Rh₀(D) immune globulin intravenous administration for immune thrombocytopenic purpura. Blood 2005;106:1532–7.
21. Yu Z, Lennon VA. Mechanism of intravenous immune globulin therapy in antibody-mediated autoimmune diseases. N Engl J Med 1999;340(3):227–8.
22. Hansen RJ, Balthasar JP. Effects of intravenous immunoglobulin on platelet count and antiplatelet antibody disposition in a rat model of immune thrombocytopenia. Blood 2002;100:2087–93.
23. Hansen RJ, Balthasar JP. PK/PD modeling of the effects of intravenous immunoglobulin on the disposition of anti-platelet antibodies in a rat model of immune thrombocytopenia. J Pharm Sci 2003;92:1206–15.
24. Samuelsson A, Towers TL, Ravetch JV. Anti-inflammatory activity of IVIG mediated through the inhibitory Fc receptor. Science 2001;291:484–6.
25. Kaneko Y, Nimmerjahn F, Ravetch J. Anti-inflammatory activity of immunoglobulin G resulting from Fc sialylation. Science 2006;313:670–3.
26. Anthony R, Nimmerjahn F, Ashline D, et al. Recapitulation of IVIG anti-inflammatory activity with a recombinant IgG Fc. Science 2008;320:373–6.
27. Anthony RM, Wermeling F, Karlsson MC, Ravetch JV. Identification of a receptor required for the anti-inflammatory activity of IVIG. Proc Natl Acad Sci U S A 2008;105(50):19571–8.
28. Proulx D, Aubin E, Lemieux R, Bazin R. Inhibition of B cell-mediated antigen presentation by intravenous immunoglobulins (IVIg). Clin Immunol 2010;135:422–9.
29. Newburger JW, Takahashi M, Beiser AS, et al. A single intravenous infusion of gamma globulin as compared with four infusions in the treatment of acute Kawasaki syndrome. N Engl J Med 1991;324:1633–9.
30. Durongpisitkul K, Gururaj VJ, Park JM, Martin CF. The prevention of coronary artery aneurysm in Kawasaki disease: a meta-analysis on the efficacy of aspirin and immunoglobulin treatment. Pediatrics 1995;96(6):1057–61.
31. Son MB, Gauvreau K, Burns JC, et al. Infliximab for intravenous immunoglobulin resistance in Kawasaki Disease: a retrospective study. J Pediatr 2011;158:644–9.
32. Tsai M-H, Huang Y-C, Yen M-H, et al. Clinical responses of patients with Kawasaki Disease to different brands of intravenous immunoglobulin. J Pediatr 2006;148:38–43.
33. Leung DYM. Immunologic aspects of Kawasaki syndrome. J Rheumatol 1990;(Suppl. 24):15–8.
34. Leung DY. Kawasaki syndrome: immunomodulatory benefit and potential toxin neutralization by intravenous immune globulin. Clin Exp Immunol 1996;104(Suppl. 1):49–54.
35. Vassilev TL, Kazatchkine MD, Van Huyen JPD, et al. Inhibition of cell adhesion by antibodies to Arg-Gly-Asp (RGD) in normal immunoglobulin for therapeutic use (intravenous immunoglobulin, IVIg). Blood 2004;93(11):3624–31.
36. Gill V, Doig C, Knight D, et al. Targeting adhesion molecules as a potential mechanism of action for intravenous immunoglobulin. Circulation 2005;112:2031–9.
37. Chang J, Shi P, Chiang E, Frenette P. Intravenous immunoglobulins reverse acute vaso-occlusive crises in sickle cell mice through rapid inhibition of neutrophil adhesion. Blood 2008;111:915–23.
38. Furuno K, Yuge T, Kusuhara K, et al. CD25+CD4+ regulatory T cells in patients with Kawasaki disease. J Pediatrics 2004;145:385–90.
39. Ephrem A, Chamat S, Miquel C, et al. Expansion of CD4+CD25+ regulatory T cells by intravenous immunoglobulin: a critical factor in controlling experimental autoimmune encephalomyelitis. Blood 2008;111:715–22.
40. Kessel A, Ammuri H, Peri R, et al. Intravenous immunoglobulin therapy affects T regulatory cells by increasing their suppressive function. J Immunol 2010;179:5571–5.
41. Maddur MS, Vani J, Hegde P, Lacroix-Desmazes S, et al. Inhibition of differentiation, amplification, and function of human TH17 cells by intravenous immunoglobulin. J Allergy Clin Immunol 2011;127:823–30.
42. Dalakas MC. Intravenous immunoglobulin in autoimmune neuromuscular diseases. J Am Med Assoc 2004;2004:2367–75.
43. Fergusson D, Hutton B, Sharma M, et al. Use of intravenous immunoglobulin for treatment of neurologic conditions: a systematic review. Transfusion 2005;45:1640–57.
44. Members of the Task Force. Elovaara I, Apostolski S, van Doorn P. EFNS guidelines for the use of intravenous immunoglobulin in treatment of neurological diseases. Eur J Neurol 2008;15:893–908.
45. Hughes RA, Raphael JC, Swan AV, Doorn PA. Intravenous immunoglobulin for Guillain-Barré syndrome. [update of Cochrane Database Syst Rev 2001;(2) CD002063; PMID: 11406030]. Cochrane Database Syst Rev 2004.
46. Yuki N, Ang CW, Koga M, et al. Clinical features and response to treatment in Guillain-Barré syndrome associated with antibodies to GM1b ganglioside. Ann Neurol 2000;47:314–21.
47. van Schaik IN, Winer JB, de Haan R, Vermeulen M. Intravenous immunoglobuline for chronic inflammatory demyelinating polyradiculoneuropathy. Cochrane Database Syst Rev 2004;2: CD001797.
48. Hughes RAC, Donofrio P, Bril V, et al. Intravenous immune globulin (10% caprylate-chromatography purified) for the treatment of chronic inflammatory demyelinating polyradiculoneuropathy (ICE study): a randomised placebo-controlled trial. Lancet Neurol 2008;7:136–44.
49. Sater RA, Rostami A. Treatment of Guillain-Barré Syndrome with intravenous immunoglobulin. Neurology 1998;51(Suppl. 5):S9–S15.
50. Gajdos P, Tranchant C, Clair B, et al. Treatment of myasthenia gravis exacerbation with intravenous immunoglobulin - a randomized double-blind clinical trial. Arch Neurol 2005;62:1689–93.
51. Zinman L, Ng E, Bril V. IV immunoglobulin in patients with myasthenia gravis - a randomized controlled trial. Neurology 2007;68:837–41.
52. Gajdos P, Chevret S, Clair B, et al. Plasma exchange and intravenous immunoglobulin in autoimmune myasthenia gravis. Ann N Y Acad Sci 1998;841:720–76.
53. Dalakas MC, Illa I, Dambrosia JM, et al. A controlled trial of high-dose intravenous immunoglobulin infusions as treatment for dermatomyositis. N Engl J Med 1993;329:1993–2000.
54. Dalakas MC. Mechanism of action of intravenous immunoglobulin and therapeutic considerations in the treatment of autoimmune neurologic diseases. Neurology 1998;51(6 Suppl. 5):S2–S8.
55. Sorensen PS, Fazekas F, Lee M. Intravenous immunoglobulin G for the treatment of relapsing-remitting multiple sclerosis: a meta-analysis. Eur J Neurol 2002;9:557–63.

56. Fazekas F, Strasser-Fuchs S, Hommes OR. Intravenous immunoglobulin in MS: promise or failure? J Neurol Sci 2007;259:61–6.

57. Malik U, Oleksowicz L, Latov N, Cardo LJ. Intravenous γ-globulin inhibits binding of anti-GM1 to its target antigen. Ann Neurol 1996;39:136–9.

58. Liblau R, Gajdos PH, Bustarret A, et al. Intravenous γ-globulin in myasthenia gravis: interaction with anti-acetylcholine receptor autoantibodies. J Clin Immunol 1991;11:128–31.

59. Buchwald B, Ahangari R, Weishaupt A, Toyka KV. Intravenous immunoglobulins neutralize blocking antibodies in Guillain-Barré syndrome. Ann Neurol 2002;51:673–80.

60. Basta M. Modulation of complement-mediated immune damage by intravenous immune globulin. Clin Exp Immunol 1996;104(Suppl. 1):21–5.

61. Dalakas M. Intravenous immunoglobulin in the treatment of autoimmune neuromuscular diseases: present status and practical therapeutic guidelines. Muscle Nerve 1999;22:1479–97.

62. Arumugam TV, Tang S-C, Lathia JD, et al. Intravenous immunoglobulin (IVIG) protects the brain against experimental stroke by preventing complement-mediated neuronal cell death. Proc Natl Acad Sci U S A 2007;104(35):14104–9.

63. Giannini EH, Lovell DJ, Silverman ED. Intravenous immunoglobulin in the treatment of polyarticular juvenile rheumatoid arthritis: a phase I/II study. Pediatric Rheumatology Collaborative Study Group. J Rheumatol 1996;23:919–24.

64. Kivity S, Katz U, Daniel N, et al. Evidence for the use of intravenous immunoglobulins—A review of the literature. Clinic Rev Allerg Immunol 2010;38:201–69.

65. Mouthon L, Kaveri SV, Spalter SH, et al. Mechanisms of action of intravenous immune globuline in immune-mediated diseases. Clin Exp Immunol 1996;104:3–9.

66. Gergely J, Sarmay G. Fc gamma RII-mediated regulation of human B cells. Scand J Immunol 1996;44:1–10.

67. von Gunten S, Simon H-U. Natural anti-Siglec autoantibodies mediate potential immunoregulatory mechanisms: Implications for the clinical use of intravenous immunoglobulins (IVIg). Autoimmun Rev 2008;7:453–6.

68. St-Amour I, Laroche A, Bazin R, Lemieux R. Activation of cryptic IgG reactive with BAFF, amyloid beta peptide and GM-CSF during the industrial fractionation of human plasma into therapeutic intravenous immunoglobulins. Clin Immunol 2009;133:52–60.

69. Jordan SC, Vo AA, Tyan D, et al. Current approaches to treatment of antibody-mediated rejection. Pediatr Transplant 2005;9:408–15.

70. Vo AA, Lukovsky M, Toyoda M, et al. Rituximab and intravenous immune globulin for desensitization during renal transplantation. N Engl J Med 2008;359(3):242–51.

71. Basta M, Kirshbom P, Frank MM, Fries L. Mechanism of therapeutic effect of high-dose intravenous immunoglobulin: attenuation of acute, complement-dependent immune damage in a guinea pig model. J Clin Invest 1989;84:1974–81.

72. Basta M, Van Goor F, Luccioli S, et al. F(ab)′2-mediated neutralization of C3a and C5a anaphylatoxins: a novel effector function of immunoglobulins. Nature Med 2003;9:431–8.

73. Shehata N, Palda VA, Meyer RM, et al. The use of immunoglobulin therapy for patients undergoing solid organ transplantation: an evidence-based practice guideline. Transfus Med Rev 2010;24(Suppl. 1):S7–S27.

74. Kaul R, McGeer A, Norrby-Teglund A, et al. Intravenous immunoglobulin therapy for streptococcal toxic shock syndrome—a comparative observational study. Clin Infect Dis 1999;28:800–7.

75. Abe R, Horiuchi A, Miyake M, Kimura S. Anti-cytokine nature of natural human immunoglobulin: one possible mechanism of the clinical effect of intravenous immunoglobulin therapy. Immunol Rev 1994;139:5–19.

76. Amemiya K, Dalakas MC. Cytokine mRNA expression in the muscle of patients with inclusion body myositis (IBM) before and after treatment with steroids and intravenous immunoglobulin [Abstract]. Neurology 1997;48:126.

77. Amemiya K, Semino-Mora C, Granger RP, Dalakas MC. Downregulation of TGF-β1 mRNA and protein in the muscles of patients with inflammatory myopathies after treatment with high-dose intravenous immunoglobulin. Clin Immunol 2000;94:99–104.

78. Ankrust P, Muller F, Svenson M, et al. Administration of intravenous immunoglobulin (IVIg) in vivo downregulatory effects on the IL-1 system. Clin Exp Immunol 1999;115:136–43.

79. Le Pottier L, Bendaoud B, Dueymes M, et al. BAFF, a new target for intravenous immunoglobulin in autoimmunity and cancer. J Clin Immunol 2007;27(3):257–65.

80. Letko E, Papaliodis DN, Papaliodis GN, et al. Stevens-Johnson syndrome and toxic epidermal necrolysis: a review of the literature. Ann Allergy Asthma Immunol 2005;94:419–36.

81. Viard I, Wehrli P, Bullanim R, et al. Inhibition of toxic epidermal necrolysis by blockade of CD95 with human intravenous immunoglobulin. Science 1998;282:490–3.

82. Faye O, Rouheau JC. Treatment of epidermal necrolysis with high-dose intravenous immunoglobulins (IVIg). Drugs 2005;65:2085–90.

83. Gurcan HM, Jeph S, Ahmed AR. Intravenous immunoglobulin therapy in autoimmune mucocutaneous blistering diseases—A review of the evidence for its efficacy and safety. Am J Clin Dermotol 2010;11:315–26.

84. Jolles S. High-dose intravenous immunoglobulin (hdIVIg) in the treatment of autoimmune blistering disorders. Clin Exp Immunol 2002;129:385–9.

85. Mydlarski PR, Ho V, Shear NH. Canadian consensus statement on the use of intravenous immunoglobulin therapy in dermatology. J Cutaneous Med Surg 2006;10(5):205–21.

86. Amagai M, Ikeda S, Shimizu H, et al. A randomized double-blind trial of intravenous immunoglobulin for pemphigus. J Am Acad Dermatol 2009;60:595–603.

87. Jolles S, Hughes J, Whittaker S. Dermatological uses of high-dose intravenous immunoglobulin. Arch Dermatol 1998;134:80–6.

88. Li N, Zhao M, Hilario-Vargas J, et al. Complete FcRn dependence for intravenous Ig therapy in autoimmune skin blistering diseases. J Clin Invest 2005;115:3440–50.

89. Mimouni D, Blank M, Payne AS, et al. Efficacy of intravenous immunoglobulin (IVIG) affinity-purified anti-desmoglein anti-idiotypic antibodies in the treatment of an experimental model of pemphigus vulgaris. Clin Exp Immunol 2010;162:543–9.

90. Spahn JD, Leung DYM, Chan MTS, et al. Mechanisms of glucocorticoid reduction in asthmatic subjects treated with intravenous immunoglobulin. J Allergy Clin Immunol 1999;103:421–6.

91. Zhuang Q, Mazer B. Inhibition of IgE production in vitro by intact and fragmented intravenous immunoglobulin. J Allergy Clin Immun 2001;108:229–34.

92. Wasserman RL, Melamed I, Stein M, et al. Tolerability and efficacy of facilitated-subcutaneous infusion of immune globulin (human), 10% and recombinant human hyaluronidase (IGHy) in a subset of study patients with primary immunodeficiency disease (PIDD). J Allergy Clin Immunol 2012;129(2):AB15. (Supplement.)

93. Anthony RM, Kobayashi T, Wermeling F, Ravetch JV. Intravenous gammaglobulin suppresses inflammation through a novel T(H)2 pathway. Nature 2011;475:110–13.

Christine Rivat,
Adrian J.
Thrasher,
H. Bobby Gaspar

Gene therapy

The concept of gene therapy emerged in the late 1960s and early 1970s with the identification of genetic defects responsible for inherited diseases. But it is the discovery of cell transformation mechanism by viruses, and the development of sophisticated genetic engineering techniques and efficient methods of gene delivery to mammalian cells that has made possible the technical implementation of gene therapy.

In 1980, in the light of surprisingly encouraging results showing β-globin expression in mice injected with transiently transduced bone marrow cells, Dr Martin Cline, from UCLA, conducted the first unauthorized gene therapy trial using a similar experimental procedure on two patients suffering from β-thalassemia, a blood disorder characterized by a reduced production of haemoglobin.[1] Unfortunately, no therapeutic effect was observed, and the trial was highly criticized both scientifically and ethically by the scientific community.[2] Nevertheless, the Cline study brought gene therapy and its technical and ethical challenges to public light, marking the start of a new chapter in genetics research and medicine.

In the following years, successful cases of stable phenotypic correction of inherited deficiencies by gene transfer to mammalian cells were reported, presenting gene therapy as a potential alternative therapeutic strategy for single gene disorders, and justifying the start of clinical studies.[3,4] The first approved clinical trial was a non-therapeutic control experiment conducted in 1989 by Dr Steven Rosenberg at the National Institute of Health and aiming to track autologous T lymphocytes marked *ex vivo* with a neomycin resistance reporter gene in five patients with metastatic melanoma. Two months after injection, modified T cells could be detected in both peripheral blood and tumor biopsies, making it the first case of successful retroviral gene transfer in patients.[5]

Eventually, in 1990 at the NIH's Clinical Center in a study led by Dr. W. French Anderson, the first patient to show success following gene therapy was a four-year-old girl suffering from adenosine deaminase (ADA) deficiency.[6] In this trial, peripherally harvested autologous T cells were transduced with a retroviral vector expressing ADA and then reinfused to the patient on a number of occasions. The restoration of ADA enzymatic activity in circulating T cells was still detectable up to 12 years after initiation of the treatment. However, the benefits of gene therapy in that case were not clear, as the correction of the disease after transfer of the modified cells was only temporary, and the patient required ongoing enzyme replacement therapy.

Considerable technical progress has been made since this proof-of-principle case, allowing improvements in the practicality and safety of gene therapy and extending its range of possible clinical applications. As a result, between 1989 and 2010, 1644 clinical trials have been approved worldwide for conditions as varied as cancers (64%), cardiovascular diseases (9%), monogenic disorders (8%), or infectious diseases (8%) (Table 86.1). This chapter focuses mainly on the development of gene therapy for primary immunodeficiencies and other hematological disorders.

Gene therapy

Gene therapy is a novel therapeutic approach, and can be defined as "the treatment of disease by replacing, altering, or supplementing a gene that is absent or abnormal and whose absence or abnormality is responsible for disease". Most frequently, a functional copy of the gene is inserted in the genome to overcome the deleterious effects of the faulty gene. Gene therapy can further be categorized in a number of ways depending on the cellular target, mode of delivery, and the eventual objective. With regard to delivery, two different approaches can be considered: *in vivo* gene therapy, in which vectors carrying the therapeutic gene are injected systemically or targeted to specific tissues to allow modification of target cells; and *ex vivo* gene therapy, which involves the removal of the target cells from the patient and their reintroduction following genetic modification. Ultimately, successful gene therapy requires the safe administration of the gene and its appropriate expression at therapeutic levels in specific tissues. The choice of vector and mode of delivery are therefore crucial, and often driven by the cell type targeted.

Methods for gene delivery

Gene delivery into target cells can be achieved using a number of different vectors but these can be broadly categorized into viral and non-viral vectors, both of which present benefits and risks. Virus-derived vectors, which represent approximately 70% of all clinical trials, are the system of choice, as they allow effective delivery to most tissues.[7] However, the proteins of the viral coat are potentially immunogenic, and the integration characteristics of the vectors themselves can lead to insertional mutagenesis. Plasmid-derived vectors appear to be safer, but are prone to gene silencing and give lower and less sustainable levels of gene expression and therefore decreased efficacy. They can also be recognized as foreign and subjected to immune clearance (Table 86.1).

Viral vectors

Natural viruses behave as cellular parasites, unloading their encapsulated DNA or RNA to a target cell and taking advantage of the existing cellular machinery to propagate their own genes.

Table 86.1 Summary of the conditions addressed and vector systems used in gene therapy clinical trials worldwide

Conditions (%)		Vectors (%)	
Cancer diseases	64.6	Adenovirus	24.3
Cardiovascular diseases	8.5	Retrovirus	20.7
Monogenic diseases	8.3	Naked DNA	18.7
Infectious diseases	8.1	Vaccinia virus	8.1
Neurological diseases	2	Liposomes	6.4
Ocular diseases	1.3	Pox virus	5.5
Inflammatory diseases	0.8	Adeno-associated virus	4.7
Other diseases	1.1	Herpes simplex virus	3.3
Gene marking	2.9	Lentivirus	2.3
Healthy volunteers	2.3	Other	6.0

Data from Gene Therapy Clinical Trials Worldwide, provided by the Journal of Gene Medicine, Wiley

But if the virus genomes are manipulated to replace pathogenic sequences with genes of interest, they can be used very efficiently *in vitro* and *in vivo* as DNA carriers. In the past two decades, various types of recombinant viral vectors, such as adenoviruses, adeno-associated viruses, herpes-simplex viruses, and retroviruses have been engineered to transfer genetic material (Table 86.2).

Adenoviruses, adeno-associated viruses, and herpes simplex virus-1

Adenoviruses are a class of viruses with double-stranded DNA genomes that do not integrate into the host DNA but replicate as episomes in the nucleus of the target cell. Adenoviral vectors are able to transduce both dividing and non-dividing cells with significant efficiency and have high tropism for specific tissues including the lung. The main limitation in using adenoviruses for gene therapy is their capability to induce a potent host immune response, leading to an inflammatory response and the clearance of the administered vectors. Adeno-associated viruses (AAV) are non-pathogenic single-stranded DNA viruses that can infect dividing and non-dividing cells and have the ability to integrate at high frequency into the human genome at chromosome 19. Recombinant AAV vectors used for gene therapy

have lost their capacity to integrate site-specifically in the genome, and form episomal concatamers lost through cell division. Residual integration is random throughout the genome. With their ability to infect quiescent cells and low immunogenicity, and despite their limited packaging capacity, AAVs have been used successfully in trials targeting non-dividing cells in tissues such as brain, retina, muscle, or liver.[8-11] Herpes simplex virus-1 (HSV-1) is a neurotropic DNA virus, therefore used mainly as a vector for gene therapy targeting the nervous system, but has also been used for immunotherapy.

Retroviruses and lentiviruses

Retroviruses are a class of RNA viruses that can produce double-stranded DNA copies of their genome that then integrate into the chromosome of the host cell. In recombinant retroviral vectors designed for gene therapy, the genome required for replication and packaging of the virus is replaced with an expression cassette containing the gene of interest under the control of a chosen promoter, rendering the virus replication deficient. The viral genes are expressed separately on plasmids in the packaging cells. Vectors derived from murine gammaretroviruses, such as the Moloney murine leukemia virus (MoMLV), were the first to be developed and used successfully in clinical trials.

Table 86.2 Comparison of the properties of gene therapy viral vectors

	Adenovirus	AAV	Retro/lentivirus
Genome	dsDNA	ssDNA	ssRNA
Coat	Naked	Naked	Enveloped
Integration profile	Non-integrating	Non-integrating	Integrating
Packaging capacity	7.5 kb	4.5 kb	8 kb
Expression	Transient	Transient	Stable
Immunogenicity	Moderate	Low	Low

Data from www.genetherapynet.com

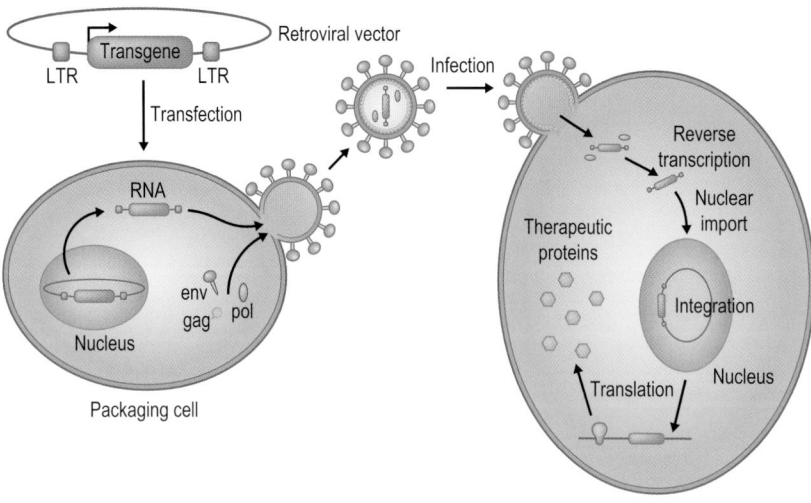

Fig. 86.1 Mechanism of retroviral gene delivery. Retroviral particles are generated in packaging cells, where viral proteins assemble to package the viral RNA and reverse transcriptase. After infection of a target cell, the reverse-transcribed DNA molecule inserts into the host genome, leading to the synthesis by the target cell machinery of therapeutic proteins encoded by the viral genome.

However, lately, interest has moved to lentiviral vectors, such as those derived from the human immunodeficiency virus (HIV)-1. Unlike gammaretroviruses, which require cell division for their reverse-transcribed DNA to access the nucleus, lentiviruses use an active transport system that allows them to transduce even quiescent cells (Fig. 86.1).

Current progress in gene therapy: clinical applications

The first obvious application for gene therapy was the treatment of patients with severe recessive monogenic diseases, as it is possible to cure the disease by transferring only one copy of the gene per cell, especially if the corrected cells have a survival advantage over the deficient patient cells. Inherited recessive single gene disorders only represent 30% of all genetic diseases, affecting less than 2% of the population. Among these, primary immunodeficiencies have become a model of choice for gene therapy for a number of reasons. These include restriction of the therapeutic gene to haematopoietic cells, the known ability of allogeneic bone marrow transplantation to correct the immunological phenotype, and the extensive experience with haematopoietic stem cell harvest and manipulation *ex vivo* (Table 86.3).

Gene therapy for primary immunodeficiencies

Primary immunodeficiencies (PIDs) arise from a mutation in a gene affecting the differentiation or function of specific blood cell populations. They vary in severity and range from those with minor antibody deficiencies to severe combined immunodeficiency where there is a profound defect in cellular and humoral immunity. Because all hematopoietic cells derive from one common pluripotent stem cell in the bone marrow, severe forms of PID can be corrected by the transfer of normal or corrected stem cells into the patient (Fig. 86.2). A few remarkable cases of spontaneous genetic reversions have been reported, where a new mutation in a stem cell or single lymphoid progenitor compensates for the mutated alleles and leads to partial reconstitution of the immune system, demonstrating that

wild-type or corrected progenitor cells can have a strong selective advantage.[12,13] Conventional treatment for severe forms of PID is allogeneic hematopoietic stem cell transplant (HSCT) and currently HSCT is the preferred option when a fully matched donor is available, despite the risks of graft-versus-host disease and the possible complications due to the conditioning regimen. Where a fully matched donor is unavailable, gene therapy now offers a valid therapeutic option.

KEY CONCEPTS

Gene therapy for PIDs as an alternative to BMT in the absence of a matched HLA donor

- SCID-X1: First successful gene therapy trial achieving sustained restoration of cellular and humoral immune functions by transfer of gene corrected autologous HSCs.
- ADA-SCID: Effective immune reconstitution and metabolic detoxification following gene therapy with mild conditioning and in the absence of PEG-ADA.
- CGD: Transient functional correction of neutrophil microbial killing activity and clinical improvement in patients.
- WAS: Restored T/B/NK and monocyte functions and improved clinical condition in patients receiving modified autologous HSCs after non-myeloablative conditioning.

X-linked SCID (SCID-X1)

The most common form of severe combined immunodeficiency (SCID) is the X-linked form SCID-X1 (40-50% of all cases) (Chapter 35). SCID-X1 results from mutations in the *IL2RG* gene situated on the X chromosome, and defective expression of its protein product, the common gamma chain (γc), a subunit shared by multiple cytokine receptors, including the IL-2, IL-4, IL-7, IL-9, IL-15, and IL-21 receptor complexes, which are involved in the development and function of lymphocytes. As a consequence, patients show profound cellular and humoral defects, resulting from the low number or absence of T and natural killer (NK) lymphocytes, and the loss of function of B lymphocytes (T⁻B⁺NK⁻ SCID).[14]

Preclinical studies with a conventional γ-retroviral vector, in which the *IL2RG* gene is under the transcriptional control of the viral LTR (long terminal repeat sequence — the γ-retroviral

Table 86.3 Selected gene therapy trials worldwide

	Centres	Vector	Conditioning	Patients	Outcome	References
SCID-X1	France	γ-retrovirus	None	10	Most patients have significant clinical benefit; 4/10 patients developed T-ALL and one patient died of T-ALL	(16,20)
	UK	γ-retrovirus	None	10	Most patients have significant clinical benefit; one patient developed T-ALL	(17,21)
	US	γ-retrovirus	None	3	Clinical benefit	(22)
	France, UK, US	SIN γ-retrovirus; mammalian promoter	None	4	Trial initiated in 2010	
ADA-SCID	Italy	γ-retrovirus	Busulfan 4 mg/kg	17	Clinical benefit; 14/17 patients off ERT	(28)
	UK	γ-retrovirus	Melphalan 140 mg/m²	8	Clinical benefit; 4/8 patients off ERT	(29)
	US	γ-retrovirus	Busulfan 4 mg/kg	11	Clinical benefit; 7/11 patients off ERT	Candotti F and Kohn DB (personal communication)
CGD	US	γ-retrovirus	None	5	No clinical benefit	(31)
	Germany, Switzerland	γ-retrovirus	Busulfan 4 mg/kg/day (×2)	3	Transient clinical benefit; all patients developed myelodysplasia; one patient died of sepsis	(32,33), Seger R (personal communication)
	UK	γ-retrovirus	Melphalan 140 mg/m²	4	Transient clinical benefit	Thrasher, A (personal communication)
	US	γ-retrovirus	Busulfan 5 mg/kg/day (×2)	3	Transient clinical benefit	(34)
	Korea	γ-retrovirus	Busulfan 3.2 mg/kg/day (×2) + fludarabine 40 mg/m² (×3)	2	Transient clinical benefit	(35)
WAS	Germany	γ-retrovirus	Busulfan 4 mg/kg/day (×2)	10	Significant clinical benefit; one patient developed T-cell leukemia	(36)
	Italy, France, UK, US	SIN-Lentivirus, *WAS* gene promoter	Busulfan 4 mg/kg/day (×2) + fludarabine 40 mg/m² (×3)	5	Trials initiated 2010	
β-thalassemia	France	SIN-lentivirus, β-globin promoter	Busulfan 3.2 mg/kg/day (×4)	1	Significant clinical benefit but evidence of clonal dominance	(44)
X-ALD	France	SIN-lentivirus, modified MND promoter	Fully myeloablative; busulfan + cyclophosphamide	2	Significant clinical benefit	(45)

gene regulatory region), showed restoration of lymphoid function in SCID-X1 patient cells and in relevant murine models.[15] Using a similar experimental framework, two clinical trials with a total of 20 subjects were conducted at Hopital Necker in Paris and at the UCL Institute of Child Health in London.[16–19] In both studies, hematopoietic stem cells were transduced *ex vivo* with a clinical grade MFG-γc vector and reinfused to the patients without preconditioning, with the expectation that the high survival advantage of transduced cells and the T lymphopenic status of the patient would allow the expansion of gene-corrected cells. Overall, the outcome of these trials was very positive, with a rapid and sustained increase in T-cell numbers, and to a lesser extent in NK cells. T cells showed normal proliferation to mitogenic stimulation and phenotypic analysis demonstrated naïve T-cell markers,

suggesting engraftment of gene corrected pre-thymic precursors. B-cell reconstitution was variable with 50% of patients continuing immunoglobulin replacement therapy. Gene marking was 100% in T cells and low (<1%) in other cell lineages, reflecting very low levels of engraftment of transduced hematopoietic stem cells as would be expected from an unconditioned procedure.

Regrettably, two to five years after the treatment, five patients who were clinically well developed a T-cell acute lymphoblastic leukemia resulting from mutagenic retroviral insertions. They were all treated with standard chemotherapy, but one patient died of refractory leukaemia. The other four are now in remission with sustained restored immunity.

One disadvantageous feature of murine leukemia virus γ-retroviruses is their tendency to integrate into sites of active

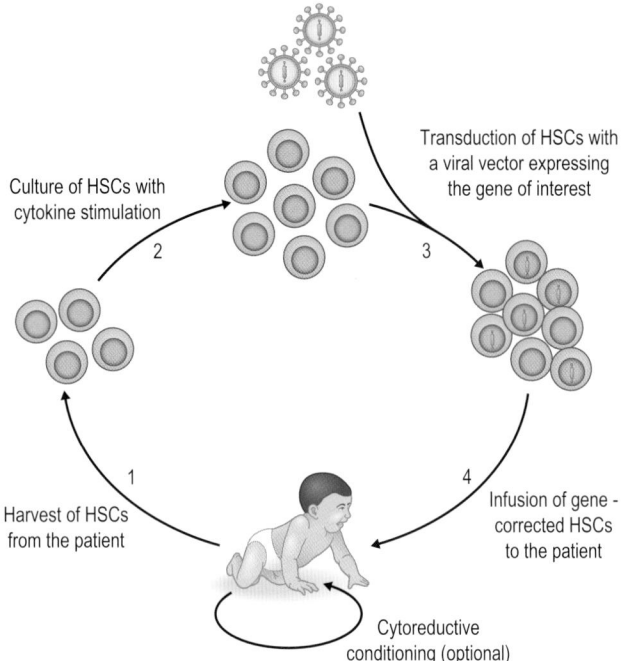

Fig. 86.2 Treatment of primary immunodeficiencies by *ex vivo* gene therapy. Autologous hematopoietic stem cells (HSCs) are reinfused into the patient after being genetically modified to express a functional protein.

chromatin, resulting in a higher probability of insertion near the transcription start sites (TSS) of genes that are highly expressed in early hematopoietic precursors (Fig. 86.3A). Leukemia is the direct consequence of the clonal expansion of a transformed T-cell

population. The mapping of the viral insertion sites in the Paris and London studies revealed insertion of the vector near the TSS of the proto-oncogene LIM domain only-2 (LMO-2) in four cases, as well as insertion in the vicinity of the cell cycle regulators BMI1 and CCND2, all of which have leukemogenic properties. Insertion into these sites led to aberrant and non-physiological transcription of the proto-oncogenes through transactivation from the enhancer elements of the viral LTR (Fig. 86.3B). Accumulation of other genetic and chromosomal abnormalities were also detected in the blast populations of these patients, including gain of function *NOTCH1* mutations and deletion of the tumor suppressor gene *CDKN2A* (cyclin dependent kinase 2A).[20,21]

A third trial was conducted at NIH, involving preadolescent subjects aged 10 to 14 years, who had previously been treated unsuccessfully by bone marrow transplant. The protocol was similar to that used in the Paris and London trials, but despite good marking of all hematological lineages, the immune reconstitution was limited, with a slight improvement of T-cell function in the youngest child only. This reduced efficacy of gene therapy in older children may be related to age-related decreased plasticity and loss of thymopoietic capacity.[22]

Adenosine deaminase (ADA)-SCID

Adenosine deaminase deficiency (ADA-SCID) represents approximately 20% of SCID cases, and was the first form of SCID to be characterized at a molecular level (Chapter 35). It is caused by mutations in the gene encoding ADA, an enzyme involved in purine metabolism. In the absence of ADA, the accumulation of toxic metabolites (especially deoxy-ATP and deoxyadenosine) in

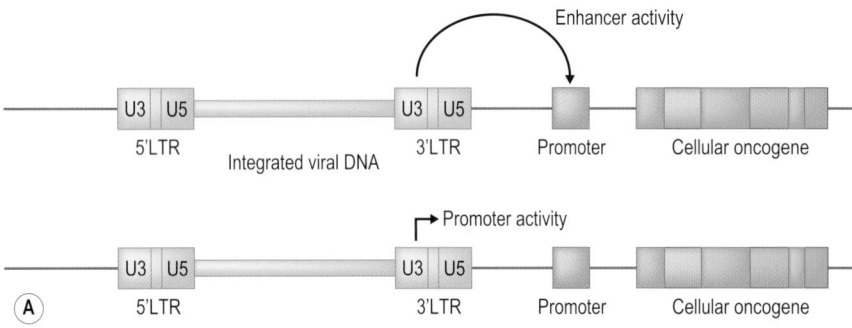

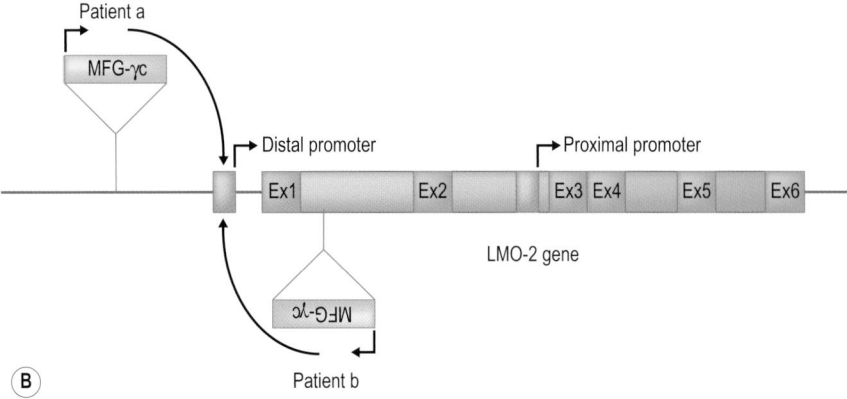

Fig. 86.3 Insertional mutagenesis: mechanism of LTR-mediated gene activation. (A) Viral LTRs can transactivate nearby genes by generating transcripts that read through the adjacent gene or by acting as enhancers for endogenous promoters. (B) Example of insertional transactivation of the *LMO-2* oncogene in the first SCID-X1 clinical trial.

the thymus has deleterious effects on lymphocyte development and function. ADA-deficient patients have a characteristic immunological profile with T⁻B⁻NK⁻ SCID. The clinical manifestations of ADA-SCID are similar to SCID-X1 with recurrent infections and failure to thrive, but because ADA is ubiquitously expressed, ADA-deficient patients also show skeletal, lung, liver, gastrointestinal tract, and neural abnormalities.

Unlike other forms of SCID, there are a number of therapeutic options available for the management of ADA-SCID. Direct intramuscular injections of pegylated bovine ADA (PEG-ADA) allow metabolic detoxification and subsequent lymphocyte development with partial restoration of T-cell function. PEG-ADA is generally well tolerated, and the survival rate is high. In most cases, there is a decline in lymphocyte counts and thymic output,[23] which raises concern on the level of long-term reconstitution and potential for infective problems.[24,25] A further important limitation of enzyme replacement therapy is its cost as weekly or twice-weekly injections are required to maintain sufficient levels of enzyme in the bloodstream. Therefore, if a fully matched donor is available, allogeneic hematopoietic stem cell transplant is the treatment of choice. The survival following matched family donor transplants, which can be performed without chemotherapy conditioning, is high, and transplanted patients develop mixed T-cell chimerism where the metabolic detoxification exerted by donor cells is sufficient to compensate the lack of ADA in endogenous T cells and leads to sustained immune recovery.

In the absence of a suitable donor, and if enzyme replacement therapy is unsuccessful or inaccessible, gene therapy is an option to treat patients. Following the first inconclusive trials targeting peripheral blood T cells in the 1990s, Bordignon and colleagues at the San Raffaele Hospital in Milan used retroviral gene transfer to transduce both bone marrow stem cells and peripheral blood lymphocytes *in vitro*, followed by reinfusion into patients without conditioning. No adverse reaction to the procedure occurred, but only low levels of marked cells were detectable in peripheral blood, and there was no evidence of clinical benefit to the patients.[26]

In a new generation of gene therapy trials, the protocol was modified to improve the culture conditions and transduction efficiency of the stem cells. In addition, a mild conditioning regime was used to facilitate engraftment in the bone marrow, and the enzyme replacement therapy was halted in order to restore the selective advantage of the corrected cells.[27]

Several trials using variations of this improved protocol have now treated over 30 patients in Italy, the United Kingdom, and the United States. Data from 10 patients treated in Milan reported that in the majority of patients a long-term engraftment with high levels of gene marking was achieved, especially in lymphoid lineages, with evidence of restored thymic activity and efficient systemic detoxification.[28]

These positive results were confirmed in a study at the Institute of Child Health, UK, and in a joint NIH-UCLA study in the USA.[19,29,30] After treatment, the majority of patients (70%) showed sufficient levels of immune reconstitution and metabolic detoxification to justify continued cessation of enzyme replacement therapy. However, failure of gene therapy was observed in 30% of patients and was predominantly related to poor stem cell harvest and the return of low numbers of gene corrected cells. In addition, in a preliminary NIH study, two patients treated in the absence of chemotherapy showed lower numbers of marked cells and reduced immune recovery, outlining the importance of a myelosuppressive conditioning regime before gene therapy.

No serious events of insertional leukemogenesis have been encountered so far following gene therapy for ADA-SCID. In five patients treated with gene therapy, integration sites were analyzed in stem cells before infusion and in bone marrow and peripheral cells up to four years after treatment. Integration hotspots were identified in transcriptionally active regions, including sites near the proto-oncogenes *LMO2*, *BCL2*, and *CCND2*, but to date there has been no evidence of clonal dominance.[31]

Chronic granulomatous disease (CGD)

CGD is a rare inherited immunodeficiency associated with mutations in genes encoding the NADPH oxidase enzymatic complex that catalyses the respiratory burst during phagocytosis. The majority of patients have an X-linked form of the disease due to mutations in GP91^{phox}, a membrane-bound component of the NADPH oxidase complex. NADPH oxidase deficiency results in a defect in the microbial killing activity of phagocytic neutrophils, leading to recurrent bacterial and fungal infections.[32] As in most severe primary immunodeficiencies, allogeneic hematopoietic stem cell transplant is curative, and is the first option if a fully HLA-matched donor is available. The initial attempt to develop gene therapy for CGD took place in the United States in the late 1990s.[33] This first trial using a standard protocol without bone marrow conditioning demonstrated the technical feasibility of gene therapy for CGD. However, the very low levels of corrected granulocytes (<0.1%) in the peripheral blood were insufficient to promote any long-term therapeutic effect.

CGD corrected stem cells are not predicted to have any selective advantage. Therefore, the clinical trial protocol initiated in 2004 in Germany included a low-dose myelosuppressive conditioning regime in order to enable the engraftment of larger numbers of stem cells.[34] In two adult patients treated, high levels of gene marking (about 20%) associated with restored superoxide production and phagocytic activity were achieved, and correlated with the clearance of pre-existing infections. But in the following months, the number of gene-corrected granulocytes in peripheral blood rose unexpectedly, as a result of insertional transactivation of *MDS1/EVI1*, *PRDM16*, and *SETBP1*, three genes involved in myeloid proliferation. One of the two patients died later of sepsis and multi-organ failure, while the other underwent successful stem cell transplant. In both cases, gp91^{phox} expression became almost undetectable, due to gene silencing through CpG methylation of the viral LTRs.[35] Similar outcomes were seen in two patients treated in Switzerland.

More patients were treated similarly in the UK, the USA, and Korea. In the majority of cases, the levels of gene-marked cells remained low and there was no evidence of clonal expansion. Despite the fact that disease correction is largely transient, the majority of patients have received some degree of clinical benefit.[36-38] Novel lentiviral vectors have recently been developed for treatment of X-CGD, which may enhance both efficacy and safety.

Wiskott–Aldrich syndrome (WAS)

Wiskott–Aldrich syndrome is an X-linked immunodeficiency characterized by microthrombocytopenia, eczema, and an increased risk of development of autoimmune disorders and hematological malignancies with age. The WAS gene product, WASP, is a cytoskeletal protein expressed in hematopoietic lineages and involved in platelet production and immune cell function. Allogeneic hematopoietic stem cell transplant can be used to treat WAS and the outcome is favorable, especially if there is a matched donor. Gene therapy is an attractive alternative therapeutic approach for this monogenic disease, and trials using retroviral and lentiviral vectors are ongoing in Europe and in the USA.

In 2010, preliminary results from a study conducted over three years on two young patients in Germany were published.[39] Sustained WASP expression was detected in all hematopoietic lineages, associated with an increase in platelet counts and correction of leukocyte functions, including NK-cell-mediated cytotoxicity, monocyte migration, immunoglobulin production, and T lymphocyte proliferation. Clinically, patients are less susceptible to infections, with resolution of eczema and autoimmune disorders. One patient has developed a T-cell leukemia, which is again associated with an insertion in the vicinity of the *LMO2* oncogene, as revealed by the mapping of viral integration sites.

Other candidate PIDs

A number of other inherited immunodeficiencies may be attractive candidates for gene therapy, in particular other forms of SCID, such as Rag 1 and Rag 2 (recombination activating proteins), Artemis, or Jak3 deficiencies. Rag1/2 and Artemis proteins participate in the V(D)J recombination, which is essential for the generation of functional B- and T-cell receptors and normal T- and B-cell development (Chapters 4, 35). Jak3 is a tyrosine kinase required for signal transduction by the γc receptor, and therefore Jak3 deficiency leads to a phenotype that is identical to SCID-X1, with an absence of circulating T and NK cells, and a loss of function of B lymphocytes. In all cases, the transfer of genetically modified hematopoietic stem cells (HSCs) can effectively reconstitute murine models of the disease.[40–43] However, further safety studies are still required before clinical translation of the vectors, especially for Jak3, which has oncogenic properties and has been linked to cancer development when overexpressed.

Leukocyte adhesion deficiency (LAD), which is caused by mutations in the CD18 integrin subunit, is a neutrophil disorder characterized by recurrent life-threatening bacterial infections. Interestingly, experience from allogeneic transplants indicates that very low numbers of normal donor neutrophils are sufficient to achieve disease control. Recently, the canine model of the disease was successfully treated using HSCs transduced with a lentiviral vector expressing CD18, which represents an important step towards the development of gene therapy for LAD patients.[44]

Other inherited conditions that could benefit from the development of gene therapy strategies include X-linked agammaglobulinemia (XLA), where a defect in the Bruton tyrosine kinase (Btk) leads to the absence of mature B cells, X-linked lymphoproliferative disease (XLP), a T and NK lymphoproliferative disorder due to mutations in the signalling adaptor SLAM-associated protein (SAP), and familial hemophagocytic lymphohistiocytosis (FHLH), a hemophagocytic disease resulting from defective NK and CD8 T-cell functions.[45] Btk and SAP are involved in multiple signalling pathways affecting proliferation, apoptosis, and differentiation, while perforin, which is the most commonly mutated protein in FHLH, is a direct effector in cytotoxic functions. Lineage-restricted expression of these genes might therefore be required to avoid deleterious effects in non-target cells. Under these conditions and those mentioned above, preclinical efficacy and safety studies using improved viral vectors are currently being undertaken, in order to determine clinical applicability and to broaden the spectrum of primary immunodeficiencies that can be successfully treated with gene transfer therapy.

Beta-thalassemia

Inherited β-globinopathies, including β-thalassemia and sickle cell anemia, are the most common monogenic disorders worldwide. β-thalassemia is caused by mutations in the β-globin gene cluster, resulting in a defective synthesis of the globin chains that form hemoglobin. Thalassemia major or Cooley disease, the most severe form of β-thalassemia, is characterized by greatly reduced or absent hemoglobin production and subsequent accumulation of iron in tissues. The ineffective erythropoiesis causes severe anemia, typically associated with erythroid hyperplasia and extramedullary hematopoiesis. Patients require chronic blood transfusions for life to survive. The only curative option is hematopoietic stem cell transplant, which has a very good outcome (90% survival) if a matched donor is available and if the patient is transfused and chelated without any iron-related organ damage.

Gene therapy for β-thalassemia is a promising alternative for patients without a matched donor, but it is particularly challenging as extremely high levels of gene expression in the erythroid lineage must be achieved for disease correction, unlike the previously described primary immunodeficiencies, where a small number of modified HSCs are able to produce sufficient numbers of long-lived lymphocytes, and limited amounts of transgene expression are sufficient to restore the cell phenotype because of the survival advantage conferred on gene corrected cells.

Extensive *in vitro* and *in vivo* studies have been performed to identify within the β-globin gene sequence the regulatory elements required to obtain high levels and specific patterns of expression. They have led to the development of a complex lentiviral vector in which the β-globin gene is placed in reverse orientation to avoid splicing of the introns during virus production and under the control of its own promoter coupled to hypersensitive sites HS-2, -3, and -4 of the locus control region. The β-globin gene is deleted of deleterious sequences in the second intron to allow stable expression, and bears a mutation at the 87th codon that confers it with anti-sickling properties. In addition, two copies of a fragment of the chicken hypersensitive site-4 insulator (cHS4) have been inserted in the vector LTRs to reduce gene silencing and position effect (Fig. 86.4).

This vector was used in a first clinical trial in France in 2007. The initial report published 3 years after the initiation of the gene therapy presented encouraging results in one patient, with good gene marking (11%), and sustained levels of hemoglobin and red blood cell production, allowing the patient to become transfusion independent by the end of the first year after transplant.[46]

However, this beneficial therapeutic effect seems to be the consequence of the proliferative advantage of a dominant erythroid clone with random integration of the vector in the *HMGA2* gene

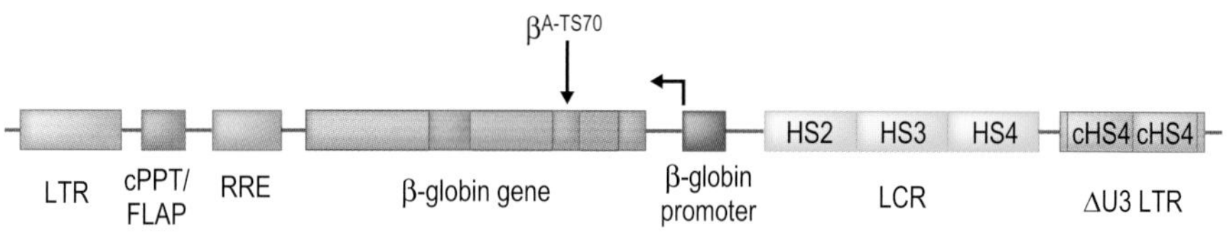

Fig. 86.4 Example of the β-thalassemia gene therapy lentiviral vector. The self-inactivating (SIN) lentiviral backbone contains a central polypurine tract/DNA flap (cPPT/flap) and a *rev*-responsive element (RRE) to enhance gene expression. The modified β-globin gene is placed under the control of its own promoter and locus control region, and position effect is reduced by the use of DNA insulators in the 3'LTR.

locus, a transcriptional co-factor with possible oncogenic activity. Interestingly, expression of a truncated form of HMGA2 was only detected in the erythroid lineage, possibly as a consequence of the transcriptional control exerted by the β-globin locus control region (LCR). The truncated form arises because the vector insertion site results in deletion of the C-terminal region of the HMGA2 protein, thereby removing miRNA target sequences that may be an additional explanation for the upregulation in gene activity. So far, this event of clonal dominance has been beneficial to the patient, allowing the rapid expansion of corrected erythroid progenitors, but it raises legitimate safety concerns regarding the use of this lentiviral vector in gene therapy.

Leukodystrophies

Leukodystrophies are a group of inherited diseases in which molecular defects of the glial cells result in the impaired development and maintenance of the myelin sheath that surrounds and insulates nerve cells within the brain, spinal cord, and peripheral nerves, causing progressive degeneration of the white matter of the brain and neurological disorders. Demyelinating leukodystrophies, which are characterized by myelin destruction, are the major group of leukodystrophies and include X-linked adrenoleukodystrophy (X-ALD), metachromatic leukodystrophy (MLD), and globoid cell leukodystrophy (GLD) or Krabbe disease.

Glial cells are non-neuronal cell populations that are crucial to maintain neuronal homeostasis and function. Among them, microglia are phagocytic macrophage-like cells derived from hematopoietic precursors that protect the central nervous system by destroying damaged neurons and infectious agents. Myelination of axons is provided by oligodendrocytes, which can also directly promote axon survival. Therefore, the irreversible loss of neuronal cells that occurs in leukodystrophies is a consequence of both demyelination and impaired oligodendrocyte function.

X-linked adrenoleukodystrophy (X-ALD)

X-ALD is a monogenic disease associated with mutations in the *ABCD1* gene, encoding a peroxisomal membrane transporter (ALDP). The loss of function of ALDP results in the accumulation of very long chain fatty acids (VLCFA) in tissues and body fluids, including oligodendrocytes and microglia, and can cause irreversible damage to the brain, adrenal gland, and peripheral nervous system. X-ALD in children is mainly characterized by the development of inflammatory cerebral demyelinating lesions, which translate into major neurological defects, such as tetraparesis, impaired vision, and speech disorders.

Hematopoietic stem cell transplantation (HSCT) can stop the progression of X-ALD if patients are treated at an early stage of the disease, when cerebral lesions and neurological defects are still limited. It is not understood how HSCT can be curative

for X-ALD, given that ALDP is not secreted, which prevents metabolic cross-correction of the oligodendrocytes. One possibility is that HSCT corrects intrinsic defects in the microglia, related or not to the accumulation of VLCFA into the brain, and that these defects are at least partially responsible for the development of X-ALD.

Despite some clinical success, the mortality risk associated with HSCT remains high, especially in the absence of a fully matched donor. Therefore, as an alternative to HSCT, gene transfer strategies using a lentiviral vector have been developed for X-ALD.

Two young male patients without any matched donor for HSCT were selected for a clinical trial started in France in 2006.[47] Because corrected stem cells are not expected to have any selective advantage, patients were submitted to a fully myeloablative conditioning regime to increase engraftment. Four years after the initiation of gene therapy, patients show long-term engraftment associated with good gene marking and sustained ALDP activity, illustrated by decreased plasma levels of VLCFA. The clinical benefits of the therapy are obvious in both patients, with a stabilization of cerebral demyelination and a positive neurologic outcome, similar to what is observed in successful HSCT with full chimerism, despite a low level of stem cell correction. The analysis of lentiviral integration sites revealed a varied clonal distribution with no emergence of a dominant clone, and no genotoxic effect has been observed so far.

Metachromatic leukodystrophy (MLD) and globoid cell leukodystrophy (GLD)

MLD is a rare inherited lysosomal storage disorder caused by a deficiency in the lysosomal enzyme arylsulfatase A (ARSA) involved in sulfatide metabolism. The absence of ARSA activity results in the accumulation of non-metabolized sulfolipids in neuronal and glial cells, leading to extensive demyelination and neurodegeneration in the central and peripheral nervous systems. The severity of the motor and cognitive deficits characteristic of MLD vary depending on the age of onset, but the prognosis is usually poor in the infantile and juvenile forms of the disease.

GLD, also known as Krabbe disease, is another demyelinating leukodystrophy caused by a deficiency in a lysosomal enzyme. In this case, the absence of functional galactocerebrosidase (GALC) impairs the catabolism of two substrates of GALC, galactoceramide (GalCer), which accumulates in macrophages to form characteristic globoid cells, and psychosin, which is toxic to oligodendrocytes and leads to demyelination. Like MLD, clinical manifestations for GLD vary and include peripheral neuropathy and alteration of mental functions. Early-onset forms of the disease are fatal in the first years of life.

Enzyme replacement has been considered for MLD and GLD, but the main limitation of this therapy is the blood–brain barrier, which restricts the access of therapeutic molecules to the brain. Hematopoietic stem cell transfer allows the direct correction of the lysosomal defect in macrophages and glial cells, and the cross-correction of oligodendrocytes thanks to the capacity of the engrafted microglia precursors in the bone marrow to migrate and settle into the brain, and secrete functional lysosomal enzyme. However, HSCT is only curative if performed in the neonatal period as the first symptoms are detected, probably because the disease progresses faster than the reconstitution of the enzymatic activity in the brain. Recent preclinical data suggesting that lentiviral gene therapy could generate supranormal levels of enzymatic activity and therefore have a better therapeutic efficacy than HSCT have led to the opening of a phase I/II gene therapy clinical trial for MLD.[48]

KEY CONCEPTS

Other successful gene therapy trials

- β-thalassemia: Restored hemoglobin and red blood cell production associated with significant clinical benefit; no genotoxic effect despite reports of erythroid clonal expansion.
- X-ALD: Stabilization of disease progression and positive neurologic outcome following lentiviral gene therapy with fully myeloablative conditioning.

Future prospects for gene therapy

Since its first steps in the 1990s, the emerging field of gene therapy has generated immense interest and hopes in the scientific community. A number of preclinical studies have demonstrated its feasibility, providing proof of principle for various therapeutic applications, and for the first time, several human gene therapy trials have been successful. However, the potential benefits of gene therapy must be weighed against the risks of genotoxicity. Events such as the death of an 18-year-old boy, who suffered multiple-organ failure after a strong immune response to the injection of an adenoviral vector, followed by the development of vector-related mutagenic events in several patients have tempered initial enthusiasm and considerably slowed down clinical progress. But despite these major setbacks, considerable amount of work has been undertaken to increase the efficiency and biosafety of therapeutic gene transfer.

Improvement of vector performances and safety profile

Viral vectors based on γ-retroviruses such as MLV were among the first to be developed and used successfully in clinical trials. However, lentiviral vectors based on the human immunodeficiency virus type 1 (HIV-1), with their capacity to transduce non-dividing cells, combined with deletion of LTR sequences and use of internal promoters with weak enhancer elements have an improved safety profile, and are promising substitutes.

In an effort to improve the performances of lentiviral vectors, new generation packaging systems have been developed. The non-essential replication and accessory viral genes were removed, leaving only the packaging plasmid, the *gag* and *pol* genes encoding the structural proteins and enzyme that surround the viral RNA, and the viral regulatory genes *tat* and *rev* (Fig. 86.5A). The *env* gene encoding the viral envelope, which is usually derived from a heterologous virus, is provided on a separate plasmid. In the third-generation packaging system, which offers

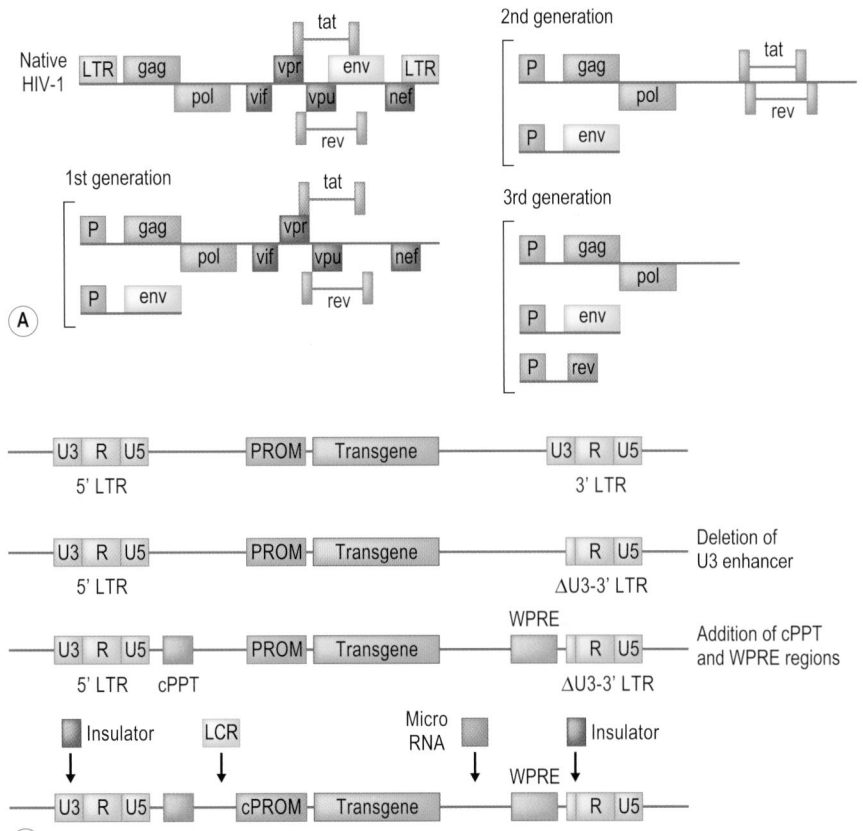

Fig. 86.5 Development of safer lentiviral expression systems. (A) Three generations of packaging systems have been derived from the native HIV-1 virus. Non-essential viral accessory genes were removed from the packaging plasmids and the viral genome was split. In the *tat*-independent third-generation system, the post-transcriptional regulator *rev* is provided on a separate plasmid. (B) The lentiviral backbone was progressively modified with the partial deletion of the 3'LTR to inactivate transcription from the LTR and the addition of cPPT and WPRE sequences to enhance transgene expression. Additional possible modifications of the lentiviral backbone include the use of a specific cellular promoter and the addition of a locus control region (LCR) or microRNA tag for a tighter regulation of gene expression, and the addition of insulator sequences to limit the risk of positional effect and insertional transactivation.

maximal biosafety, the genome was split, with the *rev* gene, encoding a post-transcriptional regulator essential for efficient gag and pol expression, being expressed from an additional fourth plasmid (Fig. 86.5A).

The enhancer/promoter unit in the U3 region of the 3'LTR was deleted to create a self-inactivating (SIN) vector, in which the LTR is transcriptionally inactive. This prevents insertional mutagenesis due to enhancer interaction and transcription from the 3'LTR, and minimizes the risk of reconstituting a replication-competent virus by producing transcripts containing the packaging psi signal. The central polypurine tract (cPPT) sequence, which is normally found in the HIV-1 genome, was added to facilitate nuclear import, together with the woodchuck hepatitis B post-transcriptional regulatory element (WPRE), which enhances gene expression by regulating post-transcriptional modifications, such as polyadenylation, RNA export, or translation (Fig. 86.5B).

More recently, to circumvent the possible mutagenesis and cell transformation due to random vector integration in the host genome, non-integrating lentiviral vectors were engineered by introducing selected mutations within the integrase coding region of the packaging plasmid. However, even though these integrase-deficient vectors retain their capacity to transduce non-dividing cells, viral DNA remains in the nucleus of the infected cell as an episome and is lost through cell divisions.

Regulation of transgene expression

In the first-generation lentiviral vectors, the transgene was often expressed under the control of viral regulatory sequences, typically derived from human cytomegalovirus (hCMV), spleen focus forming virus (SFFV), murine stem cell virus (MSCV), or myeloproliferative sarcoma virus (MPSV). Although these allow high levels of gene expression *in vitro*, they are no longer considered suitable for clinical applications, after recent reports comparing them with cellular promoters such as the phosphoglycerate kinase (PGK) and human elongation factor 1α (hEF-1α) housekeeping gene promoters showed that they were associated with a greater risk of insertional transformation.[49] In some circumstances, more regulated transgene expression is desirable, for example using tissue- or cell-specific promoters that can be associated or not with transcriptional regulators derived from genes normally expressed in the target tissue. One example of an internal promoter being used for prolonged transgene expression is the minimal *WAS* promoter driving the expression of the *WAS* gene in a new lentiviral vector designed for *WAS* gene therapy.[50] Similarly a synthetic regulatory element that directs gene expression in mature myeloid cells has been developed for treatment of CGD.[51] An increasing number of cell-specific promoters have been characterized lately in various tissues, and they will undoubtedly be used in the future to reduce the genotoxicity of lentiviral vectors in clinical applications.

Alternatively, gene expression from lentiviral vectors could be switched on and off by using inducible promoters, such as the antibiotic-dependent promoters that can be rapidly activated upon delivery of the antibiotic. The most commonly used is the tetracycline-based tet-on system, which allows dose-dependent regulated transgene expression.[52] But despite being used successfully *in vitro*, these complex systems have not yet been tried clinically.

MicroRNAs or miRNAs are short non-coding ribonucleic acids that exist naturally in human cells. There are over 1000 miRNA sequences in the genome, targeting at least 60% of human genes. It was therefore tempting to use the gene-silencing potential of miRNAs, which act as translational repressors when they bind complementary sequences on mRNA transcripts, to

regulate gene expression in the context of therapeutic cell transfer. In the case of GLD gene therapy, one of the difficulties to overcome is the toxic effect of GALC overexpression in HSC and early progenitors, even though their differentiated progeny is unaffected. Downregulation in HSCs and specific expression of GALC in mature hematopoietic cells was achieved recently using HSC-specific microRNA that act as translational repressors for the transgene when incorporated into the lentiviral vector. This successful approach allowed the correction of the disease in a murine model and gave a new rationale to consider gene therapy for GLD.[53]

Reduction of positional effects on gene expression and insertional mutagenesis

Lentiviral vectors integrate semi-randomly in the genome, and therefore transgene expression can be affected by the local genomic environment at the site of integration. To counteract this positional effect, insulator elements can be incorporated into the vector to protect silencing of the transgene, as well as to limit the long-range influence of the vector enhancers on possible neighboring genes. Chromatin insulators are short DNA elements that act as barriers between chromatin transcriptional domains (Fig. 86.6). They are characterized by either enhancer-blocking or barrier activity. Enhancer-blockers stop the communication between enhancers and distant promoters if placed between them, and therefore limit the action of enhancers to one or a few specific target promoters and suppress the undesired transactivation of other genes. Barrier elements prevent the spread of adjacent condensed heterochromatin, reducing the risk of gene silencing. Insulator elements are particularly useful in the context of lentiviral gene therapy, as the vectors integrate preferentially in transcriptionally active regions of the host genome. The cloning of a combination of an enhancer-blocker with a barrier element would probably be an even better option to increase transgene expression while reducing the genotoxic potential of vector integration. However, insulators are long DNA sequences, and their addition to the lentiviral vectors often reduces viral titers and gene expression, which has been the major limitation to their use in clinic so far. The new challenge will be to identify shorter regulatory sequences that can be included into gene therapy vectors without affecting viral production.

Homologous recombination

Although the classical approach to gene therapy is the addition into the genome of a functional copy of the mutated gene, disease correction may also be achieved by direct gene editing. A possible strategy is the use of zinc-finger nucleases (ZFN) to target

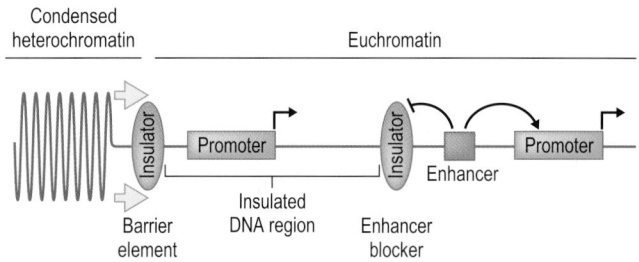

Fig. 86.6 Gene regulation by chromatin insulators. The use of a combination of barrier and enhancer-blocker insulating elements protects the inserted gene from positional effect and prevents the transactivation of neighboring genes by viral enhancers.

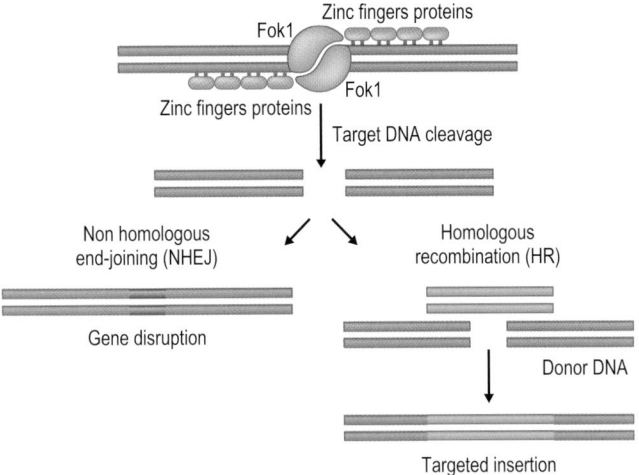

Fig. 86.7 Application of zinc finger nuclease (ZFN) technology to gene therapy. The cleavage of a target gene by specific ZFNs allows the insertion of a corrected sequence at the cleavage site when a homologous donor DNA is provided.

genomic mutations. ZFN are artificial endonucleases engineered by combining the non-specific DNA cleavage domain of the restriction enzyme FokI with zinc finger proteins, which bind specifically target DNA sequences (Fig. 86.7). The cleavage domain works as a dimer, requiring the binding of one ZFN on each strand of the DNA to introduce double-stranded DNA breaks. In the context of gene therapy, ZFNs could be used to excise fragments of DNA containing disease-causing mutations. Then, in the presence of a corrected homologous DNA template, the cellular homologous recombination machinery will repair the double stranded break and thereby replace the mutated gene with a functional copy. Using this strategy, an interesting study recently demonstrated the correction of common gamma chain (γc) mutations in cell lines and primary cells, suggesting that a similar approach could be applicable to SCID-X1 gene therapy.[54] But although manipulating the genome with custom-designed ZFNs to allow the targeted delivery of therapeutic genes is achievable *in vitro*, the requirement for multiple components to be transferred makes the technique complicated to use clinically. In addition, there is a non-negligible possibility of off-target cleavage, and the risk of triggering an immune reaction against the foreign synthetic zinc finger proteins.

● ON THE HORIZON

Improvement of the safety profile and efficacy of retro/lentiviral vectors

- Inactivation of the viral LTRs to avoid insertional mutagenesis by removing the viral enhancer elements capable of oncogene transactivation.

- Replacement of the viral promoters by more suitable cellular promoters to reduce the genotoxicity of vector insertion and provide improved transgene expression.

- Addition of miRNA sequences to the viral backbone to inhibit non-specific expression in off-target tissues.

- Use of chromatin insulator and barrier elements to reduce positional effect and block the transactivation of adjacent genes.

- Engineering of artificial ZFN to specifically target mutated genes and replace them with a functional copy using the cellular homologous recombination machinery.

● ON THE HORIZON

Improvement of safety profile of viral reactors

- Long-term follow-up of gene-transplanted patients to detect late side effects.

- Develop more sophisticated mechanisms of gene delivery:
  - Physiological promoters
  - Detargeting strategies
  - Zinc finger endonucleases for homologous recombination of gene constructs.

Translational science

Over the past decade, the promise created by technological advances in gene transfer has been translated into successful clinical trials for a number of monogenic hematopoietic disorders. At the forefront of these clinical trials have been severe primary immunodeficiencies (SCID-X1, ADA-SCID, X-CGD, and WAS) followed by other conditions such as X-ALD and β-thalassaemia. These trials have shown impressive efficacy and the overall safety profile has been impressive, especially when compared to alternatives such as mismatched HSCT. Nevertheless these initial trials have been associated with specific side effects related to the mechanisms of γ-retroviral gene transfer. Thus there has been a major effort to improve the safety profile of viral vectors and long-term follow-up in a number of current clinical trials will determine whether this has been achieved. There is also great interest in developing more sophisticated mechanisms of gene delivery including the use of physiological promoters, detargeting strategies, and use of homologous recombination mediated by zinc finger nucleases to name but a few. It is likely that these innovations will lead to the increased safe use of gene therapy for other immunodeficiencies and other monogenic hematopoietic diseases to an extent that gene therapy offers a credible alternative to allogeneic HSCT.

Acknowledgments

AJT is supported by the Wellcome Trust and GOSH Children's Charity. CR is supported by the Leukaemia Lymphoma Research Foundation. HBG is supported by Great Ormond Street Hospital Children's Charity. We are also grateful for the support given by the Jeffrey Modell Foundation to the Centre for Immunodeficiency.

References

1. Mercola KE, Stang HD, Browne J, et al. Insertion of a new gene of viral origin into bone marrow cells of mice. Science 1980;208(4447):1033–5.
2. Wade N. Gene therapy caught in more entanglements. Science 1981;212(4490):24–5.
3. Kantoff PW, Kohn DB, Mitsuya H, et al. Correction of adenosine deaminase deficiency in cultured human T and B cells by retrovirus-mediated gene transfer. Proc Natl Acad Sci U S A 1986;83(17):6563–7.
4. Willis RC, Jolly DJ, Miller AD, et al. Partial phenotypic correction of human Lesch-Nyhan (hypoxanthine-guanine phosphoribosyltransferase-deficient) lymphoblasts with a transmissible retroviral vector. J Biol Chem 1984;259(12):7842–9.
5. Rosenberg SA, Aebersold P, Cornetta K, et al. Gene transfer into humans—immunotherapy of patients with advanced melanoma, using tumor-infiltrating lymphocytes modified by retroviral gene transduction. N Engl J Med 1990;323(9):570–8.
6. Blaese RM, Culver KW, Miller AD, et al. T lymphocyte-directed gene therapy for ADA-SCID: initial trial results after 4 years. Science 1995;270(5235):475–80.
7. Edelstein ML, Abedi MR, Wixon J. Gene therapy clinical trials worldwide to 2007—an update. J Gene Med 2007;9(10):833–42.
8. Buch PK, Bainbridge JW, Ali RR. AAV-mediated gene therapy for retinal disorders: from mouse to man. Gene Ther 2008;15(11):849–57.

9. LeWitt PA, Rezai AR, Leehey MA, et al. AAV2-GAD gene therapy for advanced Parkinson's disease: a double-blind, sham-surgery controlled, randomised trial. Lancet Neurol 2011;10(4):309–19.

10. Murphy SL, High KA. Gene therapy for haemophilia. Br J Haematol 2008;140(5):479–87.

11. Tang Y, Cummins J, Huard J, Wang B. AAV-directed muscular dystrophy gene therapy. Expert Opin Biol Ther 2010;10(3):395–408.

12. Ariga T, Kondoh T, Yamaguchi K, et al. Spontaneous in vivo reversion of an inherited mutation in the Wiskott-Aldrich syndrome. J Immunol 2001;166(8):5245–9.

13. Stephan V, Wahn V, Le Deist F, et al. Atypical X-linked severe combined immunodeficiency due to possible spontaneous reversion of the genetic defect in T cells. N Engl J Med 1996;335(21):1563–7.

14. Noguchi M, Yi H, Rosenblatt HM, et al. Interleukin-2 receptor gamma chain mutation results in X-linked severe combined immunodeficiency in humans. Cell 1993;73(1):147–57.

15. Hacein-Bey H, Cavazzana-Calvo M, Le Deist F, et al. Gamma-c gene transfer into SCID X1 patients' B-cell lines restores normal high-affinity interleukin-2 receptor expression and function. Blood 1996;87(8):3108–16.

16. Cavazzana-Calvo M, Hacein-Bey S, de Saint Basile G, et al. Gene therapy of human severe combined immunodeficiency (SCID)-X1 disease. Science 2000;288(5466):669–72.

17. Gaspar HB, Parsley KL, Howe S, et al. Gene therapy of X-linked severe combined immunodeficiency by use of a pseudotyped gammaretroviral vector. Lancet 2004;364(9452):2181–7.

18. Hacein-Bey-Abina S, Hauer J, Lim A, et al. Efficacy of gene therapy for X-linked severe combined immunodeficiency. N Engl J Med 2010;363(4):355–64.

19. Gaspar HB, Cooray S, Gilmour KC, et al. Long-term persistence of a polyclonal T cell repertoire after gene therapy for X-linked severe combined immunodeficiency. Sci Transl Med 2011;3(97):97ra79.

20. Hacein-Bey-Abina S, Garrigue A, Wang GP, et al. Insertional oncogenesis in 4 patients after retrovirus-mediated gene therapy of SCID-X1. J Clin Invest 2008;118(9):3132–42.

21. Howe SJ, Mansour MR, Schwarzwaelder K, et al. Insertional mutagenesis combined with acquired somatic mutations causes leukemogenesis following gene therapy of SCID-X1 patients. J Clin Invest 2008;118(9):3143–50.

22. Chinen J, Davis J, De Ravin SS, et al. Gene therapy improves immune function in preadolescents with X-linked severe combined immunodeficiency. Blood 2007;110(1):67–73.

23. Serana F, Sottini A, Chiarini M, et al. The different extent of B and T cell immune reconstitution after hematopoietic stem cell transplantation and enzyme replacement therapies in SCID patients with adenosine deaminase deficiency. J Immunol 2010;185(12):7713–22.

24. Husain M, Gruenbaum E, Naqvi A, et al. Burkitt's lymphoma in a patient with adenosine deaminase deficiency–severe combined immunodeficiency treated with polyethylene glycol-adenosine deaminase. J Pediatr 2007;151(1):93–5.

25. Kaufman DA, Hershfield MS, Bocchini JA, et al. Cerebral lymphoma in an adenosine deaminase-deficient patient with severe combined immunodeficiency receiving polyethylene glycol-conjugated adenosine deaminase. Pediatrics 2005;116(6): e876–e879.

26. Bordignon C, Notarangelo LD, Nobili N, et al. Gene therapy in peripheral blood lymphocytes and bone marrow for ADA- immunodeficient patients. Science 1995;270(5235):470–5.

27. Aiuti A, Slavin S, Aker M, et al. Correction of ADA-SCID by stem cell gene therapy combined with nonmyeloablative conditioning. Science 2002;296(5577):2410–3.

28. Aiuti A, Cattaneo F, Galimberti S, et al. Gene therapy for immunodeficiency due to adenosine deaminase deficiency. N Engl J Med 2009;360(5):447–58.

29. Gaspar HB, Bjorkegren E, Parsley K, et al. Successful reconstitution of immunity in ADA-SCID by stem cell gene therapy following cessation of PEG-ADA and use of mild preconditioning. Mol Ther 2006;14(4):505–13.

30. Gaspar HB, Cooray S, Gilmour KC, et al. Hematopoietic stem cell gene therapy for adenosine deaminase-deficient severe combined immunodeficiency leads to long-term immunological recovery and metabolic correction. Sci Transl Med 2011;3(97):97ra80.

31. Aiuti A, Cassani B, Andolfi G, et al. Multilineage hematopoietic reconstitution without clonal selection in ADA-SCID patients treated with stem cell gene therapy. J Clin Invest 2007;117(8):2233–40.

32. Winkelstein JA, Marino MC, Johnston Jr. RB, et al. Chronic granulomatous disease. Report on a national registry of 368 patients. Medicine 2000;79(3):155–69.

33. Malech HL, Maples PB, Whiting-Theobald N, et al. Prolonged production of NADPH oxidase-corrected granulocytes after gene therapy of chronic granulomatous disease. Proc Natl Acad Sci U S A 1997;94(22):12133–8.

34. 3Ott MG, Schmidt M, Schwarzwaelder K, et al. Correction of X-linked chronic granulomatous disease by gene therapy, augmented by insertional activation of MDS1-EVI1, PRDM16 or SETBP1. Nature Med 2006;12(4):401–9.

35. Stein S, Ott MG, Schultze-Strasser S, et al. Genomic instability and myelodysplasia with monosomy 7 consequent to EVI1 activation after gene therapy for chronic granulomatous disease. Nature Med 2010;16(2):198–204.

36. Kang EM, Choi U, Theobald N, et al. Retrovirus gene therapy for X-linked chronic granulomatous disease can achieve stable long-term correction of oxidase activity in peripheral blood neutrophils. Blood 2010;115(4):783–91.

37. Kang HJ, Bartholomae CC, Paruzynski A, et al. Retroviral gene therapy for X-linked chronic granulomatous disease: results from phase I/II trial. Mol Ther 2011;19(11):2092–101.

38. Grez M, Reichenbach J, Schwable J, et al. Gene therapy of chronic granulomatous disease: the engraftment dilemma. Mol Ther 2011;19(1):28–35.

39. Boztug K, Schmidt M, Schwarzer A, et al. Stem-cell gene therapy for the Wiskott-Aldrich syndrome. N Engl J Med 2010;363(20):1918–27.

40. McCauslin CS, Wine J, Cheng L, et al. In vivo retroviral gene transfer by direct intrafemoral injection results in correction of the SCID phenotype in Jak3 knock-out animals. Blood 2003;102(3):843–8.

41. Pike-Overzet K, Rodijk M, Ng YY, et al. Correction of murine Rag1 deficiency by self-inactivating lentiviral vector-mediated gene transfer. Leukemia 2011;25(9):1471–83.

42. Benjelloun F, Garrigue A, Demerens-de Chappedelaine C, et al. Stable and functional lymphoid reconstitution in artemis-deficient mice following lentiviral artemis gene transfer into hematopoietic stem cells. Mol Ther 2008;16(8):1490–9.

43. Yates F, Malassis-Seris M, Stockholm D, Bouneaud C, et al. Gene therapy of RAG-2-/- mice: sustained correction of the immunodeficiency. Blood 2002;100(12):3942–9.

44. Hunter MJ, Tuschong LM, Fowler CJ, et al. Gene therapy of canine leukocyte adhesion deficiency using lentiviral vectors with human CD11b and CD18 promoters driving canine CD18 expression. Mol Ther 2011;19(1):113–21.

45. Kerns HM, Ryu BY, Stirling BV, et al. B cell-specific lentiviral gene therapy leads to sustained B-cell functional recovery in a murine model of X-linked agammaglobulinemia. Blood 2010;115(11):2146–55.

46. Cavazzana-Calvo M, Payen E, Negre O, et al. Transfusion independence and HMGA2 activation after gene therapy of human beta-thalassaemia. Nature 2010;467(7313):318–22.

47. Cartier N, Hacein-Bey-Abina S, Bartholomae CC, et al. Hematopoietic stem cell gene therapy with a lentiviral vector in X-linked adrenoleukodystrophy. Science 2009;326(5954):818–23.

48. Biffi A, Capotondo A, Fasano S, et al. Gene therapy of metachromatic leukodystrophy reverses neurological damage and deficits in mice. J Clin Invest 2006;116(11):3070–82.

49. Zychlinski D, Schambach A, Modlich U, et al. Physiological promoters reduce the genotoxic risk of integrating gene vectors. Mol Ther 2008;16(4):718–25.

50. Marangoni F, Bosticardo M, Charrier S, et al. Evidence for long-term efficacy and safety of gene therapy for Wiskott-Aldrich syndrome in preclinical models. Mol Ther 2009;17(6):1073–82.

51. Santilli G, Almarza E, Brendel C, et al. Biochemical correction of X-CGD by a novel chimeric promoter regulating high levels of transgene expression in myeloid cells. Mol Ther 2011;19(1):122–32.

52. Barde I, Zanta-Boussif MA, Paisant S, et al. Efficient control of gene expression in the hematopoietic system using a single Tet-on inducible lentiviral vector. Mol Ther 2006;13(2):382–90.

53. Gentner B, Visigalli I, Hiramatsu H, et al. Identification of hematopoietic stem cell-specific miRNAs enables gene therapy of globoid cell leukodystrophy. Sci Transl Med 2010;2(58):58ra84.

54. Lombardo A, Genovese P, Beausejour CM, et al. Gene editing in human stem cells using zinc finger nucleases and integrase-defective lentiviral vector delivery. Nat Biotechnol 2007;25(11):1298–306.

Frank Buttgereit,
Markus J.H.
Seibel, Johannes
W.J. Bijlsma

Glucocorticoids

Glucocorticoids exceed many other drugs in terms of numbers of patients treated, variety of applications and pharmacological experience in humans.[1] More than 60 years after their introduction into clinical practice, they still represent the most important and most frequently employed class of anti-inflammatory drug, with a steady rise in therapeutic use in recent years.[2] About 10 million new prescriptions for oral glucocorticoids are issued each year in the USA.[2] Community survey data estimate the frequency of oral glucocorticoid use as 0.5% of the general population and 1.75% of women aged over 55 years.[3,4] Between 56 and 68% of patients with rheumatoid arthritis are treated more or less continuously with glucocorticoids.[1] Glucocorticoids are relatively inexpensive, but owing to the sheer volume prescribed the total market size is about US$10 billion per year.[2]

The major reason for their widespread use is simple: glucocorticoids are the most effective (and cost-effective) anti-inflammatory and immunomodulatory drugs available. At the same time, glucocorticoids are prone to cause frequent and serious adverse effects, especially when used incorrectly.

Mechanisms of action

The basis for the use of different dosages of glucocorticoids in different clinical conditions is essentially empirical, as evidence to support preferences in specific clinical settings is scarce.[1] It is clear, however, that glucocorticoid dosages increase with clinical activity and the severity of the disease under treatment. The rationale for this (mostly successful) clinical approach is that higher dosages increase glucocorticoid receptor saturation in a dose-dependent manner (Table 87.1), which intensifies the therapeutically relevant, genomic glucocorticoid actions; and it is assumed that with increasing dosages, additional and qualitatively different, nonspecific, nongenomic actions of glucocorticoids come into play (Table 87.1).

Genomic actions of glucocorticoids

The anti-inflammatory and immunomodulatory effects of glucocorticoids (GC) are mediated predominantly by genomic mechanisms (Figs. 87.1 and 87.2). Binding to cytosolic glucocorticoid receptors (cGCR) ultimately induces ("transactivation") or inhibits ("transrepression") the synthesis of regulator proteins.[5] Between 10 and 100 genes per cell are directly regulated by glucocorticoids, but many genes are regulated indirectly through interaction with transcription factors and co-activators (see below).[6] It is estimated that glucocorticoids influence the

KEY CONCEPTS

Characteristics applying to genomic actions

- Physiologically relevant
- Therapeutically effective at all dosages, even very small ones (low-dose therapy).
- Slow; significant changes in the regulator protein concentrations are not seen within less than 30 minutes because of the time required for cGCR activation/translocation, transcription, and translation effects.
- The GC-induced synthesis of regulator proteins can be prevented by inhibitors of transcription (e.g., actinomycin D) or translation (e.g., cycloheximide).

transcription of approximately 1% of the entire genome. In the past few years, our in-depth knowledge of the genomic actions of GCs has greatly increased. Their lipophilic structure and low molecular mass allow GCs to pass easily through the cell membrane and bind to the inactive cGCR (α-form = cGCRα).

Structure of the cGCR

The unactivated cGCR is a 94-kDa protein held in the cytoplasm as a multi-protein complex consisting of several heat shock proteins (hsp), including hsp90, hsp70, hsp56, and hsp40 (chaperones) (Fig. 87.3). The cGCR interacts with immunophilins, p23 and several kinases of the mitogen-activated protein kinase (MAPK) signaling system, including Src, which also act as molecular (co)chaperones (Figs. 87.1 and 87.3).[1,7] The general function of molecular (co)chaperones is to bind and stabilize proteins at intermediate stages of folding, assembly, translocation and degradation. With regard to cGCR, they also regulate cellular signaling, which includes (i) stabilizing a specific conformational state of cGCR that binds ligand with high affinity; (ii) simultaneously opening the glucocorticoid binding cleft to access by glucocorticoids; and (iii) stabilizing the binding of GR to the promoter.[1]

The first step in assembling the multi-protein cytosolic complex is ATP- and hsp40(YDJ-1)-dependent formation of a cGCR-hsp70 complex that primes the receptor for subsequent ATP-dependent activation by hsp90, Hop, and p23.[8] The glucocorticoid receptor consists of different domains with distinct functions: an N-terminal, a DNA-binding domain (DBD) and a ligand-binding domain (LBD) (Fig. 87.3). The N-terminal harbors transactivation functions, especially within the "τ1" region. A motif common to DNA-interacting proteins, the zinc finger motif, is found twice within the DBD. The LBD consists of 12 α helices, several of which help form a hydrophobic ligand-binding

Table 87.1 Current knowledge on the relationship between clinical glucocorticoid dosing and cellular glucocorticoid actions

Terminology (mg prednisone equivalent per day)	Clinical application	Genomic actions (receptor saturation)	Unspecific nongenomic actions	cGCR-mediated nongenomic actions
Low dose (≤ 7.5)	Maintenance therapy for many rheumatic diseases	+ (< 50%)	–	?
Medium dose (>7.5– ≤30)	Initially given in primary chronic rheumatic diseases	++ (> 50– <100%)	(+)	(+)
High dose (>30– ≤100)	Initially given in subacute rheumatic diseases	++(+) (almost 100%)	+	+
Very high dose (> 100 mg)	Initially given in acute and/or potentially life-threatening exacerbations of rheumatic diseases	+++ ((almost) 100%)	++	+(+?)
Pulse therapy (≥ 250 mg for 1 or a few days)	Particularly severe and/or potentially life-threatening forms of rheumatic diseases	+++ (100%)	+++	+(++?)

From Buttgereit F, Straub RH, Wehling M, Burmester GR. Glucocorticoids in the treatment of rheumatic diseases. An update on mechanisms of action. Arthritis Rheum 2004; 50: 3408–3417, with permission.

Fig. 87.1 Mechanisms of the cellular action of glucocorticoids. As lipophilic substances, glucocorticoids pass very easily through the cell membrane into the cell, where they bind to ubiquitously expressed cytosolic glucocorticoid receptors (cGCR). This is followed by either the classic cGCR-mediated genomic effects (I) or by cGCR-mediated nongenomic effects (II). Moreover, the glucocorticoid is very likely to interact with cell membranes, either specifically via membrane-bound glucocorticoid receptors (mGCR) (III) or via nonspecific interactions with cell membranes (IV).
From Buttgereit F, Straub RH, Wehling M, Burmester GR, Glucocorticoids in the treatment of rheumatic diseases. An update on mechanisms of action. Arthr Rheum 2004; 50: 3408–3417.

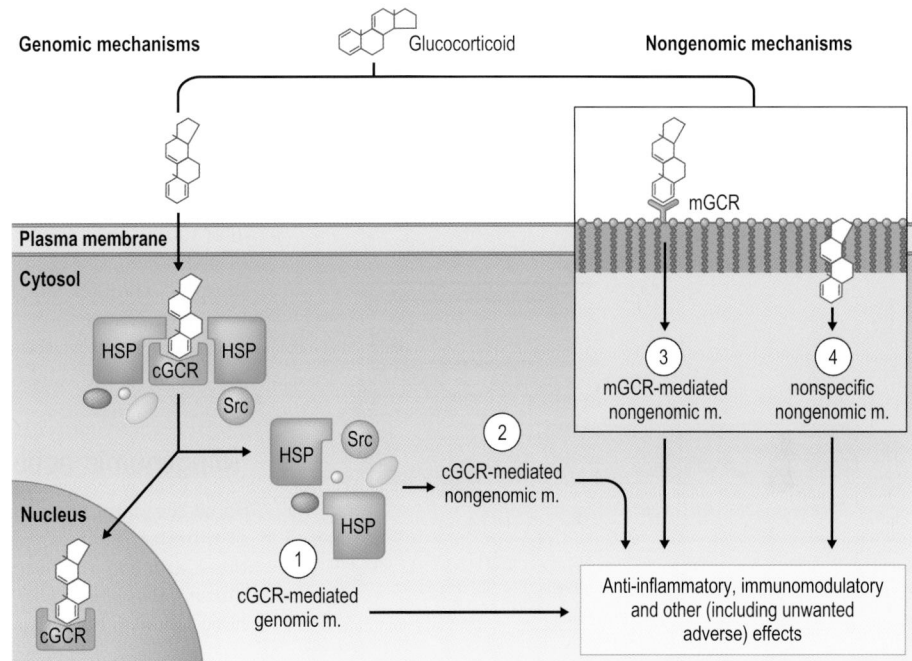

pocket.[7] The cGCR contains another major transactivation region ("τ2") that can interact with the above-mentioned cofactors (Fig. 87.3). Following glucocorticoid/receptor binding, hsp90 molecules and other chaperones are rapidly shed. This allows translocation into the cell nucleus, where the GC/cGCR complex binds as a homodimer to consensus palindromic DNA sites (GC-responsive elements—GREs).[5]

Translocation into the nucleus

Nuclear translocation of the GC/cGCR complex occurs within 20 minutes. Hormone-directed recruitment of FKBP52 and dynein to the GCR can cause its transport to the nucleus.[9] Depending on the target gene, transcription is then either activated (transactivation via positive GRE) or inhibited (transrepression via negative GRE) (Fig. 87.2A and B).

Interactions with transcription factors

Besides the interactions of GC/cGCR complexes with GREs, a further important genomic mechanism of GC action is interaction of activated cGCR monomers with transcription factors. Accordingly, although the GC/cGCR complex does not inhibit their synthesis, it modulates the activity of AP-1 (activator protein-1), NF-κB (nuclear factor-κB), and NF-AT (nuclear factor for activated T cells). This leads to inhibition of nuclear translocation and/or function of these transcription factors, and hence to inhibition of expression of many immunoregulatory and inflammatory cytokines. Possible mechanisms include:[5]

- Synthesis of IκB (a specific inhibitor of NF-κB) induced through GC/cGCR complex–GRE interaction (Fig. 87.2A).

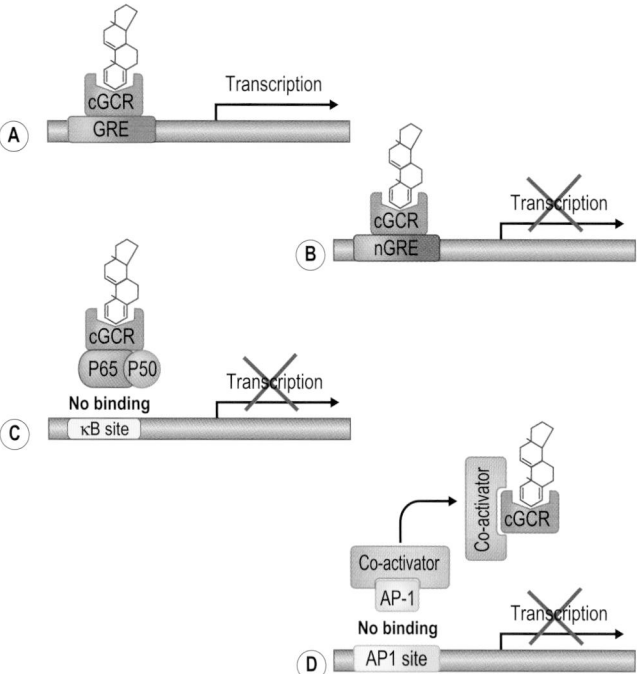

Fig. 87.2 (A–D) Genomic mechanisms of glucocorticoids. This figure illustrates the different mechanisms by which the activated glucocorticoid receptor complex leads to the induction or to the inhibition of transcription and finally translation/synthesis of specific regulator proteins. Details are given in the text.
From Buttgereit F, Straub RH, Wehling M, Burmester GR, Glucocorticoids in the treatment of rheumatic diseases. An update on mechanisms of action. Arthr Rheum 2004; 50: 3408–3417.

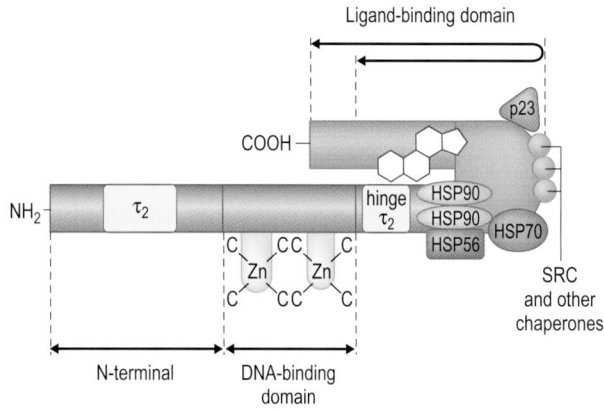

Fig. 87.3 Structure of the cytosolic glucocorticoid receptor. The unactivated (unligated) cGCR is a 94-kDa protein retained in the cytoplasm as a multi-protein complex consisting of several heat shock proteins (hsp), including hsp90, hsp70, hsp56, and hsp40 (chaperones). Furthermore, the cGCR interacts with immunophilins, p23 and several kinases of the mitogen-activated protein kinase (MAPK) signaling system, including Src, which also act as molecular (co-)chaperones. An important function of molecular (co-)chaperones is to stabilize a specific conformational state of the GC that binds ligand with high affinity (see text). The receptor protein itself consists of different domains: an N terminal, a DNA-binding domain (DBD), and a ligand-binding domain (LBD). The N-terminal harbors transactivation functions, especially within the so-called τ1 region. Another major transactivation region is τ2, which can interact with the above-mentioned cofactors.
From Buttgereit F, Straub RH, Wehling M, Burmester GR, Glucocorticoids in the treatment of rheumatic diseases. An update on mechanisms of action. Arthr Rheum 2004; 50: 3408–3417.

- Protein–protein interaction of the GC/cGCR complex with transcription factors through binding to their subunits (Fig. 87.2C), which prevents their DNA binding.
- Competition for nuclear co-activators between the GC/cGCR complex and transcription factors (Fig. 87.2D).

Inhibition of transcription factor function and the resultant inhibition of protein expression are referred to as transrepression. Numerous genes are regulated by this mechanism. Many adverse effects of GC are caused by transactivation (induced synthesis of regulator proteins), whereas most anti-inflammatory effects are mediated by transrepression (i.e., inhibited synthesis of regulator proteins). This differential molecular regulation underlies current drug-discovery programs aimed at developing dissociated cGCR-ligands.[2]

The cGCRβ isoform

An alternative splice variant of the cGCRα, the cGCRβ isoform, does not bind ligand and has been proposed to inhibit classic cGCRα-mediated transactivation. Recent structural research has shown a possible physical explanation for the lack of hormone binding and the dominant negative actions of cGCRβ.[10]

Post-transcriptional and post-translational mechanisms

Glucocorticoids also act through post-transcriptional and post-translational mechanisms, e.g., reduction of cytokine mRNA half-life and downregulation of GCR (via reduced mRNA levels and reduced stability of the GCR protein).

Glucocorticoid receptor resistance

GCR resistance is an interesting field of research. Several different mechanisms may mediate this phenomenon, among them alterations in number, binding affinity or phosphorylation status of the GCR. Other mechanisms being investigated are polymorphic changes and/or over-expression of (co-)chaperones, increased expression of inflammatory transcription factors, over-expression of the GCRβ isoform, the multidrug resistance pump, and altered mGCR expression.

Nongenomic actions of glucocorticoids

Some regulatory effects of glucocorticoids arise within seconds or minutes. These are too rapid to be explained as genomic actions, and are attributed to nongenomic mechanisms of action. Three different rapid nongenomic actions of glucocorticoids have recently been described.[1,11–13]

cGCR-mediated nongenomic actions

Croxtall et al.[11] reported that dexamethasone can rapidly inhibit epidermal growth factor-stimulated cPLA2 (cytosolic PLA2) activation with subsequent arachidonic acid release. This effect is thought to be mediated by occupation of cGCR, rather than changes in gene transcription, as the observed effect is RU486-sensitive (i.e., glucocorticoid receptor dependent), but actinomycin-insensitive (i.e., transcription independent). Chaperones or co-chaperones of the multi-protein complex can act as signaling components to mediate this effect. Following glucocorticoid binding, the cGCR is released from this complex to mediate classic genomic actions. However, there is also a rapid release of Src and other (co-)chaperones of the multi-protein complex, which may cause rapid inhibition of arachidonic acid release. Similarly, cardiovascular protective effects of dexamethasone have been reported which are neither genomic (because they occurred too quickly and were actinomycin insensitive) nor nonspecific nongenomic effects (because they occurred at a very low dosage (100 nM).[13] These may involve binding of glucocorticoids to the cGCR, leading to nontranscriptional activation of phosphatidylinositol 3-kinase, protein kinase Akt and endothelial nitric oxide synthase.

Nonspecific nongenomic actions

Glucocorticoids are sometimes administered at very high concentrations (e.g., intra-articular injection or IV pulse therapy). Systemically administered daily dosages >100 mg prednisone equivalent are regarded as "very high dose." In contrast, "pulse therapy" is the daily administration of ≥250 mg prednisone equivalent for one or a few consecutive days (Table 87.1).[14] At a daily dose of 100 mg prednisone equivalent, saturation of all cGCR is almost complete, so that specificity, i.e., the exclusivity of receptor-mediated effects, is lost at these high—but clinically relevant—glucocorticoid concentrations. Nonspecific nongenomic actions occur in the form of physicochemical interactions with biological membranes, which probably contribute to the therapeutic effect.[1] A nonspecific intercalation of glucocorticoid molecules into cell membranes is thought to alter cell function by influencing cation transport and increasing mitochondrial proton leak. The resulting inhibition of calcium and sodium cycling across the plasma membrane of immune cells is thought to contribute to rapid immunosuppression and to reduced inflammation.[1]

The use of such high glucocorticoid doses is confined to certain clinical specialties and has been criticized by endocrinologists and pharmacologists. Unfortunately, scientific evidence on this issue is lacking, as there are no randomized controlled trials. However, high-dose glucocorticoid therapy is often used with clinical success in acute exacerbations of life-threatening diseases and various clinical conditions resistant to other therapies. For example, pulsed IV methylprednisolone is effective in the treatment of systemic lupus erythematosus (SLE). However, these studies were mainly uncontrolled and retrospective in nature. A review concluded that intravenous pulses of methylprednisolone rapidly immunosuppress patients with organ- and/or life-threatening manifestations of SLE. However, the gold standard—1 g/day for 3 consecutive days—is associated with significant infectious complications, and lower doses may be just as effective.[15]

Another condition where high-dose glucocorticoids are normally (and mostly successfully) used is immune thrombocytopenia associated with SLE, although comparative studies are lacking.[16] It has been calculated that in situations like these, the concentrations achieved *in vivo* are high enough (around $10-5$ mol/L) to cause immediate nonspecific nongenomic effects on immune cells.[1] Intra-articular injections also bring high concentrations of glucocorticoids into contact with inflammatory cells, although it is difficult to assess locally achieved concentrations because crystal suspensions are most often used.

Specific nongenomic actions

Glucocorticoids can also induce specific nongenomic actions mediated through membrane-bound glucocorticoid receptors (mGCR). The existence and function of membrane-bound receptors have recently been demonstrated for various steroids (including mineralocorticoids, gonadal hormones, vitamin D and thyroid hormones).[1,17] Using immunofluorescence, small numbers of mGCR can be demonstrated on human peripheral blood mononuclear cells (monocytes and B lymphocytes) from healthy controls.[17] The monoclonal antibody used to detect mGCR also recognized cGCR, suggesting that mGCR

are probably variants of cGCR produced by differential splicing or promoter switching. It has also been found that immunostimulation with lipopolysaccharide increases the percentage of mGCR+ monocytes; this can be prevented by inhibiting the secretory pathway with brefeldin A. This suggests that mGCR are actively upregulated and transported through the cell following immunostimulation. These in vitro findings are consistent with observations that the frequency of mGCR+ monocytes is increased in patients with rheumatic disorders, and is positively correlated with disease activity in rheumatoid arthritis.[17] The function(s) of mGCR remain unclear, but this observation means that mGCR may be implicated in pathogenesis. Alternatively, and perhaps more likely, they may cause negative feedback regulation.

Glucocorticoid effects on immune cells

> ### ● KEY CONCEPTS
>
> **Glucocorticoid effects on immune cells**
>
> - Inhibit leukocyte traffic and access of leukocytes to the site of inflammation.
> - Interfere with functions of leukocytes, fibroblasts, and endothelial cells.
> - Suppress the production and actions of humoral factors involved in the inflammatory process.

Through the above mechanisms, glucocorticoids mediate a fascinating range of anti-inflammatory and immunomodulatory effects when used therapeutically, with virtually all primary and secondary immune cells affected to some extent (Table 87.2).[18]

Table 87.2 Important effects of glucocorticoids on primary and secondary immune cells

Monocytes/macrophages
↓ Number of circulating cells (↓ myelopoiesis, ↓ release)
↓ Expression of MHC class II molecules and Fc receptors
↓ Synthesis of proinflammatory cytokines (e.g., IL-2, IL-6, TNF-α) and prostaglandins

T cells
↓ Number of circulating cells (redistribution effects)
↓ Production and action of IL-2 (most important)

Granulocytes
↓ Number of eosinophil and basophil granulocytes
↑ Number of circulating neutrophils

Endothelial cells
↓ Vessel permeability
↓ Expression of adhesion molecules
↓ Production of IL-1 and prostaglandins

Fibroblasts
↓ proliferation
↓ production of fibronectin and prostaglandins

From Buttgereit F, Saag K, Cutolo M, et al. The molecular basis for the effectiveness, toxicity, and resistance to glucocorticoids: focus on the treatment of rheumatoid arthritis. Scand J Rheumatol 2005; 34: 14–21, with permission.

The role of endogenous gLUCOCORTICOIDs in inflammatory arthritis

Exogenous (i.e., therapeutic) and endogenous (i.e., physiologic) glucocorticoids differ in several respects. The most important differences relate to their mineralocorticoid and glucocorticoid (i.e., anti-inflammatory) activities. Other differences between exogenous and endogenous glucocorticoids apply to pharmacological characteristics such as plasma kinetics, metabolism, biological half-life, lipophilicity, drug-receptor interactions, and non-genomic potencies.[19]

The actions of exogenous glucocorticoids as described above are well established. In contrast, the role of endogenous glucocorticoids in, and their contribution to the susceptibility and severity of arthritis remains an area of active research. While historic dogma stipulated that glucocorticoid actions on target tissues are determined by glucocorticoid plasma concentrations and the tissue-specific density of glucocorticoid receptors only, new insights into the mechanisms of glucocorticoid action suggest that endogenous glucocorticoids are subject to extensive pre-receptor metabolism. Within target cells or tissues, glucocorticoid action depends not only on plasma hormone levels, receptor expression and receptor-effector coupling, but also on local glucocorticoid metabolism. Specifically, 11β-hydroxy-steroid dehydrogenases appear to govern access of glucocorticoids to their cognate receptors by changing the balance between active and inactive glucocorticoids within the cell (reviewed.[19] Thus, 11β-hydroxysteroid dehydrogenase *type 1* (11βHSD1) through its predominant reductase activity catalyses the formation of bioactive cortisol (in humans) and corticosterone (in rodents) from inactive cortisone and 11-dehydrocorticosterone, respectively. This $NADP^+(H)$-dependent enzyme is present in many tissues and usually increases the intracellular availability of active glucocorticoids. In contrast, 11β-hydroxysteroid dehydrogenase *type 2* (11βHSD2) only possesses dehydrogenase activity; it inactivates active glucocorticoids and therefore decreases the concentration of bioactive glucocorticoids in the cell.

Pro-inflammatory cytokines such as interleukin-1β (IL-1β) and tumor necrosis factor alpha (TNF-α) stimulate 11βHSD1 and downregulate 11βHSD2 expression. Hence, specific pro-inflammatory cytokines are able to modulate local intracellular glucocorticoid metabolism, potentially modifying their own pro-inflammatory effects. More recently, Hardy and colleagues confirmed the existence of substantial glucocorticoid metabolism in the joint by demonstrating that TNF-α and IL-1β cause a dramatic induction of 11βHSD1 activity in primary cultures of synovial fibroblasts isolated from synovial tissue biopsies from RA patients.[20]

In a rodent model of immune-mediated arthritis, targeted disruption of glucocorticoid-signalling in osteoblasts attenuates joint inflammation and cartilage destruction.[21] While somewhat unexpected, these results strongly suggest that, under the control of endogenous glucocorticoids, osteoblasts modulate immune-mediated inflammatory responses, and, as a consequence, inflammation-induced cartilage damage and bone integrity. These findings are supported by recent evidence suggesting that the effects of glucocorticoids follow a dose-response curve with permissive or even stimulatory effects at physiological concentrations, and suppressive effects at pharmacological concentrations.[20]

Therapeutic use

A wide range of GC molecules are available for clinical use; these share a common basic structure and have been modified to improve their usefulness in various clinical applications (Fig. 87.4). Despite their widespread use, the designation of GC treatment regimens is often imprecise. Recommendations for a standardized nomenclature for GC therapy are summarized below.[14]

Terminology

What term should be used to describe this class of drugs?

The term "steroids" (although very often used) is too broad, as it simply describes chemical compounds characterized by a common multiple-ring structure (including, for example, cholesterol, vitamin D and sex hormones); also, the terms "corticosteroids" or "corticoids" are not sufficiently precise, as the adrenal cortex, from which these designations are derived, synthesizes not only glucocorticoids, but also mineralocorticoids and androgens. For these reasons, the terms "glucocorticoid" or "glucocorticosteroid" are scientifically correct, but "glucocorticoid" is the more widely used.

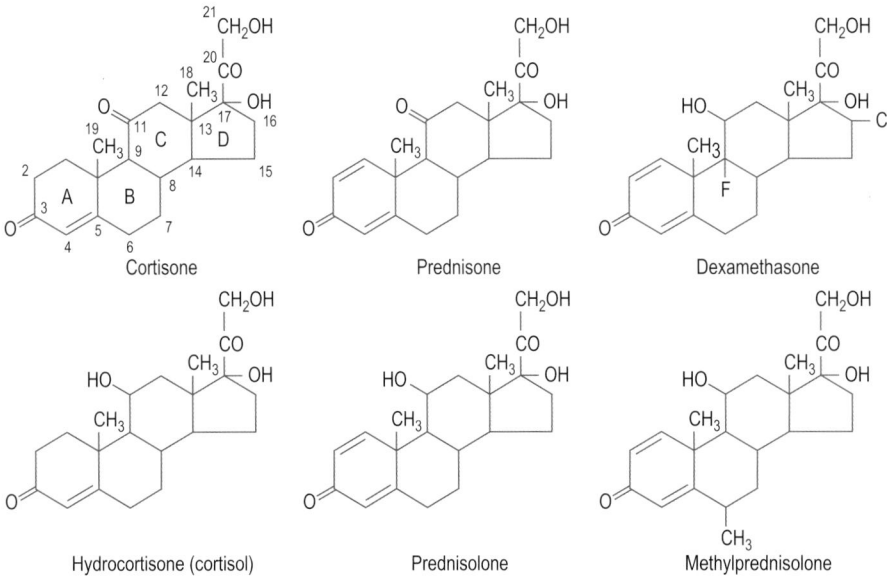

Fig. 87.4 Molecular structures of cortisone and commonly used glucocorticoids. Carbon and ring nomenclature is indicated on cortisone molecule.

How can glucocorticoid therapy schedules be described as precisely as possible?

A description has been suggested that is precise regarding the drug, the dosage, the route of administration, and the timing of administration (timing, frequency, duration, sometimes cumulative dosage where appropriate).

Of note is that different glucocorticoid drugs have different potencies. Moreover, glucocorticoids differ in their ability to produce the distinct therapeutic effects discussed above. Drug potencies are usually described by the equivalent dosages (relative potencies) to produce classic genomic effects (Table 87.3). These values have been in use for decades, although experimental and clinical evidence for their precision is weak. Nevertheless, relative potencies are useful in daily clinical practice as a general therapeutic guideline, as long as one avoids using them dogmatically. It has therefore been suggested (i) to continue to use relative potencies until more exact data are available; and (ii) to express doses of different glucocorticoids by converting them into doses of "prednisone equivalent"; the latter simply means that doses of different glucocorticoids are being expressed in milligrams of prednisone (= mg prednisolone, as the potency of prednisone is equal to that of prednisolone) by using the relative potencies mentioned above.

Recent data, however, indicate that the use of equivalent dosages is valid only if doses less than 100 mg prednisone are considered. At higher dosages nongenomic effects come into play. This is important, as the relative potencies of different glucocorticoids to produce these nongenomic effects are completely different from their classic genomic effects (Table 87.3). For instance, methylprednisolone is often preferred over prednisolone for pulse therapy of exacerbated immunologically mediated disorders in exacerbation. The two drugs have similar genomic potency, but in high-dose therapy the nonspecific nongenomic effect of methylprednisolone is more than three times stronger. This may explain the empirical clinical preference for methylprednisolone. Another example is the very low nongenomic potency of betamethasone, which may be one reason why this drug is rarely used systemically, although it has the same genomic potency as dexamethasone. In summary, the clinical usage of different glucocorticoids is clearly determined by the magnitude of their clinical efficacy, but one underlying reason for that may be their nongenomic potencies.

Glucocorticoid treatment regimens: general aspects

For decades there was some confusion in regards to glucocorticoid treatment regimens as exemplified by the many different interpretations of the various terms used to describe dosage

Table 87.3 Drug potencies of selected glucocorticoids

Cortisol	1 (per definition)
Prednyliden	3.5
Predniso(lo)ne	4.0
Methylprednisolone	5.0
Dexamethasone	25
Betamethasone	25

Drug potencies describe the potency of the respective drug to produce classical genomic (anti-inflammatory) effects relative to cortisol. These potencies provide the basis for calculating equivalent dosages.
Data from Lipworth BJ, Therapeutic implications of non-genomic glucocorticoid activity. Lancet 2000; 356: 87–89.

(very low, low, mild, mild to moderate, moderate, high, very high, ultra-high, and mega) and by the great variation in the interpretation of terms such as "low-dose therapy," "high-dose therapy," and "pulse therapy." Therefore, a clarification of this situation was needed, first for scientific conciseness and second to accommodate the fact that glucocorticoid actions are strongly dose dependent, both quantitatively and qualitatively. A 2002 consensus statement provided the following recommendations for a standardized nomenclature for glucocorticoid dosages and glucocorticoid treatment regimens.[14]

Low dose

> ### ● KEY CONCEPTS
>
> **Definition of conventional terms for glucocorticoid dosages**
>
> | | |
> | --- | --- |
> | Low dose | ≤ 7.5 mg prednisone equivalent per day |
> | Medium dose | > 7.5 mg, but ≤ 30 mg prednisone equivalent per day |
> | High dose | > 30 mg, but ≤ 100 mg prednisone equivalent per day |
> | Very high dose | > 100 mg prednisone equivalent per day |
> | Pulse therapy | ≥ 250 mg prednisone equivalent per day for 1 or a few days |

Treatment with doses of up to 7.5 mg prednisone equivalent per day is considered low-dose glucocorticoid therapy because these doses occupy less than 50% of the receptors; are frequently used for maintenance therapy; and may have relatively few adverse effects (such as osteoporosis). As there may be relative hypocortisolism in chronic inflammatory conditions such as rheumatoid arthritis and polymyalgia rheumatica, some authors regard low-dose glucocorticoids as replacement therapy for the reduced adrenal production of glucocorticoids.

Medium dose

Glucocorticoid doses of more than 7.5 mg but less than 30 mg prednisone equivalent per day are considered to represent medium-dose therapy because they lead to a significantly higher receptor engagement between 50 and <100%; are effective in modulating disease activity of various rheumatic diseases; are a "natural barrier" in the sense that most clinical rheumatologists tend to avoid doses above 30mg in the initial stages of treatment; and may have considerable and dose-dependent adverse effects if given for longer periods.

High dose

Treatment with doses of more than 30 mg and up to 100 mg of prednisone equivalent per day is considered high-dose therapy because these doses significantly increase receptor saturation in a dose-dependent manner. At approximately 100 mg prednisone equivalent per day, receptor saturation is almost complete and it is assumed that up to 100% of genomic glucocorticoid effects are exerted (Table 87.1). High-dose therapy is successfully given as initial treatment for subacute diseases such as non-life-threatening exacerbations or visceral complications of rheumatoid arthritis or other connective tissue diseases, but cannot be administered for the long-term because of the danger of severe adverse effects.

Very high dose

Doses above 100 mg of prednisone equivalent per day are considered "very high," because they cause virtually 100% saturation of cytosolic receptors. Therefore, a further increase in dose may affect the pharmacodynamics (e.g., receptor off-loading and re-occupancy), receptor synthesis and expression. Such doses may also have additional therapeutic benefit via other mechanisms, namely the above mentioned non-genomic effects. It is not yet clear whether these effects are of direct therapeutic relevance but experimental data suggest that these differential effects come increasingly into play above ~100 mg/day (Table 87.1). Doses of more than 100 mg of prednisone equivalent per day are frequently and successfully given as initial treatment for acute or life-threatening exacerbations of (rheumatic) diseases, such as connective tissue diseases, vasculitis, and rheumatoid arthritis. They cannot be administered long term because of their severe adverse effects.

Pulse therapy

"Pulse therapy" is a specific therapeutic entity involving administration of ≥250 mg prednisone equivalent per day (usually IV) for a short period of time (1–5 days, rarely longer). At such high doses, the non-genomic potencies of glucocorticoids come into play. It is likely that these are the reasons for the clinical observation that very high doses and pulse therapy are generally successful in acute exacerbations of immunologically mediated diseases. The immediate effects of very high doses could be additive to the genomic effects mediated by cytosolic GC receptors. The additional quantum of inhibition of the excessive immune processes could make a crucial contribution to the therapeutic effect by helping to terminate the acute exacerbation. In rheumatology and clinical immunology, circumstances where very high doses or pulse therapy can be successful include acute episodes or particularly severe forms of rheumatic diseases such as systemic lupus erythematosus, vasculitis, polymyositis, and rheumatoid arthritis (see below).

Alternate-day regimens

Alternate-day regimens were introduced for long-term oral GC therapy to alleviate undesirable adverse effects, such as suppression of the hypothalamo–pituitary–adrenal (HPA) axis. A single dose is administered every other morning, usually in a dose equivalent to, or somewhat higher than, twice the usual daily dose. The logic behind this regimen is that exposing the body to exogenous GC on alternate days may allow the HPA axis to remain active. This strategy, however, only works if the HPA axis is still active. Unfortunately, patients often experience breakthrough symptoms on the second day of treatment. Alternate-day regimens are used rarely these days except in patients with juvenile idiopathic arthritis (Chapter 52), in whom alternate-day glucocorticoid regimens cause less inhibition of body growth.

Glucocorticoid withdrawal regimens

Because of their significant adverse effects, GCs are generally tapered off as soon as the disease is under control. This needs to be done carefully in order to avoid a relapse in disease activity and to permit recovery of adrenal function. There are no controlled comparative studies to support a specific regimen for weaning patients off GCs as this process needs to be adjusted according to disease activity, dose/duration of therapy and clinical response. When patients with rheumatoid arthritis are treated with up to 10 mg/day of prednisone, the daily dose can be reduced by 2.5 mg every month until 5 mg/day is reached.

Thereafter, doses can often be reduced by 1 mg per month. When higher doses have been used,, a reduction by 5 mg every 1–2 weeks down to 20 mg/day is often well tolerated, followed by further reductions of 1–2.5 mg/day every 2–3 weeks. Addition of immunomodulatory drugs such as methotrexate and azathioprine may allow further dose reductions. Short courses of GC for conditions such as asthma can be ceased without tapering if the total treatment course was less than 14 days in duration. With longer periods of treatment, the dose should be reduced gradually to allow the HPA axis to recover.

Glucocorticoids in rheumatoid arthritis: an example

> ### ● KEY CONCEPTS
>
> **GC therapy in rheumatoid arthritis**
>
> - The risk–benefit ratio of low-dose GC has been shifted in the past few years:
> - GC can now be considered as disease-modifying antirheumatic drugs, especially in early RA.
> - Adverse effects of low-dose GC are less abundant and less severe than previously suggested, and some (e.g., osteoporosis) can be well managed.
> - The goal of anti-rheumatic treatment in early RA is to induce remission of disease by aggressive management; GC are part of this aggressive strategy.

Glucocorticoids are crucially important in the management of rheumatoid arthritis (RA) and are used in various dosages at different disease stages. RA (Chapter 51) is therefore a useful example to discuss GC therapy in more detail.

Low-dose maintenance therapy

In RA, GC therapy is often started and maintained at low dose, typically as additional therapy. GC in doses <10 mg are highly effective for relieving symptoms in patients with active RA; many patients are functionally dependent on this therapy and continue it long-term. A review of seven studies (253 patients in total) evaluating the symptomatic effect of GC in RA concluded that they are very effective when administered over about 6 months.[22] Improvement has been documented in all clinical parameters, including pain scales, joint scores, morning stiffness and fatigue, but also in acute inflammatory markers such as ESR and CRP. After 6 months of therapy the beneficial effects of GC seem to diminish; however, if therapy is then tapered and stopped, patients often experience an aggravation of symptoms within a few months.

The disease-modifying properties of GC were first described in 1995, in a 2-year trial of 7.5 mg prednisolone in patients with RA of short/intermediate disease duration who also were treated with NSAIDs (95%) and disease-modifying antirheumatic drugs (DMARDs, 71%).[23] Since then, other trials have confirmed the potency of GC to retard joint damage. Today, GC are considered to have disease-modifying properties in early RA, but it is less clear whether they can inhibit the progression of erosions in RA of longer duration. A recent meta-analysis reviewed 15 studies including 1 414 patients and concluded that, even on the most conservative estimate, glucocorticoids given in addition to standard therapy could substantially reduce the rate of erosion progression in rheumatoid arthritis.[24] In line with this view another recent meta-analysis of 70 randomized placebo or drug-controlled studies found similar effects of DMARDs, glucocorticoids and biologics on radiographic progression in rheumatoid arthritis.[25]

Glucocorticoid pulse therapy

GC pulse therapy is used to treat some serious complications of RA and to induce remission in active disease, often when initiating second-line anti-rheumatic treatment. Pulse therapy with methylprednisolone 1 g per day dexamethasone 200 mg per day or equivalent, given intravenously for 1–3 days, was effective in most studies; the beneficial effect generally lasts for about 6 weeks, albeit with large variations. It thus does not seem sensible to apply pulse therapy in active RA, unless the therapeutic strategy is changed (e.g., DMARD treatment introduced to maintain the remission induced by pulse therapy). A mitigated form of pulse therapy uses depot injection of 120 mg methyl prednisolone acetate.

Intra-articular glucocorticoid injections

Intra-articular injections with GC are often used in RA. The benefit achieved depends on several factors, such as the joint treated (size, weight bearing or non-weight bearing), inflammatory activity, the volume of synovial fluid in the joint, whether or not an arthrocentesis (synovial fluid aspiration) was performed before the injection, choice and dose of GC preparation, injection technique, and whether or not the joint is rested after the injection.[26] In order to prevent GC-induced joint damage, it is recommended that intra-articular GC injections should not be repeated more often than once every 3–4 weeks, and no more than 3–4 times a year in a weight-bearing joint.

Adverse effects

Studies of GC toxicity tend to be retrospective and observational.[27] This can make it difficult to differentiate unfavorable outcomes attributable to GCs from those occurring due to the underlying disease or other co-morbidities. Furthermore, there is a strong selection bias for GC use, as physicians are more inclined to use them in patients with more severe disease. Frequent, but less serious, adverse effects (e.g., skin thinning, cushingoid appearance) may be of great concern to patients, whereas more debilitating toxicities such as osteoporosis, cataracts, and GC-induced hypertension may initially go unrecognized or be asymptomatic. Interpretation of toxicity data is further confounded by the use of GCs at variable points in the disease course, limited data defining "threshold" doses for particular adverse events, and toxicity reports covering a heterogeneous group of GC-treated diseases.

Compared to other anti-rheumatic agents, GCs have a low incidence of short-term symptomatic toxicity and patients rarely discontinue therapy for these reasons. Despite over 60 years of use, we still lack robust data on the longer-term toxicities of glucocorticoids, from large randomized controlled trials with long-term follow-up. The commonest GC toxicities are summarized below, and reviewed in greater detail elsewhere.[22,27]

Clinical progress has recently been made by formulating recommendations on which adverse effects of glucocorticoid treatment should be monitored in rheumatoid arthritis, how to monitor them and how often.[28] Two levels of monitoring GC adverse events have been proposed:

(i) For daily practice, details are given on how to identify adverse events in a feasible way. This should result in preventive and therapeutic measures in order to minimize the risks of glucocorticoid therapy.

(ii) For clinical trials, recommendations are being made on how to assess accurately the frequency and severity of a larger set of adverse events.[28]

Osteoporosis

Glucocorticoid-induced osteoporosis (GIOP) is the most important potential complication of prolonged GC therapy. Chronic GC treatment results in rapid and profound reductions in bone mineral density, with most bone loss occurring during the first 6–12 months of treatment.[3,27]

GIOP initially affects trabecular bone, but with more chronic use cortical bone is also affected, at sites such as the femoral neck. Precisely how GCs affect bone remains obscure. GCs decrease calcium absorption, increase renal calcium loss, diminish sex and growth hormone production, induce muscle wasting and modulate RANKL/OPG, NF-κB and AP-1 signaling in bone.[29] All of these changes lead to enhanced osteoclast function and lifespan, and hence to increased bone resorption. Consequently, markers of bone resorption are often increased in patients treated with GCs.[23,30] However, reduced bone formation due to reduced osteoblast function is likely to be a more important effect of GCs on skeletal health. Oral doses of prednisone as low as 2.5 mg/day have been shown to suppress serum osteocalcin, a marker of bone formation. Histologically, mean wall thickness is reduced, reflecting the reduced amount of bone replaced in each remodeling unit. In vitro, osteoblasts and their precursors are highly GC responsive. Here, the predominant effect is to promote osteoprogenitor proliferation, lineage commitment and osteoblast differentiation, resulting in the formation of bone nodules of increased size and numbers. However, GCs also inhibit type I collagen expression, and reduce pre-osteoblastic replication. Finally, GCs promote apoptosis of osteoblasts and osteocytes. The inhibitory effects of GCs on bone formation may partly be due to downregulation of IGF-I expression by osteoblasts. Fortunately, we now have effective strategies for the prevention and treatment of GC-induced osteoporosis, using calcium, vitamin D and specific osteotropic agents such as bisphosphonates or parathyroid hormone.

Osteonecrosis

Osteonecrosis has long been considered an important consequence of high-dose glucocorticoid use. In a Japanese study of femoral head osteonecrosis, 35% cases were related to GC treatment. Higher average dose may be a more important predictor of avascular necrosis of bone than cumulative dose. Osteonecrosis is particularly noted in SLE, but rarely occurs in RA patients receiving low-dose therapy, affecting less than 3% of patients. Osteonecrosis rarely occurs in SLE patients on prednisone doses <20 mg/day.

Myopathy

As with osteonecrosis, GC-induced myopathy is rare in patients receiving low-dose glucocorticoids. In small studies, myopathy appears more closely associated with fluorinated GC preparations such as triamcinolone than with prednisone. Notably, myopathy has been reported after only 3 months' treatment with triamcinolone 8 mg/day. In general, myopathy attributable to prednisone only occurs after higher doses and longer durations of treatment.

Cardiovascular adverse effects

Glucocorticoid-induced hypertension seems to be at least in part mediated via fluid retention (as a result of mineralocorticoid effects); it is dose-related and less likely with medium- or low-dose therapy. Individual variation in susceptibility and other factors, such as the starting level of blood pressure, dietary salt intake, functional renal mass, associated diseases and drug therapy can also play a role.

Another troublesome potential toxicity of low-dose GCs is the development of premature atherosclerotic vascular disease. This has proved difficult to investigate; studies evaluating the effects of GCs on lipids and atherosclerosis in RA patients have yielded mixed results, with some studies suggesting that GCs may actually reverse unfavorable lipid changes. At present, there is no evidence of a strong association between low-dose glucocorticoids and cardiovascular disease in RA, even though atherosclerotic vascular disease is known to be accelerated in patients with Cushing's disease.

Dermatologic adverse effects

Even at low doses, skin thinning and ecchymoses are common adverse events with glucocorticoids. Cutaneous atrophy results from catabolic GC effects on keratinocytes and fibroblasts. Purpura and easy bruising in GC-treated patients are probably due to decreased vascular structural integrity. A Cushingoid appearance is very troubling to patients, but is uncommon at doses below the physiologic range. One study reported facial fullness ("moon facies") in 13% of patients receiving 4–12 mg triamcinolone for up to 60 days. These adverse effects are observed in over 5% of patients exposed to ≥ 5 mg prednisone equivalent for ≥ 1 year. The incidence of iatrogenic Cushing's syndrome is dose-dependent and generally becomes evident after >1 month of GC therapy. Alternate-day therapy may reduce the incidence, although there are only limited data supporting this concept. Glucocorticoid acne, hirsutism, and striae are other undesirable dermatologic effects that occur even with lower doses.

Gastrointestinal adverse effects

Glucocorticoids are considerably less toxic to the upper gastrointestinal (GI) tract than NSAIDs. If GCs independently increase the risk of GI events (e.g., gastritis, ulceration, bleeding), the effect is slight, with estimated relative risks varying from 1.1 (not significant) to 1.5 (marginally significant). There are also anecdotal reports of intestinal rupture, diverticular perforation, and pancreatitis attributed to low-dose GCs. Glucocorticoids are frequently used concurrently with NSAIDs in RA, and meta-analyses confirm that the combination of the two synergistically increases the risk of GI adverse events. In a large-scale study based on the UK General Practice Research Database, the risk of upper GI complications was 1.8 (95% CI, 1.3–2.4) times higher for GC users than for nonusers. The risk tended to be greater for higher GC doses, but the dose gradient was not statistically significant. The risk was >12 times higher for those taking both glucocorticoids and NSAIDs than for those not using either. No studies have yet looked at the GI effects of combining GCs with COX-2-selective NSAIDs.

Infectious diseases

Medium- to high-dose GC therapy, particularly when administered for prolonged periods, can increase the risk of serious infections requiring hospitalization or surgery. However, to date, no studies have explored the risk of infection in patients on lower doses. A meta-analysis showed that infection rates were not significantly increased in patients on <10 mg/day prednisone or a cumulative dose of <700 mg. in those on higher doses, the risk of infection appears to be lessened with alternate-day therapy.

In GC-treated patients, physicians should anticipate the risk of infections with both typical and atypical organisms, recognizing that GCs may blunt the classic clinical features and delay diagnosis. *Pneumocystis jiroveci* infections can occur with doses as low as 16 mg/day of prednisone for 8 weeks and an increased risk was found in one series.[31] Herpes zoster is also more common in RA patients treated with immunosuppressive agents. In one analysis.[32] eight such patients developed zoster compared with only one control ($p < 0.04$). However, it is difficult to separate the independent effects of GC use from those of other commonly used anti-rheumatic agents, such as methotrexate and anti-TNF-α agents. At present, the independent role of GCs in facilitating herpes zoster infection in patients with RA remains uncertain.

Other adverse effects

Adverse effects on the hypothalamopituitary axis and on glucose metabolism as well as neuropsychiatric and ophthalmologic adverse effects are reviewed elsewhere.[22,27]

Timing of glucocorticoid administration matters

In patients with rheumatoid arthritis, major symptoms such as pain, inflammation and stiffness vary as a function of the time of day, usually with the highest severity in the morning hours. These symptoms are preceded by elevated levels of pro-inflammatory cytokines. Based upon these considerations and given that glucocorticoids target IL-6, other humoral factors (e.g., TNF-α) as well as cellular reactions (e.g., leukocyte traffic and access of leukocytes to the site of inflammation) involved in the pathogenesis of RA, it has been proposed that improving the timing of glucocorticoid administration may help to optimize RA therapy.[19,33] A newly developed modified-release (MR) prednisone tablet releases prednisone 4 hours after ingestion, i.e., at approximately 2 a.m. if taken at bedtime. This novel formulation has been investigated in the CAPRA1 study, which had an initial 3-month double-blind phase followed by a 9-month open-label extension.[33] The new formulation was shown to be clinically superior to the conventional immediate-release preparation (IR prednisone) with respect to reducing morning joint stiffness. This beneficial effect was noted in addition to clinical control of the disease resulting from treatment with conventional prednisone. IL-6 was also decreased by MR prednisone but remained unchanged by IR prednisone. There was no difference in safety profile between the two preparations.[33] After 12 months of treatment (i.e., at the end of the open-label phase), the duration of morning stiffness was reduced by $\sim 50\%$ in patients treated with MR prednisone, and 37% of these patients achieved improvement according to the ACR20 criteria.[34] Altogether, these data support the view that optimizing the timing of glucocorticoid administration with this new drug improves the risk-benefit ratio of long-term low-dose glucocorticoid treatment in patients with RA.

New glucocorticoid receptor ligands on the horizon

The various mechanisms of GC action provide interesting opportunities for developing optimized GCs and GC-receptor ligands, which are reviewed below. More detailed information is available elsewhere.[1,27,35]

Selective glucocorticoid receptor agonists (SEGRAs)

The existence of the genomic component mechanisms of transactivation and transrepression provides a foundation for developmental research into GC-receptor ligands that predominantly cause transrepression but not transactivation. This research is based on the assumption that the anti-inflammatory properties of GCs are mostly due to repression of AP-1- and NF-κB-stimulated synthesis of inflammatory mediators, whereas most of their adverse effects are associated with transactivation of genes involved in metabolic processes. Investigators have therefore sought novel GCR ligands with high repression but low transactivation activity. One such compound, A276575, exhibits a high affinity for the GCR and potently represses IL-1α-induced IL-6 production, similarly to dexamethasone. However, unlike dexamethasone, A276575 induces little aromatase activity. Other novel nonsteroidal GCR ligands are being developed that possess high repression activities against inflammatory mediator production, but have lower transactivation activities than traditional GCs. Substances that cause a receptor conformation preferring a GCR/protein interaction and not a GCR/DNA-binding-dependent mechanism are now being called "dissociated glucocorticoids" or selective glucocorticoid receptor agonists (SEGRAs). The SEGRA concept has, however, recently been challenged by studying a mouse knock-in strain with a dimerization-deficient GR that demonstrated that some inflammatory processes can be suppressed by glucocorticoids, while others cannot.[36] Also, these mice exhibited classical adverse effects of glucocorticoids such as glucocorticoid-induced osteoporosis. Thus, depending on the process being treated, SEGRAs could be therapeutically more or less effective and not all adverse effects of glucocorticoid therapy may be reduced.[36,37] Nevertheless, from the clinical rheumatologist's point of view it is slightly disappointing that the sound underlying theory and the promising initial data have not led yet to a therapeutic breakthrough. Therefore, it remains uncertain whether SEGRAs will become clinically relevant in rheumatology in the near future.[19]

Nitro-steroids

Another new class of glucocorticoid drugs, nitro-steroids, have also been tested in RA and inflammatory bowel disease. Nitro-steroids release low levels of nitric oxide (NO) and have enhanced anti-inflammatory properties and fewer unwanted effects. The prototype of these new steroids, 21-NO-prednisolone (NCX-1015), is much more potent than prednisolone in models of acute and chronic inflammation, including collagen II-induced arthritis. In contrast, NCX-1015 did not activate primary osteoclast activity in vitro, whereas prednisolone did. This lack of adverse effect of NCX-1015 was chiefly due to NO. It has been suggested that post-translational modification of GCR (tyrosine nitration) by NCX-1015 may explain its enhanced anti-inflammatory activity. Moreover, NCX-1015 potently stimulates IL-10 production, suggesting that nitro-steroids induce regulatory T cells that negatively modulate inflammation. However, further work is needed to confirm the utility of nitro-steroids in clinical practice.

Long-circulating liposomal glucocorticoids

The anti-inflammatory efficacy of GCs can be improved by the additional benefits of nongenomic actions at high GC concentrations. This has led to the successful use of long-circulating liposomal GCs. In rats with experimental autoimmune encephalitis, GC-containing liposomes accumulate at sites of inflammation, reaching ultra-high concentrations (>10−5 mol/L for ≥18 hours). These liposomes may thus be therapeutically superior to conventional intravenous high-dose GC therapy, as evidenced by their successful use in rats with adjuvant-induced arthritis. A single injection of 10 mg/kg liposomal prednisolone phosphate resulted in complete remission of the inflammatory response for almost a week. In contrast, the same dose of unencapsulated prednisolone phosphate did not reduce inflammation, and only had a slight effect after repeated daily injections. It may be that preferential delivery of GC to the site of inflammation leads to very high GC concentrations at the inflamed joint, but lower plasma concentrations with a lower rate of adverse effects. These are very promising developments that exploit the broad spectrum of therapeutically relevant genomic and nongenomic GC actions preferentially at the site of inflammation.

The combination of prednisolone and dipyridamole

Another interesting recent development is the selective amplification of glucocorticoid anti-inflammatory activity through synergistic multi-target action of a combination drug.[19] The combination of prednisolone and the antithrombotic drug dipyridamole has been described to suppress synergistically the release of pro-inflammatory cytokines and to produce anti-inflammatory activity in acute and chronic disease models (including arthritis) that may require only a sub-therapeutic dose of prednisolone. This alternative approach may create a dissociated activity profile with an increased therapeutic window through cellular network selective amplification of glucocorticoid-mediated anti-inflammatory signalling.[19] However, the exact molecular mechanism underlying the observed synergy and multi-target action of these two drugs remains obscure.

> ### ● ON THE HORIZON
>
> **Selective glucocorticoid receptor agonists**
> - Differential effects on transrepression (anti-inflammatory) vs transactivation (associated with adverse effects)
>
> **Nitro-steroids (steroids which release low levels of nitric oxide (NO))**
> - More effective in arthritis models of arthritis
> - NO release and increased IL-10 production.
>
> **Long-circulating liposomal glucocorticoids**
> - Improved delivery of steroids to inflamed joints
> - Prolonged local action
>
> **Combinations of steroids with other drugs**
> - Synergistic multi-target action (e.g., prednisolone and dipyridamole)
> - Achieving large effects on cytokine production
> - Allowing lower doses of steroid to be used

In conclusion, recent research has greatly increased our knowledge of conventional GCs as the best anti-inflammatory agents currently available. In particular, new findings on the effects of occupation of cytosolic GCRs on intracellular signaling, transcription processes and gene expression, on the existence of membrane-bound glucocorticoid receptors, on dose–effect relationships, and on timing of glucocorticoid administration have stimulated intensive research activity aimed at translating scientific research into clinical practice as quickly as possible. MR prednisone has been already approved for the treatment of rheumatoid arthritis and the associated morning stiffness in the European Union. Further clinical developments seem likely to follow, e.g., new GCR ligands and liposome encapsulation, all with a view to improving the risk–benefit ratio of GC therapy and the well-being of patients.

References

1. Buttgereit F, Straub RH, Wehling M, Burmester GR. Glucocorticoids in the treatment of rheumatic diseases. An update on mechanisms of action. Arthritis Rheum 2004;50:3408–17.
2. Schäcke H, Döcke WD, Asadullah K. Mechanisms involved in the side effects of glucocorticoids. Pharmacol Ther 2002;96:23–43.
3. Ramsey-Goldman R. Missed opportunities in physician management of glucocorticoid-induced osteoporosis? Arthritis Rheum 2002;46:3115–20.
4. Walsh LJ, Wong CA, Pringle M, Tattersfield AE. Use of oral corticosteroids in the community and the prevention of secondary osteoporosis: a cross section study. Br Med J 1996;313:344–6.
5. Almawi WY. Molecular mechanisms of glucocorticoid effects. Mod Aspects Immunobiol 2001;2:78–82.
6. Adcock IM, Lane SJ. Mechanisms of steroid action and resistance in inflammation. Corticosteroid-insensitive asthma: molecular mechanisms. J Endocrinol 2003;178:347–55.
7. Wikström AC. Mechanisms of steroid action and resistance in inflammation. Glucocorticoid action and novel mechanisms of steroid resistance: role of glucocorticoid receptor-interacting proteins for glucocorticoid responsiveness. J Endocrinol 2003;178:331–7.
8. Murphy PJ, Morishima Y, Chen H, et al. Visualization and mechanism of assembly of a glucocorticoid receptor-Hsp70 complex that is primed for subsequent Hsp90-dependent opening of the steroid binding cleft. J Biol Chem 2003;278:34764–73.
9. Davies TH, Ning YM, Sánchez ER. A new first step in activation of steroid receptors. J Biol Chem 2002;277:4597–600.
10. Yudt MR, Jewell CM, Bienstock RJ, Cidlowski JA. Molecular origins for the dominant negative function of human glucocorticoid receptor beta. Mol Cell Biol 2003;23:4319–30.
11. Croxtall JD, Choudhury Q, Flower RJ. Glucocorticoids act within minutes to inhibit recruitment of signaling factors to activated EGF receptors through a receptor-dependent, transcription-independent mechanism. Br J Pharmacol 2000;130:289–98.
12. Falkenstein E, Norman AW, Wehling M. Mannheim classification of nongenomically initiated (rapid) steroid actions(s). J Clin Endocrinol Metab 2000;85:2072–5.
13. Hafezi-Moghadam A, Simoncini T, Yang E, et al. Acute cardiovascular protective effects of corticosteroids are mediated by nontranscriptional activation of endothelial nitric oxide synthase. Nature Med 2002;8:473–9.
14. Buttgereit F, da Silva JA, Boers M, et al. Standardised nomenclature for glucocorticoid dosages and glucocorticoid treatment regimens: current questions and tentative answers in rheumatology. Ann Rheum Dis 2002;61:718–22.
15. Badsha H, Edwards CJ. Intravenous pulses of methylprednisolone for systemic lupus erythematosus. Semin Arthritis Rheum 2003;32:370–7.
16. Vasoo S, Thumboo J, Fong KY. Refractory immune thrombocytopenia in systemic lupus erythematosus: response to mycophenolate mofetil. Lupus 2003;12:630–2.
17. Bartholome B, Spies CM, Gaber T, et al. Membrane glucocorticoid receptors (mGCR) are expressed in normal peripheral blood mononuclear cells and upregulated following in vitro stimulation and in patients with rheumatoid arthritis. FASEB J 2004;18:70–80.
18. Buttgereit F, Saag K, Cutolo M, et al. The molecular basis for the effectiveness, toxicity, and resistance to glucocorticoids: focus on the treatment of rheumatoid arthritis. Scand J Rheumatol 2005;34:14–21.
19. Buttgereit F, Burmester GR, Straub RH, et al. Exogenous and endogenous glucocorticoids in rheumatic diseases. Arthritis Rheum 2011;63:1–9.
20. Hardy R, Rabbitt EH, Filer A, et al. Local and systemic glucocorticoid metabolism in inflammatory arthritis. Ann Rheum Dis 2008;67(9):1204–10.
21. Buttgereit F, Zhou H, Kalak R, et al. Transgenic disruption of glucocorticoid signaling in mature osteoblasts and osteocytes attenuates K/BxN mouse serum-induced arthritis in vivo. Arthritis Rheum 2009;60(7):1998–2007.
22. da Silva JAP, Jacobs JWG, Kirwan JR, et al. Long-term glucocorticoid therapy in rheumatoid arthritis: An evidence-based review of potential adverse effects. Ann Rheum Dis 2006;65:285–93.
23. Shane E, Rivas M, McMahon JD, et al. Bone loss and turnover after cardiac transplantation. J Clin Endocrinol Metab 1997;82:1497–506.
24. Kirwan JR, Bijlsma JW, Boers M, Shea BJ. Effects of glucocorticoids on radiological progression in rheumatoid arthritis. Cochrane Database Syst Rev 2007; (1): CD006356.
25. Graudal N, Jurgens G. Similar effects of disease modifying anti rheumatic drugs, glucocorticoids and biologic agents on radiographic progression in rheumatoid arthritis: meta-analysis of 70 randomised placebo or drug controlled studies including 112 comparisons. Arthritis Rheum 2010;62:2852–63.
26. Gaffney K, Ledingham J, Perry JD. Intra-articular triamcinolone hexacetonide in knee osteoarthritis: factors influencing the clinical response. Ann Rheum Dis 1995;54:379–81.
27. Bijlsma JW, Saag KG, Buttgereit F, da Silva JA. Developments in glucocorticoid therapy. Rheum Dis Clin North Am 2005;31:1–17.
28. van de Goes M, Jacobs J, Boers M, et al. Monitoring adverse events of low-dose glucocorticoid therapy: EULAR recommendations for clinical trials and daily practice. Ann Rheum Dis 2010;69:1913–9.
29. O'Brien C, Jia D, Plotkin L, et al. Glucocorticoids act directly on osteoblasts and osteocytes to induce their apoptosis and reduce bone formation and strength. Endocrinology 2004;145:1835–41.
30. Seibel MJ. Markers of bone turnover in transplantation osteopathy. Clin Lab 1996;42:927–37.
31. Yale SH, Limper AH. Pneumocystis carinii pneumonia in patients without acquired immunodeficiency syndrome: associated illnesses and prior corticosteroid therapy. Mayo Clin Proc 1996;71:5–13.
32. Saag KG, Koehnke R, Caldwell JR, et al. Low dose long-term corticosteroid therapy in rheumatoid arthritis: an analysis of serious adverse events. Am J Med 1994;96:115–23.
33. Buttgereit F, Doering G, Schaeffler A, et al. Efficacy of modified-release versus standard prednisone to reduce duration of morning stiffness of the joints in rheumatoid arthritis (CAPRA-1): a double-blind, randomised controlled trial. Lancet 2008;371(9608):205–14.
34. Buttgereit F, Doering G, Schaeffler A, et al. Targeting pathophysiological rhythms: prednisone chronotherapy shows sustained efficacy in rheumatoid arthritis. Ann Rheum Dis 2010;69:1275–80.
35. Song IH, Gold R, Straub RH, et al. New glucocorticoids on the horizon. J Rheumatol 2005;32:1199–207.
36. Kleiman A, Tuckermann JP. Glucocorticoid receptor action in beneficial and side effects of steroid therapy: lessons from conditional knockout mice. Mol Cell Endocrinol 2007;275(1–2):98–108.
37. Schacke H, Zollner TM, Docke WD, et al. Characterization of ZK 245186, a novel, selective glucocorticoid receptor agonist for the topical treatment of inflammatory skin diseases. Br J Pharmacol 2009;158(4):1088–103.

Immunomodulating pharmaceuticals

Gideon P. Smith,
Edwin S.L. Chan

Excitement over biologic agents and their capacity to regulate immunological reactions that significantly impact such immunologically mediated diseases as rheumatoid arthritis and inflammatory bowel disease (IBD) has overshadowed the prior emphasis on small immunomodulating molecules. Nonetheless, some small molecules (most notably methotrexate) have proven to be nearly as effective as biologics when tested head-to-head and combining small molecule therapies with biological agents generally leads to significantly better outcomes than use of either single agent.[1] Thus, it is likely that small molecule immunomodulatory drugs will continue to be in wide use for years to come.

Methotrexate

Methotrexate (Fig. 88.1) was employed in the treatment of rheumatoid arthritis (RA) as early as 1951, but its popularity as an immunomodulatory agent in RA did not come until the 1980s. Over the years, extensive experience with its use in inflammatory diseases as diverse as RA, psoriasis, and IBD have taught us a great deal about its safety, efficacy, and toxicities, as well as its anti-inflammatory mechanisms of action.

Pharmacokinetics of methotrexate

When used as an anti-inflammatory agent, methotrexate is administered at low doses, usually 10–25 mg/week once weekly by mouth, but it can also be given subcutaneously or intramuscularly. At these doses, oral bioavailability is high (60–70%) and although transporters are required for its absorption from the gut, saturation does not occur at these doses. A small portion of methotrexate is metabolized by hydroxylation into 7-hydroxymethotrexate. Both of these compounds have a serum half-life of no more than 8 hours. The much longer anti-inflammatory action, which allows for once a week dosing, must therefore be attributable to other longer lasting metabolites, such as polyglutamates. Excretion is mainly in the urine but some goes via the biliary tract. Therefore renal function is an important consideration in methotrexate dosing, and any medication that impairs glomerular filtration can also potentiate both methotrexate's effectiveness and its toxicity.[2]

Mechanisms of action for methotrexate

Methotrexate is an analogue of folic acid, which inhibits purine and pyrimidine synthesis and thus suppresses cellular proliferation (Table 88.1). These actions depend on inhibition of dihydrofolate reductase and hence, toxicities arising from high-dose methotrexate therapy can be treated with folic acid derivatives, such as leucovorin. However, folic or folinic acid, while often given in conjunction with methotrexate in inflammatory diseases to reduce the incidence of mucositis and bone marrow suppression, do not hamper its anti-inflammatory efficacy. Decreased serum levels of purines and pyrimidines have been observed following a single dose of methotrexate, along with decreased proliferation of antigen-stimulated lymphocytes. However, these changes are transient, and are not sufficient to explain the anti-inflammatory effectiveness of once-weekly dosing. This, and the low doses of methotrexate required to produce an anti-inflammatory effect, suggest that the anti-inflammatory actions are mediated via different mechanisms.

Methotrexate also blocks intracellular transmethylation reactions and inhibits the production of S-adenosylmethionine. Since S-adenosylmethionine is necessary for formation of the toxic polyamine metabolites spermine and spermidine, their accumulation at the inflammatory site is prevented. This inhibition of transmethylation is associated with an impairment of monocyte and lymphocyte function and thus potentially the synthesis of reactive oxygen species. However, diminution of transmethylation by the S-adenosylhomocysteine hydrolase inhibitor deaza-adenosine does not have any beneficial clinical effects in RA.

Methotrexate, and its long-acting polyglutamate metabolites, also exert anti-inflammatory effects by releasing adenosine, an endogenous autocoid.[3] As potent inhibitors of the enzyme 5-aminoimidazole-4-carboxamide ribonucleotide (AICAR) transformylase, methotrexate polyglutamates promote accumulation of AICAR in tissues. Since AICAR inhibits catabolizing enzymes for both adenosine and AMP (which can be dephosphorylated to adenosine), the net effect is an intracellular and extracellular increase in adenosine levels. These metabolic pathways are pharmacologically relevant since aminoimidazole carboxamide and adenosine increase in the urine following low-dose methotrexate treatment in patients with psoriasis.[4] Adenosine causes diminution of neutrophil accumulation, adhesion, phagocytosis and generation of reactive oxygen species, inhibition of adhesion molecule expression, suppression of pro-inflammatory cytokines and induction of anti-inflammatory cytokines, and modulation of macrophage and endothelial function.[2] Indeed, blockade of adenosine receptors reversed the anti-inflammatory effects of methotrexate in animal models. It has also been suggested that caffeine, itself a non-selective antagonist of adenosine receptors, may both reduce the effectiveness of methotrexate in RA. and protect against the development of liver cirrhosis, an important side effect of methotrexate therapy.[5]

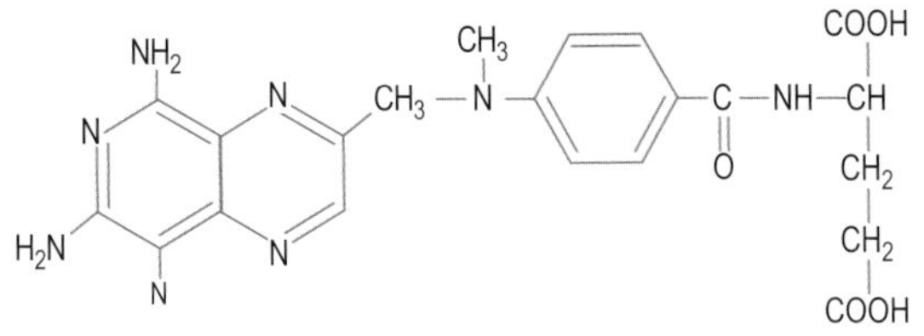

Methotrexate

Fig. 88.1 Methotrexate—chemical structure.

Table 88.1 Methotrexate: Mechanisms of action

Suggested mechanism	Rationale
Folate antagonism	Prevents purine and pyrimidine synthesis required for the proliferation of actively dividing immune cells such as lymphocytes
Inhibition of spermine and spermidine production	Reduces formation of polyamines harmful to tissues
Alteration of cellular redox state	Reversible inhibition of lymphocyte and macrophage functions
Release of adenosine	Generation of a potent endogenous anti-inflammatory mediator through inhibition of catabolism of both adenosine and AMP

Table 88.2 Methotrexate: Adverse effects

GI
Stomatitis
Anorexia
Nausea
Vomiting
Diarrhea
Cirrhosis
Pancreatitis

Hematologic
Leukopenia
Anemia
Thrombocytopenia
Hypogammaglobulinemia
Lymphoma

Cardiovascular
Pericarditis
Thrombosis

Pulmonary
Pulmonary fibrosis
Interstitial pneumonitis

Others
Skin rashes
Renal failure
Abortion
Impotence
Headache
Opportunistic infections

Adverse effects

THERAPEUTIC PRINCIPLES

Methotrexate

- Proven safety profile
- Concommitant administration of folic acid advisable
- Anti-inflammatory effects may be reduced by heavy use of caffeine
- Hepatotoxicity a rare but real concern
- Risk of hepatotoxicity increased with:
  - Alcohol use
  - Hepatitis
  - Diabetes
  - Obesity
  - Alpha-1-anttitrypsin deficiency

Over the years, methotrexate has proven to be one of the safest disease-modifying anti-rheumatic drugs (DMARDs) in use. Serious side effects such as cirrhosis are much less common than previously thought (Table 88.2), The use of folic acid has decreased the occurence of mucosal and gastrointestinal side effects, without limiting the anti-inflammatory activity, and cytopenias are managed adequately with regular blood counts While effects such as nausea and vomiting may resolve spontaneously or respond to dose reduction or folic acid supplementation, discontinuation of the medication is not needed for low-grade rises in transaminases. The risk of serious hepatotoxicity over five years of use is less than 1 in every 1000 patients with RA, but may be more common in patients with psoriasis. Risk factors such as ethanol consumption, hepatitis B and C, diabetes, obesity, and alpha-1-antitrypsin deficiency identify patients most likely to develop methotrexate-induced hepatic injury. However, other serious side effects such as pneumonitis may be overlooked, since early symptoms (mild cough or shortness of breath) are often ignored. Early identification allows for prompt discontinuation. The risk of developing solid tumors is debated, since there is an inreased risk of malignancies in some of the conditions for which methotrexate is used such as RA. Nevertheless, it is likely that this risk is real, since reports have documented tumor regression following discontinuation of methotrexate. But the absolute risk remains extremely small.

Sulfasalazine

Sulfasalazine (Fig. 88.2) was originally introduced for the treatment of RA in the late 1930s, with only limited benefit. It is now used in a wide range of inflammatory diseases, in particular, inflammatory bowel disease and the seronegative arthritides. It consists of a derivative of salicylic acid, 5-amino-salicylic acid, and the antimicrobial sulfapyridine. These two moieties are joined together by an azo bond. Which of the two is responsible for the drug's anti-inflammatory actions is unclear, but this appears to vary according to disease states. For instance, in IBD, 5-amino-salicylic acid is likely the main active component as it is poorly absorbed following metabolism by intestinal flora. But in inflammatory arthritides, sulfapyridine is likely to play a more important role, as it is relatively well absorbed and is approxmately 60% bioavailable. Since acetylation is the principal route of metabolism of sulfapyridine, acetylator status is a major determinant of the plasma half-life, and slow acetylators are also more liable to develop side effects.

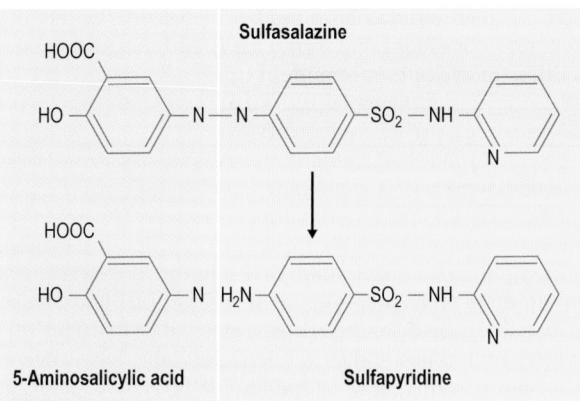

Fig. 88.2 **Sulfasalazine—chemical structure.**

Azathioprine

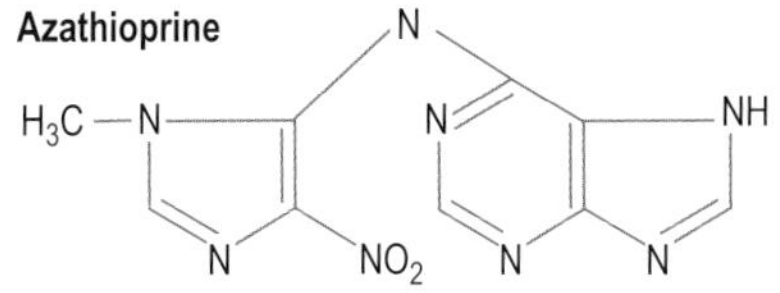

Fig. 88.3 **Azathioprine—chemical structure.**

Table 88.3 Principal enzymes involved in the metabolism of azathioprine

Enzyme	Action
Glutathione transferase	Cleaves azathioprine into 6-mercaptopurine and imidazole moieties
Thiopurine methyltransferase	Metabolism of 6-mercaptopurine
Xanthine oxidase	Conversion of 6-mercaptopurine to 6-thiouric acid

Mechanisms of action of sulfasalazine

KEY CONCEPTS

Sulfasalazine: mechanism of action

- Suppresses the proliferation of lymphocytes
- Suppresses pro-inflammatory cytokine production
- Inhibits activation of NF-κB
- Promotes adenosine accumulation

Sulfasalazine has several immunomodulatory effects. Lymphocyte proliferation is suppressed *in vitro*, and involves both B- and T-cell populations. *In vivo* a decrease in activated lymphocytes in the peripheral blood is seen. Tumor necrosis factor-α (TNF-α) production is suppressed and receptor binding is inhibited. Sulfasalazine also inhibits activation of the transcription factor, NF-κB. Like methotrexate, sulfasalazine inhibits AICAR transformylase, and thus promotes accumulation of adenosine, which has anti-inflammatory actions via the adenosine A_{2A} receptor. Indeed, treatment of animals with an adenosine A_{2A} receptor antagonist reversed the effect of sulfasalazine on reduction of leukocyte accumulation in an air-pouch model of inflammation.

Adverse effects

In a large series, a quarter of those treated over 11 years stopped treatment due to toxicity.[6] Most toxicities occurred early and were both trivial and resolved following therapy withdrawal. Most common are nausea, vomiting, anorexia, and rash. Serious cutaneous reactions such as exfoliative dermatitis or Stevens–Johnson syndrome are rare. Transaminasaemia and drug-induced hepatitis can occur. Blood dyscrasias with megaloblastic anaemia, neutropenia, aplastic anaemia, and myelodysplastic syndrome may arise. Neurologic adverse effects include headache or dizziness or more seriously peripheral neuropathy, Guillain-Barre syndrome, or transverse myelitis. Sulfasalazine should be avoided in patients with sulfonamide allergy and patients should be screened for G6PD deficiency.

Azathioprine

Azathioprine, an imidazolyl derivative of 6-mercaptopurine (Fig. 88.3), has been widely used in RA and IBD as well as solid organ transplants. Cleavage into 6-mercaptopurine and the imidazole moiety occurs rapidly within erythrocytes both enzymatically by glutathione transferase and non-enzymatically. A number of enzymes (Table 88.3) participate in the metabolism of 6-mercaptopurine into active and inactive compounds. One of these, thiopurine methyltransferase, is associated with genetic polymorphisms and inherited changes in its activity can impact patient response to azathioprine. Xanthine oxidase inactivates 6-mercaptopurine by converting it to 6-thiouric acid. Since this occurs mainly in the liver, the importance of the first pass metabolism is most marked in enzyme deficiency states, whether due to disease or to drugs such as allopurinol where toxicity from azathioprine therapy is a danger.

Proposed mechanisms of action for azathioprine

The immunomodulatory mechanism of azathioprine is still unclear. As purine analogues, the active metabolites interfere with the salvage pathway and *de novo* synthesis of purines, and are incorporated into RNA and DNA. Proliferation of both T and B lymphocytes is inhibited, and the function of natural killer cells is suppressed without a change in cell numbers. Antibody production is also suppressed although it is not known which of these effects are most clinically relevant *in vivo*. Cellular responses to chemoattractants are altered and the production of cytokines such as interleukin-6 (IL-6) is also affected.

Adverse effects

Azathioprine is generally well tolerated. The most common side effects are mild and relate to the gastrointestinal system. Pancreatitis can occur, however, as an idiosyncratic reaction. Hepatotoxicity and cholestasis are not uncommon while peliosis hepatic and nodular regenerative hyperplasia occur rarely. There have been reports of possible heightened risk for non-Hodgkin lymphoma but due to the rarity of these events, no definite link between azathioprine and malignancies has been established. Bone marrow suppression and opportunistic infections do, however, pose significant threats.

Cyclophosphamide

Alkylating agents were first used in the treatment of inflammatory diseases after promising reports with nitrogen mustard

Cyclophosphamide

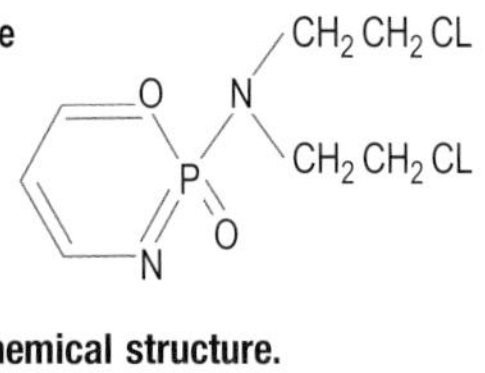

Fig. 88.4 Cyclophosphamide—chemical structure.

in RA. Cyclophosphamide (Fig. 88.4) is metabolized to produce the alkylating agent phosphorymide mustard, as well as acrolein, which though inactive as an anti-inflammatory agent, causes the hemorrhagic cystitis associated with cyclophosphamide therapy. While it can be given intravenously, oral bioavailability is high (>75%). Toxicity has severely limited its use in inflammatory diseases although it is useful in the management of lupus nephritis. The alkylating actions occur at guanine residues, principally on DNA but also on RNA, resulting in cross-linkable strands and disruption of transcription and translation.

Mechanisms of action of cyclophosphamide

This alkylating process has immunomodulating effects on resting and actively dividing cells. The number of circulating CD4 T lymphocytes are reduced, and to a lesser extent, CD8 T lymphocytes as well, thus reducing the CD4/CD8 ratio. Despite observations of an increase in immunoglobulin-secreting cells, B-cell function is suppressed and overall immunoglobulin synthesis is reduced.

Adverse effects

The best known toxicity is hemorrhagic cystitis. Since this occurs more frequently following oral dosing, this route of administration is rarely used. This may relate to continuous exposure of the bladder to acrolein, and the acrolein-neutralizing agent, 2-mercaptoethane sulfonate (Mesna), is used prophylactically along with copious hydration. Hemorrhagic myocarditis can also occur with myocardial necrosis, hemopericardium, and congestive cardiac failure as possible consequences. Survivors of acute cardiac toxicity do not, however, show any residual electrocardiographic or echocardiographic abnormalities.

As well as bone marrow suppression, reduction of fertility, and a heightened risk of infection, cyclophosphamide therapy has been associated with secondary malignancies that may occur years after cessation of the drug. Malignancies of the bladder (typically transitional cell carcinoma) tend to occur only in those patients with a history of treatment-related hemorrhagic cystitis. Myeloproliferative and lymphoproliferative disorders have also been associated with cyclophosphamide use.

Other nitrogen mustard derivatives

Chlorambucil, 4-[bis(2chlor-ethyl)amino]benzenebutanoic acid, has wide distribution in tissue and 87% oral bioavailability. Unlike cyclophosphamide, it does not require metabolism by the liver to become metabolically active.[7] The only FDA-approved indication is for treatment of chronic lymphocytic leukemia (CLL), but it has been investigated in treatment of the same wide range of inflammatory conditions as cyclophosphomide. The mechanism of action and side effect profile are similar to cyclophosphamide, but with a higher risk of permanent aplasia.[8]

Primarily used in multiple myeloma, melphalan is another phenylalanine derivative of nitrogen mustard. It has been less

widely adopted but has been used off-label in a variety of inflammatory conditions. Adverse effects and mechanism are as described for cyclophosphomide.

Leflunomide

Leflunomide is an inhibitor of *de novo* pyrimidine synthesis. Leflunomide (Fig. 88.5) is converted into the long-acting active compound A77 1726 (2-cyano-3-hydroxy-N-[4-trifluoromethyl]-butenamide) (Fig. 88.6), which is a reversible inhibitor of the pyrimidine synthesis enzyme dihydroorotate dehydrogenase. A77 1726 is highly plasma protein bound, and undergoes enterohepatic recirculation. Because of its long half-life, leflunomide therapy is usually started with a loading dose so that therapeutic levels can be rapidly achieved.

Mechanisms of action of leflunomide

By inhibiting pyrimidine synthesis, the availability of pyrimidine nucleotides becomes insufficient for proliferation of immune response cells. This deficiency is inadequately replenished by the salvage pathways, rendering cell proliferation inefficient and limiting the clonal expansion of T cells. B-cell proliferation is similarly suppressed with reduction of Cdk2, a cyclin-dependent kinase. Leflunomide also inhibits NF-κB activation. While the effects of moderate concentrations are reversed by uridine *in vitro*, this reversal does not occur at higher concentrations, suggesting that at higher concentrations, other mechanisms may be important. At higher concentrations, leflunomide is known to inhibit tyrosine kinase activity, although the relevance of this effect to therapeutically achievable concentrations *in vivo* remains questionable.

Adverse effects

Although similar to the toxicity profile of methotrexate, clinical trials have shown that these agents can be safely and effectively given together in patients with RA. However, transaminasaemia occurs more often than with methotrexate alone.[9,10] The most important toxicity of leflunomide is fulminant liver failure, which is rare but can be fatal. Gastrointestinal symptoms are more common but less serious. Most skin reactions are minor, but more serious manifestations such as Stevens–Johnson syndrome and toxic epidermal necrolysis occur occasionally.

Leflunomide

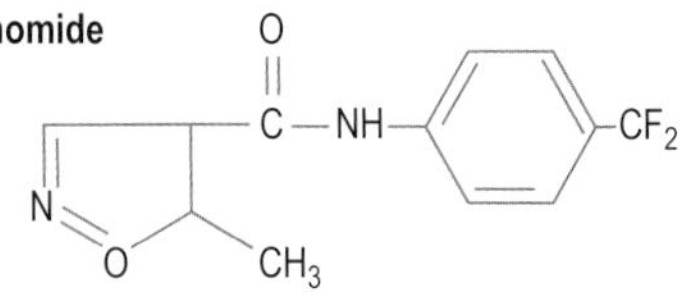

Fig. 88.5 Leflunomide—chemical structure.

A77 1726

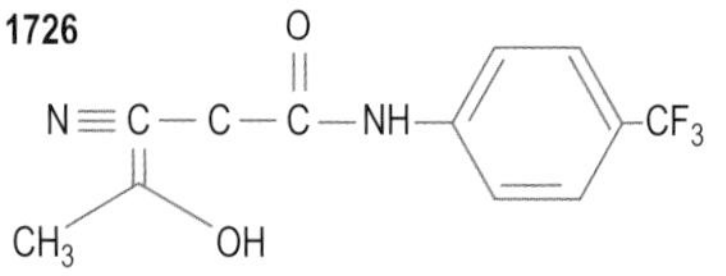

Fig. 88.6 A77 1726—chemical structure.

Mycophenolate mofetil

Mycophenolate mofetil (Fig. 88.7), widely used in solid organ transplantation, has also been increasingly successfully employed in treatment of autoimmune diseases. It is rapidly absorbed and hydrolyzed into the active compound mycophenolic acid, which is a reversible inhibitor of inosine monophosphate dehydrogenase. Since inosine monophosphate dehydrogenase is a key enzyme in the *de novo* synthesis of guanine nucleotides, its inhibition mainly affects T and B lymphocytes, which rely on this pathway as they lack the hypoxanthine-guanine phosphoribosyl transferase salvage pathway. The immunological effects are many-fold. DNA synthesis in lymphocytes requires the incorporation of guanine nucleotides and so proliferation of lymphocytes is suppressed. Antibody production and natural killer cell activity are also reduced and *in vitro* cytokine production by activated human mononuclear cells is affected.[11] In addition delayed-type hypersensitivity responses are suppressed. Although effective in a subset of psoriasis and RA patients, mycophenolate mofetil is not widely used for these indications due to the availability of other, more effective medications. It is, however, being used more often to treat diseases such as myositis, systemic contact dermatitis, severe atopic dermatitis, chronic urticaria, refractory pyoderma gangrenosum, bullous pemphigoid, pemphigoid vulgaris, and pemiphigoid foliaceus, and has a low-risk side-effect profile.

Adverse effects

Absolute contraindications for mycophenolate mofetil are drug allergy and pregnancy (Category C). Relative contraindications include lactation, renal, hepatic, or cardiopulmonary disease, and peptic ulcer. It is generally well tolerated when used in autoimmune diseases such as RA. The most common side effects are nausea, vomiting, abdominal discomfort, diarrhea, fever, headache, skin rash, back pain or tremor, but these do not often require drug discontinuation. Rarely, leukopenia and other cytopenias, cutaneous and non-cutaneous malignancies, and pancreatitis have been reported. Toxic doses have not been established for this medication. One patient suffered only moderate leukopenia with no significant gastrointestinal side effects after ingesting an overdose of 25 g of mycophenolate mofetil. Up to 4 g/day have been used in cardiac transplantation and up to 5 g/day in liver transplant patients. However, at doses above 2 g/day no increased efficacy was observed and patients were more likely to experience gastrointestinal symptoms and neutropenia. For this reason a maximum dose of 2 g/day is usually adopted in inflammatory conditions.

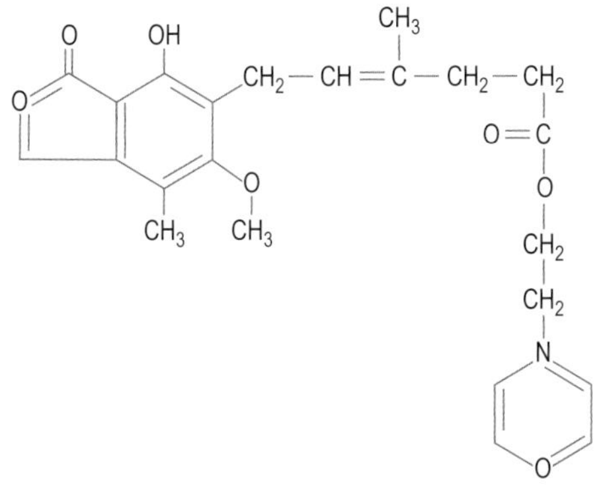

Fig. 88.7 Mycophenolate mofetil—chemical structure.

Hydroxyurea

Hydroxyurea inhibits the enzyme ribonucleotide reductase, which catalyzes the reduction of ribonucleotides to deoxyribonucleotides, and is thus essential in DNA synthesis. It is effective in the treatment of psoriasis.[12] Hydroxyurea is well tolerated with the most common side effects being hematological, usually megaloblastic anaemia, but also leukopenia and thrombocytopenia. Other significant but rare adverse effects include renal and GI toxicity, a dermatomyositis-like syndrome, leg ulcers, radiation recall, and leukemias.

Oral cyclosporine and tacrolimus (FK506)

● KEY CONCEPTS

Cyclosporine: mechanism of action

- Association with cyclophilin
- Formation of cyclosporine–cyclophilin complex
- Binds calcineurin
- Inactivates calcineurin
- Regulatory proteins unable to translocate into nucleus
- Transcription of pro-inflammatory genes affected

Cyclosporine (Fig. 88.8) and tacrolimus (Fig. 88.9) are structurally similar drugs that have been widely used in solid organ transplantation as well as immunological diseases. Cyclosporine has potent inhibitory effects in dampening the production of pro-inflammatory mediators such as IL-2 by immunocompetent cells, most importantly T lymphocytes. It does so through binding cyclophilin, which produces a cyclosporine–cyclophilin complex. This complex binds the serine/threonine phosphatase calcineurin[13] and disrupts the phosphorylation of regulatory proteins for which the transcription factor NF-AT is a critical component, thereby preventing these proteins from translocating into the nucleus. Thus, the transcription of genes such as IL-2, which induces mitogenesis in activated T cells, cannot be effectively activated. A number of other cytokines are affected, including IL-3, IL-6,

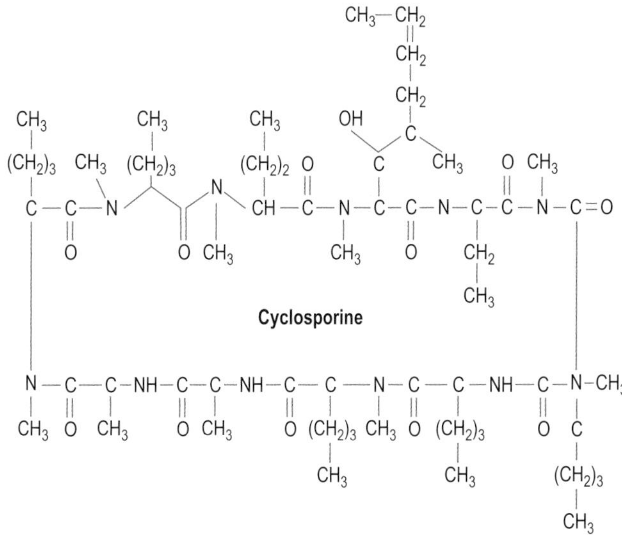

Fig. 88.8 Cyclosporine—chemical structure.

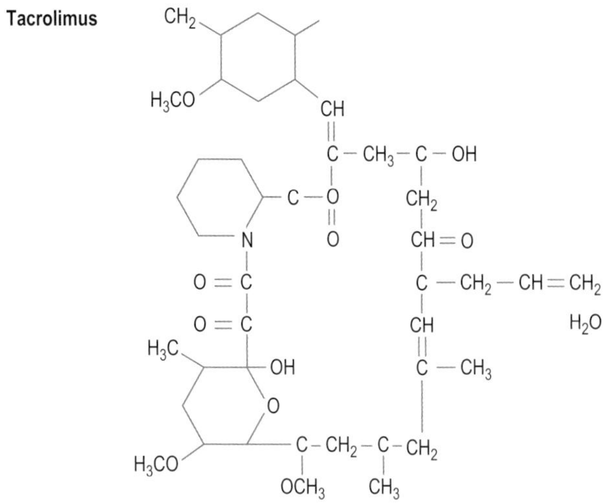

Tacrolimus

Fig. 88.9 Tacrolimus—chemical structure.

transforming growth factor-β, and interferon-γ (IFN-γ). Tacrolimus binds another T-cell-specific immunophilin (FK506-binding protein, FKBP), to form a tacrolimus–FKBP complex that inhibits calcineurin in much the same way as cyclosporine.[14]

Adverse effects

The most common side effects of cyclosporine are hypertension, hyperkalemia, hypomagnesemia, and hyperlipidemia. More importantly, cyclosporine has well-documented adverse effects on short- and long-term kidney function.[15] These data come from solid organ transplant patients, most notably renal transplant patients. In such patients, initial doses of 15–25 mg/kg/day led to a reduction in glomerular filtration rate and rise in serum creatinine in a percentage of patients, and histologically proven nephropathy.[16] The pathogenic mechanism of kidney damage is poorly understood but is believed to consist of two phases.[17] The first is a period of partial ischemia secondary to vascular contraction, which is reversible with dose reduction or drug discontinuation. The later, irreversible phase is due to chronic scarring of the glomeruli. Dosage recommendations in diseases such as psoriasis have therefore been at much lower daily doses of 5 mg/kg/day, with a reduction in dose if creatinine rises 30% above baseline. Otherwise healthy patients treated at these dosage levels have been successfully managed for multiple years on cyclosporine with no effect on glomerular filtration rate.[18] Nephrotoxicity has also been a concern during therapy with tacrolimus. Other adverse effects include increased rate of infections, malignancy, hepatotoxicity, gastrointestinal upset, rash, tremor, headache, and insomnia.

Topical pimecrolimus and tacrolimus

Tacrolimus is also available in topical formulation. Pimecrolimus is an alternative topical calcineurin inhibitor with similar structure and identical mechanisms of action. While the cyclosporine molecule is too large to penetrate skin (1203 Da), tacrolimus and pimecrolimus are much smaller molecules (804 and 80 Da, respectively) and can penetrate the skin. Both are FDA approved for the treatment of atopic dermatitis, but have found widespread use in many other conditions (psoriasis, oral and cutaneous lichen planus, vitiligo, pemphigoid and pemphigus).

They are most commonly utilized when long-term topical corticosteroids are contraindicated.

Adverse effects

The most common side effect is local irritation at the site of application in severely inflamed skin. Short-term combination with topical steroids is thus often initially used. An association with malignancy remains controversial. In 2005, 17 case reports of malignancy in patients using these topical agents resulted in a black-box warning. However, further studies suggested that the rate of lymphoma from these case reports was lower than the rate observed in the US general population. In 2006, the FDA revised the wording, but rightly or wrongly a black box warning remains in place on these products.

Sirolimus

Sirolimus is a macrolide that binds the cytosolic protein FK-binding protein 12 (FKBP12). In contrast to the tacrolimus–FKBP12 complex, which inhibits calcineurin, the sirolimus–FKBP12 complex directly binds the mammalian target of rapamycin (mTOR) complex 1 (mTORC1), thereby inhibiting the mTOR pathway. Thus, it inhibits the response to IL-2, blocking activation of T and B cells. It has shown promise in treating SLE, Sjögren's syndrome,[19] RA,[20] psoriasis, genetic disorders such as tuberous sclerosis, and neoplastic disorders such as Kaposi's sarcoma.[21] The principal advantage of sirolimus over tacrolimus or cyclosporine is reduced renal toxicity.

Imiquimod

Imiquimod (Fig. 88.10) is an imidazoquinoline drug that activates Toll-like receptor-7 and possesses both anti-viral and anti-tumor activities.[22] It is effective in the treatment of external genital warts due to human papillomavirus. Immune amplification responses are induced through stimulation of inflammatory cytokines.[23,24] Production of IFN-α is stimulated, which suppresses replication of viruses in infected keratinocytes. Natural killer cell activity is also increased, partly through the induction of oligoadenylate synthase. The increase of dermal IFN-α transcript levels is rapid and dramatic.[25] Other cytokines modulated by imiquimod include TNF-α and IL-12, with peripheral blood monocytes being most affected.[26,27] The overall effect is a shift from a Th2 toward a Th1-cytokine predominant profile. Other conditions where imiquimod is effective include actinic keratosis, herpes simplex, basal cell carcinoma, and molluscum contagiosum.

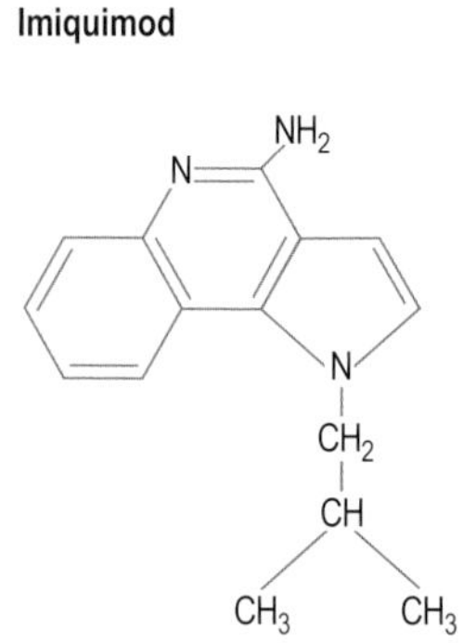

Imiquimod

Fig. 88.10 Imiquimod—chemical structure.

Adverse effects

Inflammation at the site of application is the most common adverse reaction. Other non-dermatological side effects such as fever, fatigue, myalgia, and headache have also been described.

5-Fluorouracil

5-Fluorouracil is a uracil analogue with two distinct modes of action. First, it inhibits cell proliferation via direct incorporation into RNA causing abnormal base pairing. Second, it binds thymidylate synthetase, blocking conversion of deoxyuridine monophosphate to deoxythymidine monophosphate, which is essential to DNA synthesis. It may also increase expression of p53, a gene often mutated in non-melanoma skin cancers.[28] It can be administered topically, intramuscularly, or intravenously. In topical form its primary indications are in the treatment of actinic keratosis, superficial basal cell carcinoma, Bowen's disease, keratoacanthoma, porokeratosis, and verruca vulgaris. However, it has also been used intravenously to treat recalcitrant psoriasis, mycosis fungoides, and scleroderma.

Adverse effects

The topical application is associated with an irritant dermatitis but this is sometimes seen as a marker of clinical efficacy. Adverse effects from parenteral administration are more severe and include bone marrow suppression, gastrointestinal toxicity, and cutaneous reactions. Partly because of this, parenteral administration has not been widely used for inflammatory conditions.

Glatiramer

Glatiramer acetate is a random polymer of glutamic acid, lysine, tyrosine, and alanine, four amino acids that are found in myelin basic protein (MBP). The mechanism of action for glatiramer is unknown, but its structural similarity to MBP may allow it to act as a decoy to immune targeting of myelin. It may also induce expression of glatiramer acetate-specific suppressor T cells that have been shown to be present in animal models. In contrast to imiquimod, glatiramer shifts the population of T cells from pro-inflammatory Th1 cells to regulatory Th2 cells that suppress the inflammatory response. Glatarimer is FDA approved for the treatment of adults with relapsing-remitting multiple sclerosis, even after only one event.

Adverse effects

Absolute contraindications include allergy to glatiramer, or to mannitol. It is unknown whether the drug is secreted during lactation. The most common adverse effects after subcutaneous injection are local injection site reactions, flushing, rash, dyspnea, and transient chest pain.

Fingolimod (FTY720)

Fingolimod is a relatively new immunomodulator for treating multiple sclerosis. It is a structural analogue of sphingosine and is phosphorylated intracellularly by sphingosine kinases.[29]

When signaled via one of the sphingosine-1-phosphate receptors, S1PR1, it is believed to prevent migration of lymphocytes from the lymph nodes. However, fingolimod has also been reported to act as a cPLA2 inhibitor,[30] a cannabinoid receptor antagonist,[31] and a ceramide synthase inhibitor.[32] Thus far fingolimod has only been FDA-approved for use in multiple sclerosis. However, it has also shown promise in murine models of SLE[33] and RA.[34] It could also have a role in the treatment of cutaneous inflammatory conditions such as psoriasis and atopic dermatitis.[35]

Adverse effects

The most common side effects are headache and fatigue but these are relatively minor. However, it has also been associated with serious infections, an increased rate of skin cancers, bradycardia, and one case of focal haemorrhagic encephalitis.

Conclusions

There is a wide range of new and traditional small molecule immunomodulators. The "traditional" molecules come with a long history of efficacy and known side effects that allows their safe and accurate use. Despite the introduction of biologics, traditional small molecule therapies such as methotrexate and cyclosporine remain both clinically efficacious and cost effective and thus continue to be useful tools on the pharmaceutical armamentarium. However, as our understanding of the pathways involved in inflammation has evolved, our therapeutics have been refined, allowing for the production of topically effective calcineurin inhibitors such as tacrolimus and pimecrolimus that avoid the adverse effects of systemic cyclosporine or topical steroids, and reduction of toxicity profiles of systemic FKBP2-signaling agents with the introduction of sirolimus. Newer agents, such as glatiramer and fingolimod, are being used to treat multiple sclerosis, a disease resistant to more traditional therapies, and although not in current clinical use in other inflammatory disorders, these have shown promise in animal models of SLE and RA. The field of small molecule immunomodulators therefore remains one of both current clinical relevance and continuing, exciting new developments.

● ON THE HORIZON

- Refinement of our understanding of the pathways and actions of receptors targeted by our current medications is the key to producing more elegant therapies.
- Separating therapeutic effects from the pathways leading to side effects would enable much safer and more tolerable small molecule medications.
- Better understanding of the dysregulation that occurs in inflammatory conditions, and the activation of the immune system will be essential to ensuring the efficacy of such new modalities.

The challenge in the next 5–10 years is to continue this refinement in the targeting of small molecules. Many of the agents in current use target early parts of pathways or indiscriminately trigger multiple receptors. This results in a greater range of side effects and limits the achievement of adequate dosing levels. A prime example of this is methotrexate, which leads to increased adenosine levels and thus triggers all four adenosine receptors. By developing molecules targeting, for instance, just the adenosine A_{2A} receptor, not only would we avoid the side effects attributable to other adenosine receptors, but we might also avoid the adverse effects of methotrexate on bone marrow and mucous membranes via its inhibition of dihydrofolate reductase. More specific targeting of pathways may similarly reduce side effects of other agents and make for more effective therapeutics. This will require both a better understanding of the immune system, and its dysregulation in disease, as well as the development and application of clinically relevant models in which to test new agents.

References

1. Pincus T, Furer V, Sokka T. Underestimation of the efficacy, effectiveness, tolerability, and safety of weekly low-dose methotrexate in information presented to physicians and patients. Clin Exp Rheumatol 2010;28(5 Suppl. 61):S68–S79.
2. Chan ES, Cronstein BN. Molecular action of methotrexate in inflammatory diseases. Arthritis Res 2002;4(4):266–73.
3. Cronstein BN, Naime D, Ostad E. The antiinflammatory mechanism of methotrexate. Increased adenosine release at inflamed sites diminishes leukocyte accumulation in an in vivo model of inflammation. J Clin Invest 1993;92(6):2675–82.
4. Baggott JE, Morgan SL, Sams WM, Linden J. Urinary adenosine and aminoimidazolecarboxamide excretion in methotrexate-treated patients with psoriasis. Arch Dermatol 1999;135(7):813–7.
5. Chan ES, Montesinos MC, Fernandez P, et al. Adenosine A(2A) receptors play a role in the pathogenesis of hepatic cirrhosis. Br J Pharmacol 2006;148(8):1144–55.
6. Amos RS, Pullar T, Bax DE, et al. Sulphasalazine for rheumatoid arthritis: toxicity in 774 patients monitored for one to 11 years. Br Med J (Clin Res Ed) 1986;293(6544):420–3.
7. Lind MJ, Ardiet C. Pharmacokinetics of alkylating agents. Cancer Surv 1993;17:157–88.
8. Wolverton SE, Remlinger K. Suggested guidelines for patient monitoring: hepatic and hematologic toxicity attributable to systemic dermatologic drugs. Dermatol Clin 2007;25(2):195–205 vi–ii.
9. Kremer JM, Genovese MC, Cannon GW, et al. Concomitant leflunomide therapy in patients with active rheumatoid arthritis despite stable doses of methotrexate. A randomized, double-blind, placebo-controlled trial. Ann Intern Med 2002;137(9):726–33.
10. Weinblatt ME, Kremer JM, Coblyn JS, et al. Pharmacokinetics, safety, and efficacy of combination treatment with methotrexate and leflunomide in patients with active rheumatoid arthritis. Arthritis Rheum 1999;42(7):1322–8.
11. Nagy SE, Andersson JP, Andersson UG. Effect of mycophenolate mofetil (RS-61443) on cytokine production: inhibition of superantigen-induced cytokines. Immunopharmacology 1993;26(1):11–20.
12. Menter A, Korman NJ, Elmets CA, et al. Guidelines of care for the management of psoriasis and psoriatic arthritis: section 4. Guidelines of care for the management and treatment of psoriasis with traditional systemic agents. J Am Acad Dermatol 2009;61(3):451–85.
13. Liu J, Farmer Jr JD, Lane WS, et al. Calcineurin is a common target of cyclophilin-cyclosporin A and FKBP-FK506 complexes. Cell 1991;66(4):807–15.
14. Baughman G, Wiederrecht GJ, Campbell NF, et al. FKBP51, a novel T-cell-specific immunophilin capable of calcineurin inhibition. Mol Cell Biol 1995;15(8):4395–402.
15. Wilkinson A, Ross EA, Hawkins R, Danovitch G. Measurement of true glomerular filtration rate in renal transplant patients receiving cyclosporine. Transplant Proc 1987;19(1 Pt 2):1739–41.
16. Mihatsch MJ, Antonovych T, Bohman SO, et al. Cyclosporin A nephropathy: standardization of the evaluation of kidney biopsies. Clin Nephrol 1994;41(1):23–32.
17. Gaston RS. Chronic calcineurin inhibitor nephrotoxicity: reflections on an evolving paradigm. Clin J Am Soc Nephrol 2009;4(12):2029–34.
18. Kessel A, Toubi E. Cyclosporine-A in severe chronic urticaria: the option for long-term therapy. Allergy 2010;65(11):1478–82.
19. Perl A. Emerging new pathways of pathogenesis and targets for treatment in systemic lupus erythematosus and Sjogren's syndrome. Curr Opin Rheumatol 2009;21(5):443–7.
20. Laragione T, Gulko PS. mTOR regulates the invasive properties of synovial fibroblasts in rheumatoid arthritis. Mol Med 2010;16(9–10):352–8.
21. Paghdal KV, Schwartz RA. Sirolimus (rapamycin): from the soil of Easter Island to a bright future. J Am Acad Dermatol 2007;57(6):1046–50.
22. Hemmi H, Kaisho T, Takeuchi O, et al. Small anti-viral compounds activate immune cells via the TLR7 MyD88-dependent signaling pathway. Nat Immunol 2002;3(2):196–200.
23. Dahl MV. Imiquimod: an immune response modifier. J Am Acad Dermatol 2000;43(1 Pt 2):S1–S5.
24. Skinner Jr. RB. Imiquimod. Dermatol Clin 2003;21(2):291–300.
25. Imbertson LM, Beaurline JM, Couture AM, et al. Cytokine induction in hairless mouse and rat skin after topical application of the immune response modifiers imiquimod and S-28463. J Invest Dermatol 1998;110(5):734–9.
26. Gibson SJ, Imbertson LM, Wagner TL, et al. Cellular requirements for cytokine production in response to the immunomodulators imiquimod and S-27609. J Interferon Cytokine Res 1995;15(6):537–45.
27. Tyring S. Imiquimod applied topically: A novel immune response modifier. Skin Therapy Lett 2001;6(6):1–4.
28. Ceilley RI. Mechanisms of action of topical 5-fluorouracil: Review and implications for the treatment of dermatological disorders. J Dermatolog Treat 2012;23(2):83–9. Epub 2010 Oct 31.
29. Billich A, Bornancin F, Devay P, et al. Phosphorylation of the immunomodulatory drug FTY720 by sphingosine kinases. J Biol Chem 2003;278(48):47408–15.
30. Payne SG, Oskeritzian CA, Griffiths R, et al. The immunosuppressant drug FTY720 inhibits cytosolic phospholipase A2 independently of sphingosine-1-phosphate receptors. Blood 2007;109(3):1077–85.
31. Paugh SW, Cassidy MP, He H, et al. Sphingosine and its analog, the immunosuppressant 2-amino-2-(2-[4-octylphenyl]ethyl)-1,3-propanediol, interact with the CB1 cannabinoid receptor. Mol Pharmacol 2006;70(1):41–50.
32. Berdyshev EV, Gorshkova I, Skobeleva A, et al. FTY720 inhibits ceramide synthases and up-regulates dihydrosphingosine 1-phosphate formation in human lung endothelial cells. J Biol Chem 2009;284(9):5467–77.
33. Ando S, Amano H, Amano E, et al. FTY720 exerts a survival advantage through the prevention of end-stage glomerular inflammation in lupus-prone BXSB mice. Biochem Biophys Res Commun 2010;394(3):804–10.
34. Tsunemi S, Iwasaki T, Kitano S, et al. Effects of the novel immunosuppressant FTY720 in a murine rheumatoid arthritis model. Clin Immunol 2010;136(2):197–204.
35. Herzinger T, Kleuser B, Schafer-Korting M, Korting HC. Sphingosine-1-phosphate signaling and the skin. Am J Clin Dermatol 2007;8(6):329–36.

89

Protein kinase antagonists as therapeutic agents for immunological and inflammatory disorders

Arian Laurence, Kamran Ghoreschi, Mary Byrne, John J. O'Shea

Reversible phosphorylation is one of the major mechanisms controlling protein activity in all eukaryotic cells and, as such, is involved in all fundamental cellular processes including: cell cycle and cell growth, cell shape and movement, metabolism, differentiation, and apoptosis. This covalent modification is a major means for transmitting information from outside the cell and between subcellular components within the cell. Phosphorylation is a major mechanism underlying normal signaling, as exemplified by insulin and other growth factors, but in addition, the importance of protein phosphorylation is supported by evidence that mutations and dysregulation of protein kinases play causal roles in human disease. This is especially true in cancer, in which mutant protein kinases or their upstream activators function as oncogenes.

From the point of view of an immunologist, protein phosphorylation is also the major mechanism by which immune receptors including the T-cell receptor, B-cell receptor, and NK and Fc receptors trigger signaling. The first step in signaling by multi-chain immune recognition receptors (such as the aforementioned receptors) is tyrosine phosphorylation of the receptor itself and adapter molecules like LAT, mediated by Src family protein tyrosine kinases (PTK). This leads to the recruitment of PTK members Syk and Zap70 followed by phosphorylation of adapters like SLP-76 and the activation of Tec family PTKs. These initial steps lead to activation of serine-threonine kinases including the mitogen-activated protein kinases (MAPKs) and protein kinase C (PKC) family (Fig. 89.1). We now know a great deal about details through which the cascade of protein phosphorylation links events at the plasma membrane to calcium modulation, cytoskeletal rearrangement, gene transcription, and other canonical features of lymphocyte action (Chapter 12).

Similarly, a critical first step in signaling by many cytokine receptors is the activation of phosphorylation (Table 89.1). The receptors for some cytokines, like stem cell factor and platelet-derived growth factor (PDGF), are receptor tyrosine kinases (RTKs), whereas the receptors for transforming growth factor family cytokines are receptor serine-threonine kinases. Type I and II cytokine receptors signal via the activation of receptor-associated Janus kinases (JAKs, see below, Table 89.2) (Chapter 9). Other cytokines like interleukin (IL)-1 and tumor necrosis factor (TNF) initiate signaling in a kinase-independent manner, but nonetheless signal through kinase cascades to exert their effects. It is clear that many aspects of protein phosphorylation are of major importance in immune and inflammatory mechanisms.

The non-redundant functions of various kinases in different immune cell protein kinases are well exemplified by different knock-out mice and humans with mutations. Based on these findings, targeting protein kinases has been proposed as a useful strategy in the development of novel immunosuppressant drugs. As will be discussed, the targeting of protein kinases is one of the most active areas of pharmaceutical drug development (Table 89.3), much of the impetus coming from oncology. The field is so vast that it is impractical to comprehensively review all this information in one chapter; therefore, we will both focus on important historical precedents in the field and then discuss drugs and targets that are most immunologically relevant. We will start by briefly reviewing some of the basics of kinase biochemistry.

Structure and function of protein kinases

● KEY CONCEPTS

Kinase families

- 518 kinases in the genome
- 90 protein tyrosine kinases (e.g., Jak's)
- 400 protein serine/ threonine kinases:
- AGC kinase family (e.g., protein kinase B/ Akt)
- CAMK kinase family (e.g., calmodulin-dependent kinase)
- CMGC kinase family (e.g., MAP kinases: ERK, JNK, p38)
- STE kinase family (e.g., MAPK kinases, MAPKK kinases)
- TKL kinase family (e.g., IRAK)
- Others: casein kinase family, GYC kinase family, IKK family

Protein kinases or phosphotransferases catalyze the transfer of γ phosphate of a purine nucleotide triphosphate (i.e., ATP and GTP), to the hydroxyl groups of their protein substrates. They generate phosphate monoesters using protein alcohol groups (on serine and threonine residues) and/or protein phenolic groups (on tyrosine residues) as phosphate acceptors. Thus, protein kinases can be classified by the amino acid substrate preference: serine/threonine kinases, tyrosine kinases, and dual kinases (meaning that both serine/threonine and tyrosine residues can be phosphorylated). Almost all protein kinases have catalytic domains that belong to a single eukaryotic protein kinase (ePK) superfamily. The common evolutionary ancestry of the kinase domain (also known as the catalytic domain), which consists of 250–300 amino acid residues, manifests as a highly conserved three-dimensional structure. There are 518 kinases in the human genome divided into eight major groups, which in totality represent 1.7% of the human genome. The PTK family has 90 members, one-third of which RTKs and the remainder are cytoplasmic proteins that typically function in close proximity to, and downstream of receptor–ligand complexes.

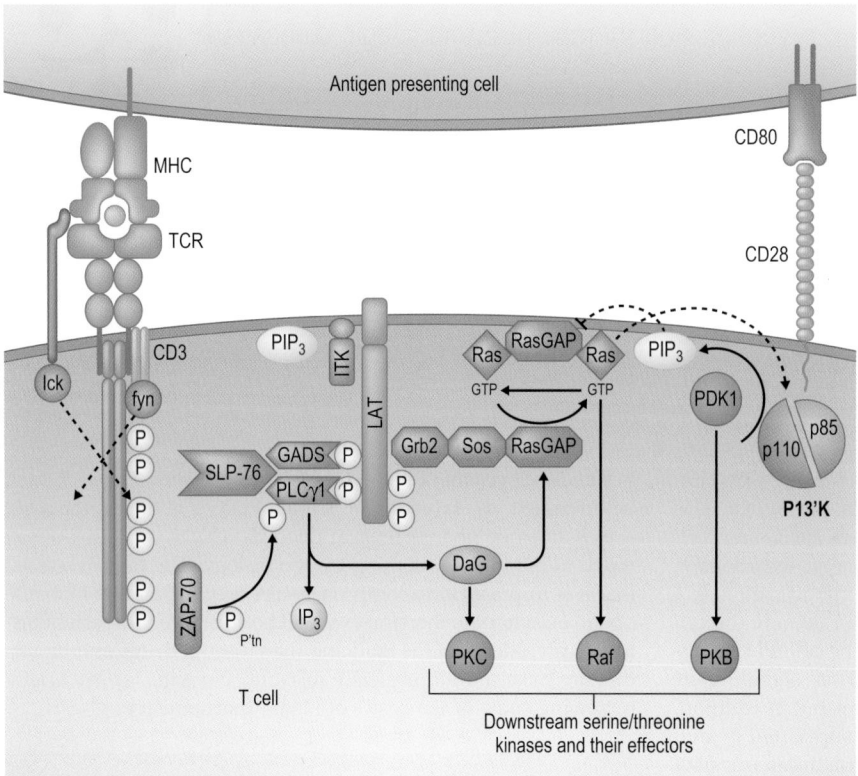

Fig. 89.1 The proximal signaling events in response to T-cell receptor activation by antigen presented by an antigen-presenting cell. Tyrosine and lipid kinases are indicated in red, serine/threonine kinases indicated in blue.

Table 89.1 The common gamma chain receptor family of cytokine receptors

Cytokine receptor	IL-2R	IL-4R	IL-7R	IL-9R	IL-15R	IL-21R
Functions	Control of peripheral self tolerance (mice)	Regulation of B-cell function (in concert with IL-21 and IL-25)	Thymocyte survival and development factor	Goblet cell hyperplasia	CD8⁺ memory T-cell survival and proliferation factor	T- and B-cell proliferation factor
	Development and maintenance of T regulatory cells. Inhibition of Th17 differentiation	Immunoglobulin class switching	Peripheral T-cell survival factor. Mediates homeostatic reconstitution of lymphopenic animals	Mucus production	Peripheral T-cell survival factor. Mediates homeostatic reconstitution of lymphopenic animals	Regulates immunoglobulin production (with IL-4)
	Differentiation of helper and cytotoxic T cells	Differentiation of helper T cells (Th2 lineage)	B-cell progenitor survival factor (mice)		NK-cell development, differentiation and survival factor	NK-cell proliferation and activation factor. Differentiation of helper T cells (Th17 and T follicular helper cell lineages)
	In vitro expansion and differentiation of antigen-selected T and NK cells	Co-stimulant for growth in T, B, and mast cells				
		Inhibition of Th1 differentiation and macrophage activation				
Downstream signaling pathways	PI3K, Ras MAPK, STAT1,3,5	PI3K, Ras MAPK, STAT6,5	PI3K, STAT(1), (3), 5	PI3K, Ras MAPK, STAT1,3,(5)	PI3K, Ras MAPK, STAT1,3,5	PI3K, Ras MAPK, STAT1,3,(5)

Table 89.2 The Jak family of tyrosine kinases

Gene	Murine phenotype associated with gene deletion	Associated receptor
Jak1	Perinatal lethality, block in thymocyte development	Many including IL-7R and IFN R's
Jak2	Embryonic lethality due to anemia	Epo receptor
Jak3	T-, B-, NK-cell lymphopenia, SCID phenotype	Common gamma chain receptor
Tyk2	Failure to clear *Toxoplasma*, reduced arthritis	IL-12/23 receptor

In terms of its catalytic role, the kinase domain has three functions: the binding of the ATP (or GTP) phosphate donor as a complex with a divalent cation (usually Mg^{2+} or Mn^{2+}), the binding of the protein substrate, and the transfer of the γ-phosphate from ATP or GTP to the protein substrate. Despite the huge number of serine/threonine and tyrosine kinases there is evidence of a common ancestor and this is reflected in structural similarities particularly in the active (ATP bound) confirmation. The major kinase domains of all typical protein kinases consists of two lobes (N- and C-lobe) that surround the nucleotide binding site (Fig. 89.2).[1] The smaller N-lobe consists of a cluster of β-pleated sheets with a single α-helix. The larger C-lobe is made up of α-helices. Within the C-lobe lies the substrate-binding site, typically a groove on the surface. A hinge region connects the two lobes. The hinge, together with two loops emerging from each lobe, forms the ATP binding pocket: the primary target for most kinase inhibitors. In many protein kinases a loop emerging from the C-lobe must be phosphorylated in order for the kinase to be fully active. This is known as the activation loop. Substrates of PTKs often include the activation loop of downstream kinases, creating signaling cascades of proteins that in turn phosphorylate each other; examples include the MAPKs (Fig. 89.3).

A short history of the generation of kinase inhibitors

Given that protein kinases bind ATP, the notion that therapeutically useful kinase inhibitors could be generated initially met with some skepticism. First, as there are more than 500 human kinases, many of which serve critical cellular functions, would it really be possible to attain the specificity needed? Second, protein kinases are not the only kinases—there are lipid kinases and nucleotide kinases, in addition to numerous other types of ATP binding proteins. Third, despite the many potential ways of designing a small molecule kinase inhibitor, in practice, the existing successful inhibitors all work by sitting within the ATP binding pocket.[2] A priori then, one might conclude that it would be impossible to generate an antagonist that did not target some other essential ATP-dependent process. Fortunately though, this dismal view does not reflect reality.

●THERAPEUTIC PRINCIPLES

- Drugs can inhibit protein tyrosine kinases with a high degree of specificity.
- Multikinase inhibitors can be well tolerated and be more efficacious than single kinase inhibitors.

Imatinib and other first-generation protein tyrosine kinase inhibitors

The first FDA-approved protein kinase inhibitor is imatinib (Table 89.3). The mutated form of the ABL tyrosine kinase, BCR-ABL, represents a fusion protein that is the result of a chromosomal translocation (Philadelphia chromosome) observed in patients suffering from chronic myeloid leukemia (CML). The pathognomonic presence of BCR-ABL in CML has led to it becoming one of the most intensively studied protein tyrosine kinases. The fusion protein consists of an oligomerization domain, a pleckstrin homology (PH) domain, and a DBL/CDC24 guanine nucleotide exchange factor homology domain that contains the *N*-terminal breakpoint cluster region (BCR) of the protein. The ABL half of the fusion protein contains a tyrosine kinase domain, a Src homology 2 (SH2) domain, and a DNA-binding domain together with nuclear localization and nuclear export motifs. The ABL kinase is constitutively active within the fusion protein and has been implicated in initiating numerous signaling pathways that mediate cell survival and proliferation. In view of this and the essential requirement for BCR-ABL kinase activity in CML it was thought to be an ideal target despite the aforementioned caveats with targeting protein kinases. As predicted, imatinib has revolutionized the treatment of CML. This inhibitor has been remarkably successful in arresting the progression of the CML, but is also well tolerated with minimal side effects.[3]

While conservation of the kinase ATP binding pocket has posed a potential problem for designing kinase inhibitors, in practice this has not happened for a number of reasons. It has been been argued that although different kinases are structurally similar in an active ATP-bound confirmation, the inactive confirmation is more unique and can be used to generate selective inhibitors.[4] The ATP binding region is made up of six polar amino acid residues that are invariant across whole families of kinases; similarly there are a number of lipophilic residues that are highly conserved. In addition, this critical region contains an amino acid whose amide carbonyl binds to N-6 of adenine in the active confirmation. The side chain of this amino acid sticks into the reaction pocket in the inactive state and for this reason is referred to as "the gate keeper residue."[5] As the side chain is not involved in direct ATP binding it varies across kinases, and variation of this gatekeeper residue is exploited by a number of inhibitors that are able to bind the inactive confirmation of specific kinases. In the case of ABL kinase the gatekeeper residue is threonine, which binds directly to a methyl group of the phenyl ring of the ABL kinase inhibitor imatinib.[4] Across the collective kinase superfamily almost any amino acid can appear as the gatekeeper, although in practice it is typically a bulky non-polar residue (methionine, tyrosine, phenylalanine, lysine).[5] Clearly, as more detailed structural information emerges from the many protein kinases, capitalizing upon subtle differences in structure would, in principle, be expected to improve potency and specificity. For instance, cyclin-dependent kinase 2 (CDK2) contains an additional pocket on its C-lobe next to the ATP binding pocket.[6] A number of CDK2-specific inhibitors exploit this by binding to both pockets.

Of further structural significance is the emergence of tumor drug resistance in response to the chronic use of protein kinase inhibitors. Mutant forms of BCR-ABL, KIT, and EGFR have been associated with loss of drug activity and disease relapse. Interestingly one of the commonest sites of mutation is the otherwise conserved "gatekeeper residue." The appearance of such mutations that lead to imatinib resistance has led to the need for other drugs with broader activity against a number of kinases. Thus, in the setting of oncology, "multikinase" inhibitors, including

Table 89.3 Selected developing/marketing kinase inhibitors and related drugs

Mechanism	Compound	Kinase inhibited	Comments
Direct binding to the kinase	Imatinib	KIT, PDGFR, and Bcr-Abl.	Approved for treatment of CML, eosinophilic leukemia, and gastric stromal tumors. Under evaluation in multiple types of cancer and in combination with other cancer drugs.
	Vandetanib	VEGFR-2, EGFR, RET, and ErbB-1 tyrosine kinases	Approved in 2011 for certain types of progressive medullary thyroid cancer. In Phase II trials for treatment of advanced non-small-cell lung cancer; has completed Phase II trials for breast cancer. Also in clinical development for treatment of additional cancers.
	Erlotinib	HER1/EGFR tyrosine kinase; mechanism of anti-tumor action is not fully characterized	Approved for treatment of pancreatic cancer and certain categories of NSCLC. In Phases II and III trials for various other cancers.
	Gefitinib	EGFR tyrosine kinases	Approved for use in NSCLC after failure of platinum-based and docetaxel regimens. In Phase II & III trials for various other cancers.
	Nilotinib	Inhibits multiple RTKs including Bcr-abl, C-kit, platelet-derived growth factor receptor kinase	Approved for Philadelphia chromosome-positive CML; in Phase III trials for GI (stromal) cancer and melanoma, Phase II trials for pulmonary HTN
	Sorafenib	Dual specific inhibitor blocking both tyrosine and serine/threonine kinases including: RAF kinase, VEGFR-2, VEGFR-3, PDGFR-B, KIT, FLT-3, and RET.	FDA-approved for treatment of advanced renal cell carcinoma and hepatocellular cancer. In Phase III clinical trials for NSCLC, thyroid and breast cancer.
	Dasatinib	Multiple Src family tyrosine kinases including BCR-Abl	Approved for treatment of adult chronic myelogenous leukemia (CML) and Philadelphia chromosome positive acute lymphoblastic leukemia (ALL). May circumvent imatinib resistance in CML patients due to less stringent binding requirements. In Phase III trials for prostate cancer.
	Lapatinib	ErbB-2 and EGFR kinases.	Approved for treatment of breast cancer. Also in development for treatment of renal, gastric, and head and neck cancers.
	Sunitinib	Inhibits multiple RTKs including PDGFR3-alpha, PDGFR-beta, VEGFR1 VEGFR2, VEGFR3, Kit, FLT3, CSF-1R, and RET.	For treatment of gastrointestinal stromal tumor after disease progression on or intolerance of imatinib mesylate, and for treatment of advanced renal cell carcinoma and pancreatic neuroendocrine tumors. In Phases I & II trials for various other cancers.
	Pazopanib	Inhibits multiple RTKs including PDGFR3-alpha, PDGFR-beta, VEGFR1 VEGFR2, VEGFR3, cKIT, Lck, c-FMS, FGFR-1, and FGFR-3	Approved for treatment of advanced renal cell cancer. An eyedrop formulation is under development for age-related macular degeneration.
	Axitinib	VEGFR1, 2 and 3, PDGFR-ß and KIT	In the USA pre-approval process for renal cancer; has orphan drug status for follicular, medullary, and anaplastic thyroid carcinoma and metastatic or locally advanced papillary thyroid cancer
	Brivanib	VEGF receptor-2, FGF receptor-1	In Phase III clinical trials for colorectal and liver cancers. Results expected in 2011. In Phase II trials for various other cancers.
	Bosutinib	Src, Bcr-Ab	In Phase III clinical trials for CML; in Phase I & II trials for various other cancers
	Intedanib	VEGFR-2, PDGF, FGF	In Phase III clinical trials for ovarian cancer, NSCLC, and idiopathic pulmonary fibrosis; in Phase I & II trials for various other cancers
	Linifanib	All members of the VEGF and PDGF receptor families, including FLT-3 and c-kit	In Phase III trials for liver cancer with results expected in Feb 2012; in Phase I & II trials for various other cancers
	Tivozanib	VEGF	In the EU pre-approval process for renal cancer, in Phase III studies in the USA for renal cancer
	Crizotinib	ALK, c-Met	Has orphan drug status in the USA for treatment of ALK-positive NSCLC; in Phase III trials for lung cancer
Receptor-associated tyrosine kinases	Tofacitinib	Janus kinase (JAK) 3	Recommended for FDA approval for the treatment of rheumatoid arthritis (RA). Efficacy shown in animal models of solid organ transplantation and chronic graft-versus-host disease

(Continued)

Table 89.3 Selected developing/marketing kinase inhibitors and related drugs—cont'd

Mechanism	Compound	Kinase inhibited	Comments
			In Phase II trials for IBD, Crohn's, UC and transplant rejection; Phase III trials underway in the treatment of psoriasis
	VX-509		Phase II trials underway for RA, results expected in third quarter of 2011
	R-348		In Phase I trials for RA and psoriasis; in the preclinical phase for Sjögren's syndrome
	PS-608504		In preclinical stage as treatment for RA and psoriasis
	R-333		In preclinical stage as treatment for cutaneous lupus erythematosus
	Ruxolitinib	JAK1 and JAK 2	FDA approved for idiopathic myelofibrosis; Phase II & III trials for cancer and myeloproliferative disorders, respectively; no longer being studied for RA
	Baracitinib		In Phase II trials for rheumatoid arthritis, and is 100 times more selective for JAKs 1 & 2 than JAK 3
	CYT-387		In Phase II trials for myelofibrosis; Phase III study expected to begin in first half of 2012; in preclinical trials for pulmonary HTN and polycythemia vera
	GLPG-0634		Shown to reduce joint-destroying enzymes in mouse RA model. Phase I trial complete; Phase II proof-of-concept trial results for RA expected in December 2011.
	LY-2784544	JAK 2	In Phase II clinical trials for myeloproliferative disorders
	AC-430		In Phase I clinical trials for RA and lymphoma
	SB-1317	CDK, Flt3, JAK2	In Phase I clinical trials for ALL, AML, CML, and myelodysplastic syndrome
	SAR-302503	JAK2, Flt3, Ret	In Phase II clinical trials for polycythemia vera, idiopathic myelofibrosis, thrombocytopenia
	AT-9283	JAK1, JAK3, aurora A/B kinase, highly active against the Gleevec-resistant T315I abl mutation	In Phase II trials for AML, ALL, CML, and myelodysplastic syndrome
	Lestaurtinib	FLT3, TrkA, and JAK2	In Phase III clinical trials for treatment of acute myelogenous leukemia patients who have an FLT3-activating mutation at first relapse from standard induction chemotherapy. In Phase II trials for psoriasis and pancreatic cancer
Cytoplasmic tyrosine kinases	Fostamatinib	Syk, Flt3	In various Phase III clinical trials for RA and Phase II trials for various cancers
	Excellair	Syk	In Phase II trials for asthma, in preclinical status for COPD and immunosuppressive potential
	R-343		Blocks IgE production in respiratory mast cells. In Phase I clinical trials for asthma, preclinical status for COPD
	PRT-062607		In Phase I clinical trials for RA, CLL, non-Hodgkin's lymphoma; preclinical for SLE
Indirect binding to kinase	Sirolimus (Rapamycin)	mTOR	Licensed for use in solid organ and bone marrow transplantation.
	Everolimus		Licensed for use with cyclosporine in cardiac and renal transplantation. Clinical trials are assessing potential for use in RA
Monoclonal antibodies binding to receptor tyrosine kinases	Trastuzumab	EGFR-2	Approved for use in HER2/neu positive breast carcinoma and metastatic gastric cancer
	Cetuximab	EGFR	Approved for use in relapsed colorectal and head/neck cancers
	Bevacizumab	VEGF – prevents binding to its receptor (FLT-1)	Approved for use in metastatic breast and colorectal cancers, glioblastoma and NSCLC (nonsquamous cell histology) in combination with traditional chemotherapy. In December 2010, the FDA recommended removal of the breast cancer indication, citing lack of sufficient survival benefit to outweigh risks of treatment (MI, HTN, GI perforation, heart failure)
Other mechanisms of action	Barasertib	Aurora kinase B (functions in the attachment of the mitotic spindle to the centromere)	Disrupts mitosis and cellular division in tumor cells; in Phase III clinical trials for AML

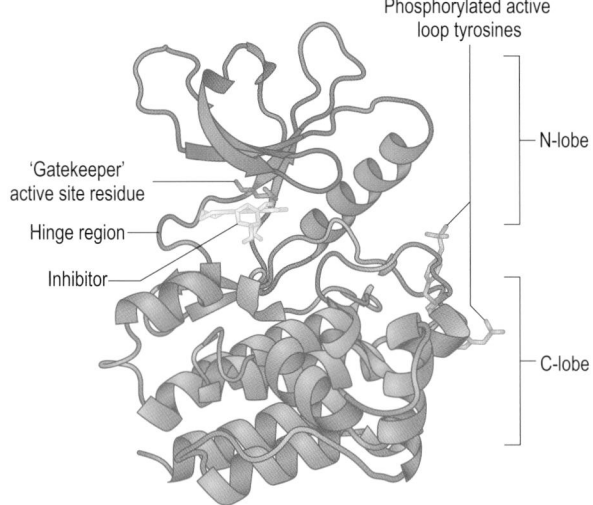

Phosphorylated active
loop tyrosines

'Gatekeeper'
active site residue

Hinge region

Inhibitor

N-lobe

C-lobe

Fig. 89.2 Crystal structure of the JAK3 kinase domain complexed with staurosporine (pdb accession code 1YVJ). This structure captures the active conformation of JAK3 with both active loop tyrosine residues phosphorylated (green). The molecule can be described in two halves, with the *N*-terminal lobe presented in blue and the *C*-terminal domain in red. These are linked by a hinge region that forms part of the active site. Highlighted in magenta within the active site is the gatekeeper residue. Bound within this site is an analog of the inhibitor staurosporine, and its proximity to the "gatekeeper" residue highlights why this residue and this region are critical for the specificity of inhibitors for individual protein kinases.

through its effects on KIT and PDGFR-FIPIL1 kinases, respectively. Despite efforts to develop highly specific kinase inhibitors, there is increasing evidence that a partial inhibition of multiple kinases is potentially less toxic than originally feared and may be important for the efficacy of many inhibitors. The recently approved ABL inhibitor dasatinib is less selective than imatinib; this lack of specificity may contribute to its improved response rates in the treatment of CML.[7] With respect to immune-mediated disease, the possibility of using imatinib in fibrotic disease is being actively pursued. At the time of writing, there are more than ten FDA-approved small molecule kinase inhibitors, all of which are approved for oncologic indications. In addition there are numerous other kinase inhibitors in clinical trial or development (summarized in Table 89.3). Aside from small molecule inhibitors of kinases, another strategy for inhibiting transmembrane receptor kinases is the generation of monoclonal antibodies (mAbs) that inhibit ligand-dependent activation. These mAbs include and target the designated RTK: bevacizumab (VEGFR), ranibizumab (VEGFR), cetuximab (EGFR), pertuzumab (HER), and trastuzumab (HER2/neu).

Targeting cytokine signaling by inhibiting Janus kinases: tofacitinib, ruxolitinib, and related compounds

Cytokines regulate growth, survival, development, and differentiation of immune cells. Their importance in driving inflammatory and immunological responses has already made them attractive targets as anti-inflammatory and immunosuppressive agents. As indicated above, a large subset of cytokines (roughly 60) signal through Janus kinases (Table 89.2).[8] The essential function of JAKs was documented by knockout mice and by patient mutations. Specifically, mutation of *JAK3* results in a severe combined immunodeficiency, characterized by an almost complete absence of T cells and natural killer cells with defective B cells (Chapter 35). This phenocopies deficiency of the cognate receptor that associates with JAK3, the IL-2 receptor common γ chain cγc (encoded by *IL2RG*), mutation of which underlies X-SCID (Table 89.1 and Fig. 89.4). The profound, but selective phenotype associated with JAK3-deficiency led to the suggestion that targeting JAKs might be a strategy for the development of a new class

dasatinib and sunitinib, have now entered clinical practice and have been approved by the FDA. Although a major problem in the treatment of malignancy this is less likely to be an issue in the treatment of autoimmune disease; nonetheless, drugs used for oncologic indications often end up being quite useful in the treatment of autoimmunity. Such precedents include cyclophosphamide, azathioprine, and methotrexate. So it is not unreasonable to speculate that a number of the kinase inhibitors developed as anti-cancer agents might ultimately be used to treat inflammatory or immunologic disease.

Though clinically well-tolerated, imatinib has activity against several other PTKs.[3] Consequently, it has been found to be useful in the treatment of a number of cancers that do not have abnormal ABL kinase activity. Imatinib has been used to treat gastrointestinal stromal tumor and hypereosinophilic syndrome

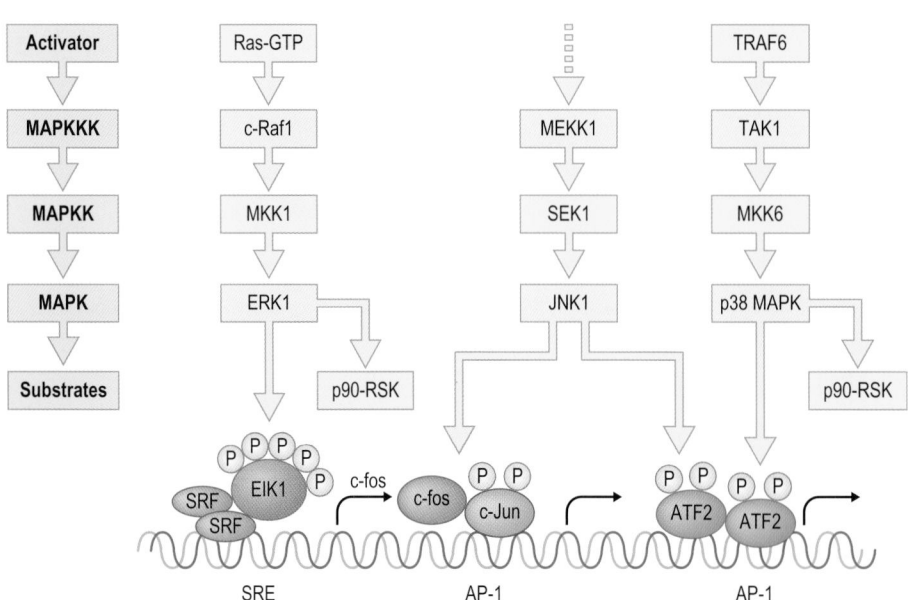

Activator	Ras-GTP		TRAF6
MAPKKK	c-Raf1	MEKK1	TAK1
MAPKK	MKK1	SEK1	MKK6
MAPK	ERK1	JNK1	p38 MAPK
Substrates	p90-RSK		p90-RSK

SRF SRF Elk1 c-fos c-fos c-Jun ATF2 ATF2

SRE AP-1 AP-1

Fig. 89.3 A summary of the MAPK signal transduction pathways. Examples of receptors that activate RAS include the IL-2 receptor and TCR; examples of receptors that activate TRAF6 include the IL-1 receptor.

Fig. 89.4 Signal transduction pathways stemming from the IL-2 receptor in T cells culminating in the activation of the mTOR serine/threonine kinase. Tyrosine kinases are indicated in red and serine/threonine kinases are indicated in blue.

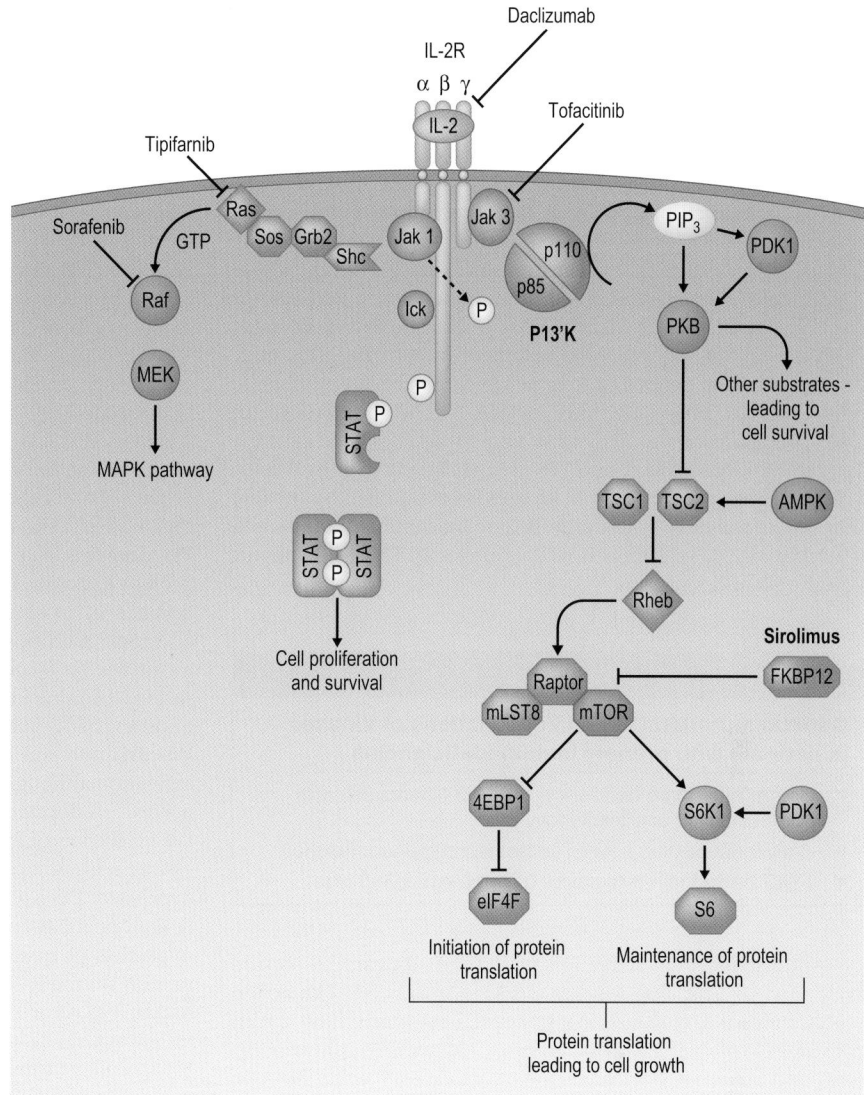

of immunomodulatory drugs. In fact, there are now many JAK inhibitors in clinical trials and under development. A number of these compounds have been found to be efficacious in preclinical models of autoimmune disease and allograft rejection.

Tofacitinib, formerly designated CP-690,550, was one of the first JAK inhibitors to enter the clinic. It inhibits JAK3 and JAK1 and to a lesser extent JAK2, but has little effect on TYK2.[9] Consequently, tofacitinib potently inhibits cγc cytokines, but also blocks IFN-γ, IL-6, and to a lesser extent IL-12 and IL-23. Functionally, tofacitinib inhibits Th1 cells and Th2 differentiation, as well as pathogenic Th17 cells.[9] In addition to inhibiting adaptive immune responses, tofacitinib also appears to inhibit innate immune responses.[9] A Phase II clinical trial investigating the role of tofacitinib in rheumatoid arthritis demonstrated rapid clinical improvement[10] and Phase III trials in rheumatoid arthritis have been completed and the drug has been recommended for approval by the FDA. Tofacitinib is also under clinical investigation for psoriasis, inflammatory bowel disease and prevention of transplant rejection. A variety of additional inhibitors that target JAK3 are under development or in clinical trials (Table 89.3).

As gene targeting of *Jak2* in mice was embryonically lethal, it was initially thought that inhibition of JAK2 should be avoided. However, the discovery that gain-of-function mutations of *JAK2* underlie polycythemia vera and myelofibrosis led to the idea

that pharmacologically targeting JAK2 could be useful. The Phase II study of patients with myelofibrosis showed clinical improvement on ruxolitinib for which the drug is now FDA approved; in addition, the drug was relatively safe in this setting.[11] As cγc cytokines employ both JAK1 and JAK3 for signaling, it might be expected that ruxolitinib and tofacitinib might block some of the same cytokines. It is therefore of interest to note that in a Phase II study in rheumatoid arthritis, ruxolinitib had efficacy that was not dissimilar from that of tofacitinib.[12]

Side effects of JAK inhibitors include anemia and leukopenia, presumably related to JAK2 inhibition and interference with cytokines such as erythropoietin and colony stimulating factors.[13] Little reduction in CD4 T cells has been seen, but significant reduction in NK cells and CD8 T cells does occur; just how significant this will be in terms of infection risk remains to be determined.[14]

Targeting antigen receptor signaling

The first event in T-cell receptor signaling is activation of Src family kinase LCK (Fig. 89.1). This has made it an attractive target as a therapy for autoimmune disease and transplant organ rejection.[15] Several Lck inhibitors have been developed and have shown promise in preclinical models of allograft rejection and autoimmunity[16] although at a cost of inducing a progressive lymphopenia. This is consistent with the finding that induced deficiency of Lck in mice leads to a progressive lymphopenia.[17] Despite considerable effort, the discovery of a selective Lck inhibitor suitable for use as an immunosuppressive agent remains elusive. Activation of LCK leads to the recruitment of a second round of tyrosine kinases to the T-cell receptor complex; these include ZAP70 or SYK (spleen tyrosine kinase). Deficiency of ZAP70 causes severe combined immunodeficiency and preferential loss of CD8 T cells (Chapter 35), but curiously, a successful ZAP70 inhibitor has yet to be obtained. In contrast, SYK inhibitors have been generated, one of which has been found to be efficacious in Phase II study in RA.[18] The recruitment of ZAP70/SYK results in activation of another class of PTKs, the Tec family kinases, RLK and ITK in T cells and BTK in B cells. The importance of this class of kinases is exemplified by the fact that mutations of *BTK* underlie Bruton's agammaglobulinemia (Chapter 34). PCI-32765 is a BTK inhibitor in Phase I trials for lymphoma and leukemia.[19]

● CLINICAL PEARLS

Genetic mutations reveal key functions of kinases in patients with primary immunodeficiencies

- Common γ-chain deficiency, JAK3 deficiency: severe combined immunodeficiency
- ZAP70 deficiency: severe combined immunodeficiency
- TYK2 deficiency: rare cause of hyper-IgE syndrome

Antigen receptor activation of PLC γ1 appears to require LCK, ZAP70, and TEC kinases working in concert. The action of PLC γ1 leads to elevation in intracellular calcium, which in turn activates the phosphatase calcineurin. Calcineurin dephosphorylates and activates nuclear factor of activated T cells (NFAT), which translocates to the nucleus and in cooperation with AP-1 transcription factors regulate transcription of IL-2 and other key lymphocyte activation genes.[20] A number of potent clinically successful immunosuppressive drugs inhibit calcineurin, including cyclosporine and tacrolimus, drugs that have revolutionized organ transplantation.[21] Despite their success these drugs are limited by renal toxicity that limits their long-term use.

Protein kinase C family

TCR signaling also leads to the activation of members of the PKC family, which in turn activate the transcription factor complex NF-κB that controls genes involved in cellular activation and resistance to apoptosis.[24] Genetic studies in mice have identified the importance of one member, PKC-θ in TCR signaling. More recent work has identified PKC-θ as an inhibitor of regulatory T-cell function.[22] Regulatory T cells (Treg), unlike conventional effector T cells, act to constrain the immune system (Chapter 15). Their use and induction have been suggested in a number of autoimmune diseases.[23] For this reason, targeting PKC-θ seems promising. In T cells, PKC-θ is the main isoform responsible for NF-κB activation. The novel PKC inhibitor AEB071 (Novartis) is currently undergoing Phase II trials for the treatment of psoriasis. It is a potent inhibitor of the PKC-θ, β, and α isoforms.[25] Early clinical testing on patients with psoriasis has demonstrated that the drug is well tolerated and was able to

inhibit T-cell proliferation, and IL-2 and IFN-γ secretion. These changes were associated with a significant suppression of inflammatory activity.[25]

Lipid kinases and downstream signaling

Kinases are also important in phosphorylating lipids and these modifications are very relevant in signal transduction through both the TCR and cytokine receptors. In addition to the production of inositol triphosphate by the action of PLC γ1, there is a second pathway of inositol lipid metabolism regulated by the T-cell receptor that is a response shared by co-stimulatory molecules such as CD28, cytokines, and chemokines. This response is mediated by the class I group of phosphatidyl-inositol 3 kinases (PI3'Ks), of which there are four isoforms (PI3'Kα to δ), which phosphorylate the 3'-OH position of the inositol ring of phosphatidyl-inositol (4,5) biphosphate (PI(4,5)P$_2$) to produce PI(3,4,5)P$_3$.[26] This lipid and its metabolite PI(3,4)P$_2$ bind to the PH domains of proteins and either induce localization of the protein to defined areas of the plasma membrane where activation can occur or induce conformational changes that allow for allosteric modifications of activity. Targets for D-3 phosphoinositides in T cells include a number of downstream protein serine/threonine kinases and the Rac-1 and RhoA guanine nucleotide exchange proteins. The small molecule PI3'K inhibitors, Wortmannin and LY294002, are both potent inhibitors of T-cell activation although toxicity prevents either from being clinically useful.[27] A derivative compound, PX-866, is being used in Phase I clinical trials of treatment of patients with advanced metastatic cancer with acceptable toxicity. In contrast to the more widely expressed PI3'Kα and β, PI3'Kγ and δ are only expressed in hematopoetic tissue[28] and deletion of PI3'Kγ results in defective migration of neutrophils and macrophages to sites of inflammation without other pathology.[29] This limited expression makes PI3'Kγ a potentially useful target and selective PI3'Kγ inhibitors have shown to be effective in mouse models of inhibiting collagen-induced arthritis.[30]

One PI(3,4,5)P$_3$-regulated kinase activated by the T-cell receptor is protein kinase B (PKB).[26] T cells stimulated in the presence of the PI3'K inhibitors Wortmannin or LY-294002 fail to activate and proliferate. The ability of cells to take up nutrients and switch on glycolysis is essential for lymphocyte activation; PKB is proposed to be the main effector that mediates the action of PI3'K on these fundamentally important metabolic pathways.[31] There are three PKB isoforms (PKB-α, -β, -γ, or Akt1, 2, 3, respectively) and T cells lacking both *Akt1*$^{-/-}$ and *Akt2*$^{-/-}$ are greatly impaired.[32] Specific inhibitors of PKB are entering clinical trials and it remains to be seen whether either of these drugs has useful immunosuppressive functions.

In addition to glucose metabolism, the PI3'K regulated serine/threonine kinase mammalian target of rapamycin (mTOR) regulates protein synthesis in response to cellular nutrient and energy levels.[33] It is activated by a number of growth factor receptors but also by cytokines like IL-2. Many signaling pathways link growth factor receptors with activation of mTOR including the AMP-dependent kinase (AMPK) and phosphatidyl inositol 3' kinase (PI3'K) (Fig. 89.4). mTOR promotes cell growth by activation of p70 S6K1 and inactivation of 4E-BP1,[34] which are critical for translation of new protein.

As its name suggests, mTOR is inhibited by the macrolide rapamycin, now licensed for the treatment of graft rejection as the drug sirolimus. Sirolimus does not inhibit mTOR by direct binding to the ATP binding pocket but acts indirectly, associating with FK506 binding protein 12 (FKBP12). This in turn inhibits the kinase complex made up of mTOR, mLST8, and raptor (mTORC1).[34] Sirolimus was hoped to be a potent anti-cancer drug but has met with limited success in this regard. In contrast, it has been successfully used as an immunosuppressant typically as part of a combination regimen for allograft rejection prophylaxis.[35] In view of the ubiquitous expression of mTOR and its role in protein translation, it is not surprising that sirolimus would be associated with varied side effects; these include hyperlipidemia, hyper-triglyceridemia, myelosuppression, and delayed wound healing. There is some evidence of renal toxicity but this is minor compared with the calcineurin inhibitors cyclosporine and tacrolimus. Myelosuppression associated with sirolimus is typically dose related and rapidly reversible even in patients receiving the drug for chronic graft-versus-host disease.[36]

There are currently three rapamycin derivatives undergoing clinical trials, namely temsirolimus, everolimus, and AP23573. Everolimus is licensed for use in the management of cardiac and renal transplantation in conjunction with cyclosporine; it is being investigated in the treatment of rheumatoid arthritis. Temsirolimus is licensed for the treatment of renal cell carcinoma and is being explored for the management of rheumatoid arthritis and multiple sclerosis where Phase II trials have reported a 50% reduction in development of lesions on MRI over a 9-month period.[37]

MAP kinase pathways

The MAPK family constitute a complex phospho-relay system of signal transduction, composed of three sequentially activated kinases that are themselves modulated by phosphorylation.[38] Substrates of MAPK pathways include transcription factors, phospholipases, cytoskeletal proteins, and other protein kinases. Three main MAPK cascades have been identified in mammalian cells: the ERK1,2 cascade, the JNK1/2 cascade, and the p38 MAPK cascade. All start with a membrane-localized activator followed by three MAPKs that sequentially phosphorylate each other (Fig. 89.3). The top level of kinases is termed MAPK kinase kinases (MAPKKKs, MKKKs, or Map3Ks). The middle level, MAPK kinases (MAPKKs, MKKs, or Map2Ks), phosphorylate a common Thr-Xaa-Tyr motif where Xaa is any amino acid. The lowest tier consists of the MAPKs that phosphorylate Ser/Thr-Pro motifs. Each pathway terminates in the phosphorylation of substrate proteins.

The extracellular signal regulated kinase (ERK) 1,2 cascade

ERK1 and 2 were identified as kinases that were activated in response to growth factor stimulation, which are mimicked by expression of constitutively active Ras. The link between active Ras and subsequent phosphorylation of the ERKs was made by both the discovery of the MAPK kinase, MEK1, and its phosphorylation by the known Ras effector RAF1, now known as a MAPK kinase kinase (M3K). The ERK1,2 cascade is ubiquitous in mammalian cells and is generally considered to be one of the main effector pathways regulated by the GTPase p21ras. Activation of the T-cell receptor or the IL-2 receptor is able to trigger ERK signaling in T cells.[38] Two small molecule inhibitors of this serine/threonine kinase pathway are undergoing clinical trials: the farsenyl inhibitor of RAS, tipifarnib, in the management of myelodysplasia, and the multi-kinase inhibitor sorafenib, which is FDA approved for the treatment of renal cell carcinoma.[39] Sorafenib is relatively well tolerated despite its ability to inhibit numerous kinases, including the M3K RAF, as well as receptor

tyrosine kinases including PDGFR, VEGFR, Kit, and FLT-3. Its role as an immunosuppressant has yet to be explored.

Downstream of RAF lie the M2K MEK1 and the MAPK ERK1. Selective inhibitors of both are being developed; the MEK1 inhibitor selumetinib has just completed Phase II trials in hepatocellular carcinoma with limited results[40] and the MEK1 inhibitor ARRY-438162 has completed Phase I trials in healthy volunteers to assess its suitability as a treatment for inflammatory disease. Selective inhibitors of ERK are being developed: FR180204 has been shown to inhibit the development of collagen-induced arthritis in mice and is being considered as an agent in the treatment of rheumatoid arthritis.[41]

The Jun kinase (JNK) cascade

Another limb of the MAPK pathway is the Jun kinase (JNK pathway). Many inflammatory agents including LPS, TNF-α, and IL-1 are able to activate the JNK pathway.[38] In synoviocytes this results in secretion of proteases implicated in joint destruction in RA.[42] A number of small molecule inhibitors of Jun kinases have been identified and are currently being investigated in animal models of autoimmune and inflammatory disease.[43]

The p38 MAPK cascade

This cascade was originally identified as part of a drugs screen looking for inhibitors of TNF-α-mediated inflammatory responses.[44] TLR-dependent production of IL-1 and TNF-α is p38 MAPK dependent. The success of TNF-α-blocking antibodies in the treatment of rheumatoid arthritis has led to much interest in the development of p38 MAPK inhibitors. However, although many p38 inhibitors have been reported, their development into therapeutic drugs has been frustrated by either unacceptable toxicity (AMG 548, BIRB 796) or poor efficacy (SCIO-469, VX-702).[45]

Conclusions

● ON THE HORIZON

- Many kinase inhibitors, initially designed as anti-tumor agents, may also be used as anti-inflammatory agents.
- Further understanding of the pathophysiology of autoimmune disease may lead to the increased use of kinase inhibitors.
- Increasing use of specific kinase inhibitors may improve our understanding of the pathophysiology of autoimmune disease.

The scientific advances in the 1990s have led to the discovery of many novel intracellular signaling pathways that link receptor and cytokine signaling with alteration of gene expression and cellular activation necessary to trigger an immune cell response. Many of these pathways are interlinked to make up a complex array of networks made up of enzymes, adaptor proteins, and transcription factors, all of which are potential targets for drug discovery. Now more than a decade since the identification of many new targets, the first generation of drugs designed to interfere with specific immune cell signals are being brought to the clinic. The success of the anti-cancer BCR-ABL inhibitor imatinib and the immunosuppressive mTOR inhibitor sirolimus has placed the protein kinases center stage as targets of future drug discovery. As many of the key steps in the activation of an immune cell are often shared with those that allow a cancer cell to proliferate, many of these agents are being tested as anticancer drugs rather than as immunosuppressants. Despite this, agents such as the mTOR inhibitors, originally intended for the treatment of cancer, have been far more successful in the field of immunology and this may continue to be true for future modifiers of cell signaling. Conversely JAK inhibitors could potentially be used in the treatment of leukemia. Either way, we are likely to see a large number of novel immunosuppressants appear both serendipitously and intentionally as new protein kinase inhibitors are licensed for a wide range of debilitating illnesses.

References

1. Hanks SK, Quinn AM, Hunter T. The protein kinase family: conserved features and deduced phylogeny of the catalytic domains. Science 1988;241:42–52.
2. Noble ME, Endicott JA, Johnson LN. Protein kinase inhibitors: insights into drug design from structure. Science 2004;303:1800–5.
3. Druker BJ, Lydon NB. Lessons learned from the development of an abl tyrosine kinase inhibitor for chronic myelogenous leukemia. J Clin Invest 2000;105:3–7.
4. Schindler T, Bornmann W, Pellicena P, et al. Structural mechanism for STI-571 inhibition of abelson tyrosine kinase. Science 2000;289:1938–42.
5. Adams J, Huang P, Patrick D. A strategy for the design of multiplex inhibitors for kinase-mediated signalling in angiogenesis. Curr Opin Chem Biol 2002;6:486–92.
6. Davies TG, Pratt DJ, Endicott JA, et al. Structure-based design of cyclin-dependent kinase inhibitors. Pharmacol Ther 2002;93:125–33.
7. Kantarjian H, Shah NP, Hochhaus A, et al. Dasatinib versus imatinib in newly diagnosed chronic-phase chronic myeloid leukemia. N Engl J Med 2010;362:2260–70.
8. Pesu M, Candotti F, Husa M, et al. Jak3, severe combined immunodeficiency, and a new class of immunosuppressive drugs. Immunol Rev 2005;203:127–42.
9. Ghoreschi K, Jesson MI, Li X, et al. Modulation of innate and adaptive immune responses by tofacitinib (CP-690,550). J Immunol 2011;186:4234–43.
10. Coombs JH, Bloom BJ, Breedveld FC, et al. Improved pain, physical functioning and health status in patients with rheumatoid arthritis treated with CP-690,550, an orally active Janus kinase (JAK) inhibitor: results from a randomised, double-blind, placebo-controlled trial. Ann Rheum Dis 2010;69:413–6.
11. Verstovsek S, Kantarjian H, Mesa RA, et al. Safety and efficacy of INCB018424, a JAK1 and JAK2 inhibitor, in myelofibrosis. N Engl J Med 2010;363:1117–27.
12. Mesa RA. Ruxolitinib, a selective JAK1 and JAK2 inhibitor for the treatment of myeloproliferative neoplasms and psoriasis. IDrugs 2010;13:394–403.
13. Borie DC, Changelian PS, Larson MJ, et al. Immunosuppression by the JAK3 inhibitor CP-690,550 delays rejection and significantly prolongs kidney allograft survival in nonhuman primates. Transplantation 2005;79:791–801.
14. Paniagua R, Si MS, Flores MG, et al. Effects of JAK3 inhibition with CP-690,550 on immune cell populations and their functions in nonhuman primate recipients of kidney allografts. Transplantation 2005;80:1283–92.
15. Molina TJ, Kishihara K, Siderovski DP, et al. Profound block in thymocyte development in mice lacking p56lck. Nature 1992;357:161–4.
16. Martin MW, Machacek MR. Update on lymphocyte specific kinase inhibitors: a patent survey. Expert Opin Ther Pat 2010;20:1573–93.
17. Zamoyska R, Basson A, Filby A, et al. The influence of the src-family kinases, Lck and Fyn, on T cell differentiation, survival and activation. Immunol Rev 2003;191:107–18.
18. Weinblatt ME, Kavanaugh A, Genovese MC, et al. An oral spleen tyrosine kinase (Syk) inhibitor for rheumatoid arthritis. N Engl J Med 2010;363:1303–12.
19. Honigberg LA, Smith AM, Sirisawad M, et al. The Bruton tyrosine kinase inhibitor PCI-32765 blocks B-cell activation and is efficacious in models of autoimmune disease and B-cell malignancy. Proc Natl Acad Sci U S A 2010;107:13075–80.
20. Muller MR, Rao A. NFAT, immunity and cancer: a transcription factor comes of age. Nat Rev Immunol 2010;10:645–56.
21. Calne RY. Organ transplantation has come of age. Sci Prog 2010;93:141–50.
22. Zanin-Zhorov A, Ding Y, Kumari S, et al. Protein kinase C-theta mediates negative feedback on regulatory T cell function. Science 2010;328:372–6.
23. Riley JL, June CH, Blazar BR. Human T regulatory cell therapy: take a billion or so and call me in the morning. Immunity 2009;30:656–65.
24. Altman A, Villalba M. Protein kinase C-theta (PKCtheta): it's all about location, location, location. Immunol Rev 2003;192:53–63.
25. Manicassamy S. Sotrastaurin, a protein kinase C inhibitor for the prevention of transplant rejection and treatment of psoriasis. Curr Opin Investig Drugs 2009;10:1225–35.
26. Cantrell DA. Phosphoinositide 3-kinase signalling pathways. J Cell Sci 2001;114:1439–45.
27. Knight ZA. Small molecule inhibitors of the PI3-kinase family. Curr Top Microbiol Immunol 2010;347:263–78.
28. Okkenhaug K, Vanhaesebroeck B. PI3K in lymphocyte development, differentiation and activation. Nat Rev Immunol 2003;3:317–30.
29. Hirsch E, Katanaev VL, Garlanda C, et al. Central role for G protein-coupled phosphoinositide 3-kinase gamma in inflammation. Science 2000;287:1049–53.
30. Camps M, Rückle T, Ji H, et al. Blockade of PI3Kgamma suppresses joint inflammation and damage in mouse models of rheumatoid arthritis. Nat Med 2005;11:936–43.
31. Edinger AL, Thompson CB. Antigen-presenting cells control T cell proliferation by regulating amino acid availability. Proc Natl Acad Sci U S A 2002;99:1107–9.
32. Juntilla MM, Wofford JA, Birnbaum MJ, et al. Akt1 and Akt2 are required for alphabeta thymocyte survival and differentiation. Proc Natl Acad Sci U S A 2007;104:12105–10.
33. Edinger AL, Thompson CB. Akt maintains cell size and survival by increasing mTOR-dependent nutrient uptake. Mol Biol Cell 2002;13:2276–88.
34. McManus EJ, Alessi DR. TSC1-TSC2: a complex tale of PKB-mediated S6K regulation. Nat Cell Biol 2002;4:E214–16.
35. Kreis H, Cisterne JM, Land W, et al. Sirolimus in association with mycophenolate mofetil induction for the prevention of acute graft rejection in renal allograft recipients. Transplantation 2000;69:1252–60.
36. Pérez-Simón JA, Sureda A, Fernández-Aviles F, et al. Reduced-intensity conditioning allogeneic transplantation is associated with a high incidence of extramedullary relapses in multiple myeloma patients. Leukemia 2006;20:542–5.
37. Kappos L, Barkhof F, Desmet A. The effect of oral temsirolimus on new magnetic resonance imaging scan lesions, brain atrophy, and the number of relapses in multiple sclerosis: results from a randomised, controlled clinical trial. J Neurol 2005;252.
38. Dong C, Davis RJ, Flavell RA. MAP kinases in the immune response. Annu Rev Immunol 2002;20:55–72.
39. Josephs DH, Ross PJ. Sorafenib in hepatocellular carcinoma. Br J Hosp Med (Lond) 2010;71:451–6.
40. O'Neil BH, Goff LW, Kauh JS, et al. Phase II study of the mitogen-activated protein kinase 1/2 inhibitor selumetinib in patients with advanced hepatocellular carcinoma. J Clin Oncol 2011;29:2350–6.
41. Ohori M, Takeuchi M, Maruki R, et al. FR180204, a novel and selective inhibitor of extracellular signal-regulated kinase, ameliorates collagen-induced arthritis in mice. Naunyn Schmiedebergs Arch Pharmacol 2007;374:311–6.
42. Gum R, Wang H, Lengyel E, et al. Regulation of 92 kDa type IV collagenase expression by the jun aminoterminal kinase- and the extracellular signal-regulated kinase-dependent signaling cascades. Oncogene 1997;14:1481–93.
43. Manning AM, Davis RJ. Targeting JNK for therapeutic benefit: from junk to gold? Nat Rev Drug Discov 2003;2:554–65.
44. Lee JC, Laydon JT, McDonnell PC, et al. A protein kinase involved in the regulation of inflammatory cytokine biosynthesis. Nature 1994;372:739–46.
45. Dominguez C, Powers DA, Tamayo N. p38 MAP kinase inhibitors: many are made, but few are chosen. Curr Opin Drug Discov Devel 2005;8:421–30.

Vaccines

Alan R. Shaw,
Mark B. Feinberg

Vaccines represent one of the most effective and cost-effective medical and public health achievements of all time. Worldwide,[1] vaccination programs are currently estimated to save over 3 million lives each year. In addition to having a major beneficial impact on vaccine-preventable disease morbidity and mortality, the direct and indirect impacts of vaccination programs translate into economic savings of many billions of dollars each year. In what is considered to be one of history's most significant medical successes, a collaborative and comprehensive vaccination campaign against smallpox resulted in the global eradication of the disease in 1979.[2] Similarly, efforts to eradicate poliomyelitis have made tremendous progress in reducing the global disease burden, and will hopefully soon overcome certain residual societal and programmatic obstacles to provide the second successful example of elimination of a major health threat by vaccination. Concerted global efforts to provide measles vaccine have resulted in the control and elimination of the disease in many countries, including substantial reductions in mortality in a number of developing countries where the residual disease burden is greatest. These and other examples provide clear evidence of the power of vaccines in favorably manipulating host immunity to confer dramatic public health benefits, at both the individual and population level.

Vaccines are administered to healthy individuals (often to entire age cohorts or populations), to prevent diseases caused by infectious agents to which they might be exposed in the future. Thus, they differ in important ways from pharmacologic agents that are used to treat individuals in whom a disease process is already manifest (or who display predispositions to disease). For this reason, vaccines are unique in the way that they impact on societies and in the way that societal commitment to vaccination determines their ultimate impact. As a result, vaccination efforts provide an informative window on challenges that need to be successfully navigated at the interface between scientific opportunity and societal capacity and commitment. Indeed, current limitations in realizing the full global potential of available vaccines relate more to existing inadequacies in health care financing and infrastructure (especially as they are manifest in developing countries), and the relative value that societies place on disease prevention, than they do to any inherent biological limitations of vaccines themselves. Following the initiation of the Expanded Programme on Immunization (EPI) in 1974, global coverage for routine vaccines (such as three doses of the diphtheria–tetanus–pertussis vaccine (DPT3)) has progressively increased, but many children in resource-limited countries still fail to receive all recommended childhood immunizations. Fortunately, recent acceleration of new vaccine introductions in developing countries through public and private initiatives (such as the GAVI Alliance and UNICEF) to build immunization

infrastructure and provide funding of vaccine purchase (including novel funding mechanisms for vaccine procurement such as the Advanced Market Commitment (AMC) for pneumococcal conjugate vaccines and the International Financing Facility for Immunization (IFFIm)) offers hope that vaccines will one day be equitably available to all who need them. Achieving this aspiration represents the focus of a recently launched initiative referred to as the Decade of Vaccines Collaboration (http://www.dovcollaboriation.org).

The importance of vaccines extends beyond their use as public health tools to include their role as drivers of immunologic discovery. The history of vaccine development is rich with immunologic insights that emerged from careful observations of how diseases spread in populations and how such spread differs in disease-naïve and experienced populations, as well as of how innovative experimental approaches revealed fundamental aspects of immune system function. The general concept of immunity induced by prior exposure to a disease (including its specificity and potential lifelong duration) was appreciated by the ancient Greeks. Use of the word "immunity" in the context of human health dates to the fourteenth century when it was applied to describe the relative susceptibility and resistance of populations to plague. The subsequent successes of Edward Jenner and Louis Pasteur in the development of effective smallpox and fowl cholera immunization strategies, respectively, provided a foundation for modern immunology; Pasteur himself coined the term "vaccine" in recognition of Jenner's use of vaccinia virus. Jenner's smallpox immunization studies also provided early experimental support for the concept of immune memory. Pasteur's efforts provided the first demonstration of the attenuation of pathogens by their propagation in culture (or by passage in nonnatural animal hosts), while Robert Koch demonstrated that killed pathogens could also engender immunity. The discovery of bacterial exotoxins by Emile Roux and Alexandre Yersin facilitated the discovery of antibodies and their potential use in passive immunotherapy with antitoxin antibodies by Emil von Behring and Shibasaburo Kitasato. These discoveries enabled the development of active immunization against diphtheria and tetanus using toxin–antitoxin mixtures. Paul Ehrlich's development of accurate methods for antibody quantitation made passive immunotherapy and active toxin–antitoxin immunization far more reliable and effective, and provided a stimulus for significant advances in immunologic theory. In each of these instances, vaccine development illuminated central mechanisms of immune system biology.

Vaccine development today has transitioned from an approach that was once largely empirical to one that is based on the hypothesis-driven application of techniques in molecular biology and immunology. Evidence for this synergy can be seen in recent studies of vaccine-elicited immune responses to illuminate the determinants of activation of innate immune responses and how these determine the magnitude and persistence of primary and memory T- and B-cell responses in humans. It also provides a strong discovery stimulus provided by ongoing efforts to develop new vaccines for major infectious diseases for which vaccines are not currently available.

Vaccine development today faces a number of significant challenges. There exist tremendous public health needs to address major well-known pandemic diseases, including acquired immunodeficiency syndrome (AIDS), tuberculosis, and malaria, for which no effective vaccines currently exist and for which natural immunity does not provide a helpful guide for vaccine development. Furthermore, there exists a need to confront effectively newly emerging and re-emerging diseases, ranging from the well-known, but constantly changing, threats from influenza pandemics to the appearance of previously unknown zoonotic infections such as the coronavirus that causes severe acute respiratory syndrome (SARS). With changes in population density, mobility, and social constructs, along with alterations in the global climate, ecological circumstances, and the proximity of humans to animal reservoirs for previously confined infectious agents, the concept of new infectious agents entering human populations and spreading rapidly around the world is no longer novel. In confronting prevalent or newly emerging diseases, vaccines are looked to as the most promising line of defense. However, the speed at which new infectious disease threats emerge and spread, and the fact that the pathogens that now need to be confronted may display tremendous genetic variability (e.g., human immunodeficiency virus (HIV)) or an identity that cannot now be predicted in advance (e.g., avian influenza or emerging zoonotic infectious agents like the SARS coronavirus) places unprecedented demands on the vaccine development process.

In addition to these new challenges, there remain unmet needs in the derivation of vaccines that can achieve the greatest public health benefit. These needs include the development of new ways to achieve more effective vaccine-elicited immune responses in neonates, whose immune systems are immature (or are impacted by maternal antibodies) (Chapter 32)[3] and in the elderly whose immune system function may be waning as a result of immune senescence (Chapter 33). Fortunately, the scientific foundation provided by basic and applied immunology and the use of new methods for pathogen identification, antigen discovery, vaccine production, adjuvant development, and novel vector derivation afford important opportunities for vaccine development; additionally they present the possibility of improving on natural immunity.

Success in vaccine development will be predicated on continuing the historical synergy between advances in vaccine technology and basic immunologic discovery. Toward that end, this chapter focuses on preventive vaccines for infectious diseases and how they are developed. Although current routine vaccine recommendations are reviewed, given the active state of new vaccine introduction and evolving vaccine recommendations, as well as differences in recommendations in different countries, readers are encouraged to refer to up-to-date national resources for the most current information. While vaccine approaches are also being actively explored to treat specific malignant and immunologic diseases (autoimmunity and allergy), these are beyond the scope of the current discussion.

Impact of vaccination programs

Unlike other medical interventions, vaccines confer benefits to both individuals and populations.[4,5] While individuals can be protected from infection or disease by vaccine-induced immune responses, decreasing the number of susceptible hosts in a population also helps break the chain of transmission that pathogens require to spread and persist in human populations through induction of "herd immunity." The benefits of herd immunity depend on achieving sufficiently high immunization rates in a population to impact pathogen transmission dynamics (including the potential for extinction of ongoing interhost transmission). The requisite level of vaccination coverage of a population needed to compromise pathogen spread significantly varies between pathogens, and is influenced both by vaccine efficacy (and its duration) and by the reproductive characteristics and infectiousness of the pathogen.

Analysis of the impact of vaccination programs in the USA provides an example of the beneficial impact of vaccines when used routinely and when high coverage levels are achieved.[6] Numerous vaccines targeting important infectious diseases have been developed since tetanus toxoid—the first vaccine licensed in the USA—was introduced in 1943. Once these vaccines were introduced into routine vaccination programs in the USA the annual morbidity of many vaccine-preventable diseases dramatically decreased (Table 90.1). In many instances, the disease

Table 90.1 Comparison of annual morbidity from vaccine-preventable diseases during the 20th century and 2010

Disease	20th Century[a]	2010[b]	% Reduction
Diphtheria	21 053	0	100
Hepatitis A	117 333	8 493[c]	93
Hepatitis B, acute	66 232	9 419[c]	86
Haemophilus influenzae type b in children aged <5 years	20 000	240[d]	99
Measles	530 217	63	>99
Mumps	162 344	2 612	98
Pertussis	200 752	27 538	86
Pneumococcus, invasive			
All ages	63 607	44 000[e]	30
<5 years	16 069	4 700[e]	72
Poliomyelitis, paralytic	16 316	0	100
Rotavirus, hospitalizations	62 500[d]	28 125[c]	55
Rubella	47 745	5	>99
Congenital rubella syndrome	152	0	100
Smallpox	29 005	0	100
Tetanus	580	26	96
Varicella	4 085 120	408 572[c]	90

[a]Estimate annual average number of cases in the prevaccine era for each disease. Source: The Journal of the American Medical Association 2007; 298: 2155–2163.
[b]Source: Morbidity and Mortality Weekly Report 2011; 60(32): 1088–1101.
[c]2009 estimate.
[d]23 type b and 223 unknown serotype (among children <5 years of age).
[e]Source: Morbidity and Mortality Weekly Report 2009; 58(No. RR-2).
Adapted from Hinman AR, Orenstien WA, Schuchat A 2011 Vaccine-preventable diseases, immunizations, and MMWR – 1961–2011. Morbidity and Mortality Weekly Report 60(4); 49–57.

burden from several vaccine-preventable diseases of childhood has been reduced by over 99% since vaccine introduction (e.g., diphtheria, tetanus, measles, mumps, rubella, and polio). The somewhat lower rate of decline of pertussis (the annual morbidity of which has been reduced by a nonetheless impressive 86%) relates to the limited duration of vaccine-induced immunity, which is estimated to wane within 5–10 years after childhood vaccination. It is anticipated that recent availability of pertussis booster vaccines for use in adolescents and adults will lead to significant further declines in pertussis morbidity. Even for diseases targeted by vaccines that have been in widespread use for less time, impressive decreases in disease morbidity have been seen (e.g., varicella, hepatitis A, pneumococcal and rotavirus diseases). In a notable recent demonstration of the population benefits of vaccines, introduction of the 7-valent pneumococcal conjugate vaccine (PCV-7) resulted in a decrease of 94% in rates of invasive pneumococcal disease (IPD) in children under 5 years of age within the first 7 years of its introduction, with infections caused by antibiotic-resistant *Streptococcus pneumoniae* also falling dramatically in this age group.[7] In a striking related finding illustrating how vaccines can impact pathogen transmission dynamics, IPD rates also decreased significantly in non-vaccinated children, as well as in individuals over the age of 65 who had not received the vaccine. Thus, direct protection by vaccination of children who represent a reservoir of infection provided, via herd immunity, significant indirect benefits to those who did not themselves receive the vaccine. In another manifestation of the impact of vaccination on the dynamics of pathogen transmission, rates of IPD caused by serotypes not included in PCV-7 (especially 19A) have increased, but remain low compared to the decreases in PCV-7-type IPD. To address this dynamic and provide even broader protection against pneumococcal disease, vaccines of higher valency (10-valent and 13-valent PCVs) have been introduced recently.

In addition to their benefits in preventing disease morbidity and mortality, routine vaccination programs are also impressively cost-effective. Evaluation in the USA of the impact of ten vaccines routinely given as part of the childhood immunization schedule (diphtheria, tetanus, pertussis, *Haemophilus influenzae* b (Hib), polio; measles, mumps, rubella, hepatitis B and varicella) found that more than 20 million cases of disease and more than 42 000 deaths were averted over the lifetime of the immunized birth cohort of children. When the cost of the vaccination program was compared to the economic impact of diseases prevented, these vaccines alone are estimated to save nearly $14 billion each year. When including indirect economic benefits (such as the time parents take off from work to care for sick children), the annual savings to society exceed $69 billion. When 30 preventive services were ranked based on clinically preventable disease burden and cost-effectiveness, childhood immunization received the highest score.[8]

Progress in the development of new vaccines accelerated significantly towards the end of the twentieth century, with the development of vaccines against diseases that were not previously preventable by vaccination, but also with the development of improved versions of existing vaccines. Thus, the number of diseases that can be prevented by vaccines included in the US Centers for Disease Control and Prevention's (CDC) routine childhood and adolescent immunization schedules grew from 7 in 1985 to 16 by 2007 (Table 90.2 and Appendix A5, and see http://www.cdc.gov/vaccines/default.htm). While expanded recommendations for some of these vaccines in children and adolescents have been introduced since 2007 (such as broader use of the quadrivalent meningococcal conjugate vaccine (MCV4), and the recommendation for routine use of the quadrivalent

Table 90.2 Number of diseases prevented by vaccines included in the US Centers of Disease Control and Prevention's routine childhood and adolescent immunization schedules

Year	1985	1995	2007
Disease	Measles Rubella Mumps Diphtheria Tetanus Pertussis Polio	Measles Rubella Mumps Diphtheria Tetanus Pertussis Polio *Haemophilus influenzae* b (infant) Hepatitis B Varicella	Measles Rubella Mumps Diphtheria Tetanus Pertussis Polio *Haemophilus influenzae* b Hepatitis B Varicella Pneumococcal disease Influenza Meningococcal disease Hepatitis A Rotavirus Human papillomavirus
Number of vaccine-preventable diseases	7	10	16

human papilloma virus vaccine (HPV4) in males), the number of targeted diseases remains constant for these age groups as of 2012. Moreover, in the past several years, new vaccines have been introduced for adolescents and young adults (e.g., pertussis booster (Tdap), meningococcal conjugate, and human papillomavirus (HPV) vaccines), and older adults (e.g., Tdap and zoster vaccines) have shown that the value of vaccines extends across the human lifespan. New combination vaccines have been developed to increase the simplicity and acceptability of vaccination regimens, as well as to improve overall compliance with the recommended series of vaccines. Such combinations include either those that contain multiple inactivated or recombinant antigens (such as a combination diphtheria, pertussis, tetanus, Hib, and hepatitis B vaccine) or multiple live attenuated viruses (such as a combination measles, mumps, rubella, and varicella vaccine (MMRV)). The development of a combination vaccine is often more complicated than simply combining individual antigens, for when antigens are administered in combination, immunologic interference is sometimes seen. This necessitates titration of antigen combinations (and in the case of combinations of inactivated and/or recombinant antigens, adjuvant selection) to achieve immune responses that are not inferior to each of the antigens administered individually.

Despite their readily demonstrable public health impact, the value of vaccines is often not appreciated, for when vaccine programs are successful the diseases that they cause become less prevalent and may disappear. However, to prevent resurgence of an infectious disease that has been brought under control, vaccination programs need to be continued. The difficulties facing current efforts to eradicate poliomyelitis have demonstrated that failure to maintain high immunization coverage rates can lead to prompt re-emergence and spread of the disease. Even in developed countries, maintenance of strong immunization programs with high degree of coverage is needed where infectious diseases can travel with remarkable speed—and do so even before the extent of spread is evident.

Principles of immunization

The terms *vaccination* and *immunization* are often used interchangeably. However, vaccination specifically refers to efforts to induce protective immune responses by administration of a vaccine, whereas immunization more generically refers to interventions—either active or passive—that seek to confer immune protection. Active immunization describes the induction of immune responses by administration of a specific antigen or antigens, while passive immunization involves the administration of exogenous immunologically active substances (historically, antibodies present in sera obtained from immune individuals or animals) to confer temporary protection from an infectious pathogen or toxin. Although the approaches for passive immunization waned in the later half of the twentieth century, the advent and increasing robustness of monoclonal antibody technology have led to a resurgence of interest in passive immunization.

Vaccines seek to engender immune responses similar to those that confer immunity to re-infection in individuals who experience (and survive) natural infection with a given pathogen. In lieu of formal demonstration of a specific type of antibody or cellular immune response that contributes to prevention or accelerated clearance of an infection, most often vaccine efficacy is demonstrated first in the course of a placebo-controlled trial. In some instances, specific immune effector mechanisms, such as a specific level or type of antibody response, can be identified that correlate with immune protection. In this case, the "correlate of immunity" provides a benchmark against which similar vaccines can be compared.[9]

In the case of most inactivated vaccines, subunit vaccines, and recombinant vaccines that produce antibody responses, but generally limited, if any, CD8 T-cell responses, it is likely that humoral immune responses are the primary or sole protective immune mechanism. In the case of live attenuated vaccines that induce both cellular and humoral immune responses against the pathogen, it is likely that both arms of the immune system act in concert to confer immunity. However, the actual mechanisms of immune protection induced by either a natural infection or a vaccine are generally not understood in detail for many infectious diseases.

Similarly, although vaccines depend on the induction of immunologic memory, the magnitude, character, and duration of immune memory differ between vaccines, as can the actual mechanism of immune protection. For certain vaccines, such as those that protect against bacterial diseases induced via production of toxins (e.g., diphtheria or tetanus), protection induced by toxoid-based vaccines is clearly dependent on persistent antibody (IgG) and memory B-cell responses, ensuring that sufficient antitoxin antibodies are present at the time of toxin exposure to inactivate and clear the toxin. In other cases, such as long-lived protection against hepatitis B, if sufficient levels of antibodies are achieved in the initial immunization period, even hosts who may with time lose detectable levels of antibody responses remain protected.[10] In this instance, given the relatively long incubation period of hepatitis B, memory antiviral B-cell responses induced by the vaccine can be activated, facilitating neutralization and clearance of the infection before clinical disease is manifest. Although it is popularly believed that vaccines confer protection by inducing "sterilizing immunity"—wherein an infectious agent is blocked from even infecting one cell in an exposed host—this is clearly not the case for a number of vaccines. For example, the inactivated poliovirus and live attenuated rotavirus vaccines do not prevent some degree of local replication of their pathogenic counterparts in the gastrointestinal tract of exposed hosts. However, they are both effective in preventing clinical disease. In the case of poliovirus vaccine, this is mediated by elicitation of antibody responses that block dissemination of the infection to the central nervous system; while in the case of rotavirus, as yet unidentified immune effectors limit local virus replication so that significant gastrointestinal damage does not occur following infection.[11,12]

With the advent of new tools of systems biology, studies to more definitively illuminate the determinants of the magnitude and duration of vaccine-elicited immune responses (such as those that examine patterns of global gene expression induced after vaccination), as well to reveal novel correlates that predict the later development of protective immune responses, now represent a very active and promising area of research.[13,14] In addition to providing new approaches to elucidate the nature of vaccine-mediated immune protection, these new methodologies are already providing windows into a much improved understanding of immune system function in humans and will also hopefully facilitate the development of safe and effective vaccines for diseases (such as for HIV, TB, RSV and others) for which vaccines are not currently available.

As described below, the major types of vaccines licensed for use include live attenuated organisms, killed or inactivated organisms, subunit vaccines consisting of purified (or partially purified) components of an organism, and subunit vaccines produced by recombinant DNA technologies.

Live attenuated vaccines

The use of live attenuated vaccines dates back to the early work of Jenner and Pasteur on smallpox and fowl cholera vaccines, respectively.[15,16] The fundamental concept of live attenuated vaccines is to mimic the effective host immune responses that follow natural infections. Most live attenuated vaccines currently in use were derived by propagation of initially pathogenic organisms in culture on cells from different (nonhuman) species, or at nonphysiologic temperatures, for prolonged periods. Driving pathogen evolution in culture to select for variants adapted to growth in heterologous cell types *ex vivo* often leads to the derivation of pathogen variants that grow poorly *in vivo* in humans and are unable to cause clinical symptoms.

Vaccines developed via this approach include those used to prevent a number of viral and bacterial infections, including yellow fever, measles, mumps, rubella, polio (the "Sabin vaccine"), varicella-zoster (used both for the prevention of chickenpox and shingles) and rotavirus (one version of the available vaccines), tuberculosis, and cholera. More recent technologies being applied to live attenuated vaccine development include the application of reverse genetic strategies (Fig. 90.1) and those involving genetic reassortment with attenuated viral variants, as have been used to develop polyvalent live attenuated vaccines against influenza and rotavirus (Fig. 90.2).[11,12]

The live attenuated vaccines currently in use are highly efficacious (> 90%) and protection is frequently durable. The efficacy of many live attenuated vaccines likely reflects the ability of the attenuated vaccine to replicate within vaccinated hosts, and to expose the immune system to pathogen-derived antigens in a manner that closely resembles the nature, location, and effects of natural infection. Because live attenuated vaccines replicate within vaccinated individuals, they can induce both cellular

(CD4 and CD8) and humoral (B cell) effector responses and immunologic memory. In addition, as the live attenuated vaccines likely activate the host innate system in a manner similar to their pathogenic parents, they provide inherent adjuvant effects in augmenting adaptive immune responses.

A key consideration in the development of any live attenuated vaccine relates to the relative balance between the ability to induce sufficient immune responses *in vivo* to confer protection (often associated with level of preserved replicative ability *in vivo*), and the ability to cause symptoms (which may also relate to the extent of *in vivo* replication). As such, an effective but also safe and well-tolerated vaccine needs to strike a specific balance between level of attenuation and level of immunogenicity. In addition, depending on the nature and number of genetic mutations responsible for the attenuated phenotype, a potential risk of reversion to a pathogenic form exists for certain vaccines. For most live attenuated vaccines, this has not been observed to be a problem in clinical practice — likely because the attenuating mutations are sufficiently numerous or genetically stable. One vaccine where reversion to pathogenic form was seen involved specific components of the live attenuated oral poliovirus vaccine (OPV; the "Sabin vaccine"). In this instance, vaccine reversion to wild-type was shown to lead rarely to cases of paralytic polio (approximately one case per million doses administered).[17] Based on these observations and the elimination of endogenous polio transmission in many developed countries, the inactivated polio vaccine (IPV; the "Salk vaccine") was substituted for OPV. However, in light of a favorable cost–

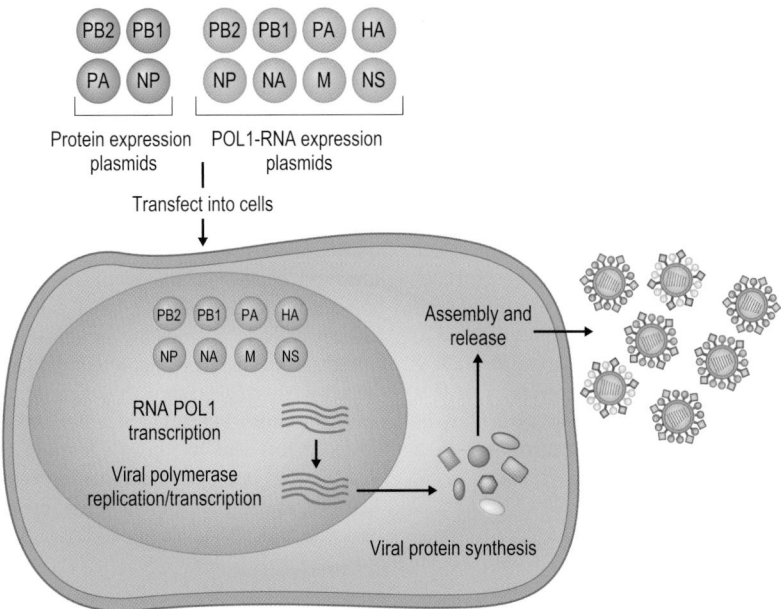

Fig. 90.1 New vaccine strategies: reverse genetic approaches. The term "reverse genetics" refers to the use of recombinant DNA methods to generate infectious viruses possessing genomes derived from cloned cDNAs. Such cDNAs can be modified to study the impact of specific genetic modifications to viral phenotype, providing a new approach for the generation of live attenuated vaccines via either introduction of targeted mutations or, in the case of segmented viruses, the preparation of vaccines via genetic reassortment (see Fig. 90.4). Reverse genetic methods provide promising tools for the study and defined manipulation of both nonsegmented and segmented negative-strand RNA viruses (such as the respiratory syncytial virus (RSV) and influenza viruses, respectively). The use of reverse genetic strategies to generate infectious viral progeny from cloned cDNAs is shown above. Influenza virus genomes are comprised of eight single-stranded (negative-sense) RNA segments. Initiation of influenza virus RNA (vRNA) transcription from negative-sense genomic RNAs, and the replication of the virus genome, depends on the viral ribonucleoprotein (RNP) complex (which includes viral RNA, the nucleoprotein (NP) and three polymerase proteins (PB1, PB2, and PA)). To generate infectious influenza virus from cDNAs of the vRNA genome segments, cells are cotransfected with all eight segments of vRNA under the control of RNA polymerase promoters. Cellular polymerase I (pol 1) synthesizes vRNAs that are then replicated and transcribed by the viral polymerase and NP proteins that comprise the RNP complex. Reverse genetics strategies are expected to facilitate the generation of novel flu vaccines by enabling preparation of well-defined vaccine preparations comprised of donor "backbone" viral segments (see Fig. 90.4) that harbor specific attenuating mutations with vRNA segments encoding the hemagglutinin (HA) and neuraminidase (NA) proteins obtained via reverse transcription of vRNA genes from circulating viruses (including those prepared from pandemic strains that may be difficult and/or unsafe to propagate in large manufacturing scale).

(Adapted from Marsh GA, Tannock GA. The role of reverse genetics in the development of vaccines against respiratory diseases. Exp Opin Biol Ther 2005; 5: 369–380, with permission from Expert Opinion.)

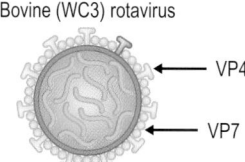

Bovine (WC3) rotavirus

Human-bovine reassortant rotavirus vaccine strains

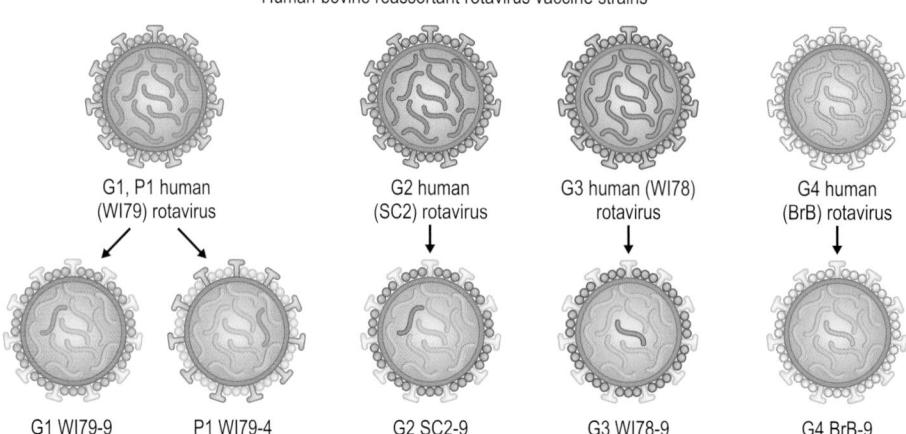

G1, P1 human
(WI79) rotavirus

G2 human
(SC2) rotavirus

G3 human (WI78)
rotavirus

G4 human
(BrB) rotavirus

G1 WI79-9   P1 WI79-4   G2 SC2-9   G3 WI78-9   G4 BrB-9

Fig. 90.2 New vaccine strategies: genetic reassortment approaches. Viruses with segmented genomes provide a new approach for the generation of attenuated vaccines via Mendelian genetic reassortment. If two such segmented viruses with different genetic characteristics are used to infect one cell, the progeny viruses from this mixed infection will carry a range of mixtures of the genes of the two parent viruses. Using either genetic or immunologic screening methods, reassorted viruses carrying the precise gene composition of interest can be selected. This approach has recently been employed to generate live attenuated vaccines against rotavirus and influenza virus. The strategy for generation of the pentavalent bovine–human reassortment rotavirus vaccine is shown above. Rotaviruses have a segmented double-stranded RNA genome comprising 11 independent RNA elements. The outer shell of the virus comprises two proteins VP4 and VP7 that are involved in cell binding and entry and that specify the viral serotype (P type for VP4 and G type for VP7). VP4 and VP7 also represent the targets of virus-neutralizing antibodies. The pentavalent bovine–human reassortment rotavirus vaccine was generated by a "modified Jennerian" approach in which the bovine rotavirus WC3 (which is attenuated in humans as a result of host range restriction) serves as the gene donor for the backbone on to which gene segments encoding four common human rotavirus G types (G1–4) as well as one very common P type (P8) (derived from individual rotavirus isolates) were reassorted via a process of cell co-infection and subsequent selection of the recombinant viruses with the desired composition of bovine and human gene segments. An analogous genetic reassortment approach has also been used to generate live attenuated influenza vaccines. In this instance, three attenuated "cold-adapted" viral strains (two A types and one type B) are used in co-infections in tissue culture with recent circulating wild-type influenza strains to derive vaccine strains that include the two relevant hemagglutinin (HA) and neuraminidase (NA)-encoding gene segments admixed with the six "backbone" genes from the attenuated master donor virus for use in annual influenza vaccines.

benefit ratio, high degree of efficacy, and ease of administration, OPV continues to be the mainstay of polio vaccination efforts in developing countries. Yet, should efforts to eradicate polio continue to advance, new solutions for polio vaccination will need to be developed that do not depend on currently available OPV (which can revert to pathogenic form at low frequency) or IPV (which is produced by inactivation of pathogenic polioviruses strains that will require high levels of biocontainment in a post-eradication environment) vaccines.

Killed or inactivated organisms

The use of physical or chemical methods to kill or otherwise inactivate a pathogenic organism represents a second major approach to vaccine production.[18,19] In most cases, treatment with chemical agents such as β-propiolactone or formaldehyde is used to eliminate pathogen infectivity. While this approach has the benefit of presenting most of a pathogen's antigenic repertoire to the immune system of the immunized host, it can only be used in instances where the inactivated pathogen does not possess constituents that would confer significant toxicity. Vaccines based on killed pathogens are believed to exert their protective effects via elicitation of pathogen-neutralizing antibodies and the induction of memory B-cell responses (likely in concert with CD4 T-cell memory). However, because inactivated

pathogens cannot accomplish *de novo* synthesis of pathogen-derived gene products in antigen-presenting cells (APCs), they do not typically induce CD8 T-cell responses (Chapter 6). In addition, killed vaccines are generally less immunogenic than live attenuated vaccines. As a result, they are commonly administered with an adjuvant (most often aluminium salts: see section on Adjuvants, below) to augment their immunogenicity. A number of viral and bacterial vaccines currently in use are killed/inactivated vaccines, including whole-cell *Bordetella pertussis* vaccine and the influenza virus, rabies virus, and hepatitis A virus vaccines.

Purified subunit vaccines

A number of bacteria produce toxins that represent the major pathogenic components responsible for disease in infected humans. Examples include *Corynebacterium diphtheriae* and *Clostridium tetani*. Detoxified versions of these toxins are referred to as "toxoids," and represent the purified components of vaccines preventing diphtheria and tetanus, respectively. Toxoids have historically been produced by chemical inactivation of toxins, but more recently, genetic inactivation via targeted mutagenesis has been employed. The acellular pertussis vaccine is also a purified subunit vaccine composed of a defined set of protein constituents prepared from cultured *Bordetella pertussis*. The mechanism of immune protection conferred by purified subunit vaccines is the antibody response elicited by vaccination.

Antibodies directed against the capsular polysaccharides present on encapsulated bacteria also confer protective immunity in a number of important instances by inducing antibodies that exert opsonophagocytic effects (promoting phagocytosis of antibody-coated bacteria) and, in some instances, bactericidal effects.[20] Initial successful vaccine efforts against *Streptococcus pneumoniae* and *Neisseria meningitidis* utilized purified preparations of capsular polysaccharides. Although such purified polysaccharides can induce protective levels of antibody responses in adults, they are poorly immunogenic in children under 2 years of age (as a function of the relative immaturity of their immune systems). In addition, T-independent antibody responses elicited by purified capsular polysaccharides are less durable than those that are produced in the presence of CD4 T-cell help. As a means of both augmenting antibody responses against polysaccharide antigens in young children and facilitating their persistence, the development of conjugate vaccines represented an important advance.[21] In this approach, purified polysaccharides are chemically conjugated to a carrier protein (such as diphtheria toxoid or an outer-membrane protein complex (OMPC) derived from *N. meningitidis*). The carrier protein augments CD4 T-cell helper responses to the polysaccharide antigens, and enables elicitation of durable protective antibody responses even in young children. Polysaccharide-conjugate vaccines have been produced that protect against *Haemophilus influenzae* b, *Streptococcus pneumoniae*, and *N. meningitidis* infections.

Recombinant protein subunit vaccines

The advent of recombinant DNA technologies provided a transformational event in the history of vaccine development. In addition to facilitating the identification and expression of pathogen-derived protective antigens, techniques were developed that enabled their large-scale manufacture as vaccines. Recombinant DNA technologies provided a new path to develop vaccines against pathogens, such as hepatitis B virus (HBV)

or HPV, that could not be grown in culture. In addition, recombinant methods provided the potential to derive even safer versions of available vaccines.

The first recombinant vaccine developed, the recombinant hepatitis B surface antigen (HBsAg) prepared in yeast, was developed in hopes of avoiding safety concerns related to the plasma-derived HBsAg vaccine.[22] The knowledge that immune sera could provide protection by passive immunization of naïve hosts, and that purified inactivated plasma-derived HBsAg vaccine could elicit protective antibodies, laid the groundwork for development of this recombinant vaccine.[23] The recombinant vaccine, when combined with adjuvant (aluminium salts), elicits favorable immune responses, is highly efficacious and is well tolerated — all features that recombinant vaccines are now expected to deliver. The second recombinant vaccine developed targeted prevention of *Borrelia burgdorferi* infection (the cause of Lyme disease), and was based on a purified recombinant version of the OspA protein. This vaccine, although conferring some degree of efficacy, faced implementation challenges, and was not widely embraced. As a result, it was withdrawn from the market.

More recently, recombinant technology-derived purified subunit vaccines have been developed that consist of virus-like particles (VLPs) that self-assemble when the L1 protein of HPV is produced in isolation of other viral proteins (Fig. 90.3).[24] The L1 protein is the target of virus-neutralizing antibodies and vaccines consisting of a mixture of types 16 and 18 (the cause of ~70% of cases of cervical cancer) and 6 and 11 (the cause of ~90% of cases of genital warts) or of HPV types 16 and 18 alone are highly efficacious and well tolerated.[25] Interestingly, HPV VLPs induce antibody responses that exceed those that follow natural HPV infections.[26]

In light of these successes, and the power and versatility of recombinant antigen production methods, a major proportion of new vaccine development efforts involves the use of protein subunit vaccines produced by recombinant technologies. Vaccines produced by this method are those that depend largely or exclusively on the induction of antibodies against individual or a selected subset of pathogen proteins. Because a number of proteins produced in isolation by recombinant methods have been

Prophylactic HPV Vaccines:
L1 Virus-like Particles (VLPs)

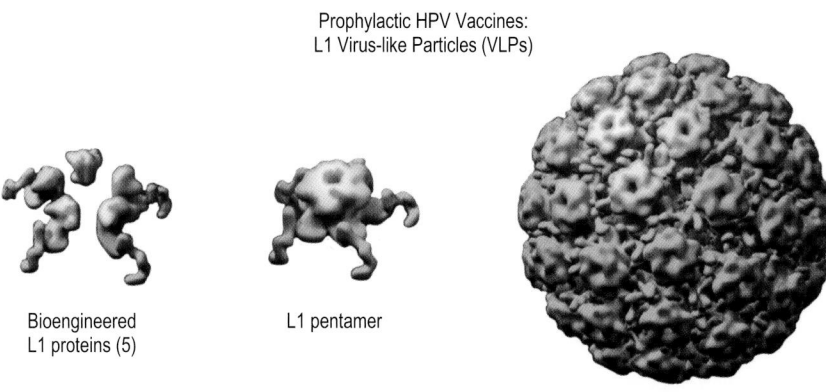

Bioengineered L1 proteins (5)　　　L1 pentamer

Self-assembled virus-like particle

Fig. 90.3 New vaccine strategies: recombinant virus-like particle (VLP) approaches. In specific instances, VLPs can be produced via a process of self-assembly of individual viral capsid proteins produced by recombinant DNA methods in cell culture systems. This approach has a number of attractive aspects, including the ability to produce VLPs that accurately display conformationally correct epitopes recognized by neutralizing antibodies and the absence of pathogen-derived nucleic acids. In addition, recombinant VLPs have been employed to derive safe and effective vaccines for pathogens, such as hepatitis B virus (HBV) and human papillomavirus (HPV), that cannot be grown in culture (and are thus refractory to standard vaccine approaches of attenuation or inactivation). The generation of the VLPs that comprises newly developed HPV vaccines is shown. The HPV L1 proteins (which represent the major capsid protein and target of virus-neutralizing, protective antibodies), derived from HPV types of interest (e.g., types 16, 18, 6, and 11) are produced via recombinant methods. Under appropriate conditions, individual bioengineered L1 proteins first self-assemble into pentamers, and then into VLPs that are comprised of 72 pentamers and that are almost identical, both morphologically and antigenically, to infectious HPV virus particles. VLPs prepared from individual HPV types are then combined with specific adjuvants to prepare the final vaccine products.

observed to elicit lower immune responses than do natural infections or live attenuated vaccines, the development and use of adjuvants to optimize recombinant vaccine immunogenicity represent an important parallel area for future exploration (see below).

Vaccine development and evaluation

KEY CONCEPTS

Considerations guiding vaccine development

The development of new vaccines depends on the convergence of public health need, biological plausibility, and practical feasibility. Vaccine development programs are influenced by multiple considerations, including:

- What are the major unmet medical and public health needs today?
- What is known about the natural history and pathogenic mechanisms of the infection of interest?
- Is immunity to a given antigen associated with protection against disease following re-exposure in the context of natural infection?
- If natural immunity capable of preventing re-infection follows an initial infection, can a specific host immune effector mechanism (e.g., antibody, CD8 T cell) be identified as the likely agent (or "correlate") of immune protection?
- Can the pathogen be grown in culture? If so, does the pathogen cause such a life-threatening disease that an attenuated version of the virus would face an impossible barrier for demonstration of safety?
- Can a specific antigen (or antigens) be identified that represents the target of protective host immune responses?
- If the protective immune response is mediated by antibodies, can the target antigen be produced in scalable quantities in a form that mimics its native structure so that it can effectively elicit antibody responses that can block the key functional role(s) of the target molecule in the pathogen or otherwise lead to pathogen clearance?
- Having chosen an antigen and presentation system, what is the best way to produce it on a large scale?
- What is the most effective way to present the antigens of the pathogen of interest to the immune system?
- Is the antigen of interest sufficiently immunogenic on its own, or is augmentation of the desired immune response by conjugation to a specific carrier or addition of an adjuvant necessary for vaccination?
- What potential safety concerns can be anticipated for the vaccine in question?
- What is the attack rate of the infection in the general population? If the infection occurs relatively rarely in an overall population, can a subset of the population be identified that has a higher risk of infection so as to accelerate the achievement of statistically significant protection?
- What tests to evaluate vaccine immunogenicity will need to be carried out on clinical samples obtained from participants in the clinical trials? Will measurement of antibody titers, T-cell responses, pathogen presence and quantity, pathogen serotype, and any other parameter peculiar to the disease in question represent the primary criteria for vaccine effect? Development and validation of these tests represent an essential component for the feasibility and success of a vaccine clinical study.

As a necessary prelude to clinical evaluation of candidate vaccines in humans, extensive preclinical research and development activities are undertaken to establish that the vaccine candidate has the desired properties. Toward this end, a number of key issues need to be addressed. First, animal studies must show that the vaccine candidate raises the desired type and magnitude of immune response against the infectious agent. Second, the vaccine needs to protect animals against death or disease in an appropriate challenge model, when feasible. Ideally, in the course of these studies, a specific type or level of immune response, referred to as a correlate of immune protection, can be identified. Third, the vaccine should be relatively free of serious discernible toxicities and side effects in animals when administered by the route intended for humans. Fourth, it is necessary to demonstrate that the vaccine can be produced in a consistent manner by a process that follows the current good manufacturing practices (cGMP) process by which the first clinical trial materials will be produced (http://www.fda.gov/cber/gdlns/indcgmp.pdf).

Even before preclinical studies are completed, vaccine developers typically begin an initial dialog with regulatory authorities (such as the Food and Drug Administration (FDA) or the European Medicines Agency (EMEA)) to set expectations about what will be necessary and sufficient for advancement to clinical studies in humans (http://www.fda.gov/cber/genetherapy/isct092506sh.pdf).

Phase I studies primarily focus on detailed assessment of the safety and tolerability of a vaccine, but evaluation of its immunogenicity is also frequently conducted. Generally, a phase I study includes fewer than 100 healthy volunteers divided unequally between those who receive vaccine or placebo (2 or 3 vaccinees per placebo recipient). Phase I studies typically employ escalating doses of the candidate vaccine, with a dose range progressively increasing in steps of three- to fivefold often being used. Blood samples are taken at prescribed intervals and analyzed for laboratory evidence of potential toxicity, as well as for evidence of vaccine-elicited immune responses. A phase I study is considered successful if it demonstrates that the candidate vaccine is well tolerated or identifies any immediate safety concerns that will need to be closely monitored in potential future clinical studies. Ideally, phase I studies also provide an initial indication of the optimal dose level and number of doses required.

A phase II study typically includes several hundred to a few thousand volunteers (randomized between vaccine and placebo) and can assume two general design types. Phase IIa studies provide additional safety data on a larger number of individuals of the intended age who receive the intended vaccine dose (who are more representative of the general population intended for vaccine use than the very healthy individuals included in the phase I study), as well as provide additional data on vaccine immunogenicity. Even larger phase IIb studies can provide additional data on vaccine safety and immunogenicity in subjects generally representative of those for whom the vaccine might be recommended, but importantly, also provide the first opportunity to address to answer the question, "Does this vaccine work in humans?" The size of a phase IIb study needed to detect a signal of vaccine efficacy depends on the attack rate of the infection being targeted by the vaccine.

Phase II studies also present the first opportunity to identify a potential laboratory immunological correlate of protection from disease — if nature and prior experience have not already done so. In order to do so, the placebo recipients in the phase II trial must experience a sufficient number of cases of disease while vaccine recipients need to exhibit significant evidence of decreased risk of infection or disease. In addition, immunological measurements in the vaccinees need to capture the relevant protective immune responses (e.g., the type and level of antibody and/or cellular immune response that predict protection) and measure them with sufficient precision and reliability. If laboratory measurements of immunity correlate with clinical protection, subsequent refinements of the vaccine, its adjuvant, its manufacturing process, or its regimen may be assessed by simple immunogenicity studies, rather than repeating efficacy studies. Once efficacy is established for a vaccine, it is very difficult ethically to carry out a double-blinded, placebo-controlled efficacy study.

Vaccines that have been shown to be immunogenic and well tolerated in phase II studies can then advance to pivotal phase III studies required for vaccine licensure by regulatory authorities. Phase III studies are intended to expand further the safety database in a larger number of individuals (who are representative of the specific populations for which the vaccine will ultimately be used), establish definitive evidence of protective efficacy, and to establish clinical consistency of the vaccine made by the process run in the facility intended for licensure and commercialization (http://www.fda.gov/cber/genetherapy/isct092506jcr.htm). Typically, phase III studies include 10 000 or more subjects in a blinded, placebo-controlled design. This size trial allows the identification of less frequent safety events. It also provides an opportunity to capture data on health care utilization, cost, and impact of the vaccine on these parameters. As a new vaccine will ultimately be included in a vaccine program where multiple vaccines may be administered at the same time, it is also necessary to conduct concomitant-use studies. The developer of the new vaccine must show that the new vaccine does not impact on the immunogenicity of the existing vaccines, and that the existing vaccines do not impact on the immunogenicity of the new vaccine.

Licensure and recommendation of vaccines

In contrast to drugs, where licensure by the FDA is the primary determinant of how a new product is implemented in medical practice, vaccine use in the USA includes an additional process that evaluates how best to employ a new vaccine to optimize its implementation and public health impact. The US CDC has responsibility for making recommendations about the use of licensed vaccines, and it relies on its Advisory Committee on Immunization Practices (ACIP) for guidance. The ACIP considers several aspects in addition to a vaccine's safety and efficacy, including the anticipated cost-effectiveness and practical feasibility of potential alternative vaccine deployment strategies and consideration of how a new vaccine can be successfully implemented in clinical practice to achieve the greatest public health impact. Once the CDC has received, reviewed, and accepted the recommendation of the ACIP (http://www.cdc.gov/vaccines/recs/ACIP), the recommendation is published in its final official form in *Morbidity and Mortality Weekly Report* (MMWR; http://www.cdc.gov/vaccines/default.htm). General recommendations concerning vaccine storage, handling and administration as well as Vaccine Information Statements (VISs) that explain both the benefits and risks of each recommended vaccine and that are to be provided to all vaccine recipients (or their parents or guardians) can also be found at this CDC website.

The approach to developing vaccine recommendations in the European Union (EU) is somewhat more complicated, as multiple sovereign countries are involved. At present, vaccines are evaluated for registration through a centralized procedure by the European Medicines Agency (http://www.ema.europa.eu) and its Committee on Medicinal Products for Human Use (CHMP). Vaccines are reviewed by a country representing the EU as a whole, and ultimately registered through a mutual recognition procedure based upon endorsement by member states, or occasionally by individual countries. In contrast, for vaccine policy determination, each member country retains its own national advisory committee with responsibility for national recommendations. As a result, there is significant heterogeneity in vaccine recommendations within the EU.

As many developing and middle-income countries lack the regulatory infrastructure and technical expertise to conduct their own formal review of new vaccines, they commonly rely on the assessments made by the World Health Organization (WHO) through its prequalification procedure (available at http://www.who.int/vaccines-documents as document WHO/IBV/05.19). The prequalification process assesses a candidate vaccine's manufacturing standards, quality, safety, efficacy, as well as its overall acceptability for procurement by UN agencies (such as UNICEF). In addition to the WHO's role related to the prequalification process, the WHO Strategic Advisory Group of Experts (SAGE) provides recommendations for vaccine use to inform national policies for countries that lack their own national vaccine policy body.

Vaccines for routine use and in special populations

The recommended immunization schedules for US children and adolescents and for adults (Appendix A5) are updated on an annual basis and can be accessed at http://www.cdc.gov/vaccines/default.htm and http://www.cdc.gov/nip/recs/adult-schedule.htm, respectively. The recommended adult immunization schedule includes information concerning use in special populations (such as health care workers and pregnant women) and individuals with specific conditions associated with altered or impaired immune function (such as individuals with congenital and acquired immunodeficiency syndromes, recipients of immunosuppressive therapies, malignancies, asplenia, liver disease, and renal disease). Readers are encouraged to check to ensure that they are following current recommendations.

Recommendations concerning the use of specific vaccines in travelers to countries were vaccine-preventable diseases may be present can be found at http://www.cdc.gov/travel/vaccinations.htm.

Pregnancy registries exist for a number of vaccines in the USA, and contact information about them can be found at http://www.fda.gov/scienceresearch/specialtopics/womenshealthresearch/ucm134848.htm. Health care professionals are encouraged to report exposures of pregnant women to the appropriate registry: HBV vaccine (800-670-6126), HPV vaccine (800-986-8999), meningococcal vaccine (800-822-2463), and varicella vaccine (800-986-8999).

Vaccine safety

Unlike drugs that are utilized to treat individuals suffering from a given disease state, vaccines are administered to normal, healthy infants, adolescents, and adults. Consequently, standards for the safety and tolerability of vaccines are set at a very high level. When developing a new vaccine, a graded process of clinical studies is employed that involves increasingly larger numbers of volunteers and that typically progresses from individuals who are selected to be free of any identifiable health problems to those who are selected to be representative of the overall population for whom the vaccine is being developed. If phase I studies reveal no evidence of safety concerns and the desired evidence of immunogenicity, a major focus of the series of larger randomized double-blind, phase II placebo-controlled studies that are then conducted is to explore the safety and tolerability of a vaccine in increasingly vulnerable populations (such as those who may have identified pre-existing health problems or asymptomatic abnormalities detected on screening laboratory studies).

Reflecting the importance of documenting the safety of a new vaccine, phase III studies to assess the safety and efficacy of a new vaccine now typically involve large numbers of volunteers. Indeed, as a result of needing to provide evidence for safety, it is now common to have the size of the phase III trial be significantly larger than would be necessary to document vaccine efficacy. The ability of a study to identify an increased risk of any given adverse event with sufficient statistical power is directly related to the size of the population in the study. As a general rule, a study of 300–400 subjects is needed to measure the risk of an event that happens in one out of 100 individuals. For one in 1000 events, 3000–4000 subjects are needed. Even in studies of this size, very rare events may not be identified, and if a specific safety concern exists substantially larger trials may be needed.

The recent experience with the development of rotavirus vaccines provides an illustrative example of the importance placed on documenting vaccine safety.[27] Rotavirus is an important cause of serious gastroenteritis in infants and young children, and the associated diarrhea and vomiting can lead to life-threatening dehydration. In developing countries where health care resources and effective rehydration options are limited, over 600 000 infants die of rotavirus gastroenteritis each year.[28] Given the global importance of rotavirus gastroenteritis, the first licensure of an orally administered rotavirus vaccine in 1998 was a very welcome advance. However, as the vaccine entered routine pediatric practice, it was recognized that a low, but increased incidence of intestinal intussusception was seen after the first and second doses (with about one case of intussusception seen per 10 000 vaccinees).[29] Upon recognition of this association, the vaccine was withdrawn from the market.[30]

With the evident public health need for a safe and effective rotavirus vaccine, it was hoped that alternative rotavirus vaccines then in development (both oral vaccines based either on a combination of bovine–human reassortant viruses (Fig. 90.2) or an attenuated human rotavirus strain) might differ from the first licensed rotavirus vaccine and not result in an increased rate of intussusception. However, to demonstrate that these alternative rotavirus vaccines were safe, and that an increased risk of intussusception was not inherent to rotavirus vaccines as a class, very large-scale safety studies were required. Toward this end, the safety of each of these vaccines was evaluated in studies involving about 70 000 infants — just to evaluate whether the rate of intussusception in vaccinees was discernibly increased compared to the normal background rates seen in the placebo recipients.[11,12] Fortunately, both vaccines were found to be well tolerated and no increase in intussusception was observed in vaccine as compared to placebo recipients. In light of the documented efficacy of these vaccines determined in earlier and significantly smaller phase III trials, both have now been licensed in a number of countries. However, even with the large phase III studies conducted for these newer rotavirus vaccines, they have been and continue to be studied in large postlicensure active surveillance safety studies and closely monitored in active and passive vaccine safety surveillance systems (see below).

Following vaccine licensure, safety is tracked via a number of means, including both active and passive surveillance studies of adverse events. Active surveillance includes phase IV postmarketing studies of vaccine safety in larger populations in real-world use. Formal postmarketing studies can include tens of thousands of individuals or more.

An alternative type of postmarketing safety monitoring is carried out by the US FDA and the CDC within the context of the Vaccine Adverse Event Reporting System (VAERS) database (http://www.vaers.hhs.gov or by telephone: 800-822-7967). The VAERS database accepts spontaneous reports of adverse experiences from health care providers, patients, parents, vaccine manufacturers, and other sources.[31] The best use of the VAERS database is to identify signals in a population that may appear following the introduction of a new vaccine.

A newer vaccine safety surveillance system, known as the Vaccine Safety Database (VSD), has been developed by the CDC in cooperation with seven large health maintenance organizations (HMOs) around the USA.[32] The VSD contains the complete medical records of all the members from the participating HMOs, and the information used to populate the database is entered by health care professionals using relatively consistent terminology, improving the quality, uniformity, and usefulness of the data. Particularly important is that the VSD construct allows comprehensive epidemiological analyses to determine if the incidence rate of a specific adverse event is higher among vaccinees than nonvaccinees. In addition to VAERS and the VSD, the CDC has also created a Clinical Immunization Safety Assessment Network that reviews patterns of clinical syndromes that may follow vaccination.

While the safety profile of a vaccine can be relatively well defined through the efforts described above, confidence in vaccination programs has often been challenged by public perceptions, either real or unsubstantiated, about vaccine safety.[33,34] In some instances, specific vaccines have been associated with increased incidence of a specific adverse experience, such as the association between the first-generation rotavirus vaccine and an increased risk of intussusception following vaccination. However, a number of other safety concerns that have emerged are not supported by scientific evidence.[35] An example of this can be found in the case of concerns about the association of whole-cell pertussis vaccines with permanent brain damage — concerns that were later shown to be unfounded. Nevertheless, public concerns about the safety of the whole-cell pertussis vaccine resulted in decreased levels of pertussis vaccination coverage that were soon followed by epidemics of whooping cough in the UK and Japan.[36] Another example is the allegation that certain vaccines, such as the combination measles, mumps, rubella (MMR) vaccine, are associated with autism. Highlighting how perceptions of temporal association can give rise to public concerns, MMR vaccines are generally given around 1 year of age, and autism is generally diagnosed in the second year of life. Although the alleged causal association between MMR and autism has been refuted by multiple extensive scientific analyses, reports in the popular media in the UK resulted in a dramatic drop in vaccination rates, followed by an increased rate of new infections.[37,38] The original publication in *The Lancet* was subsequently disavowed by the majority of the manuscript's authors[39] and then formally retracted by *The Lancet*'s editors as a result of factual misrepresentations and ethical violations.[40,41] While the purported association between MMR and autism has now been thoroughly discredited, this claim resulted in decreased MMR vaccination rates in a number of countries as a result of some parents delaying or refusing measles vaccination. With an increase in the number of geographic clusters of unvaccinated children, rates of endemic measles infections have recently increased in several countries in Europe (with a spill-over effect of nearly all of the rare cases of measles reported in the USA having originated from US travelers visiting endemic countries or immigrants from them).

Vaccines not yet available

Although an impressive armamentarium of vaccines is now available, safe and effective vaccines have yet to be developed for a number of very important infectious diseases. The reasons underlying the lack of effective vaccines for an array of important pathogens include biological considerations, safety concerns, and practical constraints. Of these, the biological considerations are often the most important barrier. As discussed above, vaccines have been successfully developed for pathogens whose natural infections give rise to natural immunity wherein the infected host (at least those who survive initial infection) is no longer susceptible to re-infection (such as measles, yellow fever virus, or smallpox) or who experiences significantly less severe clinical sequelae upon re-infection (such as rotavirus). In instances where natural immunity follows natural infection, not only is a precedent for immune protection established, but the nature of protective host responses can be studied, providing a correlate of protection to guide vaccine development efforts. However, for many of the pathogens for which vaccines remain elusive, natural immunity does not follow natural infection. In the absence of natural immunity, not only is a precedent for successful immune containment lacking, but no potential correlates of protection are available to inform vaccine development. In some instances where natural immunity does not follow natural infection, persistent infections are established and maintained by active virus replication that cannot be controlled or cleared by host immune responses (such as HIV and hepatitis C).

Alternatively, other pathogens are able to persist in the host through establishment, via diverse mechanisms, of latent infections that are resistant to host immune clearance (such as tuberculosis or herpes viruses (e.g., herpes simplex virus (HSV) or Epstein–Barr virus (EBV)). In other instances, even when the host is cleared of an infection via drug treatment, the host remains susceptible to re-infection and disease in the future (e.g., malaria). Although different pathogens have evolved diverse strategies for evasion of host immune responses — ranging from manifestation of tremendous genetic diversity and propensity for immune escape; to sequestration of critical structural domains that might be susceptible to antibody neutralization; to the utilization of specific mechanisms to evade host innate and adaptive immune effectors — the common end result is frustration of vaccine development.

While failure of host clearance of an infection is a common theme underlying the lack of vaccines, additional obstacles to vaccine development include other immunologically related considerations as well as both practical and safety considerations. Examples of immunologically related obstacles include instances where prior exposure to a given pathogen predisposes the host to more severe disease manifestations upon re-infection (as has been proposed in the case of dengue virus) or where earlier vaccine development efforts inadvertently led to severe adverse events following infection with the targeted pathogen (such as respiratory syncytial virus (RSV)). In each of these cases, the adverse events that follow a secondary immune exposure are believed to be the result of immunopathologic responses that result from the nature of the immune response elicited by the initial exposure to pathogen-derived antigens (by either infection or vaccination). Given that the mechanisms underlying these immunopathologic processes are incompletely understood, the development of vaccines that are highly immunogenic but not similarly inclined to elicit immune-mediated adverse consequences represents a substantial challenge (especially given the very high expectations for vaccine safety). An additional immunologically related challenge relates to the observation that certain organisms encode antigens that resemble constituents of the human host. For example, in the case of *Neisseria meningitidis* group B, the bacterial polysaccharide resembles those found on certain human cell lineages, thus raising concerns about whether polysaccharide-based vaccines successfully developed for group B *N. meningitidis* might yield undesirable autoimmune responses.[42]

An additional distinct, but important, practical barrier to new vaccine development relates to the prevention of diseases that are threats to pregnant women or their offspring (where immunization of the pregnant woman might be able to protect the neonate). Although a number of inactivated vaccines are either routinely recommended for use in pregnant women (e.g., inactivated influenza vaccine) or can be used in pregnant women for pre- or postexposure prophylaxis for those at risk of infection (e.g., inactivated hepatitis A vaccine and recombinant HBsAg vaccine), the development of new vaccines specifically for use in pregnant women or the study of new vaccines in pregnant women has been impeded by concerns arising from potential litigation that might follow the appearance of a congenital abnormality in a child born to a mother who was vaccinated while pregnant.[43] Given the 2–3% prevalence of congenital abnormalities, the practical difficulties in proving the safety of a new vaccine specifically administered to pregnant women, and the current litigious environment surrounding vaccines, the development of new vaccines to address important infections of pregnant women and their neonates (e.g., group B streptococcus: GBS) faces significant challenges. However, recently strengthened recommendations for vaccination of pregnant women with influenza vaccine, and compelling evidence of its benefits, may help to foster increased attention to overcoming existing obstacles to the development and appropriate use of vaccines for pregnant women.

There remain a number of important infectious diseases for which no effective preventive vaccines exist. Below, we list the major "missing" vaccines, comment on why they are not yet available, and highlight the major approaches currently being explored to develop them.

Improved Influenza vaccines

Given the importance of seasonal influenza as a serious, if frustratingly unpredictable, global health threat, and concerns about the potential emergence of highly virulent pandemic strains of influenza (which is more a question of "what and when" rather than "whether"), a tremendous effort is now being devoted to the development of novel strategies for the production of influenza vaccines to significantly improve upon limitations of the influenza vaccines currently in use. Current research and development efforts are focusing on the derivation of flu vaccine approaches that would have much greater speed and reliability of production soon after recognition of emergence of a new strain; that would be more readily produced at a scale to enable global access; that would engender increased breadth of coverage to protect against diverse influenza strains; and that would be more immunogenic and efficacious in vulnerable populations (such as the elderly) who often respond poorly to currently available vaccines. In addition to efforts to develop novel influenza vaccines, efforts to increase the immunogenicity of the flu vaccines in populations that typically respond poorly (including the elderly) and to accomplish dose-sparing benefits (that would be useful in pandemic settings where vaccine supply is limited) via the use of novel adjuvants or alternative delivery approaches (such as intradermal administration) are being actively explored.

Influenza virus was first isolated and characterized in the early 1930s by groups working in parallel in the UK and in the US. In 1935, it was demonstrated that influenza virus could grow productively in minced chick embryo tissue and in embryonated hen's eggs, and that the virus could be collected from the allantoic fluid. Shortly thereafter, the original approach to influenza vaccine production was developed that involved chemical inactivation of the virus with formalin, followed by its disruption with detergent–yielding non-infectious, but immunogenic viral fragments. Most of the currently deployed influenza vaccines continue to be manufactured according to this 60–70 year old process. More recently, based on the recognition that influenza virus also grows well in certain cultivated mammalian cells, some vaccine manufacturers are looking toward this somewhat more controlled method for producing virus that can then be inactivated by the traditional methods above.

In the late 1950s in Russia and the early 1960s in Michigan, two groups developed attenuated live-influenza vaccines, referred to as Live Attenuated Influenza Vaccines (LAIVs), that were selected to grow at low temperatures in the nasopharynx and not at the higher temperatures of the lung. As a result, they are able to engender protective immunity without disease. Both of these vaccines are currently produced in eggs.

Influenza viruses, and the vaccines made to protect against influenza type A are characterized by serotypes of the two major surface antigens, hemagglutinin (HA) and neuraminidase (NA). Type B influenza viruses do not yet have a similar serotyping system, but they share the same general structures of the type A viruses. Given the segmented genome of the virus and the relatively low-fidelity replication system, influenza viruses can mutate and swap gene segments very efficiently, requiring constant worldwide virus surveillance and an annual updating of the vaccine components based on surveillance data.

Vaccine production strains are now produced by "reverse genetics" as shown in Fig. 90.1, rather than classical co-infection and selection methods. Either way, the goal is to make vaccine viruses that display the relevant HA and NA antigens.

Until recently, influenza vaccination campaigns have been largely targeted to persons over 65 years of age and to people with immunocompromising medical conditions. The vaccines described above work well in younger healthy persons, but their immunogenicity drops off sharply above about 60 years of age. There are numerous efforts to make vaccines that perform better in these older populations. Current strategies include higher doses of flu antigen and the inclusion of adjuvants based on oil-water emulsion formulations of existing vaccines (as well as exploration of novel, more potent adjuvants (see below)).

In the late 1990s there were multiple outbreaks of avian influenza of the flu A H5N1 lineage in poultry markets in China and later in Viet Nam and Indonesia. There were numerous lethal primary infections in humans who had contact with infected chickens, leading to great concern about the spread of H5 type viruses in humans. Humans rarely have any detectable immunity against H5 viruses. This prompted numerous programs to increase capacity for making influenza vaccines rapidly in order to curtail or prevent an H5, or other novel influenza, pandemic.

In April of 2009 a large and unexpected number of cases of influenza emerged in Mexico off-season. Mexican and US CDC authorities quickly isolated the H1N1 virus responsible for this initial outbreak and showed that it had an unusual constellation of human, swine and avian gene segments. This novel H1N1 strain quickly spread to become a global pandemic. Vaccine production began soon after the initial recognition of the new flu strain, and by October of 2009 vaccine deliveries began. Unfortunately, as a result of difficulties in producing the vaccine strains in eggs, the majority of vaccine produced only arrived in late October 2009 after the peak of virus circulation had already passed, leaving 70-80 million doses wasted.

As a consequence of this experience, there is a renewed interest in modern, more efficient, influenza vaccines that perform well in all target populations. Given the need to update the composition of the flu vaccine, research attention is turning to conserved antigens that might provide broad protection against a range of influenza strains. Targets for this type of "universal" vaccine include:

- The M2 ion channel ectodomain present on type A viruses[44]
- The nucleoprotein as a cytotoxic T-cell antigen[45,46]
- The cleavage site on the stalk of the HA molecule[47]
- A conserved HA stalk structure fusion intermediate[48]

Because the major rate-limiting element of influenza vaccine production is the rate of growth of influenza virus in either eggs or cells, several laboratories have developed methods for making HA in recombinant DNA based systems, thus bypassing the need to grow the virus in eggs or on cultured cell lines. The most advanced methods include bacteria,[49] insect cells,[50,51] and tobacco plants.[52,53] A comprehensive spreadsheet that tracks the progress of pandemic influenza vaccine development can be found on the WHO website at http://www.who.int/vaccine_research/diseases/influenza/flu_trials_tables/en/index.html.

Human immunodeficiency virus (Chapter 37)

At the end of 2010, an estimated 34 million people worldwide were living with HIV infection, and in the preceding year approximately 2.7 million people became newly infected, and approximately 1.8 million individuals died of AIDs).[54] As the most promising biomedical intervention to contain the AIDS pandemic, the development of an HIV vaccine is a top global health priority. Yet, HIV infection represents a vexing challenge to vaccine development.[55,56] HIV establishes a chronic, persistent infection that cannot be cleared by host immune responses. Following infection of target cells, the genome of HIV—a retrovirus—is transcribed into a DNA copy via the action of reverse transcriptase. The newly formed DNA copy of the HIV genome then integrates into the host cell chromosomes (referred to as a provirus) as a requisite step in the viral lifecycle. Once integrated into the chromosome of an infected cell, the HIV provirus can alternatively be actively transcribed, leading to the synthesis of viral mRNAs and subsequently to production of new virus particles, or it can remain in a transcriptionally silent, functionally latent state in a small percentage of infected cells. As infected cells harboring latent HIV proviruses do not produce HIV protein antigens, they cannot be recognized by host antiviral immune responses and can thereby persist undetected. Upon subsequent activation of latently infected cells at some later time, viral RNA transcription can be coincidently activated leading to production of progeny virions.

As HIV targets activated CD4 T cells for infection and consequent depletion, the host's ability to mount both HIV-specific and non-HIV-specific immune responses is progressively impaired. The ability of the host to clear HIV infection is further complicated by the extensive genetic diversity of virus populations that emerge, and progressively diverge, within infected individuals as a function of a replicative cycle that is accomplished by the inherently error-prone reverse transcriptase and the numerous cycles of replication that occur in infected individuals. As a result of these influences, genetically diverse populations of HIV variants are established in infected persons that facilitate the outgrowth of genetic variants that can escape from selective pressures—be they effective host cellular or humoral immune responses, or the inhibitory effects of antiretroviral drugs.[57] An extraordinary degree of genetic diversity is also manifest in the HIV variants seen in different individuals and in different geographic regions. As successful vaccines for other infectious agents have historically had to protect against pathogens exhibiting only limited genetic diversity, HIV represents an unprecedented challenge to vaccine development.

As many successful vaccines protecting against viral infections are predicated on the induction of neutralizing antibody responses against the viral surface proteins that mediate attachment to and entry into target cells, significant efforts have focused on the potential of the HIV surface envelope (Env) glycoprotein, Gp120, to elicit infection-neutralizing antibodies.[58] Unfortunately, HIV gp120 is highly resistant to the neutralizing action of antibodies by virtue of its heavy glycosylation and its native conformation that shields functionally critical structural domains from antibody binding. As a result, candidate gp120-based vaccines have, to date, failed to elicit meaningful levels of neutralizing antibodies in immunized human volunteers and have not protected from HIV infection in two large phase III studies.

Given the inability, to date, of candidate HIV Env-based vaccines to elicit appreciable levels of neutralizing antibodies and the failure of initial Phase III studies of gp120-based vaccines, vaccine strategies subsequently became largely focused on the induction of CD8 cytotoxic T-cell responses against the more constrained and conserved antigens, such as *gag, pol,* and *nef.* It was hypothesized that induction of high levels of HIV-specific CD8 T-cell responses prior to infection may not prevent infection, but may enable infected individuals to control virus replication better. Should this hypothesis be valid, individuals immunized with such vaccines may exhibit lower levels of ongoing HIV replication, progress to AIDS more slowly, and potentially be less likely to transmit HIV infection to others. Much of this work targeting elicitation of CD8 T cell responses against HIV involves vectored gene delivery systems (such as adenoviral vectors, described below). However, the results of the first phase IIb "test of concept study"[59] (The Step Study) to examine this hypothesis failed to demonstrate a beneficial effect on either prevention of infection or reduction of viral load among volunteers who received the vaccine despite the induction of appreciable levels of HIV-specific CTL responses by the recombinant adenovirus-based (Ad5) vaccine employed (and was accompanied by a suggestion of increased risk of HIV acquisition in uncircumcised men with evidence of prior Ad5 infection). While this study result does not, in and of itself, refute the "CTL hypothesis", it represented a significant disappointment for the AIDS vaccine research effort, and raised important questions about the ability of vaccine-elicited cell mediated immune responses to favorably alter the outcome of HIV infection.[60]

While the test of concept study above was in progress, a Phase III study in Thailand, the RV144 study[61] was under way. This vaccine based on priming with a canarypox vector (ALVAC) encoding the gag-pol-rev-nef antigens followed by boosting with a recombinant gp120 Env glycoprotein yielded an approximately 31% reduction in infection. The vaccine had no impact on levels of post-infection viral load. The level of vaccine efficacy in this study was quite modest, and appeared to diminish with time. Realization of even this modest protective effect was unexpected, given that the gp120 immunogen used does not elicit neutralizing antibodies and had failed when delivered alone in two previous efficacy trials, and that the ALVAC-HIV vector had been found to elicit only low levels of cellular immune responses in immunized volunteers. To date, a clear correlate of protective immune responses has not been identified in the RV144 study, but its results have raised the possibility of protective effects of non-neutralizing antibodies and a preponderance of IgG antibody over IgA.[62] Efforts are currently underway to initiate additional trials seeking to replicate the results of the RV144 study, and to help identify a potential correlate of protection in regions of the world where a greater degree of viral genetic diversity is seen and where the incidence rate of HIV infection is higher.

Alternative approaches seeking to elicit both humoral (even if not neutralizing) immune responses and cellular immune responses (using viral vectors such as rare serotype adenoviruses) are also being advanced towards proof-of-concept clinical trials. There are also efforts under way to utilize the recently solved three-dimensional structure of the HIV gp120 Env glycoprotein to guide the derivation of non-native structures that might serve as better immunogens to elicit broadly cross-reactive neutralizing antibodies.[63] In addition, relatively conserved and functionally essential sequences of the extracellular domain of the HIV transmembrane Env protein, gp41, are being explored as immunogens to elicit broadly neutralizing antibodies. The recent derivation of potent, broadly neutralizing monoclonal antibodies (and the molecular cloning of the genes that encode them) from HIV-infected individuals has demonstrated that antibody neutralization of diverse HIV strains may be possible. However, it remains unclear whether and how such potent, broadly neutralizing antibodies might be elicited in humans vaccinated with defined HIV immunogens.[64] This challenge represents the fundamental goal of the next stage of HIV vaccine development efforts.

Malaria (Chapter 28)

Malaria is the world's most common vector-borne disease—estimated to cause approximately 225 million clinical cases and 780 000 deaths annually.[65,66] The disease hits hardest in Africa, and is especially severe in children under 5 years of age. In addition to direct morbidity and mortality, malaria is responsible for debilitating illness with enormous social and economic consequences. Of the four malaria-associated protozoal species, *Plasmodium flaciparum* and *P. vivax* represent the two major agents. These parasites have a three-stage lifecycle taking place both within the mosquito, and in the liver and blood of the infected host, and each cycle is largely distinct from the others from an immunological perspective. As a result of the multiple strategies for evasion of host immune response that the parasite has evolved, parasite replication proceeds at high levels despite active host immune responses.[67,68] Either as a result of these specific immune evasion strategies or the inability of the infected human host to mount immune responses that clear the parasite, prior infection does not protect an individual from repeated subsequent infections. Although the severity of disease is often attenuated following repeated infection, the mechanism of disease modulation is incompletely understood, and the limited relative immunity engendered by prior infection is easily lost if an individual leaves a malaria-endemic region. As such, the limited impact and duration of host immune responses to malaria parasites suggest that any successful vaccine strategy will need to do far better than natural immune responses—a high bar for efforts to develop an effective vaccine.

Roughly two dozen antigens have been cloned and tested as potential vaccine immunogens, and with a few exceptions, the results have been disappointing.[69] In addition, an alternative approach based on immunization by injection with irradiated or genetically attenuated sporozoites,[70,71] failed in its first large scale test. In contrast, one recombinant antigen, the circumsporozoite (CSP) antigen, when presented as a fusion molecule with HBsAg (RTS,S) and combined with a novel adjuvant formulation (AS01), has demonstrated modest promise in early human studies.[72] Two excellent reviews of this effort are available.[73] In the recently reported interim results of a large Phase III study of the RTS,S vaccine conducted in children in seven African countries, protective efficacy against malaria was 55%, while the overall reduction of severe malaria was 35%.[74] The final results of the ongoing efficacy trial of RTS,S will determine if the magnitude of protection and the safety profile will justify large-scale implementation efforts. Should the ongoing study proceed to successful conclusion, the earliest registration and WHO guidance for vaccine use might be available in 2015. While the results of this study represent an important advance, the partial protective efficacy of the RTS,S vaccine (and the now uncertain duration of protection), suggests that this vaccine will need to be but one component of a broader solution for the control and elimination of malaria.

While "proof of concept" for RTS,S seems to be supported by ongoing studies, the absolute magnitude of efficacy may be insufficient for a standalone vaccine. As such, future malaria vaccine development efforts will likely focus on the identification of additional protective antigens (expressed at specific stages of the parasite lifecycle) to include in combination vaccines and potential novel adjuvants to improve the magnitude, duration and protective efficacy of vaccine-elicited immune responses. Given the variety of antigens potentially available now that the genomes of plasmodia are fully sequenced, there is an enormous effort to find additional effective antigens that might be employed. The WHO has an impressive spreadsheet of malaria vaccine programs (http://www.who.int/vaccine_research/links/Rainbow/en/index.html).

Tuberculosis (Chapter 25)

Mycobacterium tuberculosis is an intracellular mycobacterial pathogen that represents one of the world's most common and most serious infectious diseases.[75] Over 2 billion people are believed to harbor latent *M. tuberculosis* infections, and approximately 8 million active cases of tuberculosis and over 2 million deaths occur each year. Furthermore, the interface of HIV infection and its attendant immune system damage both increases the severity of *M. tuberculosis* infection and increases the infectiousness of infected individuals. The emergence and dissemination of *M. tuberculosis* isolates that are resistant to multiple antimicrobial drugs represent a growing public health threat. However, while the need for a vaccine to prevent tuberculosis is clear, a significant number of challenges face vaccine development efforts.[76]

Most individuals infected with *M. tuberculosis* can control the acute phase of mycobacterial replication, and mount vigorous innate and adaptive immune responses to the infection. However, the infection is often not cleared by the host's immune response, and the mycobacteria are able to persist and multiply within vacuoles inside macrophages. Long-term latency is established in fibrotic cysts in the lung. The recrudescence and dissemination of *M. tuberculosis* occur at a later time in a number of infected individuals, likely as a result of waning host immune control. Although the ability of *M. tuberculosis* to persist despite active immune responses represents a major challenge to vaccine development, the fact that most individuals can contain (if not clear) *M. tuberculosis* infection suggests that a vaccine that can alter the course of the natural infection by limiting early

dissemination and decreasing the risk of later recrudescence could provide major public health benefits.

Efforts to develop a vaccine against tuberculosis date back many decades. Bacille Calmette-Guérin (better known as BCG), based on *Mycobacterium bovis*, was first introduced in 1921.[77] Currently, BCG is provided as a component of the routine Expanded Programme for Immunization (EPI) schedule and is administered to a significant majority of the world's children. Although some protective efficacy (50–80%) has been reported against miliary infection and *M. tuberculosis* meningitis in children, conflicting results have been obtained in different studies regarding the ability of BCG to protect against pulmonary tuberculosis in adults. One explanation for the overall limited efficacy of BCG emerges from formal genome sequencing studies that have disclosed significant differences between *M. tuberculosis* and of the vaccine strain of BCG. The variability in the results of BCG efficacy studies in different populations and geographies may derive from variations in the geographic prevalence of cross-reactive mycobacterial species (that may themselves confer partial protection), or the fact that BCG vaccines used throughout the world do not represent a homogenous preparation—with the root strain of BCG having been widely distributed and passaged extensively under diverse conditions.

Vaccine efforts against tuberculosis have primarily focused on the evaluation of specific mycobacterial antigens (e.g., ESAT6, Ag85, and HSP60) that have been tested as vaccines in animal models with variable success.[78,79] Some of these strategies are now being advanced into human clinical trials. A number of these antigens are being explored, often delivered by viral vectors, as ways of boosting the protective efficacy of BCG in individuals who have previously been vaccinated with BCG. The results of one such "proof of concept" study of a modified vaccinia Ankara (MVA) vector encoding the *M. tuberculosis* antigen 85A as a booster immunization in infants who had received the BCG vaccine are slated to be available in late 2012. An alternative vaccine strategy is based on improving the performance of the BCG vaccine by insertion of genes encoding specific potential protective antigens that it normally lacks. In addition, the development of auxotrophic mutants of *M. tuberculosis* is being explored as a potential immunogenic and specifically attenuated live vaccine. The determination of the sequence of the *M. tuberculosis* genome nearly a decade ago helped identify numerous previously unknown gene products, and increased the repertoire of antigens to be evaluated for their ability to induce protective immune responses.[80] The pathogen sequence is also being used to elucidate virulence determinants and thereby help guide efforts to attenuate *M. tuberculosis* rationally.

Respiratory syncytial virus (RSV) and parainfluenza virus (PIV)

Together with influenza virus, RSV and PIV account for a substantial majority of pediatric upper respiratory illness and consequent acute otitis media. A variety of influenza vaccines are licensed for pediatric use, but vaccines to prevent infection with the paromyxoviruses RSV and PIV remain elusive. A significant impediment to vaccine development for RSV and PIV traces back to unanticipated untoward results obtained in clinical studies of inactivated RSV vaccines in the early 1960s.[81] These early-generation RSV vaccines—based on cultured virus that had been inactivated with formalin—raised a potent antibody response in immunized children. However, on subsequent natural exposure to RSV, vaccine recipients exhibited more frequent and significantly more severe lower respiratory tract RSV infections than did unimmunized children. As a similar phenomenon was also seen with a formalin-inactivated measles vaccine in the same era, a common immunopathologic mechanism may be operative.[82] While the mechanism of exacerbation of RSV disease by the early inactivated vaccines is incompletely understood, it has been suggested that chemical inactivation of RSV and measles virus resulted in modification of a critical neutralizing structure on the surfaces of these viruses, thereby limiting the induction of the most potent neutralizing antibodies and favoring nonneutralizing and potentially immunopathologic antibody responses. (Passive protection against RSV is available for premature infants in the form of monoclonal antibodies that target the RSV F protein (one of the viral envelope glycoproteins); as such, certain anti-RSV antibody responses can clearly mediate protective as opposed to deleterious effects.[70]) Alternatively, or in addition, it has been proposed that inactivated RSV vaccines may have preferentially induced a Th2-type immune response when a Th1-type response may be needed to effect protection of the lower respiratory tract from RSV infection and damage.

While excellent live attenuated measles vaccines have been developed, RSV and PIV have so far resisted the approach used for measles and mumps (these are all members of the Paramyxoviridae family of viruses). Nevertheless, based on the successful precedent provided by the live attenuated measles vaccine and the desire to induce a Th-1-biased immune response, an attenuated or reverse genetics-engineered RSV, is still considered the most promising approach. However, stable attenuation of RSV has been difficult to achieve and vaccine safety concerns arising from earlier chapters in RSV vaccine development result in their cautious advancement through clinical evaluation.[83] More recently, attempts have been launched to develop hybrid attenuated recombinant RSV-PIV vaccines as well as to develop recombinant protein based RSV vaccines (in combination with specific adjuvants seeking to drive a Th-1-biased immune response).

Neisseria meningitidis

Effective vaccines for meningococcus serogroups A, C, Y, and W135 are available as simple capsular polysaccharides and as polysaccharides conjugated to a protein carrier.[84] However, as previously described, the group B polysaccharide shares chemical similarity with a shorter sugar found on the surface of neuronal tissue.[85] While it is possible to make highly immunogenic conjugates with the group B polysaccharide, theoretical concerns about cross-reactivity with self antigens has impeded the development of this type of vaccine. Current work to develop a Men B vaccine centers on a handful of relatively well-conserved surface proteins of meningococcus.[86,87] Many of these antigens have been identified by "reverse vaccinology", and indeed, a Men B vaccine candidate currently in the late stages of clinical testing may prove to be the first vaccine to be licensed that was discovered using reverse vaccinology methods (see section on antigen discovery). In addition to the combined A-C-Y-W conjugated polysaccharide vaccines that is available in many wealthier countries, a monovalent men A conjugate vaccine, has recently been developed specifically for sub-Saharan Africa where outbreaks of group A meningoccus epidemics are common. Through a novel public-private effort, development of this vaccine successfully targeted the regional need for an effective Men A vaccine and to provide the vaccine at a low price.[88] On the heels of this success, a novel mengingococcal serogroup X, once a very rare species, is now emerging as a new strain with prevalence similar to that of serogroup A ((WHO Intercountry Support Team http://www.who.int). To address this challenge, a second, independent vaccine development effort has been initiated.

Group B streptococcus

GBS is a common component of the flora of the female genital tract, and transfer to the neonate is the cause of severe infections that are fatal or have serious sequelae.[89] Short-course intrapartum antibiotics are recommended for culture-positive women, and this approach has cut the incidence of neonatal infections by about two-thirds, thus reducing somewhat the urgency of vaccine development. However, short-course antibiotics could ultimately drive the emergence of antibiotic-resistant GBS. Candidate vaccines have been shown to elicit a protective response.[43] However, aside from a reduced market, a significant impediment to development of a GBS vaccine is concern over vaccination of pregnant women or women of childbearing age. Any birth defect might be attributed to the vaccine, and in a litigious society, this would be problematic for a vaccine producer.

Hepatitis C virus (HCV)

Prior to the advent of effective polymerase chain reaction methods for screening blood donations, HCV was a significant cause of transfusion-related hepatitis. Currently, transmission of HCV among the normal population is quite low; transmission among injection drug users remains high. HCV is another pathogen where infection does not typically result in an immune response that eliminates the infection. However, a minority of HCV patients do spontaneously clear their infection, suggesting that an appropriate immune response can be generated in at least some individuals that is able to clear a nascent infection. Current vaccine work is concentrated on vectored gene delivery vaccines, primarily adenoviruses, intended to raise antiviral cytotoxic T-cell responses.[90,91] However, recent success (and tremendous ongoing efforts) in developing oral antiviral drugs that are able to control and clear HCV infections (potentially in interferon-free regimens) may decrease the public health need, as well as limit the scientific momentum and commercial impetus, to develop a HCV vaccine.

Herpes simplex virus

With the exception of the live attenuated varicella-zoster virus (VZV) vaccine used for the primary prevention of chickenpox and reactivation of latent VZV infections (the cause of shingles and postherpetic neuralgia in older individuals), there are no other vaccines available for use in humans to prevent infection with members of the herpes virus family.[92] HSV types 1 and 2 cause recurrent vesicular eruptions "above or below the belt," respectively. Like other herpes viruses, HSV infections are not cleared by the immune system and the virus can persist, remaining in a latent state that is functionally inaccessible to immune recognition and clearance. In addition, like other herpes viruses, HSV encodes a number of gene products that promote evasion of host immune responses (Chapter 27). Recent attempts to make HSV-2 vaccines have used virus glycoproteins (particularly HSV-2 glycoprotein D [gD]) produced by recombinant DNA methods. An earlier clinical efficacy trial of this approach showed partial protection of women, but not men, who were seronegative for HSV1.[93] The reasons for this curious result are not clear. However, the results of a subsequent clinical trial of an adjuvanted HSV-2 gD vaccine recently demonstrated the inability of the vaccine to protect women from HSV-2 infection or disease, in contrast to the earlier results (although modest protection [35% efficacy] was reported against HSV-1 infection).[94] In addition to recombinant gD-based approaches, a number of preclinical studies are exploring the ability of cell-mediated immune responses to HSV antigens induced by recombinant vaccine vectors (e.g., adenoviruses: see novel vaccine vectors, below) to prevent or ameliorate HSV infections. Genetically engineered attenuated HSV variants have also been studied in experimental animal models. It is not clear whether or when these new strategies will advance to clinical evaluation in humans.

Cytomegalovirus (CMV)

Another herpes virus, CMV is a very common infection in humans, with 50–80% of individuals being infected by adulthood. CMV is a cause of severe infections in neonates, causing debilitating neurological sequelae. Following initial infection, CMV persists in infected humans, despite the fact that anti-CMV antibodies are present and that a very sizeable proportion of the overall host CD4 and CD8 immune responses are specific for CMV antigens. Ongoing virus persistence and replication in the face of active host immune responses are likely explained by CMV's sophisticated repertoire of host immune evasion functions (including those that inhibit antigen presentation mechanisms and immune effector responses) (Chapter 27). For these reasons, to be successful, vaccine development efforts will need to elicit immune responses that are significantly more effective than the quantitatively impressive, but functionally limited, immune responses that are generated in the course of natural CMV infections—unless they prove to be able to prevent initial CMV infection.

Live attenuated vaccines have been investigated sporadically since the 1970s.[95] An attenuated strain, the Towne strain, showed some effect, but was judged to be insufficiently immunogenic. Hybrids of the attenuated Towne strain and the virulent Toledo strain remain in development. Of note, a recent phase II study of a recombinant CMV glycoprotein B subunit antigen combined with the MF59 adjuvant in seronegative women of childbearing age provided promising proof of concept for CMV vaccine development, with the demonstration of 50% vaccine efficacy (with a primary endpoint of time to CMV infection in the women[96]). While this result is encouraging, it is unclear if prevention of infection in women will be considered as an acceptable basis for licensure of a CMV vaccine (that is ultimately intended to protect against congenital CMV disease in their offspring) by regulatory authorities. Phase III efficacy trials to demonstrate successful prevention of congenital CMV infection would need to be significantly larger than the recently reported proof of concept study, and those demonstrating protection against congenital CMV disease even larger. Alternative CMV vaccine strategies currently in preclinical development include recombinant DNA (rDNA)-derived proteins (via either DNA vaccine approaches or recombinant viral vectors, such as attenuated poxviral vectors).[97–99]

Epstein–Barr virus (EBV)

EBV is a herpes virus that represents the causative agent of infectious mononucleosis and is widespread among the human population. In concert with incompletely understood environmental (and perhaps additional host) factors, EBV is also etiologically associated with Burkitt's lymphoma. The ability of EBV to establish persistent infections in humans (along with latent infections at the cellular level) despite readily detectable antiviral immune responses suggests that, like other herpes viruses, the development of effective EBV vaccine will likely be challenging. EBV vaccines have been in development since the 1980s with the coat protein, gp220/350, as the most common vaccine antigen studied.[100]

Dengue fever virus

Dengue fever virus is a mosquito-borne flavivirus (the virus family that includes Japanese encephalitis virus and yellow fever virus (YFV)—for which successful vaccines exist). Dengue virus is endemic in a substantial portion of tropical and subtropical areas and causes febrile disease as well as hemorrhagic fever. There are four distinct serotypes of dengue fever virus. Prior infection with one serotype has been implicated in predisposing for more severe disease following infection with a second dengue fever virus serotype, although the evidence supporting this concept has been questioned and the underlying pathogenic mechanisms are incompletely understood.[101] One hypothesis proposes that antibodies against the initial infecting serotype bind to the surface of virus particles of the novel infecting serotype, but do not neutralize the infection. In a process referred to as "immune enhancement" of infection, still infectious complexes of antibody-virus particles are envisioned to be preferentially taken up by cells of the reticuloendothelial system that represent primary target cells for virus replication. Although the veracity of this hypothesis is not established, it presents theoretical concerns about what type of antibody responses will need to be induced by vaccines to exert beneficial rather than detrimental effects.

The general belief is that a vaccine eliciting the equivalent magnitude and duration of immune responses against all four serotypes will be required. Vaccines based on inactivated virus, engineered chimeric viruses based on the yellow fever virus vaccine platform, engineered deletion mutant viruses, and rDNA-derived proteins are in various stages of development.[102] The most advanced vaccine candidate, now in phase III clinical studies, is based on four recombinant yellow fever vaccine (YF-17D) virus genomes that carry the genes encoding the surface proteins of the four serotypes of dengue fever virus (in place of the native YFV genes). An up-to-date review of the dengue fever vaccine effort is available.[103]

Staphylococcus aureus

Staphylococcus aureus infection has become a major public health threat as the species continues to acquire resistance to multiple antibiotics.[104] This need has driven the development of several new vaccines against *S. aureus* infections. One approach is based on an essential iron binding protein,[105] and the other is based on a clumping factor.[106] The iron binding protein antigen, was identified via reverse vaccinology approaches and had shown promise in preclinical studies. Based on these preclinical results, a Phase II/III clinical trial was initiated to evaluate the ability of this vaccine candidate to prevent infectious complications following surgery due to *S. aureus*. In early 2011, the sponsors of this vaccine trial terminated the study based upon data indicating that vaccine was unlikely to demonstrate a statistically significant clinical benefit. As a result, new approaches for the development of a safe and efficacious vaccine against *S. aureus* infection will be needed.

Clostridium difficile

Clostridium difficile is a Gram-positive, spore-forming rod-shaped bacterium that is the cause of a growing number of cases of severe diarrhea and colitis, primarily in hospitalized patients or long term care residents. Disease is typically triggered by antibiotic treatment for any number of reasons, resulting in a turnover of the gut flora and subsequent overgrowth by *C. difficile* and in some cases, a membranous overgrowth. Once established, *C. difficile* is difficult to clear. A vaccine,[107] based on two high molecular weight toxins secreted by the bacterium, is in early clinical trials.[104]

New antigen discovery methods

Historically, vaccine antigens were not discovered in the literal sense. Rather, whole organisms were inactivated by either heat or chemistry or organisms were attenuated by forcing growth in nonphysiological conditions. The entire antigenic repertoire of the organism was delivered to the immune system. The isolation of tetanus, diphtheria, and pertussis toxins, along with chemical detoxification schemes, allowed the production of more refined vaccines. The isolation and purification of polysaccharide capsules from a range of important bacterial pathogens enabled the development of additional vaccines.

With the advent of molecular biology in the late 1970s, a new set of tools allowed a more directed approach for the discovery of pathogen virulence factors, vaccine antigen discovery, and vaccine development. The tools of molecular biology allowed the development of vaccines against pathogens that could not be propagated in culture, including the successful development of recombinant HBV and HPV vaccines. Development of these vaccines was enabled by clinical and animal model studies showing that antibodies directed against a specific viral target antigen (e.g., the HBV surface antigen or the HPV L1 protein) were implicated in protection. In addition, molecular biologic approaches enabled the derivation of fully recombinant vaccine antigens (such as those developed using a limited set of defined antigens of *Bordetella pertussis*), including genetically modified versions of bacterial toxins that maintain their proper antigenic structures but are no longer toxic. However, for many of the pathogens for which vaccines do not currently exist, application of these recombinant DNA technology-enabled strategies are insufficient due to incomplete understanding of the pathogen antigens that would elicit a protective host immune response. As such, the development of additional techniques to discover protective antigens was needed. Fortunately, several important technological advances that facilitate discovery of previously unknown protective antigens from even very complex microorganisms have opened a new era in vaccine development.

The earliest rDNA technology-enabled methods of antigen discovery involved the expression of individual pathogen-derived gene products (or fragments thereof) in bacterial hosts (typically *Escherichia coli*) using rDNA expression vectors. Here, the genome of a pathogen is broken up, and the fragments are inserted into a plasmid or a viral vector, typically a lambda bacteriophage.[108] Colonies, or plaques, are spread on a membrane, allowed to grow, and hopefully express the cloned gene fragments. The ability of these recombinant gene products to react with antibodies present in the serum of individuals who had recovered from infection with that pathogen could then be directly assessed. Antibodies present in the immune sera are assessed for their ability to identify antigens by immunochemical reactivity. In this way, the entire genome of a given pathogen could be scanned for potential immunoreactivity.[109] Such reactivity would both indicate the *in vivo* expression of that gene product, as well as document its antigenicity. However, additional studies are needed to demonstrate whether antibody responses against a newly defined antigen have any protective potential. To document the ability of an antigen to elicit protective immune responses, it is necessary to immunize an experimental animal (most commonly, mice) and then, following experimental pathogen challenge, evaluate infection outcomes in immunized versus nonimmunized animals. As this approach has most often been used to identify antigens recognized by host humoral responses, sera from animals immunized with a candidate antigen can then be transferred to a naïve host to provide evidence that the antibody response to the antigen represents the relevant agent of immune protection.

More recently, as DNA sequencing became more efficient and scalable, determining the entire sequence of the genomes of viruses, bacteria, and parasites has become routine,[110,111] allowing identification of previously unknown genes (and predicted gene products) that can be evaluated as vaccine immunogens. Scanning the entire pathogen genome via computer programs, genes that exhibit specific characteristics can be identified (e.g., predicted expression on the cell surface by virtue of possession of a leader sequence for secretion or membrane anchor sequences).[112] In addition, the relative conservation of the gene within the pathogen population can be determined by assessment of gene sequences from multiple distinct isolates. Once potential vaccine antigens are identified, each candidate gene is expressed in an appropriate rDNA system, and the protein product is tested in an animal model.[113] The first bacterial genome sequenced in its entirety was that of *Haemophilus influenzae*, marking the beginning of a new approach to vaccine antigen discovery.[114] Since this initial bacterial genome sequence determination, genomic sequencing of pathogens has advanced exponentially. Over 300 bacterial genomes have now been sequenced, and hundreds more are currently in process. Genome-based antigen discovery is being applied to a wide range of bacteria, including streptococci, pneumococci, staphylococci and *Chlamydia*, as well as nonbacterial pathogens such as *Plasmodium falciparum*.[115] This general technique is now called "reverse vaccinology" (Fig. 90.4).

An alternate and complementary, promising approach to novel antigen discovery has been built on technological advances in proteomics.[116,117] These advances include development of high-resolution two-dimensional gel electrophoresis and mass spectrometry that enable separation, identification, and purification of individual proteins from a complex mixture of pathogen proteins. In proteomic analyses, a small culture of bacteria, preferably taken directly from an infected person, or otherwise grown in physiologically similar conditions, is subjected to physical or enzymatic treatment with specific proteases to generate peptide fragments that are then fractionated by micro-high-performance liquid chromatography and sequenced by molecular spectrometry. An overlapping set of peptides of approximately 8–10 amino acids is sufficient to identify an antigen and provides the means to find the gene.[118,119] A combination of proteomic and serologic methods to select potential novel vaccine immunogens, called serological proteome analysis, or SERPA,[120,121] can be used to screen the pathogen proteome for expressed proteins that are recognized by antibodies present in sera obtained from individuals who have recovered from an infection with the pathogen.

Translational research opportunities and challenges in vaccine development

The processes of vaccine development have changed significantly in recent years—a process facilitated by improvements in understanding of human immune system function, as well as the advent of powerful new technologies for vaccine development. Vaccine development is therefore now commonly pursued in a hypothesis-driven manner. However, at the same time, the infectious diseases for which no effective vaccines currently exist represent more challenging targets. Furthermore, global changes that influence the emergence and rate of spread of infectious diseases place unprecedented challenges on the productivity and pace of new vaccine development.

Current opportunities

- Improved understanding of human immunology (including the biology of innate immune system function, antigen presentation, and the generation and maintenance of T- and B-cell memory).
- Improved technologies to measure human cellular and humoral immune responses.
- The advent of genomic and proteomic technologies for new antigen discovery.
- The wealth of recombinant DNA methodologies that enable isolation of protective antigens from diverse pathogens and the derivation of novel vaccine vectors to elicit immune responses to pathogen-derived antigens.
- The development of recombinant and synthetic approaches for the large-scale production of precisely defined vaccine antigens (including the ability to produce immunogens that accurately recapitulate the conformational structure of native antigens, or that, alternatively, alter them so that they serve as more effective immunogens.
- The development of synthetic consensus antigens able to elicit broader immune responses than would sequences obtained from individual isolates from highly diverse pathogens (e.g., HIV, influenza).
- The emergence of new mechanism-based adjuvants to enhance immunogenicity of vaccine antigens.
- The use of novel methods to shift relative immunodominance of specific pathogen gene products to increase the immunogenicity of conserved antigens from otherwise diverse pathogen genomes that are typically poorly immunogenic in the course of natural infections.

Current challenges

- The need to develop vaccines for infections where natural immunity does not often or ever develop following natural infection (e.g., HIV, malaria, hepatitis C).
- The need to develop vaccines that protect against genetically diverse pathogen variants with a limited number of vaccine immunogens (e.g., HIV, malaria, and influenza).
- The need to develop vaccines for infections where concerns exist about vaccine elicitation of potentially autoimmune (*Neisseria meningitidis* group B) or immunopathologic (e.g., RSV) responses.
- The challenge of responding rapidly and effectively, with powerful new technologies, to newly emerging infections—including those that haven't been seen in humans before (e.g., SARS) or for which novel antigenic variants are anticipated but cannot be predicted (e.g., pandemic influenza).
- Maximizing the value of innovative new approaches while ensuring the safety of new vaccines so derived.

The proteomic approach to antigen discovery has been applied to identify novel vaccine candidates for a number of human pathogens, including *Helicobacter pylori*, *Chlamydia pneumoniae*, *Staphylococcus aureus*, *Bacillus anthracis*, *Haemophilus influenzae*, *Neisseria meningitidis* group B and *Plasmodium falciparum*. Of these vaccine candidates, the *N. meningitidis* group B vaccine is in the late stages of clinical evaluation, which if successful, will provide the first successful example of a vaccine antigen discovered by the methods of reverse vaccinology. As in new genomic methods for antigen discovery, having identified a gene encoding a candidate antigen by proteomic methods, it is then necessary to show that an immune response of the desired type can be raised against the protein. In addition, it is necessary to show that immune responses elicited following immunization with the candidate antigen engender some degree of protection.

Adjuvants

The term "adjuvant" (derived from the Latin *adjuvare*, to help) refers to any substance added as a component of a vaccine preparation—in addition to the vaccine antigens themselves—that improves the immunological response to the antigen. As such, "adjuvant" is a catch-all term including a broad range of molecular entities that act via diverse—and, in a number of instances, yet to be elucidated—pathways. Until recently, most adjuvants were derived empirically and the mechanisms by which they augmented immune responses were unknown. As a result, there were few, if any, principles available to guide the improvement of known adjuvants or the development of new ones. However, recent advances in understanding of the mechanisms by which dendritic cells sense the presence of pathogens and their constituents, and translate this information to shape the quantity, quality, and durability of host cellular and humoral adaptive immune responses, have transformed adjuvant discovery and optimization. What was once a process of trial and error now represents an area of hypothesis-driven research and mechanism-based discovery.

A particularly promising advance emerged from the discovery that pathogen sensing by the innate immune system is mediated by recognition of specific pathogen-associated molecular patterns (PAMPs) by pathogen recognition receptors (PRRs) such as the Toll-like receptors (TLRs) that are expressed on dendritic cells (DCs) and other hemato-lymphoid and some epithelial cells (Chapter 3).[122] The pathogen-derived PAMPS recognized by TLRs consist of structures that are found only in or on pathogens (including bacteria, viruses, and parasites) and are not part of normal vertebrate biology. Following binding of a specific PAMP to a specific PRR, a specific cellular activation and response cascade is triggered that can directly confront an intruding pathogen and/or lead to the activation of specific host adaptive immune response mechanisms. These breakthroughs in basic immunology have been readily translated into what can now be considered the science of adjuvant biology.[123,124]

Such progress has occurred at an especially opportune time as new vaccine development strategies have transitioned from traditional approaches using attenuated or killed pathogens to highly defined and purified recombinant proteins (so-called "subunit" vaccines) or nonreplicating vectored antigens. Although these newer approaches are promising from the perspective of vaccine safety and the opportunity they afford to design the structures of vaccine immunogens, recombinant or synthetic vaccines are often inherently less immunogenic than traditional vaccines based on attenuated live viruses or intact killed organisms. In the context of current vaccine development

Fig. 90.4 The genome of a bacterium is scanned by an algorithm that identifies genes (as open reading frames). Individual genes are analyzed for the presence of putative structures that should be present on the surface of the bacterium (membrane anchors, certain types of secretion signals, etc) that could be vaccine targets (upper two drawings). In many cases, these initial candidate genes will be re-scanned against the genomes of alternate isolates of the same species in order to identify conserved surface antigens. Candidate genes that satisfy these criteria are then expressed as recombinant proteins that are then used to vaccinate animals. Antigens that raise the desired immune response are taken forward for further development. In parallel, a proteomic exercise may be carried out to confirm the presence of a selection of antigens on the surface of the bacterium, preferably taken from a patient sample with minimal *in vitro* culturing (lower two drawings). The bacterium is treated with a protease mixture that cleaves off surface proteins. The cleavage products are collected and analyzed by mass spectrometry. The cleavage products are broken down to small peptides as part of the spectrometry process, and their sequences are imputed from their molecular weights compared against the predicted sequences from the genome. This extra proteomics step can reduce the number of candidates to be screened in more expensive animal studies.

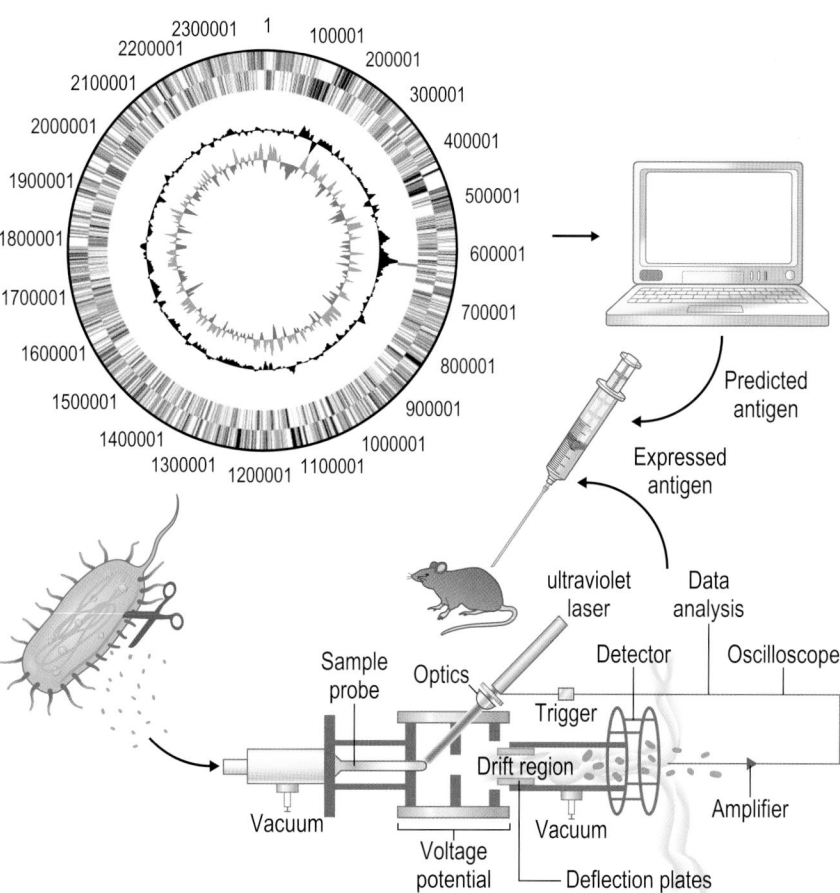

and regulatory approval processes, an adjuvant is developed as part of a vaccine, not as an independent product. Consequently, there are currently no adjuvants licensed by regulatory authorities as stand-alone products.

Most contemporary efforts to develop novel adjuvants are focused on the targeted activation of TLRs that are expressed on specific cells critical for the generation of innate and adaptive host responses to specific pathogens.[125] A family consisting of 10 distinct TLRs has been identified to date in humans (Chapter 3). TLRs are expressed in a number of innate immune cells, including DCs, macrophages, neutrophils, endothelial cells, and fibroblasts. Given the importance of DCs as critical antigen-presenting cells, most studies of the biology of TLR signaling have focused on these cells. Different TLRs are expressed on distinct subpopulations of DCs, and, depending on the TLR, in distinct cellular compartments. TLRs expressed on the surface of human myeloid DCs include TLR2 (which is heterodimerized with TLR 1 or 6), as well as TLRs 4, 5, 6, and 10 (Fig. 90.5), while these same cells express TLRs 3 and 8 within endoplasmic reticulum (ER) and phagolysosomes. Plasmacytoid DCs (pDCs) express TLR7 and 9 within ER/phagolysosomes. The TLRs expressed on the cell surface are primarily activated by PAMPs encountered in the extracellular environment, while TLRs expressed in the ER/phagolysosomes are activated by PAMPs (including viral pathogen-derived RNA or DNA) that tend to be routed through these endosomal compartments. Activation of TLRs on innate immune cells leads to their production of specific cytokines, as well as their expression of co-stimulatory molecules, leading to induction of adaptive immune responses. Given that different DCs express different TLRs, and that signaling via different TLRs

results in the expression of a distinct pattern of cytokines, it is believed that activation of specific TLRs can variously favor the induction of Th1- or Th2-biased immune responses, or can differentially augment either direct or cross-presentation pathways for antigen presentation (Fig. 90.5). Although most data on induction of specific types of immune responses by engagement of specific TLRs have emerged from murine studies (and have not yet been validated in humans), the ability to tailor an adjuvant preparation to achieve a desired type of immune response with a specific vaccine immunogen is a promising notion. Naturally occurring ligands for TLRs include lipopolysaccharide (LPS) from bacterial cell walls (recognized by TLR4), triacyl lipopeptides (recognized by TLRs 1), diacyl lipopeptides (recognized by TLRs 1), peptidoglycan (recognized by TLR2), flagellin (the monomer that makes up flagella, recognized by TLR5), single-stranded RNA (recognized by TLR7), double-stranded RNA (recognized by TLR3), and unmethylated DNA containing the dinucleotide pair CpG[126] (recognized by TLR9). Based on these insights, a variety of approaches to develop adjuvants predicated to activation of specific TLR pathways are being actively pursued.

One interesting aspect of adjuvant development is how it is revealing the mechanisms of action of adjuvants that were originally identified via a process of trial and error, as well as delineating important aspects by which certain empirically derived vaccines are able to induce high-level, long-lasting immune responses. An illustrative example is complete Freund's adjuvant (CFA), which has long served as the benchmark for laboratory studies of adjuvants. CFA is a mixed emulsion of mineral oil, mannide monooleate, and killed mycobacteria. However, it is far too reactogenic for use in humans, causing significant pain

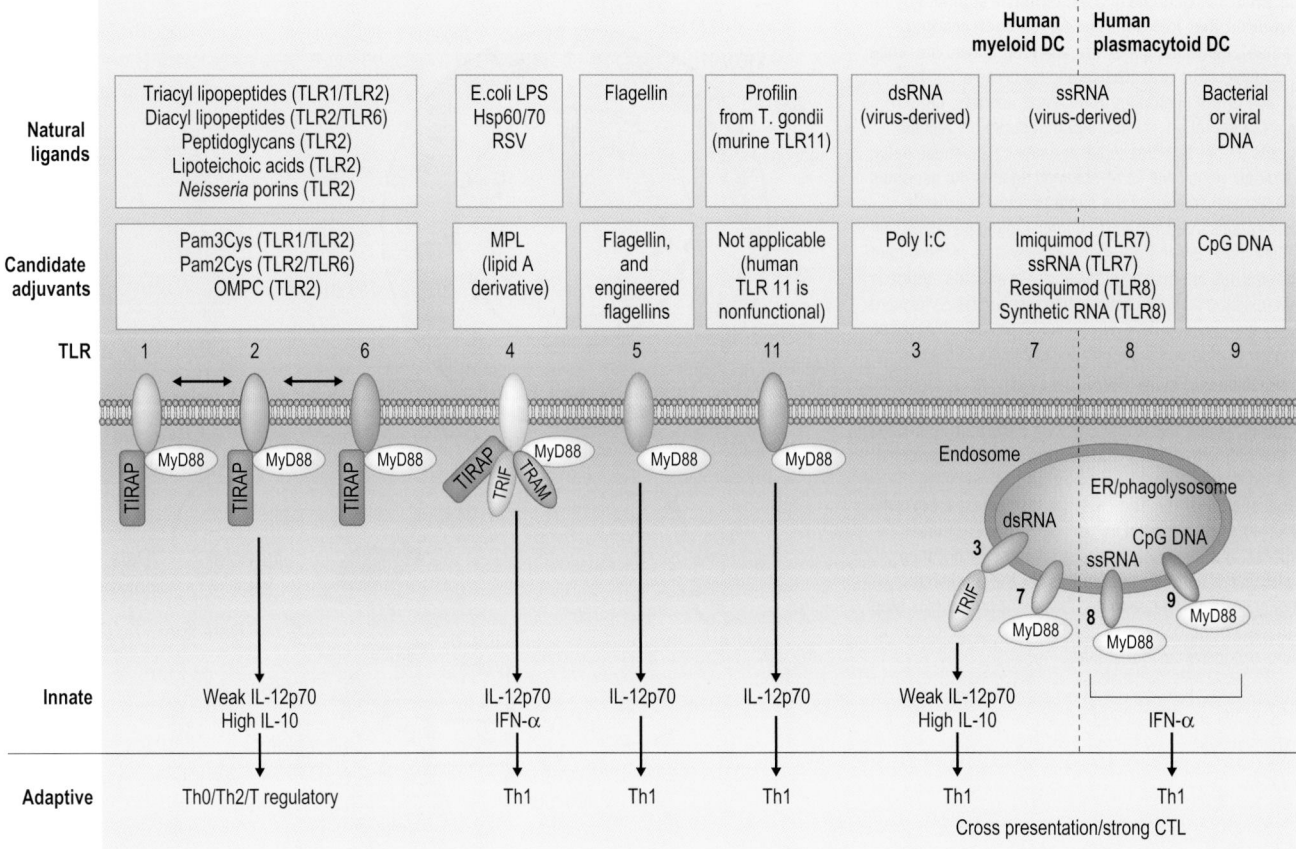

Fig. 90.5 Toll-like receptor (TLR) signaling pathways and mechanism-based adjuvants. The targeted activation of specific dendritic cell (DC) populations via engagement of specific TLRs to initiate innate and adaptive immune responses represents a very promising approach for the development of novel adjuvants based on natural or synthetic versions of the pathogen-associated molecular patterns (PAMPs) that trigger specific TLRs. Specific TLRs and their natural activating ligands are shown above. Different TLRs are associated with different adaptor proteins that propagate intracellular signaling along distinct pathways which favor specific immune responses (e.g., Th1, Th2, cross-presentation or CTL priming). The character of responses from specific TLR engagement illustrated is based on animal and *ex vivo* studies. In humans, TLRs 7 and 9 are expressed in the endoplasmic reticulum (ER)/phagolysosomes of plasmacytoid DCs (pDCs) that represent the major sources of type I interferon production (e.g., IFN-α). Human myeloid DCs (mDCs) express TLR3 (in the ER/phagolysosomes); and TLR2 (heterodimerized with TLRs 1 or 6), and TLRs 4, 5, 8, and 11 on the cell surface.
(Adapted from Pulendran B, Ahmed R. Translating innate immunity into immunologic memory: implications for vaccine development. Cell 2006; 124: 849–863, with permission from Elsevier.)

and abscesses at the site of injection—reactions that would be exacerbated if CFA were to be used repeatedly. An alternative preparation termed incomplete Freund's adjuvant (IFA) lacks the mycobacterial component, but it too is associated with injection site reactions that are severe enough to limit its use to experimental therapeutic cancer vaccines. Although CFA's toxicity precludes its use as a vaccine adjuvant in humans, many of its constituents (including liposaccharides, DNA, and specific bacterial cell wall components) are now understood to exert their adjuvant effects on vaccine-induced immune responses via engagement of specific TLRs. Similarly, the live attenuated *Mycobacterium bovis* strain, BCG, long widely employed as a vaccine for the prevention of tuberculosis, includes cell wall, peptidoglycan, and DNA components that activate specific TLRs. Interestingly, the highly effective yellow fever vaccine 17D has been shown to activate multiple TLRs as part of its induction of antiviral immune responses.[127] One version of the Hib polysaccharide conjugate vaccines now licensed for use in children for the prevention of invasive Hib disease includes the meningococcal outer-membrane protein complex (OMPC) as its protein carrier; OMPC conjugates have favorable immunogenic properties that correlate with the ability of OMPC to activate DCs via TLR2.[128]

Major classes of adjuvants now available and in development include: (1) alum; (2) liposomes; (3) immune-stimulating complexes (ISCOMs); (4) virosomes; (5) emulsions; (6) cytokines; and (7) Toll-receptor agonists.[129]

Aluminium salts

Aluminium salts (sometimes referred to generally as alum), the classical adjuvant most often used in vaccines in humans, includes a range of salts of aluminum precipitated under basic conditions, usually aluminum sulfate mixed with sodium or potassium hydroxide plus a variable amount of phosphate.[130] The composition of alum used as an adjuvant varies in currently available vaccines and can influence vaccine immunogenicity. Alum is utilized as an adjuvant in many of the currently available vaccines composed of inactivated toxins or recombinant proteins (live attenuated vaccines do not include alum or other adjuvants).

Alum serves two main purposes as an adjuvant. First, it acts as an antigen depot. Vaccine antigens adsorb to alum and elute from it following injection into the host. Second, alum acts a mild irritant, causing the recruitment of leukocytes necessary for generation of an immune response to the site of injection. Adsorption of antigens on to alum routinely improves immunogenicity, particularly the antibody response. Alum does not typically enhance CD8 T-cell responses. Alum has been a component of many vaccines for decades and has an excellent safety record, although its mechanism of action is only now being defined in detail. Recent work implicates the active binding of alum to the membranes of dendritic cells (DCs) resulting in alteration of lipid membranes structures as a key process in alum's adjuvant effect.[131] As new adjuvants are developed, alum may remain as a component of combination adjuvant mixtures (as is the case with some newer adjuvants now approaching clinical use), or it may eventually be supplanted by other agents that more effectively provide depot and local inflammatory responses to accentuate host immune responses.

Liposomes

Using lipids with polar head groups (e.g., triglycerides) and differing types of hydrophobic tails, one can form either micelles (spheres) or multilamellar sheets in aqueous environments.[132] Under the right conditions, antigens can be incorporated into the spheres or between layers of the sheets, providing a potential slow-release depot system. Immunopotentiators such as QS21 or detoxified LPS derivatives (such as monophosphoryl lipid A (MPL)) can be added to the lipid mix.[72]

Immune-stimulating complexes

Immune-stimulating complexes (ISCOMs) represent proprietary forms of liposomes made of cholesterol, saponins from quillaia bark (various members of the QS-X family of triterpene glycosides), and phospholipids that form cage-like structures into which antigens can be entrapped or intercalated.[126] ISCOM complexes can provide a depot function, as well as facilitating the delivery, uptake, and processing of vaccine immunogens by APCs.

Virosomes

Purified influenza virus hemagglutinin (HA) and neuraminidase mixed with phosphatidyl choline and phosphatidyl ethanolamine (polar lipids) will form empty particles that have the surface properties of influenza virus. Adding an antigen in solution before mixing the lipids results in the incorporation of the antigen inside the particle. This provides a vehicle for delivering antigens to the interior of a cell, via the influenza HA membrane fusion process, thereby enabling antigen processing and presentation via both major histocompatibility complex (MHC) class 1 and 2 pathways.[133]

Emulsions

Numerous oil-in-water and water-in-oil emulsions have been tested as adjuvants. One such emulsion, MF59, is used in a licensed influenza vaccine. MF59 consists of squalane, a metabolizable shark oil and two surfactants, polyoxyethylene sorbitan monooleate and sorbitan trioleate, in an oil-in-water emulsion.[134]

Cytokines

Cytokines are host-produced immunomodulators that regulate immune cell action (Chapter 9). Several cytokines are being tested as potential vaccine adjuvants, including granulocyte–macrophage colony-stimulating factor (GM-CSF), interleukin-2 (IL-2), and IL-12.

Toll-receptor agonists

Of the defined TLR agonists being explored as vaccine adjuvants, LPS and its partially detoxified form, MPL, which activate TLR 4, have been most thoroughly explored in clinical trials. With evidence of enhanced ability to increase the percentage of individuals responding with protective antibody levels to hepatitis B as compared to a standard hepatitis B vaccine, one hepatitis

B vaccine that employs an adjuvant formulation (termed AS04) consisting of a combination of alum and MPL[135] has been licensed for use in high-risk individuals, and one of the two licensed HPV vaccines (HPV2) also includes this adjuvant formulation.

A wide variety of TLR9-specific agonists consisting of oligodeoxynucleotides containing unmethylated CpG motifs (CpG-ODN) are being evaluated in preclinical studies. These CpG-ODNs resemble bacterial DNA, modified to include a phosphorothioate backbone to increase their stability. Two CpG-ODN adjuvants have been evaluated in recent phase I and II trials and shown to increase the timing and magnitude of induction of protective antibody levels, as well as the proportion of responding individuals, to recombinant HBSAg vaccine.[136] One of these CpG-ODN adjuvants also elicits protective antibody responses in immunized HIV-infected individuals who had previously failed to respond to the hepatitis B vaccine. This approach is now being studied as a way of inducing protective immune responses to hepatitis B earlier after initiation of the vaccination regimen or with fewer doses of the vaccine, and in individuals who would be predicted, as a result of specific chronic medical conditions (such as renal failure) to respond poorly to standard hepatitis B vaccines.

In addition to the CpG-ODN-based TLR9 adjuvants described above, small chemical compounds with structures that resemble nucleic acid bases have been identified that activate TLR7 (e.g., imiquimod) or both TLR7 and 8 (e.g., resiquimod). These compounds are being evaluated as vaccine adjuvants in preclinical studies. Flagellin, a TLR5 agonist, is also being explored as an adjuvant.

Recently, attention has also been focused on coupling TLR agonists to antigens, rather than merely mixing them together before injection. CpG oligonucleotides conjugated to antigens have been tested in preclinical studies of hepatitis B vaccines[137] and in human clinical trials for treatment of allergy.[138] Ligands for TLR7/8 have been coupled to HIV antigens,[139] and the ligand for TLR5 (flagellin) has been fused to a variety of antigens.[140,141] In some instances, coupling a TLR ligand to an antigen resulted in a substantial improvement of the immune response compared to mixtures—potentially the result of enabling the antigen and the TLR ligand to co-locate in the same DC compartments.

Numerous preclinical studies have confirmed that many natural and synthetic TLR agonists possess adjuvant activity. Importantly, early human clinical trials of TLR-predicated adjuvants have supported the promise of this approach to mechanism-based strategies to augment vaccine immunogenicity. An important challenge is to define the most potent and best-tolerated variants, and to define rules by which activation of specific TLR pathways might translate into predictable augmentation of desired types of immune responses. It is hoped that general rules will emerge to suggest which of an increasing number of novel adjuvants in development performs best with which type of vaccine immunogen, and if results obtained with a specific type of immunogen–adjuvant combination can be extrapolated to predict the likelihood of enhanced immunogenicity with other vaccines.

However, important challenges remain. A primary challenge for next-generation adjuvant development is finding a combination that retains immunopotentiating action while minimizing vaccine-associated adverse experiences. Short-term adverse experiences, such as local injection site reactions, represent undesirable side effects that may disqualify candidate adjuvants early in clinical development. But given that vaccines are administered to healthy people to prevent potential future infectious diseases, the potential for rarer adverse experiences (such as autoimmunity), which may only be manifest with much longer latency from the time of vaccine adjuvant administration, will undoubtedly be important considerations for use in prophylactic vaccines.

Novel vaccine vectors

As induction of cell-mediated immune responses is considered an important component of vaccine strategies for many diseases for which no vaccines are currently available (many of which are caused by intracellular pathogens), there is a need to develop safe and readily scalable approaches to elicit durable CD8 T-cell responses in immunized humans. Further, given the critical role that CD4 T cells play in induction, differentiation, and maintenance of CD8 T-cell responses, any such novel vaccine strategy will likely also require appropriate CD4 T-cell responses. As elicitation of CD8 T-cell responses against a foreign antigen usually depends on the *de novo* expression of the antigen within a host cell and its subsequent processing and presentation via class I MHC pathways (Chapter 6), most novel vaccine strategies are predicated on the need to achieve synthesis of pathogen-derived antigens within APCs of immunized human hosts. With an increasing appreciation of the role that cross-presentation pathways can play in elicitation of class I-restricted CD8 T-cell responses, such *de novo* antigen synthesis may not need to occur within APCs themselves.

One of the many attractive attributes of effective live attenuated vaccines is their ability to recapitulate (to various degrees) many of the processes that lead to the generation of potent immune responses following natural infection. These processes include the fact that replication of all viruses depends on gaining access to host cells for genome replication and for the synthesis of essential components of virus particles that permit further propagation of the infection within and between hosts. One immunologic benefit of this requirement is that *de novo* synthesis of viral gene products within infected cells provides a key opportunity for viral antigen presentation (via MHC class I pathways) and elicitation of antiviral cellular immune responses. Along with the processing and presentation of intact virus proteins via MHC class II pathways leading to production of antiviral antibody responses, live attenuated viral vaccines have a strong track record for induction of broad cellular and humoral immune responses. However, despite their track record of success, it is likely that few, if any, new live attenuated viral vaccines will be derived in a manner that resembles previous successful efforts (e.g., the empiric derivation of live attenuated polio, yellow fever, or varicella-zoster vaccines). Important reasons for this change include the desire for safe and well-characterized vaccines whose mechanisms of attenuation are defined and that can be monitored in the course of vaccine production and use. Indeed, most of the recently developed live attenuated vaccines were derived using new approaches for genetic reassortment (Fig. 90.2).[142] Although such approaches have proven successful, they are limited in that they can only be applied to homologous viruses (e.g., those derived from the same virus type) whose genomes are segmented and capable of ready genetic reassortment in culture, or to viruses that can be manipulated by reverse genetics.

In response to the desire to produce vaccines that can safely and reliably elicit desired immune responses, especially T-cell responses, several approaches are being explored to develop novel vector systems that permit the expression of pathogen-derived antigens. As many of these approaches are based on viruses distinct from the viral pathogen targeted for induction of host immune responses, the inserted pathogen-derived gene products are expressed via recombinant methods as heterologous antigens. Alternatively, in nonviral expression systems, such as DNA vaccines, the pathogen-derived antigen is expressed in isolation and does not depend on virus-mediated antigen delivery to APCs following host inoculation.

Collectively, such recombinant heterologous expression systems are commonly referred to as "vaccine vectors." In some instances, such recombinant vectors express only a specific antigen (in the case of DNA vaccines or certain viral vectors, e.g., adenovirus), while in others both the inserted pathogen-derived antigens and antigens encoded by the viral vector "backbone" are expressed (e.g., poxvirus vectors). Most new approaches employ expression systems that are inherently nonreplicating (e.g., DNA vaccines) or that employ viral vectors that can replicate at high levels in tissue culture but not *in vivo* (e.g., complemented adenovirus deletion variants or host range-restricted poxviruses). While numerous approaches are being pursued to develop novel vaccine vectors, they will all need to meet certain common criteria to emerge as vaccine approaches applicable for widespread use. In particular, any successful approach must be safe in healthy and immunodeficient humans, desirably immunogenic (including in individuals who may have been previously exposed to the virus from which the vector was derived, e.g., vaccinia or adenovirus), and able to be produced in large quantities and in a stable manner.

Several novel vaccine vectors currently being studied in preclinical studies and human clinical trials are described below, all of which depend on the delivery and expression of a candidate pathogen-derived gene sequence. In a number of ways, DNA vaccines represent the simplest approach to deliver pathogen-derived genes. Viral vectors similarly serve to deliver pathogen gene sequences to host APCs, either directly or indirectly, but do so in a manner that depends on and takes advantage of the lifecycle and tropism of the virus that is being adapted to express the exogenous pathogen gene products.

DNA vaccines

The ability of purified plasmid DNA containing heterologous antigens expressed under the control of eukaryotic transcriptional regulatory and RNA processing signals to elicit immune responses when injected into experimental animals was discovered serendipitously.[143] However, since initial description, the development of so-called DNA vaccines has become an active area of preclinical and clinical vaccine development.[144] Reasons for this enthusiasm include the attractive simplicity and facile preparation of vectors that encode only the defined antigen of interest, a reasonably straightforward method for vaccine production, the inherent stability to temperature and the avoidance of induction of anti-vector immune responses that affect recombinant viral vaccine vector approaches now in development. Although the DNA vector is most commonly injected intramuscularly, the generation of specific immune responses depends on the uptake of the vector DNA by APCs followed by the expression, processing, and presentation of vector-encoded antigens. As tissue and tissue fluids present a hostile environment for purified DNA, and the process of DNA uptake by APCs appears to be relatively inefficient, much of the dose of injected DNA is degraded before it can be reached by an APC that can initiate the desired immune response.

Most early DNA vaccine research was pursued in mice, although studies have been performed in numerous animal species more recently. Studies have usually utilized intramuscular injection of vaccine vector DNA, but various intradermal and transdermal approaches have also been explored. Murine studies have shown that administration of antigen-encoding plasmid DNA can elicit appreciable cellular and humoral immune responses that can confer protection against experimental challenge. However, translation of these promising results to humans has proven frustrating. While DNA vaccines have been generally well tolerated in immunized volunteers, in most human studies of DNA vaccines to date, administration of even substantial quantities of DNA vaccine vectors has elicited relatively low-level immune responses. It is not yet known whether these disappointing results reflects fundamental differences in the immunogenic behavior of DNA vaccines in humans and mice, or the fact that the DNA doses administered to humans do not match those administered to mice (DNA per weight of the immunized host). As such, a variety of approaches are being explored to prolong DNA survival in tissue, promote more efficient targeting of DNA to APCs, or to develop novel adjuvants that might specifically amplify immune responses to DNA vaccines.[145,146] In addition, novel DNA delivery approaches, such as in situ electroporation, have shown promise in increasing DNA vaccine immunogenicity in early clinical studies in humans.[147]

DNA vaccines are currently being used as candidate preventive vaccines for a wide variety of infectious diseases, including HIV, tuberculosis, malaria, and CMV.

Poxviruses

Poxviruses represent the family of viruses that are physically the largest viruses and that possess the largest genomes. Much of the poxvirus genome encodes gene products that serve to evade host immune responses, and that are not required for virus replication in tissue culture. Further, facile techniques for the insertion and deletion of specific viral genes have been developed. The ability to accommodate sizeable foreign gene inserts is, in part, a function of the large size of the poxvirus genome (and the large packaging capacity of poxvirus virions). As a result of these favorable attributes, poxviruses have been utilized extensively in laboratory studies of virus biology, recombinant protein production, and host immune responses.[148] Although poxviruses encode multiple gene products that help the virus evade host immune responses, they are, nevertheless, potent immunogens. Studies of individuals immunized decades ago with vaccinia virus (in the course of smallpox eradication efforts) have shown that this virus induces long-lasting memory T- and B-cell immune responses.

In contrast to most of the other viral vectors currently being developed, poxviruses can replicate readily in culture and do not require an engineered host cell to support propagation ex vivo. One important limitation of all poxvirus vectors developed to date is that, given the large size of the poxvirus genomes and the multitude of gene products they naturally express, even large inserts derived from foreign pathogens of interest will present only a minority of the vaccine vector antigens delivered to and recognized by the host immune system. To be effective, approaches to focus immune responses on the antigen of interest will need to be developed. Toward this end, a variety of so-called "prime–boost"[149] approaches are being explored where the host immune response is primed with one type of recombinant vaccine vector (such as a DNA vaccine or adenovirus vector) and then boosted with subsequent delivery of poxvirus vectors encoding the same antigen. In this manner, immune responses to antigens of interest have been significantly augmented in a number of preclinical studies.

Vaccinia virus represents the prototypic poxvirus vector. This virus is the same one that was employed in the successful smallpox eradication campaign, and has been used as a laboratory tool for decades. However, given current high expectations for vaccine safety, and the increased number of immunodeficient individuals present in the population, the original vaccinia strains used in smallpox eradication efforts are not considered safe for general use. However, studies of vaccinia-based vaccine vectors have provided a strong basic foundation for research on other more highly attenuated poxvirus variants.

Modified vaccinia Ankara (MVA) is an attenuated vaccinia virus that was originally derived by prolonged passage of a vaccinia virus isolate on chicken embryo fibroblasts in culture. In the course of extensive passage in culture, a viral variant emerged that had fortuitously deleted large sections of the viral genome, including those that encode important poxvirus immune evasion genes and those that determine the ability of the virus to replicate on cells obtained from different animal species. Specifically, while MVA grows well on chicken cells, it cannot replicate in human cells in culture or *in vivo*, conferring an inherent safety feature.

MVA was safely administered to over 100 000 individuals at high risk of adverse consequence for vaccinia immunization toward the end of the smallpox eradication effort. More recently, it has garnered renewed interest as a potential safer smallpox vaccine in the wake of concerns about bioterrorism threats. Even though MVA cannot replicate in mammalian cells, the virus demonstrates favorable immunogenic properties. MVA has been used as a vector expressing genes for a wide variety of genes, including HIV, TB and malaria antigens either alone or in "prime-boost" regimens, where MVA has been administered following initial priming immunizations with other vaccine vectors (or in the case of TB vaccines with BCG.[150] A concerted effort is under way to improve further the performance of MVA by manipulating a series of poxvirus genes that dampen the human immune response to the virus (and to any antigens inserted in it).[151]

Avipox is a family of poxviruses that infect birds and cause respiratory diseases in poultry. Canarypox, a member of the avipox group, has been adapted as a vaccine vector. Canarypox replicates well on avian cells in culture but cannot replicate on human cells in culture or in humans *in vivo*. As a result, canarypox, like MVA, provides an interesting vector system with inherent safety features.[152] Canarypox vectors (most commonly ALVAC) have been tested in several clinical studies, either alone, or in "prime–boost" regimens following priming with adenovirus vectors and recombinant protein antigens. Indeed, an ALVAC vector encoding HIV antigens provided the priming immunizations (that were boosted with recombinant HIV gp120 Env antigen) in the previously described RV144 phase III HIV vaccine trial in Thailand.[61,153] To date, the results from other human clinical trials of canarypox vectors have been disappointing, with only low-level specific immune responses generated in human volunteers.[154]

Adenoviruses

Adenoviruses, one of the common causes of upper respiratory and gastrointestinal infections, have seen extensive use in clinical trials and were one of the first gene therapy vectors.[155] Most adenovirus vectors currently being studied in preclinical and clinical settings are disabled by deletion of the early E1 genes that are necessary for replication in an immunized host. Most adenovirus vaccine vectors developed have used the well-characterized and readily produced adenovirus serotype 5 (Ad5) as the vector "backbone." Disabled adenovirus vectors are grown in cells that express the E1 genes artificially inserted into the cell's genome.[156] Once these disabled vectors, encoding a heterologous pathogen-derived antigen of interest, enter a cell, the pathogen gene product is expressed, processed, and presented by host APCs. As adenoviruses can directly infect dendritic cells, they promise to provide efficient vaccine vectors. Robust antibody and CD8 T-cell responses to heterologous antigen genes expressed by adenovirus vectors have been observed in preclinical animal models. Furthermore, in early-phase human clinical trials, adenovirus vectors have been generally well tolerated, and proven to be the most effective of any recombinant vector system studied to date in eliciting high-level CD8 T-cell responses.

The main potential drawback to widespread use of adenovirus vectors in humans is that, depending on the adenovirus type and the geographic location, variable levels of pre-existing immunity are found in humans as a result of prior naturally acquired adenovirus infections. High levels of antibody against the adenovirus vector might blunt the immunogenicity and efficacy of an adenovirus vector-based vaccine, but it remains to be seen if this will be a significant limitation.[157] Should pre-existing immunity to adenovirus vectors derived from epidemiologically prevalent serotypes (e.g., Ad5) limit vaccine immunogenicity, current efforts to develop vaccine vectors based on serotypes that are rare in human populations or novel adenovirus vectors specifically designed to avoid pre-existing antibody responses may yield effective alternative approaches. Adenovirus vectors are currently used in clinical trials for vaccines against HIV,[158] malaria, influenza, and a range of other pathogens.

Alphaviruses

Alphaviruses are RNA viruses that cause zoonotic diseases, such as Venezuelan equine encephalitis. These viruses do not normally circulate in humans, so immunity to these viruses is quite rare in humans. Alphaviruses have a strategy for overexpressing the proteins that make up the virion by making a separate subgenomic RNA specifically encoding these gene products. Current recombinant alphavirus vaccine vector strategies take advantage of this subgenomic transcript, replacing the viral genes with selected genes for other antigens, but maintaining the signals for translation and protein production. In addition, through use of genetic complementation, it is possible to generate virus particles that only contain this heterologous antigen-encoding expression cassette. Such virus particles can efficiently mediate infection of host cells, but because they lack other alphavirus genes needed for virus replication cannot spread beyond the initial target cell infected.[159,160] Alphavirus vectors rival the adenoviruses in efficiency of protein production in tissue culture and have induced robust antibody and T-cell responses in preclinical studies.[161] One current limitation of the alphavirus vector system is the difficulty of scaling the production system; however, this is a technical matter that should be addressable. In addition, ample safety data will be needed before widespread use of alphavirus vaccines achieves endorsement by regulatory authorities for use in healthy populations.

Adeno-associated virus

Adeno-associated viruses (AAV) belong to a family of small single-stranded DNA viruses (parvoviruses) that include the B19 parvovirus that causes a rash in children known as "fifth disease" (measles, mumps, rubella, and varicella make up the first four). AAV is transmitted in conjunction with adenovirus infection, and is not known to cause any significant disease. It is poorly immunogenic in the course of natural infections.[162] AAV can integrate into the genome of the infected cell, usually in a particular place on chromosome 19, although integration does not appear to be efficient or site-specific when replication-defective adeno-associated viruses of the type being developed as vaccine vectors are used. Although encouraging results have been reported in preclinical studies, phase I studies in humans have demonstrated disappointing immunogenicity. While the poor immune response to the virus may make AAV a less attractive vaccine vector, it has made it a good candidate for gene therapy wherein prolonged production of a gene might accrue without the immune system killing the infected cell. Indeed, positive results were recently reported demonstrating a clinical benefit in individuals with hemophilia B who received an AAV vector encoding human factor IX.[163] Recently, efforts have been made to adapt replication-defective AAV encoding a neutralizing monoclonal antibody against HIV as a novel strategy (termed vectored immunoprophylaxis) has demonstrated a promising ability to protect humanized mice against experimental challenge with HIV.[164] Should this approach prove similarly effective in human studies in the future, it will provide an interesting bridge between the previously distinct historical concepts of active and passive immunization approaches.

Summary

The challenges to optimizing the full public health potential of existing vaccines largely relate to programmatic considerations. In contrast, the terrible impact of infectious diseases that cannot now be prevented by vaccines (such as the "big three" killers of HIV, tuberculosis, and malaria) pose direct challenges to the scientific community to develop new generations of vaccines that overcome the largely biological obstacles to control and elimination of these diseases. The nature of the challenges posed by such pathogens necessitates that future vaccine efforts will not simply recapitulate the immune responses engendered by natural infection (as has been the premise of traditional vaccine development efforts), but rather, substantially improve upon them.

As the development of vaccines to prevent infections with the so-far refractory pathogens is pursued, improved understanding of the immune response to natural infection, as well as delineation of the reasons why host immune responses fail either to clear incipient infections or prevent future new ones, will be essential. Fortunately, early empiric approaches have now been replaced with hypothesis-driven strategies enabled by improved insight into the functioning of the human immune system, as well as new technologies, including higher-resolution tools to describe and quantitate pathogen-specific immune responses; novel methods for antigen discovery and targeted optimization of immunogenicity; the development of new, mechanism-based adjuvants; and the advent of innovative methods for vaccine vector-mediated antigen delivery. Thus, although the challenges may be vexing, the scientific and technical foundations on which vaccine development efforts rest have never been stronger.

References

1. Koppaka R. Ten great public health achievements. MMWR Morb Mortal Wkly Rep 2011;60(19):619–23.
2. Henderson DA. Principles and lessons from the smallpox eradication programme. Bull World Health Organ 1987;65:535–46.
3. PrabhuDas M, Adkins B, Gans H, et al. Challenges in infant immunity: implications for responses to infection and vaccines. Nat Immunol 2011;12(3):189–94.
4. Heymann DL, Aylward RB. Mass vaccination: when and why. Curr Top Microbiol Immunol 2006;304:1–16.
5. Anderson RM, May RM. Immunisation and herd immunity. Lancet 1990;335:641–5.
6. Hinman AR, Orenstein WA, Schuchat A. Vaccine-preventable diseases, immunizations, and MMWR—1961–2011. MMWR Surveill Summ 2011;60(Suppl. 4):49–57.
7. Pilishvili T, Lexau C, Farley MM, et al. Sustained reductions in invasive pneumococcal disease in the era of conjugate vaccine. J Infect Dis 2010;201(1):32–41.

8. Coffield AB, Maciosek MV, McGinnis JM, et al. Priorities among recommended clinical preventive services. Am J Prev Med 2001;21:1–9.

9. Plotkin SA. Correlates of protection induced by vaccination. Clin Vaccine Immunol 2010;17(7):1055–65.

10. Cross AS, Opal S, Cook P, et al. Development of an anti-core lipopolysaccharide vaccine for the prevention and treatment of sepsis. Vaccine 2004;22:812–7.

11. Ruiz-Palacios GM, Perez-Schael I, Velazquez FR, et al. Safety and efficacy of an attenuated vaccine against severe rotavirus gastroenteritis. N Engl J Med 2006;354:11–22.

12. Vesikari T, Matson DO, Dennehy P, et al. Safety and efficacy of a pentavalent human-bovine (WC3) reassortant rotavirus vaccine. N Engl J Med 2006;354:23–33.

13. Germain RN. Vaccines and the future of human immunology. Immunity 2010;33(4):441–50.

14. Pulendran B, Li S, Nakaya HI. Systems vaccinology. Immunity 2010;33(4):516–29.

15. Stewart AJ, Devlin PM. The history of the smallpox vaccine. J Infect 2006;52:329–34.

16. Tizard I. Grease, anthraxgate, and kennel cough: a revisionist history of early veterinary vaccines. Adv Vet Med 1999;41:7–24.

17. Dowdle WR, De Gourville E, Kew OM, et al. Polio eradication: the OPV paradox. Rev Med Virol 2003;13:277–91.

18. Falk LA, Chandler DK, Richman P. Review of current preclinical testing strategies for bacterial vaccines. Dev Biol Stand 1998;95:25–9.

19. Kreeftenberg JG. Standardization of acellular pertussis vaccines. Biologicals 1999;27:115–7.

20. Lesinski GB, Westerink MA. Vaccines against polysaccharide antigens. Curr Drug Targets Infect Disord 2001;1:325–34.

21. Lockhart S. Conjugate vaccines. Exp Rev Vaccines 2003;2:633–48.

22. Hilleman MR. Newer directions in vaccine development and utilization. J Infect Dis 1985;151:407–19.

23. Zuckerman AJ. The development of novel hepatitis B vaccines. Biochem Soc Symp 1987;53:39–49.

24. Kirnbauer R, Booy F, Cheng N, et al. Papillomavirus L1 major capsid protein self-assembles into virus-like particles that are highly immunogenic. Proc Natl Acad Sci USA 1992;89:12180–4.

25. Garland SM, Hernandez-Avila M, Wheeler CM, et al. Quadrivalent vaccine against human papillomavirus to prevent anogenital diseases. N Engl J Med 2007;356:1928–43.

26. Villa LL, Ault KA, Giuliano AR, et al. Immunologic responses following administration of a vaccine targeting human papillomavirus types 6, 11, 16, and 18. Vaccine 2006;24:5571–83.

27. Shaw AR. The rotavirus vaccine saga. Annu Rev Med 2006;57:167–80.

28. Parashar UD, Hummelman EG, Bresee JS, et al. Global illness and deaths caused by rotavirus disease in children. Emerg Infect Dis 2003;9:565–72.

29. Simonsen L, Morens D, Elixhauser A, et al. Effect of rotavirus vaccination programme on trends in admission of infants to hospital for intussusception. Lancet 2001;358:1224–9.

30. Matson DO. RotaShield: the ill-fated rhesus-human reassortant rotavirus vaccine. Pediatr Ann 2006;35:44–50.

31. Geier DA, Geier MR. A review of the Vaccine Adverse Event Reporting System database. Exp Opin Pharmacother 2004;5:691–8.

32. Verstraeten T, DeStefano F, Chen RT, et al. Vaccine safety surveillance using large linked databases: opportunities, hazards and proposed guidelines. Exp Rev Vaccines 2003;2:21–9.

33. Offit PA, Moser CA. The problem with Dr Bob's alternative vaccine schedule. Pediatrics 2009;123(1):e164.

34. Offit PA. New book about vaccine safety. Pediatrics 2008;122(4):871–2.

35. Stratton K, Ford A, Rusch E, Wright Claton E. Institute of Medicine Review of Adverse Effects of Vaccines 2011.

36. Griffith AH. Permanent brain damage and pertussis vaccination: is the end of the saga in sight? Vaccine 1989;7:199–210.

37. Afzal MA, Ozoemena LC, O'Hare A, et al. Absence of detectable measles virus genome sequence in blood of autistic children who have had their MMR vaccination during the routine childhood immunization schedule of UK. J Med Virol 2006;78:623–30.

38. Burgess DC, Burgess MA, Leask J. The MMR vaccination and autism controversy in United Kingdom 1998–2005: inevitable community outrage or a failure of risk communication? Vaccine 2006;24:3921–8.

39. Wakefield AJ, Murch SH, Anthony A, et al. Ileal-lymphoid-nodular hyperplasia, non-specific colitis, and pervasive developmental disorder in children. Lancet 1998;351(9103):637–41.

40. Deer B. Secrets of the MMR scare. How the vaccine crisis was meant to make money. BMJ 2011;342:c5258.

41. Deer B. How the case against the MMR vaccine was fixed. BMJ 2011;342:c5347.

42. Tsai CM. Molecular mimicry of host structures by lipooligosaccharides of Neisseria meningitidis: characterization of sialylated and nonsialylated lacto-N-neotetraose (Galbeta1-4GlcNAcbeta1-3Galbeta1-4Glc) structures in lipooligosaccharides using monoclonal antibodies and specific lectins. Adv Exp Med Biol 2001;491:525–42.

43. Healy CM, Baker CJ. Prospects for prevention of childhood infections by maternal immunization. Curr Opin Infect Dis 2006;19:271–6.

44. Neirynck S, Deroo T, Saelens X, et al. A universal influenza A vaccine based on the extracellular domain of the M2 protein. Nat Med 1999;5(10):1157–63.

45. Zhou D, Wu TL, Lasaro MO, et al. A universal influenza A vaccine based on adenovirus expressing matrix-2 ectodomain and nucleoprotein protects mice from lethal challenge. Mol Ther 2010;18(12):2182–9.

46. Webster RG, Kawaoka Y, Taylor J, et al. Efficacy of nucleoprotein and haemagglutinin antigens expressed in fowlpox virus as vaccine for influenza in chickens. Vaccine 1991;9(5):303–8.

47. Bianchi E, Liang X, Ingallinella P, et al. Universal influenza B vaccine based on the maturational cleavage site of the hemagglutinin precursor. J Virol 2005;79(12):7380–8.

48. Bommakanti G, Citron MP, Hepler RW, et al. Design of an HA2-based Escherichia coli expressed influenza immunogen that protects mice from pathogenic challenge. Proc Natl Acad Sci U S A 2010;107(31):13701–6.

49. Treanor JJ, Taylor DN, Tussey L, et al. Safety and immunogenicity of a recombinant hemagglutinin influenza-flagellin fusion vaccine (VAX125) in healthy young adults. Vaccine 2010;28(52):8268–74.

50. Cox MM, Hollister JR. FluBlok, a next generation influenza vaccine manufactured in insect cells. Biologicals 2009;37(3):182–9.

51. Pushko P, Kort T, Nathan M, et al. Recombinant H1N1 virus-like particle vaccine elicits protective immunity in ferrets against the 2009 pandemic H1N1 influenza virus. Vaccine 2010;28(30):4771–6.

52. Shoji Y, Chichester JA, Bi H, et al. Plant-expressed HA as a seasonal influenza vaccine candidate. Vaccine 2008;26(23):2930–4.

53. Landry N, Ward BJ, Trepanier S, et al. Preclinical and clinical development of plant-made virus-like particle vaccine against avian H5N1 influenza. PLoS ONE 2010;5(12):e15559.

54. McElrath MJ, Haynes BF. Induction of immunity to human immunodeficiency virus type-1 by vaccination. Immunity 2010;33(4):542–54.

55. Johnston MI, Fauci AS. An HIV vaccine—evolving concepts. N Engl J Med 2007;356:2073–81.

56. Garber DA, Silvestri G, Feinberg MB. Prospects for an AIDS vaccine: three big questions, no easy answers. Lancet Infect Dis 2004;4:397–413.

57. Johnson VA, Brun-Vezinet F, Clotet B, et al. Update of the drug resistance mutations in HIV-1: 2004. Top HIV Med 2004;12:119–24.

58. HIV gp120 vaccine—VaxGen: AIDSVAX, AIDSVAX B/B, AIDSVAX B/E, HIV gp120 vaccine—Genentech, HIV gp120 vaccine AIDSVAX—VaxGen, HIV vaccine AIDSVAX—VaxGen. Drugs R D 2003;4:249–53.

59. Shiver JW, Emini EA. Recent advances in the development of HIV-1 vaccines using replication-incompetent adenovirus vectors. Annu Rev Med 2004;55:355–72.

60. Steinbrook R. One step forward, two steps back — will there ever be an AIDS vaccine? N Engl J Med 2007;357:2653–5.

61. Rerks-Ngarm S, Pitisuttithum P, Nitayaphan S, et al. Vaccination with ALVAC and AIDSVAX to prevent HIV-1 infection in Thailand. N Engl J Med 2009;361(23):2209–20.

62. Haynes BF, Gilbert PB, McElrath MJ, et al. Immune-correlates analysis of an HIV-1 vaccine efficacy trial. N Engl J Med 2012;366(14):1275–86.

63. Ekiert DC, Wilson IA. Broadly neutralizing antibodies against influenza virus and prospects for universal therapies. Curr Opin Virol 2012;2(2):134–41.

64. McLellan JS, Pancera M, Carrico C, et al. Structure of HIV-1 gp120 V1/V2 domain with broadly neutralizing antibody PG9. Nature 2011;480(7377):336–43.

65. Smith TA, Leuenberger R, Lengeler C. Child mortality and malaria transmission intensity in Africa. Trends Parasitol 2001;17:145–9.

66. Snow RW, Trape JF, Marsh K. The past, present and future of childhood malaria mortality in Africa. Trends Parasitol 2001;17:593–7.

67. Malaguarnera L, Musumeci S. The immune response to Plasmodium falciparum malaria. Lancet Infect Dis 2002;2:472–8.

68. Achtman AH, Bull PC, Stephens R, et al. Longevity of the immune response and memory to blood-stage malaria infection. Curr Top Microbiol Immunol 2005;297:71–102.

69. Ballou WR. Malaria vaccines in development. Exp Opin Emerg Drugs 2005;10:489–503.

70. Wizel B, Houghten RA, Parker KC, et al. Irradiated sporozoite vaccine induces HLA-B8-restricted cytotoxic T lymphocyte responses against two overlapping epitopes of the Plasmodium falciparum sporozoite surface protein 2. J Exp Med 1995;182:1435–45.

71. Hoffman SL, Billingsley PF, James E, et al. Development of a metabolically active, non-replicating sporozoite vaccine to prevent Plasmodium falciparum malaria. Hum Vaccin 2010;6(1):97–106.

72. Bojang KA. RTS, S/AS02A for malaria. Exp Rev Vaccines 2006;5:611–5.

73. Wiley SR, Raman VS, Desbien A, et al. Targeting TLRs expands the antibody repertoire in response to a malaria vaccine. Sci Transl Med 2011;3(93):93ra69.

74. Regules JA, Cummings JF, Ockenhouse CF. The RTS, S vaccine candidate for malaria. Expert Rev Vaccines 2011;10(5):589–99.

75. Maher D, Raviglione M. Global epidemiology of tuberculosis. Clin Chest Med 2005;26:167–82. v.

76. Skeiky YA, Sadoff JC. Advances in tuberculosis vaccine strategies. Nat Rev Microbiol 2006;4:469–76.

77. Fine PE, Rodrigues LC. Modern vaccines. Mycobacterial diseases. Lancet 1990;335:1016–20.

78. Orme IM. Tuberculosis vaccines: current progress. Drugs 2005;65:2437–44.

79. Orme IM. Preclinical testing of new vaccines for tuberculosis: a comprehensive review. Vaccine 2006;24:2–19.

80. de Jonge MI, Brosch R, Brodin P, et al. Tuberculosis: from genome to vaccine. Exp Rev Vaccines 2005;4:541–51.

81. Fulginiti VA, Eller JJ, Sieber OF, et al. Respiratory virus immunization. I. A field trial of two inactivated respiratory virus vaccines; an aqueous trivalent parainfluenza virus vaccine and an alum-precipitated respiratory syncytial virus vaccine. Am J Epidemiol 1969;89:435–48.

82. Wilson S, Aprile MA. Sensitizing versus immunizing properties of inactivated measles vaccine. Prog Immunobiol Stand 1970;4:657–60.

83. Schmidt AC, McAuliffe JM, Murphy BR, et al. Recombinant bovine/human parainfluenza virus type 3 (B/HPIV3) expressing the respiratory syncytial virus (RSV) G and F proteins can be used to achieve simultaneous mucosal immunization against RSV and HPIV3. J Virol 2001;75:4594–603.

84. Pichichero ME. The new meningococcal conjugate vaccine. A profile of its safety, efficacy, and indications for use. Postgrad Med 2006;119:47–54 64.

85. Finne J, Leinonen M, Makela PH. Antigenic similarities between brain components and bacteria causing meningitis. Implications for vaccine development and pathogenesis. Lancet 1983;2:355–7.

86. Serruto D, Spadafina T, Ciucchi L, et al. Neisseria meningitidis GNA2132, a heparin-binding protein that induces protective immunity in humans. Proc Natl Acad Sci U S A 2010;107(8):3770–5.

87. Murphy E, Andrew L, Lee KL, et al. Sequence diversity of the factor H binding protein vaccine candidate in epidemiologically relevant strains of serogroup B Neisseria meningitidis. J Infect Dis 2009;200(3):379–89.

88. LaForce FM, Okwo-Bele JM. Eliminating epidemic Group A meningococcal meningitis in Africa through a new vaccine. Health Aff (Millwood) 2011;30(6):1049–57.

89. Schrag S, Gorwitz R, Fultz-Butts K, et al. Prevention of perinatal group B streptococcal disease. Revised guidelines from CDC. MMWR Recomm Rep 2002;51:1–22.

90. Mikkelsen M, Bukh J. Current status of a hepatitis C vaccine: encouraging results but significant challenges ahead. Curr Infect Dis Rep 2007;9:94–101.

91. Roohvand F, Kossari N. Advances in hepatitis C virus vaccines, part two: advances in hepatitis C virus vaccine formulations and modalities. Expert Opin Ther Pat 2012;22(4):391–415.

92. Ferenczy MW. Prophylactic vaccine strategies and the potential of therapeutic vaccines against herpes simplex virus. Curr Pharm Des 2007;13:1975–88.

93. Stanberry LR. Clinical trials of prophylactic and therapeutic herpes simplex virus vaccines. Herpes 2004;11(Suppl. 3):161A–169A.

94. Cohen J. Immunology. Painful failure of promising genital herpes vaccine. Science 2010;330(6002):304.

95. Plotkin SA, Huygelen C. Cytomegalovirus vaccine prepared in WI-38. Dev Biol Stand 1976;37:301–5.

96. Pass RF, Zhang C, Evans A, et al. Vaccine prevention of maternal cytomegalovirus infection. N Engl J Med 2009;360(12):1191–9.

97. Adler SP, Plotkin SA, Gonczol E, et al. A canarypox vector expressing cytomegalovirus (CMV) glycoprotein B primes for antibody responses to a live attenuated CMV vaccine (Towne). J Infect Dis 1999;180:843–6.

98. Zhong J, Khanna R. Vaccine strategies against human cytomegalovirus infection. Exp Rev Anti Infect Ther 2007;5:449–59.

99. Sung H, Schleiss MR. Update on the current status of cytomegalovirus vaccines. Expert Rev Vaccines 2010;9(11):1303–14.

100. Moutschen M, Leonard P, Sokal EM, et al. Phase I/II studies to evaluate safety and immunogenicity of a recombinant gp350 Epstein–Barr virus vaccine in healthy adults. Vaccine 2007;25:4697–705.

101. Stephenson JR. Understanding dengue pathogenesis: implications for vaccine design. Bull World Health Organ 2005;83:308–14.

102. Whitehead SS, Blaney JE, Durbin AP, et al. Prospects for a dengue virus vaccine. Nat Rev Microbiol 2007;5:518–28.

103. Murphy BR, Whitehead SS. Immune response to dengue virus and prospects for a vaccine. Annu Rev Immunol 2011;29:587–619.

104. Kaslow DC, Shiver JW. *Clostridium difficile* and methicillin-resistant *Staphylococcus aureus*: emerging concepts in vaccine development. Annu Rev Med 2011;62:201–15.

105. Kuklin NA, Clark DJ, Secore S, et al. A novel Staphylococcus aureus vaccine: iron surface determinant B induces rapid antibody responses in rhesus macaques and specific increased survival in a murine S. aureus sepsis model. Infect Immun 2006;74(4):2215–23.

106. Nanra JS, Timofeyeva Y, Buitrago SM, et al. Heterogeneous in vivo expression of clumping factor A and capsular polysaccharide by *Staphylococcus aureus*: implications for vaccine design. Vaccine 2009;27(25–26):3276–80.

107. Sougioultzis S, Kyne L, Drudy D, et al. Clostridium difficile toxoid vaccine in recurrent C. difficile-associated diarrhea. Gastroenterology 2005;128(3):764–70.

108. Ramos BV. A method for the screening of fusion protein expression by lambda-GT11 recombinant clones without the preparation of lysogens. Nucleic Acids Res 1989;17:6421.

109. Jones P. Antibody screening of bacteriophage lambda gt-11 DNA expression libraries. Methods Mol Biol 1998;80:439–47.

110. Wack A, Rappuoli R. Vaccinology at the beginning of the 21st century. Curr Opin Immunol 2005;17:411–8.

111. Rappuoli R. Reverse vaccinology, a genome-based approach to vaccine development. Vaccine 2001;19:2688–91.

112. Muzzi A, Masignani V, Rappuoli R. The pan-genome: towards a knowledge-based discovery of novel targets for vaccines and antibacterials. Drug Discov Today 2007;12:429–39.

113. Grandi G. Genomics and proteomics in reverse vaccines. Methods Biochem Anal 2006;49:379–93.

114. Tang CM, Hood DW, Moxon ER. *Haemophilus* influence: the impact of whole genome sequencing on microbiology. Trends Genet 1997;13:399–404.

115. Gardner MJ, Hall N, Fung E, et al. Genome sequence of the human malaria parasite *Plasmodium falciparum*. Nature 2002;419:498–511.

116. Nilsson CL. Bacterial proteomics and vaccine development. Am J Pharmacogenomics 2002;2:59–65.

117. Klade CS. Proteomics approaches towards antigen discovery and vaccine development. Curr Opin Mol Ther 2002;4:216–23.

118. Hillen N, Stevanovic S. Contribution of mass spectrometry-based proteomics to immunology. Exp Rev Proteomics 2006;3:653–64.

119. Strong M, Goulding CW. Structural proteomics and computational analysis of a deadly pathogen: combating *Mycobacterium tuberculosis* from multiple fronts. Methods Biochem Anal 2006;49:245–69.

120. Chitlaru T, Gat O, Grosfeld H, et al. Identification of in vivo-expressed immunogenic proteins by serological proteome analysis of the *Bacillus anthracis* secretome. Infect Immun 2007;75:2841–52.

121. Klade CS, Voss T, Krystek E, et al. Identification of tumor antigens in renal cell carcinoma by serological proteome analysis. Proteomics 2001;1:890–8.

122. Janeway Jr. CA, Medzhitov R. Innate immune recognition. Annu Rev Immunol 2002;20:197–216.

123. Blander JM, Medzhitov R. On regulation of phagosome maturation and antigen presentation. Nat Immunol 2006;7:1029–35.

124. Pulendran B, Ahmed R. Translating innate immunity into immunological memory: implications for vaccine development. Cell 2006;124:849–63.

125. Medzhitov R, Janeway Jr. CA. Innate immune induction of the adaptive immune response. Cold Spring Harb Symp Quant Biol 1999;64:429–35.

126. Kersten GF, Crommelin DJ. Liposomes and ISCOMs. Vaccine 2003;21:915–20.

127. Querec TD, Pulendran B. Understanding the role of innate immunity in the mechanism of action of the live attenuated yellow fever vaccine 17D. Adv Exp Med Biol 2007;590:43–53.

128. Latz E, Franko J, Golenbock DT, et al. *Haemophilus influenzae* type b-outer membrane protein complex glycoconjugate vaccine induces cytokine production by engaging human Toll-like receptor 2 (TLR2) and requires the presence of TLR2 for optimal immunogenicity. J Immunol 2004;172:2431–8.

129. Blander JM, Medzhitov R. Toll-dependent selection of microbial antigens for presentation by dendritic cells. Nature 2006;440(7085):808–12.

130. Hem SL, White JL. Structure and properties of aluminum-containing adjuvants. Pharm Biotechnol 1995;6:249–76.

131. Flach TL, Ng G, Hari A, et al. Alum interaction with dendritic cell membrane lipids is essential for its adjuvanticity. Nat Med 2011;17(4):479–87.

132. Desjardins R, Krzystyniak K, Therien HM, et al. Immunoactivating potential of multilamellar liposome vesicles (MLV) in murine popliteal lymph node (PLN) test. Int J Immunopharmacol 1995;17:367–74.

133. Gluck R, Burri KG, Metcalfe I. Adjuvant and antigen delivery properties of virosomes. Curr Drug Deliv 2005;2:395–400.

134. Atmar RL, Keitel WA, Patel SM, et al. Safety and immunogenicity of nonadjuvanted and MF59-adjuvanted influenza A/H9N2 vaccine preparations. Clin Infect Dis 2006;43:1135–42.

135. Kundi M. New hepatitis B vaccine formulated with an improved adjuvant system. Exp Rev Vaccines 2007;6:133–40.

136. Cooper CL, Davis HL, Angel JB, et al. CPG 7909 adjuvant improves hepatitis B virus vaccine seroprotection in antiretroviral-treated HIV-infected adults. Aids 2005;19:1473–9.

137. Payette PJ, Ma X, Weeratna RD, et al. Testing of CpG-optimized protein and DNA vaccines against the hepatitis B virus in chimpanzees for immunogenicity and protection from challenge. Intervirology 2006;49:144–51.

138. Broide DH. Immunostimulatory sequences of DNA and conjugates in the treatment of allergic rhinitis. Curr Allergy Asthma Rep 2005;5:182–5.

139. Wille-Reece U, Flynn BJ, Lore K, et al. HIV Gag protein conjugated to a Toll-like receptor 7/8 agonist improves the magnitude and quality of Th1 and CD8$^+$ T cell responses in nonhuman primates. Proc Natl Acad Sci U S A 2005;102:15190–4.

140. Huleatt JW, Jacobs AR, Tang J, et al. Vaccination with recombinant fusion proteins incorporating Toll-like receptor ligands induces rapid cellular and humoral immunity. Vaccine 2007;25:763–75.

141. McDonald WF, Huleatt JW, Foellmer HG, et al. A west nile virus recombinant protein vaccine that coactivates innate and adaptive immunity. J Infect Dis 2007;195:1607–17.

142. Clark HF, Offit PA, Ellis RW, et al. The development of multivalent bovine rotavirus (strain WC3) reassortant vaccine for infants. J Infect Dis 1996;174(Suppl. 1):S73–S80.

143. Wells DJ. Intramuscular injection of plasmid DNA. Mol Cell Biol Hum Dis Ser 1995;5:83–103.

144. Ulmer JB, Donnelly JJ, Parker SE, et al. Heterologous protection against influenza by injection of DNA encoding a viral protein. Science 1993;259:1745–9.

145. Liu MA, Wahren B, Karlsson Hedestam GB. DNA vaccines: recent developments and future possibilities. Hum Gene Ther 2006;17:1051–61.

146. Laddy DJ, Weiner DB. From plasmids to protection: a review of DNA vaccines against infectious diseases. Int Rev Immunol 2006;25:99–123.

147. Ferraro B, Morrow MP, Hutnick NA, et al. Clinical applications of DNA vaccines: current progress. Clin Infect Dis 2011;53(3):296–302.

148. Franchini G, Gurunathan S, Baglyos L, et al. Poxvirus-based vaccine candidates for HIV: two decades of experience with special emphasis on canarypox vectors. Exp Rev Vaccines 2004;3(Suppl):S75–S88.

149. Kent S, De Rose R, Rollman E. Drug evaluation: DNA/MVA prime-boost HIV vaccine. Curr Opin Invest Drugs 2007;8:159–67.

150. Verreck FA, Vervenne RA, Kondova I, et al. MVA.85A boosting of BCG and an attenuated, phoP deficient M. tuberculosis vaccine both show protective efficacy against tuberculosis in rhesus macaques. PLoS One 2009;4(4):e5264.

151. Abaitua F, Rodriguez JR, Garzon A, et al. Improving recombinant MVA immune responses: potentiation of the immune responses to HIV-1 with MVA and DNA vectors expressing Env and the cytokines IL-12 and IFN-gamma. Virus Res 2006;116:11–20.

152. Taylor J, Tartaglia J, Riviere M, et al. Applications of canarypox (ALVAC) vectors in human and veterinary vaccination. Dev Biol Stand 1994;82:131–5.

153. McEnery R. Researchers unveil plans for follow-up trials to RV144. IAVI Rep 2010;14(3):18–9.

154. Goepfert PA, Horton H, McElrath MJ, et al. High-dose recombinant Canarypox vaccine expressing HIV-1 protein, in seronegative human subjects. J Infect Dis 2005;192:1249–59.

155. McConnell MJ, Imperiale MJ. Biology of adenovirus and its use as a vector for gene therapy. Hum Gene Ther 2004;15:1022–33.

156. Graham FL, Prevec L. Adenovirus-based expression vectors and recombinant vaccines. Biotechnology 1992;20:363–90.

157. Schulick AH, Vassalli G, Dunn PF, et al. Established immunity precludes adenovirus-mediated gene transfer in rat carotid arteries. Potential for immunosuppression and vector engineering to overcome barriers of immunity. J Clin Invest 1997;99:209–19.

158. Casimiro DR, Wang F, Schleif WA, et al. Attenuation of simian immunodeficiency virus SIVmac239 infection by prophylactic immunization with DNA and recombinant adenoviral vaccine vectors expressing Gag. J Virol 2005;79:15547–55.

159. Caley IJ, Betts MR, Davis NL, et al. Venezuelan equine encephalitis virus vectors expressing HIV-1 proteins: vector design strategies for improved vaccine efficacy. Vaccine 1999;17:3124–35.
160. Perri S, Greer CE, Thudium K, et al. An alphavirus replicon particle chimera derived from Venezuelan equine encephalitis and sindbis viruses is a potent gene-based vaccine delivery vector. J Virol 2003;77:10394–403.
161. Riezebos-Brilman A, de Mare A, Bungener L, et al. Recombinant alphaviruses as vectors for anti-tumour and anti-microbial immunotherapy. J Clin Virol 2006;35:233–43.
162. un JY, Anand-Jawa V, Chatterjee S, et al. Immune responses to adeno-associated virus and its recombinant vectors. Gene Ther 2003;10:964–76.
163. Buchlis G, Podsakoff GM, Radu A, et al. Factor IX expression in skeletal muscle of a severe hemophilia B patient 10 years after AAV-mediated gene transfer. Blood 2012;119(13):3038–41.
164. Balazs AB, Chen J, Hong CM, et al. Antibody-based protection against HIV infection by vectored immunoprophylaxis. Nature 2012;481(7379):81–4.

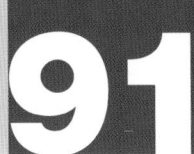
Anthony J. Frew

Immunotherapy of allergic disease

Various forms of allergic disease (involving type I hypersensitivity) can be treated by specific allergen immunotherapy (SIT)—also known as allergen desensitization. SIT involves the administration of allergen extracts to modify or abolish symptoms associated with exposure to relevant allergens. SIT is used for three distinct types of condition: anaphylaxis, rhinoconjunctivitis and asthma. In anaphylaxis, the patient is completely well between episodes; exposure is infrequent and unexpected, but provokes an immediate and potentially catastrophic response. However, since exposure only occurs occasionally, it can be difficult to know whether the treatment has been effective until an accidental exposure event occurs. Allergic rhinoconjunctivitis is clearly driven by allergen exposure, which is low level and can be either continuous or intermittent. Exposure and clinical relevance are most obvious for seasonal rhinitis (due to pollens or molds), occupational rhinitis, and for rhinitis due to animal danders. In perennial rhinitis, without seasonal variation, it is more difficult to be sure that allergen exposure drives symptoms—in some cases it clearly does, but in others there may be non-allergic or structural causes for the symptoms. The value of SIT for rhinoconjunctivitis is generally clearer when exposure is predictable, but assessing efficacy is complicated by year-to-year variations in pollen exposure due to weather patterns and individual activity. The third indication for SIT is asthma, where the role of allergen exposure is different from that in rhinoconjunctivitis. As discussed elsewhere, allergen sensitization is a risk factor for developing asthma in childhood, but it is less clear whether allergen exposure has a role in ongoing disease. At the very least, the fact that allergen avoidance measures are not usually effective in asthma begs the question whether modifying the response to allergen will influence established disease. It is inherently more risky to use SIT to treat patients with asthma than those who do not have asthma, so the physician needs to weigh the benefits and risks very carefully when considering the use of SIT to treat asthma.

The general principles of managing any allergic condition are to make an accurate diagnosis, to identify relevant trigger factors, and to institute appropriate interventions that reduce the impact of those triggers and that control symptoms and disease progression. Allergen avoidance measures may be helpful, but can be difficult to implement and are rarely sufficient to allow patients to do without other therapy. Drug treatments can be very effective, but only work as long as they are taken, so there is clearly a need for additional and long-lasting therapy. SIT is the only current therapy that modifies the immune response to allergens. The process is specific, in that the treatment is targeted at those allergens recognized by the patient and physician as responsible for symptoms. While claims have been made for bystander benefits on unrelated allergens, there is little convincing evidence that treating for one allergy will alleviate symptoms caused by a different allergen. Before deciding to use SIT it is therefore essential to assess the patient's condition carefully, with particular emphasis on the role of allergic triggers.

SIT was pioneered over 100 years ago, and developed as an empirical science of pollen vaccination, based on the concept that hay fever was a form of infection.[1] Early studies found that giving large doses of pollen would trigger allergic reactions, so regimes were developed that involve a gradual build-up from extremely low doses to a maintenance dose that can then be given every few weeks. More recently a great deal has been learned about the immunological events associated with clinically successful SIT, but some uncertainties remain about which of these events is truly important. New and modified forms of SIT have been developed to deliver these immunological effects more efficiently but none of these has yet reached a point where they are likely to replace the standard approach.

Following initial reports from the UK, SIT was taken up and developed in the 1920s–30s in North America, where some differences in practice developed compared to European practice. In particular, American allergists tend to treat for all sensitivities identified on skin testing, using a personalized mixture of extracts prepared from bulk vials, whereas in Europe patients are normally only treated with a single allergen, which is supplied direct from the manufacturer. Mixed allergen extracts are available and used in some parts of Europe, but only as custom mixes from manufacturers. Different approaches are taken to standardization of extracts: allergen extracts used in Europe are standardized according to their ability to elicit a wheal, while in the USA, standardization is based on ability to elicit erythema rather than wheal.

Whichever form of extract is chosen, patients are started on a very low dose of allergen, and the dose is then increased, usually at weekly intervals until a plateau or maintenance dose is achieved. The maintenance dose is then given at 4- to 6-weekly intervals for 3 to 5 years. Alternative induction regimes may give several doses on each day, or may give the whole series of incremental injections in a single day (rush protocols). The main drawback to rush and semi-rush protocols is the risk of adverse reactions, which are much commoner than in conventional protocols. On the other hand, full protection can be attained in a few days as compared to the three months required in the conventional regime. Normally the doses are given by subcutaneous injection, but in the past two decades there has been increasing interest in SIT by the sublingual route, which is more convenient for patients and has some advantages in terms of safety.

Mechanisms of SIT

● KEY CONCEPTS

Possible mechanisms of immunotherapy

- Induction of IgG (blocking) antibodies
- Reduction in specific IgE (long-term)
- Reduced recruitment of effector cells
- Altered T-cell cytokine balance (shift to Th1 from Th2)
- T-cell anergy
- B-cell suppression

The primary reason for studying the mechanisms of SIT is to seek out the features that are biologically important and hence devise new forms of immunotherapy that improve efficacy, increase safety margins, shorten treatment courses or achieve more durable results. At least three distinct phases can be identified in SIT, each with a distinct set of immunological mechanisms.[2] Initially there is a phase of pharmacological desensitization, in which basophils and mast cells are rendered tolerant of the allergen. This is achieved quickly, within a few days if the rush protocol is followed. Clinically, this allows the patient to tolerate the maintenance dose of allergen, but also protects against acute exposure to allergen (e.g., a wasp sting). This state of pharmacological tolerance is not permanent, and will be rapidly lost if SIT is stopped. During the first year of maintenance SIT, a state of T-cell tolerance is achieved, with abrogation of late-phase responses to allergen exposure, and the induction or regulatory T cells. Finally, with prolonged treatment, B-cell tolerance develops, and the level of sensitizing antibodies decreases.

Following subcutaneous injection of allergen extracts, a small proportion of the allergenic material is taken up by phagocytic cells and carried to the regional lymph nodes. The process is quite inefficient and less than 1% of a radiolabelled dose actually reaches the lymph nodes. Almost all studies have shown that SIT induces allergen-specific IgG antibodies, which increase progressively over the course of treatment. This led to suggestions that SIT might work by inducing antibodies that intercept the allergen and "block" the allergic response. In patients treated for venom anaphylaxis, the development of allergen-specific IgG antibody correlates with clinical efficacy, but for other allergens the magnitude of the IgG response is not closely related to the degree of efficacy. Moreover, the rise in IgG follows rather than precedes the onset of clinical benefit. Initially there is an increase in allergen-specific IgE antibodies, but the usual rise in IgE seen during natural seasonal exposure is blunted.[3] Over the course of several years, the amount of allergen-specific IgE declines, but it does not disappear. In keeping with this there is little effect on immediate skin test responses to allergen. In contrast, the late-phase skin test response is virtually abolished after successful SIT. Similar patterns are observed for late-phase nasal and airway responses.[4]

SIT also has affects allergen-specific T cells. Both in the skin and in the nose, successful SIT is accompanied by a reduction in T-cell and eosinophil recruitment in response to allergen challenge. In parallel, there is a shift in the balance of Th1 and Th2 cytokine expression in the allergen-challenged site. Th2 cytokine expression is not affected, but an increased proportion of the recruited T-cells express the Th1 cytokines IL-2, IFN-γ, and IL-12.[5,6] In addition there is induction of allergen-specific CD4 T-regulatory (Treg) cells that express CD25, FOXP3 and IL-10.[2] IL10 is induced within a few days of starting SIT and has a number of biologic effects that could explain the beneficial effects of immunotherapy. These include modulation of IL4-induced B-cell IgE production in favor of IgG4, inhibition of IgE-dependent mast cell activation, inhibition of human eosinophil cytokine production and survival, suppression of IL5, and induction of antigen-specific anergy (Fig. 91.1). Taken together, these findings suggest that SIT modulates allergen-specific T cells, which may explain why the clinical and late-phase responses are attenuated without much effect on allergen-specific antibody levels. Further work in this area is concentrating on finding more efficient ways of inducing allergen-specific Treg cells.

SIT for venom anaphylaxis

Anaphylaxis to Hymenoptera venom is relatively rare, but can be fatal (Chapter 41). Venom-specific IgE antibodies can be found in 30–40% of adults for a few months following a sting, but these usually disappear in a few months. Some individuals react more vigorously with high concentrations of venom-specific antibodies,

Fig. 91.1 Immunological mechanisms of specific immunotherapy.

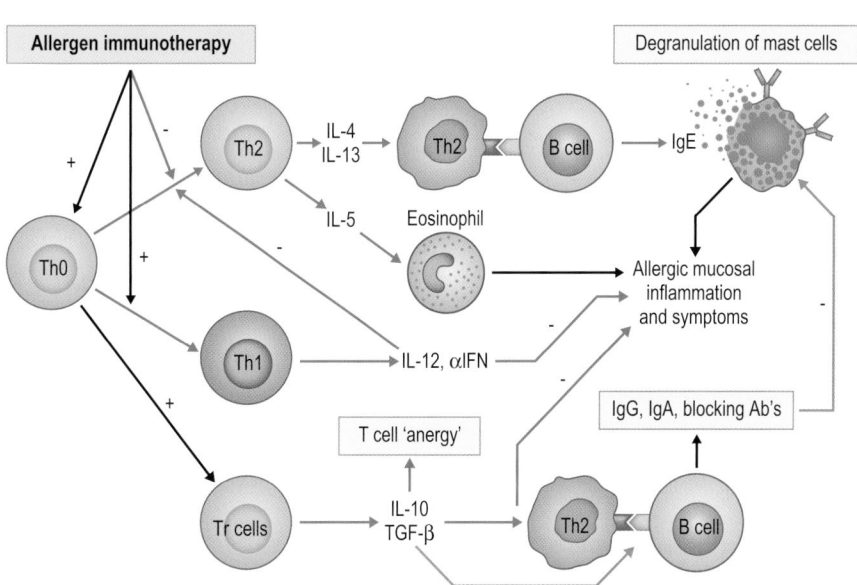

which may persist for many years without further exposure to stings. This group of patients is at risk of anaphylaxis to subsequent stings and a small number die from anaphylaxis each year. Estimates are hard to come by, but a figure of 10–20 deaths per year in the USA has been cited.

Before embarking on venom immunotherapy the patient needs to be carefully assessed and some account taken of the natural history of venom allergy.[7] Patients who have experienced systemic symptoms after a sting are at much greater risk of anaphylaxis on subsequent stings, as compared to patients who have only had large local reactions. The frequency of systemic reactions to stings in children and adults with a history of large local reactions is about 5–10%, whereas the risk in patients with a previous systemic reaction is between 30 and 70%. In general, there is a lower risk of repeated systemic reactions in children, and in those with a history of milder reactions. In adults the risk of systemic reaction to field stings diminishes over 10–20 years towards 15–30% (Fig. 91.2) but does not seem to return to the background prevalence in the general population (3%). Children with a history of cutaneous systemic reactions had less than 5% risk of anaphylaxis during observation for 10–20 years. There is no test that accurately predicts the outcome of the next sting. Live sting challenges have been used as a research tool but are not generally practical or acceptable in clinical practice. Unfortunately, even if sting challenges are performed, they are not absolutely predictive, since patients who do not react to a laboratory challenge sting may go on to react to a subsequent field sting.

In making a decision whether to recommend venom SIT, the physician should also take account of occupational and geographic factors that can affect the likelihood of future stings. Bee stings are much commoner in beekeepers, their families and neighbors, while wasp stings tend to be sporadic, but are an occupational hazard for bakers, gardeners, outdoor caterers and greengrocers. Other factors to be considered are the potential risks of emergency treatment with epinephrine and the various medical contraindications to SIT (see below). Large local reactions to stings have not historically been regarded as indications for SIT as they are not life-threatening and do not predict future problems, but there is now clinical evidence that they can be attenuated by SIT.[8]

Immunization with venom accelerates the process of risk reduction and confers rapid protection against both field and laboratory stings. There appears to remain a low risk of systemic reaction (10%) for many years after discontinuing venom immunotherapy. Although reactions to stings after completing SIT are

rarely severe, some fatalities have been reported in patients with other risk factors (mastocytosis, severe historical reactions, systemic reaction during VIT). This raises the question whether SIT should be life-long, but this also alters the cost-benefit analysis. In children, the chance of systemic reaction to a sting remains <5% for up to 20 years after discontinuing venom SIT.

In summary, desensitization with venom preparations provides protection against field and laboratory stings, but a minority of patients will react despite completing their course of SIT. The residual risk of systemic reactions after completing SIT is about 10%, but these are usually mild. Patients undergoing SIT for venom anaphylaxis are usually offered injectable epinephrine and other anti-allergic medication for use in the event of a sting during their course of SIT.

Assessing effectiveness in clinical trials of SIT for asthma and rhinitis

The two main keys to success in designing any clinical trial are the application of appropriate criteria for subject recruitment and the selection of appropriate clinical endpoints (Table 91.1). In allergic rhinitis, efficacy is generally assessed in terms of symptom scores, recorded on a daily basis on a diary card or a personal organizer.[9] Several symptom scales are in use, which all rely on a categorical grading system (e.g., 1 = mild, 2 = moderate, 3 = severe, etc.). These measures carry the implicit assumption that the step from 1 to 2 is equivalent to the step from 2 to 3 for the purposes of statistical analysis. By assigning numerical values to non-parametric variables, one may either overestimate or underestimate the true effects of therapy. Reduction in rescue medication use is also measured, as in theory patients may improve their symptoms because they use more medication. In practice most studies that show improved symptom scores show parallel reductions in medication usage, but some studies show reductions in medication usage without a statistically significant reduction in symptoms. Combining symptom and medication scores is fraught with difficulty. It is almost impossible to agree on equivalences between different drugs, let alone the relative value of one antihistamine tablet versus one day when symptoms are moderate rather than mild.

When assessing improvement in asthma, it is important to remember that the majority of patients with atopic asthma have relatively mild disease and are usually easy to control with standard doses of conventional anti-asthma drugs. Cases of severe asthma are relatively few in number and the role of allergy in

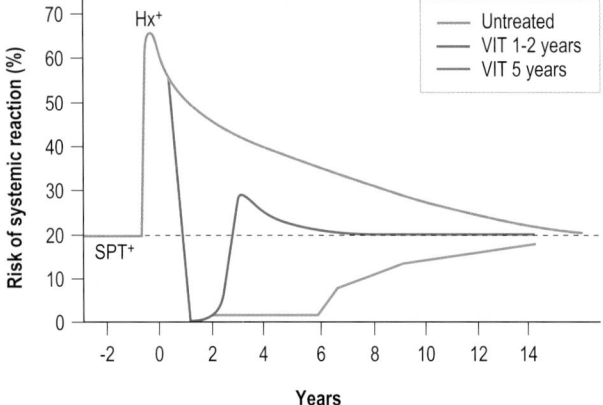

Fig. 91.2 Risk of systemic reaction (SR) from wasp stings over time after an anaphylactic event, and the effect of SIT after 1-2 years or 5 years on the natural history.
Adapted from Golden DB et al, J Allergy Clin Immunol 2000; 105:385-90.

Table 91.1 Endpoints for trials of specific immunotherapy in asthma

Spirometry	Airflow obstruction (FEV_1, PEFR) Bronchial irritability (histamine/methacholine PC_{20})
Symptoms	Wheeze, nocturnal waking, cough, breathlessness, time off work/school (diary cards or visual analogue scales)
Drug use	Bronchodilator use as surrogate for symptoms
Cost: benefit	Reduction in other drugs, lost work etc., compared to costs of SIT and time lost due to SIT
Safety	Frequency of local and systemic adverse events
Immunology	Allergen-specific IgG4 Skin test responses Nasal allergen challenge responses Inhalation allergen challenge responses

their disease is often less obvious than in mild cases. In mild cases, resting spirometry will usually be close to predicted values so there is little scope for improvement in simple spirometric measures such as FEV_1. Peak expiratory flow rates (PEFR) can show improvement, especially the early morning values that are more likely to be reduced below the patient's best possible value than evening peak flow rates. Objective measures of bronchial irritability are more useful markers and a shift in the concentration of histamine or methacholine needed to induce a 20% fall in FEV_1 (PC_{20}) is commonly used. This measurement can be quite variable within individuals, so the minimum change that would be clinically significant is a change of at least one doubling dilution in the PC_{20}. Other bronchial challenge tests such as exercise challenge or adenosine inhalation may provide additional insights into the ability of an anti-asthma treatment to prevent acute attacks. Both these parameters depend indirectly on the PC_{20} so again it is important to consider statistical and biological significance separately.

Although these challenge models are useful surrogates for evaluating anti-asthma treatment, more credence is placed on improvements in the symptoms or progression of the disease than on protection against laboratory challenges. Lately there has been a move to assess efficacy in terms of improvements in quality of life or as health gain per unit cost. These analyses are becoming increasingly sophisticated but require careful validation to ensure that the quality-of-life instrument is sensitive to the illness being studied and that the economic model is realistic.

Finally, many trials of SIT for asthma and rhinitis have studied laboratory surrogate markers such as changes in IgG subclasses, T-cell function, or skin test responses. While such paraclinical measures do change during SIT, and can shed light on the mechanisms of successful SIT, they cannot be used to provide direct evidence of clinical efficacy. Studies that show antibody or T-cell changes without direct clinical evidence of efficacy neither support nor undermine the established evidence that SIT works, albeit in mysterious ways, to improve the symptoms of appropriately selected patients.

SIT for allergic rhinitis

Allergic rhinitis is the main indication for SIT worldwide. As with all uses of SIT, it is important to select patients appropriately. The allergic basis of the rhinitis should be carefully assessed on history and skin or blood tests for IgE, while other relevant causes should be excluded. Tests of nasal sensitivity are not used in routine clinical practice but may be useful for assessing effectiveness in clinical trials.

The effectiveness of SIT in seasonal allergic rhinitis has been confirmed in many trials, using grass, ragweed and birch pollen. Moreover, SIT has been shown to be clinically effective even in patients with severe seasonal rhinitis that is resistant to conventional drug therapy.[10] In this, the largest double-blind placebo-controlled study of SIT to date, SIT was used to treat patients whose grass pollen rhinitis was resistant to standard drug therapy. The active group showed a 30–40% decrease in symptoms and medication use in the first year of treatment, which was accompanied by reduced rescue medication usage. Although they were only treated with grass pollen, patients with multiple allergic sensitization responded at least as well as those who were monosensitized to grass pollen. Limited data are available regarding the long-term efficacy of SIT for allergic rhinitis, but formal studies have shown that the effects last for at least 3 years after discontinuing therapy.[11] Longer term studies are difficult to conduct, but efficacy has been shown for up to ten years in

open studies. The benefits of SIT for perennial rhinitis are less well established than for seasonal rhinitis. In part this reflects the difficulty in determining the extent to which allergy is responsible for perennial symptoms. Allergy to house dust mite is common and does not always cause symptoms. Conversely, there are other causes of perennial rhinitis including vasomotor instability, infection, aspirin sensitivity, etc. Nevertheless, clinical trials have shown a definite benefit provided the subjects are appropriately selected.[12] Clearer evidence of efficacy has been obtained in rhinitis due to pet allergy. Several studies have shown a marked improvement in tolerance of cat exposure after SIT, confirmed both on challenge tests and simulated natural exposure.[13]

As with any therapy, the risks and cost-effectiveness of SIT need to be assessed on a case-by-case basis. Current drug therapy for rhinitis can be very effective, but about 60% of patients with seasonal allergic rhinitis report inadequate symptom control, even when taking maximal doses of antihistamines and intranasal glucocorticoids. Others experience nose bleeds from intranasal steroids and drowsiness from antihistamines. Moreover, we are now more aware of the adverse effects of rhinitis on quality of life. SIT offers a useful option for these patients as well as a logical approach to dealing with the underlying problem.

SIT for asthma

Immunotherapy was widely used to treat allergic asthma in the UK prior to 1986 but evidence of severe adverse reactions, including a small number of fatalities, has led to SIT being abandoned for asthma treatment in the UK, although asthma remains a common indication for SIT in North America and continental Europe.[12,14] There is no doubt that SIT is effective on asthma symptoms and protects against specific and non-specific triggers. However, the role of allergic sensitization in ongoing asthma is less clear than for rhinitis, and the risks of therapy are undoubtedly greater in asthma. Current drug therapies for asthma aim to suppress the airways inflammation and smooth muscle contraction that are characteristic features of asthma (Chapter 39). None of these treatments are curative and asthma recurs rapidly on ceasing treatment. Moreover, none of the current drug therapies is directed against agents that might cause asthma. Allergen avoidance has been proposed as a potentially useful maneuver in those with allergic asthma, but while asthma control can be improved by extreme forms of allergen avoidance (e.g., admission to hospital, sending children to holiday homes at altitude), there is little evidence that similar benefits can be achieved using the type of allergen avoidance that can be achieved in suburban homes. There is thus scope for improving asthma care and for identifying allergen-specific therapies. SIT offers the possibility of deviating the immune response away from the allergic pattern and towards a more protective or less damaging response.

The efficacy of SIT in adult asthma has been assessed in many trials over the past 50 years. The results of these studies have often been difficult to interpret, either because poor quality allergen extracts were used or because of poor study design. Many trials were not placebo-controlled; they were either open or single blind, and in most cases, only small numbers of patients were treated. A recently updated meta-analysis[14] has reviewed all relevant papers published between 1954 and 2008. Many of the earlier trials had methodological flaws but there are sufficient data for general conclusions to be drawn. Symptom scores improved in the treated groups—it was necessary to treat four patients to prevent one from exacerbating, and to treat five to prevent one from needing an increase in medication. SIT reduced the airways response to inhalation of specific allergen and also improved non-specific bronchial reactivity.

In double-blind placebo-controlled trials in patients with grass pollen asthma, active treatment led to a 60–75% reduction in symptom scores as compared to placebo-treated patients. Similar results were found in ragweed allergy with improved peak flow rates during the pollen season as well as reduced hay fever symptoms and reduced sensitivity to laboratory challenge with ragweed pollen extracts. However, the associated economic analysis indicated that the cost-saving in asthma drugs was less than the costs of SIT. The value of SIT thus depends on its ability to improve symptoms and quality of life rather than to reduce the costs of other medications.

In asthmatic patients sensitive to cats, SIT with standardized aqueous extracts reduces the early asthmatic response to inhaled allergen and attenuates responses to cat room exposure. Interestingly these studies showed a clear delay in onset of symptoms and an overall reduction in symptoms and peak flow recordings after exposure to cats in a "cat room," but there was no protection against allergen-induced increases in non-specific bronchial hyperresponsiveness. Another study of cat IT for asthma used a depot preparation and found a reduction in both specific and non-specific bronchial reactivity (to cat extract and histamine respectively). There is, however, no hard evidence of benefit from treating asthma due to dog allergy.

Several double-blind, placebo-controlled studies have examined the effects of SIT in asthmatic patients sensitive to house dust mite. Early series used tyrosine-adsorbed or depot preparations that yielded conflicting results, with reductions in drug requirements in children, but no improvement in asthma control in adults. Subsequent studies using more modern extracts have found beneficial effects on symptoms, anti-asthma drug use and bronchial hyperresponsiveness.

Comparison of SIT with other therapies

The majority of clinical trials of SIT for asthma have compared SIT either with untreated historical controls or with a matched placebo-treated group. To date, the effectiveness of SIT in asthma has rarely been compared with conventional management (avoidance measures and inhaled or oral anti-asthma drugs).

Effects of SIT on the natural history of allergic disease

In recent years there has been increasing interest in the possibility that SIT may have additional disease modifying or preventive effects. These are important not just in their own right as desirable outcomes, but as factors in any economic evaluation of SIT.

Children often start with a limited range of allergic sensitivities and progress over time to develop IgE against a wider range of inhaled allergens. Treatment with SIT may limit this tendency to acquire new sensitizations although the clinical benefit of this preventive effect is not clear. In the most widely cited study, asthmatic children who were sensitized only to house dust mite (HDM) were treated with HDM-SIT. Ten out of 19 treated children did not develop new sensitizations while all 22 untreated children acquired new sensitivities, in many cases to more than one new allergen.[15] A long-term study of treatment with a grass pollen allergoid has confirmed this observation, with 50% fewer new sensitizations 12 years after completion of the course of SIT.[16] Similar results have been found in a study of children treated with

sublingual immunotherapy, in which 3% of SLIT-treated children and 34% of control subjects developed new sensitizations within 3 years.[17] It seems probable that this effect is indirect. In other words it is unlikely that SIT with house dust mite directly affects B cells that recognize cat or grass pollen, but by treating the HDM allergy, SIT may reduce inflammation in the nose, and hence modify the likelihood of exposure to other allergens proceeding to sensitization.

A proportion of patients with allergic rhinitis go on to develop asthma each year. This annual rate of progression has been estimated at 5% in college students,[18] but this remains, perhaps surprisingly, an area of considerable uncertainty. Several long-term epidemiological studies are now in progress, under the auspices of the International Study of Asthma and Allergies in Childhood (ISAAC) and these should eventually shed light on the rate of progression at different ages and the extent of regional and international variation. It has been suggested that SIT may modify the natural history of asthma in children who have allergic rhinitis but have not yet developed asthma. Only limited data are available to support this proposition. In the key study, a group of 205 children aged 6–14 with birch and/or grass pollen allergy but without previously diagnosed asthma were treated with SIT for the appropriate pollen allergy in an open randomized design. Three years after completing treatment 45% of the untreated group had progressed to development of asthma while only 26% of the treated group had asthma. These results have been sustained out to seven years after completing therapy. Thus four children had to be treated to prevent one case of asthma, which makes this an extremely effective therapy.[19] Similar results have been reported with sublingual immunotherapy (SLIT): after 3 years of SLIT, 8 of 45 SLIT-treated children and 18 of 44 control subjects had developed asthma, representing a relative risk of 3.8 for untreated subjects compared to the actively treated group.[20]

SIT may also modify the progression of established asthma. An early open study using uncharacterized mixed allergen extracts supported this view, with about 70% of treated children losing their asthma after four years therapy, compared to about 19% of untreated controls, a result that was sustained up to the age of 16 years. The proportion of children whose asthma was severe at age 16 was also much lower in the treated group.[21] In this period, when clinical trials were conducted differently, well before the days of ethics committees, Johnstone and Dutton randomized all children attending their clinic between August 1953 and January 1955 to one of four treatments. Neither the subjects nor their parents were aware of the treatment being given. Compared with those who received placebo or very dilute allergens, those treated with the two higher doses of SIT were much more likely to lose their asthma after four years, and among those whose asthma persisted, the likelihood of having severe disease was much lower in those who had received active treatment. While it would be very difficult to conduct such a study today, the data are useful in confirming the dose-response of SIT, and its potential for reducing the duration and severity of asthma. A prospective, non-randomized open label study of SLIT has reported that children with asthma who received SLIT had less asthma than those on standard medication after 4–5 years, and this difference persisted for 5 years after cessation of treatment.[22]

In contrast there is no current evidence that SIT influences the evolution of established asthma in adults. In part this reflects the reluctance of physicians to use SIT to treat severe asthma. Studies that have investigated withdrawal of therapy have reported rapid recurrence of asthma symptoms although rhinitis symptoms seem to show much more sustained relief after SIT.[23]

In summary, there is persuasive evidence that both subcutaneous and sublingual immunotherapy can modify the course of allergic disease, by reducing the incidence of new sensitizations, and by preventing or slowing the development of clinical asthma. The mechanisms that underlie these observations are not fully understood. It is likely that a combination of immunological and structural alterations is involved. Economic evaluations of the benefits of SIT and SLIT need to take into account these preventive effects, in order to arrive at a full cost-benefit analysis.

Safety

> ### CLINICAL PEARLS
>
> **Factors associated with adverse reactions to specific allergen immunotherapy**
>
> - Dosage errors
> - Asthma, especially uncontrolled/severe
> - Highly sensitive patients
> - Concurrent treatment with β-adrenergic blockers
> - Accelerated regimens (rush, ultra-rush)
> - Injections from new vials (especially with nonstandardized extracts)
> - Injections during periods of exacerbation of symptoms
> - Injections given during active viral or bacterial respiratory tract infections

The main factor preventing the wider adoption of SIT is the risk of serious adverse reactions. In general, SIT is quite safe in patients who do not have asthma, but significant numbers of deaths have been reported in the UK and the US when SIT has been used to treat patients whose asthma is unstable.[24] The incidence of systemic reactions in patients receiving SIT for asthma varies between series and has been reported to range from 5 to 35%. In contrast, serious systemic reactions occur after about 1 in 500 injections in patients with rhinitis. Some adverse events are due to giving the wrong dose, emphasizing the need to check doses carefully before each injection. Others occur when patients change over from one vial to another. Most allergists therefore cut back on the dose when changing vials to minimize this risk. Systemic reactions are much more likely if the patient has an intercurrent viral illness so doses should be delayed if the patient is unwell or has any signs of active asthma. In balancing risks versus benefits, where alternative therapies exist that carry differential risks, the more risky therapy can only be justified if that therapy offers substantial additional benefit over the safer therapy. The science of assessing risk-benefit ratios is still in its infancy and we need to recognize that even when faced with the same facts, different patients and agencies can come to widely varying assessments.

Separately, it is generally agreed that immunomodulatory treatments should not be used in patients with autoimmune disorders or malignant disease. While there is no hard evidence that SIT is actually harmful in these groups, it seems unwise to attempt manipulation of the immune system in such patients, not least because of the risk that spontaneous and unrelated variations in the autoimmune disorder or cancer may be blamed on SIT. Other medical contraindications to SIT include significant coexistent cardiac disease, which may be exacerbated by any adverse reactions to SIT. Patients on beta-blockers should also not receive SIT. Although they are not at increased risk of adverse reactions, their physiological response to the cardiovascular

component of anaphylaxis will be impaired, and they will not respond to the epinephrine that is used to treat adverse reactions to SIT.

> ### CLINICAL PEARLS
>
> **Contraindications to specific allergen immunotherapy (SIT)**
>
> - Active autoimmune disease
> - Malignancy
> - Severe asthma/uncontrolled asthma
> - Pregnancy—do not start SIT, but it can be continued in a patient in whom treatment is well established
> - Patients taking regular:
>   - β-Adrenergic blockers
>   - Angiotensin-converting enzyme inhibitors
>   - Tricyclic antidepressants

Sublingual immunotherapy (SLIT)

High dose topical immunotherapy regimes were used in the first half of the twentieth century, but then lost ground to injection immunotherapy in conventional medical practice. Over the past 20 years, there has been a resurgence of interest in SLIT,[25] which is based on the concept that allergens given via the mucosal surface can induce immunological tolerance, without carrying the same risk of systemic reactions that is found with injection SIT. In animal models, IgE responses to allergens can be reduced or prevented by oral administration of allergen. Most of these models involve feeding in early life to prevent subsequent acquisition of sensitivity, so this is a different scenario from the general clinical context of treating established allergic disease. The precise mechanisms by which "oral tolerance" is induced remain unclear, but it seems likely that the route of allergen processing and presentation is a critical determinant of the consequent T-cell response. In mice, locally administered allergen is taken up by mucosal dendritic cells and then presented to T cells together with IL-12, biasing the response towards a Th1-like profile and away from the pro-IgE Th2 profile (Chapter 16). In contrast to the animal models, the immunological response to SLIT in human studies has been relatively modest. Some changes have been found in skin sensitivity but most studies have not found any change in systemic parameters such as specific IgE, specific IgG or T-cell cytokine balance.[26]

Nevertheless, a body of evidence has accumulated from well conducted clinical trials, indicating that SLIT can be effective, with up to 30–40% reductions in symptom scores and rescue medication usage in seasonal allergic rhinitis.[27] Treatment regimes typically involve a rapid build-up phase followed by treatment about three times per week with rapidly dissolving tablets containing allergen extracts. Some preparations are supplied in liquid form, with a calibrated dropper. Several large clinical trials of have shown clinically and statistically significant reductions in symptom and medication scores, supporting the conclusions of earlier meta-analyses of SLIT that looked at all the earlier, less well designed studies, which were individually small and inconclusive. The meta-analysis estimated the efficacy of SLIT as being about two-thirds of that seen in comparable studies of injection SIT, but the more recent studies have shown levels of efficacy that are equal to the best recent multi-center trials of injection SIT. Local side-effects are common with SLIT, but generally well tolerated. Systemic side effects of SLIT are very rare, but have been reported, especially in patients who have systemic reactions to injection SIT. SLIT is now being used routinely in some parts of Europe (especially Italy and France), but the doses and regimes being prescribed are often different from those that were used in the clinical trials. Overall SLIT should widen the scope of SIT and allow additional patients to be treated. As with all forms of immunotherapy, patient selection remains the key to ensuring that therapy is targeted to those who are likely to benefit from it.

Future directions

There is clearly scope to improve conventional SIT. Possible avenues include the use of recombinant allergens, which would make it much easier to standardize allergen vaccines, and might allow fine tuning of vaccines for patients with unusual patterns of reactivity. Most allergic patients react to the same components of an allergen extract, the so-called major allergens, which are defined as those allergens recognized by over 50% of sera from a pool of patients with clinically significant allergy to the material in question. However, not all patients recognize all major allergens and some patients only recognize allergens that are not recognized by the majority of allergic patient sera. This latter group may not respond to standard extracts, but might be better treated by a combination of allergens to which they are sensitive. Until the advent of molecular cloning, this has been impossible to achieve. Now that recombinant allergens for SIT are available, the range of sensitivities can be better characterized, and this may lead to patient-tailored vaccine products. Thus far, clinical trials have confirmed the efficacy of recombinant allergen cocktails but have not yet shown superiority to conventional vaccines.[28] The major barrier to this development is regulatory: under current regulations, each combination of allergen components would have to be developed as a freestanding pharmaceutical. Until a different regulatory framework is agreed, this means that recombinant allergens will only be tested as fixed combination cocktails.

Another alternative approach is to inject allergens directly into lymph nodes, under ultrasound guidance. Proponents of this approach argue that after subcutaneous injection, less than 1% of the injected material reaches the lymphatic system, and therefore if it is the dose that reaches the lymph node that drives the benefit of SIT, then direct intranodal administration should be more efficient and also safer. Early studies with doses of about 1% of standard SIT have shown immunological efficacy, with some signs of clinical efficacy and reduced risks of side-effects.[29]

Novel forms of allergenic molecules can be created: for example, a recombinant trimer consisting of three covalently linked copies of the major birch pollen allergen, Bet v 1 has been made. This trimer is much less allergenic even though it contains the same B-cell and T-cell epitopes as the native molecule, and induces Th1 cytokine release and IgG antibodies, analogous to the antibody response to standard SIT.[30] Folding variants and other modifications of the physical structure may also improve the safety of SIT.[31]

Since the epitopes recognized by IgE molecules are usually three dimensional while the epitopes recognized by T cells are short linear peptide fragments of the antigen, it should be possible to distort allergens or create peptide fragments that will modulate T cells without risking anaphylaxis. Several distinct approaches have been tested. Cross-linking allergen proteins with aldehydes reduces their ability to bind antibodies. Such allergoids do not degranulate the basophils of sensitized individuals *in vitro*, but are recognized by allergen-specific T cells. Clinically, allergoids have been shown to be effective in rhinitis due to grass pollen or house dust mite.[32]

Short peptide sequences can also be used as vaccines that should not be recognized by IgE antibodies.[33] Peptide vaccines can either be natural sequences or altered peptide ligands. If high doses of natural peptides are given, they can direct the T-cell response into high dose tolerance. Altered peptide ligands induce anergy by providing an incomplete activation signal. Both approaches will be affected by the MHC type of the individual undergoing treatment. By sequential alteration of Der p peptides, it is possible to suppress proliferation of T-cell clones recognizing native Der p peptides, as well as suppressing their expression of CD40 ligand and their production of IL-4, IL-5, and IFN-γ. These anergic T cells do not provide help for B cells for class switching to IgE, and importantly this anergy cannot be reversed by providing exogenous IL-4. In humans, the main focus has been on cat allergen (Fel d1) peptides, which can reduce the level of symptoms on exposure to cat dander.[34] Similar work has also been reported with peptides of phospholipase A2 (PLA2—a major allergen in bee venom). However, to date peptide vaccines have not shown any greater efficacy than conventional vaccines.

In an animal model, intranasal application of genetically produced hypoallergenic fragments of Bet v 1 produced mucosal tolerance with significant reduction of IgE and IgG1 antibody responses, as well as reduced cytokine production *in vitro* (IL-5, IFN-γ, IL-10). These reduced immunological responses were accompanied by inhibition of the cutaneous and airway responses that were seen with the complete Bet v 1 allergen. The mechanisms of immunosuppression seemed to be different for the allergen fragments and the whole molecule, in that tolerance induced with the whole Bet v1 molecule was transferable with spleen cells whereas that induced by the fragments was not.[35]

From epidemiological and experimental studies, we know that vaccination with mycobacteria has anti-allergic properties. In Japan, early vaccination with BCG was associated with a substantial reduction in the risk of developing allergy,[36] although similar associations were not evident in Sweden.[37] In an animal model, it has been shown that administration of BCG before or during sensitization to ovalbumin reduces the degree of airway eosinophilia that follows subsequent challenge with ovalbumin. This effect is not mediated through any direct effect on IgE production, or blood eosinophil numbers, but is mediated through IFN-γ and can be reversed by exogenous IL-5.[38]

Two new approaches using DNA vaccines are also undergoing serious consideration. The first of these is a general approach, using CpG oligodeoxynucleotides (ODN), which mimic bacterial

DNA, binding to TLR-9 and stimulating a Th1-type cytokine response. This technology is essentially a refinement of vaccination adjuvant technology, since CpG ODN have been shown to be the principal activity from complete Freund's adjuvant. In a mouse model of asthma, pre-administration of CpG ODN prevented both airways eosinophilia and bronchial hyperresponsiveness.[39] Moreover, these effects were sustained for at least 6 weeks after CpG ODN administration.[40] An alternative approach is to couple CpG ODN to the allergenic protein, which enhances immunogenicity in terms of eliciting a Th1-type response to the allergen but reduces its allergenicity[41] and stimulates Th1 cytokine expression in cultured human peripheral blood mononuclear cells.[42] Initial clinical trials confirmed that the hybrid vaccine elicits a Th1-pattern response,[43] but subsequent trials have been inconclusive. A contrasting approach is to use allergen-specific naked DNA sequences as vaccines. This technology is still in its infancy, but preliminary data suggest that giving naked DNA leads to production of allergens from within the airways epithelial cells.[44,45] Due to the different handling pathways for endogenous and exogenous allergens, it seems that the endogenously produced allergen elicits a Th1-type response and if this can be reproduced in allergic humans, it is hoped that this may overcome the existing Th2-pattern response and eliminate the allergy. However, the potential for generating a powerful Th1-type response to ubiquitous agents means that this approach will need careful evaluation in animal models before it can be pursued in man.

The recent introduction of monoclonal antibodies directed against IgE offers another alternative. Treatment with anti-IgE reduces immediate and late-phase responses to inhaled allergen[46] and should also reduce the risk of adverse effects from SIT injections. Moreover, when anti-IgE is combined with conventional SIT, the effects are additive against seasonal allergic rhinitis.[47] However, the high cost of anti-IgE and the need for regular infusions are likely to limit its use to patients with severe allergic disease that cannot be managed by other means.

Conclusions

SIT is established as a treatment for allergic rhinitis and for venom hypersensitivity, but is more controversial when used to treat allergic asthma. When used in appropriately selected patients, SIT is effective and acceptably safe, but care is needed to recognize and treat adverse reactions. Appropriate training of allergists and SIT clinic support staff is essential. Despite a century of use, the precise mechanisms of action of SIT remain uncertain. Current emphasis on the role of T regulatory cells is leading to renewed attempts to simplify SIT regimes and reduce its risks. Future directions in SIT include the development of vaccines that are better standardized, and the use of recombinant allergens, both of which should improve the safety profile of SIT. In parallel, and perhaps the longer term, we should look for the development of general immunomodulatory therapies, which would be particularly advantageous for those patients sensitized to multiple allergens.

References

1. Frew AJ. 100 years of immunotherapy. Clin Exp Allergy 2011;41:1221–5.
2. Jutel M, Akdis CA. Immunological mechanisms of allergen-specific immunotherapy. Allergy 2011;66:725–32.
3. Creticos P, Van Metre TE, Mardiney MR, et al. Dose-response of IgE and IgG antibodies during ragweed immunotherapy. J Allergy Clin Immunol 1984;73:94–104.
4. Iliopoulos O, Proud D, Adkinson NF, et al. Effects of immunotherapy on the early, late and rechallenge nasal reaction to provocation with allergen: changes in inflammatory mediators and cells. J Allergy Clin Immunol 1991;87:855–66.
5. Durham SR, Ying S, Varney VA, et al. Grass pollen immunotherapy inhibits allergen-induced infiltration of CD4 + T-lymphocytes and eosinophils in the nasal mucosa and increases the number of cells expressing mRNA for interferon-gamma. J Allergy Clin Immunol 1996;97:1356–65.
6. Ebner C, Siemann U, Bohle B, et al. Immunological changes during specific immunotherapy of grass pollen allergy: reduced lymphoproliferative responses to allergen and shift from Th2 to Th1 in T-cell clones specific for Phl p1, a major grass pollen allergen. Clin Exp Allergy 1997;27:1007–15.
7. Golden DB, Moffitt J, Nicklas RA, et al. Stinging insect hypersensitivity: a practice parameter update 2011. J Allergy Clin Immunol 2011;127:852–4.
8. Golden DB, Kelly D, Hamilton RG, Craig TJ. Venom immunotherapy reduces large local reactions to insect stings. J Allergy Clin Immunol 2009;123:1371–5.
9. Bousquet J, Schünemann HJ, Bousquet PJ, et al. How to design and evaluate randomized controlled trials in immunotherapy for allergic rhinitis: an ARIA-GA(2) LEN statement. Allergy 2011;66:765–74.
10. Frew AJ, Powell RM, Corrigan CJ, Durham SR. Efficacy and safety of specific immunotherapy with SQ allergen extract in treatment-resistant seasonal allergic rhinoconjunctivitis. J Allergy Clin Immunol 2006;117:319–25.
11. Durham SR, Walker SM, Varga EM, et al. Long-term clinical efficacy of grass pollen immunotherapy. N Engl J Med 1999;341:468–75.
12. Cox L, Esch RE, Corbett M, et al. Allergen immunotherapy practice in the United States: guidelines, measures, and outcomes. Ann Allergy Asthma Immunol 2011;107:289–99.
13. Varney VA, Edwards J, Tabbah K, et al. Clinical efficacy of specific immunotherapy to cat dander: a double blind placebo controlled trial. Clin Exp Allergy 1997;27:860–7.
14. Abramson MJ, Puy RM, Weiner JM. Injection allergen immunotherapy for asthma. Cochrane Database Syst Rev 2010 Aug 4.
15. Des Roches A, Paradis L, Menardo JL, et al. Immunotherapy with a standardized Dermatophagoides pteronyssinus extract. VI. Specific immunotherapy prevents the onset of new sensitizations in children. J Allergy Clin Immunol 1997;99:450–3.
16. Eng PA, Borer-Reinhold M, Heijnen IA, Gnehm HP. Twelve-year follow-up after discontinuation of preseasonal grass pollen immunotherapy in childhood. Allergy 2006;69:198–201.
17. Marogna M, Tomassetti D, Bernasconi A, et al. Preventive effects of sublingual immunotherapy in childhood: an open randomized controlled study. Ann Allergy Asthma Immunol 2008;101:206–11.
18. Horak F. Manifestation of allergic rhinitis in latent sensitised patients. A prospective study. Arch Otorhinolaryngol 1985;242:242–9.
19. Niggemann B, Jacobsen L, Dreborg S, et al. Five-year follow-up on the PAT study: specific immunotherapy and long-term prevention of asthma in children. Allergy 2006;61:855–9.
20. Novembre E, Galli E, Landi F, et al. Coseasonal sublingual immunotherapy reduces the development of asthma in children with allergic rhinoconjunctivitis. J Allergy Clin Immunol 2004;114:851–7.
21. Johnstone DE, Dutton A. The value of hyposensitization therapy for bronchial asthma in children. A 14 year study. Pediatrics 1968;42:793.
22. Di Rienzo V, Marcucci F, Puccinelli P, et al. Long-lasting effect of sublingual immunotherapy in children with asthma due to house dust mite: a 10-year prospective study. Clin Exp Allergy 2003;33:206–10.
23. Shaikh WA. Immunotherapy vs inhaled budesonide in bronchial asthma: an open, parallel, comparative trial. Clin Exp Allergy 1997;27:1279–84.
24. Bernstein DI, Wanner M, Borish L, Liss GM. Twelve-year survey of fatal reactions to allergen injections and skin testing: 1990-2001. J Allergy Clin Immunol 2004;113:1129–36.
25. Frew AJ. Sublinugal immunotherapy. N Engl J Med 2008;358:2259–64.
26. Scadding G, Durham SR. Mechanisms of sublingual immunotherapy. Immunol Allergy Clin North Am 2011;31:191–209.
27. Calderon MA, Penagos M, Sheikh A, et al. Sublingual immunotherapy for allergic conjunctivitis: Cochrane systematic review and meta-analysis. Clin Exp Allergy 2011;41:1263–72.
28. Pauli G, Larsen TH, Rak S, et al. Efficacy of recombinant birch pollen vaccine for the treatment of birch-allergic rhinoconjunctivitis. J Allergy Clin Immunol 2008;122:951–60.
29. Senti G, Prinz Vavricka BM, Erdmann I, et al. Intralymphatic allergen administration renders specific immunotherapy faster and safer: a randomized controlled trial. Proc Natl Acad Sci U S A 2008;105:17908–12.
30. Valenta R, Niederberger V. Recombinant allergens for immunotherapy. J Allergy Clin Immunol 2007;119:826–30.
31. Purohit A, Niederberger V, Kronqvist M, et al. Clinical effects of immunotherapy with genetically modified recombinant birch pollen Bet v1 derivatives. Clin Exp Allergy 2008;38:1514–25.
32. Corrigan CJ, Kettner J, Doemer C, et al. Efficacy and safety of preseasonal-specific immunotherapy with an aluminium-adsorbed six-grass pollen allergoid. Allergy 2005;60:801–7.
33. Larche M. Peptide immunotherapy. Immunol Allergy Clin North Am 2006;26:321–32.
34. Norman PS, Ohman JL, Long AA, et al. Treatment of cat allergy with T-cell reactive peptides. Am J Respir Crit Care Med 1996;154:1623–8.
35. Wiedermann U, Herz U, Baier K, et al. Intranasal treatment with a recombinant hypoallergenic derivative of the major birch pollen allergen Bet v 1 prevents allergic sensitization and airway inflammation in mice. Int Arch Allergy Immunol 2001;126:68–77.
36. Shirakawa T, Enomoto T, Shimazu SI, Hopkin JM. The inverse association between tuberculin responses and atopic disorder. Science 1997;275:77–9.

37. Strannegaard IL, Larsson LO, Wennergren G, Strannegaard O. Prevalence of allergy in children in relation to prior BCG vaccination and infection with atypical mycobacteria. Allergy 1998;53:249–54.

38. Erb KJ, Holloway JW, Sobeck A, et al. Infection of mice with mycobacterium bovis-BCG suppresses allergen-induced airways eosinophilia. J Exp Med 1998;187:561–9.

39. Kline JN, Waldschmidt TJ, Businga TR, et al. Modulation of airway inflammation by CpG oligodeoxynucleotides in a murine model of asthma. J Immunol 1998;160:2555–9.

40. Sur S, Wild JS, Choudury BK, et al. Long-term prevention of allergic lung inflammation in a mouse model of asthma by CpG oligodeoxynucleotides. J Immunol 1999;162:6284–93.

41. Tighe H, Takabayashi K, Schwartz D, et al. Conjugation of immunostimulatory DNA to the short ragweed allergen Amb a1 enhances its immunogenicity and reduces its allergenicity. J Allergy Clin Immunol 2000;106:124–34.

42. Marshall JD, Abtahi S, Eiden JJ, et al. Immunostimulatory sequence DNA linked to the Amb a 1 allergen promotes Th1 cytokine expression while downregulating Th2 cytokine expression in PBMCs from human patients with ragweed allergy. J Allergy Clin Immunol 2001;108:191–7.

43. Creticos PS, Eiden JJ, Broide D, et al. Immunotherapy with immunostimulatory oligonucleotides linked to purified ragweed Amb a 1 allergen: effects on antibody production, nasal allergen provocation and ragweed seasonal rhinitis. J Allergy Clin Immunol 2002;109:743–4.

44. Hsu CH, Chua KY, Tao MH, et al. Immunoprophylaxis of allergen-induced IgE synthesis and airway hyperresponsiveness in vivo by genetic immunisation. Nat Med 1996;2:540–4.

45. Hartl A, Hochreiter R, Stepanoska T, et al. Characterisation of the protective and therapeutic efficiency of a DNA vaccine encoding the major birch pollen allergen Bet v1a. Allergy 2004;59:65–73.

46. Fahy J, Fleming HE, Wong HH, et al. The effect of an anti-IgE monoclonal antibody on the early and late-phase responses to allergen inhalation in asthmatic subjects. Am J Respir Crit Care Med 1997;155:1828–34.

47. Rolinck-Werninghaus C, Hamelmann E, Keil T, et al. The co-seasonal application of anti-IgE after preseasonal specific immunotherapy decreases ocular and nasal symptom scores and rescue medication use in grass pollen allergic children. Allergy 2004;59:973–9.

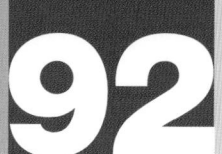

Biologic modifiers of inflammatory diseases

Pim Jetanalin,
Susan J. Lee,
Arthur
Kavanaugh

The immune system is composed of a complex array of diverse immunocompetent cells and pro- and anti-inflammatory mediators that exist in complex networks. These components interact through cascades and positive and negative feedback circuits to maintain normal inflammation and immunity. In various autoimmune and allergic diseases, a foreign or auto-antigen may upset this fine balance leading to dysregulated inflammation and ultimately pathologic findings characteristic of disease. In recent years, there has been tremendous progress delineating the specific components of the immune system that contribute to various aspects of normal immunity and to specific disease states. With progress in biotechnology, these components have become targets for more specific immunomodulatory therapies.

Traditionally, the treatment for most autoimmune diseases consisted largely of potent nonspecific immunosuppressive agents. While effective, these immunosuppressive agents rarely achieved the full extent of clinical response desired and were associated with significant toxicities such as infections and malignancies. These considerations provided the thrust for the development of a new class of target-specific therapeutic agents called "biologic agents" (Table 92.1). The notable potential for these agents derives from their ability to inhibit targets, for example particular components of the immune system, with exquisite specificity. This has the potential both to optimize outcomes by more thorough modulation of specific parts of the dysregulated immune response, as well as to minimize potential adverse events related to more broad methods of immunosuppression.

Many of these biologic agents inhibit the function of a target molecule, either soluble or cell surface, by binding to it, and thereby preventing ligation with its counter-receptor. The potential targets are myriad, and include specific molecules on B cells, T cells, and other immunocompetent cells. Various soluble inflammatory mediators such as cytokines, chemokines, complement proteins, enzymes, immunoglobulin molecules or their surface receptors can also be targeted. The effects of such inhibition most directly derive from the removal of a particular interaction, for example, blocking of an inflammatory cytokine from binding to its cell surface receptor, thereby preventing transduction of a signal. Such inhibition may interfere with the normal function of the target molecule, such as binding of a cell surface adhesion molecule. Simple competitive inhibition of a key receptor/counter-receptor pair could induce diverse downstream effects, as has been seen for the inhibitors of tumor necrosis factor (TNF)-α. Alternatively, biologic agents can alter cell populations by binding a target on a specific cell, and then engaging effector functions, such as activation of the complement cascade or antibody dependent cellular cytotoxicity (ADCC). Most biologic agents developed to date also have IgG Fc pieces as part of their construct. If such Fc pieces remain functional, then these effector mechanisms can be utilized if the binding characteristics of the target are appropriate. Because the regions of the Fc piece mediating the processes are distinct, biologic agents can be developed that predominantly affect complement ligation or ADCC. Cell depletion could also be induced by apoptosis related to ligation of an appropriate cell surface target. Relevant targets for cell-depleting therapy would include lineage-specific molecules or activation molecules. Some of the biologic agents are recombinant proteins that mimic inherent anti-viral and anti-inflammatory proteins, such as interferons.

Cytokines are small proteins that regulate diverse aspects of the immune system and the inflammatory response (Chapter 9). In a susceptible patient, an imbalance in the cytokine cascade can initiate and propagate the inflammation characteristic of autoimmune diseases. Cytokines have been explored as adjuvants to enhance immune responses in the treatment of infectious diseases and malignancies. Immunomodulatory cytokines considered of significance in various autoimmune diseases include interferon (IFN) type I (α and β), IFN-γ, IL-2, and IL-7.

Agents with anti-inflammatory effects

Interferons (IFNs)

Interferons are proteins that are released by lymphocytes upon pathogen stimulation; they can have a wide array of immunomodulating effects including regulation of angiogenesis, cell differentiation, and major histocompatibility complex antigen expression. Currently, there are three types of interferons available for the treatment of autoimmune diseases: IFN-α, IFN-β, and IFN-γ. IFN-α and IFN-β bind to the same cell surface receptor and are called type 1 IFNs, while IFN-γ binds to a different receptor and is called type 2 IFN.

IFN-α is produced by the cells of the immune system in response to the presence of double-stranded RNA viruses, inducing macrophages and NK cells activation, and enhancing antigen presentation. Both type 1 IFN-α2a and IFN-α2b have been used extensively for the treatment of chronic viral hepatitis (hepatitis B and C).[1] IFN-α, most commonly in combination with ribavarin, has been effective in the treatment of hepatitis C-associated mixed cryglobulinemia through its inhibition of viral replication. IFN-α has also been used to treat resistant Behçet's disease, familial Mediterranean fever, and Churg-Strauss vasculitis.[1] IFN-α has been shown to improve survival of several malignancies including advanced renal cell carcinoma and melanoma.[2,3]

Table 92.1 US FDA-approved therapeutic biologics*

Drugs	Description	Indications
Abciximab	Chimeric monoclonal Fab fragment to platelet IIb/IIIa	Acute MI; post- PTCA
Adalimumab	Human mAb to TNF-α	RA, psoriasis, PsA, AS, Crohn's, UC, JIA
Agalsidase beta	Recombinant human α-galactosidase A enzyme	Fabry disease
Aldesleukin	Recombinant IL-2	Metastatic renal cell cancer
Alefacept	Recombinant LFA-3 / IgG Fc construct	Psoriasis
Alemtuzumab	Humanized mAb to CD52	Chronic lymphocytic leukemia
Alteplase	Recombinant tPA	Acute MI, massive PE
Anakinra	Recombinant IL-1R antagonist	RA, CAPS
Anti-thymocyte globulin (ATG)	Horse anti-human T-cell Ig	Acute renal transplant rejection, aplastic anemia
Basiliximab	Chimeric mAb to IL-2R	Acute renal transplant rejection
Becaplermin	Recombinant human PDGF gel	Diabetic ulcer
Belimumab	Recombinant mAb to B-lymphocyte stimulator (BLys)	SLE
Bevacizumab	Humanized mAb to VEGF	Metastatic colorectal cancer, non-small cell lung cancer
Certolizumab	Pegylated Fab' fragment of human mAb to TNF-α	Crohn's disease, RA
Cetuximab	Chimeric mAb to EGFR	Metastatic cancer
Daclizumab	Humanized mAb to IL-2R	Acute renal transplant rejection
Darbepoetin alpha	Recombinant erythropoietin	Anemia related to chemotherapy
Denileukin diftitox	Recombinant diphtheria toxin / IL-2 construct	Cutaneous T-cell lymphoma
Digoxin immune Fab	Fab against digoxin	Digoxin toxicity
Drotrecogin alfa	Recombinant activated protein C	Severe sepsis
Efalizumab	Humanized mAb to LFA-1 (CD11a)	Psoriasis
Etanercept	Recombinant soluble TNF-R/IgG Fc construct	RA, JIA, PsA, AS, psoriasis
Filgrastim	Recombinant G-CSF	Neutropenia
Galsulfase (rhASB)	Recombinant N-acetylgalactosamine 4-sulfatase	Mucopolysaccharidosis VI
Gemtuzumab ozogamicin	Humanized mAb to CD33	Acute myelocytic leukemia
Golimumab	Human mAb to TNF-α	RA, PsA, AS
Ibritumomab	Murine mAb to CD20	NHL
Infliximab	Chimeric mAb to TNF-α	RA, Crohn's, UC, PsA, AS
IFN-α (2a, 2b, etc)	Recombinant IFN-α	Hepatitis B and C, hairy cell leukemia, Kaposi sarcoma, condyloma, melanoma, NHL
IFN-β (1a,1b)	Recombinant IFN-β	Multiple sclerosis
IFN-γ	Recombinant IFN-γ	Chronic granulomatous disease, osteopetrosis
Laronidase	Recombinant human α-1-iduronidase	Mucopolysaccharidosis I
Natalizumab	Humanized mAb to α4β1 integrin	Multiple sclerosis, Crohn's
Omalizumab	Humanized mAb to IgE	Severe allergic asthma
Oprelvekin	Recombinant IL-11	Thrombocytopenia
Palivizumab	Humanized mAb to RSV	Severe RSV
Rasburicase	Recombinant uricase	Post-chemotherapy hyperuricemia
Reteplase	Recombinant tPA	Acute MI
Rilonacept	Recombinant IL-1 accessory protein, IL-1R/IgG Fc construct	CAPs
Rituximab	Chimeric mAb to CD20	NHL, RA, ANCA-associated vasculitis
Tenecteplase	Recombinant tPA	Acute MI
Tocilizumab	Recombinant mAb to IL-6 receptor	RA
Tositumomab	Murine mAb to CD20	NHL refractory to rituximab
Trastuzumab	Humanized mAb to HER-2	Metastatic breast cancer
Ustekinumab	Human mAb to p40 subunit of IL12/23	Plaque psoriasis

*Accessed May 2011: http://www.fda.gov/cder/biologics and http://www.drugs.com
ANCA = anti-neutrophil cytoplasmic antibody; AS= ankylosing spondylitis; CAPS = cryopyrin-associated periodic syndrome; EGFR = epidermal growth factor receptor; Fab = fragment, antigen-binding; Fc = fragment, crystallizable; FDA = Food and Drug Administration; G-CSF = granulocyte-colony stimulating factor; HER = human epidermal growth factor receptor 2; IFN = interferon; IgE, G = immunoglobulin E, G; IL-2 = interleukin 2; JIA = juvenile idiopathic arthritis; LFA = leukocyte function antigen; mAb = monoclonal antibody; MI = myocardial infarction; NHL = non-Hodgkin's lymphoma; PDGF = platelet derived growth factor; PE = pulmonary embolism; PsA = psoriatic arthritis; PTCA = percutaneous transluminal coronary angiogram; RA = rheumatoid arthritis; RSV = respiratory syncytial virus; SLE = systemic lupus erythematosus; TNF = tumor necrosis factor; tPA = tissue plasminogen activator; UC = ulcerative colitis; VEGF = vascular endothelial growth factor.

Among patients with resected Stage III melanoma, pegylated IFN-α2b improved four-year relapse-free survival compared to observation alone (45.6 vs 39.8% with hazard ratio 0.82, $p = 0.01$), but not the overall survival rate.[3] The most common adverse events are flu-like symptoms, arthralgia, injection-site reaction, cytopenias, and potentially severe neuropsychiatric disorders. All patients with major depression should be well controlled prior to treatment with IFN-α as they are at risk of worsening depression and suicide ideation. Due to their immunodulatory properties, patients receiving IFN-α should be monitored for the development of autoimmune autoantibodies and diseases including autoimmune hepatitis, thyroiditis, immune-complex-mediated vasculitis, and rarely systemic lupus erythematosus.[1]

IFN-β is produced by fibroblasts and is 45% identical to IFN-α, sharing similar antiviral activity against double-stranded RNA viruses. Three IFN-β preparations are approved for use in the treatment of relapsing remitting multiple sclerosis (MS): IFN-β 1b, liquid IFN-β1a, and lypophilized IFN-β1a. IFNs have been effective in both relapsing-remitting as well as primary, progressive MS with minimum of 2 silent brain lesions on magnetic resonance imaging (MRI).[4,5] IFN-β use improved cognitive function and reduced annual relapse rate, number of new active brain lesions on MRI, and conversion rate to clinically definite MS over a 5-year period.[4–6] IFN-β also reduced the disability rate from 35% to 22% after 2 years of treatment.[6] IFN-β is associated with similar adverse events as IFN-α but fewer neuropsychiatric disorders and more hepatotoxicity.

IFN-γ is produced by activated leukocytes (T, NK cells) and induces macrophage activation and increases oxidative burst. Mycobacterial infections activate T and NK cells to release IFN-γ in an attempt to kill intracellular mycobacteria. Subsequently, IFN-γ therapy has been tried for the treatment of multiple mycobacterial infections including leprosy, leishmaniasis, and non-tuberculosis infections but with mixed responses.[7,8]

IFN-γ, in combination with anti-bacterial and anti-fungal prophylaxis, has also been shown to decrease the number and severity of infections in patients with chronic granulomatous disease (CGD).[9,10] CGD patients have defective phagocyte NADPH oxidase activity and are prone to recurrent bacterial, fungal infections with granuloma formation (Chapter 21). With the success of IFN-γ in patients with CGD patients, it has been successful in children with congenital malignant osteopetrosis, which is characterized by defective leukocyte superoxide formation, decreased bone resorption, and increased infections.[11] It is also used in some patients with the rare deficiency of the IFN-γ/IL-12 axis, caused by a deficiency of either of these cytokines, expecting that the administration of this cytokine would reduce the susceptibility to severe mycobacterial disease. Despite its ability to potently inhibit collagen synthesis, the effectiveness of IFN-γ has been disappointing in fibrosing conditions such as systemic sclerosis and pulmonary fibrosis.[12] Potential side effects include fever, hypotension and flu-like symptoms.

KEY CONCEPTS

Efficacy and safety of interferons (IFN)

- INF-α is commonly used for the treatment of hepatitis C in combination with ribavirin.
- INF-β is commonly used for the treatment of multiple sclerosis.
- IFN use can be associated with flu-like symptoms, cytopenias, and neuropsychiatric disorders.

Interleukin-2 (IL-2)

Recombinant IL-2 has been approved by the US Food and Drug Administration (FDA) for the treatment of metastatic renal cell carcinoma[2] and malignant melanoma.[13] It has also been used in other malignancies such as neuroblastoma, cutaneous T-cell lymphoma, and breast cancer with some clinical benefit.[14] IL-2 promotes the activation of T cells and NK cells, enhancing their anti-tumor activity. It also induces the differentiation of regulatory T cells, to control inflammatory responses. The administration of IL-2 to HIV patients[15] has resulted in an increase of CD4 T-cell counts. When used in combination with highly active anti-retroviral treatment (HAART) drugs, it did not increase HIV viremia and did reduce the occurrence of AIDS-defining infections. Earlier studies have shown PEG IL-2 therapy increased IgA and IgM levels and decreased infection rates in patients with common variable immunodeficiency and defective T-cell.[9] Side effects seem dose-related and include hypotension, flu-like symptoms, behavioral changes, and renal impairment.

Interleukin-7 (IL-7)

Due to its biological activity in the homeostasis of T cells, which includes the expansion of naïve and memory T cells in the setting of lymphopenia, IL-7 has been suggested as an adjuvant in the treatment of HIV infection, and in lymphopenia after chemotherapy. Reports of its administration in HIV-infected patients showed less significant side effects than IL-2 treatment, with sustained dose-dependent expansion of both naïve and central memory CD4+ and CD8+ T cells.[16]

Agents that inhibit pro-inflammatory cytokines

Th1 predominant cytokines such as TNF-α and interleukin-1 (IL-1) have been shown to play a central role in disease pathogenesis and sustenance in inflammatory arthritides such as rheumatoid arthritis (RA), psoriatic arthritis (PsA) and ankylosing spondylitis (AS). Among its sundry pro-inflammatory and immune regulating activities, TNF activates immunocompetent cells at sites of inflammation through activation of the vascular endothelium and upregulation of adhesion molecules. TNF-α also stimulates synthesis of other pro-inflammatory cytokines (e.g., IL-1, IL-6, GM-CSF, etc.), chemokines (IL-8, etc.), and other inflammatory mediators. IL-1 stimulates production of other pro-inflammatory cytokines, angiogenic factors and endothelial adhesion molecules. Both TNF and IL-1 activate macrophages to release mediators destructive to bone and cartilage, including matrix metalloproteinases such as collagenase and prostaglandins. In allergic diseases such as asthma, allergic rhinitis, and atopic eczema, Th2 predominant cytokines (IL-4, IL-5, IL-9, IL-13) play a central role. Several studies have investigated novel pharmacological agents that target these cytokines and are described below. Immunomodulatory and immunoglobulin therapies in allergic diseases are described in detail in other chapters in Section 10.

TNF inhibitors (Table 92.2)

There are five currently available TNF inhibitors: infliximab, a chimeric monoclonal anti-TNF-α antibody approved by the US FDA in 1998; etanercept, a recombinant soluble p75 TNF-receptor (CD120b)-IgG Fc fusion protein approved in 1998;

adalimumab, a human monoclonal anti-TNF-α antibody approved in 2002; certolizumab pegol, a pegylated Fab' fragment of a human anti-TNF-α antibody approved in 2008; and golimumab, a human monoclonal anti-TNF-α antibody approved in 2009. Although not all 5 TNF-inhibitors are approved for all of the following conditions, TNF-inhibitors are most commonly used for the treatment of RA, PsA, AS, Crohn's disease, juvenile idiopathic arthritis, and psoriasis. To date, while the monoclonal antibodies against TNF inhibitors have been effective in inflammatory bowel disease (Crohn's disease and ulcerative colitis), the fusion protein construct has not been effective.

All five TNF inhibitors have been shown to substantially improve the signs and symptoms of disease, functional status and quality of life, and to retard radiographic progression in patients with RA.[17-21] Several studies have demonstrated an even greater clinical and radiographic response and the probability of disease remission among early RA patients.[22] Interestingly, the inhibition of radiographic progression of disease seemed to be dissociated from clinical efficacy as measured by the typically utilized composite scoring measures, such as the American College of Rheumatology 20% improvement criteria (ACR20). Thus, some patients who did not achieve an ACR20 response still experienced inhibition of radiographic damage.[23] Although they can be given as monotherapy, all TNF inhibitors appeared to be more effective when used in combination with disease modifying anti-rheumatic drugs (DMARDs), commonly methotrexate (MTX). Combination therapy with MTX has beneficial pharmacokinetic effects for some TNF inhibitors, in addition to clinical synergy for the treatment of RA.

Etanercept and adalimumab have been approved for the treatment of juvenile idiopathic arthritis (JIA).[24,25] Children who received TNF inhibitors either with or without MTX had better clinical outcome as measured by the Rheumatology Pediatric (ACR Pedi) 30 score, which represents a 30% or greater improvement in JIA signs and symptoms.

Psoriatic arthritis (PsA) is characterized by the association of inflammatory arthritis with skin psoriasis. The treatment of patients with PsA requires consideration of peripheral arthritis, axial arthritis, skin and nail involvement, dactylitis, and enthesitis. TNF-α levels are notably increased in biopsy samples of skin and synovial tissues from patients with PsA, providing rationale for TNF inhibitors in the treatment of PsA and psoriasis. TNF inhibitors have been shown to be highly effective in improving the signs and symptoms of arthritis, functional status, and quality of life among patients with PsA. Similar to RA, TNF inhibitors also attenuated the progression of radiographic joint damage.[26,27] Moreover, dramatic improvements in skin psoriasis were achieved, as were improvements in extra-articular involvement characteristic of PsA, such as dactylitis and enthesitis. Improvement in skin psoriasis with TNF inhibitors has likewise been noted in patients without arthritis. While improvements in joints and skin often occur in parallel, there may be discordance between dermatologic and articular outcomes in individual patients, suggesting potential heterogeneity to pathophysiologic mechanisms underlying different clinical manifestations.

Until the advent of TNF inhibitors, non-steroidal anti-inflammatory agents (NSAIDs) were the only agents shown to alleviate axial symptoms related to ankylosing spondylitis (AS). In recent years, TNF inhibitors have demonstrated their ability to substantially decrease signs and symptoms of spinal inflammation.[28-30] Paralleling data from RA, TNF inhibitors provided rapid clinical improvement, often as early as 2 weeks. Patients with elevated acute phase reactants at study entry or with evidence for spinal inflammation on magnetic resonance

imaging (MRI) tended to respond more favorably to TNF inhibitors. Because MTX is not effective for spinal inflammation in AS, it has not been utilized in studies of the TNF inhibitors. A goal in

Table 92.2 Characteristics of therapeutic biologics: dosing and half-life

Agent	Dosing	Mode of delivery	Half-life
Cytokine inhibitors			
Adalimumab	40 mg per week to per 2 weeks	SQ	12-14 days
Anakinra	100 mg daily	SQ	4-6 hours
Certolizumab	400 mg per 2 weeks at wk 0, 2, 4 then 200 mg per 2 weeks or 400 mg per 4 weeks	SQ	14 days
Etanercept	25 mg biweekly or 50 mg per week; 0.4 mg/kg biweekly for children	SQ	4-5 days
Golimumab	50 mg per week	SQ	14 days
Infliximab	3–10 mg/kg per 4–8 weeks	IV	8-9.5 days
Rilonacept	160 mg × 2 doses on the first day then 160 mg per week; 4.4 mg/kg on the first day then 2.2 mg/kg per week for children	SQ	6.3-8.6 days
Tocilizumab	4–8 mg/kg per 4 weeks	IV	11-13 days
B-cell modulators			
Belimumab	10 mg/kg per 2 weeks × 3 doses then per 4 weeks	IV	19 days
Rituximab	NHL/ANCA vasculitis: 375 mg/M² qweek × 4 doses RA: 500–1000 mg per 2 weeks × 2 doses, ~per 6 months	IV	60-170 hours
T-cell modulators			
Abatacept	<60 kg: 500 mg IV week 0, 2, 4 then q4weeks; 60-100 kg: 750 mg IV week 0, 2, 4 then q 4 weeks; >100 kg: 1000 mg IV week 0, 2, 4 then q4 weeks weight-based dose (<60 kg: 500 mg; 60–100 kg: 750 mg; >100 kg: 1000 mg) IV loading then 125 mg SQ within 24 hours then q week	IV SQ	14.7 days 14.3 days
Alefacept	15 mg IM per week × 12 weeks (can be repeated after 12 weeks observation period)	IM	270 hours
Ustekinumab	40–90 mg at weeks 0, 4, then every 12 weeks	SQ	14-45 days
Adhesion cell modulators			
Efalizumab	1–2 mg/kg per week × 12 weeks	SQ	3-5 days
Natalizumab	300 mg per 4 weeks	IV	11 days

treating AS would be to stop the progression of spinal ankylosis. Despite their ability to attenuate spinal inflammation on a sensitive imaging modality such as MRI, TNF inhibitors have not altered radiographic progression when compared to historical controls of TNF-inhibitor-naïve AS patients.[28]

The levels of TNF-α are increased in the mucosa of inflamed intestine and thought to exert deleterious effects relevant to the pathophysiology of inflammatory bowel disease (Crohn's disease and ulcerative colitis). Treatments with infliximab, adalimumab, and certolizumab have shown improvement in both clinical and endoscopic luminal fistulas and bowel mucosal inflammation associated with Crohn's disease.[31–33] Certolizumab has also been effective for patients who have failed infliximab.[34] Initially, treatment of Crohn's disease with TNF inhibitors was reserved for the most severe, refractory fistulae as a single course. Following the success in this group of patients, repeated treatments and more chronic dosing regimens are being utilized. Intermittent usage of infliximab, commonly employed in the treatment of Crohn's disease, has been associated with a greater propensity for the development of antibodies to infliximab and can be attenuated by the concomitant use of immunosuppressives such as corticosteroids, azathioprine, methotrexate, and 6-mercaptopurine.[35] The use of infliximab in combination with immunosuppressives (e.g., MTX, azathioprine), has been shown to enhance efficacy and decrease immunogenicity.[35] TNF inhibitor monoclonal antibodies are also being studied and used in ulcerative colitis. To date, etanercept has not been shown to be effective in inflammatory bowel disease.[35] While both adalimumab and infliximab have been effective for extraintestinal manifestations of inflammatory bowel disease, such as spondyloarthropathy and pyoderma gangrenosum, only infliximab has been approved for treatment of moderate-severe ulcerative colitis.[35]

Several studies have demonstrated that switching from one TNF inhibitor to another can be effective and restore clinical response in patients who have lost therapeutic efficacy to one.[36] While the success of TNF inhibitors in these autoimmune conditions has been remarkable, it is worth noting that almost uniformly, treatment failed to induce long-term treatment-free remission or immunological tolerance. Thus, maintenance of clinical response required continuous therapy. Also, TNF inhibitors have not proven effective in other conditions, including several in which there was pathophysiologic evidence of a role for this cytokine in the disease process, such as sjögren's syndrome and Wegener's granulomatosis, and polymyalgia rheumatica/ temporal arteritis. In congestive heart failure (CHF), data from animal models of ischemic cardiomyopathy implicated TNF as a key mediator of deteriorating cardiac function, and hence an attractive target. However, TNF inhibitors have failed to improve patients with CHF in clinical trials, and sometimes resulted in worsened clinical outcome. Although they were limited, there have been studies of TNF inhibitors that had negative results in multiple sclerosis, along with anecdotal reports of the development or worsening of demyelinating symptoms among RA patients treated with these agents. TNF inhibitors are still being actively investigated in a variety of other diseases.

TNF inhibitors: safety considerations

In general, TNF inhibitors have been well tolerated in clinical trials. *In vitro* studies suggested that TNF inhibitors selectively decrease pro-inflammatory cytokines while preserving both the humoral and cell-mediated arms of the immune response. However, a number of relevant safety issues regarding the use of TNF inhibitors have emerged in post-marketing pharmacovigilance assessments.[37] Adverse events associated with TNF inhibitors can be broadly classified as target/class-related or agent-related. Target-related adverse events include those potentially attributable to the immunosuppression inherent in blocking a key component of the immune system, such as an inflammatory cytokine that may lead to increased susceptibility to infections and malignancies. In addition, specific inhibition of TNF can predispose patients to increased susceptibility to tuberculosis (TB), autoantibody production, hepatotoxicity, demyelinating disease, and clinical worsening CHF. Agent-related adverse events such as allergic reactions and antigenicity are idiosyncratic reactions that relate to the particular agent used.

Safety data from clinical trials and registries have shown a small but consistent increase in infections among TNF inhibitor treated patients compared to those treated with DMARDs, most commonly MTX (relative risk, RR up to 2). However, the risk of infection with TNF inhibitors increased significantly when TNF inhibitors were combined with other biologic agents. For example, combination therapy of etanercept and the interleukin-1 receptor antagonist (IL-1Ra), anakinra, resulted in a higher rate of serious infections in RA patients without any additive clinical benefit. Data particularly from pharmacovigilance, have noted a number of opportunistic infections (e.g., listeriosis, histoplasmosis, coccidioidomycosis) among those patients treated with TNF inhibitors. Due to the increased baseline risk of infections among RA patients, without a control group, it is difficult to ascertain if the excess infection risk is specifically attributable to TNF inhibitors in RA. Another potential sequel of immunosuppression is malignancy. With a few notable exceptions, the bulk of data do not support an increased risk of solid tumors related to TNF inhibitor therapy. However, greater numbers of hematological malignancies, particularly non-Hodgkin's lymphoma, have been observed in some registries. Complicating the assessment of the risk attributable to TNF inhibitors is the increased baseline risk of lymphoma among RA patients, especially among those with higher disease activity. This introduces bias toward observing cases among patients treated with TNF inhibitors, as the most severe and active RA patients are also often the most common type of patients treated. The relative impact of dose and duration of therapy and host factors, such as co-morbidities, relevant genetic polymorphisms, and concomitant medications, on the risk of infections and malignancy remain incompletely defined. Due to potential immunosuppression, vaccination with live vaccines is not recommended while receiving TNF inhibitors.

In addition, inhibition of TNF may predispose patients to a variety of untoward effects that seem to be specific to inhibition of the TNF molecule. There is a fair amount of animal and *ex vivo* data supporting the important role played by TNF in controlling TB. In contrast to typical presentation of acute TB as pneumonia, about half of the cases of TB related to TNF inhibitors have presented as extra-pulmonary or disseminated TB. The majority of these TB cases appear to be reactivation of latent TB, with infection occurring within the first few months of therapy; however, newly acquired cases have also been described. The incidence of cases may be greater with monoclonal anti-TNF antibodies than with the fusion protein inhibitor etanercept. Fortunately, screening for latent TB before initiating TNF inhibitor therapy has been an effective strategy with a reduction in incidence of new TB cases by approximately 85%. Latent TB can be screened using either a tuberculin skin test with purified protein derivative (PPD) or *ex vivo* tests that quantify IFN-γ release from sensitized lymphocytes in blood incubated with TB antigens. Treatment with TNF inhibitors has also been associated with development of autoantibodies. While the mechanism of this is unknown, it does not appear to result from inhibition of TNF itself, but possibly through induction of apoptosis. The autoantibodies typically generated include antinuclear antibody (ANA; which develops in about half of RA patients treated with TNF inhibitors), antibodies to double-stranded DNA (anti-dsDNA; which develops in approximately 10-15% of patients treated with TNF inhibitors), and anticardiolipin antibodies. Although rare, progression to a lupus-like illness can occur in patients treated with TNF inhibitors. Also, mild to moderate liver function tests (LFTs) elevation (generally <3 times the upper limit of normal) has been observed with TNF inhibitors. Many of these cases were confounded by concomitant use of potentially hepatotoxic drugs and underlying medical conditions. However, in light of liver failure of unidentifiable etiology in several cases, clinicians should be aware of these rare events and consider monitoring LFTs. Lastly, several cases of multiple sclerosis (MS) and other demyelinating conditions have been identified among patients treated with TNF inhibitors, although the true impact of TNF inhibitors on the development of MS remains undefined.

Despite their shared ability to inhibit TNF, there are some notable differences between the five approved TNF inhibitors. Infliximab, adalimumab, golimumab, and certolizumab are IgG1 mAb that are specific for TNF-α; etanercept is a fusion protein of the type II TNF receptor and binds both TNF-α and lymphotoxin-α (also known as TNF-β). The clinical relevance of this distinction is unknown. In addition, the binding characteristics of the monoclonal antibody and the fusion protein differ slightly. While all agents bind soluble TNF with high affinity, the monoclonal antibodies have slightly higher affinity for membrane bound TNF, presumably related to the physical constraints of the binding domains of the soluble TNF receptor, compared to that of monoclonal antibodies. Whether these differences may account variability in efficacy and safety remains to be seen.

KEY CONCEPTS

Efficacy and safety of TNF inhibitors

- Most commonly used for the treatment of RA, PsA, AS, IBD, JIA, and psoriasis.
- Substantial improvement seen in signs and symptoms of disease, functional status, and quality of life.
- Treatment can inhibit progression of joint damage assessed radiographically.
- Switching from one TNF inhibitor to another can be effective and restore clinical response in patients who have lost therapeutic efficacy to one.
- TNF inhibitor therapy rarely induces long-term remission and continuous therapy is typically required to maintain clinical response.
- Treatment with a TNF inhibitor plus methotrexate appears to have additive or synergistic efficacy, particularly as regards joint damage.
- TNF inhibitors: target-related effects derive from inhibition of the target; for immunomodulatory therapies, this often includes immunosuppression and its potential sequelae (e.g., infections, malignancies).
- TNF inhibitors: agent-related adverse effects relate to the specific agent; they may be mechanistic (e.g., cell lysis) or idiosyncratic (e.g., immunogenicity).
- Combination of two or more biologicals is not recommended due to an increased risk of infection without additive beneficial effect.
- Live vaccines are not recommended in patients receiving biological therapy.

The efficacy of certolizumab pegol in many autoimmune diseases suggests that the ultimate mechanism of action of TNF inhibitors may not appear to require Fc fragment related activities.

Interleukin-1 (IL-1) Inhibitors

IL-1 is synthesized as an inactive precursor. Upon cleavage by IL-1β-converting enzyme (ICE), IL-1 activates a variety of cells that can then release mediators destructive to bone and cartilage. Although there is an increase in the naturally occurring IL-1 receptor antagonist (IL-1Ra) that prevents the binding of IL-1 to its receptor, IL-1R, the levels in the RA synovium are apparently insufficient to counteract the effects of IL-1.

Anakinra, approved in 2001 for the treatment of RA, is a recombinant IL-1 receptor antagonist (IL-1ra) that differs from the endogenous IL-1Ra by a single amino acid addition at the amino terminus (Table 92.1). Compared to the TNF inhibitors, the clinical responses achieved by anakinra are generally more modest. Moreover, the cost and the need for daily injections has led to its relatively infrequent use in the treatment of RA. However, it has been gaining renewed interest and shown to be effective in the treatment of cryopyrin-associated periodic syndromes (CAPS), including familial cold autoinflammatory syndrome (FCAS) and Muckle-Wells syndrome (MWS) characterized by gain-of-function mutation in cryopyrin gene (*CIASI, NLRP3*).[38] These rare autosomal dominant disorders are associated with over-secretion of IL-1β, rash, arthralgia, and fever. Rilonacept (previously known as IL-1-Trap), approved in 2008 for the treatment of CAPS, is a fusion protein comprised of extracellular domain of IL-1 accessory protein and IL-1 receptor type 1 attached to the Fc portion of IgG1. Rilonacept binds to IL-1α and IL-1β with high affinity, and was generally well tolerated with injection site reactions being the most common adverse events.[39] Physicians should remain vigilant about infections with any IL-1 inhibitor. Studies evaluating the role of anakinra and rilonacept in other diseases associated with IL-1 over-secretion, such as chronic gout and adult-onset Still's disease, are ongoing with promising early results.

KEY CONCEPTS

Efficacy and safety of IL-1 inhibitors

- Anakinra is used for the treatment of RA, Still's disease, and CAPS (FCAS, MWS).
- Rilonacept is being investigated for the treatment of Still's disease and gout.
- Generally well tolerated with injection site reaction, infection, and neutropenia being the most common adverse events.

Interleukin-4 (IL-4) inhibitors

Despite high levels of IL-4 in patients with asthma, antagonizing IL-4 alone has not been shown effective in the management of reactive airway disease. This may reflect the redundant role of IL-13 in sustaining the pro-inflammatory response that is initiated by IL-4. Pitrakinra is a recombinant human IL-4 variant that inhibits the IL-4Rα receptor complex and interferes with the actions of both IL-4 and IL-13. Unlike traditional IL-4 inhibitors, nebulized pitrakinra for 4 weeks was significantly associated with less reduction of FEV1 4-10 hours after allergen challenge and decreased the frequency of rescue treatment with β2-agonists when compared to placebo.[40] Studies are ongoing to assess the long-term clinical benefit of pitrakinra.

Interleukin-5 (IL-5) inhibitors

Interleukin-5 (IL-5) is a growth factor and chemoattractant for eosinophils and is thought to play an essential role in allergic rhinitis, eosinophilic esophagitis and idiopathic hypereosinophilic syndrome.[41] Despite substantial reduction in blood and sputum eosinophil levels, mepolizumab, humanized anti-IL5 monoclonal antibody, in combination with inhaled corticosteroids failed to improve asthma symptoms or pulmonary function.[42] In a subset of asthma patients who are prednisone-dependent with sputum eosinophilia, mepolizumab decreased the number of asthma exacerbations, overall prednisone dose, and sputum and blood eosinophil counts. These patients also demonstrated sustained improvement in their FEV1 after bronchodilator treatment compared to their baseline.[43]

Anti-IL 5 monoclonal antibody has also been used for the treatment of *FIP1L1-PDGFRA* fusion-gene-negative hypereosinophilic syndrome. Mepolizumab significantly decreased peripheral eosinophilia and overall steroid dose, with some patients completely discontinuing prednisone[44]

Interleukin 6 (IL-6) inhibitors (Table 92.2)

IL-6 is a multifunctional cytokine that is involved in the acute inflammatory response, regulation of immune responses, and hematopoiesis. IL-6 induces the terminal proliferation and differentiation of B-cells, osteoclastogenesis, and acute phase proteins production in the liver. Tocilizumab is a humanized anti-human IL-6 receptor mAb that blocks the binding of IL-6 with its receptor. It was approved in 2010 for the treatment of moderate to severe RA patients who have failed one or more anti-TNF inhibitors. Tocilizumab has been shown to improve the signs and symptoms of disease and functional status, and to slow radiographic progression in RA patients. The clinical improvement was rapid and evident within the first 2 weeks of treatment.[45–47] Similarly, among patients with systemic onset juvenile idiopathic arthritis, 90% of the patients treated with tocilizumab achieved an American College of Rheumatology pediatric score of 70% improvement with no major safety issues.[48] Although it can be given as monotherapy, tocilizumab appeared to be more effective when used in combination with DMARDs. Tocilizumab was well tolerated, with most common adverse events of upper respiratory tract infections, headache, hypertension, hyperlipidemia (total cholesterol, HDL, LDL), and increased liver enzymes. These side effects were generally mild and reversible.[45–47]

Agents that inhibit T cells

There is a large body of evidence suggesting that autoreactive T cells, especially CD4 Th1 T cells, serve a key role orchestrating the immune-driven inflammatory responses in autoimmune diseases such as RA, Crohn's disease, PsA and psoriasis. Productive CD4 T-cell responses require two signals: binding of specific antigen associated MHC Class II molecule to the T-cell receptor complex and a second signal from costimulatory molecules (Chapter 12). If T cells fail to receive the second signal, then tolerance or ignorance of the antigen ensues, and a productive immune response is not generated. Among the most important costimulatory molecules is CD28, which binds CD80 and CD86. CD28 and its natural inhibitor, cytotoxic T lymphocyte-associated antigen 4 (CTLA-4; CD152) are present on T cells and bind to CD80 and CD86 on antigen presenting cells. CD28 ligation results in stimulation of T cells while CTLA-4 serves an inhibitory role. CTLA-4, which binds CD80 and CD86 with substantially higher affinity than CD28, inhibits the stimulatory effects of CD28 by competitively binding to CD80 and CD86.

⬤ CLINICAL RELEVANCE

Safety issues with TNF inhibitors

	Target related	Agent related
Definite		Injection site reactions, infusion reactions, immunogenicity (e.g., serum sickness, anaphylaxis)
Probable	Infections, serious infections, opportunistic infections (e.g., coccidioidomycosis), TB, autoantibodies, lupus-like syndromes, hepatotoxicity	
Possible	Malignancies (lymphoma), demyelinating disorders (MS), hematologic abnormalities, CHF	

CHF = congestive heart failure; MS = multiple sclerosis; TB = tuberculosis.

Abatacept (Table 92.2)

Abatacept, approved initially for intravenous use in 2005 and for subcutaneous injection in 2011 for the treatment of RA, is a soluble protein consisting of the extracellular domain of CTLA-4 linked to the Fc portion of IgG1. Abatacept has been shown to improve the signs and symptoms of disease, functional status and quality of life, and to slow radiographic progression in RA patients.[49–52] Abatacept was well tolerated in clinical trials with a slight increase in the incidence of infections, especially among those with underlying chronic obstructive pulmonary disease. In one study, abatacept appeared to have efficacy comparable to a TNF inhibitor in RA patients on MTX.[50] As with other biological agents, live vaccines should be avoided when receiving abatacept. A safety study assessing the combination of abatacept and TNF inhibitor therapy observed a higher incidence of serious adverse effects, including infections, at 1-year follow-up in comparison to those on monotherapy.[51] Given similar findings of increased infections with TNF inhibitors and IL-1ra combination therapy, combination therapy with abatacept and other biologics is also discouraged.

Alefacept (Table 92.2)

Alefacept, approved in 2003 for the treatment of chronic plaque psoriasis, is a fusion protein of a soluble form of the extracellular domain of LFA-3 attached to the Fc portion of an IgG1 molecule. It binds to CD2$^+$ T cells and is thought to improve psoriasis by inducing memory T-cell apoptosis, inhibiting inflammatory gene expression, and preventing T-cell migration into psoriatic plaques. The interaction of LFA-3 on antigen-presenting cells and CD2 on T cells is thought to be important in T-cell activation and in the development of cells into memory T cells. Alefacept, either as monotherapy or in combination with other psoriasis therapy (e.g., MTX), has been shown to be effective for skin psoriasis.[53] T-cell depletion related to therapy did not correlate nor predict the response rate during treatment or follow-up. Despite its effectiveness in the treatment of psoriasis, alefacept appears to be only modestly effective for PsA.[54] With the availability and effectiveness of TNF-I in the treatment of PsA, alefacept is therefore rarely used for the treatment of PsA.

> ### ● KEY CONCEPTS
>
> **Efficacy and safety of T-cell inhibitors**
>
> - Abatacept has been shown to improve the signs and symptoms of disease, functional status, and quality of life, and to slow radiographic progression in RA patients.
> - Alefacept and ustekinumab have been approved for the treatment of psoriasis.
> - These agents have been well-tolerated with only slightly increased rate of infection.

Interleukin-2 (IL-2) Inhibitors

Daclizumab, a humanized IgG1, and basiliximab, a chimeric IgG1, are monoclonal antibodies directed against CD25, the α-chain of the IL-2 receptor, on the surface of activated T lymphocytes.[55] Their therapeutic effect is based on blocking IL-2 binding to T and B cells, inhibiting their activation and development of an immune response, and inducing anergy. They are indicated for the prevention of organ transplant rejection, particularly kidney grafts; and have been suggested for the management of autoimmune disorders. Daclizumab in phase II trials for the treatment of multiple sclerosis has been shown to decrease the frequency of relapses. These agents induce a state of immunosuppression, which results in increased frequency of urinary tract infections and respiratory tract infections; however, opportunistic infections have not been observed.[55,56] Other side effects are paresthesias, transient elevations in liver enzyme and bilirubin levels and skin rash.

Anti-p40 agents

Another approach to modulating the function of T cells in autoimmune and inflammatory diseases targets cytokines relevant to the development of certain T cells subsets. IL-12, a cytokine central to the development of Th1 T cells, and IL-23, a cytokine that helps sustain Th17 T cells, share a common p40 subunit. Agents that target the p40 subunit common to IL-12 and IL23 can be expected to attenuate inflammatory processes driven by Th1 and Th17 T cells. Ustekinumab, a fully human IgG1κ monoclonal antibody against the p40 subunit, was approved by the FDA in 2009 for the treatment of moderate to severe plaque psoriasis (Table 92.2). Ustekinumab substantially improved skin lesions as measured by the psoriasis area and severity index (PASI)[57,58] and studies are ongoing to assess its efficacy in patients with PsA.[59] Interestingly, the duration of clinical benefit after a few injections is prolonged, and appears to far exceed the pharmacokinetic profile of the drug. ATB 874 (briakinumab) is another monoclonal antibody against IL12/23.[60]

Agents that inhibit B cells

Recent data suggest that B cells may contribute significantly to the initiation and perpetuation of the immune response in various autoimmune diseases including RA and systemic lupus erythematosus (SLE). Not only can B cells produce potentially pathologic autoantibodies (e.g., rheumatoid factor, antinuclear antibody) and pro-inflammatory cytokines, but they can also present antigens to T cells and provide co-stimulatory signals essential for T-cell activation, clonal expansion, and effector function.

CD-20 inhibitor: rituximab (Table 92.2)

Rituximab is a chimeric monoclonal IgG1 antibody directed against the B lymphocyte surface antigen, CD20. It was initially approved in 1997 for the treatment of CD20-positive B-cell non-Hodgkin's lymphoma (NHL). Rituximab was approved for the treatment of RA in 2006 and for anti-neutrophil cytoplasmic antibody (ANCA)-associated vasculitis (Wegener's granulomatosis and microscopic polyangiitis) in 2011. CD20 is a cell-surface molecule with expression restricted to the surface of pre-B through activated mature B cells. Rituximab induces lysis of CD20+ B cells by several mechanisms including complement activation, antibody-dependent cell-mediated cytotoxicity, and induction of apoptosis. Depletion of B cells can last up to 9 months or longer after a single course of therapy. Rituximab has improved overall response rate and survival outcome for patients with non-Hodgkin's lymphoma, particularly follicular and diffuse large B-cell lymphoma. Rituximab-based therapies are now included in the treatment guidelines by the National Comprehensive Cancer Network (NCCN) for treatment of follicular NHL and diffuse large B-cell lymphoma and are considered optional for the treatment of other subtypes of NHL.[61]

Rituximab has been shown to improve the signs and symptoms of disease, functional status and quality of life, and to slow radiographic progression of disease in RA patients.[62,63] Repeated treatment in patients who did not respond to an initial cycle did not induce a clinical response.[64] In addition, fixed retreatment at 6 months among clinically responsive patients, regardless of their disease activity at the time of retreatment, did not confer additional benefit.[65] Optimal treatment schedules are currently under investigation, but repeated treatment is generally recommended after 6 months for patients in whom the disease flares in association with normalization of B-cell counts and who had initially responded to rituximab therapy. Although rituximab can be used alone or in combination with DMARDs, the combination therapy yielded better clinical outcome. Also, patients who are seropositive for rheumatoid factor (RF) had greater clinical responses compared to RF seronegative patients.

In a double-blind, non-inferiority trial, 4 weekly rituximab plus glucocorticoid therapy was shown to be equally efficacious as cyclophosphamide in the treatment of ANCA-associated vasculitis. In a subgroup of patients with relapsing disease, rituximab was superior to cyclophosphamide in inducing remissions.[66]

Rituximab has also shown promising results in the treatment of other autoimmune diseases such as SLE, primary Sjögren's syndrome, inflammatory myopathy, idiopathic thromboctyopenic purpura (ITP), chronic inflammatory demyelinating polyneuropathy (CIDP), multiple sclerosis, pemphigus, and cryoglobulinemia.[67] Patients with hepatitis C-associated cryoglobulinemia treated with rituximab noted significant improvement in their extra-hepatic manifestations such as skin ulcers, glomerulonephritis, peripheral neuropathy, arthritis, and hyperviscosity syndrome.[68] Rituximab also appears to be effective in a subset of solid organ transplant patients who developed acute graft rejection or underwent ABO incompatible transplantation.[67] Additional trials are underway that should answer questions regarding dosing, treatment intervals, safety, and tolerability of rituximab in these conditions.

Although there are ongoing clinical trials assessing the role of rituximab in RA and SLE, the largest safety experience comes from oncology patients, mainly those with NHL.[69] Despite the potential for immunodeficiency related to depletion of mature B cells, only small increases in infections, either serious or opportunistic, were reported in both RA and NHL patients treated with rituximab. The overall levels of serum immunoglobulins generally remained stable during treatment. This could be related to preserved function of plasma cells, which lack CD20 and are, therefore, not depleted by rituximab. However, if rituximab is used as a recurrent or maintenance therapy for autoimmune conditions, this may become a safety concern, as plasma cells may not be replenished by memory B cells. Thus far, some patients have undergone more than 6 cycles of rituximab without an apparent increased risk of serious infection or adverse events.[70] In 2006, the safety warning on rituximab was amended to highlight an increased risk of certain viral infections including cytomegalovirus, herpes simplex virus, varicella zoster virus, hepatitis B virus, and JC virus.[71] JC virus, latent in more than 80% of the general population, can be reactivated in immunosuppressed patients to cause a fatal demyelinating disease of the central nervous system called progressive multifocal leukoencephalopathy (PML). Although more common among patients with hematologic malignancies, cases of PML have been reported among SLE and RA patients who were treated with rituximab.[72] The exact role of rituximab in the development of PML remains unknown given its rare occurrence, but it highlights the importance of pharmacovigilance and potential unforeseen long-term adverse effects related to biological agents.

Other notable adverse events include rare neutropenia and thrombocytopenia that can occur up to 5 months after therapy.[37] In general, rituximab has been well tolerated with infusion reactions being the most common adverse events. Infusion reactions are more common during the first infusion and among patients with lymphoma rather than RA.[37] Rituximab has also been associated with Stevens-Johnson syndrome and type III hypersensitivity reactions (serum sickness), occurring more commonly among patients with underlying autoimmune conditions rather than hematological malignancies.[37] In NHL, rituximab infusions have been associated with a severe, potentially life-threatening condition referred to as cytokine release syndrome. Patients often present with fever, nausea, rash, multiple laboratory abnormalities (e.g., elevated liver function tests, uric acid, lactate dehydrogenase, thrombocytopenia, prolonged coagulation time), and high cytokine levels (e.g., TNF-a, IL-6). Seventy percent of cases occur during the first infusion and more frequently in those with higher baseline lymphocyte counts ($> 50 \times 10^6$/L). Although the exact mechanism is unknown, it is hypothesized to be related to complement activation by leukostasis and apoptosis of CD20-positive cells, similar to tumor-lysis syndrome.[37] Lastly, every effort should be taken to give vaccinations before initiating rituximab therapy, as a suboptimal response to some vaccines has been seen with rituximab.

Belimumab (Table 92.2)

Belimumab is a recombinant human monoclonal antibody to soluble forms of B-lymphocyte stimulator (BLys) that was approved by the FDA in 2011 and is the first biologic agent to be approved for the treatment of SLE in over 50 years. BlyS is a member of the TNF cytokine family and is an important survival and growth factor for B cells. It can bind to 3 different receptors on B cells: TACI (transmembrane activator and calcium-modulator and cyclophilin ligand interactor), Blys-receptor 3 (BAFF-R), and BCMA (B-cell maturation protein). BlyS interaction with BAFF-R is important in the generation and maintenance of mature B-cells, induction of T-cell independent B-cell activation, immunoglobulin class switching, and B-cell homeostasis. BAFF interaction with BCMA is important for the differentiation and survival of plasma cells.[73]

Several studies including two pivotal phase III trials (BLISS-52, BLISS-76) have shown that patients treated with belimumab had less SLE disease activity as measured by the SLE Response Index and required lower doses of prednisone. Belimumab-treated patients also had a longer time to lupus flare than placebo-treated patients. No significant increases in adverse events were noted.[74-76]

KEY CONCEPTS

Efficacy and safety of B-cell inhibitors

- Rituximab, an anti-CD20 chimeric monoclonal antibody, is approved for the treatment of NHL, RA, and ANCA-associated vasculitis (Wegener's granulomatosis and MPA).
- Rituximab has been associated with cytopenias and an increased risk of viral infection (e.g. HSV/VZV, HBV, JC virus/PML) with PML occurring more frequently among patients with underlying hematological malignancies.
- Belimumab was recently approved for the treatment of mild/moderate SLE and marks the first biologic agent approved for the treatment of SLE in over 50 years.

Anti-IgE antibody: omalizumab

This antibody was developed to aid in the management of severe asthma with an allergic component. Omalizumab binds IgE with high affinity, considerably reducing levels of free IgE and inhibiting its interaction with the IgE receptor. The clinical improvement correlated well with the measurement of biological markers.[77] Its administration to severe asthmatics with low to moderately elevated serum IgE results in a 26% decrease in the frequency of asthma exacerbations and a 50% decrease in severe exacerbations and emergency room visits, as well as a reduction in systemic corticosteroid use.[78] It has also been shown to be useful to reduce symptoms in corticosteroid-resistant chronic urticaria.

Agents that inhibit cell adhesion and/or migration

Activated T lymphocytes must migrate to sites of inflammation and lymphatic tissue to exert their diverse effects. The entry of lymphocytes into specific sites occurs through several specific interactions between the adhesion molecules on lymphocytes, including the integrins, and their ligands on endothelial cells. Particularly important for lymphocyte migration and homing are LFA-1 and its counter-receptors intercellular adhesion molecule-1 (ICAM-1) and ICAM-2, and very late antigen-4 (VLA-4) and its counter-receptor vascular cell adhesion molecule-1 (VCAM-1).

Integrin inhibitors (Table 92.2)

Natalizumab, approved in 2004 for the treatment of multiple sclerosis, is a recombinant humanized IgG4 mAb directed against the α_4 subunit of $\alpha_4\beta_1$; it also binds to and inhibits the function of the $\alpha_4\beta_7$ integrins, whose ligand is mucosal addressin-cell adhesion molecule-1 (MadCAM-1). $\alpha_4\beta_1$ integrin, an adhesion molecule present on leukocytes, has been implicated in the pathogenesis of MS by facilitating migration of lymphocytes into the site of disease. In addition to blocking the migration of lymphocytes into the CNS and intestinal parenchyma, natalizumab induces T-cell apoptosis and anergy. It also prevents T-cell binding to osteopontin and fibronectin, thereby attenuating T-cell-mediated inflammation. Natalizumab, either alone or in combination with IFN-β-1a, was associated with significantly lower relapse rates, disability, and fewer new multiple sclerosis lesions on MRI.[79,80] However, shortly after FDA approval, natalizumab was temporarily withdrawn from the market after three cases of PML were reported. It has been reintroduced to the market and additional cases of PML have been observed. Similar to rituximab, the exact role of natalizumab in the development of PML remains unknown.

● KEY CONCEPTS

Efficacy and safety of integrins

- Natalizumab, alone or in combination with IFN-γ, is used for the treatment of multiple sclerosis.
- Natalizumab has been associated with several cases of PML.

CD11a inhibitor (Table 92.2)

Efalizumab, approved in 2003 for the treatment of psoriasis, is a humanized IgG1 mAb directed against the cell adhesion molecule CD11a. CD11a is the α-subunit of the LFA-1 molecule on T cells that binds to ICAM-1 on APCs and endothelial cells. In addition to inhibiting activation of T cells, efalizumab also blocks trafficking of lymphocytes into skin by blocking LFA-1/ICAM-1 interaction. Efalizumab was shown to provide greater improvement in skin psoriasis after three months of therapy, with continued increase in response, if therapy was continued for another 3-month cycle.[81] However, the development of PML among patients treated with efalizumab led to its withdrawal in 2009.

Future directions of translational research

The factors that drove the initial introduction of the biologic agents: a clinical need for better outcomes, greater delineation of pathophysiology allowing definition of various targets, and progress in biotechnology allowing development of agents will no doubt continue to fuel progress in this area. It can be expected that additional monoclonal antibodies and fusion receptors, both directed at existing targets as well as against novel targets, will continue to be developed and brought to the clinic. Along with the increased number of biological agents, it is anticipated that the conditions for which these agents are utilized will also expand. For existing biological agents, a number of questions remain in defining the optimum treatment paradigms (e.g., the sequence of biological agents) and the most appropriate patient populations for their use, considerations that will be germane for newer agents as well. As always, the balance between achieving higher levels of efficacy, with disease remission being the ultimate goal, need to be balanced against safety considerations. For macromolecules, such as monoclonal antibodies and soluble receptors, there is the potential for optimizing their characteristics, including ease of use, immunogenicity, and cost. For certain targets, it is possible that small molecule inhibitors may be developed that can address some of these issues. However, as these molecules can be anticipated to have pharmacokinetic, mechanistic, and other important differences from their macromolecular counterparts, this may translate into variable safety and efficacy concerns. Therefore, newer agents of a different class, even those whose putative target is the same as existing therapies, will need to be assessed with the same rigor as the currently available agents.

● ON THE HORIZON

- Production of monoclonal antibodies using non-mammalian cells, plants, and cell lines are being developed to decrease production costs.
- Several biosimilar biological products, which contain active substances highly similar to currently FDA-approved biological products, are being evaluated by the FDA.
- Small molecules (e.g., specific kinase inhibitors) that may have comparable efficacy to currently approved biologic agents are being studied.

References

1. Kotter I, Hamuryudan V, Ozturk ZE, et al. Interferon therapy in rheumatic diseases: state-of-the-art 2010. Curr Opin Rheumatol 2010;22(3):278–83.
2. Coppin C, Le L, Porzsolt F. Targeted therapy for advanced renal cell carcinoma. Cochrane Database Syst Rev 2008;(2) CD006017.
3. Okuyama S, Gonzalez R, Lewis KD. Pegylated interferon alpha-2b as adjuvant treatment of stage III malignant melanoma: an evidence-based review. Core Evid 2010;21(5):39–48.
4. Kappos L, Freedman MS, Polman CH, et al., for the BENEFIT study group. Long-term effect of early treatment with interferon beta-1b after a first clinical event suggestive of multiple sclerosis: 5-year active treatment extension of the phase 3 BENEFIT trial. Lancet Neurol 2009;8:987–97.
5. Freedman MS. Long-term follow-up of clinical trials of multiple sclerosis therapies. Neurology 2011;76(Suppl. 1):S26–S34.
6. Durelli L, Conti L, Clerico M, et al. T-helper 17 cells expand in multiple sclerosis and are inhibited by interferon-beta. Ann Neurol 2009;65:499–509.
7. Reljic R. IFN-gamma therapy of tuberculosis and related infections. J Interferon Cytokine Res 2007;27(5):353–64.
8. Amato VS, Tuon FF, Siqueira AM, et al. Treatment of mucosal leishmaniasis in Latin America: systematic review. Am J Trop Med Hyg 2007;77(2):266–74.
9. Roy-Ghanta S, Orange JS. Use of cytokine therapy in primary immunodeficiency. Clin Rev Allergy Immunol 2010;38:39–53.
10. Holland SM. Chronic granulomatous disease. Clin Rev Allergy Immunol 2010;38(1):3–10.
11. IFN gamma-1b: new indication. Severe malignant osteopetrosis: too many unknowns. Prescrire Int 2006;15(85):175–80.
12. Phumethum V, Jamai S, Johnson SR. Biologic therapy for systemic sclerosis: a systematic review. J Rheumatol 2011;38(2):289–96.
13. Tarhini AA, Kirkwood JM, Gooding WE, et al. A phase 2 trial of sequential temozolomide chemotherapy followed by high-dose interleukin 2 immunotherapy for metastatic melanoma. Cancer 2008;113:1632–40.
14. Manoukian G, Hagemeister F. Denileukin diftitox: a novel immunotoxin. Expert Opin Biol Ther 2009;9(11):1445–51.
15. Mitsuyasu R, Gelman R, Cherng DW, et al., AIDS Clinical Trials Group 328 Study Team. The virologic, immunologic, and clinical effects of interleukin 2 with potent antiretroviral therapy in patients with moderately advanced human immunodeficiency virus infection: a randomized controlled clinical trial–AIDS Clinical Trials Group 328. Arch Intern Med 2007;167(6):597–605.
16. Levy Y, Lacabaratz C, Weiss L, et al. Enhanced T cell recovery in HIV-1-infected adults through IL-7 treatment. J Clin Invest 2009;119:997–1007.
17. Maini RN, Breedveld FC, Kalden JR, et al. Sustained improvement over two years in physical function, structural damage, and signs and symptoms among patients with rheumatoid arthritis treated with infliximab and methotrexate. Arthritis Rheum 2004;50:1051–65.

18. van der Heijde D, Klareskog L, Rodriguez-Valverde V, et al. Comparison of etanercept and methotrexate, alone and combined, in the treatment of rheumatoid arthritis: two-year clinical and radiographic results from the TEMPO study, a double-blind, randomized trial. Arthritis Rheum 2006;54:76–81.
19. van der Heijde D, Breedveld FC, Kavanaugh A, et al. Disease activity, physical function, and radiographic progression after longterm therapy with adalimumab plus methotrexate: 5-year results of PREMIER. J Rheumatol 2010;37(11):2237–46.
20. Keystone E, van der Heijde D, Mason Jr. D, et al. Certolizumab pegol plus methotrexate is significantly more effective than placebo plus methotrexate in active rheumatoid arthritis. Arthritis Rheum 2008;58:3319–29.
21. Kay J, Matteson EL, Dasgupta B, et al. Golimumab in patients with active rheumatoid arthritis despite treatment with methotrexate. Arthritis Rheum 2008;58:964–75.
22. Breedveld FC, Weisman MH, Kavanaugh AF, et al. The PREMIER study: A multicenter, randomized, double-blind clinical trial of combination therapy with adalimumab plus methotrexate versus methotrexate alone or adalimumab alone in patients with early, aggressive rheumatoid arthritis who had not had previous methotrexate treatment. Arthritis Rheum 2006;54:26–37.
23. Landewe R, van der Heijde D, Klareskog L, et al. Disconnect between inflammation and joint destruction after treatment with etanercept plus methotrexate: results from the trial of etanercept and methotrexate with radiographic and patient outcomes. Arthritis Rheum 2006;54:3119–25.
24. Lovell DJ, Ruperto N, Goodman S, et al. Adalimumab with or without methotrexate in juvenile rheumatoid arthritis. N Engl J Med 2008;359:810–20.
25. Ruperto N, Lovell DJ, Cuttica R, et al. A randomized, placebo-controlled trial of infliximab plus methotrexate for the treatment of polyarticular-course juvenile rheumatoid arthritis. Arthritis Rheum 2007;59:3096–106.
26. Antoni CE, Kavanaugh A, van der Heijde D, et al. Two-year efficacy and safety of infliximab treatment in patients with ative psoriatic arthritis: findings of the Infliximab Multinational Psoriatic Arthritis Controlled Trial (IMPACT). J Rheumatol 2008;35:869–76.
27. Rozenblit M, Lebwohl M. New biologics for psoriasis and psoriatic arthritis. Dermatol Ther 2009;22:56–60.
28. van der Heijde D, Landewe R, Baraliakos X, et al. Radiographic findings following two years of infliximab therapy in patients with ankylosing spondylitis. Arthritis Rheum 2008;58:3063–70.
29. van der Heijde D, Pangan AL, Schiff MH. ATLAS Study Group. Adalimumab effectively reduces the signs and symptoms of active ankylosing spondylitis in patients with total spinal ankylosis. Ann Rheum Dis 2008;67:1218–21.
30. Inman RD, Davis Jr. JC, Heijde D, et al. Efficacy and safety of golimumab in patients with ankylosing spondylitis: results of a randomized, double-blind, placebo-controlled, phase III trial. Arthritis Rheum 2008;58:3402–12.
31. Rutgeerts P, Sandborn WJ, Feagan BG, et al. Infliximab for induction and maintenance therapy for ulcerative colitis. N Engl J Med 2005;353:2462–76.
32. Hanauer SB, Sandborn WJ, Rutgeerts P, et al. Human anti-tumor necrosis factor monoclonal antibody (adalimumab) in Crohn's disease: the CLASSIC-I trial. Gastroenterology 2006;130:323–33.
33. Schreiber S, Khaliq-Kareemi M, Lawrence IC, et al. Maintenance therapy with certolizumab pegol for Crohn's disease. N Engl J Med 2007;357:239–50.
34. Sandborn WJ, Feagan BG, Stoinov S, et al. PRECISE 1 Study Investigators. Certolizumab pegol for treatment of Crohn's disease. N Engl J Med 2007;357(3):228–38.
35. Leso V, Leggio L, Armuzzi A, et al. Role of the tumor necrosis factor antagonists in the treatment of inflammatory bowel disease: an update. Eur J Gastroenterol Hepatol 2010;22(7):779–86.
36. Hyrich KL, Lunt M, Watson KD, et al., British Society for Rheumatology Biologics Register. Outcomes after switching from one anti-tumor necrosis factor a agent to a second anti-tumor necrosis factor a agent in patients with rheumatoid arthritis. Arthritis Rheum 2007;56:13–20.
37. Lee SJ, Kavanaugh A. Biologic agents in rheumatology: safety considerations. Rheum Dis Clin North Am 2006;32(Suppl. 1):3–10.
38. Ross JB, Finlayson LA, Klotz PJ, et al. Use of anakinra (Kineret) in the treatment of familial cold autoinflammatory syndrome with a 16-month follow-up. J Cutan Med Surg 2008;12:8–16.
39. Hoffman HM, Throne ML, Amar NJ, et al. Efficacy and safety of rilonacept (Interleukin-1 trap) in patients with cryopyrin-associated periodic syndrome. Arthritis Rheum 2008;58:2443–52.
40. Wenzel S, Wilbraham D, Fuller R, et al. Effect of an interleukin-4 variant on late phase asthmatic response to allergen challenge in asthmatic patients: result of two phase 2a studies. Lancet 2007;370(9596):1422–31.
41. Broide DH. Immunomodulation of allergic disease. Annu Rev Med 2009;60:279–91.
42. Flood-Page P, Swenson C, Faiferman I, et al. A study to evaluate safety and efficacy of mepolizumab in patient with moderate persistent asthma. Am J Respir Crit Care Med 2007;176:1062–71.
43. Nair P, Pizzichini MM, Kjarsgaard M, et al. Mepolizumab for prednisone-dependent asthma with sputum eosinophilia. N Engl J Med 2009;360(10):985–93.
44. Rothenberg ME, Klion AD, Roufosse FE, et al. Treatment of patients with the hypereosinophilic syndrome with mepolizumab. N Engl J Med 2008;359:1215–27.
45. Smolen JF, Beaulieu A, Rubbert-Roth A, et al. Effect of interleukin-6 receptor inhibition with tocilizumab in patients with rheumatoid arthritis (OPTION study): a double-blind, placebo-controlled, randomized trial. Lancet 2008;371:987–97.
46. Genovese MC, McKay JD, Nasonov EL, et al. Interleukin-6 receptor inhibition with tocilizumab reduces diseae activity in rheumatoid arthritis with inadequate response to disease-modifying antirheumatic drugs. Arthritis Rheum 2008;58:2968–80.
47. Nishimoto N, Hashimoto J, Miyasaka N, et al. Study of active controlled monotherapy used for rheumatoid arthritis, an IL-6 inhibitor (SAMURAI): evidence of clinical and radiographic benefit from an x ray reader-blinded randomized controlled trial of tocilizumab. Ann Rheum Dis 2007;66:1162–7.
48. Yokota S, Imagawa T, Mon M. Efficacy and safety of tocilizumab in patients with systemic-onset juvenile idiopathic arthritis: a randomized, double-blind, placebo-controlled, withdrawal phase III trial. Lancet 2008;371:998–1006.
49. Genovese MC, Schiff M, Luggen M, et al. Efficacy and safety of the selective co-stimulation modulator abatacept following 2 years of treatment in patients with rheumatoid arthritis and an inadequate response to anti-tumour necrosis factor therapy. Ann Rheum Dis 2008;67:547–54.
50. Schiff M, Keiserman M, Codding C, et al. Efficacy and safety of abatacept or infliximab vs placebo in ATTEST: a phase III, multi-centre, randomised, double-blind, placebo-controlled study in patients with rheumatoid arthritis and an inadequate response to methotrexate. Ann Rheum Dis 2008;67:1096–103.
51. Weinblatt M, Combe B, Covucci A, et al. Safety of the selective costimulation modulator abatacept in rheumatoid arthritis patients receiving background biologic and nonbiologic disease-modifying antirheumatic drugs: a one-year randomized, placebo-controlled study. Arthritis Rheum 2006;54:2807–16.
52. Genovese M, Covarrubias A, Leon G, et al. Subcutaneous abatacept versus intravenous abatacept: A phase IIIb non-inferiority study in patients with an adequate response to methotrexate. Arthritis Rheum 2011;63:2854–64.
53. Sugiyama H, McCormick TS, Cooper KD, et al. Alefacept in the treatment of psoriasis. Clin Dermatol 2008;26:503–8.
54. Mease PJ, Gladman DD, Keysteone EC, et al. Alefacept in combination with methotrexate for the treatment of psoriatic arthritis. Arthritis Rheum 2006;54:1638–45.
55. Waldmann TA. Anti-Tac (daclizumab, Zenapax) in the treatment of leukemia, autoimmune diseases, and in the prevention of allograft rejection: a 25-year personal odyssey. J Clin Immunol 2007;27:1–18.
56. Wang XF, Li JD, Peng Y, et al. Interleukin-2 receptor antagonists in liver transplantation: a meta-analysis of randomized trials. Transplant Proc 2010;42(10):4567–72.
57. Leonardi CL, Kimball AB, Papp KA, et al., PHOENIX1 study investigators. Efficacy and safety of ustekinumab, a human interleukin-12/23 monoclonal antibody, in patients with psoriasis: 76-week results from a randomised, double-blind, placebo-controlled trial (PHOENIX1). Lancet 2008;371(9625):1665–74.
58. Papp KA, Langley RG, Lebwohl M, et al., PHOENIX2 study investigators. Efficacy and safety of ustekinumab, a human interleukin-12/23 monoclonal antibody, in patients with psoriasis: 52-week results from a randomised, double-blind, placebo-controlled trial (PHOENIX2). Lancet 2008;371(9625):1675–84.
59. Gottlieb A, Menter A, Mendelsohn A, et al. Ustekinumab, a human interleukin 12/23 monoclonal antibody, for psoriatic arthritis: randomized, double-blind, placebo-controlled, crossover trial. Lancet 2009;373:633–40.
60. Kimball AB, Gordon KB, Langley RG. ABT-874 study investigators. Efficacy and safety of ABT-874, a monoclonal anti-interleukin 12/23 antibody, for the treatment of chronic plaque psoriasis: 36-week observation/retreatment and 60-week open-label extension phases of a randomized phase II trial. J Am Acad Dermatol 2011;64(2):263–74.
61. Molina A. A decade of rituximab: Improving survival outcomes in non-Hodgkin's lymphoma. Annu Rev Med 2008;59:237–50.
62. Emery P, Fleischmann R, Filipowicz-Sosnowska A, et al. The efficacy and safety of Rituximab in patients with active rheumatoid arthritis despite methotrexate treatment: results of a phase IIB randomized, double-blind, placebo-controlled, dose-ranging trial. Arthritis Rheum 2006;54:1390–400.
63. Cohen SB, Emery P, Greenwald MW, et al. Rituximab for rheumatoid arthritis refractory to anti-tumor necrosis factor therapy: Results of a multicenter, randomized, double-blind, placebo-controlled, phase III trial evaluating primary efficacy and safety at twenty-four weeks. Arthritis Rheum 2006;54:2793–806.
64. Thurlings RM, Vos K, Gerlag DM, et al. Disease activity-guided rituximab therapy in rheumatoid arthritis. Arthritis Rheum 2009;58:3657–64.
65. Teng YKO, Tekstra J, Breedveld FC, et al. Rituximab fixed retreatment versus on-demand retreatment in refractory rheumatoid arthritis: comparison of two B cell depleting treatment strategies. Ann Rheum Dis 2009;68:1075–7.
66. Stone JH, Merkel PA, Spiera R, et al. Rituximab versus cyclophosphamide for ANCA-associated vasculitis. N Engl J Med 2010;363:221–32.
67. McDonald V, Leandro M. Rituximab in non-haematological disorders of adults and its mode of action. Br J Haematol 2009;146(3):233–46.
68. Pietrogrande M, DeVita S, Zignego AL, et al. Recommendations for the management of mixed cryoglobulinemia syndrome in hepatitis C virus-infected patients. Autoimmun Rev 2011;10(8):444–54.
69. Winter MC, Hancock BW. Ten years of rituximab in NHL. Expert Opin Drug Saf 2009;8(2):223–35.
70. Van Vollenhoven RF, Emery P, Bingham III CO. Long-term safety of rituximab: long-term follow-up of the RA clinical trials and retreatment population. Arthritis Rheum 2009;60(10 Suppl) Abstract 1952.
71. Aksoy S, Dizdar O, Hayran M, et al. Infectious complications of rituximab in patients with lymphoma during maintenance therapy: a systematic review and meta-analysis. Leuk Lymphoma 2009;50:357–65.
72. Calabrese LH, Molloy ES. Progressive multifocal leucoencephalopathy in the rheumatic disease: assessing the risks of biological immunosuppressive therapies. Ann Rheum Dis 2008;67(Suppl. II):iii64–65.
73. Benson MJ, Dillon SR, Castigli E, et al. Cutting edge: the dependence of plasma cells and independence of memory B cells on BAFF and APRIL. J Immunol 2008;180:3655–9.
74. Petri M, Furie R, Merrill J, et al. Four-year experience of belimumab, a BLyS-specific inhibitor, in systemic lupus erythematosus (SLE) patients. Arthritis Rheum 2009;60(10 Suppl.):S774.
75. Thanou-Stavraki A, Sawalha AH. An update on belimumab for the treatment of lupus. Biologics 2011;5:33–43.
76. Navarra S, Guzman R, Gallacher AE, et al. Efficacy and safety of belimumab in patients with active systemic lupus erythematosus: a randomized, placebo-controlled, phase 3 trial. Lancet 2011;377(9767):721–31.

77. Slavin RG, Ferioli C, Tannenbaum SJ, et al. Asthma symptom re-emergence after omalizumab withdrawal correlates well with increasing IgE and decreasing pharmacokinetic concentrations. J Allergy Clin Immunol 2009;123(1):107–13.

78. Humbert M, Beasley R, Ayres J, et al. Benefits of omalizumab as add-on therapy in patients with severe persistent asthma who are inadequately controlled despite best available therapy (GINA 2002 step 4 treatment): INNOVATE. Allergy 2005;60:309–16.

79. Hutchinson M, Kappos L, Calabresi PA, et al. The efficacy of natalizumab in patients with relapsing multiple sclerosis: subgroup analyses of AFFIRM and SENTINEL. J Neurol 2009;256:405–45.

80. Radue EW, Stuart WH, Calabresi PA, et al., SENTINEL Investigators. Natalizumab plus interferon beta-1a reduces lesion formation in relapsing multiple sclerosis. J Neurol Sci 2010;292(1–2):28–35.

81. Toth DP, Papp K, Gratton D. Long-term efficacy of up to 15 months' efalizumab therapy in patients with moderate-to-severe chronic plaque psoriasis. Dermatol Ther 2008;21(Suppl. 3):S6–S14.

PART ELEVEN
Diagnostic immunology

Assessment of proteins of the immune system

Roshini Sarah Abraham, David R. Barnidge, Ian R. Lanza

It would not be an understatement to note that proteins form the backbone of the immune system, as critical products of both the innate and adaptive immune responses. A variety of analytical methods are used to detect, quantify and measure these proteins, some of which have been in use for decades while others are more recent and part of a rapidly expanding and advancing technological armamentarium. The focus of this chapter is restricted to a few notable proteins of the immune system as examples, and the techniques used to evaluate them. Well-established yet currently used methods for protein detection and quantitation are only briefly described. The clinical versus research utility of these applications are provided where appropriate. This chapter also includes sections on proteomics and metabolomics due to the rapid growth in these disciplines.

Immunoglobulins

Immunoglobulins are an integral component of the humoral (antibody) immune response but also act to facilitate cellular immune responses. They are glycoproteins capable of binding antigens and are divided into distinct classes (isotypes) — IgM, IgD, IgG, IgA, and IgE based on structural, functional and biological characteristics (Chapters 4 and 14). The IgG and IgA immunoglobulins are further subdivided into four (G_1, G_2, G, and G_4) and two (A_1 and A_2) subclasses, respectively, based on structural and molecular differences.[1]

IgG, IgA, and IgM levels show an increase with age, from infancy to adulthood (Table 93.1). Immunoglobulins as proteins of interest and clinical relevance are quantitated using other immunoglobulins (reagent antibodies), which recognize epitopes in the constant regions of immunoglobulin isotypes and subclasses.

Quantitation of immunoglobulins is relevant when the levels are either decreased (hypogammaglobulinemia) or increased (hypergammaglobulinemia). The former is typically seen in certain primary immunodeficiencies (Chapter 34) as well as secondary to protein loss or iatrogenic causes (including medication) (Chapter 38). The latter could be related to an universal increase in one or more isotypes (non-antigen-specific) — polyclonal hypergammaglobulinemia (seen in chronic inflammatory diseases, including infectious diseases, autoimmune diseases and chronic liver diseases), in contrast to the increase observed in one or more immunoglobulin isotypes, seen in the monoclonal gammopathies (Chapter 80). In addition to intact monoclonal immunoglobulin observed in the plasma cell dyscrasias, the light chain component of the immunoglobulin molecule can be secreted independently resulting in elevated free light chains (FLC). In addition to the quantitative assessment, monitoring of the M-protein requires the use of other qualitative methods,[2] which will be described briefly.

● KEY CONCEPTS

Immunoglobulin assessment

- Quantitation of immunoglobulins (Igs) most commonly performed by nephelometry.
- Useful for measuring total immunoglobulin isotypes, isotype subclasses, free light chains, and intact heavy–light chain pairs.
- Greater sensitivity and less variability compared to immunodiffusion methods.
- Protein electrophoresis helpful for qualitative/semi-quantitative analysis of immunoglobulins in body fluids, particularly monoclonal Igs (M-proteins).
- Protein electrophoresis is useful for serial monitoring of M-protein concentrations.
- Immunofixation electrophoresis (IFE) useful for characterizing type (heavy and light chains) of M-proteins, and capable of identifying low concentration M-proteins that may be undetectable by standard protein electrophoresis.

Quantitation of immunoglobulins as analytes

Accurate interpretation of quantitative immunoglobulin analysis in serum by any method requires correlation with reference ranges developed from age-matched, healthy (non-diseased) individuals representative of both genders (Table 93.1) and since there can be variation depending on the platform used, each laboratory must generate its own reference values.

Radial immunodiffusion

Among the many quantitative methods used, radial immunodiffusion (RID) is an older method based on the classic precipitin reaction in which antigen and antibodies react and precipitate in liquid or semifluid media.[2] Under conditions of antibody excess (in the supporting media), the quantity of the precipitate is directly related to the quantity of antigen in the test sample occurring at the point of antibody-antigen equivalence. The major limitations include the duration of time required, the relative imprecision of the assay, with coefficients of variation often greater than 10%, relative insensitivity, and dependence on antigen quantity and configuration.

Nephelometry

Nephelometry has largely replaced RID in most clinical laboratories as the preferred method for measuring intact immunoglobulins, immunoglobulin light chains, immunoglobulin

Table 93.1 Immunoglobulin levels

Age of healthy donors	IgG g/L	IgG1 g/L	IgG2 g/L	IgG3 g/L	IgG4 g/L	IgA g/L	IgA1 g/L	IgA2 g/L	IgM g/L
0– <5 months	1.0–1.34	0.56–2.15	≤0.82	0.07.6–8.23	≤ 0.198	0.07–0.37	0.10–0.34	0.004–0.055	0.26–1.22
5– <9 months	1.64–5.88	1.02–3.69	≤ 0.89	0.119–0.740	≤ 0.208	0.16–0.50	0.14–0.41	0.015–0.062	0.32–1.32
9– <15 months	2.46–9.04	1.60–5.62	0.24–0.98	0.173–0.637	≤ 0.220	0.27–0.66	0.20–0.50	0.028–0.070	0.40–1.43
15– <24 months	3.13–11.70	2.09–7.24	0.35–1.05	0.219–0.550	≤ 0.230	0.36–0.79	0.24–0.58	0.039–0.077	0.46–1.52
2– <4 years	2.95–11.56	1.58–7.21	0.39–1.76	0.170–0.847	0.004–0.491	0.27–2.46	0.16–1.62	0.013–0.311	0.37–1.84
4– <7 years	3.86–14.70	2.09–9.02	0.44–3.16	0.108–0.949	0.008–0.819	0.29–2.56	0.17–1.87	0.011–0.391	0.37–2.24
7– <10 years	4.62–16.82	2.53–10.19	0.54–4.35	0.085–10.26	0.010–1.087	0.34–2.74	0.21–2.21	0.014–0.480	0.38–2.51
10– <13 years	5.03–15.80	2.80–10.30	0.66–5.02	0.115–10.53	0.010–1.219	0.42–2.95	0.27–2.50	0.026–0.534	0.41–2.55
13– <16 years	5.09–15.80	2.89–9.34	0.82–5.16	0.200–10.32	0.007–1.217	0.52–3.19	0.36–2.75	0.047–0.551	0.45–2.44
16– <18 years	4.87–13.27	2.83–7.72	0.98–4.86	0.313–0.976	0.003–1.110	0.60–3.37	0.44–2.89	0.066–0.543	0.49–2.01
≥18 years	7.67–15.90	3.41–8.94	1.71–6.32	0.184–10.60	0.024–1.210	0.61–3.56	0.50–3.14	0.097–1.560	0.37–2.86

Immunoglobulin levels were assessed in serum by nephelometry and data were statistically analyzed for the mid-95% confidence interval. For total IgG and IgG subclass quantitation, data from 156 pediatric and 92 adult donors; for total IgA quantitation, data from 201 pediatric and 99 adult donors; for IgA subclasses, data from 119 pediatric and 99 adult donors; for IgM quantitation, data from 212 pediatric and 401 adults was used.

heavy–light chain pairs, and many other proteins in body fluids.[2,3] Nephelometry is a modification of the basic precipitin reaction that relies upon light-scattering by soluble immune complexes in solution. The amount of light scatter produced by soluble immune complexes is measured in a photoelectric cell as optical density. As the concentration of antigen increases, scattered light increases. In contrast to the standard precipitin reaction, which requires the concentrations of antigen and antibody to be at equivalence, nephelometry often performs best with excess antibody. In a typical nephelometric assay for immunoglobulin, a standard curve is developed by reacting increasing concentrations of the antigen (protein) of interest with a constant, large quantity of specific antiserum. Increasing amounts of immune complexes scatter more light, and the intensity of scattered light is directly related to the concentration of antigen (protein). Antigen can be measured accurately in the antibody-excess portion of the precipitin curve and, to maintain this relationship, increased antigen concentration requires additional dilutions of the sample. *End-point (or fixed-time) nephelometry* measures the maximum scattered light after an antigen-antibody reaction has reached equilibrium, or after a fixed reaction time, while *rate or kinetic nephelometry* is an alternative method in which the peak rate of immune-complex formation is measured.[2,3] The coefficient of variation for measurements of intact immunoglobulins and free immunoglobulin light chains are typically in the range of 5%.

Some disadvantages of nephelometry include increased costs for instruments and reagents although these are compensated for by savings in personnel costs. Other potential problems include reagent antisera in settings of M proteins, i.e., poor reactivity of certain commercial antisera with unusual M-proteins; poor linearity of measurement of some M-proteins leading to inaccurate quantitation; and temperature maintenance problems with measurements of cryoglobulins. In general, from a clinical perspective, it is preferable to monitor the quantity of an M-protein during therapy of a plasma cell proliferative disease by electrophoresis with densitometric quantitation (Chapter 80).[2] Nephelometric methods may also be subject to interferences caused by particles or pigments in serum (e.g., lipemic or icteric samples) that increase background light scatter and make interpretation difficult or impossible. Nephelometry has been used effectively for quantitation of serum free light chains for monoclonal gammopathies, as well as more recently to quantitate ratios of intact immunoglobulin heavy and light chain pairs (e.g., IgGκ to IgGλ ratios) using new polyclonal antibodies specific for the junctional epitopes between heavy and light chains (HevyLite, The Binding Site, UK).[4]

The assessment of monoclonal immunoglobulins (M-protein) is best achieved using the following qualitative and semi-quantitative methods. However, it is important to note that these methods only provide an approximate quantitation of individual immunoglobulins. The analysis of body fluids other than serum may require the use of concentrated samples, e.g., 50- to 100-fold for urine or cerebrospinal fluid.

Electrophoresis

The migration of immunoglobulins on agarose electrophoresis is evidence of their diversity.[2,5] The size and shape of a protein molecule, the ionic strength of the buffer, the frictional resistance of the supporting medium, the applied current, the temperature of the reaction and the duration of the applied current all influence the migration of proteins in a typical electrophoresis assay.[2,6] Once proteins are resolved on the gel by application of an electric current, they are visualized with a marker dye and semi-quantitated by densitometry.[2] Since most proteins display a net charge in an electrical field they can be separated electrophoretically.

Serum protein electrophoresis

In the serum protein electrophoresis (SPEP) depicted in Fig. 93.1, the stained protein bands representing albumin, α_1-, α_2-, and β-globulins are easily demonstrated. It is important to note that several of the most abundant protein bands, such as albumin, are sharply delineated; whereas, the area representing the immunoglobulins (the γ-region) is broad and diffuse. The lack of resolution in the γ region is due to the presence of many electrophoretically heterogeneous immunoglobulins that migrate in the same region of the electrophoregram. Small differences in the amino acid composition of immunoglobulins from healthy individuals account for the expected polyclonal display of γ-globulins. As many as 12 discrete regions may be visualized with higher resolution protein electrophoresis using agarose and controlled voltage and temperatures. These are shown in Fig. 93.1, along with the serum proteins in each region. Serum protein electrophoresis can be used to qualitatively or semi-quantitatively identify by visual and densitometric analysis patients with monoclonal immunoglobulins, hypogammaglobulinemia, nephrotic syndrome and polyclonal hypergammaglobulinemia (Fig. 93.2).

Besides serum analysis, other body fluids are evaluated in the clinical laboratory by electrophoresis. Urine samples are routinely tested in patients with serum M-proteins to identify the M-protein components, particularly light chains; and cerebrospinal fluid can be tested for oligoclonal immunoglobulins suggestive of certain inflammatory disorders such as multiple sclerosis.

SPEP is the most common technique used to assess serum samples for the presence of monoclonal and/or polyclonal immunoglobulins.[7] Hypogammaglobulinemia can be detected as well, but SPEP is not particularly sensitive and is not the preferred method unless other methods are not readily available. A monoclonal M-protein should be further evaluated by other methods and hypogammaglobulinemia should be confirmed by quantifying the levels of IgG, IgM and IgA. Densitometric analysis of stained proteins after SPEP is an acceptable method for following the response to therapy of diseases characterized by M-proteins once the specific diagnosis has been established (Chapter 80).

Immunofixation electrophoresis

Immunofixation electrophoresis (IFE) has largely replaced immunoelectrophoresis (IEP) for establishing the presence and isotype of a monoclonal immunoglobulin M-protein in serum and urine (Fig. 93.3).[2,7] IFE is easier to perform, somewhat more sensitive, and easier to interpret than IEP. The procedure usually includes antisera to the heavy chains of IgG, IgA, and IgM, and κ and λ light chains with one lane reserved for SPEP analysis (without detection antisera). The quality of antisera used to stain the separated immunoglobulins is critical in that they must be specific for the intended targets and of high titer. The protein band and its antiserum form a precipitate on the gel at the region of antibody–antigen equivalence (Fig. 93.3). A marker dye is used for visual analysis of the monoclonal protein. The location of the immunoprecipitate depends on

Fig. 93.1 Schematic representation of key proteins in plasma and their migration pattern by agarose gel electrophoresis.

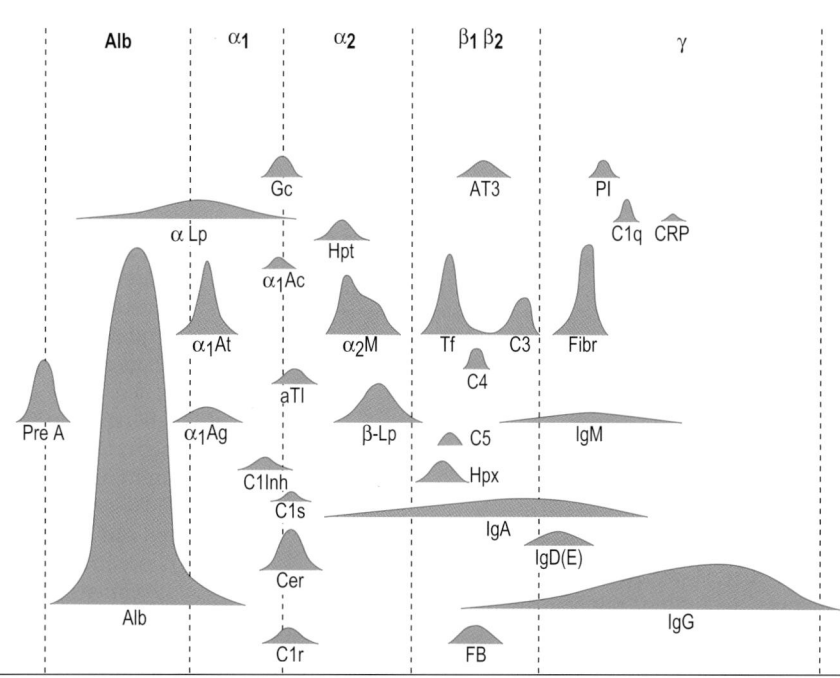

α₁Ac	α₁-antichymotrypsin	Cer	Ceruloplasmin	Pre A	Prealbumin
α₁Ag	α₁-acid glycoprotein	CRP	C-reactive protein	Tf	Transferrin
α₁At	α₁-antitrypsin	Gc	Gc-globulin (vitamin	Complement	As designated
α₂M	α₂-macroglobulin		D-binding protein)	components:	
α-LP	α-lypoprotein	FB	Factor B	C1q, C1r, C1s	
Alb	albumin	Fibr	Fibrinogen	C3, C4, C5	
At3	antihrombin III	Hpt	Haptoglobin	Immunoglobulins:	As designated
α-Lp	α-lipoprotein	Hpx	Hemopexin	IgA, IgD, IgE, IgM6	
C1lnh	C1 esterase inhibitor	PI	Plasminogen		

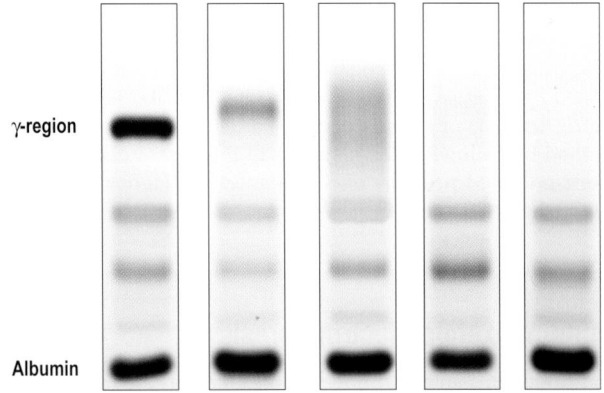

Fig. 93.2 High-resolution serum protein electrophoresis (SPEP) of serum from 5 patients. The albumin and immunoglobulin-migrating (γ) regions are indicated. The patient samples include examples of (from left to right): monoclonal gammopathy with a large M-protein, monoclonal gammopathy with a quantitatively smaller M-protein, polyclonal hypergammaglobulinemia, hypogammaglobulinemia with low serum albumin (nephrotic syndrome), and hypogammaglobulinemia with normal serum albumin.

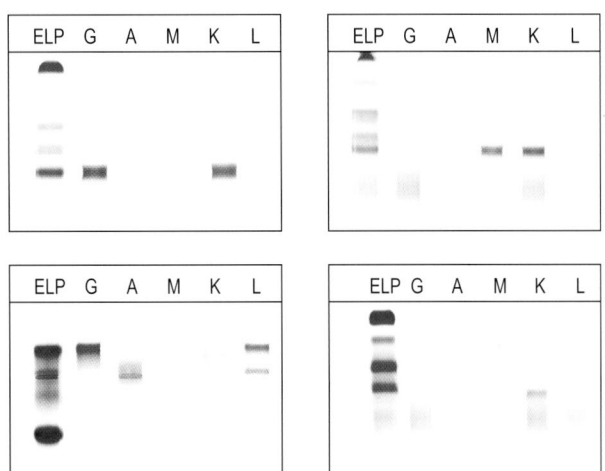

Fig. 93.3 Immunofixation electrophoresis (IFE) on serum from 4 patients. The immunofixation gels include a standard SPEP lane (without antibodies) and 5 individual lanes, one for each major immunoglobulin heavy chain isotype (G, A, and M) and one each for the light chains, κ and λ. Examples of serum IFE include (clockwise from top left): a Gκ monoclonal protein, a Mκ monoclonal protein, a Gλ + Mκ biclonal gammopathy, and a free κ light chain monoclonal gammopathy.

the electrophoretic mobility of the specific M-protein. Most clinical laboratories use IFE after screening samples with the SPEP test and/or quantitative immunoglobulin measurements.[2] Although serum is the most common sample source, urine or cerebrospinal fluid may also be examined to detect and/or characterize M-proteins or their fragments. IFE has several advantages, including: rapid turn-around time (2 hours versus overnight incubation); increased sensitivity; better resolution; and ease of interpretation compared to IEPs. IFE is particularly useful for characterizing small M-proteins and non-IgG M-proteins.

However, the IFE method is not without its disadvantages, which include the increased quality, quantity and cost of antisera required. Optimal resolution requires that the amounts of antisera be determined for each patient sample to avoid either excess dilution or excess antibody. In addition, because of the increased sensitivity of IFE, smaller bands are more frequently identified. These may be of uncertain clinical significance, leading to some difficulties in clinical interpretation.

Identification and quantitation of specific antibodies and auto-antibodies

Diagnostic testing for specific antibodies and autoantibodies is clinically relevant to screen for disease, to establish a specific diagnosis, and to monitor the clinical course of disease. This includes clinical contexts where the antibody is directly pathogenic, e.g., immediate hypersensitivity diseases, or where the antibody merely serves as a surrogate marker for disease or, alternatively, as an independent prognostic indicator.

Detection and measurement of specific antibodies is routinely performed by a variety of immunoassay methods. In virtually all cases, the methods rely upon the use of antigens as analytical reagents. Reagent antigens can be complex mixtures of molecules, e.g., an allergen mixture in a test for IgE antibodies or highly purified "native" or recombinant molecules, e.g. small nuclear ribonucleoproteins in a test for IgG autoantibodies to extractable nuclear antigens. Many reagent antigens of clinical interest are large molecules with multiple antigenic sites (epitopes) that react with antibodies of clinical interest in patients' specimens.[2] The nature of the reagent antigen also influences the precision and accuracy of antibody measurements.

Clinical applications of tests for specific antibodies are directly related to the nature of the reagent antigens. For example, tests that employ crude or complex antigen preparations, like the tissue substrates used in the test for antinuclear antibodies are useful primarily as screening tests; whereas, tests that employ highly purified or recombinant antigens, such as tests for antibodies to some microbial antigens or extractable nuclear antigens, detect antibodies that are disease-specific markers.[2]

Immunoprecipitation methods
Double immunodiffusion

A modification of the basic immunoprecipitation technique, called double immunodiffusion, is commonly used in both research and clinical laboratories to detect specific antibodies.[2] The double-immunodiffusion method while simple to perform is qualitative in nature and sensitive only to concentrations of antibodies greater than approximately 0.1 μg/ml. The relative lack of sensitivity of this method limits its application in the clinical laboratory to situations in which patients' sera contain relatively high concentrations of specific antibodies. The results of double-immunodiffusion tests are also subject to errors of interpretation. False-negative results may occur if the concentration of antigen is not carefully adjusted to produce a zone of equivalence with the concentration of antibodies usually encountered in patients' specimens. Despite these limitations, the double immunodiffusion method is still in widespread use in many clinical laboratories for the qualitative detection of autoantibodies, including antibodies to small nuclear ribonucleoproteins (e.g., SSA/Ro, SSB/La, Sm, and SmRNP) and enzymes (e.g., topoisomerase 1 and RNA synthetases) in patients with systemic rheumatic diseases.

Agglutination methods

The basic immunological principle of agglutination reactions is the same as previously described for precipitin reactions.[2] Agglutination assays for specific antibodies can be performed using insoluble native antigens such as bacterial cells, antigen-coated particles such as latex beads, or red blood cells to which antigens have been attached by chemical coupling. Most commercially available agglutination tests that are designed to detect antibodies specify the use of serum (not plasma) or cerebrospinal fluid. The sensitivity and specificity of these tests are determined by the purity of the antigens coupled to the insoluble indicator particles. Agglutination techniques are utilized routinely in the diagnosis of infectious diseases, in transfusion medicine for typing of blood cells, and in commercial assays for the detection of autoantibodies in patients with autoimmune diseases.[2]

Immunofluorescence methods

Indirect immunofluorescence

Indirect immunofluorescence (IF) is the most commonly used technique in clinical laboratories to screen for specific antibodies that react with cellular antigens. IF is more sensitive than immunodiffusion methods and faster to perform. The increased sensitivity of IF enables detection of human antibodies in concentrations less than 0.1 µg/mL. The technique is semi-quantitative, with results expressed in titers, and is readily adaptable to detection and measurement of many clinically important antibodies.[8,9] IF is routinely used in clinical laboratories to detect and measure antibodies associated with immune-mediated inflammatory diseases and antibodies to some bacteria and spirochetes in infectious diseases.

Immunometric methods

Enzyme-linked immunosorbent assay

Enzyme-linked immunosorbent assay (ELISA) currently is the most widely used immunometric assay.[2,10] There are several variations of the basic ELISA method, which include both competitive and non-competitive formats. ELISA is a sensitive method capable of measuring proteins in nanogram or picogram amounts, without the use of radioactive isotopes. ELISA methods may be used to detect specific antibodies qualitatively or to make semi-quantitative measurements of specific antibodies by use of a standard curve calibrated in arbitrary units. There are limitations to the accuracy and precision of semi-quantitative tests performed by ELISA. Microtiter ELISA methods are inherently quite variable and inter-assay coefficients of variation for positive sera may exceed 15%. In addition, the standard curve of absorbance versus antibody level is usually nonlinear. Consequently, even though results are reported on a continuous numerical scale in units, the results must be considered semi-quantitative. Results are often interpreted as falling within ranges, e.g., negative, borderline, weakly positive and strongly positive, with each category defined by a range of values expressed in units. Truly quantitative applications of the basic ELISA method are less common.

In general, immunometric assays have excellent sensitivity, reasonable precision with coefficients of variation in the range of 10% for measurements of proteins, and may be used to measure antigens of all types in human body fluids. Immunoglobulins present in serum in low abundance such as IgE, can be effectively measured using these techniques.

Very recently, single protein molecule detection by ELISA has been reported using a novel modification of the standard ELISA technique.[11] This method involves the use of a capture antibody immobilized to a matrix of thousands of microspheres. As in the usual "sandwich" ELISA format, the protein target is bound to the capture antibody and detected by a second antibody labeled with an enzyme. The novelty of this approach lies in both the large number of microspheres used (ensures capture of the large majority of the target protein) for the solid support, as well as the placement of the "antibody-target-antibody sandwich" in femtoliter-sized wells, where only a small fraction of the total beads are trapped; the sequestered target molecules are "revealed" by the addition of a fluorescent substrate, with restriction of fluorescence only to the immediate vicinity of the beads containing the "target sandwich," creating detectable dots of fluorescence that can be counted. This assay format results in the discrete measurement of individual target molecules making it particularly useful to quantify low-abundance proteins, in contrast to the measurement of a collective signal generated in a conventional ELISA of all target molecules detected. However, it remains an open question as to whether this approach will find broad applicability in the diagnostic laboratory, especially since other analytical parameters besides limit of detection (sensitivity) have to be considered for a clinically robust assay, and in all probability, the overall prize for diagnostic potential and utility will go to multiplexed, microarray assays.

Multiplex methods for protein detection and quantitation

There has been a burgeoning interest in newer methods to detect proteins in smaller samples, while simultaneously measuring multiple analytes, leading to advances in technologies for multiplex protein analysis. Though the advantages of using these approaches are self-evident, such as simultaneous detection of multiple analytes in relatively small volumes in a quantitative manner,[12–14] there are several limitations that need to be considered carefully, especially when contemplating introduction into the clinical diagnostic laboratory. The concerns include the potential that exists for artifacts in quantitation due to simultaneous detection of multiple analytes, a product of "the matrix effect." Further, there are data to suggest that there can be cross-reactivity between various capture and/or detecting antibodies across analytes, as has been reported for multiplex cytokine analysis.[15] While many of the commercially available multiplex assays come with standardized reference material for quantitation, as well as being provided in a kit format, as an optimized assay, it is nonetheless apparent from practical experience that lot-to-lot variability continues to be a significant deterrent, if a really robust approach to assay design and validation is followed. The precision of multiplex assays can also be influenced by the platform used for analysis, for example, multipurpose flow cytometers compared with smaller, relatively less versatile, but more specialized instrumentation, exemplified by the Luminex-xMAP platforms.

As a model example of performing multiplex assays with different instrumentation, one could consider cytokine analysis, in a biological sample, such as plasma. Several cytokines can be simultaneously detected and quantified using either the flow cytometry approach—Cytometric Bead Array (CBA) or the specialized instrument approach—the Luminex-xMAP technology. Both the CBA and Luminex methods use a fluorescent detection system for analyte quantitation; however, the key difference between the two lies in the fact that the former uses different fluorescent intensities of a single fluorochrome to

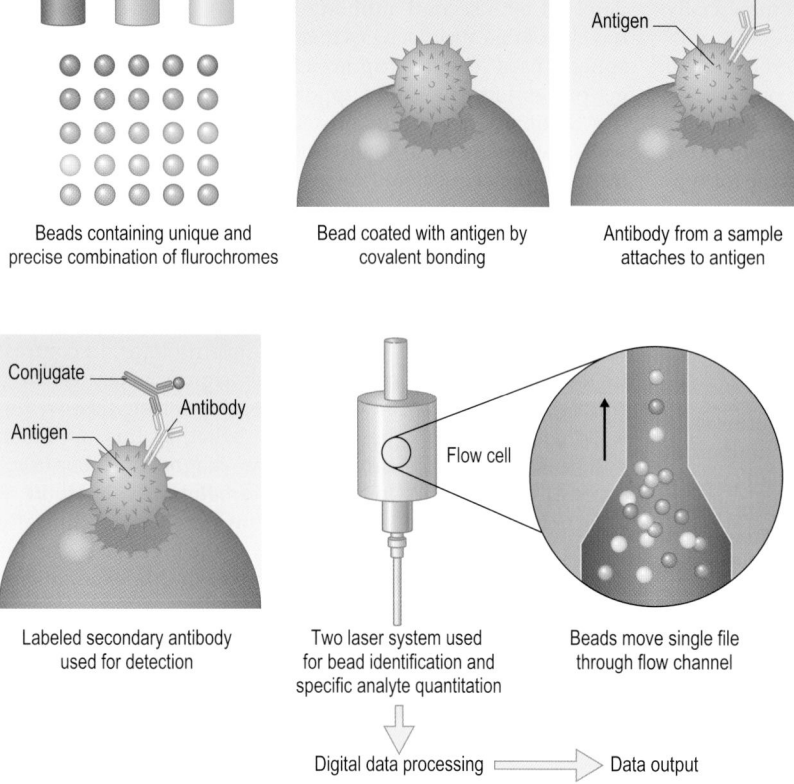

CL1   CL2   CL3

Beads containing unique and precise combination of flurochromes

Bead coated with antigen by covalent bonding

Antibody from a sample attaches to antigen

Antigen

Antibody

Fig. 93.4 Bead-based multiplex assay for protein detection. The bead-based multiplex assays can be used to quantitate antigen-specific antibodies, cytokines, or other proteins of interest, by either flow cytometry or fluorescence imaging techniques. See text for a detailed explanation of the method and utility.

Conjugate

Antibody

Antigen

Flow cell

Labeled secondary antibody used for detection

Two laser system used for bead identification and specific analyte quantitation

Beads move single file through flow channel

Digital data processing ⟹ Data output

accomplish the multiplexing, while the latter uses a combination of fluorochromes (Fig. 93.4), which provides a greater range of analyte availability. The Luminex-xMAP method uses microspheres that have a unique "spectral identity" due to precise and proportionate mixtures of fluorochromes in each bead (Fig. 93.4), theoretically permitting up to 500 different analytes to be simultaneously assessed, depending on the specific platform used within this broad technology (e.g., Luminex-100, Luminex-200, FLEXMAP 3D, and MAGPIX). The Luminex instrumentation utilizes a system with two lasers, one of which activates the fluorescent dyes that identify the specific beads used in the assay, while the second laser activates the fluorescent detector molecule. The use of digital data-processing provides the means to obtain quantitative data specific for an analyte. The MAGPIX technology is the most recent within the Luminex-xMAP repertoire, and in contrast to other Luminex systems, which utilize the underlying principle of flow cytometry, it uses fluorescent imaging for multiplex analysis. MAGPIX uses magnetic microspheres that are fluorescently color-coded, permitting simultaneous quantitation of 50 unique analytes in a single sample well. It offers significant sensitivity with detection of protein analyte in the single-digit picogram levels with a relatively large dynamic range and rapid throughput. However, this approach requires dedicated instrumentation, which incorporates both a magnet to capture the magnetic beads, along with a CCD (charge-couple device) camera to obtain images after exposure of the beads to both red and green light-emitting diodes, for bead detection and analyte quantitation, respectively.

The demonstration of accuracy of multiplex cytokine analysis methods has been made based on comparisons with standard ELISA methods. While several studies have shown relatively good correlations, it is quite evident that this does not extend to the quantitative component.[15] This is not surprising, based on the use of different capture and detection antibodies as well as other ancillary reagents between the two methods. Therefore, arguably better quantitative correlation could be obtained by using identical reagents and standardizing experimental conditions to the extent possible. Nonetheless, since both assays often use commercially available kits, which may or may not contain identical reagents, serial monitoring of cytokines or any other analyte in patients should be undertaken using only a single method, platform and set of reagents. This is a principle that would hold true for a variety of protein assays in the clinical laboratory.

The multiplex bead-based assays have the advantage over ELISA in that it uses direct fluorescent detection of the analyte providing greater sensitivity compared to enzyme-mediated colorimetric detection. Further, the capture reagents are developed by covalent coupling of antibodies or antigens to the beads, as opposed to passive adherence to plastic wells in the ELISA method, which results in greater density of the capture molecule with no concerns of washing it away during the appropriate steps of the assay. ELISA is also associated with a higher background due to the greater surface area provided in a microtiter well, in contrast to beads, especially if the blocking step of the assay is not performed correctly. The overall cost is less with the multiplex bead assays because the amount of capture reagent used is proportionately less compared to ELISA. Therefore, multiplex bead assays have become popular in the diagnostic setting, although it has by no means supplanted ELISA-based methods. The spectrum of clinical applications of multiplex bead assays is well described by Elshal and McCoy.[15]

Aptamers for protein identification

The ability to accurately identify and quantitate proteins of interest necessitates a high-affinity, high-specificity detection approach. For several years, antibodies were the undisputed kings of this universe; however, aptamers are emerging on the forefront as not only viable, but even superior candidates to antibodies for protein detection. Aptamers are oligonucleotide ligands (single-stranded nucleic acid molecules, either DNA or RNA) capable of binding to proteins and other targets with high affinity and specificity.[16,17] Aptamers can be isolated through a process called "systematic evolution of ligands by exponential enrichment (SELEX)," and can discriminate, with a high degree of specificity, surpassing that of monoclonal antibodies, between very closely related proteins or molecules, based on either relatively small structural changes or chirality. Aptamers also have additional advantages over antibodies in that they can be produced *in vitro* by chemical synthesis, possess little to no immunogenicity (valuable in therapeutic applications), and are exceedingly stable for storage (valuable for *in vitro* diagnostic reagents). These unique reagents not only bind proteins but also inhibit their effector functions. Therefore, they can be used both for identification and for functional analysis of protein targets. Besides nucleic acid aptamers, there are peptide aptamers, which are composed of peptides of variable length attached at both ends to a protein scaffold. Peptide aptamers can bind target proteins with high specificity, *in vitro* and *in vivo*, and have the capacity to selectively inhibit function of the specific protein target.[18] Nucleic acid aptamers can be used effectively in ELISA, flow cytometry and protein blotting assays. Despite the enormous potential of aptamers, these reagents are not yet widely available for use in diagnostic assays, especially in commercially available kits or reagents.[16,19] However, this may change with the overall rapid advances made in the field of *in vitro* diagnostics and the potential for aptamers in proteomics.

● KEY CONCEPTS

Multiplex protein assays

- Quantitation of multiple analytes simultaneously in a small sample volume.
- Bead-based multiplex approaches for protein analysis include use of flow cytometry or fluorescence imaging techniques.
- Cross-reactivity between reagents used for multiple analytes in a single assay must be pre-determined to ensure assay validity and robustness.
- Quantitative correlation between multiplex methods and standard ELISA is good if identical reagents and optimized experimental conditions are used.
- Greater sensitivity with multiplex methods over ELISA due to direct fluorescent detection of analyte.
- Oligonucleotide and peptide aptamers are superior to monoclonal antibodies for protein detection due to high affinity and specificity of binding to protein targets.
- Protein microarrays include standard protein arrays with recombinant antigen, antibody microarrays and reverse protein microarrays using cell lysates. Specific protein arrays offer high sensitivity of detection of low-abundance proteins (picomolar range and lower). Protein arrays offer greater flexibility in analytical design, besides multiplexing compared to ELISA.

Protein and antibody arrays

High throughput evaluation of proteins either for detection or assignment of function, beyond that which is possible using the above-described multiplex methods, requires an approach to protein analysis similar to DNA microarrays.[20] There are at least three broad formats of protein microarrays based on capture method — protein microarrays (PMA) represent a standard format utilizing purified recombinant protein, antibody microarrays (AMA) using antibodies, and reverse protein microarrays (RPMA) employing cell lysates from whole or fractionated cells.[21] With the advent of multiplex assays and the evolution of miniaturization technology, a small volume of biological sample can yield thousands or tens of thousands of data points using a protein microarray.[22,23] This approach has particular utility since proteins may be present only in small concentrations and cannot be amplified like nucleic acids. A "sandwich" approach can be used with these microarrays, where the capture and detection antibodies have known specificities and the sample is added between these two steps, combined with fluorescent scanners, which permit measurement of fluorescently labeled detection reagents (Fig. 93.5). To improve the sensitivity (limit of detection) for extremely low protein concentrations, a robust signal-enhancement method called "rolling circles amplification" (RCA) is used.[24] This modified method uses detection antibodies with DNA sequences conjugated to them, and following binding of the detection antibodies to its cognate antigen on the protein array, the DNA sequences are extended *in situ* by DNA polymerase activity, forming long DNA polymers connected to the detection antibody. Post-polymerization, the extended DNA sequences are hybridized to fluorescently labeled complementary DNA oligonucleotides. The limit of detection for this type of assay can thus be increased to detect proteins in the picomolar and subpicomolar ranges, which could represent a significant advance in the detection of proteins in biological and clinical samples. Comparison studies of microarrays with standard ELISA methods reveal comparable sensitivity between the two techniques at this juncture. Another approach to increasing sensitivity is to use bright fluorochromes for antibody detection, as well as to optimize surface chemistry and engineer antibodies to increase valency, or to use intermediate agents that have multiple binding sites, such as streptavidin or nanocrystals, such as Quantum Dots (QDots), to increase detection capacity.[21,24] Multiplex methods are of particular relevance in the field of autoimmune diseases due to several limitations with existing or standard diagnostic techniques, providing an impetus to investigate newer technologies for autoantibody detection.

An additional application of protein microarrays could include discovery of new biomarkers with the potential to be incorporated into diagnostic assays. Further, microarrays can be used to study protein function ("proteome chips"), protein–protein interactions as well as enzymatic activity.[25] In this context, phosphorylation of specific immobilized peptide substrates can be studied using an array with a protein-repellent surface, and pre-defined, homogeneously distributed, covalently bound immobilized substrates.[24] Other advances include the ability to represent membrane proteins, such as ion channel proteins, in such microarrays.[24] The use of surface plasmon resonance (SPR) technology in protein microarrays provides an ideal platform for rapid, dynamic and label-free characterization of protein interactions,[26,27]

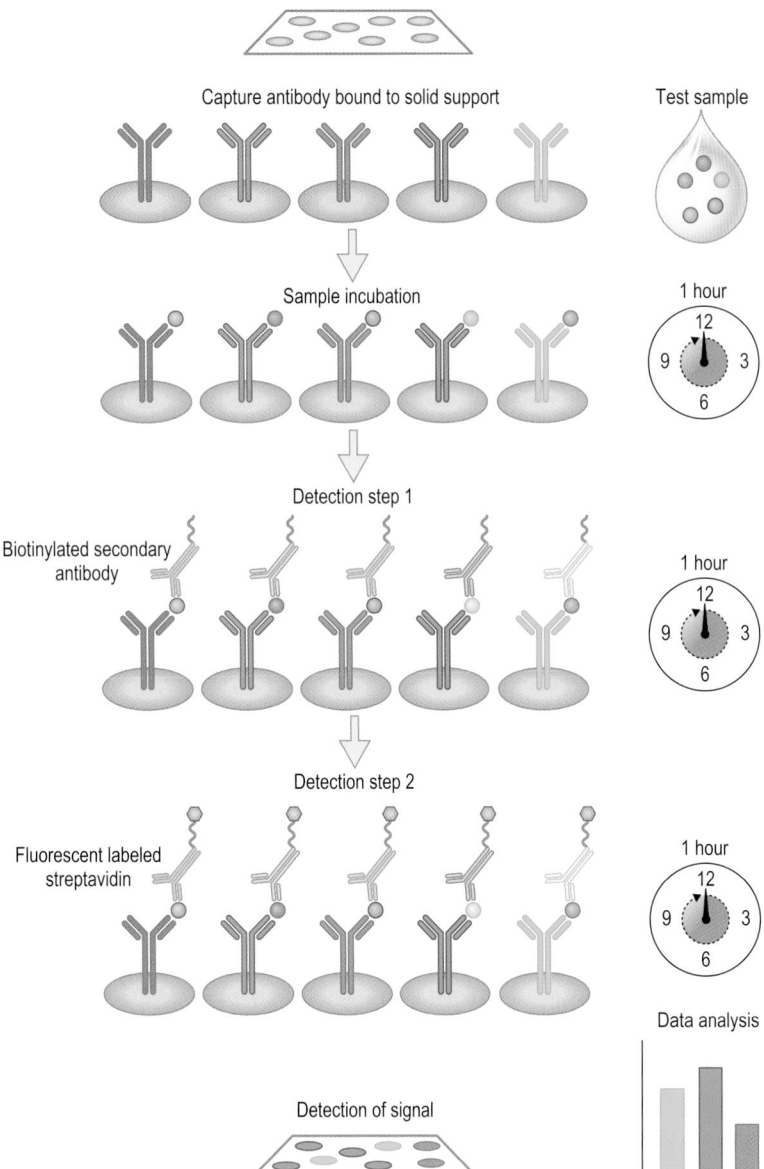

Capture antibody bound to solid support

Test sample

Sample incubation

1 hour

Detection step 1

Biotinylated secondary antibody

1 hour

Detection step 2

Fluorescent labeled streptavidin

1 hour

Data analysis

Detection of signal

Fig. 93.5 Multiplex protein array for protein detection and quantitation. Multiple proteins can be detected in a high-throughput format using antibodies, antigens or cell lysate as capture agents. Fluorescent labels are used for detection, and intensity of fluorescent signal is used for quantitation. See text for detailed explanation of technique and application.

and while these are immensely powerful tools widely used in academic and pharmaceutical industry settings, this approach has generally not been employed in diagnostic applications (although SPR immunoassays for protein hormones have been reported).

KEY CONCEPTS

Characterization of protein specificity and/or function

- Protein blotting techniques can be used to characterize the specificity of a single protein in a mixture of proteins.
- Surface plasmon resonance (SPR) can be used to assess protein–protein interactions, and in a microarray format, provides a platform for rapid, high-throughput analysis, and can be coupled to mass spectrometry.
- Phospho-flow cytometry and intracellular cytokine flow cytometry permits cellular analysis of proteins in the context of specific immunological and/or cellular pathways.
- Cytomics defines the field of study of proteins in the context of their cellular function.

Protein blotting

The resolution of proteins by gel electrophoresis as described earlier in this chapter has definite clinical utility in the immunology laboratory. However, the ability to transfer proteins separated by electrophoresis to a membrane to permit further analysis using specific immunological or molecular probes significantly enhances detection and characterization of low-abundance proteins.[28] While Western blotting is not widely used within the diagnostic laboratory setting due to its labor-intensive methodology; it is performed in specialized laboratories for in-depth characterization of proteins of interest in biological samples. A modified Western blot, the recombinant immunoblot assay (RIBA) is widely used within the clinical microbiology/immunology laboratory to identify antibodies against infectious pathogens (e.g., HIV, Lyme disease). The field of protein blotting is highly sophisticated and has evolved to include multi-antigen analysis, as well as functional protein analysis such as phosphoprotein detection. A detailed discussion of protein blotting techniques is beyond the scope of this chapter, but is well covered by Kurien and Scofield.[29]

Flow cytometry for protein detection

While the technique of flow cytometry is covered in depth in Chapter 94, a brief mention here is included as it applies to protein detection—for measuring cell-signaling proteins, such as phosphorylated proteins and cytokines. Phosphoproteins can also be detected by protein blotting or mass spectrometry techniques. However, flow cytometry provides a unique platform to measure cell-signaling pathways by assessing protein phosphorylation intracellularly after cell stimulation,[30] and allows simultaneous characterization of several phosphoproteins in different cellular subsets (Fig. 93.6). Similarly, flow cytometry provides a platform to measure products of cellular activation, such as cytokines, within the context of cells, by intracellular staining with specific antibodies. This approach offers the distinct advantage of correlation of cytokine production with other immunophenotyping parameters, which is essential in certain clinical applications.

Cytomics (the study of the proteome with associated cellular function) is yet another field that is rapidly advancing by harnessing technological development to better understand biological processes.

Proteomics

The field of proteomics incorporates many techniques to characterize and quantify proteins. New workflows have emerged that couple traditional techniques, such as electrophoresis and immunoaffinity, with newer technology, such as mass spectrometry. This section discusses mass spectrometry-based proteomics and immuno-proteomics.

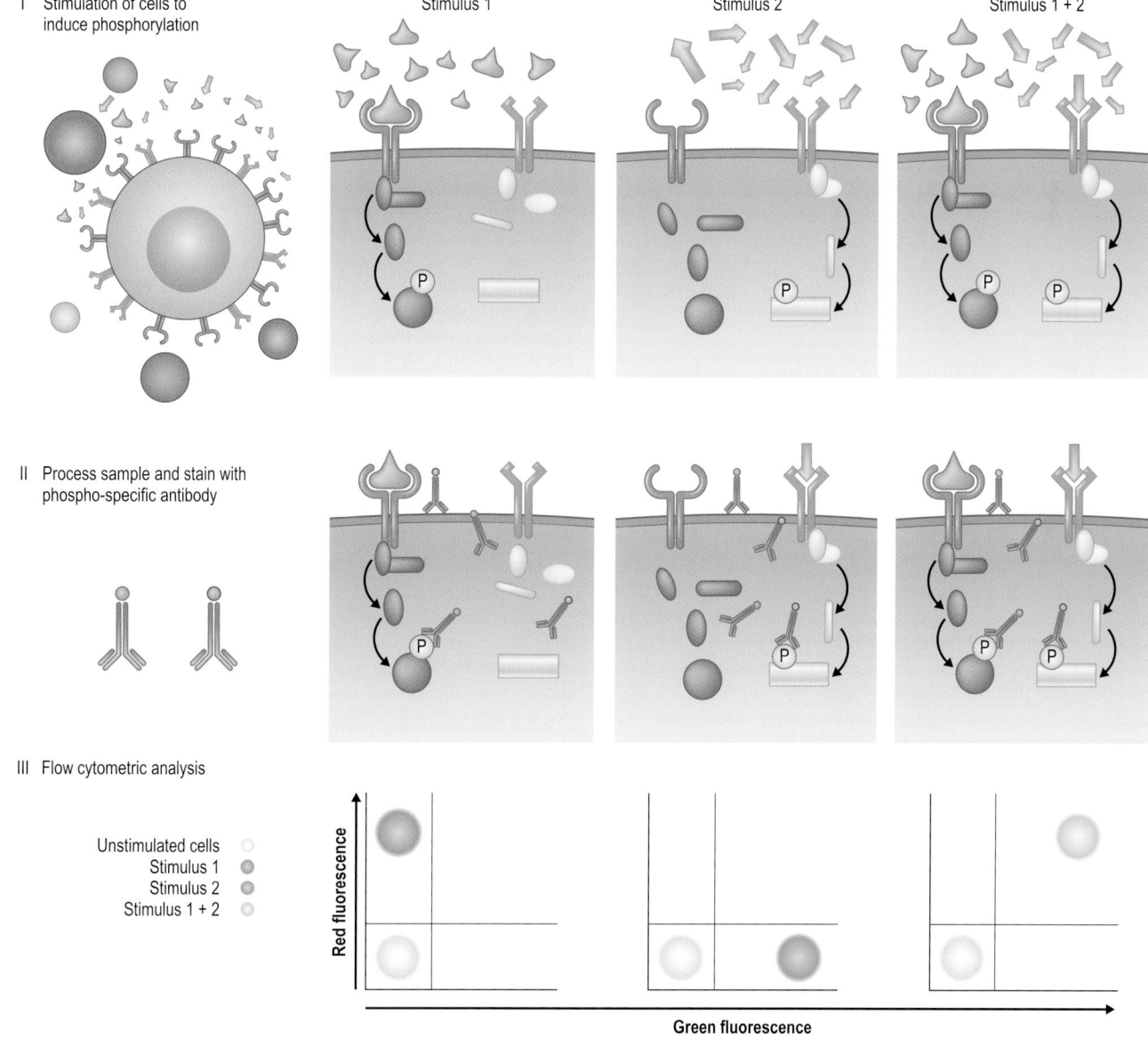

I Stimulation of cells to induce phosphorylation

Stimulus 1   Stimulus 2   Stimulus 1 + 2

II Process sample and stain with phospho-specific antibody

III Flow cytometric analysis

Unstimulated cells
Stimulus 1
Stimulus 2
Stimulus 1 + 2

Red fluorescence

Green fluorescence

Fig. 93.6 Analysis of phospho-proteins in cells by flow cytometry. Cells activated by specific stimuli can be assessed for activation and induction of specific signaling pathways by measuring phospho-proteins: single or multiple stimuli can be used that phosphorylate different proteins, and intracellular staining with phospho-specific antibodies, and subsequently analyzed by multi-color flow cytometry. See text for detailed explanation.

Modified from Fig. 2 by Krutzik P, Irish JM, Nolan GP, Perez OD, Analysis of protein phosphorylation and cellular signaling events by flow cytometry: techniques and clinical applications. Clin Immunol 2004; 110: 206-221.

Proteomics

- Mass spectrometry is a key technique used for proteomic analysis and encompasses several distinct methods.
- **MALDI: M**atrix **a**ssisted **l**aser **d**esorption **i**onization, characterized by a crystalline matrix that absorbs laser energy, and is mixed with protein sample to create ions.
- A rapid technique that uses low amount of sample, and the dried sample spots are only a few millimeters in diameter.
- **ESI: E**lectro**s**pray **i**onization, characterized by protein ions in solution that are transferred to the gas phase by a spray formed at an emitter tip held at a high electric potential.
- Ideal for complex samples that are separated by liquid chromatography in line with ESI.
- Protein identification using LC-MS/MS: involves digestion of protein with trypsin, separation of peptides by LC, fragmentation of peptide ions using MS/MS, and identification of proteins by matching MS/MS data to a protein database.

Technology and techniques

Mass spectrometry

For almost 50 years laboratories have performed gel electrophoresis as a way of identifying proteins by their size and charge. Mass spectrometry also relies on size (mass) and charge to identify proteins. The identification of two techniques more than two decades ago for ionizing large molecules to perform mass analysis changed how researchers viewed the utility of mass spectrometry.

Ionization techniques for protein analysis using mass spectrometry

The first ionization technique is electrospray ionization (ESI), whereby multiply charged analytes in solution (i.e., proteins or peptides) become multiply charged ions in the gas phase. It is called electrospray since the solution carrying the charged ions is fed through a small tube held at a high electric potential (on the order of 2–5 kV), creating a spray as the ions in the solution are repelled by the potential at the tip of the tube. Droplets formed in the spray undergo many explosions due to the charge build up and with the help of heated gas near the entrance to the mass spectrometer; ions are transferred from solution to the gas phase. The key points to remember with ESI ionization are: (1) it is a solution-based method; (2) ions in solution are transferred to the gas phase via charged droplets; and (3) it is a "soft" ionization process that produces ions with high charge states.

Laser desorption (LD) is the other ionization technique that revolutionized macromolecule mass spectrometry. This technique was developed using a matrix of ultrafine metal powder mixed with protein and glycerol. A pulsed laser beam is shot at the target containing metal particles and protein suspended in glycerol. The energy from the laser is converted to heat via the metal particles, which activates the glycerol matrix ionizing the protein. The most common form of laser desorption ionization in use today is matrix assisted laser desorption ionization, or MALDI. This technique uses a crystalline matrix consisting of organic molecules in place of metal particles to transfer laser energy in order to produce gas phase protein ions. The MALDI process produces ions with fewer charges as compared to ESI. The key points to remember with MALDI ionization are: (1) it uses a crystalline matrix method where an analyte in solution

is mixed with the matrix in solution, allowed to dry, then put into the mass spectrometer; (2) ions are made under vacuum using a laser; and (3) ions are formed by interacting with the matrix ions producing ions with low charge states.

Along with improvements in ionization sources, advances have been made in the speed, sensitivity, and robustness of mass spectrometers, making them more accessible to laboratories that would traditionally not have such instrumentation. Examples include time-of-flight (TOF), ion trap (IT), Orbitrap, and quadrupole instruments. Various combinations of these types of instruments, or hybrids, such as quadrupole time-of-flight, or Q-TOF, are also available. This chapter discusses the instrument types in relation to their function in proteomics. For further reading Yates, et al., present an excellent review on ionization techniques and mass spectrometers used in proteomics.[31]

Analysis of intact proteins using mass spectrometry

Pharmaceutical companies making therapeutic recombinant monoclonal antibodies (mAb) have chosen mass spectrometry as the analytical tool of choice for characterizing them. This decision was based on the fact that mass spectrometry can accurately determine the molecular weight of an antibody and at the same time determine amino acid sequence and post-translational modifications.[32] The term "top down" is often used in mass spectrometry-based proteomics literature to refer to the analysis of a protein in its intact form. This is the same as running an SDS-PAGE gel to determine the molecular weight of a protein. However the accuracy of the molecular weight information obtained using SDS-PAGE is poor compared to that obtained using mass spectrometry. MALDI-TOF was first used to determine the accurate mass of antibodies, and although the mass error is superior to SDS-PAGE, ($\pm$ 100 Da for an intact mAb), new ESI-TOF instruments can perform mass measurements with an accuracy of the order of $\pm$ 1.5 Da, or better, for an intact mAb with a mass of roughly 150 kDa. By using the high mass measurement accuracy of ESI-TOF, the presence of a protein modification can easily be determined. While ESI-TOF can provide highly accurate mass calculations on intact protein, it is not without its limitations. Figure 93.7 demonstrates the difference in the spectra for α and β hemoglobin using ESI (top) and MALDI (bottom). It is clear from the spectra that ESI produces a more complicated spectrum due to the fact that a single protein can produce many different ionized species while MALDI is less complicated since only low charge state ions are observed. In addition, specialized software is needed to convert ESI spectra from having many different peaks to a single peak representing the molecular weight of the protein. Therefore to deal with the increased complexity of ESI spectra, complex mixtures of proteins are typically separated first by using liquid chromatography (LC) where the LC is coupled directly to the ESI source.

Analysis of tryptic peptides using mass spectrometry

The complementary technique to the "top-down" approach is the "bottom-up" approach. The "bottom-up" approach includes a digestion step (often trypsin) breaking down proteins into smaller peptides. There are two ways that the peptides can be ionized and introduced into the mass spectrometer after digestion; either all at the same time, or first separating the various peptides from one another. In situations where a relatively small, highly pure protein (e.g., a recombinant light chain) is digested with trypsin, it is possible to quickly analyze all the peptides

Fig. 93.7 Mass spectral profiles for ESI and MALDI.
The figure demonstrates the difference in the spectra for hemoglobin using ESI (top) and MALDI (bottom). See text for detailed explanation.
Reproduced from Wada Y, Advanced analytical methods for hemoglobin variants. J Chromatogr B Analyt Technol Biomed Life Sci 2002; 781: 291-301.

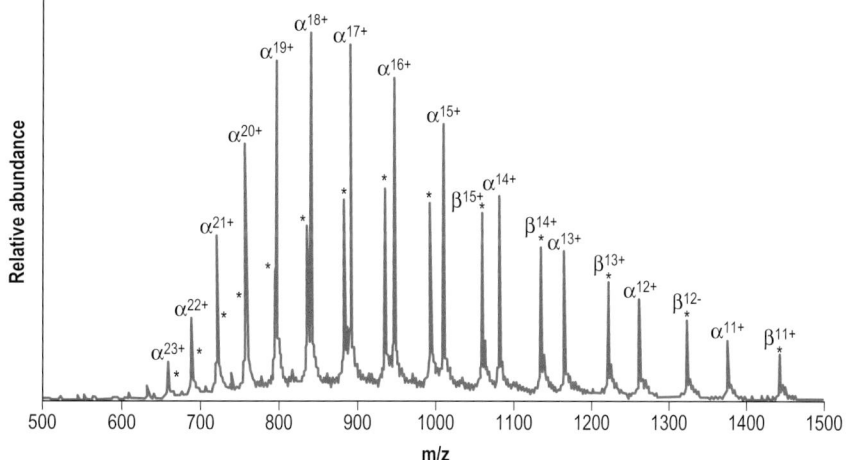

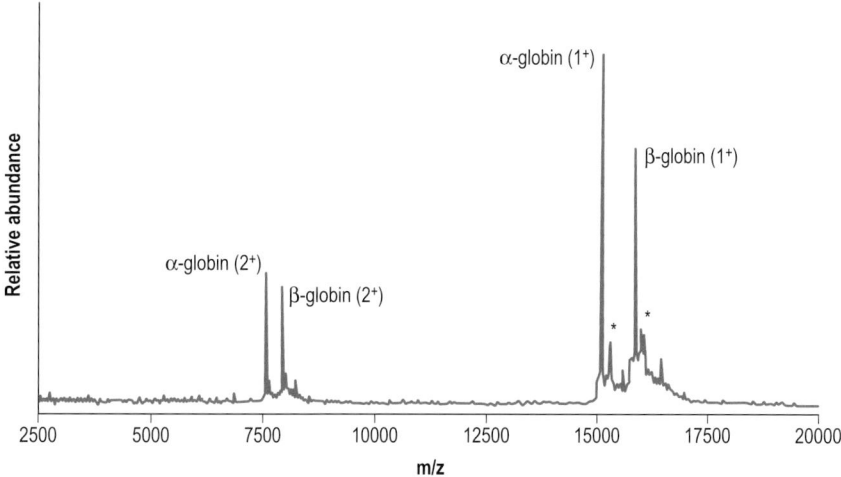

together using a MALDI-TOF instrument. Spectra acquired from the mixture of tryptic peptides can be used as a tryptic peptide map. Such a map can be compared to a digest of standard material (i.e., light chain digest from one batch versus another) to determine if modifications have taken place. The most common "bottom-up" proteomics experiment for characterizing digests of large proteins or protein mixtures involves some form of separation first, usually LC. If MALDI is going to be performed, the peptides can be fractionated off the LC, mixed with matrix and then analyzed by MALDI-TOF. Or more commonly, the peptides are separated by LC coupled to ESI then analyzed. The benefit of digestion first for LC-ESI is that the peptides are much smaller than the intact protein and have much smaller charge states making them ideal candidates for gas-phase sequencing by tandem mass spectrometry or MS/MS.

LC-MS/MS experiments are the most common form of mass spectrometry-based proteomics analysis. LC-MS/MS experiments are performed on instruments such as a Q-TOF, a triple quadrupole, an ion trap, or an Orbitrap mass spectrometer. In an LC-MS/MS experiment, peptide ions eluting from the LC are ionized by ESI and then scanned by the mass spectrometer. A spectrum is saved showing the mass peaks for the peptide ions eluting from the LC. This is called a precursor ion mass spectrum. A computer program checks the precursor mass spectrum and identifies peptides with the greatest abundance, notifying the mass spectrometer which peptide ions to select for the MS/MS experiment. The mass spectrometer then performs an

MS/MS experiment by selecting only one peptide ion which is then fragmented in the gas phase to create a product ion mass spectrum. The product ion spectrum contains fragments which can be pieced back together to identify the amino acids, and their order, in the tryptic peptide selected. Peptide sequence identification is done using a protein database search engine that matches the expected mass peaks to the mass peaks observed in the MS/MS experiment. In the case of a recombinant mAb, the amino acid sequence is known, and therefore the database is small, containing only one protein. However, there are many possible post-translational modifications or amino acid substitutions that could occur in a mAb; therefore the database search engine must be able to match any possible combination, which increases computational time.

Figure 93.8 shows a diagram with the steps involved in a "top-down" experiment where the molecular weight of an intact protein is determined using MALDI-TOF. Figure 93.9 shows a diagram with the steps involved in a "bottom-up" experiment where tryptic peptides are used to identify the proteins present in a mixture using LC-ESI-MS/MS.

Protein quantification using mass spectrometry

Recently, researchers have been using LC-MS/MS to quantify proteins. The technique is identical to the "bottom-up" approach and is based on using a tryptic peptide, often referred

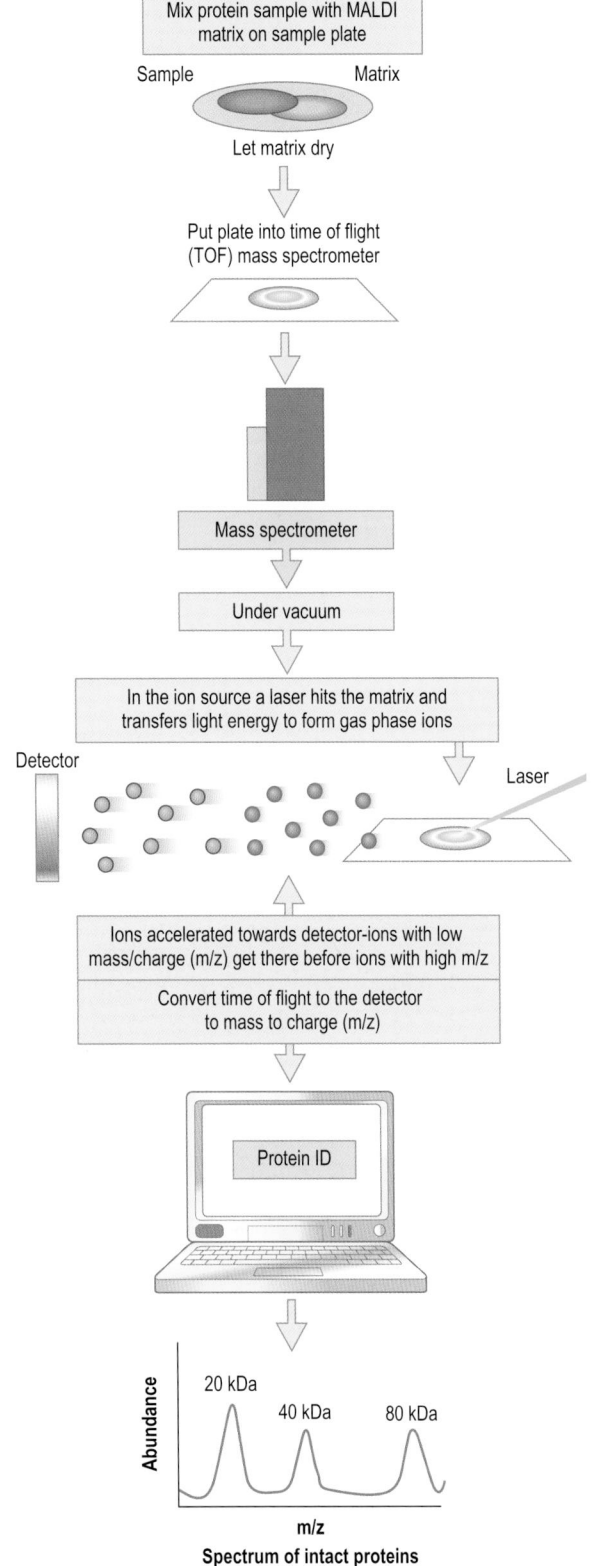

Fig. 93.8 **Schematic representation of protein analysis by MALDI-TOF.** The process involved in a "top-down" experiment where the molecular weight of an intact protein is determined using MALDI-TOF is shown.

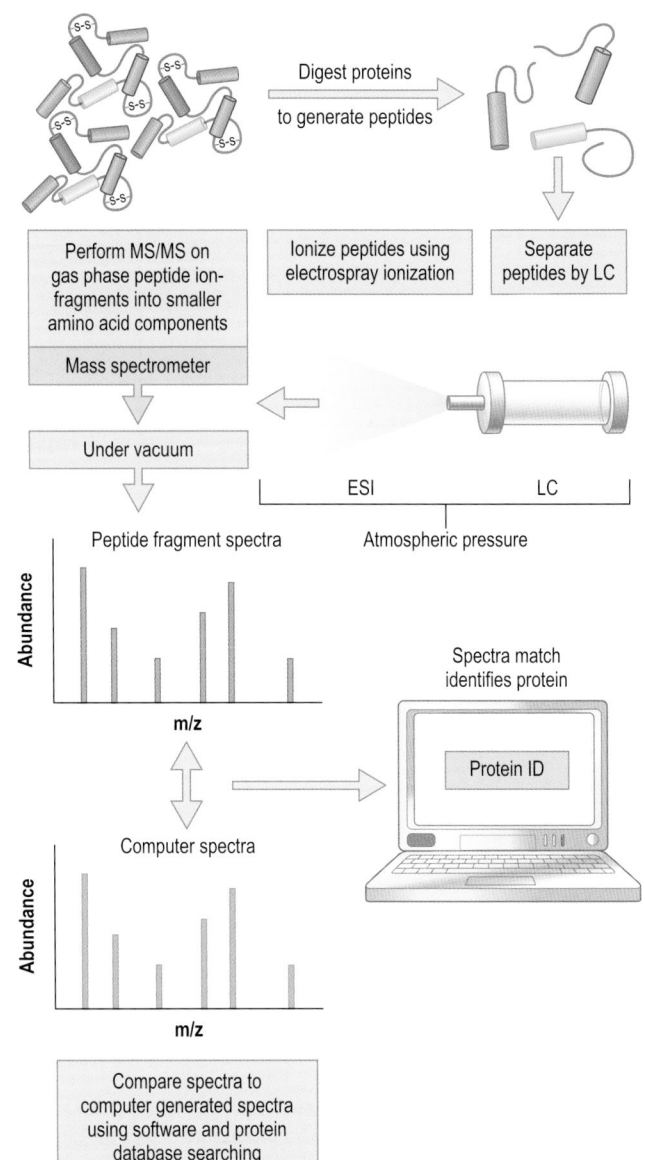

Fig. 93.9 **Schematic representation of peptide analysis by ESI-mass spectrometry.** The process involved in a "bottom-up" experiment where tryptic peptides are used to identify the proteins present in a mixture using LC-ESI-MS/MS.

to as a proteotryptic peptide, to represent the concentration of the intact protein in the sample. The sequence of the tryptic peptide selected to represent the whole protein is synthesized using stable-isotope-labeled amino acids. This synthetic peptide can then be used as an internal standard for quantitative analysis

in the same way that isotope dilution mass spectrometry is performed for small molecules. In this approach, a solution of the synthetic peptide can be introduced into the mass spectrometer and instrument conditions can be optimized specifically for that peptide. The optimized masses are programmed into a triple quadrupole mass spectrometer, which is used to perform quantification by doing a multiple-reaction-monitoring (MRM) experiment. A triple quadrupole mass spectrometer run in MRM mode allows specific peptide ions through the first region. These ions are fragmented in the second region (collision cell) and finally only specific fragments are transmitted through the third region to be detected. The ratio of the tryptic peptide from the protein digest to the known amount of internal standard can be used to quantify the protein of interest. If the unknown protein is available in pure form, a standard curve can be generated to quantify the protein more accurately.[33]

Mass spectrometry-based proteomics on proteins of the immune system

Aside from being an essential analytical methodology for characterizing therapeutic monoclonal antibodies, LC-MS/MS has been used to better understand which proteins and which post-translational modifications are important in cells of the immune system. Examples include mapping of the B-cell proteome for diseases such as multiple myeloma[34] and chronic lymphocytic leukemia[35] as well as mapping of proteins present in resting neutrophils.[36] The proteins identified in these studies were "found" by isolating cells, followed by the "bottom-up" approach with protein database review to map out the proteome of the cells. Perhaps the most intriguing use of LC-MS/MS in immunology is the mining of antigens and antibodies associated with autoimmune disease and cancer. An excellent review on this topic by Tjalsma et al. examines the concept of immunoproteomics and associated methodologies, including mass spectrometry.[37] Mapping of peptides associated with isolated soluble HLA complexes has also been performed using LC-MS/MS with protein database searching. Comparisons of HLA-peptide combinations from normal healthy donors and patients with a specific disease can be used as a filter to identify only those peptides, and therefore the parent protein, associated with the specific disease. An alternative approach is to isolate and characterize the CDR region of an antibody instead of the antigen. This approach has been successful in model systems, but may soon be an alternative way of identifying patients with autoimmune disease.[38]

Phosphoproteomics

Mass spectrometry has recently become a standard analytical tool for identifying and quantifying protein post-translational modifications (PTMs) involved in signal transduction. One of the most important post-translational modifications regulating protein function is phosphorylation, and mass spectrometry is playing a key role in mapping sites of protein phosphorylation to better understand biochemical pathways.[39] The process used to isolate phosphopeptides starts with the same "bottom-up" procedure where proteins are first isolated from tissue, cells, blood, etc., and then digested with a protease, usually trypsin. The pre-analytical portion of a phosphorylation mapping experiment focuses on ensuring that the steps in sample preparation do not alter the sites of phosphorylation, and particular caution is taken to ensure that kinases and phosphatases are inhibited. Once tryptic peptides are produced, those containing sites of phosphorylation are isolated using a variety of purification techniques. When purification is complete, the phosphorylated peptides are analyzed by LC-MS/MS.

Amino acids that contain O-phosphorylation sites such as serine, threonine, and tyrosine have a stable phosphoester-linked phosphate; however, this modification has a dramatic effect on the ionization and fragmentation pattern of the tryptic peptides. Phosphopeptides can be ionized by ESI and MALDI but the fragmentation patterns observed are more difficult to match when doing protein database searches as the intensity of the fragment ions are sometimes lower as compared to the non-phosphorylated peptide. New techniques for fragmenting phosphopeptides in the gas-phase, along with better protein database search algorithms have made the identification and quantification of phosphopeptides more efficient. This in turn has led to a better understanding of signaling pathways involving phosphorylation. Errors in these pathways that lead to disease are being mapped and quantified using mass spectrometry in the hopes of providing new prognostic markers to monitor disease progression.

Surface plasmon resonance (SPR) coupled to mass spectrometry

Surface plasmon resonance (SPR) is a label free, non-destructive way to characterize ligand binding, such as an antibody–antigen interaction. The method is based on the immobilization of a ligand capture molecule on a metal film, usually gold, layered on top of a glass slide. The ligand is introduced via liquid phase and the changes induced in the surface plasmon resonance are measured as the ligand binds to the capture molecule. Since the technique is non-destructive, the slide containing the ligand-capture molecule complex can be removed from the SPR instrument and the ligand can be isolated for analysis by mass spectrometry.[40] This approach has been useful for confirming the identity of proteins bound to immobilized antibodies.

Metabolomics

In its most elemental form, metabolomics is a systems biology discipline that deals with quantitative assessment of endogenous metabolites.[41] There are thousands of small molecular weight compounds (i.e., metabolites) involved in various aspects of cellular function. Metabolite profiling of easily obtainable tissue fluids such urine and plasma can provide insight into the biochemical phenotypes of living systems. The terms "metabolomics" and "metabonomics" have both been used to describe this concept. Metabolomics has been described as the "non-biased identification and quantitation of all metabolites in a biological system," whereas metabonomics is defined as "the quantitative measurement of the dynamic multiparametric metabolic response of living systems to pathophysiological stimuli or genetic modification."[42] There are excellent reviews that provide additional detail on metabolomics.[43,44]

The field of metabolomics is relatively new, having grown rapidly over the past 10 years because of technological advances in analytical techniques as well as methods for data mining and statistical pattern recognition. Nuclear magnetic resonance spectroscopy (NMR) and mass spectrometry (MS) are well-suited analytical methods for metabolomics because of their capacity to measure the concentrations of a large number of metabolites from tissue fluids.[42] The two platforms each boast advantages and suffer from limitations. For example, mass spectrometry

● KEY CONCEPTS

Metabolomics

- Comprises a systems biology approach focused on quantitative assessment of endogenous metabolites related to cellular function.
- Metabolite profiling performed on easily accessible biofluids.
- Uses the techniques of mass spectrometry, NMR spectroscopy, and other methods, including optical spectroscopy for data generation and metabolite analysis.
- Heavily dependent on statistical algorithms, databases, and pattern recognition analytical tools for data analysis.
- Useful for evaluating changes in metabolites over time, or under different intrinsic or extrinsic parameters.
- Of particular relevance in early detection of disease and prognosis, as well as differentiation between disease states.

has higher sensitivity and resolution than NMR, but is less reproducible and quantitative.[45] Magnetic resonance spectroscopy requires much less sample preparation than MS, but MS can be more easily automated. The choice of platform often depends on resources, skill, and practical considerations, but it is worth emphasizing that the different analytical methods often yield complementary information that can be integrated for a more complete picture.[45] Because MS features high sensitivity and specificity, and NMR is more quantitative and reproducible, it is possible to perform more comprehensive metabolic profiling with a combination of the two, than allowed by each analytical method alone.

As important as the analytical aspects of metabolomics are, the data generated by these methods requires robust statistical methods to complete the analyses (i.e., chemometrics and bioinformatics). These approaches harness the power of algorithms, databases, and multivariate pattern recognition techniques such as principal component analysis to process spectra, identify metabolites, quantitate spectral peaks, and reveal patterns in spectra from groups of individuals, patients, or experimental conditions; tasks that would be otherwise extremely time consuming or altogether impossible.

The primary focus of metabolomics is to not only to identify metabolites within a complex biological sample, but also to determine the magnitude of change (increase or decrease) that is imposed by intrinsic or extrinsic conditions, whether it be underlying disease or therapeutic interventions. In the clinical realm, metabolomics has been used extensively to understand the pathophysiology of cancer,[41] inborn errors of metabolism,[46] and other diseases. A particular utility of metabolomics is its potential not only for early detection of disease[47] but also for prognostic monitoring of disease, and differentiation between disease states. From an immunological standpoint, metabolomics (if not by that name or concept) has been part and parcel of organ transplantation practice for several decades.[48,49] One of the ongoing challenges of analyzing metabolomics data is separating the "wheat from the chaff," i.e., which changes in metabolites are irrelevant to the disease process or event being studied versus which changes are of consequence. In the field of transplantation, as in other fields of immunological interest, such as cancer or autoimmunity, the use of powerful immunomodulatory or immunosuppressive therapies, as well as chronic infection may profoundly alter the metabolomic profile, and potentially obfuscate metabolomic data analysis. A significant asset to sorting out what changes in metabolites, common or rare, are normal versus abnormal is provided by the Human Metabolome Database (http://www.hmdb.ca). Additionally, there is a database called the Small Molecule Pathway database (SMDB; http://www.smpdb.ca), which provides information on greater than 350 small molecule pathways in humans. These pathways include human metabolic pathways as well as metabolic disease pathways and more than two-thirds of this database is unique. The metabolomic databases along with advances in specific technology and data analysis are likely to facilitate ongoing development and application of metabolite profiling to clinical immunology applications in the future.

CLINICAL RELEVANCE

Proteomics, cytomics, and metabolomics

- Expanding range of techniques for assessing immunologically and clinically relevant proteins: electrophoresis, ELISA, bead-based arrays, protein arrays, protein blotting, protein detection by flow cytometry, surface plasmon resonance and mass spectrometry.

- Protein electrophoresis, immunofixation, and nephelometry widely used and relevant for diagnosis, monitoring, and prognostic assessment of patients with monoclonal gammopathies.

- ELISA-based methods used for measurement of specific antibodies and autoantibodies. Most measurements are semi-quantitative and can be variable.

- Multiplex bead-based protein assays permits quantitative assessment of disease-specific autoantibodies, cytokines, vaccine responses (antigen-specific antibodies) in small sample volumes.

- High throughput analysis on protein microarrays allows quantitation and functional characterization of proteins in various contexts—normal vs disease, identification of autoantibodies against a large panel of autoantigens, identification of potential therapeutic targets, and assessment of protein–drug interactions, as examples.

- Functional protein analysis can be performed by surface plasmon resonance or flow cytometry, though the latter is particularly useful in studying proteins in a cellular context, specific for disease or related to therapeutic drug intervention.

- Mass spectrometry used for specific identification of proteins (intact or fragments) in a complex mixture, posttranslational modifications of proteins, as well as quantitative analysis.

- Metabolite profiling useful for early detection of disease, monitoring disease activity, assessing impact of therapeutic agents on disease, measuring organ function, in cancer, transplantation, metabolic disease and other clinical contexts.

Translational research

While there are numerous methods currently available for protein detection, not all of them meet the requirements for clinical diagnostic applications, which include accuracy, speed, large dynamic range of quantitation, high-throughput, and reproducibility among other parameters. Quantitation of immunoglobulins, a mainstay of clinical immunology laboratories, is presently done in most settings by nephelometry; however, unique reagents are required for the detection of each major isotype or subclass. Early studies have revealed the promise of using the mass spectrometry, LC-MS/MS technique, for simultaneous quantitation of IgG immunoglobulin and its related four IgG subclasses using tryptic peptide generation. Initial data have revealed comparable results to nephelometry, and therefore, in the next few years, the approach to protein quantitation is likely to switch from immunoassay formats to mass spectrometry for multiple protein analysis. An additional novel and exciting technique that will emerge as a valuable clinical diagnostic tool in the foreseeable future is the use of mass cytometry, a unique technological juxtaposition of mass spectrometry and flow cytometry.[50] The versatility of flow cytometry for cellular analysis is well recognized; however, it is limited by the number of fluorochrome and laser combinations that can be used for simultaneous detection of multiple cellular proteins or parameters for immunophenotyping and/or function. Mass cytometry overcomes this limitation by using antibodies labeled with lanthanide metals that have stable and unique isotope signatures, and can be used with an Inductively Coupled Plasma-Mass spectrometer (ICP-MS) for cellular analysis by atomic mass spectrometry. This technique has already shown the potential for *ex vivo* cellular characterization in key immunological compartments of the body, as well as the ability to detect intracellular proteins and to analyze bead-arrays with high resolution, quantitative capacity, and the same breadth of dynamic range typically available with mass spectrometry.[50] These new technologies and applications will revolutionize the approach to protein analysis in the clinical immunology laboratory in the next decade.

● ON THE HORIZON

- Mass spectrometric analysis for multiple protein quantitation in the clinical diagnostic context, especially for relatively abundant proteins of immunological interest, such as IgG and subclasses.

- Replacement of immunoassays for quantitation of proteins, such as immunoglobulins, which possess an invariant component (constant region) for detection with tryptic peptides and appropriate databases.

- Enhancement of cellular analysis—phenotyping and function—using a novel combination of mass spectrometry and flow cytometry, a.k.a. mass cytometry.

- Protein detection and quantitation in cellular contexts extended from traditional flow cytometry to mass cytometry.

- Specific analytical and clinical validation design for new diagnostic technologies to facilitate rapid implementation and adoption of novel advances in the clinical immunology laboratory.

References

1. Kipps TJ. Immunoglobulin genes. In: Detrick B, Hamilton RG, Folds JD, editors. Manual of Molecular and Clinical Laboratory Immunology. 7th ed. Washington, DC: ASM Press; 2006. p. 56–68.
2. Homburger HA, Singh RJ. Assessment of proteins of the immune system. In: Rich RR, Fleisher TA, Shearer WA, et al., editors. Clinical immunology: principles and practice. 3 rd ed. Philadelphia: Mosby Elsevier; 2008. p. 1419–34.
3. Whicher JT, Price CP, Spencer K. Immunonephelometric and immunoturbidimetric assays for proteins. Crit Rev Clin Lab Sci 1983;18:213–60.
4. Bradwell AR, Harding SJ, Fourrier NJ, et al. Assessment of monoclonal gammopathies by nephelometric measurement of individual immunoglobulin kappa/lambda ratios. Clin Chem 2009;55:1646–55.
5. Keren D. Protein electrophoresis in clinical diagnosis. London: Arnold; 2003.
6. Keren D, Humphrey R. Clinical indications and applications of serum and urine protein electrophoresis. In: Detrick B, Hamilton R, Folds J, editors. Manual of molecular and clinical laboratory immunology. 7th ed. Washington, DC: ASM Press; 2006. p. 75–87.
7. Katzmann JA, Kyle RA. Immunochemical characterization of immunoglobulins in serum, urine and cerebrospinal fluid. In: Detrick B, Hamilton RG, Folds JD, editors. Manual of molecular and clinical laboratory immunology. 7th ed. Washington, DC: ASM Press; 2006. p. 88–100.
8. Collins A, Colvin R, Nousari C. Immunofluorescence methods in the diagnosis of renal and skin diseases. In: Detrick B, Hamilton R, Folds J, editors. Manual of molecular and clinical laboratory immunology. 7th ed. Washington, DC: ASM Press; 2006. p. 414–23.
9. Tampoia M, Zucano A, Antico A, et al. Diagnostic accuracy of different immunological methods for the detection of antineuronal antibodies in paraneoplastic neurological syndromes. Immunol Invest 2010;39:186–95.
10. Lequin RM. Enzyme immunoassay (EIA)/enzyme-linked immunosorbent assay (ELISA). Clin Chem 2005;51:2415–8.
11. Rissin DM, Kan CW, Campbell TG, et al. Single-molecule enzyme-linked immunosorbent assay detects serum proteins at subfemtomolar concentrations. Nat Biotechnol 2010;28:595–9.
12. Earley MC, Vogt Jr RF, Shapiro HM, et al. Report from a workshop on multianalyte microsphere assays. Cytometry 2002;50:239–42.
13. Hsu HY, Joos TO, Koga H. Multiplex microsphere-based flow cytometric platforms for protein analysis and their application in clinical proteomics—from assays to results. Electrophoresis 2009;30:4008–19.
14. Kettman JR, Davies T, Chandler D, et al. Classification and properties of 64 multiplexed microsphere sets. Cytometry 1998;33:234–43.
15. Elshal MF, McCoy JP. Multiplex bead array assays: performance evaluation and comparison of sensitivity to ELISA. Methods 2006;38:317–23.
16. Famulok M, Hartig JS, Mayer G. Functional aptamers and aptazymes in biotechnology, diagnostics, and therapy. Chem Rev 2007;107:3715–43.
17. Platt M, Rowe W, Wedge DC, et al. Aptamer evolution for array-based diagnostics. Anal Biochem 2009;390:203–5.
18. Colas P. The eleven-year switch of peptide aptamers. J Biol 2008;7:2.
19. Tombelli S, Minunni M, Mascini M. Aptamers-based assays for diagnostics, environmental and food analysis. Biomol Eng 2007;24:191–200.
20. Kersten B, Wanker EE, Hoheisel JD, et al. Multiplex approaches in protein microarray technology. Expert Rev Proteomics 2005;2:499–510.
21. Hultschig C, Kreutzberger J, Seitz H, et al. Recent advances of protein microarrays. Curr Opin Chem Biol 2006;10:4–10.
22. Hall DA, Ptacek J, Snyder M. Protein microarray technology. Mech Ageing Dev 2007;128:161–7.
23. Hartmann M, Roeraade J, Stoll D, et al. Protein microarrays for diagnostic assays. Anal Bioanal Chem 2009;393:1407–16.
24. Wilson DS, Nock S. Recent developments in protein microarray technology. Angew Chem Int Ed Engl 2003;42:494–500.
25. Korf U, Wiemann S. Protein microarrays as a discovery tool for studying protein-protein interactions. Expert Rev Proteomics 2005;2:13–26.
26. Goodrich TT, Wark AW, Corn RM, et al. Surface plasmon resonance imaging measurements of protein interactions with biopolymer microarrays. Methods Mol Biol 2006;328:113–30.
27. Maynard JA, Lindquist NC, Sutherland JN, et al. Surface plasmon resonance for high-throughput ligand screening of membrane-bound proteins. Biotechnol J 2009;4:1542–58.
28. Kurien BT, Scofield RH. Protein blotting: a review. J Immunol Methods 2003;274:1–15.
29. Kurien BT, Scofield RH. Protein blotting and detection: methods and protocols. Humana Press; 2009.
30. Perez OD, Nolan GP. Phospho-proteomic immune analysis by flow cytometry: from mechanism to translational medicine at the single-cell level. Immunol Rev 2006;210:208–28.
31. Yates JR, Ruse CI, Nakorchevsky A. Proteomics by mass spectrometry: approaches, advances, and applications. Annu Rev Biomed Eng 2009;11:49–79.
32. Zhang Z, Pan H, Chen X. Mass spectrometry for structural characterization of therapeutic antibodies. Mass Spectrom Rev 2009;28:147–76.
33. Elliott MH, Smith DS, Parker CE, et al. Current trends in quantitative proteomics. J Mass Spectrom 2009;44:1637–60.
34. Ge F, Tao S, Bi L, et al. Proteomics: addressing the challenges of multiple myeloma. Acta Biochim Biophys Sin (Shanghai) 2010;43:89–95.
35. Barnidge DR, Jelinek DF, Muddiman DC, et al. Quantitative protein expression analysis of CLL B cells from mutated and unmutated IgV(H) subgroups using acid-cleavable isotope-coded affinity tag reagents. J Proteome Res 2005;4:1310–7.
36. Tomazella GG, daSilva I, Thome CH, et al. Analysis of detergent-insoluble and whole cell lysate fractions of resting neutrophils using high-resolution mass spectrometry. J Proteome Res 2010;9:2030–6.
37. Tjalsma H, Schaeps RM, Swinkels DW. Immunoproteomics: From biomarker discovery to diagnostic applications. Proteomics Clin Appl 2008;2:167–80.
38. Dekker LJ, Zeneyedpour L, Brouwer E, et al. An antibody-based biomarker discovery method by mass spectrometry sequencing of complementarity determining regions. Anal Bioanal Chem 2010;399:1081–91.
39. Trost M, Bridon G, Desjardins M, et al. Subcellular phosphoproteomics. Mass Spectrom Rev 2010;29:962–90.
40. Nedelkov D. Integration of SPR biosensors with mass spectrometry (SPR-MS). Methods Mol Biol 2010;627:261–8.
41. Spratlin JL, Serkova NJ, Eckhardt SG. Clinical applications of metabolomics in oncology: a review. Clin Cancer Res 2009;15:431–40.
42. Dunn WB, Bailey NJ, Johnson HE. Measuring the metabolome: current analytical technologies. Analyst 2005;130:606–25.
43. Bictash M, Ebbels TM, Chan Q, et al. Opening up the "Black Box": metabolic phenotyping and metabolome-wide association studies in epidemiology. J Clin Epidemiol 2010;63:970–9.
44. Zhang S, Nagana Gowda GA, Ye T, et al. Advances in NMR-based biofluid analysis and metabolite profiling. Analyst 2010;135:1490–8.
45. Robertson DG. Metabonomics in toxicology: a review. Toxicol Sci 2005;85:809–22.
46. Shlomi T, Cabili MN, Ruppin E. Predicting metabolic biomarkers of human inborn errors of metabolism. Mol Syst Biol 2009;5:263.
47. Gowda GA, Zhang S, Gu H, et al. Metabolomics-based methods for early disease diagnostics. Expert Rev Mol Diagn 2008;8:617–33.
48. Wishart DS. Metabolomics: the principles and potential applications to transplantation. Am J Transplant 2005;5:2814–20.
49. Wishart DS. Metabolomics in monitoring kidney transplants. Curr Opin Nephrol Hypertens 2006;15:637–42.
50. Ornatsky O, Bandura D, Baranov V, et al. Highly multiparametric analysis by mass cytometry. J Immunol Methods 2010;361:1–20.

Flow cytometry

Thomas A. Fleisher, João B. Oliveira

Flow cytometry has become a standard laboratory tool in the evaluation of hematopoietic cells including the identification of leukocyte populations and subpopulations, a method referred to as immunophenotyping. The clinical application of this technology has been facilitated by the development of instruments and data analysis systems suitable for routine use in diagnostic laboratories. In addition, the expanded range of monoclonal antibodies specific for lymphocyte (and other hematopoietic cell) surface antigens directly conjugated to a number of different fluorescent indicators (fluorochromes) provide an extensive panel of reagents that facilitate multicolor (polychromatic) studies.

The clinical needs that pushed this technology relate to the emergence of absolute CD4 T-cell counts as a critical measure for disease assessment and follow-up in managing patients infected with the human immunodeficiency virus (HIV). Flow cytometry applied in the monitoring of HIV infection was followed by the routine application of cell characterization by flow cytometry in the evaluation of lymphoproliferative disorders, and more recently in the study of immunodeficiency disorders and other immune-mediated diseases.

Recent advances in instrumentation and fluorochrome chemistry now allow for routine polychromatic flow cytometry studies, with concomitant assessment of cell surface markers and intracellular parameters, including intracellular proteins, phosphoproteins and cytokines, as well as identification of changes linked to cellular activation and apoptosis. Intracellular flow cytometry also can be applied to evaluate cell cycle status (i.e., G_0-G_1, S, G_2-M) based on DNA staining, useful in evaluating tumor cells and assessing the *in vitro* lymphocyte response to various stimuli. Additonally, evaluation of lymphocyte proliferation can be performed with cell tracking dyes that allow quantitation of the rounds of cell division associated with cell activation. Finally, characterization of antigen-specific T cells following immunization or associated with normal and/or abnormal immune responses in association with disease states can be accomplished using multimer technology as well as intracellular cytokine detection following antigen exposure.

This chapter focuses on basic concepts of flow cytometry including instrument characteristics, data management, lymphocyte gating and directed use of test reagents. In addition, a brief overview of intracellular protein detection, cell activation studies, cell cycle analysis, apoptosis detection and multimer technology is provided, focusing on the appropriate application of these approaches as well as their limitations.

Instrumentation

The basic components of a flow cytometer, as shown in Fig. 94.1, include the illumination source, optical bench, fluidic system, electronics and computer.[1] Briefly, stained cells are focused and flow into single-file by the fluidic system, interrogated by a light source that generates light signals that are collected and directed by the optical system to the photodetectors, which convert light into electronic signals for storage and subsequent analysis. This process is discussed further in the section below.

The fluidic system lies at the heart of a flow cytometer and consists of isotonic sheath fluid that moves the sample stream containing the cells. This is accomplished by injecting the cell sample into the moving sheath fluid, establishing a hydrodynamically focused single-file flow of cells that move through the analysis point while maintaining this cell stream in a constant, central location.[2] The centrally focused cell stream insures that the illumination of all cells is virtually equivalent. Thus, the difference in magnitude of the emission signal(s) generated from each cell reflects biologic differences between the cells (rather than reflecting the variation in the illumination energy if the cells were not tightly focused). The use of hydrodynamic focusing has the additional advantage of producing little or no change in cell shape, although it may have an effect on cell orientation. The consistency in maintaining cell shape facilitates distinguishing "architectural" differences between specific leukocyte types (see Gating section).[3] However, this method can generate single-file cell rows with precision only up to a flow rate of 60 to 100 μl/min, which can lead to long acquisision times for the detection of very rare events. To overcome this problem, recently introduced flow cytometry instruments utilize acoustic focusing, which align cells through the use of sound waves, allowing sample flow rates of up to 1000 μl/min, without loss of signal quality.[4,5]

Illumination in standard clinical instruments is generated by two or three lasers each of which provide a specific monochromatic light source (e.g., a sapphire laser generates a 488 nm wavelength [blue] beam). Modern lasers are small and available in multiple wavelengths, including ultraviolet (350 nm), violet (405 nm), blue (488 nm), green (532 nm), yellow (560 nm), orange (610 nm), and red (633 nm), permitting the simultaneous use of multiple fluorochromes having different excitation requirements.[6,7] The point where the light illuminates the cell in analytical instruments occurs within a flow cell while in cell sorters the beam intersects cells flowing as a stream in air.

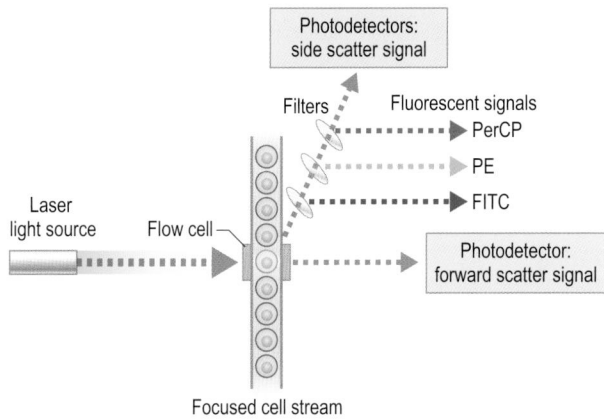

Fig. 94.1 Simplified design of a flow cytometer with one illumination source (laser) set up to collect five parameters. These include the two nonfluorescent parameters (blue light) forward and side scatter, as well as three fluorescent parameters, green (FITC), orange (PE), and red (PerCP) light.

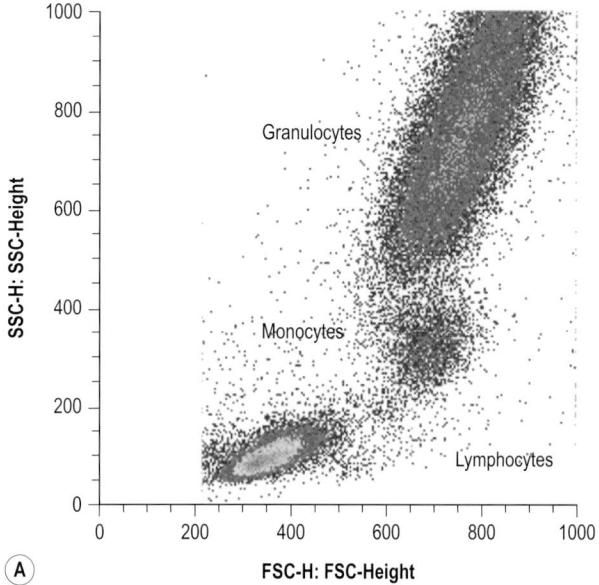

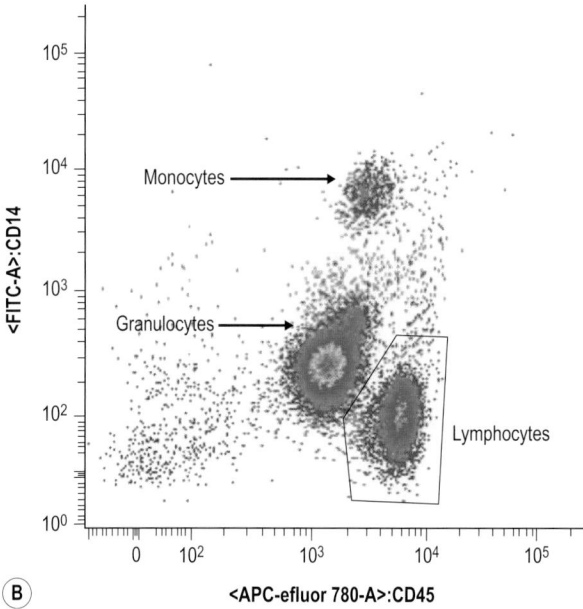

Fig. 94.2 (A) Forward- and side-scatter dot plots on a lysed whole blood sample, demonstrating the basic three-part leukocyte differential with lymphocytes, monocytes, and granulocytes. (B) Dot plot with DC45/CD14 gating reagents showing the fluorescence distribution of all the three leukocyte types identified to include lymphocytes, monocytes, and granulocytes, as well as a small number of nonlysed red blood cells and/or debris.

The optical bench contains lenses that shape and focus the illumination beam to ensure consistent excitation energy at the analysis point.

The illumination of a cell generates both nonfluorescent and fluorescent signals that are collected and measured by optically coupling the signal to a detection system consisting of filters each linked to a photodetector. The filters are chosen to allow the nonfluorescent signals to be measured at the same wavelength as the excitation signal (e.g., 488 nm from a blue light source) for the forward- and side-scatter channels (see Gating section), whereas those for the fluorescence channels specific filters only allow passage of light with wavelengths specific to each fluorochrome (e.g., green, orange or red; see Fluorochrome section). The number and arrangement of the photodetectors allows for the simultaneous evaluation of multiple colors (parameters) for each cell and a recent report described a modified clinical instrument that was capable of evaluating up to 17 colors simultaneously from each cell contained within the sample.[8]

The internal electronics in the flow cytometer provides the system for converting analog light signals (photoelectrons) received at the photodetectors into digital signals for acquisition and storage in a computer. The intensity of these converted signals is measured on a relative scale that is generally set in either 256 or 1024 equal increments (referred to as channels) for display and analysis. A number of specialized analysis programs are available and results are depicted graphically as single-parameter histograms displaying specific light (fluorescence) intensity (x-axis) versus cell number (y-axis) (Fig. 94.2), or two-color displays where the x- and y-axis reflect the light intensity of the two colors while the cell numbers are represented via dot, pseudocolor, contour or density plots (Fig. 94.3). Most analysis programs enable the operator to evaluate the number and percentage of events, mean and/or median channel fluorescence, and selected statistical measures for each identified cell and these can be aggregated into specific populations and/or subpopulations of cells. Thus, a flow cytometer provides a platform with the capacity to assess multiple pieces of discrete information (parameters) generated from each individual cell contained within a large number of cells present in the test sample and these are typically accrued at rates of 1000–2000 (or more) cells per second.

Fluorescence reagents

Standard monoclonal antibody reagents for clinical use are typically directly conjugated to a fluorochrome, a dye that absorbs and emits light of different wavelengths based on the energy lost during the return of excited electrons to their ground state associated with the illumination by a specific wavelength of light. Thus, the emitted light has a longer wavelength (lower energy) than the wavelength of the excitation beam. The number of commercially available fluorochromes has increased dramatically in the past few years, with the routine use of dye conjugates and instruments with three or more lasers.[7] Commonly used fluorochromes in

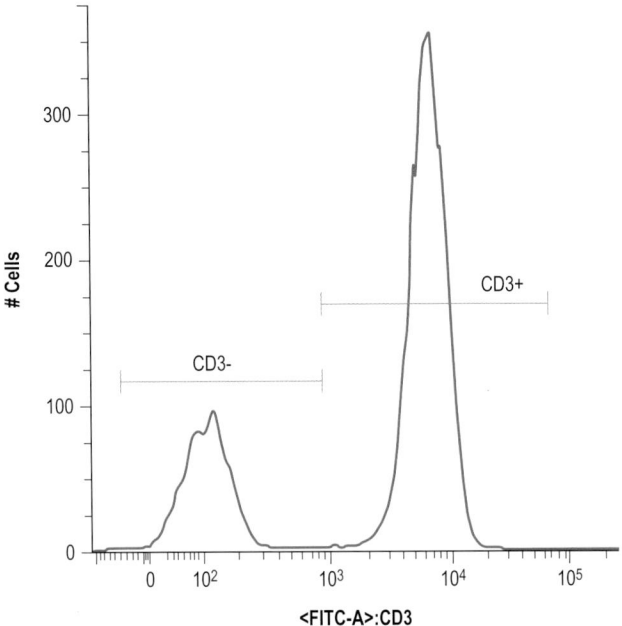

Fig. 94.3 Single-parameter histogram for CD3 expression on lymphocytes demonstrating the negative non-T-cell population (B cells, NK cells) and a positive T-cell population. Integrating the area under each curve would provide the numbers and percentage of cells present in each respective subpopulation.

Data Analysis

Gating

● KEY CONCEPTS

Gating

- Method for defining cell population of interest.
- Typically performed using forward and side scatter.
- Should be confirmed with gating reagents (anti-CD45 and anti-CD14 for lymphocytes and monocytes).

The proper assessment of specific cell types within a mixture requires initial identification of lineage-specific cells, an approach referred to as gating. In practical terms, immunophenotyping focused on lymphocytes requires minimizing the nonlymphocytes included in the evaluation and this is accomplished by lymphocyte gating. The standard sample for clinical studies is anticoagulated whole blood and directing the study to lymphocytes requires eliminating the great majority of non-lymphocytes from the collected data such that the expression of a percentage for a specific cell subpopulation is an accurate measurement. Without gating the data can also be negatively impacted by co-expression of surface antigens on different cell lineages (e.g., CD4 is found on lymphocytes and monocytes at differing density). In addition, nonspecific binding of monoclonal reagents through Fcγ receptors and the level of cytophilic human immunoglobulin varies between cell types, making appropriate gating crucial to generate valid data. These techniques are also used to focus the evaluation on other hematopoietic cells including monocytes, granulocytes, eosinophils, erythrocytes and platelets.

Initial gating to focus on a specific leukocyte population typically involves using the two nonfluorescent parameters, forward angle (low angle, FSC) and side (90°, SSC) light scatter (Fig. 94.2A).[3] Forward scatter is a reflection of cellular cross-sectional area (direct relationship to cell size) and refractile index, whereas side scatter is an indication of the cellular granularity and surface irregularity. The combination of these two nonfluorescent parameters provides a three part differential that distinguishes between normal lymphocytes, monocytes and granulocytes (in the absence of contaminating red blood cells and platelets). As can be seen in Fig. 94.2A, among leukocytes, lymphocytes have the lowest forward and side scatter, monocytes have higher forward and side scatter and granulocytes have the greatest side scatter. This method is effective in distinguishing a relatively pure population of lymphocytes under most circumstances. However, the presence of nucleated red cells, large platelets, basophils or other particulate debris can produce contaminating events (cells) within this "lymphocyte gate." Furthermore, malignant lymphoid cells may not fit into the previously outlined standard light scatter patterns.

A method for confirming the integrity of the light scatter-based lymphocyte gate uses the directly conjugated monoclonal reagents anti-CD45 and anti-CD14.[16] These "gating reagents" more accurately identify the three-part differential. Lymphocytes have the highest level of CD45 binding but are negative for CD14; granulocytes have a lower level of CD45 binding and an intermediate level of CD14 expression; and monocytes have high levels of both CD45 and CD14 expression (Fig. 94.2B). Importantly, non-leukocytes, including erythrocytes

clinical immunophenotyping include the organic dyes fluorescein isothiocyanate (FITC), phycoerythrin (PE), peridin chlorophyll protein (PerCP), and allophycocyanin (APC). Conjugations of PE and APC to cyanines (Cy5, Cy5.5, and Cy7) and Alexa Fluor dyes produce tandem dyes with additional emmission spectra, based on energy transfer from one fluorochrome to the second fluorochrome serving as the source of emitted light. This allows for the simultaneous evaluation of 6 to 8 colors in most current clinical instruments with only two or three lasers.

One recent advance in the field was the development of a new class of inorganic fluorescent semiconductor nanocrystals, named quantum dots (QDs).[9,10] These particles are perfectly suited for polychromatic flow cytometry, as they have broad excitation spectra (525-800 nm) and sharp, discrete emission spectra, that varies depending on their core size.[10] This means that quantum dots of different sizes (and consequently of different colors) can be excited by the same laser source, allowing simpler multiplexing.[11] In addition, quantum dots have high quantum yield, high molar extinction coefficients, and extraordinary resistance to photo- and chemical degradation. These qualities make them perfectly suitable for use in biological studies, including intracellular *in vivo* imaging, fluorescence resonance energy transfer (FRET) analysis and dynamic imaging of single proteins for longer periods of time.[9]

Additional dyes are available for functional studies and include calcium-sensitive dyes (e.g., fluo-3), glutathione-sensitive dyes (e.g., monochlorbimane) and H_2O_2-responsive dyes (e.g., dihydrorhodamine 123).[12,13] Assessment of DNA content can be performed with dyes that intercalate double-stranded DNA and RNA, including propidium iodide and ethidium bromide.[14] In addition there are ultraviolet-excited dyes that are highly specific for DNA, including Hoechst 33258 and 4,6-diamidino-2-phenylindole (DAPI); acridine orange is used for simultaneous staining of DNA/RNA.[15]

and platelets, are negative for these markers. In addition, malignant leukocytes that have characteristics of early precursor cells often have altered CD45 and/or CD14 expression. Gating reagents provide a reliable means of checking the light scatter-based lymphocyte gate for the frequency of nonlymphocytes within the gate as well as the extent of lymphocyte exclusion from the gate. Guidelines for an acceptable degree of contamination within the lymphocyte gate, as well as the level of lymphocyte exclusion, are contained within the US Clinical and Laboratory Standards Institute (formerly the National Committee for Clinical Laboratory Standards) guideline for lymphocyte immunophenotyping.[17] With the expanded use of polychromatic flow cytometry, some centers now include anti-CD45 in every tube to refine the gate and prevent cell contamination that cannot be excluded using the standard non-fluorescent parameters (forward and side scatter) for gating.

Data display

The simplest method for demonstrating flow cytometry data is the single-parameter histogram (Fig. 94.2), a graphic presentation of cell number on the *y*-axis versus fluorescence (light) intensity from a single fluorochrome on the *x*-axis. Integration of curve areas provides the number of cells and often there are two distinct distributions, one referred to as negative identifies cells that are not bound specifically by the monoclonal reagent and the second represents cells bound by the antibody. Negative actually reflects low-level fluorescence resulting from cellular autofluorescence together with any nonspecific binding of the monoclonal reagent(s), the magnitude of both phenomena varies between different cell types. The interpretation of the data is simplified when there are two distinct cell populations (i.e., negative

and positive) while the evaluation of two overlapping distributions is more difficult.

Multicolor data can be evaluated using a series of single-parameter histograms that consider each fluorochrome independently. However, it is more informative to present two parameters simultaneously using a correlated display (Fig. 94.4), and two-color displays are recommended for clinical flow cytometry.[18] This approach enables the simultaneous visualization of four different populations: A^+/B^-, A^-/B^+, A^+/B^+ and A^-/B^-. More recently, these displays evolved to include a mixture of logarithmic (for higher intensity expression) and linear (for lower intensity expression) intensity for each axis in order to allow for better interpretation of events with very low, zero or negative fluorescence. This combined display approach resolves the previous problem of a large number of events being displayed compacted against the axes even with properly compensated samples and will be used in the illustrations throughout this chapter.[19]

The simultaneous use of *n* monoclonal reagents can identify a total of 2^n subpopulations. These different subsets can be identified sequentially by first dividing the cells into those that are positive versus those that are negative with one reagent and then evaluating the defined subpopulations for the remaining two reagents using a two-color approach. Alternatively, more modern software can represent multiple populations as polychromatic plots, which can simplify data analysis.[20] The polychromatic approach can provide a means to further resolve subpopulations, and has been particularly useful in the evaluation of cellular differentiation, activation and functional correlates as well as clarifying overlapping cell subpopulations.

Positive–negative discrimination

The evaluation of clinical immunophenotyping data requires establishing criteria for the boundaries between negative or nonstained cells and positive (stained) cells. A commonly used approach involves using directly conjugated control monoclonal antibodies of the appropriate class or subclass (e.g., IgG1, IgG2a, IgG2b, or IgM) that do not specifically react with human lymphocyte surface antigens (commonly called "isotype controls"). The marker (discriminator) is set at the fluorescence histogram channel number such that it includes 98 to 99% of the negative cells (Fig. 94.5A).

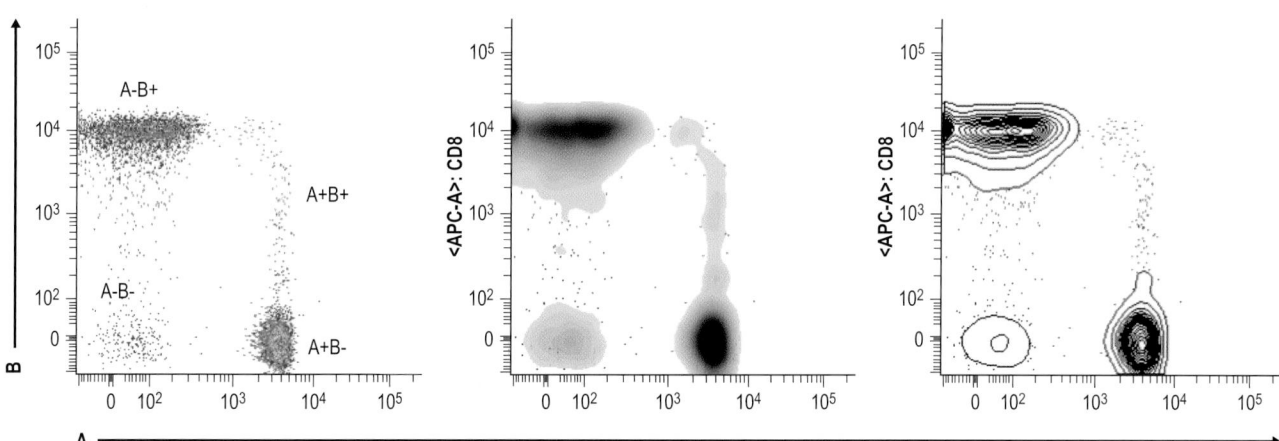

Fig. 94.4 Examples of dot pseudocolor (left), density (middle), and contour (right) displays based on the same two-color data. All three techniques enable simultaneous evaluation of both parameters, in this case evaluating the expression of markers A and B. These plots identify four populations of cells, those expressing only A or B, those expressing both A and B (very few), and those expressing neither A nor B.

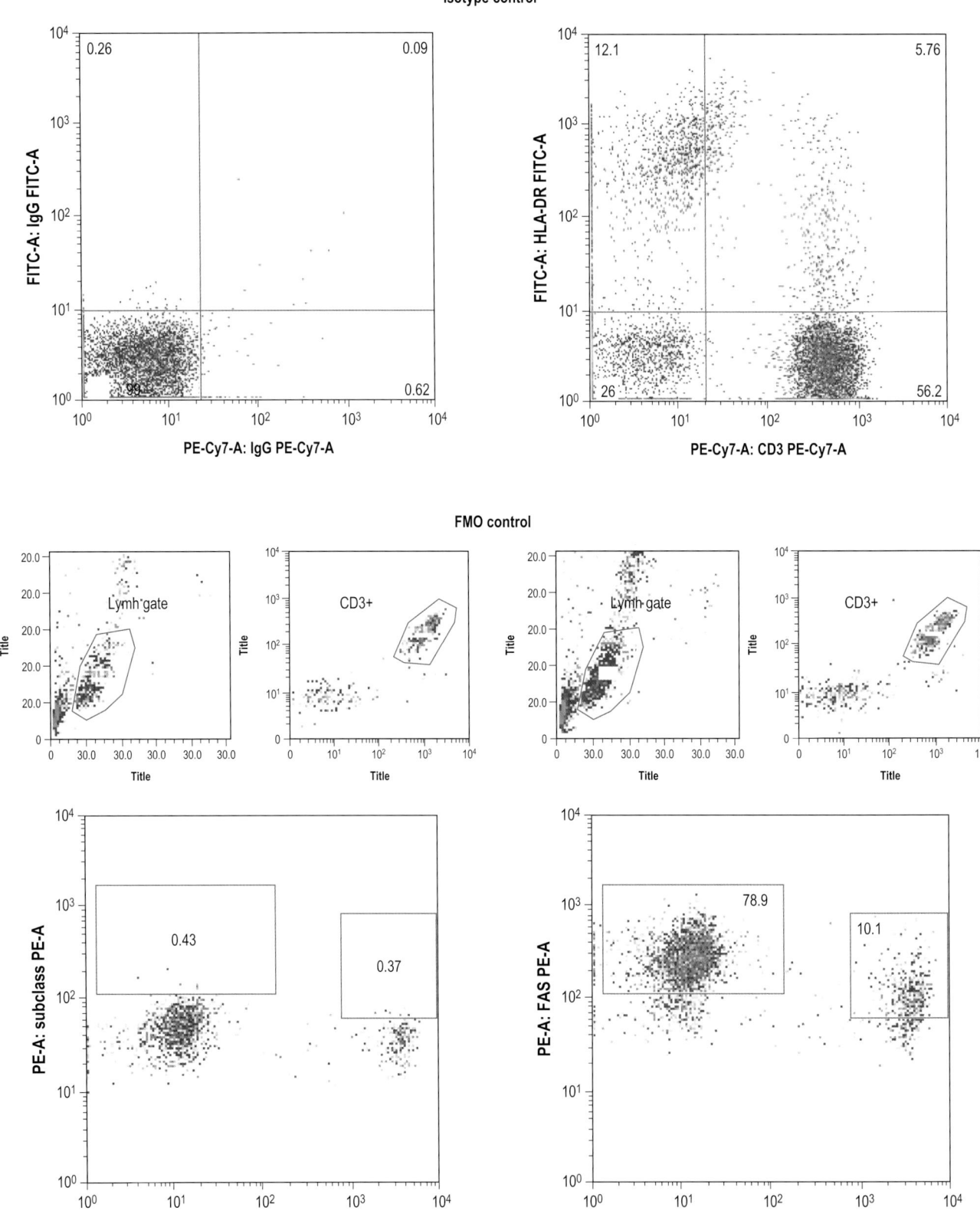

Fig. 94.5 Positive–negative discrimination strategies. (A) Non-specific antibodies (isotypes) were used to stain the sample shown on left and the positivity threshold determined and applied to the sample on the right. (B) The positivity threshold was determined by staining the sample on the left with the population-specific markers (CD3, TCRαβ, and CD8) and omitting FAS. The panel on the right contains FAS. Note that the positivity threshold is slightly different for CD8+ and CD8− cells.

As previously noted, negative refers to the aggregate of baseline cellular autofluorescence plus nonspecific reagent binding, and this can vary according to the cell type. For this reason, the use of isotype controls may not correctly identify the positive-negative threshold for specific cell types, particularly when staining dimly expressed proteins. Additionally, to perfectly mimic the specific antibody used, the isotype control would need to have the same antibody to fluorochome ratio and brightness, something that is not easily accomplished. To overcome these difficulties, an alternative method for positive-negative discrimination has been developed and called Fluorescence-minus-One (FMO).[21]

FMO involves the staining of the sample with all the antibodies of interest, except the one targeted for positive-negative threshold. As an example, if one wanted to define the negative threshold for the protein FAS (CD95) in CD8[+] and CD8[-] T cells, the FMO control tube would include the cell subset-specific markers (CD3, TCRαβ, and CD8), and omit anti-FAS. After appropriate gating on that population, the threshold can be adequately defined, and it is different for the two exemplified populations (Fig. 94.5B, right panel). One obvious limitation of this method is the higher cost, given that multiple control tubes need to be set up for each sample.

Compensation

The fluorescence signals emitted by different fluorochromes are not completely separated by the filters. This can lead to signal overlap that is corrected by electronic subtraction of the overlapping signal, a process referred to as compensation. The overlap is particularly significant when using multiple fluorochromes, each with different spectral properties.[21] The compensation process involves subtraction of the "spillover" signal detected by the photodector generated by samples stained with only one fluorochromre. Currently, most flow cytometry analysis software allows for off-line compensation, where the single reagent stained tubes are used to create a compensation matrix that is then applied to all the tubes in the experiment. This allows for much simplified compensation procedures, without the need for any hardware compensation during data collection.

Quality control

Quality control is a critical component of clinical flow cytometry to ensure optimal results.[22] This includes monitoring instrument setup and performance, optimizing sample preparation and reagents and standardizing controls and data interpretation. Quantitative flow cytometry based on a fluorescence standard curve provides quantitative data in units referred to as molecular equivalents of soluble fluorochrome (MESF). When properly constructed standard curves are used, quantitative data for different reagents can be generated and compared. Finally, participation in interlaboratory proficiency testing surveys, such as the triannual samples provided by the College of American Pathologists (CAP), is an important additional measure to monitor laboratory performance, and this is mandated in US clinical laboratories by the Clinical Laboratory Improvement Amendment of 1988 (CLIA 88).

Methods

Whole-blood lysis represents the most common technique used for sample preparation and consists of mixing a fixed volume of anticoagulated whole blood (or bone marrow) with one or more directly conjugated monoclonal antibodies, followed by incubation at a designated temperature and time.[23,24] Next the red blood cells are lysed, the sample is washed and then run into the flow cytometer, usually following fixation in paraformaldehyde to reduce the infectious risk. The nonlysed cells remaining include all peripheral blood leukocytes, as well as any nonlysed red cells, platelets and debris. The heterogeneity of the sample necessitates careful lymphocyte gating (see section above) in order to generate accurate immunophenotyping data. The advantages of the whole-blood lysis method include fewer preparation steps, less sample handling, and a lower likelihood of differential lymphocyte loss. This last point can occur when density gradient techniques are used to prepare mononuclear cells for analysis. Alternative sources of cells (e.g., bronchial alveolar lavage fluid, fine-needle aspirates) can also be evaluated with flow cytometry.[25] Patient studies must be determined with the same methods and reagents as used in the determination of the control ranges to ensure comparability. The number of events (cells) analyzed typically ranges from 10 000-20 000 in routine clinical studies but must be increased when evaluating very small subpopulations of cells in order to produce statistically relevant data necessary in rare event analysis.

The application of control ranges must take into account the fact that significant changes take place in lymphocyte distribution and development during childhood, as well as changes in lymphocytes that occur among the very elderly.[26,27] There are also immunophenotypic differences induced by drugs, including tobacco products, such that information on current medications should be obtained whenever possible.[28] Other factors can also have an impact on lymphocyte distribution, including race, gender, diurnal variation and recent or intercurrent infection.[29]

The choice of immunophenoptyping reagents depends on the cells being targeted for study and the question being asked. However, regardless of the specific set-up, the inclusion of a tube with gating reagents (anti-CD45 and anti-CD14) to confirm the integrity of the standard lymphocyte gate is recommended.[16] In addition, control reagents should be included to establish the fluorescence intensity of negative cells. Important controls that provide an internal control include a pan-T-, B-, and NK-cell marker for every sample (Table 94.1), based on the principle that the whole is the sum of its parts. Thus, the total percentage of lymphocytes in the gate determined by the gating reagents, should approximately equal the sum of the percentages for T, B, and NK cells. A technical or biological explanation must be identified when this relationship does not hold. Biological

Table 94.1 Selected lymphocyte surface antigens for immunophenotyping

T cells
Pan-T cell: CD3, CD2, CD7, CD5 Major T-cell subset: CD4, CD8 Surface antigens associated with function: CD28, CD38, CD45RA, CD45RO, CD62L Activation antigens: CD25, CD40L, CD69, CD71, HLA-DR

B cells
Pan-B cell: CD19, CD20, surface immunoglobulin Major B-cell subset: CD5, CD21 Surface antigens associated with function: CD27, CD40 Activation antigens: CD23, CD25

NK cells
Pan-NK cell: CD16, CD56 NK subset: CD2, CD8, CD57

explanations for a significant difference would include the presence of immature or malignant cells that were not identified by standard pan-T-, B-, and NK-cell reagents. In addition, if the gating reagents (CD45/CD14) had not been included, contaminating cells (e.g., myeloid precursors, nucleated red blood cells, large platelets) with forward- and side-scatter characteristics similar to those of lymphocytes could not be ruled out. Potential technical problems include reagent or fluorochrome degradation, failure to add a reagent, and a host of others. Evidence for any major technical error should result in repeating the study.

Additional data that can be used for controls depend on the set-up. For example, the availability of multiple antibodies that identify a similar cell sub-population can serve as a useful check (e.g., total T cells by comparing CD3 and CD5 or CD2; total B cells by comparing CD19 and CD20). In addition, the use of specific reagents in more than one tube enables comparison between the repeat values as a measure of consistency. The application of internal checks should be performed by the flow operator as a simple means of confirming the validity of the data. Insights regarding unusual biological findings may also be uncovered through this type of evaluation (e.g., the presence of an increased population of $CD4^-/CD8^-$ double-negative T cells).[30]

The challenge in performing immunophenotyping is to accurately identify cells with specific surface characteristics (antigens). As previously noted, the capacity to discriminate cell subpopulations is often enhanced through the directed use of antibody combinations. The typical data generated consist of the percentage of negative versus positive cells when using one reagent, and multiple subpopulations when using more than one reagent. Regardless of the experimental design, it is important to consider not only the percentage of cells within each subpopulation, but also the absolute number of cells. This is most commonly obtained by multiplying the relevant percentage from the flow cytometer by the absolute lymphocyte count obtained using a white blood count and differential. For example, when assaying for CD4 T-cell counts, the percentage of $CD4^+$ cells is multiplied by the peripheral absolute lymphocyte count to yield the absolute CD4 count. A potential problem with this approach is the requirement for two separate procedures (i.e., dual platforms) to generate the final result. This introduces the possibility of additive error, based on the inherent errors of the two different methods. It also has fueled a search for approaches that facilitate performing both tasks by flow cytometry (i.e., a single platform). One alternative involves the inclusion of a fixed number of fluorescent beads (in a defined volume) in each tube as a reference standard to generate absolute numbers without requiring the use of the complete blood count and differential to generate a lymphocyte count. A recently introduced approach involves the use of impedance based cell counting in the flow cytometer to generate an absolute lymphocyte count (dependent on a fixed volume of sample being run) and then generating both percentage and absolute number of cells in each specific population or subpopulation. Regardless of the approach, the reporting of both percentages and absolute numbers is necessary when immunophenotyping peripheral lymphocytes.

The objective of evaluating malignant cells is often to characterize the lineage and differentiation level of the abnormal cells, rather than quantifying subpopulations. The pattern of reactivity combined with fluorescence intensity is often useful in identifying leukemic patterns, whereas the absolute number of cells may not be required. However, flow cytometric detection and quantitation of rare abnormal cells can be useful in evaluating for minimal residual disease in lymphoproliferative disorders.

Practical applications of flow cytometry

Immunophenotyping studies

⬤ CLINICAL RELEVANCE

Immunophenotyping studies

- Can be used to identify cell subsets, lineage, stage of cell differentiation, state of cell activation, and clonality.
- Lymphocyte results should be checked with T cells + B cells + NK cells = 100%.
- Immunophenotyping studies are not the equivalent of lymphocyte function studies.

The majority of immunophenotyping studies are directed at quantifying specific cell subpopulations, evaluating for the presence or absence of particular surface antigens, identifying the differentiation level of specific cells, determining cell lineage, evaluating for functional correlates based on specific antigen expression, examining for evidence of cell activation, and/or establishing monoclonality.

Quantification of a particular cell subpopulation can be readily accomplished with flow cytometry. The evaluation of absolute CD4 T-cell counts has formed the basis for monitoring patients infected with HIV.[31] The quantitation of $CD34^+$ hematopoietic stem cells in donor peripheral blood or bone marrow is used in many cellular reconstitution protocols.[32] Subpopulation characterization can also be useful in the evaluation of patients with clinical history and laboratory findings suggestive of immune deficiency.[33] These studies identify the presence or absence of cells and surface proteins associated with specific functional attributes, but do not assess the actual functional status of the cells. This point is clearly illustrated by the finding of normal B-cell numbers in most patients with common variable immune deficiency despite the fact that these patients fail to produce immunoglobulins normally.[34] However, changes in the characteristics of the B cells, particularly relative to memory B cells, provides potential insight into different phenotypes of this disorder and provides additional support for heterogeneity of patients with this disorder.[34] Due to the limitations of immunophenotyping, it is common practice when evaluating the status of the immune system to perform cell function testing in parallel.

Flow cytometry can be used to test for the presence or absence of a specific cell surface antigen. An example of this type of application is in the evaluation of a patient with a history of recurrent skin infections, delayed wound healing and persistent granulocytosis, which suggests a diagnosis of leukocyte adhesion deficiency type 1.[33,35] This disorder results from a defect in the gene encoding CD18, preventing the expression of three different heterodimeric adhesion molecules (β2 integrins) each containing CD18 (Chapter 21). This disorder can usually be diagnosed by studying granulocytes (and lymphocytes) for the expression of CD18 (as well as the three isoforms of CD11). Patients often have decreased rather than absent CD18 expression and confirmation of the diagnosis can be accomplished by demonstrating a failure of CD18 (and CD11a, 11b, 11c) upregulation following granulocyte activation.[33]

The directed use of a panel of monoclonal reagents can help address questions regarding the level of cell differentiation.

Antibodies specific to proteins expressed by early (precursor) cells represent one approach, and would include evaluating for the thymocyte marker CD1, or the pre-B-cell marker CD10 (CALLA). However, many surface antigens are expressed throughout differentiation. Examples of these include CD2 and CD7 found on thymocytes and circulating T cells, or CD19 and HLA-DR found on pre-B cells as well as B cells. Thus the pattern of surface antigen expression can also help distinguish the level of differentiation. Defining the developmental level of a particular cell population or subpopulation is best accomplished using a panel of reagents that span the natural history of the cell lineage. This approach represents the standard for testing leukemias and lymphomas enabling the improved classification of the malignant cells relative to prognosis and therapy. Focusing on the presence or absence of specific antigens also involves evaluating the level of expression, which may be altered in the abnormal cells. In addition, malignant cells may express antigens associated with different lineages, such that lineage-directed studies can provide insight into shared expression of specific antigens. Malignant cells may also have altered forward- and side-scatter characteristics, as well as diminished or absent CD45 expression. Thus, the approach to gating may have to be modified when studying hematopoietic malignancies.

Issues of monoclonality can be dealt with using flow cytometry when analyzing B cells, and in some circumstances when studying T cells. Normally B cells are a heterogeneous mixture of mutually exclusive κ or λ light-chain-positive cells. The distribution of light-chain expression can be evaluated for clonal excess using a method called the Komogorov–Smirnov D value comparison.[36,37] Light-chain clonal excess will usually be accompanied by an excess in B cells expressing one particular heavy chain (α, γ, μ, or ε). The capacity to evaluate T-cell monoclonality by flow cytometry is less definitive and consists of using T-cell antigen receptor β-variable (Vβ) chain-specific reagents looking for evidence of significant over representation of one Vβ chain family. This approach currently consists of setting up a number of tubes each with three different Vβ family-specific monoclonal antibodies, one conjugated with FITC, one with PE, and the third with FITC plus PE. This combination enables distinguishing the frequency of each of the three different Vβ families per tube (green⁺, orange⁺, green⁺/orange⁺) and represents a flow cytometric method to complement PCR-based spectratyping.[38]

The state of lymphoid activation can be addressed by evaluating for the presence of surface antigens that either are found only on activated cells or are upregulated following activation. These include receptors for specific growth factors (e.g., IL-2 receptor α chain, CD25), receptors for critical elements required for cell growth (e.g., transferrin receptor, CD71), ligands that are critical for cell–cell communication following activation (CD40 ligand [CD152] on activated CD4 T cells), and surface antigens that are upregulated as a result of activation (e.g., adhesion molecules, HLA-DR, CD69). In addition, the memory status of both T cells and B cells can be assessed based on differential surface molecule expression associated with prior antigen encounter. This enables a distinction to be made between naïve T cells that express CD45RA, CD62L and CXCR7 from memory T cells that express the alternative CD45 isoform, CD45RO (and varied CD62L or CXCR7, depending on whether the cells are central or effector memory cells).[39] In addition, memory B cells can be detected by the expression of CD27 and be further divided into isotype-switched and non-switched memory cells based on their pattern of surface immunoglobulin expression.[34,40]

Intracellular evaluation

Cellular activation

> ● **CLINICAL RELEVANCE**
>
> **Intracellular flow cytometry**
>
> - Activation-directed studies:
>   - Calcium flux
>   - Intracellular protein phosphorylation
>   - Oxidative burst: neutrophils
> - Intracellular cytokine studies:
>   - Clarify the Th1/Th2/Th17 status of an immune response
>   - Can be assessed in an *in vitro* antigen-specific response
>   - Can be combined with evaluation of cell surface studies

Ligand binding and transmembrane signal transduction resulting in cellular activation can be evaluated using flow cytometry. Changes in intracellular ionic calcium concentration (Ca^{2+}) are frequently used to monitor cell activation after ligand binding. These changes are associated with the activation of phospholipase C and protein kinase C. In general, three reagents have been used to measure Ca^{2+}: quin 2, indo-1, and fluo-3. Quin 2 has a low excitation coefficient and is not useful for flow cytometry; indo-1 requires ultraviolet excitation; fluo-3 can be excited by 488 nm but does not permit ratiometric analysis. Nevertheless, because of its ease of use fluo-3 is currently the most widely used probe for intracytoplasmic Ca^{2+} evaluation by flow cytometry. Strict attention must be paid to loading conditions, the presence or absence of free Ca^{2+} in the medium, experimental temperature, baseline measurements and calibration. This approach can be combined with cell surface marker or cell cycle evaluation.[12]

Intracellular pH changes related to cellular activation also can be evaluated. The most useful probe for pH is SNARF-1.[12] This probe can be excited at 488 nm and allows for ratiometric analysis with detection wavelengths set for 575 and 640 nm. Glutathione (glutamylcysteinylglycine, GSH) is an important antioxidant generated during cell activation that can be measured by flow cytometry.[12] The fluorescent probe monochlorobimane is commonly used for this measurement, but it is complicated by the need to determine GSH by an independent method such as HPLC.

Additional approaches to evaluate cellular activation include assessment of intranuclear markers (Ki-67, PCNA) as well as surface proteins that are upregulated following cellular activation (e.g., CD69, CD25, CD71).[41] Actual cell division can be evaluated using lipophilic membrane dyes (e.g., PKH26, CFSE) also referred to as cell tracking dyes that lose 50% of their fluorescence with each round of cell division.[42] This approach has become more common in the clinical assessment of lymphocyte function due to the capacity to evaluate specific lymphocyte subpopulations responding to mitogenic and antigenic stimuli. Lipophilic membrane dyes also can be used to label target cells in cell-based cytotoxicity assays.[43] Recently, an approach to evaluate lymphocyte proliferation following cell stimulation has been described using the thymidine analog, EdU. Detection of DNA sythesis induced by the different activating agents is measured using a copper-catalyzed click chemistry, which results in EdU being covalently bonded to a fluorescent azide.[44] This approach allows the assessment of cell proliferation at the cell population or subpopulation (e.g., CD4, CD8) level and can be used in association with mitogen and recall-antigen stimulation.

Functional evaluation of cell activation can be accomplished with flow cytometry directed detection of the generation of phosphorylated intracellular proteins associated with specific activation signals. An example of this is the detection of phosphorylated STAT-1 following interferon-γ stimulation of monocytes, which has been found to be more sensitive than immunoblotting.[45] This type of assay requires fixation and permeabilization to allow the entry of the specific reagent and now has been extended to a number of additional intracellular proteins that are phosphorylated following exposure of selected cells to specific stimuli. Currently, a number of intracellular signaling proteins that undergo phosphorylation following a specific activation signal can be assessed with flow cytometry using commercially available reagents in kit form.

The assessment of oxidative burst following cell stimulation plays a central role in neutrophil function testing using the hydrogen peroxide-sensitive dye dihydrorhodamine 123 (DHR123). This procedure involves loading granulocytes with the dye, stimulating with phorbol myristate acetate (PMA), and evaluating for fluorescence by flow cytometry.[13,46] This test has proved to be extremely accurate in diagnosing patients with chronic granulomatous disease (CGD) and carriers of X-linked CGD.[46] A major advantage is its sensitivity, which allows the detection of one normal cell in a population of 1000 abnormal cells. This makes assessment of oxidative burst a useful tool in following allogeneic granulocyte survival after transfusion into patients with CGD, as well as a means of following donor chimerism in the setting of allogeneic stem cell transplantation and as a indicator of cell correction following gene therapy in CGD.[47]

Intracellular cytokine detection

Flow cytometry affords a platform to evaluate cytokine production at a single-cell level using cytokine-specific directly conjugated monoclonal antibodies following fixation and permeabilization of cells.[48] This approach allows for the simultaneous detection of two or more intracellular cytokines in combination with cell surface markers, or other intracellular markers. Important aspects of intracellular cytokine detection include the use of a protein transport inhibitor during activation, the use of proper controls and the choice of antibodies. As there is little or no spontaneous cytokine production in circulating human lymphocytes, intracellular cytokine detection requires *in vitro* activation. Initial experience was based on supraphysiological stimulation using PMA and ionomycin, but antigen-specific activation systems have also proven to be feasible. It should be emphasized that, regardless of the activation method, the duration of activation is an important variable, as individual cells reach maximum cytokine production at different times. In addition, different cytokines have different optimal periods of activation. It is recommended that a proper kinetic profile be established for the biological system or clinical condition being studied.[48]

To increase the amount of intracellular cytokines, inhibitors of intracellular protein transport (e.g., monensin or brefeldin) are commonly used, which lead to the accumulation of proteins within the cell. Nonspecific binding of the antibody reagents is an issue, as permeabilization allows access not only to the cytokine of interest, but also to other proteins present in much greater quantities than on the cell surface. In addition, fixation further increases nonspecific binding and the use of both a negative-control sample, which contains an excess of unlabeled or "cold"

anticytokine antibody, and a subclass-matched or FMO-control sample provide the optimal control. When the conjugated anticytokine is added to the negative-control sample it can only bind to other proteins in a nonspecific manner, thereby providing a measure to discriminate between specific and nonspecific binding.[39] The use of directly conjugated anticytokine antibodies not only simplifies the staining procedure, but also provides the best distinction between specific and nonspecific binding. Because the fixation agent may change the native state of certain epitopes, it is also important to use antibodies that recognize antigens after fixation when combining cell surface characterization with intracellular cytokine evaluation.

One of the main applications of intracellular cytokine detection by flow cytometry has been the study and refinement of the Th1/Th2/Th17 paradigms. It has recently become clear that the regulated secretion of cytokines can be used to study

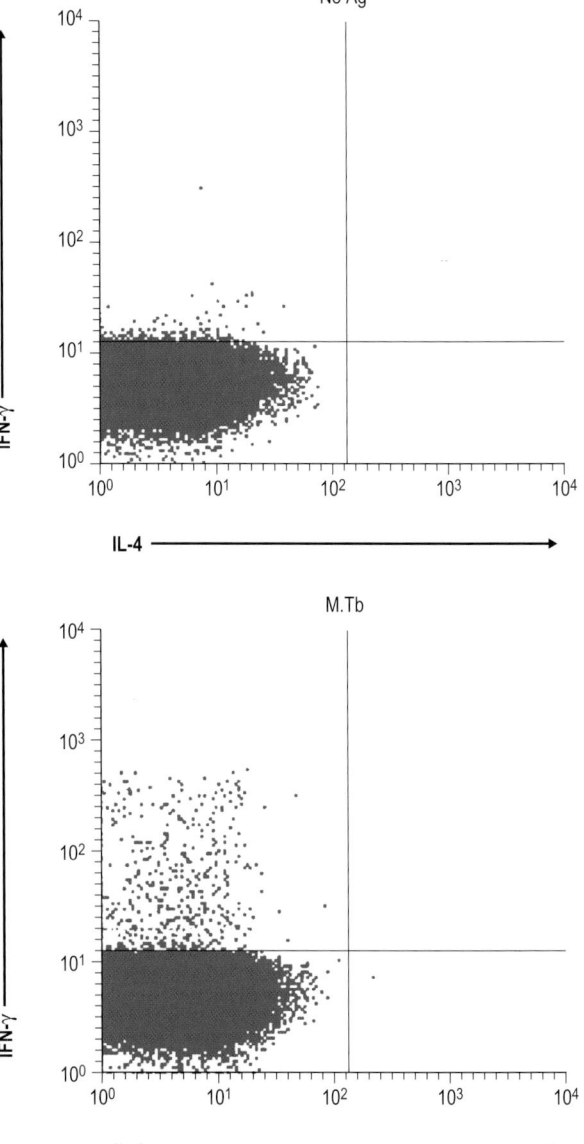

Fig. 94.6 Two-color dot plots of CD3⁺ T cells evaluated for intracytoplasmic interferon-γ and IL-4 expression. The donor had a positive skin test to PPD and demonstated a Th1 pattern of cytokine expression (interferon-γ) in response to *Mycobacterium tuberculosis* antigen, with an absence of a Th2 cytokine pattern (IL-4). Courtesy of Calman Prussin, MD.

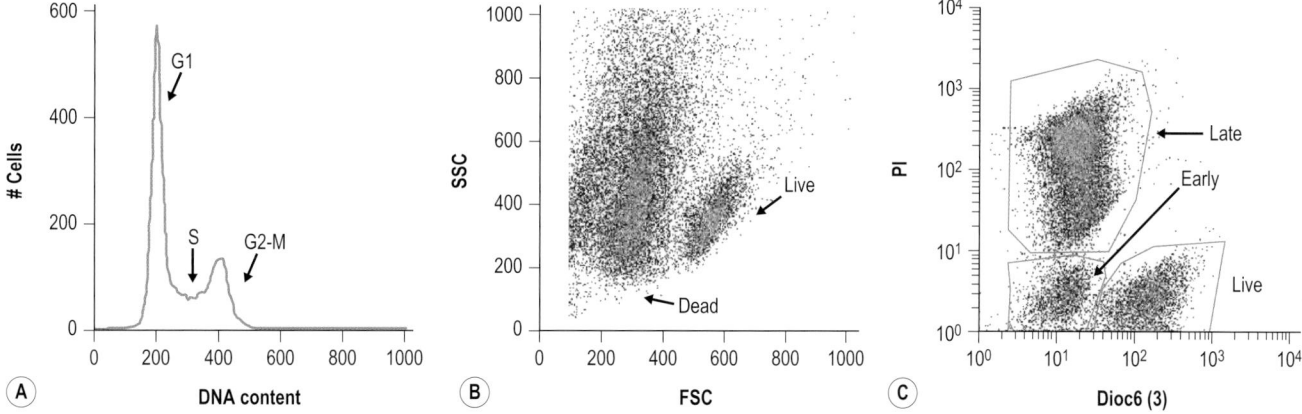

Fig. 94.7 (A) Assessment of DNA content as a reflection of cell cycle demonstrating cells in G₁, S, and G₂/M phases. (B) Assessment of live versus dead cells based on forward- and side-scatter characteristics. (C) Assessment of cell apoptosis using PI and Dioc6(3) identifying cells that recently initiated apoptosis (early), cells that are dead (late) and cells that are alive (live).

the response of individual T cells to both polyclonal stimuli and specific antigens. Measuring antigen-specific T-cell cytokine expression in response to specific antigen offers a useful alternative to the tetramer-based approach (discussed below) to quantify the frequency of antigen-specific T cells (Fig. 94.6).[49]

Cell cycle analysis

⬤ CLINICAL RELEVANCE

Cell cycle analysis

- Useful for screening percentage of S phase and aneuploidy
- Can be combined with cell surface studies
- Can be combined with markers of apoptosis

In addition to surface immunophenotyping and cytoplasmic characterization, flow cytometry is also used in cell cycle analysis. Propidium iodide (PI) is the most commonly used fluorochrome, owing to its optimal linear DNA-binding capacity in a variety of different cell types. Thus, a single-parameter histogram of DNA content using PI readily permits the determination of cell cycle compartments, expressed as the percentage of cells in G₀–G₁, S and G₂-M (Fig. 94.7A). In addition to these conventional parameters, the presence or absence of aneuploidy can be determined by inspection of the G₀–G₁ peak and/or use of a DNA index (ratio of abnormal DNA content to a diploid DNA standard). Also, elevation in the S and/or G₂-M phase can be detected. The optimal display of these data uses a combination of side scatter versus DNA content. Cells observed on the histogram in the area below the level of G₀–G₁ may be undergoing apoptosis.[50] When dealing with DNA staining, a consistent cellular source of DNA (e.g., chicken erythrocytes) should be used as an internal reference for evaluating DNA content and evaluating the cell cycle distribution.

It should be noted that several different computer algorithms have been developed to determine the relative proportion of each cell cycle compartment, and the selection of a software program is not a trivial process. The major instrument manufacturers supply cell cycle analysis programs, and there are also third-party programs available. Generally the optimal program should be capable of modeling two or more aneuploid

populations, subtracting debris (particularly if formalin-fixed paraffin-embedded archival material is used) and accurately estimating S-phase cells.[51,52] The combination of a surface marker and cell cycle has been very useful in differentiating normal cell populations from tumor cell populations. One example is the use of anti-κ, anti-λ, or B-cell reagents to separate the aneuploid B-cell clone from the remaining normal, reactive B cells in a lymphoid cell mixture. Another uses cytokeratin as a marker to distinguish between the tumor cells and the inflammatory cells that are present.

The other major event that has occurred in cell cycle analysis has been the development of technology using the incorporation of bromodeoxyuridine.[53] This thymidine analog is used to directly determine the percentage of S-phase cells. Also, when used in kinetic studies it permits a determination of the individual times for the components of the cell cycle and a determination of the growth fraction. Finally, recent developments have resulted in the availability of two anticyclin reagents to evaluate cell cycle transition points in malignant cells.[54]

Apoptosis detection

Flow cytometry has become the method of choice for the detection and quantification of cellular apoptosis.[55] This is due in part to its capacity for rapid assessment of a large number of cells and samples. Many distinct features of an apoptotic cell can be evaluated by flow cytometry based on light scatter, plasma membrane changes, mitochondrial transmembrane potential, DNA content and DNA integrity.

The light scattering properties of a cell undergoing programed cell death are the simplest attributes that can be assessed by flow cytometry. Dying cells typically shrink, producing a loss in forward light scatter (FSC) and, despite an initial transient increase in side scatter (SSC), also ultimately demonstrate a decrease in SSC (Fig. 94.7B). The use of light scatter can be combined with cell surface staining to help characterize the dying cells. However, scatter changes alone are not specific to apoptosis and should be accompanied by an additional characteristic associated with cell death. Live cells have phospholipids asymmetrically distributed in the inner and outer plasma membrane, with phosphatidylcholine and sphingomyelin on the outer surface and phosphatidylserine (PS) on the inner side. Early during apoptosis cells lose asymmetry, exposing PS on the outside. Annexin V is a protein that binds preferentially to negatively-charged phospholipids such as PS, and directly conjugated annexin V is a useful reagent for the specific detection of apoptotic cells.[55]

Another characteristic of plasma membranes associated with live cells is that they exclude charged cationic dyes such as propidium iodide (PI) and 7-amino-actinomycin-D (7-AMD). Consequently, only cells in a late stage of apoptosis, with ruptured cell membranes, will take up these dyes. Thus, the combined use of cationic dyes (e.g., PI) with annexin V allows the discrimination between live cells (annexin V negative/ PI negative), early apoptotic cells (annexin V positive/ PI negative) and late apoptotic cells (annexin V positive/ PI positive).

Assessment of mitochondrial transmembrane potential ($\Delta\psi$m) is yet another technique used to identify apoptotic cells. Cells decrease $\Delta\psi$m very early in the apoptotic process, before rupture of the plasma membrane, losing the ability to accumulate potential-dependent dyes such as rhodamine 123, JC-1 or 3,3''-dihexyloxacarbocyanine iodide (Dioc6^3). These dyes can also be used with PI to detect cells in the different stages of apoptosis (Fig. 94.7C).

Measurement of DNA content can also be employed to distinguish live from dead cells, as described above (see Cell Cycle Analysis). This kind of analysis has to be done using a linear scale, not logarithimic, in order to discriminate dying cells from debris. DNA cleavage also exposes -OH termini associated with the DNA breaks and these can be detected via the attachment of fluorochrome-conjugated deoxynucleotides, in a reaction catalysed by exogenous TdT, a technique called TUNEL.

Peptide–MHC multimers

In contrast to B cells, direct visualization of antigen-specific T cells *in vivo* has, until recently, been unsuccessful. In 1996, Altman et al. introduced a novel flow-cytometry-based methodology that enables the direct visualization and quantification of antigen-specific T cells.[56] By generating soluble peptide–MHC multimers, such that multiple TCRs are engaged at the same time, the avidity of these multimeric ligands for the peptide-specific TCR is greatly increased. The methodology involves engineering a biotinylation recognition sequence on the -COOH terminus of the extracellular domain of one chain of the MHC molecule that, after combining with a specific antigenic peptide, is bound by avidin or streptavidin. As both avidin and streptavidin have four biotin-binding sites, the result is a tetrameric peptide–MHC complex that serves as a ligand for T cells specific for both the peptide and MHC. Flow-cytometric detection is achieved by labeling streptavidin with a fluorochrome. The major pitfall to this approach is the need to know the antigen-derived peptide and its HLA-restrictions, as well as the HLA type of each subject studied. Since the initial report, an increasing number of tetramer-based studies have appeared. Most have focused on the MHC class I-mediated immune response, in both mice and humans, to a variety of infectious agents, including cytomegalovirus (CMV), HIV, Epstein–Barr virus and others. Since the initial description with class I-restricted recognition, detection of antigen-specific CD4 T cells with tetramers of soluble MHC class II molecules and covalently linked peptide has also been reported.[57]

In addition to demonstrating the feasibility of this approach, the published studies have provided several new insights into the MHC class I-mediated immune response (Chapter 5). For example, it has become clear that the extent of the MHC class I-mediated cellular response is much greater than previously estimated. Furthermore, the extensive proliferation of CD8 T cells during an acute infection is not the result of bystander activation, but represents an expansion of antigen-specific CD8 T cells. One possible explanation is that, in contrast to previously used techniques such as the limiting dilution assay, tetramer-based assays do not depend on *in vitro* cell division and survival. Peptide–MHC tetramer assays have also shown promise in the study of the kinetics of primary and secondary immune responses, as well as in a better understanding of concepts such as immunodominance and clonal exhaustion.

An obviously attractive aspect of this technology is that tetramer staining can be combined with a variety of cell surface and intracellular phenotypic and functional markers. Already there are indications that the phenotype of antigen-specific T cells varies between individuals and between different phases of the immune response. In addition, tetramer-positive T cells can be sorted for further analysis, such as cytotoxicity assays or *in vitro* expansion. The tetramer-based technology has not only proved useful for the study of the immune response to infectious agents, it has also been applied to the study of oral tolerance, autoimmune conditions and tumor immunology. It is likely that this highly sensitive and specific technology and other approaches that define antigen specific response will find many more applications and will lead to new discoveries and a reassessment of certain existing concepts.[58]

Conclusion

Flow cytometry has become readily available in clinical laboratories and the application of this technology has moved forward in parallel to significant improvements in instrumentation and the availability of an array of monoclonal reagents. Properly performed, flow cytometry can provide rapid and accurate lymphocyte subpopulation identification. The primary clinical indications of immunophenotyping remain quantifying CD4 T-cell counts in HIV infection, lineage assignment in leukemias and lymphomas, and assessing CD34 expression to identify stem cells for transplantation. Additional uses include characterizing immune deficiency disorders, evaluating immune-mediated inflammatory diseases, and assessing patients following organ transplantation. The real utility of these newer applications remains to be fully clarified and, in most settings, immunophenotyping does not represent a diagnostic procedure but rather plays a part in the evaluation and understanding of complex disorders and the longitudinal evaluation of immunomodulatory therapy.

It is critical to recognize that immunophenotyping is a means of identifying cells, but it is not directed at cell function. The expansion of flow-cytometric techniques to evaluate intracellular characteristics, assess intracellular changes associated with activation, characterize apoptosis and identify antigen-specific T cells is moving this platform into the cell function arena. These newer approaches are expanding the utility of flow cytometry as a valuable tool for the characterization of immune function.

References

1. Shapiro HM. How flow cytometers work. 4th ed. Wiley: Hoboken; 2003.
2. Kachel V. Hydrodynamic properties of flow cytometry instruments. New York: Wiley Liss; 1990.
3. Thompson JM, Gralow JR, Levy R, Miller RA. The optimal application of forward and ninety-degree light scatter in flow cytometry for the gating of mononuclear cells. Cytometry 1985;6:401–6.
4. Goddard G, Martin JC, Graves SW, Kaduchak G. Ultrasonic particle-concentration for sheathless focusing of particles for analysis in a flow cytometer. Cytometry A 2006;69:66–74.
5. Ward M, Turner P, DeJohn M, Kaduchak G. Fundamentals of acoustic cytometry. Curr Protoc Cytom 2009;49: 1.22.21–21.22.12.
6. Kapoor V, Karpov V, Linton C, et al. Solid state yellow and orange lasers for flow cytometry. Cytometry A 2008;73:570–7.
7. Chattopadhyay PK, Hogerkorp CM, Roederer M. A chromatic explosion: the development and future of multiparameter flow cytometry. Immunology 2008;125:441–9.
8. Perfetto SP, Chattopadhyay PK, Roederer M. Seventeen-colour flow cytometry: unravelling the immune system. Nat Rev Immunol 2004;4:648–55.
9. Giepmans BN, Adams SR, Ellisman MH, Tsien RY. The fluorescent toolbox for assessing protein location and function. Science 2006;312:217–24.
10. Chattopadhyay PK, Yu J, Roederer M. Application of quantum dots to multicolor flow cytometry. Methods Mol Biol 2007;374:175–84.
11. Chattopadhyay PK, Price DA, Harper TF, et al. Quantum dot semiconductor nanocrystals for immunophenotyping by polychromatic flow cytometry. Nat Med 2006;12:972–7.
12. Rabinovitch PS, June CH, Kavanagh TJ. Introduction to functional cell assays. Ann N Y Acad Sci 1993;677:252–64.
13. Vowells SJ, Sekhsaria S, Malech HL, et al. Flow cytometric analysis of the granulocyte respiratory burst: a comparison study of fluorescent probes. J Immunol Methods 1995;178:89–97.
14. Darzynkiewicz Z. Critical aspects in analysis of cellular DNA content. Curr Protoc Cytom [chapter 7]. Unit7 2.
15. Darzynkiewicz Z, Halicka HD, Zhao H. Analysis of cellular DNA content by flow and laser scanning cytometry. Adv Exp Med Biol 2010;676:137–47.
16. Loken MR, Brosnan JM, Bach BA, Ault KA. Establishing optimal lymphocyte gates for immunophenotyping by flow cytometry. Cytometry 1990;11:453–9.
17. US Clinical and Laboratory Standards Institute. Clinical applications of flow cytometry: quality assurance and immunophenotyping of peripheral blood lymphocytes. Villanova, PA: NCCLS Publication H24-T; 1992.
18. Stewart CC, Stewart SJ. Multiparameter data acquisition and analysis of leukocytes. Methods Mol Biol 2004;263:45–66.
19. Parks DR, Roederer M, Moore WA. A new "Logicle" display method avoids deceptive effects of logarithmic scaling for low signals and compensated data. Cytometry A 2006;69:541–51.
20. Roederer M, Moody MA. Polychromatic plots: graphical display of multidimensional data. Cytometry A 2008;73:868–74.
21. Roederer M. Spectral compensation for flow cytometry: visualization artifacts, limitations, and caveats. Cytometry 2001;45:194–205.
22. Owens MA, Vall HG, Hurley AA, Wormsley SB. Validation and quality control of immunophenotyping in clinical flow cytometry. J Immunol Methods 2000;243:33–50.
23. Schwartz A, Marti GE, Poon R, et al. Standardizing flow cytometry: a classification system of fluorescence standards used for flow cytometry. Cytometry 1998;33:106–14.
24. Renzi P, Ginns LC. Analysis of T cell subsets in normal adults. Comparison of whole blood lysis technique to Ficoll-Hypaque separation by flow cytometry. J Immunol Methods 1987;98:53–6.
25. Yamada M, Tamura N, Shirai T, Kira S. Flow cytometric analysis of lymphocyte subsets in the bronchoalveolar lavage fluid and peripheral blood of healthy volunteers. Scand J Immunol 1986;24:559–65.
26. Reichert T, DeBruyere M, Deneys V, et al. Lymphocyte subset reference ranges in adult Caucasians. Clin Immunol Immunopathol 1991;60:190–208.
27. Shearer WT, Rosenblatt HM, Gelman RS, et al. Lymphocyte subsets in healthy children from birth through 18 years of age: the Pediatric AIDS Clinical Trials Group P1009 study. J Allergy Clin Immunol 2003;112:973–80.
28. Tollerud DJ, Clark JW, Brown LM, et al. The effects of cigarette smoking on T cell subsets. A population-based survey of healthy caucasians. Am Rev Respir Dis 1989;139:1446–51.
29. Levi FA, Canon C, Touitou Y, et al. Seasonal modulation of the circadian time structure of circulating T and natural killer lymphocyte subsets from healthy subjects. J Clin Invest 1988;81:407–13.
30. Fleisher TA, Oliveira JB. Autoimmune lymphoproliferative syndrome. Isr Med Assoc J 2005;7:758–61.
31. Yarchoan R, Venzon DJ, Pluda JM, et al. CD4 count and the risk for death in patients infected with HIV receiving antiretroviral therapy. Ann Intern Med 1991;115:184–9.
32. Sekhsaria S, Fleisher TA, Vowells S, et al. Granulocyte colony-stimulating factor recruitment of CD34+ progenitors to peripheral blood: impaired mobilization in chronic granulomatous disease and adenosine deaminase—deficient severe combined immunodeficiency disease patients. Blood 1996;88:1104–12.
33. Oliveira JB, Notarangelo LD, Fleisher TA. Applications of flow cytometry for the study of primary immune deficiencies. Curr Opin Allergy Clin Immunol 2008;8:499–509.
34. Wehr C, Kivioja T, Schmitt C, et al. The EUROclass trial: defining subgroups in common variable immunodeficiency. Blood 2008;111:77–85.
35. Etzioni A. Defects in the leukocyte adhesion cascade. Clin Rev Allergy Immunol 2010;38:54–60.
36. Young IT. Proof without prejudice: use of the Kolmogorov-Smirnov test for the analysis of histograms from flow systems and other sources. J Histochem Cytochem 1977;25:935–41.
37. Berliner N, Ault KA, Martin P, Weinberg DS. Detection of clonal excess in lymphoproliferative disease by kappa/lambda analysis: correlation with immunoglobulin gene DNA rearrangement. Blood 1986;67:80–5.
38. Pilch H, Hohn H, Freitag K, et al. Improved assessment of T-cell receptor (TCR) VB repertoire in clinical specimens: combination of TCR-CDR3 spectratyping with flow cytometry-based TCR VB frequency analysis. Clin Diagn Lab Immunol 2002;9:257–66.
39. Sallusto F, Geginat J, Lanzavecchia A. Central memory and effector memory T cell subsets: function, generation, and maintenance. Annu Rev Immunol 2004;22:745–63.
40. Avery DT, Ellyard JI, Mackay F, et al. Increased expression of CD27 on activated human memory B cells correlates with their commitment to the plasma cell lineage. J Immunol 2005;174:4034–42.
41. Mardiney 3rd M, Brown MR, Fleisher TA. Measurement of T-cell CD69 expression: a rapid and efficient means to assess mitogen- or antigen-induced proliferative capacity in normals. Cytometry 1996;26:305–10.
42. Allsopp CE, Langhorne J. Assessing antigen-specific proliferation and cytokine responses using flow cytometry. Methods Mol Med 2002;72:409–21.
43. Slezak SE, Horan PK. Cell-mediated cytotoxicity. A highly sensitive and informative flow cytometric assay. J Immunol Methods 1989;117:205–14.
44. Yu Y, Arora A, Min W, et al. EdU incorporation is an alternative non-radioactive assay to [(3)H]thymidine uptake for in vitro measurement of mice T-cell proliferations. J Immunol Methods 2009;350:29–35.
45. Fleisher TA, Dorman SE, Anderson JA, et al. Detection of intracellular phosphorylated STAT-1 by flow cytometry. Clin Immunol 1999;90:425–30.
46. Vowells SJ, Fleisher TA, Sekhsaria S, et al. Genotype-dependent variability in flow cytometric evaluation of reduced nicotinamide adenine dinucleotide phosphate oxidase function in patients with chronic granulomatous disease. J Pediatr 1996;128:104–7.
47. Heim KF, Fleisher TA, Stroncek DF, et al. The relationship between alloimmunization and posttransfusion granulocyte survival: experience in a chronic granulomatous disease cohort. Transfusion 2001;51:1154–62.
48. Foster B, Prussin C, Liu F, et al. Detection of intracellular cytokines by flow cytometry. Curr Protoc Immunol 2007 [chapter 6]. Unit 6 24.
49. Suni MA, Picker LJ, Maino VC. Detection of antigen-specific T cell cytokine expression in whole blood by flow cytometry. J Immunol Methods 1998;212:89–98.
50. Wheeless LL, Coon JS, Cox C, et al. Measurement variability in DNA flow cytometry of replicate samples. Cytometry 1989;10:731–8.
51. Shankey TV, Rabinovitch PS, Bagwell B, et al. Guidelines for implementation of clinical DNA cytometry. International Society for Analytical Cytology. Cytometry 1993;14:472–7.
52. Braylan RC, Benson NA, Nourse V, Kruth HS. Correlated analysis of cellular DNA, membrane antigens and light scatter of human lymphoid cells. Cytometry 1982;2:337–43.
53. Rothaeusler K, Baumgarth N. Assessment of cell proliferation by 5-bromodeoxyuridine (BrdU) labeling for multicolor flow cytometry. Curr Protoc Cytom 2007 [chapter 7]. Unit7 31.
54. Gong J, Bhatia U, Traganos F, Darzynkiewicz Z. Expression of cyclins A, D2 and D3 in individual normal mitogen stimulated lymphocytes and in MOLT-4 leukemic cells analyzed by multiparameter flow cytometry. Leukemia 1995;9:893–9.
55. Telford WG, Komoriya A, Packard BZ, Bagwell CB. Multiparametric analysis of apoptosis by flow cytometry. Methods Mol Biol 699:203–27.
56. Altman JD, Moss PA, Goulder PJ, et al. Phenotypic analysis of antigen-specific T lymphocytes. Science 1996;274:94–6.
57. Mallone R, Nepom GT. MHC Class II tetramers and the pursuit of antigen-specific T cells: define, deviate, delete. Clin Immunol 2004;110:232–42.
58. Kern F, LiPira G, Gratama JW, et al. Measuring Ag-specific immune responses: understanding immunopathogenesis and improving diagnostics in infectious disease, autoimmunity and cancer. Trends Immunol 2005;26:477–84.

Jack J.H. Bleesing,
João B. Oliveira,

Assessment of functional immune responses

A comprehensive clinical evaluation of the immune system, whether to diagnose immunodeficiency or other immune-mediated disorders, ideally includes both quantitative and qualitative aspects. According to the principle: "form follows function," important clues to the functional status of the immune system are provided by the assessment of form (quantity and specific characteristics), as determined by the cellular phenotype of lymphocytes and other cell populations and by the measurement of secreted/produced factors (complement components, antibodies, cytokines, etc.).[1] This theme of interconnected determination of form and function is a central thread throughout this chapter. Rather than focusing on the technical aspects of individual assays, the emphasis is on providing a general overview in the context of indication and interpretation. For more in-depth discussions on assay procedures, the reader is referred to other sources, such as Current Protocols in Immunology and the Manual of Clinical Laboratory Immunology. In addition, an increasing amount of on-line content is available (e.g., the on-line video Journal of Visualized Experiments [JoVE], see http://www.jove.com).

Many of the assays described here are performed in specialized laboratories that often have a dual clinical/research mission. This has been somewhat artificially separated into Clinical and Research sections in this chapter. From the standpoint of the clinical laboratory, it takes considerable effort and time to translate new insights into the human immune system and associated defects into clinically applicable assays that help diagnose novel conditions. Making things more challenging, it has been recognized that immunologic conditions can defy commonly used tools of laboratory investigation, such that seemingly normal test results, in the face of data suggesting an immunological disorder, need to be regarded with appropriate suspicion. This may be due to the fact that the "wrong" populations of cells have been studied; the method of *in vitro* testing did not appropriately mimic the *in vivo* situation, and other factors.

Clinical immunology

General considerations

Since the immune system operates in a profoundly intricate manner that is difficult to define by straightforward *modi operandi*, it is generally necessary to assess immunologic function according to established models or schemes. This approach divides the immune system into compartments, such that essentially every aspect of immune function can be studied through *in vivo*, *ex vivo* or *in vitro* measurements. Focusing on the lymphoid system, functional assessment of T-, B-, and NK-cell compartments can be performed by evaluation of the different components and events required for a normal response, and by measuring the functional output (Tables 95.1 and 95.2). Finally, functional assays can be distinguished based on whether they test function *in vivo* (measured directly *ex vivo*), or after *in vitro* manipulation.

As with all laboratory studies, interpretation of abnormal immunologic assays should lead to three basic questions. *First*, does the abnormality reflect a biologically accurate and reproducible finding? It is important to confirm test results, also paying attention to correct procurement and processing of specimens. *Second*, what is its relevance? In other words, what is the underlying basis for the abnormal value(s); does it fit with the immunologic phenotype? *Third*, what are the consequences (significance) for the patient? Are (immediate) interventions indicated, such as medications, patient isolation, etc.? When dealing with pediatric patients, a *fourth* question should be asked. How do the patient's laboratory results compare to age-appropriate control values/reference ranges?

Controls (i.e., [presumed] healthy individuals) play important roles in all immunologic assays. Broadly categorized, there are assay controls and interpretation controls. Assay controls are needed to ensure that the assay is performing adequately (including shipping controls if the blood has to travel to the laboratory). In addition to a healthy control, the patient (subject) constitutes an internal assay control (i.e., intra-assay control) to distinguish between "noise" and "signal" (e.g., cells cultured in the presence [signal] and in the absence [noise] of mitogens). Thus controls are needed in the interpretation of the results by providing a framework for comparison with a healthy control analyzed in parallel with the patient together with the results from a larger group of control subjects that is captured as the reference (normal) range. As mentioned in the introduction, the use of demographics-matched controls (age [both young and old], gender, ethnicity, etc.) is important for many assays.

Guiding the appropriate choice of functional assays for immune competence, it is imperative to have an (initial) assessment of immunologic form linked to a specific question or questions posed by the patient's clinical phenotype. In most cases, clues to the nature of the functional defect are provided by abnormal form (examples are shown in Fig. 95.1). Likely explanation of abnormal results from an initial assessment should be developed in the light of the clinical findings, anticipating how the data/results of functional assays will help to explain the clinical phenotype. This approach should be balanced by keeping an open mind, especially if few clues are available, or if clues seem contradictory. An important aspect of functional testing is utilizing

Table 95.1 Lymphocyte function as reflected by events of activation or functional output

Events of activation
Expression of cell surface proteins required to respond to antigenic stimuli (TCR, BCR, CD3, CD19)
Calcium influx
Expression and/or up- or downregulation of cell surface receptors, important in early activation (CD69, CD25, CD40L)
Blastogenesis (mitogenesis) and cell division (measured by a wide range of systems)
Up- or downregulation of markers indicating chronic activation, antigen priming (CD71, CD45RO, CCR7, CD62L)
Apoptosis (cell death)

Functional output
Production of cytokines in response to polyclonal or antigen-specific stimulation (Th1/Tr1 versus Th2/Tr2)
Production of polyclonal or antigen-specific immunoglobulins
Specific and non-specific cytolytic activity (see Table 95.3)
Suppressive effects (T regulatory activity, suppression of immunoglobulin secretion)

the right assay(s) for the right scenario. For example, obtaining a proliferation assay to measure T-cell responses to recall antigens would be of no value if the antigen has not been experienced and thus cannot be "recalled."

Functional assays of T-cell immune competence

Functional assays of T cells are generally intended to determine:

1. Global immune competence;
2. Specific (selective) immune competence (e.g., in the context of specific defects in host defense);
3. *In vivo* state of immune activation;
4. Recovery of *in vivo* immune responsiveness following immunosuppression;
5. Appropriate downregulation of immune activation and induction of cell death;
6. Prior exposures to foreign antigens (through infection or immunization); and
7. HLA transplantation compatibility and evidence of prior exposure to alloantigens.

It is possible to obtain a fairly detailed assessment of the T-cell compartment with a combination of immunophenotyping and functional assays (Table 95.2). These can provide important clues to the immunologic defects underlying the clinical scenario. Depending on the complexity of the clinical circumstances, the choice of immunophenotyping can vary from a screening assessment of basic lymphocyte subsets to an extensive flow cytometric analysis of subset, activation, adhesion and many other cell surface and intracellular markers which can then be linked to functional testing. For patients with immunodeficiency states that are predominantly characterized by recurrent infections, performing a mitogen-stimulation assay, employing phytohemagglutinin (PHA), concanavalin-A (Con-A), pokeweed mitogen (PWM), immobilized anti-CD3, and/or an antigen-stimulation assay, using [3H] thymidine incorporation, are sufficient for assessment of basic T-cell immune competence.[2-5]

In patients with suspected complex cellular immunodeficiency states, combinations of functional assays that evaluate diverse cell types and/or assess different pathways and modes of activation may be helpful to develop an understanding of

Table 95.2 Methods of lymphocyte activation *in vitro*

Freq.*	Stimulator	Target	Remarks
~80-90%	*Phorbol esters*		
	- PMA	Protein kinase C	Stimulates both T and B cells (similar for ionophores)
	Ionophores		
	- Ionomycin	Ion channels	PMA + Ionomycin: Bypasses cell surface receptors and early signaling molecules
~60-70%	*Mitogens*		
	- PHA	Multiple receptors	T-cell stimulator (carbohydrate-recognizing lectin) [mitogen-stimulation assay]
	- ConA	Multiple receptors	T-cell stimulator (carbohydrate-recognizing lectin) [mitogen-stimulation assay]
	- PWM	Multiple receptors	T-cell stimulator and T-cell-dependent B-cell stimulator [mitogen-stimulation assay]
~40-50%	*Antibodies/ Ligands*		
	- anti-TCR	TCR/CD3 complex	
	- anti-CD3	TCR/CD3 complex	Mild mitogen in soluble form; potent if immobilized on membranes or beads
	- anti-CD28	CD28 on T-cells	Not mitogenic unless used in combination with TCR/CD3 stimulation
	- anti-IgM	BCR	Potent if immobilized; +/- T cells or T-cell supernatant to test regulatory T-cell effects
	- anti-CD40 or sCD40L	CD40	Polyclonal immunoglobulin secretion; isotype determined by cytokine addition
~20-30%	*Microbial antigens*		
	- SEB	TCR (non-cognate)	Superantigen, stimulates ~20% of T cells through an invariant domain of the TCR
	- SAC	BCR	SAC + IL-2: Polyclonal immunoglobulin secretion in absence of T-cells
~5-10%	*Allogeneic cells*	TCR + others	One-way, two-way mixed lymphocyte culture (MLC)
<1%	*Recall antigens*		
	- Tetanus	TCR (cognate)	Dependent on prior *in vivo* exposure to tetanus (vaccination) [antigen-proliferation assay]
	- Candida	TCR (cognate)	Dependent on prior *in vivo* exposure to candida spp. [antigen-proliferation assay]

*Estimates of frequencies of responding T cells.

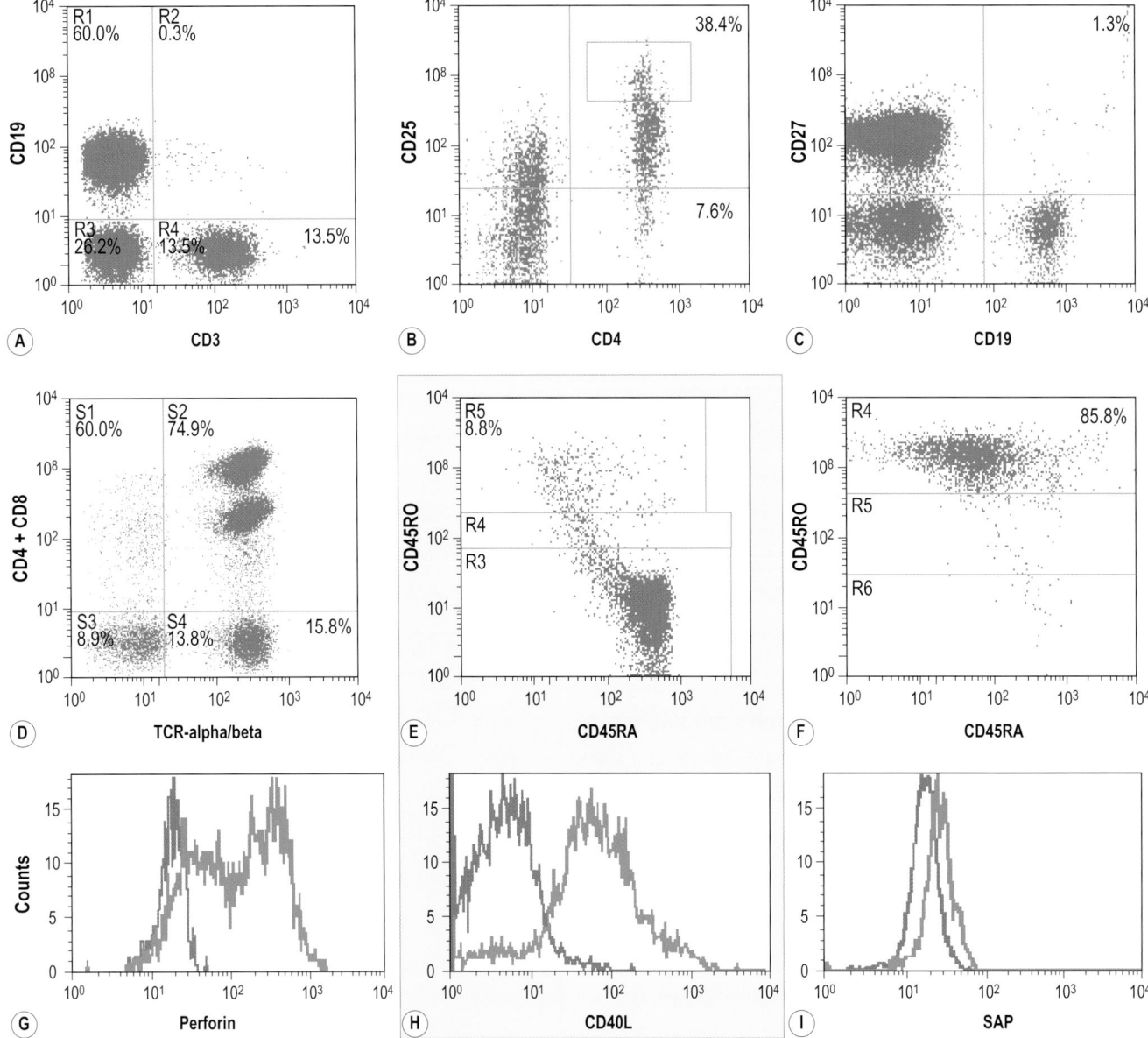

Fig. 95.1 Immunologic form follows immunologic function. Examples of abnormal immunologic form, detected by flow cytometry (dual-parameter dotplots A-F; single-parameter histograms G-I, showing patients in purple and controls in green). (A) Reduced T-cell compartment in patient with DiGeorge syndrome (gated on total lymphocytes, 13.5 vs 60-70% of lymphocytes in controls); (B) activated CD25-expressing (CD4+) T cells in patient with chronic rejection of orthotopic liver transplantation (gated on total T cells); (C) lack of memory B cells in patient with common variable immunodeficiency (CVID), as determined by CD27 expression (gated on total lymphocytes; 1.3 vs > 15% of B cells in controls); (D) presence of T cells expressing the TCR-α/β but lacking CD4 and CD8 in a patient with autoimmune lymphoproliferative syndrome (ALPS, gated on total T cells; 15.8 vs < 2% of lymphocytes in controls); (E) lack of CD45RO+ T cells in young adult with X-linked hyper-IgM syndrome (gated on total T cells, see (H) for associated functional assay); (F) lack of CD45RA+ T cells in patient 12 months post bone marrow transplantation (gated on total T cells); (G) lack of intracellular perforin in NK cells (and associated defective NK-cell function) in patient with familial form of hemophagocytic lymphohistiocytosis on the basis of mutations in the perforin gene (FHLH, gated on total NK cells); (H) lack of CD40L upregulation on (CD4+) T cells following 4-hour T-cell stimulation (gated on CD8− T cells); (I) lack of intracellular SAP expression in (CD8+) T cells in a patient with X-linked lymphoproliferative disease (XLP, gated on CD8+ T cells; cytolytic functions were abnormal in the presence of EBV infection).

the underlying defect(s). For example, PMA and ionomycin can bypass relevant cell surface receptors, such as the T-cell receptor (TCR)/CD3 complex and upstream signaling components connected to these receptors, allowing the vast majority of T cells to respond. On the other end of the spectrum is the response to specific antigens (e.g., candida or tetanus toxoid), which typically involves less than 1% of the entire T-cell repertoire Table 95.2). Adding growth factors (e.g., IL-2) to the culture system may provide additional information regarding the functional status of the cell population.[6,7]

As with most functional assays, the clinical utility of the assays described above depends on how it allows the clinician to

translate raw data into an appropriate interpretation of the results. Completely normal and completely abnormal results are relatively easy to explain; results falling in between are more difficult to interpret. Detailed functional analysis can help in making the gray zone easier to navigate. This is balanced by the added technical challenges (and potential pitfalls) of these labor-intensive assays. In the event that the results of the functional assay do not fit with the clinical phenotype, an attempt should be made to explain whether this discrepancy has a biological basis or is due to assay-related artifacts. Thus, it is crucial that adequate quality control programs are in place to ensure that data interpretation and result interpretation are valid.

Avoiding pitfalls of *in vitro* assays

What do we need to know about the patient?

- Demographic data (age, sex, ethnicity, smoking)
- Exposure history (natural infections, vaccinations)
- Medications (immunosuppression)
- Relevant (current) medical scenario (viral infection, trauma, cancer)
- Interfering factors *in vivo* (rheumatoid factor, heterophile antibodies)

What do we need to know about the assay?

- Cell source and viability (fresh, shipped, cryopreserved)
- Cell manipulation, requirement for other cells (antigen-presenting cells, interfering suppressor T cells)
- Cell nutrition, choice of serum (e.g., pooled human serum for NK-cell assays)
- Time kinetics (PHA peaks in 2-3 days, recall antigens in 6-8 days)
- Specific culture conditions (e.g., low oxygen environment if there is defective oxidative damage repair [Fanconi anemia])
- Controls (assay controls, including intra-assay, interpretation controls)
- Data scoring (ELISPOT), calculation and representation (e.g., counts-per-minute, lytic units)

An evaluation of T-cell immune competence can be achieved directly *in vivo*. Delayed-type hypersensitivity (DTH) skin tests constitute a method for determining cellular immunity based on prior exposure to certain antigens. Its major advantages are its convenience, availability and quick turn-around time (~48-72 hours). In addition, DTH skin tests measure both the afferent (e.g., antigen presentation) and efferent (e.g., T-cell and inflammatory cell infiltration) loops of the immune response. An obvious limitation is that exposures to the agents used in DTH must have taken place and the operator must have experience with this type of testing. Clinical relevance and use of DTH tests to detect diminished T-cell function is limited by the fact that the response cannot be quantified and by the fact that there are many causes of false-negative results, including young and advanced age, concurrent infections, use of immunosuppressive medications, malnutrition, atopic dermatitis, decreasing availability of reagent antigens and others. Thus, DTH tests ideally include intradermal injection of a combination of several recall antigens (e.g., tetanus toxoid, candida, mumps)

to increase the probability of a positive response (i.e., erythema and induration at 48 and 72 hours after application). Negative results for possible anergy should be interpreted with great caution, especially in young children.[8,9]

Assessment of cytolytic function

Assays that measure proliferation to mitogens, antigens, and cytokines reveal the ability of T cells to appropriately divide/proliferate in response to stimulation. However, the effector function of cytotoxic lymphocytes requires both proliferation and the ability to kill target cells. Cytolytic function pertains to subsets of T and NK cells. There are several types of cytolytic activity that differ in respect to effector cell population, specificity (e.g., MHC restriction), requirement for prior sensitization to the target, and other features (Table 95.3).[10-12] While both T-cell subsets and NK cells can function as non-MHC restricted cytolytic cells, only T cells have the ability to kill target cells via cognate (MHC/peptide) recognition, a process that requires prior exposure to the target or antigens derived from the target.[13,14] Antibody-dependent cellular cytotoxicity (ADCC) is a cytolytic process that is dependent on the cooperative interaction of several different cellular and humoral constituents of the immune system. In ADCC, effector cells with receptors for the Fc portion of antibodies (e.g., CD16) affect target cell lysis by using these Fc receptors to bind the antibodies attached to the target cells.[15,16] Lymphokine-activated killer (LAK) cells are cytotoxic cells, primarily derived from NK cells that, through activation by IL-2, acquire more potent cytolytic function against "traditional" targets, as well as a broader repertoire of potential targets (e.g., fresh tumor cells).[17,18] Cytolytic activity can be broken down into three phases starting with conjugate formation between target and effector cells, mediated by many receptor/ligand pairs. Following cellular contact, the cytolytic cells are triggered, i.e., prepared for imminent killing. This process can be measured on the basis of calcium flux or by intracellular phosphorylation events. The process is completed (and can be repeated with other targets) by lysis of target cells through membranolytic/secretory (perforin and granzymes) and by nonsecretory receptor mediated (Fas/Fas ligand) mechanisms (Chapter 17).[19-22]

Reasons for obtaining cytolytic assays broadly follow the same considerations for assays measuring T-cell immune competence. It has been long recognized that abnormal cytolytic function is found in patients with a variety of disorders that include primary and acquired immunodeficiency disorders, viral infections, cancer, trauma/burns and other conditions, some of which are

Table 95.3 Types of cytolytic function

Type of cytotoxicity	Specificity	Cell(s)	Targets	Enhancing factors
Natural killer (NK) cell function	Non-specific	NK cells (CD16$^+$, CD56$^+$)	K562 cells	Interferon
Antibody-dependent cellular cytotoxicity (ADCC)	Specificity dependent on antibody	NK cells, monocytes, macrophages, granulocytes	Chang cells, Raji cells	Opsonized IgG
Cytotoxic T-cell function	Specific, HLA-restricted	T cells	EBV-transformed B lymphoblastoid cells	Viral/tumor antigens
Cell-mediated lympholysis	Specific, HLA-restricted	T cells	Allogeneic cells	Alloantigens
Lymphokine activated killing (LAK)	Non-specific	NK cells, T cells, monocytes, macrophages	Daudi cells, patient-specific tumor cells	IL-2 (IL-12, IL-15)
Lectin-dependent cytotoxicity	Non-specific	NK cells, T cells, monocytes, macrophages	See above (killing induced by lectin interaction)	Mitogens (lectins)

better characterized than others.[12,23] From a practical standpoint, it often is difficult to translate the results of these assays into meaningful interpretations that are helpful in diagnosis and management. Development of new therapeutic options for some of these disorders (e.g., immunotherapy of cancer, novel vaccines) has invited a new look at cytolytic assays, particularly with respect to the measurement of antigen-specific cytotoxicity. Determination of cytolytic function has particular value in hemophagocytic lymphohistiocytic (HLH) disorders, including inherited forms of HLH, as well as secondary forms of HLH (e.g., viral-induced, as part of malignancies and rheumatologic disorders).[24–26] In these disorders, other measurements of function are often normal or, from an interpretation standpoint, situated in the gray zone. Again, it is the integration of the clinical phenoype that guides which cytolytic assays are most appropriate (see example in Fig. 95.1G).

In the repertoire of *in vitro* cytolytic assays, the 4-hour ^{51}Cr-release assay using the NK-cell-sensitive K562 tumor cell line is relatively straightforward from a technical and quality control aspect and has a proven track record.[27] Measuring cytotoxic T-lymphocyte (CTL) function is useful to complement other studies of T-cell immune competence and to compare with non-MHC-restricted killing (NK-cell function). CTL assays can be done by a variety of methods, including initial priming of effector T cells to irradiated target cells (e.g., Epstein–Barr virus [EBV]-transformed B cells) in a 6- to 7-day culture, followed by re-stimulation with the same, ^{51}Cr-labeled, target cells. Evaluation of ADCC capacity can be used to evaluate effector mechanisms of therapeutic monoclonal antibodies, while the LAK assay can measure cytolytic activity against patient-specific tumor cells (that can be used to generate patient-specific cancer vaccines).[10,11,28]

Common features in cytolytic assays include the use of incremental ratios between the number of effector cells and target cells (E:T ratios) that can provide potentially useful information, and can also serve quality control purposes (Fig. 95.2). Specific intra-assay controls include incubating target cells without effector cells (spontaneous lysis), target cells treated with detergent for maximum lysis, the inclusion of negative control non-relevant target cells, adding anti-HLA antibodies to block MHC-restricted killing, and using non-antibody coated target cells in ADCC assays.[22,28]

In the interpretation of the raw data, it is again important to consider the variety of assay and subject variables that can

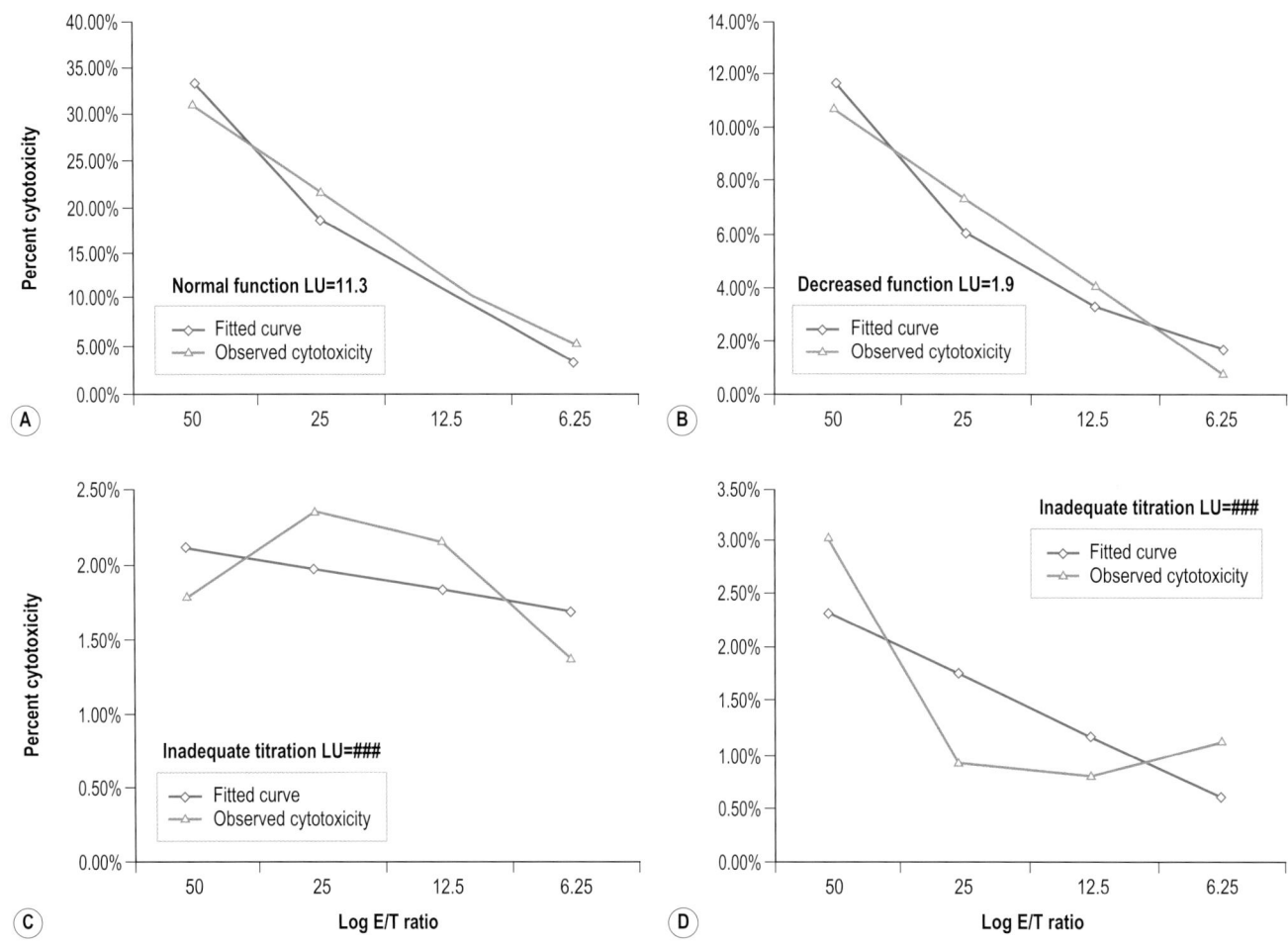

Fig. 95.2 NK-cell assays Examples of NK-cell assay data representation. First, the percentage specific lysis (cytotoxicity) is calculated for each E:T ratio by dividing the average of the experimental ^{51}Cr release (cpm)—the average spontaneous ^{51}Cr release (cpm) by the average of the maximum ^{51}Cr release (cpm)—the average spontaneous ^{51}Cr release (cpm). Next, a graph is constructed with the % lysis on the Y-axis versus the E:T ratio (50:1, 25:1, 12.5:1 and 6.25:1) on the X-axis. Using the graph, the E:T ratio, which accounts for 10% cytotoxicity (lysis) is plotted in the graph (E:T$_{10}$). To calculate the number of lytic units (LU), the number of target cells used in the assays, which is constant, is used to calculate the E_{10} (set at 1 LU). The final LU is calculated as the number of LU per a predetermined number of effector cells (e.g. 10^6; thus 10^6 divided by E_{10} = total LU). The fitted curve represents the actual, connected, data points, while the observed cytotoxicity is a "best fit" line mathematically plotted, using lysis at 50:1 and 6.25:1, the standard errors of Y-axis estimates and the degrees of freedom). Upper left shows normal NK-cell function, while the upper right shows decreased NK-cell function, based on an established normal range (LU = 3, being the lower limit of normal in this example). The graphs on the bottom show problems with the generation of fitted curves and their deviation of observed curves, making LU calculations unreliable (although percent lysis for each E:T ratio can still be shown, and, potentially used for interpretation).[28]

influence the validity of the data/results. For example, abnormal NK-cell function can be explained by absence of NK cells (detected by basic flow cytometric assessment of lymphocyte subsets), by absence of components of the cytolytic machinery (Fig. 95.1G), by predominance of regulatory (CD56-bright) NK cells that do not appear to participate in NK-cell cytotoxicity directly, and by other mechanisms.

●KEY CONCEPTS

Basic concepts of functional testing

- Immunologic form follows immunologic function
- The right assay(s) for the right clinical scenario
- An abnormal result invites several essential considerations:
  - Does it reflect a biologically accurate and reproducible finding (confirmation)?
  - What is its relevance (interpretation; pattern recognition)?
  - What is its significance (further studies, patient care issues)?
  - Is it reflective of disease and/or age (age-appropriate controls)?
- With the exception of completely normal and abnormal test results, speculation is invariably involved in data/result interpretation (the gray zone)
- *In vitro* assays that provide increasingly detailed information are also increasingly more demanding and prone to variation and artifacts, requiring rigorous quality control measures
- Contemporary T- and NK-cell testing is done mostly by *in vitro* assays
- Contemporary B-cell testing is done mostly by *in vivo* (vaccination) studies
- General considerations for vaccination studies:
  - Protein vaccines (e.g., tetanus toxoid) measure T-cell dependent responses
  - Polysaccharide vaccines (e.g. pneumovax) measure T-cell independent responses
  - Recall antigens: antigen has been experienced previously; antibody produced is typically of isotype switched subclass (e.g. IgG) when (booster) vaccine is given
  - Neo-antigens: antigen is new to immune system; antibody production is of non-isotype switched subclass (IgM) following primary (first) vaccination, and of isotype switched subclass following secondary vaccination

Assessment of B-cell function

Evaluation of defects in the B-cell compartment, underlying some of the more common immunodeficiency disorders (e.g., common variable immunodeficiency [CVID]), follows the same pathway of linking clinical observations with patterns of abnormal form, often manifested by abnormal levels of immunoglobulins, defective specific antibody responses to infectious agents and/or vaccinations, and an abnormal B-cell phenotype (Fig 95.1C).[29-31] Although similar *in vitro* assays that measure B-cell proliferation, as well as non-specific (polyclonal) and antigen-specific immunoglobulin secretion can be performed using a variety of *in vitro* culture systems, a sufficiently detailed assessment of B-cell function can generally be obtained through *in vivo* testing. Once abnormal B-cell function has been detected *in vivo*, subsequent *in vitro* testing may provide additional information. This testing may include determination of the integrity of cellular contact and signal transduction pathways, the effects of cytokines and growth factors on B-cell differentiation, and the capacity of T cells to provide help, or suppress immunoglobulin secretion. These assays are generally performed in specialized research laboratories only.

The extensive menu of contemporary vaccines provides a convenient stage to perform B-cell function analysis, as determined by the production of specific antibodies *in vivo*. In young children, a sufficient number of vaccinations have generally been administered to allow a screening assessment of B-cell function *in vivo* by measuring specific antibody levels acquired from these immunizations. In older patients and in patients with an incomplete vaccination history, functional studies typically include pre- and post-vaccination measurements of specific antibody levels, following one or more (booster) vaccinations. Functional assessment of antibody production should measure responses to both protein (e.g., tetanus toxoid) and polysaccharide antigens (e.g., *Streptococcus pneumoniae*).[29] The now routine use of conjugate-vaccines is of great benefit in providing protective immunity against certain organisms; however, from a testing perspective it should be realized that these are predominantly IgG1- (and IgG3)-mediated responses, while age-dependent maturity towards anti-polysaccharide immunity is characterized by the development of an IgG2-mediated response. Non-conjugate versions of polysaccharide-specific vaccines are needed to distinguish between immaturity of the immune system and (~ permanent) disorders of specific antibody responses to polysaccharide antigens, as well as the clinical relevance of isolated IgG2 deficiency.[29] Non-conjugate vaccines can, in general, be administered in children older than 2 to 4 years, keeping in mind that immunologic maturity is not reached at the same age by every child. Practically speaking this means that positive results (i.e., satisfactory vaccination response) points towards acquisition of anti-polysaccharide immunity, while negative results should be interpreted with care.

Antibody levels (titers) are often reported relative to protective values. These values should be regarded with caution as they are based on epidemiologic data regarding protection in large control populations. For randomly acquired antibody levels, an initial comparison to protective values can be used to decide if further vaccination studies are warranted. In other scenarios it is recommended to use the patient as his/her own (intra-assay) control and determine a change in antibody levels between pre- and post-vaccination. At least a fourfold increase can be considered a normal response to a protein antigen, and a two- to fourfold increase a normal response to a polysaccharide antigen. It has been observed that over-vaccination, as well as vaccination following (recent) exposure to the antigen via a natural infection may lead to a decreased antibody response. A recent infection represents an appropriate alternative to vaccination, but it requires that information is available regarding the responsible organism, including serotype (e.g., *S. pneumoniae* serotype).

In the workup of immunodeficiency disorders or to characterize functional immune-reconstitution following bone marrow transplantation, chemotherapy or anti-HIV viral therapy, it may be important to determine whether abnormal responses *in vivo* reflect abnormal B-cell function due to a primary B-cell defect, a primary T-cell defect, or a combination of these. Vaccinations based on recall antigens will not provide a clear, or complete, picture as to the origin(s) of abnormal B-cell function. This information can be obtained if a vaccine contains an antigen that has not previously been encountered and that induces an immune response, in which contributions by T and B cells are well characterized. For example, the T-cell-dependent neo-antigen bacteriophage phi-X174 has been extensively studied in inherited and acquired human immunodeficiency conditions;

primary and secondary antibody responses, isotype switching, and antigen clearance can be measured after primary, secondary and subsequent vaccinations, and compared to a well-established normal range.[32,33] Other potential neo-antigens that have been relatively well characterized include keyhole-limpet hemocyanin (KLH) and rabies vaccine.[34,35] An added benefit of bacteriophage and KLH is that vaccination studies can be done while the patient continues to receive intravenous immunoglobulin (IVIG) substitution but neither are FDA approved reagents so these studies must be performed via approved research protocols. Interpretation of data follows the same considerations: totally normal and totally abnormal results are relatively easy to explain, everything in between requires careful analysis. *In vitro* studies of B-cell function (Table 95.2), including the removal and addition of T cells (and other cells) and supernatant/serum may provide additional insights into the integrity of the B-cell compartment.

Research immunology

The distinction between clinical and research immunology is often rather arbitrary. In this section, attention is paid to novel methodology and applications, designed and refined in response to new basic and clinical science discoveries and/or clinical needs.

Testing linked to emerging immune disorders

NF-κB activation disorders

It has become apparent that activation of the transcription factor NF-κB constitutes an important crossroad in host defense. Several gene defects, related to abnormal activation/processing of NF-κB have been identified in individuals presenting with specific patterns of recurrent infections (Table 95.4).[41,42] NF-κB resides in cytoplasm complexed to several inhibitor proteins of NF-κB that prevent its translocation to the nucleus. Upon activation, these inhibitor proteins are targeted for degradation by the IκB kinase (IKK) complex, consisting of IKKα, IKKβ, and NEMO (NF-κB essential modulator), thereby releasing NF-κB and allowing it to translocate into the nucleus and activate its multiple gene transcription programs.[36]

NF-κB is activated by the signal transduction pathways of the TCR and the B-cell receptor (BCR), as well as tumor necrosis factor receptors (TNFR). In addition, NF-κB is part of the signal transduction pathway of the Toll-like receptor family (TLRs) and interleukin-1 receptor family (IL-1Rs). These receptors are important in specific microbial sensing, innate immunity (Chapter 3), as well as amplification of the early inflammatory response through the binding of "IL-1 family" cytokines (IL-1β, IL-18, IL-33). The TLR/IL-1R canonical signal transduction pathway is connected to NF-κB through several adaptor/sorting proteins, including MyD88, TRIF, TRAM, and SARM, which then recruit cytosolic kinases, including the IL-1R-associated kinase (IRAK) complex, containing IRAK-1 and IRAK-4. These kinases subsequently phosphorylate residues in the IKK complex, followed by ultimate release of NF-κB.[37]

Several primary immunodeficiencies involving this elaborate host defense system have been reported (Chapter 36), with mutations in *MyD88*, *IRAK4*, *NEMO*, and *IKBA*.[38] Patients with IRAK-4 and MyD88 deficiencies appear to show specific patterns of invasive pyogenic bacterial infections (meningitis, sepsis, abscesses, osteomyelitis), particularly caused by

Table 95.4 Emerging primary defects in host defense

Gene defect	Affected pathway	Functional assessment (in vitro)
MyD88	NF-κB activation	IL-1R and TLR family stimulation of cytokine production
IRAK-4	NF-κB activation	IL-1R and TLR family stimulation of cytokine production
NEMO	NF-κB activation	IL-1R, TNFR family, or TLR family stimulation of cytokine production
IκBα	NF-κB activation	IL-1R, TNFR family, or TLR family stimulation of cytokine production
IL-12 p40	Production of IL-12	Measure IL-12 production in response to IFN-γ and LPS
IL-12Rβ1	Production of IFN-γ	Measure STAT-4 phosphorylation in activated lymphocytes in response to IL-12
IFN-γR1	Response to IFN-γ	Cell surface expression of INF-γR; cytokine production and abnormal STAT-1 phosphorylation
IFN-γR2	Response to IFN-γ	Cytokine production and abnormal STAT-1 phosphorylation
STAT-1	Response to IFN-γ	Cytokine production and abnormal STAT-1 phosphorylation
STAT-3	Production/function of IL-17	T$_h$17 generation; measure production of IL-17 cytokines (IL-17A, IL-17 F, IL-22)
CARD9	Production/function of IL-17	T$_h$17 generation; measure production of IL-17 cytokines (IL-17A, IL-17 F, IL-22)
AIRE	Production/function of IL-17	Measure autoantibodies to IL-17 cytokines; T$_h$17 generation with/without patient plasma

S. pneumoniae, *Staphylococcus aureus*, and *Pseudomonas aeruginosa*, while host responses towards other bacteria, fungi, parasites, and viruses appear to be intact.[37,38] NEMO defects are associated with a variety of clinical manifestations in males, varying from recurrent bacterial, mycobacterial and viral infections (e.g., CMV), with or without ectodermal dysplasia, to cases with mild infections and severe inflammatory bowel disease. Mutation in an inhibitor of NF-κB (IκBα), reported in only one patient to date, was associated with a clinical phenotype similar to defects in NEMO, showing ectodermal dysplasia and recurrent bacterial infections. However, the patient displayed significantly depressed proliferative T-cell responses to recall antigens.[38]

Currently there is no standard immunological approach to diagnose any of these disorders other than direct genetic testing. The only functional abnormality consistently observed in boys with defects in NEMO is poor response to polysaccharide antigens, including those derived from pneumococcal species. Interestingly, the degree of impairment of the different signaling pathways depends on the nature of the mutation in NEMO. For example, T-cell function, as measured by standard techniques, can vary from being intact to being abnormal, but typically not absent (i.e., the gray zone).[38]

However, although still largely confined to research laboratories, functional assays are becoming more available. Testing the TLR/IL-1R system, to detect defects along this pathway, may offer a consistent approach to evaluate these defects. All human TLRs, except TLR3, use both MyD88 and IRAK-4 and as such should provide a method of testing the canonical pathway as it relates to defects in these two genes. There is sufficient evidence to suggest that patients with NEMO and IκBα deficiency may have abnormal signaling through TLR, IL-1R, and TNFR family members such as CD40 and TNFR.[36–38] Therefore, a clinically useful immunologic assay to capture these defects would measure the NF-κB response to stimulation in an overlapping way, using all three types of receptors (TLR, IL-1R, and TNFR).

One approach is to collect peripheral blood mononuclear cells (PBMC) from patients and controls, place cells in culture with TNF-α, IL-1β, and specific TLR agonists (including a TLR3 antagonist as an internal control), and subsequently measure cytokine secretion (IL-6, TNF-α, IL-1β) by intracellular cytokine flow cytometry (IC-FCM), ELISA or ELISPOT (Chapters 93, 94). Alternatively, a flow-based method, measuring CD62L shedding from the surface of granulocytes following TLR stimulation — with various TLR agonists — can be used.[39]

IL-12/IFN-γ axis defects

In addition to recurrent bacterial infections, patients with defects in NEMO also are at risk for developing mycobacterial infections, likely due to abnormal monocyte/macrophage function. Monocytes in patients with NEMO defects exhibit decreased IL-12 production in response to CD40 receptor activation (i.e. evidence of defective NF-κB activation).[36] IL-12 production by monocytes is required to induce lymphocytes to produce IFN-γ, creating a feedback and amplification loop of immune activation. The importance of this cooperative loop between monocytes (IL-12) and lymphocytes (IFN-γ) is underscored by another group of single gene disorders of defective production of and/or responsiveness to IL-12 and IFN-γ. Patients suffer from (non-tuberculous) mycobacterial infections, as well as infections due to other organisms (e.g. *Salmonella* species, HSV-1, HHV-8), caused by defects in several genes in the pathway, including *IL12B, IL12RB1, IFNGR1, IFNGR2, STAT1,* and *IRF8.*[40–42] The abnormal functional characteristics of these disorders are not identified by routine laboratory evaluation and require specialized (flow cytometry and ELISA-based) assays. For example, defects in response to IFN-γ stimulation due to a problem with IFN-γ receptor (IFN-γR) signaling can be tested by looking at monocyte surface IFN-γR1 expression (a constitutively expressed receptor), and functionally by stimulation of PBMC with IFN-γ and lipopolysaccharide (LPS). Response to stimulation can measure flow cytometrically by evaluating the phosphorylation of a nuclear signaling molecule, signal transducer, and activator of transcription-1 (STAT-1) or alternatively by measuring IFN-γ-induced TNF-α and IL-12 secretion (e.g., ELISA) (Fig. 95.3).[43] This approach allows screening for defects in IFN-γR1, IFN-γR2, and STAT-1 The responsiveness of activated lymphocytes to IL-12 can be measured by detection of phosphorylated STAT-4 or secretion of IFN-γ.[43] As with NEMO, IKBα, and IRAK-4, these types of functional tests are best conducted in close consultation with experts at tertiary research institutions, who also can assist in identification of gene defects that underlie these disorders.

Th17-related disorders

Pattern recognition plays an important role in host defense, but also in recognizing the existence of shared pathogenic and/or contributing factors between clinical phenotypes; even distinct immunodeficiency disorders. These patterns sometimes can be brought to visibility through *in vitro* assays linked to unique clinical phenotypes. Unraveling the nature of the mucocutaneous immune response to *Candida* species has been accelerated with the discovery of several relevant host defense mechanisms that appear to converge at the level of cytokines that are produced

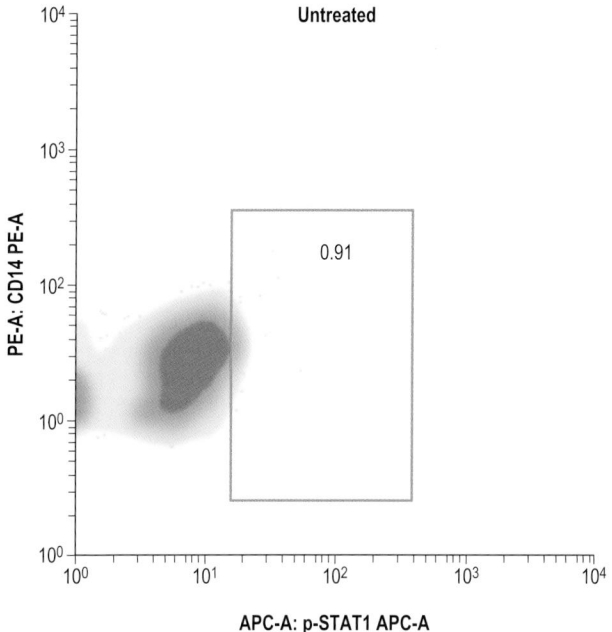

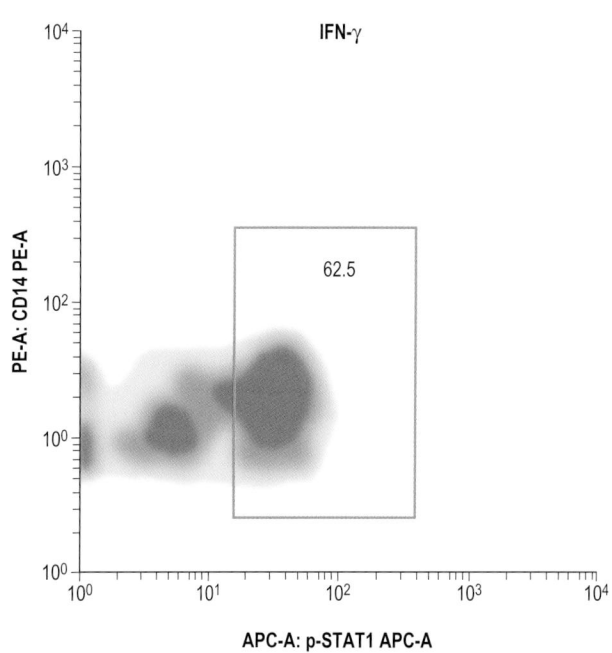

Fig. 95.3 Functional evaluation of IFN-γ signaling. Peripheral blood monocytes were either left untreated (left) or treated with IFN-γ for 15 min (right). Cells were then stained with surface anti-CD14, fixed, permeabilized and stained with an antibody specific for the phosphorylated form of STAT1 (pSTAT1). Note the very strong upregulation of pSTAT1 upon treatment (right), indicating an intact pathway.

by a subset of CD4 T effector cells that has been designated the Th17 T-cell subset. In a simplified manner, the main feature of this T-cell subset is its induction by several key cytokines, including IL-1β, IL-6, and TGF-β, that activate signal transducer and activator 3 (STAT3), to drive a transcription and differentiation program (via the retinoic acid-related orphan receptor [ROR]-γt) into Th17 T cell.[44] Antifungal immunity is mediated through the release of IL-17A, IL-17 F, and IL-22 by Th17 T cells, as well as the selective expression of chemokine receptors (CCR4 and CCR6) that direct homing to skin and mucosa. Candida-related, pathogen-associated molecular patterns (PAMPs), such as β-glucan, are recognized by TLRs and C-type lectin receptors (particularly Dectin-1 and Dectin-2). Its subsequent signal transduction pathway depends on STAT-3 phosphorylation and contains spleen tyrosine kinase (Syk) and caspase recruitment domain family member 9 (CARD9), ultimately resulting in production of IL-1β, IL-6, TGF-β, and IL-23 (important in Th17 T-cell maintenance and expansion).

Chronic/recurrent mucocutaneous candidiasis (CMC), other than caused by global T-cell deficient states, is linked to Th17 and its associated "IL-17" cytokines in several distinct conditions (Table 95.4). At the level of PAMP recognition, homozygous mutations in CARD9 have been linked to recurrent fungal infections. The patients showed reduced IL-17-expressing T cells and an almost complete lack of *in vitro* generation of Th17 T cells.[45] The importance of signaling through STAT-3 for the generation, differentiation and function of Th17 T cells is underscored by mutations in *STAT-3* that underlie the autosomal dominant form of hyper-IgE syndrome (HIES).[46] Other genetically determined defects have recently been identified that interfere with Th17 T-cell/IL-17 function that are also associated with chronic mucocutaneous candidiasis.[47]

Patients with APECED, a rare autosomal recessive disorder of multi-organ autoimmunity, often develop recalcitrant CMC. How mutations in the autoimmune regulator gene (AIRE), leading to defective negative thymic selection/deletion of autoreactive T cells, is associated with CMC has long been a mystery. The discovery of neutralizing autoantibodies to IL-17 and IL-22 provided the link between CMC and Th17 cells and IL-17 cytokines.[44] In addition to demonstrating the presence of autoantibodies, plasma derived from these patients inhibited Th17 cell proliferation and IL-17 production.

Developing *in vitro* assays that measure and quantify Th17 T-cell differentiation and generation of IL-17 cytokines ideally would detect the above-mentioned conditions, but also provide a basic assessment of a defective/dysregulated part of the immune system that can be used to explain clinical issues and perhaps point towards the existence of other emerging immunodeficiency disorders. In addition, connections between different aspects of immunity can be made, such as between the IL-17 system and the IL-12 system.[48] Methodology includes *in vitro* T-cell differentiation, such as currently used in intracellular cytokine detection of Th1- and Th2-associated cytokines, using flow cytometry, ELISA, or ELISPOT, and/or by measuring STAT-3 phosphorylation in response to specific cytokine signals. Adding patient-derived plasma to the incubation/activation step could provide clues to the existence of autoantibodies that interfere in Th17 T-cell differentiation or IL-17 activity.

Immune dysregulation disorders

Defects in immune-regulation and homeostasis are receiving more attention as clinical immunologists become increasingly cognizant that the immune response against self as well as against foreign pathogens needs to be regulated and terminated. Generally the standard menu of laboratory testing focuses on diagnosing individuals with clinical scenarios of recurrent infections, linked to abnormal T-, NK-, and B-cell function. At the other end of the clinical spectrum is an emerging field directed to studying patients with clinical scenarios characterized by lymphoproliferation, autoimmunity, allergy, or malignancy. Here again, the diagnosis is not readily discovered in the clinical immunology laboratory. In Fig. 95.1D, an example is shown of immunologic form that is not reflected in abnormal function, as measured by contemporary clinical assays of T- and NK- (and B-) cell function. Nonetheless, the presence of a markedly expanded T subpopulation that lacks expression of CD4 and CD8 but expresses TCR-α/β

(double-negative T cells) is a direct consequence of a defective immunologic function; namely, abnormal Fas-mediated apoptosis. Apoptosis assays are gaining ground in the comprehensive evaluation of the immune system: the consequence of an increasing appreciation for the importance of downregulation and termination of immunologic responses.[49] Determination of apoptosis *in vitro* is part of the evaluation of autoimmune lymphoproliferative syndrome (ALPS), linking a defined clinical phenotype with abnormal immunologic function due to a fundamental defect in Fas-mediated apoptosis.[50] For ALPS, the *in vitro* assay must approximate the *in vivo* relevance of Fas-mediated apoptosis. Resting (circulating) T cells are typically not sensitive to Fas induced apoptosis *in vivo*. Thus, PBMC (or isolated T cells) are placed in a primary culture system, similar to mitogen- or antigen-proliferation assays followed by several days of culture in the presence of exogenous IL-2. At this stage, T cells are incubated with cross-linking anti-Fas antibodies for a 24- to 48-hour period, after which T-cell apoptosis is measured, using flow cytometric readout systems (Chapter 97). Intra-assay (the patient/subject) and inter-assay (healthy subject) controls should be included. In addition, it is recommended that non-Fas-mediated apoptosis pathways be tested, for example using chemotherapeutic drugs (staurosporine), gamma irradiation, etc., to determine specificity of the defective apoptotic pathway. An example of the importance of this approach is illustrated by the discovery that patients with X-linked lymphoproliferative disease (XLP) have defective apoptosis following TCR restimulation, yet have normal Fas-mediated apoptosis.[51] This pathway may be of particular relevance in the T-cell response to (viral) antigens.

The quite different clinical phenotypes of ALPS and XLP demonstrate the far-reaching consequences and uniqueness of distinct pathways of lymphocyte apoptosis. Further development and refinement of apoptosis assays will likely uncover the existence of other defects in specific modes and pathways of apoptosis, likely to present with unique clinical phenotypes.[52]

Expression of CD25 on CD4; but within the CD25+ population is a unique subpopulation of T cells, often designated CD25^bright (Fig. 95.1B) that function as regulatory T cells (Tregs). These cells are positive for intracellular expression of cytotoxic T-lymphocyte-associated protein 4 (CTLA4) and forkhead box P3 protein (FOXP3). Tregs are found in peripheral blood, thymus, lymph nodes, and a variety of other tissues, including gut and endocrine organs.[53] The importance of Tregs is illustrated by a primary immunodeficiency disorder, designated as immune dysregulation, polyendocrinopathy, enteropathy, X-linked syndrome (IPEX). This syndrome occurs in males who are deficient in the X-linked gene encoding FOXP3.[54] Patients present with diarrhea/failure to thrive, rash, insulin dependent diabetes, and other autoimmune endocrinopathies, as well as immune-mediated cytopenias. The underlying genetic defect in IPEX is a direct result of defective generation and function of these Tregs. Their function appears to limit the immune response to selected self-antigens and probably to suppress the proliferation of activated T cells. Functional assays for Tregs have been established in research laboratories. They are based on the principle of isolating CD4/CD25bright T cells from PBMC and incubating these with the non-isolated T cells plus antigen-presenting cells and evaluating for the inhibition of by mitogens, anti-CD3, or specific antigen induced proliferation (Table 95.2). In the presence of normal Tregs, proliferation, as measured by [³H]-thymidine incorporation in dividing T cells, is reduced, while in the absence of these cells, normal proliferation is detected.

Although IPEX is a rare disorder, Tregs have fast become a well-studied cell population because of their—documented or hypothesized—impact on immune-mediated disorders and, consequently, their potential application in counteracting these disorders. It can be envisioned that clinical scenarios resulting from abnormal regulatory T-cell function will become part of contemporary clinical immunology.

Renaissance of cellular imaging

Flow cytometry is an extremely useful laboratory platform to study form as well as function of the immune system (as a "readout" platform of *in vitro* assays of T-cell/CTL function). However, it should be realized that cells such as T cells operate and interact in a spatial context with other cells, often in highly dynamic and transient interactions. Flow cytometry is not suited to provide insights into this spatial context, particularly as it pertains to the organization of the so-called immunological synapse (IS). The IS is a highly organized junction/contact zone that forms quickly after T cells engage antigen-presenting cells, resulting in T-cell activation and proliferation, through organized clustering of relevant receptors, co-stimulatory, adhesion and scaffolding molecules.[55] Using confocal microscopy, these clusters resemble a bull's eye pattern with an outer ring, the distal supramolecular activation cluster (dSMAC), a proximal (adhesion) ring, containing LFA-1 (pSMAC) and a central signaling cluster (cSMAC), containing the T-cell receptor (TCR) and its associated adaptor and transduction proteins. In CTLs, the cSMAC is divided into a signaling and secretory cluster.[56] Conformational organization into clusters applies to activated B cells as well.[57]

Although these imaging techniques have greatly advanced our understanding of T-cell function, limitations of conventional microscopy platforms prevent the translation of this basic understanding into practical (high-volume) clinical assays that can be added to the repertoire of lymphocyte function assessment. Significant recent advances in quantitative imaging flow cytometry include the development of multispectral imaging flow cytometry. This platform combines fluorescence microscopy with flow cytometry by digitally imaging cells directly in flow. The flow cytometry part can analyze and identify cells of interest, including rare cell populations and conjugates of cells that then can be evaluated by fluorescence microscopy.[55]

It is not hard to imagine that spatial visualization of T-cell function, for example with respect to IS formation, spatial organization, conjugate formation with other cells, organized vesicular trafficking of cytotoxic granules or cytokines to the IS (and target) cells, or movement and translocation of signal transduction molecules (e.g., NF-κB) within the T cell, can complement current T-cell function assays. In addition, this type of platform can be used to visualize and measure phagocytosis, DNA damage and repair, and even interactions by individual proteins through Fluorescence or Forster Resonance Energy Transfer (FRET).[58-60] It will require different and new approaches to assay development and integration of data into meaningful information for application to the clinical evaluation of patients with immunological disorders.

References

1. Bleesing JJ, Fleisher TA. Immunophenotyping. Semin Hematol 2001;38:100–10.
2. Stobo JD. Phytohemagglutin and concanavalin A: probes for murine 'T' cell activation and differentiation. Transplant Rev 1972;11:60–86.
3. Greaves M, Janossy G, Doenhoff M. Selective triggering of human T and B lymphocytes in vitro by polyclonal mitogens. J Exp Med 1974;140:1–18.
4. Vine JB, Geppert TD, Lipsky PE. T4 cell activation by immobilized phytohemagglutinin: differential capacity to induce IL-2 responsiveness and IL-2 production. J Immunol 1988;141:2593–600.
5. Geppert TD, Lipsky PE. Activation of T lymphocytes by immobilized monoclonal antibodies to CD3. Regulatory influences of monoclonal antibodies to additional T cell surface determinants. J Clin Invest 1988;81:1497–505.
6. Flomenberg N, Welte K, Mertelsmann R, et al. Immunologic effects of interleukin 2 in primary immunodeficiency diseases. J Immunol 1983;130:2644–50.
7. Chan AC, Kadlecek TA, Elder ME, et al. ZAP-70 deficiency in an autosomal recessive form of severe combined immunodeficiency. Science 1994;264:1599–601.
8. Gordon EH, Krouse HA, Kinney JL, et al. Delayed cuteneous hypersensitivity in normals: choice of antigens and comparison to in vitro assays of cell-mediated immunity. J Allergy Clin Immunol 1983;72:487.
9. Palmer DL, Reed WP. Delayed hypersensitivity skin testing. II. J Infect Dis 1974;130:138.
10. Roberts K, Lotze MT, Rosenberg SA. Separation and functional studies of the human lymphokine-activated killer cell. Cancer Res 1987;47(16):4366–71.
11. Whiteside TL, Vujanovic NL, Herberman RB. Natural killer cells and tumor therapy. Curr Top Microbiol Immunol 1998;230:221–44.
12. Sanderson CJ. The mechanism of lymphocyte-mediated cytoxicity. Biol Rev 1981;56:153–97.
13. Rees RC. MHC-restricted and nonrestricted killer lymphocytes. Blood 1990;4:204–10.
14. Greenberg AH, Shen LA. Class of specific cytotoxic cells demonstrated in vitro by arming with antigen-antibody complexes. Nat New Biol 1973;245:282–5.
15. Johnson WJ, Steplewski Z, Matthews TJ, et al. Cytolytic interactions between murine macrophages, tumor cells, and monoclonal antibodies: Characterization of lytic conditions and requirements for effector activation. J Immunol 1986;136:4707–13.
16. Melder RJ, Walker ER, Herberman RB, Whiteside TL. Surface characteristics, morphology, and ultrastructure of human adherent lymphokine-activated killer cells. J Leukoc Biol 1990;48:163–73.
17. Melder RJ, Walker E, Herberman RB, et al. Adhesion characteristics of human interleukin 2-activated natural killer cells. Cell Immunol 1991;132:177–92.
18. Berke G. The binding and lysis of target cells by cytotoxic lymphocytes: molecular and cellular aspects. Annu Rev Immunol 1994;12:735–73.
19. Russell JH, Ley TJ. Lymphocyte-mediated cytotoxicity. Annu Rev Immunol 2002;20:323–70.
20. Podack ER, Hengarner H, Lichtenheld MG. A central role of perforin in cytolysis? Annu Rev Immunol 1991;9:129–57.
21. Brunner T, Wasem C, Torgler R, et al. Fas (CD95/Apo-1) ligand regulation in T cell homeostasis, cell-mediated cytotoxicity and immune pathology. Semin Immunol 2003;15:167–76.
22. Whiteside TL, Bryant J, Day R, Herberman RB. Natural killer cytotoxicity in the diagnosis of immune dysfunction: criteria for a reproducible assay. J Clin Lab Anal 1990;4:102–14.
23. Whiteside TL, Herberman RB. Role of human natural killer cells in health and disease. Clin Diagn Lab Immunol 1994;1:125–33.
24. Sullivan KE, Delaat CA, Douglas SD, Filipovich AH. Defective natural killer cell function in patients with hemophagocytic lymphohistiocytosis and in first degree relatives. Pediatr Res 1998;44:465–8.
25. Villanueva J, Lee S, Giannini EH, et al. Natural killer cell dysfunction is a distinguishing feature of systemic onset juvenile rheumatoid arthritis and macrophage activation syndrome. Arthritis Res Ther 2005;7:R30–37.
26. Grom AA, Villanueva J, Lee S, et al. Natural killer cell dysfunction in patients with systemic-onset juvenile rheumatoid arthritis and macrophage activation syndrome. J Pediatr 2003;142:292–6.
27. Bryant J, Day R, Whiteside TL, et al. Calculation of lytic units for the expression of cell-mediated cytotoxicity. J Immunol Methods 1992;146:91–103.
28. Junghans RP, Waldmann TA, Landolfi NF, et al. Anti-Tac-H, a humanized antibody to the interleukin 2 receptor with new features for immunotherapy in malignant and immune disorders. Cancer Res 1990;50:1495–1502.
29. Sorensen RU, Moore C. Antibody deficiency syndromes. Pediatr Clin North Am 2000;47(6):1225.
30. Bleesing JJ, Fleisher TA. Human B cells express a CD45 isoform that is similar to murine B220 and is downregulated with acquisition of the memory B-cell marker CD27. Cytometry B Clin Cytom 2003;51:1–8.
31. Avanzini MA, Locatelli F, Dos Santos C, et al. B lymphocyte reconstitution after hematopoietic stem cell transplantation: functional immaturity and slow recovery of memory CD27+ B cells. Exp Hematol 2005;33:480–6.
32. Stiehm ER, Ochs HD, Winkelsein JA. Immunodeficiency disorders: general considerations. In: Stiehm ER, Ochs HD, Winkelsein JA, editors. Immunologic disorders in infants and children. 5th ed. Philadelphia, PA: Elsevier Saunders; 2004.
33. Pyuan KH, Ochs HD, Wedgwood RJ, et al. Human antibody responses to bacteriophage phiX174: sequential induction of IgM and IgG subclass antibody. Clin Immunol Immunopathol 1989;51:252–63.
34. Curtis JE, Hersh EM, Harris JE, et al. The human primary immune response to keyhole limpet haemocyanin: interrelationships of delayed hypersensitivity. Clin Exp Immunol 1970;6:473.
35. Brinkman DM, der Zijde CM Jol-van, ten Dam MM, et al. Vaccination with rabies to study the humoral and cellular immune response to a T-cell dependent neoantigen in man. J Clin Immunol 2003;23:528–38.
36. Orange JS, Levy O, Geha RS. Human disease resulting from gene mutations that interfere with appropriate nuclear factor-kappaB activation. Immunol Rev 2005;203:21–37.
37. Picard C, von Bernuth H, Ghandil P, et al. Clinical features and outcome of patients with IRAK-4 and MyD88 deficiency. Medicine (Baltimore) 2010;89:403–25.
38. Picard C, Casanova JL, Puel A. Infectious diseases in IRAK-4, MyD88, NEMO or IkBa deficiency. Clin Microbiol Rev 2011;24(3):490–7.
39. von Bernuth H, Ku CL, Rodriguez-Gallego C, et al. A fast procedure for the detection of defects in Toll-like receptor signaling. Pediatrics 2006;118:2498–2503.

40. Rosenzweig SD, Holland SM. Defects in the interferon-gamma and interleukin-12 pathways. Immunol Rev 2005;203:38–47.

41. Haverkamp MH, van Dissel JT, Holland SM. Human host genetic factors in nontuberculous mycobacterial infection: lessons from single gene disorders affecting innate and adaptive immunity and lessons from molecular defects in interferon-gamma-dependent signaling. Microbes Infect 2006;8:1157–66.

42. Hambleton S, Salem S, Bustamante J, et al. IRF8 Mutations and Human Dendritic-Cell Immunodeficiency. N Engl J Med 2011;365(2):127–38.

43. Oliveira JB, Notarangelo LD, Fleisher TA. Applications of flow cytometry for the study of primary immune deficiencies. Curr Opin Allergy Clin Immunol 2008;8:499–509.

44. Hanna S, Etzoni A. New host defense mechanisms against Candida species clarify the basis of clinical phenotypes. J Allergy Clin Immunol 2011;127(6):1433–7.

45. Glocker EO, Hennigs A, Nabavi M, et al. A homozygous CARD9 mutation in a family with susceptibility to fungal infections. N Engl J Med 2009;361:1727–35.

46. Minegishi Y, Saito M, Tsuchiya S, et al. Dominant-negative mutations in the DNA-binding domain of STAT3 cause hyper-IgE syndrome. Nature 2007;448:1058–62.

47. Puel A, Cypowyj S, Bustamante J, et al. Chronic mucocutaneous candidiasis in humans with inborn errors of interleukin-17 immunity. Science 2011;332:65–8.

48. de Beaucoudrey L, Puel A, Filipe-Santos O, et al. Mutations in STAT3 and IL12RB1 impair the development of human IL-17-producing T cells. J Exp Med 2008;205:1543–50.

49. Bidere N, Su HC, Lenardo MJ. Genetic disorders of programmed cell death in the immune system. Annu Rev Immunol 2006;24:321–52.

50. Bleesing JJ. Autoimmune lymphoproliferative syndrome (ALPS). Curr Pharm Des 2003;9:265–78.

51. Snow AL, Marsh RA, Krummey SM, et al. Restimulation-induced apoptosis of T cells is impaired in patients with X-linked lymphoproliferative disease caused by SAP deficiency. J Clin Invest 2009;119:2976–89.

52. Niemela JE, Lu L, Fleisher TA, et al. Somatic KRAS mutations associated with a human nonmalignant syndrome of autoimmunity and abnormal leukocyte homeostasis. Blood 2011;117:2883–6.

53. Chatila TA. Role of regulatory T cells in human diseases. J Allergy Clin Immunol 2005;11:949–59.

54. Wildin RS, Smyk-Pearson S, Filipovich AH. Clinical and molecular features of the immunodysregulation, polyendocrinopathy, enteropathy, X linked (IPEX) syndrome. J Med Genet 2002;39:537–45.

55. Ahmed F, Friend S, George TC, et al. Numbers matter: quantitative and dynamic analysis of the formation of an immunological synapse using imaging flow cytometry. J Immunol Methods 2009;347:79–86.

56. Bossi G, Trambas C, Booth S, et al. The secretory synapse: the secrets of a serial killer. Immunol Rev 2002;189:152–60.

57. Tolar P, Pierce SK. A conformation-induced oligomerization model for B cell receptor microclustering and signaling. Curr Top Microbiol Immunol 2010;340:155–69.

58. Maguire O, Collins C, O'Loughlin K, et al. Quantifying nuclear p65 as a parameter for NF-κB activation: Correlation between ImageStream cytometry, microscopy, and Western blot. Cytometry A 2011;79(6):461–9.

59. Ploppa A, George TC, Unertl KE, et al. ImageStream cytometry extends the analysis of phagocytosis and oxidative burst. Scand J Clin Lab Invest 2011;71(5):362–9.

60. Ouk C, Jayat-Vignoles C, Donnard M, Feuillard J. Both CD62 and CD162 antibodies prevent formation of CD36-dependent platelets, rosettes, and artefactual pseudoexpression of platelet markers on white blood cells: A study with ImageStream(®). Cytometry A 2011;79(6):477–84.

96

Assessment of neutrophil function | Douglas B. Kuhns

Neutrophils, also known as polymorphonuclear neutrophils (because of their multi-lobed nucleus) or granulocytes (because of the numerous granules found in the cytoplasm) are major contributors to the host defense against invading microorganisms, particularly bacteria and fungi. Neutrophils are bone marrow-derived, terminally differentiated cells incapable of further cellular division. They have a short life span in the circulation ($t_{1/2} = 6–8$ hours), but survive an additional 1–2 days in the surrounding tissue.[1] Neutrophils, with a diameter of 10–15 μm and a volume of 346 μm^3, have a unique morphology. The nucleus of the mature neutrophil is segmented into three to five lobes with the chromosomes randomly distributed among the lobes. Neutrophils also have an extensive array of storage granules that are defined by the biosynthesis of different granule proteins at different maturation stages of development.[2] Granules are classified into four distinct populations: azurophilic, specific, gelatinase, and secretory granules. Azurophilic granules contain myeloperoxidase, lysozyme, antimicrobial peptides, defensins, proteases, and the lysosomal acid hydrolases. The specific granules contain lactoferrin, lysozyme, and vitamin B$_{12}$-binding protein, and also serve as storage pools for CD11b/CD18 and cytochrome b$_{558}$ of the O$_2^-$-generating enzyme, NADPH oxidase or NOX2. The gelatinase granules are a subset of the specific granules that have a high content of gelatinase. The secretory granules are highly mobilizable intracellular vesicles that contain alkaline phosphatase and other surface antigens.

The primary function of neutrophils is the ingestion (phagocytosis) and subsequent killing of microorganisms. This process requires the assembly of a multi-component O$_2^-$-generating enzyme, NOX2, an enzyme complex consisting of at least two cytosolic components, p47^{phox} (phagocyte oxidase) and p67^{phox},[3] and two membrane components, p22^{phox} and gp91^{phox}, that constitute cytochrome b$_{558}$.[4,5] This enzyme reduces molecular O$_2$ to O$_2^-$ using NADPH generated by the oxidation of glucose through the pentose phosphate pathway. O$_2^-$ either spontaneously or enzymatically converts to H$_2$O$_2$. In the presence of a metal such as Fe^{2+}, H$_2$O$_2$, and O$_2^-$ can react to form the highly reactive hydroxyl radical, OH$^{\bullet}$. Alternatively, the azurophilic granule constituent, myeloperoxidase, catalyzes the formation of hypochlorous acid from H$_2$O$_2$ and Cl$^-$. The combined activities of these reactive O$_2$ intermediates (ROI), antimicrobial peptides, and lysosomal hydrolases result in the ultimate destruction of the ingested microorganism. Excess production of ROI and release of lysosomal hydrolases into the extracellular milieu can lead to tissue damage and inflammation.

Neutrophils display a diverse array of cellular functions. Abnormalities in these functions can severely compromise host defense, leading to recurrent bacterial and fungal infections (Chapter 21). To localize specific deficiencies of neutrophil function, assays have been developed that mimic these functions both *in vivo* and *in vitro*. Often, a preliminary screening of several neutrophil functions is performed to localize deficits and then more vigorous testing of specific function is performed. Assays to assess neutrophil function should address several limitations—the number of cells required for the assay, the type of cell preparation needed (isolated neutrophils versus whole blood), the overall incubation time for the assay, the complexity of the assay, and the rapidity of data collection. These issues become more critical if multiple functional assays are planned concurrently. Since neutrophils cannot be stored or frozen and maintain viability, neutrophils from a normal subject are generally assayed in parallel to validate the results, doubling the number of assays to be performed. Additionally, isolation of neutrophils can take 1–2 hours, limiting the time available for functional assays. Fluorescent probes have increased the sensitivity of many of the assays and eliminated the need for radioactive probes. The use of multi-well microplates and microplate readers has reduced the number of cells required and has facilitated the collection of data. Experience in the handling of neutrophils and the time constraints of the assays can limit the availability of this testing to laboratories that specialize in assessment of neutrophil function.

● KEY CONCEPT

Because of: (1) the short life span of neutrophils and (2) the time required to isolate neutrophils, assays of neutrophil function should have minimal complexity and rapid data collection

Isolation of neutrophils

Clinical indications and implications

Assays that avoid neutrophil isolation are preferred because of the artificial priming of neutrophils during isolation.[6] However, most assays require isolated neutrophils to eliminate any possible contributions of other leukocytes and blood components. In general, blood should be drawn using either citrate or heparin (10 units/mL) as anticoagulant and maintained at 20–25°C in polypropylene containers. Most isolation protocols require 1–2 hours to obtain purified neutrophils.

Principles and interpretation of laboratory assessment

Most neutrophil isolation protocols use differences in the cell density as the basis for the separation. The relative densities of blood cells are as follows: erythrocytes > neutrophils and eosinophils > monocytes, lymphocytes, and basophils > platelets. Ficoll-Paque is a solution of sodium diatrizoate (a dense, triiodinated compound) and Ficoll (a polysaccharide) with a density (1.077 g/cc) that falls between the density of neutrophils and that of the mononuclear cells. To isolate neutrophils,[7] whole blood is diluted with saline and underlayed with Ficoll-Paque. After centrifugation for 30 minutes at 500 g, the less-dense monocytes, lymphocytes, basophils, and platelets remain at the upper interface of the Ficoll-Paque while the denser erythrocytes and neutrophils pass through the Ficoll-Paque and pellet at the bottom. The mononuclear cells are carefully harvested and the remaining Ficoll-Paque aspirated. The erythrocyte/neutrophil pellet is resuspended with saline and mixed with 3% dextran. Dextran promotes the formation of rouleaux by the erythrocytes, causing them to sediment more rapidly than the neutrophils at 1 g. The neutrophil-enriched supernatant fluid is harvested from the bulk of the erythrocytes. Contaminating erythrocytes are removed by a brief (30-second) hypotonic lysis with 0.2% saline. The isotonicity is quickly restored with an equal volume of 1.6% saline. A second hypotonic lysis removes many of the red cell ghosts. In general, $1–2 \times 10^6$ neutrophils can be isolated per milliliter of whole blood from a normal subject with a normal white blood cell count. All procedures are performed at room temperature and the isolated cells are maintained in a balanced salt solution without divalent cations. The most common cell contaminants of the neutrophil preparation are eosinophils. Further purification of a standard neutrophil preparation with anti-CD16 magnetic immunobeads results in a neutrophil preparation that is generally ≥99% neutrophils.

KEY CONCEPT

In general, $1–2 \times 10^6$ neutrophils can be isolated per milliliter of whole blood from a normal subject with a normal white blood cell count.

A second neutrophil isolation protocol that uses a discontinuous gradient of plasma/Percoll has often been used to minimize exposure of neutrophils to trace contamination by bacterial LPS and reduce neutrophil priming.[8]

Isolated neutrophils are routinely frozen in aliquots of 5×10^6 cells/vial. For Western blot studies, neutrophils (1×10^6 cells/mL of buffer) are pretreated for 20 minutes with the cell permeant, irreversible serine protease inhibitor, diisopropylfluorophosphate (DFP, 1–5 mM). DFP is a volatile, potent neurotoxin that can irreversibly bind to and inactivate acetylcholinesterase and should be used with extreme caution. The cell suspension is then spun and the supernatant fluid removed from the cell pellet prior to freezing. Waste solutions and disposable laboratory items should be flushed with sodium hydroxide to inactivate any residual DFP. These frozen neutrophil pellets, though not viable, can also be a source of DNA for genetic analyses.

Histochemical analysis of neutrophils

Clinical indications and implications

Because of their unique morphology, microscopic examination of neutrophil preparations with a differential stain such as a Wright's stain or a histochemical stain such as Kaplow's stain for myeloperoxidase[9] remains an essential element of neutrophil study and can provide valuable insight into some genetic immunodeficiencies.

Principle and interpretation of laboratory assessment

In a Wright's stain, the nucleus of a segmented neutrophil is normally multi-lobed (usually 2–5 lobes), and each lobe connected by a narrow filament (Fig. 96.1A). The nuclear chromatin is coarsely clumped with purple staining. Nucleoli are generally not present. In a band neutrophil, the nucleus is horseshoe-shaped with no indication of constriction into lobes. The pink-violet staining of the cytosol is associated with numerous, evenly distributed, specific granules; occasionally a dark staining primary granule may be present. Kaplow's stain[9] identifies the myeloperoxidase-containing primary granules as dark blue granules uniformly distributed throughout the cytosol (Fig. 96.1B).

Neutrophils (and platelets) from patients with Chediák-Higashi syndrome have giant primary granules that are generally considered pathognomonic for the disease (Fig. 96.1 C).[10] Myeloperoxidase staining of Chediák-Higashi neutrophils is very distinctive, with staining localized to the discrete giant primary granules (Fig. 96.1D).

Neutrophils from a patient with specific granule deficiency exhibit primarily bi-lobed nuclei (pseudo-Pelger-Huët anomaly) with a paucity of specific granule staining in the cytosol (Fig. 96.1E).[11] Staining of the myeloperoxidase granules of neutrophils from a patient with specific granule deficiency appears normal, since the defect is primarily associated with the specific granules (Fig. 96.1 F).

Neutrophils from a patient with myeloperoxidase deficiency fail to stain for myeloperoxidase in the neutrophils. However, the peroxidase in the eosinophilic granules continues to stain positive (Fig. 96.1 G).[12]

Analysis of granule constituents

Clinical indications and implications

The granules of the neutrophils can be distinguished by their specific contents. Deficiency of only one granule constituent can be associated with a specific genetic defect such as myeloperoxidase deficiency; alternatively deficiency of multiple constituents of a certain granule can be associated with deficiency of an entire pool of granules such as specific granule deficiency. Both enzymatic assays and immunoassays are available to determine the cellular content of many of these granule constituents.

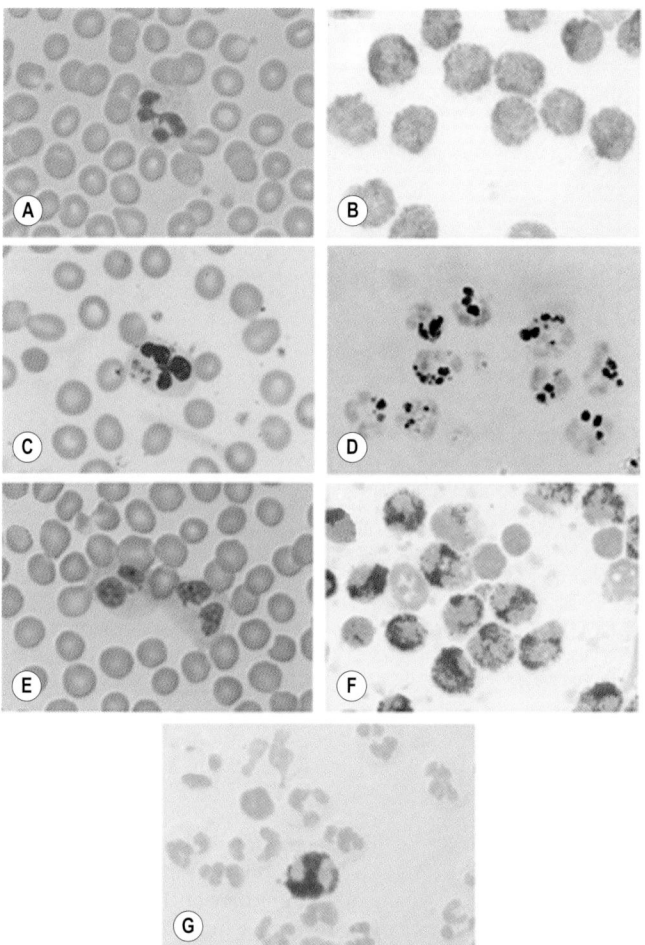

Fig. 96.1 Neutrophils stained with Wright's stain and Kaplow's stain. (A, C, and E) Blood smears stained with Wright's stain. (B, D, F, and G) Neutrophil preparations stained with Kaplow's stain. (A, B) Neutrophils from a normal subject. (C, D) Neutrophils from Chediák-Higashi. (E, F) Neutrophils from a patient with specific granule deficiency. (G) Neutrophils from a patient with myeloperoxidase deficiency. The blue positive-staining cell is an eosinophil.

Principles and interpretation of laboratory assessment

The cellular content of neutrophils can be determined by solubilization of a neutrophil pellet with 0.2% Triton X-100, followed by sonication to disrupt the cells and generate a homogeneous lysate. Analysis of the lysate using commercial immunoassays can identify deficiencies of certain granule contents. Diagnosis of myeloperoxidase deficiency can be confirmed by analysis of neutrophil lysates. Similarly, deficiency of both lactoferrin and neutrophil gelatinase (MMP-9) is indicative of specific granule deficiency, although interestingly, specific granule deficiency is also associated with a deficiency of the α-defensins (human neutrophil peptides 1–3), stored in the azurophilic granules.[13]

Neutrophil adherence

Clinical indications and implications

Adherence of neutrophils to the endothelium is a prerequisite step to the migration of neutrophils into the tissues. Neutrophils isolated from patients with leukocyte adhesion deficiency type 1

(LAD-1) who lack the common β$_2$-integrin subunit CD18 exhibit abnormal adherence to endothelium (Chapter 21),[14] and therefore are not able to migrate efficiently into the surrounding tissues, often resulting in marked granulocytosis.[15] LAD-2 is a milder form of the disease in which patients exhibit a defect in fucose metabolism and glycoprotein biosynthesis.[16] Neutrophils from patients with LAD-2 exhibit abnormal expression of the glycoprotein, L-selectin, and fail to roll along the endothelium. However, they do exhibit normal β$_2$-integrin mediated adherence.

Principles and interpretation of laboratory assessment

Adherence of neutrophils can be assessed by measuring binding to plastic using a 96-well plate either uncoated, or coated with fetal bovine serum or a specific extracellular matrix protein such as fibrinogen or fibronectin. Endothelial cell monolayers harvested from human umbilical veins may serve as a more physiological substrate for the measurement of cell adhesion. Isolated neutrophils are preloaded with the cell permeant, acetoxymethyl ester derivative of the fluorescent dye, calcein (calcein-AM). Nonspecific esterases in the cytosol cleave the ester linkage, trapping the fluorescent probe in the cytosol. The labeled neutrophils are added to each well and incubated in the absence or presence of phorbol myristate acetate (PMA) to promote adherence through activation of the integrins. At the end of the incubation, the wells are washed three times to remove non-adherent cells. The fluorescence of each well is determined with a fluorescent microplate reader and compared to the fluorescence of a control well with a fixed number of fluorescent cells. As shown in the left panel of Fig. 96.2, under control conditions, fewer than 10% of the neutrophils adhere to plastic or to plastic coated with fetal bovine serum or fibrinogen. Treatment of normal neutrophils with PMA for 30 minutes results in the adherence of >90% of the neutrophils under all conditions. This adherence assay is valuable in the diagnosis of patients with leukocyte adhesion deficiency. As shown in the right panel of Fig. 96.2, neutrophils isolated from patients with LAD-1 generally exhibit <5% adherence under control conditions and do not increase adherence after treatment with PMA.

Neutrophil chemotaxis

Clinical indications and implications

Neutrophil migration is a prerequisite for neutrophil accumulation at sites of inflammation. Patients with leukocyte chemotactic defects usually show recurrent skin abscesses and occasional life-threatening, invasive infections (Chapter 21).

Principles and interpretation of laboratory assessment

Assessment of neutrophil chemotaxis *in vivo* can be evaluated using skin windows. Skin blisters are gently raised on the volar surface of the forearm using a vacuum pump and an 8-well blister device, with little hemorrhage and vascular damage. The roof of the blister is removed and the exposed skin lesion is bathed with

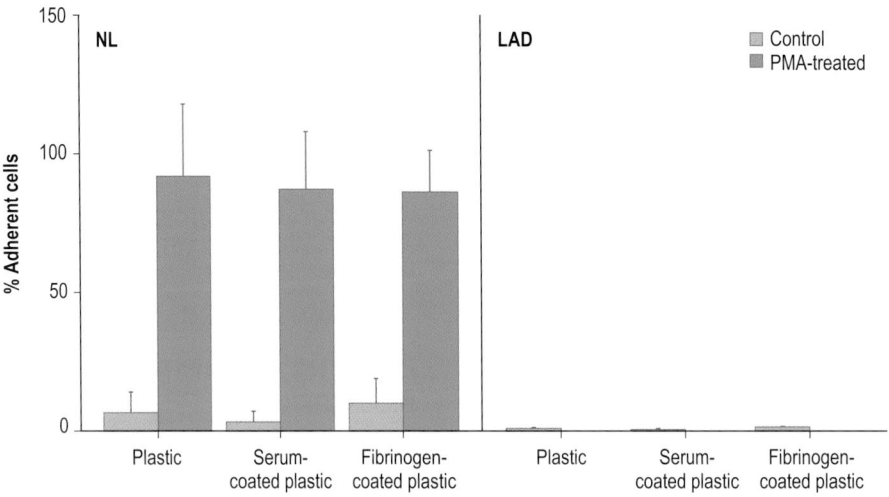

Fig. 96.2 Adherence of neutrophils to plastic: normal versus leukocyte adhesion deficiency. Neutrophils (1×10^7 cells/mL HBSS without divalent cations) were preloaded with acetoxymethyl ester derivative of calcein (calcein-AM: 5 μg/mL) for 15 minutes at 37°C. The cells were washed twice and resuspended in Hanks' balanced salt solution (HBSS)/4-(2-hydroxyethyl)-1-piperazineethanesulfonic acid (HEPES) with 2% bovine serum albumin (BSA) at a cell concentration of 2×10^6/mL. The wells of a 96-well plate were coated for 1 hour at 37°C with 32 μL of either buffer alone, fetal bovine serum, or fibrinogen (2.5 mg/mL). The wells were washed three times and then cells were added to each well (160 μL/well, 3.2×10^5/well). After a 10-minute pre-incubation at 37°C, PMA (100 ng/mL) was added and the plate was incubated for 30 minutes at 37°C. The wells were then washed three times with HBSS/HEPES to remove non-adherent neutrophils. The percentage of adherent cells was determined by the ratio of the fluorescence of the well compared to the fluorescence of a known standard well. The panel (NL) on the left represents the data (mean ± sd) from 22 normal subjects and the panel on the right represents the data from 3 patients with leukocyte adhesion deficiency.

autologous serum using a skin window chamber. In 24 hours, exudative neutrophils accumulate in the autologous serum bathing the skin lesion. The skin chamber provides a mechanism for characterizing the immune cells, as well as soluble immune mediators, that accumulate in the autologous serum during the evolution of the inflammatory response.[17]

Chemotaxis *in vitro* is generally measured using a Boyden chamber. The Boyden chamber includes three components: a lower (chemoattractant) chamber, a nitrocellulose or polycarbonate filter layer, and an upper cell chamber. The lower compartments of the Boyden chamber are filled with a chemoattractant such as fMLF (10^{-8} M) or IL-8 (10 ng/mL). Alternatively, a rapid fluorescence-based measurement of neutrophil chemotaxis has been developed that uses a 96-well disposable chemotaxis chamber[18] that can be read in a fluorescence microplate reader. The lower chamber contains the chemoattractant and is separated from the cellular compartment by a filter. However, instead of a top chamber, the filter has a hydrophobic mask around each filter site that creates surface tension in the cell suspension, and aligns the suspension on the hydrophilic filter located directly above the chemoattractant chamber. Calcein-labeled neutrophils are placed on top of the filter. The chemotaxis chamber is incubated for up to 60 minutes at 37°C. Non-migrating neutrophils atop the filter are rinsed off with buffer and then the plate is read in a fluorescence microplate reader. The number of migrating neutrophils can be determined by comparison of the fluorescence to a standard well with a known number of fluorescent neutrophils. Less than 5×10^6 fluorescent neutrophils are needed to determine neutrophil chemotaxis using several doses of the chemoattractants, fMLF, IL-8, C5a, and leukotriene B$_4$. The advantages of this assay are high sensitivity, rapid acquisition and analysis of data, and reduced labor in loading the cell suspension. The 96-well format also allows for multiple comparisons to be made under identical conditions.

New instrumentation has been developed to monitor chemotaxis temporally. Acquisition of digital images over time enables the migratory tracks of individual cells to be imaged and analyzed

by vectorial analysis, i.e., the magnitude and direction of a cell movement. Adding time as a dimension in the analysis of chemotaxis provides a mechanism to simultaneously evaluate both chemotactic and chemokinetic responses in neutrophils.

Expression of surface antigens

Clinical indications and implications

The expression of neutrophil membrane antigens is altered *in vivo* during exudation or after challenge with intravenous endotoxin. Flow cytometric analysis of adhesion molecules on the neutrophil cell surface can indirectly reflect neutrophil adhesion function. Patients with LAD-1 exhibit a deficit in the expression of the common β$_2$-integrin, CD18, resulting in deficiency in CD11a, CD11b, CD11c, and CD18 (Chapter 21).[19]

Principles and interpretation of laboratory assessment

The expression of cell surface antigens is determined on neutrophils stained with specific fluorescent monoclonal antibodies and analyzed by flow cytometric analysis (Chapter 94). Neutrophils stained with nonspecific isotype antibodies are used to determine the nonspecific background staining. To determine the expression of circulating neutrophils and avoid artifacts induced by neutrophil isolation, an aliquot of whole blood can be stained with the appropriate antibody prior to lysis of the erythrocytes. During flow cytometric analysis, the neutrophils are easily differentiated using their forward light scatter and side scatter to gate on the neutrophil population. Since very little blood is needed (100 μL) for each antigen, neutrophils can be stained with a panel of antibodies to many relevant surface antigens so that a more complete representation of surface antigen expression on neutrophils can be obtained. The panel should include the β_2 integrins (CD11a, CD11b, CD11c, and CD18), selectins (CD62L), Fcγ receptors I, II, and III (CD64, CD32 and CD16), leukosialin (CD43), the common leukocyte antigen (CD45), and distinct surface markers for the granules—carcinoembryonic antigen-related cell adhesion molecule 8 (CEACAM8 or CD66b), a GPI-anchored glycoprotein family member stored in the specific granules, and lysosomal-membrane-associated glycoprotein (LAMP-3 or CD63), stored in the azurophilic granules. During exudation, the expression of CD11b and CD18 is increased over that observed in peripheral neutrophils, while the expression of CD43 (leukosialin) and CD62L is markedly reduced.

The antibody 7D5 recognizes an extracellular epitope of gp91^{phox} and can be used to identify surface expression of gp91^{phox} as well as mobilization of latent pools of gp91^{phox} stored in the specific granules. Flow cytometric analysis of neutrophils stained with 7D5 can often be used to identify patients with X-linked CGD (no 7D5 staining) and X-linked chronic carriers of CGD (mosaic pattern of staining), particularly in patients where the number of cells available for testing is limited.

The expression of surface antigens can also be used to assess the responsiveness of neutrophils to particular ligands such as fMLF and LPS. As shown in Fig. 96.3, neutrophils isolated from a patient who has a genetic defect in IL-1 receptor-associated kinase-4 (IRAK-4, Chapter 36)[20] exhibit abnormal regulation of surface antigen expression to LPS, but exhibit normal regulation of surface antigen expression to fMLF. Antigen expression can be upregulated because of translocation of latent antigen to the plasma membrane or downregulated because of either internalization or shedding of the antigen.

Neutrophil degranulation

Clinical indications and implications

The proteases, acid hydrolases, and inflammatory mediators released from storage granules in the neutrophils can mediate bacterial killing, tissue damage, healing, and immune regulation. Lactoferrin that is released from specific granules can chelate iron, resulting in a bactericidal or bacteriostatic effect. Elevation of plasma lactoferrin is an indication of intravascular activation and degranulation of neutrophils.

Principles and interpretation of laboratory assessment

Stimulation of neutrophils with various secretagogues can result in the release of granular enzymes into the extracellular fluid. Treatment of the neutrophils with cytochalasin b (5 μg/mL)

Fig. 96.3 Upregulation of neutrophil surface antigen expression. Neutrophils (2.5×10^6/mL HBSS + 10% AB sera) isolated from a normal subject (NL) or from a patient with an interleukin-1 receptor-associated kinase-4 (IRAK-4) mutation (PT) were treated with either lipopolysaccharide (LPS: 100 ng/mL) or formyl-methionyl-leucyl-phenylalanine (fMLF: 0.1 μM) for 30 minutes at 37°C. The cells were washed and stained with C10 (an antibody that demonstrates neutrophil heterogeneity), CD18, CD11b (antibodies to β2-integrins), CD66b (a specific granule marker), CD45 (the common leukocyte antigen), and L-selectin. The green lines represent the isotype control, blue lines represent control neutrophils, and purple lines represent stimulated cells. Differences between control and stimulated cells have been shaded.
From Kuhns DB, Long Priel DA, Gallin JI. Endotoxin and IL-1 hyporesponsiveness in a patient with recurrent bacterial infections. J Immunol 1997; 158: 3959, with permission of The American Association of Immunologists, Inc.

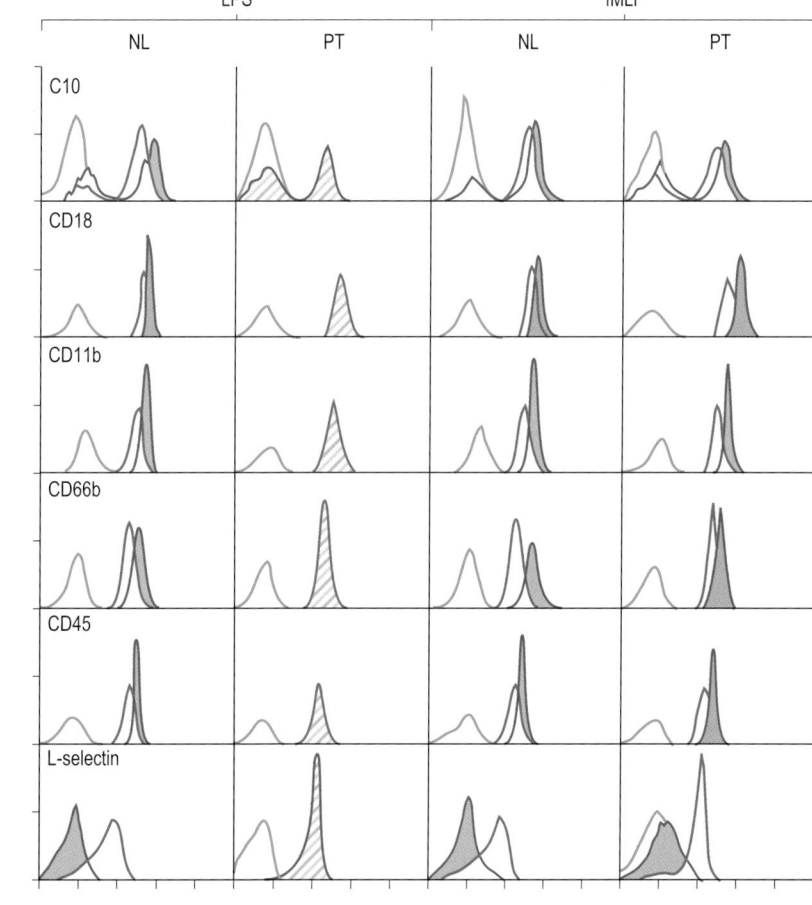

disrupts microfilament assembly and facilitates the release of both specific and azurophilic enzymes. Since stimulation of neutrophil degranulation is often accompanied by O_2^- generation and oxidative inactivation of enzymes, both the cell supernatant fluid and the cell pellet should be analyzed to determine the percentage of enzyme released. To differentiate degranulation from cell lysis, release of the cytosolic enzyme lactate dehydrogenase should be monitored simultaneously.

The release of azurophilic granules can be assessed by determination of myeloperoxidase or elastase. CD63 is also found in the membrane of azurophilic granules and migrates to the neutrophil surface after stimulation with fMLF in the presence of cytochalasin b.

The release of specific granules can be assessed by determination of lactoferrin levels using an enzyme-linked immunoassay. The carcinoembryonic antigen CD66b (formerly CD67) is found on the neutrophil surface and the specific granules, and its expression on the surface of the neutrophils is increased after stimulation with fMLF or LPS. The secretory granules usually contain proteins that are translocated into the membrane from cytosol during degranulation. Detection of the constituents of secretory granules can be assessed by flow cytometric analysis of the change in expression of surface proteins such as adhesion molecules, and cytochrome b_{558} of the NADPH oxidase.

Generation of reactive oxygen intermediates

Clinical indications and implications

The release of ROI such as O_2^- and H_2O_2 is an important component of the bactericidal machinery of a neutrophil. Neutrophils isolated from patients with chronic granulomatous disease (CGD) have a defect in the NADPH oxidase and are unable to generate ROI, resulting in an O_2-dependent bactericidal defect (Chapter 21). The production of ROI has become an important tool to perform risk assessment in patients with CGD. Patients with the lowest ROI generation (<1% of normal generation) have lower survival than patients with higher ROI generation (3–10% of normal). Moreover, survival in CGD is a continuous function of ROI production; suggesting that therapeutic interventions that result in an increase in ROI generation should incur a survival benefit to patients with CGD.[21]

● CLINICAL PEARLS

Reactive oxygen intermediates in chronic granulomatous disease

- Neutrophil ROI production, the primary determinate in diagnosis of patients with CGD, ranges from 0.1 to 27% of that observed in normal subjects.
- In addition, survival in CGD is strongly associated with residual ROI production as a continuous variable, and is independent of the specific protein defect.
- ROI production is an important, early indicator of overall risk in CGD.
- In addition, small increases (as little as 3–5% of normal) in residual neutrophil ROI production may confer a survival benefit.
- Careful monitoring with detection of even small increases in ROI may be an important indicator of clinical efficacy during therapeutic intervention.

Principles and interpretation of laboratory assessments

The production of superoxide (O_2^-) can be detected using the reduction of cytochrome c. Because O_2^- causes a one-to-one stoichiometric reduction of ferricytochrome c to ferrocytochrome c, the resultant increase in the absorption spectrum at 550 nM can be used to quantitate the production of O_2^-. Superoxide dismutase is added to an identical tube to control for the nonspecific reduction of cytochrome c. However, since cytochrome is not permeable to the cells, the detection of O_2^- is limited to that released into the extracellular milieu. Neutrophils isolated from normal volunteers produce 0.42 ± 0.67 nmol/10^6 neutrophils/10 min under resting conditions; treatment with PMA results in 35.92 ± 11.92 nmol/10^6 neutrophils/10 min (Fig. 96.4). An estimate of normal O_2^- production over 60 minutes can be obtained by reducing the number of neutrophils in the assay to 2×10^5. Neutrophils isolated from patients with CGD produce little, if any, O_2^- in response to PMA in 10 minutes (Fig. 96.4). However, some patients with autosomal forms of CGD have low, but detectable O_2^- production in 60 minutes. Neutrophils isolated from X-linked heterozygous carriers of CGD can yield a full spectrum of O_2^- production, while neutrophils from autosomal recessive carriers of CGD generally yield a normal response (Fig. 96.4). Although the detection of O_2^- by reduction of cytochrome c is useful in the diagnosis of patients with CGD, it cannot be used in the diagnosis of carriers because of the wide spectrum of responses that result from the degree of X chromosome lyonization.

Studies have shown that O_2^- determinations sufficiently reliable to diagnose CGD can be obtained from neutrophils isolated from heparinized whole blood that has been stored overnight. Hence, analyses can be performed on blood samples shipped

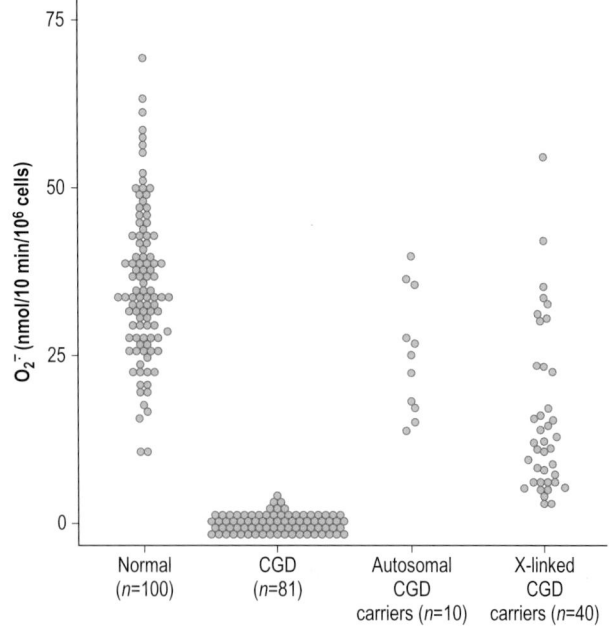

Fig. 96.4 O_2^- **generation from normal subjects, chronic granulomatous disease (CGD) patients, and CGD carriers.** Neutrophils (1×10^6/mL HBSS) were incubated in the presence of 100 μM cytochrome c with phorbol myristate acetate (PMA: 100 ng/mL) for 10 minutes at 37°C. The reaction was terminated by centrifugation at 4°C. Reduction of cytochrome c was monitored at an analytical wavelength of 549.5 nm and a micromolar extinction coefficient of 0.0211. An identical tube containing superoxide dismutase (100 μg/mL) served as a blank.

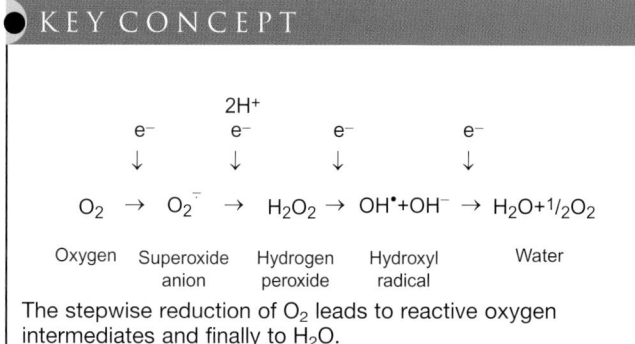

by overnight express. A normal control blood sample should accompany the sample to ensure adequate shipment handling. By 48 hours of storage, however, there are marked reductions in the PMA response and the data are no longer valid.

The extracellular release of H_2O_2 can be measured using horseradish peroxidase-induced oxidation of either phenol red or Amplex® Red. Polymorphonuclear neutrophil suspensions in the presence of horseradish peroxidase and one of the chromophores are exposed to either PMA or buffer alone. Changes in optical density of phenol red at 600 nm can be determined with a standard microplate reader. Amplex® Red is a much more sensitive fluorescent chromophore and H_2O_2-dependent changes in fluorescence can be determined with a fluorescence microplate reader.

The nitroblue tetrazolium (NBT) test is a qualitative assay of $O_2^{\bar{}}$ production. Either whole blood or isolated neutrophils are mixed with NBT in a chamber slide and stimulated with PMA for 15–30 minutes at 37 °C. The neutrophils are allowed to settle on the slide. The slide is air-dried, counterstained with 0.1% safranin, and examined under a microscope. The NBT test yields a visual record of the reduction of the NBT dye to the insoluble, blue-black deposits of formazan. Normal neutrophils, but not neutrophils from CGD patients, reduce the yellow dye to black-brown-blue aggregates in the cells. Because of the random inactivation of the X chromosome, X-linked carriers of CGD exhibit both NBT⁺ and NBT⁻ neutrophils. The percentage of NBT⁺ neutrophils in X-linked carriers of CGD ranges from 5 to 95%. The drawback of the NBT test is the manual counting necessary to obtain an accurate reflection of the percentage of positive cells.

An alternative to the NBT test is a flow cytometric assay using the dye, dihydrorhodamine-123 (Chapter 94).[22] Neutrophils are loaded with the non-fluorescent dye, and then stimulated with PMA for 15 minutes at 37 °C. The H_2O_2 produced oxidizes the dye and results in increased fluorescence, detectable with a flow cytometer. The assay is dependent on endogenous myeloperoxidase in the primary granules. Catalase is added to prevent cell-to-cell diffusion of H_2O_2. Since dye is localized to the cytoplasm, and catalase is present in the extracellular fluid, the dihydrorhodamine-123 assay detects the intracellular production of ROI. As shown in Fig. 96.5, stimulation of normal neutrophils (A) with PMA results in a two-log shift in the fluorescence intensity. Neutrophils from an X-linked carrier of CGD (B) exhibit mosaicism with a negatively stained (abnormal) population and a brightly stained positive population. Neutrophils from a patient with X-linked CGD that lack gp91^{phox} (C) express little increase in fluorescence while neutrophils from a patient with a deficiency in p47^{phox} (D) exhibit a slight increase in fluorescence. The major advantages of the dihydrorhodamine-123 assay are the sensitivity, the signal-to-noise ratio, and the ease of counting a large number of cells. Moreover, it has been shown that the dihydrorhodamine-

123 assay yields reliable results on ethylenediaminetetraacetic acid (EDTA) or heparin-treated blood samples that have been stored overnight. In general, more than 90% of the neutrophils from the control blood samples will exhibit increased dihydrorhodamine-123 fluorescence. For this same reason, however, overnight samples should not be used to rule out X-linked heterozygosity since a highly lyonized CGD carrier (>90%) could yield similar results.

Bactericidal activity

Clinical indications and implications

Assessment of bactericidal activity is a general test that encompasses a broad spectrum of neutrophil function. To show normal bactericidal activity, the neutrophil must be able to recognize and ingest bacteria, and then activate a potent microbicidal response that may include both oxidative and non-oxidative mechanisms.

Principles and interpretation of laboratory assessment

Challenging neutrophils with viable bacteria at a fixed ratio of bacteria:neutrophil is a useful assay to assess the ability of neutrophils to recognize, ingest, and kill bacteria. In our laboratory, we typically use *Staphylococcus aureus*, substrain 502A. The bacteria are suspended in trypticase soy broth and grown in a shaker water bath at 37 °C, monitoring growth until the bacteria are in log phase. In order to add a known number of bacteria, preliminary studies should be performed to determine the number of viable bacteria (i.e., colonies) versus the OD_{650nm}. In our laboratory, an OD_{650nm} of 0.250 yields $0.8–1 \times 10^8$ bacteria/mL. Since neutrophils do not directly recognize bacteria but instead recognize the opsonins (immunoglobulins, complement C3b and C3bi), the assay requires the presence of human serum to provide opsonic activity. A pool of freshly frozen AB sera isolated from at least 10 donors yields good results in our hands. Commercially available pools of AB sera have proven less satisfactory, presumably because of losses in complement and opsonic activity during processing. Neutrophils in the presence of human sera and viable bacteria are incubated at 37 °C for 90–120 minutes on an end-over-end rotator. Control reactions such as bacteria alone and bacteria with sera alone are included in the study to exclude the possibilities of serum bactericidal activity or poor bacterial viability. At specified times, an aliquot of the neutrophil suspension is lysed in distilled water to release viable bacteria. A fraction of the lysate is added to a Petri dish, mixed with warmed, liquid trypticase soy agar, and then allowed to solidify. The plates are incubated for 48 hours in a 37 °C incubator and bacterial colony formation is enumerated by either manual counting or image analysis. The data presented are percent killing of the original bacterial challenge. At a low (<4 bacteria/neutrophil) target:effector ratio, neutrophils kill >90% of the bacteria. However, increasing the bacterial challenge reduces the efficiency of bacterial killing. Challenge of neutrophils with a low target:effector ratio can be useful in identifying those patients with a marked defect in the ability to kill, while challenge with a higher ratio can be useful in identifying those patients with more subtle defects. Recently, it was reported that lysis of the neutrophils in a more basic solution results in more efficient disruption of the cells and more effective dispersion of the bacterial particles.[23] These authors suggest that much of the

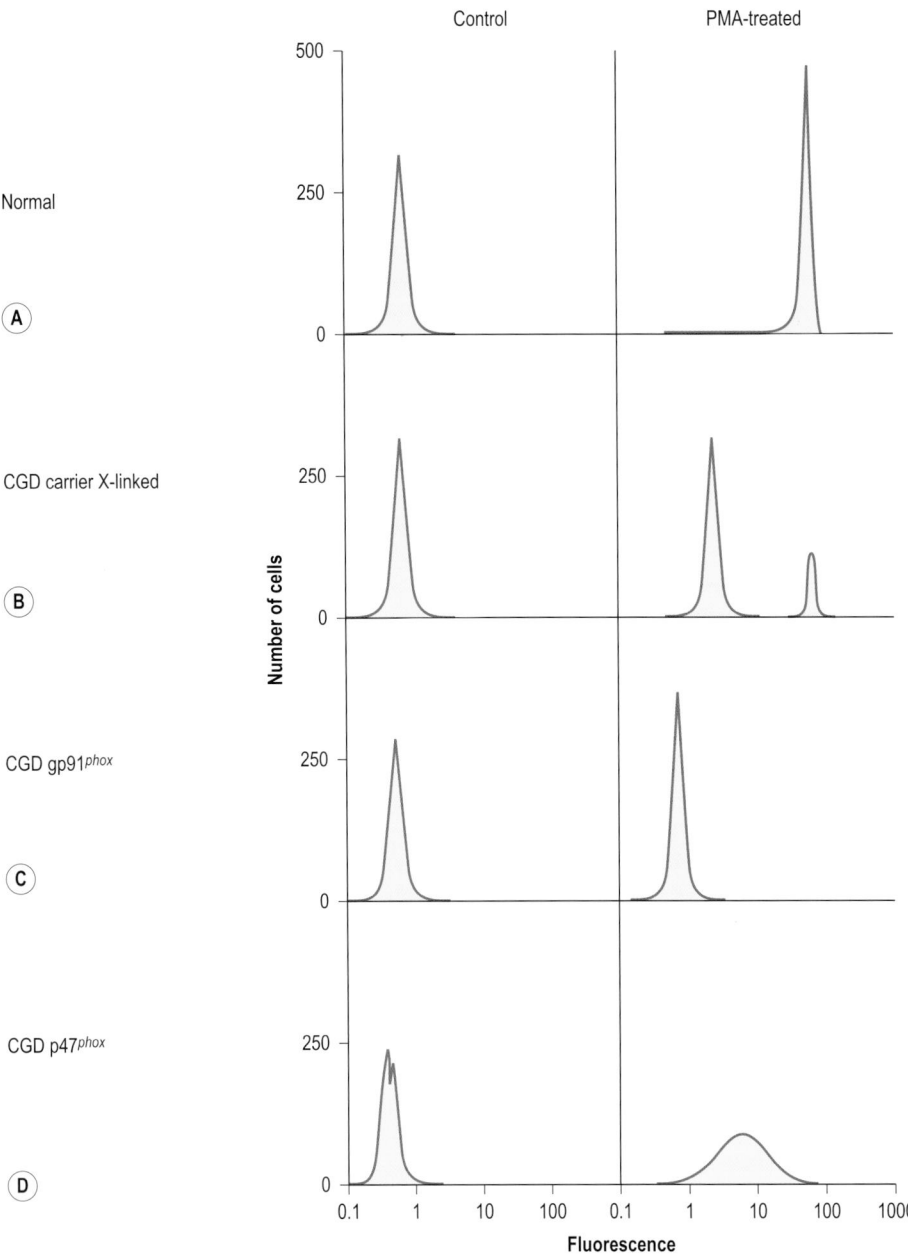

Control   PMA-treated

Normal

(A)

CGD carrier X-linked

(B)

CGD gp91^{phox}

(C)

CGD p47^{phox}

(D)

Number of cells

Fluorescence

Fig. 96.5 Flow cytometric analysis of dihydrorhodamine staining. Whole blood (1.2 mL with ethylenediaminetetraacetic acid (EDTA) as anticoagulant) collected from a normal subject (A), an X-linked chronic granulomatous disease (CGD) carrier (B), a gp91^{phox} CGD patient (C), and a p47^{phox} CGD patient (D) was lysed using an ammonium chloride–potassium bicarbonate solution. The remaining leukocytes were resuspended in HBSS and incubated with dihydrorhodamine-123 (100 μM) for 5 minutes at 37°C. The cells were then incubated an additional 15 minutes at 37°C with either buffer (control) or phorbol myristate acetate (PMA: 400 ng/mL). The cells were immediately analyzed by flow cytometric analysis. Neutrophils were gated using forward light scattering and right-angle light scattering. The analyses presented represent 5000 events within the gated area.

bactericidal activities previously reported may be overestimated and demonstrate more marked bactericidal defects in patients with CGD and myeloperoxidase deficiency.

Western blot analysis of NADPH oxidase protein subunits

Clinical indications and implications

The NADPH oxidase consists of two membrane components, p22^{phox} and gp91^{phox}, three cytosolic components, p47^{phox}, p67^{phox}, and p40^{phox}, and several guanosine triphosphate (GTP)-binding proteins. CGD is characterized by defects

in any one of four of these components – p22^{phox} (~5% of CGD patients), p47^{phox} (~25% of CGD patients), p67^{phox} (~5% of CGD patients), and gp91^{phox} (remaining 65% of CGD patients).

Principles and interpretation of laboratory assessments

The severity of CGD can be related to the specific protein defect. Determination of the specific protein defect in CGD by Western blot analysis also provides direction for determination of the specific genetic defect as well as enabling appropriate genetic counseling for the extended family. A validated normal control is included on each gel for band identification and intensity comparisons. In addition, a typical gp91^{phox} CGD is included on each blot to insure adequate development of p22^{phox}. Typical phox

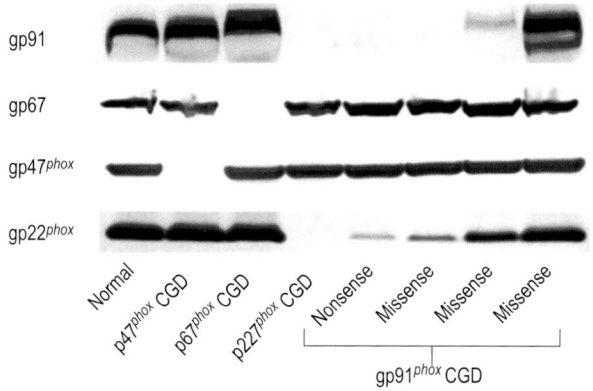

gp91

gp67

gp47^{phox}

gp22^{phox}

Normal   p47^{phox} CGD   p67^{phox} CGD   p227^{phox} CGD   Nonsense   Missense   Missense   Missense

gp91^{phox} CGD

Fig. 96.6 Determination of NADPH oxidase protein defect by Western blot analysis. Frozen, diisopropylflurophosphate (DFP)-treated neutrophil pellets (5×10^6 cells) were resuspended in polyacrylamide gel electrophoresis (PAGE) sample buffer and sonicated to break up the DNA. One million cell equivalents were loaded into each lane (10% PAGE gels for p47^{phox} and p67^{phox}, 4–12% gradient PAGE gels for p22^{phox} and gp91^{phox}). A validated normal control was run on each gel for quality control. The gels were transferred to nitrocellulose, blocked with 5% powdered milk, and incubated overnight with specific antibodies to the phox proteins. The blots were washed, incubated with peroxidase-labeled secondary antibody, and developed with a color reagent. The blots were scanned for permanent storage and a composite figure was created using the relevant bands from each blot. The lanes are identified by the specific protein defect and, for gp91^{phox}, the type of mutation.

protein band patterns are presented in Fig. 96.6. Patients with p47^{phox} CGD are Western blot-negative. Patients with p67^{phox} CGD are generally Western blot-negative; however, we have analyzed one patient with a missense mutation in p67^{phox} who is Western blot-positive. Because p22^{phox} and gp91^{phox} exist as a membrane complex, patients with a defect in p22^{phox} are generally Western blot-negative for both p22^{phox} and gp91^{phox}. In contrast, defects in gp91^{phox} yield more variable results. In general, patients with nonsense defects in gp91^{phox} exhibit low but detectable levels of p22^{phox}. Patients with missense mutations in gp91^{phox} that yield detectable gp91^{phox} protein exhibit proportionately higher levels of p22^{phox}. Neutrophils isolated from overnight samples can be used to diagnose p47^{phox} deficiency because of the stability of the protein. However, detection of other phox protein defects in overnight samples can be more problematic because of proteolysis of p67^{phox} and the gp91^{phox}:p22^{phox} complex.

Conclusion

Our understanding of neutrophil biology is undergoing significant changes. Long-standing axioms are being challenged. Pillay et al. suggested that the life span of a circulatory neutrophil is 5.4 days.[24] Chakravarti et al. suggested that treatment of neutrophils with a cocktail of cytokines can reprogram a phenotypically distinct subset of neutrophils with increased survival and altered function.[25] Rodriguez et al. have shown that patients with renal cancer have a subset of lighter density neutrophils that co-localize with mononuclear cells atop the density cushion and appear to be phenotypically "activated";[26] moreover, these lighter density neutrophils are capable of suppressing T-cell proliferation through a mechanism dependent on arginase-1 stored in the gelatinase granules, a novel function of neutrophils. Much of our current understanding of neutrophil biology has developed from the study of genetic immunodeficiencies; however, there are still gaps in our understanding of how different disease

processes can affect different "activation" states in neutrophils and alter both their function and their survival.

Acknowledgment

This project has been funded in whole or in part with federal funds from the National Cancer Institute, National Institutes of Health, under Contract HHSN261200800001E. The content of this publication does not necessarily reflect the views or policies of the Department of Health and Human Services, nor does mention of trade names, commercial products, or organizations imply endorsement by the US Government.

References

1. Bainton DF. The cells of inflammation: a general view. In: Weissman G, editor. 2nd ed New York: Elsevier/North-Holland; 1980.
2. Borregaard N, Cowland JB. Granules of the human neutrophilic polymorphonuclear leukocyte. Blood 1997;89:3503–21.
3. Volpp BD, Nauseef WM, Clark RA. Two cytosolic neutrophil oxidase components absent in autosomal chronic granulomatous disease. Science 1988;242(4883):1295–7.
4. Parkos CA, Dinauer MC, Walker LE, et al. Primary structure and unique expression of the 22-kilodalton light chain of human neutrophil cytochrome b. Proc Natl Acad Sci U S A 1988;85(10):3319–23.
5. Segal AW, Cross AR, Garcia RC, et al. Absence of cytochrome b-245 in chronic granulomatous disease—a multicenter European evaluation of Its incidence and relevance. N Engl J Med 1983;308(5):245–51.
6. Kuijpers TW, Tool ATJ, van der Schoot CE, et al. Membrane surface antigen expression on neutrophils: a reappraisal of the use of surface markers for neutrophil activation. Blood 1991;78:1105–11.
7. Böyum A. Isolation of mononuclear cells and granulocytes from human blood. Isolation of monuclear cells by one centrifugation, and of granulocytes by combining centrifugation and sedimentation at 1 g. Scand J Clin Invest Suppl 1968;97:77–89.
8. Haslett C, Guthrie LA, Kopaniak MM, et al. Modulation of multiple neutrophil functions by preparative methods or trace concentrations of bacterial lipopolysaccharide. Am J Pathol 1985;119(1):101–10.
9. Kaplow LS. Simplified myeloperoxidase stain using benzidine dihydrochloride. Blood 1965;26(2):215–9.
10. Introne W, Boissy REB, Gahl WA. Clinical, molecular, and cell biological aspects of Chediak–Higashi syndrome. Mol Genet Metab 1999;68(2):283–303.
11. Strauss RG, Bove KE, Jones JF, et al. An anomaly of neutrophil morphology with impaired function. N Engl J Med 1974;290:478–84.
12. Nauseef WM. Diagnostic assays for myeloperoxidase deficiency. In: Quinn MT, DeLeo FR, Bokoch GM, editors. Neutrophil methods and protocols. Totowa, NJ: Humana Press; 2007. p. 525–30.
13. Parmley RT, Gilbert CS, Boxer LA. Abnormal peroxidase-positive granules in "specific granule" deficiency. Blood 1989;73(3):838–44.
14. Buescher ES, Gaither T, Nath J, Gallin JI. Abnormal adherence-related functions of neutrophils, monocytes, and Epstein-Barr virus-transformed B cells in a patient with C3bi receptor deficiency. Blood 1985;65(6):1382–90.
15. Anderson DC, Schmalstieg FC, Finegold MJ, et al. The severe and moderate phenotypes of heritable Mac-1, LFA-1 deficiency: their quantitative definition and relation to leukocyte dysfunction and clinical features. J Infect Dis 1985;152(4):668–89.
16. Etzioni A, Frydman M, Pollack S, et al. Recurrent severe infections caused by a novel leukocyte adhesion deficiency. N Engl J Med 1992;327(25):1789–92.
17. Kuhns DB, DeCarlo E, Hawk DM, Gallin JI. Dynamics of the cellular and humoral components of the inflammatory response in skin blisters in humans. J Clin Invest 1992;89:1734–40.
18. Frevert CW, Wong VA, Goodman RB, et al. Rapid fluorescence-based measurement of neutrophil migration in vitro. J Immunol Methods 1998;213:41–52.
19. Anderson DC, Springer TA. Leukocyte adhesion deficiency: an inherited defect in the Mac-1, LFA-1, and p150,95 glycoproteins. Annu Rev Med 1987;38:175–94.
20. Kuhns DB, Long Priel DA, Gallin JI. Endotoxin and IL-1 hyporesponsiveness in a patient with recurrent bacterial infections. J Immunol 1997;158:3959–64.
21. Kuhns DB, Alvord WG, Heller T, et al. Residual NADPH oxidase and survival in chronic granulomatous disease. N Engl J Med 2010;363(27):2600–10.
22. Emmendörffer A, Hecht M, Lohmann-Matthes M-L, Roesler J. A fast and easy method to determine the production of reactive oxygen intermediates by human and murine phagocytes using dihydrorhodamine 123. J Immunol Methods 1990;131(2):269–75.
23. Decleva E, Menegazzi R, Busetto S, et al. Common methodology is inadequate for studies on the microbicidal activity of neutrophils. J Leukoc Biol 2006;79(1):87–94.
24. Pillay JP, den Braber I, Vrisekoop N. In vivo labeling with ^{2}H$_2$O reveals a human neutrophil lifespan of 5.4 days. Blood 2010;116(4):625–7.
25. Chakravarti A, Rusu D, Flamand N, et al. Reprogramming of a subpopulation of human blood neutrophils by prolonged exposure to cytokines. Lab Invest 2009;89:1084–99.
26. Rodriguez PC, Ernstoff MS, Hernandez C, et al. Arginase I-producing myeloid-derived suppressor cells in renal cell carcinoma are a subpopulation of activated granulocytes. Cancer Res 2009;15(4):1553–60.

Assessment of human allergic diseases

Robert G. Hamilton

Human allergic disease comprises a spectrum of IgE-mediated immediate-type hypersensitivity reactions that manifest as reactions in the skin (urticaria, dermatitis), respiratory tract (asthma or rhinitis), gastrointestinal tract and, in their most extreme condition, systemic anaphylaxis. These reactions are precipitated by exposure of a genetically-predisposed and sensitized individual to a variety of environmental substances that are ubiquitous and usually well tolerated by most healthy individuals. This chapter reviews the principles and performance characteristics of analytical methods used in the diagnosis and management of individuals with allergic disease. It examines *in vivo* and *in vitro* methods for the quantification of total and allergen-specific IgE. Other analytes used in the diagnostic work-up and management of the allergic patient are discussed including total "free" IgE, mast cell tryptase, eosinophil cationic protein, precipitating IgG antibodies, and the environmental assessment of aeroallergens in indoor environments.

Biological properties of IgE

In 1921, Prausnitz and Küstner (PK).[1] reported that an intradermal injection of serum from an allergic individual into the skin of an unsensitized (nonallergic) individual, followed 24 hours later by injection of specific antigen into the same skin site, induced local itching and swelling surrounded by a zone of erythema. This passively transferred allergic or *PK reaction* reached a maximum within 10 minutes, persisted for about 20 minutes, and gradually disappeared. The antibody mediating this reaction was shown to be thermolabile, losing its sensitizing activity after heating serum at 56°C for several hours. In 1967, this antibody was identified as a fifth human immunoglobulin isotype and designated IgE.[2–4]

Serum IgE concentrations are the lowest of the five human immunoglobulin isotypes (0–0.0001 g/L; 0.004% of the total adult serum immunoglobulin).[5] Approximately 50% of IgE is localized in the extravascular space. Its short biological half-life in peripheral blood of 1–5 days is due primarily to a relatively high fractional catabolic rate (71% of the intravascular pool catabolized/day). IgE does not pass the placenta or activate the classic complement pathway. Its reaginic (mast-cell sensitizing) activity is dependent upon its ability to bind to the α chain of the high-affinity IgE Fc-ε receptor (α-FcεRI) that resides on the membrane surface of basophils and mast cells. The interaction between IgE Fc and the α-FcεRI is blocked by the therapeutic subcutaneous administration of omalizumab (a humanized IgG$_{1-κ}$ anti-IgE Fc), as discussed below.

Total serum IgE

The concentration of IgE in the serum is highly age dependent.[5] Cord serum IgE concentrations are low, usually <2 kU/L (<4.88 µg/L; 1kU = 2.44 µg and 1 IU = 2.44 ng). Serum IgE levels progressively increase in healthy children up to the age of 10–15 years and gradually decline in an age-dependent manner from the second to the eighth decades of life. Atopic infants have an earlier and steeper rise in serum IgE levels during their early years compared to age-matched nonatopic controls.[6]

Clinically, a patient's serum IgE level should be compared to reference intervals established with sera from an age-stratified, healthy skin test-negative (nonatopic) population.[6] After age 14, serum IgE levels >333 kU/l (>800 µg/L) are considered abnormally elevated and are strongly associated with atopic disorders, such as allergic rhinitis, extrinsic or allergic asthma and atopic dermatitis. Extreme elevations in serum IgE are common in parasite infections and are necessary for the diagnosis of the hyper-IgE (Job's) syndrome. Normal or low total IgE levels in some individuals with asthma suggest that IgE-mediated mechanisms play only a minor or insignificant role in the pathogenesis of their condition. Low total serum IgE levels can thus support the diagnosis of nonallergic (intrinsic) asthma and help to exclude allergic bronchopulmonary aspergillosis. The reported overlap between IgE levels in atopic and nonatopic populations, however, is considerable.[6–8] Thus, although an elevated serum IgE can be useful in confirming the clinical diagnosis of allergic respiratory or skin diseases, a low or normal value does not eliminate the possibility of an IgE-mediated mechanism. For instance, a group of adults with allergic asthma had a mean serum IgE level of 1,589 ng/mL (range 55–12 750 ng/mL), with only about half of them having IgE concentrations >800 ng/mL. In contrast, approximately 90% of patients with atopic dermatitis had elevated total serum IgE levels (mean 978 kU/L, range 1.3–65 208 kU/L)). Parasitic infections, selected immunodeficiency states, cancer (Hodgkin disease, bronchial carcinoma), rheumatoid arthritis, liver disease and atopic dermatitis (eczema) are other disease states that have been associated with a dysregulation of total serum IgE levels. The total serum IgE must therefore be interpreted within the relevant clinical context for each patient.

Due to the overlap between atopic and nonatopic individuals, total serum IgE measurements have been largely replaced in the diagnosis of allergic disease by the quantification of allergen-specific IgE antibody. However, quantification of total serum IgE has remained important for computing the therapeutic dose of omalizumab (anti-IgE). Omalizumab is a recombinant, humanized IgG$_{1-κ}$ monoclonal anti-human IgE Fc drug that specifically binds to the region on the epsilon heavy chain that interacts with α-FcεR1. It is used to treat moderate to severe persistent allergic asthma by blocking IgE binding to the α-FcεR1 (Chapter 40). The binding of omalizumab to IgE *in vivo* reduces both the number of free IgE molecules able to interact with the α-FcεR1 and the number of FcεR1 receptors on the surface of effector cells. The consequence is a reduction in mediator release and allergy symptoms following allergen exposure.[9]

Allergen-specific IgE

In contrast to total serum IgE, the presence of allergen-specific IgE antibody on basophils or skin mast cells or in the serum is highly predictive of an individual's propensity to exhibit an allergic response upon re-exposure to that allergen. Before its identification as a novel immunoglobulin, IgE was only detectable with *in vivo* bioassays (skin test, bronchial or nasal provocation tests). Purification of IgE myeloma protein and the subsequent production of antisera specific for IgE led to the development of the first *in vitro* assay (radioallergosorbent test or RAST) for the detection of allergen-specific IgE antibody in serum.[4,10] Since then, non-isotopic autoanalyzer variants based on the original noncompetitive cellulose paper disc solid-phase radioallergosorbent test design are widely used throughout the world.[11]

A number of historical studies have compared the diagnostic sensitivity and specificity of *in vivo* and the early *in vitro* assays in the diagnosis of human allergic disease. Such inter-method comparisons have shown that the presence of IgE antibody as measured by serologic immunoassay methods usually agrees well with the presence of IgE detected in leukocyte and mast-cell histamine release assays, and provocation tests such as the skin test, food challenge and inhalation provocation test.[12] However, these early studies emphasize that the presence of IgE antibody as detected either *in vivo* or *in vitro* is at best a confirmatory measurement of sensitization. IgE antibody is necessary, but not sufficient for induction of an allergic symptom. It is considered a risk factor in the diagnosis of allergic disease that supports a patient's medical, family and environmental histories of a temporal association between allergic symptoms and allergen exposure. The clinical importance of differences in diagnostic sensitivity between skin test and serologic detection of IgE antibody may be less important for patients with allergies to inhaled (pollen, dust mite and epidermal) allergens than in those facing life-threatening anaphylactic reactions caused by Hymenoptera stings and drug administration. In these latter cases, skin tests are preferable to *in vitro* immunoassay analyses for the detection of allergen-specific IgE antibodies.[13] Immunoassay analyses of IgE antibody in serum can, however, be helpful in cases where the patient has taken antihistamines, β-receptor stimulants or high-dose steroids, which can reduce the provocation test's measured response; in children, pregnant women and elderly patients in whom skin testing may not be well tolerated; and when dealing with allergens (e.g., foods, molds) where commercial extracts can be highly variable or labile.[14]

Diagnostic methods

A combination of *in vivo* provocation and *in vitro* laboratory tests may be useful as confirmatory tests to support the clinical diagnosis of allergic disease. The actual tests selected will ultimately depend on the nature of the disease process under investigation

(e.g., allergic asthma, urticaria/angioedema, rhinitis/sinusitis or anaphylaxis).

Initial clinical laboratory tests

Following a medical history and physical examination, the patient who is suspected of having allergic disease may undergo several preliminary blood tests. A complete blood count and/or a total blood eosinophil count, if performed, should be obtained before any systemic corticosteroids or epinephrine is administered. Normal whole blood eosinophil levels range from 0 to 500 cells/mm.[3] Children generally have higher normal levels (mean 240 cells/mm;[3] 95% confidence limit = 0–740 cells/mm^3), with peak levels occurring at 4–8 years of age. Most laboratories consider a differential white blood cell count with an eosinophil level > 5–10% of the total white cell count to be abnormal. Blood, sputum and nasal secretion eosinophilia is characteristic of asthma, whether or not IgE-mediated allergic processes are present. In a bronchitic sputum specimen, neutrophils predominate. A neutrophilic nasal discharge is characteristic of sinusitis. Other laboratory tests that may be ordered as indicated include pulmonary function tests and a chest X-ray or sinus CT scan.

In vivo provocation testing

Both the skin test and nasal/bronchial/gastrointestinal provocation tests are useful diagnostic tools for the confirmation of immediate-type hypersensitivity reactions associated with allergic disease, and in the identification of offending allergens in an allergy patient's work-up for avoidance, or management with pharmacotherapy, immunotherapy or anti-IgE therapy.

Skin tests

Guerin and Watson[15] described a three-phase response that occurs in the skin during an immediate-type skin test reaction following the administration of a stimulus (allergen or histamine-positive control). First, a bluish-white area appears that involves the constriction of capillaries and that typically disappears within minutes. Second, an erythematous peripheral halo or flare appears as a result of arteriole dilatation. Finally, a circular urticarial papule or wheal is observed, as a result of extravasation of plasma into the skin, which is generally maximal by 15–20 minutes. The immediate wheal and flare reaction can be followed by a late-phase reaction 5-6 hours later that appears as a poorly defined edema-like reaction and that usually disappears by 24 hours. An allergen extract can be administered either by a prick/puncture or by intradermal injection.[16]

Puncture skin testing involves placing a drop of allergen extract on the skin of the forearm or back and the introduction of allergen into the epidermis by a needle puncture. A variety of single-point, multipoint and bifurcated needles have been used.[17] After the prick or puncture, the excess allergen is removed by blotting with tissue paper or gauze. An immediate reaction (wheal and erythema) is read at 15–20 minutes as it reaches its maximum size. Care is taken to space individual tests sufficiently far from each other as not to produce overlapping erythema. Because of the direct skin irritation, with some crude allergen extracts bleeding can produce false-positive results.

The intradermal skin test is 1000–10 000 times more sensitive by concentration than the puncture skin test. A 0.01- to 0.05-mL volume (optimally 0.02 mL) of diluted allergen extract in a 0.5- to 1.0-mL syringe is injected intracutaneously through a 26- to 27-gauge needle. A 0.02-mL injection will initially produce a superficial 2- to 3-mm-diameter bleb. Like the puncture test, the ID skin test is read at 15–20 minutes, when the reaction is maximal. Dilutions of extract greater than 1:1000 w/v are commonly used to minimize false-positive reactions due to irritation and the potential for systemic reactions. Subcutaneous administration of the allergen may lead to a false-negative result. The volume of allergen extract that is injected only slightly influences the size of the wheal and flare reaction, whereas concentration is the most important determinant of the final ID skin test results. Intradermal testing allows an investigator to perform a skin test titration to determine quantitatively the patient's skin sensitivity. For serial titration, the same volume (e.g., 0.02 mL) of three- to tenfold serial dilutions of allergen extract is injected into different sites in the skin and the concentration of allergen required to produce a wheal or erythema of a defined mean diameter (e.g., 8-mm wheal) is interpolated. The higher the concentration of allergen required to induce the defined size of wheal or erythema, the less sensitive the patient is to that allergen preparation.

Figure 97.1 shows the relationship between the ng/mL level of *Dermatophagoides pteronyssinus (Dpt,* dust mite) specific IgE antibody in sera from 30 dust mite-allergic subjects, as measured in serum by an *in vitro* assay, and the ID skin test midpoint *Dpt* allergen extract titer required to produce an 8 mm wheal in the same individual. Using the same *Dpt* extract in both tests, a higher degree of skin sensitivity (i.e., lower titer of antigen required to induce an 8 mm wheal) was strongly correlated ($r^2 = 0.77$, $p < 0.001$) with higher serum IgE antibody levels in those

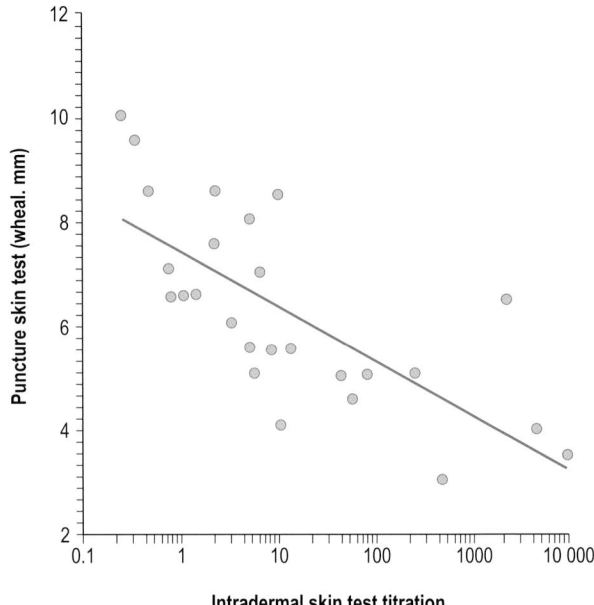

Fig. 97.2 The wheal size in millimeters at a single dose of *Dpt* allergen administered in a puncture skin test compared to the titer or ng/mL of the same *Dpt* allergen obtained in an ID skin test titration on the same 26 dust mite-allergic patients to produce an 8-mm wheal. These data indicate that the wheal size obtained with a single dose of allergen by the less labor-intensive puncture skin test is as predictive ($r^2 = 0.72$, $p < 0.001$) of relative patient sensitivity as the more technically complex intradermal skin test titration study, which involves the administration of seven increasing concentrations of the same allergen into different skin sites.

with the higher levels of skin sensitivity (<10 ng/mL midpoint). Figure 97.2 shows the strong correlation in wheal size that is observed in the same *Dpt*-allergic patients receiving the same dust mite extract in a single puncture skin test and a midpoint intradermal skin test titration.

Both the puncture and the ID skin test procedures produce a maximal wheal and flare size by 15–20 minutes, which is measured with a millimeter ruler or caliper. The maximal diameter and the midpoint perpendicular diameter are averaged to generate an index. A permanent record of the skin reaction can be made by applying adhesive cellulose tape over the wheal and flare skin area, which has previously been outlined with a felt-tip or ballpoint pen. Using a single concentration of allergen, the ID skin test can be graded according to one of several reported systems (Table 97.1).[16,17] Alternatively, a midpoint titer can be interpolated from a skin test titration including serial three- or tenfold dilutions of the allergen extract. Some investigators prefer to use the erythema (flare) size rather than the wheal size obtained during titration studies because the slope of the flare's regression line with dose is steeper.[18] The strong relationship between the size of the intradermal erythema and wheal observed with the mean of 304 duplicate skin tests is shown in Fig. 97.3. This relationship is useful to know, because the erythema is difficult to assess in many dark-skinned subjects.

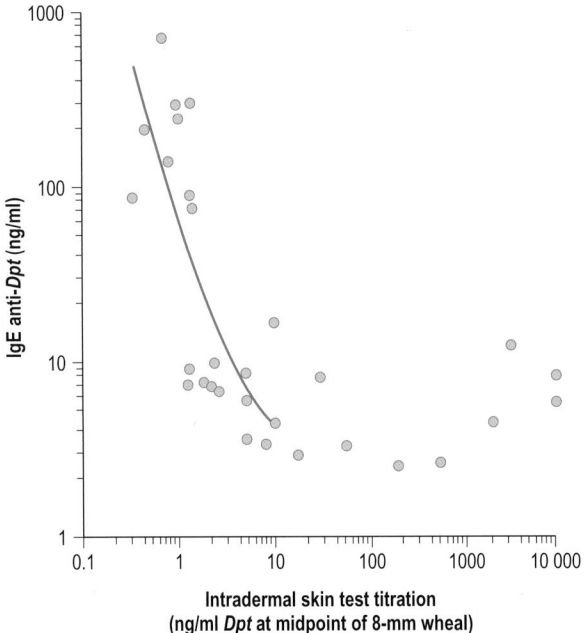

Fig. 97.1 Relationship between IgE anti-*D. pteronyssinus (Dpt)* in the skin (*x*-axis, intradermal skin test titration; ng/mL of *Dpt* required to produce an 8-mm wheal) and in the serum (*y*-axis, ng/mL of IgE anti-*Dpt* as measured by RAST; sensitivity = 2 ng/mL). These results were obtained by testing the skin and serum of 30 dust mite-allergic individuals with varying degrees of clinical sensitivity using the same *Dpt* extract in both the RAST and the ID skin test titration study. A lower "titer" of antigen required to induce an 8-mm wheal (e.g., higher degree of skin sensitivity) was strongly correlated ($r = 0.77$; $p < 0.001$) with a higher serum IgE antibody level in individuals with the higher level of skin sensitivity (<10 ng/mL midpoint). Less sensitive patients (titers >10 ng/mL *Dpt*) had lower levels of serum antibody (2–15 ng/mL) that did not relate well with skin sensitivity.

Bronchial and nasal provocation tests

Bronchial and nasal provocation challenges are performed primarily as research procedures to identify a relationship between an inhaled substance and a change in the patient's bronchial or nasal physiology. Bronchoprovocation studies with methacholine can also be useful in the diagnosis of difficult cases of asthma. The bronchoprovocation procedure involves

Table 97.1 Grading system for puncture and intradermal skin testing using histamine as a reference[a]

Grade or class	Wheal size (mm)	Erythema size (mm)
Skin testing grading system		
0	No discernible wheal	
1+	≤ 3 histamine wheal	
2+	> 3 histamine and < 1 3 histamine wheal	
3+		
4+	= size of histamine wheal ± 1 mm	
5+	> 1 3 histamine wheal and < 2 3 histamine wheal	
	> 2 3 histamine wheal	
Alternative skin test grading system for intradermal skin testing only involving interpretation of wheal and erythema responses.[b]		
0	<5	<5
+/–	5–10	5–10
1+	5–10	11–20
2+	5–10	21–30
3+	10–15	31–40
4+	> 15 with pseudopods	41–50

[a]Prick/puncture histamine (3–10 mg/mL); ID histamine (100 mg/mL). Modified from Norman PS. Skin testing. In: Middleton E, Ellis EF, Reed CE, eds. Allergy: principles and practice, 2nd edn. St Louis: CV Mosby, 1982, with permission from Elsevier.

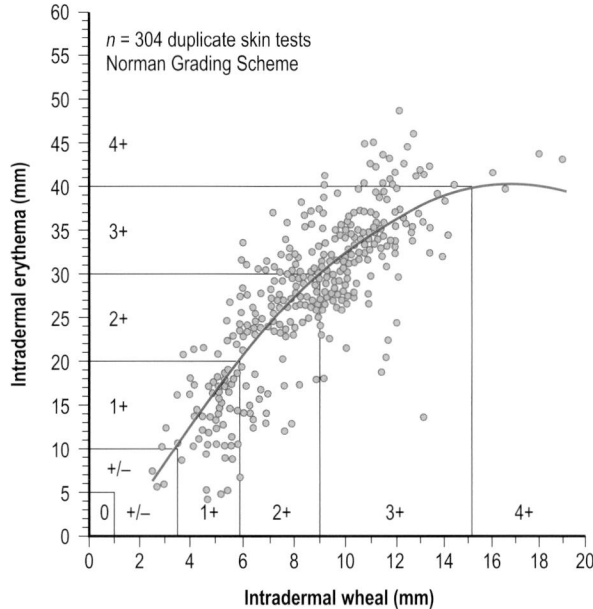

Fig. 97.3 Correlation plot of the mean wheal (x-axis) and erythema (y-axis) in millimeters for the mean of 304 duplicate intradermal skin tests to dust mite (*D. pteronyssinus*) obtained in a population of dust mite-sensitive individuals. The relationship is highly correlated ($r = 0.82$, $p < 0.001$) in grades 0–3+, indicating that either can be used to judge the degree of intradermal skin sensitivity. In highly allergic individuals (> 35 mm erythema), however, the slope declines dramatically, indicating that wheal size may be more discriminating than erythema.

the administration of either methacholine or histamine via a calibrated nebulizer, starting at doses of 0.05–0.1 mg/mL and doubling the concentration up to 10–25 mg/mL. Alternatively, allergen extracts can be administered in increasing doses. Pulmonary function is monitored after each dose. A positive response is usually defined as the concentration of agonist that results in a drop in the forced expiratory volume per second

(FEV_1) of 20% or more from the baseline (which must be >70% of that predicted for valid interpretation). More extensive details regarding the methods and interpretation of bronchial challenges are presented elsewhere.[19]

Nasal provocation in its simplest form involves the controlled administration of buffer (human serum albumin–saline) or increasing concentrations of allergen into a washed nasal passage. The symptoms (e.g., number of sneezes) induced and/or mast cell mediators released into nasal lavage fluids (e.g., TAME esterase and histamine) after each concentration of allergen indicates the relative level of sensitivity to that allergen. Nasal airway resistance is a less satisfactory end-point because of high intrinsic variations. Details of the procedure and applications can be found elsewhere.[20]

A hooded exposure chamber has been described for simultaneous nasal and bronchial challenges as a diagnostic procedure for assessing occupationally-induced latex allergy.[21,22] The challenge involves bathing the subject's conjunctiva and upper and lower airways with air alone, placebo (untreated) cornstarch, and then graded concentrations of latex cornstarch, each for 3-minute intervals separated by 15 minutes. Following each challenge the peak expiratory flow rates (PEFR) and chest and rhinoconjunctival symptoms scores are monitored. This procedure has been particularly useful in problematic diagnostic cases involving a discordant clinical history and IgE anti-latex skin test and/or serological test result.

Double-blind placebo-controlled food challenge

Food-induced gastrointestinal reactions (e.g., nausea, colic, vomiting and diarrhea) can occur minutes to hours after the consumption of food allergens by a sensitized individual (Chapter 43).[23] Commonly eaten foods that are known to contain potent allergens include cow milk (caseins, β-lactoglobulin, α-lactalbumin, lactoferrin, and bovine serum albumin), chicken egg white (ovalbumin, ovomucoid, ovotransferrin), cereal grains (wheat, rye, barley, oats), legumes (peanut, soybean, white bean), fish and seafood (shrimp, crabs, lobsters, oysters). Diagnosis of a food allergy begins with a medical history, which includes an assessment of diet diaries and elimination diets as necessary. Skin tests and serological tests for IgE antibody to extracted food allergens and open food challenges with fresh and cooked foods may be used to confirm sensitization to suspected foods. No evidence is available to indicate that food-specific IgG or IgG_4 antibody levels have any diagnostic value.[24] The double-blind placebo-controlled food challenge (DBPCFC) is considered the definitive diagnostic test for food allergy.[23] Open and single-blinded food challenges are more commonly used in clinical practice. An extensive discussion of the DBPCFC and variables influencing its outcome is presented elsewhere.[23,25]

In 2001, prospectively collected sera from 100 children and adolescents who had been previously evaluated by a skin test and DBPCFC were analyzed in the ImmunoCAP autoanalyzer (Phadia, Uppsala, Sweden) for food-specific IgE antibody.[25] The investigators were able to identify a diagnostic level of IgE antibody for egg (7 kUa/L), milk (17 kUa/L), peanut (14 kUa/L), and fish (20 kUa/L), above which they could predict clinical reactivity with more than 95% certainty. They concluded that by measuring the concentration of food-specific IgE antibody with the ImmunoCAP system, it was possible to identify a subset of children who were highly likely (>95% probability) to experience a clinical reaction to egg, milk, peanut, or fish. Quantitative serological measurements for food-specific IgE antibody may therefore be able to eliminate the need for time-consuming DBPCFCs in a significant number of children who are suspected of having food allergy. The relationship between IgE anti-chicken egg, cow's milk, and peanut as measured in the ImmunoCAP and Immulite (Siemens Healthcare Diagnostics, Tarrytown, NY, USA) has been investigated in an effort to extend published Immuno-CAP predictive values to reported Immulite measurements of IgE antibody to these foods.[26]

● KEY CONCEPTS

IgE (reaginic) antibody detection

- Allergen-specific IgE can be detected in skin test by a puncture or intradermal administration of allergen or in the serum by laboratory-based immunoassays.

- In general, the intradermal skin test is more sensitive than a puncture skin test, which is roughly comparable to the best *in vitro* methods for IgE antibody detection in serum.

- Because the results of *in vitro* tests for IgE antibody vary considerably between methods, proficiency testing surveys are essential for evaluating performance.

- Double-blind placebo-controlled food challenge is the gold standard for definitive diagnosis of food allergies.

In vitro testing

Most clinical immunology laboratories offer a variety of serological tests that can be useful in the diagnosis and management of human allergic disease. Analytes commonly measured in these laboratories include the total serum IgE, IgE antibodies to hundreds of allergen specificities, Hymenoptera venom-specific IgG, the venom-RAST inhibition test, and mast cell tryptase. IgG antibody measurements to allergens other then Hymenoptera venom have not been shown to be clinically useful. Basophil histamine release (BHR), although rarely offered as a clinical test because of the requirement for fresh blood, is a useful investigational method that is also reviewed in this section.

Total serum IgE

Of the diagnostic allergy tests that are performed in the clinical immunology laboratory, total serum IgE is currently the only analyte regulated under the US Clinical Laboratory Improvement Amendment of 1988 (CLIA-88). Currently five FDA-cleared commercial assays are used by clinical laboratories in the USA to measure the total level of IgE in serum (see College of American Pathologists [CAP] proficiency survey).[11] At present, free total IgE measurements for patients receiving omalizumab are only available with research based enzyme immunoassays.[27] and the clinical utility of free IgE levels in assessing the efficacy of omalizumab treatment needs further confirmation by prospective clinical studies.

Radioisotopes have been largely replaced by nonisotopic labels such as enzymes (horseradish peroxidase, alkaline phosphatase, β-galactosidase) or fluorophors. The minimum detectable concentration of most commercial total serum IgE assays is between 0.5 and 1 μg/L. The inter-method agreement of the different commercial IgE assays is excellent (e.g., inter-method coefficients of variation [CVs] typically <10% for serum IgE levels = 30 kIU/L).[11,28] Nonatopic age-adjusted reference intervals for total serum IgE must be used for normative interpretation.[5]

Allergen-specific IgE

Laboratories performing clinical diagnostic allergy testing need to use an FDA-cleared procedure and perform successfully in an external diagnostic allergy proficiency survey (e.g., CAP SE Survey).[11] Currently three IgE antibody assay systems are used clinically in North America. These assays have achieved unsurpassed intra-assay precision and inter-assay reproducibility and a high degree of quantification.[11] Their basic assay design can be traced back to the first IgE antibody assay, the radioallergosorbent test or RAST, reported by Wide et al. in 1967.[10]

The most highly variable component of the IgE antibody assay is the allergen-containing reagent. The Clinical and Laboratory Standards Institute has an established guideline that defines the performance characteristics of immunologic assays for human IgE antibodies to specific allergens.[29] It provides a glossary of all the allergens of clinical interest, subdividing them into extract versus component allergens and indicating whether they are well-documented, rare or undocumented allergen specificities. The latter category of undocumented allergens will be gradually eliminated from testing menus. Some allergens are known to share structurally similar or cross-reactive epitopes, and others possess unique IgE antibody-binding determinants.

Allergens have been conveniently grouped into those from weed pollen, grass pollen, tree pollen, animal epidermals, molds, house dust mites, parasites/insects, occupational allergens, drugs and venoms and foods. Among different species of a genus, such as ragweed (e.g., Canyon, Desert, Giant, Short, Silver, Southern, Western), there is extensive allergenic cross-reactivity due to structural similarity. Extensive allergenic cross-reactivity has also been documented within particular pollen groups, such as the grasses (June, Brome, Timothy, Perennial Rye, Fescue, Orchard, Red Top, Salt, Sweet Vernal, Velvet). Cross-reactivity has also been shown at the allergen component level. This is best illustrated by the PR10 family of allergens that share structural similarity (e.g., Bet v 1-birch; Cor a 1-hazelnut, Mal d 1-apple, Pru p 1-peach, Gly m 4-soybean, Ara h 8-peanut, Aln g 1-alder, Act d 8-kiwi, Api g 1-celery, and Dau c 1-carrot). Other component based cross-reactivity groups include the tropomyosins, serum albumins, parvalbumins, profilins, calcium binding proteins and lipid transfer proteins.

In contrast, certain grass pollens, such as those produced by Bermuda Grass, Johnson Grass, and cultivated corn, oat, and wheat, are minimally cross-reactive (allergenically distinct). Variations in the allergenic content of source materials, the extraction process from the raw source material, allergen-reagent manufacturing methods, differential binding to various allergosorbent supports, instability during storage, heterogeneity of internal reference allergen standards, and differences in characterization procedures (antisera, assays) make the production of reproducible allergens for *in vitro* use a challenge.

The second attribute that varies widely among commercially available IgE antibody assays is calibration methodology. All three autoanalyzers report out in the same units (kUa/L) using a reference serum that is traceable to the WHO 75/502 IgE international reference preparation. There is data that at least for one of the IgE antibody assays (ImmunoCAP), 1 kUa/L of allergen-specific IgE antibody is equivalent to 1 kU/L of total serum IgE.[30]

There is indication that IgE antibody to 10–15 aeroallergen specificities may account for the majority of aeroallergen-related disease. Although the particular allergen specificities may vary for children and adults, or for individuals in Europe, Asia and the North America, a "multiallergen" IgE antibody screening test has been developed by multiple manufacturers that is predictive of the results obtained by a panel of skin tests or *in vitro* IgE antibody tests. In these assays, 10–15 common allergen mixtures crossing the aeroallergen groups are insolubilized on a single solid phase. Alternatively, comparable purified native or recombinant allergens are adsorbed onto triplicate dots of a single solid support (silicone chip).[31] These screening assays are useful in confirming the absence of significant atopic disease in individuals suspected of having an intrinsic or non-IgE-mediated disease process. Their negative predictive value as a single test is higher than total serum IgE in identifying nonatopic individuals. Such a test can minimize the need for multiple *in vivo* or *in vitro* allergen-specific IgE measurements in patients with a low clinical probability of atopic disease. The use of such screening tests in unselected populations sometimes generates positive results of questionable clinical significance, however, as IgE antibody responses are more frequent than is symptomatic disease.

Recently, multiple crude extracts and native or recombinant allergenic components have been bound onto fluorescent-embedded particles or spotted in triplicate on glass slides or chips to provide a multi-plex matrix-based assay for IgE antibody. Alternatively, they have been adsorbed in bands onto nitrocellulose strips for use in lateral flow assay cassettes.[32] These multiplex chip-based assays and lateral flow "point of care" tests use small quantities of blood and are rapid, but they are less analytically sensitive and quantitative than single-plex autoanalyzers. Their theoretical advantage is simultaneous detection of sensitivities to cross-reactive allergenic components using minimal amounts of serum.

The quality of allergen-specific IgE antibody results reported from clinical diagnostic allergy laboratories is not uniformly equivalent.[33] For this reason, physicians requesting IgE antibody testing bear some responsibility for determining the quality of the results they receive. In the USA, testing should be performed in a clinical laboratory that is federally licensed for highly complex immunology clinical testing under CLIA-88 (verified by requesting a copy of the federal laboratory license). The requesting physician should inquire about the assay method used, the source of its reagents and how assays are quality controlled by the laboratory. As part of the formal record, the assay method used in patient analysis should be indicated on the final report.

Competitive IgE antibody inhibition assay

The competitive inhibition format of the IgE antibody assay has been widely used by researchers, allergen manufacturers and regulators to determine the relative potency of allergen extracts. One practical research application of the IgE antibody inhibition assay has been as a tool for monitoring the concentration of allergens released into environments (e.g., air sampling of airplanes for aerosolized peanut allergen). In the diagnostic allergy laboratory, the competitive IgE antibody inhibition assay has been used analytically to confirm an IgE antibody assay's minimum detectable dose (sensitivity) and nonspecific binding, and to document the extent of cross-reactivity by determining the allergen specificity of IgE antibody.

The one clinical application of the IgE antibody inhibition assay has been as an adjunct to define the appropriate therapeutic composition of venoms for insect sting-allergic

patients who have multiple potentially cross-reactive sensitivities and have elected to receive immunotherapy (Chapter 41).[34] Indications for this test include a strong skin reactivity; or a high level of serum IgE antibody to yellow jacket venom (YJV) and a weak skin reactivity; or low level of serum IgE antibody specific for *Polistes* wasp venom (PWV). The structural similarity between vespid and *Polistes* wasp phospholipase A1/B (*Ves g* I; *Pol a* I) and hyaluronidase (*Ves g* II; *Pol a* II) frequently produces IgE antibody cross-reactivity. Sera from 305 Hymenoptera venom-allergic patients with >2 ng/mL of IgE antibody to YJV and PWV were evaluated in the IgE antibody inhibition assay to document its clinical utility. The diagnostic question for these patients is whether PWV should be included in the venom immunotherapy together with yellow jacket or mixed vespid venom. Using this procedure, the venom-specific IgE antibody inhibition assay identified one-third (36.4%) of subjects with a primary YJV sensitivity who were candidates for exclusion of PWV from their immunotherapy regimen because their IgE anti-PWV was $>95\%$ cross-inhibitable with soluble YJV.[34]

● CLINICAL PEARLS

Clinical utility of hymenoptera venom rast inhibition test

- Useful in identifying venom cross-reactive IgE antibodies and selecting appropriate venoms for immunotherapy.
- One-third of venom-allergic patients with concomitant yellowjacket venom (YJV) and *Polistes* wasp venom (PWV) sensitivity can be treated with YJV alone or mixed vespid venoms, owing to $>95\%$ cross-reactive IgE anti-PWV with soluble YJV.

Allergen-specific IgG

Allergen injections during immunotherapy are known to enhance the production of specific IgG "blocking" antibodies. Quantitative measurements of total IgG antibodies or IgG subclass antibodies in studies of allergic rhinitis have not generally correlated with the control of clinical symptoms in individual patients. However, clinically successful immunotherapy is almost always accompanied by high serum levels of allergen-specific IgG.[35] In contrast, the presence or levels of IgG antibodies specific for food antigens have shown no correlation with the results of positive double-blind placebo-controlled food challenges and they are not indicated in the diagnostic work-up of a suspected food allergic patient.[24]

Allergen-specific IgG antibody measurements can be helpful in determining optimal therapy in patients with Hymenoptera venom sensitivity. In a prospective study, Hymenoptera venom-specific IgG antibodies were monitored in the serum of 109 venom-allergic patients to examine whether IgG antibody levels could predict the risk of a systemic reaction after a sting challenge in patients receiving venom immunotherapy.[36] The highest rate of allergic reactions (26%) occurred in patients who had both a venom-specific IgG antibody level <3 µg/mL and fewer than 4 years of venom immunotherapy.[36] Therefore, quantitative venom-specific IgG antibody levels appear to be useful in individualizing the dose and frequency of injections while maximizing the protective effects. However, the clinical utility of the IgG antibody measurement may be restricted to the first 4 years of venom immunotherapy.

IgG antibody measurements

- Clinically successful aeroallergen immunotherapy is almost always accompanied by high serum levels of allergen-specific IgG.
- Quantitative venom-specific IgG antibody levels can be of value in individualizing venom doses and frequencies for patients on immunotherapy for up to 4 years.
- Food-specific IgG and IgG4 assay results do not correlate with the results of double-blind placebo-controlled food challenges.

Mast-cell tryptase

Two types of mast cells have been identified in skin, respiratory, and digestive tract connective tissues based on the types of neutral proteases present in their secretory granules (Chapter 22). One group contains only tryptase, whereas the other contains both tryptase and chymase.[37] Upon activation of mast cells, these proteases are released in parallel with pre-stored histamine and newly generated vasoactive mediators. Mast-cell tryptase (MW 134 kDa) is a serine esterase with four subunits, each having an enzymatically active site. A resting mast cell contains 10–35 pg of tryptase that is stored attached to heparin. When dissociated from heparin, it rapidly degrades into its monomers and loses enzymatic activity. As basophils have ~500-fold less tryptase than mast cells, elevated tryptase levels in serum are considered a relatively specific indicator of mast cell involvement in a clinical reaction.[42]

Mast cell tryptase can be detected in the blood in both mature and immature forms. The immature form, also known as protryptase, is secreted by unstimulated mast cells and provides a measure of total mast cell number. α-Protryptase and β-protryptase represent the bulk of the immature trypase in non-anaphylactic sera. α-Protryptase remains enzymatically inactive, while some of β-protryptase is autoprocessed into a proform and then converted to the mature enzyme by a di-peptidase.[43] Total tryptase in serum from healthy humans ranges from 1 to 11.4 µg/L (average of 3-5 µg/L). A non-competitive two-site fluorescent enzyme immunoassay (Phadia, ImmunoCAP) is available to measure total tryptase in serum.[38] Elevated levels of total tryptase (>11.4 µg/L) can be detected in serum from 1 to 4 hours after the onset of systemic anaphylaxis with hypotension.[39] Baseline levels of >20 µg/L are detected in most individuals with systemic mastocytosis.[44]

The mature form of tryptase is maintained in mast cell secretory granules in an enzymatically active complex with heparin. When mast cells degranulate, mature β-tryptase is released from the cell together with histamine. Mature tryptase is normally undetectable (<1 µg/L) in serum from healthy humans who have no history of anaphylaxis during the preceding hours. An elevation in mature (β-) trypase >1 µg/L indicates mast cell (and possibly basophil) activation. Recommended serum collection times for tryptase quantification range from 30 minutes to 4 hours after the onset of an acute event. Postmortem specimens are often difficult to analyze for tryptase because of high viscosity related to gross hemolysis. However, reported mature tryptase levels in postmortem cases of fatal anaphylaxis have ranged from 12 to 150 µg/L in 9/9 Hymenoptera venom- and 6/8 food-induced fatalities.[45]

The frequency of a severe reaction to a Hymenoptera venom sting increases significantly with higher serum baseline total tryptase concentrations.[40–41] The clinical indications for and diagnostic value of tryptase as a marker of anaphylaxis and mastocytosis are reviewed elsewhere.[42]

Basophil mediator release assays

Histamine release assay

The potent vasoactive mediator histamine is stored in cytoplasmic granules of basophilic leukocytes and mast cells and released along with other mediators of inflammation in response to both immunologic and non-immunologic stimuli.[37,46] The basophil histamine release (BHR) assay has been particularly useful as a quantitative assay of allergen potency, and as an *in vitro* model for the study of triggering mechanisms of mediator release from basophils. In its most basic form, peripheral blood leukocytes are isolated from a donor and incubated with varying concentrations (e.g., three- to tenfold dilutions) of allergen extract or anti-human IgE as a positive control. Histamine release is complete within 30 minutes, and then histamine in the supernatant is measured by enzymatic, radiometric or spectrophotofluorometric techniques.[47] Details of the BHR assay are given elsewhere.[47]

Patient sensitivity for a given allergen can be determined with a positive BHR test. The results are highly correlated with those determined by skin testing[47] and bronchoprovocation.[48] Although the BHR test has been most widely used in research laboratories owing to its expense, time-consuming nature and the need for fresh blood (<24 hours old), it can be successfully applied to the clinical diagnosis of allergy in selected cases. Its results parallel those of other IgE antibody tests. BHR has also been a useful tool for clarifying discrepancies between skin test and serological IgE antibody test results.

Leukotriene C4 (LTC4) release assay

An assay method for measuring LTC4 released from allergen-activated basophils has been reported as the cellular antigen stimulation test (CAST)–ELISA.[49] The LTC4 assay is designed for use with either whole blood preparations or washed leukocytes. Using dust mite, food, Hymenoptera venoms and drugs as challenges, the observed diagnostic sensitivity of the CAST compared to the combination of a clinical history and skin test ranged from 18% with aspirin[50] to 85% for selected food allergens.[5] The reported diagnostic specificity of the CAST in the same studies ranged from 67 to 100%. These data indicate that the CAST assay is not sufficiently sensitive for effective clinical use in the diagnosis of IgE-mediated sensitivities to β-lactam or nonsteroidal anti-inflammatory drugs. Its utility in the diagnosis of sensitization to other allergen specificities appears more promising, but further documentation involving clinical studies is required.

Utility of mediator release assays as diagnostic tests

Despite their unquestioned value as research methods, the basophil histamine and LTC4 release assays are rarely used clinically in the routine diagnosis of human allergic disease and it is unlikely that this trend will change in the foreseeable future.

Flow cytometry basophil activation assays

In the late 1990s, basophils were shown to upregulate the expression of a number of surface proteins (e.g., CD45, CD63, CD69, and CD203c) when activated by allergen.[51–53] CD63 is a member of the transmembrane-4 superfamily that is expressed on basophils, mast cells, macrophages and platelets.[51,52] In resting basophils from nonatopic and allergic individuals, CD63 is attached to intracytoplasmic granules. Activated IgE-sensitized basophils express a high density of CD63 on their surface. By quantifying ~500 basophils with gated flow cytometry, the percentage of activated basophils can be identified, after correcting for spontaneous CD63 expression. A variety of criteria are used to identify an allergen-induced positive response, such as a stimulation index (allergen-induced/basal ratio) >2. One confounding variable in this analysis is the adherence of CD63-expressing platelets in basophil preparations that can sometimes generate false-positive results.

The flow assay stimulation test (FAST) using CD63 as a marker for activation was evaluated using minor determinant mixture, benzyl penicilloyl polylysine, penicillin, ampicillin amoxicillin and cephalosporin as stimulating antigens.[50] Subjects ($n = 58$) with a history of immediate-type reactions to β-lactam antibiotics or nonallergic controls ($n = 30$) were evaluated in the CD63 FAST and Phadia ImmunoCAP system for drug-specific IgE levels. Relative to the clinical history, the CD63 FAST displayed a diagnostic sensitivity and specificity of 50 and 93%, respectively. Diagnostic sensitivity was marginally increased to 66% by simultaneously using the drug-specific IgE antibody serology result. The study concluded that the CD63 basophil activation test could be helpful in supporting the diagnosis of IgE-mediated allergy to β-lactam drugs when used in conjunction with an additional diagnostic test such as IgE antibody serology.

CD203c (also known as neural cell surface differentiation antigen, E-NIPP3 PD-1β, 97A6, B10 and gp130rb13-6) is member of the ectonucleotide pyrophosphate phosphodiesterase (E-NPP) family.[54] It is expressed only on IgE-bearing basophils, mast cells and their progenitors, and is upregulated following activation of IgE-sensitized basophils with allergen or anti-IgE in a manner similar to CD63. The CD203c-based flow-assay is performed in a manner analogous to the CD63-based assay. Its advantage over CD63 is its restricted expression on basophils in peripheral blood, which minimizes concern about the adherence of platelets that may produce false-positive CD63 results. Additionally, there is no need for the use of an additional fluorescent anti-IgE reagent to gate the basophils.

Basophil activation as determined by CD203c expression was studied in Hymenoptera venom patients and healthy controls in which their basophils were activated with anti-IgE or bee/vespid venoms.[55] Fifteen minutes after stimulation, basophils from 15 wasp-sensitized patients upregulated CD203c expression from 4.2- to 13.5-fold. Moreover, basophils from six honeybee venom-allergic patients upregulated CD203c by a mean of 8.3 times. The study concluded that the CD203c-based flow assay could confirm the presence of venom-specific IgE antibody on basophils in 91% (20/22) of clinical history and skin test-positive venom-allergic patients. One false-positive was observed among 13 skin test-negative healthy controls.

Diagnostic utility of basophil activation flow cytometric assays

The utility of basophil activation flow cytometric assays is limited by a number of technical concerns.[56] First, endotoxin free whole blood must be received within 24 hours by the laboratory, where it can processed by skilled technologists. Second, the blood is pre-incubated with stimulation buffer often containing IL3 that primes the basophils. It is unclear what effect IL-3 has on altering mediator release or CD63/CD203c upregulation, and thus false-positive mediator release and/or biomarker surface expression are potential concerns.[56] Third, varying concentrations of crude allergen extract or recombinant allergen or anti-IgE need to be incubated with the cell preparation. Unfortunately, crude extracts can often be cytotoxic, and thus each stimulating allergen needs to be pre-qualified before use. Fourth, criteria for defining positive assay results vary among stimulating allergen preparations from the same manufacturer owing to their variable potency. Fifth, there is a concern about false-positive results related to platelet adherence on basophils in the CD63 assay. Possibly most important, when the performance characteristics were directly compared in clinical studies to puncture skin test results, the diagnostic sensitivity and specificity of the flow cytometric analysis of *in vitro* allergen-activated basophils is less than optimal. For these reasons, cell-based cytometry methods will most likely remain useful research techniques for the investigation of allergic disease, but have limited application to clinical diagnosis.

Other serum analytes

Several other analytes can be measured in the diagnostic allergy laboratory to support the differential diagnosis of allergies, asthma or hypersensitivity pneumonitis, and to aid in the management of asthmatic patients. These include human IgG-precipitating antibodies specific for antigens in organic dusts and aeroallergen quantification in environmental specimens (e.g., surface reservoir dust).

Precipitating IgG antibodies (precipitins)

Hypersensitivity pneumonitis (HP), also known as extrinsic allergic alveolitis, is a hypersensitivity reaction to antigenic organic dusts (e.g., molds, bird droppings) involving the lung interstitium and terminal bronchioles (Chapter 47).[57] Hours after a heavy antigenic exposure, an acute form of hypersensitivity pneumonitis can occur with chills, fever, malaise, cough, and shortness of breath. Whereas histology of the lung lesions indicates a cell-mediated pathology, most patients with hypersensitivity pneumonitis have high serum levels of IgG antibody to the offending antigen. Despite its insensitivity, the double-diffusion method (Ouchterlony) of measuring precipitating antibodies remains a means of confirming exposure but not necessarily the disease. In this assay, antigen (extract) and antibody (control or patient's serum) diffuse towards each other in an agarose gel, forming precipitin lines if high levels of antibody are present in serum. Precipitating antibodies or precipitins can be detected in the serum of nearly all ill patients, but also in the serum of as many as 50% of asymptomatic individuals who have been exposed to the relevant organic dusts.[57] Immunoassays for IgG antibody to the appropriate organic dust antigens may be less useful clinically because they are too sensitive. They typically detect IgG antibody in the sera of a higher number of non-diseased patients than do the immunodiffusion methods. Precipitin assays are currently available with specificities for the thermophilic actinomyces (*Micropolyspora faeni*, *Thermoactinomyces vulgaris*, and *Thermoactinomyces candidus*), aspergillus (*Aspergillus fumigatus*, *Aspergillus niger*, *Aspergillus flavus*), pigeon serum, *Aureobasidum pullulans*, and fecal particles from parakeets and a variety of exotic household birds (Cockatiel, Amazon).

Assessment of environmental aeroallergens

IgE-mediated diseases are currently managed using a combination of four approaches: pharmacotherapy for the treatment of symptoms, allergen-specific immunotherapy, anti-IgE therapy and allergen avoidance. Of these, avoidance or the separation of allergen and patient is potentially the least expensive, best-tolerated and most effective approach for reducing allergy symptoms and minimizing increased sensitization. The level of aeroallergens in the indoor and outdoor environments can be highly relevant for the clinical management of allergic patients.

Indoor environments

Allergen control in indoor home, school and work environments has become an important management technique for asthma. Of the known allergen specificities, aeroallergens produced by dust mites (*Dermatophagoides farinae*, *Dermatophagoides pteronyssinus*), fur-bearing pets (cats, dogs) and rodents (mice, rats), indoor insects (cockroach) and a limited number of common molds (*Penicillium*, *Aspergillus*, *Alternaria*, and *Cladosporium*) are known to produce the majority of indoor allergic diseases.[58] A number of diagnostic allergy laboratories evaluate reservoir (surface) dust collected from defined areas of allergic patients' homes, workplaces, and schools. The extracts are then analyzed in a panel of monoclonal antibody-based immunoenzymetric assays to quantify indicator indoor aeroallergens: *Der f* 1 and 2 and *Der p* 1 and 2 (allergens excreted into fecal particles by dust mites [*D. farinae*, *D. pteronyssinus*]), *Fel d* 1 (35-kDa allergen excreted by the sweat glands of the domestic cat [*Felis domesticus*]), *Bla g* 1/*Bla g* 2 (25- to 36-kDa allergens produced by the German cockroach [*Blatella germanica*]), *Mus m* 1 (19-kDa allergen excreted into urine by the mouse [*Mus musculus*]) and *Rat n* 1 (17-kDa allergen excreted in urine by the rat [*Rattus norvegicus*]). A viable mold spore analysis can also be performed on 5 mg of fine dust in a microbiological culture plate containing Sabouraud's dextrose agar.[58]

Intra- and inter-laboratory variability of aeroallergen measurements has been assessed with a multicenter proficiency study conducted by the US Department of Housing and Urban Development.[59] In this study, aliquots of homogeneous batches of house dust and filtered dust extracts were provided to eight commercial, academic and municipal laboratories. The dust preparations were each analyzed for *Der p 1*, *Der f 1*, *Fel d 1*, *Can f 1*, *Bal g 1*, and *Mus m 1* by enzyme immunoassays. Coefficients of variation on the estimated geometric means of analytical results ranged from 61 to 93%, with the dominant component of variability being variation between laboratories using different reagents. Despite this variability, it was concluded that reasonable agreement was observed between the means of allergen levels across participating laboratories. The data provided confirmation that aeroallergen results from CLIA-88-licensed reference laboratories that use enzyme immunoassay procedures display a level of accuracy and precision that is acceptable for distinguishing environments with high aeroallergen levels (e.g., expected to trigger asthma in predisposed individuals) from those with lower levels considered to be safe.

Allergens that are measured in reservoir dust can be considered "indicator" molecules because they allow the clinician and the patient to track the relative levels of associated allergen source(s) by room throughout a house, school or workplace

Levels of *Der p* 1 and/or *Der f* 1 allergen >2000 ng/g of fine dust have been associated with an increased risk of allergic symptoms in sensitized individuals, whereas levels >10 000 ng/g of fine dust have been associated with an increased risk of sensitization.[57] For cat, *Fel d* 1 levels >8000 ng/g of fine dust have been proposed as a threshold for sensitization. Any cockroach allergen, mouse and rat allergen detected in an environment identifies an indoor area that places individuals allergic to cockroach, mouse or rat at risk for symptoms and sensitization. Finally, viable mold spore levels above 25 000 colonies/g of fine dust place the mold content in the environment above the 75th percentile for homes monitored across the USA. Where these proposed threshold levels are exceeded, the allergic individual is encouraged to take action to reduce the levels. A detailed discussion of strategies for doing this can be found elsewhere.[60] Repeat household dust allergen measurements following an intervention allows monitoring and documentation of allergen reduction.

● CLINICAL PEARLS

Indoor aeroallergen analyses

- Predominant indoor aeroallergens include dust mites, cockroaches, epidermal allergens (cat, dog, mouse, rat), and a limited number of molds.
- Quantitative analysis of house dust samples enables allergic subjects to assess the individual risk for symptoms and/or sensitization in a particular home and to monitor the effects of environmental control.

Outdoor environments

In most major cities across the USA, aerobiology stations have been established to perform a daily evaluation of the outdoor air for pollen and mold spore levels. Certified pollen and mold counters who have knowledge of the morphology of the principal pollen grains and mold spores quantify them in the air from a 24-hour stained air sample that is collected on a rotorod or spore trap collector. Daily information is often transmitted to local weather stations and newspapers for public use, or posted in allergists' offices for their patients to review. An aerobiology network has been established by the American Academy of Allergy, Asthma and Immunology to certify participating laboratories and monitor their performance. This network also collates and disseminates pollen and mold data across the nation throughout the allergy season.

● ON THE HORIZON

New trends in laboratory methodology for the assessment of human allergic diseases include:

- A transition from crude allergen extract to allergenic component-based serological assays.
- The use of semi-quantitative multiplexing platforms that allow rapid simultaneous detection of IgE to many allergenic components using microliter quantities of serum.
- Qualitative "point of care" lateral-flow IgE antibody assays for use by primary care clinicians to rapidly assess sensitization to aeroallergens.

References

1. Prausnitz C, Kustner H. Studine uber die Ueberemfindlichkeil. Zentralbl Bakteriol Mikrobiol Hyg 1921;86:160.
2. Ishizaka K, Ishizaka T. Physiochemical properties of reaginic antibody. I. Association of reaginic activity with an immunoglobulin other than gamma A or gamma G globulin. J Allergy 1967;37:169.
3. Johansson SGO. Raised levels of a new immunoglobulin class (IgND) in asthma. Lancet 1967;2:951.
4. Hamilton RG. The science behind the discovery of IgE. J Allergy Clin Immunol 2005;115:648.
5. Hamilton RG. Human immunoglobulins. In: O'Gorman MRG, Donnenberg AD, editors. Handbook of human immunology. 2nd ed. Boca Raton: CRC Press; 2008. p. 63–106.
6. Barbee RA, Halomen M, Lebowitz M, et al. Distribution of IgE in a community population sample: correlations with age, sex and allergen skin test reactivity. J Allergy Clin Immunol 1981;68:106.
7. Wittig HJ, Belloit J, DeFillippi I, et al. Age-related serum IgE levels in healthy subjects and in patients with allergic disease. J Allergy Clin Immunol 1980;66:305.
8. Dati F, Ringel KP. Reference values for serum IgE in healthy nonatopic children and adults. Clin Chem 1982;28:1556.
9. Lin H, Boesel KM, Griffith DT, et al. Omalizumab rapidly decreases nasal allergic response and FcεR1 on basophils. J Allergy Clin Immunol 2004;113:297.
10. Wide L, Bennich H, Johansson SGO. Diagnosis by an in vitro test for allergen specific antibodies. Lancet 1967;2:1105.
11. Hamilton RG. Proficiency survey based evaluation of clinical total and allergen-specific IgE assay performance. Arch Pathol Lab Med 2010;134:975–82.
12. Yunginger JW, Ahlstedt S, Eggleston PA, et al. Quantitative IgE antibody assays in allergic diseases. J Allergy Clin Immunol 2000;105:1077.
13. Hamilton RG. Diagnostic methods for insect sting allergy. [Review] Curr Opin Allergy Clin Immunol 2004;4:297.
14. Eckman J, Saini SS, Hamilton RG. Diagnostic evaluation of food-related allergic diseases (review). Allergy Asthma Clin Immunol 2009;5:2–8.
15. Guerin B, Watson RD. Skin tests. Clin Rev Allergy 1988;6:211.
16. Demoly P, Piette V, Bousquet J. In vivo methods for study of allergy: Skin tests, techniques and interpretation. In: Adkinson Jr. NF, Yunginger JW, Busse WW, et al., editors. Allergy: principles and practice. 6th ed Philadelphia: Mosby; 2003. p. 631.
17. Nelson HS. In vivo testing for immunoglobulin E mediated sensitivity. In: Leung DYM, Sampson HA, Geha RS, Szefler SJ, editors. Pediatric allergy: principles and practice. Philadelphia: Mosby; 2003. p. 243.
18. Turkeltaub PC, Rastogi SC, Baer H, et al. A standardized quantitative skin test assay of allergen potency and stability. Studies on the allergen dose-response curve and effect of wheal, erythema and patient selection on assay results. J Allergy Clin Immunol 1982;70:343.
19. Fish JE, Peters SP. Bronchial challenge testing. In: Adkinson Jr. NF, Yunginger JW, Busse WW, et al., editors. Allergy: principles and practice. 6th ed Philadelphia: Mosby; 2003. p. 657.
20. Rajakulasingam K. Nasal provocation testing. In: Adkinson Jr. NF, Yunginger JW, Busse WW, et al., editors. Allergy: principles and practice. 6th ed Philadelphia: Mosby; 2003. p. 644.
21. Kurtz KM, Hamilton RG, Adkinson Jr. NF. Role and application of provocation in the diagnosis of occupational latex allergy. Ann Allergy Asthma Immunol 1999;83:634.
22. Pipkorn U, Granerus G, Proud D. The effect of a histamine synthesis inhibitor on the immediate nasal allergic reaction. Allergy 1987;42:496.
23. Sampson HA. Adverse reactions to foods. In: Adkinson Jr. NF, Yunginger JW, Busse WW, et al., editors. Allergy: principles and practice. 6th ed Philadelphia: Mosby; 2003. p. 1619.
24. Stapel SO, Asero R, Ballmer-Weber BK, Knol EF, Strobel S, Vieths S, et al. Testing for IgG4 against foods is not recommended as a diagnostic tool: EAACI Task Force Report. Allergy 2008;63:793–6.
25. Sampson HA. Utility of food specific IgE concentrations in predicting symptomatic food allergy. J Allergy Clin Immunol 2001;107:891.
26. Hamilton RG, Mudd K, White MA, Wood RA. Extension of food allergen-specific IgE ranges from the ImmunoCAP to the IMMULITE System. Ann Allergy Asthma Immunol 2011;107:139–44.
27. Hamilton RG, Marcotte GV, Saini SS. Immunological methods for quantifying free and total serum IgE in asthma patients receiving Omalizumab (Xolair) therapy. J Immunol Meth 2005;303:81–91.
28. Hamilton RG. Accuracy of Food and Drug Administration-cleared IgE antibody assays in the presence of anti-IgE (Omalizumab). J Allergy Clin Immunol 2006;117:759–66.
29. Matsson P, Hamilton RG, Homburger HA, et al. Analytical performance Characteristics and Clinical Utility of immunological assays for human immunoglobulin E (IgE) antibody of defined allergen specificities. 2nd ed. Clinical Laboratory Standards Institute 1/LA20-A; 2008.
30. Kober A, Perborn H. Quantitation of mouse-human chimeric allergen-specific IgE antibodies with ImmunoCAP technology. J Allergy Clin Immunol 2006;117:S219 [Abstract 845].
31. Jahn-Schmid B, Harwanegg C, Hiller R, et al. Allergen microarray: comparison to microarray using recombinant allergens with conventional diagnostic methods to detect allergen-specific serum immunoglobulin E. Clin Exp Allergy 2003;33:1443–9.
32. Sarratud T, Donnanno S, Terracciano L, et al. Accuracy of a point-of-care testing device in children with suspected respiratory allergy. Allergy Asthma Proc 2010;31:11–7.
33. Hamilton RG. Responsibility for quality IgE antibody results rests ultimately with the referring physician. Ann Allergy Asthma Immunol 2001;86:353–4.
34. Hamilton RG, Wisenauer JA, Golden DB, et al. Selection of Hymenoptera venoms for immunotherapy based on patient's IgE antibody crossreactivity. J Allergy Clin Immunol 1993;92:651.
35. Lichtenstein LM, Norman PS, Winkenwerder WL. A single year of immunotherapy of ragweed hay fever: immunologic and clinical studies. Ann Intern Med 1971;75:663.
36. Golden DBK, Lawrence ID, Hamilton RG, et al. Clinical correlation of the venom-specific IgG antibody level during maintenance venom immunotherapy. J Allergy Clin Immunol 1992;90:386.
37. Craig CS, Schwartz LB. Tryptase and chymase: markers of distinct types of human mast cells. Immunol Res 1989;8:130.
38. Enander I, Matsson P, Anderson AS, et al. A radioimmunoassay for human serum tryptase released during mast cell activation. J Allergy Clin Immunol 1990;85:154–9.
39. Van der Linden PW, Hack CE, Poortman J, et al. Insect sting challenge in 138 patients: relation between clinical severity of anaphylaxis and mast cell activation. J Allergy Clin Immunol 1992;90:110–8.
40. Miller JS, Schwartz LB. Tryptase levels as an indication of mast cell activation in a patient with Hymenoptera anaphylaxis and mastocytosis. N Engl J Med 1987;316:1622.
41. Ruëff F, Przybilla B, Biló MB, et al. Predictors of severe systemic anaphylactic reactions in patients with Hymenoptera venom allergy: importance of baseline serum tryptase-a study of the EAACI Interest Group on Insect Venom Hypersensitivity. J Allergy Clin Immunol 2009;124:1047–54.
42. Schwartz LB. Diagnostic value of tryptase in anaphylaxis and mastocytosis. Immunol Allergy Clin North Am 2006;26:451–63.
43. Schwartz LB, Bradford TR. Regulation of tryptase from human lung mast cells by heparin; stabilization of the active tetramer. J Biol Chem 1986;261:7372.
44. Valent P, Sperr WR, Schwartz LB, Horny HP. Diagnosis and classification of mast cell proliferative disorders: delineation of immunology diseases and non-mast cell hematopoietic neoplasms. J Allergy Clin Immunol 2004;114:3.
45. Yunginger JW, Nelson DR, Squillace DL, et al. laboratory investigation of deaths due to anaphylaxis. J Forensic Sci 1991;35:857.
46. Lichtenstein LM, Osler AG. Studies on the mechanisms of hypersensitivity phenomenon. IX. Histamine release from human leukocytes by ragweed pollen. J Exp Med 1964;120:507.
47. Siraganian RP. Automated histamine analysis for in vitro allergy testing. II. Correlation of skin test results with in vitro whole blood histamine release in 82 patients. J Allergy Clin Immunol 1977;59:214.
48. Wegner F, Hockamp R, Rutschke A, et al. Superiority of the histamine release test above case history, prick test and radioallergosorbent test in predicting bronchial reactivity to the house dust mite in asthmatic children. Klin Wochenschr 1983;61:43.
49. de Weck AL. Cellular allergen stimulation test (CAST): a new dimension in allergy diagnostics. ACI News 1993;1(5):9–14.
50. Maly FE, Marti-Wyss S, Blumber S, et al. Mononuclear blood cell sulpholeukotriene generation in the presence of interleukin 3 and whole blood histamine release in honeybee and yellow jacket venom allergy. J Invest Allergy Clin Immunol 1997;7:217–24.
51. Moneret-Vautrin DA, Sainte-Laudy J, Kanny G, Fremont S. Human basophil activation as measured by CD63 expression and LTC4 release in IgE mediated food allergy. Ann Allergy Asthma Immunol 1999;82:33.
52. Bochner BS, Sterbinsky SA, Saini SA, et al. Studies of cell adhesion and flow cytometric analyses of degranulation, surface phenotype and viability using human eosinophils, basophils and mast cells. Methods 1997;13:61–8.
53. Sanz ML, Gamboa PM, Antepara I. Flow cytometric basophil activation test by detection of CD63 expression in patients with immediate type reactions to beta lactam antibiotics. Clin Exp Allergy 2002;32:277–86.
54. Buhring HJ, Sieffert M, Giesert C. The basophil activation marker defined by antigen 97A6 is identical to ectonucleotide pyrophosphate/phosphodiesterase 3. Blood 2001;97:3303–5.
55. Platz I, Binder M, Marxer A, et al. Hymenoptera venom induced up regulation of basophil activation marker ecto-nucleotide pyrophosphatase/phosphoesterase 3 (E-NNP3, CD203c) in sensitized individuals. Int Arch Allergy Immunol 2001;126:335–42.
56. Ebo DG, Hagendorens MM, Bridts CH, et al. In vitro allergy diagnosis: should we follow the flow? [Review] Clin Exp Allergy 2004;34:332–9.
57. Fink JN, Zacharisen MC. Hypersensitivity pneumonitis. In: Adkinson Jr. NF, Yunginger JW, Busse WW, et al., editors. Middleton's allergy: principles and practice. 6th ed St Louis: Mosby; 2003. p. 1373.
58. Hamilton RG. Assessment of indoor allergen exposure. Curr Allergy Asthma Rep 2005;5:394–401.
59. Pate AD, Hamilton RG, Ashley PJ, et al. Proficiency testing of allergen measurements in residential dust. J Allergy Clin Immunol 2005;116:844–50.
60. Hamilton RG, Chapman MD, Platts-Mills TAE, Adkinson Jr. NF. House dust aeroallergen measurements in clinical practice: A guide to allergen-free home and work environments. Immunol Allergy Pract 1992;14:9.

John W. Belmont,
Luis M. Franco

Molecular methods

Molecular analysis of nucleic acids provides broad tools for the clinical laboratory and relevant information for the clinician. This chapter reviews the basic principles that underlie clinical molecular genetic testing, assesses representative standard methods that are widely employed, describes new DNA sequencing methods that are being rapidly introduced into clinical diagnostic laboratories, and suggests a multidisciplinary approach for implementation in immunological disorders.

Basic principles

Genome structure and gene expression

> **◉ KEY CONCEPTS**
>
> **Human genomics**
>
> - The human genome encompasses approximately 22 000 protein-coding genes, but each cell expresses only a subset of those genes.
> - Genetic and physical maps of the genome are essential to molecular diagnosis of immune system diseases.
> - Genetic maps depend on the co-inheritance of DNA segments—linkage—to associate DNA variants with disease.
> - Physical maps of the genome describe the exact gene locations on a chromosome. The genome DNA sequence is the finest scale physical map of the genome.

The human genome is thought to contain 20 000–25 000 protein-coding genes distributed on 23 pairs of chromosomes (http://www.ncbi.nlm.nih.gov/entrez/). The total length of one copy of the genome is $\sim 3 \times 10^9$ nucleotide bases. The protein-coding segments (exons) are split by noncoding DNA sequences (introns). The aggregate protein coding sequences, referred to as the "exome," account for about 1–1.5% of the genome. Some of the remaining DNA contains regulatory elements that direct the expression of genes, control chromatin conformation, encode regulatory RNAs, act as origins for DNA replication, and produce the large-scale chromosome structure. About 40% of the total DNA is accounted for by families of repeated sequences. These repeat elements are generally silent, but may be involved in some types of gene regulation and can become involved in mutational mechanisms of deletion, duplication, and insertion. Each cell expresses only a subset of the entire gene repertoire. "Housekeeping" genes are expressed in almost all tissues and cell types, where they perform basic metabolic and structural functions. Other genes are under very specific control and their expression is restricted to one or a few cell types. Differential gene expression specifies the unique functions of cells, e.g., immunoglobulin in B cells, and T-cell receptor in T cells. Genes that coordinate the expression of groups of tissue-specific genes primarily encode transcription factors that regulate the rate of mRNA transcription on their target genes. A few of these apparently act as "master" genes during particular developmental processes or in specific cell lineages. Some of these master genes, e.g., *PAX5*, may be involved in leukemias and lymphomas. So far, immunodeficiency genes appear to be in the category of genes that involve either innate or adaptive immunity controling cell growth, differentiation, effector functions, or apoptosis.[1]

Polymorphic variation and linkage

A genetic map relates one gene to another based on how often they are inherited together. Within a specific region of the DNA the maternal and paternal copies of the genome may be non-identical and the variants are called alleles. Protein and nucleotide differences are called polymorphisms when they are frequent enough to be found in 1–5% of the general population. Variations in single nucleotides occur in $\sim 1/200$ bases when DNA sequencing is used to survey ~ 100 chromosomes.[2] Polymorphisms arise over time in a group of individuals because of mutations in the DNA (Fig. 98.1). Some polymorphisms involve simple sequence repeats so that there is variation in the number of repeat units. These are called short tandem repeats (STR) and form the basis of the genetic marker maps that are used in forensic identification. In contrast to STRs, the most common polymorphisms involve a change in a single nucleotide position. Large databases of single nucleotide polymorphisms (SNPs, pronounced "snips") have been accumulated (http://www.ncbi.nlm.nih.gov/SNP/). It is thought that there could be ~ 20–30×10^6 SNPs with minor allele frequency $>5\%$ available across the human genome. Many STR and SNP polymorphisms are found in noncoding DNA, but functionally significant polymorphisms also occur in protein-coding and regulatory noncoding DNA sequences, and these have been shown to play a significant, albeit incomplete, role in common human diseases.

The composition of alleles within genetic loci in an individual is called the genotype. The individual's genotype interacts with the environment both in development and in maturity to create the phenotype. Some components of the phenotype, such as body weight, can be relatively simple to measure, whereas other phenotypes may be based on complex laboratory evaluation (e.g., in T-cell proliferation). A key distinction should be drawn between discrete traits and those that are represented by a quantitative continuum. Many laboratory values, which are

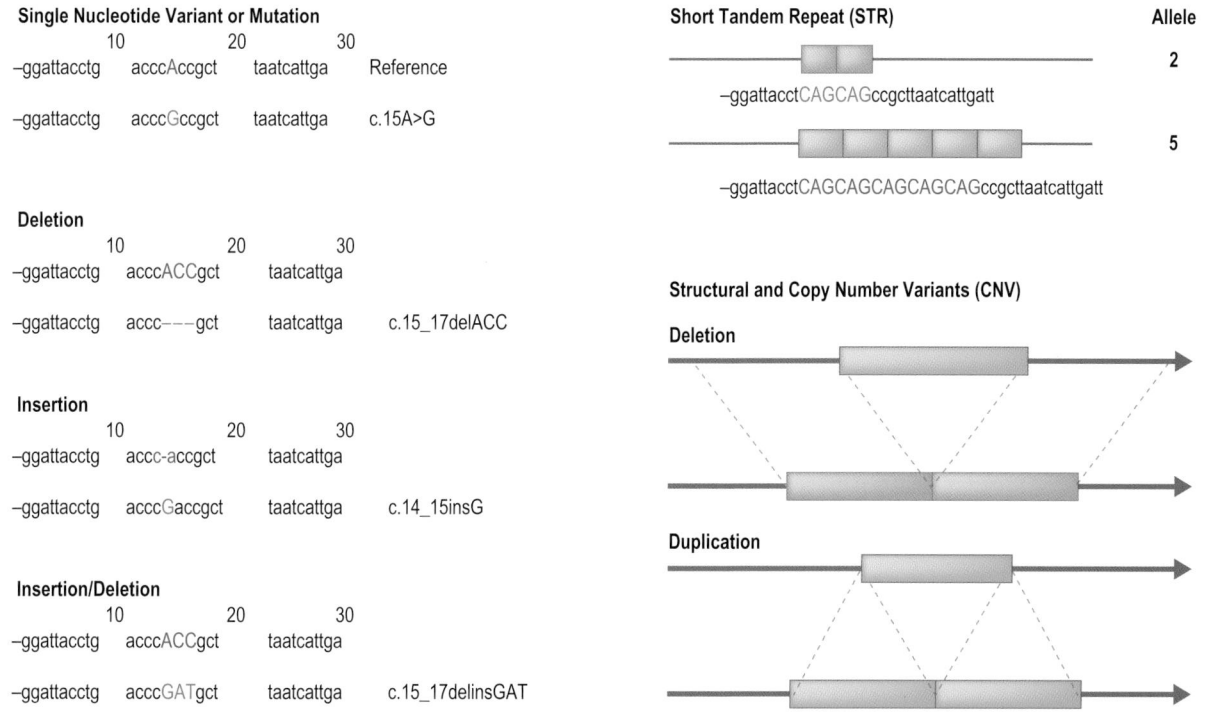

Fig. 98.1 Classes of DNA variation important for genetic testing and human genetic diseases. DNA variations can be either benign or pathogenic depending on whether they affect the underlying functions of a genetic locus and the encoded proteins. An international standard nomenclature is used to describe changes in the DNA. Structural variants have been found to be a common cause of human genetic disorders.

essentially quantitative, can be reduced to discrete traits by assigning them to "normal" or "abnormal" status. Polymorphisms account for some of the variation that is observed at the phenotype level between healthy individuals and between populations, and the cumulative percentage of the variation explained by genetic variation is called the heritability. There is a general correlation of allele frequency with the age of polymorphism, i.e., the older the polymorphism the greater the allele frequency and the greater the likelihood that it will be observed in all ethnic groups. Indeed, the more common allele is most often the ancestral form within the whole human population, in the sense that it is generally the base observed at the homologous position in chimpanzee and other primates.

Genes can be mapped in relation to one another by a *linkage* map. Genes that are physically close can be shown to be predominantly co-inherited. Linkage mapping played a large role in the identification of the X-linked immunodeficiency genes (Chapters 21, 34–36). Linkage has been much less useful for the identification of autosomal recessive genes responsible for rare immunodeficiencies because average families are not large enough to be used by themselves. Beyond small families and at the population level, the correlation of alleles among markers that are very close to each other in the genome is called linkage disequilibrium (LD). LD occurs because the mutation that creates a polymorphism occurs on a single chromosome. Then various population processes (drift, migration, and selection) cause the variant to become more frequent over time. The arrangement of alleles, however, is broken up by recombination over time as well. Hence, only markers that are relatively close to each other continue to have significant LD. A large international project (HapMap) created a dense map of SNP markers allowing a comprehensive view of LD in several reference populations.[2] This information has been efficiently exploited in genetic epidemiology projects called genome wide association studies (GWAS) that have characterized several thousand common variants that contribute to common diseases such as diabetes, rheumatoid arthritis, and lupus.

The advent of exploratory projects, such as the 1000 Genomes Project (http://www.1000genomes.org/) that assess whole exomes and genomes in normal and disease populations, has recently focused much more attention on rare genetic variation, particularly alleles with frequency of 0.01–1.0%. These variants may be equal or greater contributors to common disease compared to common variants. It is also apparent that the extent of individual genetic variation was underestimated from previous data and that each individual bears about 3.5 million simple nucleotide variants and about 1 000 structural variants.[3] Approximately 200 000–500 000 of these variants appear unique to the individual when compared to presently available data. Even given some technical reservations, the enormous extent of private variation has been clearly established. Whole exome technology promises to rapidly solve a great fraction of remaining single gene disorders including primary immune deficiencies. The biggest difficulty with these conditions is that similar clinical diseases can be caused by mutation in more than one gene locus (*locus heterogeneity*). Successful identification of pathogenic mutations, even those unique to single pedigrees, can be accomplished by combining DNA sequencing with complimentary functional technologies.

Physical maps and molecular cytogenetics

Physical maps are different from the genetic map in that they describe how genes are arranged in the DNA on a scale as large as a whole chromosome and as fine as a single nucleotide. At the coarsest level of the physical map, genes are placed in chromosome segments corresponding to the Giemsa stain banding pattern of metaphase chromosomes. A very important way to localize genes is to hybridize region-specific DNA probes directly to a chromosome spread. The technique, called fluorescence *in situ* hybridization (FISH), allows the detection of signals from the chromosome spread to directly localize genes.[4]

FISH is used for cytogenetic examination of tumors, leukemias, and lymphomas. FISH has now been largely replaced by array comparative genome hybridization (CGH), which examines many hundreds of thousands of positions using oligonucleotide probes.[5] High-density oligonucleotide arrays allow both standardization of reagents between diagnostic laboratories and extensive customization for particular disease applications. These methods are detailed below. In the DiGeorge syndrome, characteristic deletions of chromosomes 22q11 or 10p13 cannot be detected by chromosome analysis only (Chapters 35 and 84).

Mutation

> ● KEY CONCEPTS
>
> **Mutation**
>
> - Mutation can occur by deletion, insertion, or duplication of short or long DNA segments.
> - Single-base mutations can be caused by replication errors or by chemical deamination of methylcytosine.
> - Single-base mutations can affect protein coding sequence, regulatory sequences, or the RNA splice signals within a gene.
> - The parental origin of mutations (maternal or paternal) affects those mutational mechanisms most likely responsible.
> - A disease can be caused by mutations in several alternative genes (locus heterogeneity).
> - Most primary immune deficiency disease occurs because of different kinds of mutations in particular genes (allelic heterogeneity).

Mutations can involve single nucleotide substitutions, small or large deletions, insertions, inversions, or duplications. Some mutations have no measurable or functionally significant phenotypic effect. They become one of the huge pool of neutral polymorphisms in the genome. Single base substitutions in a triplet amino acid codon often disturb the normal function of proteins. These are described as *missense* (i.e., causing an amino acid substitution) or *nonsense* (i.e., terminating translation). Mutations affecting regulatory or splice signal sequences in RNA can also be deleterious. Primary mechanisms of mutation are misincorporation of nucleotides and faulty repair of chemically damaged nucleotides (e.g., 8-oxodG) during DNA replication by DNA polymerases.[6,7] Another important mechanism underlying single base or "point" mutations occurs at CpG dinucleotides.[8] The cytosine is often methylated, and chemical deamination of the methylated cytosine gives the base thymidine. At the next round of replication the CG may be changed to TG or CA, depending on which DNA strand was altered. Small insertion and deletion (indel) mutations are also very common. Indels occurring in protein coding sequence are usually deleterious as they can cause frameshifts (changing the reading frame, leading to translation termination within a few codons) and account for almost 25% of known human disease causing mutations. They result from strand slippage in repetitive sequences and misaligned intermediates during DNA synthesis.[9] An entirely different mechanism for mutation is expansion of unstable triplet repeat segments.[10] So far, no disorder that affects the immune system has been associated with this mechanism.

Heritable mutations can arise in either the male or the female germline, but the gender-related frequency is influenced by the mutational mechanism. Chromosomal nondisjunction, for example, occurs predominantly during female meiosis and has a strong maternal age effect.[11] The fact that spermatogonial proliferation occurs throughout life and involves many more cell replications than oogenesis increases the single base mutation frequency in the paternal germline. A 20-fold risk for point mutations and an 11-fold risk of mutations at CpG dinucleotides occurring in the male germline has been observed in the factor IX gene.[12]

Clinicians must cope with both locus and allele heterogeneity. Locus heterogeneity means that the same or a similar phenotype results from mutation in one of several different genes. For example, severe combined immunodeficiency (SCID) can result from mutation in the adenosine deaminase, interleukin-2 receptor γ-chain genes, *JAK3*, etc. Allelic heterogeneity, on the other hand, means that the disease is caused by different mutations in the same gene. In X-linked disorders allelic heterogeneity is typically high because affected individuals have reduced reproduction (negative evolutionary selection) and most mutations are lost in the population after a few generations. At autosomal loci some mutations have reached appreciable frequency due to demographic processes, e.g., founder effect. In the heterozygous state, recessive mutations can be weakly deleterious, neutral, or actually confer a small advantage. Because the mutant alleles are common, it is possible to test affected individuals and potential carriers directly for those mutations. This is the basis for population screening for carrier status in cystic fibrosis. However, none of the immune deficiencies, with the exception of SCID due to Artemis/*DCLRE1C* mutation seen in Native Americans of the Southwest (OMIM 602450),[13] result from common mutations that would permit efficient screening. In the autosomal recessive immune deficiencies most patients have two different very rare mutations (compound heterozygosity) at the disease locus. If there is known parental consanguinity or the family comes from an isolated population, the affected individual may be homozygous for a rare mutation.

X chromosome inactivation

Disturbances in the pattern of X inactivation are interesting phenomena in women who are carriers of X-linked disorders, including several immune deficiencies. Measurement of X chromosome activity in the blood cells of normal women shows that on average the contribution of maternal and paternal X chromosomes is approximately 50:50. Extreme skewing of X inactivation often results from abnormal proliferation of blood cells. X inactivation analysis can be used to demonstrate clonal growth of premalignant (e.g., myelodysplasia) and malignant cells. In a female carrying mutations at the X-linked severe combined immune deficiency (*XSCID*, OMIM 300400), agammaglobulinemia (*XLA*, OMIM 300300), or Wiskott–Aldrich syndrome (*WAS*, OMIM 301000) loci, cell competition and compensation mechanisms lead to a reduced contribution of cells expressing the mutant allele among affected cells.[14] In XLA, the B-cell lineage shows selective use of the nonmutant active X chromosome. In XSCID, skewing of X inactivation is observed in B cells, T cells, and NK cells. In WAS, some degree of skewing of X inactivation results from defective hematopoietic stem cell activity.[15] Historically, skewed X inactivation was very helpful in linkage mapping of these conditions. As a clinical test, X inactivation now has reduced importance compared to direct mutation analyses. There may be some role for X inactivation assays to clarify carrier status when mutation analysis is incomplete or unsuccessful.

Description and principles of DNA diagnostic techniques

The overriding theme of all DNA diagnostic techniques is the detection of variants in the DNA molecule that are associated with disease. This has historically involved a targeted search in one or a few specific segments, but the field is evolving rapidly towards techniques that allow a simultaneous survey of the entire genome. DNA copy number analysis and DNA sequencing have come to dominate individual genetic diagnostic methods. *Bioinformatics* is a necessary diagnostic laboratory discipline that must be coupled to these methods, particularly when the whole genome is surveyed.

Detection of disease-causing copy number variants: Fluorescence *in situ* hybridization and microarrays

Many genetic diseases are caused by deletions or duplications in human DNA. These conditions typically have copy number abnormalities ranging from 500 kilobases (Kb) to 5 megabases (Mb) and are commonly referred to as "genomic disorders." The most common genomic disorder with a clinically important effect on the immune system is 22q11 deletion syndrome. This disorder affects about 1 per 4000 live born infants and accounts for about 90% of DiGeorge syndrome cases. The karyotype, in which a metaphase chromosome spread was stained and visualized under the microscope, was for many decades the only clinically useful test for the detection of copy number changes. The karyotype offered a genome-wide view, but at a very low resolution: alterations smaller than 5 Mb, including those that typically cause DiGeorge syndrome, were not routinely detected. Two methods have now largely replaced conventional karyotypes for routine genetic diagnosis, and they will be described below.

Fluorescence *in situ* hybridization (FISH)

FISH provided a significant advance over older techniques that used radioactive labels for probing genes directly on chromosome spreads.[16] In its simplest form a cloned gene segment (referred to as a probe) is labelled (Fig. 98.2),[17] and allowed to hybridize to a preparation of early metaphase (condensed) chromosomes. The labelled probe hybridizes specifically to a locus and is then detected with secondary antibodies and high-sensitivity immunofluorescence techniques. The targeted locus appears as two pairs of dots corresponding to the sister chromatids from the two chromosomal homologs. Cells that are in interphase (when the DNA is largely unfolded in the nucleus) can also be probed. In the interphase cell, two single signals are observed corresponding to the two chromosomes. While FISH offered much higher resolution than a standard karyotype, it did not provide genome-wide coverage with the exception of a related technique, known as spectral karyotyping (SKY),[17,18] in which each chromosome is labelled with a differentiating pattern of fluorescent dyes. With the introduction of microarray-based methods for genome-wide copy-number analysis, the practical application of SKY has become very limited and the role of FISH has been reduced to cancer cytogenetics and as a confirmatory test for abnormalities detected by a microarray.

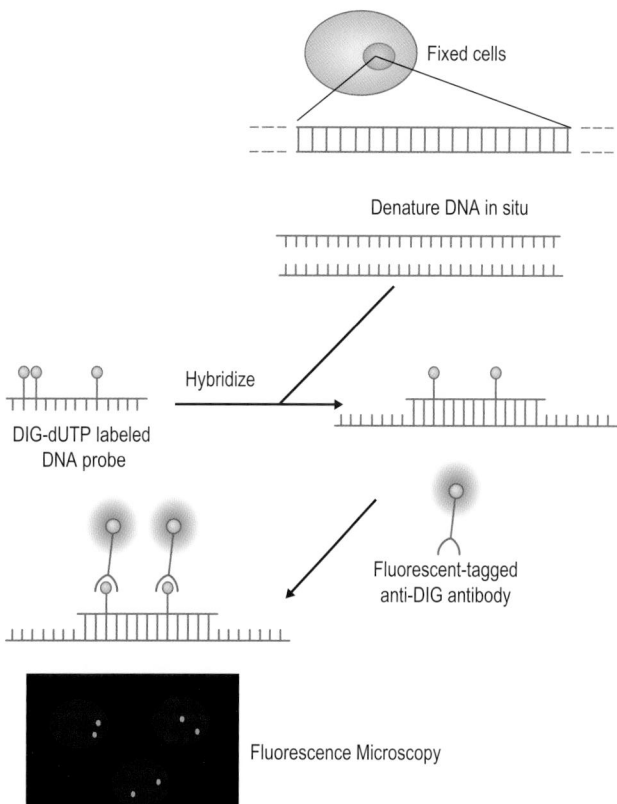

Fig. 98.2 Fluorescence *in situ* hybridization (FISH). Probes complementary to specific sites in the genome are labeled with a hapten, e.g., digoxygenin, and then hybridized to denatured DNA within cells on microscope slides. The hybridized probes are then detected by immunofluorescence microscopy.

Array-based copy number analysis

● KEY CONCEPTS

Molecular methods

- Most DNA diagnostics rely on DNA copy number analysis or DNA sequencing.

- PCR allows an exponential amplification of a DNA segment from the genome, allowing multiple analytical procedures on the single pure sequence.

- Array-based copy number analysis has become the first-line method for finding small abnormalities in the structure of chromosomes.

- New high-throughput sequencing methods which use microarrays have emerged as practical alternatives to older single analysis approaches.

- Bioinformatics is an emerging discipline relevant to molecular diagnosis. Integration of bioinformatics techniques plays a necessary role in data acquisition and interpretation.

Oligonucleotide arrays have had a revolutionary impact on molecular diagnostics, by offering high-resolution, genome-wide detection of copy-number changes. The basic principle involves synthetic oligonucleotides complementary to human nucleic acid sequences bound to a glass surface, and hybridization of fragmented, labelled human nucleic acid samples (Fig. 98.3). Array printing of activated phosphoramidite nucleotide precursors allows hundreds to thousands of oligonucleotides to be

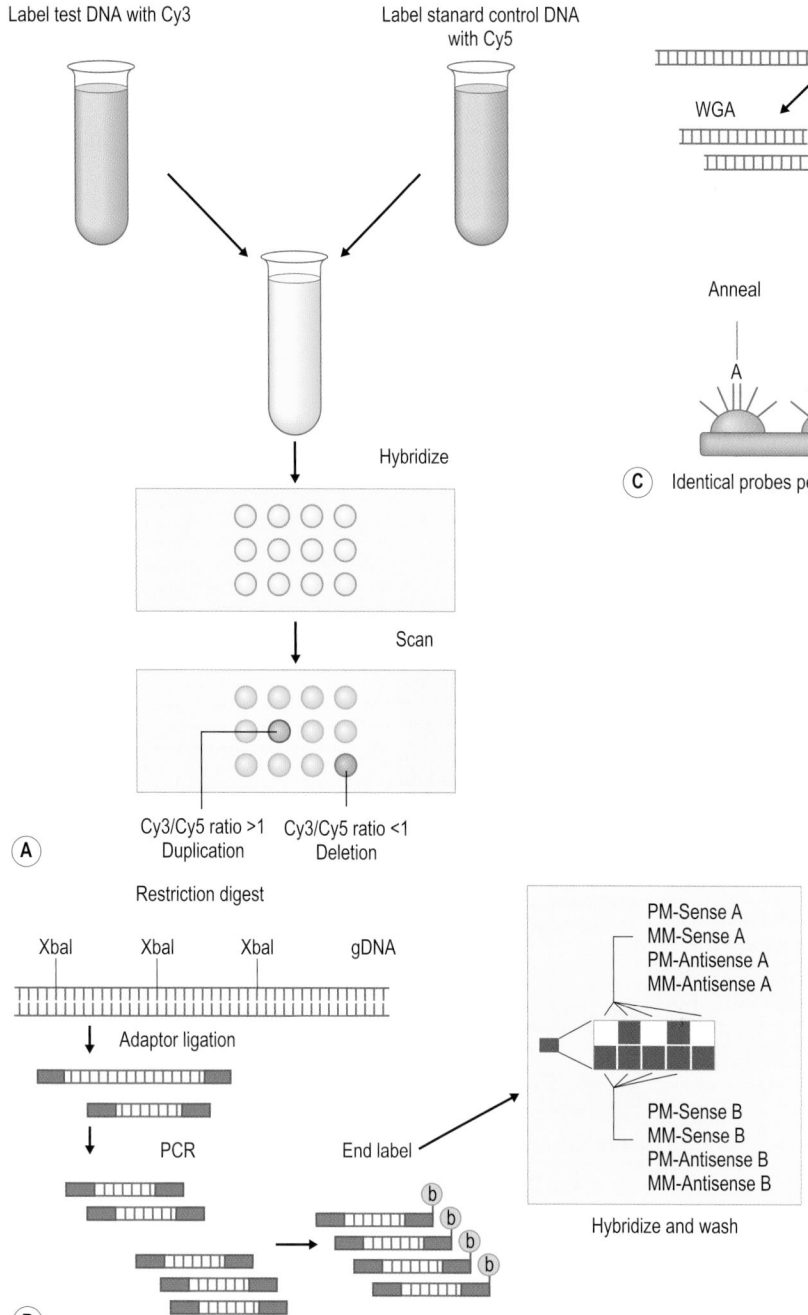

Label test DNA with Cy3

Label stanard control DNA with Cy5

Hybridize

Scan

Cy3/Cy5 ratio >1 Duplication   Cy3/Cy5 ratio <1 Deletion

(A)

Restriction digest

Xbal   Xbal   Xbal   gDNA

Adaptor ligation

PCR   End label

PM-Sense A
MM-Sense A
PM-Antisense A
MM-Antisense A

PM-Sense B
MM-Sense B
PM-Antisense B
MM-Antisense B

Hybridize and wash

(B)

gDNA

WGA

Fragment and Denature

Anneal

A   G

Scan

*TA   *CG

A   B

(C) Identical probes per bead type   Single base extension

Fig. 98.3 Array-based DNA copy number analysis. (A) Array comparative genomic hybridization (aCGH) uses a reference DNA to compare with the test DNA. The labelled DNA is hybridized to an array of oligonucleotides that are designed to be uniquely complementary to hundreds of thousands of positions in the genome. The relative intensities of the fluorescence signal from each DNA probe allow assessment of copy number. Genotyping arrays are also widely used for copy number testing (B, C). (B) Whole genome sampling and amplification (WGSA). End-labeled PCR products that constitute a sample from the genome are hybridized to oligo sets on standard chips. The oligos are organized into "probe quartets" consisting of perfect matches (PM) and single-base mismatches (MM) for each allele, A and B. Separate quartets for the sense and antisense strand of DNA help to ensure specificity and in the actual assay these quartets are repeated three to five times on the chip. This type of assay has been developed to test a standard panel of > 2 million DNA features per sample. (C) Single base extension (Illumina Infinium II). This assay uses whole genome amplification (WGA) to increase the molar concentration of target DNA. SBE on arrays of tagged microbeads allows allele discrimination and the resulting products are detected by immunostaining (signal amplification). This assay has been used for assays of up to 5 million SNPs per sample.

fabricated on activated glass surfaces (Agilent).[19–21] Light activated oligonucleotide synthesis has also been used to efficiently customize oligonucleotide arrays (Affymetrix and Nimblegen). A third approach involves synthesis of oligonucleotides on microbeads that are randomly scattered over a glass surface (Illumina).[22–24] These processes are very similar, in principle, to the fabrication of microelectronics devices, and so have given these arrays the nickname of "gene chips."

Microarrays have been used in very large scale studies to genotype common polymorphisms. Robust chemistries that can analyze standard sets of up to 5 000 000 SNPs in a single assay are now routine (Fig. 98.3). Nonamplified genomic DNA is too complex (i.e., the concentration of any particular sequence is too low) to be analyzed directly. High-throughput genotyping assays require an array-based readout and scalable, multiplex

assay chemistry. This is extremely challenging because of the complexity of the human genome; i.e., any particular unique sequence in the mixture has a low molar concentration and because of the need for exquisite specificity at the single base level. An important general principle for achieving single base specificity is the detection of physically coincident events.[25] This is exactly the route taken by the polymerase chain reaction (PCR), in which specific annealing of both primers is required for the reaction to take place (Fig. 98.4).

Whole genome sampling and amplification (WGSA) implemented in the Affymetrix SNP arrays uses parallel amplification of short DNA segments (200–1100 bp) that are then labelled and hybridized to oligonucleotide probe arrays.[26] The oligonucleotides are specific for each allele of SNPs and the resulting hybridization intensities can be used to derive the

Fig. 98.4 Polymerase chain reaction. Primers that hybridize to the target sequence are used to initiate multiple cycles of synthesis, melting, annealing, and synthesis. In practice, the potential geometric increase in DNA tapers off as reaction components become limiting.

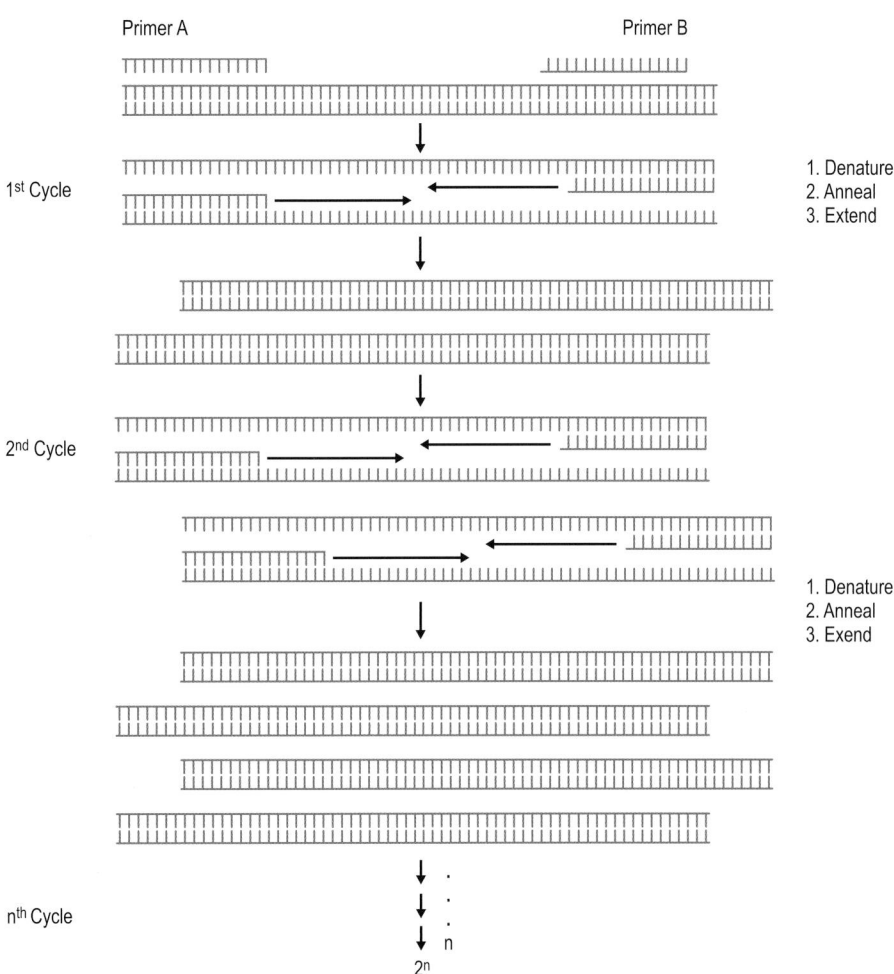

Primer A   Primer B

1st Cycle
1. Denature
2. Anneal
3. Extend

2nd Cycle
1. Denature
2. Anneal
3. Exend

nth Cycle
n
2^n

genotypes. These assays are fixed in the sense that the investigator uses the information from a standardized array but cannot add SNPs for particular purposes. An alternative approach, incorporated in the Infinium assays (Illumina), involves the detection of allele-specific primer extension or single base extension products on a self-assembling high-density microbead array.[27] In the Infinium assays genomic DNA is first subjected to whole genome amplification (WGA) and those products are hybridized to an array of locus-specific 50-mer capture probes. Either primer extension or ligation reactions on the array surface are used to accomplish allele discrimination. Signal amplification with methods familiar to users of ELISA assays are used to enhance the sensitivity. A distinct advantage of this class of assays is that the "assay conversion" (percent SNPs that actually allow inference of the genotype in the final assay mixture) is very high. This allows great latitude in the selection of SNPs, and thus proves highly useful in assays of rare variants.

For expression analysis, cDNA "target" derived from the tissue or cell source is labelled with fluorophores and used to determine complementary binding by massively parallel hybridization to the probes fixed on the array. Such arrays are extraordinarily useful for monitoring gene expression at thousands of loci in a single assay. Diagnostic and prognostic information about lymphomas,[28,29] leukemias,[30,31] and autoimmunity derived from expression arrays has already had a large impact on research.[32] However, this technology has been slow to enter clinical practice. A major challenge lies in the variation between studies in sample selection, analysis platform, and statistical

methods. Establishing criteria for clinical validity and utility are long-term challenges for this class of biomarkers.

Detection of disease causing point mutations and insertions/deletions

Methods for the detection of single-base substitutions in DNA are increasingly important in the diagnostic laboratory.[33] Although cDNA synthesized from mRNA can be used, analysis of genomic DNA is far more common. Many different methods for mutation detection have been described, but virtually all clinical diagnostic laboratories now approach an unknown mutation with DNA sequencing. When Sanger sequencing is used, the first step is to design PCR primer sets that will allow amplification of each exon. The availability of the reference human genome sequence makes determination of gene structure and amplimer design for genomic DNA straightforward. Any mutation that directly affects amplification, such as deletion or mutation in the amplimer sequence, can produce misleading results. It is always desirable to have parental specimens available to serve as a reference for proving biallelic inheritance in the affected offspring. If there is a clear clinical diagnosis and only a single gene likely to be involved, then automated fluorescent sequencing is still the preferred method. For disorders with highly complex clinical and laboratory phenotypes, like primary immune deficiencies, the problem of locus heterogeneity is very severe. In the very near future it should become routine to solve this problem by sequencing the complete exome or the complete genome in individual patients using the next generation technologies described below.

Sanger sequencing

The direct determination of a DNA sequence is fundamental to mutation identification (Fig. 98.5). The most commonly used method (called Sanger sequencing) depends on termination of DNA synthesis by chemically modified nucleotides (dideoxy-NTPs). A single-stranded DNA template is hybridized to a primer that can recognize a short known segment of DNA. The single-stranded DNA is obtained from bacterial plasmid/phage vectors, or may be produced by DNA amplification. The primer acts as a starting point for DNA synthesis by a DNA polymerase that is added to the reaction. Four separate reactions are set up, each "spiked" with one of the four possible dideoxynucleotides (ddATP, ddTTP, ddCTP, or ddGTP). As synthesis proceeds, some of the strands incorporate a dideoxynucleotide and no further extension can take place. In each reaction a family of molecules is synthesized whose unit lengths are determined by whether the reaction had been terminated by incorporation of a specific dideoxynucleotide at a given position. Either the primer or the nucleotides may be labelled. Automated instrumentation for DNA sequencing using laser scanning of fluorophore-labeled reactions has largely replaced other labeling schemes. By using four different fluorescent labels the reaction products can be analyzed together. Two classes of chemistry are popular: "dye primer," in which the primers of each reaction are tagged with different fluorophores, and "dye terminator," in which the dideoxynucleotides are themselves labelled with fluorophores. Advances in both dye primer[34] and dye terminator chemistry[35] greatly improved the accuracy of quantification and base-calling. The original instrumentation for automated fluorescent sequencing used large polyacrylamide gels, but the most recent generation of instruments exploits large renewable capillary electrophoresis arrays. These instruments (exemplified by the AB 3730xl) were crucial to completion of the reference human genome sequence.

Next-generation DNA sequencing

New technologies that promise to dramatically increase the throughput and reduce the cost of DNA sequencing are being rapidly implemented in research and diagnostic laboratories.[36] Unlike Sanger sequencing, which produces sequence data by controlled termination of the polymerase, the new techniques derive the sequence as nucleotides are sequentially added by the polymerase. Multiple chemistries have now been developed into early-stage high-throughput sequencing instruments (Fig. 98.6).

Pyrosequencing (Roche 454)

The first of these uses pyrosequencing chemistry. Pyrosequencing works by detecting the release of pyrophosphate as nucleotides are added to a DNA primer hybridized to template DNA.[37] DNA polymerase can extend the primer when there is a complementary dNTP available, but stops when only a non-complementary base is present. DNA synthesis is reinitiated following the addition of the next complementary dNTP. Pyrophosphate is released as the base is added to the growing DNA chain and detected by enzyme amplification. The sequencing instrument controls the order of dNTP addition to the reaction. The order of base addition coupled to the light emission is then decoded as the sequence. The 454 Life Sciences Corporation instrument exploits pyrosequencing on an array of about 300 000 microscopic (40 μm) wells (Fig. 98.6A). The wells each contain a single sepharose bead on which are coupled the reaction products of a single molecule of template DNA, which itself has been amplified in an oil-and-water emulsion.[38] An advantage of clonal amplification is that it deals neatly with the problem of heterozygosity. The pyrosequencing reaction is monitored in a fiberoptic system. Read lengths of about 250 nucleotides are feasible.

Sequencing by synthesis (Illumina)

One of the most widely used systems for next generation sequencing involves highly parallel imaging of single base addition on "clusters" of identical DNA molecules (Fig. 98.6B). This technology has been commercialized by Illumina, Inc. In their approach, DNA is ligated to primers that allow it to be amplified on a surface called a "flow cell".[39] The DNA templates attach to the flow cell surface by hybridization to specific primers complementary to that used to prepare the DNA library. Solid-phase bridge amplification creates many identical copies of each single template molecule in a localized cluster. The density of the clusters is extremely high and the specialized imaging system allows resolution of more than 10^9 clusters per flow cell. DNA sequence is determined in the flow cell by sequential addition of fluorescent-tagged nucleotides. A single labelled nucleotide is added to nascent DNA in each sequencing cycle. Each nucleotide has a different fluorophor so that all four are added to the mix in each cycle of base extension. The nucleotide label also terminates polymerization, i.e., only a single base is added at each cycle, and

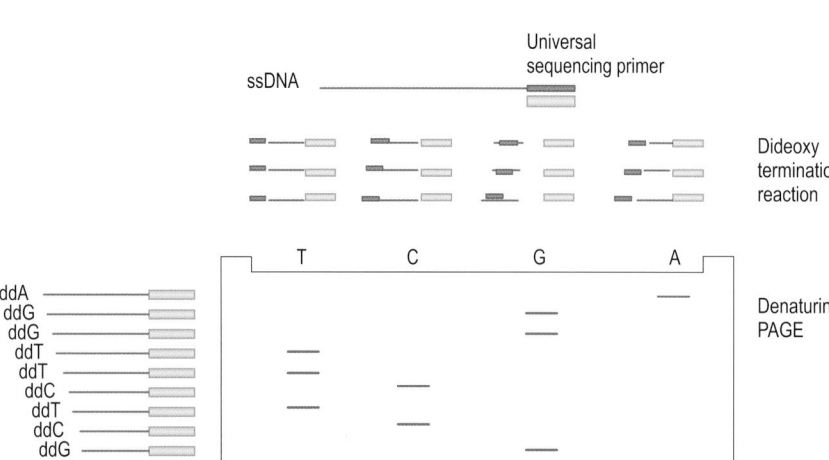

Fig. 98.5 DNA sequencing by dideoxy-NTP chain termination (Sanger). Copying of the DNA by the polymerase is terminated at specific positions when a ddNTP is incorporated. The ddNTP is added mixed with dNTPs so that, in each reaction, only some new strands terminate, whereas others continue through to the next complementary nucleotide. The sequencing products can be visualized by autoradiography or by laser scanning in an automated sequencer.

the identity of the incorporated nucleotide is determined by the fluorescent emission spectrum and intensity. Because the bases act as terminators homopolymeric segments can be resolved relatively accurately. After each dNTP incorporation, the fluorescent dye is enzymatically cleaved to allow incorporation of the next nucleotide. This class of instruments is capable of sequencing complete human genomes in a single run.

Sequencing by ligation (Life Technologies)

SOLiD (sequencing by oligonucleotide ligation and detection) is another next-generation sequencing technology that has been adapted to a sequencing instrument platform and applied in diverse research studies (Fig. 98.6C). In SOLiD sequencing[40] a DNA fragments attached to beads and clonally amplified on the bead surface so that only a single DNA sequence is associated with each magnetic bead. The fragments attached to the magnetic beads have a universal adapter sequence attached so that the starting sequence of every fragment is identical. Emulsion PCR is used to amplify the unique DNA molecules on each bead in isolation from the other beads and the PCR products attached to the beads are then covalently bound to a glass slide. After primer hybridization four fluorescently labelled di-base probes compete for ligation to the sequencing primer. The sequence of the template is inferred using the specificity of the ligation and the fluorescence signature from every first and second base.

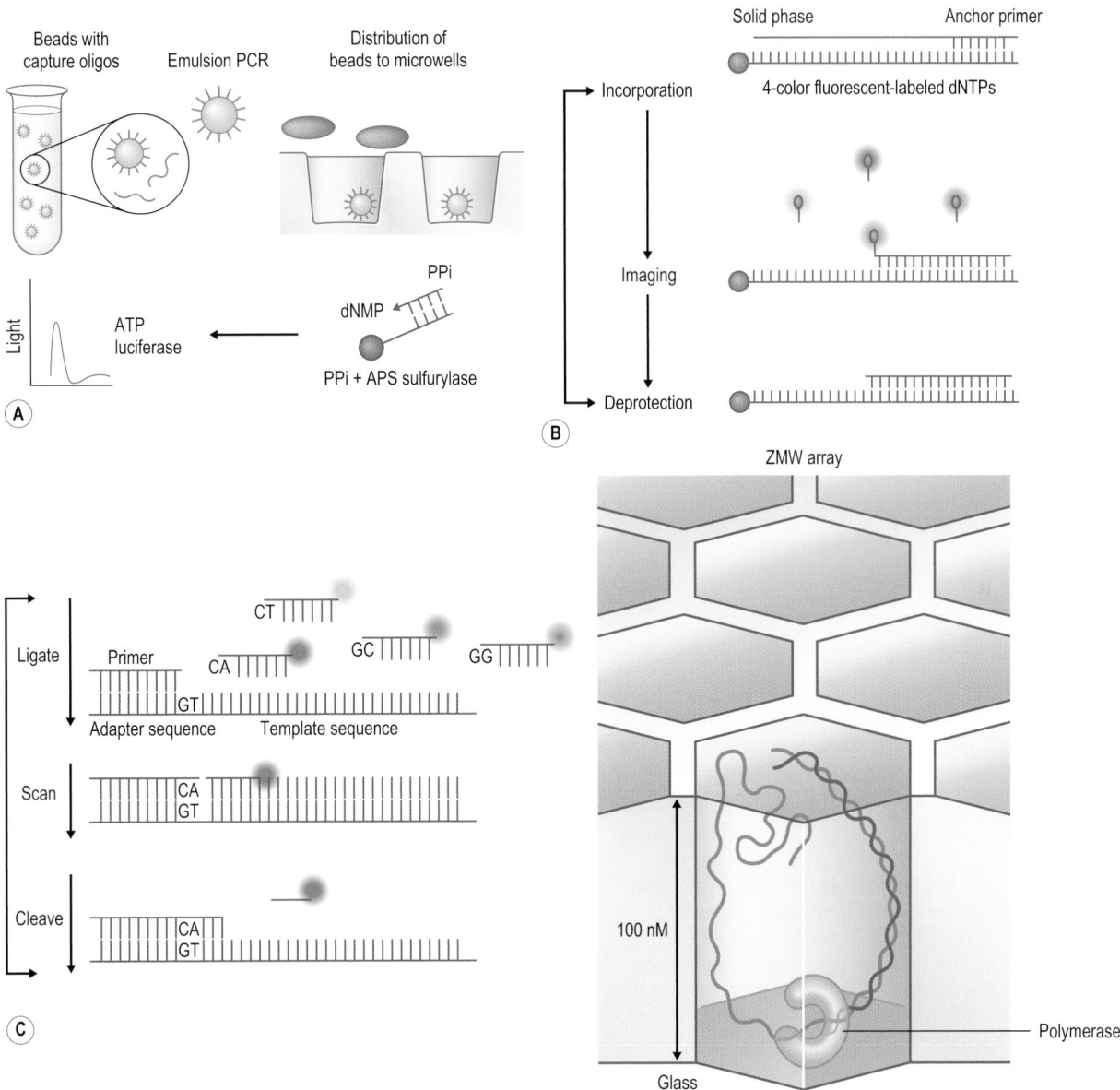

Fig. 98.6 Next generation DNA sequencing. (A) Pyrosequencing carried out in high-density picoliter reactors (Roche 454). In this method single molecules of DNA are hybridized to tagged beads and PCR is carried out in an emulsion. The beads bearing the resulting amplified products are distributed into microfabricated wells in which pyrosequencing reactions can be cycled. The release of PPi with each cycle is monitored by an enzyme-linked production of ATP, which in turn cause luciferase to emit light. An instrument that integrates these steps is produced by 454 Life Sciences. (B) Sequencing by synthesis (Illumina). This is a method in which fluorescent labelled terminator nucleotides are sequentially added and then imaged. After deprotection, another cycle of addition and imaging can take place. The currently available instrumentation allows simultaneous imaging of >1 billion "clusters" representing unique DNA elements. Approximately 100 cycles of base addition is commonly used. (C) Sequencing by ligation (SOLiD). In this method dye-labeled primers are sequentially hybridized and ligated to the template DNA. After imaging the tagged oligonucleotide is cleaved and the cycle is repeated. Currently available instrumentation allows >20 G bases per day sequence output.

(Continued)

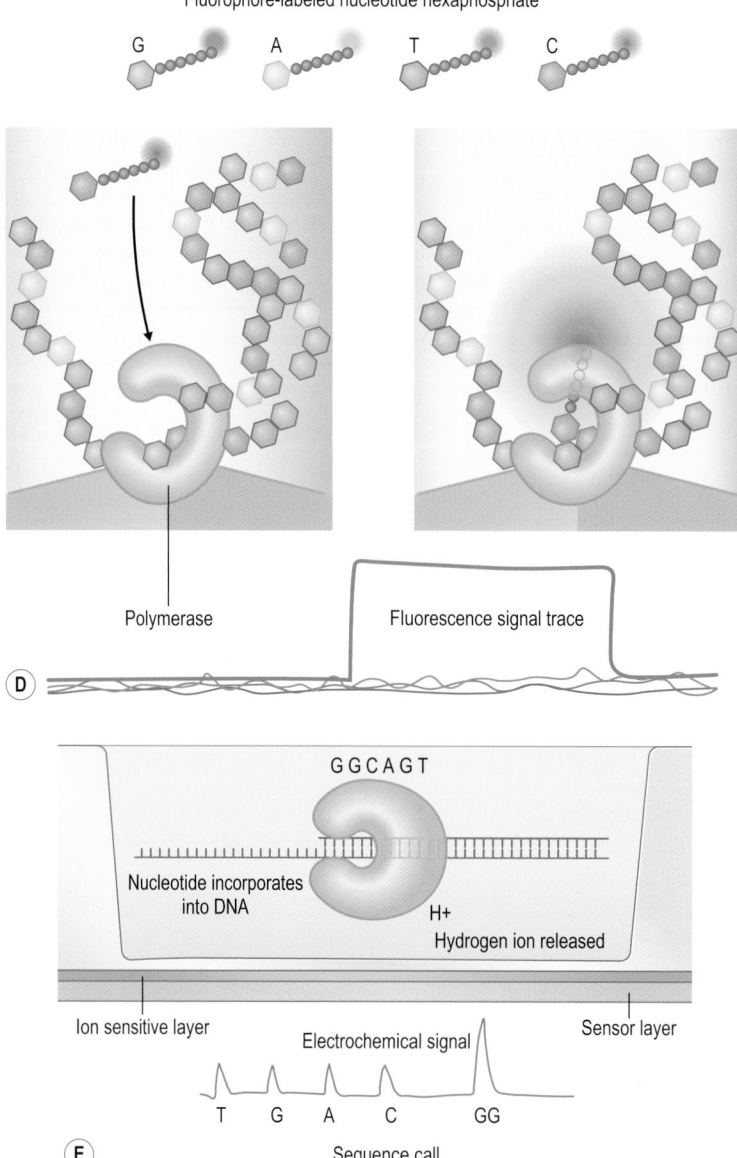

Fluorophore-labeled nucleotide hexaphosphate

G   A   T   C

Polymerase

Fluorescence signal trace

(D)

GGCAGT

Nucleotide incorporates into DNA

H+

Hydrogen ion released

Ion sensitive layer

Electrochemical signal

Sensor layer

T   G   A   C   GG

(E)   Sequence call

Fig. 98.6—cont'd (D) Single molecule sequencing (PacBio). In this method DNA polymerase is attached in a microscopic imaging unit called a zero mode wave guide (ZMW). A single DNA molecule is imaged as fluorescent nucleotides are added on the single stranded template DNA. This method distinguishes itself by the very rapid rate of reaction and the very long read length achieved. (E) Electrochemical sequencing (Ion Torrent). This method is very different from all others currently available in that it does not use any fluorescence labels or imaging. Sequences are inferred by changes in electrical conductance caused by release of hydrogen ions when bases are added to a DNA chain.

Read length is determined by the number of cycles of ligation, detection, and cleavage. Another important feature of the method is redundancy by resetting the primer to the n-1 position a process that is carried out for five rounds on each sequence tag. This allows each base to be interrogated in two independent ligation reactions by two different primers. The result is very low error rates but with some trade-off in speed and complexity of the raw data.

Single molecule sequencing (Pacific Bioscience)

A true single molecule sequencing method has been developed by Pacific Biosciences.[41] In their method DNA polymerase is immobilized in a femptoliter-sized well with special optical properties called the zero mode wave guide (ZMW)

(Fig. 98.6D). The small size of the ZMW "hole" prevents 600-nm wavelength laser light from passing entirely through and only the bottom 30 nm where the polymerase is bound is subject to the fluorescence excitation. Labelled nucleotides are flowed into the chamber and complementary bases encountering the DNA polymerase are incorporated into the growing DNA chain. During incorporation, the DNA polymerase holds the nucleotide for tens of milliseconds, orders of magnitude longer than the average diffusing nucleotide. The transient light emission is then detected and the identity of the incorporated base recorded. Nucleotides with a fluorescent dye attached to the phosphate group of the nucleotide are cleaved when the nucleotide is incorporated into the DNA strand. The label diffuses away, leaving the DNA ready for the addition of the next base. The polymerase incorporates multiple bases per second so the sequencing process is very fast with real time observation of DNA synthesis. The current configuration of the instrument uses an array of approximately

75,000 ZMWs. Each ZMW is capable of containing a DNA polymerase loaded with a different strand of DNA sample. As a result, the SMRT Cell enables the potential detection of approximately 75 000 single molecule sequencing reactions in parallel. The PacBio instrument uses four singlephoton sensitive cameras with the light pulses called as A, C, G, or T within the instrument's own software.

Electrochemical sequencing (IonTorrent)

This methodology is distinctly different from all the systems that image fluorescent tagged nucleotides or primers because the sensor is a microelectronic device (Fig. 98.6E).[42] The preparation of the DNA for sequencing is similar to that employed by 454 pyrosequencing in that the DNA is first fragmented, then ligated to adapters, and the adaptor-ligated libraries are clonally amplified by emulsion PCR onto beads. Individual beads are then loaded into single sensor wells. Nucleotides are provided in a stepwise fashion with incorporation increasing the length of the sequencing primer by one base when there is a complementary base on the template strand. Sequence determination relies on primer extension. Nucleotide incorporation into a nascent DNA strand by DNA polymerase results in hydrolysis of the nucleotide triphosphate. Hydrolysis causes production of a hydrogen ion for each nucleotide incorporated. The small shift in the pH of the surrounding solution is proportional to the number of nucleotides incorporated, which is then detected by the sensor on the bottom of each well, converted to a voltage and digitized by off-chip electronics. The chip is automatically washed and the cycle is repeated with the next nucleotide. Due to the small size of the wells diffusion into and out of the well is very fast. The sensor layer is composed of tantalum oxide, which is sensitive to proton concentration (essentially pH) allowing rapid detection of the voltage transients that follow base incorporation in each well individually. The voltage change is roughly proportion to the length of a run of the same nucleotide in the DNA so that short homopolymers can be accurately called. Chip fabrication and design are very similar to methods used for microelectronic devices. This suggests that the method will have good potential to scale up the number of molecules processed in parallel. Lacking optical components, the cost of the all-electronic detection system is far less than other sequencing instruments.

The general goal of a "$1 000 genome" articulated by the National Human Genome Research Institute no longer seems like a pipedream. Although there will be some lag in clinical application, it is highly likely that mutation scanning of large numbers of genes, or even complete genome sequencing, will be feasible in the near future.

Bioinformatics

Bioinformatics has emerged as a fundamental discipline in molecular biology as enormous DNA and protein sequence databases, gene expression patterns, and other integrated data sets have been generated by individual laboratories and international genomics projects. The growing number of genetic loci that are already known to be important in immunological disease renders it critical that both research and diagnostic laboratories make maximal use of automated processes in sample archiving, data acquisition, data analysis, and reporting.

Internal databases and data acquisition

Laboratory information management (LIM) systems are widespread and each laboratory must deal with the generic operational problems of sample accession, tracking, and reporting. DNA diagnostic laboratories have several unique problems and requirements that deserve comment. Relational databases should integrate sample accession, physical archive, quality control, and genotype information. Automated data acquisition is an important component of DNA sequencing and genotyping. Instrument-specific and secondary base-calling programs are necessary for data interpretation. More sophisticated statistical models of sequencing and genotyping data are greatly improving the ability to handle datasets per individual that would be far too large for manual analysis.[43] Automated procedures for exporting data files to analytical software and data archiving on indelible media are also important issues. The number of patient-specific data records and the complexity of relationships in family-based testing make it difficult for manual processes to achieve the required reliability.

Data interpretation and public sequence databases

Computer-based methods for genotype and DNA sequence data interpretation are necessary for efficiency and cost-effectiveness. Estimation of genetic risks based on genotype data requires a knowledge of specialized statistical procedures whose description is beyond the scope of this chapter. The development of specialized training programs in molecular genetics and molecular genetic pathology by the American Boards of Medical Genetics and Pathology[44] highlights the recognition by professional groups that this area of clinical testing is exceptionally complex. Although inferences made about disease diagnosis and carrier status based on direct detection of mutations are inherently categorical, data interpretation should incorporate known genotype–phenotype correlations, variable disease expression/ severity, incomplete penetrance, gender-specific risk, and other available data. In the future, as DNA testing is employed in the assessment of more complex traits such as autoimmune and neoplastic diseases, genotype data will perhaps be expressed as "relative risk" and incorporate gene–gene and gene–environment interactions. The reliability of these estimates will require standard data acquisition algorithms and constant updating of population-based data.

The reference human genome sequence is complete (http://genome.ucsc.edu/) and has fueled the rapid expansion of clinical sequencing and genotyping. Diagnostic laboratories must actively use information contained in the public sequence databases to interpret the biological consequences of mutations and polymorphisms. There are several broad databases that have an important role: (1) GenBank, which contains the nonredundant cDNA and protein sequences, finished human genomic sequences (http://www.ncbi.nlm.nih.gov/entrez); (2) dbSNP, which contains more than 18 000 000 common single-nucleotide polymorphisms; and (3) the Human Mutation Database, which assembles mutation information on known disease loci (http://www.hgmd.cf.ac.uk/ac/index.php). Public tools are available for DNA sequence comparisons of patient-specific data with the reference sequences (http://www.ncbi.nlm.nih.gov/BLAST/). The Smith–Waterman algorithm estimates local sequence similarity. The most common implementations employ variations on the basic alignment search tool (BLAST) that quantifies local similarity using the maximal segment pair (MSP) score. A very large database of SNPs genotyped in four reference population samples (northern Europeans from Utah; Yoruba from Ibadan, Nigeria; Han Chinese from Beijing; and Japanese from Tokyo) was produced by the International Haplotype Map Project (http://www.hapmap.org). This database is expected to enable mapping of genes that underlie complex traits such as human autoimmune diseases. The reference genotypes and their associated haplotypes give important information about the short-range correlations between markers (called linkage disequilibrium) and allow the selection of marker sets that efficiently capture most of the genetic information in a population sample.[2,45]

Interpretation of sequence and genotype information is the final output of a molecular diagnostic test. If a mutation has been observed in the proband and other family members are tested, then the expectation is that the mutation will exactly segregate with the disease. An example would be testing for a mutation in X-linked SCID in two brothers. The causal mutation will be present in both. When the proband is the only affected individual, then one may look to the research literature and locus-specific public databases (http://bioinf.uta.fi/base_root/mutationdatabases.php) to determine whether the specific mutation has previously been observed in another affected person. However, it is not uncommon to find a mutation that has not previously been observed, and as mutation analysis by DNA sequencing becomes more common this will be a frequent occurrence. Assessment of the functional consequence of a newly observed sequence variant is problematic as there is no guarantee that the variant is anything more than a rare, but neutral, polymorphism. Nonsense and frameshift mutations are relatively clear. Mutations in sites flanking coding exons known to be required for splicing are easily categorized. Missense substitutions are more difficult. Several methods based on sequence conservation and the chemical properties of amino acids have been developed. These are available in software called SIFT (Sorting Intolerant From Tolerant, http://blocks.fhcrc.org/sift/SIFT.html) and PolyPhen (http://coot.embl.de/PolyPhen/) and several others.

Recommendations for use

KEY CONCEPTS

Principles of molecular diagnostics

- DNA diagnostics can play an important role in the diagnosis of specific diseases in affected patients and in genetic risk assessment for their family members.
- Genotyping can be used to conduct prenatal diagnoses.
- Prenatal diagnosis may be used not only for elective termination of pregnancy but also for treatment planning.
- Provision of genetic testing results to patients and their families carries responsibilities for sensitivity and confidentiality.

Molecular diagnostic techniques have a wide range of potential applications in clinical immunology. DNA diagnostic procedures are used to (a) perform HLA genotyping; (b) analyze neoplastic disease; (c) provide identification or DNA "fingerprinting"; (d) monitor bone marrow engraftment; (e) establish a genetic diagnosis in a symptomatic individual; (f) determine the risk of occurrence of a disease in offspring; and (g) to establish a prenatal diagnosis. The use of DNA analysis for HLA typing is described in Chapter 5. DNA techniques are used in leukemias and lymphomas, primarily for investigation of cell lineage, proliferative

clonality, and measurement of residual abnormal cells after therapy. Molecular analysis, and especially molecular cytogenetic analysis, is important in guiding initial and follow-up therapy (see Chapters 78 and 79).

Medical genetics evaluation and counseling

There is a role for molecular testing in genetic risk assessment in primary immune deficiencies.[46] Primary immune deficiencies are genetically determined disorders and we recommend that all such children and families be referred to a medical genetics specialist. Testing is usually applied to families whose risk of recurrence has been signalled by the birth of an affected child. Almost every case has to be treated as a problem requiring initial mutation identification. The rarity of the individual disorders and the frequent occurrence of new mutations in the X-linked diseases preclude population-wide heterozygote screening.

In the recessive immune deficiencies, carrier status is assumed in the parents once an affected child has been diagnosed. A much lower risk of having an affected child is attached to other carriers in a family, as their mates are unlikely to bear a mutant disease gene allele unless they are themselves lineal relatives of the index case. In the X-linked immune deficiencies the situation is strikingly different. In those cases the origin of mutation should be investigated to ascertain the carrier status of all the at-risk women. In a family with a single affected child carrying the diagnosis of an X-linked immune deficiency, there is a substantial risk that the mother is a carrier. The risk of carrier status in such women is 67–80%, depending on the locus. After the birth of a second affected child, and if the mutation has not been directly identified, the mother would be considered an obligate carrier (although somatic mosaicism is also a less likely possibility[47,48] Women sharing a common lineage between two affected individuals in an extended pedigree, e.g., affected first cousins, would also be considered obligate carriers.

Genetic information, like any medical information, can be unsettling to patients and families. However, there are some special considerations that attach themselves to genetic testing, and practitioners need to be aware of this and appropriately cautious (http://www.ornl.gov/sci/techresources/Human_Genome/elsi/elsi.shtml). A fundamental principle of genetic testing for clinical or research purposes should be informed consent. The testing itself, as well as the plan for sample preservation or disposal, should be described in detail to the patient and family and, where appropriate, written consent obtained. An unintended consequence of genotyping may be to reveal non-paternity of the stated father. The possibility that this might emerge from genetic testing should be sensitively conveyed to the prospective clients and may be a reason for avoiding further laboratory testing. In addition, pedigree analysis may uncover unsuspected risk in other family members who may not be seeking genetic information. Some have argued for a "duty to inform" at-risk family members. Prospective testing, particularly carrier testing, in children before the age of individual consent raises troubling issues that have not been resolved. The latent possibility of employment or insurance discrimination with the incorporation of genotype information into the medical record is another area receiving a great deal of attention. It is important to emphasize in the presentation of the information that the occurrence of new mutation is a natural accident. Where possible, it is strongly preferred that genetic risk information be provided by professionals with experience and training in clinical genetics. There is currently a great deal of concern for the preservation of confidentiality relating to all genetic information.

Prenatal diagnosis

Prenatal diagnosis is accomplished either by direct measurement of the defective function, e.g., enzyme activity in ADA deficiency, or by genetic methods. Because many immune disorders affect cells of the blood system exclusively, the former would mean fetal blood sampling. This is accompanied by a higher risk of fetal loss than either amniocentesis or chorion villus sampling (CVS). DNA-based methods can be equally applied to CVS samples or amniocytes. An important technical consideration in the use of CVS is examination for maternal cell contamination, as this could lead to an erroneous diagnosis. DNA diagnosis can employ linkage analysis, in which an inference is made using neighboring DNA markers about whether the developing fetus has inherited the same mutated chromosomal segment(s) as the index case. However, direct mutation identification in the index case and then use of a direct mutation detection procedure in the developing fetus is always preferred. There is now much more experience with pre-implantation genetic diagnosis (PGD), but this remains a highly specialized and expensive procedure.[49,50] PGD involves the removal of a single blastomere at the eight-cell stage. PCR methods are used to carry out genetic analysis. Recent publications have illustrated the use of PGD to select offspring with compatible HLA types for siblings requiring hematopoietic stem cell transplantation.[51]

Prenatal diagnosis is used for either pregnancy management or treatment planning. In the case of a positive diagnosis of a primary immune deficiency, the couple should then have access to detailed information from an experienced clinical immunologist regarding the current treatment options and prognosis. The perception of the burden of disease can be colored by a previous bad therapeutic outcome caused by late diagnosis and its consequent complications. Prenatal diagnosis allows appropriate treatment planning to be carried out for isolation, prospective intravenous immunoglobulin therapy, prophylactic antibiotic therapy, and planning for bone marrow stem cell transplantation (Chapter 82).

Despite current successes in clinical management of immune deficiency, clinicians involved in providing prenatal genetic services should be prepared to be supportive toward the couple regarding decisions made to terminate an affected pregnancy. Although the ideal of genetic medicine is nondirective counseling, it has been pointed out that by offering to conduct prenatal testing, physicians are communicating a value judgment about the severity, treatability, and burden of a disease. Physicians involved in prenatal diagnosis for genetic immune deficiency should be aware of the particular couple's balance in decision making, opinions or pressures from extended family, and religious outlook.

Laboratory standards and reporting

All US laboratories providing any clinical data are subject to the regulatory requirements embodied in the Clinical Laboratory Improvement Amendments of 1988 (CLIA88).[52] Research laboratories that do not report patient-specific information are specifically exempt, but CLIA88 is clearly intended to preclude an arrangement where research laboratories perform diagnostic tests and prenatal diagnoses. CLIA88 mandates biannual laboratory inspections, quality control, quality assurance, proficiency testing, and personnel training standards. The American College of Medical Genetics has also produced guidelines for diagnostic laboratories conducting molecular genetics testing (http://www.faseb.org/genetics/acmg/stds/stdsmenu.htm). A clear argument can be made for the cost-effectiveness of prenatal diagnosis for such diseases, but it is unknown whether family analysis and carrier detection are ultimately effective in either reducing the number of affected individuals or improving their clinical outcome.

Future directions

The next decade will bring further improvements in our ability to identify family-specific mutations for all the known disease genes. Sequencing technology has moved to microscale formats, and dramatically reduced the cost of a complete genome for an individual. As our understanding of the role of polymorphisms in disease risk increases the importance of low-cost, high-throughput genotyping of standard variant panels will also increase.[53] The importance of bioinformatics in data analysis will become increasingly apparent as large amounts of individual sequence data are produced. International mutation databases will play an important role in both diagnosis and prognosis. New statistical approaches will be needed to exploit fully the potential of complete genome sequence for estimation of disease risk. Prospective screening of newborns for the T-cell immune deficiencies is now in early stage adoption.[54] Although rare, these are treatable disorders whose prognosis would be altered by early diagnosis before the onset of serious infection. In aggregate, the birth incidence is sufficient to merit screening if the techniques could be interfaced with current state screening programs. Screening for premalignant genotypic changes in peripheral blood might also be a reality one day. Careful clinical studies, including examination of the costs and benefits of mass screening programs, will be essential.

● ON THE HORIZON

- Routine diagnosis of > 150 primary immune deficiencies by complete genome sequencing.
- Rapid discovery of new primary immune deficiency genes by complete genome sequencing in individual families.
- Preconceptional screening to identify carrier status for thousands of genetic disorders.
- Non-invasive prenatal screening of fetal DNA in maternal blood for copy number abnormalities and mutations.

Translational research and clinical application

DNA sequencing technology is evolving very rapidly and we can anticipate additional technical platforms to become available over the next decade. Massive increases in sequence output, speed of sequencing, increases in read length, and more efficient bioinformatics methods will fuel dramatic reductions in cost. Complete genome sequencing will likely become a first line medical test for the diagnosis of most suspected genetic disorders including the primary immune deficiencies. Gene identification in single families with previously undescribed immune deficiencies will become routine. Personal complete genome sequencing for pre-conceptual genetic screening in the general population will become available and will impact risk counseling for thousands of autosomal recessive and X-linked disorders. By analysis of either free DNA in maternal serum or circulating fetal cells, complete genome sequencing will provide a comprehensive testing platform for non-invasive prenatal diagnosis.

References

1. International Union of Immunological Societies Expert Committee on Primary Immunodeficiencies. Notarangelo LD, Fischer A, et al. Primary immunodeficiencies: 2009 update. J Allergy Clin Immunol 2009;124:1161–78.
2. HapMap Consortium . A haplotype map of the human genome. Nature 2005;437:1299–320.
3. 1000 Genomes Project Consortium . A map of human genome variation from population-scale sequencing. Nature 2010;467(7319):1061–73.
4. de Jong H. Visualizing DNA domains and sequences by microscopy: a fifty-year history of molecular cytogenetics. Genome 2003;46:943–6.
5. Bejjani BA, Shaffer LG. Clinical utility of contemporary molecular cytogenetics. Annu Rev Genomics Hum Genet 2008;9:71–86.
6. Albertson TM, Preston BD. DNA replication fidelity: proofreading in trans. Curr Biol 2006;16:R209–211.
7. Kunkel TA. DNA replication fidelity. J Biol Chem 2004;279:16895–8.
8. Pfeifer GP. Mutagenesis at methylated CpG sequences. Curr Top Microbiol Immunol 2006;301:259–81.
9. Garcia-Diaz M, Kunkel TA. Mechanism of a genetic glissando: structural biology of indel mutations. Trends Biochem Sci 2006;31:206–14.
10. Wells RD, Dere R, Hebert ML, et al. Advances in mechanisms of genetic instability related to hereditary neurological diseases. Nucleic Acids Res 2005;33:3785–98.
11. Pellestor F, Anahory T, Hamamah S. Effect of maternal age on the frequency of cytogenetic abnormalities in human oocytes. Cytogenet Genome Res 2005;111:206–12.
12. Sommer SS, Scaringe WA, Hill KA. Human germline mutation in the factor IX gene. Mutat Res 2001;487:1–17.
13. Li L, Moshous D, Zhou Y, et al. A founder mutation in Artemis, an SNM1-like protein, causes SCID in Athabascan-speaking Native Americans. J Immunol 2002;168:6323–9.
14. Puck JM, Nussbaum RL, Conley ME. Carrier detection in X-linked severe combined immunodeficiency based on patterns of X chromosome inactivation. J Clin Invest 1987;79:1395–400.
15. Lacout C, Haddad E, Sabri S, et al. A defect in hematopoietic stem cell migration explains the nonrandom X-chromosome inactivation in carriers of Wiskott–Aldrich syndrome. Blood 2003;102:1282–9.
16. Liehr T, Claussen U. Current developments in human molecular cytogenetic techniques. Curr Mol Med 2002;2:283–97.
17. Lee C, Lemyre E, Miron PM, Morton CC. Multicolor fluorescence in situ hybridization in clinical cytogenetic diagnostics. Curr Opin Pediatr 2001;13:550–5.
18. Tchinda J, Volpert S, McNeil N, et al. Multicolor karyotyping in acute myeloid leukemia. Leuk Lymphoma 2003;44:1843–53.
19. Ylstra B, van den Ijssel P, Carvalho B, et al. BAC to the future! or oligonucleotides: a perspective for micro array comparative genomic hybridization (array CGH). Nucleic Acids Res 2006;34:445–50.
20. Chen W, Houldsworth J, Olshen AB, et al. Array comparative genomic hybridization reveals genomic copy number changes associated with outcome in diffuse large B-cell lymphomas. Blood 2006;107:2477–85.
21. Cheung SW, Shaw CA, Yu W, et al. Development and validation of a CGH microarray for clinical cytogenetic diagnosis. Genet Med 2005;7:422–32.
22. Fan JB, Oliphant A, Shen R, et al. Highly parallel SNP genotyping. Cold Spring Harb Symp Quant Biol 2003;68:69–78.
23. Gunderson KL, Steemers FJ, Lee G, et al. A genome-wide scalable SNP genotyping assay using microarray technology. Nat Genet 2005;37:549–54.
24. McGall G, Labadie J, Brock P, et al. Light-directed synthesis of high-density oligonucleotide arrays using semiconductor photoresists. Proc Natl Acad Sci U S A 1996;93:13555–60.
25. Fan JB, Chee MS, Gunderson KL. Highly parallel genomic assays. Nat Rev Genet 2006;7:632–44.
26. Kennedy GC, Matsuzaki H, Dong S, et al. Large-scale genotyping of complex DNA. Nat Biotechnol 2003;21:1233–337.
27. Peiffer DA, Le JM, Steemers FJ, et al. High-resolution genomic profiling of chromosomal aberrations using Infinium whole-genome genotyping. Genome Res 2006;16:1136–48.
28. Greiner TC. mRNA microarray analysis in lymphoma and leukemia. Cancer Treat Res 2004;121:1–12.
29. Savage KJ, Gascoyne RD. Molecular signatures of lymphoma. Int J Hematol 2004;80:401–9.
30. Ferrando AA, Look AT. DNA microarrays in the diagnosis and management of acute lymphoblastic leukemia. Int J Hematol 2004;80:395–400.
31. Margalit O, Somech R, Amariglio N, Rechavi G. Microarray-based gene expression profiling of hematologic malignancies: basic concepts and clinical applications. Blood Rev 2005;19:223–34.
32. Gladkevich A, Nelemans SA, Kauffman HF, Korf J. Microarray profiling of lymphocytes in internal diseases with an altered immune response: potential and methodology. Mediators Inflamm 2005;2005:317–30.
33. Strom CM. Mutation detection, interpretation, and applications in the clinical laboratory setting. Mutat Res 2005;573:160–7.
34. Metzker ML, Lu J, Gibbs RA. Electrophoretically uniform fluorescent dyes for automated DNA sequencing. Science 1996;271:1420–2.
35. Rosenblum BB, Lee LG, Spurgeon SL, et al. New dye-labeled terminators for improved DNA sequencing patterns. Nucleic Acids Res 1997;25:4500–4.
36. Metzker ML. Emerging technologies in DNA sequencing. Genome Res 2005;15:1767–76.
37. Ahmadian A, Ehn M, Hober S. Pyrosequencing: history, biochemistry and future. Clin Chim Acta 2006;363:83–94.
38. Margulies M, Egholm M, Altman WE, et al. Genome sequencing in microfabricated high-density picolitre reactors. Nature 2005;437:376–80.
39. Bentley DR, Balasubramanian S, Swerdlow HP, et al. Accurate whole human genome sequencing using reversible terminator chemistry. Nature 2008;456(7218):53–9.
40. McKernan KJ, Peckham HE, Costa GL, et al. Sequence and structural variation in a human genome uncovered by short-read, massively parallel ligation sequencing using two-base encoding. Genome Res 2009;19:1527–41.
41. Eid J, Fehr A, Gray J, et al. Real-time DNA sequencing from single polymerase molecules. Science 2009;323(5910):133–8.
42. Rothberg JM, Hinz W, Rearick TM, et al. An integrated semiconductor device enabling non-optical genome sequencing. Nature 2011;475(7356):348–52.
43. Stephens M, Sloan JS, Robertson PD, et al. Automating sequence-based detection and genotyping of SNPs from diploid samples. Nat Genet 2006;38:375–81.
44. Byers PH. Molecular genetic pathology: coming of age in the molecular world. J Mol Diagn 1999;1:3–4.
45. The International HapMap Project . Nature 2003;426:789–96.
46. O'Marcaigh AS, Puck JM, Pepper AE, et al. Maternal mosaicism for a novel interleukin-2 receptor gamma-chain mutation causing X-linked severe combined immunodeficiency in a Navajo kindred. J Clin Immunol 1997;17:29–33.
47. Puck JM, Pepper AE, Bedard PM, Laframboise R. Female germ line mosaicism as the origin of a unique IL-2 receptor gamma-chain mutation causing X-linked severe combined immunodeficiency. J Clin Invest 1995;95:895–9.
48. Janssen R, van Wengen A, Hoeve MA, et al. The same IkappaBalpha mutation in two related individuals leads to completely different clinical syndromes. J Exp Med 2004;200:559–68.
49. Lorusso F, Kong D, Jalil AK, et al. Preimplantation genetic diagnosis of leukocyte adhesion deficiency type I. Fertil Steril 2006;85:494 e15–e18.
50. Fiorentino F, Kahraman S, Karadayi H, et al. Short tandem repeats haplotyping of the HLA region in preimplantation HLA matching. Eur J Hum Genet 2005;13:953–8.
51. Kuliev A, Rechitsky S, Tur-Kaspa I, Verlinsky Y. Preimplantation genetics: Improving access to stem cell therapy. Ann N Y Acad Sci 2005;1054:223–7.
52. Rivers PA, Dobalian A, Germinario FA. A review and analysis of the clinical laboratory improvement amendment of 1988: compliance plans and enforcement policy. Health Care Manage Rev 2005;30:93–102.
53. Worthey EA, Mayer AN, Syverson GD, et al. Making a definitive diagnosis: successful clinical application of whole exome sequencing in a child with intractable inflammatory bowel disease. Genet Med 2011;13:255–62.
54. Routes JM, Grossman WJ, Verbsky J, et al. Statewide newborn screening for severe T-cell lymphopenia. JAMA 2009;302:2465–70.

Selected CD molecules and their characteristics

Thomas A. Fleisher

CD molecule	Predominant distribution	Identity/function
CD1a–e	Thymocytes, subset of lymphocytes, antigen-presenting cells	MHC class I-like molecules; presentation of non-peptide antigens to T cells; thymic T-cell development
CD2	T cells	Binds to LFA-3; receptor for CD48; T-cell activation; adhesion
CD3	T cells	T-cell signaling complex; associated with T-cell receptor (TCR)
CD4	T-cell subset	TCR co-receptor; interacts with MHC class II molecules on antigen-presenting cells; identifies T cells with helper function; signal transduction
CD5	Most T cells, thymocytes, B-cell subset	Binds to CD72; regulation of cell proliferation/activation; identifies B-1 B-cell subset
CD6	Thymocytes, T cells, B-cell subset	Binds CD166 (ALCAM); adhesion; mediates binding of developing thymocytes with thymic epithelial cells; thymic development; T-cell activation
CD7	Pluripotent hematopoietic cells, thymocytes, T cells	T-cell and NK-cell development
CD8	T-cell subset	TCR co-receptor; interacts with MHC class I molecules on antigen-presenting cells; identifies T cells with cytotoxic function
CD10	B cells	Neutral endopeptidase; enkephalinase; B-cell development; common acute lymphoblastic leukemia antigen (CALLA)
CD11a	Leukocytes	α-chain of LFA-1; pairs with CD18; interacts with ICAM; adhesion and cellular migration
CD11b	Monocytes, granulocytes, NK cells	α-chain of complement receptor 3 (CR3); pairs with CD18; adhesion molecule
CD11c	Monocytes, granulocytes, NK cells	α-chain of complement receptor 4 (CR4); pairs with CD18; adhesion molecule
CD13	Hematopoietic stem cells, immature and mature myeloid and monocyte elements	Appears before CD33 during myeloid differentiation
CD14	Granulocytes, monocytes/macrophages	Receptor for LPS/LPB complex; myeloid differentiation antigen; cell activation
CD15	Neutrophils, eosinophils, monocytes, basophil subset	Sialyl Lewis X antigen, plays a role in cell adhesion, defective in leukocyte adhesion deficiency type 2
CD16a,b	NK cells, monocytes/macrophages, neutrophils	$Fc\gamma$RIIIA and $Fc\gamma$RIIIB (low-affinity IgG receptors-type III); phagocytosis; ADCC
CD18	Leukocytes	β-chain of β_2-integrin molecules, including LFA-1, CR3, and CR4; pairs with CD11a, b, and c
CD19	B cells	BCR co-receptor; signal transduction; complexes with CD21
CD20	B cells	Role in B-cell activation/differentiation
CD21	B cells; follicular dendritic cells	Complement receptor type 2 (CR2): C3d receptor; B-cell co-receptor subunit; EBV receptor
CD22	B cells	Associates with BCR; signaling; regulation of B-cell activation; adhesion
CD23	B cells, macrophages, eosinophils, platelets, follicular dendritic cells	$Fc\varepsilon$RII; (low-affinity IgE receptor)
CD24	Leukocytes	Heat-stable antigen; co-stimulation; adhesion
CD25	Activated T cells and B cells	α-chain of IL-2 receptor, low-affinity IL-2 binding; signaling for cell proliferation/differentiation
CD26	Activated T cells and B cells; macrophages	Dipeptidyl peptidase; role in extracellular adhesion; cell activation
CD27	T cells; B-cell subset	Co-stimulation; T-cell proliferation, memory B cells

Continued

CD molecule	Predominant distribution	Identity/function
CD118	Broad distribution	Type 1 interferon (interferon-α/β) receptor
CD119	Broad distribution	Interferon-γ receptor
CD120a	Hematopoietic cells, nonhematopoietic cells, myeloid cells	TNF receptor-type 1; signal transduction; apoptosis
CD120b	Hematopoietic cells, nonhematopoietic cells, myeloid cells	TNF receptor-type II; signal transduction, apoptosis
CD121a	Thymocytes, T-cell subset, fibroblasts, epithelial cells, and brain cells	IL-1 receptor-type I; signal transduction
CD121b	T-cell subset, mycloid cell subsets	IL-1 receptor-type II
CD122	NK cells, T- and B-cell subset	IL-2 and IL-15 receptor β chain; signal transduction; regulation of lymphocyte development, differentiation, activation and proliferation
CD123	Bone marrow stem cells, granulocytes, monocytes, megakaryocytes	IL-3 receptor α chain; cell development and differentiation
CD124	Mature B and T cells, hematopoietic precursor cells	IL-4 receptor; signal transduction; lymphocyte development, activation, differentiation and proliferation
CD125	Eosinophils, basophils, B-cell subset	IL-5 receptor; eosinophil and B-cell growth and differentiation
CD126	Activated B cells, plasma cells, T cells, granulocytes, monocytes/macrophages; also expressed on epithelial cells, fibroblasts, hepatocytes, and neural cells	IL-6 receptor α chain; regulation of B- and T-cell differentiation and function; hematopoiesis
CD127	Bone marrow lymphoid precursors, pro-B cells, T-cell precursors, T-cell subset, monocytes	IL-7 receptor α chain; signal transduction; B- and T-cell proliferation and differentiation
CD128	Neutrophils, basophils, T-cell subset	IL-8 receptor; neutrophil activation and migration
CD129	T cells	IL-9 receptor α chain; T-cell proliferation
CD130	Broad distribution	IL-6 receptor β chain (with CD126); signal transduction
CD131	Lymphocytes, granulocytes, monocytes	IL-3, IL-5, and GM-CSF receptor; common β chain; signal transduction; see CD123 and CD125
CD132	Lymphocytes	Common γ chain of high-affinity receptor for IL-2 (with CD25 and CD122), IL-4 (with CD124), IL-7 (with CD127), IL-9 (with CD129), and IL15 (with CD122) receptors; signal transduction
CD134	Activated T cells	OX-40 antigen of TNFR superfamily (binds OX-40 ligand); T-cell–B-cell interaction and T-cell co-stimulation
CD135	Lymphoid and myeloid cell progenitor subsets	Flt3 ligand receptor; development of mycloid and lymphoid progenitors
CD137	Activated T cells	4-1BB; binds 4-1BB ligand and extracellular matrix components; T-cell–B-cell interaction and T-cell co-stimulation; extracellular adhesion; signal transduction
CD138	B-cell subset, plasma cells	Syndecan-1; binds interstitial matrix proteins; B-cell–matrix interactions
CD140a,b	Endothelial cells	PDGF receptor α and β chain; embryonic development; signal transduction; chemotaxis
CD141	Endothelium	Thrombomodulin (binds thrombin); regulates coagulation
CD142	Endothelium	Tissue factor; binds plasma factors VII/VIIa; hemostasis, coagulation, and angiogenesis
CD143	Endothelium	Angiotensin-converting enzyme (ACE); binds angiotensin 1; regulates blood pressure
CD144	Endothelium	VE-cadherin; cell–cell adhesion; maintenance of endothelium integrity
CD146	Activated T-cell subset	Mel-CAM, adhesion molecule during development
CD150	T- and B-cell subsets	Surface lymphocyte activation marker (SLAM); B-cell–T-cell interaction; co-stimulation
CD151	Not defined	PETA-3; regulates platelet aggregation and mediator release
CD152	Activated T cells	CTLA-4; binds B7-1 (CD80) and B7-2 (CD86); T-cell co-stimulation-negative signal
CD153	T cells	CD30 ligand; T-cell activation, differentiation, and regulation
CD154	Activated T cells	CD40 ligand; T-cell co-stimulation
CD156a	Leukocytes, B cells	Transmembrane glycoprotein; disintegrin and metalloproteinase domain (ADAM) family member; leukocyte adhesion and protease function; infiltration of myelomonocytic cells

CD molecule	Predominant distribution	Identity/function
CD156b	Broad distribution	TNF-α-converting enzyme (TACE); disintegrin and metalloproteinase domain (ADAM) family member; cleaves TNF and transforming growth factor-α from cell surface, thereby releasing soluble form
CD158	NK cells	Killer cell immunoglobulin (Ig)-like receptors (KIR); family of molecules that inhibit NK cytotoxic activity
CD159a	NK cells	NKG2A (killer cell lectin-like receptor)
CD161	NK cells	Natural killer cell receptor-P1; target cell recognition; NK cell activation
CD162	Granulocyte and T-cell subsets	P-selectin glycoprotein ligand-1 (PSGL-1); adhesion
CD166	Activated T cells, B cells	ALCAM; binds CD6; T-cell activation; thymocyte development
CD167a	Epithelial cells	Discoidin domain receptor 1 (DDD1); tyrosine kinase receptor; binds to collagen; cell–cell contact and adhesion
CD178	Activated T cells; various tissue cells	Fas ligand (ligand for CD95); binding to Fas triggers apoptosis
CD179a	Pro-B and pre-B cells	VpreB; forms surrogate light chain with CD179b; early B-cell differentiation
CD179b	Pro-B and pre-B cells	λ5; forms surrogate light chain with CD179a; early B-cell differentiation
CD180	B cells	RP105; toll-like receptor family; regulates B-cell recognition and signaling of LPS
CD183	Effector/memory T cells, NK cells, eos	CXCR3 receptor for interferon-inducible chemokines IP10, Mig, and I-TAC; chemotactic migration of effector T cells into areas of inflammation
CD184	Leukocytes; hematopoietic progenitors	CXCR4 receptor for chemokines such as stromal cell-derived factor-1 (SDF-1) (fusin); chemotaxis; HIV-1 co-receptor
CD195	Broad distribution; myeloid cells, lymphocytes, T lymphocytes, neurons, epithelium, endothelium	CCR5 receptor for chemokines such as macrophage inflammatory proteins, MIP-1a and MIP-1b, and RANTES; chemotaxis; HIV-1 co-receptor
CDw197	Lymphoid tissues, B cells, T-cell subset	CCR7 chemokine receptor; chemotaxis; T-cell homing and migration
CD201	Endothelial cells	Protein C receptor; coagulation
CD203c	Mast cells, basophils	Member of the ecto-nucleotide pyrophosphatase/phosphodiesterase enzymes
CD204	Myeloid cells, monocytes/macrophages	Macrophage scavenger receptor-1 (MSR1); mediates binding, internalization and processing of various negatively charged macromolecules
CD206	Dendritic cells, macrophages, myeloid cells, endothelial cells	Mannose receptor, C-type 1; binds microorganisms; phagocytosis
CD207	Dendritic cells, Langerhans' cells	Langerin; mannose receptor; phagocytosis and internalization of antigen for processing
CD208	Dendritic cells	DC-LAMP
CD209	Dendritic cells	DC-SIGN
CDw210	Broad distribution	I1-10 receptor α and β chain;
CD212	T cells, NK cells	IL-12 receptor β_1 chain;
CD213a1,a2	Lymphocytes, bronchial epithelial and smooth muscle cells	IL-13 receptor α_1 and α_2 chains
CDw217	Activated T-cell subset	IL-17; cytotoxic T-lymphocyte-associated serine esterase 8; stimulates cell activation; induces osteoclast differentiation factor (ODF)
CD220	Broad distribution	Insulin receptor; stimulates glucose uptake
CD molecule	Predominant distribution	Identity/function
CD221	Broad distribution	Insulin-like growth factor 1 receptor; cell signaling; activation, and differentiation
CD222	Broad distribution	Mannose-6-phosphate receptor; insulin-like growth factor-2 receptor
CD226	NK cells, platelets, monocytes, T-cell subset	Platelet and T-cell activation antigen 1 (PTA1); adhesion
CD233–241	Erythrocytes	Various erythrocyte membrane antigens, including blood group-associated glycoproteins
CD242	Erythrocytes	ICAM-4
CD246	T cells	TCR or CD3 ζ chain; associated with TCR and CD3; couples TCR recognition with T-cell signaling
CD247	T cells	T cells ζ chain of the TcR
CD252	Activated B cells	OX40 ligand
CD253	Activated T cells	TRAIL, death receptor

Continued

CD molecule	Predominant distribution	Identity/function
CD254	Activated T cells, LN and BM stroma	RANK ligand
CD256	Monocytes, macrophages	APRIL, binds TACI and BCMA
CD261	Activated T cells, peripheral leukocytes	TRAIL-R2, DR5, death receptor
CD262	Peripheral lymphocytes	TRAIL-R1, DR4, death receptor
CD263	Peripheral lymphocytes	TRAIL-R3, DcR1, death receptor
CD264	Peripheral lymphocytes	TRAIL-R4, DcR2, death receptor
CD265	Broad distribution	RANK
CD267	B cells, activated T cells	TACI
CD268	B cells	BAFFR, binds BLys, mature B-cell survival
CD269	Mature B cells	BCMA, binds APRIL and BAFF, B-cell survival and proliferation
CD275	B cells, dendritic cells, monocytes	ICOSL, costimulation, cytokine production
CD278	Activated T cells	ICOS, T-cell co-stimulation
CD257	Activated monocytes	BLyS, BAFF, binds TACI, BCMA, BAFFR, induces B-cell proliferation

ADCC, antibody dependent cellular cytotoxicity; ALCAM, activated leukocyte cell adhesion molecule; BCR, B-cell receptor for antigen; EBV, Epstein–Barr virus; ELAM, endothelial leukocyte adhesion molecule; G-CSF, granulocyte colony-stimulating factor; GM-CSF, granulocyte macrophage colony-stimulating factor; ICAM, intercellular adhesion molecule; LAM, leukocyte adhesion molecule; LAMP, latent membrane protein; LDL, low density lipoproteins; LECAM, lymphocyte endothelial cell adhesion molecule; LFA, lymphocyte function antigen; LPB, lipopolysaccharide binding protein; LPS, lipopolysaccharide; M-CSF, macrophage colony-stimulating factor; MHC, major histocompatibility complex; NK cells, natural killer cells; PDGF, platelet-derived growth factor; PECAM, platelet endothelial cell adhesion molecule; PETA, platelet-endothelial cell tetraspan antigen; TCR, T-cell receptor for antigen; TNF, tumor necrosis factor; TNFR, tumor necrosis factor receptor; VCAM, vascular cellular adhesion molecule; VLA, very late antigen.
This list was adapted from the results of the Eighth International Workshop on Human Leukocyte Differentiation Antigens (HLDA8) held in Adelaide, Australia, in December 2004 (Cell Immunol 2005; 236: 1–187).

Laboratory reference values

Thomas A. Fleisher

Immunoglobulin levels (age-related reference ranges; see Chapter 93)

Age of healthy donors	IgG g/L	IgG₁ g/L	IgG₂ g/L	IgG₃ g/L	IgG₄ g/L	IgA g/L	IgA₁ g/L	IgA₂ g/L	IgM g/L
0– <5 months	1.0–1.34	0.56–2.15	≤0.82	0.07.6–8.23	≤0.198	0.07–0.37	0.10–0.34	0.004–0.055	0.26–1.22
5– <9 months	1.64–5.88	1.02–3.69	≤0.89	0.119–0.740	≤0.208	0.16–0.50	0.14–0.41	0.015–0.062	0.32–1.32
9– <15 months	2.46–9.04	1.60–5.62	0.24–0.98	0.173–0.637	≤0.220	0.27–0.66	0.20–0.50	0.028–0.070	0.40–1.43
15– <24 months	3.13–11.70	2.09–7.24	0.35–1.05	0.219–0.550	≤0.230	0.36–0.79	0.24–0.58	0.039–0.077	0.46–1.52
2– <4 years	2.95–11.56	1.58–7.21	0.39–1.76	0.170–0.847	0.004–0.491	0.27–2.46	0.16–1.62	0.013–0.311	0.37–1.84
4– <7 years	3.86–14.70	2.09–9.02	0.44–3.16	0.108–0.949	0.008–0.819	0.29–2.56	0.17–1.87	0.011–0.391	0.37–2.24
7– <10 years	4.62–16.82	2.53–10.19	0.54–4.35	0.085–10.26	0.010–1.087	0.34–2.74	0.21–2.21	0.014–0.480	0.38–2.51
10– <13 years	5.03–15.80	2.80–10.30	0.66–5.02	0.115–10.53	0.010–1.219	0.42–2.95	0.27–2.50	0.026–0.534	0.41–2.55
13– <16 years	5.09–15.80	2.89–9.34	0.82–5.16	0.200–10.32	0.007–1.217	0.52–3.19	0.36–2.75	0.047–0.551	0.45–2.44
16– <18 years	4.87–13.27	2.83–7.72	0.98–4.86	0.313–0.976	0.003–1.110	0.60–3.37	0.44–2.89	0.066–0.543	0.49–2.01
≥18 years	7.67–15.90	3.41–8.94	1.71–6.32	0.184–10.60	0.024–1.210	0.61–3.56	0.50–3.14	0.097–1.560	0.37–2.86

Immunoglobulin levels were assessed in serum by nephelometry and data were statistically analyzed for the mid-95% confidence interval. For total IgG and IgG subclass quantitation, data from 156 pediatric and 92 adult donors; for total IgA quantitation, data from 201 pediatric and 99 adult donors; for IgA subclasses, data from 119 pediatric and 99 adult donors; for IgM quantitation, data from 212 pediatric and 401 adults was used at Mayo Medical Laboratories.

Total serum IgE (IU/mL)

Age	Gender	Geometric mean	Upper 95% confidence limit
6–14 years	M	42.7	527
	F	43.3	344
15–24 years	M	33.6	447
	F	18.6	262
25–34 years	M	16.8	275
	F	16.6	216
35–44 years	M	21.7	242
	F	19.3	206
45–54 years	M	19.2	254
	F	13.3	177
55–64 years	M	21.3	354
	F	11.7	148
65–74 years	M	21.2	248
	F	11.5	122
>75 years	M	18.4	219
	F	9.2	124
6–75 years	all M	22.9	317
	all F	14.7	189

Data generated using skin-prick test-negative (i.e., house dust mite, Bermuda grass, tree mix, weed mix, mold mix) individuals.
From Barbee RA, et al. J Allergy Clin Immunol 1981; 68: 106, with permission.

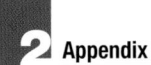

Lymphocyte immunophenotype: adult reference range (95% confidence interval)

Surface antigens	Percent positive	Cells/mm^3
T cells		
CD3	57–86	650–2108
CD5	56–84	638–2099
CD2	76–93	876–2258
CD3/CD4	29–57	358–1259
CD3/CD8	13–47	194–836
CD4/CD45RO	12–34	203–976
CD4/CD45RA	2.5–25	31–533
CD8/CD45RO	3–14	34–309
CD8/CD45RA	7–28	101–636
CD3/CD8/CD28	9.5–23	155–441
CD3/CD8/CD57	≤16	≤239
CD3/HLA–DR	≤15.1	≤291
CD3/CD25	≤37.4	≤756
B cells		
CD19	3.5–15.5	49–424
CD20	3.5–17	47–409
CD20/CD5	1.5–8.5	13–145
CD20/CD23	1.6–13.2	38–360
CD20/CD27	0.7–6.3	16–118
NK cells		
CD3$^-$/CD16$^+$CD56$^+$	4.5–30	87–505
Lymphocytes	17–41	1173–2640

Data gererated in the Flow Cytometry Section, Immunology Service, DLM, CC, NIH, Bethesda, MD. The 95% confidence interval for the WBC is 4300–9200/mm^3.

Age-dependent lymphocyte immunophenotype reference range (80% confidence interval)

	T cells					
	CD3		**CD4**		**CD8**	
Age	Percent positive	Cells/mm^3	Percent positive	Cells/mm^3	Percent positive	Cells/mm^3
0–3 mo	53–84	2500–5500	35–64	1600–4000	12–28	560–1700
3–6 mo	51–77	2500–5600	35–56	1800–4000	12–23	590–1600
6–12 mo	49–76	1900–5900	31–56	1400–4300	12–24	500–1700
1–2 yr	53–75	2100–6200	32–51	1300–4300	14–30	620–2000
2–6 yr	56–75	1400–3700	28–47	700–2200	16–30	490–1300
6–12 yr	60–76	1200–2600	31–47	650–1500	18–35	370–1100
12–18 yr	56–84	1000–2200	31–52	530–1300	18–35	330–920

	CD4 T-cell subpopulations					
	CD4/CD45RA		**CD3/CD4/CD45RO**		**CD4/HLA–DR**	
Age	Percent CD4 positive	Cells/mm^3	Percent CD3/CD4 positive	Cells/mm^3	Percent CD4 positive	Cells/mm^3
0–3 mo	64–95	1200–3700	2–22	60–900	2–6	40–180
3–6 mo	77–94	1300–3700	3–16	120–630	2–10	60–280
6–12 mo	64–93	1100–3700	5–18	160–800	2–11	50–260
1–2 yr	63–91	1000–2900	7–20	210–850	2–11	70–280
2–6 yr	53–86	430–1500	9–26	220–660	3–12	50–180
6–12 yr	46–77	320–1000	13–30	230–630	3–13	40–120
12–18 yr	33–66	230–770	18–38	240–700	4–11	30–100

	CD8 T-cell subpopulations					
	CD8/CD45RA		CD3/CD4–/CD45RO		CD8/HLA–DR	
Age	Percent CD8 positive	Cells/mm^3	Percent CD3/CD4- positive	Cells/mm^3	Percent CD8 positive	Cells/mm^3
0–3 mo	80–99	450–1500	1–9	30–330	2–20	20–160
3–6 mo	85–98	550–1400	1–7	30–290	3–17	30–170
6–12 mo	75–97	480–1500	1–8	40–330	4–27	40–290
1–2 yr	71–98	490–1700	2–12	60–570	6–33	60–600
2–6 yr	69–97	380–1100	4–16	90–440	7–37	70–420
6–12 yr	63–92	310–900	4–21	70–390	6–29	40–270
12–18 yr	61–91	240–710	4–23	60–310	5–25	30–180

	B cells and NK cells			
	CD19		CD3–/CD16–56+	
Age	Percent positive	Cells/mm^3	Percent positive	Cells/mm^3
0–3 mo	6–32	300–2000	4–18	170–1100
3–6 mo	11–41	430–3000	3–14	170–830
6–12 mo	14–37	610–2600	3–15	160–950
1–2 yr	16–35	720–2600	3–15	180–920
2–6 yr	14–33	390–1400	4–17	130–720
6–12 yr	13–27	270–860	4–17	100–480
12–18 yr	6–23	110–570	3–22	70–480

Data generated by Shearer WT, et al. J Allergy Clin Immunol 2003; 112: 973–980.

Chemokines—Cont'd

Class	Systemic name	Chemokine		Receptor(s)	Receptor(s) expressed on	Receptor class
	CCL24	Eotaxin-2		CCR3	P, Thy, T,	CC
					Ba, Eo, Plt	
	CCL25	TECK	Thymus-expressed	CCR9	P, Thy, T, DC	CC
			chemokine	CCX-CKR		
	CCL26	Eotaxin-3		CCR3	P, Thy, T,	CC
					Ba, Eo, Plt	
	CCL27	CTACK	Cutaneous T cell-attracting chemokine	CCR10	P, T	CC
		Eskine				
	CCL28	MEC	Mammary enriched chemokine	CCR3, CCR10	P, Thy, T,	CC
					Ba, Eo, Plt	
CX_3C (γ)	CX3CL1	Fractalkine		CX_3CR1	T, NK, M	CX_3C
XC (δ)	XCL1	Lymphotactin-α		XCR1	NK	XC
	XCL2	Lymphotactin-β		XCR1	NK	XC

Abbreviations for cells: B, B cells; Ba, Basophils; DC, Dendritic cells; Eo, Eosinophils; M, Macrophages/Monocytes; N, Neutrophils; NK, Natural Killer cells; NKT, NK T cells; P, plasma cells; Plt, platelets; SC, hematopoietic stem cells; T, T cells.
Other abbreviations: Antag (Antagonist)

Cytokines

Robert R. Rich

Cytokines

Cytokine	Abbreviation	Receptor	Receptor family	Signaling	Source	Target	Action	Knockout phenotype
Cardiotrophin 1	CT1		Type I (hematopoietin) gp130-utilizing	Jak1, Stat3	myocardial cells, T cells, others	myocardium	growth	Weakness, motoneuron cell death
Ciliary neurotrophic factor	CNTF	CNTFR, LIFR	Type I gp130-utilizing	Jak1, Stat3	Schwann cells, astrocytes	neuronal cells	survival	progressive atrophy and loss of motor neurons
Colony stimulating factor 1	CSF1 (M-CSF)	FMS (CSF1R)	receptor tyrosine kinases	Ras/Raf/MAPK	macrophages, endothelium, fibroblasts, other	committed myelomonocytic progenitors	differentiation, proliferation, survival	monocytopenia, osteopetrosis, female infertility
Colony stimulating factor 2	CSF2 (GM-CSF)	CSF2R	Type I βc utilizing	Jak1, Stat3	T cell, macrophages, endothelium, fibroblasts	immature and committed myelo-monocytic progenitors, mature macrophages, granulocytes, DC	growth, differentiation, survival, activation	pulmonary alveolar proteinosis
Colony stimulating factor 3	CSF3 (G-CSF)	CSF3R	Type I homodimeric	Jak2, Stat3	macrophages, endothelium, fibroblasts, other	committed progenitors	differentiation, activates mature granulocytes	neutropenia
Erythropoietin	EPO	EPOR	Type I homodimeric	Jak2, Stat5	kidney, liver	erythroid precursors	erythroid differentiation	embryonic lethal, severe anemia
FMS-related tyrosine kinase 3 ligand	FLT3 ligand	FLT3	receptor tyrosine kinases	Ras/Raf/MAPK	diverse tissues	Myeloid cells, especially DC	proliferation, differentiation	reduced repopulating hematopoietic stem cells; reduced B cell precursors
Growth hormone	GH	GHR	Type I homodimeric	Jak2, Stat5b	two GH genes, pituitary, placental	diverse tissues	growth, adipocyte differentiation, induces IGF-1	dwarfism*
Interferon-α/β	IFNα/β	IFNAR	Type II (interferons) heterodimeric	Jak1, Tyk2, Stat1, Stat2	macrophages, fibroblasts, plasmacytoid DC, other	NK cells, DC, others	antiviral, antiproliferative, increased MHC class I activation	susceptibility to viral infections
Interferon-γ	IFNγ	IFNGR	Type II heterodimeric	Jak1, Jak2, Stat1	Th1 T cells, NK cells	macrophages, endothelium, NK cells	activation, increased MHC Class II expression, increased antigen presentation	susceptibility to bacterial infections*
Interleukin-1α/β	IL1α/β	IL1R	IL-1/TLR	IRAK, MyD88, TRAF6, NF-κB	many cells, especially macrophages	CNS, endothelial cells, liver, thymocytes, macrophages	fever, anorexia, activation, acute phase reactants, costimulation, activation, cytokine secretion	decreased inflammatory responses
Interleukin-2	IL2	IL2R (TAC, CD25)	Type I γc-utilizing	Jak1, Jak3, Stat5	T cells, NK cells, NKT cells	T cells, B cells, NK cells, macrophages	proliferation, cytotoxicity, IFNγ secretion, antibody production	lymphoproliferation, Impaired response to polyclonal T cell activators, inflammatory bowel disease
Interleukin-3	IL3	IL3R	Type I βc utilizing	Jak2, Stat5	T cells, macrophages, mast cells, NKT cells, eosinophils	immature hematopoietic progenitors of multiple lineages	growth, differentiation, survival	no defects in basal hematopoiesis

Name	Abbreviation	Receptor	Receptor type	Signaling	Produced by	Target	Function	Deficiency
(Interleukin-4)	IL4	IL4R	Type I γc-utilizing	Jak1, Jak3, Stat6	Th2 cells, mast cells, NKT cells, γδ T cells	T cells, B cells, macrophages	proliferation, Th2 differentiation, IgG1 and IgE production, Inhibition of cell-mediated immunity	defective Th2 differentiation and IgE production, Decreased allergic responses
Interleukin-5	IL5	IL5R	Type I βc utilizing	Jak2, Stat5	Th2 cells, activated eosinophils, NK cells, NKT cells	eosinophils, B cells, basophils, mast cells	proliferation, activation	decreased eosinophilia, defective CD5+ B1 cell development
Interleukin-6	IL6	IL6R	Type I gp130-utilizing	Jak1, Stat3	macrophage, fibroblasts, endothelium, epithelium, T cells, other	liver, B cells, T cells, thymocytes, myeloid cells, osteoclasts	acute phase reactants, proliferation, differentiation, costimulation	reduced Ig, esp IgA, T lymphopenia, impaired acute phase response and Th17 development
Interleukin-7	IL7	IL7R	Type I γc-utilizing	Jak1, Jak3, Stat5	bone marrow, thymic stromal cells, spleen, DC, keratinocytes, monocytes, macrophages	Thymocytes, T cells, B cells	growth, differentiation, survival	SCID*
Interleukin-9	IL9	IL9R	Type I γc-utilizing	Jak1, Jak3, Stat5	Th2 cells, Th9 cells, mast cells, eosinophils	T cells, B cells, mast cell precursors	Proliferation, Th1 inhibition	Not essential for Th2 pathology
Interleukin-10	IL10	IL10R	Type II heterodimeric	Jak1, Tyk2, Stat3	Th2 cells, other cells	macrophages	decreased MHC class II expression, decreased antigen presentation	exaggerated inflammatory response and autoimmune disease
Interleukin-11	IL11	IL11R	Type I gp130-utilizing	Jak1, Stat3	stromal cells, sinoviocytes, osteoblasts	hematopoietic stem cells, hepatocytes, macrophages, neurons	proliferation	female infertility
Interleukin-12	IL12	IL12R	Type I heterodimeric	Jak2, Tyk2, Stat4	macrophages, B cells, DC	T cells, NK cells	Th1 differentiation, proliferation, cytotoxicity	defective Th1 differentiation, susceptibility to bacterial infections*
Interleukin-13	IL13	IL13R	Type I heterodimeric	Jak1, Tyk2, Stat6	activated T cells, NKT cells, mast cells, basophils	B cells, macrophages, mast cells, epithelial cells, smooth muscle cells	costimulator of proliferation, IgE, increased CD23 and MHC class II, inhibits cytokine secretion and cell-mediated immunity	defective Th2 responses and IgE production, decreased allergic responses
Interleukin-15#	IL15#	IL15R	Type I γc-utilizing	Jak1, Jak3, Stat5	many cells	T cells, especially memory cells, NK cells, NKT cells	proliferation, survival and activation	absence of NK and memory cells
Interleukin-17	IL17A	IL17R	IL17	NF-κB, MAPK	Th17 helper cells, cytotoxic T cells, γδT cells	endothelium, many cells	proinflammatory	susceptibility to extracellular bacteria
Interleukin-17B, C,D	IL17B,C,D	IL17R	IL17		many cells	Monocytes, epithelial cells	Inflammation, chondrogenesis	
Interleukin-17 F	IL17F, ML1				Th17 cells, CD8 T cells, γδ T cells monocytes, other cells		induces expression of TGFB, inhibits angiogenesis	

Continued

Cytokines—cont'd

Cytokine	Abbreviation	Receptor	Receptor family	Signaling	Source	Target	Action	Knockout phenotype
Interleukin-18	IL18	IL18R	IL-1/TLR	IRAK, MyD88, TRAF6, NF-κB	Many cells, esp macrophages, keratinocytes, osteoblasts	T cells, NK cells, macrophages, epithelial cells	Promotes IFNγ production, induces NK cell cytotoxicity, inhibits osteoclast formation	Increased susceptibility to infection. Reduced arthritis
Interleukin-19	IL19		Type I γc-utilizing	Stat1, Stat3	Th2 cells, monocytes, NKT cells, melanocytes	T cells, keratinocytes, epithelial cells	production of inflammatory cytokines, Th2 responses, activation of epithelial cells	
Interleukin-20	IL20	IL20R	Type II heterodimeric	Stat1, Stat3	Th2 cells, monocytes, NKT cells	Macrophages, T cells, keratinocytes, epithelial cells	enhanced proliferation of multipotential hematopoietic progenitors, proliferation and differentiation of keratinocytes	exaggerated inflammatory response and autoimmune disease
Interleukin-21	IL21	IL21R	Type I gp130-utilizing	Jak1, Jak3, Stat3	T cells, Th17 cells, Tfh cells	T, B and NK cells, DC, macrophages, keratinocytes	isotype switching, plasma cell differentiation, enhances CD8 T cell and NK cell responses, promotes Th17 cell differentiation	Decreased Th17 cells, acts in concert with IL4
Interleukin-22	IL22	IL22R	Type I heterodimeric	Jak1, Tyk2, Stat3	macrophages, B cells	T cells, NK cells	Th1 differentiation, proliferation, cytotoxicity	defective Th1 differentiation, susceptibility to bacterial infections*
Interleukin-23	IL23	IL23R	Type I heterodimeric	Jak2, Stat3, Stat 5	macrophages, DC	T cells, macrophages	Induces IL17 production	Reduced arthritis, inflammation
Interleukin-24	IL24		Type I γc-utilizing	Stat1, Stat3	Th2 cells, NKT cells, B cells, monocytes, macrophages	skin cells, lung cells, reproductive tissues	proliferation, survival, wound healing	
Interleukin-25 (IL-17E)	IL-25 (IL-17E)	IL17RH1	Type I		mast cells, Th2 cells, various tissues	Th2 cells , MHC class II expressing non-T, non-B accessory cells	induction of proinflammatory cytokines	Increased susceptibility to helminths
Interleukin-26	IL26	IL26R	Type II heterodimeric	Stat1, Stat3	Th17 cells, NK cells	Epithelial cells		
Interleukin-27	IL27 (IL30/EBI3)	IL27R	Type I gp130-utilizing	Jak1, Stat1, Stat3, Stat4, Stat5	CD4 cells, NK T cells, DC, macrophages, epithelial cells	T and NK cells	Antiviral immunity, promotes Th1 differentiation, isotype switching by B cells, inhibits Th17 differentiation	impaired IFNγ production, increased susceptibility to intracellular pathogens
Interleukin-28	IL28	IL28R	Type II heterodimeric	Stat1, Stat2, Stat3, Stat4, Stat5	DC,, T cells, intestinal epithelial cells, virus-infected cells,	Cytotoxic T cells, NK cells, keratinocytes. melanocytes	Antiviral immunity, increased IFN production	
Interleukin-29	IL29	IL28R	Type II heterodimeric	Stat1, Stat2, Stat4, Stat5	DC, T cells, intestinal epithelial cells, virus-infected cells	Keratinocytes, melanocytes	Antiviral immunity	

Interleukin-31	IL31	IL31R (GLMR)	Type I gp130-utilizing	Jak1, Jak2, Stat3, Stat4, Stat5	Th2 cells, CD8 T cells	Monocytes, epithelial cells, keratinocytes, eosinophils, basophils,	Induces proinflammatory cytokines, chemokines, matrix metalloproteinases, PMN recruitment,	
Interleukin-32	IL32				activated T cells, NK cells		stimulates production of TNF	
Interleukin-33	IL33	ST2/IL1RAcP	IL-1/TLR heterodimeric	MyD88, NF-κB	Endothelial cells, smooth muscle cells, cardiac myocytes, keratinocytes	T cells, mast cells, nuocytes	Enhanced Th2 responses, mucosal innate immunity, anti-helminth immunity	Diminished LPS responsiveness, reduced acute allergic response
Interleukin-35	IL35		IL12R family		Treg cells	T cells	Treg proliferation, inhibition of Th17 cells	Reduced Treg activity
Leptin	LEP	LEPR	Type I homodimeric	Jak2, Stat3	adipocytes	hypothalamus, thyroid	satiety, controls metabolic rate	Obesity
Leukemia inhibitory factor	LIF	LIFR	Type I gp130-utilizing	Jak1, Stat3	uterus, macrophage, fibroblasts, endothelium, T cells	embryonic stem cells, neurons, hematopoietic cells	survival	decreased hematopoietic progenitors, defective blastocyst implantation
Lymphotoxin-α	LTA	TNFR	TNF		activated T cells and B cells	many cells	cytolysis, lymph node architecture, activation	aberrant lymph node structure
Oncostatin M*	OSM	OSMR	Type I gp130-utilizing	Jak1, Stat3	macrophage, fibroblasts, endothelium, T cells, others	myeloid cells, liver, embryonic stem cells	differentiation, acute phase induction	
Prolactin	PRL	PRLR	Type I homodimeric	Jak2, Stat5a	two Prl genes pituitary, uterus	mammary epithelium	growth, differentiation	infertility, lactation defects
Stem cell factor	SCF, c-kit ligand	c-kit	receptor tyrosine kinases	Ras/Raf/MAPK	bone marrow stromal cells	pluripotent stem cells	activation, growth	defective hematopoietic stem cell proliferation, melanocyte production and germ cell development
Thrombopoietin	THPO	THPOR	Type I homodimeric	Jak2, Stat5	liver, kidney	committed stem cells, megakaryocytes	platelet	severe thrombocytopenia
Tissue necrosis factor	TNF	TNFR	TNFR	TRAFs, TRADD, FADD, Caspases, NF-κB	macrophages, T cell	neutrophils, macrophages, endothelium, CNS, muscle, fat, many cells	adhesion, activation, adhesion, cytokines, coagulation, fever, cachexia, cytolysis	fever deregulation *
Transforming growth facto β 1, 2, 3	TGFB 1, 2, 3	TGFBR	TGF-β receptor serine kinase family	SMADs, SARA, FAST-1, TAK1	T cells, macrophages, other	T cells, macrophages, other	inhibits growth and activation	

*Asterisks denote human disease.
#note that two forms of the IL-4 and IL 15 receptor exist.

Robert R. Rich | # Vaccine schedules

Vaccine ▼ / Age ▶	Birth	1 month	2 months	4 months	6 months	9 months	12 months	15 months	18 months	19–23 months	2–3 years	4–6 years
Hepatitis B	Hep B	HepB					HepB					
Rotavirus			RV	RV	RV							
Diphtheria, tetanus, pertussis			DTaP	DTaP	DTaP		DTaP					DTaP
Haemophilus influenzae type b			Hib	Hib	Hib		Hib					
Pneumococcal			PCV	PCV	PCV		PCV					PPSV
Inactivated poliovirus			IPV	IPV			IPV					IPV
Influenza							Influenza (Yearly)					
Measles, mumps, rubella							MMR					MMR
Varicella							Varicella					Varicella
Hepatitis A							Dose 1					HepA Series
Meningococcal							MCV4					

Range of recommended ages for all children
Range of recommended ages for certain high-risk groups
Range of recommended ages for all children and certain high-risk groups

Fig. A5.1A CDC recommended immunization schedule for persons aged 0 through 6 years – United States, 2012. This schedule includes recommendations in effect as of December 23, 2011 approved by the CDC Advisory Committee on Immunization Practices, the American Academy of Pediatrics and the American Academy of Family Physicians. Any dose not administered at the recommended age should be administered at a subsequent visit, when indicated and feasible. The use of a combination vaccine generally is preferred over separate injection of its equivalent component vaccines. Vaccination providers should consult the relevant Advisory Committee on Immunization Practices (ACIP) statement for detailed recommendations, available online at http://www.cdc.gov/vaccines/pubs/acip-list.htm. Clinically significant adverse events that follow immunization should be reported to the Vaccine Adverse Event Reporting System (VAERS) online at http://www.vaers.hhs.gov or by telephone, 800-822-7967. An in-depth version of this table is available online at http://aapredbook.aappublications.org/resources/IZSchedule0-6yrs.pdf.

Vaccine ▼ / Age ▶	7–10 years	11–12 years	13–18 years
Tetanus, diphtheria, pertussis	1 dose (if indicated)	1 dose	1 dose (if indicated)
Human papillomavirus		3 doses	Complete 3-dose series
Meningococcal		Dose 1	Booster at age 16 years
Influenza	Influenza (yearly)		
Pneumococcal			
Hepatitis A	Complete 2-dose series		
Hepatitis B	Complete 3-dose series		
Inactivated poliovirus	Complete 3-dose series		
Measles, mumps, rubella	Complete 2-dose series		
Varicella	Complete 2-dose series		

Range of recommended ages for all children
Range of recommended ages for catch-up immunization
Range of recommended ages for certain high-risk groups

Fig. A5.1B CDC recommended immunization schedule for persons aged 7 through 18 years – United States, 2012. This schedule includes recommendations in effect as of December 23, 2011, approved by the CDC Advisory Committee on Immunization Practices, the American Academy of Pediatrics, and the American Academy of Family Physicians. Any dose not administered at the recommended age should be administered at a subsequent visit, when indicated and feasible. The use of a combination vaccine generally is preferred over separate injections of its equivalent component vaccines. Vaccination providers should consult the relevant Advisory Committee on Immunization Practices statement for detailed recommendations available online at: http://www.cdc.gov/vaccines/pubs/acip-list.htm. Clinically significant adverse events that follow immunization should be reported to the Vaccine Adverse Event Reporting System (VAERS) at http://www.vaers.hhs.gov or by telephone, 800-822-7967. An in-depth version of this table is available online at http://aapredbook.aappublications.org/resources/IZSchedule7-18yrs.pdf.

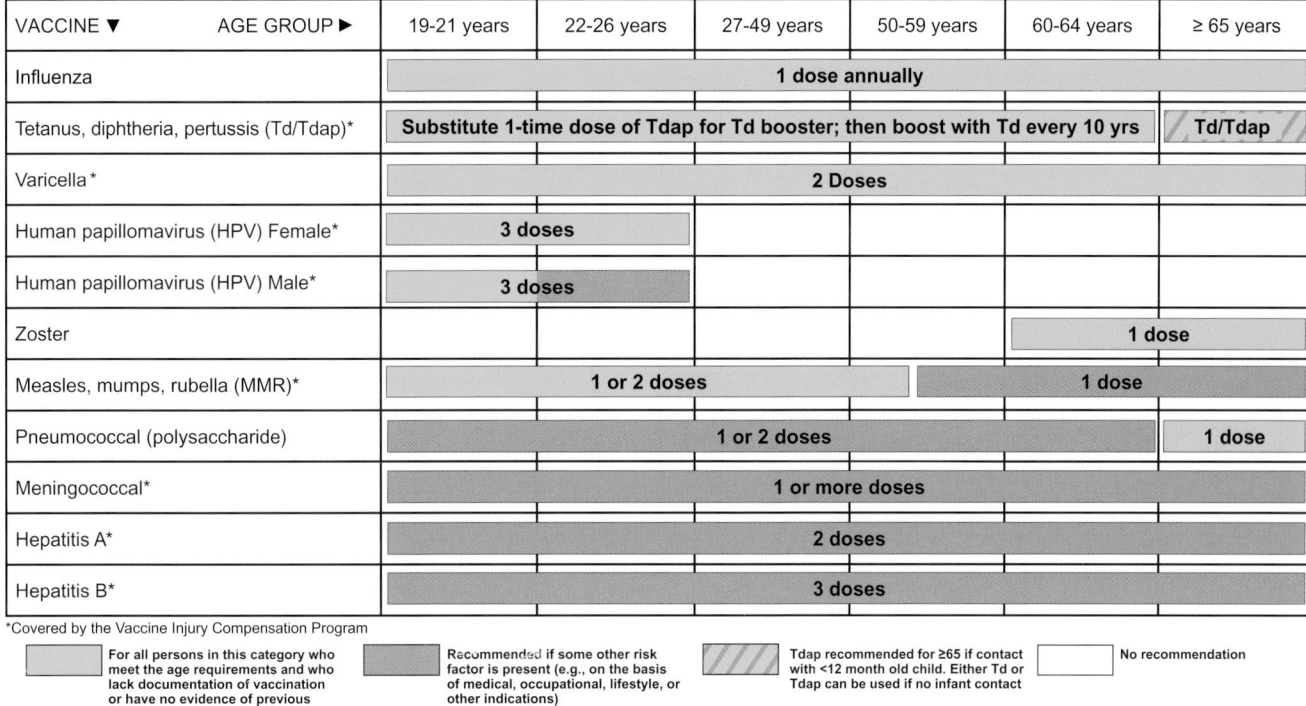

VACCINE ▼ AGE GROUP ▶	19-21 years	22-26 years	27-49 years	50-59 years	60-64 years	≥ 65 years
Influenza	1 dose annually					
Tetanus, diphtheria, pertussis (Td/Tdap)*	Substitute 1-time dose of Tdap for Td booster; then boost with Td every 10 yrs					Td/Tdap
Varicella*	2 Doses					
Human papillomavirus (HPV) Female*	3 doses					
Human papillomavirus (HPV) Male*	3 doses					
Zoster					1 dose	
Measles, mumps, rubella (MMR)*	1 or 2 doses				1 dose	
Pneumococcal (polysaccharide)	1 or 2 doses					1 dose
Meningococcal*	1 or more doses					
Hepatitis A*	2 doses					
Hepatitis B*	3 doses					

*Covered by the Vaccine Injury Compensation Program

For all persons in this category who meet the age requirements and who lack documentation of vaccination or have no evidence of previous infection

Recommended if some other risk factor is present (e.g., on the basis of medical, occupational, lifestyle, or other indications)

Tdap recommended for ≥65 if contact with <12 month old child. Either Td or Tdap can be used if no infant contact

No recommendation

Fig. A5.2 CDC recommended adult immunization schedule, by vaccine and age group – United States, 2012. This schedule indicates the recommended age groups for routine administration of currently licensed vaccines for persons aged 19 years or older, as of January 1, 2012 and approved by the CDC Advisory Committee on Immunization Practices, the American Academy of Family Physicians, the American College of Physicians, the American College of Obstetricians and Gynecologists, and the American College of Nurse-Midwives. For detailed recommendations on all vaccines, including those primarily for travelers or that are issued or updated over time, consult the manufacturers' package inserts and the complete statements of the Advisory Committee on Immunization Practices (ACIP) for additional details available online at: http://www.cdc.gov/vaccines/recs/schedules/downloads/adult/adult-schedule.pdf. Recently issued, provisional ACIP recommendations can be found at http://www.cdc.gov/vaccines/recs/provisional/default.htm. Clinically significant adverse events that follow immunization should be reported to the Vaccine Adverse Event Reporting System (VAERS) at http://www.vaers.hhs.gov or by telephone, 800-822-7967. An in-depth version of this table is available online at http://www.cdc.gov/vaccines/recs/schedules/downloads/adult/adult-schedule.pdf.

VACCINE ▼ INDICATION ►	Pregnancy	Immunocompromising conditions (excluding human immunodeficiency virus [HIV])	HIV infection CD4+ T lymphocyte count		Men who have sex with men (MSM)	Heart disease, chronic lung disease, chronic alcoholism	Asplenia (including elective splenectomy and persistent complement component deficiencies)	Chronic liver disease	Diabetes, kidney failure, end-stage renal disease, receipt of hemodialysis	Health-care personnel
			< 200 cells/μL	≥ 200 cells/μL						
Influenza	1 dose TIV annually				1 dose TIV or LAIV annually	1 dose TIV annually				1 dose TIV or LAIV annually
Tetanus, diphtheria, pertussis (Td/Tdap)*	Substitute 1-time dose of Tdap for Td booster; then boost with Td every 10 yrs									
Varicella*	Contraindicated			2 doses						
Human papillomavirus (HPV) Female*	3 doses through age 26 yrs					3 doses through age 26 yrs				
Human papillomavirus (HPV) Male*	3 doses through age 26 yrs					3 doses through age 21 yrs				
Zoster	Contraindicated			1 dose						
Measles, mumps, rubella (MMR)*	Contraindicated			1 or 2 doses						
Pneumococcal (polysaccharide)	1 or 2 doses									
Meningococcal*	1 or more doses									
Hepatitis A*	2 doses									
Hepatitis B*	3 doses									

*Covered by the Vaccine Injury Compensation Program

For all persons in this category who meet the age requirements and who lack documentation of vaccination or have no evidence of previous infection	Recommended if some other risk factor is present (e.g., on the basis of medical, occupational, lifestyle, or other indications)	Contraindicated	No recommendation

Fig. A5.3 CDC recommended adult immunization schedule for adults based on medical and other indications, United States, 2012. This schedule indicates the recommended schedules based upon certain medical or other situational indications for persons aged 19 years or older, as of January 1, 2012 and approved by the CDC Advisory Committee on Immunization Practices, the American Academy of Family Physicians, the American College of Physicians, the American College of Obstetricians and Gynecologists, and the American College of Nurse-Midwives. For detailed recommendations on all vaccines, including those primarily for travelers or that are issued or updated over time, consult the manufacturers' package inserts and the complete statements of the Advisory Committee on Immunization Practices (ACIP) for additional details available online at: http://www.cdc.gov/vaccines/recs/schedules/downloads/adult/adult-schedule.pdf. Recently issued, provisional ACIP recommendations can be found at http://www.cdc.gov/vaccines/recs/provisional/default.htm. Clinically significant adverse events that follow immunization should be reported to the Vaccine Adverse Event Reporting System (VAERS) at http://www.vaers.hhs.gov or by telephone, 800-822-7967.

Index